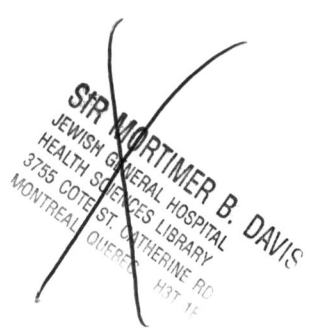

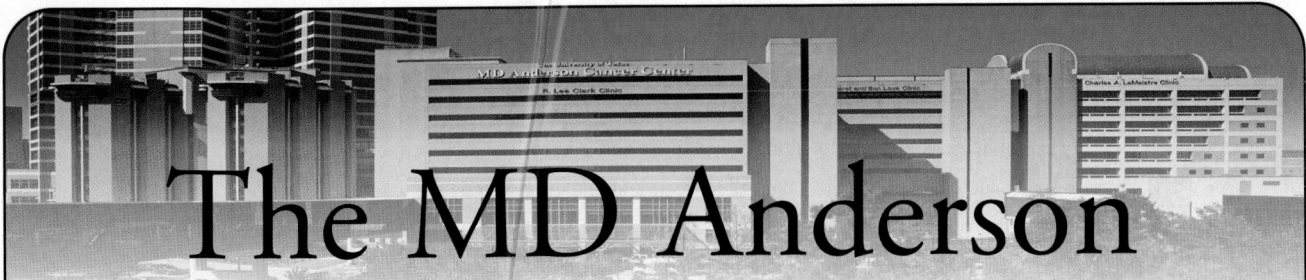

The MD Anderson
Manual *of*
MEDICAL
ONCOLOGY

NOTICE

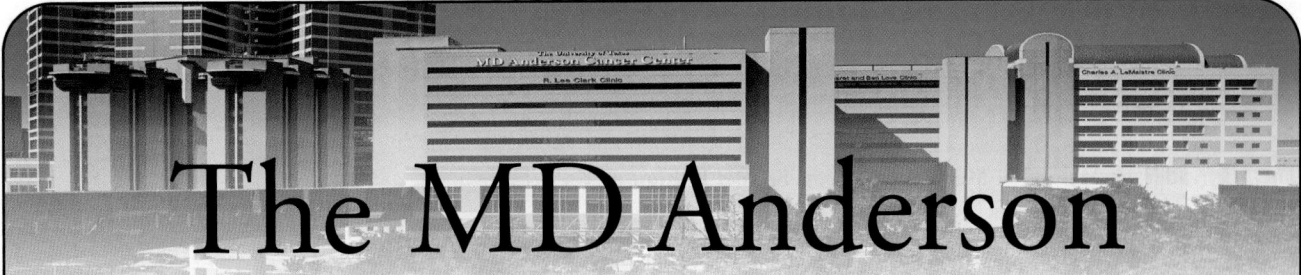

The MD Anderson
Manual *of*
MEDICAL
ONCOLOGY

Second Edition

Hagop M. Kantarjian, MD

Professor of Medicine
Chair, Department of Leukemia
The University of Texas MD Anderson Cancer Center
Houston, Texas

Robert A. Wolff, MD

Professor of Medicine
Department of Gastrointestinal Medical Oncology
The University of Texas MD Anderson Cancer Center
Houston, Texas

Charles A. Koller, MD

Professor of Medicine
Department of Leukemia
The University of Texas MD Anderson Cancer Center
Houston, Texas

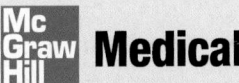 **Medical**

NewYork / Chicago / San Francisco / Lisbon / London / Madrid / Mexico City
Milan / New Delhi / San Juan / Seoul / Singapore / Sydney / Toronto

1 2 3 4 5 6 7 8 9 0   CTP/CTP   15 14 13 12 11

ISBN 978-0-07-170106-8
MHID 0-07-170106-0

This book was set in Times by Glyph International.
The editors were James Shanahan and Cindy Yoo.
The production supervisor was Sherri Souffrance.
Project management was provided by Deepti Narwat, Glyph International.
The designer was Marsha Cohen/Parallelogram; the cover designer was
Anthony Landi.
China Translation & Printing, Ltd., was printer and binder.

Cover Photo: Main Campus of MD Anderson. © 2010 The University of
Texas MD Anderson Cancer Center.

The authors wish to acknowledge the exceptional administrative and organizational contributions of Ann M. Sandler, without whom this project would not
have been completed.

Library of Congress Cataloging-in-Publication Data

Kantarjian, Hagop, 1952–
    The MD Anderson manual of medical oncology / Hagop M. Kantarjian,
Robert A. Wolff, Charles A. Koller. —2nd ed.
        p. ; cm.
    Manual of medical oncology
    Medical oncology
ISBN-13: 978-0-07-170106-8 (hardcover : alk. paper)
ISBN-10: 0-07-170106-0 (hardcover : alk. paper)
    1. Cancer--Handbooks, manuals, etc. 2.   Oncology—Handbooks, manu-
als, etc. I.   Wolff, Robert A., 1957- II.   Koller, Charles A. III.   University
of Texas M.D. Anderson Cancer Center. IV.   Title. V.   Title: Manual of
medical oncology. VI.   Title: Medical oncology.
    [DNLM: 1.   Neoplasms. QZ 200]
RC262.5.K36 2011
616.99'4—dc22
                                                                2010051541

CONTENTS

CONTRIBUTORS

Hesham Amin, MD
Associate Professor
Department of Hematopathology
The University of Texas MD Anderson Cancer Center
Houston, Texas

Eddie K. Abdalla, MD
Associate Professor
Department of Surgical Oncology
The University of Texas MD Anderson Cancer Center
Houston, Texas

Joann L. Ater, MD
Professor
Department of Pediatrics-Patient Care
The University of Texas MD Anderson Cancer Center
Houston, Texas

Tiffany P. Avery, MD, MPH
Clinical Fellow
Division of Cancer Medicine
The University of Texas MD Anderson Cancer Center
Houston, Texas

Rony Avritscher, MD
Assistant Professor
Department of Diagnostic Radiology
The University of Texas MD Anderson Cancer Center
Houston, Texas

Agop Y. Bedikian, MD
Professor
Department of Melanoma Medical Oncology
The University of Texas MD Anderson Cancer Center
Houston, Texas

Nishin A. Bhadkamkar, MD
Clinical Fellow
Division of Cancer Medicine
The University of Texas MD Anderson Cancer Center

Heather D. Brooks, MD
Clinical Fellow
Division of Cancer Medicine
The University of Texas MD Anderson Cancer Center
Houston, Texas

Carlos Bueso-Ramos, MD, PhD
Professor
Department of Hematopathology
The University of Texas MD Anderson Cancer Center
Houston, Texas

Nita R. Burrer, RN, MSN, ANP, CNS
Retired Nurse Practitioner in the Long-Term Follow-Up Clinic
Robin Bush Child and Adolescent Center
Department of Pediatrics-Patient Care
The University of Texas MD Anderson Cancer Center
Houston, Texas

Naifa Lamki Busaidy, MD
Assistant Professor
Department of Endocrine Neoplasia and Hormonal Disorders
The University of Texas MD Anderson Cancer Center
Houston, Texas

Aman U. Buzdar, MD
Professor
Department of Breast Medical Oncology
The University of Texas MD Anderson Cancer Center
Houston, Texas

Richard E. Champlin, MD
Professor and Chair
Department of Stem Cell Transplantation and Cellular Therapy
The University of Texas MD Anderson Cancer Center
Houston, Texas

Mariana Chavez-MacGregor, MD, MSc
Clinical Fellow
Division of Cancer Medicine
The University of Texas MD Anderson Cancer Center
Houston, Texas

Roy F. Chemaly, MD, MPH, MBA
Associate Professor
Department of Infectious Diseases, Infection Control, and Employee Health
The University of Texas MD Anderson Cancer Center
Houston, Texas

Hubert H. Chuang, MD, PhD
Assistant Professor
Department of Nuclear Medicine
The University of Texas MD Anderson Cancer Center
Houston, Texas

Anthony Conley, MD
Clinical Fellow
Division of Cancer Medicine
The University of Texas MD Anderson Cancer Center
Houston, Texas

Carlo M. Contreras, MD
Former Clinical Fellow
Division of Surgery
The University of Texas MD Anderson Cancer Center
Houston, Texas
Assistant Professor
Surgical Oncology
The University of South Alabama Mitchell Cancer Institute
Mobile, Alabama

Paul Corn, MD, PhD
Assistant Professor
Department of Genitourinary Medical Oncology
Genitourinary Medical Oncology
The University of Texas MD Anderson Cancer Center
Houston, Texas

Jorge Cortes, MD
Professor and Deputy Chair
Department of Leukemia
The University of Texas MD Anderson Cancer Center
Houston, Texas

Christopher H. Crane, MD
Professor
Department of Radiation Oncology
The University of Texas MD Anderson Cancer Center
Houston, Texas

Massimo Cristofanilli, MD
Former Professor
Department of Breast Medical Oncology
The University of Texas MD Anderson Cancer Center
Houston, Texas
Professor and Chairman
Department of Medical Oncology
Fox Chase Cancer Center
Philadelphia, Pennsylvania

Bogdan A. Czerniak, MD, PhD
Professor and Chair Ad Interim
Department of Pathology
The University of Texas MD Anderson Cancer Center
Houston, Texas

Bouthaina S. Dabaja, MD
Associate Professor
Department of Radiation Oncology
The University of Texas MD Anderson Cancer Center
Houston, Texas

Michael A. Davies, MD, PhD
Assistant Professor
Department of Melanoma Medical Oncology
The University of Texas MD Anderson Cancer Center
Houston, Texas

Windy Marie Dean-Colomb, MD, PhD
Clinical Fellow
Division of Cancer Medicine
The University of Texas MD Anderson Cancer Center
Houston, Texas

Colin P.N. Dinney, MD
Professor and Chair
Department of Urology
The University of Texas MD Anderson Cancer Center
Houston, Texas

Madeleine Duvic, MD
Professor
Department of Dermatology
The University of Texas MD Anderson Cancer Center
Houston, Texas

George A. Eapen, MD
Associate Professor
Department of Pulmonary Medicine
The University of Texas MD Anderson Cancer Center
Houston, Texas

Ahmed Elsayem, MD
Associate Professor
Department of Palliative Care and Rehabilitation Medicine
The University of Texas MD Anderson Cancer Center
Houston, Texas

Cathy Eng, MD
Associate Professor
Department of Gastrointestinal Medical Oncology
The University of Texas MD Anderson Cancer Center
Houston, Texas

Stefan Faderl, MD
Associate Professor
Department of Leukemia
The University of Texas MD Anderson Cancer Center
Houston, Texas

Michelle Fanale, MD
Assistant Professor
Department of Lymphoma/Myeloma
The University of Texas MD Anderson Cancer Center
Houston, Texas

Luis E. Fayad, MD
Associate Professor
Department of Lymphoma/Myeloma
The University of Texas MD Anderson Cancer Center
Houston, Texas

Michael J. Fisch, MD, MPH, FACP
Associate Professor and Chair
Department of General Oncology
The University of Texas MD Anderson Cancer Center
Houston, Texas

Keith F. Fournier, MD
Assistant Professor
Department of Surgical Oncology
The University of Texas MD Anderson Cancer Center
Houston, Texas

Nathan Fowler, MD
Assistant Professor
Department of Lymphoma/Myeloma
The University of Texas MD Anderson Cancer Center
Houston, Texas

Jack Fu, MD
Assistant Professor
Department of Palliative Care and Rehabilitation Medicine
Section of Physical Medicine and Rehabilitation
The University of Texas MD Anderson Cancer Center
Houston, Texas

Weijun Fu, MD, PhD
Visiting Associate Professor
Department of Lymphoma/Myeloma
The University of Texas MD Anderson Cancer Center
Houston, Texas

Amber Fullmer, PharmD, BCOP
Clinical Pharmacy Specialist
Division of Pharmacy
The University of Texas MD Anderson Cancer Center
Houston, Texas

Guillermo Garcia-Manero, MD
Professor
Department of Leukemia
The University of Texas MD Anderson Cancer Center
Houston, Texas

Ravin J. Garg, MD
Clinical Fellow
Division of Cancer Medicine
The University of Texas MD Anderson Cancer Center
Houston, Texas

Don Gibbons, MD, PhD
Assistant Professor
Department of Thoracic/Head and Neck Medical Oncology
The University of Texas MD Anderson Cancer Center
Houston, Texas

Sergio Giralt, MD
Former Professor
Department of Stem Cell Transplantation and Cellular Therapy
The University of Texas MD Anderson Cancer Center
Houston, Texas
Professor
Adult Bone Marrow Transplant Service
Memorial Sloan-Kettering Cancer Center
New York, New York

Bonnie S. Glisson, MD
Professor and Deputy Chair
Department of Thoracic/Head and Neck Medical Oncology
The University of Texas MD Anderson Cancer Center
Houston, Texas

Kathryn A. Gold, MD
Clinical Fellow
Division of Cancer Medicine
The University of Texas MD Anderson Cancer Center
Houston, Texas

Bruno P. Granwehr, MD, MS
Assistant Professor
Department of Infectious Diseases, Infection Control and Employee
Health
The University of Texas MD Anderson Cancer Center
Houston, Texas

G. Brandon Gunn, MD
Assistant Professor
Department of Radiation Oncology
The University of Texas MD Anderson Cancer Center
Houston, Texas

Sanjay Gupta, MD
Associate Professor
Department of Diagnostic Radiology
The University of Texas MD Anderson Cancer Center
Houston, Texas

Mouhammed Amir Habra, MD
Assistant Professor
Department of Endocrine Neoplasia and Hormonal Disorders
The University of Texas MD Anderson Cancer Center
Houston, Texas

Fredrick B. Hagemeister, MD
Professor
Department of Lymphoma/Myeloma
The University of Texas MD Anderson Cancer Center
Houston, Texas

Karin M.E. Hahn, MD, MSc, MPH, MSc (EBHC)
Associate Professor
Department of General Oncology
The University of Texas MD Anderson Cancer Center
Houston, Texas

Bryan T. Hennessy
Former Assistant Professor
Department of Gyncologic Oncology
The University of Texas MD Anderson Cancer Center
Houston, Texas

Sigmund H. Hsu, MD
Former Assistant Professor
Department of Neuro-Oncology
The University of Texas MD Anderson Cancer Center
Houston, Texas
Assistant Vice President
Susquehanna Resources and Environment
Binghamton, New York

Tzu-chuan Jane Huang, MD
Clinical Fellow
Division of Cancer Medicine
The University of Texas MD Anderson Cancer Center
Houston, Texas

Kelly K. Hunt, MD
Professor
Department of Surgical Oncology
The University of Texas MD Anderson Cancer Center
Houston, Texas

Patrick Hwu, MD
Professor and Chair
Department of Melanoma Medical Oncology
The University of Texas MD Anderson Cancer Center
Houston, Texas

Elias Jabbour, MD
Assistant Professor
Department of Leukemia
The University of Texas MD Anderson Cancer Center
Houston, Texas

Norman Jaffe, MD
Professor Emeritus
Department of Pediatrics-Patient Care
The University of Texas MD Anderson Cancer Center
Houston, Texas

Nitin Jain, MD
Former Clinical Fellow
Division of Cancer Medicine
The University of Texas MD Anderson Cancer Center
Houston, Texas
Fellow
Section of Hematology Oncology
The University of Chicago Medical Center
Chicago, Illinois

John Andrew Jakob, MD, PhD
Clinical Fellow
Division of Cancer Medicine
The University of Texas MD Anderson Cancer Center
Houston, Texas

Milind M. Javle, MD
Associate Professor
Department of Gastrointestinal Medical Oncology
The University of Texas MD Anderson Cancer Center
Houston, Texas

Faye Johnson, MD, PhD
Associate Professor
Department of Thoracic/Head and Neck Medical Oncology
The University of Texas MD Anderson Cancer Center
Houston, Texas

Eric Jonasch, MD
Associate Professor
Department of Genitourinary Medical Oncology
The University of Texas MD Anderson Cancer Center
Houston, Texas

Hagop M. Kantarjian, MD
Professor and Chair
Department of Leukemia
The University of Texas MD Anderson Cancer Center
Houston, Texas

Ahmed O. Kaseb, MD
Assistant Professor
Department of Gastrointestinal Medical Oncology
The University of Texas MD Anderson Cancer Center
Houston, Texas

John J. Kavanagh, MD
Former Professor
Department of Gynecologic Medical Oncology
The University of Texas MD Anderson Cancer Center
Houston, Texas
Professor
Faculty of Medicine
Chulalongkorn University
Bangkok, Thailand

Merrill S. Kies, MD
Professor
Department of Thoracic/Head and Neck Medical Oncology
Deputy Head
Division of Cancer Medicine
The University of Texas MD Anderson Cancer Center
Houston, Texas

Eric S. Kim, MD
Clinical Fellow
Division of Cancer Medicine
The University of Texas MD Anderson Cancer Center
Houston, Texas

Kevin B. Kim, MD
Associate Professor
Department of Melanoma Medical Oncology
The University of Texas MD Anderson Cancer Center
Houston, Texas

Sergej Konoplev, MD, PhD
Assistant Professor
Department of Hematopathology
The University of Texas MD Anderson Cancer Center
Houston, Texas

Dimitrios P. Kontoyiannis, MD, MS, ScD
Professor and Deputy Chair
Department of Infectious Diseases, Infection Control, and Employee Health
The University of Texas MD Anderson Cancer Center
Houston, Texas

Charles A. Koller, MD
Professor
Department of Leukemia
The University of Texas MD Anderson Cancer Center
Houston, Texas

Scott Kopetz, MD, PhD
Assistant Professor
Department of Genitourinary Medical Oncology
The University of Texas MD Anderson Cancer Center
Houston, Texas

Sunil Krishnan, MD
Associate Professor
Department of Radiation Oncology
The University of Texas MD Anderson Cancer Center
Houston, Texas

Maria Jimena Lange, MD
Former Clinical Fellow
Department of Gynecological Medical Oncology
The University of Texas MD Anderson Cancer Center
Houston, Texas
Hospital de Clinicas Jose de San Martin
Universidad de Buenos Aires
Buenos Aires, Argentina

Jeffrey E. Lee, MD
Professor and Chair
Department of Surgical Oncology
The University of Texas MD Anderson Cancer Center
Houston, Texas

Christopher Lieu, MD
Clinical Fellow
Division of Cancer Medicine
The University of Texas MD Anderson Cancer Center
Houston, Texas

Zita Dubauskas Lim, PA-C
Physician Assistant
Department of Genitourinary Medical Oncology
The University of Texas MD Anderson Cancer Center
Houston, Texas

Pei Lin, MD
Associate Professor
Department of Hematopathology
The University of Texas MD Anderson Cancer Center
Houston, Texas

Nina Liu, MD
Former Clinical Fellow
Division of Cancer Medicine
The University of Texas MD Anderson Cancer Center
Houston, Texas
Kaiser Permanente
San Diego, California

Christopher Logothetis, MD
Professor and Chair
Department of Genitourinary Medical Oncology
The University of Texas MD Anderson Cancer Center
Houston, Texas

Gabriel Lopez, MD
Former Clinical Fellow
Department of Palliative Care and Rehab Medicine
The University of Texas MD Anderson Cancer Center
Houston, Texas
Clinical Fellow
Hematology/Oncology
East Carolina University
Brody School of Medicine
Leo W. Jenkins Cancer Center
Greenville, North Carolina

Gary Lu, MD
Assistant Professor
Department of Hematopathology
The University of Texas MD Anderson Cancer Center
Houston, Texas

Anita Mahajan, MD
Professor
Department of Radiation Oncology
The University of Texas MD Anderson Cancer Center
Houston, Texas

Ellen F. Manzullo, MD
Professor and Deputy Chair
General Internal Medicine
The University of Texas MD Anderson Cancer Center
Houston, Texas

Maurie Markman, MD
Former Chair
Department of Gynecologic Medical Oncology
The University of Texas MD Anderson Cancer Center
Houston, Texas
Vice President of Patient Oncology Services
Cancer Treatment Centers of America
Philadelphia, Pennsylvania

Jessica Masterson, MD
Clinical Fellow
Division of Cancer Medicine
The University of Texas MD Anderson Cancer Center
Houston, Texas

Surena F. Matin, MD
Associate Professor
Department of Urology
The University of Texas MD Anderson Cancer Center
Houston, Texas

David J. McConkey, PhD
Professor
Deparment of Urology
The University of Texas MD Anderson Cancer Center
Houston, Texas

Peter McLaughlin, MD
Clinical Professor
Department of Lymphoma/Myeloma
The University of Texas MD Anderson Cancer Center
Houston, Texas

L. Jeffrey Medeiros, MD
Professor and Chair
Department of Hematopathology
The University of Texas MD Anderson Cancer Center
Houston, Texas

Randall E. Millikan, MD, PhD
Associate Professor
Department of Genitourinary Medical Oncology
The University of Texas MD Anderson Cancer Center
Houston, Texas

Susan O'Brien, MD
Professor
Department of Leukemia
The University of Texas MD Anderson Cancer Center
Houston, Texas

Bruno C. Odisio, MD
Clinical Fellow
Department of Diagnostic Radiology
The Univeristy of Texas MD Anderson Cancer Center
Houston, Texas

Michael J. Overman, MD
Assistant Professor
Department of Gastrointestinal Medical Oncology
The University of Texas MD Anderson Cancer Center
Houston, Texas

Lance C. Pagliaro, MD
Associate Professor
Department of Genitourinary Medical Oncology
The University of Texas MD Anderson Cancer Center
Houston, Texas

Sameer A. Parikh, MD
Clinical Fellow
Department of Leukemia
The University of Texas MD Anderson Cancer Center
Houston, Texas

Min S. Park, MD
Instructor
Department of Sarcoma Medical Oncology
The University of Texas MD Anderson Cancer Center
Houston, Texas

Sapna P. Patel, MD
Clinical Fellow
Division of Cancer Medicine
The University of Texas MD Anderson Cancer Center
Houston, Texas

Shreyaskumar Patel, MD, MS
Professor and Deputy Chair
Department of Sarcoma Medical Oncology
The University of Texas MD Anderson Cancer Center
Houston, Texas

Naveen Pemmaraju, MD
Clinical Fellow
Division of Cancer Medicine
The University of Texas MD Anderson Cancer Center
Houston, Texas

Alexandria T. Phan, MD
Associate Professor
Department of Gastrointestinal Medical Oncology
The University of Texas MD Anderson Cancer Center
Houston, Texas

Katherine M. Pisters, MD
Professor
Department of Thoracic/Head and Neck Medical Oncology
The University of Texas MD Anderson Cancer Center
Houston, Texas

Louis L. Pisters, MD
Professor
Department of Urology
The University of Texas MD Anderson Cancer Center
Houston, Texas

Jenny Pozadzides, MD
Clinical Fellow
Division of Cancer Medicine
The University of Texas MD Anderson Cancer Center

Sujit Prabhu, MD
Associate Professor
Department of Neurosurgery
The University of Texas MD Anderson Cancer Center
Houston, Texas

Barbara Pro, MD
Former Associate Professor
Department of Lymphoma/Myeloma
The University of Texas MD Anderson Cancer Center
Houston, Texas
Associate Professor
Department of Medical Oncology
Fox Chase Cancer Center
Philadelphia, Pennsylvania

Muzaffar H. Qazilbash, MD
Associate Professor
Department of Stem Cell Transplantation and Cellular Therapy
The University of Texas MD Anderson Cancer Center
Houston, Texas

Pedro T. Ramirez, MD
Associate Professor
Department of Gynecologic Oncology
The University of Texas MD Anderson Cancer Center
Houston, Texas

Ronald P. Rapini, MD
Professor and Chair
Department of Dermatology
Professor of Pathology
The University of Texas MD Anderson Cancer Center
Houston, Texas

Suresh K. Reddy, MD
Professor
Department of Palliative Care and Rehabilitation Medicine
The University of Texas MD Anderson Cancer Center
Houston, Texas

Valerie K. Reed, MD
Assistant Professor
Department of Radiation Oncology
The University of Texas MD Anderson Cancer Center
Houston, Texas

Adan Rios, MD
Former Assistant Professor
Department of Clinical Immunology and Biological Therapy
Associate Professor
Department of Internal Medicine
The University of Texas Medical School at Houston
Houston, Texas

Miguel A. Rodriquez-Bigas, MD
Professor
Department of Surgical Oncology
The University of Texas MD Anderson Cancer Center
Houston, Texas

M. Alma Rodriguez, MD
Professor
Department of Lymphoma/Myeloma
Vice President of Medical Affairs
The University of Texas MD Anderson Cancer Center
Houston, Texas

Kenneth V.I. Rolston, MD
Professor
Department of Infectious Diseases, Infection Control and Employee Health
The University of Texas MD Anderson Cancer Center
Houston, Texas

Pamela N. Schultz, PhD, RN
Former Research Nurse
The Department of Endocrine Neoplasia and Hormonal Disorders
The University of Texas MD Anderson Cancer Center
Houston, Texas
Professor and Interim Associate Dean
Director of the School of Nursing
New Mexico State University
La Cruces, New Mexico

Nina Shah, MD
Assistant Professor
Department of Stem Cell Transplantation and Cellular Therapy
The University of Texas MD Anderson Cancer Center
Houston, Texas

Ki Y. Shin, MD
Assistant Professor
Department of Gastrointestinal Medical Oncology
The University of Texas MD Anderson Cancer Center
Houston, Texas

Nicole A. Shonka, MD
Clinical Fellow
Department of Neuro-Oncology
The University of Texas MD Anderson Cancer Center
Houston, Texas

Rachna T. Shroff, MD
Assistant Professor
Department of Gastrointestinal Medical Oncology
The University of Texas MD Anderson Cancer Center
Houston, Texas

Arlene Siefker-Radtke, MD
Associate Professor
Department of Genitourinary Medical Oncology
The University of Texas MD Anderson Cancer Center
Houston, Texas

Charles J. Stava, MHSA
Program Manager, Internal Medicine
Department of Endocrine Neoplasia: and Hormonal Disorders
The University of Texas MD Anderson Cancer Center
Houston, Texas

William S. Stevenson, MBBS, PhD
Former Research Fellow
Department of Leukemia
The University of Texas MD Anderson Cancer Center
Houston, Texas
Clinical Senior Lecturer
Department of Haematology
Royal North Shore Hospital
Sydney, Australia

Grace K. Suh, MD
Clinical Fellow
Division of Cancer Medicine
The University of Texas MD Anderson Cancer Center
Houston, Texas

Siriwan Tangjitgamol, MD
Former Clinical Fellow
Department of Gynecologic Oncology
The University of Texas MD Anderson Cancer Center
Houston, Texas
Department of Obstetrics and Gynecology
Bangkok Metropolitan Administration Medical College and Vajira Hospital
Bangkok, Thailand

Nizar M. Tannir, MD
Associate Professor
Department of Genitourinary Medical Oncology
The University of Texas MD Anderson Cancer Center
Houston, Texas

Jeffrey J. Tarrand, MD, MS
Professor
Department of Laboratory Medicine
The University of Texas MD Anderson Cancer Center
Houston, Texas

Rachel L. Theriault, MD
Clinical Fellow
Division of Cancer Medicine
The University of Texas MD Anderson Cancer Center
Houston, Texas

Jonathon C. Trent, MD, PhD
Associate Professor
Department of Sarcoma Medical Oncology
The University of Texas MD Anderson Cancer Center
Houston, Texas

Vicente Valero, MD
Professor and Deputy Chair
Department of Breast Medical Oncology
The University of Texas MD Anderson Cancer Center
Houston, Texas

Gauri R. Varadhachary, MD
Associate Professor
Department of Gastrointestinal Medical Oncology
The University of Texas MD Anderson Cancer Center
Houston, Texas

Rena Vassilopoulou-Sellin, MD
Clinical Professor
Department of Endocrine Neoplasia and Hormonal Disorders
The University of Texas MD Anderson Cancer Center
Houston, Texas

Srdan Verstovsek, MD, PhD
Associate Professor
Department of Leukemia
The University of Texas MD Anderson Cancer Center
Houston, Texas

Michael Wang, MD
Associate Professor
Department of Lymphoma/Myeloma
The University of Texas MD Anderson Cancer Center
Houston, Texas

Donna M. Weber, MD
Associate Professor
Department of Lymphoma/Myeloma
The University of Texas MD Anderson Cancer Center
Houston, Texas

Jason Westin, MD
Clinical Fellow
Division of Cancer Medicine
The University of Texas MD Anderson Cancer Center
Houston, Texas

William Nassib William Jr., MD
Assistant Professor
Department of Thoracic/Head and Neck Oncology
The University of Texas MD Anderson Cancer Center
Houston, Texas

Robert A. Wolff, MD
Professor
Department of Gastrointestinal Medical Oncology
The University of Houston MD Anderson Cancer Center
Houston, Texas

Christopher G. Wood, MD
Professor
Department of Urology
The University of Texas MD Anderson Cancer Center
Houston, Texas

James C. Yao, MD
Associate Professor
Department of Gastrointestinal Medical Oncology
The University of Texas MD Anderson Cancer Center
Houston, Texas

Sai-Ching Jim Yeung, MD, PhD
Associate Professor
Department of General Internal Medicine
The University of Texas MD Anderson Cancer Center
Houston, Texas

Carrie Yuen, MD
Clinical Fellow
Department of Stem Cell Transplantation and Cellular Therapy
The University of Texas MD Anderson Cancer Center
Houston, Texas

W.K. Alfred Yung, MD
Professor and Chair
Department of Neuro-Oncology
The University of Texas MD Anderson Cancer Center
Houston, Texas

PREFACE

When we first envisioned *The MD Anderson Manual of Medical Oncology*, we hoped it would fill an important void in oncology reference material by serving as a hands-on resource for the practicing oncologist. The first edition, published in 2006, was written exclusively by our faculty and fellows with the idea of giving a bird's eye view of how multidisciplinary care was practiced at our institution. We were proud of that initial effort and pleased that the book received very positive reviews from several high-impact journals, including the *JAMA*, *Lancet*, and the *New England Journal of Medicine*. In addition, feedback from our broad multinational readership inspired us to move forward with an enhanced second edition.

In the second edition, we have remained faithful to the guiding principles of our first effort, providing a visually stimulating, practice-oriented reference which articulates our unique multidisciplinary approach to cancer care. We have also continued the tradition of including evidence-based management algorithms in the form of flowcharts and diagrams shaped by the clinical experience of our world-class faculty to provide readers with a practical guide to the diagnostic and therapeutic strategies used at MD Anderson.

Importantly, our new version is not merely an update of the first, but contains new chapters on myelodysplastic syndrome, myeloproliferative neoplasms, T-cell lymphomas, small bowel and appendiceal cancers, inflammatory breast cancer, and penile cancer. In addition, some chapters now provide embedded comments sharing the perspective of other experts at MD Anderson, including our colleagues in surgical oncology, radiotherapy, pulmonology, and pathology. Also in this edition, we have asked our authors to discuss future directions with special emphasis on personalized cancer care.

We hope this edition serves to help oncologists everywhere provide high-quality, state-of-the-art cancer care to their patients, who deserve nothing less.

Hagop M. Kantarjian, MD
Robert A. Wolff, MD
Charles A. Koller, MD

FOREWORD

The MD Anderson Manual of Medical Oncology, Second Edition articulates the personalized, multidisciplinary approach to cancer management pioneered by The University of Texas MD Anderson Cancer Center. This approach has contributed to our ranking as number one in cancer care in 8 of the past 10 years in the *U.S. News & World Report's* "America's Best Hospitals" survey. Our unique perspective has evolved from decades of clinical practice and research with more than 800,000 patients treated. This volume is designed to bring a pragmatic approach to cancer management that may serve as a guide for oncologists around the world. The text reflects how MD Anderson currently operates, including many patient care practices that would not have been recognized by practitioners just a decade ago. In a single year, 96,500 people with cancer—33,200 of them new patients—seek care at MD Anderson. Many of them participate in the largest clinical research program in the nation exploring novel therapies as well as our personalized approach to treatment evident in the nearly 12,000 patients enrolled in therapeutic clinical trials. Since the first edition, we have improved our ability to identify biomarkers that are predictive for survival, a major triumph in medical oncology that is demonstrated throughout the text.

The current edition emphasizes and discusses recent developments in diagnostic procedures, which include the incorporation of new molecular markers and revised staging systems. This edition also emphasizes how imaging and molecular profiling can prevent administration of overly aggressive, toxic treatment regimens, or invasive surgery to treat superficial or indolent tumors.

Two major advances in therapeutic approaches over the past decades are emphasized in *The MD Anderson Manual of Medical Oncology*, Second Edition: (1) better timing of therapeutic modalities to enhance response and (2) a growing capacity to individualize treatment to target-specific patterns of genomics, proteomics, growth factors, and cell signaling pathways identifiable today through high-throughput microarray and other advanced technologies. Most chapters offer a thorough review of relevant signaling pathways as well as major clinical studies of potential therapeutic agents that target components of these pathways.

The Manual emphasizes new therapies that have emerged from progress in our understanding of the biology of various cancers. As the genetic and epigenetic events driving carcinogenesis, invasion, metastasis, and the interaction of the tumor cells with host's microenvironment are elucidated, the development and testing of targeted molecules have mushroomed, resulting in a wider selection of therapeutic drug combinations. Discussion of new therapeutic agents used alone or in combination with preexisting therapies is expanded in the new edition. Case examples illustrate successful treatment strategies throughout the text, often using a personalized approach to selecting appropriate targeted therapies.

Reflecting new advances in our approach to cancer management, the second edition of *The MD Anderson Manual of Medical Oncology* features several new chapters. For example, special chapters on myelodysplastic syndromes and Philadelphia chromosome-myeloproliferative neoplasms have been added to be based on the 2008 changes in the WHO classification of these disorders as neoplasms, as well as significant new advances in their diagnosis, risk assessment, and management. In the new edition, aggressive B-cell and peripheral T-cell lymphomas now warrant separate focused chapters to enable greater attention to novel treatment strategies for T-cell lymphomas. Likewise, pancreatic cancer and hepatobiliary malignancies are now covered separately to devote more attention to promising novel strategies that have the potential to improve the prognosis for pancreatic cancer. A new chapter on neoplasms of the small bowel and appendix has also been added. Inflammatory breast cancer, previously mentioned briefly alongside locally advanced breast cancers, now has its own expanded chapter. In addition, this edition now contains a chapter on penile cancer.

Also new to the second edition are special commentaries invited from other subspecialists from fields such as pulmonary medicine, radiation oncology, and surgery to discuss other perspectives on management:

- A radiation oncologist discusses new strategies to reduce the long-term toxic effects of treatment of the Hodgkin lymphoma such as the risk of future secondary cancers.
- A new, minimally invasive technology for tissue sampling is recommended to improve the diagnostic accuracy of mediastinal lymph node staging in non–small cell lung cancer.
- Surgical perspectives are added to the chapter on appendiceal carcinoma, including how the surgical plan is individualized for patients whose cancer treatment began outside of MD Anderson.
- A pathologist contributes discussion of immunohistochemical markers shared by all neuroendocrine carcinomas regardless of their anatomic location.

- A special discussion of surgical options after neoadjuvant chemotherapy is embedded within the chapter on early-stage and locally advanced breast cancer.
- A research scientist adds his assessment of how a personalized medicine approach to the management of urothelial cancers would dramatically improve patient outcomes.
- Two commentaries on the role of radiation therapy and surgical management of brain tumors are introduced in the chapter on tumors of the central nervous system.
- A microbiologist comments on specific adaptations, laboratories need to make to provide adequate microbiological diagnosis of mold and viral infections in cancer patients.
- A surgeon adds his perspective on how he integrated referral to palliative care services into management of his patient with pancreatic cancer.

While the Manual discusses special considerations in the treatment of populations such as the elderly and those with comorbidities, the book stresses the many ways that recent progress in reducing treatment-associated toxicity has made advanced age less of a contraindication to many effective therapeutic regimens. Morbidity associated with surgery and radiation therapy has greatly decreased over the past decade, and many of the new, targeted oral agents have little or no toxicity.

To help clinicians quickly assess cancer management options, every chapter includes abundant tables, diagrams, and imaging photos. These include, for example, treatment algorithms and decision trees developed at MD Anderson for specific cancers or disease subtypes; promising novel therapy targets and the latest clinical trial phase of drugs targeting them; and new molecular therapies recommended to overcome resistance to previously effective therapies.

The new era of novel personalized, targeted therapeutics has also sparked the recent evolution of another crucial advancement in management of metastatic disease: the transition from sequential care culminating in the sole delivery of palliative care, to integration of ongoing active disease treatment with simultaneous interdisciplinary symptom control, palliative care, and rehabilitation to improve quality of life. Clinicians at MD Anderson no longer approach advanced metastatic disease management with palliative care goals alone; now these patients are often offered frontline cancer treatment and the opportunity to participate in clinical trials for investigational drugs. The chapter on defining palliative care in oncology starts with a traditional case vignette of a patient with metastatic pancreatic cancer who did not receive palliative care until he/she had discontinued chemotherapy, then explains the various ways in which integration of palliative and symptom care earlier in the treatment could have benefited him/her and his/her family.

In recognition of the growing pool of patients who are surviving their cancer, MD Anderson has greatly expanded programs for cancer survivors since publication of the first edition. Chapters on long-term survival and follow-up demonstrate the additional utility of this book for clinicians outside the specialty of oncology, as a high proportion of the growing number of cancer survivors will be followed by a primary care physician, cardiologist, or other specialist in their home community. The text's description of the results from MD Anderson's survey of cancer survivors serves as an essential guide to typical long-term health problems both physicians and rehabilitation specialists can expect to manage.

Over the past decade, the practice of medical oncology at MD Anderson has truly evolved to epitomize the translational research concept of "bench to bedside and back," along with an increasingly personalized approach that considers the "molecular fingerprint" of the patient's cancer in treatment decisions—a paradigm shift that this volume pertinently exhibits.

Waun Ki Hong, MD
American Cancer Society Professor
Samsung Distinguished University Chair in Cancer Medicine
Division Head, Cancer Medicine
Professor, Thoracic/Head and Neck Medical Oncology
The University of Texas MD Anderson Cancer Center
Houston, Texas
May 2011

Leukemia

ACUTE LYMPHOBLASTIC LEUKEMIA

Elias Jabbour
Amber Fullmer
Stefan Faderl

■ EPIDEMIOLOGY AND ETIOLOGY

Acute lymphoblastic leukemia (ALL) is characterized by the expansion and proliferation of lymphoid cells in the bone marrow, blood, and other organs. ALL occurs with an incidence of 1 to 1.5 per 100,000 population, although with a bimodal distribution: an early peak at around the age of 4 to 5 years where the incidence may be as high as 4 to 5 per 100,000 population, followed by a second gradual increase at around age 50 years where it reaches up to 2 per 100,000 population. ALL represents the most common childhood pediatric leukemia representing about 80% of acute leukemias, while it comprises only 20% of adult leukemias. The median age of ALL patients in most registry studies is between 25 and 35 years. ALL is the most common type of cancer in children aged 0 to 14 years and is relatively uncommon in late childhood, adolescence, and young adulthood (1-4).

The etiology of ALL remains unknown (5,6). Chromosomal translocations occurring in utero during fetal hematopoiesis have been suggested as the primary cause for pediatric ALL, whereas postnatal genetic events are suggested as secondary contributors. A higher incidence of ALL is noted among mono and dizygotic twins of patients with ALL, reflecting possible genetic predisposition (7-9). Patients with trisomy 21, Klinefelter syndrome, and inherited diseases with excessive chromosomal fragility such as Fanconi anemia, Bloom syndrome, and ataxia-telangiectasia have a higher risk of developing ALL (10-14). Implications have also been made toward infectious etiologies (15,16). Associations between human T-cell lymphotropic virus type 1 and adult T-cell leukemia/lymphoma, as well as HIV and lymphoproliferative disorders have been established (17,18). In addition, associations with varicella and influenza viruses have also been suggested (19).

■ CLINICAL PRESENTATION AND LABORATORY ABNORMALITIES

Clinical presentation of ALL is usually nonspecific. Symptoms typically include fatigue, lack of energy, easy bruising or obvious bleeding, dyspnea, dizziness, and infections. "B-symptoms" such as fever, night sweats, or weight loss can occur. Extremity and joint pain may be the only presenting symptoms in children. Whereas symptoms related to hyperleukocytosis can occur in acute myeloid leukemia (AML), they are rare in ALL, even in the presence of high white cell counts. Central nervous system (CNS) involvement (cranial neuropathies, meningeal infiltration) at presentation, common in mature B-ALL (Burkitt leukemia) occurs in 5 to 8% of patients (20). Abdominal masses and significant spontaneous tumor lysis syndrome are more likely with mature B-ALL. Lymphadenopathy and hepatosplenomegaly, rarely symptomatic, are noted in 20% of the patients, with a higher incidence in T-cell ALL and mature B-cell ALL. The combination of hypercalcemia and lytic bone lesions is suggestive of adult T-cell leukemia/lymphoma (ATLL). Chin numbness (mental nerve involvement), when elicited in the history or exam, is suggestive or mature B-cell ALL (Burkitt).

■ DIAGNOSIS

The diagnosis of ALL relies on assessment of morphology, flow cytometry immunophenotyping, and identification of cytogenetic-molecular abnormalities (Fig. 1-1). Defining ALL subtypes with different response to therapy and prognosis, that are only partially discriminated by current diagnostic tools, may be further determined by genomic profiling.

MORPHOLOGY

The French–American–British (FAB) Cooperative Group distinguishes three ALL groups (L1-L3) based on morphologic criteria (cell size, cytoplasm, nucleoli,

basophilia, and vacuolation) (21). The morphologic distinction between L1 and L2 has lost its prognostic significance. L3 morphology is associated with mature B-cell ALL (Burkitt leukemia) and is characterized by a high rate of cell turnover giving rise to the "starry sky" pattern on marrow biopsies. ALL blasts are negative for myeloperoxidase, although low-level MPO positivity (3-5%) may occur in rare cases that otherwise lack expression of myeloid markers by flow cytometry (22-24). Terminal deoxynucleotidyl transferase (TdT), albeit not specific for ALL, remains a useful marker to separate malignant lymphocytosis from reactive processes, and to distinguish L3 ALL (TdT-negative) from other ALL subtypes (25-28).

The World Health Organization (WHO) proposed new guidelines for the diagnosis of neoplastic diseases of hematopoietic and lymphoid tissues or lymphomas (29,30). In addition to lowering the blast count to ≥20% as sufficient for an ALL diagnosis, the morphologic distinction of L1, L2, and L3 morphologies is abandoned as no longer relevant. Both FAB and WHO classification systems continue to rely heavily on morphological assessment (31).

IMMUNOPHENOTYPING

Identification of the immunophenotype has become a major part of ALL diagnosis (32-34). Three broad groups can be distinguished: precursor B-cell, mature

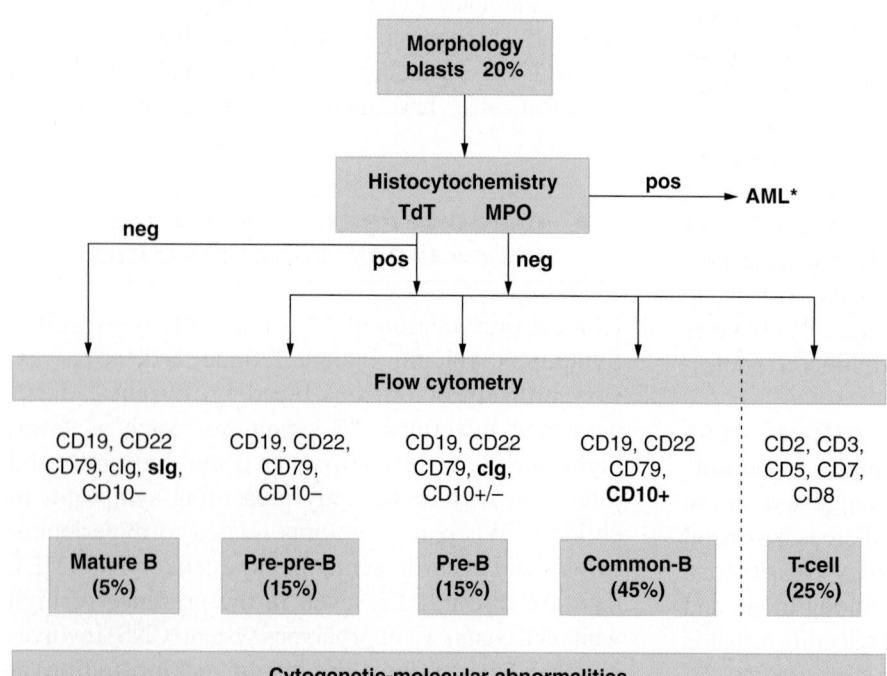

FIGURE 1-1. Diagnosis of ALL. *Low-level MPO positivity (3-5%) may occur in rare cases that otherwise lack expression of myeloid markers by flow cytometry.

TABLE 1-1	IMMUNOPHENOTYPIC CLASSIFICATION OF ALL			
B LINEAGE			**T LINEAGE**	
CD19/CD79a/CD22			*CD3 (surface/cytoplasmic)*	
Pre-pre-B ALL (pro–B-ALL)	—		Precursor T-ALL	CD1a, CD2, CD5, CD7, CD8, cCD3
Common ALL	CD10 (CALLA)		Mature T-ALL	Surface CD3 (plus any other T-cell markers)
Pre–B-ALL	Cytoplasmic IgM			
Mature B-ALL	Cytoplasmic or surface Igκ or λ			

B-cell, and T-cell ALL (Table 1-1). Precursor B-ALL blasts are positive for TdT, HLA-DR, CD19, and CD79a. Different stages of maturation have been defined as pre-pre-B ALL (pro–B-ALL), common ALL, and pre–B-ALL. Whereas pre-pre-B ALL blasts are positive for CD19, CD79a, or CD22, but no other B-cell differentiation antigens; common ALL (cALL, early pre–B-ALL) is characterized by expression of CD10 (common ALL antigen, CALLA), and pre–B-ALL by expression of cytoplasmic immunoglobulins with or without CD10. Mature B-cell ALL (Burkitt leukemia) blasts are positive for surface immunoglobulins (sIg, usually IgM), are clonal for κ or λ light chains, and are negative for TdT. Similar to B lineage ALL, T-ALL can be further stratified into subtypes based on different stages of intrathymic differentiation (35,36). Surface CD3 (sCD3) is the most lineage-specific marker for T-cell differentiation and is typically positive in mature T-ALL. Mature T-ALL is also positive for either CD4 or CD8 but not for both. Blasts in pre–T-ALL are negative for sCD3, but may still express cytoplasmic CD3 (37). Pre–T-ALL is negative for both CD4 and CD8. A different and arguably more practical classification divides T-ALL in early T-ALL (sCD3 negative, CD1a negative), thymic T-ALL (sCD3 negative or positive, but CD1a positive), and mature T-ALL (both sCD3 and CD1a positive). In a recent study, thymic T-ALL had excellent outcome with chemotherapy alone, whereas prognosis of early and mature T-ALL improved with stem cell transplantation.

Co-expression of markers from more than one lineage can be demonstrated in 15 to 50% in adult ALL and 5 to 35% in children (38-42). Using flow cytometry, lineage can be assigned in more than 95% of cases and truly biphenotypic leukemias are rare (43,44). Co-expression of markers from more than one lineage have not been found to be prognostically significant.

CYTOGENETIC-MOLECULAR ABNORMALITIES

Recurrent cytogenetic-molecular abnormalities are common in adult ALL (Table 1-2) (45-49). In addition to their prognostic significance, they provide insights into the molecular events underlying the leukemic phenotype. Differences in the frequency with which good and poor prognosis karyotypes occur in childhood versus adult ALL partly explain differences in outcome among children and adults. Oligonucleotide or cDNA microarray technologies are being investigated to identify previously unrecognized molecular ALL subtypes (50-54).

Epigenetic phenomena have emerged as a distinct molecular pathway for the definition of the leukemic phenotype (55). Hypermethylation occurs at a high frequency in ALL at presentation and at relapse (56-57). Analysis of the methylation status of several genes has identified subsets of ALL with a particular "hypermethylator" phenotype. Frequently involved genes include p73, the cyclin-dependent kinase inhibitors p15, and p57^{KIP2}, all of which play a crucial role in cell cycle regulatory pathways. Whereas methylation of a single gene did not affect outcome, simultaneous methylation of two or more has been associated with worse outcome (56-59). These observations have potential therapeutic consequences, as patients with a defined methylator phenotype may benefit from treatment with hypomethylating agents such as 5-aza-2'deoxycytidine (decitabine). Identification of genetic and epigenetic changes in adult ALL thus paves the road to the development of risk-adapted therapies.

■ THERAPY

FRONTLINE THERAPY

Therapy of ALL is among the most complex therapies of anticancer programs. Multiple drugs are molded into regimen-specific sequences of dose and time intensity

TABLE 1-2 | CYTOGENETIC AND MOLECULAR ABNORMALITIES IN ALL

Category	Cytogenetics	Involved Genes	FREQUENCY (%)	
			Adults	Children
Hyperdiploid			2-15	10-26
Hypodiploid			5-10	5-10
Pseudodiploid	t(9;22)(q34;q11)	BCR-ABL1	15-25	2-6
	del(9)(q21-22)	p15, p16	6-30	20
	t(4;11);t(9;11); t(11;19); t(3;11)	MLL	5-10	<5
	del(11)(q22-23)	ATM	25-30*	15*
	t(12;21)(p12;q22)	TEL-AML1	<1[†]	20-25[†]
	t(1;19)	E2A-PBX1	<5	<5
	t(17;19)	E2A-HLF	<5	<5
	t(1;14)(p32;q11)	TAL1	10-15	5-10
	t(7;9)(q34;q32)	TAL2	<1	<1
	t(10;14)(q24;q11)	HOX11	5-10	<5
	t(5;14)(q35;q32)	HOX11L2	1	2-3
	t(1;14)(p32;q11)	TCR	20-25[‡]	20-25[‡]
	del(13)(q14)	miR15/ miR16	<5	<5
	t(8;14); t(8;22); t(2;8)	C-MYC	5	2-5
	+8	?	10-12	2
	del(7p)	?	5-10	<5
	del(5q)	?	<2	<2
	del(6q); t(6;12)	?	5	<5

*As determined by LOH (loss of heterozygosity).
[†]As determined by PCR (polymerase chain reaction).
[‡]In T-cell ALL, overall incidence <10%.

with the goal to reconstitute normal hematopoiesis, prevent emergence of resistant subclones, provide adequate prophylaxis of sanctuary sites (eg, central nervous system [CNS], testicles), and eliminate minimal residual disease through postremission consolidation and maintenance (60). Three distinct phases and four components are distinguished: induction, intensified consolidation, maintenance, and CNS prophylaxis as the fourth component that accompanies induction and consolidation.

The combination of vincristine, corticosteroids, and anthracyclines represents the backbone of ALL induction regimens. This combination achieves complete remission (CR) rates of 72 to 92% with median remission durations of around 18 months (61). Dexamethasone is often substituted for prednisone because of better in vitro antileukemic activity and achievement of higher drug levels in the cerebrospinal fluid (CSF) (62,63). Although L-asparaginase is an important agent in the treatment of pediatric ALL, its role in adult ALL is not entirely well defined. Hematopoietic growth

factors during induction accelerate recovery from myelosuppression and allow timely administration of dose-intense treatment regimens (64). Consolidation represents a repetition of a modified induction schedule, rotational consolidation programs, or stem cell transplantation. Novel strategies try to emphasize subtype- and risk-oriented approaches of consolidation programs.

Daily 6-mercaptopurine, weekly methotrexate, and monthly pulses of vincristine and prednisone, given over 2 to 3 years are the mainstay of maintenance therapy. Extension of maintenance beyond 3 years, as well as omission or shortening of therapy is not beneficial. No maintenance therapy is given in mature B-cell ALL as these patients have a high cure rate with short-term dose-intense regimens, and relapses beyond the first year in remission are rare. The best maintenance for patients with Philadelphia (Ph)-positive ALL remains disputed, but should incorporate effective BCR-ABL tyrosine kinase inhibitors (TKIs).

Although CNS disease is uncommon at diagnosis (<10%), it can increase to as high as 50 to 75% at 1 year without CNS-directed therapy (65-67). Standard prophylaxis for CNS malignancy can involve radiation therapy, systemic chemotherapy, intrathecal (IT) chemotherapy, or a combination thereof. Cranial irradiation is associated with adverse effects such as secondary neoplasms, endocrinopathy, neurocognitive dysfunction, and neurotoxicity (68-70). Combining early intensive systemic and IT chemotherapy can lower the CNS relapse rate in patients with ALL and provide the opportunity to omit prophylactic cranial irradiation (71). High-dose cytarabine (1-7.5 mg/m^2) and methotrexate (5-8 g/m^2) have the ability to penetrate the blood brain barrier (BBB) and can serve as CNS prophylaxis (72-75). However, it is difficult to maintain prolonged therapeutic concentrations of drug in the CSF using only systemic chemotherapy. Furthermore, systemic therapy is associated with widespread toxicities. High-dose cytarabine is associated with hepatic toxicities, cerebellar dysfunction, mucositis, diarrhea, rash, and fever (76). High-dose methotrexate is associated with renal dysfunction, transient hepatitis, mucositis, and (rarely) neurotoxicity (77). The inclusion of IT chemotherapy in CNS prophylaxis protocols aims to improve the efficacy of systemic therapy while circumventing their limitations. IT chemotherapy allows direct intra-CSF treatment and potentially sustained therapeutic drug concentration in the CSF. Commonly used IT therapies include methotrexate, cytarabine, liposomal cytarabine, and thiotepa. In the absence of IT therapy, isolated CNS recurrence can account for 10 to 16% of relapses, warranting the inclusion of IT chemotherapy in CNS prophylactic regimens. The use of IT chemotherapy in combination with the hyper-CVAD regimen reduced the incidence of CNS relapse to 4% (65).

Hyper-CVAD

Our group at MD Anderson Cancer Center (MDACC) has adapted the hyper-CVAD regimen, a dose-intensive regimen with significant activity in childhood Burkitt disease, for therapy of adult patients with ALL. The regimen is composed of fractionated cyclophosphamide, vincrisine, doxorubicin, and dexamethasone (hyper-CVAD) alternating with methotrexate and high doses of cytarabine for a total of eight cycles of induction and consolidation (Table 1-3) (65). The principles of this regimen include: (1) dose intensive systemic chemotherapy to induce remission quickly followed by intensified consolidation; (2) prolonged maintenance therapy; (3) effective CNS prophylaxis; and (4) accompanying supportive care measures including use of hematopoietic growth factors and prophylactic antibiotics. The number

of IT injections depends on the risk of CNS relapse (two IT treatments per course). Our group has established mature B-cell ALL, elevated levels of serum lactate dehydrogenase (LDH), and a high proportion of bone marrow cells in a proliferative state (>14% of cells in S+G2M phase of the cell cycle) to be associated with a higher risk of CNS disease in adults (78). We have therefore adapted the following strategy: patients with low-risk CNS disease receive six IT treatments, those with undetermined risk receive eight, and those with high-risk disease receive 16 IT treatments including all patients with mature B-cell ALL (79).

Over the years, we have incorporated further modifications into the hyper-CVAD regimen for disease-specific management (Table 1-4). (1) Rituximab is included for CD20 positive patients; (2) TKIs are combined with hyper-CVAD for Ph-positive ALL; and (3) nelarabine has been included for T-cell ALL.

- Expression of CD20 is detected in 35% of adult ALL and has been associated with a worse prognosis. Expression is higher in ALL subsets; up to 55% in Ph-positive ALL and almost ubiquitous in mature B-cell ALL. We have recently shown that the addition of rituximab 375 mg/m^2 administered twice per cycle with the first four cycles of hyper-CVAD improved rates of remission and survival for younger patients (<60 years) (80). Of 23 evaluable patients with non-HIV related mature B-cell ALL treated with the combination of hyper-CVAD and rituximab, 91% achieved CR (81,82). Compared with a historical control of 48 patients treated with hyper-CVAD alone, the 2-year rates for survival were superior for the hyper-CVAD plus rituximab combination (89% versus 58%, $p < .001$), especially for those patients over age 60 years (89% versus 19%, $p < .01$).

- The Philadelphia chromosome is the most common cytogenetic abnormality in adults with ALL, occurring in 20 to 30% of patients. The outcome of patients with Ph-positive ALL with conventional chemotherapy remains poor with long-term disease-free survival rates of <10%. Allogeneic stem cell transplant (SCT) is therefore currently recommended for all patients with Ph-positive ALL who achieve CR. Incorporation of targeted therapy using TKIs has altered the outcome of this ALL subset. Synergistic effects are possible with the addition of TKIs to chemotherapy including anthracyclines, vincristine, and cytarabine. Although the optimal schedule of TKIs has yet to be determined in ALL, early initiation and prolonged treatment courses

TABLE 1-3	DOSES AND SCHEDULE OF THE HYPER-CVAD REGIMEN

Therapy Segment	*Dose and Schedule*
Induction and intensified consolidation	Hyper-CVAD (courses 1, 3, 5, and 7) • Cyclophosphamide 300 mg/m^2 IV over 3 h every 12 h for 6 doses on days 1-3 • Mesna 600 mg/m^2 as an IV continuous infusion over 24 h daily on days 1-3 (starting approximately 1 hour prior to cyclophosphamide and finishing 12 h after the last dose) • Doxorubicin 50 mg/m^2 IV continuous infusion over 24 h on day 4 • Vincristine 2 mg IV on days 4 and 11 • Dexamethasone 40 mg daily on days 1-4 and 4-11 Methotrexate (MTX) and high-dose cytarabine (courses 2, 4, 6, and 8) • MTX 200 mg/m^2 IV over 2 h followed by 800 mg/m^2 IV over 22 h on day 1 • Leucovorin rescue 15 mg every 6 h for eight doses (starting 12 h after completion of MTX) • Cytarabine 3 g/m^2 IV over 2 h every 12 h for 4 doses on days 2 and 3 • Methylprednisolone 50 mg IV twice daily on days 1-3
CNS prophylaxis	IT MTX 12 mg (6 mg if via Omaya reservoir) on day 2 and cytarabine 100 mg on day 7 of each course Low risk: 6 IT High risk: 8 IT Mature B-cell : 16 IT
Maintenance therapy	POMP • 6-mercaptopurine 50 mg orally three times per day • MTX 20 mg/m^2 orally weekly • Prednisone 200 mg orally days 1-5 every month • Vincrisine 2 mg IV every month • Intensification with four additional courses of hyper-CVAD plus MTX/cytarabine
Supportive care	• Antibiotic prophylaxis (levofloxacin, fluconazole, valacyclovir) • Hematopoietic growth factor support during induction and consolidation • Laminar air flow rooms (for patients ≥60 years of age)

MTX, methotrexate; IT, intrathecal.

have been implicated to provide the best outcomes. Imatinib mesylate has shown encouraging results in Ph-positive ALL with CR rates of 96% (83,84). Our group was among the first who have combined imatinib with an ALL induction regimen. Hyper-CVAD administered concurrently with imatinib improved remission duration and disease-free survival in comparison with the hyper-CVAD regimen alone in Ph-positive ALL (85). During induction and consolidation therapy, imatinib 400 mg/day was administered

TABLE 1-4	HYPER-CVAD MODIFICATIONS

Feature	*Original*	*Modification*
CD20-positive ALL	Hyper-CVAD	Hyper-CVAD plus rituximab
Ph-positive ALL	Hyper-CVAD	Hyper-CVAD plus imatinib/dasatinib
T-cell ALL	Hyper-CVAD	Hyper-CVAD plus nelarabine

for 14 days concurrently with hyper-CVAD (86). Imatinib, 600 mg/day administered continuously, combined with vincristine and prednisone comprised the maintenance regimen, with higher dose imatinib owing to the absence of myelosuppressive chemotherapy. All patients with active disease at start of therapy achieved CR, of which 93% were reported after one cycle. Fifty percent of patients underwent allogeneic SCT in first CR, with 90% in CR 1-year post SCT. Similar results have been reported with other studies of imatinib and dose-intense chemotherapy programs.

• The role of second-generation tyrosine kinase inhibitors in ALL is under investigation. The dual *src* and ABL inhibitor dasatinib has clinical activity in patients with imatinib-resistant chronic myeloid leukemia (CML) and Ph-positive ALL. We have recently combined hyper-CVAD with dasatinib and reported a 95% CR in newly diagnosed Ph-positive ALL patients (87). Dasatinib 100 mg daily was included for 14 days of each cycle of induction and consolidation. Continuous daily dasatinib was included in the maintenance phase of treatment. Of 39 patients evaluable, complete cytogenetic remission was documented in 79% after one treatment cycle and 56% of patients have achieved a complete molecular remission.

- Nelarabine, a prodrug of guanosine arabinoside, demonstrates antineoplastic activity in patients with relapsed/refractory T-cell ALL, as evidenced through reported CR rates of 31% (88). Our group is currently evaluating the impact of nelarabine 650 mg/m^2 daily for 5 days after completion of eight cycles of hyper-CVAD on disease-free and overall survival (89).

- Elderly patients, those above 60 to 65 years of age, have a poorer prognosis compared with younger patients when treated with similar regimens and long-term survival rates remain low. Regimens must be designed for age-specific factors including organ function and performance status, as well as causes of treatment failures. In our experience, the use of the hyper-CVAD regimen in these patients has decreased the incidence of resistant disease compared with pre–hyper-CVAD regimens (27% versus 5%, $p < 0.001$) (90). However, the primary cause of failure in elderly patients has now shifted from resistant disease to myelosuppression-associated complications. Although the induction mortality rate was 12% for elderly patients treated with the hyper-CVAD regimen, administering induction therapy in a protected environment reduced mortality to 5%. Induction therapy in the protected environment establishes our current approach to minimize mortality during induction therapy for patients over 60 years of age.

Augmented Berlin–Frankfurt–Münster (BFM) Regimen

Young adults with ALL under age 40 may benefit from chemotherapy modeled after pediatric regimens. Although significant toxicity may limit the usefulness of these regimens in older adults, outcomes in younger patients indicate the benefit of pediatric-based therapy. Of 48 newly diagnosed patients, remission was achieved in 95% after 29 days when treated with the Berlin–Frankfurt–Munster (BFM) regimen (Table 1-5) (91). Minimal residual disease (MRD) was negative for 62% of patients following completion of induction therapy, and 85% of patients after 12 weeks of therapy. The median duration of CR was 57 weeks, whereas overall survival reported after 2 years was 82%. Infection and fever requiring admission were common,

as well as elevations in liver enzymes. Most toxicity was reversible and not limiting treatment with this regimen.

Stem Cell Transplant

The outcome with SCT versus continuation of chemotherapy in ALL continues to be debated. Traditionally, SCT has been reserved for patients with Ph-chromosome positive ALL or in patients considered high risk (age >35 years, B lineage with white blood cell count $\geq 100 \times 10^9/L$, T lineage with white blood cell count $\geq 30 \times 10^9/L$) (92). Autologous SCT has not been shown to be of more benefit than chemotherapy in first CR (93-95). In high-risk patients, survival at 5 years was not significantly different between patients treated with a matched related donor SCT and those treated with continued chemotherapy or autologous SCT. However, in patients not considered high risk, improvements in survival at 5 years were significantly greater in patients treated with a matched related donor SCT. In both risk groups of patients, allogeneic SCT reduced the rate of relapse compared with chemotherapy or autologous SCT. For patients without a suitable donor, chemotherapy is favored rather than autologous SCT.

Salvage Therapy

Prognosis of adult patients with relapsed ALL remains poor. In the MRC UKALL12/ECOG 2993 study, overall survival at 5 years after relapse was only 7% (96). Factors predicting for better 5-year survival rates (10-15%) included younger age (<20 years) and longer first remission durations (>2 years). Treatment during first CR had no impact on outcome. Although there is no standard approach to salvage therapy, there is general consensus that allogeneic SCT should be the first choice. For patients who have achieved a second remission, long-term leukemia-free survival rates of 14 to 43% have been reported with subsequent SCT (97).

However, most patients will not undergo SCT for lack of a donor, other comorbid conditions, or persistent disease. Most nontransplant salvage attempts are modeled after frontline therapy: (1) combinations of vincristine, steroids, and anthracyclines; (2) asparaginase and methotrexate combinations; or (3) high-dose cytarabine. Based on recent studies in adolescents and young adults demonstrating better results using intensified postremission therapy, our group at MDACC has designed the augmented hyper-CVAD regimen (98). In it, doses of vincristine and dexamethasone are intensified and asparaginase is used from the start. Of 55 released/refractory patients who were treated, 45% achieved CR. Although short-lasting, it proved sufficient

TABLE 1-5 | **DOSES AND SCHEDULE OF THE AUGMENTED BERLIN-FRANKFURT-MÜNSTER (BFM) REGIMEN**

Therapy Segment	*Dose and Schedule*
Induction (4 weeks)	IT cytarabine 100 mg within 3 days prior to start of induction
	Daunorubicin 25 mg/m^2 IV weekly for four doses
	Vincristine 2 mg IV weekly for four doses
	Prednisone 60 mg/m^2/day orally in divided doses on days 1-28
	PEG-asparaginase 2500 international units/m^2 IV during week 1
	IT Methotrexate 12 mg during weeks 2 and 5
Extended induction (2 weeks)	Daunorubicin 25 mg/m^2 IV during week 1
	Vincristine 2 mg IV weekly for two doses
	Prednisone 60 mg/m^2/day orally in divided doses for 14 days
	PEG-asparaginase 2500 international units/m^2 IV during week 1
Consolidation 1 (8 weeks)	Cyclophosphamide 1 g/m^2 IV during weeks 1 and 5
	Cytarabine 75 mg/m^2 subcutaneously or IV on days 1-4 and 8-11 of each month
	6-Mercaptopurine 60 mg/m^2/day orally on days 1-14 of each month
	Vincristine 2 mg IV during weeks 3 and 4 of each month
	PEG-asparaginase 2500 international units/m^2 IV during weeks 3 and 6
	IT methotrexate 12 mg weekly for 4 weeks
Consolidation 2 (7 weeks)	Vincristine 2 mg IV every 10 days for five doses
	Methotrexate, starting at 100 mg/m^2 and escalating by 50 mg/m^2/dose every 10 days for five doses
	PEG-asparaginase 2500 international units/m^2 IV during weeks 1 and 4
	IT methotrexate 12 mg during weeks 1 and 5
Consolidation 3-part A (4 weeks)	Vincristine 2 mg IV weekly for three doses
	Dexamethasone 10 mg/m^2/day orally in divided doses on days 1-7 and days 15-21
	Doxorubicin 25 mg/m^2 IV weekly for three doses
	PEG-asparaginase 2500 international units/m^2 IV during week 1
	IT methotrexate 12 mg during week 1
Consolidation 3-part B (4 weeks)	Cyclophosphamide 1 g/m^2 IV during week 1
	Cytarabine 75 mg/m^2 subcutaneously or IV for 4 consecutive days during weeks 1 and 2
	Thioguanine 60 mg/m^2/day orally for 14 days
	Vincristine 2 mg IV during weeks 3 and 4
	PEG-asparaginase 2500 international units/m^2 IV during week 3
	IT methotrexate 12 mg during weeks 1 and 2
Maintenance (24 months)	Vincristine 2 mg IV monthly
	Dexamethasone 6 mg/m^2/day orally for 5 days every month
	6-Mercaptopurine 75 mg/m^2/day in divided doses
	Methotrexate 20 mg/m^2 orally weekly
	IT methotrexate 12 mg every 3 months for the first 12 months of maintenance
Supportive care	Antibiotic prophylaxis (levofloxacin, trimethoprim/sulfamethoxazole (start week 2 of induction), fluconazole, valacyclovir)

Slow early responders repeat consolidation 2 and consolidation 3A and 3B prior to maintenance therapy. If CNS disease at start of therapy, then methotrexate 12 mg IT weekly until negative for blasts, then methotrexate 12 mg IT every other week for 8 doses, then methotrexate 12 mg IT monthly for 6 months.

for some patients to serve as a bridge for SCT. Comparisons between regimens are inherently difficult because of differences in patient characteristics, prior drug exposure and sensitivity, number of salvage attempts, variations in dose and schedule of agents, the use of SCT as consolidation in some patients, and not least because of the overall poor outcome.

Exploration of new agents is a major cornerstone of clinical research in ALL therapy. Rituximab, a chimeric monoclonal antibody against the cell surface protein CD20, has been combined with chemotherapy and improved outcome in non-Hodgkin's lymphoma and subsets of patients with ALL (80). The role of alemtuzumab, a humanized CD52-directed monoclonal antibody, in CD52-positive ALL and in combination with chemotherapy in aggressive T-lymphocytic malignancies is being explored (99). Other monoclonal antibodies are in earlier stages of their clinical assessment. A continuous source of active drugs in leukemias are nucleoside analogs. Clofarabine is a new generation purine nucleoside modeled after fludarabine and cladribine, but with different mechanisms of action and spectrum of activity (100). In a phase 2 trial of 61 children with relapsed or refractory ALL, 30% responded including seven patients with complete remissions, five with marrow remissions but lack of platelet recovery (CRp), and six children with partial remissions (101). Sustained remissions for up to 64 weeks have been reported in some patients. Nelarabine is a soluble prodrug of 9-β-D-arabinofuranosylguanine (ara-G) with activity predominantly in relapsed T-lineage lymphoid malignancies and approval by the FDA for this indication in October, 2005. Response rates of 33% and up to 41% have been achieved in a group of 121 children and 39 adults with relapsed T-lineage leukemia/lymphoma, respectively (102,103). Median overall survival in the adult group was 20 weeks (103). Neurotoxicity is the major adverse event of nelarabine, which is both dose and schedule dependent and can be limited with every other day administration rather than daily. Of further interest are other compounds which have been modified to improve their pharmacokinetic properties: pegylated asparaginase, liposomal doxorubicin, or liposomal vincristine. Experience of 52 patients who have been treated with liposomal vincristine on two different studies demonstrated an overall response rate 21% with another 23% of the patients achieving hematologic improvement (104,105). Among what is considered small molecular targeted therapies, TKIs inhibitors have had the biggest impact in Ph-positive ALL.

■ **SUMMARY**

Historically, remission rates for ALL in adults have been comparable to that in children, however long-term survival remains a challenge. Progress in adults has been marked by utilization of intensive regimens proven beneficial in pediatric patients as well as the inclusion of new targeted therapy. Future therapy with ALL will incorporate novel agents to already active regimens. Inclusion of asparaginase products into regimens like hyper-CVAD and BFM may improve long-term survival. Determination of high-risk patients through molecular testing will allow for personalized

therapy, whereas the detection of early MRD will help select patients requiring further therapy. In Ph-positive ALL, advanced generation TKIs may improve response rates and allow for more patients to proceed to SCT. Developments in supportive care, such as prophylactic medications, growth factors, and granulocyte transfusions enable more patients to tolerate intensive regimens. Although significant discoveries have been observed in the treatment of patients with ALL, long-term survival in adults is still inferior to that in children. Through continuous investigation, comparable outcomes may soon be achieved in adults.

References

1. Jemal A, Siegel R, Ward R, et al. Cancer statistics 2008. *CA Cancer J Clin* 2008;58:71-96.
2. Parkin DM, Kramarova E, Draper GJ, et al. (eds). *International Incidence of Childhood Cancer*. Lyon: International Agency for Research on Cancer; 1998.
3. Groves FD, Linet MS, Devasa SS. Epidemiology of leukemia: Overview of patterns of occurrence. In: Henderson ES, Lister TA, Greaves MF (eds): *Leukemia*, 6th ed. Philadelphia: WB Saunders; 1996:145.
4. Ries LAG, Smith MA, Gurney JG, et al. (eds). *Cancer Incidence and Survival Among Children and Adolescents: United States SEER Program 1975-1995*. Bethesda: National Cancer Institute; 1999.
5. Bunin GR. Nongenetic causes of childhood cancers: Evidence from international variation, time trends, and risk factor studies. *Toxicol Appl Pharmacol* 2004;199:91-103.
6. Lightfood TJ, Roman E. Causes of childhood leukaemia and lymphoma. *Toxicol Appl Pharmacol* 2004;199:104-117.
7. Pombo de Oliveira MS, Awad el Seed FE, Foroni L, et al. Lymphoblastic leukaemia in Siamese twins: Evidence for identity. *Lancet* 1986;2:969-970.
8. Schmitt TA, Degos L. Leucemies Familiase. *Bull Cancer* 1978;65:83.
9. Li FP. Epidemiology of cancer in childhood. In: Nathan DG, Oski FA (eds): *Hematology of Infancy and Childhood*, 4th ed. Philadelphia: WB Saunders;1993:1102.
10. Mertens AC, Wen W, Davies SM, et al. Congenital abnormalities in children with acute leukemia: A report from the Children's Cancer Group. *J Pediatr* 1998;133:617.
11. Chessells JM, Harrison G, Richards SM, et al. Down's syndrome and acute lymphoblastic leukaemia: Clinical features and response to treatment. *Arch Dis Child* 2001; 85:321.
12. Toledano SR, Lange BJ. Ataxia-telangiectasia and acute lymphoblastic leukemia. *Cancer* 1980;45:1675.
13. Shaw MP, Eden OB, Grace E, Ellis PM. Acute lymphoblastic leukemia and Klinefelter's syndrome. *Pediatr Hematol Oncol* 1992;9:81.
14. Janik-Moszat A, Bubala H, Stojewska M, et al. Acute lymphoblastic leukemia in children with Fanconi anemia. *Wiad Lek* 1998;51(Suppl 4):285.
15. Greaves MF, Alexander FE. An infectious etiology for common acute lymphoblastic leukemia in childhood? *Leukemia* 1993;7:349.

16. Timonen TT. A hypothesis concerning deficiency of sunlight, cold temperature, and influenza epidemics associated with the onset of acute lymphoblastic leukemia in northern Finland. *Ann Hematol* 1999;78:408.

17. Mahieux R, Gessain A. HTLV-1 and associated adult T-cell leukemia/lymphoma. *Rev Clin Exp Hematol* 2003;7: 336-361.

18. Lombardi L, Newcomb EW, Dalla-Favera R. Pathogenesis of Burkitt's lymphoma: Expression of an activated c-myc oncogene causes the tumorigenic conversion of EBV-infected B lymphoblasts. *Cell* 1987;49:161.

19. Vianna NJ, Polan AK. Childhood lymphatic leukemia: Prenatal seasonality and possible association with congenital varicella. *Am J Epidemiol* 1976;103:321-332.

20. Cortes J. Central nervous system involvement in adult acute lymphocytic leukemia. *Hematol Oncol Clin North Am* 2001;15: 145-162.

21. Bennett JM, Catovsky D, Daniel MT, et al. Proposals for the classification of acute leukemia. French-American-British Cooperative Group. *Br J Haematol* 1976;33:451-458.

22. Ferraro S, Mariano MT, Tagliafico E, et al. Myeloperoxidase gene expression in blast cells with a lymphoid phenotype in cases of acute lymphoblastic leukemia. *Blood* 1988;72:873.

23. Serrana J, Roman J, Sanches J, et al. Myeloperoxidase gene expression in acute lymphoblastic leukemia. *Br J Haematol* 1997;97:841.

24. Wright S, Chucrallah A, Chong YY, et al. Acute lymphoblastic leukemia with myeloperoxidase activity. *Am J Hematol* 1996;51:147-151.

25. McCaffrey R, Harrison TA, Parkman P, et al. Terminal deoxynucleotidyl transferase activity in human leukemic cells and in normal thymocytes. *N Engl J Med* 1975;292:775.

26. Meenan B, Heavey C, Lichtensetin A, et al. Terminal transferase expression in the differential diagnosis of acute leukemias. Easter Cooperative Oncology Group. *Leuk Lymphoma* 1996;22:265.

27. Huh YO, Smith TL, Collins P, et al. Terminal deoxynucleotidyl transferase expression in acute myelogenous leukemia and myelodysplasia as determined by flow cytometry. *Leuk Lymphoma* 2000;37:319.

28. Faber J, Kantarjian H, Roberts MW, et al. Terminal deoxynucleotidyl transferase-negative acute lymphoblastic leukemia. *Arch Pathol Lab Med* 2000;124:92-97.

29. Harris NL, Jaffe ES, Diebold J, et al. World Health Organization classification of neoplastic diseases of the hematopoietic and lymphoid tissues: Report of the Clinical Advisory Committee Meeting-Airlie House, Virginia, November 1997. *J Clin Oncol* 1999;17:3835-3849.

30. WHO. In: Jaffe ES, Harris NL, Stein H, et al. (eds): *World Health Organization Classification of Tumours, Pathology and Genetics of Tumours of Haematopoietic and Lymphoid Tissues*. Lyon: IARC Press; 111-187.

31. Foa R, Vitale A. Towards an integrated classification of adult acute lymphoblastic leukemia. *Rev Clin Exp Hematol* 2002; 6:181.

32. Bene MC, Castoldi G, Knapp W, et al. Proposals for the immunological classification of acute leukemias. *Leukemia* 1995;9:1783.

33. Huh YO, Ibrahim S. Immunophenotypes in adult acute lymphoblastic leukemia. Role of flow cytometry in diagnosis and monitoring of disease. *Hematol Oncol Clin North Am* 2000; 14:1251.

34. Paredes-Aguilera R, Romero-Guzman L, Lopez-Santiago N, et al. Flow cytometric analysis of cell-surface and intracellular antigens in the diagnosis of acute leukemia. *Am J Hematol* 2001;38:69.

35. Terstappen LWMM, Huang S, Picker LJ. Flow cytometric assessment of human T-cell differentiation in thymus and bone marrow. *Blood* 1992;79:666.

36. Onciu M, Lai R, Vega F, et al. Precursor T-cell acute lymphoblastic leukemia in adults: Age-related immunophenotypic, cytogenetic, and molecular subsets. *Am J Clin Pathol* 2002;117:252.

37. Gores SD, Kastan MG, Civin CI. Normal human bone marrow precursors that express terminal deoxynucleotidyl transferase include T-cell precursors and possible lymphoid stem cells. *Blood* 1991;77:1681.

38. Borowitz MJ. Immunologic markers in childhood acute lymphoblastic leukemia. *Hematol Oncol Clin North Am* 1990;4:743.

39. Pui CH, Rubnitz JE, Hancock ML, et al. Reappraisal of the clinical and biological significance of myeloid-associated antigen expression in childhood acute lymphoblastic leukemia. *J Clin Oncol* 1998;16:3768.

40. Den Boer ML, Kapaun P, Pieters R, et al. Myeloid antigen co-expression in childhood acute lymphoblastic leukaemia: Relationship with in vitro drug resistance. *Br J Haematol* 1999;105:876.

41. Putti MC, Rondelli R, Cocito MG, et al. Expression of myeloid markers lacks prognostic impact in children treated for acute lymphoblastic leukemia: Italian experience in AIEOP-ALL 88-91 studies. *Blood* 1998;92:795.

42. Preti HA, Huh YO, O'Brien SM, et al. Myeloid markers in adult acute lymphoblastic leukemia: Correlations with patient and disease characteristics and with prognosis. *Cancer* 1995;76:1564-1570.

43. Matutes E, Morilla R, Farahat N, et al. Definition of acute biphenotypic leukemia. *Haematologica* 1997;82:64-66.

44. Cascavilla N, Musto P, Melillo L, et al. Is the scoring system an effective clinico-biological tool in myeloid antigen positive adult acute lymphoblastic leukemia? Results of a long-term study. *Hematol J* 2002;3:251.

45. Faderl S, Kantarjian HM, Talpaz M, et al. Clinical significance of cytogenetic abnormalities in adult acute lymphoblastic leukemia. *Blood* 1998;91:3995-4019.

46. The Groupe Francais de Cytogenetique Hematologique. Cytogenetic abnormalities in adult acute lymphoblastic leukemia: Correlations with the hematologic findings and outcome. A collaborative study of the Groupe Francais de Cytogenetique Hematologique. *Blood* 1996;3135-3142.

47. Wetzler M, Dodge RK, Mrozek K, et al. Prospective karyotype analysis in adult acute lymphoblastic leukemia: The Cancer and Leukemia Group B experience. *Blood* 1900;93:383.

48. Secker-Walker LM, Prentice HG, Durrant J, et al. Cytogenetics adds independent prognostic information in adults with acute lymphoblastic leukemia on MRC trial UKALL XA. *Br J Haematol* 1997;96:601-610.

49. Mancini M, Scappaticci D, Cimino G, et al. A comprehensive genetic classification of adult acute lymphoblastic leukemia (ALL): Analysis of the GIMEMA 0496 protocol. *Blood* 2005;3434-3441.

50. Chiaretti S, Li X, Gentlman R, et al. Gene expression profile of adult T-cell acute lymphocytic leukemia identifies distinct subsets of patients with different response to therapy and survival. *Blood* 2004;103:2771-2778.

51. Yeoh E-J, Ross ME, Surtleff SA, et al. Classification, subtype, discovery, and prediction of outcome in pediatric acute lymphoblastic leukemia by gene expression profiling. *Cancer Cell* 2002;1:133-143.

52. Ferrando A, Neuberg D, Staunton J, et al. Gene expression signatures define novel oncogenic pathways in T cell acute lymphoblastic leukemia. *Cancer cell* 2002;1:75-87.

53. Kohlman A, Schoch C, Schnittger S, et al. Pediatric acute lymphoblastic leukemia (ALL) gene expression signatures classify an independent cohort of adults ALL patients. *Leukemia* 2004;18:63-71.

54. Hanash SM, Madoz-Gurpide J, Misek DE. Identification of novel targets for cancer therapy using expression proteomics. *Leukemia* 2002;16:478-485.

55. Santini V, Kantarjian HM, Issa J-P. Changes in DNA methylation in neoplasia: Pathophysiology and therapeutic implications. *Ann Intern Med* 2001;134:573-586.

56. Garcia-Manero G, Bueso-Ramos C, Daniel J, et al. DNA methylation patterns at relapse in adult acute lymphoblastic leukemia. *Clin Cancer Res* 2002;8:1897-1903.

57. Garcia-Manerao G, Daniel J, Smith TL, et al. DNA methylation of multiple promoter-associated CpG islands in adult acute lymphoblastic leukemia. *Clin Cancer Res* 2002;8:2217-2224.

58. Shen L, Toyota M, Kondo Y, et al. Aberrant DNA methylation of p57KIP2 identifies a cell-cycle regulatory pathway with prognostic impact in adult acute lymphoblastic leukemia. *Blood* 2003;101:4131-4136.

59. Roman-Gomez J, Jimenez-Velasco A, Castijello JA, et al. Promoter hypermethylation of cancer-related genes: A strong independent prognostic factor in acute lymphoblastic leukemia. *Blood* 2004;104:2492-2498.

60. Jabbour EJ, Faderl S, Kantarjian HM. Adult acute lymphoblastic leukemia. *Mayo Clin Proc* 2005;80:1517-1527.

61. Kantarjian HM, O'Brien S, Smith T, et al. Acute lymphocytic leukaemia in the elderly: Characteristics and outcome with the vincristine-adriamycin-dexamethasone (VAD) regimen. *Br J Haematol* 1994;88:94-100.

62. Jones B, Freeman Aik, Shuster JJ, et al. Lower incidence of meningeal leukemia when prednisone is replaced by dexamethasone in the treatment of acute lymphocytic leukemia. *Med Pediatr Oncol* 1991;19:269-275.

63. Hurwitz CA, Silverman LB, Schorin MA, et al. Substituting dexamethasone for prednisone complicates remission induction in children with acute lymphoblastic leukemia. *Cancer* 2000;88:1964-1969.

64. Ottman OG, Hoelzer D, Gracien E, et al. Concomitant granulocyte colony-stimulating factor and induction chemoradiotherapy in adult acute lymphoblastic leukemia: A randomized phase III trial. *Blood* 1995;86:444-450.

65. Kantarjian HM, O'Brien S, Smith TL, et al. Results of treatment with hyper-CVAD, a dose-intensive regimen, in adult acute lymphocytic leukemia. *J Clin Oncol* 2000;18:547-561.

66. Cortes J, O'Brien SM, Pierce S, et al. The value of high-dose systemic chemotherapy and intrathecal therapy for central nervous system prophylaxis in different risk groups of adult acute lymphoblastic leukemia. *Blood* 1995;86:2091-2097.

67. Mahmoud DH Jr, Rivera GK, Hancock ML, et al. Low leukocyte counts with blast cells in cerebrospinal fluid of children with newly diagnosed acute lymphoblastic leukemia. *N Engl J Med* 1993;329:314-319.

68. Laack NN and Brown PD. Cognitive sequelae of brain radiation in adults. *Semin Oncol* 2004;31:702-713.

69. Pui C-H, Cheng C, Leung W, et al. Extended follow-up of long-term survivors of childhood acute lymphoblastic leukemia. *N Engl J Med* 2003;349:640-649.

70. Tucker J, Prior PF, Green CR, et al. Minimal neuropsychological sequelae following prophylactic treatment of the central nervous system in adult leukemia and lymphoma. *Br J Cancer* 1989;60:775.

71. Pui C-H. Central nervous system disease in acute lymphoblastic leukemia: Prophylaxis and treatment. *Hematol. Am Soc Hematol Educ Program* 2006;142-146.

72. Rudnick SA, Cadman EC, Capizzi RL, et al. High dose cytosine arabinoside (HDARAC) in refractory acute leukemia. *Cancer* 1979;44:1189-1193.

73. Capizzi RL, Yang JL, Cheng E, et al. Alteration of the pharmocokinetics of high-dose araC by its metabolite, high araU in patients with acute leukemia. *J Clin Oncol* 1983;1:L763-L771.

74. Hande KR, Stein RS, McDonough DA, et al. Effects of high-dose cytarabine. *Clin Pharmacol Ther* 1982;31:669-674.

75. Ackland SP, Schilsky RL. High-dose methotrexate: A critical reappraisal. *J Clin Oncol* 1987;5:2017-2031.

76. Wellwood J, Taylor K. Central nervous system prophylaxis in hematological malignancies. *Int Med J* 2002;32:252-258.

77. Gokbuget N, Hoelze D. High-dose methotrexate in the treatment of adult lymphoblastic leukemia. *Ann Hematol* 1996;72:194-201.

78. Kantarjian HM, Walters RS, Smith TL, et al. Identification of risk groups for development of central nervous system leukemia in adults with acute lymphocytic leukemia. *Blood* 1988;72:1784-1787.

79. Kantarjian H, Thomas D, O'Brien S, et al. Long-term follow-up results of hyperfractionated cyclophosphamide, vincristine, doxorubicin, and dexamethasone (hyper-CVAD), a dose-intensive regimen, in adult acute lymphocytic leukemia. *Cancer* 2004;101:2788-2801.

80. Thomas DA, O'Brien S, Jorgensen JL, et al. Prognostic significance of CD20 expression in adults with de novo precursor B-lineage acute lymphoblastic leukemia. *Blood* 2009;113:6330-6337.

81. Thomas DA. Cortes J, Faderl S, et al. Hyper-CVAD and rituximab therapy in HIV-negative Burkitt (BL) or Burkitt-like (BLL) leukemia/lymphoma and mature B-cell acute lymphocytic leukemia (B-ALL). *ASCO Annual Meeting Proc* 2005;23:567s.

82. Thomas DA, Cortes J, O'Brien S, et al. Hyper-CVAD program in Burkitt's-type adult acute lymphoblastic leukemia. *J Clin Oncol* 1999;17:2461-2470.

83. Thomas DA, Kantarjian HM, Cortes J, et al. Outcome with Hyper-CVAD and imatinib mesylate regimen as frontline therapy for adult Philadelphia (Ph) positive acute lymphocytic leukemia. *Blood* 2006;108:Abstract 284.

84. Thomas DA, Faderl S, Cortes J, et al. Update of the hyper-CVAD and imatinib mesylate regimen in Philadelphia (ph) positive acute lymphocytic leukemia (ALL). *Blood* 2004;104:748a.

85. Thomas DA, Faderl S, Cortes J, et al. Update of the hyper-CVAD and imatinib mesylate regimen in Philadelphia (ph) positive acute lymphocytic leukemia (ALL). *Blood* 2004; 104:748a.

86. Thomas DA, Faderl S, Cortes J, et al. Treatment of Philadelphia chromosome-positive acute lymphocytic leukemia with hyper-CVAD and imatinib mesylate. *Blood* 2004;103: 4396-4407.

87. Ravandi F, Kantarjian H, Thomas DA, et al. Phase II study of combination of the hyper-CVAD regimen with dasatinib in the front line therapy of patients with Philadelphia chromosome (Ph) positive acute lymphoblastic leukemia (ALL). *Blood* 2009;114:Abstract 837.

88. DeAngelo DJ, Yu D, Johnson JL, et al. Nelarabine induces complete remission in adults with relapsed or refractory T-lineage acute lymphoblastic leukemia or lymphoblastic lymphoma: Cancer and Leukemia Group B study 19801. *Blood* 2007;109:5136-5142.

89. Faderl S, Thomas DA, Koller CA. Hyper-CVAD plus nelarabine: A pilot study for pateints with newly diagnosed T cell acute lymphoblastic leukemia (ALL)/lymphoblastic lymphoma (LL). *Blood* 2008;112:Abstract 3960.

90. O'Brien S, Thomas DA, Ravandi F, et al. Results of the hyperfractionated cyclophosphamide, vincristine, doxorubicin, and dexamethasone regimen in elderly patients with acute lymphocytic leukemia. *Cancer* 2008;113:2097-2101.

91. Rytting M, Thomas DA, Franklin AR, et al. Pediatric-based therapy for young adults with newly diagnosed lymphoblastic leukemia. *Blood* 2009;114:Abstract 2037.

92. Goldstone AH, Richards SM, Lazarus HM, et al. In adults with standard-risk acute lymphoblastic leukemia, the greatest benefit is achieved from a matched sibling allogeneic transplantation in first complete remission, and an autologous transplantation is less effective than conventional consolidation/maintenance chemotherapy in all patients: Final results of the International ALL Trial (MRC UKALL XII/ECOG 2993). *Blood* 2008;111:1827-1833.

93. Thiebaulty A, Vernanat JP, Degos L, et al. Adult acute lymphocytic leukemia study testing chemotherapy and autologous and allogeneic transplantation. A follow-up report of the French protocol LALA 87. *Hematol Oncol Clin North Am* 2000;14:1353-1366.

94. Thomas X, Boiron J-M, Huguet F, et al. Outcome of treatment in adults with acute lymphoblastic leukaemia: Analysis of the LALA-94 trial. *J Clin Oncol* 2004;22:4075-4086.

95. Attal M, Blaise D, Marit G, et al. Consolidation treatment of adult acute lymphoblastic leukemia: A prospective randomized trial comparing allogeneic versus autologous bone marrow transplantation and testing the impact of recombinant interleukin-2 after autologous bone marrow transplantation. *Blood* 1995;86:1619-1628.

96. Fielding AK, Richards SM, Chopra R, et al. Outcome of 609 adults after relapse of acute lymphoblastic leukemia (ALL): An MRC UKALL 12/ECOG 2993 study. *Blood* 2007;109: 944-950.

97. Kebriaei P, Champlin R. The role of allogeneic stem cell transplantation in the therapy of adult acute lymphoblastic leukemia (ALL). In: Estey EH, Faderl S, Kantarjian H (eds): *Acute Leukemias*, 1st ed. Berlin: Springer, 2008; 215-228.

98. Ayoubi M, Thomas DA, Kantarjian H, et al. Augmented hyper-CVAD in adult ALL salvage therapy: The MDACC experience of hyper-CVAD using dose-intense vincristine, dexamethasone, and pegaspargase. *Blood* 2009;114:Abstract 802.

99. Parnes A, Bifulco C, Vanasse GJ. A novel regimen incorporating the concomitant administration of fludarabine and alemtuzumab for the treatment of refractory adult acute lymphoblastic leukaemia: A report of three cases. *Br J Haematol* 2007;139:164-165.

100. Jeha S, Kantarjian H. Clofarabine for the treatment of acute lymphoblastic leukemia. *Expert Rev Anticancer Ther* 2007; 7:113-118.

101. Jeha S, Gaynon PS, Razzouk BI, et al. Phase II study of clofarabine in pediatric patients with refractory or relapsed acute lymphoblastic leukemia. *J Clin Oncol* 2006;24:1917-1923.

102. Berg SL, Blaney SM, Devidas M, et al. Phase II study of nelarabine (compound 506U78) in children and young adults with refractory T-cell malignancies: A report from the Children's Oncology Group. *J Clin Oncol* 2005;23:3376-3382.

103. DeAngelo DJ, Yu D, Johnson JL, et al. Nelarabine induces complete remissions in adults with relapsed or refractory T-lineage acute lymphoblastic leukemia or lymphoblastic lymphoma: Cancer and Leukemia Group B Study 19801. *Blood* 2007;109:5136-5142.

104. Thomas DA, Sarris AH, Cortes J, *et al.* Phase II study of sphingosomal vincristine in patients with recurrent or refractory adult acute lymphocytic leukemia. *Cancer* 2006;106:120-127.

105. Thomas DA, Kantarjian HM, Stock W, et al. Phase 1 multicenter study of vincristine sulfate liposomes injection and dexamethasone in adults with relapsed or refractory acute lymphoblastic leukemia. *Cancer* 2009;115:5490-5498.

ADULT ACUTE MYELOID LEUKEMIA

Sameer A. Parikh
Elias Jabbour
Charles A. Koller

Acute myelogenous leukemia (AML) is a group of several different diseases, the treatment and outcome of which are dependent on several factors including leukemia karyotype, patient age, and comorbid conditions. Despite advances in understanding the molecular biology of AML, its treatment remains challenging. Standard regimens using cytarabine and anthracyclines for induction followed by some form of postremission therapy produce response rates of 60% and 5-year survival rates of 25%. New therapies are emerging based on the definition of specific cytogenetic-molecular abnormalities. Such targeted therapies offer the promise of better antileukemic activity in adult AML.

■ INTRODUCTION

Acute leukemias are clonal malignant hematopoietic disorders, resulting from genetic alterations in normal hematopoietic stem cells. These alterations induce differentiation arrest and/or excessive proliferation of abnormal "leukemic" cells or "blasts."

Acute myelogenous leukemia (AML; acute non-lymphocytic leukemia) is heterogeneous. Over the past several decades, improvements in chemotherapeutic regimens and supportive care have resulted in significant but modest progress in treating AML. Better understanding of the biology of AML has resulted in the identification of new therapeutic targets. Despite current optimism, most patients with AML still die of their disease. With better molecular definition and elucidation of the physiopathology of AML subtypes, and development of new and targeted therapies, a better outcome of AML may be achievable in the future.

■ EPIDEMIOLOGY, ETIOLOGY, AND RISK FACTORS

About 13,000 individuals are diagnosed annually in the United States with AML. The incidence of AML is 2.7 per 100,000 (1,2). The median age at presentation is about 65 years. The incidence of AML, along with its precursor, myelodysplasia, appears to be rising, particularly in the population over age 60. In adults, AML is by far the most common type of acute leukemia. The incidence of AML is slightly higher in males and in populations of European descent. Acute promyelocytic leukemia (APL), a distinct subtype of AML, is more common among populations of *Latino* or *Hispanic* background (3,4).

An increased incidence of AML is seen in patients with disorders associated with excessive chromatin fragility such as Bloom syndrome, Fanconi anemia, Kostmann syndrome, and with Wiskott–Aldrich syndrome or ataxia–telangiectasia. Other syndromes such as Down (trisomy of chromosome 21), Klinefelter (XXY and variants), and Patau (trisomy of chromosome 13) have also been associated with a higher incidence of AML (5-8).

Survivors of the atomic bombs in Japan had an increased incidence of myeloid leukemias that peaked 5 to 7 years following exposure (7). Therapeutic radiation increases AML risk, particularly if given with alkylating agents. There are two main types of therapy-related AML. The "classic" alkylating-agent type (eg, cyclophosphamide, melphalan, nitrogen mustard) has a latency period of 4 to 8 years, and is often associated with abnormalities of chromosomes 5 and/or 7. Exposure to agents that inhibit the DNA repair enzyme topoisomerase II (eg, etoposide, teniposide) is associated with secondary AML with a shorter latency period, usually 1 to 3 years, with chromosome 11q23 at the location of the MLL gene, and with an M4 or M5 morphology (7,9,10).

Drugs such as chloramphenicol, phenylbutazone, chloroquine, and methoxypsoralen can induce marrow damage that may later evolve into AML. Benzene, smoking, dyes, herbicides and pesticides have been implicated as potential risk factors for development of AML (6,8). AML may also be secondary to progression of a myelodysplastic process or of a chronic bone marrow "stem cell" disorder, such as polycythemia vera, chronic myelogenous leukemia, essential thrombocythemia and myelofibrosis.

■ CLINICAL PRESENTATION

Fatigue, bruising or bleeding, fever and infection, reflecting a state of bone marrow failure, are common in AML. Only 10% of patients present with white blood cell (WBC) counts greater than 100×10^9/L (1,11). These patients are at higher risk of tumor lysis syndrome, CNS involvement, and leukostasis. Leukostasis may manifest as dyspnea, chest pain, headaches, altered mental status, cranial nerve palsies, or priapism (12,13). Leukostasis and tumor lysis syndrome are oncologic emergencies and require prompt recognition and management.

Physical findings other than bleeding and infection may include organomegaly, lymphadenopathy, sternal tenderness, retinal hemorrhages, infiltration of gingivae, skin, soft tissues, or meninges (more common with monocytic variants, M4 or M5). Disseminated intravascular coagulopathy (DIC) with bleeding diathesis is a common presentation in APL.

■ DIAGNOSIS AND CLASSIFICATION

The diagnosis of AML is often demonstrated by increased number of myeloblasts in the bone marrow or peripheral blood. By the French–American–British (FAB) Cooperative Group criteria, acute leukemia is diagnosed when a 200-cell differential reveals the presence of 30% or more blasts in a marrow aspirate (14). The minimal criterion has recently been changed to 20% by the World Health Organization (WHO) (15). Patients with the cytogenetic abnormalities t(8;21)(q22;q22), inversion (16)(p13q22) or t(16;16)(p13;q22), and t(15;17)(q22;q12) should be considered to have AML regardless of the blast percentage. After establishing the diagnosis, the blasts lineage (myeloid, lymphoid, or undifferentiated) is determined. The distinction is important and dictates specific therapy. Lineage determination is made using cytochemical stains. If 3% or more blasts stain positive for myeloperoxidase (MPO) or Sudan Black B, the diagnosis is AML. If the blasts are MPO negative, but stain for butyrate or nonspecific esterase, acute monocytic leukemia is diagnosed. If not, lineage determination is based on the blasts expressing surface antigens associated with the myeloid (equivalently monocytic, erythroid, or megakaryocytic), or lymphoid immunophenotype. Myeloid antigens are CD13,

CD33, c-kit, CD 14, CD64 (the latter 2 are monocytic markers), glycophorin A (an erythroid marker), and CD41 (a megakaryocytic marker). Lymphoid markers are CD10, CD19, CD20 (pre-B or B cells) and CD2, CD3, CD4, CD5, and CD8 (T cells) (16,17). A minority of MPO negative and Sudan Black B-negative cases are AML, and may include minimally differentiated (M0), and megakaryocytic leukemias (M7) that require flow cytometry for characterization (18,19). If the blasts are peroxidase and butyrate negative and express none of the myeloid or lymphoid antigens noted earlier, the diagnosis is acute undifferentiated leukemia, which is treated like AML.

The initial marrow aspirate may be a "dry tap," reflecting marrow fibrosis. In this case, a biopsy is needed to exclude acute megakaryocytic leukemia or hairy cell leukemia. If the marrow contains >50% normoblasts and pronormoblasts, the blast percent is based only on the nonerythroid cells; in these cases, the diagnosis is typically acute erythroid leukemia (M6), which can be confirmed if glycophorin A expression on the surface of the blasts. The WHO classification incorporates molecular, cytogenetic, and clinical features (prior hematological disorder) to the morphologic characteristics to better recognize the diversity of the disease, and its response to therapy (15). For example, AML with multilineage dysplasia by the WHO classification has no exact counterpart in the FAB classification.

■ TREATMENT OF AML

In the 1960s, Freireich et al. demonstrated the significance of achieving a complete remission (CR) to improve survival (20). Since then, the objective of therapy is to produce and maintain CR, the only currently accepted approach to AML cure. Criteria for CR are a platelet count $\geq 100 \times 10^9$/L, a neutrophil count $\geq 1 \times 10^9$/L, and a bone marrow with $\leq 5\%$ blasts (21). After 3 years in CR, the probability of AML recurrence sharply declines to less than 10% (22), and patients in continuous CR for 3 or more years can be considered "potentially cured." In recent years other response criteria have been proposed, such as "CR with incomplete platelet recovery" (CRp), where the platelet count is $>30 \times 10^9$/L, but less than 100×10^9/L.

Once AML is diagnosed and the decision to treat is made, the need for emergency therapy must be assessed. Emergency treatment is required (a) in cases of APL, (b) if the circulating blast count is $>50–100 \times 10^9$/L, (c) in the presence of DIC or organ dysfunction (especially pulmonary) attributed to leukemic infiltration (mostly seen in patients with $>10 \times 10^9$/L circulating blasts and/or M4 or M5 FAB morphology). In the latter situation, it is important to initiate immediate chemotherapy. Leukapheresis for severe leukocytosis and/or leukostasis should also be considered (23).

■ STANDARD THERAPY

Conventional treatment for AML, divided into remission induction and postremission therapy, has been with combinations of anthracyclines and cytosine arabinoside (Ara-C). At MD Anderson Cancer Center (MDACC), patients less than 60 years of age undergo induction therapy with an IA-based regimen with or without an investigational agent. The dose of idarubicin (IDA) is 12 mg/m^2 for 3 days and Ara-C is given as a continuous infusion at a dose of 1.5 g/m^2 for 4 days. An alternative is the "3+7 regimen," where the anthracycline (ie, IDA or daunorubicin [DNR]) is usually given daily for 3 days, and Ara-C is given at 100 to 200 mg/m^2 daily for 7 days by continuous infusion. In clinical practice, a bone marrow aspirate is usually obtained 2 to 3 weeks after beginning therapy. A biopsy is needed only if the quality of the aspirate does not permit determination of cellularity. If the day 21 marrow is hypoplastic, therapy is usually delayed until it is clear that leukemia has reappeared, at which time the second course begins. A second repeated course of therapy can produce remissions, but these are usually of shorter duration than remissions produced after one course of therapy, although this is controversial. The timing of a second course with persistent AML is controversial. Several cooperative group studies advocate starting a second course if there is persistent AML on day 10 to 15 of chemotherapy. With high-dose cytarabine (HDAC), a delay of a second course with persistent disease on day 21 to 28 may be indicated if the blasts are decreasing because most (90%) CRs are obtained after the first course, and response to a second course is poor. It is important to recognize that the initial marrow obtained after a period of hypoplasia may demonstrate up to 30 to 50% blasts as a reflection of the regeneration of normal, not "leukemic," marrow recovery. In this circumstance, follow-up (eg, at 1-2 week intervals) marrows show reduction in blast percentages concomitant with a rise in neutrophils and platelets.

Typically, once in remission after treatment with the induction course, patients receive maintenance therapy, with the same drugs administered at approximately monthly intervals for 4 to 12 months. The need for a prolonged duration of maintenance therapy may depend on the intensity of induction and postremission therapy (24). For example, a randomized German AML Cooperative Group (AMLCG) trial noted that addition of 3 years of maintenance improved the probability of 3-year relapse-free survival (RFS) from 7 to 30% (25). However, a similar randomized trial by the same group found no difference in RFS or survival when patients in the no maintenance arm received a more intensive induction treatment and one intense postremission course (2,26). Some maintenance therapy may be needed if intensive postremission therapy is not contemplated (27). However, any benefit from traditional maintenance after the administration of 3 to 4 months of consolidation is relatively small, and perhaps nonexistent, with respect to survival (28).

■ PROGNOSTIC FACTORS WITH STANDARD THERAPY

Standard therapy (ie, 3 + 7 followed by varying lengths of consolidation or maintenance therapy) results in CR rates of 60 to 70% with median remission durations of approximately 1 year, and with less than 20% of all patients achieving long-term RFS (Fig. 2-1) (29). This dictates, depending on prognosis (based on age, karyotype, performance status, and comorbid conditions), whether a particular patient should receive palliative care, standard therapy, or (much more frequently) be considered for a clinical trial involving investigational therapies.

Prognostic factors can be divided into those primarily associated with early death and those primarily associated with resistance to chemotherapy (30-32). Rates of therapy-induced mortality increase with

TABLE 2-1	OUTCOME OF AML THERAPY BY AGE AND PERFORMANCE STATUS			
Age (Years), Performance Status (Ecog)	Patients	% Complete Remission	% Death	% Estimated 2-Year Survival
<50, 0-2	587	74	9	46
<50, 3-4	43	47	44	23
>50, 0-2	1483	52	20	23
>50, 3-4	161	29	64	7

increasing age, abnormal organ function, and poor performance status. An ambulatory (Zubrod performance status <3) younger adult (age <50 years) would be expected to have an induction mortality rate of less than 5-10%. Poor performance (Zubrod performance status 3-4) in a younger adult is associated with mortality rates of 40% versus 60% if age is 70 years or older (Table 2-1).

The primary cause of treatment failure with 3 + 7 is resistant AML in most patients (failure to achieve CR or AML relapse). The principal predictor of resistant AML following 3 + 7 is the leukemia karyotype (Table 2-2) (33). Three groups can be distinguished. A *better prognosis group* (favorable karyotype) consists of patients with a pericentric inversion of chromosome 16 (inversion 16; associated with FAB subtype M4EO) or a translocation between chromosomes 8 and 21 (t[8;21]; associated with FAB subtype M2). Each of these abnormalities disrupt the function of a transcription factor (so-called core-binding factor, CBF), regulating the expression of genes important in hematopoietic differentiation. About 10% of unselected patients (typically younger) have CBF AML. At MDACC, all newly diagnosed patients with CBF AML are treated with the

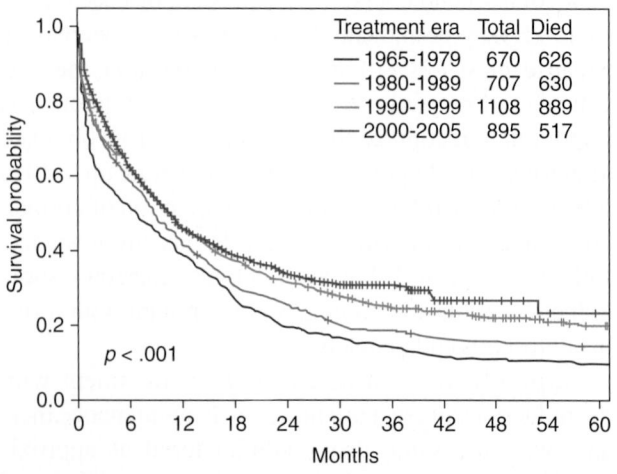

FIGURE 2-1. Overall survival in AML patients.

TABLE 2-2	AML CYTOGENETIC RISK GROUP		
Karyotype	% Frequency	% Complete Remission	% Event-Free Survival
A. Favorable			
t(8;21)	5-10	90	60-70
inv(16)	5-10	90	60-70
t(15;17)	5-10	80-90	70
B. Intermediate			
Diploid, -Y	40-50	70-80	30-40
C. Unfavorable			
−5/−7	20-30	50	5-10
+8	10	60	10-20
11q23, 20q, other	10-20	60	10

fludarabine (30 mg/m^2/day days 1-5) and high-dose Ara-C (2 g/m^2/day days 1-5) containing regimens with or without the addition of granulocyte colony stimulating factor (G-CSF). This is followed by up to six courses of high-dose Ara-C containing regimen (2 g/m^2). A CR rate of 93% and an event-free survival of 20 months in 114 newly diagnosed CBF AML patients was previously reported (34). The addition of gemtuzumab ozogamicin to this regimen (FLAG-GO protocol) was shown to have a better clinical and molecular response. Time-to-event parameters from this study are eagerly awaited (35).

A *worse prognosis group* (poor risk karyotype) comprises patients with monosomies of chromosomes 5 and/or 7 (−5, −7) or deletions of the long arms of these chromosomes (5q-, 7q-), or with abnormalities involving ≥3 chromosomes ("complex abnormalities"). These patients constitute about 30 to 40% of all patients, are usually older (>50-60), and often have either a history of abnormal blood counts prior to the diagnosis of AML (antecedent hematologic disorder [AHD]) or "secondary AML." The remaining 50 to 60% of patients fall into an *intermediate prognosis group*. Independent of karyotype, resistance is also more common with an AHD (36), with internal tandem duplication of the FLT3 gene (FLT3–ITD) (37,38), with the multidrug resistant (MDR1) phenotype (39,40), with high expression of the BAALC (brain and acute leukemia, cytoplasmic) gene (41), with the expression of RAS mutations in patients with intermediate karyotype and no FLT3 changes (42), or with partial tandem duplication within the MLL gene (MLL-PTD) found in 9% of patients with intermediate karyotype (43). Mutations of the CEBPA gene, mostly belonging to the intermediate cytogenetic risk group, confer better survival ($p = .03$) (42.44). Finally, mutation in the cytoplasmic nucleophosmin (NPM1), found in about 60% of patients with AML and normal karyotype, is associated with responsiveness to induction therapy and better survival. However, the presence of FLT3-ITD mutation trumps the better prognosis associated with NPM1 mutation. In other words, NPM1 +ve/FLT3-ITD +ve patients have a worse prognosis compared to patients with NPM1 +ve/FLT3-ITD −ve patients (45) (Table 2-3).

■ VARIANTS OF THE 3 + 7 REGIMENS

CHOICE OF ANTHRACYCLINES

Randomized trials have attempted to identify which anthracycline (eg, IDA, DNR, mitoxantrone [MTZ], aclarubicin) is better (46-48). Based on several such

| TABLE 2-3 | PROGNOSTIC FACTORS IN AML |

	Relapse Rate	Survival
↑ *BAACL*	NS	↓
FLT3 ITD/mutation	↑	↓
MLL PTD	↑	NS
↑ *BCL2* and *WT1* mRNA	↑	↓
↑ *EVI1* mRNA	↑	↓
p53 mutation	NS	↓
CEBPA mutation	↓	↑
c-kit mutation	↑	↓
NPM1(sole)	↓	↑

BAACL, brain and acute leukemia cytoplasmic; FLT3, Fms-like tyrosine kinase 3; MLL, mixed lineage leukemia; BCL2, B-cell CLL lymphoma 2; WT1, Wilms tumor 1; EVI1, ecotropic viral integration site 1; CEBPA, CCAAT/enhancer binding protein-alpha; NPM1, nucleophosmin; NS, not significant.

randomized studies, IDA (12 mg/m^2 daily days 1-3) has been proposed as the anthracycline of choice (49). This may be because the anthracyclines (IDA versus DNR) were not administered at equally toxic doses (48). Mitoxantrone is an anthraquinone rather than an anthracycline. In several studies, standard-dose Ara-C plus MTZ 12 mg/m^2 daily three times has been compared with Ara-C plus DNR at 45 mg/m^2 daily three times. Overall, the CR rates with the two regimens were similar, and there were no significant differences in the incidence or the severity of toxicities. In a three-arm randomized study comparing DNR, IDA, and MTZ as part of the induction regimen for older patients; there was no advantage for any one arm (50). In contrast, in a three-arm randomized trial conducted by the EORTC and GIMEMA comparing the same three agents, the 5-year disease-free survival (DFS) and overall survival (OS) were significantly better for patients receiving IDA and MTZ ($p = .03$ and .02, respectively). The recovery time was longer with IDA and MTZ ($p < .0001$) (51).

In two recently published reports, an escalated dose of DNR (90 mg/m^2 daily for 3 days) was compared to standard dose DNR (45 mg/m^2 daily for 3 days) in addition to standard dose cytarabine (100 or 200 mg/m^2 daily for 7 days). Both studies showed higher CR rates and OS in patients receiving higher dose of DNR, without any additional toxicity. The beneficial effect was mostly seen in patients less than 50 years of age and in those with predominantly diploid cytogenetics (52,53).

"HIGH-DOSE" ARA-C (HDAC)

Several randomized trials assessed the efficacy of HDAC (1-3 g/m^2) versus standard dose Ara-C (SDAC) (100-200 mg/m^2). The Cancer and Leukemia Group B

(CALGB) and the Eastern Cooperative Oncology Group (ECOG) restricted their analysis to patients in CR, whereas the Southwestern Oncology Group (SWOG) compared HDAC with SDAC during induction and randomized SDAC patients to SDAC or HDAC once the patients were in CR (54-56). See Figs. 2-2 and 2-3. Finally, the ALSG randomized patients to HDAC or SDAC during induction only (Table 2-4) (57). These trials concluded that: (1) the toxicity of HDAC (eg, cerebellar) outweighs the anti-AML effect in patients >65 years; (2) patients >60 years benefit from HDAC given during induction (SWOG, ALSG), in CR (CALGB, ECOG), and perhaps both (SWOG); (3) HDAC potentially increase the cure rates to 70 to 80% in patients with inversion 16 or t(8;21), and to 30 to 40% in patients with normal karyotype, but very little, if at all, in patients with prognostically worse karyotypes. In a meta-analysis of three trials in 1691 patients, induction with HDAC was compared to SDAC. Although there was no difference in CR rates, the 4-year RFS ($p = .03$), 4-year survival ($p = .0005$), and 5-year event free survival (EFS) ($p < .0001$) were better with HDAC (58).

■ STEM CELL TRANSPLANTATION

High-dose chemotherapy with or without radiation followed by SCT is increasingly used as therapy for AML in first CR. In prospective trials in Europe and the United States, patients younger than age 55 years in first CR with human leucocyte antigen (HLA)-matched sibling were assigned to allogeneic transplantation or, if no donor, randomized to autologous transplantation or one further course of HDAC (with daunorubicin in the European study) (Table 2-5) (59-67). The European trial found superior DFS in patients assigned to either type of transplant (allogeneic: 168, autologous: 127) versus chemotherapy (127), but there was no effect on survival. The US study found no difference in DFS and somewhat better overall survival with chemotherapy.

In a meta-analysis of 24 prospective clinical trials involving more than 6000 patients with AML in first CR, Koreth et al. showed that compared with nonallogeneic SCT therapies (including autologous transplant and intensive chemotherapy), allogeneic SCT has

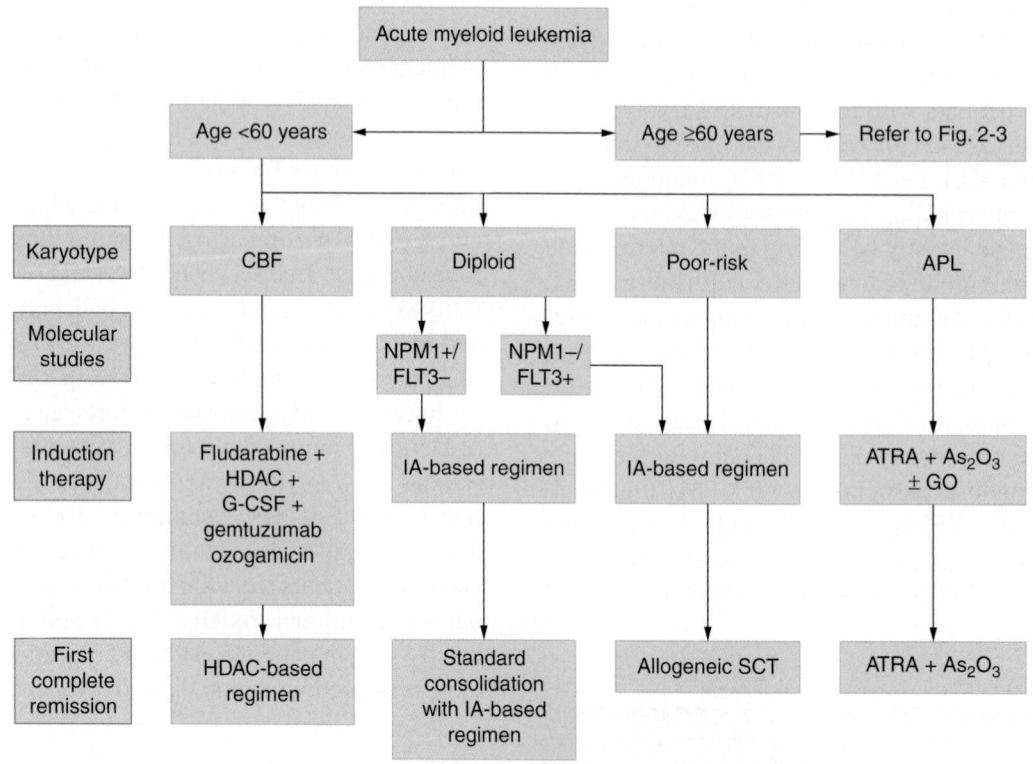

FIGURE 2-2. A proposed approach to the management of newly diagnosed adult acute myeloid leukemia. CBF, core-binding factor leukemias (including inv[16], t[8;21]); HDAC, high-dose cytarabine; NPM1, nucleophosmin; FLT3, fms-like tyrosine kinase 3; G-CSF, granulocyte-colony stimulating factor; APL, acute promyelocytic leukemia; ATRA, all-*trans* retinoic acid; SCT, stem cell transplantation; As₂O₃, arsenic trioxide; GO, gemtuzumab ozogamicin; IA, idarubicin and Ara-C.

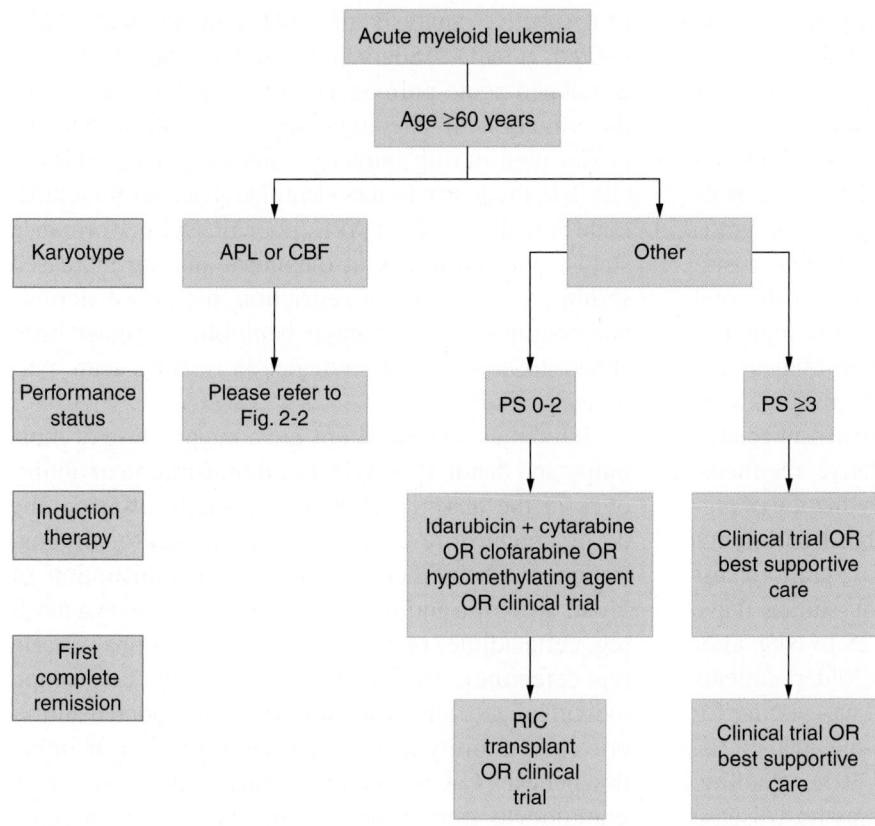

FIGURE 2-3. A proposed approach to the management of newly diagnosed adult acute myeloid leukemia in patients >60 years. APL, acute promyelocytic leukemia; CBF, core-binding factor leukemias (including inv[16], t[8;21]); PS, performance status according to the Eastern Cooperative Oncology Group (ECOG); ATRA, all-*trans* retinoic acid; RIC transplant, reduced-intensity conditioning transplant.

significant survival benefit in patients with intermediate and poor-risk AML but not with good-risk AML, based on cytogenetics (68). This finding contrasts with the retrospective review of 999 patients by Ferrant et al. that observed similar benefit with allogeneic and autologous transplantation for patients with poor-risk karyotype, and a benefit to allogeneic SCT only in patients with good and intermediate-risk cytogenetics (69). However, further stratification of risk groups based on molecular markers within individual karyotypes suggests that only specific subsets of patients may benefit from allo-SCT. Schlenk et al. demonstrated superior OS with allogeneic SCT compared to intensive chemotherapy in only the following groups of normal

TABLE 2-5	ALLOGENEIC STEM CELL TRANSPLANTATION (ASCT) VERSUS CHEMOTHERAPY IN AML IN FIRST COMPLETE REMISSION (62–70)			
Study	*N*	*% Match*	*% ASCT in CR*	*Significant Difference Favoring ASCT*
Reiffers	135	NA	NA	LFS*
Archimbaud	58	74	34	No
Schiller	82	89	30	No
Zittoun	294	63	23	LFS
Hewlett	163	65	12	No
Cassileth	238	88	23	No
Burnett	656	58	23	No

*LFS, Leukemia-free survival.

karyotype de novo AML patients: (a) FLT3-ITD +ve and (b) NPM1–ve/CEBPA–ve/FLT3-ITD–ve (45). Power et al. showed no difference in the outcomes of patients with mutant FLT3–ITD and wild-type FLT3 undergoing allogeneic SCT in first CR, thereby suggesting that allogeneic SCT abrogated the inferior outcome typically associated with the presence of mutant FLT3–ITD (70). Patients with inversion 16, or t(8;21) do better with chemotherapy (60). Patients with AML younger than 20 years have

TABLE 2-4	STANDARD VERSUS HIGH-DOSE ARA-C (HDAC) IN NEWLY DIAGNOSED AML		
Study	*HDAC during*	*N*	*Beneficial Effect of HDAC*
ALSG	Induction	279	CR duration
SWOG	Induction and/or consolidation	723	Event-free survival
ECOG	Consolidation	170	If age <60 years
CALGB	Consolidation	596	If age <60 years

relatively low transplant-related mortality and may do better with allogeneic stem cell transplantation.

New concepts in both transplantation and chemotherapy are emerging (71-74). These include the use of blood rather than marrow as the source of stem cell transplantation, the use of nonmyeloablative regimens to allow engraftment and take advantage of the graft-versus-leukemia effect, and the use of intravenous busulfan to overcome the erratic pharmacology of the oral form (75). In particular, nonmyeloablative regimens (reduced-intensity conditioning or "mini-transplant") have gained particular traction in elderly patients who have traditionally experienced high treatment-related mortality with conventional myeloablative regimens. The principles of this approach include reduction of regimen-related toxicities and shifting the burden of tumor cell kill from high-dose cytotoxic therapy to graft-versus-leukemia effects. A number of recent studies have reported 2- to 5-year survival rates of 25 to 64% after nonmyeloablative allogeneic SCT for older patients with high-risk MDS and AML. Survival was similar for recipients of related and unrelated HLA-matched grafts. The nonrelapse mortality was 16 to 39%, resulting mainly due to complications of graft-versus-host disease and comorbidities preceding SCT. Relapse rates ranged from 16 to 53%, and were influenced both by disease burden and cytogenetics at the time of SCT (76-79).

■ SUPPORTIVE CARE

Adequate and close supportive care is extremely important in the care of acute leukemia. Both G-CSF and granulocyte-macrophage colony stimulating factor (GM-CSF) have reduced the median time to neutrophil recovery by an average of 5 to 7 days (80). From existing randomized studies, G-CSF appears to be better and safer than GM-CSF (81,82). Antileukemic therapeutic efficacy is not compromised by these agents. Therapy of acute leukemia often results in rapid reduction of elevated white blood cell counts. This is often associated with the development of tumor lysis, characterized by hyperuricemia, hyperkalemia, hyperphosphatemia, hypocalcemia, acidosis, and renal failure. Prevention of tumor lysis syndrome requires administration of intravenous fluids and allopurinol (or rasburicase) if the blast count is above 10×10^9/L (83). Saline or steroid eye drops daily should be given to patients undergoing high-dose Ara-C therapy until 24 h after completion of chemotherapy. In these patients, neurologic assessments for cerebellar neurotoxicity should be performed before each dose of HDAC.

Acute pulmonary failure during induction therapy for AML is a serious complication. In a large retrospective analysis of 1541 patients with AML treated at MD Anderson Cancer Center, 120 (8%) developed acute pulmonary failure within 2 weeks of the initiation of chemotherapy; 87 of these patients (73%) died during induction and 17 (14%) achieved CR (84). Predictive factors identified at diagnosis include: male sex, diagnosis of APL, poor ECOG performance status, lung infiltrates at diagnosis, and an increased serum creatinine. Fluid restriction, high-dose steroids and continuous veno-venous hemofiltration have been shown to be effective strategies in treating acute pulmonary failure.

Infectious complications are a major cause of morbidity and death. Prophylactic administration of antibiotics in the absence of fever is usually offered. The development of fever (>101°F), unrelated to administration of chemotherapy, calls for administration of broad-spectrum antibiotics, such as imipenem or a third- (eg, ceftazidime) or a fourth-generation cephalosporin (eg, cefepime). Antibiotic selection should be prompt, individualized, and in accordance to the updated antibiotic susceptibility profile of each institution. If infection persists, G-CSF should be started and, if indicated, granulocyte transfusions, using G-CSF to increase the donors' granulocyte counts, should be given. Close fluid balance is critical as fluid retention is common, can radiologically mimic pneumonia, and may increase the risk of diffuse alveolar hemorrhage during induction.

Another controversial area is whether adherence to a neutropenic diet (avoidance of fresh fruits and vegetables) during induction chemotherapy decreases the risk of infection (85). One hundred and fifty-three patients with AML diagnosed at MDACC were admitted to a high-efficiency particulate air-filtered room for induction chemotherapy. They were randomized to receive a diet containing no raw fruits or vegetables (cooked diet) or to a diet containing fresh fruit and fresh vegetables (raw diet). Twenty-nine percent of patients in the cooked group and 35% of patients in the raw group developed a major infection ($p = .60$). Time to major infection and survival time were similar in the two groups, thereby suggesting that a neutropenic diet did not prevent major infection or death.

■ TREATMENT OF RELAPSED/ REFRACTORY AML

Although the outcome of patients with AML has improved with Ara-C and anthracycline-based chemotherapy regimens in addition to advances in supportive care, relapse remains frequent and constitutes the leading cause of mortality (Fig. 2-4). Ten to fifty percent of newly diagnosed patients may not achieve CR ("primary

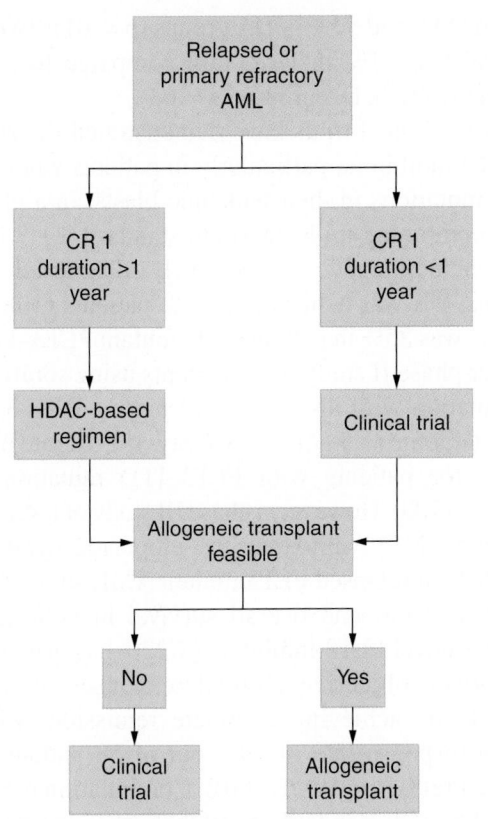

FIGURE 2-4. A proposed algorithm for management of relapsed/refractory AML. CR1, first complete remission; HDAC, high-dose cytarabine.

refractory"). In a study of 243 patients with relapsed/refractory AML conducted at MD Anderson Cancer Center in the 1980s; 33% patients obtained a CR, 24% died before achieving a response and 43% were resistant to their first salvage regimen (86). The median survival was 18 weeks and 5-year survival was only 5%. Whereas prior therapy with Ara-C or SCT did not influence prognosis, duration of first remission (CRD1) was significantly associated with subsequent outcome. In a more recent article, Breems et al. defined a prognostic score for patients with AML in first relapse based on the following variables: (a) relapse-free interval from first complete remission; (b) cytogenetics at diagnosis; (c) age at first relapse; and (d) SCT before first relapse (87). In an analysis of 594 patients who underwent second salvage therapy for relapsed AML at MDACC, 13% achieved CR (median CR duration: 7 months) and 1-year survival was 8% (88).

Allogeneic transplant appears superior to HDAC- or IDAC-containing regimens in patients with CRD1 less than 1 year; the great majority of these transplants were from HLA-matched sibling donor (26, 89-91). However, because very few patients are cured with conventional therapy, all patients with relapsed or refractory

AML should be treated in clinical trials. Gemtuzumab ozogamycin (GO), a conjugate composed of a humanized anti-CD33 antibody linked to the antitumor antibiotic calicheamicin was the only approved treatment for relapsed AML in patients older than 60 years of age with CRD1 of 3 months or longer. Complete response rates of 30% were reported with this agent. Veno-occlusive disease was observed in 5-10% of patients. GO is no longer commercially available after failing to demonstrate improvement in clinical benefit and resulting in a greater number of deaths when used in combination with chemotherapy versus chemotherapy alone. A number of investigational agents, as mentioned in the next section, targeting cytogenetic-molecular aberrations are being actively pursued in the treatment of patients with relapsed/refractory AML.

■ INVESTIGATIONAL AGENTS

Current investigational approaches include targeted therapy against surface antigens (eg, with monoclonal antibodies such as GO) (93), signal transduction targeting (FLT3, methylation, angiogenesis, inhibition of bcl-2 with antisense therapy) (94), novel nucleoside analogs, and new formulations of established drugs (eg, liposomal formulations, pegylated formulations) (95,96).

Clofarabine (2-chloro-2′-fluro-deoxy-9-β-D-arabinofuranosyladenine), in a phase I trial, induced a response rate of 16% among 32 patients with refractory/relapsed AML. The maximum tolerated dose was 55 mg/m^2 administered IV daily for 5 days (97). In a subsequent phase II study in 62 patients, clofarabine 40 mg/m^2 daily for 5 days induced a CR rate of 58% (98). In a study with 30 newly diagnosed elderly patients with AML, the response rate to clofarabine was 56% (99). The combination of clofarabine and Ara-C in relapsed AML induced a response rate of 40% (CR rate 24%), and 60% (CR rate 52%) in newly diagnosed AML (100). A multicenter phase III trial is currently ongoing in which patients >55 years with primary refractory AML or AML in first relapse are randomized to receive either clofarabine (40 mg/m^2 IV × 5 days) and Ara-C (1g/m^2 IV × 5 days) or placebo and Ara-C.

In contrast to altering the sequence of base pairs in genes, epigenetic modifications affect gene expression by two mechanisms: DNA hypermethylation and histone modification. Both alter gene expression via architectural remodeling of chromatin and are pharmacologically reversible. DNA demethylating agents and histone deacetylase inhibitors (HDACi) induce reexpression of tumor suppressor and proapoptotic genes and are now widely used in patients with myelodysplastic syndrome (MDS). Decitabine (5-aza-2′-deoxycitidine) and 5-azacitidine are hypomethylating agents approved by the FDA for treatment of high-risk MDS. In a phase I study, decitabine induced an overall response rate of 32% (nine CRs and seven PRs) among 50 patients with recurrent-refractory hematologic malignancies (101). In a final analysis of three sequential CALBG trials (N = 309) with azacitidine (75 mg/m^2/day IV or SQ × 7 days, repeated every 28 days), 35 to 48% of patients in the azacitidine group with WHO AML (N = 103) experienced CR, PR, or hematologic improvement (102). Among the 33 WHO AML responders in the three studies, the median duration of response was 7.3 months (range, 2.2-25.9 months). Median survival time for the 27 WHO AML patients in the azacitidine group was 19.3 months compared with 12.9 months for the 25 WHO AML patients randomly assigned to observation. In a more recent study comparing azacitidine with conventional care regimens (CCR) in 358 patients (113 with AML), survival at 2 years was 50% for patients in the azacitidine arm versus 16% in the CCR arm (p = .0007) with similar CR rates (103). A large multicenter phase III study comparing decitabine (20 mg/m^2 IV daily × 5 days every 4 weeks for 2 years) and best supportive care or low-dose cytarabine (20 mg/m^2 SQ daily × 5 days every 4 weeks for 2 years) has completed accrual and results are anticipated soon.

Hypomethylating agents have been combined with HDACi, such as valproic acid and vorinostat (suberoyllanilide hydroxamic acid [SAHA]), to improve response rates. In phases I to II studies using a combination of decitabine and valproic acid, a CR rate of 22% was achieved (104). Another study using a combination of azacitidine (75 mg/m^2 IV daily), valproic acid (50 mg/kg orally daily), and all-*trans* retinoic acid (45 mg/m^2 orally) in 53 patients showed a CR of 33% (105). HDACi have also been combined with conventional chemotherapy showing promising results. In a phase II study of IDA (12 mg/m^2 × 3 days) and cytarabine (1.5 g/m^2 × 4 days) combined with vorinostat (500 mg orally thrice daily) in 22 patients with high-risk MDS and AML, a CR rate of 82% was achieved (106).

A randomized phase III trial was conducted comparing three regimens in 673 patients with newly diagnosed AML in Poland: (1) DA regimen (N = 224): DNR (60 mg/m^2 IV daily × 3 days) and cytarabine (200 mg/m^2 IV daily for 7 days); (2) DAC regimen (N = 224): cladribine (5 mg/m^2 IV daily × 5 days) in addition to DNR and cytarabine; and (3) DAF regimen (N = 225): fludarabine (25 mg/m^2 IV daily for 5 days) in addition to DNR and cytarabine (107). The median age of patients enrolled was 47 years (range, 18-60 years). Sixty-eight percent patients in the DAC arm achieved a CR compared to 60% in DAF and 57% in DA groups (p = .01). Two-year survival was 51% in DAC arm compared to 36% in DAF and 39% in DA groups (p = .03).

Early clinical trials have demonstrated the activity of FLT3 inhibitors, particularly in patients who harbor FLT3 mutations in their leukemic blasts. In a phase II study combining midostaurin to standard 3 + 7 induction chemotherapy in 53 newly diagnosed AML patients, CR was achieved in 67% patients (108). The CR rate was 85% in patients with mutant FLT3–ITD. In another phase II study of 38 patients using sorafenib in combination with idarubicin (12 mg/m^2 IV × 3 days) and cytarabine (1.5 g/m^2 IV × 4 days); a CR rate of 83% (100% for patients with FLT3–ITD mutation) was achieved (109). However, a phase III study of lestaurtinib with either MEC (mitoxantrone, etoposide, cytarabine) or HDAC in relapsed FLT3 mutant AML showed similar rates of CR and overall survival in both groups. Another novel FLT3 inhibitor, AC220, has been shown to produce objective clinical responses, including six patients achieving complete remission, with an overall response rate of 29% out of 58 patients with relapsed/refractory AML (110). Combination regimens of AC220 with standard chemotherapy in the frontline setting are currently ongoing.

In a phase I study of 47 patients with refractory AML, a novel liposomal drug delivery system of cytarabine and DNR (in a fixed ratio of 5:1) called CPX-351, was shown to induce CR in 23% of patients, with minimal toxicity (111). It is currently being tested in phases II to III clinical trials comparing it with the conventional 3 + 7 regimen in both frontline and relapsed AML. In another phase I study of 26 patients with relapsed AML, voreloxin (SNS 595, 10 mg/m^2 IV on days 1 and 4) combined with cytarabine (400 mg/m^2 daily for 5 days) resulted in CR in seven (27%) patients and was well tolerated.

Other agents such as aurora kinase inhibitors (AZD 1152), kinesin spindle protein inhibitors (ARRY520 and AZD4788), X-linked inhibitor of apoptosis protein antisense oligonucleotide (AEG35156), MEK pathway inhibitors, and mTOR inhibitors (temsirolimus and everolimus) are being actively investigated in both newly diagnosed and relapsed/refractory AML.

■ ACUTE PROMYELOCYTIC LEUKEMIA

This is a distinct subtype of AML accounting for 5 to 15% of cases, with unique clinical, morphologic, and cytogenetic features. It results from a translocation between the retinoic acid α (RARα) locus on chromosome 17 and the "promyelocytic leukemia" protein (PML) locus located on chromosome 15 (112,113). This *PML–RAR*α fusion is responsible for the 15;17 translocation (t[15;17]), demonstrable in 95 to 100% of cases. Independent risk factors for a diagnosis of APL in a patient with AML are younger age, Hispanic background, and obesity (4). The main clinical presentation is bleeding diathesis resulting both from plasmin-dependent primary fibrinolysis and disseminated intravascular coagulation (114). Cytogenetic analysis detects the distinctive t(15;17). In the rare case where such analysis does not show the t(15;17), but the clinical or morphologic picture is suggestive, the molecular "POD" test, which can be performed in few hours, can detect the characteristic disruption of PML in virtually all cases. Recognition of APL is crucial because appropriate treatment is different than for other types of AML and is curative in most patients with APL (115,116). A stratification system has been developed that distinguishes newly diagnosed patients with APL into low, intermediate, or high risk. Low-risk patients present with WBC count less than $10 \times 10^9/L$ and platelet count above $40 \times 10^9/L$; a WBC count above $10 \times 10^9/L$ identifies high-risk patients. Others are at intermediate risk. Anticipated cure rates are close to 100, 90, and 70%, respectively.

Several findings have contributed recently to these increased cure rates in APL. Anthracyclines were historically the first effective treatment inducing a cure rate of 30 to 40% in APL. The role of Ara-C is questionable, and probably beneficial only in the setting of suboptimal anthracycline therapy (117,118). Addition of all-*trans* retinoic acid (ATRA), 45 mg/m^2 twice daily to chemotherapy (eg, idarubicin 12 mg/m^2 days 2, 4, 6, and 8) increases CR rate, and more dramatically the cure rate from 40 to 70% (133-136). The major toxicity of ATRA is a potentially fatal leukocytosis syndrome (APL differentiation syndrome) characterized by fever and leakage of fluid into the extravascular space producing fluid retention, effusions, dyspnea, and hypotension; it is effectively treated with dexamethasone (10 mg IV bid for 3-5 days, with a rapid taper) (119). A molecular test (*PML–RARA*α fusion transcript by PCR) that detects molecular evidence of the t(15;17) provides a relatively sensitive and highly specific means to document minimal residual disease negativity and detect impending relapse (120,121).

Arsenic trioxide (As_2O_3) is the treatment of choice for relapsed APL (either molecular or hematologic) (122,123). As_2O_3 investigated as part of postremission therapy, and together with ATRA and GO induction, in newly diagnosed patients is showing promising results (124-126). The combination of ATRA and As_2O_3 for induction and consolidation of newly diagnosed APL (without chemotherapy) was used at our institution. GO was used for patients who were at high risk for development of differentiation syndrome (WBC count >30K). This combination led to a 92% response rate and an estimated 3-year survival of 85% among 82 patients (127).

Tamibarotene is a new synthetic retinoid drug recently approved for relapsed or refractory APL in Japan. It is a specific agonist for retinoic acid receptor alpha/beta. Compared to ATRA, tamibarotene is chemically more stable and several times more potent as an inducer of differentiation in PL cells (128). A phase II clinical study (STAR-1) is currently accruing patients to assess the safety, efficacy, and pharmacokinetics of tamibarotene in relapsed/refractory APL.

■ AML IN THE OLDER ADULT

AML in older adults (≥60 years) is considered a biologically and clinically distinct entity. Factors contributing to worse outcome in elderly AML are: age >75 years, unfavorable karyotype (mostly complex), poor performance status, organ dysfunction, and a longer duration of an AHD. In general, patients with three or more of these factors have expected CR rates of less than 20%, 8-week mortality rates above 50%, and 1-year survival rates of less than 10%. These patients constitute 25 to 30% of elderly patients with AML. About 20% of elderly patients have none or one of these adverse factors and have a reasonable outcome with expected CR rates above 60%, 8-week mortality rates of 10%, and 1-year survival rates of 50% or more (129-131).

Low-dose Ara-C was superior to hydroxyurea in a randomized trial enrolling 204 elderly AML patients (132). The CR rates were 15% with low-dose Ara-C and 1% with hydroxyurea ($p = .0003$). The 1-year survivals were 27% versus 3% ($p = .0004$). GO was approved by FDA for the treatment of relapsed AML in older patients; its role as single agent and in combination therapy was under investigation prior to removal from the market. In a phase II study of 112 elderly AML patients who were unlikely to benefit from standard 3 + 7 chemotherapy, single-agent clofarabine (30 mg/m^2 IV daily for 5 days) achieved a CR rate of 46% (133). A randomized phase II study compared clofarabine (30 mg/m^2 IV × 5 days) versus clofarabine and cytarabine (20 mg/m^2 SQ daily × 14 days) in 70 elderly patients with AML (100). Combination therapy achieved a better CR (63% versus 31%; $p = .025$), better event-free survival (7.1 months versus 1.7 months; $p = .04$), but did not improve overall survival (11.4 months versus 5.8 months; $p = 0.1$).

In a retrospective analysis of 847 elderly patients with AML, lomustine (CCNU, 10 mg/m^2 orally on day 1) added to IDA (8 mg/m^2 IV daily for 5 days) and cytarabine (100 mg/m^2 IV daily for 7 days) was compared to IDA and cytarabine alone (134). Sixty-seven percent patients achieved CR and the median survival was 12.7 months in the lomustine arm compared to CR rate of 57% ($p = .002$) and median survival of 8.7 months ($p = .004$) in the comparison arm. Investigational treatment or palliative care options become more plausible in poorer-prognosis elderly AML, and the patients and their families should be involved in discussions of treatment decisions.

■ MINIMAL RESIDUAL DISEASE

Minimal residual disease (MRD) detection is a critical diagnostic tool to assess the quality of response after induction therapy and to outline postremission programs based on the individual risk of relapse. As mentioned in the section on APL, the detection of *PML–RARAα* fusion transcript after achieving CR and its subsequent monitoring to detect early relapse has become the standard of care for patients with APL. The following paragraphs describe the application of MRD in the setting of non-APL AML, where its importance is recently being recognized.

Konopleva et al. reported that in patients with newly diagnosed AML who have abnormal cytogenetics at presentation, determination of cytogenetics in the marrow at day 21 of induction chemotherapy predicts RFS independent of the number of blasts (135). Another method of quantitative detection of MRD in AML is real-time PCR (RT-PCR) (136,137). RT-PCR rapidly quantifies PCR products by RT fluorescent signals during exponential amplification. The sensitivity of molecular detection of fusion transcripts ranges from 1 leukemic cell in 1000 to 100,000 normal cells, that is, 0.1 to 0.001% (137). The fusion transcripts most extensively used to monitor MRD in AML (in addition to PML–RARα for APL) are AML1-ETO, CBFβ-MYH11, and MLL-AF9, which are present in approximately one third of non-APL AML cases (136). The Wilm's tumor 1 gene (*WT1*) is highly expressed in most acute leukemias, and its detection in bone marrow has been associated with the presence, persistence, or relapse of leukemia (138-139). In a recent report, investigators from Turin, Italy, systematically applied their best performing *WT1* RT-PCR assay on 620 patient samples and demonstrated that application of a standardized WT1 assay can indeed provide independent prognostic information in AML (140).

Leukemic cells express abnormal patterns of cellular markers, and these aberrant immunophenotypes can be identified by multiparameter flow cytometry (141). An advantage of flow cytometry-based studies of MRD is that they can accurately quantify residual leukemic cells and can also distinguish viable from apoptotic cells. Published adult AML studies report identifying abnormal phenotypes in approximately 70 to 75% of patients (142,143). However, immunophenotypic changes during the course of the disease and lack of adequate expertise make it difficult to interpret results.

In general, a lack of standardization among different laboratories, identification of thresholds and timepoints during follow-up represent the major subjects of controversy for the routine implementation of MRD detection in non-APL AML at this time.

■ CONCLUSION

Following a period of paucity in discoveries, new strategies are finally evolving that may help patients with AML. The biology of the disease is now better understood. Patients with CBF AML have high cure rate with HDAC. Patients with APL have benefited from newer treatment with ATRA and arsenical derivatives. Better definition of the complex process initiating and sustaining the leukemic process will lead to a better definition of targets for therapeutic intervention that may translate into improved cure rates. Specific attention must be given to prognostic factors that identify subsets of AML in which specific tailored therapies will be helpful.

References

1. Foon KACD. Acute leukemia. In: Casciato DA LB (ed): *Manual of Clinical Oncology*, 3rd ed. Little, Brown and Company, New York, NY; 1995:431-445.
2. Abraham JMB. The acute leukemias. In: Abraham JAC (ed): *Bethesda Handbook of Clinical Oncology*, 1st ed. Lippincott, Williams and Wilkins, Philadelphia, PA; 2001:271-285.
3. Douer D, Preston-Martin S, Chang E, et al. High frequency of acute promyelocytic leukemia among Latinos with acute myeloid leukemia. *Blood* 1996;87(1):308-313.
4. Estey E, Thall P, Kantarjian H, et al. Association between increased body mass index and a diagnosis of acute promyelocytic leukemia in patients with acute myeloid leukemia. *Leukemia* 1997;11(10):1661-1664.
5. Crane MM, Strom SS, Halabi S, et al. Correlation between selected environmental exposures and karyotype in acute myelocytic leukemia. *Cancer Epidemiol Biomarkers Prev* 1996;5(8):639-644.
6. Dong F, Brynes RK, Tidow N, et al. Mutations in the gene for the granulocyte colony-stimulating-factor receptor in patients with acute myeloid leukemia preceded by severe congenital neutropenia. *N Engl J Med* 1995;333(8):487-493.

7. Pedersen-Bjergaard J, Christiansen DH, Andersen MK, et al. Causality of myelodysplasia and acute myeloid leukemia and their genetic abnormalities. *Leukemia* 2002;16(11): 2177-2184.

8. West RR, Stafford DA, White AD, et al. Cytogenetic abnormalities in the myelodysplastic syndromes and occupational or environmental exposure. *Blood* 2000;95(6):2093-2097.

9. Armstrong SA, Staunton JE, Silverman LB, et al. MLL translocations specify a distinct gene expression profile that distinguishes a unique leukemia. *Nat Genet* 2002;30(1):41-47.

10. Ayton PM, Cleary ML. Transformation of myeloid progenitors by MLL oncoproteins is dependent on Hoxa7 and Hoxa9. *Genes Dev* 2003;17(18):2298-2307.

11. Appelbaum FR. Acute myeloid leukemia in adults. In: Abeloff MD, Armitage JO, Niederhuber JE, et al. (eds): *Clinical Oncology*, 3rd ed. Philadelphia: Elsevier Science; 2004:2825-2848.

12. Novotny JR, Muller-Beissenhirtz H, Herget-Rosenthal S, et al. Grading of symptoms in hyperleukocytic leukaemia: A clinical model for the role of different blast types and promyelocytes in the development of leukostasis syndrome. *Eur J Haematol* 2005;74(6):501-510.

13. Tan D, Hwang W, Goh YT. Therapeutic leukapheresis in hyperleukocytic leukaemias—The experience of a tertiary institution in Singapore. *Ann Acad Med Singapore* 2005; 34(3):229-234.

14. Bennett JM, Catovsky D, Daniel MT, et al. Proposals for the classification of the acute leukaemias. French-American-British (FAB) Co-operative Group. *Br J Haematol* 1976; 33(4):451-458.

15. Vardiman JW, Harris NL, Brunning RD. The World Health Organization (WHO) classification of the myeloid neoplasms. *Blood* 2002;100(7):2292-2302.

16. Klobusicka M, Kusenda J, Babusikova O. Myeloid enzymes profile related to the immunophenotypic characteristics of blast cells from patients with acute myeloid leukemia (AML) at diagnosis. *Neoplasma* 2005;52(3):211-218.

17. Wang XB, Zheng JE, Gu JX, et al. Correlation of immunophenotype to cytogenetics and clinical features of adult acute myeloid leukemia. *Ai Zheng* 2005;24(6):667-671.

18. Roumier C, Eclache V, Imbert M, et al. M0 AML, clinical and biologic features of the disease, including AML1 gene mutations: A report of 59 cases by the Groupe Francais d'Hematologie Cellulaire (GFHC) and the Groupe Francais de Cytogenetique Hematologique (GFCH). *Blood* 2003;101(4): 1277-1283.

19. Tallman MS, Neuberg D, Bennett JM, et al. Acute megakaryocytic leukemia: The Eastern Cooperative Oncology Group experience. *Blood* 2000;96(7):2405-2411.

20. Freireich EJ, Gehan EA, Sulman D, et al. The effect of chemotherapy on acute leukemia in the human. *J Chronic Dis* 1961;14:593-608.

21. Cheson BD, Bennett JM, Kopecky KJ, et al. Revised recommendations of the International Working Group for diagnosis, standardization of response criteria, treatment outcomes, and reporting standards for therapeutic trials in acute myeloid leukemia. *J Clin Oncol* 2003;21(24):4642-4649.

22. de Lima M, Strom SS, Keating M, et al. Implications of potential cure in acute myelogenous leukemia: Development of subsequent cancer and return to work. *Blood* 1997;90(12): 4719-4724.

23. Giles FJ, Shen Y, Kantarjian HM, et al. Leukapheresis reduces early mortality in patients with acute myeloid leukemia with high white cell counts but does not improve long-term survival. *Leuk Lymphoma* 2001;42(1-2):67-73.

24. Preisler HD, Anderson K, Rai K, et al. The frequency of long-term remission in patients with acute myelogenous leukaemia treated with conventional maintenance chemotherapy: A study of 760 patients with a minimal follow-up time of 6 years. *Br J Haematol* 1989;71(2):189-194.

25. Buchner T, Urbanitz D, Hiddemann W, et al. Intensified induction and consolidation with or without maintenance chemotherapy for acute myeloid leukemia (AML): Two multicenter studies of the German AML Cooperative Group. *J Clin Oncol* 1985;3(12):1583-1589.

26. Buckner CD, Sanders J, Appelbaum FR. Allogeneic marrow transplantation for acute non-lymphoblastic leukemia: First remission versus after first relapse. *Bone Marrow Transplant* 1989;4(Suppl 1):244-246.

27. Rees JK, Gray RG, Wheatley K. Dose intensification in acute myeloid leukaemia: Greater effectiveness at lower cost. Principal Report of the Medical Research Council's AML9 Study. MRC Leukaemia in Adults Working Party. *Br J Haematol* 1996;94(1):89-98.

28. Sauter C, Berchtold W, Fopp M, et al. Acute myelogenous leukaemia: Maintenance chemotherapy after early consolidation treatment does not prolong survival. *Lancet* 1984;1(8373): 379-382.

29. Estey EH. Therapeutic options for acute myelogenous leukemia. *Cancer* 2001;92(5):1059-1073.

30. Estey E, Smith TL, Keating MJ, et al. Prediction of survival during induction therapy in patients with newly diagnosed acute myeloblastic leukemia. *Leukemia* 1989;3(4):257-263.

31. Estey EH, Keating MJ, McCredie KB, et al. Causes of initial remission induction failure in acute myelogenous leukemia. *Blood* 1982;60(2):309-315.

32. Sekeres MA, Peterson B, Dodge RK, et al. Differences in prognostic factors and outcomes in African Americans and whites with acute myeloid leukemia. *Blood* 2004;103(11): 4036-4042.

33. Grimwade D, Walker H, Oliver F, et al. The importance of diagnostic cytogenetics on outcome in AML: Analysis of 1612 patients entered into the MRC AML 10 trial. The Medical Research Council Adult and Children's Leukaemia Working Parties. *Blood* 1998;92(7):2322-2333.

34. Borthakur G, Kantarjian H, Wang X, et al. Treatment of core-binding-factor in acute myelogenous leukemia with fludarabine, cytarabine, and granulocyte colony-stimulating factor results in improved event-free survival. *Cancer* 2008;113(11):3181-3185.

35. Borthakur G, Faderl S, Verstovsek S, et al. Clinical and molecular response in core binding factor acute myelogenous leukemia with fludarabine, cytarabine, G-CSF and gemtuzumab ozogamicin. *ASH Annual Meeting Abstracts* 2009; 114(22):2056.

36. Estey E, Thall P, Beran M, et al. Effect of diagnosis (refractory anemia with excess blasts, refractory anemia with excess blasts in transformation, or acute myeloid leukemia [AML]) on outcome of AML-type chemotherapy. *Blood* 1997;90(8): 2969-2977.

37. Kiyoi H, Naoe T, Nakano Y, et al. Prognostic implication of FLT3 and N-RAS gene mutations in acute myeloid leukemia. *Blood* 1999;93(9):3074-3080.

38. Kottaridis PD, Gale RE, Frew ME, et al. The presence of a FLT3 internal tandem duplication in patients with acute myeloid leukemia (AML) adds important prognostic information to cytogenetic risk group and response to the first cycle of chemotherapy: Analysis of 854 patients from the United Kingdom Medical Research Council AML 10 and 12 trials. *Blood* 2001;98(6):1752-1759.

39. Leith CP, Kopecky KJ, Chen IM, et al. Frequency and clinical significance of the expression of the multidrug resistance proteins MDR1/P-glycoprotein, MRP1, and LRP in acute myeloid leukemia: A Southwest Oncology Group Study. *Blood* 1999;94(3):1086-1099.

40. Leith CP, Kopecky KJ, Godwin J, et al. Acute myeloid leukemia in the elderly: Assessment of multidrug resistance (MDR1) and cytogenetics distinguishes biologic subgroups with remarkably distinct responses to standard chemotherapy. A Southwest Oncology Group study. *Blood* 1997;89(9):3323-3329.

41. Baldus CD, Tanner SM, Ruppert AS, et al. BAALC expression predicts clinical outcome of de novo acute myeloid leukemia patients with normal cytogenetics: A Cancer and Leukemia Group B Study. *Blood* 2003;102(5):1613-1618.

42. Radich JP, Kopecky KJ, Willman CL, et al. N-ras mutations in adult de novo acute myelogenous leukemia: Prevalence and clinical significance. *Blood* 1990;76(4):801-807.

43. Schnittger S TC, Kern W, et al. Partial tandem duplication of the MLL-gene (MLL-PTD): A meta-analysis of 2885 AML patients enrolled into the german AMLCG99 and AML96 SHG trials. *Blood* 2003;102:100a (Abstract 340).

44. Frohling S, Schlenk RF, Stolze I, et al. CEBPA mutations in younger adults with acute myeloid leukemia and normal cytogenetics: Prognostic relevance and analysis of cooperating mutations. *J Clin Oncol* 2004;22(4):624-633.

45. Schlenk RF, Dohner K, Krauter J, et al. Mutations and treatment outcome in cytogenetically normal acute myeloid leukemia. *N Engl J Med* 2008;358(18):1909-1918.

46. Berman E, Heller G, Santorsa J, et al. Results of a randomized trial comparing idarubicin and cytosine arabinoside with daunorubicin and cytosine arabinoside in adult patients with newly diagnosed acute myelogenous leukemia. *Blood* 1991;77(8):1666-1674.

47. Vogler WR, Velez-Garcia E, Weiner RS, et al. A phase III trial comparing idarubicin and daunorubicin in combination with cytarabine in acute myelogenous leukemia: A Southeastern Cancer Study Group Study. *J Clin Oncol* 1992;10(7):1103-1111.

48. Wiernik PH, Banks PL, Case DC, Jr., et al. Cytarabine plus idarubicin or daunorubicin as induction and consolidation therapy for previously untreated adult patients with acute myeloid leukemia. *Blood* 1992;79(2):313-319.

49. Wheatley K. On behalf of the AML Collaborative Group L. Meta-analysis of randomized trials of idarubicin (IDAR) or mitoxantrone (MITO) versus daunorubicin (DNR) as induction therapy for acute myeloid leukemia (AML). *Blood* 1995;86: 434a (Abstract 1274).

50. Rowe JM ND, Friedenberg W, et al. A phase III study of daunorubicin vs idarubicin vs mitoxantrone for older adult patients (>55 yrs) with acute myelogenous leukemia (AML): A study of the Eastren Cooperative Oncology Group (E3993). *Blood* 1998;92:313a (Abstract 1284).

51. Vignetti M DWT, Suciu S, et al. Daunorubicin (DNR) vs Mitoxantrone (MTZ) vs Idarubicin administered during induction and consolidation in acute myelogenous leukemia (AML) followed by autologous or allogeneic stem cell transplantation (SCT): Results of the EORTC-GIMEMA. *Blood* 2003;102:175a (Abstract 611).

52. Fernandez HF, Sun Z, Yao X, et al. Anthracycline dose intensification in acute myeloid leukemia. *N Engl J Med* 2009;361(13):1249-1259.

53. Lowenberg B, Ossenkoppele GJ, van Putten W, et al. High-dose daunorubicin in older patients with acute myeloid leukemia. *N Engl J Med* 2009;361(13):1235-1248.

54. Cassileth PA, Lynch E, Hines JD, et al. Varying intensity of postremission therapy in acute myeloid leukemia. *Blood* 1992;79(8):1924-1930.

55. Mayer RJ, Davis RB, Schiffer CA, et al. Intensive postremission chemotherapy in adults with acute myeloid leukemia. Cancer and Leukemia Group B. *N Engl J Med* 1994;331(14):896-903.

56. Weick JK, Kopecky KJ, Appelbaum FR, et al. A randomized investigation of high-dose versus standard-dose cytosine arabinoside with daunorubicin in patients with previously untreated acute myeloid leukemia: A Southwest Oncology Group study. *Blood* 1996;88(8):2841-2851.

57. Bishop JF, Matthews JP, Young GA, et al. Intensified induction chemotherapy with high dose cytarabine and etoposide for acute myeloid leukemia: A review and updated results of the Australian Leukemia Study Group. *Leuk Lymphoma* 1998;28(3-4):315-327.

58. Kern WEE. High-dose cytosine arabinoside in induction treatment of acute myeloid leukemia: Meta-analysis of three trials involving 1691 randomized patients. *Blood* 2002;100;(255a) (Abstract 581).

59. Archimbaud E, Thomas X, Michallet M, et al. Prospective genetically randomized comparison between intensive postinduction chemotherapy and bone marrow transplantation in adults with newly diagnosed acute myeloid leukemia. *J Clin Oncol* 1994;12(2):262-267.

60. Burnett AK. Transplantation in first remission of acute myeloid leukemia. *N Engl J Med* 1998;339(23):1698-1700.

61. Burnett AK, Goldstone AH, Stevens RM, et al. Randomised comparison of addition of autologous bone-marrow transplantation to intensive chemotherapy for acute myeloid leukaemia in first remission: Results of MRC AML 10 Trial. UK Medical Research Council Adult and Children's Leukaemia Working Parties. *Lancet* 1998;351(9104):700-708.

62. Cassileth PA, Harrington DP, Appelbaum FR, et al. Chemotherapy compared with autologous or allogeneic bone marrow transplantation in the management of acute myeloid leukemia in first remission. *N Engl J Med* 1998;339(23):1649-1656.

63. Hewlett J, Kopecky KJ, Head D, et al. A prospective evaluation of the roles of allogeneic marrow transplantation and low-dose monthly maintenance chemotherapy in the treatment of adult acute myelogenous leukemia (AML): A Southwest Oncology Group study. *Leukemia* 1995;9(4):562-569.

64. Reiffers J, Stoppa AM, Rigal-Huguet F, et al. Allogeneic versus autologous bone marrow transplantation versus chemotherapy for treatment of acute myeloid leukemia in first complete remission (BGM 84 and BGMT 87 studies). The BGMT Group. *Bone Marrow Transplant* 1991;7(Suppl 2):36.

65. Schiller GJ, Nimer SD, Territo MC, et al. Bone marrow transplantation versus high-dose cytarabine-based consolidation chemotherapy for acute myelogenous leukemia in first remission. *J Clin Oncol* 1992;10(1):41-46.

66. Woods WG, Neudorf S, Gold S, et al. A comparison of allogeneic bone marrow transplantation, autologous bone marrow transplantation, and aggressive chemotherapy in children with acute myeloid leukemia in remission. *Blood* 2001;97(1):56-62.

67. Zittoun RA, Mandelli F, Willemze R, et al. Autologous or allogeneic bone marrow transplantation compared with intensive chemotherapy in acute myelogenous leukemia. European Organization for Research and Treatment of Cancer (EORTC) and the Gruppo Italiano Malattie Ematologiche Maligne dell'Adulto (GIMEMA) Leukemia Cooperative Groups. *N Engl J Med* 1995;332(4):217-223.

68. Koreth J, Schlenk R, Kopecky KJ, et al. Allogeneic stem cell transplantation for acute myeloid leukemia in first complete remission: Systematic review and meta-analysis of prospective clinical trials. *JAMA* 2009;301(22):2349-2361.

69. Ferrant A, Labopin M, Frassoni F, et al. Karyotype in acute myeloblastic leukemia: Prognostic significance for bone marrow transplantation in first remission: A European Group for Blood and Marrow Transplantation study. Acute Leukemia Working Party of the European Group for Blood and Marrow Transplantation (EBMT). *Blood* 1997;90(8):2931-2938.

70. Power MDSG, Brooks-Wilson A, et al. Allogeneic stem cell transplant in first complete remission overcomes the poor prognosis associated with the FLT-3 internal tandem duplication in acute myeloid leukemia. *Blood* 2007;107 (Abstract 3491).

71. Giralt S, Estey E, Albitar M, et al. Engraftment of allogeneic hematopoietic progenitor cells with purine analog-containing chemotherapy: Harnessing graft-versus-leukemia without myeloablative therapy. *Blood* 1997;89(12):4531-4536.

72. McSweeney PA, Niederwieser D, Shizuru JA, et al. Hematopoietic cell transplantation in older patients with hematologic malignancies: Replacing high-dose cytotoxic therapy with graft-versus-tumor effects. *Blood* 2001;97(11):3390-3400.

73. Ringden O, Labopin M, Bacigalupo A, et al. Transplantation of peripheral blood stem cells as compared with bone marrow from HLA-identical siblings in adult patients with acute myeloid leukemia and acute lymphoblastic leukemia. *J Clin Oncol* 2002;20(24):4655-4664.

74. Slavin S, Nagler A, Naparstek E, et al. Nonmyeloablative stem cell transplantation and cell therapy as an alternative to conventional bone marrow transplantation with lethal cytoreduction for the treatment of malignant and nonmalignant hematologic diseases. *Blood* 1998;91(3):756-763.

75. Andersson BS, Kashyap A, Couriel D, et al. Intravenous busulfan in pretransplant chemotherapy: Bioavailability and patient benefit. *Biol Blood Marrow Transplant* 2003;9(11):722-724.

76. Gyurkocza B, Storb RF, Storer B, et al. Nonmyeloablative allogeneic hematopoietic cell transplantation in patients with de novo and secondary acute myeloid leukemia. *Blood* 2008;112 (Abstract 149).

77. Luger SRO, Pere'z WS. Similar outcomes using myeloablative versus reduced intensity and nonmyeloablative allogeneic transplant preparative regimens for AML or MDS: From the Center for International Blood and Marrow Transplant Research. *Blood* 2008;112 (Abstract 136).

78. McClune B, Weisdorf DJ, DiPersio JF, et al. Nonmyeloablative hematopoietic stem cell transplantation in older patients with AML and MDS: Results from the Center for International Blood and Marrow Transplant Research (CIBMTR). *Blood* 2008;112 (Abstract 346).

79. Mohty M, Labopin M, Milpied NJ, et al. Impact of cytogenetics risk on outcome after reduced intensity conditioning (RIC) allogeneic stem cell transplantation (allo-SCT) from an HLA identical sibling for patients with acute myeloid leukemia (AML) in first complete remission (CR1). *Blood* 2008;112:Abstract 345.

80. Godwin JE, Kopecky KJ, Head DR, et al. A double-blind placebo-controlled trial of granulocyte colony-stimulating factor in elderly patients with previously untreated acute myeloid leukemia: A Southwest oncology group study (9031). *Blood* 1998;91(10):3607-3615.

81. Heil G, Hoelzer D, Sanz MA, et al. A randomized, double-blind, placebo-controlled, phase III study of filgrastim in remission induction and consolidation therapy for adults with de novo acute myeloid leukemia. The International Acute Myeloid Leukemia Study Group. *Blood* 1997;90(12):4710-4718.

82. Moore JO, Dodge RK, Amrein PC, et al. Granulocyte-colony stimulating factor (filgrastim) accelerates granulocyte recovery after intensive postremission chemotherapy for acute myeloid leukemia with aziridinyl benzoquinone and mitoxantrone: Cancer and Leukemia Group B study 9022. *Blood* 1997;89(3):780-788.

83. Jeha S. Tumor lysis syndrome. *Semin Hematol* 2001;38 (4 Suppl 10):4-8.

84. Al Ameri A, Koller C, Kantarjian H, et al. Acute pulmonary failure during remission induction chemotherapy in adults with acute myeloid leukemia or high-risk myelodysplastic syndrome. *Cancer* 2010, 116:93-97.

85. Gardner A, Mattiuzzi G, Faderl S, et al. Randomized comparison of cooked and noncooked diets in patients undergoing remission induction therapy for acute myeloid leukemia. *J Clin Oncol* 2008;26(35):5684-5688.

86. Keating MJ, Kantarjian H, Smith TL, et al. Response to salvage therapy and survival after relapse in acute myelogenous leukemia. *J Clin Oncol* 1989;7(8):1071-1080.

87. Breems DA, Van Putten WL, Huijgens PC, et al. Prognostic index for adult patients with acute myeloid leukemia in first relapse. *J Clin Oncol* 2005;23(9):1969-1978.

88. Giles F, O'Brien S, Cortes J, et al. Outcome of patients with acute myelogenous leukemia after second salvage therapy. *Cancer* 2005;104(3):547-554.

89. Biggs JC, Horowitz MM, Gale RP, et al. Bone marrow transplants may cure patients with acute leukemia never achieving remission with chemotherapy. *Blood* 1992;80(4):1090-1093.

90. Estey E, Kornblau S, Pierce S, et al. A stratification system for evaluating and selecting therapies in patients with relapsed or primary refractory acute myelogenous leukemia. *Blood* 1996;88(2):756.

91. Forman SJ, Schmidt GM, Nademanee AP, et al. Allogeneic bone marrow transplantation as therapy for primary induction failure for patients with acute leukemia. *J Clin Oncol* 1991;9(9):1570-1574.

92. Sievers EL, Larson RA, Stadtmauer EA, et al. Efficacy and safety of gemtuzumab ozogamicin in patients with CD33-positive acute myeloid leukemia in first relapse. *J Clin Oncol* 2001;19(13):3244-3254.

93. Giles F, Estey E, O'Brien S. Gemtuzumab ozogamicin in the treatment of acute myeloid leukemia. *Cancer* 2003;98(10):2095-2104.

94. Hussong JW, Rodgers GM, Shami PJ. Evidence of increased angiogenesis in patients with acute myeloid leukemia. *Blood* 2000;95(1):309-313.

95. Cortes J, Kantarjian H, Albitar M, et al. A randomized trial of liposomal daunorubicin and cytarabine versus liposomal daunorubicin and topotecan with or without thalidomide as initial therapy for patients with poor prognosis acute myelogenous leukemia or myelodysplastic syndrome. *Cancer* 2003;97(5):1234-1241.

96. Ravandi F, Kantarjian H, Giles F, et al. New agents in acute myeloid leukemia and other myeloid disorders. *Cancer* 2004;100(3):441-454.

97. Kantarjian HM, Gandhi V, Kozuch P, et al. Phase I clinical and pharmacology study of clofarabine in patients with solid and hematologic cancers. *J Clin Oncol* 2003;21(6):1167-1173.

98. Kantarjian H, Gandhi V, Cortes J, et al. Phase II clinical and pharmacologic study of clofarabine in patients with refractory or relapsed acute leukemia. *Blood* 2003;102(7):2379-2386.

99. Burnett AKRN, Kell JW, Milligan D, et al. A phase II evaluation of single agent clofarabine as first line treatment for older patients with AML who are not considered fit for intensive chemotherapy. *Blood* 2004;104:248a (Abstract 869).

100. Faderl S, Ravandi F, Huang X, et al. A randomized study of clofarabine versus clofarabine plus low-dose cytarabine as front-line therapy for patients aged 60 years and older with acute myeloid leukemia and high-risk myelodysplastic syndrome. *Blood* 2008;112(5):1638-1645.

101. Issa JP, Garcia-Manero G, Giles FJ, et al. Phase I study of low-dose prolonged exposure schedules of the hypomethylating agent 5-aza-2′-deoxycytidine (decitabine) in hematopoietic malignancies. *Blood* 2004;103(5):1635-1640.

102. Silverman LR, McKenzie DR, Peterson BL, et al. Further analysis of trials with azacitidine in patients with myelodysplastic syndrome: Studies 8421, 8921, and 9221 by the Cancer and Leukemia Group B. *J Clin Oncol* 2006;24(24):3895-3903.

103. Fenaux P, Mufti GJ, Hellstrom-Lindberg E, et al. Efficacy of azacitidine compared with that of conventional care regimens in the treatment of higher-risk myelodysplastic syndromes: A randomised, open-label, phase III study. *Lancet Oncol* 2009;10(3):223-232.

104. Garcia-Manero G, Kantarjian H, Sanchez-Gonzalez B, et al. Results of a phase I/II study of the combination of 5-aza-2′-deoxycytidine (DAC) and valproic acid (VPA) in patients (pts) with leukemia. *Blood* 2004;104:abstract 263.

105. Soriano AO, Yang H, Faderl S, et al. Safety and clinical activity of the combination of 5-azacytidine, valproic acid, and all-trans retinoic acid in acute myeloid leukemia and myelodysplastic syndrome. *Blood* 2007;110(7):2302-2308.

106. Jabbour E, Faderl S, Ravandi F, et al. Phase II study of vorinostat (V) in combination with idarubicin and high-dose cytarabine (IA) as front-line therapy in patients (pts) with high-risk myelodyplsatic syndrome (MDS) or acute myeloid leukemia (AML). *J Clinical Oncol.,* 2009;27;Abstract 7004.

107. Holowiecki J, Grosicki S, Kyrcz-Krzemien, et al. Addition of cladribine to the standard daunorubicine-cytarabine (DA 3+7) remission induction protocol (DAC) contrary to adjunct of fludarabine (DAF) improves the overall survival in untreated adults with acute myeloid leukemia aged up to 60Y: A multicenter, randomized, phase III PALG AML 1/2004 DAF/DAC/DA study in 673 patients. *Blood* 2008;112:abstract 133.

108. Stone RM, Fischer T, Paquette R, et al. Phase IB study of PKC412, an oral FLT3 kinase inhibitor, in sequential and simultaneous combinations with daunorubicin and high-dose cytarabine (DA) induction and high-dose cytarabine consolidation in newly diagnosed adult patients (pts) with acute myeloid leukemia (AML) under age 61. *Blood* 2006;108:abstract 157.

109. Ravandi F, Cortes J, Faderl S, et al. Combination of sorafenib, idarubicin, and cytarabine has a high response rate in patients with newly diagnosed acute myeloid leukemia (AML) younger than 65 years. *Blood* 2008;112:Abstract 768.

110. Cortes JE, Ghirdaladze D, Foran JM, et al. Phase 1 AML study of AC220, a potent and selective second generation FLT3 receptor tyrosine kinase inhibitor. *Blood* 2008;112:Abstract 767.

111. Feldman EJ, Lancet J, Kolitz JE, et al. Phase I study of a liposomal carrier (CPX-351) containing a synergistic, fixed molar ratio of cytarabine (Ara-C) and daunorubicin (DNR) in advanced leukemias. *Blood* 2008;112:Abstract 2984.

112. Lo Coco F, Diverio D, Falini B, et al. Genetic diagnosis and molecular monitoring in the management of acute promyelocytic leukemia. *Blood* 1999;94(1):12-22.

113. Melnick A, Licht JD. Deconstructing a disease: RARalpha, its fusion partners, and their roles in the pathogenesis of acute promyelocytic leukemia. *Blood* 1999;93(10):3167-3215.

114. Tallman MS, Kwaan HC. Reassessing the hemostatic disorder associated with acute promyelocytic leukemia. *Blood* 1992;79(3):543-553.

115. Dyck JA, Warrell RP, Jr., Evans RM, et al. Rapid diagnosis of acute promyelocytic leukemia by immunohistochemical localization of PML/RAR-alpha protein. *Blood* 1995;86(3):862-867.

116. Golomb HM, Rowley JD, Vardiman JW, et al. "Microgranular" acute promyelocytic leukemia: A distinct clinical, ultrastructural, and cytogenetic entity. *Blood* 1980;55(2):253-259.

117. Avvisati G, Petti MC, Lo Coco F, et al. Induction therapy with idarubicin alone significantly influences event-free survival duration in patients with newly diagnosed hypergranular acute promyelocytic leukemia: Final results of the GIMEMA randomized study LAP 0389 with 7 years of minimal follow-up. *Blood* 2002;100(9):3141-3146.

118. Estey E, Thall PF, Pierce S, et al. Treatment of newly diagnosed acute promyelocytic leukemia without cytarabine. *J Clin Oncol* 1997;15(2):483-490.

119. Tallman MS, Andersen JW, Schiffer CA, et al. Clinical description of 44 patients with acute promyelocytic leukemia who developed the retinoic acid syndrome. *Blood* 2000;95(1):90-95.

120. Diverio D, Rossi V, Avvisati G, et al. Early detection of relapse by prospective reverse transcriptase-polymerase chain reaction analysis of the PML/RARalpha fusion gene in patients with acute promyelocytic leukemia enrolled in the GIMEMA-AIEOP multicenter "AIDA" trial. GIMEMA-AIEOP Multicenter "AIDA" Trial. *Blood* 1998;92(3):784-789.

121. Jurcic JG, Nimer SD, Scheinberg DA, et al. Prognostic significance of minimal residual disease detection and PML/RAR-alpha isoform type: Long-term follow-up in acute promyelocytic leukemia. *Blood* 2001;98(9):2651-2656.

122. Shao W, Fanelli M, Ferrara FF, et al. Arsenic trioxide as an inducer of apoptosis and loss of PML/RAR alpha protein in acute promyelocytic leukemia cells. *J Natl Cancer Inst* 1998;90(2):124-133.

123. Soignet SL, Frankel SR, Douer D, et al. United States multicenter study of arsenic trioxide in relapsed acute promyelocytic leukemia. *J Clin Oncol* 2001;19(18):3852-3860.

124. Estey E. Therapeutic research in untreated acute promyelocytic leukemia. *Leukemia* 2005;19(6):913-915.

125. Niu C, Yan H, Yu T, et al. Studies on treatment of acute promyelocytic leukemia with arsenic trioxide: Remission induction, follow-up, and molecular monitoring in 11 newly diagnosed and 47 relapsed acute promyelocytic leukemia patients. *Blood* 1999;94(10):3315-3324.

126. Shen ZX, Shi ZZ, Fang J, et al. All-trans retinoic acid/As2O3 combination yields a high quality remission and survival in newly diagnosed acute promyelocytic leukemia. *Proc Natl Acad Sci USA* 2004;101(15):5328-5335.

127. Ravandi F, Estey E, Jones D, et al. Effective treatment of acute promyelocytic leukemia with all-trans-retinoic acid, arsenic trioxide, and gemtuzumab ozogamicin. *J Clin Oncol* 2009;27(4):504-510.

128. Miwako I, Kagechika H. Tamibarotene. *Drugs Today (Barc)* 2007;43(8):563-568.

129. Johnson PR, Ryder WD, Yin JA. Validation of a model to predict survival in elderly patients with acute myeloid leukaemia. *Br J Haematol* 1995;90(4):954-956.

130. Johnson PR, Yin JA. Prognostic factors in elderly patients with acute myeloid leukaemia. *Leuk Lymphoma* 1994;16(1-2):51-56.

131. Kantarjian H, O'Brien S, Cortes J, et al. Results of intensive chemotherapy in 998 patients age 65 years or older with acute myeloid leukemia or high-risk myelodysplastic syndrome: Predictive prognostic models for outcome. *Cancer* 2006;106(5):1090-1098.

132. Burnett AK, Milligan D, Prentice AG, et al. Low dose ara-C versus hydroxyurea with or without retinoid in older patients not considered fit for intensive chemotherapy: the UK NCRI AML 14 trial. *Blood* 2004;104:Abstract 872.

133. Erba HP, Kantarjian H, Claxton DF, et al. Phase II study of single agent clofarabine in previously untreated older adult patients with acute myelogenous leukemia (AML) unlikely to benefit from standard induction chemotherapy. *Blood* 2008;112:Abstract 558.

134. Pigneux A, Witz F, Sauvezie M, et al. Improved outcome by addition of lomustine (CCNU) to idarubicin and cytarabine in elderly patients with de novo acute myeloid leukemia. A report from the GOELAMS Group. *Blood* 2008;112 (Abstract 761).

135. Konopleva M, Cheng SC, Cortes JE, et al. Independent prognostic significance of day 21 cytogenetic findings in newly diagnosed acute myeloid leukemia or refractory anemia with excess blasts. *Haematologica* 2003;88(7):733-736.

136. van der Velden VH, Hochhaus A, Cazzaniga G, et al. Detection of minimal residual disease in hematologic malignancies by real-time quantitative PCR: Principles, approaches, and laboratory aspects. *Leukemia* 2003;17(6):1013-1034.

137. Yin JA, Grimwade D. Minimal residual disease evaluation in acute myeloid leukaemia. *Lancet* 2002;360(9327):160-162.

138. Bergmann L, Miething C, Maurer U, et al. High levels of Wilms' tumor gene (WT1) mRNA in acute myeloid leukemias are associated with a worse long-term outcome. *Blood* 1997; 90(3):1217-1225.

139. Jacobsohn DA, Tse WT, Chaleff S, et al. High WT1 gene expression before haematopoietic stem cell transplant in children with acute myeloid leukaemia predicts poor event-free survival. *Br J Haematol* 2009;146(6):669-674.

140. Cilloni D, Renneville A, Hermitte F, et al. Real-time quantitative polymerase chain reaction detection of minimal residual disease by standardized WT1 assay to enhance risk stratification in acute myeloid leukemia: A European LeukemiaNet study. *J Clin Oncol* 2009;27(31):5195-5201.

141. Shook D, Coustan-Smith E, Ribeiro RC, et al. Minimal residual disease quantitation in acute myeloid leukemia. *Clin Lymphoma Myeloma* 2009;9(Suppl 3):S281-S285.

142. Kern W, Voskova D, Schoch C, et al. Determination of relapse risk based on assessment of minimal residual disease during complete remission by multiparameter flow cytometry in unselected patients with acute myeloid leukemia. *Blood* 2004;104(10):3078-3085.

143. San Miguel JF, Martinez A, Macedo A, et al. Immunophenotyping investigation of minimal residual disease is a useful approach for predicting relapse in acute myeloid leukemia patients. *Blood* 1997;90(6):2465-2470.

CHRONIC LYMPHOCYTIC LEUKEMIA AND ASSOCIATED DISORDERS

Ravin J. Garg
Carlos Bueso-Ramos
Susan O'Brien

Chronic lymphocytic leukemia (CLL) is an indolent lymphoid disorder involving a clonal expansion of CD5-positive B cells. Nucleoside analogs in combination with alkylating agents and/or monoclonal antibodies have produced marked improvement in remission rates. There is now evidence of an improvement in survival with chemoimmunotherapy.

■ EPIDEMIOLOGY

CLL is the most common leukemia in the Western hemisphere, accounting for 20% of all leukemias in the United States. This disease is uncommon in the Asian population, and accounts for only 2.5% of all leukemias in Japan. The incidence is age-dependent, with an increase from 5.2 per 100,000 persons older than 50 years to 30.4 per 100,000 persons older than 80 years. The male-to-female ratio is 1.5:1.

■ BIOLOGY

CELL OF ORIGIN

Surface Antigen Phenotype

CLL is a clonal B-cell lymphoid leukemia. Morphologically, CLL cells resemble small mature lymphocytes arrested in an intermediate stage of the B-cell differentiation pathway. The hallmark of CLL cells are that they express CD5, an antigen commonly found on T cells. CD5-positive B cells can be found in the mantle zone of lymphoid follicles, but they constitute a minor fraction of the B-cell population. CD19, CD20, and CD23 are other B-cell markers expressed on CLL cells. Surface immunoglobulin, FMC7, CD22, CD11c, and CD79b are either weakly expressed or negative in CLL. Based on the antigen expression profile, CLL appears to arise from an "activated" B cell (1).

Somatic Hypermutation of Immunoglobulin Variable Gene

Assessment for somatic hypermutation of immunoglobulin variable gene (IgV) defines two subsets of CLL. Recombination of variable (V), diversity (D), and joining (J) genes and insertion of nontemplated nucleotides at the V–D and D–J junction occurs in the pregerminal phase of B-cell development. Somatic hypermutations are introduced in the V(D)J rearrangement in normal B cells in the germinal center in response to antigen presented by follicular dendritic cells (2). Approximately, 50% of CLL cases have somatic hypermutation of the IgV gene (3) and thus appear to arise from postgerminal B cells, while the subset of CLL lacking IgV gene hypermutation appear to arise from naive B cells. The mutation status of CLL cells seems fixed, and mutational status is not gained or lost during the course of disease. It has been demonstrated that the mutational status provides significant prognostic information.

CYTOGENETICS

Using conventional chromosome banding techniques, cytogenetic abnormalities can be detected in up to 50% of CLL cases. These techniques are hampered by the low mitotic activity of CLL cells; B-cell mitogens may be used to enhance this activity. In addition, metaphases obtained for karyotyping may also arise from normal T cells in the sample, as indicated by sequential immuno-typing followed by karyotypic analysis (4).

Fluorescent in situ hybridization (FISH) using genomic DNA probes has greatly enhanced the ability to detect molecular abnormalities in malignant cells. This technique can detect aberrations in interphase cells. FISH has demonstrated that molecular abnormalities occur in up to 80% of cases of CLL (5).

13q deletion is the most common genetic aberration found in CLL by FISH (55%), followed by 11q deletion (18%), 12q trisomy (16%), and 17p deletion (7%) (6). Prior to the use of FISH, trisomy 12 was the most frequently detected chromosomal abnormality in CLL by conventional cytogenetic methods (7). Structural abnormalities of 13q were often missed by Giemsa banding, presumably because of the small size of the deletion. The prognosis of CLL varies with the chromosomal abnormality. When divided into five prognostic categories—17p deletion, 11q deletion, 12q trisomy, normal karyotype, and 13q deletion (as sole abnormality)—the survival times were 32, 79, 114, 111, and 133 months, respectively. Patients with 11q deletion have more significant lymphadenopathy. Patients with 17p and 11q deletion have more advanced disease and respond poorly to conventional therapy.

RESISTANCE TO APOPTOSIS

Resistance to apoptosis is a feature of CLL cells, and many mechanisms have been proposed for this resistance (8,9). Recent experiments have described a subset of peripheral blood mononuclear cells in patients with CLL that differentiate into "nurse-like" cells (NLC) in vitro and can protect CLL cells from apoptosis (10).

■ CLINICAL FEATURES

At diagnosis, most patients are older than 60 years, with more than 90% being over 50 years. The diagnosis of CLL is often incidental; routine blood counts may reveal an elevated absolute lymphocyte count (ALC). In symptomatic patients, fatigue and infections may be presenting features. B symptoms (fever, weight loss) can also occur but are uncommon. A small percentage of patients may present with autoimmune hemolytic anemia (AIHA) or autoimmune thrombocytopenia (AIT). Physical examination may reveal cervical, axillary, and/or inguinal lymphadenopathy. Splenomegaly and hepatomegaly are not uncommon.

■ LABORATORY FEATURES

Laboratory findings invariably show lymphocytosis. The ALC can range from 5×10^9/L to 500×10^9/L. CLL cells resemble mature lymphocytes; they have dense chromatin as well as scant cytoplasm and lack nucleoli (Fig. 3-1). Smear preparation from peripheral blood may damage these fragile lymphocytes and produce "smudge" cells. The extent of bone marrow infiltration varies in terms of the percentage of marrow involved as well as in the pattern of involvement, which may be nodular (Figs. 3-2A and B) to diffuse. Erythroid, myeloid, and megakaryocytic precursors may be normal or decreased. Anemia or thrombocytopenia may result from marrow infiltration or from immune destruction. Findings of microspherocytes in peripheral blood smear (Fig. 3-3) and demonstration of IgG and/or complement on red cells support the diagnosis of immune-hemolytic anemia. Pure red cell aplasia has been described in 1 to 6% of cases (11).

Patients often develop hypogammaglobulinemia, which can progress in severity with advancing disease. Monoclonal gammopathy may also develop and detection depends on methods used for diagnosis. Other laboratory abnormalities include elevated serum β_2 microglobulin (β_2-M); LDH is rarely elevated.

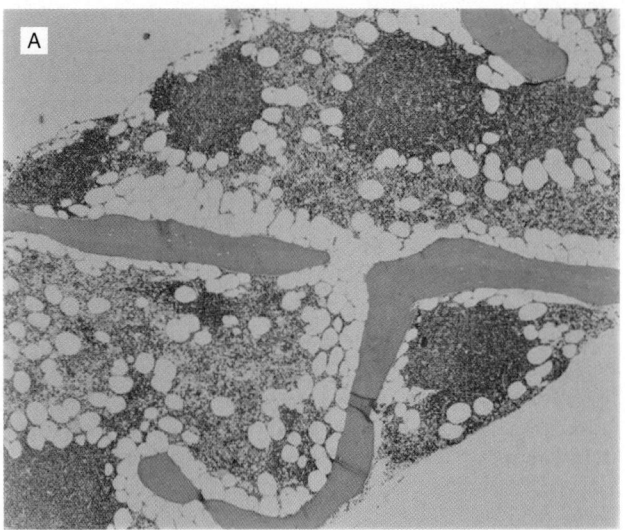

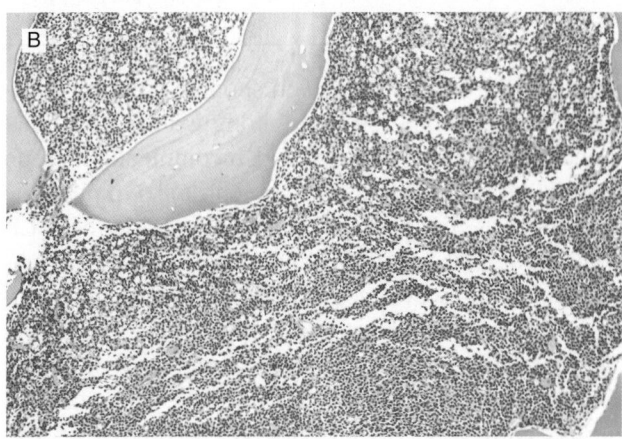

FIGURE 3-2. (**A, B**) Chronic lymphocytic leukemia. Bone marrow biopsies showing nodular, diffuse, and interstitial patterns of involvement.

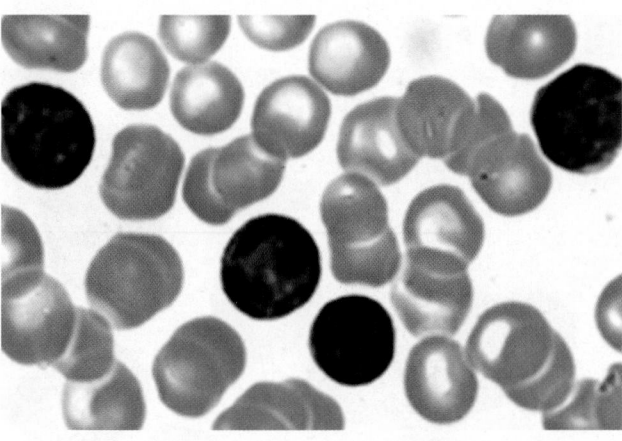

FIGURE 3-1. Chronic lymphocytic leukemia. Peripheral blood smear showing mature-appearing lymphocytes. Note dense chromatin, scant cytoplasm, absence of nucleoli, and smudge cells.

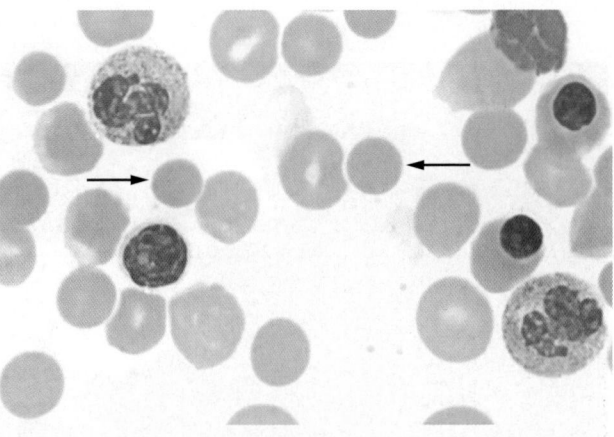

FIGURE 3-3. Immune hemolytic anemia. Presence of microspherocytes (*arrows*) and nucleated red cells indicates immune destruction of red cells. Diagnosis is confirmed by demonstrating the presence of IgG and/or complement on red cells.

TABLE 3-1	DIAGNOSTIC CRITERIA FOR CLL	

Parameter	NCI-IWCLL*
Diagnosis	
Lymphocytes (×10⁹/L)	≥5 B lymphocytes in peripheral blood
Clonality	Flow cytometry to confirm clonality
Duration of lymphocytosis	Not stated
Bone marrow lymphocytes (%)	Not necessary to make a diagnosis†‡

*National Cancer Institute—International Workshop Group on CLL (Ref. 12).
†Bone marrow aspirate and biopsy can be evaluated for factors contributing to cytopenias that may not be due to leukemia infiltration of the marrow.

■ DIAGNOSIS

In 2008, the International workshop on Chronic Lymphocytic Leukemia (IWCLL) along with the National Cancer Institute (NCI) updated recommendations on the diagnosis and treatment of chronic lymphocytic leukemia (12) (Table 3-1). The diagnosis of CLL requires at least 5×10^9 B lymphocytes/L in the peripheral blood. Flow cytometry is used to confirm the clonality of the circulating B lymphocytes, including demonstrating light-chain restriction on CLL cells. CLL cells coexpress the T-cell antigen CD5 and B-cell surface antigens CD19, CD20, CD23. ZAP-70 (Fig. 3-4) expression in CLL cells has prognostic implication (see section "Prognosis"). Distinguishing CLL from mantle cell lymphoma (Figs. 3-5A and B) (see section "Differential Diagnosis") and large granular (LG) leukemia (Fig. 3-6) is of utmost importance.

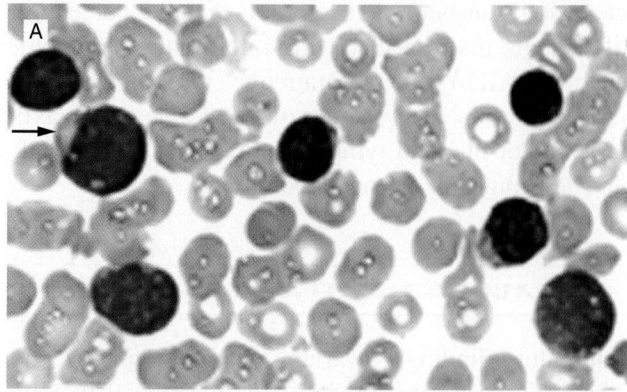

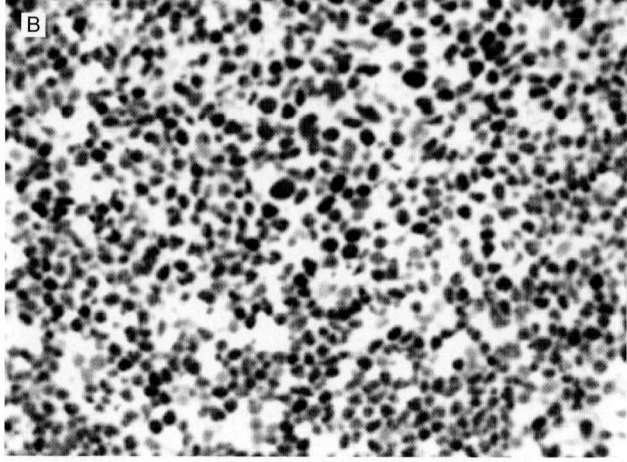

FIGURE 3-5. **A**. Mantle cell lymphoma (MCL) in leukemic phase. MCL cells (*arrow*) are larger than mature lymphocytes (center) with speckled chromatin; some show nuclear cleft. **B**. Nuclear cyclin D1 staining in mantle cells.

The presence of more than 55% of prolymphocytes would favor a diagnosis of prolymphocytic leukemia. Prolymphocytes (<55%) can be seen in peripheral blood or bone marrow of patients with CLL (Figs. 3-7A and B). A bone marrow aspirate and biopsy are not required to

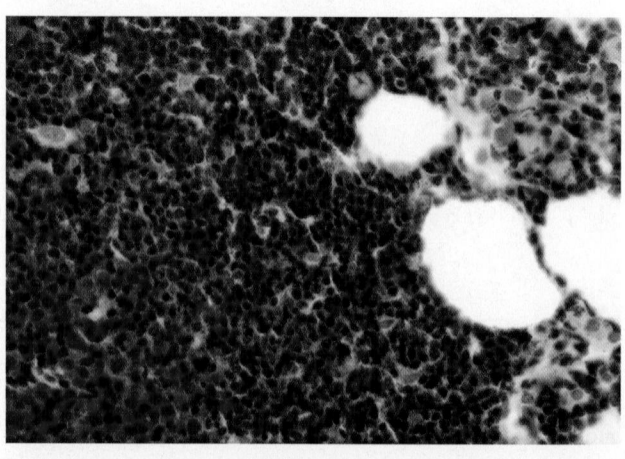

FIGURE 3-4. ZAP-70 expression in CLL cells indicates poor prognosis. Immunohistochemistry (*above*) or flow cytometry can be used to detect ZAP-70 expression.

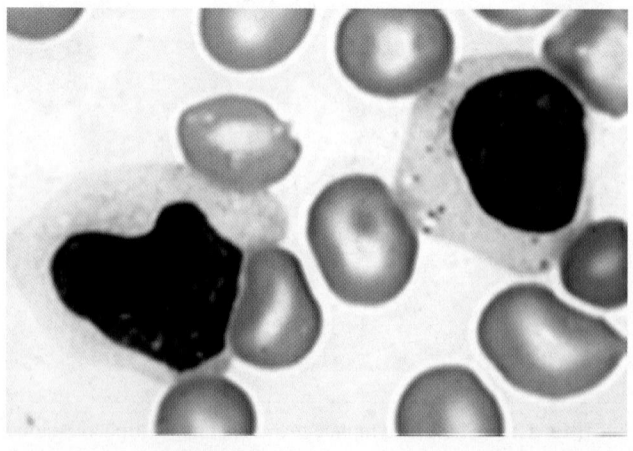

FIGURE 3-6. Large granular lymphocytes with cytoplasmic azurophilic granules.

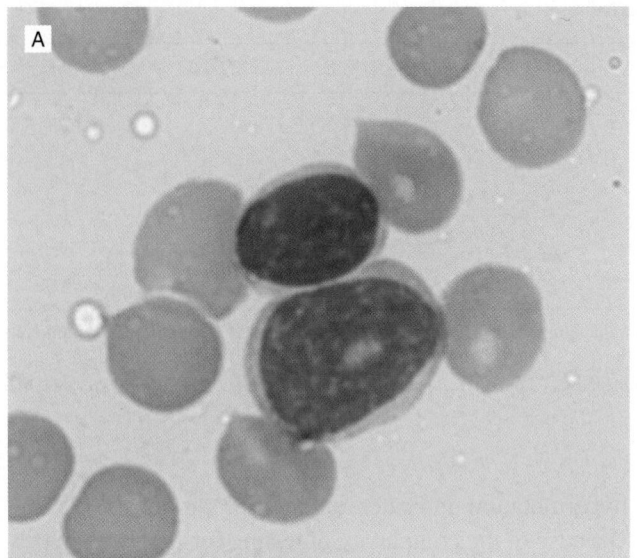

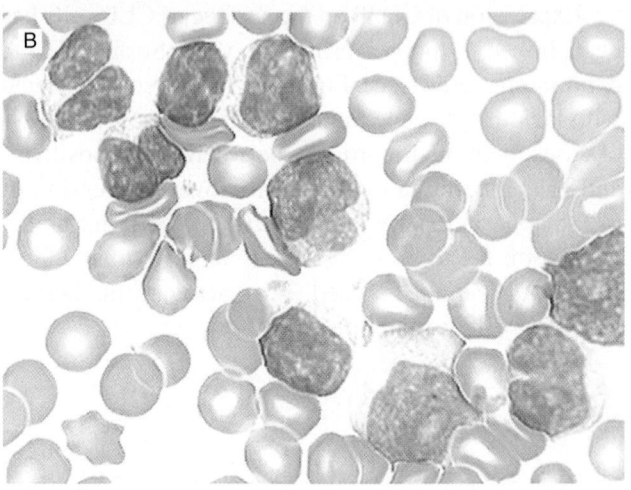

FIGURE 3-7. **A**. High-power view of a prolymphocyte juxtaposed with a mature-appearing lymphocyte. Note larger size, less condensed chromatin, and prominent nucleolus in prolymphocyte. **B**. Peripheral blood smear of patient with CLL showing cleaved cells and prolymphocytes. Note cleaved nuclei, presence of nucleoli, and more abundant cytoplasm in prolymphocytes. Presence of up to 55% of prolymphocytes is compatible with a diagnosis of CLL.

make the diagnosis of CLL. While the type of marrow infiltration (diffuse versus nondiffuse) reflects the tumor burden and can provide prognostic information, recent data suggests that new prognostic markers may be more reflective of disease trajectory (13).

■ DIFFERENTIAL DIAGNOSIS

Clinical, morphologic, immunophenotypic, and cytogenetic methods help to distinguish between B-CLL and other diseases such as T-PLL, the leukemic phase of non-Hodgkin lymphoma (mantle cell, follicular, or others), PLL, hairy cell leukemia (HCL), marginal zone lymphoma, and Waldenstrom's macroglobulinemia. Table 3-2 summarizes the immunophenotypic features of these disorders. Distinguishing CLL from mantle cell lymphoma is important as both can express CD5 (see Fig. 3-5A). Two differences, however, are that mantle cell lymphoma cells are CD23-negative and have strong surface immunoglobulin staining. Confirmation of mantle cell lymphoma can be made by detection of the t(11;14) translocation and/or positive nuclear cyclin D1 staining (see Fig. 3-5B).

Based on immunophenotyping data using five to six markers, Matutes et al. devised a scoring system to aid in differentiating CLL from other chronic B-cell disorders (14).

■ STAGING

The well-described staging systems for CLL include Rai (15) and Binet (16) staging (Table 3-3). The original Rai classification defined five stages from 0 to 4; this has been modified to three stages by defining Rai stage 0 as low-risk, joining stage 1 with 2 to form an intermediate-risk group, and stage 3 with 4 to form a high-risk group, with a median survival of >12.5, 7, and 1.5 years for each risk group, respectively (17). Similarly in Binet stages A, B, and C, median survivals are >10, 6, and 2 years, respectively. The diagnostic workup that is undertaken in CLL patients at initial presentation at the University of Texas MD Anderson Cancer Center (MDACC) is listed in Table 3-4.

■ PROGNOSIS

Both CLL staging systems confer significant prognostic information; however, they are limited by their inability to identify which patient with early-stage disease will develop disease progression. An analysis of the French Cooperative Group trial of Binet stage A patient has demonstrated that a subgroup (designated "A'") of patients with a hemoglobin ≥12 g/dL, a lymphocyte count <30 × 10^9/L, and fewer than 80% lymphocytes in the bone marrow aspirate, was less likely to progress than other stage A patients (18). A lymphocyte doubling time of >12 months, Rai stage 0 disease, nondiffuse bone marrow pattern, hemoglobin ≥13 g/dL, and ALC <30 × 10^9/L similarly define a group of "smoldering CLL" with an excellent prognosis (19). Age and response to treatment are also prognostic factors. Women fare better than men, independently of stage and age (20).

TABLE 3-2 | IMMUNOPHENOTYPIC ANALYSIS IN CHRONIC B-CELL DISORDERS

Disease	CD5	CD10	CD20	CD22	CD23	CD79B	CD103	FMC7
CLL	++	–	+	–/+	++	–/+	–	–/+
B-PLL	–/+	–/+	++	+	–/+	++	–	++
HCL	–	–	++	++	–	+	+	++
SLVL	–/+	–	++	++	–/+	++	–	++
FL	–/+	++	++	++	–/+	++	–	++
MCL	++	–	++	++	–	++	–	++

B-PLL, prolymphocytic leukemia; CLL, chronic lymphocytic leukemia; FL, follicular lymphoma; HCL, hairy cell leukemia; MCL, mantle cell lymphoma; SLVL, splenic lymphoma with villous lymphocytes.
Cyclin D1 negative in CLL, positive in MCL. If atypical immunophenotype [CD23 dim/negative, CD20 bright, sIg bright]: send for cyclin D1 IHC or FISH for t(11;14).

Several serum factors have been identified as prognostic indicators in early-stage CLL. Patients with early-stage CLL with serum thymidine kinase (TK) levels >7.0 U/L had a significantly shorter progression-free survival (PFS) compared to those with TK levels below that (21). Elevated serum β_2-M level is also an adverse prognostic feature that has been shown to correlate with clinical stage and disease progression (22). Serum soluble CD23 segregates Binet stage B disease into more or less aggressive forms (23). High serum LDH levels indicate a poor prognosis (24).

IgV gene somatic hypermutation in the leukemic cells is present in 50% of patients with CLL (3). Lack of somatic hypermutation indicates an inferior prognosis (25,26). Because of the complexity of testing for IgV gene hypermutation, a search for surrogate markers ensued (27).

Expression of CD38 on the surface of CLL cells has been linked to poorer prognosis (25). Surface CD38 expression >30% (see Fig. 3-6) has been associated with lack of IgV gene mutation (25). However, in 30% of cases, there is discordance between CD38 positivity and IgV gene mutation (28). Moreover, expression of CD38 appears to vary in some cases of CLL during the course of the disease. Thus, it appears that CD38 expression cannot be used as a surrogate marker for lack of IgV gene mutation.

TABLE 3-3 | STAGING OF CLL

Rai Stage	Modified Rai Stage	Description	Binet Stage	Description	Median Survival
0	Low risk	Lymphocytosis only	A	Hemoglobin ≥10 g/dL and platelets ≥100 × 10^9/L and <3 enlarged lymphoid bearing areas	>10 years
1	Intermediate risk	Lymphocytosis and lymphadenopathy	B	Hemoglobin ≥10 g/dL and platelets ≥100 × 10^9/L and ≥3 enlarged lymphoid bearing areas	5-7 years
2	Intermediate risk	Lymphocytosis and splenomegaly and/or hepatomegaly with/without lymphadenopathy			
3	High risk	Lymphocytosis and anemia (hemoglobin <11 g/dL)	C	Hemoglobin <10 g/dL and platelets <100 × 10^9/L and any number of lymphoid bearing areas	2-3 years
4	High risk	Lymphocytosis and thrombocytopenia (platelets <100 × 10^9/L			

TABLE 3-4	EVALUATION AND MONITORING OF PATIENTS WITH CLL AT MDACC

Initial evaluation

History and physical (close attention to lymph node areas, liver/spleen size)

  Constitutional symptoms (fever, chills, weight loss, night sweats)

    Assessment of performance status

    CBC, electrolytes, BUN, creatinine, LFT, LDH, quantitative immunoglobulins, Coombs test β_2 microglobulin

  Examination of peripheral blood smear

    Bone marrow aspiration and biopsy

    Immunophenotyping* of bone marrow lymphocytes

    Flow cytometry[†] for CD38

    Immunostaining of bone marrow for ZAP-70

    Cytogenetics/FISH for ATM gene region of chromosome 11, *p53* region of chromosome 17, the alpha satellite centromeric region of chromosome 12, the D13S319 locus in the 13q14.3 region of chromosome 13, and the LAMP1 gene on chromosome 13q34

    Mutation status of light- and heavy-chain gene rearrangements

Response assessment

  Physical examination[‡]

  CBC, differential

  Bone marrow aspirate and biopsy

  Immunophenotype

  Molecular studies (PCR for light and heavy chain gene rearrangement)

*Immunophenotyping: Recommend panel for paraffin section IHC: CD3, CD5, CD10, CD20, CD23, Cyclin D1.
[†]Flow cytometry: Kappa/lambda, CD19, CD20, CD5, CD23, CD10.
[‡]Many clinical trials are now incorporating CT scans as per new guidelines, but these are not standard of care outside a clinical trial.

TABLE 3-5	ESTABLISHED POOR PROGNOSTIC FACTORS IN CLL

Male gender

Advanced Rai or Binet staging

Cytogenetic abnormalities 11q-, 17p-, *p53* abnormalities

Lymphocyte doubling time <12 months

Initial lymphocyte count >50 × 10^9/L

Elevated serum TK

Elevated β_2 microglobin

Elevated serum-soluble CD23

CD38 expression >30% (negative is favorable, positive is unfavorable)

Expression of ZAP-70

Diffuse pattern of marrow involvement

Lack of IgV gene somatic mutation: ≤2% mutation (unfavorable)

TK, thymidine kinase.

Expression of zeta-associated protein 70 (ZAP-70) can be more useful in predicting time to progression than mutational status (29). In addition, it was found to correlate inversely with IgV gene mutation (30,31). Interestingly, this protein with tyrosine kinase activity is normally found in T lymphocytes, where it transduces signals from the T-cell receptor. Expression of ZAP-70 was shown to be associated with absence of IgV gene mutation, shorter time to progression, and worse survival (32,33). However, evaluation of ZAP-70 expression can be difficult.

Abnormal expression of *p53* detected in bone marrow biopsies by immunohistochemistry has been associated with inferior survival (34). Dysfunctional *p53* seems to coexist with a low incidence of IgV gene mutation (35). Deletion or mutation of *p53* is also associated with resistance to fludarabine (36).

Interphase FISH has identified structural chromosomal abnormalities in 80% of CLL cases. Deletion of 13q as the sole chromosomal abnormality and normal karyotype confers better prognosis, whereas 17p and 11q deletions indicate worse prognosis (6). In addition, 17p deletion can often predict resistance to chemotherapy. Analysis of correlation between chromosomal abnormalities and IgV somatic hypermutation indicated that 13q deletion as a sole chromosomal abnormality is more frequent among patients with IgV somatic hypermutation. Within the group of patients lacking somatic hypermutation, the presence of high-risk genomic abnormalities such as 17p or 11q deletion was linked with worse prognosis. Thus, IgV mutational status and chromosomal analysis provide additive prognostic information (37). These genetic lesions can evolve, thus FISH analysis should be repeated prior to each treatment. The established prognostic factors in CLL indicating poorer outcome are listed in Table 3-5.

■ TREATMENT

INDICATIONS FOR TREATMENT

Early treatment of asymptomatic CLL with chlorambucil has not been shown to prolong survival (38,39) and may be associated with increased frequency of epithelial cancers. The NCI- IWCLL-recommended criteria for treatment of CLL are summarized in Table 3-6.

ALKYLATING AGENTS

Alkylating agents such as chlorambucil or cyclophosphamide either alone or in combination with corticosteroids were the cornerstone of treatment of CLL for some decades. The combination of prednisone with chlorambucil did not improve survival compared to that

TABLE 3-6	INDICATIONS FOR TREATMENT IN CLL (NCI- IWCLL) (12)

Active disease should be confirmed prior to initiating treatment.

1. Evidence of progressive marrow failure as manifest by the development or worsening of anemia and/or thrombocytopenia
2. Massive (ie, >6 cm below the left costal margin) or progressive or symptomatic splenomegaly
3. Massive nodes or clusters (ie, at least 10 cm in longest diameter) or progressive or symptomatic lymphadenopathy
4. Progressive lymphocytosis with an increase of more than 50% over a 2-month period or an anticipated doubling time of less than 6 months*
5. Autoimmune anemia and/or thrombocytopenia poorly responsive to corticosteroid therapy or other standard therapy
6. Constitutional symptoms, defined as any one or more of the following disease-related symptoms or signs:
   a. Unintentional weight loss ≥10% within the previous 6 months
   b. Significant fatigue (ie, ECOG PS 2 or worse; cannot work or unable to perform usual activities)
   c. Fevers greater than 100.5°F or 38.0°C for ≥2 weeks without evidence of infection
   d. Night sweats for more than 1 month without evidence of infection

*In patients with a lymphocyte count of less than 30×10^9/L, lymphocyte doubling time should not be used as a single parameter to define treatment indication. Factors contributing to lymphocytosis or lymphadenopathy other than CLL (ie, infections) should be excluded.

seen with chlorambucil alone (40). Comparison of chlorambucil with or without steroids to combination regimens with cyclophosphamide, vincristine, and prednisone (CVP or COP) indicated similar outcomes (40).

ANTHRACYCLINES

The French Cooperative group reported improved 2-year survival with cyclophosphamide, vincristine, doxorubicin, and prednisone with reduced-dose of doxorubicin (mini-CHOP) in Binet stage C patients when compared with CVP (41). The survival advantage with mini-CHOP was maintained in long-term follow-up studies (42). A later report by the same group confirmed the absence of a survival advantage with mini-CHOP compared to chlorambucil plus prednisone in patients with Binet stage B disease (43). Two anthracycline-containing regimens have been tested at MDACC. The first was CAP, which was comprised of cyclophosphamide 750 mg/m^2 on day 1, doxorubicin 50 mg/m^2 on day 1, and prednisone 100 mg/day for 5 days. Maintenance was with cyclophosphamide and prednisone. Thirty-three percent of patients achieved CR (included

persistence of nodules in bone marrow) and 23% achieved partial remission (PR). The POACH program added vincristine and cytosine arabinoside (Ara-C) to CAP; this yielded responses in 56% of patients, with 21% achieving CR (44).

PURINE ANALOGS (FLUDARABINE AND CLADRIBINE)

In 1988–1989 Grever et al. (45) and the MDACC group published the first positive results in the management of CLL with fludarabine (46). In the MDACC study, a 5-day schedule of fludarabine in previously treated patients with CLL produced a CR rate of 15% and an overall response rate (ORR) of 44%. This report proposed a separate response category of nodular CR (NCR). Prior to this, patients with lymphoid nodules in the bone marrow biopsy were considered to be in CR if the lymphocyte percentage in the aspirate was <30%. The NCI-IWCLL put forth a new response criteria; patients in CR were required to have no residual nodules and those with residual nodules were considered to be in nodular PR (NPR). A large number of patients treated with fludarabine through the group C mechanism of the NCI had an overall response rate of 32% (3% CR, 29% PR) (47). When previously untreated patients received fludarabine, the ORR was 78% (33% CR [which included NPR patients at that point in time], 39% PR, and 6% PR) (48). The French Cooperative group reported an ORR of 70% with fludarabine as frontline therapy (49). Different fludarabine regimens including the addition of prednisone (50), a 3-day schedule of fludarabine (51), and a once-a-week schedule of fludarabine (52) have been studied at MDACC. Addition of prednisone to fludarabine did not improve response rates or survival. The incidence of opportunistic infections was increased. The response rates seen with the 3-day schedule of fludarabine were slightly less than that seen with the 5-day schedule but was associated with less immunosuppression and lower morbidity. The once-a-week schedule had an inferior response rate. Myelosuppression, febrile episodes, and infections are the common toxicities noted with fludarabine (46).

Cladribine, another purine analog, has also been studied as both salvage and frontline therapy for CLL. Overall response rates are comparable to those seen with fludarabine (53,54).

Comparative Trials With Fludarabine

Fludarabine, when compared to chlorambucil, produced significantly higher response rates in previously untreated patients with CLL (55). In the CALGB 9011 study, 509 patients were randomized to receive either fludarabine, chlorambucil, or both in combination. The combination arm was stopped early due to excessive toxicity. Among patients treated with fludarabine, 20% had a CR and 43% had a PR compared to 4 and 33% corresponding values for patients treated with chlorambucil ($p < .001$ for both comparisons). The median duration of remission and the median progression-free survival in the fludarabine group were 25 and 20 months, respectively, whereas both values were 14 months in the chlorambucil group ($p < .001$ for both comparisons). Patients in both the fludarabine and chlorambucil arm had the same OS during the initial 5 years following randomization. However, long-term outcome of patients on this study was recently reported (56) and showed that on longer follow-up, patients treated with fludarabine had a continued longer PFS than those treated with chlorambucil ($p < .001$) along with a better OS ($p = .04$; unadjusted for covariates).

The French Cooperative group compared fludarabine with two different alkylating-based combination regimens (French mini-CHOP and CAP) in previously untreated patients with advanced CLL (57). Fludarabine and CHOP produced a comparable remission rate (71%) that was better than that seen with CAP (58%). Although overall survival was not different, the ORR was higher with fludarabine in Binet stage B disease (fludarabine 94%, mini-CHOP 75%, CAP 72%). Fludarabine was better tolerated than CHOP, and thus emerged as the treatment of choice in CLL.

Fludarabine and Cyclophosphamide

Fludarabine in combination with cyclophosphamide (FC) has been shown to be an effective regimen in CLL. E2997 was a phase III randomized trial comparing FC versus fludarabine alone in patients with CLL receiving their first chemotherapy regimen (58). A total of 278 patients were randomly assigned. FC was associated with a higher CR (23.4% versus 4.6%; $p < .001$) and higher ORR (74.3% versus 59.5%; $p = .013$) than treatment with fludarabine as a single agent. Progression-free survival (PFS) was significantly better for patients treated with FC compared to fludarabine alone (31.6 versus 19.2 months; $p < .0001$). The FC combination caused more hematologic toxicity (thrombocytopenia, $p = .046$), but did not lead to a significantly increased number of severe infections.

Another study verified the superiority of FC compared to fludarabine alone or chlorambucil (59). A total of 777 patients with CLL requiring treatment were enrolled on study and randomly assigned to three different treatment groups: fludarabine alone (N = 194),

FC (N = 196), or chlorambucil (N = 387). Both the complete response rate (CR) and ORR were better for FC compared to fludarabine (CR 38% versus 15%, $p < .0001$; ORR 94% versus 80%, $p < .0001$). FC and fludarabine both led to a significantly better response rate than chlorambucil (CR 7%, $p = .006$; ORR 72%, $p = .04$). The 5-year PFS was significantly better with FC (36%) compared to fludarabine (10%) and chlorambucil (10%; $p < .00005$). FC was the best regimen for all patients including those older than 70 years. FC led to more neutropenia and days in the hospital, but had less hemolytic anemia (5%) compared to fludarabine (11%) and chlorambucil (12%).

A German study compared FC with fludarabine monotherapy in first-line treatment of younger patients with CLL, with most having advanced disease (60). The study enrolled 375 patients, all of whom were younger than 66 years of age. The FC combination resulted in a higher CR (24% versus 7%; $p < .001$) and ORR (94% versus 83%; $p = .001$). FC also led to a longer PFS (48 months versus 20 months; $p = .001$) and longer treatment-free survival (37 months versus 25 months; $p < .001$). Although FC led to more thrombocytopenia and leukopenia, there was no increase in the number of severe infections. Another study from Italy also demonstrated the efficacy of FC (61). Thus, three randomized trials have all shown an increased response rate and PFS with FC.

BENDAMUSTINE

Bendamustine is an alkylating agent that has structural similarities to a purine analog. It consists of both a nitrogen mustard core and purine-like side group. This agent has little cross-resistance with other alkylating agents. A pivotal phase III study comparing bendamustine to chlorambucil in patients with CLL led to its FDA approval (62). This was a randomized, open-label, multicenter study comparing the safety and efficacy of bendamustine versus chlorambucil in previously untreated patients with advanced stage CLL. A total of 319 patients were randomly assigned (162 patients to bendamustine, 157 patients to chlorambucil). Bendamustine led to a significantly higher level of ORR (110 of 162 patients, 68%) compared to chlorambucil (48 of 157, 31%; $p < .0001$). Patients in the bendamustine arm had a higher level of CR (31% versus 2%), along with a longer PFS (21.6 months versus 8.3 months; $p < .0001$) and duration of remission (21.8 months versus 8.0 months). The toxicity profile of bendamustine was manageable with grade 3/4 infections occurring in 8% of the bendamustine-treated patients. Bendamustine has also shown efficacy in the relapsed and refractory setting (63).

MONOCLONAL ANTIBODIES

Rituximab

CD20 is a B-cell-specific surface antigen that is expressed on 95% of B cells (64). It is tightly bound to the cell surface and is not shed or internalized upon antibody binding. Rituximab is a chimeric antibody that targets the CD20 antigen. It can mediate cell kill by various mechanisms, including antibody-dependent cell-mediated cytotoxicity (ADCC), complement-mediated cytotoxicity, and direct induction of apoptosis (65,66). The pivotal phase III trial of rituximab in relapsed low-grade or follicular CD20 + lymphoma was published by McLaughlin et al. (67). Rituximab given weekly for 4 weeks at a dose of 375 mg/m^2 produced an ORR of 44%; 6% of patients achieved CR. Out of 166 patients enrolled in this study, 33 had the diagnosis of small lymphocytic lymphoma; the ORR in this group was 13%, with no CR. Subsequent trials with rituximab in previously treated patients with CLL/SLL have reported response rates of 6% (1 of 15 patients) (68) to 25% (69) with no CR observed. O'Brien et al. (70) conducted a dose-escalation study with rituximab; patients received an initial dose of 375 mg/m^2 and the dose was then escalated in cohorts to a maximum of 2250 mg/m^2. Response rates were 36% in patients with CLL and 60% in those with other B-cell lymphoid leukemias. Response was correlated with dose: 22% for patients treated at 500 to 825 mg/m^2, 43% for those treated at 1000 to 1500 mg/m^2, and 75% for those treated at the highest dose of 2250 mg/m^2 ($p = .007$). This study indicated that an increased dose of rituximab correlates with a higher response rate. Another dose-intensification strategy with administration of rituximab three times a week for 4 weeks yielded an ORR of 45% in patients with CLL (71).

Combination Therapy With Rituximab

A phase II trial (CALGB study 9712) of sequential versus concurrent administration of rituximab and fludarabine in previously untreated patients with CLL has been recently updated (72). Patients were randomized to receive either (1) 6 monthly courses of fludarabine concurrently with rituximab followed 2 months later by 4 weekly doses of rituximab as consolidation or (2) fludarabine alone for 6 months followed 2 months later by the same rituximab consolidation therapy. A total of 104 patients were randomized to the concurrent (N = 51) and sequential regimens (N = 53). With median follow-up of 92 months (range 60-107), the ORR with the concurrent regimen was 90% (47% CR, 43% PR) compared to an ORR of 77% in the sequential arm

(28% CR, 49% PR). The median OS was 85 months, with 71% of patients alive at 5 years. The median PFS was 37 months with 27% progression-free at 5 years. The estimated median OS and PFS for the concurrent group were 84 and 32 months compared to 91 and 40 months, respectively in the sequential group. This trial confirmed that rituximab and fludarabine in patients with CLL has significant clinical activity with acceptable toxicity.

A chemoimmunotherapy protocol developed at MDACC demonstrated the efficacy of combining rituximab (R) with fludarabine and cyclophosphamide (FC) (73). Fludarabine was 25 mg/m^2 per day for 3 days, cyclophosphamide 250 mg/m^2 per day for 3 days, and rituximab 375 to 500 mg/m^2 on day 1 (FCR). This was a single-arm study of FCR as initial therapy in 300 patients with progressive or advanced CLL. At a median follow-up of 6 years, the ORR was 95% (CR was 72%, nodular PR was 10%, partial remission rate was 13%). The 6-year OS and failure-free survival (FFS) rate were 77 and 51%, respectively. The median time to progression was 80 months. Of note, patients who attained a CR with negative flow cytometry had a superior time to progression (TTP) (85 months versus 49 months) and OS (84% versus 65% at 6 years).

The FCR regimen has also demonstrated efficacy in the relapsed and refractory setting. In this study, 177 patients with previously treated CLL were evaluated. The ORR was 73%; CR was achieved in 25% of 177 patients, nodular PR in 16%, and PR in 32%. Twelve of 37 (32%) patients with CR also achieved molecular remission on bone marrow analysis. Overall, FCR in the pretreated population was found to be very active and well tolerated. On retrospective analysis, the FCR regimen induced a higher CR and OS for patients with relapsed and refractory CLL compared to FC (74).

The German CLL study group (GCLLSG) initiated a multicenter, phase III trial to evaluate the efficacy of FCR versus FC in the frontline treatment of patients with advanced CLL (75). A total of 817 patients were randomized to receive six courses of either FC (409 patients) or FCR (408 patients). Both treatment arms were well balanced with regard to sex, age, stage, genomic aberrations and IgV gene mutational status. With a median observation time of 25.5 months, the ORR (95% versus 88%; $p = .001$), the CR (52% versus 27%; $p < .0001$), and the 2-year PFS (76.6% versus 62.3%; $p < .0001$) were all significantly better for the FCR arm compared to FC. Although FCR led to more neutropenia/leukopenia, it did so without increasing the incidence of severe infections. Updated results of this study with longer median observation time (37.7 months) have recently been reported (76). The OS was significantly better with FCR (84.1% versus 79%; $p = .01$).

Alemtuzumab (Campath-1H)

CD52 is a surface antigen abundantly present on the surface of lymphocytes. Alemtuzumab (Campath-1H) is a humanized antibody targeting CD52 that mediates cell lysis by ADCC, complement-mediated cytotoxicity, and direct induction of apoptosis. Alemtuzumab is most effective in clearing malignant CD52-bearing cells from the blood and bone marrow (77).

The pivotal trial of alemtuzumab in previously treated patients with CLL was conducted by Keating et al. (78). Ninety-three patients, all of whom were refractory to fludarabine, received alemtuzumab in 21 centers worldwide. Alemtuzumab was given intravenously over 2 h three times weekly for a maximum of 12 weeks. The ORR in the intent-to-treat population (N = 93) was 33% (CR 2%, PR 31%). The median time to response was 1.5 months (range 0.4-3.7 months). The median time to progression was 4.7 months (9.5 months for responders). At data cut-off, 27 patients (29%) were alive and the overall median survival was 16 months (OS 32 months in responders). Grade 3/4 infections were reported in 25 patients (27%). Major antitumor response was seen in blood (97%), followed by spleen (71%) and lymph nodes (62%). Response rates were lower among patients with bulky disease. This led to FDA approval of this agent for fludarabine-refractory patients with CLL.

In a trial of alemtuzumab as initial therapy for CLL in which the antibody was administered subcutaneously three times a week (up to a maximum of 18 weeks), an ORR of 87% was reported; CR was achieved in 19% of the patients (79). Alemtuzumab in combination with rituximab has been studied at MDACC in relapsed and refractory CLL. In this study, 32 patients with CLL were treated and 20 had a response (63%) including 2 CR and 16 PR (80).

Studies have suggested that alemtuzumab may be effective for patients who harbor *p53* mutations. One study evaluated the efficacy of alemtuzumab in 36 patients with fludarabine-refractory CLL, 15 (42%) of whom had *p53* mutations or deletions. Six of 15 patients (40%) with *p53* mutations/deletions had a clinical response compared to 4 of 21 (19%) who did not carry this mutation. The median response duration for this subset of patients was 8 months (range 3-17 months). This is intriguing as the presence of *p53* mutation or deletion often portends a suboptimal response to conventional treatment (81).

Another study demonstrated the superiority of alemtuzumab over chlorambucil in the first-line treatment of patients with CLL (82). In this trial, 297 patients were randomized, 149 to alemtuzumab and 148 to chlorambucil. Alemtuzumab was found to produce a higher ORR (83% versus 55%; $p < .0001$) and CR rate (24% versus 2%; $p < .0001$). It led to a superior PFS with a 42% reduction in risk of progression or death (HR = 0.58; $p = .0001$) and an increased median time to alternative treatment compared to chlorambucil (23.3 months versus 14.7 months) (HR = 0.54; $p = .0001$). In addition, the elimination of minimal residual disease (MRD) occurred in 11 of 36 patients in alemtuzumab who attained CR compared to none of the patients treated with chlorambucil. Alemtuzumab was overall well tolerated, but did lead to a higher risk of CMV infection. Somewhat disappointingly, patients with 17p deletion, although faring better with alemtuzumab than chlorambucil, had a median PFS of only 10.8 months with alemtuzumab.

In an attempt to improve upon the efficacy of FCR, a combination of alemtuzumab and FCR (CFAR) was evaluated. A phase II study in 78 patients with relapsed CLL produced an OR of 65% (CR 24%) with a median PFS of 27 months for the 19 patients attaining CR and median PFS of 10 months in 32 patients achieving PR (83). Another study used frontline CFAR in previously untreated patients with CLL and high-risk features (84). Of 48 patients evaluated, the OR was 94% (CR 69%) including an OR of 77% (CR 54%) in 13 patients carrying del(17p).

Ofatumumab

Ofatumumab (HuMax-CD20) is a fully humanized, monoclonal IgG1 antibody that binds to a different epitope of CD20 than rituximab. It has a higher affinity to CD20 compared to rituximab and activates complement-dependent cytotoxicity more effectively, leading to killing of B-cell lines with low CD20 expression. One phase I/II study of 33 patients with relapsed CLL gave weekly ofatumumab for 4 weeks with a 50% ORR (85). Another Phase II study evaluated ofatumumab in patients with relapsed CLL who were refractory to both fludarabine and alemtuzumab (N = 59) or patients with bulky lymphadenopathy refractory to fludarabine (N = 79) (86). The ORR and OS for each cohort was 51%/13.7 months and 44%/15.4 months, respectively. These findings led to FDA approval of this agent for refractory CLL. A treatment algorithm (Table 3-7) for patients with CLL is listed.

NOVEL AGENTS IN DEVELOPMENT

Several novel agents are now being studied in CLL. Lenalidomide is an immunomodulatory drug, which is

TABLE | **TREATMENT ALGORITHM**
3-7

Clinical Scenario	Decision-Making Algorithm	Treatment
SLL/localized (Ann Arbor stage I)	If disease is locoregional	Consider RT or observation
CLL (Rai –II)	Evaluate for treatment indications*	If no tx indication: observe
CLL (Rai III–IV) or progressive disease	Likely will start treatment	FCR
Richter's transformation Transformation to DLBCL	Workup for DLBCL	Treat as aggressive DLBCL Consider transplantation

DLBCL, diffuse large B-cell lymphoma; RT, radiation treatment.
*Disease-related symptoms: constitutional symptoms, end-organ dysfunction, bulky lymph nodes >10 cm, spleen >6 cm below costal margin, lymphocyte doubling time ≤6 months, worsening anemia, platelet count <100,000 cells/mm^3

an analog of thalidomide. It has shown efficacy in patients with relapsed CLL who carry high-risk cytogenetic features. In one phase II study, lenalidomide was administered at 25 mg orally daily on days 1 to 21 every 28 days to 45 patients with relapsed CLL (87). The ORR was 47% (9% CR) and responses were seen in patients who were refractory to fludarabine and those who carried deletions of 11q and 17p. In another phase II study from MDACC, lenalidomide was administered at 10 mg oral daily continuously (with 5 mg incremental dose escalation with maximum dose of 25 mg) to 44 patients with relapsed CLL (88). The ORR was 32% (CR=7%) with a 31% ORR in patients with high-risk cytogenetic features.

Flavopiridol has shown clinical activity in patients with relapsed CLL. Flavopiridol is a synthetic flavone that inhibits cyclin-dependent kinases. A phase II study evaluated flavopiridol in 64 patients with relapsed CLL, all of whom had received prior purine analog therapy (89). Thirty-four patients (53%) achieved a response including 30 PR (47%), 3 NPR (5%), and 1 CR (1.6%). Twelve of 21 (57%) patients with deletion 17p and 14 of 28 (50%) patients with deletion 11q responded irrespective of lymph node size. The median PFS among responders was 10 to 12 months across all cytogenetic-risk groups. Other CDK inhibitors in clinical trials include SNS-032 and SCH 727965.

Oblimersen is an antisense oligonucleotide that targets the mRNA of BCL-2. A phase III trial of 241 patients with relapsed/refractory CLL who had received at least 1 prior round of chemotherapy compared FC to FC with oblimersen (90). There was a significantly higher CR and nodular PR rate (17% versus 7%; $p = .025$) in the patients treated with FC plus oblimersen. The median responses were durable (not reached versus 22 months) and OS at 54 months was 10% versus 2%. The combination was well tolerated.

Other interesting agents in clinical trials include BH-3 mimetics (ABT-263), inhibitors of phosphatidylinositol-3-kinase (CAL-101), Bruton's tyrosine kinase (BTK), and CD37 (Tru016).

STEM CELL TRANSPLANTION

Autologous transplantation has been shown to produce high CR rates in patients with CLL (91) but is associated with high relapse rates (92). Allogeneic transplantation has demonstrated more durable remissions albeit at the expense of higher attendant toxicity. The results of myeloablative allogeneic stem cell transplant in 30 patients (20 related, 10 unrelated donors) have been reported. The median interval from diagnosis to transplantation was 4.8 years and the median number of prior therapies was 3. After a median follow-up of 4.3 years, 14 of 30 (47%) patients were alive and in CR. The 5-year OS and EFS were both 39% (OS for related donors 48% versus 20% unrelated donor). The occurrence of graft-versus-host disease significantly decreased the relapse risk (93). To improve the tolerability of allogeneic transplantation, especially for older patients with refractory disease, while also preserving the graft-versus-leukemia effect (GVHD), reduced-intensity conditioning (RIC) is now being offered. These non-myeloablative strategies have also been used with success in CLL (94). A study using RIC in 30 patients with advanced CLL showed promising results (95). After a median follow-up of 2 years, 23 patients were still alive with 40% achieving a CR and 53% and a PR. Chronic GVHD was observed in 75% of patients.

Another study looked at 82 patients with advanced CLL who were treated with nonmyeloablative conditioning (TBI with fludarabine) from related and unrelated donors (96). The ORR was 70% with 55% CR. The OS and PFS were 50 and 39%. Lymphadenopathy greater than 5 cm predicted for relapse. The 5-year cumulative incidence of GVHD was 49% for related and 53% for unrelated recipients.

Despite the improved tolerability of transplantation in CLL, it can lead to treatment-related mortality that needs to be discussed with the patient. Generally speaking, transplantation should be discussed for a patient with previously treated, poor-risk CLL. Poor-risk disease is considered with a lack of response or recurrence of disease within 24 months of purine-based combination therapy and in patients with 17p deletion.

MINIMAL RESIDUAL DISEASE

Despite major advances in the treatment of CLL, a significant proportion of patients relapse after achieving CR. Persistence of MRD after treatment is associated with higher probability of relapse (97,98). With the availability of newer approaches—such as monoclonal antibodies, vaccine strategies, etc.—there may be an opportunity to eradicate MRD in CLL and improve long-term outcome. After achieving CR as defined by NCI-IWCLL, immunophenotypic analysis of bone marrow aspirate with flow cytometry and amplification of complementarity-determining region (CDR III) of immunoglobulin heavy or light chain (IgV) by polymerase chain reaction (PCR) can be used to detect MRD. Indeed, many studies have found that patients with no detectable disease via flow cytometry or PCR have a longer EFS (99), TFS (100), PFS (101), and OS (99,100). One trial confirmed that the median PFS depended on the ability to eradicate MRD in the peripheral blood, while also demonstrating that eradicating MRD in the marrow in younger, poor-risk patients confers improved survival (102). Evaluating MRD at the end of treatment is now being incorporated as an endpoint in most clinical trials.

MAINTENANCE THERAPY IN CLL/ERADICATION STRATEGY FOR MRD

Rituximab has been used as induction/maintenance therapy in previously untreated patients with CLL (103). The response rate after 4 weekly doses of rituximab was 51%, with a 4% CR rate. With additional doses of rituximab at 6-month intervals, the ORR was similar at 58%. Thus, unlike the case in indolent lymphoma (104), continued maintenance therapy with rituximab did not increase responses over those seen with the initial 4-week treatment. The use of interferon alpha (IFN-α) as maintenance therapy after fludarabine failed to prolong survival or eradicate MRD (105). Alemtuzumab has been used to treat persistent disease prior to hematopoietic stem cell transplant (HSCT) (106); its role in eradicating MRD after conventional therapy or HSCT is under evaluation. Montillo et al. (107) reported immunophenotypic and molecular CR with alemtuzumab in patients initially treated with fludarabine. In a study reported from MDACC, alemtuzumab administered after chemotherapy produced molecular remission in 38% of patients (108). Response criteria for CLL is defined (Table 3-8).

TABLE 3-8 | DEFINITION OF RESPONSE

Parameter	Complete Response	Partial Response	Progressive Disease
Group A			
Lymphadenopathy	None >1.5 cm	Decrease ≥50%	Increase ≥50%
Hepatomegaly and splenomegaly	Normal size	Decrease ≥50%	Increase ≥50%
Blood lymphocytes	$<4 \times 10^9$/L	Decrease ≥50% from baseline	Increase ≥50% from baseline
Bone marrow	Normocellular <30% lymphocytes, no B-lymphoid nodules	50% reduction in marrow infiltrate, or B-lymphoid nodules	
Group B			
Neutrophils	$>1.5 \times 10^9$/L	$>1.5 \times 10^9$/L or 50% improvement from baseline	Increase ≥50%
Platelet count	$>100 \times 10^9$/L	$>100 \times 10^9$/L or increase ≥50% over baseline	Decrease ≥50% over baseline secondary to CLL
Hemoglobin	>11 g/dL	>11 g/dL or increase ≥50% over baseline	Decrease of >2 g/dL from baseline secondary to CLL

Group A criteria define tumor load, group B criteria define function of marrow.

Modified, with permission, from Hallek M, Cheson BD, Catovsky D, et al. Guidelines for the diagnosis and treatment of chronic lymphocytic leukemia: A report from the International Workshop on Chronic Lymphocytic Leukemia updating the National Cancer Institute—Working Group 1996 Guidelines. *Blood* 2008;111(12):5446-5456.

TABLE 3-9	SUPPORTIVE CARE FOR PATIENTS WITH CLL
Situation	**Treatment Regimen**
Antibiotic prophylaxis	Acyclovir for herpes virus Sulfamethoxazole and trimethoprim for PCP If getting alemtuzumab: Valganciclovir during and 2 months after treatment
Autoimmune conditions	Pure red cell aplasia: rule out Parvovirus B19 Treatment: steroids or cyclosporine
Blood transfusions	Blood products should be irradiated (prevents graft-versus-host disease)
Recurrent infections	Antibiotics, antifungals, anti-viral agents If IgG <500 mg/dL, start IVIG every month (0.5 g/kg)

PCP, pneumocystis carinii pneumonia.

SUPPORTIVE CARE

Patients with CLL can have a host of complications ranging from hematologic to infectious. Supportive care maneuvers are delineated in Table 3-9.

AUTOIMMUNE COMPLICATIONS OF CLL

Autoimmune hemolytic anemia (AIHA), autoimmune thrombocytopenia (AIT), and pure red cell aplasia (PRCA) develop in some patients with CLL. The incidence of AIHA is 4 to 11% (109-113) and that of AIT 2 to 3%. PRCA is least common. Prednisone is the usual treatment for AIHA and AIT, with a high likelihood of response initially. However, more than 60% of patients relapse when treatment is stopped. Intravenous immunoglobulin produces response in 40% of patients (111), but these responses tend to be transient. Cyclosporine is another option for treatment of immune-mediated cytopenias and can produce responses even in patients with steroid-refractory immune cytopenias (114). Rituximab and alemtuzumab have also been used to treat autoimmune complications of CLL (115,116).

HYPOGAMMAGLOBULINEMIA

Hypogammaglobulinemia is a frequent complication of CLL. Because of the high cost of therapy and its limited activity in preventing serious infections, monthly intravenous gamma globulin replacement therapy is usually limited to hypogammaglobulinemic patients who experience repeated sinopulmonary bacterial infections.

■ TRANSFORMATIONS

RICHTER SYNDROME

The term *Richter syndrome* (RS) refers to the development of aggressive large cell lymphoma (LCL) during the course of CLL. RS is usually associated with worsening systemic symptoms, including B symptoms, elevated LDH, rapid tumor growth, and/or extranodal involvement (117). Diagnosis requires tissue biopsy. High-dose gallium and PET scans help identify sites to direct tissue biopsy (118). Gene rearrangement studies and isotype analysis suggest that the CLL and LCL cells frequently share identical clonal origins. The LCL is usually resistant to therapy, and the median survival of patients who develop RS is approximately 6 months (119).

PROLYMPHOCYTIC TRANSFORMATION

The NCI-IWCLL criteria allow a diagnosis of CLL to be made in the presence of ≤55% prolymphocytes. The presence of prolymphocytes >55% indicates prolymphocytic transformation.

■ HAIRY CELL LEUKEMIA

HCL is an uncommon B-cell lymphoproliferative disorder affecting adults and represents 2% of all leukemia. There is a marked male preponderance. Most patients have cytopenias; splenomegaly is also frequent at presentation. Hairy cells can be seen in peripheral blood, but their numbers vary. Hairy cells are twice as large as normal lymphocytes, with the nuclei showing a loose chromatin pattern and villus-like cytoplasmic projections (Fig. 3-8) (best viewed under phase-contrast microscopy). Hairy cells typically show positive staining for tartrate-resistant acid phosphatase (TRAP) (Fig. 3-9). Hairy cells infiltrate the bone marrow in an interstitial or focal pattern, with clear zones between cells ("fried-egg" appearance) (Fig. 3-10). Marrow reticulin is increased and aspirates may result in "dry taps."

Immunophenotypic analysis of hairy cells shows the presence of CD19, CD20, CD22, CD25, and CD103; in contrast to CLL, hairy cells are negative for CD5 and CD23. Hairy cells also stain strongly for surface immunoglobulin and FMC-7. Whenever a diagnosis of HCL is entertained, a panel of four antibodies consisting

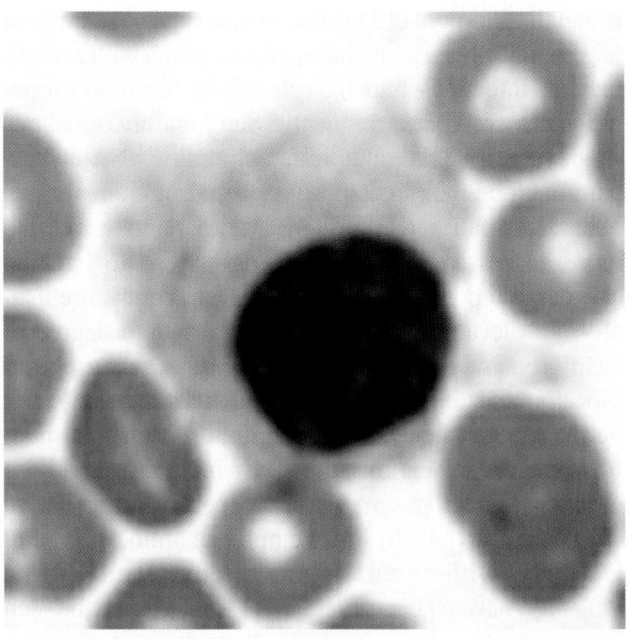

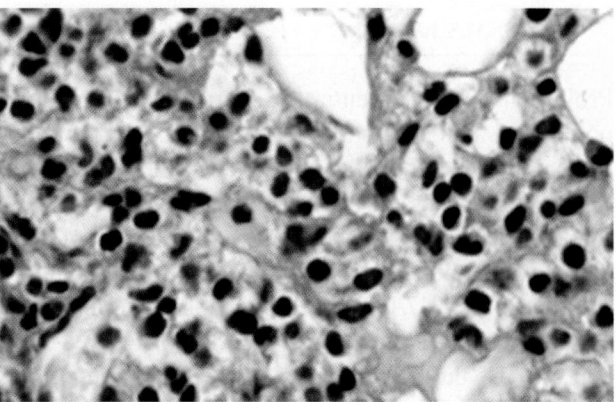

FIGURE 3-10. Bone marrow involvement by hairy cell leukemia showing "fried-egg" appearance (H&E stain).

FIGURE 3-8. Hairy cell in peripheral blood with cytoplasmic projections.

of CD11c, CD25, CD103, and HC2 should be applied. Hairy cells express three to four of these antigens (14). The use of CD103 antibody in flow-cytometric analysis is an alternative to the cytochemical staining for TRAP.

There is no staging system for HCL. Treatment decisions are usually based on the degree of cytopenia and accompanying complications (eg, bleeding, infections, anemia). Pentostatin (2-deoxycoformycin) and cladribine (2-chlorodeoxyadenosine; 2-CDA) are the nucleoside analogs that are the mainstay of treatment of HCL. Pentostatin is administered at 4 mg/m^2 every

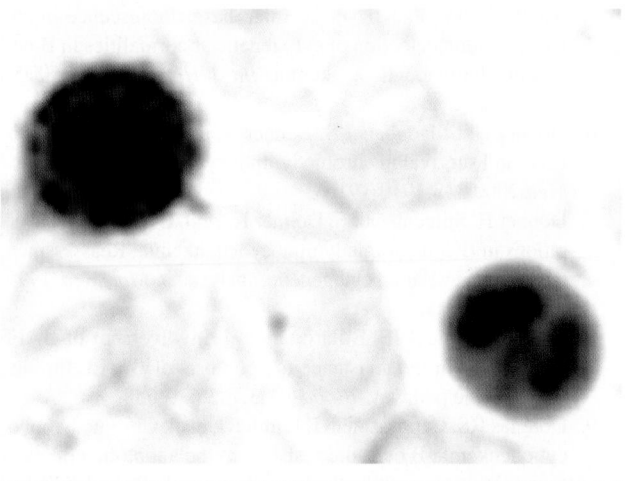

FIGURE 3-9. Hairy cell staining for tartrate-resistant acid phosphatase (*left*). Note the absence of orange-brown staining in a neutrophil.

2 weeks until maximum response and 2-CDA is given at 0.1 mg/kg/day as a continuous IV infusion for 7 days, or the same total dose can be administered as a 2-h infusion over 5 days. Because 2-CDA involves a single course of therapy and produces remission rates comparable to those achieved with pentostatin, 2-CDA is used more frequently in the United States for the treatment of HCL. Estey et al. reported a CR rate of 78% with 2-CDA in patients who had newly diagnosed or previously treated HCL (120). Hoffman et al. reported similar response rates (121) with 2-CDA, with 80% of patients remaining in remission at median follow-up of 4 years. Complications of treatment include fever, infections, neutropenia, and CD4+ lymphopenia. The majority of relapsed patients achieve second remission when retreated with pentostatin or 2-CDA. The choice of agent may depend on the duration of the first remission: if <3 years, use an alternate agent; if >5 years, use the same agent. Splenectomy, although performed infrequently, can induce hematologic remission. The use of IFN-α is currently limited to patients unresponsive to nucleoside analogs. Rituximab can play a role in patients with relapsed or primary refractory HCL after purine analogs (122). In patients receiving rituximab 375 mg/m^2 weekly × 8 planned doses (with additional four doses to responders not achieving a CR), the ORR was 80%. Eight patients (53%) achieved CR, two (13%) a CR with residual marrow disease, and two (13%) PR. Of the 12 responders followed for a median of 32 months, 5 (42%) had disease progression. One trial evaluated a strategy to improve the initial response to nucleoside analog therapy by adding additional doses of rituximab (123). This study demonstrated that eradication of MRD is possible; more data is needed to see if this generates a longer relapse-free survival.

■ PROLYMPHOCYTIC LEUKEMIA

Prolymphocytic leukemia is characterized by splenomegaly, a high number of circulating prolymphocytes, minimal lymphadenopathy, and a median survival of less than 3 years. Prolymphocytes are larger and less homogenous than CLL cells; they have abundant clear cytoplasm, clumped chromatin, and a prominent nucleolus (see Figs. 3-7A and B). Prolymphocytes can be of either B- or T-cell type. B-PLL cells usually do not express CD5 but stain strongly for surface immunoglobulin and FMC-7 (see Table 3-2). Approximately, 20% of cases of PLL are of T-cell phenotype.

Splenectomy and lymphoma-like regimens have been used to treat PLL without much success. In a study at MDACC, a 38% ORR (18% CR) was seen with a 5-day schedule of fludarabine administered every 4 weeks (124). Dearden et al. reported an ORR of 48% with pentostatin (2′deoxycoformycin) (125). Alemtuzumab (Campath-1H) has shown promising activity in T- and B-PLL, with an ORR of 51% (126,127), CR rates of up to 39.5%, and median survival of 7.5 months. In a study from Royal Marsden Hospital, alemtuzumab (Campath-1H) was administered intravenously three times weekly to patients with previously treated T-PLL until maximal response. The ORR was 76%, with 60% CR and 16% PR (128). Alemtuzumab has also been preliminarily investigated in 11 treatment-naive patients (129). All 11 patients (100%) achieved a CR, with seven out of 11 patients still alive at the median follow-up of 12 months (range 4-17 months)

■ LARGE GRANULAR LYMPHOCYTE LEUKEMIA

LG lymphocytes are larger than normal lymphocytes and contain azurophilic granules in their cytoplasm (see Fig. 3-6). LG lymphocytes comprise 10 to 15% of peripheral blood mononuclear cells and are predominantly of NK-cell phenotype, a smaller fraction being of T-cell phenotype. LG lymphoma (LGL) consists of four distinct entities: reactive/transient LG lymphocyte expansion, chronic LG lymphocytosis, indolent LGL, and aggressive LGL (130). Clonal expansion of LG lymphocytes can arise from either of the normal cellular counterparts and so may have an NK- or T-cell phenotype; the T-cell phenotype comprises 80% of LGL leukemias. T-LGL cells have a CD3+/CD57+/CD56− immunophenotype and NK-LGL are CD3−/CD56+/CD57−. Clonality of T-LGL can be established by T-cell receptor gene rearrangement studies. The clinical presentation of LGL is usually indolent (131). The median age of patients is 55 years. Cytopenias including neutropenia with accompanying infections, pure red cell aplasia, thrombocytopenia, and anemia occur frequently. Serologic abnormalities such as positive rheumatoid factor and/or ANA, hypergammaglobulinemia, and high β_2-microglobin are frequent. A small percentage of LGL patients develop a more aggressive course; these cases tend to have an NK-cell phenotype. Since lymphocyte counts are usually not elevated, diagnosis requires a high degree of suspicion and a careful examination of the peripheral blood smear and bone marrow. Although LGL may be indolent, many patients eventually need treatment for cytopenias. Various therapies including low-dose methotrexate (10 mg/m^2 PO once weekly), cyclosporine (2 mg/kg PO q 12 h), or cyclophosphamide (100 mg PO daily) with or without oral prednisone (1 mg/kg PO daily) have all been effective (132). CRs may be seen in up to 50% of cases (133). Lymphoma-type regimens (eg, CHOP) have not been effective for aggressive disease.

References

1. Damle RN, Ghiotto F, Valetto A, et al. B-cell chronic lymphocytic leukemia cells express a surface membrane phenotype of activated, antigen-experienced B lymphocytes. *Blood* 2002;99:4087-4093.
2. Kuppers R, Klein U, Hansmann ML, Rajewsky K. Cellular origin of human B-cell lymphomas. *N Engl J Med* 1999;341: 1520-1529.
3. Fais F, Ghiotto F, Hashimoto S, et al. Chronic lymphocytic leukemia B cells express restricted sets of mutated and unmutated antigen receptors. *J Clin Invest* 1998;102:1515-1525.
4. Autio K, Elonen E, Teerenhovi L, Knuutila S. Cytogenetic and immunologic characterization of mitotic cells in chronic lymphocytic leukaemia. *Eur J Haematol* 1987;39:289-298.
5. Xu W, Li JY, Pan JL, et al. Interphase fluorescence in situ hybridization detection of cytogenetic abnormalities in B-cell chronic lymphocytic leukemia. *Int J Hematol* 2007;85(5); 430-436.
6. Dohner H, Stilgenbauer S, Benner A, et al. Genomic aberrations and survival in chronic lymphocytic leukemia. *N Engl J Med* 2000;343:1910-1916.
7. Dohner H, Stilgenbauer S, Dohner K, et al. Chromosome aberrations in B-cell chronic lymphocytic leukemia: Reassessment based on molecular cytogenetic analysis. *J Mol Med* 1999; 77:266-281.
8. Kern C, Cornuel JF, Billard C, et al. Involvement of BAFF and APRIL in the resistance to apoptosis of B-CLL through an autocrine pathway. *Blood* 2003;103:679-688.
9. Douglas RS, Capocasale RJ, Lamb RJ, et al. Chronic lymphocytic leukemia B cells are resistant to the apoptotic effects of transforming growth factor-beta. *Blood* 1997;89:941-947.
10. Tsukada N, Burger JA, Zvaifler NJ, et al. Distinctive features of "nurselike" cells that differentiate in the context of chronic lymphocytic leukemia. *Blood* 2002;99:1030-1037.

11. Chikkappa G, Zarrabi MH, Tsan MF. Pure red-cell aplasia in patients with chronic lymphocytic leukemia. *Medicine (Baltimore)* 1986;65:339-351.

12. Hallek M, Cheson BD, Catovsky D, et al. Guidelines for the diagnosis and treatment of chronic lymphocytic leukemia: A report from the International Workshop on Chronic Lymphocytic Leukemia updating the National Cancer Institute—Working Group 1996 Guidelines. *Blood* 2008;111(12):5446-5456.

13. Bergmann MA, Eichhorst BF, Busch R, et al. Prospective evaluation of prognostic parameters in early stage chronic lymphocytic leukemia (CLL): Results of the CLL1-Protocol of the German CLL Study Group (GCLLSG). *Blood* (ASH Annual Meeting Abstracts) 2007;110:625.

14. Matutes E, Polliack A. Morphological and immunophenotypic features of chronic lymphocytic leukemia. *Rev Clin Exp Hematol* 2000;4(1):22-47.

15. Rai KR, Sawitsky A, Cronkite EP, et al. Clinical staging of chronic lymphocytic leukemia. *Blood* 1975;46:219-234.

16. Binet JL, Auquier A, Dighiero G, et al. A new prognostic classification of chronic lymphocytic leukemia derived from a multivariate survival analysis. *Cancer* 1981;48:198-206.

17. Rai KR, Han T. Prognostic factors and clinical staging in chronic lymphocytic leukemia. *Hematol Oncol Clin North Am* 1990;4:447-456.

18. The French Cooperative Group on Chronic Lymphocytic Leukemia. Effects of chlorambucil and therapeutic decision in initial forms of chronic lymphocytic leukemia (stage A): Results of a randomized clinical trial on 612 patients. *Blood* 1990;75:1414-1421.

19. Montserrat E, Vinolas N, Reverter JC, et al. Natural history of chronic lymphocytic leukemia: On the progression and progression and prognosis of early clinical stages. *Nouv Rev Fr Hematol* 1988;30:359-361.

20. Catovsky D, Fooks J, Richards S. Prognostic factors in chronic lymphocytic leukaemia: The importance of age, sex and response to treatment in survival. A report from the MRC CLL 1 Trial. MRC Working Party on Leukaemia in Adults. *Br J Haematol* 1989;72:141-149.

21. Hallek M, Langenmayer I, Nerl C, et al. Elevated serum thymidine kinase levels identify a subgroup at high risk of disease progression in early, nonsmoldering chronic lymphocytic leukemia. *Blood* 1999;93:1732-1737.

22. Ibrahim S, Keating M, Do KA, et al. CD38 expression as an important prognostic factor in B-cell chronic lymphocytic leukemia. *Blood* 2001;98:181-186.

23. Molica S, Levato D, Dell'Olio M, et al. Cellular expression and serum circulating levels of CD23 in B-cell chronic lymphocytic leukemia. Implications for prognosis. *Haematologica* 1996;81:428-433.

24. Lee JS, Dixon DO, Kantarjian HM, et al. Prognosis of chronic lymphocytic leukemia: A multivariate regression analysis of 325 untreated patients. *Blood* 1987;69:929-936.

25. Damle RN, Wasil T, Fais F, et al. IgV gene mutation status and CD38 expression as novel prognostic indicators in chronic lymphocytic leukemia. *Blood* 1999;94:1840-1847.

26. Hamblin TJ, Davis Z, Gardiner A, et al. Unmutated IgV(H) genes are associated with a more aggressive form of chronic lymphocytic leukemia. *Blood* 1999;94:1848-1854.

27. Montillo M, Hamblin T, Hallek M, et al. Chronic lymphocytic leukemia: Novel prognostic factors and their relevance for risk-adapted therapeutic strategies. *Haematologica* 2005;90(3):391-399.

28. Hamblin TJ, Orchard JA, Ibbotson RE, et al. CD38 expression and immunoglobulin variable region mutations are independent prognostic variables in chronic lymphocytic leukemia, but CD38 expression may vary during the course of the disease. *Blood* 2002;99:1023-1029.

29. Rassenti LZ, Huynh L, Toy TL, et al. ZAP-70 compared with immunoglobulin heavy-chain gene mutation status as a predictor of disease progression in chronic lymphocytic leukemia. *N Engl J Med* 2004;351(9):893-901.

30. Crespo M, Bosch F, Villamor N, et al. ZAP-70 expression as a surrogate for immunoglobulin-variable-region mutations in chronic lymphocytic leukemia. *N Engl J Med* 2003;348:1764-1775.

31. Durig J, Nuckel H, Cremer M, et al. ZAP-70 expression is a prognostic factor in chronic lymphocytic leukemia. *Leukemia* 2003;17:2426-2434.

32. Del Principe MI, Del Poeta G, Bussisano F, et al. Clinical significance of ZAP-70 protein expression in B-cell chronic lymphocytic leukemia. *Blood* 2006;108(3):853-861.

33. Vener C, Gianelli U, Cortelezzi A, et al. ZAP-70 immunoreactivity is a prognostic marker of disease progression in chronic lymphocytic leukemia. *Leuk Lymphoma* 2006;47(2):245-251.

34. Giles FJ, Bekele BN, O'Brien S, et al. A prognostic model for survival in chronic lymphocytic leukaemia based on *p53* expression. *Br J Haematol* 2003;121:578-585.

35. Lin K, Sherrington PD, Dennis M, et al. Relationship between *p53* dysfunction, CD38 expression, and IgV(H) mutation in chronic lymphocytic leukemia. *Blood* 2002;100:1404-1409.

36. Wattel E, Preudhomme C, Hecquet B, et al. p53 mutations are associated with resistance to chemotherapy and short survival in hematologic malignancies. *Blood* 1994;84:3148-3157.

37. Krober A, Seiler T, Benner A, et al. V(H) mutation status, CD38 expression level, genomic aberrations, and survival in chronic lymphocytic leukemia. *Blood* 2002;100:1410-1416.

38. The French Cooperative Group on Chronic Lymphocytic Leukemia. Effects of chlorambucil and therapeutic decision in initial forms of chronic lymphocytic leukemia (stage A): Results of a randomized clinical trial on 612 patients. *Blood* 1990;75:1414-1421.

39. Shustik C, Mick R, Silver R, et al. Treatment of early chronic lymphocytic leukemia: Intermittent chlorambucil versus observation. *Hematol Oncol* 1988;6:7-12.

40. CLL Trialists' Collaborative Group. Chemotherapeutic options in chronic lymphocytic leukemia: A meta-analysis of the randomized trials. *J Natl Cancer Inst* 1999;91:861-868.

41. French Cooperative Group on Chronic Lymphocytic Leukaemia. Effectiveness of "CHOP" regimen in advanced untreated chronic lymphocytic leukaemia. *Lancet* 1986;1:1346-1349.

42. French Cooperative Group on Chronic Lymphocytic Leukaemia. Long-term results of the CHOP regimen in stage C chronic lymphocytic leukaemia. *Br J Haematol* 1989;73:334-340.

43. French Cooperative Group on Chronic Lymphocytic Leukaemia. Is the CHOP regimen a good treatment for advanced CLL? Results from two randomized clinical trials. *Leuk Lymph* 1994;13:449-456.

44. Keating MJ, Scouros M, Murphy S, et al. Multiple agent chemotherapy (POACH) in previously treated and untreated patients with chronic lymphocytic leukemia. *Leukemia* 1988;2:157-164.

45. Grever MR, Kopecky KJ, Coltman CA, et al. Fludarabine monophosphate: A potentially useful agent in chronic lymphocytic leukemia. *Nouv Rev Fr Hematol* 1988;30:457-459.

46. Keating MJ, Kantarjian H, Talpaz M, et al. Fludarabine: A new agent with major activity against chronic lymphocytic leukemia. *Blood* 1989;74:19-25.

47. Sorensen JM, Vena DA, Fallavollita A, et al. Treatment of refractory chronic lymphocytic leukemia with fludarabine phosphate via the group C protocol mechanism of the National Cancer Institute: Five-year follow-up report. *J Clin Oncol* 1997;15:458-465.

48. Keating MJ, Kantarjian H, O'Brien S, et al. Fludarabine: A new agent with marked cytoreductive activity in untreated chronic lymphocytic leukemia. *J Clin Oncol* 1991;9:44-49.

49. Johnson S, Smith AG, Loffler H, et al. Multicentre prospective randomized trial of fludarabine versus cyclophosphamide, doxorubicin, and prednisone (CAP) for treatment of advanced-stage chronic lymphocytic leukaemia. The French Cooperative Group on CLL. *Lancet* 1996;347:1432-1438.

50. O'Brien S, Kantarjian H, Beran M, et al. Results of fludarabine and prednisone therapy in 264 patients with chronic lymphocytic leukemia with multivariate analysis-derived prognostic model for response to treatment. *Blood* 1993;82:1695-1700.

51. Robertson LE, O'Brien S, Kantarjian H, et al. A 3-day schedule of fludarabine in previously treated chronic lymphocytic leukemia. *Leukemia* 1995;9:1444-1449.

52. Kemena A, O'Brien S, Kantarjian H, et al. Phase II clinical trial of fludarabine in chronic lymphocytic leukemia on a weekly low-dose schedule. *Leuk Lymph* 1993;10:187-193.

53. Juliusson G, Liliemark J. Long-term survival following cladribine (2-chlorodeoxyadenosine) therapy in previously treated patients with chronic lymphocytic leukemia. *Ann Oncol* 1996;7:373-379.

54. Robak T, Blonski JZ, Kasznicki M, et al. Cladribine with or without prednisone in the treatment of previously treated and untreated B-cell chronic lymphocytic leukaemia—updated results of the multicentre study of 378 patients. *Br J Haematol* 2000;108:357-368.

55. Rai KR, Peterson BL, Appelbaum FR, et al. Fludarabine compared with chlorambucil as primary therapy for chronic lymphocytic leukemia. *N Engl J Med* 2000;343:1750-1757.

56. Rai KR, Peterson BL, Appelbaum FR, et al. Long-Term survival analysis of the North American Intergroup Study C9011 comparing fludarabine and chlorambucil in previously untreated patients with chronic lymphocytic leukemia. Blood (ASH Annual Meeting Abstracts) 2009;114:536.

57. French Cooperative Group on Chronic Lymphocytic Leukaemia. Comparison of fludarabine, cyclophosphamide/doxorubicin/prednisone, and cyclophosphamide/doxorubicin/vincristine/prednisone in advanced forms of chronic lymphocytic leukemia: Preliminary results of a controlled clinical trial. *Semin Oncol* 1993;20:21-23.

58. Flinn IW, Neuberg DS, Grever MR, et al. Phase III trial of fludarabine plus cyclophosphamide compared with fludarabine for patients with previously untreated chronic lymphocytic leukemia: US Intergroup Trial E2997. *J Clin Oncol* 2007;25(7):793-798.

59. Catovsky D, Richards S, Matutes E, et al. Assessment of fludarabine plus cyclophosphamide for patients with chronic lymphocytic leukaemia (the LRF CLL4 Trial): A randomized controlled trial. *Lancet* 2007;370(9583):230-239.

60. Eichhorst BF, Busch R, Hopfinger G, et al. Fludarabine plus cyclophosphamide versus fludarabine alone in first-line therapy of younger patients with chronic lymphocytic leukemia. *Blood* 2006;107(3):885-891.

61. Schiavone EM, De Simone M, Palmieri S, et al. Fludarabine plus cyclophosphamide for the treatment of advanced chronic lymphocytic leukemia. *Eur J Haematol* 2003;71:23-28.

62. Knauf WU, Lissichkov T, Aldaoud A, et al. Phase III randomized study of bendamustine compared with chlorambucil in previously untreated patients with chronic lymphocytic leukemia. *J Clin Oncol* 2009;27(26):4378-4384.

63. Bergmann MA, Goebeler ME, Herold M, et al. Efficacy of bendamustine in patients with relapsed or refractory chronic lymphocytic leukemia: Results of a phase I/II study of German CLL Study Group. *Haematologica* 2005;90(10):1357.

64. Nadler LM, Ritz J, Hardy R, et al. A unique cell surface antigen identifying lymphoid malignancies of B cell origin. *J Clin Invest* 1981;67:134-140.

65. Reff ME, Carner K, Chambers KS, et al. Depletion of B cells in vivo by a chimeric mouse human monoclonal antibody to CD20. *Blood* 1994;83:435-445.

66. Hofmeister JK, Cooney D, Coggeshall KM. Clustered CD20 induced apoptosis: Src-family kinase, the proximal regulator of tyrosine phosphorylation, calcium influx, and caspase 3-dependent apoptosis. *Blood Cells Mol Dis* 2000;26:133-143.

67. McLaughlin P, Grillo-Lopez AJ, Link BK, et al. Rituximab chimeric anti-CD20 monoclonal antibody therapy for relapsed indolent lymphoma: Half of patients respond to a four-dose treatment program. *J Clin Oncol* 1998;16:2825-2833.

68. Nguyen DT, Amess JA, Doughty H, et al. IDEC-C2B8 anti-CD20 (rituximab) immunotherapy in patients with low-grade non-Hodgkin's lymphoma and lymphoproliferative disorders: Evaluation of response on 48 patients. *Eur J Haematol* 1999;62:76-82.

69. Huhn D, von Schilling C, Wilhelm M, et al. Rituximab therapy of patients with B-cell chronic lymphocytic leukemia. *Blood* 2001;98:1326-1331.

70. O'Brien SM, Kantarjian H, Thomas DA, et al. Rituximab dose-escalation trial in chronic lymphocytic leukemia. *J Clin Oncol* 2001;19:2165-2170.

71. Byrd JC, Murphy T, Howard RS, et al. Rituximab using a thrice weekly dosing schedule in B-cell chronic lymphocytic leukemia and small lymphocytic lymphoma demonstrates clinical activity and acceptable toxicity. *J Clin Oncol* 2001;19:2153-2164.

72. Woyach JA, Ruppert AS, Heerema NA, et al. Treatment with fludarabine and rituximab produces extended overall survival and progression-free survival in chronic lymphocytic leukemia without increased risk of second malignancy: Long-term follow up of CALGB study 9712. Blood (ASH Annual Meeting Abstracts) 2009;114:Abstract 539.

73. Tam CS, O'Brien S, Wierda W, et al. Long-term results of the fludarabine, cyclophosphamide, and rituximab regimen as initial therapy for chronic lymphocytic leukemia. *Blood* 2008;112(4):975-980.

74. Wierda W, O'Brien S, Wen S, et al. Chemoimmunotherapy with fludarabine, cyclophosphamide, and rituximab for relapsed and refractory chronic lymphocytic leukemia. *J Clin Oncol* 2005;23(18):4070-4080.

75. Hallek M, Fingerle-Rowson G, Fink A-M, et al. Immunochemotherapy with fludarabine, cyclophosphamide, and rituximab versus fludarabine and cyclophosphamide improves response rates and progression-free survival of previously untreated patients with advanced chronic lymphocytic leukemia. *Blood* (ASH Annual Meeting Abstracts) 2008;112:325.

76. Hallek M, Fingerle-Rowson G, Fink A-M, et al. First-line treatment with fludarabine, cyclophosphamide, and rituximab improves overall survival in previously untreated patients with advanced chronic lymphocytic leukemia: Results of a randomized phase III trial on behalf of an International Group of Investigators and the German CLL Study Group. *Blood* (ASH Annual Meeting Abstracts) 2009;114:535.

77. Osterborg A, Mellstedt H, Keating M. Clinical effects of alemtuzumab (Campath-1H) in B-cell chronic lymphocytic leukemia. *Med Oncol* 2002;19(Suppl):S21-S26.

78. Keating MJ, Flinn I, Jain V, et al. Therapeutic role of alemtuzumab (Campath-1H) in patients who have failed fludarabine: Results of a large international study. *Blood* 2002;99:3554-3561.

79. Lundin J, Kimby E, Bjorkholm M, et al. Phase II trial of subcutaneous anti-CD52 monoclonal antibody alemtuzumab (Campath-1H) as first-line treatment for patients with B-cell chronic lymphocytic leukemia (B-CLL). *Blood* 2002;100:768-773.

80. Faderl S, Thomas DA, O'Brien S, et al. Experience with alemtuzumab plus rituximab in patients with relapsed and refractory lymphoid malignancies. *Blood* 2003;101:3413-3415.

81. Lozanski G, Heerema NA, Flinn IW, et al. Alemtuzumab is an effective therapy for chronic lymphocytic leukemia with p53 mutations and deletions. *Blood* 2004;103(9):3278-3281.

82. Hillmen P, Skotnicki AB, Robak T, et al. Alemtuzumab compared with chlorambucil as first-line therapy for chronic lymphocytic leukemia. *J Clin Oncol* 2007;25(35):5616-5623.

83. Wierda WG, O'Brien S, Faderl S, et al. Combined cyclophosphamide, fludarabine alemtuzumab, and rituximab (CFAR), an active regimen for heavily treated patients with CLL. *Blood* 2006;108:14a.

84. Wierda WG, O'Brien SM, Faderl S, et al. CFAR, an active frontline regimen for high-risk patients with CLL, including those with del 17p. *Blood* 2008;112:729.

85. Coiffier B, Lepretre S, Pedersen LM, et al. Safety and efficacy of ofatumumab, a fully humanized monoclonal anti-CD20 antibody, in patients with relapsed or refractory B-cell chronic lymphocytic leukemia: A phase 1-2 study. *Blood* 2008;111:1094-1100.

86. Osterborg A, Kipps TJ, Mayer J, et al. Ofatumumab (HuMax-CD20), a novel CD20 monoclonal antibody, is an active treatment for patients with CLL refractory to both fludarabine and alemtuzumab or bulky fludarabine-refractory disease: Results from the planned interim analysis of an international pivotal trial. *Blood* 2008;112:126-127.

87. Chanan-Khan A, Miller KC, Musial L, et al. Clinical efficacy of lenalidomide in patients with relapsed or refractory chronic lymphocytic leukemia: Results of a phase II study. *J Clin Oncol* 2006;24:5343-5349.

88. Ferrajoli A, Lee BN, Schlette EJ, et al. Lenalidomide induces complete and partial remissions in patients with relapsed and refractory chronic lymphocytic leukemia. *Blood* 2008;111:5291-5297.

89. Lin TS, Ruppert AS, Johnson AJ, et al. Phase II study of flavopiridol in relapsed chronic lymphocytic leukemia demonstrating high response rates in genetically high-risk disease. *J Clin Oncol* 2009;27(35):6012-6018.

90. O'Brien S, et al. Randomized phase III trial of fludarabine plus cyclophosphamide with or without oblimersen sodium (Bcl-2 antisense) in patients with relapsed or refractory chronic lymphocytic leukemia. *J Clin Oncol* 2007;25(9):1114-1120.

91. Khouri IF, Keating MJ, Vriesendorp HM, et al. Autologous and allogeneic bone marrow transplantation for chronic lymphocytic leukemia: Preliminary results. *J Clin Oncol* 1994;12:748-758.

92. Pavletic ZS, Bierman PJ, Vose JM, et al. High incidence of relapse after autologous stem cell transplantation for B-cell chronic lymphocytic leukemia or small lymphocytic lymphoma. *Ann Oncol* 1998;9:1023-1026.

93. Toze CL, Galal A, Barnett MJ, et al. Myeloablative allografting for chronic lymphocytic leukemia: Evidence for a potent graft-versus-leukemia effect associated with graft-versus-host disease. *Blone Marrow Transplant* 2005;36(9):825-830.

94. Khouri IF, Keating M, Korbling M, et al. Transplant-lite: Induction of graft-versus-malignancy using fludarabine-based nonablative chemotherapy and allogeneic blood progenitor-cell transplantation as treatment for lymphoid malignancies. *J Clin Oncol* 1998;16:2817-2824.

95. Schetelig J, Thiede C, Bornhauser M, et al. Evidence of a graft-versus-leukemia effect in chronic lymphocytic leukemia after reduced intensity conditioning and allogeneic stem cell transplantation: The Cooperative German Transplant Study Group. *J Clin Oncol* 2003;21:2747-2753.

96. Sorror ML, Storer BE, Sandmaier BM, et al. Five-year follow-up of patients with advanced chronic lymphocytic leukemia treated with allogeneic hematopoietic cell transplantation after nonmyeloablative conditioning. *J Clin Oncol* 2008;26:4912-4920.

97. Robertson LE, Huh YO, Butler JJ, et al. Response assessment in chronic lymphocytic leukemia after fludarabine plus prednisone: Clinical, pathologic, immunophenotypic, and molecular analysis. *Blood* 1992;80:29-36.

98. Provan D, Bartlett-Pandite L, Zwicky C, et al. Eradication of polymerase chain reaction-detectable chronic lymphocytic leukemia cells is associated with improved outcome after bone marrow transplantation. *Blood* 1996;88:2228-2235.

99. Rawstron AC, Villamor N, Ritgen M, et al. International standardized approach for flow cytometric residual disease monitoring in chronic lymphocytic leukaemia. *Leukemia* 2007;21(5):956-964.

100. Moreton P, Kennedy B, Lucas G, et al. Eradication of minimal residual disease in B-cell chronic lymphocytic leukemia after alemtuzumab therapy is associated with prolonged survival. *J Clin Oncol* 2005;23(13):2971-2979.

101. Wendtner CM, Ritgen M, Schweighofer CD, et al. Consolidation with alemtuzumab in patients with chronic lymphocytic leukemia in first remission-experience on safety and efficacy within a randomized multicenter phase III trial of the German CLL Study Group (GCLLSG). *Leukemia* 2004;18(6):1093-1101.

102. Boettcher S, Fischer K, Stilgenbauer S, et al. Quantitative MRD assessments predict progression free survival in CLL patients treated with fludarabine and cyclophosphamide with or without rituximab-a prospective analysis in 471 patients form the randomized GCLLSG CLL8 trial. *Blood* 2008;112:125-126.

103. Hainsworth JD, Litchy S, Barton JH, et al. Single-agent rituximab as first-line and maintenance treatment for patients with chronic lymphocytic leukemia or small lymphocytic lymphoma: A phase II trial of the Minnie Pearl Cancer Research Network. *J Clin Oncol* 2003;21:1746-1751.

104. Hainsworth JD. Rituximab as first-line and maintenance therapy for patients with indolent non-Hodgkin's lymphoma: Interim follow-up of a multicenter phase II trial. *Semin Oncol* 2002;29:25-29.

105. O'Brien S, Kantarjian H, Beran M, et al. Interferon maintenance therapy for patients with chronic lymphocytic leukemia in remission after fludarabine therapy. *Blood* 1995;86:1298-1300.

106. Dyer MJ, Kelsey SM, Mackay HJ, et al. In vivo "purging" of residual disease in CLL with Campath-1H. *Br J Haematol* 1997;97:669-672.

107. Montillo M, Cafro AM, Tedeschi A, et al. Safety and efficacy of subcutaneous Campath-1H for treating residual disease in patients with chronic lymphocytic leukemia responding to fludarabine. *Haematologica* 2002;87:695-700.

108. Ferrajoli A, Thomas DA, Albitar M, et al. Alemtuzumab for minimal residual disease in CLL. *Proc Am Soc Clin Oncol* 2003;22:569(Abstract 2290).

109. Lischner M, Prokocimer M, Zolberg A, et al. Autoimmunity in chronic lymphocytic leukaemia. *Postgrad Med J* 1988; 64:590-592.

110. Mauro FR, Foa R, Cerretti R, et al. Autoimmune hemolytic anemia in chronic lymphocytic leukemia: Clinical, therapeutic, and prognostic features. *Blood* 2000;95:2786-2792.

111. Diehl LF, Ketchum LH. Autoimmune disease and chronic lymphocytic leukemia: Autoimmune hemolytic anemia, pure red cell aplasia, and autoimmune thrombocytopenia. *Semin Oncol* 1998;25:80-97.

112. Weiss RB, Freiman J, Kweder SL, et al. Hemolytic anemia after fludarabine therapy for chronic lymphocytic leukemia. *J Clin Oncol* 1998;16:1885-1889.

113. Leach M, Parsons RM, Reilly JT, et al. Autoimmune thrombocytopenia: A complication of fludarabine therapy in lymphoproliferative disorders. *Clin Lab Haematol* 2000;22: 175-178.

114. Cortes J, O'Brien S, Loscertales J, et al. Cyclosporin A for the treatment of cytopenia associated with chronic lymphocytic leukemia. *Cancer* 2001;92:2016-2022.

115. Hegde UP, Wilson WH, White T, et al. Rituximab treatment of refractory fludarabine-associated immune thrombocytopenia in chronic lymphocytic leukemia. *Blood* 2002;100:2260-2262.

116. Rodon P, Breton P, Courouble G. Treatment of pure red cell aplasia and autoimmune haemolytic anaemia in chronic lymphocytic leukaemia with Campath-1H. *Eur J Haematol* 2003;70:319-321.

117. Robertson LE, Pugh W, O'Brien S, et al. Richter's syndrome: A report on 39 patients. *J Clin Oncol* 1993;11:1985-1989.

118. Partyka S, O'Brien S, Podoloff D, et al. The usefulness of high dose (7-10 mci) gallium (67Ga) scanning to diagnose Richter's transformation. *Leuk Lymph* 1999;36:151-155.

119. Giles FJ, O'Brien SM, Keating MJ. Chronic lymphocytic leukemia in (Richter's) transformation. *Semin Oncol* 1998; 25:117-125.

120. Estey EH, Kurzrock R, Kantarjian HM, et al. Treatment of hairy cell leukemia with 2-chlorodeoxyadenosine (2-CdA). *Blood* 1992;79:882-887.

121. Hoffman MA, Janson D, Rose E, Rai KR. Treatment of hairy-cell leukemia with cladribine: Response, toxicity, and long-term follow-up. *J Clin Oncol* 1997;15:1138-1142.

122. Thomas DA, O'Brien, Bueso-Ramos C, et al. Rituximab in relapsed or refractory hairy cell leukemia. *Blood* 2003; 102(12):3906-3911.

123. Ravandi F, Jorgensen JL, O'Brien SM. Eradication of minimal residual disease in hairy cell leukemia. *Blood* 2006; 107(12):4658-4662.

124. Kantarjian HM, Childs C, O'Brien S, et al. Efficacy of fludarabine, a new adenine nucleoside analogue, in patients with prolymphocytic leukemia and the prolymphocytoid variant of chronic lymphocytic leukemia. *Am J Med* 1991;90:223-228.

125. Dearden C, Matutes E, Catovsky D. Deoxycoformycin in the treatment of mature T-cell leukaemias. *Br J Cancer* 1991; 64:903-906.

126. Ferrajoli A, O'Brien SM, Cortes JE, et al. Phase II study of alemtuzumab in chronic lymphoproliferative disorders. *Cancer* 2003;98:773-778.

127. Keating MJ, Cazin B, Coutre S, et al. Campath-1H treatment of T-cell prolymphocytic leukemia in patients for whom at least one prior chemotherapy regimen has failed. *J Clin Oncol* 2002;20:205-213.

128. Dearden CE, Matutes E, Cazin B, et al. High remission rate in T-cell prolymphocytic leukemia with Campath-1H. *Blood* 2001;98:1721-1726.

129. Dearden C, Matutes E, Cazin B, et al. Very high response rates in previously untreated T-cell prolymphocytic leukemia patients receiving alemtuzumab (Campath-1H) therapy. *Blood* 2003;102(Abstract 2378).

130. Lamy T, Loughran TP Jr. Clinical features of large granular lymphocyte leukemia. *Semin Hematol* 2003;40:185-195.

131. Loughran TP Jr, Starkebaum G. Large granular lymphocyte leukemia. Report of 38 cases and review of the literature. *Medicine (Baltimore)* 1987;66:397-405.

132. Greer JP, Kinney MC, Loughran TP Jr. T cell and NK cell lymphoproliferative disorders (American Society of Hematology Education Program). Hematology 2001. (American Society of Hematology Education Program). 259-281.

133. Loughran TP Jr., Kidd PG, Starkebaum G. Treatment of large granular lymphocyte leukemia with oral low-dose methotrexate. *Blood* 1994;84:2164-2170.

CHAPTER
4

CHRONIC MYELOID LEUKEMIA

Naveen Pemmaraju
Sameer A. Parikh
Elias Jabbour
Hagop M. Kantarjian
Jorge Cortes

■ INTRODUCTION

Chronic myeloid leukemia (CML) is a pluripotent hematopoietic stem cell disorder leading to myeloproliferation and its attendant consequences. The BCR–ABL rearrangement, the pathognomonic molecular abnormality in CML, imparts a proliferative and survival advantage to the malignant clone leading to accumulation of leukemic cells. Patients may present with characteristic clinical findings caused by large numbers of circulating and bone marrow myeloid cells, such as splenomegaly, leukocytosis, or even isolated thrombocytosis. Often, patients are asymptomatic at diagnosis and are discovered only incidentally to have the disease in the setting of a routine complete blood count performed for an unrelated reason. A plethora of exciting discoveries have taken place in the understanding of the biology of the disease and in advancement of therapy for CML.

The elucidation of this disease entity at the molecular level and the dramatic impact of the first truly targeted therapy, imatinib mesylate, has served to single out the CML story as the model for modern molecular medicine and the era of personalized targeted therapy.

■ EPIDEMIOLOGY AND ETIOLOGY

In 2010, in the United States, an estimated 4870 cases of CML will be diagnosed and 440 patients will die of the disease; there has been little change in the incidence of CML over the preceding decades, but the mortality has been greatly reduced. CML is exceedingly rare in children, with a median age at diagnosis of 67 years and the incidence increasing with age (1). There is a mild male predominance in incidence of the disease with a ratio of 1.3-2.2:1 (2). There are no known hereditary, familial, geographic, or ethnic associations.

The exact mechanism that initiates and induces the translocation represented by the Philadelphia (Ph) chromosome, the initiating molecular event in CML, is incompletely understood. BCR–ABL is only present in hematopoietic cells, but it has been found using very sensitive PCR methods in the hematopoietic cells of 25 to 30% of healthy normal volunteers (3,4). This raises interesting questions about the role of the gene product in the development of the disease, and the need for a yet unknown "second hit" (5). There does not appear to be any chemical or infectious associations with the development of the disease, although an increased risk has been noted with exposure to ionizing radiation (6).

■ BIOLOGY OF CML

CML is the paradigm of a neoplastic process defined by one cytogenetic or molecular abnormality—the Ph chromosome. This is a balanced translocation between the long arms of chromosomes 9 and 22, t(9,22)(q34,q11.2) (7). The Ph chromosome is detectable in 90 to 95% of patients with the clinical and laboratory features of CML. Among the remaining 5 to 10%, the molecular rearrangement characteristic of CML (BCR–ABL) can be identified in 30 to 50% by sensitive methods of detection. The remaining cases, collectively referred to as true Ph-negative CML or atypical CML, are a heterogeneous group of disorders of unknown biology and with poor prognosis. The Ph chromosome has been identified in myeloid, erythroid, megakaryocytic, and B cells, which indicates that the abnormality in CML originates in a pluripotent stem cell. The Ph chromosome juxtaposes the proto-oncogene c-abl from chromosome 9 to the breakpoint cluster region (BCR) gene in chromosome 22. This results in the generation of a fusion gene, the product of which is a chimeric protein with constitutively activated tyrosine kinase activity. Depending on the breakpoint site in BCR, protein products of 190, 210, or 230 kD molecular weight are produced. Multiple downstream pathways are activated by these fusion proteins and produce the phenotypic features of the disease (8) Downstream signal transduction pathways activated via BCR–ABL include JAK/STAT, RAS, RAF, MYC, JNK, ERK, PI-3kinase, and NF-κB.

Additional chromosomal abnormalities are found in some of patients with CML, typically those with advanced disease. These most frequently include trisomy 8, monosomy 7, chromosome 17 abnormalities, and a double Ph chromosome. The occurrence of chromosomal abnormalities in addition to the Ph chromosome is known as clonal evolution and is considered a criterion of accelerated phase, particularly when it occurs during the course of the disease. Molecular abnormalities resulting from these changes include derangement of p53, RB1, C-MYC, and AML-EVI1.

CML has been classified as part of the myeloproliferative neoplasms (MPN) since the original report of Dameshak in the 1950s. This disease category includes a group that in addition to CML, includes polycythemia vera (PV), essential thrombocytosis (ET), and idiopathic myelofibrosis (IMF). In 2005, five independent groups identified the JAK2 V617F mutation, a constitutively active kinase mutation in the pseudokinase domain of the JAK2 gene, as a molecular abnormality common to PV, ET, and IMF. This discovery, with few exceptions, effectively separates the classical MPDs into BCR/ABL negative/JAK2 V617F mutation positive diseases (PV, ET, IMF) with CML as a separate category (BCR/ABL positive/JAK2 V617F negative).

■ CLINICAL FEATURES AND NATURAL HISTORY

CML can generally be divided into three separate phases of disease: a chronic phase, an intermediate or accelerated phase, and an end-stage blast phase. It is important to note that the natural course of the disease may not always include all of these phases or necessarily follow this specific order. Approximately 90% of patients are diagnosed in the chronic phase at the time of diagnosis and frequently while asymptomatic (2). When symptoms are present, they typically are due to splenomegaly (abdominal pain, abdominal mass, increased satiety). Less commonly, patients may present with catabolic symptoms of hyperuricemia, anorexia, unintentional weight loss, unexplained fevers, or consequences of thrombocytopenia such as petechiae, ecchymoses, or hemorrhage, or symptoms of anemia such as fatigue. Patients in chronic phase are usually not more susceptible to infection than healthy individuals. Leukocytosis is commonly found with white blood cell counts that can be higher than $1000 \times 10^9/L$ and could, in rare instances, lead to the catastrophic consequences of hyperleukostatis including retinal hemorrhage and signs of hyperviscosity (priapism, cerebrovascular accidents, tinnitus, confusion, stupor), but this occurrence is less common in the modern era. Historically, prior to the imatinib era, the median survival for patients in chronic phase was 4 to 5 years, with an estimated 15-20% risk of transformation to the blast phase per year. Accelerated phase CML is characterized by increasing arrest of maturation heralding transformation to the blast phase. Criteria derived from multivariate analysis that indicate progression to the accelerated phase include 15% or more blasts, 30% or more blasts plus promyelocytes, 20% or more basophils, platelets lower than $100 \times 10^9/L$ unrelated to therapy, or cytogenetic clonal evolution (9). Other criteria have been proposed (Table 4-1) but some of these classifications, such as the WHO proposal (10), have not yet been clinically validated. The criteria used to classify patients in the accelerated phase impacts the expected outcome of patients. When less strict criteria are used, such as those proposed by the IBMTR or the WHO, the expected outcome is significantly better, perhaps as a result of patients with less adverse clinical features being selected (11). Median survival for patients in accelerated phase is 1 to 2 years (12), and a significant

number of patients may die during this phase of the disease without transforming to the blast phase. Recent evidence suggests that imatinib is changing the natural history of advanced stage CML (13).

Blast phase CML is the most advanced stage of the disease. This stage is defined by the presence of at least 30% blasts present in the peripheral blood or the bone marrow, or the presence of extramedullary disease (chloroma, granulocytic sarcoma). The WHO classification has proposed that this be changed to ≥20% blasts, but this proposal has not yet been fully tested and applied clinically (14). Clinically, the blast phase is associated with anemia, an increased risk for infections and/or bleeding and constitutional symptoms (night sweats, weight loss, fever, bone pain). The phenotype of the blasts is lymphoid in 25%, myeloid in 50%, and undifferentiated in 25% (2). Median survival in blast phase CML is 3 to 6 months, with patients with lymphoid blast phase exhibiting a slightly better prognosis than for those with myeloid phenotype. For full details of treatment options for all three disease phases, please refer to section "Treatment Guidelines."

■ DIAGNOSIS AND INITIAL CLINICAL WORKUP

Initial evaluation includes history and physical examination. Symptoms may include abdominal discomfort or pain, fevers, night sweats, weight loss, early satiety, left shoulder pain (Kehr sign/indicative of splenomegaly and possible splenic rupture), anorexia, or joint pain. Particular attention should be directed to any complaints of bleeding, abnormal fatigue, petechiae or other

TABLE 4-1	CRITERIA FOR ACCELERATED PHASE ACCORDING TO MDACC, IBMTR, AND WHO		
	MDACC	*IBMTR*	*WHO*
Blasts	≥15%	≥10%	10-19[†]
Blasts+Pro's	≥30%	≥20%	NA
Basophils	≥20%	≥20%[*]	≥20%
Platelets ($\times 10^9/L$)	<100	Unresponsive ↑, persistent ↓	<100 or >1000 unresponsive
Cytogenetics	CE	CE	CE not at diagnosis
WBC	NA	Difficult to control, or doubling <5 days	NA
Anemia	NA	Unresponsive	NA
Splenomegaly	NA	Increasing	NA
Other	NA	Chloromas, myelofibrosis	Megakaryocyte proliferation, fibrosis

NA, not applicable; CE, clonal evolution.
[*]Basophils + eosinophils.
[†]Blast phase ≥20% blasts (≥30% for MDACC and IBMTR).

skin lesions, easy bruisability, or visual changes. The family and social histories are of particular importance as the documentation of existence of siblings and details of their health status should be noted, as allogeneic stem cell transplant might be an option at some point during the treatment of a CML patient.

Physical examination should note the presence of organomegaly and other signs of extramedullary hematopoiesis. Skin should be assessed for signs of cutaneous involvement, although this is infrequent. Signs of anemia (eg, pallor, dyspnea) and thrombocytopenia (ie, ecchymoses, petechiae) should be noted. Otherwise, a complete physical examination should be undertaken.

Initial laboratory workup includes complete blood count with differential and platelets, complete metabolic panel including liver function tests, BUN and creatinine, and measurement of serum uric acid level. A bone marrow aspiration and biopsy is mandatory for all patients in whom CML is being considered. This will provide information needed to confirm diagnosis (eg, cytogenetic analysis) and for stage classification. Although a FISH or PCR done in peripheral blood can confirm the presence of the Ph chromosome or the BCR–ABL rearrangement, only cytogenetics can provide evidence of additional chromosomal abnormalities that are an important element of initial diagnosis and staging.

The differential diagnosis of CML includes infection (especially mycobacterial such as tuberculosis), leukemoid reaction, other (Ph-negative/BCR/Abl negative) myeloproliferative disorders (eg, polycythemia vera, essential thrombocythemia, idiopathic myelofibrosis), Ph negative/atypical CML and myelomonocytic leukemia. In all cases, the presence of the Ph chromosome will establish the diagnosis of CML. In few instances, a patient may be diagnosed with Ph-positive acute myeloid leukemia (AML) or acute lymphoblastic leukemia (ALL). It may be impossible to determine if these cases represent de-novo Ph-positive acute leukemias or a blast phase of a previously unrecognized CML.

■ LABORATORY FEATURES

Leukocytosis is the most common laboratory characteristic seen in the chronic phase of CML with white blood counts greater than $100 \times 10^9/L$ in some patients (15). Myeloid cells in all stages of maturation are seen in the peripheral blood, frequently also with an increase of basophils and eosinophils. Historically, the leukocyte alkaline phosphatase score is low and levels of vitamin B_{12} are elevated; however, these laboratory tests are seldom

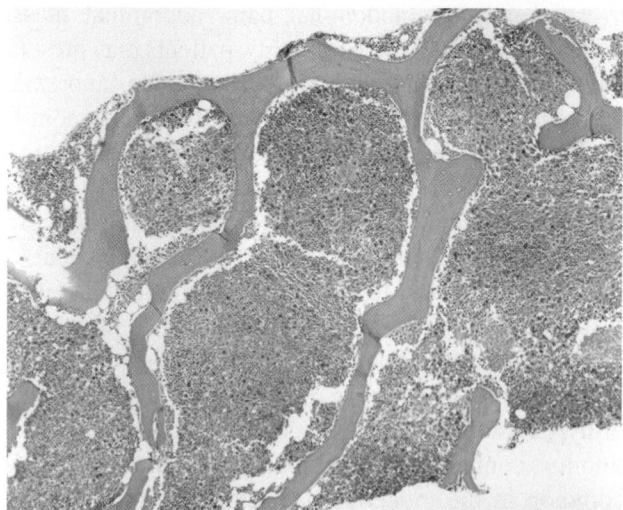

FIGURE 4-1. Chronic myeloid leukemia, chronic phase. The bone marrow biopsy is 100% cellular with granulocytic and megakaryocytic hyperplasia.

ordered in the modern era of CML diagnosis. The bone marrow is markedly hypercellular with the myeloid to erythroid ratio significantly increased (Figs. 4-1–4-5) (16). Megakaryocytosis is frequently seen in the bone marrow, and some degree of myelofibrosis may be seen in up to 40% of patients (17).

A standard cytogenetic analysis (karyotype) is needed in all cases at diagnosis and this requires a bone marrow aspiration. This will not only identify the presence of the Ph chromosome, but it also provides information on the other chromosomes to determine the

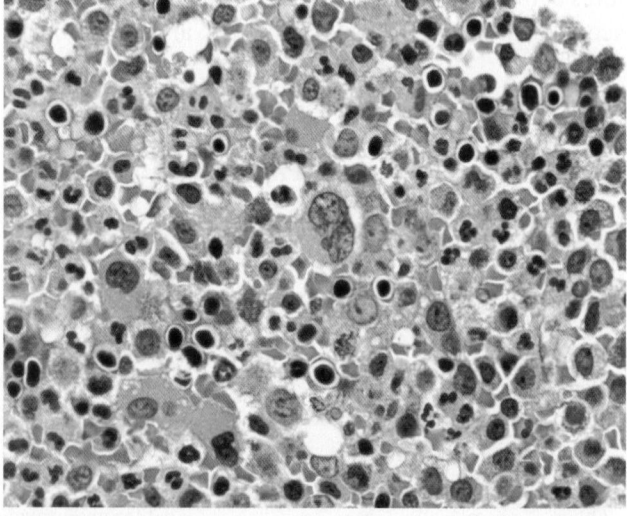

FIGURE 4-2. Chronic myeloid leukemia, chronic phase. Myeloid progenitors with increased immature cells in a hypercellular bone marrow.

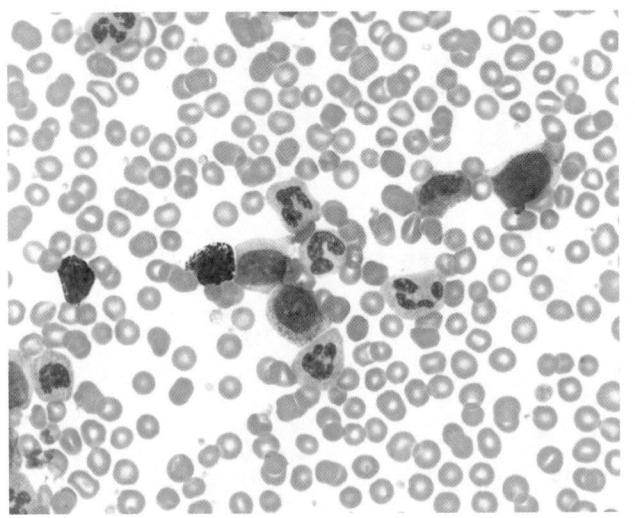

FIGURE 4-3. Chronic myeloid leukemia in accelerated phase. Aspirate smear shows increased blasts and basophils.

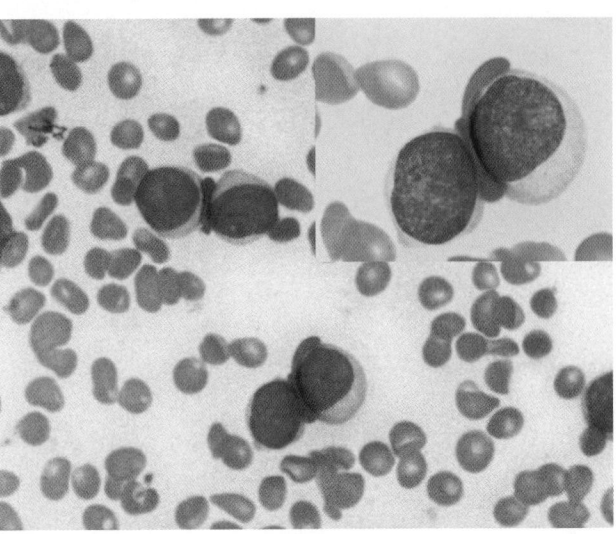

FIGURE 4-5. Chronic myeloid leukemia in blast phase. The majority of evaluable white cells are immature (blasts)

presence of clonal evolution (Fig. 4-6). Fluorescent in situ hybridization (FISH) may also identify the presence of the BCR–ABL rearrangement, even in cases where the Ph chromosome cannot be identified by conventional cytogenetic analysis. Other advantages of FISH are that it can be performed on the peripheral blood and that it can be done in interphase (Fig. 4-7). However, it has a background positivity of 0.5 to 1%, which complicates evaluation during treatment as a patient approaches a complete cytogenetic response, and it does not provide information on other chromosomes. Quantitative

PCR (usually real-time PCR) is also done at diagnosis to have a baseline measure of the BCR–ABL transcript levels prior to the start of therapy. Table 4-2 presents the proposed evaluation at diagnosis and during follow-up for patients with CML.

■ PROGNOSIS

Prognostic and staging models are important in the initial evaluation of patients. Pretreatment clinical characteristics historically associated with poor outcome include older age, hepatomegaly, splenomegaly, increased peripheral blood or bone marrow blast and basophil counts, marrow fibrosis, cytogenetic clonal evolution, anemia, and thrombocytosis or thrombocytopenia. Several models have been proposed for staging and determining prognosis in CML (18-22). From a historical standpoint, the most used model traditionally has been the one proposed by Sokal et al. (20). In this system, the hazard ratio function is derived from the following formula: $\lambda_i(+)/\lambda_o(t) = $ Exp 0.0116 (age − 43.4) + 0.0345 (spleen − 7.51) + 0.188([platelets/700]^2 − 0.563) + 0.0887 (blasts − 2.10). This classification defines three prognostic risk-groups with hazard ratios of <0.8, 0.8 to 1.2, and >1.2. A simpler prognostic model was proposed at MDACC and it appeared to have similar clinical validity as the Sokal system (19). Both of these models were developed in the preinterferon (IFN) era. The European Collaborative CML Prognostic Factors Project Group proposed a model that would be better

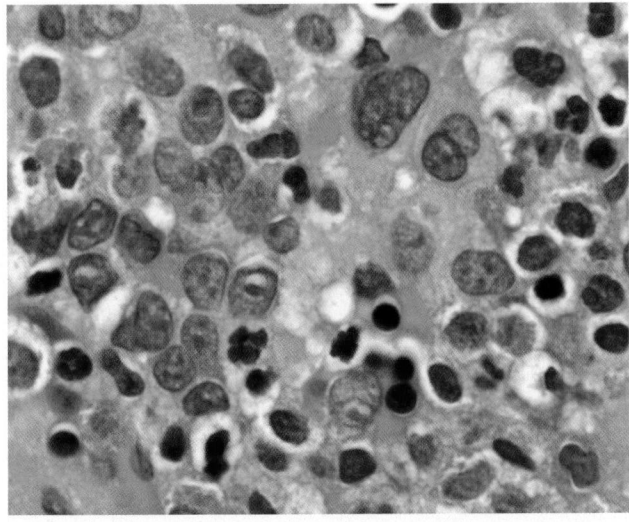

FIGURE 4-4. Chronic myeloid leukemia, accelerated phase. Bone marrow biopsy section demonstrate foci of blasts.

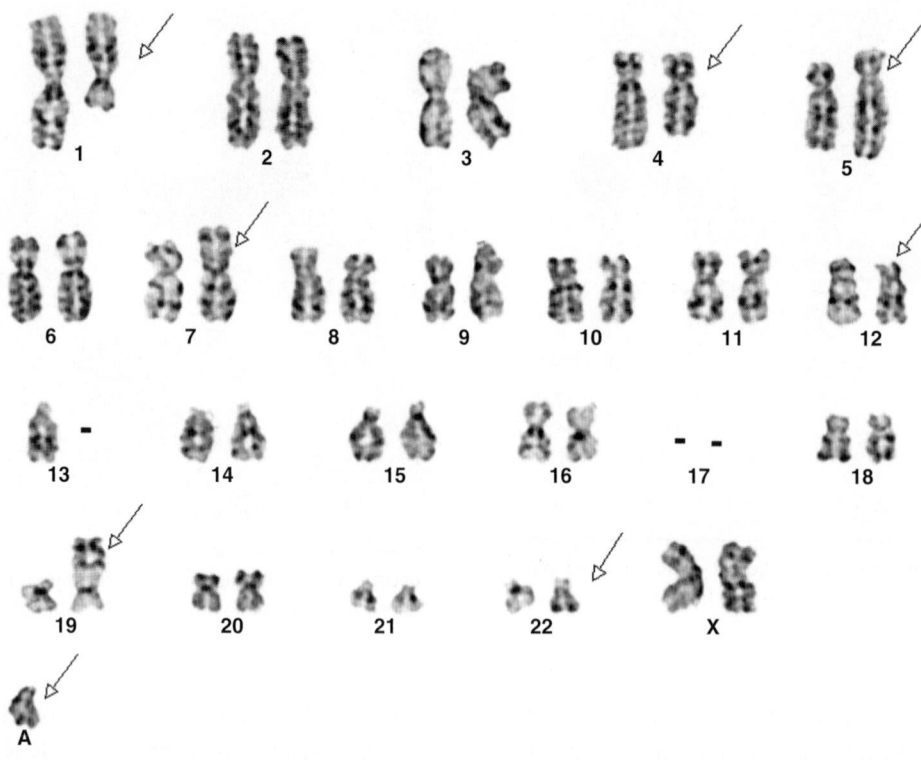

FIGURE 4-6.   Chronic Myeloid Leukemia, karyotype from a patient with blast-phase CML demonstrating clonal evolution. Reciprocal translocation involving chromosomes 9 and 22 has occurred. Additional chromosomal abnormalities are present indicating clonal evolution.

predictive of prognosis for patients treated with IFN-α (23). Both the Sokal and Euro score have been found to correlate with the probability of response to imatinib. In the seminal trial establishing imatinib as the new front-line treatment of choice in CML, the IRIS trial, the Sokal

risk classification was predictive of probability of achieving a cytogenetic response and progression-free survival (24). During therapy, achieving a cytogenetic response is the most important prognostic factor for long-term survival. Among patients treated with IFN-α who achieve

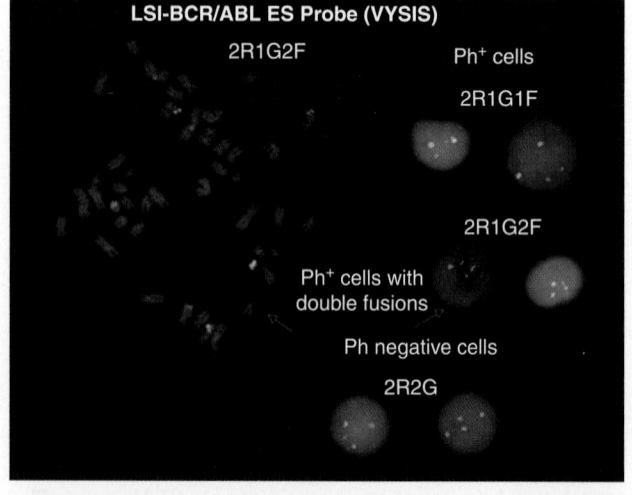

FIGURE 4-7.   FISH (in metaphase in left panel; in interphase in right panel) image showing the BCR-ABL rearrangement.

TABLE 4-2	MONITORING OF CML PATIENTS
Status	*Diagnostic Testing*
At diagnosis	• Cytogenetics • Quantitative (real-time) PCR (peripheral blood or bone marrow) • FISH
During therapy	• Cytogenetics every 3-6 months for the first year, then every 6-12 months. Once the patient achieves a stable MMR, every 12-24 months • FISH if insufficient metaphases or to monitor cytogenetic response in between bone marrow aspirations • Quantitative (real-time) PCR FISH every 3-6 months for the first year, then every 6 months

a complete cytogenetic response, the 10-year survival probability is 78%, compared to 45% for those who achieve partial cytogenetic response, and approximately 25% for those with minor or no cytogenetic response (25). Although the follow-up is still short, it is becoming evident that achieving a cytogenetic response, particularly when this is accomplished early during the course of therapy (ie, within the first 3-6 months from the start of therapy) translates into the best probability of long-term progression-free survival (26,27). Thus, achieving a complete cytogenetic remission and particularly an early cytogenetic remission should be the minimum acceptable goal of therapy for all patients with CML.

The prognostic significance of certain clinical characteristics has changed with improved therapy. In the imatinib-era older age has lost much of its prognostic significance. Although found to correlate with lower incidence of cytogenetic response in a univariate analysis, age was not found to be an independent risk factor in a multivariate analysis for survival (28). Approximately, 10 to 15% of patients present with a deletion of the derivative chromosome 9. These patients had a significantly worse prognosis when treated with chemotherapy, IFN-α or SCT (29,30). Early reports suggested that patients with deletion of derivative chromosome 9 may still have an inferior outcome even when treated with imatinib (31). More recent reports suggest that the outcome is similar regardless of the deletion status (32).

Clonal evolution in patients treated with imatinib remains an adverse prognostic characteristic, particularly when developing during the course of therapy (compared to present at the time of diagnosis) (26,33). The development of myelosuppression during treatment with imatinib has adverse prognostic implications for patients who failed prior IFN therapy (34). This has not been confirmed among patients who never received IFN.

Molecular markers that have been investigated for their impact on prognosis in CML include the breakpoint location and corresponding messages detected (b3a3 or b2a2), methylation of the PA promoter of c-ABL, elevated plasma levels of VEGF (35), and telomere length. The significance of some of these markers in the imatinib era is uncertain and ongoing studies are underway to determine the clinical value of these and a host of other molecular markers for prognostic value in CML. One recent analysis suggests that the few patients with e1a2 rearrangement (translating into a p190$^{BCR-ABL}$) have an inferior outcome compared to those with the more common b2a2 or b3a2 transcripts (36).

■ RESPONSE AND EVALUATION OF MINIMAL RESIDUAL DISEASE (TABLE 4-3)

Response to therapy is measured initially by hematologic criteria. A complete hematologic response (CHR) is defined as normalization of WBC counts to $<10 \times 10^9$/L with a normal differential, platelet count $<450 \times 10^9$/L, and disappearance of splenomegaly and other symptoms of leukemia. Patients who achieve a CHR are further classified according to their cytogenetic response.

Cytogenetic responses can be divided into major (complete or partial) and minor. Complete cytogenetic response corresponds to 0% of all metaphases remaining Ph-positive. Partial cytogenetic response is defined as 1 to 35% of metaphases being Ph-positive. A minor cytogenetic response corresponds to 35 to 95% Ph-positive metaphases. A routine cytogenetic analysis where at least 20 metaphases are analyzed is necessary to evaluate a cytogenetic response. Although results obtained with FISH correlate well with those achieved with cytogenetic analysis, cytogenetic response criteria have not been validated with FISH.

Molecular response is assessed by quantitative PCR (usually real-time PCR) in the peripheral blood or bone marrow (37). A major molecular response is considered when the BCR–ABL/ABL ratio is ≤0.1% in the international scale (IS). A complete molecular

TABLE 4-3	RESPONSE CRITERIA IN CML
Hematologic remission	
Complete	Normalization of peripheral counts and differential, and disappearance of all signs and symptoms of CML including splenomegaly
Cytogenetic remission*	
Complete	0% Ph(+) metaphases
Partial	1-35% Ph(+) metaphases
Minor	36-95% Ph(+) metaphases
None	>95% Ph+ metaphases
(Complete and partial remissions together constitute major cytogenetic remissions, ie, 0-34% Ph+ metaphases)	
Molecular remission†	
Complete	Undetectable BCR–ABL transcripts‡
Major	BCR–ABL/ABL ratio of <0.1% (International scale)

*Cytogenetic response is based on a routine karyotype analyzing at least 20 metaphases.
†Molecular responses is based on quantitative PCR (usually real-time PCR).
‡PCR with a sensitivity of at least 4.5-log.

response represents achievement of undetectable transcripts of BCR–ABL in an assay with a sensitivity of at least 4.5-logs.

■ THERAPY

STEM CELL TRANSPLANTATION

Allogeneic Stem Cell Transplant

Allogeneic stem cell transplantation (allo-SCT) was for many years the treatment of choice for younger patients because of its potential for cure. However, with the introduction of imatinib and second-generation tyrosine kinase inhibitors, there has been a paradigm shift in this thinking with an allo-SCT no longer recommended as first-line therapy, and frequently reserved for third-line or special circumstances. Transplant carries significant risks such as GVHD, veno-occlusive disease, life-threatening infections, risk of secondary malignancy, and poorer overall quality of life, although recent advances have resulted in significant reduction in some of these risks (38). Current recommendations for an allo-SCT are restricted to only those patients in accelerated and blast phase of CML, particularly if they respond to initial therapy with tyrosine kinase inhibitors, and for those patients in chronic phase who have failed imatinib and possibly one second generation TKI (such as nilotinib or dasatinib). The only exception to this is the rare patient with T315I mutation, where a transplant may be considered first-line. For younger patients with optimal donors, a transplant can also be considered as second-line therapy after failure to imatinib, particularly if this is due to resistance and the patient never achieved a cytogenetic response. Because HLA typing of an identical sibling or an unrelated donor can take time, even in cases where an allo-SCT is the treatment of choice, patients should receive either imatinib (if TKI naïve) or a second-generation TKIs (if imatinib resistant) prior to transplant. Prior treatment with imatinib does not negatively impact the outcome of allo-SCT, and patients heading to transplant with a better response may have a better outcome (39-41). This has not been definitively established for patients treated with dasatinib or nilotinib, although preliminary data does not suggest an increased toxicity when pretreated with these agents (42,43).

Nonmyeloablative Transplant

Nonmyeloablative stem cell transplant (NST) is one in which the conditioning regimen is significantly less intense with the proposed modulation of immune graft-versus-leukemia mechanisms employed to achieve remission. The advantage of this approach is increased tolerability and a decrease in morbidity and mortality, extending this option to older patients and patients with comorbidities who would otherwise have been ineligible. One caveat with this approach is the possibility of higher rates of relapse. In a study of 64 patients with advanced-phase CML who underwent NST with fludarabine-based regimens at MD Anderson Cancer Center, OS and PFS were 33 and 20%, respectively, at 5 years (44). Incidence of treatment-related mortality (TRM) was 33, 39, and 48% at 100 days, and 2 and 5 years after NST, respectively. In multivariate analysis, only disease stage at time of NST was significantly predictive for both OS and PFS.

Relapse After Transplant

The risk of relapse after bone marrow transplantation varies depending on several factors including the type of donor, manipulation of the graft (eg, T-cell depletion) and others. Patients should be followed after transplant with RT-PCR as a predictor of relapse. Patients with minimal residual disease documented by PCR after 12 months from the time of transplant have a risk of recurrence of 30 to 40% compared to <5% for patients with negative RT-PCR (45).

Patients who relapse after transplant can frequently be effectively reinduced into remission with donor lymphocyte infusion (DLI). In patients who relapse in the chronic phase, a complete remission is achievable in 70%, and may be higher if treated at the time of molecular relapse (compared to cytogenetic or hematologic relapse) (46). The response rate is 20% for those who relapse in accelerated phase and <10% for patients in blastic phase. Toxicity includes myelosuppression in 20 to 30%, GVHD in 40% as the major toxicity, and a mortality of 10 to 20%. The risks of these adverse events are lower if the DLI is used after 12 months from the initial transplant.

Imatinib is an alternative for patients who relapse after transplant (47-49). A complete hematologic remission can be achieved in most patients treated in chronic phase after relapse from transplant, and in 80 to 40% of those treated in accelerated or blast phase, respectively. A complete cytogenetic remission can be achieved in over 40% of patients treated in the chronic phase. The risks of myelosuppression and GVHD are considerably lower with imatinib. Interestingly, recurrence of GVHD was observed in 11% of patients treated with imatinib in this setting (49). These modalities can be used together or in sequence tailored to the extent of residual disease. One such approach included 38 patients who received a

NST (fludarabine-based) at MD Anderson Cancer Center. Patients with residual disease by RT-PCR analysis for *BCR-ABL* 3 months after transplant received imatinib, and those who did not achieve molecular CR within 3 months received escalating doses of DLI (50). Out of the 38 patients enrolled, 16 were in chronic phase and 17 had advanced disease, and all were previously treated with imatinib. At 3 months, all 16 early patients and 12 of the 17 advanced patients achieved CCyR. Eighteen patients with residual molecular residual disease after 3 months received imatinib; molecular CR was achieved in eight of nine early patients and two of nine with advanced CML. Of the eight patients who required DLI, four achieved a molecular CR. After a median of 6 months, 94% in chronic phase are alive, all currently in cytogenetic CR, and 58% with advanced disease are alive, 8/17 in cytogenetic CR.

NONTRANSPLANT THERAPY

Imatinib Mesylate

For many years CML was treated with busulfan or hydroxyurea, and was associated with a poor prognosis (51). These agents controlled the hematologic manifestations of the disease, but did not delay disease progression. Treatment with IFN-α changed the outcome of the disease by eliminating the Ph-chromosome positive clone in a subset of patients. A CCyR was achieved in 5 to 25% of patients with CML in CP treated with IFN-α. Importantly, achievement of a CCyR, and to some extent, PCyR, was associated with an improved survival, establishing CCyR as the primary goal of therapy (52,53). Combining IFN-α with cytarabine improved the probability of response and, in some series, the long-term survival (54,55).

Imatinib mesylate (STI-571), a 2-phenylaminopyrimidine, is a selective and potent inhibitor of Bcr-Abl and few other tyrosine kinases, including c-kit, PDGF-R α and β, and abl-related gene (ARG) (56,57). It is orally administered with 98% bioavailability and a half-life of 13 to 16 hours. Imatinib was first used in CML in patients who had developed resistance or intolerance to IFN-α (58,59). Among 532 such patients treated with imatinib, a CCyR was achieved in 60%. The estimated 5-year survival rate was 76% (59).

Based on these favorable results, a large, randomized trial was initiated among patients with CML in CP who had received no prior therapy. In this study, known as the IRIS trial, patients were randomized to receive imatinib or IFN and Ara-C, which was the standard therapy at the time (24). Treatment with imatinib was significantly better in nearly all outcomes measured,

including hematologic and cytogenetic response, toxicity and progression-free survival. In the most recent update of this series, 82% of patients achieved a CCyR with at least three fourths of these responses being sustained at the time of last follow-up (60). The 7-year EFS, PFS, and OS rates were 81, 92, and 85%, respectively. The curves seem to plateau after the fourth year and yearly event rates have ranged from 0.3 to 2%. With an annual mortality of 2%, the estimated survival of a newly diagnosed patient with CML may be in the range of 20 to 30 years. Results from a single-institution study from MDACC in 50 patients in early chronic phase treated with the standard dose of 400 mg daily reported nearly identical results, with a complete cytogenetic response rate of 78% (61). Unfortunately, the results from the IRIS study suffer from heavy censorship as many patients discontinued study drug even when they may have continued therapy with imatinib. In another study, using an intention-to-treat analysis accounting for the outcome of all patients, the event-free survival at 5 years is 63% (62).

Management of the Patient Treated With Imatinib

There are important considerations in the management of patients treated with imatinib that need to be emphasized to optimize therapy and increase the probability of a favorable outcome.

Imatinib dose

The phase I study performed in patients who had failed prior IFN therapy established a clear relationship between dose and response (58). Minimal responses were seen among patients treated with the lowest doses (below 100 mg daily), and only 50% of patients achieved a hematologic response (10% cytogenetic response) at doses of 140 to 250 mg daily. Only at doses of 300 mg daily or higher were hematologic responses seen in nearly all patients and cytogenetic responses in half of them. Thus, it is not recommended to use doses below 300 mg daily if one is to offer patients the best probability of response. Less than 5% of patients are unable to tolerate these doses with proper and opportune management of toxicity when it occurs. The dose selected for phase II studies, which has become standard in chronic phase, was 400 mg daily. However, this dose was selected somehow arbitrarily considering that there was no dose-limiting toxicity at doses of up to 1000 mg daily and a maximum tolerated dose was not defined. Several single-arm phase II studies suggested that higher doses might be associated with higher response rates and earlier responses. In a recently reported study,

The Rationale and Insight for Gleevec High-Dose Therapy (RIGHT) trial, investigators studied imatinib 400 mg twice a day as initial therapy in 115 patients (70% Sokal low risk) with newly diagnosed CML (63). Eighty-three patients (72%) completed the study, 10 patients (9%) discontinued the study because of adverse events, and six patients (5%) discontinued because of unsatisfactory therapeutic effect. The rate of complete cytogenetic response was 85% at 12 months and 83% at 18 months. The corresponding rates of major molecular response were 54% at 12 months and 63% at 18 months.

These results led to a randomized Phase III open-label study (The *T*yrosine kinase inhibitor *OP*timization and *S*electivity trial, TOPS) comparing 400 and 800 mg imatinib in 476 patients. In this study, a significant superiority for 800 mg was shown on the major molecular response rate at 3 months (3% vs. 12%), 6 months (17% vs. 34%), and 9 months (33% vs. 45%) but not at 12 months (40% vs. 46%) (64). There was a trend for fewer events and transformations during the first year for patients treated with the higher dose. However, in a recent update of the TOPS study, there was no significant difference in rates of major molecular response at 24 months also (54% vs. 51%) (65). However, patients who were able to maintain the higher doses had the best probability of achieving an MMR. Another study by the European Leukemia of reported no benefit with a higher dose (800 mg) of imatinib compared to 400 mg in 216 patients with high-risk Sokal CML. The rates of complete cytogenetic response and major molecular response in the 800 mg versus 400 mg dose were 64 and 58%, and 40 and 33%, respectively (66).

Although a number of aforementioned studies have shown improved complete cytogenetic and major molecular responses with a higher dose of imatinib, the follow-up of these studies is short to evaluate for EFS and OS. Hence, at the writing of this chapter, imatinib at a dose of 400 mg daily is still the preferred regimen of choice in newly diagnosed patients with chronic phase CML. However, it has become apparent that patients who maintain adequate dose intensity with minimal treatment interruptions and dose reductions have the best outcome. Thus, even (and particularly) when using standard dose an effort should be made to maintain the optimal dose and minimize unnecessary dose reductions and treatment interruptions.

Management of toxicity

Imatinib is overall well tolerated. Although some adverse events may occur in 30 to 40% of patients, these are usually not severe and do not require treatment interruptions or decreasing the dose. A list of some of the most frequently encountered side effects and suggestions for

TABLE 4-4	RECOMMENDED MANAGEMENT OF THE MOST COMMON ADVERSE EVENTS ASSOCIATED WITH IMATINIB
Adverse Events	**Management**
Nausea/vomiting	Take with food, fluids
	Antiemetics
Diarrhea	Loperamide
	Diphenoxylate atropine
Peripheral edema	Diuretics
Periorbital edema	Steroid-containing cream
Skin rash	Avoid sun exposure
	Topical steroids
	Systemic steroids
	(Early intervention important)
Muscle cramps	Tonic water or quinine
	Electrolyte replacement as needed
	Calcium gluconate
Arthralgia, bone pain	Nonsteroidal antiinflamatory agents
Elevated transaminases (uncommon)	Hold therapy and monitor closely
	Dose reduction upon resolu
Myelosuppression	
Anemia	Treatment interruption/dose reduction usually not indicated
	Erythropoietin or darbepoetin
Neutropenia	Hold therapy if grade ≥3 (ie, ANC $<1 \times 10^9$/L)
	Restart at lower dose if recovery takes >2 weeks
	Consider G-CSF if recurrent/persistent, or sepsis
Thrombocytopenia	Hold therapy if grade ≥3 (ie, platelets $<50 \times 10^9$/L)
	Restart at lower dose if recovery takes >2 weeks
	Consider IL-11 10 mcg/kg 3-7 days/week

management are included in Table 4-4. Grade 3 or 4 toxicity that is thought to be related to imatinib requires treatment interruption. Therapy is resumed when the toxicity resolves to grade 1 or less, and it is recommended that the doses be reduced. However, as discussed earlier, doses below 300 mg daily are not recommended. Only 2 to 3% of patients are truly intolerant to imatinib and will require permanent discontinuation of therapy. Early identification and intervention when toxicity occurs will greatly reduce the need for unnecessary treatment interruptions and dose reductions.

Myelosuppression is a more common adverse event. Dose interruptions are not recommended unless the patient develops grade 3 neutropenia or thrombocytopenia (ie, neutrophils $<1 \times 10^9$/L, platelets $<50 \times 10^9$/L).

No interruptions or dose adjustments are usually recommended for anemia alone. Treatment is restarted when counts recover above this threshold. When treatment is interrupted peripheral blood counts should be monitored at least once weekly. If recovery occurs within 2 weeks, treatment is resumed with the same dose being used when myelosuppression occurs. If recovery takes longer than 2 weeks, the dose can be reduced (eg, from 800-600 mg, from 600-400 mg, or from 400-300 mg). Myelosuppression most frequently occurs within the first 2 to 3 months from the start of therapy, is generally self-limited, and generally does not lead to clinical consequences. For patients with recurrent or prolonged myelosuppression, the use of hematopoietic growth factors may be beneficial. Both erythropoietin (67) and darbepoetin have been shown to improve the anemia in the majority of patients who develop this complication; however, these drugs may be considered only as indicated. Filgrastim may promote improvement of neutropenia and has been reported to improve the response to imatinib, probably because it helps deliver uninterrupted full doses of imatinib (68). Patients with thrombocytopenia may respond to oprelvekin (interleukin-11) (69).

Monitoring patients on imatinib

Patients should be closely monitored for response to imatinib. Monitoring involves routine blood counts and differentials, cytogenetics, and molecular testing for BCR-ABL transcript levels and for BCR–ABL kinase domain mutations. In general, routine blood counts should be performed every 2 weeks until a patient achieves CHR, and at least every 3 months after or more frequently as clinically indicated (70). Bone marrow cytogenetics should be obtained at 6 and 12 months after the initiation of therapy. Controversy exists if routine cytogenetic testing is indicated to assess response to therapy. Cytogenetic testing is the only study that gives reliable information regarding the presence of other chromosomal abnormalities. The presence of additional chromosomal abnormalities may reduce the probability of response to imatinib and overall survival (26). Approximately, 10% of patients who respond to imatinib may develop chromosomal abnormalities in the Ph-negative metaphases (71,72). The long-term implications of these abnormalities are still uncertain and most subsequently disappear. Transformation into myelodysplasia and acute leukemia can occur, but is considered to be uncommon. Thus, appearance of some of these abnormalities is not necessarily an indication of failure or progression, and may not always warrant a change of therapy. Once a patient achieves a stable CCyR, particularly if associated with MMR, bone marrow aspirations with cytogenetics are recommended only every 1 to 3 years, or if there is a significant change in the transcript levels or peripheral blood counts.

Once a complete cytogenetic response has been achieved, measurement of molecular response becomes particularly relevant. BCR-ABL transcript levels must be measured by quantitative PCR in the peripheral blood every 3 to 6 months to document the molecular response (defined as transcript levels <0.1% in the IS) (73). The significance of molecular monitoring in CML was first documented with SCT. Patients who had BCR–ABL detectable by polymerase chain reaction (PCR) 6 months after transplant have a significantly higher probability of relapse; those with the highest level of transcripts had the highest risk (74). Among patients who achieve a complete cytogenetic response, those who have a major molecular response have a significantly improved CR duration and progression-free survival compared to those who have a lesser improvement (73).

Although achieving the lowest possible levels of transcripts, and ideally undetectable, is desirable, persistence of detectable transcript levels in the context of a CCyR is not an indication of failure to therapy, even if above the levels corresponding to MMR. In some patients, transcript levels may increase. Some studies have suggested that an increase in transcript levels may increase the risk of developing mutations or failure to therapy. The magnitude of the increase that may predict for such events is variable, in part due to the variability of the testing in different laboratories. A single elevation in transcript levels should first be confirmed in a subsequent determination 1 to 3 months later and the magnitude of the increment should be determined to be greater than the variability of the test in the laboratory where it is being tested. In addition, compliance with therapy should be revisited with the patient. Still, most studies have demonstrated that the risk of relapse (or association with mutations) is mostly present when a sizeable increase (two- to tenfold) is associated with a loss of MMR (or occurs in a patient who never achieved a MMR), while increments in patients who are still below the level of MMR have little if any prognostic significance. ABL kinase domain mutation screening may be performed in those patients who have an inadequate initial response (defined as failure to achieve CHR at 3 months, partial cytogenetic response at 6 months and major cytogenetic response at 12 months) or in patients who show loss of response (hematologic relapse, Ph positivity, sustained 1-log increase in BCR–ABL transcript ratio) (70). All patients who progress to the accelerated or blast phase CML should have ABL kinase mutations tested.

Peripheral blood FISH can be used to monitor the cytogenetic response between marrow analyses. FISH has expanded the sensitivity of the standard karyotype because it can survey many more cells. This technique can be applied to peripheral blood, and is useful if cytogenetic studies are unsuccessful because of insufficient metaphases (10-20% of cases) as it can be done in interphase. FISH does carry some disadvantages: (1) even with the newest probes there is a small percentage of false positivity with FISH; (2) routine FISH does not provide information on every chromosome; and (3) although it surveys more cells for the Ph chromosome than a cytogenetic analysis, it is not as sensitive as PCR (75,76). A 100% negative FISH test corresponds to only approximately a 2-log reduction in transcript levels (similar to a CCyR by routine cytogenetic analysis), whereas with PCR the limit of detection extends to approximately 4.5 to 5 logs. A 3-log reduction of PCR is equivalent to an absolute PCR value of 0.1% on the IS. Table 4-5 summarizes the main features and differences of these three monitoring techniques utilized in CML.

Treatment discontinuation

There have been a few studies addressing the issue of discontinuing therapy with imatinib in patients after achieving a complete molecular response. In one of the earliest studies, 12 patients who had achieved a complete molecular response and had maintained it for greater than 2 years were closely monitored for relapse following discontinuation of therapy with imatinib (77). Six (50%) patients experienced a relapse at a median of 3 months; however, all of them responded very well to reintroduction of imatinib. Interestingly, these six patients were not treated with IFN previously. In more recent reports, relapses after discontinuation of therapy occurred frequently (approximately 50-60%) regardless of the prior use of IFN, they happened early (all within 7 months), were usually only molecular relapses with no cytogenetic or hematologic manifestations, and most responded to reintroduction of imatinib (78,79). Although these results suggest that some patients may maintain durable molecular responses after discontinuation of imatinib, the current recommendation is to continue therapy indefinitely. Several strategies are currently being investigated to increase the rate of sustained complete molecular responses (currently occurring in only approximately 30% of patients), and to achieve the goal of safe treatment discontinuation in more patients.

■ IMATINIB RESISTANCE

Despite the favorable results with imatinib, a subset of patients treated with imatinib will develop resistance. Among those treated in chronic phase, the rate of resistance is less than 4% per year and decreases after the first 3 years to approximately 0.5 to 1% per year; for those who achieve a CCyR, the rate of resistance beyond year 3 of imatinib therapy is less than 1%, suggesting the durable stability of a complete cytogenetic response on imatinib and the predictability of the CML course once such a response is obtained.

Several mechanisms of resistance to imatinib have been described. These can be classified into two categories: BCR–ABL dependent and BCR–ABL independent. The first group includes amplification or overexpression of BCR–ABL or its protein product (80), and point mutations of the *ABL* sequence (81). The second group includes multidrug-resistance (MDR) expression (82) and overexpression of Src kinases (82). BCR-ABL-dependent mechanisms are more common, particularly point mutations which have been identified in approximately 50% of patients who develop clinical resistance to imatinib (83,84). More than 90 different mutations have been described and occur in any of the different relevant domains of the kinase, including the ATP-binding domain (also known as P-loop), the catalytic domain, the activation loop, and amino acids that make direct contact with imatinib. The significance of these mutations varies. Although some retain sensitivity to imatinib at concentrations similar to those of the wild-type sequence, others, particularly T315I, are nearly completely insensitive to imatinib (85). Clinically, the P-loop mutations have been suggested to carry an increased risk of rapid blastic transformation and short survival (83), although the MDACC experience does not support this notion (86).

TABLE 4-5	MAIN FEATURES OF THE MONITORING TECHNIQUES AVAILABLE FOR CML		
Parameter	*Cytogenetics*	*FISH*	*PCR*
No cells evaluated	20	200	>10,000
Rapidity (days)	14-21	1-3	7-10
Source	BM	BM/PB	BM/PB
Clonal evolution	Yes	No	No
False negativity	NA	Yes	Yes
False positivity	No	≤10%	NA

Different mutations have considerable variability with respect to resistance to imatinib. Some mutations are inhibited by slightly higher concentrations of imatinib than required to inhibit the unmutated form while others are completely insensitive to imatinib. Up to now, more than 100 different mutants of Bcr–Abl have been described. Most of the clinically relevant mutations develop in a few residues in the P-loop (G250E, Y253F/H, and E255K/V), the contact site (T315I), and the catalytic domain (M351T and F359V) (87). In some patients, more than one mutation may be present at the same time. This phenomenon appears to increase in frequency after treatment with more than one tyrosine kinase mutation. Mutational analysis is useful in patients with imatinib resistance for several reasons (88-90): (1) it can identify patients with the T315I mutant that do not respond to imatinib or the second-generation TKIs (dasatinib, nilotinib, bosutinib) and who should be considered for allogeneic SCT or therapy with new agents with activity against T315I; (2) it can identify mutants with different sensitivity to the different available agents, thus guiding the selection of therapy. A list of such mutations with their IC50 values is shown in Table 4-6. The long-term outcome of patients with chronic myeloid leukemia treated with

second-generation tyrosine kinase inhibitors after imatinib failure has been shown to be predicted by the in vitro sensitivity of BCR–ABL kinase domain mutations (91). Mutations are quantified by direct sequencing and the sensitivity of such assay varies between 10 and 25% (92,93). Other methods, such as denatured high-performance liquid chromatography (93,94) increase the sensitivity to 1 to 10%. However, it is unclear at this time if identification of small mutated clones with these highly sensitive methods is clinically relevant (95,96). Mutation analysis should be carried out only in instances of failure to imatinib by standard criteria. Investigation of mutations in patients with a CCyR carries a very low yield (<5%) and may antecede cytogenetic resistance by approximately 18 months. Some studies have suggested that a mutation analysis should be performed in patients with a doubling of the transcript levels if they do not have or have lost an MMR. There is no indication that intervention at the time of mutation detection in these instances improves the outcome compared to intervening at the time of cytogenetic response.

■ TREATMENT OPTIONS AFTER FAILURE OF IMATINIB

IMATINIB DOSE ESCALATION

Dose escalation can improve the response in a subset of patients with resistance to standard dose imatinib and was the main option for managing suboptimal responses and treatment failures before the introduction of second-generation TKIs. In a retrospective analysis of patients enrolled in the IRIS trial, Kantarjian et al. reported that among 106 patients who required dose escalation due to resistance to standard-dose therapy, freedom-from-progression and overall survival rates were 89 and 84%, respectively, at 3 years from dose escalation (97). In another study from MDACC, 84 patients with chronic phase CML were dose escalated to imatinib 600 to 800 mg/day after developing hematologic failure (n = 21), or cytogenetic failure (n = 63) to standard dose imatinib (91). Among patients who met the criteria for cytogenetic failure, 75% (47/63) responded to imatinib dose escalation. In contrast, in patients where imatinib was dose escalated because of hematologic failure, 48% achieved a complete hematologic response and only 14% (3/21) achieved a cytogenetic response. Patients more likely to respond to imatinib dose increase are those that have previously achieved a cytogenetic response and then lost it and who have not developed any mutations unresponsive to imatinib. Even in these cases, a switch to a second-generation TKI is preferable unless the patient has no access to these agents (Fig. 4-8).

| TABLE 4-6 | IN VITRO SENSITIVITY OF DIFFERENT BCR-ABL MUTANTS TO DIFFERENT TYROSINE KINASE INHIBITORS |

	IC50-FOLD INCREASE (WT=1)			
	Imatinib	*Bosutinib*	*Dasatinib*	*Nilotinib*
WT	1	1	1	1
L248V	3.54	2.97	5.11	2.80
G250E	6.86	4.31	4.45	4.56
Q252H	1.39	0.31	3.05	2.64
Y253F	3.58	0.96	1.58	3.23
E255K	6.02	9.47	5.61	6.69
E255V	16.99	5.53	3.44	10.31
D276G	2.18	0.60	1.44	2.00
E279K	3.55	0.95	1.64	2.05
V299L	1.54	26.10	8.65	1.34
T315I	17.50	45.42	75.03	39.41
F317L	2.60	2.42	4.46	2.22
M351T	1.76	0.70	0.88	0.44
F359V	2.86	0.93	1.49	5.16
L384M	1.28	0.47	2.21	2.33
H396P	2.43	0.43	1.07	2.41
H396R	3.91	0.81	1.63	3.10
G398R	0.35	1.16	0.69	0.49
F486S	8.10	2.31	3.04	1.85

Mutations can be classified as sensitive (IC50 fold increase ≤2), resistant (between 2.01 and 10), or highly resistant (>10; T315I mutation).

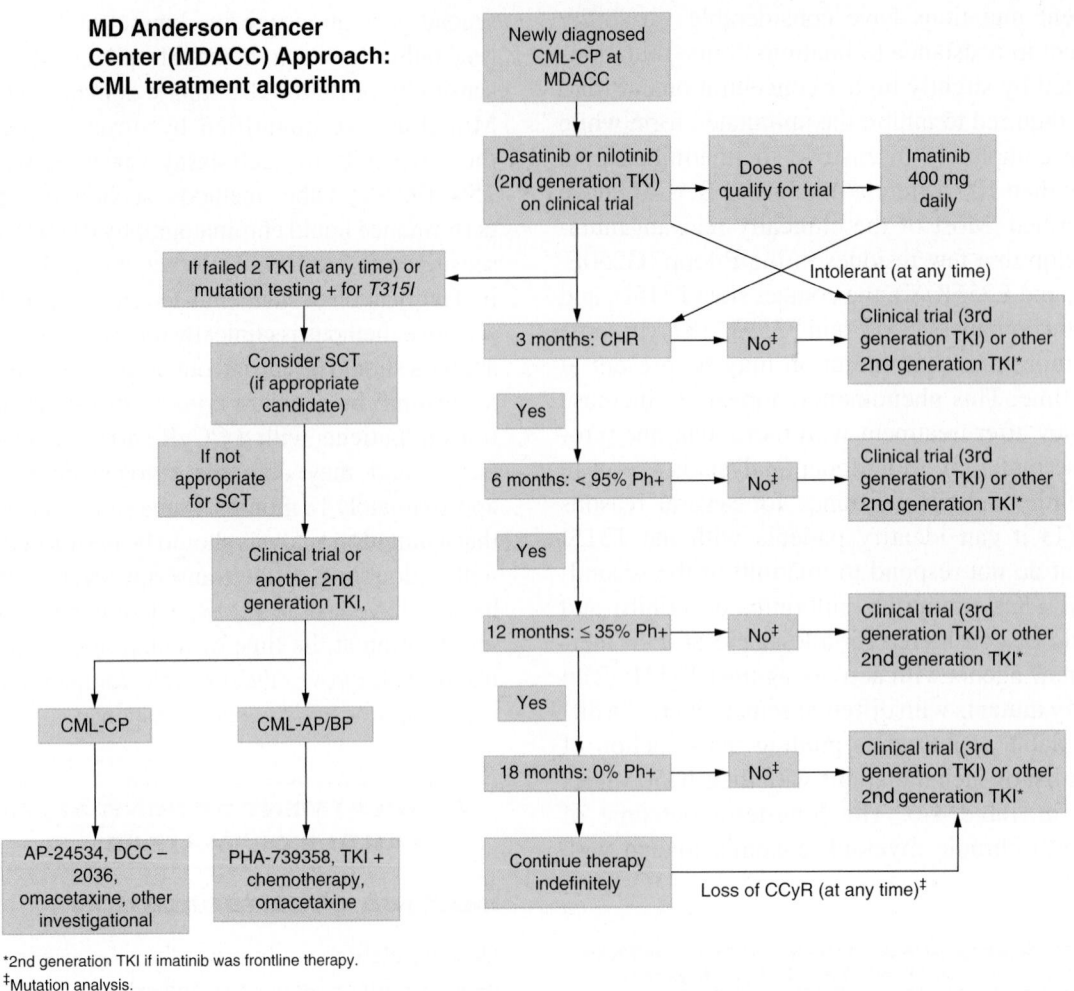

FIGURE 4-8. MD Anderson Cancer Center Approach: Chronic myeloid leukemia treatment algorithm. CP, chronic phase; AP, accelerated phase; BP, blast phase; TKI, Tyrosine kinase inhibitors (dasatinib, nilotinib, bosutinib); SCT, Allogeneic stem cell transplant.

DASATINIB

Dasatinib is a piperazinyl derivative that targets many TKs. Dasatinib was selected for study in CML for its potent inhibitory activity against *SRC* and *ABL* kinases, including the active conformation of BCR–ABL and a number of its mutants (98,99). Dasatinib has excellent oral bioavailability and exhibits 300-fold greater in vitro potency for unmutated *BCR-ABL* compared with imatinib, and significant activity against most imatinib-resistant BCR–ABL mutants, with the notable exception of T315I, and a few others mutations (eg, V299L, F317L) (100). In contrast to imatinib, dasatinib can bind to both the active and inactive conformations of BCR–ABL.

Dasatinib, at a dose of 70 mg orally twice daily, was approved by the FDA on the basis of its efficacy and safety profiles shown in a series of phase II trials in patients in all stages of CML (and those with Ph-positive

ALL) who were resistant or intolerant to imatinib therapy (101-103). Over 50% of patients treated with dasatinib in chronic phase after imatinib failure achieved a complete cytogenetic response. The response to dasatinib among patients in chronic, accelerated, and blast phase (myeloid and lymphoid) after imatinib failure are summarized in Table 4-7. A randomized trial of dasatinib versus dose increase of imatinib (to 800 mg daily) among patients who had failed prior therapy with imatinib (400-600 mg) demonstrated a significantly higher rate of response and progression-free survival for patients receiving dasatinib, particularly among those who were already receiving imatinib 600 mg, those with BCR–ABL mutations, and those who had never achieved a cytogenetic response with imatinib, establishing second-generation tyrosine kinase inhibitors as the preferred approach after failure to imatinib standard-dose therapy (97).

Dasatinib is overall well tolerated. Myelosuppression occurs frequently, with grade 3 or 4 neutropenia or thrombocytopenia occurring in nearly 50% of patients treated at a dose of 70 mg twice daily. The most common nonhematologic grade 3 to 4 toxicities at a dose of 70 mg twice daily were pleural effusion (9%), dyspnea (6%), bleeding (4%), diarrhea (3%), and fatigue (3%). In an open-label phase III trial, 670 patients with imatinib-resistant or -intolerant CP-CML were randomly assigned between four dasatinib treatment schedules: 100 mg once daily, 50 mg twice daily, 140 mg once daily, or 70 mg twice daily (104). Results of this trial showed that 100 mg once daily retained its activity and was associated with less toxicity, particularly pleural effusion and myelosuppression, with grade 3 to 4 neutropenia or thrombocytopenia occurring in approximately 30% each. Based on these results, the standard dasatinib dose for patients in chronic phase is 100 mg. Similar results among patients in advanced stage disease established 140 mg once daily as the preferred dose in advanced stage disease.

Based on the significant activity of dasatinib used as second-line therapy, a phase 2 single-arm study using dasatinib as initial therapy for patients with newly diagnosed chronic phase CML was initiated. In a recent update, 62 patients received 100 mg dasatinib daily (either 50 mg twice daily or 100 mg once daily) (105). Among 50 patients followed for at least 3 months, 49 (98%) achieved CCyR. MMR was achieved in 35 (70%), including 5 (10%) with complete molecular response. Responses occurred early, with over 90% of patients achieving CCyR already after 6 months of therapy, and MMR in 45% by 12 months and 71% by 24 months. These results compared favorably with historical controls treated with 400 and 800 mg imatinib. Responses and toxicity profile favored the 100 mg daily arm and further accrual on this dose is ongoing.

NILOTINIB

Nilotinib is an aminopyrimidine derivative that inhibits the TK activity of the unmutated and most mutated forms of BCR–ABL more potently and more selectively than imatinib (106,107). It is approved at a dose of 400 mg twice daily for patients with CML in chronic or accelerated phase who have resistance or intolerance to imatinib. Nilotinib should be administered on an empty stomach (no food for 2 h prior to and 1 h after administration) as food may significantly increase absorption increasing the plasma concentrations in an unpredictable fashion. Among patients previously treated with imatinib who received nilotinib while still in the chronic phase, a complete cytogenetic response was achieved in over 40% of patients.

Nilotinib is overall well tolerated. Grades 3 and 4 myelosuppression is the most common adverse event, with neutropenia or thrombocytopenia observed in 20 to 30%. Nonhematologic toxicity includes liver function abnormalities in 10 to 15%, and elevated (usually asymptomatic) lipase and amylase levels in 10 to 15%. Rare cases (<1%) of pancreatitis have been reported. Nilotinib (and to some extent dasatinib) has the potential for QTc prolongation, and an EKG is required prior to the start of therapy. Patients with significant QTc prolongation that is not correctable with electrolyte replacement or elimination of other agents with this potential, should not be treated with nilotinib. Drugs that prolong the QTc should be used with extreme caution in patients treated with nilotinib.

Considering the significant efficacy of nilotinib in patients treated after imatinib failure, studies using nilotinib 400 mg twice daily as initial therapy in early chronic phase have been initiated. Two recently reported single-arm, phase II studies have reported CCyR rates of over 90% as early as 6 months from the start of therapy, with an MMR rate of nearly 80% by 12 months of therapy (108,109). The preliminary results of a randomized phase III trial comparing two different dose schedules of nilotinib (300 and 400 mg bid) to imatinib as initial therapy for patients with early chronic phase CML confirmed the superiority of nilotinib, with significantly higher rates at 12 months of CCyR (78-80% with nilotinib vs. 65% with imatinib; $p < .001$) and MMR (43-44% with nilotinib vs. 22% with imatinib; $p < .001$). More important, the rate of transformation to accelerated or blast phase by 12 months of therapy was significantly lower with nilotinib (<1%) compared to imatinib (4%). These results, if maintained with longer follow-up, could establish second-generation tyrosine kinase inhibitors as the standard of care for patients with newly diagnosed CML in early chronic phase.

BOSUTINIB

Bosutinib (SKI606), an orally available dual Src/Abl inhibitor, is 30 to 50 times more potent than imatinib against unmutated BCR–ABL, with activity against most imatinib-resistant BCR–ABL mutants with the notable exception of T315I. In contrast to all other available TKIs, bosutinib has minimal inhibitory activity against C-Kit and PDGFR. It has been suggested that the decreased off-target effects may lead to decreased toxicity, particularly myelosuppression and fluid retention (89). Response to bosutinib after imatinib failure are comparable to those achieved with other inhibitors, with CCyR

TABLE 4-7 | **RESPONSES TO TKIS**

PERCENT RESPONSE

	Dasatinib				Nilotinib				Bosutinib		
	CP N=387	AP N=174	MyBP N=109	LyBP N=48	CP N=321	AP N=137	MyBP N=105	LyBP N=31	CP N=146	AP N=51	BP N=38
Median follow-up (mo)	15	14	12	12	24	9	3	3	7	6	3
% Resistant to imatinib	74	93	91	88	70	80	82	82	69	NR	NR
% Hematologic Response		79	50	40	94	56	22	19	85	54	36
CHR	91	45	27	29	76	31	11	13	81	54	36
NEL	–	19	7	6	–	12	1	0	–	0	0
% Cytogenetic Response	NR	44	36	52	NR	NR	NR	NR	NR	NR	NR
Complete	49	32	26	46	46	20	29	32	34	27	35
Partial	11	7	7	6	15	12	10	16	13	20	18
% Survival (at 12 months)	96 (15)	82 (12)	50 (12)	50 (5)	87 (24)	67 (24)	42 (12)	42 (12)	98 (12)	60 (12)	50 (10)

CP, chronic phase CML; AP, accelerated phase CML; BP, blast phase CML; MyBP, myeloid blast phase CML; LyBP, lymphoid blast phase CML; NR, not reported.

rates on over 40% among patients treated in chronic phase. Results of response to bosutinib in chronic, accelerated, and blast phase after imatinib resistance are summarized in Table 4-7. Treatment with bosutinib has been generally well tolerated with no pleural effusions and modest myelosuppression. The most common adverse events were gastrointestinal (nausea, vomiting, diarrhea) that were usually grade 1 to 2, manageable and transient, diminishing in frequency and severity after the first 3 to 4 weeks of treatment (110).

OTHER MULTIKINASE INHIBITORS

MK-0457, a potent aurora kinase inhibitor, was the first agent to demonstrate clinical activity against the T315I mutation. In a study of 14 evaluable patients with CML, 11 had an objective (hematologic, cytogenetic, and/or molecular) response, including nine patients with T315I (111). However, clinical development of MK-0457 was recently halted over toxicity concerns.

One of the most promising agents for treatment of T315I mutation in clinical trials is AP24534, an orally available multi-TKI designed using a structure-based approach as a pan-BCR-ABL inhibitor (112) AP24534 potently inhibits the enzymatic activity of BCR–ABL-T315I, the native enzyme and all other tested mutants. Importantly, AP24534 prevents the emergence of resistant mutants at concentrations of 40 nM. AP24534 also inhibits FLT3 and c-SRC. In a phase I clinical trial of

AP24534 at doses from 2 to 60 mg in 27 patients with CML (19 with chronic phase, 4 accelerated phase, and 4 blast phase), complete hematologic response was achieved or maintained in 83% of patients treated in chronic phase; major hematologic responses were also achieved in 38% of patients treated in advanced stages of the disease. More important, 9 of 20 patients treated in chronic phase achieved a major cytogenetic response (5 CCyR), including 3 of 7 with T315I (2 CCyR). The most common drug-related adverse events were elevations of lipase and amylase at a dose of 60 mg daily. Other toxicities were mostly grade 1 to 2. Grade 3 or 4 thrombocytopenia occurred in 9% of patients, with no grade 3 to 4 drug-related neutropenia.

XL228 (Exelixis Inc., San Francisco, USA) is a potent, multitargeted kinase inhibitor with potent activity against wild-type and T315I isoforms of BCR–ABL (wild-type ABL kinase, IC_{50} = 5 nM; ABL T315I, 1.4 nM), Aurora A (3.1 nM), IGF-1R (1.6 nM), SRC (6.1 nM), and LYN (2 nM). In a prelim phase I clinical study, XL228 was administered to 27 patients in six cohorts with a once-weekly dosing schedule (dose range from 0.45-10.8 mg/kg). All patients were resistant or intolerant to at least two prior standard therapies (including imatinib, dasatinib, and nilotinib) or had a known BCR–ABL-T315I mutation. Preliminary evidence of clinical activity was observed in patients treated at doses of 3.6 mg/kg and higher, including stable or decreasing white blood cell and/or platelet count within 2 months (in 14 patients, 5 with T315I), and/or >1-log reduction in BCR–ABL transcript levels by RT-PCR within 3 months (in 3 patients, 2 with T315I). XL 228 has been generally well tolerated. Dose-limiting toxicities observed with once-weekly dosing included grade 3 syncope and hyperglycemia in two patients dosed at 10.8 mg/kg. The most commonly reported grade 2 adverse effects were hyperglycemia, fatigue, nausea, vomiting, and bradycardia.

IMATINIB COMBINATIONS WITH OTHER AGENTS IN FIRST-LINE THERAPY FOR CML

The use of IFN in combination with TKI is attractive because IFN induced durable responses, and even some cures, in a small subset of patients. In a single-arm study of imatinib 400 mg daily and pegylated IFN-α in 76 patients with chronic phase CML, 81% patients were in continuous CCyR and 80% patients were in MMR after 5 years of follow-up (113). However, 50% of patients discontinued IFN after 1 year and 87% after 2 years, thereby making interpretation of the data difficult. In the recently reported randomized French Spirit Study, 636 patients with chronic phase CML were randomly assigned to receive imatinib 400 or 600 mg, or 400 mg imatinib with pegylated IFN-α or 400 mg imatinib with low-dose Ara-C (114). The best response was observed in the arm with imatinib plus IFN with a CCyR of 71% versus 57% for imatinib 400 alone at 12 months and an MMR rate of 61% versus 40% for imatinib 400 alone at 12 months. However, 46% of the patients discontinued IFN during the first year of therapy, and no difference in progression-free survival was identified. In another study, the combination of pegylated IFN (PEG-IFN-α-2b) with high-dose imatinib did not result in any difference in response rate or long-term event-free or overall survival (115). A third randomized study exploring this combination showed and advantage for imatinib 800 mg daily compared to standard dose, but no significant benefit with the use of IFN combined with imatinib (116).

NON-TYROSINE KINASE INHIBITORS

Homoharringtonine is a plant alkaloid that has been used in China for many years in the treatment of patients with AML. Before the introduction of imatinib, it was the best treatment option for patients who failed IFN-α and were not transplant candidates, with cytogenetic responses in approximately 30% of patients (116-118).

Omacetaxine mepesuccinate, a cephalotaxine ester and a derivative of homoharringtonine that has excellent bioavailability through the subcutaneous route, is a multitargeted protein synthase inhibitor that has been in clinical development for several years. Omacetaxine shows clinical activity against CML (119,120) with a mechanism of action independent of tyrosine kinase inhibition and is thus not affected by the presence of mutations. In a recently reported phase II/III clinical study of omacetaxine administered at a dose of 1.25 mg/m^2 sc twice daily for 7 days (every 28 days) to 89 patients with CML (44 chronic phase, 25 accelerated phase, and 20 blast phase) who are either intolerant or resistant to at least two TKIs (imatinib, dasatinib, or nilotinib), the rates of CHR and MCyR were 82 and 23% in chronic phase, respectively (121). In a similar trial enrolling 81 patients (49 chronic phase, 17 accelerated phase, and 15 blast phase) with T315I mutation who did not respond to imatinib, omacetaxine led to a CHR in 86% and MCyR in 27% among patients treated in CCyR (122). These responses were durable. The most commonly reported events were thrombocytopenia (58%), anemia (36%), and neutropenia (33%). Nonhematologic toxicities were primarily grade 1/2 with the most frequently reported events of diarrhea (44%), fatigue (35%), pyrexia (32%), nausea (26%), and asthenia (21%). Recent reports suggest that omacetaxine is able to affect the leukemic stem cell compartment, which would make it attractive for the potential of total elimination of the leukemic cells and potential cure.

■ TREATMENT RECOMMENDATIONS

CHRONIC PHASE

The standard of care for patients with newly diagnosed chronic-phase CML is imatinib 400 mg orally once daily. Patients should be carefully monitored for response while on imatinib, with an emphasis on patient compliance, treating associated side effects to minimize unnecessary treatment interruptions and dose reductions, and adequate monitoring and follow-up. Response definitions of chronic phase patients on imatinib as recommended by the European Leukemia Net guidelines are summarized in Table 4-8. Patients with suboptimal response to standard-dose imatinib can be offered higher doses of imatinib, usually with a doubling of the dose. In patients who are imatinib intolerant or meet the definition of failure to imatinib, second-generation TKIs, either dasatinib or nilotinib, constitute the treatment of choice. The presence of specific mutations and side-effect profiles may help in choosing one over another. In patients who have resistance to dasatinib or nilotinib, they may be

TABLE 4-8	RESPONSE DEFINITIONS TO IMATINIB IN CHRONIC PHASE CML (EUROPEAN LEUKEMIA NET GUIDELINES)		
EVALUATION TIME	**RESPONSE**		
	Optimal	*Suboptimal*	*Failure*
3 months	CHR and at least minor CyR	No CyR	No CHR
6 months	At least partial CyR	Less than partial CyR	No CyR
12 months	CCyR	Partial CyR	Less than partial CyR
18 months	MMR	Less than MMR	Less than CCyR
Any time	Stable or improving MMR	Loss of MMR, presence of mutations	Loss of CHR, loss of CCyR, clonal evolution

switched to the alternative agent. However, although some patients may respond, these responses are usually not durable (123). Thus, these patients should be considered for an allogeneic stemcell transplant (SCT) if they are good candidates, or for clinical trials if not good candidates for SCT. Similarly, patients who develop a T315I mutation or who progress to accelerated phase or blast phase, should be considered for allo-SCT or for clinical trials with one of the several options under development.

ACCELERATED AND BLAST PHASE

Options for first line therapy for patients in accelerated phase include imatinib (at a starting dose of 600 mg daily) versus a 2nd generation TKI versus consideration of allo-SCT as indicated. Options for treatment for patients with blast phase CML include TKI plus or minus chemotherapy (Hyper-CVAD for lymphoid blast phase and AML-type induction chemotherapy for myeloid blast phase, along with evaluation and consideration of allo-SCT ideally in second chronic phase. TKI plus or minus chemotherapy as indicated (ALL-type chemotherapy for lymphoid blast crisis or AML-type chemotherapy for myeloid blast crisis. Young patients with an adequate donor should be considered for SCT, particularly if they return back to chronic phase. Consideration may be given to frontline dasatinib or nilotinib if mutations poorly responsive to imatinib are detected. In patients who have been previously treated with TKIs, allo-SCT is the treatment of choice.

■ FUTURE DIRECTIONS

Imatinib has changed the understanding, management, and natural history of CML, and constitutes today the standard of care. However, it is possible to consider that we will need combination therapy to prevent the development of resistance and to increase the probability of achieving complete molecular remissions and eventually cure. For this purpose, the many molecular events that occur in CML are being targeted for development of drugs that may affect them. These drugs in turn may be combined with imatinib. In addition, the next generation of more potent tyrosine kinase inhibitors will be increasingly used. Whether their right place will be replacing imatinib, in instances when imatinib fails, or in combination with imatinib to improve responses and prevent development of resistance will be defined in the near future.

References

1. Jemal A, Siegel R, Ward E, et al. Cancer statistics, 2009. *CA Cancer J Clin* 2009;59(4):225-249.
2. Cortes JE, Talpaz M, Kantarjian H. Chronic myelogenous leukemia: A review. *Am J Med* 1996;100(5):555-570.
3. Biernaux C, Loos M, Sels A, et al. Detection of major bcr-abl gene expression at a very low level in blood cells of some healthy individuals. *Blood* 1995;86(8):3118-3122.
4. Bose S, Deininger M, Gora-Tybor J, et al. The presence of typical and atypical BCR-ABL fusion genes in leukocytes of normal individuals: Biologic significance and implications for the assessment of minimal residual disease. *Blood* 1998; 92(9):3362-3367.
5. Fialkow PJ, Martin PJ, Najfeld V, et al. Evidence for a multi-step pathogenesis of chronic myelogenous leukemia. *Blood* 1981;58(1):158-163.
6. Corso A, Lazzarino M, Morra E, et al. Chronic myelogenous leukemia and exposure to ionizing radiation—A retrospective study of 443 patients. *Ann Hematol* 1995;70(2): 79-82.
7. Kurzrock R, Gutterman JU, Talpaz M. The molecular genetics of Philadelphia chromosome-positive leukemias. *N Engl J Med* 1988;319(15):990-998.
8. Deininger MW, Goldman JM, Melo JV. The molecular biology of chronic myeloid leukemia. *Blood* 2000;96(10): 3343-3356.
9. Kantarjian HM, Dixon D, Keating MJ, et al. Characteristics of accelerated disease in chronic myelogenous leukemia. *Cancer* 1988;61(7):1441-1446.
10. Vardiman JW, Harris NL, Brunning RD. The World Health Organization (WHO) classification of the myeloid neoplasms. *Blood* 2002;100(7):2292-2302.
11. Savage DG, Szydlo RM, Goldman JM. Clinical features at diagnosis in 430 patients with chronic myeloid leukaemia seen at a referral centre over a 16-year period. *Br J Haematol* 1997;96(1):111-116.
12. Cortes J, Kantarjian H. Advanced-phase chronic myeloid leukemia. *Semin Hematol* 2003;40(1):79-86.

13. Cortes J, Talpaz M, O'Brien S, et al. Survival advantage for patients (pts) with chronic myeloid leukemia (CML) in accelerated phase (AP) treated with imatinib. *Blood* 2004;104(11):1006 (ASH Annual Meeting Abstracts).

14. Cortes J, O'Brien S, Garcia-Manero G, et al. Is the proposed World Health Organization (WHO) classification for chronic myeloid leukemia (CML) of clinical value in the imatinib era? *Blood* 2004;104(11):1014 (ASH Annual Meeting Abstracts).

15. Faderl S, Talpaz M, Estrov Z, et al. Chronic myelogenous leukemia: Biology and therapy. *Ann Intern Med* 1999;131(3):207-219.

16. Knox WF, Bhavnani M, Davson J, et al. Histological classification of chronic granulocytic leukaemia. *Clin Lab Haematol* 1984;6(2):171-175.

17. Dekmezian R, Kantarjian HM, Keating MJ, et al. The relevance of reticulin stain-measured fibrosis at diagnosis in chronic myelogenous leukemia. *Cancer* 1987;59(10):1739-1743.

18. Cervantes F, Rozman C. A multivariate analysis of prognostic factors in chronic myeloid leukemia. *Blood* 1982;60(6):1298-1304.

19. Kantarjian HM, Keating MJ, Smith TL, et al. Proposal for a simple synthesis prognostic staging system in chronic myelogenous leukemia. *Am J Med* 1990;88(1):1-8.

20. Sokal JE, Cox EB, Baccarani M, et al. Prognostic discrimination in "good-risk" chronic granulocytic leukemia. *Blood* 1984;63(4):789-799.

21. Tura S, Baccarani M, Corbelli G. Staging of chronic myeloid leukaemia. *Br J Haematol* 1981;47(1):105-119.

22. Kantarjian HM, Keating MJ, Smith TL, et al. Proposal for a simple synthesis prognostic staging system in chronic myelogenous leukemia. *Am J Med* 1990;88(1):1-8.

23. Hasford J, Pfirrmann M, Hehlmann R, et al. A new prognostic score for survival of patients with chronic myeloid leukemia treated with interferon alfa. Writing Committee for the Collaborative CML Prognostic Factors Project Group. *J Natl Cancer Inst* 1998;90(11):850-858.

24. O'Brien SG, Guilhot F, Larson RA, et al. Imatinib compared with interferon and low-dose cytarabine for newly diagnosed chronic-phase chronic myeloid leukemia. *N Engl J Med* 2003;348(11):994-1004.

25. Kantarjian HM, O'Brien S, Cortes JE, et al. Complete cytogenetic and molecular responses to interferon-alpha-based therapy for chronic myelogenous leukemia are associated with excellent long-term prognosis. *Cancer* 2003;97(4):1033-1041.

26. Cortes JE, Talpaz M, Giles F, et al. Prognostic significance of cytogenetic clonal evolution in patients with chronic myelogenous leukemia on imatinib mesylate therapy. *Blood* 2003;101(10):3794-3800.

27. Kantarjian HM, Cortes JE, O'Brien S, et al. Long-term survival benefit and improved complete cytogenetic and molecular response rates with imatinib mesylate in Philadelphia chromosome-positive chronic-phase chronic myeloid leukemia after failure of interferon-alpha. *Blood* 2004;104(7):1979-1988.

28. Cortes J, Talpaz M, O'Brien S, et al. Effects of age on prognosis with imatinib mesylate therapy for patients with Philadelphia chromosome-positive chronic myelogenous leukemia. *Cancer* 2003;98(6):1105-1113.

29. Huntly BJ, Bench A, Green AR. Double jeopardy from a single translocation: Deletions of the derivative chromosome 9 in chronic myeloid leukemia. *Blood* 2003;102(4):1160-1168.

30. Huntly BJ, Reid AG, Bench AJ, et al. Deletions of the derivative chromosome 9 occur at the time of the Philadelphia translocation and provide a powerful and independent prognostic indicator in chronic myeloid leukemia. *Blood* 2001;98(6):1732-1738.

31. Huntly BJ, Guilhot F, Reid AG, et al. Imatinib improves but may not fully reverse the poor prognosis of patients with CML with derivative chromosome 9 deletions. *Blood* 2003;102(6):2205-2212.

32. Quintas-Cardama A, Kantarjian H, Talpaz M, et al. Imatinib mesylate therapy may overcome the poor prognostic significance of deletions of derivative chromosome 9 in patients with chronic myelogenous leukemia. *Blood* 2005;105(6):2281-2286.

33. O'Dwyer ME, Mauro MJ, Kurilik G, et al. The impact of clonal evolution on response to imatinib mesylate (STI571) in accelerated phase CML. *Blood* 2002;100(5):1628-1633.

34. Sneed TB, Kantarjian HM, Talpaz M, et al. The significance of myelosuppression during therapy with imatinib mesylate in patients with chronic myelogenous leukemia in chronic phase. *Cancer* 2004;100(1):116-121.

35. Verstovsek S, Lunin S, Kantarjian H, et al. Clinical relevance of VEGF receptors 1 and 2 in patients with chronic myelogenous leukemia. *Leuk Res* 2003;27(7):661-669.

36. Verma D, Kantarjian HM, Jones D, et al. Chronic myeloid leukemia (CML) with P190 BCR-ABL: Analysis of characteristics, outcomes, and prognostic significance. *Blood* 2009;114(11):2232-2235.

37. Guo JQ, Lin H, Kantarjian H, et al. Comparison of competitive-nested PCR and real-time PCR in detecting BCR-ABL fusion transcripts in chronic myeloid leukemia patients. *Leukemia* 2002;16(12):2447-2453.

38. Baker KS, Gurney JG, Ness KK, et al. Late effects in survivors of chronic myeloid leukemia treated with hematopoietic cell transplantation: Results from the Bone Marrow Transplant Survivor Study. *Blood* 2004;104(6):1898-1906.

39. Deininger M, Schleuning M, Greinix H, et al. The effect of prior exposure to imatinib on transplant-related mortality. *Haematologica* 2006;91(4):452-459.

40. Lee SJ, Kukreja M, Wang T, et al. Impact of prior imatinib mesylate on the outcome of hematopoietic cell transplantation for chronic myeloid leukemia. *Blood* 2008;112(8):3500-3507.

41. Oehler VG, Gooley T, Snyder DS, et al. The effects of imatinib mesylate treatment before allogeneic transplantation for chronic myeloid leukemia. *Blood* 2007;109(4):1782-1789.

42. Jabbour E, Kantarjian HM, Abruzzo LV, et al. Chromosomal abnormalities in Philadelphia chromosome negative metaphases appearing during imatinib mesylate therapy in patients with newly diagnosed chronic myeloid leukemia in chronic phase. *Blood* 2007;110(8):2991-2995.

43. Shimoni A, Leiba M, Schleuning M, et al. Prior treatment with the tyrosine kinase inhibitors dasatinib and nilotinib allows stem cell transplantation (SCT) in a less advanced disease phase and does not increase SCT toxicity in patients with chronic myelogenous leukemia and philadelphia positive acute lymphoblastic leukemia. *Leukemia* 2009;23(1):190-194.

44. Kebriaei P, Detry MA, Giralt S, et al. Long-term follow-up of allogeneic hematopoietic stem-cell transplantation with reduced-intensity conditioning for patients with chronic myeloid leukemia. *Blood* 2007;110(9):3456-3462.

45. Radich JP, Gehly G, Gooley T, et al. Polymerase chain reaction detection of the BCR-ABL fusion transcript after allogeneic marrow transplantation for chronic myeloid leukemia: Results and implications in 346 patients. *Blood* 1995;85(9):2632-2638.

46. Porter DL, Collins RH, Jr., Hardy C, et al. Treatment of relapsed leukemia after unrelated donor marrow transplantation with unrelated donor leukocyte infusions. *Blood* 2000; 95(4):1214-1221.

47. DeAngelo DJ, Hochberg EP, Alyea EP, et al. Extended follow-up of patients treated with imatinib mesylate (gleevec) for chronic myelogenous leukemia relapse after allogeneic transplantation: Durable cytogenetic remission and conversion to complete donor chimerism without graft-versus-host disease. *Clin Cancer Res* 2004;10(15):5065-5071.

48. Kantarjian HM, O'Brien S, Cortes JE, et al. Imatinib mesylate therapy for relapse after allogeneic stem cell transplantation for chronic myelogenous leukemia. *Blood* 2002;100(5):1590-1595.

49. Olavarria E, Craddock C, Dazzi F, et al. Imatinib mesylate (STI571) in the treatment of relapse of chronic myeloid leukemia after allogeneic stem cell transplantation. *Blood* 2002;99(10):3861-3862.

50. Champlin RE, Giralt S, Shpall E, et al. Nonmyeloablative allogeneic transplantation in the imatinib era: Three chances to achieve molecular remission in CML. *Blood* 2007;110(11):1028 (ASH Annual Meeting Abstracts).

51. Faderl S, Talpaz M, Estrov Z, et al. The biology of chronic myeloid leukemia. *N Engl J Med* 1999;341(3):164-172.

52. Allan NC, Shepherd PC, Brackenridge I, et al. United Kingdom Medical Research Council Randomized Trial of interferon alfa in chronic-phase chronic myelogenous leukemia. *Semin Hematol* 1993;30(3 Suppl 3):20-21.

53. Ozer H, George SL, Schiffer CA, et al. Prolonged subcutaneous administration of recombinant alpha 2b interferon in patients with previously untreated Philadelphia chromosome-positive chronic-phase chronic myelogenous leukemia: Effect on remission duration and survival: Cancer and Leukemia Group B study 8583. *Blood* 1993;82(10):2975-2984.

54. Guilhot F, Chastang C, Michallet M, et al. Interferon alfa-2b combined with cytarabine versus interferon alone in chronic myelogenous leukemia. French Chronic Myeloid Leukemia Study Group. *N Engl J Med* 1997;337(4):223-229.

55. Kantarjian HM, O'Brien S, Smith TL, et al. Treatment of Philadelphia chromosome-positive early chronic phase chronic myelogenous leukemia with daily doses of interferon alpha and low-dose cytarabine. *J Clin Oncol* 1999;17(1):284-292.

56. Beran M, Cao X, Estrov Z, et al. Selective inhibition of cell proliferation and BCR-ABL phosphorylation in acute lymphoblastic leukemia cells expressing Mr 190,000 BCR-ABL protein by a tyrosine kinase inhibitor (CGP-57148). *Clin Cancer Res* 1998;4(7):1661-1672.

57. Druker BJ, Tamura S, Buchdunger E, et al. Effects of a selective inhibitor of the Abl tyrosine kinase on the growth of Bcr-Abl positive cells. *Nat Med* 1996;2(5):561-566.

58. Druker BJ, Talpaz M, Resta DJ, et al. Efficacy and safety of a specific inhibitor of the BCR-ABL tyrosine kinase in chronic myeloid leukemia. *N Engl J Med* 2001;344(14):1031-1037.

59. Kantarjian H, Sawyers C, Hochhaus A, et al. Hematologic and cytogenetic responses to imatinib mesylate in chronic myelogenous leukemia. *N Engl J Med* 2002;346(9):645-652.

60. O'Brien SG, Guilhot F, Goldman JM, et al. International randomized study of interferon versus STI571 (IRIS) 7-year follow-up: Sustained survival, low rate of transformation and increased rate of major molecular response (MMR) in patients (pts) with newly diagnosed chronic myeloid leukemia in chronic phase (CMLCP) treated with imatinib (IM). *Blood* 2008;112(11):186 (ASH Annual Meeting Abstracts).

61. Kantarjian HM, Cortes JE, O'Brien S, et al. Imatinib mesylate therapy in newly diagnosed patients with Philadelphia chromosome-positive chronic myelogenous leukemia: High incidence of early complete and major cytogenetic responses. *Blood* 2003;101(1):97-100.

62. de Lavallade H, Apperley JF, Khorashad JS, et al. Imatinib for newly diagnosed patients with chronic myeloid leukemia: Incidence of sustained responses in an intention-to-treat analysis. *J Clin Oncol* 2008;26(20):3358-3363.

63. Cortes JE, Kantarjian HM, Goldberg SL, et al. High-dose imatinib in newly diagnosed chronic-phase chronic myeloid leukemia: High rates of rapid cytogenetic and molecular responses. *J Clin Oncol* 2009;27(28):4754-4759.

64. Cortes JE, Baccarani M, Guilhot F, et al. Phase III, randomized, open-label study of daily imatinib mesylate 400 mg versus 800 mg in patients with newly diagnosed, previously untreated chronic myeloid leukemia in chronic phase using molecular end points: Tyrosine kinase inhibitor optimization and selectivity study. *J Clin Oncol*;28(3):424-430.

65. Baccarani M, Druker BJ, Cortes-Franco J, et al. 24 Months update of the TOPS study: A phase III, randomized, open-label study of 400 mg/d (SD-IM) versus 800 mg/d (HD-IM) of imatinib mesylate (IM) in patients (Pts) with newly diagnosed, previously untreated chronic myeloid leukemia in chronic phase (CML-CP). *Blood* 2009;114(22):337 (ASH Annual Meeting Abstracts).

66. Baccarani M, Rosti G, Castagnetti F, et al. Comparison of imatinib 400 mg and 800 mg daily in the front-line treatment of high-risk, Philadelphia-positive chronic myeloid leukemia: A European LeukemiaNet Study. *Blood* 2009;113(19):4497-4504.

67. Cortes J, O'Brien S, Quintas A, et al. Erythropoietin is effective in improving the anemia induced by imatinib mesylate therapy in patients with chronic myeloid leukemia in chronic phase. *Cancer* 2004;100(11):2396-2402.

68. Quintas-Cardama A, Kantarjian H, O'Brien S, et al. Granulocyte-colony-stimulating factor (filgrastim) may overcome imatinib-induced neutropenia in patients with chronic-phase chronic myelogenous leukemia. *Cancer* 2004;100(12):2592-2597.

69. Ault P, Kantarjian H, Welch MA, et al. Interleukin 11 May improve thrombocytopenia associated with imatinib mesylate therapy in chronic myelogenous leukemia. *Leuk Res* 2004;28(6):613-618.

70. Baccarani M, Cortes J, Pane F, et al. Chronic myeloid leukemia: An update of concepts and management recommendations of European LeukemiaNet. *J Clin Oncol* 2009;27(35):6041-6051.

71. Jabbour E, Cortes J, Kantarjian H, et al. Novel tyrosine kinase inhibitor therapy before allogeneic stem cell transplantation in patients with chronic myeloid leukemia: No evidence for increased transplant-related toxicity. *Cancer* 2007;110(2):340-344.

72. Medina J, Kantarjian H, Talpaz M, et al. Chromosomal abnormalities in Philadelphia chromosome-negative metaphases appearing during imatinib mesylate therapy in patients with Philadelphia chromosome-positive chronic myelogenous leukemia in chronic phase. *Cancer* 2003;98(9):1905-1911.

73. Cortes J, Talpaz M, O'Brien S, et al. Molecular responses in patients with chronic myelogenous leukemia in chronic phase treated with imatinib mesylate. *Clin Cancer Res* 2005;11(9): 3425-3432.

74. Radich JP, Gooley T, Bryant E, et al. The significance of bcr-abl molecular detection in chronic myeloid leukemia patients "late," 18 months or more after transplantation. *Blood* 2001; 98(6): 1701-1707.

75. Dewald GW, Wyatt WA, Juneau AL, et al. Highly sensitive fluorescence in situ hybridization method to detect double BCR/ABL fusion and monitor response to therapy in chronic myeloid leukemia. *Blood* 1998;91(9):3357-3365.

76. Lesser ML, Dewald GW, Sison CP, et al. Correlation of three methods of measuring cytogenetic response in chronic myelocytic leukemia. *Cancer Genet Cytogenet* 2002;137(2):79-84.

77. Rousselot P, Huguet F, Rea D, et al. Imatinib mesylate discontinuation in patients with chronic myelogenous leukemia in complete molecular remission for more than 2 years. *Blood* 2007;109(1):58-60.

78. Mahon F-X, Huguet F, Guilhot F, et al. Is it possible to stop imatinib in patients with chronic myeloid leukemia? An update from a French Pilot Study and first results from the multicentre << Stop Imatinib >> (STIM) Study. *Blood* 2008; 112(11):187 (ASH Annual Meeting Abstracts).

79. Ross DDM, Grigg A, Schwarer A, et al. The majority of chronic myeloid leukaemia patients who cease imatinib after achieving a sustained complete molecular response (CMR) remain in CMR, and any relapses occur early. *Blood* 2008; 112(11):1102 (ASH Annual Meeting Abstracts).

80. le Coutre P, Tassi E, Varella-Garcia M, et al. Induction of resistance to the abelson inhibitor STI571 in human leukemic cells through gene amplification. *Blood* 2000;95(5):1758-1766.

81. Gorre ME, Mohammed M, Ellwood K, et al. Clinical resistance to STI-571 cancer therapy caused by BCR-ABL gene mutation or amplification. *Science* 2001;293(5531):876-880.

82. Weisberg E, Griffin JD. Mechanism of resistance to the ABL tyrosine kinase inhibitor STI571 in BCR/ABL-transformed hematopoietic cell lines. *Blood* 2000;95(11):3498-3505.

83. Branford S, Rudzki Z, Walsh S, et al. Detection of BCR-ABL mutations in patients with CML treated with imatinib is virtually always accompanied by clinical resistance, and mutations in the ATP phosphate-binding loop (P-loop) are associated with a poor prognosis. *Blood* 2003;102(1):276-283.

84. Hochhaus A, Kreil S, Corbin AS, et al. Molecular and chromosomal mechanisms of resistance to imatinib (STI571) therapy. *Leukemia* 2002;16(11):2190-2196.

85. Corbin AS, La Rosee P, Stoffregen EP, et al. Several Bcr-Abl kinase domain mutants associated with imatinib mesylate resistance remain sensitive to imatinib. *Blood* 2003;101(11): 4611-4614.

86. Jabbour E, Kantarjian H, Jones D, et al. Long-term incidence and outcome of BCR-ABL mutations in patients (pts) with chronic myeloid leukemia (CML) treated with imatinib mesylate—p-loop mutations are not associated with worse outcome. *Blood* 2004;104(11):1007 (ASH Annual Meeting Abstracts).

87. Soverini S, Colarossi S, Gnani A, et al. Contribution of ABL kinase domain mutations to imatinib resistance in different subsets of Philadelphia-positive patients: By the GIMEMA Working Party on chronic myeloid leukemia. *Clin Cancer Res* 2006;12(24):7374-7379.

88. Kantarjian H, Schiffer C, Jones D, et al. Monitoring the response and course of chronic myeloid leukemia in the modern era of BCR-ABL tyrosine kinase inhibitors: Practical advice on the use and interpretation of monitoring methods. *Blood* 2008;111(4):1774-1780.

89. Redaelli S, Piazza R, Rostagno R, et al. Activity of bosutinib, dasatinib, and nilotinib against 18 imatinib-resistant BCR/ABL mutants. *J Clin Oncol* 2009;27(3):469-471.

90. O'Hare T, Eide CA, Deininger MW: Bcr-Abl kinase domain mutations, drug resistance, and the road to a cure for chronic myeloid leukemia. *Blood* 2007;110(7):2242-2249.

91. Jabbour E, Jones D, Kantarjian HM, et al. Long-term outcome of patients with chronic myeloid leukemia treated with second-generation tyrosine kinase inhibitors after imatinib failure is predicted by the in vitro sensitivity of BCR-ABL kinase domain mutations. *Blood* 2009;114(10):2037-2043.

92. Jabbour E, Kantarjian H, Jones D, et al. Frequency and clinical significance of BCR-ABL mutations in patients with chronic myeloid leukemia treated with imatinib mesylate. *Leukemia* 2006;20(10):1767-1773.

93. Soverini S, Martinelli G, Amabile M, et al. Denaturing-HPLC-based assay for detection of ABL mutations in chronic myeloid leukemia patients resistant to Imatinib. *Clin Chem* 2004;50(7):1205-1213.

94. Deininger MW, McGreevey L, Willis S, et al. Detection of ABL kinase domain mutations with denaturing high-performance liquid chromatography. *Leukemia* 2004;18(4):864-871.

95. Quintas-Cardama A, Cortes J. Molecular biology of bcr-abl1-positive chronic myeloid leukemia. *Blood* 2009;113(8): 1619-1630.

96. Willis SG, Lange T, Demehri S, et al. High-sensitivity detection of BCR-ABL kinase domain mutations in imatinib-naive patients: Correlation with clonal cytogenetic evolution but not response to therapy. *Blood* 2005;106(6):2128-2137.

97. Kantarjian H, Pasquini R, Levy V, et al. Dasatinib or high-dose imatinib for chronic-phase chronic myeloid leukemia resistant to imatinib at a dose of 400 to 600 milligrams daily: Two-year follow-up of a randomized phase 2 study (START-R). *Cancer* 2009;115(18):4136-4147.

98. Burgess MR, Skaggs BJ, Shah NP, et al. Comparative analysis of two clinically active BCR-ABL kinase inhibitors reveals the role of conformation-specific binding in resistance. *Proc Natl Acad Sci USA* 2005;102(9):3395-3400.

99. Shah NP, Tran C, Lee FY, et al. Overriding imatinib resistance with a novel ABL kinase inhibitor. *Science* 2004;305(5682): 399-401.

100. Lombardo LJ, Lee FY, Chen P, et al. Discovery of N-(2-chloro-6-methyl- phenyl)-2-(6-(4-(2-hydroxyethyl)- piperazin-1-yl)- 2-methylpyrimidin-4- ylamino)thiazole-5-carboxamide (BMS-354825), a dual Src/Abl kinase inhibitor with potent antitumor activity in preclinical assays. *J Med Chem* 2004; 47(27): 6658-6661.

101. Cortes J, Rousselot P, Kim DW, et al. Dasatinib induces complete hematologic and cytogenetic responses in patients with imatinib-resistant or—intolerant chronic myeloid leukemia in blast crisis. *Blood* 2007;109(8):3207-3213.

102. Guilhot F, Apperley J, Kim DW, et al. Dasatinib induces significant hematologic and cytogenetic responses in patients with imatinib-resistant or—intolerant chronic myeloid leukemia in accelerated phase. *Blood* 2007;109(10):4143-4150.

103. Hochhaus A, Baccarani M, Deininger M, et al. Dasatinib induces durable cytogenetic responses in patients with chronic myelogenous leukemia in chronic phase with resistance or intolerance to imatinib. *Leukemia* 2008;22(6): 1200-1206.

104. Shah NP, Kantarjian HM, Kim DW, et al. Intermittent target inhibition with dasatinib 100 mg once daily preserves efficacy and improves tolerability in imatinib-resistant and -intolerant chronic-phase chronic myeloid leukemia. *J Clin Oncol* 2008; 26(19):3204-3212.

105. Cortes JE, Jones D, O'Brien S, et al. Results of dasatinib therapy in patients with early chronic-phase chronic myeloid leukemia. *J Clin Oncol*;28(3):398-404.

106. Golemovic M, Verstovsek S, Giles F, et al. AMN107, a novel aminopyrimidine inhibitor of Bcr-Abl, has in vitro activity against imatinib-resistant chronic myeloid leukemia. *Clin Cancer Res* 2005;11(13):4941-4947.

107. Weisberg E, Manley PW, Breitenstein W, et al. Characterization of AMN107, a selective inhibitor of native and mutant Bcr-Abl. *Cancer Cell* 2005;7(2):129-141.

108. Cortes JE, Jones D, O'Brien S, et al. Nilotinib as front-line treatment for patients with chronic myeloid leukemia in early chronic phase. *J Clin Oncol*;28(3):392-397.

109. Rosti G, Palandri F, Castagnetti F, et al. Nilotinib for the frontline treatment of Ph(+) chronic myeloid leukemia. *Blood* 2009;114(24):4933-4938.

110. Cortes J, Kantarjian HM, Kim D-W, et al. Efficacy and safety of bosutinib (SKI-606) in patients with chronic phase (CP) Ph+ chronic myelogenous leukemia (CML) with resistance or intolerance to imatinib. *Blood* 2008;112(11):1098 (ASH Annual Meeting Abstracts).

111. Giles FJ, Cortes J, Jones D, et al. MK-0457, a novel kinase inhibitor, is active in patients with chronic myeloid leukemia or acute lymphocytic leukemia with the T315I BCR-ABL mutation. *Blood* 2007;109(2):500-502.

112. Cortes J, Talpaz M, Deininger M, et al. A Phase 1 Trial of oral AP24534 in patients with refractory chronic myeloid leukemia and other hematologic malignancies: First results of safety and clinical activity against T315I and resistant mutations. *Blood* 2009;114(22):643 (ASH Annual Meeting Abstracts).

113. Palandri F, Iacobucci I, Castagnetti F, et al. Front-line treatment of Philadelphia positive chronic myeloid leukemia with imatinib and interferon-alpha:5-year outcome. *Haematologica* 2008;93(5):770-774.

114. Guilhot F, Mahon F-X, Guilhot J, et al. Randomized comparison of imatinib versus imatinib combination therapies in newly diagnosed chronic myeloid leukaemia (CML) patients in chronic phase (CP): First results of the phase III (SPIRIT) trial from the French CML Group (FI LMC). *Blood* 2008; 112(11):183 (ASH Annual Meeting Abstracts).

115. Quintas-Cardama A, Kantarjian HM, Ravandi F, et al. Immune modulation of minimal residual disease (MRD) in patients (pts) with chronic myelogenous leukemia (CML) in early chronic phase (CP): A randomized trial of frontline high-dose (HS) imatinib mesylate (IM) with or without pegylated-interferon (PEG-IFN) and GM-CSF. *Blood* 2006;108(11):2207 (ASH Annual Meeting Abstracts).

116. Hehlmann R, Jung-Munkwitz S, Lauseker M, et al. Randomized comparison of imatinib 800 Mg vs. imatinib 400 Mg+/- IFN in newly diagnosed BCR/ABL positive chronic phase CML: Analysis of molecular remission at 12 months. The German CML-Study IV. *Blood* 2009;114(22):339 (ASH Annual Meeting Abstracts).

117. O'Brien S, Kantarjian H, Koller C, et al. Sequential homoharringtonine and interferon-alpha in the treatment of early chronic phase chronic myelogenous leukemia. *Blood* 1999; 93(12): 4149-4153.

118. O'Brien S, Talpaz M, Cortes J, et al. Simultaneous homoharringtonine and interferon-alpha in the treatment of patients with chronic-phase chronic myelogenous leukemia. *Cancer* 2002;94(7):2024-2032.

119. Kantarjian HM, Talpaz M, Santini V, et al. Homoharringtonine: History, current research, and future direction. *Cancer* 2001;92(6):1591-605.

120. O'Brien S, Kantarjian H, Keating M, et al. Homoharringtonine therapy induces responses in patients with chronic myelogenous leukemia in late chronic phase. *Blood* 1995;86(9): 3322-3326.

121. Cortes-Franco J, Raghunadharao D, Parikh P, et al. Safety and efficacy of subcutaneous-administered omacetaxine mepesuccinate in chronic myeloid leukemia (CML) patients who are resistant or intolerant to two or more tyrosine kinase inhibitors—Results of a multicenter phase 2/3 study. *Blood* 2009;114(22):861 (ASH Annual Meeting Abstracts).

122. Cortes-Franco J, Khoury HJ, Nicolini FE, et al. Safety and efficacy of subcutaneous-administered omacetaxine mepesuccinate in imatinib-resistant chronic myeloid leukemia (CML) patients who harbor the BCR–ABL T315I mutation—Results of an ongoing multicenter phase 2/3 study. *Blood* 2009;114(22):644 (ASH Annual Meeting Abstracts).

123. Garg RJ, Kantarjian H, O'Brien S, et al. The use of nilotinib or dasatinib after failure to 2 prior tyrosine kinase inhibitors: Long-term follow-up. *Blood* 2009;114(20):4361-4368.

MYELODYSPLASTIC SYNDROMES: THE MD ANDERSON CANCER CENTER APPROACH

William S. Stevenson
Carlos Bueso-Ramos
Guillermo Garcia-Manero

Myelodysplastic syndromes (MDS) refer to a group of hematopoietic disorders characterized by ineffective hematopoiesis and increased risk of transformation to acute myelogenous leukemia (AML). Median age of patients with MDS is 70 to 75 years and it is likely that environmental factors play an important role in the pathogenesis of this disease. MDS is classified according to WHO criteria and a number of prognostic scores can be used to calculate survival and risk of transformation. Cytogenetic alterations, more frequently involving chromosomes 5 and 7, are common in MDS and help in the prediction of prognosis. Over the last decade we have witnessed significant improvements in supportive care and therapeutic modalities for patients with MDS. These include growth factors, immune modulatory agents, such as lenalidomide, and hypomethylating agents including 5-azacitidine and decitabine. In this chapter, we summarize our knowledge of MDS and the treatment approach we use at MD Anderson Cancer Center.

■ THE MD ANDERSON APPROACH TO THE PATIENT WITH MDS

Every year approximately 250 to 300 patients are referred to our center with a diagnosis of MDS. Although percentages vary from month to month, nearly 30% of patients referred to us with a diagnosis of MDS receive a different diagnosis in our center. In most instances, the final diagnosis is that of AML but other benign and malignant conditions are often observed. Therefore, it is critical to confirm the morphological diagnosis of the patient referred and it is usually important to repeat a bone marrow aspiration and biopsy at the time of initial reevaluation of the patient.

Once the diagnosis is confirmed, the next more important step is to calculate the "risk" of the patient. Most clinicians and investigators use the IPSS (1) score to perform such analysis but newer potentially more precise models have been developed (2-4). In general, patients with low or intermediate-1 risk by the IPSS or those with less than 10% blasts in the bone marrow are considered as having "lower" risk disease whereas those with excess blasts or intermediate-2 or high-risk disease are considered as having "higher" risk disease.

Patients with lower risk disease can be candidates for a wide range of interventions, depending on their specific characteristics and transfusion needs. Patients with minimal cytopenias, transfusion independent, low percentage of blasts in the bone marrow and diploid cytogenetics are more frequently observed as their 4-year survival is close to 80% (3). At the end of the spectrum, older patients with significant cytopenias and transfusion needs can have very poor prognosis particularly if their cytogenetics are abnormal (3). The median survival of these patients is less than 12 months. Despite the fact that probably around 60 to 70% of patients with MDS are in this category, there are very few interventions known to alter the natural history of these patients. Transfusion and growth factor support are usually started on these patients. Interventions such as lenalidomide have significant activity in improving red cell counts in patients with deletion of chromosome 5 (5) but are significantly less active in patients without this alteration (6). The role of the hypomethylating agents, 5-azacitidine or decitabine, is less clear in this situation although are frequently used. Finally, allogeneic stem cell transplantation (alloSCT) is not frequently used up front in patients with lower risk disease. It is currently accepted that delaying transplantation until the time of progression is associated with longer survival even if transplant outcomes per se are poorer when performed at that time.

Treatment decisions are relatively simpler for patients with higher-risk MDS. The data with the hypomethylating agents, in particular 5-azacitidine, indicate that treatment with these agents improves significantly the survival of these patients when compared to supportive care or low-dose chemotherapy approaches. That said it is currently not known what is the optimal approach for younger (those less than 60 to 65 years) patients with MDS. These patients can be treated with either a hypomethylating agent, an AML-like induction therapy, or can be considered for up-front alloSCT. No study has compared one treatment versus the other in younger patients. An approach followed by our group is to stratify patients based on cytogenetics. Diploid younger patients are usually offered induction therapy with an AML-like approach followed when possible by alloSCT. In contrast, younger patients with abnormal karyotypes are offered hypomethylating agent-based therapy followed by alloSCT. It is not our routine to proceed with transplant up-front in patients with excess blasts. It should be noted that older patients benefit significantly from the use of hypomethylating agents and there is basically no upper age limit that may contraindicate their use (7).

Below we provide a comprehensive review of current knowledge in MDS. Current areas of intense research are the development of newer forms of therapy for patients with newly diagnosed disease and strategies for patients that have relapsed or not responded to hypomethylating based therapy.

■ EPIDEMIOLOGY AND ETIOLOGY

The incidence of MDS increases with age. Most patients diagnosed with this condition are more than 60 years old with a median age at diagnosis of 75 years (8). Incidence is higher in males than females with a 2:1 ratio (8). The incidence in the United States is 30 to 35 individuals per million per year with a relative yearly increase in the reported incidence, probably related to increase awareness of the disease and reporting efforts (9).

The risk of developing MDS is related to the individual's racial background. In the United States, MDS incidence is highest in the white population (8). MDS patients from Asia present a younger age (10). The underlying cause of this phenomenon is not known but may reflect genetic differences between different racial groups. Populations of MDS patients in Asia have a similar frequency of karyotype abnormality as European and American cohorts, although they may have less frequent alterations of chromosomes 5 and 7 (10-14). This combination of younger age at diagnosis and lack of chromosome 7 alterations can explain the longer survival observed in patients from Asia.

There is no known cause of MDS. A small number of patients appear to have either genetic or environmental risk factors. Genetic syndromes such as Down syndrome, Bloom syndrome, and Fanconi anemia are associated with an increased risk of an MDS, which often presents earlier in life (15,16). Genetic polymorphisms that influence the activity of enzymes responsible for metabolizing toxic chemicals or chemotherapy drugs, for instance, may influence an individual's predisposition to MDS. Polymorphisms have been described in the cytochrome p450 3A, glutathione-S-transferase and NAD(P)H quinine oxidoreductase enzyme systems that increase the risk of developing myeloid malignancy (17-19).

Environmental agents may contribute to the development of MDS by causing toxic damage to hematopoietic stem cells. A causal relationship between occupational exposures to benzene and radiation and the development of myeloid malignancy has been demonstrated (20). Exposure to organic solvents and pesticides has also been implicated in the development of MDS (21-23) and an occupational history of exposure to these chemicals may be associated with an increased incidence of cytogenetic abnormalities associated with a poor prognosis (24). There is no correlation between MDS and socioeconomic status (22).

The most significant risk factor for the development of a myelodysplastic syndrome is previous exposure to chemotherapy or radiotherapy used to treat antecedent hematological malignancy or solid organ cancer. Treatment-related MDS (t-MDS) constitutes a minority of MDS diagnoses but may be increasing in prevalence with improved survival rates after successful cancer therapies for solid tumors. T-MDS usually presents 5 to 6 years after initial cancer treatment and generally has a poor prognosis (25). Patients treated for lymphoma are at risk of this long-term complication with up to 2% of survivors from Hodgkin's disease developing treatment-related myeloid malignancy (26,27). Lymphoma patients who undergo autologous hematopoietic stem cell transplantation appear to be at particularly high risk of treatment-related MDS or AML with incidence rates in some centers of up to 10% (28,29).

■ CLINICAL AND LABORATORY FEATURES

At the present time, most patients with MDS are diagnosed incidentally while performing a CBC analysis either as routine or because of nonspecific symptomatology. Anemia is the most common cytopenia in MDS and is associated with progressive fatigue. A lower percentage of patients present for investigation of bleeding or bruising secondary to thrombocytopenia or infection related to neutropenia. Physical examination is often normal with hepatosplenomegaly present in patients with chronic myelomonocytic leukemia (CMML) or overlap myeloproliferative neoplasms. During follow-up of a patient, a change in the severity of cytopenia or rapid worsening of symptoms may indicate disease transformation. Patients suspected of transformation require prompt investigation as 20% of patients develop acute leukemia throughout their disease course (30).

Initial assessment of a patient suspected to have MDS should include a complete blood count (CBC), reticulocyte count, and complete serum chemistry including B12, folate, iron studies (ferritin), and erythropoietin level. A bone marrow aspirate and biopsy with samples taken for an iron stain and cytogenetic studies are required. MDS still requires morphological assessment of the disease. Cytogenetic studies may confirm the presence of clonal hematopoiesis and provide additional important prognostic information. Analysis of specific gene mutations such as JAK2, Ras, or Flt-3 is probably not indicated in all patients at the present time but may in time allow for the use of targeted interventions using respective inhibitors that are now in clinical trials. In general, no patient should be diagnosed as having MDS without knowledge of the clinical and drug history and no case should be classified while the patient is on growth factor therapy, including erythropoietin.

MORPHOLOGICAL FEATURES OF MDS

Morphological classification of MDS is based on a 500 cell differential count on the bone marrow aspirate and leukocyte differential performed on the blood smear (31). Table 5-1 shows the different subsets of MDS under the new revised World Health Organization MDS classification. This analysis determines the percentage of blasts present in the blood and bone marrow, provides an assessment of the number of myeloid lineages involved in the dysplastic process, and the iron stain determines the presence and number of ring sideroblasts (Fig. 5-1) (31).

Blood cell abnormalities on the peripheral blood smear are variable (31,32) (see Fig. 5-1). Red cells may be macrocytic and frequently display anisopoikilocytosis. Polychromasia or basophilic stippling may be present. Dysplastic granulocytes may show abnormal folding of the nucleus and cytoplasmic granules are often reduced or absent. Platelets are of variable size and may also be hypogranular. The presence of circulating blast

TABLE 5-1	CLASSIFICATION OF MDS ACCORDING TO WORLD HEALTH ORGANIZATION CRITERIA

- Refractory cytopenia with unilineage dysplasia (RCUD)
  - Refractory anemia (RA)
  - Refractory neutropenia (RN)
  - Refractory thrombocytopenia (RT)
- Refractory anemia with ring sideroblasts (RARS)
- Refractory cytopenia with multilineage dysplasia (RCMD)
- Refractory anemia with excess blasts (RAEB-1, -2)
- Myelodysplastic syndrome with isolated del(5q)
- Myelodysplastic syndrome, unclassifiable (MDS,U)
- Childhood myelodysplastic syndrome
- Refractory anemia with ring sideroblasts (RARS)
  - Refractory cytopenia of childhood (RCC)

Data from Vardiman JW, Thiele J, Arber DA, et al. The 2008 revision of the World Health Organization (WHO) classification of myeloid neoplasms and acute leukemia: Rationale and important changes. *Blood* 2009;114(5):937-951.

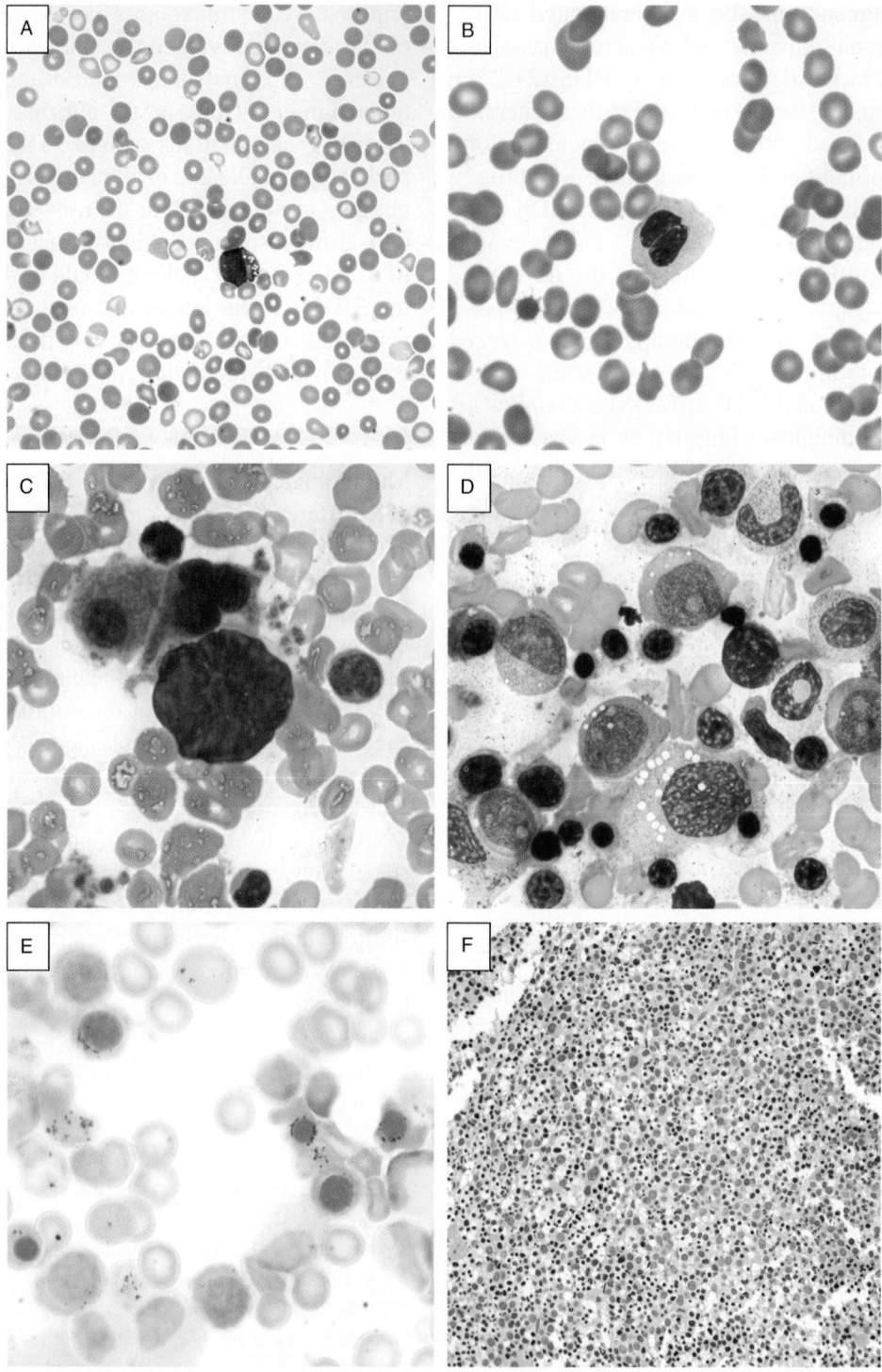

FIGURE 5-1.   Morphological features of peripheral blood and bone marrow in the myelodysplastic syndromes. Panel A shows a peripheral blood film from a patient with refractory anemia with excess blasts-1. The erythrocytes show hypochromasia, anisocytosis, and macroovalocytes. There is also an occasional blast (center). Panel B shows a peripheral blood film from a patient with refractory cytopenia with multilineage dysplasia, demonstrating pseudo-Pelger-huet cell (center) with hypercondensed chromatin and bilobed nuclei and hypogranular cytoplasm. Panel C shows dysplastic small megakaryocytes some with monolobated or with separated nuclei and mature granular cytoplasm in the bone marrow aspirate from a patient with refractory anemia with excess blasts. Panel D shows increased blasts, dysgranulopoiesis, and dyserythropoiesis in the bone marrow aspirate from a patient with refractory anemia with excess blasts. Panel E shows ring sideroblasts and pappenheimer bodies from a patient with refractory anemia with ring sideroblasts. Panel F shows a hypercellular (100%) bone marrow biopsy with increased immature cells and dysplastic megakaryocytes in a 70-year-old male with refractory anemia with excess blasts.

cells or an excess of monocytes are important for the classification of high-risk MDS and monocytic leukemias, respectively.

Definitive diagnosis requires a bone marrow aspirate and biopsy. The bone marrow is usually normocellular or hypercellular, reflecting that hematopoiesis is ineffective. Abnormal maturation of hematopoietic cells results in a variable proportion of myeloblasts that are significantly increased in the more aggressive forms of the disorder. Morphological abnormalities found in the nucleus of erythroblasts include nuclear budding, internuclear bridging, karyorrhexis, multinuclearity, and megaloblastoid changes (see Fig. 5-1). Cytoplasmic features include the presence of ring sideroblasts and abnormal vacuolization. Abnormal or absent granulation is a common feature of dysplastic granulocyte series. Aberrant nuclear folding of the neutrophil precursor can produce a dysplastic bilobed nucleus, the pseudo–Pelger-Huet anomaly. Megakaryocytes may have a very variable morphology and a small dysplastic form called the micromegakaryocyte is a very typical finding in myelodysplasia. A normal megakaryocyte has a polyploid nucleus that can be altered with dysplasia to produce hypolobulation or nuclei that are dispersed throughout the cell. The bone marrow biopsy provides the best assessment of the overall cellularity of the bone marrow and allows examination of the architecture of the marrow and surrounding bone (Fig. 5-2). The presence of fibrosis can be assessed on the biopsy with specific stains for reticulin and collagen. In normal bone marrow, the immature blast cells are frequently located near the endosteal surface. In MDS, these cells may be distant to this site and form aberrant clusters referred to as abnormal localization of immature precursors (ALIPs). Immunohistochemical staining of biopsies can aid diagnosis with CD34 staining to identify blast and progenitor cells and CD42 or CD62 for quantitation and assessment of megakaryocytes (33) (see Fig. 5-2).

Non-clonal diseases may cause dysplastic morphological changes in blood cells and these secondary causes of dysplasia should be excluded in the initial assessment of a patient and can potentially complicate the diagnosis of the disease. Blood cell dysplasia is seen with exposure to heavy metals or anti-tuberculous therapies, B12 and folate deficiency, HIV infection, excessive alcohol consumption (31), and occasionally with normal ageing (34). Dysplastic features on blood cells are very commonly observed after chemotherapy or with the therapeutic use of granulocyte-colony stimulating factor (G-CSF). These alternate diagnoses should be assessed in the history and may require exclusion with further

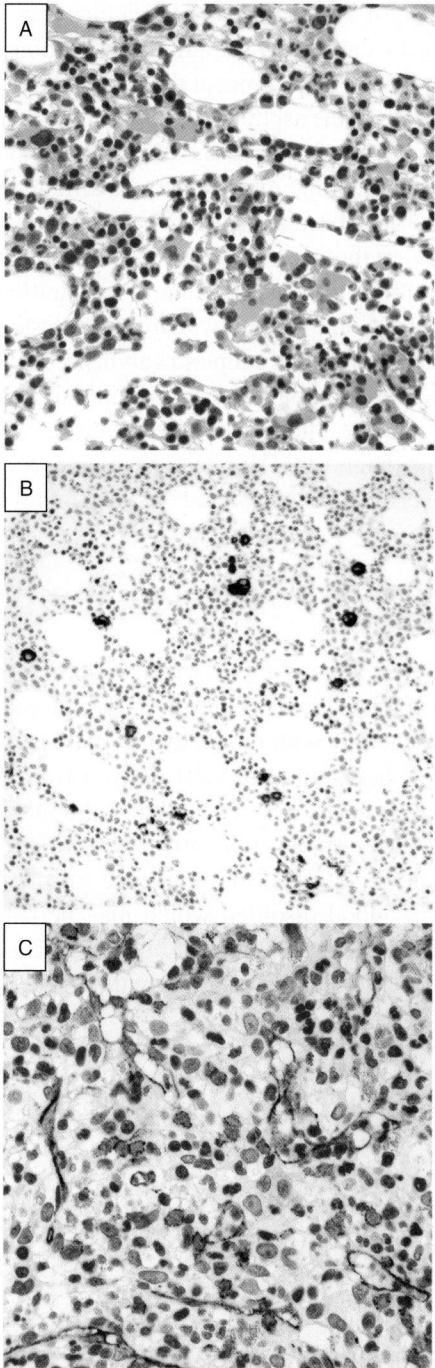

FIGURE 5-2. Morphological and immunohistochemical feature of bone marrow biopsy in the myelodysplastic syndromes. Panel A shows a trephine bone marrow biopsy with numerous dysplastic monolobated megakaryocytes in a 60-year-old female patient with refractory anemia with excess blasts type 1. Panel B shows CD61 immunohistochemical stain highlighting many dysplastic micromegakaryocytes. CD61 may be very helpful in detecting dysplastic micromegakaryocytes to aid in confirming dysmegakaropoiesis and abnormal translocation of megakaryocytes to endosteal surfaces. Panel C shows CD34 immunohistochemical staining highlighting the presence of an increased number of blasts and increased blood vessels.

laboratory testing. Diagnostic difficulties may occur in patients with marked hypocellularity of the bone marrow and in patients with prominent fibrosis as there are often very few cells in the aspirate sample to allow morphological assessment of dysplasia. Patients with prominent hypocellularity of the marrow may be difficult to distinguish from aplastic anemia where morphological dysplasia of the erythroid lineage may also be observed. In cases of marked fibrosis, bone marrow aspiration is often unsuccessful. Some patients with mild dysplastic changes in the bone marrow and a diploid karyotype may be difficult to definitively diagnose at their initial presentation and may require a period of observation to confirm the underlying diagnosis. These patients require review with repeat investigations performed for 3 to 6 months.

CYTOGENETIC AND MOLECULAR ANALYSIS

A cytogenetic abnormality is found in 40 to 50% of primary MDS in patients with lower-risk disease and is higher in patients with more advance risk. Cytogenetic analysis of hematopoietic cells derived from the bone marrow aspirate provides important additional information in the assessment of a patient with MDS. A karyotypic abnormality provides evidence for the presence of a clonal blood disorder, which may be particularly important if the morphological changes are not clear. Typically, cytogenetic analysis will assess 20 bone marrow metaphases (33). MDS are very heterogeneous and multiple different cytogenetic abnormalities have been described (35). The most common karyotype abnormalities involve loss of genetic material. These are summarized in Table 5-2. There are no specific cytogenetic abnormalities that characterized MDS. Unlike AML and chronic myeloid leukemia, genetic translocations are rare in MDS but deletions are common.

The presence or absence of a cytogenetic abnormality has a marked influence on the overall prognosis of a patient (35). Median survival of diploid patients is approximately 53 months, compared to less than 12 months for patients with three or more cytogenetic abnormalities (complex). Del(5q) and del(20q) are associated with a favorable prognosis. However, when these abnormalities are present in association with other cytogenetic abnormalities, especially as a component of a complex karyotype, the prognosis for the patient is poor. Abnormalities of chromosome 7, usually deletions, are associated with a poor prognosis regardless of the presence or absence of other abnormalities. Complex cytogenetic abnormalities are more frequently observed in patients with increased marrow blasts. Median survival with one karyotypic abnormality is 35 months, two abnormalities is 38 months, three abnormalities is 17 months, and then a progressively worse prognosis is observed with increasing complexity with patients having greater than six abnormalities, exhibiting a very poor median survival of 5 months (35).

TABLE 5-2	FREQUENCY OF COMMON KARYOTYPIC ABNORMALITIES AMONG WHO AND FAB SUBGROUPS (35)

		KARYOTYPE, NO. (%)					
Classification	*No.*	*Normal*	*del(5q)*	*−7/del(7q)*	*+8*	*−20/del(20q)*	*Complex*
All FAB	1949	942 (48.3)	295 (15.1)	209 (10.7)	162 (8.3)	86 (4.4)	282 (14.5)
RA	573	267 (46.6)	139 (24.3)	30 (5.2)	37 (6.5)	31 (5.4)	47 (8.2)
RARS	252	147 (58.3)	23 (9.1)	24 (9.5)	14 (5.6)	9 (3.6)	20 (7.9)
RAEB	415	179 (43.1)	71 (17.1)	60 (23.8)	39 (9.4)	21 (5.1)	98 (23.6)
RAEB-t	305	132 (43.3)	38 (12.5)	50 (16.4)	30 (9.8)	16 (5.2)	68 (22.3)
CMML	272	170 (62.5)	4 (1.5)	23 (8.5)	18 (6.6)	2 (<1)	12 (4.4)
MDS-AL	132	47 (30.9)	20 (15.2)	22 (16.7)	25 (18.9)	7 (5.3)	37 (28.0)
All WHO	595	285 (47.8)	110 (18.5)	53 (8.9)	40 (6.7)	22 (3.7)	71 (11.9)
5q- syndrome	61	0 (0.0)	61 (100.0)	0 (0.0)	0 (0.0)	0 (0.0)	0 (0.0)
RA	56	38 (67.9)	3 (6.5)	5 (10.9)	1 (2.2)	1 (2.2)	6 (13.0)
RARS	26	23 (88.5)	0 (0.0)	0 (0.0)	1 (3.8)	0 (0.0)	0 (0.0)
RCMD	164	88 (53.7)	11 (6.7)	20 (12.2)	12 (7.3)	8 (4.8)	18 (11.0)
RSCMD	77	34 (44.2)	8 (10.4)	8 (10.4)	8 (10.4)	3 (3.9)	12 (15.6)
RAEB-I	90	42 (45.7)	16 (17.8)	10 (11.1)	5 (5.6)	4 (4.4)	15 (16.7)
RAEB-II	121	60 (49.6)	11 (9.1)	8 (6.6)	13 (10.7)	5 (4.1)	19 (15.7)

Data from Haase D, Germing U, Schanz J, et al. New insights into the prognostic impact of the karyotype in MDS and correlation with subtypes: Evidence from a core dataset of 2124 patients. *Blood* 2007;110(13):4385-4395.

T-MDS has a particularly high incidence of cytogenetic abnormalities with karyotypic changes observed in 70 to 90% of cases (25,35,36). There is a high incidence of abnormalities associated with an unfavorable prognosis, contributing to the overall poor outlook for this group of patients. Abnormalities of chromosomes 5 and 7 are frequently observed after exposure to alkylating agents (36,37) and a variety of translocations involving 11q23 are seen after treatment with topoisomerase II inhibitors (36).

Chromosomal deletions are the most frequent cytogenetic abnormality observed in MDS, suggesting that loss of tumor suppressor function may be important in the development and progression of the disease. Despite the identification of sites in the genome of frequent deletion in MDS, specific gene defects that are causative of dysplastic cell maturation in the bone marrow have not been identified. Mutations in *RAS* genes and the transcription factor *RUNX1* are frequent mutations identified in MDS and occur in up to 10% of patients (38-40). These gene defects occur almost exclusively in MDS patients with increased marrow blast counts and *RUNX1* mutations are more frequent in t-MDS and AML. Mutations in other genes associated with AML occur very infrequently in MDS, with only small numbers of patients described with mutations in *FLT3*, *KIT*, *MLL*, or *NPM1* (40,41). Recently mutations in *TET2* have been reported to occur in approximately 20% of patients with MDS. Prognostic significance of this event is not currently understood (42).

The low frequency of genetic alterations so far reported and the high frequency of chromosomal deletions have prompted interest in the identification of epigenetic repressive alterations such as aberrant DNA methylation in MDS. Although large-scale methylation studies are yet to be reported, it is likely that these alterations are also common in MDS. Recently, aberrant DNA methylation of multiple promoter CpG islands have been associated with poor prognosis in MDS (43). Because of relative lack of numbers in the identification of frequent dominant genetic lesions in MDS, several groups have used large-scale single nucleotide polymorphisms (SNPs) arrays in MDS (44). This has allowed the identification of areas of microdeletions and uniparenteral disomy in MDS (45). It is likely that these genomic regions harbor important genes in this disease as has been recently shown for c-CBL (46).

An association between a genetic abnormality and disease phenotype is reported in a few specific MDS. An example is the 5q- syndrome. A minority of patients with an interstitial deletion of chromosome 5q display an indolent anemia with relative preservation of the platelet count associated with hypolobated megakaryocytes in the bone marrow. This array of findings is called the 5q- syndrome (47) and is recognized as a separate diagnostic entity in the current World Health Organization (WHO) classification. The genetic defect within the deleted region that is responsible for the disease is not known, however, recent research has focused on one candidate gene, *SPARC*, that may potentially contribute to the malignant phenotype (48). *CTNNA1* is another gene on chromosome 5q that has been identified to be important in MDS and AML patients with deletion of the long arm of this chromosome but without specific features of the 5q- syndrome (49). More recently, Ebbert et al. have reported the identification of RPS14 as haploinsufficient in 5q- MDS. RPS14 is involved in ribosomal biogenesis and its deficiency has a role in anemia in this syndrome (50). It is likely that a complex network of genes cooperate in the pathogenesis of this syndrome. Indeed, recently microRNA 145 and 146a have been found to be involved in the biology of 5q- syndrome (51).

A small number of patients have been described with a deletion of 17p associated with abnormalities in the *p53* gene. This specific disorder has a poor prognosis and may be suspected when morphological characteristics of prominent dysgranulopoiesis including neutrophils exhibiting the Pelger-Huet anomaly and abnormal vacuolization are present (52,53). Acquired hemoglobin H disease produces red cell changes on the blood smear reminiscent of α-thalassemia. This red cell phenotype is secondary to decreased expression of α-globin within the bone marrow MDS clone and is associated with a mutation in the *ATRX* gene in most cases (54,55). These rare syndromes represent a small minority of patients with MDS and specific gene defects are not identified in most patients.

OTHER LABORATORY STUDIES

Flow cytometry is not required for the routine diagnosis of a myelodysplastic syndrome but it may sometimes provide valuable supplementary information. Flow cytometry can confirm the presence of specific myeloid lineages within the marrow and may also identify aberrant expression of cell surface markers that are indicative of a clonal cell population. This may have diagnostic significance in confirming abnormal hematopoiesis, particularly in the setting of a normal diploid karyotype and inconclusive morphological changes (33). Quantitation of the number of CD34 positive cells in the bone marrow may also assist in the differentiation of hypoplastic MDS from aplastic anemia. In MDS, the number of CD34 cells is usually normal or increased, compared to aplastic anemia where it is frequently reduced (56).

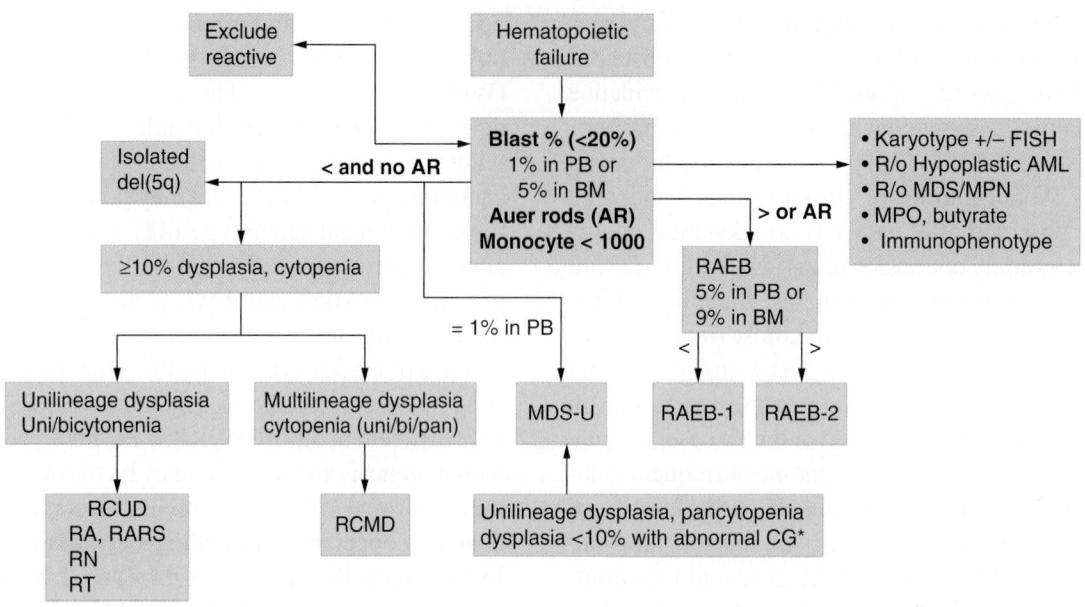

FIGURE 5-3. Algorithm for the classification of adult-onset primary myelodysplastic syndromes (MDS). This classification system is based on the 2008 criteria of the World Health Organization. AML, acute myeloid leukemia; RAEB, refractory anemia with excess blasts; RARS, refractory anemia with ring sideroblasts that are equal to or greater than 15% of bone marrow erythroid precursors; RCMD, refractory cytopenia with multilineage dysplasia; RCUD, refractory cytopenia with unilineage dysplasia.

The use of fluorescent in situ hybridization (FISH) techniques using probes specific for specific chromosomes (ie, covering chromosomes 5, 7, 20, 8) have not been fully standardized in MDS, and their use should not be consider standard of care in MDS, and cannot yet replace conventional cytogenetics.

DIAGNOSIS

The classification systems used to group different MDS has evolved over time with increased understanding of the biology and genetics of the disease. The first widely accepted classification system was that proposed by the French–American–British (FAB) study group (57). The FAB categorized MDS primarily on the percentage of blasts in the peripheral blood and bone marrow with disease entities defined by increased numbers of blasts associated with a more aggressive clinical course. In this system, patients with a bone marrow blast percentage greater than 30% were considered to have acute myeloid leukemia. This classification system used only morphological criteria to define disease groups and provided a framework that allowed the study of the natural history of MDS and its response to therapy.

The World Health Organization classification of MDS was developed with the objective of using all features of disease biology including morphology, cytogenetics, immunophenotype, and clinical behavior (31, 58).

This classification was recently updated in 2008 (59) (see Table 5-1). Figure 5-3 shows an algorithm for the morphological diagnosis of MDS. In the original WHO classification, the importance of morphological assessment of blast percentage within the bone marrow and peripheral blood was retained although the threshold level for the diagnosis of acute leukemia was altereds. So patients with more than 20% bone marrow blasts are now considered to have AML. Patients with 20 to 29% blasts have a similar prognosis as patients with greater than 30% blasts (60). Within the WHO MDS categories with an increased blast percentage, the magnitude of the blast elevation was quantified between RAEB-1 and RAEB-2, reflecting the worse prognosis of patients with an elevated blast count (30). In patients with a normal proportion of blast cells within the bone marrow, the relatively indolent refractory anemia (RA) and RA with ring sideroblasts (RARS) introduced in the FAB system were further delineated by assessment for the presence of multilineage dysplasia. Patients with dysplastic maturation limited to the erythroid lineage have a more favorable prognosis than patients with cytopenia and dysplasia present in multiple myeloid lineages. WHO also introduced the 5q- syndrome as a separate diagnostic entity primarily on the basis of a genetic abnormality rather than morphological features alone. Deletions involving chromosome 5q are relatively common in MDS and the WHO classification tightly defined

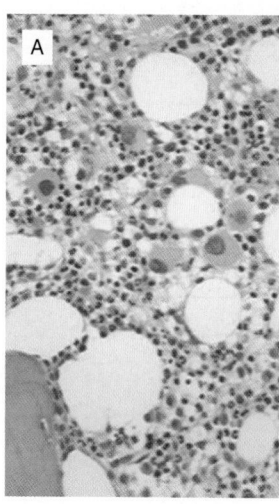
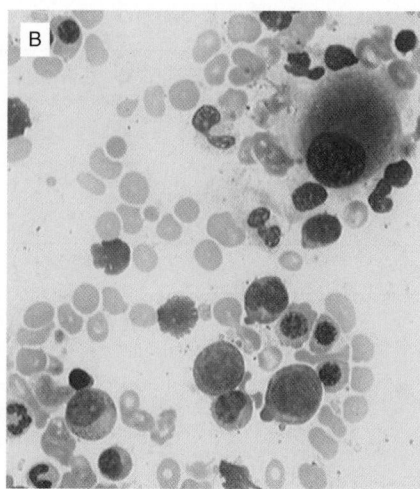

FIGURE 5-4.   Bone marrow morphology of MDS with deletion of chromosome 5.

the syndrome as an isolated del(5q) associated with anemia, a preserved or increased platelet count and hypolobated megakaryocytes on the bone marrow biopsy (Fig. 5-4). The WHO classification has been widely accepted and validated by a number of independent groups (61-63). The most recent WHO classification (59) includes the following changes: (1) specific guidelines for the requirement of specimen collection, blast and blast lineage assessment as well as for the analysis of genetic alterations; (2) there was also an effort to report new changes in the diagnosis and classification of MDS/MPN; (3) major changes specific for MDS included the inclusion of patients with cytopenias but not clear morphological evidence of MDS in the bone marrow as presumptive MDS; (4) the inclusion of refractory cytopenia with unilineage dysplasia; and (5) disappearance of the category of refractory cytopenia with multilineage dysplasia and ring sideroblasts (RCMD-RS) (59).

PROGNOSIS

The prognosis of patients with MDS is very heterogeneous. The development of clinical systems that allow accurate prognostication of individual patients into low- and high-risk categories has proven essential to guide rational management decisions and allow the introduction of investigational drug protocols. The International Prognostic Scoring System (IPSS) (30) is the most widely used system for assessment of prognosis and treatment planning. It provides an assessment of the prognosis of primary MDS patients at the time of initial diagnosis. It was designed by the retrospective analysis of a large pool of 816 MDS patients and followed the natural history of the disease to determine important factors related to patient outcome. Overall

survival and the risk of transformation to acute leukemia were found to be related to the number of blood cytopenias, the percentage of myeloblasts in the bone marrow, and the presence of specific cytogenetic abnormalities. The risk associated with cytogenetic abnormalities was determined to be good if a normal diploid karyotype, isolated del(5q), isolated del(20q), or isolated -Y were present. Poor risk abnormalities were defined as abnormalities involving chromosome 7 or complex karyotypes with the presence of three or more karyotypic abnormalities. All other cytogenetic abnormalities were considered intermediate risk. The IPSS weights these different variables to produce a score that stratifies patients into four separate risk groups: low, intermediate-1, intermediate-2, and high risk (Table 5-3). Patient survival and the risk of transformation to acute leukemia are then predicted from cohorts of different ages as illustrated in Table 5-3B. IPSS low and intermediate-1 patients are generally considered low-risk MDS and intermediate-2 and IPSS high patients are grouped into high-risk MDS.

Low-risk MDS are typically treated more conservatively than higher risk MDS. Prognostication in this low-risk group may be particularly important as it is unclear at this time whether some low-risk patients may benefit from early therapeutic intervention. To determine which low-risk patients should be considered for treatment protocols investigating early intervention, low-risk MDS patients at the MD Anderson were analyzed to further stratify prognosis in low and intermediate-1 IPSS groupings (3). Factors associated with a worse prognosis in this low-risk group include: thrombocytopenia (platelets <50 × 10^9/L), anemia (hemoglobin concentration <10 g/dL), age (>60 years), blast count >4%, and a karyotype that was not diploid or del(5q). This model stratified low-risk patients into three subgroups with a median survival of 80, 27, and 14 months,

TABLE 5-3 | THE INTERNATIONAL PROGNOSTIC SCORING SYSTEM (1)

A: IPSS score is the sum of the three listed prognostic factors

Score	0	0.5	1	1.5	2
BM blasts (%)	<5	5-10	–	11-20	21-30
Karyotype*	Good	Intermediate	Poor		
Cytopenias	0/1	2/3			

B: Prognosis determined by IPSS score

RISK GROUP	IPSS SCORE	MEDIAN SURVIVAL (YEARS)			
Age		≤60 years	>60 years	≤70 years	>70 years
Low	0	11.8	4.8	9	3.9
Intermediate-1	0.5-1.0	5.2	2.7	4.4	2.4
Intermediate-2	1.5-2.0	1.8	1.1	1.3	1.2
High	≥2.5	0.3	0.5	0.4	0.4

*Good: normal, -Y, del(5q), del(20q); Poor: complex (≥3 abnormalities) or chromosome 7 anomalies; Intermediate: other abnormalities.
Cytopenias defined as hemoglobin concentration <10 g/dL, neutrophils $<1.5 \times 10^9$/L, and platelets $<100 \times 10^9$/L.

respectively. Increased ferritin and β2 microglobulin were also associated with worse survival in these patients but these factors were not included in the prognostic model. As patient survival was significantly different between these low-risk categories, investigation of early intervention protocols in these low-risk patients with relatively poor survival may be warranted (Table 5-4). Recently, we have described the cause of death of patients with lower risk MDS (64). Approximately, 80% of patients died from a complication intrinsic to MDS and not due to disease progression that only occurs in 10 to 20% of patients. The most frequent cause of death was infection followed by bleeding. Patients with increased percentage of blasts and a monosomy 7 have an increased risk of transformation to AML (64).

The IPSS determines risk at the time of initial diagnosis but it does not provide information regarding changes in risk as patients progress through the course of their disease. A dynamic prognostication system has been developed to address this deficiency and provides a score that is predictive of survival and leukemic transformation over time. The WHO classification-based prognostic scoring system (WPSS) weights three variables: WHO diagnostic classification, karyotype abnormalities categorized according to the IPSS criteria, and transfusion requirement (2). This stratifies patients into five disease groups that demonstrate different survival and risk of evolution to acute leukemia over time. Very low-risk patients in this classification were found to have an overall mortality rate that was not different to the general population. This model incorporates changes in the disease risk profile over time, allowing further refinement in prediction of survival and leukemic progression as the disease progresses. Finally, a model

has been developed by the MD Anderson group that accounts for both de novo and secondary disease and includes CMML. The characteristics of this model are shown in Tables 5-5, 5-6, and 5-7.

TABLE 5-4 | A LOW-RISK MDS SPECIFIC MODEL

A

Adverse Factor	Coefficient	p Value	Assigned Score
Unfavorable cytogenetics*	0.203	<0.0001	1
Age ≥60 years	0.348	<0.0001	2
Hgb < 10 (g/dL)	0.216	<0.0001	1
Plt $<50 \times 10^9$/L	0.498	<0.0001	2
$(50\text{-}200) \times 10^9$/L	0.277	0.0001	1
BM blasts ≥4%	0.195	0.0001	1

B

Score	No. of Patients	Median Survival (Month)	4-year Survival (%)
0	11	NR	78
1	58	83	82
2	113	51	51
3	185	36	40
4	223	22	27
5	166	14	9
6	86	16	7
7	13	9	NA

The score is calculated in patients with MDS and an IPSS score of low or intermediate-1. *A.* Significant characteristics by multivariate analysis. Each one has an assigned score. The calculated total score can then be used in *B* to predict median and 4-year survivals (3).

| TABLE 5-5 | MDACC MODEL—SIMPLIFIED MYELODYSPLASTIC SYNDROME RISK SCORE | | |

Prognostic Factor	Coefficient	Points
Performance status		
≥2	0.267	2
Age (y)		
60-64	0.179	1
≥65	0.336	2
Platelets (×10⁹/L)		
<30	0.418	3
30-49	0.270	2
50-199	0.184	1
Hemoglobin <12 g/dL	0.274	2
Bone marrow blasts (%)		
5-10	0.222	1
11-29	0.260	2
WBC >20 × 10⁹/L	0.258	2
Karyotype: Chromosome 7 abnormality or complex ≥3 abnormalities	0.479	3
Prior transfusion, yes	0.107	1

Score points were obtained by dividing the coefficients by 0.15 and rounding to the nearest integer.

The presence of fibrosis on the bone marrow biopsy occurs in a minority of patients with MDS but this pathological feature is not incorporated into routine diagnostic classifications or prognostic systems. Fibrosis is more frequently observed in patients with multilineage dysplasia or with karyotype abnormalities and when present it is associated with a more rapid progression to severe bone marrow failure and shortened survival (65). In younger patients, it may warrant early consideration of transplant therapies.

| TABLE 5-6 | MDS MDACC MODEL—ESTIMATED OVERALL SURVIVAL BY PROGNOSTIC SCORE | | | |

| | | SURVIVAL | | |
Score	No. of Patients (%)	Median (Months)	% At 3 Years	% At 6 Years
Low				
0-4	157 (16)	54	63	38
Int-1				
5	111 (12)	30	40	14
6	116 (12)	23	29	14
Int-2				
7	127 (13)	14	19	8
8	106 (11)	13	13	4
High				
9	97 (10)	10	10	2
≥10	244 (25)	5	2	0

Int, intermediate.

| TABLE 5-7 | MDS MDACC MODEL—ESTIMATED OVERALL SURVIVAL BY FOUR LEVELS OF PROGNOSTIC SCORE POINTS* | | | |

| | | SURVIVAL | | |
Score	No. of Patients (%)	Median (Months)	Score	No. of Patients (%)
0-4	157 (16)	54	63	38
5-6	227 (24)	25	34	13
7-8	233 (24)	14	16	6
≥9	341 (36)	6	4	0.4

Adapted, with permission, from Kantarjian H, O'Brien S, Ravandi F, et al. Proposal for a new risk model in myelodysplastic syndrome that accounts for events not considered in the original International Prognostic Scoring System. *Cancer* 2008;113(6):1351-1361.

THERAPY

The number of effective drug treatments available to treat MDS has increased in recent years, providing the clinician with a range of management alternatives. Some of these treatments improve hematopoietic function and alleviate symptoms related to blood cytopenia, whereas other therapies alter the natural history of the disease and improve survival. Both approaches may be appropriate in different clinical contexts and many patients receive different combinations of treatments throughout their disease course.

The goals of therapy in MDS vary in different patient populations and a management plan should consider the patient's age, comorbidities, and disease risk. Patients with low-risk MDS most commonly experience problems related to chronic anemia and the disease may remain stable for prolonged periods. If these patients are elderly, they may best be managed with relatively nontoxic therapies that aim to maintain quality of life. Treatment options include transfusions of blood products, growth factor therapies (erythropoietin with or without colony-stimulating factors), and non-growth factor therapies with immunomodulators (lenalidomide) and epigenetic drug treatment (azacytidine and decitabine). High-risk MDS has a poor prognosis and forms a continuum with acute myeloid leukemia. Aggressive therapies may be warranted in these high-risk patients to eradicate the malignant clone and improve survival. Intensive therapies may include high-dose chemotherapy and consideration of alloSCT in younger patients. Intensive treatment protocols are not suitable for all patients because they expose the patient to significant risks of treatment-related morbidity and mortality. An algorithm for treatment approaches at MD Anderson Cancer Center is shown in Fig. 5-5.

Assessing response to treatment in MDS can be complex as treatment goals in low- and high-risk disease may be different. Clinical response criteria in low-risk

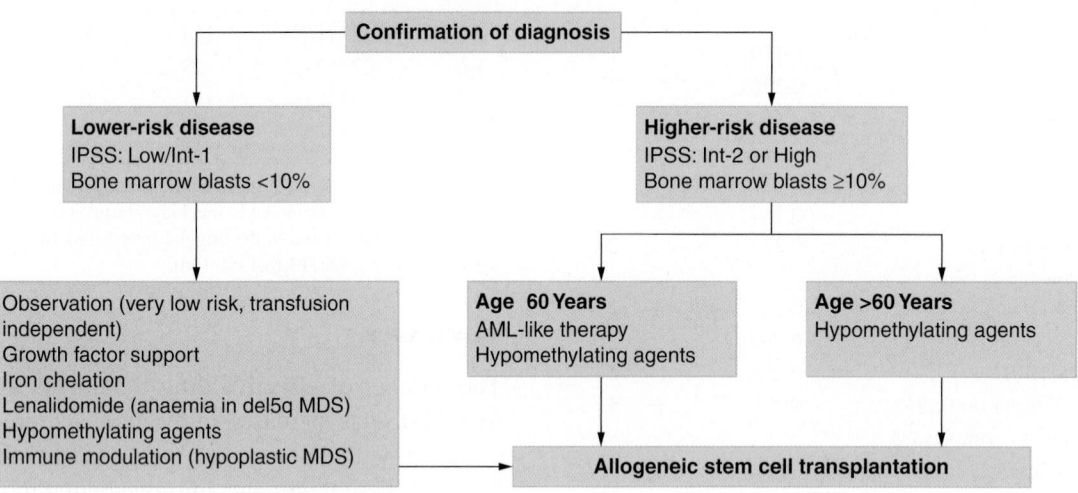

FIGURE 5-5. An approach to the management of MDS.

disease usually measure improvements in peripheral blood cell counts and quality of life factors. Response in high-risk disease is typically more stringent with measures of resolution of bone marrow changes by morphological and cytogenetic criteria. Standardized criteria are available to assess response to treatment in MDS and are particularly useful to allow comparisons between drug trials (66, 67).

Supportive Care

Chronic blood cytopenia is a principal characteristic of the MDS, so therapies aimed at alleviating problems related to anemia, neutropenia, and thrombocytopenia are an essential component of management. Bacterial infections require aggressive treatment with antibiotics. Platelet transfusions are administered for episodes of bleeding or for prophylaxis in patients with severe thrombocytopenia. Transfusion thresholds at MD Anderson include a hemoglobin level of 8 g/dL (unless the patient is otherwise symptomatic) and a platelet count of less than 10 K/UL unless bleeding. Additional hemostatic support with the use of antifibrinolytic agents may be considered for problematic mucosal bleeding or for surgical procedures. The role of prophylactic antibiotics is less established in neutropenic patients. It is our practice at MD Anderson to use triple therapy (antibacterial with a quinolone, antiviral, and antifungal) in all patients with severe neutropenia that are receiving therapy for their disease.

Symptomatic anemia is often the major clinical problem in patients with low-risk MDS. In this group, red cell transfusion is effective symptomatic therapy but a prolonged transfusion program may cause problems with transfusion-related hemosiderosis, alloantibody formation, and volume overload in patients with impaired cardiac function. Deposition of iron in body tissues is treated with iron chelation. The efficacy of iron chelation therapy is best demonstrated in thalassemia major where regular deferoxamine therapy reduces iron deposition in organs and improves survival (68,69). In MDS it is hypothesized to have similar advantages (70). This needs to be confirmed in randomized clinical trials. The parenteral administration of deferoxamine is inconvenient for patients and the development of effective oral iron chelating drugs, such as deferasirox, has allowed iron chelation to be performed more easily (71-73). Iron chelation should start with parenteral deferoxamine or oral deferasirox after 20 to 40 units of red cells have been administered, particularly if there is an expectation of prolonged survival and continued transfusion therapy (35). Serum ferritin may be used as a guide to chelation therapy with a ferritin concentration greater than 1000 µg/L typically attained after transfusion of 20 red cell units (63). Iron chelation therapy should also be considered in a younger patient who may be a candidate for allogeneic transplantation. An elevated pretransplant ferritin has been associated with a lower overall survival after allogeneic transplantation and an increase in the hepatic transplant complication of veno-occlusive disease (74).

Hematopoietic Growth Factors

Hematopoietic growth factors are the primary regulators of blood progenitor cell proliferation and are used therapeutically to promote effective hematopoiesis from myelodysplastic bone marrow. Erythropoietin therapy has been explored as an alternative to red cell transfusion in patients with low-risk MDS. Recombinant erythropoietin (rEPO) in various forms including epoetin α, epoetin β, and the long-acting darbepoetin have been studied in different cohorts of patients. Overall, erythroid responses in unselected MDS patients are modest in the range of 10 to 20% (75). Within these cohorts, the best responses were identified in patients with low-risk MDS, a low serum EPO level (<200 IU/L), and no red cell transfusion requirement (75,76). In this favorable subgroup of MDS patients, an erythroid response to rEPO therapy is observed in 40 to 60% of patients (75-77). The median duration of response is approximately 2 years and therapy is associated with improved quality of life (77). Recent data suggest that patients who respond to growth factor therapy have better survival than historical control cohorts who received supportive care alone (76).

EPO in combination with G-CSF is also an effective treatment for anemia with response rates of approximately 40 to 50% in selected cohorts (78-80). The combination of these two hematopoietic cytokines appears to offer synergistic benefit in promoting effective erythropoiesis and allow improvements in hemoglobin concentration in some patients who fail to respond to EPO monotherapy (78,81). There is some evidence that the benefit of this combination therapy is most marked in the diagnostic categories of RARS and RCMD, however, this has not been confirmed in all studies (76). Disease transformation is a theoretical risk in patients receiving chronic hematopoietic growth factor therapy but long-term observation of these patients suggest that these cytokines do not promote leukemic transformation (76,80). Hematopoietic growth factor therapy should be considered to treat anemia in patients with low-risk MDS associated with a low serum EPO. EPO can be initiated as monotherapy with the addition of G-CSF if there is no objective response in 2 to 3 months.

Thrombopoietin has been used to promote platelet production and minimize the bleeding complications related to severe thrombocytopenia. Initial trials with recombinant thrombopoietin were disappointing (82) and new second generation thrombomimetic agents are now being tested in the clinic to improve hemostatic function in patients with MDS. Initial trial data for one agent, AMG 531, are encouraging with sustained improvements in platelet counts in about 40% of patients treated for severe thrombocytopenia related to MDS (83). Despite these early results we do not recommend their use outside the setting of a clinical trial. This is due to potential concerns of increased blasts and fibrosis in patients with MDS treated with this agent.

Lenalidomide

Lenalidomide is a chemical analogue of thalidomide with diverse biological actions that encompass immune modulation and anti-angiogenic effects. Selective activity of lenalidomide against MDS associated with an interstitial deletion on the long arm of chromosome 5 was first suggested in a single center study examining the effects of this drug on anemia in patients with low-risk MDS (84). Erythroid responses were noted in 56% of the cohort with the most significant response found in the subgroup with a del(5q) abnormality. This observation was then confirmed in a larger multicenter phase II study of lenalidomide (5). This second trial demonstrated an overall erythroid response in 76% of patients with the del(5q) abnormality. Responses were prolonged and occurred rapidly with a median time to a hematologic response of 4 to 5 weeks. A cytogenetic response was documented in 73% of patients with almost half of this group developing a cytogenetic remission. Cytogenetic responses were observed in patients with the del(5q) abnormality alone and in patients with the del(5q) abnormality associated with additional cytogenetic defects. This clearly demonstrated that the activity of lenalidomide was not limited to patients with the 5q- syndrome as classified by WHO, but was observed in low-risk MDS patients with a variety of WHO classifications associated with a del(5q) abnormality on cytogenetic studies.

Lenalidomide therapy is usually started at 10 mg daily to treat MDS. A favorable response is typically characterized by normalization of anemia and cytogenetic response (5). The most important early side effect of therapy with lenalidomide is myelosuppression that may necessitate dose reduction in patients with persistent thrombocytopenia and neutropenia. Interestingly, the degree of myelosuppresion has been associated with response. Thrombocytopenia at diagnosis (platelet count $<100 \times 10^9$/L) has been associated with a worse response to lenalidomide treatment in published drug trials. This may reflect repeated or prolonged treatment interruption of the drug therapy secondary to myelosuppression.

Lenalidomide and thalidomide also demonstrate activity in low-risk MDS without the del(5q) abnormality. Lenalidomide has been studied in a group of 214 patients with low-risk MDS (IPSS low and int-1) and predominantly a normal karyotype (85). In this cohort, 26% of patients achieved transfusion independence with a further 17% developing a reduction in transfusion requirement. The median duration of transfusion independence while on therapy was 41 weeks and cytogenetic responses were documented in 19% of patients with karyotypic abnormalities.

Hypomethylating Agents

5-azacytidine and 5-aza-2'-deoxycytidine (decitabine) are chemically related drugs with a spectrum of activity that includes both low- and high-risk MDS. The mechanism of action of these drugs is uncertain, although both agents reverse abnormal promoter DNA methylation that surrounds the promoter of some tumor-suppressor genes in cancer cells. Aberrant promoter methylation is associated with transcriptional repression, or silencing, and may contribute to the loss of tumor-suppressor gene function in MDS. Decitabine and 5-azacytidine are both cytidine analogues that incorporate into DNA and form covalent bonds with DNA methyltransferase enzymes. Depletion of methyltransferase activity within the cell then causes newly synthesized DNA to be hypomethylated compared to the parent strand. After at least two cycles of cell division, DNA becomes globally hypomethylated with alteration in gene expression within the leukemic cell. Both agents display cytotoxicity at high doses while hypomethylating activity remains prominent at lower doses. These biochemical changes are an attractive target for drug therapy as normal tissues have little gene promoter methylation, so hypomethylating therapy may have some degree of specificity for the malignant clone.

5-azacytidine was the first drug that demonstrated broad spectrum activity in the MDS. Comparison of azacytidine (75 mg/m^2 subcutaneously for 7 days every 28 days) to best supportive care in a randomized control trial demonstrated an overall response rate of 48% for the hypomethylating drug compared to 5% in the supportive care arm (86,87). In this trial, therapy with azacytidine was associated with a prolongation in the time to leukemic transformation and better quality of life with improvement in symptoms of fatigue and physical function. The median time to response was three cycles after starting 5-azacytidine and response rates were independent of MDS classification. Complete responses were observed in relatively few patients (10%) with most patients in the trial experiencing hematologic improvement. A report of a multicenter phase III study of azacytidine in high-risk MDS patients has demonstrated an increase in overall survival of approximately

9 months for patients receiving azacytidine compared to other standard therapies (88). This is a particularly significant finding as it is the first drug trial that has demonstrated a survival advantage in MDS. Of interest, a subset analysis of this trial data suggests that 5-azacitidine may have significant activity in MDS associated with abnormalities in chromosome 7. This observation is important and will need to be confirmed in other studies as this cytogenetic abnormality is usually associated with a very poor outcome.

Decitabine has similar clinical activity to azacytidine and has been studied in various dose regimes in predominantly high-risk MDS and AML. Comparison of decitabine (45 mg/m^2 in three divided doses administered for 3 consecutive days every 6 weeks) to best supportive care in a randomized control trial demonstrated an overall response rate of 17% with complete remissions observed in 9% of patients with predominantly high-risk MDS (89). Subgroup analysis revealed that patients who received decitabine had a longer median time to transformation to AML or death if they were treatment naïve or had high-risk MDS. Myelosuppression was the major drug toxicity. Data from this trial may underestimate the efficacy of the drug as a significant proportion of patients on the therapy arm received a small number of treatment cycles that may have been insufficient to demonstrate a response. This notion is supported by previous phase II trial data that suggest decitabine has an overall response rate similar to azacytidine (90). Subsequent clinical trial development with decitabine has focused on improving response rates by lowering the daily dose and lengthening administration schedules. One such schedule of intravenous administration of decitabine for 5 days every 4 weeks demonstrated a complete response rate of 39% in a high-risk MDS cohort (91,92). It is recognized that improvements in hematopoietic function are often delayed after the initiation of azacytidine or decitabine therapy and drug treatment should continue for four to six cycles before cessation because of poor response. Early problems of myelosuppression may resolve over this time period and should not necessarily initiate dose reduction. Recently, a preliminary report of a randomized study of decitabine did not show any improvement in survival.

Chemical modification of histone proteins by acetylation contribute to the regulation of gene expression and probably interact with abnormal DNA methylation to cause transcriptional suppression of tumor-suppressor genes. Histone deacetylase inhibitors alter chromatin structure to promote gene transcription and their combination with hypomethylating agents demonstrates significant in vitro synergy (93). Clinical drug trials in MDS and AML are starting to examine this potentially exciting combination of drugs. Trials initiated at the MD Anderson Cancer Center have examined decitabine with valproic acid (94) and 5-azacytidine with the combination of valproic acid and all-*trans* retinoic acid (95). Other investigators have examined 5-azacytidine with sodium phenylbutyrate (96). All of these early trials demonstrate activity of combined hypomethylating drugs and HDAC inhibition with favorable response rates of up to 50% in elderly patients with low induction-related mortality. Significant decreases in global DNA methylation and increases in histone acetylation were observed in these studies but these changes did not correlate with clinical response to drug therapy.

Cytotoxic Chemotherapy

The relatively poor prognosis associated with high-risk MDS has initiated intensive treatment strategies incorporating high-dose chemotherapy in the same protocols used to treat acute myeloid leukemia. In patients diagnosed with high-risk MDS, AML-type treatment protocols produce a complete response rate of about 40 to 60%, although remissions are usually brief (60,97-100). Unfortunately, these MDS patients also experience a shorter period of survival after intensive chemotherapy compared to patients treated for AML. This poor response to high-dose chemotherapy is due, at least in part, to the relatively greater proportion of patients diagnosed with RAEB having poor prognosis cytogenetics involving complex changes of chromosomes 5 and 7 (60). Selection of patients for this treatment approach is important as elderly patients with significant comorbidities tolerate high-dose chemotherapy poorly.

Patients with high-risk MDS have been administered a variety of intensive chemotherapy regimens in the clinical trial setting at the MD Anderson Cancer Center (100,101). Clinical trial protocols have examined using intermediate to high-dose cytosine arabinoside (ara-C)(A) in various combinations with idarubicin (I), cyclophosphamide (C), fludarabine (F), and topotecan (T), as regimens: IA, FA, FAI, TA, and CAT. The overall complete response rate for these antileukemic chemotherapy protocols was 55 to 58% with activity demonstrated against all high-risk MDS diagnostic categories. A short antecedent history of hematological disorder, a normal karyotype, performance status, age, and treatment in a laminar air flow environment were all predictive of attaining a complete response. This intensive approach is beneficial in some patients as those who developed

a complete response within 6 weeks of commencing chemotherapy obtained a survival advantage. However, these regimens were toxic with significant treatment-related mortality in the first 6 weeks, ranging from 5% with TA to 21% with FAI. Consolidation chemotherapy was used in most cases where a remission was achieved with a regimen containing the drugs used in induction but at a reduced intensity of 50 to 66% of the initial dose. Survival of patients treated with IA and TA therapies were comparable and superior to those patients treated with FA, FAI, and CAT regimens but prognosis with this intensive treatment approach remains poor with a 5-year overall survival rate of 8% (25). Nevertheless, this approach does benefit some patients with younger individuals (<65 years) with a normal karyotype achieving an encouraging 5-year survival rate of 27% with intensive treatment. For older patients, the TA combination can be considered as it has a relatively low treatment-related mortality and it does not contain anthracycline drugs that are relatively contraindicated in the presence of heart disease.

Investigation of new agents as monotherapy or incorporated into protocols with other cytotoxic agents promises improved outcomes for MDS patients in the future. Clofarabine is a nucleoside analog with significant activity in AML and MDS and is currently being explored in drug trials (102). Other agents that target specific oncogenic pathways are also being investigated. Tipifarnib, a farnesyltransferase inhibitor that modulates Ras signaling, has demonstrated overall responses of 32% in high-risk MDS (103).

Immunosuppressive Therapy

Immune dysfunction contributes to blood cytopenia in some patients with a myelodysplastic syndrome, producing a clinical overlap with aplastic anemia (104). Immunosuppressive therapy with antithymocyte globulin (ATG) with or without the addition of cyclosporine has been explored in small numbers of MDS patients to determine if modulation of the immune system can improve hematopoietic function as demonstrated in therapy for aplastic anemia. Disease response rates of 30 to 50% have been observed in selected cohorts of patients with low-risk MDS administered a course of ATG with a minority of patients experiencing a prolonged remission (105-107). A range of features have been described that predict a good response to immunosuppressive therapy, including younger age, HLA-DR status, shorter duration of red cell transfusion, low-risk IPSS, and bone marrow hypocellularity (107-109). Selection of appropriate patients for immunosuppression is important as ATG therapy is poorly tolerated in an older population with low-risk MDS (107,110).

Hematopoietic Stem Cell Transplantation

AlloSCT is a potentially curative treatment modality for MDS but the therapy carries significant risk associated with treatment toxicity, prolonged cytopenia, infection and graft versus host disease. In the small proportion of MDS patients that are young with a suitable donor the transplant procedure offers the best chance of cure with a long-term disease free survival of 30 to 50% (111-115). Given the risks associated with this procedure, patient suitability and timing of the transplant are important issues to consider.

Allogeneic transplantation with myeloablative conditioning has been examined exclusively in younger patients with a median age in the mid-thirties in most studies. Patients with low-risk disease (RA/RARS) have experienced the best survival rate, however, this is also the subgroup of patients that are predicted to experience prolonged survival without aggressive therapies. This procedure is associated with significant mortality risk with a treatment-related mortality of up to 30 to 50% in some studies (113,114). Relapse of the disease after transplantation occurs in approximately 20% of cases and the relapsed disease has a relatively poor response to donor lymphocyte infusion (113,114,116). Increased risk of allogeneic transplantation in MDS has been associated with older age, poor risk cytogenetics, particularly abnormalities of chromosome 7 or a complex karyotype, the presence of excess blasts in the bone marrow and longer duration of disease (113,117,118). Patients with treatment-related MDS are also recognized to have a poor transplant outcome but analysis of this subgroup suggests that this poor survival is related to the frequency of high-risk cytogenetic changes in this group and does not specifically reflect the underlying treatment-related etiology of the disease (118,119).

The development of nonmyeloablative allogeneic transplantation with reduced intensity conditioning has allowed allogeneic transplantation to be considered in older patients with MDS and in patients whose comorbidities or organ dysfunction would exclude them from myeloablative treatment (120,121). This procedure has reduced the transplant-related mortality related to allogeneic transplantation that has been the major problem limiting the availability of this potentially curative therapy to older MDS patients. This therapy aims to minimize organ toxicity related to initial chemo- or radiotherapy but allow stable engraftment of donor cells that provide curative potential by the graft versus leukemia effect. Comparison of reduced intensity conditioning

transplantation with standard myeloablative conditioning has found reduced transplant-related mortality but increased relapse rate resulting in comparable rates of overall survival between the two transplantation strategies (117,122,123). Considering that the patients that have received nonmyelablative conditioning have been older with more significant comorbidities this result is encouraging and has allowed the possibility of cure via allogeneic transplantation to be extended to a greater proportion of the MDS population.

Statistical modeling based on historical allogeneic transplantation outcomes for matched sibling transplantation suggests that the maximal overall survival is achieved by different transplant strategies in different MDS risk groups (124). Patients with low-risk disease (IPSS low and intermediate-1 groups) maximize overall survival by delaying transplantation after diagnosis until a time when there is evidence of disease progression but before the development of overt acute leukemia. This delayed transplant approach provided greatest survival benefit to younger patients aged less than 40 years. Specific features of disease progression have not been defined but evidence of new cytogenetic abnormalities, progressive cytopenia, and increasing blast percentage in the bone marrow are suggested as potential triggers for transplantation. Patients with high-risk disease (IPSS intermediate-2 and high) should ideally receive the transplant as soon as possible after diagnosis. The presence of bone marrow fibrosis delays engraftment in allogeneic transplantation and its presence is an additional risk factor in transplant outcome in high-risk MDS. In this group, fibrosis considerably increases transplantation risk and therefore early consideration of transplantation is suggested in a younger patient with significant MDS associated fibrosis (125).

SPECIFIC CLINICAL SITUATIONS

Despite the clinical activity of several agents described earlier, most patients with MDS will eventually succumb to their disease (64) and therefore the need to develop better strategies both up-front and in patients that have failed prior therapies.

Treating Patients With Lower-Risk Disease and Poor Prognosis

It is now demonstrated that the prognosis of patients with lower-risk MDS is very heterogeneous with a significant subset of patients having poor prognosis (3). Because most of these patients will die as a consequence of MDS (64), it is possible that introducing therapy early in this selected group of patients. This has significant implications for the role of alloSCT in MDS but also for the incorporation of disease modifying strategies. We are currently studying the role of very low dose or oral schedules of hypomethylating agents and histone deacetylase inhibitors in this setting.

Treating Patients With Higher-Risk Disease: The Problem of the Hypermethylator Failure

Results from the randomized studies of 5-azacitidine have indicated that this class of compound can have a significant impact in the survival of patients with MDS, but the response rates are relatively low. Therefore, we need strategies to improve response rates and duration. The next step will be to use agents in combination. Data described above with hypomethylating agents suggest that response rates could be higher. This needs to be explored in randomized clinical trials. Other agents to combine include lenalidomide, TNF-α inhibitors, and potentially NF-kB inhibitors.

One of the main problems right now is the treatment of patients that have failed therapy with a hypomethylating agent. Data from MD Anderson (Jabbour et al., 2010) indicate that prognosis is very poor with a median survival of less than 5 months (126). This group of patients is generally refractory to most conventional antileukemia agents available such as cytarabine. These patients should be treated with investigational new agents or be considered for alloSCT as soon as possible. Agents currently being studied include nucleoside analogs clofarabine and sapacitabine and the multikinase inhibitor ON1910 among several.

References

1. Greenberg P, Cox C, LeBeau MM, et al. International scoring system for evaluating prognosis in myelodysplastic syndromes. *Blood* 1997;89(6):2079-2088.
2. Malcovati L, Germing U, Kuendgen A, et al. Time-dependent prognostic scoring system for predicting survival and leukemic evolution in myelodysplastic syndromes. *J Clin Oncol* 2007; 25(23):3503-3510.
3. Garcia-Manero G, Shan J, Faderl S, et al. A prognostic score for patients with lower risk myelodysplastic syndrome. *Leukemia* 2008;22(3):538-543.
4. Kantarjian H, O'Brien S, Ravandi F, et al. Proposal for a new risk model in myelodysplastic syndrome that accounts for events not considered in the original International Prognostic Scoring System. *Cancer* 2008;113(6):1351-1361.
5. List A, Dewald G, Bennett J, et al. Lenalidomide in the myelodysplastic syndrome with chromosome 5q deletion. *N Engl J Med* 2006;355(14):1456-1465.
6. Raza A, Reeves JA, Feldman EJ, et al. Phase 2 study of lenalidomide in transfusion-dependent, low-risk, and intermediate-1 risk myelodysplastic syndromes with karyotypes other than deletion 5q. *Blood* 2008;111(1):86-93.
7. Fenaux P, Mufti GJ, Hellstrom-Lindberg E, et al. Azacitidine prolongs overall survival compared with conventional care regimens in elderly patients with low bone marrow blast count acute myeloid leukemia. *J Clin Oncol* 2010;28(4): 562-569.
8. Ma X, Does M, Raza A, et al. Myelodysplastic syndromes: Incidence and survival in the United States. *Cancer* 2007; 109(8):1536-1542.
9. Rollison DE, Howlader N, Smith MT, et al. Epidemiology of myelodysplastic syndromes and chronic myeloproliferative disorders in the United States, 2001-2004, using data from the NAACCR and SEER programs. *Blood* 2008;112(1): 45-52.
10. Matsuda A, Germing U, Jinnai I, et al. Difference in clinical features between Japanese and German patients with refractory anemia in myelodysplastic syndromes. *Blood* 2005;106(8): 2633-2640.
11. Morel P, Hebbar M, Lai JL, et al. Cytogenetic analysis has strong independent prognostic value in de novo myelodysplastic syndromes and can be incorporated in a new scoring system: a report on 408 cases. *Leukemia* 1993;7(9): 1315-1323.
12. Chen B, Zhao WL, Jin J, et al. Clinical and cytogenetic features of 508 Chinese patients with myelodysplastic syndrome and comparison with those in Western countries. *Leukemia* 2005;19(5):767-775.
13. Toyama K, Ohyashiki K, Yoshida Y, et al. Clinical implications of chromosomal abnormalities in 401 patients with myelodysplastic syndromes: A multicentric study in Japan. *Leukemia* 1993;7(4):499-508.
14. Sole F, Luno E, Sanzo C, et al. Identification of novel cytogenetic markers with prognostic significance in a series of 968 patients with primary myelodysplastic syndromes. *Haematologica* 2005;90(9):1168-1178.
15. Poppe B, Van Limbergen H, Van Roy N, et al.: Chromosomal aberrations in Bloom syndrome patients with myeloid malignancies. *Cancer Genet Cytogenet* 2001;128(1):39-42.
16. Luna-Fineman S, Shannon KM, Atwater SK, et al. Myelodysplastic and myeloproliferative disorders of childhood: A study of 167 patients. *Blood* 1999;93(2):459-466.
17. Allan JM, Wild CP, Rollinson S, et al. Polymorphism in glutathione S-transferase P1 is associated with susceptibility to chemotherapy-induced leukemia. *Proc Natl Acad Sci USA* 2001;98(20):11592-11597.
18. Felix CA, Walker AH, Lange BJ, et al. Association of CYP3A4 genotype with treatment-related leukemia. *Proc Natl Acad Sci USA* 1998;95(22):13176-13181.
19. Larson RA, Wang Y, Banerjee M, et al. Prevalence of the inactivating 609C→T polymorphism in the NAD(P)H:quinone oxidoreductase (NQO1) gene in patients with primary and therapy-related myeloid leukemia. *Blood* 1999;94(2):803-807.
20. Descatha A, Jenabian A, Conso F, et al. Occupational exposures and haematological malignancies: Overview on human recent data. *Cancer Causes Control* 2005;16(8):939-953.
21. West RR, Stafford DA, Farrow A, et al. Occupational and environmental exposures and myelodysplasia: a case-control study. *Leuk Res* 1995;19(2):127-139.
22. Rigolin GM, Cuneo A, Roberti MG, et al. Exposure to myelotoxic agents and myelodysplasia: Case-control study and correlation with clinicobiological findings. *Br J Haematol* 1998; 103(1):189-197.
23. Nagata C, Shimizu H, Hirashima K, et al. Hair dye use and occupational exposure to organic solvents as risk factors for myelodysplastic syndrome. *Leuk Res* 1999;23(1):57-62.

24. Golomb HM, Alimena G, Rowley JD, et al. Correlation of occupation and karyotype in adults with acute nonlymphocytic leukemia. *Blood* 1982;60(2):404-411.

25. Kantarjian HM, Keating MJ, Walters RS, et al. Therapy-related leukemia and myelodysplastic syndrome: Clinical, cytogenetic, and prognostic features. *J Clin Oncol* 1986;4(12): 1748-1757.

26. Josting A, Wiedenmann S, Franklin J, et al. Secondary myeloid leukemia and myelodysplastic syndromes in patients treated for Hodgkin's disease: A report from the German Hodgkin's Lymphoma Study Group. *J Clin Oncol* 2003;21(18): 3440-3446.

27. Devereux S, Selassie TG, Vaughan Hudson G, et al. Leukaemia complicating treatment for Hodgkin's disease: The experience of the British National Lymphoma Investigation. *BMJ* 1990;301(6760):1077-1080.

28. Traweek ST, Slovak ML, Nademanee AP, et al. Clonal karyotypic hematopoietic cell abnormalities occurring after autologous bone marrow transplantation for Hodgkin's disease and non-Hodgkin's lymphoma. *Blood* 1994;84(3):957-963.

29. Stone RM, Neuberg D, Soiffer R, et al. Myelodysplastic syndrome as a late complication following autologous bone marrow transplantation for non-Hodgkin's lymphoma. *J Clin Oncol* 1994;12(12):2535-2542.

30. Greenberg P, Cox C, LeBeau MM, et al. International scoring system for evaluating prognosis in myelodysplastic syndromes. *Blood* 1997;89(6):2079-2088.

31. Jaffe ES, Harris NL, Stein R, et al. *Pathology and Genetics of Tumours of Haematopoietic and Lymphoid Tissues.* Lyon: IARC Press, 2001.

32. Gralnick HR, Galton DA, Catovsky D, et al. Classification of acute leukemia. *Ann Intern Med* 1977;87(6):740-753.

33. Valent P, Horny HP, Bennett JM, et al. Definitions and standards in the diagnosis and treatment of the myelodysplastic syndromes: Consensus statements and report from a working conference. *Leuk Res* 2007;31(6):727-736.

34. Bain BJ. The bone marrow aspirate of healthy subjects. *Br J Haematol* 1996;94(1):206-209.

35. Haase D, Germing U, Schanz J, et al. New insights into the prognostic impact of the karyotype in MDS and correlation with subtypes: Evidence from a core dataset of 2124 patients. *Blood* 2007;110(13):4385-4395.

36. Pedersen-Bjergaard J, Pedersen M, Roulston D, et al. Different genetic pathways in leukemogenesis for patients presenting with therapy-related myelodysplasia and therapy-related acute myeloid leukemia. *Blood* 1995;86(9):3542-3452.

37. Rowley JD, Golomb HM, Vardiman JW. Nonrandom chromosome abnormalities in acute leukemia and dysmyelopoietic syndromes in patients with previously treated malignant disease. *Blood* 1981;58(4):759-767.

38. Harada H, Harada Y, Niimi H, et al. High incidence of somatic mutations in the AML1/RUNX1 gene in myelodysplastic syndrome and low blast percentage myeloid leukemia with myelodysplasia. *Blood* 2004;103(6):2316-2324.

39. Harada H, Harada Y, Tanaka H, et al. Implications of somatic mutations in the AML1 gene in radiation-associated and therapy-related myelodysplastic syndrome/acute myeloid leukemia. *Blood* 2003;101(2):673-680.

40. Bacher U, Haferlach T, Kern W, et al. A comparative study of molecular mutations in 381 patients with myelodysplastic syndrome and in 4130 patients with acute myeloid leukemia. *Haematologica* 2007;92(6):744-752.

41. Caudill JS, Sternberg AJ, Li CY, et al. C-terminal nucleophosmin mutations are uncommon in chronic myeloid disorders. *Br J Haematol* 2006;133(6):638-641.

42. Langemeijer SM, Kuiper RP, Berends M, et al. Acquired mutations in TET2 are common in myelodysplastic syndromes. *Nat Genet* 2009;41(7):838-842.

43. Shen L, Kantarjian H, Guo Y, et al. DNA methylation predicts survival and response to therapy in patients with myelodysplastic syndromes. *J Clin Oncol* 2010;28(4):605-613.

44. Maciejewski JP, Mufti GJ. Whole genome scanning as a cytogenetic tool in hematologic malignancies. *Blood* 2008; 112(4):965-974.

45. Heinrichs S, Kulkarni RV, Bueso-Ramos CE, et al. Accurate detection of uniparental disomy and microdeletions by SNP array analysis in myelodysplastic syndromes with normal cytogenetics. *Leukemia* 2009;23(9):1605-1613.

46. Dunbar AJ, Gondek LP, O'Keefe CL, et al. 250K single nucleotide polymorphism array karyotyping identifies acquired uniparental disomy and homozygous mutations, including novel missense substitutions of c-Cbl, in myeloid malignancies. *Cancer Res* 2008;68(24):10349-10357.

47. Sokal G, Michaux JL, Van Den Berghe H, et al. A new hematologic syndrome with a distinct karyotype: The 5q-chromosome. *Blood* 1975;46(4):519-533.

48. Pellagatti A, Jadersten M, Forsblom AM, et al. Lenalidomide inhibits the malignant clone and up-regulates the SPARC gene mapping to the commonly deleted region in 5q-syndrome patients. *Proc Natl Acad Sci USA* 2007;104(27): 11406-11411.

49. Liu TX, Becker MW, Jelinek J, et al. Chromosome 5q deletion and epigenetic suppression of the gene encoding alpha-catenin (CTNNA1) in myeloid cell transformation. *Nat Med* 2007;13(1):78-83.

50. Ebert BL, Pretz J, Bosco J, et al. Identification of RPS14 as a 5q-syndrome gene by RNA interference screen. *Nature* 2008;451(7176):335-339.

51. Starczynowski DT, Kuchenbauer F, Argiropoulos B, et al. Identification of miR-145 and miR-146a as mediators of the 5q- syndrome phenotype. *Nat Med* 16(1):49-58.

52. Lai JL, Preudhomme C, Zandecki M, et al. Myelodysplastic syndromes and acute myeloid leukemia with 17p deletion. An entity characterized by specific dysgranulopoiesis and a high incidence of P53 mutations. *Leukemia* 1995;9(3):370-381.

53. Soenen V, Preudhomme C, Roumier C, et al. 17p Deletion in acute myeloid leukemia and myelodysplastic syndrome. Analysis of breakpoints and deleted segments by fluorescence in situ. *Blood* 1998;91(3):1008-1015.

54. Gibbons RJ, Pellagatti A, Garrick D, et al. Identification of acquired somatic mutations in the gene encoding chromatin-remodeling factor ATRX in the alpha-thalassemia myelodysplasia syndrome (ATMDS). *Nat Genet* 2003;34(4):446-449.

55. Steensma DP, Gibbons RJ, Higgs DR. Acquired alpha-thalassemia in association with myelodysplastic syndrome and other hematologic malignancies. *Blood* 2005;105(2): 443-452.

56. Matsui WH, Brodsky RA, Smith BD, et al. Quantitative analysis of bone marrow CD34 cells in aplastic anemia and hypoplastic myelodysplastic syndromes. *Leukemia* 2006;20(3):458-462.

57. Bennett JM, Catovsky D, Daniel MT, et al. Proposals for the classification of the myelodysplastic syndromes. *Br J Haematol* 1982;51(2):189-199.

58. Vardiman JW, Harris NL, Brunning RD. The World Health Organization (WHO) classification of the myeloid neoplasms. *Blood* 2002;100(7):2292-2302.

59. Vardiman JW, Thiele J, Arber DA, et al. The 2008 revision of the World Health Organization (WHO) classification of myeloid neoplasms and acute leukemia: Rationale and important changes. *Blood* 2009;114(5):937-951.

60. Estey E, Thall P, Beran M, et al. Effect of diagnosis (refractory anemia with excess blasts, refractory anemia with excess blasts in transformation, or acute myeloid leukemia (AML)) on outcome of AML-type chemotherapy. *Blood* 1997;90(8):2969-2677.

61. Germing U, Gattermann N, Strupp C, et al. Validation of the WHO proposals for a new classification of primary myelodysplastic syndromes: A retrospective analysis of 1600 patients. *Leuk Res* 2000;24(12):983-992.

62. Howe RB, Porwit-MacDonald A, Wanat R, et al. The WHO classification of MDS does make a difference. *Blood* 2004;103(9):3265-3270.

63. Malcovati L, Porta MG, Pascutto C, et al. Prognostic factors and life expectancy in myelodysplastic syndromes classified according to WHO criteria: A basis for clinical decision making. *J Clin Oncol* 2005;23(30):7594-7603.

64. Dayyani F, Conley AP, Strom SS, et al. Cause of death in patients with lower-risk myelodysplastic syndrome. (64)*Cancer*, 2010;116(9):2174-2179.

65. Buesche G, Teoman H, Wilczak W, et al. Marrow fibrosis predicts early fatal marrow failure in patients with myelodysplastic syndromes. *Leukemia* 2008;22(2):313-322.

66. Cheson BD, Bennett JM, Kantarjian H, et al. Report of an international working group to standardize response criteria for myelodysplastic syndromes. *Blood* 2000;96(12):3671-3674.

67. Cheson BD, Greenberg PL, Bennett JM, et al. Clinical application and proposal for modification of the International Working Group (IWG) response criteria in myelodysplasia. *Blood* 2006;108(2):419-425.

68. Olivieri NF, Nathan DG, MacMillan JH, et al. Survival in medically treated patients with homozygous beta-thalassemia. *N Engl J Med* 1994;331(9):574-578.

69. Brittenham GM, Griffith PM, Nienhuis AW, et al. Efficacy of deferoxamine in preventing complications of iron overload in patients with thalassemia major. *N Engl J Med* 1994;331(9):567-573.

70. Jensen PD, Heickendorff L, Pedersen B, et al. The effect of iron chelation on haemopoiesis in MDS patients with transfusional iron overload. *Br J Haematol* 1996;94(2):288-299.

71. Nisbet-Brown E, Olivieri NF, Giardina PJ, et al. Effectiveness and safety of ICL670 in iron-loaded patients with thalassaemia: A randomised, double-blind, placebo-controlled, dose-escalation trial. *Lancet* 2003;361(9369):1597-1602.

72. Cappellini MD, Cohen A, Piga A, et al. A phase 3 study of deferasirox (ICL670), a once-daily oral iron chelator, in patients with beta-thalassemia. *Blood* 2006;107(9):3455-3462.

73. Neufeld EJ. Oral chelators deferasirox and deferiprone for transfusional iron overload in thalassemia major: New data, new questions. *Blood* 2006;107(9):3436-3441.

74. Armand P, Kim HT, Cutler CS, et al. Prognostic impact of elevated pretransplantation serum ferritin in patients undergoing myeloablative stem cell transplantation. *Blood* 2007;109(10):4586-4588.

75. Hellstrom-Lindberg E. Efficacy of erythropoietin in the myelodysplastic syndromes: A meta-analysis of 205 patients from 17 studies. *Br J Haematol* 1995;89(1):67-71.

76. Park S, Grabar S, Kelaidi C, et al. Predictive factors of response and survival in myelodysplastic syndrome treated with erythropoietin and G-CSF: The GFM experience. *Blood* 2008;111(2):574-582.

77. Hellstrom-Lindberg E, Gulbrandsen N, Lindberg G, et al. A validated decision model for treating the anaemia of myelodysplastic syndromes with erythropoietin + granulocyte colony-stimulating factor: Significant effects on quality of life. *Br J Haematol* 2003;120(6):1037-1046.

78. Negrin RS, Stein R, Doherty K, et al. Maintenance treatment of the anemia of myelodysplastic syndromes with recombinant human granulocyte colony-stimulating factor and erythropoietin: Evidence for in vivo synergy. *Blood* 1996; 87(10):4076-4081.

79. Casadevall N, Durieux P, Dubois S, et al. Health, economic, and quality-of-life effects of erythropoietin and granulocyte colony-stimulating factor for the treatment of myelodysplastic syndromes: A randomized, controlled trial. *Blood* 2004;104(2):321-327.

80. Jadersten M, Montgomery SM, Dybedal I, et al. Long-term outcome of treatment of anemia in MDS with erythropoietin and G-CSF. *Blood* 2005;106(3):803-811.

81. Hellstrom-Lindberg E, Ahlgren T, Beguin Y, et al. Treatment of anemia in myelodysplastic syndromes with granulocyte colony-stimulating factor plus erythropoietin: Results from a randomized phase II study and long-term follow-up of 71 patients. *Blood* 1998;92(1):68-75.

82. Kuter DJ, Begley CG. Recombinant human thrombopoietin: Basic biology and evaluation of clinical studies. *Blood* 2002; 100(10):3457-3469.

83. Kantarjian H, Fenaux P, Sekeres MA, et al. Phase 1/2 study of AMG 531 in thrombocytopenic patients with low-risk myelodysplastic syndrome (MDS): Update including extended treatment. American Society of Hematology, Atlanta, 2007.

84. List A, Kurtin S, Roe DJ, et al. Efficacy of lenalidomide in myelodysplastic syndromes. *N Engl J Med* 2005;352(6):549-557.

85. Raza A, Reeves JA, Feldman EJ, et al. Phase II study of lenalidomide in transfusion-dependent, low- and intermediate-1-risk myelodysplastic syndromes with karyotypes other than deletion 5q. *Blood* 2008;111:86-93.

86. Silverman LR, Demakos EP, Peterson BL, et al. Randomized controlled trial of azacitidine in patients with the myelodysplastic syndrome: A study of the cancer and leukemia group B. *J Clin Oncol* 2002;20(10):2429-2940.

87. Silverman LR, McKenzie DR, Peterson BL, et al. Further analysis of trials with azacitidine in patients with myelodysplastic syndrome: Studies 8421, 8921, and 9221 by the Cancer and Leukemia Group B. *J Clin Oncol* 2006;24(24):3895-3903.

88. Fenaux P, Mufti GJ, Hellstrom-Lindberg E, et al. Efficacy of azacitidine compared with that of conventional care regimens in the treatment of higher-risk myelodysplastic syndromes: A randomised, open-label, phase III study. *Lancet Oncol* 2009;10(3):223-232.

89. Kantarjian H, Issa JP, Rosenfeld CS, et al. Decitabine improves patient outcomes in myelodysplastic syndromes: Results of a phase III randomized study. *Cancer* 2006;106(8):1794-1803.

90. Wijermans P, Lubbert M, Verhoef G, et al. Low-dose 5-aza-2¢-deoxycytidine, a DNA hypomethylating agent, for the treatment of high-risk myelodysplastic syndrome: A multicenter phase II study in elderly patients. *J Clin Oncol* 2000; 18(5):956-962.

91. Issa JP, Garcia-Manero G, Giles FJ, et al. Phase 1 study of low-dose prolonged exposure schedules of the hypomethylating agent 5-aza-2'-deoxycytidine (decitabine) in hematopoietic malignancies. *Blood* 2004;103(5):1635-1640.

92. Kantarjian H, Oki Y, Garcia-Manero G, et al. Results of a randomized study of 3 schedules of low-dose decitabine in higher-risk myelodysplastic syndrome and chronic myelomonocytic leukemia. *Blood* 2007;109(1):52-57.

93. Cameron EE, Bachman KE, Myohanen S, et al. Synergy of demethylation and histone deacetylase inhibition in the re-expression of genes silenced in cancer. *Nat Genet* 1999; 21(1):103-107.

94. Garcia-Manero G, Kantarjian HM, Sanchez-Gonzalez B, et al. Phase 1/2 study of the combination of 5-aza-2'-deoxycytidine with valproic acid in patients with leukemia. *Blood* 2006; 108(10):3271-3279.

95. Soriano AO, Yang H, Faderl S, et al. Safety and clinical activity of the combination of 5-azacytidine, valproic acid, and all-trans retinoic acid in acute myeloid leukemia and myelodysplastic syndrome. *Blood* 2007;110(7):2302-2308.

96. Maslak P, Chanel S, Camacho LH, et al. Pilot study of combination transcriptional modulation therapy with sodium phenylbutyrate and 5-azacytidine in patients with acute myeloid leukemia or myelodysplastic syndrome. *Leukemia* 2006;20(2): 212-217.

97. Wattel E, De Botton S, Luc Lai J, et al. Long-term follow-up of de novo myelodysplastic syndromes treated with intensive chemotherapy: Incidence of long-term survivors and outcome of partial responders. *Br J Haematol* 1997;98(4): 983-991.

98. Parker JE, Pagliuca A, Mijovic A, et al. Fludarabine, cytarabine, G-CSF and idarubicin (FLAG-IDA) for the treatment of poor-risk myelodysplastic syndromes and acute myeloid leukaemia. *Br J Haematol* 1997;99(4):939-944.

99. Bernasconi C, Alessandrino EP, Bernasconi P, et al. Randomized clinical study comparing aggressive chemotherapy with or without G-CSF support for high-risk myelodysplastic syndromes or secondary acute myeloid leukaemia evolving from MDS. *Br J Haematol* 1998;102(3):678-683.

100. Kantarjian H, Beran M, Cortes J, et al. Long-term follow-up results of the combination of topotecan and cytarabine and other intensive chemotherapy regimens in myelodysplastic syndrome. *Cancer* 2006;106(5):1099-1109.

101. Beran M, Shen Y, Kantarjian H, et al. High-dose chemotherapy in high-risk myelodysplastic syndrome: Covariate-adjusted comparison of five regimens. *Cancer* 2001;92(8):1999-2015.

102. Kantarjian H, Gandhi V, Cortes J, et al. Phase 2 clinical and pharmacologic study of clofarabine in patients with refractory or relapsed acute leukemia. *Blood* 2003;102(7): 2379-2386.

103. Fenaux P, Raza A, Mufti GJ, et al. A multicenter phase 2 study of the farnesyltransferase inhibitor tipifarnib in intermediate-to high-risk myelodysplastic syndrome. *Blood* 2007; 109(10): 4158-4163.

104. Sloand EM, Mainwaring L, Fuhrer M, et al. Preferential suppression of trisomy 8 compared with normal hematopoietic cell growth by autologous lymphocytes in patients with trisomy 8 myelodysplastic syndrome. *Blood* 2005;106(3): 841-851.

105. Molldrem JJ, Caples M, Mavroudis D, et al. Antithymocyte globulin for patients with myelodysplastic syndrome. *Br J Haematol* 1997;99(3):699-705.

106. Killick SB, Mufti G, Cavenagh JD, et al. A pilot study of antithymocyte globulin (ATG) in the treatment of patients with 'low-risk' myelodysplasia. *Br J Haematol* 2003;120(4):679-684.

107. Lim ZY, Killick S, Germing U, et al. Low IPSS score and bone marrow hypocellularity in MDS patients predict hematological responses to antithymocyte globulin. *Leukemia* 2007;21(7):1436-1441.

108. Saunthararajah Y, Nakamura R, Nam JM, et al. HLA-DR15 (DR2) is overrepresented in myelodysplastic syndrome and aplastic anemia and predicts a response to immunosuppression in myelodysplastic syndrome. *Blood* 2002;100(5): 1570-1574.

109. Saunthararajah Y, Nakamura R, Wesley R, et al. A simple method to predict response to immunosuppressive therapy in patients with myelodysplastic syndrome. *Blood* 2003;102(8): 3025-3027.

110. Steensma DP, Dispenzieri A, Moore SB, et al. Antithymocyte globulin has limited efficacy and substantial toxicity in unselected anemic patients with myelodysplastic syndrome. *Blood* 2003;101(6):2156-2158.

111. Arnold R, de Witte T, van Biezen A, et al. Unrelated bone marrow transplantation in patients with myelodysplastic syndromes and secondary acute myeloid leukemia: An EBMT survey. European Blood and Marrow Transplantation Group. *Bone Marrow Transplant* 1998;21(12):1213-1216.

112. Runde V, de Witte T, Arnold R, et al. Bone marrow transplantation from HLA-identical siblings as first-line treatment in patients with myelodysplastic syndromes: Early transplantation is associated with improved outcome. Chronic Leukemia Working Party of the European Group for Blood and Marrow Transplantation. *Bone Marrow Transplant* 1998;21(3):255-261.

113. Sierra J, Perez WS, Rozman C, et al. Bone marrow transplantation from HLA-identical siblings as treatment for myelodysplasia. *Blood* 2002;100(6):1997-2004.

114. Castro-Malaspina H, Harris RE, Gajewski J, et al. Unrelated donor marrow transplantation for myelodysplastic syndromes: outcome analysis in 510 transplants facilitated by the National Marrow Donor Program. *Blood* 2002;99(6):1943-1951.

115. Deeg HJ, Storer B, Slattery JT, et al. Conditioning with targeted busulfan and cyclophosphamide for hemopoietic stem cell transplantation from related and unrelated donors in patients with myelodysplastic syndrome. *Blood* 2002; 100(4): 1201-1207.

116. Campregher PV, Gooley T, Scott BL, et al. Results of donor lymphocyte infusions for relapsed myelodysplastic syndrome after hematopoietic cell transplantation. *Bone Marrow Transplant* 2007.

117. Martino R, Iacobelli S, Brand R, et al. Retrospective comparison of reduced-intensity conditioning and conventional high-dose conditioning for allogeneic hematopoietic stem cell transplantation using HLA-identical sibling donors in myelodysplastic syndromes. *Blood* 2006;108(3):836-846.

118. Armand P, Kim HT, DeAngelo DJ, et al. Impact of cytogenetics on outcome of de novo and therapy-related AML and MDS after allogeneic transplantation. *Biol Blood Marrow Transplant* 2007;13(6):655-664.

119. Chang C, Storer BE, Scott BL, et al. Hematopoietic cell transplantation in patients with myelodysplastic syndrome or acute myeloid leukemia arising from myelodysplastic syndrome: Similar outcomes in patients with de novo disease and disease following prior therapy or antecedent hematologic disorders. *Blood* 2007;110(4): 1379-1387.

120. Giralt S, Estey E, Albitar M, et al. Engraftment of allogeneic hematopoietic progenitor cells with purine analog-containing chemotherapy: Harnessing graft-versus-leukemia without myeloablative therapy. *Blood* 1997;89(12): 4531-4536.

121. Giralt S, Thall PF, Khouri I, et al. Melphalan and purine analog-containing preparative regimens: Reduced-intensity conditioning for patients with hematologic malignancies undergoing allogeneic progenitor cell transplantation. *Blood* 2001;97(3):631-637.

122. Scott BL, Sandmaier BM, Storer B, et al. Myeloablative vs nonmyeloablative allogeneic transplantation for patients with myelodysplastic syndrome or acute myelogenous leukemia with multilineage dysplasia: A retrospective analysis. *Leukemia* 2006;20(1):128-135.

123. Sorror ML, Sandmaier BM, Storer BE, et al. Comorbidity and disease status based risk stratification of outcomes among patients with acute myeloid leukemia or myelodysplasia receiving allogeneic hematopoietic cell transplantation. *J Clin Oncol* 2007;25(27):4246-4254.

124. Cutler CS, Lee SJ, Greenberg P, et al. A decision analysis of allogeneic bone marrow transplantation for the myelodysplastic syndromes: Delayed transplantation for low-risk myelodysplasia is associated with improved outcome. *Blood* 2004;104(2):579-585.

125. Scott BL, Storer BE, Greene JE, et al. Marrow fibrosis as a risk factor for posttransplantation outcome in patients with advanced myelodysplastic syndrome or acute myeloid leukemia with multilineage dysplasia. *Biol Blood Marrow Transplant* 2007;13(3):345-354.

126. Jabbour E, Garcia-Manero G, Batty N, et al. Outcome of patients with Myelodysplastic syndrome after failure of decitabine failure. *Cancer* 2010;116(16):3830-4.

PHILADELPHIA CHROMOSOME-NEGATIVE MYELOPROLIFERATIVE NEOPLASMS

Nitin Jain
Hesham M. Amin
Srdan Verstovsek

The field of myeloproliferative disorders (MPDs) has evolved considerably since the sentinel observations made by William Dameshek in 1951. He had commented in an editorial in the journal *Blood:* "To put together such apparently dissimilar diseases as chronic granulocytic leukemia, polycythemia, myeloid metaplasia and di Guglielmo's syndrome may conceivably be without foundation, but for the moment at least, this may prove useful and even productive. What more can one ask of a theory?" (1).

The central feature among the MPDs is effective clonal myeloproliferation without dysplasia. Other features shared by most MPDs include involvement of a multipotent hematopoietic progenitor cell, marrow hypercellularity, predisposition to thrombosis, hemorrhage, and marrow fibrosis, and more recently, mutations in different tyrosine kinases (TK), for example, JAK2 (Janus kinase 2), platelet-derived growth factor receptor (PDGFR), and KIT (2-5). When the concept of MPDs was first proposed, it consisted of five disorders: chronic myelogenous leukemia (CML), polycythemia vera (PV), essential thrombocythemia (ET), chronic idiopathic myelofibrosis (CIMF), and erythroleukemia. Over the years, erythroleukemia was reclassified under acute myeloid leukemia (AML). The remaining four (CML, PV, ET, CIMF) are recognized as classic MPDs.

The World Health Organization (WHO) 2001 classification assigned the classic MPDs to a broader category of chronic MPDs that also included atypical MPDs, namely, chronic neutrophilic leukemia (CNL), chronic eosinophilic leukemia/hypereosinophilic syndrome (CEL/HES), and chronic MPD, unclassifiable (MPD-U). The MPDs were, in turn, classified among one of the five categories of myeloid neoplasms, the others being: (1) AML, (2) myelodysplastic syndromes (MDS), (3) MDS/MPD, and (4) mast cell disease (MCD).

In the revised 2008 WHO classification system for chronic myeloid neoplasms, the phrase *disease* in both MPD and MDS/MPD has been replaced by *neoplasm,* reflecting the neoplastic nature of these conditions, so that MPD is now referred to as myeloproliferative neoplasm (MPN) (6). In addition, MCD is now included within the MPN category (Table 6-1). Also, CIMF has recently been renamed as primary myelofibrosis (PMF). CML, characterized by the reciprocal translocation of chromosomes 9 and 22, is discussed in detail elsewhere. Here we discuss classic MPNs, as well as CEL/HES and MCD, for which important advances have been made, both in the understanding of the disease pathology and clinical management.

TABLE 6-1	THE 2008 WORLD HEALTH ORGANIZATION CLASSIFICATION SCHEME FOR MYELOID NEOPLASMS

1. Acute myeloid leukemia
2. Myelodysplastic syndromes (MDS)
3. Myeloproliferative neoplasms (MPN)
   3.1 Chronic myelogenous leukemia
   3.2 Polycythemia vera
   3.3 Essential thrombocythemia
   3.4 Primary myelofibrosis
   3.5 Chronic neutrophilic leukemia
   3.6 Chronic eosinophilic leukemia, not otherwise categorized
   3.7 Hypereosinophilic syndrome
   3.8 Mast cell disease
   3.9 MPNs, unclassifiable
4. MDS/MPN
   4.1 Chronic myelomonocytic leukemia
   4.2 Juvenile myelomonocytic leukemia
   4.3 Atypical chronic myeloid leukemia
   4.4 MDS/MPN, unclassifiable
5. Myeloid neoplasms associated with eosinophilia and abnormalities of PDGFRA, PDGFRB, or FGFR1
   5.1 Myeloid neoplasms associated with PDGFRA rearrangement
   5.2 Myeloid neoplasms associated with PDGFRB rearrangement
   5.3 Myeloid neoplasms associated with FGFR1 rearrangement (8p11 myeloproliferative syndrome)

■ POLYCYTHEMIA VERA

PV is a clonal disorder involving a multipotent hematologic progenitor cell in which there is an accumulation of phenotypically normal red cells, granulocytes, and platelets. The word "polycythemia" is composed of the Greek words "poly" (many), "cyt" (cells), and "hemia" (blood), indicating too many blood cells (red, white, and platelets). The term "vera" is from the Latin word meaning true, making a distinction between PV and host of other conditions that can result in an increase in the number of red blood cells. The main feature of the disease is elevated red cell mass (RCM) associated with predisposition to thrombosis. PV is a disease of the elderly. In a large observational study of 1638 patients

with PV, median age at diagnosis was 62.1 years (7). Only 4% were <40 years old in this patient cohort. The median survival is long, approximately 20 years (although inferior to the general population).

JAK2–STAT (signal transducers and activators of transcription) pathway has been known to play an important role in the signaling pathways for erythropoietin (EPO) receptors. In 2005, four different groups identified an activating mutation in the JAK2 pathway in up to 97% of patients with PV (2-5). JAK proteins are expressed on the cytoplasmic domains of EPO receptors and the binding of EPO causes dimerization and phosphorylation of the JAKs (8). This leads to phosphorylation of the cytoplasmic domains of the EPO receptor. JAK2 is involved in the same manner with a number of other receptors for growth factors and cytokines. STATs bind to these phosphorylated receptor sites and in turn are phosphorylated by the JAKs. These phosphorylated and activated STATs molecules regulate the transcription of the target genes in the nucleus. JAK2 has 2 domains: JH1 (the active kinase domain) and JH2 (pseudokinase domain: inhibits kinase activity of JAK2). The most common mutation in PV is the guanine to thymine substitution at the position 617 of exon 14 of the JH2 domain (JAK2V617F) leading to valine to phenylalanine substitution. This is a gain of function mutation allowing JAK2 to be constitutively active and cause proliferation of erythroid precursors, in the absence of EPO. The pathologic nature of this mutation has been illustrated by many studies. Mice who receive bone marrow cells expressing JAK2 mutation develop erythrocytosis (3). Similarly, in contrast to wild-type JAK2-mutated JAK2 allows for in vitro EPO-independent growth of cultures cell lines (3-5). JAK2V617F mutation is present in approximately 95 to 97% of PV patients and is not present in secondary polycythemia (9). Mutations in exon 12 of JAK2 have been recently identified in the remaining patients with PV who are negative for JAK2V617F mutation (10). Therefore, with current sensitive testing, it is believed that all patients with PV should have either exon 14 or exon 12 mutation in JAK2.

CLINICAL FEATURES

Presenting constitutional symptoms (seen in 30 to 50% patients) include headache, weakness, pruritus, fatigue, dizziness, and sweating. Thrombosis and hemorrhage are the most common serious complication of this disease. Splenomegaly is seen in 70% patients and hepatomegaly in approximately 33% patients. Mild leukocytosis can occur with PV as can thrombocytosis. Thrombocytosis can lead to ocular migraine and erythromelalgia (burning pain in feet or hands associated with warmth and erythema). Some patients are asymptomatic and are discovered on routine blood counts. Bone marrow is typically hypercellular with megakaryocyte pleomorphism. In the PVSG01 study, cellularity of the pretreatment bone marrows (n = 281)

ranged from 36 to 100% (mean 82%) with the absence of stainable iron in 94% patients (11). Cytogenetic abnormalities are infrequent. In a large retrospective study of PV patients (n = 137), cytogenetics were abnormal in only 11% (trisomy 8 being the most common) and had no impact on either thrombosis risk or survival (12).

THROMBOSIS AND BLEEDING

Thrombosis is the most serious complication of this disease (Table 6-2). In a large study of 1213 patients with PV, thrombosis (both arterial and venous) occurred in 41% patients overall (64% thrombosis were at presentation or before diagnosis; 36% during follow-up) (13). Thrombosis is presenting manifestation in 15 to 20% patients (11,13). Ischemic stroke and transient ischemic attacks account for majority of arterial thromboses at diagnosis (13). Arterial thrombosis is more common overall than the venous thrombosis. The overall rate of thrombotic events was 3.4/100 patients per year and the rate of thrombotic events increased with age (1.8/100 patients per year for <40 years age group to 5.1/100 patients per year for those >70 years) (13). Older age and previous history of thrombosis have been established as risk factors for thrombosis in many large studies (13). In the PVSG studies, one-third of the individuals who survived the initial thrombotic event had recurrent thrombosis (14). Budd–Chiari syndrome (BCS) can be a presenting manifestation of PV. PV is the underlying cause for up to 50% of patients with BCS (15) and JAK2 mutation has been found in 40 to 58% of BCS patients (16).

Development of myelofibrosis (MF; called post-PV MF) and AML are the two major late complications of this disease. Post-PV MF develops in 10 to 20% of PV patients and is characterized by clinical features similar to PMF (anemia, cytopenias, leukoerythroblastosis,

TABLE 6-2 | **THROMBOSIS AND BLEEDING IN POLYCYTHEMIA VERA (AT DIAGNOSIS AND AT FOLLOW-UP)**

			AT DIAGNOSIS		AT FOLLOW-UP			
Study	*No. of Patients*	*Asymptomatic*	*Major Thrombosis (%) (Arterial %, Venous %)*	*Bleeding (%)*	*Major Thrombosis (%) (Arterial %, Venous %)*	*Bleeding (%)*	*Deaths From Thrombosis (%)*	*Deaths From Bleeding (%)*
PVSG01	431	NR	13.9 (61,39)	14.9	27.6 (NR, NR)	2.7	31	5
GISP	1213	NR	34 (66.6,33.3)	NR	19 (62.5, 37.5)	NR	29.7	2.6
ECLAP	1638	NR	35.8 (75, 25)	8.1	10.3 (69.8, 30.2)	7.1	26	3.7
Passamonti (2000)	163	37	34 (64,36)	3	18 (80, 20)	NR	19	6

and progressive splenomegaly). Trisomy 1q is the most common chromosome abnormality in post-PV MF patients. The longer disease duration (>10 years) predicted for increased risk of post-PV MF ($p < .0001$) (17). Passamonti et al. reported outcomes on a large series of 647 patients with PV of which 68 patients developed post-PV MF after a median of 13 years (18). The median survival for post-PV MF was 5.7 years (18). In the ECLAP study, 22 of the 1638 patients (1.3%) developed AML after a median of 8.4 years from the diagnosis of PV. Older age and exposure to chemotherapy (^{32}P, busulphan, and pipobroman; $p = .002$), but not HU alone was associated with increased risk of AML (7).

Most common fatal complication in PV is thrombosis, accounting for 19 to 31% of deaths during follow-up (see Table 6-2). In a large study of 1213 patients, the most frequent fatal complications were thrombosis (30%) and cancer (15% AML, 15% other cancers) (13). In the ECLAP study (n = 1638), the most common cause of death were cardiovascular diseases, AML, and solid tumors in 45, 13, and 19.5%, respectively (17). As is the case with thrombotic risk, older age and history of thrombosis are associated with increased mortality (17). Recently, leukocytosis (WBC count $>15 \times 10^9$/L) at diagnosis of PV has been correlated with increased risk of thrombosis (especially myocardial infarction) (19), leukemic transformation (20), development of post-PV MF (18), and survival (20).

DIAGNOSIS

As our understanding of this disease has improved with development of newer molecular markers such as JAK2 mutation, so have been the diagnostic criteria for PV (Table 6-3). As JAK2V617F or similar activating mutations such as exon 12 mutations are present in almost 100% of PV patients, the 2008 WHO classification appropriately incorporates JAK2 mutation as a major criterion for the PV diagnosis. In addition, as compared to the PVSG criteria where RCM measurement was mandatory, the WHO criteria's have placed less reliance on direct RCM measurement and have established hemoglobin (Hb) cutoffs (Hb >18.5 g/dL in men or Hb >16.5 g/dL in women; Hb >17 g/dL in men and >15 g/dL in women if associated with a documented and sustained increase of at least 2 g/dL from an individual's baseline value that cannot be attributed to correction of iron deficiency) for diagnostic purposes. This view point is not universally held and many experts still advocate use of direct RCM measurement (21). For patients suspected to have PV (based on elevated Hb/hematocrit (Hct), presence of symptoms or

TABLE 6-3	2008 WORLD HEALTH ORGANIZATION DIAGNOSTIC CRITERIA FOR POLYCYTHEMIA VERA

WHO (2008)

Major criteria
- Hb >18.5 g/dL in men or Hb >16.5 g/dL in women or other evidence of increased red cell volume
- Presence of JAK2V617F or other functionally similar mutations such as JAK2 exon 12 mutation

Minor criteria
- Bone marrow biopsy showing hypercellularity for age with panmyelosis with prominent erythroid, granulocytic, and megakaryocytic proliferation
- Serum erythropoietin level below the reference range for normal
- Endogenous erythroid colony formation in vitro

Diagnosis: Both major criteria with one minor or first major with any two minor criteria

Reproduced, with permission, from Tafferi A, Thiele J, Orazi A, et al. Proposals and rationale for revision of the World Health Organization diagnostic criteria for polycythemia vera, essential thrombocythemia, and primary myelofibrosis: Recommendations from an ad hoc international expert panel. *Blood* 2007;110(4):1092-1097.

thrombotic/hemorrhagic complications), initial evaluation should include peripheral blood JAK2 mutation analysis and measurement of serum EPO (Fig. 6-1). As red cell proliferation is autonomous in PV, serum EPO is generally low and erythroid colonies can grow in in vitro cultures without addition of exogenous EPO. For patients who have not received prior chemotherapy, endogenous (EPO-independent) erythroid colony formation test has sensitivity and specificity approaching 100%; however, the test is not commercially available. Classical morphologic features seen in bone marrow biopsies from PV and post-PV MF patients are shown in Figs. 6-2 to 6-4.

TREATMENT

The main goal of therapy is to prevent thrombotic events. Cornerstone of therapy is phlebotomy. This was established by the PVSG01 trial in which patients were randomized to phlebotomy alone, phlebotomy plus chlorambucil and phlebotomy plus ^{32}P. Incidence of thrombosis during the first 2 years of the trial was significantly higher in the phlebotomy arm (23%) compared to 16% in the ^{32}P arm. However, median survival was significantly higher in the phlebotomy alone arm (12.6 years versus 10.9 years in the ^{32}P arm and 9.1 in the chlorambucil arm). In addition, AML risk was 1.5, 9.6, and 13.2% in the phlebotomy alone, ^{32}P and chlorambucil arm, respectively. Incidence of MF was similar

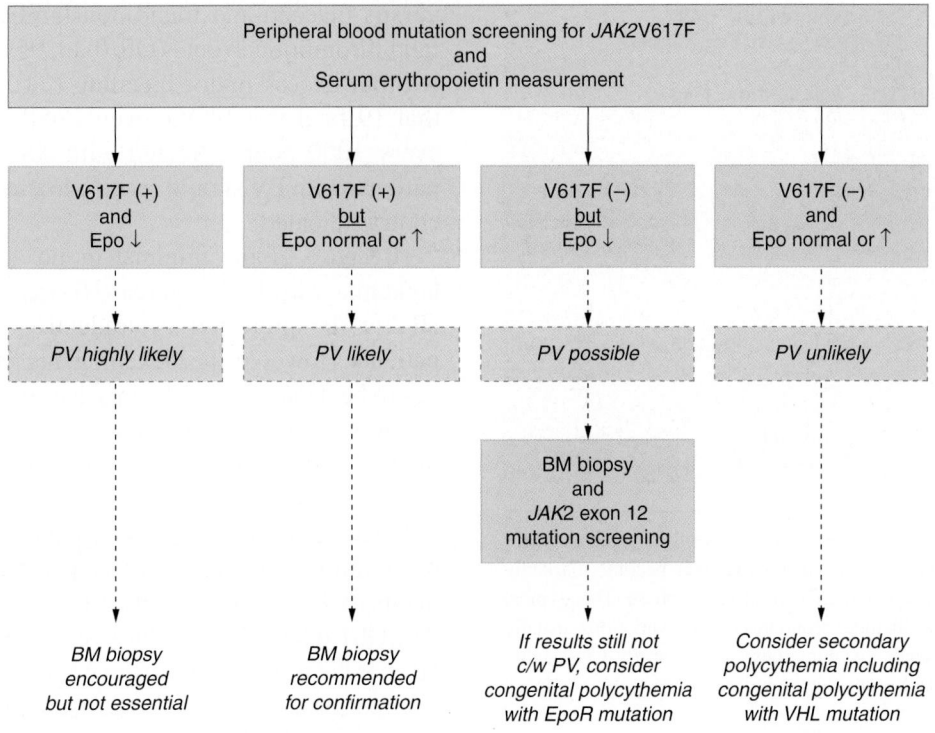

FIGURE 6-1. Diagnostic algorithm for suspected polycythemia vera. *(Reproduced, with permission, from Tefferi A, Vardiman JW. Classification and diagnosis of myeloproliferative neoplasms: The 2008 World Health Organization criteria and point-of-care diagnostic algorithms. Leukemia 2008;22:14-22.)*

in all three arms. Given the increased risk of AML in chlorambucil arm along with decreased survival, further use of chlorambucil in PV was abandoned. This trial also provided the evidence for regular use of phlebotomy in these patients. The desired goal of Hct is ≤45% for males and ≤42% for females. Regular phlebotomy induces iron deficiency, which has not been shown to be detrimental in the absence of anemia. PV patients who become iron deficient due to phlebotomy use should not receive any iron supplementation.

FIGURE 6-2. Bone marrow biopsy from a patient with PV shows remarkable hypercellularity because of myeloid hyperplasia and markedly increased megakaryocytes. Although morphologically some of the megakaryocytes demonstrate slight size variations, most of the megakaryocytes are unremarkable (200×).

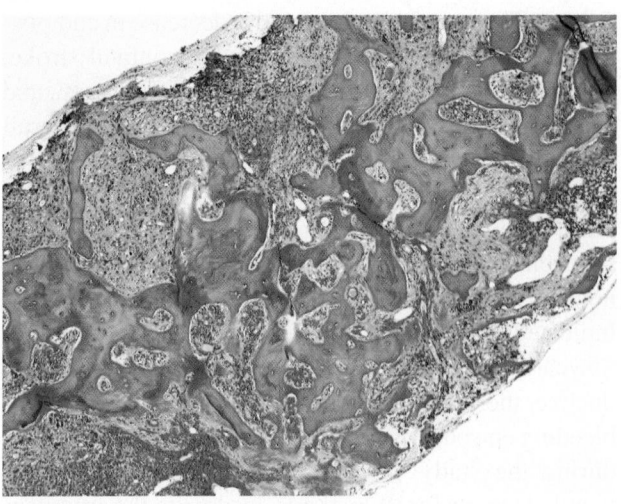

FIGURE 6-3. Extensive bone remodeling and osteosclerosis are occasionally encountered features in bone marrow biopsies during the post-polycythemic myelofibrosis phase of PV (40×).

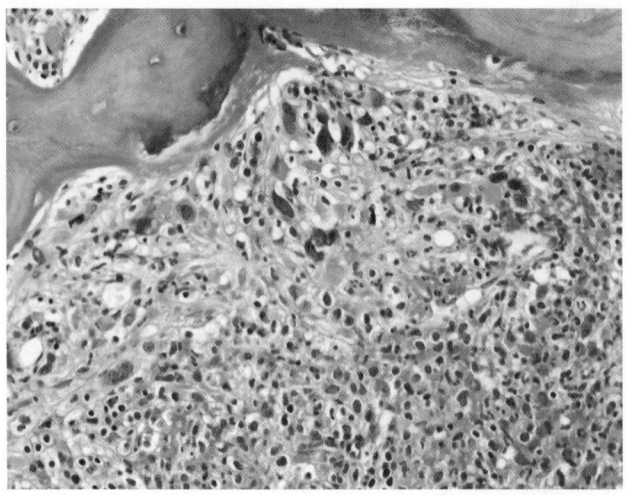

FIGURE 6-4. In contrast to the relatively normal megakaryocytes seen during early stages of PV, megakaryocytes become markedly atypical during post-polycythemic myelofibrosis phase. The atypical morphologic features include pronounced size variations usually because of the presence of numerous small forms. Classically, megakaryocytes nuclei become hyperchromatic during this advanced stage of PV (200×).

High-dose aspirin (ASA) (900 mg daily), studied by PVSG, was found to have increased risk of gastrointestinal bleeding in PV patients and was not pursued further (22). Based on pilot data that increase in thromboxane synthesis occurs in PV, predisposing to thrombosis and that ASA at low doses effectively suppress the production of thromboxane, Landolfi et al. randomized 518 patients with PV to low-dose ASA (100 mg daily) or placebo (ECLAP study) (23). All patients were previously treated with phlebotomy or cytoreductive therapy or both. The use of ASA led to 60% decrease in composite primary endpoint of nonfatal MI, nonfatal stroke, pulmonary embolism, major venous thrombosis, and death from cardiovascular standpoint ($p = .03$). Overall mortality, cardiovascular mortality, major venous thrombosis, pulmonary embolism was not statistically different between the two groups. Major cerebrovascular events were decreased from 3.8 to 1.2%, although not statistically significant ($p = .08$). Subgroup analysis indicated ASA was more effective in disease duration ≤5 years, platelets count $<334 \times 10^9$/L, no use of cytoreductive therapy and Hct ≥48%. Incidence of major bleeding episodes was similar. The median Hct achieved during the study was 46%, higher than the recommended targets for PV patients, leading to the argument that effective Hct control may lessen the beneficial effects of ASA. Recent Cochrane analysis studied 630 patients of PV randomized to low-dose ASA

versus placebo and found nonsignificant lowering of fatal thrombotic events (OR 0.20, 95% CI 0.03-1.14), without excess major bleeding (24). They predicted that 19 fatal thrombotic events will be prevented for every 1000 people treated with ASA. Therefore, all patients with PV should receive low-dose ASA, unless contraindicated.

Because of the minimal or no additional risk of leukemia with hydroxyurea (HU) use in PV patients, HU is the preferred cytoreductive therapy for PV patients. However, the leukemogenic risk of HU continues to be debated (25). Aggressive chemotherapy is not recommended. In a large study with 1213 PV patients, the risk of death due to cancer was four times higher in patients who had received ^{32}P or myelosuppressive (alkylating or nonalkylating) agents compared to those receiving phlebotomy or other pharmacological treatments (6.7% compared with 1.6%; $p = .06$) supporting PVSG01 data (13). Similarly, combination of ^{32}P and HU has been shown to worsen AML risk.

Interferon-alpha (IFN-α), first reported in 1988, has been reported to be effective on suppressing erythrocytosis in 82% of patients with a similar number reporting reduction in spleen size and alleviation of pruritus (26). IFN-α is not teratogenic and therefore the cytoreductive therapy of choice in pregnancy. It is also not leukemogenic (7). However, up to one-third of patients discontinue treatment due to side-effects such as fever, malaise, depression.

Longer-acting pegylated forms of IFN-α (PEG-IFN-α-2a) have also been studied in PV patients. Kiladjian et al. reported the results of a phase 2 multicenter French study of PEG-IFN-α-2a in 40 PV patients (27). The primary end point was hematologic response at 12 months. Complete hematologic response (CHR) was defined by a Hct <45% in males and <42% in females, without phlebotomy, absence of splenomegaly, and normal white blood cell (WBC) and platelet counts. At 12 months, all 37 evaluable patients had hematologic response, including 94.6% CHR. Sequential samples for JAK2V617F allele burden showed decrease in 26 (89.6%) patients. Complete molecular response (CMR, undetectable JAK2V617F) was achieved in seven (24.1%) patients. Our group reported results on 40 patients with PV treated with (PEG-IFN-α-2a) (28). The overall hematologic response was 80% including CHR rate of 70%. An important difference between the two trials was that the French trial treated patients early in their diagnosis with the median time between PV diagnosis and trial inclusion of 5 months as compared to 54 months in MD Anderson study. Both trials showed PEG-IFN-α-2a to be safe, with most side effects being grade 1 to 2, in less than 10% of patients. Novel therapies, targeting the JAK2 mutation are being developed for PV patients and clinical trials exploring such agents are currently underway. For example, a recent phase 2 clinical trial evaluated INCB018424, a potent, orally available JAK1/JAK2 inhibitor, in 34 patients with PV refractory to HU (29). Inclusion criteria included Hct >45% or dependence on phlebotomies. JAK2V617F mutation was present in 100% of the patients. The initial part of the trial determined the best dose schedule of 10 mg twice daily, which was then expanded with more patients in the second part of the study. The median follow-up was 10.4 months. Therapy with INCB018424 resulted in rapid and durable normalization of the Hct in 97% of the patients. There was also rapid and sustained normalization of WBC and platelet counts, reduction in spleen size and improvement in systemic symptoms (pruritus, bone pain, night sweats). Overall response rate (ORR) was 100%, including a complete response (CR) rate of 62%. CR was defined as: normalization of Hct (<45% males, <42% females), WBC counts, platelets, spleen size; no phlebotomies, and no thrombotic events. Most common side effect was anemia (grade 2: 12%), and most common grade 3 side effect was thrombocytopenia (3%). No grade 4 toxicities were recorded. These initials results were encouraging, and further studies with this compound are planned for patients with PV.

TREATMENT CONCLUSIONS

All patients with PV should undergo phlebotomy. All patients should receive low-dose ASA, unless contradicted. Patients who are at high risk for thrombosis (age >60 years or history of thrombosis) should receive cytoreductive therapy (HU is the preferred agent; however IFN-α can be considered, especially PEG-IFN-α-2a). The goal Hct is $\leq$45% for males and $\leq$42% for females. Those resistant/intolerant to standard therapies should be considered for inclusion in clinical studies with JAK2 inhibitors.

■ ESSENTIAL THROMBOCYTHEMIA

ET is characterized by persistent thrombocytosis with a predisposition to thrombosis and bleeding. ET is not a cytogenetically or a morphologically defined disease entity and remains a diagnosis of exclusion. It is a disease of the elderly and the median age of diagnosis is 55 to 60 years with a female-to-male ratio of 2:1.

It is important to exclude reactive causes of thrombocytosis. Most of times the underlying cause is apparent (post splenectomy, acute infection, blood loss). Other

MPNs such as PV or CML can present with thrombocytosis and therefore, it is important to exclude these before a diagnosis of ET is made. In a population-based study (ages 18 to 65 years), 99 of the 9998 persons studied (1%) had platelet count >400 × 10^9/L at baseline of which only 8 (0.1% of the population studied) had persistent thrombocytosis at >6 months (30). Three of these 8 patients were confirmed to have ET at baseline with one additional ET diagnosis after 5 years of follow-up. In another study of 732 patients with thrombocytosis (>500 × 10^9/L), ET was present in 5.5% and reactive thrombocytosis in 87% patients (31). Height of the elevation of the platelet count does not distinguish between reactive and clonal thrombocytosis. In 280 consecutive patients (both outpatients and inpatients) with extreme thrombocytosis (platelet count >1 million), reactive thrombocytosis was seen in 82% patients, with 14% representing MPNs including 4% ET (32). Reactive thrombocytosis, irrespective of degree of elevation of platelet count, does not per se increase the risk of thromboembolic or bleeding complications. Such complications, if seen, are results of underlying disease condition (malignancy, iron deficiency from gastrointestinal bleeding) rather than elevated platelets.

PATHOPHYSIOLOGY

Thrombopoietin (TPO) regulates the differentiation and proliferation of megakaryocytes. It is produced primarily by the liver parenchymal cells and the gene for TPO is located on chromosome 3q27-28. It binds to the c-Mpl receptors on platelets and megakaryocytes. When platelet count is low, more of free TPO is available to bind to megakaryocytes to stimulation proliferation, leading to rise in platelet count and vice-versa. In most cases of reactive thrombocytosis, TPO is increased in amount via acute phase reactants such as interleukin-6. Unlike PV where EPO levels are generally low, TPO levels are high normal or abnormally increased in ET (33). This may be due to the increased bone marrow stromal production of TPO or decreased clearance as expression on platelet c-Mpl is markedly reduced in ET patients (33). The discovery of JAK2V617F mutation ushered a new era in the understanding of ET. JAK2V617F mutation is present in approximately 50% of ET patients. More recently, MPLW515L (guanine to thymidine substitution in MPL at nucleotide 1544 resulting in a tryptophan to leucine substitution at codon 515) mutation have been reported in 1% of ET patients (34,35). In the murine model, animals with MPLW515L-transduced bone marrow developed significant thrombocytosis, leukocytosis, and bone marrow fibrosis, indicating ET/MF phenotype (35).

CLINICAL FEATURES

With the increasing use of automated blood counters and routine blood count screenings, more patients with ET are being diagnosed in asymptomatic stage. Constitutional symptoms are uncommon in ET. Vasomotor manifestations such as dizziness, lightheadedness, acral paresthesia, livedo reticularis, erythromelalgia were noted in 34% of patients in one series of 147 ET patients (36). Mild splenomegaly (<5 cm) can be seen in up to 40% patients. Leukocytosis can be seen in 30 to 40% patients and mild anemia in 10 to 20% patients. Thromboembolic and bleeding complications are the major cause of morbidity and mortality in ET. Fenaux et al. reported 18% thrombosis (15% arterial thrombosis, 3% venous thrombosis) and 4% major bleeding at diagnosis (36). Recent study by Tefferi et al. reported 26% incidence of major thrombosis and 11% incidence of major bleeding at diagnosis in a series of 322 ET patients (37). Hemorrhagic complications increase with extreme thrombocytosis (platelet count >1.5 million/μL) and with the use of antiplatelet therapy such as ASA.

Most serious late complications of ET include transformation to AML and MF (post-ET MF). In a large study of 605 patients with ET, Tefferi et al. reported risk of AML transformation to be 3.3% with the median time to transformation at 11.5 years (38). Risk factors for transformation included anemia, platelet count >1000 × 10⁹/L and increasing age (38). JAK2 mutational status or the type of therapy (including HU) did not influence the risk of leukemic transformation (38). In a series of 195 patients with ET, the median time to transform to post-ET MF was 8 years with actuarial probability of 2.7% at 5 years, 8.3% at 10 years, and 15.3% at 15 years (39).

DIAGNOSIS

ET remains a diagnosis of exclusion. Reactive thrombocytosis must be ruled out. An important change in the new 2008 WHO classification is the lowering of the platelet count for ET diagnosis from 600×10^9/L to 450×10^9/L (Table 6-4). Bone marrow biopsy is mandatory for ET diagnosis and it characteristically shows large but mature appearing megakaryocytes with deeply lobulated or hyperlobulated nuclei (Fig. 6-5). The peripheral smear is mostly significant for markedly increased platelets (Fig. 6-6). Reticulin staining should be done to rule out any underlying fibrosis. CML should be ruled out by testing for Bcr-Abl. JAK2 mutation testing should be done because if present, it establishes the clonal nature of the disease (Fig. 6-7).

TABLE 6-4	2008 WHO CRITERIA FOR DIAGNOSIS OF ESSENTIAL THROMBOCYTHEMIA

1. Sustained platelet count $\geq 450 \times 10^9$/L
2. Bone marrow biopsy specimen showing proliferation mainly of the megakaryocytic lineage with increased numbers of enlarged, mature megakaryocytes; no significant increase or left-shift of neutrophil granulopoiesis or erythropoiesis
3. Not meeting WHO criteria for PV, PMF, CML, MDS, or other myeloid neoplasm
4. Demonstration of JAK2V617F or other clonal marker, or in the absence of a clonal marker, no evidence for reactive thrombocytosis

Diagnosis of ET requires meeting all four criteria

Reproduced, with permission, from Tafferi A, Thiele J, Orazi A, et al. Proposals and rationale for revision of the World Health Organization diagnostic criteria for polycythemia vera, essential thrombocythemia, and primary myelofibrosis: Recommendations from an ad hoc international expert panel. *Blood* 2007;110(4):1092-1097.

PROGNOSIS

Like PV, thrombosis and hemorrhage are the main complications of ET. Carobbio et al. studied 1063 patients with ET and reported the risk of major thrombosis at 2.3% patients/year and of major bleeding (gastrointestinal bleeding in 80%) at 0.76% patients/year (40). Older age and history of prior thrombosis has been shown to predict for future thrombotic events in majority of the studies, whereas cardiovascular risk factors

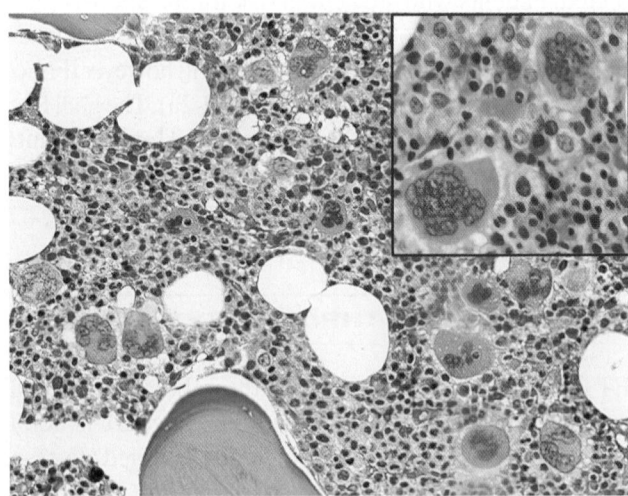

FIGURE 6-5. ET is characterized by increased bone marrow cellularity, myeloid hyperplasia, and notably increased megakaryocytes (200X). The megakaryocytes in ET tend to display larger than normal size and they also contain large hyperlobulated nuclei (insert; 400X).

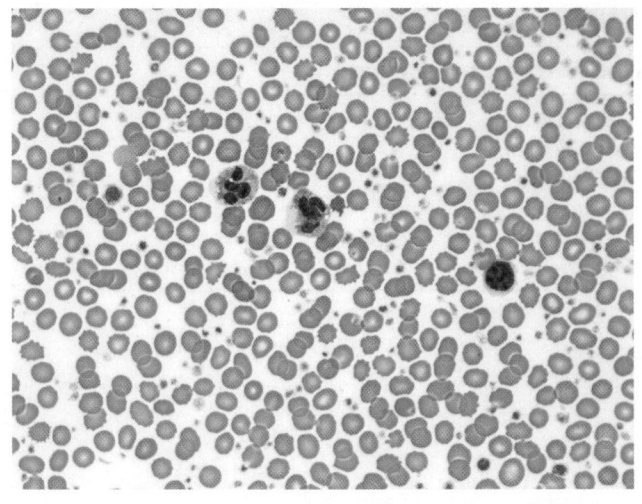

FIGURE 6-6. Peripheral blood smear from a patient with ET shows markedly increased platelets with scattered large forms (400×).

have been predictive in only some (Table 6-5). In a retrospective analysis by De Stefano et al. of 259 ET patients with prior thrombosis, there was 31.2% recurrence risk with the risk being 5.3% patient/year (41). The recurrence of either arterial or venous thrombosis depended on whether the first event was arterial or venous. Older patients (age >60) were more likely to get recurrent thrombosis. Cytoreduction reduced the risk of recurrence by 47% ($p = .0002$) (41). Antiplatelet

therapy alone reduced the risk by 28% (borderline statistically significance, $p = .07$).

Platelet count has never been shown to correlate with thrombotic risk in ET (see Table 6-5). On the contrary, recent studies have found an inverse relation between the platelet count and the thrombotic risk. This is thought to be due to acquired Von Willebrand factor (vWF) disease with elevated platelet counts, predisposing to more bleeding and protection from thrombosis. As in PV, increased WBC count is now being recognized as a risk factor for thrombosis. Carobbio et al. reported that the risk of thrombosis increased from 1.59% patients/year in patients presenting with WBC $<11 \times 10^9$/L and platelet $>1000 \times 10^9$/L to 2.95% patients/year in those presenting with WBC $>11 \times 10^9$/L and platelet $<1000 \times 10^9$/L (40).

Presence of JAK2V617F mutation is associated with older age, increased Hb, increased WBC, and lower platelet count in majority of studies in ET patients. Presence of JAK2V617F does not appear to influence either survival (42) or disease transformation rates to either AML or MF (42,43). Patients who are homozygous for JAK2V617F are at higher risk of thrombosis that in wild-type JAK2 or heterozygous patients (44). JAK2V617F homozygosity is also associated with occurrence of major cardiovascular events (hazard risk 3.97, $p = .013$ compared with wild-type ET patients) (44). JAK2 mutation has also been identified as an independent predictor of pregnancy

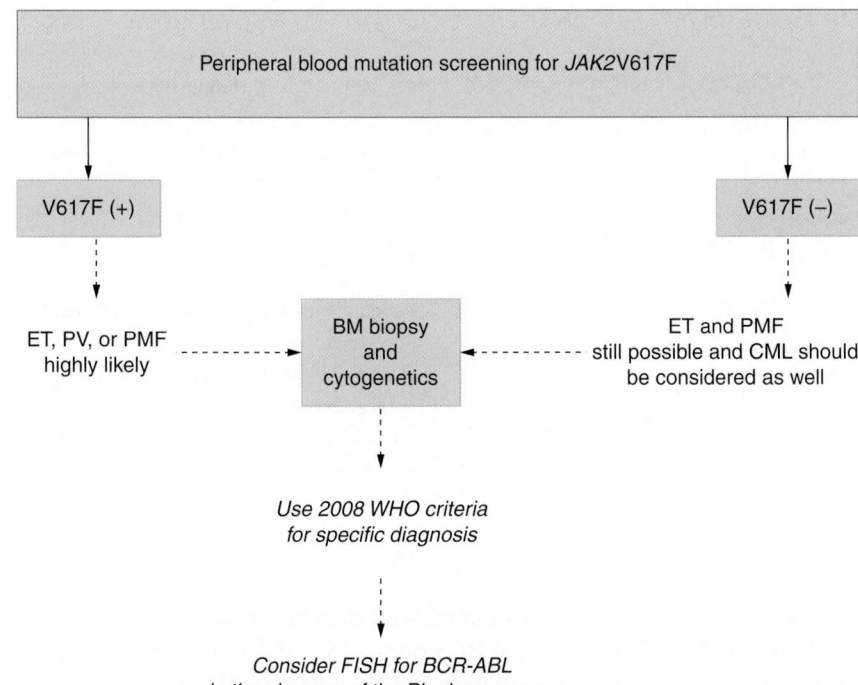

FIGURE 6-7. Diagnostic algorithm for suspected essential thrombocytosis. *(Reproduced, with permission, from Tefferi A, Vardiman JW. Classification and diagnosis of myeloproliferative neoplasms: The 2008 World Health Organization criteria and point-of-care diagnostic algorithms. Leukemia 2008; 22:14-22.)*

TABLE 6-5   RISK FACTORS FOR THROMBOSIS IN ET PATIENTS

RISK FACTORS STUDIED

Study	No. of Patients	Age >60 Years, Odds Ratio/ Hazard Ratio/ Significance Level	History of Thrombosis	Risk Factors for CV Events (Smoking, Diabetes, Hypertension, Hyperlipidemia)	Platelet Count	Leukocytosis	JAK-2 Status
Colombi (1991)	103	NS	$p < .001$	–	NS	–	–
Cortelazzo (1990)	100	10.3	13	NS	NS	–	–
Besses (1999)	148	3.3	3.0	4.7	NS	–	–
Bazzan (1999)	187	NS	–	NS	NS	–	–
Jantunen (2001)	132	NS	–	$p = .01$	NS	–	–
Chim (2005)	231	$p = .01$	NS	–	NS	–	–
Wolanskyj (2006)	322	1.51	2.3 (arterial only)	NS	–	1.74 (WBC > 15,000)	NS
Carobbio (2007)	439	2.3 (age and previous thrombosis evaluated together)	2.3	–	NS	2.3 (WBC > 8700)	NS
Alvarez-Larran (2007)	126 (<40 yrs)	NA	NS	Smoking	NS	–	NS
Radaelli (2007)	306	NS	7.6	$p < .05$	NS	–	–
Tefferi (2007)	605	NS	$p < .001$	NS	–	WBC (≥15,000) $p < .01$ for thrombosis at baseline (NS for thrombosis on follow-up)	NS
Passamonti (2008)	605	$p < .001$	$p = .03$	NS	NS	NS	–
Carobbio (2008)	1063	1.7 (age and previous thrombosis evaluated together)	1.7	–	Patients with WBC less than 11,000 and platelet < 1000: most likely to have JAK-2 mutation and highest risk of thrombosis		

NS, nonsignificant; (–), not studied.

complications (45). Cytogenetic abnormalities are uncommon in ET (<10% at diagnosis) and have not been correlated with survival or transformation risk (46). The survival in ET is similar to general population.

Factors associated with decreased survival include age ≥60 years, WBC count ≥15 × 10^9/L, low Hb (<12 g/dL in women, <13.5 g/dL in men), smoking, diabetes, and prior venous thrombosis (38).

TABLE
6-6
TREATMENT OF ESSENTIAL THROMBOCYTHEMIA

Risk Category	*Intervention*
High risk (age <60 years or history of thrombosis)	Cytoreduction* and low-dose ASA
Intermediate risk (age <60 years and no h/o thrombosis) with cardiovascular risk factors, especially smoking and/or platelet count > 1000×10^9/L	Low-dose ASA (caution ASA use with extreme thrombocytosis, rule out von Willebrand disease first)
	Cytoreduction* if bleeding present; role of cytoreduction in absence of bleeding unclear
Low risk (age <60 years and no h/o thrombosis)	Observation or low-dose ASA

*Cytoreduction: HU first choice; low-dose aspirin (ASA) indicated for microvascular symptoms for any risk group.

TREATMENT

The goal of therapy in ET is to prevent the major cause of morbidity and mortality: thromboembolic events. At the same time, as the survival in ET is considered similar to general population, excess treatment with potential dangerous side effects should be avoided. Cardiovascular risk factors should be aggressively managed in all patients. Smoking has been shown to be an important risk factor for thrombosis in many studies and therefore all patients should be advised smoking cessation. The two major classes of drugs used in ET are antiplatelet therapy and the cytoreductive therapy (Table 6-6).

ANTIPLATELET THERAPY

Antiplatelet therapy with ASA is very useful in treating the microvascular symptoms of ET, especially erythromelalgia. Role of antiplatelet therapy in reducing thrombotic episodes in ET is less clear as no placebo-controlled randomized trial is available. In a retrospective study, Van Genderen et al. showed decreased thrombosis risk with ASA monotherapy (47). Extrapolating from the ECLAP study results in PV (23), the general consensus is to use low-dose ASA (75-100 mg daily) in patients with ET, unless contraindicated by bleeding history. Caution should be exercised in using ASA in patients with very high platelet count (>1500×10^9/L) due to increased risk of bleeding due to acquired von Willebrand disease (48). In the UK MRC PT-1 trial comparing HU and anagrelide in ET, all patients received antiplatelet therapy, unless contraindicated (49). In this trial, possibly because of the synergistic effect of ASA with anagrelide, an increased risk of bleeding was noted in the anagrelide arm compared to HU.

CYTOREDUCTIVE THERAPY

HU and anagrelide are the two main cytoreductive agents currently used in patients with ET. HU is a nonspecific, cytotoxic, and myelosuppressive drug, whereas anagrelide has selective effect on megakaryocyte lineage. Two large randomized studies in ET patients have established the role of HU. In the Italian study by Cortelazzo et al., 114 patients with high-risk ET (age >60 years or history of thrombosis or both) were randomized to receive either placebo or HU with a goal platelet count to <600×10^9/L (50). After a median follow up of 27 months, 3.6% in the HU had thrombotic episodes compared to 24% in the placebo ($p = .003$). This study established the antithrombotic effect of HU in ET patients. Harrison et al. reported UK MRC PT-1 study with 809 high-risk ET patients randomized to receive HU plus ASA or anagrelide plus ASA (49). The goal platelet count was <400×10^9/L. Anagrelide group had higher rate of composite endpoint of thrombosis, serious hemorrhage or death from these complications compared to HU arm. Anagrelide arm had significantly higher arterial thrombosis with lower venous thrombosis rate compared to HU arm. Serious hemorrhage was seen more frequently in anagrelide arm, likely due to synergistic effect with ASA. Risk of MF was significantly higher in anagrelide arm (5-year risk 7% versus 2% in HU arm) and significantly more patients withdrew from the study because of side effects in the anagrelide arm compared to HU (22% versus 11%, $p = .001$). Risk of development of MDS/AML was similar in the two arms. Based on this trial, HU is now considered the standard first-line treatment for ET patients needing cytoreduction. However, the debate over the long-term safety of HU (especially potential leukemogenic risk) coupled with the recently reported ANAHYDRET study showing noninferiority of anagrelide monotherapy compared to HU monotherapy, have reignited the debate about the optimal first line therapy of ET patients (51).

IFN-α has been used with >75% hematological response rate in various series. Average starting dose is 3 to 5 million units SQ daily. Side effects such as depression and flu-like symptoms limit frontline use in ET patients. Because of nonteratogenetic nature, IFN-α is mainly used in pregnant women and in high-risk women of child bearing age. PEG-IFN-α-2a, providing once weekly dosing has been evaluated in 39 ET patients at our center (28). CHR (defined as normalization of platelet count in the absence of thromboembolic events) was noted in 76% patients. Of the 16 patients with available serial samples for JAK2 allele burden, 38% were noted to have some decease in JAK2 allele with 6% achieving CMR. The majority of side effects were grade 1 to 2 with neutropenia being the most common toxicity observed. This result establishes PEG-IFN-α-2a as an important therapeutic option for ET patients.

SPECIAL ISSUES

Management of Extreme Thrombocytosis (Platelet Count >1.5 million/μL)

ASA should be avoided due to risk of bleeding secondary to acquired von Willebrand disease. Use of cytoreductive agents is recommended, especially when bleeding is present. Many experts regard extreme thrombocytosis as a high-risk category and treat all patients in this category with cytoreduction while others reserve it for bleeding complications only.

Management of Young Patients with ET

Ruggeri et al. prospectively studied 65 asymptomatic ET patients who were <60 years age and with platelet count $<1500 \times 10^9$/L (52). No prophylactic cytoreduction was given and ASA was used only for erythromelalgia symptoms. Risk of thromboembolic complications was found to be similar to control population. The occurrence of pregnancy or minor surgical intervention was not associated with an increased risk of thrombosis. Cytoreductive therapy was needed in 27% patients at a median of 34 months. Tefferi et al. studied 74 young female ET patients <50 years of age (53). Risk of thrombosis and major hemorrhage was lower (7% at diagnosis and 18% at follow-up for thrombosis; 4% major hemorrhage at diagnosis and follow-up) than general ET patients. Patients with history of thrombosis had 45% rethrombosis rate compared to 13% in those without prior thrombosis, indicating the need for cytoreduction with history of thrombosis, even at young age. None of the 34 pregnancies in this patient population were associated with a major thrombotic complication.

■ PRIMARY MYELOFIBROSIS

PMF is a clonal disorder of a multipotent hematopoietic progenitor cell of unknown etiology, characterized by myeloid cell proliferation, megakaryocytic atypia, marrow fibrosis, leukoerythroblastic peripheral blood picture, extramedullary hematopoiesis (EMH), and splenomegaly. PMF was previously called CIMF, MF with myeloid metaplasia (MMM), or agnogenic myeloid metaplasia (AMM). The disease can occur either de novo or as a late complication of PV or ET. In either case it represents stem cell–derived clonal myeloproliferation that is accompanied by intense bone marrow stromal reaction including collagen fibrosis, osteosclerosis, and angiogenesis. Both fibrogenesis and angiogenesis are considered to develop consequent to the release of various growth-promoting factors (such as vascular endothelial growth factor [VEGF], PDGF, basic fibroblast growth factor [bFGF] and transforming growth factor β [TGF-β]) from proliferating atypical megakaryocytes in the bone marrow.

PMF is a heterogeneous disorder with variable age of onset, presenting features, phenotypic manifestations, and prognosis. The incidence increases with age. In a recent large series of 1054 patients, the median age at diagnosis was 64 years with 17% patients younger than 50 years and 5% patients younger than 40 years (54). Clinical presentation can range from no/minimal symptoms where disease is discovered during workup of leukocytosis or splenomegaly, to severe symptoms. Severe fatigue is the most common presenting symptom. Constitutional symptoms (fatigue, weight loss, pruritus, low-grade fever, night sweats) are a prominent feature of the disease and can be very debilitating. Myeloproliferation is one of the major features of the disease and can lead to sequestration of immature cells and production of blood cells in sites other than the bone marrow, a phenomenon known as EMH. This commonly manifests as marked hepatosplenomegaly, with associated pain, early satiety, portal hypertension, and anemia and thrombocytopenia. Splenomegaly is present in about 80% of patients and may extend into the pelvis. Hepatomegaly is seen in 40 to 70% of patients. EMH might cause symptoms in various other organs leading to respiratory distress, pulmonary hypertension, ascites, pericardial tamponade, cord compression, and paralysis. Peripheral smear generally provides the first clue toward PMF diagnosis by the presence of characteristic tear-drop red cells and leukoerythroblastic picture (presence of immature myeloid cells including blasts in the peripheral blood). Progressive anemia generally develops requiring transfusions. Some patients may present with leukocytosis and thrombocytosis; however, most develop leukopenia and thrombocytopenia in later stages of the disease. Among the most feared complications of PMF is transformation to AML, occurring in 10 to 20% of patients in the first 10 years from diagnosis. The outcome after transformation is very poor, with a median survival of only approximately 5 months. Risk factors for leukemic transformation include peripheral blood blast percentage $\geq 3\%$, thrombocytopenia (platelet count $<100 \times 10^9/L$), and high number of circulating CD34+ cells (55). JAK2 mutational status was not correlated with leukemic transformation (55).

DIAGNOSIS

JAK2V617F mutation has been identified in 37 to 63% of patients with PMF (54,56). Prognostic relevance of JAK2 mutation remains unclear in PMF. Tefferi et al. studied 199 PMF of which 58% were JAK2V617F positive (57). Presence of JAK2 mutation did not affect the incidence of thrombosis, leukemia free survival, or overall survival (OS). In the International Working Group for Myelofibrosis Research and Treatment (IWG-MRT) series (n = 1054), JAK2 mutation was associated with age >65 years ($p = .002$) and had no effect on survival (54). However, other studies have shown JAK2 mutation to be associated with poor survival (58). JAK2 mutation has been associated with older age, higher WBC count, higher Hb, less need for blood transfusions during follow up and pruritus (54,56,58). Barosi et al. reported association of JAK2V617F mutation with large splenomegaly, need of splenectomy, and leukemic transformation (56). Other molecular events recently identified include mutations in c-MPL (c-MPL W515L/K), occurring in 5% of PMF patients and additional mutations in exon 12 of JAK2 among patients not expressing the JAK2V617F mutation (10,34,35).

Taking these new molecular developments in mind, the 2008 WHO criteria were devised for diagnosis of PMF (Table 6-7) (6,59). Morphologic features of the bone marrow during the prefibrotic (cellular) phase of PMF are shown in Fig. 6-8, and those during the fibrotic phase are depicted in Figs. 6-9 to 6-11. Classical morphological features consistent with PMF and seen in the peripheral blood smear are demonstrated in Fig. 6-12. Bone marrow histology, especially megakaryocyte morphology is a critical diagnostic criterion for PMF (Fig. 6-13). All patients suspected of PMF should undergo bone marrow biopsy with reticulin staining and testing for JAK2V617F mutation. CML should be ruled out by Bcr-Abl testing.

PROGNOSIS

The median survival is around 5 years. In a recent review of 1054 patients with PMF, the median survival was 69 months (54). Younger patients with good prognostic features may have a life expectancy exceeding 10 years.

| TABLE 6-7 | 2008 WHO CRITERIA FOR DIAGNOSIS OF PRIMARY MYELOFIBROSIS (PMF) |

Major criteria

1. Presence of megakaryocyte proliferation and atypia, usually accompanied by either reticulin and/or collagen fibrosis, or, in the absence of significant reticulin fibrosis, the megakaryocyte changes must be accompanied by an increased bone marrow cellularity characterized by granulocytic proliferation and often decreased erythropoiesis (ie, prefibrotic cellular-phase disease)

2. Not meeting WHO criteria for PV, CML, MDS, or other myeloid neoplasm

3. Demonstration of JAK2617VF or other clonal marker (eg, MPL515WL/K), or in the absence of a clonal marker, no evidence of bone marrow fibrosis due to underlying inflammatory or other neoplastic diseases

Minor criteria

1. Leukoerythroblastosis
2. Increase in serum lactate dehydrogenase level
3. Anemia
4. Palpable splenomegaly

Diagnosis of PMF requires meeting all three major criteria and at least two minor criteria

Reproduced, with permission, from Tafferi A, Thiele J, Orazi A, et al. Proposals and rationale for revision of the World Health Organization diagnostic criteria for polycythemia vera, essential thrombocythemia, and primary myelofibrosis: Recommendations from an ad hoc international expert panel. *Blood* 2007;110(4):1092-1097.

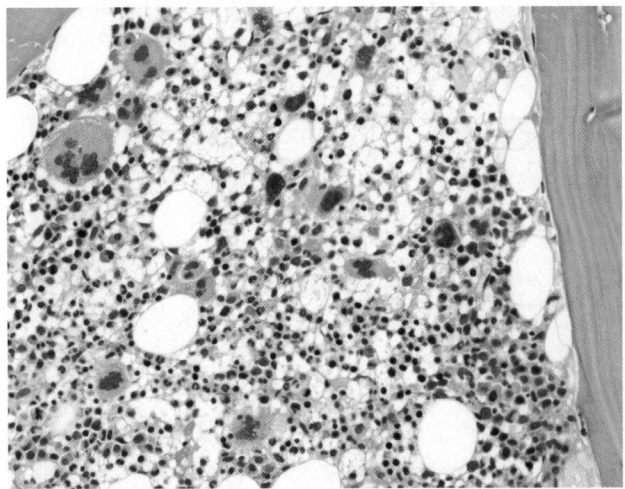

FIGURE 6-8. It is difficult to distinguish prefibrotic (cellular) phase of PMF from other types of chronic myeloproliferative neoplasms based on morphological criteria alone. However, careful microscopic examination of the bone marrow biopsy usually reveals scattered atypical megakaryocytes with morphological criteria classical for PMF in fibrotic phase. As shown, some of the megakaryocytes in this bone marrow biopsy are remarkably variable in size and shape and characteristically contain markedly hyperchromatic nuclei (200X).

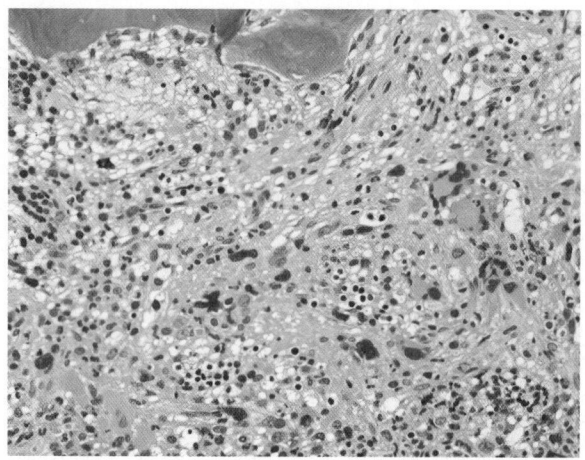

FIGURE 6-9. During the fibrotic phase of PMF, bone marrow hematopoietic cellular elements tend to decrease in number with interstitial infiltration of the bone marrow by fibroblasts that lead to streaming effect. Characteristically, the megakaryocytes demonstrate variability in size and shape, and megakaryocytes containing hyperchromatic and hyperlobulated nuclei are frequently encountered during the fibrotic phase of PMF (200×).

The most commonly used prognostic scoring system is Lille score, which is based on peripheral blood parameters (Hb <10 g/dL and WBC <4 or >30 × 10⁹/L). Based on these two parameters, patients were separated into three prognostic groups: low risk (0 factor), intermediate risk (1 factor), and high risk (2 factors), associated with a median survival of 93, 26, and 13 months, respectively. Tefferi et al. added thrombocytopenia and monocytosis to the Lille score variables to improve the prognostic

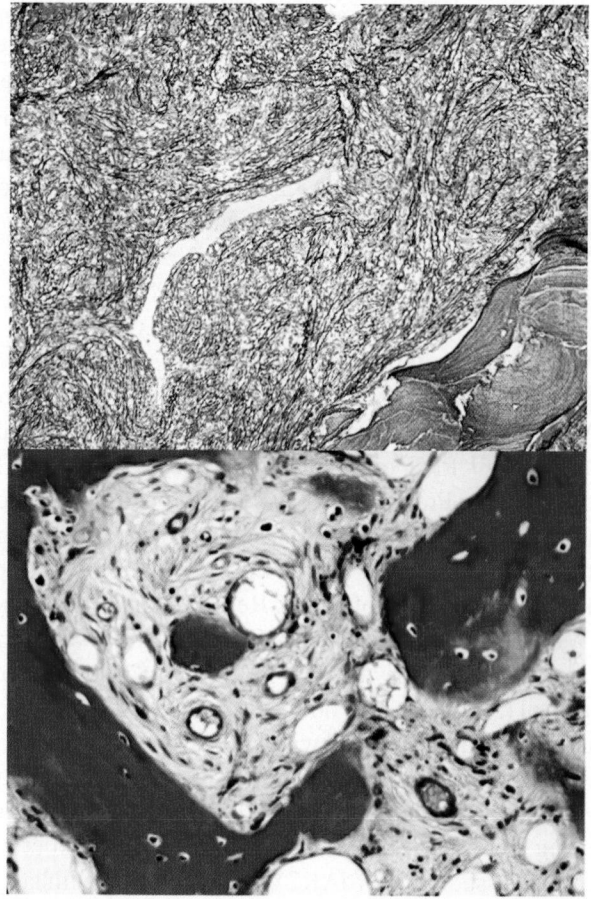

FIGURE 6-11. During the fibrotic phase of PMF the bone marrow is characterized by increased interstitial reticulin fibrosis (upper panel; 100×), which might be associated with the abnormal presence of collagen fibers that are detected by trichrome staining (lower panel; 200×).

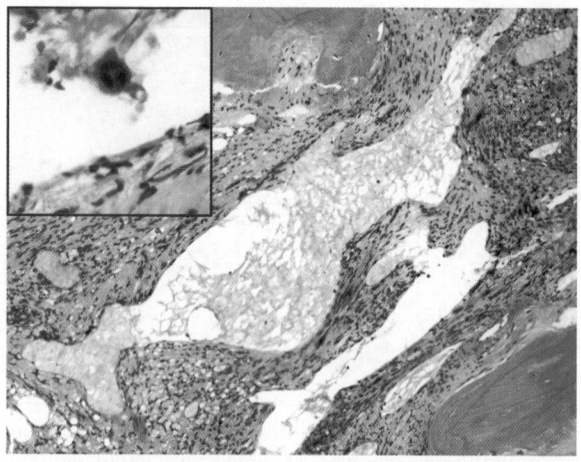

FIGURE 6-10. Another common feature of the bone marrow during the fibrotic phase is marked expansion of bone marrow sinusoids, which are usually rudimentary under normal conditions (100×). Hematopoietic cellular elements can be detected within the bone marrow sinuses; a megakaryocyte is shown, comprising what is known as intrasinusoidal hematopoiesis (insert; 400×).

accuracy (Mayo prognostic scoring system). Thrombocytopenia, monocytosis, circulating blasts, and constitutional symptoms may be prognostic in younger patients. Cervantes et al. reported a large study of 1054 patients for the IWG-MRT looking at the prognostic variables in PMF patients (54). They identified five prognostic variables for decreased survival (age >65 years, constitutional symptoms, Hb <10 g/dL, WBC count >25 × 10⁹/L, and blood blasts ≥1%). Based on the number of prognostic variables present, patients were divided into low (0 variable), intermediate-1 (1 variable), intermediate-2 (2 variables), and high (≥3 variables) groups with a median survival of 135, 95, 48, and 27 months, respectively (54). Hb <10 g/dL at diagnosis was associated with the highest impact on survival (54). Transformation to AML is the most common cause of death in MF, followed by MF progression without acute transformation, thrombosis, and cardiovascular complications, infection, bleeding, and portal hypertension.

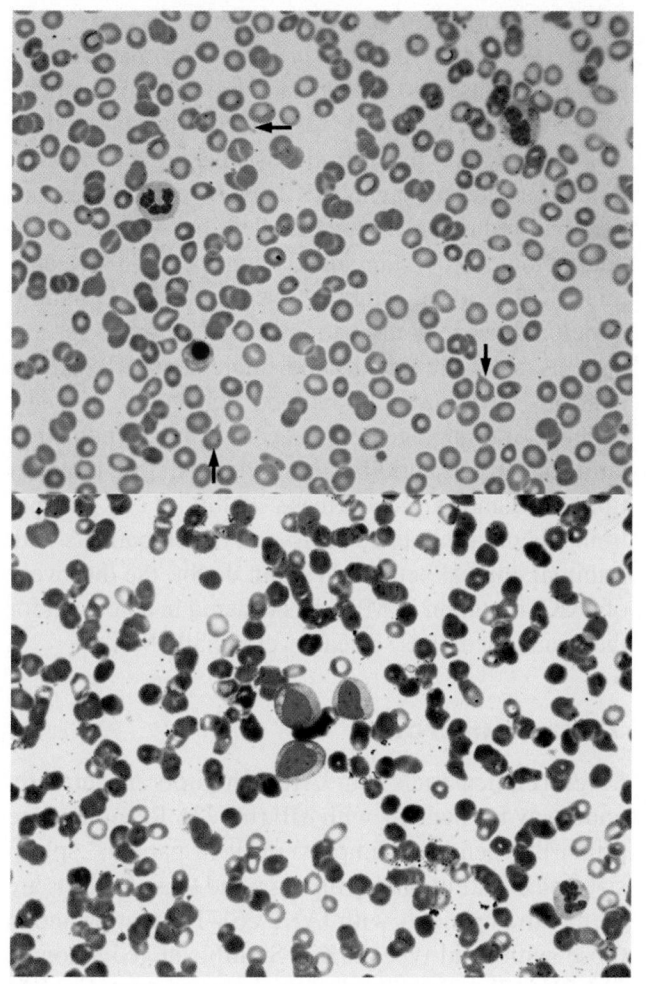

FIGURE 6-12. Careful examination of peripheral blood smears from PMF patients usually reveals teardrop red blood cells (arrows, upper panel; 400×). In addition, nucleated red blood cells (upper panel) and left-shifted granulopoiesis (lower panel; 400×) are seen; two morphologic criteria collectively described as leukoerythroblastosis.

Tam et al. analyzed 256 patients with PMF, of which 36% had chromosomal abnormality (60). They categorized patients into favorable cytogenetics (sole deletion of 13q or 20q, trisomy 9 ± one other abnormality), diploid cytogenetics, unfavorable cytogenetics (abnormalities of chromosomes 5 or 7, or complex [≥3] cytogenetics) and very unfavorable cytogenetics (abnormality of chromosome 17) with a median survival (for patients with assessment at diagnosis) of 63, 46, 15, and 5 months, respectively (60). Any chromosome abnormality of chromosome 17 was associated with worst prognosis with median survival of only 5 months (60).

TREATMENT

Treatment of MF remains unsatisfactory. No medication is approved as a specific therapy for this disease. Corticosteroids and danazol have proven helpful in treatment of the anemia in some patients. For patients with massive splenomegaly, splenectomy, splenic radiation, and chemotherapeutic agents such as busulphan and HU have been used. Anagrelide is used to control thrombocytosis. IFN-α has also been used occasionally with some success, primarily in prefibrotic stage of the disease. Allogeneic stem cell transplant (ASCT) remains the only curative modality for such patients, however most patients are not eligible for ASCT due to increased age or severe comorbidities.

The group from Seattle reported 104 patients with PMF/post-PV MF/post-ET MF who underwent ASCT (61). Day 100 transplant-related mortality (TRM) was 13% with 5-year survival of 61%. Use of targeted busulphan/cyclophosphamide, high platelet count at transplantation (for post-PV and post-ET MF patients only),

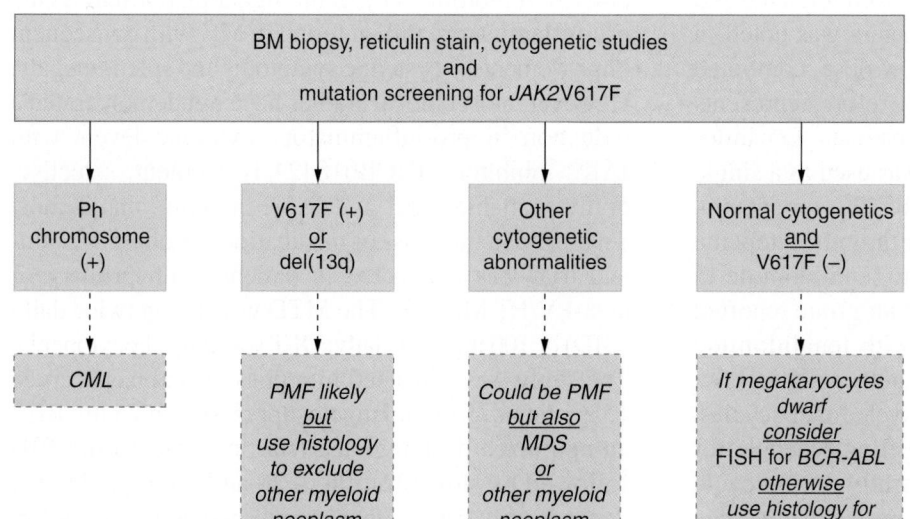

FIGURE 6-13. Diagnostic algorithm for suspected primary myelofibrosis. *(Reproduced, with permission, from Tefferi A, Vardiman JW. Classification and diagnosis of myeloproliferative neoplasms: The 2008 World Health Organization criteria and point-of-care diagnostic algorithms. Leukemia 2008;22:14-22.)*

younger age, and decreased co-morbidity score were associated with improved survival (61). As MF is a disease of the elderly who might not be suitable candidates for myeloablative ASCT, many investigators have explored use of reduced intensity conditioning in such patients. Rondelli et al. used reduced-intensity conditioning for 21 patients with MF and reported day 100 TRM of 10% with OS of 86% at 2.7 years (62). To add to the debate of the role of the ASCT in MF patients, Siragusa et al. reported survival data on young (age <60 years) patients with MF with high- or intermediate-risk disease who did not undergo transplant (63). The 1 and 3 year survival was reported ranging from 71 to 95% and 55 to 77% (depending on the center studied), similar to the data on the myeloablative or reduced-intensity conditioning ASCT, underscoring the need for controlled studies to accurately assess the role of ASCT in this setting (63). Newer prognostic models and current research will help identify patients best suited for ASCT.

New findings regarding the molecular pathogenesis of this disease along with better understanding of the bone marrow microenvironment has led to many novel treatment strategies for this disease. The immunomodulatory cytokine inhibitory and antiangiogenic drugs (IMIDs) such as thalidomide, lenalidomide, and pomalidomide have been explored in MF. Thomas et al. treated 44 patients with MF with thalidomide at a dose of 200 mg daily with escalation by 200 mg weekly until the best tolerated dose was reached (64). Improvement in anemia and thrombocytopenia was noted in approximately 20% patients and reduction in splenomegaly was noted in 31% patients. Mesa et al. reported on the use of combination therapy of thalidomide at low doses (50 mg/daily) with 3-month oral prednisone taper (starting at 0.5 mg/kg/day) in 21 symptomatic patients with MF (65). This combination was well tolerated and an objective clinical response in anemia was noted in 62% patients. Thalidomide at the low dose, combined with tapering doses of prednisone, therefore, represents active therapeutic regimen for MF patients. Lenalidomide, a derivative of thalidomide, was used as a single in 68 patients with MF with ORRs of 22% for anemia, 33% for splenomegaly, and 50% for thrombocytopenia (66). Prednisone has been added to lenalidomide in an attempt to increase the efficacy. Our group reported on 40 patients with MF treated with lenalidomide 10 mg/day (5 mg/day if baseline platelet count <100 × 10^9/L) on days 1 to 21 of a 28-day cycle for six cycles, combined with prednisone on a tapering schedule for the first three cycles (30 mg/day orally during cycle 1, 15 mg/day during cycle 2, and 15 mg every other day during cycle 3) (67). Lenalidomide therapy was continued indefinitely in responding patients. ORRs were

30% for anemia and 42% for splenomegaly. According to the IWG-MRT response criteria, 7.5% patients had partial response and 22.5% had clinical improvement. Majority of the assessable responders who started therapy with grade 4 reticulin fibrosis had at least 2 score reductions and all eight JAK2V617F-positive responders had reduction in mutant allele burden. Grade ≥3 hematologic toxicity included neutropenia (58%), anemia (42%), and thrombocytopenia (13%). Lenalidomide/prednisone combination is active therapy for MF patients but caution must be implemented regarding possible lowering of the blood cell count in many patients. Anti-angiogenic agent bortezomib, hypomethylating agent 5-azacitidine, farnesyl transferase inhibitor tipifarnib, and tyrosine kinase inhibitors (TKIs) imatinib and dasatinib have been used in MF patients with minimal clinical benefit. Without doubt, the discovery of JAK2 mutation in MPN has ushered in a new era for the treatment of these diseases, especially MF.

JAK2 INHIBITORS

Several clinical trials with JAK2 inhibitors are currently underway for patients with MF (68-73). Responses are primarily seen as an improvement in patients' spleen size and constitutional symptoms and these benefits are seen both in patients with JAK2V617F mutation and in those with wild-type JAK2. Significant reduction in JAK2V617F allele burden or improvements in BM fibrosis and cytopenias have not been seen so far. It has been proposed that these medications may work through the inhibition of cell proliferation by blocking both mutated- and wild-type-JAK2, and/or by blocking the pro-inflammatory cytokines' signaling through the inhibition of closely related JAK1 tyrosine kinase (74,75). Inhibition of cytokine signaling normalizes the pro-inflammatory milieu found in MF, with consequent improvements in systemic symptoms and splenomegaly. However, most clinical studies have not demonstrated a reduction in pro-inflammatory cytokine levels with JAK2 inhibitors. INCB018424 is a potent, selective, orally available JAK1 and JAK2 inhibitor, that is most developed in this class of medications. A phase 1/2 clinical trial was conducted in patients with primary or post-PV/ET MF (76). The MTD was 25 mg twice daily (BID) or 100 mg once daily; DLT was thrombocytopenia. The study was expanded into phase 2 and has accrued 153 patients. To avoid myelosuppression at 25 mg BID, an optimized dose regimen (starting dose 15 mg BID followed by slow titration to 20 and 25 mg BID over 2 months in patients without myelosuppression and unsatisfactory response) was developed. Use of this optimized dose regimen significantly decreased the rate of myelosuppression (grade 3 to 4 anemia 8.3%; grade 3 to 4 thrombocytopenia 2.9%) compared with 25 mg BID (grade 3 to 4 anemia 26.3%; grade 3 to 4 thrombocytopenia 29.4%). Therapy with INCB018424 led to significant reduction in spleen size (>50%) in 52% of patients as early as 1 month after start of treatment. There was also significant improvement in systemic symptoms and exercise capacity. Responses were not correlated to disease subtype (primary or post-PV/ET MF) or JAK2V617F mutational status. Responders had a significant decrease in plasma levels of proinflammatory cytokines (IL-1, TNF-α, and VEGF). Reduction in JAK2 V617F allelic burden was seen in a minority of patients and there was no improvement in BM fibrosis. After median follow up of 15 months 75% of patients are still on the therapy; early results suggest that INCB018424 therapy may lower the incidence of transformation of MF to AML and possibly extend patients life. Currently, two randomized phase III trials of INCB018424 versus best supportive care or placebo are underway for patients with MF.

TREATMENT CONCLUSIONS

MF is a disease for which there is no effective therapy that would change the natural progression of the disease and premature death. Although therapies exist that may help temporarily with particular aspects of the disease (eg, danazol for anemia, HU for splenomegaly, prednisone for fatigue and weakness), the outcome of the patients does not differ. With the discovery of new abnormalities in MF that may have significant role in the pathophysiology of the disease, new therapies are being developed. Several JAK2 inhibitors are in clinical studies and showing promise in controlling the disease such that clinical status of patients markedly improves, with the decrease of splenomegaly and improvement in quality of life, and early indications of an impact on the natural progression of the disease. Therefore, in general, patients with MF are encouraged to participate in clinical trials with novel agents because standard therapies have no potential to improve the outcome.

■ CHRONIC EOSINOPHILIC LEUKEMIA/ HYPEREOSINOPHILIC SYNDROME

HES is characterized by chronic eosinophil overproduction in the absence of obvious reactive or clonal causes of eosinophilia. Eosinophilic tissue infiltration may involve the heart, skin, central and peripheral nervous systems, lungs, spleen, liver, and gastrointestinal tract. A diagnosis of HES requires the presence of an absolute eosinophil count of >1.5 × 10^9/L for at least 6 months and evidence of end-organ damage. Patients with hypereosinophilia who are found to have clonal disease (ie, cytogenetic or molecular abnormality proving the existence of malignant clone) or have peripheral blood blasts >2% or bone marrow blasts >5% are said to have CEL (77). HES and CEL have similar clinical presentations, and distinguishing between the two can be difficult unless proper testing for a molecular/cytogenetic marker is done. As most common causes of eosinophilia are reactive, conditions such as infections (especially parasitic), atopy, drug reactions, connective tissue disorders, or vasculitis must be ruled out.

In 2003, Cools et al. described a karyotypically occult but fluorescent in situ hybridization; a (FISH)-apparent molecular aberrancy in a subset of patients diagnosed as having HES/CEL (78). This abnormality consisted of an interstitial deletion of chromosome 4q12, leading to the fusion of the FIP1-like 1 (FIP1L1) gene to the platelet-derived growth factor-α (PDGFRα) gene. The resultant product, FIP1L1–PDGFRα, is a constitutively active TK highly amenable to inhibition by imatinib, thus providing the rationale for the use of this TKI (78,79). Other molecularly defined HES/CEL include mutations involving the genes that encode for PDGFRβ (located on chromosome 5q31-q33) and fibroblast growth factor receptor 1 (FGFR1; located on chromosome 8p11) (80). All such patients have been reclassified in the new 2008 WHO classification into separate groups, as the resulting rearranged genes have become markers of disease clonality (see Table 6-1): "myeloid neoplasms associated with eosinophilia and abnormalities of PDGFRα, PDGFRβ, or FGFR1."

HES is much more common in men than women, and patients with this disease usually present between the ages of 20 and 50 years. Continuous presence of high number of eosinophils in blood can eventually cause multiple organ tissue damage due to tissue infiltration. The disease can range from minimal symptoms with a long survival probability to rapidly fatal due to sudden, severe heart failure or acute leukemia. Clinical manifestations include pruritus, urticaria, angioedema, erythematous papules, valvular heart disease, mural thrombi, cardiomyopathy, polyneuropathies, optic neuritis, pulmonary infiltrates, and pleural effusion.

DIAGNOSIS

All patients suspected to have HES must undergo bone marrow evaluation, cytogenetic analysis, and testing for FIP1L1-PDGFRα as treatment modalities for patients with this mutation is different. Figs. 6-14 and 6-15 illustrate the morphological findings in HES/CEL patients, respectively. The incidence of the FIP1L1–PDGFRα

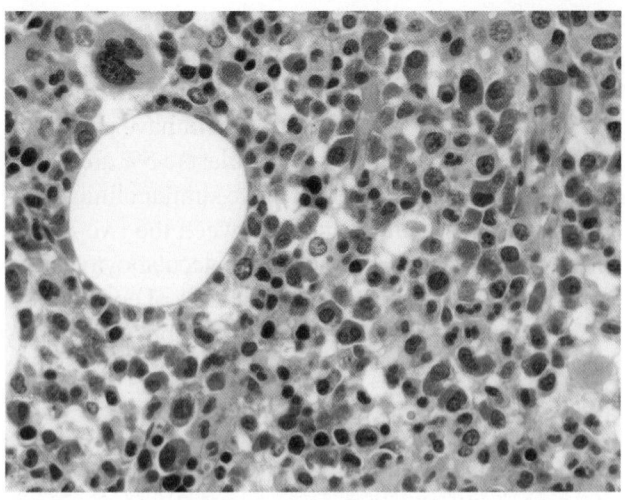

FIGURE 6-14. In CEL/HES, bone marrow typically shows increased cellularity with striking interstitial infiltration by eosinophils (400×).

rearrangement is low in patients with hypereosinophilia. In the initial study by Cools et al., FIP1L1–PDGFRα was found in 56% of the patients studied (78). Other studies have reported this abnormality at frequencies ranging from 3 to 88%, likely reflecting the intrinsic heterogeneity amongst patients with hypereosinophilia, and the impact of referral bias (78,79,81,82). In the largest study to date FISH analysis, aimed at detecting a deletion/excision of the CHIC2 locus at chromosome 4q12 (indirect test for FIP1L1-PDGFRα abnormality), was performed in 741 unselected patients with eosinophilia and only 21 (3%) were positive (82). In another study of 376 patients with persistent unexplained eosinophilia,

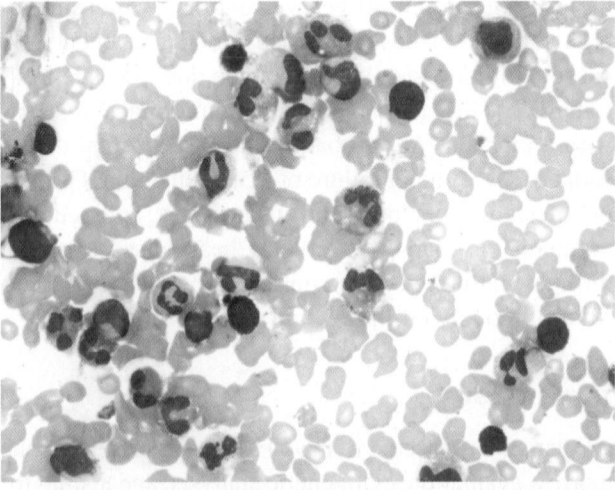

FIGURE 6-15. Markedly increased, morphologically unremarkable eosinophils are typically detected in the bone marrow aspirate smears from patients with CEL/HES (400×).

40 patients (11%) were FIP1L1–PDGFRα positive (83). T-cell immunophenotyping and T-cell receptor gene rearrangement analysis should be performed in all patients and if either clonal or immunophenotypically aberrant T cells are identified, a diagnosis of lymphoproliferative variant of HES is preferred. Chest x-ray, pulmonary function tests, echocardiogram, and measurement of serum troponin levels should be done at diagnosis. An increased level of serum cardiac troponin has been shown to correlate with the presence of cardiomyopathy in HES. Diagnostic algorithm for primary eosinophilia is presented in Fig. 6-16.

TREATMENT

For asymptomatic patient with HES with no organ damage and normal troponin, no active HES therapy is recommended. However, these patients should be closely followed. For patients with symptomatic disease or evidence of end-organ damage, therapy for HES generally entails the use of corticosteroids, IFN-α, and/or the use of cytoreductive agents such as HU, vincristine, or cyclosporine. The first-line treatment of HES is usually prednisone (starting dose of 1 mg/kg/day), with a response rate of nearly 70%. However, relapses often occur on cessation of therapy, requiring alternative drug options, such as IFN-α or HU. Vincristine is especially useful for acute reductions when total eosinophil count is very high ($\geq 50 \times 10^9$/L).

For patients who are refractory to conventional therapies, use of monoclonal antibody therapy should be considered. Two drugs are currently available: mepolizumab that targets interleukin-5 and alemtuzumab that targets the CD52 antigen that is expressed by eosinophils but not neutrophils. Rothenberg et al. conducted a randomized placebo-controlled trial evaluating the safety and efficacy of mepolizumab in patients with stable HES on steroids, without life-threatening complications, as a steroid sparing agent (84). The primary endpoint (reduction of the prednisone dose to ≤10 mg/day for ≥8 consecutive weeks) was achieved in 84% of patients in the mepolizumab group compared to 43% of patients in the placebo group ($p < .001$). Significantly more patients had suppression of absolute eosinophil count in the mepolizumab group. Verstovsek et al. treated 11 HES/CEL patients (nine previously treated) with alemtuzumab (85). Ten patients (91%) achieved CHR (defined as the reduction of the absolute eosinophil count and the percentage of eosinophils in peripheral blood to normal values [$\leq 0.4 \times 10^9$/L and ≤4%, respectively]) after a median of 2 weeks and symptoms completely resolved in nine patients. Bone marrow eosinophilia resolved in four of

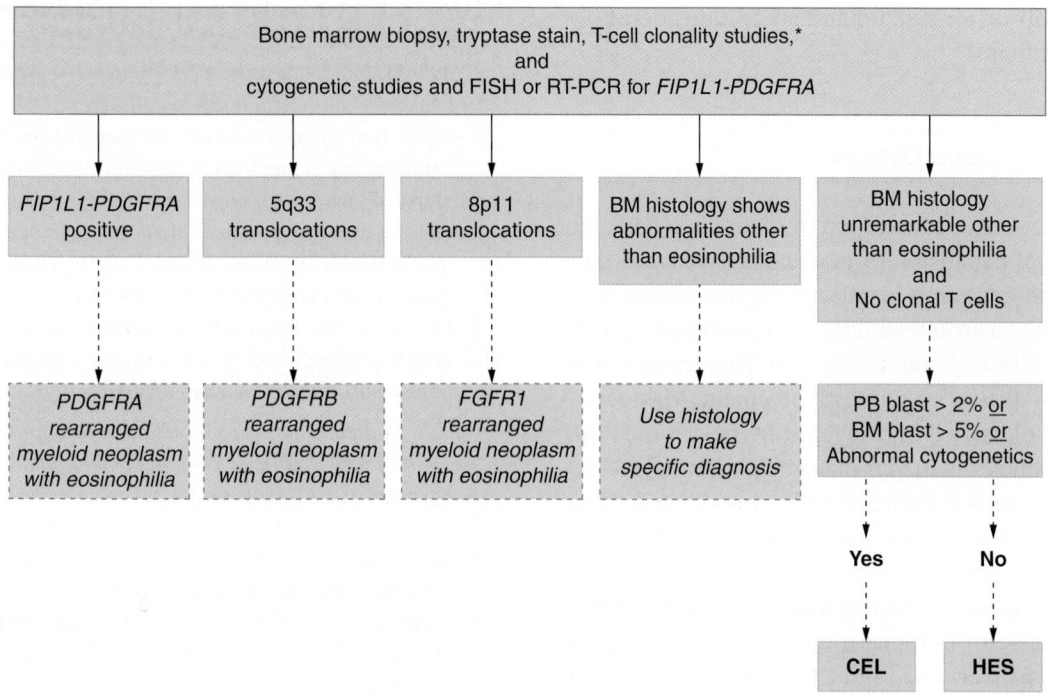

FIGURE 6-16.   Diagnostic algorithm for suspected primary eosinophilia. *(Reproduced, with permission, from Tefferi A, Vardiman JW. Classification and diagnosis of myeloproliferative neoplasms: The 2008 World Health Organization criteria and point-of-care diagnostic algorithms. Leukemia 2008;22:14-22.)*

the seven evaluable patients. The median duration of CHR was short-lived (3 months) and 7 of the 10 CHR patients relapsed. Two patients achieved second CHR upon alemtuzumab rechallenge. Although very effective in eliminating the disease in short order, therapy with alemtuzumab requires maintenance phase, where alemtuzumab is given periodically every few weeks or months, upon first signs of recurrent symptoms and signs of the disease, to provide optimal benefit.

Imatinib mesylate is a moderately potent, ATP-competitive TKI highly active against ABL, PDGFR and KIT protein kinases. Encouraged by the impressive activity of imatinib in patients with CML, imatinib was tried in patients with HES with good outcomes. The efficacy of imatinib therapy for patients with eosinophilia carrying the FIP1L1–PDGFRα has been established in multiple studies (78,86). For instance, Baccarani et al. reported a CHR of 99% in patients carrying FIP1L1–PDGFRα compared to 19% in patients without this mutation (86). Imatinib has therefore become standard of care for this subset of patients with hypereosinophilia to the point that therapy with this TKI is recommended even in the absence of symptoms to prevent the risk of end-organ damage. In the United States, imatinib is approved for the treatment of adults

with HES/CEL associated with the FIP1L1–PDGFRα kinase (starting dose of 100 mg daily with dose increase to 400 mg daily if suboptimal response and lack of side effects), and for patients with HES/CEL whose FIP1L1-PDGFRα status is negative or unknown (recommended dose is 400 mg daily). However, as the response to imatinib in FIP1L1–PDGFRα negative patients is limited, frontline therapy with imatinib for patients with HES should not be indiscriminate and should be reserved for patients who fail conventional therapy. Imatinib is also approved therapy for CEL patients with PDGFRβ involvement, which is usually discovered on cytogenetic testing, as it involves chromosomal abnormalities involving 5q31-q33.

TREATMENT CONCLUSIONS

All patients suspected of primary eosinophilia should undergo testing for a PDGFRα fusion gene. This is usually done using PCR technique for PDGFRα expression. Patients with this rearranged gene should be initiated on imatinib at 100 mg daily. For PDGFRα-negative patients, prednisone should be the first line of treatment. For patients refractory to steroids or relapsing on steroids, IFN-α/HU can be used as second-line agents.

Mepolizumab or alemtuzumab can be considered for refractory patients.

■ MAST CELL DISEASE

MCD is a heterogeneous group of disorders characterized by clonal expansion of mast cells (MC) and their excessive accumulation in various organs such as skin, bone marrow, gastrointestinal tract, lymph nodes, liver, and spleen. Clinical course can vary from no/minimal symptoms to diffuse systemic involvement. Mastocytosis has been classified into seven subtypes by the 2001 WHO guidelines: cutaneous mastocytosis, indolent systemic mastocytosis (ISM), SM with an associated clonal hematological non-MC-lineage disease (SM-AHNMD), aggressive SM (ASM), MC leukemia, MC sarcoma, and extra-cutaneous mastocytoma (87). SM is defined by the presence of one major and one minor, or three minor diagnostic criteria (Table 6-8) (87). Patients with SM are further characterized with regard to the presence of so-called "B and C findings" (assessing disease burden and disease aggressiveness, respectively) (Table 6-9). SM patients with no findings are identified as ISM, those with B findings as Smoldering SM (SSM, a subtype of ISM with possibly more aggressive clinical course) and those with C findings as ASM. The 2008 WHO guidelines redefine mastocytosis as "mast cell disease," reclassifying it as an MPNs with SM a subtype with bone marrow involvement.

TABLE 6-8 | WORLD HEALTH ORGANIZATION DIAGNOSTIC CRITERIA FOR SYSTEMIC MASTOCYTOSIS

Major criteria
1. Multifocal, dense infiltrates of mast cells (≥15 mast cells in aggregates) in bone marrow biopsy sections and/or in other extracutaneous organ(s)

Minor criteria
1. Greater than 25% mast cells in bone marrow or other extracutaneous organ(s) show an atypical morphology (typically spindle-shaped)
2. c-*kit* mutation at codon 816 is present in extracutaneous tissues
3. Mast cells in bone marrow coexpress CD117 and either CD2, CD25, or both (by flow cytometry)
4. Serum tryptase persistently is ≥20 ng/mL (not accounted for in patients with an associated, clonal, hematologic, nonmast cell disorder)

Diagnosis requires the meeting either one major criteria and one minor criteria or three minor criteria

Reproduced, with permission, from Valent P, Horny HP, Escribano L, et al. Diagnostic criteria and classification of mastocytosis: A consensus proposal. *Leukemia Res.* 2001. 25;7:23.

TABLE 6-9 | B FINDINGS AND C FINDINGS IN SYSTEMIC MASTOCYTOSIS

B findings: Indication of high MC burden and expansion of the genetic defect into various myeloid lineages
1. Infiltration grade of mast cells in bone marrow >30% on histology and serum total tryptase levels >200 ng/mL
2. Hypercellular bone marrow with loss of fat cells, discrete signs of dysmyelopoiesis without substantial cytopenias, or World Health Organization criteria for myelodysplastic syndrome or myeloproliferative disorder
3. Organomegaly: Palpable hepatomegaly, splenomegaly, or lymphadenopathy (>2 cm on computed tomography or ultrasound) without impaired organ function

C findings: Indication of impaired organ function because of MC infiltration (confirmed by biopsy in most patients)
1. Cytopenia(s): Absolute neutrophil count <1000/μL, or hemoglobin <10 g/dL, or platelets <100,000/μL
2. Hepatomegaly with ascites and impaired liver function
3. Palpable splenomegaly with hypersplenism
4. Malabsorption with hypoalbuminemia and weight loss
5. Skeletal lesions: Large osteolyses and/or severe osteoporosis causing pathologic fractures
6. Life-threatening organomegaly in other organ systems that definitively is caused by an infiltration of the tissue by neoplastic mast cells

CLINICAL FEATURES

Symptoms of mastocytosis can be divided into those due to MC mediator release or to those due to MC organ infiltration. Vasoactive mediators (histamine, leukotrienes, prostaglandins) released from MC can lead to itching, flushing, lightheadedness, syncope, palpitations, diarrhea, heartburn, fatigue, and headache and can be exacerbated by infections, alcohol, exercise, and medications. Common sites of organ infiltration include skin and gastrointestinal tract. Urticaria pigmentosa is the most common skin manifestation characterized by reddish-brown macules and papules. Scratching of affected skin characteristically leads to development of urticaria and erythema (Darier sign). Gastrointestinal involvement can present as chronic diarrhea, steatorrhea, malabsorption, and ascites. Anemia is the most common hematological abnormality due to bone marrow infiltration and peripheral eosinophilia is seen in around 20% patients. Bone pain and fractures can also occur.

DIAGNOSIS

Diagnosis relies primarily on the identification of neoplastic MC in various organs (see Table 6-8). Bone marrow examination is imperative for SM diagnosis as most adults with mastocytosis have underlying bone marrow involvement. Figs. 6-17 and 6-18 illustrate a

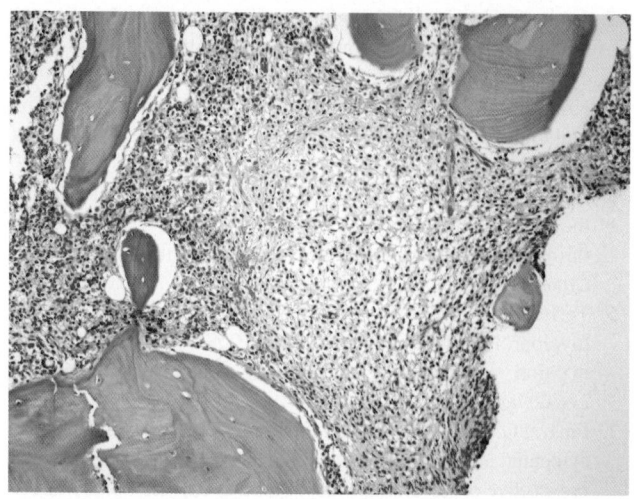

FIGURE 6-17. Bone marrow biopsy from a patient with SM demonstrates total focal replacement of the normal cellular elements by mast cells (100X). Immunohistochemical staining performed on this specimen demonstrated that the neoplastic mast cells aberrantly expressed CD2 and CD25.

case of SM detected in the bone marrow. Neoplastic MC are characteristically spindle shaped and present in multifocal aggregates and unlike normal MC, neoplastic MC express surface markers CD2 and/or CD25. Serum tryptase level and urinary histamine levels are generally increased. KIT gene D816V mutation screening should be considered for all patients. KIT is a TK receptor, encoded by the c-kit gene located on chromosome 4q12 in humans. Binding of stem cell factor (SCF) to KIT leads to receptor dimerization and phosphorylation

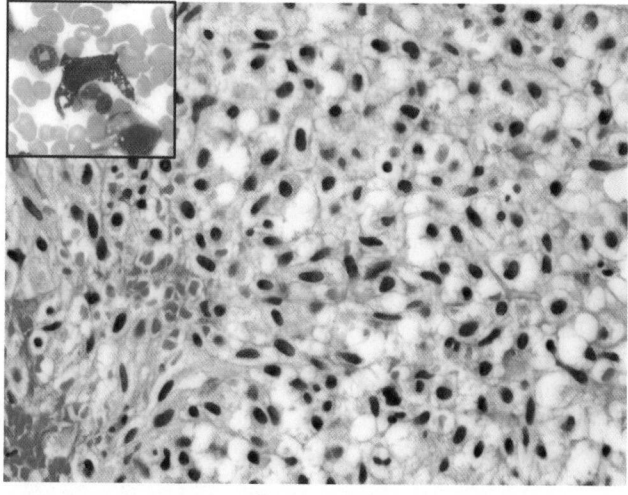

FIGURE 6-18. In SM, mast cells tend to have abundant, colorless cytoplasm and contain elongated to oval nuclei (400X). In the bone marrow aspirate smears, the mast cells are increased in number and size and attain spindle shape (insert; 400X).

of the downstream signaling molecules (88). KIT plays an important role in normal hematopoiesis and its expression declines in hematopoietic cell lines with maturation, except in MC. Furitsu et al. were first to show that KIT was constitutively activated and expressed in the absence of SCF in a MC line derived from an MC leukemia patient (89). A point mutation D816V (substitution of valine for aspartate at codon 816, Asp816Val) in the TK domain of the KIT receptor (first described by Nagata et al.) (90) has been described in >90% adult patients with SM using sensitive PCR based assay (91). Recently, TET2 mutation (candidate tumor suppressor gene at chromosome 4q24) was reported in 29% of SM patients and correlated with presence of KITD816V mutation, monocytosis, and female gender (92).

TREATMENT

There is a lack of effective treatment for SM. Symptomatic treatments include use of oral antihistamines and MC stabilizers such as cromolyn sodium (93). Patients should avoid factors which can trigger MC degranulation such as emotional stress, cold exposure, alcohol use, strenuous exercise, and use of nonsteroidal anti-inflammatory drugs. Both sedating and nonsedating H1 antihistamines can be used to alleviate pruritus and itching. Randomized controlled trials evaluating the comparative efficacy of antihistamines in SM are lacking. Cetrizine has been shown to be equivalent to hydroxyzine in relieving pruritus in patients with chronic urticaria with the advantage of lack of sedation (94). Therefore, most patients initially are treated with nonsedating H1 antihistamines. Higher doses of sedating antihistamines could be used for those with severe symptoms. As both H1 and H2 receptors are present in skin (85% cutaneous histamine receptors are H1 and 15% are H2), addition of an H2 blocker should be considered for those not responding to H1 antihistamines alone (94). Cromolyn sodium has been shown to be beneficial in patients with gastrointestinal symptoms (diarrhea, vomiting, abdominal pain). Short courses of prednisone can be considered for patients with severe symptoms, especially malabsorption and ascites. ASA can cause MC degranulation although may also help with flushing. Therefore, patients should be on H1 and H2 antihistamine therapy before starting ASA therapy (93). Patients with history of anaphylaxis or cardiovascular collapse should carry an epinephrine pen. Omalizumab (humanized murine monoclonal antibody that inhibits IgE binding to MC and basophils) has been shown to be effective in SM patients with syncopal episodes and skin manifestations. For patients with osteoporosis, bisphosphonate therapy should be considered. Cytoreductive therapies (IFN-α and cladribine) are used for severe disease symptoms. In a multicenter trial in 20 patients with SM, IFN-α-2b use led to partial or minor response in 13 patients (95). Major side effects leading to treatment discontinuation included depression and cytopenias. Combination of IFN-α-2b plus prednisone has also been studied. Use of cladribine in 33 patients with mastocytosis led to a major response in 24 patients with myelosuppression being the main side effect (96). Cladribine appears to be the best therapy for patients with ASM and is able to control the signs and symptoms of the disease in majority of patients.

Various TKI targeting KIT are now being studied in clinical trials. Imatinib is a potent inhibitor of various TK including wild-type KIT. However, imatinib is not effective against the most common KIT mutation in SM, D816V (97). This is probably due to the fact that imatinib is able to bind KIT only in inactive configuration and D816V mutation leads to stabilization of the active open configuration of KIT. The clinical experience with imatinib has corresponded to the in vitro data, with no significant responses in patients with KITD816V mutation (98,99). An important subgroup of SM patients with imatinib responsiveness is the one with FIP1L1–PDGFRα mutation. Peripheral blood eosinophilia is seen in approximately 20% of SM patients (SM-eos) and bone marrow eosinophilia has been reported in approximately 25% of SM patients. In a study by Pardanani et al., 56% of SM patients with eosinophilia had FIP1L1–PDGFRα fusion oncogene (81). In this study, all treated SM-eos patients with FIP1L1–PDGFRα mutation responded to imatinib 100 mg daily, while those SM-eos patients without FIP1L1–PDGFRα mutation did not respond (irrespective of KITD816V mutation status). All patients with SM and eosinophilia should undergo testing for FIP1L1-PDGFRα mutation. Imatinib is currently approved by FDA for adult patients with ASM without KITD816V mutation or unknown KIT mutation status (at 400 mg daily) and for ASM associated with eosinophilia (starting dose 100 mg daily with dose escalation to 400 mg daily if insufficient response and absence of side effects). Other TKI currently under investigation as therapy for SM patients with KITD816v mutation are dasatinib, nilotinib, and PKC412, however, the results of clinical studies so far have been disappointing.

References

1. Dameshek W. Some speculations on the myeloproliferative syndromes. *Blood* 1951;6(4):372-375.
2. Baxter EJ, Scott LM, Campbell PJ, et al. Acquired mutation of the tyrosine kinase JAK2 in human myeloproliferative disorders. *Lancet* 2005;365(9464):1054-1061.
3. James C, Ugo V, Le Couedic JP, et al. A unique clonal JAK2 mutation leading to constitutive signalling causes polycythaemia vera. *Nature* 2005;434(7037):1144-1148.
4. Kralovics R, Passamonti F, Buser AS, et al. A gain-of-function mutation of JAK2 in myeloproliferative disorders. *N Engl J Med* 2005;352(17):1779-1790.
5. Levine RL, Wadleigh M, Cools J, et al. Activating mutation in the tyrosine kinase JAK2 in polycythemia vera, essential thrombocythemia, and myeloid metaplasia with myelofibrosis. *Cancer Cell* 2005;7(4):387-397.
6. Tefferi A, Vardiman JW. Classification and diagnosis of myeloproliferative neoplasms: The 2008 World Health Organization criteria and point-of-care diagnostic algorithms. *Leukemia* 2008;22(1):14-22.
7. Finazzi G, Caruso V, Marchioli R, et al. Acute leukemia in polycythemia vera: An analysis of 1638 patients enrolled in a prospective observational study. *Blood* 2005;105(7):2664-2670.
8. Tefferi A, Levine RL, Kantarjian H. Oncogenic signals as treatment targets in classic myeloproliferative neoplasms. *Biol Blood Marrow Transplant* 2009;15(1 Suppl):114-119.
9. Scott LM, Beer PA, Bench AJ, et al. Prevalance of JAK2 V617F and exon 12 mutations in polycythaemia vera. *Br J Haematol* 2007;139(3):511-512.
10. Scott LM, Tong W, Levine RL, et al. JAK2 exon 12 mutations in polycythemia vera and idiopathic erythrocytosis. *N Engl J Med* 2007;356(5):459-468.
11. Wasserman LR. The treatment of polycythemia vera. *Semin Hematol* 1976;13(1):57-78.
12. Gangat N, Strand J, Lasho TL, et al. Cytogenetic studies at diagnosis in polycythemia vera: Clinical and JAK2V617F allele burden correlates. *Eur J Haematol* 2008;80(3):197-200.
13. Polycythemia vera: The natural history of 1213 patients followed for 20 years. Gruppo Italiano Studio Policitemia. *Ann Intern Med* 1995;123(9):656-664.
14. Berk PD, Goldberg JD, Donovan PB, et al. Therapeutic recommendations in polycythemia vera based on Polycythemia Vera Study Group protocols. *Semin Hematol* 1986;23(2):132-143.
15. De Stefano V, Teofili L, Leone G, et al. Spontaneous erythroid colony formation as the clue to an underlying myeloproliferative disorder in patients with Budd-Chiari syndrome or portal vein thrombosis. *Semin Thromb Hemost* 1997;23(5):411-418.
16. Kiladjian JJ, Cervantes F, Leebeek FW, et al. The impact of JAK2 and MPL mutations on diagnosis and prognosis of splanchnic vein thrombosis: a report on 241 cases. *Blood* 2008;111(10):4922-4929.
17. Marchioli R, Finazzi G, Landolfi R, et al. Vascular and neoplastic risk in a large cohort of patients with polycythemia vera. *J Clin Oncol* 2005;23(10):2224-2232.
18. Passamonti F, Rumi E, Caramella M, et al. A dynamic prognostic model to predict survival in post-polycythemia vera myelofibrosis. *Blood* 2008;111(7):3383-3387.
19. Landolfi R, Di Gennaro L, Barbui T, et al. Leukocytosis as a major thrombotic risk factor in patients with polycythemia vera. *Blood* 2007;109(6):2446-2452.
20. Gangat N, Strand J, Li CY, et al. Leucocytosis in polycythaemia vera predicts both inferior survival and leukaemic transformation. *Br J Haematol* 2007;138(3):354-358.
21. Spivak JL, Silver RT. The revised World Health Organization diagnostic criteria for polycythemia vera, essential thrombocytosis, and primary myelofibrosis: an alternative proposal. *Blood* 2008;112(2):231-239.

22. Tartaglia AP, Goldberg JD, Berk PD, et al. Adverse effects of antiaggregating platelet therapy in the treatment of polycythemia vera. *Semin Hematol* 1986;23(3):172-176.

23. Landolfi R, Marchioli R, Kutti J, et al. Efficacy and safety of low-dose aspirin in polycythemia vera. *N Engl J Med* 2004; 350(2):114-124.

24. Squizzato A, Romualdi E, Middeldorp S. Antiplatelet drugs for polycythaemia vera and essential thrombocythaemia. *Cochrane Database Syst Rev* 2008(2):CD006503.

25. Tefferi A, Spivak JL: Polycythemia vera: Scientific advances and current practice. *Semin Hematol* 2005;42(4):206-220.

26. Silver RT. Recombinant interferon-alpha for treatment of polycythaemia vera. *Lancet* 1988;2(8607):403.

27. Kiladjian JJ, Cassinat B, Chevret S, et al. Pegylated interferon-alfa-2a induces complete hematologic and molecular responses with low toxicity in polycythemia vera. *Blood* 2008;112(8): 3065-3072.

28. Quintas-Cardama A, Kantarjian H, Manshouri T, et al. Pegylated interferon alfa-2a yields high rates of hematologic and molecular response in patients with advanced essential thrombocythemia and polycythemia vera. *J Clin Oncol* 2009;27(32): 5418-5424.

29. Verstovsek S, Passamonti F, Rambaldi A, et al. A Phase 2 study of INCB018424, an oral, selective JAK1/JAK2 inhibitor, in patients with advanced polycythemia vera (PV) and essential thrombocythemia (ET) refractory to hydroxyurea. *Blood* 2009;114:311 (Abstract).

30. Ruggeri M, Tosetto A, Frezzato M, et al. The rate of progression to polycythemia vera or essential thrombocythemia in patients with erythrocytosis or thrombocytosis. *Ann Intern Med* 2003;139(6):470-475.

31. Griesshammer M, Bangerter M, Sauer T, et al. Aetiology and clinical significance of thrombocytosis: Analysis of 732 patients with an elevated platelet count. *J Intern Med* 1999; 245(3):295-300.

32. Buss DH, Cashell AW, O'Connor ML, et al. Occurrence, etiology, and clinical significance of extreme thrombocytosis: A study of 280 cases. *Am J Med* 1994;96(3):247-253.

33. Horikawa Y, Matsumura I, Hashimoto K, et al. Markedly reduced expression of platelet c-mpl receptor in essential thrombocythemia. *Blood* 1997;90(10):4031-4038.

34. Pardanani AD, Levine RL, Lasho T, et al. MPL515 mutations in myeloproliferative and other myeloid disorders: A study of 1182 patients. *Blood* 2006;108(10):3472-3476.

35. Pikman Y, Lee BH, Mercher T, et al. MPLW515L is a novel somatic activating mutation in myelofibrosis with myeloid metaplasia. *PLoS Med* 2006;3(7):e270.

36. Fenaux P, Simon M, Caulier MT, et al. Clinical course of essential thrombocythemia in 147 cases. *Cancer* 1990;66(3): 549-556.

37. Wolanskyj AP, Schwager SM, McClure RF, et al. Essential thrombocythemia beyond the first decade: Life expectancy, long-term complication rates, and prognostic factors. *Mayo Clin Proc* 2006;81(2):159-166.

38. Gangat N, Wolanskyj AP, McClure RF, et al. Risk stratification for survival and leukemic transformation in essential thrombocythemia: A single institutional study of 605 patients. *Leukemia* 2007;21(2):270-276.

39. Cervantes F, Alvarez-Larran A, Talarn C, et al. Myelofibrosis with myeloid metaplasia following essential thrombocythaemia: Actuarial probability, presenting characteristics

and evolution in a series of 195 patients. *Br J Haematol* 2002;118(3):786-790.

40. Carobbio A, Finazzi G, Antonioli E, et al. Thrombocytosis and leukocytosis interaction in vascular complications of essential thrombocythemia. *Blood* 2008;112(8):3135-3137.

41. De Stefano V, Za T, Rossi E, et al. Recurrent thrombosis in patients with polycythemia vera and essential thrombocythemia: Incidence, risk factors, and effect of treatments. *Haematologica* 2008;93(3):372-380.

42. Wolanskyj AP, Lasho TL, Schwager SM, et al. JAK2 mutation in essential thrombocythaemia: Clinical associations and long-term prognostic relevance. *Br J Haematol* 2005;131(2):208-213.

43. Campbell PJ, Scott LM, Buck G, et al. Definition of subtypes of essential thrombocythaemia and relation to polycythaemia vera based on JAK2 V617F mutation status: A prospective study. *Lancet* 2005;366(9501):1945-1953.

44. Vannucchi AM, Antonioli E, Guglielmelli P, et al. Clinical profile of homozygous JAK2 617V>F mutation in patients with polycythemia vera or essential thrombocythemia. *Blood* 2007;110(3):840-846.

45. Passamonti F, Randi ML, Rumi E, et al. Increased risk of pregnancy complications in patients with essential thrombocythemia carrying the JAK2 (617V>F) mutation. *Blood* 2007; 110(2):485-489.

46. Gangat N, Tefferi A, Thanarajasingam G, et al. Cytogenetic abnormalities in essential thrombocythemia: Prevalence and prognostic significance. *Eur J Haematol* 2009;83(1):17-21.

47. van Genderen PJ, Mulder PG, Waleboer M, et al. Prevention and treatment of thrombotic complications in essential thrombocythaemia: Efficacy and safety of aspirin. *Br J Haematol* 1997;97(1):179-184.

48. Budde U, Scharf RE, Franke P, et al. Elevated platelet count as a cause of abnormal von Willebrand factor multimer distribution in plasma. *Blood* 1993;82(6):1749-1757.

49. Harrison CN, Campbell PJ, Buck G, et al. Hydroxyurea compared with anagrelide in high-risk essential thrombocythemia. *N Engl J Med* 2005;353(1):33-45.

50. Cortelazzo S, Finazzi G, Ruggeri M, et al. Hydroxyurea for patients with essential thrombocythemia and a high risk of thrombosis. *N Engl J Med* 1995;332(17):1132-1136.

51. Gisslinger H, Gotic M, Holowiecki J, et al. Final results of the ANAHYDRET-study: Non-inferiority of anagrelide compared to hydroxyurea in newly diagnosed WHO-essential thrombocythemia patients. *Blood* 2008;112:661a.

52. Ruggeri M, Finazzi G, Tosetto A, et al. No treatment for low-risk thrombocythaemia: Results from a prospective study. *Br J Haematol* 1998;103(3):772-777.

53. Tefferi A, Fonseca R, Pereira DL, et al. A long-term retrospective study of young women with essential thrombocythemia. *Mayo Clin Proc* 2001;76(1):22-28.

54. Cervantes F, Dupriez B, Pereira A, et al. A new prognostic scoring system for primary myelofibrosis based on a study of the International Working Group for Myelofibrosis Research and Treatment. *Blood* 2009;113(13):2895-2901.

55. Huang J, Li CY, Mesa RA, et al. Risk factors for leukemic transformation in patients with primary myelofibrosis. *Cancer* 2008;112(12):2726-2732.

56. Barosi G, Bergamaschi G, Marchetti M, et al. JAK2 V617F mutational status predicts progression to large splenomegaly and leukemic transformation in primary myelofibrosis. *Blood* 2007;110(12):4030-4036.

57. Tefferi A, Lasho TL, Huang J, et al. Low JAK2V617F allele burden in primary myelofibrosis, compared to either a higher allele burden or unmutated status, is associated with inferior overall and leukemia-free survival. *Leukemia* 2008;22(4):756-761.

58. Campbell PJ, Griesshammer M, Dohner K, et al. V617F mutation in JAK2 is associated with poorer survival in idiopathic myelofibrosis. *Blood* 2006;107(5):2098-2100.

59. Tefferi A, Thiele J, Orazi A, et al. Proposals and rationale for revision of the World Health Organization diagnostic criteria for polycythemia vera, essential thrombocythemia, and primary myelofibrosis: Recommendations from an ad hoc international expert panel. *Blood* 2007;110(4):1092-1097.

60. Tam CS, Abruzzo LV, Lin KI, et al. The role of cytogenetic abnormalities as a prognostic marker in primary myelofibrosis: Applicability at the time of diagnosis and later during disease course. *Blood* 2009;113(18):4171-4178.

61. Kerbauy DM, Gooley TA, Sale GE, et al. Hematopoietic cell transplantation as curative therapy for idiopathic myelofibrosis, advanced polycythemia vera, and essential thrombocythemia. *Biol Blood Marrow Transplant* 2007;13(3):355-365.

62. Rondelli D, Barosi G, Bacigalupo A, et al. Allogeneic hematopoietic stem-cell transplantation with reduced-intensity conditioning in intermediate- or high-risk patients with myelofibrosis with myeloid metaplasia. *Blood* 2005;105(10):4115-4119.

63. Siragusa S, Passamonti F, Cervantes F, et al. Survival in young patients with intermediate-/high-risk myelofibrosis: Estimates derived from databases for non transplant patients. *Am J Hematol* 2009;84(3):140-143.

64. Thomas DA, Giles FJ, Albitar M, et al. Thalidomide therapy for myelofibrosis with myeloid metaplasia. *Cancer* 2006; 106(9):1974-1984.

65. Mesa RA, Steensma DP, Pardanani A, et al. A phase 2 trial of combination low-dose thalidomide and prednisone for the treatment of myelofibrosis with myeloid metaplasia. *Blood* 2003;101(7):2534-2541.

66. Tefferi A, Cortes J, Verstovsek S, et al. Lenalidomide therapy in myelofibrosis with myeloid metaplasia. *Blood* 2006;108(4): 1158-1164.

67. Quintas-Cardama A, Kantarjian HM, Manshouri T, et al. Lenalidomide plus prednisone results in durable clinical, histopathologic, and molecular responses in patients with myelofibrosis. *J Clin Oncol* 2009;27(28):4760-4766.

68. Santos FP, Kantarjian HM, Jain N, et al. Phase II study of CEP-701, an orally available JAK2 inhibitor, in patients with primary or post polycythemia vera/essential thrombocythemia myelofibrosis. *Blood* 2010;115(6):1131-1136.

69. Hexner E, Goldberg JD, Prchal JT, et al. A multicenter, open label phase I/II study of CEP701 (Lestaurtinib) in adults with myelofibrosis; a report on phase I: A study of the Myeloproliferative Disorders Research Consortium (MPD-RC) [abstract]. *Blood* 2009;114(22) (Abstract 754).

70. Verstovsek S, Kantarjian H, Mesa RA, et al. Long-term follow up and optimized dosing regimen of INCB018424 in patients with myelofibrosis: Durable clinical, functional and symptomatic responses with improved hematological safety [abstract]. *Blood* 2009;114(22) (Abstract 756).

71. Pardanani A, Gotlib J, Jamieson C, et al. TG101348, a JAK2-selective inhibitor, is well tolerated in patients with myelofibrosis and shows substantial therapeutic activity accompanied by a reduction in JAK2V617F allele burden. *Haematologica* 2009;94(S2) (Abstract 1088).

72. Verstovsek S, Odenike O, Scott B, et al. Phase I Dose-Escalation Trial of SB1518, a novel JAK2/FLT3 inhibitor, in acute and chronic myeloid diseases, including primary or post-essential thrombocythemia/polycythemia vera myelofibrosis [abstract]. *Blood* 2009;114(22) (Abstract 3905).

73. Shah NP, Olszynski P, Sokol L, et al. A phase I study of XL019, a selective JAK2 inhibitor, in patients with primary myelofibrosis, post-polycythemia vera, or post-essential thrombocythemia myelofibrosis [abstract]. *Blood* 2008;112(11) (Abstract 98).

74. Vannucchi AM. How do JAK2-inhibitors work in myelofibrosis: An alternative hypothesis. *Leuk Res* 2009;33(12):1581-1583.

75. Mesa R, Gale RP. Hypothesis: How do JAK2-inhibitors work in myelofibrosis. *Leuk Res* 2009;33(9):1156-1157.

76. Verstovsek S, Kantarjian H, Mesa RA, et al. Long-term follow up and optimized dosing regimen of incb018424 in patients with myelofibrosis: Durable clinical, functional and symptomatic responses with improved hematological safety. *Blood* 2009;114:756 (Abstract).

77. Bain BPR, Imbert M, Vardiman JW, Brunning RD, Flandrin G. Chronic eosinophilic leukemia and the hypereosinophilic syndrome. In: al EJe (ed.): *World Health Organization of Tumours: Tumours of Haematopoietic and Lymphoid Tissues.* Lyon: IARC Press; 2001:29-31.

78. Cools J, DeAngelo DJ, Gotlib J, et al. A tyrosine kinase created by fusion of the PDGFRA and FIP1L1 genes as a therapeutic target of imatinib in idiopathic hypereosinophilic syndrome. *N Engl J Med* 2003;348(13):1201-1214.

79. Pardanani A, Ketterling RP, Brockman SR, et al. CHIC2 deletion, a surrogate for FIP1L1-PDGFRA fusion, occurs in systemic mastocytosis associated with eosinophilia and predicts response to imatinib mesylate therapy. *Blood* 2003;102(9): 3093-3096.

80. Pardanani A, Verstovsek S. Hypereosinophilic syndrome, chronic eosinophilic leukemia, and mast cell disease. *Cancer J* 2007;13(6):384-391.

81. Pardanani A, Brockman SR, Paternoster SF, et al. FIP1L1-PDGFRA fusion: Prevalence and clinicopathologic correlates in 89 consecutive patients with moderate to severe eosinophilia. *Blood* 2004;104(10):3038-3045.

82. Pardanani A, Ketterling RP, Li CY, et al. FIP1L1-PDGFRA in eosinophilic disorders: Prevalence in routine clinical practice, long-term experience with imatinib therapy, and a critical review of the literature. *Leuk Res* 2006;30(8):965-970.

83. Jovanovic JV, Score J, Waghorn K, et al. Low-dose imatinib mesylate leads to rapid induction of major molecular responses and achievement of complete molecular remission in FIP1L1-PDGFRA-positive chronic eosinophilic leukemia. *Blood* 2007; 109(11):4635-4640.

84. Rothenberg ME, Klion AD, Roufosse FE, et al. Treatment of patients with the hypereosinophilic syndrome with mepolizumab. *N Engl J Med* 2008;358(12):1215-1228.

85. Verstovsek S, Tefferi A, Kantarjian H, et al. Alemtuzumab therapy for hypereosinophilic syndrome and chronic eosinophilic leukemia. *Clin Cancer Res* 2009;15(1):368-373.

86. Baccarani M, Cilloni D, Rondoni M, et al. The efficacy of imatinib mesylate in patients with FIP1L1-PDGFRalpha-positive hypereosinophilic syndrome. Results of a multicenter prospective study. *Haematologica* 2007;92(9):1173-1179.

87. Valent P, Horny HP, Escribano L, et al. Diagnostic criteria and classification of mastocytosis: A consensus proposal. *Leuk Res* 2001;25(7):603-625.

88. Lemmon MA, Pinchasi D, Zhou M, et al. Kit receptor dimerization is driven by bivalent binding of stem cell factor. *J Biol Chem* 1997;272(10):6311-6317.

89. Furitsu T, Tsujimura T, Tono T, et al. Identification of mutations in the coding sequence of the proto-oncogene c-kit in a human mast cell leukemia cell line causing ligand-independent activation of c-kit product. *J Clin Invest* 1993;92(4):1736-1744.

90. Nagata H, Worobec AS, Oh CK, et al. Identification of a point mutation in the catalytic domain of the protooncogene c-kit in peripheral blood mononuclear cells of patients who have mastocytosis with an associated hematologic disorder. *Proc Natl Acad Sci USA* 1995;92(23):10560-10564.

91. Garcia-Montero AC, Jara-Acevedo M, Teodosio C, et al. KIT mutation in mast cells and other bone marrow hematopoietic cell lineages in systemic mast cell disorders: A prospective study of the Spanish Network on Mastocytosis (REMA) in a series of 113 patients. *Blood* 2006;108(7):2366-2372.

92. Tefferi A, Levine RL, Lim KH, et al. Frequent TET2 mutations in systemic mastocytosis: Clinical, KITD816V and FIP1L1-PDGFRA correlates. *Leukemia* 2009;23(5):900-904.

93. Worobec AS. Treatment of systemic mast cell disorders. *Hematol Oncol Clin North Am* 2000;14(3):659-687, vii.

94. Kaplan AP. Clinical practice. Chronic urticaria and angioedema. *N Engl J Med* 2002;346(3):175-179.

95. Casassus P, Caillat-Vigneron N, Martin A, et al. Treatment of adult systemic mastocytosis with interferon-alpha: Results of a multicentre phase II trial on 20 patients. *Br J Haematol* 2002; 119(4):1090-1097.

96. Lortholary OVJ, Feger F, Palmerini F, et al. Efficacy and safety of cladribine in adult systemic mastocytosis : A French Multicenter Study of 33 patients. *Blood* 2004;104:661.

97. Akin C, Brockow K, D'Ambrosio C, et al. Effects of tyrosine kinase inhibitor STI571 on human mast cells bearing wild-type or mutated c-kit. *Exp Hematol* 2003;31(8): 686-692.

98. Pardanani A, Elliott M, Reeder T, et al. Imatinib for systemic mast-cell disease. *Lancet* 2003;362(9383):535-536.

99. Vega-Ruiz A, Cortes JE, Sever M, et al. Phase II study of imatinib mesylate as therapy for patients with systemic mastocytosis. *Leuk Res* 2009;33(11):1481-1484.

Lymphoma and Myeloma

THE INDOLENT LYMPHOMAS

Peter McLaughlin
Nathan Fowler
Nina Liu
L. Jeffrey Medeiros

The indolent non-Hodgkin lymphomas (NHLs) represent approximately one third of all malignant lymphomas (1,2); most are of B-cell origin. Follicular lymphoma (FL) is the most common indolent lymphoma.

Other indolent B-cell lymphomas include small lymphocytic lymphoma/chronic lymphocytic leukemia (SLL/CLL), the marginal zone B-cell lymphomas (MZLs) (extranodal, nodal, and splenic), and lymphoplasmacytic

TABLE 7-1	INDOLENT LYMPHOMAS
Entities included	Follicular lymphoma Small lymphocytic lymphoma/chronic lymphocytic leukemia Extranodal marginal zone B-cell lymphoma (MALT lymphoma) Splenic B-cell marginal zone lymphoma Nodal marginal zone lymphoma Lymphoplasmacytic lymphoma (including Waldenström macroglobulinemia)
Age	Mostly a disease of older adults (usually over the age of 40 years)
Extent of disease	Often disseminated (except MALT lymphoma), with >80% having stage III-IV disease. Bone marrow involvement common
Natural history	Low proliferation fraction. Slow-growing; may have a waxing and waning course. Patients typically survive for many years. Transformation to large cell lymphoma can occur.
Curability	Although current therapy such as radiotherapy or chemotherapy can often control the disease, it usually fails to eradicate the tumor except for early-stage disease (including MALT lymphoma). This is reflected in a continuous downward slope of relapse-free survival curves for patients with these lymphomas.

lymphoma (LPL), most cases of which are more specifically classified as Waldenström macroglobulinemia (Table 7-1) (2). Mantle cell lymphoma can morphologically resemble indolent B-cell lymphomas, but it is clinically more aggressive and therefore is not covered in this chapter. Indolent T-cell NHLs, such as mycosis fungoides, are also not covered in this chapter.

■ FOLLICULAR LYMPHOMAS

FL represents 22% of all NHLs (1) and 80% of indolent B-cell lymphomas. FL occurs almost exclusively in adults, with an equal frequency in men and women. FL patients typically have a relatively long survival, with a median of 8 to 10 years in the pre-rituximab era (2-4). Outcomes are improving in recent years (5-7).

CLINICAL FEATURES

Patients with FL most often present with asymptomatic lymphadenopathy (1-4). Constitutional symptoms such as fever, drenching night sweats, and significant weight loss occur in approximately 15% of patients. Patients may have symptoms related to lymph node enlargement, especially when there are bulky masses in the retroperitoneum. Other symptoms can include fatigue and, occasionally, end-organ consequences such as obstructive uropathy or bone marrow compromise. Central nervous system (CNS) disease is rare. Urgent situations, such as the superior vena cava syndrome or spinal cord compression are rare, in part related to the usual slow pace of growth of lymphadenopathy in FL. Spontaneous regression of lymphadenopathy can occur in FL. Such regressions, however, are usually partial and are typically short-lived. The potential of FL to wax and wane provides one of several clues that suggest that the host immune system can play an important role in the disease course in FL. Consequently, FL has been a prime focus for immunotherapy approaches.

Approximately 80 to 90% of FL patients present with advanced-stage disease (stage III or IV) with generalized lymphadenopathy. The bone marrow is involved in approximately 50% of patients (3,4).

FL patients can ultimately develop histologic transformation to diffuse large B-cell lymphoma (DLBCL) (8), at a rate of about 1-3% per year. Clinical features suspicious for transformation include rapidly progressive lymphadenopathy, systemic (B) symptoms, localized pain, and a rise in serum lactate dehydrogenase (LDH) level.

HISTOLOGIC, IMMUNOPHENOTYPIC, AND MOLECULAR FEATURES

In FL, the normal lymph node architecture is partially or completely replaced by lymphoma, which typically forms follicles but rarely can be diffused, composed of centrocytes (small cleaved cells) and centroblasts (large noncleaved cells). The method currently recommended in the World Health Organization (WHO) classification to grade FL is based on a count of the centroblasts (2,9). In grade 1 FL, centroblasts are rare, <5 per 400× microscopic field. Grade 2 FL contains ≥5 but <15 centroblasts per 400× microscopic field. The current WHO classification states that there is no clinical benefit derived from distinguishing grade 1 from grade 2 cases and designates these tumors as FL grade 1-2. At least two types of grade 3 FL are described. In grade 3a, >15 centroblasts per 400× microscopic field are present. In grade 3b, sheets of centroblasts are present with rare or absent centrocytes (2). Recent data suggest that FL grade 3b has more features in common with DLBCL than with the indolent FLs (10).

Some patients with B-cell lymphoma of germinal center cell origin may have histologic discordance, for

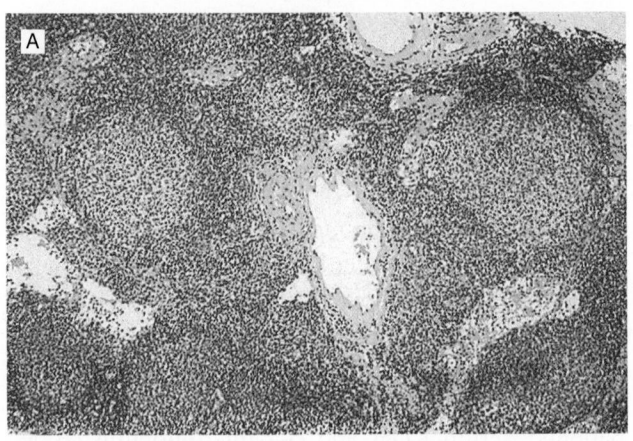
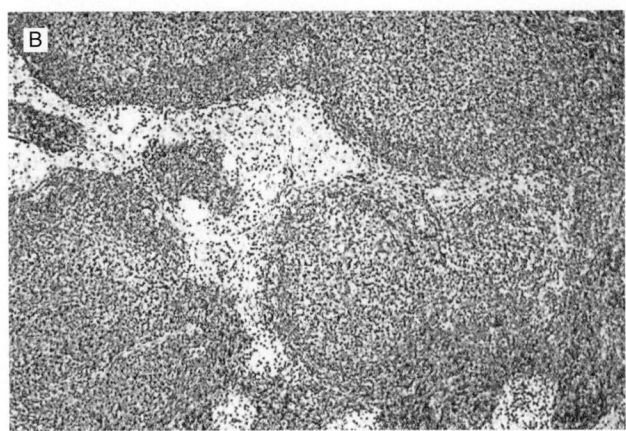

FIGURE 7-1. Follicular lymphoma, grade 1. **A.** In this needle biopsy specimen, neoplastic follicles partially replace architecture. **B.** The neoplastic cells are Bcl-2–positive, supporting lymphoma (A, H&E, 100×; B, Bcl-2 immunostain 100×).

instance with low-grade FL in the bone marrow and large B-cell lymphoma in a lymph node (11). Different lymph nodes biopsied in a given patient can also show different grades of FL.

FL is a neoplasm of mature B-cell lineage (2,12). Most grade 1 and 2 tumors express immunoglobulin, but a subset of FLs, mostly grade 3, may be immunoglobulin-negative. All FLs express pan–B-cell markers, and typically express immunoglobulin and B-cell antigens at high density ("bright" immunofluorescence by flow cytometry). These neoplasms also express the germinal center-associated markers CD10 and Bcl-6 and are negative for T-cell antigens. Bcl-2 is expressed in 80 to 90% of FLs but can be negative, most often in grade 3 neoplasms (2). Because Bcl-2 is negative in reactive germinal centers, this marker is helpful in differential diagnosis (Fig. 7-1).

Using conventional cytogenetic analysis, approximately 75% of FL cases grow in culture and can be successfully karyotyped (13). The cytogenetic hallmark of FL is the t(14;18)(q32;q21), which is identified in 80 to 90% of cases. A small subset of FLs lack the t(14;18), suggesting that a minor pathway of follicular lymphomagenesis may exist that is independent of t(14;18). This appears to apply particularly to grade 3b nodal FL, FLs arising in extranodal sites such as skin, and rare FLs that occur in children, which commonly lack the t(14;18) (2,14-16).

Other cytogenetic abnormalities have been reported in FL. Of these, trisomy 7 and 18, abnormalities of 3q27-28 and 6q23-26, and 17p deletions are most frequent. Abnormalities of 3q27-28 involve the *bcl*-6 gene and most often occur in the form of translocations (13,16,17). Secondary cytogenetic and molecular genetic abnormalities have also been extensively studied,

including in the context of transformation of FL to DLBCL (18-20).

The importance of the immunologic microenvironment in the clinical behavior of FL has been an area of intensive recent study. Gene expression profiling methods have shown molecular signatures attributable to subsets of T-cells and macrophages in FLs that influence the risk of disease progression and prognosis (21-24).

THE t(14;18) AND Bcl-2

As a result of the t(14;18), the bcl-2 oncogene on chromosome 18q21 is translocated to the joining region of the immunoglobulin heavy chain (IgH) gene on chromosome 14q32. The *bcl*-2 gene is deregulated, by being placed under the influence of IgH gene regulatory elements (enhancer region) (17,25). Insights about the role of the *bcl*-2 gene in FL were a gateway to the identification of a large family of pro-apoptotic and anti-apoptotic genes, which play a role in a wide variety of hematopoietic and solid neoplasms (26-28).

The breakpoints on chromosome 18 are primarily clustered at two sites, the major (MBR) and minor (mcr) breakpoint cluster regions, involved in 50 to 60% and 10 to 20% of cases, respectively (29). Other breakpoint clusters have also been described, for example, the intermediate cluster region (ICR). The ICR is involved in approximately 5% of cases; there may be geographic variations in the frequencies of t(14;18) breakpoints (30).

The high frequency of t(14;18) in FL provides the opportunity, using polymerase chain reaction (PCR) techniques, to monitor FL patients for minimal residual disease (MRD) (31).

The Bcl-2 protein is a 25-kD molecule that is over-expressed in FL and protects cells from programmed cell death (apoptosis) (26-28). Inhibition of apoptosis prolongs cell life, resulting in an expanded compartment of B cells, thereby providing more opportunity for additional molecular defects, which presumably are involved in histologic transformation (22-24,27). The presence of the t(14;18) alone appears not to be sufficient for neoplastic transformation. The t(14;18) has been identified in rare cells in the tonsils and lymph nodes of normal individuals without clinical evidence of lymphoma (32).

DIAGNOSTIC WORKUP AND STAGING

The physical examination should include evaluation of all lymph node sites, including epitrochlear and occipital lymph nodes, and assessment of the abdomen for splenomegaly or hepatomegaly.

The diagnosis is best established by an excisional lymph node biopsy, to provide adequate tissue for assessment of the nodal architecture. The most easily accessible lymph node may not be the most informative or representative one. For example, if a small peripheral lymph node shows grade 1 FL, but the patient has a large abdominal mass, a high serum LDH level, and other features suggestive of transformation, then an additional biopsy to exclude higher grade disease should be considered, because this would influence the selection of appropriate therapy. Core needle biopsies guided by radiographic or imaging techniques may be performed on masses that are not easily accessible. Fine-needle aspiration (FNA) can be misleading for initial diagnosis, because complete classification may not be possible because the limited tissue sample prevents

the assessment of architecture, and there is the possibility of sampling error (33,34). In the initial staging evaluation, FNA can play a role in documenting and defining sites of involvement. FNA can also be very useful for restaging or to document relapse.

Once the diagnosis of FL has been established, patients should undergo testing to determine the stage, assess prognostic risk factors, and evaluate their general health. A CBC may show anemia or thrombocytopenia, which can result from bone marrow involvement, or occasionally from hypersplenism or autoimmune problems. Leukemic involvement can occur in 10% of patients. Serum LDH and β-2-microglobulin (B2M) levels may be elevated and are of prognostic significance. Bilateral bone marrow biopsies with unilateral aspiration are recommended for the staging workup because of the patchy nature of involvement. In FL, the bone marrow characteristically shows a paratrabecular pattern of involvement (Fig. 7-2). Because the lymphoma cells are associated with stroma and are not easily aspirated, bone marrow aspirate smears assessed by routine light microscopy may not be informative. Flow cytometry and molecular assessment (eg, PCR) of aspirate material can increase the sensitivity of bone marrow assessment, but in the absence of morphologic abnormalities, positive PCR or flow findings are traditionally not taken as evidence to warrant assignment of stage IV (35). For example, it is well established that Ann Arbor stage I or II patients can have cells with the t(14;18) detected in the peripheral blood or bone marrow by PCR (36).

Imaging studies should include a chest radiograph; chest computed tomography (CT) is also useful, including for delineation of axillary lymphadenopathy. Abdominal and pelvic CT scans are essential, and a

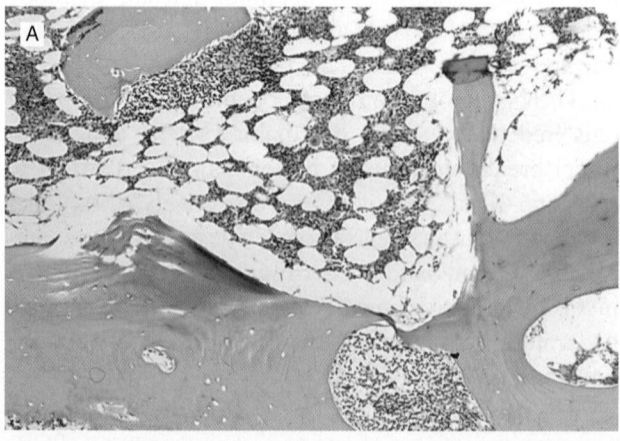
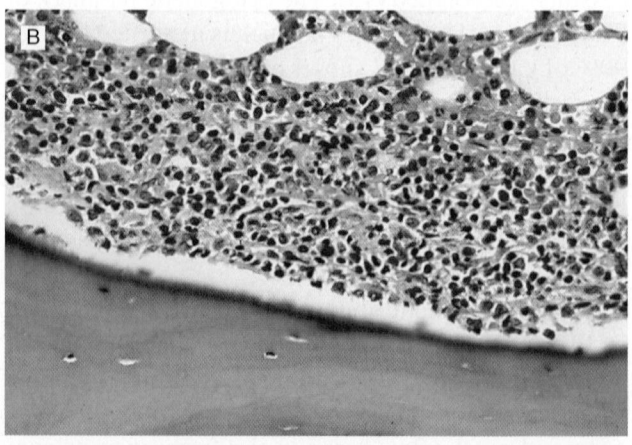

FIGURE 7-2. Follicular lymphoma involving bone marrow. **A.** The neoplasm is infiltrating the bone marrow with a paratrabecular pattern. **B.** Neoplastic small-cleaved cells adjacent to bone are seen in this field (A, B, H&E; A, 100×; B, 400×).

head-and-neck CT is also useful. Positron emission tomography (PET) using fluorine-18 fluorodeoxyglucose (18F-FDG) has emerged as a useful tool for assessing patients with aggressive lymphoma and Hodgkin's lymphoma. PET imaging is also useful in patients with indolent B-cell lymphoma (37-39). There can be low FDG uptake in indolent lymphomas, however, so the utility of PET scanning for the monitoring of patients with indolent lymphoma has not been embraced to the same extent that it has for DLBCL and Hodgkin's lymphoma (40).

PROGNOSTIC FACTORS

The prognostic importance of histologically distinguishing grade 1-2 (indolent) FL from the more aggressive grade 3 (large cell) FL is well accepted. However, most investigators have not found a clear difference in long-term survival between patients with grades 1 and 2 FL, although older literature suggested that FL grade 2 (nodular mixed cell lymphoma, in older nomenclature) was more prone to early progression than grade 1, if therapy was deferred (41). Higher degrees of nodularity have been associated in some reports with improved outcome. An increased proliferation rate is associated with a poorer prognosis (42,43).

Variables that have been shown to correlate with survival in patients with FL include tumor burden, host factors, and response to therapy. Tumor burden can be estimated by assessing stage of disease, size of nodal disease, bone marrow involvement, serum B2M and LDH levels, and number of nodal sites. Adverse host factors include advanced age, B symptoms, low hemoglobin level, male gender, and poor performance status. The background cells in the diagnostic lymph node biopsy can also provide prognostic information, as shown in gene expression profiling studies (21,22).

The International Prognostic Index (IPI) was devised for aggressive lymphomas and consists of five variables: age, performance status, Ann Arbor stage, extranodal involvement, and serum LDH level (44). Lopez-Guillermo et al. and others have shown that the IPI is also a useful predictor of survival in patients with indolent B-cell lymphomas (45). One important limitation of this system is that only 11% of the patients fell into the high-risk group, and most of these patients had poor performance status and would be poor candidates for aggressive therapy. Partly for that reason, a Follicular Lymphoma International Prognostic Index (FLIPI) was developed. Initially, an eight-parameter model including age ≥60 years, male gender, Ann Arbor stages III and IV, nodal sites ≥5, BM involvement, serum LDH

level >normal, hemoglobin level <12 g/dL, and lymphocytes ≥1000/µL was proposed (46). A simplified version of this model was found to be comparably predictive, using the five parameters of age, Ann Arbor stage, serum LDH, hemoglobin, and number of nodal sites (47). This prognostic model separates patients into three prognostic groups: good risk with 0 to 1 factors, intermediate risk with 2 factors, and poor risk with ≥3 factors. The overall 5-year survival was 90% for the good-risk group, 78% for the intermediate-risk group, and 53% for the poor-risk group (47). The validity of the FLIPI model has been demonstrated in rituximab-treated patients (48). Recently, a FLIPI-2 (F-2) model was developed through the prospective collection of prognostic factor data, producing a five-factor model that incorporates: age (>60 years adverse); hemoglobin (<12 adverse); serum B2M level (adverse if above normal range); bone marrow (adverse if involved); and size of lymphadenopathy (>6 cm adverse) (49). There are more similarities than differences in these models. For instance, the importance of serum B2M was shown in the univariate analyses of both the IPI and FLIPI data sets, but the B2M data was collected prospectively only in the F-2 report. The importance of sampling the bone marrow, as shown in the F-2 report, deserves particular emphasis, because recent practice patterns indicate that this important data is often not being collected (50). Easily applied models such as the IPI, FLIPI, or F-2 can provide a framework for selecting the timing or intensity of therapy, and can facilitate the interpretation of clinical trials, by providing a tool to assess for disparities in patient selection when results of various trials are being compared.

At the time of relapse, favorable predictors for survival in patients with FL include having achieved a complete response with initial therapy, having had a durable remission of more than 1 year following initial therapy, and being less than 60 years of age (51).

POSTTREATMENT MONITORING

An international working group has recommended standard response criteria for NHL (35). These criteria have recently been updated, with important modifications that incorporate PET scan findings; these changes pertain mostly to patients with DLBCL and Hodgkin's lymphoma (40). For indolent lymphoma, CT scans remain the standard for the evaluation of nodal disease. Bone marrow re-evaluation is performed to confirm clinical remission if the bone marrow was initially positive. Ideally, patients in clinical trials should be reassessed after completion of therapy about every 3 to 4 months for 2 years, then every 6 months for 3 years, and then annually for at least 5 years. PET scans, as mentioned earlier, are not currently a standard tool for posttreatment monitoring for indolent lymphoma patients.

Although the monitoring of patients with molecular studies is not currently considered standard practice, the presence of the t(14;18) translocation by PCR techniques has been useful in the monitoring of subclinical disease. "Molecular remission," the disappearance of cells with the t(14;18) detected by PCR, used to be considered a rarity in FL patients treated with standard therapy. Gribben et al. (52) reported that only 1 of 212 (0.5%) patients achieved molecular remission following conventional chemotherapy. With high-dose therapy and stem cell transplantation, however, molecular remissions could be attained, and those with molecular remission experienced more durable remissions. Improvements in therapy have changed this picture. Even before the advent of anti-CD20 monoclonal antibody therapy, more potent chemotherapy regimens were capable of inducing molecular remission in over half of patients (53-57). With the availability of rituximab, which can largely eradicate B cells from the blood and bone marrow, it is now common to see molecular remission. Some recent studies continue to show that molecular remission correlates with more durable clinical remission (58, 59), but other studies do not (60).

Real-time PCR techniques provide the additional benefit of quantitative information, which show a nice correlation of PCR-detectable cells with pretreatment tumor burden, in some studies (58, 59). However, these promising approaches are still research tools rather than standard tests, partly because of lack of standardization of techniques (61, 62), and other ongoing controversies in the literature.

TREATMENT OF LIMITED STAGE FL

At diagnosis, approximately 15 to 20% of FL patients have limited-stage disease (stages I and II). This stage of disease is associated with a favorable outcome, and up to half of these patients may be curable. Consequently, seizing the opportunity for cure should be strongly considered, even though some advocate deferral of therapy (63). Several series have reported long-term disease-free survival of approximately 35 to 50% for stage I to II patients treated with involved-field radiotherapy (RT), so it appears that many of these patients are cured (64-67). Studies with extended-field or total lymphoid RT, in an attempt to increase cure rates, have not shown convincing additional benefit.

The integration of chemotherapy with involved-field RT has shown promising results in some trials. Investigators

TABLE 7-2	PROGNOSTIC MODELS FOR LYMPHOMA		
	MODEL		
Prognostic Factor	*IPI*	*FLIPI*	*F-2*
Age	√	√	√
PS	√		
Stage	√	√	
No. of E sites	√		
Bone marrow			√
No. of nodal sites		√	
Size of nodes			√
LDH	√	√	
Hgb		√	√
B2M			√

PS, performance status; B2M, serum β-2-microglobulin.

at MDACC prospectively treated 85 patients with stage I-II FL with 10 cycles of COP-Bleo (cyclophosphamide, vincristine, prednisone, and bleomycin) or CHOP-Bleo (COP-Bleo plus doxorubicin) and involved-field RT "sandwiched" after the third cycle. The disease-free survival at 5 and 10 years was 80 and 72%, respectively—an apparent improvement over results with RT alone (68). The role of rituximab in stage I-II disease is not clearly defined, except by extrapolation from the stage III-IV literature.

In summary, patients with limited-stage FL appear to be potentially curable. The role of RT in these patients is well established, so involved-field RT remains the standard treatment (Table 7-2). Despite the established role of involved field RT, and its endorsement by experts (69), RT appears to be under-utilized in practice (50). Total lymphoid RT and combined-modality therapy approaches remain controversial and are seldom used.

MANAGEMENT OF ADVANCED STAGE FL

For decades, the treatment of patients with advanced stage FL has been built on two pillars that lean in opposite directions. First, there are numerous effective therapeutic options that can induce remission (Table 7-3); and second, relapse appears to be inevitable.

If and when therapeutic advances lead to more comprehensive control of FL, then there may be consensus about early intervention, because a smaller tumor burden would presumably be more easily treatable, analogous to the stage I-II situation. Until then, it is still the case that deferral of therapy is a common consideration for many asymptomatic patients.

TABLE 7-3	MANAGEMENT STRATEGIES FOR FOLLICULAR LYMPHOMA AND OTHER INDOLENT LYMPHOMAS
Stages I-II	IF RT
	RT and CT*
Stages III-IV	Deferral of therapy (if no threatening disease)
	Single-agent alkylators
	Single-agent MoAb
	COP and variants, with MoAb
	CHOP and variants,* with MoAb
	FND and variants,* with MoAb
	RT (stage III)
	CT and RT* (stage III)
	Consolidation (see text)
	Maintenance (see text)

COP, cyclophosphamide, vincristine, and prednisone; CHOP, COP and doxorubicin; CT, chemotherapy; FND, fludarabine, mitoxantrone, and dexamethasone; IF, involved field; MoAb, monoclonal antibody; RT, radiation therapy.
*MDACC protocol approaches over the years (see text).

The deferral-of-therapy issue has at times diverted the focus of clinical research in FL away from the important incremental gains that have occurred in recent years. There have been advances in the efficacy of chemotherapy, including intensified approaches with or without stem cell transplant (SCT), and the introduction of agents such as the purine nucleoside analogs. The development of biological therapy approaches, most notably anti-CD20 monoclonal antibodies (70,71), has revolutionized therapy for many B-cell lymphomas. The introduction of rituximab has led to broad and renewed interest in designing therapeutic strategies with the aim of attaining durable remissions.

The range of therapy options for patients with advanced stage FL is broad (Table 7-3). The therapeutic aim can be palliative for selected patients, with the focus on minimizing toxicity. More definitive therapy approaches have the goal of attaining durable complete remission.

Recent front-line therapy trials for indolent lymphoma have focused on: (a) the role of rituximab in conjunction with chemotherapy; (b) the role of consolidation of remission, for example, with radioimmunotherapy (RIT); (c) the role of maintenance biological therapy; (d) the impact of vaccines; and (e) the role of therapy approaches with biological agents alone.

RITUXIMAB PLUS CHEMOTHERAPY

Several trials have shown convincingly that the addition of rituximab to chemotherapy leads to improved outcomes (Table 7-4; references 72-78). Rituximab has become a standard part of induction therapy. Suitable partners for rituximab in induction regimens include three regimens that were studied in randomized trials (CVP, CHOP, and MCP) (72-75), and numerous others such as FND, FN, FCM, and bendamustine (76-78). The latter (B–R) has recently been compared with R-CHOP in a randomized trial, and the simpler B–R combination is less toxic and also modestly more effective than R-CHOP.

CONSOLIDATION THERAPY

A crossover strategy has been reported, which utilized rituximab after chemotherapy on a selective basis, for patients who did not attain molecular remission following induction chemotherapy (Table 7-5). FL patients who initially had PCR evidence of cells with t(14;18)/IgH-bcl-2 in the peripheral blood were reassessed by PCR after chemotherapy with either CHOP or FN (fludarabine plus mitoxantrone) (79, 80). About half of patients attained molecular response after the induction therapy, that is, their IgH-bcl-2 status in the peripheral blood reverted to negative after chemotherapy; those

TABLE 7-4	FRONT-LINE RITUXIMAB-PLUS-CHEMOTHERAPY TRIALS IN INDOLENT LYMPHOMA					
Regimen	Trial Design	% CR	% PR	% FFS (@ Time)	% Survival @ Time
R-CVP*	Phase III	41*	40	52 (3 years)*	89 (30 months)
R-CHOP*	Phase III	20	77	75 (3 years)*	96 (2 years)
R-MCP*	Phase III	50*	42	71 (4 years)*	87 (4 years)*
R-Bendamustine*†	Phase III	40*	53	58 (4 years)*	–
R-FND‡	Phase III	88	12	76 (3 years)	96 (3 years)
R-FCM	Phase II	83	11	58 (5 years)	89 (5 years)

*Significantly better than comparator arm. For R-CVP, survival benefit noted in 2008 update.
†Comparator arm R-CHOP.
‡Comparator arm FND, followed by rituximab (maintenance).

TABLE
7-5   **CONSOLIDATION THERAPY APPROACHES**

Induction	Consolidation	% CR After Induction	% CR After Consolidation	% CR + PR	% FFS (@ Times)
CHOP	Rituximab*	57	*	94	44 (3 years)
FN	Rituximab*	68	*	96	63 (3 years)
CHOP	Tositumomab	39	69	98	67 (5 years)
Various	Ibritumomab/Y-90	51[†]	87[†]	100[†]	53 (3 years*)
R-FND	Ibritumomab/Y-90	69	89	89	73 (3 years)
Fludarabine	Tositumomab/I-131	9	86	100	60 (5 years)

*In these trials, rituximab crossover only for subset who did not attain molecular response: conversion to molecular remission occurred in 74% and 61% in the two trials.
[†]Trial design accepted only CR and PR patients for RIT. FFS measured from study entry, before RIT but after induction chemotherapy.

patients were followed with no further therapy. Patients who still had cells with detectable IgH-bcl-2 fusion sequences were treated with rituximab after chemotherapy. In two such trials, the additional therapy with rituximab resulted in attainment of molecular remission in about half of rituximab-treated patients. This appears to be an important incremental gain, because failure to attain molecular remission has been shown by several investigators to correlate with short duration of clinical remission.

A large multicenter randomized trial of RIT consolidation therapy has shown a significant failure-free survival benefit, when used after a variety of induction therapy regimens (81). Notably, the induction therapy included rituximab in only a minority of the patients. Still, the feasibility and impact of such a strategy is noteworthy. Prolongation of disease control was significant in subset analyses of both complete and partial responders to the induction therapy. Patients who attained only partial remission (PR) after chemotherapy commonly attained complete remission (CR) after RIT (77%).

Other small trials have also studied RIT consolidation (82,83). At MDACC, patients with high-risk features by the FLIPI model received a rituximab-containing induction regimen (R-FND) followed by Zevalin. Preliminary results are encouraging (83). A Southwest Oncology Group trial of RIT after CHOP therapy (84) was encouraging enough to prompt a randomized comparison of CHOP followed by RIT, versus R-CHOP; that large randomized trial has completed accrual, but no outcome results are yet available because of short follow-up.

MAINTENANCE BIOLOGICAL THERAPY

Interferon-alpha (IFN-α) has been utilized both in conjunction with chemotherapy, and as a maintenance strategy (85-87). It has been shown to be an effective approach, but IFN has fallen into disuse, partly because of nuisance toxicity issues such as fatigue.

Rituximab maintenance (Table 7-6) has been widely utilized after front-line chemo-immunotherapy, even

TABLE
7-6   **MAINTENANCE RITUXIMAB**

		INDUCTION RESPONSE		↑ FFS WITH
	Induction	% CR	% PR	Maintenance*
A. Front-line trials	Rituximab	9	58	Yes
	CVP	13	60	Yes
	Various + R	–	–	Yes
B. Salvage	Rituximab	0	28	Yes[†]
	R-CHOP	30	55	Yes
	R-FCM	41	54	Yes

*Maintenance schedules and duration variable (see text).
[†]Benefit of maintenance was matched by re-treatment at time of progression.

| TABLE 7-7 | **PHASE III Id-KLH + GM-CSF VACCINE APPROACHES IN FOLLICULAR LYMPHOMA** |

Trial	Induction Therapy	Patients Randomized to Vaccine	Vaccination	DFS
NCI/Biovest	PACE	CR/CRu	Id-KLH + GM-CSF	↑
Genitope	CVP	CR/PR	Id-KLH + GM-CSF	NS
Favrille	Rituximab	CR/PR/SD	Id-KLH + GM-CSF	NS

CR, complete remission; PR, partial remission; SD, stable disease; NS, not significant.

though data from the most pertinent clinical trial is still only preliminary (88). The widespread acceptance of this strategy has been based on extensive data using rituximab maintenance after single-agent rituximab induction (89,91), data using rituximab maintenance after front-line chemotherapy that did not include rituximab (91), and compelling data using rituximab maintenance after salvage therapy that did include rituximab (77,92).

VACCINES

Three long-awaited trials using a post-therapy anti-idiotype vaccination approach have been reported recently (93-95). In each, a patient-specific anti-idiotype vaccine was prepared from biopsy material obtained pretreatment. There were minor differences in the vaccine preparation. There were major differences in the intensity of the induction therapy pre-vaccination, and corresponding important differences in the quality of remission that each trial required prior to entering the vaccination phase of the trial (Table 7-7).

In each of these trials, the induction therapy was chosen with the intention of minimizing immunosuppression, for example, as might occur if a nucleoside analog were included. The outcomes of the trials may be partly explained by the trade-offs that are implicit in the selection of the induction therapy. With the two mildest induction therapies, no benefit from vaccination was seen. Notably, these trials were (necessarily) less stringent about the degree of cytoreduction that was acceptable prior to the vaccination phase. The only trial of the three that demonstrated a benefit of vaccination was the one that utilized a more potent induction regimen, and demanded excellent CR before vaccination. Notably, rituximab was not included in the induction chemotherapy regimen.

One take-home message from these vaccine trials is that, although there are hints of efficacy, there is still much work to be done in this area. Another important observation is that the quality of remission, that is, the

attainment of CR, appears to be an important goal prior to a vaccination approach.

BIOLOGICAL THERAPY

The efficacy of single-agent rituximab has been demonstrated reproducibly. Although most responses to salvage rituximab are PR rather than CR, a higher fraction of CR is seen with front-line rituximab therapy (96).

With the aim of improving the CR percentage, but preserving the purely biological therapy approach, many investigators have explored biological combination approaches (Table 7-8). These include rituximab (R) + cytokines, R + other monoclonal antibodies, and R + other categories of biological or targeted therapy (97,98). Results have been encouraging but mostly preliminary. This is a promising area of investigation.

The utility of RIT was first established in the salvage setting. There are currently two approved RIT agents: both target CD20. One delivers yttrium-90 (Zevalin); the other delivers iodine-131 (Bexxar). A randomized controlled trial of Zevalin versus rituximab for relapsed or refractory low grade B-cell lymphomas revealed an 80% response rate for patients treated with Zevalin compared with a 50% response rate for patients treated with rituximab (99). A pivotal study of Bexxar for chemotherapy-refractory low grade B-cell lymphomas showed a response rate of 65% in extensively pretreated patients (100). Also impressive are results in a small

| TABLE 7-8 | **NOVEL THERAPY APPROACHES** |

A.	Rituximab + biological agents
	• Cytokines: GM-CSF; G-CSF, interferon; IL-2; others
	• Monoclonal antibodies: anti-CD22; anti-CD80
	• Other: lenalidomide; bcl-2 antisense
B.	Rituximab + other targeted therapy
	• Immunotoxin: CMC-544
	• Proteasome inhibitor: bortezomib
C.	Rituximab + other chemotherapy
	• bendamustine

cohort of patients who received RIT alone as front-line therapy (101).

Newer anti-CD20 monoclonal antibodies (MAbs) are being investigated, with modifications that theoretically represent enhancements over rituximab, such as: fully humanized MAbs as opposed to a chimeric mouse–human construct; MAbs with enhanced capacity for mediation of complement-dependent cytotoxicity; MAbs with enhanced mediation of antibody-dependent cellular cytotoxicity; and other modifications. MAbs that target antigens other than CD20 have been developed. CD19 and CD22 are B-cell-specific antigens which internalize, so the development of therapeutic Abs against these targets has included their use both alone, and as immunotoxins, that is, as delivery systems for toxins, analogous to the delivery of isotopes with RIT. One example of an immunotoxin that is of current interest is an anti-CD22/calicheamicin construct (102). There has been extensive prior study of other immunotoxins as well, for both B-cell and T-cell lymphomas (103-105).

Immunotoxin agents are not limited to MAbs. Denileukin diftitox is a combination of the enzymatically active domain of diphtheria toxin and IL-2, which targets cells that express the IL-2 receptor. Its utility is most logically and clearly demonstrated in T-cell lymphomas, but efficacy has also been seen in B-cell lymphomas, which also express CD25 (106).

Many therapeutic options under study in the past decade have been developed against specific cell growth regulatory pathways. These include inhibitors of the proteasome (eg, bortezomib), inhibitors of the mammalian target of rapamycin, or mTOR (eg, temsirolimus), inhibitors of protein kinase C (eg, enzastaurin), agents that work in part by inhibition of angiogenesis (eg, lenalidomide), and others (107-109). With some of these agents, their categorization as "biological" or "targeted" therapy, rather than conventional cytotoxic therapy, may be arguable. Some of these targeted therapies are associated with myelosuppressive toxicity, as is seen with conventional chemotherapy.

OTHER SALVAGE THERAPY

Numerous non–cross-resistant chemotherapeutic agents can be effective in indolent lymphomas (Table 7-9). Those not chosen for a patient's front-line treatment are candidates for salvage use.

Because initial MAb therapy approaches are often selected, it is notable that retreatment of previously responsive patients is a legitimate option, for example, with rituximab (110). Likewise with some chemotherapies, long-term follow-up studies have shown that

TABLE 7-9	SELECTED SALVAGE CHEMOTHERAPY REGIMENS
Ara C – Cisplatin backbone	
	ESHAP (etoposide; methylprednisone, ara C; cisplatin)
	ASHAP* (doxorubicin; methylprednisone; ara C; cisplatin)
Fludarabine-based	
	FND (fludarabine; mitoxantrone; dexamethasone)
	R-FCM (rituximab; fludarabine; cyclophosphamide; mitoxantrone)
Others	
	MINE (mesna; ifosfamide; mitoxantrone; etoposide)
	R-GemOx* (rituximab; gemcitabine; oxaliplatin)
	ICE* (ifosfamide; carboplatin; etoposide)
	B-R (bendamustine; rituximab)

*Most extensive literature in aggressive lymphoma, and/or as lead-in to stem cell transplant.

second and later responses can be attained, even with the same agents, for example, with chlorambucil; but the ensuing clinical remissions become progressively more brief (111).

Because some physicians advocate the avoidance of the toxicities of certain agents (eg, doxorubicin or the nucleoside analogs) in the front-line setting, their role in the salvage setting is an important consideration. Selected salvage chemotherapy regimens are listed in Table 7-9 (112-117). Particularly notable are the results with fludarabine-containing regimens, and the recent emergence in the West of bendamustine as a potent option, after years of positive experience in Eastern Europe.

SCT approaches can be arduous, but deserve strong consideration in patients with recurrent FL. Autologous SCT strategies result in substantially more durable remissions than conventional-dose salvage therapy (118). Allogeneic SCT is a strategy that is contingent on availability of a donor, and it is a complex undertaking that includes real risks of treatment-related mortality. Nonetheless, allogeneic SCT can result not only in long-term remission but also can potentially lead to cure, presumably through its graft-versus-lymphoma effect (119). Recent data suggests that non–myeloablative allogeneic SCT is associated with less toxicity than conventional myeloablative allogeneic SCT (120), but this is an area of controversy that has not been studied prospectively (121).

Palliative treatment for FL can include involved field RT to sites of problematic disease, for example, for obstructive uropathy. Among chemotherapy options, one of the historically mildest options is chlorambucil.

Observation without therapy is of course also an option, even at the time of initial diagnosis, in patients with active disease but no threatening or symptomatic disease. The approach of deferral of therapy is common. It should be done thoughtfully and with monitoring. Because elderly patients are often selected for the "watch and wait" strategy, that option should be weighed against the observation that elderly patients with FL have a 10-fold increased risk of dying within 1 year, compared with age-matched controls (51).

■ SMALL LYMPHOCYTIC LYMPHOMA/CHRONIC LYMPHOCYTIC LEUKEMIA

SLL represents approximately 7% of all NHLs (1,3). The WHO classification restricts SLL to tumors involving lymph nodes with the same B-cell immunophenotype as chronic lymphocytic leukemia (CLL) without leukemic involvement, and considers SLL to be the nodal or tissue counterpart of CLL (2).

CLINICAL FEATURES AND MANAGEMENT

Patients with SLL often present with asymptomatic lymphadenopathy. B symptoms are uncommon and are observed in less than 10% of patients. Splenomegaly is common. Bone marrow is often involved, in approximately 70% of patients (1-4). Although the traditional staging systems for SLL and CLL are different, these systems share common features and the prognosis of patients with SLL is similar to those with CLL (122).

Management strategies for patients with FL and CLL are often applicable to patients with SLL, but there are some caveats. For instance, as CD20 is usually dimly expressed by SLL/CLL, anti-CD20 antibody therapy for SLL may be better modeled on the results in the CLL literature rather than the results of patients with FL. Conversely, the response to anti-CD52 antibody therapy (alemtuzumab) seems to depend greatly on tissue penetration, and response is often inadequate at sites of bulky disease in SLL/CLL patients (123).

HISTOLOGIC, IMMUNOPHENOTYPIC, AND MOLECULAR FEATURES

The lymph node architecture is diffusely and usually totally effaced by SLL/CLL (2,125). The neoplastic cells are predominantly small, round lymphocytes. Vague pale areas composed of lymphocytes, prolymphocytes, and paraimmunoblasts are usually present and are diagnostic of this neoplasm. In 5 to 10% of SLL/CLL cases, residual reactive lymphoid follicles are present, surrounded by neoplasm; this represents the so-called interfollicular pattern of SLL/CLL. In this morphologic variant, proliferation centers can surround benign follicles, mimicking nodal MZL.

SLL/CLL cells express monotypic immunoglobin light chain, IgM, usually IgD, pan–B-cell antigens, and Bcl-2 (2,124). CD23 is usually positive in 90 to 95% of cases, and CD22, CD79B, and FMC7 are negative in most cases. The density of Ig and CD20 antigen expression on the surface of SLL/CLL cells is characteristically low ("dim" immunofluorescence by flow cytometry). These neoplasms almost invariably express the CD5 antigen, a pan–T-cell antigen that is not expressed on normal B cells. Other T-cell antigens are negative. CD38 and ZAP 70 are expressed by a subset of cases, and expression correlates with unmutated Ig genes and poorer prognosis (125). The neoplastic cells are negative for CD10 and Bcl-6 (2).

Conventional cytogenetic analysis has shown chromosomal abnormalities in 50 to 60% of SLL/CLL cases (126). This low frequency is partly attributable to poor cell growth in culture. The t(14;19)(q32;q13) involving the *bcl-3* gene at 19q13 is present in <5% of SLL/CLL cases and is associated with atypical morphologic or immunophenotypic features and a poorer prognosis (127).

Fluorescence in situ hybridization (FISH) analysis has shown a higher frequency of abnormalities in SLL/CLL, as this technique can assess interphase as well as metaphase nuclei and does not require cell growth in culture (128). At MDACC, SLL/CLL cases are routinely assessed by FISH with a panel of probes, including those specific for 6q, 11q (ATM), trisomy 12, 13q14, and 17p (*p53*). Deletion of the 13q14 locus is the most common abnormality in SLL/CLL. Trisomy 12 is detected in approximately 15 to 20% of cases and appears to be a secondary event, as it is usually found in only a subset of the neoplastic cells (128). Both del (11q) and trisomy 12 have been correlated with poorer prognosis. Abnormalities of the *p53* or *MYC* genes correlate with increased risk of histologic transformation (Richter's syndrome) and poorer prognosis (129).

■ MARGINAL ZONE B-CELL LYMPHOMAS

Although their names are similar, the MZLs are not closely related at the genetic level and have different pathogeneses. The MZLs include extranodal MZL of mucosa-associated lymphoid tissue (MALT lymphoma), nodal marginal zone lymphoma, and splenic B-cell marginal zone lymphoma (SMZL). Prior to the advent of immunophenotypic and molecular methods, MALT lymphomas were often classified as *pseudolymphomas.* Immunophenotypic and gene rearrangement studies showed that most pseudolymphomas express monotypic immunoglobin light chain or carry monoclonal immunoglobulin gene rearrangements.

MALT lymphomas represent 7 to 8% of all NHLs (1,3). Nodal marginal zone lymphomas represent approximately 2% of all NHLs (130). Splenic B- SMZL is rare, representing less than 1% of all NHLs (1). SMZL can be associated with circulating lymphocytes with villous cytoplasmic projections. The entity previously described as splenic lymphoma with villous lymphocytes is, in most cases, SMZL (131).

EXTRANODAL MARGINAL ZONE B-CELL LYMPHOMA

Clinical Features

Patients with MALT lymphoma present with extranodal disease that is often localized (stage I-E or II-E). There may be a history of infection or autoimmune disease and the disease is usually indolent. The bone marrow is involved in only 10 to 20% of patients, and peripheral lymph node involvement is uncommon (132,133). The most common site of involvement is the stomach, but numerous other extranodal locations can be involved including: lung, skin, orbit, salivary glands, other parts of the gastrointestinal tract, thyroid gland, and other rare sites (132). Dissemination occurs in up to 30% of cases, most often in patients with non-gastric MALT lymphoma, often to other extranodal sites. In patients with non-gastric MALT lymphomas, subclinical gastric involvement is not uncommon (133).

The stomach is the best-studied site of involvement. Patients often present with signs and symptoms suggestive of peptic ulcer disease, such as epigastric pain and dyspepsia. Anemia, weight loss, and gastrointestinal bleeding can be seen in patients with more advanced disease. *Helicobacter pylori* is present in the gastric mucosa of many patients with MALT lymphoma (134). Antibiotic eradication of *H pylori* has resulted in regression of MALT lymphoma in over half of treated patients (135,136). Thus, *H pylori* is thought to be essential to lymphomagenesis in gastric MALT lymphoma.

In non-gastric MALT lymphomas, symptoms are related to the anatomic site involved. Disseminated disease is generally more common in these patients than in patients with gastric MALT lymphoma (137,138). Despite the higher frequency of stage IV disease, the 5-year survival is 90% with a variety of therapies (132).

Histologic Features

Four findings are present in most MALT lymphomas: a population of neoplastic small lymphoid (centrocyte-like) cells that may have monocytoid features, occasional large lymphoid cells (blasts), lymphoepithelial lesions, and reactive lymphoid follicles (Figs. 7-3 to 7-5) (139).

The neoplastic small lymphoid cells exhibit a range of cytologic appearances. In some cases, the cells resemble small lymphocytes with or without plasmacytoid differentiation. In other cases, the neoplasm appears biphasic: one component is a population of small lymphoid cells and the other is a population of cells with extensive plasmacytoid differentiation, resembling mature plasma cells (see Fig. 7-5). In other cases, the cells have markedly irregular nuclear contours and resemble small-cleaved cells. All of these cell types may have abundant pale cytoplasm imparting a monocytoid appearance. In most MALT lymphomas, occasional large lymphoid cells (blasts) are also present. However, when large cells are numerous and form confluent sheets, the neoplasm has evolved to diffuse large B-cell lymphoma.

The small neoplastic cells have a marked tendency to infiltrate epithelium, forming so-called lymphoepithelial lesions (see Fig. 7-4). In well-formed lesions, aggregates of neoplastic cells are found within the epithelium. Reactive lymphoid follicles are also usually present in MALT lymphomas, generally surrounded by neoplastic small lymphoid cells. Neoplastic cells can

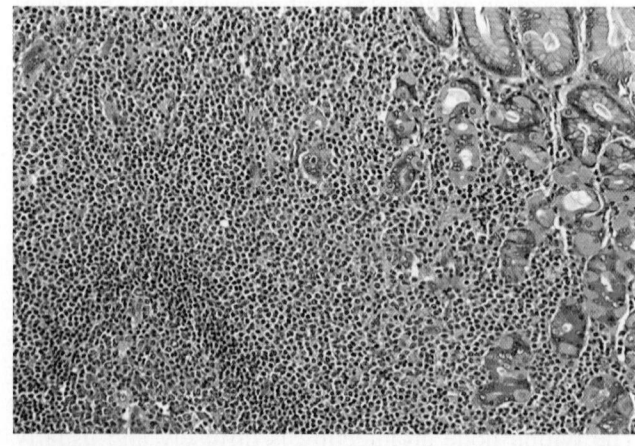

FIGURE 7-3. Extranodal marginal zone B-cell lymphoma of MALT (MALT lymphoma) involving the stomach. The neoplasm partially replaces gastric mucosa and infiltrates epithelium. A reactive follicle is present at the bottom left of the field.

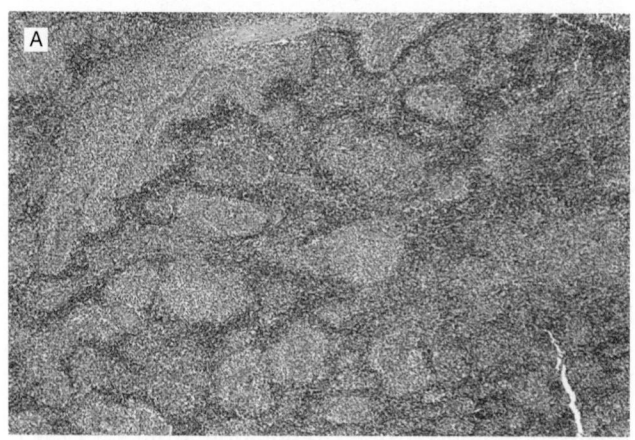
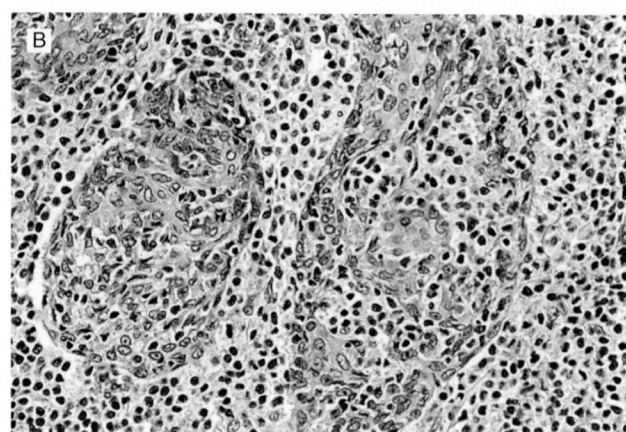

FIGURE 7-4. MALT lymphoma of salivary gland. **A.** The neoplastic cells have a pale (monocytoid) low-power appearance and surround ducts. **B.** Lymphoepithelial lesions are prominent in this case (A, B, H&E; A, 20×; B, 400×).

also accumulate in these follicles (termed *colonization*), imparting a vaguely nodular appearance at low-power magnification.

Anatomic site-specific histologic findings are also observed in MALT lymphomas, involving chronic antigenic stimulation as a result of either an infectious organism or autoimmune disease. For example, normal lymphoid tissue is not usually present in the stomach. However, benign MALT is acquired, probably in response to *H pylori* infection (134,139). *Chlamydia psittaci*, *Borrelia burgdorferi*, and *Campylobacter jejuni* are other infectious agents that have been associated with orbital, skin, and small intestinal MALT lymphomas, respectively, although the data linking

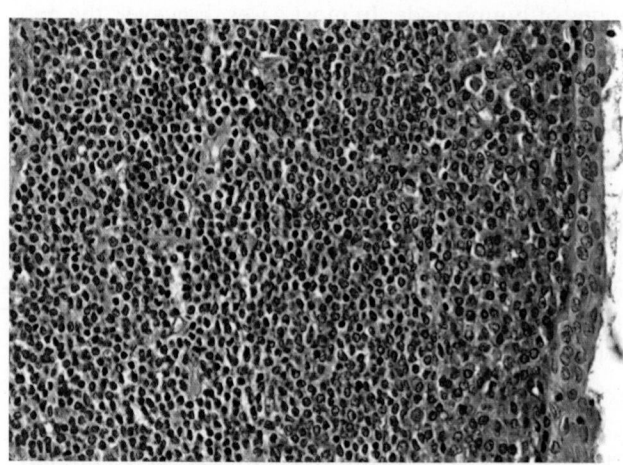

FIGURE 7-5. MALT lymphoma of conjunctiva. In this field, the neoplasm has a biphasic pattern, with the subepithelial portion exhibiting extensive plasmacytoid differentiation (periodic acid–Schiff, 400×).

B burgdorferi to skin lymphomas does not appear to be strong (140-142). Like the stomach, normal lymphoid tissue is also poorly developed in the lung. However, two inflammatory diseases are frequently associated with lung MALT lymphoma: Sjögren syndrome and lymphoid interstitial pneumonia. Similarly, MALT lymphomas of the salivary gland are usually associated with Sjögren syndrome, and Hashimoto's thyroiditis usually precedes MALT lymphoma of the thyroid gland (139).

Immunophenotypic, Cytogenetic, and Molecular Features

MALT lymphomas express monotypic immunoglobulin light chain, pan–B-cell antigens, and Bcl-2 (139). These tumors typically do not express IgD, CD10, CD21, CD23, Bcl-6, cyclin D1, or T-cell antigens, including CD5. Four chromosomal translocations are well characterized in MALT lymphomas: the t(11;18), t(14;18), t(1;14) and t(3;14) (139,143,144).

The t(11;18)(q21;q21) has been identified in approximately 20 to 30% of MALT lymphomas. In this translocation, the *api2* gene on 11q21 and the *malt*1 gene on chromosome 18q21 are disrupted and recombine to form a novel *api2–malt*1 fusion gene. The *api2* gene belongs to the inhibitor of apoptosis protein (IAP) gene family that is evolutionary conserved and plays a role in regulating apoptosis. *Malt*1 is a novel gene that is critical to the function of API2–MALT1. The t(11;18) is most common in MALT lymphomas of the lung and stomach (139,143).

The t(14;18)(q32;q21) has been identified in approximately 10 to 20% of MALT lymphomas. In this translocation, the MALT1 gene is juxtaposed next to the immunoglobulin heavy chain gene on the derivative chromosome 14. As a result, MALT1 is overexpressed. The t(14;18) appears to be most common in MALT lymphomas arising in the ocular adnexal region and liver (143).

The t(1;14)(p22;q32) is an uncommon translocation in MALT lymphomas, occurring in less than 5% of cases; it juxtaposes the *bcl-10* gene at 1p22 adjacent to the immunoglobulin heavy chain gene. This translocation truncates *bcl*-10, and thus Bcl-10 protein loses its proapoptotic function. Bcl-10 gene mutations also occur outside the context of the t(1;14) in 7 to 10% of MALT lymphomas. These mutations consist predominantly of deletions or insertions and are predicted to result in truncated proteins (139).

The t(3;14)(p14;q32) has also been described in MALT lymphomas. This translocation juxtaposes the *foxp1* gene at 3p14.1 with the immunoglobulin heavy chain gene. The t(3;14) appears to be most common in MALT lymphomas arising in the thyroid gland, ocular adnexal region, and skin (144).

Vinatzer et al. (145) have identified additional chromosomal translocations or partner genes in MALT lymphomas including: t(1;14)/IgH-CNN3, t(5;14)/IgH-ODZ2, t(3;14/IgH-Bcl6, t(9;14)/IgH-JMJD2C, and t(6;7)(q25;q11).

Activation of NF-κB may be a final common pathway in MALT lymphomas. API2–MALT1 is known to activate NF-κB. Similarly, overexpression of MALT1 or Bcl-10, by binding with each other, can form a complex in the cell and act to activate NF-κB (139).

Workup and Management

The diagnosis of gastric MALT lymphoma is established by endoscopy with multiple biopsies of abnormal and normal mucosa (136). Endoscopic ultrasound may also be helpful in the staging. Early-stage disease can be successfully treated initially with antibiotic therapy, with complete regression in 35 to 100% of patients and a low rate of recurrence (139,146). Therefore, the recommended therapy for stage I or II disease is a standard regimen of antibiotic therapy for *H pylori* with follow-up endoscopy 2 to 3 months later to document *H pylori* eradication. If patients remain *H pylori*–positive, a second-line anti-*Helicobacter* regimen is administered until they are *H pylori*–negative. The time between *H pylori* eradication and complete remission of gastric MALT lymphoma varies and can take longer than 1 year (146). More extensive disease, as documented by endoscopic ultrasound and other studies, is less likely to respond to antibiotic therapy (136). Lack of response has been correlated with the presence of the t(11;18).

Surgery, RT, chemotherapy, and anti-CD20 MAb therapy have been used for both MALT lymphomas and other MZLs. The treatment of choice is dependent on the site of disease, the stage, and the patient's clinical presentation. Surgery and RT are prime therapeutic approaches for localized MALT lymphoma, including gastric MALT lymphoma that does not respond adequately to antibiotic therapy. Chemotherapy and MAb therapy are also options, especially for widespread disease. Conconi et al. (147) have studied rituximab in patients with MALT lymphoma and have found significant activity in both untreated and relapsed patients. By extrapolation from CLL/SLL data, combinations that include nucleoside analogs have been explored (148). The best systemic treatment option is not clear (137). A multicenter trial is currently ongoing (138).

NODAL MARGINAL ZONE LYMPHOMA

Clinical Features and Management

Patients with nodal MZL typically present with peripheral and/or paraaortic lymphadenopathy and bone marrow involvement (130,131). The 5-year overall and failure-free survivals are lower for patients with nodal MZL compared with patients with MALT lymphoma (56% versus 81% and 28% versus 65%, respectively) (130). The treatment and outcome of patients with nodal MZL is similar to that of patients with advanced FL (149).

Histologic, Immunophenotypic, and Molecular Features

Nodal MZLs have a propensity to involve the marginal zones of lymph node. In most cases, however, the neoplasm also expands into the perifollicular compartments with sparing of germinal centers, or it completely replaces lymph node architecture (2,130). The cytologic features of nodal MZL are the most distinctive aspect of this neoplasm. The tumor cell cytoplasm is relatively abundant and pale, with well-delineated cell borders. The tumor cell nuclei are small, chromatin is relatively clumped, and mitotic figures are infrequent. Rare large cells are also present.

Nodal MZLs are mature B-cell neoplasms that express monotypic immunoglobulin, pan–B-cell antigens, and Bcl-2 (2,130). These tumors do not express CD10, CD21, CD23, Bcl-6, cyclin D1, or T-cell antigens, including CD5.

Conventional cytogenetics and FISH studies have identified a variety of abnormalities, most often trisomy 3 (149,150). However, there are no unique recurrent chromosomal abnormalities in nodal MZL. The t(11;18), t(14;18), and t(1;14) have *not* been identified.

SPLENIC B-CELL MARGINAL ZONE LYMPHOMA

Clinical Features and Management

Patients with SMZL usually present with splenomegaly. They commonly have modest abdominal lymphadenopathy and bone marrow involvement. Monoclonal gammopathy can be seen in 10 to 20% of patients. Peripheral lymphadenopathy and B-type symptoms are uncommon. The clinical course is indolent, with 5-year overall survival ranging from 65 to 78% (131,151).

Approximately one-third of patients with SMZL will never require therapy. Splenectomy is indicated in patients with symptomatic splenomegaly or cytopenias secondary to hypersplenism. If splenectomy is contraindicated, splenic irradiation may be an alternative. Alkylating agents have been used, but responses are usually partial and not durable (152). Patients treated with fludarabine demonstrate a higher response rate and longer-lasting remission than those treated with alkylating agents (153,154). Rituximab has significant activity in SMZL.

Histologic, Immunophenotypic, and Molecular Features

In SMZL, the white pulp is expanded by a neoplasm that initially replaces the marginal and mantle zones, and then eventually replaces the white pulp (131,151, 155). Lesser red pulp involvement is also usually present. At high-power magnification, the neoplastic cells are small lymphocytes with abundant pale (monocytoid) cytoplasm. The neoplastic cells may exhibit plasmacytoid differentiation. Occasional large lymphoid cells are present. In a peripheral blood smear, the neoplastic cells can have villous cytoplasmic projections.

Splenic MZL is a mature B-cell neoplasm that expresses monotypic immunoglobin, pan–B-cell antigens, and Bcl-2 (2,155). A subset of cases is positive for IgD or CD5 (dim intensity by flow cytometry). These neoplasms are negative for CD10, Bcl-6, cyclin D1, and T-cell antigens (other than CD5).

Conventional cytogenetics and FISH analysis have identified a variety of abnormalities, most often trisomy of chromosomes 3 and 7 (150). Deletion of 7q is present in approximately 50% of cases. A recent study using array-based comparative genomic hybridization has shown del(7q36.2) involving the sonic hedgehog (SHH) gene and del(7q31.32) involving the protection of telomere 1 (POT1) genes in SMZL (156).

■ LYMPHOPLASMACYTIC LYMPHOMA AND WALDENSTRÖM MACROGLOBULINEMIA

In the current version of the WHO classification (2), LPL is defined as a neoplasm composed of small lymphocytes, plasmacytoid lymphocytes, and plasma cells that most often involves the bone marrow, but can also involve lymph nodes and spleen. LPL is often associated with a serum IgM paraprotein, but this feature is *not* required for the diagnosis of LPL. Patients with LPL also can have a serum paraprotein composed of IgA or IgG, and the relationship of these cases to WM is not clear. In contrast, patients with Waldenström macroglobulinemia (WM) have LPL involving the bone marrow associated with a serum IgM paraprotein of any level (157,158). Using these definitions, all patients with WM have LPL, but not all patients with LPL have WM.

Patients with LPL not meeting the criteria for WM are rare and poorly characterized. Furthermore, a serum IgM paraprotein can be observed in patients with other types of indolent B-cell lymphoma (159) and there is morphologic, and immunophenotypic overlap with MZLs (160). For these reasons, our focus here is on WM.

CLINICAL FEATURES

Some patients with WM can be asymptomatic, but many have symptoms of anemia, which is a common presenting feature. Only about 15% of patients have splenomegaly, hepatomegaly, and/or lymphadenopathy (2,158). The hyperviscosity syndrome—characterized by mucosal hemorrhage, visual disturbances, neurologic changes, and cardiac failure—is dramatic and classic, but occurs in only a minority of WM patients. Other even less common manifestations include cryoglobulinemia, cold-agglutinin hemolysis, autoimmune thrombocytopenia, amyloidosis, and light-chain nephropathy (157,158).

HISTOLOGIC, IMMUNOPHENOTYPIC, AND MOLECULAR FEATURES

The bone marrow is always involved in WM (157). Bone marrow aspirate smears show increased small lymphocytes, plasmacytoid small lymphocytes, and mature plasma cells, in varying proportions. Mast cells are commonly increased. In the so-called polymorphous type of WM, large lymphoid cells are increased, 5 to 10% (161). Although the large cells do not form sheets and thus the criteria for large B-cell lymphoma are not met, patients with the polymorphous type have a poorer prognosis, suggesting that this is an early stage of large cell transformation (161).

The cells of WM are composed of essentially two immunophenotypically distinct cell populations corresponding to lymphocytes and plasma cells. The lymphocytes cells express monotypic surface immunoglobulin light chain, IgM, pan–B-cell antigens such as CD19 and CD20, and Bcl-2, and are negative for CD3 and Bcl-6 (162,163). In most cases, the lymphocytes are negative for CD5, CD10, and CD23 by immunohistochemical staining, however, dim expression of CD5 and CD23 is not uncommon when assessed by flow cytometry. The plasma cells express CD19, CD38, and CD138, and are negative for CD20 (162).

Conventional cytogenetics has shown no characteristic chromosomal abnormalities in WM. The most common cytogenetic abnormality is deletion (6q) (164). The t(9;14)(p13;q32) is a rare abnormality reported in a subset of nodal small B-cell lymphomas with plasmacytoid differentiation, previously presumed to be LPL/WM. However, studies using conventional cytogenetics or FISH have not detected the t(9;14) in any case of WM (164,165).

MANAGEMENT

A prognostic scoring system for patients with WM based on age, albumin, and number of cytopenias has been developed that stratifies patients into low-, intermediate-, and high-risk groups. Other prognostic variables include performance status and serum β_2-microglobulin level (166). Patients in the low-risk group can be observed.

Alkylating agents such as chlorambucil, nucleoside analogs such as cladribine or fludarabine, and the anti-CD20 antibody rituximab have been used as initial therapy for the treatment of patients with WM (167), either as single agents or in various combinations. An important new option is the proteasome inhibitor bortezomib (166). Individual patient characteristics need to be weighed in choosing therapy, including the age of the patient, the need for rapid disease control, and consideration of the patient's later candidacy for an autologous transplant approach. For patients with relapsed or refractory disease whose initial remission lasted more than 1 year, retreatment with the same therapy can be considered. Transplantation, both autologous and allogeneic, can be considered for patients with relapsed or primary refractory disease who have good performance status.

Plasmapheresis is indicated for the management of hyperviscosity syndrome and may be helpful for other IgM-related disorders, such as cryoglobulinemia, neuropathy, amyloidosis, and light-chain nephropathy (167,168). Plasmapheresis is typically used on a short-term basis until chemotherapy takes effect. In patients with autoimmune conditions or clinical symptoms from cryoglobulinemia, corticosteroids may be helpful.

■ CONCLUSION

To date, most advanced-stage indolent B-cell lymphomas remain incurable. Novel approaches to therapy are continuing to be explored, including monoclonal antibodies, radioimmunoconjugates, and immunotoxins. These and other biological approaches to therapy will likely play an increasingly important role in the management of patients with indolent lymphoma. Allogeneic transplantation in indolent B-cell lymphomas continues to be an area of heightened interest, especially with the development of the better-tolerated mini-allogeneic transplant strategies. The importance of the graft-versus-lymphoma effect reflects our growing knowledge that the host's immune response is a potentially powerful tool that we have not yet fully exploited. Vaccine strategies are also of considerable interest. As emerging biological therapies become integrated with the best of conventional therapies, it is hoped that curative therapy will be found for more patients with indolent B-cell lymphomas.

References

1. The Non-Hodgkin's Lymphoma Classification Project. A clinical evaluation of the International Lymphoma Study Group classification of non-Hodgkin's lymphoma. *Blood* 1997;89:3909-3918.
2. Swerdlow SH, Campo E, Harris NL, et al. (eds.) WHO Classification of Tumours of Haematopoietic and Lymphoid Tissues. Lyon, France: IARC Press; 2008.
3. Armitage JO, Weisenburger DD. New approach to classifying non-Hodgkin's lymphomas: Clinical features of the major histologic types. Non-Hodgkin's Lymphoma Classification Project. *J Clin Oncol* 1998;16:2780-2795.
4. National Cancer Institute sponsored study of classifications of non-Hodgkin's lymphomas: Summary and description of a working formulation for clinical usage. The Non-Hodgkin's Lymphoma Pathologic Classification Project. *Cancer* 1982; 49:2112-2135.
5. Liu Q, Fayad L, Cabanillas F, et al. Improvement of overall and failure-free survival in stage IV follicular lymphoma: 25 years of treatment experience at the University of Texas M.D. Anderson Cancer Center. *J Clin Oncol* 2006;24: 1582-1589.
6. Fisher RI, LeBlanc M, Press OW, et al. New treatment options have changed the survival of patients with follicular lymphoma. *J Clin Oncol* 2005;23:8447-8452.

7. Swenson WT, Wooldridge JE, Lynch CF, et al. Improved survival of follicular lymphoma patients in the United States. *J Clin Oncol* 2005;23:5019-5026.

8. Bastion Y, Sebban C, Berger F, et al. Incidence, predictive factors, and outcome of lymphoma transformation in follicular lymphoma patients. *J Clin Oncol* 1997;15:1587-1594.

9. Mann RB, Berard CW. Criteria for the cytologic subclassification of follicular lymphomas: A proposed alternative method. *Hematol Oncol* 1983;1:187-192.

10. Bosga-Bouwer AG, van den Berg A, Haralambieva E, et al. Molecular, cytogenetic, and immunophenotypic characterization of follicular lymphoma grade 3B; a separate entity or part of the spectrum of diffuse large B-cell lymphoma? *Human Pathol* 2006;37:528-533.

11. Conlan MG, Bast M, Armitage JO, et al. Bone marrow involvement by non-Hodgkin's lymphoma: The clinical insignificance of morphologic discordance between the lymph node and bone marrow. *J Clin Oncol* 1990;8:1163-1172.

12. Picker LJ, Weiss LM, Medeiros LJ, et al. Immunophenotype criteria for the diagnosis of non-Hodgkin's lymphoma. *Am J Pathol* 1987;128:181-201.

13. Offit K, Jhanwar SC, Ladanyi M, et al. Cytogenetic analysis of 434 consecutively ascertained specimens of non-Hodgkin's lymphoma: Correlations between recurrent aberrations, histology, and exposure to cytotoxic treatment. *Genes Chromosomes Cancer* 1991;3:189-201.

14. Golling P, Cozzio A, Dummer R, et al. Primary cutaneous B-cell lymphomas – clinicopathological, prognostic, and therapeutic characterisation of 54 cases according to the WHO-EORTC classification and the ISCL/EPRTC TNM classification system for primary cutaneous lymphomas other than mycosis fungoiudes and Sezary syndrome. *Leuk Lymphoma* 2008;40:1094-1103.

15. Lorsbach RB, Shay-Seymore D, Moore J, et al. Clinicopathologic analysis of follicular lymphoma occurring in children. *Blood* 2002;99:1959-1964.

16. Ott G, Katzenberger T, Lohr A, et al. Cytomorphologic, immunohistochemical, and cytogenetic profiles of follicular lymphoma: 2 types of follicular lymphoma grade 3. *Blood* 2002;99:3806-3812.

17. Yunis JJ, Frizzera G, Oken MM, et al. Multiple recurrent genomic defects in follicular lymphoma. A possible model for cancer. *N Engl J Med* 1987;316:79-84.

18. Cheung KJ, Shah SP, Steidl C, et al. Genome-wide profiling of follicular lymphoma by array comparative genomic hybridization reveals prognostically significant DNA copy number imbalances. *Blood* 2009;113:137-148.

19. Berglund M, Enblad G, Thunberg U, et al. Genomic imbalances during transformation from follicular lymphoma to diffuse large B-cell lymphoma. *Modern Pathol* 2007;20:63-75.

20. Glas AM, Knoops L, Delahaye L, et al. Gene-expression and immunohistochemical study of specific T-cell subsets and accessory cell types in the transformation and prognosis of follicular lymphoma. *J Clin Oncol* 2007;25:390-398.

21. Dave SS, Wright G, Tan B, et al. Prediction of survival in follicular lymphoma based on molecular features of tumor-infiltrating immune cells. *N Engl J Med* 2004;351:2159-2169.

22. DeJong D. Molecular pathogenesis of follicular lymphoma: A cross talk of genetic and immunologic factors. *J Clin Oncol* 2005;23:6358-6363.

23. Farinha P, Al-Tourah A, Gill K, et al. The architectural pattern of FOXP3-positive T cells in follicular lymphoma is an independent predictor of survival and histologic transformation. *Blood* 2010;115:289-295.

24. Bende RJ, Smit LA, van Noesel JM. Molecular pathways in follicular lymphoma. *Leukemia* 2007;21:18-29.

25. Tsujimoto Y, Finger LR, Yunis J, et al. Cloning of the chromosome breakpoint of neoplastic B cells with the t(14;18) chromosome translocation. *Science* 1984;226:1097-1099.

26. Reed JC. Bcl-2-family proteins and hematologic malignancies: History and future prospects. *Blood* 2008;111: 3322-3330.

27. Baliga BC, Kumar S. Role of Bcl-2 family of proteins in malignancy. *Hematol Oncol* 2002;20:63-74.

28. Danial NN and Korsmeyer SJ. Cell death: Critical control points. *Cell* 2004;116:205-219.

29. Cleary ML, Galili N, Sklar J. Detection of a second t(14;18) breakpoint cluster region in human follicular lymphomas. *J Exp Med* 1986;164:315-320.

30. Albinger-Hegyi A, Hochreutener B, Abdou MT, et al. High frequency of t(11;18)-translocation breakpoints outside of major breakpoint and minor cluster regions in follicular lymphomas: Improved polymerase chain reaction protocols for their detection. *Am J Pathol* 2002;160:823-832.

31. Lee MS, Chang KS, Cabanillas F, et al. Detection of minimal residual cells carrying the t(14;18) by DNA sequence amplification. *Science* 1987;237:175-178.

32. Ladetto M, Drandi D, Compagno M, et al. PCR-detectable nonneoplastic Bcl-2/IgH rearrangements are common in normal subjects and cancer patients at diagnosis but rare in subjects treated with chemotherapy. *J Clin Oncol* 2003;21: 1398-1403.

33. Hehn ST, Grogan TM, Miller TP. Utility of fine-needle aspiration as a diagnostic technique in lymphoma. *J Clin Oncol* 2004;22:3046-3052.

34. Sandhaus LM. Fine-needle aspiration cytology in the diagnosis of lymphoma. The next step. *Am J Clin Pathol* 2000;113:623-627.

35. Cheson BD, Horning SJ, Coiffier B, et al. Report of an international workshop to standardize response criteria for non-Hodgkin's lymphomas. NCI Sponsored International Working Group. *J Clin Oncol* 1999;17:1244-1253.

36. Berinstein NL, Reis MD, Ngan BY, et al. Detection of occult lymphoma in the peripheral blood and bone marrow of patients with untreated early-stage and advanced-stage follicular lymphoma. *J Clin Oncol* 1993;11:1344-1352.

37. Juweid ME, Stroobants S, Hoekstra OS, et al. Use of positron emission tomography for response assessment of lymphoma: Consensus of the imaging subcommittee of the international harmonization project in lymphoma. *J Clin Oncol* 2007;25: 571-578.

38. Blum R, Seymour JF, Wirth A, et al. Evaluation of 18-FDG-PET in the staging of patients with indolent non-Hodgkin's lymphoma. *Ann Oncol* 2002;13(Suppl 2):44.

39. Jerusalem G, Beguin Y, Najjar F, et al. Positron emission tomography (PET) with 18F-fluorodeoxyglucose (18F-FDG) for the staging of low-grade non-Hodgkin's lymphoma (NHL). *Ann Oncol* 2001;12:825-830.

40. Cheson BD, Pfistner B, Juweid ME, et al. Revised response criteria for malignant lymphoma. *J Clin Oncol* 2007;25:579-586.

41. Portlock CS, Rosenberg SA. No initial therapy for stage III and stage IV non-Hodgkin's lymphoma of favorable histologic type. *Ann Intern Med* 1979;90:10-13.

42. Koster A, Tromp HA, Raemaekers JM, et al. The prognostic significance of the intra-follicular tumor cell proliferative rate in follicular lymphoma. *Haematologica* 2007;92: 184-190.

43. Martin AR, Weisenburger DD, Chan WC, et al. Prognostic value of cellular proliferation and histologic grade in follicular lymphoma. *Blood* 1995;85:3671-3678.

44. Shipp MA, Harrington DP, Anderson JR, et al. A predictive model for aggressive non-Hodgkin's lymphoma. The International Non-Hodgkin's Lymphoma Prognostic Factors Project. *N Engl J Med* 1993;329:987-994.

45. Lopez-Guillermo A, Montserrat E, Bosch F, et al. Low-grade lymphoma: Clinical and prognostic studies in a series of 143 patients from a single institution. *Leuk Lymph* 1994;15:159-165.

46. Solal-Celigny P. International prognostic index for follicular lymphomas. *Proc Am Soc Clin Oncol* 2002;21:281(Abstract).

47. Solal-Celigny P, Roy P, Colombat P, et al. Follicular lymphoma international prognostic index. *Blood* 2004;104:1258-1265.

48. Buske C, Hoster E, Dreyling M, et al. The follicular lymphoma international prognostic index (FLIPI) separates high-risk form intermediate- or low-risk patients with advanced stage follicular lymphoma treated front-line with rituximab and the combination of cyclophosphamide, doxorubicin, vincristine, and prednisone (R-CHOP) with respect to treatment outcome. *Blood* 2006;108:1504-1508.

49. Federico M, Bellei M, Marcheselli L, et al. Follicular lymphoma international prognostic index 2: A new prognostic index for follicular lymphoma developed by the international follicular lymphoma prognostic factor project. *J Clin Oncol* 2009;27:4555-4562.

50. Friedberg JW, Taylor MD, Cerhan, et al. Follicular lymphoma in the United States: First report of the national LymphoCare study. *J Clin Oncol* 2009;27:1202-1208 [LymphoCare].

51. Weisdorf DJ, Andersen JW, Glick JH, et al. Survival after relapse of low-grade non-Hodgkin's lymphoma: Implications for marrow transplantation. *J Clin Oncol* 1992;10:942-947.

52. Gribben JG, Neuberg D, Barber M, et al. Detection of residual lymphoma cells by polymerase chain reaction in peripheral blood is significantly less predictive for relapse than detection in bone marrow. *Blood* 1994;83:3800-3807.

53. McLaughlin P, Hagemeister FB, Swan F, et al. Intensive conventional-dose chemotherapy for stage IV low-grade lymphoma: High remission rates and reversion to negative of peripheral blood bcl-2 rearrangement. *Ann Oncol* 1994;5(Suppl 2): 73-77.

54. Lopez-Guillermo A, Cabanillas F, McLaughlin P, et al. The clinical significance of molecular response in indolent follicular lymphomas. *Blood* 1998;91:2955-2960.

55. Tsimberidou AM, McLaughlin P, Younes A, et al. Fludarabine, mitoxantrone, dexamethasone (FND) compared with an alternating triple therapy (ATT) regimen in patients with stage IV indolent lymphoma. *Blood* 2002;100:4351-4357.

56. McLaughlin P, Rodriguez MA, Hagemeister FB, et al. Stage IV indolent lymphoma: A randomized study of concurrent vs. sequential use of FND chemotherapy (fludarabine, mitoxantrone, dexamethasone) and rituximab (R) monoclonal antibody therapy, with interferon maintenance. *Proc Am Soc Clin Oncol* 2003;22:564(Abstract).

57. Montoto S, Domingo-Domenech E, Estany C, et al. High clinical and molecular response rates with fludarabine, cyclophosphamide, and mitoxantrone in previously untreated patients with advanced stage follicular lymphoma. *Haematologica* 2008;93:207-214.

58. Rambaldi A, Carlotti E, Oldani E, et al. Quantitative PCR of bone marrow BCL2/IgH+ cells at diagnosis predicts treatment response and long-term outcome in follicular non-Hodgkin lymphoma. *Blood* 2005;105:3428-3433.

59. Zohren F, Bruns I, Barth J, et al. Quantitative real-time PCR of peripheral blood t(14;18) positive cells predicts treatment response and long-term outcome in patients with follicular lymphoma. *Blood* 2009;114(Suppl):183 (Abstract 441).

60. Van Oers MHJ, Tonnissen E, Van Glabbeke M, et al. BCL2/IgH polymerase chain reaction status at the end of induction therapy is not predictive for progression-free survival in relapsed/resistant follicular lymphoma: Results of a prospective randomized EORTC 20981 Phase II intergroup study. *J Clin Oncol* 2010;28:2246-2252.

61. Johnson PWM, Swinbank K, MacLennan S, et al. Variability of polymerase chain reaction detection of the bcl-2—IgH translocation in an international multicentre study. *Ann Oncol* 1999;10:1349-1354.

62. Darby AJ, Lanham S, Soubeyran P, Johnson PW. Variability of quantitative polymerase chain reaction detection of the bcl-2-IgH translocation in an international study. *Haematologica* 2005;90:1706-1707.

63. Soubeyran P, Eghbali H, Trojani M, et al. Is there any place for a wait-and-see policy in stage I-0 follicular lymphoma? A study of 43 consecutive patients in a single center. *Ann Oncol* 1996;7:713-718.

64. MacManus MP, Hoppe RT. Is radiotherapy curative for stage I and II low-grade follicular lymphoma? Results of a long-term follow-up study of patients treated at Stanford University. *J Clin Oncol* 1996;14:1282-1290.

65. Gospodarowicz MK, Bush RS, Brown TC, et al. Prognostic factors in nodular lymphomas: A multivariate analysis based on the Princess Margaret Hospital experience. *Int J Radiat Oncol Biol Phys* 1984;10:489-497.

66. Peterson PM, Gospodarowicz M, Tsang R, et al. Long-term outcome in stage I and II follicular lymphoma following treatment with involved field radiation therapy alone. 2004 ASCO Annual Meeting Proceedings. p. 563s (Abstract 6521).

67. Wilder RB, Jones D, Tucker SL, et al. Long-term results with radiotherapy for stage I-II follicular lymphomas. *Int J Radiat Oncol Biol Phys* 2001;51:1219-1227.

68. Seymour JF, Pro B, Fuller LM, et al. Long-term follow-up of a prospective study of combined modality therapy for stage I-II indolent non-Hodgkin's lymphoma. *J Clin Oncol* 2003;21:2115-2122.

69. Zelenetz AD, Abramson JS, Advani RH, et al. Non-Hodgkin's lymphoma. *J Natl Compr Cancer Netw* 2010;8;288-334.

70. Maloney DG, Grillo-Lopez AJ, White CA, et al. IDEC-C2B8 (rituximab) anti-CD20 monoclonal antibody therapy in patients with relapsed low-grade non-Hodgkin's lymphoma. *Blood* 1997;90:2188-2195.

71. McLaughlin P, Grillo-Lopez AJ, Link BK, et al. Rituximab chimeric anti-CD20 monoclonal antibody therapy for relapsed indolent lymphoma: Half of patients respond to a four-dose treatment program. *J Clin Oncol* 1998;16:2825-2833.

72. Marcus R, Imrie K, Belch A, et al. CVP chemotherapy plus rituximab compared with CVP as first-line treatment for advance follicular lymphoma. *Blood* 2005;105:1417-1423.

73. Marcus R, Imrie K, Solal-Celigny P, et al. Phase III study of R-CVP compared with cyclophosphamide, vincristine, and prednisone alone in patients with previously untreated advanced follicular lymphoma. *J Clin Oncol* 2008;26:4579-4586.

74. Hiddemann W, Kneba M, Dreyling M, et al. Frontline therapy with rituximab added to the combination of cyclophosphamide, doxorubicin, vincristine, and prednisone (CHOP) significantly improves the outcome for patients with advanced-stage follicular lymphoma compared with therapy with CHOP alone: Results of a prospective randomized study of the German Low Grade Lymphoma Study Group. *Blood* 2005; 106:3725-3732.

75. Herold M, Haas A, Srock S, et al. Rituximab added to first-line mitoxantrone, chlorambucil, and prednisolone chemotherapy followed by interferon maintenance prolongs survival in patients with advanced follicular lymphoma: An East German study group hematology and oncology study. *J Clin Oncol* 2007;25:1986-1992.

76. McLaughlin P, Hagemeister FB, Rodriguez MA, et al. Safety of fludarabine, mitoxantrone, and dexamethasone combined with rituximab in the treatment of stage IV indolent lymphoma. [R-FND] *Semi Oncol* 2000;27(6 Suppl 12):37-41.

77. Forstpointner R, Unterhalt M, Dreyling M, et al. Maintenance therapy with rituximab leads to a significant prolongation of response duration after salvage therapy with a combination of rituximab, fludarabine, cyclophosphamide, and mitoxantrone (R-FCM) in patients with recurring and refractory follicular and mantle cell lymphoma: Results of a prospective randomized study of the German Low Grade Lymphoma Study Group. *Blood* 2006;108:4003-4008.

78. Rummel MJ, Niederle N, Maschmeyer G, et al. Bendamustine plus rituximab is superior in respect of progression free survival an CR rate when compared to CHOP plus rituximab as first-line treatment of patients with advanced follicular, indolent, and mantle cell lymphomas: Final results of a randomized Phase III study of the StiL (Study Group Indloent Lymphoma Germany). *Blood* 2009;114(Suppl):168 (Abstract 405).

79. Rambaldi A, Lazzari M, Manzoni C, et al. Monitoring of minimal residual disease after CHOP and rituximab in previously untreated patients with follicular lymphoma. *Blood* 2002;99:856-862.

80. Zinzani PL, Pulsoni A, Perrotti A, et al. Fludarabine plus mitoxantrone with and without rituximab versus CHOP with and without rituximab as front-line treatment for patients with follicular lymphoma. *J Clin Oncol* 2004;22:2654-2661.

81. Morschhauser F, Radford J, Van Hoof A, et al. Phase III trial of consolidation with yttrium-90-ibritumomab tiuxetan compared with no additional therapy after first remission in advanced follicular lymphoma. *J Clin Oncol* 2008;26:5156-5164.

82. Leonard JP, Coleman M, Kostakoglu L, et al. Abbreviated therapy with fludarabine followed by tositumomab and iodine 131 tositumomab for untreated follicular lymohoma. *J Clin Oncol* 2005;23:5696-5704.

83. McLaughlin P, Neelapu S, Fanale M, et al. R-FND followed by radioimmunotherpay for high-risk follicular lymphoma. *Blood* 2008;112(Suppl):1050a (Abstract 3056).

84. Press O, Unger JM, Braziel RM, et al. Phase II trial of CHOP chemotherapy followed by tositumomab/iodine I-131 tositumomab for previously untreated follicular non-Hodgkin's lymphoma: Five-year follow-up of Southwest Oncology Group protocol S9911. *J Clin Oncol* 2006;24:4143-4149.

85. Solal-Celigny P, Lepage E, Brousse N, et al. Doxorubicin-containing regimen with or without interferon alfa 2b for advanced follicular lymphomas: Final analysis of survival and toxicity in the Groupe d'Etude des Lymphomes Folliculaires 86 Trial. *J Clin Oncol* 1998;16:2332-2338.

86. McLaughlin P, Cabanillas F, Hagemeister FB, et al. CHOP-Bleo plus interferon for stage IV low grade lymphoma. *Ann Oncol* 1993;4:205-211.

87. Rohatiner AZS (old 87). Allen IE, Ross SD, Borden SP, et al. Meta-analysis to assess the efficacy of interferon-alpha in patients with follicular non-Hodgkin's lymphoma. *J Immunother* 2001;24:58-65.

88. Salles GA, Seymour JF, Feugier P, et al. Rituximab maintenance for 2 years in patients with untreated high tumor burden follicular lymphoma after response to immunochemotherapy. Proceedings of the ASCO 2010 (Abstract 8004).

89. Hainsworth JD, Litchy S, Shaffer DW, et al. Maximizing therapeutic benefit of rituximab: Maintenance therapy versus re-treatment at progression in patients with indolent non-Hodgkin's lymphoma – a randomized phase II trial of the Minnie Pearl Cancer Research Network. *J Clin Oncol* 2005; 23:1088-1095.

90. Ghielmini M, Schmitz SF, Cogliatti SB, et al. Prolonged treatment with rituximab in patients with follicular lymphoma significantly increases event-free survival and response duration compared with the standard weekly X 4 schedule. *Blood* 2004;103:4416-4423.

91. Hochster H, Weller E, Gascoyne RD, et al. Maintenance rituximab after cyclophosphamide, vincristine, and prednisone prolongs progression-free survival in advance indolent lymphoma: Results of the randomized phase III ECOG1496 study. *J Clin Oncol* 2009;27:1607-1614.

92. Van Oers MHJ, Klasa R, Marcus R, et al. Rituximab maintenance improves clinical outcome of relapsed/resistant follicular non-Hodgkin lymphoma in patients both with and without rituximab during induction: Results of a prospective randomized phase 3 intergroup trial. *Blood* 2006;108: 3295-3301.

93. Freedman A, Neelapu SS, Nichols C, et al. Placebo-controlled phase III trial of patient-specific immunotherapy with mitumprotimut-T and granulocyte-macrophage colony-stimulating factor after rituximab in patients with follicular lymphoma. *J Clin Oncol* 2009;27:3036-3043.

94. Levy R, Robertson M, Ganjoo K, et al. Results of a Phase 3 trial evaluating safety and efficacy of specific immunotherapy, recombinant idiotype conjugated to KLH (Id-KLH) with GM-CSF, compared to non-specific immunotherapy, KLH with GM-CSF, in patients with follicular non-Hodgkin's lymphoma. AACR Meeting Abstracts, April 2008; 2008: LB-204.

95. Schuster SJ, Neelapu SS, Gause BL, et al. Idiotype vaccine therapy (BiovaxID) in follicular lymphoma in first complete remission: Phase III clinical trial results. 2009 ASCO Annual Meeting Proceedings. p. 5s (Abstract 2).

96. Colombat P, Salles G, Brousse N, et al. Rituximab (anti-CD20 monoclonal antibody) as single first-line therapy for patients with follicular lymphoma with a low tumor burden: Clinical and molecular evaluation. *Blood* 2001;97:101-106.

97. Schuster SJ, Venugopal P, Kern J, McLaughlin P. GM-CSF plus rituximab immunotherapy: Translation of biologic mechanisms into therapy for indolent B-cell lymphoma. *Leuk Lymphoma* 2008;49:1681-1692.

98. Kimby E, Jurlander J, Geisler C, et al. Long-term molecular remission in patients with indolent lymphoma treated with rituximab as a single agent or in combination with interferon alpha-2a: A randomized phase II study from the Nordic Lymphoma Group. *Leuk Lymphoma* 2008;49:102-112.

99. Witzig TE, Gordon LI, Cabanillas F, et al. Randomized controlled trial of yttrium-90-labeled ibritumomab tiuxetan radioimmunotherapy versus rituximab immunotherapy for patients with relapsed or refractory low-grade, follicular, or transformed B-cell non-Hodgkin's lymphoma. *J Clin Oncol* 2002;20:2453-2463.

100. Kaminski MS, Zelenetz AD, Press OW, et al. Pivotal study of iodine I 131 tositumomab for chemotherapy-refractory low grade or transformed low-grade B-cell non-Hodgkin's lymphomas. *J Clin Oncol* 2001;19:3918-3928.

101. Kaminski MS, Tuck M, Estes J, et al. 131-I tositumomab therapy as initial treatment for follicular lymphoma. *N Engl J Med* 2005;352:441 [Updated in *Blood* 2009 (Abstarct)].

102. Dang NH, Smith MR, Offner F, et al. Anti-CD22 immunoconjugate inotuzumab ozogamicin (CMC-544) + rituximab: Clinical activity including survival in patients with recurrent/refractory follicular or aggressive lymphoma. *Blood* 2009;114(Suppl):242 (Abstract 584).

103. Kreitman RJ, Pastan I. Immunotoxins in the treatment of hematologic malignancies. *Curr Drug Targets* 2006;7: 1302-1311.

104. Waldmann TA, Morris JC. Development of antibodies and chimeric molecules for cancer immunotherapy. *Adv Immunol* 2006;90:83-131.

105. Multani PS, O'Day S, Nadler LM, Grossbard ML. Phase II clinical trial of bolus infusion anti-B4 blocked ricin immunoconjugate in patients with relapsed B-cell non-Hodgkin's lymphoma. *Clin Cancer Res* 1998;4:2599-2604.

106. Dang NH, Fayad L, McLaughlin P, et al. Phase II trial of the combination of denileukin diftitox and rituximab for relapsed/refractory B-cell non-Hodgkin lymphoma. *Br J Haematol* 2007;138:502-505.

107. De Vos S, Goy A, Dakhil SR, et al. Multicenter randomized phase II study of weekly or twice-weekly bortezomib plus rituximab in patients with relapsed or refractory follicular or marginal zone B-cell lymphoma. *J Clin Oncol* 2009;27: 5023-5030.

108. Fowler N, McLaughlin P, Hagemeister FB, et al. A biologic combination of lenalidomide and rituximab for front-line therapy of indolent B-cell lymphoma. *Blood* 2009;114(Suppl): 683 (Abstract 1714).

109. Fowler N, Horowitz S, McLaughllin P. Therapy of B-cell lymphoproliferative disorders. In: Jones D (ed.): *Neoplastic Hematopathology: Contemporary Hematology*. Totowa, NJ: Humana Press; 2010.

110. Davis TA, Lopez-Grillo A, White C, et al. Rituximab anti-CD20 monoclonal antibody therapy in non-Hodgkin's lymphoma: Safety and efficacy of re-treatment. *J Clin Oncol* 2000;18:3135-3143.

111. Gallagher CJ, Gregory WM, Jones AE, et al. Follicular lymphoma: Prognostic factors for response and survival. *J Clin Oncol* 1986:4:1470-1480.

112. Velasquez WS, McLaughin P, Tucker S, et al. ESHAP—An effective chemotherapy regimen in refractory and relaplsin lymphoma: A 4-year follow-up study. *J Clin Oncol* 1994; 12:1169-1176.

113. Rodriguez J, Rodriguez MA, Fayad L, et al. ASHAP: A regimen for cytoreduction of refractory or recurrent Hodgkin's disease. *Blood* 1999;93:3632-3636.

114. Rodriguez MA, Cabanillas FC, Velasquez W, et al. Results of a salvage treatment program for relapsing lymphoma: MINE consolidated with ESHAP. *J Clin Oncol* 1995;13: 1734-1741.

115. McLaughlin P, Hagemeister FB, Romaguera JE, et al. Fludarabine, mitoxantrone, and dexamethasone: An effective new regimen for indolent lymphoma. *J Clin Oncol* 1996; 14:1262-1268.

116. El Gnaoui T, Dupuis J, Belhadj K, et al. Rituximab, gemcitabine and oxaliplatin: An effective salvage regimen for patients with relapsed or refractory B-cell lymphoma not candidates for high-dose therapy. *Ann Oncol* 2007;18:1363-1368.

117. Cheson BD, Rummel MJ. Bendamustine: Rebirth of an old drug. *J Clin Oncol* 2009;27:1492-1501.

118. Rohatiner A, Nadler L, Davies A, et al. Myeloablative therapy with autologous bone marrow transplantation for follicular lymphoma at the time of second or subsequent remission: Long-term follow-up. *J Clin Oncol* 2007;25: 2554-2559.

119. Van Besien K, Sobocinski KA, Rowlings PA, et al. Allogeneic bone marrow transplantation for low-grade lymphoma. *Blood* 1998;92:1832-1836.

120. Khouri I, McLaughlin P, Saliba R, et al. [Nonablative allogeneic hematopoietic transplantation]. *Blood* 2008;111: 5530-5536.

121. Hari P, Carreras J, Zhang MJ, et al. Allogeneic transplants in follicular lymphoma: Higher risk of disease progression after reduced-intensity compared to myeloablative conditioning. *Biol Blood Marrow Transplant* 2008;14:236-245.

122. Tsimberidou AM, Wen S, O'Brien S, et al. Assessment of chronic lymphocytic leukemia and small lymphocytic lymphoma by absolute lymphocyte counts in 2,126 patients: 20 years of experience at the University of Texas M.D. Anderson Cancer Center. *J Clin Oncol* 2007;25:4648-4656.

123. Ferrajoli A, O'Brien S, Keating MJ. Alemtuzumab: A novel monoclonal antibody. *Exp Opin Biol Ther* 2001;1:1059-1065.

124. Schlette E, Medeiros LJ, Keating M, et al. CD79b expression in chronic lymphocytic leukemia. Association with trisomy 12 and atypical immunophenotype. *Arch Pathol Lab Med* 2003;127:561-566.

125. Admirand JH, Rassidakis GZ, Abruzzo LV, et al. Immunohistochemical detection of ZAP-70 in 341 cases of non-Hodgkin and Hodgkin lymphoma. *Mod Pathol* 2004;17: 954-961.

126. Juliusson G, Merup M. Cytogenetics in chronic lymphocytic leukemia. *Semin Oncol* 1998;25:19-26.

127. Huh YO, Abruzzo LV, Rassidakis GZ, et al. The t(14;19)(q32;q13)-positive small B-cell leukaemia: A clinicopathologic analysis of seven cases. *Br J Haematol* 2007; 136:220-228.

128. Aoun P, Blair HE, Smith LM, et al. Fluorescence in situ hybridization detection of cytogenetic abnormalities in B-cell chronic lymphocytic leukemia/small lymphocytic lymphoma. *Leuk Lymph* 2004;45:1595-1603.

129. Huh YO, Lin KIC, Vega F, et al. MYC translocation in chronic lymphocytic leukaemia is associated with increased prolymphocytes and a poor prognosis. *Br J Haematol* 2008; 142:36-44.

130. Nathwani BN, Anderson JR, Armitage JO, et al. Marginal zone B-cell lymphoma: A clinical comparison of nodal and mucosa-associated lymphoid tissue types. Non-Hodgkin's Lymphoma Classification Project. *J Clin Oncol* 1999;17: 2486-2492.

131. Isaacson PG, Matutes E, Burke M, et al. The histopathology of splenic lymphoma with villous lymphocytes. *Blood* 1994;84:3828-3834.

132. Thieblemont C, Bastion Y, Berger F, et al. Mucosa-associated lymphoid tissue gastrointestinal and nongastrointestinal lymphoma behavior: Analysis of 108 patients. *J Clin Oncol* 1997;15:1624-1630.

133. Liao Z, Ha CS, McLaughlin P, et al. Mucosa-associated lymphoid tissue lymphoma with initial supradiaphragmatic presentation: Natural history and patterns of disease progression. *Int J Radiat Oncol Biol Phys* 2000;48:399-403.

134. Wotherspoon AC, Ortiz-Hidalgo C, Falzon MR, et al. *Helicobacter pylori*–associated gastritis and primary B-cell gastric lymphoma. *Lancet* 1991;338:1175-1176.

135. Wotherspoon AC, Doglioni C, Diss TC, et al. Regression of primary low-grade B-cell gastric lymphoma of mucosa-associated lymphoid tissue type after eradication of *Helicobacter pylori*. *Lancet* 1993;342:575-577.

136. Steinbach G, Ford R, Glober G, et al. Antibiotic treatment of gastric lymphoma of mucosa-associated lymphoid tissue. An uncontrolled trial. *Ann Intern Med* 1999;131:88-95.

137. Coiffier B, Thieblemont C, Felman P, et al. Indolent nonfollicular lymphomas: Characteristics, treatment, and outcome. *Semin Hematol* 1999;36:198-208.

138. Zucca E, Conconi A, Martelli M, et al. Interim analysis of the IELSG-19 randomized study of chlorambucil alone versus chlorambucil plus rituximab versus rituximab alone in extranodal marginal zone lymphomas of mucosa-associated lymphoid tissue (MALT lymphoma). *Blood* 2009;114(Suppl): 1514 (Abstarct 3939).

139. Isaacson PG, Du MQ. MALT lymphoma: From morphology to molecules. *Nat Rev Cancer* 2004;8:644-653.

140. Ferreri AJ, Guidoboni M, Ponzoni M, et al. Evidence for an association between *Chlamydia psittaci* and ocular adnexal lymphomas. *J Natl Cancer Inst* 2004;96:586-594.

141. Takino H, Li C, Hu S, et al. Primary cutaneous marginal zone B-cell lymphoma: A molecular and clinicopathological study of cases from Asia, Germany, and the United States. *Mod Pathol* 2008;21L:1517-1526.

142. Lecuit M, Abachin E, Martin A, et al. Immunoproliferative small intestinal disease associated with *Campylobacter jejuni*. *N Engl J Med* 2004;350:239-248.

143. Streubel B, Simonitsch-Klupp I, Mullauer L, et al. Variable frequencies of MALT lymphoma-associated genetic aberrations in MALT lymphomas of different sites. *Leukemia* 2004; 18:1722-1726.

144. Streubel B, Vinatzer U, Lamprecht A, et al. t(3;14) (p14.1;q32) involving IgH and FOXP1 is a novel recurrent chromosomal aberration in MALT lymphoma. *Leukemia* 2005;19:652-658.

145. Vinatzer U, Gollinger M, Mullauer L, et al. Mucosa-associated lymphoid tissue lymphoma: Novel translocations including rearrangements of ODZ2, JMJD2C, CNN3. *Clin Cancer Res* 2008;14:6426-6431.

146. Savio A, Zamboni G, Capelli P, et al. Relapse of low-grade gastric MALT-lymphoma after *Helicobacter pylori* eradication: True relapse or persistence? Long-term post-treatment follow-up of a multicenter trial in the northeast of Italy and evaluation of the diagnostic protocol's adequacy. *Recent Results Cancer Res* 2000;156:116-124.

147. Conconi A, Martinelli G, Thieblemont C, et al. Clinical activity of rituximab in extranodal marginal zone B-cell lymphoma of MALT type. *Blood* 2003;102:2741-2745.

148. Samaniego F, Fanale M, Pro B, et al. Pentostatin, cyclophosphamide, and rituximab (PCR) achieves high response rates in indolent B-cell lymphoma without prolonged myelosuppression. *Blood* 2008;112(Suppl):309a (Abstract 835).

149. Arcaini L, Lucioni M, Boveri E, et al. Nodal marginal zone lymphoma: Current knowledge and future directions of an heterogeneous disease. *Eur J Hematol* 2009;83:165-174.

150. Brynes RK, Almaguer PD, Leathery KE, et al. Numerical cytogenetic abnormalities of chromosomes 3, 7, and 12 in marginal B-cell lymphomas. *Mod Pathol* 1996;9:995-1000.

151. Matutes E, Oscier D, Montalban C, et al. Splenic marginal zone lymphoma: Proposals for a revision of diagnostic, staging, and therapeutic criteria. *Leukemia* 2008;22:487-495.

152. Franco V, Florena AM, Iannitto E. Splenic marginal zone lymphoma. *Blood* 2003;101:2464-2472.

153. Lefrere F, Hermine O, Belanger C, et al. Fludarabine: An effective treatment in patients with splenic lymphoma with villous lymphocytes. *Leukemia* 2000;14:573-575.

154. Bolam S, Orchard J, Oscier D. Fludarabine is effective in the treatment of splenic lymphoma with villous lymphocytes. *Br J Haematol* 1997;99:158-161.

155. Wu CD, Jackson CL, Medeiros LJ. Splenic marginal zone cell lymphoma. An immunophenotypic and molecular study of five cases. *Am J Clin Pathol* 1996;105:277-285.

156. Vega F, Cho-Vega JH, Lennon PA, et al. Splenic marginal zone lymphomas are characterized by loss of interstitial regions of chromosome 7q, 7q31.32 and 7q36.2 that include the protection of telomere 1 (POT1) and sonic hedgehog (SHH) genes. *Br J Haematol* 2008;142:216-226.

157. Owen RG, Treon SP, Al-Katib A, et al. Clinicopathological definition of Waldenström's macroglobulinemia: Consensus panel recommendations from the Second International Workshop on Waldenström's Macroglobulinemia. *Semin Oncol* 2003;30:110-115.

158. Dimopolous MA, Gertz MA, Kastritis E, et al. Update on treatment recommendations from the Fourth International Workshop on Waldenstrom's macroglobulinemia. *J Clin Oncol* 2009;27:120-126.

159. Lin P, Hao S, Handy BC, et al. Lymphoid neoplasms associated with IgM paraprotein: A study of 382 patients. *Am J Clin Pathol* 2005;123:200-205.

160. Lin P, Bueso-Ramos C, Wilson CS, et al. Waldenström macroglobulinemia involving extramedullary sites: Morphologic and immunophenotypic findings in 44 patients. *Am J Surg Pathol* 2003;27:1104-1113.

161. Lin P, Mansoor A, Bueso-Ramos C, et al. Diffuse large B-cell lymphoma occurring in patients with lymphoplasmacytic lymphoma/Waldenström macroglobulinemia. Clinicopathologic features of 12 cases. *Am J Clin Pathol* 2003;120: 246-253.

162. Morice WG, Chen D, Kurtin PJ, et al. Novel immunophenotypic features of marrow lymphoplasmacytic lymphoma and correlation with Waldenstrom's macroglobulinemia. *Mod Pathol* 2009;22:807-816.

163. Konoplev S, Medeiros LJ, Bueso-Ramos CE, et al. Immunophenotypic profile of lymphoplasmacytic lymphoma/Waldenstrom macroglobulinemia. *Am J Clin Pathol* 2005;124: 414-420.

164. Mansoor A, Medeiros LJ, Weber DM, et al. Cytogenetic findings in lymphoplasmacytic lymphoma/Waldenström macroglobulinemia. Chromosomal abnormalities are associated with the polymorphous subtype and an aggressive clinical course. *Am J Clin Pathol* 2001;116:543-549.

165. Schop RF, Kuehl WM, Van Wier SA, et al. Waldenström macroglobulinemia neoplastic cells lack immunoglobulin heavy chain locus translocations but have frequent 6q deletions. *Blood* 2002;100:2996-3001.

166. Kyle RA, Treon SP, Alexanian R, et al. Prognostic markers and criteria to initiate therapy in Waldenström's macroglobulinemia: Consensus panel recommendations from the Second International Workshop on Waldenström's Macroglobulinemia. *Semin Oncol* 2003;30:116-120.

167. Gertz MA, Anagnostopoulos A, Anderson K, et al. Treatment recommendations in Waldenström's macroglobulinemia: Consensus panel recommendations from the Second International Workshop on Waldenström's Macroglobulinemia. *Semin Oncol* 2003;30:121-126.

168. Treon SP. How I treat Waldenstrom macroglobulinemia. *Blood* 2009;114:2375-2385.

AGGRESSIVE AND HIGHLY AGGRESSIVE B-CELL LYMPHOMAS

Luis E. Fayad
Sergej Konoplev
Hubert H. Chuang
M. Alma Rodriguez
Commentary: Bouthaina S. Dabaja

Although not a part of the current classification system for non-Hodgkin lymphomas (NHL), it is clinically useful to divide NHL into indolent, aggressive, and highly aggressive tumors (1). Patients with indolent NHL typically have a survival of several years, even if untreated, but paradoxically are usually incurable. Patients with aggressive NHL have a survival time measured in months if untreated, whereas patients with highly aggressive NHL have a survival of only weeks to a few months if untreated. However, both aggressive and highly aggressive NHLs are chemosensitive and are frequently curable. In this chapter, we focus on the clinical characteristics, pathology, and treatment of aggressive and highly aggressive NHL.

■ EPIDEMIOLOGY

The incidence of NHL has increased significantly over the last five decades, as reported by United States and international registries (2-5). During the years 1993 to 1995, the age-adjusted incidence increased by 3% per year according to data from the Surveillance, Epidemiology, and End Results program of the National Cancer Institute (SEER) (3). There was also a concomitant increase in mortality during the same period. Some of this increased incidence can be attributed to the advent of the acquired immunodeficiency syndrome (AIDS), but that does not explain the increase of NHL prior to 1980. There has also been a marked increase of NHL in the elderly population (5). However, it is indolent NHLs that have increased most substantially in this group. These are discussed in another chapter.

An estimated 65,980 new cases of NHL will be diagnosed in the United States in 2009, and 20,790 NHL-related deaths will occur. These are estimated to be the ninth largest cause of death among US men, and

the sixth in women in 2009 (3 and 4% of cancer-related deaths, respectively) (6). There is a higher incidence among Caucasians than African Americans in the United States, especially among the elderly, but recent increases in the incidence among younger cohorts of African Americans have been noted (5). A lower incidence is also seen among other American racial subgroups. Although almost all histologic types of NHL have increased in incidence over the last 20 years, the relative frequency of aggressive and highly aggressive NHL has remained relatively stable.

■ ETIOLOGY

The causes or risk factors for NHL can generally be divided into four groups: immune suppression (both acquired and primary), infectious agents, toxic exposure, and familial (Table 8-1).

The strongest association is with immune suppression, both primary and acquired (7-9). Examples of primary immunodeficiency include inherited immune disorders, such as Wiskott–Aldrich syndrome, severe combined immune deficiency (SCID), common variable immune deficiency, and ataxia–telangiectasia. These diseases and other inherited disorders are associated with an increased lifetime risk of developing NHL, with aggressive B-cell NHL being the most common.

Patients who are immunosuppressed for therapeutic reasons—for example, after organ or bone marrow transplantation—are also at increased risk of NHL, especially if treated with cyclosporine, azathioprine, prednisone, or monoclonal antibodies for the removal of T cells (10). A loose association can be drawn between the level of immune suppression and the level of lymphoma risk. It has been noted that transplant patients treated with the highest doses of immunosuppressive

TABLE 8-1	RISK FACTORS ASSOCIATED WITH AGGRESSIVE NON-HODGKIN LYMPHOMAS

Inherited and acquired immune deficiency
   Wiskott–Aldrich syndrome
   Ataxia–telangiectasia
   Chédiak–Higashi syndrome
   X-linked immunoproliferative disorder
   Severe combined immunodeficiency
   Common variable immune deficiency
   Iatrogenic immune suppression
   Solid organ or bone marrow transplant
Toxic exposures
   Prior chemotherapy
   Phenoxyherbicides
   Dioxin
   Radiation or radiation therapy
Infectious exposures
   Epstein–Barr virus
   Human T-cell leukemia/lymphoma virus
   Human herpesvirus type 8 (HHV-8)
   Human immunodeficiency virus (HIV)
Autoimmune disorders
   Sjögren syndrome
   Celiac sprue
   Systemic lupus erythematosus
   Rheumatoid arthritis

agents, such as heart transplant recipients, are at greater risk of developing lymphomas. These lesions are also more likely to be aggressive, extranodal forms. Individuals treated with pharmacologic immune suppression for autoimmune disorders—such as systemic lupus erythematosus, Sjögren syndrome, Felty syndrome, or rheumatoid arthritis—are also at increased risk for NHL over their lifetimes (11-13). A subset of these NHLs is histologically aggressive and associated with Epstein–Barr virus (EBV). These lesions may regress following withdrawal of the immunosuppressive agent (12).

Infectious agents associated with development of the aggressive NHL include human immunodeficiency virus (HIV), EBV, human herpesvirus 8 (HHV-8), and human T-cell leukemia virus (HTLV) (13). The greatest factor involved in the worldwide increase in NHL, at least prior to the advent of highly effective antiretroviral therapy (HAART), is HIV infection (13-15). The risk of NHL is increased by as much as 300% in HIV-infected patients, rising in proportion to the duration of the HIV infection. Although the risk of NHL in HIV-infected patients appears to be decreased by HAART,

their relative risk of NHL continues to be much higher than that for those not infected with HIV. Aggressive NHL can occur in HIV-infected patients at any stage of infection, but the risk goes up dramatically as CD4 counts drop to $<100 \times 10^3/\text{mm}^3$.

EBV also plays a role in lymphomagenesis. In cases of NHL associated with EBV, infection appears to be related to chronic antigenic stimulation by the virus (16). EBV is virtually always present in some types of NHL, such as endemic (African) Burkitt lymphoma (BL) and extranodal T/NK lymphoma of nasal type. Other NHL types are infected by EBV in a subset of cases. Many HIV-related lymphomas are also infected by EBV, and primary central nervous system (CNS) lymphoma, an uncommon late-stage complication of HIV infection, is infected by EBV in essentially 100% of cases (14). HHV-8 is associated with primary effusion lymphoma (PEL), which tends to occur in HIV-infected patients. HTLV-I is associated with adult T-cell lymphoma/leukemia.

Environmental and occupational exposures to toxins have been associated with an increased risk of NHL (17,18). Herbicides, especially phenoxyacetic acid derivatives, are associated with NHL, especially in the farming belts of the United States (17). Occupations reported to be at increased risk for NHL include farming, metalworking, forestry, woodworking, and dry cleaning. One of the common exposures in these industries is the use of organic solvents. With long-term follow-up, aircraft maintenance workers who used multiple solvents were also found to be at increased risk for NHL (18).

Familial history of NHL is also a risk factor. Individuals who have relatives with NHL also have a slightly higher risk of developing NHL. In one study, the risk was higher for siblings and for male relatives (19). The genetic causes that explain familial lymphoma are poorly understood.

■ CLINICAL PRESENTATION

The clinical presentation of aggressive NHL varies substantially based on histologic type and anatomic site of disease. Approximately, 50% of patients present with "B" symptoms: fever greater than 38°C, night sweats, or weight loss greater than 10% of body weight in the preceding 6 months. The likelihood of B symptoms increases with the aggressiveness of NHL. Fatigue and malaise are less frequent than B symptoms and pruritus is unusual.

More than 60% of patients present with painless peripheral lymphadenopathy. Often, the patients with localized nodes are first treated with antibiotics for a presumed diagnosis of infection, which proves to be an incorrect diagnosis when the nodes fail to regress. Both external and internal lymph nodes are commonly involved by NHL. Symptoms vary with the anatomic site of lymphadenopathy. Those patients presenting with mediastinal adenopathy frequently experience cough, chest pain, and sometimes superior vena cava syndrome, although this is much less frequent than with solid tumors. Those patients presenting with large nodal masses in the abdomen or retroperitoneum frequently experience pain, abdominal fullness, or early satiety. Retroperitoneal tumors can cause back pain and discomfort. More frequently, peripheral lymph nodes are discovered before internal lymph nodes cause symptoms. Peripheral lymph nodes are not usually painful until they have become massively enlarged.

Extranodal disease is common in patients with aggressive and highly aggressive NHL. Larger tumors, especially in the gastrointestinal (GI) tract, can present with obstruction, blood loss with subsequent anemia, or diarrhea. Classically, the most common extranodal site of lymphoma is the stomach, followed by the intestines, tonsils, and skin, although the published frequency of involvement of these sites varies across reports. Other extranodal sites include liver, lung, testis, bones, CNS, and spleen. Pulmonary lesions can present in a lymphangitic, nodular, or alveolar pattern, sometimes with cavitary lesions reminiscent of lung cancer (20). Primary bone lesions are typically quite painful. Aggressive extranodal disease may invade almost any tissue or organ system.

■ CLINICOPATHOLOGIC CHARACTERISTICS

DIFFUSE LARGE B-CELL LYMPHOMA, NOT OTHERWISE SPECIFIED (NOS)

Diffuse large B-cell lymphoma (DLBCL) is the most common type of NHL (21,22). It occurs mainly in adults, with a median age in the sixth decade. Men are affected slightly more often than women (22). B-type symptoms or bulky disease occurs in one-third of patients. Although much less common in children, DLBCL represents 15 to 20% of childhood NHL. Nodal presentation is most common, but extranodal sites are involved in approximately 40% of patients (21-23) (Figs. 8-1 and 8-2). More than one extranodal site is involved in one-third of patients. Approximately, half of

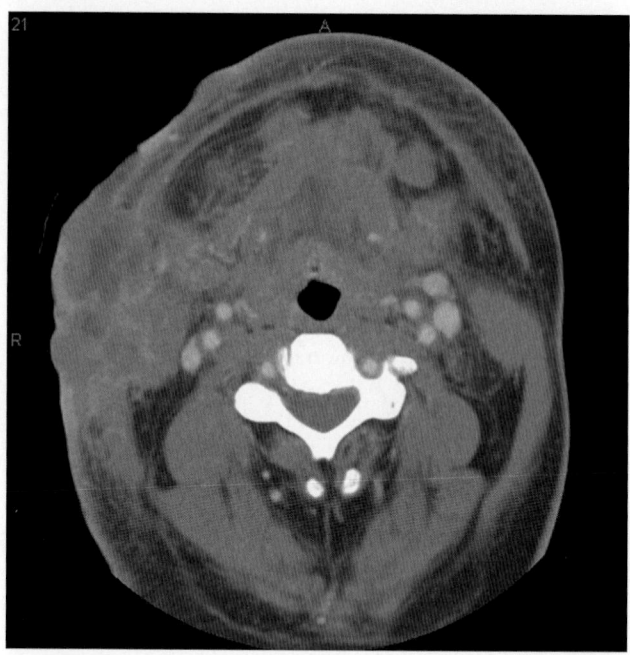

FIGURE 8-1. CT scan showing diffuse large B-cell lymphoma with extensive lymph node involvement in the neck.

affected patients present with clinical stage III or IV disease (21). Bone marrow involvement is unusual, occurring in approximately 10% of patients. DLBCLs uncommonly involve privileged sites, such as the testis and CNS. CNS involvement portends a poor prognosis.

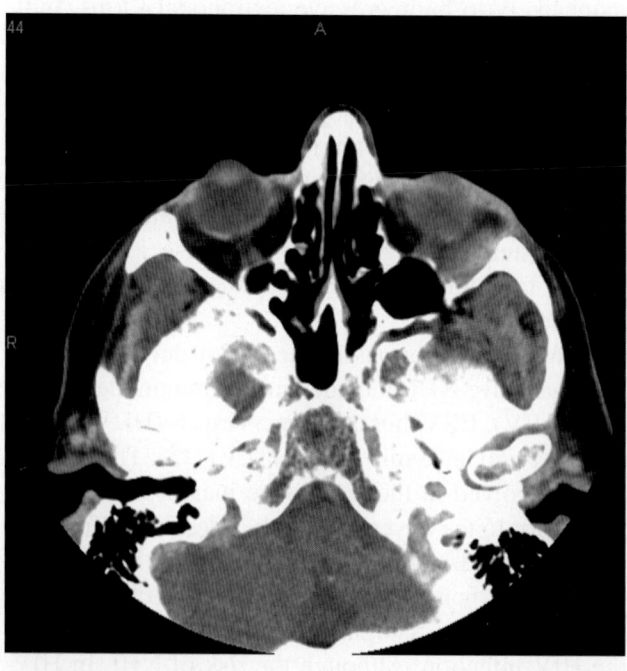

FIGURE 8-2. CT scan showing diffuse large B-cell lymphoma as a periorbital mass.

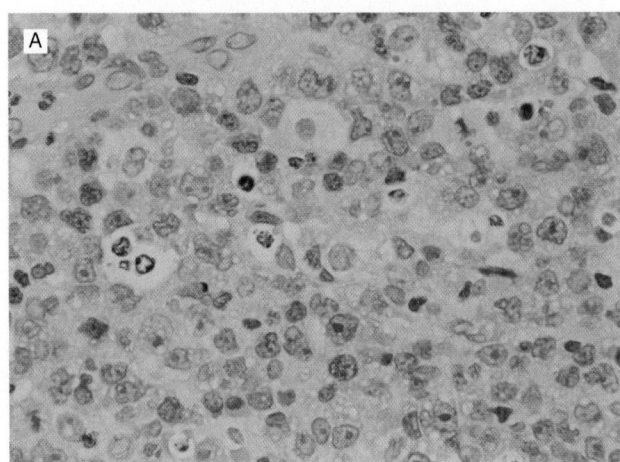
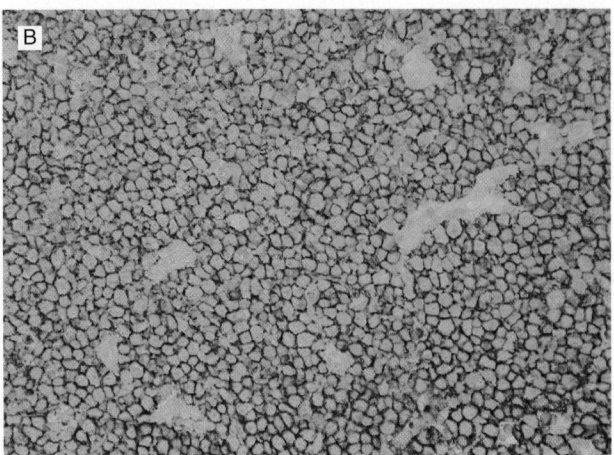

FIGURE 8-3. Diffuse large B-cell lymphoma. **A.** The neoplastic cells are large with vesicular chromatin and are arranged in a diffuse pattern. **B.** The neoplastic cells are positive for CD20. (A, hematoxylin-eosin, 1000×; B, immunohistochemistry, 400×.)

If untreated, DLBCL is invariably fatal; most patients survive <2 years. However, these neoplasms are susceptible to chemotherapy, with a significant chance for cure, particularly in patients with localized disease (23-25). With newer chemotherapy regimens, high rates of complete response have been reported. DLBCL is a curable disease with overall 5-year survival of approximately 50 to 80% (24). Overall survival correlates well with the International Prognostic Index (IPI) score. The 5-year progression-free, disease-specific, and overall survival rates for DLBCL patients with an IPI of 0 to 2 were 73, 84, and 82%, respectively, as opposed to an IPI of 3 to 4 with 37 and 32%, respectively (25).

DLBCL has a diffuse pattern on routinely stained sections and composed of neoplastic large cells. Mitotic figures are usually numerous (21). Cytologically, the neoplastic cells can be subdivided as large cleaved cells (large centrocytes), large noncleaved cells (centroblasts), and immunoblasts (26). Large cleaved cells range from 13 to 30 μm in size and have irregular or cleaved nuclear contours, relatively small, indistinct nucleoli, and a thin rim of eosinophilic cytoplasm. Large noncleaved cells are 20 to 30 μm in size and have round or oval vesicular nuclei with two or three nucleoli and more abundant amphophilic cytoplasm (Figs. 8-3 and 8-4). Often one nucleolus is centrally located and one or two nucleoli are peripherally apposed adjacent to the nuclear membrane. Neoplastic immunoblasts resemble transformed lymphocytes; they are larger than large noncleaved cells, with an eccentrically located vesicular round or oval nucleus containing a prominent target-like central nucleolus and relatively abundant amphophilic

cytoplasm (Fig. 8-5). These cells commonly exhibit plasmacytoid differentiation. In general, the cytologic features of DLBCL do not influence prognosis (26). In one large study, however, patients with the immunoblastic type of DLBCL had a poorer overall and relapse-free survival (27).

Although these descriptions of large cleaved and noncleaved cells and immunoblasts are distinctive and many neoplastic large B cells fit within these descriptions, it is also true that neoplastic large cells exhibit a spectrum of differentiation and often have intermediate cytologic features. Furthermore, DLBCLs are commonly composed of a mixture of these cell types (21).

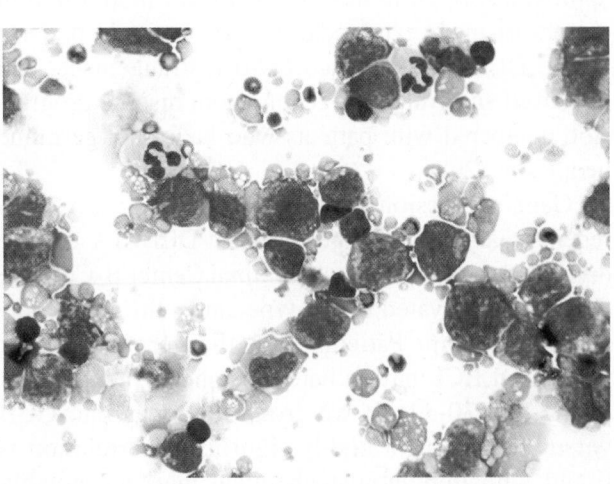

FIGURE 8-4. Diffuse large B-cell lymphoma. Fine needle aspiration of cervical lymph node. The neoplastic cells are large (compared with neutrophils in field) with abundant basophilic cytoplasm (Wright-Giemsa, 1000×).

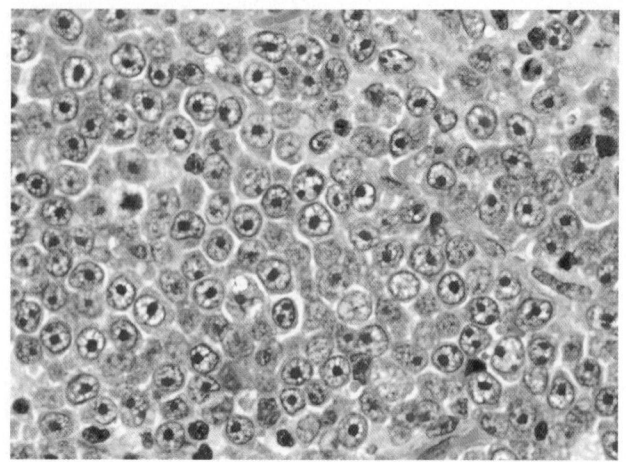

FIGURE 8-5. Diffuse large B-cell lymphoma, immunoblastic variant. The neoplastic cells are large with prominent central nucleoli imparting a "target-like" appearance (hematoxylin–eosin, 1000×).

Immunophenotypic studies have shown that DLBCLs are of mature B-cell lineage (21). Approximately, two-thirds of cases express monotypic immunoglobulin (Ig); approximately one-third of DLBCLs are Ig-negative. These tumors express pan-B-cell antigens, 60 to 70% express BCL-2, and a subset is positive for CD10 and BCL-6. Most DLBCLs have a high proliferation rate.

DLBCLs are heterogeneous at the molecular level. A subset of cases carries the t(14;18) involving the *bcl*-2 gene, as shown by conventional cytogenetic or molecular studies (28). Another subset of DLBCLs has translocations or other abnormalities involving the *bcl*-6 gene at chromosome 3q27. The *bcl*-6 gene is rearranged in approximately 20 to 40% of DLBCLs, more often in tumors arising in extranodal sites. In one study, patients whose DLBCLs contained *bcl*-6 rearrangements had improved survival and freedom from disease progression compared with patients who had *bcl*-6 germline neoplasms (29).

Gene-expression profiling studies performed in recent years have suggested that DLBCLs can be divided into three groups: Germinal Center B-Cell like (GCB), an activated B-cell type, and a third noncharacteristic group. Patients with the germinal center type of DLBCL have a better prognosis independent of the IPI (30-32). If we group the types into GCB versus non-GCB, a highly significant correlation is found with immunohistochemical markers, notably the CD10 marker identifies the germinal center type, while CD10 negativity coupled with MUM-1 and/or FOXP1 expression are indicative of the nongerminal center subtypes (33).

Diffuse Large B-Cell Lymphoma Clinicopathologic Subtypes

T-Cell/Histiocyte-Rich B-Cell Lymphoma

This variant of DLBCL is clinically indistinct from the majority of DLBCL. It is the histology that is unique. T-cell/histiocyte-rich variant of DLBCL represents a significant challenge for pathologist as most of the cells in the biopsy specimen are reactive T cells (21). Numerous benign histiocytes may also be present. Within this infiltrate, the large, neoplastic B cells represent <10% of all cells in the infiltrate (Fig. 8-6).

Primary DLBCL of the CNS

This entity includes all primary intracerebral or intraocular lymphomas. Although these lymphomas are remarkable

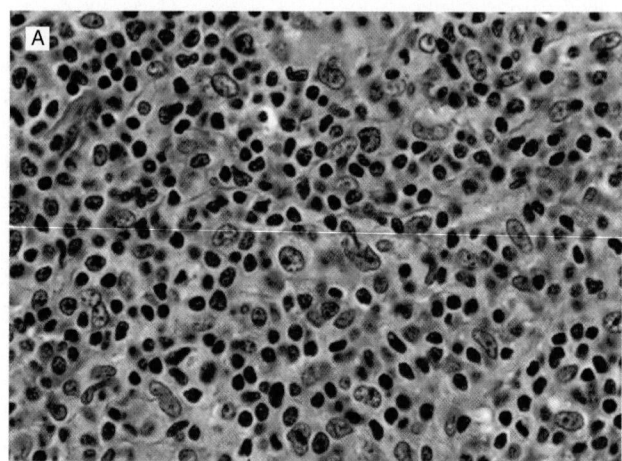

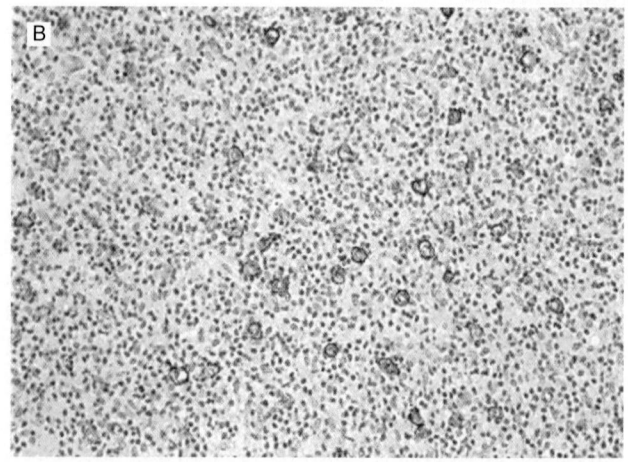

FIGURE 8-6. T-cell/histiocyte-rich large B-cell lymphoma. **A.** Scattered large neoplastic lymphoid cells in a background of numerous small lymphocytes. **B.** The large neoplastic cells are positive for CD20 and the small lymphocytes are T cells (immunostain not shown [A, hematoxylin-eosin, 630×]; B, immunohistochemistry, 200×).

for their unique clinical presentation, histologically these neoplasms represent typical DLBCL. The neoplastic cells usually express CD20, CD22, and CD79a. In many cases, the neoplastic cells strongly express BCL6 and MUM1; CD10 expression is significantly rare (34-37). The neoplastic cells also often express BCL-2. Approximately, one third of the cases demonstrate translocations involving BCL6 gene; it was demonstrated that translocations t(14;18) (q32;q21), and t(8;14)(q24;q32) are extremely rare in this category.

Primary Cutaneous DLBCL, Leg Type

Clinically, as the name suggests, the lymphoma lesions present in the lower extremities, and typically involve primarily the skin. Lesions can be ulcerated, and the clinical course is aggressive. The pathology is characteristically indicative of a non-follicle center origin. Histologic sections show diffuse sheets of monotonous neoplastic cells with centroblastic or immunoblastic morphology with often mitotic figures (38). The neoplastic cells are positive for CD20, CD79a, BCL-2, BCL-6, and monotypic immunoglobulin, and are usually negative for CD10 (39). Fluorescent in situ hybridization (FISH) studies often detect rearrangement of *BCL-6*, *IGH*, and *c-MYC* genes (40).

EBV Positive DLBCL of the Elderly

The clinical presentation of this subtype of DLBCL is in the elderly, and usually has an advanced stage at presentation. The neoplasm has a diffuse pattern and contains numerous large immunoblasts, Hodgkin and Reed-Sternberg (HRS)-like giant cells; large areas of geographical necrosis are often detected. Two morphologic variants are recognized: a polymorphous variant, with a broad range of B-cell maturation in the reactive background, and a large-cell lymphoma variant, which contains mostly transformed cells (41). The neoplastic cells usually express CD20, CD30, CD79a, MUM1, and are negative for CD10, CD15, and BCL6 (41,42).

Primary Effusion Lymphoma

PEL, also known as body cavity-based lymphoma, is a very rare neoplasm of large B cells that involves a body cavity (21,43). Usually, only one body cavity is involved. Most affected patients are homosexual men infected with HIV. The prognosis for patients with PEL is poor.

Morphogically, the neoplastic cells resemble immunoblasts or plasmablasts with prominent nucleoli and abundant basophilic cytoplasm. The tumor cells are found within body cavity fluid but may adhere to and invade body cavity surfaces.

Immunophenotypic studies of PEL are ambiguous (21,43). The neoplastic cells express CD30, CD38, CD45 (LCA), and CD138, but they are usually negative for Ig- and B-cell antigens. No characteristic chromosomal abnormalities are known. HHV-8 (also known as Kaposi sarcoma–associated herpesvirus) is present in virtually all cases of PEL, and its presence selects for a distinct cellular gene expression profile (44). EBV is also present in most cases of PEL.

Other Lymphomas of Large B Cells

Primary Mediastinal (thymic) Large B-Cell Lymphoma (PMLBCL)

At diagnosis, PMLBCLs usually are localized to the thoracic cavity. They occur more frequently in young women, with a 2:1 ratio compared to men. They can present with superior vena cava syndrome, although more frequently they present with cough, and shortness of breath, mimicking a respiratory infection. PMLBCL are diffuse and are composed of large lymphoid cells that exhibit a spectrum of cytologic appearances: most commonly large noncleaved cell (centroblastic) and less often large cleaved cell or immunoblastic (21, 45-47). Sclerosis is common, mitotic figures are usually numerous, and the tumor cells can have clear cytoplasm.

Immunophenotypic studies have shown that primary mediastinal large B-cell lymphomas are frequently Ig-negative. All tumors express pan-B-cell antigens and are usually negative for CD21; a subset of cases may lack MHC class II antigens (48). Others have suggested that these tumors may arise from B cells normally present in small numbers in the thymic medulla of the thymus. One study has shown that the *mal* gene is overexpressed in PMLBCL, but not nodal DLBCL (49). Gene profiling studies indicate that the profile of PMBCL is more like that of Hodgkin lymphoma than DLBCL (50).

Lymphomatoid Granulomatosis

Lymphomatoid granulomatosis (LyG), originally described by Liebow and colleagues, was first thought to have features that overlapped with both malignant lymphoma and Wegener granulomatosis, leading to its name (51). Many investigators now consider LyG to be neoplastic at onset.

Patients with LyG are usually of middle age and present with pulmonary and systemic symptoms. Chest radiographs typically show discrete round masses, most often bilateral. Other common sites of involvement by LyG include the kidney, CNS, and skin. The upper respiratory tract is rarely involved. Many patients with

LyG have evidence of immune dysfunction, and LyG may arise in immunodeficient patients.

LyG is characterized by an angiocentric and angiodestructive infiltrate of lymphocytes, associated with plasma cells and histiocytes. Granulocytes are rare. Necrosis can be prominent. The lymphoid cells range in size from small with minimal atypia to large, and the natural history of LyG is to accrue large cells and evolve into a process that resembles large B-cell lymphoma.

Immunophenotypic studies of LyG have shown that the majority of lymphoid cells are nonneoplastic T cells. In most cases of LyG, a small number of larger B cells can be identified; these represent the malignant cell population. Assessment of Ig expression is difficult in LyG because of the small number of large B cells, but it has been shown in a subset of cases. These large B cells express pan-B-cell antigens and commonly carry EBV (52). It is also possible that some cases of LyG may be of T-cell lineage (or peripheral T-cell lymphoma in lung can closely mimic LyG).

Intravascular Large B-Cell Lymphoma

Intravascular lymphoma, also known as angiotropic lymphoma and originally described as malignant angioendotheliomatosis, is an unusual variant of large cell lymphoma that has a predominantly intravascular distribution (53). Although rare cases are of T- or NK-cell lineage, over 90% of intravascular lymphomas are B-cell neoplasms (54).

Patients with intravascular large B-cell lymphoma (IVLBL) are typically middle-aged or elderly and present with systemic symptoms as well as symptoms attributable to specific organs that result from vascular occlusion and ischemia. These tumors most commonly affect the CNS, skin, and kidney, but any site may be involved (53). Bone marrow involvement, although difficult to appreciate morphologically, is relatively common when the bone marrow is assessed using immunophenotypic methods (54). Lymphadenopathy is uncommon. The prognosis is often poor due to the late detection of disease, but patients respond to appropriate chemotherapy.

Intravascular lymphoma is characterized by the presence of large lymphoid cells filling and/or distending vascular lumina (Fig. 8-7). The neoplastic cells are found primarily within capillaries or small blood vessels (53). Extravascular involvement occurs; although not prominent clinically, it is commonly found at autopsy.

With the advent of immunophenotypic studies, IVLBL was shown to be a variant of large B-cell lymphoma in most cases (53,54). These tumors express pan-B-cell

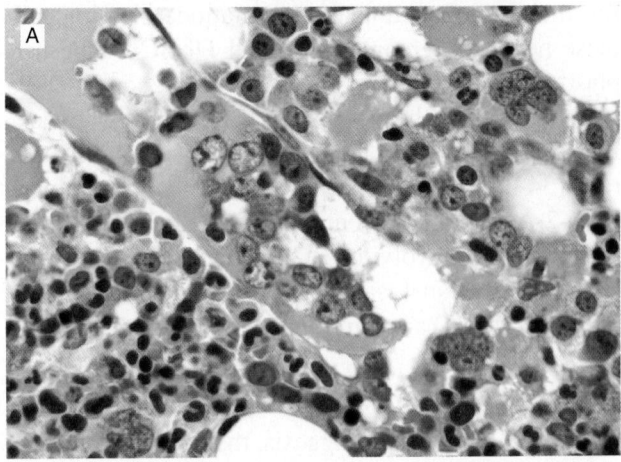

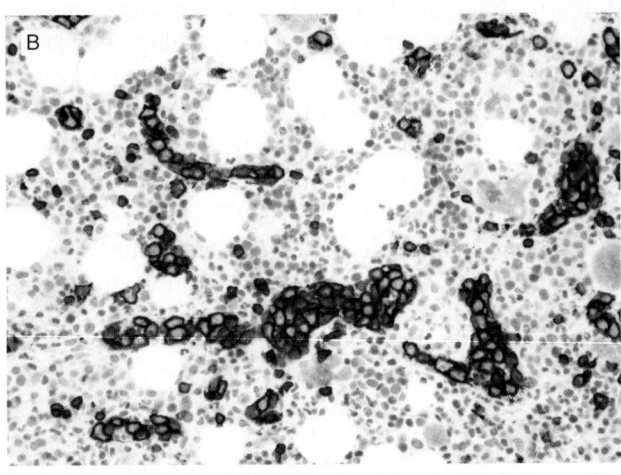

FIGURE 8-7. Intravascular large B-cell lymphoma involving bone marrow. **A.** Large neoplastic cells are present with a small blood vessel. **B.** The anti-CD20 antibody highlights numerous large neoplastic cells within many blood vessels. (A, hematoxylin–eosin, 1000×; B, immunohistochemistry, 400×.)

antigens and a subset express monotypic immunoglobulin. These neoplasms appear to be heterogeneous. Two or possibly three groups have been identified: CD5– CD10+, consistent with follicle-center cell origin; CD5+ CD10–; and CD5– CD10–. These groupings are similar to DLBCL (55).

MANTLE CELL LYMPHOMA

The term *mantle cell lymphoma* (MCL) is the currently accepted name in the WHO classification for a neoplasm previously known as malignant lymphoma, intermediate lymphocytic type, lymphocytic lymphoma of intermediate differentiation, centrocytic lymphoma, and mantle zone lymphoma. MCL represents approximately 6% of all NHLs (21-23).

Clinically, patients with MCL are usually elderly men with a median age in the seventh decade. The male/female ratio is approximately 3:1 (56-58). Most patients present with clinical stage III or IV disease and generalized lymphadenopathy. Systemic symptoms occur in approximately 40% of patients. Bone marrow is involved in approximately 60% of patients (59). An absolute peripheral blood lymphocytosis of more than 4000/mm^3 is infrequent, but low-level involvement of the peripheral blood is common when searched for morphologically or if sensitive molecular techniques are used (57). Overt leukemia may be associated with a poorer prognosis. The GI tract is commonly involved in patients with MCL (85-90%), although only one-fourth of patients have GI tract symptoms (60). A small subset of patients may present with numerous polyps involving the GI tract, a syndrome known in the literature as *multiple lymphomatous polyposis* (21).

Although a small subset of patients have clinically indolent disease (58), most patients with MCL have a poor prognosis. In a study by Fisher et al. (56), after 10 years of clinical follow-up, only 8% of patients were alive after treatment with cyclophosphamide, doxorubicin, vincristine, and prednisone (CHOP). In many studies, patient survival correlates with the pattern of involvement in lymph nodes. Patients with a mantle zone pattern of lymph node involvement have better survival than do patients with diffusely involved lymph nodes.

Histologically, the lymph node architecture is replaced by a diffuse or vaguely nodular neoplasm (Fig. 8-8). In a subset of cases, a mantle zone pattern results when the neoplasm selectively involves the follicular mantle

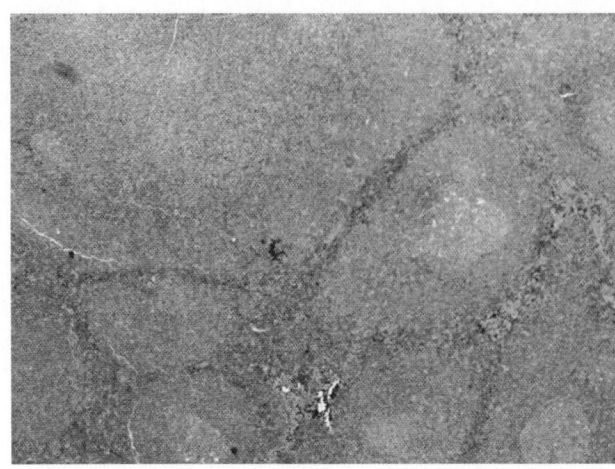

FIGURE 8-9. Mantle cell lymphoma, mantle zone pattern (hematoxylin–eosin, 50×).

zones surrounding normal or reactive germinal centers (Fig. 8-9). Cytologically, MCL is composed of a monotonous population of small lymphoid cells with slightly to clearly irregular nuclear contours (Fig. 8-10). Large nucleolated lymphoid cells are rare. Other histologic findings common in MCL include numerous eosinophilic epithelioid histiocytes and germinal centers completely surrounded by tumor without a normal lymphoid cuff (so-called naked germinal centers).

Blastoid variants of MCL occur and can be divided into two types: classic and pleomorphic (21). Classic blastoid MCL is characterized by slightly larger lymphoid cells with finely dispersed nuclear chromatin and numerous mitotic features that resemble lymphoblastic lymphoma. Pleomorphic variants of MCL are composed

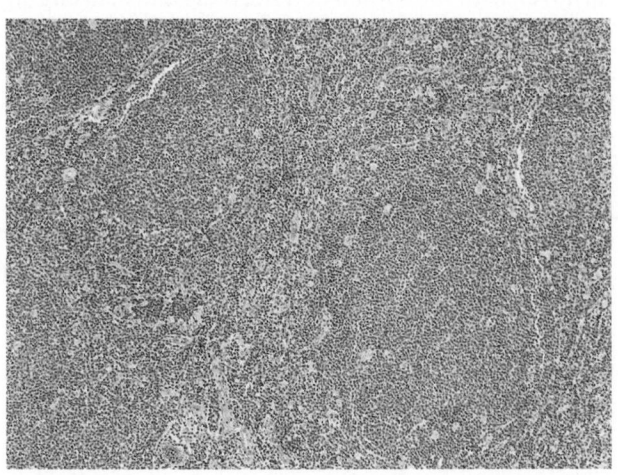

FIGURE 8-8. Mantle cell lymphoma, nodular pattern (hematoxylin–eosin, 50×).

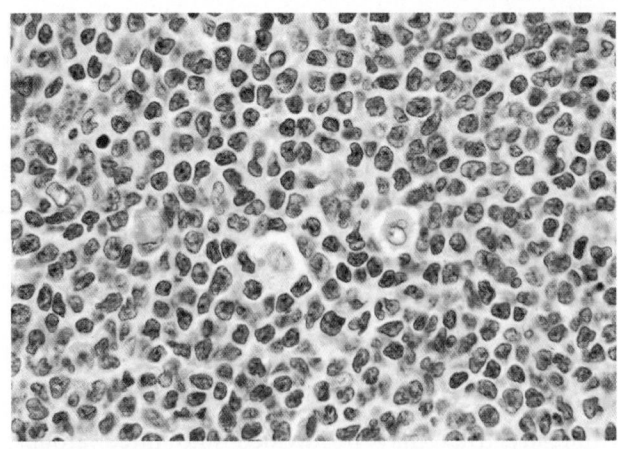

FIGURE 8-10. Mantle cell lymphoma. In this field, a uniform population of small, irregular lymphoid cells can be seen (hematoxylin–eosin, 400×).

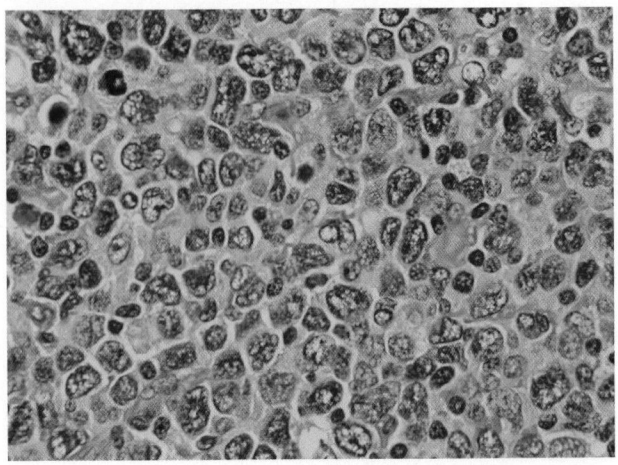

FIGURE 8-11. Mantle cell lymphoma, blastoid variant. The neoplastic cells are large and pleomorphic and were cyclin D1 positive (immunostain not shown) (hematoxylin–eosin, 1000×).

of large cells that resemble, in part, large cell lymphoma (Fig. 8-11). Blastoid MCLs have a more aggressive clinical course. In the peripheral blood, MCL can sometimes resemble prolymphocytic leukemia (61).

Immunophenotypic studies have shown that MCLs express monotypic Ig light chain (more often Ig λ), IgM, IgD, pan-B-cell antigens, BCL-2, alkaline phosphatase, and CD5 (21). Unlike CLL/SLL, MCL is often positive for CD79B and FMC-7 and typically is negative for CD10, CD23, and BCL-6. However, approximately 10% of MCLs can be CD23-positive.

The t(11;14)(q13;q32) is present in virtually all cases of MCL (62). In this translocation, the *ccnd*-1 gene (also known as *PRAD*1 and *bcl*-1) on 11q13 is juxtaposed with the Ig heavy chain gene on 14q32, resulting in overexpression of cyclin D1. Cyclin D1 facilitates cell cycle transition from G1 to S phase (63). Although the t(11;14) is central to the pathogenesis of MCL, the t(11;14) is not sufficient to cause lymphomagenesis. Other molecular abnormalities are also required. Conventional cytogenetic studies have shown a number of additional abnormalities (64,65), and mutations in the *atm*, *p16*, and *p53* genes have been detected, with *p16* and *p53* mutations more common in blastoid variants.

BURKITT LYMPHOMA

Clinically, BLs may be divided into three groups: endemic (African), sporadic (nonendemic), and AIDS-associated (21,66). A leukemic form of BL also occurs, designated by the French–American–British group as

acute lymphoblastic leukemia, L3, now recognized in the WHO classification as leukemic phase.

Endemic BL was first described in equatorial Africa (Uganda). Evidence of EBV infection is present in 95% of patients (66). The median age of patients with endemic BL is 7 years, with a boy/girl ratio of 3:1. The jaw is the best-known site of disease, involving either the maxilla or mandible in 60% of patients, but large abdominal masses involving retroperitoneal structures, the GI tract, or the gonads are also commonly present.

Sporadic BLs occur in industrialized nations and represent <1% of all NHLs (23). EBV infection is present in a subset of patients, approximately 25%. Patients affected are usually in the second or third decades of life, with a male/female ratio of 3:1. The jaw is infrequently involved, and most patients present with large abdominal masses, frequently involving the ileocecal region of the bowel (66). Other sites commonly involved include abdominal and peripheral lymph nodes, pleura, and pharynx. In patients with either endemic or sporadic BL, bone marrow and CNS involvement are uncommon at presentation in approximately 10 to 20% of cases, but they are frequent sites of subsequent dissemination.

BL can also occur in the clinical setting of HIV infection. These neoplasms are associated with EBV infection in 30 to 40% of cases and commonly involve lymph nodes or extranodal sites (67).

BL grow as expansile masses that diffusely infiltrate contiguous tissues. Reactive histiocytes are scattered throughout the tumor. The relatively clear cytoplasm of the histiocytes in a background of blue neoplastic cells imparts a "starry sky" appearance (Fig. 8-12A). This pattern results from rapid cell turnover with individual cell necrosis and scavenging of debris by macrophages. The neoplastic cells are round to ovoid, uniform in shape, and approximately the size of benign histiocyte nuclei. The chromatin is coarse, with two to five prominent basophilic nucleoli. Mitotic figures are numerous. Histologically, the endemic, sporadic, and AIDS-associated types of BL are indistinguishable (21).

BL of endemic, sporadic, and AIDS-associated types are of mature B-cell lineage and express Ig, pan-B-cell antigens, CD10, and BCL-6 (23). BL have a very high proliferation rate, >99%, using an antibody specific for Ki-67 (Fig. 8-12B,C). These tumors are negative for IgD, CD21, CD23, BCL-2, lymphocyte homing receptors, and T-cell antigens.

C-*myc* translocations are characteristic of BL. Approximately, 80% of cases carry the t(8;14)(q24;q32),

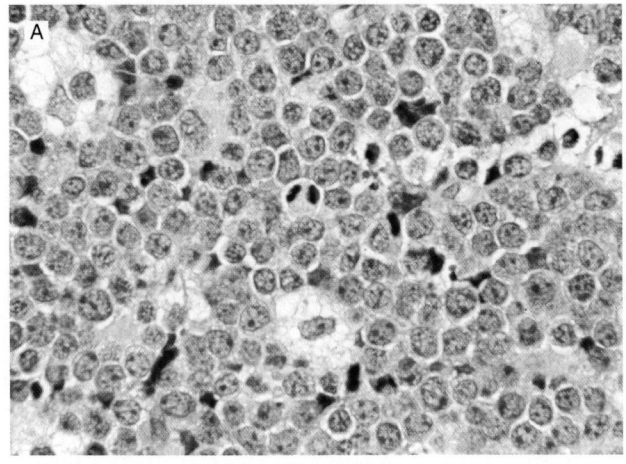

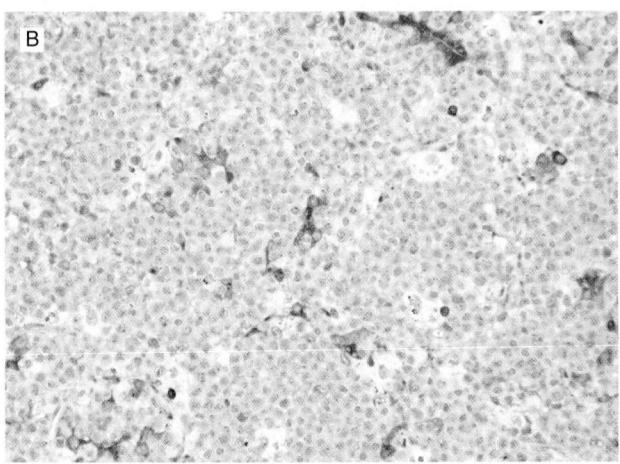

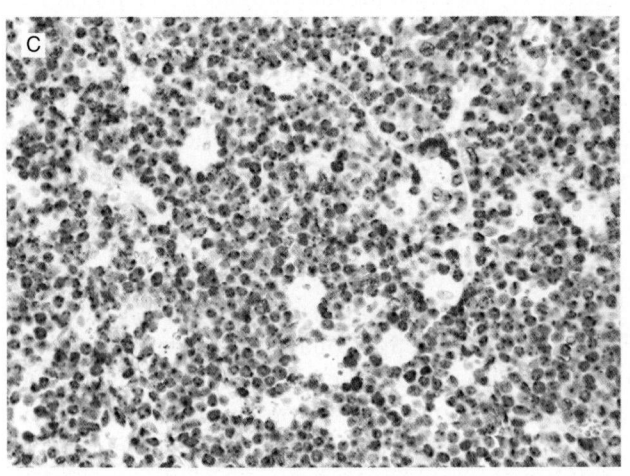

FIGURE 8-12. Burkitt lymphoma. **A.** The neoplastic cells are intermediate in size, similar to that of benign histiocyte nuclei, with multiple small nucleoli. A starry-sky pattern is also seen in this field. **B,C.** The neoplastic cells are negative for BCL-2 (B), and are >99% positive for Ki-67 (C). (A, hematoxylin–eosin, 1000×; B,C, immunohistochemistry, 400×.)

with the remaining cases having one of two variant translocations, the t(2;8)(p11;q24) or t(8;22) (q24;q11) (67-69). Common to each of these translocations is involvement of chromosome region 8q24, the site of the c-*myc* gene, which is deregulated. Via these translocations, c-*myc* is juxtaposed with the Ig heavy chain on the derivative chromosome 14, or with the IgK and Ig λ genes on the derivative chromosome 8. The breakpoints of the t(8;14) are distinctive in endemic and sporadic BL (69).

B-Cell Lymphomas With Features Intermediate Between Diffuse Large B-Cell Lymphoma and BL

This entity was recently introduced in the new 2008 edition of WHO classification of hematopoietic neoplasms. As the name implies, this category is designed for cases, which do not fit either DLBCL or BL. In the past, some of these cases were designated as atypical Burkitt/Burkitt-like lymphoma; others were also diagnosed as "High grade B-cell lymphoma," or "B-cell lymphoma with high grade features." This group is quite heterogeneous, and both morphologic and immunophenotypic deviation from typical cases of BL and DLBCL could result into placing a particular case in this category. Virtually all cases show diffuse pattern with prominent starry-sky pattern. In so-called morphologic deviants, the neoplastic cells are significantly larger than cells of BL, have irregular shape and significant degree of pleomorphism; chromatin is usually open, and numerous mitotic figures are seen (Fig. 8-13). Occasionally, neoplastic cells demonstrate prominent nucleoli. The neoplastic cells express B-cell markers such as CD19, CD20, CD22, CD79a, and show surface immunoglobulin restriction; so-called immunophenotypic deviants demonstrates deviation from classical BL phenotype (CD10+/BCL2–/BCL6+/MUM1–/TdT–). Proliferation rate as detected by Ki-67 stain is always high, at least 50%, but there is no consistency among pathologists as to what is the lowest Ki-67 level they would accept to place a particular case in this category (70-71). A significant number of cases demonstrate c-*MYC* rearrangement, although in some of the cases c-*MYC* rearrangement involves one of non-Ig partners, such as the t(8;9)(q24;p13) (72). Many cases demonstrate both c-*MYC* and *BCL-2* rearrangement, which is referred to as "double-hit lymphoma." These cases usually demonstrate strong BCL-2 expression and show dismal prognosis (73). Conventional cytogenetic studies usually demonstrate complex karyotype with numerous abnormalities (72).

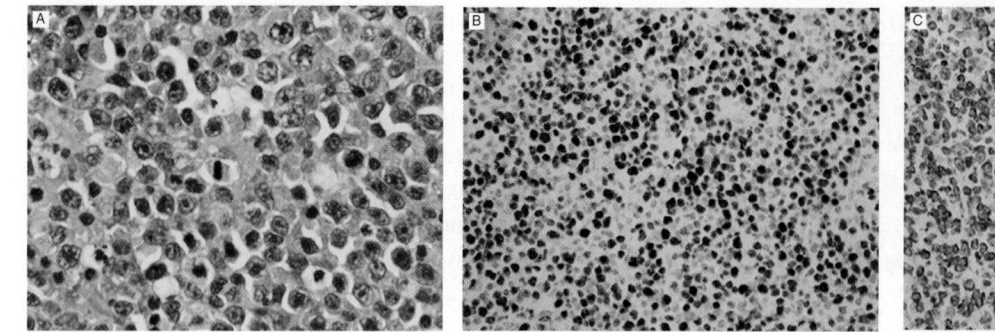

FIGURE 8-13. B-cell lymphomas with features intermediate between diffuse large B-cell lymphoma and Burkitt lymphoma. Similar to Burkitt lymphoma, the neoplastic cells are intermediate-sized and demonstrate brisk mitotic activity, but, unlike Burkitt lymphoma, cells have prominent single nucleoli (A). While proliferative rate is similar to Burkitt lymphoma (B), the neoplastic cells strongly express Bcl-2 (C). In this case, FISH detected both translocations t(8;14) and t(14;18), so-called double-hit lymphoma (Lymph node, A. H&E, x 1000; B. Ki-67 (Mib-1), x400. C. Bcl-2, x400. Courtesy of Dr. L. Jeffrey Medeiros.)

■ STAGING AND INITIAL EVALUATION

The Ann Arbor Staging system (74), developed in 1971 and used originally for Hodgkin lymphoma (disease), is widely used as the staging system for NHL (Table 8-2). It takes into account the number and locations of lymph node groups and extranodal sites involved by NHL as well as the presence or absence of systemic symptoms. Typically, NHLs are disseminated at time of diagnosis, unlike the case in Hodgkin lymphoma, for which the system was designed. This means that noncontiguous lymph node groups are frequently involved. In addition, the Ann Arbor system fails to take into account other more recently

discovered prognostic information, such as serum LDH, β_2-microglobulin levels, and genetic abnormalities.

Because aggressive NHLs very frequently present with stage III or IV disease, and there does not appear to be any meaningful difference in the treatment of patients in these two stages, the purpose of staging is to identify the patients with localized NHL that can be treated aggressively with radiation or other locally delivered therapy. Although other staging systems have been proposed for specific disease entities, the Ann Arbor system is widely used. Given the complexity of NHL classification, it may not be possible to provide a comprehensive and meaningful staging system that adequately incorporates the prognostic factors for all lymphoma types.

The initial approach to the patient with aggressive NHL requires a careful history and physical examination. Especially important in the history is the presence or absence of systemic symptoms, because they are adverse indicators in patients with aggressive NHL. Any symptoms that may point to focal lesions should be elicited. History of EBV infection, HIV, hepatitis B or C infection, therapeutic immunosuppression, occupational exposures to toxins (especially pesticides and petroleum products), and inherited immunologic disorders should be noted. Performance status should be assessed, because the ability to receive combination chemotherapy is vital to treatment. Comorbid conditions should be carefully noted and taken into account during the planning of therapy.

Physical examination should include a complete survey of all external lymph node groups including cervical,

TABLE 8-2	ANN ARBOR STAGING SYSTEM FOR NON-HODGKIN LYMPHOMAS*
Stage I	Involvement of a single nodal group or extranodal site (I$_E$)
Stage II	Involvement of two or more nodal groups on the same side of the diaphragm or localized involvement of an extranodal site or organ (II$_E$) and one or more nodal groups on the same side of the diaphragm
Stage III	Involvement of nodal groups on both sides of the diaphragm, which may be accompanied by localized involvement of an extranodal region or site (III$_E$) of spleen (III$_S$) or both (III$_{SE}$)
Stage IV	Diffuse or disseminated involvement of one or more distant extranodal sites

*Temperature >38°C, weight loss >10% of body weight in the last 6 months, night sweats preceding diagnosis are defined as "B" symptoms and designated by the suffix B. Others are designated by the suffix A.

supraclavicular, axillary, epitrochlear, femoral, popliteal, and inguinal areas. In men, the testes should be examined. Complete examination of the skin and assessment of the abdomen for hepatomegaly or splenomegaly is necessary. Examination of Waldeyer ring should be performed, with endoscopy if tonsillar lymphoma is suspected. A complete neurologic examination must also be performed. The physical examination should include a search aimed at the discovery or evaluation of comorbid conditions that might interfere with therapy.

Laboratory evaluation is guided by the pathologic findings but always includes a complete blood count with differential, peripheral blood smear, and serum studies, including LDH, β_2-microglobulin, kidney, and liver function tests, albumin, calcium, and uric acid. In some patients, serology for hepatitis is helpful or indicated. Testing for hepatitis B is indicated prior to rituximab therapy, as the virus may reactivate during or after this treatment. Testing for HIV should always be performed, as should bone marrow aspiration and biopsy (bilateral biopsies for certain NHL types; also see comments on FDG-PET and marrow findings below). Serum protein electrophoresis is helpful, at least initially, to rule out the presence of paraproteins. Examination of the CSF should be undertaken for patients with highly aggressive NHL, DLBCL associated with spinal, or paraspinal masses, skull lesions, bone marrow involvement, testicular lymphoma, nasal or sinus lymphomas, or any patient with clinical symptoms leading to suspicion of CNS involvement.

Additional clinical evaluation is guided by the histologic type of NHL, symptoms, and anatomic sites involved by NHL. GI lymphomas, especially in the stomach, require endoscopy for diagnosis unless other disease sites can be found to biopsy. It is especially important that multiple biopsies of different areas of the stomach be obtained, as sampling error is frequent. There is no utility to gastrectomy. Other types of aggressive NHL can involve the GI tract, especially MCL (58). Evaluation of primary CNS lymphoma requires biopsy of the lesion, but a vigorous search for additional disease sites should be undertaken first, with a view toward avoiding brain biopsy if other sites of disease are more easily accessible.

Imaging Studies for Initial Staging

The use of imaging studies for evaluating lymphoma patients has increased since the original Ann Arbor Staging system was formulated (74). Multidetector computer tomography (CT) scans have become the standard for anatomic imaging. These advances in

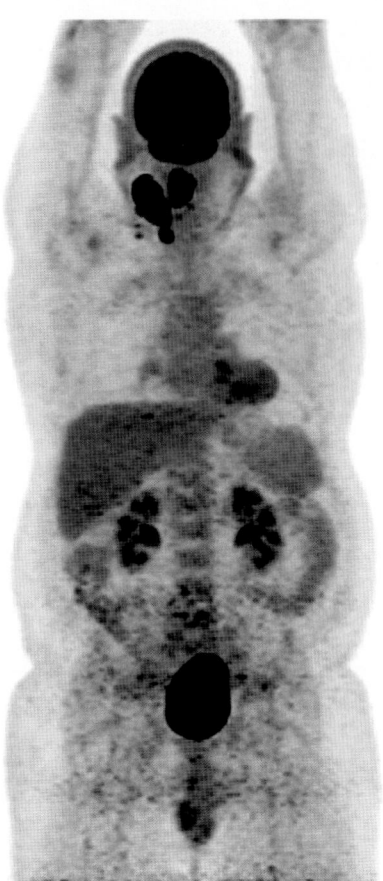

FIGURE 8-14. Positron emission tomography (PET) scan showing right cervical lymph nodes involved by diffuse large B-cell lymphoma.

imaging technology have improved detection of lymphoma, and provide prognostic information and response to therapy. Imaging studies for the initial evaluation of patients with NHL includes CT of the abdomen and pelvis and chest radiography. CT of the chest is frequently done and is mandatory if abnormalities are seen on the chest radiograph. A neck CT is commonly performed if lymph nodes are palpated in that region or related symptoms are noted. Additional imaging techniques used include fluorodeoxyglucose positron emission tomography (FDG-PET) scanning (Fig. 8-14) (75). FDG-PET imaging complements CT scanning, and multiple studies have found that its addition leads to not only changes in stage assignment, but also frequent alteration in patient management (76-79). FDG-PET adds additional information by detecting disease in nonenlarged lymph nodes and in extranodal sites (Fig. 8-15). Recently, the International Working Group recommended the routine use of FDG-PET as part of the pretreatment workup for patients entering clinical trials with DLBCL and HL (80).

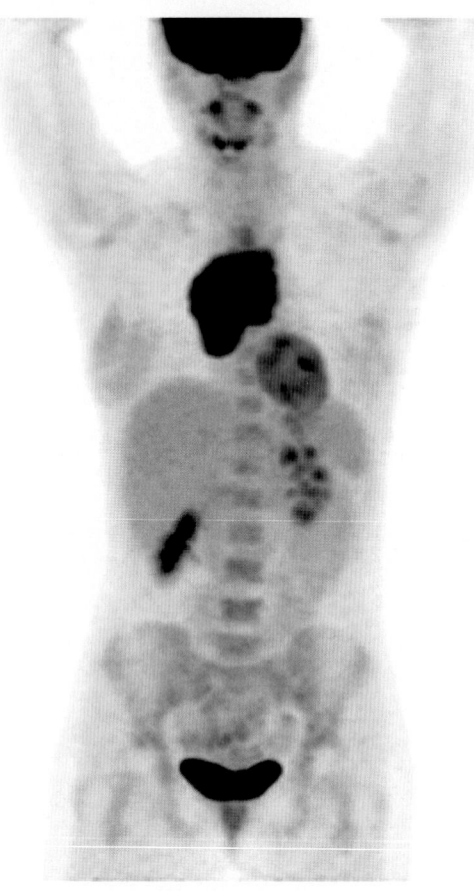

FIGURE 8-15. Extranodal lymphoma on FDG-PET/CT. The patient presented with mediastinal lymphoma; this is easily seen on maximum intensity projection (MIP) image from FDG-PET/CT. However, an additional focus is present in the right kidney: although not confirmed by biopsy, the renal lesion disappeared after chemotherapy and the stage was changed from stage I to stage IV.

Unlike CT scanning, which relies entirely on anatomic changes to detect disease, the FDG-PET is functional in nature. FDG uptake has been shown to correlate with increasing aggressiveness of NHL and the presence of large cell histology (81). Radiologic experience in the use of this technique is critical, as several other conditions can cause FDG uptake, including inflammation and infection. Pretreatment scans should be performed to ensure the usefulness of the scan, with posttreatment scanning to detect viable tumor in treated masses that require therapy.

There are several limitations to the use of FDG-PET or FDG-PET/CT alone for staging evaluation. Combined PET/CT scanners are most common, but some centers may still use PET-only machines, and even a few places still use coincidence detection on a gamma camera instead of a dedicated PET machine. This can lead to dramatic variations in the quality of the study. There is also wide variation in image reconstruction technique and in the use of oral and intravenous contrast when CT is performed as part of the FDG-PET study. There is also considerable variation in physiologic activity on FDG-PET. Variable activity can be seen in the oropharynx, heart, and bowel, and reactive lymph nodes are commonly seen in many regions. Familiarity with normal variants in uptake in with routes of tumor spread is often helpful in interpreting FDG-PET and FDG-PET/CT, and there is a wide range of experience and training as more and more radiologists and nuclear medicine physicians start to read FDG-PET. As FDG-PET continues to expand in its use, the level of expertise will continue to rise, and greater standardization in technique will be established. For now, it should not be considered a replacement for evaluation with contrast enhanced CT.

Uptake of FDG is also not specific to tumors, and infection and inflammatory processes are common false-positive findings on PET, so an unexpected FDG-avid lesion that will result in significant change in management may be confirmed before acting upon it. This will be discussed further later. In general, aggressive lymphomas are usually positive on FDG-PET, particularly when they present as a mass lesion. False-negative results are common with a low concentration of tumor cells, such as in PEL, or with low-volume disease, for example, with leptomeningeal or cutaneous involvement. The presence of high normal background activity in an organ, for example, in the kidneys or testes, may also make it difficult to identify abnormal FDG sites in that region. Although there is usually high normal metabolic activity within the brain, CNS lymphomas are often positive on FDG-PET scans, showing greater metabolic activity than the adjacent brain.

Bone Marrow Evaluation

Bone marrow aspiration and biopsy should always be performed as part of the initial evaluation of patients, as involvement suggests widespread disease (stage IV) that affects treatment and prognosis. Bilateral iliac crest biopsy is preferred, as studies have shown better detection of involvement than with unilateral biopsy (82,83). Although several studies found high accuracy of FDG-PET for predicting bone marrow involvement (84,85), a meta-analysis in 2005 concluded that although good, the performance of FDG-PET in detecting marrow involvement was not sufficient to replace bone marrow aspiration and biopsy (86). Of note, the pattern of uptake within the marrow spaces on FDG-PET is important, as a diffuse pattern is commonly seen with marrow activation (eg, with underlying anemia or

A

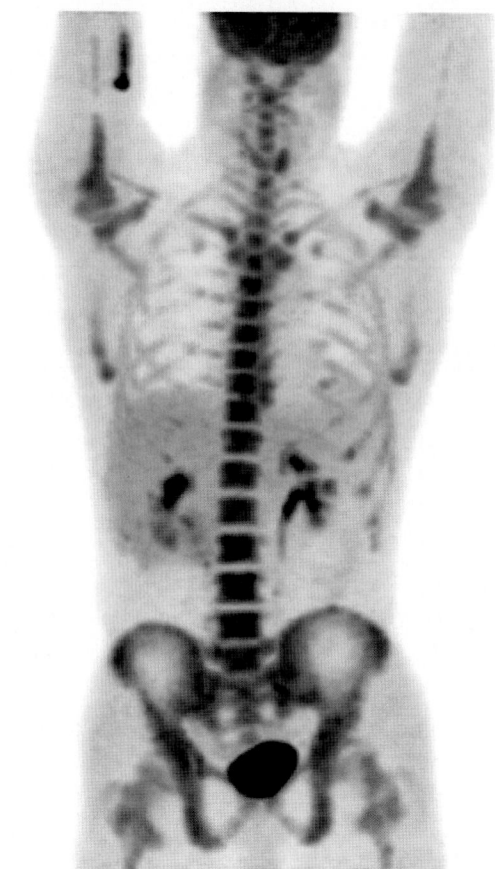

B

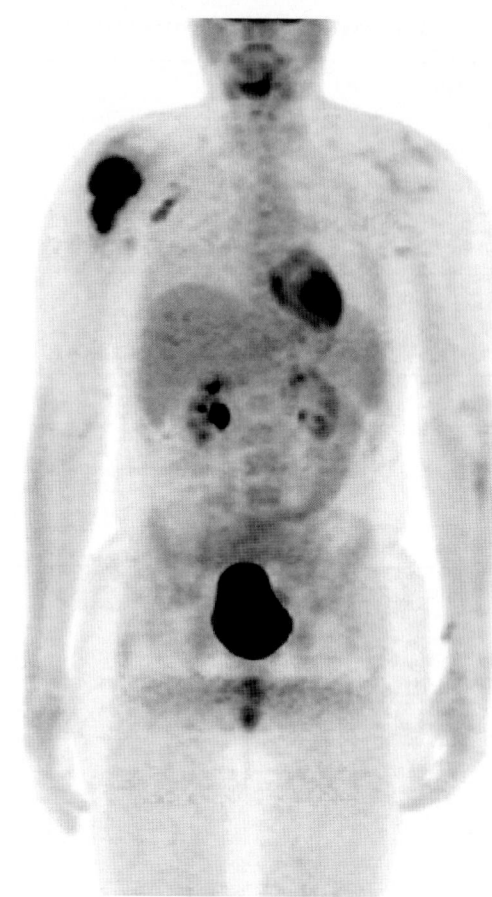

FIGURE 8-16. Bone and bone marrow uptake on FDG-PET/CT. **A.** Typical pattern of marrow activation, commonly seen after chemotherapy or with growth factor treatment. This is diffuse but homogenous. In contrast (**B**), another patient has negative bilateral iliac crest biopsies, but had focal activity in a destructive lesion involving the right humerus. Directed biopsy of this site was positive for bone involvement.

infection, or after chemotherapy or growth factor treatment), and caution should be taken in interpreting this as diffuse bone marrow involvement by tumor. In contrast, focal or nodular uptake within osseous structures is suspicious (Fig. 8-16).

■ PROGNOSTIC FACTORS

PRETREATMENT

Prognostic factors in patients with aggressive NHL can be broadly grouped into pretreatment (tumor-related) and treatment-related characteristics. Tumor-related genetic characteristics of importance in aggressive and highly aggressive lymphomas, as noted in the clinicopathologic descriptions of the various subtypes, include germinal (GCB) or non-GCB origin genetic profile, the "double-hit" genetic changes of c-myc and bcl-2

translocations. Other tumor-related characteristics reported to be of prognostic value include a complex karyotype shown by conventional cytogenetics, high proliferation rate (high Ki-67 expression), as well as BCL-2 and BCL-6 expression shown by immunohistochemical staining (23). The negative effect in prognostic of DLBCL of non GCB origin, and other markers, maybe ameliorated with the use of rituximab in the frontline combination chemotherapy treatments.

High serum LDH level is a measure of cell turnover and tumor bulk and is associated with a lower probability of complete remission and poorer long-term survival in patients with aggressive NHL. Other pretreatment prognostic factors include serum β₂-microglobulin level, stage, number of disease sites, bulky disease, presence of bone marrow involvement, poor performance status, and age (87-89). Of these pretreatment factors, age appears to be the most important, with patients over the

| TABLE 8-3 | INTERNATIONAL PROGNOSTIC INDEX WITH AGE-ADJUSTED INDEX |

FACTORS

Age	≤60 versus >60
Serum LDH	Normal versus high
Performance status	0 or 1 versus 2-4
Extranodal disease	≤1 or less versus >1
Stage	I or II versus III or IV

INTERNATIONAL INDEX

GROUP	RISK FACTORS	RELAPSE-FREE SURVIVAL		SURVIVAL	
		2 Years (%)	*5 Years (%)*	*2 Years (%)*	*5 Years (%)*
All ages	0-1	79	70	84	73
	2	66	50	66	51
	3	59	49	54	43
	4-5	52	40	34	26
Age adjusted ≤60	0	88	86	90	83
	1	74	66	79	69
	2	62	53	59	46
	3	61	58	37	32
Age adjusted >60	0	75	46	80	56
	1	64	45	68	44
	2	60	41	48	37
	3	47	37	31	21

age of 60 having lower response rates and a higher rate of relapse (90).

Currently, the most commonly used system to provide pretreatment prognostic information in patients with aggressive NHL is the IPI (Table 8-3). In 1993, the International NHL Prognostic Factors Project reported the results of a 16-center study in Canada, the United States, and Europe in which a series of clinical features were used to stratify patients into survival groups (87). A cohort of 2031 patients treated with doxorubicin-containing regimens was analyzed for the presence of factors that independently predicted survival. The most commonly used doxorubicin-based regimen was CHOP (cyclophosphamide, doxorubicin, vincristine, and prednisone) (Table 8-4). Significant prognostic factors were serum LDH (abnormal versus normal), age (≤60 versus >60), number of extranodal sites (<2 versus >2), performance status (ECOG 0-1 versus 2-4), and stage (I and II versus III and IV). Each of the five factors had an equal impact on survival. Risk groups identified were low (0-1 factor), low/intermediate (2 factors), high/intermediate (3 factors), and high (4-5 factors), with 5-year survival rates of 73, 51, 43, and 26%, respectively (87). Stage, serum LDH level, and performance status were independent predictive prognostic factors in a

simplified subanalysis of 1274 subjects ≤60 years of age in the same study. In this subgroup, the 5-year survival rate was 83% for 0 risk factors, 69% for 1 risk factor, and 46% for 2 risk factors, and 32% for 3 risk factors. In patients over 60 years of age, the 5-year survival rates were 56, 44, 37, and 21%, respectively. This further points out the prognostic significance of age on the survival of patients with aggressive NHL.

The IPI has been broadly applied as the standard for prognosis in patients with aggressive and highly aggressive NHL, although corrections or changes to the IPI have been proposed for both early stage presentations of DLBCL (modified IPI), and, most recently, with the addition of rituximab to the frontline treatment of DLBCL, Sehn et al. proposed a new revised-IPI (RIPI) in patients treated with R-CHOP. In this proposal, there are only three groups, low-risk with 0 risk factors, intermediate group with 1 and 2, and high-risk with 3 or more, for a 4-year progression-free survival (PFS) of 94, 80, and 53%, respectively (91).

Prognostic Factors in MCL

The same prognostic factors in the IPI for aggressive lymphomas are of utility in MCL. Other adverse prognostic

TABLE 8-4 | MOST COMMONLY USED CHEMOTHERAPEUTIC REGIMENS IN DIFFUSE LARGE B-CELL LYMPHOMAS

Regimen	Dose/Route	Days	Interval
FRONTLINE			
R-CHOP			
Cyclophosphamide	750 mg/m^2 IV	1	21 days
Doxorubicin	50 mg/m^2 IV	1	
Prednisone	100 mg PO	1-5	
Vincristine	1.4 mg/m^2 IV	1	
Rituximab	375 mg/m^2 IV	1	
SALVAGE (first salvage, preautologous SCT)			
RICE			
Rituximab	375 mg/m^2 IV	1	14-21 days
Ifosfamide	5 g/m^2 IV CI	2	
Mesna concurrent with Ifosfamide	5 g/m^2 IVCI 2 over 24 h, then 2 g/m^2 over 12 h	2-3	
Carboplatin*	Maximum 800 mg	2	
Etoposide	100 mg/m^2 IV	2-4	
GCSF	5 mcg/kg/day SC	7-14	

*Calculate Carboplatin dose using Calvert equation: AUC = 5 g/mL/min; dose = 5 × [25+Cl$_{cr}$] capped at 800 mg.

factors include p53 mutations or deletion, elevated Ki-67, and blastic histology. Most recently, a prognostic model in new patients with MCL treated with chemotherapy followed by high-dose chemotherapy followed by autologous stem cell transplant (MIPI) was proposed using age, performance status, LDH, and leucocyte count. Patients were divided in low, intermediate, and high risk, for a overall survival not reached, 51 months, and 29 months, respectively (92). In patients receiving R-HCVAD alternating with rituximab-methotrexate and cytarabine, this model could not be reproduced (93). However, it was reproducible in patients treated with CHOP-rituximab-like regimens consolidated with high-dose chemotherapy with stem cell transplant (94).

Prognostic Factors in Primary CNS Lymphoma

Age and LDH are important prognostic factors in patients with HIV-negative primary CNS lymphoma. Probably the most important one is performance status at the time of treatment. Elevated LDH, CSF protein, and tumor mass location(s) are also contributors to prognosis (95). Many patients can improve their condition by using steroids, and thus be candidates to high-dose methotrexate-containing regimens, which are potentially curative, instead of receiving palliative radiation therapy.

POSTTREATMENT

An important posttreatment prognostic indicator is tumor response to induction chemotherapy. In patients with aggressive and highly aggressive NHL, dramatic response to induction with early complete remission (by the third cycle of therapy) is associated with a superior outcome (96). Time to complete remission is the most reliable predictor of overall survival. FDG-PET has been found to be highly sensitive for the detection of aggressive NHL in posttreatment residual masses (76,77). Patients who fail to achieve at least a good partial response to induction chemotherapy have primary refractory disease and a very short survival despite aggressive efforts. Another important indicator of prognosis is the duration of remission obtained after induction chemotherapy, as patients with relapses occurring at <1 year have a worse outcome.

■ APPROACH TO THERAPY

EARLY-STAGE AGGRESSIVE NHL

Early-stage (localized) aggressive NHL (stages I/Ie and II/IIe) was historically treated with radiation therapy (RT) alone, and the results were highly variable (97,98). The 5-year survival with involved-field RT for stage I/II disease was approximately 50%. Patients with bulky disease (>5 cm) suffered a higher relapse rate. Although many studies were subsequently undertaken to improve the results by adjusting dosages and field coverage, it was the addition of combination chemotherapy to RT regimens that improved outcome most dramatically. To date, four randomized trials were conducted in early-stage aggressive NHL, all of them were before the era of anti-CD 20 rituximab therapy being incorporated in CHOP chemotherapy. The first of the four is a study by the Southwest Oncology Group (SWOG), eight cycles of CHOP was compared to three cycles of CHOP followed by involved-field RT (40-55 Gy) in limited-stage DLCBL. The combined modality arm achieved an overall survival of 82%, versus 72% for the CHOP arm alone (99). The Eastern Cooperative Oncology Group (ECOG) randomized patients with bulky stage I/Ie or II/IIe disease to eight cycles of CHOP with or without involved-field RT (100). Patients achieving a complete remission were randomized to involved-field RT (30 Gy) or no further therapy. Patients achieving partial remission received involved-field RT at a higher dose (40 Gy). Disease-free survival at 5 years was higher in patients who received radiation (73% versus 58%) after achieving complete remission. In addition, 28% of patients who received 40 Gy involved-field radiation therapy after partial remission then attained complete remission (100). The GELA conducted a similar study comparing aggressive chemotherapy (dose-intensified doxorubicin, cyclophosphamide, vindesine, bleomycin, and prednisone [ACVBP]) alone versus abbreviated chemotherapy (three cycles of CHOP) followed by involved-field radiation therapy for stage I or II mostly low-risk aggressive lymphoma. All patients in this study were younger than 60 years. Both the 5-year event-free (82%) and overall survival (90%) rates were significantly better in the chemotherapy group than in the combined modality group (74 and 81%, respectively). Although the addition of radiation therapy reduced relapses at the initial disease sites, this was not enough to overcome the excessive number of relapses in the abbreviated chemotherapy group (101). The MD Anderson approach to the treatment of DLBCL is shown in Fig. 8-17.

Despite these results indicating the inability of abbreviated chemotherapy plus radiation to prevent out-of-field relapses, the GELA group conducted another trial GELA LNH 93-4 comparing CHOP with CHOP plus involved-field radiation therapy to 40 Gy, this time for patients older than 60 years (102). The use of ACVBP had been dropped by the time this trial was undertaken because of excessive toxicity. At a median follow-up time of 7 years, no significant differences were evident in 5-year event-free survival rates (61% for chemotherapy alone versus 64% for chemoradiation) or overall survival rates (72% versus 68%, respectively). The results in the chemotherapy-only group were similar to those results from the group that received eight cycles of CHOP in the SWOG trial discussed in the previous paragraph. However, because

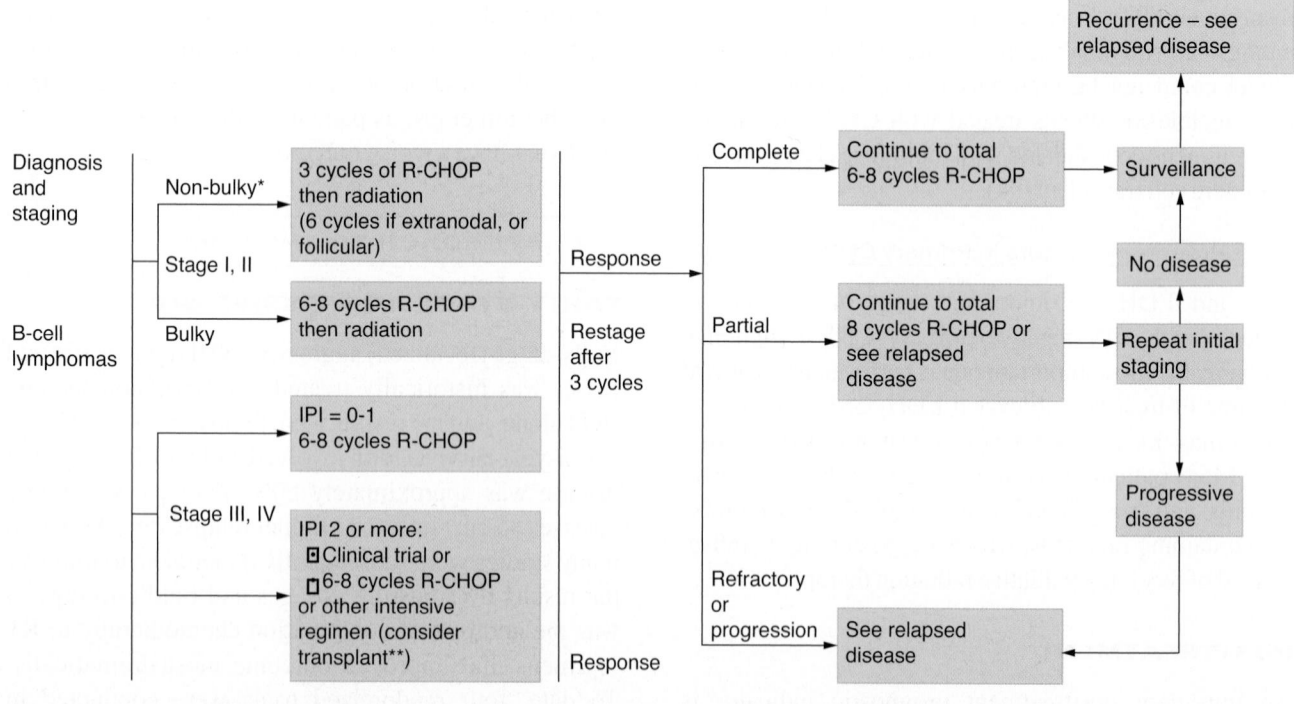

FIGURE 8-17. Algorithm for treatment of DLBCL. *Bulky disease is >5 cm by definition at MD Anderson Cancer Center; **Especially if bone marrow disease is present.

relapses could appear beyond 5 years, another 5 to 10 years should be allowed to elapse before any approach is widely adopted. Localized MCL in general has been treated in the same way as extensive disease, but the use of radiation therapy with or without chemotherapy has been reported by investigators in British Columbia to be an effective treatment as well (103).

ADVANCED-STAGE AGGRESSIVE NHL

Initial cures using chemotherapy for patients with large cell lymphoma were reported in the early to mid-1970s (104,105). The SWOG initially reported that CHOP induced complete response in 50% of patients, with long-term disease-free survival in 35%. CHOP has since represented the standard of care in the treatment of aggressive NHL despite intensive research into newer regimens. Variations of CHOP have included different prednisone schedules and doses, day 1 and day 8 vincristine, and hyperfractionated cyclophosphamide. Subsequent trials of combination chemotherapy over the last 25 years can be thought of as "generations" (105-110). The first generation included CHOP, CHOP + procarbazine (C-MOPP), CHOP + bleomycin (BACOP), and COMLA (cyclophosphamide, vincristine, methotrexate, leucovorin, and cytosine arabinoside), but follow-up studies have shown that these regimens are equivalent or inferior to CHOP.

Second and third generation more intensive chemotherapy combinations include M-BACOD (methotrexate, bleomycin, doxorubicin, cyclophosphamide, etoposide, and leucovorin), BACOD, ProMACE-MOPP (addition of etoposide), ProMACE-CytaBOM (addition of cytosine arabinoside), and MACOP-B. These regimens showed an increased rate of complete remission of nearly 80% in early studies with greater than 60% long-term disease-free survival. The SWOG undertook a landmark phase III trial comparing CHOP, MACOP-B, M-BACOD, and ProMACE-CytaBOM, which showed that, despite early reports of improved response, overall survival at 3 years varied from 50 to 54%, with disease-free survival ranging from 41 to 46% (111). There was no apparent advantage to increased intensity of therapy. Subsequent studies have shown that regimens with increased intensity add toxicity but not survival benefit. Another finding noted in the 1980s was that inclusion of an anthracycline in the chemotherapy regimen was important to long-term disease-free survival. Other approaches have included alternating regimens, higher-dose therapy, and dose-dense therapy. The first two have not been shown to have a survival benefit, whereas the third is still under scrutiny.

Escalated doses of CHOP were studied by several groups in 2002 (112,113). Their work has shown that dose intensification can be achieved with growth factor support. An Italian study (112) reported in 2002 showed that intensification to a "maximum tolerated dose" was achievable with a complete response rate of 74% in all risk groups and failure-free progression of 58% at 12 months in IPI risk categories 3 and 4. This represents an improvement over rates with standard CHOP regimens, but no head-to-head of trial of CHOP versus dose-escalated CHOP with mature data was published. Difficulties with the dose-escalated CHOP regimens are a high rate of grade 3 to 4 neutropenia and the necessity for blood product support in many cases (112,113). As a result of toxicity, dose escalation of CHOP actually results in dose reduction in some patients.

Dose-dense therapy was reported to be feasible in 2003 by the German High-Grade NHL Study Group (DSHNHL) (114). Three variants of CHOP-like therapy were evaluated, including CHOP-14, CHOEP-14 (addition of etoposide 100 mg/m^2 on days 1-3), and CHOP-21, each with hematopoietic growth factor support. An interim analysis of 959 patients showed that adherence to the dose-dense regimens was excellent, although dose reductions were more frequently required for the addition of etoposide. Recently more mature data were reported by the DSHNHL for both elderly and younger patients (115,116). To evaluate the therapies in younger patients, 710 patients with good-prognosis aggressive NHL aged 18 to 60 years were randomized to receive six cycles of CHOP-21, CHOP-14, CHOEP-21, or CHOEP-14. Patients in the 2-weekly regimens received granulocyte colony-stimulating factor (G-CSF) from day 4. Initial sites of bulky or extranodal disease were treated with 36 Gy of radiation. Patients receiving CHOEP achieved a higher complete response rate (87.6 versus 79.4%) and 5-year event-free survival (69.2 versus 57.6%) than patients treated with CHOP. Dose density (the 2-week regimens) improved overall survival in a multivariate analysis. Patients receiving CHOEP had a higher rate of myelosuppression, but generally the regimen was well tolerated.

While the German group was exploring dose density, the GELA reported their results of trial LNH98-5 in which 399 DLBCL were randomized to receive rituximab with CHOP every 21 days, versus standard CHOP alone for a total of eight cycles. Patients with DLBCL stage II to IV that were between 60 and 80 years old were eligible for this trial. No radiation therapy or intrathecal chemotherapy was administered. The complete responses (76 versus 63%), and the 5-years PFS, DFS, and overall survival, was better in the rituximab arm (117).

Commentary: On the Role of Radiation Therapy in Aggressive B-Cell Lymphomas

We can draw several conclusions from the trials for limited stage (I/II) DLBCL, which are noted in this chapter. First, combined modality therapy should be still considered the standard of care for early-stage diffuse large B-cell lymphoma. Second, abbreviated chemotherapy should be used in highly selected patients with low-risk disease, because of the pattern of relapse outside the field of radiation seen in the above trials. Third, randomized trials comparing rituximab plus CHOP with and without radiation should be conducted to address the two most pressing unresolved issues: the benefit of rituximab and the optimal number of chemotherapy cycles. It should also be noted that patients with stage II bulky tumor masses have generally not fared well, or have been excluded, from these trials.

We have conducted at MDACC a retrospective study on 469 patients with DLBCL lymphoma, stage I-IV in the era of treatment with Rituximab(1). Multivariate analysis showed that the addition of radiation therapy ($p < 0.0001$), response to therapy ($p = 0.001$) and the use of 6-8 cycles of R-CHOP ($p < 0.001$) influenced the overall survival (OS) and progression-free survival (PFS). Matched-pair analysis of patients who received 6-8 cycles of R-CHOP indicated that radiation improved OS (hazard ratio = 0.52 for stages I,II and 0.29 for stages III,IV) as well as PFS (HR = 0.45 for stages I,II, and 0.24 for stages III/IV). Although it is a retrospective study, it does show that the addition of Rituximab does not substitute for radiation.

In a retrospective study from MD Anderson Cancer Center, we analyzed outcomes of patients with aggressive non-Hodgkin lymphomas (NHL) of any stage at diagnosis, who achieved a partial or confirmed remission to CHOP-based chemotherapy, who were treated with salvage involved-field radiation therapy (RT) or salvage chemotherapy alone. The median number of cycles of CHOP was six. Local control (86 versus 53%) and progression-free survival (67 versus 8%) were significantly better in patients receiving salvage radiotherapy (2). This adds to the body of evidence on the benefit of a combined modality approach, although it was preceding the use of rituximab in the frontline treatment.

Whether RT has a role in the treatment of bulky stage III or IV large B-cell lymphoma remains a matter of debate, with some groups seeing no benefit (3-5). Others, however, suggest that delivery of involved-field radiation to lymphomas measuring 4 cm or more before induction chemotherapy may improve disease-free and overall survival rates (6-8). As noted, Phan, et al. (1) confirmed the benefit of radiation in stages III/IV in terms of OS and PFS. However, most if not all of these studies were done retrospectively; the only prospective randomized study conducted to date demonstrated that RT could benefit those patients with bulky (defined as larger than 10 cm) stage IV diffuse large B-cell lymphoma. In that study, patients who experienced a complete response to anthracycline-based chemotherapy were randomly assigned to receive or not receive involved-field RT (40-50 Gy) to initially bulky sites of disease. The addition of RT produced significant improvements in both disease-free survival rates (5-year rates 72 versus 35%, $p < .01$) and overall survival rates (5-year rates 81 vs. 55%, $p < .01$) (9). In conclusion, modern radiation therapy has improved the therapeutic ratio by better targeting the disease with fewer side effects. The use of RT in aggressive lymphoma, based on the available data, is reasonable and it is associated with an improvement in the outcome of patients with aggressive lymphoma in all stages.

Bouthaina S. Dabaja

References

1. Phan J, Mazloom A, Medeiros LJ, et al. Benefit of Consolidative Radiation Therapy in Patients With Diffuse Large B-Cell Lymphoma Treated With R-CHOP Chemotherapy. Journal of Clinical Oncology 2010, 28(27);4170-4176.
2. Wilder RB, Rodriguez MA, Tucker SL, et al. Radiation therapy after a partial response to CHOP chemotherapy for aggressive lymphomas. *Int J Radiat Oncol Biol Phys* 2001; 50:743-749.
3. Danieu L, Wong G, Koziner B, et al. Predictive model for prognosis in advanced diffuse histiocytic lymphoma. *Cancer Res* 1986;46:5372-5379.
4. Shipp MA, Klatt MM, Yeap B, et al. Patterns of relapse in large-cell lymphoma patients with bulk disease: Implications for the use of adjuvant radiation therapy. *J Clin Oncol* 1989; 7:613-618.
5. Coiffier B. Treatment of aggressive non-Hodgkin's lymphoma. *Semin Oncol* 1999;26:12-20.
6. Schlembach PJ, Wilder RB, Tucker SL, et al. Impact of involved field radiotherapy after CHOP-based chemotherapy on stage III-IV, intermediate grade and large-cell immunoblastic lymphomas. *Int J Radiat Oncol Biol Phys* 2000;48:1107-1110.
7. Crowther D. New approaches to the management of patients with non-Hodgkin's lymphoma of high-grade pathology. First Gordon Hamilton-Fairley memorial lecture. *Br J Cancer* 1981; 43:417-435.
8. Ferreri AJ, Dell'Oro S, Reni M, et al. Consolidation radiotherapy to bulky or semibulky lesions in the management of stage III-IV diffuse large B cell lymphomas. *Oncology* 2000; 58:219-226.
9. Avilés A, Delgado S, Nambo MJ, et al. Adjuvant radiotherapy to sites of previous bulky disease in patients stage IV diffuse large cell lymphoma. *Int J Radiat Oncol Biol Phys* 1994;30:799-803.

Based on the GELA LNH98-5 results and their own data, the DSHNHL designed a four arms randomized study in patients older than 60 years (RICOVER-60). Comparison of CHOP-14 with or without rituximab for six cycles versus CHOP-14 for eight cycles with or without rituximab (in the six cycles R-CHOP arm, the patients received a total of eight doses of rituximab). The CHOP alone group was inferior, and six cycles of R-CHOP + 2 rituximab, was as good as eight cycles of R-CHOP (118). Posterior to this study, preliminary results of two other studies addressing the question of R-CHOP every 21 days versus every 14 days in DLBCL, one from UK and the other from the GELA, have not shown any benefit in the dose-dense group compared to standard R-CHOP every 21 days. Final results, however, are pending.

Finally, another multicenter randomized study evaluated the addition of rituximab to standard chemotherapy in patients with DLBCL with IPI 0-1 (MINT Trial). This study demonstrated improvement in 3-year event-free-survival (79 versus 59%, $p < .0001$), and 3-year OS (93 versus 84%, $p = .0001$) (119).

SPECIAL TYPES AND SITUATIONS IN DLBCL

Primary CNS and Occular Lymphoma

The treatment of patients with primary CNS lymphoma is limited to drugs that can cross the blood–brain barrier. Standard chemotherapies such as rituximab-CHOP do not cross to the brain and they have limited activity in this condition. The initial evaluation must include slit lamp evaluation of the eyes, and MRI of the brain, in addition to the standard studies for any other lymphoma, to rule out concomitant systemic disease. The most common histology in primary CNS lymphoma is DLBCL, and the treatment's most important drug is high-dose methotrexate, in general at doses higher than 3.0 g/m^2. Investigators at Memorial Sloan Kettering Cancer Center have reported good results with the combination of chemoimmunotherapy using rituximab, high-dose methotrexate, procarbazine, and vincristine. The patients received consolidation with low-dose radiation therapy, if in complete remission. The low dose of radiation decreased the long-term neurotoxicity seen in prior studies (120,121). After the radiation therapy, the patients received consolidation with high-dose cytarabine. The use of intrathecal chemotherapy is controversial in patients with no evidence of leptomeningeal involvement, but it is used in patients with CSF disease. Radiation fields should include the eyes if those are thought to be involved.

Testicular Lymphomas

Most patients with testicular lymphoma involvement have DLBCL, but other histologies can be seen. Testicular lymphomas often have a worse prognosis compared to other DLBCL without testicular involvement. The treatment in this group of patients should include prophylaxis of CNS relapses with intrathecal chemotherapy, and radiation to the contralateral testicle to decrease the risk for localized relapses.

Intravascular Lymphomas

These lymphomas are traditionally considered to have poor prognosis. They have better outcomes with the addition of rituximab to the standard chemotherapy regimen. They have a high incidence of CNS relapse, but there are no standard CNS prophylaxis recommendations in this group of patients (122-124).

Primary Mediastinal Lymphomas

This condition can present with a rapid growing mediastinal mass causing difficulty breathing, as well as pleural and/or pericardial effusions, or superior vena cava syndrome. When possible, chemotherapy should start immediately upon diagnosis. This tumor is usually CD20+, and although there are many publications using CHOP and MACOP-B, recently the addition of rituximab to the frontline chemotherapy has become standard of care. Regimens using high-dose alkylating agents are reported (125,126). Consolidation after chemotherapy with radiation therapy is a common practice, but the benefit of this modality of treatment is unclear, and should be weighed individually against long-term toxicities, especially cardiac long-term effects and risk for secondary malignancies.

TREATMENT OF ADVANCED MANTLE CELL LYMPHOMA

MCL is considered a special case because of its recognized aggressiveness and frequent refractory behavior (Fig. 8-18). In many studies of patients with MCL, the disease has been shown to be the NHL type with the poorest prognosis overall, with complete and partial response rates of 29 and 45%, respectively, when treated with a CHOP-like regimen. Investigators at MDACC have investigated hyper-CVAD, a regimen of fractionated cyclophosphamide and continuous infusion doxorubicin, vincristine, and dexamethasone alternating with methotrexate and cytosine arabinoside, which

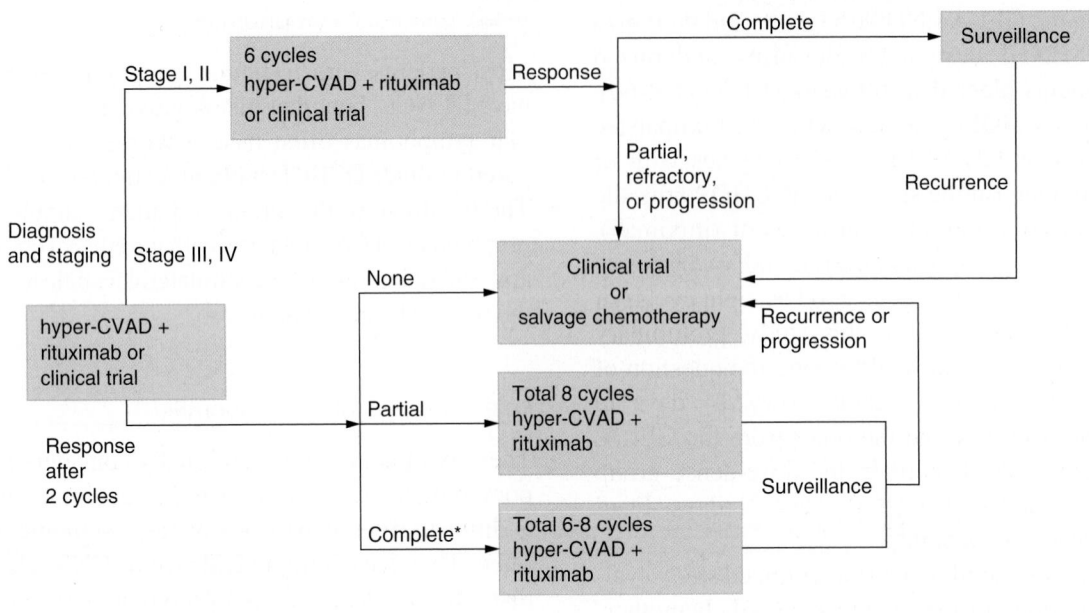

FIGURE 8-18. Algorithm for treatment of mantle cell lymphoma. *Confirm complete response by BM biopsies, upper endoscopy, and colonoscopy (with biopsies).

TABLE 8-5	R-HCVAD REGIMEN USED IN MANTLE CELL LYMPHOMA AND HIGHLY AGGRESSIVE LYMPHOMAS*		
Regimen	*Dose/Route*	*Days*	*Interval*
Hyper-CVAD/Methotrexate/ Ara-C			21-28 days
Cycles 1,3,5,7			
Rituxan	375 mg/m² IV by slow infusion	1	
Cyclophosphamide	300 mg/m²/dose over 3 h q 12 h × 6 doses	1-3	
Mesna	600 mg/m²/day CIV over 24 h daily	1-3	
	(Start 1 h prior to cyclophosphamide and complete by 12 h after last dose of cyclophosphamide)		
Doxorubicin	25 mg/m²/day CIV over 24 h daily	4-5	
	(Begin at 12 h after last dose of cyclophosphamide)		
Vincristine	1.4 mg/m² IV (max 2 mg)	4 and 11	
	(Give 12 h after last dose of cyclophosphamide and on day 11)		
Dexamethasone	40 mg PO daily	1-4 and 11-14	
Cycles 2, 4, 6, 8			
Methotrexate	200 mg/m² IV over 2 h then 800 mg/m² IV over 22 h	1	
Solumedrol	50 mg IV q 12 h × 6 doses	1-3	
Ara-C	3 g/m² IV over 2 h every 12 h × 4 doses	2-3	
Leucovorin	50 mg IV followed by 15 mg IV q 6 h × 8 doses		
	(Start 12 h after completion of methotrexate)		
Intrathecal therapy†			
Ara-C	100 mg	2	
Methotrexate	12 mg (6 mg if Ommaya reservoir)	7	

*Dose reductions for renal insufficiency, age, and previous toxicity are required. Intrathecal chemotherapy is more frequent for proven CNS disease.
†Mantle cell lymphoma is not typically treated with intrathecal therapy.

had previously been used for patients with acute lymphoblastic leukemia (Table 8-5) (127,128). In a study published in 2000, a total of 45 patients (25 untreated, 20 previously treated) were treated with the hyper-CVAD/methotrexate/cytosine arabinoside regimen with complete and partial remissions of 38 and 55%, respectively, after four cycles. Subsequently, 26 of these patients received autologous ($n = 18$) or allogeneic ($n = 8$) transplants. Overall survival at 3 years in previously untreated patients was 92%, with event-free survival of 72%—much superior to the rates for CHOP without transplantation (127). Another study by Romaguera et al. reported on the same regimen in untreated, elderly MCL patients not receiving transplants. Complete and partial remission rates were 68 and 34%, respectively (128). These results suggest that intensification of chemotherapeutic regimens may be beneficial for patients with some types of aggressive NHL. At MD Anderson Cancer Center, Romaguera et al. reported a high ORR and complete responses adding rituximab to standard HCVAD alternating with methotrexate-cytarabine. Responses in more than 90% were obtained, with 50% of the patients remaining failure-free more than 7 years in patients younger than 65 years. In the older group, the median FFS was of 3 years (129,130). Because the most toxic portion of this treatment is the high-dose methotrexate-cytarabine cycle, Kahl et al. used a modified R-HCVAD with maintenance rituximab for 2 years, obtaining a 77% ORR, a CR of 64%, and a median PFS of 37 months. This regimen did not add transplant (131). Many other groups have incorporated a consolidation with autologous stem cell transplant, after induction chemotherapy with various regimens with remarkable results (132,133). Bendamustine with rituximab has been reported to have durable responses in patients with MCL, with no cardiac toxicity. Hence, this could be an option for patients with underlying heart problems or elderly patients who are not candidates for aggressive therapies (134).

SPECIAL CONSIDERATIONS

Those patients with double hit lymphomas, that is simultaneous mutations for BCL-2 and c-myc, have a very poor outcome even with aggressive treatments. Consolidation with transplant in first response should be considered, even though transplant outcomes data is lacking due to the rarity of this condition. DLBCL with mutations of c-myc have poor results with standard R-CHOP, and treatment regimens for Burkitt should be considered (135-137).

CNS prophylaxis remains controversial. However, it is recommended in patients with high-grade lymphomas or Burkitt, bone marrow involvement with DLBCL, two or more extranodal sites, testicular involvement, and disease involvement in areas close to the CNS.

Patients with HIV-associated lymphomas, should be treated when possible. Standard treatments with rituximab containing regimens such as R-CHOP, dose-adjusted R-EPOCH, continuous infusional CDE, reported acceptable results, especially in the era of the HAART. It is important to notice, however, that when EPOCH-based treatments are used, it is recommended that HAART be stopped while on treatment. Rituximab must be used with caution in patients with low CD4 counts. Intrathecal chemoprophylaxis should be used in patients with stage IV disease, high-grade lymphomas, and in those patients with EBV-positive tumors.

■ REFRACTORY OR RELAPSED AGGRESSIVE NHL

TREATMENT OF RECURRENT/REFRACTORY DLBCL

Approximately 10% of patients treated for aggressive NHL fail to achieve a complete remission after induction therapy; their disease is termed *primary refractory* (Fig. 8-19). Although some of these patients are sensitive to a second chemotherapy regimen and patients with recurrent disease frequently still have chemosensitive disease, the majority of these patients relapse and have a poor prognosis. Conventional salvage therapy includes chemotherapeutic regimens containing ifosfamide, etoposide, taxanes, and platinum compounds. Among the most commonly used are DICE (dexamethasone, ifosfamide, cisplatin, and etoposide), ICE (carboplatin replacing cisplatin), MINE (mesna, ifosfamide, mitoxantrone, and etoposide), and ESHAP (etoposide, methylprednisolone, cytarabine, and cisplatin) (138-141). The salvage regimens tend to have higher toxicity and require greater support for administration, often including hospitalization.

Because of the poor prognosis in patients with relapsed disease, the purpose of many of the chemotherapy regimens offered in this clinical setting is to attain remission followed by high-dose chemotherapy with stem cell support. The Parma trial examined autologous bone marrow transplantation versus salvage chemotherapy in patients with relapsed, chemotherapy-sensitive NHL (142). Patients younger than 60 years who had attained a complete remission after frontline chemotherapy with no evidence of bone marrow or CNS disease

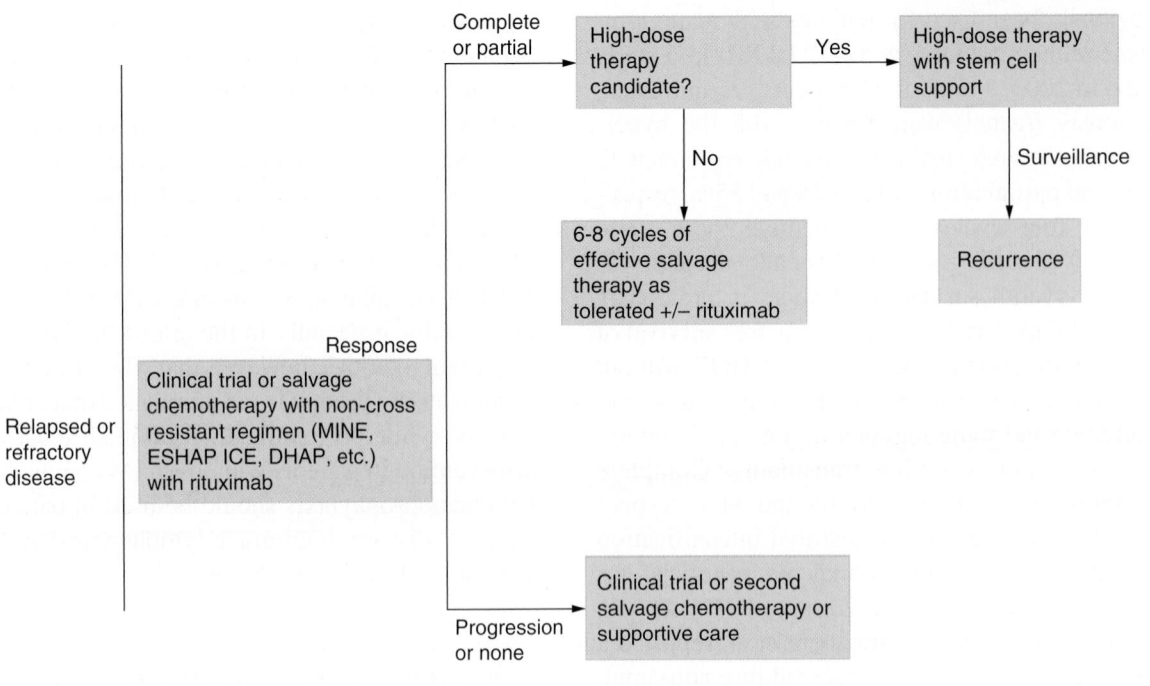

FIGURE 8-19. Algorithm for treatment of relapsed aggressive lymphomas (except high-grade or MCL).

were treated with two courses of salvage chemotherapy with DHAP (dexamethasone, high dose ara-C, and cisplatin). Those who responded were randomized to four more cycles of DHAP versus high-dose therapy with stem cell support. Event-free survival was 46% in the high-dose arm but only 12% in the conventional chemotherapy arm. This is considered strong evidence that high-dose therapy with stem cell support is the treatment of choice for patients with chemosensitive relapsed or primary refractory aggressive NHL.

Most recently, rituximab was incorporated to the salvage regimens, in an attempt to improve responses and to use it as an in vivo purging. Gisselbretch et al. reported preliminary results in a GELA study for second-line treatment for 400 recurrent/refractory CD20+ DLBCL patients who were younger than 65, and had at least a partial response to the first-line treatment. In this trial, patients were randomized to receive R-DHAP versus RICE, and if the disease responded, the patients were chemomobilized for stem cell collection, and transplanted with rituximab-BEAM. A second randomization using maintenance rituximab is part of the trial. In the preliminary report, responses were similar in both arms, in the range of 60%, failures to collect stem cells were similar and around 10%, and toxicities were similar. No difference in the PFS and OS was noted between the R-ICE and R-DHAP group. Adverse factors for outcome were IPI>1 at the time

to start the salvage therapy, prior rituximab treatment, and time to treatment failure from diagnosis <12 months (143).

Patients who are not responding to a second-line treatment should be offered palliative treatment, or investigational therapies. Patients who are responding to the second-line treatment but are unable to mobilize stem cell treatment, should be considered for alternative donor transplant. Treatment response failure beyond second relapse indicate an incurable disease. A few patients, however, can probably be rescued with salvage chemotherapy and a second stem cell transplant, often of allogeneic donor origin.

Patients who have transformed follicular lymphomas, to diffuse large B-cell lymphomas, and had prior doxorubicin-based treatment, should be treated with salvage therapy as recurrent DLBCL. Consolidation with high-dose chemotherapy and ASCT or allogeneic SCT should be considered if the patient is a candidate for such treatment.

TREATMENT OF RECURRENT MCL

The decision about what kind of salvage regimen to use in patients with recurrent MCL should be individualized, depending on their candidacy for SCT. Single agent bortezomib was approved for the treatment of recurrent MCL, based on the PINNACLE study (144). In this study,

155 patients with MCL received bortezomib 1.3 mg/m^2 on days 1, 4, 8, and 11 of a 21-day cycle, for up to 17 cycles. The overall response rate was 33% with 8% complete response rate, and the TTP was of 6.7 months (145).

At MD Anderson Cancer Center, 29 patients with recurrent MCL, were treated with R-HCVAD alternating with R-methotrexate-cytarabine. The overall response rate was 93% with 45% complete responses. The median duration of response was of 11 months. The ultimate goal in those patients who respond to salvage chemotherapy is to consolidate their response with high-dose chemotherapy followed by ASCT (most studies suggest no plateau with this treatment modality in the relapsing setting), or allogeneic transplantation including non-myeloablative regimens (136).

These patients are also candidates for new investigational agents (146). Other possible treatments including combination chemotherapy such as platinum-containing regimens, gemcitabine-containing regimens, radioimmunoisotopes, thalidomide (in combination with rituximab), lenalidomide-containing regimens are also possible alternatives.

RECURRENT PRIMARY CNS AND OCCULAR LYMPHOMA

The treatment of recurrent primary CNS lymphoma is limited because the lack of many drugs with penetration to the CNS. Retreatment with high-dose methotrexate can be attempted if there was a long duration of the first remission. Patients with prior whole brain radiation may be in high risk for methotrexate inducing encephalopathy.

Reports using temazolamide in combination with rituximab have been encouraging. Responder patients may benefit with consolidation with high-dose chemotherapy (especially with preparative regimens including thiotepa), followed by autologous stem cell transplant.

■ HIGHLY AGGRESSIVE (HIGH-GRADE) NHL

Patients with highly aggressive NHL have largely benefited from the successful application of pediatric therapy regimens to the adult population, with long-term remissions approaching 80 to 90% in some series (Fig. 8-20). The most important principle for treating patients with highly aggressive NHL is prompt systemic therapy, as these are medical emergencies. Attempts should be made to maintain dose intensity and density using supportive therapies, such as growth factor support, prophylaxis for tumor lysis syndrome, and CNS prophylaxis.

Patients with BLs should not be treated with older CHOP-like regimens because those who are so treated have poor long-term disease-free survival (147). In the past, some centers have used CNS irradiation for prophylaxis and therapy, a practice that can no longer be supported by the weight of evidence. Combined modality therapy appears to add toxicity without any proven benefit. Patients at MDACC have been treated with the hyper-CVAD/methotrexate/ara-C regimen, with intrathecal methotrexate/ara-C CNS prophylaxis with some success (148) (Table 8-5). Eight cycles are typically given and have

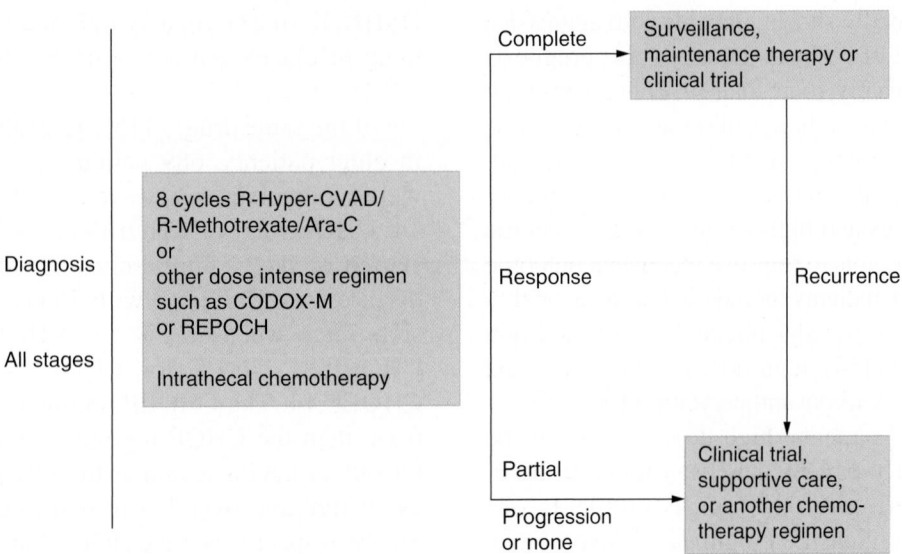

FIGURE 8-20. Algorithm for treatment of Burkitt and Burkitt-like lymphoma.

resulted in a complete remission rate of 81%, with 3-year overall survival of 49%. CNS prophylaxis is given on days 2 and 7 of each cycle and increased to twice weekly if CNS disease is actually diagnosed. The National Cancer Institute has developed an alternating regimen of cylosphosphamide, doxorubicin, vincristine, methotrexate, leucovorin, and ifosfamide, etoposide, and cytosine arabinoside (ara-C) with intrathecal ara-C and methotrexate called CODOX-M/IVAC (149). This is administered for four cycles, with CODOX-M as cycles 1 and 3 and IVAC as cycles 2 and 4. A severe neurologic syndrome can occur with this regimen, apparently related to the use of colony-stimulating factors with successive high doses of vincristine. Therefore, day 15 vincristine of the first CODOX-M cycle was eliminated. A complete remission rate of 92% was reported, with a 3-year event-free survival of 85% (149). Major toxicities were hematologic problems, mucositis, and infections. A phase II study using a slightly modified CODOX/IVAC regimen was reported in 2002, with low-risk BL patients being treated with three cycles of CODOX-M and high-risk patients receiving the full four cycles of CODOX-M/IVAC. Patients with low-risk disease had a 2-year event-free survival of 83.8%; this figure was 59.5% for patients with high-risk disease (149). Finally, at MD Anderson Cancer Center, rituximab was added to standard HCVAD alternating with methotrexate-cytarabine, (Table 8-5) resulting in disease-free survival in more than 80% of the patients. Adverse risk for those patients include elevated LDH, age, and leukemic presentation (150).

■ THERAPY IN ELDERLY PATIENTS

As has been repeatedly shown, patients with aggressive NHL over the age of 60 years have a worse prognosis (90,151). Unfortunately, more than 50% of patients with aggressive NHL are over the age of 60, and most of these patients do not experience extended long-term survival. Treatment of older patients is complicated by higher overall toxicity rates and higher rates of organ-specific damage. Some attempts to improve the dismal outcome of therapy in older patients include lower-dose weekly therapy (152,153), dose adjustment (128), the addition of immunotherapy (154), high-dose therapy (155), and the use of regimens without anthracycline (156,157).

As in younger patients, high-dose therapy in the treatment of elderly patients has been found to be of questionable benefit given the toxicity profile. In one study, ACVBP, an intensified regimen of doxorubicin, cyclophosphamide, videsine, bleomycin, prednisone, and intrathecal methotrexate induction followed by consolidation with methotrexate/leucovorin, ifosfamide, etoposide, and cytarabine, was compared to standard CHOP (155). Although overall survival at 5 years was significantly greater (46 versus 38%) in the ACVBP group, grades 3 and 4 hematologic toxicity and treatment-related deaths were higher. The increased toxicities correlated with performance status and age >65. Use of a lower-dose CHOP regimen administered at weekly intervals has been shown to lead to similar complete remission rates but inferior overall survival rates (152). Dose adjustment of CHOP chemotherapy in the elderly, although sometimes necessary because of comorbid conditions, also leads to inferior remission and overall survival (153). The hyper-CVAD regimen with the dose of cytarabine reduced to 1 g/m^2 was studied at MDACC for the treatment of elderly patients with MCL (128). Hematologic toxicity was significant, but given the poor prognosis in the elderly, use of the regimen was felt to be justified. The use of regimens without anthracycline, such as CNOP (mitroxantrone replacing doxorubicin), has been shown to be associated with decreased rates of overall survival and complete remission when compared to CHOP, but with similar rates of toxicity. In a study reported in 2003, CNOP in the elderly was found to have a similar complete remission rate but inferior overall survival when compared to CHOP (157). Coiffier et al., in a study of 399 patients, reported that the addition of rituximab to CHOP in the treatment of elderly patients with DLCBL significantly increased event-free and overall survival without an increase in clinically relevant toxicity. The complete remission rate was 76 versus 63% (CHOP + rituximab versus CHOP alone) (154).

Recently, more mature data were reported by the DSHNHL (the German lymphoma group) in the treatment of elderly patients with 2-weekly regimens of CHOP versus CHOEP and 3-weekly regimens consisting of the same drugs (115). To evaluate the therapies in older patients, 689 patients aged 61 to 75 years were randomized to six cycles of CHOP-21, CHOP-14, CHOEP-21, or CHOEP-14. G-CSF support was started on day 4. Initial sites of bulky or extranodal disease were irradiated with 36 Gy. Complete remission rates were 60.1% for CHOP-21, 70.0% for CHOEP-21, 76.1% for CHOP-14, and 71.6% for CHOEP-14. The CHOEP regimens were much more toxic than the CHOP regimens, with CHOP-14 and CHOP-21 having a similar toxicity profile. Five-year event-free and overall survival rates were 32.5 and 40.6%, respectively, for CHOP-21 and 43.8 and 53.3%, respectively, for CHOP-14. CHOP-14 appears to represent a substantial improvement for elderly patients, on a par with the addition of rituximab to CHOP, although additional studies are necessary to confirm the benefit.

Although it is sometimes necessary to reduce the doses of chemotherapeutic regimens, including CHOP, to treat elderly patients with comorbid conditions, CHOP is generally well tolerated by patients without contraindications to doxorubicin. Growth factor support should be used. Unfortunately, patients with a contraindication to doxorubicin also frequently have contraindications to other therapies, such as platinum-containing regimens. A rule of thumb is that CHOP, with the inclusion of rituximab, should remain the standard therapy in elderly patients with most types of aggressive NHL. The new evidence regarding CHOP-14 must be assimilated into this rule after additional study. Other more aggressive regimens, such as hyper-CVAD, may need to be dose-reduced, and therapies without doxorubicin may need to be considered.

■ NEW DRUGS

Many new drugs are investigated in the frontline setting and in relapsing patients with DLCBLs. Multicenter randomized studies are ongoing using bevacizumab, maintenance enzastaurin (a PKCβ inhibitor), everolimus (mTOR inhibitor). Phase II studies adding radioimmunotherapy such as ibritumomab-tioxetan as consolidation in patients achieving a complete remission after standard R-CHOP showed encouraging results.

Many other promising agents are currently under study in recurrent diseases, including as of today, 18 different histone deacetylation inhibitors divided in four groups (depsipeptide, vorinostat, etc.); new monoclonal antibodies, targeting CD20 (ofatumumab, GA-101, veltuzumab, ocrelizumab); anti-CD22 naked (epratuzumab), or conjugated to calicheamicin (CMC-544); anti-TRAIL death receptors (APO2L; Mapatumumab); anti-CD40 (SGN-40, HCD122); anti-BLyS (belimumab); anti-CD19 immunoconjugates (SAR3419). B-cell inhibitors pathways fostamatiniba spleen tyrosine kinase inhibitor [syk]; *PCI-32765* a burton tirosyne kinase inhibitor [BTK]. Immunomodulatory drugs (IMiDs) are an emerging class of oral anti-neoplastic agents. Although the mechanism of action is not completely understood, it likely relates to the drugs' ability to alter characteristics of the underlying tumor microenvironment, including inhibition of angiogenesis, stromal cell–cell interactions and pro-tumor cytokines, and enhancement of immune cell function and many others (thalidomide, lenalidomide).

Many of these promising drugs will be hopefully increasing the arsenal of drugs that can be used against different aggressive lymphomas.

■ RESPONSE AND FOLLOW-UP

DEFINITIONS OF RESPONSE

Response to therapy is assessed according to criteria based on the shrinkage or disappearance of previously observed nodal and extranodal masses (158). The classical definition of response has in recent years been evolving to include findings in FDG-PET studies (80) (Table 8-6). In the absence of PET studies pretreatment, complete remission requires a normal physical examination, normal lymph nodes or the disappearance of masses by CTs, a normal bone marrow biopsy (if initially involved by disease). If baseline FDG-PET activity was noted, posttreatment disappearance of FDG-PET hypermetabolic uptake, and normalization of marrow (if initially abnormal) will constitute complete remission, despite possible residual masses on CTs. Partial remission requires a decrease in the size of the liver and spleen after therapy, a >50% decrease in the lymph nodes involved, and >50% decrease in nodal masses; residual active FDG-PET (biopsy of site of residual activity recommended), or active residual bone marrow disease. Relapse or progression is defined as enlarging organomegaly, increasing lymph nodes and/or nodal masses, and/or the reappearance of bone marrow disease.

RESTAGING

FDG-PET has proven very useful in assessing responses to therapy. Early studies showed that a positive scan after therapy predicts treatment failure, and that FDG-PET is better at predicting response compared to conventional radiologic studies such as CT (159,160). These results prompted changes to the International Working Group response criteria (80), with the inclusion of PET criteria and the elimination of the unconfirmed complete response (CRu) category.

Although anatomic imaging plays an important role in assessing responses to therapy, these changes take time to occur and abnormalities may not completely resolve. It was estimated that 40 to 60% of patients have an anatomic abnormality that persists after therapy; however, only 10 to 20% of these patients actually have residual lymphoma (161,162). Under the new guidelines, after completion of therapy, if an FDG-PET positive mass becomes negative,

TABLE 8-6 | **RESPONSE DEFINITIONS FOR CLINICAL TRIALS**

Response	Definition	Nodal Masses	Spleen, Liver	Bone Marrow
CR	Disappearance of all evidence of disease	(a) FDG-avid or PET positive prior to therapy; mass of any size permitted if PET is negative (b) Variably FDG-avid or PET negative; regression to normal size on CT	Not palpable, nodules disappeared	Infiltrate cleared on repeat biopsy; if indeterminate by morphology, immunohisto-chemistry should be negative
PR	Regression of measurable disease and no new sites	≥50% decrease in SPD of up to six largest dominant masses; no increase in size of other nodes (a) FDG-avid or PET positive prior to therapy; one or more PET positive at previously involved site (b) Variably FDG-avid or PET negative; regression on CT	≥50% decrease in SPD of nodules (for single nodule in greatest transverse diameter); no increase in size of liver or spleen	Irrelevant if positive prior to therapy; cell type should be specified
SD	Failure to attain CR/PR or PD	(a) FDG-avid or PET positive prior to therapy; PET positive at prior sites of disease and no new sites on CT or PET (b) Variably FDG-avid or PET negative; no change in size of previous lesions on CT		
Relapsed disease or PD	Any new lesion or increase by ≥50% of previously involved sites from nadir	Appearance of a new lesion(s) >1.5 cm in any axis, ≥50% increase in longest diameter of a previously identified node >1 cm in short axis Lesions PET positive if FDG-avid lymphoma or PET positive prior to therapy	>50% increase from nadir in the SPD of any previous lesions	New or recurrent involvement

CR, complete remission; FDG, [^{18}F]fluorodeoxyglucose; PET, positron emission tomography; CT, computed tomography; PR, partial remission; SPD, sum of the product of the diameters; SD, stable disease; PD, progressive disease.
Reprinted, with permission, from Cheson BD, Pfistner B, Juweid ME, et al. Revised response criteria for malignant lymphoma. *J Clin Oncol* 2007;25: 579-586. ©2008 American Society of Clinical Oncology. All rights reserved.

this is considered a complete response (CR) even if there is a residual soft tissue abnormality (Fig. 8-21). However, if it remains positive on FDG-PET scan, this is considered a partial response (PR) when smaller anatomically, and stable disease (SD) if similar in size. If the staging FDG-PET scan is negative, then anatomic measurements are used to determine response to therapy.

SURVEILLANCE

Follow-up of patients with aggressive NHL after complete remission and cessation of therapy is typically done every 3 to 4 months for 2 years, then every 6 months for the next 2 years, then annually until year 5, as noted in the NCCN guidelines (163). CT of the abdomen and pelvis is performed, along with chest radiography and CT if the patient had disease at that site. Other sites are imaged based on previous sites of disease. Complete laboratory workup is also performed, and these studies include serum LDH, electrolytes, renal and liver function tests, and complete blood count with differential.

Because of the well-recognized ability of FDG-PET to identify cancer, its use has been proposed in

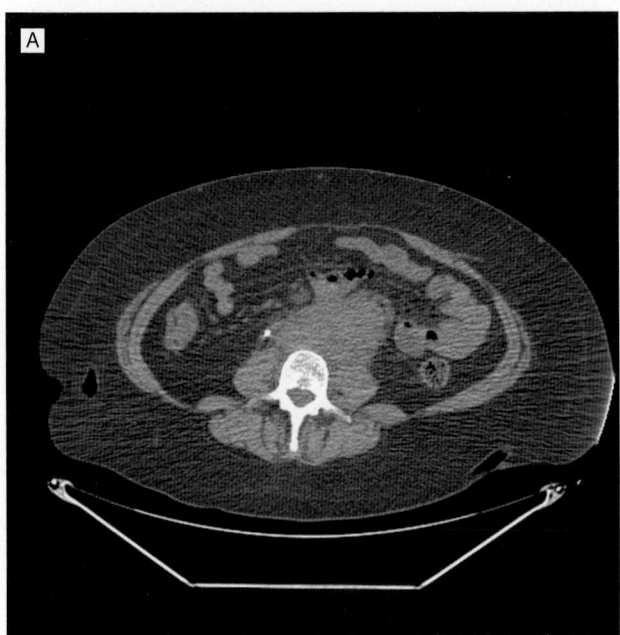 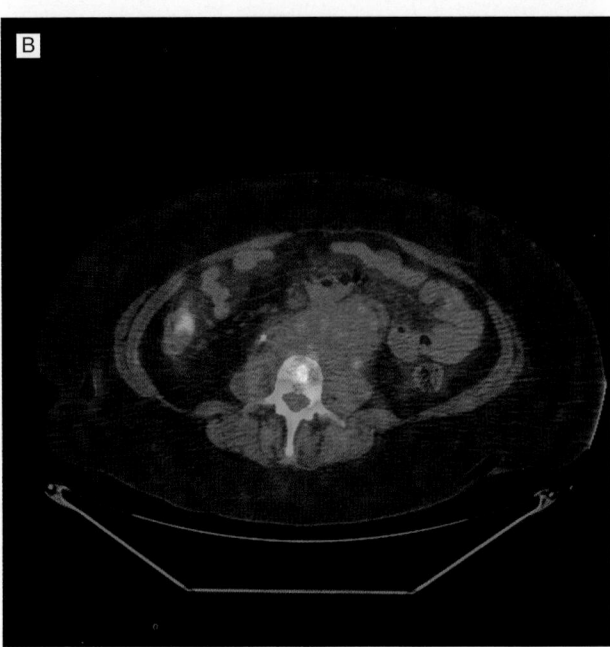

FIGURE 8-21. Residual mass, not residual lymphoma. After completing chemotherapy, this patient had a residual soft tissue abnormality in the retroperitoneum. **A.** This was previously positive on FDG-PET, but now does not have activity above background levels and is considered negative. **B.** Biopsy of this mass was negative, and it was stable on follow-up studies. Previously, this would be considered a partial response (PR) or unconfirmed complete response (CRu). Under the revised criteria, taking into account the FDG-PET findings, this is considered a complete response (CR).

surveillance after achieving clinical remission, or even for routine screening of individuals (164,165). Cheson pointed out that in the Zinzani study, the chance of relapse became insignificant after 12 to 18 months in patients with aggressive lymphomas (166). In those circumstances, a positive FDG-PET is more likely to represent a false-positive finding, requiring additional evaluation to demonstrate this, and so FDG-PET may not be useful as a routine screening modality in patients with low pretest probability for disease. In the absence of an active cancer, FDG-PET may best be used in an adjunct role, when there is clinical suspicion for recurrence or other indeterminate findings. In these situations, it provides metabolic characterization of known abnormalities, and identifies additional targets for biopsy.

The time frame for discontinuation of CT surveillance is not clearly established, although the benefit of studies perhaps even beyond year 2, as shown in the study by Zinzani, is minimal. Furthermore, the costs from the health care system and increased radiation exposure from medical imaging have come under increasing scrutiny. This is an important question to address for long-term survivors.

RELAPSE OR RECURRENCE

The presence of a new lesion, either by anatomic criteria or on FDG-PET scan, is considered relapsed or progressive disease (PD). Good clinical judgment, however, and often the assistance of a pathologist, is necessary in verifying relapsed or progressive disease, particularly when there are contradictory clinical or imaging findings. As noted earlier, FDG-PET is nonspecific, and uptake may occur in both benign and malignant tumors, in inflammatory or infectious lesions, and with normal physiologic processes. Sarcoidosis and fungal infections may mimic lymphoma, and biopsy is often necessary to exclude recurrence (Fig. 8-22). A single persistent or new focus of activity, with paradoxical response at other sites of disease, requires further evaluation. Large studies report that 1 to 3% of FDG-PET scans have an incidental clinically significant finding. This may be a premalignant lesion, such as a thyroid or colonic adenoma, but

A

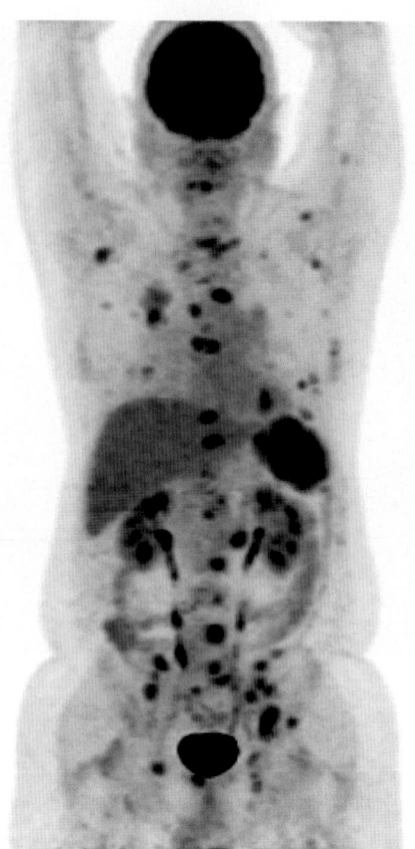

B

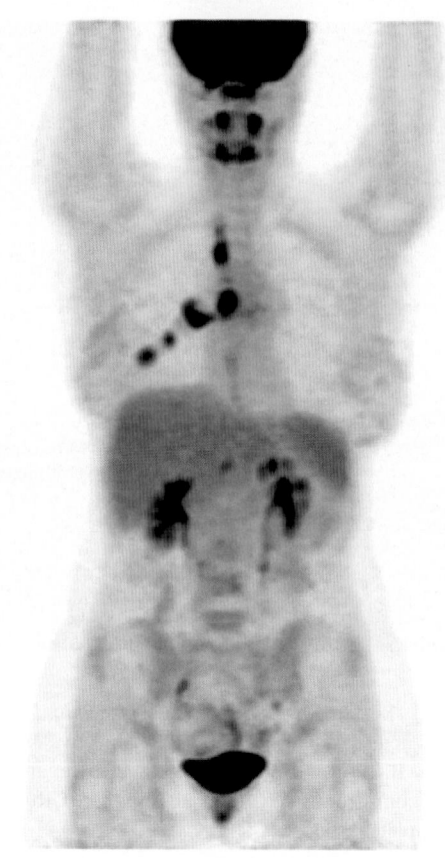

FIGURE 8-22. Examples of false-positive FDG-PET. Restaging study is suspicious for recurrent lymphoma (**A**), with predominantly osseous involvement; however, biopsy revealed non-necrotizing granulomas thought to be due to sarcoidosis. 2 months later nearly all the FDG avid sites resolved without any therapy. (**B**) A second patient presented over 10 years after successful treatment for lymphoma, with new lymphadenopathy and lung opacities, that were positive on FDG-PET. Biopsy revealed fungal lymphadenitis.

incidental second malignant tumors are not uncommon (167-169) (Fig. 8-23).

UNRESOLVED QUESTIONS

The addition of FDG-PET imaging has had an enormous impact upon patient management in a relatively short period of time. Although PET existed as a concept in the 1950s, 18F-FDG was not synthesized and used until the 1970s. Medicare approved coverage for FDG-PET for lung cancer began in 1998, coverage for lymphoma was first added in 1999, then broadened in 2001. Incorporation of FDG-PET in response assessment criteria was in 2007. However, its impact upon clinical practice is much greater, although its cost-effectiveness remains largely unaddressed. Perhaps ironically, Cheson who helped lead the inclusion of FDG-PET in response criteria argues against overuse of FDG-PET in a 2009 editorial (166). It is important to make the distinction between what is recommended, based upon good clinical trial or consensus expert opinion, and what is still under investigation, even though there may be many publications supporting the idea.

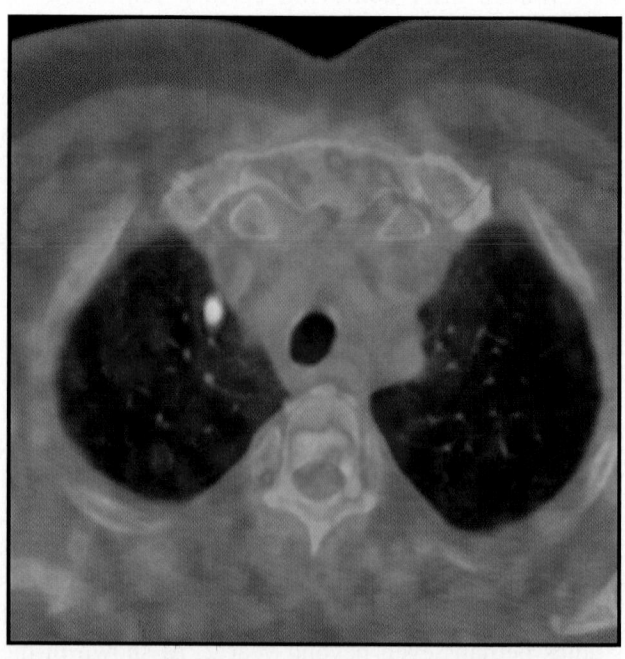

FIGURE 8-23. Incidental significant finding on FDG-PET/CT. An enlargening metabolically active lung nodule is seen. Biopsy revealed non-small cell lung cancer, and the patient went on to have lobectomy for stage I lung cancer.

Although commonly reported in clinical practice, the use of standard uptake units (SUVs) remains controversial. A semiquantitative measure of the fraction of the injected FDG dose that accumulates at a tumor site compared to the rest of the body, it is commonly used in the research setting as an objective measurement to help distinguish, for example, between benign and malignant pulmonary nodules, or to help discriminate between aggressive and indolent lymphomas (81,170). Caution should be used before applying those criteria to clinical practice, because although studies have shown that SUV measurements can be quite reproducible under controlled circumstances, in a more realistic practice-based setting, there are many more variables that must be accounted for. Short differences in time between radiopharmaceutical administration and FDG-PET imaging may result in large differences in SUVs. Tumor location and shape may also impact measurements, and there are even subtle differences in how this value is calculated and reported (171-173).

Although there is good evidence for use of FDG-PET imaging before and after completion of therapy to assess responses, there are also reports showing that FDG-PET performed after a few cycles of chemotherapy can also predict response, perhaps even better than FDG-PET performed after completion of therapy (174,175). However, there is little guidance in what to do with a positive early FDG-PET scan. Risk-adaptive therapy based upon early FDG-PET has been proposed by several groups, and variations on this theme are under investigation, focusing upon patients with aggressive NHL or HL (166,176). Given the present lack of clear guidance of what to do with results of FDG-PET scan performed before the completion of therapy, the use of early FDG-PET scan is best reserved for patients prospectively enrolled in a clinical trial.

Although metabolic activity as suggested by FDG uptake has been very successful in adding information to cancer staging and responses to therapy, FDG is not the only PET imaging agent. Flourine-18 is usable as a bone-imaging agent. Flourothymidine is under investigation as a marker of DNA synthesis (and cellular proliferation).

■ NEW DIRECTIONS

Over the last 20 years, remarkable advances have been made in the diagnosis, characterization, and treatment of patients with aggressive NHL. Most of the advances in therapy have been in the realm of chemotherapy and RT, but new technologies such as monoclonal antibodies have

made a significant impact. Although advances in the area of traditional chemotherapy remain to be discovered, it is likely that new therapeutic modalities will become more important. Research areas likely to be important in the near future are bioimmunotherapy with vaccines, newer monoclonal antibodies, and novel agents that target-specific genetic lesions. Some of these approaches (eg, lymphoma vaccines and targeted molecular technologies) are currently undergoing clinical trials. Although success to date is not confirmed and additional studies are required, the initial results are promising.

References

1. National Cancer Institute sponsored study of classifications of non-Hodgkin lymphomas: Summary and description of a working formulation for clinical usage. The Non-Hodgkin's Lymphoma Classification Project. *Cancer* 1982;49:2112-2135.
2. Baris D, Zahm SH. Epidemiology of lymphomas. *Curr Opin Oncol* 2000;12:383-394.
3. Groves FD, Linet MS, Travis LB, et al. Cancer Surveillance Series: Non-Hodgkin's lymphoma incidence by histologic subtype in the United States from 1978 through 1995. *J Natl Cancer Inst* 2000;92:1240-1251.
4. Greiner TC, Medeiros LJ, Jaffe ES. Non-Hodgkin's lymphoma. *Cancer* 1995;75(1 Suppl):370-380.
5. Clarke CA, Glaser SL. Changing incidence of non-Hodgkin lymphomas in the United States. *Cancer* 2002;94:2015-2023.
6. Jemal H, Siegel R, Ward E, et al. Cancer Statistics, 2009 *CA Can J Clin* 2009;59:225-249.
7. Filipovich AH, Mathur A, Kamat D, et al. Primary immunodeficiences: Genetic risk factors for lymphoma. *Cancer Res* 1992;52:5465s-5467s.
8. Mueller N. Overview of the epidemiology of malignancy in immune deficiency. *J Acquir Immune Defic Syndr* 1999;21: S5-S10.
9. Cunningham-Rundles C, Bodian C. Common variable immunodeficiency: Clinical and immunological features of 248 patients. *Clin Immunol* 1999;92:34-48.
10. Opelz G, Dohler B. Lymphomas after solid argon transplantation: A collaborative transplant study report. *Am J Transplant* 2004;4:222-230.
11. Kamel OW, Holly EA, van de Rijn M, et al. A population based, case control study of non-Hodgkin's lymphoma in patients with rheumatoid arthritis. *J Rheumatol* 1999;26:1676-1680.
12. Salloum E, Cooper DL, Howe G, et al. Spontaneous regression of lymphoproliferative disorders in patients treated with methotrexate for rheumatoid arthritis and other rheumatic diseases. *J Clin Oncol* 1996;14:1943-1949.
13. Lyons SF, Liebowitz DN. The roles of human viruses in the pathogenesis of lymphoma. *Semin Oncol* 1998;25:461-475.
14. Goedert JJ. The epidemiology of acquired immunodeficiency syndrome malignancies. *Semin Oncol* 2000;27:390-401.
15. Cote TR, Biggar RJ, Rosenberg PS, et al. Non-Hodgkin's lymphoma among people with AIDS: Incidence, presentation, and public health burden. AIDS/Cancer Study Group. *Int J Cancer* 1997;73:645-650.
16. Young LS, Murray PG. Epstein-Barr virus and oncogenesis: From latent genes to tumours. *Oncogene* 2003;22:5108-5121.

17. McDuffie HH, Pahwa P, McLaughlin JR, et al. Non-Hodgkin's lymphoma and specific pesticide exposures in men: Cross-Canada study of pesticides and health. *Cancer Epidemiol Biomarkers Prev* 2001;10:1155-1163.

18. Blair A, Harge P, Stewart PA, et al. Mortality and cancer incidence of aircraft maintenance workers exposed to trichloroethylene and other organic solvents and chemicals: Extended follow-up. *Occup Environ Med* 1998; 55:161-171.

19. Chatterjee N, Hartge P, Cerhan JR, et al. Risk of non-Hodgkin's lymphoma and family history of lymphatic, hematologic, and other cancers. *Cancer Epidemiol Biomarkers Prev* 2004;13:1415-1421.

20. Mentzer SJ, Reilly JJ, Skarin AT, et al. Patterns of lung involvement by malignant lymphoma. *Surgery* 1993;113:507-514.

21. Jaffe ES, Harris NL, Stein H, et al. (eds). *World Health Organization Classification of Tumours. Pathology and Genetics of Tumours of Hematopoeitic and Lymphoid Tissues.* Lyon, France: IARC Press; 2001:121-253.

22. Armitage J, Weisenburger D. New approach to classifying non-Hodgkin's lymphomas: Clinical features of the major histologic subtypes. *J Clin Oncol* 1998;16:2780-2795.

23. The Non-Hodgkin's Lymphoma Classification Project: A clinical evaluation of the International Lymphoma Study Group Classification of Non-Hodgkin's Lymphoma. *Blood* 1997;89:3909-3918.

24. Coiffier B. Diffuse large cell lymphoma. *Curr Opin Oncol* 2001;13:325-334.

25. Shipp MA. Prognostic factors in aggressive non-Hodgkin's lymphoma: Who has "high-risk" disease? 1994;83:1165-1173.

26. Kwak LW, Wilson M, Weiss LM, et al. Clinical significance of morphologic subdivision in diffuse large-cell lymphoma. *Cancer* 1991;68:1988-1993.

27. Engelhard M, Brittinger G, Huhn D, et al. Subclassification of diffuse large B-cell lymphomas according to the Kiel classification: Distinction of centroblastic and immunoblastic lymphomas is a significant prognostic factor. *Blood* 1997;89: 2291-2297.

28. Jacobson JO, Wilkes BM, Kwiatkowski DJ, et al. *bcl-2* rearrangements in *de novo* diffuse large cell lymphoma: Association with distinctive clinical features. *Cancer* 1993; 72:231-236.

29. Offit K, Lo Coco F, Louie DC, et al. Rearrangement of the *bcl-6* gene as a prognostic marker in diffuse large-cell lymphoma. *N Engl J Med* 1994;331:74-80.

30. Rosenwald A, Staudt LM. Gene expression profiling of diffuse large B-cell lymphoma. *Leuk Lymph* 2003;44(Suppl 3): S41-S47.

31. Shipp MA, Ross KN, Tamayo P, et al. Diffuse large B-cell lymphoma outcome prediction by gene-expression profiling and supervised machine learning. *Nat Med* 2002;8:68-74.

32. Monti S, Savage KJ, Kutok JL. Molecular profiling of diffuse large B-cell lymphoma identifies robust subtypes including one characterized by host inflammatory response. *Blood* 2005;105:1851-1861.

33. Hans CP, Weisenburger DD, Greiner TC, et al. Confirmation of the molecular classification of diffuse large B-cell lymphoma by immunohistochemistry using a tissue microarray. *Blood* 2004;103:275-282.

34. Braaten KM, Betensky RA, de Leval L, et al. BCL-6 expression predicts improved survival in patients with primary central nervous system lymphoma. *Clin Cancer Res* 2003;9:1063-1069.

35. Camilleri-Broet S, Criniere E, Broet P, et al. A uniform activated B-cell-like immunophenotype might explain the poor prognosis of primary central nervous system lymphomas: Analysis of 83 cases. *Blood* 2006;107:190-196.

36. Lin CH, Kuo KT, Chuang SS, et al. Comparison of the expression and prognostic significance of differentiation markers between diffuse large B-cell lymphoma of central nervous system origin and peripheral nodal origin. *Clin Cancer Res* 2006;12:1152-1156.

37. Cobbers JM, Wolter M, Reifenberger J, et al. Frequent inactivation of CDKN2A and rare mutation of TP53 in PCNSL. *Brain Pathol* 1998;8:263-276.

38. Grange F, Bekkenk MW, Wechsler J, et al. Prognostic factors in primary cutaneous large B-cell lymphomas: A European multicenter study. *J Clin Oncol* 2001;19:3602-3610.

39. Hoefnagel JJ, Vermeer MH, Jansen PM, et al. Bcl-2, Bcl-6 and CD10 expression in cutaneous B-cell lymphoma: Further support for a follicle centre cell origin and differential diagnostic significance. *Br J Dermatol* 2003;149:1183-1191.

40. Hallermann C, Kaune KM, Gesk S, et al. Molecular cytogenetic analysis of chromosomal breakpoints in the IGH, MYC, BCL6, and MALT1 gene loci in primary cutaneous B-cell lymphomas. *J Invest Dermatol* 2004;123:213-219.

41. Oyama T, Yamamoto K, Asano N, et al. Age-related EBV-associated B-cell lymphoproliferative disorders constitute a distinct clinicopathologic group: A study of 96 patients. *Clin Cancer Res* 2007;13:5124-5132.

42. Gibson SE, Hsi ED. Epstein-Barr virus-positive B-cell lymphoma of the elderly at a United States Tertiary Medical Center: An uncommon aggressive lymphoma with a nongerminal center B-cell phenotype. *Human Pathol* 2009;40:653-661.

43. Nador RG, Cesarman E, Chadburn A, et al. Primary effusion lymphoma: A distinct clinicopathologic entity associated with the Kaposi's sarcoma-associated herpes virus. *Blood* 1996;88:645-656.

44. Fan W, Bubman D, Chadburn A, et al. Distinct subsets of primary effusion lymphoma can be identified based on their cellular gene expression profile and viral association. *J Virol* 2005;79:1244-1251.

45. Falini B, Venturi S, Martelli M, et al. Mediastinal large B-cell lymphoma: Clinical and immunohistological findings in 18 patients treated with different third-generation regimens. *Br J Haematol* 1995;89:780-789.

46. Cazals-Hatem D, Lepage E, Brice P, et al. Primary mediastinal large B-cell lymphoma. A clinicopathologic study of 141 cases compared with 916 nonmediastinal large B-cell lymphomas, a GELA ("Groupe d'Etude des Lymphomas de l'Adulte") study. *Am J Surg Pathol* 1996;20:877-888.

47. Van Besien K, Kelta M, Bahaguna P. Primary mediastinal B-cell lymphoma: A review of pathology and management. *J Clin Oncol* 2001;19:1855-1864.

48. Medeiros LJ, Gelb A, Wolfson K, et al. Major histocompatibility complex class I and class II antigen expression in diffuse large cell and large cell immunoblastic lymphomas: Absence of a correlation between antigen expression and clinical outcome. *Am J Pathol* 1993;143:1086-1097.

49. Copie-Bergman C, Gaulard P, Maouche-Chretien L, et al. The MAL gene is expressed in primary mediastinal large B-cell lymphoma. *Blood* 1999;94:3567-3575.

50. Barth TF, Leithauser F, Joos S, et al. Mediastinal (thymic) large B-cell lymphoma: Where do we stand? *Lancet Oncol* 2002;3:229-234.

51. Katzenstein AL, Carrington CB, Liebow AA. Lymphomatoid granulomatosis: A clinicopathologic study of 152 cases. *Cancer* 1979;43:360-373.

52. Guinee D, Jaffe ES, Kingma D, et al. Pulmonary lymphomatoid granulomatosis. Evidence for a proliferation of Epstein-Barr virus infected B-lymphocytes with a prominent T-cell component and vasculitis. *Am J Surg Pathol* 1994;18:753-764.

53. Sheibani K, Battifora H, Winberg CD, et al. Further evidence that "malignant angioendotheliomatosis" is an angiotropic large-cell lymphoma. *N Engl J Med* 1986;314:943-948.

54. Estalilla OC, Koo CH, Brynes RK, et al. Intravascular large B-cell lymphoma. A report of five cases initially diagnosed by bone marrow biopsy. *Am J Clin Pathol* 1999;112:248-255.

55. Khalidi HS, Brynes RK, Browne P, et al. Intravascular large B-cell lymphoma: The CD5 antigen is expressed by a subset of cases. *Mod Pathol* 1998;11:983-988.

56. Fisher RI, Dahlberg S, Nathwani BN, et al. A clinical analysis of two indolent lymphoma entities: Mantle cell lymphoma and marginal zone lymphoma (including the mucosa-associated lymphoid tissue and monocytoid B-cell subcategories): A Southwest Oncology Group Study. *Blood* 1995;85: 1075-1082.

57. Weisenburger DD, Duggan MJ, Perry DA, et al. Non-Hodgkin's lymphomas of mantle zone origin. *Pathol Ann* 1991;26:139-158.

58. Majlis A, Pugh WC, Rodriguez MA, et al. Mantle cell lymphoma: Correlation of clinical outcome and biologic features with three histologic variants. *J Clin Oncol* 1997;15:1664-1671.

59. Cohen PL, Kurtin PJ, Donovan KA, et al. Bone marrow and peripheral blood involvement in mantle cell lymphoma. *Br J Haematol* 1998;101:302-310.

60. Romaguera JE, Medeiros LJ, Hagemeister FB, et al. Frequency of gastrointestinal involvement and its clinical significance in mantle cell lymphoma. *Cancer* 2003;97:586-591.

61. Schlette E, Bueso-Ramos C, Giles F, et al. Mature B-cell leukemias with more than 55% prolymphocytes: A heterogeneous group that includes an unusual variant of mantle lymphoma. *Am J Clin Pathol* 2001;11:571-581.

62. Vaandrager JW, Schuuring E, Zwikstra E, et al. Direct visualization of dispersed 11q23 chromosomal translocations in mantle cell lymphoma by multicolor DNA fiber fluorescence in situ hybridization. *Blood* 1996;88:1177-1182.

63. Bertoni F, Zucca E, Cotter FE. Molecular basis of mantle cell lymphoma. *Br J Haematol* 2004;124:130-140.

64. Wlodorska I, Pittaluga S, Hagemeijer A, et al. Secondary chromosome changes in mantle cell lymphoma. *Haematologica* 1999;84:594-599.

65. Onciu M, Schlette E, Medeiros LJ, et al. Cytogenetic findings in mantle cell lymphoma cases with a high level of peripheral blood involvement have a distinct pattern of abnormalities. *Am J Clin Pathol* 2001;116:886-892.

66. Magrath IT. African Burkitt's lymphoma: History, biology, clinical features, and treatment. *Am J Pediatr Hematol Oncol* 1991;13:222-246.

67. Ioachim HL, Dorsett B, Cronin W, et al. Acquired immunodeficiency syndrome-associated lymphomas: Clinical pathologic, immunologic, and viral characteristics of 111 cases. *Hum Pathol* 1991;22:659-673.

68. Berard CW, O'Conor GT, Thomas LB, et al. Histopathological definition of Burkitt's tumour. *Bull WHO* 1969;40: 601-607.

69. Hecht JL, Aster JC. Molecular biology of Burkitt's lymphoma. *J Clin Oncol* 2000;18:3707-3721.

70. Braziel RM, Arber DA, Slovak ML, et al. The Burkitt-like lymphomas: A Southwest Oncology Group Study delineating phenotypics, genotypic, and clinical features. *Blood* 2001;97: 3713-3720.

71. Haralambieva E, Boerma EJ, van Imhoff GW, et al. Clinical immunophenotypic, and genetic analysis of adult lymphoma with morphologic features of Burkitt lymphoma. *Am J Surg Pathol* 2005;29:1086-1094.

72. Le Gouill S, Talmont P, Touzeau C, et al. The clinical presentation and prognosis of diffuse large B-cell lymphoma with t(14;18) and 8q24/c-MYC rearrangement. *Haematologica* 2007;92:1335-1342.

73. Kamingo A, Medeiros LJ, Abruzzo LV, et al. Lymphoid neoplasms associated with concurrent t(14;18) and 8q24/c-MYC translocation generally have a poor prognosis. *Mod Pathol* 2006;19:25-33.

74. Carbone PP, Kaplan HS, Musshoff K, et al. Report of the Committee on Hodgkin's Disease Staging Classification. *Cancer Res* 1971;31:1860-1861.

75. Elstrom R, Guan L, Baker G, et al. Utility of FDG-PET scanning in lymphoma by WHO classification. *Blood* 2003;101: 3875-3876.

76. Mikhaeel NG, Timothy AR, Hain SF, et al. 18-FDG-PET for the assessment of residual masses on CT following treatment of lymphomas. *Ann Oncol* 2000;11(Suppl 1):147-150.

77. Paul R. Comparison of fluorine-18-2-fluorodeoxyglucose and gallium-67 citrate imaging for detection of lymphoma. *J Nucl Med* 1987;28:288-292.

78. Becherer A, Jaeger U, Szabo M, et al. Prognostic value of FDG-PET in malignant lymphoma. *Q J Nucl Med* 2003;47:14-21.

79. Spaepen K, Stroobants S, Dupont P, et al. Early restaging positron emission tomography with (18)F-fluorodeoxyglucose predicts outcome in patients with aggressive non-Hodgkin's lymphoma. *Ann Oncol* 2002;13:1356-1363.

80. Cheson BD, Pfistner B, Juweid ME, et al. Revised response criteria for malignant lymphoma. *J Clin Oncol* 2007;25: 579-586.

81. Schöder H, Meta J, Yap C, et al. Effect of whole-body ^{18}F-FDG PET imaging on clinical staging and management of patients with malignant lymphoma. *J Nucl Med* 2001;42:1139-1143.

82. Brunning RD, Bloomfield CD, McKenna RW, et al. Bilateral trephine bone marrow biopsies in lymphoma and other neoplastic diseases. *Ann Int Med* 1975;82:365-366.

83. Coller BS, Chabner BA, Gralnick HR. Frequencies and patterns of bone marrow involvement in Non-Hodgkin lymphomas: Observations on the value of bilateral biopsies. *Am J Hematol* 1977;3:105-119.

84. Carr R, Barrington SF, Madan B, et al. Detection of lymphoma in bone marrow by whole-body positron emission tomography. *Blood* 1998;91(9):3340-3346.

85. Moog F, Bangerter M, Kotzerke J, et al. 18-F-fluorodeoxyglucose-positron emission tomography as a new approach to detect lymphomatous bone marrow. *J Clin Oncol* 1998;16(2): 603-609.

86. Pakos EE, Fotopoulos AD, Ioannidis JPA. ^{18}F-FDG PET for evaluation of bone marrow infiltration in staging of lymphoma: A meta-analysis. *J Nucl Med* 2005;46:958-963.

87. A predictive model for aggressive non-Hodgkin's lymphoma: The International Non-Hodgkin's Lymphoma Prognostic Factors Project. *N Engl J Med* 1993;329:987-994.

88. Cabanillas F, Burke JS, Smith TL, et al. Factors predicting for response and survival in adults with advanced non-Hodgkin's lymphoma. *Arch Intern Med* 1978;138:413-418.

89. Wilder RB, Rodriguez MA, Medeiros LJ, et al. International prognostic index-based outcomes for diffuse large B-cell lymphomas. *Cancer* 2002;94:3083-3088.

90. Vose J, Armitage AJ, Weisenburger DD, et al. The importance of age in survival of patients treated with chemotherapy for aggressive non-Hodgkin's lymphoma. *J Clin Oncol* 1988;6:1838-1844.

91. Sehn LH, Berry B, Chhanabhai M, et al. The Revised International Prognostic Index (R-IPI) is a better predictor of outcome than the standard IPI for patients with diffuse large b-cell lymphoma treated with R-CHOP. *Blood* 2007;109(5):1857-1861 [Epub 2006 Nov 14].

92. Hoster E, Dreyling M, Klapper W, et al. A New Prognostic Index (MIPI) for patients with advanced-stage mantle cell lymphoma. *Blood* 2008;111(2):558-565 [Epub 2007 Oct 25].

93. Shah JJ, Fayad L, Romaguera J. Mantle Cell International Prognostic Index (MIPI) not prognostic after R-Hyper-CVAD. *Blood* 2008;112(6):2583 (Author reply 2583-2584).

94. Geisler CH, Kolstad A, Laurell A, et al. The Mantle Cell Lymphoma International Prognostic Index (MIPI) is superior to the International Prognostic Index (IPI) in predicting survival following intensive first-line immunochemotherapy and autologous stem cell transplantation (ASCT). *Blood* 2010;115(8):1530-1533 [Epub 2009 Dec 23].

95. Ferreri AJ, Abrey LE, Blay JY, et al. Summary statement on primary central nervous system lymphomas from the Eighth International Conference on Malignant Lymphoma, Lugano, Switzerland, June 12 to 15, 2002. *J Clin Oncol* 2003;21(12):2407-2414.

96. Armitage J, Weisenburger D, Hutchins M, et al. Chemotherapy for diffuse large cell lymphoma: Rapidly responding patients have more durable remission. *J Clin Oncol* 1986;4:160-164.

97. Sweet DL, Kinzie J, Gaeke ME, et al. Survival of patients with localized diffuse histiocytic lymphoma. *Blood* 1981;58:1218-1223.

98. Chen MG, Prosnitz LR, Gonzalez-Serva A, et al. Results of radiotherapy in control of stage I and II non-Hodgkin's lymphoma. *Cancer* 1979;43:1245-1254.

99. Miller TP, Dahlberg S, Cassady JR, et al. Chemotherapy alone compared with chemotherapy plus radiotherapy for localized intermediate- and high-grade non-Hodgkin's lymphoma. *N Engl J Med* 1998;339:21-26.

100. Glick J, Kim K, Earle J, et al. An ECOG randomized phase III trial of CHOP v. CHOP + radiotherapy for intermediate grade early stage non-Hodgkin's lymphoma. *Proc Am Soc Clin Oncol.* 1995;14:391. abstr #C-1221.

101. Reyes F, Lepage E, Ganem G, et al. ACVBP versus CHOP plus radiotherapy for localized aggressive lymphoma. *N Engl J Med* 2005;352:1197-1205.

102. Bonnet C, Fillet G, Mounier N, et al. CHOP alone compared with CHOP plus radiotherapy for localized aggressive lymphoma in elderly patients: A study by the Groupe d'Etude des Lymphomes de l'Adulte. *J Clin Oncol* 2007;25:787-792.

103. Leitch HA, Gayscoyne RD, Chhanabhai M, et al. Limited-stage mantle-cell lymphoma. *Ann Oncol* 2003;14(10): 1555-1561.

104. DeVita VT, Canellos GP, Chabner B, et al. Advanced diffuse histiocytic lymphoma, a potentially curable disease. *Lancet* 1975;1:248-250.

105. Skarin AT, Rosenthal DS, Maloney WC, et al. Combination chemotherapy of advanced non-Hodgkin lymphoma with bleomycin, adriamycin, cyclophosphamide, vincristine, and prednisone. (BACOP). *Blood* 1977;49:759-770.

106. Gaynor ER, Ultmann J, Golomb HM, et al. Treatment of diffuse histiocytic lymphoma (DHL) with COMLA (cylophosphamide, Oncovin, methotrexate, leucovorin, cytosine arabinoside): A 10-year experience in a single institution. *J Clin Oncol* 1985;12:1596-1604.

107. Skarin AT, Canellos G, Rosenthal D, et al. Moderate dose methotrexate (m) combined with bleomycin (B), Adriamycin (A), cyclophosphamide (C), Oncovin (O), and dexamethasone (D), m-BACOD, in advanced diffuse histiocytic lymphoma. *Proc Am Soc Clin Oncol.*1983;2:220. abstr #C-861.

108. Armitage JO, Fyfe MA, Lewis J. Long-term remission durability and functional status of patients treated for diffuse histiocytic lymphoma with the CHOP regimen. *J Clin Oncol* 1984;2:898-902.

109. Fisher RI, Longo DL, DeVita VT Jr, et al. Long-term follow-up of ProMACE-CytaBOM in non-Hodgkin's lymphomas. *Ann Oncol* 1991;2(Suppl 1):33-35.

110. Shipp MA, Harrington DP, Klatt MM, et al. Identification of major prognostic subgroups of patients with large-cell lymphoma treated with m-BACOD or M-BACOD. *Ann Intern Med* 1986;104:757-765.

111. Fisher RI, Gaynor ER, Dahlberg S, et al. Comparison of a standard regimen (CHOP) with three intensive chemotherapy regimens for advanced non-Hodgkin's lymphoma. *N Engl J Med* 1993;328:1002-1006.

112. Balzarotti M, Spina M, Sarina B, et al. Intensified CHOP regimen in aggressive lymphomas: Maximal dose intensity and dose density of doxorubicin and cyclophosphamide. *Ann Oncol* 2002;13:1341-1346.

113. Itoh K, Ohtsu T, Fukuda H, et al. Randomized phase II study of biweekly CHOP and dose-escalated CHOP with prophylactic use of lenograstim (glycosylated G-CSF) in aggressive non-Hodgkin's lymphoma: Japan Clinical Oncology Group Study 9505. *Ann Oncol* 2002;13:1347-1355.

114. Wunderlich A, Kloess M, Reiser M, et al. German high-practicability and acute haematological toxicity of 2- and 3-weekly CHOP and CHOEP chemotherapy for aggressive non-Hodgkin's lymphoma: Results from the NHL-B trial of the German High-Grade Non-Hodgkin's Lymphoma Study Group (DSHNHL). *Ann Oncol* 2003;14:881-893.

115. Pfreundschuh M, Trumper L, Kloess M, et al. Two-weekly or 3-weekly CHOP chemotherapy with or without etoposide for the treatment of elderly patients with aggressive lymphomas: Results of the NHL-B2 trial of the DSHNHL. *Blood* 2004;104:634-641.

116. Pfreundschuh M, Trumper L, Kloess M, et al. Two-weekly or 3-weekly CHOP chemotherapy with or without etoposide for the treatment of young patients with aggressive lymphomas: Results of the NHL-B1 trial of the DSHNHL. *Blood* 2004;104:626-633.

117. Feugier P, Van Hoof A, Sebban C, et al. Long-term results of the R-CHOP Study in the treatment of elderly patients with diffuse large b-cell lymphoma: A study by the Groupe D'Etude des Lymphomes de l'Adulte. *J Clin Oncol* 2005;23(18):4117-4126.

118. Pfreundschuh M, Schubert J, Ziepert M, et al. Six versus eight cycles of bi-weekly CHOP-14 with or without rituximab in elderly patients with aggressive CD20+ B-cell lymphomas: A randomized controlled trial (RICOVER-60). *Lancet Oncol* 2008;9(2):105-116.

119. Pfreundschuh M, Trümper L, Osterborg A, et al. CHOP-like chemotherapy plus rituximab versus CHOP-like chemotherapy alone in young patients with good-prognosis diffuse large-B-cell lymphoma: A randomized controlled trial by the MabThera International Trial (MInT) Group. *Lancet Oncol* 2006;7(5):379-391.

120. Shah GD, Yahalom J, Correa DD, et al. Combined immunochemotherapy with reduced whole-brain radiotherapy for newly diagnosed primary CNS lymphoma. *J Clin Oncol* 2007; 25(30):4730-5, with erratum in 2008; 26(2):340.

121. Correa DD, Rocco-Donovan M, DeAngelis LM, et al. Prospective cognitive follow-up in primary CNS lymphoma patients treated with chemotherapy and reduced-dose radiotherapy. *N Neurooncol* 2009;91(3):315-321.

122. Shimada K, Matsue K, Yamamoto K, et al. Retrospective analysis of intravascular large B-cell lymphoma treated with rituximab-containing chemotherapy as reported by the IVL Study Group in Japan. *J Clin Oncol* 2008;26(19):3189-3195.

123. Ferreri AJ, Dognini GP, Bairey O, et al. The addition of rituximab to anthracycline-based chemotherapy significantly improves outcome in 'western' patients with intravascular large B-cell lymphoma. *Br J Haematol* 2008;143(2): 253-257.

124. Ferreri AJ, Dognini GP, Govi S, et al. Can Rituximab change the usually dismal prognosis of patients with intravascular large B-cell lymphoma? *J Clin Oncol* 2008;26(31):5134-5136 [Author reply 5136-5137].

125. Zinzani PL, Martelli M, Bertini M, et al. Induction chemotherapy strategies for primary mediastinal large B-cell lymphoma with sclerosis: A retrospective multinational study on 426 previously untreated patients. *Haematologica* 2002; 87(12):1258-1264.

126. Hamlin PA, Portlock CS, Straus DJ, et al. Primary mediastinal large B-cell lymphoma: Optimal therapy and prognostic factor analysis in 141 consecutive patients treated at Memorial Sloan Kettering From 1980 to 1999. *Br J Haematol* 2005; 130(5):691-699.

127. Khouri IF, Romaguera J, Kantarjian H, et al. Hyper-CVAD and high dose methotrexate/cytarabine followed by stem-cell transplantation: An active regimen for aggressive mantle-cell lymphoma. *J Clin Oncol* 1998;16:3803-3809.

128. Romaguera JE, Khouri IF, Kantarjian HM, et al. Untreated aggressive mantle cell lymphoma: Results with intensive chemotherapy without stem cell transplant in elderly patients. *Leuk Lymph* 2000;39:77-85.

129. Romaguera JE, Fayad L, Rodriguez MA, et al. High rate of durable remissions after treatment of newly diagnosed aggressive mantle-cell lymphoma with rituximab plus Hyper- CVAD alternating with rituximab plus high-dose methotrexate and cytarabine. *J Clin Oncol* 2005;23(28): 7013-7023 [Epub 2005 Sep 6]. Erratum in: *J Clin Oncol* 2006;24(4): 724.

130. Fayad L, Thomas D, Romaguera J. Update of the M.D. Anderson Cancer Center experience with Hyper-CVAD and Rituximab for the treatment of mantle cell and Burkitt-Type lymphomas. *Clin Lymph Myel* 2007;8(Suppl 2):S57-S62.

131. Kahl BS, Longo WL, Eickhoff JC, et al. Maintenance Rituximab following induction chemotherapy may prolong progression-free survival in mantle cell lymphoma: A pilot study from the Wisconsin Oncology Network. *Ann Oncol* 2006; 17(9):1418-1423.

132. Sweetenham JW. Review: Stem cell transplantation for mantle cell lymphma: Not yet the standard of care. *Clin Adv Hematol Oncol* 2009;7(5):323-324.

133. Geisler CH, Kolstad A, Laurell A, et al. Long-term progression-free survival of mantle cell lymphoma after intensive front-line immunochemotherapy with in vivo-purged stem cell rescue: A nonrandomized phase 2 multicenter study by the Nordic Lymphoma Group. *Blood* 2008;112(7):2687-2693.

134. Rummel MJ, Niederle N, Maschmeyer G, et al. Bundamustine plus rituximab is superior in respect of progression free survival and CR rate when compared to CHOP plus rituximab as first-line treatment of patients with advanced follicular, indolent, and mantle cell lymphomas: Final results of a randomized phase III study of the StiL (Study Group Indolent Lymphomas, Germany). *Blood* (ASH Annual Meeting Abstracts), 2009;114:405.

135. Johnson NA, Savage KJ, Ludkovski O, et al. Lymphomas with concurrent BCL2 and MYC translocations: The critical factors associated with survival. *Blood* 2009;114(11): 2273-2279.

136. Savage KJ, Johnson NA, Ben-Neriah S, et al. MYC gene rearrangements are associated with a poor prognosis in diffuse large B-cell lymphoma patients treated with R-CHOP chemotherapy. *Blood* 2009;114(17):3533-3537.

137. Klapper W, Stoecklein H, Zeynalova S, et al. Structural aberrations affecting the MYC locus indicate a poor prognosis independent of clinical risk factors in diffuse large B-cell lymphomas treated within randomized trials of the German High-Grade Non-Hodgkin's Lymphoma Study Group (DSHNHL). *Leukemia* 2008;22(12):2226-2229.

138. Velasquez WS, Cabanillas F, Salvador P, et al. Effective salvage therapy for lymphoma with cisplatin in combination with high-dose Ara-C and dexamethasone (DHAP). *Blood* 1988;71:117-122.

139. Rodriguez-Monge EJ, Cabanillas F. Long-term follow-up of platinum-based lymphoma salvage regimens: The M.D. Anderson Cancer Center experience. *Hematol Oncol Clin North Am* 1997;11:937-947.

140. Rodriguez MA, Cabanillas FC, Velasquez W, et al. Results of a salvage treatment program for relapsing lymphoma: MINE consolidated with ESHAP. *J Clin Oncol* 1995;13: 1734-1741.

141. Kewalramani T, Zelenetz AD, Nimer SD, et al. Rituximab and ICE as second-line therapy before autologous stem cell transplantation for relapsed or primary refractory diffuse large B-cell lymphoma. *Blood* 2004;103(10):3684-3688 [Epub 2004 Jan 22].

142. Philip T, Guglielmi C, Hagenbeek A, et al. Autologous bone marrow transplantation as compared with salvage chemotherapy in relapses of chemotherapy-sensitive non-Hodgkin's lymphoma. *N Engl J Med* 1995;333:1540-1545.

143. Gisselbrecht S, Glass B, Mounier D, et al. R-ICE versus R-DHAP in relapsed patients with CD20 diffuse large B-cell lymphoma (DLBCL) followed by autologous stem cell transplantation: CORAL study. *J Clin Oncol* 2009;27:15s (suppl; abstr 8509).

144. Fisher RI, Bernstein SH, Kahl BS, et al. Multicenter phase II study of bortezomib in patients with relapsed or refractory mantle cell lymphoma. *J Clin Oncol* 2006;24(30): 4867-4874.

145. Goy A, Bernstein SH, Kahl BS, et al. Bortezomib in patients with relapse or refractory mantle cell lymphoma: Updated time-to-event analyses of the multicenter phase 2 PINNA-CLE Study. *Ann Oncol* 2009;20(3):520-525.

146. Wang M, Fayad L, Cabanillas F, et al. Phase 2 trial of rituximab plus Hyper-CVAD alternating with rituximab plus methotrexate-cytarabine for relapsed or refractory aggressive mantle cell lymphoma. *Cancer* 2008;113(10):2734-2741.

147. Evens AM, Gordon LI. Burkitt's and Burkitt-like lymphoma. *Curr Treat Options Oncol* 2002;3:291-305.

148. Kantarjian HM, O'Brien S, Smith TL, et al. Results of treatment with hyper-CVAD, a dose-intensive regimen, in adult acute lymphocytic leukemia. *J Clin Oncol* 2000;18:547-561.

149. Mead GM, Sydes MR, Walewski J, et al. An international evaluation of CODOX-M and CODOX-M alternating with IVAC in adult Burkitt lymphoma: Results of United Kingdom Lymphoma Group LY06 study. *Ann Oncol* 2002;13:1264-1274.

150. Thomas DA, Faderl S, O'Brien S, et al. Chemoimmunotherapy with Hyper-CVAD plus rituximab for the treatment of adult Burkitt and Burkitt-type lymphoma or acute lymphoblastic leukemia. *Cancer* 2006;106(7):1569-1580.

151. The Non-Hodgkin's Lymphomas Classification Project: Effect of age on the characteristics and clinical behaviour of non-Hodgkin's lymphoma patients. *Ann Oncol* 1997;8:973-978.

152. Meyer RM, Browman GP, Samosh ML, et al. Randomized phase II comparison of standard CHOP with weekly CHOP in elderly patients with non-Hodgkin's lymphoma. *J Clin Oncol* 1995;13:2386-2393.

153. Dixon DO, Neilan B, Jones SE, et al. Effect of age on therapeutic outcome in advanced diffuse histiocytic lymphoma: The Southwest Oncology Group experience. *J Clin Oncol* 1986;4:295-305.

154. Coiffier B, Lepage E, Briere J, et al. CHOP chemotherapy plus rituximab compared with CHOP alone in elderly patients with diffuse large B-cell lymphoma. *N Engl J Med* 2002;346:235-242.

155. Tilly H, Mounier N, Coiffier B, et al. ACVBP regimen vs. CHOP in the treatment of advanced aggressive non-Hodgkin's lymphoma (NHL). Results of the LNH93-5 study with a median follow-up of 5 years. *Proc Am Soc Clin Oncol* 2003;22:574 (Abstract 2307).

156. Sonneveld P, de Ridder M, van der Lelie H. Comparison of doxorubicin and mitoxantrone in the treatment of elderly patients with advanced diffuse non-Hodgkin's lymphoma using CHOP versus CNOP chemotherapy. *J Clin Oncol* 1995;13:2530-2539.

157. Osby E, Hagberg H, Kvaloy S, et al. CHOP is superior to CNOP in elderly patients with aggressive lymphoma while outcome is unaffected by filgrastim treatment: Results of a Nordic Lymphoma Group randomized trial. *Blood* 2003;101:3840-3848.

158. Cheson BD, Horning SJ, Coiffier B, et al. Report of an international workshop to standardize response criteria for non-Hodgkin's lymphomas. NCI Sponsored International Working Group. *J Clin Oncol* 1999;17:1244-1253.

159. Spaepen K, Stroobants S, Dupont P, et al. Prognostic value of positron emission tomography (PET) with fluorine-18 fluorodeoxyglucose ([18F]FDG) after first-line chemotherapy in non-Hodgkin's lymphoma: Is [18F]FDG-PET a valid alternative to conventional diagnostic methods? *J Clin Oncol* 2001; 19(2):414-419.

160. Juweid ME, Cheson BD. Role of positron emission tomography in lymphoma. *J Clin Oncol* 2005;23(21):4577-4580.

161. Radford JA, Cowan RA, Flanagan M, et al. The significance of residual mediastinal abnormality on the chest radiograph following treatment for Hodgkin's disease. *J Clin Oncol* 1988; 6(6):940-946.

162. Canellos G. Residual mass in lymphoma may not be residual disease. *J Clin Oncol* 1988;6(6):931-933.

163. Zelenetz AD, Abramson JS, Advani RH, et al. The NCCN clinical practice guidelines in oncology: Non-Hodgkin's lymphomas. Version 1.2010. *JNCCN* 2010;8(3):288-334.

164. Zinzani PL, Stefoni V, Tani M, et al. Role of [18F] fluorodeoxyglucose positron emission tomography scan in the follow-up of lymphoma. *J Clin Oncol* 2009;27(11):1781-1787.

165. Nishizawa S, Kojima S, Teramukai S, et al. Prospective evaluation of whole-body cancer screening with multiple modalities including [18F] fluorodeoxyglucose positron emission tomography in a healthy population: A preliminary report. *J Clin Oncol* 2009;27(11):1767-1773.

166. Cheson B. The case against heavy PETing. *J Clin Oncol* 2009;27(11):1742-1743.

167. Agress, H Jr, Cooper BZ. Detection of clinically unexpected malignant and premalignant tumors with whole-body FDG PET: Histopathologic comparison. *Radiology* 2004;230(2): 417-422 [Epub 2003 Dec 29].

168. Kamel EM, Thumshirn M, Truninger K, et al. Significance of incidental 18F-FDG accumulations in the gastrointestinal tract in PET/CT: Correlation with endoscopic and histopathologic results. *J Nucl Med* 2004;45:1804-1810.

169. Ishimori T, Patel PV, Wahl RL. Detection of unexpected additional primary malignancies with PET/CT. *J Nucl Med* 2005;46:752-757.

170. Gould MK, Maclean CC, Kuschner WG, et al. Accuracy of positron emission tomography for diagnosis of pulmonary nodules and mass lesions: A meta-analysis. *JAMA* 2001; 285(7):914-924.

171. Keyes JW Jr. SUV: Standard uptake or silly useless value? *J Nucl Med* 1995;36(10):1836-1839.

172. Shankar LK, Hoffman JM, Bacharach S, et al. Consensus recommendations for the use of 18F-FDG PET as an indicator of therapeutic response in patients in National Cancer Institute Trials. *J Nucl Med* 2006;47:1059-1066.

173. Huang S-C. Anatomy of SUV. *Nucl Med Biol* 2000;27(7): 643-646.

174. Gallamini A, Hutchings M, Rigacci L, et al. Early interim 2-[18F] fluoro-2-deoxy-D-glucose positron emission tomography is prognostically superior to international prognostic score in advanced-stage Hodgkin's lymphoma: A report from a joint Italian-Danish study. *J Clin Oncol* 2007;25(24):3746-3752.

175. Kasamon YL, Jones RJ, Wahl RL. Integrating PET and PET/CT into the risk-adapted therapy of lymphoma. *J Nucl Med* 2007;48:19S-27S.

176. Kasamon YL, Wahl RL, Ziessman HA. Phase II study of risk-adapted therapy of newly diagnosed, aggressive non-Hodgkin lymphoma based on midtreatment FDG-PET scanning. *Biol Blood Marrow Transplant* 2009;15:242-248.

T-CELL LYMPHOMAS

Jenny Pozadzides
Madeleine Duvic
Barbara Pro

■ PERIPHERAL (MATURE) T-CELL LYMPHOMAS

The term *peripheral T-cell lymphoma* (PTCL) is used to describe lymphoid neoplasms of mature T-cell lineage, as opposed to tumors of thymic origin. The terms post-thymic and mature T-cell lymphoma also have been used to describe these tumors. PTCLs represent approximately 10% of all NHLs in most European and US studies but are more common in other parts of the world (1-3). Incidences are higher in Asian populations, possibly related to a high prevalence of human T-cell lymphotrophic virus type 1 (HTLV-1) and Epstein–Barr virus.

■ CLASSIFICATION

The International Lymphoma Study Group (ILSG) incorporated morphologic, phenotypic, molecular, and clinical information in the REAL (Revised European American Lymphoma) classification. The revision provided the basis for WHO (World Health Organization) classification with the following changes: PTCLs were divided into nodal, extranodal, and leukemic types; cutaneous and systemic anaplastic large-cell lymphomas (ALCL); updated terminology with subcutaneous panniculitis-type and hepatosplenic gd T-cell lymphomas were recognized as separate entities (Table 9-1) (1).

The most common histologic subtype is classified as PTCL not "otherwise specified" and accounts for approximately 55% of all PTCL. The second most common PTCL, ALCL, accounts for 17% of all PTCL, and angioimmunoblastic T-cell lymphoma (AITL) accounts for 13%. Other types of PTCL are rare, each <5% of all cases. Unlike B-cell lymphomas, the classification of T-cell neoplasms requires much more clinicopathologic correlation.

■ PRESENTATION

Patients with T-cell lymphomas are usually adults with generalized lymphadenopathy as well as frequent involvement of the skin, spleen, bone marrow, and blood. Although the subtypes of PTCL are histologically distinct, they share a very aggressive clinical course and, with the exception of ALK-positive ALCL, a poor response to conventional therapy.

The pathologic appearance and immunophenotype may vary within a given subtype. Therefore, diagnosis

TABLE 9-1	WORLD HEALTH ORGANIZATION CLASSIFICATION OF T-CELL LYMPHOMAS

Nodal
  Peripheral T-cell lymphoma, unspecified
  Anaplastic large cell lymphoma
  Angioimmunoblastic T-cell lymphoma
Extranodal
  Extranodal NK/T cell lymphoma, nasal type
  Enteropathy-type T-cell lymphoma
  Hepatosplenic T-cell lymphoma
  Subcutaneous panniculitis-like T-cell lymphoma
Leukemic/disseminated
  T-cell prolymphocytic leukemia
  T-cell large granular lymphocytic leukemia
  Aggressive NK-cell leukemia
  Adult T-cell leukemia/lymphoma
Cutaneous
  Mycosis fungoides/Sézary syndrome
  Primary cutaneous CD30-positive T-cell lymphoproliferative disorders
  Primary cutaneous anaplastic large cell lymphoma
  Lymphomatoid papulosis
  Borderline lesions

Reproduced, with permission, from Jaffe ES, Harris NL, Stein H, et al. *World Health Organization Classification of tumours. Pathology and genetics of tumours of hematopoeitic and lymphoid tissues.* Lyon, France: IARC Press; 2001:121–253.

is usually based on a combination of clinical presentation, pathology, molecular findings, and factors that may be unique to each subtype. T-cell receptor rearrangements are found in a majority of lymphomas, but can be inconsistent.

■ PROGNOSIS

Prognosis varies according to the subtype of PTCL. With the exception of patients with ALK+ ALCL who can be successfully treated with standard anthracycline-based chemotherapy and patients with stage I nasal natural killer/T-cell lymphomas who may do well with radiotherapy or combined-modality therapy, most will have a significantly poorer prognosis than their B-cell counterparts.

The International Prognostic Index (IPI) provides a prognostic score based on clinical and laboratory factors but was developed in aggressive lymphomas before routine immunophenotyping was utilized. Recently, IPI for T-cell lymphoma was developed based on a retrospective review of a large cohort of individuals with PTCL-U following poor prognostic features: older than 60 years, Eastern Cooperative Oncology Group score 2 or higher, elevated LDH, and bone marrow involvement. Five-year overall survival ranged from 62% for those with a score of 0 to 18% for a score of 3 or 4. This was felt to be more predictive than IPI. It is less clear how these indices apply to the less common extranodal and leukemic PTCLs. Independent prognostic factors included B symptoms, stage III/IV, LDH greater than normal, and local lymph node involvement.

PERIPHERAL T-CELL LYMPHOMA, UNSPECIFIED

PTCL-U represents the largest subtype in North America (5). In the WHO classification (1), unspecified PTCL includes all mature T-cell lymphomas that do not have unique clinical or pathologic features that allow more specific classification. Unspecified PTCLs represent approximately 6% of all NHLs and 55% of PTCLs (1-3). Due to the biological heterogeneity, PTCL-U is believed to be made up of more than one disease type but how to differentiate them is unknown.

Most patients with unspecified PTCLs are adults who present with generalized lymphadenopathy (6,7). Extranodal sites including skin, liver, Waldeyer ring, and lung are also commonly involved. Advanced stage has elevated LDH and B symptoms (5). PTCL-Us are diffuse, aggressive neoplasms that require combination chemotherapy (7). The 5-year overall and failure-free survival are 26% and 20%, respectively, for patients treated with doxorubicin-containing chemotherapy regimens (5-9).

Histologically, in most cases of unspecified PTCL, the lymph node architecture is diffusely effaced (1,10). However, in a subset of cases, the neoplasm has a paracortical distribution sparing lymphoid follicles. Cytologically, the neoplastic lymphoid cells exhibit a spectrum of cell sizes including small, medium-sized, and large and can have abundant clear cytoplasm (Figs. 9-1 and 9-2). Reed-Sternberg–like cells may be found. Mitotic figures are usually easily identified and are often numerous. Blood vessels (epithelioid venules) may be prominent.

Immunophenotypic studies have shown that PTCL-Us are of mature T-cell lineage. The neoplastic cells express pan-T-cell antigens such as CD2, CD3, and CD5, usually TCR αβ, and are either CD4+ CD8– or CD4– CD8+ (1). Approximately, 75% of cases will demonstrate an aberrant T-cell immunophenotype. Cytotoxic proteins and CD56 are expressed by a subset of cases (1,11). Approximately, one-third may be CD30+ or EBV+ but relevance is unknown.

Cytogenetic abnormalities in PTCLs are common, and karyotypes are often complex. Both numerical and structural abnormalities are reported, with structural rearrangements of chromosome 6 being most common (12).

ANAPLASTIC LARGE-CELL LYMPHOMA

In the WHO classification, two types of systemic ALCL are recognized, those with translocations involving the anaplastic lymphoma kinase (alk) gene at 2p23 and those without. The latter group does not appear to be a distinct clinicopathologic entity and is more akin to unspecified PTCL. Studies have shown that tumors with ALK-pos have a 5-year survival that is superior to

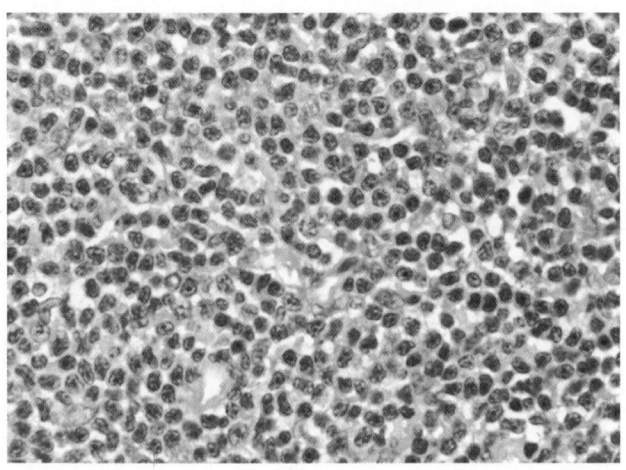

FIGURE 9-1. Peripheral T-cell lymphoma unspecified. The neoplastic cells in this case are predominantly small (hematoxylin-eosin, 1000×).

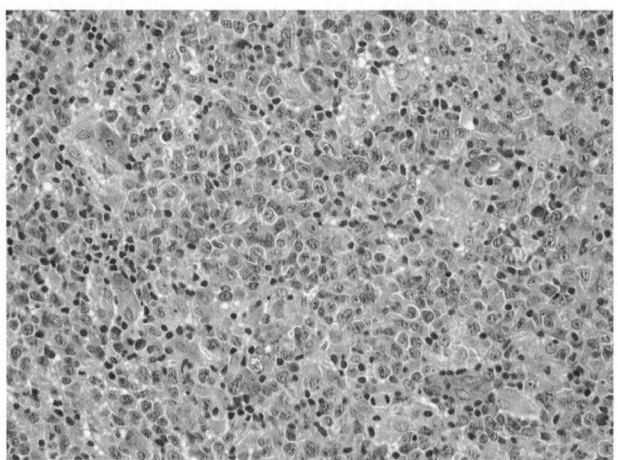

FIGURE 9-2. Peripheral T-cell lymphoma unspecified. The neoplastic cells in this case are small and large (hematoxylin-eosin, 1000×).

those that are ALK-neg (13). Here we focus on ALCL with alk gene rearrangements that express ALK. ALK-positive ALCLs represent 2 to 3% of all NHL in adults, with a higher frequency in children (1).

Patients with ALK-positive ALCL are often younger, in the first three decades of life, with a male predominance (1,14). Extranodal sites of disease, B-type symptoms, a high serum lactate dehydrogenase (LDH) level, and a high IPI are common. Peripheral blood and CNS involvement is uncommon; when present, however, they portend a poor prognosis. ALK-positive ALCLs are clinically aggressive but responsive to anthracycline-based chemotherapy; patients with these neoplasms have a better prognosis than those with other types of PTCL (14,15).

Histologically, ALK-positive ALCLs exhibit a wide histologic spectrum (Fig. 9-3). In the most common or classic cases, ALK-positive ALCLs preferentially involve lymph nodes sinuses, particularly in lymph nodes not involved extensively (1,14). With greater involvement, ALK-positive ALCL replaces the paracortical regions or may diffusely replace lymph node architecture. Cytologically, the neoplastic cells are large and bizarre, irregularly shaped, and often have horseshoe-shaped nuclei with a paranuclear hof (so-called hallmark cells) (see Fig. 9-3). The nuclear chromatin is vesicular, with prominent nucleoli. The tumor cell cytoplasm is abundant and usually basophilic. Other histologic variants of ALK-positive ALCL are described, the most common being lymphohistiocytic and small cell, with other variants being very rare (1,14). The lymphohistiocytic variant is composed of relatively few neoplastic cells associated with numerous lymphocytes and histiocytes. In the small cell variant, large anaplastic neoplastic cells are infrequent and many small neoplastic cells are present.

Immunophenotypic studies have shown that virtually all cases express CD30 (1,14). However, CD30 antigen expression is not specific for ALCL. All tumors discussed

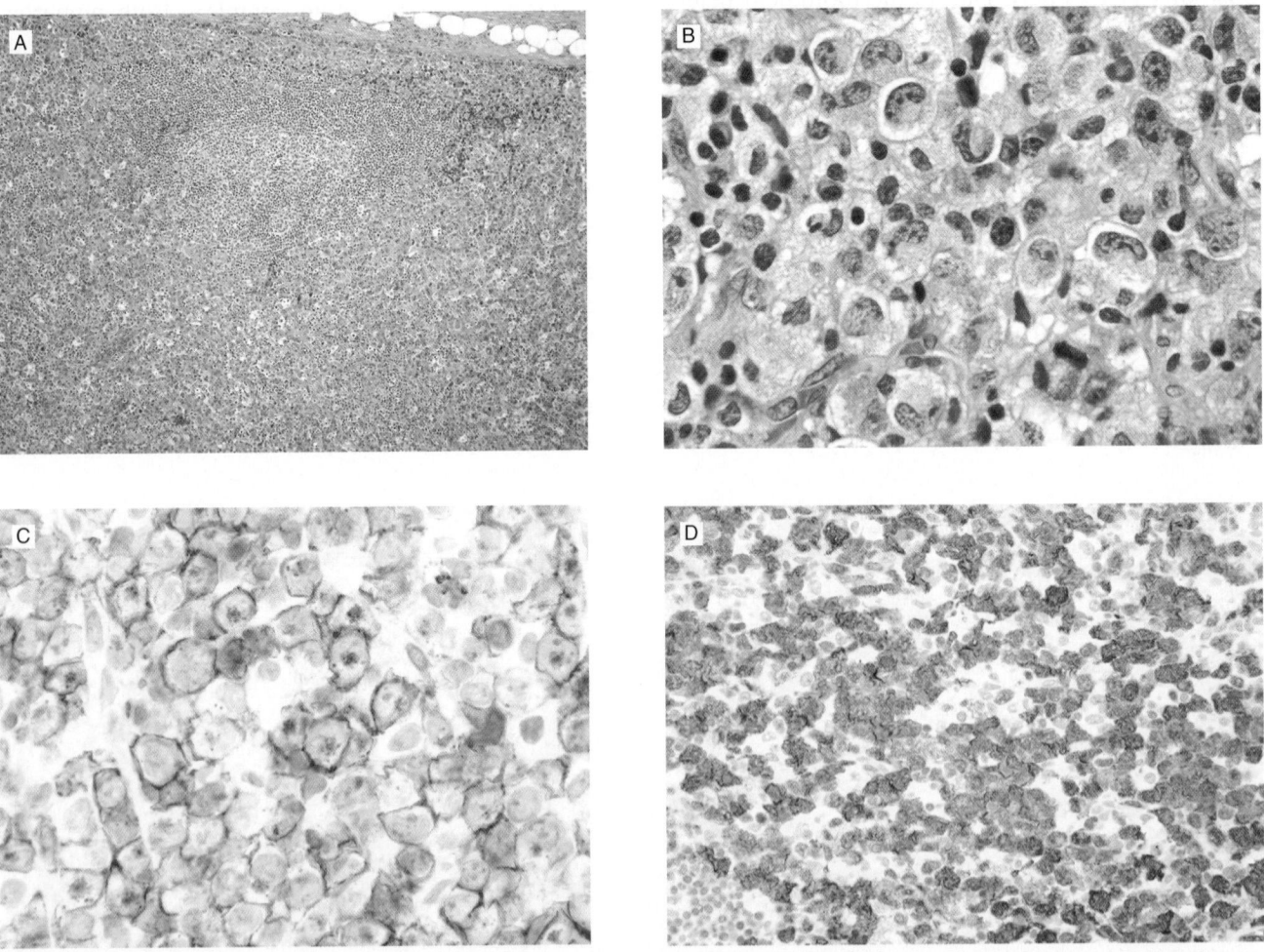

FIGURE 9-3.   ALK-positive anaplastic large cell lymphoma. **A.** In this field the neoplasm is paracortical and spares a central lymphoid follicle. **B.** The neoplastic cells are large with horseshoe-shaped nuclei. **C,D.** The neoplastic cells express CD30 (C) and ALK (D). (A,B, hematoxylin-eosin; A, 100×; B, 1000×; C,D, immunohistochemistry; C, 1000×; D, 400×.)

here also overexpress ALK. Most ALK-positive ALCLs are of mature T-cell lineage and express T-cell antigens, are most often CD4+ CD8–, and lack B-cell antigens. Most cases are negative for CD3; absence of CD5 is also common (16). Approximately, half of ALK-positive ALCLs lack leukocyte common antigen (CD45). Null-cell neoplasms lack immunophenotypic evidence of lineage. Most ALK-positive ALCLs express epithelial membrane antigen and cytotoxic proteins such as TIA-1 and perforin and are negative for BCL-2 (17,18). Both T- and null-cell ALK-positive ALCLs have T cell–receptor gene rearrangements.

Chromosomal translocations (or rarely inversions) involving chromosome 2p23, most commonly the t(2;5) (p23;q35), are characteristic of ALCL (14,19). This translocation juxtaposes the alk gene on chromosome 2p23 with the nucleophosmin (npm) gene on 5q35. Other abnormalities that result in fusion genes involving alk are also reported in a small subset of ALCL cases; all result in overexpression of ALK. The prognosis of patients with ALK-positive ALCL is similar regardless of the fusion gene that causes ALK overexpression (20).

ANGIOIMMUNOBLASTIC T-CELL LYMPHOMA

AITL was first described in the English literature as angioimmunoblastic lymphadenopathy with dysproteinemia (AILD) in 1974 (21). This entity has also been named immunoblastic lymphadenopathy and lymphogranulomatosis X in the literature. Originally, AILD was thought to be preneoplastic, but it is now considered to be a specific type of PTCL and is designated as AITL in the WHO classification (1).

Clinically, patients with AITL are elderly, with a median age in the seventh decade, and have advanced-stage disease with multiple extranodal sites of involvement at onset (22,23). Many patients have constitutional symptoms such as fever, chills, night sweats, and malaise. Physical examination reveals generalized lymphadenopathy, fever, hepatomegaly, splenomegaly, and skin rash. Various laboratory abnormalities are common, including polyclonal hypergammaglobulinemia, anemia (often with a positive direct Coombs test), cold agglutinins, circulating immune complexes, cryoglobulins, antinuclear antibodies, and eosinophilia (22). Bone marrow involvement is common. The outcome of AILT is poor with a 5-year overall survival of 30% and median survival of 3 years (5). Infection is the most common cause of death, followed by the development of malignant lymphoma.

Histologically, the diagnosis of AITL is based on a constellation of findings, including (1) partial to complete obliteration of lymph node architecture, based initially in the paracortical region (Fig. 9-4); (2) a polymorphous infiltrate of neoplastic small and medium-sized lymphoid cells, often with clear cytoplasm, associated with plasma cells, eosinophils, and immunoblasts; (3) arborizing small blood vessels corresponding to epithelioid venules; and (4) absence (in most cases) of reactive lymphoid follicles (21,24). In many cases small and atrophic (so-called burned-out) germinal centers are present. In rare instances, however, cases of AITL display prominent reactive lymphoid follicles (25).

Immunophenotypic studies of AITL have shown that these lesions are composed predominantly of mature T cells that are usually of T-helper cell lineage (1). Expansion of interfollicular regions of CD3+, usually CD4+, cells are found. AILT has prominent vascularization by arborizing venules, expansion of CD21+ follicular dendritic cell (FDC) networks (26). CXCL13, a chemokine up-regulated in germinal center T-helper cells, may also be a useful marker in AILT (27,28). An aberrant T-cell immunophenotype is often identified and the neoplastic cells can express CD10 and BCL-6 in a subset of cases (24). Numerous follicular dendritic reticulum cells are common in AITL. B cells may be common in AITL, unlike most other types of PTCL, and can be numerous in early lesions.

Nonrandom chromosomal abnormalities have been identified in AITL (12,29). Trisomy 3 and trisomy 5 are most common, having been found in 15 to 20% of cases in one study (12). EBV is commonly associated with AITL, as shown by a variety of molecular methods (30).

Patients with AITL are at risk for developing diffuse large B-cell lymphoma (1). Diffuse large B-cell lymphomas arising in the setting of AITL express B-cell antigens, carry Ig gene rearrangements, and usually have abundant EBV (31). One hypothesis to explain this finding is that immunosuppression associated with AITL predisposes to EBV infection of B cells, increasing the likelihood of secondary molecular aberrations in B cells that result in DLBCL.

RARE TYPES OF T-CELL LYMPHOMA

A number of other types of mature T-cell lymphoma are described, each type being rare and representing <5% of all T-cell lymphomas.

Adult T-Cell Lymphoma/Leukemia

Adult T-cell lymphoma/leukemia (ATLL) is a distinct clinicopathologic entity associated with infection by the

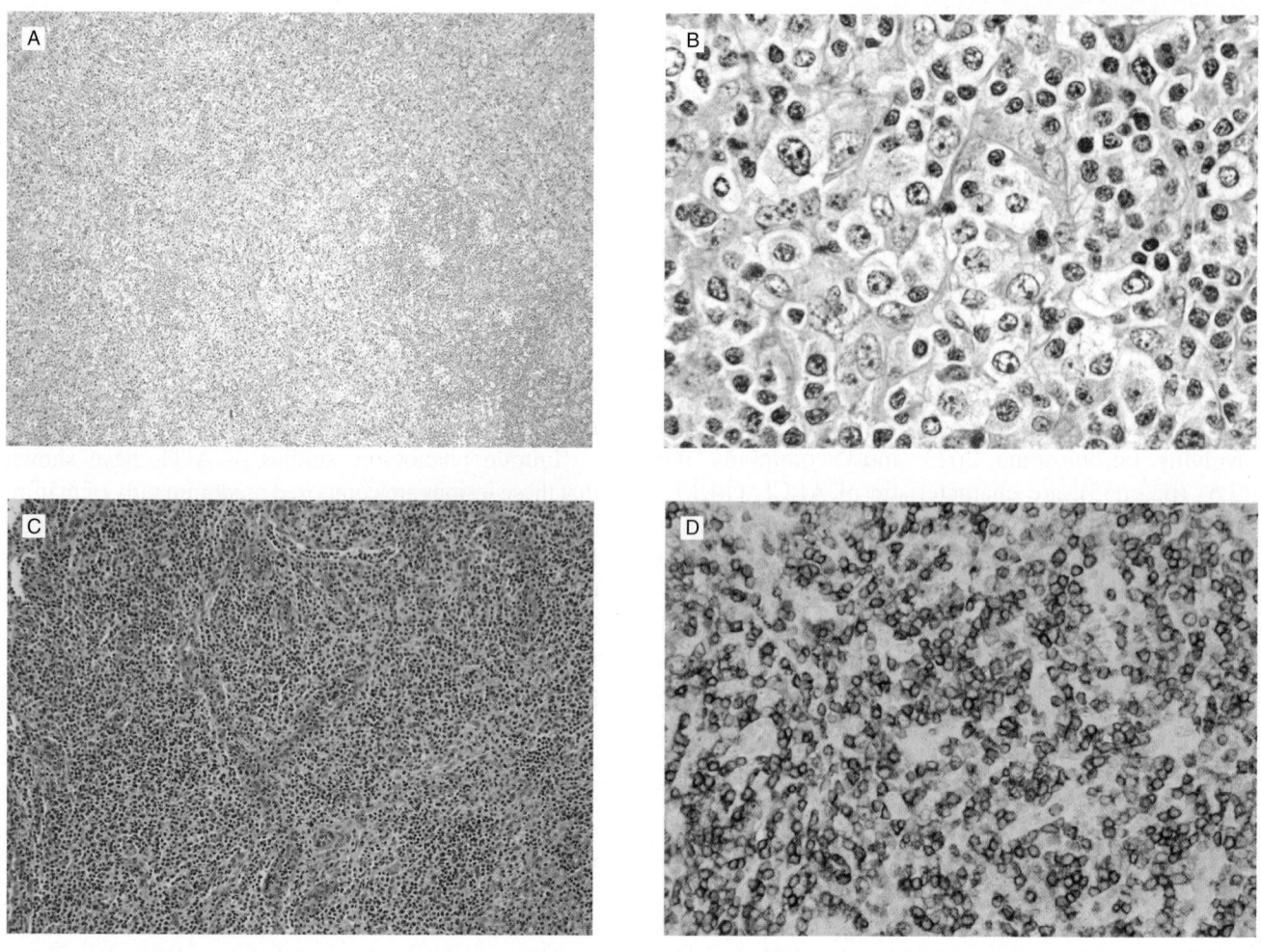

FIGURE 9-4. Angioimmunoblastic T-cell lymphoma. **A.** The neoplasm has a paracortical distribution. **B.** The neoplasm is composed of numerous cells with clear cytoplasm. **C.** In this field arborizing blood vessels are shown. **D.** The neoplastic cells are positive for CD3. (A -C, hemotoxylin-eosin; A, 100×; B, 1000×; C, 200×; D, immunohistochemistry, 400×.)

human T-cell leukemia/lymphoma retrovirus (HTLV-I) (1). HTLV-I is a single-stranded RNA retrovirus that is lymphotropic for T lymphocytes (32). ATLL develops in only 2 to 4% of patients who are carriers of the HTLV-1 virus (33). The virus is transmitted by sexual intercourse, breast milk, shared needles among intravenous drug users, and transfusion of blood products. The incubation period for development of ATLL ranges from 20 to 40 years. Patients with ATLL are usually adults, with a median age in the sixth decade (34). ATLL accounts for the high incidence of T-cell lymphoma in Japan. Clusters of cases have also been reported in Pacific Ocean islands, the Caribbean, Europe, and the southeastern United States.

ATLL is classified into four subtypes based on clinicopathologic features and prognosis: acute, lymphoma, chronic, and smoldering. Patients with acute ATLL, the most common form of the disease, have generalized lymphadenopathy, hepatosplenomegaly, skin lesions, peripheral blood involvement, lytic bone lesions, and hypercalcemia. Hypercalcemia may also develop in the absence of bone lesions, secondary to secretion of parathyroid hormone–related peptide (with activation of osteoclasts) by the neoplastic cells (35) (Fig. 9-5). The cerebrospinal fluid (CSF) is commonly involved. Patients with acute type had a median survival time of approximately 6 months. Lymphomatous ATLL is the second most common form of the disease. Patients present with prominent lymphadenopathy and tumors in other organs without hepatosplenomegaly or hypercalcemia or peripheral blood involvement. The prognosis of these patients is better than that of patients with acute ATLL with a median survival time of 10 months. Patients may also present with chronic ATLL, with an absolute lymphocytosis and cytologically abnormal cells in the peripheral blood. Skin lesions, lymphadenopathy,

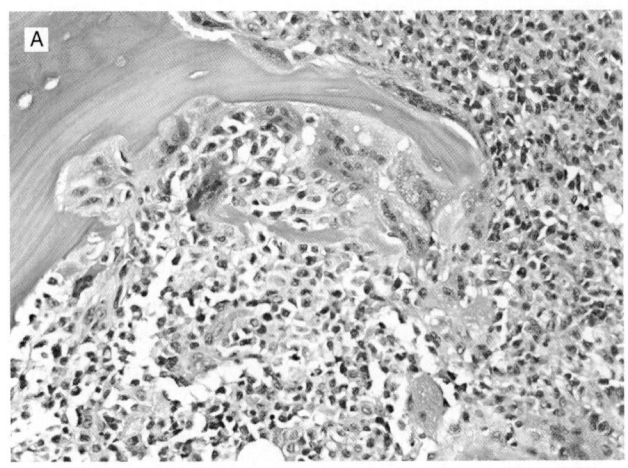

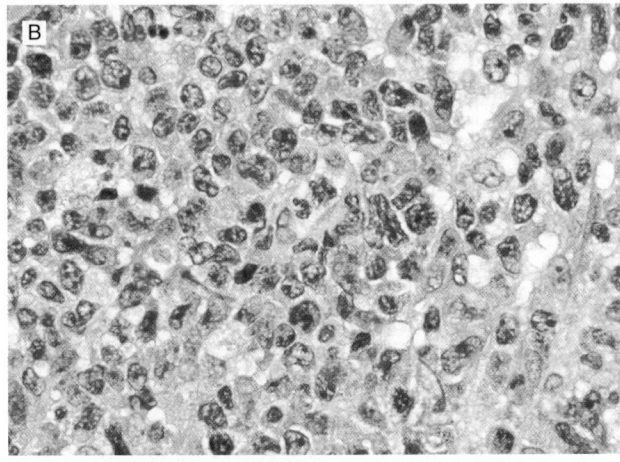

FIGURE 9-5. Adult T-cell leukemia/lymphoma involving bone. **A.** In this field, numerous osteoclasts are surrounding and resorbing bone. **B.** The neoplastic cells are large. (**A,B**, hematoxylin-eosin; **A**, 400×; **B**, 1000×.)

and involvement of other viscera may occur. These patients had a median survival time of 24 months. Finally, patients have been described with smoldering ATLL. These patients have chronic disease for years, usually skin lesions, with minimal peripheral blood involvement; the viscera are usually spared. The median survival time of patients with the smoldering type had not yet been reached.

In the peripheral blood, the neoplastic cells are medium-sized, with basophilic cytoplasm and markedly irregular, multilobulated nuclei, including cloverleaf shapes (also known as flower cells) (36). The neoplastic cells in lymph nodes and viscera involved by ATLL exhibit a spectrum of cell sizes, including small, medium-sized, and large, with relatively round or markedly irregular nuclear contours. Histologic findings do not correlate with survival (36).

Immunophenotypic studies have shown that ATLLs have a mature T-cell immunophenotype (1,34). The tumor cells express pan-T-cell antigens and TCR αβ and are CD4+ CD8−. Characteristically, the neoplastic cells intensely express the CD25 antigen.

A study done by Itoyama et al (37) examined the cytogenetic abnormalities in 50 patients with newly diagnosed ATLL. All had abnormal karyotypes and almost all chromosomes were affected. Multiple chromosomal breaks (more than 6) and aneuploidy were significantly more frequent in patients with the combined acute and lymphoma subtypes than in those with chronic ATLL. These results suggest a multistep pathogenesis for ATLL. The hallmark of ATLL is the demonstration of HTLV-1, either serologically by detection of serum antibodies or by molecular detection of the virus. The virus integrates clonally into the host cell genome in random fashion (32). HTLV-1 proteins, such as TAX, may stimulate cell growth by interacting with cell cycle proteins (38).

Extranodal NK/T-Cell Lymphoma, Nasal-Type

The term extranodal NK/T-cell lymphoma, nasal-type, is used in the WHO classification for a neoplasm previously designated as lethal midline granuloma, polymorphic reticulosis, midline malignant reticulosis, angiocentric immunoproliferative lesion, and angiocentric lymphoma (1,39,40).

Clinically, extranodal NK/T-cell lymphomas of nasal-type have a propensity for involving extranodal sites, most commonly the nasal cavity, nasopharynx, and palate (39). However, these tumors can involve other extranodal sites such as skin, soft tissue, gastrointestinal tract, and testis at time of diagnosis, and relapses commonly involve extranodal sites (41). Lymph node and bone marrow are rarely involved. These neoplasms can be associated with a hemophagocytic syndrome clinically characterized by fever, hepatosplenomegaly, pancytopenia, and laboratory evidence of hemolysis (40). EBV is thought to play a role in tumor pathogenesis, but the mechanism is unknown. NK/TCLs are dominant PTCL type in Asian populations (42). It has an aggressive course with 5-year overall survival ranging from 25 to 50% (43).

Histologically, extranodal NK/T-cell lymphomas of nasal-type are composed of a mixture of atypical lymphoid cells admixed with reactive lymphocytes and histiocytes (1,39). Eosinophils and neutrophils are rare or absent. In the early stages of disease, relatively few neoplastic cells are present, and they may be of small size. Over time, these neoplasms accrue greater numbers of large atypical cells and the diagnosis is

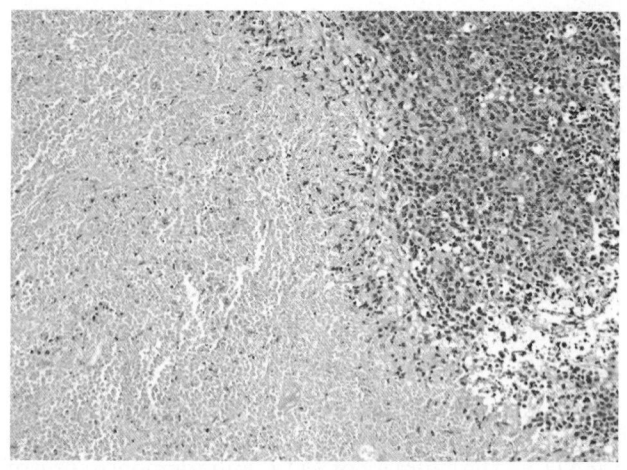

FIGURE 9-6. Extranodal NK/T-cell lymphoma, nasal-type, involving nasopharynx. Extensive necrosis (left of field) is common in these neoplasms (hematoxylin-eosin, 200×).

more easily established. These neoplasms can display a marked propensity for invading and destroying blood vessels, but angiocentricity is not a universal feature (1). Necrosis is common (Fig. 9-6).

Immunophenotypic studies of extranodal NK/T-cell lymphomas of nasal type suggest that most neoplasms are of NK-cell origin, although rare cases are of T-cell lineage. Thus, most neoplasms express the NK cell–associated antigen CD56 and NK/T cell–associated antigens such as CD2, CD7, and CD8. These tumors also express cytoplasmic CD3 but are negative for T cell–specific antigens such as surface CD3, CD5, and T-cell receptors. CD16 and CD57 are often negative.

Molecular studies of extranodal NK/T-cell lymphomas of nasal type have demonstrated an absence of TCR and Ig gene rearrangements in most cases studied (36). EBV genomes have been identified in the neoplastic cells (44,45). Comparative genomic hybridization studies have shown chromosomal losses at 1p, 12q, and 17p and chromosomal gains at 2q, 10q, and 13q in subsets of tumors (46).

Enteropathy-Type T-Cell Lymphoma

These neoplasms are rare and have been designated previously as enteropathy-associated T-cell lymphoma and intestinal T-cell lymphoma (1). Patients with enteropathy-type T-cell lymphoma (ETL) present with abdominal pain or weight loss (47). Although initially described in patients with a history of gluten-sensitive enteropathy or celiac disease, who are known to have an increased incidence of lymphoma, these tumors also arise commonly in patients without a known history of celiac disease

(47,48). Clinically, it affects older males presenting with abdominal pain, diarrhea, and intestinal perforation or obstruction. Dissemination to the liver, spleen, lung, skin, and bone marrow can occur. Survival is extremely poor (49).

Grossly, the involved intestine demonstrates multiple ulcers (Fig. 9-7); a distinct mass may not be found. The ulcers may extend deeply into the bowel wall, often resulting in perforation. The jejunum is the most common site of involvement. Histologically, the intestine not involved by neoplasm may exhibit blunting of villi as is seen in celiac disease (48). These neoplasms are diffuse and the neoplastic cells are a mixture of small, medium-sized, and large lymphoid cells (Fig. 9-7).

Immunophenotypic studies have shown that ETLs express pan-T-cell antigens, are often CD4– CD8– or CD4– CD8+, and usually have a cytotoxic profile, positive

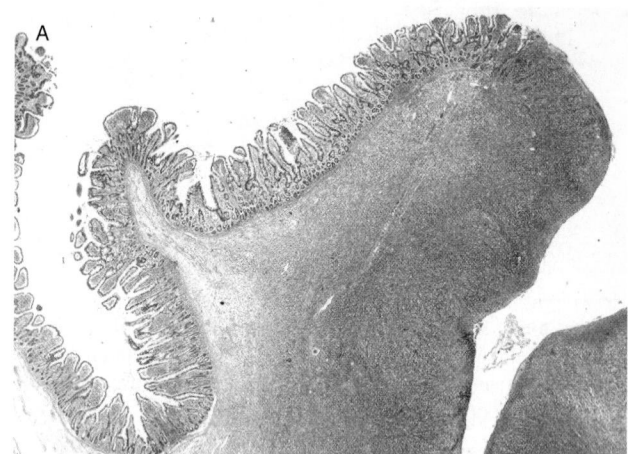

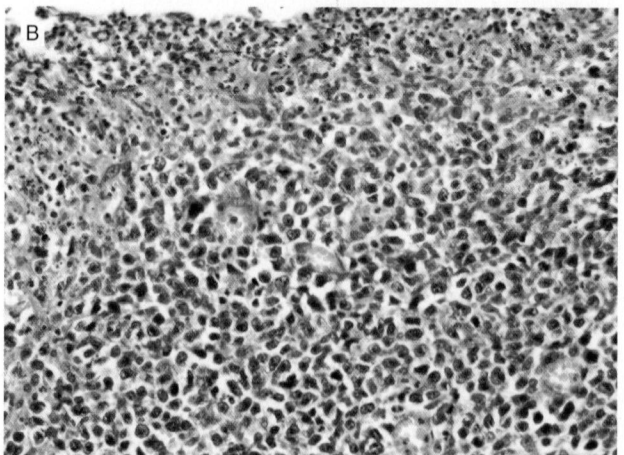

FIGURE 9-7. Enteropathy-type T-cell lymphoma. **A.** This field shows the transition from benign mucosa (left of field) to lymphoma and ulcer. **B.** The neoplastic cells are large. (**A,B**, hematoxylin-eosin; **A**, 20×; **B**, 400×.)

for TIA-1, granzyme B, and perforin. A subset of tumors is positive for EBV, CD30, CD56, or CD103 (48,50).

Hepatosplenic T-Cell Lymphoma

Hepatosplenic T-cell lymphoma (HSTCL) is a rare neoplasm that most commonly affects young adults, who present with marked hepatosplenomegaly and minimal or absent lymphadenopathy; there is a male predominance (51,52). Bone marrow involvement is common but often subtle (53). Skin lesions may occur. B symptoms such as fever, weight loss, and night sweats were frequently reported, as well as fatigue, arthralgia, myalgia, and abdominal pain (54-56). These tumors were originally called hepatosplenic γ/δ lymphoma (51). However, as a subset of cases may express the TCR α/β, the WHO classification designates these neoplasms as HSTCLs (1).

Fewer than 200 cases of HSTCL reported in the literature (1). Although the majority of these cases seem to have developed de novo, approximately a third have been associated with immunosuppressive therapy for various reasons, mostly for organ transplantations and other conditions that require immune-modifying agents; most cases involving thiopurines (54,57). Several immunocompromised conditions described in the literature include renal transplantation, heart transplantation, Hodgkin lymphoma, acute myelogenous leukemia, inflammatory bowel disease, and malaria infection (58-62). Cases of HSTCL are also associated with viral infections, including human herpes virus 6, hepatitis B virus, and Epstein–Barr virus (63,64).

HSTCL has a very aggressive clinical course. The long-term outcome is poor as many patients die within 1 year after diagnosis (8). A variety of therapeutic options have been explored, including splenectomy, CHOP-like combination of cytotoxic regimens, purine analogues, monoclonal antibodies, and autologous and allogeneic stem cell transplantation. However, no treatment option seems to improve life expectancy (65).

Histologically, these neoplasms are diffuse and composed of medium-sized lymphoid cells with slightly irregular nuclear contours, condensed chromatin, and small nucleoli (51). In the liver, HSTCL infiltrates sinusoids and spares portal tracts. In the spleen, the red pulp is involved and the white pulp spared (Fig. 9-8). In the bone marrow, the neoplastic cells can resemble blasts in aspirate smears and are commonly intrasinusoidal in core biopsy specimens (53).

Immunophenotypic studies have demonstrated that HSTCLs have a mature but aberrant T-cell immunophenotype. Most cases are negative for CD4 and CD8, but a

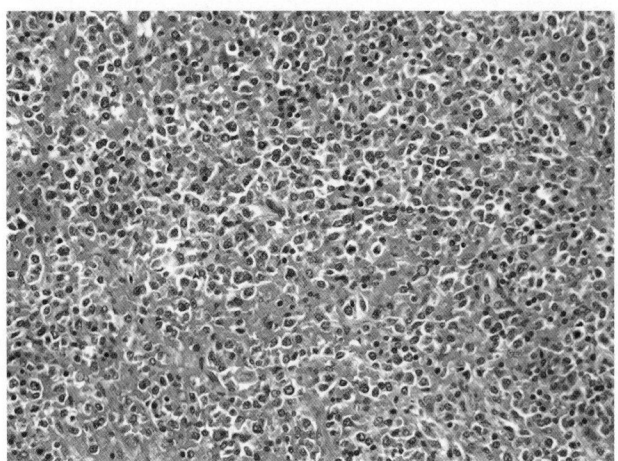

FIGURE 9-8. Hepatosplenic T-cell lymphoma involving spleen (hematoxylin-eosin, 400×).

subset may express CD8. CD5 is usually absent. CD56 is usually positive, a subset may express CD16, and CD57 is negative. These neoplasms commonly have a nonfunctional (or immature) cytotoxic profile, positive for TIA-1 but negative for granzyme B and perforin (66). At the cytogenetic level, HSTCLs often carry a characteristic cytogenetic abnormality, isochromosome (7q), and trisomy of chromosome 8 (67).

Subcutaneous Panniculitis-Like T-Cell Lymphoma

Subcutaneous panniculitis-like T-cell lymphoma (SPTCL) is the least well-defined and rarest type of PTCL. Patients with SPTCLs are usually adults, who present with multiple subcutaneous nodules, resembling lipomas (1,68). Approximately, one-third of patients present with a hemophagocytic syndrome, causing systemic symptoms with pancytopenia, fever, and hepatosplenomegaly. Additional patients develop hemophagocytic syndrome at some point in the course of their disease.

Histologically, SPTCLs involve subcutaneous tissue, with minimal involvement of overlying dermis (1). The neoplastic cells infiltrate the septa of adipose tissue and surrounding fat cells; marked coagulative necrosis and fat necrosis are common, resembling panniculitis (Fig. 9-9). Nevertheless, at high power, the tumor cells are cytologically atypical and may be a mixture of small and large cells or predominantly large cells. Large cells accrue over time. Karyorrhexis is often prominent and mitotic figures are easily identified.

Immunophenotypic studies have shown that SPTCLs have a mature T-cell immunophenotype (1,69). Most cases of SPTCL express TCR α/β. A subset of cases of SPTCL that express TCR γ/δ have been reported.

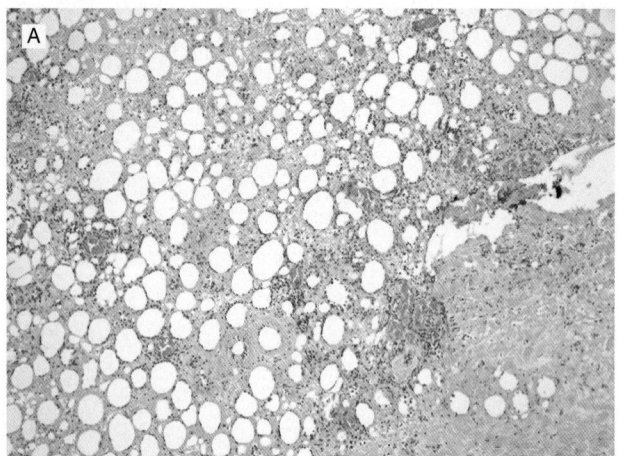

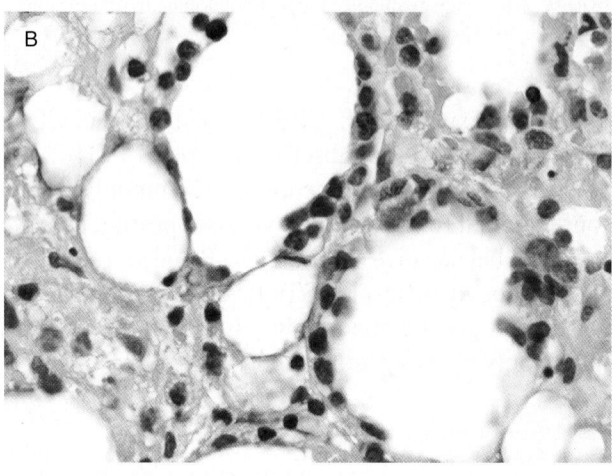

FIGURE 9-9. Subcutaneous panniculitis-like T-cell lymphoma. **A.** The neoplasm involves adipose tissue and is associated with extensive fat necrosis in this field. **B.** The neoplastic lymphocytes surround fat spaces. (Hematoxylineosin; **A**, 100×; **B**, 1000×.)

These cases have a more aggressive clinical course, and a consensus is building for considering these neoplasms a distinct disease (70). SPTCLs have a cytotoxic T-cell profile, positive for TIA-1, perforin, and granzyme B. SPTCLs are usually BCL-2–negative (69).

■ APPROACH TO THERAPY

PTCLs are generally treated much the same as other aggressive B-cell non-Hodgkin lymphomas where most patients will receive the CHOP regimen. In one study, the complete response rate reported for PTCL was about 19% with the overall response rate about 20 to 25% (71). A recent retrospective analysis of T-NHL patients treated at MD Anderson Cancer Center showed that patients treated with CHOP had similar survival

outcome as those treated with more intensive regimens (73). Given the poor outcome with conventional chemotherapy, increasingly more and more patients are being referred to stem cell transplant in first remission. However, due to lack of randomized or prospective data, this approach should be considered investigational. Retrospective data from Memorial Sloan Kettering Cancer Center showed that less than 20% of patients remained in long-term remission after salvage therapy with ifosfamide, carboplatin, and etoposide (ICE), followed by autologous stem cell transplant. To improve the outcome in this patient population, new agents need to be investigated to find an effective treatment regimen.

PRIMARY TREATMENT IN PTCLS

Nodal PTCL

For ALK-positive ALCL, CHOP-like chemotherapy is effective with complete response rates similar to diffuse large B-cell lymphoma and failure-free survival of 58% at 5 years (7). However, CHOP is inadequate therapy for most patients with ALK-negative ALCL PTCL (5). Intensifying chemotherapy by using dose-dense etoposide-containing therapy (cyclophosphamide, doxorubicin, vindesine, etoposide, and prednisone [CHOEP-14]) does not seem to have had a significant impact with one study reporting CR in only 31 (40%) of 77 patients after three cycles and with 25% either failing to respond or relapsing before reaching planned autologous stem cell transplant (ASCT) (72). In addition, neither hyperCVAD (cyclophosphamide, vincristine, doxorubicin, dexamethasone, cytarabine, and methotrexate) regimen (73) nor intensive anthracycline-based chemotherapy ACVBP (doxorubicin, cyclophosphamide, vindesine, bleomycin, and prednisone) (74) has improved outcome in PTCL patients.

Extranodal PTCL

Patients with IE nasal disease may be successfully treated with radiotherapy alone provided that doses of 50 to 55 Gy are used (75,76). Five-year overall survival and progression free survival were 78% and 63%, respectively (76). For invasive disease beyond the nasopharynx, local nodal involvement, stage IIE disease, and possibly Ki67 50% or higher, outcome is better when radiotherapy is administered before chemotherapy. Patients with stage III/IV disease or nasal type natural killer/T-cell disease outcome is poor with median overall survival less than 1 year when conventional dose chemotherapy is used.

The use of anthracycline based regimens for hepatosplenic PTCL is associated with short-duration responses and overall 5-year survival rates of 12 to 20%

(54). Patients with enteropathy-type PTCLs are frequently malnourished and have poor performance status. Median survival is 7.5 months (77) with standard chemotherapy. Patients with subcutaneous panniculitis-like PTCL presented with hemophagocytic syndrome in 37%. Anthracycline-based regimens produced durable CR in 30% of patients (78) but presence of HPS or γ/δ TCR was associated with poor survival.

Adult T-cell Leukemia/Lymphoma

Eighty-seven percent of patients fall into the lymphoma subtype. Five-year overall and failure-free survivals were 14 and 12%, respectively, in the 126 patients diagnosed in the International T-cell Lymphoma Project (79). A variety of standard treatment modalities were used, none of which proved to be superior. Although response rates to interferon-α and zidovudine have been high, remissions have not been durable. Chemotherapy plus zidovudine and interferon in one study was associated with a median survival of 17 months (80).

Hematopoietic Stem Cell Transplant

There is limited experience using either autologous or allogeneic stem cell transplant in patients with PTCL. Much of the data comes from small trials or anecdotal reports. Although autologous SCT appears to be effective salvage for some and might be recommended in the first remission for patients with nodal PTCL (excluding ALK-positive ALCL), outcome is highly dependent on complete response status at transplant and most of these studies are overwhelmed by suboptimal complete response rates to induction therapy, inclusion of patients with ALK-positive ALCL and under-representation of adult T-cell lymphoma and extranodal PTCLs. The allogeneic stem cell transplant experience for PTCL is more limited. This modality may be of greatest importance for the more chemo-resistant extranodal tumors such as the nasal-type natural killer/T-cell lymphomas and ATLL.

NOVEL TREATMENT

Table 9-2 shows the new agents used to treat peripheral T-cell lymphoma (81).

Gemcitabine

Gemcitabine is a nucleoside analog with significant activity in lymphoid malignancies. Gemcitabine has been shown to be a highly active agent as salvage therapy in both CTCL and PTCL with single-agent activity of 60 to 70% in both types (82). It competes with the nucleotide deoxycytidine and inhibits DNA synthase and ribonucleotide reductase. Combination chemotherapy incorporating gemcitabine has been of interest given the single-agent activity of this agent in T-cell lymphoma.

TABLE 9-2 NEW AGENTS IN PERIPHERAL T-CELL LYMPHOMA

Study	Target	Subtype, N	ORR (Complete Response) (%)
Nucleoside analog			
Gemcitabine	Nucleoside analog	PTCL, 10	60 (20)
Gemcitabine + cisplatin + dexamethasone	Nucleoside analog	TCL, 5	40
Gemcitabine + cisplatin + methylprednisolone	Nucleoside analog	PTCL, 16	69 (19)
Immunotoxins			
Denileukin diftitox	Interleukin-2 receptor	PTCL, 27	48 (22)
Folate analog			
Pralatrexate	Folate analog	PTCL, 109	27 (9)
Monoclonal antibodies			
MDX-060	CD30	ALCL, 7	29 (26)
SGN-30	CD30	ALCL, 39	21 (5)
SGN-35	CD30	ALCL, 2	100
Zanolimumab	CD4	PTCL, 21	23 (9)
Histone deacetylase inhibitor			
Depsipeptide	Histone deacetylation	PTCL, 48	31 (18)
Belinostat	Histone deacetylation	PTCL, 11	18

Abbreviations: ALCL, anaplastic large-cell lymphoma; ORR, overall response rate; PTCL, peripheral T-cell lymphoma; CTCL, cutaneous T-cell lymphoma. (Reproduced, with permission, from Pro B. Novel agents in peripheral T-cell lymphomas. In: *American Society of Clinical Oncology Education Booklet* 2009;486-489.)

Several studies were conducted with gemcitabine-based combinations. Twenty-six patients with PTCL in a study were treated with a regimen consisting of CHOP combined with gemcitabine and etoposide (83). The complete response rate was 62% at a median follow-up duration of 383 days. Estimated overall survival at 1 year was 70%. A study at the Royal Marsden Hospital showed the overall response rate was 69% in 16 patients treated for refractory PTCL with gemcitabine, cisplatin, and methylprednisolone. Three patients (19%) had complete remission. The 1-year overall survival was 68% and median time to progression was 123 days. However, hematologic toxicity was significant and two patients developed bowel perforation (84).

Denileukin Diftitox (Ontak)

Denileukin diftitox is a recombinant cytotoxic protein comprising the interleukin-2 (IL-2) ligand genetically fused to the membrane translocation domains of the diphtheria toxin. Once bound to the IL-2 receptor, the toxin is endocytosed and cleaved, releasing the toxin that inhibits protein synthesis, leading to apoptosis. IL2-receptor (IL-2R) is a marker of T-cell differentiation and the CD25 subunit of this receptor is expressed in a subset of patients with PTCL-U and CD30+ ALCL.

In a phase II trial, the overall response rate was 48 and 22% of 27 patients with relapsed PTCL achieved a complete remission. Twenty-nine percent of patients had stable disease. Patients with CD-25 positive status had higher response rate (61%) than patients with CD25 negative status (45%). Median progression-free survival was 6 months. Adverse events were generally mild. The most common were hypoalbuminemia, transaminase elevation, edema, and skin reaction (85). Studies are ongoing combining this agent with CHOP.

Pralatrexate

Pralatrexate is a novel folate antagonist with a high affinity for the reduced folate carrier (RFC-1) and is more efficiently internalized and retained than methotrexate. At a dose of 30 mg/m^2 weekly for 6 of 7 weeks, the overall response rate was 63% in 16 patients with PTCL and included nine complete responses and one partial response (86).

A multicenter registration phase II study of pralatrexate (PDX 008) in patients with relapsed or refractory PTCL completed accrual. Study design included supplementation with vitamin B12 and folic acid to reduce the risk of mucositis. Patients were heavily pretreated and had failed a median of three prior regimens. The overall response rate was 27%, with 9% patients achieving complete response and 17% partial response. The most common grades 3 to 4 toxicities were thrombocytopenia and mucositis (87). Furthermore, pralatrexate and gemcitabine synergize in a schedule-dependent manner in cell lines in vitro and lymphoma xenografts (88). This combination is currently being evaluated in a phases I to II study.

FDA granted accelerated approval in September 2009 to pralatrexate injection (Fotolyn) for the treatment of patients with relapsed or refractory PTCL based on the PDX 008 trial. As a condition of the accelerated approval, randomized controlled trials are required after approval to verify the clinical benefit.

Histone Deacetylase Inhibitors

Histone deacetylase inhibitors (HDAC inhibitors) are inducers of acetylation of histones and other nonhistone proteins. HDAC inhibition results in accumulation of acetylated nucleosomal histones and induces differentiation and/or apoptosis in transformed cells.

Vorinostat (suberoylanilide hydroxamic acid) is the first FDA approved HDAC inhibitor for the treatment of refractory cutaneous T-cell lymphoma (CTCL) in October 2006. The overall response rate was 30% and the median duration of response was not reached but estimated to be at least 185 days (89). It is currently under investigation in combination with other agents for the treatment of PTCLs. Romidepsin, previously known as depsipeptide or FK228, has been shown to induce cell cycle arrest and apoptosis in many cell lines. It demonstrated activity in relapsed PTCL patients with an ORR 26%. Romidepsin was recently approved in September 2009 for treatment of CTCL. Belinostat (PDX101) is another pan-HDAC inhibitor being tested in PTCL. Ongoing phase II study reported two complete responses and five cases of stable disease in 11 patients with PTCL.

IMMUNOTHERAPY

Alemtuzumab

Alemtuzumab, a humanized monoclonal antibody directed against the CD52 antigen, present on most malignant T cells, making it an attractive target for PTCL. As a single agent in heavily pretreated patients with PTCL the overall response rate with alemtuzumab was 36% in one report (90).

Zanolimumab

Zanolimumab is a fully human immunoglobulin G1 κ monoclonal antibody that targets the CD4 antigen present on T-helper lymphocytes. It inhibits CD4 positive T-cell by combining signaling inhibition with the induction of Fc-dependent effector mechanisms. Preliminary result of a phase II study in 21 patients demonstrated activity of 23%, with two complete responses, one in a patient with PTCL-U and another in a patient with AITL. Toxicities include transient myelosuppression and infusion-related adverse events (91).

Anti-CD30 Monoclonal Antibodies

CD30 is uniformly expressed in ALCL and in 30% of unspecified PTCL. It is minimally expressed on normal cells. SGN-30 is a CD30-specific chimeric antibody constructed from the variable regions of the anti-CD30 murine monoclonal AC10 and the human γ 1 heavy chain and κ light chain constant regions (81).

A multicenter, single-arm phase II trial enrolled 39 patients with refractory or relapsed ALCL treated with SGN-30 at a planned dose of 6 mg/kg per week for 6 weeks. Nine patients had received prior stem cell transplants, and 85% had ALK-negative tumors. Two patients achieved complete remission and six had a partial remission, for an overall response rate of 21% (92).

MDX-60 is a human anti-CD30 immunoglobulin G1 κ monoclonal antibody that has been shown to inhibit the growth of CD30-expressing tumor cells in preclinical models. Ansell et al. reported results of a phases I to II study in patients with recurrent HL and ALCL (93). The treatment was well tolerated. Of the seven patients with ALCL, two (28%) achieved complete remission. Ongoing trials are investigating the effect of MDX-060 in systemic or cutaneous ALCL as single agent (93).

SGN-35 is an antibody drug conjugate consisting of the chimeric antibody SGN-30 chemically conjugated to a synthetic analog of the naturally occurring antitubulin agent dolastatin 10. The mechanism is initiated by binding to CD30 and internalization with subsequent release of monomethylauristatin E, leading to G2/M phase cell cycle arrest and apoptosis. A phase I single arm study of SNG-35 has been conducted in patients with relapsed CD30-positive lymphomas. Most patients achieved best clinical response within 12 weeks, and treatment was well tolerated (94).

Other Agents

Bortezomib, a proteasome inhibitor, showed significant activity in various lymphomas. A recent phase II study demonstrated 67% response rate in 12 patients with recurrent CTCL or PTCL and isolated skin relapse. Patients received bortezomib at a dose of 1.3 mg/m^2 IV on days 1, 4, 8, and 11 every 21 days. This agent is currently being evaluated in PTCL as single agent and in combination with chemotherapy (95).

Lenalidomide is a structural analog of thalidomide with demonstrated activity in multiple myeloma and myelodysplastic syndrome. Early results from an ongoing phase II multicenter clinical trial demonstrated some evidence of clinical activity. Among nine evaluable patients, the reported response rate was 44%, with four patients achieving partial response. The most common toxicities were hematological and infectious complications (96).

■ CUTANEOUS T-CELL LYMPHOMAS

CTCLs are a clinically heterogeneous group of post-thymic lymphomas, accounting for the majority of all lymphomas arising in skin. Mycosis fungoides (MF) and Sézary syndrome (SS) are defined by their cutaneous lesions that result from the accumulation of a T-helper memory/effector subset with a CD4+, CD8−, CD45RO+CLA+ phenotype in skin and blood (97). Most commonly, MF starts as an indolent and chronic dermatitis in the sun shielded areas. A diagnostic biopsy is difficult to obtain in early MF because there are similarities with eczema or contact dermatitis.

■ CLASSIFICATION

MFs is staged using the Tumor Nodes Metastasis classification schema for the purpose of predicting disease prognosis (Fig. 9-10). MFs and SS, the most common variants, are still rare with an annual incidence of three to four new cases per million or 1200 new cases per year

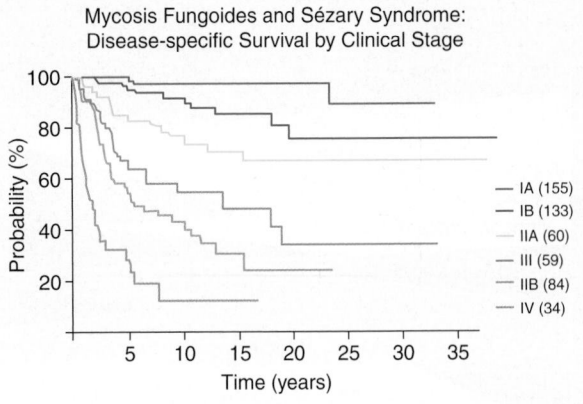

FIGURE 9-10. Mycosis fungoides and Sézary syndrome: disease-specific survival by clinical stage. Disease-specific survival of 525 patients with MF and Sézary syndrome was measured according to clinical stage at diagnosis. *(Reproduced, with permission, Kim YH, Liu HL, Mraz-Gernhard S, et al. Long-term outcome of 525 patients with mycosis fungoides and Sézary Syndrome. Arch Dermatol. 2003; 139:857-866. Copyright © 2003 American Medical Association. All rights reserved.)*

in the United States (98,99). The next most common entities are the CD30+ lymphoproliferative disorders: lymphomatoid papulosus and ALCL. Subcutaneous panniculitic T-cell lymphoma and NK-T-cell lymphomas are quite rare and more aggressive (Table 9-1).

PRESENTATION AND DIAGNOSIS

The ISCL has developed an algorithm to diagnose early stage MF. The clinical diagnosis is based on two points from the following: a chronic, persistant dermatitis, or poikilodermatous changes or heterogeneous lesions appearing on sun-shielded areas. Histological factors include atypical lymphocytes within the epidermis (epidermotropism) and a predominance of CD4+CD8+ cells with loss of other T-cell markers. The finding of clonality with respect to the T-cell receptor gene rearrangement is not diagnostic but helps to support (one point) the diagnosis of lymphoma over reactive process. MF may progress to a leukemic and erythrodermic condition called SS. SS is defined by erythroderma of >80% of the body plus the presence of >1000 per μL of atypical circulating cells found in the peripheral blood. By flow cytometry, most patients have increased numbers of CD4+CD26− cells. In the skin of SS patients, the atypical cells have lost epidermotropism and are found around the dermal vessels rather than in the epidermis. Sézary cells secrete Th2 cytokines,

IL-4, and IL-10, causing loss of cellular immunity due to decreased production of Th1 cytokines, interferon-γ, and IL-2 (100). This results in atopy characterized by erythroderma and staphylococcus colonization, peripheral eosinophilia, increased IgE production, and intractable pruritus. Molecular methods have shown that in MF there is emergence of one or more T-cell clones of skin-homing CD4+ cells and that with progression to SS, these appear in the blood and can be detected by flow cytometry (101).

PROGNOSIS

The predictive factors for survival are the T classification, extracutaneous manifestation, and age of the patient (102). Independent adverse prognostic factors are large-cell transformation, follicular mucinosis, thickness of tumor infiltrate, elevated LDH, and β_2-microglobulin (103,104). Patients with SS have worse prognosis. A high Sézary cell count, loss of T-cell subset markers such as CD5 and CD7, and chromosomal abnormalities in T cells are also associated with a poor outcome (105).

APPROACH TO THERAPY

Figure 9-11 summarizes the primary treatment map for CTCL.

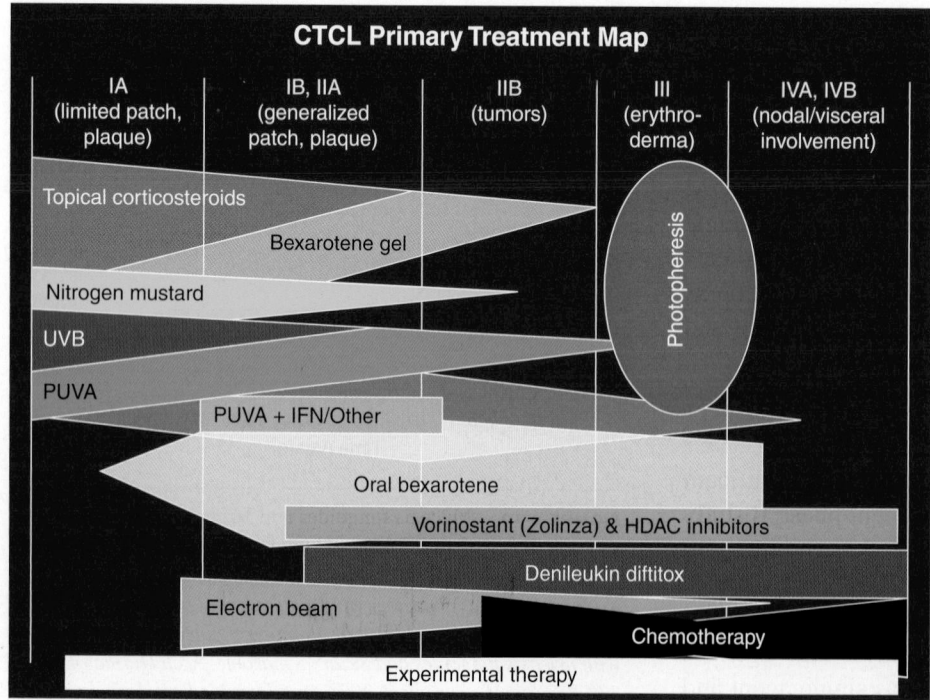

FIGURE 9-11. CTCL primary treatment map.

Current Treatment for Early Mycosis Fungoides

There are a limited number of FDA-approved therapies available to treat patients with MF/SS. However, topical agents used for eczema, psoriasis, and other forms of lymphoma and phototherapy are used and represent the standard of care for early MF.

Early MF (stage IA) is characterized by eczematous or psoriasiform dermatitis limited to less than 10% of the body surface. Early MF lesions are treated with one or more of the available skin-directed therapies. Combination therapy is the norm. The first therapy is usually topically applied corticosteroids of increasing potency. For thicker or hypertrophic lesions, the topical retinoid gels or creams may help to restore normal epidermal differentiation and reduce the time of clearing with phototherapy. The response rate of targretin gel 1% was 76% in patients not previously treated and this agent is the only topical therapy approved for MF (106). We have also found this gel to be useful for MF of the hands or feet (107), for aborting lymphomatoid papulosis lesions (108) or tumors of MF. Nitrogen mustard (mustargen) is also widely used for the topical treatment of stage I MF. Although it is not yet approved by the FDA, a randomized, two arm multicenter trial has recently been completed.

Current Treatment for Intermediate or Refractory/Transformed MFs and SS

Patients with <10% involvement (IA) who do not respond to first-line topical therapies or who have >10% of the body surface area (IB) or dermatopathic nodes (IIA) often need more extensive therapies such as topical chemotherapy with mustargen, BCNU, or with a combination of skin directed therapy plus one or more biological response modifiers. Agents that are not specifically approved for MF/SS are commonly used as the standard of care: topical steroids and mustargen, phototherapy, interferons, and chemotherapies (Table 9-3). For patch disease, narrow band UVB is effective and can be effectively combined with topical steroids, retinoids, or interferon. Thick plaque lesions or folliculotropic MF lesions are more difficult to clear and are treated with PUVA plus interferon or an oral retinoid (bexarotene, soriatane, or accutane) but often require radiation. Total electron beam radiation is reserved for patients who need skin palliation or who have extensive skin involvement and have failed to respond to skin-directed therapies, and should be followed with a form of maintenance therapy such as mustargen, PUVA, or oral bexarotene.

Intravenous denileukin diftitox (Ontak) and oral bexarotene have received FDA approval in 1998 and

TABLE 9-3	OVERVIEW OF CURRENT THERAPEUTIC OPTIONS FOR MF/SS

Skin directed therapy
- Topical corticosteroids
- Topical chemotherapy (eg, nitrogen mustard, carmustine)
- Topical retinoids (bexarotene, tazarotene)
- Topical imiquimod
- Phototherapy (UVB, NbUVB, PUVA)
- Electron beam therapy

Biological therapy
- RXR retinoid (bexarotene)
- RAR retinoid (isotretinoin)
- Interferons
- Granulocyte-macrophage colony-stimulating factor
- Extracorporeal photopheresis
- Fusion protein/toxin (denileukin difitox)

Other systemic therapies
- Cytotoxic chemotherapy (methotrexate, doxil, gemcitabine, etoposide, pentostatin)
- Bone marrow/stem cell transplantation

Experimental therapies
- HDAC inhibitors (vorinostat, depsipeptide)
- Transimmunization extracorporeal photopheresis
- Targeted monoclonal antibodies (CD52, CCR4, CD4)
- Cytokines (IL-I2, IL-2)
- TLR agonists (CpG oligodeoxynucleotides)
- Tumor vaccines

UVB, ultraviolet B light; NbUVB, narrow-band ultraviolet B light; PUVA, psoralen plus ultraviolet A light; RXR, retinoid X receptor; RAR, retinoic acid receptor; TLR, toll-like receptor 9; IL, interleukin. (Data from Kim EJ, Hess S, Richardson SK, et al. Immunopathogenesis and therapy of cutaneous T cell lymphoma. *J Clin Invest* 2005;115:798-812.)

1999, respectively, for treatment of the cutaneous manifestations of CTCL. Both are used in the setting of more advanced skin disease. Ontak received FDA approval for treatment of CTCL of all stages based on a randomized two dose arm controlled multicenter trial showing a response rate of 30% (109). Complete responses were seen in 10% of the patients enrolled (109). Capillary leak syndrome is seen in 20 to 30% of patients but may be decreased with hydration and acute fusion reactions are blocked by steroid pre-medication. Our study suggested that high expression of CD25+ in >20% of the tumor cells was associated with higher response rates 60% compared to 20% of the low expressing patient and 30% in the pivotal trial. Bexarotene and steroids may increase CD25 expression on T cells as measured by flow and could suggest synergism (110). Bexarotene monotherapy has a response rate of 54% at a dose of 300 mg/m^2 in early patients and 45% in more advanced patients (111). Its dose-limiting toxicity is hypertriglyceridemia but can often be controlled with addition of an HMG-coA reductase and/or a statin (112).

Patients with transformed MF, tumors, or nodal disease respond to local radiation, denileukin diftitox (Ontak), nucleoside analogues (gemcitabine, pentostatin), doxil, histone deacetylase inhibitors, or combination chemotherapy but often the duration of response is limited. Various chemotherapy combinations, while effective for a limited time, can also induce further immunosuppression leading to line induced sepsis or other opportunistic infections.

Generalized exfoliative erythroderma (EE) is found in patients with blood involvement (SS). Extracorporeal photopheresis was approved in 1987 for the treatment of CTCL patients and significant responses were seen in erythrodermic patients (113). Photopheresis is usually combined with biological response modifiers, especially interferon α or γ, and retinoids, for responses approaching 60 to 70% (114).

■ NOVEL TREATMENTS

The recent FDA-approved HDAC inhibitors, vorinostat (Zolinza) in 2006, and depsipeptide (Romidepsin) in 2009, represent a new strategy for targeted therapy of CTCL and were effective in patients who were highly refractory to chemotherapy and other agents. Their mechanism of action, like retinoids, involves inducing transcription of genes that control differentiation and apoptosis selectively in malignant cells. Oral Vorinostat was well tolerated at a dose of 400 mg daily and had a rapid onset of action. Vorinostat had an overall response rate of about 30% and had a higher response rate (36%) in patients with SS compared to other stages. The drug also improved skin, nodal, and blood involvement as well as reducing pruritus (115). Romidepsin, previously known as depsipeptide or FK228, was recently approved for treatment of CTCL in patients who have received at least one prior systemic therapy. The overall response rate was 35% and complete response was 6%. The recommended dose and schedule of romidepsin is 14 mg/m^2 intravenously over 4 hours on days 1, 8, and 15 of a 28-day cycle. Furthermore, most (63%) patients with moderate to severe pruritus at baseline experienced significant pruritus relief, which significantly impacted quality of life in SS and MF patients (116).

The novel therapies used for PTCL are often active for MF and SS and are employed for patients with tumors or nodal disease. Gemcitabine has an overall response rate of 70% and doxil, 80%. A phase I dose escalation trial combined gemcitabine, doxil, and velcade with four of five patients responding and several episodes of neutropenic fever.

Pralatrexate has also been investigated in MF patients at decreasing dose schedules. It was found to be active with a response rate of 57% and a dose of 15 mg/m^2 (117).

Targeted therapy with antibodies against T-cell molecules are under investigation. HuMax CD4 is being studied in a multicenter trial and is significantly active and able to deplete the peripheral T cells. Alemtuximab (campath-H) targeting CD52 is especially active in SS and can be used subcutaneously to induce remissions but it is immunosuppressive. Diptheria fusion protein coupled to CD3 is also under investigation. Forodesine is a nucleoside analogue, which inhibits PNP and build up of d-GTP causing T-cell apoptosis. A multicenter randomized trial has been conducted but the results are not available.

Other agents which have been in trials for MF patients include CpGs which activate Toll-like receptors, oral lenolidamide, sapacitabine (oral nucleoside inhibitor), and enzastaurin (AKT inhibitor).

■ FUTURE DIRECTION FOR T-CELL LYMPHOMAS

T-cell lymphomas represent a heterogenous group of diseases with poor prognosis. Therapeutic progress has been slow due to the rarity of the disease. It is strongly recommended that patients with non-ALK positive ALCL PTCLs and CTCLs receive treatment on clinical trials so that progress can be made in the management of these uncommon neoplasms. Therefore, future studies will require a multi-institution collaboration.

References

1. Jaffe ES, Harris NL, Stein H, et al. *World Health Organization classification of tumours. Pathology and genetics of tumours of hematopoeitic and lymphoid tissues.* Lyon, France: IARC Press; 2001:121-253.
2. Armitage J, Weisenburger D. New approach to classifying non-Hodgkin's lymphomas: Clinical features of the major histologic subtypes. *J Clin Oncol* 1998;16:2780-2795.
3. The Non-Hodgkin's Lymphoma Classification Project: A clinical evaluation of the International Lymphoma Study Group Classification of Non-Hodgkin's Lymphoma. *Blood* 1997;89:3909-3918.
4. Gallamini A, Stelitano C, Calvi R, et al. Peripheral T-cell lymphoma unspecified (PTCL-U): a new prognostic model from a retrospective multicentric clinical study. *Blood* 2004; 103(7):2474-2479.
5. Savage KJ, Chhanabhai M, Gascoyne RD, et al. Characterization of peripheral T-cell lymphomas in a single North American institution by the WHO classification. *Ann Oncol* 2004;15(10):1467-1475.

6. Lopez-Guillermo A, Cid J, Salar A, et al. Peripheral T-cell lymphomas: Initial features, natural history, and prognostic factors in a series of 174 patients diagnosed according to the REAL Classification. *Ann Oncol* 1998;9:849-855.

7. Gisselbrecht C, Gaulard P, Lepage E, et al. Prognostic significance of T-cell phenotype in aggressive non-Hodgkin's lymphomas. Groupe d'Etudes des Lymphomes de l'Adulte (GELA). *Blood* 1998;92:76-82.

8. Gallamini A, Stelitano C, Calvi R, et al. Peripheral T-cell lymphoma unspecified (PTCL-U): A new prognostic model from a retrospective multicentric clinical study. *Blood* 2004; 103(7):2474-2479.

9. Melnyk A, Rodriguez A, Pugh WC, et al. Evaluation of the revised European-American lymphoma classification confirms the clinical relevance of immunophenotype in 560 cases of aggressive non-Hodgkin's lymphoma. *Blood* 1997;89(12): 4514-4520.

10. Suchi T, Lennert K, Tu L-Y. Histopathology and immunohistochemistry of peripheral T-cell lymphomas: A proposal for their classification. *J Clin Pathol* 1987;40:995-1015.

11. Yamashita Y, Yatabe Y, Tsuzuki T, et al. Perforin and granzyme expression in cytotoxic T-cell lymphomas. *Mod Pathol* 1998; 11:313-323.

12. Lepretre S, Buchonnet G, Stamatoullas A, et al. Chromosome abnormalities in peripheral T-cell lymphoma. *Cancer Genet Cytogenet* 2000;117:71-79.

13. Ten Berge RL, Oudejans JJ, Ossenkoppele GJ, et al. ALK expression in extranodal anaplastic large cell lymphoma favours systemic disease *i*th (primary) nodal involvement and a good prognosis and occurs before dissemination see comments. *J Clin Pathol* 2000;53(6):445-450.

14. Falini B. Anaplastic large cell lymphoma: Pathological, molecular, and clinical features. *Br J Haematol* 2001;114: 741-760.

15. ten Berge RL, de Bruin PC, Oudejans JJ, et al. ALK-negative anaplastic large-cell lymphoma demonstrates similar poor prognosis to peripheral T-cell lymphoma, unspecified. *Histopathology* 2003;43:462-469.

16. Bonzheim I, Geissinger E, Roth S, et al. Anaplastic large cell lymphomas lack the expression of T-cell receptor molecules or molecules of proximal T-cell receptor signaling. *Blood* 2004;104:3358-3360.

17. Krenacs L, Wellmann A, Sorbara L, et al. Cytotoxic cell antigen expression in anaplastic large cell lymphomas of T- and null-cell type and Hodgkin's disease: Evidence for distinct cellular origin. *Blood* 1997;89:980-989.

18. Rassidakis GZ, Sarris AH, Herling M, et al. Differential expression of BCL-2 family proteins in ALK-positive and ALK-negative anaplastic large cell lymphoma of T/null-cell lineage. *Am J Pathol* 2001;159:527-535.

19. Duyster J, Bai RY, Morris SW. Translocations involving anaplastic lymphoma kinase (ALK). *Oncogene* 2001;20: 5623-5637.

20. Falini B, Pulford K, Pucciarini A, et al. Lymphomas expressing ALK fusion protein(s) other than NPM-ALK. *Blood* 1999;94:3509-3515.

21. Frizzera G, Moran EM, Rappaport H. Angioimmunoblastic lymphadenopathy with dysproteinemia. *Lancet* 1974;1: 1070-1073.

22. Siegert W, Nerl C, Agthe A, et al. Angioimmunoblastic lymphadenopathy (AILD)-type T-cell lymphoma: Prognostic impact of clinical observations and laboratory findings at presentation. The Kiel Lymphoma Study Group. *Ann Oncol* 1995;6:659-664.

23. Pautier P, Devidas A, Delmer A, et al. Angioimmunoblastic-like T-cell non-Hodgkin's lymphoma: Outcome after chemotherapy in 33 patients and review of the literature. *Leuk Lymph* 1999; 32:545-552.

24. Dogan A, Attygalle AD, Kyriakou C. Angioimmunoblastic T-cell lymphoma. *Br J Haematol* 2003;121:681-691.

25. Ree HJ, Kadin ME, Kikuchi M, et al. Angioimmunoblastic lymphoma (AILD-type T-cell lymphoma) hyperplastic germinal centers. *Am J Surg Pathol* 1998;22:643-655.

26. Attygalle A, Al-Jehani R, Diss TC, et al. Neoplastic T cells in angioimmunoblastic T-cell lymphoma express CD10. *Blood* 2002;99(2):627-633.

27. Dupuis, J, Boye K, Martin N, et al. Expression of CXCL13 by neoplastic cells in angioimmunoblastic T-cell lymphoma (AITL): a new diagnostic marker providing evidence that AITL derives from follicular helper T cells. *Am J Surg Pathol* 2006; 30(4):490-494.

28. Grogg, K L, Attygalle AD, Macon WR, et al. Expression of CXCL13, a chemokine highly upregulated in germinal center T-helper cells, distinguishes angioimmunoblastic T-cell lymphoma from peripheral T-cell lymphoma, unspecified. *Mod Pathol* 2006;19(8):1101-1107.

29. Schlegelberger B, Feller A, Godde E, et al. Stepwise development of chromosomal abnormalities in angioimmunoblastic lymphadenopathy. *Cancer Genet Cytogenet* 1990;50:15-29.

30. Weiss LM, Jaffe E, Liu X, et al. Detection and localization of Epstein-Barr viral genomes in angioimmunoblastic lymphadenopathy and angioimmunoblastic lymphadenopathy-like lymphoma. *Blood* 1992;79:1789-1795.

31. Abruzzo LV, Schmidt K, Weiss LM, et al. B-cell lymphoma following angioimmunoblastic lymphadenopathy: A case with oligoclonal gene rearrangements associated with Epstein-Barr virus. *Blood* 1993;82:241-246.

32. Franchini G. Molecular mechanisms of human T-cell leukemia/lymphotropic virus type I infection. *Blood* 1995;86:3619-3639.

33. Taylor GP. The epidemiology of HTLV-1 in Europe. *J Acquir Immune Defic Syndr Hum Retrovirol* 1996;13(Suppl 1):S8-S14.

34. Shimoyama M, Members of the Lymphoma Study Group. Diagnostic criteria and classification of clinical subtypes of adult T-cell leukemia-lymphoma. *Br J Haematol* 1991;79: 428-437.

35. Ejima E, Rosenblatt J, Massari M, et al. Cell-type–specific transactivation of the parathyroid hormone–related protein gene promoter by the human T-cell leukemia virus type I(HTLV-I) tax and HTLV-II tax proteins. *Blood* 1993;81: 1017-1024.

36. Ohsawa M, Nakatsuka S, Kanno H, et al. Immunophenotypic and genotypic characterization of nasal lymphoma with polymorphic reticulosis morphology. *Int J Cancer* 1999;81: 865-870.

37. Itoyama T, Chaganti RS, Yamada Y, et al. Cytogenetic analysis and clinical significance in adult T-cell leukemia/lymphoma: A study of 50 cases from the human T-cell leukemia virus type-1 endemic area, Nagasaki. *Blood* 2001;97:3612-3620.

38. Iwanaga R, Ohtani K, Hayashi T, et al. Molecular mechanism of cell cycle progression induced by the oncogene product Tax of human T-cell leukemia virus type I. *Oncogene* 2001; 20:2055-2067.

39. DeRemee RA, Weiland LH, McDonald TJ, et al. Polymorphic reticulosis, lymphomatoid granulomatosis: Two diseases or one? *Mayo Clinic Proc* 1978;53:634-640.

40. Medeiros LJ, Jaffe ES, Chen YY, et al. Localization of Epstein–Barr viral genomes in angiocentric immunoproliferative lesions. *Am J Surg Pathol* 1992;16:439-447.

41. Nakamura S, Suchi T, Koshikawa T, et al. Clinicopathologic study of CD56 (NCAM)-positive angiocentric lymphoma occurring in sites other than the upper and lower respiratory tract. *Am J Surg Pathol* 1995;19:284-296.

42. Banks PM, Warnke RA. Mature T-cell and NK-cell neoplasms. In: Jaffe ES, Harris NL, Stein H, et al. (eds.). *World Health Organization Classification of Tumours: Pathology and Genetics of Tumours of Hematopoetic and lymphoid Tissues.* Lyon: IARC Press; 2001:189-230.

43. Kwong, YL. Natural killer-cell malignancies: Diagnosis and treatment. *Leukemia* 2005;19(12):2186-2194.

44. Medeiros LJ, Peiper SC, Elwood L, et al. Angiocentric immunoproliferative lesions: A molecular analysis of 8 cases. *Hum Pathol* 1991;22:1150-1157.

45. Kanavaros P, Lescs MC, Briere J, et al. Nasal T-cell lymphoma: A clinicopathologic entity associated with peculiar phenotype and with Epstein-Barr virus. *Blood* 1993;81:2688-2695.

46. Ko YH, Choi KE, Han JH, et al. Comparative genomic hybridization study of nasal-type NK/T-cell lymphoma. *Cytometry* 2001;46:85-91.

47. Gale J, Simmonds PD, Mead GM, et al. Enteropathy-type intestinal T-cell lymphoma: Clinical features and treatment of 31 patients in a single center. *J Clin Oncol* 2000;18:795-803.

48. Murray A, Cuevas EC, Jones DB, et al. Study of the immunohistochemistry and T cell clonality of enteropathy-associated T cell lymphoma. *Am J Pathol* 1995;146:509-519.

49. Savage KJ. Aggressive peripheral T-cell lymphomas (specified and unspecified types). *Hematology Am Soc Hematol Educ Program* 2005;267-277.

50. Katoh A, Ohsima K, Kanda M, et al. Gastrointestinal T cell lymphoma: Predominant cytotoxic phenotypes, including alpha/beta, gamma/delta and natural killer cells. *Leuk Lymph* 2000;39:97-111.

51. Farcet JP, Gaulard P, Marolleau JP, et al. Hepatosplenic T-cell lymphoma: Sinusal/sinusoidal localization of malignant cells expressing the T-cell receptor gamma delta. *Blood* 1990;75: 2213-2219.

52. Weidmann E. Hepatosplenic T cell lymphoma. A review on 45 cases since the report describing the disease as a distinct lymphoma entity in 1990. *Leukemia* 2000;14:991-997.

53. Vega F, Medeiros LJ, Bueso-Ramos C, et al. Hepatosplenic gamma/delta T-cell lymphoma in bone marrow: A sinusoidal neoplasm with blastic cytologic features. *Am J Clin Pathol* 2001;116:410-419.

54. Shale M, Kanfer E, Panaccione R, et al. Hepatosplenic T cell lymphoma in inflammatory bowel disease. *Gut* 2008;57(12): 1639-1641.

55. Hanson MN, Morrison VA, Peterson PA, et al. Posttransplant T-cell lymphoproliferative disorders—An aggressive, late complication of solid-organ transplantation. *Blood* 1996; 88(9):3626-3633.

56. Roelandt PR, Maertens J, Vandenberghe P, et al. Hepatosplenic gammadelta T-cell lymphoma after liver transplantation: report of the first 2 cases and review of the literature. *Liver Transpl* 2009;15(7):686-692.

57. Ghobrial IM, Habermann TM, Maurer MJ, et al. Prognostic analysis for survival in adult solid organ transplant recipients with post-transplantation lymphoproliferative disorders. *J Clin Oncol* 2005;23(30):7574-7582.

58. Thayu M, Markowitz JE, Mamula P, et al. Hepatosplenic T-cell lymphoma in an adolescent patient after immunomodulator and biologic therapy for Crohn disease. *J Pediatr Gastroenterol Nutr* 2005;40(2):220-222.

59. Belhadj K, Reyes F, Farcet JP, et al. Hepatosplenic gammadelta T-cell lymphoma is a rare clinicopathologic entity with poor outcome: Report on a series of 21 patients. *Blood* 2003;102(13):4261-4269.

60. Rosh JR, Gross T, Mamula P, et al. Hepatosplenic T-cell lymphoma in adolescents and young adults with Crohn's disease: a cautionary tale? *Inflamm Bowel Dis* 2007;3(8):1024-1030.

61. Khan WA, Yu L, Eisenbrey AB, et al. Hepatosplenic gamma/ delta T-cell lymphoma in immunocompromised patients. Report of two cases and review of literature. *Am J Clin Pathol* 2001;116(1):41-50.

62. Wu H, Wasik MA, Przybylski G, et al. Hepatosplenic gamma-delta T-cell lymphoma as a late-onset posttransplant lymphoproliferative disorder in renal transplant recipients. *Am J Clin Pathol* 2000;113(4):487-496.

63. Ohshima K, Haraoka S, Harada N, et al. Hepatosplenic gammadelta T-cell lymphoma: relation to Epstein-Barr virus and activated cytotoxic molecules. *Histopathology* 2000;36(2): 127-135.

64. Beigel F, Jurgens M, Tillack C, et al. Hepatosplenic T-cell lymphoma in a patient with Crohn's disease. *Nat Rev Gastroenterol Hepatol* 2009;6(7):433-436.

65. Rossbach HC, Chamizo W, Dumont DP, et al. Hepatosplenic gamma/delta T-cell lymphoma with isochromosome 7q, translocation t(7;21), and tetrasomy 8 in a 9-year-old girl. *J Pediatr Hematol Oncol* 2002;24(2):154-157.

66. Salhany KE, Feldman M, Kahn MJ, et al. Hepatosplenic gammadelta T-cell lymphoma: Ultrastructural, immunophenotypic, and functional evidence for cytotoxic T lymphocyte differentiation. *Hum Pathol* 1997;28:674-685.

67. Alonsozana EL, Stamberg J, Kumar D, et al. Isochromosome 7q: The primary cytogenetic abnormality in hepatosplenic gammadelta T cell lymphoma. *Leukemia* 1997;11:1367-1372.

68. Weenig RH, Ng CS, Perniciaro C. Subcutaneous panniculitis-like T-cell lymphoma: An elusive case presenting as lipomembranous panniculitis and a review of 72 cases in the literature. *Am J Dermatopathol* 2001;23:206-215.

69. Sen F, Rassidakis GZ, Jones D, et al. Apoptosis and proliferation in subcutaneous panniculitis-like T-cell lymphoma. *Mod Pathol* 2002;15:625-631.

70. Willemze R, Jaffe ES, Burg G, et al. WHO-EORTC classification for cutaneous lymphomas. *Blood* 2005;105:3768-3785.

71. Merck: Vorinostat Investigator's Brochure; 2006.

72. D'Amore F, Relander T, Laureitzsen G, et al. Dose-dense induction followed by autologous stem cell transplant as 1st line treatment in peripheral T-cell lymphomas. *Blood* 2006;108:401.

73. Escalon MP, Liu NS, Yang Y, et al. Prognostic factors and treatment of patients with T-cell non-Hodgkin lymphoma: The M. D. Anderson Cancer Center experience. *Cancer* 2005; 103(10):2091-2098.

74. Mourad N, Mounier N, Birere J, et al. Angioimmunoblastic T-cell lymphoma: kA clinicopathologic study of 158 patients treated in GELA trials. *Blood* 2006;108:397.

75. You JY, Chi KH, Yang MH, et al. Radiation therapy versus chemotherapy as initial treatment for localized nasal natural killer (NK)/T-cell lymphoma: A single institute survey in Taiwan. *Ann Oncol* 2004;15(4):618-625.

76. Li Y, Yao B, Jin J, et al. Radiotherapy as primary treatment for stage IE and IIE nasal natural killer/T-cell lymphoma. *J Clin Oncol* 2006;24:181-189.

77. Gale J, Simmonds PD, Mead GM, et al. Enteropathy-type intestinal T-cell lymphoma: Clinical features and treatment of 31 patients in a single center. *J Clin Oncol* 2000;18(4):795-803.

78. Go RS, Wester SM. Immunophenotypic and molecular features, clinical outcomes, treatments and prognostic factors associated with subcutaneous panniculitis-like T-cell lymphoma. *Cancer* 2004;101:1404-1413.

79. Suzumiya J, Ohshima K, Tamura K, et al. Treatment of adult T-cell leukemia-lymphoma: A clinicopathologic study of 126 cases from the International T-cell Lymphoma Project. *Blood* 2006;108:2059.

80. Besson C, Panelatti G, Delaunay C, et al. Treatment of adult T-cell leukemia-lymphoma by CHOP followed by therapy with antinucleosides, alpha interferon and oral etoposide. *Leuk Lymphoma* 2002;43(12):2275-2279.

81. Pro B. Novel agents in peripheral T-cell lymphomas. *American Society of Clinical Oncology Education Booklet*; 2009:486-489.

82. Sallah S, Wan JY, Nguyen NP. Treatment of refractory T-cell malignancies using gemcitabine. *Br J Haematol* 2001;113(1):185-187.

83. Kim JG, Sohn SK, Chae YS, et al. CHOP plus etoposide and gemcitabine (CHOP-EG) as front-line chemotherapy for patients with peripheral T cell lymphomas. *Cancer Chemother Pharmacol* 2006;58(1):35-39.

84. Arkenau HT, Chong G, Cunningham D, et al. Gemcitabine, cisplatin and methylprednisolone for the treatment of patients with peripheral T-cell lymphoma: the Royal Marsden Hospital experience. *Haematologica* 2007;92(2):271-272.

85. Dang NH, Pro B, Hagemeiser FB, et al. Phase II trial of denileukin diftitox for relapsed/refractory T-cell non-Hodgkin lymphoma. *Br J Haematol* 2007;136(3):439-447.

86. O'Connor OA, Hamlin PA, Gerecitano J, et al. Pralatrexate (PDX) produces durable complete remissions in patients with chemotherapy resistant precursor and peripheral T-cell lymphomas: Results o the MSKCC phase I/II experience. *Blood* 2006;108 (Abstract 400).

87. O'Connor OA, Pro B, Pinter-Brown L, et al. PROPEL: A multi-center phase II open label study of pralatrexate (PDX) with vitamin B12 and folic acid supplementation in patients with relapsed or refractory peripheral T cell lymphoma. *Blood* 2008;112 (Abstract 261).

88. Toner LE, Vrhovac R, Smith EA, et al. The schedule-dependent effects of the novel antifolate pralatrexate and gemcitabine are superior to methotrexate and cytarabine in models of human non-Hodgkin's lymphoma. *Clin Cancer Res* 2006; 12(3 Pt 1):924-932.

89. Olsen EA, Kim YH, Kuzel TM, et al. Phase IIb multicenter trial of vorinostat in patients with persistent, progressive, or treatment refractory cutaneous T-cell lymphoma. *J Clin Oncol* 2007;25(21):3109-3115.

90. Enblad G, Hagberg H, Erlanson M, et al. A pilot study of alemtuzumab (anti-CD52 monoclonal antibody) therapy for patients with relapsed or chemotherapy-refractory peripheral T-cell lymphomas. *Blood* 2004;103(8):2920-2924.

91. d'Amore F, Radford J, Jerkeman M, et al. Zanolimumab (HuMax-CD4TM) a fully human monoclonal antibody: Efficacy and safety in patients with relapsed or treatment-refractory non-cutaneous CD4+ T-cell lymphoma. *Blood* 2007;110 (Abstract 3409).

92. Forero-Torres A, Leonard JP, Younes A, et al. A Phase II study of SGN-30 (anti-CD30 mAb) in Hodgkin lymphoma or systemic anaplastic large cell lymphoma. *Br J Haematol* 2009;146(2):171-179.

93. Ansell SM, Horwitz SM, Angert A, et al. Phase I/II study of an anti-CD30 monoclonal antibody (MDX-060) in Hodgkin's lymphoma and anaplastic large-cell lymphoma. *J Clin Oncol* 2007;25(19):2764-2769.

94. Younes A, Forero-Torres A, Barlett NL, et al. Multiple complete responses in a Phase I dose-escalation study of the antibody-drug conjugate SGN-35 in patients with relapsed or refractory CD-30 positive lymphomas. *Blood* 2008;112 (Abstract 1006).

95. Zinzani, PL, Musuraca G, Tani M, et al. Phase II trial of proteasome inhibitor bortezomib in patients with relapsed or refractory cutaneous T-cell lymphoma. *J Clin Oncol* 2007;25(27):4293-4297.

96. Reiman T, Finch D, Chua N, et al. First report of a phase II clinical trial of lenalidomide oral therapy for peripheral T-cell lymphoma. *Blood* 2007;110 (Abstract 2579).

97. Heider U, Kaiser M, Sterz J, et al. Histone deacetylase inhibitors reduce VEGF production and induce growth suppression and apoptosis in human mantle cell lymphoma. *Eur J Haematol* 2006;76:42-50.

98. Giardi M, Heald PW, Wilson LD. The pathogenesis of mycosis fungoides. *N Engl J Med* 2004;350:1978-1988.

99. Kazakov DV, Burg G, Kempf W. Clinicopathological spectrum of mycosis fungoides. *J Eur Acad Dermatol Venereol* 2004;18:397-415.

100. Kim EJ, Hess S, Richardson SK, et al. Immunopathogenesis and therapy of cutaneous T cell lymphoma. *J Clin Invest* 2005;115:798-812.

101. Vega F, Luthra R, Medeiros LJ, et al. Clonal heterogeneity in mycosis fungoides and its relationship to clinical course. *Blood* 2002;100:3369-3373.

102. Kim YH, Liu HL, Mrz-Gernhard S, et al. Long-term outcome of 525 patients with mycosis fungoides and Sézary syndrome: Clinical prognostic factors and risk for disease progression. *Arch Dermatol* 2003;139:857-866.

103. Diamandilou E, Colome M, Fayad L, et al. Prognostic factor analysis in mycosis fungoides/Sézary syndrome. *J Am Acad Dermatol* 1999;40:914-924.

104. Diamandilou E, Colome-Grimmer M, Fayad L, et al. Transformation of mycosis fungoides/Sézary syndrome: Clinical characteristics and prognosis. *Blood* 1998;92:1150-1159.

105. Scarisbrick JJ, Whittacker S, Evans AV, et al. Prognostic significance of tumor burden in the blood of patients with erythrodermic primary cutaneous T-cell lymphoma. *Blood* 2001;97:624-630.

106. Breneman D, Duvic M, Kuzel T, et al. Phase 1 and 2 trial of bexarotene gel for skin-directed treatment of patients with cutaneous T-cell lymphoma. *Arch Dermatol* 2002;138(3):325-332.

107. Lain T, Talpur R, Duvic M. Long-term control of mycosis fungoides of the hands with topical bexarotene. *Int J Dermatol* 2003;42(3):238-241.

108. Kraken WA, Ward SR, Duvic M. Bexarotene is a new treatment option for lymphomatoid papulosis. *Dermatology* 2003;206(2):142-147.

109. Olsen E, Duvic M, Frankel A, et al. Pivotal phase III trial of two dose levels of denileukin diftitox for the treatment of cutaneous T-cell lymphoma. *J Clin Oncol* 2001;19(2): 376-388.

110. Foss F, Demierre MF, DiVenuti G, et al. A phase-1 trial of bexarotene and denileukin diftitox in patients with relapsed or refractory cutaneous T-cell lymphoma. *Blood* 2005;106(2): 454-457.

111. Duvic M, Martin AG, Kim Y, et al. Phase 2 and 3 clinical trial of oral bexarotene (Targretin capsules) for the treatment of refractory or persistent early-stage cutaneous T-cell lymphoma. *Arch Dermatol* 2001;137(5):581-593.

112. Assaf C, Bagot M, Dummer R, et al. Minimizing adverse side-effects of oral bexarotene in cutaneous T-cell lymphoma: an expert opinion. *Br J Dermatol* 2006;155(2):261-266.

113. Lim HW, Edelson RL. Photopheresis for the treatment of cutaneous T-cell lymphoma. *Hematol Oncol Clin North Am* 1995;9(5):1117-1126.

114. McGinnis KS, Ubriani R, Newton S, et al. The addition of interferon gamma to oral bexarotene therapy with photopheresis for Sézary syndrome. *Arch Dermatol* 2005;141(9): 1176-1178.

115. Duvic M, Vu J. Vorinostat: A new oral histone deacetylase inhibitor approved for cutaneous T-cell lymphoma. *Expert Opin Investig Drugs* 2007;16(7):1111-1120.

116. Piekarz RL, Frye R, Turner M, et al. Phase II multi-institutional trial of the histone deacetylase inhibitor romidepsin as monotherapy for patients with cutaneous T-cell lymphoma. *J Clin Oncol* 2009;27(32):5410-5417.

117. Hortwitz SM, Duvic M, Kim Y, et al. Pralatrexate is active in cutaneous T-cell lymphoma (CTCL): Results of a Multicenter, Dose-Finding Trial. *Blood* 2009;114:919 (ASH Annual Meeting Abstracts).

HODGKIN LYMPHOMA

Jason Westin
Fredrick B. Hagemeister
Valerie K. Reed
Michelle Fanale

FOREWORD

The management of Hodgkin lymphoma continues to change. Before the widespread use of modern poly-chemotherapy, radical radiation therapy alone cured many patients. However, reliance on radiation alone required extensive radiation portals to treat nearly the entire lymphatic system with radiation doses up to 44 Gy. With long-term follow-up, many of these patients developed heart toxicity and second malignancies.

Over the past 10 to 20 years, efforts have been made to reduce the long-term toxicities of treatment for Hodgkin lymphoma, while maintaining excellent cure rates. With modern chemotherapy, multiple randomized studies have shown that radiation portals can be safely reduced from extended-field radiation to involved-field radiation. This is very important to reduce the risk of secondary breast cancers in young women. The majority of breast exposure to radiation is from treating the axillary nodes with large mantle fields. Because most women with early stage Hodgkin lymphoma do not present with axillary adenopathy, eliminating radiation to the axilla will decrease the risk of secondary breast carcinomas. In addition, several centers are using novel treatment techniques, such as innovative patient positioning systems to move the breasts out of the field, intensity-modulated radiation therapy and proton radiation to further reduce exposure of normal tissues to radiation. Currently, the European Organization for Research and Treatment of Cancer (EORTC) has further reduced the radiation portals from involved-field to involved-nodal radiation, where the portal is tailored to the involved node only and not the entire lymph node region. In addition, studies are also currently underway to determine if it is possible to reduce the radiation dose after chemotherapy from 30 to 20 Gy. Thus, the radiation portals are much smaller, more conformal, and the doses are lower than those 20 to 40 years ago.

In multiple studies in patients with early-stage Hodgkin lymphoma, the complete omission of radiation therapy resulted in an inferior outcome. In the future, functional imaging such as positron emission tomography may allow the identification of patients in whom radiotherapy can be eliminated, but this is still being examined in carefully controlled clinical trials. However, radiation therapy with greatly revised techniques and lower doses will likely continue to play an important role in the management of Hodgkin lymphoma.

■ TYPES OF HODGKIN LYMPHOMA

Over the past decade, investigators have made significant progress in the diagnosis, classification, staging, prognosis, and treatment of Hodgkin lymphoma (HL). In past years, the true lineage of the neoplastic cells in HL was unknown, hence the term "Hodgkin disease" was used. It is now recognized that almost all cases of HL are of B-cell lineage, hence the name change to HL.

The classification of HL has remained relatively stable over the past 40 years and the World Health Organization (WHO) classification of lymphoid neoplasms was

TABLE 10-1	WHO CLASSIFICATION OF HODGKIN LYMPHOMA
Nodular lymphocyte predominant	
Classical Hodgkin lymphoma	
Nodular sclerosis	
Lymphocyte-rich	
Mixed cellularity	
Lymphocyte depleted	

updated recently in 2008 (1) (Table 10-1). The current WHO classification recognizes that nodular lymphocyte predominant HL (NLPHL) is distinct from the other types that can be grouped together under the rubric of classical HL (cHL) (1).

In 2009 it is estimated that 8,510 Americans will be diagnosed with HL and classical HL makes up to 95% of the cases (2). HL has been traditionally defined as a hematopoietic neoplasm composed of diagnostic Hodgkin and Reed-Sternberg (HRS) cells within a reactive cell background. A HRS cell is large, 30 to 60 μm, containing a bilobed, vesicular nucleus, with each lobe containing a prominent, round, eosinophilic nucleolus surrounded by a clear zone or halo; it also has abundant cytoplasm. However, HRS cells often comprise less than 1% of the involved tumor tissue and are absent in the nonclassical NLPHL. HRS cells are believed to be derived from germinal center (GC) B cells that have unfavorable immunoglobulin V gene mutations. Whereas, lymphocyte predominant (LP) cells that were previously termed lymphocytic and histiocytic (LH) cells are thought to originate from antigen-selected GC B cells (3).

NODULAR LYMPHOCYTE PREDOMINANT HODGKIN LYMPHOMA

Clinical Features

Approximately 5% of patients with HL have the lymphocyte predominant (NLPHL) type. This disease is usually localized and most often involves cervical or axillary lymph nodes (1,4). The disease affects patients of all ages, males more often than females, and is clinically indolent (Table 10-2). Systemic symptoms—such as fever, weight loss, and night sweats (also known as B symptoms)—are infrequent. Patients with NLPHL often relapse over time in a manner analogous to low-grade non-HL (4). Patients with NLPHL are at risk for developing diffuse large B-cell lymphoma (DLBCL) or T-cell/histiocyte-rich large B-cell lymphoma with the risk being approximately 5 to 6% (1).

TABLE 10-2 | COMPARISON OF CLINICAL FEATURES OF NODULAR LYMPHOCYTE PREDOMINANT (NLPHL) AND CLASSICAL HODGKIN LYMPHOMA

Clinical Feature	NLPHL	Classical HL
Frequency	5%	95%
Age distribution	Unimodal: equal in children and adults	Bimodal: peak in second and third decades
Male	70%	50%
Sites involved	Lymph nodes with sparing mediastinum	Mediastinum, cervical lymph nodes
Stage at diagnosis*	I	II or III
B symptoms	<20%	40%
Clinical course	Indolent, late relapses	Aggressive, curable

*Most common stage at time of diagnosis.

Histologic Features

NLPHL is characterized by effacement of nodal architecture by variably sized, vague nodules composed of numerous small lymphocytes, histiocytes, and characteristic neoplastic LP cells (Fig. 10-1A) (1,5). The typical description for these cells is that they are large, with pale cytoplasm and polyploid, vesicular nuclei containing inconspicuous nucleoli resembling kernels of popped corn, hence the nickname popcorn cells (Fig. 10-1B). However, LP cells can exhibit a range of cytologic appearances. These cells can be round and/or have relatively prominent nucleoli. Eosinophils, neutrophils, and plasma cells are usually absent in NLPHL, and there is no associated necrosis or fibrosis.

Cases of NLPHL can also have diffuse areas. When diffuse areas are large, their presence often correlates with more aggressive disease. To reflect this change in clinical behavior, many pathologists diagnose such cases as NLPHL with progression to T-cell/histiocyte-rich large B-cell lymphoma, also described as T-cell-rich B-cell lymphoma (TCRBCL). Other pathologists use the term NLPHL with large diffuse areas and suggest that the diffuse areas may represent the beginning stages of progression to diffuse large B-cell lymphoma. The boundary between NLPHL with diffuse areas and TCRBCL remains blurred. Most cases previously designated as diffuse LPHL, as defined previously (6), are now classified differently. With appropriate workup, these cases are usually classified as either NLPHL with large diffuse areas, lymphocyte-rich classical (LRC) HL, or T-cell-rich B-cell lymphoma.

Gene expression profiling of NLPHL has been done to determine the origin and pathogenesis of LP cells, and found significant similarities between NLPHL, TCRBCL, and classical HL (7). Overall LP cells are thought to derive from antigen-selected GC B cells (3). LP cells also demonstrate deregulation of numerous apoptosis regulators and putative oncogenes and a partial loss of their B-cell phenotype. In addition, there is constitutive activation of nuclear factor-κB (NF-κB), Janus kinases/signal transducers and activator of transcription (JAK/STAT) pathway, and aberrant extracellular-regulated kinase signaling.

Immunophenotypic Findings

NLPHL is immunophenotypically distinct from other types of HL. The LP cells usually express LCA (CD45), immunoglobulin J chain, B-cell antigens (CD19, CD20, CD22, CD79A, and BCL-6), and epithelial membrane antigen (EMA) and are negative for CD15 and CD30 (Fig. 10-1C and D). These results suggest that the LP cells are B cells that arise from the GC. The LP cells are negative for T-cell antigens but are often surrounded by a rosette of small, reactive T cells that may be positive for pan-T-cell antigens and CD57 (Fig. 10-1E). Epstein–Barr virus (EBV) is almost always absent in the LP cells of NLPHL.

LYMPHOCYTE-RICH CLASSICAL HODGKIN LYMPHOMA

In recent years, cases of HL have been recognized that resemble NLPHL histologically but are classical HL immunophenotypically (1,4,5). The frequency of this type of HL is not well known but is most likely low, below 5%. Clinically, patients with LRC HL are similar to patients with other subtypes of classical HL or have clinical findings intermediate between NLPHL and cHL. Unlike patients with NLPHL, late relapse is uncommon in patients with LRCHL.

Histologically, these tumors are rich in small lymphocytes and histiocytes. Granulocytes and plasma cells are usually infrequent. Necrosis is usually not present. LRCHL may be either nodular or diffuse. The nodular type closely resembles NLPHL. Vague nodules of numerous small lymphocytes are present and the nodules may have a small compressed GC (Fig. 10-2A and B). The neoplastic cells are present in the mantle zones of the nodules. These neoplastic cells usually

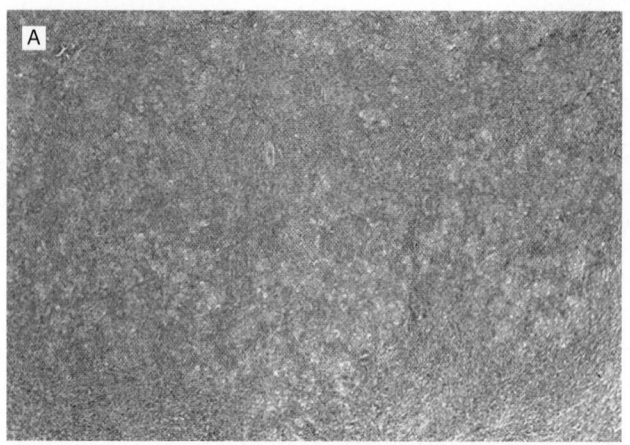

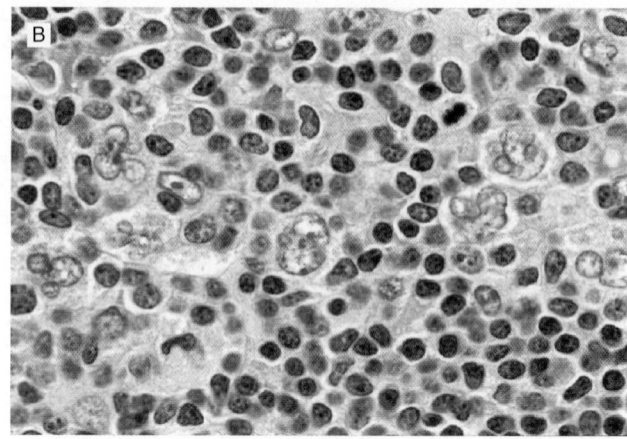

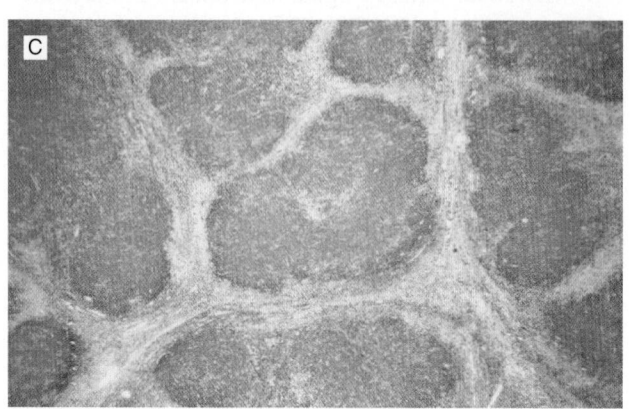

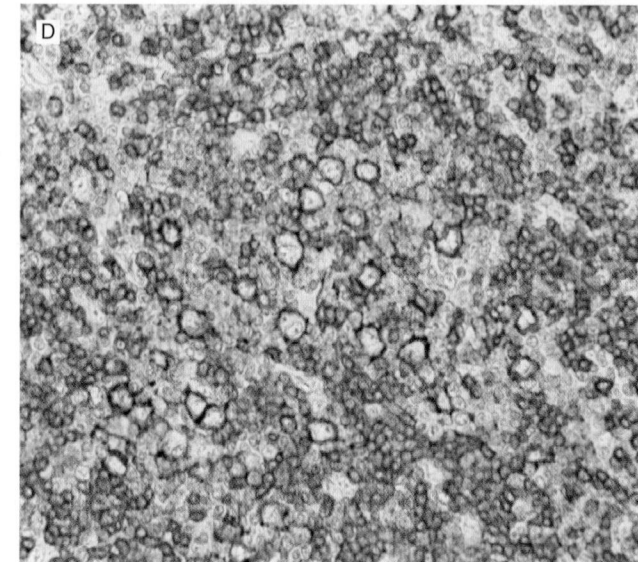

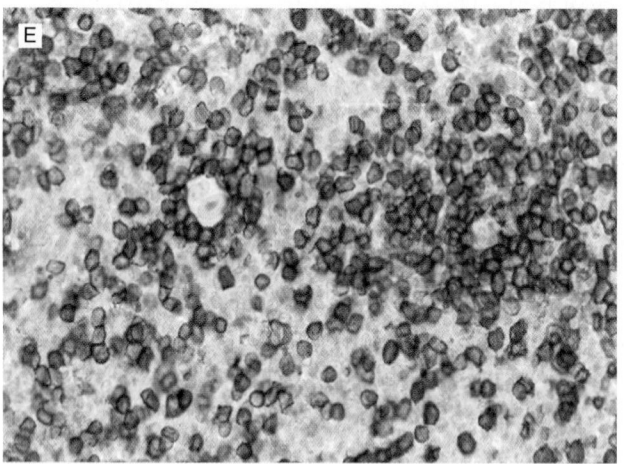

FIGURE 10-1. Nodular lymphocyte predominant Hodgkin lymphoma. **A.** At low-power magnification, the neoplasm is vaguely nodular. **B.** At high-power magnification, large L&H cells, resembling popped kernels of corn, are identified in a background of reactive lymphocytes and histocytes. **C** and **D.** Immunohistochemical stain for CD20. **C.** At low-power magnification, this immunostain highlights the nodular pattern and shows numerous B cells in the nodules. **D.** At high-power magnification, large L&H cells and small reactive B cells are positive for CD20. **E.** Immunohistochemical stain for CD3. Scattered small reactive T cells are present and focally surround the L&H cells (so-called rosetting).

resemble Reed-Sternberg and typical mononuclear variant cells (so-called Hodgkin cells) rather than LP cells. The cell composition is similar in diffuse cases of LRCHL, but nodularity is minimal or absent. Immunohistochemical studies of LRCHL show that the large neoplastic cells have an immunophenotype similar to that of all classical HL cases, positive for

CD15 and CD30 and negative for LCA (CD45) (Fig. 10-2C to E).

In a recent study of NLPHL by the European Task Force on Lymphoma (5), a large number of tumors that had been classified as NLPHL were reviewed; the diagnosis was confirmed in only half of these cases. Most of those excluded were reclassified as LRCHL.

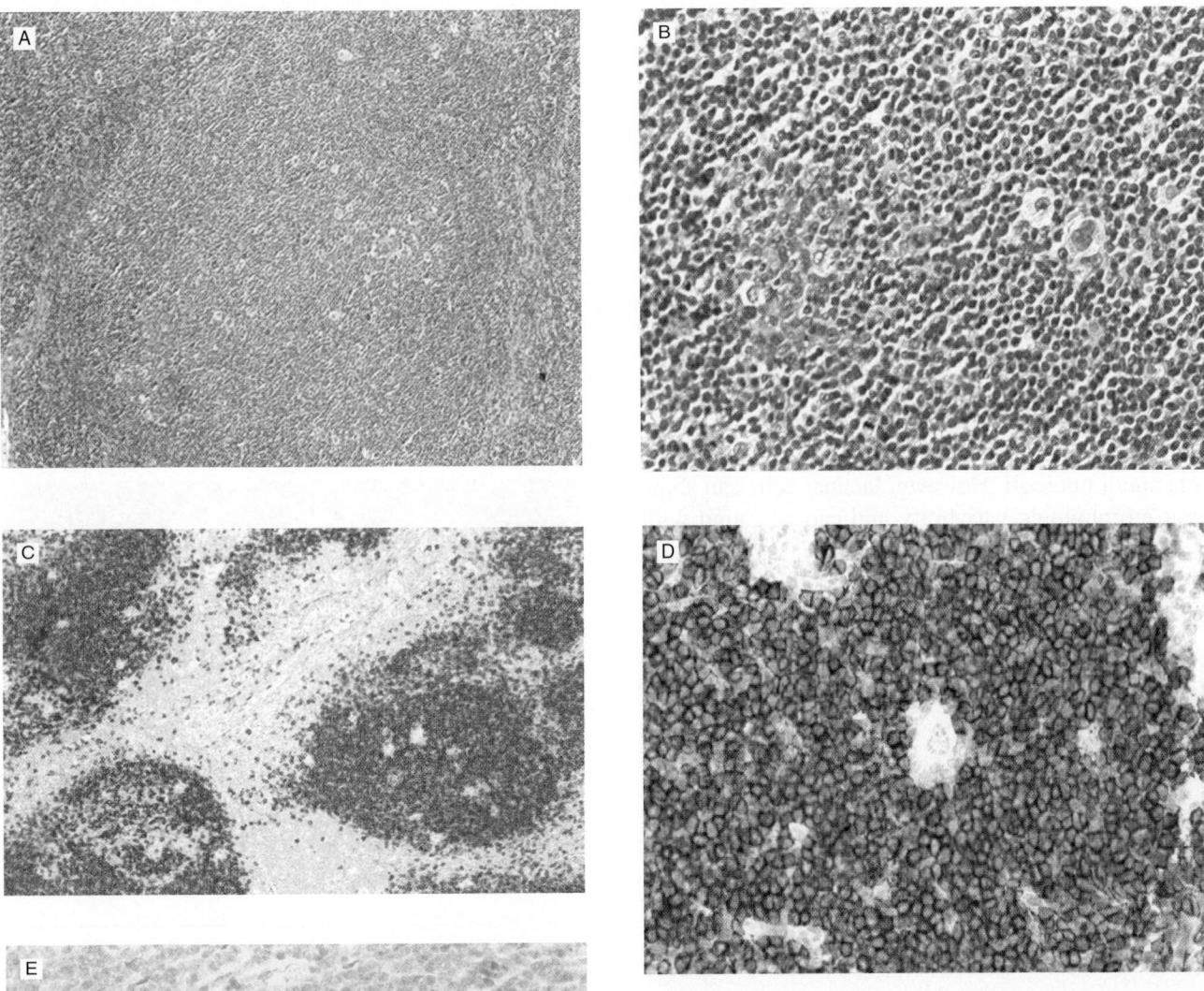

FIGURE 10-2. Lymphocyte-rich classical Hodgkin lymphoma, nodular variant. **A.** At low-power magnification, the neoplasm has a nodular pattern and is rich in reactive small lymphocytes (resembling nodular lymphocyte predominant Hodgkin lymphoma). **B.** At high-power magnification, large neoplastic cells (so-called Hodgkin cells) are identified in the mantle zone of the follicle (note reactive germinal center to left of field). **C** and **D.** Immunohistochemical stain for CD20. **C.** The nodules contain numerous small reactive B-cells. **D.** The Hodgkin cells are negative for CD20. **E.** Immunohistochemical stain for CD30. The Hodgkin cells are positive.

NODULAR SCLEROSIS HODGKIN LYMPHOMA

Clinical Features

Nodular sclerosis (NS) is the most common form of cHL, representing approximately 60 to 70% of all cases in western countries; it is also the most common type of cHL in patients below the age of 50 years. Nodular sclerosis HL is much less frequent in developing countries. The age-adjusted incidence rate of NSHL is increasing in the United States according to the National Cancer Institute (NCI) Statistics, Epidemiology, and End Results (SEER) data (8). The increase is greatest for adolescents and young adults between the ages of 15 and 45 years. The male/female ratio is approximately equal. Whites are affected more often than others. NSHL has a marked predilection for involving mediastinal, supraclavicular, and cervical lymph nodes. A mediastinal mass is very common and the thymus may be involved.

Histologic Features

Nodular sclerosis HL is characterized by a triad of findings: (1) a nodular pattern, (2) broad bands of fibrosis that outline the nodules, and (3) characteristic mononuclear cell variants known as lacunar cells (Fig. 10-3). A lacunar cell has abundant clear cytoplasm with a sharply demarcated cell membrane. In formalin-fixed tissue, a characteristic artifact occurs. The cell cytoplasm retracts, leaving a clear space or lacuna surrounding the cell; thus the name. The typical lacunar cell has a polylobulated nucleus with one or multiple small nucleoli. However, lacunar cells can show great morphologic variability and can be round with

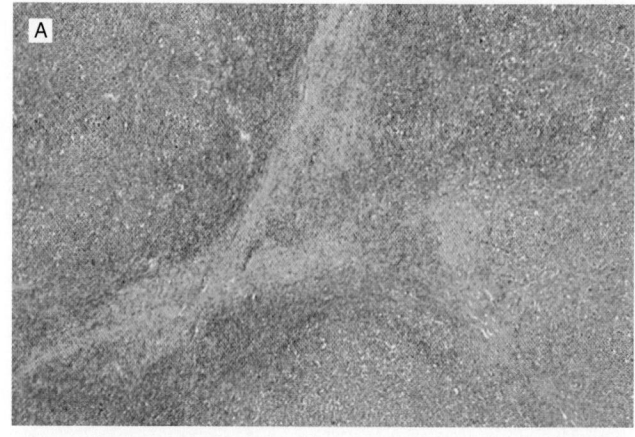

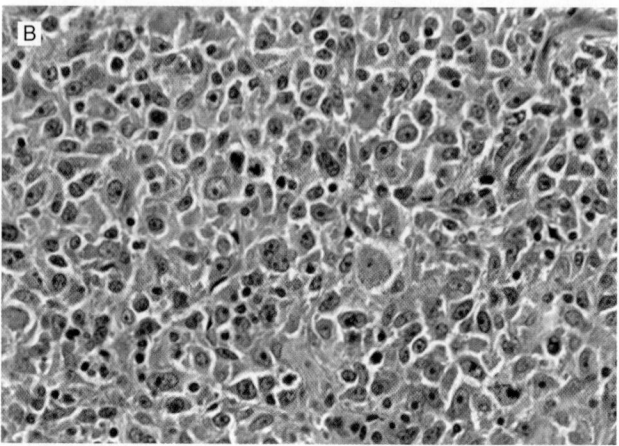

FIGURE 10-4. Syncytial variant of nodular sclerosis Hodgkin lymphoma. **A.** Nodularity and a fibrous bond can be appreciated in this field. **B.** The nodules are composed of many neoplastic cells with depletion of small lymphocytes.

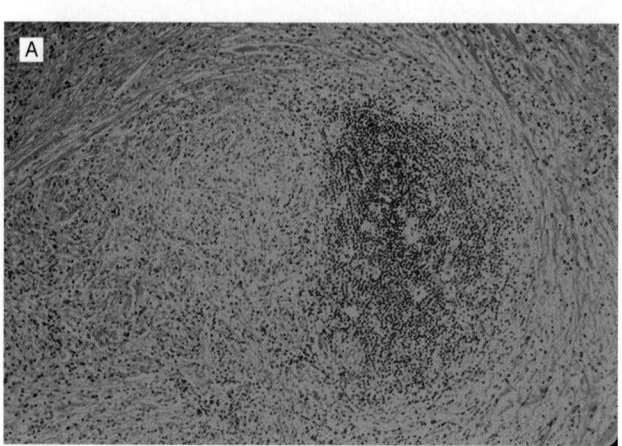

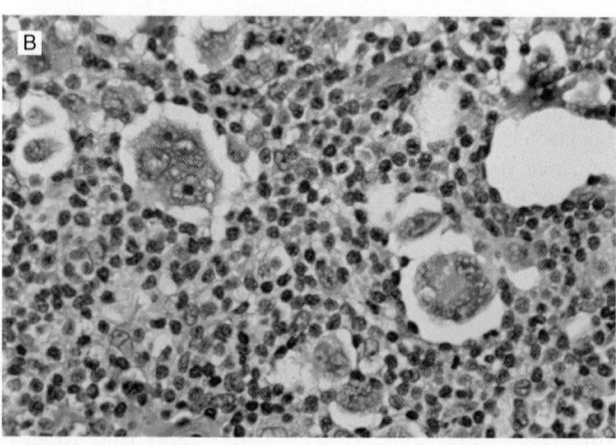

FIGURE 10-3. Nodular sclerosis Hodgkin lymphoma. **A.** The neoplasm is nodular and the nodules are surrounded by dense fibrous bands. **B.** The large neoplastic cells (lacunar cells) lie within lacunar spaces and many are multinucleated in this field. Reactive cells are present in the background.

prominent nucleoli, or they may resemble large non-cleaved cells. A heterogeneous mixture of reactive cells may be seen in HL, including small lymphocytes, histiocytes, eosinophils, neutrophils, and plasma cells in variable numbers.

Nodular sclerosis HL has been graded (as 1 or 2) by the British National Lymphoma Investigation (BNLI) group (9) according to the numbers of neoplastic cells and reactive cells present, and this grading system has been adopted by the WHO Classification (1). Grade 2 cases of NSHL show numerous neoplastic (lacunar) cells and depletion of reactive lymphocytes. Lymphocyte depleted and syncytial variants (Fig. 10-4) of NSHL have been described; these cases are the outermost examples of grade 2 NSHL. The syncytial variant of NSHL is composed of sheets of neoplastic cells and necrosis.

MIXED CELLULARITY HODGKIN LYMPHOMA

Clinical Features

The mixed cellularity variant of HL (MCHL), the second common type, affects 15 to 25% of all patients with the disease and is the most common form in patients above 50 years of age (1,8). Males are affected more often than females. According to NCI SEER data, MCHL is relatively more common in blacks and Hispanics than in whites in the United States. A substantial percentage of patients with MCHL have clinical stage III or stage IV disease and B symptoms.

Histologic Features

MCHL is characterized by a large number of Reed–Sternberg cells and Hodgkin cells in a background of numerous eosinophils, plasma cells, histiocytes, and granulocytes in varying proportions (1) (Fig. 10-5). The lymph node architecture is usually diffusely replaced. Partially involved lymph nodes show selective paracortical infiltration. Disorderly fibrosis may be seen, but the broad fibrous bands and capsular fibrosis characteristic of NSHL are absent.

Two variants of MCHL can be relatively more difficult to diagnose. In the interfollicular variant, which most likely represents partial involvement of lymph node by HL, the tumor is located in the interfollicular region and is often associated with reactive follicular hyperplasia and marked plasmacytosis. In the epithelioid histiocyte-rich variant, numerous epithelioid histiocytes, and granulomas are present; these can be so numerous as to obscure the neoplastic cells. The importance of these variants of MCHL lies in their unusual histologic findings.

LYMPHOCYTE DEPLETED HODGKIN LYMPHOMA

Clinical Features

Lymphocyte depleted HL (LDHL) is the least common type, representing 1% of all cases (8). In the NCI SEER study, the age-adjusted incidence rate for LDHL has decreased. This decrease is most likely explained by the recognition by pathologists that many tumors previously classified as LDHL are, in fact, non-HLs (such as anaplastic large-cell lymphoma). Improved classification is the result of application of immunohistochemical and molecular methods to the study of these tumors.

Patients with LDHL are usually elderly, and LDHL is rare in individuals younger than 40 years old (8).

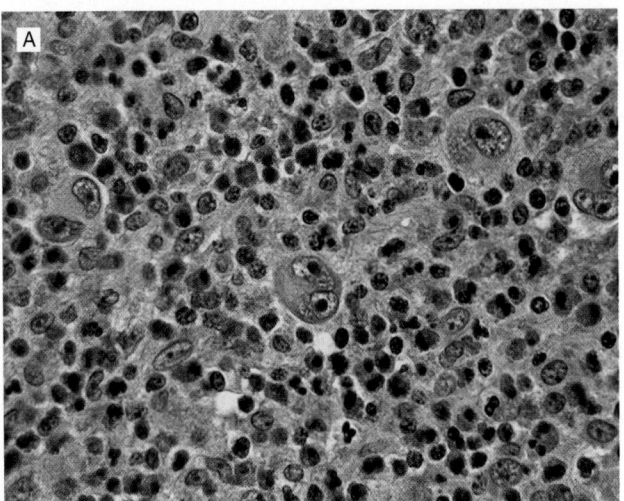

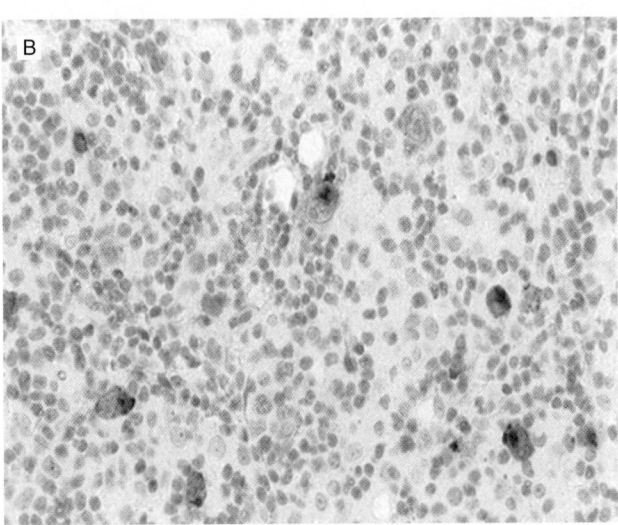

FIGURE 10-5. Mixed cellularity Hodgkin lymphoma. **A.** Classic Reed-Sternberg cell (center of field) and mononuclear Hodgkin cells can be appreciated in a background of reactive lymphocytes, histiocytes, and eosinophils. **B.** Immunostain for Epstein-Barr virus latent membrane protein type 1. The neoplastic cells are positive.

There is a slight male predominance. Whites and blacks populations are equally affected. Most patients have disease of an advanced clinical stage and B symptoms. Patients commonly have a large contiguous mass of matted lymph nodes or diffuse visceral involvement. The diffuse fibrosis type of LD commonly has a subdiaphragmatic distribution. LDHL has the poorest prognosis of all types of HL (8).

Histologic Features

The LDHL category includes two variants originally recognized by Lukes and Butler: diffuse fibrosis and

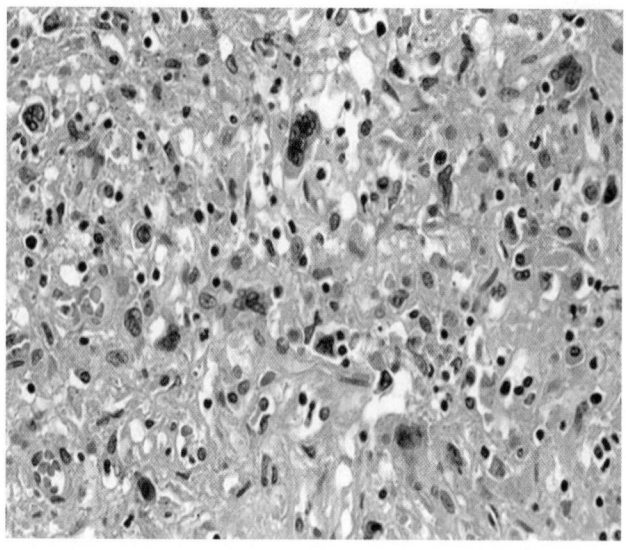

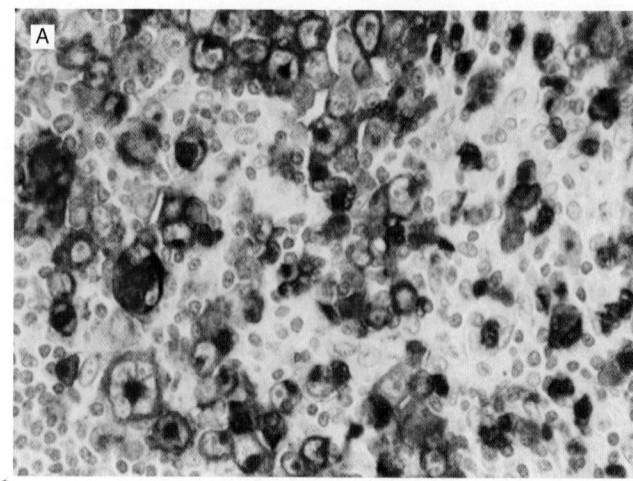

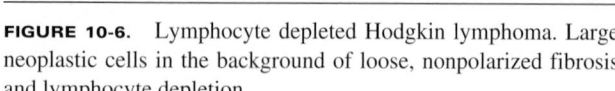

FIGURE 10-6. Lymphocyte depleted Hodgkin lymphoma. Large neoplastic cells in the background of loose, nonpolarized fibrosis and lymphocyte depletion.

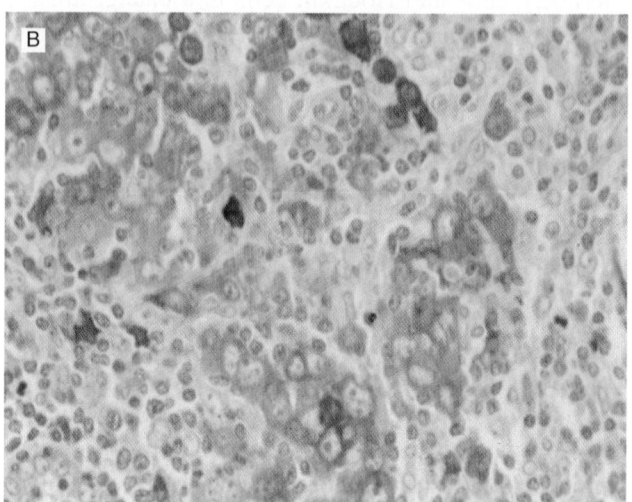

reticular (Fig. 10-6). The diffuse fibrosis variant of LDHL is characterized by an extensive proliferation of disordered, hypocellular fibrosis. Diagnostic HRS cells can be difficult to find and may be spindled within dense collagen. Reactive inflammatory cells are relatively few. The reticular variant of LDHL has numerous HRS cells and bizarre variants that have been termed pleomorphic variants. These cells may exhibit marked variations in nuclear number and shape, often with giant nucleoli. Normal small lymphocytes are infrequent compared with the other subtypes of HL. Necrosis is common and may be extensive. HRS cells and pleomorphic variants may be found in sheets. Mitotic figures are usually numerous.

IMMUNOPHENOTYPIC FINDINGS IN CLASSICAL HODGKIN LYMPHOMA

Overall the mature B-cell origin of the HRS cells is not readily apparent because HRS cells have a very unusual phenotype and have expression of genes which are seen on many hematopoietic cell types. The neoplastic cells are positive for CD15 and CD30 and negative for LCA (CD45) (Fig. 10-7) and EMA (1). B-cell antigens—such as CD20, CD79A, PAX-5/BSAP, and MUM1/IRF4—are expressed in a subset of cases. CD20 expression is often weak. T-cell antigens are usually not expressed by the neoplastic cells. BCL-2 is positive in up to half the cases and has been correlated with poorer prognosis (10). EBV is relatively common

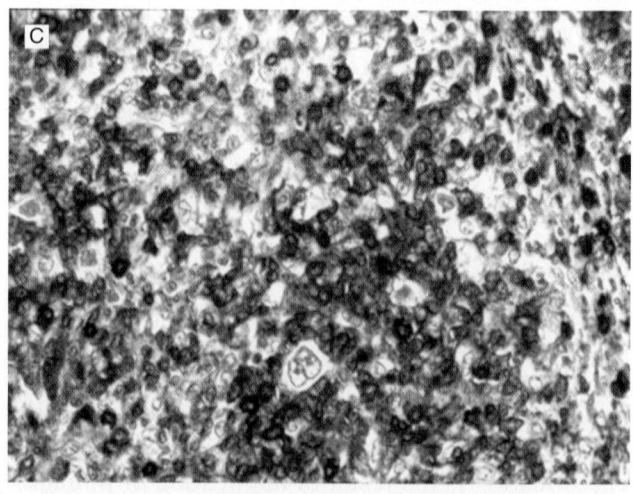

FIGURE 10-7. Typical immunohistochemical findings in classic Hodgkin lymphoma. The Hodgkin cells are positive for CD15 (**A**) and CD30 (**B**). The Hodgkin cells in (**C**) are negative for LCA (CD45RB).

in classical HL, but its frequency varies greatly among different types.

HODGKIN LYMPHOMA CELL LINEAGE, NF-κB ACTIVATION, AND MICROENVIRONMENT

In the past decade, molecular studies and particularly studies using the single-cell polymerase chain reaction (PCR) have shown that in most cases of HL, both NLPHL and classical types of HL, the neoplastic cells arise from B-cell precursors (10). These studies have shown that the neoplastic cells of HL carry monoclonal immunoglobulin (Ig) gene rearrangements. In NLPHL, the Ig gene rearrangements are usually functional, and Ig mRNA transcripts can be identified in most LP cells. The Ig gene variable regions also carry somatic mutations. As the process of somatic mutation is restricted to the GC of secondary lymphoid follicles, the presence of somatic mutations suggests that NLPHL arises from GC B cells.

In classical HL, single-cell PCR studies also have shown that over 95% of cases carry monoclonal Ig gene rearrangements, with somatic mutations in the variable regions suggesting GC B-cell origin. However, unlike the case in NLPHL, there are defects in Ig transcription, and thus Ig mRNA transcripts are often absent. In 25% of cases, the mutations are extensive or involve stop codons, so-called "crippling mutations." In the remainder of cases, one would predict that the Ig gene rearrangements should be functional, but blocks occur in transcription; these are poorly understood. In a very small subset of classical HL cases, T-cell receptor gene rearrangements have been identified (1).

NF-κB is a transcription factor. When proteasomal degradation occurs its dimers then move into the nucleus and can activate target genes. High activity of NF-κB is seen in both HRS and LP cells. NF-κB is usually only transiently activated in normal B cells. However, in HRS cells the receptors expressed on the cell surface including the tumor necrosis family (TNF) proteins CD30, CD40, BCMA (B-cell maturation antigen), TACI (transmembrane activator and CAML-interactor) result in constitutive activation of NF-κB through both the classical and alternative pathways (11). Other mutational changes including to the negative NF-κB regulator A20 in HRS cells can also lead to the constitutive activation (12).

The microenvironment has an important role in promoting the growth of HRS cells and is composed of many different cell types including B and T cells and macrophages. These surrounding cells are needed for HRS cell survival and this likely contributes to the difficulty seen of growing HRS cells in culture (13). The TNF superfamily of proteins has a key role in the microenvironment cross-signaling with the HRS cells and is composed of APRIL (A proliferation-inducing ligand), BLyS (B lymphocyte stimulator), CD30L/CD30, and CD40L/CD40. Although not a TNF protein, CC thymus and activation-related cytokine (TARC) is a protein produced by the HRS cells and attracts T cells by stimulating the CC chemokine receptor 4 (CCR4). Thus, TARC is thought to be a mechanism by which HRS cells provide positive feedback to the microenvironment T cells. Serum levels of BLyS, soluble CD30, and TARC have been found to correlate with rates of classical HL relapse and survival (14-16).

EPSTEIN-BARR VIRUS AND HODGKIN LYMPHOMA

For many years EBV has been known to be associated with HL, although the role of the virus in the pathogenesis of HL was not elucidated until more recently (1). The virus is known to be the cause of infectious mononucleosis, and adolescents who have recovered from infectious mononucleosis have an increased risk of subsequent HL. Patients with HL are known to have high-titer serum antibodies directed against EBV antigens, such as early antigen and viral capsid antigen. The presence of antibodies specific for EBV early antigen suggests that virus infection is active. Also, Mueller et al. (17), using serum obtained from blood donors, have shown that high EBV antibody titers are often present before the onset of HL. Direct proof of EBV in HL was not available until in situ hybridization studies demonstrated EBV within HRS cells (1).

In EBV positive HL nearly all of the HRS cells are found to be positive for the virus. This suggests that EBV infection likely is an early event in the development of these cases of HL. EBV has been shown to rescue preapoptotic GC B cells from apoptosis, and render them independent from survival signals normally provided by the B-cell receptor (18). EBV nuclear antigen (EBNA) as well as latent membrane proteins (LMP) 1 and 2 are expressed in EBV positive HL cells (Fig. 10-5B). Studies have shown that LMP1 acts to mimic a CD40 receptor while LMP2 can mimic BCR, and by doing so provides necessary survival signaling to the HRS cells (19, 20).

Latent EBV infection is present in approximately 40% of cHL (1). The virus is also more common in HL arising in young patients. Almost all HL cases arising in the setting of human immunodeficiency virus (HIV) infection are EBV-positive (1).

■ HODGKIN LYMPHOMA IS LIKELY TWO DIFFERENT DISEASES

MacMahon suggested that HL is heterogeneous and represents at least two diseases (21). This initial "two-disease hypothesis," based primarily on epidemiologic data, considered the NS and MC types of HL as two different diseases. Treatment advances have made the clinical difference between these two types largely irrelevant.

Although the age-adjusted incidence rates, sites of disease, and the role of EBV exposure vary among subtypes of cHL, the clinical behavior is similar, and thus we consider it one disease. NLPHL has a distinct clinical course, and the histologic and immunophenotypic findings indicate that this type of HL is second type of HL (1).

■ HODGKIN LYMPHOMA: STAGING AND THERAPY

The MD Anderson Cancer Center diagnostic and treatment algorithms for Hodgkin Lymphoma are shown in Figure 10-8.

STAGING OF THE PATIENTS

The Ann Arbor system for staging patients with HL at the time of initial presentation forms the basis for the treatment of disease and has allowed comparison of results achieved by different investigators for almost two decades. Important modifications of the Ann Arbor system were developed at the Cotswold Conference in 1989 (Table 10-3) (22). At this meeting, attendees recommended that patients who had bulky disease, including masses larger than 10 cm in greatest dimension or mediastinal masses greater than one-third the chest wall diameter, have a stage designated with the suffix "X," and that patients achieving a greater than 90% partial response with stable adenopathy be designated as having achieved "CRu" (complete response uncertain). This CRu criteria has now been eliminated by the more recent revised response criteria (23). Other recommendations included recognizing the importance of computed tomography (CT) in evaluating liver and spleen involvement and designating abdominal disease substages III_1, and III_2. Patients with stage III_1 disease have splenic involvement or lymphadenopathy involving the splenic hilar, celiac, or portal lymph nodes. Disease involving the paraaortic, iliac, or mesenteric lymph nodes is designated as III_2.

PATIENT EVALUATION

The initial evaluation of patients with HL has both prognostic and therapeutic significance (Fig. 10-8). Routine studies that should be performed include a complete blood cell count with differential, electrolytes, blood urea nitrogen (BUN), creatinine, liver function tests,

TABLE 10-3	ANN ARBOR STAGING SYSTEM WITH COTSWOLD MODIFICATIONS FOR HODGKIN LYMPHOMA
Stage I	Involvement of a single lymph node region or lymphoid structure (eg, spleen, thymus, Waldeyer's ring) or a single extralymphatic site.
Stage II	Involvement of two or more lymph node regions on the same side of the diaphragm; localized contiguous involvement of only one extralymphatic organ or site and lymph node region on the same side of the diaphragm (IIE). The number of anatomic regions involved should be indicated by a subscript (eg, II_3).
Stage III	Involvement of lymph node regions on both sides of the diaphragm (III), which may also be accompanied by spleen involvement (IIIS) or by localized contiguous involvement of only one extralymphatic organ or site (IIIE) or both (IIISE).
III_1	With involvement of splenic, hilar, celiac, or portal lymph nodes.
III_2	With involvement of paraaortic, iliac, and mesenteric lymph nodes.
Stage IV	Diffuse or disseminated involvement of one or more extranodal organs or tissues, with or without associated lymph node involvement.

MODIFYING FEATURES	
A	No symptoms
B	Fever (>38°C), drenching night sweats, unexplained weight loss of >10% body weight within the preceding 6 months
X	Bulky disease: greater than one-third widening of the mediastinum, greater than 10 cm maximum diameter of a nodal mass
E	Involvement of a single extranodal site that is contiguous or proximal to the known nodal site
CS	Clinical stage
PS	Pathologic stage (as determined by laparotomy)

Diagnosis

- FNA alone is generally insufficient
- Core needle biopsy may be adequate if diagnostic, but recommend excisional nodal biopsy
- Recommend immunohistochemistry:
  - Classical HL is usually CD15+, CD30+, CD3–, CD45–, CD20+/–
  - LPHL is usually CD20+, CD45+, CD3–, CD15–, CD30–
- EBV proteins (ie, LMP1) testing can be considered for classical HL nodular sclerosis grade 2 or anaplastic variants

Workup

A

- History and physical including:
  - B symptoms
  - ETOH intolerance
  - Pruritis
  - Fatigue
  - Performance status
  - Exam of nodes
  - Spleen, liver
- CBC with differential
- LDH, Liver function tests including alkaline phosphatase, SGOT, SGPT, and albumin
- BUN, creatinine
- HIV
- Chest x-ray
- CT neck, chest, abdomen, pelvis
- PET/CT
- Bilateral bone marrow biopsies
- Pulmonary function tests if ABVD or BEACOPP is planned
- MUGA or echocardiogram
- Counseling: Fertility, psychosocial if clinically indicated

Useful in selected cases:
- Pregnancy test: women of childbearing age
- Semen cryopreservation: If chemotherapy or pelvic radiotherapy indicated
- Consideration of IVF or oocyte/ovarian preservation if BEACOPP is planned

Clinical Presentation

B

Primary Treatment

Note: Clinical trials are preferred initial therapy for eligible patients

Clinical Presentation	Primary Treatment
Classic Hodgkin lymphoma Clinical stage IA-IIB Favorable	• Clinical trial • ABVD 4 cycles with IFRT • Consider ABVD 2 cycles with IFRT
Classic Hodgkin lymphoma Clinical stage IA-IIB Unfavorable	• Clinical trial • Non-bulky mediastinal disease: ABVD 4 cycles with IFRT • Bulky mediastinal disease: ABVD 6 cycles with IFRT
Nodular lymphocyte Predominant Hodgkin lymphoma	• Clinical trial • Early stage, no B symptoms: IFRT • Early stage, B symptoms: R-CHOP with IFRT • Advanced stage: R-CHOP 6 cycles
Classic Hodgkin lymphoma Clinical stage III-IV	• Clinical trial • ABVD 6-8 cycles • Consider IFRT if initial bulky mass converts to PET negative but remains present

ABVD: Doxorubicin, bleomycin, vinblastine, dacarbazine
IFRT: Involved field radiation
Favorable/Unfavorable: See prognostic factors

FIGURE 10-8. MD Anderson Cancer Center algorithms for Hodgkin lymphoma (A–I).

Restaging at Completion of Treatment
Clinical stages IA, IB, IIA, IIB
Classical Hodgkin lymphoma

Repeat PET/CT

PET/CT scan

Positive

- Recommend biopsy to confirm refractory disease
- Clinical trial preferred
- Second line or salvage chemotherapy followed by ASCT

Negative

- Treatment completed
- Enter into follow up

Restaging at Completion of Treatment
Clinical Stages III and IV
Classical Hodgkin lymphoma

Repeat PET/CT

PET/CT scan

Positive

- Recommend biopsy to confirm refractory disease
- Clinical trial preferred
- Second line or salvage chemotherapy followed by ASCT

Negative

- If bone marrow was initially involved at time of diagnosis confirm negative by repeat bone marrow biopsy
- Treatment completed
- Enter into follow up

C

Follow up after Completion of Treatment
- Follow up with an oncologist is recommended
- Interim H&P, laboratory studies, radiographic tests: every 3 to 4 months for year 1, every 4 to 6 months for year 2, then every 6 months for year 3-5, then annually
  - Laboratory studies: CBC with differential, chemistry profile, TSH every 6 months if radiation to the neck
  - Radiographic tests: CT scans of neck, chest, abdomen/pelvis
- Pneumoccocal and meningoccoal revaccination every 6 years if treated with splenic radiotherapy
- Annual influenza vaccine (especially if treated with bleomycin or chest radiotherapy)

- Annual mammographic screening: initiate 8-10 years post completion of therapy or at age 40, whichever comes first
- Counseling: reproduction, health habits, psychosocial, cardiovascular, breast self-exam, other cancer screening studies as recommended for age.

If relapse would be suspected recommend repeat staging similar to initial work-up and biopsy to confirm disease relapse.

D

Salvage Treatment for Classical Hodgkin Lymphoma
Note: Clinical trials are preferred initial therapy for eligible patients.

- Clinical trial preferred
- Second-line chemotherapy followed by ASCT

Relapse/Refractory after ASCT

- Clinical trial preferred
- Salvage chemotherapy including gemcitabine containing regimens
- Consideration of allogeneic SCT in select patients

FIGURE 10-8. *(Continued)*

Prognostic Factors for Classical Hodgkin Lymphoma

E

European Organization for the Research and Treatment of Cancer

Unfavorable CS I-II

Any of the following:

1. Age >50
2. No B symptoms with ESR >50 or B symptoms with ESR >30
3. Large mediastinal mass
4. Stage II
5. At least 4 nodal regions involved

German Hodgkin Study Group

Unfavorable CS I-II

Any of the following:

1. Large mediastinal mass
2. At least 3 nodal regions involved
3. No B symptoms with ESR >50 or B symptoms with ESR >30
4. Extranodal lesions

International Prognostic Score

Unfavorable Advanced Disease

Assign 1 point per factor

- Albumin <4g/dL
- Hemoglobin <10.5 g/dL
- Male
- Age ≥45 years
- Stage IV disease
- WBC ≥15,000/mm^3
- Lymphocytopenia (ALC less than 8% of total WBC or <600/mm^3)

International Prognostic Score

Score	5-year FFP, percent	5-year OS, percent
0	84	89
1	77	90
2	67	81
3	60	78
4	51	61
5 or more	42	56

FIGURE 10-8. (*Continued*)

lactate dehydrogenase (LDH), albumin, pregnancy test in women of childbearing age, erythrocyte sedimentation rate (ESR), pulmonary function test (PFT) with carbon monoxide diffusing capacity (DLCO), evaluation of cardiac ejection fraction, chest x-ray and CT of neck, chest, abdomen and pelvis, and positron emission tomography (PET)/CT (Table 10-4). Other diagnostic procedures should be ordered depending upon the disease presentation and planned treatment. Bilateral bone marrow biopsies should be routinely performed, although these are more likely to yield positive results in patients with B symptoms.

Gallium scans were introduced prior to the advent of PET, and served a similar role in distinguishing complete versus partial metabolic responses to therapy. At the time of initial staging evaluation, the ^{67}Ga scan was found to not replace CT, but to be complementary. Hagemeister et al. (24) retrospectively reviewed 240 gallium scans from 165 patients with HL. In untreated disease, the sensitivity of this test was only 64%, with a specificity of 95%. In untreated patients or those in whom disease had recurred, gallium uptake was predictive for disease in specific sites. Unfortunately,

95% of relapses were not predicted by this study during routine follow-up. Nevertheless, there are abundant reports showing that ^{67}Ga scans before and after therapy are valuable in monitoring the HL disease status (25). The usefulness of the ^{67}Ga scan, therefore, may be limited to confirming the diagnosis of HL in new patients and in treated patients who have new or residual lesions.

Magnetic resonance imaging (MRI) has not superseded CT scanning of the chest and abdomen in the evaluation of HL. It is largely restricted to the assessment of specific situations such as bony involvement and spinal cord compression as well as in lieu of CT scans in pregnant patients.

PROGNOSTIC FACTORS

In HL patients at a low clinical stage (CS)—that is, CS I or CS II, several prognostic factors, based largely on patients treated only with radiotherapy, have been identified through retrospective studies. These adverse factors are (1) advanced age, which correlates with the presence of occult abdominal disease and with poor

TABLE 10-4	RECOMMENDED PROCEDURES FOR STAGING OF HODGKIN LYMPHOMA
History and examination	Identification of B symptoms
Radiologic and other assessments	Chest radiograph
	Computed tomographic (CT) scans including neck, chest, abdomen, and pelvis whole-body positron emission tomography (PET) scan
	Gallium scanning if PET scan is not available
	Echocardiogram or multi gated acquisition (MUGA) scan
	Pulmonary function tests
	HIV serology
	Pregnancy test in women of childbearing age
Hematologic procedures	Complete blood count with differential
	Erythrocyte sedimentation rate (ESR)
	Bilateral bone marrow aspiration and biopsy
Biochemical procedures	Liver function tests
	Serum albumin
	Lactate dehydrogenase
Procedures for use under special circumstances	Ultrasound scanning
	Magnetic resonance imaging

TABLE 10-5	PROGNOSTIC CLASSIFICATION OF THE EORTC AND GHSG GROUPS FOR CLINICAL STAGE I/II HODGKIN LYMPHOMA

EORTC

Unfavorable (presence of *any* of the following):
   Age ≥50 years
   ESR >50 mm/h without B symptoms, ESR >30 mm/h with B symptoms
   ≥4 nodal sites of involvement
   Bulky mediastinal mass

GHSG

Unfavorable (presence of *any* of the following):
   ESR >50 mm/h without B symptoms, ESR >30 mm/h with B symptoms
   ≥3 nodal sites of involvement
   Bulky mediastinal mass
   Extranodal involvement

EORTC, European Organization for the Research and Treatment of Cancer; ESR, erythrocyte sedimentation rate; GHSG, German Hodgkin Lymphoma Study Group.

factors: (1) large mediastinal mass, (2) at least three nodal regions involved, (3) no symptoms present with ESR >50 mm/h or B symptoms with ESR >30 mm/h, or (4) localized extranodal infiltration (so-called E lesions) (Table 10-5) (29). In advanced disease, the International Prognostic Score (IPS) was developed on the basis of an analysis of 5141 patients treated initially with an anthracycline-containing chemotherapy regimen. Seven factors were identified, as shown in Table 10-6 (30).

PET SCAN

Whole-body PET is as good as or slightly better than CT at time of initial diagnostic work-up, as demonstrated by several studies (31, 32). Interim PET obtained after two cycles of therapy (PET-2) has been shown to have a stronger prediction of outcome than the IPS with 2-year progression-free survival for patients with positive

TABLE 10-6	INTERNATIONAL PROGNOSTIC SCORE (IPS) FOR HODGKIN LYMPHOMA

Hemoglobin <10.5 g/dL
Age ≥45 years
Male gender
Lymphocyte count <600/mm^3 or <8% of white blood cell count
Serum albumin <4 g/dL
White blood cell count ≥15,000/mm^3
Stage IV disease (Ann Arbor system)

Reproduced, with permission, from Hasenclever D, Diehl V. A prognostic score for advanced Hodgkin lymphoma disease: International Prognostic Factors Project on Advanced Hodgkin Disease. *N Engl J Med* 1998;339: 1506-1514.

results of salvage therapy; (2) male gender; (3) MC histologic type, which is associated with the presence of occult abdominal disease; (4) B symptoms, also associated with the presence of occult abdominal disease; (5) large mediastinal mass, defined as a mass measuring greater than one-third the chest diameter on a standard chest radiograph; (6) a larger number of involved nodal regions; (7) an elevated ESR; (8) anemia; and (9) a low serum albumin level (26, 27).

Internationally based organizations have defined various systems that calculate the risk of recurrence of disease or, in some cases, death, following treatment for HL. The European Organization for the Research and Treatment of Cancer (EORTC) has defined CS I and CS II patients as having an unfavorable risk of development of recurrence if any of the following factors apply: (1) age >50 years, (2) no symptoms present with ESR >50 mm/h or B symptoms with ESR >30 mm/h, (3) large mediastinal mass, (4) stage II, or (5) at least four nodal regions involved (28). The German Hodgkin Study Group (GHSG) has assigned CS I and CS II patients to the category of unfavorable disease with any of the following adverse

PET-2 of 13% as compared to 95% for those with a negative PET-2 (33). PET-2 also strongly predicts treatment failure (34). In a recent meta-analysis, a positive PET after two cycles of therapy in low-intermediate risk advanced HL patients was shown to be a reliable predictor of poor response (35). The recently opened S0816 Phase II Intergroup trial is evaluating interim PET in stage III or stage IV cHL patients treated with two cycles of ABVD (doxorubicin, bleomycin, vinblastine, dacarbazine) (36). Patients who have negative PET would receive four additional cycles of ABVD, whereas PET positive patients would receive BEACOPP (bleomycin, etoposide, adriamycin, cyclophosphamide, vincristine, procarbazine, prednisone) baseline if HIV positive and BEACOPP escalated if HIV negative.

The HD15 trial showed a negative predictive value of 94% for PET after BEACOPP-based therapy in advanced stage HL (37). The PFS at 12 months was 96% for PET negative patients and 86% for PET positive patients. At the time of posttreatment examination, PET has higher diagnostic and prognostic value than conventional CT (38-40). Studies have shown that PET performs better than the gallium scan in predicting treatment response and disease-free survival (DFS) as well (41, 42). The role of PET prior to transplant has recently been evaluated in a small study, which found a negative PET prior to autologous transplant yielded a 76% continuous complete response (CCR) (43). In the same study, a positive pretransplant PET resulted in an 18% CCR.

RESPONSE ASSESSMENT

Prior to 1999, the criteria used to assess response to therapy were not routinely standardized. The International Working Group (IWG) formulated guidelines for the assessment of response to therapy (44). These criteria were widely used but with time several components arose as being recommended for revision including the lack of assessment of extranodal disease, the somewhat subjective CRu term, and the introduction of PET in place of gallium scans. Thus, the IWG criteria were updated in 2007 and serve as the current standard for response assessment (23). These current response definitions eliminate the CRu term, incorporate PET scan response for FDG-avid lymphomas like HL, and clearly define the routine clinical endpoints used in clinical trials.

TREATMENT OF HODGKIN LYMPHOMA

The common practice for treatment and participation in clinical trials is to divide HL patients into three treatment groups: early-stage favorable, early-stage unfavorable, and advanced stage.

Favorable, Early-Stage Hodgkin Lymphoma

Radiotherapy alone

Treatment of favorable early-stage HL is evolving. Historically, wide or extended-field radiotherapy (RT) was the standard of care as a result of the study by Rosenberg et al. (45). Extended-field RT (EFRT) produced superior overall survival (OS) and disease-free survival (DFS) as compared with involved-field RT (IFRT). These findings were validated in other trials and in a meta-analysis conducted by Specht et al. (46). The analysis was of combined data from almost 2000 patients with early-stage HL obtained from eight randomized trials. In comparing treatment with more versus less extensive RT, it was found that more extensive RT significantly reduced the risk of failure at 0 to 4, 5 to 9, and 10 or more years. There was a trend toward fewer HL deaths in the more extensive RT arm, although the difference was not statistically significant. Moreover, there was a trend of higher risk of dying from causes other than HL with more extensive RT.

The EORTC H5F trial randomized patients with favorable pathologic stage I/stage II HL into mantle-field plus paraaortic RT versus mantle-field RT alone and detected no significant difference in failure-free and OS at 15 years follow-up (47). However, this approach required staging by laparotomy, a practice not commonly used today. The GHSG HD4 trial treated favorable early-stage HL patients with EFRT alone and randomized them to 40 Gy of EFRT versus 30 Gy of EFRT plus an additional 10 Gy to the involved field. Seven-year relapse-free survival rates were 78% in the 40-Gy arm and 83% for the 30-Gy arm; OS rates were 91% for the 40-Gy arm and 96% in the 30-Gy arm. These differences favored the low-dose EFRT group but did not reach statistical significance (48).

EFRT was found to have considerable long-term side effects. In a large prospective analysis of over 15,000 HL patients, the actuarial risk of developing a solid tumor was 21.9% at 25 years after HL diagnosis, with the absolute risk being nearly 50%. Common secondary solid tumors were female breast and lung cancers (49). The Stanford group (50) reported a 15% 15-year actuarial risk of developing a second cancer. Treatment-related deaths began to surpass HL-related deaths at 15 years of follow-up (50). With the recognition of notable long-term side effects as well as high relapse rates, EFRT monotherapy has now been abandoned in favor of combined-modality therapy.

Combined-modality therapy

Combined-modality therapy has evolved over the last 20 years, based on the premise that this approach results in high freedom from recurrence in early-stage HL and that efficacy can be maintained using less toxic chemotherapy and RT regimens. There are many completed and ongoing trials addressing issues of the best modality, best RT field, optimal dose of RT, optimal combination of drugs, number of cycles, and optimal timing of chemotherapy with the goal being to maintain efficacy and minimize toxicities (Table 10-7).

In a meta-analysis that combined 12 trials including 1666 early-stage HL patients, combined chemotherapy plus RT was compared with RT alone (46). This study demonstrated that combined chemotherapy plus

TABLE 10-7	KEY TRIALS FOR PATIENTS WITH FAVORABLE, EARLY-STAGE HODGKIN LYMPHOMA
Trial	**Trial Design**
Milan 1990 to 1997	ABVD × 4 → STLI
	ABVD × 4 → IFRT
Stanford	Stanford V × 8 weeks → IFRT
EORTC/GELA H9F	EBVP × 6 → 20 Gy IFRT
	EBVP × 6 → 30 Gy IFRT
	EBVP × 6 alone
GHSG HD10	ABVD × 2 → 2 Gy IFRT
	ABVD × 4 → 20 Gy IFRT
	ABVD × 2 → 30 Gy IFRT
	ABVD × 4 → 30 Gy IFRT
GHSG HD13	ABVD × 2 → 30 Gy IFRT
	ABV × 2 → 30 Gy IFRT
	AVD × 2 → 30 Gy IFRT
	AV × 2 → 30 Gy IFRT
EORTC/GELA H10F	ABVD × 3 → INRT
	ABVD × 2 → then PET scan
	• If PET negative → ABVD × 2
	• If PET positive → BEACOPP escalated × 2 → INRT
GHSG HD16	ABVD × 2 → IFRT
	ABVD × 2 → then PET scan
	• If PET negative → stop treatment
	• If PET positive → IFRT

EORTC, European Organization for Research and Treatment of Cancer; GELA, Groupe d'Etude des Lymphomes de l'Adulte; GHSG, German Hodgkin Lymphoma Study Group; SWOG, Southwest Oncology Group; STLI, subtotal lymphoid irradiation; IFRT, involved field radiotherapy; INRT, involved nodal radiotherapy; ABVD, doxorubicin, bleomycin, vinblastine, dacarbazine; Stanford V, mechlorethamine, doxorubicin, vinblastine, vincristine, bleomycin, etoposide, prednisone; EBVP, epirubicin, bleomycin, vinblastine, prednisone.

RT significantly reduced the risk of failure by 53% at 10 years, from approximately one-third to approximately one-sixth. The absolute benefit appeared greatest in years 0 to 4, with significantly fewer recurrences also in years 5 to 9. The reduction in the risk of failure was similar among trials that used combined chemotherapy plus IFRT versus more extensive RT, such as EFRT, subtotal nodal RT, or total lymphoid irradiation (TLI). This highly significant reduction in failure translated into only a borderline significant improvement in OS at 10 years. After year 10, due to non-HL-related deaths, there were slightly more deaths in those who had received chemotherapy. However, the chemotherapy regimen most often used in this study was MOPP (mechlorethamine, vincristine, procarbazine, prednisone) or a variant of this combination.

Multiple studies have shown that chemotherapy followed by RT provides better freedom-from-failure rates than RT alone in patients with CS I to CS II disease. The EORTC H7F trial evaluated six cycles of EBVP (epirubicin, bleomycin, vinblastine, prednisone) followed by IFRT versus subtotal nodal irradiation (STNI). The 6-year failure-free survival was significantly higher following combined chemotherapy and IFRT (92 versus 81%), but OS rates were not significantly different (51). The Stanford group compared six cycles of a novel combination of agents called VBM (vinblastine, bleomycin, methotrexate) followed by IFRT versus STNI or TLI alone (52). The actuarial freedom-from-progression (FFP) at 5 years was 70% after STNI or TLI and 95% after VBM plus IFRT. The data for VBM combined with IFRT appear superior to previous actuarial results at 5 years using IFRT alone (FFP = 35%) and compare favorably with prior results reported with MOPP and IFRT (FFP = 80% at 5 years). The SWOG 9133/CALGB 9391 trial evaluated treatment of CS IA to CS IIA patients with either doxorubicin and vinblastine for three cycles followed by STLI versus STLI alone (53). The 3-year FFS was 94 versus 81%, and a 10-year relapse free survival update continued to show a significant difference (88 versus 78%). The Milan group performed a landmark study comparing four cycles of ABVD followed by IFRT or the same chemotherapy and subtotal nodal RT in early-stage HL. At 10 years of follow-up, ABVD plus IFRT yielded results equivalent to those obtained with ABVD plus STNI (54). In the EORTC H8F trial, favorable early-stage HL patients received either three cycles of MOPP/ABV hybrid and IFRT versus mantle-field and paraaortic/splenic RT. MOPP/ABV plus IFRT was more effective than STNI and provided a 5-year event-free survival (EFS) of 98% (55).

At MD Anderson Cancer Center, from 1980 to 1995, investigators performed a retrospective analysis of a group of 286 patients with early-stage HL treated with chemotherapy followed by IFRT or EFRT with a median dose of 40 Gy. Five-year relapse-free and OS were 88 and 93%, respectively, with a mean of 7.4 years of follow-up. The type and number of chemotherapy cycles used did not significantly affect relapse-free survival (RFS) and OS. However, the 5-, 10-, and 15-year cumulative risks of developing solid tumors in patients treated with chemotherapy and IFRT were 0, 6.9, and 11.4%, respectively. These results were strikingly more favorable than those of patients treated with chemotherapy plus EFRT (2.7, 11.1, and 28.7%, respectively) (56).

It has become clear that the longer HL patients live, the less likely it is that they will die of HL and the more likely it becomes that their deaths will be due to causes other than HL. Investigators have therefore tried to limit the amount or extent of RT in the management of these patients. In a study of HL in children, combined chemotherapy with low-dose RT (<25 Gy) or high-dose RT (30-40 Gy) provided the same 10-year and failure-free survival rates of 88 and 67%, respectively (57). A phase III trial for early-stage HL conducted by the GHSG confirmed that 20 Gy is sufficient therapy when extended IFRT of early-stage HD is being used following four cycles of COPP (cyclophosphamide, vincristine, procarbazine, prednisone)/ABVD hybrid (58).

In a landmark trial for advanced HL conducted by Santoro et al. (59), six cycles of ABVD versus six cycles of MOPP followed by EFRT were tested. Seven-year follow-up results revealed that ABVD was superior to MOPP in terms of FFP rates (80.8 versus 62.8%; $p < .002$), RFS (87.7 versus 77.2%; $p = .06$), and OS (77.4 versus 67.9%; $p = .03$). Moreover, ABVD was less toxic than MOPP. Subsequently, the EORTC H6U trial for early-stage HL randomized six cycles of ABVD versus six cycles of MOPP followed by mantle field RT; it confirmed that the ABVD arm had superior freedom from progression (FFP) at 6 years of follow-up (88 versus 76%; $p = .01$), although OS rates were not statistically different (91 versus 85%; $p = .22$) (60). Based on these results, the ABVD regimen has replaced MOPP and has become the standard chemotherapy regimen.

The EORTC H9F trial was a three-arm trial comparing six cycles of EBVP with six cycles of EBVP followed by IFRT, either 20 or 36 Gy. In this trial the EBVP alone arm was closed emphasizing the role for CMT. However, EBVP is believed by many to be an inferior regimen to ABVD (61).

In the Stanford G4 trial 87 patients with non-bulky, above the diaphragm stages I and IIA disease were treated with 8 weeks of the Stanford V regimen (mechlorethamine, doxorubicin, vinblastine, vincristine, bleomycin, etoposide, prednisone) followed by 30 Gy of IFRT. According to the GHSG criteria 54% of patients had unfavorable risk factors. FFP and OS are 94 and 96% at a median of 9 years of follow-up, with FFP being 100% for patients with early-stage favorable disease. No late cardiopulmonary toxicities were seen (62).

The recently completed GHSG HD10 trial had four arms testing two versus four cycles of ABVD followed by 20 versus 30 Gy of IFRT in patients with favorable, early-stage HL (63). This trial addressed both the optimal dose of RT and the optimal number of cycles of chemotherapy. The ABVD two- and four-cycle arms both had CR rates of 97%. The 20 and 30 Gy IFRT groups had CR rates of 97 and 98%, respectively. With a median follow up of 7 years, there was no difference between the four groups in PFS, FFTF, and OS. The four ABVD and 30 Gy IFRT treatment groups had more toxicity than the less intensive treatment groups. Based on these data, the GHSG standard approach for early favorable stage HL is two ABVD cycles and 20 Gy IFRT.

In the GHSG HD13 trial, the aim is to omit bleomycin or dacarbazine from the chemotherapy. This four-arm trial investigates ABVD, AVD, ABV, and AV plus 30 Gy of IFRT. In this ongoing trial, the ABV and AV plus IFRT arms have been closed because of safety concerns (64).

The British Columbia Cancer Agency recently published their data on combined chemotherapy and either extended field, involved field, or involved nodal radiation therapy in limited stage Hodgkins patients from 1989 to 2005 (65). They found that reduction in the radiation field did not lead to increased local regional failure and thus appears safe.

Chemotherapy alone

In early-stage HL, the risk of mortality from causes other than HL, including second tumors and cardiac disease, increases over time and remains elevated more than 20 years after treatment (49,66). The relative risk for second tumor is significantly higher among patients receiving combined chemotherapy plus RT or RT alone; this risk increases with increasing size of the radiation field in patients who receive combined-modality therapy (67). Therefore, there is interest in potentially determining whether patients with early-stage favorable HL could potentially be treated with chemotherapy alone.

In a randomized trial conducted by Biti et al. (68), six cycles of MOPP were compared with mantle-field RT for patients with favorable, early-stage HL. Eight-year relapse-free survivals were similar, but 8-year OSs favored the mantle-field RT group due to less successful salvage treatment in the chemotherapy arm. The Grupo Argentino de Tratamiento de la Leucemia Aguda (GATLA) conducted another randomized trial comparing six cycles of CVPP (cyclophosphamide, vinblastine, procarbazine, and prednisone) versus six cycles of CVPP plus IFRT for favorable early-stage HL. DFS rates (77 versus 70%) and OS rates (92 versus 91%) at 84 months for these two arms were similar. However, the chemotherapy regimens used in these two trials are outdated by today's standards.

At Memorial Sloan–Kettering, a prospective randomized clinical trial was done to assess ABVD alone followed by radiation therapy versus ABVD alone. A total of 152 patients were enrolled with stage of disease ranging from IA to IIIA. Radiation therapy given ranged from IFRT for 11 patients and modified EFRT for the remaining patients. For patients treated with ABVD plus RT, the complete remission (CR) was 94%. At 5 years, the FFP and OS for the ABVD plus RT versus the ABVD alone were 91 versus 87% and 86 versus 81% and significant differences were not seen. However, this trial was not powered to detect small differences in outcomes (69).

However, the randomized GHSG HD16 and the EORTC H10F trials are further investigating the role of chemotherapy alone for early-stage favorable patients. Both of these trials utilize PET scan response to determine radiation treatment by having patients in the experimental arms have radiation therapy omitted if PET negative after two cycles of ABVD (70).

MD Anderson approach

In summary, the treatment for favorable early-stage HL is still evolving. Patients are typically screened for clinical protocol options if available. As standard therapy at MD Anderson Cancer Center, we have utilized four cycles of ABVD plus IFRT for this group of patients. Based on the recently reported GHSG HD10 trial we are now considering two cycles of ABVD plus IFRT for this group of patients.

Unfavorable Early-Stage Hodgkin Lymphoma

Among major centers and study groups, the type and number of cycles of chemotherapy and dose of radiation used in the treatment of patients with unfavorable early-stage HL is controversial.

Extended to involved field radiotherapy

Multiple trials have shown that reduction of radiation field does not lead to inferior clinical outcomes. The EORTC H8U trial evaluated six versus four cycles of MOPP/ABV and IFRT versus STLI and found four cycles of MOPP/ABV followed by IFRT to have a 88% EFS at 5 years and 85% OS at 10 years with no difference noted as compared to the other treatment arms (55). Bonadonna et al. also compared STLI to IFRT after four cycles of ABVD and showed similar outcomes in both arms (54). The GHSG HD8 trial evaluated two cycles of alternating COPP/ABVD with either IFRT versus EFRT and reported no significant relapse rates or survival but higher toxicity in those treated with EFRT (71). At MD Anderson Cancer Center 286 patients with early-stage HL were treated with chemotherapy followed by IFRT or EFRT. Of these patients 58% had unfavorable early-stage disease, and the median dose of RT was 40 Gy. The 5-year relapse-free and OS were 88 and 93%, respectively. The type and number of chemotherapy regimens used did not significantly affect relapse-free and OS. However, 5-, 10-, and 15-year risks of developing solid tumors in patients treated with chemotherapy plus IFRT were 0, 6.9, and 11.4%, respectively with a trend toward higher risks of secondary tumors in the EFRT group (56). The optimal dose of RT to be used following chemotherapy also remains controversial. In early studies of RT for HL, 40 Gy was necessary for 98% in-field disease control (72). In a reanalysis of the dose–response data for HL, there was no evidence of an increased response to doses above 32.5 Gy and most current trials of the GHSG and EORTC use 30 Gy of IFRT (73).

The optimal chemotherapy regimen

As similar to early-stage favorable HL, ABVD alone has been found to be as more effective than MOPP and equally as effective as the alternating regimen MOPP/ABVD and less toxic (74). However, given the relapses that occur with ABVD combined modality therapy there has been international interest in evaluating alternative more intensive regimens (Table 10-8).

At Stanford patients with early-stage unfavorable disease secondary to bulky disease were treated with 12 weeks of the Stanford V regimen followed by 36 Gy of IFRT to bulky disease. The FFP was 92% at 8 years for those with stages I and II bulky disease (75). Data from Memorial Sloan-Kettering Cancer Center and Italy has shown similar outcomes (76, 77). To address whether ABVD or Stanford V would be the best approach for patients with early-stage bulky unfavorable *HL*, the intergroup SWOG (Southwest Oncology Group)/ECOG

TABLE
10-8

KEY TRIALS FOR PATIENTS WITH UNFAVORABLE, EARLY-STAGE HODGKIN LYMPHOMA

Trial	Trial Design
SWOG/ECOG 2496	ABVD × 6 → 36 Gy IFRT to >5 cm disease
	Standord V × 12 weeks → 36 Gy IFRT to >5 cm disease
EORTC/GELA H9U	ABVD × 6 → IFRT
	ABVD × 4 → IFRT
	BEACOPP × 4 → IFRT
GHSG HD11	ABVD × 4 → 30 Gy IFRT
	ABVD × 4 → 20 Gy IFRT
	BEACOPP baseline × 4 → 30 Gy IFRT
	BEACOPP baseline × 4 → 20 Gy IFRT
GHSG HD14	ABVD × 4 → 30 Gy IFRT
	BEACOPP escalated + ABVD × 2 → 30 Gy IFRT
EORTC/GELA H10F	ABVD × 4 → INRT
	ABVD × 2 → then PET scan
	• If PET negative → ABVD × 4
	• If PET positive → BEACOPP escalated × 2 → INRT

SWOG, Southwest Oncology Group; ECOG, Eastern Cooperative Oncology Group; GELA, Groupe d'Etude des Lymphomes de l'Adulte; EORTC, European Organization for Research and Treatment of Cancer; GHSG, German Hodgkin Lymphoma Study Group; IFRT, involved field radiotherapy; INRT, involved nodal radiotherapy; ABVD, doxorubicin, bleomycin, vinblastine, dacarbazine; Stanford V, mechlorethamine, doxorubicin, vinblastine, vincristine, bleomycin, etoposide, prednisone BEACOPP, bleomycin, etoposide, doxorubicin, cyclophosphamide, vincristine, procarbazine, prednisone.

(Eastern Cooperative Oncology Group) 2496 was conducted. In this recently completed trial, early-stage bulky unfavorable patients were randomized to six cycles of ABVD followed with IFRT at 36 Gy to bulk greater than 5 cm versus 12 weeks of Stanford V followed by the same IFRT plan of care. Results of this trial are pending release.

The BEACOPP at both baseline and escalated doses has been evaluated in trials compared to ABVD by both the GHSG and the EORTC. In the EORTC H9U trial, patients were randomized to receive either six cycles of ABVD followed by IFRT, four cycles of ABVD followed by IFRT, or four cycles of BEACOPP baseline followed by IFRT. All patients received 30 Gy of IFRT. At a median follow-up of four years EFS and OS remain statistically equivalent in all arms with EFS ranging from 87 to 91% and OS ranging from 93 to 95% (78). The GHSG HD 11 randomized patients to four arms of therapy and evaluated four cycles of ABVD followed by 30 versus 20 Gy of IFRT and compared outcomes to four cycles of BEACOPP baseline followed by 30 versus

20 Gy of IFRT. Current data available from the interim analysis at 3 years of follow-up shows in general no differences across the four arms of therapy with a freedom from treatment failure (FFTF) of 87% (79).

Given the continued level of relapses in the trials above the GHSG is now conducting the HD14 trial which randomizes patients to two arms of treatment. Patients receive four cycles of ABVD followed by 30 Gy of IFRT or two cycles of BEACOPP escalated followed by two cycles of ABVD and then 30 Gy of IFRT. The GHSG HD17 trial which is currently in development will examine whether radiation field can be decreased to an involved node and also whether it is possible to perform RT or no RT according to the PET scan response after two cycles of ABVD. In the EORTC's current trial, H10U PET scan response is incorporated into a risk-adapted treatment plan with patients in the experimental arm receiving two cycles of ABVD and if repeat PET scan shows negativity then four cycles further of ABVD without IFRT if given. A preliminary report has been released for the EORTC H10F/U trials. A total of 1097 patients were treated and a baseline PET was available for 93% of the patients overall and centralized PET review is performed after cycle two of ABVD. Six nuclear medicine physicians provide the assessment of PET scan response within 72 hours. In the unfavorable early-stage patients, 24% were found to have a positive PET scan result after two cycles of ABVD (80).

MD Anderson approach

In summary, ABVD plus IFRT is presently a standard of care option for unfavorable early-stage HL pending the results of ongoing trials. We screen our patients for any available clinical protocols. As our standard therapy we typically use four cycles of ABVD plus IFRT for patients with early-stage unfavorable disease including those with nonbulky mediastinal disease. If a patient has a bulky mediastinal mass of 10 cm or greater then we typically treat with six cycles of ABVD followed by involved field radiation therapy.

Advanced-Stage Hodgkin Lymphoma

Chemotherapy

Despite the fact that therapy with ABVD alone or a combination of MOPP (or MOPP-like therapy) and ABVD appears better than treatment with MOPP alone, 20% of patients with advanced-stage HL will still fail to achieve CR and one-third of patients entering CR will ultimately develop relapse, resulting in a long-term FFS rate of only 60 to 70%. Various chemotherapy regimens have been developed in an attempt to improve on these results, with varying degrees of success in both patients with low- and high-risk disease as defined by the IPS (30) (see Table 10-6).

A Stanford trial evaluated 108 patients with stages III and IV disease. They received 12 weeks of Stanford V followed by 36 Gy of IFRT to sites of initial disease with bulk greater than 5 cm. With 12 years now of follow-up, the FFP was 83% with a 95% OS (75). These results mirror similar positive results seen from evaluation of this regimen for early-stage unfavorable patients. A multicenter Intergroup Italian randomized trial showed that Stanford V is potentially inferior to ABVD; however, this is thought to be potentially accounted for by suboptimal levels of radiation delivered (81).

The GHSG HD9 trial evaluated in a three-arm randomized trial four cycles of COPP/ABVD versus eight cycles of BEACOPP baseline versus eight cycles of BEACOPP escalated. At 10 years of follow-up, FFTF respectively was 64, 70, and 82% and OS was respectively 75, 80, and 86%. This data shows superior results with BEACOPP escalated.

The following GHSG HD12 trial investigated whether the number of cycles of BEACOPP escalated could be de-escalated by evaluating eight BEACOPP escalated versus four BEACOPP escalated plus four BEACOPP baseline and what the potential added benefit of consolidation radiation treatment would be in treating sites of initial bulk or residual disease. Currently with 4 years of follow-up there is not a statistically significant difference in FFTF or OS, with FFTF of 88% for eight cycles of BEACOPP escalated and 86% for four BEACOPP escalated plus four BEACOPP baseline (82) (Table 10-9).

The next GHSG trial assessed the role of PET scan response in assessing need for IFRT and also the role of dose dense BEACOPP standard delivered every 14 days (BEACOPP-14). In HD15 patients were randomized to three arms using eight cycles of BEACOPP escalated, six cycles of BEACOPP escalated, and eight cycles of BEACOPP-14. In addition, patients with PET scan residual disease of 2.5 cm or greater received IFRT. Results in regards to the overall long-term outcomes for patients treated on each of the three arms of chemotherapy are awaited, however PET at completion of frontline chemotherapy was found to have a high negative predictive value of 94% at 1 year (83).

A Cochrane meta-analysis of trials compared ABVD and BEACOPP regimens in intermediate to advanced HL evaluated data from the HD9 and HD14 trials from Germany, and the HD2000 and GSM-HD

TABLE 10-9	KEY TRIALS FOR ADVANCED-STAGE HODGKIN LYMPHOMA
Trials	**Design**
GHSG HD12	BEACOPP escalated × 8
	BEACOPP escalated × 8
	BEACOPP escalated × 4 + BEACOPP baseline × 4 → IFRT to bulk/residual mass
	BEACOPP escalated × 4 + BEACOPP baseline × 4
GHSG HD15	BEACOPP escalated × 8 → IFRT to PET positive residual masses ≥2.5 cm
	BEACOPP escalated × 6 → IFRT to PET positive residual masses ≥2.5 cm
	BEACOPP-14 × 8 → IFRT to PET positive residual masses ≥2.5 cm
EORTC 20012 IPS >2	ABVD × 8
	BEACOPP escalated × 4 + BEACOPP baseline × 4
GHSG HD18	BEACOPP escalated × 2 → then PET scan
	• If PET negative
	• BEACOPP escalated × 6
	• BEACOPP escalated × 2
	• If PET positive
	• BEACOPP escalated × 6
	• BEACOPP escalated × 6 + rituximab

GHSG, German Hodgkin Lymphoma Study Group; EORTC, European Organization for Research and Treatment of Cancer; IFRT, involved field radiotherapy; ABVD, doxorubicin, bleomycin, vinblastine, dacarbazine; BEACOPP, bleomycin, etoposide, doxorubicin, cyclophosphamide, vincristine, procarbazine, prednisone.

trials from Italy (84). This found the BEACOPP regimen had higher incidence of toxicities, but demonstrated prolonged PFS and a nonsignificant trend toward improved OS. At the time of the analysis, the GHSG HD 9 had the longest follow-up at greater than 5 years and thus the results of this review are strongly influenced by this trial. The Intergroup trial 20012, which was initiated by the EORTC, is currently evaluating eight cycles of ABVD versus four cycles of BEACOPP escalated plus four cycles of BEACOPP baseline. It is hoped that results of this trial can best define an answer as to whether BEACOPP escalated is superior to ABVD.

Another approach is to intensify ABVD and this was assessed by Russo et al. in intermediate and advanced cHL (85). Patients with intermediate cHL received ABVD on a 21-day cycle with chemotherapy delivered on days 1 and 11 (dose dense), and patients with advanced HL received dose dense ABVD with increased doxorubicin dose of $70 \, mg/m^2$ (dose intense) during cycles 1 to 4. Total cycles of ABVD were 6 and 70 patients overall were treated. At a 12 month minimum follow up, they demonstrated a 5-year EFS of 93% in the combined experimental groups, compared with 73% for standard ABVD. Based on these data, a randomized trial is being considered to prospectively assess intensified versus baseline ABVD.

PET results after cycle two of therapy (PET-2) can also be used to stratify which patients would have highest chance of benefiting from BEACOPP and also minimize exposure to potential toxicities of BEACOPP by only treating patients who are predicted to have poor long-term outcomes with continued ABVD therapy. In the ongoing SWOG 0816 trial, patients with stages III and IV disease are enrolled and undergo a baseline PET scan. They then receive two cycles of ABVD and PET scan is repeated. If the PET-2 scan is negative then four further cycles of ABVD are given. If the PET-2 scan, however, is positive then treatment is changed and intensified to BEACOPP escalated for six cycles if patient is HIV negative and to BEACOPP standard for six cycles for patients who are HIV positive. This trial is also the first American study to use centralized real-time intergroup review (SWOG, ECOG, CALGB [Cancer and Leukemia Group B]) of the PET scan results for treatment decisions. PET-2 response has also been incorporated into GHSG HD18 trial in which advanced stage patients receive two cycles of BEACOPP escalated. If PET-2 is negative patients are then randomized to receive six more cycles of BEACOPP escalated versus two more cycles of BEACOPP escalated. If PET-2 is positive then patients are randomized to receive six more cycles of BEACOPP escalated versus six more cycles of BEACOPP escalated plus rituximab (see section "Novel Agents"). The PET-2 positive patients they will only receive radiation treatment if they have residual disease of 2.5 cm or greater at the end of chemotherapy treatment which remains PET scan positive and PET-2 negative patients will not receive radiation treatment.

It is currently unclear whether the risks of dose-intensive therapy are justified by the improvement in survival rates except in patients who are at high risk for death (IPS ≥3). In the GHSG HD9 trial, BEACOPP escalated induced an approximately 50% improvement in the 5-year FFS and OS rates for the high-risk group when compared to COPP/ABVD (86). A pilot study from Italy also initially demonstrated that high-dose chemotherapy (HDCT) followed by autologous stem cell transplantation (ASCT) for high-risk patients produced an OS rate of 77% at a median of 7 years of follow-up, compared with 33% in a comparable group that did not undergo SCT (87). However, a subsequent randomized trial did not support autologous SCT for patients with high-risk disease (88).

Radiotherapy

The role of radiation used after chemotherapy for consolidation in patients with advanced stage HL is controversial. The potential role of RT in patients with advanced-stage HL was initially demonstrated by a study in which relapse usually occurred at initially involved sites and RT lowered the rate of relapse (89). The GHSG conducted a trial that compared two additional cycles of chemotherapy versus adjuvant IFRT in patients with CR after six cycles of chemotherapy. There was no benefit of IFRT in this stud (90). The CALGB also has demonstrated that adjuvant RT had no advantage following chemotherapy (91).

In a meta-analysis of 1740 patients on 14 trials, Loeffler et al. (92) found that adjuvant RT offered no benefit for OS at 10 years of follow-up, even though there was an 11% improvement in disease control, because of deaths due to non-HL-related causes. This observation was confirmed by a large phase III trial in which adjuvant IFRT in patients with CR after six to eight cycles of MOPP/ABV did not improve FFS or OS rates at 5 years (93). However, RT did increase the incidence of late toxicity, including second malignancy (4.0% cumulative rate at 5 years without IFRT versus 7.8% with IFRT) (94).

In a randomized SWOG study in the treatment of patients with bulky disease in CR after chemotherapy, adjuvant IFRT resulted in a 75% 5-year FFS rate, compared to only 57% for the group that received no further treatment ($p = .05$). However, there was no difference in OS between the two groups (95). In an EORTC and Group Pierre-et-Marie-Curie phase III trial for advanced-stage HL, adjuvant IFRT after MOPP/ABV-induced partial remission (PR) produced excellent 5-year FFS and OS rates (75 and 87%, respectively) (96). A Dutch study also demonstrated that the 5-year OS rate following IFRT in patients with PR after chemotherapy was comparable to that of patients in CR who did not receive adjuvant IFRT (87 versus 91%). The French H89 trial reported long-term follow up of nearly 10 years (97), with no difference seen in OS or DFS between patients who achieved a CR or PR (of at least 75%) and were consolidated with additional chemotherapy or radiation therapy.

In the GHSG HD12 trial, half of the patients enrolled received IFRT treatment to initial areas of bulk or residual disease after completion of BEACOPP chemotherapy (82). The GHSG HD15 trial takes an alternative approach of using PET scan response at the completion of front-line chemotherapy to stratify which patients might potentially benefit from radiation therapy and only gives patients IFRT after BEACOPP chemotherapy is they have a residual PET scan positive mass that is 2.5 cm or greater (37). Using this approach many fewer patients are receiving radiation and a high negative predictive value was seen for PET scan negativity at completion of chemotherapy. Longer follow-up of both of these trials will better help to determine the role of radiation for advanced stage HL patients who receive intensive chemotherapy.

MD Anderson approach

In summary, at MD Anderson we screen patients for our available protocols for initial treatment of advanced stage disease. This includes our current SWOG 0816 and our randomized rituximab plus ABVD versus ABVD (see section "Novel Agents") protocols. As our standard approach off clinical protocol we generally treat these patients with six to eight cycles of ABVD. Although the data supporting IFRT for advanced stage patients is controversial, we consider IFRT for patients who have presented with an initial bulky mass who continue to have a residual mass at the end of therapy with PET negative status.

Refractory or Relapsed Hodgkin Lymphoma

Although many patients with HL are cured with front-line therapy, approximately up to 15% of early-stage disease with unfavorable risk factors and 40% of patients with advanced stage disease with high-risk factors can develop disease relapse. Also approximately 10 to 15% of patients can develop refractory disease (74, 98).

Status of disease at relapse as a prognostic factor

Refractory or relapsed HL can be divided into four subgroups: relapse after primary RT; early relapse within 12 months of CR after first-line chemotherapy; late relapse after CR, >12 months after firstline chemotherapy; and primary refractory HL (ie, patients who never achieve a CR). Prognostic factors may vary among these groups, and studies that have evaluated these prognostic features often group patients in these various categories together, making comparisons of results from different studies difficult.

In the Royal Marsden study, adverse factors identified in patients with relapse after RT alone were age >40 years, unfavorable histology, and extranodal relapse (99). The OS at 10 years after relapse was 63%. In the GHSG study, adverse prognostic factors at the time of relapse were analyzed in a group of 4754 patients registered in

the GHSG database between 1988 and 1999. The outcomes of these patients were strongly dependent on the type of initial treatment and time to relapse. Additional prognostic factors at time of relapse were age, performance status, clinical stage, B symptoms, and anemia. The time to relapse, clinical stage, and anemia at time of relapse could be used to form a prognostic score to distinguish patients with a different rate of freedom from second treatment failure and OS (100). The GHSG also analyzed the results of therapy for 206 patients with primary refractory HL. The 5-year OS was 26%. Significant adverse prognostic factors were age >50 years, ECOG performance status >1, and failure to achieve a temporary remission to initial chemotherapy. The 5-year OS rate for patients with no risk factors was 55%, compared with 0% for those with all three risk factors (101). Moksowitz et al. identified three prognostic factors associated with EFS in patients undergoing ICE (ifosfamide, carboplatin, etoposide chemotherapy), followed by an HDCT and ASCT as: CR less than 1 year, extranodal disease, presence of B symptoms. In patients with 0 to 1 factors, the 5-year EFS was 83% compared to 10% if all three factors were present (102).

Chemotherapy for relapsed or refractory Hodgkin lymphoma

Generally, given current standards of care radiation treatment alone is generally no longer used for front-line treatment. However, some patients who previously received radiation treatment alone can develop late relapse and present currently for additional treatment. Overall up to 35% of patients who had stage I or stage II disease and received radiation treatment alone at time of initial diagnosis have disease relapse (99). These patients should be treated with according to current algorithms of management for newly diagnosed patients with chemotherapy. They can also be considered for consolidative IFRT after chemotherapy if they have relapsed with limited disease as long as planned IFRT radiation fields would not overlap with prior IFRT fields and result in higher risks for radiation associated toxicities. In general, these patients have favorable outcomes with a described 10-year OS of 90% (103).

For patients with relapsed or refractory disease after standard front-line management additional salvage chemotherapy followed by HDCT plus ASCT is the standard approach. One of the key goals of salvage chemotherapy is to achieve CR prior to HDCT plus ASCT. Multiple salvage regimens are used (Table 10-10). It is difficult to directly compare these regimens as they have not been evaluated in randomized clinical trials.

TABLE 10-10	SALVAGE CHEMOTHERAPY REGIMENS FOR HODGKIN LYMPHOMA	
Regimen	*ORR (%)*	*CR (%)*
DHAP	88	21
ASHAP	70	34
ESHAP	73	41
MINE	73	34
ICE	85	26
IGEV	81	54
GND	70	19
GDP	62	10

ASHAP, doxorubicin, methylprednisolone, cytarabine, cisplatin; DHAP, dexamethasone, cytarabine, cisplatin; ESHAP, etoposide, methylprednisolone, cytarabine, cisplatin; MINE, mitoguazone, ifosfamide, vinorelbine, etoposide; ICE, ifosfamide, carboplatin, etoposide; IGEV, ifosfamide, gemcitabine, vinorelbine; GND, gemcitabine, vinorelbine, pegylated liposomal doxorubicin; GDP, gemcitabine, dexamethasone, cisplatin.

The most common salvage chemotherapy options are the platinum-containing regimens ICE, ESHAP (etoposide, methylprednisolone, cytarabine, cisplatin), DHAP (cisplatin, cytarabine, dexamethasone), and ASHAP (doxorubicin, solumedrol, cytarabine, and cisplatin). When given to 56 patients with relapsed or refractory HL ASHAP induced a ORR of 70% with 34% CR (104). ESHAP was evaluated in 22 HL patients with relapsed or refractory disease and resulted in a ORR of 73% with 41% CR (105). DHAP showed similar also favorable results with 89% ORR and 21% CR (106). ICE induced an ORR of 84% with 26% CR. Gemcitabine-containing regimens have also been shown to be effective. GND (gemcitabine, vinorelbine, pegylated liposomal doxorubicin) was evaluated in 91 relapsed or refractory HL patients and induced an ORR of 70% with a CR of 19%. GDP (gemcitabine, dexamethasone, platinum) induced similar results with an ORR of 62% and 10% CR. A recent evaluation of IGEV (ifosfamide, gemcitabine, vinorelbine) was evaluated in 91 patients with an ORR of 81% and a high CR of 54% with 60% of primary refractory patients responding to IGEV (107).

Radiotherapy for relapsed Hodgkin lymphoma

Salvage radiation therapy is not commonly used for relapsed or refractory HL. This is because of the belief that relapsed or refractory HL is generally a systemic disease. Two studies support potential use in certain circumstances.

For patients who relapse with localized disease and who are not good candidates for systemic chemotherapy, clinical protocols, or transplant salvage radiation treatment can be considered. In a retrospective study, patients with relapsed localized HL without significant risk factors were treated with RT alone with CR of 77% and 51% 5-year OS (108). IFRT has also been evaluated in combined modality salvage treatment. Sixty-five patients received two cycles of ICE followed by IFRT to nodal disease greater than 5 cm or sites of residual disease present after ICE. ORR to ICE paired with IFRT was 88% and EFS at 43 months was 68% with nearly all patients undergoing successful HDCT plus ASCT. In patients who developed further relapse after this treatment only 18% relapsed in the field of RT (102).

HDCT with ASCT for relapsed Hodgkin lymphoma

For patients with chemotherapy-sensitive disease, the treatment of choice after relapse is HDCT followed by ASCT. This recommendation is based on reports from two randomized clinical trials. In the British National Lymphoma Investigation (BNLI) study, patients with relapsed or refractory HL received BEAM (carmustine, etoposide, cytarabine, and melphalan) at high doses (BEAM) followed by an ASCT or at lower doses (mini-BEAM) without an ASCT. The 3-year freedom from second treatment failure was significantly better for patients who received HDCT (53 versus 10%) (109). The GHSG/EBMT (European Group for Blood and Bone Marrow Transplantation) conducted another randomized trial to compare four cycles of Dexa-BEAM (dexamethasone plus BEAM) or two cycles of Dexa-BEAM followed by autologous SCT. At 3 years, the FFTF in the high-dose therapy group was 55%, better than that for the arm receiving an additional two cycles of chemotherapy, which was 34% (110). Notably neither of these trials showed a survival benefit for transplant which could be accounted by generally short follow-up or cross-over of patients on the chemotherapy alone arms to ultimately receive an ASCT.

Multiple studies have shown that level of remission to salvage chemotherapy is a strong predictor of long-term outcomes after ASCT. This level of stratification in long-term outcomes based on pre-ASCT response has been shown recently with 5-year PFS of 79, 59, and 17%, respectively, for patients in CR, PR, and for those with resistant disease (111). For primary refractory patients with overall chemosensitive disease, pre-ASCT had 39% improvement in PFS compared to those with chemoresistant disease (112). Recent studies have also shown the impact of pre-ASCT PET scan results on EFS, with patients with negative pre-ASCT PET scans having significantly higher EFS and failure-free survival (FFS) compared to patients with positive pre-ASCT PET scans with a range of improvement of 16 to 47% (113-115).

Tandem ASCT has been investigated as an approach for patients who have poor-risk relapsed disease or primary refractory disease. The GELA (Groupe d' Etude des Lymphomes de l' Adulte)/SFGM (Société Française de Greffe de Moelle) evaluated a risk-adapted transplantation approach in 245 patients (116). Patients were assessed by the presence of the risk factors of relapse within 12 months, stage III or stage IV disease at relapse, or relapse to previously irradiated sites. The 150 patients who had primary refractory disease or poor-risk relapsed HL as defined by the presence of 2 of the above risk factors underwent tandem ASCT, while the remaining 95 intermediate-risk patients with one or more factor present at relapsed underwent a single ASCT. The 5-year FFTF and OS were 73 and 85% for the intermediate-risk patients and 46 and 57% for the poor-risk patients. Additional patients with chemotherapy resistant disease experience a 16% improvement in OS at 5 years to 46% when compared to previous studies. Overall these results suggested a possible benefit for patients with chemotherapy-resistant disease or those in partial remission after salvage chemotherapy.

Treatment of Relapse After Autologous Stem Cell Transplant

In patients who relapse after an ASCT their survival is highly predicted by their time to relapse. A recent international multicenter retrospective study demonstrated that patients who relapse within 6 to 12 months after an ASCT have a median OS of 2.4 years (117). Although patients who relapse within 3 months of an ASCT have a very short OS of 8 months, thus emphasizing the high need for additional treatment options.

Allogeneic Stem Cell Transplant

The main advantage of an allogeneic stem cell transplant (allo-SCT) is its graft-versus-HL effect. Retrospective studies have shown this benefit by documenting lower relapse rates in allo-SCT patients who have chronic graft-versus-host disease (GHVD) and that donor lymphocyte infusion (DLI) can induce relatively long-lasting remissions (118). Initial studies of allo-SCT in HL patients described high rates of transplant-related mortality (TRM) up to 61%, thus more recent studies have evaluated reduced-intensity conditioning (RIC) and have shown decreases in TRM (119-122). Overall RIC allo-SCT induces modest long-term remissions with PFS in the mid-30% range (123-126).

The German Cooperative Transplantation Study Group has recently conducted a retrospective review of HL patients who have undergone allo-SCT from sibling and unrelated donors (127). A total of 79 patients were reviewed at 18 centers with 82% of the patients having undergone a prior ASCT. At time of allo-SCT 18% were in CR and 54% in PR. TRM was 21% and 2 year PFS and OS were respectively 42 and 51%, and contrary to other studies within this review remission status at time of allo-SCT did not impact PFS or OS. The lymphoma group of the European Group for Blood and Marrow Transplantation (EBMT) reviewed 49 patients who had undergone RIC allo-SCT using a fludarabine-melphalan conditioning regimen. Eighty-one percent had undergone a prior ASCT and 67% had chemosensitive disease. At 3 years of follow-up, the OS was 43 and 59% of patients had experienced further relapse. Sensitivity to chemotherapy though improved outcomes with a 42% decrease in relapse for those with chemosensitive disease at 2 years of follow-up (128).

At MD Anderson Cancer Center we have reviewed the outcomes of 58 patients who received an RIC regimen of fludarabine-melphalan in preparation for allo-SCT (129). Overall 83% had undergone a prior ASCT and 52% had chemotherapy-sensitive disease at time of allo-SCT. TRM at 2 years was 15% with nearly half of the TRM occurring within the first 100 days after allo-SCT. The incidence of chronic GHVD was 73%. The calculated 2-year PFS and OS were, respectively, 32 and 64% with a trend toward improvement in PFS for those with chemotherapy-sensitive disease but not for OS.

Novel Agents

Advances in our understanding of HL pathology and biology have led to the development of targeted agents that are now undergoing clinical trial investigations. It is hopeful that these current investigations will lead to approval of new drugs for HL by the Food and Drug Administration (FDA).

Antibodies and immunotherapies

CD30 has highly restricted and dense expression on HRS cells and anaplastic large cell lymphoma (ALCL) cells. Two unconjugated CD30 antibodies were evaluated in clinical trials. The chimeric SGN-30 induced stable disease (SD) in four HL patients but treatment did not result in PRs or CRs (130). MDX-060 was a humanized anti-CD30 antibody and treatment resulted in an ORR of 8% with a 4% CR (131). Given these modest clinical results there was a strong desire to further optimize anti-CD30 directed therapies. One approach taken was by improving antigen and Fcγ receptor IIIA binding in the generation of XmAb2513. Relapsed HL and ALCL patients were treated in a phase I study. Patients were treated with infusions every other week with doses of 0.3 to 12 mg/kg with overall good tolerability. Final results of trial are pending release (132,133).

Another approach to increase efficacy is through conjugation. SGN-35 (brentuximab) is an anti-CD30 antibody that is conjugated to a microtubule agent, monomethyl auristatin E (MMAE). The linker in SGN-35 is stable in plasma but is broken down in the presence of lysosomal enzymes. Thus, the anti-CD30 component of SGN-35 allows for targeting of HL cells and once internalized MMAE is released and exerts an antitubulin effect.

SGN-35 has been evaluated in two phase I studies. In the first phase I study, SGN-35 treatment was given intravenously every 3 weeks. A total of 45 patients were treated with 93% HL patients and 73% of patients had relapsed disease after a prior ASCT. Patients received treatment intravenously every 21 days at dose levels ranging from 0.1 to 3.6 mg/kg with the maximum tolerated dose (MTD) defined at 1.8 mg/kg. The ORR was 39% with a 50% ORR and 25% CR at the 1.8 mg/kg MTD level with median duration of response of at least 10 months (134, 135). In a second phase I study, weekly dosing of SGN-35 was evaluated. Forty-four patients were treated with 86% of those enrolled being HL patients and 68% having undergone a prior ASCT. Similar to the every 3-week trial SGN-35 was generally well tolerated with the MTD established at 1.2 mg/kg. There was a trend toward higher incidence of peripheral neuropathy with weekly as compared to every 3-week dosing with an ORR for HL patients of 52% and a CR of 27% (136,137). Given the promising level of clinical activity and overall tolerability SGN-35 has been evaluated in a phase II pivotal relapsed HL trial and results from this trial are anticipated to be release soon. A second pivotal trial for patients with relapsed ALCL is also ongoing. Furthermore, SGN-35 is also being evaluated as a maintenance therapy for HL patients who have a high risk of disease relapse after ASCT.

CD20 is expressed on less than 20% of HRS cells, however it is nearly always expressed by B cells which surround the HRS cells and make up the microenvironment. Thus, treating with a CD20 antibody is believed to deplete B cells from the microenvironment and thus then potentially decrease the survival of HRS cells. In a pilot trial at MD Anderson Cancer Center 22 patients with relapsed HL were treated with 6 weekly doses of rituximab 375 mg/m^2. The ORR was 22% with all patients responding having nodal disease (138).

Tumor necrosis factor apoptosis-inducing ligand (TRAIL) has four receptors. TRAIL-R1 (DR4) and TRAIL-R2 (DR5) are the receptors that stimulate the death pathways (139). HL cells express both TRAIL-R1

and TRAIL-R2 as well as the decoy receptor TRAIL-R4 (140). In cell culture TRAIL-R1 and TRAIL-R2 agonistic antibodies are able to induce HL cell death, and TRAIL-R1 agonistic antibodies have been shown to have good activity for treating relapsed follicular lymphoma (141).

The immunomodulatory drug lenalidomide which is FDA approved for relapsed/refractory multiple myeloma and myelodysplastic syndrome with deletion 5 q abnormality has also been investigated as therapy for relapsed HL. Activity has been seen in two separate trials which treated patients with 25 mg/day of lenalidomide for 21 days out of a 28 day cycle (142, 143). ORR ranged from 13 to 33% with a time to progression of 3.2 months reported by Kuruvilla et al. As anticipated the most common side effects were myelosuppression and skin rash.

EBV-positive HRS cells express proteins including LMP2 that allow the development of targeted T-cell therapies. Bollard et al. in a recent trial produced cytotoxic T lymphocytes (CTL) that targeted the LMP2 EBV viral antigen in 14 lymphoma patients. Eighty-three percent of patients who received this therapy after prior chemotherapy or transplantation remained in remission up to 22 months (144). Building from this approach gene transfer into antigen-presenting cells (APC) is used to increase the rate of occurrence of CTLs that are specific for LMP2. Using this technology 90% of patients treated with high risk of relapse remained in remission and 83% of those with relapsed lymphoma responded (145). CTL therapies are also currently being developed for EBV negative HL as only approximately 30% of HL tumors are EBV positive. Another target being evaluated is the cancer/testis antigen (CTA) MAGE-A4, which has been shown to be feasible in preclinical studies (146).

Inhibitors of survival pathway

Gene transcription is in part regulated by posttranscriptional histone modification. Histone deacetylases (HDAC) act on lysine amino acid groups on multiple proteins including many transcription factors. HDAC are grouped into four classes with classes I, II, and IV being zinc-dependent. Several HDAC inhibitors are being investigated as therapies for relapsed/refractory HL. MGCD0103 is an oral class I or isotype selective HDAC inhibitor. In a phase II trial relapsed HL patients received doses of 85 or 110 mg three times per week. In the 110 mg dose cohort, the ORR was 38% with a 10% CR, however the higher dose was not well tolerated and thus modification were made to allow enrollment to the 85 mg dose level. At the 85 mg level, the ORR was 30% (147). Two patients within this trial developed pericardial effusions that resulted in discontinuation of MGCD0103, overall for the 437 patients with solid tumors and hematologic malignancies that have been treated with MGCD0103 4.3% developed a pericardial serious adverse event (148). Serum concentration of TARC which is highly expressed by HRS cells was found to decrease by at least 40% in patients who responded to therapy, and preclinical studies have also demonstrated down regulation of CD30 and activation of NF-κB (149, 150). Entinostat (SNDX-275) is another oral class I HDAC inhibitor that has been shown preclinically to upregulate CTAs which is proposed to potentially facilitate CTLs ability to eradicate HL cells (151). Clinical phase II trials for patients with relapsed HL are ongoing. Panobinostat (LBH589) is an HDAC classes I and II or pan-HDAC inhibitor. Given the ORR of 38% seen in a phase I trial for patients with hematologic cancers, panobinostat has been evaluated in a phase II relapsed/refractory HL trial (152). In this trial patients received panobinostat given orally 40 mg three times a week for 21 day cycles. For the first 51 patients who had completed at least two cycles of therapy the ORR was 21% with one CR. Overall treatment was well tolerated with the most common grade 3 to 4 adverse event being thrombocytopenia (151). A SWOG phase II trial of vorinostat reported a 4% PR and 16% SD rate, however was closed early due to not meeting prespecified efficacy benchmarks (153).

The Janus kinase 2 (JAK2) has a key role in the proliferation of hematologic cancers, and somatic activating point mutations are know to occur in myeloproliferative disorders. The oral JAK2 inhibitor SB1518 has been evaluated in a phase I trial in patients with relapsed lymphoma including HL. Preliminary data from patients treated on this trial have shown that for the first 15 patients treated at escalating dose levels starting at 100 mg daily that 73% had SD and no dose limiting toxicities (DLT) (154).

Bendamustine which acts as a bifunctional alkylating agent is FDA approved for treatment of chronic lymphocytic leukemia and indolent B-cell non-HL that is refractory to rituximab-containing therapies. Given its activity in other lymphoma subtypes it has recently been evaluated in a phase II trial for relapsed HL with bendamustine given at a dose of 120 mg/m^2 on days 1 and 2 every 28 days. For the first 18 patients enrolled the ORR was 75% with a 38% CR and a significant portion of patients were able to undergo an allo-SCT (155).

The role of nuclear factor-κB (NF-κB) signaling was first identified in multiple myeloma and led to the development and approval of the proteasome inhibitor bortezomib (156). Activation of NF-κB allows for transcription of proteins that drive cell survival and decrease apoptosis. Bortezomib was shown in relapsed/refractory B-cell non-HL to have ORR ranging from 19 to 58%, and the strong activity in relapsed mantle cell lymphoma lead to its FDA approval for this indication (157, 158). In HL cells, bortezomib was found to induce apoptosis by activation of the caspase cascade and decrease Bcl-2 (159). Given these findings a pilot trial was conduced at MD Anderson Cancer Center. In this study, 14 patients with relapsed/refractory HL were treated with bortezomib at doses of 1.3 mg/m^2 on days 1, 4, 8, and 11 of a 21-day cycle. One patient had a PR and two patients had SD (160). These results were supported by three separate clinical trials (161-163).

Novel agents in combination with each other or chemotherapy

An important strategy to improve HL patient outcomes is the early investigation of targeted agents in combination with each other or with chemotherapy. Given the promising activity of SGN-35 in HL it is now being evaluated in a phase I clinical study in combination with ABVD. Patients with stage IIA bulky or stage IIB to stage IV disease are treated with six cycles of ABVD. SGN-35 is then given as escalating dose levels of 0.6 to 1.2 mg/kg on days 1 and 15 of the 28-day cycle.

The single-agent activity of rituximab in HL lead to trials evaluating the level of benefit that can be potentially gained through combining with chemotherapy. A phase II study treated patients with relapsed/refractory HL with gemcitabine plus rituximab 33 patients were enrolled and received rituximab 375 mg/m^2 weekly for 6 weeks with gemcitabine at a dose of 1250 mg/m^2 IV on days 1 and 8 of a 21-day cycle for a maximum of six cycles. ORR was 48% and the median FFS was 2.7 months (164). In a follow-up study conducted at MD Anderson Cancer Center, rituximab was combined with ABVD for front-line treatment of HL. The IPS was used to stratify patients according to risk of relapse. Patients received 6 weekly doses of rituximab, which was added to the standard dose schedule of ABVD (R-ABVD). An interim analysis performed in 70 patients showed that with a median follow-up of 32 months the estimated EFS was 85% with an EFS of 77% for those with an IPS >2. In addition, 55 patients had a PET performed after two to three cycles (PET-2/3) of R-ABVD. The 5-year EFS was 93 versus 75%, respectively, for those with a negative versus positive PET-2/3 (165). Compared with historical data, the outcomes were improved in each IPS group, with the most striking difference in the patients with IPS >2. A recent update with a median of 5 years of follow-up showed a 25%

improvement in EFS for HL patients with an IPS >2 treated with R-ABVD as compared to historical outcomes for ABVD (166). A randomized multicenter phase II trial comparing R-ABVD versus ABVD in advanced stage HL patients with IPS >2 is ongoing. An international multicenter noninferiority phase III trial lead through Fondazione Michelangelo is currently comparing four cycles of R-ABVD versus four cycles of ABVD followed by IFRT for patients with stage I to stage IIA nonbulky HL. Furthermore, the GHSG ongoing HD18 is treating stage III/stage IV patients with escalated BEACOPP for two cycles and then assessing PET-2 response. Patients who are PET-2 negative are randomized to receive six versus two more cycles of escalated BEACOPP and patients who are PET-2 positive are randomized to receive six more cycles of escalated BEACOPP versus six more cycles of escalated BEACOPP plus rituximab. If there is residual disease after end of treatment ≥2.5 cm patients receive IFRT if the disease is still PET positive.

Given the preclinical data of TRAIL-R2 presence on HL cells and clinical efficacy in NHL AMG 655 (conatumumab), an agonistic antibody of TRAIL-R2 was given in combination with bortezomib or the pan-HDAC inhibitor vorinostat because both agents enhance death receptor stimulated apoptosis. Patients with relapsed NHL and HL were enrolled, and an interim analysis done after 27 patients were treated documented one CR in an HL patient who received AMG 655 5 mg/kg IV every 3 weeks plus vorinostat 400 mg orally daily (167).

The oral mammalian target of rapamycin (mTOR) inhibitor everolimus was shown to induce a 47% ORR in patients with relapsed HL (168). Also preclinical data have shown that mTOR inhibitors can synergize with HDAC inhibitors (169). Thus, a phase I trial is ongoing for relapsed HL and NHL patients which combines the oral HDAC inhibitor panobinostat with the oral mTOR inhibitor everolimus. Furthermore, given the positive data seen for single-agent activity of panobinostat in relapsed HL future additional combination clinical trials are being planned.

Although the single-agent responses for bortezomib in HL was low, nonhematologic malignancy trials suggested that bortezomib could have a role in overcoming chemotherapy resistance (170,171). Thus, at MD Anderson Cancer Center we conducted a trial in which bortezomib was combined with standard ICE chemotherapy (BICE) for relapsed HL. Patients received bortezomib ranging from 1 to 1.5 mg/m^2 on days 1 and 4 of each cycle of ICE. Almost half of the patients had primary refractory disease and after three cycles of ORR

was 75% with all patients becoming PET scan negative. Treatment was well tolerated and all responding patients underwent successful stem cell collection in preparation for ASCT. The most common side effects were reversible neutropenia and thrombocytopenia (172). A randomized phase II trial comparing second-line treatment with BICE versus ICE is currently enrolling relapsed HL patients. A second trial evaluated bortezomib 1 mg/m^2 on days 1, 4, 8, and 11 in combination with gemcitabine 800 mg/m^2 on days 1 and 8 in every 21-day cycles. The ORR was low at 22% and hepatotoxicity was observed (173).

MD Anderson approach

In summary, at MD Anderson patients with relapsed/refractory HL are planned for second-line or salvage chemotherapy followed by an ASCT. We screen patients who have relapsed/refractory HL for our current clinical trial options including our current randomized phase II clinical trial of bortezomib plus ICE (BICE) versus ICE. Patients who respond to salvage chemotherapy are recommended to proceed onto an ASCT. We screen patients with relapsed HL after an ASCT for our novel agent clinical trial options as our first preference. If they have previously not received gemcitabine-containing chemotherapy they can also be considered for regimens such as GND. Given the benefits versus risks of allogeneic stem cell transplant a subset of patients can be potentially considered for this approach.

Special Cases of Hodgkin Lymphoma

Nodular Lymphocyte Predominant Hodgkin Lymphoma

LPHL is a rare hematologic malignancy with only 400 to 600 cases per year in the United States. In a GHSG retrospective analysis of 394 patients, 63% of patients had early-stage favorable disease, 16% had early-stage unfavorable, and 21% had advanced stage disease. Outcomes at 50 months showed better outcomes for patients with LPHL as compared to classical HL (174).

Early-stage

Data supports overall positive outcomes for patients treated with IFRT alone. Patients with stage IA LPHL treated with radiation treatment alone have favorable 5-year relapse free survival (RFS) of 95% and OS of 100% (175). The Australasian Radiation Oncology Group reported long-term follow-up at 15 years and showed that for patients treated with radiation therapy alone had FFP respectively of 84% and 73% for stages I and II (176). Data from the GHSG further supports the use of radiation for stage IA patients with CR of 100% and generally equivalent FFTF for patients treated with RT as compared to CMT (177). The EORTC-GELA also describes similar outcomes at 9.3 years for stage I or stage II patients treated with CMT as compared to RT alone. A recent large single institution report from Boston's Joint Center for Radiation Therapy reinforces RT alone for LPHL patients with stage I or stage II disease. In this review, 113 patients were followed who received treatment spanning over 35 years. Overall 93 patients received RT alone with 29% receiving limited-field RT. Ten-year PFS were respectively 85 and 61% for stages I and II patients. Furthermore, OS and PFS was similar among patients treated with different fields (limited, regional, or extended) of radiation (178). Excellent outcomes were also seen in a British Colombia retrospective review. For the 92 patients with stage I or stage II disease, reviewed the 10-year PFS and OS were 71% and 84% for RT alone versus 100% and 100% for ABVD +/− RT (179).

Advanced-stage

Patients with advanced-stage LPHL have overall poorer long-term outcomes than their early-stage LPHL counterparts. The European Task Force on Lymphoma (ETFL) has reported for patients treated mostly with MOPP or ABVD-like regimens +/− RT that the FFTF at 8 years was 41 and 24%, respectively, for those respectively with stages III and IV disease (4). Although RT for advanced stage is viewed to be inadequate, no trial has established in which chemotherapy regimen would be preferred. In general, regimens often considered are ABVD, CHOP, or CVP with or without rituximab given the CD20 positivity in LPHL and data as described later. A case report provides support for consideration of R-CHOP for advanced stage LPHL and the two patients treated had CR lasting up to 40 months (180). We performed a retrospective review at MD Anderson Cancer Center of newly diagnosed LPHL treated at our institution over a decade. Thirty-one patients were treated with 12 patients having advanced stage disease. Overall nine patients received R-CHOP with a CR of 100% and lack of relapses during a median of 23 months of follow-up (181). There was also a trend toward overall improvement in outcomes compared to other chemotherapy regimens given. To further evaluate R-CHOP we are designing a phase II trial in conjunction with SWOG.

Relapsed/refractory

Rituximab has been evaluated for treatment of relapsed LPHL. In a study which enrolled 14 patients by the

GHSH rituximab therapy resulted in an ORR of 100%, CR of 57%, and median TTP of 33 months (182). Stanford has examined the benefit of limited versus extended rituximab therapy in the frontline and relapsed setting. Twenty-one patients including seven patients with stage III disease were treated with 4 weeks of rituximab. An amendment to the protocol then allowed for maintenance rituximab given every 6 months for 2 years. Higher CR was seen in the extended treatment as compared to the limited treatment at respectively 88 versus 41%. In addition at 30 months, the estimated FFP was 88% for extended rituximab compared with 52% for limited rituximab (183).

Transformation at time of relapse can also occur. Patients with LPHL are generally viewed as having a higher risk of transformation to aggressive NHL as compared to patients with HL. In a recent retrospective study by the British Columbia Cancer Agency (BCCA), 95 patients were identified as being diagnosed with LPHL over a 40-year time period. Median time of follow-up was 6.5 years and 14% experienced transformation. Median time to transformation was 8.1 years and with 80 to 20% ratio of diffuse large B-cell lymphoma (DLBCL) to T-cell-rich B-cell lymphoma (TCRBCL). In the 10 patients with transformed lymphoma their 10-year PFS and OS were respectively 52 and 62% (184).

Overall the rarity of the disease makes it difficult to prospectively evaluate the role of ASCT for patients with relapsed or refractory LPHL. A recent MD Anderson Cancer Center retrospective study reviewed the outcomes for 26 patients who underwent ASCT. At time of transplantation many had transformation to TCRBCL. Overall at time of ASCT 85% were in remission with 35% in CR. At a median of 50 months of follow-up there were seven patients who relapsed with a 69% EFS (185).

MD Anderson approach

At MD Anderson, we treat stage IA and stage IIA LPHL patients with IFRT. It is rare for a stage I or stage II patient to present with B symptoms but if patient does we generally favor, particularly for stage IIB patients, combined modality therapy with an anthracycline-containing chemotherapy regimen followed by IFRT. Our preferred regimen is R-CHOP. For advanced stage patients we treat with R-CHOP for six cycles. Patients who relapse can be considered for extended rituximab therapy. Although patients with evidence of transformation to DLBCL or TCRBCL are generally treated with salvage chemotherapy with regimens such as rituximab-ICE (RICE) followed by ASCT.

Hodgkin Lymphoma in the Elderly Patient

Although many elderly patients are in good health, age is an IPS risk factor. About 20% of patients diagnosed with HL are greater than 60 year olds and 7% are older than 70 (186). Most studies consider patients to be elderly if they are above 60 years old. In general, elderly patients are at higher risk presenting with advanced stage disease, having comorbidities, inability to receive full dose intensity, higher treatment-related toxicities, and decreased survival after relapse. A retrospective review of elderly patients performed by the GHSG highlights these concerns (187). Overall elderly patients should be considered for standard therapy if they do not have any significant comorbidities. The GHSG study compared advanced HL patients aged 66 to 75 treated with BEACOPP against COPP–ABVD (188). They demonstrated no difference in OS or disease-related survival, however, treatment-related mortality with BEACOPP was 21%. The GHSG has also performed a trial to evaluate PVAG (prednisone, vinblastine, doxorubicin, gemcitabine) in patients 60 to 75 years old. A trial goal was to minimize risks of treatment toxicity by eliminating bleomycin and dacarbazine as given traditionally in ABVD. A total of 61 patients were enrolled with a median age of 69 years old. ORR was 81% with DLT occurring in four patients (186).

Hodgkin Lymphoma in Adolescent and Young Adults

Prior studies have highlighted potential improved outcomes for adolescents treated on pediatric protocols citing reductions in anthracycline and alkylator doses as having positive long-term benefits (189). However, recently the GHSG analyzed the treatment and outcomes for adolescents (15-20 years) and young adults (21-45 years) in trials HD4–HD9 (190). They identified 557 adolescents and 3228 young adults treated on the various protocols. Six-year FFTF estimates were 80.2 and 79.7%, 6-year OS estimates were 93.6 and 90.9% in adolescents and young adults, respectively. The risk factors and occurrence of secondary malignancies was not significantly different between the two groups. They concluded that adolescents could safely and effectively be treated on adult protocols.

Hodgkin Lymphoma during Pregnancy

HL occurs rarely in pregnant women. Estimates have ranged from one per 1000 to 6000 deliveries, making it the fourth most common cancer diagnosed during pregnancy (191). Pregnancy does not appear to have a negative effect on HL outcomes (192). Although the clinical presentation of HL is not influenced by pregnancy; the staging workup is significantly limited. CT scanning should be avoided because it exposes the fetus to ionizing radiation. PET scans are contraindicated. Ultrasonography, which is without known adverse fetal effects, can be helpful for assessing fetal development and may also detect the presence of lymphadenopathy. However, the absence of lymphadenopathy should not be taken as evidence that there is no abdominal nodal involvement. MRI can be used for evaluating lymph nodes, liver, and spleen (193). Decisions about the need for a chest radiograph should be made on the basis of clinical examination, but this is generally safe, especially with appropriate shielding.

Because implantation and embryogenesis occur during the first trimester, chemotherapy drug exposure can result in spontaneous abortions and fetal malformation. Overall effects of chemotherapy on the fetus are less pronounced in the second and third trimesters (194). Currently most pregnant patients receive therapy while pregnant, although some groups have cited evidence supporting consideration of deferring therapy for patients presenting with stage IA or stage IIA disease who present late in the second or third trimester (195). It is imperative that all pregnant HL patients are comanaged by a high-risk obstetrician.

Chemotherapy administered during the second and third trimesters is associated with a low risk of fetal malformation that approximates the incidence in the general population (196). It is well known that MOPP has significant teratogenic potential, carrying significant fetal toxicity (197). However, ABVD appears to be safe for fetal development, based on a small series with an 18-year follow-up (198). Because chemotherapeutic agents reach significant levels in milk, mothers should be advised to avoid breast-feeding during treatment.

Several series including from MD Anderson Cancer Center have documented that radiation therapy during the second and third trimesters is effective for management of HL (199). The overall goal is for partial therapy and the fetal dose should be limited to a maximum of 0.10 Gy. With these guidelines followed there does not appear to be a higher rate of fetal malformations or spontaneous abortions (199, 200).

Hodgkin Lymphoma in HIV-Positive Patients

There is an increased incidence of HL in patients with HIV type I infection and acquired immunodeficiency syndrome (AIDS). However, HL is not an AIDS-defining illness. Characteristics of HL in HIV-infected patients include the predominance of unfavorable histologic types, advanced-stage disease, extranodal involvement, and a high frequency of EBV infection (201-203). Patients with IPS >2 may also have a much worse outcome than those with IPS ≤2. Treatment also may increase the risk of opportunistic infections by inducing further immunosuppression.

In an AIDS Clinical Trials Group (ACTG) study of patients with HL and HIV from Italy, ABVD without highly active antiretroviral therapy (HAART) resulted in a 43% CR rate and a median OS of 18 months, associated with a 29% incidence of opportunistic infections (204). The same group tested the EVBP regimen plus HAART and G-CSF in similar patients and obtained a 74% CR and 53% 3-year OS rate, with only an 8% incidence of opportunistic infection (205). The Stanford V regimen plus HAART and G-CSF support were used in another phase II study (206). The estimated 3-year OS and FFP rates were 51 and 60%, respectively, which may be better than those obtained with ABVD or EVBP. Opportunistic infections during chemotherapy or within 3 months of completion of chemotherapy were significantly lower (7%) than those occurring during the ACTG study (29%) (204). The GHSG studied the BEACOPP regimen in HIV-infected HL patients, achieving a 100% CR rate, however, 16% (2/16) died of opportunistic infections (207).

A recent meta-analysis of HL in the HAART era demonstrated a CR rate of 72% and 2-year OS of 69% (208), however, only 59% of patients were treated with HAART. Advanced stage disease was present in 63%, and histology other than nodular sclerosis was seen in 76%. Another study recently analyzed the outcomes for advanced stage HL HIV-positive patients treated with HAART and ABVD. The CR occurred in 87% and 5-year EFS was 71% and supported that HIV patients can receive and do well with standard ABVD therapy (209).

Overall appropriate management of an HIV positive HL patient requires a combination of chemotherapy, antiretroviral agents, prophylaxis of opportunistic infections, and hematopoietic growth factors.

COMPLICATIONS OF TREATMENT

Second Malignancies

The treatment of HL appears to predispose patients to second malignancies (Table 10-11). The most common second malignancies are acute nonlymphocytic leukemia, myelodysplastic syndrome, non-HLs, and solid tumors. After 15 and 20 years, there is a 2.3 and 4.0% excess risk of second malignancy per person per year, with a cumulative risk of 15% (210). Risk factors associated with the development of acute leukemia include prolonged exposure to alkylating agents and advanced

patient age. Non-HLs are most often diffuse aggressive B-cell lymphomas, and the cumulative 10-year risk is 4 to 5% (211-213).

Unlike hematologic malignancies, the occurrence of solid tumors in patients with HL appears to be related to RT (213, 214). This is supported by a meta-analysis that highlights that the risk of secondary malignancies was lower when CMT as compared to RT alone was used as the initial HL therapy (215). The incidence of secondary solid tumors appears to begin to rise approximately 7 years after treatment and continues to rise with time and the patient's age (214). The cumulative incidence of solid tumors is 9% at 10 years (216). Solid tumors with a significantly increased incidence include sarcomas, carcinomas of the lung, breast and head and neck, and melanomas (217-222).

Overall lung cancer and breast cancer are the most common secondary cancers in HL patients. Women with HL who have received chest or axillary radiation are recommended to undergo routine annual mammogram or MRI of the breast starting 8 to 10 years after completion of treatment.

Endocrine Complications

Patients who receive treatment for HL may experience endocrine abnormalities (216). These are primarily limited to thyroid and gonad dysfunction. Patients may develop thyroid hyperplasia as well as hypothyroidism. Patients who have received neck or upper mediastinal radiation should undergo year thyroid function tests and a thyroid exam. The latter occurs in 6 to 25% of patients treated with mantle-field or cervical RT in some studies, although the rate of subclinical hypothyroidism may be much higher. Chemotherapy has little or no role in the development of thyroid dysfunction. Thyroid malignancy may develop in patients treated for HL, especially children and adults who receive partial thyroid ablation with radiation.

Because some patients with HL attain prolonged DFS, preservation of fertility is also an important issue (216). Radiotherapy or its scatter may affect testicular function. Recovery of that function and the length of time to recovery are related to RT dose. Alkylating agents are the most important chemotherapeutic agents that affect male fertility. These agents include cyclophosphamide, chlorambucil, mechlorethamine, and procarbazine. Twelve cycles of MOPP therapy results in prolonged testicular dysfunction in 80% of men. Only 10% of patients will show partial recovery within 1 to 7 years after treatment. Patients who receive fewer than four cycles of MOPP have a more rapid recovery. Studies of ABVD have shown that 54% of treated men have

TABLE
10-11 **LONG-TERM COMPLICATIONS IN PATIENTS CURED OF HODGKIN LYMPHOMA**

Complication	Etiology/Risk Factors	Management and Prevention
Immune dysfunction	HL; treatment	Appropriate vaccinations
Herpes zoster/varicella	HL; treatment	Systemic antiviral therapy; zoster immune globulin
Pneumococcal sepsis	Splenectomy; asplenia following radiotherapy	Pretreatment pneumococcal vaccine; selected antibiotic prophylaxis; avoid unnecessary splenectomy
Acute nonlymphocytic leukemia	Treatment; age above 40	Low-dose or aggressive antileukemic treatment
Myelodysplastic syndrome	Treatment; age above 40	Same as above
Non-Hodgkin lymphoma	Treatment	Aggressive chemotherapy
Solid tumors	Treatment	Conventional management
Thymic hyperplasia	HL; treatment	Resection
Hypothyroidism	Direct/indirect RT	Hormone replacement
Thyroid cancer	Direct/indirect RT chronic TSH stimulation	Conventional management
Male infertility	Treatment	Attempt sperm storage; testicular shielding during RT; possible suppression of spermatogenesis during chemotherapy
Male impotence	Treatment	Counseling; trial of testosterone
Female infertility	Treatment	Oophoropexy; possible ovarian suppression during treatment; cyclic estrogen replacement
Female impotence	Treatment	Counseling; cyclic estrogen replacement
Pericarditis, acute	Mediastinal treatment; chemotherapy; recall postirradiation	Appropriate treatment technique; avoid doxorubicin post-RT; anti-inflammatory medication
Pericarditis, chronic	Mediastinal RT	Appropriate RT technique; pericardiectomy
Cardiomyopathy	Mediastinal RT; recall postirradiation	Appropriate RT technique; avoid doxorubicin post-RT; limit cumulative doxorubicin dosage; provide medical support

Adapted, with permission, from Bookman MA, Longo DL. Concomitant illness inpatients treated for Hodgkin lymphoma disease. *Cancer Treat Rev* 1986;13:77-111.

impaired spermatogenesis, but they all recover adequate function within 2 years. However, azoospermia rates are high for patients treated with BEACOPP escalated or baseline and range from 87 to 93% (223).

Fertility in women is also affected by chemotherapy. Ovarian dysfunction may be heralded by irregular or anovulatory cycles. However, even with preexisting ovarian damage, pregnancy can occur; thus, pregnancy should not be considered a sign of completely normal ovarian function (216). As with the testis, the ovary appears to be more affected by alkylating agents and rates of infertility after BEACOPP for women are similar to men. ABVD is believed to induce a low rate of infertility and a recent study found that the fertility ratio as determined by a questionnaire among HL female survivors is similar to their matched controls (224,225). In a update on the Stanford V regimen documented that posttreatment conceptions occurred in 25% of patients treated (75). In general, the ovary tolerates RT better than the testis does. Patients nearer to menopause will experience primary amenorrhea at lower RT doses than

will others. Ovarian shielding may be useful for preventing excessive radiation to the ovary if RT to the abdomen is being considered.

Men being planned to start HL therapy should be considered for sperm banking. Gonadotropin-releasing hormone (GnRH) agonists have been evaluated as ovarian protectants in multiple small studies. A recent meta-analysis of 579 women found overall positive outcomes for those treated with GnRH agonists but the results remain controversial as in many trials the GnRH and control groups had different characteristics and follow-up was not equal (226). Alternatively for female patients planned to receive regimens with a high risk of infertility cryopreservation of embryos or oocytes with ovarian stimulation should be considered (227).

Cardiovascular Complications

Both RT and chemotherapy can have deleterious effects on the heart. Overall mediastinal radiation and doxorubicin-based chemotherapy are the highest risks for developing cardiac complications (228). The cardiac toxicity associated with RT develops about 5 to 10 years or greater after initial treatment. Decreases in radiation field size should further decrease the risks of developing cardiac disease.

Pericarditis is a common cardiovascular side effect resulting from mantle-field irradiation. Its incidence is related to the dose, rate, and anatomic volume treated. The frequency of the observation of this side effect has become significantly lower because mantle-field radiation fields are now infrequently used. Use of anterior–posterior ports contributed significantly to cardiac toxicity in early trials. The highest incidence of pericarditis occurs 5 to 9 months after completion of mantle-field RT (229). Most patients with pericarditis are asymptomatic, but others may present with cardiomegaly, friction rub, effusion, tamponade, fever, electrocardiographic changes, and pleuritic pain. Multiple modes of therapy for acute pericarditis exist, depending upon symptomatology. For symptomatic relief, nonsteroidal agents, digoxin, and diuretics have been used. Patients with hemodynamic compromise may require pericardiocentesis or pericardiectomy.

Myocardial damage also may occur after RT. Brosius et al. (230) conducted a postmortem study of 16 patients who received greater than 35 Gy to the heart. Fifteen of these patients had signs of myocardial damage. Utilizing radionuclide ventriculography, Burns et al. (231) examined ventricular function after RT in 12 of 21 asymptomatic patients and 10 historical controls. Right-ventricular ejection fraction dysfunction was the most common finding. The authors concluded that the right ventricle may experience more damage because of its anatomic location. Other studies of HL in patients who underwent RT with various cardiac-shielding techniques suggest that newer techniques may decrease the severity of myocardial damage.

Valvular abnormalities have been seen in HL patients following RT. These abnormalities include aortic valve or mitral valve regurgitation, both of which occur in the setting of myocardial fibrosis (232). Atherosclerosis accelerated by RT has also resulted in myocardial infarction in otherwise healthy patients (233).

Various chemotherapeutic agents have been implicated in the development of cardiac toxicity. The most important agent in the treatment of patients with HL is doxorubicin. At cumulative doses below 400 mg/m^2, the incidence of cardiomyopathy is less than 2% (234). In addition to the chronic effects of doxorubicin, patients may experience severe acute side effects such as myocarditis and arrhythmias (234). The mortality rate from doxorubicin-induced cardiomyopathy is 50%. Sequential endocardial biopsy may be helpful in predicting whether patients can continue to receive doxorubicin. Potential factors associated with increased risk of cardiomyopathy, including advanced patient age, uncontrolled hypertension, and previous RT. The combination of RT with doxorubicin has been associated with "radiation recall," an inflammatory endothelial reaction. In addition, cyclophosphamide may act synergistically with doxorubicin to produce cardiac damage (236).

Patients treated for HL should undergo blood pressure monitoring at a minimum of once per year. Certain panels including the National Comprehensive Cancer Network (NCCN) recommend a baseline stress test or echocardiogram a decade after completion of treatment. The utility of stress testing is supported by a Stanford study in which 294 patients who had received mediastinal radiation doses of 35 Gy were assessed for cardiac disease (237). Patients underwent stress echocardiography and perfusion imaging. On stress testing, 14% were found to have asymptomatic perfusion defects. Follow-up coronary angiography identified coronary artery stenosis of at least 50% in 22 patients and ultimately bypass graft surgery was conducted in seven patients. Thus, potentially stress testing can identify patients at risk for cardiac complication after mediastinal radiation and prevent later events including acute myocardial infarction.

Pulmonary Complications

The pulmonary system is also subject to the side effects of HL therapy. The effects secondary to RT can be categorized as acute or chronic changes. Acute radiation pneumonitis is the most common side effect. This phenomenon is related to the total radiation dose, dose rate, and volume of lung treated (238). Acute radiation pneumonitis may present with shortness of breath, cough, fever, pain, and wheezing. Chest radiograph will most often show paramediastinal densities and interstitial pneumonitis. Pleural effusions may occur.

Some patients require little or no therapy, whereas others may need treatment with corticosteroids (216). Rapid discontinuation of corticosteroids after steroid therapy may precipitate acute radiation pneumonitis (239). There may be synergy between RT and certain drugs (bleomycin, cyclophosphamide, and methotrexate) in producing acute radiation pneumonitis. Doxorubicin, bleomycin, and dactinomycin have also been implicated in the radiation recall phenomenon, previously mentioned, which is characterized by clinical signs and symptoms of chronic restrictive fibrosis occurring 9 to 12 months after the completion of therapy. Chest radiography shows findings consistent with chronic fibrosis, and spirometry shows evidence of restrictive airways disease (216).

Chemotherapeutic agents associated with pulmonary toxicity include bleomycin and carmustine (BCNU). Bleomycin toxicity most commonly presents as interstitial pneumonitis (216). Martin et al. recently described that bleomycin-related pulmonary toxicity is significantly increased by 17% for patients receiving growth factors with chemotherapy (240). Also two separate trials have shown that full dose chemotherapy can be delivered for HL patients without growth factor support (241,242). Evens et al. showed that although the absolute neutrophil count was $0.5 \times 10^9/L$ on 26% of treatment days with ABVD only 0.44% treatments were complicated by febrile neutropenia (242). Pulmonary fibrosis has been associated with carmustine and hypersensitivity pneumonitis with procarbazine (243,244). Increased pulmonary toxicity has also been associated with multiple-agent regimens (245).

Patients who are planned to receive ABVD or BEA-COPP should undergo a baseline pulmonary function test (PFT) with calculation of diffusing capacity of the lung for carbon monoxide (DLCO). In addition, the GHSG HD13 trial is currently evaluating whether bleomycin can be omitted from initial therapy for patients with early-stage favorable HL.

Miscellaneous Complications

Patients with HL may experience musculoskeletal complications, such as avascular necrosis of bone. The incidence is increased with RT to bone (246). Children who receive RT to bone may also experience growth asymmetry secondary to premature closure of the epiphyseal plates (216). This risk may warrant lowering the dose of RT administered. Patients who receive RT to soft tissues may develop fibrosis with edema, venous thrombosis, and nerve entrapment.

Patients treated with mantle field or cervical RT may experience transient or permanent xerostomia, with an increased risk of dental caries (229).

■ CONCLUSION

HL remains one of the most treatable human malignancies. A wide range of therapeutic modalities is available, including chemotherapy, RT, and combinations of the two. Many new and promising therapeutic agents are currently under investigation. Controversies remain as to the appropriate treatment of HL at different stages, but this debate may be resolved with future studies. Finally, the improved outcome of patients with HL makes it imperative to consider the acute and long-term side effects of each therapeutic modality in treatment planning and future clinical trials.

References

1. Swerdlow SHCE, Harris NL, et al. (eds). *WHO Classification of Tumours of Haematopoietic and Lymphoid Tissues* (4th ed.). Lyon, France: International Agency for Research on Cancer; 2008.
2. National Cancer Institute Surveillance Research Program. Available at http://seer.cancer.gov/statfacts/html/hodg.html. Accessed on 4/9/2010.
3. Schmitz R, Stanelle J, Hansmann M-L, et al. Pathogenesis of classical and lymphocyte-predominant Hodgkin lymphoma. *Ann Rev. Pathol.: Mech Disease* 2009;4:151-174.
4. Diehl V, Sextro M, Franklin J, et al. Clinical presentation, course, and prognostic factors in lymphocyte-predominant Hodgkin's disease and lymphocyte-rich classical Hodgkin's disease: Report from the European Task Force on Lymphoma Project on lymphocyte-predominant Hodgkin's disease. *J Clin Oncol* 1999;17:776-783
5. Anagnostopoulos I, Hansmann M-L, Franssila K, et al. European Task Force on Lymphoma Project on lymphocyte predominance Hodgkin disease: Histologic and immunohistologic analysis of submitted cases reveals 2 types of Hodgkin disease with a nodular growth pattern and abundant lymphocytes. *Blood* 2000;96:1889-1899.
6. Lukes RJ, Butler JJ. The pathology and nomenclature of Hodgkin's disease. *Cancer Res* 1966;26:1063-1081.
7. Brune V, Tiacci E, Pfeil I, et al. Origin and pathogenesis of nodular lymphocyte-predominant Hodgkin lymphoma as revealed by global gene expression analysis. *J Exp Med* 2008;205:2251-2268.
8. Medeiros LJ. Hodgkin's disease. *Cancer* 1995;1:357-369.
9. Maclennan KA, Bennett MH, Tu A, et al. Relationship of histopathologic features to survival and relapse in nodular sclerosing Hodgkin's disease. A study of 1659 patients. *Cancer* 1989;64:1686-1693.
10. Küppers R. Molecular biology of Hodgkin's lymphoma. *Adv Cancer Res* 2002;84:277-312.
11. Fiumara P, Snell V, Li Y, et al. Functional expression of receptor activator of nuclear factor kappa B in Hodgkin disease cell lines. *Blood* 2001;98:2784-2790.
12. Schmitz R, Hansmann ML, Bohle V, et al. TNFAIP3 (A20) is a tumor suppressor gene in Hodgkin lymphoma and primary mediastinal B cell lymphoma. *J Exp Med* 2009;206:981-989.
13. Kuppers R. The biology of Hodgkin's lymphoma. *Nat Rev Cancer* 2009;9:15-27.
14. Oki Y, Georgakis GV, Migone TS, et al. Elevated serum BLyS levels in patients with non-Hodgkin lymphoma. *Leuk Lymphoma* 2007;48:1869-1871.
15. Nadali G, Tavecchia L, Zanolin E, et al. Serum level of the soluble form of the CD30 molecule identifies patients with Hodgkin's disease at high risk of unfavorable outcome. *Blood* 1998;91:3011-3016.
16. Weihrauch MR, Manzke O, Beyer M, et al. Elevated serum levels of CC thymus and activation-related chemokine (TARC) in primary Hodgkin's disease: Potential for a prognostic factor. *Cancer Res* 2005;65:5516-5519.

17. Mueller N, Evans A, Harris NL, et al. Hodgkin's disease and Epstein-Barr virus. Altered antibody pattern before diagnosis. *N Engl J Med* 1989;320:689-695.

18. Bechtel D, Kurth J, Unkel C, et al. Transformation of BCR-deficient germinal-center B cells by EBV supports a major role of the virus in the pathogenesis of Hodgkin and post-transplantation lymphomas. *Blood* 2005;106:4345-4350.

19. Kilger E, Kieser A, Baumann M, et al. Epstein-Barr virus-mediated B-cell proliferation is dependent upon latent membrane protein 1, which simulates an activated CD40 receptor. *EMBO J* 1998;17:1700-1709.

20. Mancao C, Hammerschmidt W. Epstein-Barr virus latent membrane protein 2A is a B-cell receptor mimic and essential for B-cell survival. *Blood* 2007;110:3715-3721.

21. MacMahon B. Epidemiology of Hodgkin's disease. *Cancer Res* 1966;26:1189-1201.

22. Lister T, Crowther D, Sutcliffe S, et al. Report of a committee convened to discuss the evaluation and staging of patients with Hodgkin's disease: Cotswolds meeting [published erratum appears in *J Clin Oncol* 1990;8(9):1602]. *J Clin Oncol* 1989;7:1630-1636.

23. Cheson BD, Pfistner B, Juweid ME, et al. Revised response criteria for malignant lymphoma. *J Clin Oncol* 2007;25: 579-586.

24. Hagemeister FB, Fesus SM, Lamki LM, et al. Role of the gallium scan in Hodgkin's disease. *Cancer* 1990;65:1090-1096.

25. Delcambre C, Reman O, Henry-Amar M, et al. Clinical relevance of gallium-67 scintigraphy in lymphoma before and after therapy. *Eur J Nucl Med* 2000;27:176-184.

26. Tubiana M, Henry-Amar M, van der Werf-Messing B, et al. A multivariate analysis of prognostic factors in early stage Hodgkin's disease. *Int J Radiat Oncol Biol Phys* 1985;11: 23-30.

27. Mauch P, Tarbell N, Weinstein H, et al. Stage IA and IIA supradiaphragmatic Hodgkin's disease: Prognostic factors in surgically staged patients treated with mantle and paraaortic irradiation. *J Clin Oncol* 1988;6:1576-1583.

28. EORTC Lymphoma Cooperative Group and GELA. Trial H9 protocol: Prospective controlled trial in clinical stages I–II supradiaphragmatic Hodgkin's disease—Evaluation of treatment efficacy, (long term) toxicity and quality of life in two different prognostic subgroups. Brussels: EORTC Lymphoma Cooperative Group and GELA, 1999: EORTC Protocol 20982. Available at http://www.eortc.be. Accessed 4/1/2010.

29. Diehl V, Brilliant C, Engert A. HD10: Investigating reduction of combined modality treatment intensity in early stage Hodgkin's lymphoma. Interim analysis of a randomized trial of the German Hodgkins Study Group (GHSG). *Proc Am Soc Clin Oncol* 2005. ASCO Meeting Abstracts. May 28, 2005:6506.

30. Hasenclever D, Diehl V. A prognostic score for advanced Hodgkin's disease. International Prognostic Factors Project on Advanced Hodgkin's Disease. *N Engl J Med* 1998;339: 1506-1514.

31. O'Doherty MJ, Macdonald EA, Barrington SF, et al. Positron emission tomography in the management of lymphomas. *Clin Oncol (R Coll Radiol)* 2002;14:415-426.

32. Hutchings M, Loft A, Hansen M, et al. Position emission tomography with or without computed tomography in the primary staging of Hodgkin's lymphoma. *Haematologica* 2006;91:482-489.

33. Gallamini A, Hutchings M, Rigacci L, et al. Early interim 2-[18F]fluoro-2-deoxy-d-glucose positron emission tomography is prognostically superior to International Prognostic Score in advanced-stage Hodgkin's lymphoma: A report from a Joint Italian-Danish Study. *J Clin Oncol* 2007;25: 3746-3752.

34. Hutchings M, Loft A, Hansen M, et al. FDG-PET after two cycles of chemotherapy predicts treatment failure and progression-free survival in Hodgkin lymphoma. *Blood* 2006; 107:52-59.

35. Terasawa T, Lau J, Bardet S, et al. Fluorine-18-fluorodeoxyglucose positron emission tomography for interim response assessment of advanced–stage Hodgkin's lymphoma and diffuse large B-cell lymphoma: A systematic review. *J Clin Oncol* 2009;27:1906-1914.

36. Southwest Oncology Group Lymphoma Committee 2009. http://swog.org/Visitors/ViewProtocolDetails.asp?ProtocolID=2141.

37. Kobe C, Dietlein M, Franklin J, et al. Positron emission tomography has a high negative predictive value for progression or early relapse for patients with residual disease after first-line chemotherapy in advanced-stage Hodgkin lymphoma. *Blood* 2008;112:3989-3994.

38. Jerusalem G, Beguin Y, Fassotte MF, et al. Whole-body positron emission tomography using 18F-fluorodeoxyglucose for posttreatment evaluation in Hodgkin's disease and non-Hodgkin's lymphoma has higher diagnostic and prognostic value than classical computed tomography scan imaging. *Blood* 1999;94:429-433.

39. Devizzi L, Maffioli L, Bonfante V, et al. Comparison of gallium scan, computed tomography, and magnetic resonance in patients with mediastinal Hodgkin's disease. *Ann Oncol* 1997;8(Suppl 1):53-56.

40. de Wit M, Bohuslavizki KH, Buchert R, et al. 18FDG-PET following treatment as valid predictor for disease-free survival in Hodgkin's lymphoma. *Ann Oncol* 2001;12:29-37.

41. Van Den Bossche B, Lambert B, De Winter F, et al. 18FDG PET versus high-dose 67Ga scintigraphy for restaging and treatment follow-up of lymphoma patients. *Nucl Med Commun* 2002;23:1079-1083.

42. Kostakoglu L, Leonard JP, Kuji I, et al. Comparison of fluorine-18 fluorodeoxyglucose positron emission tomography and Ga-67 scintigraphy in evaluation of lymphoma. *Cancer* 2002;94:879-888.

43. Pulsoni A, Cavalieri E, Capria S, et al. Prognostic role of PET-FDG before autologous stem cell transplantation in advanced Hodgkin's lymphoma. *ASH Ann Meeting Abstr* 2009;14:1548.

44. Cheson BD, Horning SJ, Coiffier B, et al. Report of an International Workshop to standardize response criteria for non-Hodgkin's lymphomas. *J Clin Oncol* 1999;17:1244-1253.

45. Rosenberg SA, Kaplan HS. The evolution and summary results of the Stanford randomized clinical trials of the management of Hodgkin's disease: 1962-1984. *Int J Radiat Oncol Biol Phys* 1985;11:5-22.

46. Specht L, Gray RG, Clarke MJ, et al. Influence of more extensive radiotherapy and adjuvant chemotherapy on long-term outcome of early-stage Hodgkin's disease: A meta-analysis of 23 randomized trials involving 3,888 patients. International Hodgkin's Disease Collaborative Group. *J Clin Oncol* 1998; 16:830-843.

47. Carde P, Burgers JM, Henry-Amar M, et al. Clinical stages I and II Hodgkin's disease: A specifically tailored therapy according to prognostic factors. *J Clin Oncol* 1988;6:239-252.

48. Duhmke E, Franklin J, Pfreundschuh M, et al. Low-dose radiation is sufficient for the noninvolved extended–field treatment in favorable early-stage Hodgkin's disease: Long-term results of a randomized trial of radiotherapy alone. *J Clin Oncol* 2001;19:2905-2914.

49. Dores GM, Metayer C, Curtis RE, et al. Second malignant neoplasms among long–term survivors of Hodgkin's disease: A population-based evaluation over 25 years. *J Clin Oncol* 2002;20:3484-3494.

50. Hoppe RT. Hodgkin's disease: Complications of therapy and excess mortality. *Ann Oncol* 1997;8(Suppl 1):115-118.

51. Noordijk EM, Carde P, Mandard AM, et al. Preliminary results of the EORTC–GPMC controlled clinical trial H7 in early-stage Hodgkin's disease. EORTC Lymphoma Cooperative Group. Groupe Pierre-et-Marie-Curie. *Ann Oncol* 1994; 5(Suppl 2):107-112.

52. Horning SJ, Hoppe RT, Hancock SL, et al. Vinblastine, bleomycin, and methotrexate: An effective adjuvant in favorable Hodgkin's disease. *J Clin Oncol* 1988;6:1822-1831.

53. Press OW, LeBlanc M, Lichter AS, et al. Phase III randomized intergroup trial of subtotal lymphoid irradiation versus doxorubicin, vinblastine, and subtotal lymphoid irradiation for stage IA to IIA Hodgkin's disease. *J Clin Oncol* 2001; 19:4238-4244.

54. Bonadonna G, Bonfante V, Viviani S, et al. ABVD plus subtotal nodal versus involved-field radiotherapy in early-stage Hodgkin's disease: Long-term results. *J Clin Oncol* 2004;22:2835-2841.

55. Ferme C, Eghbali H, Meerwaldt JH, et al. Chemotherapy plus involved-field radiation in early-stage Hodgkin's disease. *N Engl J Med* 2007;357:1916-1927.

56. Chronowski GM, Wilder RB, Tucker SL, et al. Analysis of in-field control and late toxicity for adults with early-stage Hodgkin's disease treated with chemotherapy followed by radiotherapy. *Int J Radiat Oncol Biol Phys* 2003;55:36-43.

57. Maity A, Goldwein JW, Lange B, et al. Comparison of high-dose and low-dose radiation with and without chemotherapy for children with Hodgkin's disease: An analysis of the experience at the Children's Hospital of Philadelphia and the Hospital of the University of Pennsylvania. *J Clin Oncol* 1992;10:929-935.

58. Loeffler M, Diehl V, Pfreundschuh M, et al. Dose-response relationship of complementary radiotherapy following four cycles of combination chemotherapy in intermediate-stage Hodgkin's disease. *J Clin Oncol* 1997;15:2275-2287.

59. Santoro A, Bonadonna G, Valagussa P, et al. Long-term results of combined chemotherapy-radiotherapy approach in Hodgkin's disease: Superiority of ABVD plus radiotherapy versus MOPP plus radiotherapy. *J Clin Oncol* 1987;5: 27-37.

60. Carde P, Hagenbeek A, Hayat M, et al. Clinical staging versus laparotomy and combined modality with MOPP versus ABVD in early-stage Hodgkin's disease: The H6 twin randomized trials from the European Organization for Research and Treatment of Cancer Lymphoma Cooperative Group. *J Clin Oncol* 1993;11:2258-2272.

61. Eghbali H, Brice P, Creemers G-Y, et al. Comparison of three radiation dose levels after EBVP regimen in favorable supradiaphragmatic clinical stages (CS) I-II Hodgkin's lymphoma (HL): Preliminary results of the EORTC-GELA H9-F trial. *ASH Ann Meeting Abstr* 2005;106:814.

62. Advani RH, Hoppe RT, Baer DM, et al. Efficacy of abbreviated Stanford V chemotherapy and involved field radiotherapy in early stage Hodgkin's disease: Mature Results of the G4 Trial. *ASH Ann Meeting Abstr* 2009;114:1670.

63. Engert A, Diehl V, Pluetschow A, et al. Two cycles of ABVD followed by involved field radiotherapy with 20 gray (Gy) is the new standard of care in the treatment of patients with early-stage Hodgkin lymphoma: Final analysis of the randomized German Hodgkin Study Group (GHSG) HD10. Study supported by the Deutsche Krebshilfe and in part by the Competence Network Malignant Lymphoma. *ASH Ann Meeting Abstr* 2009;114:716.

64. Klimm B, Engert A. Combined modality treatment of Hodgkin's lymphoma. *Cancer J* 2009;15(2):143-149.

65. Campbell BA, Voss N, Pickles T, et al. Involved-nodal radiation therapy as a component of combination therapy for limited-stage Hodgkin's lymphoma: A question of field size. *J Clin Oncol* 2008;26:5170-5174.

66. Ng AK, Bernardo MP, Weller E, et al. Long-term survival and competing causes of death in patients with early-stage Hodgkin's disease treated at age 50 or younger. *J Clin Oncol* 2002;20:2101-2108.

67. Ng AK, Mauch PM. The impact of treatment on the risk of second malignancy after Hodgkin's disease. *Ann Oncol* 2006; 17:1727-1729.

68. Biti GP, Cimino G, Cartoni C, et al. Extended-field radiotherapy is superior to MOPP chemotherapy for the treatment of pathologic stage I-IIA Hodgkin's disease: Eight-year update of an Italian prospective randomized study. *J Clin Oncol* 1992;10:378-382.

69. Straus DJ, Portlock CS, Qin J, et al. Results of a prospective randomized clinical trial of doxorubicin, bleomycin, vinblastine, and dacarbazine (ABVD) followed by radiation therapy (RT) versus ABVD alone for stages I, II, and IIIA nonbulky Hodgkin disease. *Blood* 2004;104:3483-3489.

70. Raemaekers JM, van der Maazen RW. Hodgkin's lymphoma: News from an old disease. *Neth J Med* 2008;66:457-466.

71. Engert A, Schiller P, Josting A, et al. Involved-field radiotherapy is equally effective and less toxic compared with extended-field radiotherapy after four cycles of chemotherapy in patients with early-stage unfavorable Hodgkin's lymphoma: Results of the HD8 trial of the German Hodgkin's Lymphoma Study Group. *J Clin Oncol* 2003;21:3601-3608.

72. Vijayakumar S, Myrianthopoulos LC. An updated dose-response analysis in Hodgkin's disease. *Radiother Oncol* 1992;24:1-13.

73. Brincker H, Bentzen SM. A re-analysis of available dose-response and time-dose data in Hodgkin's disease. *Radiother Oncol* 1994;30:227-230.

74. Canellos GP, Anderson JR, Propert KJ, et al. Chemotherapy of advanced Hodgkin's disease with MOPP, ABVD, or MOPP alternating with ABVD. *N Engl J Med* 1992;327: 1478-1484.

75. Horning SJ, Hoppe RT, Advani R, et al. Efficacy and late effects of stanford V chemotherapy and radiotherapy in untreated Hodgkin's disease: Mature data in early and advanced stage patients. *ASH Ann Meeting Abstr* 2004;104:308.

76. Aversa SM, Salvagno L, Soraru M, et al. Stanford V regimen plus consolidative radiotherapy is an effective therapeutic program for bulky or advanced-stage Hodgkin's disease. *Acta Haematol* 2004;112:141-147.

77. Edwards-Bennett SM, Jacks LM, Moskowitz CH, et al. Stanford V program for locally extensive and advanced Hodgkin lymphoma: The Memorial Sloan-Kettering Cancer Center experience. *Ann Oncol* 2010 Mar;21(3):574-581.

78. Ferme C, Divine M, Vranovsky A, et al. Four ABVD and involved-field radiotherapy in unfavorable supradiaphragmatic clinical stages (CS) I-II Hodgkin's lymphoma (HL): Preliminary results of the EORTC-GELA H9-U trial. *ASH Ann Meeting Abstr* 2005;106:813.

79. Diehl V, Brillant C, Engert A, et al. Recent interim analysis of the HD11 trial of the GHSG: Intensification of chemotherapy and reduction of radiation dose in early unfavorable stage Hodgkin's lymphoma. *ASH Ann Meeting Abstr* 2005; 106:816.

80. Andre MPE, Reman O, Federico M, et al. First report on the H10 EORTC/GELA/IIL randomized intergroup trial on early FDG-PET scan guided treatment adaptation versus standard combined modality treatment in patients with supra-diaphragmatic stage I/II Hodgkin's lymphoma, for the Groupe d'Etude Des Lymphomes De l'Adulte (GELA), European Organisation for the Research and Treatment of Cancer (EORTC) Lymphoma Group and the Intergruppo Italiano Linfomi (IIL). *ASH Ann Meeting Abstr* 2009;114:97.

81. Gobbi PG, Levis A, Chisesi T, et al. ABVD versus modified Stanford V versus MOPPEBVCAD with optional and limited radiotherapy in intermediate- and advanced-stage Hodgkin's lymphoma: Final results of a multicenter randomized trial by the Intergruppo Italiano Linfomi. *J Clin Oncol* 2005;23: 9198-9207.

82. Engert A, Franklin J, Mueller R-P, et al. HD12 randomised trial comparing 8 dose-escalated cycles of BEACOPP with 4 escalated and 4 baseline cycles in patients with advanced stage Hodgkin lymphoma (HL): An Analysis of the German Hodgkin Lymphoma Study Group (GHSG), University of Cologne, D-50924 Cologne, Germany. *ASH Ann Meeting Abstr* 2006;108:99.

83. Kobe C, Dietlein M, Franklin J, et al. Positron emission tomography has a high negative predictive value for progression or early relapse for patients with residual disease after first–line chemotherapy in advanced-stage Hodgkin lymphoma. *Blood* 2008;112:3989-3994.

84. Brillant C, Bauer K, Herbst C, et al. Escalated BEACOPP versus ABVD-like chemotherapy for Hodgkin lymphoma patients: A Cochrane review. *ASH Ann Meeting Abstr* 2009; 114:3705.

85. Russo F, Corazzelli G, Lastoria S, et al. Dose-dense(dd) ABVD and dose-dense/dose-intense(dd-di) ABVD in newly diagnosed patients (pts), intermediate- and advanced-stage with classical Hodgkin's lymphoma (cHL): Final results. *ASH Ann Meeting Abstr* 2009;114:715.

86. Diehl V, Franklin J, Pfreundschuh M, et al. Standard and increased-dose BEACOPP chemotherapy compared with COPP-ABVD for advanced Hodgkin's disease. *N Engl J Med* 2003;348:2386-2395.

87. Carella AM, Prencipe E, Pungolino E, et al. Twelve years experience with high-dose therapy and autologous stem cell transplantation for high-risk Hodgkin's disease patients in first remission after MOPP/ABVD chemotherapy. *Leuk Lymphoma* 1996;21:63-70.

88. Federico M, Bellei M, Brice P, et al. High-dose therapy and autologous stem-cell transplantation versus conventional

therapy for patients with advanced Hodgkin's lymphoma responding to front-line therapy. *J Clin Oncol* 2003;21: 2320-2325.

89. Yahalom J, Ryu J, Straus DJ, et al. Impact of adjuvant radiation on the patterns and rate of relapse in advanced-stage Hodgkin's disease treated with alternating chemotherapy combinations. *J Clin Oncol* 1991;9:2193-2201.

90. Diehl V, Loeffler M, Pfreundschuh M, et al. Further chemotherapy versus low-dose involved-field radiotherapy as consolidation of complete remission after six cycles of alternating chemotherapy in patients with advance Hodgkin's disease. German Hodgkins' Study Group (GHSG). *Ann Oncol* 1995;6:901-910.

91. Coleman M, Rafla S, Propert KJ, et al. Augmented therapy of extensive Hodgkin's disease: Radiation to known disease or prolongation of induction chemotherapy did not improve survival—Results of a Cancer and Leukemia Group B study. *Int J Radiat Oncol Biol Phys* 1998;41:639-645.

92. Loeffler M, Brosteanu O, Hasenclever D, et al. Meta-analysis of chemotherapy versus combined modality treatment trials in Hodgkin's disease. International Database on Hodgkin's Disease Overview Study Group. *J Clin Oncol* 1998;16: 818-829.

93. Aleman BM, Raemaekers JM, Tirelli U, et al. Involved-field radiotherapy for advanced Hodgkin's lymphoma. *N Engl J Med* 2003;348:2396-2406.

94. Doria R, Holford T, Farber LR, et al. Second solid malignancies after combined modality therapy for Hodgkin's disease. *J Clin Oncol* 1995;13:2016-2022.

95. Fabian CJ, Mansfield CM, Dahlberg S, et al. Low-dose involved field radiation after chemotherapy in advanced Hodgkin disease: A Southwest Oncology Group Randomized Study. *Ann Internal Med* 1994;120:903-912.

96. Raemaekers J, Burgers M, Henry-Amar M, et al. Patients with stage III/IV Hodgkin's disease in partial remission after MOPP/ABV chemotherapy have excellent prognosis after additional involved-field radiotherapy: Interim results from the ongoing EORTC-LCG and GPMC phase III trial. The EORTC Lymphoma Cooperative Group and Groupe Pierre-et-Marie-Curie. *Ann Oncol* 1997;8(Suppl 1):111-114.

97. Ferme C, Mounier N, Casasnovas O, et al. Long-term results and competing risk analysis of the H89 trial in patients with advanced-stage Hodgkin lymphoma: A study by the Groupe d'Etude des Lymphomes de l'Adulte (GELA). *Blood* 2006; 107:4636-4642.

98. Oza AM, Ganesan TS, Leahy M, et al. Patterns of survival in patients with Hodgkin's disease: Long follow up in a single centre. *Ann Oncol* 1993;4:385-392.

99. Horwich A, Specht L, Ashley S. Survival analysis of patients with clinical stages I or II Hodgkin's disease who have relapsed after initial treatment with radiotherapy alone. *Eur J Cancer* 1997;33:848-853.

100. Josting A, Franklin J, May M, et al. New prognostic score based on treatment outcome of patients with relapsed Hodgkin's lymphoma registered in the database of the German Hodgkin's lymphoma study group. *J Clin Oncol* 2002;20:221-230.

101. Josting A, Rueffer U, Franklin J, et al. Prognostic factors and treatment outcome in primary progressive Hodgkin lymphoma: A report from the German Hodgkin Lymphoma Study Group. *Blood* 2000;96:1280-1286.

102. Moskowitz CH, Nimer SD, Zelenetz AD, et al. A 2-step comprehensive high-dose chemoradiotherapy second-line program for relapsed and refractory Hodgkin disease: Analysis by intent to treat and development of a prognostic model. *Blood* 2001;97:616-623.

103. Ng AK, Li S, Neuberg D, et al. Comparison of MOPP versus ABVD as salvage therapy in patients who relapse after radiation therapy alone for Hodgkin's disease. *Ann Oncol* 2004; 15:270-275.

104. Rodriguez J, Rodriguez MA, Fayad L, et al. ASHAP: A regimen for cytoreduction of refractory or recurrent Hodgkin's disease. *Blood* 1996;93:3631-3632.

105. Aparicio J, Segura A, Garcera S, et al. ESHAP is an active regimen for relapsing Hodgkin's disease. *Ann Oncol* 1999; 10:593-595.

106. Josting A, Raemakers JM, Diehl V, et al. New concepts for relapsed Hodgkin's disease. *Ann Oncol* 2002;13(Suppl 1): 117-121.

107. Santoro A, Magagnoli M, Spina M, et al. Ifosfamide, gemcitabine, and vinorelbine: A new induction regimen for refractory and relapsed Hodgkin's lymphoma. *Haematologica* 2007;92:35-41.

108. Josting A, Nogova L, Franklin J, et al. Salvage radiotherapy in patients with relapsed and refractory Hodgkin's lymphoma: A retrospective analysis from the German Hodgkin Lymphoma Study Group. *J Clin Oncol* 2005;23:1522-1529.

109. Linch DC, Winfield D, Goldstone AH, et al. Dose intensification with autologous bone-marrow transplantation in relapsed and resistant Hodgkin's disease: Results of a BNLI randomised trial. *Lancet* 1993;341:1051-1054.

110. Schmitz NSM, Pfistner B. HDR-1: High-dose therapy (HDT) followed by hematopoietic stem cell transplantation (HSCT) for relapsed chemosensitive Hodgkin's disease (HD): Final results of a randomized GHSG and EBMT trial (HDR1). *Proc Am Soc Clin Oncol Suppl* 1999:18a.

111. Sirohi B, Cunningham D, Powles R, et al. Long-term outcome of autologous stem-cell transplantation in relapsed or refractory Hodgkin's lymphoma. *Ann Oncol* 2008;19:1312-1319.

112. Moskowitz CH, Kewalramani T, Nimer SD, et al. Effectiveness of high dose chemoradiotherapy and autologous stem cell transplantation for patients with biopsy-proven primary refractory Hodgkin's disease. *Br J Haematol* 2004;124: 645-652.

113. Filmont JE, Gisselbrecht C, Cuenca X, et al. The impact of pre- and post-transplantation positron emission tomography using 18-fluorodeoxyglucose on poor-prognosis lymphoma patients undergoing autologous stem cell transplantation. *Cancer* 2007;110:1361-1369.

114. Schot BW, Zijlstra JM, Sluiter WJ, et al. Early FDG-PET assessment in combination with clinical risk scores determines prognosis in recurring lymphoma. *Blood* 2007;109: 486-491.

115. Svoboda J, Andreadis C, Elstrom R, et al. Prognostic value of FDG-PET scan imaging in lymphoma patients undergoing autologous stem cell transplantation. *Bone Marrow Transplant* 2006;38:211-216.

116. Morschhauser F, Brice P, Ferme C, et al. Risk-adapted salvage treatment with single or tandem autologous stem-cell transplantation for first relapse/refractory Hodgkin's lymphoma: Results of the prospective multicenter H96 trial by the GELA/SFGM Study Group. *J Clin Oncol* 2008;26:5980-5987.

117. Horning S, Fanale M, deVos S, et al. Defining a population of Hodgkin lymphoma patients for novel therapeutics: An international effort. In: *Proceedings of the 10th International Conference on Malignant Lymphoma (10–ICML)118*; 2008. Lugano, Switzerland.

118. Laport GG. Allogeneic hematopoietic cell transplantation for Hodgkin lymphoma: A concise review. *Leuk Lymphoma* 2008;49:1854-1859.

119. Milpied N, Fielding AK, Pearce RM, et al. Allogeneic bone marrow transplant is not better than autologous transplant for patients with relapsed Hodgkin's disease. European Group for Blood and Bone Marrow Transplantation. *J Clin Oncol* 1996;14:1291-1296.

120. Akpek G, Ambinder RF, Piantadosi S, et al. Long-term results of blood and marrow transplantation for Hodgkin's lymphoma. *J Clin Oncol* 2001;19:4314-4321.

121. Jones RJ, Ambinder RF, Piantadosi S, et al. Evidence of a graft-versus-lymphoma effect associated with allogeneic bone marrow transplantation. *Blood* 1991;77:649-653.

122. Anderson JR, Jenkin RD, Wilson JF, et al. Long-term follow-up of patients treated with COMP or LSA2L2 therapy for childhood non-Hodgkin's lymphoma: A report of CCG-551 from the Children's Cancer Group. *J Clin Oncol* 1993;11:1024-1032.

123. Thomson KJ, Peggs KS, Smith P, et al. Superiority of reduced-intensity allogeneic transplantation over conventional treatment for relapse of Hodgkin's lymphoma following autologous stem cell transplantation. *Bone Marrow Transplant* 2008;41:765-770.

124. Sureda A, Robinson S, Canals C, et al. Reduced-intensity conditioning compared with conventional allogeneic stem-cell transplantation in relapsed or refractory Hodgkin's lymphoma: An analysis from the Lymphoma Working Party of the European Group for Blood and Marrow Transplantation. *J Clin Oncol* 2008;26:455-462.

125. Peggs KS, Hunter A, Chopra R, et al. Clinical evidence of a raft-versus-Hodgkin's-lymphoma effect after reduced-intensity allogeneic transplantation. *Lancet* 2005;365:1934-1941.

126. Alvarez I, Sureda A, Caballero MD, et al. Nonmyeloablative stem cell transplantation is an effective therapy for refractory or relapsed Hodgkin Lymphoma: Results of a Spanish prospective cooperative protocol. *Biol Blood Marrow Transplant* 2006;12:172-183.

127. Scheid C, Dreger P, Beelen DW, et al. Allogeneic stem cell transplantation for Hodgkin's disease from sibling and unrelated donors: The German Cooperative Transplantation Study Group Experience. *ASH Ann Meeting Abstr* 2009;114:2293.

128. Sureda A. Autologous and allogeneic stem cell transplantation in Hodgkin's lymphoma. *Hematol Oncol Clin North Am* 2007;21:943-960.

129. Anderlini P, Saliba R, Acholonu S, et al. Fludarabine-melphalan as a preparative regimen for reduced-intensity conditioning allogeneic stem cell transplantation in relapsed and refractory Hodgkin's lymphoma: The updated M.D. Anderson Cancer Center experience. *Haematologica* 2008;93:257-264.

130. Bartlett NL, Younes A, Carabasi MH, et al. A phase 1 multidose study of SGN-30 immunotherapy in patients with refractory or recurrent CD30+ hematologic malignancies. *Blood* 2008;111:1848-1854.

131. Ansell SM, Horwitz SM, Engert A, et al. Phase I/II study of an anti-CD30 monoclonal antibody (MDX-060) in Hodgkin's lymphoma and anaplastic large-cell lymphoma. *J Clin Oncol* 2007;25:2764-2769.

132. Younes A, Zalevsky J, Blum KA, et al. Evaluation of the pharmacokinetics, immunogenicity, and safety of XmAb(R)2513 in the ongoing study XmAb2513-01: A phase 1 study of every other week XmAb2513 to evaluate the safety, tolerability, and pharmacokinetics in patients with Hodgkin lymphoma or anaplastic large cell lymphoma. *ASH Ann Meeting Abstr* 2008; 112:5012.

133. Blum KA, Smith M, Fung H, et al. Phase I study of an anti-CD30 Fc engineered humanized monoclonal antibody in Hodgkin lymphoma (HL) or anaplastic large cell lymphoma (ALCL) patients: Safety, pharmacokinetics (PK), immunogenicity, and efficacy. *J Clin Oncol* 2009;27:8531 (Meeting Abstracts).

134. Younes A, Forero-Torres A, Bartlett NL, et al. Multiple complete responses in a phase 1 dose-escalation study of the antibody-drug conjugate SGN-35 in patients with relapsed or refractory CD30-positive lymphomas. *ASH Ann Meeting Abstr* 2008;112:1006.

135. Younes A, Forero-Torres A, Bartlett NL, et al. Robust antitumor activity of the antibody-drug conjugate SGN-35 when administered every 3 weeks to patients with relapsed or refractory CD30 positive hematologic malignancies in a phase I study. In: *Proceedings of the 14th Congress of the European Hematology Association 503*; 2009. Berlin, Germany.

136. Fanale M, Bartlett NL, Forero-Torres A, et al. The antibody-drug conjugate brentuximab vedotin (SGN-35) induced multiple objective responses in patients with relapsed or refractory CD30-positive lymphomas in a phase 1 weekly dosing study. *ASH Ann Meeting Abstr* 2009;114:2731.

137. Bartlett N, Forero-Torres A, Rosenblatt J, et al. Complete remissions with weekly dosing of SGN-35, a novel antibody-drug conjugate (ADC) targeting CD30, in a phase I dose-escalation study in patients with relapsed or refractory Hodgkin lymphoma (HL) or systemic anaplastic large cell lymphoma (sALCL). *J Clin Oncol* 2009;27:8500 (Meeting Abstracts).

138. Younes A, Romaguera J, Hagemeister F, et al. A pilot study of rituximab in patients with recurrent, classic Hodgkin disease. *Cancer* 2003;98:310-314.

139. Ashkenazi A. Targeting death and decoy receptors of the tumour-necrosis factor superfamily. *Nat Rev Cancer* 2002;2: 420-430.

140. Zheng B, Fiumara P, Li YV, et al. MEK/ERK pathway is aberrantly active in Hodgkin disease: A signaling pathway shared by CD30, CD40, and RANK that regulates cell proliferation and survival. *Blood* 2003;102:1019-1027.

141. Younes A, Vose JM, Zelenetz AD, et al. Results of a phase 2 trial of HGS-ETR1 (Agonistic Human Monoclonal Antibody to TRAIL Receptor 1) in subjects with relapsed/refractory non-Hodgkin's lymphoma (NHL). *ASH Ann Meeting Abstr* 2005;106:489.

142. Fehniger TA, Larson S, Trinkaus K, et al. A phase II multicenter study of lenalidomide in patients with relapsed or refractory classical Hodgkin lymphoma (cHL): Preliminary results. *ASH Ann Meeting Abstr* 2008;112:2595.

143. Kuruvilla J, Taylor D, Wang L, et al. Phase II trial of lenalidomide in patients with relapsed or refractory Hodgkin lymphoma. *ASH Ann Meeting Abstr* 2008;112:3052.

144. Bollard CM, Huls MH, Buza E, et al. Administration of latent membrane protein 2-specific cytotoxic T lymphocytes to patients with relapsed Epstein-Barr virus-positive lymphoma. *Clin Lymphoma Myeloma* 2006;6:342-347.

145. Bollard CM, Gottschalk S, Leen AM, et al. Complete responses of relapsed lymphoma following genetic modification of tumor-antigen presenting cells and T-lymphocyte transfer. *Blood* 2007;110:2838-2845.

146. Cruz CRY, Leen AM, Gerdemann U, et al. Immune-based therapies targeting mage-A4 for relapsed/refractory Hodgkin's lymphoma after stem cell transplant. *ASH Ann Meeting Abstr* 2009;114:4089.

147. Bociek RG, Kuruvilla J, Pro B, et al. Isotype-selective histone deacetylase (HDAC) inhibitor MGCD0103 demonstrates clinical activity and safety in patients with relapsed/refractory classical Hodgkin Lymphoma (HL). *J Clin Oncol* 2008; 26:8507 (Meeting Abstracts).

148. Martell RE, Garcia–Manero G, Younes A, et al. Clinical development of MGCD0103, an isotype-selective HDAC inhibitor: Pericarditis/pericardial effusion in the context of overall safety and efficacy. *ASH Ann Meeting Abstr* 2009; 114:4756.

149. Younes A, Pro B, Fanale M, et al. Isotype-selective HDAC inhibitor MGCD0103 decreases serum TARC concentrations and produces clinical responses in heavily pretreated patients with relapsed classical Hodgkin lymphoma (HL). *ASH Ann Meeting Abstr* 2007;110:2566.

150. Buglio D, Mamidipudi V, Khaskhely NM, et al. The histone deacetylase inhibitor MGCD0103 down regulates CD30, activates NF-κB, and synergizes with proteasome inhibitors by HDAC6 independent mechanism in Hodgkin lymphoma. *ASH Ann Meeting Abstr* 2009;114:3735.

151. Khaskhely NM, Buglio D, Shafer J, et al. The histone deacetylase (HDAC) inhibitor entinostat (SNDX-275) targets Hodgkin lymphoma through a dual mechanism of immune modulation and apoptosis induction. *ASH Ann Meeting Abstr* 2009;114:1562.

152. DeAngelo D, Spencer A, Ottman O, et al. Panobinostat has activity in treatment-refractory Hodgkin lymphoma. In: *The proceedings of the 14th Congress of the European Hematology Association 505*; 2009. Berlin, Germany.

153. Kirschbaum MH, Goldman BH, Zain JM, et al. Vorinostat (suberoylanilide hydroxamic acid) in relapsed or refractory Hodgkin lymphoma: SWOG 0517. *ASH Ann Meeting Abstr* 2007;110:2574.

154. Younes A, Fanale M, McLaughlin P, et al. Phase-I study of the novel oral JAK-2 inhibitor SB1518 in patients with relapsed lymphoma: Evidence of clinical and biologic activity. *ASH Ann Meeting Abstr* 2009;114:588.

155. Moskowitz AJ, Hamlin PA, Jr., Gerecitano J, et al. Bendamustine is highly active in heavily pre-treated relapsed and refractory Hodgkin lymphoma and serves as a bridge to allogeneic stem cell transplant. *ASH Ann Meeting Abstr* 2009; 114:720.

156. Richardson PG, Barlogie B, Berenson J, et al. A phase 2 study of bortezomib in relapsed, refractory myeloma. *N Engl J Med* 2003;348:2609-2617.

157. Goy A, Bernstein S, Kahl B, et al. Bortezomib in patients with relapsed or refractory mantle cell lymphoma (MCL): Preliminary results of the PINNACLE study. *J Clin Oncol* 2005;23:6563 (Meeting Abstracts).

158. O'Connor OA, Wright J, Moskowitz C, et al. Phase II clinical experience with the novel proteasome inhibitor bortezomib in patients with indolent non-Hodgkin's lymphoma and mantle cell lymphoma. *J Clin Oncol* 2005;23:676-684.

159. Zheng B, Georgakis GV, Li Y, et al. Induction of cell cycle arrest and apoptosis by the proteasome inhibitor PS–341 in Hodgkin disease cell lines is independent of inhibitor of nuclear factor-κB mutations or activation of the CD30, CD40, and RANK receptors 10.1158/1078-0432.CCR-03-0494. *Clin Cancer Res* 2004;10:3207-3215.

160. Younes A, Pro B, Fayad L. Experience with bortezomib for the treatment of patients with relapsed classical Hodgkin lymphoma. *Blood* 2006;107:1731-1732.

161. Trelle S, Sezer O, Naumann R, et al. Bortezomib is not active in patients with relapsed Hodgkin's lymphoma: Results of a prematurely closed phase II study. *ASH Ann Meeting Abstr* 2006;108:2477.

162. Blum KA, Johnson JL, Niedzwiecki D, et al. A phase II study of bortezomib in relapsed Hodgkin lymphoma: Preliminary results of CALGB 50206. *J Clin Oncol* 2006;24:7576 (Meeting Abstracts).

163. Strauss SJ, Maharaj L, Hoare S, et al. Bortezomib therapy in patients with relapsed or refractory lymphoma: Potential correlation of in vitro sensitivity and tumor necrosis factor alpha response with clinical activity. *J Clin Oncol* 2006;24: 2105-2112.

164. Oki Y, Pro B, Fayad LE, et al. Phase 2 study of gemcitabine in combination with rituximab in patients with recurrent or refractory Hodgkin lymphoma. *Cancer* 2008;112:831-836.

165. Wedgwood AR, Fanale MA, Fayad LE, et al. Rituximab + ABVD improves event-free survival (EFS) in patients with classical Hodgkin lymphoma in all International Prognostic Score (IPS) groups and in patients who have PET positive disease after 2-3 cycles of therapy. *ASH Ann Meeting Abstr* 2007;110:215.

166. Copeland AR, Cao Y, Fanale M, et al. Final report of a phase-II study of rituximab plus ABVD for patients with newly diagnosed advanced stage classical Hodgkin lymphoma: Results of long follow up and comparison to institutional historical data. *ASH Ann Meeting Abstr* 2009;114:1680.

167. Younes A, Kirschbaum M, Sokol L, et al. Safety and tolerability of conatumumab in combination with bortezomib or vorinostat in patients with relapsed or refractory lymphoma. *ASH Ann Meeting Abstr* 2009;114:1708.

168. Johnston PB, Ansell SM, Colgan JP, et al. mTOR inhibition for relapsed or refractory Hodgkin Lymphoma: Promising single agent activity with everolimus (RAD001). *ASH Ann Meeting Abstr* 2007;110:2555.

169. Yazbeck VY, Buglio D, Georgakis GV, et al. Temsirolimus downregulates p21 without altering cyclin D1 expression and induces autophagy and synergizes with vorinostat in mantle cell lymphoma. *Exp Hematol* 2008;36:443-450.

170. Fanucchi MP, Fossella FV, Belt R, et al. Randomized phase II study of bortezomib alone and bortezomib in combination with docetaxel in previously treated advanced non-small-cell lung cancer. *J Clin Oncol* 2006;24:5025-5033.

171. Davies AM, Lara PN, Lau DH, et al. The proteasome inhibitor, bortezomib, in combination with gemcitabine (Gem) and carboplatin (Carbo) in advanced non-small cell lung cancer (NSCLC): Final results of a phase I California Cancer Consortium study. *ASCO Meeting Abstr* 2004;22:7106.

172. Fanale MA, Fayad LE, Pro B, et al. A phase I study of bortezomib in combination with ICE (BICE) in patients with relapsed/refractory classical Hodgkin lymphoma. *ASH Ann Meeting Abstr* 2008;112:3048.

173. Mendler JH, Kelly J, Voci S, et al. Bortezomib and gemcitabine in relapsed or refractory Hodgkin's lymphoma. *Ann Oncol* 2008;19:1759-1764.

174. Nogova L, Reineke T, Brillant C, et al. Lymphocyte-predominant and classical Hodgkin's lymphoma: A comprehensive analysis from the German Hodgkin Study Group. *J Clin Oncol* 2008;26:434-439.

175. Schlembach P, Wilder R, Jones D, et al. Radiotherapy alone for lymphocyte-predominant Hodgkin's disease. *Cancer J* 2002;8:377-383.

176. Wirth A, Yuen K, Barton M, et al. Long-term outcome after radiotherapy alone for lymphocyte-predominant Hodgkin lymphoma: A retrospective multicenter study of the Australasian Radiation Oncology Lymphoma Group. *Cancer* 2005;104:1221-1229.

177. Nogova L, Reineke T, Eich HT, et al. Extended field radiotherapy, combined modality treatment or involved field radiotherapy for patients with stage IA lymphocyte-predominant Hodgkin's lymphoma: A retrospective analysis from the German Hodgkin Study Group (GHSG) 10.1093/annonc/mdi323. *Ann Oncol* 2005;16:1683-1687.

178. Chen RC, Chin MS, Ng AK, et al. Early-stage, lymphocyte-predominant Hodgkin's lymphoma: Patient outcomes from a large, single-institution series with long follow-up. *J Clin Oncol* 2010;28:136-141.

179. Savage K, Hoskins P, Klasa R, et al. ABVD chemotherapy is essential for optimal treatment of limited stage nodular lymphocyte predominant Hodgkin lymphoma. *Haematologica* 2007;92(s5):27.

180. Unal A, Sari I, Deniz K, et al. Familial nodular lymphocyte predominant Hodgkin lymphoma: Successful treatment with CHOP plus rituximab. *Leuk Lymphoma* 2005;46:1613-1617.

181. Fanale MA, Fayad L, Romaguera J, et al. Experience with R-CHOP in patients with lymphocyte predominant Hogdkin lymphoma (LPHL). *Haematologica* 2007;92(s5):57.

182. Schulz H, Rehwald U, Morschhauser F, et al. Rituximab in relapsed lymphocyte-predominant Hodgkin lymphoma: Long-term results of a phase 2 trial by the German Hodgkin Lymphoma Study Group (GHSG). *Blood* 2008;111:109-111.

183. Horning SJ, Bartlett NL, Breslin S, et al. Results of a prospective phase II trial of limited and extended rituximab treatment in nodular lymphocyte predominant Hodgkin's disease (NLPHD). *ASH Ann Meeting Abstr* 2007;110:644.

184. Al-Mansour M, Connors JM, Gascoyne RD, et al. Transformation to aggressive lymphoma in nodular lymphocyte-predominant Hodgkin's lymphoma. *J Clin Oncol* 2010;28: 793-799.

185. Popat U, Hosing C, Fanale M, et al. Autologous transplantation for nodular lymphocyte-predominant Hodgkin lymphoma (NLPHL). *ASH Ann Meeting Abstr* 2009;114:2310.

186. Bredenfield H, Borchmann P, Engert A. PVAG-A new regimen in elderly patients with Hodgkin lymphoma. *Ann Oncol* 2008;19(s4):iv136.

187. Engert A, Ballova V, Haverkamp H, et al. Hodgkin's lymphoma in elderly patients: A comprehensive retrospective analysis from the German Hodgkin's Study Group. *J Clin Oncol* 2005;23:5052-5060.

188. Ballova V, Ruffer J-U, Haverkamp H, et al. A prospectively randomized trial carried out by the German Hodgkin Study Group (GHSG) for elderly patients with advanced Hodgkin's disease comparing BEACOPP baseline and COPP-ABVD (study HD9elderly). *Ann Oncol* 2005;16:124-131.

189. Yung L, Smith P, Hancock BW, et al. Long term outcome in adolescents with Hodgkin's lymphoma: Poor results using regimens designed for adults. *Leuk Lymphoma* 2004;45: 1579-1585.

190. Eichenauer DA, Bredenfeld H, Franklin J, et al. Hodgkin lymphoma in adolescents treated with adult protocols: An analysis from the German Hodgkin Study Group (GHSG). *ASH Ann Meeting Abstr* 2009;114:719.

191. Haas JF. Pregnancy in association with a newly diagnosed cancer: A population-based epidemiologic assessment. *Int J Cancer* 1984;34:229-235.

192. Lishner M, Zemlickis D, Degendorfer P, et al. Maternal and fetal outcome following Hodgkin's disease in pregnancy. *Br J Cancer* 1992;65:114-117.

193. Pelsang RE. Diagnostic imaging modalities during pregnancy. *Obstet Gynecol Clin North Am* 1998;25:287-300.

194. Barnicle MM. Chemotherapy and pregnancy. *Semin Oncol Nurs* 1992;8:124-132.

195. Gelb AB, van de Rijn M, Warnke RA, et al. Pregnancy-associated lymphomas. A clinicopathologic study. *Cancer* 1996;78:304-310.

196. Doll DC, Ringenberg QS, Yarbro JW. Antineoplastic agents and pregnancy. *Semin Oncol* 1989;16:337-346.

197. Ebert U, Loffler H, Kirch W. Cytotoxic therapy and pregnancy. *Pharmacol Ther* 1997;74:207-220.

198. Aviles A, Neri N. Hematological malignancies and pregnancy: A final report of 84 children who received chemotherapy in utero. *Clin Lymphoma* 2001;2:173-177.

199. Woo SY, Fuller LM, Cundiff JH, et al. Radiotherapy during pregnancy for clinical stages IA–IIA Hodgkin's disease. *Int J Radiat Oncol Biol Phys* 1992;23:407-412.

200. Jacobs C, Donaldson SS, Rosenberg SA, et al. Management of the pregnant patient with Hodgkin's disease. *Ann Intern Med* 1981;95:669-675.

201. Franceschi S, Dal Maso L, Arniani S, et al. Risk of cancer other than Kaposi's sarcoma and non-Hodgkin's lymphoma in persons with AIDS in Italy. Cancer and AIDS Registry Linkage Study. *Br J Cancer* 1998;78:966-970.

202. Tirelli U, Errante D, Dolcetti R, et al. Hodgkin's disease and human immunodeficiency virus infection: Clinicopathologic and virologic features of 114 patients from the Italian Cooperative Group on AIDS and Tumors. *J Clin Oncol* 1995;13: 1758-1767.

203. Tsimberidou AM, Sarris AH, Medeiros LJ, et al. Hodgkin's disease in patients infected with human immunodeficiency virus: Frequency, presentation and clinical outcome. *Leuk Lymphoma* 2001;41:535-544.

204. Levine AM, Li P, Cheung T, et al. Chemotherapy consisting of doxorubicin, bleomycin, vinblastine, and dacarbazine with granulocyte-colony-stimulating factor in HIV-infected patients with newly diagnosed Hodgkin's disease: A prospective, multi-institutional AIDS clinical trials group study (ACTG 149). *J Acquir Immune Defic Syndr* 2000;24:444-450.

205. Errante D, Gabarre J, Ridolfo AL, et al. Hodgkin's disease in 35 patients with HIV infection: An experience with epirubicin, bleomycin, vinblastine and prednisone chemotherapy in combination with antiretroviral therapy and primary use of G-CSF. *Ann Oncol* 1999;10:189-195.

206. Spina M, Gabarre J, Rossi G, et al. Stanford V regimen and concomitant HAART in 59 patients with Hodgkin disease and HIV infection. *Blood* 2002;100:1984-1988.

207. Hartmann P, Rehwald U, Salzberger B, et al. BEACOPP therapeutic regimen for patients with Hodgkin's disease and HIV infection. *Ann Oncol* 2003;14:1562-1569.

208. Sunil M, Mixon T, Reid E, et al. HIV related Hodgkin's lymphoma in the HAART Era: A comprehensive review and meta-analysis of response and survival rates. *ASH Ann Meeting Abstr* 2009;114:1652.

209. Xicoy B, Ribera JM, Miralles P, et al. Results of treatment with doxorubicin, bleomycin, vinblastine and dacarbazine and highly active antiretroviral therapy in advanced stage, human immunodeficiency virus-related Hodgkin's lymphoma. *Haematologica* 2007;92:191-198.

210. Ng AK, Bernardo MV, Weller E, et al. Second malignancy after Hodgkin disease treated with radiation therapy with or without chemotherapy: Long-term risks and risk factors. *Blood* 2002;100:1989-1996.

211. Kim HD, Bedetti CD, Boggs DR. The development of non-Hodgkin's lymphoma following therapy for Hodgkin's disease. *Cancer* 1980;46:2596-2602.

212. Zarate-Osorno A, Medeiros LJ, Longo DL, et al. Non-Hodgkin's lymphomas arising in patients successfully treated for Hodgkin's disease. A clinical, histologic, and immunophenotypic study of 14 cases. *Am J Surg Pathol* 1992;16:885-895.

213. Munker R, Grutzner S, Hiller E, et al. Second malignancies after Hodgkin's disease: The Munich experience. *Ann Hematol* 1999;78:544-554.

214. Glicksman AS, Pajak TF, Gottlieb A, et al. Second malignant neoplasms in patients successfully treated for Hodgkin's disease: A cancer and leukemia group B study. *Cancer Treat Rep* 1982;66:1035-1044.

215. Franklin J, Pluetschow A, Paus M, et al. Second malignancy risk associated with treatment of Hodgkin's lymphoma: Meta-analysis of the randomised trials. *Ann Oncol* 2006;17: 1749-1760.

216. Bookman MA, Longo DL. Concomitant illness in patients treated for Hodgkin's disease. *Cancer Treat Rev* 1986;13:77-111.

217. Halperin EC, Greenberg MS, Suit HD. Sarcoma of bone and soft tissue following treatment of Hodgkin's disease. *Cancer* 1984;53:232-236.

218. List AF, Doll DC, Greco FA. Lung cancer in Hodgkin's disease: Association with previous radiotherapy. *J Clin Oncol* 1985;3: 215-221.

219. Wallner KE, Leibel SA, Wara WM. Squamous cell carcinoma of the head and neck after radiation therapy for Hodgkin's disease. A report of two cases and a review of the literature. *Cancer* 1985;56:1052-1055.

220. Tucker MA, Misfeldt D, Coleman CN, et al. Cutaneous malignant melanoma after Hodgkin's disease. *Ann Intern Med* 1985;102:37-41.

221. Thar TL, Million RR. Complications of radiation treatment of Hodgkin's disease. *Semin Oncol* 1980;7:174-183.

222. Carey RW, Linggood RM, Wood W, et al. Breast cancer developing in four women cured of Hodgkin's disease. *Cancer* 1984;54:2234-2236.

223. Sieniawski M, Reineke T, Nogova L, et al. Fertility in male patients with advanced Hodgkin lymphoma treated with BEACOPP: A report of the German Hodgkin Study Group (GHSG). *Blood* 2008;111:71-76.

224. Hodgson DC, Pintilie M, Gitterman L, et al. Fertility among female Hodgkin lymphoma survivors attempting pregnancy following ABVD chemotherapy. *Hematol Oncol* 2007;25:11-15.

225. Kulkarni SS, Sastry PS, Saikia TK, et al. Gonadal function following ABVD therapy for Hodgkin's disease. *Am J Clin Oncol* 1997;20:354-357.

226. Beck-Fruchter R, Weiss A, Shalev E. GnRH agonist therapy as ovarian protectants in female patients undergoing chemotherapy: A review of the clinical data. *Hum Reprod Update* 2008;14: 553-561.

227. Roberts JE, Oktay K. Fertility preservation: A comprehensive approach to the young woman with cancer. *J Natl Cancer Inst Monogr*. 2005;(34):57-59.

228. Aleman BM, van den Belt-Dusebout AW, De Bruin ML, et al. Late cardiotoxicity after treatment for Hodgkin lymphoma. *Blood* 2007;109:1878-1886.

229. Carmel RJ, Kaplan HS. Mantle irradiation in Hodgkin's disease. An analysis of technique, tumor eradication, and complications. *Cancer* 1976;37:2813-2825.

230. Brosius FC, 3rd, Waller BF, Roberts WC. Radiation heart disease. Analysis of 16 young (aged 15 to 33 years) necropsy patients who received over 3,500 rads to the heart. *Am J Med* 1981;70:519-530.

231. Burns RJ, Bar-Shlomo BZ, Druck MN, et al. Detection of radiation cardiomyopathy by gated radionuclide angiography. *Am J Med* 1983;74:297-302.

232. Morton DL, Glancy DL, Joseph WL, et al. Management of patients with radiation-induced pericarditis with effusion: A note on the development of aortic regurgitation in two of them. *Chest* 1973;64:291-297.

233. McReynolds RA, Gold GL, Roberts WC. Coronary heart disease after mediastinal irradiation for Hodgkin's disease. *Am J Med* 1976;60:39-45.

234. Minow RA, Benjamin RS, Lee ET, et al. Adriamycin cardiomyopathy-risk factors. *Cancer* 1977;39:1397-1402.

235. Von Hoff DD, Layard MW, Basa P, et al. Risk factors for doxorubicin-induced congestive heart failure. *Ann Intern Med* 1979;91:710-717.

236. Billingham ME, Bristow MR, Glatstein E, et al. Adriamycin cardiotoxicity: Endomyocardial biopsy evidence of enhancement by irradiation. *Am J Surg Pathol* 1977;1:17-23.

237. Heidenreich PA, Schnittger I, Strauss HW, et al. Screening for coronary artery disease after mediastinal irradiation for Hodgkin's disease. *J Clin Oncol* 2007;25:43-49.

238. Hellman S, Mauch P, Goodman RL, et al. The place of radiation therapy in the treatment of Hodgkin's disease. *Cancer* 1978;42:971-978.

239. Castellino RA, Glatstein E, Turbow MM, et al. Latent radiation injury of lungs or heart activated by steroid withdrawal. *Ann Intern Med* 1974;80:593-599.

240. Martin WG, Ristow KM, Habermann TM, et al. Bleomycin pulmonary toxicity has a negative impact on the outcome of patients with Hodgkin's lymphoma. *J Clin Oncol* 2005;23: 7614-7620.

241. Boleti E, Mead GM. ABVD for Hodgkin's lymphoma: Full-dose chemotherapy without dose reductions or growth factors. *Ann Oncol* 2007;18:376-380.

242. Evens AM, Cilley J, Ortiz T, et al. G-CSF is not necessary to maintain over 99% dose-intensity with ABVD in the treatment of Hodgkin lymphoma: Low toxicity and excellent outcomes in a 10-year analysis. *Br J Haematol* 2007;137:545-552.

243. Weiss RB, Poster DS, Penta JS. The nitrosoureas and pulmonary toxicity. *Cancer Treat Rev* 1981;8:111-125.

244. Cersosimo RJ, Licciardello JT, Matthews SJ, et al. Acute pneumonitis associated with MOPP chemotherapy of Hodgkin's disease. *Drug Intell Clin Pharm* 1984;18:609-611.

245. Levi JA, Wiernik PH, Diggs CH. Combination chemotherapy of advanced previously treated Hodgkin's disease with streptozotocin, CCNU, adriamycin and bleomycin. *Med Pediatr Oncol* 1977;3:33-40.

246. Engel IA, Straus DJ, Lacher M, et al. Osteonecrosis in patients with malignant lymphoma: A review of twenty-five cases. *Cancer* 1981;48:1245-1250.

CHAPTER
11

MULTIPLE MYELOMA AND OTHER PLASMA CELL DYSCRASIAS

Tiffany P. Avery
Nina Shah
Weijun Fu
Donna M. Weber
Gary Lu
Pei Lin
Muzaffar H. Qazilbash
Michael Wang

Plasma cell dyscrasias are a group of diseases with malignant proliferation of a monoclonal population of plasma cells. These cells may or may not secrete detectable levels of the monoclonal immunoglobulin or paraprotein commonly referred to as M protein. Although the most common plasma cell dyscrasia is monoclonal gammopathy of undetermined significance (MGUS), closely related disorders include multiple myeloma, solitary plasmacytoma of bone, extramedullary plasmacytoma, Waldenström macroglobulinemia (WM), primary amyloidosis, and heavy-chain disease. The spectrum of MGUS, solitary plasmacytoma of bone, and asymptomatic and symptomatic multiple myeloma may actually represent a natural progression of the same disease. This chapter focuses on the etiology, diagnosis, clinical features, and current therapy for multiple myeloma and other plasma cell disorders.

Since the publication of the first edition in 2006, there has been much progress in our understanding of the biology of multiple myeloma (MM) and in its treatments. New diagnostic criteria have been developed, and an International Staging System has replaced the Durie-Salmon Staging System. The role of single and double autologous stem cell transplantation has been clarified by randomized trials. Most importantly, thalidomide, bortezomib, lenalidomide, and liposomal doxorubicin have emerged as new active agents and are rapidly being incorporated into the treatment of both newly-diagnosed and relapsed MM.

■ MULTIPLE MYELOMA

Multiple myeloma (MM) is a malignant proliferation of monoclonal plasma cells that produces a monoclonal immunoglobulin. The immunoglobulin secreted in the majority of cases is IgG (60%). Immunoglobulin A (IgA) is secreted in 20%, IgD in 2%, and IgE in <0.1%; biclonal secretion (<1%) is rare. Secretion of light chain only is noted in 18%, and <5% of patients do not secrete an M protein (nonsecretory MM) (1).

■ EPIDEMIOLOGY

The National Cancer Institute estimates that 20,580 people will be diagnosed with multiple myeloma in the United States in 2009, and there will be 10,580 deaths from the disease (2). The median age of diagnosis is 70 years. The incidence is highest in the age range of 75 to 84 years (27.6%), followed by the 65 to 74 year-old range (26.5%). The annual age-adjusted incidence of the disease per 100,000 populations is 6.6 among white men and 4.1 in white women. Among African Americans, the frequency doubles to 14.3 in men and 10.0 in women. Similarly, there is a difference in mortality by racial group. The annual age-adjusted mortality rate per 100,000 is 4.3 and 2.7 in white men and women, respectively. This rate increases to 8.2 and 5.8 in African-American men and women, respectively (3).

■ ETIOLOGY

No predisposing events appear to be important in the etiology of MM. Some events that have been suggested include radiation exposure (in radiologists and radium-dial workers); occupational exposure (in agricultural, chemical, metallurgical, rubber plant, pulp, paper workers, and leather tanners); and chemical exposure to benzene, formaldehyde, epichlorohydrin, hair dyes, paint spray, and asbestos; most of these associations have been countered by negative correlations (4).

Initially, it was reported that survivors of the atomic bombing of Hiroshima had a greater risk of developing myeloma, but longer follow-up data now refute any evidence of increased risk among survivors (5). Some reports suggest that a lower level of prolonged radiation exposure over many years may have caused some cases of MM among radiologists and radium watch-dial painters (6,7). However, no relationship has been shown between the incidence of MM and exposure to diagnostic x-rays or therapeutic irradiation (4,8).

Another factor previously thought to be associated with myeloma was intense, prolonged exposure to benzene, such as was experienced by unprotected workers in the rubber industry (9). Although the relationship of benzene and its metabolites to the occurrence of leukemia has been accepted, benzene's relationship with myeloma remains unproven (10).

Although myeloma is not an inherited disease, there have been numerous case reports and studies of MM occurring in the same family (4). Lynch et al. reported a family with five cases of myeloma, three cases of MGUS, and five cases of prostate cancer in two generations (11). A case-controlled study of over 37,000 first-degree relatives of multiple myeloma patients in Sweden found that these relatives had a twofold increase in the risk of developing myeloma compared to controls (12). Similarly, an increased risk of myeloma was also found in first-degree relatives of 218 myeloma cases in a family registry study conducted in Iceland (13). Although these studies are suggestive, no clear genetic alteration has been demonstrated among patients with myeloma, and the role of genetics in the development of myeloma is evolving (14).

■ BIOGENETICS

Multiple myeloma may be the result of mutations in terminally differentiated B cells or even from early but committed B cells, such as germinal center B cells, that manifest clinically as more differentiated plasma cells (15-18). The expression of multiple markers of different cell lineages (B and T) by plasma cells supports the possibility of either an aberrant expression of unexpected phenotypes, as in other malignancies, or a stem cell precursor from which all hematopoietic cells arise (15-18). A listing of various types and subtypes of plasma cell disorders is presented in Table 11-1.

In light of the fact that plasma cell dyscrasia is the prototype for monoclonal malignancies of plasma cells, characterized by the proliferation of malignant immunoglobulin-producing plasma B-cells in the bone marrow (19,20), the marked genetic heterogeneity in plasma cells plays important roles in tumorigenesis and disease development.

Different genomic abnormalities have been found involved in different pathways in the development of

TABLE 11-1	PLASMA CELL DISORDERS: SUBTYPES AND VARIANTS

Monoclonal gammopathy of undetermined significance (MGUS)

Plasma cell myeloma variants
    Asymptomatic myeloma
    Symptomatic myeloma
    Plasma cell leukemia

Plasmacytoma variants
    Solitary plasmacytoma of bone
    Extramedullary plasmacytoma
    Light or heavy chain deposition diseases
    Waldenström's macroglobulinemia

POEMS syndrome

Amyloidosis

POEMS, polyneuropathy, organomegaly, endocrinopathy, M component, skin changes.
Reproduced, with permission, from Hoffbrand AV, Moss PAH, Pettit JE. Essential Haematology. 5th ed. Wiley-Blackwell, 2006: p. 368.

plasma cell dyscrasia. So far four genomic pathways have been proposed (21-31). These include (1) pathway characterized by chromosomal aneuploidy, (2) pathway involving immunoglobin heavy-chain (IGH) mapped to chromosome 14q32 region, (3) pathway with −13/del(13q), and (4) pathway of rearrangements in chromosome 1 (Fig. 11-1). Genetic interaction or correlation occurs amongst the four genomic pathways in the myeloma development. Mutations in oncogenes, usually present in the advanced stages, play important roles in disease progression. The most commonly known oncogenes include *RAS, p18INK4c, TP53,* and *c-MYC*. The *MYC* rearrangement is most commonly observed in plasma cell leukemia, an aggressive malignancy of multiple myeloma (32-38).

Almost all the multiple myeloma tumors and most cases of monoclonal gammopathy of undetermined significance (MGUS), a premyeloma entity, are aneuploid and can be revealed by flow cytometry with DNA content measurements and FISH analysis (39-41). Aneuploid can either indicate a hyperdiploid or non-hyperdiploid state, with the former being the most common. Numerical chromosome gains represent the majority of hyperdiploid, characterized by trisomies for chromosomes 3, 5, 7, 9, 11, 15, 19, and 21 that can be frequently observed in MGUS(42,43). Myeloma develops from MGUS with increase in the frequency of chromosome gains, which represents about 10% of the cases, indicating the important role of the chromosome gains in tumor development (23). However, the specific genomic mechanism for the chromosome gains is undefined. Hypodiploid represents non-hyperdiploid, and it is usually observed in the course of disease progression, and more common

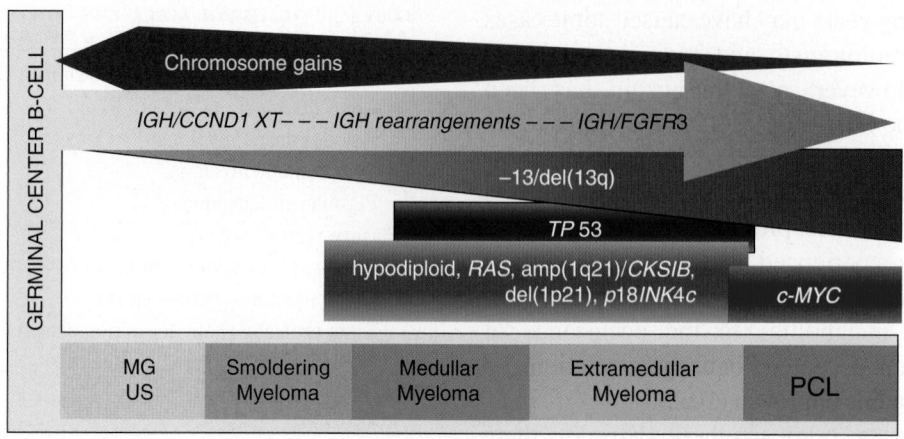

FIGURE 11-1. Genomic pathways in the development of multiple myeloma. *IGH* rearrangements include t(11;14)(q13;q32)/*IGH/CCND1 XT*, t(6;14)(p21;q32)/*IGH/CCND3*, t(14;20)(q32;q11.2)/*IGH/MAFB*, (14;16)(q32;q23)/*IGH/MAF*, t(4;14) (p16;q32)/*IGH/FGFR3*, and others. Chromosome gains mainly include trisomies for chromosomes 3, 5, 7, 9, 11, 15, 19, and 21. Hypodiploid mainly includes monosomies for chromosomes 13, 14, 16, and 22. *RAS* includes both *K-RAS* and *N-RAS*. MGUS, monoclonal gammopathy of undetermined significance; PCL, plasma cell leukemia.

in cases that show *IGH* rearrangements (22,44-46). This indicates the interaction between the aneuploidy and IgH rearrangement in the development of multiple myeloma.

Rearrangements involving *IGH* locus are the most important and common abnormalities in myeloma development (22,44). A combined prevalence of the *IGH* rearrangements in multiple myeloma can be up to 70%. The most common partners of the 14q32/*IGH* translocation are chromosomes 11, 4, 16, 6, and 20, with an incidence of approximately 15-20%, 20-25%, 2-10%, 3-5%, and 2%, respectively. The *IGH* translocations are all believed to be primarily genetic events occurring during the course of myeloma development (22,44) in that several regulators in the cell cycle are involved.

Translocation t(11;14)(q13;q32), resulting in *IGH/ CCND1 XT* fusion gene, is one of the most common translocations involving the *IGH* locus. The fusion gene typically results in deregulation of cyclin D1, which is an important cell cycle regulator. It is typically seen in cases with lymphoplasmablastic morphology of plasma cells, CD20 expression, and in oligo-secretory or light-chain-only myeloma. Translocation t(4;14) (p16.3;q32) leads to upregulation of oncogenes *MMSET* and *FGFR3* on chromosome 4p. The oncogene *FGFR3* is a growth factor receptor tyrosine kinase, whereas *MMSET* is a regulator of transcription. Translocation t(14;16) (q32;q23) results in the upregulation of *c-MAF*, also a transcription factor, and subsequently affects cyclin D2 functioning in the cell cycle. Another *IGH* rearrangement

that deregulates a cell cycle factor is t(6;14)(p21;q32) that involves cyclin D3 mapped to 6p21 (47). So far *IGH* rearrangements directly or indirectly deregulate three major cell cycle regulators, cyclin D1, D2, and D3. Deregulation of the three cell cycle regulators directly affects the proliferation of plasma cells or even of earlier B cells in the germinal center. Translocation of t(14;16)(q32;q23) and t(14;20)(q32;q11.2) are the other abnormalities involving *c-MAF* and *MAFB*, respectively (22,44,48-50). Oncogene *C-MAF* is a leucine zipper-containing transcription factor whereas *MAFB* is a regulator of hindbrain segmentation and interacts with the ICD through a leucine zipper domain (51,52). However, the role of *c-MAF* and *MAFB* in myeloma development is unclear. Similar to other tumors, their deficiency or their interaction with other pathogenetic factors may be present (53).

IgH translocation involving chromosomes 8q24/*c-MYC* is considered as secondary change, and has been revealed at a much lower incidence. The *c-MYC* oncogene rearrangement is often found in advanced tumors or myeloma cell lines and is associated with unfavorable prognosis.

Monosomy 13 and interstitial 13q deletion can be observed in about 70% of myeloma cases (23,54,55). As a primary change, the −13/del(13q) frequency rises along with an increase in chromosome gains in MGUS and myeloma, or in the course of disease progression from MGUS to myeloma. Evidence shows that the frequency of −13/del(13q) increases with the plasma cell count in the development of myeloma. This indicates that a chromosome 13 abnormality may be a prerequisite for clonal expansion of myeloma. However, the −13/del(13q) abnormality frequently interacts with other genomic changes, in particular IGH rearrangements with the t(11;14)(q13;q32) most commonly involved. Loss of heterozygosity has been proposed as the mechanism of the −13/del(13q) in tumor development. Tumor suppression gene *RB1* is mapped to 13q14 region. Loss of the *RB1* gene often leads to dysregulation of the cell cycle, affecting plasma cell proliferation. With a new technique using Array CGH, numerous loci that are deleted along the long arm of chromosome 13 have been identified (56), indicating that additional pathogenic genes are involved, directly or indirectly, in the deletion genomic pathway.

Genomic rearrangements in chromosome 1 are common in myeloma. Recently a 17-gene model has been proposed and most of them are mapped to chromosome 1 (31). Del(1p21) and amp(1q21) in chromosome 1 are the two most common changes involving *CDC14C* and *CKS1B*, respectively(29-31). Both the del(1p21) and amp(1q21) are frequently detected in disease progression. The del(1p21) is found rarely in MGUS patients, but has the highest incidence, at about 30%, in PCL. Amplification in the chromosome 1q21 region increases during the course of disease development from MGUS to myeloma (57). The molecular mechanism for the role of del(1p21) and amp(1q21) is currently under further study.

In addition to *c-MYC*, mutated with *IgH* rearrangement, other genomic markers involving myeloma progression include del(17p13), with an incidence of 10% in myeloma (57), and *RAS* and *p18INK4c* as well (34-36,58).

Deletion of 17p13 involving oncogene *TP53* is a secondary independent risk genomic marker in myeloma and can be observed in 40% of advanced myeloma cases including plasma cell leukemia (38,59). It is well known that inactivation of *TP53* directly alters cell cycle, which plays an important role in myeloma progression. As an inhibitor against cyclin-dependent kinases (CDK) in the cell cycle, *p18INK4c* has been shown to be required for cell-cycle termination and final differentiation of nonsecreting plasmacytoid cells to antibody-secreting plasma cells. Deletion of *p18INK4c* can be observed in myeloma (34,35). Finally, mutations in *RAS* mostly involving the *N-RAS* can be detected in 20% of patients. The mutations usually do not correlate with the presence of chromosome 13q deletion, trisomy of chromosome 11, 1q amplification, or hyperdiploidy. This indicates an independent entity of the *RAS* gene in myeloma development. *RAS* can be activated by genomic instability (36,37).

In addition to the roles in tumorigenesis or development of myeloma, genomic abnormalities demonstrate prognostic significance. The t(11;14) is the only abnormality involving IGH locus clearly associated with a good prognosis. Patients harboring the t(4;14) usually have the IgA isotype, aggressive clinical features, and poor prognosis even after high-dose therapy, (60,61) whereas patients with the translocation t(6;14) often respond well to intensive therapy (62). Myeloma patients with 17p/*P53* deletion have a significantly poorer prognosis (63,64). The prognosis associated with t(14;16) is considered poor with short survival, even when treated with high-dose melphalan (65,66). All the genomic markers involving disease progression, including del(17p)/*TP53*, del(1p21), amp(1q21), *c-MYC*, *p18INK4c,* and *RAS* are considered unfavorable in prognosis.

In conclusion, three genomic pathways are involved in the development of plasma cell dyscrasia. Several factors in cell cycle, mainly including cyclin D1, D2, and D3, *RB1, TP53*, and *p18INK4c* are mutated due to the genomic abnormalities in the pathways. Dysregulation of the cell cycle results in aberrant proliferation and differentiation of plasma cells, leading to the development of the tumors. Genomic abnormalities that play roles in disease progression are heterogeneitic.

■ CLINICAL FEATURES

The clinical presentation of MM is quite variable. Bone pain, especially from compression fractures of vertebrae or ribs, is the most common symptom. Findings that suggest a diagnosis of MM include lytic bone lesions, anemia, azotemia, hypercalcemia, and recurrent infections. However, approximately 20% of patients with MM are free of symptoms.

BONE DISEASE

Bone lesions are due to accelerated osteoclast activity with increased resorption of areas infiltrated by plasma cells (lytic bone lesions) (Fig. 11-2). Interactions between myeloma cells and bone marrow stromal cells stimulate stromal cells to produce cytokines, including IL-6, IL-11, and IL-1β. The myeloma cells produce cytokines, including macrophage inflammatory protein 1α (MIP1α), hepatocyte growth factor, and osteopontin. These cytokines activate osteoclasts and lead to increased bone resorption (67).

In addition to direct stimulation by cytokines, osteoclast activation is also regulated by the balance between the receptor activator of NFkB ligand (RANKL) and

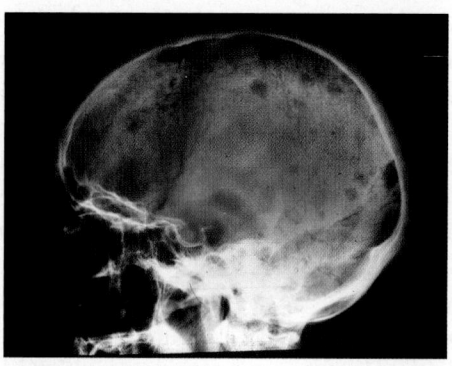

FIGURE 11-2. Radiographic image of the skull showing "punched out" osteolytic lesions characteristic of multiple myeloma.

osteoprotegerin (OPG) (68). The osteoblast–stromal cell complex produces RANKL, which binds to RANK on osteoclasts and activates them. Normally, this is balanced by marrow stromal cell production of OPG, an inhibitor of RANKL, allowing for normal bone remodeling. Myeloma cells induce RANKL overexpression and inhibit OPG production, resulting in uncontrolled activation of osteoclasts (68). Myeloma cells also inhibit osteoblast activity by production of DKK-1 and sFRP-2, which further contributes to bone loss (67). Although studies are underway to determine the clinical role of the manipulation of RANKL and OPG, currently bisphosphonates remain the standard of care for myeloma bone disease.

Bisphosphonates (pamidronate, zoledronic acid) have been shown to reduce the amount of skeletal-related events in myeloma when compared with placebo (69,70). A total of 392 patients with Durie-Salmon stage II myeloma were randomized to receive pamidronate 90 mg intravenously each month or placebo. Patients were assigned to stratum 1 if they were receiving first-line chemotherapy or stratum 2 if receiving second-line chemotherapy (69). Skeletal-related events at 9 months were significantly less in the pamidronate group (24%) as compared with the placebo group (41%; $p = .001$) (69). Zoledronic acid is a bisphosphonate that is approximately 100 to 1000 times more potent and can be administered more rapidly than pamidronate. In a phase II study of zoledronic acid, 109 patients with myeloma (with more than one osteolytic lesion and at least one prior skeletal event or failure after initial therapy) were randomized to receive monthly pamidronate (90 mg) or 0.4, 2, or 4 mg of zoledronic acid for nine cycles. The number of skeletal events for both the groups receiving 2 or 4 mg of zoledronic acid was comparable with that of those receiving pamidronate (70). An increased

incidence of renal failure and osteonecrosis of the jaw has been reported in patients receiving zoledronic acid and studies are necessary to clarify toxicity and dosing schedules (71,72). Bisphosphonate therapy with either pamidronate or zoledronic acid for 2 years in patients with lytic bone lesions or spinal compression fractures from osteopenia is the current recommendation for treatment of bone disease in myeloma (73). If, after 2 years, disease response or stability has been attained, bisphosphonate therapy should end, due to the increased risk of adverse events with continued treatment. In patients who have active or progressive disease, therapy should continue; however, there is no consensus regarding the duration of treatment (67).

A full skeletal survey remains the standard of care for evaluation of bone disease. At diagnosis, nearly 70% of patients with myeloma have lytic bone lesions with or without pathologic fracture. Patients who are asymptomatic, but have radiologic bone disease of at least one lytic lesion, are at high risk for progression of myeloma (74). One drawback of using x-rays to detect lytic bone lesions is that lytic lesions may only become evident when 30% of trabecular bone loss has already occurred (75). Another disadvantage of the skeletal survey is that patients' ability to tolerate the extensive examination, which requires approximately 20 views, may be diminished by pain (74). CT imaging is an alternative for those patients who cannot undergo full skeletal surveys due to pain. It is also useful for radiation therapy planning, surgical planning, and to identify lesions in patients that are symptomatic, but have negative skeletal surveys (74). Magnetic resonance imaging (MRI) provides greater detail of bone disease, paraspinal involvement, and epidural components; abnormalities are noted on MRI scans even when x-rays are normal, and they appear to be predictive of early disease progression in asymptomatic patients (76). MRI is also indicated in evaluating patients with solitary plasmacytoma of bone, urgent evaluation of suspected cord compression, and in patients with disease progression and bone pain with negative skeletal survey (74). Nuclear bone imaging is less sensitive, because bone scan isotopes are not taken up by lytic lesions. This modality is generally not used in the evaluation of bone disease.

Painful vertebral compression fractures, with or without cord pressure, may require radiation therapy, but this should be used judiciously because of its effects on stem cell collection. Decompressive laminectomy is rarely necessary for cord compression, but surgery may be required for radioresistant myeloma, retropulsed bone fragments, or intervertebral disk disease when severe pain and/or disability result. Fractures of the femora or humeri require intramedullary rod fixation. For disabling pain, secondary to vertebral compression fractures, vertebroplasty or kyphoplasty (in which the vertebral body height is restored through an inflatable bone tamp), followed by instillation of a highly viscous bone cement, may be useful in appropriate cases (77). Frequently, this will relieve pain related to nerve root pressure or vertebral instability. Occasionally, surgical procedures to stabilize the spine may be necessary.

HYPERCALCEMIA

Hypercalcemia (defined as a corrected serum calcium level >11.5 mg/dL) occurs in approximately 20% of patients with newly diagnosed MM and results from progressive bone destruction. Treatment includes generous hydration and prompt combination chemotherapy, which should always include a glucocorticoid that produces a rapid response. Bisphosphonate therapy is used in addition to hydration and chemotherapy, and if further therapy is needed, treatment with calcitonin should be considered (67).

High-dose pulse dexamethasone alone remains an alternative for patients who require palliative radiotherapy for the spine. If possible, radiation should be avoided in patients who are candidates for stem cell transplant. This is especially true when radiation fields involve the pelvis femurs. Maximum physical activity should be encouraged, because prolonged immobility exacerbates hypercalcemia.

RENAL FAILURE

Approximately 20% of patients with myeloma present with renal insufficiency, and another 20% will develop this complication during the course of their disease (78). Casts of Bence Jones protein in the distal tubule are the most common cause of renal failure (79,80), but hypercalcemia, dehydration, and hyperuricemia are also contributing factors (78). Uncommonly, amyloidosis or light-chain deposition disease may also contribute to renal failure.

Treatment includes hydration, sodium bicarbonate for acidosis, allopurinol for hyperuricemia, and hemodialysis if necessary. Plasmapheresis has been proposed by some researchers, but controlled studies have not shown that it yields any improvement in survival. In approximately 50% of previously untreated patients with renal failure, kidney function normalizes with chemotherapy for the myeloma (80). Vincristine,

doxorubicin, dexamethasone (VAD) therapy for myeloma does not require dose adjustments for renal failure, since none of the drugs are metabolized by the kidneys. Bortezomib is also safe and efficacious for use in patients with renal failure (81,82). Ludwig et al. reported reversibility of renal failure with bortezomib therapy in five patients (83). Bortezomib and dexamethasone with or without dose adjustments is an effective therapy in this scenario.

ANEMIA

A normocytic, normochromic anemia is present in up to 60% of patients at diagnosis. Anemia is due to a variety of factors, including decreased erythropoietin levels, decreased responsiveness of red cells to erythropoietin, impaired iron utilization, direct apoptotic effects of erythroid precursors, and a shortened lifespan of red cells (67). The serum M protein at high concentrations can lead to rouleaux formation of the red blood cells.

Patients with myeloma, with or without renal failure, could also have decreased levels of erythropoietin, which may worsen the degree of anemia (84). Use of erythropoiesis-stimulating agents (ESAs) is the treatment of choice for anemia. Smith et al. found that cancer patients not undergoing active treatment who received ESAs had a poorer rate of survival (85). Therefore, ESAs should be used only in patients who are undergoing active treatment for myeloma (67). Use of parenteral iron can also be considered for patients who are iron deficient while being treated with ESAs.

INFECTION

Many patients with myeloma develop bacterial infections that may be quite serious. In the past, gram-positive organisms (eg, *Streptococcus pneumoniae* and *Staphylococcus aureus*) and *Haemophilus influenzae* have been the most common pathogens, although more recently gram-negative organisms have become an increasing problem (86). The increased susceptibility of patients with myeloma to bacterial infection has been attributed to impairment of host-defense mechanisms, which includes depressed levels of uninvolved immunoglobulins, impaired antibody response (87), decreased numbers and adherence of polymorphonuclear leukocytes (88), decreased surface immunoglobulin expression (89,90), poor opsonic activity (90), depressed lysozyme levels (91), and decreased complement levels (92). Use of high-dose immunoglobulins in the management of infection could be considered on a case by case basis. Myeloma patients should receive pneumo-coccal vaccination, and antibiotic prophylaxis can be considered during the first 2 months of therapy in high-risk patients (67,93).

ACQUIRED FACTOR DEFICIENCIES

Rarely the M protein will function as an inhibitor to a coagulation protein, leading to a bleeding diathesis. The most common is an inhibitor to factor VIII.

■ DIAGNOSIS

A diagnosis of MM (Table 11-2) (94) requires at least 15% clonal plasmacytosis on bone marrow examination or biopsy-proven clonal plasmacytoma, M protein in serum or urine (except in nonsecretory myeloma), and evidence of end-organ damage attributable to myeloma involvement (hypercalcemia, renal insufficiency, ane-mia, or bone disease, known as CRAB) (Figs. 11-3 to 11-4). Smoldering myeloma is diagnosed when mon-oclonal protein (IgG or IgA) of at least 3g/dL is detected

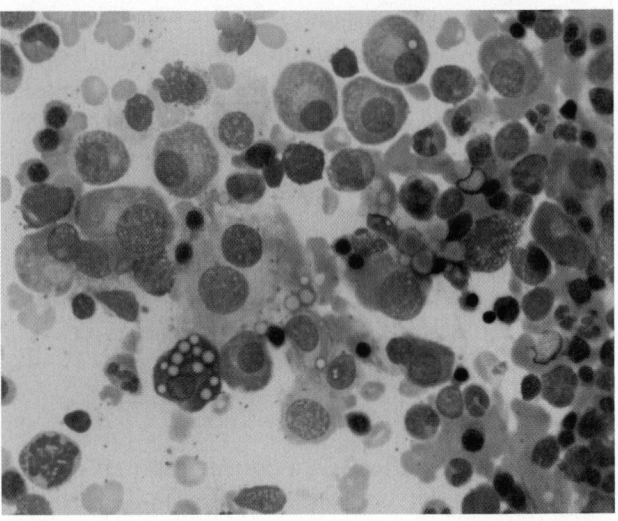

FIGURE 11-3. Multiple myeloma of low-grade cytology. Some plasma cells have cytoplasmic immunoglobulin inclusions. (Wight-Giemsa, × 500).

in the serum, and/or there is at least 10% clonal plas-macytosis on bone marrow, and absence of end-organ damage.

In myeloma, one class of immunoglobulins is pro-duced in excess, and the other immunoglobulin (Ig) classes are depressed. Biclonal elevations of myeloma protein levels occur in less than 1% of cases. The types of monoclonal protein produced are IgG (60%), IgA (20%), IgD (2%), IgE (<0.1%), and light-chain kappa or lambda only (18%) (1). Patients lacking heavy-chain expression are classified as having light-chain disease. In these patients, M protein may not be detected in serum, but is detectable in urine. Therefore, serum and

TABLE 11-2	COMMON LABORATORY FEATURES OF PLASMA CELL DYSCRASIAS

Multiple myeloma
   Marrow plasmacytosis >15%
   Monoclonal immunoglobulin peak (usually >3.0 g/dL)
   Decreased levels of uninvolved immunoglobulins
   Bence Jones protein
   Lytic bone lesions
Asymptomatic myeloma
   Same as multiple myeloma but without symptoms
   Hemoglobin >10.5 g/dL
   Normal serum calcium level
   Monoclonal immunoglobulin peak (<4.5 g/dL)
   No lytic bone lesions
Solitary plasmacytoma of bone
   Solitary bone lesion due to plasma cell tumor
   Negative skeletal survey and spinal MRI
   Negative bone marrow
   No anemia, hypercalcemia, or renal disease
   Preserved levels of uninvolved immunoglobulins
Monoclonal gammopathy of unknown significance (MGUS)
   Monoclonal immunoglobulin level of <3.0 g/dL
   Bone marrow plasma cells ≤10%
   No bone lesions
   Asymptomatic
   Usually preserved levels of uninvolved immunoglobulins
Amyloidosis without myeloma
   Same as MGUS + evidence of amyloidosis on biopsy

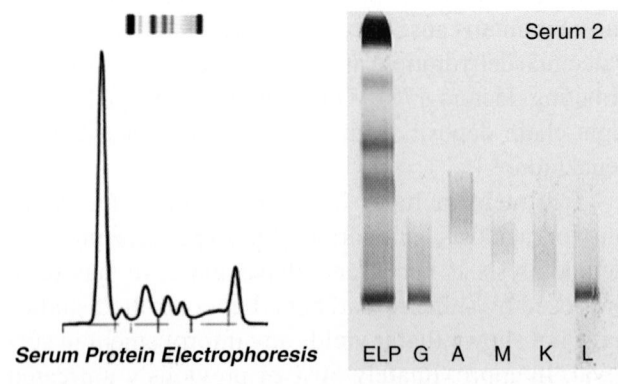

Serum Protein Electrophoresis   ELP G A M K L

FIGURE 11-4. Serum protein electrophoresis demonstrates an M-protein peak (left). Immunofixation electrophoresis confirms it to be monoclonal IgG lambda type.

urine protein electrophoresis and immunofixation (IFE) must be performed in all patients suspected of having multiple myeloma (95). Fewer than 5% of patients with myeloma are unable to secrete or synthesize light- or heavy-chain immunoglobulins, a condition categorized as nonsecretory myeloma. The serum free light-chain assay, which measures the levels of unbound κ and λ light chains, aids in diagnosis and monitoring of these cases (95).

Katzmann et al. examined whether serum free light-chain assay could replace urine immunofixation in the diagnosis of plasma cell disorders. In a study of 428 patients with positive urine IFEs, serum protein electrophoreses with IFE, and free light-chain assays, they reported that serum electrophoresis with IFE alone would have missed diagnoses of myeloma, amyloidosis, plasmacytoma, smoldering myeloma, and MGUS in 28 patients. In contrast, free light-chain assays would have missed diagnoses in 14% of patients. In patients with positive urine immunofixation, serum immunofixation in combination with free light-chain assay identified 99.5% of patients (96). The free light-chain assay is indicated in screening for plasma cell disorders, in combination with serum protein electrophoresis and immunofixation, and in monitoring of patients with nonsecretory myeloma or light-chain disease. It is also required to document a stringent complete response by International Response Criteria for monitoring myeloma patients (97).

After chemotherapy has been instituted, serum and 24-h urine measurements of abnormal proteins should be evaluated serially to confirm that the myeloma protein or proteins have been markedly reduced and that the patients have responded to treatment.

THE MD ANDERSON APPROACH FOR DIAGNOSIS AND STAGING WORKUP (FIG. 11-5)

In addition to the history and physical, the initial workup of a patient with myeloma at MD Anderson includes a CBC, complete metabolic and hepatic panel, LDH beta-2 microglobulin, electrophoresis with immunofixation of both serum and 24-hour urine, quantitiative immunoglobulins, serum free light-chain assay, skeletal survey and unlilateral bone marrow aspirate biopsy. The bone marrow aspirate should be sent for flow cytometry, cytogenetics, and FISH for t(4:14), t(14:16), t(11:14), del13, del 17p, and 1p gains. We order additional tests as necessary, including MRI of relevant structures (particularly if there is question of spinal cord compression), biopsy of any suspected plasmacytoma, serum viscosity, and bone densitometry prior to initiation of

INITIAL DIAGNOSTIC WORKUP

History and physical
- CBC, differential, platelets
- BUN, creatinine, electrolytes
- LDH
- Calcium/albumin
- Beta-2-microglobulin
- Quantitative immunoglubulins
- 24-h urine total protein
- Serum free light chain assay
- Skeletal survey
- Unilateral bone marrow aspirate and biopsy
- Bone marrow flow cytometry

Cytogenetics
- FISH (t(4:14), t(14:16), t(11:14), Del13, Del 17p; 1 gains)

If indicated:
- MRI (avoid Gadolinium if creatinine greater than 2)
- CT scan (avoid intravenous contrast, particularly with elevated creatinine)
- PET/CT scan
- Tissue biopsy to diagnose extraossecous plasmacytoma
- Bone densitometry
- Staining of marrow and fat pad for amyloid (Congo Red with or without EM)
- Serum viscosity
- HLA typing

FIGURE 11-5. The MD Anderson approach for diagnosis and staging workup of multiple myeloma. (*Adapted with permission from The University of Texas MD Anderson Cancer Center.*)

bisphosphonate therapy. If there are symptoms concerning amyloidosis, we usually arrange for a fine-needle aspiration of abdominal wall fat pad aspirate for Congo red stain.

- CBC with differential and platelets, chemistry
- Unilateral bone marrow aspiration and biopsy
- Complete bone survey with long bones
- MRI of cervical, thoracic, and lumbar spine if needed

■ STAGING AND PROGNOSIS

In staging myeloma, the lack of standard definitions and consistency among investigators has resulted in different criteria being used at different institutions (Tables 11-3 and 11-4) (1,15,16).

The level of serum beta microglobulin (β_2M) is an important and convenient prognostic indicator because it reflects the extent of disease in a single measurement. This protein is a catabolic product of the histocompatibility leukocyte antigen present on the surface of all nucleated cells and found in higher concentrations on lymphoid and plasma cells (17). In a study of three staging systems and other variables by Bataille et al., β_2M

TABLE 11-3	DURIE-SALMON STAGING SYSTEM FOR MULTIPLE MYELOMA	
Stage	**Criteria**	**Myeloma Cell Mass** $(\times 10^{12}/m^2)$
I	Hemoglobin >10 g/dL	<0.6 (low)
	Serum calcium ≤12 mg/dL (normal)	
	Normal bone or solitary plasmacytoma on X-ray	
	Low production rates of M component:	
	IgG <5 g/dL	
	IgA <3 g/dL	
	Urine light chain	
	M component <4 g/24 h	
II	Not fitting stage I or III	0.6-1.20 (intermediate)
III	Hemoglobin <8.5 g/dL	>1.20 (high)
	Serum calcium >12 mg/dL	
	Multiple lytic bone lesions on X-ray	
	High production rates of M component:	
	IgG <7 g/dL	
	IgA <5 g/dL	
	Urine light chain	
	M component <12 g/24 h	
Subclassification	**Criterion**	
A	Normal renal function (serum creatinine level <2.0 mg/dL)	
B	Abnormal renal function (serum creatinine level ≥2.0 mg/dL)	

Reproduced, with permission, from Durie BG, Salmon SE. A clinical staging system for multiple myeloma. Correlation of measured myeloma cell mass with presenting clinical features, response to treatment, and survival. Cancer. 1975;36:842-854.

was the single most important indicator of prognosis (18,98). An International Staging System (ISS) was proposed by the International Myeloma Working Group (IMWG), it separates patients into three stages based on β_2M and albumin (Table 11-4) (99). Because β_2M is excreted by the kidneys, high levels of it are present when renal failure occurs, which complicates the interpretation of a high value.

High levels of lactate dehydrogenase (LDH) in serum have also been associated with shortened survival (9 months), as well as with drug resistance, in both treated and untreated patients with myeloma

(18,100). Other features associated with an elevated LDH level include lymphoma-like extra osseous disease, plasma cell leukemia, and plasma cell hypodiploidy (100,101).

Shortened survival also has been noted in patients with DNA hypodiploidy (102), low plasma cell RNA levels (103), high plasma cell labeling indices (104,105), and plasmablastic histology (106). Cytogenetic prognostic factors include poor prognosis in patients with deletion of chromosome 13, translocations of (4:14) or (14;16), and deletion 17p identified by FISH.

■ RESPONSE CRITERIA

Because the criteria of response to treatment have varied among institutions, response rates have been difficult to compare. Blade et al. proposed response criteria of a 50% reduction in serum M protein and a 90% reduction in Bence Jones protein for partial remission (PR); in addition, they defined criteria for minimal response (MR) and stable disease (SD) (107,108). To achieve a complete remission (CR) of disease (by either Blade), there must be disappearance of the M protein

TABLE 11-4	INTERNATIONAL STAGING SYSTEM FOR MULTIPLE MYELOMA
Stage 1	β_2M <3.5 mg/L
	Albumin ≥3.5 g/dL
Stage 2	β_2M 3.5-5.5 mg/L
	or
	β_2M <3.5 mg/L and
	Albumin <3.5 g/dL
Stage 3	β_2M >5.5 mg/L

β_2M, beta-2 microglobulin.

and/or Bence Jones protein by immunofixation and no monoclonal plasma cells in the bone marrow as assessed by the most sensitive techniques.

The International Myeloma Working Group has proposed guidelines for uniform response criteria to standardize response criteria and facilitate comparison of results between centers. The criteria include four response categories, including stringent complete response (which requires CR plus a normalized free light-chain ratio and absence of clonal cells in bone marrow by immunohistochemistry or immunofluorescence), complete response (negative serum and urine immunofixation, less than 5% plasmacytosis in marrow, and disappearance of plasmacytomas), very good partial response (detectable M-protein on immunofixation, but not on electrophoresis, or 90% reduction in M protein with urine M-protein less than 100 mg/day), partial response, stable disease, and

relapse criteria (108). At MD Anderson we use the IMWG guidelines.

■ TREATMENT OF NEWLY DIAGNOSED MYELOMA (FIG. 11-6)

Concurrent with the management of specific complications, chemotherapy should be instituted promptly in symptomatic myeloma to reduce the number of malignant plasma cells. Induction chemotherapy followed by autologous stem cell transplantation is the standard of care for treatment of newly diagnosed myeloma in eligible patients. Because some chemotherapeutic agents affect outcomes in autologous stem cell transplantation, the regimen chosen for initial treatment of newly diagnosed multiple myeloma depends upon whether or not the patient is a candidate for stem cell transplantation.

Note: If available, clinical trials should be considered as preferred treatment options for eligible patients.

A

*Note on Induction: High-risk translocation t(4:14), t(14:16), Del 17p, Del 13, chromosome 1 gains, consider induction therapy with novel agents and/or autologous followed by mini-allogeneic stem cell transplant.

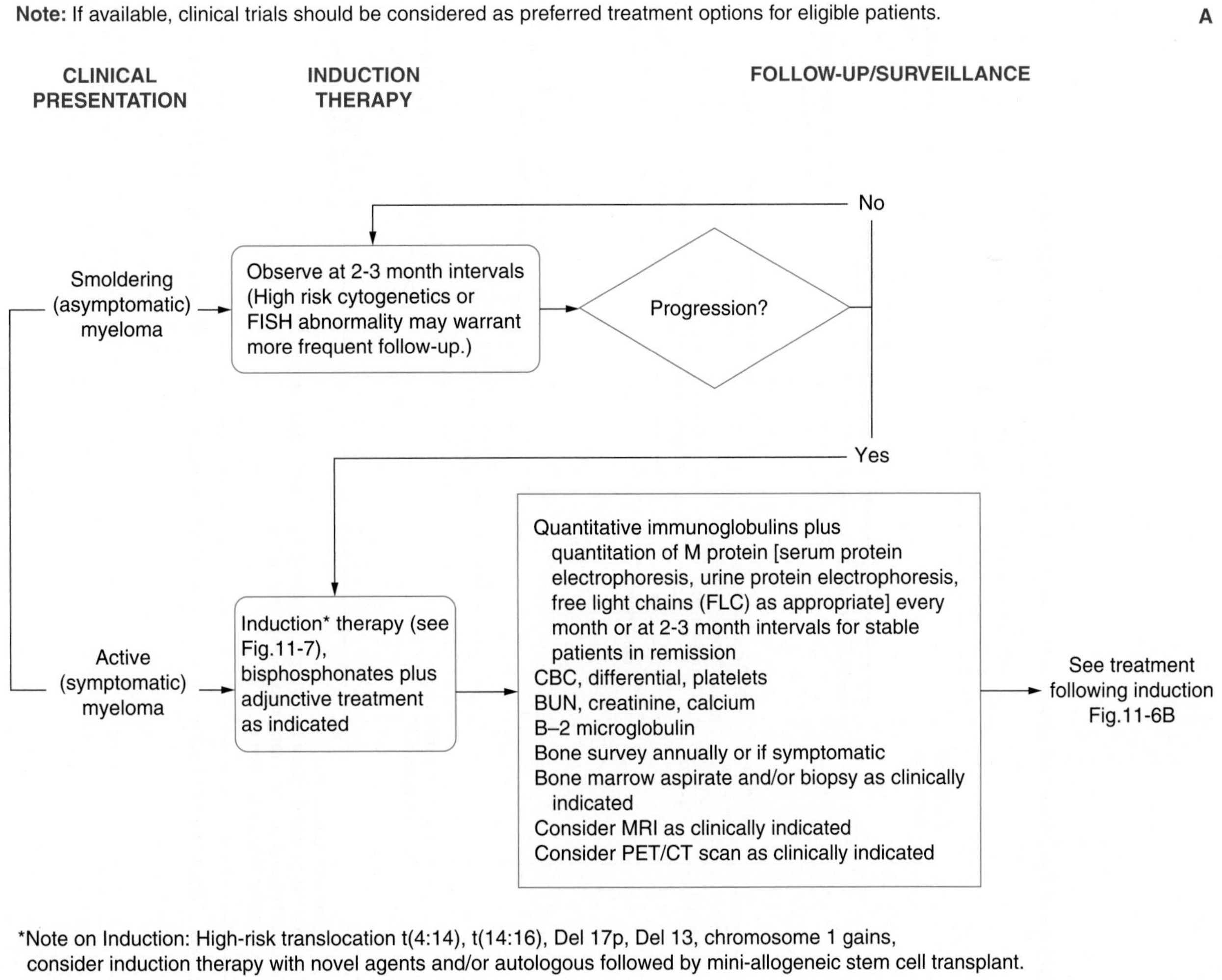

FIGURE 11-6A. Treatment of newly diagnosed multiple myeloma. (*Adapted with permission from The University of Texas MD Anderson Cancer Center.*)

Note: If available, clinical trials should be considered as preferred treatment options for eligible patients.

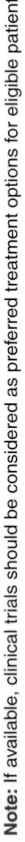

B

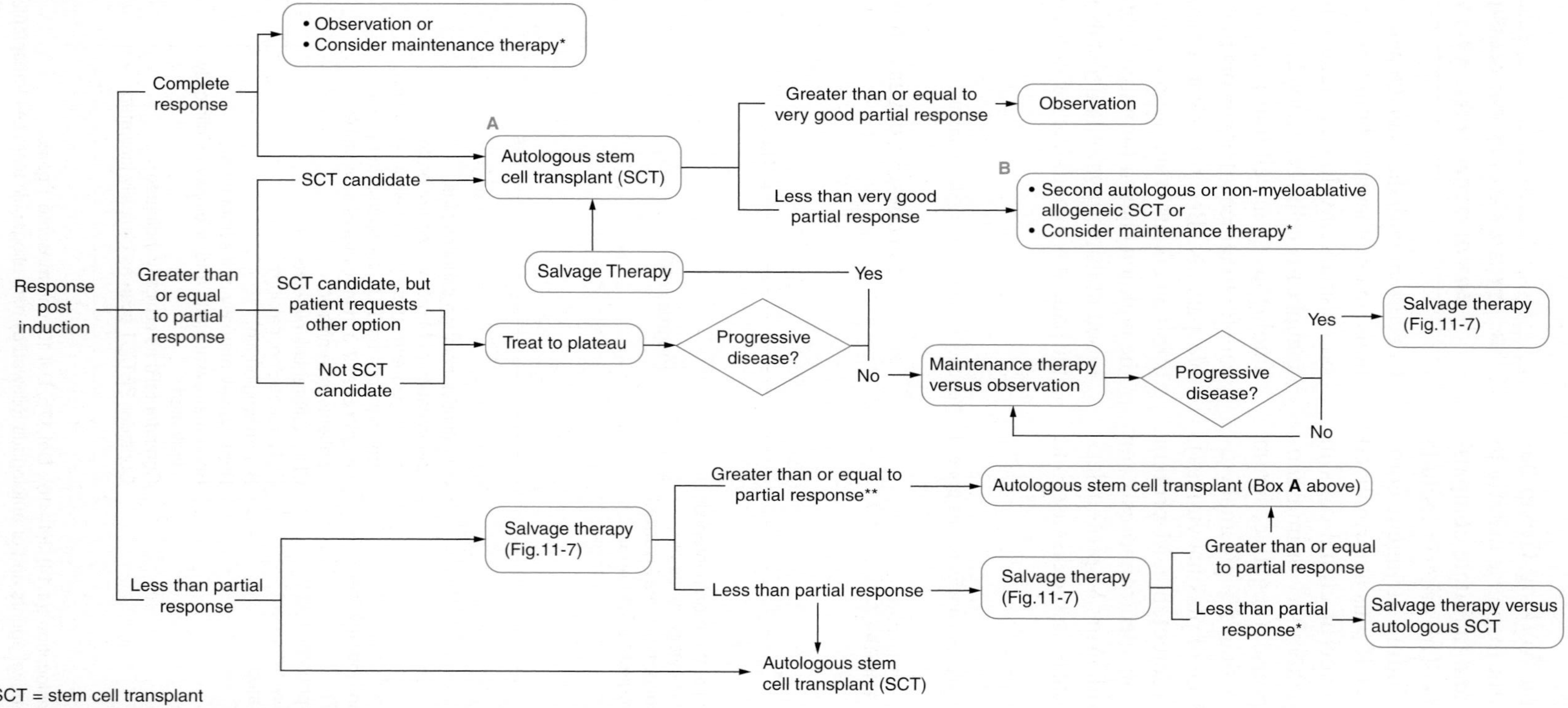

Response post induction

Complete response → • Observation or
• Consider maintenance therapy*

Greater than or equal to partial response

SCT candidate → Autologous stem cell transplant (SCT)

  A

  Greater than or equal to very good partial response → Observation

  B

  Less than very good partial response → • Second autologous or non-myeloablative allogeneic SCT or
  • Consider maintenance therapy*

SCT candidate, but patient requests other option → Salvage Therapy → Autologous stem cell transplant (SCT)

Not SCT candidate → Treat to plateau → **Progressive disease?**

  Yes → Maintenance therapy versus observation → **Progressive disease?** → Yes → Salvage therapy (Fig.11-7)

  No → Maintenance therapy versus observation

  Progressive disease? No → Autologous stem cell transplant (Box **A** above)

Less than partial response → Salvage therapy (Fig.11-7)

  Greater than or equal to partial response** → Autologous stem cell transplant (SCT)

  Less than partial response → Salvage therapy (Fig.11-7) → Greater than or equal to partial response → Salvage therapy versus autologous SCT

  Less than partial response*

SCT = stem cell transplant

*The best role for maintenance therapy has not been determined. Could consider for all not acheiveing complete response, but not mandatory.

**Required for Medicare patients.

FIGURE 11-6B. Treatment of multiple myeloma after induction. (*Adapted with permission from The University of Texas MD Anderson Cancer Center.*)

256

■ TREATMENTS

INDUCTION THERAPY FOR TRANSPLANT CANDIDATES (FIG. 11-7)

Induction chemotherapy followed by autologous stem cell transplantation in eligible candidates is the standard of care for myeloma treatment. Generally, patients who are under 65-75 years and without renal failure are eligible for transplant. However, individual patient factors must be considered when deciding whether a patient is a transplant candidate. If the patient is a transplant candidate, induction regimens with alkylating agents, such as melphalan, should be avoided due to the effects on stem cell reserve and subsequent ability to harvest stem cells.

Dexamethasone used as a single agent or in combination with vincristine and doxorubicin (VAD) has been used for induction therapy (109,110). However, this practice is being used less and less because the use of novel agents, including bortezomib, thalidomide, and lenalidomide in the frontline setting has resulted in improved response rates; they are now considered to be the first choices for induction therapy in transplant-eligible candidates.

It is important to keep in mind that all FDA-approved agents have been shown to have single-agent activity in MM. But generally, they should be used in combination for better efficacy. Choice of induction therapy should be individualized based upon coexisting clinical conditions such a neuropathy, diabetes, infections, thrombocytopenia, deep venous thrombosis, thrombocytopenia, bone marrow suppression, and so on, and the preferred route of administration (intravenous versus oral, and in the future, subcutaneous). Single agents could be considered in special clinical settings, such as in an elderly, frail patient whose myeloma has not caused acute symptoms. There should be a plan to add sequential agents later.

Thalidomide and Dexamethasone as Induction Therapy

Thalidomide in combination with dexamethasone (TD) has been extensively studied in newly diagnosed patients. In a phase III randomized, double-blind, placebo-controlled trial, thalidomide, 50-200 mg/day, with dexamethasone, 40 mg days 1-4, 9-12, and 17-20 in 4-week cycles, was compared to single agent dexamethasone. The thalidomide group showed a significantly greater response rate compared to the placebo group (63% versus 46%, $p < .01$). Time to progression was significantly longer in the thalidomide group (median, 22.6 versus 6.5 months, $p < .001$), and grade 4 adverse events were more frequent in the thalidomide group (111). A second phase III study of thalidomide, 200 mg/day, with dexamethasone versus dexamethasone alone was performed by the Eastern Cooperative Oncology Group (ECOG), with 207 patients randomized between the two arms. The response rate with thalidomide with dexamethasone was 63% versus 41% in the dexamethasone arm. Grade 3 toxicities were significantly higher in the thalidomide group (109). Another randomized trial produced higher VGPR rate of TD when compared to VAD before auto-SCT. At 6 months posttransplant, the benefit of TD was not further observed with VGPR rates of 44.4% in the TD arm and 41.7% in the VAD arm ($p = .87$) (112).

Data exist that TD is not as good as triple-drug induction therapies and that thalidomide with pulsed dexamethasone is not good for elderly patients due to dexamethasone-related toxicities.

The main toxicities of thalidomide in combination with dexamethasone include venous thromboembolism, peripheral neuropathy, constipation, and fatigue. Prophylaxis with warfarin or low-molecular-weight heparin is advised for use in patients being treated with thalidomide. Aspirin is an alternative for patients who cannot take warfarin or heparin (113). Peripheral neuropathy may limit the duration of therapy, and, in patients with preexisting neuropathy, other drugs may be preferable to thalidomide (113).

Lenalidomide and Dexamethasone as Induction Therapy

Lenalidomide is a second-generation immunomodulatory drug that is structurally related to thalidomide, but was developed as an alternative to thalidomide with fewer side effects and improved efficacy (114). Lenalidomide was first approved in the setting of relapsed and refractory myeloma; however, subsequent trials proved its activity in newly diagnosed myeloma. In a phase II trial of 34 patients, 56% attained a CR or VGPR. Lenalidomide was given 25 mg daily on days 1-21 of a 28-day cycle and dexamethasone was given 40 mg on days 1-4, 9-12, 17-20. Impressively, 91% percent of patients achieved an objective response. Four cycles of treatment were given and patients could then proceed to stem cell transplantation or continue on therapy at the discretion of their oncologist. Forty-seven percent of patients had grade 3 or higher nonhematologic side effects, most commonly fatigue (115,116). Thirteen patients proceeded to autologous stem cell transplant. Two-year progression-free survival (PFS) rates were 83% for patients who went on to transplant and 59% for patients remaining on

Note: If available, clinical trials should be considered as preferred treatment options for eligible patients.

Induction therapy for stem cell transplant candidates:	Primary treatment for non-stem cell transplant candidates:
Preferred treatments: • Bortezomib/steroid containing therapy • Lenalidomide/steroid containing therapy • Thalidomide/steroid containing therapy • Bortezomib plus liposomal doxorubicin with or without steroid • Bortezomib plus thalidomide with steriod • Bortezomib plus lenalidomide with steroid **Alternative choices:** • Dexamethasone • VAD (vincristine, dexamethasone, doxorubicin) • HyperCVAD (cyclophosphamide, mesna, doxorubicin, vincristine, dexamethasone) **Special considerations:** • If neuropathy, consider lenalidomide/dexamethasone containing therapy • If renal impairment, and creatinine greater than or equal to 2.5 mg/dL, avoid lenalidomide (if no other options, dose reduce according to guidelines, [Chen, et all) or low dose dexamethasone schedule • If diabetes, consider low-dose dexamethasone-based combination therapy or bortezomib/liposomal doxorubicin or bortezomib/lenalidomide salvage	Consider treatments as indicated for stem cell transplant candidates plus the addition of melphalan-based therapy such as: • MPT (melphalan, prednisone, and thalidomide) • VMP (bortezomib, melphalan, and prednisone) • MPR (melphalan, prednisone, and lenalidomide) **Maintenance therapy:** • Steroids • Thalidomide **Salvage therapy:** • If greater than 6 months post initial therapy, may repeat induction treatment **If not previously used:** • Bortezomib alone or in combination (combination preferable) • Bortezomib plus liposomal doxorubicin • Lenalidomide with steroid • Thalidomide in combination • Cyclophosphamide or melphalan-based regimen • HyperCVAD (cyclophosphamide, mesna, doxorubicin, vincristine, dexamethasone) • DT PACE (dexamethasone, thalidomide, cisplatin, doxorubicin, cyclophosphamide, and etoposide) • DCEP (dexamethasone, cyclophosphamide, etoposide, cisplatin) • VAD (vincristine, dexamethasone, doxorubicin)

FIGURE 11-7. Treatment strategy for patients with multiple myeloma. (*Adapted with permission from The University of Texas MD Anderson Cancer Center.*)

lenalidomide and dexamethasone. Overall survival rates were 92% at years 2 and 3 in the transplant group, and 92% and 85% in years 2 and 3 in the group that remained on treatment (111).

A randomized phase III non-inferiority trial of lenalidomide with high-dose or low-dose dexamethasone was reported by ECOG. Patients were treated with lenalidomide, 25 mg/day on days 1-21 for 28 days, and either dexamethasone, 40 mg on days 1-4, 9-12, and 17-20 or dexamethasone, 40 mg on days 1, 8, 15, and 22. Four hundred forty-five patients were randomized. At one year, overall survival was significantly better in the low-dose dexamethasone group compared to the high-dose group (96% versus 87%). The 2-year survival data was 87% in the low-dose group compared to 75% in the high-dose group. Further analysis examined outcomes at 3 years based on whether or not patients proceeded to stem cell transplant. Overall survival was 55% among patients who did not progress to transplant and was not different between the high and low-dose groups. Of the patients who underwent transplantation, 3-year survival was 92% in both groups. Increased mortality in the high-dose arm was due to higher rates of toxicity in the first four months and increased risk of thromboembolic events, particularly in patients over age 65 (117).

The main side effect of lenalidomide is myelosuppression, with thrombocytopenia and neutropenia the most common causes of delay in lenalidomide treatment. Lenalidomide is renally excreted and its dosage should be adjusted in patients with creatinine >2.5. Thromboembolism is also a risk with lenalidomide, and prophylaxis for thromboembolism is required. Pregnancy in female patients must be avoided, as lenalidomide is teratogenic (103). Finally, difficulties with stem cell mobilization with G-CSF alone have been reported; therefore, early collection of stem cells is recommended to avoid later problems with stem cell collection (118).

Although this is an acceptable induction therapy, the efficacy and time to response shall be challenged by triple or quadruple regimens in the near future in the authors' personal opinion.

Bortezomib and Dexamethasone and Other Combinations in Induction Therapy

Bortezomib is a first-in-class proteosome inhibitor which interferes with proteosomal degradation of a number of proteins, and exerts its antiproliferative and antiangiogenic effects on myeloma tumor cells through this mechanism (113). The clinical activity of bortezomib in myeloma was first demonstrated in the relapsed/refractory setting. However, a number of trials have tested bortezomib alone or in combination in the frontline setting.

Bortezomib has also been studied in combination with dexamethasone in the frontline setting. Harousseau et al. reported results of a phase II study of bortezomib, 1.3 mg/m^2 on days 1, 4, 8, 11, and dexamethasone, 40 mg on days 1-4, 9-12 of first two cycles, then days 1-4 for remaining cycles. Four cycles were given. Fifty-two patients accrued to the trial, and of the 48 evaluable patients, 67% showed an objective response. Twenty-one percent had a CR/nCR. After transplantation, 90% showed a response, with 33% of those as CR/nCR (119). Fifty patients were accrued in a similar phase II study of bortezomib compared to bortezomib/dexamethasone. Bortezomib, 1.3 mg/m^2, was administered for 6 cycles, and patients who did not achieve at least a PR after 2 cycles or CR after 4 cycles were given dexamethasone, 40 mg/day. Of the 40 patients evaluable, 85% showed objective response. Dexamethasone was added for 28 patients, and an improvement in response was observed in 19 patients (120).

Bortezomib/dexamethasone was compared to VAD for induction chemotherapy in transplant-eligible patients in a phase III trial by the Intergroupe Francophone du Myelome (IFM). The trial randomized 482 patients to four cycles of either therapy. Consolidation with dexamethasone, cyclophosphamide, etoposide, and platinum (DCEP) was also evaluated, but found not to add any benefit. The CR and near-CR rate was improved in the bortezomib group compared to VAD (67% response rate prior to transplant in 48 evaluable patients). Of the 42 patients who proceeded to transplant, the posttransplant response rate was 90%, with 33% CR/nCR. The bortezomib group had a lower rate of adverse events overall, but a higher rate of neuropathy. Stem cell collection was adequate in both groups (110).

Bortezomib has been evaluated in combination with immunomodulatory agents. In a retrospective study of 36 patients at MDACC, Wang et al. reported a 78% response rate with a CR rate of 19% with the combination of bortezomib, thalidomide, and dexamethasone. After stem cell transplantation, the total percentage of responders increased to 89% with 31% of patients in CR (121). A study of bortezomib, thalidomide, and dexamethasone was conducted by the GIMEMA Italian Multiple Myeloma Network. This combination was compared to thalidomide and dexamethasone (TD), followed by double autologous stem cell transplant and consolidation with the same regimen used for induction. The bortezomib group showed improved CR, near CR, and VGPR rates compared to TD, in both the pre- and posttransplant setting. At 15 months, PFS was significantly longer in the bortezomib group, and this benefit was also seen in poor prognostic groups. Grade 3 or 4 peripheral neuropathy was higher in the bortezomib group (122).

The main toxicity of bortezomib is the development of peripheral neuropathy, which is generally reversible upon discontinuation of treatment; thrombocytopenia, neutropenia, and fatigue have also been associated with bortezomib treatment (113). When thalidomide is combined with dexamethasone or bortezomib or with chemotherapeutic agents such as doxorubicin, the majority of clinical trials showed increased rate of deep venous thrombosis and pulmonary embolism. In these combinations, anticoagulation with warfarin (INR 2-3) or therapeutic low-molecular-weight heparin should be considered. Risks of bleeding and benefits of decreased rate of DVT/PE, and risks of fall should be carefully weighed.

Other Combination Trials

Further trials have evaluated bortezomib in combination with chemotherapeutic agents. Phase II trials were done to evaluate the activity of bortezomib with doxorubicin and dexamethasone. Oakervee et al. reported a trial of bortezomib, 1.3 mg/m^2 on days 1, 4, 8, 11, and doxorubicin 0, 4.5, or 9 mg/m^2 on days 1-4, with dexamethasone, 40 mg on days 1-4, 8-11, 15-18 for cycle 1 and days 1-4 for cycles 2-4. Twenty-one patients were enrolled, and an overall response rate of 95% was observed with 29% CR/nCR (123). A trial by Popat et al. studied a lower dose of bortezomib, 1.0 mg/m^2, with doxorubicin, 9 mg/m^2, and dexamethasone. Overall response rate was 89% with low toxicities. There was a 100% response rate after transplant (124). The phase III trial, HOVON-65/GMMG-HD4, compared bortezomib, doxorubicin, and dexamethasone (PAD) to VAD. Patients were randomized to undergo three cycles of either arm of therapy. Autologous stem cell transplant was planned for all patients, followed by maintenance therapy with bortezomib or thalidomide for 2 years. The first analysis showed significant improvement in CR+PR+VGPR in the PAD arm (125). Two additional studies have been reported using bortezomib in combination with pegylated liposomal doxorubicin and dexamethasone with overall response rates of approximately 80% (113).

It is important to realize that the quality of initial therapy is important to a patient with newly diagnosed myeloma. The quality of the therapies is at best defined by the most current and the most stringent criteria for complete remission. It might be controversial with debates, but it is the author's belief that time will eventually prove true that the most stringent complete remission is a major surrogate marker for long-term survival and cure in myeloma. It is also important to calculate the cost of achieving complete remission based on comorbidities and toxicity profiles on an individualized basis. As the golden rule in medicine states, benefits should outweigh the risks and treatment choices should be explained to the patients patiently. The judgment of the oncologist is critical.

The MD Anderson Approach for Induction Therapy for the Transplant Candidates

At MD Anderson, our first choice for induction therapy is a clinical trial. Outside of a trial, for transplant-eligible patients, we prefer triple combination therapy that includes either bortezomib, lenalidomide, or thalidomide with low-dose dexamethasone (40 mg weekly). For those patients who are unable to tolerate steroids, we may instead choose bortezomib plus liposomal doxorubicin or use low-dose steroids. There are some patients for whom thalidomide is more appropriate than lenalidomide (eg, those patients with renal dysfunction or unexplained cytopenias). For other patients, (eg, those with neuropathy) lenalidomide is more appropriate than thalidomide. Additionally, patients with significant neuropathy may not be candidates for bortezomib therapy at full doses. For highly aggressive disease with large tumor burden, we may also consider hyper-CVAD or modified CVAD. Those patients who have active bony disease receive intravenous bisphosphonates monthly for 2 years.

CLINICAL TRIALS

- Bortezomib-cyclophosphamide-dexamethasone
- Bortezomib-lenalidomide-dexamethasone
- Bortezomib-thalidomide-dexamethasone
- Bortezomib-dexamethasone
- Lenalidomide-dexamethasone

INDUCTION THERAPY FOR NON-TRANSPLANT CANDIDATES

A patient's candidacy for stem cell transplant could be limited due to patient choice, insurance, comorbidities, and other issues. The age limit is varied: 65 years in Europe and 75 years in the United States, although data show that transplants could be safely done in elderly patients with MM (126). The introduction of novel agents with activity in multiple myeloma during the last decade has affected the treatment paradigm in nontransplant candidates. Dating back to the 1960s, melphalan/prednisone (MP) given in intermittent courses has been the standard chemotherapy for all patients (127,128). The MP combination induces a remission in approximately 40-60% of previously untreated patients (129). The median duration of remission for these patients is approximately 2 years, and the median survival is approximately 3 years. The low frequency of CR (10%) and the inevitable relapse indicate that inherent drug resistance represents the major impediment to long-term remission or cure.

Recently, the MP combination was studied in combination with immunomodulatory agents in patients who were not transplant candidates. The first trial, reported by Palumbo et al., randomized 255 patients to MP or MP with thalidomide (MPT). This trial showed PR rates of 76% and 47.6% in the MPT and MP groups, respectively (130,131). Updated results showed a longer PFS in the MPT group compared to the MP group (38.1 months versus 21.8 months, respectively) but no difference in overall survival (131).

Hulin et al. reported a randomized, phase III trial comparing melphalan, 0.2 mg/kg, and prednisone, 2 mg/kg on days 1-4, with melphalan, prednisone, and thalidomide, 100 mg daily. All patients were age 75 or older. Overall and progression free survival were significantly longer in the thalidomide group, but neutropenia and neuropathy were more common (132). Three additional trials comparing MP to MPT produced similar results, with improved overall response rates and progression free survival observed with MPT. Overall survival was improved in two of the trials with the MPT combination. These trials enrolled different patient populations, and used different durations of treatment, but taken together, the results support the use of MPT as first-line therapy for non-transplant candidates (133-136).

One trial comparing MP to MP plus bortezomib (MPB) has been reported. In this trial of 682 nontransplant eligible patients, MPB showed increased progression-free survival, time to next treatment, and complete response compared to MP. The 3-year overall survival rate was also significantly increased in the MPB group compared to the MP group, (72% versus 59%, $p = .003$). Notably, poor prognostic indicators, including complex cytogenetics, advanced age, and impaired renal function did not impact outcomes in this trial. Grade 3 non-hematologic toxicity and peripheral neuropathy were more common in the MPB group (137).

The thalidomide and dexamethasone combination has been compared to melphalan and prednisolone in nontransplantable, elderly patients. A group of 289 patients was randomized to either thalidomide, 200 mg, with dexamethasone, 40 mg on days 1-4 and 15-18 during even cycles and days 1-4 on odd cycles; or melphalan,

0.25 mg/kg, and prednisolone, 2 mg/kg on days 1-4. Patients with stable disease or those who got better on either therapy then went onto maintenance with either interferon alpha alone or in combination with thalidomide. Thalidomide and dexamethasone resulted in a significantly higher percentage of overall responses, but overall survival was shorter due to increased non-myeloma deaths in patients over 75. The main causes of death in these cases were infectious and cardiovascular causes. Additionally, there was more neuropathy and constipation in the thalidomide, dexamethasone group. Leukopenia and thrombocytopenia were increased in the melphalan group (138). Outcomes in the two maintenance groups were also similar and not statistically different. Randomized Phase III Trials in Patients with Newly Diagnosed Myeloma which are ineligible for ASCT are listed in Table 11-5.

At MD Anderson, myeloma patients who are not eligible for transplant receive either MPT, bortezomib, melphalan and prednisone (VMP) or melphalan prednisone and lenalidomide (MPR). This is based on the above data and more recent data suggesting an additive effect of any of the novel agents over standard melphalan and prednisone. Again, these patients tend to be older with a greater number of comorbidities and thus, overall tolerability of the regimen should be considered on an individual basis.

Summary of Induction Chemotherapy Options in Transplant and Nontransplant Candidates

- Melphalan and prednisone plus a novel agent (either thalidomide or bortezomib) produce superior results for elderly patients with newly diagnosed myeloma.
- Immunomodulatory-derivative regimens containing multiple high doses of dexamethasone per month produce excessive toxicity in older patients, without an improved antimyeloma effect.
- Autologous stem cell transplantation is currently considered the standard of care in patients younger than 65 with multiple myeloma without renal failure.
- Thalidomide after autologous stem cell transplantation improves the complete remission/very good partial remission, progression-free survival, and overall survival rates.
- Bortezomib plus dexamethasone increases the complete remission/very good partial remission rate both before and after autologous stem cell transplantation.
- Reduced-intensity conditioning allergenic stem cell transplantation should not be offered to good-risk patients with multiple myeloma and should be used for other patients only as part of a clinical trial.

TABLE 11-5	RANDOMIZED PHASE III TRIALS IN PATIENTS WITH NEWLY DIAGNOSED MYELOMA WHICH ARE INELIGIBLE FOR ASCT				
Author	*Treatment*	*ORR (≥nCR) (%)*	*PFS/EFS (mo)*	*OS (mo)*	*2-y OS (%)*
Facon et al.[133]	MPT	76 (18)*	27.5*	51.6*	78
	MP	35 (2)	17.8	33.2	60
Palumbo et al.[130,131]	MPT	76 (27.9)*	21.8*	45	82
	MP	47.9 (7.1)	14.5	47.6	65
Hulin et al.[132]	MPT	61 (71)*	24.1*	45.3*	~70
	MP	31 (1)	19	27.7	~60
Waage et al.[135]	MPT	57 (13)	15	30	~62
	MP	38 (4)	14	30	~60
Wijermans et al.[134]	MPT	66 (2)*	13*	37	–
	MP	47 (2*)	9	30	–
San Miguel et al.[137]	MP+B	71 (35)*	24*	NYR	83*
	MP	30 (4)	16.6	NYR	70
Rajkumar et al.[111]	TD	63 (7.7)*	14.9*	–	71
	Dex	46 (2.6)	6.5	–	~64
Ludwig et al.[138]	TD	68 (2)*	16.7	41.5*	61
	MP	50 (2)	20.7	49.4	70
Rajkumar et al.[117]	Len+HDdex	79	–	NYR	~84
	Len+LDdex	69	–	NYR	93

ORR, overall response rate; nCR, near-complete remission; PFS, progression-free survival; EFS, event-free survival; OS, overall survival; Dex, dexamethasone; PLD, pegylated liposomal doxorubicin; NYR, not yet reached; MPT, melphalan, prednisone, thalidomide; B, bortezomib; Len+HDdex, lenalidomide + high-dose dexamethasone; LDdex, low-dose dexamethasone.
*Statistically significant.

- Therapy can be individualized based on biologic risk profiling as proposed by the Mayo Clinic at www.msmart.org (Stratification for Myeloma And Risk-Adapted Therapy).
- High-risk myeloma is defined by t(4;14), t(14;16), del(17p), or a plasma cell labeling index of more than 3%.
- Stem cells should be collected in all eligible patients, but may be cryopreserved for use as a salvage regimen.
- Bortezomib appears to overcome the adverse prognostic effect of unfavorable genetics and can be used safely with serum creatinine greater than 2.5 mg/dL.
- Lenalidomide, combined with low-dose dexamethasone induction, reduced early mortality for older patients with myeloma.

Follow-up

For follow-up, we recommend serum and urine electrophoresis with immunofixation, serum free light chains, and quantitative immunoglobulins in addition to a standard CBC and chemistries every month initially and every 2-3 months as the disease stabilizes with treatment. Some patients may also require frequent reimaging with MRI, depending on the location or imminent danger of any lesions. After disease has stabilized we perform serum analysis as above every 6 months. Bone imaging via skeletal survey (or MRI or PET/CT if indicated) and bone marrow biopsy are performed annually for restaging.

REMISSION MAINTENANCE

When myeloma has a maximal response, as defined by a low, constant myeloma level (plateau), residual plasma cells have less proliferative activity and increased resistance to chemotherapy (128). Continued therapy with alkylating agents may induce repeated myelosuppression and the risk of acute leukemia and does not prolong survival compared with no maintenance therapy followed by resumption of alkylating agents at relapse.

A meta-analysis by the Myeloma Trialists' Collaborative Group of 4012 patients in 24 randomized trials evaluating maintenance with interferon alpha (IFN-α) demonstrated a similar gain in median remission duration of 6 months and a minor gain in median survival of 4 months (139). The survival benefit was mainly noted in smaller trials and was generally unconfirmed by large studies. While interferon may be useful for some patients, this modest gain in remission duration must be balanced against the side effects and cost of interferon and lack of overall survival benefit (140). The Southwest Oncology

Group (SWOG) evaluated VAD with or without chemosensitizers (verapamil, quinine) followed by the randomization of 89 patients to maintenance therapy with 3 million units of IFN-α three times weekly or IFN-α plus 50 mg prednisone (IFN/P) on the morning after IFN-α until relapse (141). Patients who received IFN/P had an improved progression-free survival rate (median 19 versus 9 months for IFN; $p = .008$), although the median survival rate was not significantly different (IFN/P 57 months versus IFN 46 months, $p = .36$).

At MD Anderson, 172 consecutive previously untreated patients were given induction therapy with melphalan and intermittent high-dose dexamethasone (MD) (142). Within 5 months, 84 patients were randomized to receive IFN-β or dexamethasone 20 mg/m^2 for 4 days each month until relapse. The median duration of first remission of 10 months was identical in both arms; however, more patients responded to the resumption of MD after disease relapse in the IFN-α arm (82%) than in the dexamethasone arm (44%; $p = .001$). The median remission from randomization to melphalan-resistant second relapse was 32 months for patients treated with IFN-α compared with 19 months for patients treated with dexamethasone ($p = .01$).

The benefit of steroids is unclear from the SWOG and MD Anderson trials, both of which were randomized and included similar numbers of patients. All of these studies support a modest gain in remission duration with little or no survival benefit for maintenance therapy, regardless of the agent used.

Thalidomide has been investigated as maintenance therapy after induction chemotherapy with thalidomide, dexamethasone, and Doxil. A group of 103 patients were randomized either to undergo maintenance with interferon and pulsed dexamethasone or thalidomide and pulsed dexamethasone. Overall survival was significantly better in the thalidomide arm (84% versus 68%), and 2-year event-free survival was also significantly improved in the thalidomide group. Notably, at 3 years, likelihood of discontinuation was 44% in the interferon group and 21% in the thalidomide group (143).

The role of maintenance therapy after autologous stem cell transplant (ASCT) has been investigated in a few trials and will continue to evolve as more trials are completed. Lokhorst et al. reported a trial of 556 patients randomly assigned to induction therapy with thalidomide, doxorubicin, and dexamethasone (TAD) or VAD. Patients in both arms then underwent ASCT, and, if at least a partial response was obtained, maintenance with IFN-α or thalidomide was started until relapse or progression. Treatment with thalidomide as induction chemotherapy or maintenance resulted in

significantly improved overall response rates; the highest response rate of all arms was 88%. Thalidomide induction and maintenance also resulted in a longer progression-free and event-free survival (34 months in both instances). Overall survival was better in the thalidomide group, but this was not statistically significant (144). Attal et al. reported a trial of 597 patients who underwent ASCT and were then randomly assigned to maintenance with pamidronate alone, pamidronate with thalidomide 200 mg/day, or no maintenance. Overall response, probability of 3-year event-free survival, and 4-year probability of survival were all significantly increased in the thalidomide arm. The greatest benefit was observed in patients who were not in CR or VGPR at the beginning of maintenance. Skeletal events were not reduced with pamidronate. Results from this trial suggest that thalidomide is a viable alternative for maintenance therapy after ASCT (145).

In a recent trial of 269 patients who underwent ASCT were randomly assigned to indefinite maintenance with prednisolone (control group) or to indefinite prednisolone with 12 months of thalidomide (treatment group). Overall survival rates were 85% and 76% in the thalidomide group and the control group, respectively. Progression-free survival was 42% and 23% in the thalidomide group versus the control group (146). The benefits of thalidomide were observed in patients who had achieved CR and VGPR after ASCT. Results from this trial support the role of thalidomide as maintenance therapy after ASCT. The role of maintenance therapy in myeloma is under active investigation and will continue to evolve.

At MD Anderson, we consider maintenance therapy with thalidomide, lenalidomide, or dexamethasone after induction therapy if the patient has achieved a CR and will not be proceeding to transplant imminently. In the posttransplant setting, we have moved from thalidomide to lenalidomide for maintenance. This is based on interim results from CALGB 100104, which preliminarily showed a decrease in risk of disease progression for those patients who received lenalidomide maintenance versus those patients who received placebo. Other maintenance options commonly used at MD Anderson, either in the posttransplant or postinduction setting, include dexamethasone and thalidomide. For those patients who have been previously refractory to thalidomide or lenalidomide we consider weekly bortezomib for maintenance therapy. In the posttransplant setting, we typically offer maintenance therapy to those patients who have only achieved a PR, though arguments can also be made to offer this to those who achieve a VGPR.

RELAPSING AND REFRACTORY DISEASE

Despite the unprecedented advances in the treatment of multiple myeloma, nearly all patients relapse at some point after frontline or salvage treatment. Fortunately, the advent of novel therapeutics has afforded physicians greater choice in therapeutic options so that patients with relapsed or refractory disease can experience meaningful survival times. Among the numerous therapeutic choices, the superiority of any one novel combination has not been definitely established (13). To date, the best choice for each patient continues to depend both on the existing data for each agent or its combinations with others and the individual clinical scenario such as age, physical condition, prior toxicity, availability of an HLA-matched sibling donor, and patient's preferences. The approved therapies are bortezomib, thalidomide, and lenalidomide, alone and in combination with each other, and conventional antineoplastic agents, as well as other agents in active clinical development. The key randomized phase III trials are listed in Table 11-6.

Single-agent high-dose dexamethasone has been used in patients with relapsed disease but has fallen out of favor in the era of novel therapeutics. Pulse-dosed dexamethasone can yield a response rate of about 20% but it is usually short-lived, between 3 and 5 months (147-149). However, it should be noted that steroids are a relatively benign intervention in comparison with the more active agents and thus provide an option for palliative intent or to acutely manage complications (eg, bony disease). The majority of applications for steroids in the relapsed/refractory setting are in conjunction with other anti-myeloma agents, as detailed below.

The International Myeloma Working Group (IMWG) divides refractory myeloma into two groups: primary refractory and relapsed-refractory. Primary refractory disease is defined by a failure to achieve a minor response (MR) with any therapy while relapsed-and-refractory disease is defined by nonresponsive disease while on salvage therapy or disease progression within 60 days of last therapy in patients who have achieved MR. Relapsed disease is progression of disease in patients who have been treated, who are now more than 60 days off therapy (150).

Perhaps the most important factor to consider is the length of response to prior therapy. In patients whose response has been <1 year, an alternative regimen should be considered. In those patients who have had a longer progression-free interval (3-4 years), one may choose retreatment with the previously successful regimen. Equally important in this decision is the patient's overall performance status and co-morbidities. A patient with long-standing neuropathy may be served best by avoiding re-treatment with bortezomib while a patient with significant cytopenias may not be an appropriate candidate for lenalidomide. In addition, the highly sensitive measures of disease detection (electrophoresis combined with serum free light-chain quantification) can often herald the relapse before any clinically significant sequelae. In this case the physician may choose to initiate low-dose thalidomide, lenalidomide, or bortezomib maintenance therapy to prolong the development of overt relapse.

Thalidomide-Dexamethasone

Thalidomide monotherapy in relapsed/refractory multiple myeloma (MM) has a response rate of 30%. The combination of thalidomide with dexamethasone (Thal/Dex) is expected to improve responses. In the initial study of Thal/Dex combination from The MD Anderson Cancer Center, the response rate (CR and PR) was approximately 45% of patients with relapsed or refractory

TABLE 11-6	RANDOMIZED PHASE III TRIALS OF PATIENTS WITH RELAPSED/REFRACTORY MULTIPLE MYELOMA			
Author	**Treatment**	**ORR (CR) (%)**	**TTP (mo)**	**OS**
Richardson et al.[147]	Bortezomib	38 (6)*	6.2*	80% at 1 year*
	Dex	18 (1)	3.5	66% at 1 year
Orloswki et al.[172]	Bortezomib	41 (2)	6.5*	65% at 15 months*
	Bortezomib + PLD	44 (4)	9.3	76% at 15 months
Weber et al.[149]	Lenalidomide + dex	61 (14.1)*	11.1*	29.6*
	Dex	19.9 (0.6)	4.1	20.2
Dimopoulos et al.[148]	Lenalidomide + dex	60.2 (15.9)*	11.3*	NYR*
	Dex	24 (3.4)	4.7	20.6

ORR, overall response rate; CR, complete remission; TTP, time to progression; OS, overall survival; Dex, dexamethasone; PLD, pegylated liposomal doxorubicin; NYR, not yet reached.
*Statistically significant

myeloma, while 30% of patients who had no response to thalidomide monotherapy responded after dexamethasone was added (151). The efficacy of Thal/Dex was confirmed by several other clinical studies (152,153). In a systematic review of 12 trials of Thal/Dex in relapsed/refractory MM that included 451 patients (154), the response rate (CR and PR) was 46% (95% CI 42-51%). Therapy-related toxicity was comparable to thalidomide monotherapy and included somnolence (26%, 95% CI 22-31%), constipation (37%, 95% CI 32-42%), and peripheral neuropathy (27%, 95% CI 23-32%). Only venous thromboembolism appeared to occur more often with Thal/Dex (5%, 95% CI 3-8%). Thus, using Thal/Dex results in an improved response rate in relapsed/refractory MM, with a toxicity rate comparable to thalidomide monotherapy (154).

Lenalidomide-Dexamethasone

Two major trials have established the combination of lenalidomide-dexamethasone ("len-dex") as a regimen superior to dexamethasone alone for relapsed or refractory multiple myeloma (148,149). In these multi-center, randomized double-blind phase III studies, patients were assigned to either lenalidomide (25 mg po daily for first 21 of 28-day cycle) plus high-dose dexamethasone (40 mg on days 1-4, 9-12, and 17-20) versus high-dose dexamethasone alone. Outcomes in the two trials were similar: in the MM-009 trial the overall response rate (ORR) was 61% in the len-dex group versus 20% in the placebo group ($p < .001$) and in the MM-010 trial the ORR was 60.2% versus 24% ($p < .001$). Both trials demonstrated a significant benefit in TTP and OS for the patients treated with len-dex. Interestingly, further analysis showed that this benefit was seen in patients who had received prior thalidomide or bortezomib. In both trials myelosuppression and thromboembolic events were more common in the len-dex group. Because the combination of lenalidomide and high-dose dexamethasone appears to be more thrombogenic than lenalidomide alone, appropriate prophylactic measure are indicated in certain populations (155).

Lenalidomide has been combined with doxorubicin and dexamethasone (RAD) in relapsed/refractory MM with a response rate of 73%, including 15% CR. The main side effects were hematological toxicity and infections (156). Combination lenalidomide with low-dose oral cyclophosphamide and prednisone has also demonstrated a high activity (CR in 14.3% and $\geq$ minimal response in 64.3%) with good tolerability in relapsed patients who were refractory to the lenalidomide-dexamethasone regimen (157).

Bortezomib

As with the other novel agents, bortezomib's first successes were in the relapsed/refractory setting. Initial phase II studies showed the ORR to be 34 to 35%, in previously heavily treated patients (158,159). A subsequent phase III trial compared bortezomib with high-dose dexamethasone in relapsed/refractory paptients (147). The ORR was 38% for bortezomib and 18% for dexamethasone ($p < .001$), and median TTP was 6.22 months and 3.49 months, respectively ($p < .001$). A most recent analysis of this trial showed a survival of 29.8 months for bortezomib versus 23.7 months for dexamethasone, though many patients had crossed-over to bortezomib at the time of this analysis (160). Another analysis of this trial showed that while patients with prior thalidomide exposure had worse outcomes overall, the superiority of bortezomib over dexamethasone was maintained regardless of either prior thalidomide or prior autologous stem cell transplantation (161).

Bortezomib-Dexamethasone

A retrospective analysis of 21 relapsed myeloma patients treated with bortezomib-dexamethasone found an ORR of 70% and a PFS of 12 months (162). Several small phase II studies have examined the combination of bortezomib and dexamethasone and have found ORRs of 64% to 73% (163-165). Finally, the addition of dexamethasone to bortezomib in relapsed/refractory patients who had had a suboptimal response to single-agent bortezomib resulted in improved responses in 22% of patients, without significantly worsened toxicity, suggesting that steroids do add to the effect of this proteasome inhibitor (166).

Bortezomib-Chemotherapy Combinations

The combination of vincristine, doxorubicin, and dexamethasone (VAD) has yielded positive results in patients previously treated with alkylating agents. This was first reported in 1984 by Barlogie et al. (167) but reflected treatment in the era before autologous stem cells transplant and novel agents. In that trial, responses were achieved in 14 of 20 patients whose disease was resistant to alkylating agents and in 3 of 9 patients who had a history of resistance to doxorubicin. In subsequent studies of VAD in relapsed or refractory myeloma patients, the overall response rate (ORR) ranged from 40 to 60% with a CR rate of as high as 10% (168-170). This was an improvement in response rates typically seen with single-agent dexamenthasone (148,149).

Though anthracyclines are active in multiple myeloma, the risk of cardiotoxicity is notable. Pegylated liposomal formulation of doxorubicin (PLD) is known to cause less cardiotoxicity than doxorubicin (171) and thus is an attractive option. In a randomized phase III study, the combination of pegylated liposomal doxorubicin (PLD) and bortezomib was compared with bortezomib alone. Though the ORR was similar between the 2 arms (44% for PLD + bortezomib versus 41% for bortezomib), median TTP was 9.3 months with the PLD-bortezomib versus 6.5 months for bortezomib ($p = .000004$). As expected there were more grade 3/4 adverse events in the combination group (80% versus 64%), with increases in myelosuppression, asthenia, fatigue, diarrhea, and hand-foot syndrome (172). Liposomal doxorubicin in combination with bortezomib is indicated for the treatment of patients with multiple myeloma who have not previously received bortezomib and have received at least one previous therapy.

Bortezomib has also been combined with low-dose melphalan. In 46 evaluable patients, the ORR was 70%, with 4% CR, 11% near-CR, 35% PR, and 20% minor response (MR). Response rates were similar in patients with prior melphalan or bortezomib exposure, and the median progression-free survival and overall survival in this study were 9 months and 32 months, respectively (173). Bortezomib and dexamethasone have also been combined with oral or IV cyclophosphamide in several phase I/II trials, with response rates of 75 to 95% (including minor responses) (174-176). The combination of bortezomib with bendamustine has also shown significant activity in heavily pretreated patients (177).

Combining Novel Agents

Bortezomib-Thalidomide–Based Regimens

The positive results of bortezomib in patients previously treated with thalidomide have led to efforts to combine the novel agents in the hopes of further improvements in response. In addition, preclinical data suggest that immunomodulatory agents may potentiate the activity of proteosome inhibitors (178).

A phase I/II trial of bortezomib, thalidomide, and dexamethasone (VTD) in 85 patients with advanced and refractory myeloma showed a PR of 63% with a 4-year EFS and OS of 6% and 23%, resectively (179). This therapy was relatively well-tolerated, with fatigue as the most prevalent toxicity at the MTD. Based on two other studies, adding melphalan to this type of regimen (VMPT or VDMT) may improve these response rates (66-67%) with a greater proportion of patients achieving a VGPR (180,181). Addition of other agents, such as

doxorubicin or liposomal doxorubicin, to the bortezomib/thalidomide combination also resulted in significant responses (182,183). These trials suggest that novel agents can be safely combined and may be an option for patients who were previously treated with either bortezomib or an immunomodulatory agent.

Lenalidomide-Thalidomide-Based Regimens

In a phase II trial by Palumbo et al., lenalidomide, thalidomide, melphalan, prednisone combinations produced a PR rate of 82%, including VGPR 36% in 44 patients with relapsed and/or refractory myeloma. The 1-year progression-free survival was 49%. Grade 3-4 hematological adverse events included neutropenia (67%), thrombocytopenia (36%), and anemia (30%). Grade 3-4 nonhematological adverse events included infections (21%), neurologic toxicity, and fatigue (9%). No thromboembolic events were reported (184).

Bortezomib-Lenalidomide-Based Regimens

In a phase I, dose-escalation trial of lenalidomide-bortezomib in relapsed or refractory myeloma patients (185), the maximum tolerated dose (MTD) was lenalidomide 15 mg/day plus bortezomib 1.0 mg/m^2. The majority of these patients had been previously treated with thalidomide, lenalidomide, or bortezomib. Of note, patients who were progressing after two cycles were also treated with dexamethasone. Of the 36 evaluable patients, 61% achieved minimal response (MR) or better. Of the 18 patients who also received dexamethasone, 83% achieved stable disease or better. Median overall survival was 37 months. Myelosuppression was the most common grade 3-4 toxicity. The results of a phase II study of this regimen with dexamethasone (VRD) have been reported in abstract form: the ORR was 79% with 33% achieving a VGPR or CR (186).

Although prognostic factors of relapsed/refractory disease remain to be comprehensively defined the condition of patients with t(4;14) or t(14;16) translocation(s), deletion of chromosomes 17 or 13, hypodiploidy, high beta-2 microglobulin, and low serum albumin and renal failure, which have been identified as poorer risks for newly diagnosed myeloma, should also be taken into account before choosing a regimen. For patients with abnormal cytogenetics, thalidomide treatment has been associated with a poor outcome (187,188).

Retrospective studies indicated that bortezomib is effective for patients with t(4;14) and 13q deletion (189,190). One analysis has shown that len+dex is also efficacious in these unfavorable subsets, although this has not been confirmed in other studies; patients with del(17p), however, had poorer results (191). In patients with myeloma-related renal failure, both bortezomib- and thalidomide-based combinations have been shown to be safe and effective, and are also associated with a significant probability of renal function improvement in some patients with relapsed/refractory disease (81-83,192). In practice, most patients with myeloma receive a therapeutic trial of all available agents at some point during the multiple relapses that characterize this disease.

New Agents

The success of the IMiDs and proteosome inhibitors in myeloma has prompted a swell in the investigations of novel compounds. A phase II study of a the IMiD pomalidomide (in combination with weekly dexamethasone) showed an ORR of 63%; notably, responses occurred in patients previously refractory to thalidomide, lenalidomide, and bortezomib (193). Other novel agents including the second-generation proteasome inhibitors carfilzomib (PR-171) (194), Hsp90 inhibitor tanespimycin (195), AKT inhibitor Perifosine, (196) and defibrotide (197) alone or in combination with chemotherapy also showed considerable activity in phase I/II trials in relapsed and/or refractory MM. Clinical trials are the future of advances in the treatment of myeloma.

The MD Anderson Approach

If patients have a >6 month history of response from their previous treatment, retreatment with the induction regimen is acceptable. Otherwise we favor addition of a new agent not previously used (lenalidomide, bortezomib, or liposomal doxorubicin). Cyclophosphamide, in combination with steroids, is also an option, as is a melphalan-based regimen if the patient is not a transplant candidate or if enough cells have been stored before a previous transplant. For aggressive disease we favor a hyper-CVAD–based regimen or the combination of dexamethasone, thalidomide, cisplatin, doxorubicin, cyclophosphamide, and etoposide (DT-PACE). Dexamethasone, cyclophosphamide, etoposide, cisplatin (DHEP) is also an option, as is VAD.

HEMATOPOIETIC STEM CELL TRANSPLANTATION (HCT)

Autologous HCT

High-dose melphalan without autologous HCT was first reported in 1983 by McElwain et al. from the Royal Marsden Hospital (198). When compared with chemotherapy alone, intensified chemotherapy followed by autologous HCT appears to prolong both event-free and overall survival in previously untreated patients

with myeloma. One comparative study and two randomized trials showed the autologous HCT provided survival benefits of approximately 12 months (199-201).

In the French IFM 90 trial, high-dose chemotherapy supported by autologous HCT was compared with conventional chemotherapy in 200 previously untreated patients with myeloma and less than 65 years of age (199). The results showed a higher CR rate (22% versus 5%), a higher rate of 5-year event-free (28% versus 10%), and overall (52% versus 12%) survival in the autologous HCT group. The median duration of overall survival in patients assigned to the HCT arm was 13 months longer (57 versus 44 months).

The Medical Research Council Myeloma VII trial compared conventional dose chemotherapy with high-dose therapy and autologous HCT in 401 previously untreated patients with myeloma aged <65 years (201). The rates of complete response were higher in the autologous HCT group than in the standard therapy group (44% versus 8%, $p < .001$). Intention-to-treat analysis showed a higher rate of overall survival ($p = .04$) and progression-free survival ($p < .001$) in the HCT group than in the standard-therapy group. As compared with standard therapy, autologous HCT increased median survival by almost 1 year (54.1 versus 42.3 months). There was a trend toward a greater survival benefit in the group of patients with a poor prognosis, as defined by a high (more than 8 mg/L) beta-2-microglobulin level.

In three other randomized studies, however, there has been no survival benefit to autologous HCT (202-204). Comparison among these trials is difficult due to the variability in patient eligibility including age, induction chemotherapy, the conditioning regimen for HCT, and the definitions of response.

Many different preparative regimens have been assessed over the last 20 years, but only one prospective, randomized trial, by a French Cooperative group, has directly compared two different preparative regimens. In 282 newly diagnosed symptomatic patients under 65 years of age, high-dose melphalan at 200 mg/m^2 was shown to be superior to a combination of melphalan 140 mg/m^2 + 8 Gy of total body irradiation (TBI), mainly due to reduced toxicity including mucositis and transplant-related mortality (205).

Several nonrandomized trials have suggested that double autologous HCT may be associated with a better outcome (101,206). A French randomized trial of 399 previously untreated patients under 60 years of age found significantly improved 7-year EFS (20% versus 10%) and overall survival (42% versus 21%) in recipients of double versus single autologous HCT (207). The beneficial effect of the second HCT was seen mainly in patients with less than a VGPR to the first autologous HCT. Cavo et al. reported on 321 patients, randomly assigned to receive either a single course of high-dose melphalan, 200 mg/m^2, or melphalan, 200 mg/m^2 followed, after 3 to 6 months by melphalan at 120 mg/m^2 and busulfan, 12 mg/kg (208). Patients in the tandem autologous HCT arm had a significantly increased probability of attaining at least a near complete response (nCR; 33% versus 47%, respectively; $p = .008$), prolonged relapse-free survival (median, 24 versus 42 months, respectively; $p < .001$), and prolonged EFS (EFS; median, 23 versus 35 months, respectively; $p = .001$). Tandem transplantations, however, failed to significantly prolong overall survival. The administration of a second transplantation and of novel agents to treat sequential relapses in up to 50% of patients randomly assigned to receive a single autologous HCT likely contributed to the prolonged survival duration of the whole group, whose 7-year rate (46%) was similar to that of the double autologous HCT group (43%; $p = .90$). Benefits offered by double autologous HCT were particularly evident among patients who failed at least nCR after one autologous HCT.

The potential shortcomings of the tandem approach are an increased duration of hospitalization and overall health care costs, and the potential lack of additional benefit for patients who had already achieved CR with a first autologous HCT. Based on the two randomized trials cited above, a patient who fails to achieve a VGPR after the first autologous HCT should be offered a second autologous transplantation.

At MD Anderson, we offer a single autologous HCT to all eligible patients after induction therapy regardless of their age. We use a preparative regimen of melphalan 200 mg/m^2 unless the patient is treated on a clinical trial for a novel preparative regimen. In selected patients (>70 years or dialysis-dependent), we lower the melphalan dose to 140 mg/m^2. As mentioned above, in view of recent data, we are offering maintenance therapy with lenalidomide, 10 to 15 mg daily, approximately 3 months after autologous HCT to most of our patients. We offer tandem autologous HCT only in the setting of a clinical trial, or if the patient has had significant residual disease after first autologous HCT. A second, salvage transplant is an option for patients with relapsed disease; we tend to offer this mainly to those patients whose benefit from transplant was >1 year and whose disease burden can be significantly reduced by salvage chemotherapy.

Allogeneic HCT

The curative potential of allogeneic HCT comes from a graft-versus-tumor effect and dose-intense therapy

rescued with a tumor-free graft. This latter observation is supported by the analysis of the syngeneic transplantation series reported to date (209). The existence of a graft-versus-myeloma effect was first documented by Tricot et al., and later confirmed in large single- and multi-institutional series of donor lymphocyte infusions (210-213).

Although high-dose therapy has been associated with high rates of nonrelapse mortality, the achievements of molecular remissions, as well as the lack of relapses in a significant proportion of patients who achieved CR after this therapy, suggest that this therapy is potentially curative (214). In order to overcome toxicity from high-dose regimens and to extend the applicability of this procedure to older patients with significant comorbidities, allogeneic HCT with reduced-intensity conditioning regimens has been attempted in patients with multiple myeloma.

Two prospective trials looking at the tandem autologous plus reduced-intensity allogeneic HCT approach as part of the initial therapy for multiple myeloma have reported conflicting results (215,216). Recently, the IFM group has reported on the outcomes of patients with high-risk disease (defined by high levels of beta-2 microglobulin or deletion of chromosome 13 as detected by FISH), who received an initial autologous HCT with melphalan, 200 mg/m^2. Sixty-five patients had an HLA-identical sibling donor, of which 46 received a reduced intensity conditioning regimen consisting of fludarabine, busulfan, and anti-thymocyte globulin (ATG). Patients without an HLA sibling donor received a second autologous HCT prepared with melphalan, 220 mg/m^2. On an intent-to-treat basis, the OS and the EFS did not differ significantly between the two groups (median 35 and 25 months in the allogeneic HCT patients versus 41 and 30 months in the autologous HCT patients). There was a trend toward a better OS in patients treated with tandem autologous HCT, (median 47.2 months versus 35 months, $p = .07$) for patients who actually received a reduced intensity allogeneic HCT (216). The Italian Cooperative Group performed a similar study reported by Bruno et al. After a median follow up of 3 years, nonrelapse mortality was 11% for the autologous-plus-allogeneic group versus 4% for the tandem autologous group ($p = .09$). CRs were significantly higher in the autologous-plus-allogeneic group than the tandem autologous group (46% versus 16%, $p = .0001$), as were OS (84% versus 62%, $p = .003$) and EFS (75% versus 41%, $p = .00008$) (215). A clinical trial sponsored by the Bone Marrow Transplant Clinical Trials Network (BMT CTN) has recently been concluded, and its findings should provide valuable information that will allow patients and physicians make informed decisions regarding this treatment option.

Our group at MD Anderson only performs reduced intensity allogeneic HCT. We use the tandem autologous + allogeneic HCT approach only in the setting of a clinical trial. Most of our allogeneic HCTs are offered to patients with relapsed, chemosensitive disease, who are younger than 70, have an HLA-identical sibling or unrelated donor, and are in good general physical condition. Our preparative regimen is a combination of fludarabine and melphalan (100 or 140 mg/m^2), with anti-thymocyte globulin added for unrelated donor HCT.

■ OTHER PLASMA CELL DYSCRASIAS

Other plasma cell dyscrasias include monoclonal gammopathy of unknown significance, solitary plasmacytoma of bone, asymptomatic myeloma, Waldenström macroglobulinemia, amyloidosis, and immunoglobulin heavy-chain diseases.

MONOCLONAL GAMMOPATHY OF UNKNOWN SIGNIFICANCE

Monoclonal gammopathy of unknown significance (MGUS), or benign monoclonal gammopathy, occurs in 3.2% of normal individuals older than 50 years (217). This disorder is defined by the presence of a monoclonal paraprotein of <3g/dL, bone marrow biopsy with <10% plasma cells, and the absence of any clinically significant end-organ sequelae (boney lesions, renal insufficiency, hypercalcemia, or anemia) related to the paraprotein. The frequency of this disorder rises progressively with age and the risk of progression to clinically significant multiple myeloma is about 1% per year (218). Furthermore, recent evidence suggests that nearly all patients with symptomatic myeloma had a preceding MGUS (219).

Initial evaluation of a patient with MGUS should include complete blood count, serum chemistries, serum and urine electrophoresis (with immunofixation), serum free light-chain assay, quantitative immunoglobulins, and bone survey. Risk factors for these patients predict disease course and include abnormal serum free light-chain ratio, non-immunoglobulin G (IgG) MGUS, and an elevated serum M protein ≥15g/L. In one study, progression to clinically significant disease occurred in 58% of patients with all 3 risk factors, 37% with two risk factors present, 21% with one risk factor present, and 5% with none of the risk factors present (220).

Based on this data, a patient with any of these risk factors should undergo bone marrow biopsy at initial evaluation.

Though MGUS itself does not require treatment, it is a harbinger of future clinically significant disease and requires close follow-up. Patients with IgG or IgA MGUS are at risk for developing a plasma cell disorder such as multiple myeloma, primary amyloidosis, or plasma cell leukemia. Those with IgM MGUS may develop a lymphoproliferative disorder, such as Waldenström macroglobulinemia.

In a study of 1384 patients with MGUS, 115 (22%) developed MM, macroglobulinemia, amyloidosis, or another malignant lymphoproliferative disorder (median follow-up, 15.4 years) (218). The cumulative probability of progression was 10% at 10 years, 21% at 20 years, and 26% at 25 years. For patients who developed MM, the course of the disease and the response to therapy were similar to those of other patients treated promptly after diagnosis. This study demonstrates that MGUS usually does not progress to a malignant disorder. The long period of stability supports the value of indefinite periodic observation for such patients. Based on the above data, patients with the aforementioned three risk factors should be followed at least annually while those with no risk factors can likely be followed less frequently (221). Patients with one to two risk factors should be followed regularly at the discretion of the provider. At MD Anderson we follow these guidelines, though the bulk of our patients have progressed beyond MGUS at the time of their initial evaluation here.

SOLITARY PLASMACYTOMA OF BONE

A solitary plasmacytoma of bone is defined by the presence of a plasmacytoma without bone marrow evidence of monoclonal plasma cells, lytic bony lesions, or other clinically significant sequelae of multiple myeloma. Approximately 5% of patients with plasma cell disorders have a solitary plasmacytoma of bone (222) and approximately 24 to 72% demonstrate a monoclonal protein in serum or urine (223). MRI may reveal abnormalities not detected by bone survey and may cause patients who were previously classified as having solitary plasmacytoma to be staged upward to MM (224). Initial workup should include all of the aforementioned serum and urine laboratory studies used in evaluation of multiple myeloma. In addition, an MRI of the spine and pelvis is recommended to rule out other high-risk sites of disease. Treatment should include radiation therapy of at least 40 Gy, though for lesions greater than 5 cm one may consider a dose of up to 50 Gy (222). At MD Anderson we treat lesions less than 5cm with 45 Gy and we treat lesions greater than 5cm with 50 Gy. After radiation we perform a complete serological staging and full imaging. If there is residual paraprotein or other signs of active myeloma, we follow the algorithm for primary treatment of myeloma. If there is no further disease activity, we follow the patient closely, initially every 3 months and then less frequently per the discretion of the clinician.

While there is no evidence to support the use of adjuvant chemotherapy for solitary plasmacytomas that are not responding to radiation therapy, the role of bisphosphonates in currently under investigation. Patients with solitary plasmacytoma of bone often progress to MM within 2 to 4 years (225), with a median OS of 7.5 to 12 years (223). As mentioned, when disease progression does occur, treatment algorithms should follow those detailed above for multiple myeloma.

ASYMPTOMATIC MYELOMA

Asymptomatic (smoldering) myeloma is defined as having a serum IgG or IgA monoclonal protein of ≥3.0 g/dL and/or ≥10% more plasma cells in the bone marrow without evidence of end-organ damage. In comparison with MGUS, this premyeloma condition appears to carry a higher risk of progression to overt disease with median time to progression of 2-5 years (226,227). In one study of 279 patients with asymptomatic myeloma over a 26-year period, the risk of progression to myeloma was 10% per year for the first 5 years, 3% per year for the next 5 years, and 1% per year for the last 10 years. In this study the cumulative probability of progression was 73% at 15 years (227).

Similar to MGUS, the risk for disease progression depends on several factors which reflect burden of disease, most notably bone marrow involvement by plasma cells of ≥10% and serum monoclonal protein of ≥3 g/dL. A recent prognostic model was developed using these criteria: at 15 years, 87% of patients with both risk factors progressed to myeloma or amyloidosis, while 70% of patients with ≥10% bone marrow plasma cells (but monoclonal protein of <3 g/dL) and 39% of patients with monoclonal protein of ≥3 g/dL (but <10% bone marrow plasma cells) progressed ($p < .001$) (227). More recently, serum free light chains have been suggested as an independent prognostic factor for disease progression and have been incorporated to this prognostic model (228). In addition, cytogenetic abnormalities may also be emerging as an independent prognostic factor (229), though larger studies are needed to confirm this.

As with MGUS, active treatment for asymptomatic myeloma is currently not recommended. A 2003 meta-analysis examined the effect of early versus deferred (at progression) chemotherapy (230). The analysis included three randomized trials with a total of 262 patients. The conclusions of this study were that early treatment delayed disease progression (odds ratio of 0.16, 95% CI 0.09-0.29), but did not impact mortality or response rate. It should be noted that the therapies offered in these clinical trials were melphalan-based and thus did not incorporate novel agents. Because of the significant activity of thalidomide in refractory myeloma, thalidomide-dexamethasone has been studied in patients with asymptomatic myeloma (151,231). ORR in these trials ranged between 64% and 73% but given the long period of disease stability for asymptomatic disease, any impact on time to progression or survival will take many years to determine. In a multicenter, randomized trial comparing zoledronic acid versus observation in patients with asymptomatic myeloma, the monthly use of zoledronic acid for 1 year reduced the development of skeletal-related events when patients progressed, but did not impact TTP or development of nonskeletal complications of disease (232).

In summary, because of the high risk of developing multiple myeloma, particularly in the time most immediate to diagnosis, clinical evaluation every 4 months is recommended (226). Since early treatment of asymptomatic patients with other agents has not previously improved survival, use of thalidomide and other agents in asymptomatic disease should be restricted to clinical trials until the benefits and long-term side effects are established.

The MD Anderson Approach

At MD Anderson, we tend to follow patients with asymptomatic myeloma very closely, at 2 to 3 months intervals. Patients with high-risk cytogenetics may need more frequent follow-up. In addition we obtain an MRI of the spine based on our findings that patients with an abnormal MRI had a significantly shorter time to progression of disease.

WALDENSTRÖM MACROGLOBULINEMIA

Waldenström macroglobulinemia (WM) is an uncommon, low-grade lymphoid malignancy composed of mature plasmacytoid lymphocytes with monoclonal IgM production (233). It usually affects older persons and may cause symptoms due to tumor infiltration (marrow, lymph nodes, and/or spleen), circulating IgM (hyperviscosity, cryoglobulinemia, and/or cold agglutinin anemia), and tissue deposition of IgM (neuropathy, glomerular disease, and/or amyloidosis). With hyperviscosity syndrome, patients may have visual disturbances, dizziness, cardiopulmonary symptoms, decreased consciousness,

Waldenström Macroglobulinemia-Initial Workup and Indications for Treatment.

Initial work-up at MD Anderson
- History and physical
- CBC, differential and platelets
- BUN, creatinine, electrolyte
- Quantitative immunoglobulins
- Serum protein electrophoresis (SPEP), serum immunofixation electrophoresis (SIFE), urine immunofixation electrophoresis (UIFE)
- Liver function tests
- Serum viscosity
- Hepatitis serology
- Cryocrit
- Cold agglutinins
- PT/PTT
- Unilateral bone marrow aspirate and biopsy
- Chest x-ray
- Chest/abdominal/pelvis CT

Indications for treatment:
- Symptomatic hyperviscosity (eye grounds, neurologic changes)
- Anemia (Hgb less than 10 g/dL), pancytopenia (due to marrow involvement/hypersplenism)
- Bulky adenopathy
- Symptomatic organomegaly
- Symptomatic cryoglobulinemia

FIGURE 11-8. Waldenström macroglobulinemia: initial workup and indications for treatment.

and a bleeding diathesis. Neuropathy usually is caused by an IgM antibody reacting with a myelin-associated glycoprotein (MAG) and can be treated with rituximab (single-agent or as part of a combination regimen, as detailed below).

Initial evaluation (Fig. 11-8) of the patient suspected of having WM should include a complete blood count, serum chemistries, liver function tests, hepatitis serology, serum protein electrophoresis (SPEP), beta-2 microglobulin, serum viscosity level, and quantitative immunoglobulin levels. Patients who may have cryoglobulinemia should have a warm bath collection to assess serum IgM levels. Patients can also present with cold or warm autoimmune hemolytic anemia, iron deficiency anemia or dilutional anemia. A bone marrow biopsy can help determine the cause of an existing anemia and demonstrate infiltration by lymphoplasmacytic cells. Flow cytometry will typically show a pattern of sIgM⁺, CD19⁺, CD20⁺, CD22⁺, CD79⁺ (234). Patients should also have baseline CT scans of the chest, abdomen, and pelvis to evaluate the presence of extramedullary disease. Finally, an ophthalmologic examination should be obtained for patients with suspected hyperviscosity syndrome to evaluate retinal changes (235).

Asymptomatic patients (those without anemia, thrombocytopenia, bulky lymphadenopathy, hyperviscosity,

peripheral neuropathy, amyloidosis, cyroglybulinemia, cold-agglutinin disease) can be observed closely. These patients can be followed every 3 months with longer follow-up intervals after the first year if their disease is stable. One study suggests that the risk of developing symptomatic disease is approximately 4% per year (236). In this study, IgM levels, hemoglobin, and gender were each associated with risk of progression. At MD Anderson, therapy is initiated for symptomatic hyperviscosity (eye grounds, neurologic changes), anemia (Hgb <10 g/dL), pancytopenia (due to marrow involvement/hypersplenism), bulky adenopathy, symptomatic organomegaly, or symptomatic cryoglobulinemia.

Therapy for hyperviscosity consists of plasmapheresis followed by chemotherapy to control the malignant proliferation. Like myeloma, one may want to avoid oral alkylators or nucleoside analogs for patients who are eligible for stem cell transplantation. Cyclophosphamide-containing regimens include R-CHOP, R-CVP, and R-cyclophosphamide-dexamethasone and may be an alternative in the up-front setting. ORR with these regimens ranges from 77 to 96% (237-240). Thalidomide-rituximab is also an option with one study showing an ORR of 70% and a median PFS of 3 years (241). Rituximab may be used as a single agent for patients with less aggressive disease and, in various dosing durations has yielded and ORR between 20-50% (235).

For those patients who are candidates for nucleoside analog therapy, options include fludarabine and 2-chlorodeoxyadenosine (2-CdA, cladribine)-containing regimens. Single agent fludarabine has demonstrated activity, with a 10-year EFS rate of 20% (242). Fludarabine-rituximab has also been studied; a trial by the WMCTG demonstrated an ORR of 96% and median PFS of 51.2 months (243). Cladribine alone or in combination with prednisone, cyclophsphamide, or rituximab, yielded an ORR of 60 to 94% in 90 previously untreated patients (222). Preliminary data from 18 previously untreated WM patients who received a combination of cladribine, cyclophosphamide, and rituximab shows an ORR of 94% with a median duration of response of 58.6 months (244). Another, newer option for initial treatment is bortezomib-dexamethasone-rituximab (BDR). In a recent phase II trial conducted by the Waldenström macroglobulineamia clinical trials Group (WMCTG), the ORR to BDR was 96%, including a CR rate of 22% (245). Though rituximab is often a part of the treatment regimen, it should be used with caution in patients with highly elevated IgM levels, due to the potential for a rituximab-mediated IgM flare. In these cases it may be most prudent to avoid rituximab for the first one or two cycles. At MD Anderson we prefer either bortezomib-based or 2-CdA–based chemotherapy with rituximab. We collect stem cells from patients before they receive nucleoside analogs.

For relapsed WM, patients may be re-treated with a previously successful regimen, if they are more than 2 years from initial treatment. With a shorter disease-free-interval, one may consider the other first-line regimens detailed above. Patients who have been treated with several different regimens may also be considered for alemtuzumab, as WM cells express CD52 (246,247). In a study of alemtuzumab and rituximab in 28 previously treated patients with lymphoplasmacytic lymphoma or WM, the ORR was 76% (248). As mentioned, bortezomib is active in WM. A multicenter trial of this single agent in 27 relapsed/refractory WM patients demonstrated an ORR of 85% with median TTP of 7.9 months (249). For progressive disease, we recommend a clinical trial (including trials of transplant, see below). Otherwise, we recommend treatment with agents not initially used (alkylators, bortezomib, monoclonal antibodies). We have also used thalidomide- or lenalidomide-based therapy in this setting.

The role of stem cell transplantation in WM is still being defined. A retrospective review of 201 WM patients (14% of who had relapsed or refractory disease) treated with high-dose chemotherapy and autologous stem cell transplantation (auto-SCT) found a 5-year PFS and OS of 33% and 61%, respectively (250). Several groups have also studied allogeneic SCT in WM. Overall, there appears to be some evidence for a graft-versus-tumor effect, with 5-year PFS between 48% and 61% but with a notable treatment-related mortality (251).

Based on the above data, the Consensus Panel from the Fourth International Workshop on Waldenström Macroglobulinemia has made the following recommendations: for up-front treatment, one may choose a combination of rituximab and alkylators and/or nucleoside analogues, depending on auto-SCT eligibility. Thalidomide and rituximab may also be used. For salvage therapy one can reuse previously active therapies or move on to a new combination of agents recommended for first-line treatment. In addition, one may also consider bortezomib, alemtuzumab, and auto- or allo-SCT (251). Given the recent promising data with bortezomib in the front-line setting, this agent may eventually be recommended in for initial treatment of WM.

AMYLOIDOSIS

Amyloidosis (AL) is a plasma cell proliferative process that results from organ deposition of amyloid fibrils that consist of the NH_2-terminal amino acid residues of the variable portion of the light-chain immunoglobulin molecule (252). This disease occurs in 10% of patients with MM and may produce nephrotic syndrome, cardiomyopathy, hepatomegaly, neuropathy, macroglossia, anemia, carpal tunnel syndrome, and periorbital purpura. Serum immunoelectrophoresis shows a monoclonal immunoglobulin in serum or urine in 89% of patients with amyloidosis; lambda light chains are noted more frequently than kappa light chains. Diagnosis can be made in many patients by a Congo red–stained sample of bone marrow, subcutaneous fat aspirate, or rectal biopsy that exhibits apple-green birefringence with polarized light (Fig.11-5) (252).

The median survival is approximately 25 months for all patients (253), and the presence of congestive heart failure, renal failure, hepatomegaly, and/or significant weight loss worsens the prognosis. In a study of 147 patients with primary amyloidosis, factors associated with a poor prognosis were peripheral blood plasma cell count >500,000/L, circulating plasma cell percentage >1%, beta-2 microglobulin ≥2.7 μg/mL, bone marrow plasma cell percentage >10%, and significant cardiac involvement (232). In addition, elevated NT-pro-BNP (a cleavage by-product of the prohormone pro-brain natriuetic peptide) and cardiac troponin T levels have also been found to have an adverse effect on prognosis (253,254). More recently, a prognostic model has been developed which includes uric acid >8.0 mg/dL, NT-pro-BNP >332 ng/L, and troponin T >0.035 microg/L. This model is based on a study of 1977 patients, including 293 patients who had undergone SCT (255).

According to the National Comprehensive Cancer Network (NCCN) the optimal therapy for amyloidosis is still under investigation and therefore, a clinical trial should be considered for all patients with this disease. Otherwise, one may choose between variations of melphalan-prednisone, dexamethasone-interferon alpha, or regimens containing the newer agents thalidomide, lenalidomide, or bortezomib (256). In one study, treatment with melphalan and high-dose dexamethasone yielded an ORR of 67% and 5-year PFS and OS of 33% and 67%, respectively (257). As in the case of myeloma, this regimen is reserved for patients who are not candidates for SCT.

A SWOG study of dexamethasone-interferon alpha demonstrated a CR rate of 24% and median OS of 31 months. Because of its success in myeloma, thalidomide-dexamethasone (TD) has also been tried. In a study of 31 relapsed or refractory patients, 48% of patients responded to this combination (258). In another study of patients with advanced amyloidosis, the addition of cyclophosphamide to TD yielded an ORR of 74% with a median OS of 41 months (259). Of note, one must exercise caution in using thalidomide-based regimens, as the risk of peripheral neuropathy is significant in patients with amyloidosis. Lenalidomide-dexamethasone has also been studied with ORR ranging between 43 and 67% (260,261).

The role of SCT is still being investigated. One randomized trial which compared SCT to conventional chemotherapy (melphalan-prednisone) suggested that there was no benefit of SCT (262). However, a significant proportion of the patients in this study had involvement of at least three organ systems and therefore may have had a worse outcome. When employed in a more selective manner, auto-SCT may be beneficial, especially in patients with less advanced disease. For example, in one study of 312 patients who had adequate cardiopulmonary status and underwent auto-SCT, the CR rate was 40%, with a median survival of 4.6 years (263). A case-controlled study compared similarly highly-selected patients who underwent auto-SCT versus those who did not and found a significant survival advantage for the auto-SCT group (264). A recent meta-analysis of high-dose chemotherapy and auto-SCT for primary systemic amyloidosis reviewed 12 studies and concluded that auto-SCT was not superior to conventional chemotherapy for amyloidosis (265). However the authors of this study admitted that the number of high-quality studies is limited and therefore, this conclusion will have to be verified with more randomized controlled trials.

Finally, the benefits of high-dose chemotherapy must be balanced against the potential risks of this procedure in a relatively ill population. The treatment-related mortality for auto-SCT in amyloidosis has thus been reported to be 11% to 25% in various studies (266). In summary, there is likely a benefit of auto-SCT for selected patients with adequate organ function. However, in the absence of phase III trials to support this claim, auto-SCT is best performed within the framework of a clinical trial.

At MD Anderson we are moving toward treatment with bortezomib-based regimens for patients with symptomatic amyloidosis. For patients with significant neuropathy, lenalidomide can also be an option. If the patients are transplant candidates we do offer this option and consider maintenance therapy (as detailed above) in the transplant setting.

IMMUNOGLOBULIN HEAVY-CHAIN DISEASE

Heavy-chain diseases are plasma cell dyscrasias characterized by the production of heavy-chain immunoglobulin

molecules (gamma, alpha, mu) that lack light chains. Alpha-chain disease is the most common variant and can be thought of as an extranodal marginal-zone lymphoma of mucosa-associated lymph-node tissue. The disease results from lymphocyte and plasma cell infiltration of the mesenteric nodes and small bowel and has features of malabsorption, such as diarrhea, weight loss, abdominal pain, edema, and clubbing. The heavy-chain molecule may be detected in serum, jejunal secretions, and urine (267). These patients may be treated with antibiotics or occasionally surgery. If symptoms persist or if a lymphoma is suspected, chemotherapy may be used.

Gamma heavy-chain disease is similar to lymphoplasmacytoid non-Hodgkin lymphoma (268). Patients may present with fever, weakness, lymphadenopathy, hepatosplenomegaly, and Waldeyer right involvement. Eosinophilia, leukopenia, and thrombocytopenia are common. Treatment with regimens similar to those used for non-Hodgkin lymphoma may be effective (267).

Mu heavy-chain disease is extremely rare and is often seen in patients with chronic lymphocytic leukemia, though it has been described in patients with underlying Waldenström's macroglobulinemia or myeloma (269). Vacuolated plasma cells are common in the marrow, and many patients have lambda light chains in urine. Though no standard treatment is recommended, therapy choice should follow existing recommendations for the underlying primary disease.

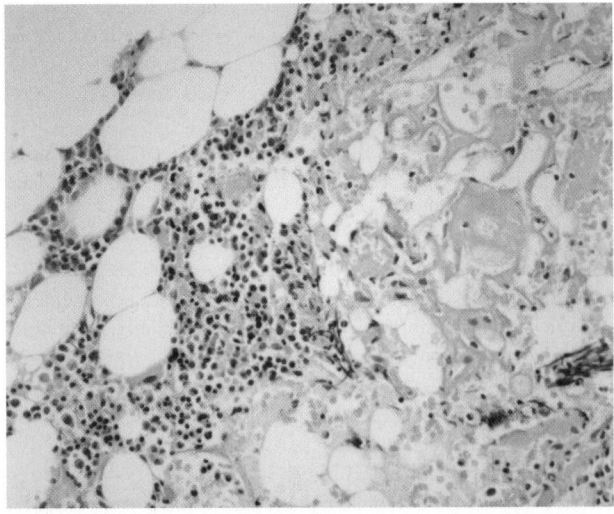

FIGURE 11-9. Amyloid deposits in the bone marrow medullary space (Congo red stain). The amorphous material is apple-green birefringent when viewed with polarized light.

■ CONCLUSION

There have been many recent advances in the understanding of plasma cell dyscrasias. The origin of myeloma from a primordial stem cell is suggested by the phenotypic expression of early precursors. Various cytokines are produced that may serve as myeloma cell growth factors or osteoclast-activating factors.

Better understanding of the prognostic factors of myeloma, markers of drug resistance (ie, LDH and chromosome 13 deletion), and measures of tumor cell mass (ie, β_2M) has helped to identify patients who may benefit from novel therapeutic approaches. Recently, the addition of several novel therapeutic agents—including thalidomide, bortezomib, and ImiDs—have added new hope for an improved survival in MM. In addition, synergy of new and old agents, despite prior resistance, and myeloablative therapy with autologous stem cell support, provide many options for effective treatment of MM.

Waldenström macroglobulinemia and mu heavy-chain disease have been treated with alkylating agents, but cladribine appears promising for superior long-term results. Further studies are needed to understand the etiology and biology of plasma cell dyscrasias, in order to develop more effective agents and regimens for controlling these disorders and to justify immunologic and other procedures for sustaining long-term control.

Reference

1. The International Myeloma Working Group: Criteria for the classification of monoclonal gammopathies, multiple myeloma and related disorders: A report of the International Myeloma Working Group. *Br J Hematol* 2003;121:749-757.
2. American Cancer Society. Cancer Facts and Figures 2009. Atlanta, GA: 2009.
3. Horner MJ, Ries LA. RL, Krapcho M, et al. (eds). SEER Cancer Statistics Review, 1975-2006. Bethesda, MD: National Cancer Institute; 2009.
4. Riedel DA, Pottern LM. The epidemiology of multiple myeloma. *Hematol Oncol Clin North Am* 1992;6:225-247.
5. Preston DL, Kusumi S, Tomonaga M, et al. Cancer incidence in atomic bomb survivors. Part III. Leukemia, lymphoma and multiple myeloma, 1950-1987. *Radiat Res* 1994;137: S68-S97.
6. Lewis EB. Leukemia, Multiple Myeloma, and Aplastic Anemia In American Radiologists. *Science* 1963;142:1492-1494.
7. Stebbings JH, Lucas HF, Stehney AF. Mortality from cancers of major sites in female radium dial workers. *Am J Ind Med* 1984;5:435-459.
8. Boffetta P, Stellman SD, SS, Garfinkel L, et al. A case control study of multiple myeloma in the American Cancer Society prospective study. *Int J Cancer* 1989;43:554-559.

9. Rinsky RA, Hornung RW, Silver SR, et al. Benzene exposure and hematopoietic mortality: A long-term epidemiologic risk assessment. *Am J Ind Med* 2002;42:474-480.
10. Bergsagel DE, Wong O, Bergsagel PL, et al. Benzene and multiple myeloma: appraisal of the scientific evidence. *Blood* 1999;94:1174-1182.
11. Lynch HT, Ferrara K, Barlogie B, et al. Familial myeloma. *N Engl J Med* 2008;359:152-157.
12. Kristinsson SY, Bjorkholm M, Goldin LR, et al. Patterns of hematologic malignancies and solid tumors among 37,838 first-degree relatives of 13,896 patients with multiple myeloma in Sweden. *Int J Cancer* 2009;125:2147-2150.
13. Ogmundsdottir HM, Haraldsdottirm V, Johannesson GM, et al. Familiality of benign and malignant paraproteinemias. A population-based cancer-registry study of multiple myeloma families. *Haematologica* 2005;90:66-71.
14. Bourguet CC, Grufferman S, Delzell E, et al. Multiple myeloma and family history of cancer. A case-control study. *Cancer* 1985;56:2133-2139.
15. Durie BG, Salmon SE. A clinical staging system for multiple myeloma. Correlation of measured myeloma cell mass with presenting clinical features, response to treatment, and survival. *Cancer* 1975;36:842-854.
16. Greipp P, San Miguel J, Fonseca R, et al. Development of an international prognostic index for myeloma: Report of the international myeloma working group (abstr). *Eur J Hematol* 2004;4:s42.
17. Alexanian R, Barlogie B, Fritsche H. Beta 2 microglobulin in multiple myeloma. *Am J Hematol* 1985;20:345-351.
18. Bataille R, Durie BG, Grenier J, Sany J. Prognostic factors and staging in multiple myeloma: a reappraisal. *J Clin Oncol* 1986;4:80-87.
19. Bataille R, Harousseau JL. Multiple myeloma. *N Engl J Med* 1997;336:1657-1664.
20. Greenlee RT, Murray T, Bolden S, Wingo PA. Cancer statistics, 2000. *CA Cancer J Clin* 2000;50:7-33.
21. Chiecchio L DG, White HE, Towsend MR, et al. Frequent upregulation of MYC in plasma cell leukemia. *Genes Chromosomes Cancer* 2009;48:624-636.
22. Bergsagel PL, Kuehl WM. Chromosome translocations in multiple myeloma. *Oncogene* 2991:20:5611-5622.
23. Liebisch P, Dohner H. Cytogenetics and molecular cytogenetics in multiple myeloma. *Eur J Cancer* 2006;42: 1520-1529.
24. Hideshima T, Bergsagel PL, Kuehl WM, Anderson KC. Advances in biology of multiple myeloma: clinical applications. *Blood* 2004;104:607-618.
25. Avet-Loiseau H, Facon T, Grosbois B, et al: Intergroupe Francophone du Myélome. Oncogenesis of multiple myeloma: 14q32 and 13q chromosomal abnormalities are not randomly distributed, but correlate with natural history, immunological features, and clinical presentation. *Blood* 2002;99: 2185-2191.
26. Kaufmann H, Ackerman J, Baldia C, et al. Both IGH translocations and chromosome 13q deletions are early events in monoclonal gammopathy of undetermined significance and do not evolve during transition to multiple myeloma. *Leukemia* 2004;18:1879-1882.
27. Fonseca R, Bergsagel P, Drach J, et al. International Myeloma Working Group molecular classification of multiple myeloma: spotlight review. *Leukemia* 2009;23:2210-2221.

28. Rasillo A, Tabernero D, Sánchez ML, et al. Fluorescence in situ hybridization analysis of aneuploidization patterns in monoclonal gammopathy of undetermined significance versus multiple myeloma and plasma cell leukemia. *Cancer* 2003;97: 601-609.

29. Chesi M, Kuehl W, Bergsagel PL. Recurrent immunoglobulin gene translocations identify distinct molecular subtypes of myeloma. *Ann Oncol* 2000;11:131-135.

30. Terpos E, Eleutherakis-Papaiakovou V, Dimopoulos MA. Clinical implications of chromosomal abnormalities in multiple myeloma. *Leuk Lymphoma* 2006;47:803-814.

31. Chng WJ, Glebov O, Bergsagel PL, et al. Genetic events in the pathogenesis of multiple myeloma. *Best Pract Res Clin Haematol* 2007;20:571-596.

32. Tasaka T, Berenson J, Vescio R, et al. Analysis of the p16INK4A, p15INK4B and p18INK4C genes in multiple myeloma. *Br J Haematol* 1997;96:98-102.

33. Chen Kiang S. Cell-cycle control of plasma cell differentiation and tumorigenesis. *Immunol Rev* 2003;194:39-47.

34. Intini D, Agnelli L, Ciceri G, et al. Relevance of Ras gene mutations in the context of the molecular heterogeneity of multiple myeloma. *Hematol Oncol* 2007;25:6-10.

35. Kastrinakis NG, Gorgoulis VG, Foukas PG, et al. Molecular aspects of multiple myeloma. *Ann Oncol* 2000;11:1217-1228.

36. Avet Loiseau H. Role of genetics in prognostication in myeloma. *Best Pract Res Clin Haematol* 2007;20:625-635.

37. Chang H, Qi X, Jiang A, et al. 1p21 deletions are strongly associated with 1q21 gains and are an independent adverse prognostic factor for the outcome of high-dose chemotherapy in patients with multiple myeloma. *Bone Marrow Transplant* 2010;45:117-121.

38. Chang H, Ning, Y, Qi X, et al. Chromosome 1p21 deletion is a novel prognostic marker in patients with multiple myeloma. *Br J Haematol* 2007;139:51-54.

39. San Miguel JF, Gutierrez NC, Mateo G, et al. Review. Conventional diagnostics in multiple myeloma. *Eur J Cancer* 2006 Jul;42(11):1510-1519.

40. Chng WJ, Winkler JM, Greipp PR, et al. Ploidy status rarely changes in myeloma patients at disease progression. *Leuk Res* 2006;30:266-271.

41. Chng WJ, Van Wier SA, Ahmann GJ, et al. A validated FISH trisomy index demonstrates the hyperdiploid and nonhyperdiploid dichotomy in MGUS. *Blood* 2005;106: 2156-2161.

42. Kyle RA, Rajkumar SV. Monoclonal gammopathy of undetermined significance. *Br J Haematol* 2006;134:573-589.

43. Tabernero D, San Miguel JF, Garcia-Sanz M, et al. Incidence of chromosome numerical changes in multiple myeloma: fluorescence in situ hybridization analysis using 15 chromosome-specific probes. *Am J Pathol* 1996;149:153-161.

44. Liebisch P, Dohner H. Cytogenetics and molecular cytogenetics in multiple myeloma. *Eur J Cancer* 2006;42: 1520-1520.

45. Debes-Marun CS, Dewald GW, Bryant S, et al. Chromosome abnormalities clustering and its implications for pathogenesis and prognosis in myeloma. *Leukemia* 2003;17: 427-436.

46. Rafael Fonseca, Carina S. Debes-Marun, Elisa B. Picken, et al. The recurrent IgH translocations are highly associated with nonhyperdiploid variant multiple myeloma. *Blood* 2003; 102:2562-2567.

47. Shaughnessy J, Jr., Gabrea A, Qi Y, et al. Cyclin D3 at 6p21 is dysregulated by recurrent chromosomal translocations to immunoglobulin loci in multiple myeloma. *Blood* 2001;98: 217-223.

48. van Stralen E, van de Wetering M, Agnelli L, et al. Identification of primary MAFB target genes in multiple myeloma. *Exp Hematol* 2009;37:78-86.

49. Stralen E, Leguit RJ, Begthel H, et al. MafB oncoprotein detected by immunohistochemistry as a highly sensitive and specific marker for the prognostic unfavorable t(14;20) (q32;q12) in multiple myeloma patients. *Leukemia* 2009; 23:801-803.

50. Bergsagel PL, Kuehl WM. Molecular pathogenesis and a consequent classification of multiple myeloma. *J Clin Oncol* 2005;23:6333-6338.

51. Petersen HH, Hilpert J, Jacobsen C, et al. Low-density lipoprotein receptor-related protein interacts with MafB, a regulator of hindbrain development. *FEBS Lett* 2004;565:23-27.

52. Natkunam Y, Tedoldi S, Paterson JC, et al. Characterization of c-Maf transcription factor in normal and neoplastic hematolymphoid tissue and its relevance in plasma cell neoplasia. *Am J Clin Pathol* 2009;132:361-371.

53. Aziz A, Soucie E, Sarrazin S, et al. MafB/c-Maf deficiency enables self-renewal of differentiated functional macrophages. *Science* 2009;326:867-871.

54. Avet-Loiseau H, Li JY, Morineau N, et al. Monosomy 13 is associated with the transition of monoclonal gammopathy of undetermined significance to multiple myeloma. Intergroupe Francophone du Myelome. *Blood* 1999;94:2583-2589.

55. Fonseca R, Oken MM, Harrington D, et al. Deletions of chromosome 13 in multiple myeloma identified by interphase FISH usually denote large deletions of the q arm or monosomy. *Leukemia* 2001;15:981-986.

56. Lennon PA, Zhuang Y, Pierson D, et al. Bacterial artificial chromosome array-based comparative genomic hybridization using paired formalin-fixed, paraffin-embedded and fresh frozen tissue specimens in multiple myeloma. *Cancer* 2009; 115:345-354.

57. Hanamura I, Stewart JP, Huang Y, et al. Frequent gain of chromosome band 1q21 in plasma-cell dyscrasias detected by fluorescence in situ hybridization: incidence increases from MGUS to relapsed myeloma and is related to prognosis and disease progression following tandem stem-cell transplantation. *Blood* 2006;108:1724-1732.

58. Kastrinakis NG, Gorgoulis, VG, Foukas PG, et al. Molecular aspects of multiple myeloma. *Ann Oncol* 2000;11:1217-1228.

59. Kumar V, Varma N, Varma S, et al. Flow cytometric analysis of DNA indices, expression of p53 and multidrug resistance genes in multiple myeloma patients. *Anal Quant Cytol Histol* 2004;26:271-277.

60. Chng WJ, Kuehl WM, Bergsagel PL, et al. Translocation t(4;14) retains prognostic significance even in the setting of high-risk molecular signature. *Leukemia* 2008;22: 459-461.

61. Jaksic W, Trudel S, Chang H, et al. Clinical outcomes in t(4;14) multiple myeloma: a chemotherapy-sensitive disease characterized by rapid relapse and alkylating agent resistance. *J Clin Oncol* 2005;23:7069-7073.

62. Fonseca R, Bergsagel PL, Drach J, et al. International Myeloma Working Group molecular classification of multiple myeloma: spotlight review. *Leukemia* 2009;23: 2210-2221.

63. Bergsagel PL, Kuehl WM. Chromosome translocations in multiple myeloma. *Oncogene* 2001;20:5611-5622.

64. Kumar V, Varma N, Varma S, et al. Flow cytometric analysis of DNA indices, expression of p53 and multidrug resistance genes in multiple myeloma patients. *Anal Quant Cytol Histol* 2004;26:271-277.

65. Takimoto M, Ogawa K, Kato Y, et al. Close relation between 14q32/IGH translocations and chromosome 13 abnormalities in multiple myeloma: a high incidence of 11q13/CCND1 and 16q23/MAF. *Int J Hematol* 2008;87:260-265.

66. Yeung J, Chang H. Genomic aberrations and immunohisto-chemical markers as prognostic indicators in multiple myeloma. *J Clin Pathol* 2008;61:832-836.

67. Terpos E, Cibeira MT, Blade J, et al. Management of complications in multiple myeloma. *Semin Hematol* 2009;46:176-189.

68. Sezer O, Heider U, Zavrski I, et al. RANK ligand and osteoprotegerin in myeloma bone disease. *Blood* 2003;101:2094-2098.

69. Berenson JR, Lichtenstein A, Porter L, et al. Efficacy of pamidronate in reducing skeletal events in patients with advanced multiple myeloma. Myeloma Aredia Study Group. *N Engl J Med* 1996;334:488-493.

70. Berenson JR. New advances in the biology and treatment of myeloma bone disease. *Semin Hematol* 2001;38:15-20.

71. Chang JT, Green L, Beitz J. Renal failure with the use of zoledronic acid. *N Engl J Med* 2003;349:1676-1679; discussion 1676-1679.

72. Ruggiero SL, Mehrotra B, Rosenberg TJ, et al. Osteonecrosis of the jaws associated with the use of bisphosphonates: a review of 63 cases. *J Oral Maxillofac Surg* 2004;62:527-534.

73. Kyle RA, Yee GC, Somerfield MR, et al. American Society of Clinical Oncology 2007 clinical practice guideline update on the role of bisphosphonates in multiple myeloma. *J Clin Oncol* 2007;25:2464-2472.

74. Dimopoulos M, Terpos E, Comenzo RL, et al. International myeloma working group consensus statement and guidelines regarding the current role of imaging techniques in the diagnosis and monitoring of multiple Myeloma. *Leukemia* 2009;23:1545-1556.

75. Edelstyn GA, Gillespie PJ, Grebbell FS. The radiological demonstration of osseous metastases. Experimental observations. *Clin Radiol* 1967;18:158-162.

76. Alexanian R, Dimopoulos MA. Management of multiple myeloma. *Semin Hematol* 1995;32:20-30.

77. Berenson JR, Pflugmacher R, Jarzem P, et al. Final Results of the First Randomized Trial Comparing Balloon Kyphoplasty (BKP) to Non-Surgical Management Among Cancer Patients with Vertebral Compression Fractures: Marked Improvement in Back Function, Quality of Life and Pain in the BKP Arm. *Blood* (ASH Annual Meeting Abstracts) 2009;114:2873.

78. Johnson WJ, Kyle RA, Pineda AA, et al. Treatment of renal failure associated with multiple myeloma. Plasmapheresis, hemodialysis, and chemotherapy. *Arch Intern Med* 1990;150:863-869.

79. Rota S, Mougenot B, Baudouin B, et al. Multiple myeloma and severe renal failure: a clinicopathologic study of outcome and prognosis in 34 patients. *Medicine (Baltimore)* 1987;66:126-137.

80. Alexanian R, Barlogie B, Dixon D. Renal failure in multiple myeloma. Pathogenesis and prognostic implications. *Arch Intern Med* 1990;150:1693-1695.

81. San-Miguel JF, Richardson PG, Sonneveld P, et al. Efficacy and safety of bortezomib in patients with renal impairment: results from the APEX phase 3 study. *Leukemia* 2008;22:842-849.

82. Chanan-Khan AA, Kaufman JL, Mehta J, et al. Activity and safety of bortezomib in multiple myeloma patients with advanced renal failure: a multicenter retrospective study. *Blood* 2007;109:2604-2606.

83. Ludwig H, Drach J, Graf H, et al. Reversal of acute renal failure by bortezomib-based chemotherapy in patients with multiple myeloma. *Haematologica* 2007;92:1411-1414.

84. Ludwig H, Fritz E, Kotzmann H, et al. Erythropoietin treatment of anemia associated with multiple myeloma. *N Engl J Med* 1990;322:1693-1699.

85. Smith RE, Jr., Aapro MS, Ludwig H, et al. Darbepoetin alpha for the treatment of anemia in patients with active cancer not receiving chemotherapy or radiotherapy: results of a phase III, multicenter, randomized, double-blind, placebo-controlled study. *J Clin Oncol* 2008;26:1040-1050.

86. Savage DG, Lindenbaum J, Garrett TJ. Biphasic pattern of bacterial infection in multiple myeloma. *Ann Intern Med* 1982;96:47-50.

87. Fahey JL, Scoggins R, Utz JP, et al. Infection, Antibody Response And Gamma Globulin Components In Multiple Myeloma And Macroglobulinemia. *Am J Med* 1963;35:698-707.

88. MacGregor RR, Negendank WG, Schreiber AD. Impaired granulocyte adherence in multiple myeloma: relationship to complement system, granulocyte delivery, and infection. *Blood* 1978;51:591-599.

89. Chen Y, Bhoopalam N, Yakulis V, et al. Changes in lymphocyte surface immunoglobulins in myeloma and the effect of an RNA-containing plasma factor. *Ann Intern Med* 1975;83:625-631.

90. Cheson BD, Plass RR, Rothstein G. Defective opsonization in multiple myeloma. *Blood* 1980;55:602-606.

91. Karle H, Hansen NE, Plesner T. Neutrophil defect in multiple myeloma. Studies on intraneutrophilic lysozyme in multiple myeloma and malignant lymphoma. *Scand J Haematol* 1976;17:62-70.

92. Spitler LE, Spath P, Petz L, et al. Phagocytes and C4 in paraproteinaemia. *Br J Haematol* 1975;29:279-292.

93. Oken MM, Pomeroy C, Weisdorf D, et al. Prophylactic antibiotics for the prevention of early infection in multiple myeloma. *Am J Med* 1996;100:624-628.

94. Kyle RA, Rajkumar SV. Criteria for diagnosis, staging, risk stratification and response assessment of multiple myeloma. *Leukemia* 2009;23:3-9.

95. Rajkumar SV, Kyle RA. Multiple myeloma: diagnosis and treatment. *Mayo Clin Proc* 2005;80:1371-1382.

96. Katzmann JA, Dispenzieri A, Kyle RA, et al. Elimination of the need for urine studies in the screening algorithm for monoclonal gammopathies by using serum immunofixation and free light chain assays. *Mayo Clin Proc* 2006;81:1575-1578.

97. Dispenzieri A, Kyle R, Merlini G, et al. International Myeloma Working Group guidelines for serum-free light chain analysis in multiple myeloma and related disorders. *Leukemia* 2009;23:215-224.

98. Bataille R, Boccadoro M, Klein B, et al. C-reactive protein and beta-2 microglobulin produce a simple and powerful myeloma staging system. *Blood* 1992;80:733-737.

99. Greipp PR, San Miguel J, Durie BG, et al. International staging system for multiple myeloma. *J Clin Oncol* 2005;23: 3412-3420.

100. Dimopoulos MA, Barlogie B, Smith TL, et al. High serum lactate dehydrogenase level as a marker for drug resistance and short survival in multiple myeloma. *Ann Intern Med* 1991; 115:931-935.

101. Barlogie B, Smallwood L, Smith T, et al. High serum levels of lactic dehydrogenase identify a high-grade lymphoma-like myeloma. *Ann Intern Med* 1989;110:521-525.

102. Kantarjian HM, Keating MJ, Walters RS, et al. Acute promyelocytic leukemia. M.D. Anderson Hospital experience. *Am J Med* 1986;80:789-797.

103. Barlogie B, Alexanian R, Gehan EA, et al. Marrow cytometry and prognosis in myeloma. *J Clin Invest* 1983;72:853-861.

104. Greipp PR, Kyle RA. Clinical, morphological, and cell kinetic differences among multiple myeloma, monoclonal gammopathy of undetermined significance, and smoldering multiple myeloma. *Blood* 1983;62:166-171.

105. Kyle RA. Prognostic factors in multiple myeloma. *Hematol Oncol* 1988;6:125-130.

106. Greipp PR, Raymond NM, Kyle RA, et al. Multiple myeloma: significance of plasmablastic subtype in morphological classification. *Blood* 1985;65:305-310.

107. Blade J, Samson D, Reece D, et al. Criteria for evaluating disease response and progression in patients with multiple myeloma treated by high-dose therapy and haemopoietic stem cell transplantation. Myeloma Subcommittee of the EBMT. European Group for Blood and Marrow Transplant. *Br J Haematol* 1998;102:1115-1123.

108. Durie BG, Harousseau JL, Miguel JS, et al. International uniform response criteria for multiple myeloma. *Leukemia* 2006;20:1467-1473.

109. Rajkumar SV, Blood E, Vesole D, et al. Phase III clinical trial of thalidomide plus dexamethasone compared with dexamethasone alone in newly diagnosed multiple myeloma: a clinical trial coordinated by the Eastern Cooperative Oncology Group. *J Clin Oncol* 2006;24:431-436.

110. Harousseau JL CM, Attal M, et al. Bortezomib/dexamethasone versus VAD as induction prior to autologous stem cell tranplantation (ASCT) in previously untreated multiple myeloma (MM): Updated data from IFM 2005/01 trial [abstract]. *J Clin Oncol*, ASCO Annual Meeting Proceedings (Post Meeting Edition) 2008;26(15S):8505.

111. Rajkumar SV, Rosinol L, Hussein M, et al. Multicenter, randomized, double-blind, placebo-controlled study of thalidomide plus dexamethasone compared with dexamethasone as initial therapy for newly diagnosed multiple myeloma. *J Clin Oncol* 2008;26:2171-2177.

112. Macro M DM, Uzunhan Y, et al. Dexamethasone+Thalidomide (Dex/Thal) Compared to VAD as a Pre-Transplant Treatment in Newly Diagnosed Multiple Myeloma (MM): A Randomized Trial. *Blood (ASH Annual Meeting Abstracts)* 2006;108:22a, Abstract 57.

113. Richardson PG, Mitsiades C, Schlossman R, et all. New drugs for myeloma. *Oncologist* 2007;12:664-689.

114. Dimopoulos MA, Kastritis E, Rajkumar SV. Treatment of plasma cell dyscrasias with lenalidomide. *Leukemia* 2008;22: 1343-1353.

115. Rajkumar SV, Hayman SR, Lacy MQ, et al. Combination therapy with lenalidomide plus dexamethasone (Rev/Dex) for newly diagnosed myeloma. *Blood* 2005;106:4050-4053.

116. Lacy MQ, Gertz MA, Dispenzieri A, et al. Long-term results of response to therapy, time to progression, and survival with lenalidomide plus dexamethasone in newly diagnosed myeloma. *Mayo Clin Proc* 2007;82:1179-1184.

117. Rajkumar SV, Jacobus S, Callander NS, et al. Lenalidomide plus high-dose dexamethasone versus lenalidomide plus low-dose dexamethasone as initial therapy for newly diagnosed multiple myeloma: an open-label randomised controlled trial. *Lancet Oncol* 2010;11:29-37.

118. Kumar S, Dispenzieri A, Lacy MQ, et al. Impact of lenalidomide therapy on stem cell mobilization and engraftment post-peripheral blood stem cell transplantation in patients with newly diagnosed myeloma. *Leukemia* 2007;21: 2035-2042.

119. Harousseau JL, Attal M, Leleu X, et al. Bortezomib plus dexamethasone as induction treatment prior to autologous stem cell transplantation in patients with newly diagnosed multiple myeloma: results of an IFM phase II study. *Haematologica* 2006;91:1498-1505.

120. Jagannath S, Durie B, Wolf J, et al. Bortezomib therapy alone and in combination with dexamethasone for patients with previously untreated multiple myeloma. *Blood (ASH Annual Meeting Abstracts)* Nov 2005;106:783.

121. Wang M, Delasalle K, Giralt S, Raymond Alexanian. Rapid control of previously untreated multiple myeloma with bortezomib-thalidomide-dexamethasone followed by early intensive therapy. *Blood* (ASH Annual Meeting Abstracts) Nov 2005;106:784.

122. Cavo M, Tacchetti P, Patriarca F, et al. Superior complete response rate and progression-free survival after autologous transplantation with up-front velcade-thalidomide-dexamethasone compared with thalidomide-dexamethasone in newly diagnosed multiple myeloma. *Blood (ASH Annual Meeting Abstracts,* Nov 2008;112:158.

123. Oakervee HE, Popat R, Curry N, et al. PAD combination therapy (PS-341/bortezomib, doxorubicin and dexamethasone) for previously untreated patients with multiple myeloma. *Br J Haematol* 2005;129:755-762.

124. Popat R, Oakervee H, Curry N, et al. Reduced dose pad combination therapy (ps-341/bortezomib, adriamycin and dexamethasone) for previously untreated patients with multiple myeloma. *Blood* (ASH Annual Meeting Abstracts) Nov 2005; 106:2554.

125. Sonneveld P, van der Holt B, Schmidt-Wolf IGH, et al. First analysis of HOVON-65/GMMG-HD4 Randomized Phase III Trial Comparing Bortezomib, Adriamycine, Dexamethasone (PAD) Vs VAD as Induction Treatment Prior to High Dose Melphalan (HDM) in Patients with Newly Diagnosed Multiple Myeloma (MM). *Blood* (ASH Annual Meeting Abstracts) Nov 2008;112:653.

126. Qazilbash MH, Saliba RM, Hosing C, et al. Autologous stem cell transplantation is safe and feasible in elderly patients with multiple myeloma. *Bone Marrow Transplant* 2007;39: 279-283.

127. Alexanian R, Haut A, Khan AU, et al. Treatment for multiple myeloma. Combination chemotherapy with different melphalan dose regimens. *JAMA* 1969;208:1680-1685.

128. Boccadoro M, Pileri A. Standard chemotherapy for myelomatosis: an area of great controversy. *Hematol Oncol Clin North Am* 1992;6:371-382.

129. McLaughlin P, Alexanian R. Myeloma protein kinetics following chemotherapy. *Blood* 1982;60:851-855.

130. Palumbo A, Bringhen S, Caravita T, et al. Oral melphalan and prednisone chemotherapy plus thalidomide compared with melphalan and prednisone alone in elderly patients with multiple myeloma: randomised controlled trial. *Lancet* 2006; 367:825-831.

131. Palumbo A, Bringhen S, Liberati AM, et al. Oral melphalan, prednisone, and thalidomide in elderly patients with multiple myeloma: updated results of a randomized controlled trial. *Blood* 2008;112:3107-3114.

132. Hulin C, Facon T, Rodon P, et al. Efficacy of melphalan and prednisone plus thalidomide in patients older than 75 years with newly diagnosed multiple myeloma: IFM 01/01 trial. *J Clin Oncol* 2009;27:3664-3670.

133. Facon T, Mary JY, Hulin C, et al. Melphalan and prednisone plus thalidomide versus melphalan and prednisone alone or reduced-intensity autologous stem cell transplantation in elderly patients with multiple myeloma (IFM 99-06): a randomised trial. *Lancet* 2007;370:1209-1218.

134. Wijermans P, Schaafsma M, van Norden Y, et al. Melphalan + Prednisone Versus Melphalan + Prednisone + Thalidomide in Induction Therapy for Multiple Myeloma in Elderly Patients: Final Analysis of the Dutch Cooperative Group HOVON 49 Study. *Blood* (ASH Annual Meeting Abstracts) Nov 2008;112:649.

135. Waage A, Gimsing P, Juliusson G, et al. Melphalan-Prednisone-Thalidomide to Newly Diagnosed Patients with Multiple Myeloma: A Placebo Controlled Randomised Phase 3 Trial. *Blood* (ASH Annual Meeting Abstracts) Nov 2007; 110:78.

136. Reece D, Harousseau JL, Gertz M A, et al. Nontransplant therapy of myelom, high-dose therapy for myeloma, and a personalized care plan for treatment of myeloma. In: R G, (ed.): ASCO 2009 Educational Book. Orlando: Curzio J; 2009;502-509.

137. San Miguel JF, Schlag R, Khuageva NK, et al. Bortezomib plus melphalan and prednisone for initial treatment of multiple myeloma. *N Engl J Med* 2008;359:906-917.

138. Ludwig H, Hajek R, Tothova E, et al. Thalidomide-dexamethasone compared with melphalan-prednisolone in elderly patients with multiple myeloma. *Blood* 2009;113: 3435-3442.

139. The Myeloma Trialists' Collaborative Group. Interferon as therapy for multiple myeloma: an individual patient data overview of 24 randomized trials and 4012 patients. *Br J Haematol* 2001;113:1020-1034.

140. Alexanian R, Weber D. Whither interferon for myeloma and other hematologic malignancies? *Ann Intern Med* 1996;124: 264-265.

141. Salmon SE, Crowley JJ, Balcerzak SP, et al. Interferon versus interferon plus prednisone remission maintenance therapy for multiple myeloma: a Southwest Oncology Group Study. *J Clin Oncol* 1998;16:890-896.

142. Alexanian R, Weber D, Dimopoulos M, Delasalle K, Smith TL. Randomized trial of alpha-interferon or dexamethasone as maintenance treatment for multiple myeloma. *Am J Hematol* 2000;65:204-209.

143. Offidani M, Corvatta L, Polloni C, et al. Thalidomide-dexamethasone versus interferon-alpha-dexamethasone as maintenance treatment after ThaDD induction for multiple myeloma: a prospective, multicentre, randomised study. *Br J Haematol* 2009;144:653-659.

144. Lokhorst HM, van der Holt B, Zweegman S, et al. A randomized phase 3 study on the effect of thalidomide combined with adriamycin, dexamethasone, and high-dose melphalan, followed by thalidomide maintenance in patients with multiple myeloma. *Blood* 115:1113-1120.

145. Attal M, Harousseau JL, Leyvraz S, et al. Maintenance therapy with thalidomide improves survival in patients with multiple myeloma. *Blood* 2006;108:3289-3294.

146. Spencer A, Prince HM, Roberts AW, et al. Consolidation therapy with low-dose thalidomide and prednisolone prolongs the survival of multiple myeloma patients undergoing a single autologous stem-cell transplantation procedure. *J Clin Oncol* 2009;27:1788-1793.

147. Richardson PG, Sonneveld P, Schuster MW, et al. Bortezomib or high-dose dexamethasone for relapsed multiple myeloma. *N Engl J Med* 2005;352:2487-2498.

148. Dimopoulos M, Spencer A, Attal M, et al. Lenalidomide plus dexamethasone for relapsed or refractory multiple myeloma. *N Engl J Med* 2007;357:2123-2132.

149. Weber DM, Chen C, Niesvizky R, et al. Lenalidomide plus dexamethasone for relapsed multiple myeloma in North America. *N Engl J Med* 2007;357:2133-2142.

150. Kyle RA, Rajkumar SV. Criteria for diagnosis, staging, risk stratification and response assessment of multiple myeloma. *Leukemia* 2009;23(1):3-9.

151. Weber D, Rankin K, Gavino M, et al. Thalidomide alone or with dexamethasone for previously untreated multiple myeloma. *J Clin Oncol* 2003;21:16-19.

152. Palumbo A, Giaccone L, Bertola A, et al. Low-dose thalidomide plus dexamethasone is an effective salvage therapy for advanced myeloma. *Haematologica* 2001;86:399-403.

153. Dimopoulos MA, Zervas K, Kouvatseas G, et al. Thalidomide and dexamethasone combination for refractory multiple myeloma. *Ann Oncol* 2001;12:991-995.

154. von Lilienfeld-Toal M, Hahn-Ast C, Furkert K, et al. A systematic review of phase II trials of thalidomide/dexamethasone combination therapy in patients with relapsed or refractory multiple myeloma. *Eur J Haematol* 2008;81:247-252.

155. Palumbo A, Rajkumar SV, Dimopoulos MA, et al. Prevention of thalidomide- and lenalidomide-associated thrombosis in myeloma. *Leukemia* 2008;22:414-423.

156. Knop S, Gerecke C, Liebisch P, et al. Lenalidomide, adriamycin, and dexamethasone (RAD) in patients with relapsed and refractory multiple myeloma: a report from the German Myeloma Study Group DSMM (Deutsche Studiengruppe Multiples Myelom). *Blood* 2009;113:4137-4143.

157. van de Donk NW, Wittebol S, Minnema MC, et al. Lenalidomide (Revlimid) combined with continuous oral cyclophosphamide (endoxan) and prednisone (REP) is effective in lenalidomide/dexamethasone-refractory myeloma. *Br J Haematol* 2010;148: 335-337.

158. Jagannath S, Barlogie B, Berenson J, et al. A phase 2 study of two doses of bortezomib in relapsed or refractory myeloma. *Br J Haematol* 2004;127:165-172.

159. Richardson PG, Barlogie B, Berenson J, et al. A phase 2 study of bortezomib in relapsed, refractory myeloma. *N Engl J Med* 2003;348:2609-2617.

160. Richardson PG, Sonneveld P, Schuster M, et al. Extended follow-up of a phase 3 trial in relapsed multiple myeloma: final time-to-event results of the APEX trial. *Blood* 2007; 110:3557-3560.

161. Vogl DT, Stadtmauer EA, Richardson PG, et al. Impact of prior therapies on the relative efficacy of bortezomib compared with dexamethasone in patients with relapsed/refractory multiple myeloma. *Br J Haematol* 2009;147:531-534.

162. Khosravi Shahi P, Sabin Dominguez P, Encinas Garcia S, et al. [Efficiency of bortezomib and dexamethasone in relapsed multiple myeloma treatment: retrospective study in consecutive cases]. *Ann Med Interna* 2008;25:73-77.

163. Kropff MH, Bisping G, Wenning D, et al. Bortezomib in combination with dexamethasone for relapsed multiple myeloma. *Leuk Res* 2005;29:587-590.

164. Ozaki S, Tanaka O, Fujii S, et al. Therapy with bortezomib plus dexamethasone induces osteoblast activation in responsive patients with multiple myeloma. *Int J Hematol* 2007;86: 180-185.

165. Yuan ZG, Hou J, Zhou F, et al. [Bortezomib in combination with dexamethasone for the treatment of relapsed or refractory multiple myeloma]. *Zhonghua Xue Ye Xue Za Zhi* 2006;27: 653-655.

166. Jagannath S, Richardson PG, Barlogie B, et al. Bortezomib in combination with dexamethasone for the treatment of patients with relapsed and/or refractory multiple myeloma with less than optimal response to bortezomib alone. *Haematologica* 2006;91:929-934.

167. Barlogie B, Smith L, Alexanian R. Effective treatment of advanced multiple myeloma refractory to alkylating agents. *N Engl J Med* 1984;310:1353-1356.

168. Anderson H, Scarffe JH, Ranson M, et al. VAD chemotherapy as remission induction for multiple myeloma. *Br J Cancer* 1995;71:326-330.

169. Lokhorst HM, Meuwissen OJ, Bast EJ, et al. VAD chemotherapy for refractory multiple myeloma. *Br J Haematol* 1989;71:25-30.

170. Phillips JK, Sherlaw-Johnson C, Pearce R, et al. A randomized study of MOD versus VAD in the treatment of relapsed and resistant multiple myeloma. *Leuk Lymphoma* 1995;17:465-472.

171. Safra T, Muggia F, Jeffers S, et al. Pegylated liposomal doxorubicin (doxil): reduced clinical cardiotoxicity in patients reaching or exceeding cumulative doses of 500 mg/m2. *Ann Oncol* 2000;11:1029-1033.

172. Orlowski RZ, Nagler A, Sonneveld P, et al. Randomized phase III study of pegylated liposomal doxorubicin plus bortezomib compared with bortezomib alone in relapsed or refractory multiple myeloma: combination therapy improves time to progression. *J Clin Oncol* 2007;25:3892-3901.

173. Berenson JR, Yang HH, Vescio RA, et al. Safety and efficacy of bortezomib and melphalan combination in patients with relapsed or refractory multiple myeloma: updated results of a phase 1/2 study after longer follow-up. *Ann Hematol* 2008;87:623-631.

174. Davies FE, Wu P, Jenner M, et al. The combination of cyclophosphamide, velcade and dexamethasone induces high response rates with comparable toxicity to velcade alone and velcade plus dexamethasone. *Haematologica* 2007;92:1149-1150.

175. Kropff M, Bisping G, Schuck E, et al. Bortezomib in combination with intermediate-dose dexamethasone and continuous low-dose oral cyclophosphamide for relapsed multiple myeloma. *Br J Haematol* 2007;138:330-337.

176. Reece DE, Rodriguez GP, Chen C, et al. Phase I-II trial of bortezomib plus oral cyclophosphamide and prednisone in relapsed and refractory multiple myeloma. *J Clin Oncol* 2008; 26:4777-4783.

177. Fenk R, Michael M, Zohren F, et al. Escalation therapy with bortezomib, dexamethasone and bendamustine for patients with relapsed or refractory multiple myeloma. *Leuk Lymphoma* 2007;48:2345-2351.

178. Mitsiades N, Mitsiades CS, Poulaki V, et al. Apoptotic signaling induced by immunomodulatory thalidomide analogs in human multiple myeloma cells: therapeutic implications. *Blood* 2002;99:4525-4530.

179. Pineda-Roman M, Zangari M, van Rhee F, et al. VTD combination therapy with bortezomib-thalidomide-dexamethasone is highly effective in advanced and refractory multiple myeloma. *Leukemia* 2008;22:1419-1427.

180. Palumbo A, Ambrosini MT, Benevolo G, et al. Bortezomib, melphalan, prednisone, and thalidomide for relapsed multiple myeloma. *Blood* 2007;109:2767-2772.

181. Terpos E, Kastritis E, Roussou M, et al. The combination of bortezomib, melphalan, dexamethasone and intermittent thalidomide is an effective regimen for relapsed/refractory myeloma and is associated with improvement of abnormal bone metabolism and angiogenesis. *Leukemia* 2008;22: 2247-2256.

182. Chanan-Khan A, Miller KC. Velcade, Doxil and Thalidomide (VDT) is an effective salvage regimen for patients with relapsed and refractory multiple myeloma. *Leuk Lymphoma* 2005;46:1103-1104.

183. Ciolli S, Leoni F, Casini C, et al. The addition of liposomal doxorubicin to bortezomib, thalidomide and dexamethasone significantly improves clinical outcome of advanced multiple myeloma. *Br J Haematol* 2008; 141:814-819.

184. Palumbo A, Patrizia F, Sanpaolo G, et al. Combination of lenalidomide, melphalan, prednisone and thalidomide (RMPT) in relapsed/refractory multiple myeloma: results of a multicenter phase II clinical trial. Abstract 868. In: American Society of Hematology Annual Meeting 2008.

185. Richardson PG, Weller E, Jagannath S, et al. Multicenter, phase I, dose-escalation trial of lenalidomide plus bortezomib for relapsed and relapsed/refractory multiple myeloma. *J Clin Oncol* 2009;27:5713-5719.

186. Richardson P, Jagannath S, Raje N, et al. Lenalidomide, Bortezomib, and Dexamethasone (Rev/Vel/Dex) as Front-Line Therapy for Patients with Multiple Myeloma (MM): Preliminary Results of a Phase 1/2 Study. *Blood* (ASH Annual Meeting Abstracts). 2007;110:187.

187. Barlogie B, Desikan R, Eddlemon P, et al. Extended survival in advanced and refractory multiple myeloma after single-agent thalidomide: identification of prognostic factors in a phase 2 study of 169 patients. *Blood* 2001;98:492-494.

188. van Rhee F, Dhodapkar M, Shaughnessy JD, Jr., et al. First thalidomide clinical trial in multiple myeloma: a decade. *Blood* 2008;112:1035-1038.

189. Chang H, Trieu Y, Qi X, et al. Bortezomib therapy response is independent of cytogenetic abnormalities in relapsed/refractory multiple myeloma. *Leuk Res* 2007;31:779-782.

190. Jagannath S, Richardson PG, Sonneveld P, et al. Bortezomib appears to overcome the poor prognosis conferred by chromosome 13 deletion in phase 2 and 3 trials. *Leukemia* 2007; 21:151-157.

191. Reece D, Song KW, Fu T, et al. Influence of cytogenetics in patients with relapsed or refractory multiple myeloma treated with lenalidomide plus dexamethasone: adverse effect of deletion 17p13. *Blood* 2009;114:522-525.

192. Tosi P, Zamagni E, Cellini C, et al. Thalidomide alone or in combination with dexamethasone in patients with advanced, relapsed or refractory multiple myeloma and renal failure. *Eur J Haematol* 2004;73:98-103.

193. Lacy MQ, Hayman SR, Gertz MA, et al. Pomalidomide (CC4047) plus low-dose dexamethasone as therapy for relapsed multiple myeloma. *J Clin Oncol* 2009;27:5008-5014.

194. Jagannath S, Ravi V, Stewart A, et al. Phase II Study of Carfilzomib (CFZ) in Patients with Relapsed and Refractory Multiple Myeloma (MM). *Blood* (ASH Annual Meeting Abstracts) 2008;112:864.

195. Richardson P, Alban A, Khan C, et al. A multicenter phase I clinical trial of tanespimycin (KOS-953)+bortezomib (BZ): encouraging activity and manageable toxicity in heavily pre-treated patients with relapsed refractory multiple myeloma (MM). American Society of Hamatology Annual Meeting Abstract 406. 2006.

196. Ghobrial I, Leleu X, Rubin N, et al. Final Results of a Phase II Trial of the Novel Oral Akt Inhibitor Perifosine in Relapsed and/or Refractory Waldenström Macroglobulinemia (WM). *Blood* (ASH Annual Meeting Abstracts) 2008;112:1010.

197. Palumbo A, Larocca A, Genuardi M, et al. Melphalan, prednisone, thalidomide and defibrotide in relapsed/refractory multiple myeloma: results of multicenter phase I/II trial. *Haematologica* 2010;95(7):1144-1149.

198. McElwain TJ, Powles RL. High-dose intravenous melphalan for plasma-cell leukaemia and myeloma. *Lancet* 1983;2:822-824.

199. Attal M, Harousseau JL, Stoppa AM, et al. A prospective, randomized trial of autologous bone marrow transplantation and chemotherapy in multiple myeloma. Intergroupe Francais du Myelome. *N Engl J Med* 1996;335:91-97.

200. Barlogie B, Jagannath S, Vesole DH, et al. Superiority of tandem autologous transplantation over standard therapy for previously untreated multiple myeloma. *Blood* 1997;89:789-793.

201. Child JA, Morgan GJ, Davies FE, et al. High-dose chemotherapy with hematopoietic stem-cell rescue for multiple myeloma. *N Engl J Med* 2003;348:1875-1883.

202. Barlogie B, Kyle RA, Anderson KC, et al. Standard chemotherapy compared with high-dose chemoradiotherapy for multiple myeloma: final results of phase III US Intergroup Trial S9321. *J Clin Oncol* 2006;24:929-936.

203. Blade J, Rosinol L, Sureda A, et al. High-dose therapy intensification compared with continued standard chemotherapy in multiple myeloma patients responding to the initial chemotherapy: long-term results from a prospective randomized trial from the Spanish cooperative group PETHEMA. *Blood* 2005;106:3755-3759.

204. Fermand JP, Katsahian S, Divine M, et al. High-dose therapy and autologous blood stem-cell transplantation compared with conventional treatment in myeloma patients aged 55 to 65 years: long-term results of a randomized control trial from the Group Myeloma-Autogreffe. *J Clin Oncol* 2005;23:9227-9233.

205. Moreau P, Facon T, Attal M, et al. Comparison of 200 mg/m(2) melphalan and 8 Gy total body irradiation plus 140 mg/m(2) melphalan as conditioning regimens for peripheral blood stem cell transplantation in patients with newly diagnosed multiple myeloma: final analysis of the Intergroupe Francophone du Myelome 9502 randomized trial. *Blood* 2002;99:731-735.

206. Barlogie B, Shaughnessy J, Tricot G, et al. Treatment of multiple myeloma. *Blood* 2004;103:20-32.

207. Attal M, Harousseau JL, Facon T, et al. Single versus double autologous stem-cell transplantation for multiple myeloma. *N Engl J Med* 2003;349:2495-2502.

208. Cavo M, Tosi P, Zamagni E, et al. Prospective, randomized study of single compared with double autologous stem-cell transplantation for multiple myeloma: Bologna 96 clinical study. *J Clin Oncol* 2007;25:2434-2441.

209. Bensinger WI, Demirer T, Buckner CD, et al. Syngeneic marrow transplantation in patients with multiple myeloma. *Bone Marrow Transplant* 1996;18:527-531.

210. Lokhorst HM, Schattenberg A, Cornelissen JJ, et al. Donor lymphocyte infusions for relapsed multiple myeloma after allogeneic stem-cell transplantation: predictive factors for response and long-term outcome. *J Clin Oncol* 2000;18:3031-3037.

211. Lokhorst HM, Wu K, Verdonck LF, et al. The occurrence of graft-versus-host disease is the major predictive factor for response to donor lymphocyte infusions in multiple myeloma. *Blood* 2004;103:4362-4364.

212. Salama M, Nevill T, Marcellus D, et al. Donor leukocyte infusions for multiple myeloma. *Bone Marrow Transplant* 2000;26:1179-1184.

213. Tricot G, Vesole DH, Jagannath S, et al. Graft-versus-myeloma effect: proof of principle. *Blood* 1996;87:1196-1198.

214. Corradini P, Cavo M, Lokhorst H, et al. Molecular remission after myeloablative allogeneic stem cell transplantation predicts a better relapse-free survival in patients with multiple myeloma. *Blood* 2003;102:1927-1929.

215. Bruno B, Rotta M, Patriarca F, et al. A comparison of allografting with autografting for newly diagnosed myeloma. *N Engl J Med* 2007;356:1110-1120.

216. Garban F, Attal M, Michallet M, et al. Prospective comparison of autologous stem cell transplantation followed by dose-reduced allograft (IFM99-03 trial) with tandem autologous stem cell transplantation (IFM99-04 trial) in high-risk de novo multiple myeloma. *Blood* 2006;107:3474-3480.

217. Kyle RA, Therneau TM, Rajkumar SV, et al. Prevalence of monoclonal gammopathy of undetermined significance. *N Engl J Med* 2006;354:1362-1369.

218. Kyle RA, Therneau TM, Rajkumar SV, et al. A long-term study of prognosis in monoclonal gammopathy of undetermined significance. *N Engl J Med* 2002;346:564-569.

219. Landgren O, Kyle RA, Pfeiffer RM, et al. Monoclonal gammopathy of undetermined significance (MGUS) consistently precedes multiple myeloma: a prospective study. *Blood* 2009;113:5412-5417.

220. Kyle RA, Rajkumar SV. Monoclonal gammopathy of undetermined significance and smouldering multiple myeloma: emphasis on risk factors for progression. *Br J Haematol* 2007;139:730-743.

221. Blade J, Rosinol L, Cibeira MT, de Larrea CF. Pathogenesis and progression of monoclonal gammopathy of undetermined significance. *Leukemia* 2008;22:1651-1657.

222. Dores GM, Landgren O, McGlynn KA, Curtis RE, Linet MS, Devesa SS. Plasmacytoma of bone, extramedullary plasmacytoma, and multiple myeloma: incidence and survival in the United States, 1992-2004. *Br J Haematol* 2009;144:86-94.

223. Dimopoulos MA, Moulopoulos LA, Maniatis A, Alexanian R. Solitary plasmacytoma of bone and asymptomatic multiple myeloma. *Blood* 2000;96:2037-2044.

224. Dimopoulos MA, Hamilos G. Solitary bone plasmacytoma and extramedullary plasmacytoma. *Curr Treat Options Oncol* 2002;3:255-259.

225. Soutar R, Lucraft H, Jackson G, et al. Guidelines on the diagnosis and management of solitary plasmacytoma of bone and solitary extramedullary plasmacytoma. *Br J Haematol* 2004; 124:717-726.

226. Blade J, Rosinol L. Smoldering multiple myeloma and monoclonal gammopathy of undetermined significance. *Curr Treat Options Oncol* 2006;7:237-245.

227. Kyle RA, Remstein ED, Therneau TM, et al. Clinical course and prognosis of smoldering (asymptomatic) multiple myeloma. *N Engl J Med* 2007;356:2582-2590.

228. Dispenzieri A, Kyle RA, Katzmann JA, et al. Immunoglobulin free light chain ratio is an independent risk factor for progression of smoldering (asymptomatic) multiple myeloma. *Blood* 2008;111:785-789.

229. Depil S, Leleu X, Micol JB, et al. Abnormal cytogenetics and significant bone marrow plasmacytosis are predictive of early progression and short survival in patients with low tumor mass asymptomatic multiple myeloma. *Leuk Lymphoma* 2004; 45:2481-2484.

230. He Y, Wheatley K, Clark O, et al. Early versus deferred treatment for early stage multiple myeloma. *Cochrane Database Syst Rev* 2003: CD004023.

231. Rajkumar SV, Dispenzieri A, Fonseca R, et al. Thalidomide for previously untreated indolent or smoldering multiple myeloma. *Leukemia* 2001;15:1274-1276.

232. Musto P, Petrucci MT, Bringhen S, et al. A multicenter, randomized clinical trial comparing zoledronic acid versus observation in patients with asymptomatic myeloma. *Cancer* 2008;113:1588-1595.

233. Dimopoulos MA, Panayiotidis P, Moulopoulos LA, et al. Waldenström's macroglobulinemia: clinical features, complications, and management. *J Clin Oncol* 2000;18:214-226.

234. San Miguel JF, Vidriales MB, Ocio E, et al. Immunophenotypic analysis of Waldenström's macroglobulinemia. *Semin Oncol* 2003;30:187-195.

235. Treon SP. How I treat Waldenström macroglobulinemia. *Blood* 2009;114:2375-2385.

236. Baldini L, Goldaniga M, Guffanti A, et al. Immunoglobulin M monoclonal gammopathies of undetermined significance and indolent Waldenström's macroglobulinemia recognize the same determinants of evolution into symptomatic lymphoid disorders: proposal for a common prognostic scoring system. *J Clin Oncol* 2005;23:4662-4668.

237. Buske C, Hoster E, Dreyling M, et al. The addition of rituximab to front-line therapy with CHOP (R-CHOP) results in a higher response rate and longer time to treatment failure in patients with lymphoplasmacytic lymphoma: results of a randomized trial of the German Low-Grade Lymphoma Study Group (GLSG). *Leukemia* 2009;23: 153-161.

238. Dimopoulos MA, Anagnostopoulos A, Kyrtsonis MC, et al. Primary treatment of Waldenström macroglobulinemia with dexamethasone, rituximab, and cyclophosphamide. *J Clin Oncol* 2007;25:3344-3349.

239. Treon SP, Hunter Z, Barnagan AR. CHOP plus rituximab therapy in Waldenström's macroglobulinemia. *Clin Lymphoma* 2005;5:273-277.

240. Ioakimidis L PC, Hunter ZR, Soumerai JD, et al. Comparative outcomes following CP-R, CVP-R, and CHOP-R in Waldenström's macroglobulinemia. *Clin Lymphoma Myeloma* 2009;9:62-66.

241. Treon SP, Soumerai JD, Branagan AR, et al. Thalidomide and rituximab in Waldenström macroglobulinemia. *Blood* 2008;112:4452-4457.

242. Dhodapkar MV, Hoering A, Gertz MA, et al. Long-term survival in Waldenström macroglobulinemia: 10-year follow-up of Southwest Oncology Group-directed intergroup trial S9003. *Blood* 2009;113:793-796.

243. Treon SP, Branagan AR, Ioakimidis L, et al. Long-term outcomes to fludarabine and rituximab in Waldenström macroglobulinemia. *Blood* 2009;113:3673-3678.

244. Thomas SK, Delassalle KB, Gavino M, et al. DM. 2-CDA-cyclophosphamide +/- Rituximab for symptomatic Waldenström's Macroglobulinemia. *Haematologica* 2007; 92:1227a.

245. Treon SP, Ioakimidis L, Soumerai JD, et al. Primary therapy of Waldenström macroglobulinemia with bortezomib, dexamethasone, and rituximab: WMCTG clinical trial 05-180. *J Clin Oncol* 2009;27:3830-3835.

246. Treon SP, Kelliher A, Keele B, et al. Expression of serotherapy target antigens in Waldenström's macroglobulinemia: therapeutic applications and considerations. *Semin Oncol* 2003; 30:248-252.

247. Santos DD, Hatjiharissi E, Tournilhac O, et al. CD52 is expressed on human mast cells and is a potential therapeutic target in Waldenström's Macroglobulinemia and mast cell disorders. *Clin Lymphoma Myeloma* 2006;6: 478-483.

248. Hunter ZR, Boxer M, Kahl B, et al. Phase II study of alemtuzumab in lymphoplasmacytic lymphoma: Results of WMCTG trial 02-079. *J Clin Oncol* 2003;24:7523a.

249. Treon SP, Hunter ZR, Matous J, et al. Multicenter clinical trial of bortezomib in relapsed/refractory Waldenström's macroglobulinemia: results of WMCTG Trial 03-248. *Clin Cancer Res* 2007;13:3320-3325.

250. Kyriakou C, Canals C, Taghipour G, et al. Allogeneic stem cell transplantation (ALLO-SCT) in Waldenström macroglobulinemia (WM): An analysis of 106 cases from the European Bone Marrow Registry (EBMT). *Haematologica* 2007;92(6, Suppl. 2):92.

251. Dimopoulos MA, Gertz MA, Kastritis E, et al. Update on treatment recommendations from the Fourth International Workshop on Waldenström's Macroglobulinemia. *J Clin Oncol* 2009;27:120-126.

252. Gertz MA, Rajkumar SV. Primary systemic amyloidosis. *Curr Treat Options Oncol* 2002;3:261-271.

253. Pardanani A, Witzig TE, Schroeder G, et al. Circulating peripheral blood plasma cells as a prognostic indicator in patients with primary systemic amyloidosis. *Blood* 2003; 101:827-830.

254. Palladini G, Campana C, Klersy C, et al. Serum N-terminal pro-brain natriuretic peptide is a sensitive marker of myocardial dysfunction in AL amyloidosis. *Circulation* 2003;107: 2440-2445.

255. Kumar S, Dispenzieri A, Lacy MQ, et al. Serum uric acid: novel prognostic factor in primary systemic amyloidosis. *Mayo Clin Proc* 2008;83:297-303.

256. National Comprehensive Cancer Network. NCCN Clinical Practice Guidelines in Oncology: Multiple Myeloma. 2010;v. 2:AL-1.

257. Palladini G, Russo P, Nuvolone M, et al. Treatment with oral melphalan plus dexamethasone produces long-term remissions in AL amyloidosis. *Blood* 2007;110:787-788.

258. Palladini G, Perfetti V, Perlini S, et al. The combination of thalidomide and intermediate-dose dexamethasone is an effective but toxic treatment for patients with primary amyloidosis (AL). *Blood* 2005;105:2949-2951.

259. Wechalekar AD, Goodman HJ, Lachmann HJ, et al. Safety and efficacy of risk-adapted cyclophosphamide, thalidomide, and dexamethasone in systemic AL amyloidosis. *Blood* 2007; 109:457-464.

260. Dispenzieri A, Lacy MQ, Zeldenrust SR, et al. The activity of lenalidomide with or without dexamethasone in patients with primary systemic amyloidosis. *Blood* 2007; 109:465-470.

261. Sanchorawala V, Wright DG, Rosenzweig M, et al. Lenalidomide and dexamethasone in the treatment of AL amyloidosis: results of a phase 2 trial. *Blood* 2007;109:492-496.

262. Jaccard A, Moreau P, Leblond V, et al. High-dose melphalan versus melphalan plus dexamethasone for AL amyloidosis. *N Engl J Med* 2007;357:1083-1093.

263. Skinner M, Sanchorawala V, Seldin DC, et al. High-dose melphalan and autologous stem-cell transplantation in patients with AL amyloidosis: an 8-year study. *Ann Intern Med* 2004; 140:85-93.

264. Dispenzieri A, Kyle RA, Lacy MQ, et al. Superior survival in primary systemic amyloidosis patients undergoing peripheral blood stem cell transplantation: a case-control study. *Blood* 2004;103:3960-3963.

265. Mhaskar R, Kumar A, Behera M, et al. Role of high-dose chemotherapy and autologous hematopoietic cell transplantation in primary systemic amyloidosis: a systematic review. *Biol Blood Marrow Transplant* 2009;15:893-902.

266. Gertz MA, Lacy MQ, Dispenzieri A, et al. Transplantation for amyloidosis. *Curr Opin Oncol* 2007; 19:136-141.

267. Witzig TE, Wahner-Roedler DL. Heavy chain disease. *Curr Treat Options Oncol* 2002;3:247-254.

268. Wahner-Roedler DL, Kyle RA. Heavy chain diseases. *Best Pract Res Clin Haematol* 2005;18:729-746.

269. Wahner-Roedler DL, Kyle RA. Mu-heavy chain disease: presentation as a benign monoclonal gammopathy. *Am J Hematol* 1992;40:56-60.

Stem Cell
Transplantation

ALLOGENEIC TRANSPLANTATION

Carrie Yuen
Sergio Giralt

Allogeneic hematopoietic cell transplantation was first explored in humans in the late 1950s and early 1960s based on observations in animal models that the lethal myelosuppression induced by total-body irradiation (TBI) could be overcome by the infusion of unirradiated bone marrow (1). The initial experience was limited to patients with terminal leukemia or with severe marrow failure states resulting from radiation exposure or disease. Almost all of these early patients died from complications of graft failure, graft-versus-host disease (GVHD), infections, or their primary disease (2). The first successful allogeneic bone marrow transplant was reported in 1968 in a patient with severe combined immunodeficiency (3). Because of this result and the pioneering work of the group in patients with refractory leukemia, the number of allogeneic transplants has increased dramatically over the last decades (4).

Since these initial experiences, allogeneic stem cell transplantation has been used to treat thousands of patients with historically incurable diseases. In the early days of the field, it was thought that the curative effect of allogeneic transplant was provided primarily by the high doses of chemoradiotherapy administered and that the donor bone marrow simply allowed for hematopoietic recovery in an adequate period of time. It is now apparent that the true success of transplantation

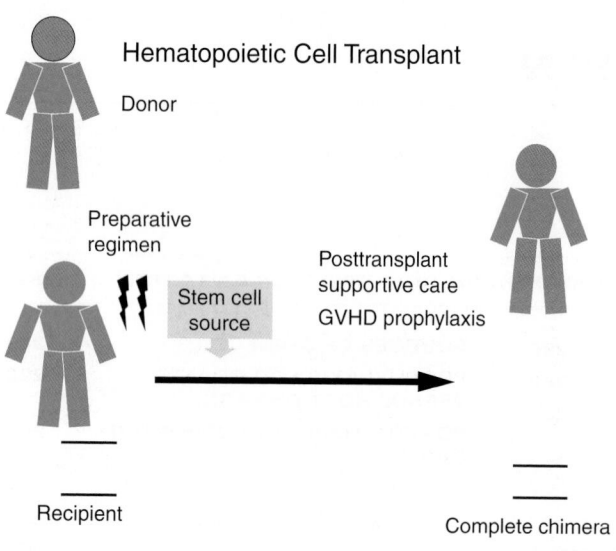

FIGURE 12-1. Components of allogeneic hematopoietic transplantation.

relies on a powerful donor immune response against the host malignancy, a phenomenon known as the graft-versus-tumor (GVT) effect.

The primary components of all allogeneic hematopoietic transplants are schematically represented in Fig. 12-1 and include:

1. Recipient
2. Donor
3. Preparative regimen
4. Stem cell source
5. Prophylaxis against graft-versus-host disease (GVHD) (including posttransplant immune suppression)
6. Posttransplant supportive care

Successful allografting depends on careful consideration of all these components in an effort to minimize the risks of potentially fatal posttransplant complications.

Despite the known curative potential of allogeneic transplantation, this procedure is performed in only a minority of potentially eligible patients. Broader application of allogeneic stem cell transplantation has been limited by donor availability and the intensity and toxicity associated with the procedure. This chapter reviews the current state of the major components of allogeneic stem cell transplantation, with particular attention to strategies being utilized and evaluated at the MD Anderson Cancer Center (MDACC). The specific role of allogeneic stem cell transplantation with regard to the treatment

of specific conditions is reviewed in the chapters dealing with them.

■ COMPONENTS OF ALLOGENEIC PROGENITOR CELL TRANSPLANTATION

TRANSPLANT RECIPIENT

It is estimated that over 20,000 allogeneic transplants have been performed worldwide for a variety of malignant and nonmalignant disorders (5). The International Bone Marrow Transplant Registry (IBMTR), an invaluable resource that collects data from over 400 centers worldwide, allows transplant physicians to see current transplant trends, compare outcomes of different transplant strategies, and do retrospective and prospective studies in hematopoietic stem cell transplantation.

According to data submitted to the IBMTR, the most common diagnoses for which allogeneic progenitor cell transplantation is being performed are, in decreasing order, (a) acute myelogenous leukemia (AML), (b) acute lymphocytic leukemia (ALL), (c) chronic myelogenous leukemia (CML), and (d) myelodysplastic syndromes (MDS). The indications for transplantation have changed over time, as—since the advent of imatinib mesylate—CML is no longer the most commonly transplanted hematologic malignancy. Likewise, the maximum age of transplant candidates has increased over time. Over the last 5 years, the proportion of patients receiving allografts over the age of 50 years is approaching 15%. This trend is related to nonmyeloablative conditioning regimen, which allows treatment to be more tolerable with lower treatment-related mortality.

Recipient factors are important in predicting transplant outcomes. Among the most important are:

1. Disease stage at transplant
2. Recipient age
3. Recipient performance status
4. Comorbidities

Although there is no specific parameter except very poor performance status that precludes allografting in an individual patient, all potential transplant recipients undergo an extensive pretransplant evaluation. At a minimum, this workup includes a complete history and physical examination in addition to evaluation of cardiac, pulmonary, hepatic, and renal function. Thus, the decision to proceed to transplant depends on a careful assessment and discussion of the risks and benefits of the procedure when contrasted with the natural history of the disease.

TRANSPLANT DONOR

Most allografts are performed using hematopoietic progenitor cells obtained from a human leukocyte antigen (HLA)-identical sibling. However, transplants using cells procured from volunteer donors, mismatched family members, and even cord blood are rapidly becoming more common. The most important factor to consider in selecting an allogeneic donor is HLA compatibility, which is determined by HLA typing. HLA compatibility is the single most important determinant for the occurrence of severe GVHD.

The HLA system is encoded by a series of genes on chromosome 6. For stem cell transplantation, HLA-A, HLA-B, and HLA-DR are routinely evaluated (6-8). In its strictest sense, *HLA identity* means that the donor and recipient are matched for the amino acid sequence encoded by all HLA loci. Identity is assumed in the setting of related transplant when segregation analysis demonstrates that the donor and recipient have inherited the same maternal and paternal haplotypes (genotypic HLA identity) (6). Otherwise, HLA identity can be verified only by sequencing all HLA loci (phenotypic HLA identity), which is impractical and rarely done.

It is important to note that conventional typing techniques detect a limited number of HLA polymorphic sequences. Therefore, "HLA-matched" may not actually be "HLA-identical." Conventional serologic typing is based on the complement-dependent microlymphocytotoxicity test and uses selected HLA-specific alloantisera or monoclonal antibodies to identify HLA antigens (6). A mismatch between cross-reactive antigens is considered minor, whereas a mismatch between non-cross-reactive antigens is considered major. For related patient–donor pairs, a single minor mismatch may be of little biological significance. Molecular typing relies on polymerase chain reaction (PCR) amplification of specific gene segments and can be performed (a) at a level corresponding to the specificities identified by serology (low resolution), (b) at a level where a limited number of alleles are possible (intermediate resolution), or (c) at a level where the specific allele is identified (high resolution). Sequence-based HLA typing is the most precise technique available.

At MDACC, we perform HLA-A and HLA-B serologic typing or molecular typing at the low-resolution level for most sibling-related transplants. Intermediate- and high-resolution typing is reserved for unrelated donor transplants and for cases where initial results are ambiguous.

Once identified, the donor must undergo a thorough medical evaluation to determine that (a) he or she may donate safely, (b) his or her cells will be adequate for the recipient, and (c) he or she understands the risks and benefits of the procedure and is providing cells voluntarily (9). Careful donor evaluation and attention to detail has resulted in only a handful of serious complications after more than 100,000 bone marrow or peripheral blood stem cell harvests (10).

PREPARATIVE REGIMENS

Standard Regimens

Preparative regimens in the setting of allogeneic transplant serve the dual purpose of eradicating the underlying malignancy as well as inducing a state of immune tolerance that allows the donor cells to engraft and expand. It is this second effect that ultimately gives rise to the powerful GVT effect, mediated by donor T cells (11-15). Allogeneic transplant conditioning regimens can generally be divided into chemotherapy-based protocols or TBI-based protocols.

TBI is both immunosuppressive and myeloablative. Single-dose TBI is associated with greater organ toxicity, particularly pulmonary, when compared with fractionated regimens (16,17). Therefore, most modern regimens deliver a total dose of 1000 to 1500 cGy using a variety of fractionation schedules. There is some evidence that higher total doses of TBI may be more effective at preventing relapse, but these benefits have been offset by increased nonrelapse mortality in the first 6 months after treatment (18-20). High-dose cyclophosphamide, a potent immunosuppressive agent, is often given as 60 mg/kg IV on two consecutive days prior to fractionated TBI. Other chemotherapy regimens with demonstrated efficacy in conjunction with TBI include high-dose etoposide (60 mg/kg) and the combination of etoposide and cyclophosphamide. The efficacy of these regimens appears similar, with the combination of etoposide and cyclophosphamide showing increased toxicity in patients with advanced disease (21,22). Although efficacious, TBI is associated with a number of short- and long-term complications, including secondary malignancies, cataracts, and endocrine dysfunction (23).

The toxicities of TBI-based strategies led to the development of radiation-free conditioning regimens. Of these, the most commonly used chemotherapy is the combination of busulfan and cyclophosphamide. Busulfan is traditionally administered orally as 4 mg/kg divided into four daily doses and given on each of four successive days (total dose, 16 mg/kg). More recently, an intravenous formulation of busulfan has become available that allows for once- or twice-daily dosing with more predictable drug delivery (24,25). Compared with standard cyclophosphamide-TBI regimens for the treatment of chronic-phase CML patients, the combination of busulfan and cyclophosphamide was found to be better tolerated, with comparable relapse and survival times (26,27). Of note, in AML, some randomized trials have shown a potential survival benefit for TBI-based regimens. Also, ALL registry analysis suggests that TBI-based regimens are superior (28). With these exceptions, there are currently no data confirming the superiority of one specific regimen over another. At MDACC, only patients with ALL or selected patients with low-grade lymphomas or who are refractory AML undergo allografting with a TBI-based conditioning regimen preferentially. Although intravenous busulfan is the most effective way of delivering this agent, many centers continue to use oral busulfan. Optimal use of oral busulfan requires pharmacologic monitoring to target busulfan levels in the blood, due to inter- and intrapatient variability in absorption (29,30).

It has been recently determined that cyclophosphamide and its metabolites contribute not only to the development of hemorrhagic cystitis posttransplant, but also, significantly, to the liver toxicity of the preparative regimen (31). Fludarabine has been used instead of cyclophosphamide in many modern myeloablative regimens. Initial studies with the combination of fludarabine and busulfan have produced high engraftment rates with low levels of toxicity (32-34). Results of the three largest series using fludarabine and busulfan combinations are summarized in Table 12-1.

Nonmyeloablative Regimens

The substantial toxicities associated with traditional conditioning regimens have limited the application of this modality to relatively young patients with good performance status. Patients with a history of extensive pretransplantation chemotherapy, prior radiotherapy to the chest or abdomen, or underlying dysfunction of heart, lung, liver, or kidneys are at particularly high risk for transplant-related morbidity. The development of strategies that minimize treatment-related toxicities is essential in broadening the scope of potential patients, improving overall survival rates, and enhancing the quality of life in long-term survivors.

There is now abundant evidence that the efficacy of allogeneic transplantation in effecting long-term cures resides in the potent alloimmune effect exerted by donor lymphocytes against tumor cells: the GVT effect (35-37). Thus, development of immunosuppressive conditioning regimens that would permit the engraftment of the donor graft while sparing the patient many of the toxicities related to traditional high-dose therapy could allow allografting in older and medically debilitated patients. Studies at MDACC for the treatment of chronic lymphocytic leukemia (CLL), lymphoma, and AML have contributed to initial reports demonstrating the efficacy of such nonmyeloablative strategies (38,39). Other chemotherapy-based reduced-intensity conditioning regimens have included the use of purine analogs with alkylating agents as well as the addition of monoclonal antibodies (40,41).

In addition to chemotherapy-based regimens, the role of TBI has been revisited in the setting of

TABLE 12-1	RESULTS OF FLUDARABINE/BUSULFAN CONDITIONING REGIMENS				
Reference	*N/Median Age Diagnosis*	*NRM*	*OS*	*EFS*	*Comments*
Bornhauser (33)	42/52	7% at D100	42% at 18 months	35% at 18 months	Six cases of pneumonitis
	CML/MDS	24% at 18 months			
De Lima (32)	41/42	0% at D100	CR patients	CR patients	
	AML/MDS		83% at 12 months	79% at 12 months	
			No CR patients	No CR patients	
			30% at 12 months	25% at 12 months	
Russell (34)	70/41	5% at D100	Low risk	Low risk	
	Various hematologic malignancies	10% at 24 months	88% at 24 months	74% at 24 months	
			High-risk AML	High-risk AML	
			37% at 24 months	26% at 24 months	
			High-risk other	High-risk other	
			71% at 24 months	65% at 24 months	

AML, acute myelogenous leukemia; CML, chronic myelogenous leukemia; CR, complete remission; D, day; EFS, event-free survival; MDS, myelodysplastic syndromes; NRM, nonrelapse mortality; OS, overall survival.

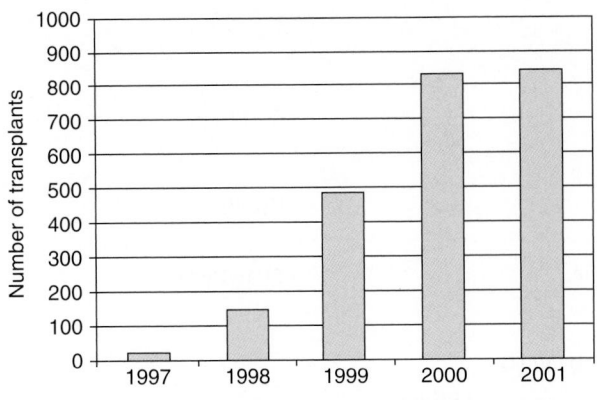

FIGURE 12-2. Number of nonmyeloablative transplants registered with the IBMTR between 1997 and 2001. Note that the data from 2000 to 2001 are incomplete (155).

nonmyeloablative transplantation. Preclinical work in a canine model established that doses as low as 2 Gy were sufficient to allow engraftment of donor stem cells when used in conjunction with postgrafting immunosuppression consisting of cyclosporine and mycophenolate mofetil (MMF) (42). A similar regimen piloted in human patients with hematologic malignancies who were more than 50 years old or had significant medical contraindications to standard transplantation demonstrated a very low degree of treatment-related toxicity and a high rate of mixed chimerism by day 28 (43). A substantial proportion (20%) of patients experienced graft rejection using this regimen; however, a later modification to the conditioning regimen included fludarabine, which resulted in a substantial decrease in the incidence of graft rejection (3%).

The number of nonmyeloablative transplants being performed has increased dramatically over the last 5 years, as evidenced by data reported to the IBMTR and summarized in Fig. 12-2. The great variety of regimens as well as their relative intensity is schematically represented in Fig. 12-3. This variety as well as the lack of controlled trials have made it impossible to determine the superiority of one nonmyeloablative regimen over another and should provide impetus for the design and implementation of well-designed clinical trials.

SOURCES OF STEM CELLS

Historically, hematopoietic stem cells used for transplantation were obtained through the harvest of bone marrow cells from the posterior iliac crests of normal donors. As approximately 150 aspirations are necessary to yield 10 to 15 mL/kg of bone marrow, this procedure is usually performed under general anesthesia. The procedure is associated with a very low incidence of complications and can generally be done on an outpatient basis (9). Common sequelae of bone marrow harvest include pain and transient postoperative fever. Life-threatening complications occur in less than 1% of patients.

In general, cell doses of 1 to 4×10^8 cells per kilogram of recipient weight are required to induce stable engraftment in patients treated with chemotherapy or TBI. Marrow cell dose has been shown to be an important prognostic factor for survival in both sibling and unrelated donor transplantation (44).

Since the early 1990s, the use of peripheral blood-derived stem cells (PBSCs) has become increasingly common. The rationale for using PBSCs is derived from studies in the autologous setting demonstrating accelerated recovery of hematopoiesis as compared with traditional BMT (45,46). Numerous studies have now confirmed the efficacy and safety of this approach (47-52). For the donors, this has eliminated the risks and morbidity associated with general anesthesia and bone marrow harvest. The recombinant growth factor granulocyte colony-stimulating factor (G-CSF), given for 4 to 6 days at doses of 6 to 16 μg/kg/day, is used to mobilize hematopoietic stem cells into the peripheral blood, where they may be collected by one or more leukapheresis procedures.

In addition to the benefits to the donor, PBSC transplantation offers a number of advantages to the recipient. G-CSF–mobilized PBSCs are enriched for pluripotent CD34+ hematopoietic progenitors when compared with marrow grafts (50). This has shortened the duration of absolute neutropenia and thrombocytopenia in recipients by approximately 5 days (49). In addition, studies at MDACC have demonstrated the potential for durable PBSC engraftment using nonmyeloablative chemotherapy, which would not be expected to result in engraftment of a comparable marrow allograft (39). Donor T cells, found in much higher concentration in PBSC grafts, likely mediate this effect. The presence of higher numbers of T cells initially raised concern for greater frequency and severity of GVHD; however, several large studies have now established that the risk of acute GVHD using PBSCs does not exceed the risk seen in traditional bone marrow grafts (42,49,53). Among patients undergoing allogeneic transplant for hematologic malignancies, a survival benefit was noted in those receiving PBSCs, due to lower nonrelapse mortality. Given the similarity in incidence of GVHD between the two groups, the survival was postulated to be due to more rapid hematologic recovery and/or earlier

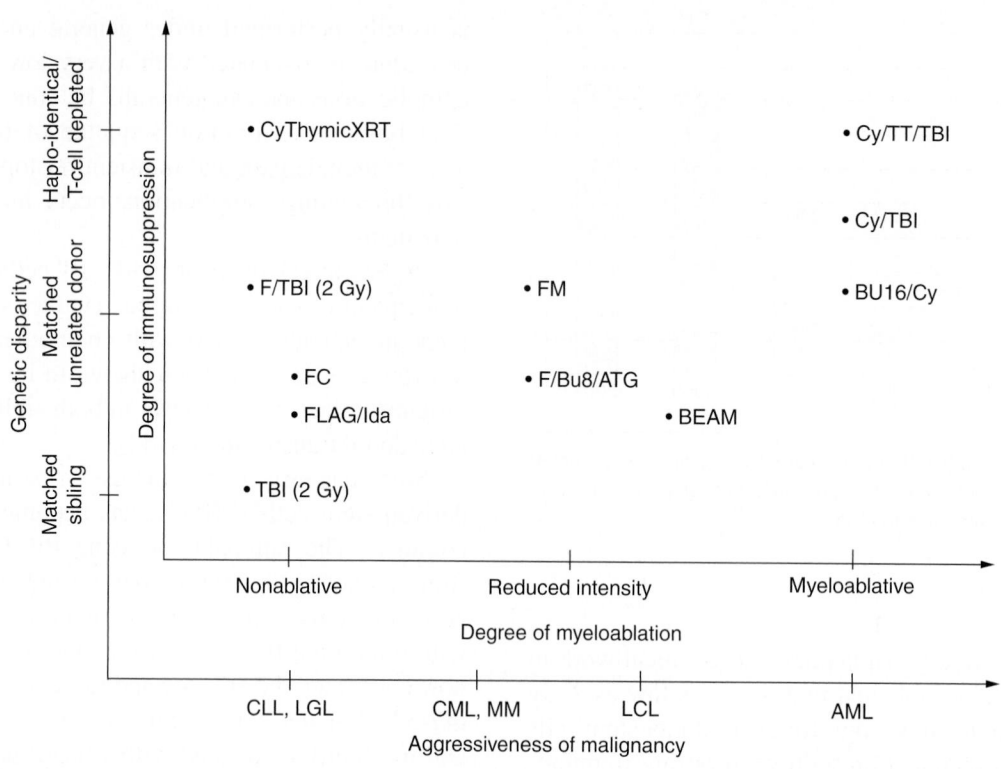

FIGURE 12-3. Relative intensity and use of most commonly reported ablative, reduced intensity, and nonablative conditioning regimens. AML, acute myelogenous leukemia; BEAM, carmustine + etoposide + cytarabine + melphalan; Bu16/Cy, busulfan, 16 mg/kg + cyclophosphamide; CLL, chronic lymphocytic leukemia; CML, chronic myelogenous leukemia; Cy/Thymic XRT, cyclophosphamide + thymic irradiation; Cy/TBI, cyclophosphamide + total body irradiation; Cy/TT/TBI, cyclophosphamide + thiotepa + total body irradiation; F/Bu8/ATG, fludarabine + busulfan, 8 mg/kg + antithymocyte globulin; FC, fludarabine + cyclophosphamide; FLAG/Ida, fludarabine + cytarabine + granulocyte colony stimulating factor + idarubicin; FM, fludarabine + melphalan; F/TBI, fludarabine + total body irradiation; LCL, large-cell lymphoma; LGL, low-grade lymphoma; MM, multiple myeloma; TBI, total body irradiation.

immune reconstitution (53). The incidence of chronic GVHD in patients receiving PBSC grafts has tended to be higher than in those receiving bone marrow grafts, and these patients will need to be followed long term to determine the impact of this observation.

Another source of hematopoietic stem cells used in allogeneic transplantation is umbilical cord blood (UCB). UCB transplants offer several potential advantages, including (1) increasing the available donor pool due to reduced HLA restriction, (2) reducing the period of time required to identify a donor, and (3) a potentially lower risk of acute GVHD compared with other unrelated donor grafts. Early results using UCB as a source of stem cells for the treatment of malignant and nonmalignant disease in pediatric patients were favorable and confirmed a low rate of acute GVHD (54). In a review of over 500 UCB transplant recipients, 80% of patients successfully engrafted and grade III/IV GVHD was reported in 9% of matched transplants, 22% of single-antigen-mismatched transplants, and 25% of two or

more mismatched transplants (55). Engraftment was mostly closely related to the total nucleated cell (TNC) dose in the graft, an issue particularly relevant to UCB grafts, as the typical stem cell dose is significantly lower than that seen with other types of transplant. Ex vivo expansion of umbilical cord blood using mesenchymal stem cells (56) or ex vivo culture of hematopoietic progenitor cells in umbilical cord blood in media containing stem cell factor, FLT-3 ligand, interleukin-6, thrombopoietin, and copper chelator tetraethylenepentamine (TEPA) result in clinically significant expansion of TNC and CD34+ cells for successful engraftment.

PROPHYLAXIS FOR GRAFT-VERSUS-HOST DISEASE

GVHD represents the undesired targeting of host tissues by immunocompetent donor cells. It continues to represent one of the major obstacles for allogeneic transplantation, especially as the use of mismatched or unrelated donor grafts increases. GVHD is often associated with and is mechanistically linked to the desired outcome of the GVT effect—a concept that is now universally accepted as a major reason for the success of allogeneic transplantation in reducing disease relapses (11,12,14,15). Although GVHD and GVT are both largely mediated by donor T cells, they are separable on the basis of antigen specificity (13). Delineating the specific antigens important for each effect is the subject of considerable interest and research. As GVHD requires immunocompetent donor T cells, it is not surprising that the severity of GVHD correlates with the number of donor T cells transfused (57). Donor T cells target tissue antigens not present in the donor. The most important of these include members of the major histocompatibility complex (MHC). An increasing number of minor histocompatibility antigens (mHA) are being identified that are also targets of GVHD (57-60). The greater the degree of disparity between donor and host, the more severe the resultant GVHD is likely to be.

Two forms of GVHD are commonly distinguished based on timing of occurrence and the clinical manifestations. Acute GVHD typically presents within the first 3 months after transplantation, while the chronic form may present more insidiously later in the posttransplant period. However, it is now known that changes characteristic of chronic GVHD may develop within 60 days of transplantation; therefore, acute and chronic GVHD are more appropriately described in terms of the clinical and histologic findings.

The incidence of acute GVHD is inversely related to the intensity of immunosuppression. The prophylactic use of cyclosporine and methotrexate is effective in reducing the incidence of acute GVHD as well as improving the survival of transplant patients (61). Methylprednisolone has also been successfully used in combination with cyclosporine for GVHD prophylaxis.

Cyclosporine is a cyclic polypeptide that prevents T-cell activation by inhibiting the production of interleukin-2 (IL-2) and the expression of IL-2 receptors. Although effective as GVHD prophylaxis, cyclosporine imparts significant toxicities, including hypertension, nephrotoxicity, hypomagnesemia, a risk for seizures, hypertrichosis, gingival hyperplasia, tremors, and anorexia. Treatment is initiated intravenously 1 to 2 days prior to stem cell infusion and converted to oral twice-daily dosing when possible. The risk of acute GVHD increases when cyclosporine blood concentrations drop below a target level (62). Cyclosporine also has a myriad of drug interactions, which may result in fluctuating levels.

Methotrexate has the potential for increased severity of regimen-related mucositis and delays in engraftment. These toxicities frequently preclude full dosing of the drug. At MDACC, a modification of the cyclosporine and methotrexate regimen using "minidose methotrexate" was found to be as effective as the full dose, with less toxicity (63).

Tacrolimus is a macrolide lactone closely resembling cyclosporine in mechanism of action, spectrum of toxicities, and pharmacologic interactions. The combination of tacrolimus and methotrexate used as prophylaxis was demonstrated to be superior to cyclosporine and methotrexate in reducing grade II to grade IV acute GVHD (64). Of note, in this study, there was a higher regimen-related death rate in patients with advanced disease who received tacrolimus, possibly related to the use of tacrolimus at levels beyond the currently recommended 5 to 15 ng/mL. The implications of this finding are unclear.

Antithymocyte globulin (ATG) has also been used effectively in the prophylactic setting (65-67). In patients with aplastic anemia who underwent transplantation using a conditioning regimen of cyclophosphamide and ATG, low rates of acute (15%) and chronic GVHD (34%) were reported. A second study in a similar group of patients found a significant survival benefit at 3 years for patients receiving cyclophosphamide and ATG compared with historic controls who received cyclophosphamide alone (92 versus 72%) (67).

In addition to the immunosuppressive agents above, T-cell depletion prior to marrow infusion has been shown to effectively reduce the incidence and severity of GVHD; however, T-cell depletion also results in increased graft rejection, infectious complications, and relapse rates in a disease-specific manner (68). Selective depletion of T-cell subsets may be a more effective means of reducing the risk of acute GVHD while preserving the GVT effect (69).

POSTTRANSPLANT SUPPORTIVE CARE

The basic principle underlying the supportive care of the transplanted patient is prevention. Most transplant complications have a temporal relation to the conditioning regimen and the transplant. The appropriate supportive care measures to employ are therefore largely dependent on what complications the patient is at risk for at any given posttransplant date. The temporal relationship of common infectious and noninfectious complications is depicted in Fig. 12-4.

The common occurrence of nausea, dehydration, and gastrointestinal symptoms associated with the

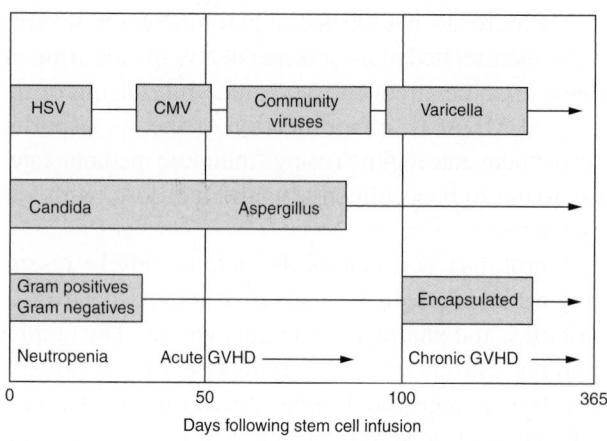

FIGURE 12-4. Time line of common infectious and noninfectious complications of allogeneic transplantation.

conditioning regimen are well managed with standard symptomatic measures and careful monitoring of fluid and electrolyte status.

Infection prophylaxis is generally provided to guard against bacterial, fungal, and viral pathogens. Based on the high risk for infectious complications and the associated significant morbidity, a number of prophylactic and surveillance strategies have been developed to protect patients in the regard. In a randomized study, the prophylactic use of fluconazole has been shown to reduce the incidence of systemic and superficial fungal infections (70). Fluconazole has not, however, been shown to affect the incidence of infections with resistant organisms such as *Candida krusei* or *Aspergillus*. Trimethoprim-sulfamethoxazole, twice weekly for a year, is given to prevent pneumococcal or pneumocystic infections. Alternatively, twice-weekly doses of penicillin and inhaled pentamidine have been shown to be efficacious in sulfa-allergic patients (71).

Viral infections continue to pose significant challenges to clinicians managing posttransplant patients. In addition to community respiratory viruses, intestinal viruses are easily transmitted through person-to-person contact and have been associated with increased morbidity and mortality (72). Because of a lack of specific therapies for these agents, the focus must be on appropriate isolation of patients and the prevention of nosocomial spread.

The routine prophylactic use of ganciclovir has largely eliminated cytomegalovirus (CMV) disease after transplantation. Historically, CMV infection tends to occur 1 to 3 months after transplantation. Randomized studies have clearly demonstrated efficacy in reducing the incidence of CMV disease by the prophylactic

treatment of all CMV-seropositive patients (73,74). However, this strategy is problematic in that 30 to 35% of treated patients develop neutropenia requiring discontinuation of therapy and placing the patients at increased risk for other infections (75). An alternative strategy is to initiate preemptive therapy when reactivation is first detected. Highly sensitive tests are now available to detect CMV reactivation prior to overt CMV disease and include direct detection of CMV pp65 antigen in peripheral blood leukocytes and detection of CMV DNA in leukocytes, plasma, or serum. When compared with universal ganciclovir prophylaxis starting at time of engraftment, patients receiving antigenemia-directed prophylaxis had similar rates of CMV-related death and survival. Patients receiving automatic prophylaxis did experience less CMV disease in the first 100 days posttransplant; however, this benefit was offset by a higher rate of invasive fungal infections and late CMV disease (74). Thus, current recommendations support close patient monitoring and the use of reactivation-based preemptive strategies. For patients who are CMV seronegative and have CMV-seronegative donors, the use of CMV-seronegative or CMV-filtered blood products is effective in preventing primary infections (76,77).

Reactivation of herpes simplex virus (HSV) occurs in greater than 70% of seropositive patients during the first 6 weeks posttransplant unless prophylaxis is administered (76). Patients in whom HSV reactivation occurs should be treated with acyclovir or valacyclovir. For patients who develop resistance after multiple episodes of HSV reactivation, foscarnet may be required. Acyclovir prophylaxis has been shown to prevent reactivation, reduce morbidity, and lower the incidence of antibiotic resistance; it is routinely administered (78,79).

■ TREATMENT-RELATED COMPLICATIONS

GENERAL CONSIDERATIONS

The transient occurrence of nausea, vomiting, stomatitis, enteritis, alopecia, erythema or rash, and diarrhea is frequent in graft recipients and can generally be managed through aggressive supportive care. Although mucosal or gastrointestinal complications are among the most prominent, less than 10% of patients experience severe toxicities in this regard (80). More serious complications include interstitial pneumonitis, hemorrhagic cystitis, heart failure or pericarditis, hepatic venoocclusive disease (VOD), or infections stemming from profound myelosuppression. The frequency of hemorrhagic cystitis associated with high-dose cyclophosphamide has been largely abrogated by the use of mesna and aggressive hydration (81). Likewise, the routine use of antiepileptic agents such as dilantin for patients receiving high-dose busulfan has dramatically reduced the incidence of grand-mal seizures (82). Life-threatening complications are seen in less than 20% of patients. Regimen-related mortality is generally considered to be between 15 and 25% using standard regimens in young patients in remission. Patients receiving grafts from compatible-related donors experience substantially less toxicity than those receiving grafts from alternative sources (80).

MYELOSUPPRESSION

Shortly after infusion, hematopoietic stem cells migrate to sites in the lungs, liver, spleen, and marrow. For most patients, a variably cellular marrow can be demonstrated within 14 days. Engraftment is defined as the first of three consecutive days on which the absolute neutrophil count is greater than 0.5×109/L and the platelet count is greater than 20×109/L. This generally occurs 14 to 24 days after stem cell infusion. Prior to engraftment, patients require aggressive hematologic support with platelet and red blood cell transfusions. All blood products are routinely irradiated to minimize the possibility of graft-versus-host reactions mediated by donor T cells (83). For patients experiencing prolonged cytopenias, growth factors may be used to shorten the duration of aplasia without increasing the risk of GVHD or relapse (84,85).

GRAFT FAILURE

The failure to recover hematologic function or the loss of marrow function after initial reconstitution constitutes graft failure. This can occur in 5 to 11% of HLA-identical recipients and may be mediated by immunologic graft rejection by the host immune system, infections, drugs, or an inadequate stem cell dose (86-88). Graft failure generally takes place within 60 days of transplantation, although late graft failure has been known to occur.

A number of factors are known to increase the risk of graft failure in allogeneic transplants. A low nucleated cell count infused, T-cell depletion, increasing HLA disparity between donor and host, and inadequate immunosuppression of the host all increase the risk of failure. In patients transplanted for aplastic anemia, allo-immunization by prior transfusions increased the risk of graft rejection (89). In these situations, the rate of graft failure may be as high as 30%. Abundant evidence now exists implicating host T cells as the mediators of an active host immune response against the minor alloantigens expressed by the donor cells (90,91). Based on this understanding, several strategies to further eliminate or inactivate host T cells have evolved. These include the use of additional or increased-intensity immunosuppressive agents such as fludarabine or thiotepa or the elimination of host T cells through the use of antithymocyte globulin or OKT3.

Treatment of graft failure depends on whether donor cells can be detected in the patient's marrow. If present, a repeat infusion of donor cells can be attempted with or without further conditioning. When no donor hematopoietic cells are detected, a second conditioning regimen may be administered, followed by donor stem cells. However, outcomes in this setting are extremely poor (86).

HEPATIC VENOOCCLUSIVE DISEASE

One of the most serious complications of high-dose chemotherapy used in preparative regimens is VOD. This comprises a constellation of findings including fluid retention with weight gain, painful hepatomegaly, and hyperbilirubinemia; it is caused by endothelial damage to the hepatic sinusoids (92,93). This, in turn, leads to obstruction of blood flow through hepatic capillaries and venules, which may cause extensive centrilobular necrosis. In severe cases, portal hypertension may result in gastrointestinal bleeding; similarly, a low-perfusion state may give rise to prerenal azotemia or overt renal failure. Mortality in such cases reaches 40 to 60% (92-95). The overall incidence of VOD varies between 5 and 70% in studies, in large part due to differences in diagnostic criteria, variable conditioning regimens, and adult versus pediatric patients. The spectrum of disease is also variable, ranging from mild and transient symptoms to multisystem organ failure and death. The diagnosis of VOD is generally made based on clinical findings, requiring two of the following three features within 20 days posttransplant: (a) hyperbilirubinemia >2 mg/dL, (b) painful hepatomegaly, and (c) weight gain >2% of baseline body weight due to fluid retention (93).

A number of factors are felt to contribute to an individual patient's risk for VOD (Table 12-1). Preexisting liver disease or elevated transaminases appear to confer an increased risk of VOD. Historically, allogeneic transplantation has been felt to be associated with higher rates of VOD; however, this may be more a function of the higher-intensity conditioning regimens used in this setting. Agents commonly used in allogeneic transplantation, including cyclophosphamide, busulfan, and TBI, have all been implicated in the pathogenesis of VOD. When used as part of GVHD prophylaxis, methotrexate has been linked to higher risk of VOD (96). Finally, patients receiving mismatched transplants or unrelated donor transplants are at increased risk (97).

The treatment of VOD remains investigational. The rate and degree of bilirubin elevation appear to correlate with outcome but have limited sensitivity early in disease, when treatments would be expected to have the greatest impact (95). Treatment of VOD with thrombolytics has shown an unacceptably high rate of bleeding complications and is therefore not recommended (92). An emerging treatment for VOD appears to involve the use of defibrotide, a polydeoxyribonucleotide with adenosine receptor agonist activity. Defibrotide increases prostaglandin and thrombomodulin on the endothelial cell surface and has the advantage of lacking any intrinsic anticoagulant properties. Favorable results in preliminary studies in patients with established VOD warrant further investigation (98,99). Until more definitive treatments for VOD are established, aggressive supportive care remains integral to treating such patients. Careful maintenance of intravascular volume must be tempered by the dangers of fluid overload. In this regard, blood products or albumin are frequently used to optimize intravascular volume. Low-dose dopamine and diuretics may be used to maintain renal perfusion. The use of additional hepatotoxic agents must obviously be minimized in this group of patients.

PULMONARY COMPLICATIONS

Following allogeneic stem cell transplant, patients are at risk for a wide range of pulmonary complications, ranging from pulmonary edema to diffuse alveolar hemorrhage to interstitial pneumonitis (IP). In fact, IP remains one of the most common sources of morbidity and mortality in the 20 to 40% of transplant patients affected (100,101). Although many cases are deemed idiopathic or related to an aberrant systemic inflammatory response, the majority are likely to be related to viral infections. In recent years, the importance of adenovirus, respiratory syncytial virus (RSV), influenza virus, and parainfluenza in the pathogenesis of interstitial pneumonias have become more apparent (102). Transplant patients experiencing pneumonia caused by one of these viruses may have a mortality rate as high as 50% (103). Risk factors for the development of IP include advanced age, a history of underlying pulmonary disease, or exposure to lung-toxic drugs such as bleomycin, GVHD, and the use of TBI (104,105).

At the MDACC, all patients undergoing allogeneic transplantation are rigorously screened for symptoms suggestive of community respiratory virus infection. When symptoms are present, transplant is delayed even if rapid-detection tests are negative. In transplant recipients who develop RSV pneumonia, early therapy is instituted with ribavirin and intravenous immunoglobulin (102).

INFECTION

Infectious complications result from profound humoral and cellular immune deficiencies that occur shortly after conditioning and may persist for more than 18 months posttransplant (106,107). Cellular deficiencies are characterized by impaired T-cell responses to alloantigens and mitogens, diminished CD4+ helper T-cell function, as well as quantitative deficiencies in the immediate posttransplant period. Even following quantitative recovery, numerous groups have shown profound deficits in the functional capacity of T-cell subsets, which may persist for months. Compromised humoral immunity is evidenced by a decrease in IgG2 and IgG4 levels as well as by impaired transitions from primary antibody production (IgM) to secondary antibody production (IgG). Immune deficiencies can be exacerbated by the routine use of immunosuppressive agents for the treatment of GVHD.

Immune deficiencies have been broadly described in three phases (108). Phase 1 represents the immediate posttransplant period until engraftment, during which profound neutropenia and mucositis are common. This increases the patient's risk of bacterial infection. In the past, gram-negative infections predominated; in modern transplantation protocols, however, the use of prophylactic antibiotics has resulted in a decrease in gram-negative bacteremia and a relative increase in the proportion of gram-positive infections. An algorithm for the initial management of neutropenic fever at MDACC is presented in Fig. 12-5. Phase 2 generally occurs between engraftment and month 4 or 5 and is noteworthy for ongoing deficits in cellular immunity and immunosuppression caused by the treatment of GVHD. During this period patients are at risk for CMV reactivation or the development of fungal infections. Finally, phase 3 lasts from month 4 until immunity is restored. Despite adequate numbers of circulating neutrophils, there may be skewed or incomplete T-cell reconstitution. Patients continue to be at risk for reactivation of latent viruses, particularly of the herpes virus family.

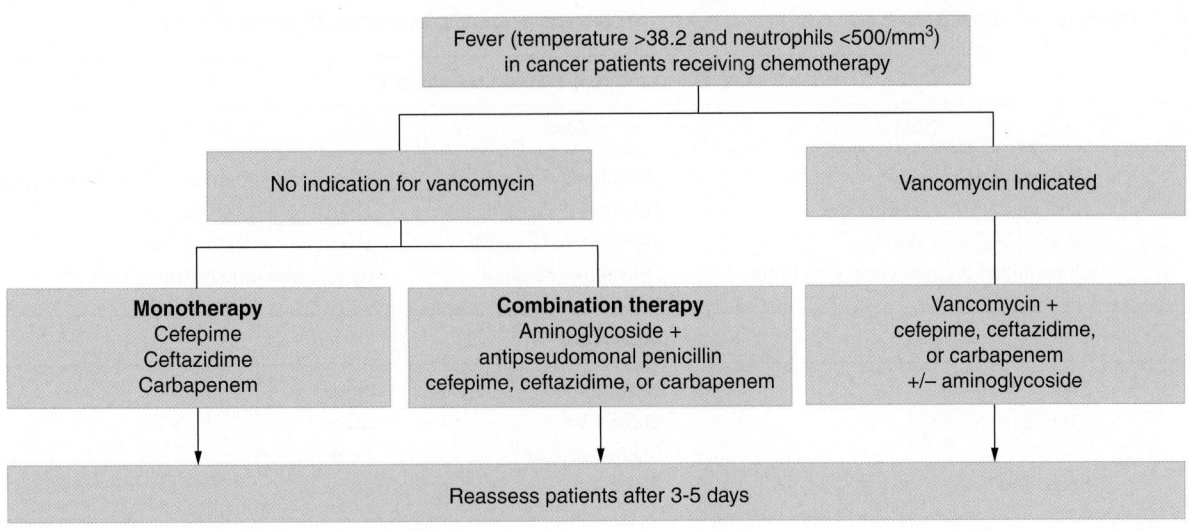

FIGURE 12-5. Algorithm for the initial management of neutropenic fever. *(Adapted with permission from Hughes WT, Armstrong D, Bodey GP, et al. 2002 guidelines for the use of antimicrobial agents neutropenic patients with cancer. Clin Infect Dis 2002;34(6):730-751.)*

The severe cellular immunodeficiency in addition to steroid therapy for GVHD increases the risk of invasive mold infection (109). Coupled with better control of CMV infection over the last decade, fungal infections have emerged as a leading cause of death among transplant patients. Although the routine use of fluconazole has dramatically reduced the rate of invasive *Candida albicans* infections, several centers have reported increases in the frequency of invasive mold infections. *Aspergillus* species are most commonly isolated. During the first-year posttransplantation, the cumulative incidence of invasive aspergillosis is approximately 10 to 14% (110-112). Moreover, the 20% survival rate for patients who develop such infections reflects their poor response to currently available therapy. Risk factors for the development of early invasive aspergillosis (before posttransplant day 40) include advanced patient age and the use of peripheral blood stem cells rather than marrow-derived cells (110). The latter risk factor is partially explained by the longer duration of neutropenia associated with bone marrow grafts. Late-onset invasive aspergillosis (beyond posttransplant day 40) occurs with increased frequency in older patients, recipients of T-cell-depleted or CD34-selected grafts, patients with CMV disease, patients with prolonged neutropenia, and patients with active GVHD who are receiving corticosteroid therapy (110). Patients receiving mismatched or unrelated donor grafts also appear to be at increased risk for invasive mold infections. Recent data suggest that itraconazole may be more effective than fluconazole for fungal prophylaxis, in part due to itraconazole's greater in vitro activity against *Aspergillus* and some fluconazole-resistant *Candida* species (113,114).

Epstein-Barr virus (EBV)–related lymphoproliferative disorder (LPD) is an uncommon but rapidly progressive lymphoma that was uniformly fatal prior to the advent of new therapies. The condition stems from the unchecked proliferation of EBV-transformed B lymphocytes in the setting of immune dysfunction and generally occurs in the first-year posttransplant (115,116). An absence of functional EBV-specific cytotoxic T cells (CTLs) is felt to be integral to the pathogenesis of this disorder. Indeed, the incidence of LPD is increased in patients receiving anti-CD3 monoclonal antibody, antithymocyte globulin, T-cell depleted grafts, or HLA-mismatched grafts (116,117). Therapies that restore circulating EBV-specific CTLs are efficacious in inducing sustained remissions. This may be accomplished through the administration of unmanipulated donor leukocytes or virus-specific lymphocytes (118-123). More recently, the anti-CD20 monoclonal antibody rituximab has been successfully used to prevent and treat EBV-LPD (124,125).

ACUTE GVHD

Clinical manifestations of acute GVHD include a maculopapular skin rash, enteritis involving the distal small bowel or colon, and hepatitis (126). Organs may be involved in isolation or simultaneously. In general, acute GVHD presents within the first 100 days posttransplant.

TABLE 12-2	CLINICAL GRADING OF ACUTE GRAFT-VERSUS-HOST DISEASE (DAYS 1-100)

EXTENT OF ORGAN INVOLVEMENT

Stage	Skin	Liver	Gut
1	Rash on <25% of skin*	Bilirubin 2-3 mg/dL[†]	Diarrhea >500 mL/d[‡] or persistent nausea[#]
2	Rash on 25-50% of skin	Bilirubin 3-6 mg/dL	Diarrhea > 1000 mL/day
3	Rash on >50% of skin	Bilirubin 6-15 mg/dL	Diarrhea > 1500 mL/day
4	Generalized erythroderma with bullae	Bilirubin >15 mg/dL	Severe abdominal pain ± ileus

GRADE[§]

I	Stage I or II	None	None
II	Stage 3 or	Stage 1 or	Stage 1
III	–	Stage 2 or 3 or	Stage 2, 3, or 4
IV[¶]	Stage 4 or	Stage 4	–

*Use the "rule of nines" or burn chart to determine extent of rash.
[†]Range given as total bilirubin. Downgrade one stage if additional causes of hyperbilirubinemia are documented.
[‡]Volume of diarrhea applies to adults. Downgrade one stage if additional causes of diarrhea are documented.
[#]Persistent nausea with histologic evidence of GVHD in the stomach or duodenum.
[§]Criteria for grading given as the minimum degree of organ involvement required to confer that grade.
[¶]Grade IV may also include lesser organ involvement but with decrease in performance status.

However, delayed de novo presentations of acute GVHD are reported. A clinical grading system allowing for quantitative estimates of disease severity and response to therapy is presented in Table 12-2. Severity is described as grade I (mild) to grade IV (severe). The incidence of clinically significant GVHD (grade II to grade IV) in recipients of HLA genotypically identical grafts (T-cell replete) and using cyclosporine and methotrexate for GVHD prophylaxis is approximately 40% (127). Increasing HLA disparity increases both the incidence and severity of resultant GVHD with recipients of phenotypically matched unrelated donor grafts experiencing a 50 to 80% incidence of grade II to grade IV GVHD (128,129). Other risk factors for acute GVHD include older age, a parous or alloimmunized donor, less intense immunosuppression, or the use of a T-cell-replete versus T-cell-depleted graft (130).

Acute GVHD can often be diagnosed on the basis of clinical findings. Histologic confirmation can be valuable in excluding other possibilities, such as infection. Mild GVHD of the skin may demonstrate vacuolar degeneration and infiltration of the basal layer by lymphocytes. With more advanced disease, histologic findings of necrotic dyskeratotic cells with acantholysis may progress to frank epidermolysis. In the liver, early GVHD may be difficult to distinguish from hepatitis of other causes.

Moderate-to-severe GVHD (grade II-IV) requires appropriate treatment. The mainstay of therapy has long been corticosteroid therapy. Methylprednisolone,

at a dose of 2 mg/kg/day, can be expected to achieve responses in 40 to 60% of patients. Higher doses of steroids have not been shown to be of greater benefit (131). Steroid-refractory GVHD responds poorly to second-line therapies and is associated with increased mortality. ATG is commonly used as a second-line treatment, with limited success. Novel treatments showing efficacy in preliminary studies include extracorporeal phototherapy and the combination of MMF and tacrolimus. Sirolimus has also been shown to be well tolerated and effective as a primary therapy for acute GVHD in patients who do not tolerate steroid therapy (132) or in steroid refractory GVHD (133). In general, acute GVHD of the skin is most responsive to treatment, whereas GVHD of the liver is least responsive. The fatality rate for acute GVHD may be as high as 50%. Recent studies showed that the combination of tacrolimus/sirolimus +/– MTX for GVHD prophylaxis in the setting of RIC HCT reduce the incidence of severe acute GVHD compared to CSA/MMF +/– MTX (134,135). The addition of alemtuzumab to an RIC regimen dramatically reduces the incidence of aGVHD and cGVHD in patients with AML and MDS undergoing allogeneic transplantation (136).

CHRONIC GVHD

Chronic GVHD occurs in 20 to 50% of long-term survivors. Risk factors include old age, prior acute GVHD, use of donor buffy coat infusions, and prior

HSV infection. In 20% of cases, there is no history of prior acute GVHD (137). Patients are at risk for developing chronic GVHD from 3 months after transplantation to 6 months after discontinuation of all immunosuppressives, although recent studies show that histologic changes consistent with chronic GVHD may be detected within 60 days of transplant. Common manifestations include the sicca syndrome, lichen planus-like skin rash, scleroderma-like skin changes, esophageal and intestinal fibrosis, obstructive lung disease with or without pneumonitis (138), and elevated alkaline phosphatase with or without hyperbilirubinemia (139). Underlying immunologic deficiencies including hypogammaglobulinemia are common, placing patients at increased risk for infectious events.

As with the acute form of the disease, the primary mediators of chronic GVHD are felt to be donor T cells. These activated T cells are capable of cytolysis and cytokine production which, in turn, give rise to the clinical manifestations. The histologic findings in chronic GVHD are best described for skin, lips, and liver. An initial cellular inflammatory phase progresses slowly to widespread fibrosis. The histologic findings of chronic GVHD can antedate clinical manifestations. When study patients were screened at day 100 after transplantation, detection of subclinical GVHD in two or more organs was predictive of eventual clinical GVHD development (140).

Chronic GVHD may be limited or extensive. Limited disease implies localized skin involvement with minimal or no liver involvement, whereas extensive disease suggests generalized skin involvement with or without other organ involvement. Patients with limited disease have a good prognosis with 60 to 70% long-term survival while those with extensive disease experience 20 to 30% long-term survival.

Treatment for chronic GVHD is guided by the extent of disease. Initiation of therapy prior to functional impairment is of critical importance. Combination therapy with every-other-day cyclosporine or tacrolimus and prednisone has demonstrated efficacy in the treatment of chronic GVHD (141). Alternatives include azathioprine, UV light, psoralen-UV-A, or thalidomide (142). For liver cGVHD, bezafibrate has shown to be efficacious even in patients who are ursodeoxycholic acid-resistant (143). MSCs may prevent the lethal cGVHD after allogeneic hematopoietic stem cell transplantation and raise the survival rate by increasing the ratio of CD4/CD8 and proportion of regulatory T cells in vivo (144). The most common cause of death in patients with chronic GVHD remains infection; therefore, all patients should receive prophylactic

trimethoprim-sulfamethoxazole with or without intravenous immunoglobulin.

LATE COMPLICATIONS

Patients at MDACC are evaluated annually for several delayed toxicities resulting from allogeneic stem cell transplantation. These include endocrine toxicities such as hypothyroidism, hypogonadism, or growth hormone deficiency in younger patients; pulmonary effects may include obstructive lung disease or pulmonary fibrosis. Other late effects include cataracts and leukoencephalopathy (23). As previously reported, late infectious complications can occur, including viral reactivation, as well as late fungal infections. These complications are more common in patients who have received T-cell-depleted grafts, long-term steroids for GVHD, or both.

Patients undergoing stem cell transplantation experience an increased risk for secondary malignancies. At 15 years posttransplant, recent retrospective analyses have demonstrated a 10 to 13% incidence of a secondary malignancy (145,146). The spectrum of malignancies reported was broad and included non-Hodgkin lymphoma, myelodysplastic syndrome, skin cancer, head and neck cancers, as well as other solid tumor malignancies. Older patient age and immunosuppressive therapy for chronic GVHD were significantly correlated with the risk of developing a secondary malignancy.

The intensive treatment and prolonged recovery from allogeneic transplant can have profound psychosocial implications for patients and their families. A pretransplant psychosocial evaluation can identify individuals who may require additional intervention after transplantation (147). Most long-term survivors, however, report good to excellent health and functional ability, with outcomes comparable to those of long-term cancer survivors who received less intensive treatments (148).

■ RELAPSE

A major benefit of allogeneic stem cell transplantation is the reduction in the relapse rate, especially when compared with relapse rates following conventional chemotherapy. More advanced disease clearly confers an increased risk of relapse for transplant recipients, as summarized in Table 12-3. As previously discussed, the rate of relapse for recipients of allografts is markedly lower than that for recipients of autologous or syngeneic transplants due to the GVT effect (37). Evidence

TABLE 12-3	INDICATIONS AND CURRENT RESULTS OF ALLOGRAFTING FOR HEMATOLOGIC MALIGNANCIES AT MD ANDERSON CANCER CENTER (MDACC)			
Disease/Stage	**Allograft Recommended**	**Current Results DFS At 5 Years**	**MDACC Approach**	**Comments**
AML CR1				
Good-risk cytogenetics	No	N/A		
Intermediate-risk cytogenetics	Yes	50-60%	Fludarabine/IV Busulfan targeted dose Reduced-intensity conditioning regimens for older patients	
Poor-risk cytogenetics	Yes	30-40%	Fludarabine/IV Busulfan targeted dose Reduced-intensity conditioning regimens for older patients Appropriate for alternative stem cell donor transplants (unrelated, mismatched, and cord blood)	
AML > CR1	Yes	30% if in remission 10-20% if active disease	Fludarabine/IV Busulfan targeted dose Reduced-intensity conditioning regimens for older patients Appropriate for alternative stem cell donor transplants (unrelated, mismatched, and cord blood)	Candidates for phase I/II transplant trials.
MDS good risk	No	N/A		
MDS poor risk	Yes	50-60% if in remission 10-30% if active disease	Fludarabine/IV Busulfan targeted dose Reduced-intensity conditioning regimens for older patients Appropriate for alternative stem cell donor transplants (unrelated, mismatched, and cord blood)	Candidates for phase I/II transplant trials
ALL CR1	Yes (high-risk disease)	40-50%	Cyclophosphamide-TBI with rituximab if CD20+ Reduced-intensity conditioning regimens for older patients	Candidate for phase II trials
ALL > CR1	Yes	30% if in remission, 10-20% if active disease	Cyclophosphamide-TBI with rituximab if CD20+ Reduced-intensity conditioning regimens for older patients	Candidates for phase I/II trials
CML CP1	Yes in Imatinib failures	60%	Fludarabine/IV Busulfan targeted dose Reduced-intensity conditioning regimens for older patients Appropriate for alternative stem cell donor transplants (unrelated, mismatched, and cord blood)	
CML > CP1	Yes	30-40% accelerated phase 10-20% blast crisis	Fludarabine/IV Busulfan targeted dose Reduced-intensity conditioning regimens for older patients Appropriate for alternative stem cell donor transplants (unrelated, mismatched, and cord blood)	Candidates for phase I/II trials

(Continued)

TABLE 12-3 | **INDICATIONS AND CURRENT RESULTS OF ALLOGRAFTING FOR HEMATOLOGIC MALIGNANCIES AT MD ANDERSON CANCER CENTER (MDACC)** (*CONTINUED*)

Disease/Stage	Allograft Recommended	Current Results DFS At 5 Years	MDACC Approach	Comments
NHL/CLL CR1	No	N/A		
NHL/CLL 1st relapse	Only if autograft not feasible	N/A	Reduced-intensity conditioning regimens with rituximab Appropriate for alternative stem cell donor transplants (unrelated, mismatched, and cord blood)	
NHL/CLL > first relapse	Yes	10-50% depending on disease status and chemosensitivity	Reduced-intensity conditioning regimens with rituximab Appropriate for alternative stem cell donor transplants (unrelated, mismatched, and cord blood)	
Hodgkin disease	Only autograft failures	20-30%	Reduced-intensity conditioning regimens for older patients Appropriate for alternative stem cell donor transplants (unrelated, mismatched, and cord blood)	
Myeloma	Yes Intermediate- and high- risk patients or autograft failures	Depends on disease stage and chemosensitivity	Auto followed by reduced-intensity conditioning regimens Alternative stem cell donor transplants (unrelated, mismatched, and cord blood) only for patients with high-risk disease	

ALL, acute lymphocytic leukemia; AML, chronic myelogenous leukemia; CLL, chronic lymphocytic leukemia; CR1, first complete remission; IV, intravenous; MDS, myelodysplastic syndromes; NHL, non-Hodgkin lymphoma.

for GVT exists in the treatment of both leukemias and lymphomas.

Among hematologic malignancies, CML appears to be particularly vulnerable to the GVT effect. Among patients undergoing allogeneic transplantation in the chronic phase, up to 75% may be long-term survivors. Disease phase at the time of transplantation also has a prominent effect on outcome. Disease-free survival for patients in first chronic phase, accelerated phase, or blast phase is 40 to 60%, 26 to 38%, and less than 15%, respectively (149,150). Long-term survivors are generally PCR-negative for the Bcr-Abl fusion protein, which characterizes CML. For those patients who relapse, donor lymphocyte infusion (DLI) is an effective strategy to reinduce complete remissions (151).

Relapse rates in acute myelogenous leukemias are also highly dependent on the status of disease at time of allogeneic transplantation. Transplantation after achievement of first remission is much more likely to be curative than transplantation performed in second remission or beyond. Except for patients with favorable cytogenetics, AML patients are at high risk for relapse and should therefore be considered for experimental therapies, including transplantation in first remission. For patients with myelodysplastic syndrome, relapse rates are highly correlated with cytogenetic subgroups, with poor risk patients having an 82% relapse rate (152).

■ CURRENT APPROACHES TO ALLOGENEIC TRANSPLANTATION AT MD ANDERSON CANCER CENTER

Table 12-3 summarizes the current approaches to allogeneic transplant in the most common hematologic disorders seen at MDACC.

■ CONTROVERSIES AND FUTURE DIRECTIONS

NONMYELOABLATIVE CONDITIONING REGIMENS

Allogeneic transplantation has been successfully used to cure a spectrum of neoplastic and hereditary diseases for which there had previously been no cure. However, the substantial toxicities associated with traditional conditioning regimens have limited the application of this modality to relatively young patients with good performance status. One of the most important controversies in allogeneic transplantation today is whether nonablative or reduced-intensity conditioning regimens should replace conventional myeloablative regimens. Theoretically, the use of less intensive regimens could improve the outcomes of these patients even further. It has been an option for patients with myeloma (153), refractory mantle cell lymphoma (154). It has also shown benefits to patients >50 years old with high-risk ALL in first complete remission (155).

As expected, toxicity profiles with nonmyeloablative regimens compare favorably to conventional regimens. Severe mucositis, VOD, and other life-threatening organ toxicities related to the treatment regimen are rare (156,157). Infectious complications, although still a significant issue, may be abrogated in the immediate post-transplantation period due to the persistence of host hematopoiesis. The occurrence of CMV disease appears substantially delayed in recipients of nonablative regimens, but the overall incidence by 1 year after transplantation has been found to be similar to that in conventional transplant patients. Therefore, after day 100, these patients should be followed in a manner similar to that used for conventional transplant recipients (157).

The rates of acute and chronic GVHD do not appear to be substantially different from those observed in the conventional setting. Numerous studies have reported the incidence of acute GVHD as between 25 and 60%. These episodes can be precipitated by DLI or withdrawal of immunosuppression, often performed in hopes of augmenting the GVT effect (158). The optimal regimens for prophylaxis and treatment of GVHD in this patient population remain to be defined.

TIMING OF TRANSPLANTATION

The other important controversy involves the optimal time for an allogeneic transplant. While allogeneic transplantation is potentially curative for a number of hematologic malignancies, the decision to proceed with it must be tempered by an evaluation of disease-specific factors (disease type, early versus advanced disease, cytogenetic prognostic factors, chemoresponsive versus refractory disease) and patient-specific factors (age, performance status, availability of a donor, and psychosocial support). Situations exist where multiple treatment modalities could reasonably be entertained as front-line therapy. For example, allogeneic transplantation is felt to be the most established therapy for CML. However, the advent of imatinib mesylate has provided some CML patients with a relatively nontoxic means of long-term disease control. In the past, delaying transplantation for CML patients undergoing short-term treatment with interferon was not associated with worse outcomes. It is currently unclear whether delaying transplantation for imatinib treatment will yield a similar result. Only long-term follow-up of such patients will provide definitive answers to these questions.

For patients with CLL, results of allogeneic transplantation are less clear. Although it is evident that such strategies can effectively produce long-term remissions, it is unclear whether allogeneic transplantation produces outcomes superior to those of conventional therapies. Studies in patients with low-grade lymphomas and Hodgkin disease have also been suggestive of a GVT effect, but early treatment-related mortality rates of 25 to 30% mitigate this finding. It is possible that reduced-intensity regimens will effectively harness a GVT effect while avoiding the early toxicities associated with conventional transplantation in these patients.

Expected long-term survival rates for HLA-identical stem cell recipients vary with disease and disease status. As with relapse rates, patients with more advanced disease have significantly higher mortality rates, in large part due to progressive disease. For leukemic patients with primary chemotherapy-refractory disease, allogeneic transplant is effective salvage therapy in less than 20% of cases. These patients remain among the most significant challenges in allogeneic transplantation today. The addition of targeted therapies (ie, monoclonal antibodies) or novel maintenance therapies is currently being explored.

ROLE OF ALLOGENEIC STEM CELL TRANSPLANT IN MULTIPLE MYELOMA

For patients who has multiple myeloma (MM) failing to achieve at least near-complete remission after a first autologous stem cell transplantation, a reduced-intensity-conditioning allograft as compared to a second autologous transplant if there is an HLA-identical sibling donor available demonstrated a higher increase in complete remission (CR) rate and a trend toward a longer progression-free survival. However, it is associated with a higher transplantation-related mortality, which offset the event-free survival and overall survival (153). Therefore, this should still be considered investigational and restricted to well-designed prospective clinical trials.

MAINTENANCE THERAPY

Acute Myelogenous Leukemia

Relapse is the major cause of treatment failure after HSCT for relapsed AML. Maintenance therapy may provide an "adjuvant" support for the allogeneic graft-versus-leukemia effect, decreasing the likelihood of recurrence. AZA is a DNA methyltransferase inhibitor that induces DNA hypomethylation, leading to leukemic cell differentiation and potentially increased tumor immunogenicity. Azacitidine has been shown to be effective in treatment of AML (159,160). A phase I study has determined the safest dose and schedule of azacitidine that can be administered to the posttransplant patients who previously had been heavily treated. We initiated a randomized, controlled study azacitidine for 1 year versus no maintenance therapy posttransplant for high-risk patients with AML/MDS to evaluate relapse.

Multiple Myeloma

For patients with multiple myeloma, diseases relapse despite autologous transplantation. Novel agents such as lenalidomide, thalidomide, and bortezomib have been effective as induction therapy in both newly diagnosed and relapsed myeloma. Thalidomide and bortezomib are indicated as consolidating agents. Because of concerns about the toxicity of thalidomide, further clinical trials using alternative novel therapeutic agents such as lenalidomide and bortezomib should be explored to better define the efficacy, toxicity, and quality of life during maintenance therapy in patients with MM (161).

■ HIGH-DOSE CYTOXAN FOR GVHD PROPHYLAXIS POSTHAPLOIDENTICAL TRANSPLANT

Haploidentical transplant (haploSCT) offers an option for patients who have high-risk hematologic diseases requiring stem cell transplant but has no HLA-compatible donors. This type of transplant carries a high risk of GVHD due to antigen mismatch. T-cell depletion prior to haploSCT can minimize GVHD but carries a high rate of disease relapse with diminished graft-versus-malignancy effect and serious infectious complications from delayed in immune reconstitution (162). HSCT are quiescent nondividing cells expressing a high level of aldehyde dehydrogenase, thus they are resistant to cytoxan, whereas T, B, and NK cells expressing low level of aldehyde dehydrogenase, thus are sensitive to cytoxan cytotoxicity (163). Thus, posttransplant high-dose cytoxan can induce donor–host tolerance to allografting and decrease GVHD by eliminating alloreactive T-cells clones without myeloablation (164). Two doses of posttransplant cytoxan reduces extensive cGVHD more effectively as compared to one dose (165,166). Posttransplant high-dose cytoxan followed nonmyeloablative conditioning regimen with fludarabine and low-dose TBI had been shown to produce durable engraftment (165,166). HaploSCT following nonmyeloablative conditioning regimen in lymphoid malignancy has shown to have a decreased incidence of relapse/progression, nonrelapse mortality (NRM), and lower rate of extensive chronic GVHD as compared to match-related and match-unrelated transplant (167). At MD Anderson, we use fludarabine, melphalan, and thiotepa as the reduced-intensity conditioning as our retrospective analysis on cord blood transplant and T-cell-depleted haploidentical transplant using this regimen showed a 95% engraftment of cord blood and haploSCT (in patients without donor-specific anti-HLA antibodies), low treatment-related mortality of less than 10%, NRM, and improved OS as compared to patients received TBI-based preparative regimen or myeloablative regimen (168-170).

References

1. Thomas ED, Storb R, Clift RA, et al. Bone marrow transplantation. *N Eng J Med* 1975;292(17):895-902.
2. Bortin MM. A compendium of reported human bone marrow transplants. *Transplantation* 1970;9(6):571-587.
3. Gatti RA, Meuwissen HJ, Allen HD, et al. Immunological reconstitution of sex-linked lymphopenic immunological deficiency. *Lancet* 1968;2(7583):1366-1369.
4. Fefer A, Buckner CD, Thomas ED, et al. Cure of hematologic neoplasia with transplantation of marrow from identical twins. *N Eng J Med* 1977;293(3):146-148.
5. *Trends in Allogeneic Transplant.* NMDP Newsletter 2009.
6. Ottinger HD, Muller CR, Goldmann SF, et al. Second German consensus on immunogenetic donor search for allotransplantation of hematopoietic stem cells. *Ann Hematol* 2001;80(12):706-714.
7. Petersdorf EW, Longton GM, Anasetti C, et al. Definition of HLA-DQ as a transplantation antigen. *Proc Natl Acad Sci USA* 1996;93(26):15358-15363.

8. Petersdorf E, Anasetti C, Servida P, et al. Effect of HLA matching on outcome of related and unrelated donor transplantation therapy for chronic myelogenous leukemia. *Hematol Oncol Clin North Am* 1998;12(1):107-121.

9. Buckner CD, Clift RA, Sanders JE, et al. Marrow harvesting from normal donors. *Blood* 1984;64(3):630-634.

10. Confer DL. Hematopoietic Cell Donors. In:Thomas Third Edition, Blume KG, Forman SJ, Appelbaum FR.(eds). Hematopoietic Cell Transplantation, 3rd ed. Blackwell Science, Malden, MA;2009.

11. Giralt SA, Kolb HJ. Donor lymphocyte infusions. *Curr Opin Oncol* 1996;8(2):96-102.

12. Molldrem J, Dermime S, Parker K, et al. Targeted T-cell therapy for human leukemia: Cytotoxic T lymphocytes specific for a peptide derived from proteinase 3 preferentially lyse human myeloid leukemia cells. *Blood* 1996;88(7):2450-2457.

13. Mavroudis DA, Dermime S, Molldrem J, et al. Specific depletion of alloreactive T cells in HLA-identical siblings: A method for separating graft-versus-host and graft-versus-leukaemia reactions. *Br J Haematol* 1998;101(3):565-570.

14. Kolb HJ, Holler E. Adoptive immunotherapy with donor lymphocyte transfusions. *Curr Opin Oncol* 1997;9(2):139-145.

15. Kolb HJ, Schattenberg A, Goldman JM, et al. Graft-versus-leukemia effect of donor lymphocyte transfusions in marrow grafted patients. *Blood* 1995;86(5):2041-2050.

16. Vriesendorp HM, Chu H, Ochran TG, et al. Radiobiology of total body radiation. *Bone Marrow Transplant* 1994; 14(Suppl 4): S4-S8.

17. Socie G, Devergie A, Girinsky T, et al. Influence of the fractionation of total body irradiation on complications and relapse rate for chronic myelogenous leukemia. The Groupe d'Etude des greffes de moelle osseuse (GEGMO). *Int J Radiat Oncol Biol Phys* 1991;20(3):397-404.

18. Gopal R, Ha CS, Tucker SL, et al. Comparison of two total body irradiation fractionation regimens with respect to acute and late pulmonary toxicity. *Cancer* 2001;92(7): 1949-1958.

19. Clift RA, Buckner CD, Appelbaum FR, et al. Long-term follow-up of a randomized trial of two irradiation regimens for patients receiving allogeneic marrow transplants during first remission of acute myeloid leukemia. *Blood* 1998;92(4): 1455-1456.

20. Clift RA, Buckner CD, Appelbaum FR, et al. Allogeneic marrow transplantation in patients with acute myeloid leukemia in first remission: A randomized trial of two irradiation regimens. *Blood* 1990;76(9):1867-1871.

21. Giralt S, LeMaistre CF, Vriesendorp H, et al. Etoposide, cyclophosphamide, total-body irradiation, and allogeneic bone marrow transplantation for hematologic malignancies. *J Clin Oncol* 1994;12(9):1923-1930.

22. Snyder DS, Negrin RS, O'Donnell MR, et al. Fractionated total-body irradiation and high-dose etoposide as a preparatory regimen for bone marrow transplantation for 94 patients with chronic myelogenous leukemia in chronic phase. *Blood* 1994;84(5):1672-1679.

23. Kolb HJ, Bender-Götze C. Late complications after allogeneic bone marrow transplantation for leukaemia. *Bone Marrow Transplant* 1990;6(2):61-72.

24. Andersson BS, Kashyap A, Gian V, et al. Conditioning therapy with intravenous busulfan and cyclophosphamide (IVbucy2) for hematologic malignancies prior to allogeneic stem cell transplantation: A phase II study. *Biol Blood Marrow Transplant* 2002;8(3):145-154.

25. Andersson BS, Madden T, Tran HT, et al. Acute safety and pharmacokinetics of intravenous busulfan when used with oral busulfan and cyclophosphamide as pretransplantation conditioning therapy: A phase I study. *Biol Blood Marrow Transplant* 2000;6(5A):548-554.

26. Devergie A, Blaise D, Attal M, et al. Allogeneic bone marrow transplantation for chronic myeloid leukemia in first chronic phase: A randomized trial of busulfan-cytoxan versus cytoxan-total body irradiation as preparative regimen: A report from the French Society of Bone Marrow Graft (SFGM). *Blood* 1995;85(8):2263-2268.

27. Clift RA, Buckner CD, Thomas ED, et al. Marrow transplantation for chronic myeloid leukemia: A randomized study comparing cyclophosphamide and total body irradiation with busulfan and cyclophosphamide. *Blood* 1994;84(6): 2036-2043.

28. Blaise D, Maraninchi D, Archimbaud E, et al. Allogeneic bone marrow transplantation for acute myeloid leukemia in first remission: A randomized trial of a busulfan-Cytoxan versus Cytoxan-total body irradiation as preparative regimen: A report from the Group d'Etudes de la Greffe de Moelle Osseuse. *Blood* 1992;79(10):2578-2582.

29. McCune JS, Gibbs JP, Slattery JT. Plasma concentration monitoring of busulfan: Does it improve clinical outcome? *Clin Pharmacokinet* 2000;39(2):155-165.

30. Hassan M, Ljungman P, Bolme P, et al. Busulfan bioavailability. *Blood* 1994;84(7):2144-2150.

31. McDonald GB, Slattery JT, Bouvier ME, et al. Cyclophosphamide metabolism, liver toxicity, and mortality following hematopoietic stem cell transplantation. *Blood* 2003;101(5): 2043-2048.

32. Russell JA, Tran HT, Quinlan D, et. al. One-daily intravenous busulfan given with fludarabine as conditioning for allogeneic stem cell transplantation: Study of pharmacokinetics and early clinical outcomes. *Biol Blood Marrow Transplant* 2002;8(9):468-476.

33. Bornhauser M, Storer B, Slattery JT, et al. Conditioning with fludarabine and targeted busulfan for transplantation of allogeneic hematopoietic stem cells. *Blood* 2003;102(3):820-826.

34. de Lima M, Couriel D, Shahjahan M. Allogeneic transplantation for acute myeloid leukemia (AML) and myelodysplastic syndrome (MDS) using a low toxicity combination of intravenous busulfan and fludarabine. *Blood* 2002;100:853a.

35. Sullivan KM, Weiden PL, Storb R, et al. Influence of acute and chronic graft-versus-host disease on relapse and survival after bone marrow transplantation from HLA-identical siblings as treatment of acute and chronic leukemia. *Blood* 1989;73(6):1720-1728.

36. Weiden PL, Flournoy N, Thomas ED, et al. Antileukemic effect of graft-versus-host disease in human recipients of allogeneic-marrow grafts. *N Engl J Med* 1979;300(19):1068-1073.

37. Horowitz MM, Gale RP, Sondel PM, et al. Graft-versus-leukemia reactions after bone marrow transplantation. *Blood* 1990;75(3):555-562.

38. Khouri IF, Keating M, Korbling M, et al. Transplant-lite: Induction of graft-versus-malignancy using fludarabine-based nonablative chemotherapy and allogeneic blood progenitor-cell transplantation as treatment for lymphoid malignancies. *J Clin Oncol* 1998;16(8):2817-2824.

39. Giralt S, Estey E, Albitar M, et al. Engraftment of allogeneic hematopoietic progenitor cells with purine analog-containing chemotherapy: Harnessing graft-versus-leukemia without myeloablative therapy. *Blood* 1997;89(12):4531-4536.

40. Khouri IF, Saliba RM, Giralt SA, et al. Nonablative allogeneic hematopoietic transplantation as adoptive immunotherapy for indolent lymphoma: Low incidence of toxicity, acute graft-versus-host disease, and treatment-related mortality. *Blood* 2001;98(13):3595-3599.

41. Branson K, Chopra R, Kottaridis PD, et al. Role of nonmyeloablative allogeneic stem-cell transplantation after failure of autologous transplantation in patients with lymphoproliferative malignancies. *J Clin Oncol* 2002;20(19):4022-4031.

42. Storb R, Yu C, Wagner JL, et al. Stable mixed hematopoietic chimerism in DLA-identical littermate dogs given sublethal total body irradiation before and pharmacological immunosuppression after marrow transplantation. *Blood* 1997;89(8):3048-3054.

43. McSweeney PA, Niederwieser D, Shizuru JA, et al. Hematopoietic cell transplantation in older patients with hematologic malignancies: Replacing high-dose cytotoxic therapy with graft-versus-tumor effects. *Blood* 2001;97(11):3390-3400.

44. Dominietto A, Lamparelli T, Raiola AM, et al. Transplant-related mortality and long-term graft function are significantly influenced by cell dose in patients undergoing allogeneic marrow transplantation. *Blood* 2002;100(12):3930-3934.

45. To LB, Roberts MM, Haylock DN, et al. Comparison of haematological recovery times and supportive care requirements of autologous recovery phase peripheral blood stem cell transplants, autologous bone marrow transplants and allogeneic bone marrow transplants. *Bone Marrow Transplant* 1992;9(4):277-284.

46. Sheridan WP, Begley CG, Juttner CA, et al. Effect of peripheral-blood progenitor cells mobilised by filgrastim (G-CSF) on platelet recovery after high-dose chemotherapy. *Lancet* 1992;339(8794):640-644.

47. Schmitz N, Bacigalupo A, Hasenclever D, et al. Allogeneic bone marrow transplantation vs filgrastim-mobilised peripheral blood progenitor cell transplantation in patients with early leukaemia: First results of a randomised multicentre trial of the European Group for Blood and Marrow Transplantation. *Bone Marrow Transplant* 1998;21(10):995-1003.

48. Blaise D, Kuentz M, Fortanier C, et al. Randomized trial of bone marrow versus lenograstim-primed blood cell allogeneic transplantation in patients with early-stage leukemia: A report from the Societe Francaise de Greffe de Moelle. *J Clin Oncol* 2000;18(3):537-546.

49. Bensinger WI, Martin PJ, Storer B, et al. Transplantation of bone marrow as compared with peripheral-blood cells from HLA-identical relatives in patients with hematologic cancers. *N Engl J Med* 2001;344(3):175-181.

50. Korbling M, Przepiorka D, Huh YO, et al. Allogeneic blood stem cell transplantation for refractory leukemia and lymphoma: Potential advantage of blood over marrow allografts. *Blood* 1995;85(6):1659-1665.

51. Link H, Arseniev L, Bahre O, et al. Transplantation of allogeneic CD34+ blood cells. *Blood* 1996;87(11):4903-4909.

52. Heldal D, Tjonnfjord G, Brinch L, et al. A randomised study of allogeneic transplantation with stem cells from blood or bone marrow. *Bone Marrow Transplant* 2000;25(11):1129-1136.

53. Couban S, Simpson DR, Barnett MJ, et al. A randomized multicenter comparison of bone marrow and peripheral blood in recipients of matched sibling allogeneic transplants for myeloid malignancies. *Blood* 2002;100(5):1525-1531.

54. Wagner JE, Rosenthal J, Sweetman R, et al. Successful transplantation of HLA-matched and HLA-mismatched umbilical cord blood from unrelated donors: Analysis of engraftment and acute graft-versus-host disease. *Blood* 1996;88(3):795-802.

55. Rubinstein P, Carrier C, Scaradavou A, et al. Outcome among 562 recipeints of placental-blood transplant from unrelated donors. *N Engl J Med* 1998;339(22):1565-1577.

56. McNiece I, Harrington J, Turney J, et al. Ex vivo expansion of cord blood mononuclear cells on mesenchymal stem cells. *Cytotherapy* 2004;6(4):311-317.

57. Kernan NA, Collins NH, Juliano L, et al. Clonable T lymphocytes in T cell-depleted bone marrow transplants correlate with development of graft-v-host disease. *Blood* 1986;68(3):770-773.

58. Perreault C, Decary F, Brochu S, et al. Minor histocompatibility antigens. *Blood* 1990;76(7):1269-1280.

59. den Haan JM, Sherman NE, Blokland E, et al. Identification of a graft versus host disease-associated human minor histocompatibility antigen. *Science* 1995;268(5216):1476-1480.

60. Wang W, Meadows LR, den Haan JM, et al. Human H-Y: A male-specific histocompatibility antigen derived from the SMCY protein. *Science* 1995;269(5230):1588-1590.

61. Storb R, Leisenring W, Deeg HJ, et al. Long-term follow-up of a randomized trial of graft-versus-host disease prevention by methotrexate/cyclosporine versus methotrexate alone in patients given marrow grafts for severe aplastic anemia. *Blood* 1994;83(9):2749-2750.

62. Przepiorka D, Shapiro S, Schwinghammer TL, et al. Cyclosporine and methylprednisolone after allogeneic marrow transplantation: Association between low cyclosporine concentration and risk of acute graft-versus-host disease. *Bone Marrow Transplant* 1991;7(6):461-465.

63. Yau JC, Dimopoulos MA, Huan SD, et al. An effective acute graft-vs.-host disease prophylaxis with minidose methotrexate, cyclosporine, and single-dose methylprednisolone. *Am J Hematol* 1991;38(4):288-292.

64. Ratanatharathorn V, Nash RA, Przepiorka D, et al. Phase III study comparing methotrexate and tacrolimus (prograf, FK506) with methotrexate and cyclosporine for graft-versus-host disease prophylaxis after HLA-identical sibling bone marrow transplantation. *Blood* 1998;92(7):2303-2314.

65. Kroger N, Zabelina T, Renges H, et al. Long-term follow-up of allogeneic stem cell transplantation in patients with severe aplastic anemia after conditioning with cyclophosphamide plus antithymocyte globulin. *Ann Hematol* 2002;81(11):627-631.

66. Storb R, Etzioni R, Anasetti C, et al. Cyclophosphamide combined with antithymocyte globulin in preparation for allogeneic marrow transplants in patients with aplastic anemia. *Blood* 1994;84(3):941-949.

67. Storb R, Leisenring W, Anasetti C, et al. Long-term follow-up of allogeneic marrow transplants in patients with aplastic anemia conditioned by cyclophosphamide combined with antithymocyte globulin. *Blood* 1997;89(10):3890-3891.

68. Marmont AM, Horowitz MM, Gale RP, et al. T-cell depletion of HLA-identical transplants in leukemia. *Blood* 1991;78(8):2120-2130.

69. Champlin R, Giralt S, Przepiorka D, et al. Selective depletion of CD8-positive T-lymphocytes for allogeneic bone marrow transplantation: Engraftment, graft-versus-host disease and graft-versus leukemia. *Prog Clin Biol Res* 1992;377:385-394; discussion 395-398.

70. Goodman JL, Winston DJ, Greenfield RA, et al. A controlled trial of fluconazole to prevent fungal infections in patients undergoing bone marrow transplantation. *N Engl J Med* 1992;326(13):845-851.

71. Przepiorka D, Selvaggi K, Rosenzweig PQ, et al. Aerosolized pentamidine for prevention of *Pneumocystis pneumonia* after allogeneic marrow transplantation. *Bone Marrow Transplant* 1991;7(4):324-325.

72. Yolken RH, Bishop CA, Townsend TR, et al. Infectious gastroenteritis in bone-marrow-transplant recipients. *N Engl J Med* 1982;306(17):1010-1012.

73. Winston DJ, Ho WG, Bartoni K, et al. Ganciclovir prophylaxis of cytomegalovirus infection and disease in allogeneic bone marrow transplant recipients. Results of a placebo-controlled, double-blind trial. *Ann Intern Med* 1993;118(3): 179-184.

74. Boeckh M, Gooley TA, Myerson D, et al. Cytomegalovirus pp65 antigenemia-guided early treatment with ganciclovir versus ganciclovir at engraftment after allogeneic marrow transplantation: A randomized double-blind study. *Blood* 1996;88(10):4063-4071.

75. Goodrich JM, Mori M, Gleaves CA, et al. Early treatment with ganciclovir to prevent cytomegalovirus disease after allogeneic bone marrow transplantation. *N Engl J Med* 1991; 325(23):1601-1607.

76. Hiemenz JW, Greene JN. Special considerations for the patient undergoing allogeneic or autologous bone marrow transplantation. *Hematol Oncol Clin North Am* 1993;7(5): 961-1002.

77. Bowden RA, Sayers M, Flournoy N, et al. Cytomegalovirus immune globulin and seronegative blood products to prevent primary cytomegalovirus infection after marrow transplantation. *N Engl J Med* 1986;314(16):1006-1010.

78. Gluckman E, Lotsberg J, Devergie A, et al. Prophylaxis of herpes infections after bone-marrow transplantation by oral acyclovir. *Lancet* 1983;2(8352):706-708.

79. Wade JC, Newton B, Flournoy N, et al. Oral acyclovir for prevention of herpes simplex virus reactivation after marrow transplantation. *Ann Intern Med* 1984;100(6):823-828.

80. Balduzzi A, Valsecchi MG, Silvestri D, et al. Transplant-related toxicity and mortality: An AIEOP prospective study in 636 pediatric patients transplanted for acute leukemia. *Bone Marrow Transplant* 2002;29(2):93-100.

81. Haselberger MB, Schwinghammer TL. Efficacy of mesna for prevention of hemorrhagic cystitis after high-dose cyclophosphamide therapy. *Ann Pharmacother* 1995;29(9):918-921.

82. De La Camara R, Tomas JF, Figuera A, et al. High dose busulfan and seizures. *Bone Marrow Transplant* 1991;7(5):363-364.

83. Anderson KC, Weinstein HJ. Transfusion-associated graft-versus-host disease. *N Engl J Med* 1990;323(5):315-321.

84. Barge AJ. A review of the efficacy and tolerability of recombinant haematopoietic growth factors in bone marrow transplantation. *Bone Marrow Transplant* 1993;11(Suppl 2):1-11.

85. Nemunaitis J, Singer JW, Buckner CD, et al. Use of recombinant human granulocyte-macrophage colony-stimulating factor in graft failure after bone marrow transplantation. *Blood* 1990;76(1):245-253.

86. Champlin RE, Horowitz MM, van Bekkum DW, et al. Graft failure following bone marrow transplantation for severe aplastic anemia: Risk factors and treatment results. *Blood* 1989;73(2):606-613.

87. Davies SM, Ramsay NK, Haake RJ, et al. Comparison of engraftment in recipients of matched sibling of unrelated donor marrow allografts. *Bone Marrow Transplant* 1994; 13(1):51-57.

88. Davies SM, Weisdorf DJ, Haake RJ, et al. Second infusion of bone marrow for treatment of graft failure after allogeneic bone marrow transplantation. *Bone Marrow Transplant* 1994; 14(1):73-77.

89. Storb R, Champlin RE. Bone marrow transplantation for severe aplastic anemia. *Bone Marrow Transplant* 1991;8(2): 69-72.

90. Voogt PJ, Fibbe WE, Marijt WA, et al. Rejection of bone-marrow graft by recipient-derived cytotoxic T lymphocytes against minor histocompatibility antigens. *Lancet* 1990; 335(8682):131-134.

91. Marijt WA, Kernan NA, Diaz-Barrientos T, et al. Multiple minor histocompatibility antigen-specific cytotoxic T lymphocyte clones can be generated during graft rejection after HLA-identical bone marrow transplantation. *Bone Marrow Transplant* 1995;16(1):125-132.

92. Bearman SI, Lee JL, Baron AE, et al. Treatment of hepatic venocclusive disease with recombinant human tissue plasminogen activator and heparin in 42 marrow transplant patients. *Blood* 1997;89(5):1501-1506.

93. Shulman HM, Hinterberger W. Hepatic veno-occlusive disease–liver toxicity syndrome after bone marrow transplantation. *Bone Marrow Transplant* 1992;10(3):197-214.

94. Jones RJ, Lee KS, Beschorner WE, et al. Venoocclusive disease of the liver following bone marrow transplantation. *Transplantation* 1987;44(6):778-783.

95. Bearman SI, Anderson GL, Mori M, et al. Venoocclusive disease of the liver: Development of a model for predicting fatal outcome after marrow transplantation. *J Clin Oncol* 1993; 11(9):1729-1736.

96. Essell JH, Thompson JM, Harman GS, et al. Marked increase in veno-occlusive disease of the liver associated with methotrexate use for graft-versus-host disease prophylaxis in patients receiving busulfan/cyclophosphamide. *Blood* 1992; 79(10):2784-2788.

97. McDonald GB, Hinds MS, Fisher LD, et al. Veno-occlusive disease of the liver and multiorgan failure after bone marrow transplantation: A cohort study of 355 patients. *Ann Intern Med* 1993;118(4):255-267.

98. Richardson PG, Elias AD, Krishnan A, et al. Treatment of severe veno-occlusive disease with defibrotide: Compassionate use results in response without significant toxicity in a high-risk population. *Blood* 1998;92(3):737-744.

99. Chopra R, Eaton JD, Grassi A, et al. Defibrotide for the treatment of hepatic veno-occlusive disease: Results of the European compassionate-use study. *Br J Haematol* 2000; 111(4):1122-1129.

100. Wingard JR, Mellits ED, Sostrin MB, et al. Interstitial pneumonitis after allogeneic bone marrow transplantation. Nine-year experience at a single institution. *Medicine* (Baltimore) 1988;67(3):175-186.

101. Granena A, Carreras E, Rozman C, et al. Interstitial pneumonitis after BMT: 15 years experience in a single institution. *Bone Marrow Transplant* 1993;11(6):453-458.

102. Champlin RE, Whimbey E. Community respiratory virus infections in bone marrow transplant recipients: The M.D. Anderson Cancer Center experience. *Biol Blood Marrow Transplant* 2001;7(Suppl):S8-S10.

103. Whimbey E, Champlin RE, Couch RB, et al. Community respiratory virus infections among hospitalized adult bone marrow transplant recipients. *Clin Infect Dis* 1996;22(5):778-782.

104. Hartsell WF, Czyzewski EA, Ghalie R, et al. Pulmonary complications of bone marrow transplantation: A comparison of total body irradiation and cyclophosphamide to busulfan and cyclophosphamide. *Int J Radiat Oncol Biol Phys* 1995;32(1):69-73.

105. Weiner RS, Bortin MM, Gale RP, et al. Interstitial pneumonitis after bone marrow transplantation. Assessment of risk factors. *Ann Intern Med* 1986;104(2):168-175.

106. Atkinson K. Reconstruction of the haemopoietic and immune systems after marrow transplantation. *Bone Marrow Transplant* 1990;5(4):209-226.

107. Lum LG. Immune recovery after bone marrow transplantation. *Hematol Oncol Clin North Am* 1990;4(3):659-675.

108. Armitage JO, Antman KH (eds). *High Dose Cancer Therapy: Pharmacology, Hematopoietin, Stem Cells*, 3rd ed. Philadelphia, PA: Lippincott, Williams & Wilkins; 2000.

109. Wald A, Leisenring W, van Burik JA, et. al. Epidemiology of Aspergillus infections in a large cohort of patients undergoing bone marrow transplantation. *J Infect Dis* 1997;175(6):1459-1466.

110. Marr KA, Carter RA, Boeckh M, et al. Invasive aspergillosis in allogeneic stem cell transplant recipients: Changes in epidemiology and risk factors. *Blood* 2002;100(13):4358-4366.

111. Martino R, Caballero MD, Canals C, et al. Reduced-intensity conditioning reduces the risk of severe infections after allogeneic peripheral blood stem cell transplantation. *Bone Marrow Transplant* 2001;28(4):341-347.

112. Junghanss C, Marr KA, Carter RA, et al. Incidence and outcome of bacterial and fungal infections following nonmyeloablative compared with myeloablative allogeneic hematopoietic stem cell transplantation: A matched control study. *Biol Blood Marrow Transplant* 2002;8(9):512-520.

113. Morgenstern GR, Prentice AG, Prentice HG, et al. A randomized controlled trial of itraconazole versus fluconazole for the prevention of fungal infections in patients with haematological malignancies. U.K. Multicentre Antifungal Prophylaxis Study Group. *Br J Haematol* 1999;105(4): 901-911.

114. Winston DJ, Maziarz RT, Chandrasekar PH, et al. Intravenous and oral itraconazole versus intravenous and oral fluconazole for long-term antifungal prophylaxis in allogeneic hematopoietic stem-cell transplant recipients. A multicenter, randomized trial. *Ann Intern Med* 2003;138(9):705-713.

115. Deeg HJ, Socie G. Malignancies after hematopoietic stem cell transplantation: Many questions, some answers. *Blood* 1998;91(6):1833-1844.

116. Curtis RE, Travis LB, Rowlings PA, et al. Risk of lymphoproliferative disorders after bone marrow transplantation: A multi-institutional study. *Blood* 1999;94(7):2208-2216.

117. Zutter MM, Martin PJ, Sale GE, et al. Epstein-Barr virus lymphoproliferation after bone marrow transplantation. *Blood* 1988;72(2):520-529.

118. Meijer E, Cornelissen JJ. Epstein-Barr virus-associated lymphoproliferative disease after allogeneic haematopoietic stem cell transplantation: Molecular monitoring and early treatment of high-risk patients. *Curr Opin Hematol* 2008;15(6):576-585.

119. Heslop HE, Slobod KS, Pule MA, et al. Long term outcome of EBV specific T-cell infusions to prevent or treat EBV-related lymphoproliferative disease in transplant recipients. *Blood* 2010;115(5):925-935.

120. Rooney CM, Smith CA, Ng CY, et al. Infusion of cytotoxic T cells for the prevention and treatment of Epstein-Barr virus-induced lymphoma in allogeneic transplant recipients. *Blood* 1998;92(5):1549-1555.

121. Leen AM, Christin A, Myers GD, et al. Cytotoxic T lymphocyte therapy with donor T cells prevents and treats adenovirus and Epstein-Barr virus infections after haploidentical and matched unrelated stem cell transplantation. *Blood* 2009;114(19):4283-4292.

122. Hanley PJ, Cruz CR, Savoldo B, et al. Functionally active virus-specific T cells that target CMV, adenovirus, and EBV can be expanded from naive T-cell populations in cord blood and will target a range of viral epitopes. *Blood* 2009;114(9):1958-1967.

123. Gerdemann U, Christin AS, Vera JF, et al. Nucleofection of DCs to generate multivirus-specific T cells for prevention or treatment of viral infections in the immunocompromised host. *Mol Ther* 2009;17(9):1616-1625.

124. Ganne V, Siddiqi N, Kamaplath B, et al. Humanized anti-CD20 monoclonal antibody (rituximab) treatment for post-transplant lymphoproliferative disorder. *Clin Transplant* 2003;17(5):417-422.

125. van Esser JW, Niesters HG, van der Holt B, et al. Prevention of Epstein-Barr virus-lymphoproliferative disease by molecular monitoring and preemptive rituximab in high-risk patients after allogeneic stem cell transplantation. *Blood* 2002;99(12):4364-4369.

126. Vogelsang GB, Hess AD, Santos GW. Acute graft-versus-host disease: Clinical characteristics in the cyclosporine era. *Medicine* (Baltimore) 1988;67(3):163-174.

127. Beatty PG, Hansen JA, Longton GM, et al. Marrow transplantation from HLA-matched unrelated donors for treatment of hematologic malignancies. *Transplantation* 1991;51(2):443-447.

128. Mickelson EM, Petersdorf E, Anasetti C, et al. HLA matching in hematopoietic cell transplantation. *Hum Immunol* 2000;61(2):92-100.

129. Anasetti C, Hansen JA. Effect of HLA incompatibility in marrow transplantation from unrelated and HLA-mismatched related donors. *Transfus Sci* 1994;15(3):221-230.

130. Gale RP, Bortin MM, van Bekkum DW, et al. Risk factors for acute graft-versus-host disease. *Br J Haematol* 1987;67(4):397-406.

131. Van Lint MT, Uderzo C, Locasciulli A, et al. Early treatment of acute graft-versus-host disease with high- or low-dose 6-methylprednisolone: A multicenter randomized trial from the Italian Group for Bone Marrow Transplantation. *Blood* 1998;92(7):2288-2293.

132. Pidala J, Kim J, Anasetti C. Sirolimus as primary treatment of acute graft-versus-host disease following allogeneic hematopoietic cell transplantation. *Biol Blood Marrow Transplant* 2009;15(7):881-885.

133. Hoda D, Pidala J, Salgado-Vila N, et al. Sirolimus for treatment of steroid-refractory acute graft-versus-host disease. *Bone Marrow Transplant* 2010;45(8):1347-1351.

134. Ho VT, Aldridge J, Kim HT, et al. Comparison of tacrolimus and sirolimus (Tac/Sir) versus Tacrolimus, Sirolimus, and mini-methotrexate (Tac/Sir/MTX) as acute graft-versus-host disease prophylaxis after reduced-intensity conditioning allogeneic peripheral blood stem cell transplantation. *Biol Blood Marrow Transplant* 2009;15(7):844-850.

135. Snyder DS, Palmer J, Gaal K, et al. Improved outcomes using tacrolimus/sirolimus for graft versus host disease prophylaxis with a reduced intensity conditioning regimen for allogeneic hematopoietic cell transplant as treatment of myelofibrosis. *Biol Blood Marrow Transplant* 2010;16(2):281-286.

136. van Besien K, Kunavakkam R, Rondon G, et al. Fludarabine-melphalan conditioning for AML and MDS: Alemtuzumab reduces acute and chronic GVHD without affecting long-term outcomes. *Biol Blood Marrow Transplant* 2009;15(5):610-617.

137. Ferrara JL, Cooke KR, Pan L, et al. The immunopathophysiology of acute graft-versus-host-disease. *Stem Cells* 1996;14(5): 473-489.

138. Chien JW, Duncan S, Williams KM, et al. Bronchiolitis obliterans syndrome after allogeneic hematopoietic stem cell transplantation—An increasingly recognized manifestation of chronic graft-versus-host disease. *Biol Blood Marrow Transplant* 2010;16(1):106-114.

139. Atkinson K. Chronic graft-versus-host disease. *Bone Marrow Transplant* 1990;5(2):69-82.

140. Loughran TP, Jr., Sullivan K, Morton T, et al. Value of day 100 screening studies for predicting the development of chronic graft-versus-host disease after allogeneic bone marrow transplantation. *Blood* 1990;76(1):228-334.

141. Sullivan KM, Witherspoon RP, Storb R, et al. Alternating-day cyclosporine and prednisone for treatment of high-risk chronic graft-v-host disease. *Blood* 1988;72(2):555-561.

142. Parker PM, Chao N, Nademanee A, et al. Thalidomide as salvage therapy for chronic graft-versus-host disease. *Blood* 1995;86(9):3604-3609.

143. Hidaka M, Iwasaki S, Matsui T, et al. Efficacy of bezafibrate for chronic GVHD of the liver after allogeneic hematopoietic stem cell transplantation. *Bone Marrow Transplant* 2010; 45(5):912-918.

144. Zhang LS, Liu QF, Huang K, et al. [Mesenchymal stem cells for treatment of steroid-resistant chronic graft-versus-host disease]. Zhonghua Nei Ke Za Zhi 2009;48(7):542-546.

145. Kolb HJ, Socie G, Duell T, et al. Malignant neoplasms in long-term survivors of bone marrow transplantation. Late Effects Working Party of the European Cooperative Group for Blood and Marrow Transplantation and the European Late Effect Project Group. *Ann Intern Med* 1999;131(10): 738-744.

146. Bhatia S, Ramsay NK, Steinbuch M, et al. Malignant neoplasms following bone marrow transplantation. *Blood* 1996;87(9): 3633-3639.

147. Meyers CA, Weitzner M, Byrne K, et al. Evaluation of the neurobehavioral functioning of patients before, during, and after bone marrow transplantation. *J Clin Oncol* 1994; 12(4):820-826.

148. Wingard JR, Curbow B, Baker F, et al. Health, functional status, and employment of adult survivors of bone marrow transplantation. *Ann Intern Med* 1991;114(2):113-118.

149. Gratwohl A, Hermans J. Allogeneic bone marrow transplantation for chronic myeloid leukemia. Working Party Chronic Leukemia of the European Group for Blood and Marrow Transplantation (EBMT). *Bone Marrow Transplant* 1996; 17(Suppl 3):S7-S9.

150. Horowitz MM, Rowlings PA, Passweg JR. Allogeneic bone marrow transplantation for CML: A report from the International Bone Marrow Transplant Registry. *Bone Marrow Transplant* 1996;17(Suppl 3):S5-S6.

151. Porter DL, Roth MS, McGarigle C, et al. Induction of graft-versus-host disease as immunotherapy for relapsed chronic myeloid leukemia. *N Engl J Med* 1994;330(2):100-106.

152. Nevill TJ, Fung HC, Shepherd JD, et al. Cytogenetic abnormalities in primary myelodysplastic syndrome are highly predictive of outcome after allogeneic bone marrow transplantation. *Blood* 1998;92(6):1910-1917.

153. Rosinol L, Perez-Simon JA, Sureda A, et al. A prospective PETHEMA study of tandem autologous transplantation versus autograft followed by reduced-intensity conditioning allogeneic transplantation in newly diagnosed multiple myeloma. *Blood* 2008;112(9):3591-3593.

154. Tam CS, Khouri IF. Autologous and allogeneic stem cell transplantation: Rising therapeutic promise for mantle cell lymphoma. *Leuk Lymphoma* 2009;50(8):1239-1248.

155. Forman SJ. Role of reduced intensity transplant in adult patients with acute lymphoblastic leukemia: If and when? *Best Pract Res Clin Haematol* 2009;22(4):557-566.

156. Niederwieser D, Maris M, Shizuru JA, et al. Low-dose total body irradiation (TBI) and fludarabine followed by hematopoietic cell transplantation (HCT) from HLA-matched or mismatched unrelated donors and postgrafting immunosuppression with cyclosporine and mycophenolate mofetil (MMF) can induce durable complete chimerism and sustained remissions in patients with hematological diseases. *Blood* 2003;101(4):1620-1629.

157. Slavin S, Nagler A, Naparstek E, et al. Nonmyeloablative stem cell transplantation and cell therapy as an alternative to conventional bone marrow transplantation with lethal cytoreduction for the treatment of malignant and nonmalignant hematologic diseases. *Blood* 1998;91(3):756-763.

158. Childs R, Clave E, Contentin N, et al. Engraftment kinetics after nonmyeloablative allogeneic peripheral blood stem cell transplantation: Full donor T-cell chimerism precedes alloimmune responses. *Blood* 1999;94(9):3234-3241.

159. Graef T, Kuendgen A, Fenk R, et al. Successful treatment of relapsed AML after allogeneic stem cell transplantation with azacitidine. *Leuk Res* 2007;31(2):257-259.

160. Fenaux P, Mufti GJ, Hellstrom-Lindberg E, et al. Azacitidine prolongs overall survival compared with conventional care regimens in elderly patients with low bone marrow blast count acute myeloid leukemia. *J Clin Oncol* 2010;28(4):562-9.

161. Magarotto V, Palumbo A. Evolving role of novel agents for maintenance therapy in myeloma. *Cancer J* 2009;15(6):494-501.

162. Powles RL, Morgenstern GR, Kay HE, et al. Mismatched family donors for bone-marrow transplantation as treatment for acute leukaemia. *Lancet* 1983;1(8325):612-615.

163. Jones RJ, Barber JP, Vala MS, et al. Assessment of aldehyde dehydrogenase in viable cells. *Blood* 1995;85(10):2742-2746.

164. Mayumi H, Umesue M, Nomoto K. Cyclophosphamide-induced immunological tolerance: An overview. *Immunobiology* 1996;195(2):129-139.

165. Luznik L, Jalla S, Engstrom LW, et al. Durable engraftment of major histocompatibility complex-incompatible cells after nonmyeloablative conditioning with fludarabine, low-dose total body irradiation, and posttransplantation cyclophosphamide. *Blood* 2001;98(12):3456-3464.

166. O'Donnell PV, Luznik L, Jones RJ, et al. Nonmyeloablative bone marrow transplantation from partially HLA-mismatched related donors using posttransplantation cyclophosphamide. *Biol Blood Marrow Transplant* 2002;8(7):377-386.

167. Burroughs LM, O'Donnell PV, Sandmaier BM, et al. Comparison of outcomes of HLA-matched related, unrelated, or HLA-haploidentical related hematopoietic cell transplantation following nonmyeloablative conditioning for relapsed or refractory Hodgkin lymphoma. *Biol Blood Marrow Transplant* 2008;14(11):1279-1287.

168. Ciurea SO, Kebriaei P, Khouri I, et al. Fludarabine, melphalan and thiotepa conditioning for unrelated donor cord blood transplantation. *Biol Blood Marrow Transpl* 2009; 15(2):48-49.

169. Ciurea SO, Saliba R, G. Rondon G, et al. Improved outcomes of patients with AML/MDS undergoing haploidentical stem cell transplantation using fludarabine, melphalan and thiotepa conditioning chemotherapy. *Biol Blood Marrow Transpl* 2009;14(2):50.

170. Ciurea SO, Saliba R, Rondon G, et al. Reduced-intensity conditioning using fludarabine, melphalan and thiotepa for adult patients undergoing haploidentical SCT. *Bone Marrow Transplant* 2010;45(3):429-436.

AUTOLOGOUS STEM CELL TRANSPLANTATION

Carrie Yuen
Richard E. Champlin

■ BASIC CONCEPTS

High-dose chemotherapy (HDCT) with autologous stem cell rescue is an effective treatment modality for a variety of hematologic malignancies and selected solid tumors. This chapter reviews the current role of autologous hematopoietic transplants in the treatment of cancer and outlines promising future directions.

The maximal dose of radiation and cytotoxic chemotherapy a patient can receive is limited by its toxicity to normal tissues. The dose of many effective agents is limited by toxicity to the bone marrow. The dose can be substantially escalated to more effective levels if followed by autologous or allogeneic transplantation of hematopoietic stem cells to restore hematopoiesis.

Pluripotent hematopoietic stem cells present in the transplant graft proliferate and differentiate into the mature elements of the blood and immune system, including neutrophils, lymphocytes, platelets, and erythrocytes. Autologous transplantation involves collection and cryopreservation of the patient's own hematopoietic cells. Allogeneic transplantation involves transplantation from another person, a normal donor.

GENERAL PROCEDURES FOR AUTOLOGOUS TRANSPLANTATION

The following steps are involved in the general procedure for autologous stem cell transplantation (ASCT). The process is summarized in Fig. 13-1.

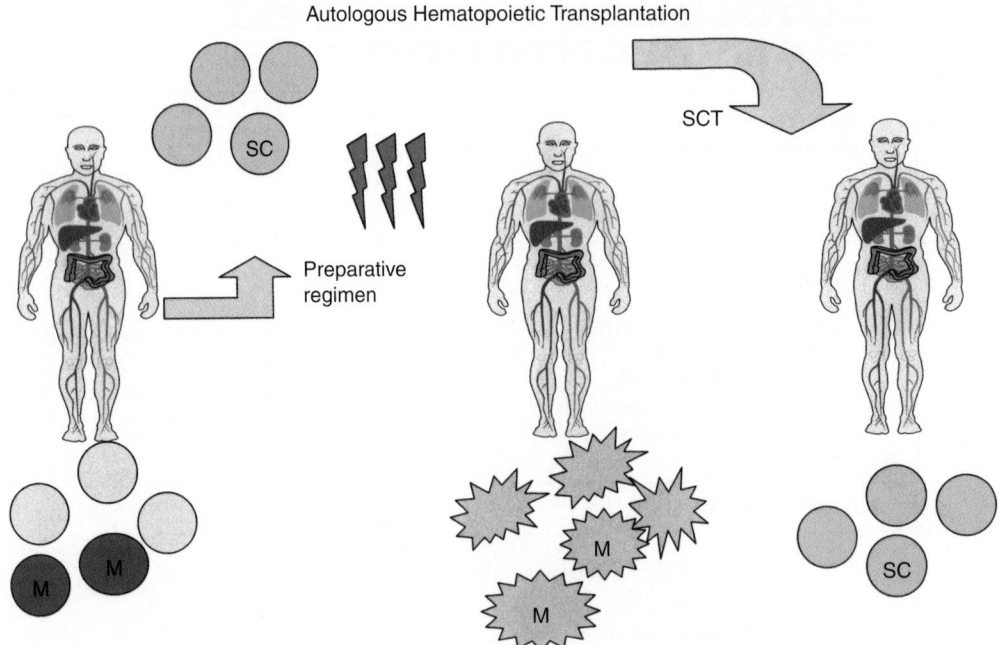

Autologous Hematopoietic Transplantation

FIGURE 13-1. The procedure for autologous stem cell transplantation (ASCT). Patients with malignancy have normal and malignant cells (M) sensitive to myeloablative chemotherapy and/or radiation. They undergo the collection of bone marrow or peripheral blood containing hematopoietic stem cells (SC), which are then cryopreserved. In some cases, the harvested cells are treated in the laboratory to enrich the stem cell number or deplete contaminating malignant cells. Patients later receive a high-dose preparative regimen of chemotherapy alone or with total-body irradiation designed to eradicate the malignant cells. This treatment also destroys the normal bone marrow, but it can be administered if followed by the infusion of the stored stem cells to restore hematopoiesis.

Assessment of Patients

Transplant physicians evaluate potential candidates to determine their appropriateness for high-dose therapy and their risk for major complications. This consists of a complete history and physical examination, review of past treatment and response, baseline laboratory data, and restaging of the malignancy. If the patient is felt to be an appropriate candidate, additional testing is performed to fully evaluate the function of all organ systems. In general, autologous transplants are generally most effective against chemosensitive malignancies with low-bulk disease. Patients must be in sufficiently good general medical condition in order to tolerate the high-dose myelosuppressive therapy.

Induction Chemotherapy

Standard chemotherapy is usually given to reduce the tumor burden prior to proceeding to stem cell transplantation. The success of transplantation depends on whether the patient's tumor is chemosensitive; the best outcomes are, in general, in patients who are in remission or with minimal tumor load at time of transplantation.

Stem Cell Collection

After patients undergo stem cell collection, the bone marrow or peripheral blood progenitor cells (PBPC) are cryopreserved and stored. Bone marrow is collected via multiple aspirations from the posterior-superior iliac crest in a sterile environment (usually a surgical operating room) while the patient is under anesthesia. Ideally, stem cells should be collected while the patient's marrow is normocellular and uninvolved by the malignancy. Hematopoietic stem cells can also be collected from peripheral blood. Stem cells are normally infrequent in the blood but are mobilized into the blood during the recovery after chemotherapy and following treatment with hematopoietic growth factors such as granulocyte colony-stimulating factor (G-CSF) and granulocyte-macrophage colony-stimulating factor (GM-CSF). These are termed peripheral blood progenitor cells (PBPC). PBPC are collected after mobilization using apheresis and continuous-flow cell separation. One to four daily leukapheresis sessions are usually required to achieve a sufficient collection (at least 2×10^6/kg, and preferably 5×10^6/kg).

Multiple factors have been shown to be predictors of result of stem cell mobilization and collection, which include age, diagnoses, duration of preceding chemotherapy, the presence of marrow infiltrating disease or history of radiation, low premobilization platelet counts, short intervals from last chemotherapy cycle to mobilization, a low premobilization bone marrow CFU-GM level and inadequate chemopriming regimens and/or low-dose G-CSF (1), and previous treatment with lenalidomide (2). Peripheral blood CD34 >10/μL is necessary for an adequate collection; most centers will not attempt to collect PBPCs with less than this level. Plerixafor (formerly known as AMD 3100) has recently become available as a stem cell mobilizing agent. This is a bicyclam molecule which inhibits the SDF-1 alpha/CXCR4 binding between the CD34+ stem cells and the marrow stroma, resulting in the release of CD34+ stem cells into the blood stream. Plerixafor is synergistic with G-CSF for stem cell mobilization (3-6) and has been approved by FDA to be used in combination with G-CSF. A risk-adapted approach has been designed by the Mayo Clinic to enhance the success of stem cell collection and cost-effectiveness for use of plerixafor. If CD34<10/μL after 4 days of G-CSF at 10 μg/kg/day, then plerixafor is indicated for initiation to allow successful collection of CD34 stem cells for autologous transplantation. An increase by 2.6 fold in CD34 stem cells was collected with addition of plerixafor (7).

High-Dose Therapy

Autologous transplants are most effective in diseases with a steep dose response curve, in which escalated doses of myelosuppressive drugs or radiation lead to a markedly increased cytotoxic effect on the malignancy. The most commonly used drugs are alkylating agents and platinum compounds alone or in combination with total-body radiation therapy. Many commonly used regimens escalate the doses of the combination three to five times higher than would be tolerable without transplantation.

The most common cause of failure after autologous transplantation is relapse of the underlying malignancy. This may occur because of inadequate systemic cytoreduction or from reinfusion of malignant cells contaminating the transplant infusion. The optimal preparative regimen has yet to be determined, and various approaches are being studied to improve the final outcomes, including novel chemotherapy agents (8,9), monoclonal antibodies (10), chemoradiotherapy (11,12), and targeted radiation treatments; "tandem" or serial transplants have

been studied (13). In chemosensitive malignancies, increasing the total dose of myelosuppressive therapy may markedly improve the tumor response, but this also increases the severity of side effects. Preparative regimens must be optimally designed in phases I, II, and III studies to provide the optimal therapeutic index. However, using plerixafor has not been shown to increase peripheral blood tumor cells (7).

Reinfusion of Collected Stem Cells

The bone marrow or PBPC transplant is infused intravenously after the high-dose therapy is eliminated from the patient's bloodstream, usually 1 to 3 days after completion of the chemotherapy treatment. The cells circulate transiently and home to the bone marrow. Hematopoiesis is restored within a few weeks. Hematopoietic recovery is most rapid with infusion of high doses of CD34+ cells. Most centers require a minimum of 0.5×10^6 CD34+ cells per kilogram from bone marrow and 2×10^6 CD34+ cells per kilogram from peripheral blood (14). Peripheral blood counts generally recover after 2 to 3 weeks of cell infusion.

Supportive Care

Patients usually receive G-CSF or other hematopoietic growth factors to accelerate marrow recovery, shortening neutrophil recovery by 3 to 7 days. Hematopoietic growth factors are usually administered until the absolute neutrophil count (ANC) exceeds 1000/mm^3. The available hematopoietic growth factors do not accelerate recovery of red blood cell line or platelets. Recombinant human erythropoietin (rhuEPO) has not substantially accelerated erythroid recovery (15), and no agent has been shown to accelerate platelet recovery posttransplant (16).

Patients are routinely placed on prophylactic antibiotic, antiviral, and antifungal therapy for prevention of infection during the initial phase of marrow engraftment and hematologic recovery.

■ CONTROVERSIES

Autologous Versus Allogeneic Transplants

The relative role of allogeneic versus autologous stem cell transplant is debated for most hematologic malignancies. Autologous transplantation is a process that carries less overall morbidity and mortality because the reinfused cells are not subject to immunologic rejection and will not produce graft-versus-host disease (GVHD). On the other hand, there is a risk that the collected autologous stem cells may be contaminated by malignant cells. Moreover, the immune-mediated graft-versus-tumor effect associated with allogeneic stem cell transplantation does not occur with autologous transplants.

Peripheral Blood Versus Bone Marrow Transplantation

In the recent years, PBPCs have largely replaced bone marrow stem cells for autologous transplantation. PBPCs have come to be preferred because larger numbers of CD34+ cells can generally be collected, resulting in more rapid recovery of neutrophils and platelets compared to bone marrow transplants. This approach also avoids the discomfort of the multiple aspirations required for a bone marrow harvest. The use of PBPC requires treatment with growth factor injections, insertion of a large-bore central venous catheter, and frequently bone pain related to treatment with G-CSF (17).

Purging

One of the major concerns with autologous stem cell transplantation is the possibility of PBPC or marrow contamination with malignant cells at the time of the collection. Tumor cells can be detected by a number of methods, including light microscopy, flow cytometry, and immunohistochemical, clonogenic, and molecular assays (18).

Some clinical studies have shown that autograft contamination is correlated with shortened disease-free survival (DFS) (19) and that the presence of tumor cells or their inadequate purging in autologous samples may correlate with the extent of the disease. Gene-marking studies have shown that cells in the autograft can contribute to systemic relapse.

A variety of procedures have been proposed to deplete contaminating malignant cells from the graft, most frequently including ex vivo treatment with monoclonal antibodies or drugs. Despite these findings, there is no conclusive evidence that any purging method can improve the clinical outcome of autologous transplantation (18). However, if improved preparative treatment can eliminate systemic disease, purging may still be important to prevent relapse of the malignancy.

■ COMPLICATIONS OF HIGH-DOSE CHEMOTHERAPY

HDCT produces profound pancytopenia that usually lasts from 10 to 28 days, until the infused stem cells restore hematopoiesis. The nadir of the absolute neutrophil count represents the highest risk for infectious complications, ranging from febrile neutropenia to life-threatening septic episodes.

High doses of chemotherapy and radiation produce major toxicities in many nonhematopoietic tissues. Drug and radiation toxicities may occur and can be life-threatening. The oral mucosa and the gastrointestinal tract are generally the most sensitive tissues to these effects. The lungs, heart, liver, kidneys, and bladder are often affected by these toxicities. This is particularly true in patients who have been heavily pretreated by previous chemotherapy or have comorbid conditions with organ dysfunction. Overall, 3 to 5% of patients die of treatment-related complications, including these toxic effects and infections. The rate of complications is substantially lower with autologous transplant than that seen with allogeneic transplantation.

Pneumonitis secondary to the pulmonary toxicity of the preparative regimens occurs in up to 16% (20) of patients undergoing high-dose therapy. It has been described with a number of different chemotherapy agents (21,22) and with total-body irradiation (TBI) (20). It is particularly common in patients who have received high-dose carmustine (BCNU) following prior mediastinal radiotherapy (23,24). Different therapies have been tried on an empiric basis for the prophylaxis (23,25) or treatment (23,26) of acute pulmonary complications, but none have been documented to be beneficial.

Cardiac toxicity is common with regimens containing high doses of cyclophosphamide or anthracyclines, especially in combination with carmustine. Prior radiation therapy to the mediastinum or left chest wall and advanced age are also predictors of an increased risk of cardiac complications (27). Central nervous system complications are relatively rare, but dementia and leukoencephalopathy have been described as a complication of high-dose chemotherapy. Hypothyroidism frequently occurs 6 months to 2 years after therapy.

Bladder toxicity may produce hemorrhagic cystitis, particularly with regimens containing high-dose cyclophosphamide. It has a complex pathophysiology that involves direct toxicity by acrolein, a cyclophosphamide metabolite, and infection by polyomavirus (BK virus). This adverse side effect may occur during high-dose chemotherapy but is more typically a delayed complication, developing after weeks to months. Concurrent treatment with mesna (Mesnex), an uroprotective agent (28,29), has been reported to reduce the bladder toxicity of high-dose cyclophosphamide. There is also evidence that aminoguanidine can prevent cyclophosphamide-induced urotoxicity and lead to better tolerance of the drug (30).

■ RESULTS OF AUTOLOGOUS TRANSPLANTATION

This section discusses outcomes and current controversies regarding autologous transplantation for specific malignancies.

ACUTE MYELOGENOUS LEUKEMIA

Autologous stem cell transplants have been used to consolidate a chemotherapy-induced first or second remission in patients with acute myelogenous leukemia (AML), but results are controversial. Encouraging results have been reported in phase II studies, but autologous transplants have not been shown to improve survival in controlled studies or in a recent meta-analysis (31). Patients with high-risk factors—that is, poor cytogenetics or failure to achieve complete remission (CR) with induction chemotherapy, relapsed disease—should be considered for allogeneic stem cell transplantation from the best suitable donor (32). Patients younger than 60 years should be considered to have an allogeneic transplantation at first complete remission for improved relapse-free survival unless they have good-risk cytogenetics without cKIT mutation or intermediate-risk category with mutant CEBPA or NPM1$^+$FLT3-ITD negative (33,34). For patients who lack an HLA-identical donor for allogeneic transplantation, a double umbilical cord blood transplant can be considered because it has been shown to give the same degree of disease-free survival as match unrelated donor transplant (35).

ACUTE LYMPHOBLASTIC LEUKEMIA

Treatment for adult acute lymphoblastic leukemia (ALL) has considerably improved, with newer treatment modalities with complete remission rates as high as 91%, with 5-year survival rates of 38% in a median follow-up of 63 months (36). Relapse remains a major cause of treatment failure, particularly in patients with high-risk factors such as age >50, white cell count >30,000, prolonged time to achieve CR, and high-risk cytogenetics, including t(9;22) and t(4;11). Minimal residual disease (MRD) after induction was predictive for relapse at various follow-up time points (37).

Autologous transplantation has been most effective for childhood ALL and is considered for patients in second remission (38). It has been less effective in adult ALL (39) and has poorer overall survival and disease-free survival as compared to allogeneic transplantation (40). Thus, its routine use has been questioned. Several different studies in high-risk patients have been reported.

Conclusive statements regarding the outcomes have been limited owing to the small number of patients or the short period of follow-up (41).

CHRONIC MYELOGENOUS LEUKEMIA

The management of chronic myelogenous leukemia (CML) has dramatically changed with the advent of imatinib and other tyrosine kinase inhibitors as front-line therapy (42). Imatinib has induced a high rate of complete cytogenetic and molecular responses in patients in chronic-phase CML (43). The National Comprehensive Cancer Network has modified its CML treatment guidelines so that they now include the use of imatinib as first-line therapy, and second generation of tyrosine kinase inhibitors have been effective second line of therapy to regain control of the disease when there is a failure to imatinib therapy (44,45).

Allogeneic stem transplantation is an effective form of treatment and is still the only proven curative therapy of CML (46). However, it has substantial risks and suitable donors are not available for every patient in need of therapy.

Autologous transplantation for CML is an investigational approach for patients with CML. It involves collection and cryopreservation of marrow or PBPC during the chronic phase of the disease (47). Patients may subsequently receive intensive chemotherapy alone or in combination with total-body irradiation (TBI), followed by the infusion of autologous cells (48). A major limitation for autologous transplant for CML in accelerated or blastic phase is the resistance of acute-phase cells to intensive chemotherapy and radiotherapy. Even though most of these patients return to a chronic phase, this is usually brief, with median duration of just 4 months; only a small number of patients survive as long as 1 year.

Relapse following autologous transplantation may be due to the presence of leukemic cells in the autologous infusion or to the persistence of resistant leukemic cells systemically despite high-dose chemotherapy. The ability of autografting to achieve durable remissions will depend on the development of improved methods for graft purging and also of active antileukemia agents to consolidate patients in remission (49). Combination of autologous stem cell transplantation with tyrosine kinase inhibitors is being studied.

CHRONIC LYMPHOCYTIC LEUKEMIA

Chronic lymphocytic leukemia (CLL) is an incurable hematologic malignancy, but it is a chronic disorder with a long natural history. The recent advances in autologous transplantation technology and the low risk of transplant-related-mortality (TRM) have supported evaluation of autologous stem cell transplantation for consolidation of chemotherapy-induced responses in young patients with good performance status (50). Poor-risk patients may be defined as those with advanced-stage, symptomatic disease, short doubling time, high lymphocyte counts, a diffuse pattern of marrow infiltration (51), unmutated Ig VH genes (52-54), chromosomal abnormalities (55), and Zap 70 expression (56).

High-dose therapy and autologous stem cell transplantation can produce complete remission in CLL (50,57), but patients followed for prolonged periods continue to relapse and no study has demonstrated improvement in overall survival (51,52,58). Allogeneic stem cell transplantation is more effective and a substantial fraction of patients achieve durable disease-free survival. Allogeneic transplants should be considered for patients with high-risk features or recurrent disease (59).

Innovative approaches for allogeneic and autologous stem cell transplantation are under investigation. Monoclonal antibodies have been used to increase the likelihood of elimination of MRD prior to autologous SCT. Alemtuzumab was used after fludarabine induction chemotherapy in fludarabine-responsive disease for purging to eradicate MRD in the conditioning regimen for autologous SCT in one arm of the German CLL Study Group CLL3 trial. When alemtuzumab was used at modified dose (10 mg subcutaneously three times per week for 6 weeks) in 34 patients who had had a clinical response to a fludarabine-based regimen, the CR rate improved from 35 to 79.5% with 56% achieving eradication of MRD. Peripheral blood stem cell (PBSC) collection was subsequently successfully performed in 92%. Eighteen patients underwent auto-SCT with 17 remaining in CR at a median follow-up of 14.5 months post-SCT (10).

NON-HODGKIN LYMPHOMA

Autologous transplantation has been extensively studied in patients with non-Hodgkin lymphoma (NHL). Most of these patients have been treated for high- or intermediate-grade lymphoma and failed to respond or have relapsed after an initial CR following standard chemotherapy.

Intermediate- and High-Grade Lymphoma

High-dose chemotherapy and autologous stem cell transplant are the standard of care for patients with recurrent intermediate-grade lymphoma (diffuse large cell lymphoma). This was initially confirmed by a large randomized trial, the Parma study (60). In a recent multicenter

trial for patients with aggressive lymphoma treated in first relapse or second CR, the 3-year survival rate was as high as 44%. This study found that factors such as chemotherapy resistance, increased lactic dehydrogenase (LDH) at diagnosis, CR of <12 months, age <40, and the use of growth factors were adverse predictors of survival (61).

There is considerable interest in the role of high-dose therapy in patients with high-risk features in first remission (62-65). Conflicting results have been reported, but several studies (62-64) demonstrated an improvement in progression-free survival (PFS) using high-dose therapy with ASCT during first-line treatment of patients with poor-prognosis aggressive lymphoma in first complete remission.

The best results for autologous transplant in aggressive lymphoma have been noted in patients transplanted in first or second CR, who have no bone marrow involvement, with good performance status at relapse, a prolonged first CR, normal LDH, few prior chemotherapy regimens, and a low International Prognostic Index (IPI) rating at relapse. Patients with evidence of residual disease by positron emission tomography (PET) scan have a poor prognosis with autologous stem cell transplant (66,67).

Low-Grade Lymphoma

The role of autologous transplantation is controversial in the management of patients with low-grade lymphoma (LGL). The high-dose cyclophosphamide (68) and TBI preparative regimen have been most frequently used (69); 20 to 60% of patients with relapsed disease will survive 3 to 5 years free of recurrence, depending on prognostic features. This is an indolent disease, however, and it is controversial whether autologous stem cell transplantation prolongs overall survival. Autologous stem cell transplants have been most promising in patients with chemosensitive recurrent disease after a relatively long first remission (70).

The major problem is potential contamination of the autologous graft by malignant cells (71). Several purging techniques have been proposed to eliminate this difficulty without damaging the hematopoietic stem cells needed for engraftment. Monoclonal antibodies have been used for selective elimination of malignant cells because of their specificity (72). Polymerase chain reaction amplification of the t(14;18) has been used to detect residual lymphoma cells in bone marrow before and after purging in patients undergoing autologous transplant to assess the efficiency of the purging on disease-free survival (DFS) (73). Systemic treatment with rituximab reduces the numbers of circulating lymphoma cells and acts as in vivo purging to reduce contamination of autologous PBPC grafts (74,75).

Recent studies including rituximab in the preparative regimen have improved the results of autologous stem cell transplantation (75). Rituximab has been shown to improve 4-year event-free survival in patients with poor-risk diffuse large B-cell lymphoma when given as maintenance therapy for four doses between 45 and 65 days posttransplant (76).

Non-Hodgkin lymphoma is a highly radiosensitive malignancy. Radioimmunotherapy (RIT) has become an attractive approach to improve the outcome of autologous transplantation in relapsed or refractory lymphomas (77). RIT is composed of a monoclonal antibody targeting a tumor-specific cell-surface antigen, conjugated to a radionuclide as a means of delivering radiotherapy within the tumor. Two radioconjugates have been evaluated for RIT for non-Hodgkin lymphoma: Yttrium-90 (^{90}Y)-ibritumomab (Zevalin) and iodine-131(^{131}I)-tositumomab (Bexxar). In contrast to TBI, RIT (conventional and high dose) has been better tolerated and can be effectively used in the preparative regimen in elderly patients and those with comorbidities (11,12). In addition, addition of RIT has also been shown to improve response rate as compared to chemotherapy alone when used as a consolidation regimen (78).

HODGKIN LYMPHOMA

The majority of the patients with Hodgkin lymphoma (HL) are curable with first-line therapy; however, 10 to 20% of patients with advanced HL will not enter into a durable CR and approximately 30% will relapse after an initial response (79,80).

Patients with systemic relapse within 12 months of CR despite aggressive first-line therapy with standard regimens such as ABVD [Adriamycin (doxorubicin), bleomycin, vinblastine, dacarbazine] can be retreated with salvage chemotherapy regimens; this may lead to a response in up to 85%, including CR rates ranging from 26 to 62% (81). Unfortunately these remissions are usually transient, particularly in those who are refractory to first-line therapy or who relapsed shortly after the initial CR. Autologous stem cell transplants can produce durable remissions in patients with recurrent, chemosensitive disease (80,82). Most studies have described results in patients with primary refractory or relapsed HL. Clinical distinction between the two sets of patients is not always clear. Patients with primary refractory HL have early TRM of 12 to 16% and a long-term DFS and PFS expectation of 30 to 40% (83). Patients with relapsed HL have a TRM of 4 to

7% and long-term DFS/PFS expectation as high as 40 to 65% (83).

Controversy remains regarding the selection of optimal patients and the most effective conditioning regimen. The most commonly used include BECM (BCNU [carmustine], etoposide, cytarabine, melphalan); CBV (cyclophosphamide, BiCNU [carmustine], VePesid [etoposide]) (83); and ICE (ifosfamide, carboplatin, etoposide) (84).

Favorable prognostic features for autologous transplant include first remission of greater than 1 year, good performance status, limited number of nodal sites, absence of visceral disease, and absence of B symptoms. Patients with all favorable prognostic features have a DFS of more than 70% at 4 years, compared with 20% in patients with adverse features (85). PET scan uptake has major prognostic importance; patients with a negative PET scan have improved disease-free survival (86,87).

Patient selection and disease-related factors have such a major impact on response and survival rates that it is very difficult to compare phase II studies treatment regimens among institutions or in different subgroups of patients, where prognostic features vary or are not well defined.

The optimal interactions of salvage chemotherapy and autologous transplantation are still uncertain although multiple prognostic factors have shown to be related to the success of HDC/ASCT (88,89). Some institutions have performed autologous transplantation as first treatment of relapsed disease (90), whereas most have utilized salvage chemotherapy to achieve a minimal disease state (91-95) with consolidation with high-dose chemotherapy and PBSC transplant.

MULTIPLE MYELOMA

High-dose therapy with autologous stem cell transplantation is an established treatment for multiple myeloma (MM). High-dose melphalan chemotherapy with autologous stem cell transplantation is a standard therapy used in consolidating an initial chemotherapy response. A large randomized trial documented improved time to progression and survival in patients receiving autologous stem cell transplantation (96-99). Overall survival with high-dose chemotherapy followed by autologous stem cell transplant has reached up to 40 to 50% (96).

A number of studies have evaluated novel preparative regimens, but, to date, none have proven superior to high-dose melphalan 200 mg/m^2 (100). The addition of TBI or additional chemotherapeutic agents have increased toxicity but not disease response. Use of a second course of high-dose melphalan and autologous transplantation (tandem autologous transplants) was reported superior to a single transplant in some, (100-102) but not in all studies (103). One of the studies reported that a CR or very good partial response was achieved by 50% of patients in the double-transplant group, against 42% of patients in the single-transplant arm. Also, the estimated event-free survival at 7 years was 20% in the double-transplant group versus 10% in the single-transplant group. Last, the overall 7-year survival rate was 42% in the tandem arm versus 21% in the single-transplant arm (102).

Bortezomib, a proteosome inhibitor, has a synergistic effect with melphalan. Bortezomib (1 mg/m^2 × 4) and melphalan (200 mg/m^2) as conditioning regimen (Bor-HDM) resulted in 70% of patients achieving at least very good partial response (VGPR), including 17 patients with CR (32%) after ASCT versus 11% in a cohort of patients treated with high-dose melphalan only prior to autologous transplant in a matched control analysis, and there was no increased hematologic toxicity with bortezomib (8).

There is considerable interest in the use of posttransplant maintenance therapy with thalidomide or lenalidomide. A recent study reported prolonged survival with lenalidomide and prednisolone given for 12 months after a single high-dose therapy with ASCT in patients with newly diagnosed MM (104). The role of tandem transplants and posttransplant maintenance therapy is the subject of active investigation.

The goal of treatment is to induce a complete remission (105). It is controversial whether patients with complete remission to induction treatment will benefit from an autologous stem cell transplant in first remission. Presence of poor prognostic markers predicts poor outcome (106,107) and thus would favor SCT. Nevertheless, trials are needed to determine the clinical benefit of early SCT in patients who have already achieved a high quality of response.

An expert panel concluded that autologous stem cell transplantation (ASCT) with melphalan is the treatment of choice in patients younger than 65 years, and induction therapy including new drugs seems the most suitable preparatory regimen before ASCT. In patients who fail to achieve at least a VGPR after transplant, a consolidation with a second transplant is of clinical benefit. Also, there is evidence that maintenance with thalidomide or lenalidomide after ASCT in young patients failing to reach at least VGPR could prolong survival. In elderly patients who are poor candidates for high-dose chemotherapy and autologous transplant, the combination of an alkylating drug with a novel agent should be considered as standard approach. Relapsed MM should be retreated after the reappearance of symptoms and signs

of organ and tissue damage. Salvage regimens should include corticosteroids plus bortezomib, thalidomide, or lenalidomide (108,109).

BREAST CANCER AND OTHER SOLID TUMORS

High-dose therapy has also been evaluated for a range of chemotherapy-sensitive solid tumors. This approach improves response rates, but its use is controversial in adult nonhematologic malignancies. The most encouraging data have been reported in patients with breast cancer. Numerous controlled trials have been reported. In several studies, progression-free survival was improved in some studies involving high-risk stages II and III disease, but overall survival has not been improved (110). Long-term remissions have been reported in selected patients with low-bulk, chemosensitive metastatic disease, but controlled studies have not demonstrated a survival benefit (111).

The most encouraging results for breast cancer have come from a large study from the Netherlands. In this study the investigators randomized 885 young women with stage II or III high-risk breast cancer (with four or more positive axillary lymph nodes). After a 57-month follow-up, the 5-year relapse-free survival rates were 59% in the conventional group versus 65% in the autologous transplant group. Furthermore, in the subgroup with 10 or more positive axillary nodes, the relapse-free survival rates were 51% in the conventional group versus 61% in the transplant group (112). A recent meta-analysis failed to demonstrate a statistically significant benefit with high-dose chemotherapy and autologous stem cell transplantation (113).

Inflammatory breast cancer (IBC) is a rare clinicopathologic entity with a poor prognosis, and has made minimal progress with current chemotherapy in long-term outcome. There are recent phase II trials showing promising data on progression-free survival, event-free survival, and overall survival in a 6-year follow-up after high-dose melphalan followed by autologous stem cell transplant (114). High-dose chemotherapy followed by autologous transplant has been shown to be effective among triple-negative breast cancer based on retrospective subsets analysis (115). Currently, the use of autologous transplantation for breast cancer is not recommended outside a clinical trial.

High dose chemotherapy has been successful in inducing prolonged disease free survival in relapsed testicular germ cell carcinomas (116-118), most commonly utilizing ICE chemotherapy and given for one or two courses. There is debate regarding the specific indications for transplantation and its role versus alternative forms of salvage chemotherapy (119).

High-dose chemotherapy and autologous SCT has also been studied in ovarian cancer (120); phase II studies have reported a high rate of durable remissions (121), and controlled trials are needed to determine the role of autologous transplantation in this disease. Concern is medullar toxicity with high-dose chemotherapy. Autologous transplants have also been studied for other solid tumors, lung carcinomas (122), and melanoma (123). The results of these treatment modalities have not been encouraging in these diseases, and their use is not recommended outside a clinical trial.

■ FUTURE DIRECTIONS

The collection of marrow or PBPC offers the potential for ex vivo genetic therapy to hematopoietic stem cell or lymphocytes to improve treatment results. Transfection of genes for drug resistance, such as multidrug resistance 1 (MDR1), into normal hematopoietic stem cells may allow better tolerance to subsequent chemotherapy with agents such as doxorubicin, vinca alkaloids, and paclitaxel. Patients with rapid recovery of lymphocyte counts have had the best progression-free survival after autologous stem cell transplantation. Following myeloablative therapy and autologous transplantation, there is homeostatic expansion of lymphocytes; this provides an opportunity for active vaccination or infusion of antigen-specific tumor-reactive lymphocytes or to infuse genetically modified lymphocytes to enhance antitumor effects. One recent approach utilizes redirecting the specificity of T cells using a chimeric T-cell receptor, targeting tumor-related antigens such as CD19 or CD20 in lymphomas (124).

Improvement in the results of autologous transplantation for solid tumors requires the development of more effective treatment regimens that are not excessively toxic to normal tissues. Further phases I and II clinical trials with pharmacokinetic and pharmacodynamic studies are required to develop regimens with the optimal therapeutic index. Candidate drugs should have documented efficacy in standard dosage, have toxic effects limited primarily to the bone marrow, and should lack substantial nonhematopoietic toxicity.

Novel classes of drugs including immunomodulatory drugs (IMIDs), proteasome inhibitors, antiangiogenic agent, and molecularly targeted therapy (such as epidermal growth factor receptor [EGFR] inhibitor, tyrosine kinase receptor [TRK] inhibitor) have activity against many cancers and may be important components

of future high-dose combination chemotherapeutic regimens. It may be possible to improve results further using strategies to overcome drug resistance mechanisms, such as the administration of inhibitors to glycoprotein or chemoprotectant agents.

High-dose therapy with autologous stem cell transplantation is a highly effective modality to achieve major antitumor cytoreduction. Autologous transplants need to be integrated into the multimodality management of hematologic malignancies and solid tumors. Many current studies focus on posttransplant strategies to prevent regrowth of minimal residual disease, including molecularly targeted approaches and angiogenesis inhibition. Further clinical trials will be needed to optimize the use of stem cell transplantation in the overall treatment of cancer.

References

1. Ikeda K, Kozuka T, Harada M. Factors for PBPC collection efficiency and collection predictors. *Transfus Apher Sci* Dec 2004;31(3):245-259.
2. Popat U, Saliba R, Thandi R, et al. Impairment of filgrastim-induced stem cell mobilization after prior lenalidomide in patients with multiple myeloma. *Biol Blood Marrow Transplant* Jun 2009;15(6):718-723.
3. Flomenberg N, Devine SM, Dipersio JF, et al. The use of AMD3100 plus G-CSF for autologous hematopoietic progenitor cell mobilization is superior to G-CSF alone. *Blood* Sep 1 2005;106(5):1867-1874.
4. Grignani G, Perissinotto E, Cavalloni G, et al. Clinical use of AMD3100 to mobilize CD34+ cells in patients affected by non-Hodgkin's lymphoma or multiple myeloma. *J Clin Oncol* Jun 1 2005;23(16):3871-3872; author reply 3872-3873.
5. Cashen AF. Plerixafor hydrochloride: A novel agent for the mobilization of peripheral blood stem cells. *Drugs Today (Barc)* Jul 2009;45(7):497-505.
6. Rosenbeck LL, Srivastava S, Kiel PJ. Peripheral blood stem cell mobilization tactics. *Ann Pharmacother* Jan 2010;44(1):107-116.
7. Fruehauf S, Ehninger G, Hubel K, et al. Mobilization of peripheral blood stem cells for autologous transplant in non-Hodgkin's lymphoma and multiple myeloma patients by plerixafor and G-CSF and detection of tumor cell mobilization by PCR in multiple myeloma patients. *Bone Marrow Transplant* Feb 2010;45(2):269-275.
8. Roussel M, Moreau P, Huynh A, et al. Bortezomib and high dose melphalan as conditioning regimen before autologous stem cell transplantation in patients with de novo multiple myeloma: A phase II study of the Intergroupe Francophone du Myelome (IFM). *Blood* Jan 7 2010;115(1):32-37. Epub Nov 2 2009.
9. Barlogie B. Thalidomide and CC-5013 in multiple myeloma: The University of Arkansas experience. *Semin Hematol* Oct 2003;40(4 Suppl 4):33-38.
10. Montillo M, Tedeschi A, Miqueleiz S, et al. Alemtuzumab as consolidation after a response to fludarabine is effective in purging residual disease in patients with chronic lymphocytic leukemia. *J Clin Oncol* May 20 2006;24(15):2337-2342.

11. Vose JM, Bierman PJ, Enke C, et al. Phase I trial of iodine-131 tositumomab with high-dose chemotherapy and autologous stem-cell transplantation for relapsed non-Hodgkin's lymphoma. *J Clin Oncol* Jan 20 2005;23(3):461-467.

12. Krishnan A, Nademanee A, Fung HC, et al. Phase II trial of a transplantation regimen of yttrium-90 ibritumomab tiuxetan and high-dose chemotherapy in patients with non-Hodgkin's lymphoma. *J Clin Oncol* Jan 1 2008;26(1):90-95.

13. Mehta J. Re: Tandem vs single autologous hematopoietic cell transplantation for the treatment of multiple myeloma: A systematic review and meta-analysis. *J Natl Cancer Inst* Oct 21 2009;101(20):1430-1431; author reply 1431-1433.

14. Ketterer N, Salles G, Raba M, et al. High CD34(+) cell counts decrease hematologic toxicity of autologous peripheral blood progenitor cell transplantation. *Blood* May 1 1998; 91(9):3148-3155.

15. Miller CB, Lazarus HM. Erythropoietin in stem cell transplantation. *Bone Marrow Transplant* May 2001;27(10): 1011-1016.

16. Schuster MW, Beveridge R, Frei-Lahr D, et al. The effects of pegylated recombinant human megakaryocyte growth and development factor (PEG-rHuMGDF) on platelet recovery in breast cancer patients undergoing autologous bone marrow transplantation. *Exp Hematol* Sep 2002;30(9):1044-1050.

17. Favre G, Beksac M, Bacigalupo A, et al. Differences between graft product and donor side effects following bone marrow or stem cell donation. *Bone Marrow Transplant* Nov 2003; 32(9):873-880.

18. Shimoni A, Korbling M. Tumor cell contamination in re-infused stem cell autografts: Does it have clinical significance? *Crit Rev Oncol Hematol* Feb 2002;41(2):241-250.

19. Kopp HG, Yildirim S, Weisel KC, et al. Contamination of autologous peripheral blood progenitor cell grafts predicts overall survival after high-dose chemotherapy in multiple myeloma. *J Cancer Res Clin Oncol* Apr 2009;135(4): 637-642.

20. Chen CI, Abraham R, Tsang R, et al. Radiation-associated pneumonitis following autologous stem cell transplantation: Predictive factors, disease characteristics and treatment outcomes. *Bone Marrow Transplant* Jan 2001;27(2):177-182.

21. Fassas A, Gojo I, Rapoport A, et al. Pulmonary toxicity syndrome following CDEP (cyclophosphamide, dexamethasone, etoposide, cisplatin) chemotherapy. *Bone Marrow Transplant* Aug 2001;28(4):399-403.

22. Williams L, Beveridge RA, Rifkin RM, et al. Increased pulmonary toxicity results from a 1-day versus 2-day schedule of administration of high-dose melphalan. *Biol Blood Marrow Transplant* 2002;8(6):334-335.

23. Alessandrino EP, Bernasconi P, Colombo A, et al. Pulmonary toxicity following carmustine-based preparative regimens and autologous peripheral blood progenitor cell transplantation in hematological malignancies. *Bone Marrow Transplant* Feb 2000;25(3):309-313.

24. Cao TM, Negrin RS, Stockerl-Goldstein KE, et al. Pulmonary toxicity syndrome in breast cancer patients undergoing BCNU-containing high-dose chemotherapy and autologous hematopoietic cell transplantation. *Biol Blood Marrow Transplant* 2000;6(4):387-394.

25. McGaughey DS, Nikcevich DA, Long GD, et al. Inhaled steroids as prophylaxis for delayed pulmonary toxicity syndrome in breast cancer patients undergoing high-dose chemotherapy and autologous stem cell transplantation. *Biol Blood Marrow Transplant* 2001;7(5):274-278.

26. Zappasodi P, Vitulo P, Volpini E, et al. Successful therapy with high-dose steroids and cyclosporine for the treatment of carmustine-mediated lung injury. *Ann Hematol* Jun 2002; 81(6):347-349.

27. Nieto Y, Cagnoni PJ, Bearman SI, et al. Cardiac toxicity following high-dose cyclophosphamide, cisplatin, and BCNU (STAMP-I) for breast cancer. *Biol Blood Marrow Transplant* 2000;6(2A):198-203.

28. Frustaci S, Foladore S, De Pascale A, et al. Feasibility and efficacy of arginine 2-mercaptoethanesulfonate (ARGIMESNA) in the prevention of hemorragic cystitis from ifosfamide (IFO). *Ann Oncol.* Apr 1992;3(Suppl 2):S115-S118.

29. Khojasteh NH, Zakerinia M, Ramzi M, et al. A new regimen of MESNA (2-mercaptoethanesulfonate) effectively prevents cyclophosphamide-induced hemorrhagic cystitis in bone marrow transplant recipients. *Transplant Proc* May 2000; 32(3):596.

30. Abraham P, Rabi S, Kulothungan P. Aminoguanidine, selective nitric oxide synthase inhibitor, ameliorates cyclophosphamide-induced hemorrhagic cystitis by inhibiting protein nitration and PARS activation. *Urology* Jun 2009;73(6): 1402-1406.

31. Nathan PC, Sung L, Crump M, et al. Consolidation therapy with autologous bone marrow transplantation in adults with acute myeloid leukemia: A meta-analysis. *J Natl Cancer Inst* Jan 7 2004;96(1):38-45.

32. Hamadani M, Awan FT, Copelan EA. Hematopoietic stem cell transplantation in adults with acute myeloid leukemia. *Biol Blood Marrow Transplant* May 2008;14(5):556-567.

33. Schlenk RF, Dohner K, Krauter J, et al. Mutations and treatment outcome in cytogenetically normal acute myeloid leukemia. *N Engl J Med* May 1 2008;358(18):1909-1918.

34. Slovak ML, Kopecky KJ, Cassileth PA, et al. Karyotypic analysis predicts outcome of preremission and postremission therapy in adult acute myeloid leukemia: A Southwest Oncology Group/Eastern Cooperative Oncology Group Study. *Blood* Dec 15 2000;96(13):4075-4083.

35. Barker JN, Weisdorf DJ, DeFor TE, et al. Transplantation of 2 partially HLA-matched umbilical cord blood units to enhance engraftment in adults with hematologic malignancy. *Blood* Feb 1 2005;105(3):1343-1347.

36. Kantarjian H, Thomas D, O'Brien S, et al. Long-term follow-up results of hyperfractionated cyclophosphamide, vincristine, doxorubicin, and dexamethasone (Hyper-CVAD), a dose-intensive regimen, in adult acute lymphocytic leukemia. *Cancer* Dec 15 2004;101(12):2788-2801.

37. Bruggemann M, Raff T, Flohr T, et al. Clinical significance of minimal residual disease quantification in adult patients with standard-risk acute lymphoblastic leukemia. *Blood* Feb 1 2006;107(3):1116-1123.

38. Maldonado MS, Diaz-Heredia C, Badell I, et al. Autologous bone marrow transplantation with monoclonal antibody purged marrow for children with acute lymphoblastic leukemia in second remission. Spanish Working Party for BMT in Children. *Bone Marrow Transplant* Dec 1998;22(11):1043-1047.

39. Goldstone AH, Richards SM, Lazarus HM, et al. In adults with standard-risk acute lymphoblastic leukemia, the greatest benefit is achieved from a matched sibling allogeneic transplantation in first complete remission, and an autologous transplantation is less effective than conventional consolidation/maintenance chemotherapy in all patients: Final results of the International ALL Trial (MRC UKALL XII/ECOG E2993). *Blood* Feb 15 2008;111(4):1827-1833.

40. Willemze R, Labar B. Post-remission treatment for adult patients with acute lymphoblastic leukemia in first remission: Is there a role for autologous stem cell transplantation? *Semin Hematol* Oct 2007;44(4):267-273.

41. Egerer G, Goldschmidt H, Zoz M, et al. Autologous bone marrow transplantation in adult patients with acute lymphoblastic leukemia. *Leuk Lymphoma* Jan 2003;44(1):9-14.

42. Schiffer CA, Hehlmann R, Larson R. Perspectives on the treatment of chronic phase and advanced phase CML and Philadelphia chromosome positive ALL(1). *Leukemia* Apr 2003;17(4):691-699.

43. Talpaz M, Silver RT, Druker BJ, et al. Imatinib induces durable hematologic and cytogenetic responses in patients with accelerated phase chronic myeloid leukemia: Results of a phase 2 study. *Blood* Mar 15 2002;99(6):1928-1937.

44. Kantarjian H, Cortes J. BCR-ABL tyrosine kinase inhibitors in chronic myeloid leukemia: Using guidelines to make rational treatment choices. *J Natl Compr Canc Netw* Mar 2008; 6(Suppl 2):S37-S42; quiz S43-S44.

45. Kantarjian HM, Cortes J, La Rosee P, et al. Optimizing therapy for patients with chronic myelogenous leukemia in chronic phase. *Cancer* Mar 15;116(6):1419-1430.

46. Gratwohl A, Heim D. Current role of stem cell transplantation in chronic myeloid leukaemia. *Best Pract Res Clin Haematol* Sep 2009;22(3):431-443.

47. Gordon MK, Sher D, Karrison T, et al. Successful autologous stem cell collection in patients with chronic myeloid leukemia in complete cytogenetic response, with quantitative measurement of BCR-ABL expression in blood, marrow, and apheresis products. *Leuk Lymphoma* Mar 2008;49(3): 531-537.

48. Olavarria E. Autologous stem cell transplantation in chronic myeloid leukemia. *Semin Hematol* Oct 2007;44(4):252-258.

49. Klyuchnikov E, Kroger N, Brummendorf TH, et al. Current status and perspectives of tyrosine kinase inhibitor treatment in the post-transplant period in patients with chronic myeloid leukemia (CML). *Biol Blood Marrow Transplant* Mar 2010;16(3):301-310. Epub Sep 7 2009.

50. Milligan DW, Fernandes S, Dasgupta R, et al. Results of the MRC pilot study show autografting for younger patients with chronic lymphocytic leukemia is safe and achieves a high percentage of molecular responses. *Blood* Jan 1 2005;105(1): 397-404.

51. Dreger P, Montserrat E. Autologous and allogeneic stem cell transplantation for chronic lymphocytic leukemia. *Leukemia* Jun 2002;16(6):985-992.

52. Gribben JG, Zahrieh D, Stephans K, et al. Autologous and allogeneic stem cell transplantations for poor-risk chronic lymphocytic leukemia. *Blood* Dec 15 2005;106(13):4389-4396.

53. Dreger P, Stilgenbauer S, Benner A, et al. The prognostic impact of autologous stem cell transplantation in patients with chronic lymphocytic leukemia: A risk-matched analysis based on the VH gene mutational status. *Blood* Apr 1 2004;103(7):2850-2858.

54. Hamblin TJ, Davis Z, Gardiner A, et al. Unmutated Ig V(H) genes are associated with a more aggressive form of chronic lymphocytic leukemia. *Blood* Sep 15 1999;94(6):1848-1854.

55. Dohner H, Stilgenbauer S, Benner A, et al. Genomic aberrations and survival in chronic lymphocytic leukemia. *N Engl J Med* Dec 28 2000;343(26):1910-1916.

56. Crespo M, Bosch F, Villamor N, et al. ZAP-70 expression as a surrogate for immunoglobulin-variable-region mutations in chronic lymphocytic leukemia. *N Engl J Med* May 1 2003; 348(18):1764-1775.

57. Jantunen E, Itala M, Siitonen T, et al. Autologous stem cell transplantation in patients with chronic lymphocytic leukaemia: The Finnish experience. *Bone Marrow Transplant* Jun 2006; 37(12):1093-1098.

58. Esteve J, Villamor N, Colomer D, et al. Stem cell transplantation for chronic lymphocytic leukemia: Different outcome after autologous and allogeneic transplantation and correlation with minimal residual disease status. *Leukemia* Mar 2001;15(3):445-451.

59. Tam CS, Khouri I. The role of stem cell transplantation in the management of chronic lymphocytic leukaemia. *Hematol Oncol* Jun 2009;27(2):53-60.

60. Philip T, Guglielmi C, Hagenbeek A, et al. Autologous bone marrow transplantation as compared with salvage chemotherapy in relapses of chemotherapy-sensitive non-Hodgkin's lymphoma. *N Engl J Med* Dec 7 1995;333(23):1540-1545.

61. Vose JM, Rizzo DJ, Tao-Wu J, et al. Autologous transplantation for diffuse aggressive non-Hodgkin lymphoma in first relapse or second remission. *Biol Blood Marrow Transplant* Feb 2004;10(2):116-127.

62. Sweetenham JW, Proctor SJ, Blaise D, et al. High-dose therapy and autologous bone marrow transplantation in first complete remission for adult patients with high-grade non-Hodgkin's lymphoma: The EBMT experience. Lymphoma Working Party of the European Group for Bone Marrow Transplantation. *Ann Oncol* 1994;5(Suppl 2):155-159.

63. Jackson GH, Lennard AL, Taylor PR, et al. Autologous bone marrow transplantation in poor-risk high-grade non-Hodgkin's lymphoma in first complete remission. Newcastle and Northern Lymphoma Group. *Br J Cancer* Sep 1994;70(3):501-505.

64. Vranovsky A, Ladicka M, Lakota J. Autologous stem cell transplantation in first-line treatment of high-risk aggressive non-Hodgkin's lymphoma. *Neoplasma* 2008;55(2):107-112.

65. Tarella C, Gianni AM. Bone marrow transplantation for lymphoma CR1. *Curr Opin Oncol* Mar 2005;17(2):99-105.

66. Poulou LS, Thanos L, Ziakas PD. Unifying the predictive value of pretransplant FDG PET in patients with lymphoma: A review and meta-analysis of published trials. *Eur J Nucl Med Mol Imaging* Jan;37(1):156-162.

67. Johnston PB, Wiseman GA, Micallef IN. Positron emission tomography using F-18 fluorodeoxyglucose pre- and post-autologous stem cell transplant in non-Hodgkin's lymphoma. *Bone Marrow Transplant* Jun 2008;41(11):919-925.

68. Horning SJ, Negrin RS, Hoppe RT, et al. High-dose therapy and autologous bone marrow transplantation for follicular lymphoma in first complete or partial remission: results of a phase II clinical trial. *Blood* Jan 15 2001;97(2):404-409.

69. Freedman AS, Ritz J, Neuberg D, et al. Autologous bone marrow transplantation in 69 patients with a history of low-grade B-cell non-Hodgkin's lymphoma. *Blood* Jun 1 1991;77(11): 2524-2529.

70. Wrench D, Gribben JG. Stem cell transplantation for non-Hodgkin's lymphoma. *Hematol Oncol Clin North Am* Oct 2008;22(5):1051-1079, xi.

71. Gribben JG. Autologous hematopoietic transplantation for low-grade lymphomas. *Cytotherapy* 2002; 4:205-215.

72. Gisselbrecht C. In vivo purging and relapse prevention following ASCT. *Bone Marrow Transplant* Feb 2002;29(Suppl 1): S5-S9.

73. Gribben JG, Freedman AS, Neuberg D, et al. Immunologic purging of marrow assessed by PCR before autologous bone marrow transplantation for B-cell lymphoma. *N Engl J Med* Nov 28 1991;325(22):1525-1533.

74. Kato H, Taji H, Ogura M, et al. Favorable consolidative effect of high-dose melphalan and total-body irradiation followed by autologous peripheral blood stem cell transplantation after rituximab-containing induction chemotherapy with in vivo purging in relapsed or refractory follicular lymphoma. *Clin Lymphoma Myeloma* Dec 2009;9(6):443-448.

75. Cerny J, Trneny M, Slavickova A, et al. Rituximab based therapy followed by autologous stem cell transplantation leads to superior outcome and high rates of PCR negativity in patients with indolent B-cell lymphoproliferative disorders. *Hematology* Aug 2009;14(4):187-197.

76. Haioun C, Mounier N, Emile JF, et al. Rituximab versus observation after high-dose consolidative first-line chemotherapy with autologous stem-cell transplantation in patients with poor-risk diffuse large B-cell lymphoma. *Ann Oncol* Dec 2009; 20(12):1985-1992.

77. Gisselbrecht C, Vose J, Nademanee A, et al. Radioimmunotherapy for stem cell transplantation in non-Hodgkin's lymphoma: In pursuit of a complete response. *Oncologist* 2009;14(Suppl 2):41-51.

78. Hainsworth JD, Spigel DR, Markus TM, et al. Rituximab plus short-duration chemotherapy followed by Yttrium-90 Ibritumomab tiuxetan as first-line treatment for patients with follicular non-Hodgkin lymphoma: A phase II trial of the Sarah Cannon Oncology Research Consortium. *Clin Lymphoma Myeloma* Jun 2009;9(3):223-228.

79. Viviani S, Bonadonna G, Santoro A, et al. Alternating versus hybrid MOPP and ABVD combinations in advanced Hodgkin's disease: Ten-year results. *J Clin Oncol* May 1996;14(5):1421-1430.

80. Champlin R. Bone marrow transplantation for Hodgkin's disease–recent advances and current issues. *Leuk Lymphoma* 1993;10(Suppl):103-108.

81. Avivi I, Goldstone AH. Autologous stem cell transplantation in Hodgkin's disease. *Ann Oncol* 2002;13(Suppl 1):122-127.

82. Lavoie JC, Connors JM, Phillips GL, et al. High-dose chemotherapy and autologous stem cell transplantation for primary refractory or relapsed Hodgkin lymphoma: Long-term outcome in the first 100 patients treated in Vancouver. *Blood* Aug 15 2005;106(4):1473-1478.

83. Anderlini P. Hematopoietic stem-cell transplantation for Hodgkin's disease (HD): Current status. *Cytotherapy* 2002; 4(3):241-251.

84. Moskowitz CH, Nimer SD, Zelenetz AD, et al. A 2-step comprehensive high-dose chemoradiotherapy second-line program for relapsed and refractory Hodgkin disease: Analysis by intent to treat and development of a prognostic model. *Blood* Feb 1 2001;97(3):616-623.

85. Jagannath S, Armitage JO, Dicke KA, et al. Prognostic factors for response and survival after high-dose cyclophosphamide, carmustine, and etoposide with autologous bone marrow transplantation for relapsed Hodgkin's disease. *J Clin Oncol* Feb 1989;7(2):179-185.

86. Castagna L, Bramanti S, Balzarotti M, et al. Predictive value of early 18F-fluorodeoxyglucose positron emission tomography (FDG-PET) during salvage chemotherapy in relapsing/refractory Hodgkin lymphoma (HL) treated with high-dose chemotherapy. *Br J Haematol* May 2009;145(3):369-372.

87. Jabbour E, Hosing C, Ayers G, et al. Pretransplant positive positron emission tomography/gallium scans predict poor outcome in patients with recurrent/refractory Hodgkin lymphoma. *Cancer* Jun 15 2007;109(12):2481-2489.

88. Sureda A, Constans M, Iriondo A, et al. Prognostic factors affecting long-term outcome after stem cell transplantation in Hodgkin's lymphoma autografted after a first relapse. *Ann Oncol* Apr 2005;16(4):625-633.

89. Constans M, Sureda A, Terol MJ, et al. Autologous stem cell transplantation for primary refractory Hodgkin's disease: Results and clinical variables affecting outcome. *Ann Oncol* May 2003;14(5):745-751.

90. Schmitz N, Pfistner B, Sextro M, et al. Aggressive conventional chemotherapy compared with high-dose chemotherapy with autologous haemopoietic stem-cell transplantation for relapsed chemosensitive Hodgkin's disease: A randomised trial. *Lancet* Jun 15 2002;359(9323):2065-2071.

91. Bartlett NL, Niedzwiecki D, Johnson JL, et al. Gemcitabine, vinorelbine, and pegylated liposomal doxorubicin (GVD), a salvage regimen in relapsed Hodgkin's lymphoma: CALGB 59804. *Ann Oncol* Jun 2007;18(6):1071-1079.

92. Santoro A, Magagnoli M, Spina M, et al. Ifosfamide, gemcitabine, and vinorelbine: A new induction regimen for refractory and relapsed Hodgkin's lymphoma. *Haematologica* Jan 2007;92(1):35-41.

93. Kuruvilla J, Nagy T, Pintilie M, et al. Similar response rates and superior early progression-free survival with gemcitabine, dexamethasone, and cisplatin salvage therapy compared with carmustine, etoposide, cytarabine, and melphalan salvage therapy prior to autologous stem cell transplantation for recurrent or refractory Hodgkin lymphoma. *Cancer* Jan 15 2006;106(2):353-360.

94. Rodriguez J, Rodriguez MA, Fayad L, et al. ASHAP: A regimen for cytoreduction of refractory or recurrent Hodgkin's disease. *Blood* Jun 1 1999;93(11):3632-3636.

95. Aparicio J, Segura A, Garcera S, et al. ESHAP is an active regimen for relapsing Hodgkin's disease. *Ann Oncol* May 1999;10(5):593-595.

96. Attal M, Harousseau JL, Stoppa AM, et al. A prospective, randomized trial of autologous bone marrow transplantation and chemotherapy in multiple myeloma. Intergroupe Francais du Myelome. *N Engl J Med* Jul 11 1996;335(2):91-97.

97. Child JA, Morgan GJ, Davies FE, et al. High-dose chemotherapy with hematopoietic stem-cell rescue for multiple myeloma. *N Engl J Med* May 8 2003;348(19):1875-1883.

98. Lenhoff S, Hjorth M, Holmberg E, et al. Impact on survival of high-dose therapy with autologous stem cell support in patients younger than 60 years with newly diagnosed multiple myeloma: A population-based study. Nordic Myeloma Study Group. *Blood* Jan 1 2000;95(1):7-11.

99. Palumbo A, Triolo S, Argentino C, et al. Dose-intensive melphalan with stem cell support (MEL100) is superior to standard treatment in elderly myeloma patients. *Blood* Aug 15 1999;94(4):1248-1253.

100. Barlogie B, Shaughnessy J, Tricot G, et al. Treatment of multiple myeloma. *Blood* Jan 1 2004;103(1):20-32.

101. Barlogie B, Jagannath S, Desikan KR, et al. Total therapy with tandem transplants for newly diagnosed multiple myeloma. *Blood* Jan 1 1999;93(1):55-65.

102. Attal M, Harousseau JL, Facon T, et al. Single versus double autologous stem-cell transplantation for multiple myeloma. *N Engl J Med* Dec 25 2003;349(26):2495-2502.

103. Giralt S, Vesole DH, Somlo G, et al. Re: Tandem vs single autologous hematopoietic cell transplantation for the treatment of multiple myeloma: a systematic review and meta-analysis. *J Natl Cancer Inst* Jul 1 2009;101(13):964; author reply 966-967.

104. Spencer A, Prince HM, Roberts AW, et al. Consolidation therapy with low-dose thalidomide and prednisolone prolongs the survival of multiple myeloma patients undergoing a single autologous stem-cell transplantation procedure. *J Clin Oncol* Apr 10 2009;27(11):1788-1793.

105. Harousseau JL, Attal M, Avet-Loiseau H. The role of complete response in multiple myeloma. *Blood* Oct 8 2009; 114(15):3139-3146.

106. Fassas AB, Spencer T, Sawyer J, et al. Both hypodiploidy and deletion of chromosome 13 independently confer poor prognosis in multiple myeloma. *Br J Haematol* Sep 2002; 118(4):1041-1047.

107. Jacobson J, Barlogie B, Shaughnessy J, et al. MDS-type abnormalities within myeloma signature karyotype (MM-MDS): only 13% 1-year survival despite tandem transplants. *Br J Haematol* Aug 2003;122(3):430-440.

108. Patriarca F, Petrucci MT, Bringhen S, et al. Considerations in the treatment of multiple myeloma: A consensus statement from Italian experts. *Eur J Haematol* Feb 2009;82(2): 93-105.

109. Lonial S, Cavenagh J. Emerging combination treatment strategies containing novel agents in newly diagnosed multiple myeloma. *Br J Haematol* Jun 2009;145(6):681-708.

110. Zander AR, Schmoor C, Kroger N, et al. Randomized trial of high-dose adjuvant chemotherapy with autologous hematopoietic stem-cell support versus standard-dose chemotherapy in breast cancer patients with 10 or more positive lymph nodes: Overall survival after 6 years of follow-up. *Ann Oncol* Jun 2008;19(6):1082-1089.

111. Lotz JP, Cure H, Janvier M, et al. High-dose chemotherapy with haematopoietic stem cell transplantation for metastatic breast cancer patients: Final results of the French multicentric randomised CMA/PEGASE 04 protocol. *Eur J Cancer* Jan 2005;41(1):71-80.

112. Rodenhuis S, Bontenbal M, Beex LV, et al. High-dose chemotherapy with hematopoietic stem-cell rescue for high-risk breast cancer. *N Engl J Med* Jul 3 2003;349(1):7-16.

113. Farquhar CM, Marjoribanks J, Lethaby A, et al. High dose chemotherapy for poor prognosis breast cancer: Systematic review and meta-analysis. *Cancer Treat Rev* Jun 2007;33(4): 325-337.

114. Sportes C, Steinberg SM, Liewehr DJ, et al. Strategies to improve long-term outcome in stage IIIB inflammatory breast cancer: Multimodality treatment including dose-intensive induction and high-dose chemotherapy. *Biol Blood Marrow Transplant* Aug 2009;15(8):963-970.

115. Nieto Y, Shpall EJ. High-dose chemotherapy for high-risk primary and metastatic breast cancer: Is another look warranted? *Curr Opin Oncol* Mar 2009;21(2):150-157.

116. Muller AM, Ihorst G, Waller CF, et al. Intensive chemotherapy with autologous peripheral blood stem cell transplantation during a 10-year period in 64 patients with germ cell tumor. *Biol Blood Marrow Transplant* Mar 2006;12(3): 355-365.

117. Ayash LJ, Clarke M, Silver SM, et al. Double dose-intensive chemotherapy with autologous stem cell support for relapsed and refractory testicular cancer: The University of Michigan experience and literature review. *Bone Marrow Transplant* May 2001;27(9):939-947.

118. Schmoll HJ, Kollmannsberger C, Metzner B, et al. Long-term results of first-line sequential high-dose etoposide, ifosfamide, and cisplatin chemotherapy plus autologous stem cell support for patients with advanced metastatic germ cell cancer: An extended phase I/II study of the German Testicular Cancer Study Group. *J Clin Oncol* Nov 15 2003;21(22):4083-4091.

119. Hara I, Miyake H, Yamada Y, et al. High-dose chemotherapy for male germ cell tumor. *Int J Urol* Aug 2006;13(8):1037-1044.

120. Donato ML, Gershenson D, Ippoliti C, et al. High-dose ifosfamide and etoposide with filgrastim for stem cell mobilization in patients with advanced ovarian cancer. *Bone Marrow Transplant* Jun 2000;25(11):1137-1140.

121. Tiersten A, Selleck M, Smith DH, et al. Phase I/II study of tandem cycles of high-dose chemotherapy followed by autologous hematopoietic stem cell support in women with advanced ovarian cancer. *Int J Gynecol Cancer* Jan-Feb 2006;16(1): 57-64.

122. Rizzo JD, Elias AD, Stiff PJ, et al. Autologous stem cell transplantation for small cell lung cancer. *Biol Blood Marrow Transplant* 2002;8(5):273-280.

123. Schrader AJ, Atzpodien J. High-dose chemotherapy with autologous stem-cell transplantation in patients with pretreated advanced malignant melanoma. *Ann Oncol* Oct 2000;11(10): 1361-1362.

124. Singh H, Serrano LM, Pfeiffer T, et al. Combining adoptive cellular and immunocytokine therapies to improve treatment of B-lineage malignancy. *Cancer Res* Mar 15 2007;67(6): 2872-2880.

Lung Cancer

CHAPTER 14

SMALL CELL CARCINOMA OF THE LUNGS

Kathryn A. Gold
Bonnie S. Glisson
Commentary: Cesar Moran

■ INTRODUCTION

Small cell lung cancer (SCLC) is a highly aggressive malignant epithelial tumor. Patients typically present with rapidly growing, symptomatic disease, and distant metastases at diagnosis are common. Most cases are highly sensitive to chemotherapy, but the disease frequently recurs, and most patients will die of their disease. SCLC remains a therapeutic challenge.

■ EPIDEMIOLOGY

Approximately 219,440 patients in the United States are diagnosed with lung cancer every year, and approximately 159,390 will die of their disease (1). Small cell lung cancer currently accounts for approximately 13% of all lung cancers in the United States, compared to its incidence in the 1980s when it represented 18% of cases (2). Historically, a majority of patients with SCLC were male, but recent analyses show that equal numbers of men and women are affected, probably due to increasing use of tobacco among women starting in the 1960s (2).

■ RISK FACTORS

Cigarette smoking is the single most important risk factor for development of SCLC. It has been estimated that well over 90% of small cell lung cancers are attributable to cigarette smoking (3), and in our experience, it is rare to see a nonsmoking patient diagnosed with small cell lung cancer. The risk is related to both the duration and intensity of tobacco use, and the risk for former smokers is lower than that for current smokers, though still far higher than that of nonsmokers (4). Some studies suggest that the risk of small cell lung cancer is greater for smoking women than for men (3). Other than the association of tobacco, exposure to asbestos, benzene, coal tar, and radon gas has been associated with risk, usually as co-carcinogens with tobacco. Smoking cessation counseling is a widely accepted method of primary prevention. Even after diagnosis of SCLC, smoking cessation should be encouraged, as there is evidence of worse outcomes in patients who continue to smoke through and after treatment (5).

■ NATURAL HISTORY AND PROGNOSTIC FACTORS

The natural history of SCLC was documented in the placebo arm of an early randomized trial from the Veterans Administration Lung Cancer Study Group which tested the effect of three doses of intravenous cyclophosphamide (6). In this trial, the median survival time for patients in the placebo arm was 6 weeks for patients with obvious metastatic disease, known as extensive disease, and 12 weeks for patients who appeared to have disease limited to one hemithorax, known as limited disease. Given the era, staging in this trial was rudimentary and, thus, outcomes in both groups would probably be better today because of stage shift. Cyclophosphamide treatment increased the median survival time by 75 days in both groups of patients, tripling the survival of patients with metastases and doubling that of patients with chest-confined disease. This was the first observation foretelling the important role chemotherapy would come to play in management of small cell lung cancer.

The use of effective combination chemotherapy and, in the case of patients with tumor amenable to definitive radiation, combined modality treatment has increased the median survival rate of patients with SCLC. According to a recent SEER (Surveillance, Epidemiology, and End Results) database analysis, the 2-year survival for patients with extensive disease is now 4.6%, and the 5-year survival for patients with limited disease is 10%, improved from 1.5 to 4.9%, respectively, in 1973 (2).

There are a number of known prognostic factors. Stage is of course a powerful prognostic factor, with patients with limited-stage disease having improved survival over patients with extensive disease. Among patients with limited disease, good performance status, age younger than 70, female sex, and normal lactate dehydrogenase (LDH) were found to be predictive of a favorable outcome. In extensive disease, normal LDH, treatment with a multidrug regimen, and a single metastatic lesion predicted better outcomes (7). Other studies report that paraneoplastic phenomena may also predict a worse outcome (8). Models to assist clinicians with prognostication have been published (7).

■ PATHOLOGY

According to the World Health Organization lung cancer classification of 1999, small cell carcinoma is "a malignant epithelial tumor consisting of small cells with scant cytoplasm, ill-defined cell borders, finely granular nuclear chromatin, and absent or inconspicuous nucleoli. The cells are round, oval, and spindle-shaped and nuclear molding is prominent. The mitotic count is high" (9). Please see Fig. 14-1 for pathologic images of SCLC. Differentiation between SCLC and non–small cell lung cancer (NSCLC) is most frequently accomplished using light microscopy with immunohistochemical markers (10). Since surgery is rarely performed for SCLC, diagnoses are often made with small pathologic specimens.

A variant of SCLC, combined small cell carcinoma, includes tumors with at least 10% of the tumor consisting of any other non–small cell component (11). SCLC is most aggressive of a spectrum of neuroendocrine

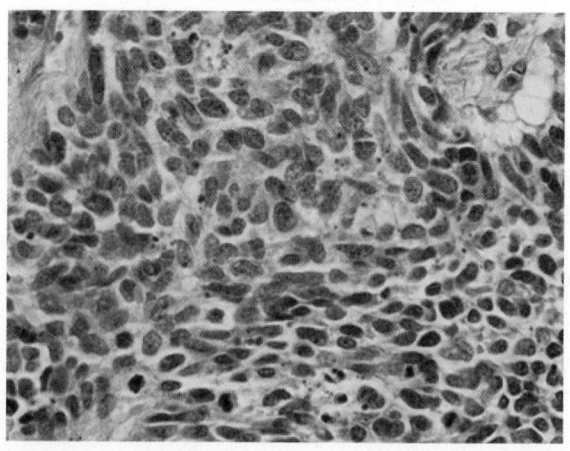

FIGURE 14-1. Light microscopic images of SCLC. Note the small round and spindle-shaped cells with hyperchromic nuclei and scant cytoplasm.

tumors of the lungs, including typical carcinoid tumors, atypical carcinoids, and large cell neuroendocrine carcinoma (9). Large cell neuroendocrine carcinoma (LCNEC) is classified as a non–small cell lung cancer but has similar biology, behavior, and natural history as SCLC (11).

SCLC is a "small round blue cell tumor," and the differential diagnosis includes other small round blue cell tumors: lymphomas, small-celled sarcomas such as Ewing sarcoma and primitive neuroectodermal tumors and Merkel cell carcinoma, a high-grade neuroendocrine carcinoma of the skin. Histologically, identical tumors can arise in other organs, for example, prostate, cervix, and larynx, and these are termed extrapulmonary small cell carcinomas. Their behavior is typically similar to that of SCLC. Useful immunohistochemical markers include chromogranin and synaptophysin, though SCLC is a high-grade neuroendocrine tumor and does not typically express these proteins as highly as would be seen in a low-grade

TABLE 14-1	GENETIC ALTERATIONS ASSOCIATED WITH SMALL CELL LUNG CANCER	
Tumor Suppressor Genes		*Protooncogenes*
RASSF1A		*Myc*
FHIT		*Bcl-2*
Retinoic acid receptor-beta		*c-Kit*
p53		*c-Met*
RB		*IGF-1*
Telomeres		*TGF-B*
		G protein–coupled receptors

IGF-1, Insulin-like growth factor 1; *TGF-B*, transforming growth factor beta.

neuroendocrine tumor, such as a carcinoid tumor. Keratin markers can be useful to identify a tumor of epithelial origin and exclude lymphomas and sarcomas (9). Table 14-1 describes some of the genes whose expression is altered in SCLC.

Commentary: The Spectrum of Pulmonary Neuroendocrine Carcinomas

The term *neuroendocrine carcinoma* encompasses tumors of low, intermediate-, and high-grade histology. By far, the tumors are more common in the gastrointestinal system where they account for more than 50% in occurrence. Although in the past it has been stated that these tumors behave more favorably in certain anatomic location, it is very likely that the behavior of these tumors will be determined not only by their clinical and surgical stage but also by the grade of differentiation. One important observation that requires special attention is the fact that the histopathological features of these tumors regardless of their anatomic location are identical. Therefore, in many circumstances the determination of a primary site will require careful clinical evaluation.

From the histopathological point of view, great controversy has existed regarding the best way to determine behavior in these tumor and many histopathological schemas have been presented. In addition, the grading system that is ascribed to these tumors has some differences based on the anatomic location of the tumor. Although more recent work is being done to implement a more universal nomenclature for these tumor, currently that is still on review. However, it is this pathological grading system that is currently used to determine not only treatment but also behavior and prognosis. (see Table 14-2 for grading criteria for these tumors) The conventional and more common immunohistochemical markers used to determine the neuroendocrine nature of these tumors are

essentially shared by all of these tumors regardless of the anatomic location. In some cases, there are some immunohistochemical studies that appear to be more specific for tumors in certain locations; an example of it would be the use of the immunohistochemical study for TTF-1 (thyroid transcriptase factor-1) and the use of CDX-2. These markers may in some cases be of aid as TTF-1 is commonly positive in thoracic tumors while CDX2, a transcription factor frequently expressed in intestinal neoplasia, is more commonly seen positive in gastrointestinal tumors.

One important point that requires attention is the fact that on limited biopsies a definitive grading of the tumor may prove impossible mainly in tumors of low and intermediate grade. In addition, in cases such as large cell neuroendocrine carcinoma, such diagnosis requires immunohistochemical proof by showing positive staining for neuroendocrine markers (chromogranin, synaptophysin, etc.). Needless to say, there is a wide spectrum of tumors that may share either similar histological or immunohistochemical features that will require careful analysis and proper exclusion.

Cesar Moran

References

Moran CA, Suster S, Coppola D, et al. Neuroendocrine tumors of the lung: A reappraisal. *Am J Clin Pathol* 2009;131:206-221.

TABLE 14-2	GRADING CRITERIA FOR NEUROENDOCRINE CARCINOMAS	
Grade	*Histology*	*Conventional Nomenclature*
Low-grade NE Ca	<3 mitotic figures × 10 hpf Absent necrosis	Carcinoid tumor
Intermediate-grade NE Ca	>3 but <10 mitoses × 10 hpf Necrosis	Atypical carcinoid
High-grade NE Ca		
Small cell type	>10 mitoses × 10 hpf Necrosis	Small cell carcinoma
Large Cell NE Ca	> 10 mitoses ×10 hpf Necrosis	Large cell NE Ca

Ca, carcinoma; hpf, high power fields; NE, neuroendocrine.
*This grading system is based on surgical resections.

■ CLINICAL PRESENTATION AND DIAGNOSTIC EVALUATION

Because SCLC is a rapidly growing and aggressive tumor, patients will often develop symptoms over a short period of time and are usually diagnosed within 3 months from onset of symptoms (6). SCLC typically arises in the central airways and infiltrates the submucosa, in contrast to the polypoid luminal occlusion seen with squamous cancers. The tumor gradually obstructs the bronchial lumen through extrinsic or endobronchial spread. Patients most frequently present with symptoms of dyspnea and persistent cough. Hemoptysis and postobstructive pneumonia are relatively uncommon due to the submucosal growth pattern of the tumor. Spread to the mediastinal lymph nodes is a hallmark of SCLC, and syndromes resulting from mass effect are commonly seen, including superior vena caval obstruction, hoarseness (resulting from recurrent laryngeal nerve compression), phrenic nerve palsy, dysphagia (resulting from esophageal compression), and stridor (resulting from tracheal compression). SCLC is the most common malignant cause of superior vena caval obstruction. SCLC is often metastatic at presentation, and patients may present with symptoms of metastatic disease: bone or right upper quadrant abdominal pain, headache, seizures, fatigue, and anorexia. Occasionally, patients with SCLC present with a paraneoplastic syndrome, which will be discussed in detail later.

Initial radiographic images often show a large hilar mass with bulky mediastinal lymphadenopathy

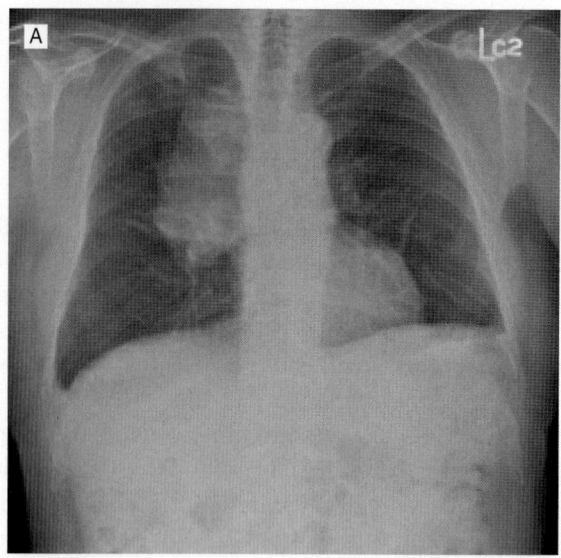
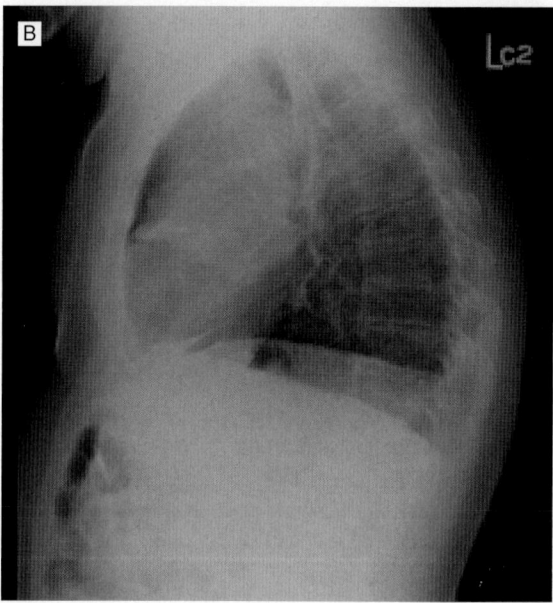

FIGURE 14-2. Chest radiograph of a patient with SCLC. The right upper lobe mass appears contiguous with the right hilum.

(Fig. 14-2). SCLC tumors are usually centrally located, although occasional peripheral satellite nodules are found.

The initial clinical evaluation should include a chest radiograph, history and physical examination, pathologic review, chest x-ray, computed tomography (CT) scans of the chest and abdomen, a magnetic resonance imaging (MRI) or CT scan of the brain, a bone scan, and baseline laboratory tests. In the presence of obvious extensive disease (eg, metastasis to liver), staging may be clinically directed. The goal of complete staging is to identify the limited-stage patient who is a candidate for definitive therapy. It may also be preferable to image the brain in all

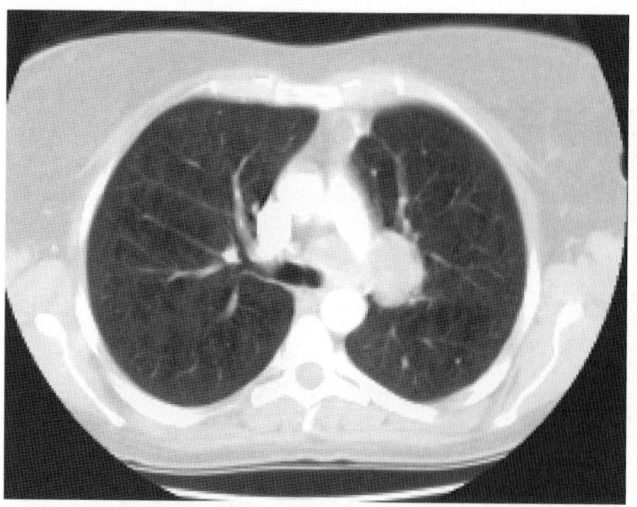

FIGURE 14-3. Chest CT scan of a patient with extensive-stage SCLC. A left hilar mass and paratracheal and subcarinal lymphadenopathy are present.

patients given the morbidity of uncontrolled disease in the central nervous system (CNS). Baseline laboratory evaluations should include complete blood count, platelet count, and comprehensive metabolic profile. Figures 14-3 through 14-5 depict typical radiographic images from SCLC patients.

Additional studies may be necessary if clinical findings demonstrate other abnormalities. If a pleural effusion is the only indicator of extensive stage, a thoracentesis should be performed and fluid sent for cytologic testing. If the fluid is exudative or if malignant cells are present, the patient is diagnosed with extensive-stage disease and chemoradiation is not indicated. Sampling of cerebrospinal fluid is indicated if there is suspicion of leptomeningeal spread. Pulmonary function tests should be performed in patients who are candidates for definitive chemoradiation.

Positron emission tomography (PET) imaging is frequently performed but is not yet part of the standard workup. There is some evidence that PET imaging may help to upstage some patients who were otherwise thought to have limited disease; however, more research is necessary before PET scans are recommended for all patients (12).

Treatment should be initiated as quickly as is feasible after diagnosis, given the typically rapid progression of disease. In many cases, it is necessary to initiate therapy before completion of staging.

■ STAGING

SCLC is commonly staged using a modified version of the two-stage Veterans Administration Lung Cancer Study Group (VALCSG) system, which classifies SCLC

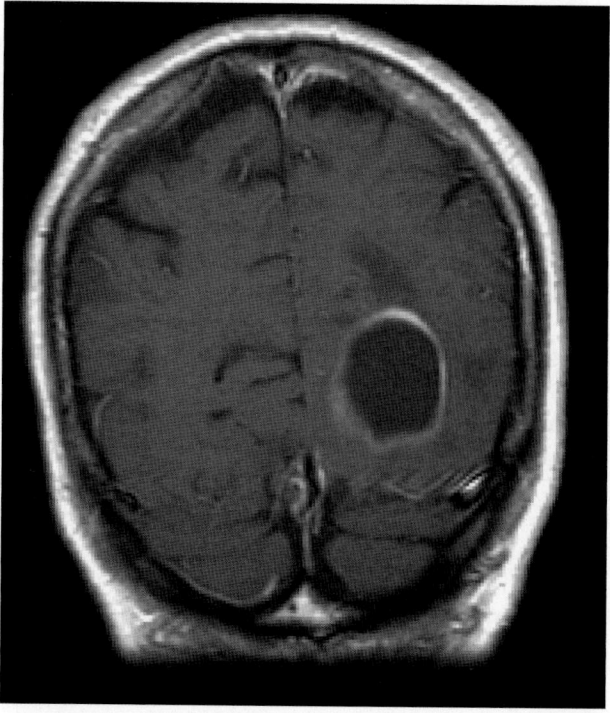
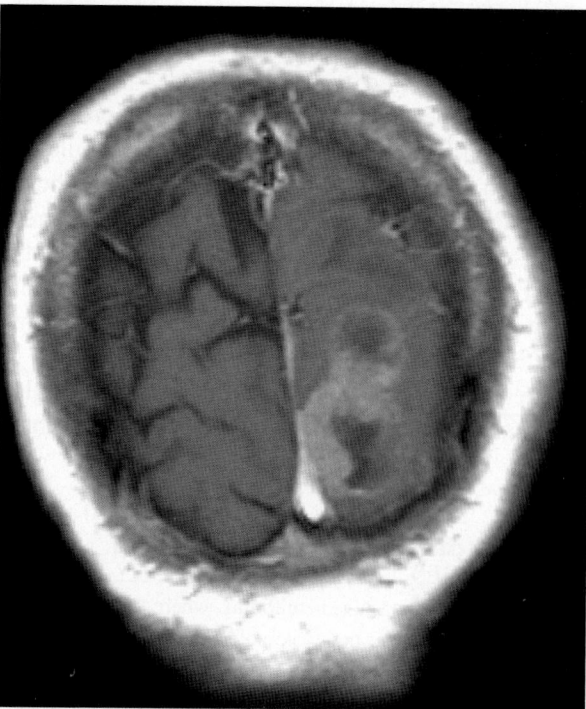

FIGURE 14-4. Brain MRI of a patient with extensive-stage small cell lung cancer. There is a left occipital lobe mass with a cystic component.

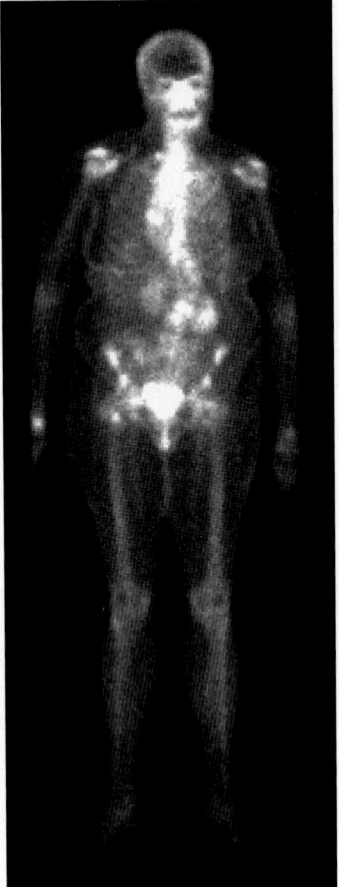

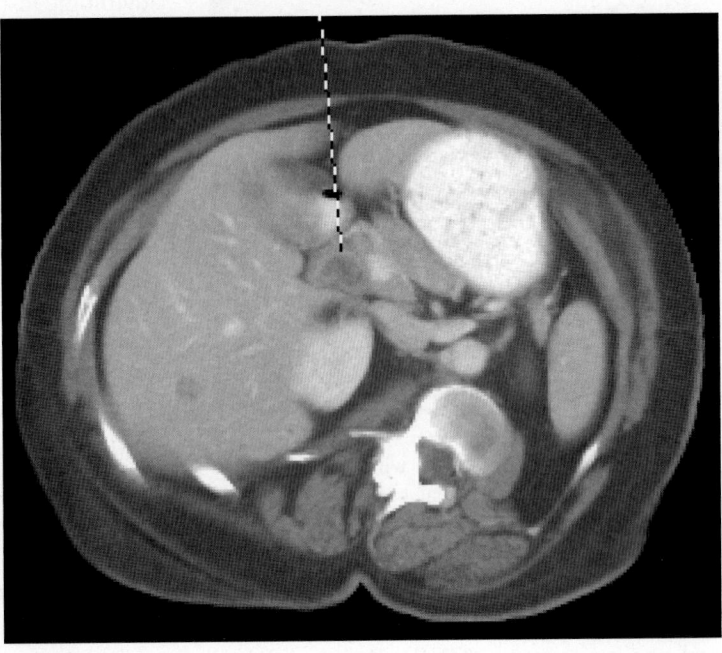

FIGURE 14-5. Radiographic studies of a patient with extensive-stage SCLC with liver, brain, and bone metastases. The images shown are a bone scan and abdominal CT.

as limited- or extensive-stage disease (Table 14-3) (6,13). The International Association for the Study of Lung Cancer, however, has suggested that small cell lung cancer should be staged by the tumor-nodes-metastases (TNM) system, because it provides important prognostic information. They suggest that this staging should be incorporated into clinical trials (14). Despite these recommendations, the VALCSG system is still frequently used clinically. Approximately 40% of patients with SCLC will have limited-stage disease on initial presentation; the remainder will have extensive-stage disease (2,15).

Limited-stage disease is confined to a single hemithorax that can be encompassed within one tolerable radiotherapy port, excluding the presence of pleural or pericardial effusion (6,16). In the era of definitive chemoradiation, limited stage may exclude patients with lymphadenopathy in the contralateral hilum and/or the contralateral supraclavicular fossa due to the large size of the required radiation port. Patients with malignant pericardial or pleural effusion or disease beyond what is described in limited-stage disease are considered as having extensive-stage disease.

■ **TREATMENT**

LIMITED-STAGE DISEASE

▋ Surgery

Surgery is an option for very few patients with SCLC. An autopsy series from the National Cancer Institute (NCI) revealed that, 30 days following resection of SCLC, 90% of patients had evidence of mediastinal disease, and almost two-thirds of patients had distant metastases (17). In a trial where patients thought to have operable SCLC were randomized to surgery or to

TABLE 14-3	STAGING OF SMALL CELL LUNG CANCER

Limited: Confined to a single hemithorax, where the tumor can be encompassed by a single tolerable radiation port
Extensive: Malignant pleural or pericardial effusion or disease that extends beyond limited stage

radiation therapy, patients in the radiation group had significantly longer overall survival (18). These results show that, even when metastatic disease cannot be documented, surgery alone is insufficient treatment for SCLC.

For patients with a T1 or T2 primary and no nodal involvement, designated very limited disease, surgery may play a role in multimodality treatment. In one trial, patients with very limited disease had a 5-year survival of 48% when treated with surgery followed by adjuvant chemotherapy (19). In an analysis of the SEER database, TNM staging was found to be prognostic in patients with resected SCLC (20). Preoperative mediastinal staging with mediastinoscopy or endoscopic bronchial ultrasound is recommended for patients with apparent stage I SCLC. Resection is indicated in the absence of nodal involvement. All patients should be considered for adjuvant chemotherapy. If nodal involvement is found at the time of surgery, chemoradiation, similar to management of limited disease, is recommended.

Combined Chemoradiation

Based on the results of a British Medical Research Council trial demonstrating surgery to be inferior to radiation therapy for the treatment of limited-stage SCLC (18), radiation became standard of care for local control for these patients. Though early studies indicated that radiation therapy could increase local control compared to chemotherapy alone, these studies did not consistently show significant survival benefits to combination therapy over chemotherapy (21). Because of this controversy, two meta-analyses were performed that showed a significant survival benefit of 5.4% at 2 years with the addition of radiation therapy to systemic chemotherapy for patients with limited disease SCLC (21,22). It is noteworthy that the best outcomes from these older trials included concurrent as opposed to sequential approaches; in addition, the regimens used in this era were anthracycline- and alkylator-based and were associated with excessive in-field toxicity when administered with concurrent radiation. The development of the etoposide/cisplatin (EP) regimen was critical to improving the tolerance and feasibility of concurrent chemoradiation and, at least in part because full doses of these drugs can be given with full-dose thoracic radiation, disease control is also improved. Please see Fig. 14-6 for radiographic images of postradiation changes in a patient who has undergone concurrent chemoradiation for limited-stage SCLC.

An anthracycline-based regimen (cyclophosphamide, epirubicin, and vincristine, [CEV]) was directly compared to EP in a phase III trial (23). Patients with limited-stage disease received thoracic radiotherapy concurrently with the third cycle of chemotherapy, and prophylactic cranial irradiation (PCI) was administered to those with a complete response. The results showed that in patients with limited-stage disease, EP was superior to CEV for survival rates at 2 and 5 years (14 and 5% versus 6 and 2%, respectively; p = .0001), as well as median

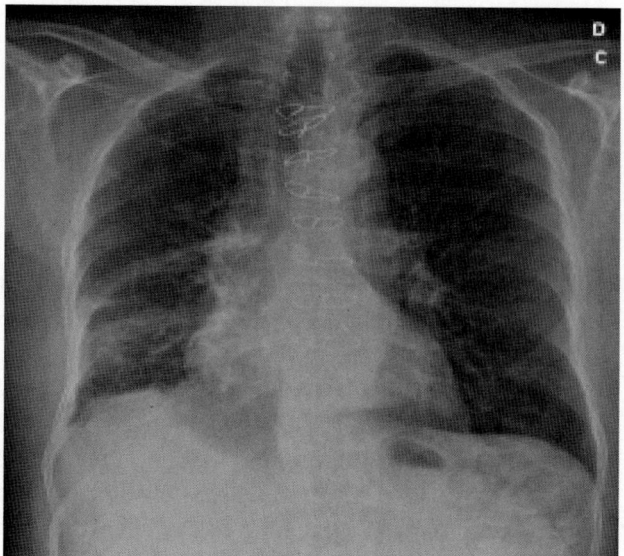
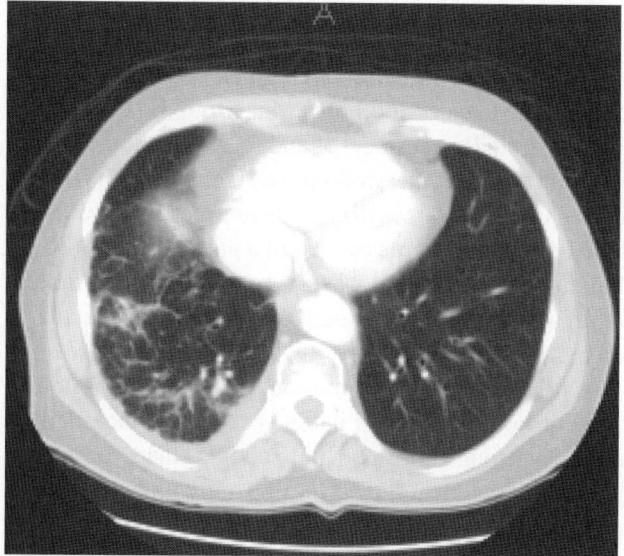

FIGURE 14-6. Chest CT and x-ray showing radiation changes and a pleural effusion in a patient with limited-stage SCLC treated with concurrent chemotherapy and radiotherapy.

overall survival (14.5 versus 9.7 months; $p = .001$). In patients with extensive-stage disease, no survival difference was noted.

The addition of other cytotoxins to the EP regimen—either as a triplet with paclitaxel or alternating therapy with cyclophosphamide, doxorubicin, and vincristine—has also been studied, but to date a new standard in the treatment of limited-stage SCLC has not emerged (15,24-27).

Radiation Intensity

Based on the radiobiology of SCLC, Intergroup (INT) trial 0096 studied accelerated hyperfractionated radiation compared to conventional fractionation in a phase III trial (28). Over 400 patients were randomized between the two arms. All patients received four cycles of EP. Radiation therapy was administered concurrently, starting with the first cycle of chemotherapy. All patients received 45 Gy, either in once-daily 1.8 Gy fractions for 5 weeks or twice-daily 1.5 Gy fractions for 3 weeks. Patients in the twice-daily radiation group had an improved overall median survival (23 versus 19 months) and 5-year survival (26 versus 16%), at the cost of increased weight loss and grade 3 esophagitis (27 versus 11%). Local failure rates were lower in the twice-daily radiation therapy arm, presumably the major reason for improved survival (28).

INT 0096 convincingly showed an overall survival benefit to concurrent chemoradiation with hyperfraction; however, this regimen is rarely used in the community (29). Reasons for this include concerns for side effects as well as the logistical difficulties involved in twice-daily treatment. The control arm of the INT 0096 study used a relatively low total dose, and since the results of INT 0096 have become available, conventionally fractionated radiation in higher doses has been studied. The Cancer and Leukemia Group B (CALGB) trial has tested a regimen of induction paclitaxel and topotecan for two cycles, followed by radiation with 70 Gy in 35 daily fractions with concurrent carboplatin and etoposide (total of three cycles) in a phase II study (30). Median overall survival was 22.4 months, comparable to that found with accelerated hyperfractionated radiation in INT 0096.

Another schedule of radiation therapy tested is concomitant boost, in which patients received once-daily radiation through most of their course, then received hyperfractionated therapy at the end of treatment, so that treatment is accelerated without the need for twice-daily therapy throughout the treatment course. Radiation Therapy Oncology Group (RTOG) trial 0239 tested this approach in a phase II trial. Patients received 61.2 Gy over 5 weeks, with twice-daily treatment in the final

9 days (31). Radiation therapy started on day 1 of chemotherapy with four cycles of EP. Although survival at 2 years was only 37%, somewhat less than that found in both INT 0096 and the CALGB trial (41 and 48% survival at 2 years, respectively) (28,30), local control at 2 years was excellent.

There is an ongoing study to resolve this controversy. An Intergroup study is comparing the experimental arms of 70 Gy once-daily radiation and 61.2 Gy concomitant boost therapy with the standard from INT 0096, 45 Gy twice-daily radiation. All three arms will receive concurrent etoposide and cisplatin, and radiation therapy will commence with the first cycle of chemotherapy.

Timing of Chemotherapy

Sequential, concurrent, and alternating chemotherapy have all been tested with thoracic radiation therapy. Early studies did not show a survival benefit to concurrent chemotherapy; however, this was likely due to the increased toxicity when using cyclophosphamide- or doxorubicin-based chemotherapy. EP is far better tolerated than these earlier regimens when administered concurrently with radiation.

The National Cancer Institute of Canada reported a phase III trial of alternating CAV/EP with radiation therapy in either the second or sixth cycle of chemotherapy (32). The patients receiving early radiation therapy had improved overall survival (21.2 versus 16 months). The Japanese Clinical Oncology group led by Takada compared radiation therapy (45 Gy in twice-daily 1.5 Gy fractions) starting with either cycle 1 of EP or following completion of the chemotherapy course (33). More myelosuppression was noted in the patients in the concurrent arm, but there was a significant reduction in risk of death for early concurrent therapy with a hazard ratio of 0.70 ($p = 0.02$) (33).

Although not all trials have consistently shown a benefit for concurrent chemoradiation, the data are quite strongly in support of this and its early integration in treatment when the regimen is EP, as contrasted with anthracyline or alkylator based. Further, efficacy outcomes are consistently better with EP in the treatment of limited stage SCLC.

Given that small cell lung cancer is such a rapidly dividing malignancy, it has been hypothesized that accelerated proliferation of tumor clonogens can affect outcome, and that treatment should be delivered in a condensed fashion (34). A meta-analysis examined the influence of a novel measure, the start of any treatment to the end of thoracic radiation (SER), on overall survival in limited-stage SCLC. A shorter SER was found to be a significant predictor of better outcome. For each week that the SER was lengthened, overall survival at 5 years showed an absolute decrease of almost 2% (34). The data from INT 0096 had a strong influence on this result.

Carboplatin has often been substituted for cisplatin in clinical practice, especially for patients with extensive-stage disease (35). Skarlos et al. performed a randomized study comparing EP to carboplatin and etoposide in 147 patients with limited- or extensive-stage SCLC (36). In this trial, no significant differences were seen in response rate or median survival time (12.5 months for EP versus 11.8 months for carboplatin and etoposide), but less toxicity was reported in the carboplatin-containing arm. Although carboplatin is frequently used in extensive disease due to its more favorable toxicity profile, cisplatin is more frequently preferred in curative intent treatment of the limited-stage patient. Also, there are concerns regarding excess myelotoxicity when carboplatin is given concurrently with thoracic radiation. In patients with limited-stage disease who are being treated with curative intent, cisplatin should be used unless there is a contraindication.

EXTENSIVE-STAGE DISEASE

Approximately 60% of patients with SCLC have extensive-stage disease at the time of diagnosis (2). For these patients, chemotherapy represents the main treatment modality. Radiation therapy is reserved for palliation of symptoms due to local or metastatic disease, and surgery is rarely used.

Small cell lung cancer is known to be highly chemosensitive. In an early study, patients with SCLC had a highly significant improvement in survival with intravenous cyclophosphamide compared to placebo, increasing median survival from just 12 weeks to almost 5 months (37). In the 1970s, studies began to use combination therapy, and the CAV regimen (cyclophosphamide, anthracycline, vincristine) became the standard of care (23).

A new regimen, etoposide and cisplatin (EP), was first tested in patients who had recurred after or failed to respond to treatment with CAV, and was found to be active, with responses in 55% of patients (38). It was later tested as first-line therapy in patients who were unable to tolerate CAV (39). Median overall survival for patients with limited-stage disease was 63 weeks, and for patients with extensive disease, 39 weeks, results comparable to historical data for CAV.

EP (4 cycles) was directly compared to CAV (6 cycles) and to alternating EP and CAV (3 cycles of each). In a phase III trial performed by the Southeastern Cancer Study Group (Roth BJ, Johnson DH, Einhorn LH, et al.

J Clin Oncol 10:282-291, 992). Response rates and survival were essentially equivalent across all 3 arms. Further, brief therapy with EP was much better tolerated. Similar results were seen in a study of similar design in Japan. These studies led to the adoption of EP for a minimum of 4 cycles as a standard of care for the patients with extensive disease (40).

Given the chemosensitivity of SCLC, many different strategies have been tested to improve both progression-free and overall survival. Unfortunately, despite many clinical trials, no regimen has been found to be substantially better than EP, which remains our standard of care.

Increased Length of Induction and Maintenance Chemotherapy

The SEG trial discussed above established the minimum duration of induction chemotherapy to 4 cycles of EP. Additonal chemotherapy beyond this as consolidation or maintenance has not been shown to result in survival benefit when EP is given as induction (40-49). A Southeastern Cancer Study Group studied compared four cycles of EP, six cycles of CAV, and six cycles of alternating CAV/EP, and found overall survival (8.6, 8.3, and 8.1 months, respectively) and response rates (61%, 51%, and 59%, respectively) equivalent between the arms (40). Based on this trial, four cycles of EP became the standard of care, though some clinical trials include up to six cycles.

Substitutions and Additions to Induction Therapy

Adjustments to the EP regimen have been investigated. Please see earlier for a discussion of carboplatin—it is frequently used in combination with etoposide in extensive disease because of similar efficacy to cisplatin and a favorable toxicity profile.

In a phase III trial by the French Federation of Cancer Institutes, EP was compared to EP plus cyclophosphamide and 4'-epidoxorubicin (PCDE) in patients with extensive-stage SCLC (50). The patients receiving the four-drug regimen had a slight improvement in overall survival (10.5 versus 9.3 months); this regimen is not commonly used because of concern for excess toxicity and minimal survival impact. In another randomized trial comparing a four-drug combination of cisplatin, vincristine, doxorubicin, and etoposide (CODE) with alternating CAV and EP in patients with extensive-stage SCLC, CODE did not provide a survival benefit and only added toxicity (51). The addition of ifosfamide to EP led to a slight improvement in survival (9.0 versus 7.3 months, $p = .045$), but because of the greater toxicities and the modest survival benefit, this regimen is not commonly used (52). Another phase III trial comparing VIP to PE in both limited- and extensive-stage SCLC did not show any difference in response or overall survival rates (53). Addition of paclitaxel to EP did not improve overall survival in two large phase III trials (54,55).

Irinotecan (CPT-11) is a camptothecin derivative that inhibits the nuclear enzyme topoisomerase I. Single-agent irinotecan has been evaluated in patients with previously treated sensitive and refractory relapsed SCLC and has shown activity (56). The main toxicities from this agent are neutropenia and diarrhea. Irinotecan in combination with cisplatin (IP) was evaluated by the Japanese Cooperative Oncology Group (JCOG) as a multicenter phase III trial comparing IP to EP in previously untreated patients with extensive-stage SCLC (57). Although the projected accrual was set for 230 patients, a clear median survival advantage was seen in the IP group after enrollment of 154 patients (IP versus EP: 12.8 versus 9.4 months; $p = .0021$) and the study was closed early.

These results generated much excitement; however, subsequent studies have failed to confirm this benefit. Two North American trials and one German trial have not shown an improvement in survival (58-60). Another European study showed an improvement in survival with irinotecan plus carboplatin over etoposide plus carboplatin (8.5 versus 7.1 months) (61); however, this study had multiple schedule, eligibility, and design issues which may have influenced this result and which make comparison with other studies difficult.

Alternating or Sequential Combinations

SCLC has a high relapse rate despite initial chemosensitivity. Several theories have been proposed to account for this phenomenon. One theory is that resistant clones develop during induction treatment. Based on this, the Goldie and Coldman hypothesis proposed that non–cross-resistant regimens could be rapidly alternated to eliminate resistant clones (15). Several randomized phase III trials have evaluated PE and CAV regimens in direct and alternating sequences (24,40,62). Although the Fukuoka trial reported that patients with limited-stage disease benefited from alternating PE and CAV, alternating combination regimens have failed to confer a consistent survival advantage to patients with extensive-stage SCLC (24).

In another approach, rapid sequencing of several active agents over a short treatment period was evaluated. The most studied regimen comprised weekly treatments of CODE. Although early studies indicated

that CODE conferred a possible survival advantage to patients with extensive disease, subsequent phase III trials did not show that it was any better than more traditional regimens (63,64).

Altering Dose Intensity and Density

Higher-dose chemotherapy remains controversial as a solution to resistant SCLC. A 1991 meta-analysis of 60 trials showed that in patients with extensive-stage SCLC, increasing the dose-intensity of CAV and EP did not improve survival (65). Two randomized trials compared high-dose to standard dose platinum-etoposide doublets, and neither showed a survival advantage (66,67).

Dose-dense chemotherapy is another proposed means of addressing SCLC resistance. The proposed mechanism of action is to reduce the time interval between cycles of chemotherapy by using hematopoietic growth factors. Several trials evaluated this hypothesis. Steward et al. randomized patients with limited- and extensive-stage disease to ifosfamide, etoposide, carboplatin, and vincristine given every 3 (intensified) or 4 (standard) weeks (68). Patients in the dose-intense arm were found to have a longer median survival (443 versus 351 days, respectively) and a better 2-year survival rate (33 versus 18%, respectively; $p = .0014$). Generally, it was quite feasible to administer this chemotherapy in a 3-week cycle; thus, it is difficult to consider this approach dose-dense. Thatcher et al. randomized 403 patients with SCLC to doxorubicin, cyclophosphamide, and etoposide every 2 (intensified) or 3 weeks (standard) (69). A small survival advantage was seen in the dose-dense arm (10.9 versus 11.5 months, $p = .04$); however, many clinicians consider this increase not to be clinically meaningful and this regimen is rarely used.

Studies have assessed the value of autologous stem cell support and dose escalation in SCLC. Two randomized trials compared ifosfamide, carboplatin, and etoposide (ICE) every 4 weeks with ICE every 2 weeks with autologous stem cell support having been performed. One small trial enrolling 83 patients was stopped at interim analysis showed an improvement in overall survival in the high-dose regimen (30.3 versus 18.5 months), but a larger randomized phase III trial did not find a significant improvement in overall survival (14.4 months in the high-dose arm versus 13.9 months in the standard-dose arm) (70,71).

RECURRENT DISEASE

Though SCLC is chemosensitive, 80% of patients with limited-stage SCLC and virtually all patients with extensive-stage SCLC will have recurrence of their disease following initial chemotherapy (72). Historically, these recurrent tumors are less responsive and survival is poor, with median survival of approximately 14 weeks following relapse without chemotherapy (73). Studies have shown that response to initial treatment as well as time to relapse following induction chemotherapy is an important determinant of response to salvage chemotherapy (74). Patients with objective response to initial treatment and progression-free survival at least 60 to 90 days following completion of induction chemotherapy are more likely to respond to additional chemotherapy and are considered to have "sensitive" disease. Those who do not achieve disease regression with initial chemotherapy or with shorter duration of response after chemotherapy is discontinued are considered "refractory" or "resistant" (75).

Case series provided the first suggestion that some patients with prolonged progression-free survival after first-line therapy could benefit from reintroduction of similar chemotherapy following relapse. Batist et al. reported on a series of six patients who had achieved a remission of more than 2 years following induction chemotherapy. Five of these patients received chemotherapy that contained some or all of the components of their induction regimen, with four responses, lasting up to 18 months (76). Another study showed that patients frequently responded to retreatment with their induction regimen if they had either a complete response to first-line therapy or duration of response greater than 34 weeks following induction (77). Several other studies also suggested responses when first-line therapy was reintroduced at relapse (78,79). In the modern era, when many patients receive just four courses of EP as induction, it is not unreasonable to consider retreatment with EP if initial response was dramatic and unmaintained progression-free survival is greater than 3 months.

The topoisomerase I inhibitors, topotecan and irinotecan, have been studied in recurrent disease. Topotecan is the only drug for which there are several randomized trials in this setting. It showed activity as a single agent and in combination against both sensitive and refractory relapsed SCLC in a number of single-arm trials (75,80). A randomized phase III trial showed that intravenous topotecan had similar efficacy in patients with sensitive relapse to combination chemotherapy with CAV, with a 24% response rate for topotecan compared to 18% for CAV and median survival 25.0 versus 24.7 weeks (75). Oral topotecan was found to have similar efficacy to intravenous topotecan, with fewer side effects and better ease of administration (81,82). A phase III registration trial compared oral topotecan to best supportive

care in patients who were not candidates for standard intravenous chemotherapy and showed increased median survival in the topotecan group from 13.9 to 25.9 weeks (73). The experimental group also had a slower deterioration in quality of life. Notably, even in patients with a short remission after induction therapy (<60 days), topotecan was associated with a statistically significant improvement in overall survival (73). Irinotecan has not been directly compared to topotecan nor have phase III trials been performed; phase II studies suggest similar efficacy compared to topotecan in the recurrent setting (56).

Amrubicin is a novel anthracycline that has shown promising activity with response rates greater than 50% in a single-arm Japanese study, though hematologic toxicities were significant, with neutropenia in 83% of patients. One-year survival was 40% in patients with refractory disease and 46% in patients with sensitive disease (83). A randomized phase II Japanese trial compared amrubicin and intravenous topotecan in patients with relapsed disease. Patients treated with amrubicin had a statistically significant improvement in response rate (38 versus 13%) and a trend toward improved progression-free survival (3.5 versus 2.2 months) (84). Further studies involving this agent are planned.

TARGETED AGENTS

A variety of targeted agents have been tested in SCLC, both as monotherapy and in combination with cytotoxic agents. A variety of pathways have been tested as therapeutic targets.

p53

The *p53* gene is located on chromosome 17q13.1 and encodes for a transcription factor that blocks the progression of cells from the G1 phase, facilitating repair of DNA damage before DNA replication and cell division and, thus, supporting fidelity of the genome, *p53* mutation and altered expression are found in the majority of patients with SCLC. In a single-arm phase II trial presented in abstract form, patients received a vaccine against p53. Immunity was generated in the majority of patients, but there were no responses, though the investigators theorized that the vaccine sensitized patients to further chemotherapy (85). Further studies are ongoing.

Angiogenesis

Vascular endothelial growth factor (VEGF) is an important regulator of angiogenesis and has a role in many human cancers. SCLC is a highly angiogenic tumor, and elevated VEGF is associated with poor outcomes (86).

Bevacizumab is a monoclonal antibody against VEGF. It has been approved for the treatment of non–small cell lung cancer (87), as well as other tumor types. Several single-arm phase II trials have combined bevacizumab with chemotherapy—cisplatin/etoposide in one study, irinotecan/carboplatin in another—in patients with previously untreated extensive-stage SCLC. The response rates and overall survival found in these studies compare favorably to historical control; a randomized trial is pending (88,89). Bevacizumab has also been tested for limited-stage SCLC in combination with chemoradiation, but trials were stopped early due to an unacceptably high rate of tracheoesophageal fistula (90).

Thalidomide is an oral antiangiogenic agent, approved for use in multiple myeloma. It has been tested in a randomized phase III trial in patients with extensive-stage disease in combination with induction chemotherapy (PCDE). This study did not show a significant difference between the two arms, though there was a trend toward improved survival for patients receiving thalidomide (11.7 versus 8.7 months, $p = .16$) (91). A second trial evaluating thalidomide both with induction chemotherapy and as maintenance found that thalidomide was not associated with improved survival in either limited or extensive disease. Further, there was increased risk of thrombotic events on the thalidomide arm and a trend to decreased survival in extensive-stage patients (10.1 versus 10.5 months) (92).

Vandetanib is an oral small molecule tyrosine kinase inhibitor. It has activity against both VEGF-R and EGFR. It was tested in a randomized phase II trial enrolling patients with both limited- and extensive-stage SCLC who had achieved a response to induction chemotherapy. Vandetanib was administered as maintenance therapy. Unfortunately, there was no difference in progression-free or overall survival (93).

Sorafenib is another oral small molecular tyrosine kinase inhibitor. It inhibits a number of targets, including VEGF-R2. In a single-arm phase II trial reported as an abstract, patients who recurred following platinum-based chemotherapy received sorafenib 400 mg PO twice-daily until progression. Response rates were low, and overall survival was comparable to historical controls (94).

c-Kit

The c-kit is a transmembrane receptor that is overactive in a number of tumors, most notably gastrointestinal stromal tumors. Imatinib is a tyrosine kinase inhibitor that blocks c-kit signaling. Between 28 and 93% of SCLCs overexpress c-kit, and in cells lines, inhibition of c-kit can decrease growth (95). Despite multiple trials, some of which selected patients based on c-kit expression, imatinib was not shown to have activity in SCLC, either as a single agent (95,96) or in combination with chemotherapy (97).

Apoptosis

Apoptosis is altered in SCLC. Bcl-2 family members regulate cellular apoptosis, and overexpression of Bcl-2, a negative regulator of cell death, is associated with resistance to cytotoxins in preclinical models (98,99). Cell line studies suggest that inhibition of Bcl-2 may increase efficacy of chemotherapy (100). A phase II trial reported by Rudin et al. randomized patients with extensive-stage SCLC to carboplatin and etoposide with or without oblimersen, a *bcl-2* antisense oligonucleotide. They found no benefit with the addition of oblimersen and a trend toward worse outcomes (100). Other Bcl-2 antagonists, including obatoclax and ABT-263, are in early clinical testing (101).

Matrix Metalloproteinases

Matrix metalloproteinases (MMPs) are involved in the degradation of the extracellular matrix. It is thought that overexpression of these proteins facilitates metastasis. They are widely overexpressed in SCLC and correlate with poor prognosis (102). An MMP inhibitor, marimastat, was studied as a maintenance therapy following induction chemotherapy in SCLC. It did not improve survival and had significant side effects, mainly involving musculoskeletal toxicity (103).

Epidermal Growth Factor Receptor

Mutations in the epidermal growth factor receptor (EGFR) are known to be important in non–small cell lung cancer, and EGFR inhibitors are an important treatment option for these patients (104). EGFR mutations are thought to be exceedingly rare in SCLC, and studies of the EGFR inhibitor gefitinib in nonselected patients with SCLC have been negative (105). There are case reports of nonsmokers with SCLC having characteristic EGFR mutations, and those patients had disease responsive to EGFR inhibition (106). Because of the rarity of SCLC in nonsmokers, EGFR mutation analysis is not typically performed.

Insulin-like Growth Factor-1 Receptor

The insulin-like growth factor-1 receptor (IGF-1R) plays an important role in carcinogenesis, contributing to cell growth, cell division, and protection from apoptosis. Aberrant IGF-1R signaling has been seen in many tumor types (107). In vitro, antibodies against IGF-1R slow the growth of SCLC cell lines (108), and small molecule inhibitors sensitize the cells to chemotherapy (109). There are multiple antibodies and small molecular inhibitors of IGF-1R in clinical development, and this represents a promising area in SCLC research. Trials are ongoing with IGF-1R antibodies in combination with chemotherapy.

PROPHYLACTIC CRANIAL IRRADIATION

In SCLC, metastasis to the brain imparts substantial morbidity and mortality. Though only 10% of patients will have brain metastases at diagnosis, the risk of developing brain metastasis in patients alive at 2 years after diagnosis who did not receive elective cranial radiation have been reported to range between 50 and 80% (110,111). It is hypothesized that the blood–brain barrier prevents chemotherapy from effectively reaching micrometastatic disease in the brain. Therefore, PCI has been studied in an effort to treat and control metastatic disease before it becomes clinically evident. Initial trials did demonstrate reduced incidence of brain metastasis with PCI; however, a survival impact was not apparent.

In the Prophylactic Cranial Irradiation Overview Collaborative Group meta-analysis, which evaluated seven randomized trials that required patients to have designation of complete response after treatment, PCI was shown to provide a 5% improvement in survival at 3 years, as well as a decreased risk of brain metastases (112). The majority of these patients had limited disease at diagnosis (85%).

Following this study, PCI became the standard of care for patients with limited disease who achieved a complete or near-complete response to therapy; however, it was not known if PCI improved survival in patients with extensive disease. A European Organization for Research and Treatment of Cancer (EORTC) study randomized patients with extensive small cell lung cancer who responded to initial chemotherapy to either PCI or not. Baseline imaging of the brain was required only for patients with neurologic symptoms. The patients in the PCI group had a lower risk of brain metastasis (14.6 versus 40.4%) and a significantly longer overall survival from the time of randomization (6.7 versus 5.4 months) (113). Progression-free survival was similar between the groups (14.7 versus 12.0 weeks), but more patients in the PCI group received second-line chemotherapy (68 versus 45%), possibly accounting for

the improvement in overall survival. PCI was not without side effects—most notably hair loss and fatigue—but global health status and cognitive functioning were not significantly different between the groups in the first 9 months following irradiation (113,114).

Given these results, all patients with small cell lung cancer who respond to chemotherapy can be offered prophylactic cranial irradiation if there are no contraindications. It should be used with caution in the elderly and in patients with significant ischemic cerebrovascular disease due to a concern for increased acute and late brain toxicity.

It is important to separate PCI from chemotherapy and to use radiation regimens with a dose and schedule that have been documented safe as regards the incidence of late neurotoxic effects. One of the most commonly used radiation regimens used is 25 Gy in 10 daily fractions.

Please see Table 14-4 for a summary of the National Cancer Center Network recommendations for the treatment of SCLC.

SPECIAL POPULATIONS: THE ELDERLY AND INFIRM

Approximately 25% of patients with SCLC are over the age of 70 years. This population of patients has often been excluded from clinical trials because of concerns for greater toxicity due to lowered organ reserves, especially myelosuppression and frequently lowered functional status due to comorbid conditions. However, retrospective studies have shown that elderly patients with retained performance have improved outcomes with more aggressive treatment (115). In a Canadian analysis,

TABLE 14-4	NATIONAL COMPREHENSIVE CANCER NETWORK GUIDELINES FOR SMALL CELL LUNG CANCER

1. In limited-stage disease, concurrent chemoradiotherapy is recommended. Four cycles of cisplatin and etoposide combined with 45 Gy of thoracic radiotherapy is recommended. Thoracic radiotherapy should begin during either cycle 1 or 2 of chemotherapy.
2. Prophylactic cranial irradiation (PCI) is recommended for all patients who achieve a complete or partial response to first-line chemotherapy.
3. In extensive-stage disease, combination chemotherapy is recommended, most commonly a platinum in combination with either etoposide or irinotecan.
4. Patient participation in clinical trials should be encouraged.
5. Smoking cessation should be encouraged.

elderly patients of age 70 years or above who received four or more cycles of chemotherapy (CAV or EP) had a median survival time of 10.7 months (116). Elderly patients who received fewer than three cycles had a median survival time of 3.9 months, and patients with no treatment survived a median time of 1.1 months. Multivariate analysis showed that neither increasing age nor comorbid disease was an adverse prognostic factor. This review reported that performance status, stage of disease, and treatment were the most important prognostic features. Additional studies have confirmed these conclusions, whereas only one retrospective Australian review reported that the complications from therapy adversely affected outcome in the elderly population (117-122).

With regard to radiation tolerance in the case of limited-stage disease, elderly patients have been reported to have increased toxicity. Analysis of the patients above 70 years of age in the Intergroup trial 0096 (EP with conventional thoracic radiation versus hyperfractionated and accelerated treatment) showed that they experienced a higher rate of treatment-related death (>70 years versus ≥70 years: 10 versus 1%, respectively) (22). However, the 5-year overall survival rate for elderly patients in this trial was 16%, similar to the survival for the entire group of patients on the control arm. Altered fractionation did not appear to benefit the elderly subgroup.

General recommendations for this population are as follows: Patients with good performance status and no significant organ dysfunction should receive full-dose chemotherapy and radiotherapy. Their higher risk of treatment-related death implies a need for close monitoring and intense supportive care.

Patients with severe comorbid conditions, a worse performance status prior to diagnosis, or the very elderly may require a change in strategy from standard of care. However, randomized trials in patients with "poor-risk" SCLC (and generally extensive disease) have consistently shown a benefit to combination chemotherapy relative to single-agent oral etoposide (123). These trials reported that intravenous combination regimens palliated symptoms better and improved median progression-free and overall survival. It can be concluded from these trials that in patients with a poor performance status, initial treatment should be combination chemotherapy.

Previously, EP for three to four cycles was recommended over cyclophosphamide- or doxorubicin-based regimens in the elderly population because it is less myelosuppressive (115). More recent studies have evaluated the combination of carboplatin and etoposide (124-127). With the exception of the trial reported by Samantas et al. (126), which used low doses of both agents, studies using carboplatin and etoposide have

shown good response rates and tolerance in elderly patients.

In conclusion, carboplatin (AUC 5) and etoposide (100 mg/m^2 for 3 days) can be recommended for most patients with SCLC considered "high risk" on the basis of age, comorbidities, or reduced functional status. It is clear that the time of highest risk for treatment-related mortality is in the first cycle. Close monitoring and support are critical during this time. Continued research in this area, especially in the very elderly, is needed.

■ PARA-NEOPLASTIC SYNDROMES

SCLC is known to cause several paraneoplastic processes. The most common of these are hormonally mediated and include the syndrome of inappropriate antidiuretic hormone (SIADH) and Cushing syndrome. These conditions result from ectopic secretion of the polypeptide hormones vasopressin and adrenocorticotropic hormone, respectively. Patients with SIADH present with hyponatremia, sometimes with neurologic symptoms. If patients develop SIADH, treatment with fluid restriction, saline infusion for symptomatic patients, and demeclocycline is advised, as well as initiation of chemotherapy as soon as feasible.

Three to 7% of patients with SCLC will present with Cushing syndrome. The typical presentation of ectopic Cushing syndrome is edema, hypertension, weakness, hypokalemia metabolic alkalosis, and hyperglycemia (8). These patients are immunosuppressed and at high risk for opportunistic infections from hypercortisolism. It is therefore advisable to treat patients with cortisol-suppressing agents, such as metyrapone or ketoconazole, prior to initiating myelosuppressive antineoplastic therapy (128). Radiotherapy can also be used in these cases to palliate and temporize until hypercortisolism has been controlled. Endocrine syndromes parallel cancer control, subsiding with cytoreduction of tumor and recurring with progression.

Paraneoplastic disorders of neurologic origin are less common and believed autoimmune in mechanism. These disorders occur as the result of onconeuronal antibodies recognizing tumor antigens as well as neuronal cell antigens (129-134). The most common disorder is Eaton-Lambert myasthenic syndrome, which is seen in 3% of patients with SCLC. Autoantibodies impair acetylcholine release from the presynaptic motor terminal at the neuromuscular junction and cause transient cranial nerve palsies, upright presyncopal symptoms, proximal muscle weakness with lower extremity predominance, and depressed tendon reflexes (135). Additional paraneoplastic central nervous system disorders include encephalomyelitis and cerebellar degeneration resulting from anti-Hu antibodies (ANNA-1) and "stiff-man syndrome," resulting from antiamphiphysin antibodies.

Patients with paraneoplastic neurologic syndromes have been reported to have a better survival overall that may be based in part on immunity to the tumor. However, these patients frequently experience progressive neurologic decline that may not be influenced by tumor control with treatment. This is in part due to limited treatment options for the autoimmune disease, and the observation that often, by the time clinical neurologic dysfunction is observed, significant permanent damage to neuronal tissue has occurred.

■ SUMMARY

Despite much effort to identify more effective strategies for treatment, survival in small cell lung cancer has remained relatively stable over the past 20 years. The standard of care for both limited- and extensive-stage disease is etoposide and platin chemotherapy for a minimum of 4 courses. Early integration of concurrent thoracic radiation is indicated for the patient with limited disease. PCI can be offered to patients who have disease control with initial treatment.

Advances in treatment will likely require greater knowledge of this tumor's unique biology and the ability to target the abnormal phenotype. Currently, the greatest promise appears to be in combining relevant targeted agents with chemotherapy, and many such trials are ongoing.

References

1. Jemal A, Siegel R, Ward E, et al. Cancer statistics 2009. *CA Cancer J Clin* 2009;29(4):225-249.
2. Govindan R, Page N, Morgensztern D, et al. Changing epidemiology of small-cell lung cancer in the United States over the last 30 years: Analysis of the Surveillance, Epidemiologic, and End Results database. *J Clin Oncol* 2006;24(28):4539-4544.
3. Brownson RC, Chang JC, Davis JR. Gender and histologic type variations in smoking-related risk of lung cancer. *Epidemiology* 1992;3(1):61-64.
4. Barbone F, Bovenzi M, Cavallieri F, et al. Cigarette smoking and histologic type of lung cancer in men. *Chest* 1997;112(6):1474-1479.
5. Videtic GMM, Stitt LW, Dar AR, et al. Continued cigarette smoking by patients receiving concurrent chemoradiotherapy for limited-stage small-cell lung cancer is associated with decreased survival. *J Clin Oncol* 2003;21(8):1544-1549.

6. Hanna N, Einhorn L. Small cell lung cancer: State of the art. *Clin Lung Cancer* 2002;4:87-94.
7. Albain KS, Crowley JJ, LeBlanc M, et al. Determinants of improved outcome in small-cell lung cancer: An analysis of the 2,580 patient Southwest Oncology Group Data Base. *J Clin Oncol* 1990;8(9):1563-1574.
8. Yip D, Harper PG. Predictive and prognostic factors in small cell lung cancer: Current status. *Lung Cancer* 2000; 28:173-185.
9. Zakowski MF. Pathology of small cell carcinoma of the lung. *Semin Oncol* 2003;30(1):3-8.
10. Junker K, Wiethege T, Muller KM. Pathology of small-cell lung cancer. *J Cancer Res Clin Oncol* 2000;126:361-368.
11. Brambilla E, Travis WD, Colby TV, et al. The new World Health Organization classification of lung tumours. *Eur Respir J* 2001;18:1059-1068.
12. Vinjamuri M, Craig M, Campell-Fontaine A, et al. Can positron emission tomography be used as a staging tool for small-cell lung cancer? *Clin Lung Cancer* 2008;9(1):30-34.
13. Anger G, vonParis V, Schmidt R. Staging of inoperable small cell bronchial cancer. *Z Gesamte Inn Med* 1987;42:20-23.
14. Shepherd FA, Crowley J, VanHoutte P, et al. The International Association for the Study of Lung Cancer lung cancer staging project: Proposals regarding the clinical staging of small cell lung cancer in the forthcoming (seventh) edition of the tumor, node, metastasis classification of lung cancer. *J Thorac Oncol* 2007;2(12):1067-1077.
15. Sandler AB. Chemotherapy for small cell lung cancer. *Semin Oncol* 2003;30:9-25.
16. Kristjansen PE, Hansen HH. Management of small cell lung cancer: A summary of the Third International Association for the Study of Lung Cancer Workshop on Small Cell Lung Cancer. *J Natl Cancer Inst* 1990;82:263-266.
17. Matthews MJ, Kanhouwa S, Pickner J, et al. Frequency of residual and metastatic tumors in patients undergoing curative surgical resection of lung cancer. *Cancer Chemother Rep* 1973;3:63-67.
18. Fox W, Scadding JG. Medical Research Council comparative trial of surgery and radiotherapy for primary treatment of small-celled or oat-celled carcinoma of bronchus: Ten-year follow-up. *Lancet* 1973;302(7820):63-65.
19. Shepherd FA, Evans WK, Feld R, et al. Adjuvant chemotherapy following surgical resection for small-cell carcinoma of the lung. *J Clin Oncol* 1988;6(5):832-838.
20. Vallieres E, Shepherd FA, Crowley JJ, et al. The IASLC Lung Cancer Staging Project: Proposals regarding the relevance of TNM in the pathologic staging of small cell lung cancer in the forthcoming (seventh) edition of the TNM classification for lung cancer. *J Thorac Oncol* 2009;4(9):1049-1059.
21. Warde P, Payne D. Does thoracic irradiation improve survival and local control in limited-stage small-cell carcinoma of the lung? *J Clin Oncol* 1992;10(6):890-895.
22. Pignon JP, Arriagada R, Ihde DC, et al. A meta-analysis of thoracic radiotherapy for small-cell lung cancer. *N Engl J Med* 1992;327(23):1618-1624.
23. Sundstrom S, Bremnes RM, Kaasa S, et al. Cisplatin and etoposide regimen is superior to cyclophosphamide, epirubicin, and vincristine regimen in small-cell lung cancer: Results from a randomized phase III trial with 5 years' follow-up. *J Clin Oncol* 2002;20(24):4665-4672.

24. Fukuoka M, Furuse K, Saijo N, et al. Randomized trial of cyclophosphamide, doxorubicin, and vincristine versus cisplatin and etoposide versus alternation of these regimens in small-cell lung cancer. *J Natl Cancer Inst* 1991;83:855-861.

25. Levitan N, Dowlati A, Shina D, et al. Multi-institutional phase I/II trial of paclitaxel, cisplatin, and etoposide with concurrent radiation for limited-stage small-cell lung carcinoma. *J Clin Oncol* 2000;18(5):1102-1109.

26. Hainsworth JD, Gray JR, Stroup SL, et al. Paclitaxel, carboplatin, and extended schedule etoposide in the treatment of small-cell lung cancer: Comparison of sequential phase II trials using different dose-intensities. *J Clin Oncol* 1997;15:3464-3470.

27. Johnson DH. Management of small cell lung cancer: Current state of the art. *Chest* 1999;116:525s-530s.

28. Turrisi AT, Kim K, Blum R, et al. Twice-daily compared with once-daily thoracic radiotherapy in limited small-cell lung cancer treated concurrently with cisplatin and etoposide. *N Engl J Med* 1999;340(4):265-271.

29. Movsas B, Moughan J, Komaki R, et al. Radiotherapy patterns of care study in lung carcinoma. *J Clin Oncol* 2003;21:4553-4559.

30. Bogart JA, Herndon JE, Lyss AP, et al. 70 Gy thoracic radiotherapy is feasible concurrent with chemotherapy for limited-stage small-cell lung cancer: Analysis of Cancer and Leukemia Group B study 39808. *Int J Radiat Oncol Biol Phys* 2004;59(2):460-468.

31. Komaki R, Paulus R, Ettinger DS, et al. A phase II study of accelerated high-dose thoracic radiation therapy (AHTRT) with concurrent chemotherapy for limited small cell lung cancer: RTOG 0239. 2009 ASCO Annual Meeting Proceedings. *J Clin Oncol* 2009;27(152):7527.

32. Murray N, Coy P, Pater JL, et al. Importance of timing for thoracic irradiation in the combined modality treatment of limited-stage small-cell lung cancer. *J Clin Oncol* 1993;11:336-344.

33. Takada M, Fukuoka M, Kawahara M, et al. Phase III study of concurrent versus sequential thoracic radiotherapy in combination with cisplatin and etoposide for limited-stage small-cell lung cancer: Results of the Japan Clinical Oncology Group study 9104. *J Clin Oncol* 2002;20(14):3054-3060.

34. DeRuysscher D, Pijls-Johannesma M, Bentzen SM, et al. Time between the first day of chemotherapy and the last day of chest radiation is the most important predictor of survival in limited-disease small-cell lung cancer. *J Clin Oncol* 2006;24(7):1057-1063.

35. Bishop JF, Raghavan D, Stuart-Harris R, et al. Carboplatin (CBDCA, JM-8) and VP-16-213 in previously untreated patients with small-cell lung cancer. *J Clin Oncol* 1987;5:1574-1578.

36. Skarlos DV, Samantas E, Kosmidis P, et al. Randomized comparison of etoposide-cisplatin vs. etoposide-carboplatin and irradiation in small-cell lung cancer: A Hellenic Co-operative Oncology Group study. *Ann Oncol* 1994;5:601-607.

37. Green RA, Humphrey E, Close H, et al. Alkylating agents in bronchogenic carcinoma. *Am J Med* 1969;46(4):516-525.

38. Evans WK, Osoba D, Feld R, et al. Etoposide (VP-16) and cisplatin: An effective treatment for relapse in small-cell lung cancer. *J Clin Oncol* 1985;3(1):65-71.

39. Evans WK, Shepherd FA, Feld R, et al. VP-16 and cisplatin as first-line therapy for small-cell lung cancer. *J Clin Oncol* 1985;3(11):1471-1477.

40. Roth BJ, Johnson DH, Einhorn L, et al. Randomized study of cyclophosphamide, doxorubicin, and vincristine versus etoposide and cisplatin versus alternation of these two regimens in extensive small-cell lung cancer: A phase III trial of the Southeastern Cancer Study Group. *J Clin Oncol* 1992;10:282-291.

41. Maurer LH, Tulloh M, Weiss RB, et al. A randomized combined modality trial in small cell carcinoma of the lung: Comparison of combination chemotherapy-radiation therapy versus cyclophosphamide-radiation therapy effects of maintenance chemotherapy and prophylactic whole brain irradiation. *Cancer* 1980;45(1):30-39.

42. Cullen M, Morgan D, Gregory W, et al. Maintenance chemotherapy for anaplastic small cell carcinoma of the bronchus: A randomised, controlled trial. *Cancer Chemother Pharmacol* 1986;17(2):157-160.

43. Schiller JH, Adak S, Cella D, et al. Topotecan versus observation after cisplatin plus etoposide in extensive-stage small-cell lung cancer: E7593—a phase III trial of the Eastern Cooperative Oncology Group. *J Clin Oncol* 2001;19:2114-2122.

44. Ettinger DS, Finkelstein DM, Abeloff MD, et al. A randomized comparison of standard chemotherapy versus alternating chemotherapy and maintenance versus no maintenance therapy for extensive-stage small-cell lung cancer: A phase III study of the Eastern Cooperative Oncology Group. *J Clin Oncol* 1990;8:230-240.

45. Lebeau B, Chastang C, Allard P, et al. Six vs twelve cycles for complete responders to chemotherapy in small cell lung cancer: Definitive results of a randomized clinical trial. *Eur Respir J* 1992;5:286-290.

46. Giaccone G, Dalesio O, McVie GJ, et al. Maintenance chemotherapy in small-cell lung cancer: Long-term results of a randomized trial, European Organization for Research and Treatment of Cancer Lung Cancer Cooperative Group. *J Clin Oncol* 1993;11:1230-1240.

47. Beith JM, Clarke SJ, Woods RL, et al. Long-term follow-up of a randomised trial of combined chemoradiotherapy induction treatment, with and without maintenance chemotherapy in patients with small-cell carcinoma of the lung. *Eur J Cancer* 1996;32A:438-443.

48. Sculier JP, Paesmans M, Bureau G, et al. Randomized trial comparing induction chemotherapy versus induction chemotherapy followed by maintenance chemotherapy in small-cell lung cancer. European Lung Cancer Working Party. *J Clin Oncol* 1996;14(2337-2344):2337.

49. Byrne MJ, vanHazel G, Trotter J, et al. Maintenance chemotherapy in limited small cell lung cancer: A randomised controlled clinical trial. *Brit J Cancer* 1989;60(3):413-418.

50. Pujol JL, Daures JP, Riviere A, et al. Etoposide plus cisplatin with or without the combination of 4-epidoxorubicin plus cyclophosphamide in treatment of extensive small-cell lung cancer: A French Federation of Cancer Institutes multicenter phase III randomized study. *J Natl Cancer Inst* 2001;93:300-308.

51. Murray N, Livingston RB, Shepherd FA, et al. Randomized study of CODE versus alternating CAV/EP for extensive-stage small-cell lung cancer: An intergroup study of the National Cancer Institute of Canada Clinical Trials Group and the Southwest Oncology Group. *J Clin Oncol* 1999;17:2300-2308.

52. Loehrer PJ, Ansari R, Gonin R, et al. Cisplatin plus etoposide with and without ifosfamide in extensive small-cell lung cancer: A Hoosier Oncology Group study. *J Clin Oncol* 1995; 13:2594-2599.

53. Miyamoto H, Nakabayashi T, Isobe H, et al. A phase III comparison of etoposide/cisplatin with or without added ifosfamide in small-cell lung cancer. *Oncology* 1992;49: 431-435.

54. Niell HB, Herndon JE, Miller AA, et al. Randomized phase III intergroup trial of etoposide and cisplatin with or without paclitaxel and granulocyte colony-stimulating factor in patients with extensive-stage small-cell lung cancer: Cancer and Leukemia Group B trial 9732. *J Clin Oncol* 2005;23:3752-3759.

55. Mavroudis D, Papadakis E, Veslemes M, et al. A multicenter randomized clinical trial comparing paclitaxel-cisplatin-etoposide versus cisplatin-etoposide as first-line treatment in patients with small-cell lung cancer. *Ann Oncol* 2001;12: 463-470.

56. Masuda N, Fukuoka M, Kusunoki Y, et al. CPT-11: A new derivative of camptothecin for the treatment of refractory or relapsed small-cell lung cancer. *J Clin Oncol* 1992;10(8): 1225-1229.

57. Noda K, Nishiwaki Y, Kawahara M, et al. Irinotecan plus cisplatin compared with etoposide plus cisplatin for extensive small-cell lung cancer. *N Engl J Med* 2002;346(2):85-91.

58. Hanna N, Bunn PA, Langer C, et al. Randomized phase III trial comparing irinotecan/cisplatin with etoposide/cisplatin in patients with previously untreated extensive-stage disease small-cell lung cancer. *J Clin Oncol* 2006;24(13): 2038-2043.

59. Lara PN, Natale R, Crowley JJ, et al. Phase III trial of irinotecan/cisplatin compared with etoposide/cisplatin in extensive-stage small-cell lung cancer: Clinical and pharmacogenomic results from SWOG S0124. *J Clin Oncol* 2009; 27(18):2530-2535.

60. Schmittel AH, Sebastian M, Fischer von Weikersthal L, et al. Irinotecan plus carboplatin versus etoposide plus carboplatin in extensive disease small cell lung cancer: Results of the German randomized phase III trial. 2009 ASCO Annual Meeting Proceedings. *J Clin Oncol* 2009;27(15s):8029.

61. Hermes A, Bergman B, Bremnes R, et al. Irinotecan plus carboplatin versus oral etoposide plus carboplatin in extensive small-cell lung cancer: A randomized phase III trial. *J Clin Oncol* 2008;26(26):4261-4267.

62. Evans WK, Feld R, Murray N, et al. Superiority of alternating non-cross-resistant chemotherapy in extensive small cell lung cancer: A multicenter, randomized clinical trial by the National Cancer Institute of Canada. *Ann Intern Med* 1987; 107(3):451-458.

63. Murray N, Shah A, Osoba D, et al. Intensive weekly chemotherapy for the treatment of extensive-stage small-cell lung cancer. *J Clin Oncol* 1991;9:1632-1638.

64. Furuse K, Fukuoka M, Nishiwaki Y, et al. Phase III study of intensive weekly chemotherapy with recombinant human granulocyte colony-stimulating factor versus standard chemotherapy in extensive-disease small-cell lung cancer: The Japan Clinical Oncology Group. *J Clin Oncol* 1998; 16:2126-2132.

65. Klasa RJ, Murray N, Coldman AJ. Dose-intensity meta-analysis of chemotherapy regimens in small-cell carcinoma of the lung. *J Clin Oncol* 1991;9:499-508.

66. Ihde DC, Mulshine JL, Kramer BS, et al. Prospective randomized comparison of high-dose and standard-dose etoposide and cisplatin chemotherapy in patients with extensive-stage small-cell lung cancer. *J Clin Oncol* 1994;12(10):2022-2034.

67. Heigener DF, Manegold C, Jager E, et al. Multicenter randomized open-label phase III study comparing efficacy, safety, and tolerability of conventional carboplatin plus etoposide versus dose-intensified carboplatin plus etoposide plus lenograstim in small-cell lung cancer in "extensive disease" stage. *Am J Clin Oncol* 2009;32:61-64.

68. Steward WP, vonPawel J, Gatzemeier U, et al. Effects of granulocyte-macrophage colony-stimulating factor and dose intensification of V-ICE chemotherapy in small-cell lung caner: A prospective randomized study of 300 patients. *J Clin Oncol* 1998;16:642-650.

69. Thatcher N, Girling DJ, Hopwood P, et al. Improving survival without reducing quality of life in small-cell lung cancer patients by increasing the dose intensity of chemotherapy with granulocyte colony-stimulating factor support: Results of a British Medical Research Council multicenter randomized trial. *J Clin Oncol* 2000;18:395-404.

70. Lorigan P, Woll PJ, O'Brien MER, et al. Randomized phase III trial of dose-dense chemotherapy supported by whole-blood hematopoietic progenitors in better-prognosis small-cell lung cancer. *J Natl Cancer Inst* 2005;97:666-674.

71. Buchholz E, Manegold C, Pilz L, et al. Standard versus dose-intensified chemotherapy with sequential reinfusion of hematopoietic progenitor cells in small cell lung cancer patients with favorable prognosis. *J Thorac Oncol* 2007;2(1):51-58.

72. Tiseo M, Ardizzoni A. Current status of second-line treatment and novel therapies for small cell lung cancer. *J Thorac Oncol* 2007;2(8):764-772.

73. O' Brien MER, Ciuleanu TE, Tsekov H, et al. Phase III trial comparing supportive care alone with oral topotecan in patients with relapsed small-cell lung cancer. *J Clin Oncol* 2006;24(34):5441-5447.

74. Giaccone G, Donadio M, Bonardi G, et al. Teniposide in the treatment of small-cell lung cancer: The influence of prior chemotherapy. *J Clin Oncol* 1988;6(8):1264-1270.

75. vonPawel J, Schiller JH, Shepherd FA, et al. Topotecan versus cyclophosphamide, doxorubicin, and vincristine for the treatment of recurrent small-cell lung cancer. *J Clin Oncol* 1999;17(2):658-667.

76. Batist G, Ihde DC, Zabell A, et al. Small-cell carcinoma of the lung: Reinduction therapy after late relapse. *Ann Intern Med* 1983;98(1):472-474.

77. Postmus PE, Berendsen HH, vanZandwijk N, et al. Retreatment with the induction regimen in small cell lung cancer relapsing after an initial response to short term chemotherapy. *Eur J Cancer Clin Oncol* 1987;23(9):1409-1411.

78. Giaccone G, Ferrati P, Donadio M, et al. Reinduction chemotherapy in small cell lung cancer. *Eur J Cancer Clin Oncol* 1987;23(11):1697-1699.

79. Vincent M, Evans B, Smith I. First-line chemotherapy rechallenge after relapse in small cell lung cancer. *Cancer Chemother Pharmacol* 1988;21:45-48.

80. Ardizzoni A, Manegold C, Debruyne C, et al. European Organization for Research and Treatment of Cancer (EORTC) 08957 phase II study of topotecan in combination with cisplatin as second-line treatment of refractory and sensitive small cell lung cancer. *Clin Cancer Res* 2003;9:143-150.

81. vonPawel J, Gatzemeier U, Pujol JL, et al. Phase II comparator study of oral versus intravenous topotecan in patients with chemosensitive small-cell lung cancer. *J Clin Oncol* 2001; 19(6):1743-1749.

82. Eckardt JR, vonPawel J, Pujol JL, et al. Phase III study of oral compared with intravenous topotecan as second-line therapy in small-cell lung cancer. *J Clin Oncol* 2007;25(15): 2086-2092.

83. Onoda S, Masuda N, Seto T, et al. Phase II trial of amrubicin for treatment of refractory or relapsed small-cell lung cancer: Thoracic Oncology Research Group Study 0301. *J Clin Oncol* 2006;24(34):5448-5453.

84. Inoue A, Sugawara S, Yamazaki K, et al. Randomized phase II trial comparing amrubicin with topotecan in patients with previously treated small-cell lung cancer: North Japan Lung Cancer Study Group Trial 0402. *J Clin Oncol* 2008;26(33): 5401-5406.

85. Chiappori A, Sereno M, Gabrilovich D, et al. Phase II trial of patients with extensive stage small cell lung cancer immunized with p53-transduced dendritic cells: Immune sensitization to chemotherapy. 2007 ASCO Annual Meeting Proceedings. *J Clin Oncol* 2007;25(18s):3012.

86. Lucchi M, Mussi A, Fontanini G, et al. Small cell lung carcinoma (SCLC): The angiogenic phenomenon. *Eur J Cardiothorac Surg* 2002;21:1105-1110.

87. Sandler A, Gray R, Perry MC, et al. Paclitaxel-carboplatin alone or with bevacizumab for non-small-cell lung cancer. *N Engl J Med* 2006;355(24):2542-2550.

88. Spigel DR, Greco FA, Zubkus JD, et al. Phase II trial of irinotecan, carboplatin, and bevacizumab in the treatment of patients with extensive-stage small-cell lung cancer. *J Thorac Oncol* 2009;4(12):1555-1560.

89. Horn L, Dahlberg SE, Sandler AB, et al. Phase II study of cisplatin plus etoposide and bevacizumab for previously untreated, extensive-stage small-cell lung cancer: Eastern Cooperative Oncology Group Study E3501. *J Clin Oncol* 2009;27(35):6006-6011.

90. Spigel DR, Hainsworth JD, Yardley DA, et al. Tracheoesophageal fistula formation in patients with lung cancer treated with chemoradiation and bevacizumab. *J Clin Oncol* 2009;27:Epub.

91. Pujol JL, Breton JL, Gervais R, et al. Phase III double-blind, placebo-controlled study of thalidomide in extensive-disease small-cell lung cancer after response to chemotherapy: An Intergroup study FNCLCC cleo04-IFCT 00-01. *J Clin Oncol* 2007;25(25):3945-3951.

92. Lee SM, Woll PJ, Rudd R, et al. Anti-angiogenic therapy using thalidomide combined with chemotherapy in small cell lung cancer: A randomized, double-blind, placebo-controlled trial. *J Natl Cancer Inst* 2009;101:1049-1057.

93. Arnold AM, Seymour L, Smylie M, et al. Phase II study of vandetanib or placebo in small-cell lung cancer patients after complete or partial response to induction chemotherapy with or without radiation therapy: National Cancer Institute of Canada Clinical Trials Group Study BR.20. *J Clin Oncol* 2007;25(27):4278-4284.

94. Gitlitz BJ, Glisson BS, Moon J, et al. Sorafenib in patients with platinum treated extensive stage small cell lung cancer: A SWOG (S0435) phase II trial. 2008 ASCO Annual Meeting Proceedings. *J Clin Oncol* 2008;26(15s):8039.

95. Krug LM, Crapanzano JP, Azzoli CG, et al. Imatinib mesylate lacks activity in small cell lung carcinoma expressing c-kit protein. *Cancer* 2005;103(10):28-31.

96. Dy GK, Miller AA, Mandrekar SJ, et al. A phase II trial of imatinib (ST1571) in patients with c-kit expressing relapsed small-cell lung cancer: A CALGB and NCCTG study. *Ann Oncol* 2005;16:1811-1816.

97. Spigel DR, Hainsworth JD, Simons L, et al. Irinotecan, carboplatin, and imatinib in untreated extensive-stage small-cell lung cancer: A phase II trial of the Minnie Pearl Cancer Research Network. *J Thorac Oncol* 2007;2(9):854-861.

98. Ohmori T, Podack ER, Nishio K, et al. Apoptosis of lung cancer cells caused by some anti-cancer agents (MMC, CPT-11, ADM) is inhibited by BCL-2. *Biochem Biophys Res Commun* 1993;192(1):30-36.

99. Korsmeyer SJ. Regulators of cell death. *Trends Genet* 1995; 11:101-105.

100. Rudin CM, Salgia R, Wang X, et al. Randomized phase II study of carboplatin and etoposide with or without the bcl-2 antisense oligonucleotide oblimersen for extensive-stage small-cell lung cancer: CALGB 30103. *J Clin Oncol* 2008; 26(6):870-876.

101. Chiappori A, Schreeder MT, Moezi MM, et al. A phase Ib trial of Bcl-2 inhibitor obatoclax in combination with carboplatin and etoposide for previously untreated patients with extensive-stage small cell lung cancer. 2009 ASCO Annual Meeting Proceedings. *J Clin Oncol* 2009;27(15s):3576.

102. Michael M, Babic B, Khokha R, et al. Expression and prognostic significance of metalloproteinases and their tissue inhibitors in patients with small-cell lung cancer. *J Clin Oncol* 1999;17(6):1802-1808.

103. Shepherd FA, Giaccone G, Seymour L, et al. Prospective, randomized, double-blind, placebo-controlled trial of marimastat after response to first-line chemotherapy in patients with small-cell lung cancer: A trial of the National Cancer Institute of Canada Clinical Trials Group and the European Organization for Research and Treatment of Cancer. *J Clin Oncol* 2002;20(22):4434-4439.

104. Ciardiello F, Tortora G. EGFR antagonists in cancer treatment. *N Engl J Med* 2008;358(11):1160-1174.

105. Moore AM, Einhorn LH, Estes D, et al. Gefitinib in patients with chemo-sensitive and chemo-refractory relapsed small cell cancers: A Hoosier Oncology Group phase II trial. *Lung Cancer* 2006;52:93-97.

106. Zakowski MF, Ladanyi M, Kris MG. EGFR mutations in small-cell lung cancers in patients who have never smoked. *N Engl J Med* 2006;355(2):213-215.

107. Baserga R, Peruzzi F, Reiss K. The IGF-1 receptor in cancer biology. *Int J Cancer* 2003;107:873-877.

108. Yeh J, Litz J, Hauck P, et al. Selective inhibition of SCLC growth by the A12 anti-IGF-1R monoclonal antibody correlates with inhibition of Akt. *Lung Cancer* 2008;60:166-174.

109. Warshamana-Greene GS, Litz J, Buchdunger E, et al. The insulin-like growth factor-I receptor kinase inhibitor, NVP-ADW742, sensitizes small cell lung cancer cell lines to the effects of chemotherapy. *Clin Cancer Res* 2005;11:1563-1571.

110. Nugent JL, Bunn PA, Matthews MJ, et al. CNS metastases in small cell bronchogenic carcinoma: Increasing frequency and changing pattern with lengthening survival. *Cancer* 1979; 44:1885-1893.

111. Vines EF, LePechoux C, Arriagada R. Prophylactic cranial irradiation in small cell lung cancer. *Semin Oncol* 2003;30:38-46.

112. Auperin A, Arriagada R, Pignon JP, et al. Prophylactic cranial irradiation for patients with small-cell lung cancer in complete remission. *N Engl J Med* 1999;341:476-484.

113. Slotman BJ, FaivreFinn C, Kramer G, et al. Prophylactic cranial irradiation in extensive small-cell lung cancer. *N Engl J Med* 2007;357(7):664-672.

114. Slotman BJ, Mauer ME, Bottomley A, et al. Prophylactic cranial irradiation in extensive disease small-cell lung cancer: Short-term health-related quality of life and patient reported symptoms—results of an international phase III randomized controlled trial by the EORTC radiation oncology and lung cancer groups. *J Clin Oncol* 2009;27(1):78-84.

115. Johnson DH. Small cell lung cancer in the elderly patient. *Semin Oncol* 1997;24:484-491.

116. Shepherd FA, Amdemichael E, Evans WK, et al. Treatment of small cell lung cancer in the elderly. *J Am Geriatr Soc* 1994;42:64-70.

117. Dajczman E, Fu LY, Small D, et al. Treatment of small cell lung carcinoma in the elderly. *Cancer* 1996;77:2032-2038.

118. Cuttitta F, Carnery DN, Mulshine J, et al. Bombesin-like peptides can function as autocrine growth factors in human small-cell lung cancer. *Nature* 1985;316:823-826.

119. Clamon GH, Audeh MW, Pinnick S. Small cell carcinoma in the elderly. *J Am Geriatr Soc* 1982;30:299-302.

120. Poplin E, Thompson B, Whitacre M, et al. Small cell carcinoma of the lung: Influence of age on treatment outcome. *Cancer Treat Rep* 1987;71:291-296.

121. Kelly P, O'Brien AA, Daly P, et al. Small-cell lung cancer in elderly patients: The case for chemotherapy. *Age Aging* 1991;20:19-22.

122. Findlay MP, Griffin AM, Raghavan D, et al. Retrospective review of chemotherapy for small cell lung cancer in the elderly: Does the end justify the means? *Eur J Cancer* 1991; 27:1597-1601.

123. Girling DJ. Comparison of oral etoposide and standard intravenous multidrug chemotherapy for small cell lung cancer: A stopped multicentre randomised trial. *Lancet* 1996; 348:563-566.

124. Carney DN. Carboplatin/etoposide combination chemotherapy in the treatment of poor prognosis patients with small cell lung cancer. *Lung Cancer* 1995;12(Suppl 3):S77-S83.

125. Matsui K, Masuda N, Fukuoka M, et al. Phase II trial of carboplatin plus oral etoposide for elderly patients with small-cell lung cancer. *Br J Cancer* 1998;77:1961-1965.

126. Samantas E, Skarlos DV, Pectasides D, et al. Combination chemotherapy with low doses of weekly carboplatin and oral etoposide in poor risk small cell lung cancer. *Lung Cancer* 1999;23:159-168.

127. Okamoto H, Watanabe K, Nishiwaki Y, et al. Phase II study of area under the plasma-concentration-versus-time curve-based carboplatin plus standard-dose intravenous etoposide in elderly patients with small-cell lung cancer. *J Clin Oncol* 1999;17:3540-3545.

128. Dimopoulos MA, Fernandez JF, Samaan NA, et al. Paraneoplastic Cushing's syndrome as an adverse prognostic factor in patients who die early with small cell lung cancer. *Cancer* 1992;69:66-71.

129. Dalmau J, Furneaux HM, Rosenblum MK, et al. Detection of the anti-Hu antibody in specific regions of the nervous system and tumor from patients with paraneoplastic encephalomyelitis/sensory neuropathy. *Neurology* 1991;41:1757-1764.

130. Buckanovich RJ, Posner JB, Darnell RB. Nova, the paraneoplastic Ri antigen, is homologous to an RNA-binding protein and is specifically expressed in the developing motor system. *Neuron* 1993;11:657-672.

131. Peterson K, Rosenblum MK, Kotanides H, et al. Paraneoplastic cerebellar degeneration: A clinical analysis of 55 anti-Yo antibody-positive patients. *Neurology* 1992;42:1931-1937.

132. Darnell RB, Furneaux HM, Posner JB. Antiserum from a patient with cerebellar degeneration identifies a novel protein in Purkinje cells, cortical neurons, and neuroectodermal tumors. *J Neurosci* 1991;11:1224-1230.

133. Graus F, Dalmau J, Valldeoriola F, et al. Immunological characterization of a neuronal antibody (anti-Tr) associated with paraneoplastic cerebellar degeneration and Hodgkin's disease. *J Neuroimmunol* 1997;74:55-61.

134. Dalmau J, Gultekin SH, Voltz R, et al. Ma1, a novel neuron- and testis-specific protein, is recognized by the serum of patients with paraneoplastic neurological disorders. *Brain* 1999;122:27-39.

135. Vincent A, Lang B, Newsom-Davis J, et al. Autoimmunity to the voltage-gated calcium channel underlies the Lambert-Eaton myasthenic syndrome, a paraneoplastic disorder. *Trends Neurosci* 1989;12:496-502.

NON-SMALL CELL LUNG CANCER

Don Gibbons
Katherine M. Pisters
Faye Johnson
Commentary: George A. Eapen

Lung cancer is the leading cause of cancer-related deaths in the United States and worldwide (1,2). The high rate of mortality results from both the high incidence and the late stage of disease at diagnosis. It is estimated that in the year 2009, approximately 219,440 new cases will be diagnosed and 159,390 deaths due to lung cancer will occur in the United States. These numbers represent approximately 15% of all new cancer cases and 28% of cancer deaths in this population (1).

These statistics emphasize that lung cancer is a lethal disease, with poor overall survival. Only 15% of patients diagnosed with lung cancer are alive 5 years later (1,2). More than 70% of patients will be diagnosed with advanced disease that is not amenable to curative therapy (3). Even those who present with early-stage disease have a high rate of recurrence.

Lung cancer is broadly divided into small cell lung cancer (SCLC) and non-small cell lung cancer (NSCLC). Approximately 85% of lung cancer is NSCLC. This chapter briefly describes the epidemiology, etiology, histology, prevention, and molecular biology of NSCLC. The major focus of this chapter is to describe and discuss the clinical presentation, diagnosis, staging, and treatment of NSCLC based on current clinical knowledge, with an emphasis on our approach to the management of NSCLC at the University of Texas MD Anderson Cancer Center (MDACC).

■ EPIDEMIOLOGY

Lung cancer is rarely diagnosed in people less than 35 years old. Incidence and death rates rise exponentially among patients older than 35, then approximately plateau among patients greater than 75 years old (4). NSCLC accounts for the greatest number of deaths from cancer in both men and women over age 60 (1).

Analysis of the incidences of smoking and lung cancer in the United States over the past century demonstrates parallel courses, with a latency period of about 20 years between the former and latter events. The current epidemic of lung cancer began with a sharp increase in incidence among men in the 1930s, following the availability of manufactured cigarettes in the 1910s. The increase in lung cancer incidence among women did not start until the 1960s, again following an increase in exposure to tobacco (this time due to changes in smoking practices after World War II), and by 1987 lung cancer surpassed breast cancer as the leading cause of cancer-related death in women (5). In the 1990s, the incidence of lung cancer in the United States decreased among men. In women, the rates of lung cancer stabilized from 2003 to 2005. In the year 2009, the estimated ratio of male-to-female deaths due to lung cancer in the United States was 1.3:1 (1). There is some evidence that women are at a greater risk for lung cancer; however, other studies have not confirmed this finding.

Smoking behaviors might also account for socioeconomic and racial differences in lung cancer incidence. Declines in lung cancer since the 1990s have been most pronounced in individuals of all ethnic backgrounds with a college education and appear to correlate with the marked decrease between 1992 and 2007 in cigarette consumption among people in this group (6). The highest incidence of lung cancer in the United States is in African-American males. Although some of this high rate of cancer incidence is clearly attributable to smoking behaviors, evidence suggests that this population might be more susceptible than others to the carcinogenic effects of tobacco smoke.

■ ETIOLOGY

SMOKING

The causal relationship between tobacco smoke and lung cancer was established as early as the 1950s in case-control and later cohort studies; this evidence led to the 1964 report of the US Surgeon General, concluding that smoking can cause lung cancer (reviewed in Alberg and Samet [7]). Currently, it is estimated that 85 to 90% of lung cancer is due to smoking, but that nonsmokers who are exposed to secondhand smoke are also at an increased risk for lung cancer (4). Pipe and cigar smoking also increases the risk for lung cancer. The relative risk for lung cancer in current smokers is approximately 11 to 17 times higher than that for people who have never smoked (8), although there is evidence for a dose-response relationship between smoking and lung cancer (9) and risk depends upon the duration and amount smoked (Table 15-1). In addition, smoking cessation leads to a decrease in lung cancer risk over time (9,10).

Tobacco smoke is a complex mixture of several thousand chemicals that includes multiple carcinogens and growth factors (11). The N-nitrosamines and polycyclic aromatic hydrocarbons are the two major classes of tobacco-related inhaled carcinogens. N-nitrosamines are formed during tobacco processing and pyrosynthesis. They originate from nicotine and the alkaloid arecoline. Chemicals derived from tobacco smoke cause lung tumors in experimental animals. The main nitrosation products of nicotine are NNK (nicotine-derived nitrosamino ketone) and NNN (N'-nitrosonornicotine). They are considered very strong lung carcinogens. The nitrosamines are activated through hydroxylation by the P450 enzyme system and exert their action through the formation of DNA adducts. The number of DNA adducts formed is directly related to the number of cigarettes consumed. DNA adducts can remain in the system for as long as 5 years without significant change; in heavy smokers, they can be responsible for as many as 100 mutations per cell genome. The polycyclic aromatic hydrocarbons benzo(a)pyrene and dimethylbenz(a)anthracene are also significant chemical mutagenic/carcinogenic substances that lead to the formation of DNA adducts. Recent evidence has also identified the nicotine acetylcholine receptor as a

TABLE
15-1
APPROXIMATE 10-YEAR RISK OF DEVELOPING LUNG CANCER*

| | DURATION OF SMOKING | | | | | |
| | 25 YEARS | | 40 YEARS | | 50 YEARS | |
Age (Years)	Quit (%)	Still Smoking (%)	Quit (%)	Still Smoking (%)	Quit (%)	Still Smoking (%)
One-pack-per-day smokers						
55	<1	1	3	5	NA	NA
65	<1	2	4	7	7	10
75	1	2	5	8	8	11
Two-packs-per-day smokers						
55	<1	2	4	7	NA	NA
65	1	3	6	9	10	14
75	2	3	7	10	11	15

NA, not available.

*These tables assume that people who have quit smoking will continue to abstain for the next 10 years and those who are still smoking will keep smoking the same amount for the next 10 years.

Adapted, with permission, from Bach PB, Kattan MW, Thornquist MD, et al. Variations in lung cancer risk among smokers. Cancer 2003;95(1):470-478.

susceptibility locus in lung cancer (12,13), suggesting that nicotine simultaneously accounts for the addiction to smoking and is capable of driving tumorigenesis and metastasis in experimental systems (14,15).

Although smoking is clearly the largest risk factor, 10 to 15% of cases of NSCLC occur in never smokers, corresponding to approximately 20,000 deaths annually and making this category one of the top 10 causes of cancer mortality (4). Although incompletely understood, increasing focus has been placed on this category of NSCLC and several important facts are clear: first, incidence increases with age; second, no clear change in risk has occurred over time; third, no clear gender bias exists; fourth, among female never smokers, large population differences exist, with higher risk in East Asian countries, especially China. In addition to secondhand smoke exposure, several other agents have also been linked to the development of lung cancer (Table 15-2).

TABLE
15-2
RELATIVE RISK OF DEVELOPING LUNG CANCER

Risk Factor	Relative Risk	Reference
Cigarette smoking in males	17.4	8
Cigarette smoking in females	10.8	8
Passive smoking	1.5	4
Asbestos	1.2-2.6	9, 18
Asbestos and smoking	28.8	19
Mining	3-8	4, 21
Radon (residential)	1.1-2	4

ASBESTOS

Asbestos exists in many natural forms. The silicate fiber has been implicated in carcinogenesis, is chemically inert, and can remain in a person's lungs for a lifetime. Epidemiologic studies have confirmed the association between asbestos exposure and certain lung diseases, such as pulmonary fibrosis, mesothelioma, and lung cancer (16). Most asbestos exposure occurs in the workplace—for example, among shipyard workers or plumbers (Table 15-3) (17).

In a study of British asbestos workers, the relative risk of lung cancer was 1.4 to 2.6 (18). Asbestos most likely acts as a tumor promoter. As smoking is known to impair bronchial clearance, it is reasonable to assume that smoking prolongs the presence of asbestos in the pulmonary epithelium. In addition, asbestos might enhance the mutagenicity of tobacco carcinogens. When smoking is combined with asbestos exposure, the relative risk of lung cancer is strikingly increased to 28.8 (19).

RADON

Radon is a naturally occurring decay product of uranium. It is a colorless, odorless, chemically inert gas that can penetrate the earth's crust and accumulate in buildings. Radon decays to products that emit heavy ionizing alpha particles, which may damage the DNA in respiratory epithelial cells. Radon exposure increases the risk of developing lung cancer, usually the small cell type (20). Among uranium miners who smoke, the

TABLE 15-3 **OCCUPATIONS WITH SIGNIFICANT EXPOSURE TO ASBESTOS (PARTIAL LIST)**

Acoustic product installers
Asbestos cement makers, users
Asbestos grout makers, users
Asbestos millboard makers, users
Asbestos millers
Asbestos miners
Asbestos paper makers, users
Asbestos plaster makers, users
Asbestos products manufacturers
Asphalt mixers
Auto mechanics
Boiler makers
Brake lining repairers
Brake refabricators
Bricklayers
Carpenters
Chemical workers
Clay workers
Construction workers
Demolition workers
Drywall tapers
Electricians
Electrical wire makers
Firefighters
Gasket makers, users
Glass workers
Iron ore miners and millers
Insulators
Laborers
Machinery producers
Maintenance and custodial workers
Oil and gas extraction workers
Petroleum refinery workers
Primary metal industry workers
Pipecoverers
Pipefitters
Plumbers
Powerhouse workers
Railroad repair workers
Rubber makers
Reinforced plastic makers, users
Roofers
Sheet metal workers
Shipyard workers
Stationary firemen
Steamfitters
Stone workers
Talc miners
Textile workers
Tile makers, users
Transportation equipment repairers
Transportation workers
Turbine manufacturing workers

Adapted, with permission, from Levin SM, Kann PE, Lax MB, Medical examination for asbestos-related disease. Am J Ind Med, 2000. 37(1): p. 6-22.

risk of developing lung cancer is 10 times that of their nonsmoking colleagues (21). Based upon epidemiologic studies in the United States and Europe, residential exposure is clearly associated with an increased risk of lung cancer and is estimated to account for 2100-2900 cases annually in the United States (reviewed in Samet et al [4]).

DIET

Diet might also influence risk for lung cancer. Studies in this field have focused on the intake of fruits, vegetables, and specific micronutrients. The effects of smoking confound these studies in that smokers might, in the aggregate, have a less healthy lifestyle and diet than nonsmokers. Also, the detrimental effects of smoking far exceed the potential protective effect of diet or nutrition.

Many studies have examined the effect of fruit intake on lung cancer incidence. The results have not been consistent, with the majority of studies showing no protective effect. The majority of studies that examined vegetable consumption in relation to lung cancer did show a protective effect (reviewed in Alberg [7]). No studies have shown an increased incidence of lung cancer with increased fruit or vegetable consumption. These data, combined with data on other tumor types, prompted the National Cancer Institute to recommend consumption of five or more servings of fruits and vegetables daily.

The agents in fruits and vegetables that result in a decreased incidence of lung cancer remain unknown. Several studies have examined the effects of carotenoids, retinol, and vitamin C. Studies that examined the effect of dietary retinol intake on lung cancer incidence found mixed effects, with some studies showing a protective effect and others showing no effect. Several studies have demonstrated an inverse correlation between serum beta-carotene levels and the incidence of lung cancer. Increased intake of carotenoids in general and beta-carotene in particular has been linked with a decreased risk of lung cancer, although other studies did not show this protective effect. Vitamin C might also prevent lung cancer, although some studies do not confirm a protective effect (reviewed in Alberg [7]).

Surprising results, however, came from three large-scale randomized trials that examined the effects of beta-carotene on lung cancer risk. The Alpha-Tocopherol/Beta-Carotene (ATBC) trial enrolled 29,133 male smokers 50 to 69 years old and randomly assigned them to one of four regimens: alpha-tocopherol, 50 mg/day; beta-carotene, 20 mg/day; both alpha-tocopherol and beta-carotene; or placebo (22). Patients were followed up for 5 to 8 years. No reduction in the incidence of lung cancer was observed among the men receiving alpha-tocopherol. Patients receiving beta-carotene alone or in combination with alpha-tocopherol had a higher incidence of lung cancer (relative risk 1.18; 95% CI, 1.03-1.36) and 8% higher mortality from lung cancer and heart disease than did patients not receiving beta-carotene. Similar results were obtained in the Beta-Carotene and Retinol Efficacy Trial (CARET) (23). CARET was a multicenter, randomized trial that enrolled 18,314 men and women smokers who were treated with both beta-carotene and retinyl palmitate. Among the carotene and retinol-treated patients, the relative risk of lung cancer was 1.28 (95% CI, 1.04-1.57) and of death from lung cancer was 1.46 (95% CI, 1.07-2.00) compared with placebo-treated patients. The Physicians' Health Study (PHS) randomized 22,071 healthy male physicians to placebo or beta-carotene treatment arms. There were no significant differences between smokers and non-smokers in the incidence of lung cancer after 12 years of follow-up (24).

Several other large trials assessing the connection between vitamin supplements and cancer incidence have been reported. In the Physicians' Health Study II, 14,641 male physicians aged 50 years or older were randomized in a double-blind, placebo-controlled factorial trial of vitamins C and E. Running from 1997 to 2007 and with a median follow-up time of 8 years, there was no effect of vitamin C (HR = 0.97, p = .58) or vitamin E (HR = 1.01, p = .86) versus placebo on the incidence of total cancer, or of any site-specific cancer analyzed, including lung (25). A study using combined data from two large Norwegian randomized, double-blind, placebo-controlled trials of folic acid and vitamin B_{12} as homocysteine-lowering agents in cardiovascular disease demonstrated an increase in overall cancer incidence (HR = 1.21, p = .02) and mortality (HR = 1.38, p = .01), which was primarily driven by the increase in lung cancer cases (HR = 1.59, 95% CI, 0.92-2.75) (26).

The reasons for the discrepancy between the epidemiologic data and the chemoprevention studies are unclear. Certainly, fruits and vegetables contain a complex array of micronutrients that might influence cancer incidence, modulate the effects or biologic doses of various agents, including beta-carotene, alpha-tocopherol, or retinols (27).

OTHER FACTORS

Environmental or industrial exposure to arsenic, chromium, chloromethyl ether, vinyl chloride, and polycyclic aromatic hydrocarbons increases lung cancer risk (reviewed in Schottenfeld [28]). Preexisting lung disease such as tuberculosis, silicosis, and pulmonary fibrosis is also associated with an increased lung cancer incidence. The risk of lung cancer appears to be increased in individuals with chronic obstructive pulmonary disease (COPD), even when correcting for the degree of cigarette consumption. These findings are most consistent with the idea that pathophysiologic pathways common to both processes, such as chronic inflammation, can drive the tumorigenic process, providing the rationale for clinical study of agents such as the COX-2 inhibitors (29).

GENETIC PREDISPOSITION

It has been estimated that cigarette smoking is responsible for 85-90% of lung cancers occurring in the United States (4). However, only a fraction of smokers and those exposed to secondhand smoke, asbestos, radon, and other agents develop a bronchial malignancy. This suggests that cancer susceptibility differs among individuals and might have a genetic basis. Several findings support this hypothesis.

Many groups have studied familial aggregation of lung cancer, and most studies demonstrate that a family history of lung cancer is associated with an increased risk for the disease (reviewed in [30]). In general these are case-control studies that control for smoking. Tokuhata et al. conducted a case-control study that examined the frequency of lung cancer among parents and siblings of 270 lung cancer patients (31). The incidence of lung cancer was twice as great as expected among smokers and four times as great as expected among nonsmokers. Another case-control study reviewed a population of 336 deceased lung cancer patients from Louisiana. Lung cancer was much more common in first-degree relatives than in spouses of patients (32). In addition, the predisposition to developing lung cancer at an early age is inherited in a Mendelian codominant fashion (33,34).

Metabolism of tobacco smoke includes several steps that might be influenced by genetics. Variations in the ability to oxidize substances metabolically via the cytochrome P450 system may contribute to differences in susceptibility to cancer. Individuals with increased oxidative activity might be at increased risk of developing cancer because of their increased level of activated carcinogens. Two enzymes, CYP1A1 and CYP2D6, have been implicated, but results from studies regarding lung cancer risk and specific polymorphisms are conflicting and vary depending on the population. CYP2D6 is the enzyme responsible for metabolism of the antihypertensive drug debrisoquine. Increased metabolism of debrisoquine is associated with an increased risk of lung cancer. The enzyme glutathione S-transferase (GST) detoxifies tobacco carcinogens, and some studies show that increased activity of this enzyme is linked to a reduced risk of cancer (35,36), although other studies do not support this finding (37). One study showed a markedly increased risk for lung cancer in those individuals with the combination of a specific polymorphism of CYP1A1 combined with deficient GST activity (38).

Since tobacco smoke and other carcinogens induce DNA damage, differences in the ability to repair DNA damage have been examined as a potential source of cancer susceptibility. Work by Spitz and colleagues has clearly delineated a role for altered DNA repair capacity in the risk of development of NSCLC in smokers and never smokers (39,40). The increased risk with suboptimal DNA repair capacity is independent of, but able to modify, the risk of tobacco exposure, and is therefore useful as an independent variable in models of risk prediction for lung cancer (41).

Thus, although the genetic risk factors associated with lung cancer are incompletely defined, multiple studies confirm the existence of a genetic predisposition to the development of lung cancer.

■ PREVENTION OF LUNG CANCER DEATHS

SMOKING CESSATION AND PREVENTION

Clearly the most effective method of preventing lung cancer is cessation and primary prevention of smoking. In the United States, campaigns to reduce smoking rates have been successful. From 1965 to 1991, there was a 77% decline in the percentage of Americans who actively smoked (42). The subsequent decade showed a more modest change, with a decrease in the percentage of adult smokers from 25 to 23.4% from 1993 to 2000 (43). In 2008 the adult smoking rate in the United States was 20.5% (6). However, despite efforts to prevent smoking and encourage smoking cessation, there are still a significant number of smokers in the United States, former smokers still retain an increased risk of lung cancer, and the increasing use of cigarettes worldwide is expected to shift the majority of tobacco-related deaths to developing countries over the next 20 years (2). Thus, additional strategies to diminish lung cancer deaths have been devised; these include early detection and chemoprevention.

EARLY DETECTION

The goal of lung cancer screening is to detect the disease at an early stage, when cure is possible, so as to reduce deaths due to lung cancer. Thus the most meaningful endpoints of screening studies are lung cancer–specific and overall mortality. Screening studies for lung cancer have been confounded by lead time, length time, and over-diagnosis biases (reviewed in Patz et al. [44]).

Several studies have examined the role of chest x-ray, with or without cytologic analysis of sputum, to screen for lung cancer. None of these studies have clearly shown that these techniques reduce deaths due to lung cancer.

Spiral computed tomography (CT)—also called helical CT or low-dose CT—is also being studied as a screening tool. Spiral CT is appealing because it is much more sensitive than chest x-ray and can be done quickly, with minimal inconvenience to patients (45). Several nonrandomized studies have used spiral CT to screen high-risk patients for lung cancer and uniformly found a high percentage of potentially curable early-stage disease. This finding suggests that screening with CT will result in a stage shift, with more cancers diagnosed at an early stage; however, it could also represent a bias toward overdiagnosis. Therefore it is not clear whether CT screening will result in lower rates of death due to lung cancer. The National Lung Screening Trial is a multicenter trial that opened in 2002 and enrolled 53,000 current and former smokers (with a minimum history of 30 packs/year over a 2-year period) within an 18 month period. Patients were randomized to undergo screening by either chest x-ray or CT annually for 2 years. Initial results were released in November 2010 and identify 20% fewer lung cancer deaths in those who were screened with low dose helical CT. These preliminary results suggest that smokers and former smokers will benefit from screening with annual CT scans (46). There is a similar trial of approximately 15,000 high-risk patients being conducted in Belgium and the Netherlands, with an 80% power to test if there is a 25% reduction in mortality at 10 years after baseline CT screening (47). The trial is scheduled to run through the end of 2015.

No screening technique has yet been shown to clearly reduce the risk of death due to lung cancer. Despite the popularity of screening, which has been promoted by direct-to-consumer marketing, there is currently no accepted screening technique for lung cancer. In fact, routine screening of asymptomatic individuals outside of a clinical trial, regardless of smoking status, could be harmful: the costs and risks of obtaining a diagnosis for a small pulmonary nodule can be high, and there is no proven benefit of early diagnosis (reviewed in Patz et al. [44] and Mulshine [48]).

CHEMOPREVENTION

Cigarette smokers experience an increased risk of multiple types of cancer because the carcinogens in cigarette smoke affect multiple tissues. Diffuse injury to the aerodigestive tract (field cancerization) predisposes smokers to multiple cancers in this area, among them lung and head and neck squamous cell cancers (HNSCC). Those who survive lung cancer or HNSCC are at high risk to develop a second primary tumor (SPT) and are therefore an appropriate group in which to study chemoprevention strategies.

A randomized, placebo-controlled trial of high-dose 13-*cis*-retinoic acid in patients who were disease free after treatment for HNSCC showed a dramatically reduced rate of SPTs (including lung cancers) in the treatment arm (6%) compared with the placebo arm (28%) (49). Significant toxicity was associated with the high-dose 13-*cis*-retinoic acid, however, prompting a Phase III trial of low-dose 13-*cis*-retinoic acid versus placebo in the same patient population (50). Unfortunately, in this trial there was no survival advantage or reduction in the rate of second primary tumors with low-dose 13-*cis*-retinoic acid. EUROSCAN was a randomized, placebo-controlled study of retinyl palmitate and *N*-acetylcysteine in patients with early-stage lung cancer and HNSCC (51). The treatment did not affect SPT occurrence. Similarly, US Intergroup NCI 91-0001 showed no effect of low-dose 13-*cis*-retinoic acid on SPT occurrence in patients with a history of stage I NSCLC (52). The results of the ATBC, CARET, and PHS trials are outlined above. None of these studies has shown any reduction in cancer risk in patients treated with beta-carotene, alpha-tocopherol, or retinyl palmitate.

Despite the negative findings in the majority of chemoprevention studies, there is still great interest in them because of the high mortality associated with lung cancer and the large population of current and former smokers who are at risk. Given the potential connection between inflammation and tumorigenesis and epidemiologic data supporting a preventive role in patients receiving selective COX-2 inhibitors (53), phase II studies are underway to assess the efficacy of COX-2 inhibition and other anti-inflammatory agents such as iloprost in high-risk groups for NSCLC (54).

■ MOLECULAR BIOLOGY

Advances in our understanding of the biology of lung cancer, coupled with new molecular-targeted therapies have lead to progress in the diagnosis and therapy of lung cancer. Carcinogenesis of lung cancer evolves through a multistep process involving multiple changes induced by carcinogens (eg, in cigarette smoke), as the bronchial epithelium progresses from normal to hyperplastic, dysplastic, carcinoma in situ (CIS), and finally invasive cancer. These steps can include activation of oncogenes, inactivation of tumor suppressor genes, and loss of genomic stability. These changes can be genetic (eg, deletion, mutation) or epigenetic (eg, methylation), and they control diverse processes, such as cell proliferation, differentiation, and apoptosis. Mutations in multiple tumor suppressor genes and oncogenes have been associated with the development of NSCLC (Tables 15-4 and 15-5).

Cytogenetic studies of lung cancer have revealed a large number of chromosomal abnormalities, several of which are nonrandom. Allelic loss is one mechanism for loss of tumor suppressor genes. Commonly identified chromosomal deletions involve the 3p, 6p, 8p, 9p, 11p, 13q, 17p, and 19q arms, among others (55). Some of these changes are also found in the normal-appearing bronchial epithelium of smokers and former smokers, further supporting the multistep hypothesis of cancer development and a role for genes on these chromosomes in the early stages of lung cancer pathogenesis. Recent analysis of a large collection of snap-frozen resection specimens by dense single nucleotide polymorphism arrays revealed that 26 of 39 autosomal chromosome arms had consistent large-scale copy-number

TABLE 15-4	ONCOGENES COMMONLY EXPRESSED IN LUNG CANCER				
Protooncogene	*SCLC*	*NSCLC*	*Note*	*Reference*
K-*ras* mutation	Rare	15-20%	More common in adenocarcinoma	190, 191
Myc amplification	10-40%	5-10%		190, 192
HER-2/neu increased expression	30%	19-33%	Rare gene amplification	192, 193
BCL-2	90%	25%		190, 194, 195
EGFR	0%	40-80%		196, 197
Telomerase activity	100%	10-35%		198

TABLE
15-5 | **TUMOR SUPPRESSOR GENES WITH DECREASED EXPRESSION IN LUNG CANCER**

Tumor Suppressor	SCLC	NSCLC	Note	Reference
p53 mutation	80-90%	50-60%		57, 190
Rb inactivation	>90%	15-30%		190, 191
FHIT abnormal transcript	80%	42%	Candidate on chromosome 3p	199
P16 protein expression	95%	60%	Protein expression lost via methylation	190, 200
P16 protein inactivation	<10%	30-70%		
Chromosome 3p	90%	50%	Unknown tumor suppressor	190

changes (gain or loss), with 24 recurrent focal amplifications and 7 homozygous deletions (56). The majority of changes are not associated with any currently known mutations and therefore represent potential new oncogenes. These findings also highlight the significant genetic heterogeneity found in NSCLC and emphasize the need for greater stratification of patients when thinking about application of targeted therapies.

Two of the most extensively studied tumor suppressor genes are *p53* and retinoblastoma (*Rb*). The *p53* gene produces a nuclear phosphoprotein important for DNA repair, growth regulation, cell division, and programmed cell death (apoptosis). Under normal conditions, p53 production is increased when DNA damage occurs, arresting the cell in the G1 phase to allow for DNA repair. Absent DNA repair, the cell is diverted toward apoptosis. When mutation or deletion occurs in the *p53* gene, the abnormal cell is allowed to proceed to S phase, further propagating the genetic damage, which can lead to cancer. Inherited lesions of *p53* have been found in the Li-Fraumeni syndrome, which is associated with an increased incidence of brain cancer, breast cancer, soft tissue sarcomas, and lung cancer. Mutations in *p53* are found in 50 to 60% of NSCLC. The type of *p53* mutation in those exposed to cigarette smoke is different from the mutations found in those exposed to other carcinogens, such as radon (*p53* mutations are reviewed in Szak et al. [57]). The *Rb* gene codes for a nuclear phosphoprotein that is an important regulator of the cell cycle. Mutations of the *Rb* gene are very common in patients with SCLC. However, only 15 to 30% of tumor specimens from NSCLC have *Rb* inactivation.

Each member of the *ras* family of oncogenes (H-*ras*, N-*ras*, and K-*ras*) codes for a 21-kDa guanine-binding protein that mediates signal transduction pathways from cell surface receptors to intracellular molecules. The *ras* oncogene can be activated by point mutations that lead to unregulated, constitutive activation; by

overexpression; or by amplification. K-*ras* mutations are commonly found in NSCLC, especially in patients with a history of smoking and in adenocarcinoma histology. Some trials have demonstrated an adverse prognosis in patients with K-*ras* mutation after resection of lung adenocarcinoma (58,59), although there is limited evidence that K-*ras* mutation is predictive of response to conventional chemotherapy (60). Current ASCO guidelines also note that the current data are too limited to incorporate K-*ras* mutation testing into clinical decision making (61). For *ras* to function in signal transduction, it must attach to the plasma membrane. This requires a specific posttranslational modification called farnesylation. Farnesyl transferase inhibitors (FTIs) abrogate *ras* activity *in vitro*, therefore prompting clinical testing, but have failed to demonstrate benefit in three Phase II clinical trials for NSCLC (62).

Several different cell-surface receptor tyrosine kinases (RTKs) are expressed in NSCLC and might promote tumor progression by activating mutations, by overexpression, or by responding to inappropriate autocrine or paracrine growth factor production. In NSCLC, RTKs that are frequently upregulated or amplified include epidermal growth factor receptor (EGFR), *Her-2/neu*, c-*met*, insulin-like growth factor (IGF) receptor, c-*kit*, and others. Additionally, a new fusion protein (EML4-ALK) has been identified as the oncogenic driver in a subset of patients with NSCLC (63). Among the growth factors produced by tumor and stromal cells are EGF, transforming growth factor–alpha (TGF-α), TGF-β, platelet-derived growth factor (PDGF), parathyroid hormone–related protein (PTHrP), IGF, hepatocyte growth factor (HGF), and others.

The best-studied of the RTKs in NSCLC is EGFR, which is commonly expressed in NSCLC. Blockade of EGFR by specific antibodies or tyrosine kinase inhibitors leads to cell-cycle arrest and cell death *in vitro*, inhibits tumor growth *in vivo*, and has become an intensely studied area in NSCLC. EGFR as a therapeutic target is discussed in more detail later in the chapter.

■ HISTOLOGY

The majority of lung tumors arise from epithelial cells and are called bronchogenic carcinomas. Neuroendocrine tumors also arise in the lung and can appear as small cell lung cancer (SCLC), carcinoids, or large cell neuroendocrine carcinomas. Bronchogenic carcinomas include NSCLCs, a category comprising three major types: adenocarcinoma, squamous cell carcinoma (SCC), and large cell carcinoma. The proportion of adenocarcinoma cases has been increasing since the late 1960s in both smokers and never smokers. Reasons for this increase have not been established but might include changes in smoking habits and the use of low-tar or filtered cigarettes.

NSCLCs are classified according to features detectable by light microscopy (Table 15-6) (64). Immunohistochemistry is used in conjunction with light microscopy to distinguish between primary and metastatic adenocarcinoma, determine neuroendocrine features, diagnose mesotheliomas, and determine the presence of specific targets for selection of therapy (eg, EGFR mutation). Electron microscopy is rarely used. Pulmonary adenocarcinomas usually stain positive for cytokeratin 7, thyroid transcription factor 1 (TTF-1), and surfactant apoprotein A and are negative for cytokeratin 20. Metastatic adenocarcinomas from other sites except the thyroid stain negative for TTF-1. All carcinoids and most SCLCs stain positive for chromogranin and synaptophysin, whereas NSCLC is usually negative for these two markers. Mesothelioma is distinguished from adenocarcinoma by the presence of calretinin and cytokeratin 5/6 and the absence of carcinoembryonic antigen (CEA), B72.3, Ber-EP4, and MOC-31.

In some cases, the exact histologic subtype of NSCLC cannot be determined; however, as long as NSCLC can be clearly documented, therapeutic plans can proceed.

ADENOCARCINOMA

Adenocarcinoma is the most common subtype of NSCLC in the United States and constitutes 41% of all NSCLC cases (65). Although adenocarcinoma is associated with smoking, it is especially predominant among women and nonsmokers. These tumors are classically peripheral and arise from surface epithelium or bronchial mucosal glands and as peripheral scar

TABLE 15-6	THE 2004 WHO/INTERNATIONAL ASSOCIATION FOR THE STUDY OF LUNG CANCER HISTOLOGIC CLASSIFICATION OF INVASIVE MALIGNANT EPITHELIAL TUMORS

Squamous cell carcinoma
    Variants: papillary, clear cell, small cell, basaloid
Small cell carcinoma
    Variants: combined small cell carcinoma
Adenocarcinoma
    Acinar
    Papillary
    Bronchoalveolar carcinoma
        Non-mucinous (Clara cell/type II pneumocyte type)
        Mucinous (goblet cell type)
        Mixed mucinous and non-mucinous (Clara cell/type II) pneumocyte and goblet cell type) or indeterminate
    Solid adenocarcinoma with mucin formation
    Mixed
    Variants: well-differentiated fetal adenocarcinoma, mucinous ("colloid"), mucinous cystadenocarcinoma, signet ring, clear cell
Large cell carcinoma
    Variants: large cell neuroendocine carcinoma, combined large cell neuroendocine carcinoma, basaloid carcinoma, lymphoepithelioma-like carcinoma, clear cell carcinoma, large cell carcinoma with rhabdoid phenotype
Adenosquamous carcinoma
Carcinomas with pleomorphic, sarcomatoid or sarcomatous elements
    Carcinoma with spindle and/or giant cells
    Pleomorphic carcinoma
    Spindle cell carcinoma
    Giant cell carcinoma
Carcinosarcoma
    Blastoma (pulmonary blastoma)
    Others
Carcinoid tumor
    Typical carcinoid
    Atypical carcinoid
Carcinomas of salivary gland type
    Mucoepidermoid carcinoma
    Adenocystic carcinoma, others
Unclassified carcinoma

Data from The 2004 WHO/International Association for the Study of Lung Cancer Histologic Classification of Invasive Malignant Epithelial Tumors.

carcinomas. On histologic examination, adenocarcinoma demonstrates gland formation, papillary structures, or mucin production (Fig. 15-1).

Patients with adenocarcinoma frequently present with metastatic disease before symptoms of the primary cancer are evident. Pulmonary adenocarcinoma can be associated with hypertrophic pulmonary osteoarthropathy and Trousseau syndrome. The bronchoalveolar subtype

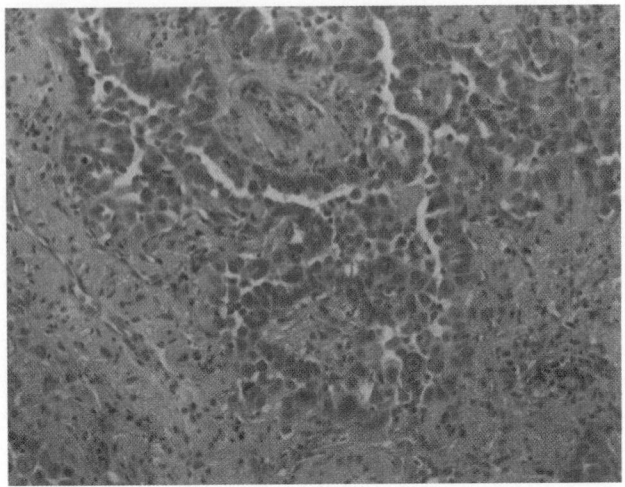

FIGURE 15-1. Adenocarcinoma. Photomicrograph of adenocarcinoma of the lung stained with hematoxylin and eosin. (*Courtesy of Cesar Moran, MD.*)

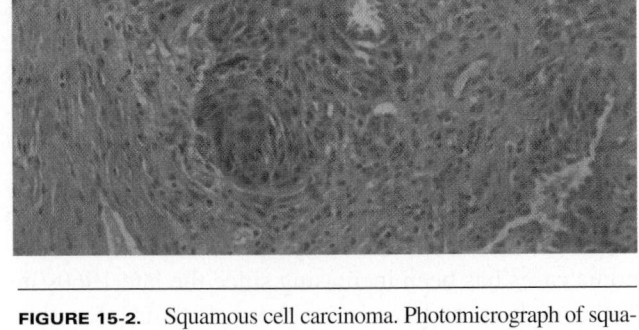

FIGURE 15-2. Squamous cell carcinoma. Photomicrograph of squamous cell carcinoma of the lung stained with hematoxylin and eosin. (*Courtesy of Cesar Moran, MD.*)

of adenocarcinoma is a distinct clinicopathologic entity. It can present as a solitary peripheral nodule, multicentric disease, or rapidly progressing pneumonic involvement. It can occur as early as the second decade of life; the characteristic clinical presentation is multiple pulmonary nodules.

SQUAMOUS CELL CARCINOMA

Squamous cell carcinoma (SCC), or epidermoid carcinoma, formerly the most common subtype of NSCLC, is now the second most frequent, accounting for 34% of NSCLC (65). This tumor arises most frequently in the proximal bronchi. Because of its central location and the tendency of these cells to exfoliate, SCC can often be detected by cytologic examination of the sputum. With time, these tumors tend to cause bronchial obstruction, with resultant atelectasis or pneumonia. They also tend to remain localized and cavitate.

Of all the subtypes of NSCLC, the squamous cell variety has the strongest association with smoking. Pathologically, it is characterized by visible keratinization, with prominent desmosomes and intercellular bridges (Fig. 15-2). Increased secretion of a PTHrP in SCC has led to the association of this subtype with hypercalcemia.

LARGE CELL CARCINOMA

The least common subtype of NSCLC, large cell carcinoma, accounts for approximately 8% of all NSCLCs

(Fig. 15-3). Refinements in histopathologic techniques have led to the diagnosis of adenocarcinoma or SCC in cases previously diagnosed as undifferentiated large cell carcinoma.

OTHER TYPES

Other, uncommon types of NSCLC are adenosquamous carcinoma and carcinoma with pleomorphic, sarcomatoid, or sarcomatous elements.

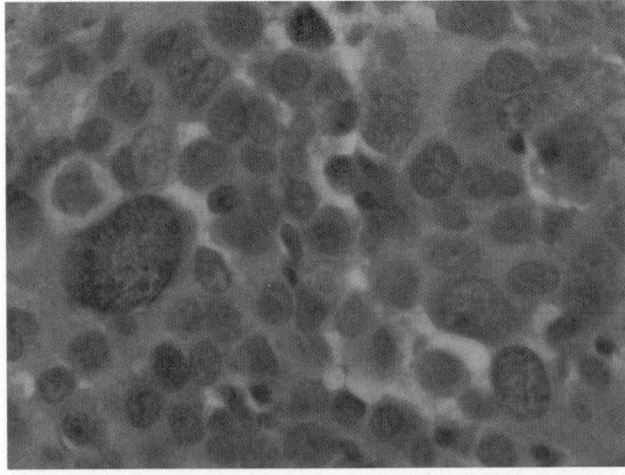

FIGURE 15-3. Large cell carcinoma. Photomicrograph of large cell carcinoma of the lung stained with hematoxylin and eosin. (*Courtesy of Cesar Moran, MD.*)

■ CLINICAL PRESENTATION

The signs and symptoms of lung cancer are related to the specific locations of tumor masses and the occurrence of paraneoplastic syndromes. Some patients present asymptomatically with a lung mass discovered on a routine chest x-ray or "screening" CT scan; the number of patients who fall into this category might increase if screening for lung cancer increases. The symptoms of centrally located lesions include cough, hemoptysis, wheezing, stridor, dyspnea, and postobstructive pneumonia. Peripheral lesions can cause pain due to pleural or chest wall invasion, cough, or restrictive dyspnea.

Lesions involving the intrathoracic nerves can cause several syndromes. Pancoast syndrome, which is characterized by shoulder pain radiating to the arm in an ulnar distribution, is caused by tumor invasion of the eighth cervical and first thoracic nerves in the superior sulcus. Horner syndrome, which consists of enophthalmos, ptosis, miosis, and ipsilateral dyshidrosis, can be caused by extension of the tumor into the paravertebral sympathetic nerves.

Because the left recurrent laryngeal nerve passes through the aorticopulmonary window, it is susceptible to injury secondary to mediastinal lymph node involvement. Such injury causes vocal cord paralysis, with subsequent hoarseness. Tumor invasion of the mediastinum can cause paralysis of the phrenic nerve, which in turn can cause elevation of the hemidiaphragm.

Patients with pleural effusions often present with dyspnea or cough. Pericardial effusions secondary to pericardial invasion can cause shortness of breath, orthopnea, tachycardia, chest pain, and physical signs of tamponade. Superior vena cava syndrome with swelling of the face and arm and superficial venous engorgement can be caused by either a central tumor in the right lung or mediastinal lymphadenopathy. Dysphagia can result from compression of the esophagus.

NSCLC is frequently metastatic, and symptoms secondary to metastases are common. The most common sites for metastases are listed in Table 15-7.

TABLE 15-7	MOST COMMON SITES OF LUNG CANCER METASTASES
Hilar and mediastinal lymph nodes	
Pleura	
Opposite lung	
Liver	
Adrenal gland	
Bone	
Central nervous system	

Bone metastases can be associated with pain, pathologic fractures, or spinal cord compression. Liver metastases are often asymptomatic but can be associated with pain or jaundice. Central nervous system metastases are often indicated by seizures, headache, nausea, vomiting, altered mental status, or focal neurologic signs. Weight loss due to tumor-related cachexia is a very common presenting symptom and an independent adverse prognostic factor.

The production of ectopic hormones or hormone-like substances is not uncommon in lung cancer and results in paraneoplastic syndromes. These have been described most commonly with SCLC but also occur in NSCLC. Cancer cachexia is the only paraneoplastic syndrome that is common in NSCLC. It is characterized by weight loss, impaired immune function, weakness, and decline in performance status. Weight loss in this setting is distinct from that due to poor nutritional intake or anorexia caused by tumor involvement of the gastrointestinal tract. The exact mechanism for development of cachexia is unknown, but tumor-elaborated cytokines have been implicated. Cancer cachexia is difficult to treat. Nutritional supplementation is generally not beneficial. Megestrol acetate therapy does lead to weight gain. Presumably, successful treatment of the underlying cancer would be the ideal treatment.

Hypercalcemia, caused by ectopic production of a PTHrP or bone metastases, is the second most frequent paraneoplastic syndrome in NSCLC. PTHrP acts on the bones to stimulate bone resorption and promotes phosphate wasting by the kidneys. Hypercalcemia is most commonly associated with the squamous cell subtype.

Hypertrophic pulmonary osteoarthropathy (HPO) is characterized by arthropathy and clubbing of the fingers and toes. Although clubbing is common in those with NSCLC, HPO is distinguished by the presence of periostitis of the long bones (Fig. 15-4). Radionucleotide bone scans are more sensitive to the periosteal changes than plain radiographs. The etiology of HPO is unknown. HPO is more common in cases of adenocarcinoma and large cell carcinoma than in SCC.

Several other paraneoplastic syndromes are seen rarely in NSCLC. The syndrome of inappropriate anti-diuretic hormone (SIADH) is more common in SCLC but also occurs in NSCLC. SIADH is characterized by hyponatremia and serum hypoosmolarity. Hematologic manifestations of NSCLC include anemia, leukocytosis, thrombocytosis, and Trousseau syndrome with deep vein thrombosis and pulmonary embolism.

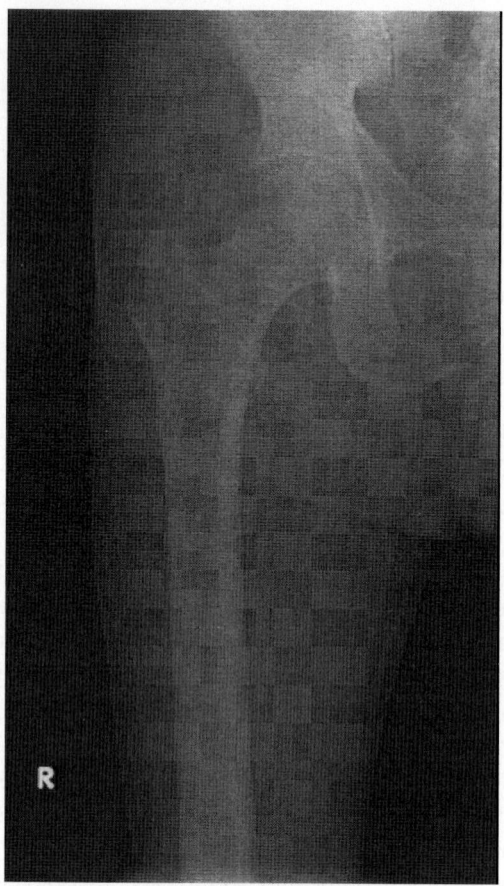 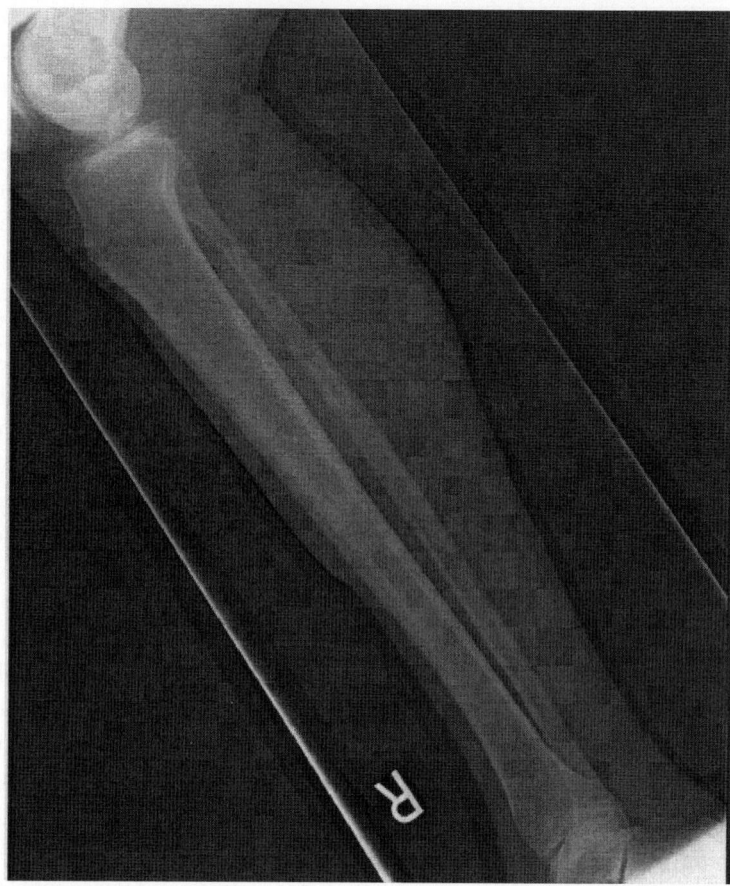

FIGURE 15-4. Hypertrophic pulmonary osteoarthropathy (HPO). This 62-year-old man with NSCLC reported a 1-month history of finger clubbing and arthritic lower extremity pain. The plain radiographs of the lower extremities show periosteal reaction in both femora as well as in bilateral tibias/fibulas that is consistent with HPO.

■ DIAGNOSIS

SOLITARY PULMONARY NODULE

A solitary pulmonary nodule (SPN) is a single mass, usually found incidentally on chest x-ray, that is surrounded by lung tissue, is well circumscribed, measures less than 3 cm, and does not show evidence of mediastinal or hilar adenopathy. Nodules which are larger than 3 cm, have associated adenopathy, invade the chest wall or hilum, or are likely to be malignant must be biopsied. The differential diagnosis of SPN must include primary cancer, metastatic cancer, infection, benign tumors (eg, hamartomas), vascular abnormalities, and inflammation (eg, granulomatous disease) (66).

SPN represents a diagnostic dilemma. Review of previous chest x-rays is the single most important step in evaluating an SPN. Lesions that are unchanged for 2 years are considered benign. A CT scan of the chest with contrast is essential to determine whether other nodules, adenopathy, or chest wall invasion is present. Among the radiologic characteristics suggesting a benign process are distinct margins, high-density on diagnostic CT scan, and certain calcification patterns, such as diffuse solid, central-core bull's eye (granuloma), "popcorn ball" (hamartoma), or concentric layers. Although radiologic tests alone are not sufficient to conclusively rule out malignancy, these calcification patterns indicate benign disease (67). Positron emission tomography (PET) using the glucose analog 18-fluorodeoxyglucose (FDG-PET) takes advantage of the fact that malignant tissues tend to take up glucose more avidly than does normal tissue. FDG-PET is used in the evaluation of SPNs. False positives are seen when inflammatory or infectious lesions are present. False negatives occur when the tumors are smaller than 1 cm and when the cancer is of a type that does not take up glucose avidly, such as carcinoid tumor or bronchoalveolar carcinoma. In a meta-analysis of 1474 focal pulmonary lesions, the mean sensitivity and specificity of FDG-PET were 96 and 73%, respectively (68). The negative and positive predictive value of PET for pulmonary nodules and masses is about 90% (69).

Pathologic diagnosis in specimens obtained by fine-needle aspiration (FNA), transbronchial biopsy, or resection is needed in any SPN that is growing. Any new lesion that does not contain benign calcifications and measures greater than 5 mm also requires pathologic diagnosis. A "watch and wait" strategy, with reimaging by CT scan at 3, 6, 12, and 24 months after PET, is reasonable in the low-risk patient (ie, age <40 years and nonsmoker) with a lesion that does not show up in FDG-PET scans and that measures less than 2 cm.

The majority of SPNs are benign. The Early Lung Cancer Action Project (ELCAP) study enrolled 1000 asymptomatic smokers and former smokers at least 60 years old (45). Baseline chest x-ray and low-dose CT were carried out on all participants. Nodules that contained benign calcifications, had smooth margins, and measured less than 2 cm were considered benign and not investigated further. Nodules that did not meet these criteria were investigated using serial CT scans (if less than 5 mm) or using surgical biopsy (if larger). Thirty-five percent of the solitary nodules detected by low-dose CT had benign calcifications. CT detected solitary noncalcified pulmonary nodules in 159 participants; 12% of these were malignant. Larger nodules were more likely to be malignant (Table 15-8). The Dutch-Belgian randomized lung cancer screening trial (Nederlands-Leuvens Longkanker Screenings Onderzoek, NELSON) also incorporated volumetric changes on a second scan of any noncalcified pulmonary nodules, which by this screening algorithm eliminated the majority of indeterminate scans (70). This study identified 196 positive scans out of 7557 participants, of which 70 were found to have lung cancer and 7 were found to have metastases from a non-lung cancer.

PULMONARY MASS

An accurate pathologic diagnosis is essential to the management of lung cancer. A complete history, physical examination, chest x-ray, and CT of the chest and upper abdomen will reveal the extent of disease in the chest and detect any disease at the most likely metastatic sites. An easily biopsied lesion in such a location as a supraclavicular lymph node might be found by physical examination or CT. In patients with a central tumor, sputum cytology may yield a diagnosis. Alternatively, flexible fiberoptic bronchoscopy is appropriate for central lesions. For lesions that can be visualized endoscopically, diagnoses are made in 97% of tumors by a combination of biopsies, bronchial washings, and bronchial brushings. Only 55% of lung cancers can be diagnosed using only bronchial brushings and washings when the lesion is peripheral and cannot be visualized. Percutaneous transthoracic FNA of pulmonary nodules can be useful in some clinical settings. It is usually performed under fluoroscopic or CT guidance. Negative results on FNA biopsy must be considered indeterminate until the diagnosis is established by another method. The diagnosis might be confirmed by results from cytologic analysis of malignant pleural effusions or FNA biopsy of metastases to lymph nodes, liver, adrenal glands, or bone. Mediastinoscopy or endobronchial ultrasound (EBUS) can be used to obtain biopsy samples from the mediastinal nodes.

STAGING

Once the histologic diagnosis of NSCLC has been established, the extent of disease must be determined (Fig. 15-5).

The stage of disease will dictate therapy. All patients must undergo a complete history and physical examination, chest x-ray, and CT scan of the chest and upper abdomen (to include the adrenal glands), a complete blood count, and blood chemistry tests that include electrolyte and liver enzyme studies. This evaluation may suggest sites of extrathoracic spread, which should be confirmed using appropriate imaging studies. For example, bone pain or elevations in serum calcium or alkaline phosphatase should prompt a radionuclide bone scan and plain radiographs of the affected area. The routine use of CT scanning or magnetic resonance imaging (MRI) of the brain in asymptomatic patients remains controversial and is probably not cost-effective. If stage IV disease is identified by this staging evaluation, then no further workup is needed. For stage I-III NSCLC,

TABLE 15-8	FREQUENCY OF MALIGNANT DISEASE BY SIZE OF SOLITARY PULMONARY NODULE				
Size of noncalcified nodule by screening CT	2-5 mm	6-10 mm	11-20 mm	21-45 mm	All sizes
Rate of malignant disease	1%	24%	33%	80%	12%

Adapted, with permission, from Detterbeck FC, Boffa DJ, Tanoue LT. The new lung cancer staging system. Chest, 2009;136(1):260-71.

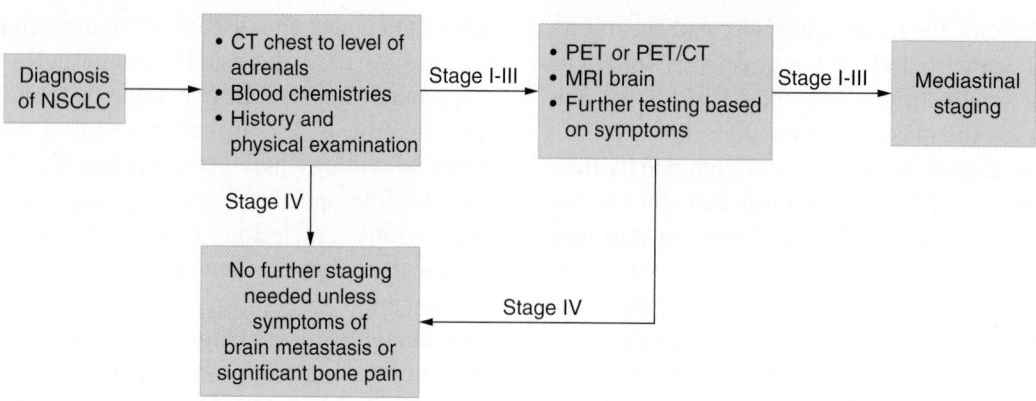

FIGURE 15-5. Staging algorithm for NSCLC. See text for details.

a ^{18}F-fluorodeoxyglucose (FDG)-positron emission tomography (PET) should be performed to evaluate mediastinal nodes and for distant metastasis.

PET can be used to identify enlarged nodes in the mediastinum that do not contain cancer and small nodes that do contain cancer. In this setting, the specificity and sensitivity of PET are 96 and 83%, respectively (69). Thus, if a false-positive result on PET would result in the patients not receiving potentially curative surgery, mediastinoscopy or endobronchial ultrasound (EBUS) is indicated to confirm the presence of cancer. PET is also used to identify distant metastasis. Again, any finding of cancer on PET must be confirmed by plain radiography, CT, or MRI or must be confirmed pathologically if the types of lesion(s) identified by PET could affect the therapeutic approach. The use of combined PET and CT might improve the accuracy of PET scanning (70). Owing to poor uptake of FDG, PET usually does not detect bronchoalveolar cancer.

The most important question that the staging evaluation must answer is whether the patient is a candidate for surgery. In patients with no evidence of distant metastasis, staging of mediastinal disease is critical in planning therapy. Mediastinoscopy can reveal unsuspected tumor spread to the mediastinal lymph nodes and thereby avoid unnecessary thoracotomy and resection. Recent evidence also indicates that endobronchial ultrasound (EBUS) with lymph node biopsies can be used for appropriate staging of the mediastinum (see Box Commentary). Routine use of mediastinoscopy or EBUS in patients with a normal-appearing mediastinum on PET-CT scans is controversial.

After the completion of staging evaluation, the disease is assigned a TNM stage (Figs. 15-6–15-13;

Tables 15-9 and 15-10). The TNM staging for NSCLC was revised in the recently updated 7th edition of the AJCC/UICC staging system (72), based upon recommendations from the International Association for the Study of Lung Cancer staging project (3). The recommendations were founded upon the compilation of outcomes from more than 100,000 cases worldwide in the decade 1990-2000, and therefore better define prognosis versus stage given modern treatment regimens (72). Additionally, in the new system there appear to be meaningful differences in the percentage of patients who may be considered to have resectable disease (73).

Clinical staging has inherent inaccuracies and therefore typically underestimates the true extent of disease. Because of this feature, clinical staging shows higher mortality rates than would be expected at the same pathologic disease stage and necessitates that in patients who undergo surgical tumor resection, surgical/pathologic staging should be done to predict recurrence and to evaluate the need for possible adjuvant therapy. Patients' 5-year survival rates by tumor stage are shown in Table 15-11.

■ TREATMENT

STAGES I AND II DISEASE

Surgery is standard treatment for stages I and II NSCLC (Figs. 15-14 and 15-15). Adjuvant therapy may be offered to patients following resection (see below).

Despite thorough investigation prior to surgery, many patients are found to have more extensive disease during thoracotomy. A complete ipsilateral mediastinal lymph node dissection or systematic sampling should

Commentary: Mediastinal Lymph Node Sampling Using Endobronchial Ultrasound and Transbronchial Needle Aspiration

Accurate mediastinal lymph node staging is a critical aspect of non–small cell lung cancer (NSCLC) management. Non-invasive staging typically relies on a combination of computed tomography (CT) and ^{18}F-fluorodeoxyglucose (FDG)–positron emission tomography (PET) data to detect mediastinal metastases. Lymph nodes are considered abnormal by CT criteria if the short-axis diameter is >10 mm, however both false negatives and false positives are possible. FDG-PET scanning has been a welcome addition to the staging armamentarium and increases diagnostic accuracy. However, limitations of non-invasive staging modalities remain and current guidelines recommend tissue sampling by invasive means to improve diagnostic accuracy among patients whose subsequent therapy is contingent on mediastinal involvement.

Multiple modalities are available for sampling mediastinal and hilar lymph nodes. These range from minimally invasive approaches such as endobronchial ultrasound–guided transbronchial needle aspiration (EBUS-TBNA), endoscopic ultrasound guided–fine-needle aspiration (EUS-FNA), and CT-guided needle aspiration to surgical approaches such as mediastinoscopy and thoracotomy.

EBUS-TBNA is a relatively new technology that adapts and miniaturizes endoscopic ultrasound for use in the tracheobronchial tree. An integrated ultrasonic bronchoscope allows for real time image–guided transbronchial needle aspiration biopsy of lymph nodes in proximity to the central airways. EBUS-TBNA is currently our preferred method for assessing mediastinal lymph node involvement. It is a minimally invasive procedure that is typically performed on an outpatient basis and often utilizes only moderate sedation. Biopsies can be taken at all lymph node stations adjacent to a major airway and as such, EBUS-TBNA can sample more lymph nodes in a single procedure than any other invasive mediastinal tissue sampling technique. Furthermore, rather than merely confirming malignancy in an enlarged or FDG-avid lymph node, true lymph node mapping can be carried out using this technology. It can be safely performed in most patients, including those that have undergone prior surgical or radiation therapy to the thorax. The risk profile is minimal and similar to the risks of standard bronchoscopy. Numerous studies have documented the safety and diagnostic accuracy of EBUS-TBNA in staging lung cancer. Importantly, EBUS-TBNA has shown significant utility even in patients with radiologically normal mediastinum.

While cervical mediastinoscopy is still considered the reference standard for invasive mediastinal lymph node sampling, it is difficult to repeat, is more invasive, and has higher associated morbidity and mortality than EBUS-TBNA, with preliminary data suggesting diagnostic equivalence.

In summary, EBUS-TBNA provides a safe, minimally invasive, and highly accurate method of mediastinal lymph node sampling and it has rapidly become part of our standard practice in the mediastinal staging of NSCLC.

George A. Eapen

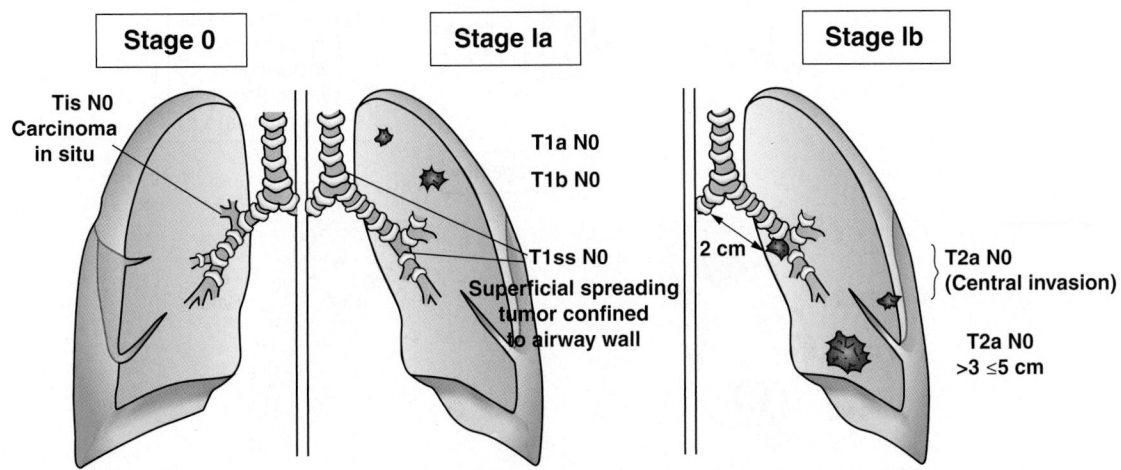

FIGURE 15-6. Stages 0-Ib. Illustration of primary tumor (T) characteristics defining the differences between stages 0, Ia, and Ib. *(Adapted, with permission, from Detterbeck FC, Boffa DJ, Tanoue LT. The new lung cancer staging system. Chest 2009;136[1]:260-71.)*

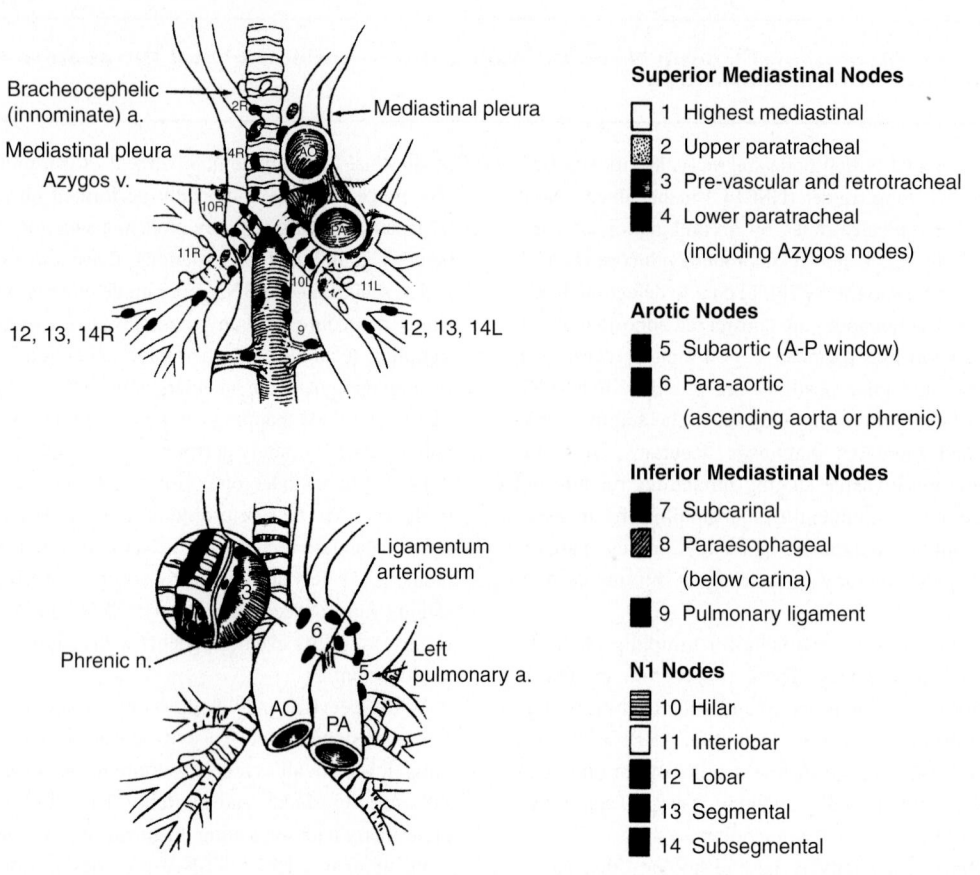

FIGURE 15-7. Classification of regional lymph nodes. *(Adapted, with permission, from Mountain CF, Libshitz HI, Hermes KE. Lung Cancer: A Handbook for Staging, Imaging, and Lymph Node Classification. Houston: Charles P. Young; 1999.)*

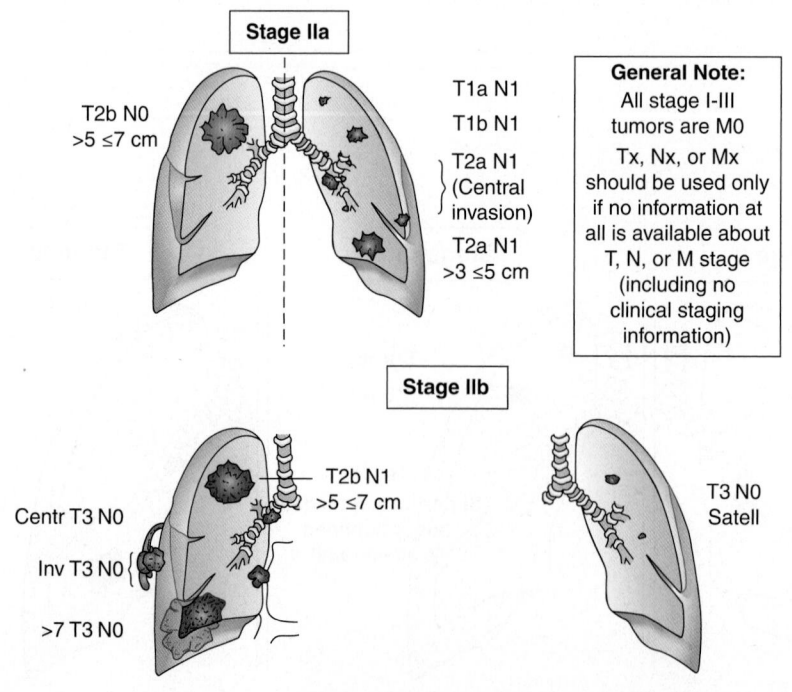

FIGURE 15-8. Stage II. Illustration of primary tumor (T) and lymph node (N) characteristics defining stages IIa and IIb. *(Adapted, with permission, from Detterbeck FC, Boffa DJ, Tanoue LT. The new lung cancer staging system. Chest 2009;136[1]:260-71.)*

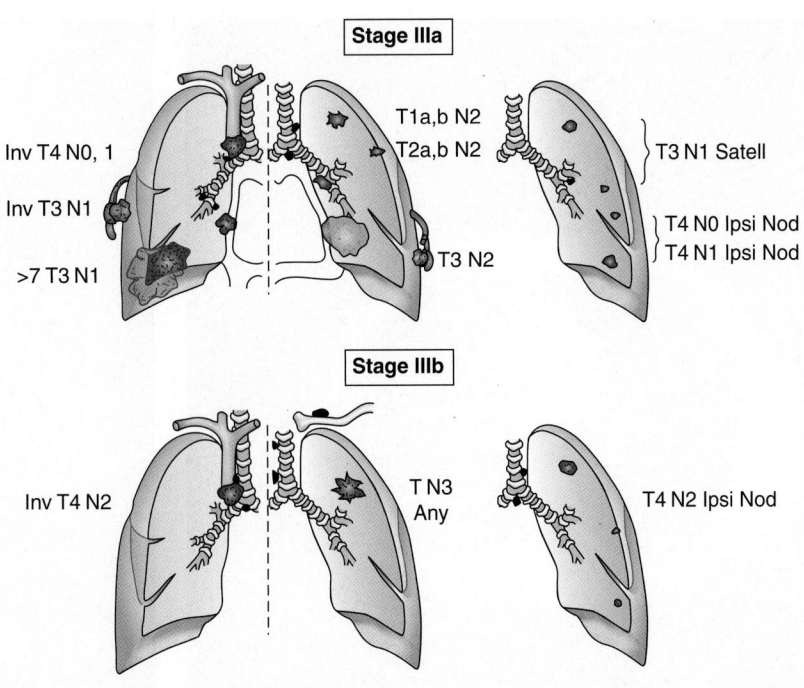

FIGURE 15-9. Stage III. Illustration of primary tumor (T) and lymph node (N) characteristics defining stages IIIa and IIIb *(Adapted, with permission, from Detterbeck FC, Boffa DJ, Tanoue LT. The new lung cancer staging system. Chest 2009;136[1]:260-71.)*

be done to stage the disease accurately (74). At MDACC, the current practice is to perform a complete lymph node dissection at the time of surgery. This provides more accurate pathologic staging. The extent of lung resection will be dictated by the size and location

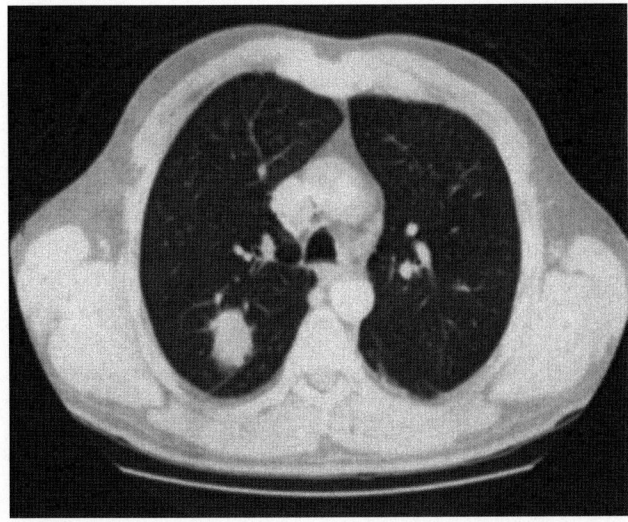

FIGURE 15-10. Stage I NSCLC. This T2, N0, M0 NSCLC was an incidental finding when the patient presented with an unrelated medical illness. The CT of the chest revealed a 3.8- by 3.1-cm right-upper-lobe mass with no hilar or mediastinal adenopathy. Pathologic staging after a right-upper lobectomy and mediastinal lymph node dissection confirmed the clinical stage.

of the tumor. The entire tumor must be resected, with margins negative for cancer. Wedge resection and segmentectomy are associated with higher rates of local recurrence than lobectomy and pneumonectomy and are not considered standard care (75).

Although a healthy individual can easily recover from a pneumonectomy, most patients with NSCLC are older smokers with COPD and compromised pulmonary reserve. Any patient who is being considered for surgery must undergo pulmonary function tests (PFTs) to assess the ability to withstand pulmonary resection. Split-lung function studies can further help to predict lung function after the planned resection. There is no one accepted value, criterion, or cutoff for pulmonary resection. Published criteria that have been shown to predict high risk for lung resection include estimated posttreatment FVC under 2 L, FEV_1 under 1 L, and DL_{CO} less than 40 to 60% (76,77).

Some patients with early-stage lung cancer cannot undergo surgery because of poor pulmonary reserve or other medical illness. These "medically inoperable" patients might be able to tolerate radiotherapy with curative intent. Historically radiotherapy outcomes are inferior to surgery for early-stage disease, resulting in a 5-year survival of approximately 20 to 40% in patients with stage I disease (78,79). However, several case series have demonstrated that stereotactic radiosurgery (SRS) is a promising new treatment modality for early

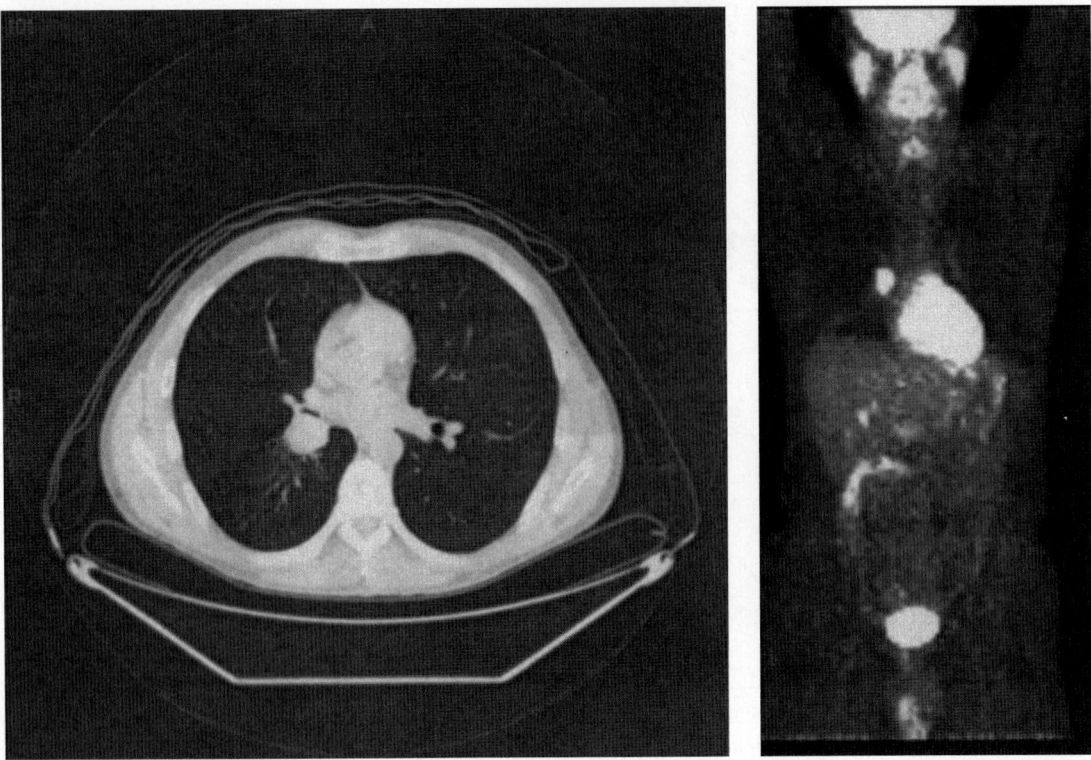

FIGURE 15-11.   Stage II NSCLC. This patient presented with symptoms of pneumonia and was found to have a right hilar mass impinging on the right-lower-lobe bronchus and a right-lower-lobe infiltrate by CT scan. PET scan showed increased uptake in the hilar mass and physiologic uptake. Staging evaluation showed no distant metastatic disease. He underwent a right-middle and lower lobectomy with a mediastinal lymph node dissection. This revealed a 3.1-cm primary squamous cell carcinoma with two positive hilar nodes and no involved mediastinal nodes (T2, N1, M0).

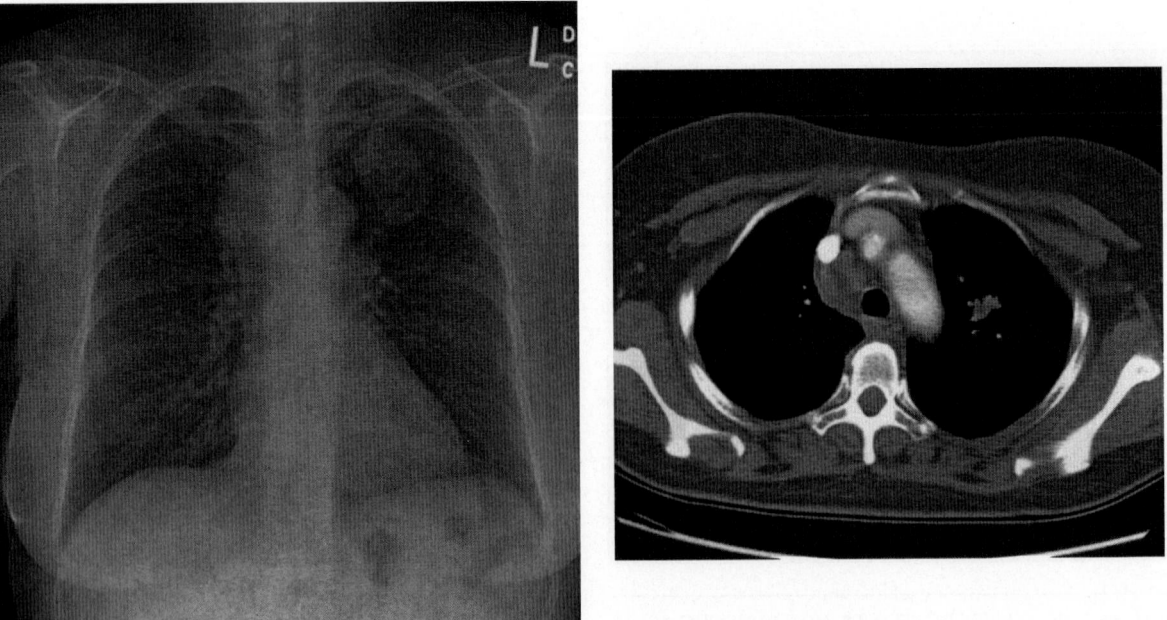

FIGURE 15-12.   Stage IIIB NSCLC. This patient presented with chest pain, and the chest x-ray (*left*) showed an approximately 4.0- by 3.0-cm mass in the left upper lobe and an additional mass in the right mediastinum. Initial CT revealed a 4.5-cm mass in the left upper lobe and a 5-cm mass in the paratracheal region. Biopsy confirmed NSCLC. Staging evaluation showed no distant metastatic disease (T2, N3, M0). The patient was treated with concurrent chemotherapy and radiotherapy. The posttreatment CT (*right*) showed significant therapeutic response.

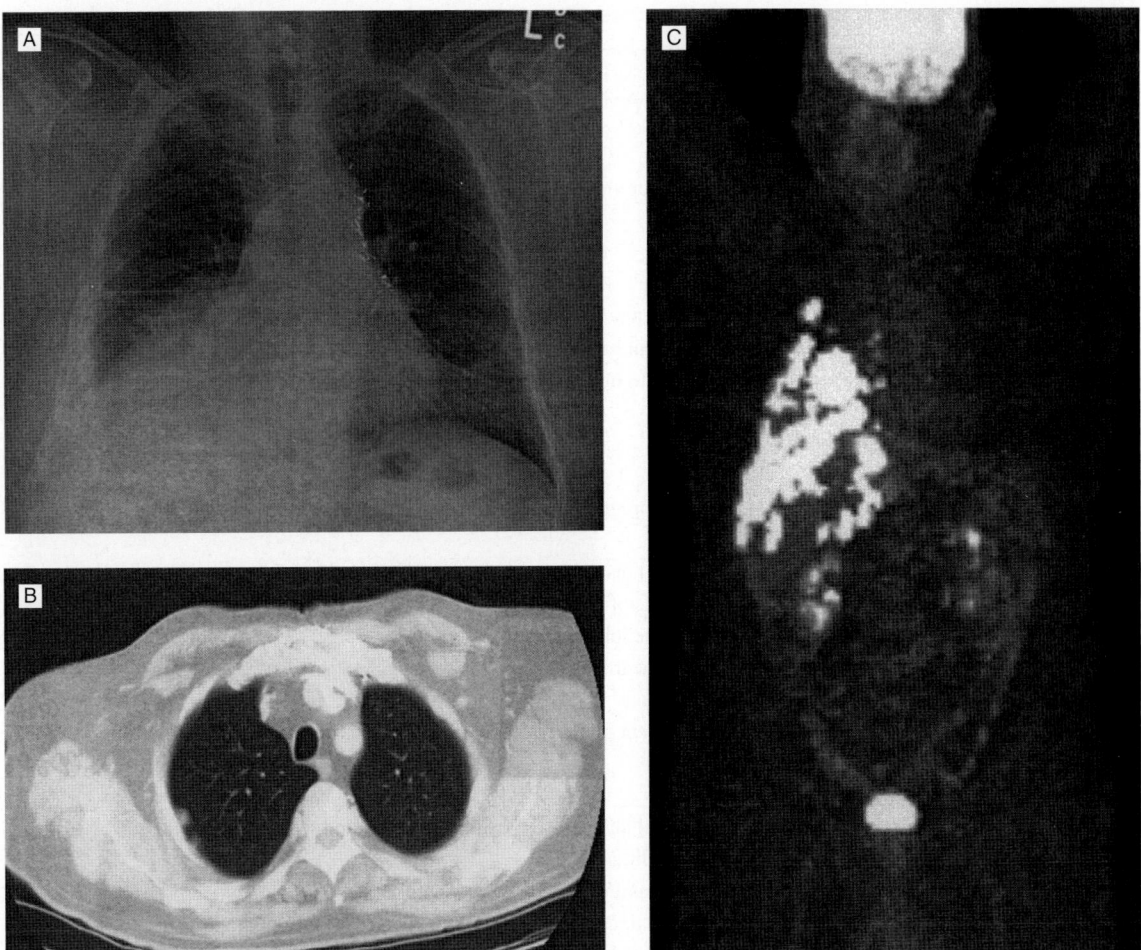

FIGURE 15-13. Stage IV NSCLC. Upon evaluation for back pain, this patient was found to have a pleural effusion, and biopsy revealed NSCLC. PET/CT revealed a 5.4- by 3.6-cm hypermetabolic mass in the right middle lobe, many small satellite FDG-avid right lung nodules, and extensive FDG-avid pleural-based masses on the right (T4, N0, M1). No disease was found outside the chest.

stage NSCLC (80, 81), and a prospective multicenter trial of SRS for patients with early-stage medically inoperable disease is underway to assess efficacy, toxicity, and impact on quality of life (82).

At MDACC, medically inoperable early-stage patients with stage I disease are treated with radiotherapy alone. Those with stage II and IIIA disease are treated with a combination of chemotherapy and radiotherapy similar to those with IIIB disease unless they are unable to tolerate combination therapy based on concurrent illness or poor performance status.

The major causes of death in patients with stage I or II disease are distant metastatic disease and second primary tumors. In a trial by the Lung Cancer Study Group, the rate of second cancers (not lung primaries) was 1.8% per year, and the rate of new lung cancers was 1.6% per year (83). A series of nearly 600 stage I

NSCLC patients with mature follow-up from Memorial Sloan Kettering Cancer Center had an overall incidence of recurrence of 27% (local or regional, 7%; systemic, 20%) and an incidence of second primary tumors of 34% (84). This finding led to current studies aimed at identifying prognostic factors for relapse and to trials of chemoprevention and adjuvant therapy.

STAGE III DISEASE

Stage III NSCLC comprises a heterogeneous patient population. These patients have locally advanced disease, and their survival is poor because of both local and distant disease recurrence. A multidisciplinary approach is appropriate for most stage III NSCLC. The recent change in lung cancer staging will most likely impact this group of patients, as the T4, N0 cases have

TABLE
15-9   **DEFINITIONS FOR T, N, M DESCRIPTORS**

Descriptors	Definitions	Subgroups*
T	**Primary tumor**	
T0	No primary tumor	
T1	Tumor ≤3 cm,[†] surrounded by lung or visceral pleura, not more proximal than the loboar bronchus	
T1a	Tumor ≤2 cm[†]	T1a
T1b	Tumor >2 but ≤3 cm[†]	T1b
T2	Tumor >3 but ≤7 cm[†] or tumor with any of the following[‡]:	
	Invades visceral pleura, involves main bronchus ≥2 cm distal to the carina, atelectasis/ obstructive pneumonia extending to hilum but not involving the entire lung	
T2a	Tumor >3 but ≤5 cm[†]	T2a
T2b	Tumor >5 but ≤7 cm[†]	T2b
T3	Tumor >7 cm;	$T3_{>7}$
	or directly invading chest wall, diaphragm, phrenic nerve, mediastinal pleura, or parietal pericardium	$T3_{inv}$
	or tumor in the main bronchus <2 cm distal to the carina[§];	$T3_{center}$
	or atelectasis/obstructive pneumonitis of entire lung;	$T3_{center}$
	or separate tumor nodules in the same lobe	$T3_{satell}$
T4	Tumor of any size with invasion of heart, great vessels, trachea, recurrent laryngeal nerve, esophagus, vertebral body, or carina;	$T4_{inv}$
	or separate tumor nodules in a different ipsilateral lobe	$T4_{ipsi\ nod}$
N	**Regional lymph nodes**	
N0	No regional node metastasis	
N1	Metastasis in ipsilateral peribronchial and/or perihilar lymph nodes and intrapulmonary nodes, including involvement by direct extension	
N2	Metastasis in ipsilateral mediastinal and/or subcarinal lymph nodes	
N3	Metastasis in contralateral mediastinal, contralateral hilar, ipsilateral or contralateral scalene, or supraclavicular lymph nodes	
M	**Distant metastasis**	
M0	No distant metastasis	
M1a	Separate tumor nodules in a contralateral lobe;	$M1a_{contr\ Nod}$
	or tumor with pleural nodules or malignant pleural dissemination[¶]	$M1a_{pl\ Dissem}$
M1b	Distant metastasis	M1b
Special situations		
TX, NX, MX	T, N, or M status not able to be assessed	
Tis	Focus of *in situ* cancer	Tis
T1[§]	Superficial spreading tumor of any size but confined to the wall of the trachea or mainstem bronchus	$T1_{ss}$

*These subgroups labels are not defined in the IASLC publications but are added here to facilitate a clear discussion.
[†]In the greatest dimension.
[‡]T2 tumors with these features are classified as T2a if ≤5 cm.
[§]The uncommon superficial spreading tumor in central airways is classified as T1.
[¶]Pleural effusions are excluded that are cytologically negative, nonbloody, transudative, and clinically judged not to be due to cancer.
Adapted, with permission, from Detterbeck, FC, Boffa DJ, Tanoue LT. The new lung cancer staging system. Chest, 2009. 136(1): p. 260-71.

been re-classified as IIIA and a recent study demonstrated stage migration from IIIB to IIIA in a meaningful number of cases (73).

Management of stage IIIA disease usually involves chemotherapy in combination with surgery or radiotherapy (Fig. 15-16). Some patients with stage III disease are candidates for complete surgical tumor resection. Surgery may be of benefit in selected patients with T4 primaries (locally invasive) and minimal ipsilateral lymph node involvement. As in early-stage cancer, patients must be assessed for their ability to tolerate surgery. For those who are candidates for surgery and

TABLE 15-10	7th EDITION AMERICAN JOINT COMMITTEE ON CANCER TNM STAGING SYSTEM FOR NSCLC			
T/M stage	*N0*	*N1*	*N2*	*N3*
T1	Ia	IIa	IIIa	IIIb
T2a	Ib	IIa	IIIa	IIIb
T2b	IIa	IIIb	IIIa	IIIb
T3	IIb	IIIa	IIIa	IIIb
T4	IIIa	IIIa	IIIb	IIIb
M1	IV	IV	IV	IV

Reproduced, with permission, from Detterbeck, FC, Boffa DJ, Tanoue LT. The new lung cancer staging system. *Chest* 2009. 136(1): p. 260-71.

have T4 or N2 disease, two to three cycles of neoadjuvant chemotherapy is utilized in most cases at MDACC in an attempt to downsize the tumor prior to surgery and improve outcome. Randomized trials have found a benefit of preoperative chemotherapy in stage IIIA NSCLC (85-87).

Patients with stage IIIB disease are not candidates for surgery and are most often treated with a combination of chemotherapeutic agents and radiation. Concurrent chemotherapy is associated with higher survival rates and increased toxicity when compared to sequential chemotherapy. Two large phase III studies have sought to determine which dosage schedule is more effective. The West Japan Lung Cancer Group randomized patients with unresectable NSCLC to receive cisplatin, vindesine, and mitomycin either prior to or concurrent with radiation (88). Survival was superior among patients in the concurrent-administration arm (16.8 versus 13.8 months, $p = .02$). RTOG 94-10 showed similar results in a trial of concurrent vinblastine and cisplatin plus radiation versus sequential therapy. Again, survival was superior among patients in the concurrent-treatment arm (17 versus 14.6 months) (89). Alternative regimens consisting of induction chemotherapy followed

TABLE 15-11	FIVE-YEAR SURVIVAL FOR NSCLC BY PATHOLOGIC AND CLINICAL STAGE	
	Clinical	*Pathologic*
Ia	50%	73%
Ib	43%	58%
IIa	36%	46%
IIb	25%	36%
IIIa	19%	24%
IIIb	7%	9%
IV	2%	13%

Reproduced, with permission, from Detterbeck, FC, Boffa DJ, Tanoue LT. The new lung cancer staging system. *Chest* 2009. 136(1): p. 260-71.

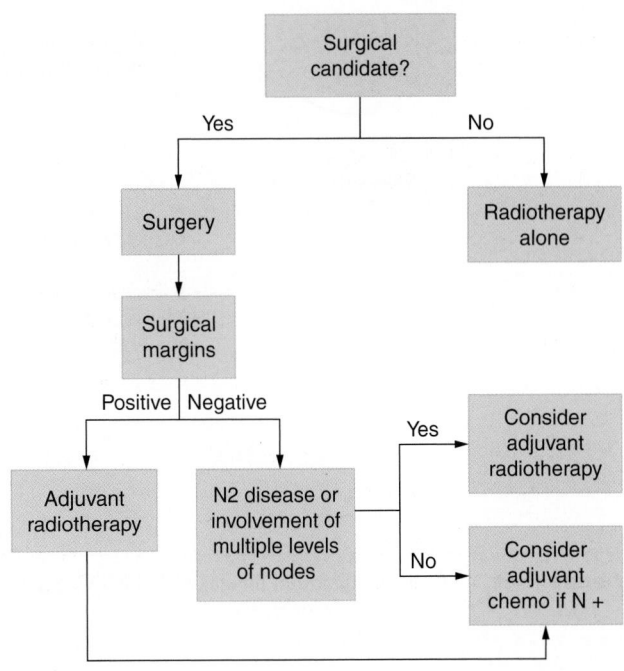

FIGURE 15-14. Treatment algorithm for stage I NSCLC. See text for details.

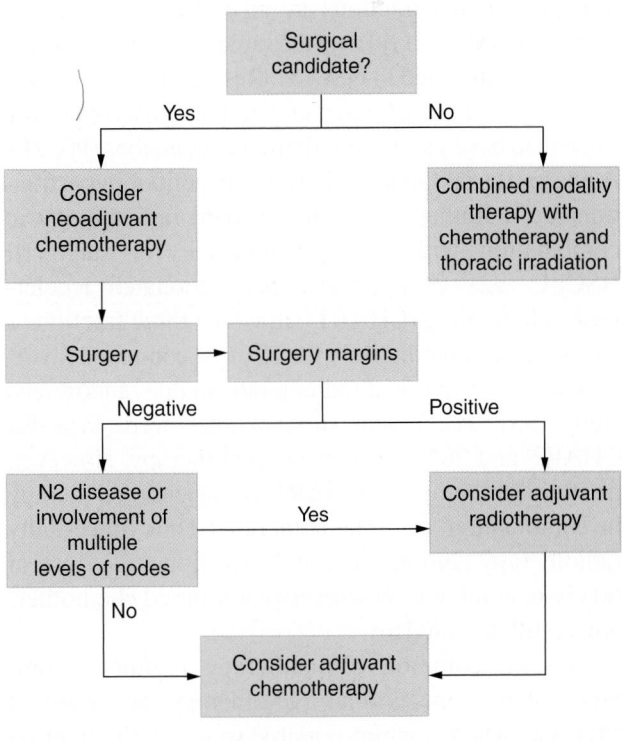

FIGURE 15-15. Treatment algorithm for stage II NSCLC. See text for details.

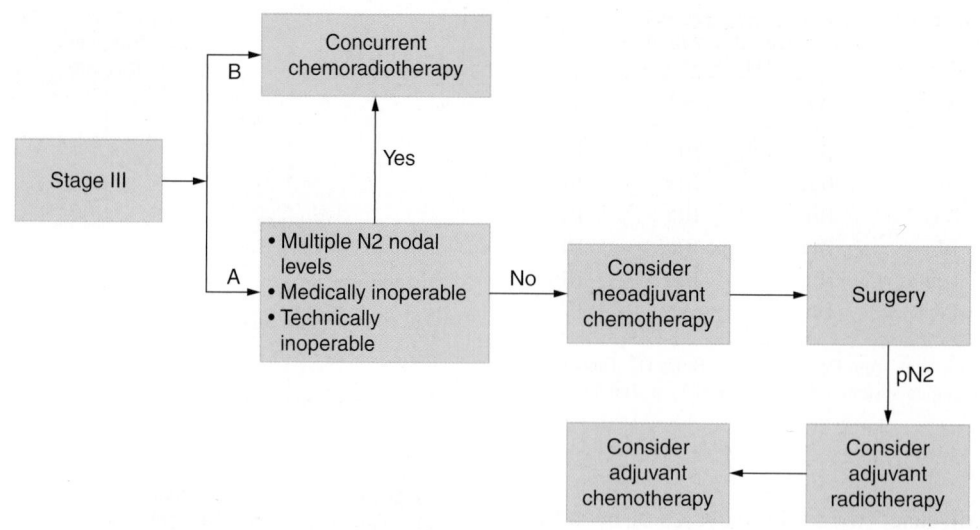

FIGURE 15-16. Treatment algorithm for stage III NSCLC. See text for details.

by concurrent therapy, concurrent therapy followed by consolidation chemotherapy, and concurrent therapy with alternative chemotherapy agents are being investigated.

Standard radiotherapy for stage IIIB NSCLC consists of radiation given once daily for 6 weeks (30 fractions) to a total dose of 60 Gy. Hyperfractionated radiotherapy, in which smaller fractions are given twice daily to the same total dose (60 Gy) over the same duration (6 weeks), has also been tested in NSCLC. Results of these studies have not been consistent, and two meta-analyses of the same data have yielded conflicting conclusions (90, 91). A phase III trial failed to show any benefit of hyperfractionated radiotherapy versus standard radiotherapy in combination with cisplatin/etoposide for stage III NSCLC (92). Continuous hyperfractionated accelerated radiotherapy (CHART), in which three fractions a day are given continuously for 12 days, compared favorably with conventional radiotherapy in one randomized study (93). The 2-year survival rates were 29% for CHART and 20% for conventional therapy. However, no study has compared CHART to conventional therapy in combination with chemotherapy. Thus, once-daily radiotherapy administered in 30 fractions to a dose of 60 Gy in combination with cisplatin-based chemotherapy is still the standard.

Several common chemotherapy regimens combined with conventional radiotherapy are used at MDACC when it is not possible to place a patient on study protocol. Two such standard regimens include the following: (1) two cycles of cisplatin and etoposide during radiotherapy followed by three cycles of adjuvant docetaxel (SWOG S9504) (94), (2) The SWOG S9504 regimen without the consolidation docetaxel (95), or (3) weekly carboplatin and paclitaxel for 6 weeks during radiotherapy followed by two cycles of adjuvant chemotherapy (96).

A tumor in the apex of the lung that invades the apical structures is a Pancoast (superior sulcus) tumor (Fig. 15-17). Because of the anatomic location of these tumors, it is impossible to obtain a wide margin during their resection and the risk of local recurrence is high. In addition, patients with Pancoast tumors have a high rate of distant metastasis and their survival is poor. Historically, these patients were treated with preoperative radiation. More recently, neoadjuvant and adjuvant chemoradiotherapy have been studied in Pancoast tumors. For T3 to T4, N0 to N1 Pancoast tumors, preoperative concurrent chemotherapy and radiotherapy followed by surgery yields high rates of tumor resectability and patient survival. For patients not on clinical trial, standard therapy at MDACC for T3 to T4, N0 to N1 Pancoast tumors is surgery followed by postoperative concurrent chemotherapy and radiotherapy. Patients with N2 to N3 disease are not candidates for surgery and should be treated with concurrent chemoradiation alone.

ADJUVANT THERAPY

Adjuvant chemotherapy and radiotherapy have been studied in NSCLC patients following surgical resection because of the poor survival of these patients relative to

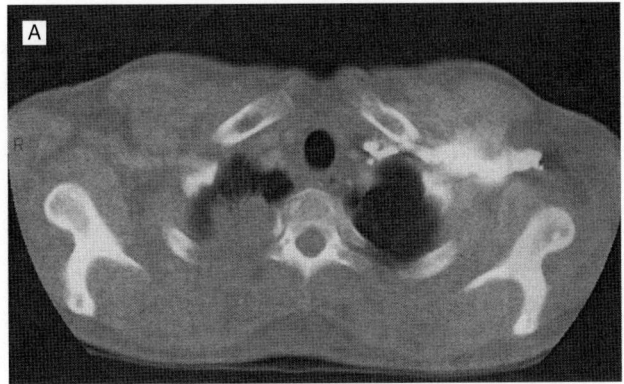

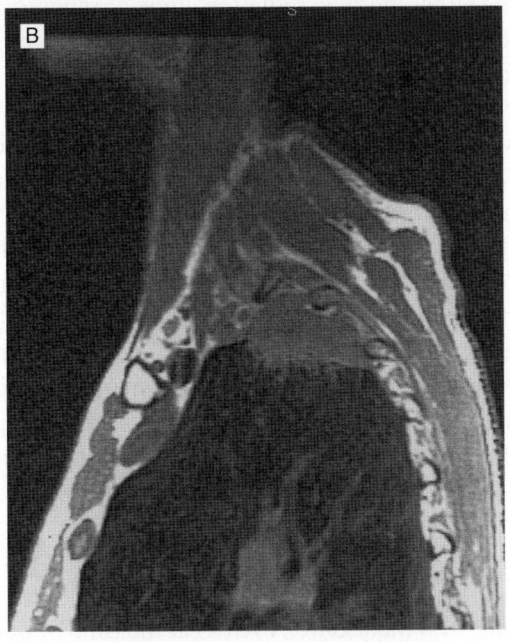

FIGURE 15-17. Pancoast tumor. By MRI, this NSCLC tumor at the right lung apex invades the second right rib and extends apically into right apical fat, with a loss of the fat plane between the tumor and the T1 nerve. The T2 nerve is also involved by the mass.

TABLE 15-12	CHEMOTHERAPY REGIMENS FOR ADJUVANT TREATMENT OF NSCLC
Trial	**Regimen**
IALT	Cisplatin 80-120 mg/m^2 every 3 of 4 weeks, for 3-4 cycles, with: Vinorelbine 30 mg/m^2 weekly; or vinblastine 4 mg/m^2 every week for 5 weeks, then every 2 weeks; or etoposide 100 mg/m^2, days 1-3 with each cisplatin
ANITA	Cisplatin 100 mg/m^2 and vinorelbine 30 mg/m^2, day 1 every 4 weeks for 4 cycles
NCIC-CTG JBR.10	Cisplatin 50 mg/m^2, days 1 and 8, every 4 weeks for 4 cycles; vinorelbine 25 mg/m^2 every week for 16 cycles

the disease stage (Table 15-11). Several recent systematic reviews have been conducted on the role of adjuvant chemotherapy after complete resection, and along with data from five large randomized controlled trials, form the basis for the joint clinical practice guidelines issued by Cancer Care Ontario and the American Society of Clinical Oncology (97-100). These guidelines are consistent with our current clinical practice at MDACC.

For patients with stage IA disease, no adjuvant treatment is recommended, as there is no evidence to suggest a benefit for adjuvant chemotherapy in this group of patients. Data on the use of adjuvant chemotherapy in stage IB are controversial. For stage IB, neither the LACE meta-analysis nor four of the

published randomized trials demonstrate a benefit for adjuvant therapy (101-105). However, the CALGB 9633 trial did demonstrate a benefit for those patients with stage IB with tumors larger than 4 cm, many of whom would be reclassified as stage IIB in the new staging system (ie, those with tumors >5 cm) (106).

For patients with completely resected stage II-III, adjuvant treatment is recommended with a cisplatin-based regimen, such as that used in the IALT, ANITA, or NCIC-CTG JBR.10 trials (Table 15-12). The pooled analysis for patients receiving cisplatin-based adjuvant therapy demonstrated an overall survival advantage with a hazard ratio of 0.89 (95% CI 0.82-0.96; $p = .005$). Alkylating agents should not be used in the adjuvant setting because the 1995 NSCLC Collaborative Group meta-analysis (n = 9387) demonstrated a survival disadvantage with a hazard ratio of 1.15 ($p <0.005$) (107).

In addition to trials of these platinum-based regimens, six trials using an oral uracil/tegafur combination (UFT) as the sole adjuvant chemotherapy have been conducted in Japan, and several others using UFT after two cycles of cisplatin-based chemotherapy (108). These trials have entered patients with completely resected disease and have all had a surgery-only control arm. UFT was administered orally at 400-600 mg/day for 1-2 years (depending on the study) and was well-tolerated. Although all of these studies showed a trend toward improved survival (relative to surgery only) by treatment group or subset analysis, a meta-analysis of the six trials with UFT alone, with more than 2000 patients demonstrated clear benefit to UFT with a HR = 0.74 (95% CI 0.61-0.88, $p =.001$) (109).

Confirmatory trials in Europe and North America evaluating prolonged oral administration of fluoropyrimidines are indicated.

Neoadjuvant chemotherapy offers several real and theoretical advantages over postoperative therapy: better patient compliance, improved tumor resectability, earlier treatment of micrometastatic disease, and earlier assessment of clinical and pathologic response. Two randomized trials of preoperative chemotherapy using cisplatin-based regimens in stage IIIA NSCLC showed significantly improved survival compared with surgery alone (86,87). Long-term survival rates for these studies showed the same trend toward increased survival (110,111), but these trials have been criticized for enrolling only 60 patients each. A randomized trial of preoperative chemotherapy using mitomycin, ifosfamide, and cisplatin has been conducted in early-stage (stages IB-IIIA) NSCLC (112). This trial found an 11-month increase in median survival (26 versus 37 months, $p = .15$), a significant increase in disease-free survival (27 versus 13 months, $p = .033$), and a decrease in distant metastases (hazard ratio 0.54, $p = .01$). In the patients with stage I or II disease, the HR of death was significantly decreased to 0.68 ($p = .027$). Two other large randomized trials have been reported, representing the experience of the Southwest Oncology Group in S9900 and the multinational intergroup trial (MRC LU22/NVALT2/EORTC 08012) (113,114). Although both of these trials reported results with a trend toward PFS and OS benefits to preoperative chemotherapy, they were not statistically significant. Currently, the available data favor the use of adjuvant chemotherapy in this setting.

Postoperative radiotherapy (PORT) for patients with resected NSCLC has also been studied. A meta-analysis found an adverse effect of PORT on survival, with an HR for death of 1.21 and a reduction in overall survival from 55 to 48% at 2 years (115,116). Subset analysis showed that patients with N2 disease did not suffer this adverse effect. The analysis has been criticized because it includes patients who were treated with techniques that are now considered suboptimal. Data from trials using modern equipment showed an improvement in local control among patients with N1/N2 disease but no difference in overall survival (117,118). The Lung Cancer Study Group of PORT randomly assigned patients with resected stage II or III NSCLC to postoperative radiotherapy or no adjuvant treatment and found a reduction in local recurrence, although no change in overall survival (119). Based upon the PORT meta-analysis, along with data from the ANITA trial (105) and Surveillance, Epidemiology and End Results study (SEER) (120), the CCO/ASCO practice guidelines recommend against the use of adjuvant radiation in stage I and II patients, while use in stage III patients should be guided by emerging trial data and the specifics of individual cases (100). Patients most likely to benefit from postoperative radiotherapy are those with resection margins positive for disease or multiple areas of lymph node involvement.

The combination of chemotherapy and radiotherapy has also been studied. The Eastern Cooperative Oncology Group (ECOG) randomized 488 patients with completely resected stage II or IIIA NSCLC to receive either thoracic radiation alone or radiation with concurrent cisplatin and etoposide postoperatively. There was no difference in overall survival or local recurrence between the two groups (121). Several other trials as well as meta-analysis, have confirmed the lack of benefit of postoperative adjuvant concurrent chemoradiotherapy (122-124).

The treatment of early-stage lung cancer should include surgery whenever feasible. Postoperative chemotherapy improves survival in stage II-III. Currently at MDACC, all patients who undergo surgical resection for NSCLC are referred to medical oncology to discuss adjuvant chemotherapy; such therapy is undertaken only after a thorough discussion of the relative and absolute benefits for the individual patient.

STAGE IV DISEASE

Patients with metastatic NSCLC at the time of diagnosis, including those with a malignant pleural effusion, should be assessed for the suitability of systemic cytotoxic chemotherapy or biologic/targeted therapy. Those with symptomatic brain or spinal cord metastases, hemoptysis, postobstructive pneumonia, or painful bone metastases should first be given palliative radiotherapy. Patients with poor performance status (3 or 4 by ECOG criteria) are less likely than others to respond to chemotherapy and more likely to experience toxic side effects (125). Poor performance status is an independent predictor of decreased survival (126). Based on this information, it is unlikely that those with poor performance status will benefit from currently available cytotoxic chemotherapy. Newer biological agents or alternative schedules (eg, weekly therapy) have an emerging role in this population and in fact this group of patients has become the proving ground for the multiple new therapies added to our armamentarium in NSCLC over the past several years.

Several studies have examined the potential benefit of chemotherapy over best supportive care. A meta-analysis

TABLE
15-13 **COMPARISON OF CHEMOTHERAPY REGIMENS FOR ADVANCED NSCLC**

	Median Survival (Months)	Overall Response Rate	Median 2-Year Survival	Median Time to Progression (Months)
Cisplatin 75 mg/m² on day 2; paclitaxel 135 mg/m² over 24 h on day 1: 3-week cycle	7.8	21%	10%	3.4
Cisplatin 100 mg/m² on day 1; gemcitabine 1000 mg/m² on days 1, 8, and 15: 4-week cycle	8.1	22%	13%	4.2 (p = .001 compared to cisplatin/paclitaxel)
Cisplatin 75 mg/m² on day 1; docetaxel 75 mg/m² on day 1: 3-week cycle	7.4	17%	11%	3.7
Carboplatin AUC 6 mg/mL/min on day 1; paclitaxel 225 mg/m² over 3 h on day 1: 3-week cycle	8.1	17%	11%	3.1
Overall	7.9	19%	11%	3.6

Reproduced, with permission, from Schiller JH, Harrington D, Belani CP, et al., Comparison of four chemotherapy regimens for advanced non-small-cell lung cancer. N Engl J Med 2002. 346(2): p. 92-8. Copyright © 2002 Massachusetts Medical Society. All rights reserved.

of sixteen trials enrolling 2714 patients showed that chemotherapy provided a clear improvement in survival (although modest), with an increased median survival of 1.5 months and a relative increase in survival of 23% (127). Several studies have shown an improved quality of life among patients receiving chemotherapy relative to those only receiving supportive care (128,129). The Big Lung Trial was a randomized trial comparing best supportive care with cisplatin-based chemotherapy. Results from 725 patients showed an increase in median survival (5.7 versus 8.0 months) due to the chemotherapy, with no difference in quality of life or economic outcome between the two groups (130). Newer chemotherapeutic regimens incorporating such agents as gemcitabine, vinorelbine, irinotecan, docetaxel, and paclitaxel are also superior to best supportive care in terms of patient response rates, survival, and quality of life.

Results from early phase II trials suggest that newer chemotherapeutic agents are superior to the older regimens used in the 1980s (ie, cisplatin-etoposide, mitomycin-ifosfamide-cisplatin, cisplatin-vindesine). Although randomized trials generally show that the newer agents are less toxic than the older ones, survival and quality-of-life outcomes are similar. In several trials, the survival benefits of new agents were not statistically significant (reviewed in Bunn [131]).

Randomized trials have compared several of the modern regimens to one another and have not shown any one to be clearly superior. Schiller et al. randomized 1207 patients to receive cisplatin-paclitaxel, cisplatin-gemcitabine, cisplatin-docetaxel, or carboplatin-paclitaxel (132). All combinations elicited nearly identical response rates and survival (Table 15-13). Several others have compared a variety of newer regimens and have generally found no differences in survival (133,134). Toxic effects vary with the agent: gemcitabine causes more thrombocytopenia and anemia; peripheral neuropathy is more common with paclitaxel; neutropenia and nausea are more common with vinorelbine.

The choice of platinum compound is controversial. Cisplatin confers more neurotoxicity, nausea/vomiting, and nephrotoxicity than carboplatin, which confers more myelosuppression and is easier to administer. In some studies the two platinums have shown equivalent efficacy against NSCLC (132-134), but cisplatin has been superior in others (135,136). A recent individual patient data meta-analysis of nine randomized phase II or III trials with 2968 patients demonstrated that carboplatin was inferior to cisplatin in objective response (OR for no response = 1.37, 95% CI = 1.16-1.61, p <.001) and in overall survival (HR of death = 1.07, 95% CI 0.99-1.15, p = .1), although the later was not statistically significant (137). Restriction of the analysis to patients who received third-generation platinum-based regimens (HR = 1.11, 95% CI 1.01-1.21) or with nonsquamous histology (HR = 1.12, 95% CI 1.01-1.23) demonstrated a slight superiority to cisplatin over carboplatin.

Several randomized studies have compared one-agent cytotoxic therapies with two-drug combinations and found that a two-drug combination is always superior (138-140). Comparisons of two- and three-drug combinations in multiple randomized trials have shown that no survival advantage is gained by using three cytotoxic drugs (141-143); targeted biologic agents added to cytotoxic doublets are discussed later. The three-drug combinations were, however, more toxic than the two-drug regimens. Alternating doublets has also shown no advantage over a single two- or three-drug regimen (144).

As a first-line therapy, the relatively new antifolate cytotoxic agent, pemetrexed, has been approved for use in combination with cisplatin, based upon improved survival versus a combination of cisplatin and gemcitabine in a phase III trial (145). Interestingly, analysis of the outcomes in this and other trials has clearly demonstrated that histology is a predictive marker of response to pemetrexed, with squamous cell histology predictive of poor outcome and non-squamous histology predictive of response and improved PFS and OS. This difference is attributed to the differential expression of the primary target for pemetrexed, thymidylate synthase, between adenocarcinoma and squamous cell carcinoma.

The optimal duration of first-line therapy is an area with current controversy. Prior to the addition of biologically targeted therapies, this issue had been addressed for cytotoxic therapy by a phase III randomized study in which patients received carboplatin and paclitaxel for either four courses or until disease progression (146). Extending chemotherapy beyond four cycles yielded no benefit in terms of survival, response rate, or quality of life. Another study using mitomycin, vinblastine, and cisplatin showed that six cycles of therapy were no more beneficial than three (147). Both studies showed increased cumulative toxic effects in patients receiving more courses of chemotherapy. However, as outlined in the subsequent section, the role of maintenance therapy is rapidly changing.

In an effort to attain better response rates and longer survival, new agents targeted to particular molecular processes have been developed and tested alone or in combination with traditional cytotoxic chemotherapy. Understanding the successes, failures, and best ways to use these agents clinically is a primary focus of clinical research in NSCLC today.

New blood vessel growth (angiogenesis) is essential for tumor growth and survival. Angiogenesis is controlled by an array of pro- and anti-angiogenic factors. The vascular endothelial growth factor (VEGF), a peptide growth factor, promotes angiogenesis in multiple tumor types. Bevacizumab (Avastin) is a monoclonal antibody against the vascular endothelial growth factor that has been developed to target this process. ECOG4599 demonstrated for the first time that addition of a third agent (bevacizumab) to carboplatin and paclitaxel could

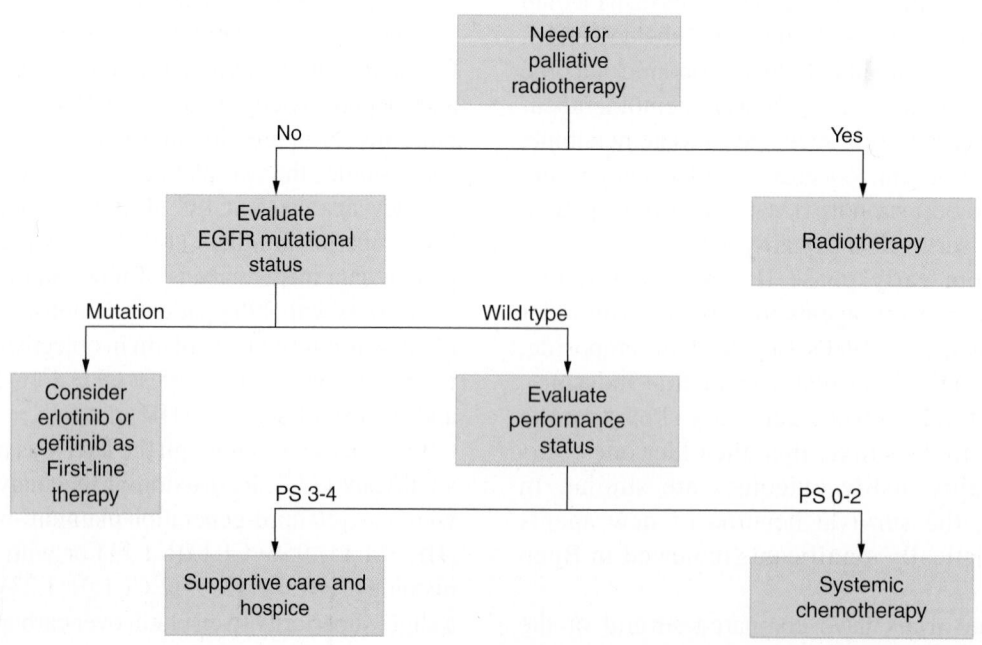

FIGURE 15-18.   Treatment algorithm for stage IV NSCLC. See text for details.

produce an overall survival benefit in selected patients with advanced or recurrent non–squamous non-small cell lung cancer (148). When given in combination with standard carboplatin and paclitaxel every 3 weeks for 6 cycles, followed by bevacizumab maintenance until disease progression, a median overall survival of 12.3 months was observed versus 10.3 months for chemotherapy alone. There was a statistically and clinically meaningful increase in the rates of bleeding for the bevacizumab arm (4.4% versus 0.7%, $p < .001$), including cases of pulmonary hemorrhage. Retrospective analysis demonstrated that patients older than 70 on the bevacizumab arm experienced much higher rates of grade 3 to 5 toxicities (87% versus 61%, $p < 0.001$), but without an increase in overall survival (149). The increased risk for hemorrhage and the questionable benefit for some subgroups highlight the need for appropriate patient selection in the use of this combination. For example, patients with squamous histology, hemoptysis, or uncontrolled hypertension are not candidates for bevacizumab.

Patients whose disease progresses after treatment with one of the above regimens, but who maintain good performance status, are candidates for second-line therapy. Two large phase III studies examined the efficacy of docetaxel in patients with advanced NSCLC who had not responded to a platinum-based regimen. Docetaxel conferred a higher response rate, a longer median survival, and a higher 1-year survival rate than best supportive care (150) or chemotherapy consisting of vinorelbine or ifosfamide (151). Prior exposure to paclitaxel did not diminish the clinical benefit of docetaxel as a second-line therapy. Pemetrexed, a multitargeted antifolate, demonstrated similar efficacy to docetaxel in the second-line setting when compared in a phase III randomized trial, but with an improved toxicity profile (152). The EGFR inhibitor erlotinib is also approved for second-line therapy, where its use can produce striking clinical responses (Fig. 15-19).

The most extensively studied molecularly targeted therapy in NSCLC is epidermal growth factor receptor (EGFR) inhibition. Among the known EGFR inhibitors are antibodies (cetuximab [C225, Erbitux] and ABX-EGF) and small-molecule tyrosine kinase inhibitors (gefitinib [ZD1839, Iressa] and erlotinib [OSI774, Tarceva]). The EGFR tyrosine kinase inhibitors (TKIs) erlotinib and gefitinib were initially evaluated as third-line therapy for advanced NSCLC in patients whose cancers were not responsive to either a platinum-containing regimen or docetaxel. Gefitinib was adopted based on its performance in two randomized phase II

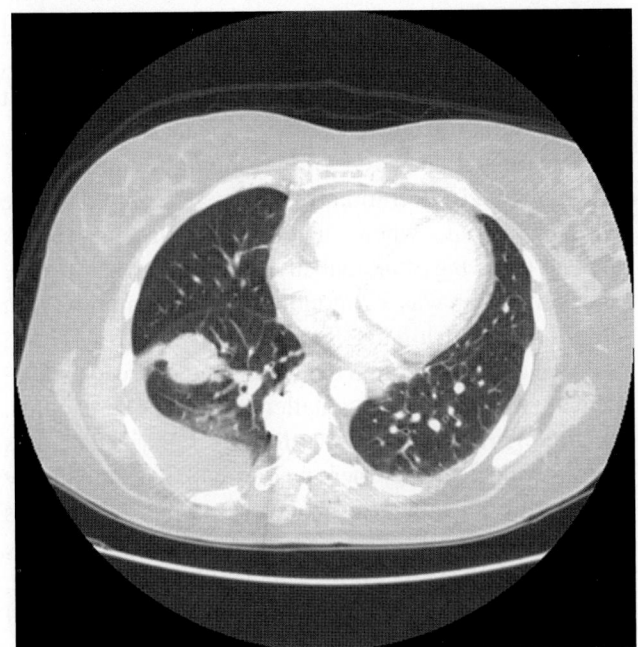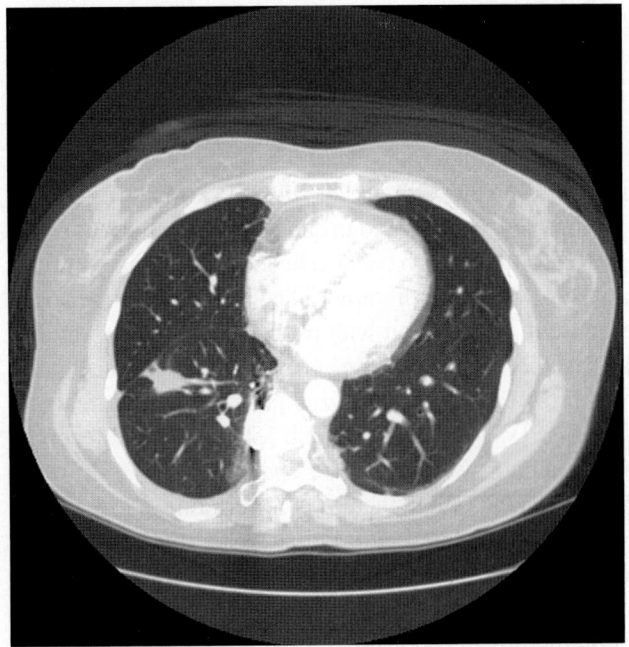

FIGURE 15-19. Treatment response to the EGFR-TKI erlotinib. This 44-year-old female patient with a smoking history of less than 200 cigarettes in her lifetime presented with back pain and was found to have a primary lung adenocarcinoma with lung and bone metastases, including a vertebral metastasis. The tumor had an exon 19 mutation in EGFR. After vertebrectomy and postoperative radiation therapy to the thoracic spine, she received oral erlotinib. The pre-treatment CT shows the primary lung tumor prior to erlotinib (*left*); CT imaging after 4 months of erlotinib therapy revealed significant response (*right*).

studies (IDEAL 1 and IDEAL 2) of patients with advanced NSCLC, after progression of disease on platinum-containing regimens, who received 250 or 500 mg daily (153,154). The response rate was approximately 19% (13.6% for those who had received two prior chemotherapy regimens) in IDEAL 1, and symptom rates were significantly reduced. Both IDEAL 1 and 2 confirmed that the dose of 250 mg/day was as effective as and less toxic than the dose of 500 mg/day. Although the subsequent ISEL trial (Iressa Survival Evaluation in Lung Cancer), which evaluated gefitinib at 250 mg/day versus BSC in 1692 patients, failed to confirm an advantage to gefitinib use (155), with loss of its FDA approval, it has continued to be used outside of the United States. With the results of the recent INTEREST trial (Iressa NSCLC Trial Evaluating Response and Survival versus Taxotere) (156), there is renewed discussion on how best to incorporate this agent into clinical practice. The multinational INTEREST trial randomized 1466 patients to directly compare gefitinib (250 mg/day) to docetaxel (75 mg/m^2 every 3 weeks) in the second-line setting after progression or recurrence with a platin-based regimen, and demonstrated non-inferior survival for gefitinib (HR = 1.020, 96% CI 0.905-1.150).

Three large phase III placebo-controlled trials of erlotinib in NSCLC have been conducted (157-159). The NCIC CTG BR.21 study randomized 731 patients with stage IIIB/IV NSCLC who had failed first-line or second-line chemotherapy to placebo or oral erlotinib 150 mg/day (159). The overall response rate in the erlotinib arm was 8.9% (95% CI 6.6-12, p <.001). There was a statistically significant difference in overall survival between the erlotinib and placebo arms (6.7 versus 4.7 months, p = .001), and in quality-of-life analyses.

EGFR inhibitors have also been evaluated in combination with chemotherapy. The TRIBUTE (Tarceva response in conjunction with paclitaxel and carboplatin) and TALENT (Tarceva Lung Cancer Investigation Trial) trials prospectively randomized patients with untreated stage IIIB/IV NSCLC to erlotinib 150 mg/day or placebo in conjunction with cytotoxic chemotherapy, followed by maintenance monotherapy with erlotinib (157,158). Both trials enrolled more than 1000 patients, and neither demonstrated statistically significant differences between the chemotherapy plus erlotinib and the chemotherapy plus placebo arms in terms of overall survival, objective responses, or response duration.

Original clinical observations indicated that several subgroups may have a better rate of response to gefitinib than others: nonsmokers, females, Asians, and those with adenocarcinoma, highlighting the need for identification

of which patient subgroups derive benefit from treatment. Multiple studies reported in 2004 demonstrated that patients whose tumors contained a mutation in the EGFR molecule achieved the best response to EGFR-TKI treatment (160-162). The recently updated ASCO guidelines for stage IV NSCLC indicate that selection of an EGFR TKI over carboplatin/paclitaxel in patients with EGFR mutation is reasonable, although they note that an improvement in PFS, toxicity, and quality of life has not translated into an improvement in overall survival in any study to date (61).

In support of this approach, the Iressa Pan-Asia Study (IPASS) was a phase III trial conducted in 87 centers in East Asia, which compared gefitinib to carboplatin plus paclitaxel in 1217 randomized chemo-naïve patients with advanced adenocarcinoma who were nonsmokers or former light smokers (163). Analysis of the data from the overall population clearly revealed two separate populations with differing responses: the patients with EGFR mutations had an objective response rate of 71.2% and prolonged PFS (HR = .48, 95% CI .36-.64, p<.001), while the patients with wild-type EGFR had an objective response rate of 1.1% and did worse with erlotinib versus chemotherapy (HR = 2.85, 95% CI 2.05-3.98, p <.001).

In the recently reported FLEX trial (First-Line ErbituX in lung cancer), the use of a monoclonal antibody against EGFR, cetuximab, in combination with cisplatin and vinorelbine, produced an overall survival benefit (11.3 versus 10.1 months; HR for death = 0.871, 95% CI 0.762-0.996, p = .044) in the first-line treatment of 1125 randomized patients with advanced or metastatic disease and positive EGFR staining by immunohistochemistry (164). Similar results were reported for the BMS-099 trial, where median overall survival in patients receiving cetuximab in combination with a taxane and carboplatin was 9.7 months, versus 8.4 months with chemotherapy alone (HR = 0.89, 95% CI 0.75-1.05, p = .17) (164). Although the results did not reach statistical significance in this smaller trial with 676 patients, the findings are consistent with the FLEX trial data. It is currently unclear why there was a small, but statistically significant advantage to cetuximab, when other trials using oral EGFR TKIs along with chemotherapy have failed to do so. It is also unclear how this regimen, which relies upon weekly infusions of cetuximab until the time of progression, will translate into community practice.

Based on these recent data, the exact use of EGFR inhibitors in NSCLC is somewhat controversial. The IPASS study suggests that those patients whose tumors have an EGFR mutation should receive front-line

EGFR TKI. However, it is also reasonable to use chemotherapy as a first-line treatment and reserve EGFR TKI therapy as a second-line treatment. The clinical data, along with our understanding of the biology of EGFR mutations, clearly demonstrates that EGFR mutant patients should receive an EGFR TKI either as first- or second-line therapy. For the majority of patients with wild type EGFR, EGFR TKIs can be used as second- or third-line therapy. Although true responses are uncommon, survival benefits have been documented. The lack of benefit of EGFR TKIs in combination with cytotoxic chemotherapy precludes their use in this setting.

For patients with bronchoalveolar carcinoma histology, EGFR-TKI treatment has high response rates, especially in the presence of EGFR mutation or increased copy number, and provides a good option for this disease with limited sensitivity to standard cytotoxic agents (166).

A rapidly changing area in the study and treatment of advanced NSCLC is the use of maintenance therapy after first-line doublet therapy has achieved disease stabilization or maximum tumor response. This approach is being tested for both cytotoxic agents and the EGFR TKIs. In a large, multinational trial, 663 patients who had not progressed on four cycles of platinum-based therapy were randomized to receive maintenance pemetrexed at 500 mg/m2 or placebo, given on day 1, every 3 weeks until disease progression. Improvement was seen in PFS and overall survival (13·4 months [11·9-15·9] versus 10·6 months [8.7-12.0]; HR 0.79, 0.65-0.95, p = .012) (167). As with the other trials of pemetrexed in NSCLC (discussed above), the patients with squamous cell carcinoma did not benefit from maintenance therapy with pemetrexed. Preliminary results have been presented for the SATURN trial of erlotinib maintenance therapy after four cycles of platinum-based chemotherapy, with no evidence of disease progression (168). In the trial, of the 1949 patients who received first-line chemotherapy, 889 were eligible for randomization to erlotinib at 150 mg/day or placebo until progression or withdrawal due to toxicity. PFS was improved (HR = .71, 95% CI 0.62-0.82, p <.0001) compared with placebo, with a response rate of 12% versus 5% for placebo. Overall survival data are not yet mature. Collectively these results suggest that maintenance therapy may play an increasingly important role in management of advanced NSCLC in the coming years.

Treatment of advanced NSCLC in the elderly has been addressed in several prospective studies and retrospective analyses (reviewed in Basche and Kelly [169]). These have shown that patients more than 70 years old with good performance status who received combination chemotherapy (two agents) have response rates and median survival times equivalent to those of younger patients. Elderly patients do experience a higher incidence of hematologic toxic effects than younger patients, but other toxic effects are not increased. Prospective trials of single agents (vinorelbine or gemcitabine) in the elderly showed good response rates and survival, improvement in symptoms, and acceptable tolerability. Currently, we recommend that elderly patients with good performance status be offered standard combination chemotherapy or single-agent therapy with gemcitabine or vinorelbine.

Clearly, more effective therapy is needed for NSCLC and, when possible and appropriate, patients are first offered therapy on an experimental protocol (see section Future Directions, later). Current standard first-line therapy for stage IV NSCLC at MDACC can consist of one of several two-drug combinations, with or without bevacizumab: a platinum with a taxane; gemcitabine with cisplatin; vinorelbine with cisplatin; or gemcitabine with a taxane. Pemetrexed plus carboplatin can also be considered for patients with non-squamous NSCLC. The choice of standard regimen is often based on expected toxicities of the therapy in an individual patient since the efficacy of these regimens is equivalent. Maintenance therapy is still investigational, but pending the final results of current studies, may quickly become a new option. Multiple agents have demonstrated efficacy in the second-line setting, including docetaxel, pemetrexed, and the EGFR TKIs, erlotinib and gefitinib.

OTHER THERAPIES FOR ADVANCED DISEASE

Although chemotherapy can be used in patients with metastatic disease, radiotherapy and surgery may be helpful in managing disease in selected patients with stage IV NSCLC. Radiotherapy is indicated for palliation of symptomatic lesions in this population. Radiotherapy to the chest may help relieve pain, hemoptysis, or obstructive symptoms. Palliative chest radiotherapy is given without concurrent chemotherapy. Radiotherapy for bone metastases can help prevent pathologic fractures and relieve pain.

In patients with a metachronous solitary brain or adrenal metastasis, surgical resection of both the metastatic lesion and the primary tumor yields 5-year survival rates of 16 to 30% in those undergoing complete tumor resection (170). The role of postoperative whole-brain radiotherapy in this setting is unclear and currently being studied (171). Likewise, the rate of

5-year survival for those who undergo complete surgical resection of an isolated adrenal metastasis and the primary lung tumor is 10 to 23% (115). In both of these scenarios, a complete staging workup must rule out distant metastasis prior to surgery.

FUTURE DIRECTIONS

There is an obvious need for better treatments for NSCLC. Recent research in the clinic and laboratory has focused on molecularly targeted therapies: strategies include inhibition of cellular signaling pathways that promote cancer cell growth, inhibition of tumor blood vessel formation (angiogenesis), and promotion of apoptosis. Cytotoxic chemotherapies and immunotherapies are also being investigated. In addition to newly developed agents, recent progress in treating patients with NSCLC has highlighted the benefit to identifying the subsets of patients who will respond to particular agents. The development of personalized medicine protocols, such as the BATTLE (Biomarker-integrated Approaches of Targeted Therapy for Lung cancer Elimination) trial, have proven the feasibility of enrolling patients in a trial to obtain sufficient material from diagnostic biopsies to broadly profile the tumor characteristics from individual patients for stratification and randomization into treatment groups (172). More efforts of this type will be needed in clinical protocols and programs like this will need to be translated into community pathology practices to facilitate treatment planning for patients and their physicians.

Ras-driven disease has been difficult to target. Farnesyltransferase inhibitors (FTIs) target the *ras* oncogene and possibly other farnesylated molecules involved in tumor progression and survival. However, given the overall poor results of these agents in clinical trials, efforts have turned toward other agents. For example, inhibitors of phosphoinositide 3-kinase have been combined with inhibitors of mitogen-activated protein kinase (MEK) with striking results in preclinical animal models of mutant Kras-driven NSCLC inhibitors (173). MEK inhibitors such as AZD6244 are currently being tested in combination with chemotherapy in phase II trials of NSCLC.

Other small molecule tyrosine kinase inhibitors targeting multiple receptors, including the VEGF receptor (eg, Vandetanib/Zactima/AstraZeneca, or Sunitinib/ Sutent/ Pfizer), are in development and clinical testing for NSCLC. A completed phase III trial (ZODIAC) of vandetanib in combination with docetaxel in second-line treatment showed an improved PFS versus chemotherapy alone (HR = .79, 97.58% CI 0.70-0.90, P <.001), although the median PFS was marginally changed (174).

The drug is currently being tested in combination with other cytotoxic agents and in the first-line setting. Sunitinib is a multi-targeted tyrosine kinase inhibitor with activity against Flt-3, VEGF receptor, PDGF receptor, and c-KIT. Results of a phase II trial of sunitinib as a single agent after progression of disease with a platinum-based doublet indicate good tolerability and activity similar to currently approved agents (175).

Many other agents targeting components of signal transduction pathways have been under development in the past few years. For example, the inhibitor of the insulin-like growth factor-1 receptor (IGF-1R), figitumumab, was tested in a phase II study in previously untreated patients with advanced disease and indicated that the inhibitor combined with paclitaxel/carboplatin had improved activity over chemotherapy alone (176). Unfortunately, the phase III trial of the figitumumab/ carboplatin/taxol combination as first-line therapy for advanced NSCLC was officially closed after an interim analysis indicated that the the experimental arm would not have a meaningful chance of superiority to standard chemotherapy with placebo. The inhibitor is still under investigation in combination with erlotinib. Agents that inhibit Raf kinase, MAPK kinase, the P13 kinase pathway, the cyclin-dependent kinases, JAK/STAT pathway, Src kinases, ALK kinase, c-Met, and other potential novel targets are also in early clinical development.

The treatment of lung cancer patients who possess an ALK gene rearrangement with the ALK inhibitor crizotinib, resulted in partial responses in 57% and stable disease in 33% (66,177)—markedly better than one would expect from chemotherapy. A phase III trial comparing crizotinib to chemotherapy in this patient population is on-going.

Despite the recent successes in treating some patients with the EGFR TKIs, drug resistance usually develops, primarily by two main mechanisms: acquisition of a second mutation that allows EGFR activation despite the presence of an inhibitor (eg, T790M) or development of dependence on an alternative signaling pathway that allows for the activation of downstream signaling pathways (eg, PI3K/AKT) despite EGFR inhibition. Based upon work from several groups, the T790M mutation is found in about 50% of the cases with acquired resistance to EGFR TKIs (178). One approach to overcoming this resistance is the use of an irreversible EGFR inhibitor. However, the response to irreversible EGFR inhibitors has been clinically unimpressive, potentially because the mechanisms of resistance are not mutually exclusive and can coexist in different tumors in the same patient, and even within the same tumor (178). Another explanation is that the irreversible EGFR inhibitors inhibit wildtype EGFR better than they inhibit mutant EGFR. Another approach is to develop agents that preferentially inhibit mutant EGFR—specifically T790M (179). As an example of the second way in which resistance develops, c-Met amplification is found in about 10% of patients with acquired resistance to EGFR TKIs. In models of acquired resistance, the combination of EGFR and c-MET inhibition strongly inhibits growth and induces apoptosis (180). Likewise preliminary data demonstrate clinical responses.

Nonsteroidal anti-inflammatory drugs (NSAIDs) might prevent cancer in humans. A prospective study of 12,668 subjects showed that the incidence of lung cancer, breast cancer, and colon cancer was lower in those who reported aspirin use (181). The mechanisms by which NSAIDs might prevent cancer are unclear, although it is likely that the inhibition of cycloxygenase-2 (COX-2) is at least partly responsible for their chemopreventive effects. COX-2 is frequently expressed in NSCLC and in premalignant lesions (182-184). COX-2 expression correlates with a worse prognosis than a lack of expression does, at least in those with early-stage disease (183,184). Histologically normal epithelium from smokers with and without known cancer shows negligible COX-2 expression (187,188). Selective COX-2 inhibitors are being studied in several settings: combined with chemotherapy for advanced NSCLC, combined with radiotherapy for locally advanced NSCLC, and for chemoprevention in patients at high risk of developing NSCLC. Although COX-2 inhibitors are well tolerated and may have the added benefit of preventing multiple types of cancer, they may also increase the risk of cardiovascular dealth which has hampered their clinical development.

■ CONCLUSIONS

NSCLC remains one of the most devastating illnesses in the United States and worldwide in terms of incidence and overall mortality rates. Primary prevention achieved by smoking cessation and smoking prevention is the only well-established mechanism of reducing the number of people affected by lung cancer. Improved screening strategies and effective chemoprevention regimens are essential, but have been frustrating and are being pursued aggressively. Surgery offers the potential for significant long-term survival in those patients who have early, localized disease. Unfortunately, 70% of all NSCLC patients have regional, nodal, or metastatic disease at the time of diagnosis. Multimodality therapies offer some hope of improving survival of patients with locally advanced disease, but current therapies are inadequate for patients with metastatic disease.

Multiple new therapeutic approaches, based upon a better understanding of the molecular heterogeneity of tumors and identification of driving genetic events, along with improved methods of identifying and selecting patients for particular therapies, have shown promise in clinical trials and further study is ongoing

References

1. Jemal A, Siegel R, Ward E, et al. Cancer statistics, 2009. *CA Cancer J Clin* 2009;59(4):225-249.
2. Kamangar F, Dores GM, Anderson WF. Patterns of cancer incidence, mortality, and prevalence across five continents: defining priorities to reduce cancer disparities in different geographic regions of the world. *J Clin Oncol* 2006;24(14): 2137-2150.
3. Goldstraw P, Crowley J, Chansky K, et al. The IASLC Lung Cancer Staging Project: proposals for the revision of the TNM stage groupings in the forthcoming (seventh) edition of the TNM Classification of malignant tumours. *J Thorac Oncol* 2007;2(8):706-714.
4. Samet JM, Avila-Tang E, Boffetta P, et al. Lung cancer in never smokers: clinical epidemiology and environmental risk factors. *Clin Cancer Res* 2009;15(18):5626-5645.
5. Devesa SS, Blot WJ, Stone BJ, et al. Recent cancer trends in the United States. *J Natl Cancer Inst* 1995;87(3):175-182.
6. Cokkinides V, Bandi P, McMahon C, et al. Tobacco control in the United States– recent progress and opportunities. *CA Cancer J Clin* 2009; 59(6):352-365.
7. Alberg AJ, Samet JM. Epidemiology of lung cancer. *Chest* 2003;123(1 Suppl):21S-49S.
8. Garfinkel L, Silverberg E. Lung cancer and smoking trends in the United States over the past 25 years. *CA Cancer J Clin* 1991;41(3):137-145.
9. Bach PB, Kattan MW, Thornquist MD, et al. Variations in lung cancer risk among smokers. *J Natl Cancer Inst* 2003; 95(6):470-478.
10. *A Report of the Surgeon General: The Health Benefits of Smoking Cessation.* 1990, US Department of Health and Human Services.
11. Hecht SS. Progress and challenges in selected areas of tobacco carcinogenesis. *Chem Res Toxicol* 2008;21(1):160-171.
12. Hung RJ, McKay JD, Gaborieau V, et al. A susceptibility locus for lung cancer maps to nicotinic acetylcholine receptor subunit genes on 15q25. *Nature* 2008;452(7187):633-637.
13. Thorgeirsson TE, Geller F, Sulem P, et al. A variant associated with nicotine dependence, lung cancer and peripheral arterial disease. *Nature* 2008;452(7187):638-642.
14. Lam DC, Girard L, Ramirez R, et al. Expression of nicotinic acetylcholine receptor subunit genes in non-small-cell lung cancer reveals differences between smokers and nonsmokers. *Cancer Res* 2007; 67(10):4638-4647.
15. Davis R, Rizwani W, Banerjee S, et al. Nicotine promotes tumor growth and metastasis in mouse models of lung cancer. *PLoS One* 2009;4(10): e7524.
16. Mossman BT, Bignon J, Corn M, et al. Asbestos: scientific developments and implications for public policy. *Science* 1990;247(4940):294-301.
17. Levin SM, Kann PE, Lax MB. Medical examination for asbestos-related disease. *Am J Ind Med* 2000;37(1):6-22.
18. Hodgson JT, Jones RD. Mortality of asbestos workers in England and Wales 1971-81. *Br J Ind Med* 1986;43(3):158-164.

19. Kjuus H, Skjaerven R, Langard S, et al. A case-referent study of lung cancer, occupational exposures and smoking. II. Role of asbestos exposure. *Scand J Work Environ Health* 1986; 12(3):203-209.

20. Samet JM. Radon and lung cancer. *J Natl Cancer Inst* 1989; 81(10):745-757.

21. Harley N, Samet JM, Cross FT, et al. Contribution of radon and radon daughters to respiratory cancer. *Environ Health Perspect* 1986;70:17-21.

22. The effect of vitamin E and beta carotene on the incidence of lung cancer and other cancers in male smokers. The Alpha-Tocopherol, Beta Carotene Cancer Prevention Study Group. *N Engl J Med* 1994;330(15):1029-1035.

23. Omenn GS, Goodman GE, Thornquist MD, et al. Effects of a combination of beta carotene and vitamin A on lung cancer and cardiovascular disease. *N Engl J Med* 1996;334(18): 1150-1155.

24. Hennekens CH, Buring JE, Manson JE, et al. Lack of effect of long-term supplementation with beta carotene on the incidence of malignant neoplasms and cardiovascular disease. *N Engl J Med* 1996; 334(18):1145-1149.

25. Gaziano JM, Glynn RJ, Christen WG, et al. Vitamins E and C in the prevention of prostate and total cancer in men: The Physicians' Health Study II randomized controlled trial. *JAMA* 2009;301(1):52-62.

26. Ebbing M, Bonaa KH, Nygard O, et al. Cancer incidence and mortality after treatment with folic acid and vitamin B12. *JAMA* 2009;302(19): 2119-2126.

27. Omenn GS. Chemoprevention of lung cancers: Lessons from CARET, the beta-carotene and retinol efficacy trial, and prospects for the future. *Eur J Cancer Prev* 2007;16(3): 184-191.

28. Schottenfeld D. Etiology and epidemiology of lung cancer. In: HI Pass HI, Mitchell JB, Johnson DH, Turrisis AT, Minna JD, (eds): *Lung Cancer: Principles and Practice*. Philadelphia: Lippincott Williams and Wilkins; 2000:367-388.

29. Lee G, Walser TC, Dubinett SM. Chronic inflammation, chronic obstructive pulmonary disease, and lung cancer. *Curr Opin Pulm Med* 2009;15(4):303-307.

30. Rudin CM, Avila-Tang E, Harris CC, et al. Lung cancer in never smokers: Molecular profiles and therapeutic implications. *Clin Cancer Res* 2009; 15(18):5646-5661.

31. Tokuhata GK, Lilienfeld AM. Familial aggregation of lung cancer in humans. *J Natl Cancer Inst* 1963;30:249-253.

32. Ooi WL, Elston RC, Chen VW, et al. Increased familial risk for lung cancer. *J Natl Cancer Inst* 1986;76(2):217-222.

33. Sellers TA, Bailey-Wilson JE, Elston RC, et al. Evidence for Mendelian inheritance in the pathogenesis of lung cancer. *J Natl Cancer Inst* 1990; 82(15):1272-1279.

34. Sellers TA, Chen PL, Potter JD, et al. Segregation analysis of smoking-associated malignancies: Evidence for Mendelian inheritance. *Am J Med Genet* 1994;52(3):308-314.

35. Nazar-Stewart V, Motulsky AG, Eaton DL, et al. The glutathione S-transferase mu polymorphism as a marker for susceptibility to lung carcinoma. *Cancer Res* 1993;53(10 Suppl):2313-2318.

36. Seidegard J, Pero RW, Markowitz MM, et al. Isoenzyme(s) of glutathione transferase (class Mu) as a marker for the susceptibility to lung cancer: A follow up study. *Carcinogenesis* 1990;11(1):33-36.

37. Brockmoller J, Kerb R, Drakoulis N, et al. Genotype and phenotype of glutathione S-transferase class mu isoenzymes mu and psi in lung cancer patients and controls. *Cancer Res* 1993;53(5):1004-1011.

38. Nakachi K, Imai K, Hayashi S, et al. Polymorphisms of the CYP1A1 and glutathione S-transferase genes associated with susceptibility to lung cancer in relation to cigarette dose in a Japanese population. *Cancer Res* 1993;53(13):2994-2999.

39. Gorlova OY, Weng SF, Zhang Y, et al. DNA repair capacity and lung cancer risk in never smokers. *Cancer Epidemiol Biomarkers Prev* 2008; 17(6):1322-1328.

40. Shen H, Spitz MR, Qiao Y, et al. Smoking, DNA repair capacity and risk of nonsmall cell lung cancer. *Int J Cancer* 2003;107(1):84-88.

41. Spitz MR, Etzel CJ, Dong Q, et al. An expanded risk prediction model for lung cancer. *Cancer Prev Res (Phila, PA)* 2008;1(4):250-254.

42. Office of Smoking and Health, Cigarette smoking among adults—United States, 1992, and changes in the definition of current cigarette smoking. US centers for Disease Control. *MMWR Morb Mortal Wkly Rep* 1994;43.

43. Cigarette smoking among adults–United States, 2000. *MMWR Morb Mortal Wkly Rep* 2002;51(29):642-645.

44. Patz EF, Jr., Goodman PC, Bepler G. Screening for lung cancer. *N Engl J Med* 2000;343(22):1627-1633.

45. Henschke CI, McCauley DI, Yankelevitz DF, et al. Early Lung Cancer Action Project: Overall design and findings from baseline screening. *Lancet* 1999; 354(9173):99-105.

46. Anonymous. Lung cancer trial results show mortality benefit with low-dose CT. http://www.cancer.gov/newscenter/press-releases/NLSTresultsRelease-Posted November 4, 2010.

47. van Iersel CA, de Koning HJ, Draisma G, et al. Risk-based selection from the general population in a screening trial: Selection criteria, recruitment and power for the Dutch-Belgian randomised lung cancer multi-slice CT screening trial (NELSON). *Int J Cancer* 2007; 120(4):868-874.

48. Mulshine JL. Screening for lung cancer: In pursuit of pre-metastatic disease. *Nat Rev Cancer* 2003;3(1):65-73.

49. Hong WK, Lippman SM, Itri LM, et al. Prevention of second primary tumors with isotretinoin in squamous-cell carcinoma of the head and neck. *N Engl J Med* 1990;323(12):795-801.

50. Khuri FR, Lee JJ, Lippman SM, et al. Randomized phase III trial of low-dose isotretinoin for prevention of second primary tumors in stage I and II head and neck cancer patients. *J Natl Cancer Inst* 2006;98(7):441-450.

51. van Zandwijk N, Dalesio O, Pastorino U, et al. EUROSCAN, a randomized trial of vitamin A and N-acetylcysteine in patients with head and neck cancer or lung cancer. For the EUropean Organization for Research and Treatment of Cancer Head and Neck and Lung Cancer Cooperative Groups. *J Natl Cancer Inst* 2000; 92(12):977-986.

52. Lippman SM, Lee JJ, Karp DD, et al. Randomized phase III intergroup trial of isotretinoin to prevent second primary tumors in stage I non-small-cell lung cancer. *J Natl Cancer Inst* 2001;93(8): 605-618.

53. Harris RE, Beebe-Donk J, Alshafie GA. Cancer chemoprevention by cyclooxygenase 2 (COX-2) blockade: Results of case control studies. *Subcell Biochem* 2007;42:193-212.

54. Lee JM, Yanagawa J, Peebles KA, et al. Inflammation in lung carcinogenesis: New targets for lung cancer chemoprevention and treatment. *Crit Rev Oncol Hematol* 2008;66(3):208-217.

55. Girard L, Zochbauer-Muller S, Virmani AK, et al. Genome-wide allelotyping of lung cancer identifies new regions of allelic loss, differences between small cell lung cancer and

non-small cell lung cancer, and loci clustering. *Cancer Res* 2000;60(17):4894-4906.

56. Weir BA, Woo MS, Getz G, et al. Characterizing the cancer genome in lung adenocarcinoma. *Nature* 2007;450(7171): 893-898.

57. Szak ST, Pietenpol JA, Carbone DP. p53. In: HI, Mitchell JB, Johnson DH, Turrisi AT, Minna JD, (eds): *Lung Cancer: Principles and Practice,*. Philadelphia: Lippincott Williams and Wilkins; 2000:120-132.

58. Rodenhuis S, Slebos RJ. Clinical significance of ras oncogene activation in human lung cancer. *Cancer Res* 199;52(9 Suppl): 2665S-2669S.

59. Slebos RJ, Kibbelaar RE, Dalesio O, et al. K-ras oncogene activation as a prognostic marker in adenocarcinoma of the lung. *N Engl J Med* 1990; 323(9):561-565.

60. Loriot Y, Mordant P, Deutsch E, et al. Are RAS mutations predictive markers of resistance to standard chemotherapy? *Nat Rev Clin Oncol* 2009;6(9):528-534.

61. Azzoli CG, Baker S, Jr., Temin S, et al. American Society of Clinical Oncology Clinical Practice Guideline update on chemotherapy for stage IV non-small-cell lung cancer. *J Clin Oncol* 2009;27(36):6251-6266.

62. Johnson BE, Heymach JV. Farnesyl transferase inhibitors for patients with lung cancer. *Clin Cancer Res* 2004;10(12 Pt 2): 4254S-4257S.

63. Shaw AT, Yeap BY, Mino-Kenudson M, et al. Clinical features and outcome of patients with non-small-cell lung cancer who harbor EML4-ALK. *J Clin Oncol* 2009; 27(26):4247-4253.

64. Travis WD, Brambilla E, Muller-Hermlink HK, et al. *World Health Organization Classification of Tumours. Pathology and Genetics of Tumours of the Lung, Pleura, Thymus and Heart.* Lyon: IARC Press; 2004.

65. Morgenszstern D, Waqar S, Subramanian J, et al. Improving survival for stage IV non-small cell lung cancer: A surveillance, epidemiology, and end results survey from 1990 to 2005. J *Thorac Oncol* 2009; 4(12):1524-1529.

66. Tang AW, Moss HA, Robertson RJ. The solitary pulmonary nodule. *Eur J Radiol* 2003;45(1):69-77.

67. Erasmus JJ, Connolly JE, McAdams HP, et al. Solitary pulmonary nodules: Part I. Morphologic evaluation for differentiation of benign and malignant lesions. *Radiographics* 2000;20(1):43-58.

68. Gould MK, Maclean CC, Kuschner WG, et al. Accuracy of positron emission tomography for diagnosis of pulmonary nodules and mass lesions: A meta-analysis. *JAMA* 2001; 285(7):914-924.

69. Fischer BM, Mortensen J, Hojgaard L. Positron emission tomography in the diagnosis and staging of lung cancer: A systematic, quantitative review. *Lancet Oncol* 2001;2(11): 659-666.

70. van Klaveren RJ, Oudkerk M, Prokop M, et al. Management of lung nodules detected by volume CT scanning. *N Engl J Med* 2009; 361(23):2221-2229.

71. Lardinois D, Weder W, Hany TF, et al. Staging of non-small-cell lung cancer with integrated positron-emission tomography and computed tomography. *N Engl J Med* 2003;348(25):2500-2507.

72. Detterbeck FC, Boffa DJ, Tanoue LT. The new lung cancer staging system. *Chest* 2009;136(1):260-271.

73. Kassis ES, Vaporciyan AA, Swisher SG, et al. Application of the revised lung cancer staging system (IASLC Staging Project) to a cancer center population. *J Thorac Cardiovasc Surg.* 2009;138(2):412-418 e1-2.

74. Keller SM. Complete mediastinal lymph node dissection— Does it make a difference? *Lung Cancer* 2002;36(1):7-8.

75. Ginsberg RJ, Rubinstein LV. Randomized trial of lobectomy versus limited resection for T1 N0 non- small cell lung cancer. Lung Cancer Study Group. *Ann Thorac Surg* 1995;60(3): 615-622; discussion 622-623.

76. Ferguson MK, Little L, Rizzo L, et al. Diffusing capacity predicts morbidity and mortality after pulmonary resection. *J Thorac Cardiovasc Surg* 1988;96(6):894-900.

77. Miller JI, Jr. Physiologic evaluation of pulmonary function in the candidate for lung resection. *J Thorac Cardiovasc Surg* 1993;105(2):347-351; discussion 351-2.

78. Bush DA, Slater JD, Bonnet R, et al. Proton-beam radiotherapy for early-stage lung cancer. *Chest* 1999;116(5):1313-1319.

79. Morita K, Fuwa N, Suzuki Y, et al. Radical radiotherapy for medically inoperable non-small cell lung cancer in clinical stage I: A retrospective analysis of 149 patients. *Radiother Oncol* 1997;42(1): 31-36.

80. Pennathur A, Luketich JD, Heron DE, et al. Stereotactic radiosurgery for the treatment of stage I non-small cell lung cancer in high-risk patients. *J Thorac Cardiovasc Surg* 2009;137(3):597-604.

81. Timmerman R, Papiez L, McGarry R, et al. Extracranial stereotactic radioablation: Results of a phase I study in medically inoperable stage I non-small cell lung cancer. *Chest* 2003;124(5):1946-1955.

82. Christie NA, Pennathur A, Burton SA, et al. Stereotactic radiosurgery for early stage non-small cell lung cancer: Rationale, patient selection, results, and complications. *Semin Thorac Cardiovasc Surg* 2008;20(4):290-297.

83. Thomas P, Rubinstein L. Cancer recurrence after resection: T1 N0 non-small cell lung cancer. Lung Cancer Study Group. *Ann Thorac Surg* 1990;49(2):242-246; discussion 246-247.

84. Martini N, Bains MS, Burt ME, et al. Incidence of local recurrence and second primary tumors in resected stage I lung cancer. *J Thorac Cardiovasc Surg* 1995;109(1):120-129.

85. Martin LW, Correa AM, Hofstetter W, et al. The evolution of treatment outcomes for resected stage IIIA non-small cell lung cancer over 16 years at a single institution. *J Thorac Cardiovasc Surg* 2005; 130(6):1601-1610.

86. Rosell R, Gomez-Codina J, Camps C, et al. A randomized trial comparing preoperative chemotherapy plus surgery with surgery alone in patients with non-small-cell lung cancer. *N Engl J Med* 1994;330(3): 153-158.

87. Roth JA, Fossella F, Komaki R, et al. A randomized trial comparing perioperative chemotherapy and surgery with surgery alone in resectable stage IIIA non-small-cell lung cancer. *J Natl Cancer Inst* 1994;86(9):673-680.

88. Furuse K, Fukuoka M, Kawahara M, et al. Phase III study of concurrent versus sequential thoracic radiotherapy in combination with mitomycin, vindesine, and cisplatin in unresectable stage III non-small-cell lung cancer. *J Clin Oncol* 1999;17(9):2692-2699.

89. Curran W, Scott C, Langer C, et al. Phase III comparison of sequential vs concurrent chemoradiation for patients (Pts) with unresected stage III non-small cell lung cancer (NSCLC): Initial Report of Radiation Therapy Oncology Group (RTOG) 9410. in *American* Society of Clinical Oncology, 2000.

90. Jett JR, Scott WJ, Rivera MP, et al. Guidelines on treatment of stage IIIB non-small cell lung cancer. *Chest* 2003;123 (1 Suppl):221S-225S.

91. Stuschke M, Thames HD. Hyperfractionated radiotherapy of human tumors: Overview of the randomized clinical trials. *Int J Radiat Oncol Biol Phys* 1997;37(2):259-267.

92. Schild SE, Stella PJ, Geyer SM, et al. Phase III trial comparing chemotherapy plus once-daily or twice-daily radiotherapy in stage III non-small-cell lung cancer. *Int J Radiat Oncol Biol Phys* 2002; 54(2):370-378.

93. Saunders M, Dische S, Barrett A, et al. Continuous, hyperfractionated, accelerated radiotherapy (CHART) versus conventional radiotherapy in non-small cell lung cancer: Mature data from the randomised multicentre trial. CHART Steering committee. *Radiother Oncol* 1999;52(2):137-148.

94. Fisher MD, D'Orazio A. Concurrent chemoradiotherapy followed by consolidation docetaxel in stage IIIB non small-cell lung cancer (SWOG 9504). *Clin Lung Cancer* 2000;2(1):25-26.

95. Bhatia S, Hanna N, Ansari R, et al. Carboplatin plus paclitaxel and sequential radiation followed by consolidation carboplatin and paclitaxel in patients with previously untreated locally advanced NSCLC. A Hoosier Oncology Group (HOG) phase II study. *Lung Cancer* 2002;38(1):85-89.

96. Hanna N, Neubauer M, Yiannoutsos C, et al. Phase III study of cisplatin, etoposide, and concurrent chest radiation with or without consolidation docetaxel in patients with inoperable stage III non-small-cell lung cancer: The Hoosier Oncology Group and U.S. Oncology. *J Clin Oncol* 2008;26(35): 5755-5760.

97. Alam N, Darling G, Evans WK, et al. Adjuvant chemotherapy for completely resected non-small cell lung cancer: A systematic review. *Crit Rev Oncol Hematol* 2006;58(2):146-155.

98. Alam N, Darling G, Shepherd FA, et al. Postoperative chemotherapy in non-small cell lung cancer: A systematic review. *Ann Thorac Surg* 2006; 81(5):1926-1936.

99. Okawara G, Ung YC, Markman BR, et al. Postoperative radiotherapy in stage II or IIIA completely resected non-small cell lung cancer: A systematic review and practice guideline. *Lung Cancer* 2004; 44(1):1-11.

100. Pisters KM, Evans WK, Azzoli CG, et al. Cancer Care Ontario and American Society of Clinical Oncology adjuvant chemotherapy and adjuvant radiation therapy for stages I-IIIA resectable non small-cell lung cancer guideline. *J Clin Oncol* 2007;25(34):5506-5518.

101. Pignon JP, Tribodet H, Scagliotti GV, et al. Lung adjuvant cisplatin evaluation: A pooled analysis by the LACE Collaborative Group. *J Clin Oncol* 2008;26(21):3552-3559.

102. Scagliotti GV, Fossati R, Torri V, et al. Randomized study of adjuvant chemotherapy for completely resected stage I, II, or IIIA non-small-cell Lung cancer. *J Natl Cancer Inst* 2003;95(19): 1453-1461.

103. Arriagada R, Bergman B, Dunant A, et al. Cisplatin-based adjuvant chemotherapy in patients with completely resected non-small-cell lung cancer. *N Engl J Med* 2004;350(4): 351-360.

104. Winton T, Livingston R, Johnson D, et al. Vinorelbine plus cisplatin vs. observation in resected non-small-cell lung cancer. *N Engl J Med* 2005; 352(25):2589-2597.

105. Douillard JY, Rosell R, De Lena M, et al. Adjuvant vinorelbine plus cisplatin versus observation in patients with completely resected stage IB-IIIA non-small-cell lung cancer (Adjuvant Navelbine International Trialist Association [ANITA]): A randomised controlled trial. *Lancet Oncol* 2006;7(9):719-727.

106. Strauss GM, Herndon JE, 2nd, Maddaus MA, et al. Adjuvant paclitaxel plus carboplatin compared with observation in stage IB non-small-cell lung cancer: CALGB 9633 with the Cancer and Leukemia Group B, Radiation Therapy Oncology Group, and North Central Cancer Treatment Group Study Groups. *J Clin Oncol* 2008;26(31): 5043-5051.

107. Chemotherapy in non-small cell lung cancer: A meta-analysis using updated data on individual patients from 52 randomised clinical trials. Non-small Cell Lung Cancer Collaborative Group. *BMJ* 1995;311(7010):899-909.

108. Vallieres E. Role of adjuvant systemic therapy for stage I NSCLC. *Thorac Surg Clin* 2007;17(2):279-285.

109. Hamada C, Tanaka F, Ohta M, et al. Meta-analysis of postoperative adjuvant chemotherapy with tegafur-uracil in non-small-cell lung cancer. *J Clin Oncol* 2005;23(22):4999-5006.

110. Rosell R, Gomez-Codina J, Camps C, et al. Preresectional chemotherapy in stage IIIA non-small-cell lung cancer: A 7-year assessment of a randomized controlled trial. *Lung Cancer* 1999;26(1):7-14.

111. Roth JA, Atkinson EN, Fossella F, et al. Long-term follow-up of patients enrolled in a randomized trial comparing perioperative chemotherapy and surgery with surgery alone in resectable stage IIIA non-small-cell lung cancer. *Lung Cancer* 1998;21(1):1-6.

112. Depierre A, Milleron B, Moro-Sibilot D, et al. Preoperative chemotherapy followed by surgery compared with primary surgery in resectable stage I (except T1N0), II, and IIIa non-small- cell lung cancer. *J Clin Oncol* 2002;20(1):247-253.

113. Gilligan D, Nicolson M, Smith I, et al. Preoperative chemotherapy in patients with resectable non-small cell lung cancer: Results of the MRC LU22/NVALT 2/EORTC 08012 multicentre randomised trial and update of systematic review. *Lancet* 2007;369(9577): 1929-1937.

114. Pisters KM, Vallieres E, Crowley JJ, et al. Surgery with or without preoperative paclitaxel and carboplatin in early-stage non-small cell lung cancer: Southwest Oncology Group Trial S9900, an intergroup, randomized, Phase III trial. *J Clin Oncol* 2010. in press.

115. PORT Meta-Analysis Trialists Group. Postoperative radiotherapy in non-small-cell lung cancer: Systematic review and meta-analysis of individual patient data from nine randomised controlled trials. PORT Meta-analysis Trialists Group. *Lancet* 1998;352(9124):257-263.

116. PORT Meta-Analysis Trialists Group. Postoperative radiotherapy for non-small cell lung cancer. *Cochrane Database Syst Rev* 2003;1.

117. Rube C, Phu Nguyen T, Fleckenstein J, et al. Postoperative radiotherapy in localized non-small cell lung cancer. *Lung Cancer* 2001;33 (Suppl 1): 29S-33S.

118. Trodella L, Granone P, Valente S, et al. Adjuvant radiotherapy in non-small cell lung cancer with pathological stage I: Definitive results of a phase III randomized trial. *Radiother Oncol* 2002;62(1): 11-19.

119. Effects of postoperative mediastinal radiation on completely resected stage II and stage III epidermoid cancer of the lung. The Lung Cancer Study Group. *N Engl J Med* 1986; 315(22):1377-1381.

120. Lally BE, Zelterman D, Colasanto JM, et al. Postoperative radiotherapy for stage II or III non-small-cell lung cancer using the surveillance, epidemiology, and end results database. *J Clin Oncol* 2006;24(19): 2998-3006.

121. Keller SM, Adak S, Wagner H, et al. A randomized trial of postoperative adjuvant therapy in patients with completely resected stage II or IIIA non-small-cell lung cancer. Eastern Cooperative Oncology Group. *N Engl J Med* 2000;343(17): 1217-1222.

122. The benefit of adjuvant treatment for resected locally advanced non- small-cell lung cancer. The Lung Cancer Study Group. *J Clin Oncol* 1988;6(1):9-17.

123. Dautzenberg B, Chastang C, Arriagada R, et al. Adjuvant radiotherapy versus combined sequential chemotherapy followed by radiotherapy in the treatment of resected nonsmall cell lung carcinoma. A randomized trial of 267 patients. GETCB (Groupe d'Etude et de Traitement des Cancers Bronchiques). *Cancer* 1995;76(5): 779-786.

124. Pisters KM, Kris MG, Gralla RJ, et al. Randomized trial comparing postoperative chemotherapy with vindesine and cisplatin plus thoracic irradiation with irradiation alone in stage III (N2) non-small cell lung cancer. *J Surg Oncol* 1994;56(4):236-241.

125. Sweeney CJ, Zhu J, Sandler AB, et al. Outcome of patients with a performance status of 2 in Eastern Cooperative Oncology Group Study E1594: A Phase II trial in patients with metastatic nonsmall cell lung carcinoma. *Cancer* 2001;92(10):2639-2647.

126. Albain KS, Crowley JJ, LeBlanc M, et al. Survival determinants in extensive-stage non-small-cell lung cancer: The Southwest Oncology Group experience. *J Clin Oncol* 1991;9(9):1618-1626.

127. Chemotherapy in addition to supportive care improves survival in advanced non-small-cell lung cancer: A systematic review and meta-analysis of individual patient data from 16 randomized controlled trials. *J Clin Oncol* 2008;26(28):4617-4625.

128. Ellis PA, Smith IE, Hardy JR, et al. Symptom relief with MVP (mitomycin C, vinblastine and cisplatin) chemotherapy in advanced non-small-cell lung cancer. *Br J Cancer* 1995;71(2):366-370.

129 Helsing M, Bergman B, Thaning L, et al. Quality of life and survival in patients with advanced non-small cell lung cancer receiving supportive care plus chemotherapy with carboplatin and etoposide or supportive care only. A multicentre randomised phase III trial. Joint Lung Cancer Study Group. *Eur J Cancer* 1998; 34(7):1036-1044.

130. Spiro SG, Rudd RM, Souhami RL, et al. Chemotherapy versus supportive care in advanced non-small cell lung cancer: Improved survival without detriment to quality of life. *Thorax* 2004;59(10):828-836.

131. Bunn PA Jr. Chemotherapy for advanced non-small-cell lung cancer: Who, what, when, why? *J Clin Oncol* 2002;20(18 Suppl): 23S-33S.

132. Schiller JH, Harrington D, Belani CP, et al. Comparison of four chemotherapy regimens for advanced non-small-cell lung cancer. *N Engl J Med* 2002;346(2):92-98.

133. Kelly K, Crowley J, Bunn PA, Jr., et al. Randomized phase III trial of paclitaxel plus carboplatin versus vinorelbine plus cisplatin in the treatment of patients with advanced non–small-cell lung cancer: A Southwest Oncology Group trial. J *Clin Oncol* 2001;19(13): 3210-3218.

134. Scagliotti GV, De Marinis F, Rinaldi M, et al. Phase III randomized trial comparing three platinum-based doublets in advanced non-small-cell lung cancer. *J Clin Oncol* 2002; 20(21):4285-4291.

135. Belani C. Phase III randomized trial of docetaxel in combination with cisplatin or carboplatin or vinorelbine plus cisplatin in advanced non–small cell lung cancer: Interim analysis. *Semin Oncol* 2001;28(3 Suppl 9):10-14.

136. Rosell R, Gatzemeier U, Betticher DC, et al. Phase III randomised trial comparing paclitaxel/ carboplatin with paclitaxel/cisplatin in patients with advanced non-small-cell lung cancer: A cooperative multinational trial. *Ann Oncol* 2002;13(10):1539-1549.

137. Ardizzoni A, Boni L, Tiseo M, et al. Cisplatin- versus carboplatin-based chemotherapy in first-line treatment of advanced non-small-cell lung cancer: An individual patient data meta-analysis. *J Natl Cancer Inst* 2007;99(11): 847-857.

138. Georgoulias V, Androulakis N, Kotsakis A, et al. Docetaxel versus docetaxel plus gemcitabine as front-line treatment of patients with advanced non-small cell lung cancer: A randomized, multicenter phase III trial. *Lung Cancer* 2008;59(1):57-63.

139. Lilenbaum RC, Herndon JE, 2nd, List MA, et al. Single-agent versus combination chemotherapy in advanced non-small-cell lung cancer: The cancer and leukemia group B (study 9730). *J Clin Oncol* 2005;23(1):190-196.

140. Sederholm C. Gemcitabine versus gemcitabine/carboplatin in advanced non-small cell lung cancer: Preliminary findings in a phase III trial of the Swedish Lung Cancer Study Group. *Semin Oncol* 2002;29(3 Suppl 9):50-54.

141. Crino L, Scagliotti GV, Ricci S, et al. Gemcitabine and cisplatin versus mitomycin, ifosfamide, and cisplatin in advanced non-small-cell lung cancer: A randomized phase III study of the Italian Lung Cancer Project. *J Clin Oncol* 1999;17(11):3522-3530.

142. Greco FA, Gray JR, Jr., Thompson DS, et al. Prospective randomized study of four novel chemotherapy regimens in patients with advanced nonsmall cell lung carcinoma: A minnie pearl cancer research network trial. *Cancer* 2002;95(6):1279-1285.

143. Souquet PJ, Tan EH, Rodrigues Pereira J, et al. GLOB-1: A prospective randomised clinical phase III trial comparing vinorelbine-cisplatin with vinorelbine-ifosfamide-cisplatin in metastatic non-small-cell lung cancer patients. *Ann Oncol* 2002;13(12):1853-1861.

144. Alberola V, Camps C, Provencio M, et al. Cisplatin plus gemcitabine versus a cisplatin-based triplet versus nonplatinum sequential doublets in advanced non-small-cell lung cancer: A Spanish Lung Cancer Group phase III randomized trial. *J Clin Oncol* 2003;21(17):3207-3213.

145. Scagliotti GV, Parikh P, von Pawel J, et al. Phase III study comparing cisplatin plus gemcitabine with cisplatin plus pemetrexed in chemotherapy-naive patients with advanced-stage non-small-cell lung cancer. *J Clin Oncol* 2008;26(21):3543-3551.

146. Socinski MA, Schell MJ, Peterman A, et al. Phase III trial comparing a defined duration of therapy versus continuous therapy followed by second-line therapy in advanced-stage IIIB/IV non-small-cell lung cancer. *J Clin Oncol* 2002;20(5):1335-1343.

147. Smith IE, O'Brien ME, Talbot DC, et al. Duration of chemotherapy in advanced non-small-cell lung cancer: A randomized trial of three versus six courses of mitomycin, vinblastine, and cisplatin. *J Clin Oncol* 2001;19(5):1336-1343.

148. Sandler A, Gray R, Perry MC, et al. Paclitaxel-carboplatin alone or with bevacizumab for non-small-cell lung cancer. *N Engl J Med* 2006;355(24):2542-2550.

149. Ramalingam SS, Dahlberg SE, Langer CJ, et al. Outcomes for elderly, advanced-stage non small-cell lung cancer patients treated with bevacizumab in combination with carboplatin and paclitaxel: Analysis of Eastern Cooperative Oncology Group Trial 4599. *J Clin Oncol* 2008;26(1):60-65.

150. Shepherd FA, Dancey J, Ramlau R, et al. Prospective randomized trial of docetaxel versus best supportive care in patients with non-small-cell lung cancer previously treated with platinum-based chemotherapy. *J Clin Oncol* 2000;18(10):2095-2103.

151. Fossella FV, DeVore R, Kerr RN, et al. Randomized phase III trial of docetaxel versus vinorelbine or ifosfamide in patients with advanced non-small-cell lung cancer previously treated with platinum-containing chemotherapy regimens. The TAX 320 Non-Small Cell Lung Cancer Study Group. *J Clin Oncol* 2000; 18(12):2354-2362.

152. Hanna N, Shepherd FA, Fossella FV, et al. Randomized phase III trial of pemetrexed versus docetaxel in patients with non-small-cell lung cancer previously treated with chemotherapy. *J Clin Oncol* 2004; 22(9):1589-1597.

153. Fukuoka M, Yano S, Giaccone G, et al. Multi-institutional randomized phase II trial of gefitinib for previously treated patients with advanced non-small-cell lung cancer (The IDEAL 1 Trial) [corrected]. *J Clin Oncol* 2003;21(12): 2237-2246.

154. Kris MG, Natale RB, Herbst RS, et al. Efficacy of gefitinib, an inhibitor of the epidermal growth factor receptor tyrosine kinase, in symptomatic patients with non-small cell lung cancer: A randomized trial. *JAMA* 2003;290(16):2149-2158.

155. Thatcher N, Chang A, Parikh P, et al. Gefitinib plus best supportive care in previously treated patients with refractory advanced non-small-cell lung cancer: Results from a randomised, placebo-controlled, multicentre study (Iressa Survival Evaluation in Lung Cancer). *Lancet* 2005;366(9496): 1527-1537.

156. Kim ES, Hirsh V, Mok T, et al. Gefitinib versus docetaxel in previously treated non-small-cell lung cancer (INTEREST): A randomised phase III trial. *Lancet* 2008;372(9652): 1809-1818.

157. Gatzemeier U, Pluzanska A, Szczesna A, et al. Phase III study of erlotinib in combination with cisplatin and gemcitabine in advanced non-small-cell lung cancer: The Tarceva Lung Cancer Investigation Trial. *J Clin Oncol* 2007;25(12): 1545-1552.

158. Herbst RS, Prager D, Hermann R, et al. TRIBUTE: A phase III trial of erlotinib hydrochloride (OSI-774) combined with carboplatin and paclitaxel chemotherapy in advanced non-small-cell lung cancer. *J Clin Oncol* 2005;23(25):5892-5899.

159. Shepherd FA, Rodrigues Pereira J, et al. Erlotinib in previously treated non-small-cell lung cancer. *N Engl J Med* 2005;353(2):123-132.

160. Lynch TJ, Bell DW, Sordella R, et al. Activating mutations in the epidermal growth factor receptor underlying responsiveness of non-small-cell lung cancer to gefitinib. *N Engl J Med* 2004;350(21): 2129-2139.

161. Paez JG, Janne PA, Lee JC, et al. EGFR mutations in lung cancer: Correlation with clinical response to gefitinib therapy. *Science* 2004; 304(5676):1497-500.

162. Pao W, Miller V, Zakowski M, et al. EGF receptor gene mutations are common in lung cancers from "never smokers" and are associated with sensitivity of tumors to gefitinib and erlotinib. *Proc Natl Acad Sci USA* 2004;101(36):13306-13311.

163. Mok TS, Wu YL, Thongprasert S, et al. Gefitinib or carboplatin-paclitaxel in pulmonary adenocarcinoma. *N Engl J Med* 2009;361(10):947-957.

164. Pirker R, Pereira JR, Szczesna A, et al. Cetuximab plus chemotherapy in patients with advanced non-small-cell lung cancer (FLEX): An open-label randomised phase III trial. *Lancet* 2009;373(9674): 1525-1531.

165. Lynch TJ, Patel T, Dreisbach L, et al. Overall survival (OS) results from the phase III trial BMS 099: Cetuximab+Taxane/carboplatin as 1st-line treatment for advanced NSCLC. *J Thorac Oncol* 2008; 3(11(S4)):305S.

166. Miller VA, Riely GJ, Zakowski MF, et al. Molecular characteristics of bronchioloalveolar carcinoma and adenocarcinoma, bronchioloalveolar carcinoma subtype, predict response to erlotinib. *J Clin Oncol* 2008;26(9):1472-1478.

167. Ciuleanu T, Brodowicz T, Zielinski C, et al. Maintenance pemetrexed plus best supportive care versus placebo plus best supportive care for non-small-cell lung cancer: A randomised, double-blind, phase 3 study. *Lancet* 2009; 374(9699):1432-1440.

168. Cappuzzo F, Ciuleanu T, Stelmakh L, et al. SATURN: A double-blind, randomized, phase III study of maintenance erlotinib versus placebo following nonprogression with first-line platinum-based chemotherapy in patients with advanced NSCLC. *J Clin Oncol* 2009; 27(15S): p. suppl; abstr 8001.

169. Basche M, Kelly K. Treatment of non-small-cell lung cancer in older persons. *Oncology (Huntingt)* 2003;17(1):31-39; discussion 43-44, 47-48.

170. Detterbeck FC, Jones DR, Kernstine KH, et al. Lung cancer. Special treatment issues. *Chest* 2003;123(1 Suppl): 244S-258S.

171. Flannery TW, Suntharalingam M, Regine WF, et al. Long-term survival in patients with synchronous, solitary brain metastasis from non-small-cell lung cancer treated with radiosurgery. *Int J Radiat Oncol Biol Phys* 2008;72(1):19-23.

172. Kim ES, Herbst RS, Lee JJ, et al. Phase II randomized study of biomarker-directed treatment for non-small cell lung cancer (NSCLC): The BATTLE (Biomarker-Integrated Approaches of Targeted Therapy for Lung Cancer Elimination) clinical trial program. *J Clin Oncol* 2009;27(15S): p. suppl; abstr 8024.

173. Engelman JA, Chen L, Tan X, et al. Effective use of PI3K and MEK inhibitors to treat mutant Kras G12D and PIK3CA H1047R murine lung cancers. *Nat Med* 2008;14(12): 1351-1356.

174. Morabito A, Piccirillo MC, Falasconi F, et al. Vandetanib (ZD6474), a dual inhibitor of vascular endothelial growth factor receptor (VEGFR) and epidermal growth factor receptor (EGFR) tyrosine kinases: Current status and future directions. *Oncologist* 2009; 14(4):378-390.

175. Novello S, Scagliotti GV, Rosell R, et al. Phase II study of continuous daily sunitinib dosing in patients with previously treated advanced non-small cell lung cancer. *Br J Cancer* 2009;101(9):1543-1548.

176. Karp DD, Paz-Ares LG, Novello S, et al. Phase II study of the anti-insulin-like growth factor type 1 receptor antibody CP-751,871 in combination with paclitaxel and carboplatin in previously untreated, locally advanced, or metastatic non-small-cell lung cancer. *J Clin Oncol* 2009;27(15):2516-2522.

177. Choi YL, Soda M, Yamashita Y, et al. EML4-ALK mutations in lung cancer that confer resistance to ALK inhibitors. *N Engl J Med.* 2010;363:1734-9.

178. Engelman JA, Janne PA. Mechanisms of acquired resistance to epidermal growth factor receptor tyrosine kinase inhibitors in non-small cell lung cancer. *Clin Cancer Res* 2008;14(10): 2895-2899.

179. Zhou W, Ercan D, Chen L, et al. Novel mutant-selective EGFR kinase inhibitors against EGFR T790M. *Nature* 2009; 462(7276):1070-1074.

180. Engelman JA, Zejnullahu K, Mitsudomi T, et al. MET amplification leads to gefitinib resistance in lung cancer by activating ERBB3 signaling. *Science* 2007;316(5827):1039-1043.

181. Schreinemachers DM, Everson RB. Aspirin use and lung, colon, and breast cancer incidence in a prospective study. *Epidemiology* 1994;5(2):138-146.

182. Hida T, Yatabe Y, Achiwa H, et al. Increased expression of cyclooxygenase 2 occurs frequently in human lung cancers, specifically in adenocarcinomas. *Cancer Res* 1998;58(17): 3761-3764.

183. Watkins DN, Lenzo JC, Segal A, et al. Expression and localization of cyclo-oxygenase isoforms in non-small cell lung cancer. *Eur Respir J* 1999;14(2):412-418.

184. Wolff H, Saukkonen K, Anttila S, et al. Expression of cyclooxygenase-2 in human lung carcinoma. *Cancer Res* 1998;58(22):4997-5001.

185. Achiwa H, Yatabe Y, Hida T, et al. Prognostic significance of elevated cyclooxygenase 2 expression in primary, resected lung adenocarcinomas. *Clin Cancer Res* 1999;5(5):1001-1005.

186. Khuri FR, Wu H, Lee JJ, et al. Cyclooxygenase-2 overexpression is a marker of poor prognosis in stage I non-small cell lung cancer. *Clin Cancer Res* 2001;7(4):861-867.

187. Hasturk S, Kemp B, Kalapurakal SK, et al. Expression of cyclooxygenase-1 and cyclooxygenase-2 in bronchial epithelium and nonsmall cell lung carcinoma. *Cancer* 2002;94(4): 1023-1031.

188. Soslow RA, Dannenberg AJ, Rush D, et al. COX-2 is expressed in human pulmonary, colonic, and mammary tumors. *Cancer* 2000;89(12):2637-2645.

189. Mountain CF, Libshitz HI, Hermes KE. *Lung Cancer: A Handbook for Staging, Imaging, and Lymph Node Classification.* Houston: Charles P Young; 1999.

190. Salgia R, Skarin AT. Molecular abnormalities in lung cancer. *J Clin Oncol* 1998;16:1207-1217.

191. Hittleman WN, Kurie JM, Swisher SG. Molecular events in lung cancer. In: Fossella FV, Komaki R, Putnam JB (eds): *Lung Cancer.* New York: Springer-Verlag; 2003: 280-298.

192. Potti A, Willardson J, Forseen C, et al. Predictive role of HER-2/neu overexpression and clinical features at initial presentation in patients with extensive stage small cell lung carcinoma. *Lung Cancer* 2002;36:257-261.

193. Hirsch FR, Franklin WA, Veve R, et al. HER2/neu expression in malignant lung tumors. *Semin Oncol* 2002; 29:51-58.

194. Yan JJ, Chen FF, Tsai YC, et al. Immunohistochemical detection of Bcl-2 protein in small cell carcinomas. *Oncology* 1996;53:6-11.

195. Jiang SX, Sato Y, Kuwao S, et al. Expression of bcl-2 oncogene protein is prevalent in small cell lung carcinomas. *J Pathol* 1995;177:135-138.

196. Ritter CA and Arteaga CL. The epidermal growth factor receptor-tyrosine kinase: A promising therapeutic target in solid tumors. *Semin Oncol* 2003;30:3-11.

197. Franklin WA, Veve R, Hirsch FR, et al. Epidermal growth factor receptor family in lung cancer and premalignancy. *Semin Oncol* 2002;29:3-14.

198. Hiyama K, Hiyama E, Ishioka S, et al. Telomerase activity in small-cell and non–small-cell lung cancers. *J Natl Cancer Inst* 1995;87:895-902.

199. Sozzi G, Veronese ML, Negrini M, et al. The FHIT gene 3p14.2 is abnormal in lung cancer. *Cell* 1996;85:17-26.

200. Yuan J, Knorr J, Altmannsberger M, et al. Expression of p16 and lack of pRB in primary small cell lung cancer. *J Pathol* 1999;189:358-362.

Head and Neck Cancer

HEAD AND NECK CANCER

Eric S. Kim
G. Brandon Gunn
William Nassib William Jr.
Merrill S. Kies

Head and neck cancers are a diverse group of diseases, each with distinct epidemiologic, anatomic, and pathologic features. The natural history and treatment considerations may vary widely. In this chapter, our focus is on the primary management of squamous cell carcinomas (SCCs) of the head and neck (SCCHN). In recent years, we have observed significant advances in diagnosis and treatment, and recognition of the human papillomavirus (HPV) as a significant causative agent for cancers of the oropharynx. Tumor imaging is increasingly precise. Primary therapy eradicates disease in a majority of patients with early-stage SCCHN, and the long-term management of these patients currently involves an emphasis on general medical care, avoiding known carcinogens such as alcohol and tobacco, and participation in chemoprevention strategies to reduce the risk of second primary tumors (SPTs). Therapy for patients with locally advanced disease has become multimodal, and success has been achieved in improving local tumor control, disease remission, organ preservation, and overall survival. The integration of chemotherapy and novel "targeting" systemic treatment approaches with surgery and/or radiotherapy is under study and is discussed.

■ EPIDEMIOLOGY

In the United States, SCCHN represented approximately 3% (48,000) of new cancer cases and 2% (11,000) of cancer deaths in 2009 (1). However, the disease is more common in many developing countries, with a worldwide annual incidence of more than 500,000 (2).

The risk of developing head and neck cancer increases with age; most patients are above age 50. There has been a clearly demonstrated association with tobacco and alcohol use. Molecular studies provide evidence that carcinogens found in these substances have a causal role. The prevalence and spectrum of *p53* mutations are greater in cancers of patients with a history of tobacco and alcohol usage than in those without (3). Cancers of the floor of the oral cavity, larynx, and hypopharynx are uncommon in persons with no smoking history.

HPV infection is now widely accepted as another etiologic factor for SCCHN. In the United States, more than 50% of cancers arising in the oropharynx, particularly in the palatine tonsils and tongue base, contain oncogenic HPV (4). It appears that the HPV-positive oropharyngeal malignancy represents a distinct clinical and pathological subgroup of SCCHN, with poorly differentiated, basaloid histopathology (5), and marked tumor responsiveness to radiation and chemotherapy. Moreover, SCCHNs with transcriptionally active HPV-16 DNA are characterized by occasional chromosomal loss, while those lacking HPV DNA typically have gross deletions, involving chromosomal arms known to be abnormal in SCCHN (6). Thus, HPV-16 infection may be an early carcinogenic event. HPV DNA-positive tumors, particularly those associated with E6 and E7 proteins, have improved survival after chemoradiotherapy when compared to HPV-negative tumors (7). A recent case-control study reported that HPV-16-positive SCCHN were independently associated with several measures of sexual behavior and exposure to marijuana but not with cumulative measures of tobacco smoking, alcohol use, or poor oral hygiene (8). These findings suggest that HPV-16–positive SCCHN and HPV-16–negative SCCHN have different risk factor profiles. Last, SCCHN patients with heavy tobacco and alcohol exposures are at high risk of developing multiple cancers, with "field cancerization" throughout the upper aerodigestive tract and bladder. Molecular evidence indicates that some multiple primary cancers within the head and neck region and the lung may derive from a common clonal progenitor cell with an early molecular alteration (9,10). The observation that treated head and neck cancer patients may have a high risk (estimated to be 3-4% per year) of metachronous tumors has driven chemoprevention trials designed to reduce the risk of SPTs.

■ MOLECULAR PATHOGENESIS

The progression of SCCHN is thought to involve multiple stepwise alteration of molecular pathways in the squamous epithelium (11). Alterations in the *p53* gene are implicated in early steps of tumor progression, whereas mutations in the *p16* gene, an inhibitor of cyclin-dependent kinase, are associated with later stages of tumor progression (12-15). Approximately half of all tumor samples from patients with SCCHN contain p53 mutations whereas about a third contain mutations in cyclin D1 (12,13,16). Notably, patients with HPV-positive tumors have been found to be less likely to harbor a p53 mutation (17).

Metastatic progression is a partially understood and complicated process that evolves from the interaction of malignant stem cells and surrounding extracellular matrix, keratins, cell-surface proteases, mesenchymal-cell markers, cell-matrix adhesion molecules, and chemokines (11,18-22). Chemokine (C-X-C motif) receptor (CXCR4), and its ligand, stromal cell–derived factor (SDF-1) may affect the development of metastases and may stimulate the secretion of vascular endothelial growth factors (VEGFs) and related receptors (11,23-28).

The epidermal growth factor receptor (EGFR) is overexpressed in invasive SCC of the head and neck in a majority of sample tumors (29). Binding to EGFR by its natural ligands, mainly epidermal growth factor or transforming growth factor alpha (TGF-α), results in a conformational change in the receptor through dimerization which results in subsequent autoactivation of the tyrosine kinase from the intracellular domain of the receptor. This process will activate an intracellular signaling pathway, leading to the inhibition of apoptosis, activation of cell proliferation and angiogenesis, as well as an increase in metastatic spread potential (30). Moreover, increased EGFR concentration is associated with advanced stage and poor prognosis following conventional therapy (31-33).

Identifying molecular mechanisms of tumor progression will facilitate discovery of new prognostic markers and therapeutic targets.

■ DIAGNOSIS AND STAGING

Optimal therapy and treatment outcomes depend on the precise identification of the primary tumor as well as the local, regional, and distant extent of disease (Fig. 16-1). Patients with early-stage disease may present with vague symptoms and minimal physical findings, which

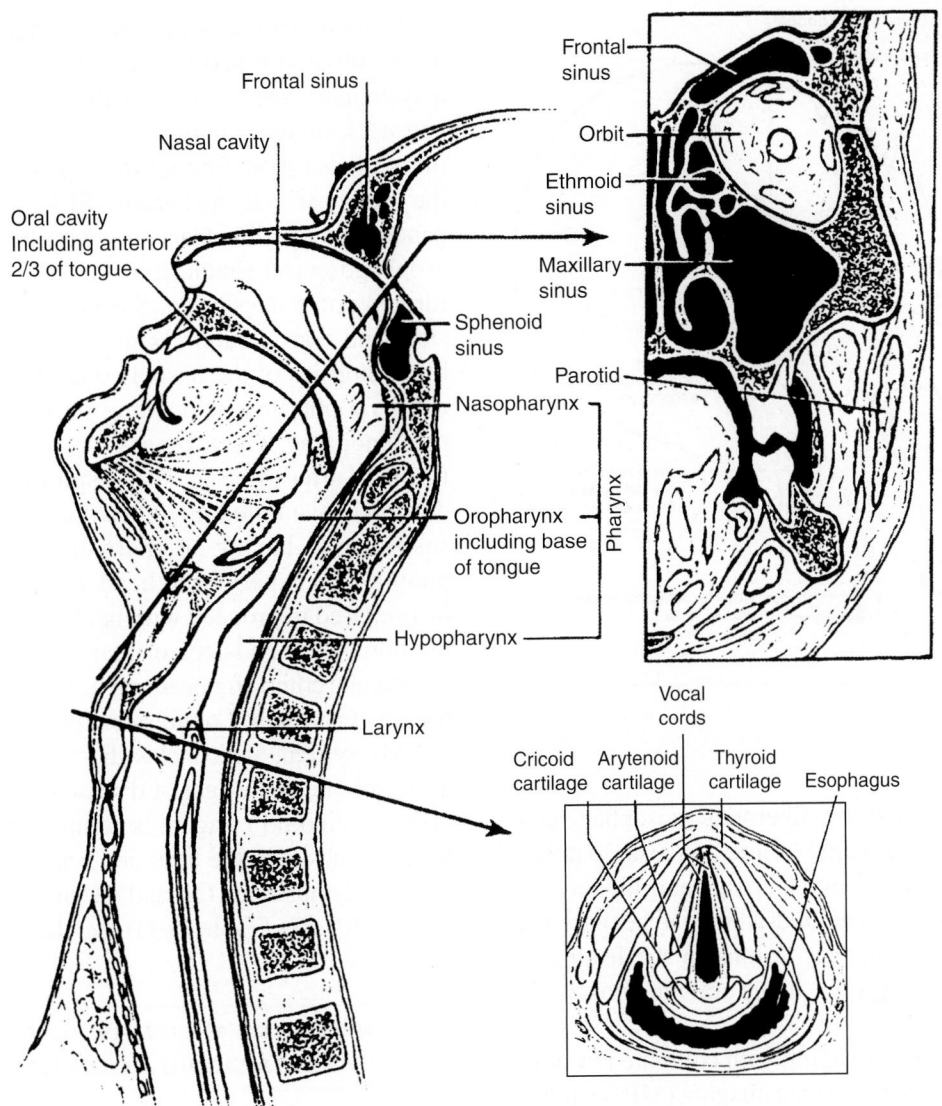

FIGURE 16-1. Head and neck anatomy.

is why a high index of suspicion for early diagnosis is needed, especially for tobacco users. A majority of patients will present with signs and symptoms of locally advanced disease, which vary according to the subsite in the head and neck. Sinusitis, unilateral nasal airway obstruction and epistaxis may be early signs of cancers of the nasal cavity or paranasal sinuses. Otitis media that is recurrent or is refractory to antibiotics is an indication for a complete ENT (ear, nose, throat) evaluation to rule out a nasopharyngeal neoplasm. Chronic otalgia, dysphagia, odynophagia (lasting ≥6 weeks), and soreness may be the presenting symptoms of oropharyngeal or hypopharyngeal cancer. Persistent hoarseness demands visualization of the larynx. However, supraglottic laryngeal neoplasms do not usually present early; in

some patients, a neck mass will be the presenting sign. Careful examination of lymph nodes in the facial, cervical, and supraclavicular regions is important because the anatomic patterns of lymphatic drainage reflect the specific subsite of a head and neck primary tumor (Fig. 16-2). Level 2/3 adenopathy, for example, suggests a primary cancer of the oral tongue or oropharynx, and posterior cervical adenopathy is frequently a result of regional spread of a nasopharyngeal tumor.

Physical examination should include careful inspection of the skin and oral/oropharyngeal mucosal surfaces; palpation of the tongue, floor of the mouth, and oropharynx; and systematic palpation of the neck. A complete examination also requires an indirect mirror examination of the oropharynx, hypopharynx, and

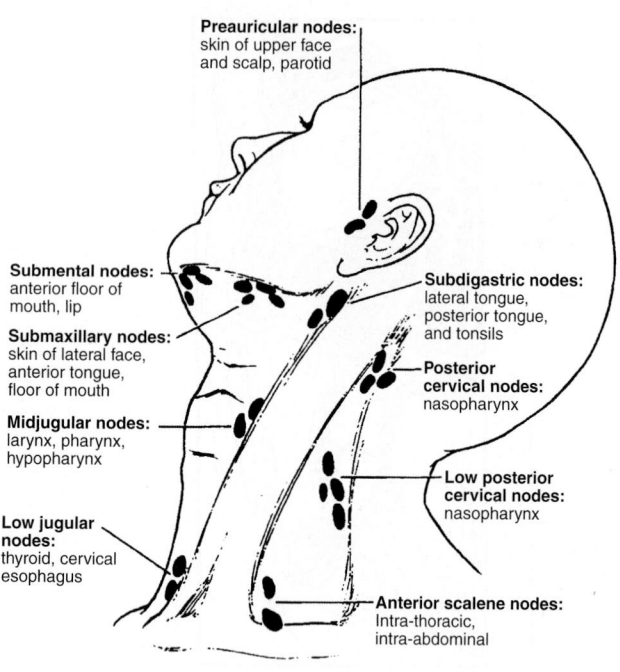

FIGURE 16-2. Nodal drainage.

larynx, complemented by fiberoptic nasopharyngolaryngoscopy. Leukoplakia (white mucosal patches that cannot be removed by scraping) and higher-risk erythroplakia (red or mixed red-white patches) are the most common premalignant lesions in the head and neck. Any suspicious surface in the oral mucosa should undergo biopsy.

Three-dimensional imaging with computed tomography (CT), magnetic resonance imaging (MRI), and/or ultrasonography is also needed to evaluate the extent of disease and to complete staging. MRI is the preferred local imaging modality for nasopharyngeal cancer. These techniques are also helpful in evaluating the response to therapy. Because the lungs are the most common sites of distant metastases, a chest x-ray should be performed as well. CT scanning of the chest should be performed for symptomatic or high-risk patients. This would include patients with nasopharyngeal cancer or those with primary tumors of other sites but presenting with N2b or greater nodal disease and low neck or supraclavicular metastases. Circulating tumor markers that would be reliable in early detection of SCCHN have not yet been identified. Epstein-Barr virus (EBV) DNA is found predominately in nasopharyngeal carcinoma (NPC) and has been identified in the serum of patients with NPC (34); thus, in patients with cervical lymphadenopathy and no obvious primary tumor, detection of EBV DNA in a lymph node may suggest a tumor of nasopharyngeal origin.

Patients who present with a suspicious neck mass and no obvious primary mucosal lesion should undergo a systematic examination of the head and neck. Head and neck imaging may be helpful. If no obvious primary site is found, fine-needle aspiration may establish the diagnosis. If metastatic SCC is demonstrated, panendoscopy (direct laryngoscopy, bronchoscopy, and esophagoscopy) should follow. This procedure is performed under anesthesia. Suspicious lesions are biopsied, and consideration is given to tonsillectomy and blind biopsies of the nasopharynx, base of the tongue and hypopharynx, depending on the pattern of lymphadenopathy. Open biopsy of a neck mass is performed after fine-needle aspiration and panendoscopy have failed to yield a diagnosis or in patients suspected of having an alternative process (eg, lymphoma). An experienced head and neck surgeon may be prepared to proceed with neck dissection if SCC of unknown head and neck primary origin is determined.

Staging criteria for head and neck cancers are based on the American Joint Commission tumor-nodes-metastasis (TNM) system, which classifies tumors according to anatomic site and extent of disease (35). Head and neck primary tumor (T) staging is complex, varying with the primary subsite in the head and neck region. Classifications for lymph node (N) and distant metastases (M) are uniform for sites (Table 16-1) other than nasopharynx.

■ NATURAL HISTORY AND IMPLICATIONS FOR THERAPY

Two-thirds of patients with SCCHN will present with stage III or IV disease. For patients with T1/2 disease (stage I/II), surgery or radiotherapy as a single modality is most often applicable and effective. Depending on the precise primary site and stage, a curative outcome will be achieved in 70 to 90% of cases. In patients with intermediate and locally advanced disease at diagnosis, combined treatment strategies have become the standard of care. Traditional surgery with postoperative radiotherapy has largely been replaced by multimodal treatment plans designed to balance competing goals of tumor eradication and organ preservation (36,37). Despite optimal local therapy, 30 to 50% of patients may develop local or regional recurrence, and nearly 20 to 30% are at risk for distant metastases. Thus, the dual goals of improved survival and decreased treatment-related morbidity have encouraged the investigation of new approaches. The addition of chemotherapy is under intense study in patients with locally advanced disease, with promising results.

TABLE
16-1A **TNM STAGING FOR THE ORAL CAVITY AND OROPHARYNX**

PRIMARY TUMOR (T)

TX	Primary tumor cannot be assessed.
T0	No evidence of primary tumor.
Tis	Carcinoma in situ.
T1	Tumor ≤2 cm in greatest dimension.
T2	Tumor >2 cm but not >4 cm in greatest dimension.
T3	Tumor >4 cm in greatest dimension.
T4(lip)	Tumor invades through cortical bone, inferior alveolar nerve, floor of mouth, or skin of face, ie, chin or nose.
T4a	Tumor invades structures adjacent to the oral cavity (eg, through cortical bone, into deep [extrinsic] muscle of tongue [genioglossus, hyoglossus, palatoglossus, and styloglossus], maxillary sinus, skin of face).
T4b	Tumor invades masticator space, pterygoid plates, or skull base and/or encases internal carotid artery.

Note: Superficial erosion alone of bone/tooth socket by gingival primary tumor is not sufficient to classify a tumor as T4.

REGIONAL LYMPH NODES (N)

NX	Regional lymph nodes cannot be assessed.
N0	No regional node metastases.
N1	Metastasis to a single ipsilateral lymph node ≤3 cm in greatest dimension.
N2	Metastasis to a single ipsilateral lymph node >3 cm but not >6 cm in greatest dimension, or to multiple ipsilateral lymph nodes none >6 cm in greatest dimension, or to bilateral or contralateral lymph nodes none >6 cm in greatest dimension.
N2a	Metastasis to a single ipsilateral lymph node >3 cm but not >6 cm in greatest dimension.
N2b	Metastasis to multiple ipsilateral lymph nodes >3 cm but not >6 cm in greatest dimension.
N2c	Metastases to bilateral or contralateral lymph nodes none >6 cm in greatest dimension.
N3	Metastasis in a lymph node >6 cm in greatest dimension.

DISTANT METASTASIS (M)

MX	Presence of distant metastasis cannot be assessed.
M0	No evidence of distant metastasis.
M1	Distant metastasis.

TABLE
16-1B **STAGE GROUPING**

Stage 0	Tis	N0	M0
Stage I	T1	N0	M0
Stage II	T2	N0	M0
Stage III	T3	N0	M0
	T1	N1	M0
	T2	N1	M0
	T3	N1	M0
Stage IVA	T4a	N0	M0
	T4a	N1	M0
	T1	N2	M0
	T2	N2	M0
	T3	N2	M0
	T4a	N2	M0
Stage IVB	Any T	N3	M0
	T4b	Any N	M0
Stage IVC	Any T	Any N	M1

NASOPHARYNX

Over 95% of endemic nasopharyngeal carcinomas (NPC) are classified as WHO type 3 and associated with EBV. NPC tends to occur in younger persons and is not associated with tobacco usage. NPC is an aggressive neoplasm with cervical lymph node metastases present in 60 to 90% of patients at diagnosis. Because of unique anatomic, biological, and clinical characteristics, therapy for NPC is distinctive. Radiotherapy is the mainstay of local therapy. The anatomy of the nasopharynx and tumor sensitivity to radiotherapy limit the role of surgery to obtaining the initial biopsy and, for selected patients, resection of residual lymphadenopathy after radiotherapy. NPCs are highly chemoradiosensitive. Intensity-modulated radiation therapy (IMRT) allows for greater conformality of the high-dose regions with relative sparing of adjacent normal tissues compared to traditional radiation techniques. Because of the proximity of the nasopharynx to normal critical structures of the central nervous system and given the propensity of NPC for skull base invasion, IMRT is the preferred radiation technique for NPC in order to improve tumor coverage and potentially reduce long-term treatment-related toxicity.

With concomitant chemoradiotherapy followed by adjuvant drug therapy, progression-free survival is 70% at 3 years in patients with locally advanced disease (37,38). In the study of Al-Sarraf et al., all histologic subtypes were included (38).

Langendijk and colleagues have published a meta-analysis indicating that concomitant chemotherapy has a substantial effect on overall survival in NPC (39). Hui and colleagues have reported a more recent randomized phase II trial of concurrent cisplatin-radiotherapy with or without neoadjuvant docetaxel and cisplatin in advanced NPC (40). Three-year progression-free survival (88 versus 60%) and overall survival (94 versus 68%) favor the sequential treatment program. A phase III study is planned.

ORAL CAVITY

The majority of oral cavity neoplasms occur in the anterior two-thirds of the tongue (oral tongue) and the floor of the mouth. Oral tongue lesions commonly arise on the lateral and ventral surfaces. Surgical resection, often with postoperative radiotherapy, is the most common and effective local treatment approach (11,37). Depending on site and tumor volume, early cancers should be resected but may be treated with radiotherapy. Small superficial lesions may be excised with little morbidity. For T2 disease, we favor surgical resection and neck dissection with postoperative concomitant chemoradiotherapy for selected patients with narrow margins or nodal metastases, particularly if there is extracapsular spread. Perineural invasion is also a significant negative prognostic sign. Forty percent of patients present with clinically evident lymph nodes. Bilateral nodal involvement is not uncommon. For primary therapy,

interstitial radiotherapy may be used in combination with external beam therapy for selected cases to achieve higher control rates than external radiation alone.

Local tumor control rates of patients with stages I and II tumors are 80 to 90% and 40 to 80%, respectively (41). For patients with locally more advanced disease (Fig. 16-3 shows an example of a patient with a retromolar trigone primary tumor invading bone, T4), surgery followed by radiation therapy (or chemoradiotherapy) is the most widely accepted approach. At the University of Texas MD Anderson Cancer Center (MDACC), neck dissection is most often performed for patients with stages II to IVa.

OROPHARYNX

We favor radiotherapy (using IMRT for parotid gland sparing to mitigate long-term xerostomia) as the principal treatment modality for oropharyngeal primary malignancies, used as a single modality for T1 and many T2 tumors. The most common cancers of the oropharynx are of the base of tongue and tonsils. Early tonsillar lesions are most often treated with radiotherapy, with quite favorable results. For T1 lesions, local control is obtained in over 90% and for T2 disease in 70 to 85%. Regional lymph nodes are treated in nearly all cases, but unilateral neck radiation is considered for

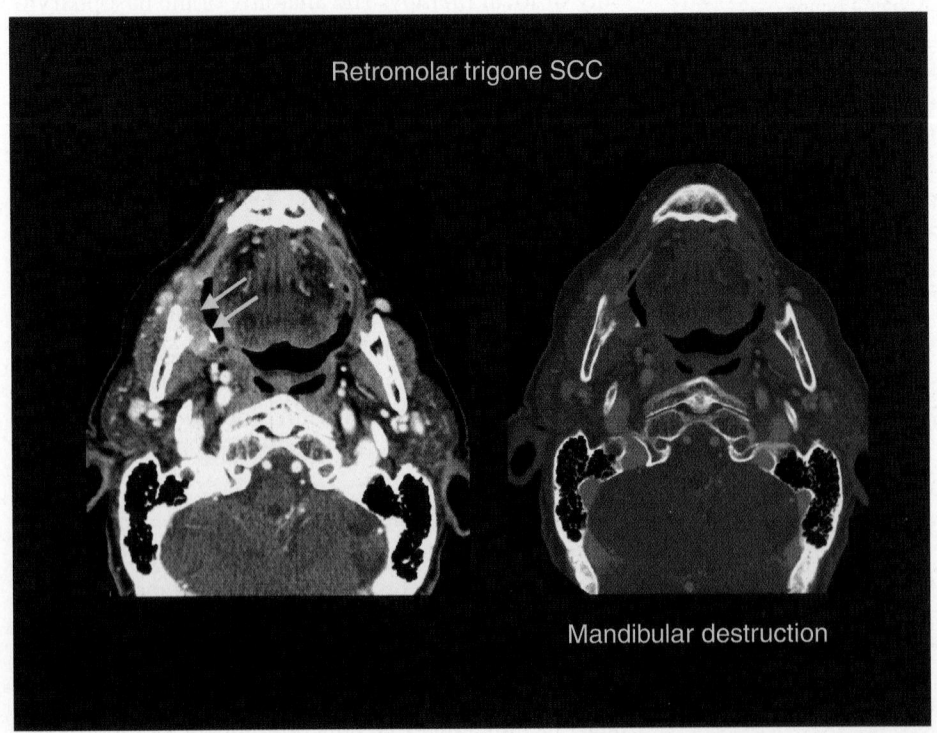

FIGURE 16-3. Retromolar trigone SCC with mandibular destruction.

well-lateralized early-stage tonsillar primaries, which reduces greatly the radiation dose to the contralateral parotid gland. Proton therapy as a radiation modality has the potential advantage of reducing the volume of normal tissue receiving radiation, but its role in head and neck cancer is not well established.

SCC of the tongue base presents a more difficult problem than tonsillar cancer because of its anatomic location, a tendency to late diagnosis, and a frequent association with nodal metastases. At presentation, 75% of patients have stage III or IV disease. Concomitant chemoradiotherapy is the current standard of care for a large majority of patients with tobacco-associated tongue base cancers.

As discussed above, an increasing percentage of tonsillar and tongue base cancers may be associated with HPV. Nodal metastases are common. Moreover, these tumors may be highly sensitive to drug or radiation therapy, and the overall prognosis for these patients appears to be superior to matched patients with HPV negative tumors (7). See the accompanying discussion.

HYPOPHARYNX

With 75% of lesions occurring in the pyriform sinus, carcinoma of the hypopharynx is relatively uncommon but virulent (Fig. 16-4). At presentation, more than 75% of patients have advanced disease (T3 and T4). Selected patients are candidates for laryngectomy; for most, consideration is given to multimodal therapy. The overall 5-year survival rate is lower than 30%. The European Organization for Research and Treatment of Cancer (EORTC), in a phase III trial, has demonstrated that laryngeal preservation with sequential chemoradiotherapy is a feasible alternative to radical surgery for many

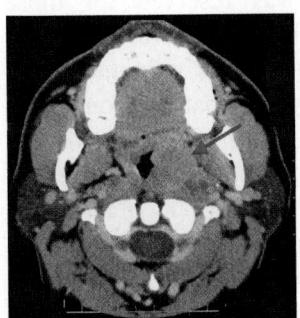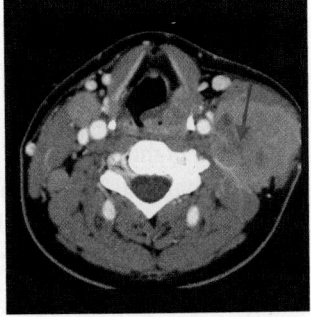

FIGURE 16-4. Axial CT, advanced SC of the pyriform sinus, T3, N3, N0.

patients with locally advanced disease (42). In a quite recent trial of patients with resectable advanced squamous cell carcinoma of the larynx or hypopharynx, Lefebvre et al. (43) compared sequential treatment with two cycles of cisplatin and 5-fluorouracil (5-FU) followed by radiotherapy with an alternating arm of four cycles of cisplatin and fluorouracil administered during weeks 1, 4, 7, and 10 alternating with radiotherapy. A total of 450 patients were entered. Survival with a functional larynx was similar in comparison of the arms, as was overall survival (4.4 versus 5.1 years, respectively). Late edema or fibrosis was observed in 16% of patients in the sequential arm and in 11% in the alternating arm.

LARYNX

Modern conservation surgical techniques are applicable for some patients with SCC of the larynx, and this subject has been reviewed (44). The most widely used treatment of T1 and T2 cancers of the larynx is radiotherapy, which has demonstrated 5-year survival rates of 96 to 98% for patients with T1 disease and 80 to 94% for those with T2 disease (45). For fixed vocal cords (T3 disease), radiotherapy has produced local control rates between 30 and 60% (46). Combined treatment with systemic chemotherapy and radiotherapy is more often the current therapeutic strategy also a nonsurgical alternative. In patients with local recurrence, salvage laryngectomy has achieved control in up to 80% of cases (47). For most patients with T4 lesions, total laryngectomy with postoperative radiation has been the standard approach.

Induction chemotherapy with cisplatin and fluorouracil has long been recognized as highly active, with clinical partial and complete responses observed in 80 to 90% of previously untreated patients (48,49). See Fig. 16-5 for examples of laryngeal cancers that are responding to chemotherapy. It was previously postulated that a substantial response to initial treatment with chemotherapy would lead to an improvement in therapeutic efficacy for surgery or radiotherapy. This led to the Department of Veterans Affairs (VA) Laryngeal Cancer Study (50), in which 332 patients with stage III or IV SCC of the larynx were randomized to receive either induction chemotherapy consisting of cisplatin and fluorouracil followed by radiotherapy or surgery and postoperative radiotherapy. Patients who experienced no tumor response to chemotherapy or those who had locally persistent or recurrent cancer underwent salvage laryngectomy. Two-year survival for both treatment

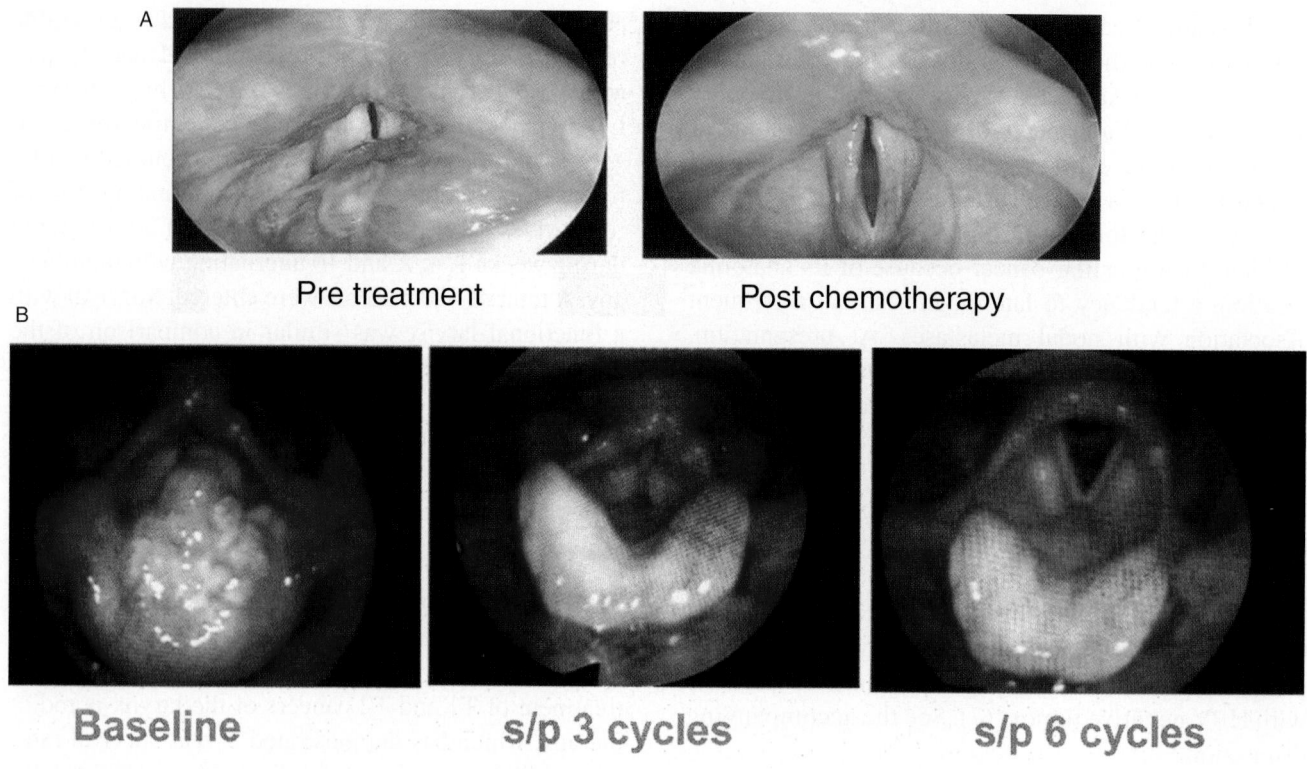

FIGURE 16-5. **A.** Videostroboscopy of a patient with SCC of the larynx—T2, N0, M0—before and after induction chemotherapy. **B.** Videostroboscopy of a patient with supraglottic larynx SCC—T2, N1, M0—before and after induction chemotherapy.

groups was 68%, and 41% of patients randomly assigned to the experimental arm were alive with a functional larynx at 2 years. Thus, the efficacy of chemotherapy followed by radiotherapy (with surgical salvage) was similar to that of surgery followed by radiotherapy and established organ preservation as a realistic goal of nonsurgical treatment administered with curative intent. Lefebvre et al. (42) later reported sequential chemotherapy and radiation could also be effective in selected patients with cancers of the hypopharynx.

In the VA study (50), trends in patterns of tumor relapse were observed with 20% of patients in the chemotherapy arm having locoregional recurrence versus 7% in the surgery arm. Distant disease recurrence was more likely in the surgical arm, affecting 17% of patients versus 11% in the chemotherapy/radiotherapy arm. Salvage laryngectomy was required more often in patients with glottic cancers than in those with supraglottic primary sites (43 versus 31%), in patients with fixed vocal cords than in those with mobile vocal cords (41 versus 29%), and in patients with gross invasion of thyroid cartilage than in patients without (41 versus 35%). Notably, salvage laryngectomy was required in

56% of patients with T4 cancers, compared with 29% of patients with smaller primary tumors (p = .001).

The VA larynx study prompted further investigations of chemotherapy and radiotherapy for the treatment of larynx cancer using the sequential administration of induction chemotherapy, consisting of cisplatin and fluorouracil followed by radiotherapy as the control arm. This was compared with concomitant cisplatin-radiotherapy and radiotherapy administered as a single treatment modality (51). For all groups, totaling 547 patients, surgical salvage was reserved for those patients with persistent or locally recurrent disease. Survival was not affected by treatment assignment. At a median follow-up of 3.8 years, patients randomly assigned to concomitant cisplatin and radiotherapy achieved a higher rate of laryngeal preservation, 84 versus 72% in patients receiving sequential chemoradiotherapy (p = .005) or radiotherapy alone 67% (p <.001). At 2 years, 80% of patients on the concomitant chemoradiotherapy arm achieved local disease control versus 64% of patients receiving sequential chemotherapy and then radiation and 58% of patients treated with radiotherapy alone. As expected, acute mucocutaneous toxic effects of treatment were greatest in the patients who received radiotherapy with concomitant cisplatin. These trials indicate that for patients with intermediate-stage SCC of the larynx, a combined treatment program with the objectives of tumor eradication and laryngeal preservation is appropriate. It is also important to recognize that patients with locally advanced, destructive primary laryngeal cancers were not included in the more recent multigroup trial. These patients may require total laryngectomy for optimal tumor control and preservation of function.

A recent phase III study (52) in 220 patients with locally advanced but resectable SCC of the larynx or hypopharynx has demonstrated that the addition of docetaxel to cisplatin and fluorouracil (TPF) may increase tumor responsiveness and lead to definitive treatment with radiotherapy and improved larynx preservation (70 versus 58% in the PF arm), with no compromise in overall survival.

IMPACT OF NONSURGICAL TREATMENT OF ADVANCED LARYNGEAL CANCER ON SPEECH AND SWALLOWING FUNCTION

As described, combinations of chemotherapy and radiation for laryngeal preservation are well-documented alternatives to ablative surgery for disease, but few studies have objectively addressed the issue of preservation of function. Radiation produces tissue changes that can result in immediate- and long-term alterations in speech and swallowing. The magnitude of the problem will frequently depend on the administered dose and duration of treatment, the extent of the treatment field, and whether concomitant chemotherapy was used.

In general, radiotherapy has a greater impact on swallowing than it does on speech, and the addition of concomitant chemotherapy can exacerbate normal tissue injury. The adverse impact of radiation may equal or exceed that associated with surgery, dependent on the treatment dose and volume, and because the sequelae may increase in severity years after the completion of treatment. Contributing factors to poor swallowing ability include tissue edema, fibrosis, and possible alterations in sensory awareness. In addition to restricting laryngeal movements, fibrosis may reduce the range of motion of the tongue and jaw and diminish pharyngeal wall motion. In our experience, 10 to 20% of patients receiving chemoradiotherapy for SCC of the oropharynx and hypopharynx may require long-term gastrostomy-tube feedings.

Radiation to the larynx often results in swallowing problems related to pharyngeal transport. Restricted laryngeal motion, impaired true vocal fold closure, and aspiration are common complications in patients who have been treated with radiation. Similarly, dysphonia is often present, but its impact on daily oral communication does not seem to be as significant as the deficits that occur with impaired swallowing.

To counteract the deleterious effects of radiation and chemoradiotherapy, there are rehabilitative options, which are best administered by a qualified speech pathologist. These interventions include exercise protocols to strengthen and maintain range of motion, precision, muscle elasticity and mobility. Also taught are compensatory strategies that should be started early, preferably at the initiation of treatment, and continued throughout the course of treatment. These maneuvers have been shown to improve pharyngeal mobility during the swallow, thereby enhancing pharyngeal clearance, airway protection, and elimination of aspiration in a majority of cases. The continuing use of exercises may be necessary to counter long-term adverse effects in patients who have received radiotherapy.

SALIVARY GLAND CANCERS

Tumors of the salivary glands constitute approximately 5000 cases per year in the United States and are distributed according to size of the gland—for example, parotid tumors versus others. Histologies are diverse. The age range of patients affected is broad. Many salivary neoplasms are benign, often involving the parotid gland and accounting for approximately 80% of parotid tumors, 50% of tumors arising in submandibular glands and 25% of tumors arising in minor salivary glands. The latter may be scattered about the mucous membranes of the upper aerodigestive tract.

Risk factors for parotid cancers are poorly defined. There has been some association of woodworking and chemical exposure in tannery workers, with anecdotal reports of paranasal sinus adenocarcinomas. Radiotherapy may be causative for salivary ductal cancers. Table 16-2 lists primary salivary malignancies.

Primary treatment depends on tumor extent and histology. After a thorough head and neck examination and consideration of the histologic diagnosis, CT staging

TABLE 16-2	SALIVARY GLANDS
Frequently observed: adenoid cystic carcinoma; adenocarcinoma not otherwise specified; mucoepidermoid carcinoma (well versus poorly differentiated)	
Less common: salivary ductal carcinoma; acinic cell carcinoma; squamous cell carcinoma	

is recommended before surgery. Notably, parotid lymphadenopathy may reflect metastatic involvement by squamous cancers of the scalp or by melanomas, and this must be borne in mind in evaluating these patients. Following a complete head and neck evaluation, consideration may be given to CT imaging of chest and a bone scan, as these are common metastatic sites.

Surgical resection is the fundamental primary treatment for most patients, and the approach will be influenced by the primary histology (53). Adenoid cystic carcinoma (ACC) tends to track along nerves and may involve structures of the skull base, an important consideration in surgical and radiation therapy planning. Lymph node metastases are uncommon. Low-grade mucoepidermoid carcinomas tend to be localized and are most often treated by surgery alone. High-grade mucoepidermoid carcinomas carry a much higher risk of lymph node and distant metastases. Salivary ductal carcinomas may be high grade and share biomarker characteristics, such as estrogen or progesterone receptor and HER2/neu overexpression, with breast cancer. In addition, c-kit is overexpressed in ACC (54). Imatinib, a small molecule targeting c-kit kinase function, has been evaluated in patients with ACCs overexpressing wild-type c-kit (55). Hotte et al. reported nine patients had stable disease after at least two cycles of therapy (56). Further study is needed. As a generalization, large tumors or those with close surgical margins will require postoperative radiotherapy. Studies are ongoing to evaluate the efficacy of photon radiotherapy versus treatment with heavy particles. Concomitant chemoradiation has not been well studied in the treatment of salivary cancers but may be a consideration for good-performance-level patients with locally advanced and unresectable disease.

For patients with recurrent disease not amenable to further local treatment or those with distant metastases, treatment with systemic chemotherapy is an option (55,57). Cisplatin, fluorouracil, cyclophosphamide, and doxorubicin are active compounds. The taxanes also have activity, although not demonstrated in patients with adenoid cystic carcinoma. Combinations may be more effective, with response rates ranging from 30 to 40%; on occasion there may be a durable response. Trials with targeted therapy such as erlotinib and imatinib (in ACC), dasatinib (all types), and trastuzumab (Her 2 positive tumors) are underway. In a phase II trial, lapatinib, a dual inhibitor of EGFR and erbB2 tyrosine kinase activity, was investigated to determine the antitumor activity in advanced malignant salivary gland tumors, including ACC. Among 19 assessable patients with ACC, 15 patients (79%) had stable disease (58).

Some patients with advanced salivary tumors will have a protracted and indolent clinical course. This has been frequently observed in patients with metastatic adenoid cystic carcinoma involving lung, so it is important to assess the pace of the disease before committing a patient to potentially hazardous systemic chemotherapy or investigational treatment.

■ COMBINED-MODALITY THERAPY

For patients who are not candidates for definitive surgery or radiotherapy, much effort has been directed toward improvements in primary management with the addition of chemotherapy to surgery, radiotherapy, or both. Toward this end, three general strategies have been undertaken: (1) induction, also known as neoadjuvant therapy, with chemotherapy given before surgery or radiation; (2) concomitant chemoradiation, with chemotherapy given simultaneously with radiation to enhance its effect; and (3) adjuvant therapy, where chemotherapy is given after surgery or radiation in an effort to decrease metastatic disease burden.

INDUCTION CHEMOTHERAPY

Theoretically, induction chemotherapy has several advantages. It allows for the delivery of systemic therapy to the host, with optimal patient compliance and better tolerance. Chemotherapy in this setting is highly active and may be administered with objectives (1) of organ preservation by obviating the need for surgery and (2) reducing risk of distant disease recurrence with treatment of "micrometastatic" regional or distant disease. There also is the potential for favorably affecting the efficacy of definitive radiotherapy, with or without concomitant chemotherapy, by reducing tumor bulk with necrotic-hypoxic centers before radiotherapy is administered. Upfront patient evaluation by a multidisciplinary team before commencing induction chemotherapy is critical to ensure that local treatment modality planning is based on the initial extent of disease.

With the introduction of cisplatin into clinical trials in the mid-1970s, combination therapy soon consisted of cisplatin-based regimens. An important combination was studied in the 1980s at Wayne State University, with cisplatin (100 mg/m^2) followed by a 5-day infusion of 5-FU (1 g/m^2/day) (48). In a phase II trial, this regimen was reported to achieve responses in 93% of patients, with a 54% clinical complete response rate, when three cycles were administered to treatment-naïve patients.

Randomized trials of induction chemotherapy before surgery or radiotherapy have shown that the approach is feasible for those with locally advanced disease and does not add to the morbidity of subsequent definitive local treatment (59,60). Approximately 30% of radiographic and clinical complete responses will be confirmed pathologically. A response to induction chemotherapy also correlates with response to subsequent radiotherapy (57,58). Thus patients who are resistant to cisplatin-based induction chemotherapy have a high likelihood of not responding well to radiotherapy. However, randomized trials are necessary to draw firm conclusions regarding disease-free survival and overall survival benefit.

Domenge and others (61) reported a phase III trial in which 318 patients with locally advanced oropharyngeal SCCs were randomized to induction chemotherapy with cisplatin and 5-FU followed by locoregional treatment or locoregional therapy alone. Overall survival was better in the chemotherapy group (median 5.1 versus 3.3 years; $p = .03$), although an improvement in locoregional tumor control was not conclusively demonstrated. Paccagnella and others (62), in a large Italian study, observed an improvement in local control, metastatic rate, and survival time for inoperable patients treated with induction cisplatin and 5-FU.

A multicenter, phase III trial (TAX 323) (63) evaluated the safety and efficacy of a combination of docetaxel, cisplatin, and fluorouracil as induction chemotherapy for patients with SCCHN. A total of 358 patients with untreated, unresectable, and locally advanced tumors were randomized to receive either docetaxel 75 mg/m^2, cisplatin 75 mg/m^2 and fluorouracil 750 mg/m^2/day for 5 days (TPF) or cisplatin 100 mg/m^2 and fluorouracil 1000 mg/m^2/day for 5 days (PF), followed by radiotherapy alone. The primary endpoint, median progression-free survival, was 11.0 months in the TPF group and 8.2 months in the PF group (hazard ratio for disease progression or death in the TPF group, 0.72; $p = .007$). Treatment with TPF resulted in a reduction in the risk of death of 27% ($p = .02$), with a median overall survival of 18.8 months, as compared with 14.5 months in the PF group. There were more grade 3 or 4 events of leukopenia and neutropenia in the TPF group. The rates of death from toxic effects were 2.3% in the TPF group and 5.5% in the PF group.

Another randomized, phase III trial (TAX 324) (64) sequenced induction chemotherapy and concomitant chemoradiotherapy in 501 patients. Previously untreated patients with locally advanced SCCHN (unresectable or candidates for organ preservation) were randomized to receive either TPF (docetaxel 75 mg/m^2 of body-surface area, cisplatin 100 mg/m^2, and fluorouracil 1000 mg/m^2/day for 4 days) or PF (cisplatin 100 mg/m^2 and fluorouracil 1000 mg/m^2/day for 5 days) administered for three cycles, and followed by concurrent chemoradiotherapy with weekly carboplatin at area under curve 1.5. The median overall survival was 71 months in the TPF group and 30 months in the PF group ($p = .006$). Notably, there was better locoregional control in the TPF group than in the PF group ($p = .04$). Risk of distant metastases was also lower in the TPF group (HR = 0.60), but the number of events was low and the difference was not statistically significant ($p = .14$). Rates of neutropenia and febrile neutropenia were higher in the TPF group. These two phase III trials led to Food and Drug Administration (FDA) approval of induction chemotherapy with docetaxel, cisplatin, and fluorouracil for patients with locally advanced SCCHN.

There are phase III trials in the United States and Italy in which patients have been randomized to TPF (with some variation in dose and schedule among the studies) or no induction chemotherapy followed by concomitant chemoradiotherapy for both groups. The American studies have completed accrual and the outcomes analyses are pending. The Italian study is ongoing.

A recent phase II trial at MDACC investigated the efficacy of combining cetuximab with paclitaxel and carboplatin as induction chemotherapy, followed by risk-based local therapy (radiation, concomitant chemoradiotherapy, or surgery) based on tumor stage and site at diagnosis. After induction chemotherapy, 9 patients (19%) achieved a complete response, and 36 patients (77%) achieved a partial response. The 3-year progression-free survival and overall survival rates were 87% and 91%, respectively (65). This strategy is to undergo further testing.

CONCOMITANT RADIOTHERAPY AND CHEMOTHERAPY

In patients with locally advanced but M0 disease, the strategy of concomitant radiotherapy and chemotherapy has led to improved local and regional tumor control (66). Interactions between cytotoxic drugs and radiation that results in additive or synergistic enhancement have been reviewed in detail (67-70). This biological phenomenon rests on several mechanisms, including (1) inhibition of DNA repair; (2) redistribution of cells to sensitive phases of the cell cycle; and (3) promoting oxygenation of anoxic tissues. The net effect is to improve cellular cytotoxicity (69-71). However, combined therapy also enhances acute mucocutaneous toxicity which may prompt subsequent dose reductions and treatment interruptions in radiotherapy. This may have deleterious overall effects. Thus, in combining these two treatment modalities, it is essential that toxicity not preclude the use of chemotherapy and radiation in an effective schedule, generally free of interruptions, particularly of radiotherapy, to avoid compromise of efficacy.

Cisplatin

The exact mechanism of interaction between cisplatin and radiation is not known. Hypoxic and aerobic cell sensitization and the inhibition of cellular repair processes for sublethally damaged cells contribute to the effects observed in vitro systems (72). In a phase II trial, the Radiation Therapy Oncology Group (RTOG) administered cisplatin (100 mg/m^2) every 3 weeks to 124 patients with locally advanced unresectable head and neck cancer (73). Sixty percent of patients completed the combined treatment per protocol, and 69% of all patients achieved a complete response. A separate analysis of the disease-free and overall survival times for those with nasopharyngeal and non-nasopharyngeal primary sites with more than 5 years of follow-up has been published (74). A comparison to RTOG patients treated with radiotherapy alone suggested improvement in survival time for the combined treatment.

Concomitant chemotherapy and radiotherapy has been effective for the treatment of patients with NPC. The Head and Neck Intergroup NPC 0099 trial completed accrual in 1995, demonstrating favorable results for the combined approach compared to radiotherapy as a single modality (38). In this study, patients received either radiotherapy alone or cisplatin (100 mg/m^2 on days 1, 22, and 43) during radiotherapy, followed by adjuvant chemotherapy with cisplatin and 5-FU (three cycles). Analysis of 147 randomized patients revealed significant differences in 3-year survival time (78 versus 47%) and progression-free survival time (69 versus 24%), favoring the chemotherapy group. These exciting results changed the standard of care for those with NPC in the United States. Patients with stage III or IV disease should be treated with concomitant chemoradiotherapy followed by adjuvant chemotherapy.

However, the results of the Head and Neck Intergroup (NPC) trial using concomitant cisplatin in patients with locally advanced nasopharyngeal cancer should not necessarily be generalized to other disease sites.

Carboplatin

There are limited data on radiosensitizing properties of carboplatin. One trial comparing cisplatin with carboplatin demonstrated similar results (75). The side effects of carboplatin are better tolerated than those observed with cisplatin. Carboplatin is commonly used in combination with paclitaxel.

Cetuximab

Cetuximab, a monoclonal antibody, is approved for use in combination with radiation in previously untreated patients. In a landmark study, patients with locoregionally advanced head and neck cancer were randomly assigned to receive either high-dose radiotherapy alone (213 patients) or high-dose radiotherapy plus weekly cetuximab (211 patients) at an initial dose of 400 mg/m^2 of body-surface area, followed by 250 mg/m^2 weekly for the duration of radiotherapy (76). The primary endpoint, median duration of locoregional control, was 24.4 months among patients treated with cetuximab plus radiotherapy and 14.9 months among those given radiotherapy alone (hazard ratio for locoregional progression or death = 0.68; p = .005). The median duration of overall survival was 49.0 months among patients treated with combined therapy and 29.3 months among those treated with radiotherapy alone (hazard ratio for death = 0.74; p = .03). Radiotherapy plus cetuximab significantly prolonged progression-free survival (hazard ratio for disease progression or death = 0.70; p = .006). However, the rates of distant metastases at 1 and 2 years were similar in both groups. With the exception of acneiform rash and infusion reactions, the incidence of grade 3 or greater toxic effects, including mucositis, did not differ significantly between the two groups.

The clinical applicability of the results from this trial remains uncertain since concurrent chemoradiotherapy was not included in the study. A large, randomized, phase III study (RTOG 0522) comparing chemoradiotherapy with chemoradiotherapy plus cetuximab is currently ongoing.

Multiple Agents

Combining several drugs with radiation will enhance acute toxicity, which may be severe. Therefore, investigators have piloted trials designed with split-course radiation to allow for healthy tissue recovery. Most of these studies have been limited to patients with stages III and IV locally advanced SCC with local control and improved survival time as the primary objectives. These regimens alternate chemotherapy and radiotherapy or use split-course radiotherapy to maximize tumor cell kill and minimize tissue toxicity. However, protracted radiation treatment times may result in decreased local control rates because of accelerated repopulation of cancer stem cells (77,78). The strategy of alternating non–cross-resistant agents may potentially eliminate not only tumor cell repopulation but also primary drug resistance.

The use of concomitant combination chemotherapy and radiation has continued to be under intense study in recent years (79). Meta-analysis (66) of prospective clinical trials demonstrates an enhancement of local tumor control and improvement of survival with combined therapy over radiation treatment alone (Table 16-3). There also has been a substantial increase in acute toxicities, especially dermatitis and mucositis; with longer follow-up, evidence of increased late toxicity has begun to emerge.

In general, patients admitted to these studies have had variable head and neck primary sites, although oropharyngeal primaries tend to predominate. Brizel and others (80) have compared a hyperfractionated radiotherapy arm to total dose 75 Gy with the same radiation schedule, to 70 Gy, and concomitant cisplatin and 5-fluorouracil. The concomitant treatment was followed by two cycles of adjuvant chemotherapy. There was a statistically significant improvement in local disease control and a strong trend toward improved

overall survival for the combined modality arm. In this trial, neck dissection was recommended in patients with N2/3 disease. Clayman and colleagues (81) have reviewed the MDACC experience, examining the indication for neck dissection in this patient population. Their report suggests that neck dissections are required only when there is radiographic evidence of residual disease 6 to 8 weeks following the completion of definitive chemoradiation. Wendt et al. (82) reported a statistically significant 3-year survival advantage after the concurrent use of cisplatin, 5-FU and leucovorin with split course radiotherapy versus radiotherapy given as a single therapeutic modality. Calais and colleagues (83) compared a more standard once-daily fractionation radiation schedule with the same radiotherapy and concurrent carboplatin and 5-FU, demonstrating a statistically significant advantage in locoregional tumor control, and overall survival at 3 years. This report is particularly germane, as the study group consisted only of patients with oropharyngeal cancer. Jeremic and colleagues (84) also investigated the value of adding cisplatin given daily to a hyperfractionated radiation therapy program versus the same radiation schedule

TABLE 16-3A | SELECTED RANDOMIZED CHEMOTHERAPY TRIALS

Study	Patient Group	Experimental Arms	Outcome
Brizel (80), 1998	"Advanced"	HFRT + CF → CF × 2 (N = 56)	Improved local control 70 versus 44%; trend to better OS 55 versus 34% ($p = .07$) at 3 years
Calais (83), 1999	Unresectable— oropharynx	RT + cbdca/FU (N = 109)	Survival improved: 51 versus 31% at 3 years
Adelstein (85), 2003	"Advanced"	RT + cisplatin (N = 87)	Survival improved: 37 versus 23% at 3 years
		RT split course + cisplatin/FU (N = 89)	No difference

TABLE 16-3B | POSTOPERATIVE CHEMOTHERAPY—RANDOMIZED TRIALS

Study	Eligibility	Experimental Arms	Outcome
Bachaud (86), 1996	Nodal ECS	RT + weekly cisplatin (N = 39)	DFS ($p < .02$) and OS ($p < .01$) better
RTOG 9501 (88), 2004	Multiple nodal metastases, ECS, or + margins	RT + cisplatin days 1, 22, 43 (N = 228)	2-year LRC (82 versus 72% $p = .01$) + PFS ($p = .04$) better
EORTC 22931 (87), 2004	Stage III/IV	RT + cisplatin days 1, 22, 43 (N = 167)	PFS ($p = .04$) + OS ($p = .02$) better

cbdca, carboplatin; CF, cisplatin/fluorouracil; DFS, disease-free survival; ECS, extracapsular spread; HFRT, hyperfractionated radiotherapy; LRC, local and regional control; OS, overall survival; PFS, progression-free survival; RT, radiotherapy.

given alone in patients with locally advanced SCCHN. In this report, locoregional and distant disease control, and overall survival were improved at 5 years. More recently, Adelstein and colleagues (85) compared standard daily radiotherapy with two schedules of concomitant chemoradiotherapy in a large intergroup study. The addition of high-dose cisplatin to conventional single-daily–dose radiotherapy improved survival from 23 to 37% at 3 years. The clearest benefit in these studies was an improvement in locoregional control, which translated into a survival advantage. Acute toxicity was increased, especially mucositis and hematologic effects, but there was no obvious escalation of long-term sequelae. However, this may need further investigation. In aggregate, overall 3-year survival exceeded 50% in these experimental programs, underscoring the potential therapeutic efficacy of concomitant chemotherapy and radiation in patients with advanced head and neck cancers.

Concomitant chemotherapy, particularly with multiple drugs, leads to a marked increase in acute toxicity. "In-field" mucositis and dermatitis can be severe, are associated with much discomfort, and may lead to increased risk of infection, poor nutritional intake, and interruption of radiotherapy or chemotherapy treatment schedules. This may compromise tumor control and ultimate survival. There is also the potential for an increase in serious long-term toxicities as survival increases after these intensive treatment programs. For optimal results, concomitant treatments should be administered in centers with sufficient training and expertise and with experienced supportive care teams.

The aggregate results of these trials indicate that improved disease-free and overall survival times have been obtained for patients with locally advanced SCCHN using concomitant chemotherapy and radiotherapy rather than radiotherapy as a single treatment modality. Well-designed clinical trials are needed to determine optimal chemotherapy and radiotherapy schedules. Randomized trials are currently in progress to help clarify these issues.

ADJUVANT CHEMORADIOTHERAPY

Adjuvant chemotherapy after primary surgery has been shown to be effective in patients with breast cancer and osteogenic sarcoma. Adjuvant chemotherapy has several potential advantages over induction treatment. First, surgery is not delayed for patients with resectable disease. Second, induction therapy can blur the margins of disease, making the objective of surgical resection less obvious. Finally, successful induction chemotherapy

can lead to symptom abatement, resulting in the patient's refusal to undergo definitive treatment (ie, surgery or radiotherapy) afterward. For patients at high risk of recurrence after surgical resection, generally defined as having narrow or involved margins at the primary site, multiple nodal metastases or extracapsular spread, concomitant chemoradiotherapy with cisplatin appears to be superior to radiotherapy used as a single modality (86-89).

Two large phase III studies conducted by RTOG 9501 (88) and EORTC 22931 (87) tested cisplatin-based concomitant chemoradiotherapy in the adjuvant setting. In both trials, patients with high-risk features (positive margin, extracapsular spread, lymphovascular invasion, perineural invasion, and multiple positive lymph nodes) were randomly assigned to receive either radiotherapy alone or radiotherapy plus cisplatin at 100 mg/m^2 every 3 weeks for three cycles.

In RTOG 9501, concomitant chemoradiotherapy significantly reduced the risk of locoregional recurrence, as compared with radiotherapy alone (hazard ratio for local or regional recurrence = 0.61; $p = 0.01$). However, no survival benefit was observed. In addition, the incidence of adverse effects of grade 3 or greater was 34% in the radiotherapy group and 77% in the combined-therapy group ($p < .001$).

In EORTC 22931, the rate of progression-free survival was significantly higher in the combined-therapy group than radiotherapy group (hazard ratio = 0.75; $p = .04$). The overall survival rate was also significantly higher in the combined-therapy group than in the radiotherapy group (hazard ratio = 0.70; $p = .02$). Severe adverse effects were more frequent in combined-therapy group (41%) than in radiotherapy group (21%).

Although postoperative concomitant chemoradiotherapy was more effective than radiotherapy alone, it was more toxic in both trials. In an analysis of the data from both studies, the two risk factors that were associated with a significant benefit from concurrent chemoradiotherapy were extracapsular extension and positive surgical margins (90). Therefore, adjuvant chemoradiotherapy should be considered in patients who have a good performance status and the high-risk features defined earlier, in particular those with extracapsular extension or positive surgical margins.

■ ORGAN PRESERVATION

Many SCCHN are diagnosed at a late stage. Stages III and IV tumors often necessitate extensive or radical surgery, which may alter organ function. Problems with radical surgery include loss of speech, loss of swallowing function, or disfigurement without a concomitant improvement in survival time. Therefore, preservation of function became one of the major challenges in the 1990s. A role for combined modality treatment in preserving organ function has already been noted for laryngeal preservation. As discussed earlier in the VA larynx study (50), neoadjuvant chemotherapy followed by radiotherapy was more successful in preserving voice function than was surgery without a loss in survival time.

In addition to the VA larynx study (50), another large randomized study of patients with hypopharynx cancers has been completed. This study (42) was performed by the EORTC beginning in 1990 and compared a larynx-preserving therapy (induction chemotherapy plus radiation) with conventional surgery plus postoperative radiation. The design of the EORTC study was similar to that of the VA larynx study, as patients were randomized to either treatment; patients receiving induction chemotherapy received cisplatin plus 5-FU. After two cycles of chemotherapy, only responders (ie, partial or complete responders) received a third cycle. Patients achieving a complete response then received definitive radiotherapy. Nonresponders or those with partial responses underwent conventional surgery followed by postoperative radiation. As in the VA study, the overall survival data were not different between the two arms, and the median duration of survival time was longer for the chemotherapy arm. Local failures occurred more commonly in the chemotherapy arm, but the rate of distant metastasis was lower. In both studies, a large number of patients were enrolled, and of the surviving patients, a significant percentage achieved larynx preservation.

The Head and Neck Intergroup study, previously discussed, further supports the concept that, for selected patients, definitive treatment with chemotherapy and radiation may allow for organ preservation with no compromise in survival. In the Head and Neck Intergroup R91-11 trial, there was a comparison between induction chemotherapy, radiotherapy alone, and radiotherapy with concomitant cisplatin. The results indicated a significant advantage for concomitant cisplatin treatment with preservation of the larynx in 88% of patients treated in the concomitant arm. It can be concluded that the option of organ preservation therapy with chemotherapy and radiation therapy is becoming a reality for many patients with SCCs of the head and neck. Certainly enrollment of patients with advanced cancers of the larynx and hypopharynx to clinical trials of multimodal therapy is encouraged.

Earlier cited, Pointreau et al. (52) compared induction chemotherapy with TPF versus PF for organ preservation in patients with hypopharynx and larynx cancer. The overall response rate was 80% in the TPF group versus 59% in the PF group, with larynx preservation in 70% of patients in the TPF arm.

RECURRENT OR METASTATIC DISEASE

Patients with recurrence after primary treatment who are not candidates for surgical salvage commonly may be offered palliative cytotoxic chemotherapy or treatment or investigational therapy. Methotrexate, cisplatin or carboplatin, bleomycin, fluorouracil, and the taxanes are drugs with single-agent activity in the range of 15 to 25%. Previous studies have consistently demonstrated response rates of 30 to 40% for combination chemotherapy, usually cisplatin-based, with a median survival 6 to 9 months. There has been no clear demonstration of a survival advantage over single-agent treatment or even best supportive care. However, in the appropriate context with the goal of reducing symptoms, combination chemotherapy with cisplatin/ 5-FU or a platinum/taxane combination has become a frequently exercised practice in the care of patients with incurable SCCHN.

Current investigations are under way in an attempt to develop effective targeted treatment approaches. SCCHN is believed to evolve as a result of cumulative molecular events, which could be potential therapeutic targets.

As previously discussed, EGFR is overexpressed in a majority of invasive SCC of the head and neck. The small-molecule inhibitors gefitinib (500 mg/day) and erlotinib (150 mg/day) downregulate the phosphorylation of tyrosine kinase residues in the cytoplasmic domain of EGFR and have demonstrated single-agent activity in 11 and 5% of patients, respectively, with advanced disease (91-93). Of note, the response rate to gefitinib was minimal at 250 mg daily which had been a standard dose for treating advanced non–small cell lung cancer (92).

Cetuximab is a chimeric murine-human monoclonal antibody directed against the extracellular domain of EGFR. Burtness and colleagues (94) conducted a prospective randomized trial in patients with recurrent SCCHN and demonstrated responses in 26% of patients treated with cetuximab and cisplatin versus 10% of patients treated with cisplatin alone. However, the primary endpoint, progression-free survival, was not significantly different. Cetuximab was tested in a phase II trial as a monotherapy in 103 patients with recurrent or metastatic SCCHN refractory to platinum-based therapy (95). The response rate was 13%, disease control rate (complete response/partial response/stable disease) was 46%, and median time to progression was 70 days. There appeared to be no benefit in adding cisplatin to these patients.

In a major phase III trial, cetuximab in combination with chemotherapy was investigated in patients with untreated recurrent or metastatic SCCHN (96). In this trial, 442 patients were randomized to receive either cisplatin or carboplatin plus fluorouracil, with or without cetuximab. The cetuximab group had longer overall survival (10.1 versus 7.4 months) and median progression-free survival (5.6 versus 3.3 months). Thus, cetuximab plus platinum-fluorouracil chemotherapy improved overall survival when given as first-line treatment in patients with recurrent or metastatic SCCHN.

■ CHEMOPREVENTION

The decades-long history of clinical and translational study of retinoids in oral premalignant lesions, or intraepithelial neoplasia (IEN), has advanced our understanding of the biology of carcinogenesis and molecular-targeted drug development, even though definitive clinical testing has not shown that retinoids can prevent oral cancer (97). One early trial in 1986 tested a high dose of the retinoid 13-*cis*-retinoic acid (13cRA) against placebo in 44 evaluable oral IEN patients for only 3 months (98). The complete-plus-partial clinical response rate in the retinoid arm was 67% (versus 10% in the placebo arm) ($p = .0002$). Histopathologic responses also favored the 13cRA arm. Over half of the responders in the 13cRA arm, however, recurred or developed new lesions within 3 months of stopping the intervention. This high-dose, short-term trial led to another early trial in oral IEN patients, which was designed to reduce the toxicity of and prolong the response to 13cRA. A short-term (3 months) course of high-dose 13cRA (1.5 mg/kg/day) was followed by a 9-month maintenance course with low-dose 13cRA (0.5 mg/kg/day) or beta-carotene (30 mg/day) in responding or stable IEN patients to the induction phase (99). The maintenance-phase progression rates were 8% in the 13cRA group and 55% in the beta-carotene group ($p < .001$). Nonetheless, on long-term follow-up (median of 66 months), the incidence of in situ or invasive cancer was not different between the two arms (23% for low-dose 13cRA versus 27% for the beta-carotene) (100).

To address the short-lived chemopreventive effects of 13cRA, Papadimitrakopoulou et al. designed a follow-up study comparing an extended, 3-year treatment period with 13cRA at lower doses (0.5 mg/kg/day for 1 year followed by 0.25 mg/kg/day orally for 2 years; control arm) to beta-carotene (50 mg/day) plus vitamin A (ie, retinyl palmitate 25,000 IU/day; experimental arm) in 162 patients with leukoplakia, using a noninferiority design (101). During the study, beta-carotene had to be dropped from the experimental arm due to emerging data demonstrating an increased risk of lung cancer incidence and mortality in other ongoing chemoprevention trials at that time. The study showed an inferior 3-month response rate in the vitamin A alone arm, lower tolerance to treatment with 13cRA, a lack of statistical significance in the test for noninferiority between the control and the experimental arm(s), and, more importantly, a similar oral cancer–free survival across all groups. This study, which is one of the longest term performed to date in patients with leukoplakia, demonstrated that 13cRA is still not well tolerated for long-term treatment, even at reduced doses, and that less toxic regimens (ie, vitamin A alone) are ineffective. Furthermore, an impact on oral cancer incidence is yet to be demonstrated with any of these regimens. In addition to trials involving oral IEN, retinoids have also been studied for prevention of second primary head and neck cancers. A randomized, placebo-controlled study of high-dose 13cRA (50-100 mg/m^2/day for 12 months) in definitively resected head and neck cancer patients demonstrated a lack of effect of the retinoid on distant, nodal, or local recurrence rates, but there was a statistically significant decrease in the incidence of second primary tumors (4 versus 24%, $p = .005$), that persisted on long-term follow-up (102,103). Unfortunately, a follow-up trial of a tolerable low dose of 13cRA (30 mg/day for 3 years) in 1190 early-stage patients did not prevent second primary tumors (104). Randomized studies in this setting with the second-generation retinoid etretinate (N = 316 patients) (105), vitamin A, and/or N-acetylcysteine (N = 2592) (106), beta-carotene (N = 264) (107), and alpha-tocopherol plus beta-carotene (N = 540) (108) also did not demonstrate any clinical benefit in terms of prevention of second primary tumors.

While the randomized retinoid trials failed to produce a chemoprevention strategy that could be considered standard of care, they were embedded with translational studies that helped to advance the overall understanding of the biology of intraepithelial carcinogenesis, molecular markers—for example, retinoic acid receptor (RAR)-beta, p53, p16, EGFR, genetic instability—for developing drugs, monitoring interventions, and assessing cancer risk and pharmacogenomics.

In terms of cancer risk assessment, cyclin D1 genotype (109,110) and loss of heterozygosity at certain chromosomal sites (111-113) have emerged in multiple studies as prognostic factors that could be potentially useful in the clinic. Building on these data, there is an ongoing, placebo-controlled trial at MDACC evaluating the effects of erlotinib (150 mg/day for 1 year) on the incidence of invasive cancer in patients with oral premalignant lesions (with or without a prior history of oral cancer) selected for high risk based on loss of heterozygosity testing—the Erlotinib Prevention of Oral Cancer (EPOC) study (114).

As the role of HPV-16 in the pathogenesis of a subgroup of SCCHN becomes substantiated, preventive strategies targeting this infectious agent could be explored as well. HPV vaccination is already being used to prevent cervical cancer. The same strategy could be applied as a potential means for preventing HPV-induced SCCHN.

■ SUMMARY

SCCHN is a major international health problem. General public health strategies such as reducing tobacco usage and increasing awareness of associated risks are of primary importance.

The demonstration of HPV as a causative agent for oropharyngeal cancers is of great importance as this will carry implications for prevention and also will influence decision making in treatment planning as well as the conduct of clinical trials.

The optimal care and treatment of head and neck cancer patients are multidisciplinary. Emerging data support the administration of chemotherapy, as a component of combined-modality treatments, especially for patients with advanced SCCHN. For patients with locally recurrent or metastatic disease, combination chemotherapy may produce response rates of 30 to 40%. However, responses tend to be brief lasting 3 to 5 months, and are associated with only a modest prolongation of survival. Thus, chemotherapy for these patients is palliative. An exception to this is for patients with NPC with higher response rates and a small proportion of long-term disease-free survivors. For patients with metastatic SCCHN of any primary site, the addition of cetuximab to platinum-fluorouracil appears to improve tumor responses and overall survival. More targeting agents are currently under investigation. Prognostic factors are needed to improve selection of those patients who are most likely to benefit from palliative treatment.

In the newly diagnosed patient with locally advanced disease, high response rates have been observed with induction chemotherapy. The addition of a taxane to the more traditional cisplatin/fluorouracil platform has increased efficacy without a notable change significant toxicity. The major objective of induction systemic therapy is to reduce the risk of distant tumor recurrence. The potential for augmentation of local control with a substantial response to chemotherapy followed by definitive surgery or radiation is also under investigation. Three large multicenter randomized trials have been successfully conducted with preservation of laryngeal function in subsets of patients. Chemotherapy administered concomitantly with radiotherapy has improved local control and survival in a sequence of studies. The increase in toxicity associated with these regimens should be carefully considered in selecting patients for combined treatment.

Patients with earlier-stage disease (ie, stage I or II) generally should receive therapy with either surgery or radiotherapy, or both. Patients with locally advanced M0 (stage III/IVa/b) disease may be considered for nonsurgical therapy, most often with chemotherapy and radiation or entered into a combined chemoradiation treatment protocol. Patients with "resectable" disease can be further divided by site. Patients with primary oral cavity tumors are best served with surgery followed by radiotherapy (or chemoradiotherapy if there are high-risk pathologic features), whereas those with oropharyngeal, hypopharyngeal, or laryngeal tumors are often treated with radiation, with or without chemotherapy, depending on precise site and stage. Patients with metastatic disease should receive systemic therapy with palliative intent, if performance status is favorable. Enrolling in investigational studies is strongly supported.

Basic and translational chemoprevention research in head and neck carcinogenesis is advancing our understanding of the molecular characteristics of carcinogenesis and cancer risk. We are studying EGFR inhibition in a prospective, controlled trial in high-risk patients. This project illustrates the convergence of prevention and therapy, as promising new approaches with molecularly targeted agents, such as cyclooxygenase-2 and EGFR inhibitors, test principles known to also have efficacy in the setting of invasive cancer.

The management of head and neck cancer is a multidisciplinary activity. The identification of effective chemotherapeutic agents and their integration into the initial therapy of head and neck cancer have the potential to improve survival time and preserve organ function. Through well-designed and executed clinical trials, coupled with basic research of the biology of upper aerodigestive tract tumors, further advances in the management and prevention of these cancers can be achieved.

References

1. Jemal A, Center MM, Ward E, et al. Cancer occurrence. *Methods Mol Biol* 2009;471:3-29.

2. Parkin DM, Bray F, Ferlay J, et al. Global cancer statistics, 2002. *CA Cancer J Clin* 2005;55:74-108.

3. Brennan JA, Boyle JO, Koch WM, et al. Association between cigarette smoking and mutation of the p53 gene in squamous-cell carcinoma of the head and neck. *N Engl J Med* 1995;332:712-717.

4. Gillison ML, Koch WM, Capone RB, et al. Evidence for a causal association between human papillomavirus and a subset of head and neck cancers. *J Natl Cancer Inst* 2000;92:709-720.

5. Gillison ML. Human papillomavirus-associated head and neck cancer is a distinct epidemiologic, clinical, and molecular entity. *Semin Oncol* 2004;31:744-754.

6. Braakhuis BJ, Snijders PJ, Keune WJ, et al. Genetic patterns in head and neck cancers that contain or lack transcriptionally active human papillomavirus. *J Natl Cancer Inst* 2004;96:998-1006.

7. Gillison M, Harris J, Westra W, et al. Survival outcomes by tumor human papillomavirus (HPV) status in stage III-IV oropharyngeal cancer (OPC) in RTOG 0129, ASCO. Orlando; 2009:301s.

8. Gillison ML, D'Souza G, Westra W, et al. Distinct risk factor profiles for human papillomavirus type 16-positive and human papillomavirus type 16-negative head and neck cancers. *J Natl Cancer Inst* 2008;100:407-420.

9. Bedi GC, Westra WH, Gabrielson E, et al. Multiple head and neck tumors: Evidence for a common clonal origin. *Cancer Res* 1996;56:2484-2487.

10. Califano J, Leong PL, Koch WM, et al. Second esophageal tumors in patients with head and neck squamous cell carcinoma: An assessment of clonal relationships. *Clin Cancer Res* 1999;5:1862-187.

11. Haddad RI, Shin DM. Recent advances in head and neck cancer. *N Engl J Med* 2008;359:1143-1154.

12. Callender T, el-Naggar AK, Lee MS, et al. PRAD-1 (CCND1)/cyclin D1 oncogene amplification in primary head and neck squamous cell carcinoma. *Cancer* 1994;74:152-158.

13. Papadimitrakopoulou VA, Izzo J, Mao L, et al. Cyclin D1 and p16 alterations in advanced premalignant lesions of the upper aerodigestive tract: Role in response to chemoprevention and cancer development. *Clin Cancer Res* 2001;7:3127-3134.

14. Weber A, Wittekind C, Tannapfel A. Genetic and epigenetic alterations of 9p21 gene products in benign and malignant tumors of the head and neck. *Pathol Res Pract* 2003;199:391-397.

15. El-Naggar AK, Hurr K, Huff V, et al. Allelic loss and replication errors at microsatellite loci on chromosome 11p in head and neck squamous carcinoma: Association with aggressive biological features. *Clin Cancer Res* 1996;2:903-907.

16. Gasco M, Crook T. The p53 network in head and neck cancer. *Oral Oncol* 2003;39:222-231.

17. D'Souza G, Kreimer AR, Viscidi R, et al. Case-control study of human papillomavirus and oropharyngeal cancer. *N Engl J Med* 2007;356:1944-1956.

18. Thompson EW, Newgreen DF, Tarin D. Carcinoma invasion and metastasis: A role for epithelial-mesenchymal transition? *Cancer Res* 2005;65:5991-5995; discussion 5995.

19. Katayama A, Bandoh N, Kishibe K, et al. Expressions of matrix metalloproteinases in early-stage oral squamous cell carcinoma as predictive indicators for tumor metastases and prognosis. *Clin Cancer Res* 2004;10:634-640.

20. O'Donnell RK, Kupferman M, Wei SJ, et al. Gene expression signature predicts lymphatic metastasis in squamous cell carcinoma of the oral cavity. *Oncogene* 2005;24:1244-1251.

21. Chung CH, Parker JS, Karaca G, et al. Molecular classification of head and neck squamous cell carcinomas using patterns of gene expression. *Cancer Cell* 2004;5:489-500.

22. Roepman P, Wessels LF, Kettelarij N, et al. An expression profile for diagnosis of lymph node metastases from primary head and neck squamous cell carcinomas. *Nat Genet* 2005;37:182-186.

23. Peled A, Petit I, Kollet O, et al. Dependence of human stem cell engraftment and repopulation of NOD/SCID mice on CXCR4. *Science* 1999;283:845-848.

24. Guleng B, Tateishi K, Ohta M, et al. Blockade of the stromal cell-derived factor-1/CXCR4 axis attenuates in vivo tumor growth by inhibiting angiogenesis in a vascular endothelial growth factor-independent manner. *Cancer Res* 2005;65:5864-5871.

25. Uchida D, Begum NM, Almofti A, et al. Possible role of stromal-cell-derived factor-1/CXCR4 signaling on lymph node metastasis of oral squamous cell carcinoma. *Exp Cell Res* 2003;290:289-302.

26. Kerbel R, Folkman J. Clinical translation of angiogenesis inhibitors. *Nat Rev Cancer* 2002;2:727-739.

27. Carmeliet P, Jain RK. Angiogenesis in cancer and other diseases. *Nature* 2000;407:249-257.

28. Bergers G, Song S, Meyer-Morse N, et al. Benefits of targeting both pericytes and endothelial cells in the tumor vasculature with kinase inhibitors. *J Clin Invest* 2003;111:1287-1295.

29. Grandis JR, Tweardy DJ. Elevated levels of transforming growth factor alpha and epidermal growth factor receptor messenger RNA are early markers of carcinogenesis in head and neck cancer. *Cancer Res* 1993;53:3579-3584.

30. Roskoski R, Jr. The ErbB/HER receptor protein-tyrosine kinases and cancer. *Biochem Biophys Res Commun* 2004;319:1-11.

31. Dassonville O, Formento JL, Francoual M, et al. Expression of epidermal growth factor receptor and survival in upper aerodigestive tract cancer. *J Clin Oncol* 1993;11:1873-1878.

32. Shin DM, Xu XC, Lippman SM, et al. Accumulation of p53 protein and retinoic acid receptor beta in retinoid chemoprevention. *Clin Cancer Res* 1997;3:875-880.

33. Chung CH, Ely K, McGavran L, et al. Increased epidermal growth factor receptor gene copy number is associated with poor prognosis in head and neck squamous cell carcinomas. *J Clin Oncol* 2006;24:4170-4176.

34. Lo YM, Chan LY, Lo KW, et al. Quantitative analysis of cell-free Epstein-Barr virus DNA in plasma of patients with nasopharyngeal carcinoma. *Cancer Res* 1999;59:1188-1891.

35. Edge SA. Head and neck sites. In: Edge, S.B.; Byrd, D.R.; Compton, C.C.; Fritz, A.G.; Greene, F.L.; Trotti, A. (eds): *American Joint Committee on Cancer Staging Manual*, 7th ed. New York: Springer, 2010.

36. Vokes EE, Weichselbaum RR, Lippman SM, et al. Head and neck cancer. *N Engl J Med* 1993;328:184-194.

37. Forastiere A, Koch W, Trotti A, et al. Head and neck cancer. *N Engl J Med* 2001;345:1890-1900.

38. Al-Sarraf M, LeBlanc M, Giri PG, et al. Chemoradiotherapy versus radiotherapy in patients with advanced nasopharyngeal cancer: Phase III randomized Intergroup study 0099. *J Clin Oncol* 1998;16:1310-1317.

39. Langendijk JA, Leemans CR, Buter J, et al. The additional value of chemotherapy to radiotherapy in locally advanced nasopharyngeal carcinoma: A meta-analysis of the published literature. *J Clin Oncol* 2004;22:4604-4012.

40. Hui EP, Ma BB, Leung SF, et al. Randomized phase II trial of concurrent cisplatin-radiotherapy with or without neoadjuvant docetaxel and cisplatin in advanced nasopharyngeal carcinoma. *J Clin Oncol* 2009;27:242-249.

41. Koch WA, Stafford E, Bajaj G. Head and neck cancer. In: Harrison LB, Sessions RB, Hong WK (eds): *Cancer of the Oral Cavity, General Principles and Management*, 3rd ed. Philadelphia, PA: Lippincott Williams & Wilkins; 2009.

42. Lefebvre JL, Chevalier D, Luboinski B, et al. Larynx preservation in pyriform sinus cancer: Preliminary results of a European Organization for Research and Treatment of Cancer phase III trial. EORTC Head and Neck Cancer Cooperative Group. *J Natl Cancer Inst* 1993;88:890-899.

43. Lefebvre JL, Rolland F, Tesselaar M, et al. Phase 3 randomized trial on larynx preservation comparing sequential vs alternating chemotherapy and radiotherapy. *J Natl Cancer Inst* 2009;101:142-152.

44. Mendenhall WM, Sulica L, Sessions RB. Early-Stage Cancer of the Larynx. In: Harrison LB, Sessions RB, Hong WK, eds., *Head & Neck Cancer: A Multidisciplinary Approach, 2nd ed.* Philadelphia, PA: Lippincott Williams & Wilkins, 2004:352-380.

45. Mendenhall WM, Parsons JT, Stringer SP, et al. Stage T3 squamous cell carcinoma of the glottic larynx: A comparison of laryngectomy and irradiation. *Int J Radiat Oncol Biol Phys* 1992;23:725-732.

46. Mendenhall WM, Hinerman RW, Stringer SP. Management of early and advanced laryngeal cancer. Updates in Head and Neck Cancer 2001; 1:1-14.

47. Weber RS, Berkey BA, Forastiere A, et al. Outcome of salvage total laryngectomy following organ preservation therapy: The Radiation Therapy Oncology Group trial 91-11. *Arch Otolaryngol Head Neck Surg* 2003;129:44-49.

48. Rooney M, Kish J, Jacobs J, et al. Improved complete response rate and survival in advanced head and neck cancer after three-course induction therapy with 120-hour 5-FU infusion and cisplatin. *Cancer* 1985;55:1123-1128.

49. Forastiere AA. Randomized trials of induction chemotherapy. A critical review. *Hematol Oncol Clin North Am* 1991;5:725-736.

50. The Department of Veterans Affairs Laryngeal Cancer Study Group. Induction chemotherapy plus radiation compared with surgery plus radiation in patients with advanced laryngeal cancer. *N Engl J Med* 1991;324:1685-1690.

51. Forastiere AA, Goepfert H, Maor M, et al. Concurrent chemotherapy and radiotherapy for organ preservation in advanced laryngeal cancer. *N Engl J Med* 2003;349:2091-2098.

52. Pointreau Y, Garaud P, Chapet S, et al. Randomized trial of induction chemotherapy with cisplatin and 5-fluorouracil with or without docetaxel for larynx preservation. *J Natl Cancer Inst* 2009;101:498-506.

53. Eisele D and Kleinberg L. Management of malignant salivary gland tumors. In: Harrison L, Sessions R, Hong W (eds): *Head and Neck Cancer—A Multidisciplinary Approach*, 2nd ed. Philadelphia, PA: Lippincott Williams & Wilkins, 2004.

54. Jeng YM, Lin CY, Hsu HC. Expression of the c-kit protein is associated with certain subtypes of salivary gland carcinoma. *Cancer Lett* 2000;154:107-111.

55. Vattemi E, Graiff C, Sava T, et al. Systemic therapies for recurrent and/or metastatic salivary gland cancers. *Expert Rev Anticancer Ther* 2008;8:393-402.

56. Hotte SJ, Winquist EW, Lamont E, et al. Imatinib mesylate in patients with adenoid cystic cancers of the salivary glands expressing c-kit: A Princess Margaret Hospital phase II consortium study. *J Clin Oncol* 2005;23:585-590.

57. Dimery IW, Legha SS, Shirinian M, et al. Fluorouracil, doxorubicin, cyclophosphamide, and cisplatin combination chemotherapy in advanced or recurrent salivary gland carcinoma. *J Clin Oncol* 1990;8:1056-1062.

58. Agulnik M, Cohen EW, Cohen RB, et al. Phase II study of lapatinib in recurrent or metastatic epidermal growth factor receptor and/or erbB2 expressing adenoid cystic carcinoma and non adenoid cystic carcinoma malignant tumors of the salivary glands. *J Clin Oncol* 2007;25:3978-3984.

59. Stell PM, Dalby JE, Strickland P, et al. Sequential chemotherapy and radiotherapy in advanced head and neck cancer. *Clin Radiol* 1983;34:463-467.

60. Ensley JF, Jacobs JR, Weaver A, et al. Correlation between response to cisplatinum-combination chemotherapy and subsequent radiotherapy in previously untreated patients with advanced squamous cell cancers of the head and neck. *Cancer* 1984;54:811-814.

61. Domenge C, Hill C, Lefebvre JL, et al. Randomized trial of neoadjuvant chemotherapy in oropharyngeal carcinoma. French Groupe d'Etude des Tumeurs de la Tete et du Cou (GETTEC). *Br J Cancer* 2000;83:1594-1598.

62. Paccagnella A, Orlando A, Marchiori C, et al. Phase III trial of initial chemotherapy in stage III or IV head and neck cancers: A study by the Gruppo di Studio sui Tumori della Testa e del Collo. *J Natl Cancer Inst* 1994;86:265-272.

63. Vermorken JB, Remenar E, van Herpen C, et al. Cisplatin, fluorouracil, and docetaxel in unresectable head and neck cancer. *N Engl J Med* 2007;357:1695-1704.

64. Posner MR, Hershock DM, Blajman CR, et al. Cisplatin and fluorouracil alone or with docetaxel in head and neck cancer. *N Engl J Med* 2007;357:1705-1715.

65. Kies MS, Holsinger FC, Lee JJ, et al. Induction chemotherapy and cetuximab for locally advanced squamous cell carcinoma of the head and neck: Results from a phase II prospective trial. *J Clin Oncol* 2010;28:8-14.

66. Pignon JP, le Maitre A, Maillard E, et al. Meta-analysis of chemotherapy in head and neck cancer (MACH-NC): An update on 93 randomised trials and 17,346 patients. *Radiother Oncol* 2009;92:4-14.

67. Fu KK. Biological basis for the interaction of chemotherapeutic agents and radiation therapy. *Cancer* 1985;55:2123-2130.

68. Steel GG, Peckham MJ. Exploitable mechanisms in combined radiotherapy-chemotherapy: The concept of additivity. *Int J Radiat Oncol Biol Phys* 1979;5:85-91.

69. Seiwert TY, Salama JK, Vokes EE. The chemoradiation paradigm in head and neck cancer. *Nat Clin Pract Oncol* 2007;4:156-171.

70. Seiwert TY, Salama JK, Vokes EE. The concurrent chemoradiation paradigm—general principles. *Nat Clin Pract Oncol* 2007;4:86-100.

71. Vokes EE, Schilsky RL, Weichselbaum RR, et al. Induction chemotherapy with cisplatin, fluorouracil, and high-dose leucovorin for locally advanced head and neck cancer: A clinical and pharmacologic analysis. *J Clin Oncol* 1990;8:241-247.

72. Dewitt L. Combined treatment of radiation and cisdiamminedichloroplatinum (II): A review of experimental and clinical data. *Int J Radiat Oncol Biol Phys* 1987;13:403-426.

73. Al-Sarraf M, Pajak TF, Marcial VA, et al. Concurrent radiotherapy and chemotherapy with cisplatin in inoperable squamous cell carcinoma of the head and neck. An RTOG Study. *Cancer* 1987;59:259-265.

74. Marcial VA, Pajak TF, Mohiuddin M, et al. Concomitant cisplatin chemotherapy and radiotherapy in advanced mucosal squamous cell carcinoma of the head and neck. Long-term results of the Radiation Therapy Oncology Group study 81-17. *Cancer* 1990;66:1861-1868.

75. Jeremic B, Shibamoto Y, Stanisavljevic B, et al. Radiation therapy alone or with concurrent low-dose daily either cisplatin or carboplatin in locally advanced unresectable squamous cell carcinoma of the head and neck: A prospective randomized trial. *Radiother Oncol* 1997;43:29-37.

76. Bonner JA, Harari PM, Giralt J, et al. Radiotherapy plus cetuximab for squamous-cell carcinoma of the head and neck. *N Engl J Med* 2006;354:567-578.

77. Amdur RJ, Parsons JT, Mendenhall WM, et al. Split-course versus continuous-course irradiation in the postoperative setting for squamous cell carcinoma of the head and neck. *Int J Radiat Oncol Biol Phys* 1989;17:279-285.

78. Pajak TF, Laramore GE, Marcial VA, et al. Elapsed treatment days—a critical item for radiotherapy quality control review in head and neck trials: RTOG report. *Int J Radiat Oncol Biol Phys* 1991;20:13-20.

79. Kies MS, Bennett CL, Vokes EE. Locally advanced head and neck cancer. *Curr Treat Options Oncol* 2001;2:7-13.

80. Brizel DM, Albers ME, Fisher SR, et al. Hyperfractionated irradiation with or without concurrent chemotherapy for locally advanced head and neck cancer. *N Engl J Med* 1998; 338:1798-1804.

81. Clayman GL, Johnson CJ, 2nd, Morrison W, et al. The role of neck dissection after chemoradiotherapy for oropharyngeal cancer with advanced nodal disease. *Arch Otolaryngol Head Neck Surg* 2001;127:135-139.

82. Wendt TG, Grabenbauer GG, Rodel CM, et al. Simultaneous radiochemotherapy versus radiotherapy alone in advanced head and neck cancer: A randomized multicenter study. *J Clin Oncol* 1998;16:1318-1324.

83. Calais G, Alfonsi M, Bardet E, et al. Randomized trial of radiation therapy versus concomitant chemotherapy and radiation therapy for advanced-stage oropharynx carcinoma. *J Natl Cancer Inst* 1999;91:2081-2086.

84. Jeremic B, Shibamoto Y, Milicic B, et al. Hyperfractionated radiation therapy with or without concurrent low-dose daily cisplatin in locally advanced squamous cell carcinoma of the head and neck: A prospective randomized trial. *J Clin Oncol* 2000;18:1458-1464.

85. Adelstein DJ, Li Y, Adams GL, et al. An intergroup phase III comparison of standard radiation therapy and two schedules of concurrent chemoradiotherapy in patients with unresectable squamous cell head and neck cancer. *J Clin Oncol* 2003;21:92-98.

86. Bachaud JM, Cohen-Jonathan E, Alzieu C, et al. Combined postoperative radiotherapy and weekly cisplatin infusion for locally advanced head and neck carcinoma: Final report of a randomized trial. *Int J Radiat Oncol Biol Phys* 1996;36: 999-1004.

87. Bernier J, Domenge C, Ozsahin M, et al. Postoperative irradiation with or without concomitant chemotherapy for locally advanced head and neck cancer. *N Engl J Med* 2004;350: 1945-1952.

88. Cooper JS, Pajak TF, Forastiere AA, et al. Postoperative concurrent radiotherapy and chemotherapy for high-risk squamous-cell carcinoma of the head and neck. *N Engl J Med* 2004;350:1937-1944.

89. Laramore GE, Scott CB, al-Sarraf M, et al. Adjuvant chemotherapy for resectable squamous cell carcinomas of the head and neck: Report on Intergroup Study 0034. *Int J Radiat Oncol Biol Phys* 1992;23:705-713.

90. Bernier J, Cooper JS, Pajak TF, et al. Defining risk levels in locally advanced head and neck cancers: A comparative analysis of concurrent postoperative radiation plus chemotherapy trials of the EORTC (#22931) and RTOG (# 9501). *Head Neck* 2005;27:843-850.

91. Cohen EE, Rosen F, Stadler WM, et al. Phase II trial of ZD1839 in recurrent or metastatic squamous cell carcinoma of the head and neck. *J Clin Oncol* 2003;21:1980-1987.

92. Cohen EE, Lingen MW, Vokes EE. The expanding role of systemic therapy in head and neck cancer. *J Clin Oncol* 2004;22:1743-1752.

93. Soulieres D, Senzer NN, Vokes EE, et al. Multicenter phase II study of erlotinib, an oral epidermal growth factor receptor tyrosine kinase inhibitor, in patients with recurrent or metastatic squamous cell cancer of the head and neck. *J Clin Oncol* 2004;22:77-85.

94. Burtness B, Goldwasser MA, Flood W, et al. Phase III randomized trial of cisplatin plus placebo compared with cisplatin plus cetuximab in metastatic/recurrent head and neck cancer: An Eastern Cooperative Oncology Group study. *J Clin Oncol* 2005;23:8646-8654.

95. Vermorken JB, Trigo J, Hitt R, et al. Open-label, uncontrolled, multicenter phase II study to evaluate the efficacy and toxicity of cetuximab as a single agent in patients with recurrent and/or metastatic squamous cell carcinoma of the head and neck who failed to respond to platinum-based therapy. *J Clin Oncol* 2007;25:2171-2177.

96. Vermorken JB, Mesia R, Rivera F, et al. Platinum-based chemotherapy plus cetuximab in head and neck cancer. *N Engl J Med* 2008;359:1116-1127.

97. Hong WK, Endicott J, Itri LM, et al. 13-cis-retinoic acid in the treatment of oral leukoplakia. *N Engl J Med* 1986;315: 1501-1505.

98. Lippman SM, Batsakis JG, Toth BB, et al. Comparison of low-dose isotretinoin with beta carotene to prevent oral carcinogenesis. *N Engl J Med* 1993;328:15-20.

99. Lotan R, Xu XC, Lippman SM, et al. Suppression of retinoic acid receptor-beta in premalignant oral lesions and its up-regulation by isotretinoin. *N Engl J Med* 1995;332:1405-1410.

100. Papadimitrakopoulou VA, Hong WK, Lee JS, et al. Low-dose isotretinoin versus beta-carotene to prevent oral carcinogenesis: Long-term follow-up. *J Natl Cancer Inst* 1997; 89:257-258.

101. Papadimitrakopoulou VA, Lee JJ, William WN, Jr., et al. Randomized trial of 13-cis retinoic acid compared with retinyl palmitate with or without beta-carotene in oral premalignancy. *J Clin Oncol* 2009;27:599-604.

102. Hong WK, Lippman SM, Itri LM, et al. Prevention of second primary tumors with isotretinoin in squamous-cell carcinoma of the head and neck. *N Engl J Med* 1990;323:795-801.

103. Benner SE, Pajak TF, Lippman SM, et al. Prevention of second primary tumors with isotretinoin in patients with squamous cell carcinoma of the head and neck: Long-term follow-up. *J Natl Cancer Inst* 1994;86:140-141.

104. Dannenberg AJ, Lippman SM, Mann JR, et al. Cyclooxygenase-2 and epidermal growth factor receptor: Pharmacologic targets for chemoprevention. *J Clin Oncol* 2005;23:254-266.

105. Bolla M, Lefur R, Ton Van J, et al. Prevention of second primary tumours with etretinate in squamous cell carcinoma of the oral cavity and oropharynx. Results of a multicentric double-blind randomised study. *Eur J Cancer* 1994;30A: 767-772.

106. van Zandwijk N, Dalesio O, Pastorino U, et al. EUROSCAN, a randomized trial of vitamin A and N-acetylcysteine in patients with head and neck cancer or lung cancer. For the European Organization for Research and Treatment of Cancer Head and Neck and Lung Cancer Cooperative Groups. *J Natl Cancer Inst* 2000;92:977-986.

107. Mayne ST, Cartmel B, Baum M, et al. Randomized trial of supplemental beta-carotene to prevent second head and neck cancer. *Cancer Res* 2001;61:1457-1463.

108. Bairati I, Meyer F, Gelinas M, et al. A randomized trial of antioxidant vitamins to prevent second primary cancers in head and neck cancer patients. *J Natl Cancer Inst* 2005;97:481-488.

109. Izzo JG, Papadimitrakopoulou VA, Liu DD, et al. Cyclin D1 genotype, response to biochemoprevention, and progression rate to upper aerodigestive tract cancer. *J Natl Cancer Inst* 2003;95:198-205.

110. Papadimitrakopoulou V, Izzo JG, Liu DD, et al. Cyclin D1 and cancer development in laryngeal premalignancy patients. *Cancer Prev Res (Phila Pa)* 2009;2:14-21.

111. Mao L, Lee JS, Fan YH, et al. Frequent microsatellite alterations at chromosomes 9p21 and 3p14 in oral premalignant lesions and their value in cancer risk assessment. *Nat Med* 1996;2:682-685.

112. Rosin MP, Cheng X, Poh C, et al. Use of allelic loss to predict malignant risk for low-grade oral epithelial dysplasia. *Clin Cancer Res* 2000;6:357-362.

113. Rosin MP, Lam WL, Poh C, et al. 3p14 and 9p21 loss is a simple tool for predicting second oral malignancy at previously treated oral cancer sites. *Cancer Res* 2002;62:6447-6450.

114. William WN, Jr., Heymach JV, Kim ES, et al. Molecular targets for cancer chemoprevention. *Nat Rev Drug Discov* 2009;8:213-225.

Gastrointestinal Carcinomas

PART

VI

Gastrointestinal
Carcinomas

GASTRIC AND ESOPHAGEAL CANCER

Alexandria T. Phan

■ INTRODUCTION

From 1944 to 2004, 11,261 patients with upper gastrointestinal carcinomas (6215 gastric; 5046 esophageal) were treated at The University of Texas MD Anderson Cancer Center. Of these, 5112 (2393 gastric; 2719 esophageal) underwent a definitive treatment at MD Anderson. Overall survival (OS) significantly improved at 5 and 10 years over this 60-year interval. Absolute OS improvements at 5 years were 20.3% for gastric cancer (11.8 versus 32.1%, $p < .0001$) and 24.9% for esophageal cancer (2.3 versus 27.2%, $p < .0001$).

■ GASTRIC CANCER

In the United States, an estimated 21,130 new cases of gastric cancer were diagnosed in 2009, with 10,620 deaths (1). According to the Surveillance Epidemiology and End Results (SEER) 17 (2000-2006) database, only 24% of gastric cancers are confined to the stomach (localized); 31 to 32% of newly diagnosed cases have spread beyond the stomach into the regional lymph nodes (regional) or other organs (distant), respectively (2). Gastric cancer predominantly affects men, at a ratio of 2:1. The median age at diagnosis is 71 years (2). The 5-year OS rate is 25.7%, which has not changed significantly over the past 30 to 40 years (2). Surgery is still the only chance for cure, and survival can be improved with multimodality therapy.

EPIDEMIOLOGIC CHARACTERISTICS

The incidence of gastric carcinoma varies widely, both worldwide and within individual country. The highest incidence (>20 per 100,000 in men) is in Japan, China, Eastern Europe, and South America, while the lowest incidence (<10 per 100,000 in men) is in North America, parts of Africa, and Southern Asia (3). In the United States, gastric cancers occur at a median age of 69 years for men and 73 for women (2). African Americans, Hispanic Americans, and Native Americans are 1.5 to 2.5 times more likely to develop gastric cancer than whites (4). On the basis of SEER 2002-2006 data, the age-adjusted incidence of gastric cancer is 7.9 per 100,000 men and women per year (2).

In the United States, the incidence of gastric cancer has been decreasing over the past several decades, reflecting a significant reduction in distal (body and antrum) disease. The reason for the decline is not known but may be related to dietary habits, food preservation, and improved surgical morbidity and mortality rates. However, the incidence of proximal stomach and gastroesophageal junction (GEJ) adenocarcinomas has steadily increased at a rate exceeding that of any other cancers except melanoma and lung cancer (5). Observational studies suggest that proximal cancers have a different pathogenesis than do distal cancers (6). Potential causes of distal gastric cancers include *Helicobacter pylori* infection or E-cadherin expression loss, whereas proximal gastric cancer may behave similarly to distal esophageal and GEJ cancers, which progresses from Barrett metaplasia to dysplasia to invasive adenocarcinoma. Only 24% of newly diagnosed gastric cancers are localized. The 5-year survival rate of patients with metastatic disease is less than 5%. Thus, even in the United States, despite decreasing incidence, gastric cancer remains a public health concern because of its high fatality rate.

ETIOLOGIC CHARACTERISTICS AND RISK FACTORS

Histology of gastric cancers is most frequently adenocarcinoma, which consists of two main histologic variants: intestinal and diffuse. Intestinal-type gastric adenocarcinoma likely begins with an *H pylori* infection that leads to multistep progression. More than 40 to 50% of distal gastric adenocarcinomas are associated with *H pylori* infection (6). Studies have shown that different strains of *H pylori* carry differential risks of gastric cancer. Infection with vacAs1-, vacAm-, and cagA-positive strains of *H pylori* are associated with an increased risk of gastric cancer (7). *H pylori* infections probably start early in childhood and have a long latency period in which the gastric mucosa progresses through a series of well-defined histopathologic steps: chronic active nonatrophic gastritis, multifocal atrophic gastritis, intestinal metaplasia, dysplasia, and invasive adenocarcinoma (8). Other environmental risk factors and inflammatory cytokines may influence and contribute to this multistep progression.

Population studies have identified certain environmental risk factors associated with gastric cancer. Low consumption of fruits and vegetables, high intake of N-nitroso compounds in salted and preserved foods, and occupational exposure in coal mining and nickel, rubber, and timber processing are commonly described

risk factors. Long-standing chronic superficial gastritis caused by a high-salt diet or conditions such as pernicious anemia eventually leads to chronic atrophic gastritis and intestinal metaplasia. Gastric atrophy is accompanied by a loss of parietal cell mass and thus a reduction in acid production (hypochlorhydria or achlorhydria), a decrease in luminal ascorbic acid (vitamin C) levels, and a compensatory increase in serum gastrin, a potent inducer of gastric epithelial cell proliferation. The increase in gastric pH would permit colonization by bacteria capable of converting dietary nitrates to potent mutagenic N-nitroso compounds. Additional notable risk factors include meat consumption, smoking, gastric surgery, and reproductive hormones. A meta-analysis estimated that the relative risk of gastric cancer associated with consumption of 30 g of processed meat per day (about one-half an average serving) was 1.15 (95% confidence interval [CI], 1.04-1.27) (9). A prospective study (10) found that smokers were at increased risk for gastric cardia (hazard ratio [HR], 2.9; 95% CI, 1.7-4.7), and gastric non-cardia cancer compared with nonsmokers (HR, 2.0; 95% CI, 1.3-3.2) (11). Two meta-analyses estimated that the relative risk of gastric cancer among gastric surgery patients was 1.5 to 3.0, depending on the type of surgery, duration of follow-up, and geographic location (12). Perhaps one explanation for the lower incidence of gastric cancer among women has to do with the protective effect of reproductive hormones. A recent prospective study from China suggested that there are associations between gastric cancer in women and age of menopause, years of fertility, years since menopause, and intrauterine device use (13).

Overall, the pathogenesis of intestinal-type gastric adenocarcinomas involves a series of events. This sequence of events—increased cell proliferation due to the promotional effects of hypergastrinemia or bile reflux, increased luminal levels of mutagens (eg, N-nitroso compounds and free radicals), and decreased luminal levels of protective factors (eg, vitamin C)—provides an ideal milieu for carcinogenesis in susceptible hosts. Furthermore, many inflammatory cytokines have been studied to determine whether they are associated with an increased risk of gastric cancer; the most significant association seems to be with interleukin-1 beta (IL-1β) (14). The molecular effect of *H pylori*–induced gastritis seems to be associated with the IL-1β pathway and other proinflammatory cytokines such as interleukin-10 (IL-10) and tumor necrosis factor-alpha (TNF-α)

The molecular effect of *H pylori*–induced gastritis seems to be associated with the IL-1β pathway and other pro-inflammatory cytokines such as interleukin-10 (IL-10) and tumor necrosis factor-α (TNF-α) (15). The effect is most likely mediated through induction of hypochorhydria and severe corpus gastritis, which leads to subsequent gastric atrophy (16). Interleukin-1 (IL-1) is unregulated in the presence of *H pylori* and is important in initiating and amplifying response to infection.

Excess nitric oxide produced by increased IL-1 expression has been shown to be the cause of chronic inflammation and contributes to *H pylori*–induced gastric cancer (17). IL-1 also has several genotypic polymorphisms, and only some specific genotypes are associated with an increased risk of gastric cancer (7,18). The alleles of the *IL-1* gene have been associated with increased risk of atrophic gastritis and gastric cancer in Eastern Asia and Europe. By conducting a comparative case-control study of 334 hospitalized atrophic gastritis or gastric cancer patients and 158 nonatrophic gastritis patients in Peru, MD Anderson investigators found that an increased risk of atrophic gastritis (odds ratio [OR] 5.60) and gastric cancer (OR 2.36) was associated with the *IL-1β-511C* allele (19). Therefore, even among different cohorts, it is likely that interplay between bacterial virulence and cytokine genotype leads to a varied spectrum of gastric carcinogenesis, ranging from pre-neoplastic lesions to overt cancer (20).

In contrast to intestinal-type gastric cancer, diffuse-type gastric adenocarcinoma results from defective intracellular adhesion molecules, which is the consequence of loss of E-cadherin protein expression, which is encoded by *CDH1*. This can occur through germline or somatic mutation, loss of heterozygosity (LOH), or epigenetic silencing of gene transcription through aberrant methylation of the *CDH1* promoter. A study by Zheng et al. showed a positive rate of E-cadherin promoter methylation in dysplasia, early cancer, and advanced cancer (21). Furthermore, 30% of hereditary diffuse gastric cancer (HDGC) families show *CDH1* germline mutations, whereas the rest remain genetically unexplained (22). Currently, many families with HDGC have *CDH1* germline mutations. Inheritance is dominant. The lifetime cumulative risk for advanced gastric cancer has been estimated to be 40 to 67% in men and 60 to 83% in women (23). Women in affected families are also at high risk for developing lobular breast carcinoma, with a cumulative risk of 52% (23).

Affected patients generally develop gastric cancer at a mean age of 38 years. The consensus criteria for diagnosing HDGC from the International Gastric Cancer Linkage (IGCL) include: (1) more than two cases of diffuse-type gastric cancer in first- or second-degree

relatives, with one aged <50 years, or (2) more than three cases of diffuse-type gastric cancer in first- or second-degree relatives of any age (24). A germline mutation in *TP53* is associated with familial gastric cancer (FGC) (22), which includes Li-Fraumeni syndrome. Another familial cancer syndrome associated with gastric cancer is hereditary non-polyposis colorectal cancer (HNPCC), resulting from defects of DNA mismatch repair genes (*hMLH1* and *hMSH2*, more frequent) (22).

Epstein-Barr virus (EBV)-associated gastric cancers have distinct clinicopathologic characteristics, including male predominance, preferential location in the gastric cardia or postsurgical gastric stump, lymphocytic infiltration, a more favorable prognosis (25,26), and a diffuse-type in most (26) but not all (25) series. Among 235 patients with surgically resected gastric cancer at MD Anderson who did not undergo preoperative therapy, the prevalence of EBV infection was 5%. Intranuclear EBV staining was exclusively seen in primary and metastatic tumor cells. The detection of EBV in tumor cells in all involved lymph nodes suggests simultaneous replication of EBV and tumor cells. Patients with EBV-associated gastric cancer were younger than were those with non-EBV–associated gastric cancer (median age, 62 versus 66 years). In this retrospective analysis, EBV-associated gastric cancer patients were predominantly male and relatively young, suggesting an association between this disease and other factors, such as lifestyle (27).

In summary, the pathogenesis of gastric cancers varied according to the histologic subtypes, intestinal and diffuse. Intestinal-type gastric cancer is most likely a result of multistep progression starting from chronic gastritis, modulated by environmental risk factors, resulting from chronic inflammation. These factors include infectious and nutritional agents and inflammatory cytokines. In contrast, diffuse-type gastric cancer results from defective intracellular adhesion molecules, which is the consequence of loss of E-cadherin protein expression, which is encoded by *CDH1*. This can occur through germline or somatic mutation, LOH, or epigenetic silencing of gene transcription through aberrant methylation of the *CDH1* promoter. Notable mutations in gastric cancer include *TP53*, *hMLH1*, and *hMSH2*, found in Li-Fraumeni and HNPCC familial syndromes, respectively, as shown in Table 17-1. Despite recent progress, the precise etiologic characteristics of gastric cancer and the relationship between the environment and host are unknown. Ongoing research promises to better elucidate the tumorigenesis of gastric cancer.

TABLE 17-1 SUMMARY OF SELECTED RECURRENT CYTOGENETIC ABNORMALITIES AND FREQUENT MOLECULAR CHANGES ASSOCIATED WITH GASTRIC CANCER (42)

Conventional cytogenetics	Simple karyotypes	Complex karyotypes
	+X, +8, +9, +19, del(7q), i(8q)	1, 3, 6, 7, 8, 11, 13, 17, 19
Molecular cytogenetics	Gains	Loss
	3q, 7p, 7q, 8q, 13q, 17q, 20p, 20q	4q, 9p, 17p, 18q

Genes	Abnormalities	Clinical Association
c-met	Amplification	Tumor invasion, lymph node metastasis, poor prognosis
K-sam	Amplification	Advanced tumor stage/poor prognosis
c-erbB2	Amplification	Advanced tumor stage, lymph node and liver metastases, poor prognosis
c-myc	Amplification	Poor clinical course/predictor of aggressiveness
TP53	Loss of heterozygosity Mutation Hypermethylation	Proliferative rate/lymph node metastasis/shortened survival
Bcl-2	Loss of heterozygosity	Depth of invasion, lymph node metastasis and survival
RUNX3	Deletion Hypermethylation Loss of expression	Metastasis
PTEN	Loss of heterozygosity Mutation	Advanced tumor stage/metastasis
E-cadherin (CDH1)	Loss of heterozygosity Mutation Hypermethylation Reduced expression	Tumor metastatic ability and poor prognosis
Cyclin E	Amplification	Disease aggressiveness/lymph node metastasis
p27	Reduced expression	Advanced tumor stage/depth of invasion/lymph node metastasis
p16	Reduced expression	Tumor invasion/metastasis
DNA repair genes/MSI	Mutation Hypermethylation Reduced expression	Age/low prevalence of lymph node metastasis/prolonged survival
syndecan-1	Reduce expression	Tumor differentiation
beta-catenin	Amplification	Lymph node metastasis
CD44s and CD44v6	Amplification	Lymph node metastasis
Sp1	Amplification	Cancer angiogenic potential, poor prognosis

CLINICAL PRESENTATION

At presentation, most symptomatic patients will likely have advanced gastric cancer. Symptoms are generally nonspecific and most frequently include weight loss, abdominal pain, and nausea. Dysphagia is more common in patients with cancer originating in the gastric cardia or GEJ. Occult gastrointestinal bleeding is also common, whereas overt bleeding is observed in only 20% of cases.

PATHOLOGIC CHARACTERISTICS

More than 95% of gastric cancers are adenocarcinoma. The remaining 5% include carcinoid, lymphoma, squamous cell carcinoma, and sarcoma. Gastric adenocarcinoma is classified using the Lauren classification system. Histologic types are also associated with differential complex of clinical characteristics of patients with gastric cancer. Lauren type 1 is intestinal, with distinctive glands and a well-differentiated columnar epithelium. Type 2 is diffuse, with poorly organized clusters of mucin-rich cells in infiltrative patterns. Type 1 is more common in high-risk populations, men, and older patients; type 2 is more often found in women and younger patients and carries a poorer prognosis (28). Figures 17-1 through 17-9 show the gross morphologic and microscopic characteristics of gastric cancer.

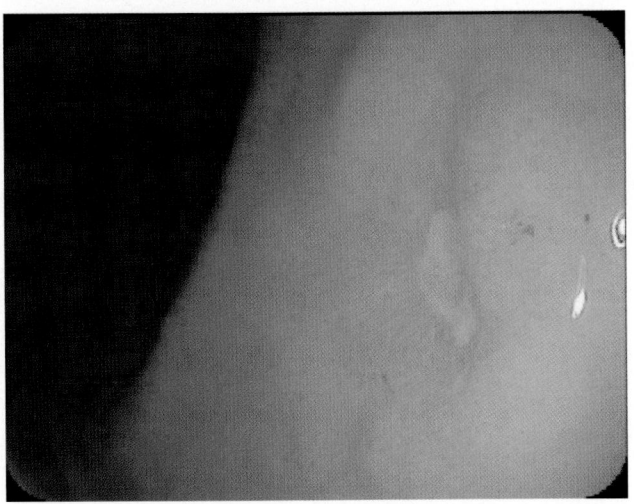

FIGURE 17-1. Gastric ulcer, benign, endoscopic view. (*Courtesy of Norio Fukami, MD, University of Texas, MD Anderson, Department of GI Medicine and Nutrition, Houston, TX.*)

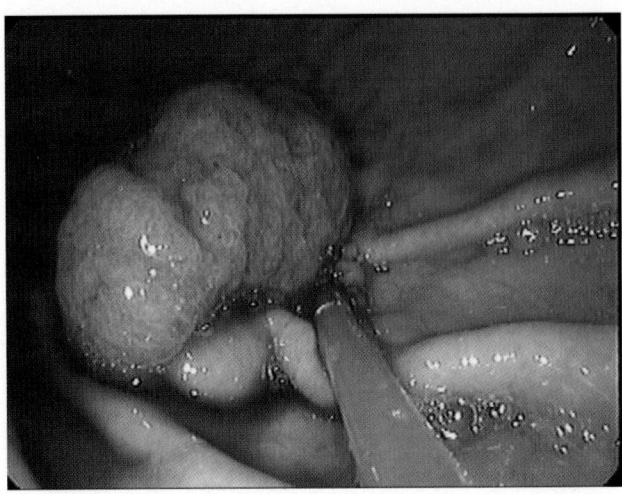

FIGURE 17-3. Gastric adenocarcinoma, endoscopic view. (*Courtesy of Norio Fukami, MD, University of Texas, MD Anderson, Department of GI Medicine and Nutrition, Houston, TX.*)

STAGING AND PROGNOSIS

Upper GI series with barium swallow and upper esophagoduodenoscopy (EGD) are mainstays for diagnosing gastric cancer and both provide complementary diagnostic information. EGD is more sensitive and specific to obtain tissue diagnosis. A single biopsy has 70% sensitivity for diagnosing gastric cancer; performing seven biopsies from the ulcer margin and base increases the sensitivity to >98% (29). In contrast, barium swallow with upper GI series can identify both malignant gastric ulcers and infiltrating lesions, including some

early gastric cancers. However, the false-negative rate with barium swallow can be as high as 50% (30) and may be even higher for early gastric cancer, and sensitivity can be as low as 14% (30).

Staging is important because treatment is based on the stage of disease at diagnosis, according to the TNM (tumor, node, metastasis) system of the American Joint Commission on Cancer (AJCC). Version 7 is the most current and is represented in Table 17-2 (31). In this newest version, GEJ and proximal gastric cancers <5 cm from the GEJ are now included in the esophageal

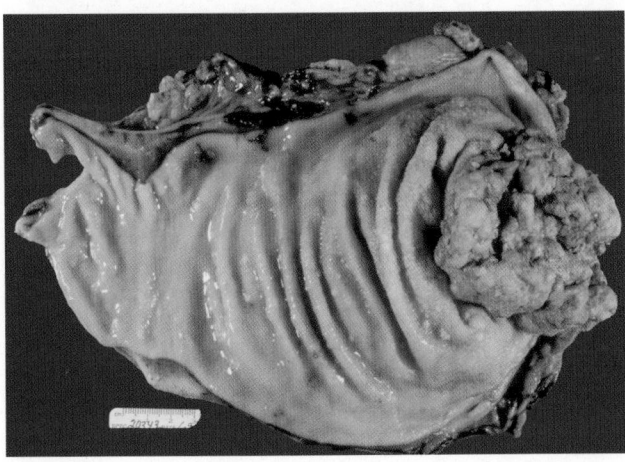

FIGURE 17-2. Gastric adenocarcinoma, gross view. (*Courtesy of Asif Rashid, MD, University of Texas, MD Anderson, Department of Pathology, Houston, TX.*)

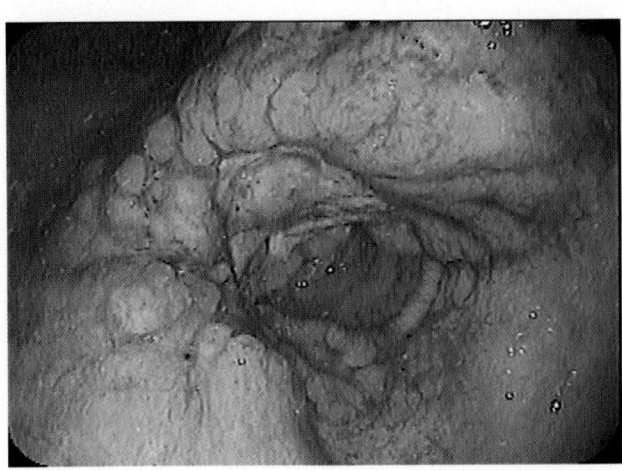

FIGURE 17-4. Gastric malignant ulcer and cancer type 3, endoscopic view. (*Courtesy of Norio Fukami, MD, University of Texas, MD Anderson, Department of GI Medicine and Nutrition, Houston, TX.*)

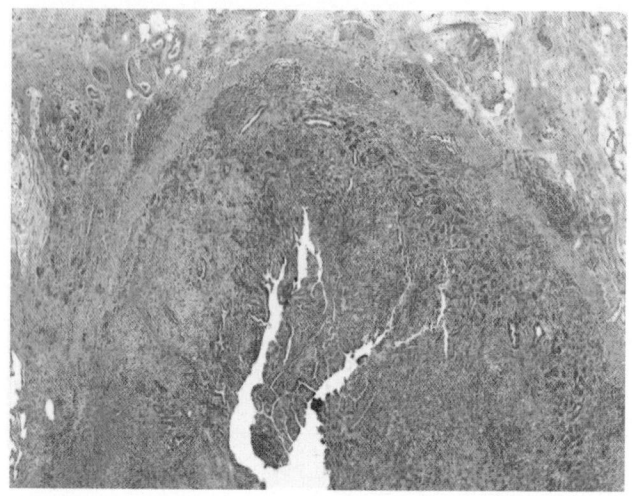

FIGURE 17-5. Gastric adenocarcinoma, low-power view. (*Courtesy of Dr. Asif Rashid, Department of Pathology, University of Texas, MD Anderson, Houston, TX.*)

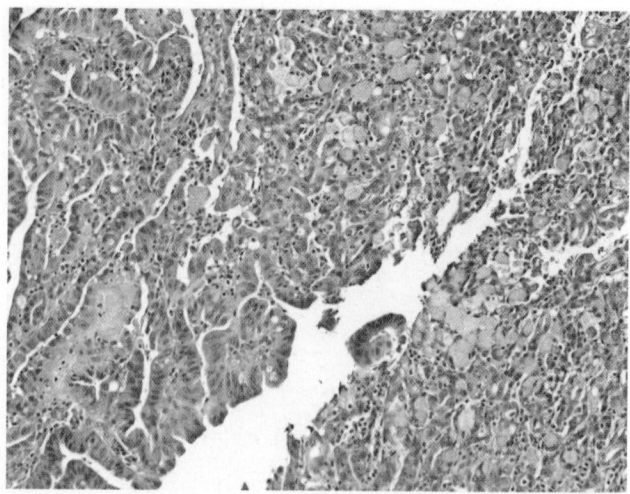

FIGURE 17-7. Gastric adenocarcinoma, high-power view. (*Courtesy of Dr. Asif Rashid, Department of Pathology, University of Texas, MD Anderson, Houston, TX.*)

cancer staging system. The T classification has been modified to harmonize with the new esophageal T classification. T1 and T4 have been further subdivided. Positive peritoneal cytologic results are classified as M1. Because of its noninvasive nature, computer-assisted tomography (CAT/CT) has become the cornerstone of gastric cancer staging, although it is not sensitive at detecting the tumor invasion depth and local and regional lymph node involvement. Currently, CT is used in conjunction with endoscopic ultrasonography (EUS) of the primary site, which provides the most

accurate data for depth of tumor invasion and locoregional lymph nodes involvement. EUS has an accuracy of 77% (versus 40-50% with CT) for staging depth and 69% for staging nodes (32). Limitations of EUS include under-staging nodal disease and its short field of vision (5-7 cm). The availability of EUS-guided biopsy of suspicious local and regional lymph nodes has circumvented its former limitation. Figures 17-10 through 17-14 show endoscopic images of gastric cancer. Laparoscopy is more invasive than CT or EUS, but it has the advantage of directly visualizing the liver surface, peritoneum,

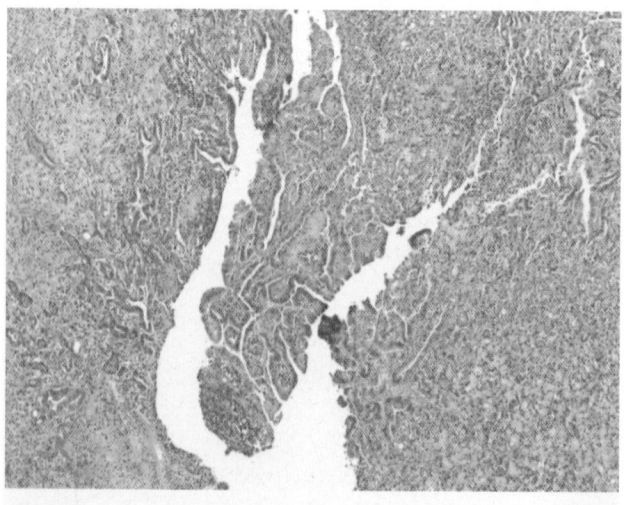

FIGURE 17-6. Gastric adenocarcinoma, medium-power view. (*Courtesy of Dr. Asif Rashid, Department of Pathology, University of Texas, MD Anderson, Houston, TX.*)

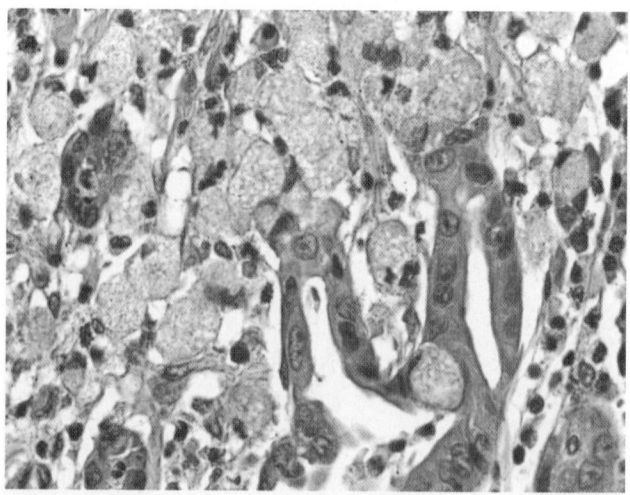

FIGURE 17-8. Gastric adenocarcinoma, signet ring cell pattern. (*Courtesy of Dr. Asif Rashid, Department of Pathology, University of Texas, MD Anderson, Houston, TX.*)

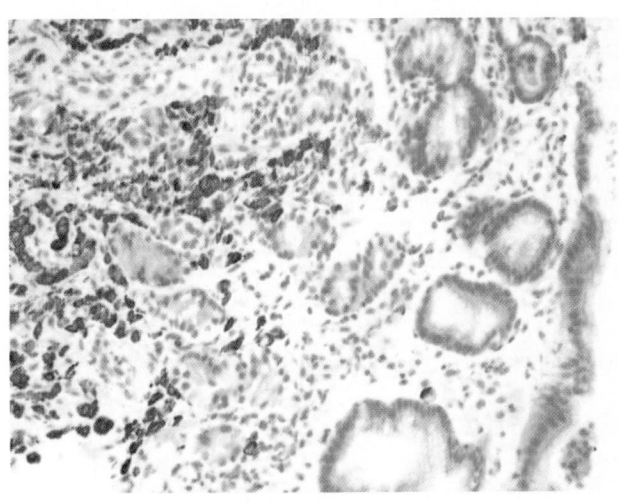

FIGURE 17-9. Gastric adenocarcinoma, IMH for cytokeratin. (*Courtesy of Dr. Asif Rashid, Department of Pathology, University of Texas, MD Anderson, Department of Pathology, Houston, TX.*)

and local lymph nodes. It is sensitive at diagnosing liver metastases; in one review, it diagnosed peritoneal metastases in 23% of patients in whom no such involvement was seen on CT (33). Diagnostic laparoscopy is usually performed when all noninvasive studies (CT and EUS) demonstrate localized or potentially resectable disease.

The effectiveness of fluorodeoxyglucose-positron emission tomography (FDG-PET) at diagnosing gastric cancer is uncertain because as many as 50% of primary tumors are FGD-negative, particularly early gastric cancers (34). Insufficient FDG uptake is mostly associated with diffuse-type gastric cancer with signet ring cells and mucinous content (35). Stahl et al. presented a prospective trial using FDG-PET scanning to predict response to preoperative chemotherapy. These investigators suggested that gastric cancer's response to preoperative therapy is associated with a metabolic response of >35% on FDG-PET scan uptake (36). Currently, FDG-PET has no role in the primary detection of gastric cancer because of its low sensitivity. On the other hand, FDG-PET shows better results in the evaluation of lymph node metastases in gastric cancer compared with CT and could thus have a role in preoperative staging. For patients with FDG-positive disease, FDG-PET can be used to predict histologic response and survival outcomes (37), similar to results seen among patients with distal esophageal and GEJ adenocarcinoma (38-40). The addition of FDG-PET to CT increase diagnostic accuracy for recurrent gastric cancer because PET/CT is as sensitive and specific as contrast CT at detecting recurrent disease, except peritoneal seeding (41).

Scientific advances have made it possible to further understand the molecular interplay between the host and the environment, but it had also led to a better understanding of other molecular abnormalities in the tumorigenesis of gastric cancer, along with the development of molecular detection or screening for patients at risk. Conventional immunohistochemistry, aided by molecular cytogenetic methods such as fluorescence in situ hybridization (FISH), comparative genomic hybridization (CGH), and multicolor karyotyping had been used to identify genetic changes in gastric cancer tumorigenesis. Molecular studies of specific genes such as proto-oncogenes, tumor suppression genes, cell-cycle regulators, cell adhesion molecules, and DNA repair genes have supplied important information about the genetic events in gastric cancer. Gastric tumorigenesis results from LOH/inactivation of tumor suppressor genes, or widespread somatic alterations in simple repetitive genomic sequences, leading to microsatellite instability. These frequent molecular changes (42) and other tumor markers with potential prognostic significance in gastric cancer, such as syndecan-1, bcl-2, RUNX3, and beta-catenin (43,44), are also listed in Table 17-1.

S-1 overexpression is directly correlated with the angiogenic potential and poor prognosis of gastric cancer (45). Gastric cancer tissues of patients with distant metastases have higher *p53* expression than those of patients without metastases. *p53* expression is significantly associated with depth of invasion, lymph node and distant metastasis, and lower 5-year survival rates (46). MD Anderson investigators studied 51 candidate genes in 7 gastric cancer cell lines and 24 samples to determine the methylation status of these genes. Epigenetic alterations, as distinct and crucial mechanisms of silencing methylated tissue-specific and imprinted genes, have been extensively studied in gastric carcinoma and play important roles in gastric carcinogenesis (47). In a study comparing the methylation profiles of tumor suppressor gene *p16*, DNA mismatch repair gene *hMLH1*, four CpG islands (MINT1, MINT2, MINT25, and MINT31), and microsatellite instability using five microsatellite markers in 83 resected gastric carcinoma patients from MD Anderson, an association was found between CIMP status and microsatellite instability. Concordant methylation of multiple genes and loci (CIMP-H) is associated with better survival but is not an independent predictor of prognosis in resected gastric cancer (47). MINT25 methylation had the best sensitivity (90%) and specificity (96%) in terms of tumor detection in gastric washes (48). By evaluating functional single nucleotide polymorphisms (SNPs) of the

| TABLE | AMERICAN JOINT CANCER COMMITTEE TNM STAGING |
| 17-2 | SYSTEM FOR GASTRIC CANCER (31) |

PRIMARY TUMOR (T)

Tx	Primary tumor cannot be assessed
T0	No evidence of primary tumor
Tis	Carcinoma in situ: intraepithelial tumor with invasion of the lamina propria
T1	Tumor invades muscularis propria or submucosa
T1a	Tumor invades lamina propria, muscularis mucosae, or submucosa
T1b	Tumor invades submucosa
T2	Tumor invades muscularis propria
T3	Tumor penetrates the subserosal connective tissue without invasion of visceral peritoneum or adjacent structures
T4	Tumor invades serosa (visceral peritoneum) or adjacent structures
T4a	Tumor invades serosa (visceral peritoneum)
T4b	Tumor invades adjacent structures

REGIONAL LYMPH NODES (N)

Nx	Regional lymph node(s) cannot be assessed
N0	No regional lymph node metastasis
N1	Metastasis in 1-2 regional lymph nodes
N2	Metastasis in 3-6 regional lymph nodes
N3	Metastasis in ≥7 regional lymph nodes
N3a	Metastasis in 7-15 regional lymph nodes
N3b	Metastasis in ≥16 regional lymph nodes

DISTANT METASTASES (M)

Mx	Distant metastasis cannot be assessed
M0	No distant metastases
M1	Distant metastases

Stage Grouping				*5-Year Survival Rates (%)*
Stage 0 (in situ)	Tis	N0	M0	>90
Stage IA	T1	N0	M0	71
Stage IB	T1	N1	M0	57
	T2	N0	M0	
Stage IIA	T1	N2	M0	46
	T2	N1	M0	
Stage IIB	T3	N0	M0	
	T1	N3	M0	33
	T2	N2	M0	
	T3	N1	M0	
	T4a	N0	M0	
Stage IIIA	T2	N3	M0	20
	T3	N2	M0	
	T4a	N1	M0	
Stage IIIB	T3	N3	M0	14
	T4a	N2	M0	
	T4b	N1	M0	
	T4b	N0	M0	
Stage IIIC	T4a	N3	M0	9
	T4b	N3	M0	
	T4b	N2	M0	
Stage IV	Any T	Any N	M1	4

Used with the permission of the American Joint Committee on Cancer (AJCC), Chicago, Illinois. The original source for this material is the AJCC Cancer Staging Manual, Seventh Edition (2010) published by Springer Science and Business Media LLC, www.springer.com.

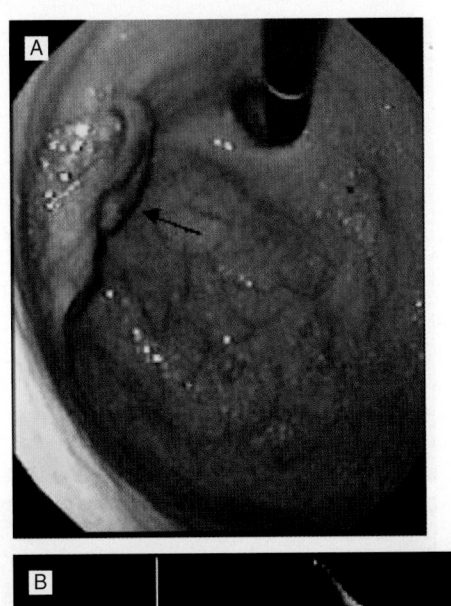

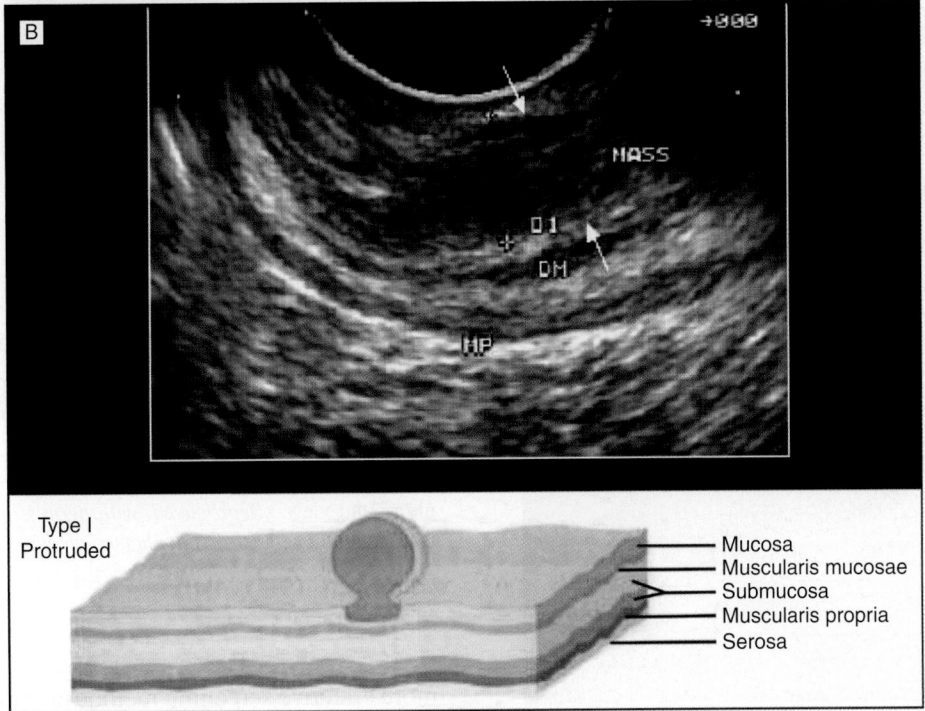

FIGURE 17-10. Gastric cancer: T1 lesion. **A.** Endoscopic view. **B.** Endoscopic ultrasound view. (*Reproduced, with permission, from http://www.massgeneral.org/gastro/endo_homepage.htm.*)

VEGF gene, other investigators at MD Anderson found that VEGF-634G>C SNP has the potential to be a marker for susceptibility to gastric cancer (49).

Currently, histologic types and stages remain the most consistent prognostic factors in gastric cancer patients who had not been to surgery. The best chance for long-lasting survival of patients with gastric cancer remains with curative resection. Patients who do not undergo resection have a poor prognosis, with survival ranging from 3 to 11 months (31). Among gastric cancer patients who had surgery, status of nodal involvement is perhaps the most powerful prognostic factor for them. Additionally, after curative resection, other factors affecting gastric cancer prognosis include tumor location, histologic grade, and lymphovascular invasion (31). Patients with proximal gastric cancer have poorer prognosis than those with distal gastric cancer, at 28.5 versus 58.6 months ($p < .02$) (50). Although associations have been found between molecular genetic changes and pathologic features and

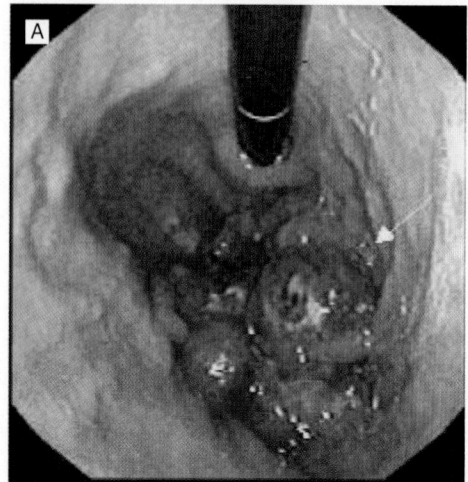

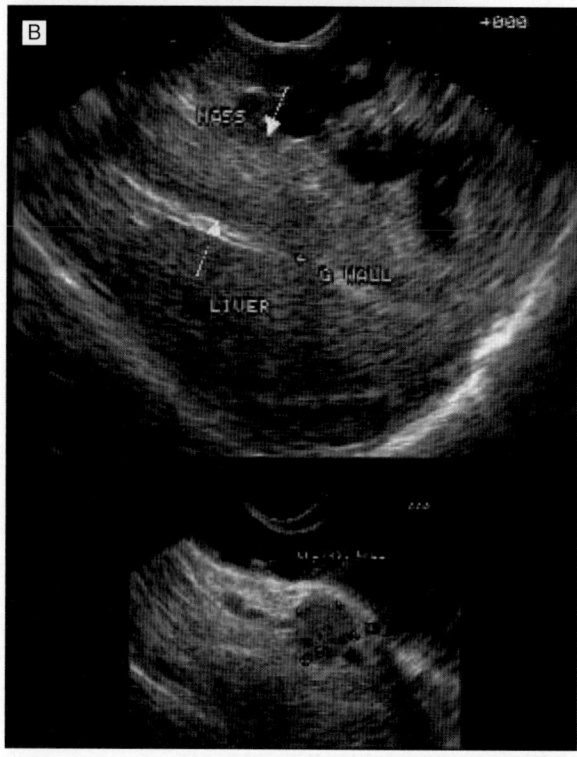

FIGURE 17-11. Gastric cancer: T2,N1 lesion. **A.** Endoscopic view. **B.** Endoscopic ultrasound view. (*Reproduced, with permission, from http://www.massgeneral. org/gastro/endo_homepage.htm.*)

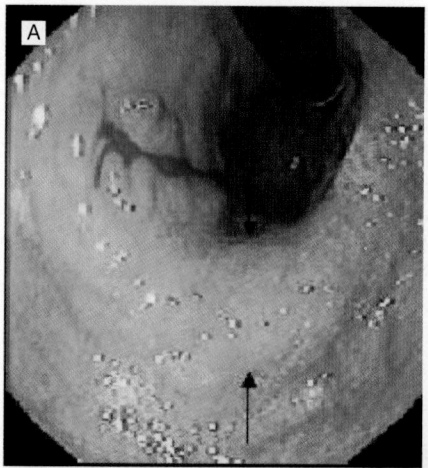

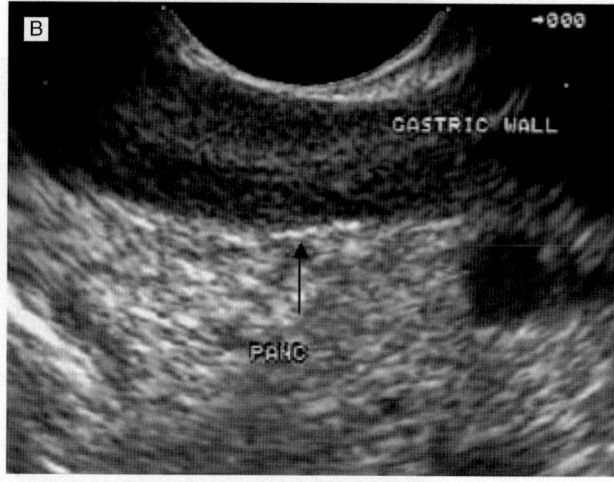

FIGURE 17-12. Linitis plastica. **A.** Endoscopic view. **B.** Endoscopic ultrasound view. (*Reproduced, with permission, from http://www. massgeneral.org/gastro/endo_homepage.htm.*)

biologic behavior and prognosis, the clinical significance of these genetic changes have not yet been established. Another word, these genetic parameters have been unable to translate into meaningful clinical diagnostic or prognostic markers. Therefore, the putative screening method for gastric cancer also remains elusive. However, with better appreciation of the complex interplay between environment and host factors leading to gastric tumorigenesis, researchers hope to produce more effective screening methods for high-risk patients, better prognostic and predictive biomarkers, and superior therapeutic indices of cancer drugs.

TREATMENT

Gastric cancer is treated according to the cancer stage at presentation. Reflecting the newest changes in the AJCC staging system, treatment for GEJ and proximal gastric adenocarcinoma <5 cm from the GEJ is discussed in the esophageal cancer section. Treatment for patients with locally advanced gastric cancer is dichotomized into resectable and unresectable disease. Surgery remains the best chance for long-term survival. Furthermore, survival outcome after surgery can be improved with the addition of other therapeutic modalities, such as chemotherapy or chemoradiotherapy.

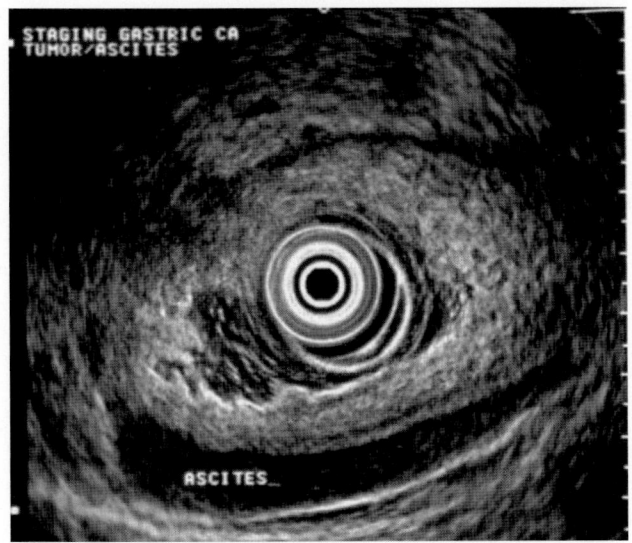

FIGURE 17-13. Gastric cancer with ascites. EUS imaging reveals a markedly thickened gastric wall (>1 cm thick; normal is 3-5 mm) with a small amount of previously undetected perigastric fluid in a patient with newly diagnosed gastric cancer. These findings are concerning for carcinomatosis, which was confirmed at the time of resection. (*Reproduced, with permission, from http://gi.ucsf.edu/ eusHistory.html.*)

Perioperative chemotherapy and postoperative chemoradiotherapy appear to be standard care for patients with locally advanced resectable gastric cancer. Ongoing clinical research into novel cytotoxic and targeted agents will continue to further improve the survival of patients with locally advanced curable gastric cancer.

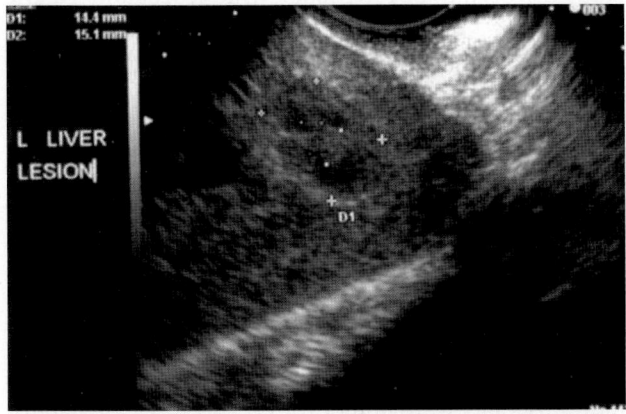

FIGURE 17-14. This image shows a small hepatic lesion, not identified on CT scan, in a patient undergoing staging for esophageal adenocarcinoma. Endoscopic ultrasound–guided fine-needle aspiration (EUS-FNA) confirmed the diagnosis of metastatic disease. (*Reproduced, with permission, from http://gi.ucsf.edu/eusHistory. html.*)

Unfortunately, the main therapeutic goal in patients with locally advanced unresectable disease is symptom palliation. The treatment of locally advanced, unresectable, and distant and metastatic gastric cancers is discussed in two separate subsections: Locally Advanced Unresectable Gastric, Gastroesophageal Junction, and Esophageal Carcinomas; and Advanced and Metastatic Gastric, Gastroesophageal Junction, and Esophageal Carcinomas. A summary of standard-of-care treatment options, based on stage of disease, is presented in Fig. 17-15 that illustrates MD Anderson approach to gastric cancer.

Resectable Disease

Surgery

Surgical resection offers the best chance for long-term survival in patients with localized disease, particularly in combination with postoperative (adjuvant) chemoradiotherapy (51) or perioperative chemotherapy (52). Even with newer staging modalities, the major barrier to accurately identifying patients with potentially resectable disease is the ability to accurately stage disease. In the United States, 67% of patients present with stage III or IV disease and only 10% present with stage I disease (53).

By definition, curative resection (also referred to as R0 resection) involves removal of the primary cancer and regional lymph nodes with free margins. The goals of surgery are twofold: (1) eradication of gastric cancer and (2) attainment of accurate pathologic staging. Considerations for surgical management of gastric cancer are the (1) extent of luminal resection (total versus partial gastrectomy) and (2) extent of lymph node dissection. Total gastrectomy is mainly reserved for proximal gastric cancer and large mid-gastric tumors or linitis plastica (wherein a large region of the stomach is extensively infiltrated by cancer, resulting in a rigid, thickened fold), whereas partial gastrectomy may be used in distal gastric tumors. Two randomized control trials have demonstrated similar survival outcomes for total and partial gastrectomy in gastric cancer (54,55). Overall survival rates improved from 5% for R2 (surgical resection with gross residual disease) to 50% for R0 (56). Five percent of primary gastric cancers are linitis plastica, mostly in younger cohorts; linitis plastica is commonly associated with a diffuse histologic type. This condition has a poor prognosis: more than 50% of newly diagnosed patients with linitis plastica will have metastatic or peritoneal metastases, and the 1- and 7-year survival rates are 50% and 8%, respectively (57). Total gastrectomy is the treatment of choice, although most

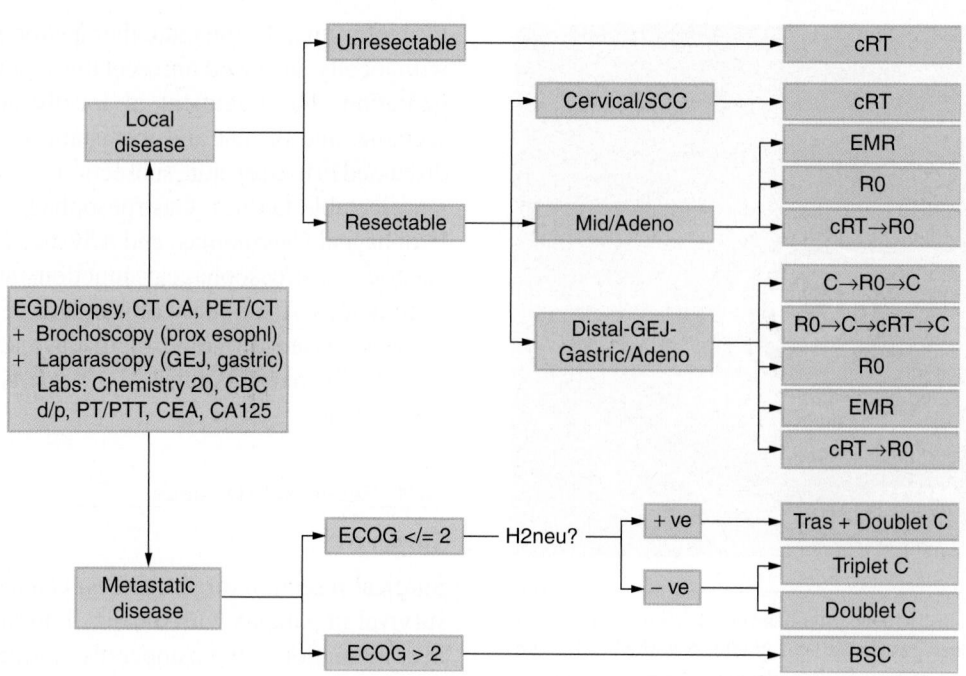

FIGURE 17-15. MD Anderson Treatment algorithms for gastroesophageal cancer. C, chemotherapy; CRT, chemoradiotherapy; O, observation; RT, radiotherapy; S, surgery; tras, trastuzumab; ECOG, Eastern Cooperative Oncology Group Performance Status Score.

surgeons consider linitis plastica as contraindication for performing curative surgery.

One of the unresolved controversies in the surgical management of gastric cancer is the extent of lymph node dissection. Japanese surgeons routinely perform extended lymphadenectomy, whereas in the United States, 54% of primary gastrectomy patients undergo less than a D1 lymphadenectomy (51). A D1 lymphadenectomy refers to a limited dissection of the perigastric lymph nodes, whereas D2 refers to the removal of nodes along the hepatic, left gastric, celiac, and splenic arteries, as well as those in the splenic hilum. A D3 lymph node dissection includes lymph nodes located within the porta hepatis and periaortic regions.

Proponents of extended lymphadenectomy argue that only with extended dissection can accurate staging be guaranteed, which also implies accurate prediction of stage-specific survival. Furthermore, with extensive nodal dissection, locoregional relapse rates are lower. From SEER 1973-2000, Schwarz and Smith (58) evaluated 1377 patients with locally advanced gastric cancer (stages IIIA, IIIB, and IV, N0). The total LN count (or number of negative LNs examined; $p < .0001$) and number of positive LNs ($p < .0001$) were independent prognostic survival predictors. Furthermore, the stage-based survival prediction depended on the total LN number and number of negative LNs. In their earlier analysis of SEER 1973-1999 data, these same investigators

demonstrated that for every 10 extra LNs dissected, survival improved by 7.6% (T1/2N0), 5.7% (T1/2N1), 11% (T3,N0), or 7% (T3,N1) (59). The results of this analysis demonstrated that for all T-stages, extensive nodal dissection affects survival outcomes. Similarly, a 5-year survival benefit was reported for patients with D2 and D3 dissections compared with D1 lymphadenectomy (60 versus 54%, $p = .041$) in a Taiwanese study involving 221 patients with resectable gastric cancer (60).

Since the initial Japanese retrospective studies demonstrated improved survival with more extensive lymphadenectomy (61), additional supporting evidence came from other retrospective studies as well as the Taiwanese prospective randomized trial. Despite the evidence, prospective studies performed in non-Asian countries were unable to confirm these findings (62-65). The Medical Research Council (MRC) randomly assigned 400 patients with resectable gastric cancer to D1 or D2 nodal dissection. Postoperative morbidity and mortality rates were higher for D2 (46%, 13%) than for D1 (28%, 6%) dissection (65). Both the initial and long-term follow-up results in the Dutch Gastric Cancer Group (DGCG) study demonstrated a significant increase in morbidity and mortality, with no survival difference, between D1 and D2 dissections (62,64). Although these large prospective studies performed in non-Asian countries could not confirm the initial findings, they went on to suggest that extended lymphadenectomy carries increased rates of morbidity and mortality, with a negligible change in survival.

In a more recent retrospective evaluation of 223 gastrectomy patients, Danielson et al. reported a hospital mortality rate of 3.7% for D2 and D3 and 1.8% for D1 (p = .438). D2 and D3 were associated with a longer postoperative hospital stay and operation time, more blood loss, and a higher need for blood transfusions compared with D1. The 5-year survival rate was not statistically different between the groups (63). Unlike the DGCG study, this later analysis suggested that perioperative mortality and survival rates were similar for D1, D2 and D3; thus, extensive lymphadenectomy may be feasible without compromising surgical mortality and disease survival. The DGCG and MRC studies were originally published in 1999, and the Finish study was published in 2007, so almost a decade separates these studies. Improved surgical techniques, postoperative hospital care, and surgical experience may have contributed to the improved surgical mortality rate reported in the later cohort.

The reason for the divergence in surgical outcomes between Asian and non-Asian countries is not readily apparent but may be that (1) earlier stages are diagnosed in Japan as a result of national screening programs; and (2) Japanese surgeons' extensive experience in gastric surgery and nodal dissection is not easily translatable. The controversy about the extent of lymph dissection continues in present time, but most experts agree that D2 dissection should be the goal in curative resection. However, it is preferred and recommended that aggressive lymphadenectomy be performed by surgeons at centers with experience in managing patients with gastric cancer. At MD Anderson, D2 nodal dissection is considered the standard of care.

Development of expertise in extended nodal dissections requires experience and training. The Nationwide Inpatient Sample for 1988-2000 reported a 20% decline in gastric resection rates. The declining number of gastric cancer resections in the United States will likely result in practicing surgeons who are less qualified to do extended nodal dissection. Proponents for extended nodal dissection rely on minimizing surgical morbidities to widen the beneficial index via minimizing surgical morbidities. Unfortunately, significant variation in mortality rates was noted between low- and high-volume hospitals (8.9 versus 6.4%, p < .001) (66). In this analysis, low-volume hospitals performed one to four gastrectomies per year, whereas high-volume hospitals performed more than nine. In a population study using national Medicare data (1994-1999), Birkmeyer et al.

reported significantly lower surgical mortality rates for gastrectomy and esophagectomy in National Cancer Institute (NCI)-designated hospitals than in non-NCI–designated hospitals: 8.0 versus 12.2%, (p < .001) for gastrectomy and 7.9 versus 10.9% (p = .027) for esophagectomy (67). In a study of 214 Texas hospitals with 1864 gastrectomy patients, treatment at high-volume hospitals decreased the odds of mortality (odd ratio [OR], 0.22; 95% CI, 0.05-0.89). Treatment failure was lower for patients at high-volume hospitals (OR, 0.53; 95% CI, 0.29-0.97) (68).

Surgical resection remains the best chance for cure. The survival outcomes of distal gastric cancer patients are not significantly different for segmental and total gastrectomies. Although conflicting data exist on lymphadenectomy (D1 versus D2), most experts agree that extensive lymphadenectomy should be performed by experienced surgeons. Gastric cancer patients require high-risk, high-skilled surgeries and thus should be referred to NCI-designated cancer centers or high-volume centers.

Postoperative Therapy

Curative resection offers the best chance for long-term survival in patients with gastric cancer, but more than 50% of newly diagnosed gastric cancers will have spread to the regional lymph nodes at resection. The 5-year survival rates are correlated with nodal involvement: 10% for patients with >15 positive lymph nodes, 30% for those with 7 to 15 positive lymph nodes, 40% for patients with <6 lymph nodes, and 50% for those without nodal metastasis (69). In addition, the 5-year survival rate of patients with completely resected node-negative gastric cancer is approximately 75% (70) whereas it is <30% (71) for those with extensive lymph node involvement. As a result, researchers had been evaluating the use of chemotherapy and chemoradiotherapy, postoperatively or preoperatively, to improve surgical outcomes. The high recurrence rate after complete surgical resection, especially in patients with nodal disease, provides even more impetus and rationale for combining surgery with other modalities.

Because resected gastric cancer tends to recur in the peritoneum, investigators have evaluated the role of intraperitoneal therapy. However, few large well-designed clinical trials have been performed; thus, the results are conflicting. Yan et al. performed a meta-analysis of 10 randomized control studies of intraperitoneal chemotherapy. A significant improvement in survival was found for hyperthermic intraperitoneal chemotherapy (HR, 0.60; 95% CI, 0.43-0.83; p = .002). There was no significant trend toward survival improvement with normothermic intraoperative intraperitoneal chemotherapy ($p = .06$). Additionally, intraperitoneal chemotherapy was found to be associated with higher risks of intra-abdominal abscess (relative risk [RR], 2.37; 95% CI, 1.32-4.26; $p = .003$) and neutropenia (RR, 4.33; 95% CI, 1.49-12.61; $p = .007$) (72). Despite demonstrating an improved outcome on meta-analysis, intraperitoneal chemotherapy is still considered investigational because of a lack of large well-designed controlled trials. Currently, intraperitoneal chemotherapy should only be performed at centers with expertise to minimize the high risk of intra-abdominal abscess.

Chemotherapy continues to play an important role in resected gastric cancer treatment. Currently, its use varies widely by geographic location (Asian versus non-Asian countries and sometimes North American versus European countries). The current practice trend is partly derived from historical data of past clinical trials. Trials have been done to evaluate various sequence and combination of additional therapy to surgery. Many randomized control clinical trials have been performed worldwide to evaluate the benefit of postoperative chemotherapy after curative gastrectomy. In ECOG study EST 3275, 180 patients were randomly assigned to 2 years of chemotherapy with 5-fluorouracil plus semustine or observation after en bloc resection. After a median follow-up of 64 months, the median OS durations were 32.7 and 36.6 months ($p = .73$). The results did not support the use of postoperative chemotherapy in patients with resectable gastric cancer (73). Other results have contradicted these, perhaps because of weaknesses in study design and variations in geography, etiology, biology, and practices. Even in trials that demonstrate survival benefit, the results have occasionally remained unconfirmed. Several meta-analyses have been performed to address conflicting results (Table 17-3) (72,74-79). Postoperative chemotherapy seems to result in a statistically significant survival benefit. However, subgroup meta-analyses have demonstrated a disparity between Asian and non-Asian studies, with more benefits seen among Asian patients (78).

These meta-analyses only include older clinical trials and thus may not reflect the more effective current regimens.

More recent clinical trials have also demonstrated a disparity between Asian and non-Asian populations. Sakuramoto et al. evaluated 529 patients with stage II or III gastric cancer after curative resection with D2-nodal dissection. Patients were randomly assigned to observation or 1 year of postoperative chemotherapy (80 mg/m^2/day of S-1, administered 4 weeks on and 2 weeks off). The trial was stopped early because a 1-year interim analysis concluded that patients receiving postoperative S-1 had a higher OS rate than did surgery-only patients ($p = .002$). The 3-year OS rates were 80.1% in the S-1 group and 70.1% in the surgery-only group. The HR for death in the S-1 group was 0.68 compared with surgery only (95% CI, 0.52-0.87; $p = .003$) (80). Meanwhile Di Costanzo et al. (81) published the negative results of 258 patients with resected gastric cancer who were randomly assigned to receive no further therapy or additional postoperative chemotherapy with cisplatin, epirubicin, leucovorin, and 5-fluorouracil (PELF). The lower doses of PELF may have contributed to the lack of effectiveness in this trial. However, the results of these two studies from Japan and Italy are consistent with those in meta-analyses. The observed benefit of postoperative chemotherapy in Asian patients does not translate into non-Asian patients.

Conflicting results in clinical studies relating to the role of postoperative chemotherapy or intraperitoneal chemotherapy may have assisted research focus toward other modality of therapy to improve survival outcome after curative surgery. Past data from early esophageal cancer trials suggested that concurrent chemoradiotherapy could improve locoregional control and OS compared with radiotherapy alone (82). Unfortunately, these early trials had inadequate numbers of patients, heterogeneous treatment groups, poor randomization schemes, high drop-out rates, and lack of proper control groups. These early studies were disappointing, and unable to

TABLE 17-3	POSTOPERATIVE THERAPY: RESULTS OF META-ANALYSES OF RANDOMIZED CONTROL CLINICAL TRIALS IN LOCALLY ADVANCED RESECTED GASTRIC CANCER			
Reference	*No. of Studies*	*N*	*OR*	*Treatment*
Hermans et al. (74)	11	2096	0.88	Chemotherapy, immunotherapy, intraperitoneal, radiotherapy
Mari et al. (76)	21	3658	0.82	Chemotherapy
Pazini et al. (77)	17	3118	0.72	Chemotherapy, R0
Janunger et al. (78)	21	3962	0.84	Chemotherapy, R0, Asian and non-Asian countries
Sun et al. (79)	12	3809	0.78	Chemotherapy, 1998-2007

N, total number of patients; OR, odds ratio; R0, margin negative-complete surgical resection.

advance the care of gastric cancer patients after curative surgery. Results that transformed care for resectable gastric cancer patients in the United States did not appear until the 21st century. In the Intergroup 0116 (INT116) trial, 603 stage IB-IV (M0) gastric cancer patients who had undergone curative resection were randomly assigned to observation (surgery alone) or additional postoperative therapy. Patients who were randomized to receive additional therapy were given chemotherapy consisted of 5-fluorouracil and leucovorin (FL) × 1 cycle, concurrent chemoradiotherapy with FL and 45 Gy/25 fractions, and then FL × 2 cycles. The 3-year OS (50 versus 41%; $p = .005$) and disease-free survival (DFS) rates (48 versus 31%; $p = .001$) in the treatment arm were significantly higher (51). A major criticism of this trial, however, was the inadequacy of the surgical procedure. Although the trial recommended D2 lymphadenectomy, fewer than 10% of patients underwent the procedure, and 54% underwent less than D1 lymphadenectomy (51). These suboptimal surgeries may have contributed to the low survival rate and high relapse rate in the surgery-alone arm. More telling is that the trial may have reflected accurately the pattern of surgical practice outside of academic centers; hence its results may be more applicable to the general

community. Regardless, the results of this large randomized, controlled trial changed practice and ultimately led to a new standard of care in the United States. In translating the results of the trial into current oncology practice, critics have pointed out that the chemotherapy regimen FL was older and likely inferior to what is available now. The same likely applies to radiotherapy techniques used in the study.

In an effort to update the results of INT116, the Cancer and Leukemia Group B (CALGB) is conducting a large phase III randomized controlled clinical trial comparing the INT116 FL regimen with epirubicin, cisplatin, and infusional 5-fluorouracil (ECF) before and after infusional 5-fluorouracil and radiotherapy. CALGB 80101 hopes to accrue 824 patients, but accrual is very slow. At the 2006 American Society of Clinical Oncology (ASCO) Gastrointestinal Cancer Symposium, Fuchs et al. presented the interim toxicity results for 113 patients. At that time, 180 patients had been enrolled. Grades 4 and 5 toxicities occurred in 35% of patients in Arm A (FL) and 25% in Arm B (ECF) (83). On the basis of the INT116 toxicity profile, the researchers suggested that postoperative ECF, before and after 5-FU, and concurrent RT was similar and possibly superior. Accrual for the trial is ongoing. Table 17-4

| TABLE 17-4 | POSTOPERATIVE THERAPY: ONGOING PHASE III RANDOMIZED CONTROL CLINICAL TRIALS IN LOCALLY ADVANCED RESECTABLE GASTRIC, GASTROESOPHAGEAL JUNCTION, AND LOWER ESOPHAGEAL CANCERS |||||

Trial	N	Treatment	Control	Status
Switzerland SWS-SAKK-43/99	240	DCF-S	S-DCF	Completed accrual
Japan JCOG 9206-2	280	S≥D2-P + UFT	S≥D2	Completed accrual
Asia/Sanofi CLASSIC	1024	S≥D2-CapeOx	S≥D2	Completed accrual
Korea/SMC ARTIST	490	S≥D2-XP	S≥D2-XP/RT	Completed accrual
United States CALGB-80101	824	S-ECF + FL/RT-ECF	S-FL-FL/RT-FL	Open not accruing
Netherlands CRITICS	788	S-CC/RT	ECC-S-ECC	Accruing
Japan TMOG-GC01	480	S≥D2-S1 + PSK	S≥D2-S1	Accruing
Hong Kong China CRE-2001.463-T	214	S (R0)-Rofecoxib	S (R0) alone	Completed accrual

ARTIST, Adjuvant RadioTherapy in gastric cancer and Systemic Therapy; CALGB, Cancer and Leukemia Group B; CapeOx, capecitabine + oxaliplatin; CC, capecitabine + cisplatin; CLASSIC, Capecitabine and Oxaliplatin Adjuvant Study in Stomach Cancer; CRITICS, ChemoRadiotherapy after Induction Chemotherapy in Cancer of the Stomach; DCF, docetaxel, cisplatin, 5-fluorouracil; ECC, epirubicin, cisplatin, capecitabine; ECF, epirubicin, cisplatin, 5-fluorouracil; FL, 5-fluorouracil, leucovorin; GC, gastric cancer; JCOG, Japanese Clinical Oncology Group; N, number of patients; PSK, protein-bound polysaccharide K (arrest cycle and induce apoptosis); R0, complete margins negative surgical resection; RT, radiotherapy; S, surgery; S≥D2, surgery with at least D2 lymphadenectomy; SMC, Samsung Medical Center; SWS-SAKK, Swiss Group for Clinical Research; TMOG, Tokyo Metropolitan Oncology Group; UFT, tegafur-uracil; XP, capecitabine, cisplatin.

summarizes several ongoing phase III postoperative trials in locally advanced resectable gastric, gastroesophageal junction, and lower esophageal cancers.

In the end, the role of systemic or intraperitoneal chemotherapy remains ill-defined. Marginally positive survival benefit in meta-analyses cannot overcome the lack of well-designed large studies to evaluate postoperative intraperitoneal chemotherapy for patients with gastric cancer, restricting intraperitoneal chemotherapy to academic centers and making it investigational therapy. Additionally, despite multiple meta-analyses demonstrating survival benefits with postoperative systemic chemotherapy, the improvement is restricted to gastric cancer patients in Asian countries and not commonly offered to patients in the non-Asian countries. On the basis of available evidence, after curative gastrectomy, chemoradiotherapy is the accepted option for standard of care in patients with resectable gastric cancer in the United States.

Preoperative and Perioperative Therapy

Since 2001, postoperative chemoradiotherapy has become frequently used to treat gastric cancer patients after curative resection. However, postoperative therapy is generally poorly tolerated; fewer than 50% of patients are able to complete treatment (51,52). Research focus had shifted to evaluating the benefit of preoperative therapy followed by curative resection. The theoretical advantages of preoperative therapy include improved tolerance, early therapy initiation, enhanced delivery of effective therapy, and down-staging the primary cancer,

with the possibility of improved cancer resectability. More than 25 clinical trials had been performed to assess the benefits of preoperative chemotherapy compared with surgery alone. Rougier et al. (84) treated 30 patients with localized gastric or GEJ adenocarcinoma with 6 cycles of continuous infusion 5-fluorouracil (5FU) and bolus cisplatin. The median survival duration was 16 months, while the R0 resection and pathological complete remission (pathCR) rates were 78% and 0%, respectively. For the most part, the results of phase II clinical trials have been consistent. After preoperative chemotherapy, the rate of R0 resection and median survival were around 75% and 16 months respectively, with the incidence of pathCR being very rare.

To date, four phase II or III randomized control trials have assessed the role of pre-and perioperative (therapy before and after surgery) chemotherapy versus surgery alone in resectable gastric cancer (Table 17-5). However, only two have been published. Kang et al. (85) evaluated 107 patients randomly assigned to receive perioperative or postoperative chemotherapy (etoposide, 5-fluorouracil, and cisplatin [EFP]). The R0 resection (79 versus 61%) and pathCR (8 versus 0%) rates were significantly higher for perioperative therapy than for postoperative therapy. Patients undergoing perioperative chemotherapy had longer median survival duration (43 versus 30 months). The only difference between the two arms was the additional preoperative chemotherapy; thus, the results suggest that preoperative chemotherapy leads to improved outcomes. In a smaller Dutch Gastric Cancer Group (DGCG) study, 56 patients were

TABLE 17-5	PRE-/PERIOPERATIVE THERAPY: RESULTS OF SELECTED COMPLETED PHASE II/III RANDOMIZED CONTROL CLINICAL TRIALS IN LOCALLY ADVANCED RESECTABLE GASTRIC AND LOWER ESOPHAGEAL CANCERS				

Trial	*N*	*Treatment*	*R0 (%)*	*pathCR (%)*	*Median Survival (Months)*
Korea phase III	53	EFP-S-EFP	79	8	43
Kang et al. (85)	54	S-EFP	61	0	30
Netherlands DGCG	27	FAMTX-S	75	N/R	18
Songun et al. (86)	29	S alone	75	N/R	30
MAGIC/MRC-ST02	250	ECF-S-ECF	74	N/R	30
Cunningham et al. (52)	253	S alone	68	N/R	18
France FNLCC/FFCD	113	CF-S	84	N/R	N/R
Boige et al. (87)	111	S alone	73	N/R	N/R

CF, cisplatin, 5-fluorouracil; CP, cisplatin, paclitaxel; DGCG, Dutch Gastric Cancer Group; ECF, epirubicin, cisplatin, and 5-fluorouracil; EFP, etoposide, 5-fluorouracil, cisplatin; FAMTX, 5-fluorouracil, doxorubicin, methotrexate; EORTC, European Organization for Research and Treatment of Cancer; FFCD, Fédération Francophone de la Cancérologie Digestive; FNLCC, Fédération Nationale des Centres de Lutte Contre le Cancer; HR, hazard ratio; MAGIC, Medical Research Council Adjuvant Gastric Infusional Chemotherapy; MRC-ST02, Medical Research Council Stomach 02; N, number of patients; N/A, not applicable; N/R, not reported or not reached; pathCR, pathological complete remission; PLF, cisplatin, leucovorin, 5-fluorouracil; R0, margins negative complete surgical resection; RT, radiotherapy; RTOG, Radiation Therapy Oncology Group; S, surgery.

randomly assigned to surgery alone or preoperative chemotherapy with 5-fluorouracil, doxorubicin, and methotrexate (FAMTX) and surgery. Curative resection rates were higher among patients who underwent preoperative chemotherapy (62 versus 56%). Among patients who underwent preoperative chemotherapy, the pathCR rate was 8% (86).

Perhaps the strongest evidence for preoperative therapy came from Europe; the United Kingdom MAGIC/MRC-ST02 (Medical Research Council Adjuvant Gastric Infusional Chemotherapy/Medical Research Council Stomach 02) and the French FNLCC ACCORD07-FFCD 9703 trials are also shown in Table 17-5. Five hundred and three patients with resectable GEJ/gastric cancer were randomly assigned to surgery alone or perioperative ECF and surgery in the MAGIC trial. After surgery, fewer than 50% of patients were able to complete the full course of chemotherapy. At 3-year follow-up, patients who received perioperative chemotherapy had a significantly higher progression-free survival (PFS) rate (HR 0.66; $p < .0001$) and were more likely to have undergone R0 resection (79 versus 69%). The 5-year OS rate was also significantly higher with treatment (36 versus 23%, $p = .0009$) (52). Although they have not been published, the results of the French FNLCC ACCORD07-FFCD 9703 trial provided additional evidence for preoperative chemotherapy. Two hundred twenty-four patients with resectable distal esophageal and proximal gastric adenocarcinoma were randomly assigned to surgery alone or preoperative chemotherapy and surgery. Patients who experienced a response to chemotherapy, had stable disease, or had lymph node involvement received two or three more cycles of

chemotherapy (5-fluorouracil and cisplatin [FP]) after surgery. At 5-year follow-up, 109 patients received preoperative FP and 54 received postoperative FP. Almost 50% of patients in the treatment arm underwent additional chemotherapy after surgery; whether or not this confounded the results remains unclear until the final results are published. R0 resection rates were 73% and 84% ($p = .04$), favoring treatment with preoperative FP. The HR of death was 0.69 (95% CI, 0.50-0.95; $p = .02$) with 3- and 5-year OS rates of 35 and 24% versus 48 and 38%, respectively (87).

On the basis of current evidence, perioperative chemotherapy improves OS when added to R0 gastrectomy. Hence, it is another acceptable standard-of-care option for patients with resectable gastric cancer. What remains unclear is which chemotherapy regimen should be used. Fewer than 40 to 50% of patients completed postoperative chemotherapy in the INT116 and MAGIC/MRC-ST02 trials; it remains unanswered whether additional chemotherapy provides additional benefit, especially in patients who have already undergone preoperative treatment. Evidence supporting preoperative chemoradiotherapy in gastric cancer is less prevalent than that for postoperative settings. The benefits of preoperative chemoradiotherapy should be similar to those of preoperative chemotherapy, but it has not been as well studied in gastric cancer as in esophageal cancer. Results from ongoing phase III studies may further improve the current evidence-based management for gastric cancer patients with resectable disease. Table 17-6 lists selected ongoing pre- or perioperative phase II or III clinical trials for patients with resectable gastric cancer. The United

TABLE 17-6	PRE-/PERIOPERATIVE THERAPY: ONGOING PHASE II/III RANDOMIZED CONTROL CLINICAL TRIALS IN LOCALLY ADVANCED RESECTABLE GASTRIC AND LOWER ESOPHAGEAL CANCERS				
Trial	*N*	*Treatment*	*Control*	*Status*
Japan/KYUHUHAGC0403	100	S1 + P-S-S1	S-S1	Completed accrual
Switzerland SWS-SAKK-43/99	240	DCF-S	S-DCF	Accruing
Netherlands CRITICS	788	S-CX/RT	ECX-S-ECX	Accruing
United Kingdom MRC ST03	1100	ECX + B × 3-S-ECX + B × 3-B × 6	ECX-S-ECX	Accruing
Japan JCOG0501	316	S1 + P-S≥D2	S≥D2	Accruing
United Kingdom QUINTETT	96	CF/RT-S	S-ECF/RT	Accruing
France TRACE	200	FOLFIRI-FL/RT-S	S-FOLFIRI-FL/RT	Not open yet

B, bevacizumab; CRITICS, ChemoRadiotherapy After Induction Chemotherapy in Cancer of the Stomach; CF, cisplatin and 5-fluorouracil; CX, cisplatin and capecitabine; DCF, docetaxel, cisplatin, 5-fluorouracil; ECF, epirubicin, cisplatin, 5-fluorouracil; ECX, epirubicin, cisplatin, capecitabine; FL, 5-fluorouracil, leucovorin; FOLFIRI, folinic acid (leucovorin), 5-fluorouracil, irinotecan; JCOG, Japanese Clinical Oncology Group; KYUHUHAGC, Kyoto University Hospital University Hospital Association Gastric Cancer; MRC-ST, Medical Research Council-Stomach; N, number of patients; P, cisplatin; QUINTETT, Quality of Life in Neoadjuvant Versus Adjuvant Therapy of Esophageal Cancer Treatment Trial; RT, radiotherapy; S, surgery; S≥D2, surgery with at least or more than D2 lymphadenectomy; SW-SAKK, Swiss Group for Clinical Research; TRACE, Adjuvant Treatment of Gastric Cancer With Chemotherapy and Chemoradiotherapy.

Kingdom MRC-ST03 study was designed to compare perioperative chemotherapy with or without bevacizumab, whereas the Dutch CRITICS (ChemoRadiotherapy After Induction Chemotherapy in Cancer of the Stomach) study was designed to compare the two current standard approaches to resectable gastric cancer, postoperative chemoradiotherapy and perioperative chemotherapy.

Until practice changing results from ongoing and future clinical trials, the current evidence-based therapeutic options to resectable gastric cancer remain: (1) surgery, particularly D2 extensive nodal dissection, performed at a large-volume center with expert trained surgeons; and (2) postoperative chemoradiotherapy or perioperative chemotherapy.

MD Anderson Approach to Resectable Gastric Cancer

All patients with newly diagnosed gastric cancer will have their staging workup completed. Patients with resectable gastric cancer are evaluated by a multidisciplinary team that consists of surgeons, radiation oncologists, and medical oncologists. Treatment recommendations are made in multidisciplinary conferences. Both standard-of-care treatment options and clinical trials are provided to patients. Patient's treatment plan is individualized to optimize outcomes for each patient. For decades, MD Anderson has been developing the practice of multimodality management in a multidisciplinary setting for all patients, but it is especially useful for those with resectable disease. Arguments for front-loading therapy before surgery include inaccuracy of clinical staging, poor tolerance and compliance to postoperative therapy, early initiation of therapy, early palliation of symptoms, opportunity for cancer downstaging, enhanced surgical resectability, and increasing rate of pathCR rates. Preoperative trimodality therapy, consisted of induction chemotherapy, followed by chemoradiotherapy then surgical resection, has been tested and evolved at MD Anderson over many years. Since the mid-1990s, it had been clinically recognized that preoperative trimodality therapy did not increase morbidity or mortality rates of subsequent surgery, and can improve pathologic response. Ajani et al. (88) reported the results of several phase II studies that demonstrated the feasibility and effectiveness of a three-step strategy. Thirty-seven patients with locally advanced resectable gastric cancer were treated with trimodality therapy on phase II clinical trial. Chemotherapy consisted of infusional 5-fluorouracil (F), cisplatin (P), and paclitaxel (T) (FPT). 45 Gy of radiotherapy was administered concurrently with FPT. R0 and pathCR rates were 95% and 30%, respectively. Fourteen

percent of patients had only microscopic residual disease. Patients who achieved pathCR or pathPR after preoperative therapy had significantly longer median survival durations than those who did not (63.9 versus 12.6 months, $p = .03$).

As a result of MD Anderson single-institution success with preoperative trimodality therapy, the Radiation Therapy Oncology Group (RTOG) sponsored a multi-institution cooperative study, RTOG 9904. The primary endpoint was pathCR rate. Forty-nine patients with localized resectable gastric cancer from 20 institutions received FLP as induction chemotherapy, followed by concurrent chemoradiotherapy with F and weekly paclitaxel. The pathCR and R0 resection rates were 26% and 77%, respectively. At 1 year, more patients who had achieved pathCR (82%) were alive than those who did not (69%) (89). A D2 dissection was performed in 50% of patients. The heterogeneity of different treating institutions minimized the selection bias typical of single institution results. Outcomes in RTOG 9904 were no better or worse than those of more recent studies, particularly the pathCR and D2 lymphadenectomy rates. Figure 17-15 summarizes the MD Anderson approach to gastric cancer.

■ ESOPHAGEAL AND GASTROESOPHAGEAL JUNCTION CANCERS

An estimated 16,470 new cases of esophageal cancer and 14,530 deaths are expected to occur in the United States in the year 2009 (2). According to the SEER 17 (2000-2006) database, only 23% of esophageal cancers are confined to the esophagus (localized); 30% and 32% have spread beyond the esophagus into the regional lymph nodes (regional) or other organs (distant), respectively (2). The incidence increases with age, as esophageal cancer is 22.3 times more common in individuals aged ≥65 years (90). Esophageal cancer is also 3.8 times more common in men than in women (1). The median age at diagnosis is 68 years of age (2). The 5-year survival rate is 16.8%, which has remained unchanged over time (2).

The incidence of GEJ adenocarcinoma has continued to increase over the past several decades. In recent years, this trend reached a new plateau, coinciding with the increased incidence of distal esophageal adenocarcinoma since the mid-1990s, a phenomenon confined to North America and other non-Asian countries. In the latest version of the AJCC TNM staging manual, esophageal cancer staging system now includes GEJ and proximal gastric less than 5 cm from the GEJ (31). Table 17-7 illustrates the latest TNM staging system for

TABLE 17-7 | **AMERICAN JOINT CANCER COMMITTEE TNM STAGING SYSTEM FOR GASTROESOPHAGEAL JUNCTION AND ESOPHAGEAL CANCERS (31)**

PRIMARY TUMOR (T)

TX	Primary tumor cannot be assessed
T0	No evidence of primary tumor
Tis	High-grade dysplasia
T1	Tumor invades lamina propria, muscularis mucosae, or submucosa
T1a	Tumor invades lamina propria or muscularis mucosae
T1b	Tumor invades submucosa
T2	Tumor invades muscularis propria
T3	Tumor invades adventitia
T4	Tumor invades adjacent structures
T4a	Resectable tumor invading pleura, pericardium, or diaphragm
T4b	Unresectable tumor invading other adjacent structures, such as aorta, vertebral body, trachea, etc.

REGIONAL LYMPH NODES (N)

Nx	Regional nodes cannot be assessed
N0	No regional nodal metastasis
N1	Metastasis in 1-2 regional lymph nodes
N2	Metastasis in 3-6 regional lymph nodes
N3	Metastasis in ≥7 regional lymph nodes

DISTANT METASTASES (M)

M0	No distant metastases
M1	Distant metastases

GRADE (G)

GX	Grade cannot be assessed—stage grouping as G1
G1	Well differentiated
G2	Moderately differentiated
G3	Poorly differentiated
G4	Undifferentiated—stage group as G3 squamous

LOCATION

Upper	15 to <20 cm
Middle	25 to <30 cm
Lower	30-45 cm

SQUAMOUS CELL CARCINOMA STAGE GROUPING

Stage	T	N	M	Grade	Tumor Location	5-Year Survival Rates (%)
0	Tis	N0	M0	1,X	Any	>80
IA	T1	N0	M0	1,X	Any	>80
IB	T1	N0	M0	2-3	Any	60
	T2-3	N0	M0	1,X	Lower, X	
IIA	T2-3	N0	M0	1,X	Upper, middle	53
	T2-3	N0	M0	2-3	Lower, X	
IIB	T1-2	N1	M0	Any	Any	40
	T2-3	N0	M0	2-3	Upper, middle	
IIIA	T1-2	N2	M0	Any	Any	25
	T3	N1	M0	Any	Any	
	T4a	N0	M0	Any	Any	
IIIB	T3	N2	M0	Any	Any	17
IIIC	T4a	N1-2	M0	Any	Any	13
	T4b	Any	M0	Any	Any	
	Any	N3	M0	Any	Any	
IV	Any	Any	M1	Any	Any	5

(Continued)

TABLE 17-7	AMERICAN JOINT CANCER COMMITTEE TNM STAGING SYSTEM FOR GASTROESOPHAGEAL JUNCTION AND ESOPHAGEAL CANCERS (31) (Continued)

ADENOCARCINOMA STAGE GROUPING

Stage	T	N	M	Grade	5-Year Survival Rates (%)
0	Tis	N0	M0	1, X	83
IA	T1	N0	M0	1-2, X	77
IB	T1	N0	M0	3	65
	T2	N0	M0	1-2, X	
IIA	T2	N0	M0	3	50
IIB	T1-2	N1	M0	Any	40
	T3	N0	M0	Any	
IIIA	T1-2	N2	M0	Any	25
	T3	N1	M0	Any	
	T4a	N0	M0	Any	
IIIB	T3	N2	M0	Any	17
IIIC	T4a	N1-2	M0	Any	15
	T4b	Any	M0	Any	
	Any	N3	M0	Any	
IV	Any	Any	M1	Any	<5

Used with the permission of the American Joint Committee on Cancer (AJCC), Chicago, Illinois. The original source for this material is the AJCC Cancer Staging Manual, Seventh Edition (2010) published by Springer Science and Business Media LLC, www.springer.com.

esophageal cancer. Overall, the prognosis of patients with esophageal/GEJ cancer remains poor. Histologic type makes a difference, as squamous cell carcinoma has a poorer prognosis than adenocarcinoma. Surgery is still the only chance for cure, and survival after surgery can be improved with multimodality therapy.

EPIDEMIOLOGIC CHARACTERISTICS

Esophageal cancer carries an ominous prognosis. It has a poor survival rate: only 17% (2) of patients in the United States and 10% (91) in Europe survive at 5 years. In the United States, esophageal cancer is estimated to be the seventh (1) most common cause of cancer death among men in the United States and the sixth (3) most common cause of cancer death worldwide. Like gastric cancer, the worldwide incidence of esophageal cancer also varies geographically. The median age at time of diagnosis for esophageal cancer is usually a decade earlier for squamous cell carcinoma than adenocarcinoma. Although squamous cell carcinoma is the most common histologic type in many parts of the world, it is relatively uncommon outside of Asian and middle-Eastern countries. Squamous cell carcinoma is 20 times more common in China than in the United States (3). The incidence of esophageal cancer has increased in recent decades, coinciding with a shift in histologic type and tumor location toward distal esophageal and GEJ adenocarcinoma (5). Squamous

cell carcinoma is more common in blacks than in whites, but adenocarcinoma is much more common in whites than in any other ethnic group (92).

ETIOLOGY AND RISK FACTORS

The most significant risk factors associated with esophageal squamous cell carcinoma are tobacco and alcohol use (93). Smoking and alcohol can synergistically increase the risk of esophageal squamous cell carcinoma. Dietary associations with esophageal squamous cell carcinoma have been uncovered in Asia. Foods containing N-nitroso compounds have long been implicated (94). These compounds are known to be animal carcinogens that may exert their mutagenic potential by inducing alkyl adducts in DNA (94). Betel nut chewing, widespread in certain regions of Asia has been implicated in the development of esophageal squamous cell carcinoma (95). In other endemic regions, such as Iran, Russia, and South Africa, the ingestion of hot foods and beverages (such as tea) has been associated with esophageal squamous cell carcinoma (96,97). In a population-based study including 1062 patients with achalasia, the risk of squamous cell carcinoma increased more than 16-fold during the first 1 to 24 years after diagnosis; cancer was detected a mean of 14 years after diagnosis of achalasia (98). On average, squamous cell carcinoma developed 41 years after ingestion of lye. Tylosis, a rare disease associated with hyperkeratosis of the palms of the hands and soles of the feet, is associated with a high rate of esophageal squamous cell carcinoma (99). The inherited type of tylosis (Howell-Evans syndrome) has been most strongly linked to esophageal squamous cell carcinoma. The disease has an autosomal dominant mode of inheritance; a gene locus has been mapped to chromosome 17q25.1, which probably contains a tumor suppressor gene (100). Evidence remains inconclusive relating to bisphosphonates use or a history of head-neck carcinoma.

Unlike squamous cell carcinoma, the risk factors for esophageal adenocarcinoma remain elusive. The strongest and most consistent risk factors include gastroesophageal reflux disorder (GERD), smoking, obesity, and dietary exposure to nitrosamines; these are found in almost 80% of cases in the United States. A high-fat, low-protein, high-calorie diet can also increase the risk. The increased prevalence of obesity in Western countries prompted a population-based study that demonstrated an association between increased body mass index and esophageal cancer risk (101). A meta-analysis of eight studies showed that the pooled adjusted OR for those with a body mass index (BMI) of 25 to 30 kg/m^2 was 1.52, while it was even higher for those with a BMI more than 30 kg/m^2, with OR 2.78 (102). More than 50% of esophageal adenocarcinoma patients have no history of symptomatic reflux disease (103). The role of GERD as an independent risk factor has not been well defined. Smoking plays a larger role in squamous cell carcinoma pathogenesis than adenocarcinoma pathogenesis. In a large population-based study, smoking was associated with only 40% of esophageal adenocarcinoma cases (104).

Much is known about the early pathologic characteristics of esophageal adenocarcinoma because of early-stage disease found during surveillance of Barrett esophagus (BE) patients. A well-recognized model for esophageal adenocarcinoma development is the sequence of events leading from BE to dysplasia and eventually carcinoma. In BE, the intestinal-type epithelium called the specialized intestinal metaplasia replaces the normal stratified squamous epithelium lining the distal esophagus. BE is generally believed to be a consequence of severe and chronic GERD. The presence of BE is associated with an increased risk of esophageal adenocarcinoma. Typically, long-segment BE (LSBE) is defined as a segment of metaplasia ≥3 cm in length, and short-segment BE (SSBE) is a segment <3 cm in length (105). The median age of BE diagnosis is 40 to 55 years, and it is most common in men (106).

The reported prevalence of BE in the United States varies widely, with higher rates found at autopsy than in population-based studies (0.9 versus 4.5); this finding suggests that most BE cases go unrecognized (107). The sensitivity of endoscopy at detecting BE is related to the length of involved mucosa, with detection being more likely in patients with a long segment (108). The overall reliability of endoscopy with biopsy at detecting specialized intestinal metaplasia in BE is approximately 80% (109). Five studies have been published that included more than 1000 patient-years of follow-up of BE. The risk of adenocarcinoma was 1/180 (110).

The transforming process leading to metaplasia in BE is still not fully understood. However, the causes depend on the location of BE. For example, SSBE may result from GEJ accumulation of noxious chemicals, such as gastric acid, and nitric oxide from dietary nitrates (111). Contrary to popular belief, BE develops over a short period of time (<1 year), not slowly over many years of extension of columnar cells replacing reflux-damaged squamous cells. BE likely develops >20 years before the mean age of clinical recognition or the development of esophageal adenocarcinoma (112). BE classification has implications for cancer risk. A population-based study reported that the prevalence of dysplasia or adenocarcinoma in patients with SSBE is lower than that in patients with LSBE (10 versus 31%) (107). However, because other studies also suggested that the risk of adenocarcinoma in SSBE is not significantly lower than that in LSBE (113), the current recommendation is to manage both types of BE similarly.

The tumorigenesis sequence of BE-dysplasia-adenocarcinoma had been proposed to be from a sequence of DNA mutations, giving abnormally replaced columnar cells a growth advantage. Genetic changes observed in BE include alterations in the tumor suppressor genes *p53* (also known as *TP53*) and *p16* (also known as *CDKN2A*) and in the cyclin D1 proto-oncogene (114). These DNA abnormalities endow cells with certain growth advantages, permitting them to hyperproliferate. During hyperproliferation, the cells acquire more genetic changes, resulting in neoplastic cells. When enough DNA abnormalities accumulate, a clone of malignant cells emerges that can invade adjacent tissues and proliferate abnormally. These additional genetic alterations develop involving LOH at chromosomes 5q, 13q, and 18q, with 18q and 17p losses occurring earlier than 5q loss (115,116). Chromosomal allelic loss rates on 3p, 5q, 9p, and 17p are not significantly different in high-grade dysplasia/T1 adenocarcinoma in LSBE or SSBE (117). The synergistic effect between altered cell-cycle regulators (caused by allelic loss) and inflammation-associated molecular effectors may play a role in progression to adenocarcinoma (118). Despite the recent increased research into BE, which has led to multiple hypotheses, the exact evolutionary genetic changes are not yet clearly understood.

Dysplasia is defined as morphologic changes resulting from DNA mutations. Depending on the severity of morphologic distortion, dysplasia is further classified as low grade (LGD) or high grade (HGD). Diagnosing and grading of dysplasia depends on the quality of endoscopic tissues obtained and the experience of the pathologist. The inter-observer agreements for LGD and HGD are 32% and 80%, respectively (119,120). Agreement rates among gastrointestinal pathologists for HGD and adenocarcinoma are 47% and 30%, respectively (121). Consequently, dysplasia is a poor surrogate marker of progression from BE to adenocarcinoma. Recent molecular profiles have been developed at MD Anderson to determine better predictive and prognostic surrogate markers of progression. Using unsupervised hierarchical clustering and class comparison analyses, researchers found that miRNA expression profiles in HGD BE tissues were significantly different from those in corresponding normal tissues. Similar findings were observed for adenocarcinoma, but not for LGD BE (122). One marker with growth-promoting and antiapoptotic functions is miRNA-196a (miR-196a) (123). All of these findings further fuel research. However, the proposed biomarkers must still be validated in large prospective studies.

CLINICAL PRESENTATION

The presenting symptoms of esophageal cancer usually include dysphagia, weight loss, bleeding, throat pain, and hoarseness. By all accounts, dysphagia is the most common complaint and becomes apparent when the esophageal lumen is narrowed to one-third of its normal diameter. For proximal esophageal tumors, increasing cough may be a sign of tracheal-esophageal fistula.

PATHOLOGY

Esophageal cancer includes adenocarcinomas, squamous cell carcinoma, mucoepidermoid, small cell carcinoma, sarcoma, adenoid, cystic, or primary lymphoma. Adenocarcinoma is now more prevalent than squamous cell carcinoma in non-Asian countries and mostly develops in the distal esophagus (124). In general, squamous cell carcinoma is found in the upper half of the esophagus, whereas adenocarcinoma predominates closer to the GEJ. Figures 17-16 through 17-21 show the gross morphologic and microscopic characteristics of BE and esophageal carcinoma.

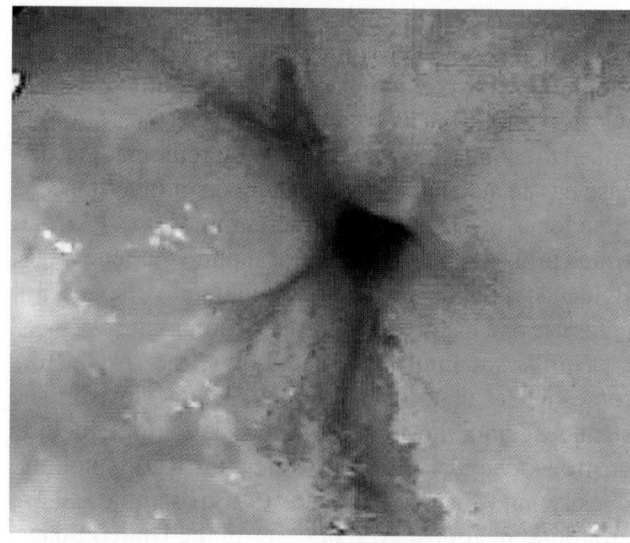

FIGURE 17-16. Barrett esophagus, endoscopic view. (*Courtesy of Klaus Monkemuller, MD, University of Alabama at Birmingham, Birmingham, AL.*)

STAGING AND PROGNOSIS

Esophageal cancer is a treatable disease but is rarely curable. Specifically, a major surgery literature review in 1980 reported a mortality rate of 29% (125). However, the overall surgical mortality rate has decreased by approximately 20 to 40% over the past 20 years (126,127). This improvement may be attributed to improved surgical, medical, and radiologic procedures. Since the mid-1990s, the histologic type and location of carcinoma of the upper gastrointestinal tract has changed. The incidences of proximal gastric, GEJ, and distal esophageal adenocarcinomas have steadily increased until the past

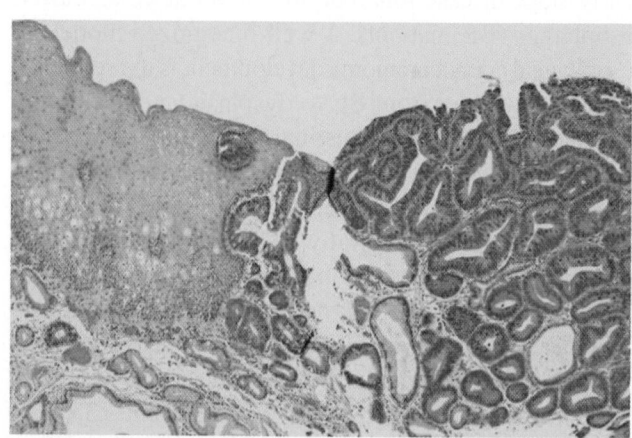

FIGURE 17-17. Barrett esophagus, microscopic view. (*Courtesy of Dr. Asif Rashid, University of Texas, MD Anderson, Department of Pathology, Houston, TX.*)

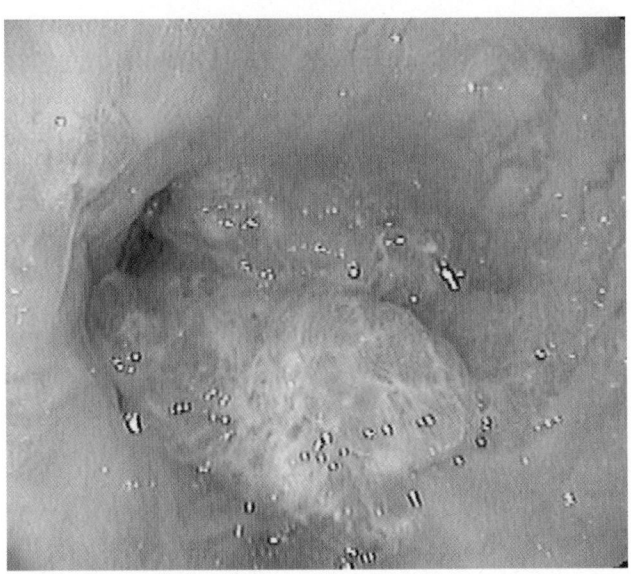

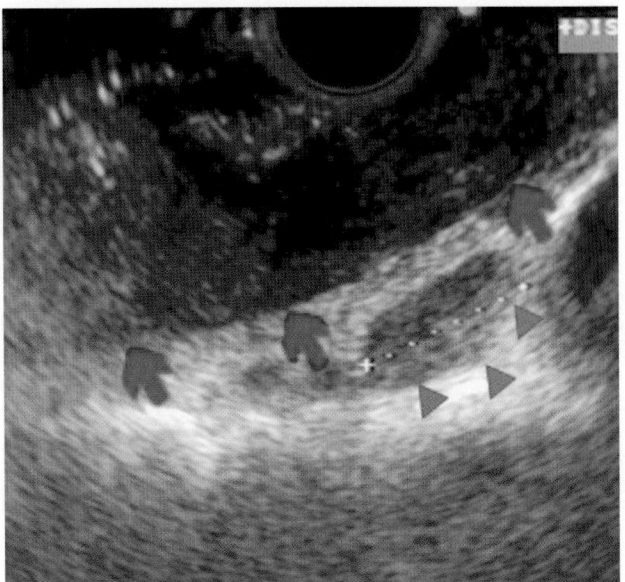

FIGURE 17-18. Barrett esophagus with adenocarcinoma endoscopy. (*Courtesy of Dr. Norio Fukami, University of Texas, MD Anderson, Department of GI Medicine and Nutrition, Houston, TX.*)

several years, where it now appears to have reached a steady state. Table 17-7 summarizes version 7 of the AJCC TNM staging system for esophageal cancer. This most current version now includes primary tumors of the GEJ or proximal gastric cancer 5 cm into the gastrium as part of esophageal cancer staging (31). It also requires clinical and pathologic information. Other noticeable changes include redefinition of Tis and subclassification of T4. Regional node involvement now depends on the number of lymph nodes. Recognizing the differences in clinical manifestation and the biologic process of esophageal squamous cell carcinoma and adenocarcinoma, each

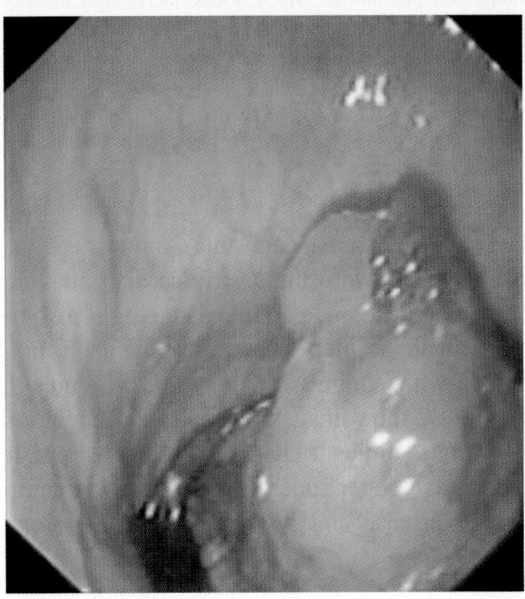

FIGURE 17-20. Esophageal squamous cell carcinoma. (*Courtesy of Adrian Saftiou, MD, University of Medicine and Pharmacy Craiova, Romania.*)

histologic type now has a separate staging system. For the squamous cell carcinoma staging system, T1-3N0 are further refined into different stages by the grade of tumor differentiation and location of the primary tumor. For the adenocarcinoma staging system, grade is only required to further differentiate T1-2N0.

Clinical staging uses EGD with EUS, CT, and FDG-PET. Special circumstances may require additional staging modalities. In patients with proximal esophageal cancer, bronchoscopy is recommended to evaluate potential tracheal invasion or document and

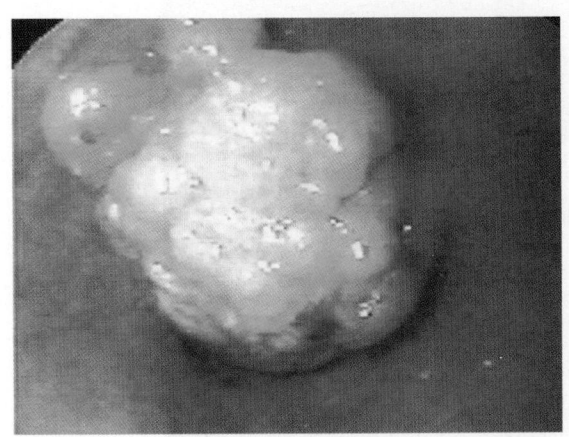

FIGURE 17-19. Esophageal mass, endoscopic view. (*Courtesy of Klaus Monkemuller, MD, University of Alabama at Birmingham, Birmingham, AL.*)

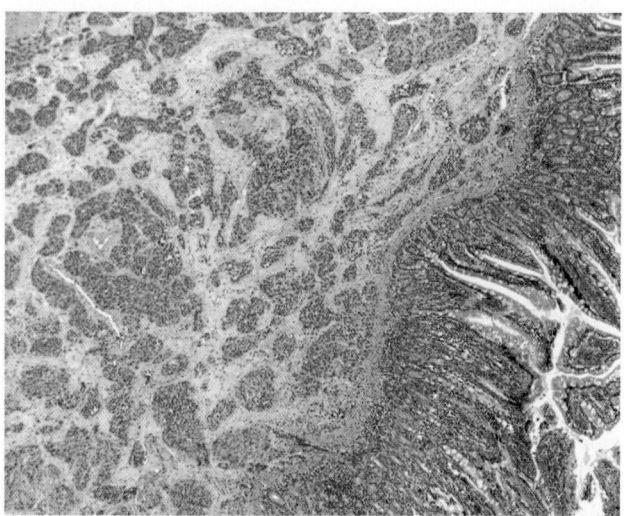

FIGURE 17-21. Submucosal jejunal metastasis of the esophageal squamous cell carcinoma (SCC). Photomicrograph of specimen showing the metastasis, associated with local submucosal venous and lymphatic infiltration. Neither the jejunal serosa nor the mucosa is affected by the carcinoma (hematoxylin and eosin × 50). (*Courtesy of Lindenmann J, Gollowitsch F, Matzi V, et al. World Journal of Surgical Oncology 200, 3:44; doi:10.1186/1477-7819-3-44.*)

palliate tracheal-esophageal fistula. Among patients with disease extending into the gastric cardia, most experts agree that laparoscopic peritoneal staging is also necessary to evaluate occult peritoneal seeding that is not well visualized with noninvasive modalities. Figures 17-22 through 17-32 show images of esophageal carcinoma.

In various studies, FDG-PET has been consistently shown to have better specificity than CT at diagnosing metastatic disease and lymph node status. However, because of variable results regarding the sensitivity of FDG-PET in diagnosing lymph node metastasis (128), it is precluded from use as a first-line method of investigation. FDG-PET can better reveal bone metastasis than can bone scans (129) and commonly reflects images of multiple foci of intense uptake. Studies have shown significant correlations between FDG uptake and tumor invasion depth and lymph node metastasis and survival rates, with a high degree of accuracy in the neck and upper thoracic and abdominal regions (130). FDG-PET had low accuracy at diagnosing locoregional metastasis than did CT and EUS combined, which was mostly due to a significant lack of sensitivity (131). The accuracy of detecting distal nodal metastases was significantly higher for FDG-PET than that for CT and EUS combined (131). It is unclear whether FDG-PET is superior at detecting esophageal cancer as a first-line diagnostic procedure, but it is superior at detecting distant metastasis. Other uses of FDG-PET scanning include early diagnosis of recurrent disease and differentiation of surgical scars from recurrence (132). It is also gaining importance for staging and follow-up. Unlike with gastric cancer, FDG-PET results have been found to be important predictors of response and prognosis. In a retrospective analysis, Swisher et al. reported the results FDG-PET use in 103 consecutive patients with locally advanced esophageal cancer who underwent preoperative chemoradiotherapy. At surgery, 58 patients (56%) had experienced a pathologic response to chemoradiotherapy (surgical pathologic results ≤10% viable residual cancer cells). Pathologic response was associated with FDG-PET standardized uptake value (SUV) (3.1 versus 5.8, $p = .01$). A post-chemoradiotherapy

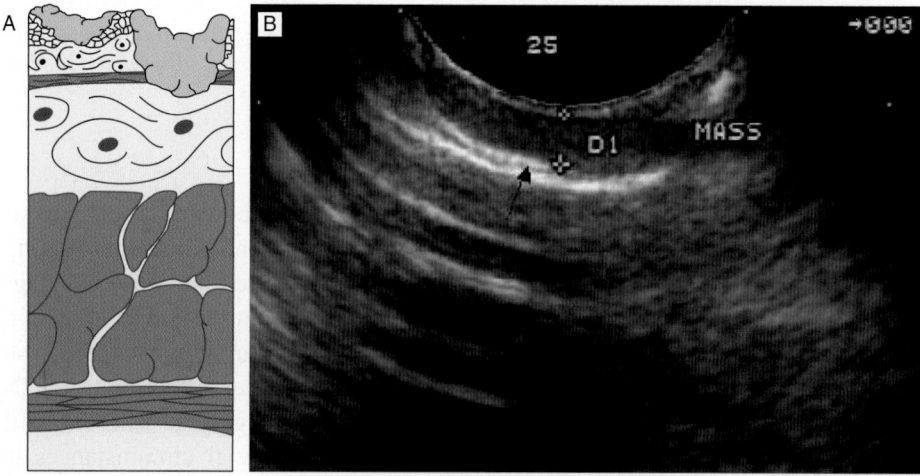

FIGURE 17-22. EUS image of T1 esophageal cancer. (*Reproduced, with permission, from http://www.massgeneral.org/gastro/endo_homepage.htm.*)

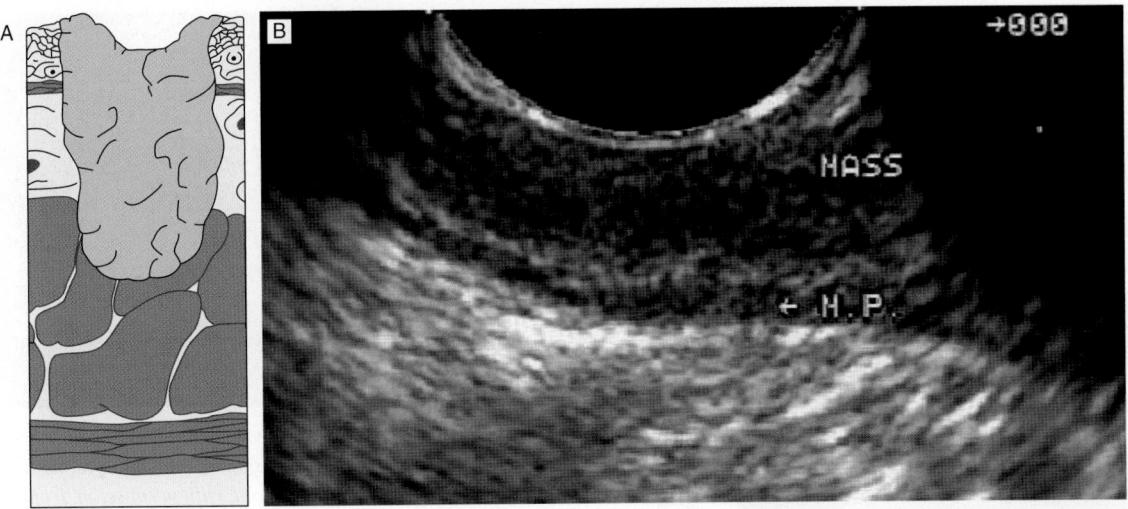

FIGURE 17-23. EUS image of T2 esophageal cancer. (*Reproduced, with permission, from http://www.massgeneral.org/gastro/endo_homepage.htm.*)

FDG-PET SUV ≥4 had the highest accuracy and was an independent predictor of survival (HR 3.5; p = .04) on multivariate analysis (133). The results of a subsequent report from the same research group suggested that FDG-PET is useful for baseline staging. FDG-PET was performed before therapy in 47 patients with locally advanced esophageal cancer. The number of FDG-PET abnormalities, SUV of the primary tumor, peak SUV, and total SUV were collected from baseline FDG-PET scans and compared with outcomes (OS and DFS) on univariate and multivariate analyses. The number of

abnormalities was significantly associated with OS (p = .04) and DFS (p = .04) and on multivariate analysis remained a strong independent prognostic factor for OS (p = .03). Patients with more than one peak abnormality had an HR of death of 4.49 (134).

Many other studies have confirmed the importance of FDG-PET scans in esophageal cancer. Studies have also proposed different uses for FDG-PET, particularly as a surrogate marker of treatment response. Investigators at Massachusetts General Hospital reported their findings of FDG-PET usage in squamous cell carcinoma

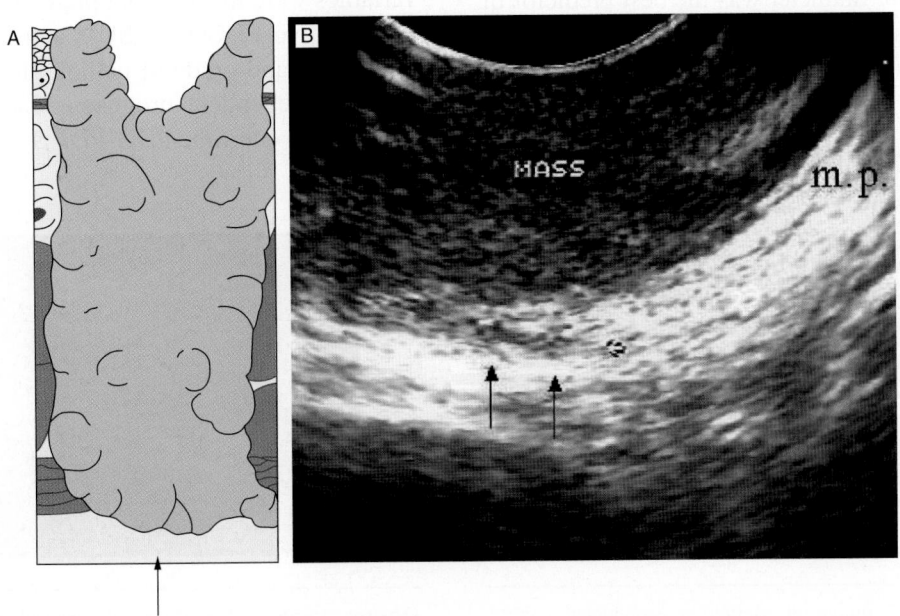

FIGURE 17-24. EUS image of T3 esophageal cancer. (*Reproduced, with permission, from http://www.massgeneral.org/gastro/endo_homepage.htm.*)

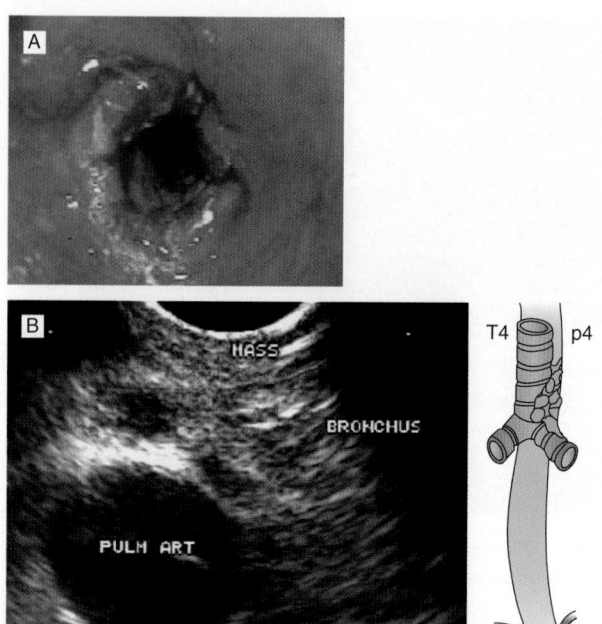

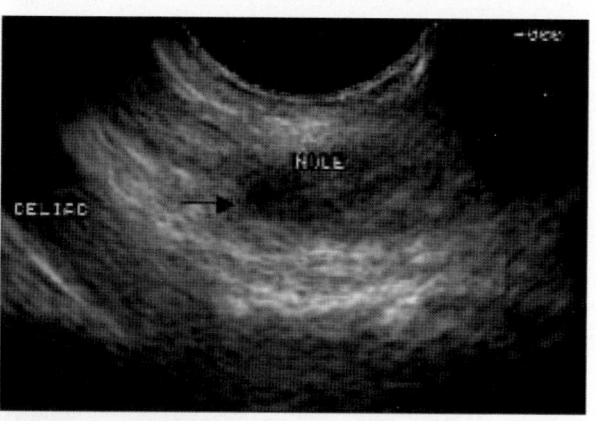

FIGURE 17-27. EUS image of celiac lymphadenopathy in esophageal cancer. (*Reproduced, with permission, from http://www. massgeneral.org/gastro/endo_homepage.htm.*)

FIGURE 17-25. **A.** Endoscopic image of T4 esophageal cancer. **B.** EUS image of the same tumor. (*Reproduced, with permission, from http://www.massgeneral.org/gastro/endo_homepage.htm.*)

and survival. A DSI decrease of ≥55% was predictive of pathologic response with a sensitivity of 91% and specificity of 93%. On common confounder in determining FDG-PET SUV activity after chemoradiotherapy is radiation-induced esophagitis, which is a frequent finding. In this study, the calculated DSI appeared to remove this confounder, allowing for the use of FDG-PET ability to predict response and survival (135). Shenfine et al. evaluated preoperative FDG-PET SUV activity in 45 patients with distal esophageal adenocarcinoma who underwent primary esophagectomy without preoperative therapy. Pathologic data were retrieved and patients were followed up for a median of 44 months. On multivariate analysis, only postoperative pathologic variables were independent predictors of DFS and OS. Preoperative FDG-PET SUV activity was associated with stage and grade of pathologic variables but was not an independent prognostic indicator of survival outcome. A one-time FDG-PET SUV value may not be

patients after chemoradiotherapy. Pre- and post-chemoradiotherapy FDG-PET scans of 49 consecutive patients with locally advanced esophageal squamous cell carcinoma were analyzed. A "diameter-SUV index" (DSI) was generated for each patient by multiplying the tumor diameter by the mean SUV. A decrease in metabolic tumor diameter was the best predictor of treatment response and tumor-free survival, but the calculated DSI was most accurate at predicting response

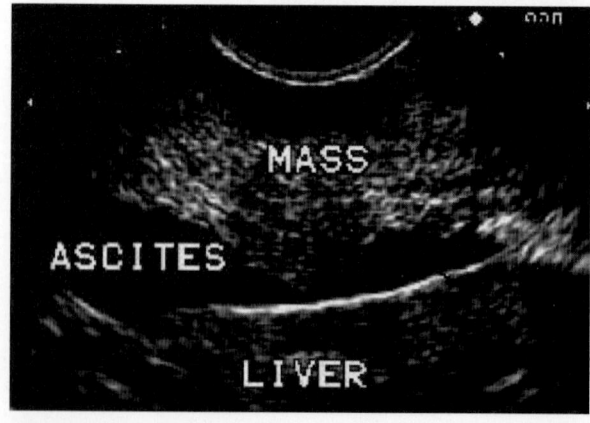

FIGURE 17-26. EUS image of ascites in esophageal cancer. (*Reproduced, with permission, from http://www.massgeneral.org/ gastro/endo_homepage.htm.*)

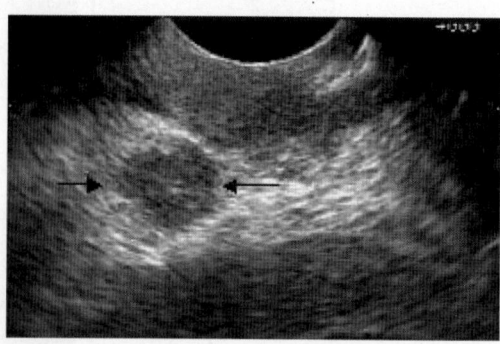

FIGURE 17-28. EUS image of gastrohepatic ligament lymphadenopathy in esophageal cancer. (*Reproduced, with permission, from http://www.massgeneral.org/gastro/endo_homepage.htm.*)

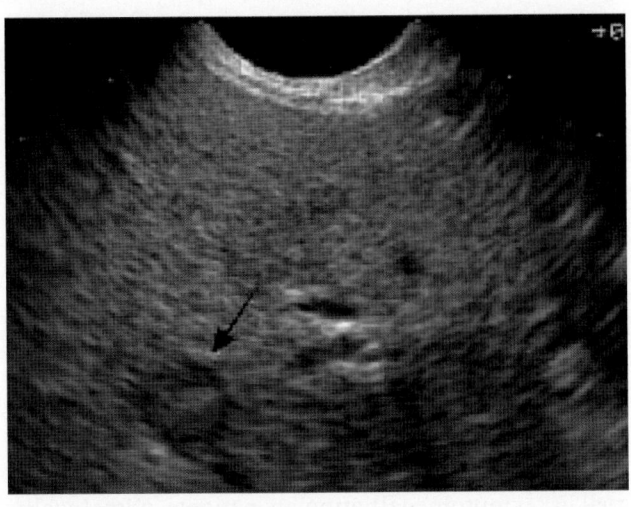

FIGURE 17-29. EUS image of hepatic metastases in esophageal cancer. (*Reproduced, with permission, from http://www.massgeneral.org/gastro/endo_homepage.htm.*)

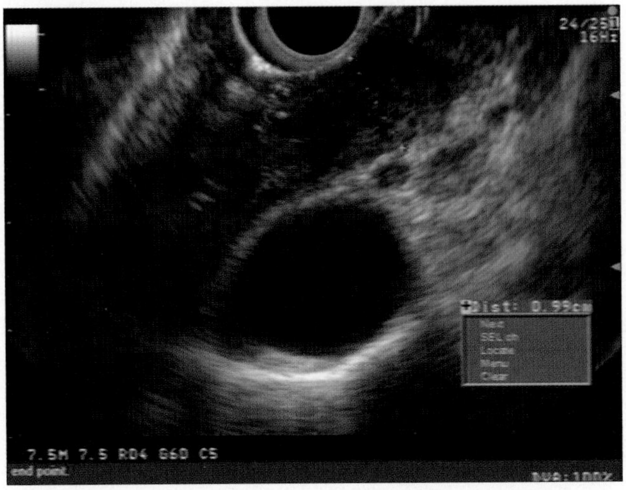

FIGURE 17-31. Endosonography of esophageal cancer shows the tumor to be circumferential and to extend through the esophageal wall. (*Reproduced, with permission, from Jeffrey H. Lee, MD.*)

prognostic or a predictor of response, but it may be used as part of staging to identify high-risk patients who may benefit from preoperative therapy (136).

Perhaps the strongest endorsement for using FDG-PET as predictor of response came from the MUNICON1 (Metabolic response evalUatioN for Individualisation of neoadjuvant Chemotherapy in oesOphageal and oesophagogastric adeNocarcinoma) trial. Lordick et al. evaluated the feasibility and applicability of FDG-PET in clinical practice in 110 evaluable patients with locally advanced esophageal adenocarcinoma, AEG types 1

and 2, who underwent 2 weeks of induction chemotherapy with 5-fluorouracil, leucovorin, and cisplatin (FLP). FDG-PET scans were obtained for all patients at baseline and after induction chemotherapy. Metabolic response was defined as an SUV decrease ≥35%. Responders underwent more chemotherapy with FLP or folinic acid, 5-fluorouracil, and oxaliplatin (FOLFOX) × 12 weeks followed by surgery. Nonresponders discontinued further chemotherapy after the 2 weeks of initial induction chemotherapy and underwent surgery. In this study, there were 54 responders (metabolic response rate, 49%).

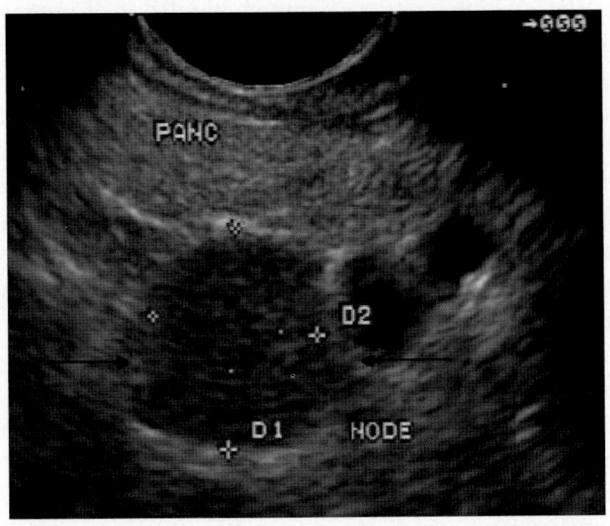

FIGURE 17-30. EUS image of peripancreatic lymphadenopathy in esophageal cancer. (*Reproduced, with permission, from http://www. massgeneral.org/gastro/endo_homepage.htm.*)

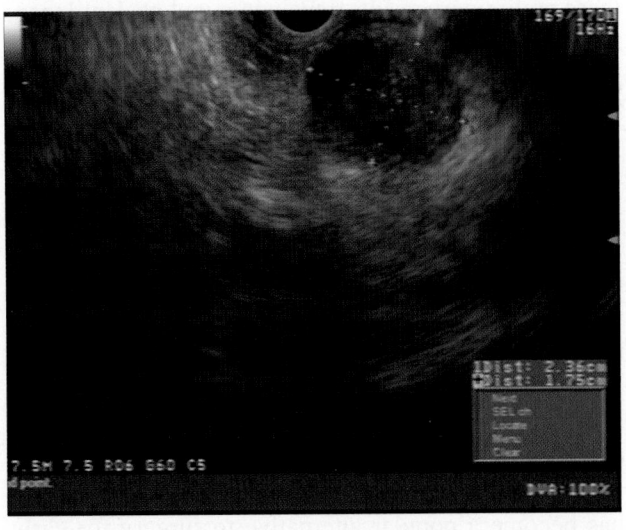

FIGURE 17-32. Endosonography shows the tumor and esophageal wall to be less thickened, likely reflecting response to chemoradiotherapy. (*Reproduced, with permission, from Jeffrey H. Lee, MD.*)

One hundred four patients (54 responders and 50 nonresponders) patients underwent surgery. At 2.3 years of follow-up, the median OS for responders was not reached and was 25.8 months (HR, 2.13; $p = .015$) for nonresponders. The median event-free survival durations for responders and nonresponders were 29.7 months and 14.1 months, respectively (HR, 2.18; $p = .002$). Major pathologic remissions (<10% residual tumor) were noted in 58% of responders and 0% of nonresponders (40). Preoperative induction therapy for locally advanced adenocarcinoma of distal esophageal cancer and GEJ has become an acceptable practice in most Western countries. In the MUNICON1 study, the response to induction therapy was valuable for stratifying patients to appropriate therapy, further establishing the clinical utility of FDG-PET in limiting exposure to unnecessary toxicity and maximizing therapeutic benefits.

The role of tumor markers and cytogenetics in esophageal cancer staging and prognosis is another subject of active investigation. Esophageal cancer has certain molecular markers that may be predictive. N-cadherin may be associated with increased tumor invasion and invasion depth (137), and activin A may mediate N-cadherin expression. NF-κB is induced by low pH and bile acid exposure to esophageal cell lines and is associated with progressive Barrett tumorigenesis (138). Other molecular factors that affect prognosis of esophageal cancer include MUC1, whose increased expression is associated with a high rate of metastasis (139), and Bcl-2, the expression of which is associated with significantly improved survival and the reduced expression of which is associated with progression of BE to adenocarcinoma (140). Large population-based studies to validate these preliminary results remain incomplete. Until then, the clinical interpretation of currently available data should be done with caution.

TREATMENT

As a result of the epidemiologic shift, distal esophageal and GEJ adenocarcinomas are the most common diagnoses in patients in non-Asian countries. Worldwide, squamous cell carcinoma is the most common histologic type. Similar to early gastric cancer, the gold standard for treating high-grade dysplasia and early or superficial esophageal cancer is esophagectomy. However, endomucosal resection/endosubmucosal resection (EMR/EMSD), with or without photodynamic therapy (PDT), has become a popular alternative to surgery for early esophageal disease. Despite the recognized epidemiologic and clinical differences between esophageal squamous cell carcinoma and adenocarcinomas, there is still

inadequate evidence that treatment for esophageal cancer should be based on histologic type. Locally advanced cervical esophageal cancer is preferably managed with definitive chemoradiotherapy. For all other esophageal carcinomas, current evidence supports the use of preoperative chemoradiotherapy and pre- or perioperative chemotherapy to enhance surgical survival outcome in patients with locally advanced resectable disease. Surgery remains the best chance for long-term survival. Ongoing international clinical research with novel cytotoxic and targeted agents will continue to further define and improve survival outcomes of patients with locally advanced curable esophageal and GEJ cancers. Unfortunately, the main therapeutic goal is symptom palliation in patients with locally advanced, unresectable disease. The treatment of locally advanced, unresectable, and distant and metastatic esophageal and gastroesophageal cancers is discussed in two separate subsections: Locally Advanced Unresectable Metastatic Gastric, Gastroesophageal Junction, and Esophageal Carcinomas; and Advanced and Metastatic Gastric, Gastroesophageal Junction, and Esophageal Carcinomas. A summary of standard treatment options based esophageal cancer stage is presented in Figure 17-15 illustrates MD Anderson approach to esophageal cancer management.

Barrett Esophagus and Esophageal Dysplasia

Barrett esophagus (BE) is a condition in which intestinal-type epithelium called specialized intestinal metaplasia replaces the normal stratified squamous epithelium lining the distal esophagus. BE results from chronic GERD, which is often asymptomatic. BE is of interest to clinicians because it is a predisposing condition for dysplasia, which is a premalignant condition for invasive adenocarcinoma. Dysplasia is further classified as LGD or HGD on the basis of the level of morphologic distortion. However, accurate grading depends on the quality of the endoscopic tissues submitted and the expertise of the pathologist. Inter-observer variability is significant. All of these barriers decrease the accuracy and value of using dysplasia grade to predict the likelihood of malignant transformation. The risks of invasive carcinoma for BE without dysplasia range from 0.5% (141) for LGD to 6% (142) for HGD. The actual risk of malignant transformation from BE to dysplasia or adenocarcinoma remains unknown because published results conflict for both short segment BE (SSBE) and long segment BE (LSBE). As a result, most experts and professional societies recommend the same management approach for SSBE and LSBE.

The first goal in BE management is treating GERD. Most authorities on GERD recommend using proton pump inhibitors (PPI) to manage symptoms. Researchers at the Palo Alto Veteran Affairs Health Care System reported on cell proliferation and differentiation in BE patients after modulating intraesophageal pH, using villin and proliferating cell nuclear antigen (PCNA) as markers, respectively. Villin and PNCA, as well as dysplasia, were assessed at baseline and then after 6 months of treatment with lansoprazole to pH normalization. Twenty-four patients achieved a normal pH and 15 did not. Despite evidence suggesting that DNA abnormalities occurred, it is not clear that treating GERD decreases the incidence of BE. While in some groups of BE patients, the incidence of dysplasia may be reduced with PPI therapy, in other groups, esophageal dysplasia may develop from other predisposed conditions and pH modulation is ineffective. GERD should be treated for symptom management.

The second goal is surveillance and monitoring of BE to detect early and curable stage adenocarcinoma. The cost-effectiveness of this approach was questioned initially. Wright et al. reviewed their experience involving 166 BE patients who underwent annual endoscopic surveillance. The screened group had a significantly earlier stage than did the unscreened control group ($p < .05$) (143). Cost per life-year saved was $4151 for adenocarcinoma versus $57,926 for breast cancer (144). Hence, not only does endoscopic surveillance has a high detection rate, in 1994, its cost-effectiveness is similar to that of mammography in women.

The current practice of endoscopic surveillance was based on data from the University of Washington (145). In their 2008 position statement on surveillance, the American Gastroenterological Association (AGA) recommended that surveillance endoscopy be performed with four random biopsies, where specimens are obtained at least every 1 to 2 cm of esophageal mucosa and additional biopsy specimens are taken of any mucosal abnormalities (146). Surveillance should be performed in patients whose reflux symptoms are not controlled with PPIs. Patients without dysplasia or mucosal abnormalities at initial evaluation should be evaluated again in 1 year to decrease the chances of sampling error. If no dysplasia is found again, surveillance can reasonably be deferred for another 5 years until the patient reaches a point at which cancer therapy is not possible or life expectancy is limited. Patients with low LGD should undergo a follow-up endoscopy within 6 months. If no abnormalities are found, yearly endoscopy is warranted until no dysplasia is present on two consecutive annual endoscopies. The finding of

HGD in flat mucosa should be confirmed by an expert gastrointestinal pathologist and a subsequent endoscopy should be performed within 3 months. Patients with HGD and mucosal irregularity should undergo EMR. Patients with confirmed HGD, even if unifocal, should be counseled regarding therapeutic options. Patients who appear to have lost their dysplasia on surveillance should be treated according to the highest degree of dysplasia previously found. The presence of multifocal HGD is associated with an increased risk of cancer, and these patients may be candidates for more aggressive treatment. However, surveillance can be offered if both the patient and physician are willing to follow a careful regimen of endoscopy every 3 months with at least eight random biopsy specimens taken every 2 cm. All mucosal abnormalities should be investigated or further staged with EUS and EMR to be certain that there is no underlying invasive carcinoma. If ablative therapy has been performed previously, surveillance is still needed in the same area of involvement at least as frequently as if ablation had not been performed.

Recently, several studies questioned the current practice of surveillance, particularly in patients who have HGD. In one study, the standard recommended biopsy protocol of four quadrant jumbo biopsies (every 1 cm) with biopsies of mucosal abnormalities (the Seattle protocol) was compared with four quadrant biopsies (every 2 cm) in 33 patients with BE. The rate of discovery of unsuspected intramucosal cancer was not significantly different between the two protocols (40 versus 30%, $p = .6$). Preoperative mucosal nodularity (50 versus 75%) and multifocal HGD (88 versus 50%) were identified less with the Seattle protocol than the new proposed surveillance method (147). Results of study need confirmation, but if confirmed, it may suggest that endoscopic surveillance can be done less stringently without losing sensitivity and accuracy. However, at present, it remains unclear whether continued surveillance is as effective as definitive therapy and whether a more intense biopsy protocol will improve the OS outcome for patients with HGD in BE. The first question will likely only be answered with a large randomized study with long-term follow-up. Perhaps the second question can be more easily addressed with more reliable and accurate endoscopic technology.

The current practice of systematically obtaining random biopsies has been criticized as time-consuming, labor-intensive, costly, and limited by sampling errors. Metaplasia and dysplasia occur at focused points; thus, quadrant samplings are likely inadequate. Over the past several years, many improvements have enhanced and expanded endoscopic abilities. Charged-couple device

(CCD) and high-definition (HD) video endoscopes are high-resolution endoscopes that allow 1080 scanning lines on a screen and can be projected onto a large screen with high image quality. Narrow-band imaging (NBI) endoscopy uses spectral narrow-band optical fibers instead of full-spectrum white light. Specifically, NBI uses the wavelength in the ranges of the hemoglobin absorption spectrum. This allows visualization of vascular patterns on surface mucosa. A recent randomized controlled crossover trial compared NBI target biopsies with HD endoscopy in 123 patients with BE. Targeted biopsies using NBI and four quadrant biopsies every 2 cm diagnosed similar numbers of patients with intestinal metaplasia (85% each) and dysplasia (71 versus 55%, $p = .15$) lesions. However, significantly fewer samples were required with NBI (3.6 versus 7.6 per procedure; $p < .0001$) (148). Finally, confocal laser endomicroscopy involves stimulating tissue with laser light, which is reflected back through a pinhole, enabling computer-aided generation of a cross-sectional microscopic image and thus allowing real-time subsurface microscopic mucosal and in vivo histologic analyses. Magnification of >1000 times can be used, and various cellular and subcellular elements, including crypt architecture, mucosal cells and goblet cells in intestinal crypts, capillaries, and red blood cells, can be visualized (149).

In addition to treating GERD with PPIs and following BE with endoscopic surveillance, the last and third goal in BE is treatment. Treatment options include esophagectomy, EMR, photodynamic therapy (PDT), and intensive endoscopic surveillance in which invasive therapies are withheld until biopsy specimens reveal adenocarcinoma. The benefits of these options are variably supported by evidence and most are associated with substantial risks, particularly esophagectomy. The follow-up duration in most studies on treatments for dysplasia in BE is considerably less than 5 years; there are no long-term results. Consequently, the efficacy of these therapies for BE in reducing cancer deaths is not established. Treatment is recommended when there is dysplasia or mucosal abnormalities. BE without dysplasia and LGD should be monitored. BE with HGD requires definitive therapy. Esophagectomy (in which the neoplastic epithelium is removed) is the only therapeutic option for HGD, although the mortality and morbidity rates are relatively high. In centers that perform high-volume esophagectomies, perioperative mortality can be as low as 2% compared with 13% in low-volume centers (150). Early reports of minimal invasive esophagectomy suggested that perioperative morbidity and mortality were similar to

traditional esophagectomy; however, there were reduced blood loss, postoperative pain, and intensive care unit (ICU) stay (151).

EMR has gained popularity in Asia for the treatment of superficial or early esophageal cancer (EEC) as well as BE with HGD. By providing large tissue specimens that can be examined to determine the characteristics and extent of the lesion and the adequacy of resection, EMR is both therapeutic and diagnostic. EMR has been reported in several small prospective case series to be effective, with an initial complete remission (CR) rate of 59 to 99% (152,153). Five-year follow-up data on 486 (288 with EEC and 61 with HGD) BE patients treated with EMR or PDT revealed a CR in 337 patients (97%); surgery was necessary in 13 (4%) because of endoscopic failure. Metachronous lesions developed in 74 patients (22%), and the 5-year survival rate was 84%. High-risk features for recurrence included piecemeal resection, LSBE, no ablative therapy after CR, time to CR of >10 months, and multifocal neoplasia (154). The ideal clinical characteristics for EMR are small (<2 cm diameter), solitary, flat lesions that are confined to the mucosa (T1a). Because EMR has a relatively high recurrence rate, it is recommended that BE and HGD or EEC patients be followed up endoscopically every 3 months during the first year and annually thereafter. Complications associated with EMR are bleeding (4-46%), perforation (1%), and stricture (20%) (155).

PDT involves prior intravenous administration of porfimer sodium, a photosensitizer drug that concentrates in dysplastic and malignant tissue. When laser light is applied to this tissue in the presence of oxygen, the drug is activated, resulting in a photochemical reaction that leads to selective tissue destruction. The two major side effects of PDT are photosensitivity and chest discomfort secondary to local swelling and inflammation of the esophagus. PDT can be used to treat multifocal early-stage esophageal cancer. The results of one small, prospective, randomized, blinded European trial of PDT demonstrated that squamous re-epithelialization requires preceding columnar mucosal injury, providing the first evidence to support PDT in BE. In this study, 36 patients with BE on omeprazole were randomly assigned to receive 5-aminolevulinic acid (ALA)-PDT versus a placebo. The percentage decreases in the area of the treated region between PDT and the placebo were 30 versus 0% ($p < .001$). No dysplasia was seen in the columnar epithelium in the treatment area of any patient in the PDT group (156). Five years later, a large randomized controlled trial involving 208 patients with BE demonstrated that PDT was superior to omeprazole alone for eradicating HGD (77 versus 39%, $p < .0001$)

and preventing invasive carcinoma (13 versus 28%, $p < .006$). However, treatment-related side effects were higher in the PDT arm (94 versus 13%), with 36% of patients developing esophageal stenosis (157).

Resectable Disease

Surgery

Only 23% of patients with esophageal cancer present with clinically resectable localized disease (2). The only chance of cure for these patients is usually primary surgical resection. However, surgical resection does not often result in durable disease remission. Recent data indicate that the overall 5-year survival rate of esophageal cancer patients after curative surgery is about 25% (51,52). Means of improving surgical outcome have been intensely studied over the past decades.

One criterion for determining whether the disease is resectable is patients' performance status. In the United States, the median age of esophageal cancer patients is 67 years (158). However, physiologic rather than chronologic age should be used to determine disease resectability. A retrospective review of 505 consecutive patients who were operated on by a single surgical team over 17 years found no difference in the perioperative mortality rate and median survival duration between patients who were older and younger than 70 years (159). Patient age should not be the lone determinant of surgical approach. Furthermore, in patients with GEJ adenocarcinoma, involvement of the celiac axis should not be designated as metastatic disease. The optimal management of patients with GEJ carcinoma has long been debated, and the Siewert classification of GEJ cancer helps in unifying surgical management of these disease. Adenocarcinoma of esophagogastric junction (AEG) has its own classification. The borders of AEG are between the esophagus and stomach (160).

No uniform surgical approaches to curative resection exist. One approach involves transhiatal esophagectomy, with anastomosis of the stomach to the cervical esophagus (161). Another, the Ivor-Lewis transthoracic esophagectomy, involves abdominal mobilization of the stomach and transthoracic excision of the esophagus, with anastomosis of the stomach to the upper thoracic or cervical esophagus. Limitations of the Ivor-Lewis procedure include a limited proximal resection margin and a higher risk of bile reflux because of the intrathoracic location of the anastomosis (162). The modified Ivor-Lewis procedure involves a left thoracoabdominal incision with a gastric pull-up into the left chest (163). Another surgical approach is tri-incisional esophagectomy, in which transhiatal and transthoracic approaches are combined, allowing for transthoracic esophagectomy with node dissection and cervical esophagogastric anastomosis (164). Special consideration applies to proximal esophageal cancer. In fact, all disciplines should be involved in the care of patients with cervical esophageal cancer. The cervical esophagus is 6 to 8 cm long, extending from the cricopharyngeus to the thoracic inlet. The incidence of cervical squamous cell carcinoma of the esophagus is likely less than 5% in the United States. The most common presenting complications are tracheal invasion and vocal cord paralysis (prevalence 35% and 24%, respectively) (165). Surgery is associated with significant morbidity because it involves removal of portions of the pharynx, larynx, thyroid gland, and proximal esophagus, resulting in a permanent terminal tracheostomy. Recent results discussed later may provide support for reevaluating esophagectomy after chemoradiotherapy (35,166).

For patients with potentially resectable disease, R0 resection is generally believed to be necessary to achieve durable survival (160). R0 resection is defined as resection of the primary tumor with negative proximal, distal, and circumferential margins. In one report, the 5-year OS after R0 resection increased from 17.5% before 1980 to 31.5% from 1984 to 1989 and 38.5% since 1990 (167). In one retrospective case-control analysis, 220 patients underwent limited transhiatal or extensive mediastinal lymphadenectomy with transthoracic esophagectomy. At a median of 4.7 years of follow-up, there was a trend toward higher DFS (39 versus 27%) and OS (39 versus 29%) rates in patients with more extensive nodal dissection (168). Despite a lack of prospective randomized studies, there is a growing consensus that more extensive nodal dissection is needed, including the removal of all cancerous tissue from the mediastinum improves DFS and OS durations through better control of locoregional recurrence. Also, aggressive lymphadenectomy is generally recommended to increase the accuracy of pathologic staging. In the latest version of AJCC staging manual, the adequate number of lymph nodes is required for defining stage of disease. In the United States, en bloc resection of the mediastinal and upper abdominal lymph nodes are considered standard for transthoracic esophagectomy, and three-field lymphadenectomy is not considered a standard treatment for patients with esophageal cancer.

Though cure is possible with R0 resection, it is a rare occurrence in esophageal cancer. With the steady improvement of surgical techniques, morbidity and complication decreased, contributing to improved survival outcomes of patients with resectable esophageal cancer through the years. Factors that influence postoperative short-term morbidity, 30-day mortality, and long-term prognosis are key areas needing to improve. Patients with esophageal cancer have a modestly poorer prognosis at low-volume hospitals or when treated by surgeons with little experience with esophageal cancer surgery. Among 232 patients who underwent esophagectomy at Swedish hospitals from 1994 to 1997, low-volume hospital (HR, 1.3; 95% CI, 1.0-1.9), inexperienced surgeon (HR, 1.4; 95% CI, 1.0-2.0), and postoperative need for respirator support (HR, 1.4; 95% CI, 1.0-1.9) were associated with a worse prognosis (169). Patients who undergo esophagectomy at high-volume hospitals have lower perioperative mortality rates and better early clinical outcomes than those who undergo surgery at low-volume hospitals (170). Other retrospective population-based analysis further illustrated that surgical outcomes significantly depend on several factors, including surgeon experience, hospital type (academic or community), and hospital surgical volume. In a multivariate analysis of more than 5000 esophageal cancer diagnoses identified from the SEER registry from 1984 to 1993, high-volume hospitals had lower mortality rates for esophagectomy ($p < .001$). For patients undergoing esophagectomy, the 30-day operative mortality rate increased to 17.3% in low-volume hospitals compared with 3.4% in high-volume hospitals (low-volume and high-volume were defined as <5 and >11 esophagectomies per year, respectively) (171). Dimick et al. (172) further elucidated the factors associated with increased surgical morbidity at low-volume hospitals. Three hundred sixty-six patients discharged from a nonfederal, acute-care hospital in Maryland after esophageal resection from 1994 to 1998 were included in their analysis. Rates of postoperative complications at high-volume and low-volume hospitals were compared. Mortality were much lower for high-volume hospitals than for low-volume hospitals (2.5 versus 15.4%; $p < .001$), with an OR of death 5.7 (95% CI, 2.0-16; $p < .001$). Increased risks of renal failure (OR, 19; 95% CI, 1.9-178; $p = .01$), pulmonary failure (OR, 4.8; 95% CI, 1.6-14; $p = .002$), septicemia (OR, 4.0; 95% CI, 1.1-15; $p = .04$), reintubation (OR, 2.9; 95% CI, 1.4-6.1; $p = .004$), surgical complications (OR, 3.3; 95% CI, 1.6-6.9; $p = .001$), and aspiration (OR 1.8; 95% CI, 1.0-3.3; $p = .04$) were observed in low-volume hospitals (172).

Results from a Swedish hospital system confirmed the relationship between hospital volume and mortality. In a multivariate analysis of 1429 patients who underwent esophagectomies and gastrectomies, Werner et al. (173) found a higher long-term survival rate among patients treated at high-volume (>15 resections/year) versus low-volume (<5 resections/year) hospitals

(5-year OS 17 versus 22%; $p = .02$). These results support the use of tertiary referral centers for complex oncologic procedures such as esophagectomies and gastrectomies. Wouters et al. (174) evaluated 555 cancer-related esophagectomy cases from 1990 to 2004, performed in 11 hospitals in the Comprehensive Cancer Center West (CCCW) region. Three hundred forty-two underwent surgery before (group 1) and 213 after (group 2) the introduction of a centralization project. In this project, patients were referred to hospitals with superior outcomes, as determined by a regional audit that compared patient, tumor, and operative details and clinical outcomes between hospitals. Patients treated at centralized hospitals had improved outcomes, along with reduced postoperative morbidity and length of stay. The mortality rate decreased from 12 to 4%, and survival improved significantly ($p = .001$). Referring patients with esophageal cancer to centers with adequate surgical experience and superior outcomes (outcome-based referral) improves quality of care.

Postoperative Therapy

More than 50% of patients with esophageal cancer will have regional node involvement. For both adenocarcinoma and squamous cell carcinoma of the esophagus, the 5-year OS rates dramatically decrease from about 80 to 40% on the basis of the number of involved nodes (0 or 1 to 3) (31). For GEJ adenocarcinoma, the 5-year OS rate for surgery alone is approximately 25% (51,52,87). To decrease the recurrence rate after surgical resection and improve OS, it is necessary to both improve combined modality therapy and develop predictors to individualize patient care. The main contributor to poor survival outcome after esophagectomy is distant disease recurrence (175).

Three randomized controlled studies and one retrospective case-control analysis have been performed of systemic chemotherapy after surgery. Reflecting the incidence of esophageal cancer during the 1980s and 1990s, these studies included more patients with squamous cell carcinoma than with adenocarcinoma; this is a shortcoming of these early studies. In a study by Pouliquen et al. of 120 patients, 116 were randomly assigned to surgery alone (N = 68) or FP (5-fluorouracil plus cisplatin) chemotherapy after surgery (N = 52) (176). Patients were subdivided into two strata. Stratum 1 encompassed patients with complete resection of the tumor with lymph node involvement (N = 62), and stratum 2 consisted of patients with incomplete resections, leaving macroscopic tumor tissue in situ, or patients with metastases (N = 54). The duration of treatment ranged from 6 to 8 months. No survival difference was noted between the two groups (median OS, 14 months) or between the strata. Conversely, significantly more patients in the treated group experienced hematologic, neurologic, and renal complications. Hence FP chemotherapy was considered toxic and not beneficial in patients with resected esophageal squamous cell carcinoma.

Two more studies further confirmed the lack of survival benefit for chemotherapy after esophagectomy. The Japanese Clinical Oncology Group (JCOG) 9204 trial was designed to determine whether postoperative chemotherapy improved outcome in patients with esophageal squamous cell carcinoma who underwent radical surgery. Two hundred forty-two patients at 17 institutions who underwent transthoracic esophagectomy with lymphadenectomy from 1992 to 1997 were randomly assigned to surgery alone (N = 122) or surgery plus postoperative chemotherapy with two courses of FP (N = 120). Adaptive stratification factors were institution and lymph node status (pN0 versus pN1), and the primary endpoint was DFS. The 5-year DFS rates favored postoperative chemotherapy group (45 versus 55%; $p = .037$). However, the 5-year OS rate remained unchanged with postoperative chemotherapy (52 versus 61%, $p = .13$). Hence postoperative chemotherapy was better able to prevent relapse than surgery alone, but unable to improve survival (177). The other study is a retrospective case-control study, designed to evaluate the effect of postoperative chemotherapy in patients who underwent R0 esophagectomy with radical lymphadenectomy. Two hundred and eleven patients with esophageal squamous cell carcinoma had R0 resection with extensive lymphadenectomy, such as three-field lymphadenectomy or total two-field lymphadenectomy, from 1988 to 2000. Ninety-four patients received postoperative chemotherapy with two courses of FP, whereas the other 117 patients had surgery alone. The OS was compared between the two groups after they were stratified by the numbers of metastasis-positive lymph nodes (LN+). In the subgroup of patients with >8 LN+, postoperative chemotherapy significantly improved the OS compared with surgery alone. Therefore, the authors suggested that postoperative chemotherapy after R0 resection with radical lymphadenectomy was beneficial only in patients with >8 metastatic lymph nodes (178), reducing the risk of relapse. However, it did not improve the OS compared with surgery alone.

Many studies have been performed to evaluate the role of postoperative radiotherapy. Unfortunately, the results have been widely inconsistent, with most revealing no improved survival compared with surgery alone. In a multicenter study by Teniere et al. (179) of patients with locally advanced resectable esophageal squamous cell carcinoma, surgery alone (N = 119) was compared with surgical treatment followed by radiation therapy (N = 102). Patients were categorized into one of three groups: N0, no lymph node invasion; N+1, invasion of paraesophageal lymph nodes; and N+2, invasion of distal lymph nodes. All patients underwent R0 resection. A total of 45 Gy to 55 Gy of radiation was delivered to the mediastinal, right, and left supraclavicular areas and to the celiac area when celiac lymph node invasion was present. Results of the analysis concluded that postoperative radiotherapy did not improve survival, regardless of node stratification. In a prospective randomized study, Zieren et al. (180) evaluated postoperative radiation therapy after R0 resection of esophageal squamous cell carcinoma. Thirty-three patients who underwent postoperative radiotherapy were compared with a control group of 35 patients who underwent surgery alone. No statistically significant differences in OS and DFS were found between the two groups. However, postoperative radiotherapy significantly increased the incidence of fibrotic strictures of the esophagogastric or esophagocolonic anastomoses. Because of the lack of benefit and a significant decrease in quality of life (QOL), the authors could not advocate postoperative radiotherapy after R0 esophagectomy.

Results from two other randomized studies revealed conflicting findings. Xiao et al. (181) demonstrated that postoperative radiotherapy improved the 5-year OS in esophageal cancer patients with stage III disease. After radical resection, 495 esophageal cancer patients were randomly assigned to surgery-alone group (N = 275) or surgery plus radiotherapy (N = 220). A total dose of 50 Gy to 60 Gy was delivered over 5 to 6 weeks. The 5-year OS rates for surgery and postoperative radiotherapy were 32% and 41%, respectively ($p = .4474$). Among LN+ patients, the 5-year OS rates were 15% and 29% ($p = .0698$) for the same two groups, respectively. The 5-year OS rates of stage III patients were 13% and 35% ($p = .0027$), respectively. In contrast, Fok et al. found shorter survival durations in patients who underwent postoperative radiotherapy (182). In this study, 130 patients were stratified according to curative or palliative resection and then randomly assigned to undergo postoperative radiotherapy or no additional treatment. Sixty patients underwent curative resection; 30 were randomly assigned to radiotherapy and 30 to the control group. Patients who underwent postoperative radiotherapy had shorter survival durations as a direct result of irradiation-related death and the early appearance of metastatic disease. Thus, the utility of postoperative radiotherapy may be limited.

To develop an optimal postoperative therapy, Malthaner et al. (183) performed a meta-analysis of 34 randomized control trials and six meta-analyses in which patients with locally advanced esophageal cancer underwent pre- or postoperative chemotherapy, radiotherapy, or chemoradiotherapy. Three randomized comparison studies of postoperative chemotherapy compared with surgery alone were pooled for analysis. No significant difference in mortality risk was found at 3 years for postoperative chemotherapy compared with surgery alone (RR, 0.94; 95% CI, 0.74-1.18; $p = .59$) (183). Five randomized studies of postoperative radiotherapy compared with surgery alone were analyzed. Again, no significant difference in the mortality risk was found for postoperative radiotherapy at 1 year (RR, 1.23; 95% CI, 0.95-1.59; $p = .11$) (183). The results of this meta-analysis suggest that after R0 esophagectomy, patients with locally advanced esophageal cancer do not benefit from additional chemotherapy or radiotherapy.

Results from the RTOG 85-01 (82) trial demonstrated that local control and OS rates improved with chemoradiotherapy. The available evidence suggests that postoperative chemotherapy or radiotherapy do not result in a benefit; thus, comparison studies of postoperative chemoradiotherapy and surgery alone were needed. However, few randomized comparisons have been performed of these two treatments. In a study by Ogoshi et al. (184), 187 patients with esophageal squamous cell carcinoma were followed up over a period of 5 years. One hundred seventy-four patients (93.1%) underwent esophagectomy and were then randomly assigned to receive radiotherapy with or without protein-bound polysaccharide (PSK) or radiotherapy (RT) plus chemotherapy (CT) with or without PSK. The 5-year OS of patients with RT, RT + PSK, RT + CT, and RT + CT + PSK were 40%, 42%, 29%, and 37%, respectively. Although it was not statistically significant, there was a trend toward longer survival among patients receiving PSK ($p = .1930$). In the Intergroup (INT) 0116 study (51), 556 patients with resected GEJ and gastric adenocarcinoma were randomly assigned to surgery plus postoperative chemoradiotherapy or surgery alone. Adjuvant treatment consisted of 5-fluorouracil plus leucovorin (FL) for 5 days, followed by 45 Gy of radiation with modified doses of FL on the first 4 and the last 3 days of radiotherapy. One month after radiotherapy, two 5-day cycles of FL were given 1 month apart. The median OS improved with postoperative chemoradiotherapy from 27 to 36 months (HR, 1.35; 95% CI, 1.09-1.66; $p = .005$), and the HR for relapse was 1.52 (95% CI, 1.23-1.86; $p < .001$). INT116

included 111 (20%) patients with GEJ or lower esophageal adenocarcinoma (51). Extrapolation of these results as supporting evidence for postoperative chemoradiotherapy in esophageal cancer should be performed with caution.

On the basis of the available evidence, patients with esophageal cancer gain limited survival benefit with postoperative chemotherapy and chemoradiotherapy after R0 resection. The limited contribution of postoperative therapy is probably due to the moderate toxicity, which leads to treatment-related complications or an inability to complete therapy. As discussed in the gastric cancer section, fewer than 50% of patients undergoing postoperative therapy completed all therapy after surgery (51,52).

Preoperative and Perioperative Therapy

Preoperative radiotherapy was studied in the early 1980s. However, in several phase III studies, a benefit similar to that of surgery alone was not shown (185). In the United States, radiotherapy alone is not frequently included in multimodality therapy. Because of historical development and entrenched regional practices, it is unlikely that studies comparing radiotherapy alone with surgery or chemoradiotherapy will be performed.

Preoperative chemotherapy theoretically increases the curative resection rates by downsizing and downstaging the primary tumor and lymph node metastases, reducing the local and distant relapse rates through suppression and elimination of micrometastases, improving tumor-related symptoms with early initiation of anti-neoplastic therapy, and appraising in vivo the chemosensitivity of the primary tumor that will influence the choice of chemotherapy in the adjuvant setting. Preoperative therapy is hypothesized to result in tumor downstaging, which allows for higher R0 resection and pathCR rates (186).

The prognostic significance of downstaging and pathCR was shown in an analysis of questionnaires from 169 Japanese advanced esophageal adenocarcinoma patients who experienced more than 1 year of clinical complete responses (cCR) after chemotherapy or radiotherapy (N = 106) or pathCR, as found in surgical specimens (N = 63). The 5-year OS rates were 62% and 64.8% for patients in cCR and pathCR, respectively. The effect of a CR on survival was significant. In esophageal carcinoma patients who experience a cCR or pathCR, the prognosis is independent of the initial stage (187). The feasibility of preoperative treatment in locally advanced upper gastrointestinal cancer has been shown in numerous phase II studies with different regimens (188). Older studies of preoperative chemotherapy used platinum-based regimens. The objective response rate (ORR) for platinum-based chemotherapy ranges from 25 to 50%. (189,190). Compared with that of historical controls, the prognosis of patients undergoing preoperative chemotherapy has improved and toxicity has decreased (188). Furthermore, treatment acceptance and compliance have been high, and a significantly higher percentage of patients are able to complete therapy. Several small randomized studies have been performed to determine the feasibility of preoperative chemotherapy and determine resection and pathCR rates. Kok et al. (191) reported significant improvement when chemotherapy was given before curative resection (median OS 18.5 versus 11.0 months). However, Ancona et al. (192) and Roth et al. (193) found no significant survival difference. It is difficult to draw conclusions from such different results. Large randomized controlled studies are needed to determine the role of preoperative chemotherapy.

In one prospective randomized study of 147 patients with resectable esophageal squamous cell carcinoma, 74 received preoperative chemotherapy with cisplatin and 5-fluorouracil (CF) and 73 underwent surgery therapy alone. The primary endpoints were cancer-and therapy-related death. Sixty-six patients (89%) in the preoperative chemotherapy group underwent resection compared with 69 (95%) in the control group (p = NS). Of the 60 patients who underwent resection after chemotherapy, four (6.7%) experienced a pathCR. The postoperative mortality rates were 8.3% and 8.7% (p = NS) for patients in the preoperative chemotherapy and surgery groups, respectively. Significant downstaging was evident with chemotherapy; R0 resections were possible in 67% of these patients compared with 35% in the surgery group (p = .0003). T3 and T4 tumors were found in 67 versus 91% of patients (p = .0002), N1 disease was found in 70 versus 88% of patients (p = .009), and the median OS durations were 16.8 versus 13 months (p = .17) in the chemotherapy versus surgery-alone groups, respectively. In addition, chemotherapy resulted in a significant reduction in locoregional disease. The results of this study further confirmed the safety, feasibility, and benefits of preoperative chemotherapy, including significant downstaging and a higher R0 resection rate. The survival rate was not higher than in the surgery group, but responders had a higher survival rate than did nonresponders (194).

The two largest studies evaluating the role of preoperative chemotherapy were the United States INT123 (195) and United Kingdom Mardsen Royal College OEO-2 randomized controlled trials (196). Four hundred forty and 802 patients were enrolled in INT123 and

OEO-2, respectively. Both studies determined the survival benefit of preoperative chemotherapy compared with surgery alone in patients with resectable esophageal squamous cell carcinoma and adenocarcinoma. CF was administered in both studies. The two studies had completely divergent findings. INT123 found no clinical, pathologic benefit or survival improvement with preoperative chemotherapy followed by surgery compared with surgery alone (195). OEO-2, on the other hand, reported a statistically significant improved R0 resection rate (78 versus 70%) and median OS (17.2 versus 13.3 months) in patients who underwent preoperative chemotherapy (196). Results of both INT123 and OEO 2 studies did not help determine the role of preoperative chemotherapy in patients with resectable esophageal cancer. In the United Kingdom and other countries in Europe, preoperative chemotherapy became the acceptable standard of care. The two most recent randomized studies of preoperative and perioperative chemotherapy, the French ACCORD7 (87) and United Kingdom MAGIC trials (52), are the strongest validations of the benefits of preoperative and perioperative chemotherapy. These two studies are described in detail in the Gastric Cancer section of this chapter. MAGIC trial assessed whether the addition of a perioperative chemotherapy regimen consisting of epirubicin, cisplatin, and 5-fluorouracil (ECF) to surgery improved OS among patients with potentially curable gastric cancer. A protocol adjustment was made later to allow the enrollment of GEJ and distal esophageal adenocarcinoma patients to improve the accrual rate. Five hundred three patients were randomly assigned to perioperative ECF and surgery (N = 250) or surgery alone (N = 253). The postoperative complication rates were similar in both groups (46 versus 45%). The perioperative chemotherapy group had a higher 5-year OS rate (36 versus 23%; HR, 0.75; 95% CI, 0.60-0.93; p = .009). The PFS was also significantly higher (HR, 0.66; 95% CI, 0.53-0.81; p < .001) (52). Only 25% of patients had GEJ or distal esophageal adenocarcinoma.

Perhaps the strongest evidence for preoperative chemotherapy in resectable esophageal cancer came from the ACCORD7 study, which was performed in Europe to evaluate the effects of two or three cycles of preoperative CF on disease-free survival (DFS) in resectable gastric and lower esophageal adenocarcinomas patients. From 1995 to 2003, 224 patients from 28 centers were randomly assigned to surgery alone (N = 111) or preoperative chemotherapy followed by surgery (N = 113). Importantly, 75% of patients had GEJ or distal esophageal adenocarcinoma. A higher R0 resection rate was found for preoperative chemotherapy (73 versus 84%; p = .04). The study met its objective of demonstrating that preoperative CF improved the 5-year DFS rate (21 versus 34%; HR, 0.65; 95% CI, 0.48-0.89; $p = .003$). The HR of death was 0.69 (95% CI, 0.50-0.95; $p = .02$), with a higher 5-year OS rate for preoperative chemotherapy than that for surgery alone (38 versus 24%) (87).

Investigators at Marsden Royal College (MRC) are currently conducting two large phase III randomized controlled studies. MRC OEO-5 is evaluating the use of preoperative chemotherapy, comparing two preoperative chemotherapy regimens—CF versus ECX (epirubicin, cisplatin, and capecitabine). Meanwhile, other researchers in the United Kingdom are evaluating the addition of targeted therapy to perioperative chemotherapy. The MRC ST03 trial will determine whether the addition of bevacizumab to perioperative ECX improves survival. Both of these trials are expected to enroll a large number of patients (1300 and 1100 patients for OEO-5 and ST03, respectively). Table 17-8 lists the ongoing studies of locally advanced resectable gastric, GEJ, and distal esophageal adenocarcinomas.

In the United States, pre- or perioperative chemotherapy is not as common as preoperative chemoradiotherapy for locally advanced esophageal and GEJ cancer on the basis of the results of several small randomized studies comparing preoperative chemoradiotherapy with surgery alone for resectable esophageal cancer. Table 17-9 shows selected randomized phases II and III studies of preoperative chemoradiotherapy. The design of the earliest studies of chemoradiotherapy for esophageal cancer was based on its success in anal carcinoma. The potential activity of chemotherapy against micrometastases and its ability to act as a radiotherapy-sensitizing agent formed the basis for combining chemotherapy and radiotherapy to treat locally advanced carcinoma.

In the RTOG 85-01 study, patients with locally advanced esophageal adenocarcinoma or squamous cell carcinoma were randomly assigned to chemoradiotherapy with CF or radiotherapy. The 5-year OS rates were 0% and 26% for radiotherapy and chemoradiotherapy, respectively (82).

A comprehensive review of the pattern of care for esophageal cancer in the United States from 1992 to 1994 surveyed 400 patients with locally advanced esophageal cancer treated at 63 institutions (197). The study confirmed that using combined concurrent chemoradiotherapy as a nonoperative strategy to achieve superior survival and local tumor control was better than radiotherapy alone (197). The report also suggested a trend toward survival improvement with chemoradiotherapy before surgery compared with chemoradiotherapy or surgery alone. Furthermore, the results of a long-term follow-up study of patients undergoing preoperative chemoradiotherapy using vinblastine plus CF demonstrated a prolonged survival benefit, with a 5-year OS approximately twice as high as expected and a pathCR rate of 20 to 30%.

Between six (198-203) randomized studies of predominantly adenocarcinoma, two (198,202) demonstrated a statistically significant improvement and one (199) showed a trend toward improvement in survival for preoperative chemoradiotherapy. Urba et al. (199) at the University of Michigan performed a randomized comparison of preoperative chemoradiotherapy (5-fluorouracil, cisplatin, and vinblastine [FAV] given concurrently with 45 Gy of radiation) and surgery and surgery alone in 100 patients with resectable esophageal cancer. At a median follow-up of 8.2 years, no significant survival difference was found for surgery versus preoperative chemoradiotherapy (17.6 versus

TABLE 17-8	PERIOPERATIVE THERAPY: ONGOING PHASE II/III RANDOMIZED CONTROL CLINICAL TRIALS IN LOCALLY ADVANCED POTENTIALLY RESECTABLE ESOPHAGEAL, GASTROESOPHAGEAL JUNCTION, AND DISTAL ESOPHAGEAL CANCERS				
Trial	*N*	*Treatment*	*Control*	*Status*
United Kingdom MRC OEO 5	1300	ECX × 4-	CF × 2-S	Accruing
United Kingdom MRC-ST03	1100	ECX + B × 3-S-ECX + B × 3-B × 6	ECX-S-ECX	Accruing
United States CALGB-80101	824	S-ECF + FL/RT-ECF	S-FL-FL/RT-FL	Open not accruing
France NCT00047112	380	CF/RT-S	S	Open not accruing
Netherlands CROSS (only SCC) ISRCTN80832026	350	Paclitaxel + carboplatin/RT-S	S	Open not accruing
Hong Kong CURE (only SCC)	80	CF/RT	S	Complete accruing

B, bevacizumab; CALGB, Cancer and Leukemia Group B; CF, cisplatin, 5-fluorouracil; CURE, Chinese University Research Group for Esophageal Cancer; ECF, epirubicin, cisplatin, 5-fluorouracil; ECX, epirubicin, cisplatin, capecitabine; FL, 5-fluorouracil (leucovorin); MRC, Mardsen Royal College; N, number of patients; OEO, Oesophageal Preoperative Chemotherapy Trial; P, cisplatin; RT, radiotherapy; S, surgery; SCC, squamous cell carcinoma; ST, stomach.

TABLE
17-9 | **PREOPERATIVE CHEMORADIOTHERAPY: RESULTS OF SELECTED RANDOMIZED CONTROL CLINICAL TRIALS IN LOCALLY ADVANCED POTENTIALLY RESECTABLE GASTROESOPHAGEAL JUNCTION AND ESOPHAGEAL CANCERS**

Study	N	Treatment	pathCR (%)	Survival*	Histology
Walsh et al. (198)	58	CDDP + 5-FU × 2 + RT, then surgery	25	32%, 16 months (p = 0.0003)	Adeno
Dublin 1996	55	Surgery	0	6%, 11 months	
Bosset et al. (299)	143	CDDP + RT, then surgery	29	38%, 19 months (NS)	SCC
France 1997	139	Surgery	0	35 %, 19 months	
Urba et al. (199)	50	CDDP + 5-FU + vinblastine + RT, then surgery	28	30%, 16.9 months (p = .09)	SCC/Adeno
UMich 2001	50	Surgery	0	16%, 17.6 months	
Burmeister et al. (200)	128	CDDP + 5-FU + RT, then surgery	N/R	33% (NS)	SCC/Adeno
Australia 2005	128	Surgery	N/R	30%	
Stahl et al. (166)	86	FLEP × 3 then PE + RT (40 Gy), then surgery	FFP 64 (p = .003)	16.4, 31% (NS)	SCC
Germany 2005	86	FLEP × 3 then PE + RT (50-60 Gy)	FFP 41	14.9, 24%	
Bedenne et al. (209)	130	CF/P-RT or CF/SC-RT	N/R	37%, 19 months (NS)	SCC
FFCD9102 2007	129	Surgery	N/R	37%, 18 months	
Crehange et al. (300)	285	CF/SC-RT, then either surgery or more CF/SC-RT then CF × 2	DFS 25	30%, 15.6 months	SCC/Adeno
FFCD9102 2007	161	CF/P-RT, then either surgery or more CF/P-RT then CF × 2	DFS 28 (p = .55)	37%, 18.4 months (p = .25)	
Kleinberg et al. (201)	42	PP + RT (45 Gy) then surgery, then PP × 3	N/R	35 months (NS)	Adeno
E1201 2008	44	IP + RT (45 Gy) then surgery, then IP × 3	N/R	21 months	
Tepper et al. (202)	30	CDDP + 5-FU + RT, then surgery	40	39%, 4.5 (p = .002)	SCC/Adeno
CALGB9781 2008	26	Surgery	0	16%, 1.8	
Stahl et al. (203)	110	PLF × 3, then surgery	2	21.1, 28%	Adeno
POET 2009	109	PLF × 2, then PE + RT, then surgery	16	33.1, 48% (p = .07)	

CALGB, Cancer and Leukemia Group B; CDDP, cisplatin; E1201, Eastern Cooperative Oncology Group; FFCD, Fédération Francophone de la Cancérologie Digestive; 5-FU, fluorouracil; IP, intraperitoneal; IP, irinotecan, cisplatin; N, number of patients; PE, cisplatin, etoposide; PLF, cisplatin, leucovorin, 5-FU; pathCR, rate of pathologic complete response; POET, Preoperative Chemoradiotherapy or Chemoradiotherapy in Esophagogastric Adenocarcinoma Trial; PP, cisplatin, paclitaxel; RT, radiotherapy; SCC, squamous cell carcinoma; VP-16, etoposide.
*Survival (%, months median survival, months disease-free survival whenever data are available) at 3 years.
†Survival (%, months median survival, months disease-free survival whenever data are available) at 2 years.

16.9 months; p = .09). The 3-year survival rates were 16% and 30% (p = .15). This study was statistically powered to detect a relatively large increase in median survival duration, from 1 to 2.2 years, with at least 80% power. The authors argued that a statistical difference may not have been detected because of the study's design. Two independent studies demonstrated a statistically significant survival improvement for preoperative chemoradiotherapy and surgery.

Investigators in Ireland conducted a phase III randomized controlled study comparing survival outcomes in esophageal adenocarcinoma patients treated with surgery alone and chemoradiotherapy followed by surgery. Walsh et al. (198) reported a modest but statistically significant survival duration benefit (16 versus

11 months) for induction chemoradiotherapy (CF and concurrent 40 Gy radiation plus surgery) compared with resection alone. The small sample size, short follow-up, early termination on the basis of the interim analysis, disproportionate number of patients withdrawn from the combined modality arm, and lack of stratification by pretreatment disease stage are some of the limitations of this trial. Furthermore, because patients in the surgical control arm had much poorer survival durations than expected, many researchers have argued that the endpoints were not accurately assessed.

The more recent CALGB 9781 trial provided additional support for preoperative chemoradiotherapy, although it was stopped early because of a slow accrual rate. Fifty-six patients were randomly assigned to surgery alone (N = 26) or CF chemotherapy and concurrent radiotherapy (N = 30). At a median follow-up of 6 years, an intent-to-treat analysis showed a median OS duration of 4.5 versus 1.8 years (p = .002) in favor of trimodality therapy. The 5-year OS rates were 39% (95% CI, 21-57%) versus 16% (95% CI, 5-33%) in favor of trimodality therapy. These results indicate that trimodality therapy results in a long-term survival advantage in esophageal cancer and support its use as a standard of care.

Hofstetter et al. (204) retrospectively reviewed 1097 consecutive patients with primary esophageal cancer who were treated at MD Anderson from 1970 to 2001. A case-control multivariate analysis of survival factors was performed in 879 patients with no systemic metastases and who survived the preoperative period. Survival and R0 rates were compared between patients who underwent only esophagectomies (N = 685) and those who underwent preoperative chemoradiotherapy followed by resection (N = 194). Preoperative chemoradiotherapy was associated with longer survival duration and an increased R0 resection rate. However, a multivariate analysis revealed that long-term survival was associated with R0 resection (HR 0.46; 95% CI, 0.35-0.61; p = .0001) and the use of EUS for staging (HR, 1.74; 95% CI, 1.22-2.50; p = .001), whereas preoperative chemoradiotherapy was associated with successful R0 resection (p = 0.04) (204).

The most current meta-analysis of randomized studies of preoperative chemotherapy or preoperative chemoradiotherapy versus surgery alone for resectable esophageal cancer included 10 of preoperative chemoradiotherapy (N = 1209) and 8 of preoperative chemotherapy (N = 1724) in patients. Gebski et al. (205) reported improved survival with preoperative chemotherapy and chemoradiotherapy. The HR for all-cause mortality with preoperative chemoradiotherapy versus surgery alone was 0.81 (95% CI, 0.70-0.93; p = .002), corresponding to a 13% absolute difference in survival at 2 years, with similar results for different histologic tumor types (squamous cell carcinoma HR, 0.84; p = .04; adenocarcinomas HR, 0.75; p = .02). The HR for preoperative chemotherapy was 0.90 (95% CI, 0.81-1.00; p = .05), which indicates a 2-year absolute survival benefit of 7%. There was no significant effect on all-cause mortality for preoperative chemotherapy in squamous cell carcinoma (HR, 0.88; p = .12), but there was a benefit in AC (HR 0.78; p = .014) (205). With chemoradiotherapy, evidence seems to suggest that treating physicians can expect a pathologic complete response (pCR) rate of 20 to 30%, a median OS duration

of 16 to 24 months, and a therapy-related mortality rate of 5 to 10%.

Evidence from Europe and the United States, as well as a retrospective analysis of 1724 patients at MD Anderson and a recent meta-analysis, suggests that both pre- and perioperative chemotherapy can contribute to the surgical outcome of esophageal cancer patients. However, which is superior is unknown. The POET (Preoperative Chemotherapy or Chemoradiotherapy in Esophagogastric Adenocarcinoma Trial) phase III study was designed to evaluate the survival outcomes of patients treated with preoperative chemotherapy (C) compared with preoperative chemoradiotherapy (CRT). Three hundred fifty-four patients were needed to detect a 10% increase in 3-year survival from 25 to 35%, but the study was prematurely closed because of slow accrual. One hundred twenty-six patients enrolled, and 119 were eligible for evaluation. The median follow-up was 3.8 years, and the primary outcome was OS. R0 resection rates did not differ between treatment groups (70 versus 72%). Patients in the CRT arm had a significantly higher probability of a pathCR (15.6 versus 2.0%) and tumor-free lymph nodes (64 versus 38%) at resection. Postoperative mortality rates did not differ (10 versus 4%; p = .26). Furthermore, the 3-year OS rate improved with radiotherapy (28 versus 47%; HR, 0.67; 95% CI, 0.41-1.07; p = .07). These results suggest that preoperative chemoradiotherapy confers a survival advantage over preoperative chemotherapy in distal esophageal and GEJ adenocarcinoma.

The limited ability to deliver therapy after surgery, as demonstrated by results from both the INT116 and MAGIC studies (51,52), suggests that all effective therapy should be administered before surgery. The use of induction chemotherapy before chemoradiotherapy and surgery has been evaluated in several small phase II studies. Ajani et al. (88) performed a feasibility study of preoperative induction combination chemotherapy with chemoradiotherapy to improve curative resection, local control, and survival in 2001. Thirty-seven potentially resectable carcinomas of the esophagus and GEJ were treated with induction chemotherapy, followed by chemoradiotherapy and curative surgery. Induction chemotherapy consisted of 2 cycles of CF plus and paclitaxel (CFP). After chemoradiotherapy, consisting of 45 Gy of radiation and concurrent CF, patients underwent surgery. Thirty-five (95%) of the 37 patients underwent surgery (R0 resection). The pathCR rate was 30% (11 of 37); an additional five patients (14%) had only microscopic carcinoma. Downstaging was significant; the prevalence of T3 before surgery and at surgery were 89% and 9%, respectively (p = .01), and the prevalence of N1 were 66% and 20%, respectively ($p = .01$) (88).

The three-step strategy was studied further in the multi-institutional RTOG 113 trial, which evaluated induction chemotherapy followed by definitive chemoradiotherapy in patients with localized unresectable esophageal cancer. The primary goal was to determine whether any approach would result in a >78% 1-year OS, surpassing the historical 66% rate from RTOG 9405. Seventy-two evaluable patients were randomly assigned to induction with CFP followed by CFP and 50.4 Gy of radiation (CFP arm, N = 37) or induction with paclitaxel plus cisplatin (PP) and PP and 50.4 Gy of radiation (PP arm, N = 35). The median OS durations for the CFP and PP arms were 28.7 and 14.9 months, respectively (18.8 months in RTOG 9405). The study did not reach its preset objective because the 1-year OS rate of CFP and PP arms did not meet or surpass 78% (CFP 1-year OS, 76%). The 2-year OS rates for the CFP and PP arms were 56% and 37%, respectively. Toxicity was quite high in both arms—43 to 54% and 27 to 40% that experienced grades 3 and 4 toxicities, respectively. Therefore, neither combination (CFP or PP) was recommended for further evaluation (206).

Since then, results from the POET trial, presented by Stahl et al. (203), provided further support for three-step preoperative therapy, although the study was closed prematurely because of slow accrual. One hundred nineteen patients were randomly assigned to chemotherapy followed by surgery (N = 60) or chemoradiotherapy followed by chemoradiotherapy and surgery (N = 59). The R0 resection rates were 70% and 72% (p = NS), the pathCR rates were 16% and 2% ($p < .001$), and the N0 rates were 64% and 38% ($p < .001$). The 3-year OS rate trended toward improvement with induction chemotherapy, chemoradiotherapy, and surgery (28-47%, $p = .07$) (203). Maximizing duration and amount of therapy before surgery theoretically could improve the ability to deliver all planned effective therapies, initiate palliative therapy early, and improve pathCR, local control, cure, and survival rates. However, patient selection is important because the current three-step strategy exchanges moderate toxicity for modest survival improvement. Ongoing studies are evaluating the combination of radiotherapy and newer agents such as docetaxel, irinotecan, and oxaliplatin. Most of these studies have yet to reach phase III. Until results from large randomized studies confirm that the survival benefits significantly outweigh the toxicities, the induction chemotherapy, chemoradiotherapy, and surgery strategy remains investigational.

Three recent meta-analyses have been performed to further support the available evidence for preoperative therapy. In 2003, Urschel et al. (207) analyzed the results of nine randomized studies, including 1116 patients with resectable esophageal cancer who were treated with surgery alone or preoperative chemoradiotherapy. The OR for chemoradiotherapy and surgery versus surgery alone were calculated. The 3-year OS rate was higher with preoperative chemoradiotherapy (OR, 0.66; 95% CI, 0.47-0.92; $p = .016$), as was the R0 resection rate (OR, 0.53; 95% CI, 0.33-0.84; $p = .007$). Finally, surgical and all-treatment mortality rates did not significantly differ between two arms (OR, 1.72; 95% CI, 0.96-3.07; $p = .07$) and (OR, 1.63; 95% CI, 0.99-2.68; $p = .053$), respectively (207).

In 2004, Malthaner et al. (208) analyzed 34 randomized studies and 6 meta-analyses, including all preoperative and postoperative therapy versus surgery alone, and calculated the RR of mortality. No statistically significant differences were found for preoperative chemotherapy, perioperative chemotherapy, or preoperative radiotherapy compared with surgery alone (RR 1.00; 95% CI, 0.83-1.19; $p = .98$; RR, 0.99; 95% CI, 0.81-1.21; $p = .93$; and RR, 1.01; 95% CI, 0.88-1.16; $p = .87$, respectively). However, a significant difference was found for preoperative chemoradiotherapy. Six randomized trials and two meta-analyses of preoperative chemoradiotherapy followed by surgery versus surgery alone were evaluated; a significant difference in mortality risk at 3 years was found for preoperative chemoradiotherapy (RR, 0.87; 95% CI, 0.80-0.96; $p = 0.004$) (208).

In 2007, Gebski et al. analyzed 10 randomized studies of preoperative chemoradiotherapy followed by surgery versus surgery alone (N = 1209) and 8 studies of preoperative chemotherapy and surgery versus surgery alone (N = 1724) in patients with locally advanced, resectable esophageal cancer. They calculated the HR for all-cause mortality. Unlike Malthaner et al. they found a significant difference for preoperative chemotherapy (HR, 0.90; 95% CI, 0.81-1.00; $p = .05$), indicating a 2-year absolute survival benefit of 7%. This improvement seemed to be more common in adenocarcinoma patients (HR, 0.78; 95% CI, 0.64-0.95; $p = .014$). Similar to the findings of Urschel et al. and Malthaner et al. preoperative chemoradiotherapy was superior to surgery alone (HR, 0.81; 95% CI, 0.70-0.93; $p = .002$), corresponding to a 13% absolute difference in survival at 2 years. This improvement was seen for both histologic tumor types: HR 0.84 (95% CI, 0.71-0.99; $p = .04$) for SCC and 0.75 (95% CI, 0.59-0.95; $p = .02$) for AC (205).

Cumulatively, these three meta-analyses determined that the most consistent significant survival benefit resulted from the combination of surgery and preoperative chemoradiotherapy, and to a lesser extent, preoperative chemotherapy. Limited evidence exists to support the use of postoperative chemotherapy or radiotherapy alone. The 20 to 25% of patients in INT116 with GEJ or distal esophageal adenocarcinoma suggest that postoperative chemoradiotherapy contributes to a survival benefit after surgery.

Finally, patients with resectable esophageal cancer are commonly treated with pre- or perioperative chemotherapy in Europe and the United Kingdom, whereas patients in the United States are more likely to undergo preoperative chemoradiotherapy. Until further results confirm the findings of the POET study, the use of preoperative chemotherapy or chemoradiotherapy therapy will remain regionally variable. Proponents of preoperative chemoradiotherapy reason that a pathCR, a surrogate marker of survival, is more likely with chemoradiotherapy than with chemotherapy alone, on the basis of the POET study results. However, although these results demonstrated significant downstaging and improved pathCR and N0 rates, they did not show a survival benefit. Furthermore, although the results of phase II studies of induction chemotherapy, chemoradiotherapy, and surgery appear promising, their use is investigational. Only large well-designed randomized comparative trials can determine which preoperative modality results in better survival outcome and less toxicity. Especially important is the ability to separate therapy-related toxicities from benefits; thus, better predictive or prognostic markers will be needed to improve patient selection.

Squamous Cell Carcinoma

It has become abundantly clear that esophageal squamous cell carcinoma and adenocarcinoma behave differently. Squamous cell carcinoma (SCC) is typically located in the cervical or mid esophagus. Although squamous cell carcinoma is still the most common histologic type in most of the world, it is rare (<5% of all esophageal cancers) (165) in the United States. The risk factors for esophageal squamous cell carcinoma are tobacco and alcohol use. The age at diagnosis is typically 10 years younger than that for esophageal adenocarcinoma. With proximal and cervical disease, bronchoscopy is indicated for staging because of the high risk of tracheoesophageal (TE) fistula. Version 7 of the AJCC staging system now classifies adenocarcinomas and squamous cell carcinoma differently. Unlike in adenocarcinoma, BE or dysplasia is not a predisposing

condition for esophageal squamous cell carcinoma. At 10 years, 2 to 5% of patients treated with chemoradiotherapy in the RTOG 85-01 trial were still alive; most of them had squamous cell carcinoma. Furthermore, in the 5-year OS rate for esophageal squamous cell carcinoma is higher than that for adenocarcinoma (21 versus 13%) (82). The treatment of locally advanced esophageal squamous cell carcinoma deserves unique consideration. Evidence from the past 5 to 10 years has resulted in an active debate as to whether surgery is necessary after chemoradiotherapy in patients with locally advanced esophageal squamous cell carcinoma.

The cervical esophagus is 6 to 8 cm long and extends from the cricopharyngeus to the thoracic inlet. Surgery in this area is a highly morbid procedure, resulting in the removal of portions of the pharynx, larynx, thyroid gland, and proximal esophagus. Patients will live with a permanent tracheostomy and esophago-cervical fistula while waiting for a jejunal interposition graft or a deltopectoral or pectoralis major myocutaneous flap. Thus, definitive chemoradiotherapy is preferred for patients with cervical esophageal carcinoma. Patients with mid- and distal esophageal squamous cell carcinoma are treated similarly to those with distal esophageal and GEJ adenocarcinoma. Patients with locally advanced but resectable disease can be treated with additional preoperative chemoradiotherapy or pre- or perioperative chemotherapy. However, the results of several large randomized studies from Europe suggest an alternative option for patients with esophageal squamous cell carcinoma.

Stahl et al. (203) performed a randomized comparison of chemotherapy, chemoradiotherapy followed by surgery (surgical arm, N = 86), and chemotherapy followed by chemoradiotherapy and no surgery (nonoperative arm, N = 86) in 172 patients with locally advanced esophageal squamous cell carcinoma. The median follow-up duration was 6 years. OS rates were similar for the surgical and nonsurgical arms ($p < .05$). The 2-year local PFS rate was higher in the surgical arm than the nonsurgical arm (64 versus 41%; HR, 2.1; 95% CI, 1.3-3.5; $p = .003$). The treatment-related mortality rate was significantly higher in the surgical arm (12.8 versus 3.5%, $p = .03$). The clinical tumor response to induction chemotherapy was the only independent prognostic factor for OS (HR, 0.30; 95% CI, 0.19-0.47; $p < .0001$). The results of this study suggested that adding surgery to chemoradiotherapy improves local tumor control but not survival in patients with locally advanced esophageal squamous cell carcinoma. Tumor response to induction chemotherapy is associated with a favorable prognostic group in these high-risk patients, regardless of treatment (166). Of course, the difficulty of incorporating these results into clinical practice is detecting residual disease or response after preoperative therapy.

Another randomized comparison in only responders to chemoradiotherapy [45 Gy conventional (C) or 60 Gy split-course (SC) radiation] was conducted by Bedenne et al. (209). Patients with resectable esophageal squamous cell carcinoma were treated with two cycles of CF along with concurrent radiotherapy (C/SC). Patients who experienced a response were then randomly assigned to surgery or more chemoradiotherapy. Two hundred fifty-nine patients were randomly assigned to undergo surgery or more chemoradiotherapy. The 2-year OS rates were 34% and 40%, respectively (HR, 0.90; p = .44), the median OS durations were 18 and 19 months (p = NS), the 2-year local control rates were 66% and 57% (p < .01), and the 3-month mortality rates were 9.3% and 0.8% (p = .002) (209). The authors concluded that in patients who experience a response to chemoradiotherapy, surgery after chemoradiotherapy results in no added benefit over continued chemoradiotherapy (209).

Most data are not yet sufficiently mature to allow conclusions about optimal therapy for locally advanced squamous cell carcinoma of the noncervical esophagus. In an ongoing phase III study (CURE [Chinese University Research Group for Esophageal Cancer]), investigators from China are comparing the survival benefits of esophagectomy versus chemoradiotherapy. From 2000 to 2004, 80 patients were randomly assigned to esophagectomy (N = 44) or chemoradiotherapy (N = 36). A two- or three-stage esophagectomy with two-field lymphadenectomy was performed. Chemoradiotherapy consisted of continuous infusional 5-fluorouracil plus cisplatin (CF) and concurrent 50-60 Gy of radiation. Tumor response was assessed by EGD, EUS, and CT. Salvage esophagectomies were performed for incomplete response or recurrence. The median follow-up was 1.4 years. No difference in the early cumulative survival rate was found between the two groups (RR, 0.89; 95% CI, 0.37-2.17; p = .45), nor was a difference in DFS. Patients treated with surgery only had a slightly higher recurrence rate in the mediastinum, whereas those treated with chemoradiotherapy had a higher rate in the cervical or abdominal region (210).

In summary, patients with locally advanced cervical esophageal cancer should undergo definitive chemoradiotherapy; surgery should only be considered for local recurrence or persistent disease. However, patients and their families should understand that surgery will result in a permanent tracheostomy and possibly a transient esophagocervical fistula. Whether or not treatment of squamous cell carcinoma will ultimately differ from adenocarcinoma remain to be seen. Evidence from a European randomized controlled trial suggests that patients who experience a response to preoperative chemoradiotherapy do not need surgery, as surgery appeared to improve local control but not OS. The final results of the Dutch CROSS and Chinese CURE randomized studies of esophageal squamous cell carcinoma have not been published. CROSS is designed to compare the survival outcomes of surgery alone and surgery after chemoradiotherapy with carboplatin plus paclitaxel; an accrual of 350 patients is expected. CURE is designed to compare surgery alone with chemoradiotherapy alone (using cisplatin and 5-fluorouracil). Preliminary data from CURE suggested no difference in early survival between the two arms.

Surgery is the foundation of treatment for locally advanced resectable esophageal cancer. Early results from European studies suggested that patients with esophageal squamous cell carcinoma will not benefit from surgery after chemoradiotherapy. The caveat of the nonsurgical approach to solid tumors is detecting minimal residual disease. Therefore, until more confirmatory evidence and clinical tools become available for detecting minimal residual disease or molecular or imaging predictive markers in patients who require surgery after preoperative therapy, the treatments for squamous cell carcinoma and adenocarcinoma will remain similar.

MD Anderson Approach to Resectable Esophageal and Gastroesophageal Junction Cancers

Because MD Anderson is a tertiary referral cancer center, BE and dysplasia are not commonly seen. BE treatment consists of three objectives: treating GERD, endoscopically monitoring BE, and administering definitive therapy with EMR/ESMR, with or without PDT or esophagectomy for HGD or invasive carcinoma. All patients with newly diagnosed invasive carcinoma, including HGD, undergo careful staging, which includes endoscopic assessment of the location and size of the primary tumor and EUS staging, CT, and PET/CT. Patients with cervical or proximal esophageal cancer also undergo bronchoscopy as part of a recommended staging workup. For distal esophageal disease or gastric cardia cancer, staging laparoscopy is performed in some patients, but the decision is made on a case by case basis. Again, as in locally advanced gastric cancer, all patients with only localized disease are further evaluated by a multidisciplinary team that includes thoracic surgeons and oncologic radiotherapists. Furthermore, patients with localized disease are discussed at the weekly

Esophageal Multidisciplinary Tumor Board. Patients are considered to have resectable or unresectable disease on the basis of pathologic, radiologic, and endoscopic findings reviewed at the conference. Patients with resectable disease have the option of enrolling in clinical trials or undergoing standard therapy.

Currently, at MD Anderson treatment modality for locally advanced resectable esophageal cancer include surgery, and chemoradiotherapy then surgery. For GEJ adenocarcinoma, postoperative chemoradiotherapy and perioperative chemotherapy are additional options available to patients. Patients with locally advanced cervical esophageal cancer are treated with primary definitive chemoradiotherapy, even those with resectable disease. Salvage surgery is considered only in patients with persistent or locally recurrent disease. Results from the RTOG 85-01 and 94-05 studies established that adding chemotherapy to radiotherapy improved survival and local relapse rates and that the optimal radiation dosage is 50.4 Gy in 28 fractions. If at all possible, all locally advanced resectable esophageal cancers are treated on protocol at MD Anderson or with preoperative chemoradiotherapy, followed by surgical resection.

MD Anderson protocols for resectable disease have evolved from a couple of decades of research that demonstrates that induction chemotherapy followed by chemoradiotherapy and surgery result in high pathCR and survival rates. This approach has been tested in other studies, including the POET trial; this study was closed because of slow accrual, but an analysis of evaluable patients demonstrated significantly improved pathCR and PFS rates for with chemotherapy followed by chemoradiotherapy and surgery. These results further support our use of induction chemotherapy followed by chemoradiotherapy. Although promising, this three-step preoperative therapy is still being investigated. Patients with GEJ carcinoma may also undergo perioperative chemotherapy or postoperative chemoradiotherapy. Figure 17-15 illustrates the MD Anderson approach to treatment and standard care for esophageal cancer, respectively.

Locally Advanced Unresectable Gastric, Gastroesophageal Junction, and Esophageal Carcinomas

Prolonged progression-free survival is possible in some patients, but durable survival without surgery is unlikely. For patients with locally advanced but unresectable gastric, GEJ, and esophageal carcinomas, the most important objective is symptom palliation rather than cure. These patients make up a heterogeneous group that includes patients with primarily unresectable disease, patients who are poor surgical candidates, and patients who decline surgery. The goal of symptom palliation is to optimize quality of life. It is important to be familiar with how to restore or maintain the ability to swallow and how to manage pain, prevent bleeding, minimize aspiration, and maintain or restore the airway. Surgical unresectability should be determined by a multidisciplinary team. Patients with primary unresectable disease include those with cervical esophageal, T4b, or local M1b disease, such as in the retroperitoneal nodes, and patients with positive peritoneal cytologic findings or brain metastases.

Current or potential signs or symptoms that affect QOL should be assessed during the initial evaluation of patients with unresectable disease. Available treatment options include external-beam radiotherapy, with or without concurrent chemotherapy; chemotherapy; endoscopic palliation with luminal dilation, stents, or laser or chemical ablation; and palliative surgery. Palliative surgery is rarely performed because it is rare that the potential benefits clearly outweigh the risks of surgery. Several special issues to consider in this group of patients include (1) problems specifically associated with local disease; (2) nutrition; (3) diagnosis and treatment of TE fistulas; and (4) management of oral secretions.

For cervical esophageal cancer in which the primary tumor is above the carina, evaluation should include bronchoscopy to evaluate for posterior membranous tracheal invasion. As discussed in the Surgery subsection of the Esophageal and Gastroesophageal Junction Cancers section, primary surgery is rarely performed because of the resulting functional deficits and impaired quality of life. Regardless of resectability, patients with cervical esophageal cancer are treated with definitive chemoradiotherapy. For patients with distal esophageal or gastric cancer, laparoscopic staging can identify 20 to 30% of patients with occult peritoneal disease.

All patients, especially those who present with more than 15% weight loss from their normal baseline, should undergo formal nutritional evaluation, and alternative nutritional support methods should be considered. Adequate nutrition and hydration are crucial to ensure that patients complete the full course of therapy. Jejunostomy feeding tubes (J-tubes), which are inserted primarily via a surgical procedure, can be considered in patients with gastric and gastroesophageal junction cancer; they can be placed during the initial laparoscopic evaluation. Percutaneous gastrostomy feeding tubes, placed by endoscopic (PEG) or radiologic (G-tube) guidance, can be considered for esophageal cancer. Nasogastric feeding tubes are an option for nutritional support, but they are rarely a practical long-term solution. Total parental nutrition (TPN) is often a nutrition choice of last resort and usually considered in patients with a life expectancy of >16 weeks. TPN requires a chronic indwelling venous catheter, which can increase the risk of infection and thrombosis. Furthermore, in patients who are moderately or severely malnourished, TPN can exacerbate problems associated with fluid retention and edema. Rather than bypassing the gastrointestinal tract, the continued use of jejunostomy, gastrostomy, or nasogastric feeding tubes is considered the first choice if nutrition cannot be supported orally. The focus of care for patients with locally advanced unresectable gastric, GEJ, and esophageal carcinomas is to improve QOL, which should be considered when choosing a nutritional support modality.

TE fistulas may result from complications of chemoradiotherapy (6%) or may be present at initial diagnosis (6%) (211). The prognosis of patients with TE fistulas is poor, with a life expectancy of less than 9 months. In one study, spontaneous fistula closure occurred in 70% of patients after chemoradiotherapy (212). Persistent TE fistulas can be addressed with a tracheal or esophageal stent, esophageal exclusion, or palliative esophageal resection. Esophageal exclusion consists of cervical esophagostomy, gastrostomy, and jejunostomy tubes for aspiration risk and nutrition. Lastly, special attention should be paid to patients with increased oral or gastrointestinal secretions. Malignant esophageal stenosis is usually the cause, in which, aspiration must be reduced using an esophageal stent to restore patency or a feeding tube to minimize stomach fullness and regurgitation.

All patients with locally advanced but primarily unresectable gastric, GEJ, and esophageal carcinomas, as well as those with locally advanced cervical esophageal cancer, are candidates for definitive chemoradiotherapy. Both the RTOG 85-01 (82) and 94-05 (213) trials demonstrated that chemoradiotherapy is better than radiotherapy alone, and the standard dose 50.4 Gy of radiation is preferred. Definitive chemoradiotherapy has a role in patients with locally advanced, unresectable gastroesophageal cancers. In a series at Fox Chase Cancer Center, radiotherapy plus chemotherapy consisting of 5-fluorouracil and mitomycin resulted in a local control rate of 75%, which was associated with improved swallowing, and an actuarial DFS rate of 30% (OS rate, 18%) at 5 years in patients with stages I and II disease (214). Furthermore, in the RTOG 85-01 study of chemotherapy plus radiotherapy resulted in a higher 5-year survival rate than did radiotherapy alone (26 versus 0%) (82). This trial established a new standard for definitive chemoradiotherapy in patients with locoregional esophageal carcinoma. Furthermore, an Eastern Cooperative Oncology Group (ECOG) trial of 135 patients also showed that chemotherapy plus radiotherapy provided a higher 2-year survival rate than did radiotherapy alone (215). Chemotherapy agents used in combination with radiotherapy included cisplatin plus 5-fluorouracil. The results of small phase II and large phase III trials have demonstrated the safety and feasibility of using other chemotherapy agents for radiosensitization. Currently accepted radiosensitizing agents include taxanes (paclitaxel and docetaxel), other platinums (carboplatin and oxaliplatin), oral fluoropyrimidines (capecitabine and S-1), and irinotecan. Recently, targeted agents have been safely used, alone or in combination with chemotherapy, as radiosensitizing agents. The most widely used targeted agent is cetuximab (216).

Patients with borderline performance status may not be candidates for definitive chemoradiotherapy, even with consistent nutritional support via feeding tubes. Therapy should be based on the patient's most pressing symptoms. Malnutrition should be addressed, whenever feasible, with gastrostomy or a jejunostomy tube. Airway compromise should be addressed via minimized aspiration and restoring airway or gastrointestinal patency with dilation, stents, or ablation. Upper gastrointestinal bleeding and pain can be palliated with radiotherapy, alone or with endoscopic cauterization. Options for treating TE fistulas are discussed above.

In newly diagnosed gastric, GEJ, and esophageal carcinomas, malignant gastroparesis results from direct tumor invasion into the stomach, such as in linitis plastica (mechanical), celiac plexus/vagus nerve (functional) or postsurgical dysmotility (functional), or outlet obstruction (mechanical). It is difficult to treat mechanical causes, but antineoplastic therapy can improve symptoms. However, in refractory disease, other therapy modalities may be used, such as duodenal stents or gastrostomy to decompress tube placement. The functional causes of gastroparesis can be treated with pharmacologic agents (erythromycin [217] or metoclopramide [218]).

Finally, effective chemotherapy can directly improve symptoms such as dysphagia and pain, as well as indirectly improve nutrition and minimize bleeding risk and aspiration. The use of brachytherapy has waned in the United States for patients with locally advanced unresectable disease and patients requiring symptom palliation. Ongoing studies are designed to clarify the role of stents, brachytherapy, and targeted therapy during definitive chemoradiotherapy or palliation of dysphagia.

Advanced and Metastatic Gastric, Gastroesophageal Junction, and Esophageal Carcinomas

The prognosis of patients with advanced or metastatic gastric, gastroesophageal junction (GEJ), and esophageal cancers is poor; thus, clinicians should be cognizant of patients' quality of life and weigh the risks and benefits of therapy. The overall 5-year survival rate of upper gastrointestinal cancer patients is less than 5%. The standard of care for advanced disease is chemotherapy. Many frontline combination chemotherapy regimens are available, but no head-to-head comparison has been performed of most of these; thus, the optimal choice is not obvious, and treatment remains regionally variable. However, with the advent of molecular targeted therapy, it may be possible to select therapy on the basis of the disease's molecular characteristics. The results of the Trastuzumab in Gastric Cancer (ToGA) study (219) raised the exciting possibility of personalized treatment for upper gastrointestinal carcinomas. Until more specific and accurate molecular markers of response and prognosis become available, however, patients' outcome with systemic therapy is best predicted by their clinical characteristics, such as performance status.

Systemic Cytotoxic Chemotherapy

More than two-thirds of patients diagnosed with gastric, GEJ, and esophageal cancers have unresectable or metastatic disease. The mean 5-year overall survival (OS) rate is less than 17%. Therapeutic decision is between a strictly supportive approach and exposing patients to the side effects of a potentially ineffective treatment.

In several small retrospective and prospective studies, chemotherapy has been found to improve the survival duration compared with best supportive care (BSC) in patients with good performance status (220-225). To further clarify the survival benefit of systemic therapy in patients with advanced upper gastrointestinal carcinoma, Wohrer et al. (223) pooled data from 101 studies. Of these studies, only four were randomized studies comparing palliative chemotherapy with BSC in 174 patients with advanced gastric cancer. Effectiveness and side effects were evaluated in 73 phase II studies and 24 randomized phase III studies. Chemotherapy was found to be superior to BSC alone. In patients with poor performance status, leucovorin-modulated 5-fluorouracil alone should be considered. However, the prognosis remained poor, as the increased survival duration with systemic chemotherapy was moderate at best (223). Two years after Wohrer et al. (223) published their findings, Wagner et al. (225) further demonstrated that chemother-

apy improved survival in patients with advanced and metastatic upper gastrointestinal carcinomas when compared with BSC, by incorporating more recent studies. On the basis of an analysis of three studies conducted before 1990 in 184 patients, an overall hazard ratio (HR) of 0.39 (95% CI, 0.28-0.52) was calculated for chemotherapy versus BSC alone, which represented a weighted mean survival benefit of chemotherapy of 6 months (226). A meta-analysis revealed that combination chemotherapy had a statistically significant advantage ($p = .001$) over single-agent chemotherapy (HR, 0.83; 95% CI, 0.74-0.93), representing a weighted mean survival benefit of 1 month (226). Although small, this benefit may be considered clinically relevant given the unfavorable prognosis of advanced and metastatic upper gastrointestinal carcinoma, which typically carried a median OS duration of 5 to 7 months after 5-fluorouracil treatment (227). Despite advanced molecular techniques, the factors that predict survival after systemic therapy are clinical characteristics, including performance status, nutritional status, histologic grade, and metastases location (228).

The treatment of advanced or metastatic upper gastrointestinal carcinomas varies regionally. S-1 is available in Japan and is being used as single agent to treat metastatic gastric cancer, despite not having demonstrated superiority over 5-fluorouracil in a large phase III study. In Europe, epirubicin is combined with fluoropyrimidine and a platinum compound (229). Meanwhile, in other parts of Asia and the United States, fluoropyrimidine and a platinum compound are combined, with or without another agent. These regional variations and a lack of direct comparisons between several first-line chemotherapy regimens hinder the identification of the optimal regimen for advanced and metastatic gastric, GEJ, and esophageal cancers. In addition, this lack of an evidence-based consensus makes designing clinical trials and advancing treatment more difficult because there is no optimal control arm or platform for the investigation of biologically targeted agents. Historically, the study and treatment of advanced gastric and esophageal cancers differed. However, because of the shift in histologic characteristics and the location of primary site, where GEJ and distal esophageal adenocarcinomas are predominant, regimens historically used for advanced gastric cancer are being used for advanced esophageal cancer, and vice versa. As a result of this epidemiologic shift and the lack of evidence that patient outcomes will differ if the diseases are treated on the basis of the primary tumor site, advanced and metastatic gastric, GEJ, and esophageal carcinomas are all treated similarly (230).

Many studies of single agents have been small and uncontrolled, making it difficult to draw firm conclusions regarding effectiveness. Classes of cytotoxic agents that have demonstrated single-agent activity include fluoropyrimidines, platinums, anthracyclines, topoisomerase I and II inhibitors, taxanes, and alkylators. 5-Fluorouracil is the most extensively studied single agent in patients with advanced upper gastrointestinal carcinoma; it results in ORR of 21% and a median OS duration of 10 months (223). Antitumor activity of single agent against upper gastrointestinal carcinomas ranges from ORRs of 0 to 49% (223). In small phase II studies, combination chemotherapy commonly resulted in a higher ORR (14-73%) and longer median OS (4.5-12.0 months) (223). However, in randomized phase III studies, combination chemotherapy has not consistently demonstrated a survival improvement (4.0-11.2 months) (223,231), despite a higher response rate (6-51%) (223) than that of single-agent chemotherapy.

The management of advanced and metastatic upper gastrointestinal carcinoma patients with combination chemotherapy regimens evolved through practice-changing results of phase III randomized controlled clinical studies. Results of the 1982 Gastrointestinal Tumor Study Group study established that 5-fluorouracil, doxorubicin, and mitomycin-C (FAM) had superior survival and efficacy to that of single-agent 5-fluorouracil (232). FAM was replaced by 5-fluorouracil, doxorubicin, and methotrexate (FAMTX) in a subsequent European Organization for Research and Treatment of Cancer (EORTC) study (233). Level 1 evidence for cisplatin and 5-fluorouracil (CF) was derived from the results of another EORTC study that showed that CF was not inferior to etoposide, leucovorin, and 5-fluorouracil and FAMTX (234). A phase II study from the United Kingdom involving 128 patients with advanced gastric cancer treated with epirubicin, cisplatin, and 5-fluorouracil (ECF) reported an ORR 71% (235). In a phase III randomized controlled study comparing ECF with FAMTX, ECF had a superior ORR (45 versus 21%) and median OS (8.9 versus 5.7 months) (236). Several more randomized studies established ECF as a standard-of-care regimen by demonstrating the superiority of ECF over mitomycin, cisplatin, and 5-fluorouracil (237) and cisplatin, epirubicin, leucovorin, and 5-fluorouracil (238). With these results, CF and ECF were established as the standards of care for advanced and metastatic gastric cancer, respectively, in the United States and United Kingdom.

In the V-325 study, Van Cutsem et al. (239) established docetaxel as a Federal Drug Administration–approved agent to be used in combination with CF for advanced and metastatic gastric and GEJ cancers. In this multi-institution international study, 445 patients with advanced gastric and GEJ cancer were randomly assigned to receive CF or docetaxel plus CF (DCF). The primary endpoint was time to progression (TTP). A superior ORR (37 versus 25%) and 2-year OS rate (18 versus 9%) were found with DCF. DCF also resulted in a 32% risk reduction in TTP ($p < .001$) and 23% risk reduction in OS compared with CF ($p = .02$) (239). Despite meeting its goal, V-325 was heavily criticized for being toxic and involving a highly selective patient cohort. Grades 3 and 4 neutropenia (82 versus 57%), stomatitis (21 versus 27%), and complicated neutropenia (29 versus 12%) were more frequently experienced by patients treated with DCF (239). Of note, this study did not allow for the primary prophylactic use of granulocyte colony–stimulating factor. A later analysis reported that quality of life was preserved longer among patients on DCF than among those on CF at all time points (240) Roth et al. (241) presented the results of a Swiss phase II randomized study comparing the effectiveness of docetaxel and cisplatin (TC), TC and 5-fluorouracil (TCF), and ECF in 119 patients with advanced and metastatic gastric cancer. The primary endpoint was ORR. The ORRs of ECF, TC, and TCF were 25.0%, 18.5%, and 36.6%, respectively. The median OS durations were 8.3, 11.0, and 10.4 months. These results further solidified the role of docetaxel in the treatment of upper gastrointestinal carcinoma. Additionally, several phase II and randomized phase II studies have been conducted to improve the side-effect profile of DCF. On behalf of the Australasian Gastro-Intestinal Trials Group (AGITG), Tebbutt et al. (242) reported the results of a randomized, noncomparative phase II study of weekly docetaxel with cisplatin plus 5-fluorouracil (wDCF) versus weekly docetaxel plus capecitabine (wDX) in advanced gastric and GEJ cancer patients. This study is commonly referred to as the ATTAX study. The premise of the study was to improve the side-effect profile of the every-3-week regimen of V-325. One hundred six therapy-naïve patients with advanced and metastatic gastric and GEJ carcinoma were randomly assigned to receive wDCF (N = 50) or wDX (N = 56). The primary endpoint was ORR. The ORRs of wDCF and wDX were 47% and 26%, respectively, and the median PFS and OS durations were 5.9 versus 11.2 months and 4.6 versus 10.1 months, respectively (242). The ORRs and OS durations of wDCF were similar to those of wDCF (ORR, 37%; median OS, 9.2 months) (239), further suggesting that DCF is an active regimen and that hematologic toxicity of the original every-3-week regimen of V-325 can be overcome with a weekly dosing modification.

For years, the results from several phase II studies suggested that irinotecan and cisplatin (IP) had robust antitumor activity against upper gastrointestinal carcinoma (243-245). IP was compared with irinotecan, 5-fluorouracil plus folinic acid in an international randomized phase II trial involving 41 centers in 13 European countries and Israel, Lebanon, Turkey, and South Africa. One hundred fifteen patients with advanced gastric and GEJ cancer were treated. The ORRs in the irinotecan, 5-fluorouracil plus folinic acid (N = 59) and IP arms (N = 56) were 42.4% and 32.1%, respectively. The median TTP and OS duration of irinotecan, 5-fluorouracil plus folinic acid were superior to those of IP (6.5 versus 4.2 months, $p < .0001$; and 10.7 versus 6.9 months, $p < .0018$, respectively). The toxicity profile was also better than that of IP (246). In a larger follow-up phase III randomized study, 333 patients with advanced and metastatic gastric or GEJ adenocarcinoma were randomly assigned to receive either irinotecan, 5-fluorouracil plus folinic acid or 5-fluorouracil and cisplatin (CF). Patients treated with irinotecan, 5-fluorouracil plus folinic acid versus CF had median TTPs and OS durations of 5.0 versus 4.2 months (HR, 1.23; $p = .088$) and 9.0 versus 8.7 months (HR, 1.08; $p = .53$) and ORRs and times to treatment failure of 31.8 versus 25.8% and 4.0 versus 3.4 months (HR, 1.43; $p = .018$), respectively. Although irinotecan, 5-fluorouracil plus folinic acid were not found to be superior, a trend toward significance was found for TTP, suggesting that these drugs combination can be used as a platinum-free regimen with improved tolerance (247).

Results from other randomized phases II and III studies have introduced new chemotherapy agents for treating patients with upper gastrointestinal tract carcinoma. REAL-2, a phase III randomized controlled study from the United Kingdom, evaluated capecitabine (X), an oral fluoropyrimidine, and oxaliplatin (O), a fourth-generation platinum compound, as alternatives to infusional 5-fluorouracil (F) and cisplatin (C), respectively. In a 2 × 2 design, 1002 patients with advanced or metastatic gastric, GEJ, and esophageal adenocarcinomas were randomly assigned into four arms of chemotherapy. Epirubicin (E) plus CF (ECF), ECX, EOF, or EOX were the four chemotherapy regimens. The primary endpoint was no inferiority in OS for the triplet therapies containing X compared with F, and for those containing O compared with C. In the capecitabine: 5-fluorouracil comparison, the HR for death was 0.86 (95% CI, 0.80-0.99); in the oxaliplatin:cisplatin comparison, the HR was 0.92 (95% CI, 0.80-1.10). For ECF, ECX, EOF, and EOX, the OS durations and 1-year survival rates were 9.9, 9.9, 9.3, and 11.2 months and 37.7%, 40.8%,

40.4%, and 46.8%, respectively (231). The study demonstrated that the efficacy of capecitabine and 5-fluorouracil as well as oxaliplatin and cisplatin was equivalent.

Oxaliplatin's equivalency to cisplatin was further confirmed in another randomized study from Asia. Two hundred twenty therapy-naïve patients with advanced or metastatic gastric and GEJ were randomly assigned to receive infusional 5-fluorouracil and leucovorin with oxaliplatin (FLO) or cisplatin (FLP). The primary endpoint was PFS duration. A trend toward a longer median PFS was found for FLO versus FLP (5.8 versus 3.9 months; $p = .077$), but no significant difference was found in the median OS duration (10.7 versus 8.8 months). FLO was associated with significantly less anemia (54 versus 72%), nausea (53 versus 70%), vomiting (31 versus 52%), renal toxicity (11 versus 34%), thromboembolic events (0.9 versus 7.8%), and serious adverse events related to treatment (9 versus 19%). FLP was associated with significantly less peripheral neuropathy (22 versus 63%). In patients older than 65 years, treatment with FLO resulted in a significantly superior ORR (41.3 versus 16.7%; $p = .012$) and longer time to treatment failure (5.4 versus 2.3 months; $p < .001$), PFS (6.0 versus 3.1 months; $p = .029$), and median OS (13.9 versus 7.2 months; $p < .001$) durations than did FLP (248). Similarly, capecitabine's noninferiority to 5-fluorouracil was confirmed in another phase III randomized study from Asia. In 2009 Kang et al. (249) reported the results of a phase III randomized controlled trial involving 316 patients with advanced and metastatic gastric cancer. The goal was to demonstrate that capecitabine and cisplatin (XP) were not inferior to 5-fluorouracil and cisplatin (FP), with PFS duration as primary endpoint. The median PFS durations of XP (N = 139) and FP (N = 137) were 5.6 versus 5.0 months (equivalent HR, 0.81; $p < 0.001$), and the median OS durations were 10.5 versus 9.3 months (equivalent HR = 0.85; $p = .008$). The most common treatment-related grades 3 and 4 adverse events in XP versus FP patients were neutropenia (16 versus 19%), vomiting (7 versus 8%), and stomatitis (2 versus 6%) (249).

A novel cytotoxic oral fluoropyrimidine known as 1 M tegafur-0.4 M 5-chloro-2,4-dihydroxypyridine-1 M potassium oxonate (S-1) was developed in Japan in the mid-1990s. S-1 is an oral formulation of the following components in a 1:0.4:1 ratio: tegafur, the prodrug for 5-fluorouracil; gimeracil (5-choloro-2,4-dihydroxypyridine), an inhibitor of dihydropyrimidine dehydrogenase that prevents its degradation in the gastrointestinal tract and prolongs its half-life; and potassium oxonate (oteracil), a specific inhibitor of orotate phosphoribosyl transferase that phosphorylates 5-fluorouracil in the intestines (250). Phosphorylation of 5-fluorouracil is thought to be the main cause of treatment-related diarrhea. The first level 1 evidence for S-1's antitumor efficacy in gastric cancer came from the results of the Japanese Clinical Oncology Group (JCOG) 9912 study. Seven hundred and four advanced or metastatic gastric cancer patients from 34 institutions in Japan were randomly assigned to receive infusional 5-fluorouracil (ci5FU) (N = 234), irinotecan plus cisplatin (IP) (N = 236), or 40 mg/m^2 twice a day (bid) of S-1 (N = 234), 4 weeks on and 2 weeks off. The primary endpoint was noninferiority of OS. The median OS durations were 10.8, 12.3, and 11.4 months, respectively, for infusional 5FU, IP, and S-1. Using infusional 5FU as the control, the HRs of IP and S-1 were 0.85 (95% CI, 0.70-1.04; $p = .0552$) and 0.83, respectively (95% CI, 0.68-1.01; $p = .0005$). S-1 was shown to be noninferior to ci5FU for gastric cancer. Interestingly, the ORR for IP was higher (38%) than that of single-agent infusional 5FU (9%) and S-1 (28%), but it did not translate into a longer OS duration (251). After the success of JCOG 9912, the S-1 plus cisplatin versus S-1 alone for first-line treatment of advanced gastric cancer (SPIRITS trial) study was conducted, in which 298 patients with advanced gastric cancers were randomly assigned to receive either S-1 plus cisplatin (SP, N = 148) or S-1 alone (N = 150). The primary endpoint was OS duration. The ORRs for SP and S-1 were 54% and 31%, with median PFS durations of 6.0 and 4.0 months, respectively ($p < .0001$). The median OS duration was significantly longer in patients treated with SP than in those on S-1 alone (13.0 versus 11.0 months; HR, 0.77; $p = .04$). More grades 3 and 4 adverse events, including leukopenia, neutropenia, anemia, nausea, and anorexia, were observed in the SP group than in the S-1 group (252). Results from the SPIRITS study established SP as frontline chemotherapy for advanced and metastatic gastric cancer in Japan. IRIS, a subsequent study of irinotecan and S-1, was not as successful as the SPIRITS study in meeting its goal. In this phase III randomized controlled trial, 315 advanced or metastatic gastric cancer patients were assigned to receive irinotecan and S-1 (IRIS, N = 160) or S-1 alone (N = 155). The primary endpoint was OS duration. At a median follow-up duration of 1.5 years, Imamura et al. (253) presented the results of this trial at the 2009 American Society of Clinical Oncology (ASCO) Gastrointestinal Cancers Symposium. The ORR was higher for IRIS than for S-1 (42 versus 27%, $p = .035$). However, no statistically significant survival difference was found; the 1-year OS rates were 52 versus 45%, and the median OS durations were 12.8 versus 10.5 months (HR, 0.86; $p = .23$). For IRIS versus S-1 alone, the most

common grades 3 and 4 toxicities were neutropenia (11 versus 27%), diarrhea (6 versus 16%), anorexia (19 versus 17%), nausea (6 versus 7%), and vomiting (2 versus 3%) (253). Despite being well tolerated and having a higher ORR, the combination of irinotecan and S-1 did not demonstrate statistically significant superiority to S-1 alone in OS.

In the process of introducing S-1 into the Western countries, S-1's dosage and tolerability were meticulously evaluated in phases I and II studies. The recommended dosage for phase III study was 25 mg/m^2 twice a day, 3 weeks on and 1 week off, which is significantly lower than that for S-1 (80 mg/m^2 bid, 4 weeks and 2 weeks off), administered to Japanese patients in both SPIRITS and IRIS studies. FLAGS (First-Line Advanced Gastric Cancer Study) was a multicenter, international randomized study comparing CF with cisplatin plus S-1 (CS) as first-line therapy in 1029 patients with advanced or metastatic gastric adenocarcinoma. The primary endpoint was OS. Patients were randomly assigned to receive either CS (N = 521) or CF (N = 508). The median OS durations for CS versus CF were 8.6 versus 7.9 months, respectively (HR, 0.92; 95% CI, 0.80-1.05 months; $p = .1983$). Statistically, significantly fewer grades 3 and 4 adverse events were found for CS versus CF, including neutropenia (19 versus 40%), febrile neutropenia (2 versus 7%), and stomatitis (1 versus 14%). Treatment-related deaths occurred in 2.5% of patients in the CS arm versus 4.9% in the CF arm ($p < .05$) (254). The results of FLAGS have not been published, but the preliminary data, presented at both the 2009 ASCO annual meeting and the ASCO 2009 Gastrointestinal Cancers Symposium, demonstrated that although S-1 plus cisplatin did not result in a significantly longer OS duration, they may be less toxic than the CF reference regimen.

Until 2009, the standard of care for advanced and metastatic upper gastrointestinal carcinoma is to treat patients with cytotoxic chemotherapy regimens, which included CF, DCF, or ECF. These regimens could be modified based on findings of phase III randomized control studies, demonstrating that efficacy of capecitabine and oxaliplatin was not inferior to that of 5-fluorouracil and cisplatin. Furthermore, results from other phase III studies also suggested that modifications to the original every-3-week DCF are possible, preserved efficacy, and much less toxicity. Arbeitsgemeinschaft Internische Onkologie (AIO) weekly infusional 5-fluorouracil plus leucovorin and irinotecan combination has been validated as a nonplatinum alternative to CF. Many phase II single-arm studies have provided level 2 evidence for several chemotherapy doublets, including paclitaxel plus carboplatin (255), docetaxel plus capecitabine (242), docetaxel plus cisplatin (241), docetaxel plus oxaliplatin (256), docetaxel plus irinotecan (257), and IP (244). Colorectal cancer chemotherapy regimens (258-260) also are common in clinical practices with supporting phase II studies. ORR of most of these regimens had been reported to be approximately greater than 60%, with median survival duration of 15 months. However, these impressive outcomes were either not maintained or have not been evaluated in randomized studies.

The indications for and benefits of second-line chemotherapy for advanced or metastatic upper gastrointestinal carcinoma remain unclear. Several studies have reported lower ORRs and increased toxicity for patients receiving second-line therapy compared with those therapy-naïve patients being treated with first-line chemotherapy. Although salvage chemotherapy has yet to demonstrate survival benefits, it is common in most oncology practice to offer further chemotherapy after first-line treatment failure. This is partly because both patients and physicians have difficulty accepting only BSC, without the possibility of systemic anticancer effects. In general, in patients with newly diagnosed advanced or metastatic upper gastrointestinal cancers, chemotherapy could be used to prolong survival and improve quality of life (QOL). While the question of whether chemotherapy beyond first line has clinically relevant benefit remained unaddressed, it is even more important that any second-line or salvage chemotherapy regimens should at least satisfy the criteria of being tolerable with beneficial effects on QOL. Currently, evidence supporting various salvage chemotherapy regimens in patients with advanced upper gastrointestinal carcinoma is from findings of single-arm phase II studies of very selected groups of patients. After failing first-line chemotherapy, not all patients are candidates for second-line or salvage chemotherapy. Patient selection and personalized treatment recommendation based on case-by-case process will be very important in ensuring relevant clinical outcomes for those receiving additional chemotherapy after their gastric, GEJ, esophageal cancers failed first-line chemotherapy. Therefore, a thorough understanding of disease-specific prognostic and predictive factors will assist with the identification of a subset of patients where salvage chemotherapy may be meaningful.

Ji et al. (261) performed a retrospective analysis of second-line treatment in 1455 patients. Seven hundred twenty-five (50%) patients received second-line chemotherapy after first-line treatment failure. The ORR with second-line chemotherapy was 16% (95%

CI, 13-19%). Patients with an ECOG performance status ≥ 2 were significantly less likely to experience a response to second-line chemotherapy (9 versus 21%; $p = .016$). Other factors associated with lack of optimal response were the presence of ascites (8 versus 20%; $p = .018$) and bone marrow involvement (0 versus 20%; $p = .038$). The response rate was not significantly influenced by age, sex, weight loss, baseline laboratory parameters, bone or liver metastases, prior response to first-line chemotherapy, or treatment-free interval. Furthermore, no relevant median OS difference was found between patients who received single-agent (6.8 months; 95% CI, 5.1-8.4 months) and combination regimens (6.7 months; 95% CI, 5.7-7.6 months; $p = .373$). The median OS duration was significantly longer in patients receiving third-line chemotherapy (11.5 months; 95% CI, 10.8-12.1 months) than in those who were not treated further (4.9 months; 95% CI, 4.5-5.4 months; $p < .001$). The median PFS duration was 2.9 months (95% CI, 2.6-3.3 months), and the median OS duration was 6.7 months (95% CI, 5.8-7.5 months). In a univariate model, the OS duration was significantly shorter for patients with a low baseline hemoglobin level, ascites, and poor performance. However, in a multivariate Cox regression analysis, only hemoglobin <9.8 g/L (HR, 0.74; 95% CI, 0.61-0.90 g/L) and ECOG performance status >2 (HR, 0.66; 95% CI, 0.52-0.83) were independent negative prognostic factors of OS duration (261). In another retrospective analysis of 1080 chemotherapy-naïve patients with gastroesophageal cancer, Chau et al. (262) reported the prognostic significance of baseline factors. Poor performance status, metastasis to the liver and peritoneum, and high alkaline phosphatase were significantly predictive of poor survival. Similarly, a retrospective analysis of 1455 patients identified no previous gastrectomy, low albumin level, high alkaline phosphatase level, bone metastasis, ascites, and poor performance status to be poor prognostic factors (263). In British Columbia, only weekly cisplatin and 5-fluorouracil is supported as first-line chemotherapy for patients with advanced or metastatic gastroesophageal cancers. All other regimens, including second-line chemotherapy, require Compassionate Access Program approval for public funding.

Survival outcomes of 85 patients with advanced or metastatic gastroesophageal cancer (53 gastric, 32 esophageal, and 10 GEJ), collected from 1999 to 2006, who experienced progression on first-line therapy, were analyzed to determine the benefit of getting salvage chemotherapy. The median OS durations of all patients, patients who had not undergone chemotherapy, and patients who had undergone chemotherapy were 9.7 (95% CI, 6.2-13.1), 11.6 (95% CI, 8.4-14.9), and 5.2 months (95% CI, 2.4-7.9 months), respectively (264). The response rates to salvage therapy in patients with advanced or metastatic upper gastrointestinal cancers are predominantly based on the results of phase II studies. The ORRs, median TTPs, and median OS durations for second-line chemotherapy are 11 to 32%, 2.5 to 4.5 months, and 5.4 to 9.3 months, respectively (265). In addition, the data suggest that patients who experience a response to second-line therapy consistently survive longer than those who do not experience a response, and perhaps more importantly, they may experience symptomatic benefits (264). Many experts agree that the lack of progress in improving the OS duration may be partly due to the lack of more effective salvage therapy.

Only one-third to one-half of patients with advanced gastroesophageal cancers can undergo second-line treatment (226). Second-line or salvage chemotherapy regimens have very narrow therapeutic index, significant therapy-related side effects and modest clinically relevant benefit. Therefore, to improve the OS of advanced upper gastrointestinal cancer patients, more effective and less toxic salvage therapies are needed. Patient selection is another important barrier to overcome. The results of the retrospective studies described above are a starting point for isolating baseline clinical selection criteria. Patients with low hemoglobin level (261,266) and poor performance status (261,264) will do poorly on salvage chemotherapy. Patient selection may become more accurate with the use of molecular predictive and prognostic markers such as epidermal growth factor receptor (EGFR) expression (267), vascular endothelial growth factor (VEGF) expression (268), her2neu amplification (269), insulin-like growth factor type 1 receptor (IGF-1R) expression (270), and excision repair cross-complementing gene 1 *(ERCC-1)* expression (270). Furthermore, the results of randomized controlled studies had not been able to elucidate on which regimens are best for second-line chemotherapy. From their retrospective analysis, Ji et al. (261) suggested that single-agent chemotherapy results in a similar survival outcome to that of combination chemotherapy. Additionally, the choice of second-line agent depends on the first-line treatment. Single-agent chemotherapy should be considered for patients who would benefit from additional therapy. Prospective clinical trials of the association between clinical outcomes and known prognostic clinical factors are warranted. Emerging scientific findings and an improved molecular knowledge of disease will further guide clinicians toward personalized management of advanced gastric, GEJ, and esophageal cancers.

Targeted Therapy

At diagnosis, most patients in non-Asian countries have advanced stage gastric, GEJ, or esophageal cancers. Chemotherapy is the standard therapeutic approach for these patients. Independent studies have demonstrated that systemic chemotherapy results in better survival outcomes for metastatic gastroesophageal cancers than does BSC. Various chemotherapy regimens have resulted in improved survival durations, from approximately 6 to 14 months, and novel therapies are being developed to improve effectiveness and reduce toxicity. Globally, advancements in our molecular and genetic understanding of cancers have translated into improved OS for patients. Specifically, agents that target VEGF and VEGFR have successfully transformed the care and survival of colorectal cancer patients. Unfortunately, improvements for metastatic gastric, GEJ, or esophageal cancer patients are modest at best; these patients' overall prognosis remains dismal, unchanged since 1973 (271).

Therapies that can result in additive survival outcome for patients with upper gastrointestinal carcinoma must satisfy two key criteria: enhanced efficacy and minimal toxicity profile. These criteria can be satisfied through gaining deeper and better understanding of the molecular pathogenesis of this disease and developing smarter and more specific cancer therapies. Whether as a single agent or in combination with chemotherapy, biologically targeted agents offer hope. The Food and Drug Administration has approved 17 new targeted therapies since 2000. However, none of them have been approved for the treatment of gastric, GEJ, or esophageal carcinomas. With the positive results of the recent ToGA study, the race is on to identify more targeted agents to manage patients with upper gastrointestinal cancers. Most definitely, results of ongoing phase III clinical trials will help to further define the benefits of and indications for these novel agents.

A better understanding of the molecular pathogenesis of gastroesophageal cancers had led to the identification of many aberrantly expressed genes that are important in gastric, GEJ, or esophageal tumorigenesis. Several developed inhibitors of different but vital cancer-promoting processes are already available for other cancers or have been developed but still looking for therapeutic indications: inhibitors to common cellular interactions or processes such as (1) the cell surface receptor, (2) the cell cycle, (3) downstream signaling pathways, (4) epigenetics, and (5) microenvironment modulation.

Judging from the early processes of successfully developed targeted agents in solid tumors, the most popular approach to cancer drug development had been to target cancer growth factors and their cell surface receptors. Aberrant signal transduction through an activated growth factor receptor is a common feature of many solid tumor types. Simply stated, blocking growth receptors inhibits tumor growth and cellular activity. Many biological agents are available that have been engineered to target these receptors to selectively attack tumor cells. These agents may be monoclonal antibodies that bind and block growth factor receptors directly or small molecular tyrosine kinase inhibitors that block many or just one specific signal transduction that is downstream of and activated by growth factors. Commonly recognized growth factors and receptors are epidermal growth factor and its receptor (EGF and EGFR), vascular endothelial growth factor and its receptor (VEGF and VEGFR), platelet-derived growth factor and its receptor (PDGF and PDGFR), insulin growth factor 1 receptor (IGF-1R), and human epidermal growth factor receptor 2 (HER2). The monoclonal antibodies against VEGF (bevacizumab), EGFR (cetuximab, panitumumab), and HER2 (trastuzumab) already have FDA approval and indications in cancers.

Some of the existing targeted agents have already demonstrated promising preclinical and early clinical antitumor activity in gastric, GEJ, or esophageal carcinomas. No targeted agents have been approved yet for the management of advanced cancers of the stomach, GEJ, or esophagus. Clinical research in upper gastroesophageal cancers had been very active. Table 17-10 lists ongoing randomized studies.

Bevacizumab is a humanized monoclonal antibody against VEGF-A. Shah et al. (272) reported the results of the first phase II study using bevacizumab. Forty-seven patients with metastatic or unresectable gastric or GEJ adenocarcinoma were treated with bevacizumab and irinotecan plus cisplatin (IP) on days 1 and 8, every 21 days. The primary goal was to demonstrate a 50% improvement in TTP over historical values (pooled from three phase II studies [244], TTP ranged 4.2-5.8 months). With a median follow-up of 12.2 months, patients

| TABLE 17-10 | FRONTLINE TARGETED THERAPY: ONGOING PHASE II/III RANDOMIZED CONTROL CLINICAL TRIALS IN ADVANCED/METASTATIC GASTRIC, GASTROESOPHAGEAL JUNCTION, AND ESOPHAGEAL CANCERS |

FRONTLINE CHEMOTHERAPY WITH TARGETED AGENTS				
Trial	*N*	*Experimental Arm*	*Control Arm*	*Status*
USA/Genetech AVAGAST	760	XP + bevacizumab (VEGFR)	XP	Completed
Australia/AGITG MAX trial	333	X + bevacizumab	X	Completed
UK/EMD Serano/MRC MATRIX EG	72	ECX + matuzumab (EGFR)	ECX	Completed
International/Merck EXPAND	870	XP + cetuximab (EGFR)	XP	Accruing
UK/MRC REAL 3	730	EOX + panitumumab (EGFR)	EOX	Accruing
International/GSK LOGiC	410	CapeOx + lapatinib (Her2neu/EGFR)	CapeOx	Accruing
China/Hoffman ML22367	200	XP + bevacizumab (VEGFR)	XP	Accruing
USA/USOnc/ImClone 06063	150	DO + cetuximab (EGFR)	DO	Accruing
International/Amgen 20060317	136	ECX + AMG102 (HGF/SF)	ECX	Accruing
NYCC-09-0356	116	FOLFOX + GDC0449 (SHH)	FOLFOX	Accruing
Rosewell/RPCI-I-106207	60	Docetaxel + vandetanib (VEGFR/EGFR)	Docetaxel	Accruing

AVAGAST, Avastin in Gastric Cancer Study; CapeOx, capecitabine, oxaliplatin; DO, docetaxel, oxaliplatin; ECX, epirubicin, cisplatin, capecitabine; EOX, epirubicin, oxaliplatin, capecitabine; EXPAND, Erbitux in Combination With Xeloda and Cisplatin in Advanced Esophagogastric Cancer; FOLFOX, folinic acid, 5-fluorouracil, oxaliplatin; LOGiC, Lapatinib Optimization Study in ErbB2 (Her2) Positive Gastric Cancer; MATRIX EG, MATuxumab, Randomized With Xeloda Epirubicin in Gastric Cancer; MAX, methotrexate, avastin, capecitabine; MRC, Medical Research Council; REAL, randomized evaluation of aloxi; SHH, sonic hedge hog; X, capecitabine; XP, capecitabine, cisplatin.

treated with IP plus bevacizumab had an 8.3 month median TTP (95% CI, 5.5-9.9 months). In 34 patients with measurable disease, the ORR was 65% (95% CI, 46-80%), and the median OS duration was 12.3 months (95% CI, 11.3-17.2 months). Grades 3 and 4 toxicities included hypertension (28%), thromboembolic events (25%), gastric perforation (6%), and myocardial infarction (2%). The study met its goal of demonstrating that TTP improved over that of the historical control by 75%, although it was criticized for using historical controls pooled from several different small phase II studies. Many available standard-of-care first-line chemotherapy regimens exist, including ECF or DCF and their derivatives. Though commonly used, IP had not been recognized as level 1 evidence-based first-line chemotherapy regimen for patients with advanced gastric, GEJ, or esophageal carcinomas. Therefore, combining bevacizumab with IP limited further development of this regimen. After the positive results of this study, the same investigators pursued their objective to assess the role of bevacizumab by combining it with docetaxel, cisplatin, plus 5-fluorouracil (DCF), a regimen that had been recognized as level 1 evidence-based chemotherapy for treating therapy-naïve patients with advanced gastric or GEJ carcinoma (239). DCF was administered every 14 days, with a 50% dose reduction in the original regimen. Kelsen et al. (273) reported that the combination of bevacizumab and a 50% reduction in DCF resulted in an ORR rate of 67% and PFS and median OS durations of 6.0 and 16.2 months, respectively. However, notable bevacizumab-related toxicities were observed among 39 patients treated, including perforation (3%), bleeding (3%), and thromboembolism (31%). No grade 3 or 4 hypertension or proteinuria was observed. The results of ongoing phase III randomized studies are expected to clarify the benefits of bevacizumab. AVAGAST (Avastin in Gastric Cancer Study) has completed its accrual of 760 patients. The study is designed to compare capecitabine plus cisplatin (XP) alone with XP plus bevacizumab. The Australian MAX study plans to accrue 333 patients and randomly assign them to one of three treatment arms (capecitabine alone, capecitabine plus bevacizumab, or capecitabine plus methotrexate and bevacizumab).

EGFR is commonly overexpressed in many human tumors, including gastrointestinal tract tumors. Mutations in the tyrosine kinase domain of the EGFR gene have been found to be correlated with the response to therapies such as erlotinib or gefitinib. In 2006, Kimura et al. (274) evaluated EGFR mutations in 11 esophageal, 6 gastric, and 12 colorectal cancer cell lines. They only observed one missense mutation and 10 single

nucleotide polymorphisms in a gastric and esophageal cancer cell lines, suggesting that mutations in the tyrosine kinase domain of the EGFR gene are rare. Another word, erlotinib and gefitinib are unlikely to be effective as single-drug therapies for gastroesophageal cancers because of the rarity of EGFR mutation among upper gastrointestinal carcinoma. This information may help to explain the negative results of Southwestern Oncology Group (SWOG) 0127 (275). Among 69 (43 GEJ and 26 gastric) therapy naïve-patients with metastatic GEJ or gastric AC who were treated with erlotinib, the ORR was 9% (PR were only observed in GEJ patients). Similarly, low activity was found for gefitinib. In Rojo et al. (276) phase II study of gefitinib (250 mg/day or 500 mg/day) in 75 advanced gastric cancer patients, there was no CR or PR, and 18% had SD.

Cetuximab is a chimeric (mouse-human) monoclonal antibody that inhibits EGFR. The combination of irinotecan, infusional 5-fluorouracil, leucovorin plus cetuximab has been reported to result in high response and disease control rates. In particular, the FOLCETUX study demonstrated that adding cetuximab to the FOLFIRI (folnic acid, 5-fluorouracil, irinotecan) regimen led to increased survival (TTP 8 months, OS 16 months) in 38 untreated patients with advanced or metastatic gastric or GEJ adenocarcinoma. The treatment was delivered for a maximum of 24 weeks, followed by cetuximab alone that was administered to patients who had experienced a CR, PR, or SD. Consequently, the ORR was 44%, with a CR in 4 patients and a PR in 11 patients. Sixteen patients had SD (277). Cetuximab has been combined with various chemotherapy regimens to treat patients with metastatic gastric, GEJ, or esophageal cancers. In addition to being combined with FOLFIRI, it was added to FUFOX, resulting in an ORR of 66% (CR, 9%; PR, 57%) and TTP and OS durations of 7.6 and 9.5 months, respectively (278). Among all cetuximab studies with published results, only one was a randomized phase II study; it compared the ORR between CF alone and CF plus cetuximab. Fifty-four chemotherapy-naïve patients were randomly assigned to receive CF or CF plus cetuximab. The primary endpoint was ORR. Lorenzen et al. (216) reported ORRs of 13% and 19% for CF and CF plus cetuximab, respectively, with PFS durations of 3.6 and 5.9 months, respectively. The combination of cetuximab and chemotherapy was well tolerated, resulting in high response rates and disease control among patients with advanced and metastatic gastric and GEJ adenocarcinoma. However, cetuximab did not result in a superior response rate. At present, cetuximab is being evaluated in three ongoing phase III randomized control studies. EXPAND

(Erbitux in Combination With Xeloda and Cisplatin in Advanced Esophagogastric Cancer) will enroll 870 patients and randomly assign them to capecitabine plus cisplatin (XP) alone or XP plus cetuximab. Another study of 150 patients will compare the combination of docetaxel and oxaliplatin, with or without cetuximab. The third phase III randomized trial is being conducted by the Cancer and Leukemia Group B (CALGB). Three recognized active chemotherapy regimens for advanced and metastatic gastric, GEJ, and esophageal carcinomas are epirubicin ECF, IP, and FOLFIRI. In a randomized controlled phase II study, CALGB-C80403 will compare the ORRs of cetuximab (plus these three regimens). The premise is that the most active regimen will be evaluated in the next Intergroup study of resectable disease. Updated results are planned to be presented at 2010 ASCO. Other monoclonal antibodies against EGFR are also already being evaluated for patients with upper gastrointestinal cancers, and these clinical studies are already in phase II or III. The REAL-3 (Randomized Trial of EOC ± Panitumumab for Advanced and Locally Advanced Esophagogastric Cancer) is a phase III randomized controlled trial; the study plan to accrue 730 therapy-naïve patients with advanced or metastatic gastric, GEJ, and esophageal adenocarcinomas, and randomly assign them to be treated with EOX or EOX plus panitumumab. In the MATRIX (MATuxumab, Randomized with Xeloda Epirubicin in Gastric Cancer), designed as a phase II randomized controlled study to evaluate the efficacy of matuzumab in therapy-naïve patients with advanced upper gastroesophageal carcinoma, 72 patients will be accrued and randomly assigned to ECX or ECX plus matuzumab.

For patients with advanced gastric and GEJ adenocarcinoma, the most exciting and important development of 2009 may be the introduction of the first targeted agent, along with its specific predictive marker for molecularly selecting patients who would be benefiting from it. HER2 (c-erbB-2) is a transmembrane tyrosine kinase receptor and a member for the human EGFR (HER) family (HER-1, 2, 3, and 4). Each receptor has an extracellular domain at which ligand-binding occurs, α-helical transmembrane segment, and an intracellular protein tyrosine kinase domain. Receptor dimerization is essential for HER2 function and signaling activity. Dimerization can occur between two different HER receptors (heterodimerization) or two molecules of the same receptor (homodimerization). After receptor dimerization, activation of the tyrosine kinase portion of the complex occurs. Phosphorylation allows the recruitment and activation of downstream proteins and initiation of the signaling cascade. HER2 functions as an oncogene. Gene amplification induces protein overexpression in cell membranes and regulates signal transduction in cellular processes, including proliferation, differentiation, and cell survival. Aberrant HER2 expression or function has been implicated in gastric carcinogenesis (279).

Trastuzumab is a recombinant humanized anti-HER2 monoclonal antibody directed against the HER2 extracellular domain. Trastuzumab's exact mechanism of action is not completely understood; however, some actions have been postulated (280), including (1) blocking HER2 receptor cleavage and inhibiting dimerization, consequently reducing HER2 signaling; (2) increasing receptor destruction by endocytosis by inducing HER2 downregulation and subsequent degradation in HER2 overexpressing cancer cells; (3) inhibiting intracellular signaling pathways such as phosphoinositide 3-kinase (PI3K) that have been linked to cellular functions such as cell growth, proliferation, differentiation, motility, survival, and intracellular trafficking; (4) producing antiangiogenesis effects by reducing VEGF and indirectly modulating proangiogenic and antiangiogenic factors; (5) inducing the cyclin-dependent kinase (CDK) inhibitor p27Kip1, resulting in cellular proliferation arrest in G1 phase; and (6) increasing tumor infiltration by lymphoid cells and modulation of antibody-dependent cell-mediated cytotoxicity, leading to cytostatic and cytotoxic activity. Trastuzumab has been available since 1998, but mainly for breast cancer treatment. The reported rates of HER2/ErbB2 overexpression and amplification in gastric cancer vary widely (6-45%) because of small sample sizes and methodologic differences among studies (281-283). In perhaps the largest dataset—3807 advanced gastric cancer samples—Bang et al. (284) reported an HER2 positivity rate of 22.1%. The investigators used an HER2-scoring system adapted from breast cancer protocols in which immunohistochemical analysis 3+ or fluorescence in situ hybridization positive was considered HER2 positive. The immunohistochemical analysis and fluorescence in situ hybridization concordance was 87.5%. The HER2 positivity rate was similar between Europe (23.6%) and Asia (23.5%). HER2 positivity rates were higher in GEJ than in gastric cancer (33.2 versus 20.9%; $p < .001$) and higher in intestinal than in diffuse or mixed cancer (32.2 versus 6.1%/20.4%; $p < .001$).

The ToGA study was designed to compare chemotherapy (5-fluorouracil or capecitabine plus cisplatin) alone versus chemotherapy and trastuzumab for 6 months in patients with HER2-positive advanced or metastatic GEJ or gastric adenocarcinoma. Trastuzumab was given until disease progression occurred. An interim analysis was planned for when 75% of patients enrolled onto the study had died and the median follow-up duration was 17.1 months. Tumors from 3807 patients were centrally tested for HER2 status; 594 HER2-positive patients were identified and randomly assigned 1:1 to the two treatment arms. The median OS duration was significantly longer in the trastuzumab plus chemotherapy group than in the chemotherapy alone group (13.5 versus 11.1 months; HR, 0.74; 95% CI, 0.60-0.91; $p = .0048$), with ORRs of 47.3% and 34.5%, respectively ($p = .0017$). The safety profiles were similar, with no unexpected adverse events. No difference was found in the rate of symptomatic congestive heart failure between the two arms. The asymptomatic left ventricular ejection fraction decreases were 4.6% and 1.1% for trastuzumab plus chemotherapy and chemotherapy alone, respectively (219). The results of this practice-changing study were presented at the 2009 ASCO annual meeting.

Several protein kinase families orchestrate the complex events that drive the cell cycle, and their activity is frequently deregulated in hyperproliferative cancer cells. Aberrant genes in cancer result from mutations or altered levels or patterns of expression. Such changes contribute to the deregulation of cell cycle kinases, which is often associated with the irregular division and uncontrolled proliferation of cancer cells. Gene products that regulate the key cell cycle machinery include the cyclin-dependent kinases (CDKs), which have been established as master regulators of cell proliferation; protein kinases, which coordinate the cellular response to DNA damage; and protein kinases, which regulate mitosis. An example of a protein kinase in cell cycle is the class of aurora kinases. Aurora kinases (A, B, and C) are serine/threonine kinases that regulate mitotic progression and control centromere maturation, separation, mitotic entry, spindle formation, and chromosome alignment. Overexpression of aurora kinase A results in chromosomal instability in gastric cancer via the AKT/hdm2 pathway (285). Furthermore, aurora kinase A overexpression prevents the release of cytochrome C from mitochondria, which leads to caspase inactivation and thus protects cells from apoptosis (286). The polo-like kinases (PLKs) are a family of four serine/threonine kinases that are involved in the signal transduction pathway that is essential for mitotic processes such as centrosome maturation and chromosome segregation. PLK-1 is the most common isoform overexpressed in gastric cancer and is associated with lymph node metastasis and a diffuse growth pattern (287). Cyclin-dependent kinases comprise a group of protein kinases (CDK1-CDK9) that are involved in cell cycle regulation via the retinoblastoma product (the tumor suppressor gene Rb).

Inactivation of the Rb pathway results from overexpression or amplification of CDKs or downregulation of negative factors such as endogenous CDK inhibitors or Rb mutations. In gastroesophageal cancers, as well as other cancers, this pathway is deregulated, resulting in a disbursed G1 to S phase of the cell cycle (288). Flavopiridol is a synthetic flavonoid that strongly inhibits CDKs, including CDK-1, -2, -4, and -7, and hypophosphorylates Rb. The results of a phase II study evaluating flavopiridol in 16 patients with advanced gastric cancer showed that it had no activity, but it did result in moderate toxicity (289). Several inhibitors of aurora kinase-A and PLK-1 are in currently in preclinical development.

The most important and relevant downstream signaling pathways in gastroesophageal cancer are heat shock protein 90 (hsp90), the ubiquitin-proteosome pathway, and the PI3K/Akt/mTOR pathway. Hsp90 is a highly expressed molecular chaperone protein capable of sensing cellular stress. It mediates the maturation and stability of a set of cancer-associated proteins, collectively referred to as "clients," including steroid receptors, EGFR family members, IGFR, MET, Raf-1, AKT, Bcr-abl, mutant p53, and CDK-4. These client proteins are involved in cell cycle regulation, signal transduction, and apoptosis, which are all commonly deregulated in cancer. Hsp90 is overexpressed in gastric cancer and is associated with lymph node metastasis (290). The ubiquitin-proteasome pathway plays an important role in the degradation of cellular proteins and cell cycle control. Disturbance in the degradation of such proteins has profound effects on tumor growth, cell proliferation, and apoptosis. Bortezomib, a boronic acid dipeptide derivative, is a potent inhibitor of proteasomes and has prominent effects in vivo and in vitro against several gastric cancer cell lines (291). In a phase II study reported by Ocean et al. (292) involving 44 therapy-naïve patients with advanced gastroesophageal cancer, 11 received irinotecan plus bortezomib and 12 received bortezomib alone. The study found ORRs of 9 versus 44%, PFS durations of 1.4 versus 1.9 months, and OS durations of 5.4 versus 4.1 months for bortezomib and irinotecan versus bortezomib alone, respectively; these results were reported at the 2007 ASCO Gastrointestinal Cancers Symposium.

Another important pathway involved in gastric carcinogenesis is the intracellular signaling machinery of the PI3K/AKT/mTOR downstream signaling pathway. Events resulting in mTOR activation involve PTEN function loss, PI3K mutation or amplification, AKT amplification, and AKT-associated mTOR-regulatory protein inactivation or mutation. A reduction in or abnormal level of PTEN expression indirectly stimulates PI3K activity, thereby contributing to oncogenesis. Abnormal PTEN expression is infrequent in gastric cancer (11%) and is related to tumor differentiation, infiltration depth, lymph node metastasis, tumor stage, and chemoresistance (293). Everolimus is an oral mTOR inhibitor that has shown activity in vitro and in vivo models of gastric cancer (294). The phase II study of 54 previously treated patients with advanced gastroesophageal cancer reported an SD rate of 55% and a PFS duration of 2.8 months for 10 mg/day everolimus (295). An ongoing international phase III study is comparing everolimus with placebo as second-line treatment for advanced and metastatic gastric and GEJ cancers.

Other ongoing clinical studies are listed in Table 17-10. Having demonstrated the benefit of combining anti-VEGF or anti-EGFR agents with chemotherapy, investigators are extending their goal into combination of targeted agents, particularly to evaluate the role of vandetanib in upper gastrointestinal cancers. Lapatinib is a dual inhibitor of the tyrosine kinase activity associated with two oncogenes, EGFR and her2neu. It is currently available for high-risk breast cancer patients. Ongoing is a phase II study evaluating the antitumor activity of lapatinib in therapy-naive patients with metastatic GEJ and gastric adenocarcinoma; eligible patients are required to have her2neu overexpression. Using a two-stage Simon's design, Iqbal et al. (296) found an ORR of 12% (PR 12%) and an SD rate of 20% in 43 HER2-positive patients treated with 1500 mg/day lapatinib. The OS and time to treatment failure durations were 2 and 5 months, respectively. The study did not reach predetermined ORR and was terminated; however, the study was able to demonstrate that when used as a single agent, lapatinib was well-tolerated, with some antitumor activity in patients with her2neu positive gastric or GEJ carcinoma. Ongoing now is the LOGiC (Lapatinib Optimization Study in ErbB2 [Her2] Positive Gastric Cancer) trial. This is an international randomized control study comparing capecitabine and oxaliplatin, with or without lapatinib, in 410 patients with her2neu-amplified metastatic or advanced gastric or GEJ adenocarcinoma. The advantage of targeting her2neu is that the status of her2neu expression in patients' cancer specimens can be used to select only patients who would benefit from therapy. However, only 22% of patients with gastric or GEJ adenocarcinoma demonstrate her2neu overexpression.

In summary, monoclonal antibodies against surface growth factors and growth factor receptors, such as bevacizumab (anti-VEGFA), cetuximab and panitumumab (anti-EGFR), and trastuzumab (anti-her2neu),

have been the most studied of all monoclonal antibodies. As discussed above, phase II studies of chemotherapy and bevacizumab or cetuximab in therapy-naïve patients demonstrated good tolerance, promising tumor activity, and durable disease control. Several phase III randomized studies of bevacizumab and cetuximab are ongoing. ToGA was the first phase III randomized study of combining chemotherapy with a targeted agent, where survival outcomes of patients with amplified her2neu metastatic gastroesophageal cancer, can be significantly improved with the addition of trastuzumab. This study was a milestone in gastroesophageal cancer clinical research because not only did it generate the first positive results for combining targeted agent with chemotherapy, but it also provided clinicians with a predictive marker for trastuzumab use. A better understanding of the molecular pathogenesis of gastroesophageal cancer will help to identify more targets for drug development. Many clinical trials are ongoing in metastatic gastroesophageal cancer to evaluate the role of targeted therapy—alone or combined with chemotherapy and as first-line or salvage treatment—and many more targeted agents are in development. More research and rational drug development will hopefully produce clinically meaningful therapy, personalized for each patient with gastric, GEJ, and esophageal cancers.

MD Anderson Approach to Advanced Gastric, Gastroesophageal Junction, and Esophageal Cancers

MD Anderson's approach to advanced or metastatic gastric, GEJ, and esophageal cancer is shown in Figure 17.15. Since the positive results of the ToGA trial were released, all patients with upper gastrointestinal carcinomas are tested for her2neu status at MD Anderson. Trastuzumab is considered as frontline therapy for patients with her2neu-positive disease (as determined by fluorescence in situ hybridization and immunohistochemical analysis). Because the 5-year survival rate of patients with advanced and metastatic gastroesophageal cancer is less than 5%, clinicians should take into consideration the risks and benefits of treatment. The goal in treating metastatic disease is to palliate symptoms to maintain patients' QOL. All patients at MD Anderson with advanced disease are assessed, and treatment recommendations will be individualized, depending on what is mostly likely to provide durable disease control for that patient. Standard-of-care chemotherapy as well as available clinical trials is offered. On the foundation of existing results from phase III randomized studies, standard-of-care chemotherapy regimens may be epirubicin-, taxane-, or irinotecan-based. S-1, a new oral fluoropyrimidine, is currently not available because it is not approved for use in the United States for upper gastrointestinal cancers. No clear survival benefit has been found for two- versus three-agent chemotherapy combinations, so chemotherapy regimen is chosen on the basis of its drug and regimen toxicity profile and the goals of therapy.

■ SUMMARY

Gastric cancer remains the second most common cause of cancer-related death worldwide. Its incidence in the United States is decreasing, resulting in a significant increase in distal esophageal and GEJ adenocarcinoma. In fact, according to the current version of the AJCC TNM staging manual, esophageal cancer now includes GEJ to 5 cm below the gastric cardia. The explanation for this epidemiologic phenomenon is unknown, because it is the putative cause of gastric cancer.

Two different pathogeneses of gastric cancer have been proposed, correlating to two histologic types, intestinal and diffuse. *H pylori* infection, chronic inflammatory state, cytokines, and host response, leading to acquisition of different genetic mutations and abnormalities, are the likely steps leading to intestinal-type invasive adenocarcinoma. On the other hand, diffuse-type gastric cancer may result from defective intracellular adhesion molecules, which is the consequence of loss of E-cadherin protein expression in gastric cancer.

Most patients with newly diagnosed gastric cancer have distant or locally advanced disease; hence, curative resection may not be possible. Because of mass-screening programs in high-risk countries such as Japan, more cases of EGC are being identified. Gastric cancer treatment is based on disease stage. EGC is cured by gastrectomy with lymphadenectomy, but similar outcomes have been reported for EMR/EMSD, which is gaining popularity in Japan and other Asian countries. Although surgery is the only chance for durable survival from gastric cancer, by itself, it is not adequate.

The results of two pivotal trials have shaped the current practice of resectable gastric cancer treatment. The INT116 study was the first to establish postoperative chemoradiotherapy as standard practice in the United States, whereas MRC ST02/MAGIC led to the use of perioperative chemotherapy as an alternative to radiotherapy. The MD Anderson approach to gastric cancer is summarized in Fig. 17-15. Despite data from Asia, postoperative chemotherapy alone after R0 resection is still considered investigational in the United States. Many ongoing large international clinical trials will likely answer some of the questions regarding the role of post- versus preoperative therapy.

Tables 17-4 and 17-6 list most of the ongoing randomized controlled clinical studies of locally advanced resectable gastroesophageal cancer (85,297). The Swiss SWS-SAKK-43/49 (Swiss Group for Clinical Research) trial will hopefully determine whether chemotherapy has a role as pre- or postoperative treatment. Meanwhile, the CLASSIC (Capecitabine and Oxaliplatin Adjuvant Study in Stomach Cancer) trial, sponsored by Sanofi-Aventis, may not only confirm the role of postoperative chemotherapy but also provide alternative chemotherapy regimens. The Korean ARTIST (Adjuvant RadioTherapy in gastric cancer and Systemic Therapy) trial will shed light on whether postoperative chemotherapy or chemoradiotherapy contributes to improved outcomes after surgery. Most interesting of all is the Dutch CRITICS study, which will compare postoperative chemoradiotherapy with perioperative chemotherapy.

Only 30 to 40% of patients with esophageal cancer have potentially resectable disease at presentation, and in many series only 5 to 20% of those undergoing surgery alone for clinically localized disease are alive at 3 to 5 years. The AJCC TNM staging system for esophageal cancer introduced several important changes: (1) disease extending ≤5 cm into the gastric cardia is now part of esophageal cancer staging, (2) the grade and number of lymph nodes involved are important in surgical staging, and (3) esophageal squamous cell carcinoma and adenocarcinoma have their own staging groups.

BE-dysplasia-carcinoma is the favored mechanism of esophageal tumorigenesis. Both LSBE and SSBE are treated by treating GERD, which is frequently associated with BE, with a proton pump inhibitor, careful surveillance and monitoring (the frequency of monitoring should be based on the presence of high-risk characteristics), and therapy for any HGD or invasive carcinoma. HGD and early esophageal carcinoma (EEC) are not common in the United States but are treated with esophagectomy or EMR/EMSD (commonly used in high-risk countries such as Japan and Korea). Although no large randomized controlled prospective studies have compared EMR/EMSD with primary esophagectomy, the results of a retrospective case-control series suggest that the initial curative resection rates are similar. Endoscopic therapy is most effective when used to treat small (<2 cm diameter) solitary, flat lesions that are confined to mucosa (T1a).

The use of EMR for diagnosis and therapy has been validated in many studies. EMR combined with PDT is the most popular treatment for patients with EEC who are not surgical candidates because of comorbidity or who decline surgery. However, surgery remains the best chance for durable survival for patients with locally advanced esophageal and GEJ carcinomas. After multidisciplinary evaluation, patients with locally advanced disease that is deemed potentially resectable should be considered for combined modality therapy. Evidence from several small randomized control studies and meta-analyses suggests that pre- or perioperative chemotherapy or preoperative chemoradiotherapy can improve surgical survival outcomes.

The results of the RTOG 85-01 trial established that chemoradiotherapy is more effective at reducing local recurrence and improving survival than radiotherapy alone. In addition, the results of the RTOG 94-05 trial established a standard dose of radiation of 50.4 Gy. Whether chemotherapy alone or chemoradiotherapy is used with surgery, therapy response and pathCR at surgery are predictive of survival outcome, independent of initial stage. Although it did not demonstrate improved survival with chemotherapy and chemoradiotherapy before surgery compared with chemotherapy alone before surgery, the POET study concluded that the addition of radiotherapy would improve pathCR rates and hence survival.

Cervical esophageal cancer staging should include bronchoscopy. Because surgery for cervical esophageal cancer includes removal of portions of several neck organs, including the voice box, most patients with localized disease undergo definitive chemoradiotherapy. The results of several randomized studies from Europe suggest that esophageal squamous cell carcinoma be treated differently than adenocarcinoma. However, until the final results of the CURE and CROSS studies are released, esophageal squamous cell carcinoma and adenocarcinoma treatments remain the same. The MD Anderson approach to treating gastric cancer is summarized in Fig. 17-15. The incidence of distal esophageal, GEJ, and proximal gastric adenocarcinoma was on a steep increase until recently. Stage for stage, esophageal cancer has a poorer prognosis than gastric cancer. Therefore, it is important that all patients with localized esophageal cancer be accurately staged and that management decisions be made by a multidisciplinary panel. Ongoing international and national randomized studies will further elucidate the role of adjuvant therapy in esophageal squamous cell carcinoma. Table 17-8 lists selected important ongoing phases II and III randomized controlled studies in resectable esophageal and GEJ carcinoma.

In summary, complete surgical resection of the tumor provides the best chance of cure; however, only a minority of patients present with resectable disease. The evidence-based approach should include perioperative chemotherapy or postoperative chemoradiotherapy for selected patients. All patients should be encouraged to enroll in clinical trials. Similarly, for resectable esophageal and GEJ cancers, adding preoperative and perioperative chemotherapy or preoperative chemoradiotherapy will enhance surgical outcomes and improve the pathCR rate.

The development of response or survival markers appears to be more advanced for esophageal cancer. PET after induction therapy and pathCR are solid predictors of response and prognosis, respectively. Tables 17-6 and 17-8 summarize important ongoing randomized phase II and III trials for resectable gastric, GEJ, and esophageal carcinomas. Advanced or metastatic gastric, GEJ, and esophageal cancers are treated similarly. More than 60% of patients who present with newly diagnosed gastric, GEJ, and esophageal cancers will have advanced unresectable or metastatic disease. Although a cure is not possible, systemic therapy can prolong survival compared with best supportive care. In recent decades, advances have been made in the treatment of gastric cancer, with expansion of effective agents in several cytotoxic classes—docetaxel, oxaliplatin, capecitabine, and S-1. So far, the only targeted therapy that has demonstrated a survival benefit is trastuzumab in patients with *her2neu*-positive disease.

Over the past 5 to 7 years, more chemotherapy combinations have been introduced for frontline treatment, including ECF and its derivatives (ECX, EOF, and EOX), DCF and its less toxic modifications (wDCX and wDX), FP and its modern derivatives (XP and FLO), and S-1 plus cisplatin. On the basis of the results of the FLAGS study, S-1 is not in use in Western countries. Unfortunately, despite the wealth of chemotherapy regimens, no clear consensus exists as to which chemotherapy regimen is best. Currently, patients in the United States are likely to undergo frontline therapy with platinum-, fluoropyrimidine-, or taxane-based chemotherapy regimens. Meanwhile, patients in Europe are likely to receive ECF or its derivatives and taxane-based chemotherapy regimens. Ongoing phase III clinical trials with cytotoxic chemotherapy for advanced or metastatic upper gastrointestinal carcinomas are listed in Table 17-11. The positive results of the ToGA trial has likely transformed frontline therapy for patients with *her2neu*-positive metastatic gastric, GEJ, and esophageal cancers. However, only 20% of gastric, GEJ, and esophageal cancers patients have *her2neu* overexpression. Both

TABLE 17-11 | FRONTLINE CHEMOTHERAPY: ONGOING PHASE II/III RANDOMIZED CONTROL CLINICAL TRIALS IN ADVANCED/METASTATIC GASTRIC, GASTROESOPHAGEAL JUNCTION, AND ESOPHAGEAL CANCERS

FRONTLINE CHEMOTHERAPY

Trial	N	Experimental Arm		Control Arm	Status
Japan JACCRO GC-03	628	Docetaxel + S1		S1	Completed accrual
France FFCD 0307	416	ECC-FOLFIRI		FOLFIRI-ECC	Completed accrual
International Sanofi-DOCOXC0082	270	DO	DF	DOX	Completed accrual
Japan/Wyett ISO-5FU-10	200	1-LV (isovorin) + F		S1	Completed accrual
Germany GC-ICE-2003	120	XP		IP	Completed accrual
Greece CT/04.18	110	IOX		FLOX	Completed accrual
Ohio OSU-0151	78	I-Mitomycin C		Mitomycin C-I	Completed accrual
Switzerland SWS-SAKK-42/99	111	DCF	DC	ECF	Completed accrual
Germany FLOT65+	140	FLO		FLOT	Completed accrual
Korea AMC SOS	622	S1 + P q5w		S1 + P q3w	Accruing
China/Roche PACLIC-C	320	X + cisplatin-X		X + paclitaxel-X	Accruing
International Sanofi-DOCET_L_02195	240	DCF		CF	Accruing
Ireland ELECT	140	EOX		ElTax	Accruing
MSKCC 06-103	120	mDCF		DCF + GCSF	Accruing
China NCT01015339	320	Paclitaxel + X		Cisplatin + X	Accruing

AMC, Asan Medical Center; CF, cisplatin, 5-fluorouracil; DC, docetaxel, cisplatin; DF, docetaxel, 5FU; DCF, docetaxel, cisplatin, 5-fluorouracil; DO, docetaxel, oxaliplatin; DOCET, docetaxel; DOX, docetaxel, oxaliplatin, capecitabine; ECC, epirubicin, cisplatin, capecitabine; ECF, epirubicin, cisplatin, 5-fluorouracil; ELECT, eloxatin, epirubicin, cisplatin, docetaxel; ElTax = oxaliplatin, docetaxel; EOX, epirubicin, oxaliplatin, capecitabine; F, 5FU; FFCD, Fédération Francophone de la Cancérologie Digestive; FLO, 5FU, leucovorin, oxaliplatin; FLOT65+, 5FU, leucovorin, oxaliplatin, docetaxel in >65 years of age; FLOX, 5FU, leucovorin, oxaliplatin; FOLFIRI, folnic acid, 5-fluorouracil, irinotecan; I, irinotecan; IOX, irinotecan, oxaliplatin, capecitabine; IP, irinotecan, cisplatin; JCCRO, Japanese Cancer Clinical Research Organization; mDCF, modified DCF; MSKCC, Memorial Sloan Kettering Cancer Center; OSU, Ohio State University; P, cisplatin; PACLIC-C, paclitaxel-cisplatin; SW-SAKK, Swiss Group for Clinical Research; SOS, S1 against S1; X, capecitabine; XP, capecitabine, cisplatin.

cetuximab and bevacizumab have demonstrated good activity when combined with cytotoxic regimens in small randomized or single-arm phase II studies. The results of ongoing randomized control phase III trials using targeted agents, in combination and alone, will transform the treatment of patients with advanced disease.

Figure 17-15 illustrates the MD Anderson approach to gastric, GEJ, and esophageal cancers. Despite the rarity of upper gastrointestinal cancers in the United States, it is still common in many other countries. Both gastric and esophageal cancers carry an ominous prognosis; thus, they are still considered a major public health problem. Advancements have been made in the areas of surgery and radiotherapy that have improved the mortality rates of upper gastrointestinal cancer patients. Many more reference chemotherapy regimens are available for the treatment of advanced disease. However, more research is needed. A multimodality approach to therapy will be the cornerstone to screening, diagnosing, staging, treating, and supporting patients with upper gastrointestinal cancers.

Metastatic gastric, GEJ, and esophageal cancers (stage IV) is not curable, but survival and cancer-related symptom control can be improved with systemic chemotherapy. Effective palliation may be achieved with various combinations of chemotherapy, radiotherapy, and therapeutic endoscopy (298). In particular, systemic chemotherapy can result in temporary palliation. Objective response rates of 30 to 50% and a median survival duration of <1 year have been reported for platinum-based combination regimens with 5-fluorouracil (5-FU), a taxane, or a topoisomerase inhibitor (236). Therefore, all patients should be offered the opportunity to participate in clinical trials. Surgery remains the treatment modality of choice for stages I and II cancers. Treatment consisting of definitive chemoradiotherapy and photodynamic therapy can also be considered for selected patients.

References

1. Jemal A, Siegel R, Ward E, et al. Cancer statistics, 2009. *CA Cancer J Clin* 2009;59(4):225-249.
2. SEER. *SEER Stats Facts Sheet*. [Cited 2009 December 27, 2009]. Available from: http://www.seer.cancer.gov/statfacts/html/stomach.html.
3. Parkin DM, Bray F, Ferlay J, et al. Global cancer statistics, 2002. *CA Cancer J Clin* 2005;**55**(2):74-108.

4. Neugut AI, Hayek M, Howe G. Epidemiology of gastric cancer. *Semin Oncol* 1996;23(3):281-291.

5. Blot WJ, McLaughlin JK. The changing epidemiology of esophageal cancer. *Semin Oncol* 1999;26(5 Suppl 15):2-8.

6. Alexander GA, Brawley OW. Association of Helicobacter pylori infection with gastric cancer. *Mil Med* 2000;165(1):21-27.

7. Figueiredo C, Machado JC, Pharoah P, et al. Helicobacter pylori and interleukin 1 genotyping: An opportunity to identify high-risk individuals for gastric carcinoma. *J Natl Cancer Inst* 2002;94(22):1680-1687.

8. Correa P. Human gastric carcinogenesis: A multistep and multifactorial process—First American Cancer Society Award Lecture on Cancer Epidemiology and Prevention. *Cancer Res* 1992;52(24):6735-6740.

9. Larsson SC, Orsini N, Wolk A. Processed meat consumption and stomach cancer risk: A meta-analysis. *J Natl Cancer Inst* 2006;98(15):1078-1087.

10. Barstad B, Sorensen TI, Tjonneland A, et al. Intake of wine, beer and spirits and risk of gastric cancer. *Eur J Cancer Prev* 2005;14(3):239-243.

11. Freedman ND, Abnet CC, Leitzmann MF, et al. A prospective study of tobacco, alcohol, and the risk of esophageal and gastric cancer subtypes. *Am J Epidemiol* 2007;165(12):1424-1433.

12. Stalnikowicz R, Benbassat J. Risk of gastric cancer after gastric surgery for benign disorders. *Arch Intern Med* 1990; 150(10):2022-2026.

13. Freedman ND, Chow WH, Gao YT, et al. Menstrual and reproductive factors and gastric cancer risk in a large prospective study of women. *Gut* 2007;56(12):1671-1677.

14. Yamanaka N, Morisaki T, Nakashima H, et al. Interleukin 1beta enhances invasive ability of gastric carcinoma through nuclear factor-kappaB activation. *Clin Cancer Res* 2004; 10(5):1853-1859.

15. Machado JC, Figueiredo C, Canedo P, et al. A proinflammatory genetic profile increases the risk for chronic atrophic gastritis and gastric carcinoma. *Gastroenterology* 2003; 125(2):364-371.

16. El-Omar EM, Carrington M, Chow WH, et al. Interleukin-1 polymorphisms associated with increased risk of gastric cancer. *Nature* 2000;404(6776):398-402.

17. Tatemichi M, Sawa T, Gilibert I, et al. Increased risk of intestinal type of gastric adenocarcinoma in Japanese women associated with long forms of CCTTT pentanucleotide repeat in the inducible nitric oxide synthase promoter. *Cancer Lett* 2005;217(2):197-202.

18. Garza-Gonzalez E, Bosques-Padilla FJ, Tijerina-Menchaca R, et al. Comparison of endoscopy-based and serum-based methods for the diagnosis of *Helicobacter pylori*. *Can J Gastroenterol* 2003;17(2):101-106.

19. Gehmert S, Velapatino B, Herrera P, et al. Interleukin-1 beta single-nucleotide polymorphism's C allele is associated with elevated risk of gastric cancer in *Helicobacter pylori*-infected Peruvians. *Am J Trop Med Hyg* 2009; 81(5):804-810.

20. Figueiredo C, Quint W, Nouhan N, et al. Assessment of *Helicobacter pylori* vacA and cagA genotypes and host serological response. *J Clin Microbiol* 2001;39(4):1339-1344.

21. Zheng ZH, Sun XJ, Ma MC, et al. (Studies of promoter methylation status and protein expression of E-cadherin gene in associated progression stages of gastric cancer). *Yi Chuan Xue Bao* 2003;30(2):103-108.

22. Oliveira C, Ferreira P, Nabais S, et al. E-Cadherin (CDH1) and p53 rather than SMAD4 and Caspase-10 germline mutations contribute to genetic predisposition in Portuguese gastric cancer patients. *Eur J Cancer* 2004;40(12):1897-1903.

23. Kaurah P, MacMillan A, Boyd N, et al. Founder and recurrent CDH1 mutations in families with hereditary diffuse gastric cancer. *JAMA* 2007; 297(21):2360-2372.

24. Caldas C, Carneiro F, Lynch HT, et al. Familial gastric cancer: Overview and guidelines for management. *J Med Genet* 1999;36(12):873-880.

25. Murphy G, Pfeiffer R, Camargo MC, et al. Meta-analysis shows that prevalence of Epstein-Barr virus-positive gastric cancer differs based on sex and anatomic location. *Gastroenterology* 2009;137(3):824-833.

26. Kusano M, Toyota M, Suzuki H, et al. Genetic, epigenetic, and clinicopathologic features of gastric carcinomas with the CpG island methylator phenotype and an association with Epstein-Barr virus. *Cancer* 2006;106(7):1467-1479.

27. Truong CD, Feng W, Li W, et al. Characteristics of Epstein-Barr virus-associated gastric cancer: A study of 235 cases at a comprehensive cancer center in U.S.A. *J Exp Clin Cancer Res* 2009;28:14.

28. Lauren P. The two histological main types of gastric carcinoma: Diffuse and so-called intestinal-type carcinoma. An attempt at a histo-clinical classification. *Acta Pathol Microbiol Scand* 1965;64:31-49.

29. Graham DY, Schwartz JT, Cain GD, et al. Prospective evaluation of biopsy number in the diagnosis of esophageal and gastric carcinoma. *Gastroenterology* 1982;82(2):228-231.

30. Moss AA, Schnyder P, Marks W, et al. Gastric adenocarcinoma: A comparison of the accuracy and economics of staging by computed tomography and surgery. *Gastroenterology* 1981;80(1):45-50.

31. Edge SB, Byrd DR, Compton C, et al. (eds). *AJCC Cancer Staging Manual*, 7th ed. New York: Springer, 2010.

32. Rosch T, Lorenz R, Zenker K, et al. Local staging and assessment of resectability in carcinoma of the esophagus, stomach, and duodenum by endoscopic ultrasonography. *Gastrointest Endosc* 1992;38(4):460-467.

33. Conlon KC, Karpeh MS, Jr. Laparoscopy and laparoscopic ultrasound in the staging of gastric cancer. *Semin Oncol* 1996;23(3):347-351.

34. Sun L, Su XH, Guan YS, et al. Clinical role of 18F-fluorodeoxyglucose positron emission tomography/computed tomography in post-operative follow up of gastric cancer: Initial results. *World J Gastroenterol* 2008;14(29):4627-4632.

35. Ott K, Lordick F, Herrmann K, et al. The new credo: Induction chemotherapy in locally advanced gastric cancer: Consequences for surgical strategies. *Gastric Cancer* 2008; 11(1):1-9.

36. Stahl A, Ott K, Schwaiger M, et al. Comparison of different SUV-based methods for monitoring cytotoxic therapy with FDG PET. *Eur J Nucl Med Mol Imaging* 2004;31(11):1471-1478.

37. Ott K, Herrmann K, Lordick F, et al. Early metabolic response evaluation by fluorine-18 fluorodeoxyglucose positron emission tomography allows in vivo testing of chemosensitivity in gastric cancer: Long-term results of a prospective study. *Clin Cancer Res* 2008; 14(7): 2012-2018.

38. Javeri H, Xiao L, Rohren E, et al. The higher the decrease in the standardized uptake value of positron emission tomography

after chemoradiation, the better the survival of patients with gastroesophageal adenocarcinoma. *Cancer* 2009;115(22): 5184-5192.

39. Swisher SG, Erasmus J, Maish M, et al. 2-Fluoro-2-deoxy-D-glucose positron emission tomography imaging is predictive of pathologic response and survival after preoperative chemoradiation in patients with esophageal carcinoma. *Cancer* 2004;101(8):1776-1785.

40. Lordick F, Ott K, Krause BJ, et al. PET to assess early metabolic response and to guide treatment of adenocarcinoma of the oesophagogastric junction: The MUNICON phase II trial. *Lancet Oncol* 2007;8(9):797-805.

41. Sim SH, Kim YJ, Oh DY, et al. The role of PET/CT in detection of gastric cancer recurrence. *BMC Cancer* 2009;9:73.

42. Panani AD. Cytogenetic and molecular aspects of gastric cancer: Clinical implications. *Cancer Lett* 2008;266(2):99-115.

43. Watari J, Saitoh Y, Fujiya M, et al. Reduction of syndecan-1 expression in differentiated type early gastric cancer and background mucosa with gastric cellular phenotype. *J Gastroenterol* 2004;39(2):104-112.

44. Abu-Elmagd KM, Mazariegos G, Costa G, et al. Lymphoproliferative disorders and de novo malignancies in intestinal and multivisceral recipients: Improved outcomes with new outlooks. *Transplantation* 2009;88(7):926-934.

45. Kanai M, Wei D, Li Q, et al. Loss of Kruppel-like factor 4 expression contributes to Sp1 overexpression and human gastric cancer development and progression. *Clin Cancer Res* 2006;12(21):6395-6402.

46. Mouridsen H, Gershanovich M, Sun Y, et al. Prognostic significance of Bcl-2 and p53 expression in gastric cancer. *Int J Colorectal Dis* 2003; 18(6):518-525.

47. An C, Choi IS, Yao JC, et al. Prognostic significance of CpG island methylator phenotype and microsatellite instability in gastric carcinoma. *Clin Cancer Res* 2005;11(2 Pt 1):656-663.

48. Watanabe Y, Kim HS, Castoro RJ, et al. Sensitive and specific detection of early gastric cancer with DNA methylation analysis of gastric washes. *Gastroenterology* 2009;136(7): 2149-2158.

49. Guan X, Zhao H, Niu J, Tang D, Ajani JA, Wei Q, et al. The VEGF -634G>C promoter polymorphism is associated with risk of gastric cancer. *BMC Gastroenterol* 2009;9:77.

50. Talamonti MS, Kim SP, Yao KA, et al. Surgical outcomes of patients with gastric carcinoma: The importance of primary tumor location and microvessel invasion. *Surgery* 2003;134(4): 720-727; discussion 727-729.

51. Macdonald JS, Smalley SR, Benedetti J, et al. Chemoradiotherapy after surgery compared with surgery alone for adenocarcinoma of the stomach or gastroesophageal junction. *N Engl J Med*. 2001;345(10):725-730.

52. Cunningham D, Allum WH, Stenning SP, et al. Perioperative chemotherapy versus surgery alone for resectable gastroesophageal cancer. *N Engl J Med* 2006;355(1):11-20.

53. Wanebo HJ, Kennedy BJ, Chmiel J, Steele G, Jr., Winchester D, Osteen R, et al. Cancer of the stomach. A patient care study by the American College of Surgeons. *Ann Surg* 1993; 218(5):583-592.

54. Bozzetti F, Marubini E, Bonfanti G, Miceli R, Piano C, Gennari L, et al. Subtotal versus total gastrectomy for gastric cancer: Five-year survival rates in a multicenter randomized Italian trial. Italian Gastrointestinal Tumor Study Group. *Ann Surg* 1999;230(2):170-178.

55. Gouzi JL, Huguier M, Fagniez PL, et al. Total versus subtotal gastrectomy for adenocarcinoma of the gastric antrum. A French prospective controlled study. *Ann Surg* 1989;209(2):162-166.

56. Martin RC, 2nd, Jaques DP, Brennan MF, Karpeh M. et al. Extended local resection for advanced gastric cancer: Increased survival versus increased morbidity. *Ann Surg* 2002;236(2):159-165.

57. Yao JC, Schnirer, II, Reddy S, et al. Effects of sex and racial/ethnic group on the pattern of gastric cancer localization. *Gastric Cancer* 2002;5(4):208-212.

58. Schwarz RE, Smith DD. Clinical impact of lymphadenectomy extent in resectable gastric cancer of advanced stage. *Ann Surg Oncol* 2007;14(2):317-328.

59. Smith DD, Schwarz RR, Schwarz RE. Impact of total lymph node count on staging and survival after gastrectomy for gastric cancer: Data from a large US-population database. *J Clin Oncol* 2005;23(28):7114-7124.

60. Wu CW, Hsiung CA, Lo SS, et al. Nodal dissection for patients with gastric cancer: A randomised controlled trial. *Lancet Oncol* 2006;7(4):309-315.

61. Noguchi Y, Imada T, Matsumoto A, Coit DG, Brennan MF, et al. Radical surgery for gastric cancer. A review of the Japanese experience. *Cancer* 1989;64(10):2053-2062.

62. Bonenkamp JJ, Hermans J, Sasako M, et al. Extended lymphnode dissection for gastric cancer. *N Engl J Med* 1999; 340(12):908-914.

63. Danielson H, Kokkola A, Kiviluoto T, et al. Clinical outcome after D1 vs D2-3 gastrectomy for treatment of gastric cancer. *Scand J Surg* 2007;96(1):35-40.

64. Hartgrink HH, van de Velde CJ, Putter H, et al. Extended lymph node dissection for gastric cancer: Who may benefit? Final results of the randomized Dutch gastric cancer group trial. *J Clin Oncol* 2004;22(11):2069-2077.

65. Cuschieri A, Weeden S, Fielding J, et al. Patient survival after D1 and D2 resections for gastric cancer: Long-term results of the MRC randomized surgical trial. Surgical Cooperative Group. *Br J Cancer* 1999;79(9-10):1522-1530.

66. Wainess RM, Dimick JB, Upchurch GR, Jr., Cowan JA, Mulholland MW. et al. Epidemiology of surgically treated gastric cancer in the United States, 1988-2000. *J Gastrointest Surg* 2003;7(7):879-883.

67. Birkmeyer NJ, Goodney PP, Stukel TA, Hillner BE, Birkmeyer JD, et al. Do cancer centers designated by the National Cancer Institute have better surgical outcomes? *Cancer* 2005;103(3):435-441.

68. Smith DL, Elting LS, Learn PA, Raut CP, Mansfield PF. et al. Factors influencing the volume-outcome relationship in gastrectomies: A population-based study. *Ann Surg Oncol* 2007;14(6):1846-1852.

69. Klein Kranenbarg E, Hermans J, van Krieken JH, van de Velde CJ et al. Evaluation of the 5th edition of the TNM classification for gastric cancer: Improved prognostic value. *Br J Cancer* 2001;84(1):64-71.

70. Middleton G, Cunningham D. Current options in the management of gastrointestinal cancer. *Ann Oncol* 1995;6(Suppl 1): 17-25; discussion 25-26.

71. Agboola O. Adjuvant treatment in gastric cancer. *Cancer Treat Rev* 1994;20(3):217-240.

72. Yan TD, Black D, Sugarbaker PH, et al. A systematic review and meta-analysis of the randomized controlled trials on adjuvant intraperitoneal chemotherapy for resectable gastric cancer. *Ann Surg Oncol* 2007;14(10):2702-2713.

73. Engstrom PF, Lavin PT, Douglass HO, Jr., Brunner KW. Postoperative adjuvant 5-fluorouracil plus methyl-CCNU therapy for gastric cancer patients. Eastern Cooperative Oncology Group study (EST 3275). *Cancer* 1985;55(9):1868-1873.

74. Hermans J, Bonenkamp JJ, Boon MC, et al. Adjuvant therapy after curative resection for gastric cancer: Meta-analysis of randomized trials. *J Clin Oncol* 1993;11(8):1441-1447.

75. Earle CC, Schrag D, Neville BA, et al. Effect of surgeon specialty on processes of care and outcomes for ovarian cancer patients. *J Natl Cancer Inst* 2006;98(3):172-180.

76. Mari E, Floriani I, Tinazzi A, et al. Efficacy of adjuvant chemotherapy after curative resection for gastric cancer: A meta-analysis of published randomised trials. A study of the GISCAD (Gruppo Italiano per lo Studio dei Carcinomi dell'Apparato Digerente). *Ann Oncol* 2000;11(7):837-843.

77. Panzini I, Gianni L, Fattori PP, et al. Adjuvant chemotherapy in gastric cancer: A meta-analysis of randomized trials and a comparison with previous meta-analyses. *Tumori* 2002;88(1):21-27.

78. Janunger KG, Hafstrom L, Glimelius B. Chemotherapy in gastric cancer: A review and updated meta-analysis. *Eur J Surg* 2002;168(11):597-608.

79. Sun P, Xiang JB, Chen ZY. Meta-analysis of adjuvant chemotherapy after radical surgery for advanced gastric cancer. *Br J Surg* 2009;96(1):26-33.

80. Sakuramoto S, Sasako M, Yamaguchi T, et al. Adjuvant chemotherapy for gastric cancer with S-1, an oral fluoropyrimidine. *N Engl J Med* 2007;357(18):1810-1820.

81. Di Costanzo F, Gasperoni S, Manzione L, et al. Adjuvant chemotherapy in completely resected gastric cancer: A randomized phase III trial conducted by GOIRC. *J Natl Cancer Inst* 2008;100(6):388-398.

82. Cooper JS, Guo MD, Herskovic A, et al. Chemoradiotherapy of locally advanced esophageal cancer: Long-term follow-up of a prospective randomized trial (RTOG 85-01). Radiation Therapy Oncology Group. *JAMA* 1999;281(17):1623-1627.

83. C. Fuchs, J. E. Tepper, D. Niedwiecki, et al. Postoperative adjuvant chemoradiation for gastric or gastroesophageal adenocarcinoma using epirubicin, cisplatin, and infusional (CI) 5-FU (ECF) before and after CI 5-FU and radiotherapy (RT): Interim toxicity results from Intergroup trial CALGB 80101. *J Clin Oncology* 2006, Gastrointestinal Cancers Symposium Proceedings, Abstr 61.

84. Rougier P, Mahjoubi M, Lasser P, et al. Neoadjuvant chemotherapy in locally advanced gastric carcinoma—a phase II trial with combined continuous intravenous 5-fluorouracil and bolus cisplatinum. *Eur J Cancer* 1994;30A(9):1269-1275.

85. Kang YK, Choi DW, Im YH, et al. A phase III randomized comparison of neoadjuvant chemotherapy followed by surgery versus surgery for locally advanced stomach cancer. 1996 Annual Meeting Proceedings. *J Clin Oncol.* 1996 (abstract 503).

86. Songun I, Keizer HJ, Hermans J, et al. Chemotherapy for operable gastric cancer: Results of the Dutch randomised FAMTX trial. The Dutch Gastric Cancer Group (DGCG). *Eur J Cancer* 1999;35(4):558-562.

87. Boige V, Pignon JP, Saint-Aubert B, et al. Final results of a randomized trial comparing preoperative 5-fluorouracil (F)/cisplatin (P) to surgery alone in adenocarcinoma of stomach and lower esophagus (ASLE): FNLCC ACCORD07-FFCD 9703 trial. 2007 ASCO Annual Meeting Proceedings. *J Clin Oncol* 2007;25(18S Suppl) (abstract 4510).

88. Ajani JA, Komaki R, Putnam JB, et al. A three-step strategy of induction chemotherapy then chemoradiation followed by surgery in patients with potentially resectable carcinoma of the esophagus or gastroesophageal junction. *Cancer* 2001; 92(2):279-286.

89. Ajani JA, Winter K, Okawara GS, et al. Phase II trial of preoperative chemoradiation in patients with localized gastric adenocarcinoma (RTOG 9904): Quality of combined modality therapy and pathologic response. *J Clin Oncol* 2006;24(24): 3953-3258.

90. Blot WJ. Esophageal cancer trends and risk factors. *Semin Onco* 1994;21(4):403-410.

91. Sant M, Aareleid T, Berrino F, et al. EUROCARE-3: Survival of cancer patients diagnosed 1990-94—results and commentary. *Ann Oncol* 2003;14(Suppl 5):v61-v118.

92. Holscher AH, Bollschweiler E, Schneider PM, Siewert JR. Prognosis of early esophageal cancer. Comparison between adeno- and squamous cell carcinoma. *Cancer* 1995;76(2): 178-186.

93. Thun MJ, Peto R, Lopez AD, et al. Alcohol consumption and mortality among middle-aged and elderly U.S. adults. *N Engl J Med* 1997;337(24):1705-1714.

94. Lin K, Wu Y, Shen W. Interaction of total N-nitroso compounds in environment and in vivo on risk of esophageal cancer in the coastal area, China. *Environ Int* 2009;35(2):376-381.

95. Wu CM, Lee YS, Wang TH, et al. Identification of differential gene expression between intestinal and diffuse gastric cancer using cDNA microarray. *Oncol Rep* 2006;15(1):57-64.

96. Islami F, Pourshams A, Nasrollahzadeh D, et al. Tea drinking habits and oesophageal cancer in a high risk area in northern Iran: Population based case-control study. *BMJ* 2009;338:b929.

97. Nasseri-Moghaddam S. Tea drinking habits and oesophagial cancer in a high-risk area in northern Iran: Population based case-control study. *Arch Iran Med* 2009;12(3):330-332.

98. Sandler RS, Nyren O, Ekbom A, Eisen GM, Yuen J, Josefsson S. The risk of esophageal cancer in patients with achalasia. A population-based study. *JAMA* 1995;274(17):1359-1362.

99. Ribeiro U, Jr., Posner MC, Safatle-Ribeiro AV, Reynolds JC. Risk factors for squamous cell carcinoma of the oesophagus. *Br J Surg* 1996;83(9):1174-1185.

100. Ruhrberg C, Williamson JA, Sheer D, Watt FM. Chromosomal localisation of the human envoplakin gene (EVPL) to the region of the tylosis oesophageal cancer gene (TOCG) on 17q25. *Genomics* 1996;37(3):381-385.

101. Lagergren J, Bergstrom R, Nyren O. Association between body mass and adenocarcinoma of the esophagus and gastric cardia. *Ann Intern Med* 1999;130(11):883-890.

102. Hampel H, Stephens JA, Pukkala E, et al. Cancer risk in hereditary nonpolyposis colorectal cancer syndrome: Later age of onset. *Gastroenterology* 2005;129(2):415-421.

103. Bytzer P, Christensen PB, Damkier P, Vinding K, Seersholm N. Adenocarcinoma of the esophagus and Barrett's esophagus: A population-based study. *Am J Gastroenterol* 1999; 94(1):86-91.

104. Gammon MD, Wolff MS, Neugut AI, et al. Temporal variation in chlorinated hydrocarbons in healthy women. *Cancer Epidemiol Biomarkers Prev* 1997;6(5):327-332.

105. Gammon MD, Wolff MS, Neugut AI, et al. Short segment Barrett's esophagus—the need for standardization of the definition and of endoscopic criteria. *Am J Gastroenterol* 1998;93(7): 1033-1036.

106. Cook MB, Wild CP, Forman D. A systematic review and meta-analysis of the sex ratio for Barrett's esophagus, erosive reflux disease, and nonerosive reflux disease. *Am J Epidemiol* 2005;162(11):1050-1061.

107. Hirota WK, Loughney TM, Lazas DJ, Maydonovitch CL, Rholl V, Wong RK. Specialized intestinal metaplasia, dysplasia, and cancer of the esophagus and esophagogastric junction: Prevalence and clinical data. *Gastroenterology* 1999;116(2):277-285.

108. Eloubeidi MA, Homan RK, Martz MD, Theobald KE, Provenzale D. A cost analysis of outpatient care for patients with Barrett's esophagus in a managed care setting. *Am J Gastroenterol* 1999;94(8):2033-2036.

109. Kim SL, Waring JP, Spechler SJ, et al. Diagnostic inconsistencies in Barrett's esophagus. Department of Veterans Affairs Gastroesophageal Reflux Study Group. *Gastroenterology* 1994;107(4):945-949.

110. van der Burgh A, Dees J, Hop WC, van Blankenstein M. Oesophageal cancer is an uncommon cause of death in patients with Barrett's oesophagus. *Gut* 1996;39(1):5-8.

111. Iijima K, Henry E, Moriya A, Wirz A, Kelman AW, McColl KE. Dietary nitrate generates potentially mutagenic concentrations of nitric oxide at the gastroesophageal junction. *Gastroenterology* 2002;122(5):1248-1257.

112. Cameron AJ, Lomboy CT. Barrett's esophagus: Age, prevalence, and extent of columnar epithelium. *Gastroenterology* 1992;103(4):1241-1245.

113. Rudolph RE, Vaughan TL, Storer BE, et al. Effect of segment length on risk for neoplastic progression in patients with Barrett esophagus. *Ann Intern Med* 2000;132(8):612-620.

114. Souza RF, Morales CP, Spechler SJ. Review article: A conceptual approach to understanding the molecular mechanisms of cancer development in Barrett's oesophagus. *Aliment Pharmacol Ther* 2001;15(8):1087-1100.

115. Wu TT, Watanabe T, Heitmiller R, Zahurak M, Forastiere AA, Hamilton SR. Genetic alterations in Barrett esophagus and adenocarcinomas of the esophagus and esophagogastric junction region. *Am J Pathol* 1998;153(1):287-294.

116. Barrett MT, Sanchez CA, Prevo LJ, et al. Evolution of neoplastic cell lineages in Barrett oesophagus. *Nat Genet* 1999;22(1):106-109.

117. Nobukawa B, Abraham SC, Gill J, Heitmiller RF, Wu TT. Clinicopathologic and molecular analysis of high-grade dysplasia and early adenocarcinoma in short- versus long-segment Barrett esophagus. *Hum Pathol* 2001;32(4):447-454.

118. Izzo JG, Luthra R, Wu TT, et al. Molecular mechanisms in Barrett's metaplasia and its progression. *Semin Oncol* 2007;34(2 Suppl 1):S2-S6.

119. Montgomery E, Bronner MP, Goldblum JR, et al. Reproducibility of the diagnosis of dysplasia in Barrett esophagus: A reaffirmation. *Hum Pathol* 2001;32(4):368-378.

120. Reid BJ, Haggitt RC, Rubin CE, et al. Observer variation in the diagnosis of dysplasia in Barrett's esophagus. *Hum Pathol* 1988;19(2):166-178.

121. Downs-Kelly E, Mendelin JE, Bennett AE, et al. Poor interobserver agreement in the distinction of high-grade dysplasia and adenocarcinoma in pretreatment Barrett's esophagus biopsies. *Am J Gastroenterol* 2008;103(9):2333-2340; quiz 2341.

122. Yang JH, Zhang YC, Qian HQ. Survivin antisense oligodeoxynucleotide inhibits growth of gastric cancer cells. *World J Gastroenterol* 2004;10(8):1121-1124.

123. Maru DM, Singh RR, Hannah C, et al. MicroRNA-196a is a potential marker of progression during Barrett's metaplasia-dysplasia-invasive adenocarcinoma sequence in esophagus. *Am J Pathol* 2009; 174(5):1940-1948.

124. Blot WJ, Devesa SS, Kneller RW, Fraumeni JF, Jr. Rising incidence of adenocarcinoma of the esophagus and gastric cardia. *JAMA* 1991;265(10):1287-1289.

125. Earlam R, Cunha-Melo JR. Oesophageal squamous cell carcinoms: II. A critical view of radiotherapy. *Br J Surg* 1980; 67(7):457-461.

126. Steup WH, De Leyn P, Deneffe G, Van Raemdonck D, Coosemans W, Lerut T. Tumors of the esophagogastric junction. Long-term survival in relation to the pattern of lymph node metastasis and a critical analysis of the accuracy or inaccuracy of pTNM classification. *J Thorac Cardiovasc Surg* 1996;111(1):85-94; discussion 94-95.

127. Altorki NK, Girardi L, Skinner DB. En bloc esophagectomy improves survival for stage III esophageal cancer. *J Thorac Cardiovasc Surg* 1997;114(6):948-955; discussion 955-956.

128. Kneist W, Schreckenberger M, Bartenstein P, Grunwald F, Oberholzer K, Junginger T. Positron emission tomography for staging esophageal cancer: Does it lead to a different therapeutic approach? *World J Surg* 2003;27(10):1105-1112.

129. Nakamoto Y, Osman M, Wahl RL. Prevalence and patterns of bone metastases detected with positron emission tomography using F-18 FDG. *Clin Nucl Med* 2003;28(4):302-307.

130. Kato H, Kuwano H, Nakajima M, et al. Comparison between positron emission tomography and computed tomography in the use of the assessment of esophageal carcinoma. *Cancer* 2002;94(4):921-928.

131. Lerut T, Flamen P, Ectors N, et al. Histopathologic validation of lymph node staging with FDG-PET scan in cancer of the esophagus and gastroesophageal junction: A prospective study based on primary surgery with extensive lymphadenectomy. *Ann Surg* 2000;232(6):743-752.

132. Skehan SJ, Brown AL, Thompson M, Young JE, Coates G, Nahmias C. Imaging features of primary and recurrent esophageal cancer at FDG PET. *Radiographics* 2000;20(3): 713-723.

133. Swisher SG, Maish M, Erasmus JJ, et al. Utility of PET, CT, and EUS to identify pathologic responders in esophageal cancer. *Ann Thorac Surg* 2004;78(4):1152-1160; discussion 1152-1160.

134. Hong D, Lunagomez S, Kim EE, et al. Value of baseline positron emission tomography for predicting overall survival in patient with nonmetastatic esophageal or gastroesophageal junction carcinoma. *Cancer* 2005;104(8):1620-1626.

135. Roedl JB, Halpern EF, Colen RR, Sahani DV, Fischman AJ, Blake MA. Metabolic tumor width parameters as determined on PET/CT predict disease-free survival and treatment response in squamous cell carcinoma of the esophagus. *Mol Imaging Biol* 2009;11(1):54-60.

136. Shenfine J, McNamee P, Steen N, Bond J, Griffin SM. A randomized controlled clinical trial of palliative therapies for patients with inoperable esophageal cancer. *Am J Gastroenterol* 2009;104(7):1674-1685.

137. Yoshinaga K, Inoue H, Utsunomiya T, et al. N-cadherin is regulated by activin A and associated with tumor aggressiveness in esophageal carcinoma. Clin Cancer Res, 2004; 10(17):5702-5707.

138. Abdel-Latif MM, O'Riordan J, Windle HJ, et al. NF-kappaB activation in esophageal adenocarcinoma: Relationship to Barrett's metaplasia, survival, and response to neoadjuvant chemoradiotherapy. *Ann Surg* 2004;239(4):491-500.

139. Song ZB, Gao SS, Yi XN, et al. Expression of MUC1 in esophageal squamous-cell carcinoma and its relationship with prognosis of patients from Linzhou city, a high incidence area of northern China. *World J Gastroenterol* 2003;9(3):404-407.

140. Raouf AA, Evoy DA, Carton E, Mulligan E, Griffin MM, Reynolds JV. Loss of Bcl-2 expression in Barrett's dysplasia and adenocarcinoma is associated with tumor progression and worse survival but not with response to neoadjuvant chemoradiation. *Dis Esophagus* 2003;16(1):17-23.

141. Bani-Hani K, Sue-Ling H, Johnston D, Axon AT, Martin IG. Barrett's oesophagus: Results from a 13-year surveillance programme. *Eur J Gastroenterol Hepatol* 2000;12(6):649-654.

142. Katz D, Rothstein R, Schned A, Dunn J, Seaver K, Antonioli D. The development of dysplasia and adenocarcinoma during endoscopic surveillance of Barrett's esophagus. *Am J Gastroenterol* 1998;93(4):536-541.

143. Wright TA, Gray MR, Morris AI, et al. Cost effectiveness of detecting Barrett's cancer. *Gut* 1996;39(4):574-579.

144. Streitz JM, Jr., Ellis FH, Jr., Tilden RL, Erickson RV. Endoscopic surveillance of Barrett's esophagus: A cost-effectiveness comparison with mammographic surveillance for breast cancer. *Am J Gastroenterol* 1998;93(6):911-915.

145. Sharma P, McQuaid K, Dent J, et al. A critical review of the diagnosis and management of Barrett's esophagus: The AGA Chicago Workshop. *Gastroenterology* 2004;127(1):310-330.

146. Wang A, Mattek NC, Corless CL, Lieberman DA, Eisen GM. The value of traditional upper endoscopy as a diagnostic test for Barrett's esophagus. *Gastrointest Endosc* 2008;68(5):859-866.

147. Kariv R, Plesec TP, Goldblum JR, et al. The Seattle protocol does not more reliably predict the detection of cancer at the time of esophagectomy than a less intensive surveillance protocol. *Clin Gastroenterol Hepatol* 2009;7(6):653-658; quiz 606.

148. Sharma VK, Jae Kim H, Das A, Wells CD, Nguyen CC, Fleischer DE. Circumferential and focal ablation of Barrett's esophagus containing dysplasia. *Am J Gastroenterol* 2009;104(2):310-317.

149. Kiesslich R, Gossner L, Goetz M, et al. In vivo histology of Barrett's esophagus and associated neoplasia by confocal laser endomicroscopy. *Clin Gastroenterol Hepatol* 2006;4(8):979-987.

150. Swisher SG, Deford L, Merriman KW, et al. Effect of operative volume on morbidity, mortality, and hospital use after esophagectomy for cancer. *J Thorac Cardiovasc Surg* 2000;119(6):1126-1132.

151. Santillan AA, Farma JM, Meredith KL, Shah NR, Kelley ST. Minimally invasive surgery for esophageal cancer. *J Natl Compr Canc Netw* 2008;6(9):879-884.

152. Ciocirlan M, Lapalus MG, Hervieu V, et al. Endoscopic mucosal resection for squamous premalignant and early malignant lesions of the esophagus. *Endoscopy* 2007;39(1):24-29.

153. Prasad GA, Wu TT, Wigle DA, et al. Endoscopic and surgical treatment of mucosal (T1a) esophageal adenocarcinoma in Barrett's esophagus. *Gastroenterology* 2009;137(3):815-823.

154. Sharma P, Falk GW, Sampliner R, Jon Spechler S, Wang K. Management of nondysplastic Barrett's esophagus: Where are we now? *Am J Gastroenterol* 2009;104(4):805-808.

155. Soetikno RM, Gotoda T, Nakanishi Y, Soehendra N. Endoscopic mucosal resection. *Gastrointest Endosc* 2003;57(4):567-579.

156. Ackroyd R, Brown NJ, Davis MF, et al. Photodynamic therapy for dysplastic Barrett's oesophagus: A prospective, double blind, randomised, placebo controlled trial. *Gut* 2000;47(5):612-617.

157. Overholt BF, Lightdale CJ, Wang KK, et al. Photodynamic therapy with porfimer sodium for ablation of high-grade dysplasia in Barrett's esophagus: International, partially blinded, randomized phase III trial. *Gastrointest Endosc* 2005;62(4):488-498.

158. Ginsberg RJ. Cancer treatment in the elderly. *J Am Coll Surg* 1998;187(4):427-428.

159. Ellis FH, Jr., Williamson WA, Heatley GJ. Cancer of the esophagus and cardia: Does age influence treatment selection and surgical outcomes? *J Am Coll Surg* 1998;187(4):345-351.

160. Rudiger Siewert J, Feith M, Werner M, Stein HJ. Adenocarcinoma of the esophagogastric junction: Results of surgical therapy based on anatomical/ topographic classification in 1,002 consecutive patients. *Ann Surg* 2000;232(3):353-361.

161. Ellis FH, Jr., Gibb SP, Watkins E, Jr. Esophagogastrectomy. Esophagogastrectomy. A safe, widely applicable, and expeditious form of palliation for patients with carcinoma of the esophagus and cardia. *Ann Surg* 1983;198(4):531-540.

162. Baba M, Aikou T, Natsugoe S, et al. Appraisal of ten-year survival following esophagectomy for carcinoma of the esophagus with emphasis on quality of life. *World J Surg* 1997;21(3):282-285; discussion 286.

163. Krasna MJ. Left transthoracic esophagectomy. *Chest Surg Clin N Am* 1995;5(3):543-554.

164. Swanson SJ, Batirel HF, Bueno R, et al. Transthoracic esophagectomy with radical mediastinal and abdominal lymph node dissection and cervical esophagogastrostomy for esophageal carcinoma. *Ann Thorac Surg* 2001;72(6):1918-1924; discussion 1924-1925.

165. Mendenhall WM, Sombeck MD, Parsons JT, Kasper ME, Stringer SP, Vogel SB. Management of cervical esophageal carcinoma. *Semin Radiat Oncol* 1994;4(3):179-191.

166. Stahl M, Stuschke M, Lehmann N, et al. Chemoradiation with and without surgery in patients with locally advanced squamous cell carcinoma of the esophagus. *J Clin Oncol* 2005;23(10):2310-2317.

167. Peracchia A, Bardini R, Ruol A, et al. Surgical management of carcinoma of the hypopharynx and cervical esophagus. *Hepatogastroenterology* 1990;37(4):371-375.

168. Lerut T, Coosemans W, De Leyn P, Van Raemdonck D, Deneffe G, Decker G. Treatment of esophageal carcinoma. *Chest* 1999;116(6 Suppl):463S-465S.

169. Sundelof M, Lagergren J, Ye W. Surgical factors influencing outcomes in patients resected for cancer of the esophagus or gastric cardia. *World J Surg* 2008;32(11):2357-2365.

170. Birkmeyer JD, Sun Y, Wong SL, Stukel TA. Hospital volume and late survival after cancer surgery. *Ann Surg* 2007;245(5):777-783.

171. Begg CB, Cramer LD, Hoskins WJ, Brennan MF. Impact of hospital volume on operative mortality for major cancer surgery. *JAMA* 1998;280(20):1747-1751.

172. Dimick JB, Pronovost PJ, Cowan JA, Lipsett PA. Surgical volume and quality of care for esophageal resection: Do high-volume hospitals have fewer complications? *Ann Thorac Surg* 2003;75(2):337-341.

173. Wenner J, Zilling T, Bladstrom A, Alvegard TA. The influence of surgical volume on hospital mortality and 5-year survival for carcinoma of the oesophagus and gastric cardia. *Anticancer Res* 2005;25(1B):419-424.

174. Wouters MW, Karim-Kos HE, le Cessie S, et al. Centralization of esophageal cancer surgery: Does it improve clinical outcome? *Ann Surg Oncol* 2009;16(7):1789-1798.

175. Ilson DH. Adjuvant therapy for noncolorectal cancers. *Curr Opin Oncol* 2001;13(4):287-290.

176. Pouliquen X, Levard H, Hay JM, McGee K, Fingerhut A, Langlois-Zantin O. 5-Fluorouracil and cisplatin therapy after palliative surgical resection of squamous cell carcinoma of the esophagus. A multicenter randomized trial. French Associations for Surgical Research. *Ann Surg* 1996;223(2):127-133.

177. Ando N, Iizuka T, Ide H, et al. Surgery plus chemotherapy compared with surgery alone for localized squamous cell carcinoma of the thoracic esophagus: A Japan Clinical Oncology Group Study—JCOG9204. *J Clin Oncol* 2003; 21(24):4592-4596.

178. Heroor A, Fujita H, Sueyoshi S, et al. Adjuvant chemotherapy after radical resection of squamous cell carcinoma in the thoracic esophagus: Who benefits? A retrospective study. *Dig Surg* 2003;20(3): 229-235; discussion 236-237.

179. Teniere P, Hay JM, Fingerhut A, Fagniez PL. Postoperative radiation therapy does not increase survival after curative resection for squamous cell carcinoma of the middle and lower esophagus as shown by a multicenter controlled trial. French University Association for Surgical Research. *Surg Gynecol Obstet* 1991;173(2):123-130.

180. Zieren HU, Muller JM, Jacobi CA, Pichlmaier H, Muller RP, Staar S. Adjuvant postoperative radiation therapy after curative resection of squamous cell carcinoma of the thoracic esophagus: A prospective randomized study. *World J Surg* 1995;19(3):444-449.

181. Xiao ZF, Yang ZY, Liang J, et al. Value of radiotherapy after radical surgery for esophageal carcinoma: A report of 495 patients. *Ann Thorac Surg* 2003;75(2):331-336.

182. Fok M, Sham JS, Choy D, Cheng SW, Wong J. Postoperative radiotherapy for carcinoma of the esophagus: A prospective, randomized controlled study. *Surgery* 1993;113(2):138-147.

183. Malthaner RA, Wong RK, Rumble RB, Zuraw L. Neoadjuvant or adjuvant therapy for resectable esophageal cancer: A clinical practice guideline. *BMC Cancer* 2004;4:67.

184. Ogoshi K, Satou H, Isono K, Mitomi T, Endoh M, Sugita M. Immunotherapy for esophageal cancer. A randomized trial in combination with radiotherapy and radiochemotherapy. Cooperative Study Group for Esophageal Cancer in Japan. *Am J Clin Oncol* 1995;18(3):216-222.

185. Gignoux M, Roussel A, Paillot B, et al. The value of preoperative radiotherapy in esophageal cancer: Results of a study of the E.O.R.T.C. *World J Surg* 1987;11(4):426-432.

186. Parker EF, Reed CE, Marks RD, Kratz JM, Connolly M. Chemotherapy, radiation therapy, and resection for carcinoma of the esophagus. Long-term results. *J Thorac Cardiovasc Surg* 1989;98(6):1037-1042; discussion 1042-1044.

187. Aoyama N, Koizumi H, Minamide J, Yoneyama K, Isono K. Prognosis of patients with advanced carcinoma of the esophagus with complete response to chemotherapy and/or radiation therapy: A questionnaire survey in Japan. Int *J Clin Oncol* 2001;6(3):132-137.

188. Ott K, Bader FG, Lordick F, Feith M, Bartels H, Siewert JR. Surgical factors influence the outcome after Ivor-Lewis esophagectomy with intrathoracic anastomosis for adenocarcinoma of the esophagogastric junction: A consecutive series of 240 patients at an experienced center. *Ann Surg Oncol* 2009;16(4):1017-1025.

189. Schlag P. Results of surgery in multimodality therapy of esophageal cancer. *Onkologie* 1991;14(1):13-14, 16, 18-20.

190. Ilson DH, Kelsen DP. Combined modality therapy in the treatment of esophageal cancer. *Semin Oncol* 1994;21(4):493-507.

191. Kok TC, Lanschot Jv, Siersema PD, Overhagen Hv, Tilanus HW. Neoadjuvant chemotherapy in operable esophageal squamous cell cancer: Final report of a phase III multicenter randomized controlled trial (meeting abstract). 1997 ASCO Annual Meeting.

192. Ancona E, Ruol A, Santi S, et al. Only pathologic complete response to neoadjuvant chemotherapy improves significantly the long term survival of patients with resectable esophageal squamous cell carcinoma: Final report of a randomized, controlled trial of preoperative chemotherapy versus surgery alone. *Cancer* 2001;91(11):2165-2174.

193. Roth JA. Esophageal cancer: Does preoperative chemotherapy make a difference? *J Surg Oncol* 1992;50(2):67-69.

194. Law S, Fok M, Chu KM, Wong J. Thoracoscopic esophagectomy for esophageal cancer. *Surgery* 1997;122(1):8-14.

195. Kelsen DP, Ginsberg R, Pajak TF, et al. Chemotherapy followed by surgery compared with surgery alone for localized esophageal cancer. *N Engl J Med* 1998;339(27):1979-1984.

196. Allum WH, Stenning SP, Bancewicz J, Clark PI, Langley RE. Long-term results of a randomized trial of surgery with or without preoperative chemotherapy in esophageal cancer. *J Clin Oncol* 2009;27(30):5062-5067.

197. Coia LR, Minsky BD, Berkey BA, et al. Outcome of patients receiving radiation for cancer of the esophagus: Results of the 1992-1994 Patterns of Care Study. *J Clin Oncol* 2000; 18(3):455-462.

198. Walsh TN, Noonan N, Hollywood D, Kelly A, Keeling N, Hennessy TP. A comparison of multimodal therapy and surgery for esophageal adenocarcinoma. *N Engl J Med* 1996;335(7):462-467.

199. Urba SG, Orringer MB, Turrisi A, Iannettoni M, Forastiere A, Strawderman M. Randomized trial of preoperative chemoradiation versus surgery alone in patients with locoregional esophageal carcinoma. *J Clin Oncol* 2001;19(2):305-313.

200. Burmeister BH, Smithers BM, Gebski V, et al. Surgery alone versus chemoradiotherapy followed by surgery for resectable cancer of the oesophagus: A randomised controlled phase III trial. *Lancet Oncol* 2005;6(9):659-668.

201. Kleinberg L, Powell ME, Forastiere A, Keller SM, Anne P, Benson A. Survival outcome of E1201: An Eastern Cooperative Oncology Group (ECOG) randomized phase II trial of neoadjuvant preoperative paclitaxel/cisplatin/radiotherapy (RT) or irinotecan/cisplatin/RT in endoscopy with ultrasound (EUS) staged esophageal adenocarcinoma. 2008 ASCO Annual Meeting Proceedings. *J Clin Oncol* 2008;26(May 20 Suppl) (abstract 4532).

202. Tepper J, Krasna MJ, Niedzwiecki D, et al. Phase III trial of trimodality therapy with cisplatin, fluorouracil, radiotherapy, and surgery compared with surgery alone for esophageal cancer: CALGB 9781. *J Clin Oncol* 2008;26(7):1086-1092.

203. Stahl M, Walz MK, Stuschke M, et al. Phase III comparison of preoperative chemotherapy compared with chemoradiotherapy in patients with locally advanced adenocarcinoma of the esophagogastric junction. *J Clin Oncol* 2009;27(6): 851-856.

204. Hofstetter W, Swisher SG, Correa AM, et al. Treatment outcomes of resected esophageal cancer. *Ann Surg* 2002; 236(3):376-384; discussion 384-385.

205. Gebski V, Burmeister B, Smithers BM, Foo K, Zalcberg J, Simes J. Survival benefits from neoadjuvant chemoradiotherapy or chemotherapy in oesophageal carcinoma: A meta-analysis. *Lancet Oncol* 2007;8(3):226-234.

206. Ajani J. Therapy of localized esophageal cancer: It is time to reengineer our investigative strategies. *Onkologie* 2008;31(7): 360-361.

207. Urschel JD, Vasan H. A meta-analysis of randomized controlled trials that compared neoadjuvant chemoradiation and surgery to surgery alone for resectable esophageal cancer. *Am J Surg* 2003;185(6):538-543.

208. Malthaner RA, Wong RK, Rumble RB, Zuraw L. Neoadjuvant or adjuvant therapy for resectable esophageal cancer: A systematic review and meta-analysis. *BMC Med* 2004;2:35.

209. Bedenne L, Michel P, Bouche O, et al. Chemoradiation followed by surgery compared with chemoradiation alone in squamous cancer of the esophagus: FFCD 9102. *J Clin Oncol* 2007;25(10):1160-1168.

210. Chiu PW, Chan AC, Leung SF, et al. Multicenter prospective randomized trial comparing standard esophagectomy with chemoradiotherapy for treatment of squamous esophageal cancer: Early results from the Chinese University Research Group for Esophageal Cancer (CURE). *J Gastrointest Surg* 2005;9(6):794-802.

211. Muto M, Ohtsu A, Miyamoto S, et al. Concurrent chemoradiotherapy for esophageal carcinoma patients with malignant fistulae. *Cancer* 1999; 86(8):1406-1413.

212. Koike R, Nishimura Y, Nakamatsu K, Kanamori S, Shibata T. Concurrent chemoradiotherapy for esophageal cancer with malignant fistula. *Int J Radiat Oncol Biol Phys* 2008;70(5): 1418-1422.

213. Minsky BD, Pajak TF, Ginsberg RJ, et al. INT 0123 (Radiation Therapy Oncology Group 94-05) phase III trial of combined-modality therapy for esophageal cancer: High-dose versus standard-dose radiation therapy. *J Clin Oncol* 2002; 20(5):1167-1174.

214. Coia LR, Engstrom PF, Paul AR, Stafford PM, Hanks GE. Long-term results of infusional 5-FU, mitomycin-C and radiation as primary management of esophageal carcinoma. *Int J Radiat Oncol Biol Phys* 1991;20(1):29-36.

215. Smith TJ, Ryan LM, Douglass HO, Jr., et al. Combined chemoradiotherapy vs. radiotherapy alone for early stage squamous cell carcinoma of the esophagus: A study of the Eastern Cooperative Oncology Group. *Int J Radiat Oncol Biol Phys* 1998;42(2):269-276.

216. Lorenzen S, Schuster T, Porschen R, et al. Cetuximab plus cisplatin-5-fluorouracil versus cisplatin-5-fluorouracil alone in first-line metastatic squamous cell carcinoma of the esophagus: A randomized phase II study of the Arbeitsgemeinschaft Internistische Onkologie. *Ann Oncol* 2009;20(10): 1667-1673.

217. Maganti K, Onyemere K, Jones MP. Oral erythromycin and symptomatic relief of gastroparesis: A systematic review. *Am J Gastroenterol* 2003;98(2):259-263.

218. Nelson KA, Walsh TD. Metoclopramide in anorexia caused by cancer-associated dyspepsia syndrome (CADS). *J Palliat Care* 1993;9(2):14-18.

219. van Cutsem E, Kang YK, Chung H, et al. Efficacy results from the ToGA trial: A phase III study of trastuzumab added to standard chemotherapy (CT) in first-line human epidermal growth factor receptor 2 (HER2)-positive advanced gastric cancer (GC). *J Clin Oncol* 2009;27(18s):LBA4509.

220. Pyrhonen S, Kuitunen T, Nyandoto P, Kouri M. Randomised comparison of fluorouracil, epidoxorubicin and methotrexate (FEMTX) plus supportive care with supportive care alone in patients with non-resectable gastric cancer. *Br J Cancer* 1995;71(3):587-591.

221. Glimelius B, Ekstrom K, Hoffman K, et al. Randomized comparison between chemotherapy plus best supportive care with best supportive care in advanced gastric cancer. *Ann Oncol* 1997;8(2):163-168.

222. Janunger KG, Hafstrom L, Nygren P, Glimelius B. A systematic overview of chemotherapy effects in gastric cancer. *Acta Oncol* 2001;40(2-3):309-326.

223. Wohrer SS, Raderer M, Hejna M. Palliative chemotherapy for advanced gastric cancer. *Ann Oncol* 2004;15(11):1585-1595.

224. Murad AM, Santiago FF, Petroianu A, Rocha PR, Rodrigues MA, Rausch M. Modified therapy with 5-fluorouracil, doxorubicin, and methotrexate in advanced gastric cancer. *Cancer* 1993;72(1):37-41.

225. Wagner AD, Grothe W, Haerting J, Kleber G, Grothey A, Fleig WE. Chemotherapy in advanced gastric cancer: A systematic review and meta-analysis based on aggregate data. *J Clin Oncol* 2006;24(18):2903-2909.

226. Pozzo C, Barone C. Is there an optimal chemotherapy regimen for the treatment of advanced gastric cancer that will provide a platform for the introduction of new biological agents? *Oncologist* 2008;13(7):794-806.

227. Bouche O, Raoul JL, Bonnetain F, et al. Randomized multicenter phase II trial of a biweekly regimen of fluorouracil and leucovorin (LV5FU2), LV5FU2 plus cisplatin, or LV5FU2 plus irinotecan in patients with previously untreated metastatic gastric cancer: A Federation Francophone de Cancerologie Digestive Group Study—FFCD 9803. *J Clin Oncol* 2004;22(21):4319-4328.

228. Rohatgi PR, Swisher SG, Correa AM, et al. Histologic subtypes as determinants of outcome in esophageal carcinoma patients with pathologic complete response after preoperative chemoradiotherapy. *Cancer* 2006;106(3):552-558.

229. Webb A, Cunningham D, Scarffe JH, et al. Randomized trial comparing epirubicin, cisplatin, and fluorouracil versus fluorouracil, doxorubicin, and methotrexate in advanced esophagogastric cancer. *J Clin Oncol* 1997;15(1):261-267.

230. Chau I, Ashley S, Cunningham D. Validation of the Royal Marsden hospital prognostic index in advanced esophagogastric cancer using individual patient data from the REAL 2 study. *J Clin Oncol* 2009;27(19):e3-e4.

231. Cunningham D, Starling N, Rao S, et al. Capecitabine and oxaliplatin for advanced esophagogastric cancer. *N Engl J Med* 2008;358(1):36-46.

232. A comparative clinical assessment of combination chemotherapy in the management of advanced gastric carcinoma: The Gastrointestinal Tumor study Group. *Cancer* 1982;49(7):1362-1366.

233. Klein HO, Wils J, Bleiberg H, Buyse M, Duez N. An EORTC gastrointestinal (GI) group randomized evaluation of the toxicity of sequential high dose methotrexate and 5-fluorouracil combined with adriamycin (FAMTX) vs 5-fluorouracil, adriamycin and mitomycin (FAM) in advanced gastric cancer. *Med Oncol Tumor Pharmacother* 1989;6(2):171-174.

234. Vanhoefer U, Rougier P, Wilke H, et al. Final results of a randomized phase III trial of sequential high-dose methotrexate,

fluorouracil, and doxorubicin versus etoposide, leucovorin, and fluorouracil versus infusional fluorouracil and cisplatin in advanced gastric cancer: A trial of the European Organization for Research and Treatment of Cancer Gastrointestinal Tract Cancer Cooperative Group. *J Clin Oncol* 2000;18(14): 2648-2657.

235. Findlay M, Cunningham D, Norman A, et al. A phase II study in advanced gastro-esophageal cancer using epirubicin and cisplatin in combination with continuous infusion 5-fluorouracil (ECF). *Ann Oncol* 1994;5(7):609-616.

236. Waters JS, Norman A, Cunningham D, et al. Long-term survival after epirubicin, cisplatin and fluorouracil for gastric cancer: Results of a randomized trial. *Br J Cancer* 1999;80(1-2): 269-272.

237. Ross P, Nicolson M, Cunningham D, et al. Prospective randomized trial comparing mitomycin, cisplatin, and protracted venous-infusion fluorouracil (PVI 5-FU) with epirubicin, cisplatin, and PVI 5-FU in advanced esophagogastric cancer. *J Clin Oncol* 2002;20(8):1996-2004.

238. Cocconi G, Carlini P, Gamboni A, et al. Cisplatin, epirubicin, leucovorin and 5-fluorouracil (PELF) is more active than 5-fluorouracil, doxorubicin and methotrexate (FAMTX) in advanced gastric carcinoma. *Ann Oncol* 2003;14(8): 1258-1263.

239. Van Cutsem E, Moiseyenko VM, Tjulandin S, et al. Phase III study of docetaxel and cisplatin plus fluorouracil compared with cisplatin and fluorouracil as first-line therapy for advanced gastric cancer: A report of the V325 Study Group. *J Clin Oncol* 2006;24(31):4991-4997.

240. Ajani JA, Moiseyenko VM, Tjulandin S, et al. Clinical benefit with docetaxel plus fluorouracil and cisplatin compared with cisplatin and fluorouracil in a phase III trial of advanced gastric or gastroesophageal cancer adenocarcinoma: The V-325 Study Group. *J Clin Oncol* 2007;25(22):3205-3209.

241. Roth AD, Fazio N, Stupp R, et al. Docetaxel, cisplatin, and fluorouracil; docetaxel and cisplatin; and epirubicin, cisplatin, and fluorouracil as systemic treatment for advanced gastric carcinoma: A randomized phase II trial of the Swiss Group for Clinical Cancer Research. *J Clin Oncol* 2007;25(22): 3217-3223.

242. Tebbutt NC, Cummins MM, Sourjina T, et al. Randomised, non-comparative phase II study of weekly docetaxel with cisplatin and 5-fluorouracil or with capecitabine in oesophagogastric cancer: The AGITG ATTAX trial. *Br J Cancer* 102(3):475-481.

243. Ajani JA, Baker J, Pisters PW, et al. Irinotecan/cisplatin in advanced, treated gastric or gastroesophageal junction carcinoma. *Oncology (Williston Park)* 2002;16(5 Suppl 5):16-18.

244. Ilson DH. Phase II trial of weekly irinotecan/cisplatin in advanced esophageal cancer. *Oncology (Williston Park)*. 2004;18(14 Suppl 14):22-25.

245. Boku N, Ohtsu A, Shimada Y, et al. Phase II study of a combination of irinotecan and cisplatin against metastatic gastric cancer. *J Clin Oncol* 1999;17(1):319-323.

246. Pozzo C, Barone C, Szanto J, et al. Irinotecan in combination with 5-fluorouracil and folinic acid or with cisplatin in patients with advanced gastric or esophageal-gastric junction adenocarcinoma: Results of a randomized phase II study. *Ann Oncol* 2004;15(12):1773-1781.

247. Dank M, Zaluski J, Barone C, et al. Randomized phase III study comparing irinotecan combined with 5-fluorouracil and folinic acid to cisplatin combined with 5-fluorouracil in chemotherapy naive patients with advanced adenocarcinoma of the stomach or esophagogastric junction. *Ann Oncol* 2008;19(8):1450-1457.

248. Al-Batran SE, Hartmann JT, Probst S, et al. Phase III trial in metastatic gastroesophageal adenocarcinoma with fluorouracil, leucovorin plus either oxaliplatin or cisplatin: A study of the Arbeitsgemeinschaft Internistische Onkologie. *J Clin Oncol* 2008;26(9):1435-1442.

249. Kang YK, Kang WK, Shin DB, et al. Capecitabine/cisplatin versus 5-fluorouracil/cisplatin as first-line therapy in patients with advanced gastric cancer: A randomised phase III noninferiority trial. *Ann Oncol* 2009;20(4):666-673.

250. Shirasaka T, Nakano K, Takechi T, et al. Antitumor activity of 1 M tegafur-0.4 M 5-chloro-2,4-dihydroxypyridine-1 M potassium oxonate (S-1) against human colon carcinoma orthotopically implanted into nude rats. *Cancer Res* 1996; 56(11):2602-2606.

251. Boku N, Yamamoto S, Fukuda H, et al. Fluorouracil versus combination of irinotecan plus cisplatin versus S-1 in metastatic gastric cancer: A randomised phase 3 study. *Lancet Oncol* 2009;10(11):1063-1069.

252. Koizumi W, Narahara H, Hara T, et al. S-1 plus cisplatin versus S-1 alone for first-line treatment of advanced gastric cancer (SPIRITS trial): A phase III trial. *Lancet Oncol* 2008; 9(3):215-221.

253. Imamura H, Ilishi H, Tsuburaya A, et al. Randomized phase III study of irinotecan plus S-1 (IRIS) versus S-1 alone as first-line treatment for advanced gastric cancer (GC0301/ TOP-002). 2008 ASCO Gastrointestinal Cancers Symposium. *J Clin Oncol* 2008 (abstract 5).

254. Ajani JA, Rodriguez W, Bodoky G, et al. Multicenter phase III comparison of cisplatin/S-1 with cisplatin/infusional fluorouracil in advanced gastric or gastroesophageal adenocarcinoma study: The FLAGS trial. *J Clin Oncol* 28(9): 1547-1553.

255. El-Rayes BF, Shields A, Zalupski M, et al. A phase II study of carboplatin and paclitaxel in esophageal cancer. *Ann Oncol* 2004;15(6):960-965.

256. Kim KH, Park YS, Chang MH, et al. A phase I/II trial of docetaxel and oxaliplatin in patients with advanced gastric cancer. *Cancer Chemother Pharmacol* 2009;64(2):347-353.

257. Park SR, Chun JH, Yu MS, et al. Phase II study of docetaxel and irinotecan combination chemotherapy in metastatic gastric carcinoma. *Br J Cancer* 2006;94(10):1402-1406.

258. Kim SG, Oh SY, Kwon HC, et al. A phase II study of irinotecan with bi-weekly, low-dose leucovorin and bolus and continuous infusion 5-fluorouracil (modified FOLFIRI) as salvage therapy for patients with advanced or metastatic gastric cancer. *Jpn J Clin Oncol* 2007;37(10):744-749.

259. Lordick F, Lorenzen S, Stollfuss J, et al. Phase II study of weekly oxaliplatin plus infusional fluorouracil and folinic acid (FUFOX regimen) as first-line treatment in metastatic gastric cancer. *Br J Cancer* 2005;93(2):190-194.

260. Cao W, Yang W, Lou G, et al. Phase II trial of infusional fluorouracil, leucovorin, oxaliplatin, and irinotecan (FOLFOXIRI) as first-line treatment for advanced gastric cancer. *Anticancer Drugs* 2009;20(4):287-293.

261. Ji SH, Lim do H, Yi SY, et al. A retrospective analysis of second-line chemotherapy in patients with advanced gastric cancer. *BMC Cancer* 2009;9:110.

262. Chau I, Norman AR, Cunningham D, Waters JS, Oates J, Ross PJ. Multivariate prognostic factor analysis in locally

advanced and metastatic esophago-gastric cancer—pooled analysis from three multicenter, randomized, controlled trials using individual patient data. *J Clin Oncol* 2004;22(12): 2395-2403.

263. Lee KW, Kim JH, Yun T, et al. Phase II study of low-dose paclitaxel and cisplatin as a second-line therapy after 5-fluorouracil/platinum chemotherapy in gastric cancer. *J Korean Med Sci* 2007; 22(Suppl):S115-S121.

264. Wilson KS, Barnett JB, Shah A, Khoo KE. The BC Cancer Agency Compassionate Access Program: Outcome analysis of patients with esophagogastric cancer. *Curr Oncol* 2009; 16(5):9-14.

265. Rosati G, Ferrara D, Manzione L. New perspectives in the treatment of advanced or metastatic gastric cancer. *World J Gastroenterol* 2009;15(22):2689-2692.

266. Lee JL, Ryu MH, Chang HM, et al. A phase II study of docetaxel as salvage chemotherapy in advanced gastric cancer after failure of fluoropyrimidine and platinum combination chemotherapy. *Cancer Chemother Pharmacol* 2008;61(4): 631-637.

267. Galizia G, Lieto E, Orditura M, et al. Epidermal growth factor receptor (EGFR) expression is associated with a worse prognosis in gastric cancer patients undergoing curative surgery. *World J Surg* 2007;31(7):1458-1468.

268. Lieto E, Ferraraccio F, Orditura M, et al. Expression of vascular endothelial growth factor (VEGF) and epidermal growth factor receptor (EGFR) is an independent prognostic indicator of worse outcome in gastric cancer patients. *Ann Surg Oncol* 2008;15(1):69-79.

269. Park DI, Yun JW, Park JH, et al. HER-2/neu amplification is an independent prognostic factor in gastric cancer. *Dig Dis Sci* 2006;51(8):1371-1379.

270. Matsubara J, Nishina T, Yamada Y, et al. Impacts of excision repair cross-complementing gene 1 (ERCC1), dihydropyrimidine dehydrogenase, and epidermal growth factor receptor on the outcomes of patients with advanced gastric cancer. *Br J Cancer* 2008;98(4):832-839.

271. Wang X, Wu CX, Zheng Y, Wang JJ. (Time trends and characteristics of gastric cancer incidence in urban Shanghai). *Zhonghua Liu Xing Bing Xue Za Zhi* 2007; 28(9):875-880.

272. Shah MA, Ramanathan RK, Ilson DH, et al. Multicenter phase II study of irinotecan, cisplatin, and bevacizumab in patients with metastatic gastric or gastroesophageal junction adenocarcinoma. *J Clin Oncol* 2006;24(33):5201-5206.

273. Kelsen D, Jhawer M, Ilson D, et al. Analysis of survival with modified docetaxel, cisplatin, fluorouracil (mDCF), and bevacizumab (BEV) in patients with metastatic gastroesophageal (GE) adenocarcinoma: Results of a phase II clinical trial. 2009 ASCO Annual Meeting Proceedings. *J Clin Oncol* 2009;27(15s) (abstract 4512).

274. Kimura T, Maesawa C, Ikeda K, Wakabayashi G, Masuda T. Mutations of the epidermal growth factor receptor gene in gastrointestinal tract tumor cell lines. *Oncol Rep* 2006;15(5): 1205-1210.

275. Dragovich T, McCoy S, Fenoglio-Preiser CM, et al. Phase II trial of erlotinib in gastroesophageal junction and gastric adenocarcinomas: SWOG 0127. *J Clin Oncol* 2006;24(30): 4922-4927.

276. Rojo F, Tabernero J, Albanell J, et al. Pharmacodynamic studies of gefitinib in tumor biopsy specimens from patients with advanced gastric carcinoma. *J Clin Oncol* 2006; 24(26):4309-4316.

277. Pinto C, Di Fabio F, Siena S, et al. Phase II study of cetuximab in combination with FOLFIRI in patients with untreated advanced gastric or gastroesophageal junction adenocarcinoma (FOLCETUX study). *Ann Oncol* 2007;18(3): 510-517.

278. Lordick F, Luber B, Lorenzen S, et al. Cetuximab plus oxaliplatin/leucovorin/ 5-fluorouracil in first-line metastatic gastric cancer: A phase II study of the Arbeitsgemeinschaft Internistische Onkologie (AIO). *Br J Cancer* 2010;102(3): 500-505.

279. Baselga J, Swain SM. Novel anticancer targets: Revisiting ERBB2 and discovering ERBB3. *Nat Rev Cancer* 2009;9(7): 463-475.

280. Valabrega G, Montemurro F, Aglietta M. Trastuzumab: Mechanism of action, resistance and future perspectives in HER2-overexpressing breast cancer. *Ann Oncol* 2007;18(6):977-984.

281. Marx AH, Tharun L, Muth J, et al. HER-2 amplification is highly homogenous in gastric cancer. *Hum Pathol* 2009;40(6): 769-777.

282. Barros-Silva JD, Leitao D, Afonso L, et al. Association of ERBB2 gene status with histopathological parameters and disease-specific survival in gastric carcinoma patients. *Br J Cancer* 2009;100(3):487-493.

283. Yu GZ, Chen Y, Wang JJ. Overexpression of Grb2/HER2 signaling in Chinese gastric cancer: Their relationship with clinicopathological parameters and prognostic significance. *J Cancer Res Clin Oncol* 2009;135(10):1331-1339.

284. Bang YJ, Chung H, Xu J, et al. Pathological features of advanced gastric cancer (GC): Relationship to human epidermal growth factor receptor 2 (HER2) positivity in the global screening programme of the ToGA trial. 2009 ASCO Annual Meeting Proceedings. *J Clin Oncol* 2009;27(15S) (abstract 4556).

285. Dar AA, Belkhiri A, El-Rifai W. The aurora kinase A regulates GSK-3beta in gastric cancer cells. *Oncogene* 2009; 28(6):866-875.

286. Macarulla T, Ramos FJ, Tabernero J. Aurora kinase family: A new target for anticancer drug. *Recent Pat Anticancer Drug Discov* 2008;3(2):114-122.

287. Weichert W, Ullrich A, Schmidt M, et al. Expression patterns of polo-like kinase 1 in human gastric cancer. *Cancer Sci* 2006;97(4):271-276.

288. Senderowicz AM. Small molecule modulators of cyclin-dependent kinases for cancer therapy. *Oncogene* 2000; 19(56):6600-6606.

289. Schwartz GK, Ilson D, Saltz L, et al. Phase II study of the cyclin-dependent kinase inhibitor flavopiridol administered to patients with advanced gastric carcinoma. *J Clin Oncol* 2001;19(7):1985-1992.

290. Zuo DS, Dai J, Bo AH, Fan J, Xiao XY. Significance of expression of heat shock protein90alpha in human gastric cancer. *World J Gastroenterol* 2003;9(11):2616-6218.

291. Fujita T, Doihara H, Washio K, et al. Antitumor effects and drug interactions of the proteasome inhibitor bortezomib (PS341) in gastric cancer cells. *Anticancer Drugs* 2007;18(6): 677-686.

292. Ocean AJ, Schnoll-Sussman F, Chen X, et al. Recent results of phase II study of PS-341 (bortezomib) with or without irinotecan in patients (pts) with advanced gastric adenocarcinomas

(AGA). 2007 Gastrointestinal Cancers Symposium. *J Clin Oncol* 2007 (abstract 45).

293. Oki E, Baba H, Tokunaga E, et al. Akt phosphorylation associates with LOH of PTEN and leads to chemoresistance for gastric cancer. *Int J Cancer* 2005;117(3):376-380.

294. Cejka D, Preusser M, Fuereder T, et al. mTOR inhibition sensitizes gastric cancer to alkylating chemotherapy in vivo. Anticancer Res 2008; 28(6A):3801-3808.

295. Yamada Y, Doi T, Muro K, et al. Multicenter phase II study of everolimus in patients with previously treated metastatic gastric cancer: Main results. 2009 Gastrointestinal Cancers Symposium. *J Clin Oncol* 2009 (abstract 77).

296. Iqbal S, Goldman H, Lenz HJ, Fenoglio CJ, Blanke CD. S0413: A phase II SWOG study of GW572016 (lapatinib) as first line therapy in patients (pts) with advanced or metastatic gastric cancer. 2007 ASCO Annual Meeting Proceedings. *J Clin Oncol* 2007;25(18S Suppl) (abstract 4621).

297. Chang AC, Ji H, Birkmeyer NJ, Orringer MB, Birkmeyer JD. Outcomes after transhiatal and transthoracic esophagectomy for cancer. *Ann Thorac Surg* 2008;85(2):424-429.

298. Bourke MJ, Hope RL, Chu G, et al. Laser palliation of inoperable malignant dysphagia: Initial and at death. *Gastrointest Endosc* 1996; 43(1):29-32.

299. Bosset JF, Gignoux M, Triboulet JP, et al. Chemoradiotherapy followed by surgery compared with surgery alone in squamous-cell cancer of the esophagus. *N Engl J Med* 1997;337(3):161-167.

300. Crehange G, Peignaux K, Bosset M, Servagi-Vernat S, Bosset JF, Maingon P. Exclusive chemoradiotherapy for patients with medically inoperable early-stage oesophageal cancer. *Clin Oncol (R Coll Radiol)* 2007;19(8):632-633.

301. Han SW, et al. Phase II study and biomarker analysis of cetuximab combined with modified FOLFOX6 in advanced gastric cancer. *Br J Cancer* 2009;100(2):298-304.

Rachna T. Shroff
Robert A. Wolff
Milind M. Javle

■ PANCREATIC CANCER

When clinicians use the term *pancreatic cancer*, they refer to adenocarcinoma of the pancreas, one of the most challenging malignancies facing oncologists today. This disease is characterized by significant morbidity and poor prognosis. During the course of illness, a variety of problems may beset the patient and confront the clinician. At The University of Texas MD Anderson Cancer Center (MDACC), we manage pancreatic cancer patients with a multidisciplinary team and view

palliation as the primary goal. However, for patients with potentially resectable disease, we take an aggressive multimodality approach whenever medically appropriate. In the setting of advanced disease, cure is not possible, but as our understanding of the underlying molecular events involved in carcinogenesis, invasion, and metastasis expands, more effective therapeutic strategies are expected to emerge. Therefore, whenever feasible, patients with advanced disease are treated in clinical trials with special emphasis on targeted therapy. This chapter reviews our current knowledge about pancreatic cancer, including its epidemiology, risk factors, molecular biology, diagnosis and staging, and clinical strategies for current and future therapies.

HARD FACTS ABOUT PANCREATIC CANCER

Pancreatic cancer, the most common pancreatic neoplasm, is an aggressive and often rapidly fatal malignancy. In the United States, it represents only 2% of all cancer cases but accounts for 5% of all cancer deaths (1). Currently, it is the fourth leading cause of cancer death, ranking only behind lung cancer, colorectal cancer, and breast cancer. While recent evidence suggests marginal improvements in 5-year survival rates over the last 25 years (2% in 1974-1976, 3% in 1983-1985, and 4% in 1992-1997), life expectancy remains short and is generally measured in months (2). Significant improvements in survival have been hampered by a number of factors, including inefficient and ineffective screening strategies, resulting in frequent presentation with advanced disease, technically challenging and often debilitating surgery (which is commonly misapplied), and minimally effective chemotherapy and radiotherapy.

Moreover, pancreatic cancer is a dynamic disease, and sudden changes in clinical status occur frequently. Patients may rapidly develop worsening pain, biliary obstruction, or stent occlusion with cholangitis, gastrointestinal bleeding, thromboembolism, gastric outlet obstruction, or peritoneal carcinomatosis with intestinal dysmotility or intractable ascites. Any of these problems may preclude the timely delivery of cytotoxic therapy and limit opportunities to alter survival. Therefore most efforts should focus on symptom control, but for patients with adequate performance status, treatment is encouraged.

EPIDEMIOLOGY

There are approximately 30,000 new cases of pancreatic cancer each year in the United States and 170,000 cases worldwide. Overall, the incidence and mortality of pancreatic cancer are similar throughout the world, but incidence rates are highest in industrialized societies and Western countries. Of particular note is the risk of pancreatic cancer among African Americans, in whom pancreatic cancer mortality rates are higher than for most other ethnic groups in the United States and considerably higher than the rates for African blacks (3). This finding mimics the epidemiology of colon cancer, a disease in which African Americans also have a substantially higher risk than American whites or African blacks. These observations implicate environmental factors conspiring with genetic background as causes of the increase in risk.

The risk of developing pancreatic cancer is low in the first three to four decades of life but increases sharply after the age of 50 years. At the time of diagnosis, most patients are between the ages of 60 and 80 years. Pancreatic cancer is uncommon in patients under 40 years of age, but apparently sporadic cases may rarely occur in patients younger than 30 years. In the past, pancreatic cancer occurred more frequently in men, but incidence and mortality rates in women have steadily increased, and now the disease is becoming more common in women, probably secondary to the increased use of tobacco by women.

RISK FACTORS FOR PANCREATIC CANCER

Surprisingly, relatively little is known about the risk factors for the development of pancreatic cancer. Table 18-1 summarizes genetic and environmental factors associated with an increased risk of pancreatic cancer.

Tobacco

Other than age, the only consistently reported risk factor for pancreatic cancer is cigarette smoking. Cigarette smoking is estimated to account for roughly 30% of all pancreatic cancer mortality (4). An etiologic role for tobacco smoke has been supported by experimental models, which have demonstrated that nitrosamines found in tobacco smoke are carcinogenic for the pancreas. Research performed at MDACC has shown that smoking-related aromatic DNA adducts and other types of DNA damage have all been detected in human pancreatic tissues and may be critical initiating events in pancreatic carcinogenesis.

Diabetes Mellitus

An association between diabetes mellitus and pancreatic cancer has long been known, although the precise mechanisms have yet to be defined and not all studies have supported diabetes as a definite risk factor. Diabetes has been implicated both as an early manifestation of pancreatic cancer and as a predisposing factor. A meta-analysis of studies published between 1975 and 1994 showed that pancreatic cancer occurred with increased frequency in patients with long-standing diabetes (diabetes diagnosed at least 5 years prior to the diagnosis of pancreatic cancer or death due to pancreatic

TABLE 18-1 | ACQUIRED AND GENETIC RISKS FACTORS ASSOCIATED WITH PANCREATIC CANCER

Acquired Risk Factors	Relative Risk	Comments
Tobacco smoking	2-5	Risk increases with increasing exposure.
Diabetes mellitus	2	Not all authorities concur; many patients have altered glucose metabolism on presentation.
High body mass index	2	
Chronic pancreatitis	13-18	Not all authorities concur with this degree of increased risk.

Inherited Disorders	Relative Risk	Known Defects
Hereditary pancreatitis	10-53	PRSS1
FAMMM syndrome	22	p16INK/CDKN2
HNPCC	8	MLH1, MSH2, MSH6
Peutz-Jeghers syndrome	13-30	LBK1/STK11
Familial adenomatous polyposis	4-5	APC
Li-Fraumeni syndrome	?	p53
Familial breast and ovarian cancer	3-5	DNA repair pathways, BRCA2

FAMMM, familial atypical mole and melanoma; HNPCC, hereditary non-polyposis colon cancer.

cancer) (5). Further, recent cohort studies have suggested that abnormal glucose metabolism is associated with an increased risk of developing pancreatic cancer. It is believed that insulin resistance and secondary hyperinsulinism may be involved in pancreatic carcinogenesis, with high insulin concentrations in the microenvironment of the pancreatic ductal cells contributing to malignant transformation.

Chronic Pancreatitis

As with diabetes, an association between pancreatitis and pancreatic cancer has been suspected, but a clear link remains uncertain. Early clinical studies have suggested that chronic forms of pancreatitis were most closely associated with the subsequent development of pancreatic cancer. For example, in a study of 715 patients with chronic pancreatitis diagnosed between 1971 and 1995, a 13- to 18-fold increase in the incidence of pancreatic cancer was demonstrated (6).

More recent studies have suggested that the type of pancreatitis may affect the risk of pancreatic cancer, in particular hereditary pancreatitis. Lowenfels and Maisonneuve obtained data on 246 patients with hereditary pancreatitis from pancreatologists in 10 countries. The estimated cumulative risk of developing pancreatic cancer by age 70 was approximately 40% in this group. Of note, the mean age at diagnosis was 57 years (7). Recent molecular data strongly suggest that mutations in the cationic trypsinogen gene *PRSS1* play an important role in hereditary and possibly acquired forms of

pancreatitis, thereby increasing the risk for pancreatic cancer (8).

Diet

Positive associations have been discovered between pancreatic cancer and meat and carbohydrate intake. However, there is no general consensus on the role of dietary fat as a factor leading to pancreatic cancer. Epidemiologic studies of pancreatic cancer have shown a protective role for diet high in fruits and vegetables. This effect may be related to dietary intake of folate and other methyl donor groups.

Body Mass Index

Recent epidemiologic studies have also implicated a high body mass index as increasing risk, and current estimates suggest that people with a high body mass index have an increased risk of developing pancreatic cancer. This may be explained by relative hyperinsulinemia, commonly observed in these individuals and thought to promote pancreatic carcinogenesis (9).

Familial Pancreatic Cancer and Other Genetic Syndromes

Another emerging risk factor for pancreatic cancer is family history. Pancreatic cancer patients who have two first-degree relatives with a history of pancreatic cancer are defined as having familial pancreatic cancer. The relative risk for other family members has been estimated to be increased 10- to 20-fold over the general population. In addition, several genetic syndromes are associated with an increased risk of pancreatic cancer, including hereditary pancreatitis, hereditary nonpolyposis colorectal cancer, ataxia-telangiectasia, Peutz-Jeghers syndrome, familial breast and ovarian cancer, and familial atypical multiple-mole melanoma (10).

Occupational Exposures

Exposure to carcinogens in the workplace has been implicated in the etiology of pancreatic cancer, but with the possible exception of formaldehyde, the available evidence is insufficient to identify any specific exposure as likely to substantially increase the risk.

Prior Gastrointestinal Surgery

Surgical procedures such as gastrectomy and cholecystectomy have been reported to increase pancreatic cancer risk and are possibly linked to elevated levels of cholecystokinin and hypergastrinemia. However, other studies have not demonstrated such a clear risk (11).

LINKING RISK FACTORS TO MOLECULAR EVENTS

Research efforts aimed at quantifying risk factors and identifying individuals at high risk are critical to the eventual prevention of and screening for this disease. To that end, there have been some major advances in understanding the interactions between the host's environment and its susceptibility to tissue injury at the molecular level that ultimately lead to human cancer, including pancreatic cancer. Studies performed at MDACC by Li et al., have identified novel associations between polymorphisms of DNA damage-repair and insulin growth factor pathway genes, Body Mass Index and ABO blood groups with risk of pancreatic cancer (12-15). Growing evidence supports the hypothesis that individuals with deficient carcinogen detoxification and DNA repair capabilities are at increased risk of pancreatic cancer (16). More studies are needed to elucidate the role of other genes and pathways critical for pancreatic carcinogenesis.

MOLECULAR EVENTS IN HUMAN PANCREATIC CARCINOGENESIS

Pancreatic carcinogenesis is a complex series of events at the molecular level, which ultimately transforms the normal ductal cells having tightly regulated growth mechanisms to normal-appearing cells with a proliferative advantage and finally to histologically abnormal cells, with inappropriate growth regulation and invasive potential.

The molecular events leading to human pancreatic cancer have not been fully elucidated, but mutations of a few specific oncogenes and tumor suppressor genes appear critical for pancreatic carcinogenesis. Recently, investigators from Johns Hopkins performed a comprehensive genetic analysis of pancreatic cancer and reported their findings in the journal *Science*. They noted that pancreatic cancers contain an average of 63 genetic alterations, the majority of which are point mutations. These alterations defined a core set of 12 cellular signaling pathways and processes that were each genetically altered in the majority of the pancreatic cancers. These included the K-*ras*, *wnt/notch*, hedgehog, *TGF-β*, integrin, and JNK signaling pathways (17).

Oncogene Mutation: The *ras* Oncogene

Pancreatic cancer has the highest frequency of K-*ras* mutation among all human cancers. Greater than 85% cases of pancreatic ductal cancer have an activating point mutation in the K-*ras* gene. The most common mutation is a G-to-T transversion at codon 12 of K-*ras* (18). This point mutation leads to constitutive activation of the RAS protein, leading to growth-promoting signal cascades propagated through the mitogen-activated protein (MAP)-kinase pathway. Preclinical models have implicated this mutation as a very early event in pancreatic carcinogenesis; this is supported by clinical findings. For example, *ras* oncogene mutations were retrospectively noted in pancreatic juice that was collected 3.5 years before the patient's diagnosis of pancreatic cancer was made (19).

Tumor Suppressor Gene Mutation and Inactivation

The *p16* tumor suppressor gene is inactivated in approximately 95% of pancreatic cancers; this typically occurs later in pancreatic carcinogenesis. The second most frequently inactivated tumor suppressor gene is *p53*, a well-characterized tumor suppressor located on chromosome 17p. Its inactivation also appears to be a late event in tumorigenesis. The *DPC4* gene (SMAD4) is inactivated in 55% of pancreatic adenocarcinomas. Inactivation of *DPC4*, like that of *p53*, is a relatively late event in pancreatic tumorigenesis. Other less common genetic alterations continue to be described in pancreatic cancer. In a recent comprehensive mutational analysis of 42 pancreatic ductal cancers, Rozenblum and colleagues found that all tumors harbored mutations in the K-*ras* oncogene. The individual mutational frequencies of tumor suppressor genes *p16*, *p53*, *DPC4*, and *BRCA2* were 82, 76, 53, and 10%, respectively (19).

The Multistep Sequence of Pancreatic Carcinogenesis

Like the adenoma-carcinoma sequence proposed for the development of colorectal cancer, current data suggest that there is a temporal sequence of molecular events in pancreatic carcinogenesis leading from an "adenomatous" or proliferative ductal cell phenotype to pancreatic intraepithelial neoplasia (Pan-IN) and finally to invasive cancer. This theory has been supported by the recognition of noninvasive proliferative ductal lesions (Pan-IN1) found within human pancreata resected for carcinoma. Furthermore, examination of the genetic changes found in these early lesions demonstrates genetic mutations commonly found in pancreatic cancer. Growing evidence suggests that the gradual accumulation of genetic and biochemical alterations in these early lesions causes progression through higher levels of dysplasia (Pan-IN2 and Pan-IN3) and ultimately to cancer. The phenotypic changes are associated with mutation of the K-*ras* oncogene as an early event and mutations of the tumor suppressor genes *p53*, *p16*, and *DPC4* as later events.

Other Molecular Events in Pancreatic Carcinogenesis, Invasion, and Metastasis

In addition to the mutations commonly found in pancreatic adenocarcinomas, there is growing appreciation for the role of other gene products in pancreatic tumor progression, invasion, and metastasis. These include overexpression of epidermal growth factor receptor (EGFR), vascular endothelial growth factor (VEGF), matrix metalloproteinases, cyclooxygenase 2 (COX-2), hedgehog signaling, and insulin-like growth factor-1 (IGF-1) pathways. Studies conducted at MDACC have also demonstrated that the nuclear transcription factor NF-κB is commonly activated in pancreatic cancer cells (20).

Hedgehog Signaling Pathway

Hedgehog signaling is an essential pathway during embryogenesis of the normal pancreas and its dysregulation has been reported in both precancerous PanIN-1 and -2 as well as in primary and metastatic pancreatic adenocarcinomas. Notably, inhibition of hedgehog signaling by cyclopamine induced apoptosis and blocked proliferation in a subset of the pancreatic cancer cell lines both *in vitro* and *in vivo* (21). Hedgehog inhibition also depletes tumor-associated stroma and may play an important role in the efficient delivery of chemotherapeutic agents like gemcitabine (22). Clinical trials of hedgehog inhibitors in combination with gemcitabine are ongoing.

IGF-1 Pathway

IGF-1 upregulates cell proliferation and invasiveness through activation of PI3K/Akt signaling pathway. IGF-1 also downregulates the tumor suppressor chromosome 10 (PTEN). Akt mediates the gemcitabine and erlotinib resistance mechanisms. Clinical investigations designed to exploit these molecular targets are now under way in an effort to improve therapy. A current study at MDACC is investigating the combination of gemcitabine, erlotinib ± MK-0646, a humanized monoclonal antibody directed against the IGF-1 receptor. Targeted therapy has been a major focus of clinical research within our pancreatic cancer working group, and these approaches have generally taken priority over the study of more conventional cytotoxic agents, particularly among patients with locally advanced or metastatic disease. Preliminary studies with agents designed to abrogate RAS function have been disappointing (23). Likewise, administration of inhibitors of matrix metalloproteinases has failed to demonstrate a meaningful clinical advantage compared to conventional chemotherapy (24). Recent studies that included the inhibitors of EGFR, VEGF, NF-κB, or COX-2 are discussed in further detail later in this chapter.

PATHOLOGY

The normal architecture of the pancreas is quite typical of the architecture of other secretory glands. Pancreatic acinar cells account for approximately 80% of the cell number and volume of the gland, with islet cell clusters accounting for 1 to 2%. The ductal system is made up of single-layered, cuboidal epithelial cells comprising 10 to 15% of the gland's structure, with a sparse interlacing network of blood vessels, lymphatics, nerves, and collagenous stroma. In carcinoma, this architecture is markedly altered: the predominant histologic feature is a dense collagenous stroma with atrophic acini, remarkably preserved islet cell clusters, and a slight to moderate increase in the number of ducts, both normal-appearing and cancerous (Fig. 18-1). The diagnosis of ductal adenocarcinoma rests on the identification of mitoses, nuclear and cellular pleomorphism, discontinuity of ductal epithelium, and evidence of perineural, vascular, or lymphatic invasion.

Almost all malignant neoplasms of pancreatic origin (95%) arise from the exocrine portion of the gland and have light microscopic features consistent with

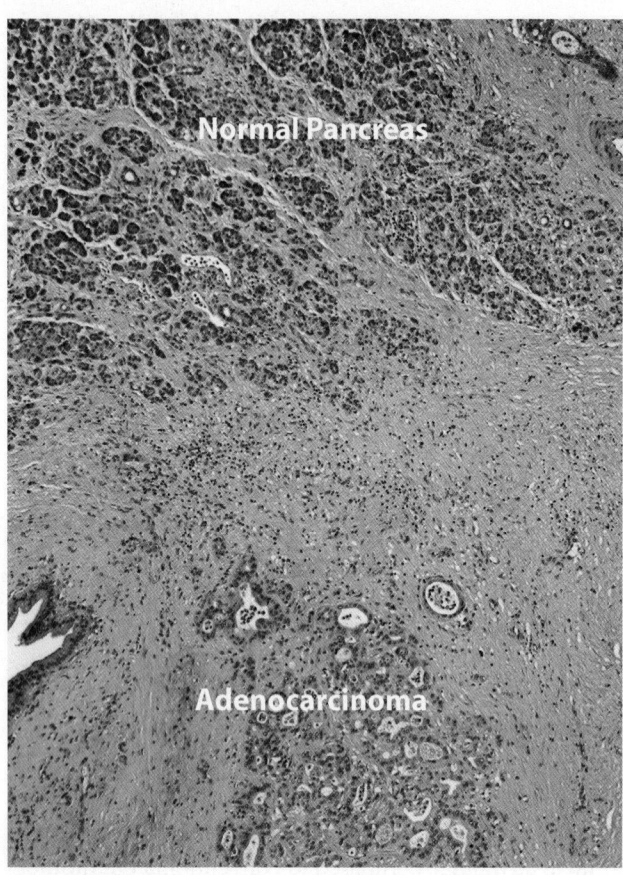

TABLE 18-2	HISTOLOGIC CLASSIFICATION OF PRIMARY EXOCRINE PANCREATIC TUMORS

Malignant
  Ductal adenocarcinoma
  Mucinous cystadenocarcinoma
  Acinar carcinoma
  Unclassified large cell carcinoma
  Small cell carcinoma
  Pancreatoblastoma
Benign
  Serous cystadenoma
Variable malignant potential
  Intraductal papillary mucinous tumor
  Mucinous cystadenoma
  Papillary cystic neoplasm

FIGURE 18-1. Photomicrograph of ductal adenocarcinoma of the pancreas with well-preserved islet cells and pancreatic architecture above and infiltrating tumor with poorly formed glandular structures below.

those of adenocarcinomas. Tumors arising from the islets of Langerhans (endocrine) cells of the pancreas are much more infrequent, and primary nonepithelial tumors of the pancreas (eg, lymphomas or sarcomas) are extremely rare. A current view of the histologic classification of exocrine pancreatic neoplasms is presented in Table 18-2. Although the origin of pancreatic adenocarcinomas from the ductal epithelium is generally accepted, the cell of origin of pancreatic adenocarcinoma remains an active area of research.

CLINICAL PRESENTATION

The clinical presentation of pancreatic cancer is primarily dependent on the location of the tumor within the pancreas. The majority (85%) of pancreatic cancers develop within the pancreatic head. About 10% are located in the pancreatic body and 5% in the tail. Nonspecific, poorly localized, epigastric or back pain of autonomic origin is the most common initial presentation of pancreatic cancer. It is usually caused by

invasion or compression of the celiac, splanchnic, or mesenteric plexi. Tumors in the head or neck of the pancreas typically cause pain in the epigastric area or in the right upper quadrant of the abdomen. Cancers of the pancreatic body may cause unremitting, severe back pain, and tumors in the pancreatic tail are associated with left-upper-quadrant pain.

Painless jaundice, another common presentation, is generally associated with tumors in the pancreatic head or uncinate process. Jaundice may be the only complaint; it usually precipitates immediate medical evaluation and subsequent diagnosis, which may result in the discovery of a small, potentially resectable primary tumor. In contrast, when the tumor does not arise in proximity to the intrapancreatic portion of the bile duct, diagnosis may be delayed and characterized by abdominal pain or back pain without jaundice.

Acute pancreatitis, while not common, can be caused by a ductal adenocarcinoma; in patients with no other reason for acute pancreatitis (lack of gallstones, no history of alcohol or other precipitating drugs), an underlying pancreatic neoplasm should be considered (25). Symptoms of chronic pancreatitis are relatively common however and include diarrhea, bloating or constipation, abdominal distention, and weight loss.

Last, patients with tail lesions often present with signs or symptoms of metastatic disease, including pain over the liver, night sweats, anorexia, and weight loss.

DIAGNOSIS AND STAGING OF PANCREATIC CANCER

While the oncologist is not usually involved in the diagnosis of pancreatic cancer, it is important for oncologists to recognize that pancreatic cancer can be difficult to diagnose, particularly in patients with nonspecific complaints. Therefore patients who present to the oncologist for treatment recommendations may harbor feelings of frustration and anger, having endured a significant delay from the onset of symptoms to diagnosis. The awareness that a patient with pancreatic cancer has often undergone a circuitous workup prior to diagnosis should provide the oncologist with some insight into the patient's frame of mind when management recommendations are being made. For example, patients with lesions of the pancreatic head or body often complain of burning abdominal pain or pressure, which is often attributed to "excess gas" or gastritis. Thus upper endoscopy may be performed to rule out peptic ulcer disease or other pathology. Endoscopy will seldom be helpful unless the pancreatic tumor has invaded the adjacent gastric or duodenal mucosa, leading to ulceration. In this uncommon situation, biopsies may demonstrate adenocarcinoma, and subsequent cross-sectional body imaging reveals an underlying pancreatic mass. Even more rarely, extrinsic compression on the gastric or duodenal wall may be appreciated endoscopically, prompting radiographic imaging. Unfortunately, upper endoscopy may be misleading and demonstrate mild esophagitis, gastritis, or duodenitis, with or without evidence of *Helicobacter pylori*. This discovery often leads to medical therapy, and when *H pylori* infection is discovered, antibiotics are usually prescribed. When symptoms do not abate, medications are commonly changed, but reassessment of the diagnosis may not occur for some time. Alternatively, patients complaining of right-upper-quadrant pain may undergo ultrasonography with attention focused on the gallbladder. This test may not be sensitive enough to visualize a pancreatic abnormality but may also reveal gallstones, prompting cholecystectomy. This procedure is usually of temporary benefit and delays the discovery of a pancreatic tumor until pain returns and worsens over time. Last, for patients presenting with complaints of back pain, a musculoskeletal evaluation commonly ensues, with the procurement of plain x-rays, myelograms, or magnetic resonance imaging (MRI) of the spine. Physical therapy or chiropractic manipulations and nonsteroidal anti-inflammatory drugs may be prescribed, which may provide temporary relief; over time, pain intensifies and becomes associated with other problems, including anorexia and asthenia. By the time a diagnosis is finally made, patients may have endured significant suffering, to the point of despondency and depression.

For those patients who present with obstructive jaundice, suspicion of pancreatic cancer is sufficiently high that the diagnostic workup usually proceeds in an orderly fashion with directed imaging studies. These usually include an abdominal ultrasound, or computed tomography (CT) scan of the abdomen, or both. In some centers, discovery of a mass in the head of the pancreas without obvious metastatic disease or evidence for unresectability will prompt an exploratory laparotomy prior to biopsy confirmation of malignancy. This approach is not embraced at MDACC for reasons outlined later.

Tissue Acquisition

With rare exception, all patients seen at MDACC who are suspected of having a pancreatic neoplasm are advised to undergo tissue confirmation. However, cross-sectional imaging (multidetector CT) should always be performed before interventional endoscopic or radiologic procedures to prevent procedure-related inflammatory changes from confounding assessment of the local tumor. For patients presenting with obstructive jaundice, tissue may be obtained at the time of endoscopic retrograde cholangiopancreatography (ERCP) via brushings of the bile duct at the level of stricture. However, if brushings are nondiagnostic and CT or MRI suggests that the tumor may be nonmetastatic, we advise endoscopic ultrasound (EUS) with EUS-guided fine-needle aspiration (FNA) biopsy (26). This procedure can be performed by experienced operators with minimal risk of duodenal perforation. Moreover, it is thought to decrease the risk of peritoneal or needle-track seeding, which has been reported among patients undergoing transcutaneous US- or CT-directed biopsies (27). Alternatively, when CT or MRI clearly demonstrates an unresectable, locally advanced cancer, CT- or ultrasound-guided transcutaneous biopsy may substitute for EUS-guided aspiration. In the situation in which a patient presents with obstructive jaundice and biliary stricture without radiographic evidence of a pancreatic mass, EUS examination is also advised. If a hypoechoic area is detected on this study, FNA may also be performed.

When there is radiographic evidence of metastatic disease and an obvious pancreatic mass, we recommend biopsy of a metastatic site, such as the liver, which can usually be performed with US guidance. This confirms both the diagnosis and the presence of metastatic disease with one procedure.

Misdiagnosis of Pancreatic Cancer

It is not uncommon for patients to be misdiagnosed with pancreatic cancer. The most common mistake we see is in the setting of bulky peripancreatic adenopathy without a parenchymal pancreatic mass. Adenocarcinomas of the pancreas do metastasize to regional lymph nodes, but these lymph nodes are typically small- or medium-sized. Bulky lymph nodes are seen in other gastrointestinal (GI) malignancies, such as tumors of the esophagus, stomach, duodenum, and, occasionally, colon. Lymphoma, non-small cell lung cancer, and carcinomas of unknown primary origin may also lead to bulky peripancreatic lymphadenopathy, thus mimicking a primary pancreatic neoplasm. Thin-cut dynamic-phase contrast-enhanced CT will usually rule out the presence of a primary mass in the pancreas in this setting. Another helpful radiographic finding may be the presence or absence of atrophy of the pancreatic body and tail. Although commonly seen in adenocarcinomas originating in the head of the pancreas, this finding is usually absent in the setting of bulky peripancreatic adenopathy, neuroendocrine tumors, and acinar cell tumors. Importantly, patients with neuroendocrine tumors of the pancreas are sometimes misdiagnosed as having a poorly differentiated carcinoma of the pancreas. Patients with well-preserved performance status out of proportion to tumor burden, normal CA19-9 measurements, or hypervascular liver lesions should have biopsy specimens reviewed with special stains for neuroendocrine markers.

Staging Evaluation

Many patients are referred to a tertiary center for further evaluation and treatment recommendations after a diagnostic workup has been completed. Unfortunately, it is common for prereferral diagnostic studies to be inadequate for treatment planning; therefore high-quality cross-sectional imaging is always part of our initial evaluation. Accurate pretreatment staging is the most important element in the development of a management plan for patients with pancreatic cancer (28,29).

High-Quality CT Imaging

The single most important imaging modality is multidetector (multislice) CT. This technique is used to objectively define (anatomically) potentially resectable disease. Although contrast-enhanced CT is widely available, accurate interpretation and reporting of the tumor-related findings remains inconsistent. For optimal pretreatment staging, a CT report in a patient with suspected periampullary or pancreatic cancer should include the following information:

1. The presence or absence of a primary tumor in the pancreas or periampullary region
2. The presence or absence of peritoneal and hepatic metastases

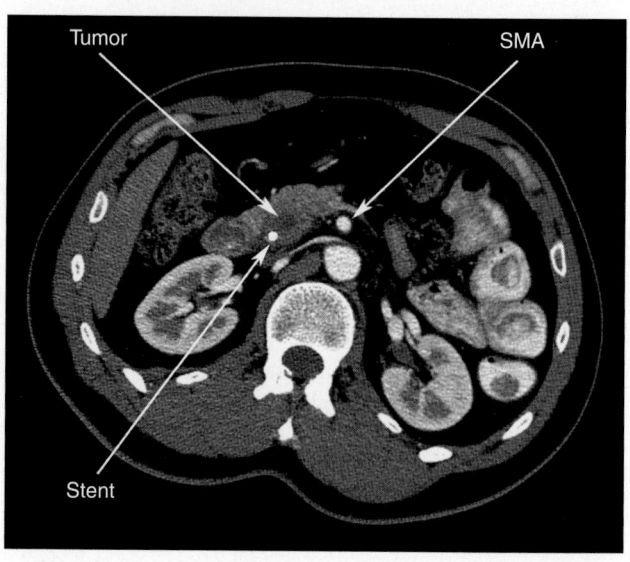

FIGURE 18-2. CT image of tumor within the pancreatic head. Note the stent in the bile duct and the subtle low-density mass within the head. The superior mesenteric artery (SMA) has a fat plane completely surrounding it. This defines a potentially resectable tumor.

3. Description of the patency of the superior mesenteric vein (SMV) and portal vein (PV) and the relationship of these veins to the tumor
4. Description of the relationship of the tumor to the superior mesenteric artery (SMA), celiac axis, and hepatic artery

Specific, objective radiographic criteria can be used to define a potentially resectable primary tumor of the pancreatic head or uncinate process (Fig. 18-2). The criteria used at our institution include (1) no extrapancreatic disease, (2) a patent SMV and PV (assuming the technical ability to resect and reconstruct this venous confluence, and (3) a definable tissue plane between the tumor and regional arterial structures, including the celiac axis and SMA. Using CT staging and objective criteria for assessment of resectability, many centers have reported resectability rates as high as 75 to 80% (30). Thus a single imaging study that is accurately interpreted can objectively define localized, potentially resectable pancreatic cancer and differentiate such tumors from locally advanced, unresectable, or metastatic cancers. Of note, CT of the chest is not routinely part of our staging workup. However, if either plain chest x-rays or CT images of the lung bases reveal pulmonary nodules or other suspicious findings, a dedicated CT scan of the chest is obtained. CT chest should also be considered in case of pancreatic tail primaries. Bone scans and brain imaging are rarely indicated and should not be part of routine staging examinations.

Positron Emission Tomography

While certain situations will prompt the acquisition of a positron emission tomography (PET) scan, this procedure is not routinely part of staging for pancreatic cancer patients seen at MDACC. However, its role is evolving and this modality is likely to be used more commonly. PET scans are occasionally obtained in the setting of equivocal radiographic findings such as indeterminate lesions in the liver or lungs. Unfortunately, many times such lesions will be subcentimeter in size, and in this setting, ^{18}F-fluorodeoxyglucose uptake not increased, even when metastatic disease is present (31). PET scanning is most commonly considered when a patient has undergone previous resection and subsequently develops a rising CA19-9 and soft tissue changes in the surgical bed with no other evidence of relapsing disease.

Serum CA19-9 Determinations

The serum tumor marker CA19-9 measures the specific carbohydrate moiety of the mucin MUC-1 (32). This is the most commonly elevated tumor marker in pancreatic cancer, but it is not specific for this disease and may be elevated in other GI tumors. Whether it should be measured prior to surgery as an independent predictor of resectability or as an adjunct to other clinical staging has not been rigorously studied. Most analyses have been performed retrospectively, but they generally suggest that a high preoperative CA19-9 level (>500-1000 IU/mL) implies more advanced disease that is not amenable to resection. We recently retrospectively analyzed pretreatment CA19-9 levels obtained from 79 patients enrolled in a trial of gemcitabine-based preoperative chemoradiation. All patients had radiographically defined, biopsy-proven, resectable pancreatic cancer without any evidence of metastatic disease. It was found that serum levels greater than 668 IU/mL predicted either the development of overt metastatic disease prior to surgery or early relapse after surgical resection (33). If these findings are validated in a larger prospective study, low serum CA19-9 levels may be incorporated into future staging criteria to define resectable disease. Alternatively, future clinical trials may stratify patients based on preoperative serum CA19-9 levels. Presently, serum CA19-9 measurements are obtained at presentation to MDACC. In patients with apparently resectable disease, elevated CA19-9 levels do not alter treatment planning. If such a patient ultimately undergoes resection, a CA19-9 level is obtained 6 to 8 weeks postoperatively to confirm the absence of persistent disease. When postoperative CA19-9 levels do not normalize within this time frame, it portends early relapse (34). Patients clinically staged as having locally advanced disease but with markedly elevated CA19-9 levels (>5000) are suspected of having occult metastatic disease. Assuming that pain is adequately controlled, these patients are usually advised to undergo a trial of systemic therapy with serial measurements of CA19-9 levels prior to considering chemoradiation. Improvement of CA19-9 levels by 50% has been correlated with an improved survival resultant from systemic therapy (35).

The Role of Laparoscopy

For patients with potentially resectable disease, some authorities have advocated laparoscopy with biopsies and peritoneal washings as part of routine staging (36,37). This procedure may confirm the presence of metastatic disease in a subset of patients; if, however, high-quality CT imaging is obtained, the yield of subsequent laparoscopy will be low. In our experience, not more than 20% of patients with tumors in the head of the pancreas will be found to harbor occult metastatic disease when this added staging procedure is performed. Given the expense and expected negative findings for 80% of patients undergoing laparoscopy, our approach has been to limit this procedure to patients with indeterminate findings on CT (38). An exception applies to the small subset of patients who present with tumors in the body or tail of the pancreas that are radiographically resectable. These patients are more likely to have occult metastatic disease, and the chances of a visible peritoneal metastasis or a positive cytology on peritoneal washing is sufficiently high to justify laparoscopy as part of staging in these patients (39).

The TNM System Versus Clinically Oriented Staging

As with other solid tumors, a TNM (tumor, node, metastasis) staging system for pancreatic cancer has been devised; it is outlined in Table 18-3. For patients undergoing resection, pathologic staging of the tumor using the TNM system is somewhat useful in providing prognostic information and, to a lesser degree, possibly in guiding adjuvant therapy. However, we normally do not utilize the TNM system in clinical decision making for patients with pancreatic cancer. Generally, patients are staged as having potentially resectable disease, locally advanced unresectable disease, or metastatic disease. While there is a subset of patients who do not fit cleanly into one of these three categories, treatment decisions are based on this stratification for the large majority of patients. For patients with resectable disease who are able to tolerate it, surgery is indicated.

TABLE 18-3 | TNM CRITERIA FOR PANCREATIC ADENOCARCINOMA

TNM DEFINITIONS

Tx:	Primary tumor cannot be assessed
T0:	No evidence of primary tumor
Tl:	Tumor <2 cm in greatest dimension
T2:	Tumor >2 cm in greatest dimension
T3:	Tumor extends directly to the duodenum, bile duct, or peripancreatic tissue
T4:	Tumor extends directly to stomach, spleen, colon, or adjacent large vessels
Nx:	Regional lymph node status cannot be assessed
N0:	No regional lymph node metastasis
N1:	Positive regional lymph node metastasis
Mx:	Distant metastasis cannot be assessed
M0:	No distant metastasis
M1:	Distant metastasis

STAGING CLASSIFICATION

Stage	T	N	M
0	Tis	N0	M0
I	T1-2	N0	M0
II	T3	N0	M0
III	T1-3	N1	M0
IVA	T4	Any N	M0
IVB	Any T	Any N	Ml

Surgery can be preceded by preoperative therapy, usually on protocol, or it may be followed by adjuvant therapy. Patients with metastatic disease and adequate performance status usually receive systemic therapy. For patients presenting with locally advanced disease, treatment should be individualized and may initially involve either chemoradiation or systemic therapy.

TREATMENT STRATEGIES FOR PANCREATIC CANCER

Resectable Pancreatic Cancer

With some exceptions, resectable pancreatic cancers are limited to small tumors in the head of the pancreas. These are removed with a Whipple procedure (40), more appropriately described as a pancreaticoduodenectomy. Occasionally, a patient will present with a pancreatic tail lesion that appears amenable to resection with distal pancreatectomy. Caution is advised when resection of a tail neoplasm is being considered, even when these tumors appear localized, they will be associated with a higher likelihood of peritoneal seeding compared to a head lesion. Body lesions are almost never amenable to surgical resection.

It is widely known that surgery holds the only hope of cure for patients with pancreatic cancer. Unfortunately, patients and oncologists are often not aware of the potential drawbacks associated with up-front surgery:

1. *Surgical morbidity and mortality is inversely correlated to experience with the procedure.* Several studies have confirmed significant differences in the risk of major perioperative complications and death between hospitals that perform the operation frequently and those that do not (41,42). Moreover, long-term survival after pancreaticoduodenectomy is also improved when the surgery takes place in a high-volume center (43). This is likely attributable to a combination of decreased operative mortality and superior patient selection. Whether quantitative or qualitative differences in the delivery of postoperative therapy between major medical centers and smaller community hospitals has a survival impact is unknown.

2. *Positive surgical margins are associated with a very poor prognosis.* Table 18-4 demonstrates that median survival for patients undergoing surgery with a positive surgical margin is quite poor. Surgical margins after pancreaticoduodenectomy can be either microscopically positive (R1 resection), or grossly positive (R2). In either circumstance, median survivals with a positive surgical margin usually range between 6 and 12 months, similar to, if not worse than, the survival of patients with locally advanced disease (44-47). Despite clear evidence that high-quality cross-sectional imaging accurately predicts resectability, it is likely that many patients undergo laparotomy for pancreatic cancer without adequate preoperative assessment. Some will be found to have unresectable tumors intraoperatively or be left with a grossly positive

TABLE 18-4 | MEDIAN SURVIVAL RATES OF PATIENTS WITH A GROSS (R2) OR MICROSCOPIC (R1) SURGICAL MARGIN AT THE TIME OF RESECTION

Author	Number of Patients	Margin Status	Median Survival (Months)
Sohn	184	R1/R2	12
Neoptolemos	101	R1	11
Nishimura	70	R1/R2	6
Millikan	22	R1	8
Richter	72	R1/R2	12
Kuhlman	80	R1/R2	16
Takai	42	R1/R2	8

surgical margin when it might have been possible to predict this prior to surgery. Laparotomy in such patients may therefore lead to a delay in the initiation of either chemoradiation or systemic therapy while the patient recovers. With the exception of patients who present with gastric outlet obstruction or biliary obstruction not amenable to endoscopic or percutaneous stenting, we discourage surgical intervention without clear high-quality radiographic evidence of resectability. If the preoperative CT and/or its interpretation have been suboptimal and the surgeon has failed to perform a complete resection, surgery may even be deleterious and compromise the patients survival.

3. *A substantial proportion of patients do not recover sufficiently to receive postoperative adjuvant therapy.* Pancreaticoduodenectomy is a major surgical procedure with removal of portions of the stomach, duodenum, pancreas, and bile duct. This operation also requires extensive reconstruction of the upper alimentary canal. Pancreatic anastomotic leaks and delayed gastric emptying are common complications. Retrospective analyses and prospective clinical trials of adjuvant therapy demonstrate that a significant percentage of people do not adequately recover to receive further postoperative therapy. For example, at Johns Hopkins University, a recent report demonstrated that of 870 patients who underwent resection for pancreatic cancer with curative intent between 1993 and 2005, only 53% received adjuvant therapy (48). Similarly, the Mayo Clinic experience demonstrated that only 58% of patients receiving an R0 resection actually received postoperative therapy (49). Furthermore, analyses of Medicare-eligible patients suggest that among patients 65 years of age or older, fewer than half receive adjuvant therapy (50). It is reasonable to assume that a substantial proportion of elderly patients have sufficient difficulty recovering from surgery and this impacts adjuvant therapy, which may be delayed or cancelled.

4. *Surgically resected patients remain at risk for local failure and metastatic disease.* Approximately 80% of resected patients will ultimately relapse and die of disease recurrence. The high risk of relapse stems from an inability to prevent locoregional failure and to eradicate microscopic metastatic disease. Factors predisposing to local recurrence have not been fully elucidated, but recent evidence implicates perineural invasion as an important mediating process. Rich neural networks surround the pancreas and are intimately associated with the

local vascular structures. Invasion of nerve sheaths draping over the vessels may occur as a pervasive superficial infiltration that cannot be appreciated intraoperatively, even by the most experienced surgeons.

In addition, the development of overt metastatic disease is common after surgery. Once patients relapse with distant disease or local failure, no curative strategy is available. Adjuvant therapy, while tending to improve median survival, has not made any significant advances over the past 20 years. This suggests that improvements in systemic therapy will be required to reduce the risk of distant disease after surgery.

The Role of Adjuvant Therapy

Adjuvant therapy for resected pancreatic cancer is intended to reduce the risk of relapse and improve long-term survival for patients undergoing surgery. Since the mid-1980s, efforts have been directed toward improving outcomes for patients with resected disease by delivering postoperative adjuvant therapy, but there is no consensus regarding the role of chemotherapy with radiation in this setting. Early retrospective analyses of patients undergoing resection have suggested local failure rates as high as 50 to 80%, which prompted many centers to advocate radiotherapy as a component of adjuvant therapy. The first randomized trial, performed by the Gastrointestinal Tumor Study Group (GITSG), demonstrated a significant survival advantage with 5-FU–based chemoradiation compared with resection alone (21 versus 11 months) (51). The 5-year survival rates were 18 versus 8%, respectively. However, 15 years later, the European Organization for Research and Treatment of Cancer (EORTC) 40891 trial produced conflicting results. In this case, 218 patients receiving 5-FU chemoradiation did not demonstrate a survival advantage over those on observation alone, though this population was more heterogeneous than GITSG since patients with periampullary cancer and those with an R1 resection were included (52).

More recently in Europe, large randomized adjuvant trials were conducted by the European Study Group for Pancreatic Cancer (ESPAC). In the ESPAC-1 trial, 289 patients were randomized to observation, chemotherapy alone, chemoradiation, or chemoradiation followed by chemotherapy in a two-by-two factorial design (53). Interestingly, chemoradiation was found to have a deleterious effect on survival in this analysis (median survival 15.9 versus 17.9 months respectively, $p = .05$). On the other hand, chemotherapy appeared beneficial with a median survival of 20.1 months versus 15.5 months in the no-chemotherapy arm ($p = .009$). As a result of these three studies, the role of radiation in adjuvant therapy became controversial. Radiation has been abandoned in the adjuvant therapy approaches for pancreatic cancer in many European centers.

After gemcitabine showed superiority to 5-FU in advanced disease, a number of randomized trials tested its role in the adjuvant setting. The Radiation Therapy Oncology Group designed RTOG 9704 to compare systemic gemcitabine with systemic 5-FU given before and after 5-FU–based chemoradiation. The use of gemcitabine demonstrated a modest, but not significant, improvement in survival over 5-FU (20.5 months compared to 16.9 months, $p = .09$) (54).

The benefit of adjuvant gemcitabine was further confirmed with the long-term data from the CONKO 001 trial. Investigators showed a significant improvement in disease-free survival and overall survival with the use of gemcitabine postoperatively (13 and 22.8 months, respectively) compared to surgery alone (6.9 and 20.2 months) (55). ESPAC-3 further explored the role of adjuvant chemotherapy by comparing postoperative gemcitabine to 5-FU (56). No statistical difference in survival was noted between the two arms after a median follow-up of 34 months, though gemcitabine appeared to be better tolerated than bolus 5-FU (Table 18-5 summarizes the adjuvant therapy trials).

Preoperative Therapy for Potentially Resectable Disease

Sadly, there has been no significant progress in adjuvant therapy for resected pancreatic cancer since the GITSG study was first reported in 1985. More recent studies have been fairly consistent with the GITSG findings: median survival for resected patients treated with postoperative therapy hovers around 20 months and remains at 12 months for patients undergoing surgery alone. As previously noted, pancreaticoduodenectomy has been associated with significant morbidity and, in less experienced centers, mortality. Of the patients who undergo potentially curative surgery for pancreatic cancer, up to 50% do not recuperate adequately to embark on postoperative chemoradiation, or they require prolonged recovery in order to consider such treatment. Moreover, rapid disease progression with early systemic relapse is not uncommon after surgery. Therefore neoadjuvant therapy followed by surgery offers some theoretical advantages over immediate surgery.

First, up-front surgery may preclude the delivery of postoperative treatment to some patients, whereas preoperative therapy allows all potential surgical candidates to receive neoadjuvant therapy. Second, patients who present with potentially resectable disease are generally physiologically fit and make attractive candidates for neoadjuvant therapy. Third, preoperative therapy allows delivery of chemotherapy or chemoradiation

TABLE 18-5	**SUMMARY OF RANDOMIZED AND NONRANDOMIZED ADJUVANT TRIALS**					
Study Year	*Number of Patients*	*Patients With R1 Resection (%)*	*Treatment A Median Survival (Months)*	*Treatment B Median Survival (Months)*	*p-Value*	*Local Failure Rate (%)*
GITSG 1985	49	0	5-FU/XRT + 5-FU 21.0	Observation 10.9	0.035	NR
EORTC 1999	114	19	5-FU/XRT 17.1	Observation 12.6	0.099	34
ESPAC-1 2004	289	18	5-FU/LV 20.1	No-5-FU/LV 15.5	0.009	60
			5-FU/XRT 15.9	No 5-FU/XRT 17.9	0.05	
RTOG 9704 2008	368	>35	Gem + 5-FU/XRT 20.5	5-FU + 5-FU/XRT 16.9	0.09	34
CONKO 001 2008	388	19	Gem 22.8	Observation 20.2	0.005	25
ESPAC-1/ESPAC-3 2009	458	25	5-FU/LV 23.2	Observation 16.8	0.003	NR
ESPAC-3 (v2) 2009	1088	35	Gem 23.6	5-FU/LV 23.0	0.39	NR

5-FU, 5-fluorouracil; Gem, gemcitabine; LV, leucovorin; NR, not reported; XRT, radiation.

| TABLE 18-6 | SUMMARY OF PREOPERATIVE TRIALS PERFORMED AT MDACC |

Author Year	Number of Patients	Preoperative Regimen	Resection Rate (%)	% R1	Median Survival Resected Patients	Local Recurrence Rate (%)
Evans, 1992	28	5-FU + XRT 50.4 Gy	61		18	
Pisters, 1998	35	5-FU + XRT 30 Gy	57	10	25	10
Pisters, 2002	37	Paclitaxel + XRT 30 Gy	54	32	19	NR
Evans, 2008	86	Gem + XRT 30 Gy	75	12	34	11
Varadhachary, 2008	90	Gem/Cis then Gem + XRT 30 Gy	58	4	31	25

5-FU, 5-fluorouracil; Gem, gemcitabine; XRT, Radiotherapy.

to a relatively well-perfused tumor bed and provides early treatment to microscopic metastases. Fourth, positive surgical margins are commonly reported after upfront resection; this is associated with poor prognosis, suggesting that surgery alone provides inadequate local control. Preoperative therapy may provide for sufficient tumor destruction, particularly at the periphery, to increase the chances of a margin-negative resection. Fifth, preoperative therapy allows for observation of the tumor's underlying biology and those with aggressive disease are spared a major surgical procedure.

Five preoperative trials have been completed at MDACC (Table 18-6) (57-61). These trials, performed in sequence, have had nearly identical inclusion criteria, with standardized radiographic criteria for resectability, surgical technique, and assessment of resection margins. Our data demonstrate that preoperative therapy is associated with a relatively low local failure rate compared to adjuvant therapy, and, over time, we have noted modest improvements in overall survival, especially with the use of gemcitabine over 5-FU or paclitaxel-based chemoradiation.

Two recent studies at MDACC involved preoperative chemoradiation with gemcitabine in patients with potentially resectable disease. In the first trial by Evans et al., a total of 86 patients received gemcitabine followed by chemoradiation and 74% of them were able to undergo pancreaticoduodenectomy (57). The median survival for these patients was 34 months compared to 7 months for those who did not receive resection. The pattern of failure favored distant metastases; thus, a second trial was designed to increase the amount of systemic therapy. This trial enrolled 90 patients to receive gemcitabine with cisplatin followed by chemoradiation and 66% underwent resection. The addition of cisplatin to gemcitabine did not improve survival beyond gemcitabine alone (31 versus 34 months). While these studies were not designed to be compared to adjuvant

trials, the median survival in both preoperative studies is notably better than that seen in the adjuvant data we have to date. In the gemcitabine-based chemoradiation trial, complete pathologic responses were observed in two surgical specimens, and the same has been observed sporadically in both gemcitabine-based and 5-FU–based neoadjuvant programs. These observations are important, and while preoperative chemoradiation has not been established as a standard approach, experience to date suggests that it may increase the likelihood of a margin-negative resection. Using preoperative therapy, negative surgical margins are reported more frequently, and while these are probably not sufficient to ensure cure, they are likely to be necessary for extended survival.

MDACC Approach to Potentially Resectable Disease

Oncologists should not become lost in the specific details of varying pre- and postoperative regimens administered to patients with resectable pancreatic cancer. Rather, the principles underlying these strategies should be kept in mind in considering treatment options (Fig. 18-3). Overall, our focus has been on the delivery of preoperative therapy prior to considering surgery, for the reasons outlined earlier. All patients being considered for surgery undergo high-quality dual-phase helical CT scans of the abdomen to define resectability before surgery, not during surgery. An attempt to prove the presence of malignancy is always advised. Patients with biopsy-proven resectable adenocarcinoma are offered protocol-based preoperative therapy as an institutional priority. For patients in whom malignancy is suspected but not confirmed with biopsy, surgical resection is recommended. When patients undergo up-front surgery, adjuvant therapy is recommended and, whenever possible, treatment on a clinical trial is encouraged.

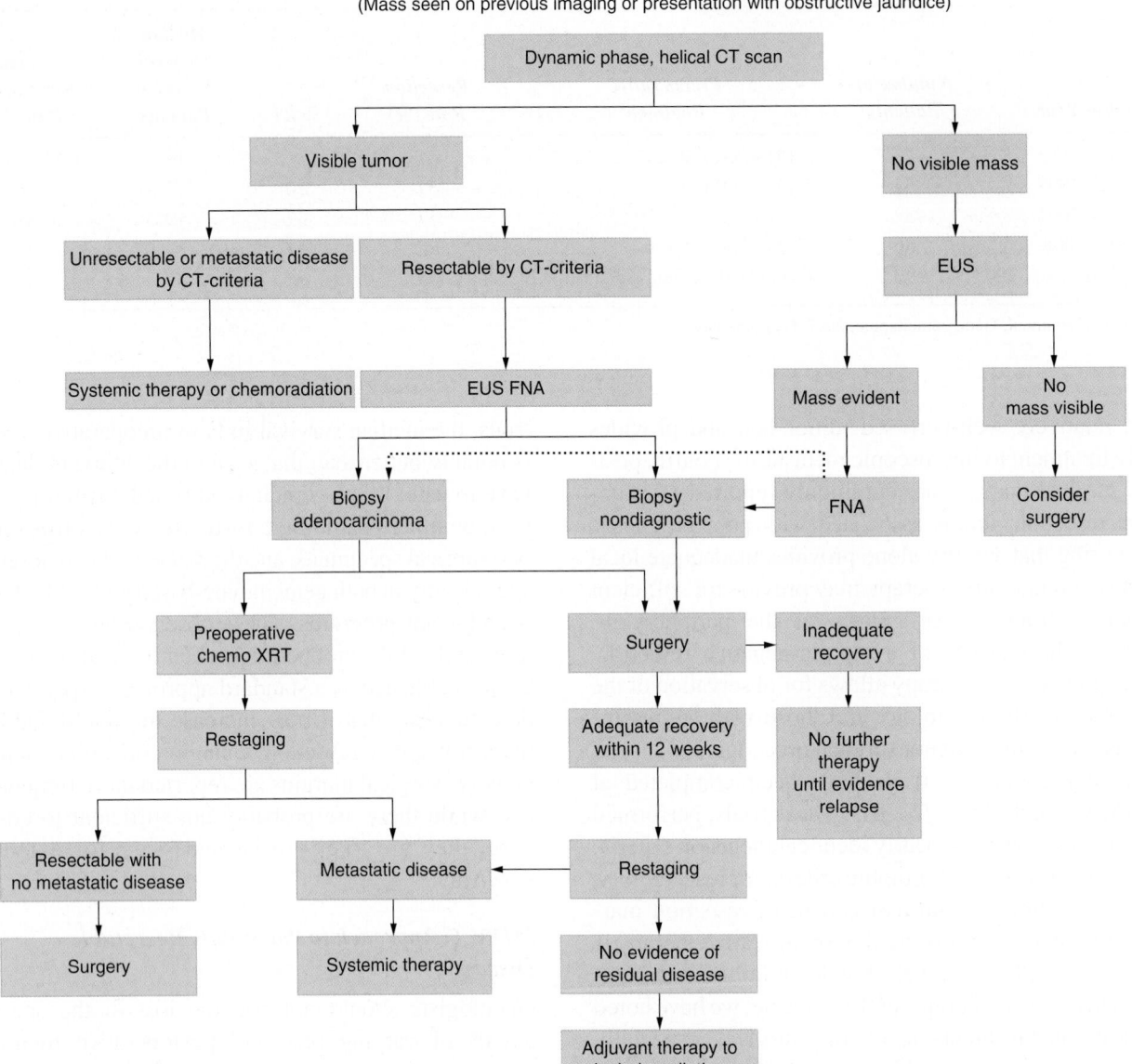

FIGURE 18-3.   General algorithm for diagnostic workup and management of newly diagnosed pancreatic cancer.

MDACC Approach to Adjuvant Therapy

One of the drawbacks of the randomized trials of adjuvant therapy performed to date is a general lack of discipline in the trial designs. For example in the GITSG, EORTC, and ESPAC-1 trials, there was no requirement for preoperative imaging to confirm the tumor's resectability. While not stated in any of the results, tumor removal was probably based on the surgeon's intraoperative assessment, and whether margins were rendered grossly negative relies purely on the surgeon's word. While ESPAC-1 encouraged central pathology review, this was not mandated as a requirement for protocol enrollment. Moreover, no strict criteria for evaluating surgical margins have ever been utilized. Based

on guidelines stemming from UICC, we ink the retroperitoneal margin (to the right of the SMA) in order to orient the pathologist and focus attention on this margin, which is most likely to be microscopically positive. Last, none of these trials required postoperative imaging or laboratory tests to ensure that eligible patients were without evidence of disease, based on CT imaging or acquisition of a postoperative CA19-9 level. Any of these factors can have a far greater impact on the survival of patients with pancreatic cancer than that of adjuvant therapy using agents with minimal activity in advanced disease.

Therefore, at MDACC, adjuvant therapy is delivered with the following principles in mind:

1. Patients must demonstrate adequate recovery from surgery to be considered for further treatment. This includes ample oral caloric intake and no significant impairment of the alimentary tract (delayed gastric emptying, dumping syndrome, uncontrolled pancreatic exocrine insufficiency). Adequate wound healing and absence of infection are also required. Patients should have a performance status of 0 to 1.

2. Patients must have adequate hepatic and renal function with sufficient hematologic parameters to undergo cytotoxic therapy.

3. Restaging CT scans are obtained just prior to initiation of adjuvant therapy. This restaging study is generally performed 6 to 10 weeks postoperatively. A serum CA19-9 level is also measured; if it is more than twice the upper limit of normal, we do not allow patients to receive adjuvant therapy on in-house protocols. Recent retrospective analysis suggests that 5 to 10% of patients who undergo surgery at MDACC will have early radiographic or serologic evidence of relapsing disease prior to initiation of adjuvant therapy. When this occurs, any further therapy is not considered adjuvant.

4. Chemotherapy followed by chemoradiation remains the foundation of adjuvant therapy.

At MDACC, patients are encouraged to enroll in postoperative trials of adjuvant therapy. Our experience with preoperative therapy has shown us that the patients have differences in disease biology, with 30% having aggressive disease for whom systemic therapy will be of more value than chemoradiation wherein the doses of chemotherapeutic agents are attenuated. Furthermore, to extrapolate from the experience in locally advanced unresectable disease, patients benefiting from chemoradiation are those who have experienced stable disease with induction chemotherapy.

Therefore, our approach at this time includes induction chemotherapy with gemcitabine or a gemcitabine-based doublet for 3 months followed by restaging scans. If no radiographic or serologic evidence of relapse is present at that time, chemoradiation with 5-FU or capecitabine is advised. Radiation is administered in a dose of 50.4 Gy in 28 fractions.

Once postoperative therapy has been completed, patients are followed with restaging CT scans, chest x-ray, physical examination, and standard laboratory tests, including CA19-9 assays every 3 months for the first 2 years, then every 6 months for the next 2 years, and annually thereafter. A rising CA19-9 after adjuvant therapy does not trigger further systemic therapy until clear evidence of relapse, based on physical examination or radiographic studies, is present. PET scanning is considered in this situation.

MDACC Approach to Preoperative Therapy

Patients with clinical and radiographic evidence of potentially resectable disease are generally advised to receive protocol-based preoperative therapy, which always involves chemoradiation. The inclusion criteria, study endpoints (hospitalization rate, resection rate, local treatment effect, and survival), surgical technique, and postoperative care have remained fairly constant, with minimal changes over the past 16 years. Chemoradiation regimens have varied, and our most encouraging results have been achieved with our gemcitabine-based regimen. Gemcitabine-based preoperative therapy will continue to be our primary focus, although future preoperative regimens will likely incorporate targeted agents. After chemoradiation had been completed, patients are allowed to recover over 4 to 5 weeks; they then undergo restaging studies, including dual-phase helical scanning. For patients with no clinical or radiographic evidence of metastatic disease and no contraindications to surgery, laparotomy proceeds. (In our experience local tumor progression precluding resection has not occurred as an isolated finding and is observed only when metastatic disease is also evident.) At the time of exploration, when no visible evidence of distant disease is encountered, pancreaticoduodenectomy is performed. After surgery, no further chemotherapy or radiation is delivered and patients are followed expectantly with periodic restaging studies as outlined earlier. Patients who relapse with adequate performance status are offered further systemic therapy on or off protocol.

It is important to emphasize that we do not deliver preoperative therapy as a means of staging the primary tumor downward. All patients enrolled in our preoperative protocols must have evidence of resectable disease on presentation. The medical literature has scattered reports of neoadjuvant therapy being used to successfully staging down patients with locally advanced disease to the point of resectability (62,63). Caution is advised in interpreting these results, since we believe it is possible to stage down patients with borderline or marginally resectable tumors (tumors that abut but do not encase the celiac artery or SMA). These tumors represent a discrete subset; their management, while similar, is more tailored. Fig. 18-4 displays an algorithmic approach for resectable pancreatic cancer.

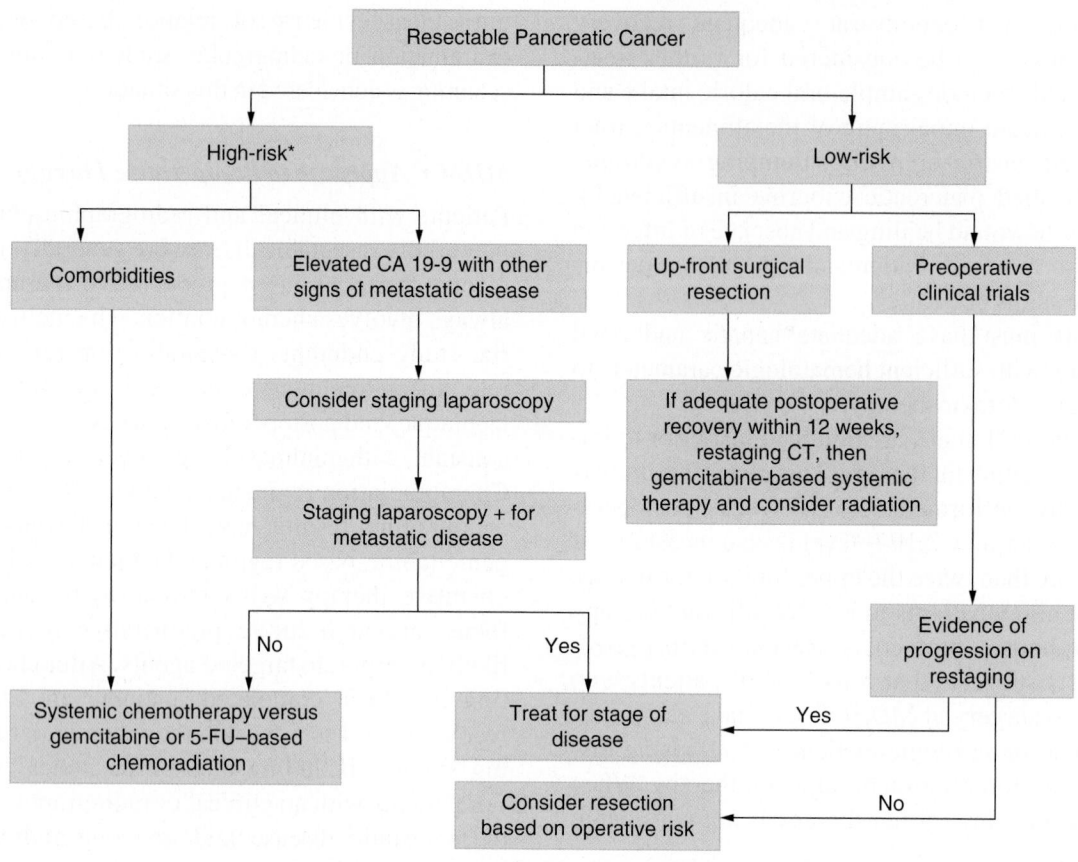

FIGURE 18-4. Treatment algorithm for the management of resectable pancreatic cancer.
*High-Risk Clinical Features: -Suspicion of metastatic disease -CA 19-9 >1000 with normal bilirubin -Comorbidities suggesting high operative risk

MDACC Approach to Patients With Borderline Resectable Pancreatic Cancer

As high-quality dynamic-phase helical CT scanning has developed, an appreciation for the existence of a distinct subset of tumors best described as borderline resectable or marginally resectable has emerged. In this situation, some authorities believe that up-front surgery is more likely to lead to an R1- or R2- rather than an R0-resection. This entity is defined as ≤180 tumor abutment of the SMA or celiac axis, short segment abutment or encasement of the common hepatic artery that is amenable to segmental resection and reconstruction, or short segment occlusion of the SMV, PV, or SMV-PV confluence with an normal SMV below and PV above the tumor to allow for reconstruction (64). Previous neoadjuvant approaches have demonstrated the ability to downstage marginally resectable pancreatic tumors to the point of resectability (65). In fact, at MDACC, this has been seen in up to 40% of patients with borderline resectable disease, and these patients have a median survival of >40 months.

At MDACC, patients with marginally resectable tumors are typically treated with gemcitabine-based chemotherapy for an indefinite period of time, with restaging studies every 2 months. Treatment is continued to maximum benefit, as defined by a nadir in the CA19-9 level or best radiographic response. Thereafter, chemoradiation is delivered and subsequent restaging studies are performed about 4 to 6 weeks after this treatment is complete. If there has been some evidence of tumor destruction, usually manifest by both a drop in CA19-9 and radiographic evidence of response, and no interval development of metastatic disease is apparent, an attempt at surgery will proceed. It remains unclear whether the staging of such tumors downward to technical resectability is of biological significance; therefore at least 6 months generally elapse at MDACC prior to the contemplation of surgery.

Management of Patients With Locally Advanced Disease

Patients are defined as having locally advanced pancreatic cancer when there is radiographic evidence of SMA or celiac artery encasement, occlusion of the SMV-portal venous confluence, or significant involvement of the common hepatic artery originating from the celiac trunk. There should be no clinical or radiographic evidence of metastatic disease. Currently, roughly half of all patients present with locally advanced disease. Symptoms are usually directly related to the primary tumor. Pain is very common and its control must be continually reassessed. Jaundice may be a presenting symptom, or it may develop during the course of illness. As with resectable pancreatic cancer, an understanding of certain principles will aid in clinical decision making.

1. Patients with locally advanced pancreatic cancer are extremely heterogeneous in terms of their symptoms and performance status. Pain is frequently present, but its severity can vary widely. Some patients have minimal constitutional symptoms and are able to maintain their caloric intake and weight. Other patients are debilitated, with poorly controlled pain and asthenia as well as weight loss. Depression is common.

2. Locally advanced pancreatic cancer typically progresses over the course of some months. Local tumor progression with worsening pain, new or recurrent biliary obstruction, and gastric outlet obstruction represent difficult management problems. Portal vein or mesenteric venous thrombosis can lead to nonmalignant ascites with generalized bowel edema and intestinal dysmotility. Development of metastatic disease is usually associated with worsening functional status and, unless preceded by a long progression-free interval, is rarely responsive to further therapy.

3. Assessment of response to therapy can be challenging. These tumors may be composed of small nests of adenocarcinoma surrounded by large areas of desmoplasia (Fig. 18-5). Even when cytotoxic therapy is effective, the desmoplastic component of the residual mass may not regress and the overall tumor mass may appear unchanged after treatment. Furthermore, distinguishing the primary tumor mass from surrounding inflammatory changes can complicate the reliable measurement of tumors.

4. All surgical interventions should be considered carefully and be based on performance status and life expectancy. Palliative nonsurgical procedures may produce results similar to those of aggressive surgery.

5. One of the primary reasons for considering chemoradiation for patients with locally advanced disease is palliation of pain. However, the clinical benefit associated with chemoradiation has not been rigorously studied. In a retrospective analysis, Minsky et al. reported significant variations in the estimation of pain relief, with 31 to 77% of patients having improvement in pain after receiving chemoradiation for unresectable pancreatic cancer (66).

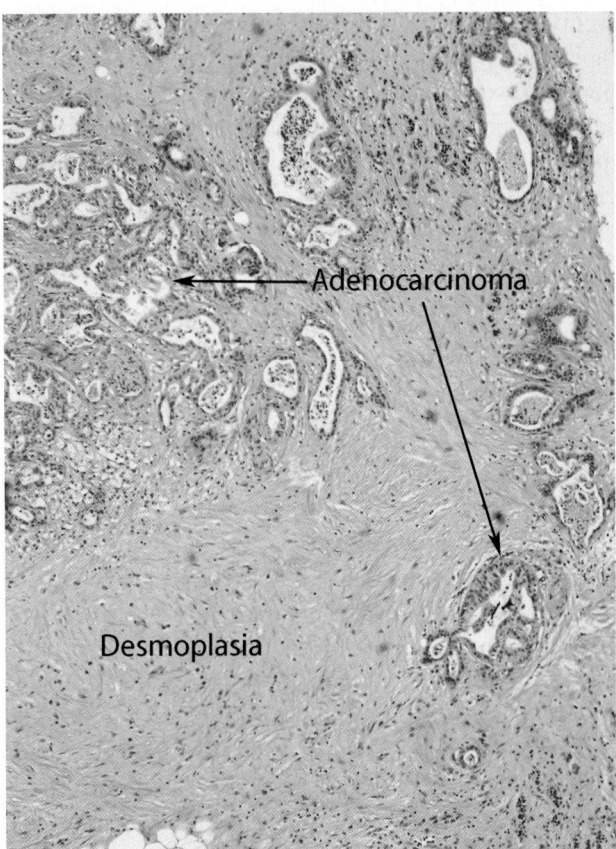

FIGURE 18-5. Photomicrograph of ductal adenocarcinoma of the pancreas with intense desmoplastic reaction. Even if the tumor cells regress in response to therapy, a residual fibrotic mass may remain. This confounds assessment of response to therapy using standard radiographic criteria.

Historically, chemoradiation has been the foundation of therapy for patients with locally advanced disease. However, with the advent of gemcitabine, which is approved for use in this setting, treatment for locally advanced pancreatic cancer is in evolution.

Data Regarding 5-FU–Based Chemoradiation

Support for chemoradiation originates from studies performed by the GITSG. In the original study, patients with locally advanced pancreatic cancer were randomly assigned to receive 40 Gy of radiation plus 5-FU, 60 Gy plus 5-FU, or 60 Gy alone. The median survival was 10 months in each of the chemoradiation groups and only 6 months for patients who received 60 Gy without 5-FU (67). Of note, these patients had undergone laparotomy and were surgically staged. Only those patients with disease confined to the pancreas and peripancreatic organs, regional lymph nodes, or regional peritoneum were eligible for the study. While this made for a more uniform study population, it also introduced significant selection bias: enrollment was limited to rapidly recovering patients. In subsequent GITSG studies, neither doxorubicin (Adriamycin) used as a radiation sensitizer nor multidrug chemotherapy with streptozocin, mitomycin, and 5-FU (SMF) alone or continued after chemoradiation was found to be superior to 5-FU–based chemoradiation (68). Additional chemotherapy after 5-FU–based chemoradiation increased toxicity without apparent therapeutic benefit.

In contrast to the results from the GITSG demonstrating better survival with 5-FU–based chemoradiation over SMF chemotherapy alone, an ECOG study suggested no benefit of chemoradiation over 5-FU alone (69). The ECOG study randomly assigned patients with locally advanced or incompletely resected pancreatic adenocarcinoma to receive chemoradiation (40 Gy and 600 mg/m^2/day 5-FU for 3 days) or 5-FU alone (600 mg/m^2/week). The chemoradiation group received weekly bolus 5-FU following chemoradiation until there was evidence of disease progression. As in the GITSG studies, all patients were surgically staged and entered in the study within 6 weeks of surgery. Patients with incomplete resections and those with limited peritoneal involvement were also allowed to participate. The median survival was 8.3 months in the group that received chemoradiation and 8.2 months in the group that received 5-FU alone.

More recent trials of chemoradiation for locally advanced pancreatic cancer have investigated continuous-infusion 5-FU in combination with EBRT. The ECOG performed a phase I study to determine the maximal tolerated dose (MTD) of prolonged infusional 5-FU when combined with EBRT to 59.4 Gy in patients with pancreatic or extrahepatic biliary tumors. The MTD of 5-FU was 250 mg/m^2/day, with gastrointestinal toxicity being the dose-limiting factor (70). A subsequent study conducted in Japan demonstrated the feasibility of utilizing low-dose continuous-infusion 5-FU (200 mg/m^2/day) over 5.5 weeks combined with a single course of EBRT to 50.4 Gy for patients with locally advanced pancreatic cancer. This was followed by weekly 5-FU treatments until disease progression was documented. The median survival of treated patients was 10 months, similar to the that of patients treated with bolus 5-FU and EBRT in the GITSG trials (71). Thus, while infusional 5-FU may provide greater radiosensitivity than bolus 5-FU, no clear survival advantage has been established for this approach. In general, for selected patients, treatment programs consisting of EBRT and chemotherapy may result in median survivals of approximately 10 to 12 months and a 2-year survival rate of 20%. Long-term survivors are rare.

Concurrent Chemoradiation Versus Systemic Chemotherapy

Chemoradiotherapy was compared with chemotherapy in a recent randomized trial by the French the Fédération Francophone de Cancérologie Digestive (FFCD) group. In this study, chemoradiotherapy was administered in a dose of 60 Gy concurrently with cisplatin and 5-FU (continuous infusion at 300 mg/m^2/day). The chemotherapy arm consisted of gemcitabine (1000 mg/m^2/week). Surprisingly, the overall survival was shorter in the chemoradiotherapy arm (72). Higher grade 3 to 4 toxicity rates were observed in the chemoradiotherapy arm compared with the chemotherapy arm (66 versus 40%, respectively) which may have at least partially accounted for the worse survival with chemoradiation.

In 2008, the results of another phase III trial (ECOG 4201) comparing chemoradiotherapy and chemotherapy alone were presented at the 44th annual ASCO meeting. In this trial, patients with locally unresectable pancreatic cancer were randomly assigned between chemoradiotherapy with concurrent gemcitabine followed by gemcitabine versus gemcitabine alone. In the chemoradiotherapy arm, the total radiotherapy dose was 50.4 Gy with concurrent gemcitabine (600 mg/m^2/week). The inclusion of 316 patients was planned, but the study closed after the inclusion of 74 patients because of low accrual rate. Median overall survival was slightly better in the chemoradiotherapy arm (11 versus 9.2 months, $p = .044$) (73). These results should be considered cautiously because of the limited number of patients included.

A recent literature-based meta-analyses concluded that overall survival was not significantly different after chemoradiotherapy or chemotherapy (74).

Integration of Novel Agents Into Concurrent Chemoradiation Strategies

Given the limited benefit noted with 5-FU–based chemoradiation, there has been an effort to incorporate alternative agents into concurrent therapies including gemcitabine, paclitaxel, capecitabine, and novel targeted agents, including bevacizumab, cetuximab, and erlotinib. Because of its role in metastatic disease, gemcitabine with EBRT has been extensively investigated for patients with localized pancreatic cancer. Several doses and schedules of gemcitabine have been combined radiation (75). Most of these studies report gastrointestinal toxicity as dose-limiting, but hematologic toxicity has also been observed. Anecdotal experience with gemcitabine-based chemoradiation suggests that objective response to gemcitabine-based chemoradiation is occasionally quite impressive.

Currently, however, there is no compelling evidence to suggest improved survival using gemcitabine-based chemoradiation over 5-FU–based programs for patients with locally advanced disease. Li et al. conducted a small randomized trial which directly compared 5-FU–based chemoradiation with gemcitabine-based chemoradiation. In that trial, median survival for the 18 patients randomized to receive gemcitabine with EBRT was 14.5 months, compared with 6.7 months in 16 patients treated with 5-FU–based radiation. The result of this trial should be interpreted with caution, given the small sample size and relatively poor outcome of patients treated with 5-FU and EBRT (76). Another prospective study compared FU with cisplatin-gemcitabine–based chemoradiation and did not demonstrate any difference in overall survival, with radiotherapy to a total dose of 50.4 Gy (77).

At present, there is no standard approach, dose, or schedule for gemcitabine combined with radiation. However, based on completed phases I and II studies, we have defined the MTD of gemcitabine, associated toxicity, the size of radiation port, and dose (78). 5-FU or capecitabine-based chemoradiation is now standard at MDACC for locally advanced pancreatic cancer. Gemcitabine is also considered in the context of clinical trials.

In general, for patients with significant pain as the primary symptom but who are maintaining adequate performance status, initial treatment with chemoradiation is reasonable. Progressive disease may be seen after completion of chemoradiation. This may take the form of local tumor progression with increasing pain, gastric outlet obstruction or recurrent biliary obstruction, or distant metastatic disease with liver or lung metastases, or peritoneal carcinomatosis. At MDACC, investigations of novel agents with potential cytostatic properties to be used after chemoradiation have been conducted. In recent RTOG 0411 study, patients with locally advanced pancreatic cancer were treated with capecitabine, bevacizumab, and radiation followed by maintenance therapy with capecitabine and bevacizumab. The overall median survival reported in this study was 11 months, which is similar to that reported in previous RTOG trials that did not include bevacizumab (79).

Systemic therapy with gemcitabine alone or in combination also represents a reasonable off-protocol alternative in patients with locally advanced pancreatic cancer. Systemic therapy alone may improve both pain control and performance status, and avoids the gastrointestinal toxicity associated with chemoradiation. For those patients with stable or responding disease after 4 to 6 months of systemic therapy, chemoradiation is often delivered to maximize locoregional tumor control. This treatment sequence has the advantage of avoiding the toxicity of chemoradiation in those patients who have evidence of metastatic disease following systemic therapy. Chemoradiation is thereby applied only to the patients most likely to benefit as defined by the absence of disease progression during systemic therapy. This strategy was validated by the Groupe Cooperateur Multidisciplinaire en Oncologie (GERCOR) group, who recently performed a retrospective analysis of patients with locally advanced pancreatic cancer who received chemoradiation. These investigators noted that 30% of patients developed metastatic disease after induction chemotherapy and are not candidates for radiation. The remaining 70% received either continued chemotherapy or consolidative chemoradiation. The overall survival in the two groups was 12 and 15 months ($p = .0009$) and the PFS was 7 and 11 months, respectively. These data support the strategy of consolidative chemoradiation following induction chemotherapy (of at least 3 months) in patients with locally advanced pancreatic cancer (80). Our retrospective data from MDACC also strongly suggest that patients who have received induction chemotherapy have a better outcome than those receiving primary chemoradiation (81).

MDACC Approach to Locally Advanced Pancreatic Cancer

For patients who have poor performance status, supportive care is encouraged and radiation is contraindicated. Adequate pain control in these patients—as in all cancer patients—is critically important. In the subgroup of patients with significant pain related to the primary tumor, aggressive use of narcotics is initiated. For patients with poor tolerance of narcotics or inadequate pain control with their administration, celiac or splanchnic nerve block is recommended. Proper pain control improves performance status and quality of life. Once pain control has improved, the patient's performance status is reassessed and therapeutic options are discussed. When possible, given the limited therapeutic options available for these patients and the modest impact of current treatments, enrollment of patients into trials of novel systemic agents is encouraged. For patients who have a good performance status, induction chemotherapy followed by chemoradiation is our preferred institutional approach. At least 3 to 4 months of induction chemotherapy with a gemcitabine-based regimen followed by capecitabine or 5-FU and radiation is the favored approach. Figure 18-6 shows the MDACC protocol for individualizing therapy for patients with locally advanced disease.

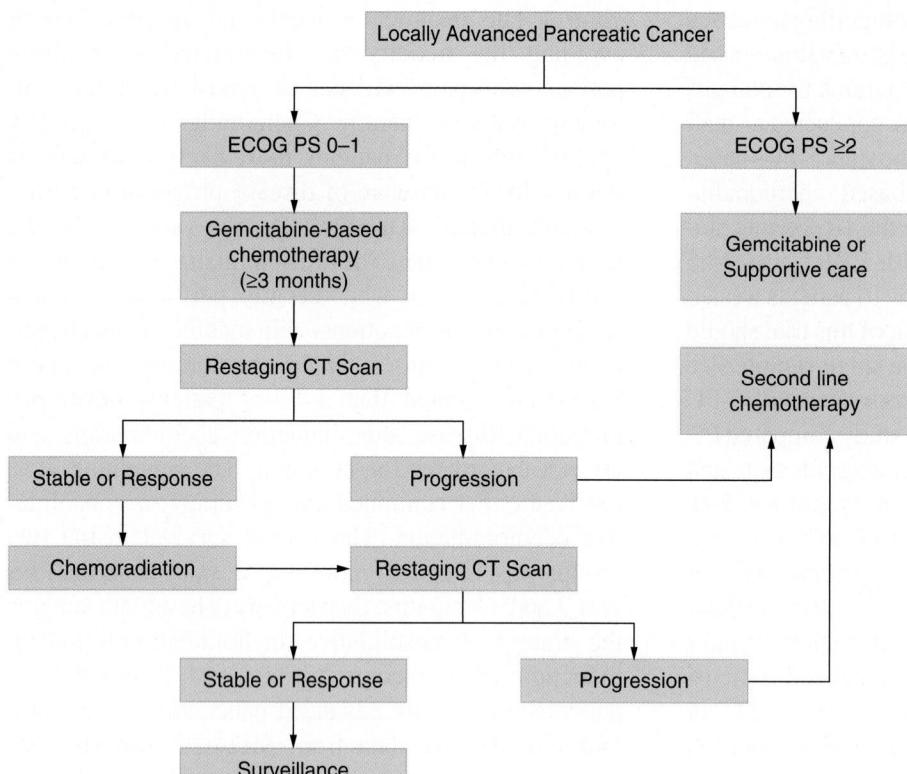

FIGURE 18-6. Treatment algorithm applied to the management of patients with locally advanced pancreatic cancer.

Management of Metastatic Disease

Progress in the treatment of metastatic pancreatic cancer has been extremely slow, and prognosis for these patients remains very poor. Compared with patients having other common malignancies, such as cancer of the colon or breast, patients with advanced pancreatic cancer are often much more debilitated. Therefore making an impact on their survival remains a challenge for oncologists. Palliation remains the primary goal of therapy, and continual reassessment of symptoms should be an important focus of care. Management of patients with metastatic disease should be guided by the following principles:

1. The disease course may be quite dynamic, and the clinical status of a patient can change quickly. Patients may develop biliary obstruction, rapidly worsening pain, stent occlusion with cholangitis, intractable ascites, gastrointestinal bleeding, or venous thromboembolism. Patients therefore require frequent reassessment, whether or not they are undergoing cytotoxic therapy.
2. Pancreatic cancer is quite resistant to systemic therapy and responses to therapy are very rarely observed in patients with poor performance status or high tumor burden.

3. Peritoneal disease is usually not responsive to chemotherapy and, in our experience, carries a particularly poor prognosis. Metastatic disease predominantly located in the liver or lung is more likely to be responsive to systemic therapy. When the disease is metastatic to the lung only, its course may be somewhat more indolent.
4. Improvement in the treatment for pancreatic cancer is desperately needed, and—whenever possible—patients with good performance status should be encouraged to participate in clinical trials.

Systemic Therapy for Metastatic Disease—Lessons From the Past

Trials of chemotherapy for pancreatic cancer date from the 1960s to the present time. Early published data frequently reported response rates to chemotherapy exceeding 20%. However, with the advent of high-quality CT and MRI, which provide better cross-sectional imaging, modern trials of chemotherapy have reported substantially lower response rates. Importantly, cooperative group studies of 5-FU–based therapies dating back to the 1980s have not clearly demonstrated any meaningful survival advantage for patients treated with single-agent chemotherapy compared with 5-FU combinations or even best supportive care. Thus, for many years, no standard drug or drug regimen had emerged as an accepted frontline therapy for metastatic pancreatic cancer.

Gemcitabine for Metastatic Pancreatic Cancer

Chemotherapy for pancreatic cancer changed with the advent of 2′difluoro, 2′deoxycytidine, better known as gemcitabine, which was developed in the 1990s. This drug has demonstrated modest activity in advanced disease and, while the response rate to the drug remains low, it is associated with reproducible clinical benefit for a subset of patients. For example, in an early multicenter trial of gemcitabine in 44 pancreatic cancer patients, 5 objective responses (11%) were documented (82). Of note, however, the investigators reported frequent subjective symptomatic benefits often in the absence of objective responses. In another study, gemcitabine again led to few objective responses (2 of 32 patients), but symptomatic improvement was also reported by patients enrolled in that trial (83). Based on these observations, two subsequent trials of gemcitabine for advanced pancreatic cancer were completed. In the randomized trial that led to gemcitabine's approval in the United States, weekly gemcitabine was compared to bolus weekly 5-FU in previously untreated patients (84). Patients treated with gemcitabine achieved a higher response rate (5.4 versus 0%) and a statistically significant improvement in median survival compared to those treated with 5-FU (5.65 versus 4.41 months, $p = .0025$). The 1-year survival rate for patients treated with gemcitabine was 18%, whereas the rate was only 2% for those treated with 5-FU. Importantly, more clinically meaningful effects on disease-related symptoms were recorded with gemcitabine than with 5-FU. These clinical benefits were also documented in patients treated with gemcitabine after experiencing disease progression with 5-FU. The clinical benefit and the modest survival advantage attributed to gemcitabine compared to bolus weekly 5-FU have helped to make it the first-line therapy for patients with advanced pancreatic adenocarcinoma. This trial enrolled a heterogeneous patient population, with patients having either locally advanced, unresectable disease or metastatic disease. About 70% of the treated patients had metastatic pancreatic cancer, and this is the basis for its use as frontline therapy in patients with disseminated disease. At MDACC, gemcitabine-based therapy remains the standard for patients with metastatic disease, and adequate performance status. While most authorities would agree that gemcitabine has led to a small incremental advance in the treatment of metastatic pancreatic cancer, it does represent the standard treatment against which other treatments may be tested.

Fixed-Dose Rate Gemcitabine

Further investigation of gemcitabine as a treatment for pancreatic cancer has attempted to improve its therapeutic index. Gemcitabine is a prodrug that must be phosphorylated to its active metabolites gemcitabine diphosphate and gemcitabine triphosphate. Gemcitabine diphosphate inhibits ribonucleotide reductase, thereby depleting intracellular pools of the triphosphate nucleotides. Gemcitabine triphosphate can incorporate into an elongating chain of DNA and lead to premature chain termination and cell death. Gemcitabine triphosphate may also inhibit normal DNA repair mechanisms. This may explain its potent radiosensitizing properties and synergy with other DNA-damaging cytotoxic agents.

Once phosphorylated, gemcitabine accumulates within cells and—based on pharmacokinetic studies—intracellular concentrations are highest when the drug is given at a fixed-dose rate (FDR) of 10 mg/m^2/min. The administration of gemcitabine at this dose rate has been shown to improve clinical outcome in a randomized phase II trial in metastatic pancreatic cancer. Results from this study demonstrated that compared to giving gemcitabine at 2300 mg/m^2 over 30 min, a dose of 1500 mg/m^2 delivered over 150 min (10 mg/m^2/min) led to a higher objective response rate (16.2 versus 2.7%) and a trend toward improved survival (6.1 versus 4.7 months) (85). Therefore when we use the drug off protocol, it is administered at fixed-dose rate.

FUTURE DIRECTIONS OF CHEMOTHERAPY IN PANCREATIC CANCER

Gemcitabine Combinations: Cytotoxic Agents

Given the growing acceptance of gemcitabine as first-line therapy for advanced pancreatic cancer, gemcitabine-based combinations have been studied. The efforts to build on gemcitabine have taken two separate pathways. One approach has been to combine gemcitabine with other cytotoxic drugs. Most trials have combined it with one other agent, such as docetaxel, oxaliplatin, 5-FU, cisplatin, or irinotecan. In addition, regimens using two to four other drugs with gemcitabine are starting to appear in the literature. These include combinations of gemcitabine, capecitabine, and docetaxel (GTX); gemcitabine, 5-FU, leucovorin, irinotecan, and cisplatin (G-FLIP). Randomized trials of gemcitabine versus gemcitabine-based doublets of cytotoxic therapy thus far have shown no statistically

TABLE 18-7	SUMMARY OF TRIALS COMBINING GEMCITABINE WITH A SECOND CYTOTOXIC AGENT				
Author Year	*Number of Patients*	*% of Pts w/ Metastatic Disease*	*Control Arm Med Surv (Months)*	*Combination Therapy Med Surv (Months)*	*p-Value*
Berlin, 2002	322	90	Gem 5.4	Gem/5-FU 6.7	0.09
Colucci, 2002	107	58	Gem 5.4	Gem/cisplatin 7.0	0.43
Heinemann, 2006	195	80	Gem 6.0	Gem/cisplatin 7.5	0.12
Rocha-Lima, 2004	342	80	Gem 6.6	Gem/irinotecan 6.3	NS
Louvet, 2004	313	70	Gem 7.0	Gem/oxaliplatin 9.0	0.13
Poplin, 2006	555	88	Gem 4.9	Gem/oxaliplatin 5.9	0.16
Abou-Alfa, 2006	349	78	Gem 6.2	Gem/exactecan 6.7	0.52
Hermann, 2007	319	80	Gem 7.2	Gem/capecitabine 8.4	0.23
Cunningham, 2009	533	71	Gem 6.2	Gem/capecitabine 7.1	0.08

5-FU, 5-fluorouracil; Gem, gemcitabine.

significant survival advantage (Table 18-7). However, gemcitabine combined with a platinum does appear to have some benefit in patients with good performance status (86).

Recent Trials Evaluating Combination Therapy

A phase II study, the Cancer and Leukemia Group B (CALGB) 89904, was a four-arm study comparing FDR gemcitabine with various gemcitabine doublets, including cisplatin, docetaxel, and irinotecan. Six-month survival, the primary endpoint, did not differ significantly between the four arms (range: 53-57%) (87). Overall survival was also similar across the groups. The combination of gemcitabine with cisplatin was further tested in a phase III trial in Germany with an improvement in progression-free and median survival over single-agent gemcitabine, but the difference was not statistically significant (median survival 7.5 versus 6.0 months, $p = .15$) (88). Similarly, a phase III trial evaluating the combination of gemcitabine and irinotecan versus gemcitabine alone failed to demonstrate a survival advantage over gemcitabine alone (89).

More recently, the combination of gemcitabine with oxaliplatin has been studied. Preclinical data suggest that this combination may be synergistic and the order in which the drugs administered may be critical to their activity. Previously, the GERCOR/GISCAD (Italian Group for the Study of Digestive Tract Cancer) phase III trial with FDR gemcitabine and oxaliplatin demonstrated a statistically significant higher response rate and progression-free survival in patients with locally advanced and metastatic disease (90). However, improvement in overall survival observed with the combination did not reach statistical significance based on the study design (9.0 versus 7.1 months, $p = .13$). These results were followed by ECOG 6201 which had three arms: FDR gemcitabine with oxaliplatin, FDR gemcitabine alone, and gemcitabine in a 30-min infusion (91). A total of 832 patients were enrolled, and the overall survival was not statistically different between the three groups: 4.9 months in the gemcitabine 30-min infusion group, 6.2 months in the FDR gemcitabine group, and 5.7 months with gemcitabine plus oxaliplatin ($p = $ N.S.).

Investigations of prolonged infusional 5-FU and the orally bioavailable fluorinated pyrimidine, capecitabine, suggest some activity with these approaches. Capecitabine, when used in combination with gemcitabine, demonstrated a modest clinical benefit over gemcitabine alone and also appeared to improve median overall survival in patients with good performance status (92). Most recently in a phase III trial, Cunningham and colleagues randomized patients to receive gemcitabine alone versus gemcitabine plus capecitabine (gemcitabine—1000 mg/m^2 IV weekly × 3 every 4 weeks; capecitabine—1660 mg/m^2/day PO for 3 weeks and 1 week's rest) (93). The addition of capecitabine to gemcitabine significantly improved overall response rate and progression-free survival ($p = .03$ and $.004$, respectively) and showed a trend toward improved OS ($p = .08$).

Gemcitabine Combinations: Molecular Therapeutics

While other cytotoxic drugs may provide some survival benefit when combined with gemcitabine, any documented improvements in patient outcome are predicted to be relatively small. Therefore, the investigation of targeted molecular therapies should be given priority. The foundation of such therapies is the recent elucidation of molecular events implicated in pancreatic carcinogenesis and chemoresistance and a greater understanding of the metastatic process, including angiogenesis. Treatment strategies being developed include interruption or modulation of known growth factors and signal-transduction pathways involved with cell growth, invasion, and angiogenesis. This is an active area of clinical investigation; a few examples are provided below.

Epidermal Growth Factor Receptor Inhibition

Antibodies to the epidermal growth factor receptor (EGFR) have been shown to compete with the growth-stimulatory ligands for binding to this receptor. Binding with specific antibodies leads to growth inhibition and, in some cases, apoptosis. Small molecular inhibitors of the tyrosine kinase activity of the EGFR have been developed and are being investigated for activity in a variety of solid tumors, including pancreatic cancer. In a large international phase III trial, erlotinib (Tarceva), an oral small molecule inhibitor of EGFR, in combination with gemcitabine led to a slightly longer median survival compared to gemcitabine alone (6.24 versus 5.91 months, $p = .038$) (94). Importantly, treatment-related toxicities were not significantly worse for the patients receiving the combination compared with those on gemcitabine monotherapy. This trial resulted in FDA approval for erlotinib in metastatic pancreatic cancer and remains the only targeted agent approved for this disease to date. A phase II trial studying the toxicity and efficacy of gemcitabine combined with cetuximab has been reported. The objective response rate to the combination was 12%, not significantly different from that reported for gemcitabine alone. Overall survival was

7.1 months (95). These data were followed by Southwest Oncology Group (SWOG) S0205, a phase III trial evaluating gemcitabine with cetuximab. Overall survival was 6 months for gemcitabine alone versus 6.5 months for the combination ($p = .14$). Progression-free survival and response rates were also similar between the two arms.

Antiangiogenic Agents

Tumor angiogenesis is important in the establishment and progression of metastatic implants, and a variety of endogenous angiogenic factors have been identified. It is now generally accepted that inhibition of these factors represents a feasible approach to impeding metastatic progression. Over the last several years, several agents with potent antiangiogenic activity have been developed and are currently being tested in the clinic. One cytokine that is believed to be central to angiogenesis in pancreatic cancer is VEGF, which is often overexpressed in pancreatic cancer. VEGF inhibition may have two roles: blocking VEGF receptors to inhibit tumor growth and impeding angiogenesis.

Bevacizumab, an anti-VEGF antibody, has been investigated in patients with advanced pancreatic cancer. Phase II data demonstrated promising response rates ranging from 11 to 24% and overall survivals of 8.1 to 9.8 months (96). Unfortunately, a randomized phase III trial, CALGB 80303, did not mirror these results. Patients were assigned to receive gemcitabine alone versus gemcitabine plus bevacizumab (10 mg/kg). Median overall survival was not different (5.2 versus 5.8 months), and there was no significant improvement in response rate or progression-free survival (97). Most recently, a randomized phase III trial with gemcitabine, bevacizumab, and erlotinib was reported. This multicenter trial included 607 metastatic patients, randomly assigned to receive gemcitabine with bevacizumab and erlotinib (dosed at 1000 mg/m^2 IV 7 out of 8 weeks, followed by 3 out of 4 weeks, 5 mg/kg IV every 14 days, and 100 mg PO daily, respectively) or gemcitabine with erlotinib plus placebo (98). Median overall survival was not significantly improved when compared to gemcitabine plus erlotinib (7.1 versus 6.0 months; HR 0.89; 95% CI, 0.74-1.07; $p = .2087$); however, there was a significant improvement in progression-free survival (4.6 versus 3.6 months; HR, 0.73; 95% CI, 0.61-0.86; $p = .0002$).

MDACC APPROACH TO THE PATIENT WITH METASTATIC DISEASE

Metastatic pancreatic cancer is a disease characterized by anorexia, cachexia, and pain. Jaundice may result from the primary tumor or intrahepatic metastases. Local tumor progression can lead to worsening pain, gastric outlet obstruction, or gastroparesis and patients with peritoneal carcinomatosis may suffer from intractable ascites, intestinal dysmotility, or mechanical obstruction. Constipation is very common. Patients are also at risk for thrombotic events, including superficial or deep venous thromboses and thromboembolism. Palliation must always be the primary goal for this group of patients and is facilitated by a multidisciplinary approach. Symptomatic relief of biliary obstruction and pain should be addressed prior to consideration of systemic therapy. Most patients with metastatic disease can achieve adequate pain control with the use of long- or short-acting narcotics, and this approach is generally preferred. However, if pain is not well controlled with oral or transdermal narcotics or if these agents are poorly tolerated, patients should undergo an evaluation with an anesthesiologist or neurologist to consider ablation of the celiac or splanchnic plexus. In addition to aggressive pain-control efforts, other supportive measures should be considered, including appetite enhancers, antidepressants, and central nervous system stimulants.

Given the poor prognosis of patients with metastatic disease, biliary obstruction should be relieved by nonsurgical means whenever possible, and we advocate the insertion of expandable metal stents rather than polyethylene biliary stents. On occasion, percutaneous biliary drainage may be required in the setting of extrahepatic biliary obstruction.

When a patient develops gastric outlet obstruction, we try to estimate the prognosis at that juncture. If his or her life expectancy is greater than 12 weeks, surgical intervention for definitive gastric bypass is usually considered. For patients with end-stage metastatic disease, the use of duodenal stents is encouraged for those with gastric obstruction in the face of stage IV disease and limited survival. For patients with intractable symptomatic ascites, it is important to realize that this may not be caused by carcinomatosis and frequently results from portal vein or SMV thrombosis. Serum-ascitic albumin gradient (SAAG) has replaced the older transudate versus exudate concept for the diagnosis of portal hypertension. In portal hypertension, the SAAG is 1.1 g/dL or higher. In other etiologies including malignancy, the SAAG is less than 1.1 g/dL (99). Ascites secondary to portal hypertension will respond to diuretics including spironolactone whereas malignant ascites requires repeated paracentesis or an indwelling peritoneal tunneled catheter. Shunting procedures for ascites should be reserved for selected patients with SMV or portal vein thrombosis as the primary cause in the face of nonmetastatic disease. Gastroparesis is another commonly occurring problem from advanced pancreatic cancer which requires promotility agents, dietary and behavioral modification.

MDACC Approach to Systemic Therapy for Advanced Pancreatic Cancer

Systemic therapy for metastatic disease should be actively discouraged in patients with poor performance status (ECOG >2) or significant metastatic tumor burden. End-of-life discussions and planning are appropriate at the time of diagnosis in the setting of metastatic disease.

Whenever possible, patients with good performance status should be treated with systemic therapy in a clinical trial. The current trial at MDACC involves the use of an antibody directed against the insulin-like growth factor receptor (IGF-1R). The IGF-1R pathway appears to play a crucial role in pancreatic cancer as it activates various downstream signaling pathways that promote tumor growth. Preclinical data suggest synergy between gemcitabine and anti–IGF-1R therapy. We are investigating the IGF-1R monoclonal antibody, MK-0646 (dalotuzumab) in combination with gemcitabine alone or with gemcitabine and erlotinib in a randomized phase II trial.

Second-line treatment can be considered in those patients with good performance status. After progression on gemcitabine, most second-line options include 5-FU–based therapies, including 5-FU, leucovorin and oxaliplatin (FOLFOX) , 5-FU, leucovorin and irinotecan (FOLFIRI), or single-agent capecitabine in patients who cannot tolerate combination treatment. Our institution reported on a phase II study with 41 patients who received Capecitabine and oxaliplatin (XELOX) as second-line therapy (oxaliplatin 130 mg/m^2, capecitabine 1000 mg/m^2 twice daily for 14-21 days) (100). Progression-free survival was 9.9 weeks and median overall survival was 23 weeks with a 6-month overall survival of 44%. The responses were especially pronounced in patients with good performance status and those who responded to first-line therapy. A recent phase II study compared Modified FOLFIRI (mFOLFIRI3) with Modified FOLFOX (mFOLFOX) as second-line therapy in gemcitabine-refractory pancreatic cancer (101). Sixty-one patients were randomized to either regimen with toxicities being similar in both arms. Six-month survival rates were 27% with FOLFIRI and 30% with FOLFOX. Median overall survival was 16.6 and 14.9 weeks, respectively. Patients who have experienced disease stability or response with gemcitabine-based first-line therapy can be considered for second-line therapy with gemcitabine-based combinations (such as gemcitabine, docetaxel, and capecitabine [GTX]) (102). However, this approach can be associated with toxicity and is best reserved for patients with good performance status.

For those patients who do not wish to enroll in a clinical trial, a course of gemcitabine as first-line therapy is reasonable. At MDACC, our off-protocol approach is to deliver fixed-dose-rate gemcitabine at a dosage of 600 mg/m^2 over 60 min (10 mg/m^2/min) in combination with cisplatin 30 mg/m^2 and erlotinib. Each cycle is administered every two weeks. Restaging studies should include CT of the abdomen and pelvis in the eighth week. When an objective response or stable disease is observed, chemotherapy is usually continued until there is radiographic or clinical evidence of disease progression, with restaging studies generally performed every 8 to 12 weeks. During this time, continuous and frequent reassessment of the patient's clinical status is recommended. Gemcitabine-platinum doublets are offered only to those patients with excellent performance status, which may justify more aggressive therapy. Importantly, patients are informed that the use of such treatment has not been shown to clearly prolong survival. Gemcitabine as a single agent in a dose of 600 or 800 mg/m^2 as an FDR infusion weekly × 3, repeated every 4 weeks is another alternative.

In summary, clinically meaningful advances in the treatment of metastatic pancreatic cancer have developed quite slowly. However, with a greater understanding of the underlying genetic and molecular abnormalities involved in pancreatic carcinogenesis, rational cytotoxic chemotherapy in combination with molecular agents and aggressive supportive methods are expected to alter the natural course of this disease in the near future. Continued efforts to enroll patients with advanced pancreatic cancer into well-designed clinical trials should remain a high priority for oncologists across all disciplines.

References

1. Jemal A, Siegel R, Ward E, et al. Cancer statistics, 2009. CA Cancer J Clin 2009;59:225-249.
2. Konner J, O'Reilly E. Pancreatic cancer: Epidemiology, genetics, and approaches to screening. Oncology (Williston Park) 2002;16:1615-1622.
3. Villeneuve PJ, Johnson KC, Mao Y, et al. Environmental tobacco smoke and the risk of pancreatic cancer: Findings from a Canadian population-based case-control study. Can J Public Health 2004;95:32-37.
4. Hassan MM, Abbruzzese JL, Bondy ML, et al. Passive smoking and the use of noncigarette tobacco products in association with risk for pancreatic cancer: A case-control study. Cancer 2007;109:2547-2556.
5. Everhart J, Wright D. Diabetes mellitus as a risk factor for pancreatic cancer: A meta-analysis. JAMA 1995;273:1605-1609.
6. Talamini G, Falconi M, Bassi C, et al. Incidence of cancer in the course of chronic pancreatitis. Am J Gastroenterol 1999;94:1253-1260.
7. Lowenfels AB, Maisonneuve P. Epidemiologic and etiologic factors of pancreatic cancer. Hematol Oncol Clin North Am 2002;16:1-16.
8. Felderbauer P, Stricker I, Schnekenburger J, et al. Histopathological features of patients with chronic pancreatitis due to mutations in the PRSS1 gene: Evaluation of BRAF and KRAS2 mutations. Digestion 2008;78:60-65.
9. Hanley AJ, Johnson KC, Villeneuve PJ, et al. Physical activity, anthropometric factors and risk of pancreatic cancer: Results from the Canadian enhanced cancer surveillance system. Int J Cancer 2001;94:140-147.
10. Hruban RH, Canto MI, Yeo CJ. Prevention of pancreatic cancer and strategies for management of familial pancreatic cancer. Dig Dis 2001;19:76-84.
11. Guo YS, Townsend CM, Jr. Roles of gastrointestinal hormones in pancreatic cancer. J Hepatobiliary Pancreat Surg 2000;7:276-285.
12. Li D, Morris JS, Liu J, et al. Body mass index and risk, age of onset, and survival in patients with pancreatic cancer. JAMA 2009;301:2553-2562.
13. Li D, Yeung SC, Hassan MM, et al. Antidiabetic therapies affect risk of pancreatic cancer. Gastroenterology 2009;137:482-488.
14. Amundadottir L, Kraft P, Stolzenberg-Solomon RZ, et al. Genome-wide association study identifies variants in the ABO locus associated with susceptibility to pancreatic cancer. Nat Genet 2009;41:986-990.
15. Suzuki H, Li Y, Dong X, et al. Effect of insulin-like growth factor gene polymorphisms alone or in interaction with diabetes on the risk of pancreatic cancer. Cancer Epidemiol Biomarkers Prev 2008;17:3467-3473.
16. Li D, Jiao L. Molecular epidemiology of pancreatic cancer. Int J Gastrointest Cancer 2003;33:3-14.
17. Jones S, Zhang X, Parsons DW, et al. Core signaling pathways in human pancreatic cancers revealed by global genomic analyses. Science 2008;321:1801-1806.
18. Grunewald K, Lyons J, Frohlich A, et al. High frequency of Ki-ras codon 12 mutations in pancreatic adenocarcinomas. Int J Cancer 1989;43:1037-1041.
19. Rozenblum E, Schutte M, Goggins M, et al. Tumor-suppressive pathways in pancreatic carcinoma. Cancer Res 1997;57:1731-1734.
20. Wang W, Abbruzzese JL, Evans DB, et al. The nuclear factor-kappa B RelA transcription factor is constitutively activated in human pancreatic adenocarcinoma cells. Clin Cancer Res 1999;5:119-127.
21. Feldmann G, Habbe N, Dhara S, et al. Hedgehog inhibition prolongs survival in a genetically engineered mouse model of pancreatic cancer. Gut 2008;57:1420-1430.
22. Olive KP, Jacobetz MA, Davidson CJ, et al. Inhibition of Hedgehog signaling enhances delivery of chemotherapy in a mouse model of pancreatic cancer. Science 2009;324:1457-1461.
23. Van CE, van de VH, Karasek P, et al. Phase III trial of gemcitabine plus tipifarnib compared with gemcitabine plus placebo in advanced pancreatic cancer. J Clin Oncol 2004;22:1430-1438.

24. Bramhall SR, Schulz J, Nemunaitis J, et al. A double-blind placebo-controlled, randomised study comparing gemcitabine and marimastat with gemcitabine and placebo as first line therapy in patients with advanced pancreatic cancer. *Br J Cancer* 2002;87:161-167.

25. Mujica VR, Barkin JS, Go VL. Acute pancreatitis secondary to pancreatic carcinoma. Study Group Participants. *Pancreas* 2000;21:329-332.

26. Raut CP, Grau AM, Staerkel GA, et al. Diagnostic accuracy of endoscopic ultrasound-guided fine-needle aspiration in patients with presumed pancreatic cancer. *J Gastrointest Surg* 2003;7:118-126.

27. Rashleigh-Belcher HJ, Russell RC, Lees WR. Cutaneous seeding of pancreatic carcinoma by fine-needle aspiration biopsy. *Br J Radiol* 1986;59:182-183.

28. Tamm EP, Silverman PM, Charnsangavej C, et al. Diagnosis, staging, and surveillance of pancreatic cancer. *AJR Am J Roentgenol* 2003;180:1311-1323.

29. Tamm E, Charnsangavej C. Pancreatic cancer: Current concepts in imaging for diagnosis and staging. *Cancer J* 2001;7:298-311.

30. Tamm EP, Loyer EM, Faria S, et al. Staging of pancreatic cancer with multidetector CT in the setting of preoperative chemoradiation therapy. *Abdom Imaging* 2006;31:568-574.

31. Kalady MF, Clary BM, Clark LA, et al. Clinical utility of positron emission tomography in the diagnosis and management of periampullary neoplasms. *Ann Surg Oncol* 2002;9:799-806.

32. Pleskow DK, Berger HJ, Gyves J, et al. Evaluation of a serologic marker, CA19-9, in the diagnosis of pancreatic cancer. *Ann Intern Med* 1989;110:704-709.

33. Fogelman DR, Pathak P, Qiao W, et al. Serum CA 19-9 level as a surrogate marker for prognosis in locally advanced pancreatic cancer (LAPC). *J Clin Oncol (Meeting Abstracts)* 2008;26:15514.

34. van den Bosch RP, van Eijck CH, Mulder PG, et al. Serum CA19-9 determination in the management of pancreatic cancer. *Hepatogastroenterology* 1996;43:710-713.

35. Ko AH, Hwang J, Venook AP, et al. Serum CA19-9 response as a surrogate for clinical outcome in patients receiving fixed-dose rate gemcitabine for advanced pancreatic cancer. *Br J Cancer* 2005;93:195-199.

36. Warshaw AL, Tepper JE, Shipley WU. Laparoscopy in the staging and planning of therapy for pancreatic cancer. *Am J Surg* 1986;151:76-80.

37. Fernandez-del Castillo CL, Warshaw AL. Pancreatic cancer. Laparoscopic staging and peritoneal cytology. *Surg Oncol Clin N Am* 1998;7:135-142.

38. Pisters PW, Lee JE, Vauthey JN, et al. Laparoscopy in the staging of pancreatic cancer. *Br J Surg* 2001;88:325-337.

39. Warshaw AL. Implications of peritoneal cytology for staging of early pancreatic cancer. *Am J Surg* 1991;161:26-29.

40. Whipple AO. The rationale of radical surgery for cancer of the pancreas and ampullary region. *Ann Surg* 1941;114:612-615.

41. Wade TP, Virgo KS, Johnson FE. Distal pancreatectomy for cancer: Results in U.S. Department of Veterans Affairs hospitals, 1987-1991. *Pancreas* 1995;11:341-344.

42. Birkmeyer JD, Siewers AE, Finlayson EV, et al. Hospital volume and surgical mortality in the United States. *N Engl J Med* 2002;346:1128-1137.

43. Birkmeyer JD, Warshaw AL, Finlayson SR, et al. Relationship between hospital volume and late survival after pancreaticoduodenectomy. *Surgery* 1999;126:178-183.

44. Chang DK, Johns AL, Merrett ND, et al. Margin clearance and outcome in resected pancreatic cancer. *J Clin Oncol* 2009;27:2855-2862.

45. Kuhlmann KF, de Castro SM, Wesseling JG, et al. Surgical treatment of pancreatic adenocarcinoma: Actual survival and prognostic factors in 343 patients. *Eur J Cancer* 2004;40:549-558.

46. Millikan KW, Deziel DJ, Silverstein JC, et al. Prognostic factors associated with resectable adenocarcinoma of the head of the pancreas. *Am Surg* 1999;65:618-623.

47. Neoptolemos JP, Stocken DD, Dunn JA, et al. Influence of resection margins on survival for patients with pancreatic cancer treated by adjuvant chemoradiation and/or chemotherapy in the ESPAC-1 randomized controlled trial. *Ann Surg* 2001;234:758-768.

48. Herman JM, Swartz MJ, Hsu CC, et al. Analysis of fluorouracil-based adjuvant chemotherapy and radiation after pancreaticoduodenectomy for ductal adenocarcinoma of the pancreas: Results of a large, prospectively collected database at the Johns Hopkins Hospital. *J Clin Oncol* 2008;26:3503-3510.

49. Corsini MM, Miller RC, Haddock MG, et al. Adjuvant radiotherapy and chemotherapy for pancreatic carcinoma: The Mayo Clinic experience (1975-2005). *J Clin Oncol* 2008;26:3511-3516.

50. Lim JE, Chien MW, Earle CC. Prognostic factors following curative resection for pancreatic adenocarcinoma: A population-based, linked database analysis of 396 patients. *Ann Surg* 2003;237:74-85.

51. Kalser MH, Ellenberg SS. Pancreatic cancer. Adjuvant combined radiation and chemotherapy following curative resection. *Arch Surg* 1985;120:899-903.

52. Smeenk HG, van Eijck CH, Hop WC, et al. Long-term survival and metastatic pattern of pancreatic and periampullary cancer after adjuvant chemoradiation or observation: Long-term results of EORTC trial 40891. *Ann Surg* 2007;246:734-740.

53. Neoptolemos JP, Stocken DD, Friess H, et al. A randomized trial of chemoradiotherapy and chemotherapy after resection of pancreatic cancer. *N Engl J Med* 2004;350:1200-1210.

54. Regine WF, Winter KA, Abrams RA, et al. Fluorouracil vs gemcitabine chemotherapy before and after fluorouracil-based chemoradiation following resection of pancreatic adenocarcinoma: A randomized controlled trial. *JAMA* 2008;299:1019-1026.

55. Javle M, Hsueh CT. Updates in Gastrointestinal Oncology—insights from the 2008 44th annual meeting of the American Society of Clinical Oncology. *J Hematol Oncol* 2009;2:9.

56. Neoptolemos J, Buchler M, Stocken DD, et al. ESPAC-3(v2): A multicenter, international, open-label, randomized, controlled phase III trial of adjuvant 5-fluorouracil/folinic acid (5-FU/FA) versus gemcitabine (GEM) in patients with resected pancreatic ductal adenocarcinoma. *J Clin Oncol (Meeting Abstracts)* 2009;27:LBA4505.

57. Evans DB, Varadhachary GR, Crane CH, et al. Preoperative gemcitabine-based chemoradiation for patients with resectable adenocarcinoma of the pancreatic head. *J Clin Oncol* 2008;26:3496-3502.

58. Pisters PW, Wolff RA, Janjan NA, et al. Preoperative paclitaxel and concurrent rapid-fractionation radiation for resectable pancreatic adenocarcinoma: Toxicities, histologic response rates, and event-free outcome. *J Clin Oncol* 2002; 20:2537-2544.

59. Varadhachary GR, Wolff RA, Crane CH, et al. Preoperative gemcitabine and cisplatin followed by gemcitabine-based chemoradiation for resectable adenocarcinoma of the pancreatic head. *J Clin Oncol* 2008;26:3487-3495.

60. Pisters PW, Abbruzzese JL, Janjan NA, et al. Rapid-fractionation preoperative chemoradiation, pancreaticoduodenectomy, and intraoperative radiation therapy for resectable pancreatic adenocarcinoma. *J Clin Oncol* 1998;16:3843-3850.

61. Crane CH, Ellis LM, Abbruzzese JL, et al. Phase I trial evaluating the safety of bevacizumab with concurrent radiotherapy and capecitabine in locally advanced pancreatic cancer. *J Clin Oncol* 2006;24:1145-1151.

62. Todd KE, Gloor B, Lane JS, et al. Resection of locally advanced pancreatic cancer after downstaging with continuous-infusion 5-fluorouracil, mitomycin-C, leucovorin, and dipyridamole. *J Gastrointest Surg* 1998;2:159-166.

63. White R, Lee C, Anscher M, et al. Preoperative chemoradiation for patients with locally advanced adenocarcinoma of the pancreas. *Ann Surg Oncol* 1999;6:38-45.

64. Varadhachary GR, Tamm EP, Abbruzzese JL, et al. Borderline resectable pancreatic cancer: Definitions, management, and role of preoperative therapy. *Ann Surg Oncol* 2006;13: 1035-1046.

65. Brown KM. Multidisciplinary approach to tumors of the pancreas and biliary tree. *Surg Clin North Am* 2009;89: 115-131, ix.

66. Minsky BD, Hilaris B, Fuks Z. The role of radiation therapy in the control of pain from pancreatic carcinoma. *J Pain Symptom Manage* 1988;3:199-205.

67. Moertel CG, Frytak S, Hahn RG, et al. Therapy of locally unresectable pancreatic carcinoma: A randomized comparison of high dose (6000 rads) radiation alone, moderate dose radiation (4000 rads + 5-fluorouracil), and high dose radiation + 5-fluorouracil: The Gastrointestinal Tumor Study Group. *Cancer* 1981;48:1705-1710.

68. The concept of locally advanced gastric cancer. Effect of treatment on outcome. The Gastrointestinal Tumor Study Group. *Cancer* 1990;66:2324-2330.

69. Klaassen DJ, MacIntyre JM, Catton GE, et al. Treatment of locally unresectable cancer of the stomach and pancreas: A randomized comparison of 5-fluorouracil alone with radiation plus concurrent and maintenance 5-fluorouracil—an Eastern Cooperative Oncology Group study. *J Clin Oncol* 1985;3: 373-378.

70. Whittington R, Neuberg D, Tester WJ, et al. Protracted intravenous fluorouracil infusion with radiation therapy in the management of localized pancreaticobiliary carcinoma: A phase I Eastern Cooperative Oncology Group Trial. *J Clin Oncol* 1995;13:227-232.

71. Ishii H, Okada S, Tokuuye K et al. Protracted 5-fluorouracil infusion with concurrent radiotherapy as a treatment for locally advanced pancreatic carcinoma. *Cancer* 1997;79: 1516-1520.

72. Chauffert B, Mornex F, Bonnetain F et al. Phase III trial comparing intensive induction chemoradiotherapy (60 Gy, infusional 5-FU and intermittent cisplatin) followed by maintenance gemcitabine with gemcitabine alone for locally advanced unresectable pancreatic cancer. Definitive results of the 2000-01 FFCD/SFRO study. *Ann Oncol* 2008;19: 1592-1599.

73. Cardenes HR, Powell M, Loehrer PJ, et al. E4201: Randomized phase II study of gemcitabine in combination with radiation therapy versus gemcitabine alone in patients with locally advanced, unresectable, pancreatic cancer (LAPC): Quality-of-life (QOL) analysis. *J Clin Oncol (Meeting Abstracts)* 2009; 27:4627.

74. Sultana A, Tudur SC, Cunningham D, et al. Systematic review, including meta-analyses, on the management of locally advanced pancreatic cancer using radiation/combined modality therapy. *Br J Cancer* 2007;96:1183-1190.

75. McGinn CJ, Zalupski MM. Combined-modality therapy in pancreatic cancer: Current status and future directions. *Cancer J* 2001;7:338-348.

76. Li CP, Chao Y, Chi KH, et al. Concurrent chemoradiotherapy treatment of locally advanced pancreatic cancer: Gemcitabine versus 5-fluorouracil, a randomized controlled study. *Int J Radiat Oncol Biol Phys* 2003;57:98-104.

77. Huguet F, Girard N, Guerche CS-E, et al. Chemoradiotherapy in the management of locally advanced pancreatic carcinoma: A qualitative systematic review. *J Clin Oncol* 2009;27: 2269-2277.

78. Crane CH, Wolff RA, Abbruzzese JL, et al. Combining gemcitabine with radiation in pancreatic cancer: Understanding important variables influencing the therapeutic index. *Semin Oncol* 2001;28:25-33.

79. Crane CH, Winter K, Regine WF, et al. Phase II study of bevacizumab with concurrent capecitabine and radiation followed by maintenance gemcitabine and bevacizumab for locally advanced pancreatic cancer: Radiation Therapy Oncology Group RTOG 0411. *J Clin Oncol* 2009;27:4096-4102.

80. Huguet F, Andre T, Hammel P, et al. Impact of chemoradiotherapy after disease control with chemotherapy in locally advanced pancreatic adenocarcinoma in GERCOR phase II and III studies. *J Clin Oncol* 2007;25:326-331.

81. Krishnan S, Rana V, Janjan NA, et al. Induction chemotherapy selects patients with locally advanced, unresectable pancreatic cancer for optimal benefit from consolidative chemoradiation therapy. *Cancer* 2007;110:47-55.

82. Casper ES, Green MR, Kelsen DP, et al. Phase II trial of gemcitabine (2,2′-difluorodeoxycytidine) in patients with adenocarcinoma of the pancreas. *Invest New Drugs* 1994;12: 29-34.

83. Carmichael J, Fink U, Russell RC, et al. Phase II study of gemcitabine in patients with advanced pancreatic cancer. *Br J Cancer* 1996;73:101-105.

84. Burris HA, III, Moore MJ, Andersen J, et al. Improvements in survival and clinical benefit with gemcitabine as first-line therapy for patients with advanced pancreas cancer: A randomized trial. *J Clin Oncol* 1997;15:2403-2413.

85. Tempero M, Plunkett W, Ruiz VHV, et al. Randomized phase II comparison of dose-intense gemcitabine: Thirty-minute infusion and fixed dose rate infusion in patients with pancreatic adenocarcinoma. *J Clin Oncol* 2003;21:3402-3408.

86. Heinemann V, Boeck S, Hinke A, et al. Meta-analysis of randomized trials: Evaluation of benefit from gemcitabine-based combination chemotherapy applied in advanced pancreatic cancer. *BMC Cancer* 2008;8:82.

87. Kulke MH, Tempero MA, Niedzwiecki D, et al. Randomized phase II study of gemcitabine administered at a fixed dose rate or in combination with cisplatin, docetaxel, or irinotecan in patients with metastatic pancreatic cancer: CALGB 89904. *J Clin Oncol* 2009;27:5506-5512.

88. Heinemann V, Quietzsch D, Gieseler F, et al. Randomized phase III trial of gemcitabine plus cisplatin compared with gemcitabine alone in advanced pancreatic cancer. *J Clin Oncol* 2006;24:3946-3952.

89. Rocha Lima CM, Green MR, Rotche R, et al. Irinotecan plus gemcitabine results in no survival advantage compared with gemcitabine monotherapy in patients with locally advanced or metastatic pancreatic cancer despite increased tumor response rate. *J Clin Oncol* 2004;22:3776-3783.

90. Heinemann V, Labianca R, Hinke A, et al. Increased survival using platinum analog combined with gemcitabine as compared to single-agent gemcitabine in advanced pancreatic cancer: Pooled analysis of two randomized trials, the GERCOR/GISCAD intergroup study and a German multicenter study. *Ann Oncol* 2007;18:1652-1659.

91. Poplin E, Feng Y, Berlin J, et al. Phase III, randomized study of gemcitabine and oxaliplatin versus gemcitabine (fixed-dose rate infusion) compared with gemcitabine (30-minute infusion) in patients with pancreatic carcinoma E6201: A trial of the Eastern Cooperative Oncology Group. *J Clin Oncol* 2009;27:3778-3785.

92. Herrmann R, Bodoky G, Ruhstaller T, et al. Gemcitabine plus capecitabine compared with gemcitabine alone in advanced pancreatic cancer: A randomized, multicenter, phase III trial of the Swiss Group for Clinical Cancer Research and the Central European Cooperative Oncology Group. *J Clin Oncol* 2007;25:2212-2217.

93. Cunningham D, Chau I, Stocken DD, et al. Phase III randomized comparison of gemcitabine versus gemcitabine plus capecitabine in patients with advanced pancreatic cancer. *J Clin Oncol* 2009;27:5513-5518.

94. Moore MJ, Goldstein D, Hamm J, et al. Erlotinib plus gemcitabine compared with gemcitabine alone in patients with advanced pancreatic cancer: A phase III trial of the National Cancer Institute of Canada Clinical Trials Group. *J Clin Oncol* 2007;25:1960-1966.

95. Philip PA. Improving treatment of pancreatic cancer. *Lancet Oncol* 2008;9:7-8.

96. Kindler HL, Friberg G, Singh DA, et al. Phase II trial of bevacizumab plus gemcitabine in patients with advanced pancreatic cancer. *J Clin Oncol* 2005;23:8033-8040.

97. Kindler HL, Niedzwiecki D, Hollis D, et al. A double-blind, placebo-controlled, randomized phase III trial of gemcitabine (G) plus bevacizumab (B) versus gemcitabine plus placebo (P) in patients (pts) with advanced pancreatic cancer (PC): A preliminary analysis of Cancer and Leukemia Group B (CALGB). *J Clin Oncol (Meeting Abstracts)* 2007;25:4508.

98. Van Cutsem E, Vervenne WL, Bennouna J, et al. Phase III trial of bevacizumab in combination with gemcitabine and erlotinib in patients with metastatic pancreatic cancer. *J Clin Oncol* 2009;27:2231-2237.

99. Runyon BA, Montano AA, Akriviadis EA, et al. The serum-ascites albumin gradient is superior to the exudate-transudate concept in the differential diagnosis of ascites. *Ann Intern Med* 1992;117:215-220.

100. Xiong HQ, Varadhachary GR, Blais JC, et al. Phase 2 trial of oxaliplatin plus capecitabine (XELOX) as second-line therapy for patients with advanced pancreatic cancer. *Cancer* 2008;113:2046-2052.

101. Yoo C, Hwang JY, Kim JE, et al. A randomised phase II study of modified FOLFIRI.3 vs modified FOLFOX as second-line therapy in patients with gemcitabine-refractory advanced pancreatic cancer. *Br J Cancer* 2009;101:1658-1663.

102. Fine RL, Fogelman DR, Schreibman SM et al. The gemcitabine, docetaxel, and capecitabine (GTX) regimen for metastatic pancreatic cancer: A retrospective analysis. *Cancer Chemother Pharmacol* 2008;61:167-175.

HEPATOBILIARY MALIGNANCIES

Nishin A. Bhadkamkar
Milind Javle
Rony Avritscher
Sunil Krishnan
Ahmed O. Kaseb

Hepatobiliary malignancies comprise a diverse group of tumors including hepatocellular carcinoma (HCC), variants such as fibrolamellar HCC and cholangiocellular carcinoma, cholangiocarcinoma, carcinoma of the gallbladder, and rare cancers such as sarcoma, angiosarcoma, and hepatoblastoma. The relative frequency of these tumors is shown in Table 19-1. The estimated new cases and deaths from liver and intrahepatic bile duct cancer in the United States in 2009 total 22,620 and 18,160, respectively (1).

The majority of primary liver tumors are HCC or cholangiocarcinoma. These tumor types have different etiologies, epidemiologies, clinical presentations, and treatment options; thus, they are discussed separately.

■ HEPATOCELLULAR CARCINOMA

Hepatocellular carcinoma (HCC) is a malignancy of worldwide significance and has become increasingly important in the United States. HCC is the most common primary liver malignancy, the sixth most common cancer, and the third most common cause of cancer-related deaths worldwide (2). Eighty percent of new

TABLE 19-1 | RELATIVE FREQUENCY OF HEPATOBILIARY TUMORS DIAGNOSED IN THE UNITED STATES

Subtype of Hepatobiliary Cancer	Frequency%
Hepatocellular	84
Cholangiocarcinoma	13
Cholangiocellular and fibrolamellar	2
Angiosarcoma, sarcoma, hepatoblastoma	1

cases occur in developing countries, but the incidence is rising in economically developed regions, including Japan, western Europe, and the United States (3-6). The worldwide distribution of HCC and its associated etiologies are summarized in Table 19-2. Liver cirrhosis is the seventh leading cause of death in the world, the tenth most common cause of death in the United States, and acknowledged as a premalignant condition for developing HCC (7-9). In the United States, hepatitis C virus (HCV), alcohol use, and nonalcoholic fatty liver disease (NAFLD) are the most common causes of cirrhosis (9). The incidence of HCC doubled during the period 1975 to 1995 and continued to rise through 1998 (10,11). This trend is expected to continue due to the estimated 4 million hepatitis C–seropositive individuals in the United States and the known latency of HCC development from the initial HCV infection, which may take two to three decades (11). It is also known that NAFLD-associated cirrhosis is on the rise in the United States (12-14). A majority of patients present with advanced disease that is not amenable to curative procedures. Overall, HCC has a very poor prognosis, with a 5-year survival rate of 5%.

EPIDEMIOLOGY

As shown in Table 19-1, HCC represents approximately 85% of all primary liver cancers (15). The distribution of HCC varies significantly by geography; it is endemic in parts of the world where hepatitis B virus (HBV) is also endemic. In Western countries, HCV infection and alcoholic cirrhosis are the principal risk factors for HCC. Due to rising incidence of HCV infection in American subpopulations, the incidence of HCC is projected to increase four-fold by 2015 (11). The incidence of HCC increases with age, with the age of peak incidence varying somewhat with population. The median age group of HCC is between the fifth and sixth decades. HCC is seen in children and young adults in areas where HBV is endemic, and most of these infections occur perinatally. In all populations worldwide, there is a strong male predominance in HCC incidence. In the United States, the male-to-female ratio is 2.7 to 1. In the United States, HCC incidence rates are higher among African Americans than Caucasians (6.1 versus 2.8 per 100,000 in men). Hispanics, Asians, Pacific Islanders, and Native Americans have a much higher HCC frequency. Independent of HBV status, a family history of HCC in first-degree relatives carries a relative risk (RR) of 2.4 and overall risk (OR) of 2.9 (16). Familial aggregation and germline mutations of the APC (adenomatous polyposis coli) gene have been reported in hepatoblastoma (17).

ETIOLOGY AND RISK FACTORS

HCC develops commonly, but not exclusively, in a setting of liver cell injury, which leads to inflammation, hepatocyte regeneration, liver matrix remodeling, fibrosis, and ultimately cirrhosis. The major etiologies of liver cirrhosis are diverse and include chronic HBV and HCV infection, alcohol consumption, certain medications or toxic exposures, and genetic metabolic diseases. The mechanisms by which these varied etiologies lead to HCC are not fully elucidated.

TABLE 19-2 | INCIDENCE OF HEPATOCELLULAR CARCINOMA (HCC) WORLDWIDE

Region	INCIDENCE*		Number of Cases	Principal Associations
	Males	Females		
Asia, sub-Saharan Africa	30-120	9-30	>500,000 cases per year	HBV, aflatoxin exposure
Japan	10-30	3-9		HCV
Southern Europe, Argentina, Switzerland	5-10	2-5		HCV
Western Europe	<5	<3		HCV
United States	<5	<3	19,000 predicted for 2004	HCV, alcohol

HBV, hepatitis B virus; HCV, hepatitis C virus.
*Cases per 100,000 population.

TABLE 19-3 | ETIOLOGIC FACTORS ASSOCIATED WITH AN INCREASED RISK OF CIRRHOSIS AND HEPATOCELLULAR CARCINOMA

Category	Specific Etiology	Comment
Infectious (77% of cases of HCC worldwide attributed to viral hepatitis)	Hepatitis B virus	Underlying etiology in a significant majority of HCC cases worldwide, primarily in Asia, sub-Saharan Africa
	Hepatitis C virus	Principal underlying etiology in Japan, the United States, western Europe, Mediterranean basin countries; may account for 20-25% HCC cases worldwide
Metabolic disorders	Hemachromatosis α_1 antitrypsin deficiency	
	Wilson disease	
	Porphyria cutanea tarda	
	Glycogen storage disease	
	Citrullinemia	
	Familial cholestatic cirrhosis	
Other	Alcohol	Significant cause of liver cirrhosis; cofactor with HCV
	Aflatoxin B	Cofactor with HBV that increases risk of developing HCC
		Relative risk varies from two- to four-fold in nonendemic regions
	Androgenic steroids Oral contraceptives Autoimmune hepatitis	Some association reported, primarily case reports, and small series
	Nonalcoholic steatohepatitis (NASH)	Increasing evidence for association with HCC with or without cirrhosis; incidence of NAFLD is rising in the United States
	Tobacco	Weak association suggested that it is independent of HBV infection, alcohol

The principal risk factors that have been associated with cirrhosis and HCC are listed in Table 19-3.

Chronic Viral Hepatitis

Chronic hepatitis B or C viral infection is the most important risk factor for developing HCC. HCV alone causes about 40% of HCCs in the United States. Chronic HBV or HCV carriers usually take 10 to 20 years to develop hepatic cirrhosis and 30 to 40 years to develop HCC. HBV is a DNA virus that commonly integrates into the host hepatocyte genome and may play a direct procarcinogenic role. HCV is an RNA virus with no insertional mutagenesis. Although HBV and HCV contain no known viral oncogene to immortalize hepatocytes, hepatitis Bx antigen (HBxAg) may inactivate p53 protein and downregulate DNA repair ability (18,19). Some of the principal differences between HBV- and HCV-associated HCC are listed in Table 19-4.

Alcohol and Cirrhosis

Excessive alcohol consumption can lead to hepatic cirrhosis and thus is a risk factor for HCC. The autopsies of patients with alcoholic cirrhosis have reported up to 10% undiagnosed HCC. In the United States, alcoholic cirrhosis is associated with about 15% of HCC and cholangiocarcinoma (20,21). In HCV carriers, alcohol increases circulating HCV viral titer and HCC risk. Other types of cirrhosis and parenchymal liver diseases—such as primary biliary cirrhosis, hemochromatosis, Wilson disease, alpha-1 antitrypsin deficiency, and glycogen storage disease—significantly increase HCC risks when alcohol is a cofactor.

Aflatoxin

Food contaminated with aflatoxin, a mycotoxin found in grains, can induce HCC in animals. There is also a strong association between aflatoxin exposure and HBV

TABLE 19-4	COMPARISON BETWEEN HEPATITIS B VIRAL INFECTION AND HEPATITIS C INFECTION AND HEPATOCELLULAR CARCINOMA	
Factor	*HBV*	*HCV*
Mean age	52-56 (20-80)	62
Highest incidence	400 million carriers in Asia and Africa	170 million infected worldwide; accounts for 50% of HCC cases in Japan, the United States, and western Europe
Cirrhosis	25-50%	>75%
Morphology	Solitary lesions	Multifocal lesions, more severe inflammation
Rate of progression to HCC	10-30 years	>30 years
Percent likely to develop HCC	4% per year	1-7% per year

carrier status. Relative risks of HCC are three-fold for aflatoxin, nine-fold for chronic HBV infection, and 59-fold for concurrent aflatoxin and chronic HBV infection. The underlying mechanism is polymorphism variants of glutathione-S-transferase M1 and epoxide hydrolase genes and G-to-T point mutation of the *p53* gene (19).

Other Environmental Factors

The use of oral contraceptive pills (OCPs) significantly increases the incidence of benign hepatic adenomas. There is some evidence that OCPs also increase HCC risk. Multiple studies on tobacco smoking and HCC risk have yielded mixed conclusions. Occupational exposure to arsenic or vinyl chloride significantly increases the risk of liver angiosarcoma. Exposure to the x-ray contrast medium thorium dioxide from 1930 to 1955 is associated with an extremely high risk of hemangiosarcoma, cholangiocarcinoma, and HCC.

CLINICAL PRESENTATION

Most cases of HCC are identified incidentally or through screening programs of high-risk individuals. It is common for patients to be asymptomatic until their disease is very far advanced; less than 30% of patients are candidates for surgery or other liver-directed therapy at presentation. Many patients present with symptoms of advanced liver dysfunction from both cirrhosis and HCC. The most common initial symptom is right upper quadrant abdominal pain. Anorexia or early satiety with weight loss is the second most common symptom. HCC may present with various paraneoplastic symptoms through the secretion of numerous hormones. Late-stage symptoms include jaundice, tumor fever, bone pain due to metastatic lesions, and

complications from portal venous hypertension, such as esophagogastric varices, hypoalbuminemia, ascites, thrombocytopenia, and coagulopathy.

On physical examination, hepatomegaly is present in over 90% of patients. A hepatic arterial bruit or a friction rub, ascites, splenomegaly, and jaundice are found in up to 50% of patients. Muscle wasting, fever, and dilated abdominal veins are also quite common. The Budd-Chiari syndrome is caused by malignant invasion and occlusion of the hepatic veins. The HCC marker alpha-fetoprotein (AFP) is often elevated to above 400 ng/mL.

PATHOLOGY

Based on the growth pattern, HCC may be classified into four major gross anatomic types: spreading, multifocal, encapsulated, and combined patterns (22). Normal liver parenchyma is shown in Fig. 19-1. The spreading type of HCC grows in nodular, pseudolobular, or invasive patterns with poorly defined margins, occurs in the setting of hepatic cirrhosis, and accounts for nearly 50% of cases in the United States. The multifocal type has numerous tumors of similar size that make it difficult to determine whether the lesions are intrahepatic metastases or second primary tumors (Fig. 19-2*A* and *B*). The encapsulated type of tumor grows by expanding, compressing, and distorting the surrounding liver tissue. Satellite or metastatic lesions are seen in late stage disease. This type is most common in Asia and Africa but seen in only 13% of cases in the United States. The combined patterns of the above three are seen in up to 25% of cases. Figure 19-3 shows a histopathology specimen of HCC.

Approximately 60 to 70% of Caucasian and 80 to 90% of Asian HCC cases show elevated AFP, which is the most useful marker for HCC. AFP is originally produced by the fetal liver and yolk sac but falls to below

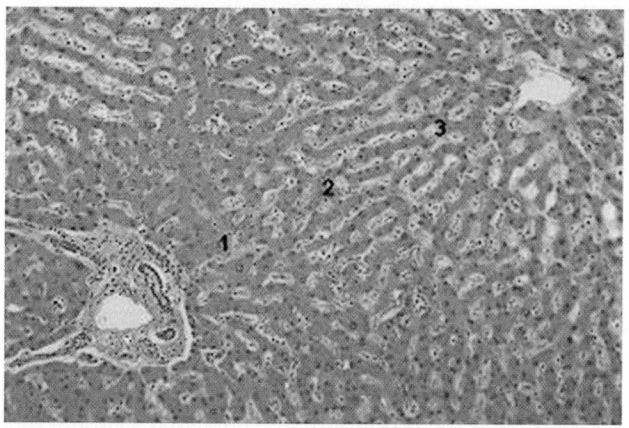

FIGURE 19-1. Photomicrograph of normal liver parenchyma. The liver is divided histologically into lobules. The center of the lobule is the central vein. At the periphery of the lobule are the portal triads. Functionally the liver can be divided into three zones, based on oxygen supply. Zone 1 encircles the portal tracts where the oxygenated blood from hepatic arteries enters. Zone 3 is located around central veins, where oxygenation is poor. Zone 2 is located in between.

10 ng/mL in adult serum. A transient elevation of AFP to 20 to 400 ng/mL may occur when there is hepatocyte regeneration, as in cirrhosis, active hepatitis, or partial hepatectomy. The HCC positive predictive value of an AFP level of 400 ng/mL is over 95%, and normal AFP levels may exist in patients with low tumor burden. The lectin-reactive isoenzyme of AFP (AFP-L3) has shown an increased sensitivity. Other markers such as gamma-glutamyl transferase (GGT) isoenzymes, alkaline phosphatase, isoferritins, and monoclonal antibodies are not more useful than AFP (23). Currently, serum AFP level and ultrasonography are the "gold standard" for HCC screening in high-risk populations (24).

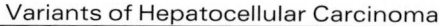 Variants of Hepatocellular Carcinoma

There are five HCC variants: HCC with biliary differentiation, clear cell HCC, cholangiocellular carcinoma (CCC), fibrolamellar hepatocellular carcinoma (FLHCC), and focal nodular hyperplasia (FNH). Cholangiocellular carcinoma is a combination of cholangiocarcinoma and hepatocellular carcinoma. It occurs in the non-cirrhotic liver and behaves like a cholangiocarcinoma; it has a male predominance. The outcome of patients with CCC is uniformly fatal.

FLHCC is predominantly seen in the right hepatic lobe, accounts for 2 to 4% of HCC, and occurs equally in men and women. FLHCC typically occurs in adolescents and young adults; the etiology is unknown. It is characterized by fibrosis arranged in lamellar fashion around HCC cells. FLHCC consists of well-circumscribed large solitary lesions without hepatic cirrhosis or elevated AFP (25). The imaging studies often show a heterogeneous mass with a central scar that is similar to FNH. In comparison to classic HCC, FLHCC demonstrates a higher resection rate and better survival, with a 3-year survival of almost 100%.

FNH occurs predominantly in young women. Liver function studies and the serum AFP level are normal. A technetium sulfur colloid radioisotope scan of the liver shows increased radioisotope uptake in FNH compared with hepatic adenomas or carcinomas. The prognosis is excellent.

Clear cell HCC has a distinguishing appearance and better prognosis. HCC with biliary differentiation has a much poorer prognosis because of its rapid growth, decreased vascularity, and resistance to embolic therapy.

Rare primary liver neoplasms include hepatoblastoma, sarcoma, angiosarcoma, rhabdomyosarcoma,

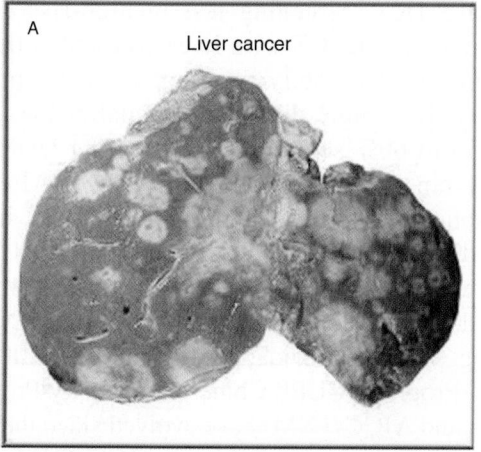

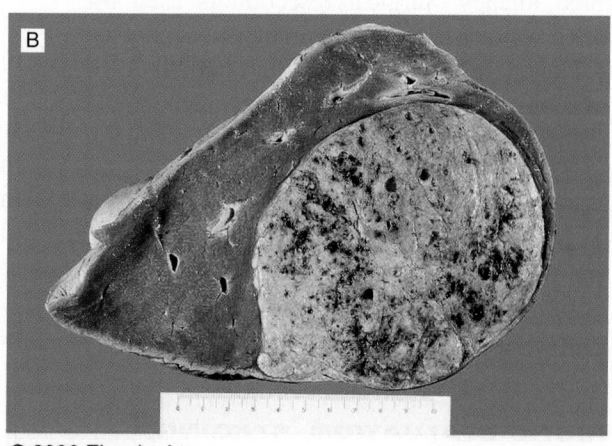

© 2006 Elsevier Inc.

FIGURE 19-2. **A.** Gross pathologic specimens of multifocal hepatocellular carcinoma. **B.** Gross appearance of liver cell carcinoma. The tumor is well circumscribed and shows numerous small hemorrhagic foci. *(Courtesy of Dr RA Cooke, Brisbane, Australia. From Cooke RA, Stewart B: Colour Atlas of Anatomical Pathology. Edinburgh, Churchill Livingstone, 2006.)*

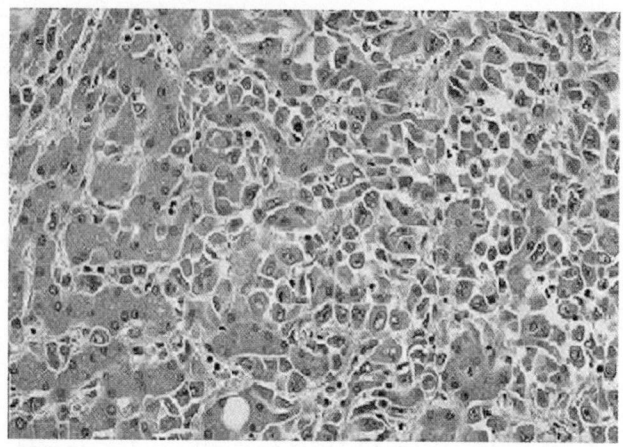

FIGURE 19-3. Photomicrograph with standard H&E stain of hepatocellular carcinoma cells in hepatic parenchyma.

and epitheloid hemangioendothelioma. Patients may present with fatigue, anorexia, weight loss, and abdominal pain. Hemorrhagic ascites is common and AFP level is normal. Angiography and contrast-enhanced CT of the liver are the best diagnostic tools. Open or percutaneous liver biopsy is needed for diagnosis. Surgical resection is still the principal means of therapy if tumors are diagnosed at relatively early stages. They are often resistant to chemotherapy and radiotherapy, and the overall prognosis is poor.

Benign Liver Tumors

Hemangiomas are the most common benign tumors of the liver. Their size ranges from a few millimeters to 25 cm. They appear as calcified solitary lesions in up to 7% of the general population. MRI is much better than CT in distinguishing HCC from hemangioma on heavily T2-weighted images. Surgical resection is used for symptomatic lesions or when malignancy cannot be excluded. Hepatic artery ligation is an alternative for large cavernous hemangiomas. Hepatic adenoma is another common benign solitary tumor seen in women who have used OCPs for more than 10 years. It is composed of sinusoids, central veins, and arteries without well-defined portal tracts or bile ducts. Hepatic angiography is the most valuable diagnostic tool. Small adenomas usually regress when OCPs are discontinued. Symptomatic lesions are treated with resection.

DIAGNOSTIC EVALUATION, STAGING, AND PROGNOSIS

In addition to performing a complete medical history and physical examination, the diagnostic workup for a

patient suspected of having HCC should include serum for complete blood count, electrolytes, liver function tests (LFTs), albumin, prothrombin time, hepatitis B and C serology, and tumor markers (AFP, CA19-9, CA125). The medical history should include a thorough review of potential HCC risk factors: transfusions, tattoos, intravenous drug abuse, high-risk sexual practices, familial syndromes, OCP and/or hormone replacement use, androgenic steroid use, and chemical exposures. Several radiographic imaging modalities are useful in evaluating a patient with HCC. Ultrasound often serves as the initial screening modality, followed by CT scan or MRI. Randomized studies have shown that hepatic ultrasonography has a 78% sensitivity and 93% specificity to detect HCC in high-risk populations, especially for patients with normal AFP levels (24,26). Color-flow Doppler can assist preoperative assessment and planning.

Abdominal CT has relatively higher sensitivity and specificity than ultrasonography. With special arterial- and venous-phase scans, CT also makes it possible to evaluate the blood supply of the normal liver parenchyma (portal vein) and neoplastic lesions (hepatic artery). MRI is useful in distinguishing benign lesions from malignant tumors by the combination of T2-weighted phase-contrast and spin-echo sequences. Also, MRI can demonstrate fatty degeneration of tumor and vascular invasion (27).

Hepatic radionuclide imaging has low spatial resolution and is only about 70% sensitive in demonstrating neoplasms. Using glucose metabolic difference between neoplastic and normal cells, positron-emission tomography (PET) is used to differentiate benign lesions from malignant tumors, detect extrahepatic metastasis, and evaluate response to therapy.

In summary, ultrasonography is the most cost-effective HCC screening test in high-risk populations. Abdominal CT with liver protocol is the most helpful in accurately staging patients prior to surgery. No single diagnostic modality has greater than 50 to 60% sensitivity in detecting lesions less than 1 cm in size. The combination of AFP level, ultrasonography, and CT provides the best hope of early diagnosis.

A variety of staging and prognostic systems have been developed to evaluate patients with HCC. Four staging systems (Okuda; CLIP, Cancer of the Liver Italian Program; CUPI, Chinese University Prognostic Index; and AJCC-TNM) have evolved since the 1980s. Currently, we use a combined AJCC-TNM staging system at MD Anderson Cancer Center (MDACC) (Table 19-5) (25). The Child-Pugh Classification

TABLE 19-5	COMBINED AJCC-TNM STAGING SYSTEM FOR HEPATOCELLULAR CARCINOMA	
Stage Group	*TNM*	*Scheme*
Stage I	T1,N0,M0	Single tumor <2 cm without vascular invasion
Stage II	T2,N0,M0	Single tumor <2 cm with vascular invasion or multiple tumors <2 cm in one lobe or single tumor 2 cm without vascular invasion
Stage IIIA	T3,N0,M0	Multiple tumors in one lobe ± vascular invasion or any tumor >5 cm or single tumor >2 cm with vascular invasion
Stage IIIB	T1-3,N1,M0	Positive regional lymph node
Stage IVA	T4,N0-1,M0	Multiple tumor in 2+ lobes or tumors involving major portal or hepatic vein
Stage IVB	T1-4,N0-1,M1	Remote metastasis
Fibrosis score		0-4, none to moderate; 5-6, severe fibrosis/cirrhosis

System (Figure 19-4, Appendix C) provides an estimate of a patient's functional liver reserve and is used principally to assist in evaluating a patient's suitability for hepatic resection.

Based on a review of the database developed at MDACC, patients with HCC had an overall 3-year survival rate of 10% and a median survival time of 7.8 months. Favorable prognostic factors are female gender, absence of cirrhosis, and resection of the tumor; these factors correlated with longer survival, especially if the tumors were located in the left hepatic lobe. For patients with unresectable HCC, systemic chemotherapy or supportive care yielded a 44% 1-year survival rate, and no patient survived for 3 years. The size and number of nodules were not determinants of survival. Poor prognostic factors included advanced stage, unresectability associated with cirrhosis, and vascular invasion.

TREATMENT

The current treatment options for HCC are summarized in Table 19-6. At present, liver transplantation is considered the only potentially "curative" treatment. The current 1- and 5-year survival rates for HCC patients undergoing orthotopic liver transplantation are 77.0 and 61.1%, respectively. The 5-year survival rate has steadily improved, from 25.3% in 1987 to 61.1% in the most recent period studied (1996-2001) (28). The authors attribute this improvement to the incorporation of the "Milan" criteria as guidelines for patient selection at most US liver transplantation centers. These criteria, as published by Mazzaferro et al., suggest that long-term survival after liver transplantation is highest in HCC patients with either a single lesion ≤5 cm or three lesions ≤3 cm each and no evidence of gross vascular invasion (29). A large number of liver transplant

candidates remain on the waiting list until they die of tumor progression or cirrhosis-related complications. Partial hepatectomy is the current standard treatment for localized T1-3, N0, M0 HCC. Resectability is determined by the extent of liver cirrhosis, the future liver remnant (FLR), and an adequate surgical margin. An FLR of 35 to 40% is considered the minimal cutoff for a safe liver remnant. Patients of Child-Pugh class B and C or with significant signs of portal hypertension are not surgical candidates. Minor or major resection is based on the following criteria: (1) minor resection: Child A, normal LFTs (bilirubin ≤1.0 mg/dL), absence of ascites, and platelet count >100,000/mm; (2) major resection: minor criteria as above, absence of portal hypertension, and portal vein embolization (PVE) for a small future remnant (30). The perioperative mortality has decreased from 20% in the 1980s to less than 5% at present (31). The median disease-free survival after partial hepatectomy is about 2 years. Tumor size <5.0 cm (0.6 RR) was associated with improved survival, while the presence of vascular invasion, AFP >2000 mg/mL, and advanced Child-Pugh classification was associated with worse outcome. Patients with cirrhosis generally are not considered good candidates for surgical resection due to the high morbidity and mortality associated with cirrhosis and its complications. For those who do undergo resection, recurrence rates are among the highest of any solid tumor and approach 75 to 100% at 5 years. Estimated 5-year survival rates are in the range of 26 to 50%, and disease-free survival is 13 to 29% (32).

Locoregional Therapy for Hepatocellular Carcinoma

Hepatocellular carcinoma derives its blood supply almost exclusively from the hepatic artery. This important

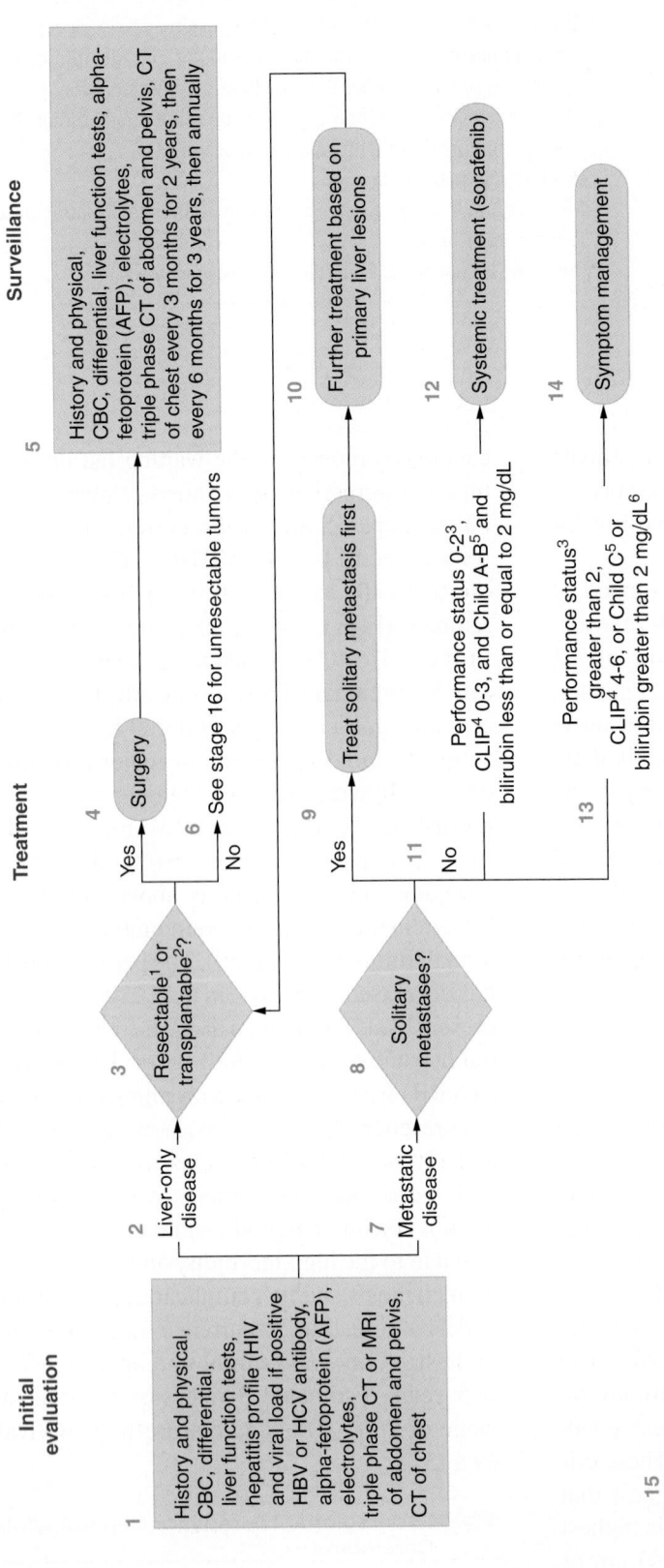

Initial evaluation

1

History and physical,
CBC, differential,
liver function tests,
hepatitis profile (HIV
and viral load if positive
HBV or HCV antibody,
alpha-fetoprotein (AFP),
electrolytes,
triple phase CT or MRI
of abdomen and pelvis,
CT of chest

2 Liver-only disease

3 Resectable[1] or transplantable[2]?

7 Metastatic disease

8 Solitary metastases?

Treatment

4 Yes → Surgery

6 No → See stage 16 for unresectable tumors

9 Yes → Treat solitary metastasis first

11 No

Performance status 0-2[3],
CLIP[4] 0-3, and Child A-B[5], and
bilirubin less than or equal to 2 mg/dL

13 Performance status[3]
greater than 2,
CLIP[4] 4-6, or Child C[5] or
bilirubin greater than 2 mg/dL[6]

Surveillance

5

History and physical,
CBC, differential, liver function tests, alpha-
fetoprotein (AFP), electrolytes,
triple phase CT of abdomen and pelvis, CT
of chest every 3 months for 2 years, then
every 6 months for 3 years, then annually

10 Further treatment based on primary liver lesions

12 Systemic treatment (sorafenib)

14 Symptom management

15

[1]Minor or major resection based on:
• Minor resection: Child A, normal liver function tests (bilirubin less than or equal 1.0 mg%), absence of ascites, and plate count greater than 100,000/mm^3
• Major resection: Idem minor plus absence of portal hypertension, portal vein embolization (PVE) for a small future remnant
[2]Milan criteria; criteria for eligibility for liver transplantation for patients with hepatocellular carcinoma and cirrhosis: the presence of a tumor 5 cm or less in diameter in patients with single hepatocellular carcinomas, or no more than three tumor: nodules, each 3 cm or less in diameter, in patients with multiple tumors, and without macrovascular invasion per imaging studies.
[3]See Appendix A for ECOG performance status
[4]CLIP: refer to Appendix A for determination of CLIP score
[5]CHILD: refer to Appendix B for CHILD scores
[6]Treatment may be considered in select cases with bilirubin 2-3 mg/dL.

Note: Consider clinical trials as treatment options for eligible patients.

FIGURE 19-4. MD Anderson management approach for a patient with gallbladder cancer or cholangiocarcinoma. (*Adapted with permission from The University of Texas MD anderson Cancer Center.*)

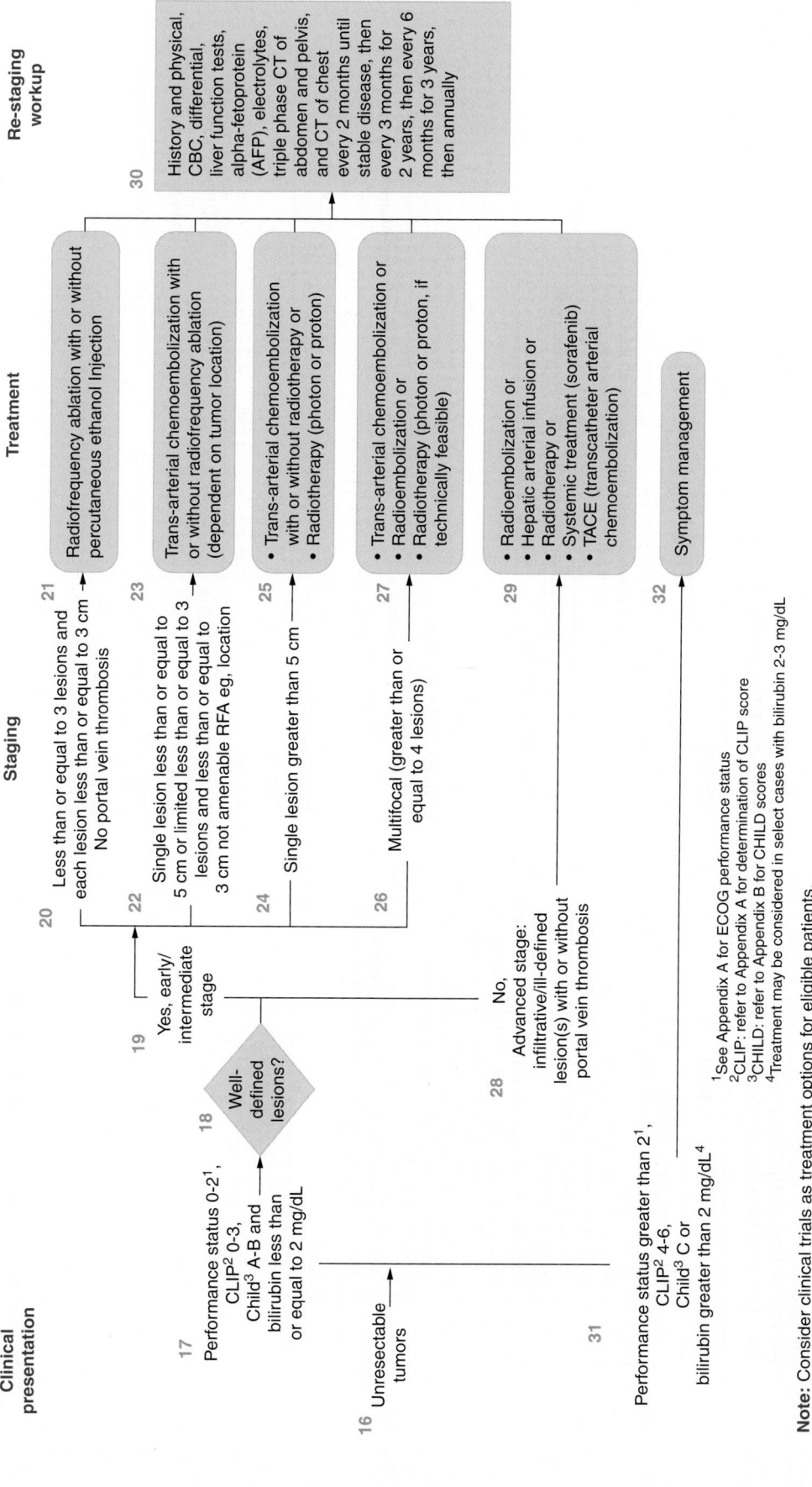

Clinical presentation

16 Unresectable tumors

17 Performance status 0-2[1], CLIP[2] 0-3, Child[3] A-B and bilirubin less than or equal to 2 mg/dL

31 Performance status greater than 2[1], CLIP[2] 4-6, Child[3] C or bilirubin greater than 2 mg/dL [4]

Staging

18 Well-defined lesions?

19 Yes, early/intermediate stage

28 No, Advanced stage: infiltrative/ill-defined lesion(s) with or without portal vein thrombosis

20 Less than or equal to 3 lesions and each lesion less than or equal to 3 cm No portal vein thrombosis

22 Single lesion less than or equal to 5 cm or limited less than or equal to 3 lesions and less than or equal to 3 cm not amenable RFA eg, location

24 Single lesion greater than 5 cm

26 Multifocal (greater than or equal to 4 lesions)

Treatment

21 Radiofrequency ablation with or without percutaneous ethanol Injection

23 Trans-arterial chemoembolization with or without radiofrequency ablation (dependent on tumor location)

25
• Trans-arterial chemoembolization with or without radiotherapy or
• Radiotherapy (photon or proton)

27
• Trans-arterial chemoembolization or
• Radioembolization or
• Radiotherapy (photon or proton, if technically feasible)

29
• Radioembolization or
• Hepatic arterial infusion or
• Radiotherapy or
• Systemic treatment (sorafenib) or
• TACE (transcatheter arterial chemoembolization)

32 Symptom management

Re-staging workup

30 History and physical, CBC, differential, liver function tests, alpha-fetoprotein (AFP), electrolytes, triple phase CT of abdomen and pelvis, and CT of chest every 2 months until stable disease, then every 3 months for 2 years, then every 6 months for 3 years, then annually

[1]See Appendix A for ECOG performance status
[2]CLIP: refer to Appendix A for determination of CLIP score
[3]CHILD: refer to Appendix B for CHILD scores
[4]Treatment may be considered in select cases with bilirubin 2-3 mg/dL

Note: Consider clinical trials as treatment options for eligible patients.

FIGURE 19-4. (*Continued*)

APPENDIX A
EASTERN COOPERATIVE ONCOLOGY GROUP (ECOG) PERFORMANCE STATUS CRITERIA

Grade	Scale
0	Fully active, able to carry on all predisease performance without restriction (Karnofsky 90-100)
1	Restricted in physically strenuous activity but ambulatory and able to carry out work of a light or sedentary nature, ie light housework, office work (Karnofsky 70-80)
2	Ambulatory and capable of all self-care but unable to carry out any work activities. Up and about more than 50% of waking hours (Karnofsky 50-60)
3	Capable of only limited self-care, confined to bed or chair more than 50% of waking hours (Karnofsky 30-40)
4	Completely disabled. Cannot carry out any self-care. Totally confined to bed or chair (Karnofsky 10-20)
5	Dead

APPENDIX B
CLIP SCORING SYSTEM

Variables	0	1	2
Child-Pugh Stage	A	B	C
Tumor morphology	Uninodular and extension less than or equal to 50%	Multinodular and extension less than or equal to 50%	Greater than 50%
AFP	Less than 400 ng/dL	Less than 400 ng/dL	
Portal vein thrombosis	No	Yes	

APPENDIX C
CHILD-PUGH SCALE

Chemical and Biochemical Parameters	Scores (Points) for Increasing Abnormality		
	1	2	3
Encephalopathy	None	1-2	3-4
Ascites	None	Slight	Moderate
Albumin	Greater than 3.5 g/dL	2.8-3.5 g/dL	Less than 2.8 g/dL
Prothrombin time prolonged	1-4 s	4-6 s	Greater than 6 s
Bilirubin	1-2 mg/dL	2-3 mg/dL	Greater than 3 md/dL
For primary biliary cirrhosis	1-4 mg/dL	4-10 mg/dL	Greater than 10 mg/dL

Class A = 5 to 6 points
Class B = 7 to 9 points
Class C = 10 to 15 points

Note: Consider clinical trials as treatment options for eligible patients.

FIGURE 19-4. *(Continued)*

TABLE
19-6 **TREATMENT OPTIONS FOR MANAGEMENT OF HEPATOCELLULAR
CARCINOMA**

Treatment Option	*Comments*
Liver transplantation	Historically low survival rates (20-36%).
	Recent improvement (61.1%, 1996-2001), likely related to adoption of "Milan" criteria at US transplant centers.
	Currently HCC represents 20+ % of liver transplants performed annually in the United States
Surgical resection	Historic 5-year survival rates 30-40%.
	Recent series indicate 5-year PFS as high as 48%. A majority of patients develop recurrence or second primary tumors.
	Resection in cirrhotic patients carries high morbidity and mortality.
Transarterial embolization/ chemoembolization (TACE)	Multiple trials show objective tumor responses and "slowed" tumor progression but questionable survival benefit compared to supportive care. Greatest benefit seen in patients with preserved liver function, absence of vascular invasion, and smallest tumors.
	Modest survival benefit demonstrated for repeated TACE (82% 1-year survival) versus supportive care (63%) in patients with preserved liver function, PS 0, small tumor burden.
	Improvement in 1-year survival from 32% in control (supportive care) to 57% for TACE shown in randomized study of 279 primarily HBV+ patients with tumors <7 cm.
Percutaneous treatments (ethanol injection, thermal ablation, cryoablation, hypertonic saline injection)	PEI well tolerated, high RR in small (<3 cm) solitary tumors. No randomized trial comparing resection to percutaneous treatments. Recurrence rates similar to postresection.
Hormonal therapy	Antiestrogen therapy with tamoxifen studied in several trials; mixed results across studies, but generally considered ineffective.
	Octreotide (somatostatin analog) showed 13-month MS versus 4-month MS in untreated patients in a small randomized study.
Chemotherapy	*Adjuvant:* No randomized trials showing benefit of neoadjuvant or adjuvant systemic therapy in HCC. Single trial showed decrease in new tumors in patients receiving oral synthetic retinoid for 12 months after resection/ablation. Results not reproduced.
	Palliative: Regimens including as single agents or combinations of doxorubicin, cisplatin, 5-fluorouracil, interferon, epirubicin, and paclitaxel have not shown any survival benefit; RR range from 0 to 25%. A few isolated major responses allowing patients to undergo partial hepatectomy. No published results from any randomized trial of systemic chemotherapy.

anatomic feature offers unique advantages for catheter-based therapies, since arterial embolization interrupts blood flow to the tumor while preserving the portal vein and normal liver parenchyma. The combination of tissue ischemia with highly concentrated chemotherapy delivered into the hepatic artery enhances tumor necrosis. Transarterial chemoembolization (TACE) was first described by Yamada and incorporates these concepts (33). It has since become one of the most commonly utilized procedures in the interventional radiology practice. Landmark prospective randomized clinical trials published in 2002 validated the use of chemoembolization for unresectable advanced hepatocellular carcinoma. In the multicenter study by Llovet et al. including 112 patients, when compared to bland embolization or best supportive therapy, patients who underwent TACE with a combination of doxorubicin and iodized oil followed by gelatin sponge demonstrated a clear

survival advantage leading to premature stoppage of the trial (34). Survival in the chemoembolization group at 1 and 2 years was 82% and 63%, respectively. Survival in the bland embolization group was 75% and 50%, respectively; in the best supportive care group, survival was 63% and 27%, respectively, and reached statistical significance. Lo et al. conducted a single center study comparing 80 patients with unresectable hepatocellular carcinoma randomized to TACE with cisplatin and iodized oil followed by gelatin sponge or best supportive care (35). Survival in the chemoembolization group at 1 and 2 years was 57% and 31%, respectively. Survival for the patients randomized to the supportive care group was 32% and 11%, respectively, also reaching statistical significance. The difference in survival rates between the Llovet and Lo studies can be attributed to the inclusion of a larger proportion of patients with more advanced stages of underlying chronic liver disease in the latter study.

Chemoembolization is contraindicated in patients with overt signs of portal hypertension and advanced underlying liver disease.

An important limitation of conventional chemoembolization using iodized oil lies in the uncontrolled washout of the cytotoxic drugs into the systemic circulation. Recently, a drug-eluting bead that allows controlled and sustained release of chemotherapic agents into the surrounding tumor was made available. This device enables delivery of higher concentration of drugs with low systemic toxicity. Initial studies demonstrated that chemoembolization using drug-eluting beads is safe with potentially increased effectiveness for patients with more advanced disease (36-38). At MD Anderson, TACE is routinely utilized for hepatocellular carcinoma patients with more than three lesions measuring up to 3 cm each or a single lesion greater than 5 cm. In patients with portal vein thrombosis, infiltrative disease, or more than four lesions, radioembolization with yttrium-90 microspheres is well tolerated and has been shown to improve outcomes. A recent study assessing the use of radioembolization in hepatocellular carcinoma showed response rates of 42% based on WHO criteria (39).

Radiofrequency ablation causes tissue necrosis by controlled deposition of thermal energy. This technique is highly effective in the treatment of small and early hepatocellular carcinoma, with outcomes similar to surgical resection (40). Radiofrequency ablation is limited by lesion proximity to adjacent structures such as colon, gallbladder, and diaphragm. In addition, vascular structures adjacent to the target lesion steal heat from the area and decrease effectiveness of the ablation. The combination of chemoembolization followed by radiofrequency ablation may improve cell death, since occlusion of blood flow leads to larger ablation zones (41,42).

Systemic Chemotherapy and Hormonal Therapy

A majority (>80%) of patients diagnosed with HCC have advanced disease at presentation and—based on the number, size, and location of lesions, as well as the severity of the underlying cirrhosis—are not candidates for transplantation, surgical resection, or liver-directed therapies. At present, systemic chemotherapy is ineffective in HCC, as evidenced by low response rates and no demonstrated survival benefit (see Table 19-6). Hepatocellular carcinomas are inherently chemotherapy-resistant (43) and known to express the multidrug-resistance gene MDR-1 (44,45). Few well-controlled, randomized chemotherapy trials have been published in HCC. The ability to conduct controlled clinical trials of systemic regimens in HCC patients has been hampered by many factors, including

TABLE 19-7	MEDICAL COMORBIDITIES COMPLICATING HCC
Problem	*Intervention*
Esophageal, gastric varices	Beta blockade for portal HTN for primary prophylaxis of GI bleeding
	Endoscopic variceal banding for clinically significant GI bleeding
Thrombocytopenia	Splenic artery embolization
Hypoalbuminemia	Nutrition, caution with protein-bound medications
Ascites	K+-sparing diuretics, fluid restriction
Chronic active hepatitis	HCV: IFN/ribavirin have antiviral, antifibrotic effects HBV: lamivudine, ±IFN
Coagulopathy	PT most sensitive indicator of liver dysfunction

HBV, hepatitis B virus; HCV, hepatitis C virus; HTN, hypertension; IFN, interferon; K, potassium; PT, protime.

the multiple comorbidities of cirrhosis (Table 19-7), the advanced nature of HCC at presentation, rapid disease progression in many instances, and the distribution of patients primarily in developing nations, where multidisciplinary treatment of HCC may not be available.

Approximately 15 to 40% of HCCs are estrogen receptor–positive. Hormonal therapy with tamoxifen or octreotide analogs has demonstrated some survival benefit (46); however, the results of other studies are conflicting.

Clinical Trials of Antiangiogenesis Agents

Several systemic targeted agents have been recently tested in clinical trials, for patients with advanced HCC, including agents targeting the VEGF pathway, either alone (47-59) or in combination with other systemic therapies (60-67). The cancer cell has been the only target of anticancer systemic therapy for more than 50 years. However, the cancer cell is genetically unstable, leading to accumulation of mutations. On the other hand, antiangiogenic therapy agents target endothelial cells that are genetically stable. The mechanism of action of thalidomide was thought to be partly based on its antiangiogenic effects. Nevertheless, several clinical trials of thalidomide showed rare responses ranging from 0 to 6.3% (57,58). Sunitinib is an oral multikinase inhibitor that exerts its antiangiogenic effect by targeting VEGFR and platelet-derived growth factor receptor (PDGFR) tyrosine kinases. Sorafenib, an oral multikinase inhibitor, exerts its antitumor effect by targeting Raf/MEK/ERK signaling at the level of Raf kinase, and possesses an antiangiogenic effect by targeting VEGFR-2/-3. Most recently, two phase III trials of sorafenib were reported (47,59). The pivotal randomized, placebo-controlled phase III trial of sorafenib in patients with advanced HCC (SHARP trial) reported modest activity with a 2.8-month improvement in median overall survival ($p = .0006$), along with an increased time to progression and disease control rate and a response rate of 2.3% as defined by RECIST criteria (47). This led to FDA approval of sorafenib for advanced HCC. Bevacizumab is a recombinant, humanized monoclonal antibody that exerts its antitumor activity by targeting VEGF and may augment chemotherapy administration by making tumor vasculature less permeable which decreases the elevated tumor interstitial pressure. Erlotinib is an oral tyrosine kinase inhibitor. It blocks phosphorylation at the intracellular domain level of the epithelial growth factor receptor (EGFR). Most recently, we reported a phase II single-arm, open-label trial of bevacizumab and erlotinib that showed improved response rate, median overall survival, and progression- free survival (60).

Collectively, application of antiangiogenesis to patients with advanced HCC has eventually led to improved survival despite surprisingly low response rates. Notably, there is a poor correlation between survival benefit and conventional methods of response assessment, namely RECIST. This poses questions regarding how best to evaluate response to antiangiogenic agents and quantify efficacy of anti-angiogenic agents. Despite tumors increasing in size sometimes, the observation of tumor necrosis in many studies is intriguing. Therefore, in 2000, a panel of experts recommended that the response criteria be amended to take into account tumor necrosis induced by targeted agent therapy (68). Although its utility in assessing efficacy of anticancer agents in HCC needs to be established, tumor necrosis is a potentially significant clinical end point that warrants further investigation in future studies.

Radiation

Advances in our understanding of partial liver tolerance of radiation therapy (RT), ability to visualize target tumors during respiration, radiation planning and delivery techniques have permitted us to escalate the dose of radiation to focal HCCs without dose-limiting toxicity. This improved ability to deliver tumoricidal doses of RT safely has led to a resurgence of interest in treatment of HCC using RT. Promising clinical data from multiple studies suggest that HCCs are indeed radiosensitive. Sustained local control rates ranging from 71 to 100% have been reported following 30 to 90 Gy delivered over 1 to 8 weeks (69,70). Investigators from Michigan have used conformal RT (1.5 Gy twice daily over 6-8 weeks)

with concurrent hepatic arterial fluorodeoxyuridine to treat HCCs safely to doses as high as 90 Gy and achieved a median survival duration of 15.2 months (71). Analysis of this data suggested that doses greater than 75 Gy resulted in more durable in-field local control than lower doses. A prospective French phase II trial administered 66 Gy in 33 fractions to HCCs ineligible for curative therapies and noted 92% tumor responses and 78% 1-year local control rates (72). Using higher doses and fewer fractions (hypofractionated RT), Canadian researchers have noted excellent local control rates ranging from 70 to 90% when the radiation beam can be directed from multiple planes (stereotactic RT) converging on the tumor, the majority of the liver can be spared from irradiation and treatment is image-guided (70,73,74). In contrast to photon irradiation where the dose delivered to the tumor is limited by the entrance and exit doses that can potentially harm normal tissues, accelerated proton beams deposit dose within the tumor without exiting through normal tissues beyond the tumor. Japanese investigators have reported mature results of the treatment of 162 patients with 192 unresectable HCCs with 72 Gy in 16 fractions of proton beam therapy (75). The 5-year local control rate of 87% and overall survival rate of 23.5% in the absence of significant toxicity are clinically noteworthy. Furthermore, an impressive 5-year survival rate of 53.5% was achieved in a subset of 50 patients with solitary tumors and Child-Pugh Class A cirrhosis. Across all partial liver radiation paradigms, the most common site of first recurrence is intrahepatic but outside the high-dose irradiated volume and toxicities are more common in Child-Pugh Class B patients. Given the excellent local control rate noted above with RT alone, RT has been combined with TACE to overcome treatment resistance. Korean researchers initially noted >60% response rates and a significant drop in tumor markers levels using this combination treatment strategy (76,77). TACE followed by RT was reported to improve overall survival over TACE alone in a retrospective analysis of this experience. Similar results have been reported by other groups as well (78-80). For the treatment of unfavorable tumors, multiple groups have reported favorable outcomes in patients with portal venous tumor thrombus (PVTT) treated with RT (81-90). Response rates range from 37.5 to 100% and median survival durations range from 3.8 to 10.7 months. Taken together, these advances have permitted the escalation of radiation dose to unresectable HCCs without causing undue toxicity. Strategies that combine RT with other therapies merit continued evaluation to maximize the relative benefits of each approach.

MDACC APPROACH TO HEPATOCELLULAR CARCINOMA

HCC and other primary liver tumors require multidisciplinary input, and patients benefit from clinical care that integrates the expertise of surgical oncology, liver transplantation, diagnostic and interventional radiology, gastroenterology and hepatology, radiation oncology, and medical oncology. New cases of HCC are reviewed at a weekly Multidisciplinary Liver Tumor Conference to develop a consensus approach to each patient's case. Careful attention is paid to precise tumor staging, histopathologic diagnosis, and each patient's performance status (PS).

HCC patients who meet current UNOS criteria are offered liver transplantation or resection if they are highly likely to benefit. Liver-directed therapies, principally RFA and TACE, are commonly employed in patients who are not candidates for surgical intervention. Good-PS patients with advanced HCC are encouraged to participate in a clinical trial of systemic therapy. Figure 19-4 depicts the general approach followed by the multidisciplinary hepatobiliary team in managing HCC patients evaluated at MDACC.

■ CARCINOMAS OF THE GALLBLADDER AND BILIARY TRACT

EPIDEMIOLOGY

There are about 8000 newly diagnosed cases of cancer of the gallbladder and bile ducts annually in the United States; this rate has remained stable or increased slightly over the past three decades (91). These cancers account for 15-20% of the primary hepatobiliary malignancies. They are most frequently diagnosed in patients in their sixties and seventies and are more common in females, with an overall female-to-male ratio of 2.5 to 1 and 15 to 1 for those under the age of 40. The incidence in American Indians is six times higher than in the remainder of the population (92). Autopsy and operative data suggested a prevalence rate of 0.5 to 2%. Cholangiocarcinomas are classified as intrahepatic, hilar, or distal extrahepatic. Intrahepatic cholangiocarcinoma is the second most common primary hepatic malignancy and is increasing in incidence in the United States; this is at least partly explained by the redesignation of liver metastasis of unknown primary to intrahepatic cholangiocarcinoma. It arises from the epithelium of the intrahepatic bile duct and consists of well-differentiated adenocarcinoma cells.

TABLE 19-8	RISK FACTORS FOR CARCINOMA OF THE GALLBLADDER
Gallbladder stones	
Chronic diarrhea	
Multiparas ≥3	
Obesity	
Chronic cholecystitis, chronic mucosal damage	
Polypoidal lesions of the gallbladder	
Genetic predisposition	
Exposure to carcinogens	

ETIOLOGY AND RISK FACTORS

Chronic cholelithiasis and cholecystitis are closely associated with gallbladder carcinoma (93). The relative risk is 2.4-fold for patients with stones of 2.0 to 2.9 cm and 10-fold for stones >3.0 cm in diameter. Chronic cholecystitis induces adenomatous polyps, which can undergo malignant transformation. Environmental carcinogens include methylcholanthrene and nitrosamines. Other risk factors are listed in Tables 19-8 and 19-9 (94,95).

CLINICAL PRESENTATION

Primary gallbladder cancer is incidentally found in 0.4 to 2% of laparoscopic cholecystectomy procedures. The most common symptoms and signs of gallbladder carcinoma are nonspecific right upper quadrant abdominal pain and tenderness, which are also frequently seen in cholelithiasis or cholecystitis. The clinical features of cholangiocarcinoma vary from hepatomegaly and upper abdominal pain with intrahepatic tumors to the rapid onset of painless, deep jaundice with hilar tumors.

Intrahepatic tumors often present at a more advanced stage due to the nonspecific nature of symptoms. Serum tumor markers, specifically CA19-9 and CA125, are

TABLE 19-9	RISK FACTORS FOR BILIARY TRACT CANCERS
Major risk factor: chronic inflammatory state	
Parasitic infections (*Clonorchis sinensis, Opisthorchis viverrini*)	
Autoimmune disease (primary biliary cirrhosis, sclerosing cholangitis, inflammatory bowel disease)	
Anatomic abnormalities (biliary atresia, congenital bile duct abnormalities)	
Cystic liver disease	
Biliary calculi (cholecystolithiasis, hepatolithiasis)	
Choledochal cysts	
Some association with cirrhosis, less so than HCC	
Carcinogens: thorotrast, oxymethalone, nitrosamines	

TABLE 19-10	RELATIVE FREQUENCIES OF GALLBLADDER MALIGNANCIES
Tumor Type	*Percent of Total*
Adenocarcinoma	75.8
Papillary	5.8
Mucinous	4.6
Adenosquamous	3.6
Oat cell	0.5
Nonspecific	7.6

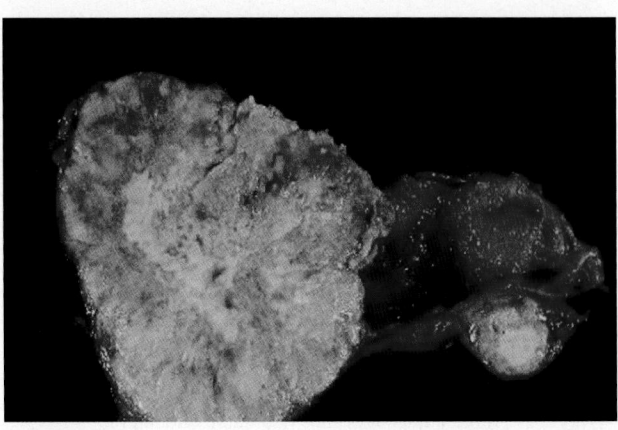

FIGURE 19-6. A specimen of gallbladder cancer filling the entire gallbladder lumen.

frequently elevated but are not pathognomonic for biliary tract cancer.

PATHOLOGY

Early-stage cancers of the gallbladder and bile duct may present as subtle mucosal abnormalities, such as plaques or ulcerations. A majority of gallbladder carcinomas are papillary or tubular adenocarcinomas with mucin-producing or signet-ring cells (Table 19-10, Fig. 19-5). Sessile or pedunculated tumors are rare. The remaining 10% are adenosquamous carcinomas, anaplastic carcinomas, and rarely carcinoid tumors or embryonal rhabdomyosarcomas (72). Only 10% of patients with gallbladder cancer have a tumor confined to the gallbladder wall (T1) at the time of diagnosis (Fig. 19-6). Most patients are found to have metastasis to the liver and contiguous organs, regional lymph nodes and nerves, or distant organs.

Early lymph node metastasis is unfortunately common in gallbladder adenocarcinoma. The local and regional draining lymph nodes are cystic, choledochal,

or pancreaticoduodenal nodes. Distant lymph nodes are the paraaortic or inferior vena cava nodes near the left renal vein (74).

The current hypothesis suggests that cancers of the gallbladder and bile duct originate from premalignant epithelial dysplasia, which gradually progresses to atypical hyperplasia and carcinoma in situ (96). Epidermal growth factor and a mutated *ras* oncogene are overexpressed during the transition from premalignant lesions to cancers (97). Mutation and abnormal expression of tumor suppressor gene *p53*, cell-cycle regulator cyclin E, and apoptosis regulator Bcl-2 are all involved in the development of invasive gallbladder cancer (98,99).

STAGING AND PROGNOSIS

Abdominal CT is the primary imaging study for biliary cancers and bile duct obstruction in symptomatic patients. With contrast enhancement, CT may detect 90 to 95% of intraluminal masses or gallbladder wall thickening of >0.5 mm (100). Gallbladder carcinomas are currently staged by the tumor-node-metastasis (TNM) staging schema developed by the American Joint Committee on Cancer (AJCC) (Table 19-11); however, there are several staging systems in clinical use (Table 19-12).

TREATMENT

Curative Surgery

Most patients are not surgical candidates due to extensive locoregional and distant metastases. The curative resection rates of gallbladder carcinoma are about 10 to 30%. The extent of resection remains a controversial issue. Simple cholecystectomy is an adequate treatment

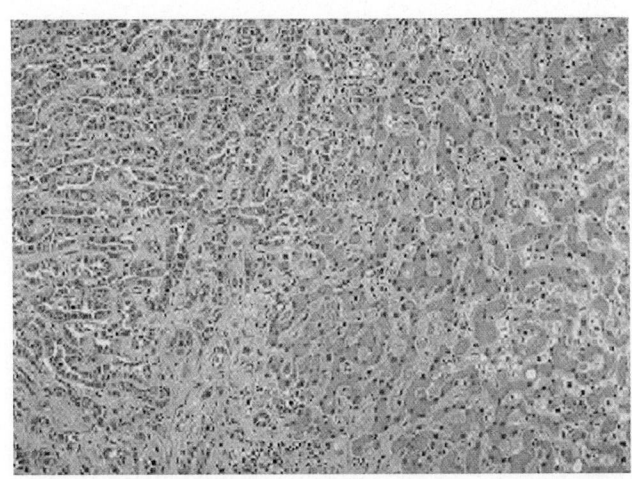

FIGURE 19-5. Photomicrograph with standard H&E stain of a cholangiocarcinoma specimen composed of cuboidal, mucin-producing adenocarcinomas with a dense fibrous stroma.

TABLE
19-11 **TNM STAGING SYSTEM FOR
GALLBLADDER CARCINOMA**

TNM DEFINITIONS

Tx	Primary tumor cannot be assessed.
Nx	Regional lymph nodes cannot be assessed.
Mx	Presence of distant metastasis cannot be assessed.
T1	Tumor invades mucosa (T1a) or muscle layer (T1b).
T2	Tumor invades perimuscular connective tissue, no extension beyond serosa or into liver.
T3	Tumor invades beyond serosa or into one adjacent organ or both (extension <2 cm into liver).
T4	Tumor extends >2 cm into liver and/or into two or more adjacent organs (stomach, duodenum, colon, pancreas, omentum, extrahepatic bile ducts).
N0	No regional lymph node metastasis.
N1	Regional lymph node metastasis.
N1a	Metastasis in cystic duct, pericholedochal, and/or gastrohepatic lymph nodes.
N1b	Metastasis in peripancreatic, periduodenal periportal, celiac, and/or superior mesenteric artery lymph nodes.

STAGING CLASSIFICATION

I	Cancer confined to subserosal layers (T1,N0,M0 and T2,N0,M0)
II	Cancer confined to the mucosa and muscularis (T1,N1,M0)
III	Cancer extends through the serosa (T2,N1,M0,T3, any N,M0)
IV	T4, any N,M0, any T, any N,M1

for T1a,N0,M0 tumors confined to the mucosa. About 15% of T1b patients have regional lymph node metastases. Extended cholecystectomy is recommended for patients with T1b,N0,M0, or stage II gallbladder carcinomas. The procedure includes cholecystectomy, wedge resection of the gallbladder fossa (including a 3- to 5-cm margin of normal liver), and cystic, pericholedochal, gastrohepatic, pancreaticoduodenal, and paraaortic lymphadenectomy (101).

The 5-year survival rate for T1a,N0,M0 patients undergoing simple cholecystectomy ranges from 57 to 100% (101). The incidence of lymph node metastases in these patients after simple cholecystectomy is less than 10%. It is further reduced to 2.5% for patients who undergo cholecystectomy and regional lymphadenectomy. However, extended resection has a mortality rate of 2 to 5% and a major postoperative morbidity rate of over 13%. The poor prognostic factors are listed in Table 19-13 (101).

Palliative Surgery

Most patients with gallbladder or bile duct carcinoma are diagnosed at advanced stages with symptomatic jaundice and gastroduodenal obstruction. Jaundice symptoms can be relieved by palliative procedures such as biliary tract bypass, intrahepatic cholangioenteric anastomosis, and percutaneous transhepatic biliary catheters. Gastroduodenal obstruction can be treated with gastrojejunostomy, intraoperative radiation, decompression gastrostomy, or jejunostomy feeding tube.

TABLE
19-12 **SUMMARY OF COMMONLY USED STAGING SYSTEMS FOR GALLBLADDER CANCER**

Stage	TNM System	Modified Nevin System	Japanese Biliary Surgical Society System	Proposed New Staging System
I	Mucosal or muscular invasion (T1,N0,M0)	In situ carcinoma	Confined to gallbladder capsule	Mucosal or muscular invasion
II	Transmural invasion (T2,N0,M0)	Mucosal or muscular invasion	N1 lymph nodes; minimal liver or bile duct invasion	Transmural invasion
III	Liver invasion <2 cm; lymph node metastases (T3,N1,M0)	Transmural direct liver invasion	N2 lymph nodes; marked liver or bile duct invasion	A: liver invasion <2 cm (T4,N0,M0) B: liver invasion >2 cm (T4,N0,M0)
IV	A: liver invasion >2 cm (T4,N0,M0,TX,N1,M0) B: distant metastasis (TX,N2,M0,TX,NX,M1)	Lymph node metastasis	Distant metastasis	A: N1 disease (TX,N1,M0) B: distant metastases (TX,NX,M1)
V		Distant metastasis		

TABLE
19-13 | **POOR PROGNOSTIC FACTORS FOR GALLBLADDER CARCINOMA**

Tumor stage T3 or T4

Regional lymph node metastases

Direct tumor invasion of the hepatic parenchyma

Microscopically positive liver resection margins

Incidental Cancers Found at Laparoscopy

Gallbladder carcinoma is incidentally found in 2% of routine cholecystectomies in the United States. Laparoscopic cholecystectomy carries a small risk of seeding cancer cells at the peritoneal surfaces and the laparoscopic port. If a patient is suspected of having a gallbladder carcinoma pre- or intraoperatively, he or she should undergo open laparotomy or percutaneous biopsy rather than laparoscopy (103).

Systemic Chemotherapy

In prior studies, 5-FU showed an objective partial response rate of less than 12%. Gemcitabine has a response rate similar to that of 5-FU. Complete remission is very rare, and the median survival is typically 11 months or less (104). The duration of response is usually 3 to 6 months.

The recent Advanced Biliary Cancer trials (ABC-01 and -02) have changed the treatment paradigm in this disease (105,106). Based on the results of the randomized phase II study (ABC-01), the MRC of United Kingdom initiated the ABC-02 study, consisting of gemcitabine plus cisplatin versus gemcitabine as a single agent (106). The study enrolled 400 patients and demonstrated a significant survival advantage with the platinum-based combination (11.7 months vs 8.1 months); the combination arm also had improved PFS (8 months vs 5 months). Similar survival figures have been reported with phase II studies of gemcitabine/capecitabine, gemcitabine/oxaliplatin, and gemcitabine/irinotecan.

Locoregional Therapy

Biliary tumors are less vascularized than hepatocellular cancers and the data regarding arterial therapy for biliary cancers are limited. Hepatic arterial infusion (HAI) chemotherapy with mitomycin resulted in a high partial response rate without any notable survival benefit (107). TACE is an evolving treatment modality for unresectable intrahepatic cholangiocarcinoma. Several single-institution studies have demonstrated its efficacy in this setting (108-110), but the lack of prospective, randomized data makes its precise role in the therapeutic

algorithm unclear. Moreover, coexistence of biliary obstruction leads to a higher risk of hepatic abscess formation. Recent studies indicate a role for radioembolization with yttrium-90 microspheres (SIR-Spheres or TheraSpheres) for metastatic colorectal cancer or neuroendocrine cancer with liver involvement. Such an approach is currently considered experimental for biliary cancer.

Radiation Therapy

Radiation therapy in biliary cancers is administered in the adjuvant setting following surgical resection or for the palliation of advanced disease. Local recurrence is the most common type of failure after surgical resection and therefore adjuvant radiation has strong rationale. Unfortunately, level one evidence regarding adjuvant radiotherapy after surgical resection is lacking as there are no randomized controlled trials. However, based on population-based registries such as SEER, regionally advanced or hepatic-invasive gallbladder cancer is treated with adjuvant radiation in the United States, which may result in survival improvement. At our institution, patients have been selectively referred for adjuvant chemoradiation when they have positive lymph nodes or positive margins. Adjuvant therapy has improved the outcome in these poor prognosis patients such that their outcome is similar to that of node-negative/margin negative patients, suggesting that treatment makes up for these poor prognostic features (111). After re-exploration for incidentally diagnosed gallbladder cancers, most studies are small and nonrandomized and do not have sufficient power to address the survival benefit of such treatment (112-115). In contrast to cholangiocarcinomas, since the patterns of failure suggest a predominantly distant pattern of failure for gallbladder cancers (116), it may be reasonable to establish that there is no unrecognized metastatic disease (over a course of systemic chemotherapy) before consolidating with chemoradiation therapy (117). In all instances of adjuvant treatment for cholangiocarcinomas and gallbladder cancers, typical doses of radiation are roughly 50 Gy administered in 5 to 6 weeks with concurrent fluoropyrimidine chemotherapy.

For the majority of nonmetastatic patients who are unable to undergo complete surgical resection with negative margins (117), multiple small studies have concluded that RT improves overall survival when compared to no treatment (or stenting alone) (118-123). However, these studies are constrained by the nonuniform criteria for determination of resectability, inclusion of patients with all extrahepatic cholangiocarcinomas (and gallbladder cancer occasionally), and/or the use of older radiographic imaging and radiation treatment techniques. In most series reporting chemoradiation outcomes for unresectable cholangiocarcinomas, the dose of external beam radiation therapy has been 50 Gy. There is also evidence that higher doses increase the efficacy of treatment, with one pretransplantation series reporting 24 to 42% pathological complete response rates (124).

External beam radiation therapy in a dose of 45 Gy may be used as palliative treatment to relieve pain, maintain biliary patency and improve survival. Endobiliary stents are associated with higher patency rates if the obstructed segment of the biliary tract is also treated with radiation; this is particularly the case with interstitial radiation using iridium-192. Higher-dose radiation therapy with radiosensitizing 5-FU has produced occasional long-term survival (125).

Targeted Therapies

Recent data indicate that EGFR and VEGF are important targets in biliary cancer. Erlotinib is an active agent that has produced an 8% response rate and a median survival of 7 months for biliary cancer patients, some of whom had received prior therapy (126). Biweekly cetuximab is combined with gemcitabine and oxaliplatin in the ongoing BINGO trial (127). The interim safety analysis of this randomized study indicated no added toxicity with the addition of cetuximab; efficacy data are awaited. Investigators from Massachusetts General Hospital in Boston have combined gemcitabine and oxaliplatin with bevacizumab and demonstrated promising efficacy of this combination. In this study, 18-fluorodeoxyglucose (FDG)-PET scan was used to assess response; this could be particularly useful in biliary tract cancers, which are often nonmeasurable by RECIST. PET responses correlated with survival, and further exploration of this imaging modality is warranted (128).

Multidisciplinary Approaches

Several nonrandomized studies suggest potential survival benefits of adjuvant or neoadjuvant chemotherapy and/or radiation therapy for patients with stage I, II, or III tumors (129,130). Intraoperative low-dose radiation therapy (20-30 Gy) relieves obstruction of extrahepatic bile ducts in the majority of unresectable patients. It improves patients' quality of life without significant survival benefit or perioperative morbidity (130). A current SWOG study is investigating gemcitabine plus capecitabine followed by capecitabine-based chemoradiation as an adjuvant strategy for resected extrahepatic cholangiocarcinoma.

Hilar cholangiocarcinomas have been treated at the Mayo Clinic with preoperative chemoradiation followed by orthotopic liver transplant. This therapeutic strategy was demonstrated to result in improved survival for this subset of patients (131,132).

GALLBLADDER CARCINOMA VERSUS CHOLANGIOCARCINOMA

Although gallbladder cancers and cholangiocarcinomas are often grouped together as "biliary tract cancers" in clinical studies and the scientific literature, these are disparate malignancies and should be recognized accordingly. Gallbladder cancers have a strong association with cholelithiasis and occur in unique high-prevalence areas (Chile, northern India, etc). Cholangiocarcinomas on the other hand are linked with sclerosing cholangitis and the association with cholelithiasis is less common. Modes of disease spread are also distinct, with gallbladder cancers carrying a higher risk of dissemination into the peritoneum and along surgical planes than cholangiocarcinomas. These clinical and epidemiological differences also lead to differences in disease biology. Therefore, gallbladder cancers and cholangiocarcinomas should be stratified accordingly in clinical trials.

MDACC APPROACH TO GALLBLADDER AND BILIARY TRACT CARCINOMAS

In contrast to patients with hepatocellular carcinoma, patients with gallbladder or biliary tract cancer are not candidates for liver transplantation unless this is performed in the context of a clinical trial. These tumors have a high incidence of early spread to regional lymph nodes, adjacent liver, and peritoneum, even with apparent low tumor volume; therefore, few patients who present with clinical symptoms are surgical candidates. Patients with T1 GB tumors are considered cured of their disease with simple cholecystectomy. Currently, there is no standard surgical approach for patients with T2 disease but, in the absence of radiographically apparent extrahepatic disease, these patients are generally offered re-resection of the GB bed and regional lymph nodes. The role of adjuvant therapy—either radiation, chemotherapy, or combined-modality therapy—has not been defined prospectively in GB and biliary tract cancers. Patients with positive margins or lymph node involvement on surgical pathology are known to be at high risk of recurrence. They are frequently offered adjuvant chemoradiation with or without additional chemotherapy, although there are no randomized, controlled trials demonstrating a survival advantage with this approach. For locally advanced biliary cancers, the use of yttrium-90 microspheres is likely to expand at centers such as MDACC where this therapy is available. Clinical trials designed to answer important questions about both adjuvant therapy

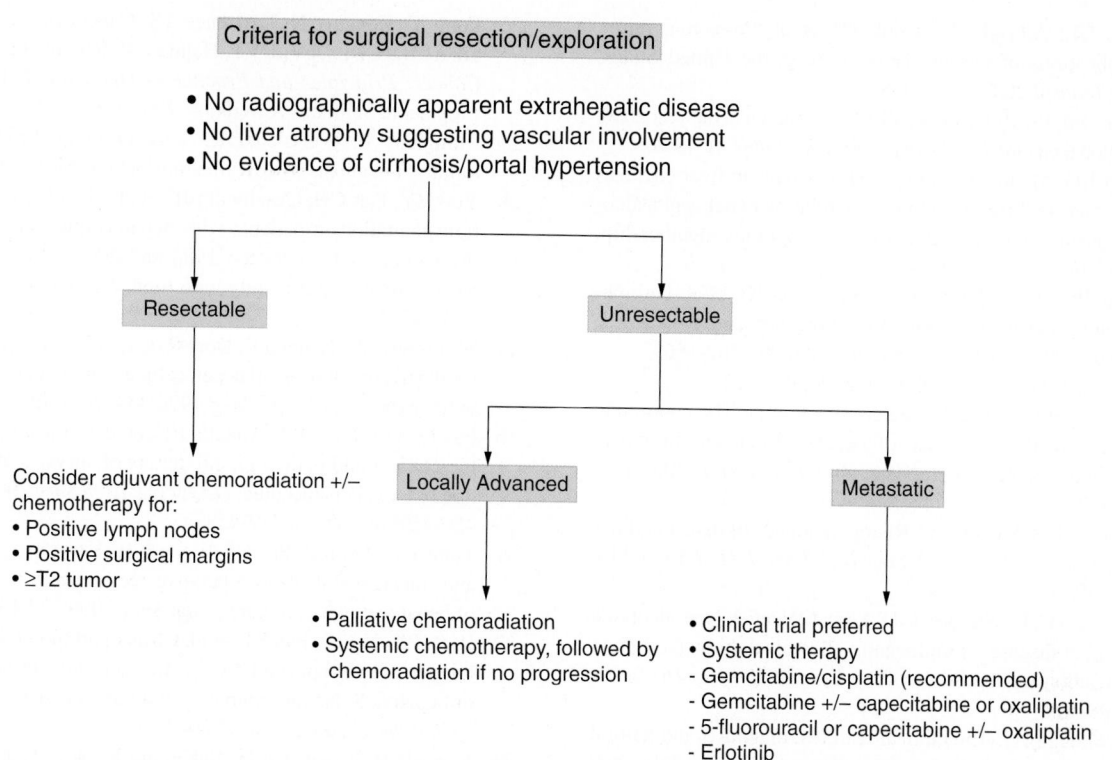

FIGURE 19-7. MD Anderson approach to HCC treatment. (*Adapted with permission from The University of Texas MD Anderson Cancer Center.*)

and systemic treatment of advanced disease are a current research priority. Figure 19-7 outlines the general approach of the MDACC hepatobiliary group in evaluating a patient with GB or biliary cancer, recognizing that each patient requires individualized care, within the confines of minimal prospective data, to optimize clinical outcomes.

PROMISING TARGETS IN HEPATOBILIARY CANCERS

While targeted therapy has yet to produce a major impact on disease-free or overall survival in hepatobiliary cancers, many signaling pathways are being explored as potential therapeutic targets. Much attention has been focused on inhibition of angiogenesis and EGFR; several ongoing clinical trials should further elucidate the role of agents targeting these pathways. The PI3K/Akt/mTOR axis may be an attractive target, since activation of this pathway occurs in 30 to 50% of HCCs and has been associated with a poor prognosis (133,134). In addition, overexpression of Akt and p-Akt has been documented in cholangiocarcinomas (95% and 65% of cases, respectively) (135). Low expression of PTEN, a negative regulator of the pathway, correlated with worse survival in a cohort of patients with extrahepatic cholangiocarcinoma (136).

The hepatocyte growth factor (HGF)/c-met pathway has also been implicated in hepatobiliary cancers.

Aberrant c-met signaling promotes tumor cell proliferation, invasiveness, and angiogenesis. C-met expression has been detected by immunohistochemistry (IHC) in >80% of surgically resected HCC specimens, and elevated postoperative HGF levels have been correlated with inferior clinical outcomes (137). C-met inhibition blunts the invasive phenotype of HCC and cholangiocarcinoma cells in vitro (138,139). The insulin-like growth factor-1 receptor (IGF-1R) and Ras/Raf/MAPK pathways may represent additional therapeutic targets.

Specific inhibitors of PI3K, Akt, HGF, c-Met, and IGF-1R are currently being investigated in early-phase clinical trials. Improved understanding of the molecular pathogenesis of hepatobiliary cancers will guide future drug development and shed light on how to best incorporate targeted agents into current treatment paradigms.

References

1. Jemal A, Siegel R, Ward E, et al. Cancer statistics, 2009. *CA Cancer J Clin* 2009;59:225-249.
2. World Health Organization. Mortality database. WHO Statistical Information System. Available at: http://www.who.int/whosis. Accessed March 22, 2010.
3. Taylor-Robinson SD, Foster GR, Arora S, et al. Increase in primary liver cancer in the UK, 1979–94. *Lancet* 1997;350:1142-1143.
4. Deuffic S, Poynard T, Buffat L, et al. Trends in primary liver cancer. *Lancet* 1998;351:214-215.

5. Davis GL, Albright JE, Cook SF, et al. Projecting future complications of chronic hepatitis C in the United States. *Liver Transpl* 2003;9:331-338.

6. Parkin DM, Bray FI, Devesa SS. Cancer burden in the year 2000. The global picture. *Eur J Cancer* 2001;37 (Suppl 8): 4S-66S.

7. Smart RG, Mann RE, Suurvali H. Changes in liver cirrhosis death rates in different countries in relation to per capita alcohol consumption and Alcoholics Anonymous membership. *J Stud Alcohol* 1998;59:245-249.

8. Wong JB, McQuillan GM, McHutchison JG, et al. Estimating future hepatitis C morbidity, mortality, and costs in the United States. *Am J Public Health* 2000;90:1562-1569.

9. *National Vital Statistics Report*. 2002;50:28-31

10. El–Serag HB, Davila JA, Petersen NJ, et al. The continuing increase in the incidence of hepatocellular carcinoma in the United States: An update. *Ann Intern Med* 2003;139: 817-823.

11. El–Serag HB, Mason AC. Rising incidence of hepatocellular carcinoma in the United States. *N Engl J Med* 1999;340: 745-750.

12. Loguercio C, De Simone T, D'Auria MV, et al. Non-alcoholic fatty liver disease: A multicentre clinical study by the Italian Association for the Study of the Liver. *Dig Liver Dis* 2004; 36:398-405.

13. McCullough AJ. The clinical features, diagnosis and natural history of nonalcoholic fatty liver disease. *Clin Liver Dis* 2004; 8:521-533.

14. Ruhl CE, Everhart JE. Epidemiology of nonalcoholic fatty liver. *Clin Liver Dis* 2004;8:501-519.

15. Parkin DM. The global burden of cancer. *Semin Cancer Biol* 1998;8:219-235.

16. Shen F-M, Lee MK, Gong H-M, et al. Complex segregation analysis of primary hepatocellular carcinoma in Chinese families: Interaction of inherited susceptibility and hepatitis B viral infection. *Am J Hum Genet* 1991;99:88-93.

17. Giardiello FM, Petersen GM, Brensinger JD, et al. Hepatoblastoma and APC gene mutation in familial adenomatous polyposis. *Gut* 1996;39:867-869.

18. Jia L, Wang XW, Harris CC. Hepatitis B virus × protein inhibits nucleotide excision repair. *Int J Cancer* 1999;80: 875-879.

19. Groisman I, Koshy R, Henkler F, et al. Downregulation of DNA excision repair by the hepatitis B virus × protein occurs in p53-proficient and deficient cells. *Carcinogenesis* 1999;3: 479-483.

20. Soresen HT, Friis S, Olsen JH, et al. Risk of liver and other types of cancer in patients with cirrhosis: a nationwide cohort study in Denmark. *Hepatology* 1998; 28:821-925.

21. DiBisceglie AM, Rustgi VK, Hoofnagle JH, et al. NIH conference: Hepatocellular carcinoma. *Ann Intern Med* 1988; 108:390-401.

22. Fong Y, Sun R, Jarnagin W, et al. An analysis of 412 cases of hepatocellular carcinoma at a western center. *Ann Surg* 1999; 229:790-800.

23. Sutton FM, Russell NC, Guinee VF, et al. Factors affecting the prognosis of primary liver carcinoma. *J Clin Oncol* 1988; 6:321-328.

24. Pateron D, Ganne N, Trinchet JC, et al. Prospective study of screening for hepatocellular carcinoma in Caucasian patients with cirrhosis. *J Hepatol* 1994;20:65-71.

25. Vauthey JN, Lauwers GY, Esnaola NF. Simplified staging for hepatocellular carcinoma. *J Clin Oncol* 2002;20:1527-1536.

26. Fong Y, Kemeny N, Lawrence TS. Cancer of the liver and biliary tract. In: DeVita VT, Hellman H, Rosenberg SA, (eds). *Cancer: Principles and Practice of Oncology*. Philadelphia: Lippincott, Williams & Wilkins; 2001:1162-1203.

27. Rummeny E, Weissleder R, Stark D, et al. Primary liver tumors: Diagnosis by MR imaging. *AJR* 1989;152:63-72.

28. Yoo HY, Patt CH, Geschwind JF, et al. The outcome of liver transplantation in patients with hepatocellular carcinoma in the United States between 1988 and 2001: 5-Year survival has improved significantly with time. *J Clin Oncol* 2003;21: 4329-4335.

29. Mazzaferro V, Regalia E, Doci R, et al. Liver transplantation for the treatment of small hepatocellular carcinomas in patients with cirrhosis. *N Engl J Med* 1996;334:693-699.

30. Pawlik TM, Poon RT, Abdalla EK, et al. Critical appraisal of the clinical and pathologic predictors of survival after resection of large hepatocellular carcinoma. *Arch Surg* 2005;140(5): 450-457; discussion 457-458.

31. Tung-Ping Poon R, Fan ST, Wong J. Risk factors, prevention, and management of postoperative recurrence after resection of hepatocellular carcinoma. *Ann Surg* 2000;232:10-24.

32. Poon RT, Ng IO, Fan ST, et al. Clinicopathologic features of long-term survivors and disease-free survivors after resection of hepatocellular carcinoma: A study of a prospective cohort. *J Clin Oncol* 2001;19:3037-3044.

33. Yamada R, Nakatsuka H, Nakamura K, et al. Hepatic artery embolization in 32 patients with unresectable hepatoma. *Osaka City Med J* 1980;26(2):81-96.

34. Llovet JM, Real MI, Montaña X, et al. Arterial embolisation or chemoembolisation versus symptomatic treatment in patients with unresectable hepatocellular carcinoma: A randomised controlled trial. *Lancet* 2002;359(9319):1734-1739.

35. Lo CM, Ngan H, Tso WK, et al. Randomized controlled trial of transarterial lipiodol chemoembolization for unresectable hepatocellular carcinoma. *Hepatology* 2002;35(5):1164-1171

36. Lammer J, Malagari K, Vogl T, et al. Prospective randomized study of doxorubicin-eluting-bead embolization in the treatment of hepatocellular carcinoma: Results of the PRECISION V study. *Cardiovasc Intervent Radiol* 2010;33(1):41-52. (epub).

37. Reyes DK, Vossen JA, Kamel IR, et al. Single-center phase II trial of transarterial chemoembolization with drug-eluting beads for patients with unresectable hepatocellular carcinoma: Initial experience in the United States. *Cancer J* 2009; 15(6):526-532.

38. Poon RT, Tso WK, Pang RW, et al. A phase I/II trial of chemoembolization for hepatocellular carcinoma using a novel intra-arterial drug-eluting bead. *Clin Gastroenterol Hepatol* 2007;5(9):1100-1108.

39. Salem R, Lewandowski RJ, Mulcahy MF, et al. Radioembolization for hepatocellular carcinoma using yttrium-90 microspheres: A comprehensive report of long-term outcomes. *Gastroenterology* 2010;138(1):52-64.

40. Chen MS, Li JQ, Zheng Y, et al. A prospective randomized trial comparing percutaneous local ablative therapy and partial hepatectomy for small hepatocellular carcinoma. *Ann Surg* 2006;243(3):321-328.

41. Veltri A, Moretto P, Doriguzzi A, et al. Radiofrequency thermal ablation (RFA) after transarterial chemoembolization (TACE) as a combined therapy for unresectable non-early hepatocellular carcinoma (HCC). *Eur Radiol* 2006;16(3): 661-669.

42. Marelli L, Stigliano R, Triantos C, et al. Treatment outcomes for hepatocellular carcinoma using chemoembolization in combination with other therapies. *Cancer Treat Rev* 2006; 32(8):594-606.

43. Huang M, Liu G. The study of innate drug resistance of human hepatocellular carcinoma Bel7402 cell line. *Cancer Lett* 1999;135:97-105.

44. Kato A, Miyazaki M, Ambiru S, et al. Multidrug resistance gene (MDR-1) expression as a useful prognostic factor in patients with human hepatocellular carcinoma after surgical resection. *J Surg Oncol* 2001;78:110-115.

45. Kuo MT, Zhao JY, Teeter LD, et al. Activation of multidrug resistance (P-glycoprotein) mdr3/mdr1a gene during the development of hepatocellular carcinoma in hepatitis B virus transgenic mice. *Cell Growth Differ* 1992;3:531-540.

46. Kouroumalis E, Skordilis P, Thermos K, et al. Treatment of hepatocellular carcinoma with octreotide: A randomized controlled study. *Gut* 1998;42:442-447.

47. Llovet JM, Ricci S, Mazzaferro V, et al. Sorafenib in advanced hepatocellular carcinoma. *N Engl J Med* 2008; 359(4):378-390.

48. Gruenwald V, Wilkens L, Gebel M, et al. A phase II open-label study of cetuximab in unresectable hepatocellular carcinoma. *J Clin Oncol* 2006;24(18S):14079.

49. O'Dwyer PJ, Giantonio BJ, Levy DE, et al. Gefitinib in advanced unresectable hepatocellular carcinoma: Results from the Eastern Cooperative Oncology Group's Study E1203. *J Clin Oncol* 2006;24(18S):4143.

50. Abou-Alfa GK, Schwartz L, Ricci S, et al. Phase II study of sorafenib in patients with advanced hepatocellular carcinoma. *J Clin Oncol* 2006;24(26):4293-4300.

51. Siegel AB, Cohen EI, Ocean A, et al. Phase II trial evaluating the clinical and biologic effects of bevacizumab in unresectable hepatocellular carcinoma. *J Clin Oncol* 2008;26(18): 2992-2998.

52. Thomas MB, Chadha R, Glover K, et al. Phase 2 study of erlotinib in patients with unresectable hepatocellular carcinoma. *Cancer* 2007;110(5):1059-1067.

53. Ramanathan RK, Belani CP, Singh DA, et al. Phase II study of lapatinib, a dual inhibitor of epidermal growth factor receptor (EGFR) tyrosine kinase 1 and 2 (Her2/Neu) in patients (pts) with advanced biliary tree cancer (BTC) or hepatocellular cancer (HCC). A California Consortium (CCC-P) Trial. *J Clin Oncol* 2006;24(18S):4010.

54. Philip PA, Mahoney MR, Allmer C, et al. Phase II study of erlotinib (OSI-774) in patients with advanced hepatocellular cancer. *J Clin Oncol* 2005;23(27):6657-6663.

55. Zhu AX, Sahani DV, di Tomaso E, et al. A phase II study of sunitinib in patients with advanced hepatocellular carcinoma. *J Clin Oncol* 2007;25(18S):4637.

56. Zhu AX, Blaszkowsky L, Enzinger PC, et al. Phase II study of cetuximab in patients with unresectable or metastatic hepatocellular carcinoma. *J Clin Oncol* 2006; 24(18S): 14096.

57. Patt YZ, Hassan MM, Lozano RD, et al. Thalidomide in the treatment of patients with hepatocellular carcinoma: A phase II trial. *Cancer* 2005;103(4):749-755.

58. Schwartz JD, Sung M, Schwartz M, et al. Thalidomide in advanced hepatocellular carcinoma with optional low-dose interferon-alpha2a upon progression. *Oncologist* 2005;10(9): 718-727.

59. Cheng A, Kang Y, Chen Z, et al. Randomized phase III trial of sorafenib versus placebo in Asian patients with advanced hepatocellular carcinoma. *J Clin Oncol* 2008; 26(15S):4509.

60. Thomas MB, Morris JS, Chadha R, et al. Phase II trial of the combination of bevacizumab and erlotinib in patients who have advanced hepatocellular carcinoma. *J Clin Oncol* 2008; 27(6):843-850.

61. Sun W, Haller DG, Mykulowycz K, et al. Combination of capecitabine, oxaliplatin with bevacizumab in treatment of advanced hepatocellular carcinoma (HCC): A phase II study. *J Clin Oncol* 2007;25(18S):4574.

62. Zhu AX, Blaszkowsky LS, Ryan DP, et al. Phase II study of gemcitabine and oxaliplatin in combination with bevacizumab in patients with advanced hepatocellular carcinoma. *J Clin Oncol* 2006;24(12):1898-1903.

63. Louafi S, Boige V, Ducreux M, et al. Gemcitabine plus oxaliplatin (GEMOX) in patients with advanced hepatocellular carcinoma (HCC): Results of a phase II study. *Cancer* 2007; 109(7):1384-1390.

64. O'Neil BH, Bernard SA, Goldberg RM, et al. Phase II study of oxaliplatin, capecitabine, and cetuximab in advanced hepatocellular carcinoma. *J Clin Oncol* 2008;26(15S):4604.

65. Abou-Alfa GK, Johnson P, Knox J, et al. *Final results from a phase II (PhII), randomized, double-blind study of sorafenib plus doxorubicin (S+D) versus placebo plus doxorubicin (P+D) in patients (pts) with advanced hepatocellular carcinoma (AHCC).* 2008 Gastrointestinal Cancers Symposium Proceedings, Abstract 128.

66. Hsu C, Yang T, Hsu C, et al. Phase II study of bevacizumab (A) plus capecitabine (X) in patients (pts) with advanced/metastatic hepatocellular carcinoma (HCC): Final report. *J Clin Oncol* 2008;26(15S):4603.

67. Shen Y, Shao Y, Hsu C. Phase II study of sorafenib plus tegafur/uracil (UFT) in patients with advanced hepatocellular carcinoma (HCC). *J Clin Oncol* 2008;26(15S):15664.

68. Bruix J, Sherman M, Llovet JM, et al. Clinical management of hepatocellular carcinoma. Conclusions of the Barcelona-2000 EASL conference. European Association for the Study of the Liver. *J Hepatol* 2001;35(3):421-430.

69. Krishnan S, Dawson LA, Seong J, et al. Radiotherapy for hepatocellular carcinoma: an overview. *Ann Surg Oncol* 2008; 15:1015-1024.

70. Hawkins MA, Dawson LA. Radiation therapy for hepatocellular carcinoma: from palliation to cure. *Cancer* 2006;106: 1653-1663.

71. Ben-Josef E, Normolle D, Ensminger WD, et al. Phase II trial of high-dose conformal radiation therapy with concurrent hepatic artery floxuridine for unresectable intrahepatic malignancies. *J Clin Oncol* 2005;23:8739-8747.

72. Mornex F, Girard N, Beziat C, et al. Feasibility and efficacy of high-dose three-dimensional-conformal radiotherapy in cirrhotic patients with small-size hepatocellular carcinoma non-eligible for curative therapies-mature results of the French Phase II RTF-1 trial. *Int J Radiat Oncol Biol Phys* 2006;66: 1152-1158.

73. Mendez Romero A, Wunderink W, Hussain SM, et al. Stereotactic body radiation therapy for primary and metastatic liver tumors: a single institution phase I-II study. *Acta Oncol* 2006;45:831-837.

74. Dawson LA, Eccles C, Craig T. Individualized image guided iso-NTCP based liver cancer SBRT. *Acta Oncol* 2006;45: 856-864.

75. Chiba T, Tokuuye K, Matsuzaki Y, et al. Proton beam therapy for hepatocellular carcinoma: a retrospective review of 162 patients. *Clin Cancer Res* 2005;11:3799-3805.

76. Seong J, Keum KC, Han KH, et al. Combined transcatheter arterial chemoembolization and local radiotherapy of unresectable hepatocellular carcinoma. *Int J Radiat Oncol Biol Phys* 1999;43:393-397.

77. Seong J, Park HC, Han KH, et al. Local radiotherapy for unresectable hepatocellular carcinoma patients who failed with transcatheter arterial chemoembolization. *Int J Radiat Oncol Biol Phys* 2000;47:1331-1335.

78. Yasuda S, Ito H, Yoshikawa M, et al. Radiotherapy for large hepatocellular carcinoma combined with transcatheter arterial embolization and percutaneous ethanol injection therapy. *Int J Oncol* 1999;15:467-473.

79. Guo WJ, Yu EX. Evaluation of combined therapy with chemoembolization and irradiation for large hepatocellular carcinoma. *Br J Radiol* 2000;73:1091-1097.

80. Chia-Hsien Cheng J, Chuang VP, Cheng SH, et al. Unresectable hepatocellular carcinoma treated with radiotherapy and/or chemoembolization. *Int J Cancer* 2001;96:243-252.

81. Tazawa J, Maeda M, Sakai Y, et al. Radiation therapy in combination with transcatheter arterial chemoembolization for hepatocellular carcinoma with extensive portal vein involvement. *J Gastroenterol Hepatol* 2001;16:660-665.

82. Yamada K, Izaki K, Sugimoto K, et al. Prospective trial of combined transcatheter arterial chemoembolization and three-dimensional conformal radiotherapy for portal vein tumor thrombus in patients with unresectable hepatocellular carcinoma. *Int J Radiat Oncol Biol Phys* 2003;57:113-119.

83. Ishikura S, Ogino T, Furuse J, et al. Radiotherapy after transcatheter arterial chemoembolization for patients with hepatocellular carcinoma and portal vein tumor thrombus. *Am J Clin Oncol* 2002;25:189-193.

84. Yamada K, Soejima T, Sugimoto K, et al. Pilot study of local radiotherapy for portal vein tumor thrombus in patients with unresectable hepatocellular carcinoma. *Jpn J Clin Oncol* 2001; 31:147-152.

85. Nakagawa K, Yamashita H, Shiraishi K, et al. Radiation therapy for portal venous invasion by hepatocellular carcinoma. *World J Gastroenterol* 2005;11:7237-7241.

86. Zeng ZC, Fan J, Tang ZY, et al. A comparison of treatment combinations with and without radiotherapy for hepatocellular carcinoma with portal vein and/or inferior vena cava tumor thrombus. *Int J Radiat Oncol Biol Phys* 2005;61: 432-443.

87. Lin CS, Jen YM, Chiu SY, et al. Treatment of portal vein tumor thrombosis of hepatoma patients with either stereotactic radiotherapy or three-dimensional conformal radiotherapy. *Jpn J Clin Oncol* 2006;36:212-217.

88. Hsu WC, Chan SC, Ting LL, et al. Results of three-dimensional conformal radiotherapy and thalidomide for advanced hepatocellular carcinoma. *Jpn J Clin Oncol* 2006; 36:93-99.

89. Kim DY, Park W, Lim DH, et al. Three-dimensional conformal radiotherapy for portal vein thrombosis of hepatocellular carcinoma. *Cancer* 2005;103:2419-2426.

90. Minagawa M, Makuuchi M. Treatment of hepatocellular carcinoma accompanied by portal vein tumor thrombus. *World J Gastroenterol* 2006;12:7561-7567.

91. de Groen PC, Gores GJ, LaRusso NF, et al. Biliary tract cancers. *N Engl J Med* 1999;341:1368-1378.

92. Barr IH. Carcinoma of the gallbladder. *Am Surg* 1984;50: 275-282.

93. Albores-Saavedra J, Acantra-Vazquez A, Cruz-Ortiz H, et al. The precursor lesions of invasive gallbladder carcinoma. Hyperplasia, atypical hyperplasia, and carcinoma in situ. *Cancer* 1980;45(5):919-927.

94. Soumiyoshi K, Nagai E, Chijiiwa K, et al. Pathology of carcinoma of gallbladder. *World J Surg* 1991;15:315-321.

95. Nagorney DM, McPherson GA. Carcinoma of the gallbladder and extrahepatic bile ducts. *Semin Oncol* 1988;15: 106-115.

96. Ohtsuka M, Miyazaki M, Itoh H, et al. Routes of hepatic metastasis of gallbladder carcinoma. *Am J Clin Pathol* 1998; 109:62-68.

97. Yukawa M, Fujimori T, Hirayama D, et al. Expression of oncogene products and growth factors in early gallbladder cancer, advanced gallbladder cancer, and chronic cholecystitis. *Hum Pathol* 1993;24:37-40.

98. Rashid A. Cellular and molecular biology of biliary tract cancers. *Surg Oncol Clin North Am* 2002;11:995-1009.

99. Mikami T, Yanagisawa N, Baba N. Association of Bcl-2 protein expression with gallbladder carcinoma differentiation and progression and its relation to apoptosis. *Cancer* 1999; 85:318-325.

100. Saini S. Imaging of the hepatobiliary tract. *N Engl J Med* 1997;336:1889-1894.

101. Gagner M, Rossi RL. Radical operations for carcinoma of the gallbladder: Present status in North America. *World J Surg* 1991;15:344-347.

102. North JH, Pack MS, Hong C, et al. Prognostic factors for adenocarcinoma of the gallbladder: An analysis of 162 cases. *Am Surg* 1998;64:437-440.

103. Pearlstone DE, Curley SA, Feig BW. The management of gallbladder cancer: Before, during, and after laparoscopic cholecystectomy. *Semin Laparosc Surg* 1998;5: 121-128.

104. Castro MP. Efficacy of gemcitabine in the treatment of patients with gallbladder carcinoma. *Cancer* 1998;82;639-641.

105. Valle JW, Wasan H, Johnson P, et al. Gemcitabine alone or in combination with cisplatin in patients with advanced or metastatic cholangiocarcinomas or other biliary tract tumours: A multicentre randomised phase II study—The UK ABC-01 Study. *Br J Cancer* 2009;101(4):621-627.

106. Valle J, Wasan H, Palmer DH, et al. Cisplatin plus gemcitabine versus gemcitabine for biliary tract cancer. *N Engl J Med* 2010;362:1273-1281.

107. Makela JT, Kairaluoma MI. Superselective intra-arterial chemotherapy with mitomycin C for gallbladder cancer. *Br J Surg* 1993;80:912-915.

108. Herber S, Otto G, Schneider J, et al. Transarterial chemoembolization (TACE) for inoperable intrahepatic cholangiocarcinoma. *Cardiovasc Intervent Radiol* 2007; 30(6):1156-1165.

109. Aliberti C, Benea G, Tilli M, et al. Chemoembolization (TACE) of unresectable intrahepatic cholangiocarcinoma with slow-release doxorubicin-eluting beads: Preliminary results. *Cardiovasc Intervent Radiol* 2008;31(5):883-888.

110. Poggi G, Amatu A, Montagna B, et al. OEM-TACE: A new therapeutic approach in unresectable intrahepatic cholangiocarcinoma. *Cardiovasc Intervent Radiol* 2009;32(6): 1187-1192.

111. Borghero Y, Crane CH, Szklaruk J, et al. Extrahepatic bile duct adenocarcinoma: patients at high-risk for local recurrence treated with surgery and adjuvant chemoradiation have an equivalent overall survival to patients with standard-risk treated with surgery alone. *Ann Surg Oncol* 2008;15:3147-3156.

112. Kresl JJ, Schild SE, Henning GT, et al. Adjuvant external beam radiation therapy with concurrent chemotherapy in the management of gallbladder carcinoma. *Int J Radiat Oncol Biol Phys* 2002;52:167-175.

113. Duffy A, Capanu M, Abou-Alfa GK, et al. Gallbladder cancer (GBC): 10-year experience at Memorial Sloan-Kettering Cancer Centre (MSKCC). *J Surg Oncol* 2008;98: 485-489.

114. Czito BG, Hurwitz HI, Clough RW, et al. Adjuvant external-beam radiotherapy with concurrent chemotherapy after resection of primary gallbladder carcinoma: a 23-year experience. *Int J Radiat Oncol Biol Phys* 2005;62:1030-1034.

115. Gold DG, Miller RC, Haddock MG, et al. Adjuvant therapy for gallbladder carcinoma: the Mayo Clinic Experience. *Int J Radiat Oncol Biol Phys* 2009;75:150-155.

116. Jarnagin WR, Ruo L, Little SA, et al. Patterns of initial disease recurrence after resection of gallbladder carcinoma and hilar cholangiocarcinoma: implications for adjuvant therapeutic strategies. *Cancer* 2003;98:1689-1700.

117. Ben-David MA, Griffith KA, Abu-Isa E, et al. External-beam radiotherapy for localized extrahepatic cholangiocarcinoma. *Int J Radiat Oncol Biol Phys* 2006;66:772-779.

118. Milella M, Salvetti M, Cerrotta A, et al. Interventional radiology and radiotherapy for inoperable cholangiocarcinoma of the extrahepatic bile ducts. *Tumori* 1998;84:467-471.

119. Foo ML, Gunderson LL, Bender CE, Buskirk SJ. External radiation therapy and transcatheter iridium in the treatment of extrahepatic bile duct carcinoma. *Int J Radiat Oncol Biol Phys* 1997;39:929-935.

120. Gonzalez Gonzalez D, Gerard JP, Maners AW, et al. Results of radiation therapy in carcinoma of the proximal bile duct (Klatskin tumor). *Semin Liver Dis* 1990;10:131-141.

121. Kamada T, Saitou H, Takamura A, Nojima T, Okushiba SI. The role of radiotherapy in the management of extrahepatic bile duct cancer: an analysis of 145 consecutive patients treated with intraluminal and/or external beam radiotherapy. *Int J Radiat Oncol Biol Phys* 1996;34:767-774.

122. Morganti AG, Trodella L, Valentini V, et al. Combined modality treatment in unresectable extrahepatic biliary carcinoma. *Int J Radiat Oncol Biol Phys* 2000;46:913-919.

123. Shinohara ET, Mitra N, Guo M, Metz JM. Radiotherapy is associated with improved survival in adjuvant and palliative treatment of extrahepatic cholangiocarcinomas. Int J Radiat Oncol Biol Phys 2009;74:1191-1198.

124. Rea DJ, Heimbach JK, Rosen CB, et al. Liver transplantation with neoadjuvant chemoradiation is more effective than resection for hilar cholangiocarcinoma. *Ann Surg* 2005;242: 451-458.

125. Smoron GL. Radiation therapy of carcinoma of gallbladder and biliary tract. *Cancer* 1977;40:1422-1424.

126. Philip PA, Mahoney MR, Allmer C, et al. Phase II study of erlotinib in patients with advanced biliary cancer. *J Clin Oncol* 2006;24(19):3069-3074.

127. Malka D, Trarbach T, Fartoux L, et al. A multicenter, randomized phase II trial of gemcitabine and oxaliplatin (GEMOX) alone or in combination with biweekly cetuximab in the first-line treatment of advanced biliary cancer: Interim analysis of the BINGO trial. *J Clin Oncol* 2009;27(15S):4520.

128. Zhu AX, Meyerhardt JA, Blaszkowsky LS, et al. Efficacy and safety of gemcitabine, oxaliplatin, and bevacizumab in advanced biliary-tract cancers and correlation of changes in 18-fluorodeoxyglucose PET with clinical outcome: A phase 2 study. *Lancet Oncol* 2010;11(1):48-54.

129. Aretxabala X, Roa I, Burgos L, et al. Preoperative chemoradiotherapy in the treatment of gallbladder cancer. *Am Surg* 1999;65:241-246.

130. Busse PM, Cady B, Bothe A, et al. Intraoperative radiation therapy for carcinoma of the gallbladder. *World J Surg* 1991; 153:352-356.

131. Heimbach JK. Successful liver transplantation for hilar cholangiocarcinoma. *Curr Opin Gastroenterol* 2008;24(3): 384-388.

132. Hassoun Z, Gores GJ, Rosen CB. Preliminary experience with liver transplantation in selected patients with unresectable hilar cholangiocarcinoma. *Surg Oncol Clin N Am* 2002; 11(4):909-921.

133. Villanueva A, Chiang DY, Newell P, et al. Pivotal role of mTOR signaling in hepatocellular carcinoma. *Gastroenterology* 2008;125:1972-1983.

134. Schmitz KJ, Wohlschlaeger J, Lang H, et al. Activation of the ERK and AKT signalling pathway predicts poor prognosis in hepatocellular carcinoma and ERK activation in cancer tissue is associated with hepatitis C virus infection. *J Hepatol* 2008; 48:83-90.

135. Javle MM, Yu J, Khoury T, et al. Akt expression may predict favorable prognosis in cholangiocarcinoma. *J Gastroenterol Hepatol* 2006;21(11):1744-1751.

136. Chung JY, Hong, SM, Choi BY, et al. The expression of phospho-AKT, phospho-mTOR, and PTEN in extrahepatic cholangiocarcinoma. *Clin Cancer Res* 2009;15: 660-667.

137. Chau GY, Lui WY, Chi CW, et al. Significance of serum hepatocyte growth factor levels in patients with hepatocellular carcinoma undergoing hepatic resection. *Eur J Surg Oncol* 2008;34:333-338.

138. Salvi A, Arici B, Portolani N, et al. In vitro c-met inhibition by antisense RNA and plasmid-based RNAi down-modulates migration and invasion of hepatocellular carcinoma cells. *Int J Oncol* 2007;31(2):451-460.

139. Leelawat K, Leelawat S, Tepaksorn P, et al. Involvement of c-Met/hepatocyte growth factor pathway in cholangiocarcinoma cell invasion and its therapeutic inhibition with small interfering RNA specific for c-Met. *J Surg Res* 2006; 136(1):78-84.

SMALL BOWEL CANCER AND APPENDICEAL TUMORS

Michael J. Overman
Christopher Lieu
Commentary: Keith F.Fournier

Part A: Small Bowel Cancer

Part B: Appendiceal Neoplasms

Small bowel cancer is a rare malignancy representing approximately 2% of gastrointestinal neoplasms (1). In 2009, it was estimated that 6230 new cases of small bowel cancer and 1110 small bowel cancer–related deaths would occur (1). Most cancers of the small intestine are adenocarcinomas. Because of the non-specific clinical presentation of small bowel adeno-carcinoma and the difficulty in imaging the small bowel, most patients with small bowel adenocarci-noma present with lymph node involvement or distant metastases. Even in patients with localized disease who undergo resection with curative intent, the prog-nosis is poor, and no studies have yet demonstrated a clear benefit from adjuvant therapy. However, there have been some recent advances in the use of chemother-apy as palliative treatment. In this chapter, the epi-demiology, diagnosis, and treatment of small bowel cancers, in particular small bowel adenocarcinoma, are reviewed.

■ EPIDEMIOLOGY

Based on an analysis of the Surveillance, Epidemiology, and End Results database, the age-adjusted incidence rate for small bowel cancers has slowly increased from 0.9 per 100,000 persons in 1973-1982 to 1.8 per 100,000 persons in 2000-2004 (2,3). The majority of this increase has been attributed to an almost three-fold increase in the incidence of carcinoid tumors (4). Among the 14,253 cases of small bowel cancer diagnosed between 1985 and 1995 in the American College of Surgeons' National Cancer Database, 35% were adenocarcinomas, 28% were carcinoid tumors, 21% were lymphomas, 10% were sarcomas, and 6% were other histologic types (5). The incidence of histologic subtypes varies in the differ-ent sections of the small intestine, with adenocarcinomas representing 80% of duodenal cancers and carcinoids representing 60% of ileal cancers (6).

The incidence of small bowel adenocarcinoma peaks in the seventh and eighth decades of life, with a mean age at diagnosis of 65 years. A slightly increased inci-dence is seen in men and blacks (7).

One of the more interesting aspects of small bowel adenocarcinoma is its rarity in comparison to large intestine adenocarcinoma. Even though the small intes-tine represents approximately 70 to 80% of the length and over 90% of the surface area of the alimentary tract, the incidence of small bowel adenocarcinoma is 30-fold less than the incidence of colon adenocarci-noma. Numerous theories have been proposed to explain the small intestine's relative protection from the devel-opment of carcinoma. Proposed protective factors have centered around two concepts. First, the rapid turnover time of small intestinal cells results in epithelial cell shedding prior to the necessary acquisition of multiple genetic defects. Second, the small bowel's exposure to the carcinogenic components of our diet are limited due to a rapid small bowel transit time, the lack of bacterial degradation activity that occurs in the small bowel, and the relatively dilute, alkaline environment of the small bowel.

■ ANATOMY

The small intestine is divided into three sections. The duodenum represents the first 25 cm of the small intes-tine and is subdivided into four anatomic segments. The proximal portion of the first (ascending) segment of the duodenum is intraperitoneal, and then the distal portion, as well as the rest of the duodenum, becomes retroperi-toneal. The second (descending) segment of the duode-num contains the ampulla of Vater, through which the pancreatic and biliary secretions exit. The third (horizontal) segment of the duodenum is the longest, and as it crosses the left border of the aorta, the fourth (ascending) seg-ment of the duodenum begins. The duodenal-jejunal junction is characterized by the attachment of the suspen-sory ligament of Treitz. The next segment of the small bowel, the jejunum, is approximately 2.5 m long, and the final segment, the ileum, is approximately 3.5 m long.

■ ETIOLOGY

Little is known about the etiology of small bowel adenocarcinoma. As seen in colorectal adenocarcinomas, adenocarcinomas of the small intestine undergo a similar phenotypic adenoma-carcinoma transformation (8-10). An increase in the size of small bowel adenomas and the presence of a villous histology are risk factors for the development of invasive adenocarcinoma (11).

Common underlying genetic or environmental factors of both large and small intestine adenocarcinomas have been suggested by studies that have demonstrated an increased risk of small bowel adenocarcinoma in patients with colon adenocarcinoma and vice versa (12). In small bowel adenocarcinoma, microsatellite instability occurs at a similar rate to that seen in colorectal cancer. In a study of 89 patients with small bowel adenocarcinoma identified from a Swedish population-based cancer registry, the rate of microsatellite instability was 18% (13). This result along with the known clinical association between hereditary nonpolyposis colorectal cancer syndrome (HNPCC) and small bowel adenocarcinoma indicates that in a subset of patients with small bowel adenocarcinoma, a germ-line mutation in one of the mismatch repair proteins contributes to carcinogenesis.

The possible role of pancreaticobiliary secretions in the development of adenocarcinoma of the duodenum has been suggested by the anatomic clustering of duodenal carcinomas in the periampullary area. For example, in patients with familial adenomatous polyposis (FAP), 80% of small intestinal adenocarcinomas will occur in the second portion of the duodenum (14). One study evaluating 213 cases of duodenal carcinomas identified from the Los Angeles County tumor registry determined that 57% of the cases originated in the second part of the duodenum (15).

ENVIRONMENT AND DIETARY RISK FACTORS

A number of case-control studies have analyzed associations between environmental and dietary factors and the development of small bowel adenocarcinoma. Two studies have demonstrated that there is an association between the ingestion of smoked or salt-cured foods and the development of small bowel adenocarcinoma (16,17). An association between tobacco use and cancer risk has also been demonstrated in two studies but other studies have suggested that there is not an increased risk of small bowel adenocarcinoma with tobacco use (16,18,19). Other case-control studies have demonstrated an association between an increased risk of small bowel adenocarcinoma and high alcohol intake, high sugar intake, high red meat intake, low fiber intake, celiac disease, peptic ulcer disease, and prior cholecystectomy (16,17,20-22). Studies on the relationship between obesity and small bowel adenocarcinoma are conflicting, with some showing an increased risk and others showing a decreased risk for obese patients (19,23-25).

GENETIC CANCER SYNDROMES

The genetic cancer syndromes HNPCC, FAP, and Peutz-Jeghers syndrome (PJS) are all associated with small bowel adenocarcinoma. The estimated lifetime risk for small bowel adenocarcinoma is 1 to 4% in patients with HNPCC, 5% in those with FAP , and 13% in those with PJS (26-29). Patients with HNPCC develop small bowel adenocarcinoma at a younger age with a median age at diagnosis of 49 years. Patients with PJS, an autosomal dominant polyposis disorder characterized by multiple hamartomatous polyps throughout the intestinal tract, have a markedly increased risk for small bowel adenocarcinoma, with one meta-analysis demonstrating a 520-fold increased relative risk (27). Duodenal adenomas are seen in approximately 80% of patients with FAP, and regular endoscopic screening for the development of adenocarcinoma is required for these patients. The optimal frequency of endoscopic screening depends on a number of factors, such as the number of polyps, polyp size, polyp histology, and amount of dysplasia present (26). With the early use of colectomy in FAP patients, duodenal adenocarcinomas and desmoid tumors are now a more common cause of death in this population than cancer arising from the colorectum (14,30).

INFLAMMATORY BOWEL DISEASE

Inflammatory bowel disease, particularly Crohn disease, is associated with the development of small bowel adenocarcinoma. The increase in risk varies depending on both the extent and duration of small bowel involvement. In one study, the cumulative risk of small bowel adenocarcinoma in patients with Crohn disease was 0.2% at 10 years and 2.2% at 25 years (31). Because Crohn disease frequently involves the ileum, 70% of the small bowel cancers in patients with Crohn disease will occur in the ileum. Patients with Crohn disease who develop small bowel adenocarcinoma appear to have a worse prognosis, with one study of 37 patients with small bowel adenocarcinoma demonstrating significantly shorter overall survival in the patients with Crohn disease (32).

■ PRESENTATION AND DIAGNOSIS

CLINICAL PRESENTATION

The symptoms associated with small bowel adenocarcinoma are nonspecific and frequently do not occur until advanced disease is present. The most commonly reported symptoms are abdominal pain (45-76% of patients), nausea and vomiting (31-52%), weight loss (22-29%), and gastrointestinal bleeding (8-34%). Delays in diagnosis are common, with one retrospective study reporting a mean delay of 7.8 months from the time of initial physician evaluation until a final diagnosis was made (33). According to the National Cancer Database, 39% of patients present with stage I/II disease, 26% present with stage III disease, and 32% present with stage IV disease (5).

DIAGNOSIS

Given the nonspecific presenting symptoms, a high index of suspicion is a crucial first step in diagnosis. Because imaging of the small intestine is difficult, multiple tests may be needed. However, with the availability of wireless capsule endoscopy, the need for older small bowel imaging techniques has declined.

A barium small bowel follow-through study has been the radiographic gold standard for small bowel evaluation. In patients with advanced-stage disease, this technique has a sensitivity of approximately 60% for diagnosing small bowel tumors (34,35). Enteroclysis, in which contrast material is infused directly into the small intestine through a nasogastric tube, provides a slightly higher sensitivity than small bowel follow-through. Endoscopic evaluation of the small intestine, or enteroscopy, requires expertise and is frequently unable to evaluate the entire small intestine.

The incorporation of wireless capsule endoscopy, which was approved by the US Food and Drug Administration in 2001, has allowed a much simpler and improved method for evaluating the lumen of the small intestine. This technique has primarily been applied to the evaluation of obscure gastrointestinal bleeding, for which it has shown superiority over other imaging and endoscopy techniques (36). In one study evaluating capsule endoscopy in 60 patients with suspected small bowel pathology but without gastrointestinal bleeding, the overall diagnostic yield of capsule endoscopy was 62% (37). In that study, all patients had undergone upper and lower gastrointestinal endoscopy, and many had undergone enteroclysis, small bowel follow-through, push enteroscopy, and abdominal computed tomography

(CT). In a large single center retrospective review of 562 patients who underwent capsule endoscopy, small bowel tumors were found in 8.9% of cases (38). The major limitations of capsule endoscopy are that no tissue sampling can be conducted and that the patients cannot have bowel obstruction, which could result in the capsule's becoming trapped in the bowel.

Three-dimensional imaging with either CT or magnetic resonance imaging is useful in identifying locoregional lymph node involvement and the presence of distant metastatic disease. For tumors of the duodenum, endoscopic ultrasonography can be useful in assessing both the tumor and nodal status. Though not directly studied for duodenal adenocarcinomas, endoscopic ultrasonography has been demonstrated to improve staging accuracy for both ampullary and pancreatic cancers (39,40).

STAGING AND PROGNOSIS

The TNM (tumor, node, metastasis) staging system for small bowel adenocarcinoma is shown in Table 20-1 (41). In a study of 4995 patients who were diagnosed with small bowel adenocarcinoma between 1985 and 1995 (identified in the National Cancer Database), the 5-year disease-specific survival rate was 65% for patients with stage I disease, 48% for patients with stage II disease, 35% for patients with stage III disease, and 4% for patients with stage IV disease (5). A multivariate analysis from this study identified age >75 years, primary duodenal tumor site, non–cancer-directed surgery, and higher-stage disease as poor prognostic factors. Though significant on a univariate analysis, a poorly differentiated histology was not a significant prognostic factor on multivariate analysis ($p = .089$). In other studies, the histopathologic factors reported to be correlated with poor survival are poorly differentiated histology, positive margins, lymphovascular invasion, lymph node involvement, and T4 tumor stage (32, 42-48). The 5-year overall survival rates from various single-institution studies for resected small bowel adenocarcinoma are presented in Table 20-2.

■ TREATMENT

SURGICAL MANAGEMENT

For patients with localized disease a complete removal of the tumor with negative surgical margins and local lymph node removal are critical for an potentially curative resection. For jejunal and ileal

TABLE 20-1	TNM STAGING FOR ADENOCARCINOMA OF THE SMALL INTESTINE

PRIMARY TUMOR (T)

TX	Primary tumor cannot be assessed
T0	No evidence of primary tumor
Tis	Carcinoma in situ
T1a	Tumor invades lamina propria
T1b	Tumor invades submucosa
T2	Tumor invades muscularis propria
T3	Tumor invades through the muscularis propria into the subserosa or into the nonperitonealized perimuscular tissue (mesentery or retroperitoneum) with extension 2 cm or less*
T4	Tumor perforates the visceral peritoneum or directly invades other organs or structures (includes other loops of small intestine, mesentery, or retroperitoneum >2 cm, and abdominal wall by way of serosa; for duodenum only, invasion of pancreas or bile bile duct)

REGIONAL LYMPH NODES (N)

NX	Regional lymph nodes cannot be assessed
N0	No regional lymph node metastasis
N1	Metastasis in 1-3 regional lymph nodes
N2	Metastasis in four or more regional lymph nodes

DISTANT METASTASIS (M)

M0	No distant metastasis
M1	Distant metastasis

STAGE GROUPING

Stage 0	Tis	N0	M0
Stage I	T1	N0	M0
	T2	N0	M0
Stage IIA	T3	N0	M0
Stage IIB	T4	N0	M0
Stage IIIA	Any T	N1	M0
Stage IIIB	Any T	N2	M0
Stage IV	Any T	Any N	M1

*The nonperitonealized perimuscular tissue is for the jejunum and ileum, part of the mesentery; and for duodenum in areas where serosa is lacking, part of the interface with the pancreas.

Used with the permission of the American Joint Committee on Cancer (AJCC), Chicago, Illinois. The original source for this material is the AJCC Cancer Staging Manual, seventh edition (2010) published by Springer Science and Business Media LLC, www.springer.com.

lesions, an oncologically successful resection requires a wide local excision with lymphadenectomy. Lesions located in the duodenum generally require a pancreaticoduodenectomy; however, for small distal lesions in the third and fourth portions of the duodenum, a wide local excision may be an option. In a surgical series of 68 patients with duodenal adenocarcinoma, no differences in the 5-year overall survival rates, local recurrence rates, or margin negative resection rates were seen between the 50 patients who underwent pancreatic resections and the 18 patients who underwent distal duodenal segmental resections (49). The presence of locoregional lymph node involvement should not deter surgical intervention, since well over one-third of patients will survive long-term (5,50,51). This is in contrast to patients with lymph node–positive pancreatic cancer, of whom only 7% survive 5 years (52).

PATTERNS OF RECURRENCE

Recurrence after potentially curative resection of small bowel adenocarcinoma occurs most commonly at distant sites. In a series of 146 patients who underwent resection for small bowel adenocarcinoma, 56 patients relapsed at a median of 25 months, with the sites of relapse reported as distant in 59%, peritoneum in 20%, abdominal wall in 7%, and local in 18% (45). In a second study of 30 patients who underwent potentially curative resection for small bowel adenocarcinoma, 21 patients experienced a relapse, with the sites of relapse being the liver in 67% of the patients, lung in 38%, retroperitoneum in 29%, and peritoneum in 25% (42).

Patients with duodenal adenocarcinoma have a higher rate of locoregional failure than jejunal and ileal adenocarcinoma, with one study reporting a 39% rate of locoregional failure among 31 patients after curative resection of duodenal adenocarcinoma (53). In that study, positive margin status was the strongest predictor of local recurrence, with 4 of the 5 patients who had a margin positive resection developing a local recurrence. However, distant recurrences are still predominant, with a retrospective review of recurrence patterns in 67 patients with resected duodenal adenocarcinoma revealing local recurrences in 33% of the patients and distant recurrences in 67% (54).

ADJUVANT THERAPY

Currently, there is no evidence demonstrating a benefit from adjuvant therapy in patients with small bowel adenocarcinoma who undergo potentially curative resection. However, owing to the rarity of small bowel adenocarcinoma, only a limited number of primarily small retrospective studies have been conducted (Table 20-3). Selection bias is the major limitation of these retrospective studies, since the patients selected to receive

| TABLE 20-2 | REPORTED OVERALL SURVIVAL OF PATIENTS WITH CURATIVELY RESECTED SMALL BOWEL ADENOCARCINOMA |

First Author	Period	Tumor Location	Number of Patients	OVERALL SURVIVAL	
				Median (Months)	5-Year (%)
Agarawal	1971-2005	Small intestine	30	56	45
Kelsey	1975-2005	Duodenum	25	NR	64
Wu	1983-2003	Small intestine	45	NR	27
Swartz	1994-2003	Duodenum	14	41	44
Dabaja	1978-1998	Small intestine	142	36	29
Czaykowski	1990-2000	Small intestine	19	39	NR
Talamonti	1977-2000	Small intestine	26	40	42
Abrahams	1978-1999	Small intestine	37	NR	52
Brucher	1985-1998	Small intestine	22	NR	45
Bakaeen	1976-1996	Duodenum	68	NR	54
Rose	1983-1994	Duodenum	42	NR	60
Cunningham	1970-1991	Small intestine	19	23	32
Frost	1960-1989	Small intestine	22	NR	32

NR, not reported.

adjuvant therapy were the patients believed to be at highest risk for disease recurrence. One prospective phase III study conducted by the European Organization for Research and Treatment of Cancer enrolled 92 patients with periampullary carcinoma, defined as adenocarcinoma of the distal common bile duct, ampulla of Vater, or duodenum. Ninety patients were randomized to receive either no adjuvant therapy or concurrent 5-fluorouracil (5-FU) and radiation therapy (55). The 5-year overall survival rates were similar in the two groups, but 30% of the patients assigned to receive adjuvant therapy did not actually receive it, and no description of the results in the duodenal adenocarcinoma subgroup were reported. In a series by Kelsey et al., no differences in the 5-year overall survival rates were seen between the patients who did or did not receive adjuvant therapy after resection of duodenal adenocarcinoma. However, in the subgroup of patients who had undergone a margin negative resection, the 5-year overall survival rate was 53% in the patients who underwent resection only and 83% in the patients who had resection and adjuvant chemoradiation therapy ($p = .07$) (53).

Limited data are available regarding a neoadjuvant (preoperative) treatment approach for duodenal adenocaricnoma. In one report in which 11 patients underwent neoadjuvant chemoradiation therapy followed by resection for duodenal adenocarcinoma, a complete pathologic response was seen in 2 patients, and none of the 11 patients had histopathologic nodal involvement at the time of surgery (53).

THE MD ANDERSON APPROACH TO NONMETASTATIC DISEASE

At the University of Texas MD Anderson Cancer Center, patients with high risk, resected small bowel adenocarcinoma are typically offered postoperative adjuvant chemotherapy. In general, patients who are considered to be at high risk are those with lymph node involvement and positive resection margins. The lack of proven benefit from adjuvant chemotherapy for this tumor type must be discussed with the patient. However, the rationale for considering adjuvant chemotherapy is based on:

1. The known poor prognosis of patients with high-risk disease
2. The predominantly systemic relapse pattern for small intestinal adenocarcinoma
3. The proven activity of chemotherapy in the treatment of metastatic small intestinal adenocarcinoma
4. The known benefit of adjuvant chemotherapy in large intestinal adenocarcinoma, which appears to have a number of similarities to small intestinal adenocarcinoma
5. The extremely limited amount of high-quality data to support or refute the role of adjuvant therapy for small bowel adenocarcinoma

Based on the substantial activity of a 5-FU and platinum combination in the metastatic disease setting, we generally utilize the combination of capecitabine and oxaliplatin (CAPOX) as adjuvant therapy for nonmetastatic small bowel adenocarcinoma. In addition

TABLE
20-3

REPORTED OVERALL SURVIVAL OF PATIENTS WHO RECEIVED ADJUVANT THERAPY AFTER RESECTION OF SMALL BOWEL ADENOCARCINOMA

First Author	Time Period	Study Type	Tumor Location	Type of Adjuvant Therapy	NUMBER OF PATIENTS			MEDIAN OVERALL SURVIVAL (MONTHS)		
					Total	No Adjuvant Therapy	Adjuvant Therapy	No Adjuvant Therapy	Adjuvant Therapy	p Value
Agrawal	1971-2005	Retrospective review	Small bowel	Not specified	30	19	11	41	56	NR
Kelsey	1975-2005	Retrospective review	Duodenum	5-FU/radiation	32	16	16	44%*	57%*	0.42
Fishman	1986-2004 review	Retrospective	Small bowel	Not specified	60	45	15	28	22	NR
Dabaja	1978-1998	Retrospective review	Small bowel	Not specified	120	62	58	36	19	0.49
Klinkenbijl	1987-1995	Randomized phase III trial	Periampullary	5-FU/radiation	93	49	44	40	40	0.74
Sohn	1984-1996	Retrospective review	Duodenum	5-FU/radiation	48	37	11	35	27	0.73

5-FU, 5-fluorouracil; NR, not reported.
*5-Year overall survival rate.

to systemic chemotherapy, radiation therapy is considered for patients with duodenal adenocarcinoma who are at high risk for a local recurrence based on the presence of positive margins or T4 disease.

METASTATIC DISEASE

In general, chemotherapy for metastatic small bowel adenocarcinoma has been based on the principles used for treating colon cancer. Several single-institution retrospective series have demonstrated a survival benefit in patients with metastatic or unresectable small bowel adenocarcinoma who received chemotherapy when compared to patients who did not receive chemotherapy (45,56,57).

Most of the studies evaluating chemotherapy for small bowel adenocarcinoma have been retrospective, with only two prospective phase II studies reported (Table 20-4). One multicenter study conducted by the Eastern Cooperative Oncology Group reported on the combination of 5-FU, doxorubicin, and mitomycin C (FAM) in 39 patients with adenocarcinomas of the duodenum, jejunum, ileum, or ampulla of Vater. The overall response rate was 18%, with a median overall

| TABLE 20-4 | REPORTED RESPONSE AND OVERALL SURVIVAL FOR PATIENTS TREATED WITH SYSTEMIC CHEMOTHERAPY FOR METASTATIC SMALL BOWEL ADENOCARCINOMA | | | | | | |

First Author	Year	Study Type	Disease Status	Number of Patients	Type of Chemotherapy	Overall Response Rate (%)	Median Overall Survival (Months)
Overman	2009	Prospective phase II trial	Metastatic, LAD	30	CAPOX	50	20.3
Overman	2008	Retrospective review	Metastatic	29	5-FU + platinum	41	14.8
				51	Various agents	16	12.0
Fishman	2007	Retrospective review	Metastatic, LAD	44	Various agents	29	18.6
Locher	2005	Retrospective review	Metastatic, LAD	20	5-FU + platinum	21	14.0
Gibson	2005	Prospective phase II trial	Metastatic	38	FAM	18	8
Enzinger	2005	Prospective phase I trial	Metastatic	4	5-FU + cisplatin + irinotecan	50	NS
Czaykowski	2007	Retrospective review	Metastatic, LAD	16	5-FU–based therapy	6	15.6
Goetz	2003	Prospective phase I trial	Metastatic, LAD	5	5-FU + oxaliplatin + irinotecan	40	NS
Polyzos	2003	Case series	Metastatic	3	Irinotecan	0	NS
Crawley	1998	Retrospective review	Metastatic, LAD	8	ECF +5-FU–based therapy	37	13
Jigyasu	1984	Retrospective review	Metastatic	14	5-FU–based therapy	7	9
Ouriel	1984	Retrospective review	Metastatic	14	5-FU–based therapy	NS	10.7
Morgan	1977	Retrospective review	Metastatic	7	5-FU–based therapy	0	NS
Rochlin	1965	Retrospective review	NS	11	5-FU	36	NS

CAPOX, capecitabine and oxaliplatin; ECF, 5-FU, epirubicin, and cisplatin; FAM, 5-FU, doxorubicin, and mitomycin C; 5-FU, 5-fluorouracil; LAD, locally advanced, unresectable disease; NS, not significant.

survival time of 8 months (58). A single-institution study conducted at MD Anderson evaluated CAPOX in 30 patients with metastatic or locally advanced small bowel or ampullary adenocarcinomas. The overall response rate was 50%, with a median time to progression of 9.8 months and an overall survival time of 20.3 months (59). An example of a response to CAPOX chemotherapy in a patient treated in that study is shown in Fig. 20-1.

Several retrospective studies have confirmed the substantial activity of 5-FU combined with a platinum agent for metastatic small bowel adenocarcinoma, with response rates of 18-46% (56, 60-62). In the largest retrospective study to date, a total of 80 patients with metastatic small bowel adenocarcinoma were treated with various regimens: 29 received 5-FU with a platinum (19 received cisplatin, 4 received carboplatin, and 6 received oxaliplatin), 41 received 5-FU–based therapy without a platinum (32 received 5-FU alone, 3 received FAM, 3 received 5-FU and mitomycin, and 3 received other 5-FU combinations), and 10 received non-platinum–based and non-5-FU–based therapy (62). Patients who received 5-FU combined with a platinum agent had a higher overall response rate (46 versus 16%; $p <.01$) and longer median progression-free survival time (8.7 versus 3.9 months; $p <.01$) than patients who received other chemotherapy regimens. Though not statistically significant, there was also a trend toward improved median overall survival times in patients who received 5-FU plus a platinum agent (14.8 versus 12.0 months; $p = .1$).

Irinotecan-based chemotherapy is also active against metastatic small bowel adenocarcinoma. One retrospective study reported that 5 of 12 patients responded to irinotecan-based therapy (three patients responded to 5-FU plus irinotecan, one responded to capecitabine plus irinotecan, and one responded to single-agent irinotecan) (56). A second study of salvage therapy with irinotecan in the second line setting noted stable disease in 4 of 8 treated patients (61). Responses to gemcitabine-based therapy have also been noted, though the number of patients treated has been small (56,62). The role of targeted therapies against the vascular endothelial growth factor or epidermal growth factor receptors has not been studied in small bowel adenocarcinoma.

THE MD ANDERSON APPROACH TO METASTATIC DISEASE

The substantial response rates and prolonged overall survival times recently reported with modern day chemotherapy combinations in small bowel adenocarcinomas strongly argue for an aggressive approach in treating patients with metastatic small bowel adenocarcinoma. Given the extremely encouraging phase II trial results

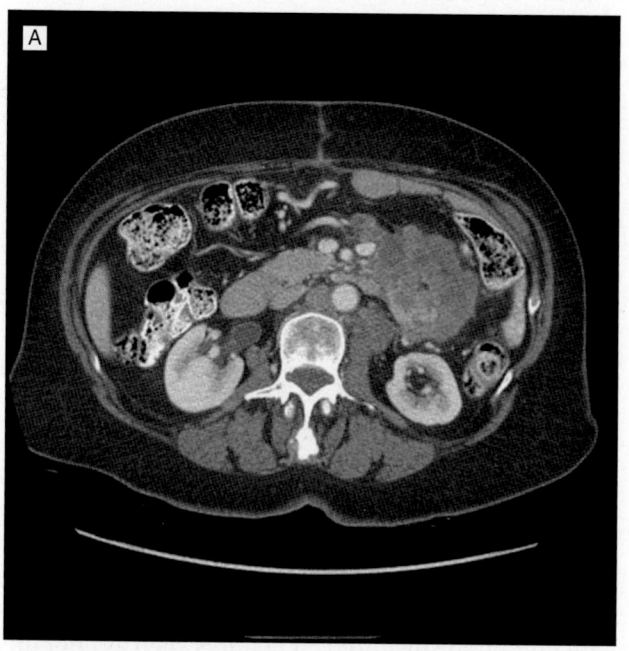
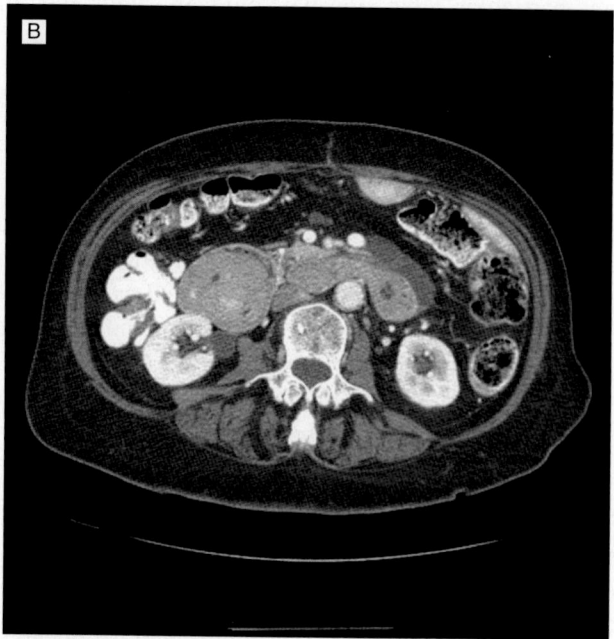

FIGURE 20-1. Radiographic response to capecitabine and oxaliplatin (CAPOX) chemotherapy in a patient with locally advanced small bowel adenocarcinoma. Pretreatment (**A**) and posttreatment (**B**) computed tomography scans shown.

with CAPOX for metastatic small bowel adenocarcinoma, we generally recommend this regimen at MD Anderson. Following frontline CAPOX chemotherapy patients are then treated with an irinotecan-based regimen. In addition, patients with limited metastatic disease who respond to initial chemotherapy are considered for surgical resection if all disease sites can be successfully excised. Investigations are ongoing at MD Anderson to evaluate the role of epidermal growth factor receptor inhibition in addition to CAPOX chemotherapy for small bowel adenocarcinoma. More effective treatments for small bowel adenocarcinoma remain needed, and participation in clinical trials for this rare tumor type is strongly encouraged.

Part B: Appendiceal Tumors

Appendiceal tumors encompass a rare and diverse group of neoplasms. With an age-adjusted incidence of about 0.12 cases per 1 million individuals per year, appendiceal tumors represent only 1% of all colorectal cancers (CRCs) diagnosed each year in the United States (63,64). Historically, appendiceal tumors have been grouped together with CRCs. However, appendiceal tumors, in which outcomes are strongly determined by histologic subtype, tend to have a biology very different from that of CRC. Appendiceal tumors comprise two types: appendiceal carcinoid tumors and appendiceal epithelial tumors. Appendiceal carcinoid tumors account for approximately 50% of all appendiceal neoplasms, and appendiceal epithelial tumors represent the remaining 50% (65). This chapter on appendiceal tumors will discuss the management of these two tumor types (carcinoid and epithelial) and in particular, the unusual clinical syndrome of pseudomyxoma peritonei.

■ INCIDENCE

Data derived from the Surveillance, Epidemiology, and End Results (SEER) database of the National Cancer Institute between 1973 and 1998 revealed that the most common histologic subtypes of malignant tumors of the appendix were adenocarcinomas (67%) and carcinoids (33%) (63). However, this analysis captured neither adenomatous tumors nor benign carcinoids. The subtypes of adenocarcinoma were mucinous type (56%), nonmucinous intestinal type (38%), and signet ring-cell type (6%). Alternatively, in a separate study of 7970 appendectomy specimens, tumors were identified in 1% of specimens, with carcinoids representing 57% of all tumors identified (65). Adenomas and adenocarcinomas represented 18% and 11% of the identified tumors, respectively.

■ PRESENTATION AND PROGNOSIS

The majority of appendiceal tumors are identified incidentally at the time of pathological review of appendectomy specimens (66). Symptoms of appendicitis are most often the presenting symptom, especially with tumors located at the base of the appendix where obstruction is more likely to occur. Other symptoms seen with more advanced appendiceal disease can reflect the nonspecific abdominal symptoms associated with peritoneal involvement: abdominal pain and distention, altered bowel motility, and early satiety. Metastatic carcinoid tumors may also present with symptoms related to the carcinoid syndrome with episodic flushing, wheezing, and diarrhea. Patient age at presentation differs depending on histologic subtype of the tumor, with the mean age for patients with carcinoid tumors of 38 years and the mean age for those with adenocarcinomas of 60 years (63).

Staging for appendiceal cancers is based on the tumor, node, metastasis (TNM) staging system for CRC (67). Prognosis for appendiceal cancer is strongly dependent on the histopathologic subtype of the tumor, with patients who have carcinoids having a significantly better survival than do patients with adenocarcinomas (Fig. 20-2) (63). In addition, early stage tumors identified incidentally at the time of appendectomy have a better prognosis than patients who are diagnosed once symptoms develop.

Prognosis for patients with epithelial tumors is also strongly dependent on histopathology of the tumor. For metastatic epithelial tumors of the appendix prognosis is excellent for those with low-grade mucinous tumors, termed disseminated peritoneal adenomucinosis, whereas appendiceal adenocarcinomas with high-grade histological features such as poor differentiation or signet ring-cell morphology have a much poorer survival.

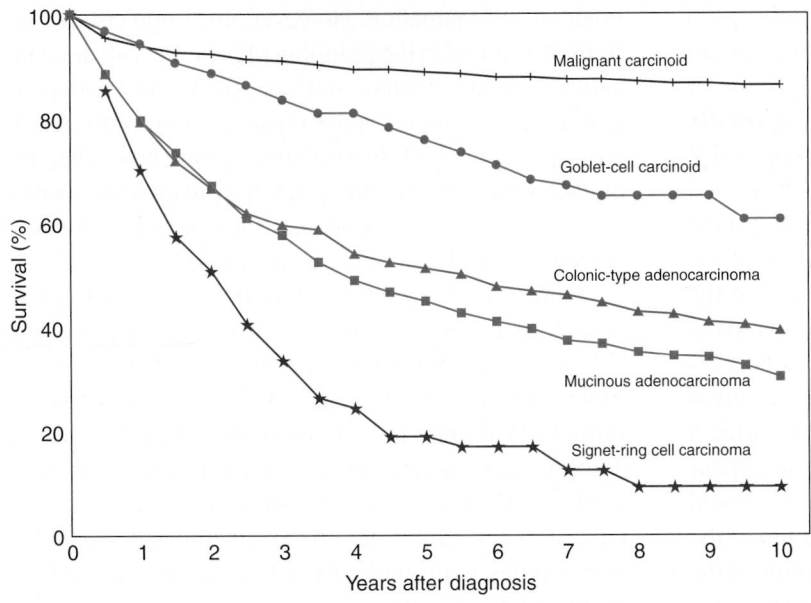

FIGURE 20-2. Overall survival of malignant appendiceal cancers according to the Surveillance, Epidemiology and End Results registry (SEER), stratified by histological subtype. (*Reproduced, with permission, from McCusker ME, Coté TR, Clegg LX, et al. Primary malignant neoplasms of the appendix. Cancer 2002;94[12]:3307-3312.*)

APPENDICEAL CARCINOID TUMORS

Similar to other intestinal carcinoid tumors, appendiceal carcinoid tumors arise from neuroendocrine cells within the lamina propria and submucosa. Appendiceal carcinoid tumors can secrete serotonin and vasoactive substances responsible for the carcinoid syndrome, though this is rarely seen in patients in the absence of extensive liver metastases. Appendiceal carcinoid tumors are usually seen in young patients and are seen slightly more common in women (68,69).

A rare histological variant of carcinoid tumors, termed goblet-cell carcinoids, or adenocarcinoids, is characterized by malignant cells that demonstrate both exocrine and neuroendocrine characteristics. This histological subtype has outcomes in between that of a carcinoid and that of an adenocarcinoma (Fig. 20-2) (70).

MANAGEMENT OF APPENDICEAL CARCINOIDS

As most appendiceal carcinoid tumors are discovered incidentally from an appendectomy specimen, a critical and somewhat controversial oncologic question relates to the need for performing a more complete surgical staging procedure. For appendiceal cancers, a complete surgical staging procedure would entail a right hemicolectomy with complete removal of the base of the appendix, mesoappendix, and draining lymph nodes.

The most useful criteria used to determine the need for a complete right hemicolectomy are tumor size (≥2 cm in diameter) or mesoappendix involvement (71). In

a retrospective study of appendiceal carcinoids, Moertel et al. reported no metastases in 127 patients with tumors <2 cm, whereas metastatic disease was seen in 3 of the 14 patients with tumors 2 to 3 cm and 4 of the 9 patients with tumors ≥3 cm (72). Patients with an adenocarcinoid histological variant are generally treated as an appendiceal adenocarcinoma.

For patients with metastatic disease, the use of somatostatin analogs can alleviate the symptoms of the carcinoid syndrome but rarely causes objective tumor regression. Given the slow-growing nature of appendiceal carcinoid tumors, local modality therapies such as hepatic embolization or surgical resection may also be beneficial in selected patients with metastatic disease. For additional information on management of this type of tumor, please refer to Chapter 23.

APPENDICEAL EPITHELIAL TUMORS

Little is known about the risk factors or etiology of epithelial tumors of the appendix. Although generally viewed as a subset of CRC, most epithelial tumors of the appendix have a markedly different biology and natural history than do adenocarcinomas of the colorectum. In particular, a subset of appendiceal epithelial tumors that have disseminated peritoneal mucinous deposits derived from a ruptured appendiceal mucinous adenoma can demonstrate excellent long-term survival with aggressive surgical cytoreduction (CRS) and hyperthermic intraperitoneal chemotherapy (HIPEC) (73,74).

Most appendiceal epithelial tumors begin as a mucinous adenoma with appendiceal distention caused by excessive mucin production. On gross inspection or radiographic evaluation, this dilated mucin-filled appendix is frequently referred to as a mucocele. With progressive growth, the appendiceal lumen can become obstructed and result in increased intraluminal pressure within the appendix, which can cause the appendix to rupture. Appendiceal rupture represents the critical step in the dissemination of the mucinous appendiceal tumor to the peritoneal cavity. For this reason, it is critical that care is taken when surgically removing an appendiceal mucocele to prevent rupture and peritoneal seeding during a routine appendectomy (75). When resecting an appendiceal mucocele, the peritoneum should be inspected closely to evaluate any evidence of dissemination to the peritoneal cavity. During pathological examination of the appendix, any fluid or mucus in the peritoneal spaces surrounding the appendix should undergo cytologic examination (71). In patients with localized disease, the presence of carcinoma requires a completion right hemicolectomy for oncologic staging.

■ PSEUDOMYXOMA PERITONEI

Pseudomyxoma peritonei (PMP), or false mucinous tumor, is a term originally described by Werth in 1884, who described the pathological findings in a patient with a ruptured ovarian cystadenoma who had copious gelatinous intraperitoneal ascites (Fig. 20-3) (76). This term has been applied broadly to include any mucinous tumor-type involving the peritoneal cavity with any histologic grade of differentiation. However, this imprecise definition has resulted in the grouping of patients with dramatically different outcomes and has generated considerable confusion for patients and even among clinicians. A better understanding of disease biology has shown that this clinical term is most appropriately applied to the pathological subtype of appendiceal tumors called disseminated peritoneal adenomucinosis (DPAM) (77).

However, the term PMP is frequently utilized to refer to the clinical syndrome of mucinous peritoneal deposits resulting from any mucinous appendiceal tumor. When used in this fashion this term encompasses both DPAM and the appendiceal epithelial tumor subtype termed peritoneal mucinous carcinomatosis (PMCA). However, the inclusion of these two histological subtypes combines two appendiceal epithelial tumor types with markedly different overall survivals (Table 20-5) (77,78).

■ HISTOPATHOLOGIC SUBTYPES OF EPITHELIAL APPENDICEAL TUMORS

DISSEMINATED PERITONEAL ADENOMUCINOSIS

Disseminated peritoneal adenomucinosis (DPAM) is characterized by peritoneal lesions composed of abundant extracellular mucin-containing scant simple to focally proliferative mucinous epithelium with little cytologic atypia or mitotic activity, with or without an associated appendiceal mucinous adenoma (77). In essence, the underlying epithelium in DPAM may have low-grade adenomatous changes but may not have any

| TABLE 20-5 | OVERALL SURVIVAL FOR APPENDICEAL EPITHELIAL TUMORS STRATIFIED BY HISTOLOGY SUBTYPE OF DISSEMINATED PERITONEAL ADENOMUCINOSIS (DPAM) OR PERITONEAL MUCINOUS CARCINOMATOSIS (PMCA) | | | | | | |

			DPAM			PMCA		
Author	*Year*	*Study*	*No. of Pts.*	*5-Year OS*	*10-Year OS*	*No. of Pts.*	*5-Year OS*	*10-Year OS*
Miner	2005	Retrospective, MSKCC	42	85%	70%	46	40%	12%
Sugarbaker	1999	Retrospective, Washington Cancer Institute	224	80%		161	28%	
Stewart	2006	Retrospective, Wake Forest University	55	68%		29	35%	
Ronnett	2001	Retrospective, Washington Cancer Institute	65	75%	68%	43	26%	9%
Smeenk*	2007	Retrospective, Netherlands Cancer Institute	66	73%*		7	0%*	

MSKCC, Memorial Sloan Kettering Cancer Center; No. of Pts, number of patients; OS, overall survival.
*Disease-specific survival.

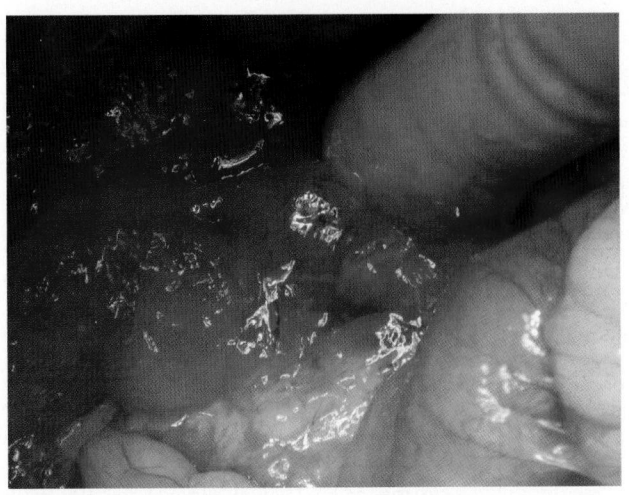

FIGURE 20-3. Peritoneal mucin in a patient undergoing surgical cytoreduction for peritoneal mucinous carcinomatosis (PMCA). (*Reproduced, with permission, from Ronnett BM, Zahn CM, Kurman RJ, et al. Disseminated peritoneal adenomucinosis and peritoneal mucinous carcinomatosis. A clinicopathologic analysis of 109 cases with emphasis on distinguishing pathologic features, site of origin, prognosis, and relationship to "pseudomyxoma peritonei." Am J Surg Pathol 1995; 19[12]:1390-408.*)

evidence of invasion or carcinoma. This subgroup of tumors (DPAMs) demonstrates the classic PMP clinical syndrome of massive amounts of benign-appearing mucinous ascites that over time slowly fill the entire peritoneal cavity (Fig. 20-4). Although spread to the peritoneal cavity is present, these tumors do not metastasize to regional lymph nodes or via hematogenous spread to the liver or other distant sites (79).

Patients with DPAM typically present with gradually increasing abdominal girth (80). For women, DPAM may present as a new ovarian mass, and for men it may present as a new-onset hernia (80). In women, secondary involvement of the ovaries is common, and since histopathological features of DPAM from a primary ovarian tumor are extremely rare, a thorough pathological examination of the appendix should be conducted (81). When molecular and immunohistochemical evaluations have been performed on cases with both appendix and ovarian involvement, these evaluations have uniformly demonstrated the primary site of disease as the appendix (82-84).

PERITONEAL MUCINOUS CARCINOMATOSIS

If evidence of invasion and carcinoma is present, then the pathological diagnosis of peritoneal mucinous carcinomatosis (PMCA) should be used (77). PMCA is characterized by peritoneal lesions composed of more abundant mucinous epithelium with the architectural

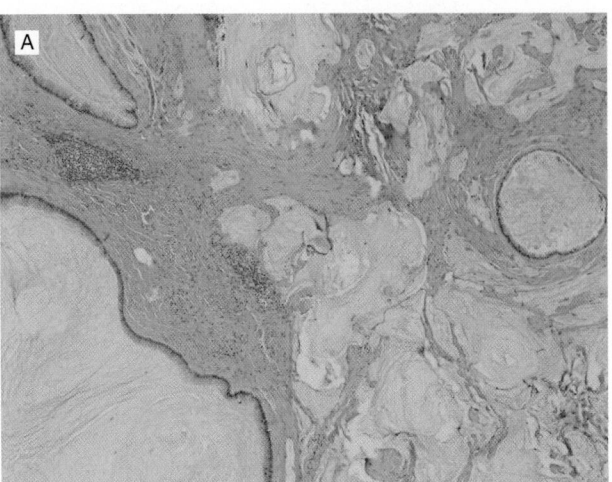

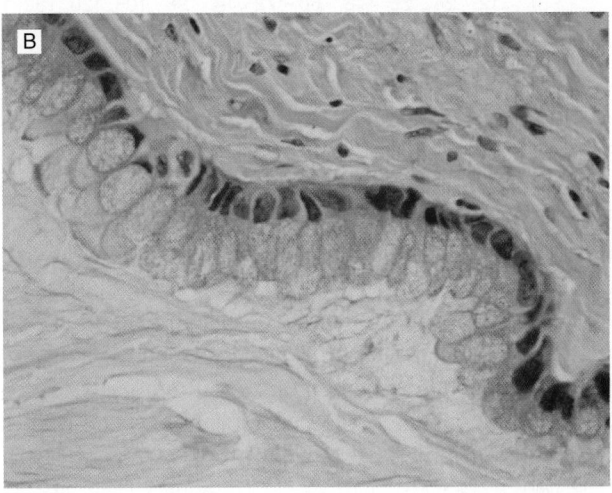

FIGURE 20-4. Histology from a patient with disseminated peritoneal adenomucinosis (DPAM) and the clinical syndrome of pseudomyxoma peritonei (PMP): (A) adenoma-like epithelium with acellular mucin pools dissecting through the fibrous stroma with chronic inflammation, 40 X magnification; (B) adenoma-like epithelium with abundant acellular mucin, 400 X magnification.

and cytologic features of carcinoma, with or without an associated primary mucinous adenocarcinoma. A subset of PMCA tumors that demonstrate features of both DPAM and PMCA have been termed PMCA with intermediate or discordant features (PMCA-I/D) (77). In an analysis of 109 patients with clinical features of PMP, 60% were classified as DPAM, 27% were classified as PMCA, and 13% were classified as PMCA-I/D (77,85). In this study, the 5- and 10-year survival rates for patient with DPAM were 75% and 68%, respectively. This was significantly higher than patients with PMCA who demonstrated 5- and 10-year survival rates of 14% and 3%. Those patients with PMCA-I/D had survival more closely associated with that of PMCA patients (Fig. 20-5).

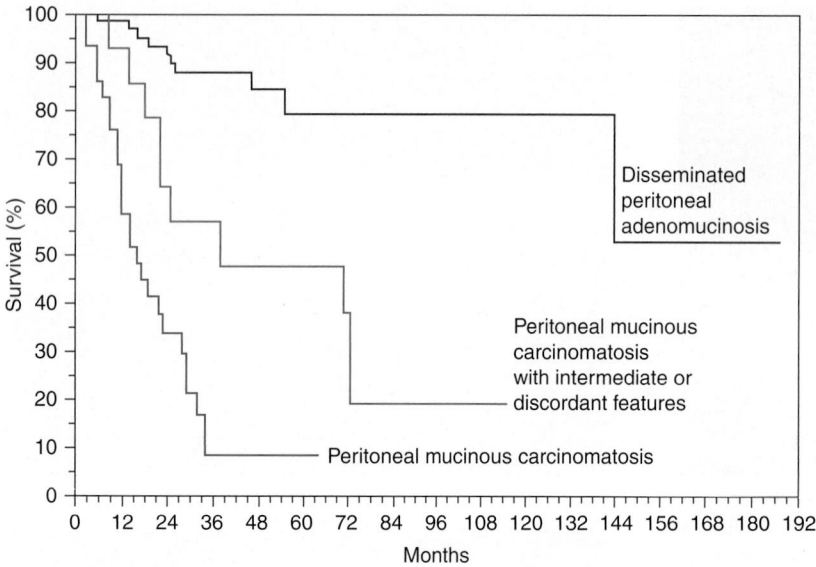

FIGURE 20-5. Overall survival for 109 cases with the clinical syndrome of pseudomyxoma peritonei (PMP) according to histological subtype.

Although appendiceal PMCAs are invasive tumors with distant metastatic potential, the majority of these tumors will remain localized to the peritoneal cavity. Even in the subset of patients with very aggressive-appearing histologies, the rate of distant hematogenous metastases remains low. In one retrospective study of 90 appendiceal adenocarcinomas with either poor differentiation or signet ring-cell morphology the rate of extraperitoneal metastases was only 17% (86).

NONMUCINOUS/COLONIC-TYPE ADENOCARCINOMA

Occurring less frequently, nonmucinous or colonic-type adenocarcinomas of the appendix demonstrate a different tumor biology than mucinous appendiceal tumors. These cancers are more aggressive and appear to behave more like colonic adenocarcinomas. In a study by Kabbani et al., 43% of patients with nonmucinous apendiceal adenocarcinoma had evidence of extraperitoneal metastases (87). The patients with nonmucinous carcinomas in this study had a significantly worse overall survival and disease-free survival than those with mucinous carcinomas.

■ TREATMENT

CYTOREDUCTIVE SURGERY

Because of the relative rarity of this disease, prospective randomized clinical trials studying the treatment of appendiceal epithelial tumors are lacking. The majority of data evaluating the various treatment modalities in this disease have been derived from retrospective, single-institution studies. Surgical cytoreduction has been the primary mode of therapy for these tumors based on the following factors:

1. Lack of extraperitoneal disease spread
2. Primarily mucinous nature of peritoneal deposits
3. Indolent growth rate
4. Limited activity of systemic chemotherapy
5. Lack of an effective systemic mucolytic agent

The goal of surgical cytoreduction is complete tumor removal from the peritoneal cavity. Because of the large surface area of the peritoneum, surgical cytoreduction to remove all visible sites of disease can be challenging. Optimal cytoreductive surgery (CRS) may involve removal of the appendix, right colon, intraperitoneal tumor debulking, resection of multiple abdominal and pelvic organs with peritoneal tumor studding, and stripping of all involved parietal peritoneum (88). Following successful surgical cytoreduction patients with the DPAM or PMCA tumors can experience re-accumulation of mucinous peritoneal implants, which may be complicated by fibrosis from prior surgery, requiring repeated surgical cytoreductive procedures.

In a 97-patient series from Memorial Sloan Kettering Cancer Center, in which surgical resection alone represented the primary treatment modality in over two-thirds of the patients, the 5-year overall survival rate was 90% for patients with DPAM and 50% for patients with PMCA (73). In the 55% of patients who underwent a complete cytoreduction of all visible tumors, 91% had recurrent disease. The average number of surgical cytoreductions that patients underwent in this study was 2.2, with a range of 1 to 6 (73).

HYPERTHERMIC INTRAPERITONEAL CHEMOTHERAPY

In an attempt to diminish the rate of disease recurrence following cytoreductive surgery, the administration of intraperitoneal chemotherapy following a surgical cytoreduction has been used to try and treat any residual microscopic disease in the peritoneal cavity. Historically a number of methods of delivering intraperitoneal chemotherapy have been utilized; although the most commonly utilized method is hyperthermic intraperitoneal chemotherapy (HIPEC) administered at the time of cytoreduction (89).

At MD Anderson, following complete cytoreductive surgery, administration of heated mitomycin C at a dose of 25 mg/m^2 for patients who are chemo-naïve or 20 mg/m^2 for patients who have received previous chemotherapy in a volume of 5 to 6.5 L of electrolyte solution at a flow rate of 3 to 3.5 L/min. Intraoperative hemodynamic monitoring and thermal monitoring are essential for optimal outcomes in these patients. The HIPEC is continued for 90 minutes with vigorous shaking of the closed abdomen. Upon completion of HIPEC, necessary bowel anastomoses are performed and gastrostomy and jejunostomy tubes are placed for postoperative management of nutritional deficiencies and prolonged gastric ileus.

Intraperitoneal administration of chemotherapy offers an advantage of providing high concentrations of drug directly to the target, while hyperthermia provides a synergistic anti-tumor effect when combined with chemotherapy (90). However, as a locally applied modality, the maximum penetration into tumor tissue is usually limited to 2 to 5 mm from the surface (91). At present, no randomized study has compared the benefit of adding HIPEC to surgical cytoreduction, although single-institution series have indirectly suggested a benefit when disease-free survival rates of patients treated with surgical cytoreduction and HIPEC (37-57%) (78,92) are compared with the historical rates of surgical cytoreduction alone (9-12%) (73,93).

Cytoreductive surgery with HIPEC represents an aggressive treatment requiring significant surgical expertise and should only be conducted at centers experienced in performing peritoneal cytoreduction. Operation time is approximately 8 to 12 h, with an average hospital stay of 20 to 25 days. The 30-day postoperative mortality

and morbidity range from 0 to 12% and 12 to 56%, respectively (92,94).

Prognosis for patients undergoing cytoreductive surgery with HIPEC is primarily dependent on two critical factors: histologic classification and completeness of surgical resection. A quantitative score, the completeness of cytoreduction score proposed by Sugarbaker and colleagues, categorizes the completeness of cytoreduction (CC) based on the size of nodules remaining at the end of surgery: CC-0 (no visible disease), CC-1 (nodules <0.25 cm), CC-2 (nodules 0.25 to <2.5 cm), and CC-3 (nodules ≥2.5 cm) (74, 95). In an analysis of 224 patients with DPAM histology, Sugarbaker et al. found that patients with complete cytoreduction (CC-0 or CC-1) had a 5-year overall survival rate of 86%, whereas patients with incomplete cytoreduction (CC-2 or CC-3) had a 5-year overall survival rate of 20% (*p* <.0001) (Fig. 20-6) (74). The importance of completeness of cytoreduction has been confirmed by other authors, though various methods of categorizing a complete cytoreduction have been used (78,92).

Additional prognostic measures include the peritoneal cancer index (PCI), a quantitative measure of the size and distribution of nodules on the peritoneal surface; the previous surgical score (PSS), a measure of the extent of prior cytoreduction; and the extent of disease on the small bowel and small bowel mesentery (73,74,96,97). The prognostic value of these different factors relates primarily to their ability to predict the likelihood of obtaining a complete cytoreduction.

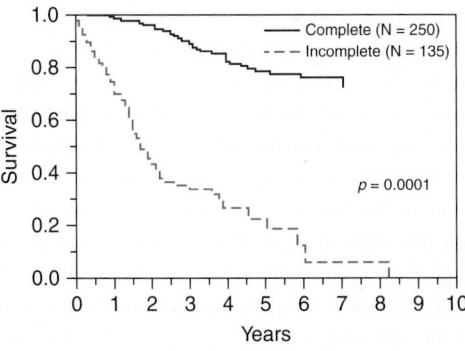

FIGURE 20-6. Overall survival for 385 cases with the mucinous epithelial tumors of the appendix (disseminated peritoneal adenomucinosis and peritoneal mucinous carcinomatosis) according to completeness of surgical cytoreduction. Complete cytoreduction defined as a completeness of cytoreduction score (CC) of CC-0 or CC-1, and an incomplete cytoreduction defined as a score of CC-2 or CC-3. (*Reproduced, with permission, from Sugarbaker PH. Results of treatment of 385 patients with peritoneal surface spread of appendiceal malignancy. Ann Surg Onc 1999;6[8].*)

For patients who cannot undergo complete cytoreductive surgery, the benefit obtained from an incomplete cytoreduction remains unknown. If complete cytoreductive surgery cannot be performed, a surgical cytoreduction is generally considered only if there are particular symptoms that can be palliated by tumor debulking. Given that HIPEC has limited tumor penetration, use of HIPEC should be limited to patients with a complete or near-complete cytoreductive surgery.

■ SYSTEMIC CHEMOTHERAPY

The role of systemic chemotherapy has not been well delineated in appendiceal epithelial tumors and has generally been utilized in patients who are not candidates for surgical cytoreduction (98). The challenges of using systemic chemotherapy to treat appendiceal

tumors relate to the slow-growing nature of the disease, the primarily mucinous component of the tumors, and the challenges in radiographically measuring disease response.

Traditionally, PMP has been considered resistant to systemic chemotherapy, although a recently completed phase II study evaluating the use of concurrent mitomycin C and capecitabine in patients with advanced, unresectable DPAM or PMCA has suggested a role for systemic chemotherapy (99). In this study of 39 patients, a clinical benefit rate of 38% was determined based on the definition of either semiquantitative reductions in mucinous deposition or stabilization of previously progressive disease (99). In this study, the 2-year cancer-related mortality rate was 39%. Elevations in tumor markers (CEA, CA 19-9, or CA-125) occurred in all patients, and a 50% reduction in one of these markers occurred in 51% of patients (99). Although limited by

---

Commentary: Surgical Perspectives in Appendiceal Carcinoma

Once the diagnosis of appendiceal carcinoma has been established, a thorough evaluation must be performed including computer tomography (CT) imaging, colonoscopy, laboratory studies, and a complete medical history to determine the potential resectability of the tumor and the appropriateness and fitness of the patient for aggressive treatment.

In our experience, patients over the age of 70 must be approached with caution because the potential risks of CRS and HIPEC may be greater than the potential benefits. A number of studies have also identified an ECOG status of <2, as essential for patients to tolerate CRS/HIPCE. Similarly, because of the sensitivity of the liver to hyperthermia, patients with evidence of cirrhosis are not offered HIPEC. Likewise, patients with renal insufficiency may prove difficult to manage postoperatively because of significant fluid shifts associated with surgery and HIPEC. Previous surgical procedures and obesity offers the same challenges as in other complex operations, but are not contraindications to surgery.

To determine the extent of the tumor and potential for complete cytoreduction, CT scans of the chest, abdomen, and pelvis appear to be the most useful. We do not use MRI or PET scanning routinely as these offer little advantage over CT alone. Imaging findings suggestive of an inability to completely cytoreduce the tumor include: a large volume of disease involving the porta hepatis and the retrohepatic vena cava, large volume of tumor involving the small bowel mesentery with a gathering together of this mesentery termed "cauliflowering," obstruction of more than one segment of small bowel, and evidence for retroperitoneal organ involvement. In these patients, consideration for systemic

chemotherapy should be given with surgery limited to palliation of symptoms.

At MD Anderson, we often see patients who have been evaluated and treated at outside institutions. Many patients have undergone an incomplete cytoreduction or combinations of therapy that we would not consider standard. The approach to these patients begins with an evaluation of the pathology, review of all operative notes to assess the amount of disease present at the time of surgery and extent of disease left behind at the completion of surgery. Repeat imaging is obtained as necessary. Upon completion of the workup, an individualized plan is developed. If the patient had what was described as a complete cytoreduction, and CT imaging demonstrates no evidence of disease, repeat imaging is performed at 6 month intervals and consideration is given to diagnostic laparoscopy at the 1 year anniversary of the original surgery. If there is disease identified during these steps, CRS/HIPEC is offered if the patient meets the selection criteria previously outline.

In patients who have clearly had and incomplete cytoreduction or have evidence of disease on baseline imaging, if the pathology is low or moderate grade appendiceal adenocarcinoma, we offer CRS/HIPEC. In the setting of high-grade/signet ring-cell appendiceal adenocarcinoma, we typically have the patient evaluated for systemic chemotherapy. If after completing systemic chemotherapy there is stability of disease and the disease is potentially resectable based on imaging studies, we may offer CRS/HIPEC in selected cases.

Keith F. Fournier

the small sample size, tumor marker response did not appear to correlate with radiographically assessed clinical benefit rate (99).

In an additional study supporting the role of systemic chemotherapy in patients with PMCA, Shapiro et al. retrospectively reviewed data collected from 54 patients who were suboptimal surgical cytoreductive candidates (98). Systemic chemotherapy in this report consisted of a fluoropyrimidine with or without a platinum agent in 69% of patients. Radiographic stabilization or response to therapy was noted in 55% of patients, median progression-free survival was 7.6 months, and median overall survival was 56 months (98). In this study, poorly differentiated histology and signet-ring histology were both negative prognostic indicators for overall survival.

The studies discussed in this section suggest a role for chemotherapy in patients who are suboptimal candidates for cytoreductive surgery, but further prospective randomized clinical trials will be needed before any definitive statement regarding the exact benefit and timing of chemotherapy use can be made.

■ THE MD ANDERSON APPROACH TO EPITHELIAL APPENDICEAL TUMORS

Unlike CRC, appendiceal epithelial malignancies have a more indolent natural history that is determined by their underlying histopathology. At MD Anderson, patients with DPAM and well-to-moderately differentiated PMCA tumors are evaluated initially for cytoreductive surgery. Patients with a complete cytoreduction (CC-0 or CC-1) are treated with HIPEC utilizing intraperitoneal mitomycin at 42°C. If a complete cytoreductive surgery is not obtained, or if radiographic imaging indicates that obtaining a complete cytoreduction is highly unlikely, or medical comorbidities preclude a surgical procedure; then patients are considered for systemic chemotherapy. HIPEC is also utilized at MD Anderson for the control of refractory ascites. We have found that the use of HIPEC in patients who have undergone an incomplete cytoreductive surgery can provide long-term control of ascites, and should be considered in patients with refractory ascites.

Given the indolent nature of well-to-moderate PMCA tumors, systemic chemotherapy is generally reserved for patients who either have clear evidence of disease progression on radiographic imaging or have significant tumor-related symptoms. Frontline chemotherapy is fluoropyrimidine-based, and additional agents may be added based on the perceived tolerance of more aggressive combinations. Given the general good prognosis of these patients, it is critical that treatment is closely aligned with quality of life and that cumulative toxicities are kept to a minimum.

The use of multiagent systemic chemotherapy, as administered in CRC, is the treatment of choice for patients who have signet-ring cells, poorly differentiated tumors, or nonmucinous tumors. Since patients with poorly differentiated or signet ring-cell appendiceal adenocarcinomas have consistently shown worse outcomes following aggressive cytoreductive surgery, our approach has been to only consider surgical cytoreduction in these patients following initial treatment with systemic chemotherapy. In a recent retrospective study from MD Anderson, Lieu et al. showed that patients with stage IV poorly differentiated or signet ring-cell morphology appendiceal adenocarcinomas had an median overall survival of 24 months, which appears very similar to the known overall survival for metastatic CRC (86).

Although trials evaluating the benefit of vascular-endothelial growth factor (VEGF) inhibitors or epidermal growth factor receptor (EGFR) inhibitors in appendiceal epithelial tumors are lacking, their effectiveness in CRC suggests a possible role for these agents in appendiceal epithelial tumors. VEGF expression has been demonstrated in appendiceal adenocarcinomas and high levels of expression have been correlated with poor outcome (100). Though not well studied, it appears that mutations in the K-ras oncogene are common with 22 of 31 tested samples demonstrating an activating mutation in K-ras (101).

Due to the rarity of appendiceal tumors, our understanding of these tumors is limited, and further research into the molecular characteristics of these tumors is needed. The role of cytoreductive surgery is well-established for appendiceal epithelial tumors. The use of systemic chemotherapy in appendiceal epithelial tumors needs further study and, in particular, the role of newer targeted therapies needs to be determined.

References

1. Jemal A, Siegel R, Ward E, et al. Cancer statistics, 2009. *CA Cancer J Clin* 2009;59(4):225-249.
2. Key C, Meisner A. Cancers of the esophagus, stomach, and small intestine. In: Ries LAG et al (eds): *SEER Survival Monograph: Cancer Survival Among Adults: U.S. SEER Program, 1988-2001, Patient and Tumor Characteristics*. National Cancer Institute, SEER Program, NIH Pub. No. 07-6215, Bethesda, MD, 2007.
3. Weiss NS, Yang CP. Incidence of histologic types of cancer of the small intestine. *J Natl Cancer Inst* 1987;78(4):653-656.

4. Haselkorn T, Whittemore AS, Lilienfeld DE. Incidence of small bowel cancer in the United States and worldwide: Geographic, temporal, and racial differences. *Cancer Causes Control* 2005;16(7):781-787.

5. Howe JR, Karnell LH, Menck HR, et al. The American College of Surgeons Commission on Cancer and the American Cancer Society. Adenocarcinoma of the small bowel: Review of the National Cancer Data Base, 1985-1995. *Cancer* 1999; 86(12):2693-2706.

6. Hatzaras I, Palesty JA, Abir F, et al. Small-bowel tumors: Epidemiologic and clinical characteristics of 1260 cases from the connecticut tumor registry. *Arch Surg* 2007; 142(3):229-35.

7. Scelo G, Boffetta P, Hemminki K, et al. Associations between small intestine cancer and other primary cancers: An international population-based study. *Int J Cancer* 2006; 118(1):189-96.

8. Sellner F. Investigations on the significance of the adenoma-carcinoma sequence in the small bowel. *Cancer* 1990;66(4): 702-715.

9. Ryan DP, Schapiro RH, Warshaw AL. Villous tumors of the duodenum. *Ann Surg* 1986;203(3):301-306.

10. Joesting DR, Beart RW, Jr., van Heerden JA, et al. Improving survival in adenocarcinoma of the duodenum. *Am J Surg* 1981;141(2):228-231.

11. Perzin KH, Bridge MF. Adenomas of the small intestine: A clinicopathologic review of 51 cases and a study of their relationship to carcinoma. *Cancer* 1981;48(3):799-819.

12. Neugut A. The association between cancers of the small and large bowel. *Cancer Epidemiol Biomarkers Prev* 1993;2.

13. Planck M, Ericson K, Piotrowska Z, et al. Microsatellite instability and expression of MLH1 and MSH2 in carcinomas of the small intestine. *Cancer* 2003;97(6):1551-1557.

14. Spigelman AD, Williams CB, Talbot IC, et al. Upper gastrointestinal cancer in patients with familial adenomatous polyposis. *Lancet* 1989;2(8666):783-785.

15. Ross RK, Hartnett NM, Bernstein L, et al. Epidemiology of adenocarcinomas of the small intestine: Is bile a small bowel carcinogen? *Br J Cancer* 1991;63(1):143-145.

16. Wu AH, Yu MC, Mack TM. Smoking, alcohol use, dietary factors and risk of small intestinal adenocarcinoma. *Int J Cancer* 1997;70(5):512-517.

17. Chow WH, Linet MS, McLaughlin JK, et al. Risk factors for small intestine cancer. *Cancer Causes Control* 1993;4(2): 163-9.

18. Chen CC, Neugut AI, Rotterdam H. Risk factors for adenocarcinomas and malignant carcinoids of the small intestine: Preliminary findings. *Cancer Epidemiol Biomarkers Prev* 1994; 3(3):205-207.

19. Negri E, Dal Maso L, Ron E, et al. Risk factors for adenocarcinoma of the small intestine. *Int J Cancer* 1999;82(2):171-4.

20. Neugut AI, Jacobson JS, Suh S, et al. The epidemiology of cancer of the small bowel. *Cancer Epidemiol Biomarkers Prev* 1998;7(3):243-251.

21. Schatzkin A, Park Y, Leitzmann MF, et al. Prospective study of dietary fiber, whole grain foods, and small intestinal cancer. *Gastroenterology* 2008;135(4):1163-1167.

22. Delaunoit T, Neczyporenko F, Limburg PJ, et al. Pathogenesis and risk factors of small bowel adenocarcinoma: A colorectal cancer sibling? *Am J Gastroenterol* 2005;100(3): 703-710.

23. Bjorge T, Tretli S, Engeland A. Height and body mass index in relation to cancer of the small intestine in two million Norwegian men and women. *Br J Cancer* 2005;93(7):807-10.

24. Wolk A, Gridley G, Svensson M, et al. A prospective study of obesity and cancer risk (Sweden). *Cancer Causes Control* 2001;12(1):13-21.

25. Samanic C, Gridely G, Chow WH, et al. Obesity and cancer risk among white and black United States veterans. *Cancer Causes Control* 2004;15(1):35-43.

26. Groves CJ, Saunders BP, Spigelman AD, et al. Duodenal cancer in patients with familial adenomatous polyposis (FAP): Results of a 10 year prospective study. *Gut* 2002;50(5):636-641.

27. Giardiello FM, Brensinger JD, Tersmette AC, et al. Very high risk of cancer in familial Peutz-Jeghers syndrome. *Gastroenterology* 2000;119(6):1447-1453.

28. Aarnio M, Mecklin JP, Aaltonen LA, et al. Life-time risk of different cancers in hereditary non-polyposis colorectal cancer (HNPCC) syndrome. *Int J Cancer* 1995;64(6):430-433.

29. Vasen HF, Wijnen JT, Menko FH, et al. Cancer risk in families with hereditary nonpolyposis colorectal cancer diagnosed by mutation analysis. *Gastroenterology* 1996;110(4): 1020-1027.

30. Jagelman DG, DeCosse JJ, Bussey HJ. Upper gastrointestinal cancer in familial adenomatous polyposis. *Lancet* 1988; 1(8595):1149-1151.

31. Palascak-Juif V, Bouvier AM, Cosnes J, et al. Small bowel adenocarcinoma in patients with Crohn's disease compared with small bowel adenocarcinoma de novo. *Inflamm Bowel Dis* 2005;11(9):828-832.

32. Abrahams NA, Halverson A, Fazio VW, et al. Adenocarcinoma of the small bowel: A study of 37 cases with emphasis on histologic prognostic factors. *Dis Colon Rectum* 2002; 45(11):1496-1502.

33. Maglinte DD, O'Connor K, Bessette J, et al. The role of the physician in the late diagnosis of primary malignant tumors of the small intestine. *Am J Gastroenterol* 1991; 86(3):304-308.

34. Bessette JR, Maglinte DD, Kelvin FM, et al. Primary malignant tumors in the small bowel: A comparison of the small-bowel enema and conventional follow-through examination. *AJR Am J Roentgenol* 1989;153(4):741-744.

35. Bruneton JN, Drouillard J, Bourry J, et al. Adenocarcinoma of the small intestine. Current state of diagnosis and treatment. A study of 27 cases and a review of the literature. *J Radiol* 1983;64(2):117-123.

36. Lewis BS, Eisen GM, Friedman S. A pooled analysis to evaluate results of capsule endoscopy trials. *Endoscopy* 2005; 37(10):960-965.

37. Sturniolo GC, Di Leo V, Vettorato MG, et al. Clinical relevance of small-bowel findings detected by wireless capsule endoscopy. *Scand J Gastroenterol* 2005;40(6):725-733.

38. Cobrin G, Pittman R, Lewis B. Diagnosing small bowel tumors with capsule endoscopy [abstract 86]. American Society of Clinical Oncology Gastrointestinal Cancers Symposium, 2005.

39. Midwinter MJ, Beveridge CJ, Wilsdon JB, et al. Correlation between spiral computed tomography, endoscopic ultrasonography and findings at operation in pancreatic and ampullary tumours. *Br J Surg* 1999;86(2):189-193.

40. Oh YS, Early DS, Azar RR. Clinical applications of endoscopic ultrasound to oncology. *Oncology* 2005;68(4-6):526-537.

41. Greene FL, Page DL,, Fleming ID, et. al. AJCC *Cancer Staging Manual*, 6th ed. New York: Springer; 2005.

42. Agrawal S, McCarron EC, Gibbs JF, et al. Surgical management and outcome in primary adenocarcinoma of the small bowel. *Ann Surg Oncol* 2007;14(8):2263-2269.

43. Bauer RL, Palmer ML, Bauer AM, et al. Adenocarcinoma of the small intestine: 21-Year review of diagnosis, treatment, and prognosis. *Ann Surg Oncol* 1994;1(3):183-188.

44. Brucher BL, Stein HJ, Roder JD, et al. New aspects of prognostic factors in adenocarcinomas of the small bowel. *Hepatogastroenterology* 2001;48(39):727-732.

45. Dabaja BS, Suki D, Pro B, et al. Adenocarcinoma of the small bowel: Presentation, prognostic factors, and outcome of 217 patients. *Cancer* 2004;101(3):518-526.

46. Ouriel K, Adams JT. Adenocarcinoma of the small intestine. *Am J Surg* 1984;147(1):66-71.

47. Talamonti MS, Goetz LH, Rao S, et al. Primary cancers of the small bowel: Analysis of prognostic factors and results of surgical management. *Arch Surg* 2002;137(5):564-570; discussion 570-1.

48. Wu TJ, Yeh CN, Chao TC, et al. Prognostic factors of primary small bowel adenocarcinoma: Univariate and multivariate analysis. *World J Surg* 2006;30(3):391-398; discussion 399.

49. Bakaeen FG, Murr MM, Sarr MG, et al. What prognostic factors are important in duodenal adenocarcinoma? *Arch Surg* 2000;135(6):635-641; discussion 641-642.

50. Sohn TA, Lillemoe KD, Cameron JL, et al. Adenocarcinoma of the duodenum: Factors influencing long-term survival. *J Gastrointest Surg* 1998;2(1):79-87.

51. North JH, Pack MS. Malignant tumors of the small intestine: A review of 144 cases. *Am Surg* 2000;66(1):46-51.

52. Jemal A, Siegel R, Ward E, et al. Cancer statistics, 2008. *CA Cancer J Clin* 2008;58(2):71-96.

53. Kelsey CR, Nelson JW, Willett CG, et al. Duodenal adenocarcinoma: Patterns of failure after resection and the role of chemoradiotherapy. *Int J Radiat Oncol Biol Phys* 2007;69(5):1436-1441.

54. Barnes G Jr, Romero L, Hess KR, et al. Primary adenocarcinoma of the duodenum: Management and survival in 67 patients. *Ann Surg Oncol* 1994;1(1):73-78.

55. Klinkenbijl JH, Jeekel J, Sahmoud T, et al. Adjuvant radiotherapy and 5-fluorouracil after curative resection of cancer of the pancreas and periampullary region: Phase III trial of the EORTC gastrointestinal tract cancer cooperative group. *Ann Surg* 1999;230(6):776-782; discussion 782-784.

56. Fishman PN, Pond GR, Moore MJ, et al. Natural history and chemotherapy effectiveness for advanced adenocarcinoma of the small bowel: A retrospective review of 113 cases. *Am J Clin Oncol* 2006;29(3):225-231.

57. Halfdanarson T, Quevedo, F, McWilliams, RR. Small bowel adenocarcinoma: A review of 491 cases (abstract). *J Clin Oncol* 2006;24:209S.

58. Gibson MK, Holcroft CA, Kvols LK, et al. Phase II study of 5-fluorouracil, doxorubicin, and mitomycin C for metastatic small bowel adenocarcinoma. *Oncologist* 2005;10(2):132-137.

59. Overman MJ, Varadhachary GR, Kopetz S, et al. Phase II study of capecitabine and oxaliplatin for advanced adenocarcinoma of the small bowel and ampulla of Vater. *J Clin Oncol* 2009;27(16):2598-2603.

60. Crawley C, Ross P, Norman A, et al. The Royal Marsden experience of a small bowel adenocarcinoma treated with protracted venous infusion 5-fluorouracil. *Br J Cancer* 1998; 78(4):508-510.

61. Locher C, Malka D, Boige V, et al. Combination chemotherapy in advanced small bowel adenocarcinoma. *Oncology* 2005;69(4):290-294.

62. Overman MJ, Kopetz S, Wen S, et al. Chemotherapy with 5-fluorouracil and a platinum compound improves outcomes in metastatic small bowel adenocarcinoma. *Cancer* 2008;113(8):2038-2045.

63. McCusker ME, Coté TR, Clegg LX, et al. Primary malignant neoplasms of the appendix. *Cancer* 2002;94(12):3307-3312.

64. Fann J, Vierra M, Fisher D, et al. Pseudomyxoma peritonei. *Surg Gynecol Obstet* 1993;177:441-447.

65. Connor SJ, Hanna GB, Frizelle FA. Appendiceal tumors: Retrospective clinicopathologic analysis of appendiceal tumors from 7,970 appendectomies. *Dis Colon Rectum* 1998;41(1):75-80.

66. Roggo A, Wood W, Ottinger L. Carcinoid tumors of the appendix. *Ann Surg* 1993;217(4):385-390.

67. Greene FL Page DL, Fleming ID, et. al. *AJCC Cancer Staging Manual*. 6th ed. New York: Springer; 2005.

68. Irvin MM, Kevin DL, Mark K. A 5-decade analysis of 13,715 carcinoid tumors. *Cancer* 2003;97(4):934-959.

69. Sandor A, Modlin I. A retrospective analysis of 1570 appendiceal carcinoids. *Am J Gastroenterol* 1998;93(3):422-428.

70. McCusker ME, Cote TR, Clegg LX, et al. Primary malignant neoplasms of the appendix: A population-based study from the surveillance, epidemiology and end-results program, 1973-1998. *Cancer* 2002;94(12):3307-3312.

71. Sugarbaker PH. Epithelial appendiceal neoplasms. SO - Cancer J 2009;15(3):225-235.

72. Moertel C, Weiland L, Nagorney D, et al.Carcinoid tumor of the appendix: Treatment and prognosis. *N Engl J Med* 1987; 317(27):1699-1701.

73. Miner TJ, Shia J, Jaques DP, et al. Long-term survival following treatment of pseudomyxoma peritonei: An analysis of surgical therapy. *Ann Surg* 2005;241(2):300-308.

74. Sugarbaker PH, Chang D. Results of treatment of 385 patients with peritoneal surface spread of appendiceal malignancy. *Ann Surg Oncol* 1999;6(8):727-731.

75. Misdraji JMD, Yantiss RKMD, Graeme-Cook FMMD, et al. Appendiceal Mucinous Neoplasms: a Clinicopathologic Analysis of 107 Cases. *Am J Surg Pathol* 2003;27(8): 1089-1103.

76. Werth R. Klinische and anatomische Unteruschungen Zur Lehre Von den Bauchgeschwilsten und der Laparotomie. *Arch Gynecol Obstet* 1884;42:100-118.

77. Ronnett BM, Zahn CM, Kurman RJ, et al. Disseminated peritoneal adenomucinosis and peritoneal mucinous carcinomatosis. A clinicopathologic analysis of 109 cases with emphasis on distinguishing pathologic features, site of origin, prognosis, and relationship to "pseudomyxoma peritonei". *Am J Surg Pathol* 1995;19(12):1390-1408.

78. Smeenk RM, Verwaal VJ, Antonini N, et al. Survival analysis of pseudomyxoma peritonei patients treated by cytoreductive surgery and hyperthermic intraperitoneal chemotherapy. *Ann Surg* 2007;245(1):104-109.

79. González-Moreno S, Sugarbaker PH. Right hemicolectomy does not confer a survival advantage in patients with mucinous carcinoma of the appendix and peritoneal seeding. *Br J Surg* 2004;91(3):304-311.

80. Esquivel J, Sugarbaker PH. Clinical presentation of the pseudomyxoma peritonei syndrome. *Br J Surg* 2000;87(10):1414-1418.

81. Ronnett BM, Kurman RJ, Zahn CM, et al. Pseudomyxoma peritonei in women: a clinicopathologic analysis of 30 cases with emphasis on site of origin, prognosis, and relationship to ovarian mucinous tumors of low malignant potential. *Hum Pathol* 1995;26(5):509-524.

82. Guerrieri C, Franlund B, Fristedt S, et al. Mucinous tumors of the vermiform appendix and ovary, and pseudomyxoma peritonei: histogenetic implications of cytokeratin 7 expression. *Hum Pathol* 1997;28(9):1039-1045.

83. Ronnett BM, Shmookler BM, Diener-West M, et al. Immunohistochemical evidence supporting the appendiceal origin of pseudomyxoma peritonei in women. *Int J Gynecol Pathol* 1997;16(1):1-9.

84. Szych C, Staebler A, Connolly DC, et al. Molecular genetic evidence supporting the clonality and appendiceal origin of Pseudomyxoma peritonei in women. *Am J Pathol* 1999; 154(6):1849-1855.

85. Ronnett BM, Yan H, Kurman RJ, et al. Patients with pseudomyxoma peritonei associated with disseminated peritoneal adenomucinosis have a significantly more favorable prognosis than patients with peritoneal mucinous carcinomatosis. *Cancer* 2001;92(1):85-91.

86. Lieu C, Lambert L, Wolff R, et al. The role of surgical cytoreduction and systemic chemotherapy in metastatic poorly differentiated or signet ring cell adenocarcinomas of the appendix. Presented at the ASCO GI Symposium 2010,Orlando, FL, January, 2010 #479.

87. Kabbani W, Houlihan PS, Luthra R, et al. Mucinous and non-mucinous appendiceal adenocarcinomas: different clinico-pathological features but similar genetic alterations. *Mod Pathol* 2002;15(6):599-605.

88. Sugarbaker P. Peritonectomy procedures. *Ann Surg* 1995; 221(1):29-42.

89. Sugarbaker PH. New standard of care for appendiceal epithelial neoplasms and pseudomyxoma peritonei syndrome? *Lancet Oncol* 2006;7(1):69-76.

90. Witkamp AJ, de Bree E, Van Goethem R, et al. Rationale and techniques of intra-operative hyperthermic intraperitoneal chemotherapy. *Cancer Treat Rev* 2001;27(6):365-374.

91. Los G, Verdegaal E, Mutsaers P, et al. Penetration of carboplatin and cisplatin into rat peritoneal tumor nodules after intraperitoneal chemotherapy. *Cancer Chemother Pharmacol* 1991;28(3):159-165.

92. Stewart JHt, Shen P, Russell GB, et al. Appendiceal neoplasms with peritoneal dissemination: Outcomes after cytoreductive surgery and intraperitoneal hyperthermic chemotherapy. *Ann Surg Oncol* 2006;13(5):624-634.

93. Gough DB, Donohue JH, Schutt AJ, et al. Pseudomyxoma peritonei. Long-term patient survival with an aggressive regional approach. *Ann Surg* 1994;219(2):112-119.

94. Sugarbaker PH, Alderman R, Edwards G, et al. Prospective morbidity and mortality assessment of cytoreductive surgery plus perioperative intraperitoneal chemotherapy to treat peritoneal dissemination of appendiceal mucinous malignancy. *Ann Surg Oncol* 2006;13(5):635-44.

95. Jacquet P, Jelinek JS, Chang D, et al. Abdominal computed tomographic scan in the selection of patients with mucinous peritoneal carcinomatosis for cytoreductive surgery. *J Am Coll Surg* 1995;181(6):530-538.

96. Glehen O, Mohamed F, Sugarbaker PH. Incomplete cytoreduction in 174 patients with peritoneal carcinomatosis from appendiceal malignancy. *Ann Surg* 2004;240(2): 278-85.

97. Yan TD, Bijelic L, Sugarbaker PH. Critical analysis of treatment failure after complete cytoreductive surgery and perioperative intraperitoneal chemotherapy for peritoneal dissemination from appendiceal mucinous neoplasms. *Ann Surg Oncol* 2007;14(8):2289-2299.

98. Shapiro JF, Chase JL, Wolff RA,et al. Modern systemic chemotherapy in surgically unresectable neoplasms of appendiceal origin: A single-institution experience. *Cancer* 2009;116(2):316-22.

99. Farquharson AL, Pranesh N, Witham G, et al. A phase II study evaluating the use of concurrent mitomycin C and capecitabine in patients with advanced unresectable pseudomyxoma peritonei. *Br J Cancer* 2008;99(4):591-596.

100. Logan-Collins J, Lowy A, Robinson-Smith T, et al. VEGF expression predicts survival in patients with peritoneal surface metastases from mucinous adenocarcinoma of the appendix and colon. *Annals Surg Oncol* 2008;15(3):738-744.

101. Catalogue of Somatic Mutations in Cancer; http://www.sanger.ac.uk/genetics/CGP/cosmic/.

CHAPTER
21

COLORECTAL CANCER

Nishin Bhadkamkar
Christopher H. Crane
Miguel Rodriguez-Bigas
Scott Kopetz
Cathy Eng

Colorectal cancer is a major cause of cancer-related mortality in the United States and many other regions of the world. It is currently the second most common cause of cancer death in the United States for men and women combined (nearly 150,000 new cases and 50,000 deaths each year), accounting for about 10% of cancer mortality (1). The incidence of colorectal cancer declined by 2.1% between 1992 and 1996, and current data suggest that mortality rates may also be declining. These trends may be attributable to increased screening efforts, early intervention with prophylactic polypectomy, and improved adjuvant therapies. This has encouraged further research in prevention, detection, and treatment of colorectal cancer.

During the recent past, investigators from a variety of disciplines have made important discoveries in the areas of carcinogenesis, screening and prevention, and anticancer therapy. Over time, these advances should contribute to continued reduction in the overall incidence and mortality of colorectal cancer. As an example, standard therapy for stages III and IV colorectal cancer, which remained stagnant for many years, has continuously evolved since 2000. The number of drugs and drug combinations available for treatment and prevention has continued to grow and now includes targeted agents.

This chapter reviews our current understanding of colorectal cancer, describes the known genetic mutations and risk factors, and outlines emerging screening, prevention, and therapeutic strategies, with particular emphasis on the approach taken at the University of Texas MD Anderson Cancer Center (MDACC).

■ EPIDEMIOLOGY AND ETIOLOGY OF COLORECTAL NEOPLASIA

GEOGRAPHIC DISTRIBUTION

Colorectal cancer is more common in Western industrialized countries (ie, the United States, Canada, Scandinavia, northern and western Europe, and New Zealand) than in Asia, most of South America, and Africa (2). Since 1978, colon cancer mortality has declined in some western

European countries and in the United States, while the incidence and mortality rates for colorectal cancer continues to rise in Japan and China (2). Individuals who migrate from known low-incidence regions assume the colon cancer risk of their adopted country, implicating interplay of environmental and genetic factors in the development of this disease. The age-specific incidence of colorectal cancer in the United States rises steadily, with more than 90% of cases diagnosed in patients 50 years of age or older. The male/female ratio for colon cancer is 1.34 while the ratio for rectal cancer is 1.73 (3).

CARCINOGENESIS: THE ADENOMA-ADENOCARCINOMA SEQUENCE

Results from numerous studies, including those of Vogelstein group (4) and the National Polyp Study (5,6), suggest that colorectal neoplasia results from sequential accumulation of genetic and molecular alterations over many years, ultimately causing normal epithelium to transform into intraepithelial neoplasia (dysplasia) and then malignant epithelium. The morphologic adenoma–adenocarcinoma sequence that was recognized over 40 years ago is now known to begin with aberrant crypt foci and includes serrated lesions as well as traditional adenomas. Many distinct genetic and epigenetic pathways can eventually lead to malignancy. While a complete overview is beyond the scope of this chapter, there appear to be at least three different pathways driving carcinogenesis: chromosomal instability, microsatellite instability (MSI), and CpG island methylation. In the chromosomal instability pathway, early mutations include inherited or acquired changes in the tumor suppressor gene *APC*, located on the long arm of chromosome 5, and the K-*ras* proto-oncogene. Later genetic events include mutations in the deleted in colon cancer (*DCC*) gene on chromosome 18q and in the tumor suppressor gene *p53* on chromosome 17p. Genetic mutations occurring in inherited colorectal cancer following the chromosomal instability pathway include those of the *APC* gene in familial adenomatous polyposis (FAP). The accumulation of genetic alterations, with structural and copy number abnormalities in numerous chromosomes, eventually leads to phenotypic alterations in the colorectal epithelium. This is associated with the development of adenomas that can progress to invasive carcinoma with eventual metastases (7,8).

Since the Vogelstein group first proposed the genetic model for colorectal carcinogenesis, subsequent investigations have recognized other important pathways. In the microsatellite instability (MSI) pathway, alterations in genes encoding a variety of DNA mismatch repair enzymes occur in the inherited form of the disease (hereditary nonpolyposis colorectal cancer syndrome [HNPCC]/Warthin-Lynch syndrome) as a result of a germline mutation. Silencing of one of these genes (hMLH1) by methylation may also be seen in the sporadic form of colorectal cancer and is reported to occur in approximately 15% of patients. The form of genomic instability associated with defective DNA mismatch repair in tumors is called microsatellite instability (MSI). Mismatch repair deficiency leads to numerous mutations in single nucleotides (mutator phenotype) and genes that have repeated nucleotide sequences (microsatellites), but chromosomal alterations are uncommon (9). A panel of five microsatellites are the reference panel for determination of MSI status: the recommended validated panel is composed of two mononucleotide repeats (BAT26 and A4725) and three dinucleotide repeats (D5S346, D2S123, and D17S250) (10). Tumors may be characterized on the basis of: high-frequency MSI (MSI-H) if two or more of the five markers show instability (ie, have insertion/deletion mutations), low-frequency MSI (MSI-L) if only one of the five markers shows instability, or MSI-stable (MSI-S), if no change in loci are noted. A diagnosis of MSI-H may impact choice of adjuvant chemotherapy (11). In the CpG island methylation pathway, epigenetic hypermethylation of DNA occurs, leading to suppression of gene expression by promoter methylation (12,13). These perturbations affect expression of important regulatory proteins controlling cell morphology, growth, and adhesion. Hypomethylation of intronic DNA accompanies hypermethylation. Abnormalities of more than one of the three recognized pathways are often evident in a single colorectal cancer, as CpG island methylation can occur in concert with both the chromosomal instability pathway and the MSI pathway (12).

Other pathways have been proposed to explain the development of colon cancer in the setting of diseases such as ulcerative colitis. In this model, the primary abnormality arises within the stromal cells of the colon, resulting in a microenvironment conducive to epithelial dysregulation. This has been termed the landscaper defect pathway (14). In general, recognition of these distinct molecular pathways may alter the clinical management of established cancers, with emerging data suggesting important differences in prognosis and response to therapy may exist among them (15). Moreover, with a greater understanding of these mechanistic differences, tailored screening and preventive strategies may be developed.

TABLE 21-1 | LIFETIME RISKS OF COLORECTAL CANCER

Characteristic	Incidence
General population	5%
Personal history of colorectal cancer	15-20%
Inflammatory bowel disease	15-40%
Adenomatous polyps: personal	Variable
Hereditary nonpolyposis colorectal cancer mutation	70-80%
Familial adenomatous polyposis	>95%

RISK FACTORS

General risk factors for the development of colorectal cancer include genetic predisposition, environmental factors, and acquired risks. These factors are involved in a stepwise progression from normal colonic mucosa to adenomatous polyps to invasive adenocarcinoma. The neoplastic process often develops in individuals who have acquired (somatic) or inherited genetic (germline) mutations, which are promoted further by environmental, dietary, or other less well understood factors.

Personal or family histories of colorectal cancer or polyps, older age, and inflammatory bowel disease (IBD) have all been associated with an increased risk of colorectal cancer (Table 21-1). Other possible risk factors include a sedentary lifestyle and a diet high in fat, low in dietary fiber, or deficient in specific micronutrients. Cigarette smoking has been implicated in the formation of colonic adenomas and carcinomas, with the relative risk correlating with total exposure and duration of smoking [16].

Diet

Some studies have shown that a "Western" diet rich in saturated fat is associated with an increased risk of colon cancer, whereas a diet that includes a high proportion of fruits and vegetables seems to protect against colorectal cancer [17]. Dietary fat has been shown to promote tumors in animal models of colorectal cancer. A high-fat diet may alter the colonic flora, leading to a predominance of anaerobic species. Certain enzymes capable of metabolizing pro-carcinogens to overt carcinogens are present in higher concentrations in the large bowel. It should be noted that the role of dietary fat has not been firmly established, and some studies have failed to demonstrate that a high-fat diet is associated with an increased risk of malignancy [18].

Fiber may provide a protective effect by decreasing the concentration of fecal carcinogens and decreasing their transit time, thus reducing the period of exposure to colonic mucosa. Some studies have suggested that fresh fruits and vegetables are protective, although whether this effect is due to the fiber content or to the presence of other protective micronutrients and antioxidants remains unclear. Moreover, the protective benefit of fiber, micronutrients, or antioxidants has not been consistently demonstrated. The Nurses Health Study, a prospective study of 88,757 women aged 34 to 59 years, found no association between fiber intake (measured in grams per day) and the risk of colorectal cancer after a median follow-up of 16 years [19].

Obesity

While diets rich in fat or low in fiber have long been implicated as risk factors for colorectal cancer, more recent analyses have suggested that an increased body mass index (BMI), and in particular central obesity, is a risk factor for colorectal cancer. Data from the Framingham Study found that a BMI >30 increased the risk of colon cancer by 50% among middle-aged (30-54 years) individuals and by 2.4-fold for those aged 55 to 79 years [20]. Of note, waist circumference was actually a stronger predictor for colon cancer risk than BMI. The link between obesity and colon cancer is not fully understood; however, insulin and leptin, an adipocyte-derived hormone, have been proposed as possible factors increasing cancer risk [21].

Adenomatous Polyps

Colorectal tumors occur more often in patients with adenomatous polyps than those without polyps. Carcinoma is present in 5% of adenomas, and, in general, the risk correlates with the histology and size of the polyp. The potential for malignant transformation is 8 to 10 times higher for villous and tubulovillous adenomas than tubular adenomas. Just over 1% of adenomatous polyps <1 cm in size are malignant, whereas up to 40% of adenomas >2 cm are malignant [3].

Recent interest has developed in serrated adenomas which have a serrated hyperplastic-like architecture and adenomatous changes or dysplasia [22]. Serrated adenomas are identified in up to 7 to 15% of colonoscopies, with most polyps occurring in the left colon. Sessile-serrated adenomas are commonly right-sided, large, and poorly circumscribed, and may be confused for a fold. The serrated polyp may also have a unique molecular signature.

Inflammatory Bowel Disease

Patients with IBD (ulcerative colitis or Crohn disease) are at increased risk of developing colorectal carcinoma [23].

TABLE 21-2	CURRENT RECOMMENDATIONS FOR COLORECTAL CANCER SCREENING
Patient Populations	*Screening Tests*
General population *AND* Patient with any distant relative with CRC or polyps	FOBT annually and sigmoidoscopy every 3-5 years or colonoscopy every 10 years, beginning at age 50.
Patient with first-degree relative CRC	FOBT annually and sigmoidoscopy every 3-5 years or colonoscopy every 10 years. Begin at age 40.
Moderate-risk patients	Polyp removal; repeat colonoscopy at 3 years; if normal extend interval to 5 years.
Patient with two first-degree relatives with CRC	Colonoscopy every 3-5 years. Begin screening at age 40 or 10 years younger than youngest affected relative.
OR Patient with one first-degree relative with colorectal cancer diagnosed at 50 years of age or younger	
Patient with HNPCC risk	Colonoscopy every 2 years, then yearly after age 40. Begin screening at age 25 or 10 years younger than the youngest affected relative. Consider genetic counseling and testing.
Patient with FAP risk	Sigmoidoscopy every 1-2 years. Begin screening at age 12 years. Genetic counseling and testing.
Patient with personal history of CRC	Total colon examination (TCE: ACBE or colonoscopy) within 1 year after resection. Repeat at 3 years. Repeat at 5 years if normal.
Patient with personal history of adenoma	Polyp removal. Repeat at 3 years. Repeat at 5 years if normal.

ACBE, air contrast barium enema; CRC, colorectal cancer; HNPCC, hereditary nonpolyposis colon cancer; FAP, familial adenomatous polyposis; FOBT, fecal occult blood test.

For patients with ulcerative colitis, the risk of colorectal cancer correlates with the duration of active disease, extent of colitis, development of mucosal dysplasia, and duration of symptoms. Colon cancer risk for patients with Crohn disease exceeds that of the general population, although to a lesser degree than patients with ulcerative colitis. Recognizing the increased risk of colorectal cancer for patients with IBD, appropriate screening should be instituted as detailed in Table 21-2.

Familial Syndromes

The estimated risk of developing colorectal cancer attributable to various hereditary syndromes is listed in Table 21-1. Most of the genetic abnormalities associated with the development of colorectal cancer involve deletion of fragments of chromosomes, a phenomenon known as allelic loss or loss of heterozygosity (LOH), or errors in DNA mismatch repair. The following molecular markers have been associated with particularly aggressive colorectal cancer: loss of expression of the *DCC* gene, p11, p27, or p53; or overexpression of thymidylate synthase (TS), Ki-67, or bcl-2.

Sporadic colon cancers comprise approximately 80% of all cases, with the remainder attributed to different inherited syndromes. FAP, Gardner syndrome, and HNPCC are all inherited in an autosomal dominant pattern. FAP represents <1% of familial colorectal cancer, while HNPCC accounts for 2 to 3% of cases (8,24,25). MUTYH-associated polyposis (MAP) is an autosomal recessive syndrome caused by biallelic mutation in the base repair gene MUTYH that may be confused with attenuated adenomatous polyposis or even familial adenomatous polyposis (26,27).

Familial Adenomatous Polyposis

This syndrome is caused by a mutation of *APC*, a tumor suppressor gene located at 5q21. When *APC* is mutated, the function of both *APC* alleles is lost; one defective allele is inherited as a germline mutation, and the other allele is mutated in individual colon cells in early childhood. Familial adenomatous polyposis (FAP) has a high penetrance, and patients who inherit the genetic disorder are very likely to develop colon cancer. In individuals with FAP, thousands of adenomatous polyps grow throughout the colon and rectum, and some of these polyps invariably progress to cancer. Once polyposis develops, a prophylactic resection of the entire colon and rectum is recommended because the adenomatous polyps in FAP are too numerous for endoscopic removal. The onset of malignancy in untreated patients occurs at an average age of 42 years; invasive cancer develops 20 to 30 years after the onset of polyposis. The multiple polyps accumulate other mutations in oncogenes and tumor suppressor genes, causing benign adenomas to become malignant tumors (28). In cases of FAP, mutations in other tumor suppressor genes, such as *p53* and *DCC*, and activation of proto-oncogenes (especially K-*ras*), occur sequentially in the neoplastic transformation of the bowel epithelium (4).

Hereditary Nonpolyposis Colorectal Cancer

The genetic penetrance of hereditary nonpolyposis colorectal cancer (HNPCC) (Lynch syndrome) is lower than that of FAP but remains significant, ranging from 30 to 70% (28). In the past, HNPCC was commonly divided into two clinical subgroups: Lynch type I, which involves tumors of the large bowel only, and Lynch type II, which includes carcinomas of the large bowel, endometrium, and ovaries, among others (29). Adenomas develop in patients with HNPCC at roughly the same rate as the general population. However, an adenoma that develops in the colon or rectum of a patient with HNPCC tends to rapidly progress to carcinoma.

Patients with HNPCC do not have the *APC* gene mutation that characterizes FAP. Rather, HNPCC is caused by defects in DNA mismatch repair. DNA replication is often imperfect, and correct transmission of the genetic code relies on the ability of the cell's DNA mismatch repair system to correct errors. Several proteins participate in the repair process and are encoded by various genes, several of which may have germline mutations in patients with HNPCC, thereby causing the HNPCC syndrome. Additional mutations involving tumor suppressor genes and oncogenes rapidly accumulate within these DNA repair–deficient cells; as a result, a benign adenoma can undergo malignant transformation in only 3 to 5 years. Recently, mutations in the human homologues of the bacterial *mut*HLS gene complex (hMSH2, hMSH6, hMLH1, hPMS1, and hPMS2) were found to predispose to the development of HNPCC; two of these genes, hMLH1 and hMSH2, are thought to account for more than 90% of HNPCC cases (30,31). Such mutations lead to genetic instability, which is reflected in DNA replication errors (32,33).

MUTYH-Associated Polyposis

MUTYH-associated polyposis (MAP) is caused by biallelic mutation in the base excision repair gene MUTYH (26). It has been reported that MUTYH base excision repair interacts with the DNA mismatch repair

MSH2-MSH6 complex to prevent 8-oxoG–mediated mutagenesis (27,34). Patients with the syndrome are characterized by oligopolyposis, usually >15 but <100 polyps. However, as mentioned previously, some patients may develop hundreds of adenomas. The onset of adenomas is older than in classic FAP, but similar to attenuated adenomatous polyposis (45-55 years of age) (27,35). Affected patients may have extracolonic manifestations seen in FAP but to a lesser extent. The most common mutations are Y179C and G396D, formerly known as G165C and G382D (36,37). Biallelic mutation carriers have been reported to have a 53-fold risk of colorectal cancer compared to the general population (35,36). A European study reported that the risk of CRC in heterozygote carriers was similar to individuals with first-degree relatives with CRC (38).

■ SCREENING FOR COLORECTAL NEOPLASIA

As with screening tests for all types of diseases, the presence of risk factors, such as genetic predisposition, or epidemiologic factors, such as high disease prevalence in a geographic area, increases the sensitivity of a test. Researchers have therefore attempted to stratify populations in order to identify individuals who are at the greatest risk of developing colorectal cancer and who would benefit most from screening and surveillance (Table 21-2). Numerous tests have been developed over the years to screen individuals at risk of colorectal cancer, and the subject of screening various populations continues to be studied and debated. The 5-year survival rate of patients diagnosed with early-stage colorectal cancer is 90%, compared with less than 15% for patients diagnosed with stage IV disease. Presently, less than 40% of cases of colorectal cancer are discovered early (39). It is therefore believed that increased detection of premalignant lesions and early-stage tumors will improve overall survival (OS) for patients with colorectal cancer. Unfortunately, despite the benefits associated with screening, a very small proportion of all colon cancers are discovered by routine screening; the majority of colon cancers continue to be diagnosed in symptomatic patients.

DETECTION METHODS

Fecal Occult Blood Testing

Among the screening modalities for colorectal cancer, fecal occult blood testing (FOBT) may be the most controversial, even though several large trials have shown an increase in the percentage of early-stage colorectal cancers discovered (40-42), and at least one large randomized trial has conclusively demonstrated that the use of FOBT-decreased colorectal cancer mortality (43). Meta-analysis of four randomized trials investigating the role of FOBT also demonstrated a reduction in mortality from colorectal cancer (44). The test is relatively inexpensive and simple to use, but the use of rehydrated slides has resulted in a high percentage of patients undergoing unnecessary colonoscopy. In addition, the relatively high number of false-negative, as well as false-positive, results has generated questions regarding the true ability of FOBT to detect colorectal cancers in a cost-effective manner. Nevertheless, the current recommendation of the American College of Physicians is that all individuals over 40 years of age undergo annual FOBT (45).

Sigmoidoscopy

The 60-cm flexible sigmoidoscope can be inserted as far as the descending colon and does not require sedation. Sigmoidoscopy is a relatively safe and inexpensive procedure. It can be performed by a primary care physician, surgeon, or a GI endoscopist and may be suitable for screening large populations at low risk, particularly when used in combination with FOBT (46). However, recent studies show that the presence or absence of adenomas in the distal colon is not necessarily indicative of the presence of proximal lesions, and sigmoidoscopy may miss nearly 50% of all colonic lesions (47). This method is not appropriate for screening patients suspected to have HNPCC, in which approximately two-thirds of the lesions are right-sided. Most oncologists would agree that any adenomatous lesion in the distal colon or rectum warrants evaluation of the entire colon. For patients with adenomas in the distal colon detected by flexible sigmoidoscopy, a full colonoscopy or an alternative method to assess the entire colon should be conducted for completeness, such as air contrast barium enema (ACBE) or CT colonography.

Air Contrast Barium Enema

In some settings, high-quality ACBE plus flexible sigmoidoscopy may be substituted for full colonoscopy. The technique is limited by its lack of sensitivity for small polyps (<1 cm in diameter) and areas within the rectosigmoid and hepatic/splenic flexures, where overlapping large bowel loops might make a single lumen difficult to identify. In addition, ACBE is unsuitable as a screening or surveillance technique for HNPCC, ulcerative colitis, or flat adenoma syndrome (48).

However, the greatest problem with ACBE may be its highly operator-dependent nature; in recent years, it has been used with less frequency.

CT Colonography (Virtual Colonoscopy)

Adherence rates for colorectal cancer screening in the United States are low compared to those for other cancers, so improved screening methods are desirable (49-52). Virtual colonoscopy (VC) is an emerging radiographic technique that involves reconstruction of three-dimensional images of the colon from the two-dimensional data obtained by a spiral CT scanner. The images can be displayed so that the entire bowel is seen from the outside, similar to that obtained by a double contrast barium enema, and from within the lumen. Bowel preparation is required, but the technique is less invasive and does not require sedation; consequently, patient acceptance of this technique is high (53-55). VC has since been adopted as one possible option for screening and has been determined to be comparable to standard colonoscopy (56,57). However, VC lacks the advantage of a colonoscopy for direct access to colonic tissue for biopsies or other interventions.

Colonoscopy

Colonoscopy not only enables full visualization of the entire colon but also allows for biopsy or removal of any suspicious lesions. It is considered the gold standard for evaluating the colon for pathology. Several recent studies suggest the increasing importance of colonoscopy in colorectal cancer screening. One study showed that more than half of all the advanced proximal neoplasms found in colonoscopic screening of a series of asymptomatic men aged 50 to 75 years would have been missed if only the distal colon had been evaluated (47). In another retrospective study, 1994 patients were examined to determine whether the size and histologic features of distal lesions are predictive of proximal lesions, as identification of these factors would help determine who should undergo full colonoscopy after sigmoidoscopic screening. The findings in the distal and proximal colon are shown in Table 21-3 (58).

In the 50 patients with advanced proximal neoplasia, no polyps were found in 23 patients (46%). Thus, the proximal neoplasms of these patients would not have been detected if a full colon evaluation was done only in patients with distal findings. The study also found that a polyp of any size or type was associated with an increased risk of histologically advanced proximal neoplasia, and that the magnitude of risk was proportional to the histologic features of the distal lesion.

TABLE 21-3	FINDINGS IN THE DISTAL AND PROXIMAL COLON IN COHORT OF 1994 PATIENTS			
	DISTAL COLON		PROXIMAL COLON	
Finding	No.	%	No.	%
No polyp	1564	78.4	1686	84.6
Hyperplastic polyp	201	10.1	72	3.6
Tubular adenoma	168	8.4	186	9.3
Advanced neoplasm	61	3.1	50	2.5

In addition to its benefits as a screening modality, colonoscopy has some promise as a preventive strategy (59). This has been suggested by findings from a variety of sources, including the National Polyp Study conducted in the United States and other data from Europe and Japan (60-62). In general, patients undergoing colonoscopy or sigmoidoscopy with polyp removal were less likely to develop colorectal cancer compared with a predefined reference group, with substantial reduction in overall risk. For example, as part of The National Polyp Workgroup, Winawer et al. followed the course of 1418 patients over a period of time averaging 5.9 years. There was a significant reduction in the expected incidence of colorectal cancer in these patients undergoing colonoscopy and polypectomy compared to three distinct reference groups who did not (60). A similar conclusion was reached by investigators in Japan, who also performed a case-control study to evaluate the benefit of colonoscopy and polypectomy (62). Using a different approach, investigators in the Veterans Administration hospital network found that veterans who had undergone an endoscopic examination up to the sigmoid colon or beyond were significantly less likely to be subsequently diagnosed with colorectal cancer compared to veterans who had not undergone a prior endoscopic examination (63). Taken together, these studies corroborate the hypothesis that colonoscopy with polyp removal reduces the risk of subsequent colorectal cancer and has utility both as a screening modality for detecting early-stage cancer in asymptomatic patients and as a preventive strategy. However, it is unlikely that a large, prospective randomized trial comparing colonoscopy and polypectomy to colonoscopy alone to reduce colorectal cancer mortality will ever be performed.

Molecular Diagnostics

DNA analysis of stool samples for mutations of *KRAS* and other genes is becoming more readily available, but its utility in the clinic has yet to be determined. Recently published data suggest that it may be more sensitive than fecal occult blood testing, but only about 40% of invasive colon cancers would be detected using these techniques (64). In time, if molecular tests have sufficient sensitivity and specificity, genomic or proteomic assays of stool or blood samples may become widely used as preferable alternatives to endoscopic or radiographic evaluations of the colon and rectum.

Genetic Testing and Counseling

Genetic testing for *APC* mutations, MUTYH mutations, and DNA mismatch repair gene mutations are now available and currently being employed to identify carriers of FAP, MUTYH, and HNPCC, respectively. Upon diagnosis of colorectal cancer, patients may be known members of FAP kindred. A diagnosis of FAP in these individuals is usually not a clinical dilemma, unless they have the attenuated form of the syndrome, which presents at an older age and with fewer polyps. However, when a newly diagnosed patient with classic FAP or with oligopolyposis is tested but has a negative APC mutation, then MUTYH mutation testing should be considered. There is a reported incidence of 7 to 29% of biallelic MUTYH in polyposis patients with negative APC testing (35,65). At MDACC, newly diagnosed patients suspected of having FAP are referred to a dedicated gastroenterologist and a genetic counselor to discuss screening recommendations, genetic testing, prevention, and surgical intervention for themselves and other potentially affected family members. These patients continue to be subjects in clinical chemoprevention trials, if available.

In HNPCC, the diagnosis is not always so obvious, as there is no pathognomonic clinical feature such as the adenomatosis that characterizes FAP. When patients with newly diagnosed colorectal cancer are referred to MDACC, careful attention is paid to a number of parameters to identify potential cases of HNPCC. Table 21-4 summarizes the Amsterdam Criteria (both original and modified), which have been developed to provide a guide to clinicians to assess the risk of HNPCC in patients from whom an accurate family history can be obtained (66). In addition, when patients proceed with surgery for primary tumor resection, pathology may suggest MSI. MSI is a hallmark of HNPCC, but it also occurs in about 15% of spontaneous colon cancers. Histology that suggests an MSI tumor may include mucinous features, poor differentiation, or the presence of tumor-infiltrating lymphocytes (TILs) (Fig. 21-1). Such features are not pathognomonic for MSI or HNPCC. However, in patients <50 years of age, female, proximal

TABLE 21-4	ORIGINAL AND REVISED ICG-HNPCC CRITERIA ("AMSTERDAM" CRITERIA I AND II)	
Original Criteria (Amsterdam Criteria I)	***Revised Criteria (Amsterdam Criteria II)***	
There should be at least three relatives with colorectal cancer; all the following criteria should be present	There should be at least three relatives with an HNPCC-associated-cancer (colorectal cancer, cancer of endometrium, small bowel, ureter, or renal pelvis)	
One should be a first-degree relative of the other two	One should be a first-degree relative of the other two	
At least two successive generations should be affected	At least two successive generations should be affected	
At least one colorectal cancer should be diagnosed before age of 50	At least one should be diagnosed before age of 50	
Familial adenomatous polyposis should be excluded	Familial adenomatous polyposis should be excluded in the colorectal in cancer case(s) if any	
Tumors should be verified by pathological examination	Tumors should be verified by pathological examination	

tumors, poorly differentiated histology, and/or mucinous tumors, HNPCC should be considered even when the patient's family history is not suggestive.

Immunohistochemical (IHC) stains are now available to assess tumors for loss of heterozygosity in hMSH2, hMSH6, or hMLH1 gene loci. Both MSI and IHC testing can easily be done on sections from the diagnostic biopsy obtained at the time of colonoscopy. This is important as it allows these evaluations to be carried out prior to surgical resection, thereby guiding the extent of colon resection at the time of definitive surgery. Currently, we are testing all surgically resected patients at MDACC for MSI status to formally evaluate it as a predictive and prognostic marker. Specific genetic testing for underlying germline mutations may proceed following an informative MSI or IHC. In carefully selected cases, mutational testing may be performed even if the MSI and IHC are not informative, but it must be emphasized that the diagnostic yield will be much lower in such cases. Moreover, it should be noted that currently unidentified mutations are likely to be present in some families, and a negative test does not exclude HNPCC. Thus, whenever genetic testing is being considered for an individual, genetic counseling prior to and after testing is strongly recommended.

■ PREVENTION STRATEGIES

PRIMARY PREVENTION

Prevention of colorectal neoplasia is usually considered primary or secondary. In primary prevention, broad-based interventions may decrease the risk of colorectal cancer for those at average risk. Primary prevention efforts are particularly beneficial in regions where the disease has a relatively high incidence. Americans currently have a 1 in 20 lifetime risk of developing colorectal cancer, with strong evidence pointing to diet as a contributor to this risk. Consequently, fairly simple alterations in our diet may have a significant impact on the overall incidence of colorectal cancer.

Diet and Micronutrients

Early epidemiologic data suggested that diets rich or supplemented with carotenoids, other antioxidants, calcium, vitamin D, folate, or multivitamins may reduce the risk of colorectal cancer. Based on a number of epidemiologic, clinical, and animal studies, there is general consensus that a diet rich in fruits and vegetables with an adequate supply of fiber and a limited amount of meat (particularly red meat) may reduce the risk of colorectal

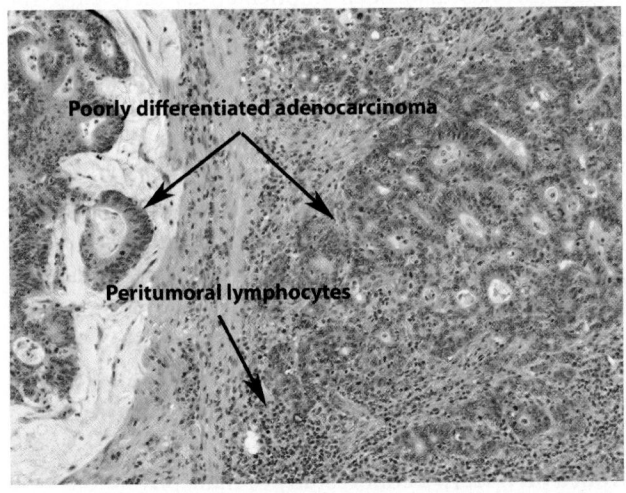

FIGURE 21-1. Photomicrograph of a tumor with microsatellite instability. Upper arrows point to poorly differentiated malignant cells with some glandular differentiation and mucin. Lower arrow shows peritumoral lymphocytes clustering near areas of malignant cells and permeating the local stroma.

cancer. Whether supplementation with enriched sources of carotenoids, folate, calcium, vitamin D, or other vitamins reduces risk further has not been established. It appears that the combination of micronutrients present in the proposed diet described earlier leads to complex, beneficial interactions that are likely responsible for risk reduction. A recent European analysis showed an inverse linear dose–response association between serum vitamin D levels and risk of colorectal cancer ($p < .001$). Low levels were associated with higher colorectal cancer risk (<25.0 nmol/L: incidence rate ratio 1.32 [95% confidence interval 0.87-2.01]; 25.0-49.9 nmol/L: 1.28 [1.05-1.56]), and higher concentrations with lower risk (75.0-99.9 nmol/L: 0.88 [0.68-1.13]; ≥100.0 nmol/L: 0.77 [0.56-1.06]). Patients in the highest quintile had a 40% reduced risk of colorectal cancer ($p < .001$). Subgroup analyses showed a strong association for colon but not rectal cancer ($p = .048$). However, there may also be significant variability in capturing vitamin D levels, as well as variability due to genetic polymorphisms in the vitamin D receptor (67,68).

Because it is not logistically feasible to conduct sufficiently powered, randomized prospective trials utilizing colorectal cancer as an endpoint of intervention efficacy, such rigorous interventions have instead focused on the more frequent cancer antecedent, the colorectal adenoma. In these trials, confirmation of the broad trends toward protection suggested by the epidemiologic studies has largely fallen short. This is probably due to insufficient power (sample size) to detect modest effects in short-term trials.

Nonsteroidal Anti-Inflammatory Drugs

For over 20 years, there have been epidemiologic and preclinical data to suggest that nonsteroidal anti-inflammatory agents slow or prevent the formation of adenomatous polyps. Animal studies, consistent with a variety of epidemiologic studies, have pointed to the chemoprotective effect of a number of anti-inflammatory drugs. These include piroxicam, sulindac, and aspirin. Small clinical studies have also demonstrated that sulindac is capable of reducing polyp burden in patients with FAP (69). Growing evidence implicates prostaglandin E_2 (PGE_2) as an important modulator of cell proliferation and malignant transformation. PGE_2 is formed by the catalytic activity of cyclooxygenases, which facilitate conversion of arachidonic acid to prostanoids (70). There are two predominant isoforms of cyclooxygenase. Cyclooxygenase 1 (COX-1) is constitutively active and expressed in a number of tissues, and it appears to regulate tissue repair and homeostasis.

COX-2 is an inducible enzyme that appears to play a role in inflammation and tumor promotion. Aspirin potently inhibits both isoforms in a dose-dependent manner, which may explain its observed beneficial effects. Epidemiologic and clinical data have shown that aspirin can protect against the development of adenomas and reduce the risk of colorectal carcinoma (71). With the advent of selective COX-2 inhibitors, there has been great interest in exploring these agents as putative chemoprevention agents in colorectal neoplasia. In a rat model, COX-2 inhibitors have been shown to reduce the number of carcinogen-induced tumors (72). Furthermore, celecoxib, a selective COX-2 inhibitor, reduced the incidence of adenocarcinoma in the same model, suggesting that this agent may be attractive for primary prevention.

In a study of FAP patients, celecoxib at a dose of 400 mg twice daily for 6 months significantly reduced the number of adenomas, when compared with placebo or a lower dose of celecoxib (73). This relatively large trial led the Food and Drug Administration (FDA) to approve celecoxib as a chemopreventive agent for patients with FAP, to be used as an adjunct to regular endoscopic surveillance/polypectomy and surgical resection. Thus, this chemopreventive strategy is considered a component of secondary prevention since all eligible patients were known to have FAP and a history of polyps.

Recent data from a variety of sources, including sporadic adenoma prevention trials, suggest that COX-2 inhibitors, notably rofecoxib, increase the risk of stroke and myocardial infarction compared to placebo (74). Celecoxib has also been implicated as increasing the risk of these events (75). Therefore, trials assessing the efficacy of celecoxib in various high-risk populations were temporarily suspended, pending development of more stringent exclusion criteria for subjects at increased risk of cardiovascular disease.

While the safety and efficacy of COX-2 inhibitors as primary chemoprevention agents remains unclear, the preponderance of epidemiologic data suggests that aspirin has primary chemopreventive properties. In a study performed through the Nurses' Health Study, the risk of colorectal cancer was substantially reduced among women who were regular users of aspirin for at least 20 years (76). Additional epidemiologic data come from a prospective cohort study of male physicians who were followed over a 4-year period. Regular users of aspirin (≥2 times per week) at the beginning of the study period had a lower risk of developing colorectal cancer during the study period compared with nonusers (RR = 0.68; 95% confidence interval [CI] 0.52-0.92).

In addition, aspirin users had a lower risk of developing advanced colorectal cancer (RR = 0.52; 95% CI 0.32-0.84) (77). Since daily aspirin is now commonly advised for patients with risk factors for cardiovascular disease, a modest reduction in the incidence of colorectal cancer may become apparent in the future.

Patients with no prior history of colorectal cancer but known to be at increased risk due to history of adenoma are encouraged to enroll in chemoprevention trials. In general, a decrease in the formation of recurrent adenomatous polyps is the primary endpoint of these studies. Otherwise, drug therapy is not routinely advised. All patients are advised to make healthy dietary choices, including high intake of fresh fruits and vegetables, limited red meat intake, and sufficient cereals and grains to provide adequate dietary fiber. Aspirin is not necessarily advised as a component of primary prevention. However, because of an observed reduction in recurrent adenomas seen in several prospective trials (see later) coupled with the increasingly liberal use of cardioprotective doses of aspirin in the aging American population, consideration of aspirin is not unreasonable.

SECONDARY PREVENTION

Outside of the clinical trial setting, patients with FAP are treated with celecoxib at a dose of 400 mg twice daily. Recognizing the potential cardiovascular risk associated with COX-2 inhibitors, patients with cardiovascular disease or risk factors need to either be excluded from COX-2 treatment or have the risk factor aggressively managed (eg, control blood pressure, diabetes, and low-density lipoprotein and total cholesterol). Finally, although the original FAP trial supported the efficacy of high-dose (400 mg twice a day) celecoxib, there may be a role for case-by-case consideration of dose reduction. The role of COX-2 inhibition as a component of secondary prevention for FAP and colorectal cancer has been outlined earlier. Whether celecoxib or other COX-2 inhibitors provide a secondary protective effect for people without FAP, such as those with HNPCC or other at-risk populations, is currently unknown.

While the role of selective COX-2 inhibitors is currently being debated, aspirin does appear to have secondary chemopreventive benefits. In a large randomized, placebo-controlled trial, aspirin has demonstrated a protective benefit for patients with a prior history of colorectal cancer. This study randomized over 600 patients with a history of colorectal cancer to receive either 325 mg of aspirin daily or a placebo. Patients randomized to aspirin had a significantly reduced risk of developing adenomatous polyps compared to the placebo group (RR = 0.65; 95% CI 0.46-0.91) (78). In a separate study, 1121 patients with a recent history of adenomatous polyp removal were randomized to receive aspirin 81 mg daily, aspirin 325 mg daily, or a placebo. Both groups receiving aspirin had a reduced risk of subsequent colorectal adenomas compared to the placebo group. Overall, the 81-mg dose appeared to be superior to the 325-mg dose (79). A prospective cohort study of 1279 patients with stage I to III colorectal cancer was recently reported. After a median follow-up of 11.8 years, participants who regularly used aspirin had a multivariate hazard ratio (HR) for colorectal cancer-specific mortality of 0.71 (95% CI, 0.53-0.95) and overall mortality of 0.79 (95% CI, 0.65-0.97). Among 719 participants who did not use aspirin before diagnosis, aspirin use initiated after diagnosis was associated with a multivariate HR for colorectal cancer-specific mortality of 0.53 (95% CI, 0.33-0.86). The benefit of aspirin was dependent on COX-2 expression ($p = .04$). Regular aspirin use after diagnosis was associated with lower risk of colorectal cancer-specific mortality in patients whose tumors overexpressed COX-2 (multivariate HR, 0.39; 95% CI, 0.20-0.76). The cooperative group, Cancer and Leukemia Group B (CALGB), is helping to lead the efforts for an intergroup trial of adjuvant chemotherapy with a second randomization to celecoxib. Thus, patients at MDACC with a history of colorectal cancer or adenomatous polyps, and no contraindications to the use of aspirin, are often advised to take 81 mg of aspirin daily.

◼ DIAGNOSTIC EVALUATION AND STAGING

CLINICAL PRESENTATION

Among the malignancies that occur in the colon itself, 60 to 70% of sporadic colorectal cancers are left-sided, whereas inherited colon cancers occur mainly in the right colon (80,81). Left-sided colorectal cancers are often associated with a change in bowel habits, constipation, small-caliber stool, fecal impaction, or obstructive symptoms. Right-sided lesions are often associated with vague abdominal pain and bloating, acute or chronic gastrointestinal bleeding, or bowel obstruction. Colonic lesions in any location can cause bleeding, which may manifest as melena, hematochezia, a positive hemoccult testing, or iron deficiency anemia. Weight loss, anorexia, and other constitutional symptoms are particularly concerning, as they may reflect the presence of metastatic disease. Any unexplained iron deficiency anemia should prompt an evaluation of the gastrointestinal tract.

Patients may attribute their symptoms to other causes such as hemorrhoids, aging, or irritable bowel syndrome and delay medical evaluation. Conversely, primary care physicians, unaware of the overall incidence of colorectal cancer, may attribute signs and symptoms to benign conditions, and several months may elapse before more intensive diagnostic procedures are performed. A delay in diagnosis may have serious consequences for the patient. Providing information to the patients and their family members about the lifetime risk of colon cancer and the current recommendations for screening is highly encouraged.

STAGING STUDIES

Proper staging provides both prognostic information and a guide to therapeutic decision making. For patients with apparently localized disease, primary tumor control is the focus of therapy. When metastatic disease is uncovered, attention to local control may be outweighed by systemic tumor burden and its consequences. At MDACC, cancers of the colon and rectum are managed with a multidisciplinary approach, and treatment planning is based on thorough staging, which is best done preoperatively. This is particularly true given the nonsurgical options that may be considered for patients with advanced disease discovered prior to surgical intervention. For the majority of patients diagnosed with a colonic or rectal neoplasm, urgent surgery is not required and should be actively discouraged. However, preoperative evaluation is not always possible, particularly in the setting of acute bowel obstruction, and the staging evaluation in these cases should be completed within several weeks of surgery. It should be noted that accurate postoperative staging may be confounded by the preceding surgery and therefore should not be obtained for at least 3 to 6 weeks after the operative procedure. When surgery is performed emergently, patients usually require additional cross-sectional imaging and a full colonoscopy. For example, if a patient has undergone an urgent left segmental colon resection for an obstructing descending colon carcinoma, a full colonoscopy in the postoperative period is necessary to assess for synchronous lesions in the colon proximal to the obstructing site. MDACC patients are advised to wait a minimum of 4 weeks after surgery before undergoing a colonoscopy, in order to minimize risk to the surgical anastomosis. The same time interval (4 weeks) holds true for the procurement of CT, MR, or PET/CT imaging, since patients need time for wound healing prior to considering further therapy. In addition, common, nonspecific postoperative radiographic findings of inflammation may mimic lymphadenopathy and peritoneal disease. An exception occurs when peritoneal disease is encountered at the time of surgery. In this situation, we usually delay postoperative imaging for up to 6 weeks to allow stranding changes in the omental fat attributable to surgery to subside.

Preoperative Staging for Colonic Neoplasms

In patients found to have a colonic neoplasm not requiring urgent or emergent surgery, a complete history and physical examination should be performed in conjunction with full colonoscopy with biopsies. For patients undergoing flexible sigmoidoscopy as their initial diagnostic procedure, a full colonoscopy to the cecum is highly recommended to exclude synchronous primary tumors that may occur in 3 to 4% of patients with colorectal neoplasms (82).

Laboratory evaluation should include at least a complete blood count with differential, electrolytes, liver function studies, carcinoembryonic antigen (CEA) level, blood urea nitrogen (BUN), and creatinine. The preoperative CEA is particularly useful in predicting extent of disease and may subsequently be used as an indicator of recurrence (83-85). Imaging studies should include at least routine posteroanterior and lateral chest radiographs, or CT of the chest, and CT scan or MRI of the abdomen/pelvis.

Importantly, rectal carcinomas commonly metastasize to the lungs by venous and lymphatic drainage via the retroperitoneum, by way of the middle and inferior hemorrhoidal veins and the inferior vena cava (IVC). On the other hand, colon cancers typically spread hematogenously to the liver through the portal circulation. Although not always, both colon and rectal cancers typically invade in a stepwise fashion, first through the mucosa, submucosa, and muscularis propria, then to the perirectal or pericolonic lymph nodes, and subsequently to the more distant lymph node groups, the liver, and the lungs.

Rectal Cancer Staging

Anatomic differences between the rectum and colon produce different patterns of spread and often prompt different treatment strategies. Rectal cancers have been variably defined as those tumors occurring below the sacral promontory, below the peritoneal reflection, or those situated less than 12 to 15 cm from the anal verge (43).

The rectum resides in a funnel below the pelvic brim and is circumscribed posteriorly by the sacrum, laterally by the pelvic sidewalls, and anteriorly by either the prostate gland or the posterior wall of the vagina. The rectum also rests below the peritoneal reflection. Therefore, while the proximal and distal margins of resection can be ascertained with some certainty, the confined anatomy creates challenges in establishing the radial margin of resection. Consequently, rectal cancers tend to recur locally, and in some older series local failure rates have been as high as 25 to 50% (86). For the majority of patients who develop a local recurrence after resection of rectal cancer, salvage surgery is not possible. Locally recurrent rectal cancer may be associated with significant morbidity. Common complications include pain, ureteral obstruction, and the development of fistulous tracts to the bladder, vagina, or skin; clinical efforts to palliate these problems require a multidisciplinary approach. Fortunately, modern studies have shown that the risk of local recurrence can be substantially reduced using improved surgical techniques such as total mesorectal excision (TME) and radiotherapy delivered either preoperatively or postoperatively (87-89). Complete clinical staging of rectal cancer is particularly important when patients are being considered for preoperative therapy (neoadjuvant therapy). In addition to the staging studies recommended earlier for colon cancer, newly diagnosed rectal cancer patients seen at MDACC are typically staged with endorectal ultrasound (EUS). This imaging modality has been found to be more accurate than CT imaging for assessing the depth of tumor invasion into or through the bowel wall and determining perirectal lymph node involvement. However, EUS may have a false-positive rate of 18 to 20%, resulting in overstaging of the patient (88). A dedicated pelvic MRI to evaluate the mesorectal planes and perirectal lymph nodes may improve the accuracy of preoperative staging (90).

The Role of Positron Emission Tomography in Staging Cancers of the Colon and Rectum

Positron emission tomographic (PET) scanning using (^{18}F)-fluorodeoxyglucose (FDG-PET) is a sensitive functional imaging study now being employed in a variety of malignancies, including colorectal cancer, and it has an approved indication for staging (91). This modality exploits a difference in glucose metabolism between normal cells and cancer cells. Tumor cells have higher levels of glucose transporters and hexokinase, but lower levels of glucose-6-phosphatase. Since FDG lacks a hydroxyl group at the 2 position that is present in glucose, it cannot be further metabolized within tumor

cells and remains trapped. Thus, areas of increased ^{18}FDG uptake detected on FDG-PET often denote sites of malignancy as small as 1 cm. On a cautionary note, sites of inflammation may also exhibit increased ^{18}FDG uptake and thus confound accurate staging of patients with colorectal cancers. FDG-PET is not part of routine MDACC staging for patients with newly diagnosed colon or rectal cancer. It is more commonly employed in patients with a rising post therapy CEA without other clinical or radiographic evidence for measurable disease or in the setting of equivocal CT findings.

PATHOLOGY

More than 95% of all colorectal malignancies are adenocarcinomas. These have been further subclassified on the basis of histology as well-differentiated, moderately differentiated, poorly differentiated, and undifferentiated. However, while tumor grade may provide additional prognostic information, it is not typically used in treatment planning (4). A small number of adenocarcinomas fall into the mucinous and signet-ring cell subtypes, which generally display atypical patterns of spread and confer a poorer prognosis. These tumors are more likely to be present in younger patients and more commonly spread to the peritoneum. Treatment, however, does not differ from the more typical adenocarcinoma subtypes.

Pathologic Staging

Throughout the years, many staging systems have been developed for colorectal cancer. The first widely accepted system was the Dukes classification system and its subsequent variations. However, the American Joint Committee on Cancer (AJCC) TNM classification system (Table 21-5) has recently been revised (version 7.0). Staging is used to provide prognostic information and to guide recommendations for treatment, particularly the use of adjuvant chemotherapy and radiotherapy.

Importance of Lymph Node Dissection and Sampling

Adequate lymph node dissection and subsequent pathologic assessment of lymph nodes are both important components of multidisciplinary care. At the time of resection, tumor removal should involve segmental resection of the involved colon or rectum along the appropriate vascular pedicles with careful removal of all regional lymph nodes. Failing to do so may lead to relapse in lymph nodes draining the affected segment of bowel, as shown in Fig. 21-2. Retrospective analyses have demonstrated that removal and inspection of fewer

TABLE 21-5	TNM STAGING OF COLORECTAL CANCER		
TNM Stage	*Primary Tumor*	*Lymph Metastasis*	*Distant Metastasis*
0	Tis	N0	M0
I	T1	N0	M0
	T2	N0	M0
II	T3	N0	M0
	T4	N0	M0
IIIA	T1,2	N1	M0
IIIB	T3,4	N1	M0
IIIC	Any T	N2	M0
IV	Any T	Any N	M1

M1, any distant metastatic site; N1, metastases to 1-3 regional lymph nodes; N2, metastases in 4 or more regional lymph nodes; Tis, tumor in situ; T1, Tumor invades submucosa; T2, tumor invades muscularis propria; T3, tumor invades through muscularis mucosa to subserosa or periolic or perirectal tissues; T4, tumor perforates the visceral peritoneum or directly invades other organs.

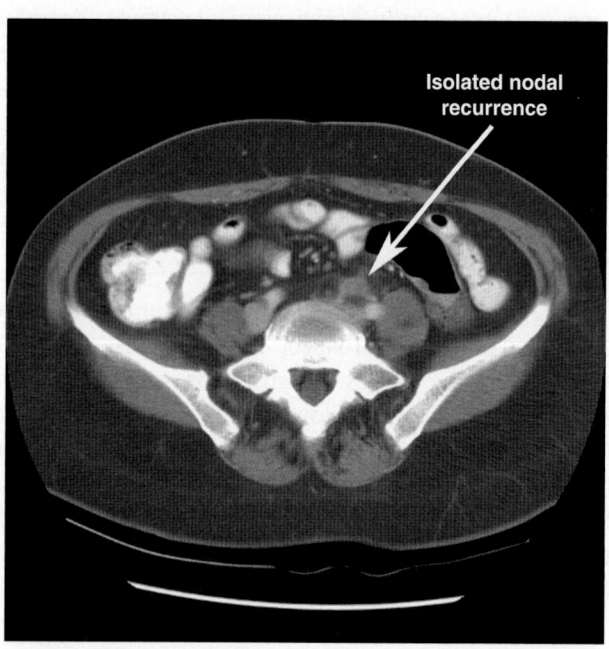

Isolated nodal recurrence

FIGURE 21-2. CT image of a 54-year-old woman with a history of T3,N0,M0 adenocarcinoma of the sigmoid colon found incidentally at the time of hysterectomy for benign disease. Surgical resection of the sigmoid mass was performed by her gynecologist. The patient received adjuvant therapy for 6 months but subsequently developed a rising serum CEA level and a nodal mass at the base of the inferior mesenteric artery (IMA). After a course of chemotherapy for metastatic disease, she underwent repeat laparotomy with the finding of an isolated nodal mass which was removed and was positive for adenocarcinoma. In retrospect, inadequate resection of the sigmoid mesentery to the level of the IMA was thought to explain the recurrence.

than 12 lymph nodes confers poorer prognosis compared to patients undergoing a more robust lymph node dissection (92). This holds true for patients with either stage II or III disease. In addition, when patients are being considered for adjuvant therapy, tumors are considered high-risk stage II (T3,N0,M0 or T4,N0,M0) unless at least 12 lymph nodes are inspected and found to be negative for metastatic disease (93). The American Society of Clinical Oncology (ASCO) consensus panel recommended that patients who had suboptimal lymph nodes analyzed should be considered to be at high risk of relapse (94). The National Quality Forum as supported by the American College of Surgeons (ACoS) Commission on Cancer (CoC), working in concert with the American Society of Clinical Oncology (ASCO) and the National Comprehensive Cancer Network (NCCN), has recommended dissection of no fewer than 12 lymph nodes (http://www.facs.org/cancer/ qualitymeasures.html, accessed, May 5, 2010).

Lymphatic Mapping

Lymphatic mapping studies suggest that lymph node metastases develop in an orderly manner from the primary site, and these studies can identify the node or nodes at highest risk for tumor involvement. Such nodes have been described as sentinel lymph nodes, and their identification has become part of pathologic staging for breast cancer and melanoma. Examination of sentinel nodes may be further refined with immunohistochemical stains for cytokeratins or molecular probes. Some studies have shown that, using such techniques, sentinel lymph node examination for micrometastases may upstage 14 to 18% of node-negative colorectal tumors to node-positive (88); long-term results from prospective studies have not been reported. In a multi-institutional study, the identification of sentinel node(s) appeared not to be predictive of nodal status in a significant number of patients, suggesting that lymphatic mapping in colon cancer surgery may not improve the accuracy of nodal staging (95,96). At MDACC, sentinel lymph node mapping is not commonly performed as part of pathologic staging for colorectal cancer.

■ THERAPEUTIC APPROACHES

LOCAL AND REGIONAL CONTROL

Most patients with colorectal cancer present at a stage at which all gross tumor can be resected. Nevertheless, almost half of the patients undergoing curative resection will ultimately die of metastatic disease, as a result of residual microscopic disease not evident at the time of surgery. If complete resection of all gross disease is achieved, the risk of relapse can be estimated based on pathologic staging. Patients identified to be at relatively high risk of relapse based on clinical or pathologic staging may also be considered for additional local therapy in the form of preoperative or postoperative radiotherapy, systemic adjuvant chemotherapy, or both.

Surgical Management of Colon Cancer

The primary management of localized colon cancer involves surgery to remove the affected segment of bowel, the adjacent mesentery, and the draining lymph nodes. In both colon and rectal cancer surgery, any attached adjacent organ(s) or structures to the tumor must be removed without violating the adhesions, as the latter have been reported to be malignant in over 40% of the cases. Pathologic staging can be completed once the surgical specimen has been removed. Asymptomatic patients with stage IV disease with their primary malignancy intact do not necessarily require surgical resection of their primary, unless there is a significant signs of impending bowel obstruction, bleeding, or other complications. Prior studies have indicated leaving a primary malignancy intact is safe without compromising any further delay in systemic chemotherapy (97). Laparoscopic colectomy has been determined to be noninferior to an open colectomy in several prospective randomized studies. Initial concerns regarding laparoscopic surgery included inadequate nodal resection, increased time, inability to palpate intra-abdominal organs, and increased risk of tumor seeding during specimen removal (98). In the United States, the COST study (Clinical Outcomes of Surgical Therapy Study Group) randomized 872 patients to open colectomy versus laparoscopic assisted colon resection. After a median follow-up of 7 years, the 5-year disease-free survival (DFS) as well as the overall survival was similar in both groups; 68.4% and 69.2% (p = .94) and 74.6% and 76.4% (p =.93), respectively. The investigators noted perioperative recovery was shorter in the laparoscopic-surgery group than in the open-colectomy group, as reflected by the median hospital stay (5 versus 6 days, p < .001), decreased duration of parenteral narcotic use (3 versus 4 days, p < .001), and oral analgesics (1 versus 2 days, p = 0.02). The rates of intraoperative complications, 30- and 60-day postoperative mortality were comparable between the two groups (99). The authors concluded that laparoscopic colon resection is a safe and effective surgical procedure for colon cancer, and there is growing acceptance of this approach in the oncology community.

Evidence Regarding Adjuvant Therapy for Colon Cancer

Patients with stages II and III colon cancer may relapse after surgical resection due to micrometastatic disease, which cannot be addressed by surgical resection alone. Systemic therapy, usually in the form of chemotherapy, has been employed in an attempt to eradicate these micrometastases. Numerous trials conducted in the 1970s and 1980s did not show a clear survival benefit for postoperative (adjuvant) chemotherapy. However, in 1988, the National Surgical Adjuvant Breast and Bowel Project (NSABP) published results of a large prospective trial comparing surgery alone with adjuvant immunotherapy using bacille Calmette-Guérin (BCG) and adjuvant chemotherapy consisting of 5-fluorouracil (5-FU), semustine, and vincristine (100). There was a small but statistically significant survival advantage for patients receiving chemotherapy compared to immunotherapy or surgery alone. Subsequently, numerous studies assessed 5-FU in combination with other modulators, such as levamisole and folinic acid (leucovorin) (101-104). Currently, for patients with stage III colon cancer (node- positive without clinically detectable metastases), adjuvant chemotherapy is provided for a total of 6 months. Controversy remains regarding the role of adjuvant chemotherapy in stage II patients. Prior studies failed to demonstrate a role for adjuvant chemotherapy for all stage II patients (105). To date, the largest study of stage II patients, QUASAR (QUick and Simple and Reliable), evaluated the role of adjuvant single-agent 5-FU versus observation following surgical resection (106). The absolute benefit in overall survival following adjuvant chemotherapy was a modest 3.6%.

Although the commonly used intravenous regimens of 5-FU and leucovorin are still considered acceptable, new regimens have largely replaced former regimens. The oral fluoropyrimidine, capecitabine, is equivalent to IV 5-FU in the adjuvant and metastatic setting (107,108). More importantly, update of the MOSAIC (Multicenter International Study of Oxaliplatin/5-Fluorouracil/Leucovorin in the Adjuvant Treatment of Colon Cancer) trial demonstrated an improvement in 5-year DFS from 67 to 73% for patients receiving a combination of infusional 5-FU, leucovorin, and oxaliplatin (FOLFOX) rather than 5-FU and leucovorin alone (109). The FOLFOX group also showed a small improvement in 6-year overall survival (79 versus 76%). The benefits in overall and disease-free survival achieved statistical significance in stage III patients only. Although a trend toward improved DFS was seen in stage II patients with high-risk features. However, oxaliplatin-based therapy is associated with neuropathic toxicities that may linger for several months (110). Recent data also support that the cumulative dose of oxaliplatin may correlate with the development of splenomegaly (111). Hence, consideration of adjuvant chemotherapy for the high-risk stage II patient needs to be discussed fully by weighing the risks and the benefits with the patient. One new diagnostic tool is the Oncotype DX 12-gene assay (Genomic Health, Redwood City, California). It is FDA approved and has been validated as a prognostic marker for recurrence risk in stage II colon cancer. However, it was not determined to be a diagnostic tool for predictive efficacy of 5-FU–based therapy (112). The role of the Oncotype DX assay in stage III disease is currently unknown.

In a similar patient population, NSABP C-07 also showed modest improvement in DFS with FLOX (weekly bolus 5-FU/LV and oxaliplatin) (113). However, FLOX is associated with significant grade 3 gastrointestinal toxicity. Therefore, FOLFOX is the preferred adjuvant regimen for resected colon cancer. Recent data support the use of capecitabine in combination with oxaliplatin (XELOX/CAPEOX) as a treatment option; this regimen was determined to be well tolerated in elderly patients (>65 years old) (114).

The role of irinotecan in the adjuvant setting remains an enigma. Irinotecan has been determined to be beneficial as a single agent and in combination for advanced colon cancer. Yet, three randomized phase III trials of approximately 4900 patients comparing irinotecan/5-FU/LV–based therapy to 5-FU and leucovorin failed to show an improvement in disease-free or overall survival in the adjuvant setting (115-117). The lack of efficacy for irinotecan in the setting of microscopic disease following hepatic metastatic resection still held true (118). An exploratory analysis of CALGB 89803 (IFL versus bolus 5-FU/LV) indicates that MSI-H patients may derive benefit in DFS from irinotecan-based therapy. MSI-H tumors had an improved 5-year DFS versus MSI-S or MSI-L tumors (0.76; 95% CI, 0.64-0.88-0.59; 95% CI, 0.53-0.64; $p = .03$).

Conversely, a retrospective analysis of an Eastern Cooperative Oncology Group (ECOG) study has suggested that adjuvant single-agent 5-FU–based therapy for patients with stage II, MSI-H tumors led to inferior survival (11). A larger pooled analysis of the Adjuvant *Colon Cancer* Endpoints (ACCENT) database validates these earlier findings indicating that MSI-H patients do not derive any benefit from single-agent 5-FU and in fact doing so may negatively impact overall survival (119). However, the role of adjuvant FOLFOX in the high-risk stage II or stage III MSI-H patient population is unknown. An ongoing ECOG trial (ECOG 5202) is utilizing molecular markers (18q deletion and MSI status) to select stage II

patients for consideration of adjuvant therapy, hoping to prospectively validate these potential prognostic and predictive markers in the stage II setting (www.cancer.gov).

Overall, few therapeutic changes appear to be on the horizon for the treatment of adjuvant colon cancer. Investigators are attempting to modify the role of chemotherapy, reduce the duration of treatment from 6 to 3 months (120), and evaluate the role of diagnostic imaging modalities to improve our approach to these patients.

The MDACC Approach to Nonmetastatic Colon Cancer

When patients present to MDACC with a diagnosis of colon cancer, a detailed history with careful attention to the family history and a physical examination are obtained. Previous endoscopic findings are reviewed, and any biopsy material is submitted for pathology review. As discussed earlier, in cases of suspected Lynch syndrome, tumor tissue can be tested for microsatellite instability (MSI) and/or for mismatch repair gene protein expression by immunohistochemistry. (This is done with informed consent and genetic counseling.) Routine laboratory data are obtained, including a baseline serum CEA level. Radiographic studies include cross-sectional imaging of the chest, abdomen, and pelvis (CT or CT chest/MRI of the abdomen/pelvis). As shown in the diagnostic and therapeutic algorithm for colon cancer, patients with no evidence of metastatic disease and no contraindications to surgery should undergo primary resection with curative intent (Fig. 21-3). Of note, patients who have not undergone full colonoscopy as part of their initial diagnostic evaluation should have a colonoscopy performed to rule out synchronous lesions. If there is an obstruction, colonoscopy is usually performed within 3 months of the primary surgery. Surgery may consist of segmental resection or subtotal colectomy, depending on the underlying colonic pathology (multifocal cancer, FAP, HNPCC, etc); pathologic staging is then determined from the surgical specimens. Patients with stage 0 or I tumors are not advised to receive further therapy. For patients determined to have stage II or III colon cancer, referral to a medical oncologist is recommended after adequate surgical recovery has occurred for discussion of adjuvant chemotherapy.

Our current approach favors individualized decision making for patients. Most stage III patients are offered FOLFOX (Table 21-6) for 6 months, while those who are considered better candidates for a fluoropyrimidine may be offered capecitabine instead of intravenous 5-FU. Adjuvant therapy should begin within 4 to 8 weeks after surgery, unless surgical complications or medical comorbidities warrant a delay.

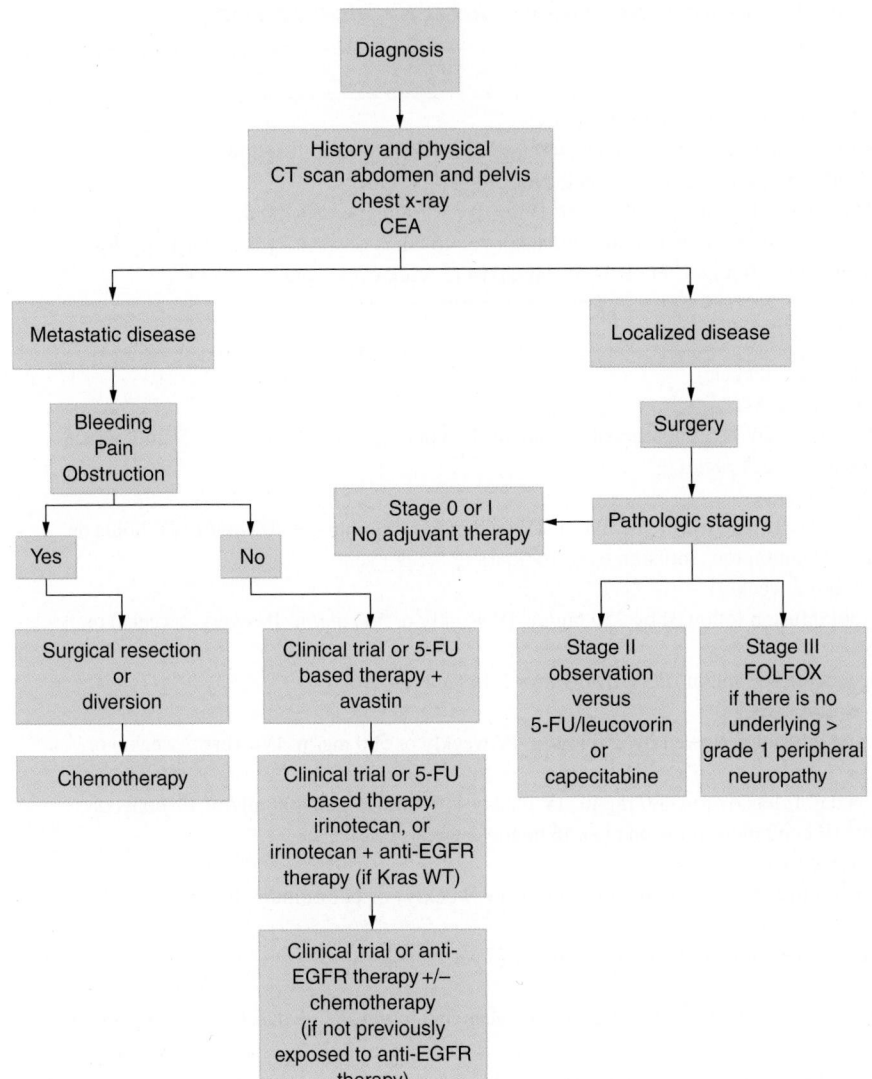

FIGURE 21-3. Diagnostic and therapeutic algorithm for colon cancer.

As stated earlier, adjuvant chemotherapy in patients with stage II colon cancer remains controversial and should be made on a case-by-case basis. Patients with stage II colon cancer have a 75 to 80% chance of long-term disease-free survival with surgical resection alone. However, as stated earlier, there is growing appreciation for the role of adequate lymph node sampling as part of risk assessment that may help clinicians decide about adjuvant therapy for these patients (92). Additional high-risk features such as bowel perforation, lymphovascular or perineural invasion, and poorly differentiated histology confer a worse prognosis and generally warrant adjuvant therapy for stage II colon cancer (94). Early data suggested that the presence of loss of heterozygosity of 18q is a poor prognostic indicator for survival (121). However, recent data contradict the significance of LOH 18q for 5-year colon cancer specific survival ($p = .54$) (122,123). Recent data also support the presence of a mutation in the proto-oncogene serine/ threonine-protein

kinase (B-RAF), also known as V-raf murine sarcoma viral oncogene homolog B1, (<10% of colorectal patients) is a poor prognostic indicator for OS (124).

Currently, at our institution in the absence of high-risk features, stage II colon cancer patients with MSI-H tumors are generally not offered adjuvant therapy. However, in the setting of the high-risk stage II or III patient, adjuvant FOLFOX-based chemotherapy is considered and discussed with the patient.

Surveillance for Patients With Resected Colon Cancer

Once all components of active therapy are completed, patients are followed carefully for evidence of relapse. Patients undergo clinical evaluations every 3 to 4 months for the first 3 years, every 6 months for the following 2 years, and annually thereafter. The highest risk of recurrence is within 3 years following surgical resection (125). Bowel and sexual functioning are assessed

TABLE 21-6 | **SUMMARY OF COMMON CHEMOTHERAPY REGIMENS USED AT MDACC FOR COLORECTAL CANCER**

Adjuvant Chemotherapy

Capecitabine: 1000 mg/m^2 PO BID on days 1-14 (3 week cycle, total 8 cycles)

5-fluorouracil/leucovorin: Leucovorin 400 mg/m^2 IV on day 1; 5-fluorouracil 400 mg/m^2 IV bolus on day 1, followed by 5-fluorouracil 2400 mg/m^2 IV continuous infusion over 46 hours (2 week cycle, total 12 cycles)

Modified FOLFOX 6: Oxaliplatin 85 mg/m^2 IV on day 1; leucovorin 400 mg/m^2 IV on day 1; 5-fluorouracil 400 mg/m^2 IV bolus on day 1, followed by 5-fluorouracil 2400 mg/m^2 IV continuous infusion over 46 hours (2 week cycle, total 12 cycles)

XELOX: Oxaliplatin 130 mg/m^2 on day 1; capecitabine 850 mg/m^2 PO BID on days 1-14 (3 week cycle, total 8 cycles)

Therapy for Metastatic Disease

Capecitabine: 1000 mg/m^2 PO BID on days 1-14 (3 week cycle)
- With or without bevacizumab (7.5 mg/kg IV every 3 weeks)

5-fluorouracil/leucovorin: Leucovorin 400 mg/m^2 IV on day 1; 5-fluorouracil 400 mg/m^2 IV bolus on day 1, followed by 5-fluorouracil 2400 mg/m^2 IV continuous infusion over 46 hours (2 week cycle)

With or without bevacizumab (5 mg/kg IV every 2 weeks)

Modified FOLFOX 6: Oxaliplatin 85 mg/m^2 IV on day 1; leucovorin 400 mg/m^2 IV on day 1; 5-fluorouracil 400 mg/m^2 IV bolus on day 1, followed by 5-fluorouracil 2400 mg/m^2 IV continuous infusion over 46 hours (2 week cycle)
- With or without bevacizumab (5 mg/kg IV every 2 weeks)
- With or without cetuximab[1] (400 mg/m^2 IV first infusion followed by 250 mg/m^2 IV weekly or 500 mg/m^2 IV every 2 weeks) or panitumumab[1] (6 mg/kg IV every 2 weeks)

XELOX: Oxaliplatin 130 mg/m^2 on day 1; capecitabine 850 mg/m^2 PO BID on days 1-14 (3 week cycle)

With or without bevacizumab (7.5 mg/kg IV every 3 weeks)
- With or without cetuximab[1] (400 mg/m^2 IV first infusion followed by 250 mg/m^2 IV weekly or 500 mg/m^2 IV every 2 weeks) or panitumumab[1] (9 mg/kg IV every 3 weeks)

Modified FOLFIRI: Irinotecan 180 mg/m^2 IV on day 1; leucovorin 400 mg/m^2 IV on day 1; 5-fluorouracil 400 mg/m^2 IV bolus on day 1, followed by 5-fluorouracil 2400 mg/m^2 IV continuous infusion over 46 hours (2 week cycle)
- With or without bevacizumab (5 mg/kg IV every 2 weeks)
- With or without cetuximab[1] (400 mg/m^2 IV first infusion followed by 250 mg/m^2 IV weekly) or panitumumab[1] (6 mg/kg IV every 2 weeks)

Irinotecan: 180 mg/m^2 IV on day 1 (2 week cycle) or 300-350 mg/m^2 IV on day 1 (3 week cycle)

Cetuximab[1]/Irinotecan:
- Cetuximab[1] 400 mg/m^2 IV first infusion followed by 250 mg/m^2 IV weekly + irinotecan 350 mg/m^2 IV on day 1 (3 week cycle) or 180 mg/m^2 IV on day 1 (2 week cycle)
- Cetuximab[1] 500 mg/m^2 IV every 2 weeks +/– irinotecan 180 mg/m^2 IV every 2 weeks

Panitumumab[1]: 6 mg/kg IV every 2 weeks or 9 mg/kg IV every 3 weeks

[1]Cetuximab and panitumumab are indicated only in patients with *KRAS* wild-type tumors.

Concurrent Chemotherapy and Radiation Therapy (Rectal Cancer)

Continuous infusion 5-fluorouracil: 250-300 mg/m^2 IV daily (Monday-Friday on days of radiation therapy only)

Capecitabine: 825 mg/m^2 PO BID (Monday-Friday on days of radiation therapy only)

---

during these clinic visits. Colonoscopy is recommended 1 year after surgery and every 3 years thereafter (some patients require more frequent examinations based on endoscopic findings or high-risk status). Laboratory studies, including CEA level, are checked every 3 to 6 months; abdominopelvic CT or MRI and a chest x-ray/CT of the chest are obtained at a minimum of 12 months and earlier if clinically indicated. At 5 years, patients are offered long-term follow-up, with their medical oncologist consisting of their surveillance colonoscopy (every 3 years) and annual physical examination, and CEA. All patients are encouraged to maintain a relationship with a primary care physician for optimal surveillance and health care (annual lipid panel, well-woman visits, etc).

Local Therapy for Rectal Cancer

Similar to colon cancer surgery, the principles of rectal cancer surgery involves removal of the primary tumor with its mesorectum and draining lymphatics. Because of the confined anatomy of the pelvis and difficulty in achieving clear tumor margins (distal and radial) while preserving sphincter function, resection of rectal tumors is generally more challenging than resection of colon tumors. In general, over two-thirds of the patients with rectal cancer will be able to have a sphincter-saving procedure whether it is a low anterior resection with a primary handsewn or stapled anastomosis or a proctectomy with a coloanal anastomosis (CAA). An abdominoperineal resection (APR) which includes removal of the rectum, anus, sphincter muscles, and a permanent colostomy is reserved most of the time for patient whose sphincter muscles are involved by tumor or for patients with rectal cancer who have poor sphincter function preoperatively. Ideally, a surgical margin of at least 2 cm should be obtained. Recent evidence suggests that a margin as small as 1 cm may be sufficient, thus allowing more sphincter-saving procedures. Patients who have localized, nontransmural cancer or who receive preoperative chemotherapy and radiation therapy may be resected with lesser distal margins (126). A sharp mesorectal excision should be performed in patient with rectal cancer. There is no role for blunt dissection in the pelvis in rectal cancer surgery. Transanal excision may be considered in selected patients, but these patients must be followed closely given the risk of local recurrence (127,128). For patients with metastatic rectal cancer, systemic chemotherapy or concurrent chemoradiation therapy may be utilized. In these patients, other nonsurgical palliative measures can be considered and will be further discussed later in the chapter.

Radiotherapy

Radiotherapy has been shown to improve survival in patients with locally advanced rectal cancer. Standard radiotherapy doses are 45 Gy in 25 fractions, followed by a 5.4-Gy boost. Concurrent protracted venous infusional (PVI) 5-FU provides similar efficacy with lower gastrointestinal and hematologic toxicity rates than bolus 5-FU or a high-dose infusion of 5-FU (129). A phase III intergroup trial demonstrated inferiority for bolus 5-FU during radiation therapy versus prolonged infusional 5-FU resulted in higher overall survival rates ($p = .005$) (94). Capecitabine, is widely believed to be comparable to infusional 5-FU, and is often substituted for 5-FU as the radiation sensitizer. External-beam radiotherapy is not routinely recommended for primary tumors of the colon. However, it may be considered in cases of clinical or histologic evidence of tumor perforation or positive margins.

Adjuvant Therapy for Rectal Cancer

Since the mid-1970s, studies have shown that combined-modality therapy offers a clear benefit for patients with stage II or III rectal cancer. The Gastrointestinal Tumor Study Group (GITSG) performed a randomized trial in patients with rectal cancer undergoing surgery with curative intent. Patients were randomized to four arms: observation, chemotherapy alone, radiotherapy alone, or chemoradiotherapy. The

rates of disease-free survival and overall survival were higher in the combined-modality therapy group than in the other arms (130). A subsequent trial comparing chemoradiotherapy with radiotherapy alone also showed that combined-modality treatment conferred an advantage in terms of both disease-free and overall survival (131). Currently, standard adjuvant therapy for patients with stage II or III rectal cancer should consist of fluoropyrimidine-based chemotherapy and external-beam radiotherapy of the pelvis. Clinicians should use infusional 5-FU or oral capecitabine during the course of radiotherapy.

Preoperative Therapy for Rectal Cancer

First principles of radiotherapy have predicted that chemoradiation should be better tolerated and more efficacious when administered preoperatively rather than postoperatively in rectal cancer patients. In the postoperative setting, the small bowel is often fixed in the pelvis, increasing the irradiated bowel volume; the tumor bed is hypoxic, limiting therapeutic efficacy; and the vasculature is interrupted, compromising chemotherapy delivery. A number of phase II studies of preoperative therapy reported complete pathologic responses (pCR) to single-agent fluorouracil-based chemoradiation 5 to 20% of the time. In the United States, two cooperative groups have attempted to compare preoperative chemoradiation to postoperative chemoradiation in patients with nonmetastatic, resectable rectal cancer. However, neither the NSABP nor the CALGB could accrue a sufficient number of patients for a definitive conclusion, and both studies closed prematurely to target accrual (126). However, results from the NSABP trial suggested that patients undergoing preoperative therapy were more likely to undergo sphincter preservation. Two European studies have supported the use of preoperative therapy for resectable rectal cancer.

The German Arbeitsgemeinschaft Internistische Onkologie (AIO) trial comparing preoperative and postoperative chemoradiation has confirmed all of these hypotheses (88). In this study, more than 800 patients were staged with CT scan and endoscopic ultrasound, and those with clinical stage T3 or T4 tumors were randomly assigned to receive preoperative versus postoperative chemoradiation (50.4 Gy in 28 fractions) with concurrent high-dose infusional 5-FU (1000 mg/m^2/ day on days 1-5 and 21-25). All patients underwent TME 6 weeks after completing chemoradiation, while some patients in the postoperative arm received an additional 5.4Gy boost to the tumor bed. Patients in both arms were scheduled to receive four cycles of bolus 5-FU (500 mg/m^2/day, five times weekly, every 4 weeks), either after surgery (preoperative arm) or after chemoradiation (postoperative arm). Results showed a lower pelvic recurrence rate in the preoperative chemoradiation arm (6 versus 13% postoperative, respectively, $p = .0006$), despite 25% more patients than in the postoperative arm had low-lying tumors. In addition, patients receiving preoperative therapy had lower rates of grade 3 or 4 acute (27 versus 40%, $p = .001$) and late (14 versus 24%, $p = .01$) toxicities. The most striking toxicity difference between the arms was the incidence of anastomotic strictures (4 versus 12%, $p < .003$). Overall survival was unchanged. In patients who, based on pretreatment clinical evaluation, were believed to require APR chemoradiation also led to increased sphincter preservation rates (39 versus 19%, $p = .004$) and fewer anastomotic strictures.

The reasons for poorer local control in the postoperative chemoradiation group may be due to hypoxia in the tumor bed limiting efficacy, as predicted by preclinical modeling and numerous clinical studies. Moreover, poor compliance in the postoperative arm due to toxicity may have contributed to the difference. Only 54% of patients in the postoperative arm received the full radiation dose and 50% received full-dose chemotherapy, compared with 92 and 89%, respectively, in the preoperative arm ($p < .001$). Regardless of the reason for success in the neoadjuvant chemoradiotherapy arm, this trial has been widely interpreted as having defined a new standard of care in the neoadjuvant treatment of rectal cancer. One disadvantage associated with preoperative therapy is the potential overtreatment of patients whose pretreatment clinical stage is judged higher than that determined pathologically at the time of surgery. For example, 18% of patients randomized to the postoperative arm were spared adjuvant therapy because they were found to have stage I disease at the time of surgery, and another 10% of patients did not receive adjuvant treatment due to detection of metastatic disease or postoperative complications/death. This suggests that 15 to 20% of patients receiving preoperative chemoradiation may be overtreated. At MDACC, endorectal ultrasound and pelvic MRI are included in the standard workup and considered essential in the initial evaluation of patients with rectal tumors.

Studies have completed accrual to determine whether neoadjuvant single-agent 5-FU, capecitabine, ± oxaliplatin chemotherapy can decrease local recurrence rates and improve overall survival. NSABP R-04 is a phase III trial composed of four arms: (1) 5-FU, (2) capecitabine, (3) 5-FU/oxaliplatin, and (4) CapeOX. Two phase III trials (Studio Terapia Adiuvante Retto and Action Clinique Coordonnées en cancérologie Digestive [STAR and ACCORD] 12) have failed to determine an improvement in pathologic complete response (CR) with the addition of weekly oxaliplatin and resulted in increased GI toxicities (132,133).

Identified prognostic indicators for rectal cancer recurrence include pathologic tumor regression grade and molecular markers (134,135). These indicators are currently being applied to modern approach to rectal cancer treatment.

The MDACC Approach to Nonmetastatic Rectal Cancer

Preoperative Chemoradiation

The diagnostic pathway and general therapeutic approach to rectal cancer is outlined in Fig. 21-4. When patients present to MDACC, they are generally seen initially by a multidisciplinary team of radiation oncology, medical oncology, and colorectal surgery. A thorough history and physical examination are performed. Careful attention is paid to family history, including information about noncolorectal malignancies affecting other family members. Physical examination includes digital rectal examination, inguinal lymph node examination, and rigid proctoscopy. Staging studies are then obtained as previously outlined. For patients found to have metastatic disease, endoscopic ultrasound (EUS) is generally not indicated. However, it is recommended that the patency of the colonic lumen be evaluated by proctoscopy, flexible sigmoidoscopy, or colonoscopy before starting systemic chemotherapy and continued to be followed every 4 to 6 months to avoid impending obstruction/perforation while receiving chemotherapy. Rather than a surgical diversion, consideration of APC (argon plasma coagulation) or colonic/rectal stent may be viable options.

For patients with nonmetastatic disease, EUS and MRI of the pelvis are obtained as part of routine preoperative staging. Both imaging modalities are considered to optimize accuracy of pretreatment staging. Capecitabine, which is widely believed to be comparable to infusional 5-FU, is frequently substituted for 5-FU as the radiation sensitizer at MDACC (825 mg/m^2 bid, M-F, on days of radiation therapy only).

Bowel exclusion techniques such as the use of an open table top device ("belly-board") are typically used during simulation to minimize the amount of small bowel in the field. Patient education begins prior to initiation of therapy and continues through the course of treatment. Uneventful successful treatment is largely dependent on pretreatment patient education and encouragement of a patient's adherence. Radiation oncology and medical oncology evaluate patients every 1 to 2 weeks

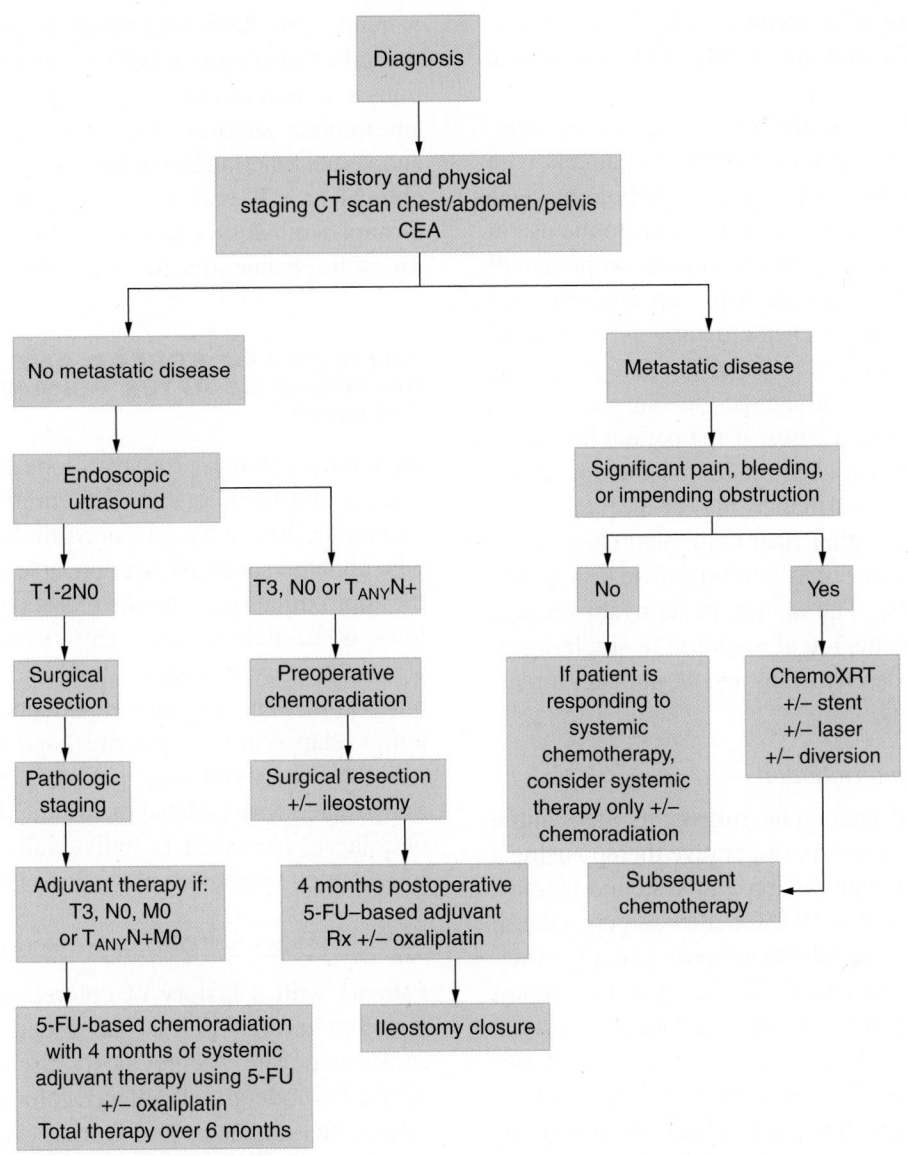

FIGURE 21-4. Diagnostic and therapeutic algorithm for rectal cancer.

during radiation therapy for nutritional status, GI toxicities, and skin and mucosal integrity. An important component of treatment tolerability is the use of appropriate supportive care with antiemetic and antidiarrheal regimens. Electrolytes, renal function, and hematologic parameters are checked weekly and more often if clinically indicated. Various topical barrier creams are prescribed for application to the perineum for patient comfort depending on the degree of radiation dermatitis; grade 1 to 3 is not uncommon and may vary based on underlying body habitus and personal hygiene. Should greater than grade 2 nonhematologic toxicity develop (excluding radiation dermatitis), concurrent chemotherapy is held until it resolves but radiation is continued.

After chemoradiation, perianal pain and ulceration, anorexia, diarrhea, and fatigue typically subside within

2 to 3 weeks (varies by the baseline physical condition of the patient at baseline). Approximately 6 weeks after completion of therapy, patients undergo repeat physical examination with proctoscopy. The patient then undergoes surgical resection. Tumors in the distal or mid-rectum may require APR or other surgical approaches, including LAR or proctectomy with coloanal anastomosis. In all cases, TME is carried out. For those patients undergoing a sphincter-sparing surgery after preoperative therapy, a diverting ileostomy is usually created and remains in place for at least 6 weeks to prevent anastomotic leak in an area of previously irradiated bowel. Ideally, we do not recommend reversal of the diverting ileostomy until after the completion of adjuvant chemotherapy due to erratic bowel managements and its potential impact on adherence with completion of adjuvant chemotherapy.

For those patients who recover fully from surgery, postoperative chemotherapy is delivered for a total of 4 months.

While the role of oxaliplatin as a component of adjuvant therapy has not been established in patients with rectal cancer, patients with clinical or pathologic stage III rectal cancer, and no contraindications to the use of oxaliplatin, are advised to receive it as a component of FOLFOX or in combination with capecitabine. Our choice of postoperative chemotherapy is commonly based on the preoperative stage of the patient and the degree of pathologic downstaging following neoadjuvant chemotherapy. In select cases, if the patient has had a pCR with 5-FU–based chemoradiation therapy alone, single-agent 5-FU–based therapy may be the preferential adjuvant treatment rather than combined chemotherapy with FOLFOX due to its potential dose liming toxicity of neuropathy. The choice of adjuvant therapy may vary based on degree of response to single-agent fluoropyrimidine-based therapy and the patient's underlying comorbidities.

Postoperative Chemoradiation

Patients who have undergone surgery as their initial intervention may require postoperative therapy using a combination of chemoradiation and systemic therapy. When patients present to MDACC after surgery, careful attention is paid to the operative report, and all pathology is internally reviewed. If the operative report describes tumor at or below the peritoneal reflection, such a tumor is considered rectal in origin for purposes of adjuvant therapy. For patients with T3,N0,M0 or T2,N1 disease, radiotherapy is often omitted if the tumor was located in the high pelvis (>10 cm from the anal verge) (136), there is a good nodal sampling (>12 lymph nodes) (137), and the radial margin is negative (>2 mm) (138) because pelvic tumor control is excellent without the use of chemoradiation (136,139). In all other stages II and III rectal cancer cases, local failure is high enough to warrant the use of chemoradiation. Additionally, 4 months of systemic therapy with either capecitabine or 5-FU/leucovorin is typically integrated with chemoradiation. Patients at higher risk of distant metastasis often receive chemotherapy first. In patients with no contraindications to the use of oxaliplatin, FOLFOX would generally be recommended as the systemic therapy.

Surveillance for Patients With Resected Rectal Cancer

Follow-up for patients with resected rectal cancer is very similar to that for colon cancer. However, rectal cancer patients who have undergone a sphincter-preserving procedure also require periodic proctoscopic examinations to look for evidence of relapsing local disease and anastomotic strictures that might compromise bowel and sexual function. A steadily rising CEA without other clinical or CT evidence of relapse is more likely to prompt acquisition of a pelvic MRI or PET/CT to look for subtle changes that may indicate local recurrence.

PATTERNS OF SPREAD AND RECURRENCE AFTER PRIMARY THERAPY

As noted previously, 70% of colon cancer patients have disease that is resectable with curative intent, and the remaining 30% have advanced disease. Among those who undergo surgical resection, at least 25% will recur; the approximate distribution of sites of relapse is as follows: 60%, multiple sites; 15%, liver metastases only; 4%, pulmonary metastases only; and 21%, local recurrence (140). The majority of patients will develop systemic relapse in multiple sites, and these patients are generally managed with palliative systemic therapy. For patients with isolated metastatic disease at the time of relapse, treatment is individualized, with surgical intervention sometimes playing a role.

Management of Locally Recurrent Disease

Patients with a history of colorectal cancer are estimated to have a 3 to 4% risk of local recurrence at the anastomotic site. As previously discussed, patients are advised to undergo surveillance colonoscopy 12 months after initial diagnosis and at least every 3 years thereafter. In some cases, tumors that recur at the anastomotic site may be resected for cure. The same pathologic staging, prognostic implications, and treatment algorithms used for the primary neoplasm apply to the anastomotic recurrence. In the case of rectal cancer, local recurrence is more common, even with TME, and may be caused either by direct submucosal extension or intramural lymphatic spread.

Locally recurrent rectal cancer with or without evidence of metastatic disease is a formidable therapeutic challenge. Surgical salvage is considered but may not be feasible for the majority of patients. Importantly, the collective experience at MDACC suggests that systemic therapy, while capable of causing regression of distant disease, is rarely active against locally recurrent disease. An occasional patient may have some symptomatic improvement with the use of chemotherapy, but objective responses are uncommon and virtually never durable. These patients are best managed in a multidisciplinary fashion, with early involvement of pain management physicians, interventional radiology, surgical oncologists, radiation oncologists, and medical oncologists. Pain in particular may be difficult to control and, whenever possible, further palliative radiation is delivered as external-beam radiotherapy or brachytherapy catheters. Aggressive use of narcotics is routine, but intrathecal analgesics or neurolytic blocks are employed for those patients with inadequate pain control or intolerance to narcotics. Aggressive bowel management must be pursued to prevent narcotic-induced ileus.

Other complications may also develop, including ureteral obstruction or fistulas to the skin, bladder, or vagina. Placement of nephrostomy tubes or indwelling ureteral stents may be required. Skin integrity and perineal hygiene is monitored in conjunction with wound care nursing specialists, and every effort is made to maximize comfort and dignity for patients who confront these challenges.

For the subset of rectal cancer patients who may be candidates for salvage surgery, careful staging and treatment planning are vetted in a multidisciplinary colorectal cancer conference held weekly at MDACC. Prior chemoradiation and surgery may lead to significant fibrosis, confounding interpretation of imaging studies in this setting. In our experience, MRI of the pelvis appears to be superior to CT imaging for distinguishing posttreatment changes from viable tumor and provides excellent detail of surrounding pelvic structures, including sacral nerve roots and vasculature. These particular anatomic details are required to define potentially resectable, locally recurrent disease. Even when imaging and other clinical parameters (worsening pelvic pain or rising CEA levels) suggest local recurrence, biopsy confirmation of recurrent disease is always recommended. While not routinely part of surgical staging, FDG-PET is employed in cases of equivocal radiographic evidence of distant disease. EUS has not been particularly useful as a staging modality for patients with locally recurrent rectal tumors.

For those patients being considered for surgical salvage, additional chemoradiation is delivered using a hypofractionated schedule to a total dose of 39 Gy (if at least 1 year has elapsed since prior pelvic radiation). Radiosensitization with 5-FU or capecitabine is also considered. Approximately 6 to 8 weeks after completion of chemoradiation, a final decision about surgery is made; this may require the participation of reconstructive plastic surgeons, urologists, and occasionally neurosurgeons to maximize tumor extirpation and minimize disfigurement and functional

impairment. In most cases, the operative strategy may also include intraoperative radiotherapy (IORT) or insertion of brachytherapy catheters for high-dose afterloading. The role of postoperative chemotherapy after aggressive preoperative chemoradiation and salvage surgery is at the discretion of the treating physician and may vary by the patient's recovery following surgical resection. However, there is broad agreement that surgery for locally recurrent disease is not indicated in those patients with unresectable metastatic disease, given the overall poor prognosis, significant morbidity, and prolonged recovery associated with this complex pelvic surgery required for recurrent disease.

SYSTEMIC THERAPY FOR METASTATIC DISEASE: A RAPIDLY CHANGING THERAPEUTIC LANDSCAPE

Since the late 1950s, systemic chemotherapy with 5-FU has been the mainstay of palliative treatment for patients with metastatic disease not amenable to surgical intervention. During the ensuing decades, a variety of 5-FU schedules have been employed, including bolus injections administered either weekly (Roswell Park regimen) or daily for 5 days (Mayo regimen) and continuous infusion given via central catheter and portable pump. Objective response rates have ranged from 15 to 25% with these schedules. When 5-FU is administered as a bolus injection, leucovorin is often added to enhance binding of 5-FU to its target, thymidylate synthase (TS). After a long period of uncertainty regarding the optimal dose and schedule of 5-FU with leucovorin, infusional 5-FU regimens have been recognized as superior to bolus regimens. However, prior to the advent of irinotecan and oxaliplatin, while infusional delivery of 5-FU led to better response rates compared with bolus therapy, no clear survival advantage was ever demonstrated. Given the barriers to delivery of infusional 5-FU, including the need for a central venous catheter and its associated risks, bolus 5-FU with leucovorin was widely accepted in the United States as frontline therapy for metastatic colorectal cancer well into the 1990s.

Since that time, therapeutic options for metastatic disease have been rapidly evolving, and oncologists now have access to several drugs with activity in the first-, second-, and even third-line settings. In addition to cytotoxic drugs, the targeted agents cetuximab, panitumumab, and bevacizumab have emerged as clinically relevant components of systemic therapy for advanced disease. It is important for oncologists to have a general understanding of these drugs and their roles in the treatment of metastatic disease.

Capecitabine: An Orally Bioavailable Fluoropyrimidine

Capecitabine is an oral fluoropyrimidine that is converted to 5-FU primarily in tumor tissues. It passes through the intestinal mucosa essentially unchanged and is subsequently metabolized by a sequential three-enzyme pathway (141). First, capecitabine is converted to 5′-deoxy-5-fluorocytidine (5′-DFCR) by carboxylesterase (primarily in the liver). 5′-DFCR is then converted to 5′-deoxy-5-fluorouridine (5′-DFUR) by cytidine deaminase, which is found in both the liver and tumor tissues. The metabolism of 5′-DFUR to the pharmacologically active agent 5-FU is mediated by thymidine phosphorylase (TP), also known as platelet-derived endothelial cell growth factor (PD-ECGF). Concentrations of TP are relatively higher in tumor tissue than normal tissue, which accounts for the preferential intratumoral release of 5-FU. Two large phase III trials compared capecitabine with a bolus regimen of 5-FU (142,143), and the results were subsequently pooled. The response rates were superior with capecitabine, and the median survival was equivalent, with less neutropenia and mucositis among those patients receiving capecitabine.

In patients with contraindications to combination chemotherapy, capecitabine monotherapy is a reasonable alternative to 5-FU and leucovorin in the metastatic setting.

Irinotecan

Irinotecan, an inhibitor of topoisomerase I, was originally developed as second-line chemotherapy for patients in whom 5-FU was ineffective (144-146). In phase II trials of irinotecan performed in the United States, response rates in 5-FU refractory patients were approximately 15% superior to those reported prior to the advent of irinotecan; this led the FDA to approve the drug as a second-line therapy in patients with advanced, 5-FU refractory disease (147). The survival benefit of second-line irinotecan was subsequently verified in a European trial, in which patients who had been previously treated with 5-FU were randomized to receive irinotecan every 3 weeks or best supportive care (BSC) (148). Patients randomized to BSC were allowed to receive infusional 5-FU. This trial demonstrated a survival advantage for patients in the irinotecan arm compared to those in the BSC arm (9.2 versus 6.5 months; $p = .0001$).

Shortly thereafter, studies were performed to investigate the potential benefit of irinotecan as a component of frontline therapy in patients with metastatic colorectal cancer. Two large, randomized trials were conducted in the United States and Europe, comparing 5-FU and leucovorin with 5-FU, leucovorin, and irinotecan as first-line treatment of metastatic colorectal cancer (149,150). Both studies demonstrated that the response and overall survival rates for the group treated with triple-drug therapy were superior to those for the group treated with 5-FU and leucovorin. The response rates for the triple-drug combination ranged from 35 to 40%, the median time to disease progression was 7 months, and median survival was prolonged by 2 months. These results prompted the FDA to approve the use of these irinotecan-based combinations for first-line treatment of colorectal cancer in 2000. For a brief period of time, the IFL regimen (bolus 5-FU at 500 mg/m^2, leucovorin 20 mg/m^2, and irinotecan 125 mg/m^2, administered weekly for 4 weeks on a 6-week cycle) became standard first-line therapy for patients with metastatic colon cancer in the United States. However, as these studies were being performed, a novel platinum analog, oxaliplatin, was also showing impressive activity in combination with 5-FU and leucovorin, generating great interest in the drug.

Oxaliplatin

Oxaliplatin is a third-generation platinum derivative that has shown additive and/or synergistic antitumor activity in combination with a variety of standard antineoplastic agents, including 5-FU; oxaliplatin is ineffective without 5-FU (151). While irinotecan was being studied in the United States, oxaliplatin was already approved in Europe. In 2000, de Gramont and colleagues reported the results of a phase III trial of infusional 5-FU/leucovorin and oxaliplatin (FOLFOX4), versus 5-FU/leucovorin alone, as first-line treatment in advanced colorectal cancer (152). Four hundred twenty patients were randomized, and progression-free survival (PFS) was the primary endpoint. Progression-free survival and response rates were significantly better for the FOLFOX arm compared to the 5-FU/leucovorin arm (9.0 months and 50% versus 6.2 months and 22%, respectively). Even though the FOLFOX arm experienced more grades 3 and 4 neutropenia, diarrhea, and neurosensory toxicity, this did not impair quality of life. The primary objective of median overall survival was not met (14.7 months for the 5-FU/leucovorin arm and

16.2 months for the FOLFOX arm, $p = .12$) and consequently initially failed to be FDA approved.

Goldberg and associates subsequently compared the activity and toxicity of three different drug combinations in untreated patients with metastatic colorectal cancer. Seven hundred ninety-five patients were randomized to receive IFL, FOLFOX, or IROX (irinotecan + oxaliplatin) (153). The results favored FOLFOX for all endpoints, including time to progression, response rate, and overall survival. Median survival in the FOLFOX, IFL, and IROX groups was 19.5, 15.0, and 17.4 months, respectively. The authors concluded that FOLFOX should be considered a standard first-line regimen for advanced colorectal cancer. A limitation of this study was that 60% of the patients treated with oxaliplatin received irinotecan in the second-line setting, but only 24% of patients in the IFL arm could get oxaliplatin as second-line treatment because it was not approved in the United States at the time of the study.

Tournigand and colleagues answered the important question of how to sequence these regimens. They reported the results of a phase III study investigating 5-FU, leucovorin, and irinotecan (FOLFIRI), followed by FOLFOX6 (see Table 21-6) upon progression of disease, versus the opposite sequence (FOLFOX6 followed by FOLFIRI) (154). The two sequences were equivalent in terms of progression-free and overall survival, although the toxicity profiles were different. Median survival was 21.5 months in the FOLFIRI-FOLFOX arm (109 patients) and 20.6 months in the FOLFOX-FOLFIRI arm (111 patients) ($p = .99$).

An aggressive approach is the combination of oxaliplatin, irinotecan, and 5-FU/leucovorin (FOLFOXIRI) (155). An impressive response rate of 66% was noted in a phase III trial of FOLFOXIRI versus FOLFIRI fulfilling the primary endpoint of PFS. However, a serious adverse toxicity associated with this regimen is severe myelosuppression. Concerns about this regimen are largely due to discussion of limited options for second-line therapy if the patient should progress. Furthermore, an earlier phase III Greek trial failed to note an improvement in OS perhaps due to the limited second-line chemotherapy options for patients treated with FOLFOXIRI (156). Common chemotherapy regimens for both colon and rectal carcinoma are listed in Table 21-6.

Monoclonal Antibodies

Therapeutic use of the immune system against cancer has been studied for decades but remained elusive until recently due to technical difficulties. The fact that tumor cells are recognized as a part of the normal host makes the development of vaccines very difficult, and the logical alternative would involve development of foreign antibodies that could be delivered to the patient. The development of those antibodies was not possible until 1975, when the hybridoma technique was perfected by Kohler and others, allowing the development of specific antibodies against antigens restricted to, or overexpressed in, tumor cells (157). Initially, the development of these antibodies was proposed as a direct immunologic and cytotoxic approach for treatment of malignant disease. While such efforts continue, this strategy has been refined to include the development of antibodies that target specific proteins critical to intracellular signaling, tumor cell function, or the host-tumor interface. Three new monoclonal antibodies have been recently approved in the United States for treatment of metastatic colorectal cancer.

Cetuximab

Cetuximab is a chimeric IgG1 monoclonal antibody directed against the epidermal growth factor receptor (EGFR), also known as ErbB-1 (158). In the colorectal cancer arena, it was primarily studied in previously treated patients. Cetuximab monotherapy yielded a response rate of 9% and median survival of 6.4 months in a small group of irinotecan-refractory patients (159). When compared to BSC in a treatment-refractory patient population, single-agent cetuximab resulted in superior overall survival (6.1 versus 4.6 months) and quality of life. Two Phase III randomized trials (Bowel Oncology and *Cetuximab* Antibody, Erbitux Plus Irinotecan for Metastatic Colorectal Cancer [BOND, EPIC]) subsequently confirmed the efficacy of cetuximab in combination with irinotecan in previously treated patients (160,161), with response rates of approximately 20%. Improvement in overall survival versus best supportive care (BSC) has since been validated in heavily pretreated patients (162). The reason for the apparent synergy between cetuximab and irinotecan is not well understood; it is known that EGFR mediates not only proliferation signals, but also a number of other processes whose inhibition may render cells more sensitive to apoptotic stimuli, such as chemotherapy.

EGFR inhibition is fraught with potential treatment-related toxicities, including a pustular acneiform rash of the upper torso and scalp. Hence, identification of a predictive marker for efficacy of anti-EGFR therapy would decrease unnecessary drug exposure and financial burden. It is now recognized that EGFR expression does not correlate with efficacy of therapy (163). However, mutation of the *KRAS* oncogene is present in 35 to 50% of all colorectal patients and has an early role in the transition of adenoma to carcinoma, with reported concordance between the primary and the metastatic site (164). The mutations are commonly G>A transitions and G>T transversions; codons 12 and 13 are the most frequently affected, and rarely codons 61 and 146. In addition to *KRAS*, mutations in *NRAS* have been recently identified as a potential predictive indicator of anti-EGFR efficacy. The *NRAS* mutation may be present in 10% of patients and was also associated with reduced response to panitumumab (165). Patients with *KRAS* wild-type (WT) and *NRAS* wild-type tumors had improved PFS (HR = 0.39, 95% CI = 0.27, 0.56) compared with those receiving BSC, whereas those with *NRAS* mutant tumors did not appear to benefit from panitumumab (HR = 1.94, 95% CI = 0.44, 8.44).

The Cetuximab combined with iRinotecan in first line therapY for metaSTatic colorectAL (CRYSTAL) phase III trial randomized nearly 1200 patients with untreated metastatic colorectal cancer to FOLFIRI with or without cetuximab. Median PFS (8.9 versus 8.0 months) and response rate (47 versus 39%) were modestly improved with cetuximab. Most importantly, however, investigators later discovered that clinical benefit was limited to those patients with *KRAS* WT tumors in an unplanned retrospective analysis. In this group of patients, the findings were impressive; cetuximab improved the response rate from 43 to 59% and median PFS from 8.7 months to 9.9 months (166). Updated results of the CRYSTAL trial were recently presented, indicating an overall survival advantage for FOLFIRI and cetuximab in the *KRAS* WT group (23.5 versus 20.0 months) (167). This is the first trial to demonstrate an improvement in OS with cetuximab in combination with chemotherapy in treatment-naïve patients. In addition, OPUS, a randomized phase II trial in treatment-naïve patients, compared FOLFOX4 plus cetuximab to FOLFOX4 alone and also showed improvement in response rate and PFS with cetuximab. Once again, analysis revealed that this benefit was restricted to patients without *KRAS* mutations (168). Neither study has indicated what percentage of specimens analyzed were from the primary versus the metastatic site and if true concordance exists. Despite the current evidence supporting *KRAS* testing, the FDA delayed mandating *KRAS* testing largely due to the retrospective unplanned analyses. Soon after, the American Society of Clinical Oncology (ASCO) released a provisional clinical opinion advising against use of EGFR monoclonal antibodies in colorectal cancer patients with *KRAS* mutant tumors (169); subsequently the

FDA revised the label of cetuximab and panitumumab in July 2009.

The most significant toxicities associated with cetuximab include diarrhea, hypomagnesemia, hypocalcemia, and an acneiform rash. Traditionally, the risk of an allergic hypersensitivity reaction is reported to be <5%. However, life-threatening anaphylactic hypersensitivity reactions have been reported in up to 30% of patients residing in select geographic locations (170). IgE antibodies against cetuximab have been discovered and may allow screening for patients at risk for this reaction.

Development of the skin rash appears to be a clinical predictor of response and survival, but the mechanisms involved in this process are poorly understood (171). The Dose-Escalation *Study* of *Cetuximab* for Metastatic Colorectal Cancer (EVEREST) study, which was undertaken to address the association between skin rash and clinical response to cetuximab, stratified patients with no or mild rash to standard-dose or dose-escalated cetuximab . Dose escalation increased the response rate from 13 to 30%. Although these results are intriguing, firm conclusions about the dose–response relationship with cetuximab cannot be drawn from this small phase II trial, and the final results have not been reported. Recent data support that the pharmacokinetics of cetuximab is not compromised with administration every 2 weeks rather than weekly (170). Furthermore, a small phase II trial indicates that preemptive dermatological care may improve patient outcome when using EGFR inhibitors (172).

Cetuximab is currently FDA-approved as monotherapy for patients with metastatic colorectal cancer who are intolerant of irinotecan-based regimens or in combination with irinotecan after progression of disease. The findings of the CRYSTAL trial will likely result in a FDA application for approval for cetuximab in the frontline setting.

Panitumumab

Panitumumab is a fully human IgG2 monoclonal antibody directed against the EGFR. In a randomized phase III trial, patients with refractory metastatic disease received BSC with or without panitumumab. The response rate and stable disease rate with panitumumab were 10% and 27%, respectively, compared to 0% and 10% with BSC alone. An overall survival difference could not be demonstrated in this trial, likely due to crossover from the BSC group (173). Subsequent analysis revealed that only patients with *KRAS* WT tumors benefited from panitumumab (174). Although cetuximab and panitumumab have not been compared head-to-head, they appear to have similar efficacy and toxicity in patients. Infusion reactions are uncommon with panitumumab, since it is a fully human monoclonal antibody. It is now FDA-approved as a single agent for patients failing irinotecan- and oxaliplatin-based chemotherapy. Two phase III trials have recently been reported of FOLFOX or FOLFIRI ± panitumumab for both treatment-naïve and previously treated patients, respectively (175,176). Both studies reported superior response and PFS for the combination and will likely also result in an application for approval in combination with chemotherapy in the front and second-line setting.

Bevacizumab

In studies dating back over 30 years, Dr. Judah Folkman demonstrated that tumors cannot grow beyond 1 mm without creating new vessels to deliver oxygen and nutrients. He therefore predicted that a drug capable of blocking angiogenesis would be able to arrest the growth of tumors (177). Among the several angiogenic factors isolated to date, vascular endothelial growth factor (VEGF) seems to be particularly important, with elevated circulating levels being associated with poor prognosis in patients with colorectal cancer (178,179). Bevacizumab is a humanized monoclonal antibody that binds all isoforms of circulating VEGF, thereby inhibiting permeability and angiogenesis mediated by this factor (180).

Bevacizumab is currently FDA-approved in multiple tumor types, including lung, breast, and colorectal cancer. A randomized phase II trial compared weekly 5-FU/leucovorin with the same chemotherapy combined with either 5 mg/kg or 10 mg/kg of bevacizumab. Both experimental arms performed better than the control 5-FU/leucovorin arm (181). However, the best results were seen with the lower dose of bevacizumab, leading the investigators to recommend a dose of 5 mg/kg for a phase III trial in colorectal cancer.

The phase III trial compared the IFL regimen, which was considered the standard regimen for metastatic colorectal cancer at that time, with IFL plus bevacizumab (5 mg/kg) (182). A third arm with 5-FU/leucovorin plus bevacizumab was added as a precaution, but it was dropped after the first 100 patients were treated safely. Patients on the exploratory arm were allowed to continue bevacizumab with their second-line chemotherapy regimen following progression of disease. When compared to IFL alone, the addition of bevacizumab resulted in a 10% increase in overall response rate (35-45%). More importantly, patients randomized to IFL plus bevacizumab had a median survival of 20.3 months, while patients randomized to IFL alone had a median survival

of 15.6 months ($p < .0004$). The absolute improvement in OS was superior to any incremental survival advantage observed using conventional combination chemotherapy alone. As a result, bevacizumab became the first drug of its class to receive FDA approval for colorectal cancer.

These promising results in the frontline setting have been confirmed in other trials. In the phase II TREE-2 study, Hochster and colleagues demonstrated the safety and efficacy of bevacizumab in combination with oxaliplatin-based chemotherapy (mFOLFOX6, bFOL, or XELOX) (183). This trial was not powered for direct comparisons among the three arms, but time to progression (9.9 and 10.3 months, respectively) and overall survival (26.1 and 24.6 months, respectively) were virtually identical in the mFOLFOX6 and XELOX arms. In the NO16966 trial, untreated patients were randomized in a 2×2 design to FOLFOX4 or XELOX (noninferiority) with or without bevacizumab (184). The pooled analysis revealed superior median PFS (9.4 versus 8.0 months, $p = .002$) in the bevacizumab containing groups, but a difference in response and overall survival did not achieve statistical significance. Surprisingly, when PFS was stratified by chemotherapy regimen, the XELOX regimen fared better. In both of these trials, bevacizumab did not increase the toxicities of chemotherapy. However, it may exist when bevacizumab is combined with an oxaliplatin-based regimen and the use of antiangiogenic therapy in conjunction with oxaliplatin-based chemotherapy is not well understood as originally believed. The most significant adverse events associated with bevacizumab were hypertension, proteinuria, thrombosis, and rare instances of bleeding (mostly epistaxis), delayed wound healing, and gastrointestinal perforation.

The Bolus, Infusional, or Capecitabine with Camptosar-Celecoxib (BICC) trial was a phase III trial that evaluated the role of bevacizumab in combination with irinotecan-based regimens (IFL, FOLFIRI, and CapeIri). During patient enrollment, bevacizumab was subsequently approved, requiring an amendment to the trial design. An expanded cohort of 117 patients randomized to IFL or FOLFIRI + bevacizumab was created. No statistical difference in PFS or response was noted, but an impressive median OS was reported for the FOLFIRI + bevacizumab arm (28.0 versus 19.2 months, $p = .037$).

The efficacy of bevacizumab as an adjunct to chemotherapy has been validated in the second-line setting as well. ECOG 3200 randomized over 800 metastatic colorectal cancer patients previously treated with 5-FU and irinotecan (but not oxaliplatin or bevacizumab) to one of three arms: FOLFOX4, bevacizumab, or the combination. The arm receiving bevacizumab as monotherapy was closed to accrual after an interim analysis revealed inferior outcomes compared to the other two arms. Ultimately, the addition of bevacizumab to chemotherapy resulted in improved PFS (median 7.3 versus 4.7 months, $p < .0001$) and OS (median 12.9 versus 10.8 months, $p = .0011$) (185).

A recent large patient registry trial (Bevacizumab Regimens: Investigation of Treatment Effects and Safety [BRiTE]) suggested that continuation of bevacizumab following first-line progression of disease will positively impact patient outcome versus no therapy or continuing second-line chemotherapy without continuing bevacizumab (186). This data is intriguing but was not collected in a prospective randomized fashion. Regardless, ongoing clinical trials have adopted this methodology of bevacizumab as the control arm. Admittedly in the *KRAS* MT tumor patient, consideration of continuing bevacizumab is an option given the limitations of biologic therapy in a *KRAS* MT tumor–type patient, but it should be considered with a note of caution given the lack of evidence-based medicine and potential toxicities associated with bevacizumab.

The role of bevacizumab in the adjuvant setting is questionable at this time. A large phase III trial (NSABP C-08) was completed in both stages II and III patients (187). Patients were randomized to FOLFOX (6 months) versus FOLFOX + bevacizumab (5 mg/kg × 12 months). After a median follow-up of 35.6 months, the investigators failed to meet their primary endpoint of DFS (HR = 0.89, $p = .15$). The AVANT trial is a three-arm randomized study FOLFOX4 (6 months) versus FOLFOX4 + bevacizumab (5 mg/kg × 12 months) versus XELOX + bevacizumab (7.5 mg/kg × 12 months) in the adjuvant treatment of patients with stage III or high-risk stage II colon cancer. Preliminary toxicities results have been reported with final efficacy results pending (188).

Unlike the EGFR inhibitors, predictive markers for efficacy of initial anti-VEGF therapy have not been identified. Intriguing data from a phase II study of bevacizumab in treatment-naïve patients has noted a possible correlation with levels of basic fibroblast growth factor (bFGF) (189).

Bevacizumab represents a significant step for the use of anti-angiogenesis agents in the treatment of colorectal cancer. It was FDA-approved for use in combination with fluorouracil-based regimens as a first- or second-line treatment for metastatic colorectal cancer. Because bevacizumab has essentially no clinical activity as monotherapy in colorectal cancer, it cannot be recommended as a single agent in colorectal cancer and should not be considered for adjuvant therapy outside of a clinical trial.

Dual Antibody Anti-VEGF and Anti-EGFR Therapy

Based on compelling preclinical data suggesting additive antitumor efficacy, the concept of dual inhibition of VEGF and EGFR has been investigated in several clinical studies. The BOND-2 trial randomized 83 irinotecan-refractory, bevacizumab-naïve patients to cetuximab plus bevacizumab with or without irinotecan (CB versus CBI). The CBI arm showed a better response rate (37 versus 20%) and time to progression (7.3 versus 4.9 months). In addition, the concurrent use of monoclonal antibodies did not result in any unexpected safety signals. This encouraging data prompted two large phase III trials (CApecitabine, IRinotecan, Oxaliplatin 2 [CAIRO2], Panitumumab Advanced Colorectal Cancer Evaluation [PACCE]) to examine the efficacy of dual biologic therapy in metastatic colorectal cancer. The CAIRO2 trial randomized 755 untreated patients to XELOX/bevacizumab with or without cetuximab. Unexpectedly, the patients receiving cetuximab experienced shorter PFS (9.4 versus 10.7 months, $p = .01$). Furthermore, in subgroup analyses, cetuximab-treated patients with *KRAS* mutant tumors had significantly inferior PFS (8.1 versus 12.5 months, $p = .003$) and OS (17.2 versus 24.9 months, $p = .03$) compared to patients with *KRAS* mutant tumors who did not receive cetuximab. Even in the subset of *KRAS* wild-type patients, the addition of cetuximab did not produce a PFS benefit (190).

The PACCE trial investigated dual biologic therapy in the first-line setting by randomizing patients receiving oxaliplatin- or irinotecan-based chemotherapy (investigator's discretion) to bevacizumab plus or minus panitumumab (191). The panitumumab arms were discontinued after a planned interim analysis of patients in the oxaliplatin cohort revealed inferior PFS (8.8 versus 10.5 months, $p = .04$) with the addition of panitumumab. The final results showed worse overall survival (19.4 versus 24.5 months) and significant excess toxicity with dual antibody therapy. The negative clinical impact of panitumumab was seen irrespective of *KRAS* status. In light of the data from PACCE and CAIRO2, dual VEGF and EGFR inhibition currently has no role in the treatment of patients with colorectal cancer and should not be pursued outside of a clinical trial.

Decision Making for Potential Surgical Resection in Patients With Metastatic Colorectal Cancer

Despite therapeutic advances, the estimated 5-year OS for a surgically unresectable patient will remain at 11%.

Therefore, when surgical resection with curative intent is a possibility for a metastatic colorectal cancer patient, it is best to initiate discussion with your colleagues in the other disciplines. It is imperative early discussion regarding each individual patient is initiated early on if there is a potential for surgical resection with curative intent to optimize patient outcomes. Maximizing diagnostic imaging capabilities has an important role when considering surgical resection such as MRI, PET/CT, and volumetric imaging. The use, choice, and duration of neoadjuvant chemotherapy should be determined by the treating medical oncologist and surgeon in a multidisciplinary fashion. Prior studies indicate that patients who have a partial response or stable disease to neoadjuvant therapy will fare better than those with progression of disease (192). Prior studies have indicated a trend in DFS and OS for adjuvant single-agent 5-FU–based chemotherapy versus observation following hepatic resection (193). Hence, clinical trials are under way to modify the neoadjuvant and adjuvant approach for candidates of hepatic resection. Challenges remain in the setting of a patient with a primary rectal cancer and the timing and role of radiotherapy.

In general, it is recommended that patients have *KRAS* testing completed early on in preparation for both immediate and subsequent chemotherapy treatment planning. When considering hepatic resection, it is crucial that patients are not treated until the point of radiographic CR. It is well known that a radiographic CR harbors microscopic disease that is only appreciated on the tissue specimen once surgically resected (194). Furthermore, if patients are not surgically resected following path CR or near path CR, progression of disease will develop. In addition, prolonged chemotherapy may negatively impact surgical mortality (195).

Follow-Up for Patients With Resected Metastatic Colorectal Cancer

Following metastasectomy, patients are followed closely with physician visits, CEA, and diagnostic imaging. Patients undergo clinical evaluations every 3 to 4 months for the first 3 years, every 6 months for the following 2 years, and annually thereafter. Colonoscopy will continue to be completed every 3 years thereafter (some patients require more frequent examinations based on endoscopic findings or high-risk status). CT of chest, abdomen, and pelvis (or MRI) is standard recommended cross-sectional imaging modality. PET/CT is completed only if inconclusive findings are noted on CT/MRI or if a rising CEA is noted without measurable disease on CT/MRI. All patients are encouraged to maintain a relationship with a primary care physician for optimal surveillance and health care.

The MDACC Approach to Patients With Metastatic Disease

It is difficult to articulate a general treatment algorithm for patients with metastatic disease, but consideration of each patient's case as an individual is always taken into account. For the majority of patients with metastatic colorectal cancer, surgical resection of metastatic disease will not be technically possible or clinically appropriate. Whenever possible, patients with good performance status and no significant problems related to local tumor are offered therapy as part of a clinical trial.

Once patients fail frontline therapy, a period of observation may ensue, or second-line therapy may be instituted. Previous analyses have suggested a survival advantage for patients treated with all three active conventional cytotoxic agents (5-FU, irinotecan, and oxaliplatin) during the course of their treatment (196), but the precise order of targeted agents in the therapeutic sequence has yet to be fully elucidated. However, *KRAS* tumor mutation status has become a core part of treatment decision making.

Broad principles have emerged as the foundation for therapeutic decisions at MDACC:

1. *Asymptomatic patients with metastatic disease are usually offered systemic chemotherapy treatment.* Systemic chemotherapy has served an integral role in our care of patients with metastatic disease with regard to quality of life, palliation of pain, and improvement in overall survival. A multidisciplinary approach is always considered when the primary malignancy remains in place. Evaluation of lumen patency is completed before initiating systemic chemotherapy. With the advent of newer agents such as irinotecan, oxaliplatin, and the monoclonal antibodies, overall survival of patients with metastatic disease has been steadily improving over the last several years. Moreover, frontline therapy is better tolerated and more likely to be beneficial in asymptomatic patients with good performance status. An exception to this principle applies to those patients with known metastatic disease that is either not evaluable or extremely low volume. In these cases, close follow-up with frequent cross-sectional imaging may be an appropriate initial

strategy. Therapy is then initiated once measurable disease is evident or, in the oncologist's judgment, further expectant follow-up is likely to lead to symptoms. Patients with a rising serum CEA level are usually not recommended to undergo treatment in the absence of clear clinical or radiographic evidence of metastatic disease and are followed closely. When deciding between an oxaliplatin- or irinotecan-containing regimen, the choice of chemotherapy is largely based on the objectives of treatment: surgical intent, borderline resectable, and unresectable for palliation. FOLFIRI and FOLFOX are comparable in terms of efficacy, but toxicities are distinctly different. When considering systemic chemotherapy for an unresectable patient, FOLFIRI is commonly selected at our institution given its lack of dose-limiting toxicities.

2. *The initial treatment for metastatic disease may depend on the timing and residual toxicities of prior adjuvant therapy.* Many patients who develop metastatic disease have received prior adjuvant therapy consisting of oxaliplatin, 5-FU, and leucovorin. When patients relapse, they should be considered refractory to this combination if fewer than 12 months have elapsed since the completion of adjuvant therapy. Irinotecan often becomes the primary cytotoxic agent in the treatment of relapsed disease after recent adjuvant therapy.

3. *Patients should be treated to maximal benefit or until therapy becomes intolerable.* When patients are receiving systemic therapy for metastatic disease, we usually continue treatment until the tumor becomes refractory to the regimen, toxicity dictates discontinuation, or patient deferment of therapy. Patients receiving oxaliplatin in conjunction with capecitabine or 5-FU, as part of a FOLFOX or XELOX regimen, may develop unacceptable peripheral neuropathy. A study performed in France suggests that there is no disadvantage to discontinuation of oxaliplatin, provided maintenance therapy with 5-FU and leucovorin continues. Oxaliplatin may be reintroduced as a component of the regimen once neuropathic symptoms subside or the tumor starts to progress (197).

This concept was analyzed in a prospective trial, Optimized 5-FU and Oxaliplatin Study (OPTIMOX1). It demonstrated that switching to a nonoxaliplatin maintenance regimen (5-FU/ leucovorin) after 6 cycles of FOLFOX, with reintroduction of oxaliplatin after 12 cycles of maintenance therapy or at disease progression, did not worsen clinical outcomes when compared to continuous FOLFOX until disease progression. In fact, patients on the maintenance arm experienced less grades 3 and 4 toxicities after the initial six cycles of treatment (198). A subsequent trial (OPTIMOX2) randomized patients to maintenance therapy (as in OPTIMOX1) or a chemotherapy holiday after six cycles of FOLFOX, with similar rules for oxaliplatin reintroduction. The maintenance arm showed superior median PFS (8.6 versus 6.6 months, $p = .0017$) and duration of disease control (13.1 versus 9.2 months, $p = .046$), with a trend toward improved overall (199). In clinical practice, however, the benefit of maintenance therapy must be weighed against potential toxicity, and patient preference must be considered as well. Therefore, a chemotherapy treatment holiday may be appropriate for patients after prolonged response or stability of disease.

4. *Once frontline therapy has been exhausted, a period of observation may be advantageous.* With newer drugs and combinations creating significant inroads as debulking agents, metastatic colorectal cancer can be viewed as a chronic illness for some patients, rather than a suddenly life-threatening disease. Therefore, immediate initiation of second- or third-line therapy after failing frontline treatment is not always necessary, and punctuating regimens with periods of observation has at least two advantages. First, it provides patients with a chemotherapy holiday, which may improve overall quality of life; second, it allows for more robust physiologic and hematopoietic recovery after prior treatment. Therefore, once a decision is made to restart cytotoxic therapy, timely delivery of full-dose therapy is more likely to proceed without interruption. As described earlier, when we follow patients expectantly, restaging studies are performed every 8 to 12 weeks, unless the clinical situation requires restaging sooner.

5. *The need for local control should always be considered.* Some patients with metastatic disease may also have intact primary tumors or locally recurrent disease. Recent experience with combination therapies suggests that the primary tumor may respond well to systemic therapy in some cases, obviating the need for local therapies. As a general rule, however, locally recurrent tumor at a site of previous surgery or radiotherapy is not particularly responsive to systemic therapy. Therefore, oncologists must continuously reassess whether local tumor control should take priority over treatment for disseminated disease. Such decisions are usually made with input from a multidisciplinary team

that may include radiotherapists, surgical oncologists, and gastroenterologists.

CHALLENGING CLINICAL MANAGEMENT PROBLEMS

The Malignant Polyp

Occasionally, an oncologist may be asked to evaluate a patient who has undergone endoscopic removal of a pedunculated polyp, which demonstrates areas of invasive adenocarcinoma arising within a villous or tubular adenoma on pathology review. Treatment recommendations in this situation should be individualized. Favorable prognostic features include free margins of resection with no evidence of invasion beyond the submucosa, well- or moderately differentiated adenocarcinoma, and no evidence of lymphatic or vascular invasion. In this setting, as long as the endoscopist expresses confidence in complete polyp removal, the risk of lymph node metastases is low (5%), and continued follow-up with periodic colonoscopic examinations is reasonable (3).

Unfortunately, when a retrieved polyp is sessile or bulky, it may require removal in a piecemeal fashion, distorting the orientation of the polyp and making pathologic examination inconclusive regarding the depth of invasion or margin status. In this situation, or when pathology demonstrates poor differentiation, invasion into the muscularis, or lymphovascular invasion, surgical resection is generally advised for patients with no contraindications to surgery. In particular, suspected T2 tumors have a 20% likelihood of concomitant lymph node metastases, so continued endoscopic follow-up without further surgical intervention is not appropriate.

When a malignant polyp is located in the distal or mid-rectum, this poses a particularly difficult problem. Further local staging is usually not possible, since endoscopic rectal polypectomy leads to unreliable EUS imaging. Definitive surgical resection should be considered for a rectal polyp initially removed without clear margins or one with adverse pathologic features as outlined earlier. In the case of equivocal margins without evidence of muscle invasion, transanal excision by an experienced surgeon may be feasible. Even when laparotomy is considered, a sphincter-preserving procedure is usually possible. However, in rare cases, a patient should be fully informed that surgical removal of the affected rectum may require creation of a permanent ostomy, and final surgical pathology may demonstrate no residual carcinoma and no lymph node metastases. Nevertheless, surgery is an appropriate recommendation because the benefit of complete resection of the affected area with subsequent pathologic staging still outweighs the risk of residual disease in situ. Occasionally, an adequately informed patient will refuse surgery, or medical comorbidities preclude surgery as an option. In these special circumstances, patients may be offered combined-modality chemoradiation as an alternative to definitive resection. Patients are advised that such an approach should not be considered the standard of care.

Nonsurgical Options for Partially Obstructing Tumors

Patients with colorectal cancer may present with evidence of metastatic disease and have signs and symptoms of bowel obstruction. Importantly, the diagnosis of bowel obstruction is usually based on clinical grounds and not endoscopic or radiographic findings. Many patients have presented to MDACC with endoscopic evidence of tumor completely obstructing the bowel lumen, but no symptoms to suggest bowel obstruction. Likewise, CT imaging may demonstrate a large colonic mass that appears to obstruct the lumen completely. Unless the CT shows significant colonic dilation proximal to the lesion or evidence of perforation, clinically significant bowel obstruction may not be present.

While surgical intervention with bowel resection or diverting ostomy may be appropriate, patients with metastatic disease may have significant tumor burden or poor performance status (commonly converging parameters); therefore, nonsurgical options to manage bowel compromise should be considered. Increasingly, gastroenterologists are capable of maintaining bowel patency with the deployment of expandable metal stents, especially in the rectosigmoid region. Obstructing sites higher in the colon can pose technical barriers to stent insertion, and other alternatives may need to be investigated. While considering other treatment options and completing the staging evaluation, relief may be temporarily afforded by an endoscopically placed colonic decompression tube *proximal* to the obstruction. If the primary tumor is predominantly polypoid or exophytic, neodymium-yttrium aluminum garnet (Nd-YAG) laser or argon plasma coagulation (APC) may provide sufficient intraluminal tumor destruction to recanalize the lumen and thus avoid the need for surgery or stent placement. Once this is accomplished, or if the tumor is less acutely obstructing, external-beam radiotherapy may be quite effective in preventing complete obstruction and alleviating partial obstruction. In the case of rectal primaries, radiotherapy may also be effective in relieving sacral plexus pain syndromes. When patients present with impending bowel obstruction, hospitalization may be advised for bowel rest, nasogastric tube decompression, and IV hydration, followed by multidisciplinary evaluation by a gastroenterologist, surgical oncologist, medical oncologist, and radiotherapist. This may facilitate the rapid development and implementation of a treatment strategy. While stent insertion, photocoagulation of intraluminal disease, or radiotherapy may all rapidly reverse impending bowel obstruction, the use of systemic therapy in a patient with tenuous bowel patency should be discouraged.

Multidisciplinary Management of Poor Bowel Function After Curative Treatment

Anticancer therapy is usually associated with both short- and long-term consequences. In the case of colorectal cancer, segmental resections of bowel can lead to permanent alterations in the frequency and character of bowel movements, a problem that can only be addressed through open communication between patient and physician. Rectal cancer therapy, in particular, can lead to major changes in stool patterns and have a significant impact on a patient's subsequent lifestyle. Since rectal cancer surgery leads to loss of the rectal vault, stool storage for any period of time is often compromised. In addition, the delivery of radiotherapy, especially postoperative radiotherapy, may promote stricture at the anastomotic site in patients undergoing a sphincter-sparing procedure. Lastly, sphincter function may not return to normal after surgery and/or chemoradiation. Some patients have anastomotic strictures that may be amenable to dilation over time, but more commonly, the problem is both functional and mechanical; patients may report small, frequent bowel movements, sometimes in clusters, with episodes of fecal incontinence.

At each follow-up visit, a detailed history of bowel habits is reviewed. In general, patients are advised that bowel habits may continue to improve for up to 1 year from the time of surgery or up to 6 months after completion of all adjuvant therapy. Thus, persistence and patience are encouraged as a routine part of oncologic follow-up; patients receive ongoing education about factors that may promote frequent stooling and interventions to reduce it. For patients with more chronic and severe problems (innumerable small bowel movements or fecal incontinence), a multidisciplinary team of surgeons, gastroenterologists, and enterostomal nursing staff is employed to evaluate individual patient factors and recommend a detailed bowel regimen. With adequate compliance, such bowel regimens can lead to major improvement in a patient's quality of

life and satisfaction with sphincter preservation. On rare occasions, however, a patient who has undergone a sphincter-preserving procedure may express unbearable dissatisfaction with bowel function after completion of anti-cancer therapy. In this situation, colostomy or ileostomy may be recommended as a last resort to improve functional status and quality of life.

Carcinoma With Neuroendocrine Features

As previously discussed, the histologic features of a colonic carcinoma may not always reflect those of a typical adenocarcinoma, and tumors occasionally demonstrate evidence of focal neuroendocrine differentiation. This type of colorectal carcinoma may be poorly differentiated and should be readily distinguished from small cell carcinomas or high-grade neuroendocrine tumors, which may be occasionally seen in the rectum. If inconclusive, additional stains for chromogranin and synaptophysin should be completed. Patients with metastatic neuroendocrine carcinomas of the gastrointestinal tract have been treated with either irinotecan/cisplatin or irinotecan/oxaliplatin at MDACC, with some observed partial responses; however, durable responses are not common. Metastatic colorectal cancer patients with stage II, III, or IV colon carcinomas with neuroendocrine features are generally offered standard chemotherapy for colorectal cancer.

■ SUMMARY

Over the last 30 years, significant advances have been made in understanding the pathogenesis of colorectal cancer, important risk factors (both acquired and genetic), and strategies for screening and prevention. Applying this knowledge should contribute to continued reduction in colorectal cancer mortality in the future. An expanded array of biologic agents is currently being investigated in phase I through phase III trials in the advanced disease setting (Table 21-7). Many of these trials include the option of tissue or blood correlatives, in the hopes of better understanding the mechanisms of action of these agents. Hence, patient enrollment in clinical trials is highly encouraged. Overall, given the increasing sophistication required to address specific problems faced by individual patients, the MDACC approach is one of multidisciplinary care to reduce risk, improve clinical outcomes, and maximize quality of life.

TABLE
21-7 | **TARGETED THERAPIES IN DEVELOPMENT FOR ADVANCED COLORECTAL CANCER**

Mechanism of Action	Example of Agents	Phase of Study*
PI3K/Akt/mTOR inhibition	Perifosine, RAD001, MK-2206, GSK690693	Phase III
FGFR inhibition	Brivanib, AZD-4547	Phase III
cMET/HGF inhibition	ARQ-197, AMG-102	Randomized Phase II
Apo2L/TRAIL inhibition	AMG-655, CS-1008	Randomized Phase II
MEK/BRAF inhibition	AS703026, Selumetinib, PLX-4032, XL281	Randomized Phase II
IGFR inhibition	MK-0646, AMG-479	Randomized Phase II
PARP inhibition	Olaparib, ABT-888	Phase II
Demethylating agent	Decitabine, Azacitadine	Phase II
Histone deacetylase	Vorinostat, Entinostat	Phase II
Notch/_-secretase inhibition	RO4929097	Phase II
PPAR-_ inhibition	CS7017	Phase II
PDGFR inhibition	Imatinib	Phase II
Src inhibition	Dasatinib	Phase II
Integrin inhibition	EMD 525797	Phase II

*For most advanced agent in development

References

1. Jemal A, Siegel R, Ward E, et al. Cancer statistics, 2009. *CA Cancer J Clin* 2009;59(4):225-249.

2. Center MM, Jemal A, Ward E. International trends in colorectal cancer incidence rates. *Cancer Epidemiol Biomarkers Prev* 2009;18(6):1688-1694.

3. Skibber JM MB, Hoff PM. Cancer of the colon, 6th ed. In: DeVita VT Jr HS, Rosenberg SA (eds): *Principles and Practice of Oncology*. Philadelphia: Lippincott-Rave; 2001.

4. Vogelstein B, Fearon ER, Hamilton SR, et al. Genetic alterations during colorectal-tumor development. *N Engl J Med* 1988;319(9):525-532.

5. Winawer SJ, Zauber AG, Ho MN, et al. The National Polyp Study. *Eur J Cancer Prev* 1993;2(Suppl 2):83-87.

6. Winawer SJ, Zauber AG, O'Brien MJ, et al. The National Polyp Study. Design, methods, and characteristics of patients with newly diagnosed polyps. The National Polyp Study Workgroup. *Cancer* 1992;70(5 Suppl):1236-1245.

7. Fodde R, Kuipers J, Rosenberg C, et al. Mutations in the APC tumour suppressor gene cause chromosomal instability. *Nat Cell Biol* 2001;3(4):433-438.

8. Houlston RS, Collins A, Slack J, et al. Dominant genes for colorectal cancer are not rare. *Ann Hum Genet* 1992;56(Pt 2):99-103.

9. Perucho M. Microsatellite instability: The mutator that mutates the other mutator. *Nat Med* 1996;2(6):630-631.

10. Boland CR, Thibodeau SN, Hamilton SR, et al. A National Cancer Institute Workshop on Microsatellite Instability for cancer detection and familial predisposition: Development of international criteria for the determination of microsatellite instability in colorectal cancer. *Cancer Res* 1998;58(22):5248-5257.

11. Ribic CM, Sargent DJ, Moore MJ, et al. Tumor microsatellite-instability status as a predictor of benefit from fluorouracil-based adjuvant chemotherapy for colon cancer. *N Engl J Med* 2003;349(3):247-257.

12. Grady WM, Markowitz SD. Genetic and epigenetic alterations in colon cancer. *Annu Rev Genomics Hum Genet* 2002;3:101-128.

13. Toyota M, Ohe-Toyota M, Ahuja N, et al. Distinct genetic profiles in colorectal tumors with or without the CpG island methylator phenotype. *Proc Natl Acad Sci U S A* 2000;97(2):710-715.

14. Kinzler KW, Vogelstein B. Landscaping the cancer terrain. *Science* 1998;280(5366):1036-1037.

15. Popat S, Hubner R, Houlston RS. Systematic review of microsatellite instability and colorectal cancer prognosis. *J Clin Oncol* 2005;23(3):609-618.

16. Pande M AC, Eng, C, Frazier ML. Interactions between cigarette smoking and selected polymorphisms in xenobiotic metabolizing enzymes in risk for colorectal cancer: A case-only analysis. 2010.

17. Slattery ML, Edwards SL, Boucher KM, et al. Lifestyle and colon cancer: An assessment of factors associated with risk. *Am J Epidemiol* 1999;150(8):869-877.

18. Jarvinen R, Knekt P, Hakulinen T, et al. Dietary fat, cholesterol and colorectal cancer in a prospective study. *Br J Cancer* 2001;85(3):357-361.

19. Fuchs CS, Giovannucci EL, Colditz GA, et al. Dietary fiber and the risk of colorectal cancer and adenoma in women. *N Engl J Med* 1999;340(3):169-176.

20. Moore LL, Bradlee ML, Singer MR, et al. BMI and waist circumference as predictors of lifetime colon cancer risk in Framingham Study adults. *Int J Obes Relat Metab Disord* 2004;28(4):559-567.

21 Jaffe T, Schwartz B. Leptin promotes motility and invasiveness in human colon cancer cells by activating multiple signal-transduction pathways. *Int J Cancer* 2008;123(11): 2543-2556.

22. Noffsinger AE. Serrated polyps and colorectal cancer: New pathway to malignancy. *Annu Rev Pathol* 2009;4:343-364.

23. Itzkowitz S. Colon carcinogenesis in inflammatory bowel disease: Applying molecular genetics to clinical practice. *J Clin Gastroenterol* 2003;36(5 Suppl):S70-S74; discussion S94-S96.

24. Lynch HT, Watson P, Smyrk TC, et al. Colon cancer genetics. *Cancer* 1992;70(5 Suppl):1300-1312.

25. Lynch HT, Smyrk TC, Lanspa SJ, et al. Upper gastrointestinal manifestations in families with hereditary flat adenoma syndrome. *Cancer* 1993;71(9):2709-2714.

26. Al-Tassan N, Chmiel NH, Maynard J, et al. Inherited variants of MYH associated with somatic G:C–>T:A mutations in colorectal tumors. *Nat Genet* 2002;30(2):227-232.

27. Sampson JR, Dolwani S, Jones S, et al. Autosomal recessive colorectal adenomatous polyposis due to inherited mutations of MYH. *Lancet* 2003;362(9377):39-41.

28. Vogelstein B. Genetic testings for cancer: The surgeon's critical role. Familial colon cancer. *J Am Coll Surg* 1999;188(1):74-79.

29. Lynch HT, Lynch J. The Lynch syndromes. *Curr Opin Oncol* 1993 Jul;5(4):687-696.

30. Liu B, Parsons R, Papadopoulos N, et al. Analysis of mismatch repair genes in hereditary non-polyposis colorectal cancer patients. *Nat Med* 1996;2(2):169-174.

31. Giardiello FM, Brensinger JD, Petersen GM. AGA technical review on hereditary colorectal cancer and genetic testing. *Gastroenterology* 2001;121(1):198-213.

32. Bronner CE, Baker SM, Morrison PT, et al. Mutation in the DNA mismatch repair gene homologue hMLH1 is associated with hereditary non-polyposis colon cancer. *Nature* 1994; 368(6468):258-261.

33. Leach FS, Nicolaides NC, Papadopoulos N, et al. Mutations of a mutS homolog in hereditary nonpolyposis colorectal cancer. *Cell* 1993;75(6):1215-1225.

34. Gu Y, Parker A, Wilson TM, et al. Human MutY homolog, a DNA glycosylase involved in base excision repair, physically and functionally interacts with mismatch repair proteins human MutS homolog 2/human MutS homolog 6. *J Biol Chem* 2002;277(13):11135-11142.

35. Lindor NM. Hereditary colorectal cancer: MYH-associated polyposis and other newly identified disorders. *Best Pract Res Clin Gastroenterol* 2009;23(1):75-87.

36. Jenkins MA, Croitoru ME, Monga N, et al. Risk of colorectal cancer in monoallelic and biallelic carriers of MYH mutations: A population-based case-family study. *Cancer Epidemiol Biomarkers Prev* 2006;15(2):312-314.

37. Nielsen M, Joerink-van de Beld MC, Jones N, et al. Analysis of MUTYH genotypes and colorectal phenotypes in patients with MUTYH-associated polyposis. *Gastroenterology* 2009; 136(2):471-476.

38. Jones N, Vogt S, Nielsen M, et al. Increased colorectal cancer incidence in obligate carriers of heterozygous mutations in MUTYH. *Gastroenterology* 2009;137(2):489-494, 494 e1; quiz 725-726.

39. August DA, Sugarbaker PH, Ottow RT, et al. Hepatic resection of colorectal metastases. Influence of clinical factors and adjuvant intraperitoneal 5-fluorouracil via Tenckhoff catheter on survival. *Ann Surg* 1985;201(2):210-218.

40. Brevinge H, Lindholm E, Buntzen S, et al. Screening for colorectal neoplasia with faecal occult blood testing compared with flexible sigmoidoscopy directly in a 55-56 years' old population. *Int J Colorectal Dis* 1997;12(5):291-295.

41. Mandel JS, Bond JH, Church TR, et al. Reducing mortality from colorectal cancer by screening for fecal occult blood. Minnesota Colon Cancer Control Study. *N Engl J Med* 1993; 328(19):1365-1371.

42. Mandel JS, Bond JH, Bradley M, et al. Sensitivity, specificity, and positive predictivity of the Hemoccult test in screening for colorectal cancers. The University of Minnesota's Colon Cancer Control Study. *Gastroenterology* 1989;97(3): 597-600.

43. Mandel JS, Church TR, Ederer F, et al. Colorectal cancer mortality: Effectiveness of biennial screening for fecal occult blood. *J Natl Cancer Inst* 1999;91(5):434-437.

44. Towler B, Irwig L, Glasziou P, et al. A systematic review of the effects of screening for colorectal cancer using the faecal occult blood test, hemoccult. *BMJ* 1998; 317(7158): 559-565.

45. Ransohoff DF, Lang CA. Screening for colorectal cancer with the fecal occult blood test: A background paper. American College of Physicians. *Ann Intern Med* 1997;126(10):811-822.

46. Atkin WS, Edwards R, Kralj-Hans I, et al. Once-only flexible sigmoidoscopy screening in prevention of colorectal cancer: A multicentre randomised controlled trial. *Lancet* 2010; 375(9726):1624-1633.

47. Lieberman DA, Weiss DG, Bond JH, et al. Use of colonoscopy to screen asymptomatic adults for colorectal cancer. Veterans Affairs Cooperative Study Group 380. *N Engl J Med* 2000; 343(3):162-168.

48. Toribara NW, Sleisenger MH. Screening for colorectal cancer. *N Engl J Med* 1995;332(13):861-867.

49. Coughlin SS, Thompson TD, Seeff L, et al. Breast, cervical, and colorectal carcinoma screening in a demographically defined region of the southern U.S. *Cancer* 2002;95(10):2211-2222.

50. Seeff LC, Shapiro JA, Nadel MR. Are we doing enough to screen for colorectal cancer? Findings from the 1999 Behavioral Risk Factor Surveillance System. *J Fam Pract* 2002;51(9): 761-766.

51. Nadel MR, Blackman DK, Shapiro JA, et al. Are people being screened for colorectal cancer as recommended? Results from the National Health Interview Survey. *Prev Med* 2002;35(3):199-206.

52. Shapiro JA, Seeff LC, Nadel MR. Colorectal cancer-screening tests and associated health behaviors. *Am J Prev Med* 2001; 21(2):132-137.

53. Angtuaco TL, Banaad-Omiotek GD, Howden CW. Differing attitudes toward virtual and conventional colonoscopy for colorectal cancer screening: Surveys among primary care physicians and potential patients. *Am J Gastroenterol* 2001; 96(3):887-893.

54. Thomeer M, Bielen D, Vanbeckevoort D, et al. Patient acceptance for CT colonography: What is the real issue? *Eur Radiol* 2002;12(6):1410-1415.

55. Svensson MH, Svensson E, Lasson A, et al. Patient acceptance of CT colonography and conventional colonoscopy: Prospective comparative study in patients with or suspected of having colorectal disease. *Radiology* 2002;222(2):337-345.

56. Pickhardt PJ, Kim DH, Meiners RJ, et al. Colorectal and extra-colonic cancers detected at screening CT colonography in 10,286 asymptomatic adults. *Radiology* 2010;255(1):83-88.

57. Pickhardt PJ, Kim DH. Colorectal cancer screening with CT colonography: Key concepts regarding polyp prevalence, size, histology, morphology, and natural history. *AJR Am J Roentgenol* 2009;193(1):40-46.

58. Imperiali G, Minoli G. Colonic neoplasm in asymptomatic patients with family history of colon cancer: Results of a colonoscopic prospective and controlled study. Results of a pilot study of endoscopic screening of first degree relatives of colorectal cancer patients in Italy. *Gastrointest Endosc* 1999; 49(1):132-133.

59. Nelson D. Colonoscopy and polypectomy. *Hematol Oncol Clin North Am* 2002;16(4):867-874.

60. Winawer SJ, Zauber AG, O'Brien MJ, et al. Randomized comparison of surveillance intervals after colonoscopic removal of newly diagnosed adenomatous polyps. The National Polyp Study Workgroup. *N Engl J Med* 1993;328(13):901-906.

61. Hoff G, Sauar J, Vatn MH, et al. Polypectomy of adenomas in the prevention of colorectal cancer: 10 years' follow-up of the Telemark Polyp Study I. A prospective, controlled population study. *Scand J Gastroenterol* 1996;31(10):1006-1010.

62. Murakami R, Tsukuma H, Kanamori S, et al. Natural history of colorectal polyps and the effect of polypectomy on occurrence of subsequent cancer. *Int J Cancer* 1990;46(2):159-164.

63. Muller AD, Sonnenberg A. Prevention of colorectal cancer by flexible endoscopy and polypectomy. A case-control study of 32,702 veterans. *Ann Intern Med* 1995;123(12):904-910.

64. Imperiale TF, Ransohoff DF, Itzkowitz SH, et al. Fecal DNA versus fecal occult blood for colorectal-cancer screening in an average-risk population. *N Engl J Med* 2004;351(26):2704-2714.

65. Sieber OM, Lipton L, Crabtree M, et al. Multiple colorectal adenomas, classic adenomatous polyposis, and germ-line mutations in MYH. *N Engl J Med* 2003;348(9):791-799.

66. Vasen HF, Watson P, Mecklin JP, et al. New clinical criteria for hereditary nonpolyposis colorectal cancer (HNPCC, Lynch syndrome) proposed by the International Collaborative group on HNPCC. *Gastroenterology* 1999;116(6):1453-1456.

67. Hofmann JN, Yu K, Horst RL, et al. Long-term variation in serum 25-hydroxyvitamin D concentration among participants in the Prostate, Lung, Colorectal, and Ovarian Cancer Screening Trial. *Cancer Epidemiol Biomarkers Prev* 2010;19(4):927-931.

68. Egan JB, Thompson PA, Ashbeck EL, et al. Genetic polymorphisms in vitamin D receptor VDR/RXRA influence the likelihood of colon adenoma recurrence. *Cancer Res* 2010;70(4):1496-1504.

69. Giardiello FM, Hamilton SR, Krush AJ, et al. Treatment of colonic and rectal adenomas with sulindac in familial adenomatous polyposis. *N Engl J Med* 1993;328(18):1313-1316.

70. Williams CS, Mann M, DuBois RN. The role of cyclooxygenases in inflammation, cancer, and development. *Oncogene* 1999;18(55):7908-7916.

71. Turini ME, DuBois RN. Primary prevention: Phytoprevention and chemoprevention of colorectal cancer. *Hematol Oncol Clin North Am* 2002;16(4):811-840.

72. Reddy BS. Studies with the azoxymethane-rat preclinical model for assessing colon tumor development and chemoprevention. *Environ Mol Mutagen* 2004;44(1):26-35.

73. Steinbach G, Lynch PM, Phillips RK, et al. The effect of celecoxib, a cyclooxygenase-2 inhibitor, in familial adenomatous polyposis. *N Engl J Med* 2000;342(26):1946-1952.

74. Topol EJ. Failing the public health—rofecoxib, Merck, and the FDA. *N Engl J Med* 2004;351(17):1707-1709.

75. Solomon SD, McMurray JJ, Pfeffer MA, et al. Cardiovascular risk associated with celecoxib in a clinical trial for colorectal adenoma prevention. *N Engl J Med* 2005;352(11):1071-1080.

76. Giovannucci E, Egan KM, Hunter DJ, et al. Aspirin and the risk of colorectal cancer in women. *N Engl J Med* 1995;333(10):609-614.

77. Giovannucci E, Rimm EB, Stampfer MJ, et al. Aspirin use and the risk for colorectal cancer and adenoma in male health professionals. *Ann Intern Med* 1994;121(4):241-246.

78. Sandler RS, Halabi S, Baron JA, et al. A randomized trial of aspirin to prevent colorectal adenomas in patients with previous colorectal cancer. *N Engl J Med* 2003;348(10):883-890.

79. Baron JA, Cole BF, Sandler RS, et al. A randomized trial of aspirin to prevent colorectal adenomas. *N Engl J Med* 2003;348(10):891-899.

80. Lynch HT, Lanspa S, Smyrk T, et al. Hereditary nonpolyposis colorectal cancer (Lynch syndromes I & II). Genetics, pathology, natural history, and cancer control, Part I. *Cancer Genet Cytogenet* 1991;53(2):143-160.

81. Lynch PM, Wargovich MJ, Lynch HT, et al. A follow-up study of colonic epithelial proliferation as a biomarker in a Native-American family with hereditary nonpolyposis colon cancer. *J Natl Cancer Inst* 1991;83(13):951-954.

82. Arenas RB, Fichera A, Mhoon D, et al. Incidence and therapeutic implications of synchronous colonic pathology in colorectal adenocarcinoma. *Surgery* 1997;122(4):706-709; discussion 709-710.

83. Moertel CG, O'Fallon JR, Go VL, et al. The preoperative carcinoembryonic antigen test in the diagnosis, staging, and prognosis of colorectal cancer. *Cancer* 1986;58(3):603-610.

84. Ratto C, Sofo L, Ippoliti M, et al. Prognostic factors in colorectal cancer. Literature review for clinical application. *Dis Colon Rectum* 1998;41(8):1033-1049.

85. Marchena J, Acosta MA, Garcia-Anguiano F, et al. Use of the preoperative levels of CEA in patients with colorectal cancer. *Hepatogastroenterology* 2003;50(52):1017-1020.

86. Rich T, Gunderson LL, Lew R, et al. Patterns of recurrence of rectal cancer after potentially curative surgery. *Cancer* 1983;52(7):1317-1329.

87. Havenga K, Enker WE, Norstein J, et al. Improved survival and local control after total mesorectal excision or D3 lymphadenectomy in the treatment of primary rectal cancer: An international analysis of 1411 patients. *Eur J Surg Oncol* 1999;25(4):368-374.

88. Sauer R, Becker H, Hohenberger W, et al. Preoperative versus postoperative chemoradiotherapy for rectal cancer. *N Engl J Med* 2004;351(17):1731-1740.

89. Wolmark N, Wieand HS, Hyams DM, et al. Randomized trial of postoperative adjuvant chemotherapy with or without radiotherapy for carcinoma of the rectum: National Surgical Adjuvant Breast and Bowel Project Protocol R-02. *J Natl Cancer Inst* 2000;92(5):388-396.

90. Taylor FG, Swift RI, Blomqvist L, et al. A systematic approach to the interpretation of preoperative staging MRI for rectal cancer. *AJR Am J Roentgenol* 2008;191(6):1827-1835.

91. Whiteford MH, Whiteford HM, Yee LF, et al. Usefulness of FDG-PET scan in the assessment of suspected metastatic or recurrent adenocarcinoma of the colon and rectum. *Dis Colon Rectum* 2000;43(6):759-767; discussion 767-770.

92. Chang GJ, Rodriguez-Bigas MA, Skibber JM, et al. Lymph node evaluation and survival after curative resection of colon cancer: Systematic review. *J Natl Cancer Inst* 2007;99(6):433-441.

93. Bilimoria KY, Bentrem DJ, Stewart AK, et al. Lymph node evaluation as a colon cancer quality measure: A national hospital report card. *J Natl Cancer Inst* 2008;100(18):1310-1317.

94. Benson AB, 3rd, Schrag D, Somerfield MR, et al. American Society of Clinical Oncology recommendations on adjuvant chemotherapy for stage II colon cancer. *J Clin Oncol* 2004; 22(16):3408-3419.

95. Bertagnolli M, Miedema B, Redston M, et al. Sentinel node staging of resectable colon cancer: Results of a multicenter study. *Ann Surg* 2004;240(4):624-628; discussion 628-630.

96. Lim SJ, Feig BW, Wang H, et al. Sentinel lymph node evaluation does not improve staging accuracy in colon cancer. *Ann Surg Oncol* 2008;15(1):46-51.

97. Poultsides GA, Servais EL, Saltz LB, et al. Outcome of primary tumor in patients with synchronous stage IV colorectal cancer receiving combination chemotherapy without surgery as initial treatment. *J Clin Oncol* 2009;27(20):3379-3384.

98. Wexner SD, Cohen SM, Johansen OB, et al. Laparoscopic colorectal surgery: A prospective assessment and current perspective. *Br J Surg* 1993;80(12):1602-1605.

99. Fleshman J, Sargent DJ, Green E, et al. Laparoscopic colectomy for cancer is not inferior to open surgery based on 5-year data from the COST Study Group trial. *Ann Surg* 2007;246(4): 655-662; discussion 662-664.

100. Wolmark N, Fisher B, Rockette H, et al. Postoperative adjuvant chemotherapy or BCG for colon cancer: Results from NSABP protocol C-01. *J Natl Cancer Inst* 1988;80(1):30-36.

101. O'Connell MJ, Mailliard JA, Kahn MJ, et al. Controlled trial of fluorouracil and low-dose leucovorin given for 6 months as postoperative adjuvant therapy for colon cancer. *J Clin Oncol* 1997;15(1):246-250.

102. Moertel CG, Fleming TR, Macdonald JS, et al. Fluorouracil plus levamisole as effective adjuvant therapy after resection of stage III colon carcinoma: A final report. *Ann Intern Med* 1995;122(5):321-326.

103. Wolmark N, Rockette H, Fisher B, et al. The benefit of leucovorin-modulated fluorouracil as postoperative adjuvant therapy for primary colon cancer: Results from National Surgical Adjuvant Breast and Bowel Project protocol C-03. *J Clin Oncol* 1993;11(10):1879-1887.

104. Moertel CG, Fleming TR, Macdonald JS, et al. Levamisole and fluorouracil for adjuvant therapy of resected colon carcinoma. *N Engl J Med* 1990;322(6):352-358.

105. Marsoni S. Efficacy of adjuvant fluorouracil and leucovorin in stage B2 and C colon cancer. International Multicenter Pooled Analysis of Colon Cancer Trials Investigators. *Semin Oncol* 2001;28(1 Suppl 1):14-19.

106. Quasar Collaborative G, Gray R, Barnwell J, et al. Adjuvant chemotherapy versus observation in patients with colorectal cancer: A randomised study. *Lancet* 2007;370(9604): 2020-2029.

107. Van Cutsem E, Hoff PM, Harper P, et al. Oral capecitabine vs intravenous 5-fluorouracil and leucovorin: Integrated efficacy data and novel analyses from two large, randomised, phase III trials. *Br J Cancer* 2004;90(6):1190-1197.

108. Scheithauer W, McKendrick J, Begbie S, et al. Oral capecitabine as an alternative to i.v. 5-fluorouracil-based adjuvant therapy for colon cancer: Safety results of a randomized, phase III trial. *Ann Oncol* 2003;14(12):1735-1743.

109. Andre T, Boni C, Mounedji-Boudiaf L, et al. Oxaliplatin, fluorouracil, and leucovorin as adjuvant treatment for colon cancer. *N Engl J Med* 2004;350(23):2343-2351.

110. Andre T, Boni C, Navarro M, et al. Improved overall survival with oxaliplatin, fluorouracil, and leucovorin as adjuvant treatment in stage II or III colon cancer in the MOSAIC trial. *J Clin Oncol* 2009;27(19):3109-3116.

111. Overman MJ, Maru DM, Charnsangavej C, et al. Oxaliplatin-mediated increase in spleen size as a biomarker for the development of hepatic sinusoidal injury. *J Clin Oncol* 28(15): 2549-2555.

112. Kerr D, Gray R, Quirke P, et al. A quantitative multigene RT-PCR assay for prediction of recurrence in stage II colon cancer: Selection of the genes in four large studies and results of the independent, prospectively designed QUASAR validation study. ASCO, Orlando, Florida. *J Clin Oncol* 2009; 27(Suppl).

113. Kuebler JP, Wieand HS, O'Connell MJ, et al. Oxaliplatin combined with weekly bolus fluorouracil and leucovorin as surgical adjuvant chemotherapy for stage II and III colon cancer: Results from NSABP C-07. *J Clin Oncol* 2007;25(16): 2198-2204.

114. Haller DG, Cassidy J, Tabernero J, et al. Efficacy findings from a randomized phase III trial of capecitabine plus oxaliplatin versus bolus 5-FU/LV for stage III colon cancer (NO16968): No impact of age on disease-free survival (DFS). 2010 GI Cancers Symposium, San Francisco, CA, 2009.

115. Saltz LB, Niedzwiecki D, Hollis D, et al. Irinotecan fluorouracil plus leucovorin is not superior to fluorouracil plus leucovorin alone as adjuvant treatment for stage III colon cancer: Results of CALGB 89803. *J Clin Oncol* 2007;25(23): 3456-3461.

116. Van Cutsem E, Labianca R, Bodoky G, et al. Randomized phase III trial comparing biweekly infusional fluorouracil/ leucovorin alone or with irinotecan in the adjuvant treatment of stage III colon cancer: PETACC-3. *J Clin Oncol* 2009; 27(19):3117-3125.

117. Ychou M, Raoul JL, Douillard JY, et al. A phase III randomised trial of LV5FU2 + irinotecan versus LV5FU2 alone in adjuvant high-risk colon cancer (FNCLCC Accord02/ FFCD9802). *Ann Oncol* 2009;20(4):674-680.

118. Ychou M, Hohenberger W, Thezenas S, et al. A randomized phase III study comparing adjuvant 5-fluorouracil/folinic acid with FOLFIRI in patients following complete resection of liver metastases from colorectal cancer. *Ann Oncol* 2009; 20(12):1964-1970.

119. Sargent DJ, Marsoni S, Thibodeau SN, et al. Confirmation of deficient mismatch repair (dMMR) as a predictive marker for lack of benefit from 5-FU based chemotherapy in stage II and III colon cancer (CC): A pooled molecular reanalysis of randomized chemotherapy trials. ASCO. *J Clin Oncol* 2008; 26(20 Suppl).

120. NCI. FOLFOX-4: 3 months versus 6 months and bevacizumab as adjuvant therapy for patients with stage II/III colon cancer, 2010, vol 2010.

121. Watanabe T, Wu TT, Catalano PJ, et al. Molecular predictors of survival after adjuvant chemotherapy for colon cancer. *N Engl J Med* 2001;344(16):1196-1206.

122. Ogino S, Nosho K, Irahara N, et al. Prognostic significance and molecular associations of 18q loss of heterozygosity: A cohort study of microsatellite stable colorectal cancers. *J Clin Oncol* 2009;27(27):4591-4598.

123. Tejpar S, Bosman F, Delorenzi M, et al. Microsatellite instability (MSI) in stage II and III colon cancer treated with 5FU-LV or 5FU-LV and irinotecan (PETACC 3-EORTC 40993-SAKK 60/00 trial). ASCO, Orlando, Florida. *J Clin Oncol* 2009; 27(Suppl).

124. Roth AD, Tejpar S, Delorenzi M, et al. Prognostic role of KRAS and BRAF in stage II and III resected colon cancer: Results of the translational study on the PETACC-3, EORTC 40993, SAKK 60-00 trial. *J Clin Oncol* 2010;28(3):466-474.

125. de Gramont A, Hubbard J, Shi Q, et al. Association between disease-free survival and overall survival when survival is prolonged after recurrence in patients receiving cytotoxic adjuvant therapy for colon cancer: Simulations based on the 20,800 patient ACCENT data set. *J Clin Oncol* 2010;28(3): 460-465.

126. Roh MS, Colangelo LH, O'Connell MJ, Yothers G, Deutsch M, Allegra CJ, Kahlenberg MS, Baez-Diaz L, Ursiny CS, Petrelli NJ, Wolmark N. *J Clin Oncol.* 2009 Nov 1;27(31): 5124-5130. Epub 2009 Sep 21. PMID: 19770376.

127. Garcia-Aguilar J, Mellgren A, Sirivongs P, et al. Local excision of rectal cancer without adjuvant therapy: A word of caution. *Ann Surg* 2000;231(3):345-351.

128. Greenberg JA, Shibata D, Herndon JE, 2nd, et al. Local excision of distal rectal cancer: An update of cancer and leukemia group B 8984. *Dis Colon Rectum* 2008;51(8):1185-1191; discussion 1191-1194.

129. Smalley SR, Benedetti JK, Williamson SK, et al. Phase III trial of fluorouracil-based chemotherapy regimens plus radiotherapy in postoperative adjuvant rectal cancer: GI INT 0144. *J Clin Oncol* 2006;24(22):3542-3547.

130. Prolongation of the disease-free interval in surgically treated rectal carcinoma. Gastrointestinal Tumor Study Group. *N Engl J Med* 1985;312(23):1465-1472.

131. Tepper JE, O'Connell MJ, Petroni GR, et al. Adjuvant postoperative fluorouracil-modulated chemotherapy combined with pelvic radiation therapy for rectal cancer: Initial results of intergroup 0114. *J Clin Oncol* 1997;15(5):2030-2039.

132. Aschele C, Pinto C, Cordio S, et al; STAR Network Investigators. Pre-operative FU-based chemoradiation +/-weekly oxaliplatin in locally advanced rectal cancer. Preliminary safety findings of the STAR (Studio Terapia Adiuvante Retto)-01 randomized trial. 2007 GI Cancers Symposium, 2007.

133. Gerard J, Azria D, Gourgou-Bourgade S, et al. Randomized multicenter phase III trial comparing two neoadjuvant chemoradiotherapy (CT-RT) regimens (RT45-Cap versus RT50-Capox) in patients (pts) with locally advanced rectal cancer (LARC): Results of the ACCORD 12/0405 PRODIGE. *J Clin Oncol* 2009;27:18S.

134. Rodel C, Martus P, Papadoupolos T, et al. Prognostic significance of tumor regression after preoperative chemoradiotherapy for rectal cancer. *J Clin Oncol* 2005;23(34): 8688-8696.

135. He Y, Van't Veer LJ, Mikolajewska-Hanclich I, et al. PIK3CA mutations predict local recurrences in rectal cancer patients. *Clin Cancer Res* 2009;15(22):6956-6962.

136. Kapiteijn E, Marijnen CA, Nagtegaal ID, et al. Preoperative radiotherapy combined with total mesorectal excision for resectable rectal cancer. *N Engl J Med* 2001;345(9):638-646.

137. Tepper JE, O'Connell MJ, Niedzwiecki D, et al. Impact of number of nodes retrieved on outcome in patients with rectal cancer. *J Clin Oncol* 2001;19(1):157-163.

138. Kapiteijn E, Marijnen CA, Nagtegaal ID, et al. Preoperative radiotherapy combined with total mesorectal excision for resectable rectal cancer. *N Engl J Med* 2001;345(9):638-646.

139. Gunderson LL, Sargent DJ, Tepper JE, et al. Impact of T and N stage and treatment on survival and relapse in adjuvant rectal cancer: A pooled analysis. *J Clin Oncol* 2004;22(10): 1785-1796.

140. August DA, Ottow RT, Sugarbaker PH. Clinical perspective of human colorectal cancer metastasis. *Cancer Metastasis Rev* 1984;3(4):303-324.

141. Eng C, Kindler HL, Schilsky RL. Oral fluoropyrimidine treatment of colorectal cancer. *Clin Colorectal Cancer* 2001; 1(2):95-103.

142. Hoff PM, Ansari R, Batist G, et al. Comparison of oral capecitabine versus intravenous fluorouracil plus leucovorin as first-line treatment in 605 patients with metastatic colorectal cancer: Results of a randomized phase III study. *J Clin Oncol* 2001;19(8):2282-2292.

143. Van Cutsem E, Twelves C, Cassidy J, et al. Oral capecitabine compared with intravenous fluorouracil plus leucovorin in patients with metastatic colorectal cancer: Results of a large phase III study. *J Clin Oncol* 2001;19(21):4097-4106.

144. Van Cutsem E, Cunningham D, Ten Bokkel Huinink WW, et al. Clinical activity and benefit of irinotecan (CPT-11) in patients with colorectal cancer truly resistant to 5-fluorouracil (5-FU). *Eur J Cancer* 1999;35(1):54-59.

145. Rothenberg ML, Cox JV, DeVore RF, et al. A multicenter, phase II trial of weekly irinotecan (CPT-11) in patients with previously treated colorectal carcinoma. *Cancer* 1999;85(4): 786-795.

146. Rothenberg ML, Eckardt JR, Kuhn JG, et al. Phase II trial of irinotecan in patients with progressive or rapidly recurrent colorectal cancer. *J Clin Oncol* 1996;14(4):1128-1135.

147. Rougier P, Bugat R, Douillard JY, et al. Phase II study of irinotecan in the treatment of advanced colorectal cancer in chemotherapy-naive patients and patients pretreated with fluorouracil-based chemotherapy. *J Clin Oncol* 1997;15(1): 251-260.

148. Cunningham D, Pyrhonen S, James RD, et al. Randomised trial of irinotecan plus supportive care versus supportive care alone after fluorouracil failure for patients with metastatic colorectal cancer. *Lancet* 1998;352(9138):1413-1418.

149. Saltz LB, Cox JV, Blanke C, et al. Irinotecan plus fluorouracil and leucovorin for metastatic colorectal cancer. Irinotecan Study Group. *N Engl J Med* 2000;343(13):905-914.

150. Douillard JY, Cunningham D, Roth AD, et al. Irinotecan combined with fluorouracil compared with fluorouracil alone as first-line treatment for metastatic colorectal cancer: A multicentre randomised trial. *Lancet* 2000;355(9209): 1041-1047.

151. Rothenberg ML, Oza AM, Bigelow RH, et al. Superiority of oxaliplatin and fluorouracil-leucovorin compared with either therapy alone in patients with progressive colorectal cancer after irinotecan and fluorouracil-leucovorin: Interim results of a phase III trial. *J Clin Oncol* 2003;21(11):2059-69.

152. de Gramont A, Figer A, Seymour M, et al. Leucovorin and fluorouracil with or without oxaliplatin as first-line treatment in advanced colorectal cancer. *J Clin Oncol* 2000;18(16): 2938-2947.

153. Goldberg RM, Sargent DJ, Morton RF, et al. A randomized controlled trial of fluorouracil plus leucovorin, irinotecan, and oxaliplatin combinations in patients with previously untreated metastatic colorectal cancer. *J Clin Oncol* 2004; 22(1):23-30.

154. Tournigand C, Andre T, Achille E, et al. FOLFIRI followed by FOLFOX6 or the reverse sequence in advanced colorectal cancer: A randomized GERCOR study. *J Clin Oncol* 2004; 22(2):229-237.

155. Falcone A, Ricci S, Brunetti I, et al. Phase III trial of infusional fluorouracil, leucovorin, oxaliplatin, and irinotecan (FOLFOXIRI) compared with infusional fluorouracil, leucovorin, and irinotecan (FOLFIRI) as first-line treatment for metastatic colorectal cancer: The Gruppo Oncologico Nord Ovest. *J Clin Oncol* 2007;25(13):1670-1676.

156. Souglakos J, Androulakis N, Syrigos K, et al. FOLFOXIRI (folinic acid, 5-fluorouracil, oxaliplatin and irinotecan) vs FOLFIRI (folinic acid, 5-fluorouracil and irinotecan) as first-line treatment in metastatic colorectal cancer (MCC): A multicentre randomised phase III trial from the Hellenic Oncology Research Group (HORG). *Br J Cancer* 2006;94(6):798-805.

157. Kohler G, Milstein C. Continuous cultures of fused cells secreting antibody of predefined specificity. *Nature* 1975; 256(5517):495-497.

158. Baselga J. The EGFR as a target for anticancer therapy—focus on cetuximab. *Eur J Cancer* 2001;37(Suppl 4):S16-S22.

159. Saltz LB, Meropol NJ, Loehrer PJ, Sr., et al. Phase II trial of cetuximab in patients with refractory colorectal cancer that expresses the epidermal growth factor receptor. *J Clin Oncol* 2004;22(7):1201-1208.

160. Sobrero AF, Maurel J, Fehrenbacher L, et al. EPIC: Phase III trial of cetuximab plus irinotecan after fluoropyrimidine and oxaliplatin failure in patients with metastatic colorectal cancer. *J Clin Oncol* 2008;26(14):2311-2319.

161. Cunningham D, Humblet Y, Siena S, et al. Cetuximab monotherapy and cetuximab plus irinotecan in irinotecan-refractory metastatic colorectal cancer. *N Engl J Med* 2004;351(4):337-345.

162. Jonker DJ, O'Callaghan CJ, Karapetis CS, et al. Cetuximab for the treatment of colorectal cancer. *N Engl J Med* 2007; 357(20):2040-2048.

163. Chung KY, Shia J, Kemeny NE, et al. Cetuximab shows activity in colorectal cancer patients with tumors that do not express the epidermal growth factor receptor by immunohistochemistry. *J Clin Oncol* 2005;23(9):1803-1810.

164. Santini D, Loupakis F, Vincenzi B, et al. High concordance of KRAS status between primary colorectal tumors and related metastatic sites: Implications for clinical practice. *Oncologist* 2008;13(12):1270-1275.

165. Peeters M, Oliner KS, Parker A, et al. Use of massively parallel, next-generation sequencing to identify gene mutations beyond *KRAS* that predict response to panitumumab in a randomized, phase 3, monotherapy study of metastatic colorectal cancer (mCRC). AACR, 2010.

166. Van Cutsem E, Kohne CH, Hitre E, et al. Cetuximab and chemotherapy as initial treatment for metastatic colorectal cancer. *N Engl J Med* 2009;360(14):1408-1417.

167. Van Cutsem E, Lang I, Folprecht G, et al. Cetuximab plus FOLFIRI in the treatment of metastatic colorectal cancer (mCRC): The influence of *KRAS* and *BRAF* biomarkers on outcome: Updated data from the CRYSTAL trial. 2010 GI Cancers Symposium, Orlando, Florida, 2010.

168. Bokemeyer C, Bondarenko I, Makhson A, et al. Fluorouracil, leucovorin, and oxaliplatin with and without cetuximab in the first-line treatment of metastatic colorectal cancer. *J Clin Oncol* 2009;27(5):663-671.

169. Allegra CJ, Jessup JM, Somerfield MR, et al. American Society of Clinical Oncology provisional clinical opinion: Testing for KRAS gene mutations in patients with metastatic colorectal carcinoma to predict response to anti-epidermal growth factor

170. Chung CH, Mirakhur B, Chan E, et al. Cetuximab-induced anaphylaxis and IgE specific for galactose-alpha-1,3-galactose. *N Engl J Med* 2008;358(11):1109-1117.

171. Susman E. Rash correlates with tumour response after cetuximab. *Lancet Oncol* 2004;5(11):647.

172. Lacouture ME, Mitchell EP, Piperdi B, et al. Skin toxicity evaluation protocol with panitumumab (STEPP), a phase II, open-label, randomized trial evaluating the impact of a preemptive skin treatment regimen on skin toxicities and quality of life in patients with metastatic colorectal cancer. *J Clin Oncol* 2010;28(8):1351-1357.

173. Van Cutsem E, Peeters M, Siena S, et al. Open-label phase III trial of panitumumab plus best supportive care compared with best supportive care alone in patients with chemotherapy-refractory metastatic colorectal cancer. *J Clin Oncol* 2007;25(13):1658-1664.

174. Amado RG, Wolf M, Peeters M, et al. Wild-type KRAS is required for panitumumab efficacy in patients with metastatic colorectal cancer. *J Clin Oncol* 2008;26(10):1626-1634.

175. Peeters M, Prince T, Hotko YS, et al. Randomized phase III study of panitumumab (pmab) with FOLFIRI versus FOLFIRI alone as second-line treatment (tx) in patients (pts) with metastatic colorectal cancer (mCRC): Patient-reported outcomes (PRO). 2010 GI Cancers Symposium, Orlando, Florida, 2010.

176. S. Siena S, Cassidy J, Tabernero J, et al. Randomized phase III study of panitumumab (pmab) with FOLFOX4 compared to FOLFOX4 alone as first-line treatment (tx) for metastatic colorectal cancer (mCRC): PRIME trial 2010 GI Cancers Symposium, Orlando, Florida, 2010.

177. Folkman J. Tumor angiogenesis: A possible control point in tumor growth. *Ann Intern Med* 1975;82(1):96-100.

178. Werther K, Christensen IJ, Brunner N, et al. Soluble vascular endothelial growth factor levels in patients with primary colorectal carcinoma. The Danish RANX05 Colorectal Cancer Study Group. *Eur J Surg Oncol* 2000;26(7):657-662.

179. De Vita F, Orditura M, Lieto E, et al. Elevated perioperative serum vascular endothelial growth factor levels in patients with colon carcinoma. *Cancer* 2004;100(2):270-278.

180. Salgaller ML. Technology evaluation: Bevacizumab, Genentech/Roche. *Curr Opin Mol Ther* 2003;5(6):657-667.

181. Kabbinavar F, Hurwitz HI, Fehrenbacher L, et al. Phase II, randomized trial comparing bevacizumab plus fluorouracil (FU)/leucovorin (LV) with FU/LV alone in patients with metastatic colorectal cancer. *J Clin Oncol* 2003;21(1):60-65.

182. Hurwitz H, Fehrenbacher L, Novotny W, et al. Bevacizumab plus irinotecan, fluorouracil, and leucovorin for metastatic colorectal cancer. *N Engl J Med* 2004; 350(23): 2335-2342.

183. Hochster HS, Hart LL, Ramanathan RK, et al. Safety and efficacy of oxaliplatin and fluoropyrimidine regimens with or without bevacizumab as first-line treatment of metastatic colorectal cancer: Results of the TREE Study. *J Clin Oncol* 2008;26(21):3523-3529.

184. Saltz LB, Clarke S, Diaz-Rubio E, et al. Bevacizumab in combination with oxaliplatin-based chemotherapy as first-line therapy in metastatic colorectal cancer: A randomized phase III study. *J Clin Oncol* 2008;26(12):2013-2019.

185. Giantonio BJ, Catalano PJ, Meropol NJ, et al. Bevacizumab in combination with oxaliplatin, fluorouracil, and leucovorin (FOLFOX4) for previously treated metastatic colorectal cancer: Results from the Eastern Cooperative Oncology Group Study E3200. *J Clin Oncol* 2007;25(12):1539-1544.

186. Grothey A, Sugrue MM, Purdie DM, et al. Bevacizumab beyond first progression is associated with prolonged overall survival in metastatic colorectal cancer: Results from a large observational cohort study (BRiTE). *J Clin Oncol* 2008; 26(33):5326-5334.

187. Wolmark W, Yothers G, O'Connell MJ, et al. A phase III trial comparing mFOLFOX6 to mFOLFOX6 plus bevacizumab in stage II or III carcinoma of the colon: Results of NSABP Protocol C-08. ASCO Chicago, IL, 2009.

188. Hoff PM, Clarke S, Cunningham D, et al. A three-arm randomized phase III trial of FOLFOX4 vs FOLFOX4 + bevacizumab vs XELOX + bevacizumab in the adjuvant treatment of patients with stage III or high-risk stage II colon cancer: Results of the interim safety analysis of the AVANT trial. ECCO 15 ESMO 34, 2010.

189. Kopetz S, Hoff PM, Morris JS, et al. Phase II trial of infusional fluorouracil, irinotecan, and bevacizumab for metastatic colorectal cancer: efficacy and circulating angiogenic biomarkers associated with therapeutic resistance. *J Clin Oncol* 2010;28(3):453-459.

190. Tol J, Koopman M, Cats A, et al. Chemotherapy, bevacizumab, and cetuximab in metastatic colorectal cancer. *N Engl J Med* 2009;360(6):563-572.

191. Hecht JR, Mitchell E, Chidiac T, et al. A randomized phase IIIB trial of chemotherapy, bevacizumab, and panitumumab compared with chemotherapy and bevacizumab alone for metastatic colorectal cancer. *J Clin Oncol* 2009; 27(5):672-680.

192. Adam R, Pascal G, Castaing D, et al. Tumor progression while on chemotherapy: A contraindication to liver resection for multiple colorectal metastases? *Ann Surg* 2004;240(6): 1052-1061; discussion 1061-1064.

193. Mitry E, Fields AL, Bleiberg H, et al. Adjuvant chemotherapy after potentially curative resection of metastases from colorectal cancer: A pooled analysis of two randomized trials. *J Clin Oncol* 2008;26(30):4906-4911.

194. Benoist S, Brouquet A, Penna C, et al. Complete response of colorectal liver metastases after chemotherapy: Does it mean cure? *J Clin Oncol* 2006;24(24):3939-3945.

195. Vauthey JN, Pawlik TM, Ribero D, et al. Chemotherapy regimen predicts steatohepatitis and an increase in 90-day mortality after surgery for hepatic colorectal metastases. *J Clin Oncol* 2006;24(13):2065-2072.

196. Grothey A, Sargent D, Goldberg RM, et al. Survival of patients with advanced colorectal cancer improves with the availability of fluorouracil-leucovorin, irinotecan, and oxaliplatin in the course of treatment. *J Clin Oncol* 2004;22(7): 1209-1214.

197. Maindrault-Goebel F, Tournigand C, Andre T, et al. Oxaliplatin reintroduction in patients previously treated with leucovorin, fluorouracil and oxaliplatin for metastatic colorectal cancer. *Ann Oncol* 2004;15(8):1210-1214.

198. Tournigand C, Cervantes A, Figer A, et al. OPTIMOX1: A randomized study of FOLFOX4 or FOLFOX7 with oxaliplatin in a stop-and-Go fashion in advanced colorectal cancer—a GERCOR study. *J Clin Oncol* 2006;24(3):394-400.

199. Chibaudel B, Maindrault-Goebel F, Lledo G, et al. Can chemotherapy be discontinued in unresectable metastatic colorectal cancer? The GERCOR OPTIMOX2 Study. *J Clin Oncol* 2009;27(34):5727-5733.

ANAL CANCER

Tzu-chuan Jane Huang
Cathy Eng
Commentary: Christopher H. Crane

Carcinoma of the anal canal is a rarely discussed malignancy representing 1.9 % of all identified gastrointestinal malignancies (1). It is estimated in the year 2009 that approximately 5290 patients will be diagnosed with carcinoma of the anal canal, resulting in 710 deaths (1). A practicing oncologist will evaluate and treat less than one such patient per year. The majority of anal carcinoma arises within the mucosa of the anus and are of squamous cell histology (2). Traditionally, 74 to 90% of carcinomas of the anal canal are cured with the combined modalities of chemoradiation, reserving an abdominoperineal resection (APR) for salvage therapy (3). As a consequence of its exceptional response to multimodality treatment and its infrequent presentation, few clinical studies on carcinoma of the anal canal have been completed. Furthermore, the majority of studies that have been recently completed are often small single-institution studies. Little has changed over the past three decades, resulting in minimal modifications in the treatment approach. Hence, the ability to redefine the standard of care of these patients exists. This chapter focuses primarily on the historical and current treatment of squamous cell carcinoma of the anal canal and the potential innovative strategies that lie ahead.

■ EPIDEMIOLOGY

A recent population-based analysis of the National Cancer Institute's Surveillance, Epidemiology, and End Results (SEER) data between the years 1973 and 2000 reported a steady overall increase of anal canal cancers in the United States with this increase more pronounced for men (4). Whereas men previously had lower incidence rates than women, that gender difference in the annual incidence has normalized with similar rates demonstrated at 2.04 per 100,000 for men and 2.06 per 100,000 for women. There has been an overall increase in the rate of in situ disease from 0.09 to 0.45 per 100,000 persons, surpassing a less pronounced increase in rate of invasive disease, with a more advanced disease stage inversely associated with overall survival. Disparities exist, in particular for black men who exhibited a 2.5-fold increase in incidence rate from 1994 to 2000 and with black patients overall having a consistently higher mortality with a poorer stage-specific relative survival at 5 years when compared with white patients. An especially high incidence of anal cancer has also been seen in the populations of men who have sex with men (MSM) and patients infected with human immunodeficiency virus (HIV) (5).

■ ANATOMY/HISTOLOGY

The anal canal is approximately 4 cm wide and is composed of the region extending from the proximal anorectal ring to the distal anal verge (margin) (Fig. 22-1). It is imperative to differentiate the borders of the rectum, anal canal, and margin. As various definitions of the normal anal canal anatomy exist, classifying these tumors by a histologic definition based on the lining mucosa offers a more consistent approach to guide diagnosis and treatment (2). The majority of anal carcinomas are of squamous cell histology.

Malignancies of the anal margin are treated as primary skin cancers and are often surgically excised. The rectal mucosa adjacent to the anorectal ring is composed

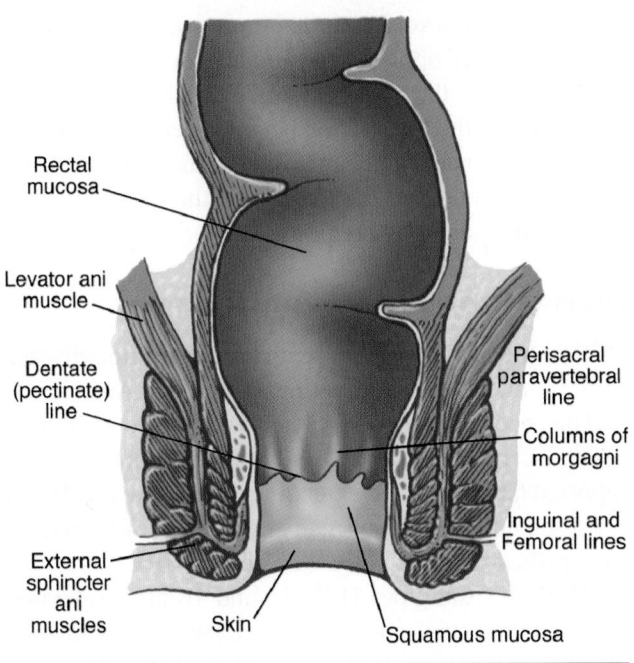

FIGURE 22-1. Anatomy of the anal canal.

(Labels on figure: Rectal mucosa, Levator ani muscle, Dentate (pectinate) line, External sphincter ani muscles, Skin, Perisacral paravertebral line, Columns of morgagni, Inguinal and Femoral lines, Squamous mucosa)

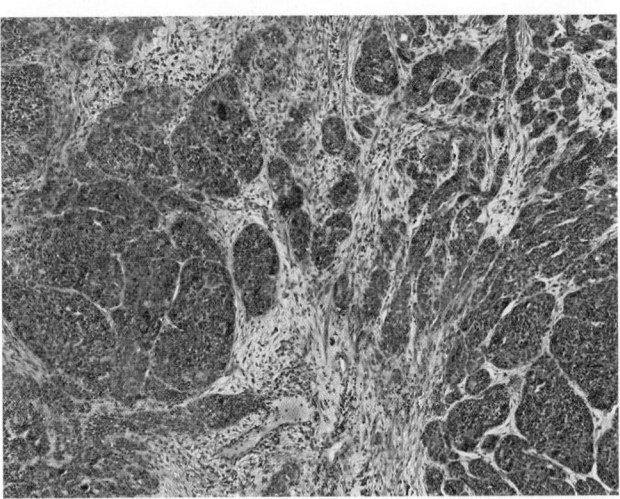

FIGURE 22-2. Nonkeratinized squamous cell carcinoma of the anal canal.

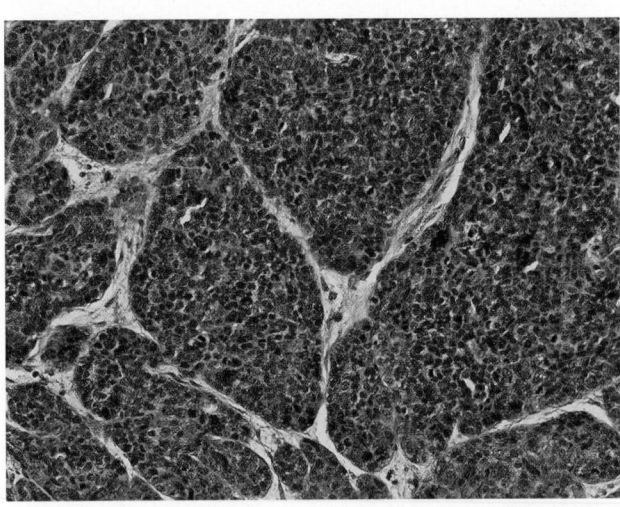

FIGURE 22-3. Magnified view of nonkeratinized squamous cell carcinoma of the anal canal.

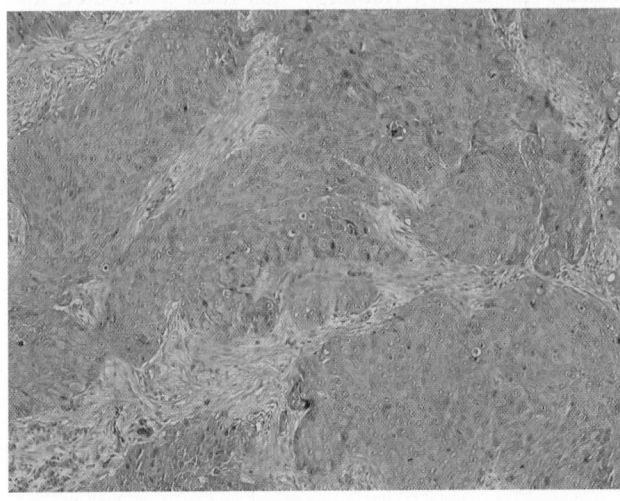

FIGURE 22-4. Keratinized squamous cell carcinoma of the anal canal.

of columnar epithelium. A transition zone of both cuboidal and columnar epithelium (6-12 mm in length) extends from the distal rectum to the dentate line. The dentate line separates the columnar epithelium (columns of Morgagni) of the proximal anal canal and the squamous epithelium of the distal canal, which extends to the anal verge. The anal verge is the convergence of squamous epithelium and the anal margin. The anal margin comprises the dermis, located within 5 cm of the anal verge.

The mucosa of the transition zone, formally referred to as the cloacogenic mucosa, represents 66% of the lesions now commonly referred to as nonkeratinizing squamous cell carcinoma (SCC) (Figs. 22-2 and 22-3) (6). Tumors distal to the dentate line are usually keratinizing SCC (Figs. 22-4 and 22-5). There appears to be little prognostic difference between nonkeratinizing and keratinizing SCC. Other rare histologic subtypes of malignancy arising in the anus include malignant melanoma, small cell carcinoma, verrucous carcinoma, basal cell carcinoma, Bowen and Paget disease.

The vascular supply of the anal canal consists of the superior, middle, and inferior rectal vessels that originate from the inferior mesenteric, internal iliac, and internal pudendal arteries, respectively. Lymphatic drainage superior to the dentate line is identical to rectal carcinomas flowing to the perirectal and paravertebral nodes. Tumors located inferior to the dentate line drain

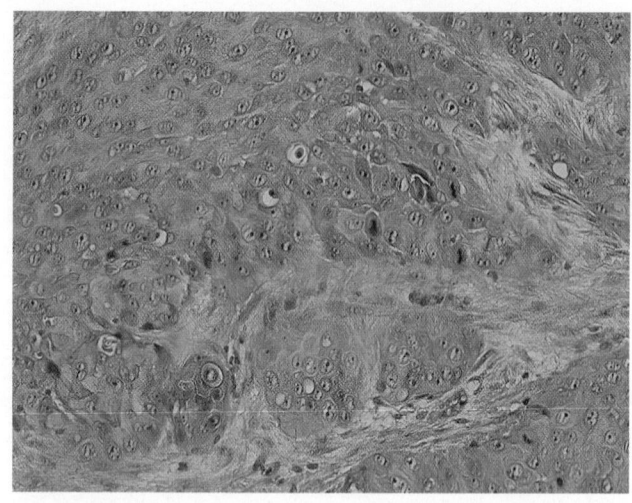

FIGURE 22-5. Magnified view of keratinized squamous cell carcinoma of the anal canal.

to the inguinal and femoral lymph nodes. A complete physical examination should include examination of the lymph nodes of the groin.

■ ETIOLOGY

Multiple risk factors have been associated with the development of carcinoma of the anal canal. Early studies implicated chronic inflammatory bowel diseases such as ulcerative colitis and Crohn disease in the development of anal carcinoma, but recent large population studies have shown these conditions do not predispose patients to a higher risk of developing anal cancer (7-9). Benign conditions such as hemorrhoids, fissures, and anal fistulas have also not been determined to be causal factors (8). Rather, it has been postulated that these benign conditions may instead represent the initial symptoms of anal cancer (8).

SEXUAL ACTIVITY

The pathogenesis of developing anal cancer is largely related to sexual practices as well as history of genital viral and bacterial sexually transmitted infections. Common risk factors associated with anal cancer include a history of more than 10 sexual partners; receptive anal intercourse before the age of 30; and sexually transmitted diseases, including condyloma acuminata (genital warts, attributed to human papillomavirus [HPV]), gonorrhea, herpes virus, hepatitis, *Chlamydia trachomatis,* or a history of infection with HIV (10-12). Women with a history of cervical, vaginal, or vulvar

cancer are three to five times more likely to develop anal cancer as opposed to stomach or colon cancer, demonstrating the link between sexual activity (13). Causality for the association between cervical, vaginal, and vulvar cancers and carcinoma of the anal canal has been attributed to exposure to and the acquisition of HPV in these anatomic regions.

HUMAN PAPILLOMAVIRUS (HPV)

HPV is the most common sexually transmitted disease in the United States, affecting 20 million Americans, and has been strongly associated with the development of anal carcinoma (14). Condyloma acuminata has a reported latency period extending up to 40 years (15). It is estimated that 75% of men and women of reproductive age have been infected with genital HPV.

High-risk subtypes HPV 16 and 18 are associated with anal cancer—as is cervical dysplasia—and may result in anal intraepithelial neoplasia (AIN). HPV subtype 16 reportedly results in a greater incidence of high-grade AIN (16). However, unlike cervical dysplasia, AIN is a premalignant condition for which standard screening methods currently have not been universally recommended and have been limited to select high-risk individuals, as no studies have yet been performed to show treatment of high-grade AIN prevents cancer (17). Progression of AIN to invasive anal carcinoma is based on the factors of HIV seropositivity, a lower CD4 count, subtype of HPV, and higher DNA levels of high-risk HPV subtypes in the anal canal (18).

A systematic literature review of all peer-reviewed studies published until July 2007 on HPV type distribution in anal cancer showed a combined HPV 16 and/or 18 with an overall prevalence of 72% in invasive anal cancer, with the prevalence of HPV subtype 16 being the highest in these cases as in cervical cancer (19). Introduction in 2006 and 2009 of prophylactic vaccines Gardasil and Cervarix, respectively, directed against primary infection by HPV in an effort to prevent cervical cancer has demonstrated efficacy in reducing precancerous anogenital lesions caused by all the targeted subtypes 6, 11, 16, and 18 (20-22). However, the overall effect of vaccination on prevention of HPV infection of the anal canal, anal cancer, and other cancers associated with HPV remains unknown and may not be determined for decades. While both vaccines were initially approved for the vaccination of adolescent females, Gardasil has subsequently been extended to males of the same age category after it was shown to be efficacious and may offer a promising primary prevention strategy in both genders (23).

HUMAN IMMUNODEFICIENCY VIRUS

HIV may be the risk factor with the largest global impact. The annual incidence of anal cancer among all men in the United States is estimated to be 1.55 per 100,000 men, but in MSM the incidence may rise to 25 to 37 per 100,000 (5). The World Health Organization estimates that 33.4 million people were living with HIV in 2008, with 2.7 million people becoming newly infected and 2.0 million deaths from AIDS-related illnesses (24). Africa continues to be the continent most heavily affected by HIV, accounting for 67% of HIV infections worldwide and 68% of new HIV infections among adults.

Although a direct relationship between HIV and carcinoma of the anal canal has not been clearly established, a strong correlation exists between HIV and HPV. Compared with HIV-negative patients, HIV-positive patients are two to six times more likely to be diagnosed with HPV regardless of sexual practices and are also more likely to have a persistent infection (25-26). HIV-positive men and women are less likely to become HPV negative (26-27). For patients who are infected with HIV, the prevalence of anal carcinoma is greater and presents at a younger age of onset than HIV-positive patients versus HIV-negative (28). HIV-positive women are also five times as likely to have a lower genital tract neoplasm (29).

Recent data indicate the introduction of highly active antiretroviral therapy (HAART) has not affected the incidence of anal cancer in contrast to other common malignancies affecting HIV-positive individuals (30-31). According to a recent analysis among 4506 HIV-infected men, the rate of anal cancer (per 100,000 person-years) increased from 11 in the pre-HAART era to 55 in the HAART era ($p = 0.02$); and increased further to 128 in 2006 to 2008. Furthermore, being HIV-positive for >15 years resulted in a 12-fold higher incidence rate than those with <5 years (348 versus 28, respectively, $p < .01$). Whether the CD4 lymphocyte count has any bearing on the prognosis in carcinoma of the anal canal remains controversial (27-28, 31). However, a CD4 cell count <200/µL has been associated with persistent HPV infection (27).

The AIDS-Cancer Match Registry Study Group has completed a US analysis of 309,365 HIV-positive patients to determine whether the incidence of HPV-associated cancers in HIV patients was increased due to lifestyle risk factors or a result of the chronic immuno-suppressed state of the HIV patient (32). Patients were studied for 5 years prior to the onset of AIDS and 5 years thereafter. Surprisingly, although overall risks were increased for anal cancer, the relative risk of invasive carcinoma changed little over the 10-year span. Based on these findings, the authors concluded that the immune system has minimal effect on the development of invasive carcinoma in HIV-positive patients.

CHRONIC IMMUNOSUPPRESSION

Solid-organ transplantation has been associated with a 10-fold increased risk of developing anal cancer and a 20-fold increased risk for vulvar and vaginal cancers (33). Renal transplant recipients appear to be at increased risk for developing HPV, which may place these patients at greater risk for anal cancer relative to those receiving other organ transplants (34). A recent population-based cohort study conducted using the Danish National Patient Registry and the Danish Cancer Registry (DCR) from 1978 to 2005 found HIV infection, solid organ transplantation, hematological malignancies, and a range of specific autoimmune diseases strongly associated with increased risk of anal SCC (35).

TOBACCO USE

Prior case-control studies have indicated that chronic tobacco use may result in a two- to five-fold increased likelihood of developing anal cancer (36). A Danish and Swedish case-control study found an increased risk of anal carcinoma among premenopausal women who currently smoke tobacco (multivariate OR, 5.6; 95% confidence interval [CI], 2.4-12.7); increasing linearly by 6.7% per pack-year smoked (one pack-year is equivalent to one pack of cigarettes smoked per day for 1 year) ($p < .001$). Smoking was not statistically significantly associated with anal cancer risk in postmenopausal women (37). In contrast, a more recent case-control study associated an increased risk of anal carcinoma for both male and female smokers independent of age and other risk factors (OR, 3.9 [95% CI, 1.9-8.0] and OR, 3.8 [95% CI, 2.4-6.2], respectively) (12). Moreover, tobacco smoking appears to be associated with recurrence of anal carcinoma and is related to increased mortality; thus, smoking cessation should be encouraged once a diagnosis of anal carcinoma is made (38).

■ PRESENTATION AND DIAGNOSIS

The mean age of diagnosis is approximately 61.8 years (39). Men tend to present at a younger age in the third to fifth decade, in contrast to a higher rate of diagnosis seen

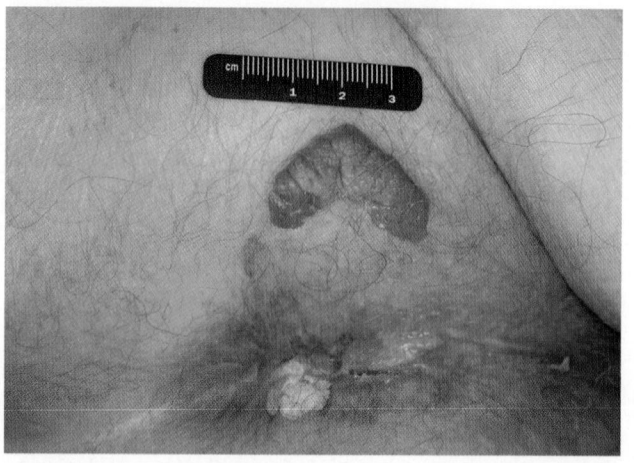

FIGURE 22-6. Perianal mass.

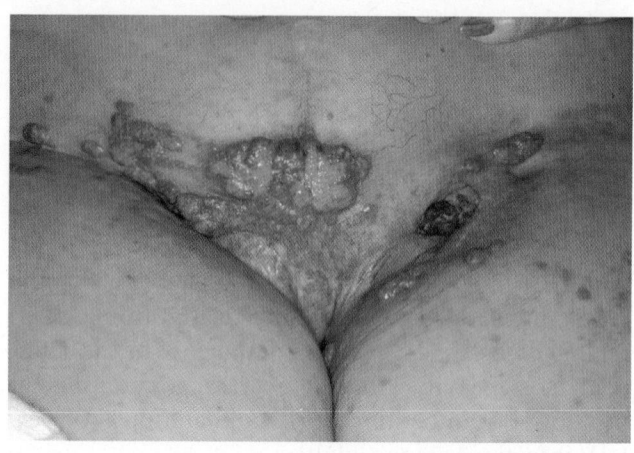

FIGURE 22-7. Multiple verrucous lesions originating from squamous cell carcinoma of the anal canal.

in the seventh decade for women (4). The most common presenting complaint is rectal bleeding. Other symptoms may include tenesmus, pain, local irritation, discharge, or a change in bowel habits. Clinically enlarged lymph nodes are present in 15 to 25% of patients at presentation (40). Extreme case presentations may include a fungating perianal mass or a verrucous mass, as seen in Figs. 22-6 and 22-7.

A diagnostic evaluation should consist of a complete physical examination including examination of the inguinal lymph nodes, a digital rectal examination (DRE), and evaluation of the surrounding mucosa of the anus. Diagnostic studies should include proctosigmoidoscopy or anoscopy, chest x-ray, and computed tomography (CT) chest, abdomen, or pelvis, or magnetic resonance imaging (MRI) of the abdomen and pelvis to rule out distant disease. Though not validated for staging or treatment planning, a positron emission tomography (PET/CT) scan may provide additional

staging information particularly in the evaluation of pelvic lymph nodes (40, 41). A transrectal or transvaginal ultrasound may be of added benefit in accurate disease staging (42-45). Histologic confirmation is recommended, with a tissue biopsy of the suspected area and/or fine-needle aspiration of any palpable inguinal lymph nodes since this may impact the radiation fields. An HIV test should be completed in all patients at risk for HIV, given the potential impact on future treatment, tolerance, concomitant medications, and outcome (Fig. 22-8). The role of HPV testing following the diagnosis of anal carcinoma is not clear.

■ STAGING AND PROGNOSIS

In 1958, the International Union against Cancer, or Union Internationale Contre le Cancer (UICC), created the concept of a classification scheme that would

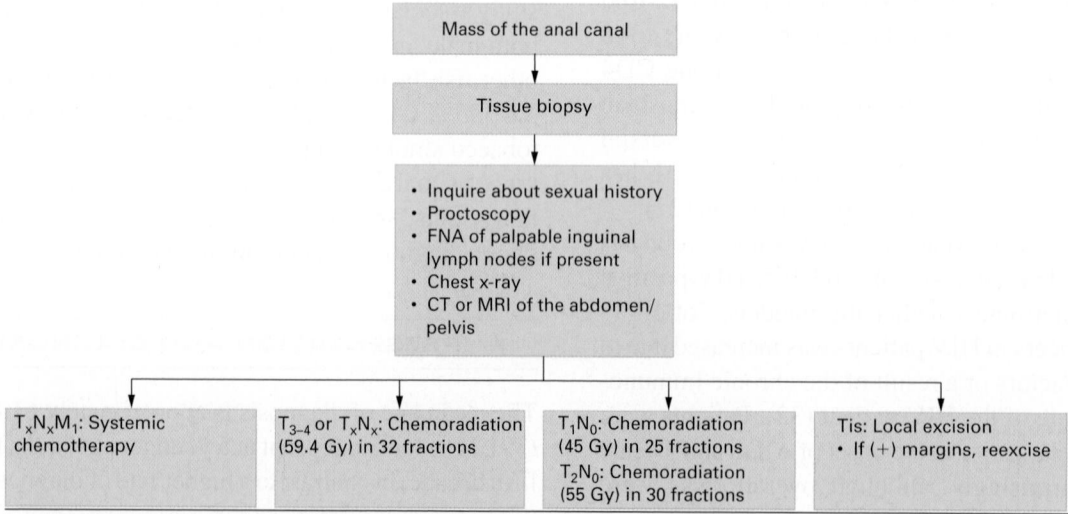

FIGURE 22-8. Diagnostic evaluation for anal canal mass.

encompass all aspects of cancer distribution in terms of primary tumor (T), regional lymph nodes (N), and distant metastasis (M). The UICC classification was adopted by the American Joint Commission on Cancer (Fig. 22-9). The T stage, unlike most gastrointestinal

---

DEFINITION OF T,N,M

PRIMARY TUMOR (T)

TX	Primary tumor cannot be accessed
T0	No evidence of primary tumor
Tis	Carcinoma in situ
T1	Tumor 2 cm or less in greatest dimension
T2	Tumor .2 cm but not .5 cm in greatest dimension
T3	Tumor .5 cm in greatest dimension
T4	Tumor of any size invades adjacent organ(s), eg, vagina, urethra, bladder*

* Note: Direct invasion of the rectal wall, perirectal skin, subcutaneous tissue, or the sphincter muscle(s) is not classified as T4.

REGIONAL LYMPH NODES (N)

NX	Regional lymph nodes cannot be assessed
N0	No regional lymph node metastasis
N1	Metastasis in perirectal lymph node(s)
N2	Metastasis in unilateral internal iliac and/or inguinal lymph node(s)
N3	Metastasis in perirectal and inguinal lymph nodes and/or bilateral internal iliac and/or inguinal lymph nodes

DISTANT METASTASIS (M)

MX	Distant metastasis cannot be assessed
M0	No distant metastasis
M1	Distant metastasis

STAGE GROUPING

Stage 0	Tis	N0	M0
Stage I	T1	N0	M0
Stage II	T2	N0	M0
	T3	N0	M0
Stage IIIA	T1	N1	M0
	T2	N1	M0
	T3	N1	M0
	T4	N0	M0
Stage IIIB	T4	N1	M0
	Any T	N2	M0
	Any T	N3	M0
Stage IV	Any T	Any N	M1

FIGURE 22-9. Definition of primary tumor (T), regional lymph nodes (N), and distant metastasis (M) and group staging. *(Used with the permission of the American Joint Committee on Cancer (AJCC), Chicago, Illinois. The original source for this material is the AJCC Cancer Staging Manual, seventh edition (2010) published by Springer Science and Business Media LLC, www.springer.com.)*

malignancies, is not dependent on the degree of tumor tissue penetration but rather on the size of the primary tumor site.

Carcinomas of the anal margin are commonly excised with complete resolution of the tumor. SCCs of the anal canal behave less aggressively than adenocarcinomas of the anal canal (46). Independent poor prognostic features include tumor size (T stage) with a clear distinction in prognosis between T2 and T3 tumors ($p < .0001$) (28-30). Patients with T1 to T2 tumors have an expected 5-yr survival of 80%, versus those with T3 to T4 tumors, with an expected median 5-year survival of <20% (39). Inguinal lymph node involvement may reduce the cure rate by 50%, with increased nodal stage being a significant prognostic factor (46-49). Multivariate analysis of the results from RTOG 98-11, in which 682 patients were randomized to receive either radiotherapy with concurrent 5-fluorouracil (5-FU) and mitomycin C, or induction chemotherapy with 5-FU and cisplatin, followed by radiotherapy with concurrent 5-FU and cisplatin, indicates that tumor-related prognosticators for poorer overall survival included node-positive status ($p = .0001$), large tumor diameter >5 cm ($p = .01$), and male sex ($p = .016$) (50). Combined analysis of both prospective arms of RTOG 98-11 revealed that tumor diameter >5 cm is the only pretreatment variable that independently predicts an increased likelihood of colostomy (51).

Review of the Surveillance, Epidemiology, and End Results (SEER) Program, a system of population-based tumor registries in the United States for the period 1997 to 2004 revealed squamous cell histology to be a favorable prognostic factor (4).

■ TREATMENT PARADIGMS

SURGERY

Prior to the 1970s, conventional treatment for anal cancer was an APR, resulting in a permanent end-colostomy. With this as the only treatment modality, the estimated 5-year probability of survival is 40 to 70% (24). An APR is a surgical procedure where the surgeon performs an en bloc resection of the rectum, including the anal sphincter and the surrounding mesentery. Perioperative complications may include significant bleeding due to the proximal veins in the presacral plexus (6). Immediate postoperative complications may include poor wound healing and urinary dysfunction. The chronic sequelae of an APR may be physically, socially, and psychologically debilitating. Immediate postoperative concerns following a permanent colostomy include educating patients regarding colostomy care and potential psychosocial stigma. Chronic psychological sequelae may include sexual dysfunction and depression. Therefore equivalent or superior alternative treatment modalities are preferred if a permanent colostomy can be avoided.

RADIATION AS A SINGLE MODALITY

Radiation therapy was initially evaluated as an alternative to an APR. It has been utilized in the treatment of anal cancer since the early 1900s (52). Radiation therapy allows preservation of the anal sphincter with the potential for long-term survival. Compared with APR, it has been reported that the overall survival (OS) after radiation therapy is equivalent if not better, with a complete response (CR) being achieved in approximately 75% of patients (Table 22-1) (53-56).

To date, the largest analysis of patients treated with definitive irradiation is a retrospective study of 305 patients completed over a 25-year period (57). The majority of patients (81%) had T2 to T3 tumors; the tumor size was ≥5 cm in 52% of patients. Regional lymph-adenopathy was identified in 16% of patients. External-beam radiation therapy (EBRT) was provided, with concomitant chemotherapy in 19 patients (6%) or interstitial brachytherapy in 17 patients (6%). The median dose of EBRT was 45 Gy. A radiation boost of 20 Gy was provided after a median delay of 37 days (median cumulative dose of 63 Gy) in 279 patients (92%). All palpable lymph nodes received a booster dose of 10 to 15 Gy. All patients were evaluated for response 4 and 8 weeks after completion of radiation. After a median follow-up of 103 months, a complete response was achieved in 79 to 96% of T1 to T3 tumors but markedly less for T4 tumors (44%). Radiation as a single modality resulted in local control in only 68% of all patients: T1 to T2, 78 to 81%; T3, 63%; and T4, 33%. Overall, the local control rate following salvage surgery or brachytherapy was 84% and varied by stage: 92% for T1 to T2 tumors, 82% for T3 tumors, and 50% for T4 tumors. If these patients were further substratified, a total of 186 patients (61%) sustained both local control and preservation of the anal sphincter: T1, 81%; T2, 68.5%; T3, 58%, and T4, 24%. The estimated 5- and 10-year overall survival rates were 66.7% and 55.4%, respectively. The development of distant metastatic disease occurred in 31 patients (10%).

The investigators concluded that independent prognostic factors by multivariate analysis included tumor size ≥4 cm, tumor depth, the use of concomitant chemotherapy with radiation, and initial response after the first course of EBRT. A treatment delay >38 days during radiation therapy had a negative impact on disease-free survival ($p = 0.0025$). At the time this study was initiated, a rest period between two courses of radiation therapy was commonplace ("split-course" radiation therapy). Results from the Radiation Therapy Oncology Group (RTOG 92-08) confirmed that split-course radiation therapy increases the risk of locoregional recurrence and concluded that treatment interruptions in anal canal treatment should be kept to a minimum (58).

TABLE 22-1	RADIATION AS A SINGLE MODALITY IN THE TREATMENT OF ANAL CANCER					
Author	*Radiation Dose (Gy)*	*N*	*Complete Response*	*Locoregional Control*	*5-Year Overall Survival*	
Cummings et al. (52), 1982	45-50	51	65%	57% 73%[*]	71%	4% palliative colostomy 8% perineal fibrosis 14% anal stricture
Eschwege et al. (55), 1985	60	64	—	T1-T2 (91.8%) T3 (76%) T4 (66%)	46% T1-T2 (72%) T3-T4 (35%)	14% with grade 3 treatment-related toxicities
Martenson et al. (53), 1993	45-50	18	—	100%	94%	11% required palliative colostomy for rectovaginal fistula and anal ulcer
Deniaud-Alexandre et al. (57), 2003	45 + 20 Gy (boost)	305	80%	84%[*] T1-T2 (92%) T3 (82%) T4 (50%)	77%	6% necrosis of the anal canal resulting in incontinence, stenosis, pain, and rectovaginal fistulas

[*]Salvage surgery.

CHEMORADIATION—NIGRO REGIMEN

A pivotal approach by investigators at Wayne State University led to the anecdotal finding that surgery may not be necessary for curative intent in the treatment of SCC of the anal canal (59). The benefits of combined chemoradiation in other gastrointestinal malignancies prompted Nigro and colleagues to consider the use of 5-FU as a radiation sensitizer. In this clinical study, patients received neoadjuvant concomitant continuous infusion of 5-FU (1000 mg/m^2/day, on days 1-4 and 28-31) and mitomycin C (15 mg/m^2 on day 1), which was administered along with EBRT (30 Gy). The pathologic specimens in 3 of 3 patients failed to demonstrate any viable tumor. This observation culminated in the use of chemoradiation as the primary treatment modality for the treatment of anal cancer and revolutionized the approach to its treatment. The Nigro approach of chemoradiation has subsequently been evaluated in several other small phase II studies with radiation doses ranging from 30 to 60 Gy.

A retrospective analysis from the Princess Margaret Hospital reviewed the charts of 192 patients who had been treated with (1) radiation alone, (2) 5-FU/mitomycin C, (3) split-course 5-FU/mitomycin C, or (4) split-course 5-FU (60). The total dose of radiation was 45 to 55 Gy. The 5-year disease-free survival (DFS) was significantly improved in the 5-FU/mitomycin C arms versus 5-FU alone (76 versus 64%). Nodal disease was controlled in 33 of 38 patients (87%) at the conclusion of their treatment. Clinically node-positive disease did not have a bearing on overall survival of these patients. Although the combination of 5-FU/mitomycin C was superior in locoregional control (LRC) with the addition of mitomycin C (86 versus 60%), the use of split-course radiation resulted in decreased morbidity, notably acute skin toxicities. Overall, the anorectal sphincter was preserved in 64% of patients. Therefore prospective studies were created to validate these findings.

■ PHASE III CLINICAL TRIALS

The United Kingdom Coordinating Committee on Cancer Research (UKCCCR) and the European Organization for Research and Treatment of Cancer Radiotherapy and Gastrointestinal Cooperative Groups (EORTC) have completed two fundamental studies that have permanently altered the treatment of anal carcinoma, thereby establishing the role of concomitant chemoradiation as the standard of care.

■ RADIATION VERSUS CHEMORADIATION: THE ROLE OF MITOMYCIN C

UKCCCR

The UKCCCR created the phase III anal cancer trial (ACT I). Patients (N = 585) were randomized between 1987 and 1991 to radiation alone (45 Gy) versus continuous infusion 5-FU (1000 mg/m^2 on days 1 to 4 or 750 mg/m^2 on days 1-5) during the first and last weeks of radiation (45 Gy) with mitomycin C (12 mg/m^2 on day 1) (61). Patients of all stages were accrued including metastatic patients. Patients with significant comorbidities or ≥70 years of age were provided a reduced dose of 5-FU (750 mg/m^2 on days 1-4) and mitomycin C (10 mg/m^2 on day 1). All patients were evaluated for clinical response to treatment 6 weeks after the completion of their radiation therapy. Salvage surgery was offered to all patients with <50% response rate. If the response was ≥50%, a boost of radiation therapy was offered, 20 Gy of EBRT or 25 Gy for iridium implants. The primary objective was the observation of local failure rate. Patient demographics were equivalent between the two arms.

After a median follow-up of 42 months, it was determined that the 3-year local failure rate was significantly reduced in the chemoradiation arm versus the radiation-alone arms (39% versus 61%, $p < 0.0001$), most developing recurrence within the first 18 months. The majority of local failures (69%) were treated with surgery; those remaining were determined to be surgically unresectable. A benefit in overall survival could not be determined ($p = .25$) (Table 22-2).

Notably, the 3-year mortality rate in the radiation-only arm was greater than that of the chemoradiation arm (39 versus 28%, $p = 0.02$). Twenty patients (3%) required a palliative colostomy or anorectal excision due to treatment-related morbidities. Early morbidity was significant in the chemoradiation arm ($p = 0.03$), with 6 deaths attributed to chemotherapy, two as a result of sepsis. Subsequently, dose reduction of mitomycin C was recommended if the patient was ≥70 years of age or if deemed medically necessary. Further dose reduction to 8 mg/m^2 was recommended for any patient ≥80 years of age. Late morbidity complications were equivalent between the two arms ($p = 0.39$). The authors concluded that chemoradiation provided a 46% reduction in local recurrence compared with radiation alone ($p < 0.0001$). Forty percent of deaths were a result of distant disease. A recent update after a median follow-up of 13.1 years noted that combined modality

TABLE 22-2	RANDOMIZED PHASE III STUDIES OF RADIATION THERAPY VERSUS CHEMORADIATION	
	RADIATION	**CHEMORADIATION**
UKCCCR	*N = 285*	*N = 292*
Complete response	76 (30%)	100 (39%)
Partial response (>50%)	157 (62%)	138 (53%)
Minimal response (<50%)	22 (9%)	21 (8%)
Three-year local failure	164 (61%)	101 (39%)
Three-year overall survival	58%	65%, p = .25
EORTC	*N = 52*	*N = 51*
Complete response	54%	80%
Five-year locoregional control		p = .02
Five-year colostomy-free interval	—	p = .002
Three-year overall survival	65%	72% (p = .17)

Data from UKCCCR. Epidermoid anal cancer: Results from the UKCCCR randomised trial of radiotherapy alone versus radiotherapy, 5-fluorouracil, and mitomycin. UKCCCR Anal Cancer Trial Working Party. UK Co-ordinating Committee on Cancer Research. Lancet 1996;348:1049–1054.

Bartelink H, Roelofsen F, Eschwege F, et al. Concomitant radiotherapy and chemotherapy is superior to radiotherapy alone in the treatment of locally advanced anal cancer: Results of a phase III randomized trial of the European Organization for Research and Treatment of Cancer Radiotherapy and Gastrointestinal Cooperative Groups. J Clin Oncol 1997;15:2040-2049.

therapy resulted in a risk reduction of relapsing or dying (HR, 0.70; 95% CI, 0.58-0.84; p < .001); the absolute risk difference for death or relapse at 5 yrs was -13% (62). Combined modality therapy resulted in a risk reduction of relapse or death (HR = 0.61, 95% CI 0.49-0.76, p < .001). The absolute risk difference remained the same at 2 years versus 12 years (−18%). The median OS was 7.6 years versus 5.4 years in favor for the combined modality arm.

EORTC

A smaller study completed by the European Organization for Research and Treatment of Cancer (EORTC) explored the role of chemoradiation and its potential benefit in LRC and colostomy-free interval (63). Between 1987 and 1994, a total of 110 patients were randomized to radiation (45 Gy) or continuous infusion 5-FU (750 mg/m^2 on days 1-5 and 29-33)/mitomycin C (15 mg/m^2 on day 1). If inguinal lymphadenopathy was present, a boost of radiation was provided to the involved region. Patients were evaluated for response at 6 weeks, with a boost of 15 or 20 Gy provided for complete and partial responses, respectively. If there was evidence of progression or stable disease, salvage surgery was recommended.

No significant differences in acute or late toxicities of treatment were noted. One patient died of neutropenic sepsis during the third week of treatment. Event-free survival was superior in the combined-modality arm (p = 0.03). Ironically, tumor size was not determined to be a poor prognostic indicator in this study, but any nodal involvement was a poor prognostic

factor. The overall 5-year survival was 56% in this patient population. In contrast to the UKCCCR study, this clinical trial was limited to T3 to T4 or node-positive tumors. Chemoradiation contributed 18% actuarial improvement in 5-year LRC and an increase in colostomy-free survival (CFS) (36%).

In summary, the phase III UKCCCR and EORTC studies established combined chemoradiation as superior to radiation alone for LRC and CFS. Unfortunately neither study was able to provide a difference in OS.

THE ROLE OF MITOMYCIN C

Clinical investigators proceeded to ascertain the true benefit of mitomycin C in combination with 5-FU. A prospective nonrandomized study of 110 patients concluded that mitomycin C improved the local control rate from 58 to 87% (p = .005) and improved 4-year actuarial cause-specific survival (80% versus 64%, p = .02) (64). Hematologic toxicity was the primary adverse effect.

The RTOG initiated a phase III Intergroup study (RTOG 87-04) in 310 patients (65) (Table 22-3). The primary objective was to determine the incidence of negative tissue biopsy, LCR, DFS, OS, and toxicity. Between 1988 and 1991, patients were stratified before randomization by nodal status, histology, and tumor size. They were then randomized to radiotherapy (45 Gy) and continuous infusion 5-FU (1000 mg/m^2 on days 1-5 and 28-33) or the same regimen of radiotherapy and continuous infusion of 5-FU with the addition of mitomycin C (10 mg/m^2 on days 1 and 28). If the patient had node-positive disease, a boost of 5.4 Gy was

TABLE 22-3	**RTOG STUDY OF 5-FU/RADIATION VERSUS 5-FU/MITOMYCIN C/RADIATION**		
	5-FU/Radiation (N = 145)	*5-FU/Mitomycin C/Radiation* (N = 146)	*p Value*
Complete response	115 (86)	119 (92)	*p* = .135
Tumor size >5 cm	42 (81)	42 (86)	*p* = .02
Tumor size <5 cm	73 (90)	77 (96)	*p* = .002
Time to colostomy (4 years)	32 (22)	13 (9)	*p* = .002
Colostomy-free survival	89 (61)	109 (75)	*p* = .014
Four-year DFS	71 (51)	98 (73)	*p* = .0003
Four-year OS	42 (29)	32 (22)	*p* = 31

DFS, disease-free survival; OS, overall response.
Data from Flam M, John M, Pajak TF, et al. Role of mitomycin in combination with fluorouracil and radiotherapy, and of salvage chemoradiation in the definitive nonsurgical treatment of epidermoid carcinoma of the anal canal: Results of a phase III randomized intergroup study. J Clin Oncol 1996;14:2527-2539.

provided. A full-thickness biopsy was obtained 4 to 6 weeks after the treatment was completed for evaluation of response. If the biopsy was positive, patients underwent salvage chemoradiation therapy (9 Gy) with concomitant 5-FU (1000 mg/m^2 on days 1-5)/cisplatin (100 mg/m^2 on day 2). A biopsy was repeated after 6 weeks. If residual disease remained, patients were recommended to proceed with salvage surgery.

Ninety percent of patients enrolled were evaluable for response. The median follow-up was for 3.01 years. The single poor prognostic factor identified was tumor size ≥5 cm (*p* = .02). Furthermore, mitomycin C appeared to have the greatest impact on the colostomy rate reduction in T3 to T4 tumors (*p* = 0.014), but it provided no added benefit in T1 to T2 tumors (*p* = 0.14). Acute grade 4 toxicities were prominent in the 5-FU/mitomycin C arm versus the 5-FU—only arm (23 versus 7%), resulting in neutropenia, thrombocytopenia, and infection. Unfortunately, failure to reduce the dose in the mitomycin C arm resulted in two deaths. The use of cisplatin in salvage chemoradiation provided a prolonged benefit in 4 of 22 (18%) patients, who continue to remain disease-free at 4 years. The investigators concluded that mitomycin C is not recommended in patients who are potentially immunosuppressed.

■ THE INTRODUCTION OF CISPLATIN

Despite the evident benefits of mitomycin C in the treatment of anal cancer, potential treatment-related toxicities may include leukopenia, thrombocytopenia, and, rarely, hemolytic uremic syndrome (HUS) and leukemia. Although a review of prior 5-FU/mitomycin C clinical trials in SCC of the anal canal suggests the potential for superior results, these often come at the cost of treatment-related morbidity and mortality, with several instances of severe myelosuppression. Therefore other agents that may reduce treatment-related toxicities without compromising efficacy would be preferable.

The radiosensitization properties of cisplatin have long been recognized in the treatment of SCCs of the head and neck, lung, esophagus and in carcinoma of the anal canal. Table 22-4 demonstrates some of the phase II studies that have been completed.

Doci and colleagues completed a phase II study of 5-FU/cisplatin (CDDP) in 35 patients with locally advanced carcinoma of the anal canal (66). Thirty-three patients (94%) achieved a CR; the remaining two demonstrated a partial response (PR) and proceeded on to salvage surgery. After a median follow-up of 37 months, 94% were disease-free and 86% remained colostomy-free. The local recurrence rate was favorable at 6%.

The Eastern Cooperative Group (ECOG 4292) attempted to evaluate the 5-FU/cisplatinum combination further (Table 22-4) (67). Nineteen patients were accrued and received a total of 59.4 Gy in 33 fractions, with a 2-week break following 36 Gy of treatment. All treatment was completed by day 60. The overall response rate (ORR) was 95%, 13 patients (68%) were determined to have a CR, and 5 (26%) had a PR. One patient with stable disease was reevaluated after 8 weeks and was determined to have had a CR. Fifteen patients (79%) experienced ≥ grade 3 toxicities. Grade 4 toxicities included diarrhea and thrombocytopenia. One patient suffered from *Clostridium difficile* pseudomembranous colitis, resulting in her demise. LRC could not be achieved in approximately one-third of patients accrued. This treatment schedule with split-course radiation was identical to that reported in RTOG 92-08. The authors concluded that the delay in radiation treatment likely accounted for the inferior LRC rate and recommended examining this combination further.

TABLE 22-4	FU/CISPLATIN CHEMOTHERAPY COMBINATIONS
Authors	**Treatment Regimen**
Doci et al. (66), 1996	Continuous infusion
	5-FU (750 mg/m^2, days 1-4, 21-25) and cisplatin (100 mg/m^2, days 1 and 4)
Martenson et al. (67), 1996	Continuous 5-FU (1000 mg/m^2/day, days 1-4, 43-46) and cisplatin (75 mg/m^2, days 1 and 43)
Gerard et al. (69), 1998	<70 years old: continuous 5-FU (800 mg/m^2/day, days 1-4 and 43-46), cisplatin (25 mg/m^2, days 1-4)
	≥70 years old: or ECOG PS = 2 (1000 mg/m^2/day, days 1-4 and 43-46), cisplatin (25 mg/m^2, days 1-4)
Hung et al. (68), 2003	Continuous infusion 5-FU (250 mg/m^2/day, Mon-Fri) and continuous infusion cisplatin (4 mg/m^2/day, Mon-Fri) for the entire duration of radiation therapy
	NEOADJUVANT CHEMOTHERAPY
Peiffert et al. (70), 2001	Neoadjuvant: continuous 5-FU (800 mg/m^2/day, days 1-4) and cisplatin (80 mg/m^2, day 1) every 28 days
	During radiation therapy: continuous 5-FU (800 mg/m^2/day, days 1 and 29-33) and cisplatin (80 mg/m^2, days 1 and 29)
Meropol et al. (71), 1999	Neoadjuvant: continuous 5-FU (1000 mg/m^2/day, days 1-5) and cisplatin (100 mg/m^2, day 1) weeks 1 and 5.
	During radiation therapy: continuous 5-FU (1000 mg/m^2/day, days 1-4) and mitomycin C (10 mg/m^2, day 1) weeks 9 and 15.

A retrospective analysis in patients with TxNxM0 SCC of the anal canal was completed at MD Anderson in 92 patients (Tables 22-4 and 22-5) (68). Patients received continuous infusion of 5-FU and cisplatin for the duration of radiation therapy (55 Gy). The majority of patients were node-negative (71%). They were followed for a median of 44 months. LRC was adversely affected by tumor >T2. Nodal stage >N1 resulted in shortened DFS, OS, and increased likelihood of distant metastases; 25% of patients with N2 to N3 disease will develop distant metastases at 5 years. All patients with a local recurrence underwent salvage APR or diverting colostomies and developed for 15 of 16 patients within 16 months; 10 of 13 patients had isolated recurrences and remain disease-free after a median follow-up of 40 months. Grade 4 acute toxicities (diarrhea, dehydration, and skin ulceration) were infrequent (5%), and one patient died of renal failure due to chronic cystitis. This study is limited since it was completed retrospectively, but it suggests that the 5-FU/cisplatin combination has

added advantages and may be potentially less toxic than the traditional 5-FU/mitomycin C regimen. Subsequently, between 1982 and 1993, Gerard and colleagues accrued 95 locally advanced patients with SCC of the anal canal (69). All patients received EBRT; the majority (85%) received 30 Gy in 10 fractions, with the remaining patients receiving 39 Gy in 13 fractions. A large portion of these patients (63%) had tumors ≥4 cm and 10 had histologically confirmed inguinal lymph nodes. Seven of the 10 patients with positive inguinal lymph node involvement received neoadjuvant chemotherapy with 5-FU/cisplatin prior to chemoradiation. Inguinal node dissection was completed if necessary, followed by 45 Gy in 15 fractions to the involved area. Following an 8-week rest period, 85 patients received an iridium-192 interstitial brachytherapy implant. Concomitant chemotherapy was provided with 5-FU/cisplatin, with dosage based upon age or World Health Organization (WHO) performance status (Table 22-4). Eight weeks after irradiation, the patients were evaluated clinically for response.

LRC was possible in 80% of patients; 43% of patients were determined to have had a complete response. After a median of 1 year, 6 of 12 patients developed local recurrences and underwent salvage APR; 2 patients progressed distally. The ultimate rate of LRC following salvage treatment was 93%. The 5-year OS, DFS, and the CFS rates were 84%, 90%, and 71%, respectively. By multivariate analysis, the only poor prognostic factor was initial response to chemoradiation therapy. The acute toxicities encountered were minor (proctitis, perianal skin reaction, and pain) and

TABLE 22-5	FIVE-YEAR RESULTS FOLLOWING CONTINUOUS INFUSION 5-FU/CISPLATIN	
Overall survival		85%
Disease-free survival		77%
Colostomy-free survival		8%
Locoregional control		83%
Distant metastases		9%

Data from Hung A, Crane C, Delclos M, et al. Cisplatin-based combined modality therapy for anal carcinoma: a wider therapeutic index. Cancer 2003;97:1195-1202.

reversible after 3 to 4 weeks if appropriately treated. Unfortunately, one elderly patient died after receiving an inappropriate dose of 5-FU. After a median of 8 months, residual treatment-related toxicities were noted in 14 patients, resulting in painful necrosis of the anus. Consequently, 5 patients received a permanent colostomy for palliation of symptoms. Nevertheless, the anal sphincter was preserved in 82% of patients. A fault of this study was the prolonged accrual period and the differences in radiation technique: Papillon (85%) versus three-field (15%).

NEOADJUVANT (INDUCTION) CHEMOTHERAPY

In place of standard chemoradiation therapy, could another treatment strategy provide an improvement in overall survival and decrease the risk of distant disease development? Rather than simply substituting cisplatin for mitomycin C, French investigators proceeded to investigate the role of neoadjuvant chemotherapy in patients with T ≥ 4 cm and/or positive lymph nodes (Table 22-4) (70). Over a 3-year period, 80 patients were accrued. Two cycles of 5-FU/cisplatin with an additional two cycles during radiation therapy (45 Gy in 25 fractions) were followed by a radiation boost of 15 Gy for involved inguinal lymph nodes. Response rates (RR) following neoadjuvant chemotherapy appeared promising (CR, 10%; PR, 51%). The RR was enhanced further following chemoradiation therapy (CR, 67%; PR, 28%), with an ultimate complete response rate of 93% after salvage surgery. Chemotherapy dose reductions were required in 21% of patients who completed all four cycles of proposed chemotherapy. Overall, the treatment was tolerated very well except for one patient who died unexpectedly of a pulmonary embolism; no other deaths occurred. After a median follow-up of 29 months, 21 patients relapsed; 10 patients failed locally. At 3 years the OS, DFS, and CFS were 86%, 73%, and 67%, respectively for these poor-prognosis patients.

Investigators of the Cancer and Leukemia Group B (CALGB) proceeded slightly differently (71). Forty-five patients with T3 to T4 or node-positive disease received two cycles of neoadjuvant 5-FU/cisplatin followed by 5-FU/mitomycin C during chemoradiation (Table 22-4). A third cycle of 5-FU/cisplatin with radiation boost was given to patients with persistent primary site disease or bulky N2 or N3 disease at presentation. Split-dose radiation therapy occurred after 30.6 Gy with a 19-day break, for a total of 45 Gy. An early response to neoadjuvant chemotherapy was noted: 8 CRs

(18%), 21 PRs (47%), and 13 SDs (29%). One patient succumbed to pneumonia while during treatment and another progressed. At the conclusion of chemoradiation, the response rate remained favorable: 37 CRs (82%), 4 PRs (9%), and 2 SDs (4%). One patient had progression of disease. Grade 3 to 4 treatment-related toxicities included neutropenia (60%), thrombocytopenia (41%), stomatitis (38%), and infection (18%). After a follow-up of 4 years, DFS was 61%, CFS 50%, and 68% of patients were still alive. The results of this prospective phase II trial demonstrated that this combined-modality approach was tolerable, active, and may result in long-term disease control in poor-risk patients comparable to that of radiotherapy without induction therapy.

Based on similar treatment principles, the phase III Intergroup/ACCORD 03 Trial created a 2 × 2 factorial design to compare standard-dose (45 Gy/25 fractions + boost of 15 Gy) versus high-dose radiation therapy (boost of 20-25 Gy) and the potential benefits of induction chemotherapy with 5-FU (800 mg/m^2 days 1-4)/cisplatin (80 mg/m^2, day 1) × 2 cycles in locally advanced SCCA of the anal canal (72). Patients were required to have T2 > 4 cm or node-positive disease. The primary objective was to detect an increase from 70 to 85% of CFS at 3 years. Three hundred and six patients were allocated to one of four treatment arms: (1) induction with standard-dose radiation therapy, (2) induction with high-dose radiation therapy, (3) control arm of 5-FU/cisplatin + standard boost, and (4) control arm of 5-FU/cisplatin + high-dose boost. The results were compared in terms of CFS. The preliminary results with a median follow-up of 43 months did not show benefit with intensification of radiation therapy or with induction chemotherapy. After a median follow-up of 43 months, no difference in CFS was noted for the induction arm (NS) or the higher dose radiation therapy arm ($p = .67$) versus the control arm. Overall, no statistical differences were noted across all arms for local control, CFS, event-free survival, or overall survival. Analysis of these results are ongoing, with final results pending publication. A prospective quality of life (QOL) assessment subsequently has been reported on a subgroup of these patients before and after conservative treatment demonstrating that induction chemotherapy and/or high-dose radiotherapy did not provide a negative impact on QOL (73).

RTOG 98-11

The RTOG was a large phase III multiinstitutional randomized trial (98-11) for locally advanced squamous cell carcinoma of the anal canal (50). On the premise of the promising results from the CALGB study, this non-blinded study randomized 682 patients with category T2 to T4 tumors and any nodal status to receive 5-FU/mitomycin C and concurrent radiation (control arm) or induction 5-FU/cisplatin followed by concurrent 5-FU/cisplatin and radiation. Patients were enrolled over a 7-year period; HIV-positive patients were excluded. All patients received 45-50 Gy of radiation doses, with an additional 10-14 Gy in 2 Gy fractions given to patients with residual evidence of disease, tumors >5 cm or tumor invasion of adjacent organs. Patients were assessed for response at 8 weeks after the completion of therapy. At the conclusion of a median follow-up of 2.51 years, there was no statistically significant difference in OS between the two treatment arms, with the 3-year- and 5-year OS of 84% and 75% for the control group, versus 76% and 71% for the induction plus cisplatin group ($p = .10$), respectively. The estimated 3-year- and 5-year DFS also was comparable at 67% and 60% for the control group, versus 61% and 54% for the induction and cisplatin group, respectively ($p = .17$). While the rate of acute non-hematologic grade 3 or 4 toxicity was 74% in both therapeutic arms, there was a significantly higher rate of acute grade 3 or 4 hematologic toxicity in the control group at 61 versus 42% ($p < 0.001$). The investigational induction cisplatin arm demonstrated an increased 5-year rate of colostomy at 19 versus 10% for the control ($p = 0.02$). This study has since been criticized for the inequality of the two treatment schedules, making a direct comparison of mitomycin C and cisplatin difficult due to the confounding factor of induction chemotherapy in the investigational arm (74). As a result of this limitation in trial design, the question whether cisplatin is a viable alternative to mitomycin C cannot be answered (75).

MITOMYCIN VERSUS CISPLATIN AND THE ROLE OF ADJUVANT THERAPY

The UK ACT II trial is the largest phase III trial conducted in SCCA of the anal cancer and is the first direct analysis of 5-FU/mitomycin C versus 5-FU/cisplatin with concurrent radiation therapy. ACT II also evaluated whether maintenance (adjuvant) chemotherapy following completion of chemoradiotherapy reduces recurrence-free survival (RFS) (76). Using a 2×2 factorial design, 940 patients with T1 to T4 node negative and positive disease were randomly assigned between 5-FU (1000 mg/m^2 days 1-4, 29-32)/mitomycin C (12 mg/m^2 day 1) or 5-FU(1000 mg/m^2 days 1-4, 29-32)/cisplatin (60 mg/m^2, days 1 and 29) administered

concurrently with continuous radiotherapy of 50.4 Gy. The second randomization was two courses of 5-FU/cisplatin (same schedule) consolidation chemotherapy or no further treatment. There were greater incidences of acute grade 3/4 hematologic toxicity on the MMC arm (24.7% versus 13.4%, $p < 0.001$), but no statistical differences in grade 3/4 non-hematologic toxicities ($p = .17$). Preliminary results after a median follow-up of 3 years demonstrate no statistically significant differences for the endpoint of 6-month CR rate for concurrent chemoradiation with 5-FU/MMC versus 5-FU/cisplatin (94.5 versus 95.4%) no difference in RFS, and no difference in colostomy rates (13.7 versus 11.7%), respectively. The role of maintenance (adjuvant) 5-FU/cisplatin chemotherapy has no added benefit for RFS or OS. To date, final results have not been published.

Although the investigators failed to fulfill the primary endpoint of superiority for the cisplatin-based regimen, the final results indicate that 5-FU/cisplatin is non-inferior to 5-FU/MMC in achieving a CR, but is associated with unique treatment-related toxicities that are different from MMC. At MD Anderson Cancer Center, 5-FU/cisplatin remains our favored regimen due to its efficacy, decreased myelosuppression, and minimal toxicities allowing optimal treatment of HIV-positive and elderly patients.

EORTC-22011: IS 5-FU REQUIRED AS THE FOUNDATION OF THERAPY?

European investigators have evaluated the role of a non—5-FU-based regimen. Rather than comparing mitomycin C to cisplatin, they have analyzed the additive effects of a cisplatin/MMC combination in a randomized phase II trial (77). In this trial, only patients with T2N0 equal to or greater than 4 cm in largest dimension were included, with 88 patients enrolled. Patients were randomized to one of two arms: the first was radiation therapy (weeks 1-4, 7-8, and part of week 9), continuous infusion 5-FU (days 1-26 and 43-59) and mitomycin C (days 1 and 43). The second arm was comprised of radiation therapy (weeks 1-4 and 7-8 as well as part of week 9), cisplatin (days 1, 8, 15, 22, 43, 50, and 57) and mitomycin C (days 1 and 43). The doses are as follows: MMC 10 mg/m^2 day 1 of each sequence; 5-FU 200 mg/m^2/daily; cisplatin 25mg/m^2 weekly. The primary endpoint assessment occurred at week 16. The investigators reported an impressive ORR of 79.5% for the control arm versus 91.9% for the investigational arm. However, two patients discontinued therapy in the control arm versus 11 patients (30%) in the investigational arm. The primary treatment-related toxicity was hematological; nine grade 3 hematologic toxicities occurred in the investigational arm versus none in the control arm. While the median event-free, overall and progression-free survivals (PFS) have not yet been reached, the 1-year PFS was 94.2% for cisplatin/mitomycin C and 76.3% for 5-FU/mitomycin C. A QOL analysis will be reported.

OTHER NOVEL APPROACHES

A single institution phase II study completed at MD Anderson evaluated capecitabine (825 mg/m^2 bid, M-F) and (oxaliplatin 60 mg/m^2, weekly) with concurrent radiation therapy with the option of IMRT (78). Twenty patients were enrolled; all patients were evaluable for toxicity and 19 were evaluable for response. Increased grade 3 diarrhea was noted with the weekly oxaliplatin regimen and the regimen was since modified to omit chemotherapy for weeks 3 and 6. All 19 patients had a complete response at the primary site. The final results are to be reported shortly.

■ RADIATION TECHNIQUE

Currently, the most commonly used approach in the combined-modality treatment of carcinoma of the anal canal is continuous-course radiation (45 Gy in 1.8-Gy fractions using opposed anterior and posterior treatment fields with a boost to the primary tumor to 5.4 Gy) plus two cycles of concurrent continuous infusion 5-FU plus mitomycin C. This regimen is considered by most to be the standard of care. This technique was adopted from the vulvar cancer technique. However, the genitalia is not part of the pattern of failure in anal cancer and this technique unfortunately results in severe acute and late morbidity related to the unnecessary high dose to the genitalia. The advantage of the technique in clinical trials is its simplicity. The significant disadvantage is that it includes full dose to the genitalia and bowel resulting in severe acute skin toxicity leading to treatment breaks that compromise tumor control and universal sexual dysfunction in females and contributes to impotence in males.

Between 1988 and 2004, at the University of Texas, MD Anderson Cancer Center (MDACC), all patients were treated with a 3D conformal technique designed to spare the genitalia and small bowel—areas that are not at risk for tumor recurrence (Fig. 22-10). Using this technique, patients are positioned supine in the frog leg position with upper and lower immobilization. A composite 3D CT plan is then generated without need for

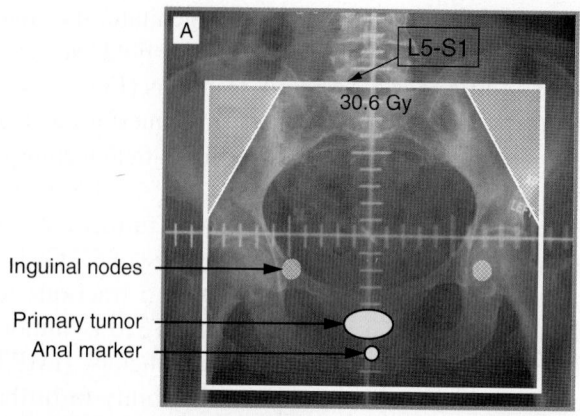

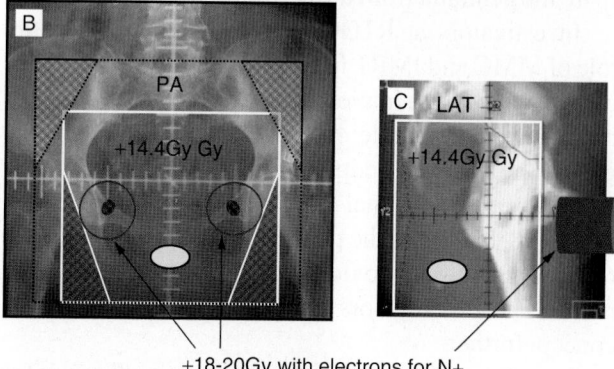

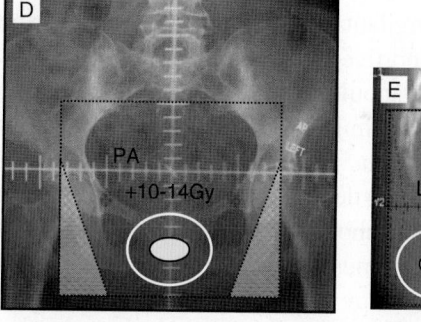
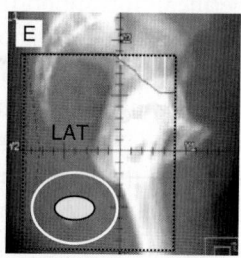

FIGURE 22-10. The MD Anderson Cancer Center 3D anal cancer technique was designed to spare unnecessary radiation dose to the genitalia and bowel. The initial 30.6 Gy is administered via anteroposterior-posteroanterior portals (**A**). An additional 14.4 Gy is given to the pelvis, for a total dose of 45 Gy, in a posterior three-field approach, using posteroanterior and two lateral fields. Clinically involved inguinal nodes simultaneously receive a boost of 18-20 Gy with electrons (**B** and **C**). Finally, a localized boost field is given an additional 10-14 Gy, for a total dose of 55-59 Gy depending on the T stage, also using a posterior three-field approach (**D** and **E**). *(This article was published in Cox JD, Ang KK. Radiation Oncology: Rationale, Technique, Results. 9th ed. Copyright Elsevier 2009.)*

resimulation. Initially opposed anterior and posterior fields are used encompassing the primary tumor, pararectal, inguinal, external, internal, and common iliac lymph nodes—for a total dose of 30.6 Gy in 17 fractions (Fig. 22-10A). That is followed by a reduction of the superior border and a switch to a posterior three-field technique that spares the genitalia and small bowel. Posterior, right, and left lateral fields are used for an additional 14.4 Gy in 8 fractions (Fig. 22-10*B* and *C*). A boost of 18-20 Gy using anterior electron fields is started with the posterior three-field technique to grossly involved inguinal nodes Fig. 22-10*C*). Following that, the three-field technique is further reduced to treat gross disease only for a final boost of 5.4 Gy in 3 fractions for Tx/T1 tumors, 10 Gy in 5 fractions for T2 tumors, and 14 Gy in 7 fractions for T3 to T4 tumors. Since 2004, intensity-modulated radiotherapy (IMRT) has been used exclusively due to its ability to further spare the genitalia from the high-dose region.

Investigators at RTOG have recently reported the role of MMC and IMRT in a phase II trial (RTOG 0529) of anal carcinoma patients with ≥T2. A total of 52 patients were evaluable; HIV-positive patients were eligible. The primary endpoint was a 15% reduction in grade-2 gastrointestinal (GI) toxicities compared to RTOG 98-11. While the primary endpoint was not met, reduced grade-3 GI toxicities and skin toxicities were noted. The investigators are planning to explore this concept further.

It would not be unusual during radiation therapy for patients to develop grade 2-3 radiation dermatitis. Patients require vigilant evaluations of the perianal and perineal for supportive skin care recommendations. Strict instructions should be provided by the radiation oncology team regarding emollients for the day versus the evening since some may potentially serve as a barrier. Grade 4 radiation dermatitis will warrant a delay in radiation therapy but should only be for a brief period. If any treatment delays must occur, it is best to temporarily defer the chemotherapy rather than the radiation since treatment delays may compromise patient outcome.

MANAGEMENT OF INGUINAL LYMPHADENOPATHY

Advanced lymphadenopathy at presentation has been correlated with an increased risk of distant recurrence. The American Joint Committee on Cancer (AJCC) staging system (see Fig. 22-8) classifies unilateral inguinal lymphadenopathy as N2 and bilateral inguinal adenopathy or a combination of unilateral adenopathy and mesorectal or iliac adenopathy, or bilateral iliac adenopathy as N3. Advanced lymphadenopathy is a poor prognostic indicator (79,80,50). Some investigators have taken novel approaches to the diagnosis and staging of these high-risk patients, such as incorporating sentinel lymph node biopsy (81,82), but the only value of this approach is accurate pathologic staging of

subcentimeter nodes. Lymphadenopathy <2 cm is readily controlled with standard chemoradiation.

Cummings had suggested that the inguinal region should be prophylactically treated with radiation (45-50 Gy) regardless of clinical indication (52). However, in 1984, Cummings concluded that radiation or combined chemoradiation provided LRC in 87% of patients with regional lymph node involvement without the necessity of an inguinal node dissection (83).

French investigators have conducted a focal retrospective analysis regarding the clinical significance of inguinal lymph nodes metastases in 270 patients with SCC of the anal canal (84). The patients had been treated between the years 1980 and 1996 with radiation. Concomitant chemoradiation, usually with a regimen of 5-FU/cisplatin, was provided in 159 patients. Patients with inguinal nodes suspected to be clinically involved underwent inguinal lymph node dissection and adjuvant radiation therapy to inguinal region (50 Gy/5 weeks). Elective inguinal nodal irradiation was not used for patients with clinically negative nodes. Inguinal nodes were pathologically confirmed to be positive at presentation in 10% of patients overall (N = 270) and in 16% of T3/T4 lesions (N = 27). Inguinal nodal recurrence developed in 19 of the N0 patients (7.8%), and the 5-year OS for these patients was 41.4% demonstrating the relatively low risk of nodal recurrence in patient with initially clinically uninvolved nodes that are not treated and the value of salvage therapy in these patients. Another interesting finding from this series was that lymphadenopathy occurred in the ipsilateral inguinal region for single lateral located lesions (36 of 36 cases).

The opposed anterior and posterior radiation technique to 45 Gy that has been used in clinical trials encompasses the pararectal, inguinal, external, internal, and common iliac lymph nodes. A boost dose of 5.4 Gy is typically given to grossly involved lymph nodes. Using the the MD Anderson 3D technique, a total dose of 55 Gy is used for nodes that are greater than 1 cm but less than 5 cm and 59 Gy for nodes greater than 5 cm. Similar total doses are used when intensity-modulated radiation therapy (IMRT) is used.

■ WHAT IS THE CORRECT DOSE OF RADIATION THERAPY?

Review of the literature has shown the gradual increase in radiation from 30 Gy to 59.4 Gy in recent studies. Prior studies have indicated that there is a dose-response relationship between treatment and outcome. An analysis completed at MDACC from 1979 to 1987 revealed a dramatic difference in LRC for those patients who received 45 to 49 Gy (50%) versus ≥55 Gy (90%) (85). Investigators at Massachusetts General Hospital and Boston University Medical Center retrospectively analyzed 50 patients with all T and N stage M0 disease (86). After a median of 43 months, patients who had received a radiation dose of ≥54 Gy fared better than those who had received <54 Gy; the resultant impact on survival ($p = .02$), DFS ($p = .09$), and local control ($p = .04$) was significant.

At MDACC, our initial experience of 55 Gy for all patients indicated that the local failure rate was 25 to 30% in patients with T3-4 tumors (68). In 1999 based on this data, the dose was increased to 59 Gy for T3-4 tumors. Definitive evidence that the higher dose improves local tumor control will eventually be determined. It should be noted that radiation dosages >60 Gy result in an unacceptably high risk of anal canal and urethral stricture, ulceration, and fistula formation.

■ EVALUATION OF RESPONSE

Earlier studies typically evaluated a patient's response with tissue biopsy as early as 4 weeks following completion of chemoradiation therapy. However, the effects of radiation vary per individual and may be appreciated as far as 8 to 12 weeks following the conclusion of radiation therapy. When Deniaud-Alexandre and colleagues evaluated the single modality of radiation therapy, they noted that at 4 weeks following radiation therapy, only 36 of 299 patients (12%) had a clinical complete response (57). However, a reevaluation at 8 weeks revealed that 244 of 305 patients (80%) were considered to have a complete clinical response. Clonogenically inactive cells may be present as long as 3 months treatment and can result in a false-positive biopsy. A drawback to a tissue biopsy is the potential for ulceration and fistula formation in the irradiated tissue occasionally resulting in an APR for pallation of symptoms. Of particular concern are anterior lesions in female patients that are at risk for fistulas of the rectovaginal

Commentary: Improved Radiation Techniques Spare Acute Skin Reactions and Preserve Sexual Functioning

The treatment of anal cancer is on one hand a story of a pioneering organ preservation strategy that serves as a model for other disease sites and on the other hand a sad commentary about the failure of oncology leadership to identify, understand, and address the ruinous effect that a treatment can have one of the most important aspects of a patient's quality of life: sexual function. The fact that the *de facto* standard radiation treatment technique for anal cancer (identical to the one used for vulvar cancer) involves the delivery of as much radiation dose to the genitalia as the primary tumor is unconscionable. The vagina, urethra and small bowel are not part of the pattern of tumor recurrence. Genital moist desquamation, diarrhea, and urethritis become intolerable during the fifth week of treatment in most patients treated with the vulvar technique. The long-term function of the vagina and vulva are particularly vulnerable to the effects of radiation. Vaginal dryness, fibrosis, and stenosis result in dysparunia and permanently end the sex life of the majority of the women treated this way. Yet, this vulvar technique has been the recommended technique for all phase III trials in the past.

Within this chapter we describe and illustrate an alternative 3D technique that we have used for decades. The use of this technique allows partial sparing of the vulva and total sparing of the penis and scrotum from the high radiation dose, which makes chemoradiation much better tolerated than the vulvar technique. We have since moved forward to an even better

way to spare the genitalia: intensity-modulated radiation therapy (IMRT). Using IMRT with a radioopaque vaginal dilator in place, we are able to safely deliver high doses to the gross disease while sparing the genitalia, urethra, and bowel like never before. (For guidelines: http://rtog.org/pdf_file2.html?pdf_document=AnorectalContouringGuidelines.pdf) The typical patient only experiences perianal moist desquamation during treatment and treatment breaks and hospitalizations are a thing of the past. This advance has trivialized the argument about whether to use cisplatin instead of mytomycin to reduce toxicity. The improved avoidance of the genital skin and small bowel makes it a mute point. All patients should be treated this way, but there is a learning curve that most practitioners will never climb.

Additional advances that would address the limitations of therapy include the further study of adjuvant chemotherapy in patients at high risk for distant recurrence (N1 >3cm, N2 and N3 disease) and of improved local treatment effect (radiosensitization) in patients at high risk for local recurrence (T3 and T4 patients). It is reasonable to consider 4 months of adjuvant chemotherapy in patients with advanced nodal presentations and the use of 59 Gy for T3 and T4 tumors because we know both are tolerable and that these approaches address the risk and pattern of recurrence.

Christopher H. Crane

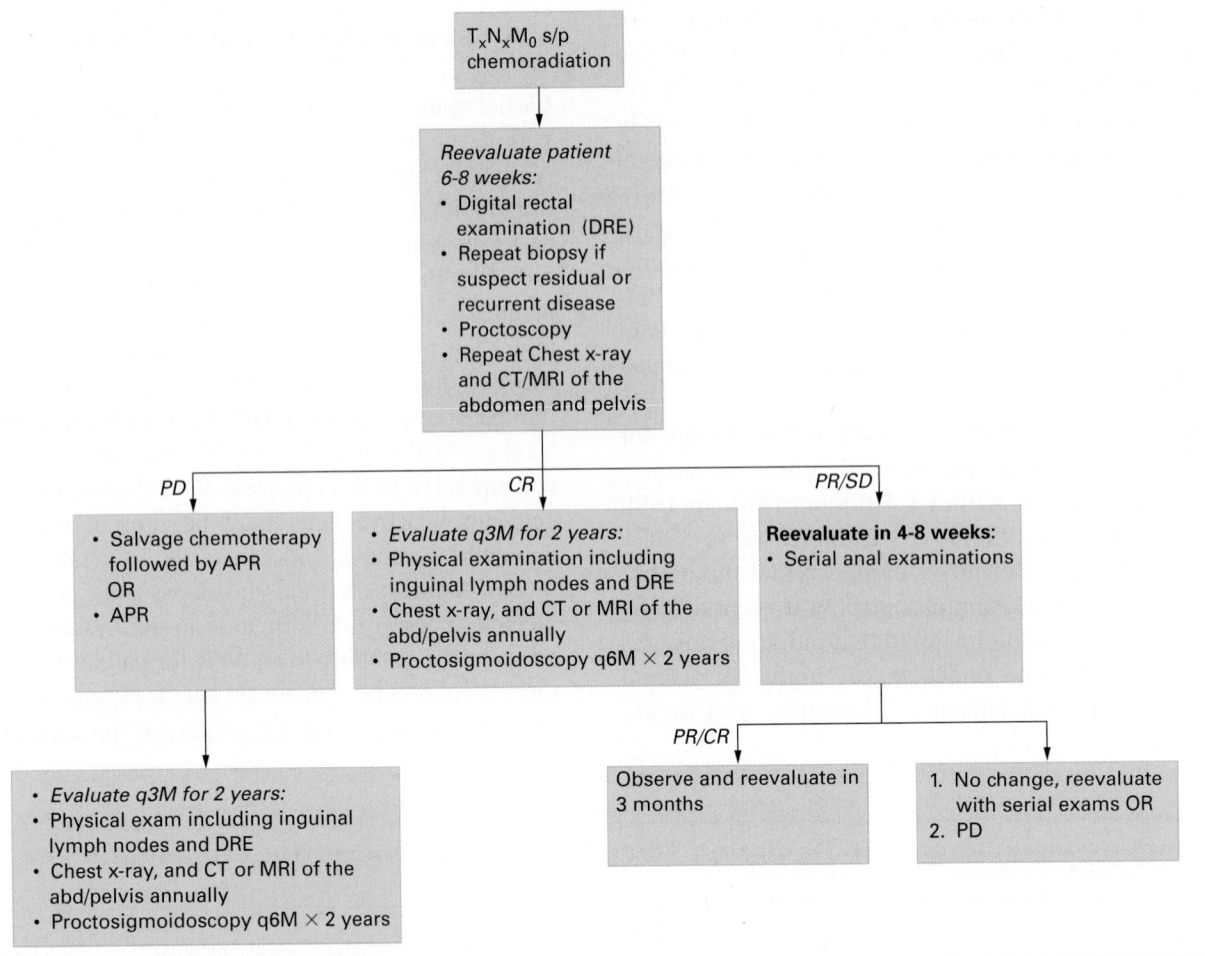

FIGURE 22-11.   Postchemoradiation evaluation and surveillance.

septum. Currently, tissue biopsies are no longer recommended to confirm complete response to therapy. Response is largely based on clinical examination. A tissue biopsy should only be pursued if there is clinical evidence of progression or significant residual disease despite an adequate surveillance period. Since anal cancer tends to remain locoregionally confined, the opportunity will not typically be missed for salvage APR with curative intent even if a clinically concerning area is followed closely without biopsy. Recent treatment guidelines suggest that a tumor biopsy be performed only if recurrent or persistent disease is suspected after serial DRE (Fig. 22-11) (87).

(88). The use of chemoradiation resulted in increased treatment-related morbidity; late complications occurred in 49% of patients. The authors could not determine added benefit in LRC with the addition of chemotherapy and recommended restricting elderly patients to radiation only. However, these recommendations should be viewed with caution. As in the treatment of other malignancies, physiologic age rather than actual age should be the determining factor. Age has not been clearly defined as a negative prognostic indicator in the treatment of SCCA of the anal canal. Furthermore, given the latency of HPV, the median age of the patient population may be rising.

■ SHOULD AGE BE A LIMITING FACTOR?

Chauveinc and colleagues noted that patient age was a determining factor in pursuing radiation as a single modality versus combined chemoradiation therapy

■ ANAL CANCER AND HIV

SCC of the anal canal is one of several malignancies linked with HIV. Unlike cervical carcinoma, SCC of the anal canal is not considered an AIDS-defining malignancy. A diagnosis of HIV and chronic immunosuppression is a peril that physicians will face in treating a patient. Hesitancy to consider full-dose chemotherapy or radiation therapy in these patients is understandable. However, with the advances and advent of highly active antiretroviral therapy (HAART), the CD4 cell count may not be affected in even the most advanced immunosuppressive states (89). An outcome analysis of 73 patients with SCC of the anal canal has been completed, 23 of whom were HIV-positive, with a mean CD4 cell count of 222/µL (90). The 1- and 5-year mortality rates were 40% and 80%, respectively. Patients on HAART were less likely to develop treatment complications or to require treatment breaks. The mean presenting CD4 cell count for those patients who died was 133/µL versus 261/µL for those who remained alive ($p = 0.03$). However, investigators at University of California San Francisco (UCSF) have completed a retrospective unpublished analysis in a small group of patients on HAART (91). Of their 11 patients, 8 (72%) developed $\geq$ grade-3 toxicities, resulting in moist desquamation and neutropenia. The high rate of acute and chronic toxicities witnessed suggest that HAART cannot prevent the unavoidable challenges in the treatment of these patients.

Overall, acute treatment toxicities appear to be greater in HIV-positive patients who undergo chemoradiation therapy with curative intent ($p < 0.01$) (92). Should a surgical approach be preferred, wound healing in HIV-positive patients may be delayed and may be dependent on the CD4 count (93-94). Vatra and colleagues completed a retrospective analysis in 20 HIV-positive patients versus 24 HIV-negative patients noting an increased likelihood of lymph node metastases (60% versus 17%, respectively) (95). The overall survival of the HIV-positive patients was determined to be significantly less (18 versus 28 months, $p < 0.01$). However, patients who were HIV-positive were less likely to have received combined-modality therapy (54 versus 25%), possibly accounting for the inferior results. More recently, studies specifically evaluating HIV-associated squamous cell carcinoma of the anus in the era of HAART demonstrate similar survival between HIV-positive and HIV-negative individuals (96-99).

Annual Pap smear screening in women has become commonplace in the arsenal against cervical cancer in diagnosing HPV and carcinoma in situ (CIS). Modifications of the screening procedures used for cervical cancer have been applied in screening efforts for AIN, a premalignant condition to anal carcinoma. One means to aid in the earlier diagnosis of HIV-positive patients

may be incorporating anal cytology screening as a preventive measure in these high-risk patients. Screening with anal cytology has been proven to be cost-effective among HIV-positive men and in men who engage in homosexual activity regardless of their CD4 cell count (100). Screening was also cost-effective in HIV-negative men (101). Barriers to the implementation of its use may be largely due to the lack of education of physicians, lack of large randomized prospective clinical studies, and concerns regarding reimbursement for services rendered. High-resolution anoscopy, a colposcopic evaluation of the anus, may further be useful in the diagnosis of AIN.

Review of the few clinical studies available suggests that in patients with a CD4 cell count >200/µmL who do not have signs or symptoms of other HIV-related diseases combined modality therapy is appropriate. However, patients must be followed closely. A recent retrospective analysis performed on 21 HIV-positive patients who were receiving HAART were treated with concurrent chemoradiotherapy with 5-FU and mitomycin C for invasive anal carcinoma between 1997 and 2008 suggests that HIV-related anal cancer can be treated with standard CRT without dose reductions (102). For these patients, 38% experienced acute grade-3 toxicity though there was only one death due to treatment-related toxicity. A CR was achieved in 81% and the 5-year local control, cancer-specific, and overall survival rate was 59%, 75%, and 67%, respectively. Though the median CD4 count significantly decreased during the course of therapy from 374.5 cells/µ pretreatment to 125 cells/µ 3 to 7 weeks after chemoradiation therapy completion ($p < .001$), for those patients with a CD4 cell count <200/µL or who have signs or symptoms of other HIV-related diseases, attenuated doses of radiation and/or chemotherapy are recommended at the start of treatment with close observation.

RECURRENT DISEASE

SALVAGE OF RECURRENT DISEASE

APR is the only effective treatment option for localized recurrent or residual primary disease following chemoradiation for SCC of the anal canal. Fifty to 70% of patients are cured who undergo APR for recurrence at the primary site (103,104). There is no role for definitive re-irradiation for an in-field recurrence, but neoadjuvant chemoradiation (39 Gy in 26 fx twice daily with chemotherapy) may be used in cases where there are concerns about the radial margin.

The management of nodal recurrences should be individualized based on the extent of disease, prior radiation delivered to the area of recurrence, and performance status of the patient. In cases where patients have been referred to MDACC with nodal recurrence outside of or at the margin of a prior radiation field, salvage chemoradiation has been effective provided a full dose of re-irradiation is possible. For in-field nodal recurrences, we typically use preoperative chemoradiation to 39 Gy in 26 fractions bid followed by surgical resection.

Since the risk of distant disease recurrence is significant in patients with recurrent disease, adjuvant systemic chemotherapy may be considered, particularly for patients with nodal recurrences. However, the choice of adjuvant chemotherapy would be at the discretion of the treating physician due to the lack of published data using such an approach.

■ ADENOCARCINOMA OF THE ANAL CANAL

Anal adenocarcinoma has been reported to represent 16.5% of all anal cancers (39). However, most of the reports overestimate the incidence of adenocarcinoma of the anal canal because they do not exclude contamination by the more common distal rectal cancer. The true incidence is likely less than 10%. Its etiology remains unclear but, like its squamous cell counterpart, it has been linked in the past to chronic inflammatory conditions and HPV (46,103). The most appropriate management remains to be defined, with no large prospective studies completed to date. The most striking difference between adenocarcinoma and SCC of the anal canal is the high distant metastasis rate, which tends to undermine the impact of local tumor control.

The largest study is a retrospective European analysis of 82 patients. Patients were separated into three treatment groups: (1) surgery plus radiation; (2) chemoradiotherapy; or (3) APR (46). The 10-year DFS was 20% and did not improve between approaches. The authors concluded from their analysis that chemoradiation with APR for salvage was their preferred approach (Table 22-6).

At MD Anderson Cancer Center, we initially reported a high distant failure rate and an exceedingly high local recurrence rate of 54% among 16 patients treated between the period of 1976 to 1998 (105). The 5-year actuarial disease-free survival and overall survival rates were 19% and 64%, respectively. An updated cohort was recently published of 34 patients treated during the period of 1983 to 2004 (106). Twenty-eight

TABLE 22-6	RETROSPECTIVE COMPARISON OF TREATMENT MODALITIES IN ANAL ADENOCARCINOMAS (N = 82)			
	N	5-Year LCR	5-Year OS	5-Year DFS
Radiation/surgery	45	37% (NS)	29% (p = .027)	25% (p = .038)
Chemoradiation	31	36%	58%	54%
APR	6	20%	21%	22%

APR, abdominoperineal resection; DFS, disease-free survival; LCR, locoregional recurrence; OS, overall survival.
Data from Belkacemi Y, Berger C, Poortmans P, et al. Management of primary anal canal adenocarcinoma: A large retrospective study from the Rare Cancer Network. Int J Radiat Oncol Biol Phys 2003;56:1274-1283.

patients were considered evaluable. After a median follow-up of 37 months, 13 patients (46%) were treated with local excision followed by radiotherapy or chemoradiotherapy and 15 patients (54%) underwent radical surgery and preoperative or postoperative chemoradiotherapy. The median DFS was 13 months after local excision and 32 months after radical surgery (p = .055). The 5-year OS was 43% for patients treated with local excision and 63% for patients treated with radical surgery (p = .3). Tumor grade (p = .04) and recurrence (p = .046) was predictive for OS. Multivariate analysis demonstrated that the type of surgical treatment was an important predictor of OS (p = .045) and DFS (p = .004). These two studies indicate the benefit of neoadjuvant chemoradiation followed by APR with the consideration of adjuvant chemotherapy analogous to the treatment of rectal cancer.

■ METASTATIC ANAL CARCINOMA

Though the majority of patients with squamous cell carcinoma of the anal canal will be cured with chemoradiation, a minority of patients will develop distant metastatic disease. Overall, 5% of patients initially present with extrapelvic metastases, 10 to 20% of patients treated with curative intent will develop metastatic disease. Due to the rarity of this disease, a universally accepted treatment paradigm has not been established, with choice and duration of therapy largely based on individual case studies and small case series (107). It is reasonable to consider treatment advances for other more common squamous cell carcinomas (head and neck, lung cancer, etc) in the treatment of this rare malignancy. 5-FU- and platinum-based chemotherapy appears to be the most commonly utilized systemic chemotherapy in the metastatic disease setting (107).

Our retrospective analysis of experience at MD Anderson has demonstrated the majority of patients with metastatic anal carcinoma receive a fluorouracil- and cisplatin-based regimen as first-line therapy. Thirty patients were identified to be treatment-naïve from the period of 2000 to 2009 (107). Patients received a median of 3 lines of cytotoxic chemotherapy. The median PFS was 7.4M and the overall survival was 38M. Further data are pending at this time. Thus, systemic treatment should be considered in any patient demonstrating a good performance status, with duration of therapy continued indefinitely for maximal outcome if tolerated well. Consideration of surgical resection with curative intent should be encouraged for patients if surgically resectable or borderline resectable. As a need for novel treatment approaches exists for this rare malignancy, advances made in more common squamous cell carcinomas (lung cancer, head and neck, cervial cancer, etc) may form the basis of establishing a new therapeutic paradigm in anal cancer.

■ SURVEILLANCE

When patients are treated with chemoradiation therapy with curative intent, patients should be evaluated every 6 to 8 weeks until a maximal clinical response is achieved. Biopsy should not be performed before 12 weeks following chemoradiation therapy unless there is clear evidence of residual disease or progression is suspected. If clinical complete response is achieved then patients should be evaluated quarterly until 2 years after diagnosis. Typical signs and symptoms of local recurrence include enlarging mass, ulcerated mucosa, bleeding, tenesmus, and pain. Quality-of-life assessment should include questions about sexual function, bowel continence, and pelvic pain. Physical examination must include a digital rectal examination, and assessment for any palpable inguinal lymph nodes. Vaginal dilators may be used three times a week if needed. The critical time for the prevention of vaginal stenosis is 3 to 6 months following completion of chemoradiation therapy. Vaginal hormonal creams and suppositories are also useful for treatment of vaginal dryness and dysparunia. Proctosigmoidoscopy should be performed biannually following a CR for 2 years. Chest x-ray and CT chest, abdomen, and pelvis, or MRI of the abdomen and pelvis should be completed annually for 2 years (Fig. 22-10). Pap smears should continue to be performed annually.

Anal adenocarcinoma patients should be followed for a more extensive period with the surveillance period analogous to a rectal carcinoma patient with regular physical examinations, DRE, and inguinal lymph node evaluation for a minimum of 5 years due to the high risk of recurrent disease. Cross-sectional imaging should be completed annually (unless clinically indicated sooner) for a minimum of 5 years.

■ FUTURE DIRECTIONS AND CHALLENGES

It is likely that additional chemotherapy agents other than 5-FU, mitomycin C, or cisplatin may provide benefit to patients with SCC of the anal canal. The large majority of these agents have an adjunctive role as radiation sensitizers.

Rather than focusing our efforts solely on the type and dosage of cytotoxic chemotherapy, methods to decrease chemotherapy but yet enhance the efficacy of radiation should be considered. The outcome and treatment of other SCCs may lead the way to future development in evaluating the microenvironment of anal canal cancers. Prior studies have examined the prognostic significance of anemia in association with radiation response and outcome (108-110). Tumor hypoxia as a prognostic indicator of radiation resistance has been extensively studied in head and neck, lung, and cervical carcinomas, with inconclusive results (111-114). Other investigators have evaluated proapoptotic (p53, Bax) and antiapoptotic (Bcl-2) protein expression in carcinogenesis as well as a potential determinant of LCR and DFS (115,116). Recent data suggest not only a history of HPV but HPV viral load may also be determinants of outcome (117).

BIOLOGIC AGENTS

Recent developments in advanced colorectal carcinoma have included incorporating "targeted" therapy against the epidermal growth factor receptor (EGFR) and the vascular endothelial growth factor receptor (VEGF) for improved efficacy. The use of these targeted therapies will likely serve as a prototype for clinical trials—in combination with chemotherapy and/or radiation therapy—in other solid tumor malignancies. The role of bevacizumab in SCCA of the anal canal has not been reported. Yet, some supportive data in cervical carcinoma may provide a precedence for the possible role for bevacizumab in the treatment of metastatic disease (118,119). The serine threonine kinase tumor suppressor gene, *KRAS*, is mutated in 35 to 50% of colorectal cancer patients. The presence of the mutation is predictive for anti-EGFR efficacy. A series of small retrospective analyses have not demonstrated the presence of the *KRAS* mutation in SCCA of the anal canal (120-122). Treatment with cetuximab, a chimeric antibody against EGFR, in 5 patients with K-ras wild type metastatic anal cancer has shown the ability to induce remission and stable disease (119). However, recent phase III data in metastatic NSCLC indicate the benefit of cetuximab when combined with carboplatin/paclitaxel may not be beneficial for PFS and OS but only response ($p < .007$) (123). In contrast, a second phase III trial with navelbine/cisplatin/cetuximab demonstrated improvement in median OS for treatment of naïve-advanced NSCLC patients (11.3 versus 10.1 months; HR for death 0.871 [95% CI, 0.762-0.996], $p = .044$) (124). Therefore, treatment objectives are best to be identified prior to consideration of a biologic agent whether it being neoadjuvant, borderline resectable, or for palliation.

ROLE OF HPV VACCINE

As mentioned earlier, the HPV vaccine is currently approved for the prevention of high-risk subtypes of HPV namely 16 and 18 in adolescent girls and has just recently approved for boys. It is presumed with the reduction of the incidence of HPV, the development of HPV associated malignancies will eventually decrease (125). However, it should be kept in mind that HPV is not the only single risk factor accountable for the development of anal carcinoma. It is not known if the HPV vaccine will have any role in sexually active individuals with no prior history of HPV, individuals who are HIV positive but HPV negative, or in those with a known prior history of high risk of HPV in preventing secondary HPV-associated malignancies.

■ CONCLUSION

In short, several challenges remain in the treatment of carcinoma of the anal canal. The literature is fraught with small phase II studies with significant variability in chemotherapy dose as well as radiation therapy dose and technique. The rarity of this disease and low accrual rates hamper modifications in treatment approaches. Furthermore, the landmark trials of the past were initiated at a time when patient and physician education regarding HIV was rarely discussed and often considered ineligible. Discussion regarding sexual practices and history of sexually transmitted diseases was considered taboo. However, we are now aware that these matters are lucrative components of a patient's past medical history.

Based on the original design of RTOG 98-11, two phase II studies have been created utilizing induction followed by chemoradiation therapy. ECOG 3205 and AMC (AIDS Medical Consortium) 045 are two cooperative group trials for both HIV-negative and HIV-positive patients, respectively, with the intent of two cycles of induction 5-FU/cisplatin/cetuximab followed by the same chemotherapy combined with radiation therapy (www.clinicaltrials.gov, accessed 2/18/10). The objective of the ECOG 3205 study is to reduce the 3-year local failure rate from 35 to 18%. Both trials have since been amended to remove the induction component following the final results of RTOG 98-11 continues to accrue patients. The RTOG cooperative group also intends to proceed with a biologic agent as a chemoradiation sensitizer with the inclusion of HIV-positive patients.

The challenges in treating anal carcinoma patients require a collective effort on behalf of a multidisciplinary group of surgeons, radiation oncologists, pathologists, diagnostic radiologists, and medical oncologists. The use of the HPV vaccine may make significant differences in the prevention of HPV-associated malignancies, but it is likely we will not see any significant reductions until several years from now. In the interim, large cooperative group studies or intergroup studies will help expedite the modification of the treatment approach which has remained unchanged for greater than three decades. Furthermore, given the prevalence of HPV and increased incidence of patients living longer with HIV, it is presumed the number of individuals diagnosed with carcinoma of the anal canal will continue to rise. In conclusion, carcinoma of the anal canal is a unique malignancy where chemoradiation therapy is provided with curative intent or failure to respond to therapy will result in an APR. Hence, it is recommended that all patients diagnosed be initially evaluated at a tertiary cancer center or the equivalent, with a multidisciplinary team with significant expertise in this rare malignancy.

■ ACKNOWLEDGMENT

The authors would like to acknowledge Dr. Stanley Hamilton, and the anal carcinoma patients at the University of Texas MD Anderson Cancer Center who allowed their photographs to be taken as a contribution to this chapter.

References

1. Jemal A, Siegel R, Ward E, et al. Cancer statistics, 2009. *CA Cancer J Clin* 2009;59:225-249.

2. Rickert RR, Compton CC. Protocol for the examination of specimens from patients with carcinomas of the anus and anal canal: a basis for checklists. Cancer Committee of the College of American Pathologists. *Arch Pathol Lab Med* 2000;124: 21-25.

3. Bendell JC, Ryan DP. Current perspectives on anal cancer. *Oncology (Williston Park)* 2003;17:492-497, 502-503; discussion 503, 507-509.

4. Johnson L, Madeleine M, Newcomer L, et al. Anal Cancer Incidence and Survival: The Surveillance, Epidemiology, and End Results Experience, 1973-2000. *Cancer* 101(2): 281-288.

5. Daling JR, Weiss NS, Klopfenstein LL, et al. Correlates of homosexual behavior and the incidence of anal cancer. *JAMA* 1982;247:1988-1990.

6. Gervasoni JE Jr, Wanebo HJ. Cancers of the anal canal and anal margin. *Cancer Invest* 2003;21:452-464.

7. Daly JJ, Madrazo A. Anal Crohn's disease with carcinoma in situ. *Dig Dis Sci* 1980; 25:464-466.

8. Frisch M, Olsen JH, Bautz A, et al. Benign anal lesions and the risk of anal cancer. *N Engl J Med* 1994;331:300-302.

9. Frisch M, Johansen C. Anal carcinoma in inflammatory bowel disease. *Br J Cancer* 2000;83:89-90.

10. Frisch M, Glimelius B, van den Brule A, et al. Sexually transmitted infection as a cause of anal cancer. *N Engl J Med* 1997;337(19):1350-1358.

11. Patel P, Hanson MS, Sullivan P, et al. Incidence of types of cancer among HIV-infected persons compared with the general population in the United States, 1992-2003. *Ann Int Med* 2008;148(10):728-736.

12. Daling JR, Madeleine M, Johnson LG, et al. Human papillomavirus, smoking, and sexual practices in the etiology of anal cancer. *Cancer* 2004;101(2):270-280.

13. Melbye M, Sprogel P. Aetiological parallel between anal cancer and cervical cancer. *Lancet* 1991;338:657-659.

14. Naomi J, Moscicki A. Human papilloma virus infection in women. In: Goldman MH (ed): *Women & Fitness*. San Diego, CA: Academic Press; 2000.

15. zur Hausen H. Human papillomaviruses and their possible role in squamous cell carcinomas. *Curr Top Microbiol Immunol* 1977;78:1-30.

16. Critchlow CW, Surawicz CM, Holmes KK, et al. Prospective study of high grade anal squamous intraepithelial neoplasia in a cohort of homosexual men: Influence of HIV infection, immunosuppression and human papillomavirus infection. *AIDS* 1995;9:1255-1262.

17. Palefsky J, Rubin M. The epidemiology of anal human papillomavirus and related neoplasia. *Obstet Gynecol Clin N Am* 2009;36:187-200.

18. Palefsky JM, Holly EA, Hogeboom CJ, et al. Virologic, immunologic, and clinical parameters in the incidence and progression of anal squamous intraepithelial lesions in HIV-positive and HIV-negative homosexual men. *J Acquir Immune Defic Syndr Hum Retrovirol* 1998;17(4):314-319.

19. Hoots BE, Palefsky JM, Pimenta JM, et al. Human papillomavirus type distribution in anal cancer and anal intraepithelial lesions. *Int J Cancer* 2009;124(10):2375-2385.

20. Kahn JA. HPV vaccination for the prevention of cervical intraepithelial neoplasia. *N Engl J Med* 2009;361: 271-280.

21. Garland S, Hernandez-Avila M, Wheeler C, et al. Quadrivalent vaccine against human papillomavirus to prevent anogenital disease. *N Engl J Med* 2007;356:1928-1943.

22. Approval letter—Cervarix. Rockville: U.S. Food and Drug Administration. Available at: http://www.fda.gov/Biologics-BloodVaccines/Vaccines/ApprovedProducts/ucm186959.htm. Accessed November 30, 2009.

23. Approval letter—Gardasil. Rockville: U.S. Food and Drug Administration. Available at: http://www.fda.gov/Biologics-BloodVaccines/Vaccines/ApprovedProducts/ucm186991.htm. Accessed November 30, 2009.

24. Global summary of the HIV/AIDS epidemic, December 2008. Geneva: World Health Organization. Available at: http://www.who.int/hiv/data/2009 global_summary.gif. Accessed November 30, 2009.

25. Piketty C, Darragh TM, Da Costa M, et al. High prevalence of anal human papillomavirus infection and anal cancer precursors among HIV-infected persons in the absence of anal intercourse. *Ann Intern Med* 2003;138:453-459.

26. Sun XW, Kuhn L, Ellerbrock TV, et al. Human papillomavirus infection in women infected with the human immunodeficiency virus. *N Engl J Med* 1997;337:1343-1349.

27. Critchlow CW, Hawes SE, Kuypers JM, et al. Effect of HIV infection on the natural history of anal human papillomavirus infection. *AIDS* 1998;12:1177-1184.

28. Sobhani I, Vuagnat A, Walker F, et al. Prevalence of high-grade dysplasia and cancer in the anal canal in human papillomavirus-infected individuals. *Gastroenterology* 2001;120:857-66.

29. Ferenczy A, Coutlee F, Franco E, Hankins C. Human papillomavirus and HIV coinfection and the risk of neoplasias of the lower genital tract: A review of recent developments. *CMAJ* 2003;169:431-434.

30. D'Souza G, Wiley DJ, Li X, et al. Incidence and epidemiology of anal cancer in the multicenter aids cohort study. *J Acquir Immune Defic Syndr* 2008;48:491-499.

31. Crum-Cianflone NF, Hullsiek KH, Marconi VC, et al. Anal Cancers among HIV-infected persons: HAART is not slowing rising incidence. *AIDS* 2010; 20; 24 (4): 535-543.

32. Frisch M, Biggar RJ, Goedert JJ. Human papillomavirus-associated cancers in patients with human immunodeficiency virus infection and acquired immunodeficiency syndrome. *J Natl Cancer Inst* 2000;92:1500-1510.

33. Adami J, Gabel H, Lindelof B, et al. Cancer risk following organ transplantation: A nationwide cohort study in Sweden. *Br J Cancer* 2003;89:1221-1227.

34. Arends MJ, Benton EC, McLaren KM, et al. Renal allograft recipients with high susceptibility to cutaneous malignancy have an increased prevalence of human papillomavirus DNA in skin tumours and a greater risk of anogenital malignancy. *Br J Cancer* 1997;75:722-728.

35. Sunesen KG, Nørgaard M, Thorlacius-Ussing O, et al. Immunosuppressive disorders and risk of anal squamous cell carcinoma: A nationwide cohort study in Denmark, 1978-2005. *Int J Cancer* 2009 Dec 3. [Epub ahead of print].

36. Daling JR, Sherman KJ, Hislop TG, et al. Cigarette smoking and the risk of anogenital cancer. *Am J Epidemiol* 1992;135: 180-189.

37. Frisch M, Glimelius B, Wohlfahrt J, et al. Tobacco smoking as a risk factor in anal carcinoma: An antiestrogenic mechanism. *J Natl Cancer Inst* 1999;91:708-715.

38. Ramamoorthy S, Luo L, Luo E, Carethers J. Tobacco smoking and risk of recurrence for squamous cell cancer of the anus. *Cancer Detect Prev* 2008;32:116-120.

39. Myerson RJ, Karnell LH, Menck HR. The National Cancer Data Base report on carcinoma of the anus. *Cancer* 1997;80: 805-815.

40. Khatri VP, Chopra S. Clinical presentation, imaging, and staging of anal cancer. *Surg Oncol Clin N Am* 2004 Apr;13(2): 295-308.

41. Trautmann TG, Zuger JH. Positron emission tomography for pretreatment staging and posttreatment evaluation in cancer of the anal canal. *Mol Imaging Biol* 2005;7:309-313.

42. Cotter S, Grigsby P, Siegel B, et al. FDG-PET/CT in the evaluation of anal carcinoma. *Int J Radiation Oncology Biol Phys* 2006;65(3):720-725.

43. Mackay SG, Pager CK, Joseph D, et al. Assessment of the accuracy of transrectal ultrasonography in anorectal neoplasia. *Br J Surg* 2003;90:346-350.

44. Tarantino D, Bernstein MA. Endoanal ultrasound in the staging and management of squamous-cell carcinoma of the anal canal: Potential implications of a new ultrasound staging system. *Dis Colon Rectum* 2002;45:16-22.

45. Berton F, Gola G, Wilson S. Perspective on the role of transrectal and transvaginal sonography of tumors of the rectum and anal canal. *AJR* 2008;19:1495-1504.

46. Belkacemi Y, Berger C, Poortmans P, et al. Management of primary anal canal adenocarcinoma: A large retrospective study from the Rare Cancer Network. *Int J Radiat Oncol Biol Phys* 2003;56:1274-1283.

47. Touboul E, Schlienger M, Buffat L, et al. Epidermoid carcinoma of the anal canal. Results of curative-intent radiation therapy in a series of 270 patients. *Cancer* 1994;73:1569-1579.

48. Esiashvili N, Landry J, Matthews RH. Carcinoma of the anus: Strategies in management. *Oncologist* 2002;7:188-199.

49. Hill J, Meadows H, Haboubi N, et al. Pathological staging of epidermoid anal carcinoma for the new era. *Colorectal Dis* 2003;5:206-213.

50. Ajani J, Winter K, Gunderson L, et al. Fluorouracil, mitomycin, and radiotherapy versus fluorouracil, cisplatin and radiotherapy for carcinoma of the anal canal. *JAMA* 2008; 299(16):1914-1921.

51. Ajani J, Winter K, Gunderson L, et al. US intergroup anal carcinoma trial. Tumor diameter predicts for colostomy. *J Clin Oncol* 2009;27(7):1116-1121.

52. Cummings BJ, Thomas GM, Keane TJ, et al. Primary radiation therapy in the treatment of anal canal carcinoma. *Dis Colon Rectum* 1982;25:778-782.

53. Martenson JA Jr, Gunderson LL. External radiation therapy without chemotherapy in the management of anal cancer. *Cancer* 1993;71:1736-1740.

54. Svensson C, Goldman S, Friberg B. Radiation treatment of epidermoid cancer of the anus. *Int J Radiat Oncol Biol Phys* 1993;27:67-73.

55. Eschwege F, Lasser P, Chavy A, et al. Squamous cell carcinoma of the anal canal: Treatment by external beam irradiation. *Radiother Oncol* 1985;3:145-150.

56. Dubois JB, Garrigues JM, Pujol H. Cancer of the anal canal: Report on the experience of 61 patients. *Int J Radiat Oncol Biol Phys* 1991;20:575-580.

57. Deniaud-Alexandre E, Touboul E, Tiret E, et al. Results of definitive irradiation in a series of 305 epidermoid carcinomas of the anal canal. *Int J Radiat Oncol Biol Phys* 2003;56: 1259-1273.

58. Konski A, Garcia M, Madhu J, et al. Evaluation of planned treatment breaks during radiation therapy for anal cancer: Update of RTOG 92-08. *Int J Radiation Oncology Biol Phys* 2008;72(1):114-118.

59. Nigro ND, Vaitkevicius VK, Considine B Jr. Combined therapy for cancer of the anal canal: A preliminary report. *Dis Colon Rectum* 1974;17:354-356.

60. Cummings BJ, Keane TJ, O'Sullivan B, et al. Epidermal anal cancer: Treatment by radiation alone or by radiation and 5-fluorouracil with and without mitomycin C. *Int J Radiat Oncol Biol Phys* 1991;21:1115-1125.

61. UKCCCR. Epidermoid anal cancer: Results from the UKCCCR randomised trial of radiotherapy alone versus radiotherapy, 5-fluorouracil, and mitomycin. UKCCCR Anal Cancer Trial Working Party. UK Co-ordinating Committee on Cancer Research. *Lancet* 1996;348:1049-1054.

62. Northover J, Glynne Jones R, Sebag-Montefiore D, et al. Chemoradiation for the treatment of epidermoid anal cancer: 13 year follow-up of the first randomized UKCCCR Anal Cancer Trial (ACT I). *British J of Can* 2010;102 (7):1123-1128.

63. Bartelink H, Roelofsen F, Eschwege F, et al. Concomitant radiotherapy and chemotherapy is superior to radiotherapy alone in the treatment of locally advanced anal cancer: Results of a phase III randomized trial of the European Organization for Research and Treatment of Cancer Radiotherapy and Gastrointestinal Cooperative Groups. *J Clin Oncol* 1997;15:2040-2049.

64. Cummings BJ, Keane TJ, O'Sullivan et al. Mitomycin in anal canal carcinoma. *Oncology* 1993;50(suppl 1):63-69.

65. Flam M, John M, Pajak TF, et al. Role of mitomycin in combination with fluorouracil and radiotherapy, and of salvage chemoradiation in the definitive nonsurgical treatment of epidermoid carcinoma of the anal canal: Results of a phase III randomized intergroup study. *J Clin Oncol* 1996;14:2527-2539.

66. Doci R, Zucali R, La Monica G, et al. Primary chemoradiation therapy with fluorouracil and cisplatin for cancer of the anus: Results in 35 consecutive patients. *J Clin Oncol* 1996;14: 3121-3125.

67. Martenson JA, Lipsitz SR, Wagner H Jr, et al. Initial results of a phase II trial of high dose radiation therapy, 5-fluorouracil, and cisplatin for patients with anal cancer (E4292): An Eastern Cooperative Oncology Group study. *Int J Radiat Oncol Biol Phys* 1996;35:745-749.

68. Hung A, Crane C, Delclos M, et al. Cisplatin-based combined modality therapy for anal carcinoma: a wider therapeutic index. *Cancer* 2003;97:1195-1202.

69. Gerard JP, Ayzac L, Hun D, et al. Treatment of anal canal carcinoma with high dose radiation therapy and concomitant fluorouracil-cisplatinum. Long-term results in 95 patients. *Radiother Oncol* 1998;46:249-256.

70. Peiffert D, Giovannini M, Ducreux M, et al. High-dose radiation therapy and neoadjuvant plus concomitant chemotherapy with 5-fluorouracil and cisplatin in patients with locally advanced squamous-cell anal canal cancer: Final results of a phase II study. *Ann Oncol* 2001;12:397-404.

71. Meropol NJ, Niedzwiecki D, Shank B, et al. Induction therapy for poor-prognosis anal canal carcinoma: A phase II study of the cancer and leukemia group B (CALGB 9281). *J Clin Oncol* 2008;26(19):3229-3234.

72. Conroy T, Ducreux M, Lemanski E, et al. Treatment intensification by induction chemotherapy (ICT) and radiation dose escalation in locally advanced squamous cell anal canal carcinoma (LAAC): Definitive analysis of the intergroup ACCORD 03 trial. *J Clin Oncol* 2009; 27:15s(suppl; abstr 4033).

73. Tournier_Rangeard L, Mercier M, Peiffert D, et al. Radiochemotherapy of locally advanced anal canal carcinoma: Prospective assessment of early impact on the quality of life (randomized trial ACCORD 04). *Radiother Oncol* 2008; 87:392-397

74. Glynne-Jones R, Mawdsley S. Anal cancer: The end of the road for neoadjuvant chemoradiotherapy? *J Clin Oncol* 2008; 26(22):3669-3671.

75. Eng C, Crane C, Rodriguez-Bigas M. Should cisplatin be avoided in the treatment of locally advanced squamous cell carcinoma of the anal canal? *Nat Clin Pract Gastr* 2009; 6(1):16-17.

76. James R, Wan S, Glynne-Jones R, et al. A randomized trial of chemoradiation using mitomycin or cisplatin, with or without maintenance cisplatin/5FU in squamous cell carcinoma of the anus (ACT II). *J Clin Oncol* 2009;27(18s) (abstr LBA 4009).

77. Matzinger O, Roelofsen F, Mineur L, et al. Mitomycin C with continout fluorouracil or with cisplatin in combination with radiotherapy for locally advanced anal cancer (European Organisation for Research and Treatment of Cancer phase II study 22011-40014). *Eur J Cancer* 2009;45:2782-2791.

78. Eng C, Chang GJ, Das P, et al. Phase II study of capecitabine and oxaliplatin with concurrent radiation therapy (XELOX-XRT) for squamous cell carcinoma of the anal canal. *J Clin Oncol* 2009; 27:15s (suppl; abstr 4116).

79. Shepherd NA, Scholefield JH, Love SB, et al. Prognostic factors in anal squamous carcinoma: A multivariate analysis of clinical, pathological and flow cytometric parameters in 235 cases. *Histopathology* 1990;16:545-555.

80. Stearns MW Jr, Quan SH. Epidermoid carcinoma of the anorectum. *Surg Gynecol Obstet* 1970;131:953-957.

81. Ulmer C, Bembenek A, Gretschel S, et al. Sentinel node biopsy in anal cancer: A promising strategy to individualize therapy. *Onkologie* 2003;26:456-460.

82. Damin DC, Rosito MA, Schwartsmann G. Sentinel lymph node in carcinoma of the anal canal: A review. *Eur J Surg Oncol* 2006 Apr;32(3):247-252.

83. Cummings B, Keane T, Thomas G, et al. Results and toxicity of the treatment of anal canal carcinoma by radiation therapy or radiation therapy and chemotherapy. *Cancer* 1984;54: 2062-2068.

84. Gerard JP, Chapet O, Samiei F, et al. Management of inguinal lymph node metastases in patients with carcinoma of the anal canal: Experience in a series of 270 patients treated in Lyon and review of the literature. *Cancer* 2001;92:77-84.

85. Hughes LL, Rich TA, Delclos L, et al. Radiotherapy for anal cancer: Experience from 1979-1987. *Int J Radiat Oncol Biol Phys* 1989;17:1153-1160.

86. Constantinou EC, Daly W, Fung CY, et al. Time-dose considerations in the treatment of anal cancer. *Int J Radiat Oncol Biol Phys* 1997;39:651-657.

87. The NCCN Clinical Practice Guidelines in Oncology" Anal Carcinoma (Version V.I.2010). © 2009 National Comprehensive Cancer Network, Inc. Available at: NCCN.org. Accessed December 5, 2009. To view the most recent and complete version of the NCCN Guidelines, go online to NCCN.org.

88. Chauveinc L, Buthaud X, Falcou MC, et al. Anal canal cancer treatment: Practical limitations of routine prescription of concurrent chemotherapy and radiotherapy. *Br J Cancer* 2003;89:2057-2061.

89. Anastos K, Barron Y, Cohen MH, et al. The prognostic importance of changes in CD4+ cell count and HIV-1 RNA level in women after initiating highly active antiretroviral therapy. *Ann Intern Med* 2004;140:256-264.

90. Place RJ, Gregorcyk SG, Huber PJ, Simmang CL. Outcome analysis of HIV-positive patients with anal squamous cell carcinoma. *Dis Colon Rectum* 2001;44:506-512.

91. Klencke BJ, Palefsky JM. Anal cancer: An HIV-associated cancer. *Hematol Oncol Clin North Am* 2003;17:859-872.

92. Kim JH, Sarani B, Orkin BA, et al. HIV-positive patients with anal carcinoma have poorer treatment tolerance and outcome than HIV-negative patients. *Dis Colon Rectum* 2001; 44:1496-1502.

93. Consten EC, Slors FJ, Noten HJ, et al. Anorectal surgery in human immunodeficiency virus-infected patients. Clinical outcome in relation to immune status. *Dis Colon Rectum* 1995;38:1169-1175.

94. Consten EC, van Lanschot JJ, Henny CP, et al. General operative aspects of human immunodeficiency virus infection and acquired immunodeficiency syndrome. *J Am Coll Surg* 1995; 180:366-380.

95. Vatra B, Sobhani I, Aparicio T, et al. Anal canal squamous-cell carcinomas in HIV positive patients: Clinical features, treatments and prognosis. *Gastroenterol Clin Biol* 2002;26: 150-156.

96. Chiao E, Giordano T, Richardson P, et al. Human immunodeficiency virus-associated squamous cell cancer of the anus: Epidemiology and outcomes in the highly active antiretroviral therapy era. 2008;26(3):474-479.

97. Oehler-Janne C, Seifert B, Lutolf UM, et al. Local tumor control and toxicity in HIV-associated anal carcinoma treated with radiotherapy in the era of antiretroviral therapy. *Radiat Oncol* 2006;1:20.

98. Stadler RF, Gregorcyk SG, Euhus DM, et al. Outcome of HIV-infected patients with invasive squamous-cell carcinoma of the anal canal in the era of highly active antiretroviral therapy. *Dis Colon Rectum* 2004;47:1305-1309.

99. Blazy A, Hennequin C, Gornet JM, et al. Anal carcinomas in HIV-positive patients: High-dose chemotherapy is feasible in the era of highly active antiretroviral therapy. *Dis Colon Rectum* 2005;48:1176-1181.

100. Goldie SJ, Kuntz KM, Weinstein MC, et al. The clinical effectiveness and cost-effectiveness of screening for anal squamous intraepithelial lesions in homosexual and bisexual HIV-positive men. *JAMA* 1999;281:1822-1829.

101. Goldie SJ, Kuntz KM, Weinstein MC, et al. Cost-effectiveness of screening for anal squamous intraepithelial lesions and anal cancer in human immunodeficiency virus—negative homosexual and bisexual men. *Am J Med* 2000;108:634-641.

102. Fraunholz I, Weiss C, Eberlein K, et al. Concurrent chemoradiotherapy with 5-fluorouracil and mitomycin C for invasive anal carcinoma in human immunodeficiency virus-positive patients receiving highly active antiretroviral therapy. *Int J Radiat Oncol Biol Phys* 2009 Sept 8. [Epub ahead of print]

103. Nilsson PJ, Svensson C, Goldman S, et al. Salvage abdominoperineal resection in anal epidermoid cancer. *Br J Surg* 2002;89:1425-1429.

104. Tarazi R, Nelson RL. Anal adenocarcinoma: A comprehensive review. *Semin Surg Oncol* 1994;10:235-240.

105. Papagikos M, Crane CH, Skibber J, et al. Chemoradiation for adenocarcinoma of the anus. *Int J Radiat Oncol Biol Phys* 2003;55:669-678.

106. Chang GJ, Gonzalez RJ, Skibber JM, et al. A twenty-year experience with adenocarcinoma of the anal canal. *Dis Colon Rectum* 2009;52(8):1375-1380.

107. Eng C, Pathak P. Treatment options in metastatic squamous cell carcinoma of the anal canal. *Curr Treat Options Oncol* 2008 Dec;9(4-6):400-407s.

108. Pirker R, Wiesenberger K, Pohl G, Minar W. Anemia in lung cancer: Clinical impact and management. *Clin Lung Cancer* 2003;5:90-97.

109. Abels RI. Use of recombinant human erythropoietin in the treatment of anemia in patients who have cancer. *Semin Oncol* 1992;19:29-35.

110. Harrison LB, Shasha D, Homel P. Prevalence of anemia in cancer patients undergoing radiotherapy: Prognostic significance and treatment. *Oncology* 2002;63(Suppl 2):11-18.

111. Bachtiary B, Schindl M, Potter R, et al. Overexpression of hypoxia-inducible factor 1alpha indicates diminished response to radiotherapy and unfavorable prognosis in patients receiving radical radiotherapy for cervical cancer. *Clin Cancer Res* 2003;9:2234-2240.

112. Dachs GU, Patterson AV, Firth JD, et al. Targeting gene expression to hypoxic tumor cells. *Nat Med* 1997;3:515-520.

113. Adam MF, Gabalski EC, Bloch DA, et al. Tissue oxygen distribution in head and neck cancer patients. *Head Neck* 1999; 21:146-153.

114. Jeremic B, Machtay M. Concurrent radiochemotherapy in the treatment of locally advanced non-small cell lung cancer. *Hematol Oncol Clin North Am* 2004;18:91-100.

115. Allal AS, Waelchli L, Brundler MA. Prognostic value of apoptosis-regulating protein expression in anal squamous cell carcinoma. *Clin Cancer Res* 2003;9:6489-6496.

116. Allal AS, Brundler MA, Gervaz P. Differential expression of anti-apoptotic protein Bcl-2 in keratinizing versus non-keratinizing squamous cell carcinoma of the anus. *Int J Colorectal Dis* 2005;20(2):161-164.

117. Kim JY, Park S, Nam BH, et al. Low initial human papilloma viral load implicates worse prognosis in patients with uterine cervical cancer treated with radiotherapy. *J Clin Onc* 2009; 27:5088-5093.

118. Takano M, Kikuchi Y, Kita T et al. Complete remission of metastatic and relapsed uterine cervical cancers using weekly administration of bevacizumab and paclitaxel/carboplatin. *Onkologie* 2009 Oct;32(10):595-597. Epub 2009 Sep 11.

119. Monk BJ, Sill MW, Burger RA, et al. Phase II trial of bevacizumab in the treatment of persistent or recurrent squamous cell carcinoma of the cervix: A gynecologic oncology group study. *J Clin Oncol* 2009 Mar 1;27(7):1069-1074. Epub 2009 Jan 12.

120. Zampino MG, Magni E, Sonzogni A, et al. K-ras status in squamous cell anal carcinoma: It's time for target-oriented treatment? *Cancer Chemother Pharmacol* 2009;65(1):197-199.

121. Lukan N, Strobel P, Willer A, et al. Cetuximab-based treatment of anal cancer: Correlation of response with KRAS mutational status. *Oncology* 2009;77(5):293-299.

122. Van Damme N, Van Roy N, Speleman A, et al. EGFR and K-RAS gene status evaluation in anal canal squamous cell carcinoma. *J Clin Oncol* 2008;26: (May 20 suppl, #155569).

123. Lynch TJ, Patel T, Dreisbach L et al. Cetuximab and first-line taxane/carboplatin chemotherapy in advanced non-small-cell lung cancer: Results of the randomized multicenter phase III trial BMS099. *J Clin Oncol* 2010 Feb 20;28(6): 911-917. Epub 2010 Jan 25.

124. Pirker R, Pereira JR, Szczesna A et al. Cetuximab plus chemotherapy in patients with advanced non-small-cell lung cancer (FLEX): An open-label randomised phase III trial. *Lancet* 2009 May 2;373(9674):1525-1531.

125. Francheschi S, De Vuyst H. Human papillomavirus vaccines and anal carcinoma. *Curr Opin HIVAIDS* 2009;4:57-63.

NEUROENDOCRINE TUMORS

John Andrew Jakob
Carlo M. Contreras
Bruno C. Odisio
Sanjay Gupta
Eddie K. Abdalla
James C. Yao

■ INTRODUCTION

Neuroendocrine tumors (NETs) originate from neuroendocrine cells located throughout the body. This chapter focuses on low- to intermediate-grade NETs, though the term "neuroendocrine tumor" also denotes diseases such as small cell carcinomas of pulmonary and extrapulmonary origin, thyroid medullar carcinoma, neuroblastoma, and Merkel cell tumor. Islet cell carcinomas, also known as pancreatic endocrine tumors, pancreatic NETs, or pancreatic carcinoid, arise from the islets of Langerhans. Low- to intermediate-grade NETs arising from other sites are generally called carcinoids and are localized most often in the gastrointestinal tract or bronchopulmonary tree. These tumors share the capacity for hormone production and usually have an indolent clinical course. Presenting symptoms, when present, are caused by excess hormones, local tumor growth, and/or metastasis. Surgical resection is the curative approach for localized disease. In unresectable and/or metastatic disease, long-acting somatostatin analogues such as octreotide have significantly improved quality of life. The roles of newer targeted agents are under investigation in phase III trials discussed in this chapter. This chapter also presents sample clinical cases from the MD Anderson Cancer Center to illustrate the challenges of caring for the NET patient and the utility of the multi-disciplinary approach.

■ EPIDEMIOLOGY

The overall incidence of NET in the United States is estimated at 5.25 cases per 100,000 (1). Most NETs progress slowly and may remain undiagnosed for many years. Of note, carcinoid tumors were found in 0.65 to 1.2% of patients during unselected small intestine necropsy (2,3). These tumors are usually diagnosed in the sixth and seventh decades of life. NETs have been described as more common among African Americans owing to a higher diagnosed incidence of rectal carcinoid (1,4). The gastrointestinal tract is the most common primary site of NETs, accounting for 58% of all carcinoid tumors (1). The distribution of NETs is illustrated in Table 23-1.

■ PROGNOSIS

The overall prognosis for patients with NET varies by histologic grade, extent of disease, and site of primary tumor. High-grade NETs have high metastatic potential and an aggressive growth pattern, and the treatment

TABLE
23-1

ORGAN DISTRIBUTION OF NEUROENDOCRINE TUMORS (CARCINOIDS AND PANCREATIC ISLET CELL TUMORS)	
Organ Site	*Distribution (%)*
Pulmonary	27
Gastrointestinal	58
Stomach	6
Small intestine	17
Appendix	3
Colon	4
Rectum	17
Pancreas	6
Unknown/other	15

Data from analysis of SEER 17 Registry, 2000-2004 (1).

strategy is similar to that for small cell carcinoma of the lungs. Most low- to intermediate-grade NETs have a more favorable prognosis than adenocarcinoma of the same primary site. The median overall survival duration of patients with localized low- to intermediate-grade NET is 223 months, according to a recent analysis of the Surveillance Epidemiology and End Results (SEER) database of patients registered from 1973 to 2004. For patients with regional disease, defined as involvement of regional lymph nodes or extension to adjacent tissue or both, the median overall survival duration is 111 months. For metastatic disease, the median overall survival plummets to 33 months (1). The prognoses of NETs by anatomical site are discussed in depth in subsequent sections, Carcinoid Clinical Behavior by Site and Clinical Features of Islet Cell Tumors.

■ PATHOGENESIS AND MOLECULAR BIOLOGY

Neuroendocrine tumors occur both sporadically and in the context of an inherited disorder. Little is known about the pathogenesis of sporadic NETs. The *MEN1* gene, mutated in *Multiple Endocrine Neoplasia*, type I, whose germ-line mutation predisposes to inherited islet cell carcinomas, does manifest mutation (20%) and loss of heterozygosity (70%) in sporadic islet cell carcinomas (5). Menin, the protein product of the *MEN1* gene, appears to suppress tumorigenesis and growth by multiple mechanisms, including transcription regulation/chromatin remodeling via interaction with histone methyltransferases, direct regulation of cell cycle progression via interaction with the genetic loci of the cyclin dependent kinase inhibitors p18ink4c and p27kip1, and

facilitation of apoptosis by increased production of caspase 8 (6). Cell culture–based experiments have implicated transcription factor Hoxc6 in the control of growth of human NET cells via an interaction with activator protein-1 component JunD (7).

The two most frequently mutated tumor suppressors in human cancer, p53 and PTEN, are not altered in NETs of the gastroenteropancreatic system. p53 mutations have been reported in atypical pulmonary carcinoids (8). PTEN protein expression was not altered in a limited sample of nine assayed carcinoid lesions, although expression was lost in poorly differentiated neuroendocrine carcinomas (9).

The expression of various angiogenesis and tumor growth factors, such as vascular endothelial growth factor (VEGF), epidermal growth factor (EGF) transforming growth factor (TGF), platelet-derived growth factor (PDGF), and their receptors, is elevated in carcinoid tumors (10-12). Somatostatin receptors also are expressed in the majority of carcinoids.

Investigators have employed positional cloning techniques to identify novel candidate tumor suppressor or oncogene loci for sporadic NETs. In a series of 12 foregut tumors (mostly islet cell carcinomas) and 14 midgut tumors (mostly carcinoids of the ileum), comparative genomic hybridization identified gain of chromosome arm 20q as the most common chromosome imbalance in the foregut tumors (58%) and gains of 17p and 19q as the most common imbalances in midgut tumors (57% each). This study also demonstrated loss of chromosome arm 18q in 43% of midgut carcinoid tumors (13). A separate investigation of 18 midgut carcinoids with comparative genomic hybridization revealed loss of 18q22-qter as the most common chromosomal abnormality (14). Higher-resolution single nucleotide polymorphism–based array technology has recently confirmed frequent loss of chromosome 18 (34%) (15).

A significant minority of NETs, 5 to 10%, occur in the context of multiple endocrine neoplasia, type I (MEN1), an autosomal dominant disorder characterized by pituitary tumors, hyperparathyroidism, and islet cell carcinomas. Neuroendocrine tumors related to MEN1 syndrome differ from sporadic disease insofar as they comprise a unique pattern of symptomatic and nonsymptomatic lesions. Symptomatic lesions include duodenal gastrinoma, which causes Zollinger-Ellison syndrome, a condition that afflicts nearly 60% of MEN1 patients with peptic ulcers, gastroesophageal reflux, and diarrhea. Characteristic nonsymptomatic lesions include small duodenal foci of somatostatin expression and pancreatic microadenoma and macroadenoma. These pancreatic lesions tend to be asymptomatic and express glucagon or pancreatic polypeptide. Roughly 20% of MEN1-associated pancreatic macroadenomas are "insulinomas," causing hyperinsulinemic hypoglycemic syndrome. Notably, approximately 10% of pancreatic islet cell carcinomas are associated with MEN1 syndrome (16).

Other inherited disorders, such as neurofibromatosis type 1, von Hippel-Lindau syndrome, and tuberous sclerosis complex 2, predispose to NETs. Carcinoids of the ampulla of Vater, mediastinum, and duodenum are seen in roughly 1% of patients with neurofibromatosis type 1; islet cell carcinomas are associated with 5 to 17% and <1% of von Hippel-Lindau and tuberous sclerosis complex 2 cases, respectively. However, these diseases account for far fewer cases of NET disease than sporadic and MEN1-related tumors (16).

PATHOLOGIC CLASSIFICATION

Neuroendocrine tumors are derived from neuroectodermal cells and are characterized by monotonous sheets of small round cells with uniform nuclei and cytoplasm (Fig. 23-1). Neuroendocrine cells store endocrine or paracrine substances in membrane-bound vesicles, releasing them by exocytosis. Immunohistochemical markers used to confirm a carcinoid diagnosis on tumor tissue include neuron-specific enolase, CD56, chromogranin A (CGA), and synaptophysin (Table 23-2).

Carcinoid cells have minimal mitotic activity, cytological atypia, or nuclear polymorphism. Pulmonary carcinoids with more than two mitoses per 10 high-power

TABLE 23-2	IMMUNOHISTOCHEMICAL MARKERS OF NEUROENDOCRINE CARCINOMA
Marker	*Significance*
Neuron-specific enolase	Cytoplasmic glycolytic enzyme, a less specific neuroendocrine marker
Synaptophysin	Presynaptic vesicle membrane glycoprotein, present on normal and neoplastic neuroendocrine cells
Chromogranin A	Acidic protein, universal marker for neuroendocrine tissue
CD56	Neural adhesion molecule
Cytokeratin(s)	Lack of cytokeratin expression suggests the tumor is either an anaplastic neoplasm or may not be a carcinoma

fields (HPF) are considered "atypical" and are more likely to metastasize. Tumors with high mitotic activity or necrosis are called poorly differentiated, anaplastic, or high-grade neuroendocrine carcinoma. If tumor grade cannot be determined from available tumor specimens, a repeat core needle biopsy is recommended, as the results may determine treatment. A formal histologic grading system for gastrointestinal NETs recently proposed by the American Joint Committee on Cancer (AJCC) includes three grades based on mitotic count and Ki-67 index: G1, <2 mitoses per 10 HPF or Ki-67 index ≤2%; G2, 2 to 20 mitoses per 10 HPF or Ki-67 index 3 to 20%; G3, >20 mitoses per 10 HPF or Ki-67 index >20% (17).

CLINICAL PRESENTATION, DIAGNOSTIC WORKUP, AND CLINICAL STAGING

The classic symptoms associated with hormonal overproduction in carcinoid syndrome, such as flushing and diarrhea, are typically present in the setting of metastases. These symptoms can be insidious in onset and present years before diagnosis. Symptoms of local and regional carcinoid and islet cell carcinoma disease, with the exception of hypoglycemia in insulinoma, tend to be vague. Symptoms often occur as complications of acute obstruction from primary tumor, mesenteric fibrosis, or ischemia secondary to mesenteric vascular involvement.

Multiple diagnostic procedures are typical, including computed tomography (CT) of the abdomen and pelvis, esophagogastroduodenoscopy, and colonoscopy, sometimes without achieving a diagnosis. This situation is particularly frustrating when clinical suspicion

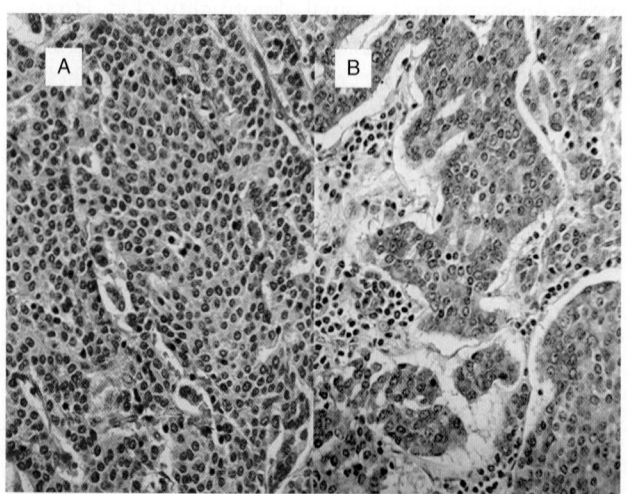

FIGURE 23-1. Histologic appearance of neuroendocrine tumors. Microscopic appearance of low-grade NET. **A.** Standard microscopy showing few mitoses, no necrosis, and large numbers of tumor vessels. **B.** Immunohistochemical staining for chromogranin A.

of carcinoid syndrome is great; fortunately, serum and urine laboratory markers, described in the next section, often are performed in parallel with more invasive testing and can confirm the diagnosis, if not localize the primary lesion.

NEUROENDOCRINE TUMOR LABORATORY TESTS AND MARKERS

Frequently measured tumor markers in carcinoid disease include serum chromogranin A and 5-hydroxyindoleacetic acid (5-HIAA) levels in a 24-hour urine sample. Tryptophan-rich foods should be avoided during urine collection for 5-HIAA levels. False-positive results occur with consumption of serotonin-rich foods such as plantain, pineapple, banana, kiwi, plums, tomatoes, butternuts, walnuts, shagbark, mockernut, pecans, and sweet pignuts. Common medications that affect urinary 5-HIAA levels include guaifenesin, acetaminophen, and salicylates.

Serum chromogranin A level is a very sensitive, but nonspecific, marker for all NETs. The level is frequently elevated among patients on a proton pump inhibitor or with poor renal function. Urine 5-HIAA and serum CGA also may serve as biochemical markers for monitoring progression of disease and treatment response.

In addition to chromogranin A and 5-HIAA, neuroendocrine tumors synthesize other bioactive amines and peptides such as 5-hydroxytryptamine (5-HTP), 5-hydroxytryptophan (5-HT), serotonin, insulin, gastrin, glucagon, somatostatin, vasoactive intestinal polypeptide (VIP), growth hormone, adrenocorticotropic hormone, melanocyte-stimulating hormone, pancreatic polypeptide, calcitonin, substance P, and pancreastatin (8).

IMAGING

Endoscopy

Endoscopic techniques localize tumors and facilitate biopsy of lesions of interest. Upper endoscopy can often locate gastric and duodenal carcinoid tumors. Colonoscopy is used in identification of colorectal carcinoids. Unfortunately, conventional endoscopy is generally not useful in localizing jejunal or ileal tumors. However, double-balloon enteroscopy and capsule endoscopy are emerging techniques that could play prominent roles in imaging tumors in these locations. The disadvantages of endoscopy include the requirement for patient sedation and the difficulty in visualizing small submucosal lesions. Endoscopic ultrasound is useful in the assessment, visualization, and biopsy of pancreatic and some small duodenal NETs.

Computed Tomography and Magnetic Resonance Imaging

Computed tomography and magnetic resonance imaging (MRI) can be used for the diagnostic workup of NETs. The utility of CT and MRI imaging for diagnosis of a typical small bowel carcinoid of the ileum is limited at best; usually the presence of such lesions can only be inferred by the presence of luminal narrowing, adenopathy, and mesenteric fibrosis. CT and MRI technologies are far more useful in detection of hepatic metastases, which frequently present convenient sites for biopsy to confirm diagnosis. CT and MRI are helpful in the detection of primary pancreatic islet cell carcinomas, for which the sensitivities of CT and MRI are 64 to 82% and 74 to 100%, respectively (18).

OctreoScan

Somatostatin receptor scintigraphy has improved the visualization of NETs. OctreoScan utilizes a somatostatin analogue, ^{111}In-labeled diethylenetriamine penta-acetic acid octreotide (DTPA-D-Phe[1]-octreotide), to visualize somatostatin receptor–positive tumors. Compared with routine CT or MRI, OctreoScan detects additional metastases in about one-third of patients. Moreover, OctreoScan may help to identify insulinoma and gastrinoma when conventional scan results are negative. The overall sensitivity of OctreoScan is 80 to 90% (19).

Positron Emission Tomography

There is little experience with positron emission tomography imaging in evaluation of NETs. Because 2-fluoro-2-deoxy-D-glucose (FDG) PET scan identifies only tumors with moderate to high proliferative activity, false-positive and false-negative results are common. ^{11}C-labeled 5-HT PET is used to image tryptophan metabolism and is superior to routine FDG PET or CT scan (20,21). Currently, ^{11}C-labeled 5-HT PET is not readily available in North America.

Other Nuclear Scintigraphy Techniques

Metaidobenzyguanidine (MIBG) is absorbed by carcinoid tumor cells. [131]Iodine-labeled MIBG (^{131}I-MIBG) has an overall sensitivity of 55 to 70% in detecting NETs (19,22-24). Although ^{131}I-MIBG is less sensitive than OctreoScan, it has the advantage that it may be used in patients who are treated by long-acting octreotide.

CLINICAL STAGING

The AJCC has proposed a traditional TNM (tumor, node, metastasis) staging system for carcinoid tumors (ie, gastrointestinal NETs excluding the pancreas). This system is site-specific, with different T classifications depending on the location of the primary lesion. The prognostic value of this system is still uncertain. The AJCC recommends determination of histologic grade of the primary lesion for purposes of prognosis and classification. High-grade NETs (ie, G3 with mitotic count >20/10 HPF or Ki-67 >20%) are excluded from this TNM staging system and are to be staged according to guidelines for carcinomas of the primary site (17). The AJCC also recommends clinical staging of pancreatic NETs with the TNM system used for exocrine pancreatic malignancies; mitotic index of the primary lesion is recommended for prognostic purposes (25).

■ CARCINOID CLINICAL BEHAVIOR BY SITE

GASTRIC CARCINOID

Gastric carcinoid tumors are divided into three distinct groups. Group 1 (75%) is associated with chronic atrophic gastritis, group 2 (5-10%) with Zollinger-Ellison syndrome (5-10%), and group 3 (15-25%) is sporadic gastric carcinoid tumors (26). Group 3 has the worst prognosis, frequently presenting with metastatic disease. Analysis of the SEER database demonstrates a median overall survival duration of just 13 months for patients with metastatic gastric carcinoid (1). Clinical features of the three groups of gastric carcinoid are summarized in Table 23-3.

SMALL INTESTINE CARCINOID

Small intestine carcinoid tumors, the carcinoid most frequently associated with typical symptoms of carcinoid syndrome, are often found in the distal ileum within 60 cm of the ileocecal valve. At diagnosis, multiple putative "primary" lesions may be present in multiple sites. Analysis of SEER data from 1973 to 2004 demonstrates that jejunum and ileum carcinoids (30%) were far more likely than rectal (5%) or appendiceal (9%) lesions to have distant metastases at diagnosis. However, only 9% of duodenal carcinoids presented with distant metastases. The median overall survival durations for duodenal and jejunum/ileum carcinoids were 107 and 111 months, respectively, for localized disease and 57 and 56 months, respectively, for metastatic disease (1).

APPENDICEAL CARCINOID

Carcinoid tumors are found incidentally in 1 of 200 to 300 appendectomies in young adults. For appendiceal carcinoids less than 1 cm in diameter, surgical resection is sufficient. For tumors more than 2 cm in diameter, the risk of metastasis is significantly higher, and a right hemicolectomy is recommended (27). Histologic subtype also influences surgical management; right hemicolectomy is recommended for tumors of goblet cell histology (which can include signet-ring cells), regardless of size of primary tumor, because of the aggressiveness of these lesions (28). The median overall survival duration for patients with carcinoid restricted to the appendix is greater than 360 months. In contrast, individuals with metastatic disease at diagnosis fare far worse, with a median overall survival duration of only 27 months (1).

RECTAL CARCINOID

Rectal carcinoid occurs most frequently in middle-aged adults. This tumor is found incidentally in approximately 1 in 2500 proctoscopies as a small yellow-gray submucosal nodule in the wall of the rectum. The majority of rectal carcinoids are less than 1 cm in diameter and do not metastasize, whereas 60 to 80% of lesions larger than 2 cm do metastasize. Local excision is adequate for rectal carcinoids smaller than 1 cm. Lesions measuring 1 to 1.9 cm without evidence of high-risk features such as muscularis, lymphovascular, or perineural invasion can be excised locally (29). A tumor displaying any of these high-risk features should prompt consideration of a more aggressive segmental rectal resection, sphincter-sparing if possible. In patients with metastatic rectal carcinoid at diagnosis, excision is performed with palliative, not curative, intent (30). The median overall survival duration of patients with metastatic rectal carcinoid is just 22 months (1).

TABLE 23-3	THE CLINICAL FEATURES OF GASTRIC CARCINOID BY GROUP			
Group	Clinical Feature	Tumor Size	Metastasis	Prognosis
Group 1	Chronic gastritis	<1 cm	10%	Good
Group 2	ZES, gastrinoma	<1.5 cm	25%	Intermediate
Group 3	Atypical carcinoid	>1 cm	Frequent	Poor

ZES, Zollinger-Ellison syndrome.

■ CLINICAL FEATURES OF ISLET CELL TUMORS

INSULINOMA

Insulinoma is the most common type of islet cell tumor. The incidence of insulinoma peaks in patients between 30 and 60 years of age, and these tumors are more frequent in women. Insulinoma is usually benign (90%), intrapancreatic (nearly 100%), solitary, and small (<2 cm). About 5% of these tumors are associated with the MEN1 syndrome; screening of the family members of an MEN1 index case should be considered (5). Hyperinsulinism causes obesity and neurologic/psychiatric disturbances in many patients. A recent series of four patients demonstrated that everolimus, which frequently causes hyperglycemia as a side effect, is effective in treatment of the hypoglycemia of metastatic, progressive insulinoma (31).

The insulinoma diagnosis is made by detection of inappropriately high concentrations of both insulin and C peptide in the blood at a blood glucose level of less than 50 mg/dL together with symptoms of hypoglycemia. Although conventional CT scan, transabdominal ultrasonography, and selective arteriography fail to localize an insulinoma in about 40% of cases, a sensitivity greater than 90% can be achieved with combinations of MRI, thin-section pancreatic protocol CT scan, and endoscopic ultrasound. OctreoScan is another noninvasive modality available to assist in localization of insulinomas. Portal venous sampling and arterial calcium stimulation are technically demanding, invasive procedures that are not widely available. When preoperative studies fail to definitively localize the insulinoma, surgical exploration with intraoperative ultrasonography can be considered (32). At the authors' institution, radiologic innovations have rendered blind surgical exploration unnecessary.

GASTRINOMA

Gastrinoma causes Zollinger-Ellison syndrome, and its clinical hallmark is multiple recurrent peptic ulcers. Most gastrinomas are located in the "gastrinoma triangle," which encompasses the duodenum, pancreatic head, and hepatoduodenal ligament. Gastrinoma of the duodenum is often a small submucosal tumor that can be missed easily during routine upper gastrointestinal endoscopy; gastrinoma of the pancreas can exceed 1 cm in size (33).

The diagnostic workup for gastrinoma often involves two steps. An elevated concentration of gastrin in a blood sample from a fasting patient and increased basal gastric acid output (>15 mEq/h) suggest the presence of gastrinoma. A secretin stimulation test is required to differentiate gastrinoma from other causes of gastrin elevation. Octreotide scan has 77% sensitivity for gastrinoma. Sixty percent of gastrinomas are malignant, and 50% of those have metastases at diagnosis. The median survival duration for patients with gastrinoma is between 3 and 6 years. Roughly one-fifth of gastrinomas occur in the context of MEN1 syndrome (33).

GLUCAGONOMA

Glucagonoma is a rare alpha-cell tumor of the pancreas that occurs in people aged 50 to 70 years. These tumors are located primarily within the pancreas; most are malignant. They penetrate the pancreatic capsule and invade the regional lymph nodes. Symptoms may not appear until the tumor is larger than 5 cm in diameter. At diagnosis, 50 to 80 % of these tumors have metastasized to liver. Serum glucagon levels are usually quite elevated (>1000 pg/mL; normal range, 150-200 pg/mL) and assist in diagnosis.

Mild glucose intolerance is the most common clinical feature of glucagonoma. A characteristic skin rash called necrolytic erythema migrans may precede the diagnosis by as long as 5 years. The initial lesion consists of red papules or pale brown macules on the face, abdomen, groin, perineum, or extremities. The erythematous areas form superficial bullae that eventually break down and become encrusted. Anemia, thromboembolic disease with venous thrombosis or pulmonary emboli, and psychiatric disturbances are other clinical features of glucagonoma. Anticoagulation therapy is recommended in individuals with glucagon excess (34).

SOMATOSTATINOMA

Somatostatinoma is very rare. Most occur in the pancreas or duodenum. Patients with this tumor often present with diabetes mellitus, cholelithiasis, diarrhea, steatorrhea, hypochlorhydria, anemia, and/or weight loss. These tumors are generally malignant and are usually diagnosed late in their course. Metastases to lymph nodes, liver, and bone may be found at diagnosis (35).

VIPOMA

VIPoma is characterized by watery diarrhea (>3 L/day), hypokalemia, and achlorhydria. These clinical features are mediated by VIP as well as other peptides secreted by malignant islet cells. VIPomas are located in the pancreas in adults and rarely in extrapancreatic sites in children. They are often metastatic at diagnosis. The stool is essentially isotonic, and the diarrhea persists even during fasting with nasogastric suction. Large amounts of potassium and bicarbonate are lost in the stool, leading to hypokalemia and metabolic acidosis. Diagnosis is made by typical clinical presentation, presence of a large pancreatic mass per imaging, and elevated plasma VIP levels. Somatostatin analogues are effective in control of the hormonal syndrome (35).

PANCREATIC POLYPEPTIDOMA

Pancreatic polypeptide is synthesized and released from pancreatic polypeptide cells in the normal pancreas. Pancreatic polypeptidoma often is found unexpectedly in patients with symptoms produced by metastases to the liver and bone (36).

■ **CARCINOID SYNDROME, CARCINOID HEART DISEASE, AND CARCINOID CRISIS**

CARCINOID SYNDROME

Carcinoid syndrome is often observed in patients with metastatic disease or when the primary tumor site allows secreted amines to escape into the enterohepatic circulation (Table 23-4). Common symptoms include flushing, diarrhea, abdominal cramping, and, less frequently, wheezing, heart valve dysfunction, and pellagra, all of which result from synergistic interactions between 5-HTP metabolites, kinins, and prostaglandins. The incidence of carcinoid syndrome ranges from 10% in localized carcinoid to 40 to 50 % in advanced tumors. As is discussed in more detail in a subsequent section, somatostatin analogues such as octreotide are the mainstay of medical therapy for carcinoid syndrome.

CARCINOID HEART DISEASE

Carcinoid heart disease is due to fibrosis of the endocardium of the right heart and occasionally leads to tricuspid regurgitation and right heart failure. However, the relationship between carcinoid heart disease and frank heart failure in the somatostatin analogue era is unclear. A recent study of 150 patients with carcinoid syndrome and a midgut lesion described a 20 % prevalence of carcinoid valve disease as determined by echocardiography. Of those with valve disease by echocardiogaphy, 53% were assessed clinically as having New York Heart Association heart failure class I or II. Twenty-seven percent of the patients with moderate or severe valvular disease by echocardiography had class I, or essentially asymptomatic, heart failure. Notably, more than 70 % of all patients in the study were maintained on a somatostatin analogue, though no relationship was demonstrated between somatostatin analogue use and presence of carcinoid heart disease or heart failure. Patients with carcinoid heart disease did exhibit increased urine 5-HIAA and serum CGA levels (37). Currently, the United States National Comprehensive Cancer Network guidelines suggest echocardiography for patients with carcinoid syndrome and clinical signs/symptoms of heart failure or in whom major surgery is planned (38).

CARCINOID CRISIS

Carcinoid crisis is caused by a massive release of bioactive products to the systemic blood, and is characterized by profuse hypotension, watery stools, and abdominal cramps. Characteristic symptoms and signs such as itching, palpitations, and facial edema are related to large amounts of circulating histamine, kinins, and prostaglandins. Carcinoid crisis is often precipitated by a surgery or procedure; treatment consists of prompt intravenous delivery of octreotide, with initiation of octreotide infusion at 50 to 100 µg/h as

TABLE 23-4	SYMPTOMS OF CARCINOID SYNDROME		
Symptom	*Frequency (%)*	*Characteristics*	*Involved Mediators*
Flushing	85-90	Foregut: long-lasting, purple	Killirein, 5-HTP
			Histamine, substance P
		Midgut: short-lasting, pink	PGs
Diarrhea	70	Secretory	Gastrin, 5-HTP, histamine, PGs, VIP
Abdominal pain	35	Progressive	Small bowel obstruction, hepatomegaly, ischemia
Telangioectasia	25	Face	Unknown
Bronchospasm	15	Wheezing	Histamine, 5-HTP
Pellagra	5	Dermatitis, diarrhea, dementia	Niacin deficiency

5-HTP, 5-hydroxytryptophan; PGs, prostaglandins; VIPs, vasoactive intestinal peptide.

needed. Premedication of carcinoid patients with additional octreotide in subcutaneous or intravenous form is often used to prevent or mitigate carcinoid crisis caused by an intervention (39).

■ GENERAL APPROACH TO TREATMENT

The indolent features of NETs and their lack of response to conventional cytotoxic chemotherapy complicate treatment decisions for patients with these tumors. Localized NET should be surgically excised whenever possible. In general, in asymptomatic or mildly symptomatic disease in patients with a low-volume but unresectable NET, treatment should be delayed and the disease monitored every 3 to 6 months. For advanced, well to moderately differentiated, and asymptomatic NET of the midgut, we recommend surgical resection of all gross disease that can be reasonably removed.

There are multiple indications for palliative surgical interventions for advanced neuroendocrine tumors. These indications extend beyond the commonly appreciated complications of refractory intestinal obstruction and bleeding. Locally advanced tumors are often associated with bulky mesenteric lymphadenopathy; these

nodes can cause mesenteric vascular compromise manifesting as visceral ischemia. Surgical intervention can also alleviate refractory hormone-mediated symptoms. Furthermore, surgical resection of a pancreatic NET can prevent pancreatitis and/or biliary obstruction. Ideally, all palliative resections should include excision of the primary tumor mass and removal of the mesenteric nodal burden. Intestinal bypass is another strategy, but this does not address bulky mesenteric lymphadenopathy.

The somatostatin analogues are the mainstays of medical treatment for symptomatic advanced carcinoid and VIPoma. When carcinoid syndrome symptoms persist with somatostatin analogue therapy, or mass effect symptoms worsen, debulking or ablation surgery, as already discussed, may be used to reduce tumor load and provide effective palliation. Interferon-alpha (IFNα), alone or in combination with a somatostatin analogue, can offer palliation after somatostatin analogue failure. For patients with unresectable disease confined to the liver, liver-directed therapy, such as hepatic artery embolization and radiofrequency ablation (discussed in subsequent subsections), should be considered for bulky disease, progression, or symptom palliation. A general approach for the therapy of unresectable disease is depicted in Fig. 23-2.

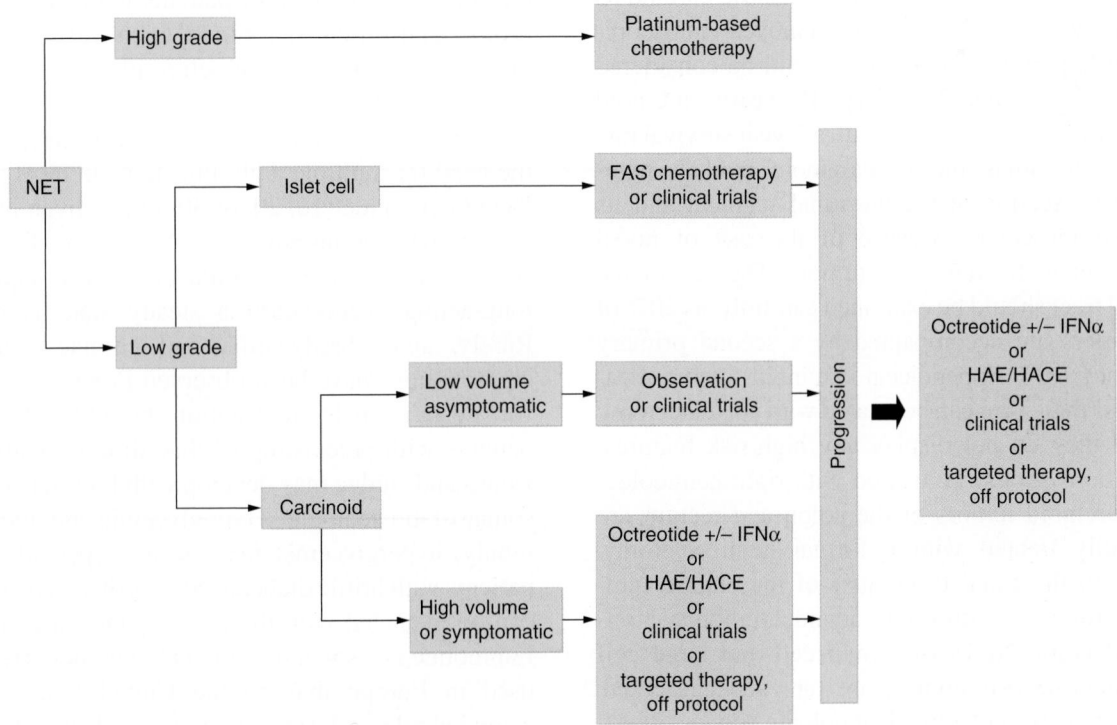

FIGURE 23-2. Approach to therapy for advanced neuroendocrine tumors. NET, neuroendocrine tumor; islet cell, islet cell carcinoma of pancreas; carcinoid, pulmonary, or gastrointestinal carcinoid; FAS chemotherapy, 5-fluorouracil, doxorubicin, streptozocin systemic chemotherapy; HAE, hepatic artery embolization; HACE, hepatic artery chemoembolization; IFNα, interferon-alfa. (*Modified, with permission, from Talamonti K, Yao J. Neuroendocrine tumors of the gastrointestinal tract: How aggressive should we be? American Society of Clinical Oncology 2004 Education Book. Alexandria, VA: American Society of Clinical Oncology, 2004; p. 206-215.*).

In general, NETs respond poorly to conventional chemotherapy. However, two situations are appropriate for initiation of cytotoxic therapy. High-grade NETs, because of their rapid rate of growth and responsiveness to platinum-based chemotherapy, are reasonable candidates for prompt initiation of systemic treatment. The second situation appropriate for cytotoxic therapy in advanced NETs is progressive, symptomatic metastatic or unresectable islet cell carcinoma. The authors' group at MD Anderson has noted radiographic response rates of nearly 40% in a series of 84 such patients, using a regimen of 5-fluorouracil, doxorubicin, and streptozocin (FAS). Importantly, several patients with a radiographic response in this series became surgical candidates for potentially curative resection after chemotherapy (40).

■ TREATMENT OF RESECTABLE NEUROENDOCRINE TUMORS

Surgery is the only treatment offering a potential cure for NET. The surgical management of gastrointestinal NET is dependent on multiple factors. The most important considerations are the site and histology of the primary tumor, the extent of detectable disease, and the clinical presentation. Types I and II gastric carcinoids measuring less than 2 cm can be removed endoscopically, while partial gastrectomy should be considered for tumors larger than 2 cm. Type III gastric carcinoid has a more aggressive course, with a 5-year survival rate less than 50%. Small intestine carcinoid should be managed with resection of the intestinal segment and its associated mesentery because of the risk of nodal involvement with even small tumors. The rest of the intestinal tract should be examined carefully, as 20% of these tumors are accompanied by a second primary malignancy (41). Appendiceal carcinoid tumors measuring less than 2 cm can be treated with appendectomy provided they do not display any high-risk features; larger lesions should be treated with right hemicolectomy. Carcinoid tumors of the colon and rectum are successfully treated with a formal hemicolectomy, adhering to the usual techniques of mesenteric lymphadenectomy as with colon adenocarcinoma. Noncarcinoid colon NETs (ie, small cell and large cell neuroendocrine carcinomas) are rare and aggressive and have a worse outcome than colonic adenocarcinomas; patients with one of these lesions have a median survival duration of approximately 10 months (42). As such, these patients rarely benefit from resection and are usually treated with chemotherapy.

■ TREATMENT OF ADVANCED NEUROENDOCRINE TUMORS

The current goal of treatment of advanced unresectable NET is amelioration of hormone-related symptoms. Reduction of tumor burden is also desirable, but the ultimate aim is palliation of symptoms. The current standard of care for hormone-related symptom control remains a somatostatin analogue. Other therapeutic methods, including the surgical resection of hepatic metastases, hepatic artery embolization/chemoembolization, and peptide receptor radionuclide therapy, an emerging technology, are occasionally useful. Identifying targeted therapies with the potential to alter the natural history of advanced NET and extend survival remains a key research effort.

SOMATOSTATIN ANALOGUES

Somatostain analogues such as octreotide, depot octreotide, and lanreotide are the frontline medications for control of symptoms associated with advanced/nonresectable carcinoid and VIPoma. Octreotide is an intermediate-acting somatostatin analogue that can be administered subcutaneously every 6 to 12 h. It provides complete resolution or partial relief of flushing or diarrhea in about 85% of patients with carcinoid syndrome, and produces a biochemical response rate of up to 72% (8). The dose of octreotide varies from 50 to 500 μg, three times a day.

Long-acting somatostatin analogues have obviated the need for multiple daily injections in most patients. Depot octreotide (10, 20, or 30 mg) is given intramuscularly once a month (43). An intermediate-acting somatostatin analogue should be used to supplement long-acting agents until a steady state is reached. Rarely, sinus bradycardia and cardiac conduction abnormalities have been observed in patients taking a somatostatin analogue. Caution should be observed in patients with preexisting cardiac disease. Gallbladder stones and sludge may develop with long-term use of a somatostatin analogue. Hypoglycemia and, more commonly, hyperglycemia may occur, especially among patients with brittle diabetes. Steatorrhea may occur but can be managed with the use of pancreatic enzymes. Lanreotide is a somatostatin analogue more frequently used in Europe than in the United States, and in extended release form, is administered subcutaneously once a month in doses of 60, 90, or 120 mg.

Somatostatin analogues may have cytostatic activity. Stabilization of growing NETs has been reported in nonrandomized phase II studies (44,45). Interim analysis of a phase III randomized trial of depot octreotide 30 mg monthly in untreated metastatic carcinoid of the midgut demonstrated that treated patients had a significantly longer time to progression than patients who received placebo (14.3 versus 6 months, $p < .001$), though this benefit was more prominent among patients with less than 10% hepatic volume replaced by tumor (46). Moreover, an international phase III trial is now under way to test the effect of lanreotide (120 mg, every 28 days) on progression-free survival in patients with a nonfunctioning NET (47).

SURGICAL RESECTION OF HEPATIC METASTASES

There are several important considerations in the evaluation of a patient with isolated hepatic metastases from a NET. In general, liver metastases are resectable if two basic criteria are satisfied: (a) all tumors in the liver can be completely resected and (b) an adequate volume of liver (20% of the standardized total liver volume) with adequate biliary drainage, arterial inflow, and venous outflow can be preserved. If the locoregional and hepatic tumor burden is completely resectable, then this is the preferred management of metastatic NETs whether functional or nonfunctional. Hepatic resection is most effective for low-grade NETs (48).

Unique to functional NETs is the concept of incomplete resection, or "debulking." Debulking at least 90% of the hepatic tumor burden in patients with functional metastases improves endocrinopathy-related symptoms and may prolong survival (49). Patients with unresectable hepatic NET metastases may benefit from liver-directed therapies such as radiofrequency ablation (alone or in combination with resection), hepatic artery infusion, bland hepatic artery embolization, or hepatic artery chemoembolization. Notably, hepatic artery embolization and surgical resection are equally effective in ameliorating pain and symptoms of hormonal excess (50).

HEPATIC ARTERIAL EMBOLIZATION AND HEPATIC ARTERIAL CHEMOEMBOLIZATION

Liver metastases from NETs are hypervascular, receiving between 80 and 100% of their blood supply via the hepatic artery; normal liver parenchyma, on the other hand, receives 60 to 70% of its perfusion from the portal vein. This feature is the rationale behind the use of transcatheter arterial embolization, which uses gelatin sponge or polyvinyl alcohol particles to treat these metastases by inducing tumor ischemia. Addition of a chemotherapeutic agent to the embolic material, also known as transcatheter arterial chemoembolization, allows delivery of relatively larger doses of chemotherapeutic agents directly to the tumor, and combines the local cytotoxic effect of chemotherapeutic agent with selective ischemia induced by embolization. Administration of an embolic agent also prolongs the intratumoral dwell time of the chemotherapeutic agent. The most frequently used chemotherapeutic agents for chemoembolization in patients with NET liver metastases include doxorubicin, cisplatin, mitomycin C, and streptozocin (51-63).

The generally accepted indications for embolization and chemoembolization in patients with NET hepatic metastases include relief of signs and symptoms related to hormonal excess or to tumor bulk, amelioration of rapid progression of liver disease, and reduction of tumor load before hepatic resection or tumor ablation. Many nonrandomized retrospective reports have shown that embolization and chemoembolization can reduce hormone levels, palliate symptoms, and reduce tumor burden in many patients with NET hepatic metastases. Review of the published clinical experience shows that use of embolization and chemoembolization can result in radiologic response in 25 to 83% and symptomatic response in 64.3 to 93% of patients with NET liver metastasis. The reported 5-year survival rates vary from 13.7 to 83% (51-63). These wide ranges in response rates and survival durations are related to the marked heterogeneity of various studies in terms of patient populations; treatment regimens used (embolization versus chemoembolization, number of sessions performed, type of chemotherapeutic agent, and embolization material); timing of embolization (ie, early or late in the clinical course); previous, concurrent, or subsequent use of octreotide and systemic chemotherapy; and the extent of liver involvement by metastatic disease.

Despite the theoretical advantages of chemoembolization over embolization, it is still unclear whether chemoembolization offers any therapeutic advantages over embolization in patients with metastatic NET to the liver. Review of results of various studies in the literature show no difference in the response rates for the two treatment methods (63). In a report from the authors' institution, Gupta et al. showed that, although chemoembolization did not show any therapeutic benefit over embolization in patients with carcinoid tumors, patients with islet cell carcinoma treated with chemoembolization had a tendency toward prolonged survival (31.5 versus 18.2 months) and an improved radiologic response rate (50 versus 25%) when compared with those treated with embolization alone (64). However, these differences didn't reach statistical significance. This was not an unexpected result, since carcinoid tumors classically have a lower response rate to systemic chemotherapy than islet cell carcinomas. Another retrospective multi-institutional review revealed that patients who underwent chemoembolization demonstrated trends toward improvements in time to progression, symptom control, and overall survival compared to patients who underwent embolization. Again, statistical significance was not achieved in this small cohort, but these results warrant further prospective randomized trials (65).

In patients with extensive liver tumor burden, only one lobe of the liver or a portion of one lobe is subjected to embolization during each session; in most cases, the hepatic lobe with the greatest tumor burden is treated first. Embolization of the whole liver in a single treatment session is not recommended because of the risk of prolonged postembolization syndrome or liver failure. Patients with extensive disease in the untreated portion of the liver, persistent symptoms, or inadequate hormonal response require additional sessions. The timing of subsequent embolizations is determined primarily by the patient's symptoms, biochemical or tumor status, and ability to tolerate the procedure.

It remains unclear whether embolization should be performed early or late in the clinical course of disease. Although some investigators advocate early embolization to reduce the tumor burden before initiation of systemic therapy, other studies suggest that late embolization can also be effective. In a randomized study, patients with carcinoid tumors treated at the time of diagnosis with liver embolization followed by IFN therapy had a higher objective response rate after 1 year (86%) than patients who received IFN only (42%). However, embolization was not shown to have any significant effect on survival (66). In a study by Eriksson et al., in which embolization or chemoembolization was performed at a median of 37 months after diagnosis, the median patient life expectancy after embolization was 80 months and the 5-year survival rate was 60%, indicating that "late" embolization is very effective (67). This is similar to the authors' experience at MD Anderson; duration of liver disease before embolization had no effect on response rates or overall or progression-free survival durations in either group of patients on univariate and multivariate analyses (64).

Involvement of more than 50% of the liver by metastatic disease has been considered an exclusion criterion in many reports because of the risk of inducing liver failure. Again, the authors' results suggest that, although median survival durations and response

rates are lower in patients with more than 75% liver disease, many of these patients can benefit from selective embolizations, if small portions of the liver are embolized in sessions that are well separated in time (68).

Postembolization syndrome is the most common adverse effect of embolization/chemoembolization; it is characterized by nausea, vomiting, abdominal pain, malaise, fever, leukocytosis, and elevation of liver function enzyme levels. Postembolization syndrome is generally self-limited, improving with conservative management, but can occasionally be severe and require prolonged hospitalization. Major complications such as liver and/or renal failure, gallbladder perforation, cholangitis, peptic ulcer hemorrhage, and abscess formation have been observed but are rare (69). Embolization/chemoembolization procedures can stimulate release of hormones by functional liver tumors, resulting in carcinoid crisis. This can be prevented by administration of a somatostatin analogue before these procedures.

Y-90 MICROSPHERE BRACHYTHERAPY, RADIOEMBOLIZATION, OR SELECTIVE INTERNAL RADIATION THERAPY

Intra-arterial radioembolization with yttrium-90 (^{90}Y) microspheres is an emerging technique that is being used increasingly in patients with unresectable primary and/or metastatic liver lesions. Yttrium-90 is a pure B emitter with a mean soft tissue penetration of 2.5 mm and a maximal depth of 1.1 cm. Two FDA-approved ^{90}Y microsphere products are in clinical use at present: TheraSphere (MDS Nordion Inc., Kanata, Ontario, Canada), a glass microsphere, and the resin-based SIR-Spheres (SIRTeX Medical Ltd., Sydney, New South Wales, Australia). The ^{90}Y micrsopheres, when selectively injected via the hepatic artery, are preferentially distributed into the tumoral and peritumoral vasculature, allowing delivery of radiation to the tumor in high enough doses to result in tumor necrosis while sparing the surrounding normal liver parenchyma. Radioembolization with ^{90}Y has a significantly lower incidence of postembolization syndrome than embolization or chemoembolization, allowing it to be performed as an outpatient procedure. However, a great degree of care must be taken with the use of ^{90}Y radioembolization in order to avoid nontarget delivery of radioactive microspheres to organs such as the stomach, duodenum, and pancreas. It is essential to perform an angiogram with selective embolization of all extrahepatic arteries before the treatment. Technetium-99 macroaggregated albumin is also injected at this moment to estimate the hepatopulmonary shunt fraction so that the risk of radiation-induced pneumonitis can be minimized.

The literature on the use of radioembolization for treatment of neuroendocrine liver metastases is limited. In a retrospective review of 148 patients with liver metastases from NET treated with 185 separate radioembolization procedures using resin ^{90}Y microspheres, Kennedy et al. observed a complete response in 3%, partial response in 66.7%, stable disease in 25%, and progressive disease in 5.3% of patients. The median survival duration was 70 months (70). In a recent prospective study that involved nine patients with unresectable liver metastases from NETs treated with ^{90}Y radioembolization, partial response was seen in six patients (66%), and survival rates were 100% and 57% for 1 and 3 years, respectively. No major complications occurred (71). These initial results suggest that ^{90}Y radioembolization represents a viable alternative therapy for patients with hepatic NET tumors, especially in those in whom traditional therapies have failed. Further investigation, long-term follow-up, and prospective clinical trials are warranted to determine the exact role of this treatment method in the management of NET hepatic metastases.

PEPTIDE RECEPTOR RADIONUCLIDE THERAPY

More recently, radiolabeled somatostatin analogues have been developed that are based on the somatostatin receptor properties of these tumors. Two recent studies have been reported in which intra-arterial administration of one of these radiolabeled somatostatin analogues has resulted in modest treatment responses. McStay et al., in a study of 23 patients with NET hepatic metastases treated with intra-arterial ^{90}Y-DOTA-lanreotide, reported a response rate of 16% and 1-year survival rate of 63% (72). More recently, Limouris et al. observed a complete or partial response in 53% and a survival duration of 32 months in 70.5% in their series of 17 patients treated with hepatic arterial infusion of ^{111}In-DTPA-D-Phe^1-octreotide (73). Currently, neither of these therapies is available in the United States.

RADIOFREQUENCY ABLATION

Local thermal ablative therapies such as radiofrequency ablation (RFA) are being used increasingly for treatment of primary and metastatic liver tumors. Radiofrequency ablation involves placement of a needle-like probe directly in the liver tumor, and can be done percutaneously or intraoperatively using image-guidance techniques. The radiofrequency waves passing through the probe increase the temperature within tumor tissue, resulting in destruction of the tumor.

Radiofrequency ablation has been used for palliative treatment of hormone-related symptoms in selected patients with NET liver metastases, alleviating those symptoms in 69 to 80% of cases (74,75). Furthermore, RFA may achieve local control of liver metastases in as many as 74% of patients. The use of RFA is generally limited to patients with five or fewer lesions in the liver, each tumor measuring less than 3 cm in size. Achieving complete necrosis with RFA in tumors larger than 3 cm in diameter is difficult. The largest reported series using RFA in patients with NET liver metastases consisted of 34 patients with 234 tumors who were treated in 42 sessions with laparoscopic RFA. The intent of therapy was palliative in 28 patients and curative in 6. The number of tumors treated in each patient ranged from 1 to 16, and the mean tumor diameter was 2.3 cm (range, 0.5-10 cm). "Complete" or "significant" symptom relief was achieved in 80% of the symptomatic patients and lasted an average of 10 months (range, 6-24 months). The mean survival duration was 1.6 years (74).

BIOTHERAPY

Interferon-alpha can induce biochemical response in most patients with carcinoid syndrome (8). The combination of octreotide and IFN$\acute{\alpha}$ may have a synergistic effect on symptom control and biochemical responses in NETs (76-78). However, IFN$\acute{\alpha}$ is more toxic than somatostatin analogues, with adverse effects such as fatigue, fever, anorexia, psychiatric disturbances, and weight loss. In the authors' academic practice at MD Anderson, the use of IFN$\acute{\alpha}$ is usually reserved for patients with symptoms refractory to single-agent somatostatin analogue therapy.

BIOCHEMOTHERAPY

The combination of chemotherapy (streptozocin and doxorubicin or 5-fluorouracil) plus IFN$\acute{\alpha}$ does not improve response rate in NETs (76,79).

EFFICACY OF CHEMOTHERAPY IN CARCINOIDS AND ISLET CELL CARCINOMAS

Carcinoids are resistant to conventional cytotoxic chemotherapy (79). As already mentioned, triple-agent therapy with 5-fluorouracil, doxorubicin, and streptozocin has activity in islet cell carcinomas (40). The FAS regimen is typically employed when islet cell carcinoma patients become symptomatic despite octreotide therapy. Scant data exist to support the use of FAS in metastatic carcinoid.

ADDITIONAL SYMPTOM CONTROL METHODS

Carcinoid symptoms may be controlled or even eliminated by avoiding stress, minimizing tryptophan-rich foods, and supplementing dietary nicotinamide. Medical management of carcinoid symptoms can include a bronchodilator for bronchospasm, loperamide or diphenoxylate for frequent, loose bowel movements, and diuretics for fluid overload secondary to valvular dysfunction. A proton pump inhibitor should be given for managing gastric hypersecretion in patients with gastrinoma.

■ TARGETED THERAPY

The identification of effective targeted therapy for NETs is an active area of research. Phase II trials of modern targeted molecular therapies as single agents are summarized in Table 23-5. A study comparing VEGF inhibitor bevacizumab and monthly depot octreotide versus pegylated IFNά-2b and depot octreotide in 44 patients with metastatic carcinoid demonstrated 95% progression-free survival at 18 weeks in the former versus 68% in the latter. A radiographic response rate of 18% was observed in the bevacizumab/depot octreotide arm, whereas there were no responses in the IFNά-2b/depot octreotide arm (81). Bevacizumab in combination with temozolimide has demonstrated a 14% radiographic response rate (all partial responses) in pancreatic NETs in a separate phase II trial (82).

Inhibition of the VEGF receptor by sunitinib has also shown promise in a phase II trial. Kulke and associates report a 16% overall response rate in advanced islet cell carcinoma as well as median times to progression of 7.7 and 10.2 months in advanced islet cell carcinomas and carcinoids, respectively (83). A planned interim analysis of an international phase III trial of oral sunitinib 37.5 mg daily versus placebo in 154 patients with advanced pancreatic NET demonstrated progression-free survival durations of 11.1 versus 5.5 months by investigator review, in favor of sunitinib ($p < .001$). These results are preliminary, however, and overall survival data from this trial are not yet available (84).

Everolimus, or RAD001, an inhibitor of the mammalian target of rapamycin (mTOR), has proven efficacious alone and in combination with depot octreotide. In a phase II study of patients with advanced carcinoid or islet cell carcinoma, an overall response rate of 22% and progression-free survival duration of 60 weeks were observed (85). Everolimus has also shown clinical

TABLE 23-5	PHASE II TRIALS OF TARGETED MOLECULAR AGENTS IN ADVANCED CARCINOID AND ISLET CELL CARCINOMA			
Agent(s)	Number of Patients	Median PFS	CR/PR/OR	Reference
Bevacizumab + octreotide LAR	22	66 weeks	0/18/18%	(81)
Bevacizumab + temozolimide	34	8.6 months	0/14/14%	(82)
Bortezomib	16	N/A	0/0/0%	(90)
Everolimus + octreotide LAR	60	60 weeks	0/22/22%	(81)
Everolimus	115 (islet cell)	9.7 months (islet cell)	0/9.6/9.6% (islet cell)	(86)
Gefitinib	37	30% at 6 months, (carcinoid) 14% at the rate of 6 months, (islet cell)	0/4/4%	(91)
Imatinib	27	24 weeks	0/3/3%	(92)
Sunitinib	107	10.2 months, carcinoid (TTP) 7.7 months, islet cell (TTP)	0/11/11% 0/16.7/16.7% (islet cell)	(83)
Temsirolimus	36	6 months (TTP)	0/5.5/5.5%	(93)

CR, complete response rate; OR, overall response rate; PFS, progression-free survival; PR, partial response rate; TTP, time to progression.

efficacy as a single agent in advanced islet cell carcinomas progressing after prior chemotherapy (86). Current, ongoing multicenter phase III studies of modern targeted agents' effects on progression-free survival include investigations of bevacizumab/octreotide versus IFNά-2b/octreotide in advanced carcinoid (87), everolimus/octreotide versus placebo/octreotide in advanced carcinoid (88), and everolimus versus placebo in islet cell carcinoma (89).

■ NEUROENDOCRINE TUMOR CASES

The following three clinical vignettes, based on actual patients in our practice, reinforce (a) the typical clinical presentations of metastatic carcinoid and islet cell carcinoma disease, (b) the symptom control modalities currently in use (medical and surgical), and (c) the prolonged natural history of metastatic carcinoid and islet cell carcinoma disease. We hope these clinical cases serve as a guide to what to expect in the patient with metastatic carcinoid for the practitioner who encounters this disease infrequently.

CASE 1: NEW DIAGNOSIS OF METASTASTIC CARCINOID OF THE SMALL INTESTINE

Patient 1 presented to our clinic to confirm diagnosis of metastatic carcinoid and discuss treatment options. For 3 years prior to our first clinical encounter, this 62-year-old man experienced frequent watery stools that disrupted his daily activities. This condition worsened progressively; he described "massive" watery bowel movements six to eight times a day in the months just before our first encounter. During this time, he first experienced flushing, as often as three times a day. His primary care physician suspected carcinoid disease and ordered a 24-hour 5-HIAA urine measurement; elevated levels demonstrated increased serotonin metabolism. Imaging ordered by his local physicians revealed bilobar hepatic metastases as well as a mesenteric nodal mass in direct contact with the ileum, the likely primary site of disease. This gentleman's primary care physician referred him to an oncologist who in turn initiated octreotide, 50 µg subcutaneously three times daily, for roughly 1 month before our initial clinical encounter. This intervention resolved his symptoms of watery diarrhea and greatly lessened his flushing. We confirmed his diagnosis with an ultrasound-guided biopsy of the liver.

Our care plan for Patient 1 focused on symptom control. We switched him to a long-acting octreotide

analogue, octreotide LAR 30 mg, for monthly intramuscular injection. We planned abdominal imaging 3 months after the initial encounter to assess the extent of disease progression; if his disease has stabilized, our surgical services may intervene and remove his mesenteric mass to prevent obstruction of the associated ileum. Nonetheless, the mainstay of this gentleman's treatment will be medical, with the ultimate goal to control symptoms.

CASE 2: METASTATIC, SYMPTOMATIC VIPOMA

Patient 2, a 63-year-old man with a nearly 10-year history of VIPoma, represents the challenge of symptom control in metastatic islet cell carcinoma that progressed after the initial treatment. His oncologic history is notable for a remote partial pancreatectomy at the time of diagnosis and resulting insulin dependence as well as liver metastases and multiple hepatic arterial embolization procedures, and, 5 years ago, eight cycles of FAS chemotherapy with a clinical response allowing discontinuation of octreotide LAR. Three or 4 months prior to our most recent clinical encounter, however, he noted an increase in frequency and volume of watery bowel movements. Reinitiation of the long-acting octreotide failed to control this symptom. His outside oncologist placed him on a shorter-acting octreotide, twice daily; his frequency and volume of stool nonetheless increased.

Patient 2 subsequently presented to an outside hospital, roughly 6 weeks before our office visit, with dehydration and diabetic ketoacidosis. A continuous infusion of octreotide controlled his bowel movements; he was discharged on short-acting octreotide, 400 µg every 8 h. This intervention never achieved adequate symptom control; within a week he presented to the MD Anderson Emergency Center in diabetic ketoacidosis caused by profound dehydration from near-constant watery bowel movements. During this admission, octreotide infusion was again started and our service was consulted. We arranged for him to see his outside oncologist and for initiation of IFNα-2b soon after discharge. Treatment with IFNα-2b, 3 million units subcutaneously three times weekly, achieved symptom control. When seen in the office a month after his most recent discharge, he reported only one to two bowel movements a day of moderate consistency; his regimen also includes long-acting octreotide (ie, octreotide LAR 30 mg intramuscularly each month) as well as short-acting octretotide 200 µg subcutaneously three times daily.

Imaging studies showed relative stability of tumor volume despite the increasing symptoms. Additional clinical options for Patient 2 are limited. Not surprisingly, this patient's pancreatic islet cell disease (VIPoma) exhibited a response to FAS chemotherapy 5 years ago. However, resumption of this regimen is risky because of the cumulative exposure to anthracycline and the low probability of major response. The current situation of Patient 2 calls for optimizing symptom control with somatostatin analogues and biological therapy with IFNα. This patient will benefit from introduction to our palliative care service.

CASE 3: METASTASTIC RECTAL CARCINOID

The case of Patient 3 presents clinical challenges and objectives different than those of Patients 1 and 2. Five years prior to our most recent encounter, a screening colonoscopy identified an asymptomatic rectal carcinoid. Subsequent imaging identified multiple metastatic lesions in the liver. At diagnosis, this individual manifested no evidence of carcinoid syndrome; his diagnosis could be characterized as an "incidentaloma." He did undergo a transanal excision of the primary lesion to prevent obstructive complications. In the year after his diagnosis, this gentleman underwent hepatic artery embolization twice, as imaging demonstrated extensive parenchymal replacement by metastasis. We elected to treat him off protocol with octreotide LAR and bevacizumab every 3 weeks for roughly 18 months. His disease burden remained stable during this period. Ultimately, progression of liver metastases prompted referral to our phase I clinic, though his disease remained asymptomatic. Over the course of the subsequent year, this gentleman's hepatic disease progressed on multiple phase I agents as well as a phase I hepatic artery chemoembolization protocol.

The first symptoms Patient 3 manifested were diplopia and vision loss, roughly 4 years after initial diagnosis. Appropriate imaging and biopsy demonstrated metastatic disease to his left orbit, and he underwent external beam radiation therapy and then surgical debulking 5 years after his initial diagnosis. When seen in the clinic recently, he reported fatigue and anorexia (related to tumor burden and mass effect) without evidence of hormonal symptoms. In this situation, best supportive care under the supervision of the palliative care service was felt to be appropriate.

■ CONCLUSION

The multidisciplinary approach to effective, efficient diagnosis and treatment of both localized and advanced NETs is paramount. The care of the patient with localized NET disease requires the expertise of both the surgeon and the pathologist. The patient with advanced NET presents the physician with different challenges, and interventional radiologists in addition to medical oncologists have a role to play in symptom control. Unfortunately, the options presently available to the medical oncologist to halt or prolong the natural history of advanced NET disease are currently limited. However, several ongoing phase III trials address the effectiveness of newer and promising targeted therapies in delaying the progression of disease in advanced NET. Specific targets include VEGF (bevacizumab), the VEGF receptor (sunitinib), and mTOR (everolimus). Notably, the clinical utility of several targeted agents is being evaluated both as single-agent therapy and in combination with depot octreotide. Furthermore, the potential of somatostatin analogues alone to alter the natural history of advanced NETs is the subject of ongoing clinical investigation. This research will, we hope, produce an evidence-based strategy, possibly employing targeted therapy and/or somatostatin analogues, to prolong overall survival in patients with advanced NET.

References

1. Yao JC, Hassan M, Phan A, et al. One hundred years after "carcinoid": Epidemiology of and prognostic factors for neuroendocrine tumors in 35,825 cases in the United States. *J Clin Oncol* 2008;26(18):3063-3072.
2. Moertel CG, Sauer WG, Dockerty MB, et al. Life history of the carcinoid tumor of the small intestine. *Cancer* 1961;14: 901-912.
3. Berge T, Linell F. Carcinoid tumours. Frequency in a defined population during a 12-year period. *Acta Pathol Microbiol Scand A* 1976;84(4):322-330.
4. Modlin IM, Lye KD, Kidd M. A 5-decade analysis of 13,715 carcinoid tumors. *Cancer* 2003;97(4):934-959.
5. Toumpanakis CG, Caplin ME. Molecular genetics of gastroenteropancreatic neuroendocrine tumors. *Am J Gastroenterol* 2008;103(3):729-732.
6. Yang Y, Hua X. In search of tumor suppressing functions of menin. *Mol Cell Endocrinol* 2007;265-266:34-41.
7. Fujiki K, Duerr EM, Kikuchi H, et al. Hoxc6 is overexpressed in gastrointestinal carcinoids and interacts with JunD to regulate tumor growth. *Gastroenterology* 2008;135(3):907-916, 916 e1-e2.
8. Schnirer, II, Yao JC, Ajani JA. Carcinoid—a comprehensive review. *Acta Oncol* 2003;42(7):672-692.
9. Wang L, Ignat A, Axiotis CA. Differential expression of the PTEN tumor suppressor protein in fetal and adult neuroendocrine tissues and tumors: Progressive loss of PTEN expression in poorly differentiated neuroendocrine neoplasms. *Appl Immunohistochem Mol Morphol* 2002;10(2): 139-146.

10. Terris B, Scoazec JY, Rubbia L, et al. Expression of vascular endothelial growth factor in digestive neuroendocrine tumours. *Histopathology* 1998;32(2):133-138.

11. Krishnamurthy S, Dayal Y. Immunohistochemical expression of transforming growth factor alpha and epidermal growth factor receptor in gastrointestinal carcinoids. *Am J Surg Pathol* 1997;21(3):327-333.

12. Chaudhry A, Papanicolaou V, Oberg K, et al. Expression of platelet-derived growth factor and its receptors in neuroendocrine tumors of the digestive system. *Cancer Res* 1992; 52(4):1006-1012.

13. Tonnies H, Toliat MR, Ramel C, et al. Analysis of sporadic neuroendocrine tumours of the enteropancreatic system by comparative genomic hybridisation. *Gut* 2001;48(4):536-541.

14. Kytola S, Hoog A, Nord B, et al. Comparative genomic hybridization identifies loss of 18q22-qter as an early and specific event in tumorigenesis of midgut carcinoids. *Am J Pathol* 2001;158(5):1803-1808.

15. Kim do H, Nagano Y, Choi IS, et al. Allelic alterations in well-differentiated neuroendocrine tumors (carcinoid tumors) identified by genome-wide single nucleotide polymorphism analysis and comparison with pancreatic endocrine tumors. *Genes Chromosomes Cancer* 2008;47(1):84-92.

16. Anlauf M, Garbrecht N, Bauersfeld J, et al. Hereditary neuroendocrine tumors of the gastroenteropancreatic system. *Virchows Arch* 2007;451(Suppl 1):S29-S38.

17. Neuroendocrine tumors. In: Edge SB, Byrd DR, Compton CC, et al. (eds): *AJCC Cancer Staging Manual*, 7th ed. Springer; 2010.

18. Tamm EP, Kim EE, Ng CS. Imaging of neuroendocrine tumors. *Hematol Oncol Clin North Am* 2007;21(3):409-432, vii.

19. Krenning EP, Kooij PP, Bakker WH, et al. Radiotherapy with a radiolabeled somatostatin analogue, [111In-DTPA-D-Phe1]-octreotide. A case history. *Ann N Y Acad Sci* 1994;733:496-506.

20. Eriksson B, Bergstrom M, Lilja A, et al. Positron emission tomography (PET) in neuroendocrine gastrointestinal tumors. *Acta Oncol* 1993;32(2):189-196.

21. Eriksson B, Bergstrom M, Sundin A, et al. The role of PET in localization of neuroendocrine and adrenocortical tumors. *Ann N Y Acad Sci* 2002;970:159-169.

22. Vinik AI, Thompson N, Eckhauser F, et al. Clinical features of carcinoid syndrome and the use of somatostatin analogue in its management. *Acta Oncol* 1989;28(3):389-402.

23. Feldman JM. Carcinoid tumors and the carcinoid syndrome. *Curr Probl Surg* 1989;26(12):835-885.

24. Hanson MW, Feldman JM, Blinder RA, et al. Carcinoid tumors: Iodine-131 MIBG scintigraphy. *Radiology* 1989;172(3): 699-703.

25. Exocrine and endocrine pancreas. In: Edge SB, Byrd DR, Compton CC, et al. (eds) *AJCC Cancer Staging Manual*, 7th ed. 2010.

26. Nilsson O. Gastrointestinal carcinoids—aspects of diagnosis and classification. *APMIS* 1996;104(7-8):481-492.

27. Stinner B, Rothmund M. Neuroendocrine tumours (carcinoids) of the appendix. *Best Pract Res Clin Gastroenterol* 2005; 19(5):729-738.

28. Goede AC, Caplin ME, Winslet MC. Carcinoid tumour of the appendix. *Br J Surg* 2003;90(11):1317-1322.

29. Kwaan MR, Goldberg JE, Bleday R. Rectal carcinoid tumors: Review of results after endoscopic and surgical therapy. *Arch Surg* 2008;143(5):471-475.

30. Wang AY, Ahmad NA. Rectal carcinoids. *Curr Opin Gastroenterol* 2006;22(5):529-535.

31. Kulke MH, Bergsland EK, Yao JC. Glycemic control in patients with insulinoma treated with everolimus. *N Engl J Med* 2009;360(2):195-197.

32. Tucker ON, Crotty PL, Conlon KC. The management of insulinoma. *Br J Surg* 2006;93(3):264-275.

33. Fendrich V, Langer P, Waldmann J, et al. Management of sporadic and multiple endocrine neoplasia type 1 gastrinomas. *Br J Surg* 2007;94(11):1331-1341.

34. Doherty GM. Rare endocrine tumours of the GI tract. *Best Pract Res Clin Gastroenterol* 2005;19(5):807-817.

35. Schonfeld WH, Eikin EP, Woltering EA, et al. The cost-effectiveness of octreotide acetate in the treatment of carcinoid syndrome and VIPoma. *Int J Technol Assess Health Care* 1998; 14(3):514-525.

36. Sakai H, Kodaira S, Ono K, et al. Disseminated pancreatic polypeptidioma. *Intern Med* 1993;32(9):737-741.

37. Bhattacharyya S, Toumpanakis C, Caplin ME, et al. Analysis of 150 patients with carcinoid syndrome seen in a single year at one institution in the first decade of the twenty-first century. *Am J Cardiol* 2008;101(3):378-381.

38. NCCN. Neuroendocrine Tumors. 2009. http://www.nccn.org/professionals/physician_gls/PDF/neuroendocrine.pdf.Accessed 10/25/2010.

39. Dierdorf SF. Carcinoid tumor and carcinoid syndrome. *Curr Opin Anaesthesiol* 2003;16(3):343-347.

40. Kouvaraki MA, Ajani JA, Hoff P, et al. Fluorouracil, doxorubicin, and streptozocin in the treatment of patients with locally advanced and metastatic pancreatic endocrine carcinomas. *J Clin Oncol* 2004;22(23):4762-4771.

41. Memon MA, Nelson H. Gastrointestinal carcinoid tumors: Current management strategies. *Dis Colon Rectum* 1997; 40(9):1101-1118.

42. Bernick PE, Klimstra DS, Shia J, et al. Neuroendocrine carcinomas of the colon and rectum. *Dis Colon Rectum* 2004; 47(2):163-169.

43. Rubin J, Ajani J, Schirmer W, et al. Octreotide acetate long-acting formulation versus open-label subcutaneous octreotide acetate in malignant carcinoid syndrome. *J Clin Oncol* 1999; 17(2):600-606.

44. Saltz L, Trochanowski B, Buckley M, et al. Octreotide as an antineoplastic agent in the treatment of functional and nonfunctional neuroendocrine tumors. *Cancer* 1993;72(1):244-248.

45. Arnold R, Benning R, Neuhaus C, et al. Gastroenteropancreatic endocrine tumours: Effect of Sandostatin on tumour growth. The German Sandostatin Study Group. *Digestion* 1993;54(Suppl 1): 72-75.

46. Rinke A, Muller HH, Schade-Brittinger C, et al. Placebo-controlled, double-blind, prospective, randomized study on the effect of octreotide LAR in the control of tumor growth in patients with metastatic neuroendocrine midgut tumors: A report from the PROMID Study Group. *J Clin Oncol* 2009; 27(28):4656-4663.

47. Clincaltrials.gov. Phase III, randomised, double-blind, stratified comparative, placebo controlled, parallel group, multi-centre study to assess the effect of deep subcutaneous injections of lanreotide autogel 120 mg administered every 28 days on tumour progression free survival in patients with non-functioning entero-pancreatic endocrine tumour, 2006. http:// www.clinicaltrials. gov/ ct2/show/ NCT00353496? term= lanreotide+autogel+120+ mg&rank=7.

48. Cho CS, Labow DM, Tang L, et al. Histologic grade is correlated with outcome after resection of hepatic neuroendocrine neoplasms. *Cancer* 2008;113(1):126-134.

49. Que FG, Nagorney DM, Batts KP, et al. Hepatic resection for metastatic neuroendocrine carcinomas. *Am J Surg* 1995; 169(1):36-42; discussion 42-43.

50. Chamberlain RS, Canes D, Brown KT, et al. Hepatic neuroendocrine metastases: Does intervention alter outcomes? *J Am Coll Surg* 2000;190(4):432-445.

51. Liu DM, Kennedy A, Turner D, et al. Minimally invasive techniques in management of hepatic neuroendocrine metastatic disease. *Am J Clin Oncol* 2009;32(2):200-215.

52. Hajarizadeh H, Ivancev K, Mueller CR, et al. Effective palliative treatment of metastatic carcinoid tumors with intra-arterial chemotherapy/chemoembolization combined with octreotide acetate. *Am J Surg* 1992;163(5):479-483.

53. Ruszniewski P, Rougier P, Roche A, et al. Hepatic arterial chemoembolization in patients with liver metastases of endocrine tumors. A prospective phase II study in 24 patients. *Cancer* 1993;71(8):2624-2630.

54. Therasse E, Breittmayer F, Roche A, et al. Transcatheter chemoembolization of progressive carcinoid liver metastasis. *Radiology* 1993;189(2):541-547.

55. Kim YH, Ajani JA, Carrasco CH, et al. Selective hepatic arterial chemoembolization for liver metastases in patients with carcinoid tumor or islet cell carcinoma. *Cancer Invest* 1999; 17(7):474-478.

56. Dominguez S, Denys A, Madeira I, et al. Hepatic arterial chemoembolization with streptozotocin in patients with metastatic digestive endocrine tumours. *Eur J Gastroenterol Hepatol* 2000;12(2):151-157.

57. Carrasco CH, Chuang VP, Wallace S. Apudomas metastatic to the liver: Treatment by hepatic artery embolization. *Radiology* 1983;149(1):79-83.

58. Roche A, Girish BV, de Baere T, et al. Trans-catheter arterial chemoembolization as first-line treatment for hepatic metastases from endocrine tumors. *Eur Radiol* 2003;13(1): 136-140.

59. Drougas JG, Anthony LB, Blair TK, et al. Hepatic artery chemoembolization for management of patients with advanced metastatic carcinoid tumors. *Am J Surg* 1998;175(5): 408-412.

60. Gupta S, Yao JC, Ahrar K, et al. Hepatic artery embolization and chemoembolization for treatment of patients with metastatic carcinoid tumors: The M.D. Anderson experience. *Cancer J* 2003;9(4):261-267.

61. Mavligit GM, Pollock RE, Evans HL, et al. Durable hepatic tumor regression after arterial chemoembolization-infusion in patients with islet cell carcinoma of the pancreas metastatic to the liver. *Cancer* 1993;72(2):375-380.

62. Loewe C, Schindl M, Cejna M, et al. Permanent transarterial embolization of neuroendocrine metastases of the liver using cyanoacrylate and lipiodol: Assessment of mid- and long-term results. *AJR Am J Roentgenol* 2003;180(5):1379-1384.

63. Madoff DC, Gupta S, Ahrar K, et al. Update on the management of neuroendocrine hepatic metastases. *J Vasc Interv Radiol* 2006;17(8):1235-1249; quiz 1250.

64. Gupta S, Johnson MM, Murthy R, et al. Hepatic arterial embolization and chemoembolization for the treatment of patients with metastatic neuroendocrine tumors: Variables affecting response rates and survival. *Cancer* 2005;104(8): 1590-1602.

65. Ruutiainen AT, Soulen MC, Tuite CM, et al. Chemoembolization and bland embolization of neuroendocrine tumor metastases to the liver. *J Vasc Interv Radiol* 2007;18(7):847-855.

66. Hanssen LE, Schrumpf E, Kolbenstvedt AN, et al. Recombinant alpha-2 interferon with or without hepatic artery embolization in the treatment of midgut carcinoid tumours. A preliminary report. *Acta Oncol* 1989;28(3):439-443.

67. Eriksson BK, Larsson EG, Skogseid BM, et al. Liver embolizations of patients with malignant neuroendocrine gastrointestinal tumors. *Cancer* 1998;83(11):2293-2301.

68. Kamat PP, Gupta S, Ensor JE, et al. Hepatic arterial embolization and chemoembolization in the management of patients with large-volume liver metastases. *Cardiovasc Intervent Radiol* 2008;31(2):299-307.

69. O'Toole D, Ruszniewski P. Chemoembolization and other ablative therapies for liver metastases of gastrointestinal endocrine tumours. *Best Pract Res Clin Gastroenterol* 2005; 19(4):585-594.

70. Kennedy AS, Dezarn WA, McNeillie P, et al. Radioembolization for unresectable neuroendocrine hepatic metastases using resin 90Y-microspheres: Early results in 148 patients. *Am J Clin Oncol* 2008;31(3):271-279.

71. Kalinowski M, Dressler M, Konig A, et al. Selective internal radiotherapy with Yttrium-90 microspheres for hepatic metastatic neuroendocrine tumors: A prospective single center study. *Digestion* 2009;79(3):137-142.

72. McStay MK, Maudgil D, Williams M, et al. Large-volume liver metastases from neuroendocrine tumors: Hepatic intraarterial 90Y-DOTA-lanreotide as effective palliative therapy. *Radiology* 2005;237(2):718-726.

73. Limouris GS, Chatziioannou A, Kontogeorgakos D, et al. Selective hepatic arterial infusion of In-111-DTPA-Phe1-octreotide in neuroendocrine liver metastases. Eur J Nucl Med Mol Imaging. 2008;35(10):1827-1837.

74. Berber E, Flesher N, Siperstein AE. Laparoscopic radiofrequency ablation of neuroendocrine liver metastases. *World J Surg* 2002;26(8):985-990.

75. Gillams A, Cassoni A, Conway G, et al. Radiofrequency ablation of neuroendocrine liver metastases: The Middlesex experience. *Abdom Imaging* 2005;30(4):435-441.

76. Janson ET, Ronnblom L, Ahlstrom H, et al. Treatment with alpha-interferon versus alpha-interferon in combination with streptozocin and doxorubicin in patients with malignant carcinoid tumors: A randomized trial. *Ann Oncol* 1992;3(8):635-638.

77. Janson ET, Kauppinen HL, Oberg K. Combined alpha- and gamma-interferon therapy for malignant midgut carcinoid tumors. A phase I-II trial. *Acta Oncol* 1993;32(2):231-233.

78. Frank M, Klose KJ, Wied M, et al. Combination therapy with octreotide and alpha-interferon: Effect on tumor growth in metastatic endocrine gastroenteropancreatic tumors. *Am J Gastroenterol* 1999;94(5):1381-1387.

79. Saltz L, Kemeny N, Schwartz G, et al. A phase II trial of alpha-interferon and 5-fluorouracil in patients with advanced carcinoid and islet cell tumors. *Cancer* 1994;74(3):958-961.

80. Strosberg JR, Nasir A, Hodul P, et al. Biology and treatment of metastatic gastrointestinal neuroendocrine tumors. *Gastrointest Cancer Res* 2008;2(3):113-125.

81. Yao JC, Phan A, Hoff PM, et al. Targeting vascular endothelial growth factor in advanced carcinoid tumor: A random assignment phase II study of depot octreotide with bevacizumab and pegylated interferon alpha-2b. *J Clin Oncol* 2008;26(8):1316-1323.

82. Kulke MH, Stuart KM, Earle CC, et al. A phase II study of temozolomide and bevacizumab in patients with advanced neuroendocrine tumors. ASCO 2006, Atlanta, Georgia, 2006.

83. Kulke MH, Lenz HJ, Meropol NJ, et al. Activity of sunitinib in patients with advanced neuroendocrine tumors. *J Clin Oncol* 2008;26(20):3403-3410.

84. Raoul JL, Niccoli P, Bang YJ, et al. Sunitinib (SU) vs placebo for treatment of progressive, well-differentiated pancreatic islet cell tumours: Results of a phase III, randomised, double-blind trial. *Eur J Cancer Suppl*;7(2):361.

85. Yao JC, Phan AT, Chang DZ, et al. Efficacy of RAD001 (everolimus) and octreotide LAR in advanced low- to intermediate-grade neuroendocrine tumors: Results of a phase II study. *J Clin Oncol* 2008;26(26):4311-4318.

86. Yao JC, Lombard-Bohas C, Baudin E, et al. Daily oral everolimus activity in patients with metastatic pancreatic neuroendocrine tumors after failure of cytotoxic chemotherapy: A phase II trial. *J Clin Oncol* 2010;28(1):69-76.

87. Clincaltrials.gov. Phase III prospective, randomized comparison of depot octreotide plus interferon alpha versus depot octreotide plus bevacizumab (NSC #704865) in advanced, poor prognosis carcinoid patients, 2007. http://www.clinicaltrials.gov/ct2/show/NCT00569127?term=octreotide+plus+bevacizumab&rank=1.

88. Clincaltrials.gov. A randomized, double-blind placebo-controlled, multicenter phase III study in patients with advanced carcinoid tumor receiving octreotide depot and everolimus 10 mg/day or octreotide depot and placebo, 2006. http://www.clinicaltrials.gov/ct2/show/NCT00412061?term=octreotide+depot+and+everolimus&rank=1.

89. Clinicaltrials.gov. A Randomized double-blind phase III study of RAD001 10 mg/d plus best supportive care versus placebo plus best supportive care in the treatment of patients with advanced pancreatic neuroendocrine tumor (NET), 2007.

90. Shah MH, Young D, Kindler HL, et al. Phase II study of the proteasome inhibitor bortezomib (PS-341) in patients with metastatic neuroendocrine tumors. *Clin Cancer Res* 2004; 10(18 Pt 1):6111-6118.

91. Hobday T, Holen K, Donehower R et al. A phase II trial of gefitinib in patients (pts) with progressive metastatic neuroendocrine tumors (NET): A Phase II Consortium (P2C) study. Atlanta, Georgia, 2006.

92. Yao JC, Zhang JX, Rashid A, et al. Clinical and in vitro studies of imatinib in advanced carcinoid tumors. *Clin Cancer Res* 2007;13(1):234-240.

93. Duran I, Kortmansky J, Singh D, et al. A phase II clinical and pharmacodynamic study of temsirolimus in advanced neuroendocrine carcinomas. *Br J Cancer* 2006;95(9): 1148-1154.

94. Talamonti MS, Stuart K, Yao J. Neuroendocrine tumors of the gastrointestinal tract: How aggressive should we be? *American Society of Clinical Oncology 2004 Education Book*. Alexandria: American Society of Clinical Oncology; 2004:206-215.

Breast Cancer

PART
VII

Breast Cancer

EARLY-STAGE AND LOCALLY ADVANCED BREAST CANCER

Sapna P. Patel
Aman U. Buzdar
Commentary: Kelly K. Hunt

■ EPIDEMIOLOGY

INCIDENCE

Breast cancer is the second most common cause of death for women and is the most common cause of death for women aged 45 to 55. In 2009, it is estimated that 192,370 American women will be diagnosed with breast cancer and that 40,170 women will die from this disease. This number of deaths would be second only to lung cancer as related to cancer-caused mortality (Figs. 24-1 and 24-2) (1).

In the early 1980s, the rates of breast cancer diagnosis rose sharply, likely related to increased mammographic screening, since it was the incidence of stage I carcinomas that rose most sharply. Data from the Surveillance, Epidemiology, and End Results (SEER) program of the National Cancer Institute demonstrate that while the incidence of breast cancer has been stable since the late 1980s, there has been an increase in the percentage of breast cancers that are hormone receptor–positive, which is contemplated to be due either to new ligand receptor assays versus an increased use of hormone replacement therapy by women (2,3).

WORLDWIDE TRENDS

Breast cancer incidence has long varied in different regions of the world. Incidence is highest in Northern Europe and North America and lowest in Asia and Africa. Data suggest that this variability is due not only to environmental factors but also to lifestyle. This is supported by the observation that breast cancer incidence is higher in second-generation Asian immigrants in the United States (4).

MORTALITY

Breast cancer overall mortality rates had been stable for more than 50 years prior to 1989. However, in the 1990s there was a steady decrease in breast cancer deaths per year. Mortality rates declined by 1.4% per year from 1989 to 1995 and thereafter by 3.2% per year. This is thought to be due in part to increased use of mammography, resulting in earlier diagnosis, and the use of effective treatments. Mortality rates continue to be higher for African-American women. This is thought to be due in part to disparities in terms of health care access that exist both for diagnosis as well as treatment (5).

■ RISK FACTORS

HEREDITARY

Family History

Although it is known that family history is an important risk factor for breast cancer, only 10% of newly

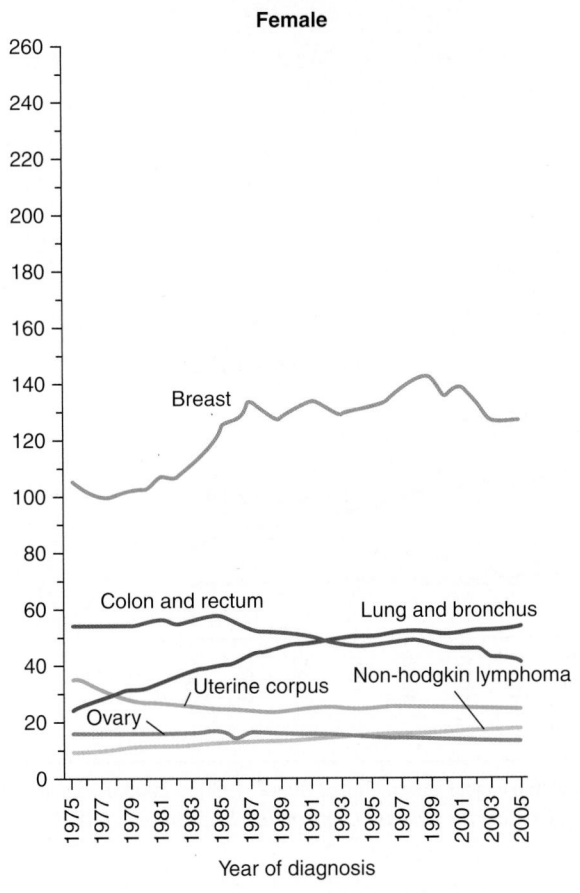

Female

Year of diagnosis

FIGURE 24-1. Annual age-adjusted cancer incidence rates among females for selected cancer types, United States, 1973 to 2005. Rates are age-adjusted for the 2005 US population. (*Surveillance, Epidemiology, and End Results [SEER] program [www.seer.cancer.gov]. Delay-adjusted incidence database, SEER Incidence Delay-Adjusted Rates, from nine registries, 1975 to 2005. National Cancer Institute, DCCPS, Surveillance Research Program, Statistical Research and Applications Branch, released April 2008, based on the November 2007 SEER data submission.*)

diagnosed breast cancer patients have a positive family history. The Gail model was the first to incorporate the number of first-degree relatives into a comprehensive model of breast cancer risk assessment (6). Claus then went on to estimate risk of breast cancer based on the number of familial cases and their ages of diagnosis (7). It is now well known that the risk for each patient with a positive family history is affected by the age of the family member at diagnosis, the total number of first-degree relatives affected, and the patient's age. Based on data from a large meta-analysis, the risk of breast cancer for one affected first-degree relative was increased 1.80-fold; if there were two affected first-degree relatives, that risk was increased 2.93-fold. This risk was then further modified by the age of the patient, such that a

women's risk of cancer prior to age 40 was increased to 5.7-fold if one relative was diagnosed prior to age 40 (8).

Genetic Mutations

It is estimated that the overall prevalence of specific genetic mutations accounting for breast cancer is rare, accounting for only 5 to 10% of all cases. Risk can be further subdivided based on a patient's history. The most commonly studied mutations are *BRAC1* and *BRAC2*, although multiple other mutations exist, such as *p53*, *ATM*, *PTEN*, *MLH1*, and *MSH2*. In a study that analyzed 10,000 individuals, it was shown that, excluding those with Ashkenazi ancestry, the prevalence of *BRAC1* and *BRAC2* mutations varied sharply, with a low of 2.9% if the patient and all first- or second-degree relatives had no prior history of breast cancer or ovarian cancer at less than 50 years of age. A maximum prevalence of 81.3% was noted if the patient and any first- or second-degree relative had breast cancer diagnosed at less than 50 years of age and ovarian cancer at any age (9). Since genetic testing often leads to complicated medical decisions both for the patient and other family members, it is very important to find a way to determine whom it is most appropriate to screen by taking into account population-dependent positive and negative predictive values of the test, using statistical models.

CONDITIONS OF THE BREAST

Ductal Carcinoma In Situ and Lobular Carcinoma In Situ

There has been a rapid increase in the literature surrounding the epidemiology, natural history, and treatment of ductal carcinoma in situ (DCIS) and lobular carcinoma in situ (LCIS). (See detailed information in Chap. 27.)

With DCIS, the 10-year risk of invasive breast cancer is 5% in the contralateral breast. LCIS has been regarded as a risk factor for ipsilateral and contralateral breast cancer. Recent research supports that LCIS is a direct precursor of both invasive lobular and ductal carcinoma. For patients diagnosed with LCIS, the risk of developing breast cancer in either breast is 1% a year (10).

NATURAL HORMONAL FACTORS

Age at Menarche

A later age of menarche is protective. One study has reported that for every 2-year delay in menarche there was a 10% reduction in breast cancer risk (11).

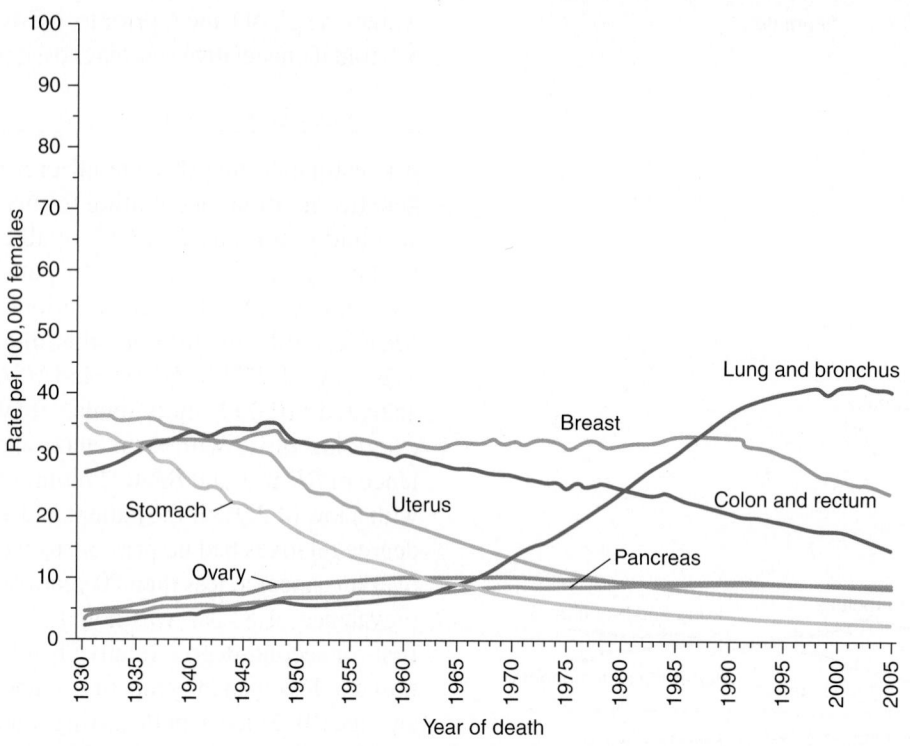

FIGURE 24-2. Annual age-adjusted cancer death rates among females for selected cancer types, United States, 1930 to 2005. Rates are age-adjusted to the 2005 U.S. population. (*National Center for Health Statistics, Centers for Disease Control and Prevention, 2008. US mortality data, 1960 to 2005, US Mortality Vol. 1930 to 1959.*)

Age at First Pregnancy

It is acknowledged that there is a favorable risk reduction associated with earlier age of pregnancy. Women who give birth for the first time at age 35 have a 1.6-fold higher risk of breast cancer than if they were 26 to 27 at time of first birth. Further, women who are over age 30 at the time of first birth are at higher risk than nulliparous women (12).

Age at Menopause

Late menopause is associated with a higher risk of breast cancer. It has been shown that oophorectomy before age 40 will decrease the lifetime risk of breast cancer up to 50% (13).

Pregnancy

Breast cancer is the second most common cancer associated with pregnancy, its incidence being 1 in 3000. The incidence of pregnancy-associated breast cancer is likely related to the delay of childbirth until after age 30. There are also controversial data, from two reports, suggesting that pregnancy might cause a transient rise in breast cancer risk. However, a clearly documented decreased risk of breast cancer occurs 10 to 15 years after childbirth (14).

EXOGENOUS HORMONAL USE

Oral Contraceptives

Most studies have not shown an increased risk of breast cancer with oral contraceptive use (15,16). However, a meta-analysis did show a significant but small increase in relative risk of breast cancer (17). A concern about the meta-analysis is that follow-up was limited in length.

Hormone Replacement Therapy

The Women's Health Initiative did show that the relative risk of breast cancer was increased to 1.26 for women who took combined treatment with estrogen and progesterone for a mean of 5.2 years as compared to placebo (18). While long-term hormone replacement therapy is associated with a higher risk of breast cancer, short-term use does not seem to significantly increase the risk of breast cancer.

■ STAGING OF BREAST CANCER

2002 TNM REVISIONS

The 2002 6th edition of the *Cancer Staging Manual* published by the American Joint Committee on Cancer (AJCC) was modified compared to the prior staging criteria, published in 1997 (Tables 24-1 and 24-2) (19).

TABLE
24-1 **TNM STAGING SYSTEM FOR BREAST CANCER**

PRIMARY TUMOR (T)

TX	Primary tumor cannot be assessed
T0	No evidence of primary tumor
Tis	Carcinoma in situ
Tis (DCIS)	Ductal carcinoma in situ
Tis (LCIS)	Labular carcinoma in situ
Tis (Paget)	Paget disease of the nipple with no tumor
	Note: Paget disease associated with a tumor is classified according to the size of the tumor.
T1	Tumor ≤20 mm in greatest dimension
T1mi	Microinvasion ≤1 mm in greatest dimension
T1a	Tumor >1 mm but ≤5 mm in greatest dimension
T1b	Tumor >5 mm but ≤10 mm in greatest dimension
T1c	Tumor >10 mm but ≤20 mm in greatest dimension
T2	Tumor >20 mm but ≤50 mm in greatest dimension
T3	Tumor >50 mm in greatest dimension
T4	Tumor of any size with direct extension to
	(a) chest wall or
	(b) skin, only as described below
T4a	Extension to chest wall, not including pectoralis muscle
T4b	Ulceration or edema (including peau d'orange) of the skin of the breast, or satellite skin nodules confined to the same breast
T4c	Both T4a and T4b
T4d	Inflammatory carcinoma with typical skin changes involving a third or more of the skin of the breast

REGIONAL LYMPH NODES (N)

NX	Regional lymph nodes cannot be assessed (eg, previously removed)
N0	No regional lymph node metastases
N1	Metastases in movable ipsilateral axillary lymph node(s)
N2	Metastases in ipsilateral axillary lymph nodes fixed or matted, or in clinically apparent ipsilateral internal mammary nodes in the absence of clinically evident axillary lymph node metastases
N2a	Metastases in ipsilateral axillary lymph nodes fixed to one another (matted) or to other structures
N2b	Metastases only in clinically apparent ipsilateral internal mammary nodes and in the absence of clinically evident axillary lymph node metastases
N3	Metastases in ipsilateral infraclavicular lymph node(s), or in clinically apparent ipsilateral internal mammary lymph node(s) and in the presence of clinically evident axillary lymph node metastases; or metastases in ipsilateral supraclavicular lymph node(s) with or without axillary or internal mammary lymph node involvement
N3a	Metastases in ipsilateral infraclavicular lymph node(s)
N3b	Metastases in ipsilateral internal mammary lymph node(s) and axillary lymph node(s)
N3c	Metastases in ipsilateral supraclavicular lymph node(s)

REGIONAL LYMPH NODES (PN)

pNX	Regional lymph nodes cannot be assessed (eg, previously removed, or not removed for pathologic study)
pN0	No regional lymph node metastases histologically
pN0(i−)	No regional lymph node metastases histologically, negative IHC
pN0(i+)	No regional lymph node metastases histologically, positive IHC cluster ≤0.2 mm
pN0(mol−)	No regional lymph node metastases histologically, negative molecular findings (RT-PCR)
pN0(mol+)	No regional lymph node metastases histologically, positive molecular findings (RT-PCR)
pN1mi	Micrometastases (>0.2 mm but not >2.0 mm)
pN1	Metastases in one to three axillary lymph nodes and/or in internal mammary nodes with microscopic disease detected by sentinel lymph node dissection but not clinically apparent
pN1a	Metastases in one to three axillary lymph nodes, at least one metastasis >2.0 mm
pN1b	Metastases in internal mammary nodes with disease detected by sentinel lymph node dissection but not clinically apparent

(Continued)

TABLE 24-1 | **TNM STAGING SYSTEM FOR BREAST CANCER (*Continued*)**

pN1c	Metastases in one to three axillary lymph nodes and in internal mammary lymph nodes with disease detected by sentinel lymph node dissection but not clinically apparent
pN2	Metastases in four to nine axillary lymph nodes, or in clinically apparent internal mammary nodes in the absence of axillary lymph node metastases
pN2a	Metastases in four to nine axillary lymph nodes (at least one tumor deposit >2.0 mm)
pN2b	Metastases in clinically apparent internal mammary lymph nodes in the absence of axillary lymph node metastases
pN3	Metastases in 10 or more axillary lymph nodes; or in infraclavicular lymph nodes, or in clinically apparent ipsilateral internal mammary lymph nodes in the presence of one or more positive axillary lymph nodes; or in more than three axillary lymph nodes with metastases in internal mammary lymph nodes detected by sentinel lymph node biopsy but not clinically apparent; or in ipsilateral supraclavicular lymph nodes
pN3a	Metastases in 10 or more axillary lymph nodes (at least one tumor deposit >2.0 mm); or metastases to infraclavicular lymph nodes
pN3b	Metastases in clinically apparent ipsilateral internal mammary lymph nodes in the presence of one or more positive axillary lymph nodes; or in more than three axillary lymph nodes and in internal mammary lymph nodes with disease detected by sentinel lymph node biopsy but not clinically apparent
pN3c	Metastases in ipsilateral supraclavicular lymph nodes

DISTANT METASTASES (M)	
MX	Distant metastases cannot be assessed
M0	No clinical or radiographic evidence of distant metastases
M0(i+)	No clinical or radiographic evidence of distant metastases, but deposits of molecularly or microscopically detected tumor cells in circulating blood, bone marrow, or other non-regional nodal tissue that are no larger than 0.2 mm
M1	Distant metastases detectable by clinical or radiographic means and/or larger than 0.2 mm

IHC, immunohistochemistry; RT-PCR, reverse transcription polymerase chain reaction.
Used with the permission from the American Joint Committee on Cancer (AJCC), Chicago, Illinois. The original source for this material is the *AJCC Cancer Staging Manual,* 7th ed. New York, NY: Springer-Verlag; 2010.

These changes were based on continuing developments in breast cancer diagnosis as well as management. One driving force behind the modifications was the knowledge that two patients both having small tumors can have very divergent outcomes. The revised staging system seeks to use histologic observations and tumor markers to further stratify the patients.

Immunochemical and molecular approaches are now used routinely in sentinel lymph node analysis. Once detected, these microscopic lesions may be used to guide therapy. Therefore the staging system was revised to capture this information so that it could be used to accurately analyze data on the outcomes of these therapies. The new staging system discriminates micrometastases from isolated tumor cells by size and uses identifiers for sentinel lymph node dissection (20).

Significant changes were made to reclassify nodal status by number of involved axillary nodes. This was done because there is strong clinical evidence that the number of positive axillary lymph nodes is the most important prognostic factor. The classification used for one to three axillary lymph nodes is pN1a, four to nine

positive axillary lymph nodes is pN2a, and ten or more is pN3a.

There has been an addition of classification of metastasis to the infraclavicular lymph node to N3, and reclassification of metastases to supraclavicular lymph nodes to N3 rather than M1. In addition, significant changes were made to the classification of internal mammary nodes. Microscopic involvement of the internal mammary nodes detected by sentinel lymph node is N1 disease, macroscopic involvement detected by imaging or clinical examination is N2 disease, and N3 disease exists if involvement of the internal mammary nodes occurs in the presence of metastases to the axillary lymph nodes. These changes were made because current data have now led to questioning of the prior significance assigned to metastases to infraclavicular (level III axillary lymph nodes) and to nonaxillary nodal basins, such as the supraclavicular and internal mammary nodes.

Although there was much discussion about whether to add histologic grade to the TNM staging system, it was finally decided against because of a dearth of uniform

TABLE 24-2 | TNM STAGE GROUPING FOR BREAST CANCER

STAGE GROUPING

0	Tis	N0	M0
IA	T1*	N0	M0
IB	T0	N1mi	M0
	T1*	N1mi	M0
IIA	T0	N1	M0
	T1*	N1	M0
	T2	N0	M0
IIB	T2	N1	M0
	T3	N0	M0
IIIA	T0	N2	M0
	T1*	N2	M0
	T2	N2	M0
	T3	N1	M0
	T3	N2	M0
IIIB	T4	N0	M0
	T4	N1	M0
	T4	N2	M0
IIIC	Any T	N3	M0
IV	Any T	Any N	M1

*T1 includes T1mi.

Used with the permission from the American Joint Committee on Cancer (AJCC), Chicago, Illinois. The original source for this material is the *AJCC Cancer Staging Manual*, 7th ed. New York, NY: Springer-Verlag; 2010.

information regarding correlation with tumor grade and outcome. However, further evidence points to using the Nottingham grading system, since it uses a semiquantitative method. The Nottingham system incorporates percent of tubule formation, degree of nuclear pleomorphism, and accurate mitotic count (21).

WILL ROGERS PHENOMENON

It is important to consider how these changes in the AJCC staging criteria from 1988 to 2002 affect stage-specific outcomes. It has been demonstrated that reclassification will result in improved outcomes. A recent study examined overall stage-specific survival using both staging systems for a total of 1350 patients. It was noted that only 55% of patients who were classified as having stage II disease according to the 1988 system had stage II according to the 2002 system. However, in direct comparison, the number of patients with stage III disease increased by 114%. Thus it is important that attention be paid to this in order to draw appropriate conclusions regarding therapeutic interventions as compared to historical controls or prior published outcome data (22).

■ PROGNOSTIC FACTORS

There has been significant interest in the assessment of prognostic factors in breast cancer. It is known that 30% of node-negative patients will die from a breast cancer–related cause. Thus there is a great thrust of research to determine markers that could further identify which patients would benefit most from available adjuvant treatment.

PREDICTIVE VERSUS PROGNOSTIC FACTORS

With the growing array of articles in this field, it has become very important to make a distinction between predictive factors and prognostic factors. A predictive factor is one that can provide information on the likelihood of response to a given therapeutic intervention, whereas a prognostic factor is one that can provide information on outcome at the time of diagnosis (23,24). Lymph node status is an example of a prognostic factor and estrogen receptor (ER) status is an example of a prognostic and predictive factor.

PATHOLOGIC FACTORS

Prognosis is still determined in largest part by pathology. It has been shown by multiple studies that the most powerful prognostic factors are the extent of disease in the axillary lymph nodes and tumor size (25-27). Other important pathologic factors are hormone receptor status, histologic grade, tumor type, and lymphovascular invasion.

Tumor Size

The SEER group correlated tumor diameter with survival in more than 13,000 patients and found that the relative overall survival (OS) rate was almost 99% in patients with tumors of 1 to 3 cm, and 85% in patients with tumors larger than 3 cm (28).

Axillary Lymph Nodes

Over 20 years ago there was significant documentation that the number of involved lymph nodes could be used to predict 5-year disease-free survival (DFS). It was noted that the 62% for one to three positive axillary lymph nodes, 58% for four to nine lymph nodes, and 29% for ten or more lymph nodes (29).

Nuclear Grade

In the early twentieth century, a formal grading system of tumors was developed. Nuclear or histologic grade describes the degree of tumor differentiation and is based on a pathologist's assessment of nuclear size and shape, number of mitoses, and degree of tubule formation. As stated earlier, although a nuclear grade of 1 (most differentiated) to 3 (least differentiated) is reported with every breast cancer pathology report, its use in predicting outcome is still heavily debated (21). This is in part secondary to interobserver variation in the classification of differentiation. The Nottingham combined grading system seems to be most useful because of its semiquantitative approach and is currently recommended by the College of American Pathologists.

Hormone Receptor Status

ER and progesterone receptor (PR) positivity correlate with prolonged DFS and OS. However, the importance of hormone receptor status has been documented more consistently in node-positive than in node-negative disease. Initially biochemical ligand-binding assays were the method of choice. Immunocytochemical assays have now become the favored approach because of their ability to be used with a variety of specimens. A "positive" specimen is usually termed to be one in which 5 to 10% of the cells stain for the hormone receptor, but one large academic center uses a cutoff of 1% for positivity (30).

Proliferative Rate

This can be evaluated by a variety of methods including mitotic figure count, S-phase fraction as determined by flow cytometry, thymidine labeling index, and monoclonal antibodies to antigens in proliferating cells. A high S-phase fraction is usually associated with poor differentiation and lack of ER positivity. In addition, some studies have found an association with a high S-phase fraction (the fraction of cells synthesizing DNA) and poor OS (31). Antibodies to Ki-67 and PCNA/cyclin can be used to determine a proliferative rate that corresponds with the S-phase fraction. The percentage of Ki-67–positive cells has been used to stratify patients according to good or bad prognosis. A report examining 371 node-negative breast cancers found that women with a high labeling index had a 20-fold greater mortality rate (32).

HER-2/Neu Overexpression

The c-*erb* B-2 (*HER-2/neu*) oncogene codes for a 185-kDa transmembrane glycoprotein that has intracellular tyrosine kinase activity, and c-*erb* B-2 is a member of the family of epidermal growth factor receptors. This group of receptors has an important role in the activation

of epidermal transduction pathways controlling for epithelial growth and differentiation. Overexpression of the *HER-2/neu* oncogene is present in up to 30% of invasive breast cancers

Several methods exist to measure activity of *HER-2/neu*. The fluorescene in situ hybridization (FISH) method can detect amplification of *HER-2/neu*. Overexpression of *HER-2/neu* RNA can be determined by Northern blotting or reverse transcription polymerase chain reaction (RTPCR). Furthermore, the protein product of *HER-2/neu* can be evaluated by Western blotting, enzyme-linked immunosorbent assay (ELISA), or immunohistochemistry (IHC).

One limitation of these various methods of detection is heterogeneity of test results. It has been noted that different techniques, especially when performed with nonstandardized methods, can yield nonuniform results. Two recent studies from United States Cooperative Groups (33,34) revealed that approximately 20% of positive assays from the community could not be confirmed by replication in a larger centralized laboratory. Also the source of specimens differs among the various testing techniques. ELISA and Western and Northern blots require fresh frozen tissue; however, IHC and FISH have the advantage that fixed, paraffin-embedded tissue can be used.

Currently the tests approved by the US Food and Drug Administration (FDA) are two FISH assays and one IHC assay. Ongoing studies are addressing the predictive capability of the varying assays. Preliminary data seem to point to FISH as being better at selecting patients with metastases who would benefit from trastuzumab (35). False-positive test results are most commonly noted for patients with a 2+ result by IHC. Therefore there is evidence that a 2+ result by IHC should be confirmed by FISH (36).

Implications and targeted therapy for *HER-2/neu* positivity have been studied predominantly in the metastatic setting. However, it has been demonstrated that overexpression of *HER-2/neu* in node-positive disease seems to correlate with a shorter DFS and OS (37). For node-negative disease, the results are more mixed. It seems that *HER-2/neu* overexpression may be useful in identifying good-risk subjects with small tumors who might have a poorer prognosis. A study that examined node-negative patients with tumors smaller than 3 cm in diameter found that the 5-year DFS was only 40% in those with overexpression of *HER-2/neu*, compared to 80% for patients without overexpression of *HER-2/neu* (38).

Preclinical data suggest that there is a possible interaction between the *HER-2/neu* and ER signal transduction pathways. In vitro work has demonstrated that transfection and overexpression of *HER-2/neu* can cause tamoxifen resistance in ER-positive human breast cancer cell lines. The exact mechanism causing this is unknown; however, possible methods include phosphorylation of the ER and other methods of regulating ER expression. Conflicting data have been reported in regard to *HER-2/neu* overexpression and response to hormonal therapy. Several studies, including the GUN-1 cooperative trial (39), have documented a negative effect in response to tamoxifen for *HER-2/neu*–positive tumors, but other trials including the Danish Breast Cooperative Group trial (40) and a CALGB trial (41) have shown that *HER-2/neu* status does not affect response to tamoxifen. Thus, at this time, *HER-2/neu* status is not used to predict response to hormonal therapies.

FACTORS UNDER INVESTIGATION

Cyclin E

Recent published data regarding cyclin E suggests promise in regard to its usefulness as an independent prognostic factor. Cyclin E regulates the transition from the G_1 to the S phase. Prior studies have yielded contradictory findings in regard to the prognostic significance of cyclin E. A recent retrospective study by Keyomarsi et al. looked at the levels of low-molecular-weight cyclin E in addition to the levels of total cyclin E. The results of this study suggest that levels of cyclin E as measured by Western blot strongly correlate with survival in breast cancer. Of special interest is the fact that the cyclin E level was useful for differentiating outcomes in stage I disease. A total of 114 patients with stage I disease were analyzed and none of the 102 patients with low levels of cyclin E died within 5 years of diagnosis, whereas all 12 patients with a high level of the low-molecular-weight form of cyclin E died within 5 years (42).

p53 Mutations

Mutations in this tumor suppressor gene have been reported in 20 to 50% of human breast cancers and are especially noted in the hereditary cancer syndromes, such as the Li-Fraumeni syndrome. The independent prognostic value of these mutations is currently being investigated (43,44).

Microvessel Density

An initial study showed microvessel density as a marker of angiogenesis to be a statistically significant independent predictor of OS for all breast cancer patients, both node-positive and node-negative patients. However, further studies have shown conflicting results (45).

VEGF Levels

Vascular endothelial growth factor (VEGF) is thought to be the most important protein in tumor angiogenesis. Preliminary data have demonstrated that high VEGF appears to predict poor OS in both node-positive and node-negative breast cancer patients (46,47).

Cathepsin D

This marker appears to be a key lysosomal proteolytic enzyme with a possible role as a surrogate marker of tumor invasion. At this point its use remains investigational; however, a meta-analysis that examined a total of 2690 patients found that the relative risk of relapse at 84 months for low versus high levels of cathepsin was 0.61 (48).

Gene Expression Profiling

The use of DNA microarrays to prognosticate is an area of intense research. The largest study to date enrolled 295 patients with either stage I or stage II breast cancer. These patients were then classified using a 70-gene profile as having a poor or good prognosis. Patients were followed for a minimum of 10 years; at that point, the OS and distant metastasis-free survival were greater in those having a good prognosis according to their molecular profile alone (49). Current research by Pusztai et al. is ongoing to evaluate the use of microarrays in determining which patients would have the highest likelihood of achieving a complete pathologic response to neoadjuvant paclitaxel followed by FAC chemotherapy (50).

Thoughts for the Future

As we gain more knowledge on the molecular level, it is important to reflect on the fact that we need to develop methods to use new knowledge in a clinically relevant manner. Clinically, it would be very beneficial if we could find a way to stratify early-stage breast cancer patients into those who would benefit from adjuvant or neoadjuvant chemotherapy and also to better define risk of recurrence for an individual patient. While it is beneficial to identify novel independent prognostic factors, it would truly be very useful to develop a method that could be used to incorporate multiple molecular and pathologic factors to determine an accurate risk score for recurrence of breast cancer for an individual patient.

■ OVERALL BENEFITS OF ADJUVANT THERAPY

Many articles have been published that try to address the question of quantifying benefits of systemic therapy for both physicians and their patients. This issue is especially important since the number of articles per issue in major journals about breast cancer therapies is steadily increasing. Often the terminology in these articles is somewhat confusing, since terms such as *annual proportional reduction* are used instead of *disease-free survival* or *overall survival*.

Loprinzi, et al. published a paper that seeks to predict this benefit (51). Information from previous studies predicts that patients with node-negative disease have a 60 to 75% 10-year DFS, whereas node-positive patients have a 25 to 30% 10-year DFS. In this study, 11 breast cancer specialists were asked to complete questionnaires in which they were asked to estimate the 10-year DFS for patients treated with locoregional therapy alone (Table 24-3).

Randomized controlled trials and meta-analysis data were then reviewed and a computer-based algorithm was developed to calculate the 10-year DFS. These outcome data were then put into easy-to-use tabular forms, which address DFS for both ER-positive and ER-negative patients (Tables 24-4 and 24-5).

The hope is that these data can be used by physicians and their patients to make better-informed decisions about therapy. This study, while influential, does have several limitations in that other prognostic markers, such as *HER-2/neu,* were not incorporated, and data regarding the outcomes from the combination of Adriamycin (doxorubicin), cyclophosphamide, and paclitaxel were from a single study.

A second study by Buchholz et al. addressed the effect of systemic therapy for node-negative disease treated with breast conservation surgery and radiation therapy. A total of 277 patients treated with systemic therapy (128 patients receiving chemotherapy with or without tamoxifen; 149 patients receiving tamoxifen alone) were analyzed, and these data were compared with those from 207 patients who received no systemic treatment. Patients treated with systemic therapy had a statistically improved 5-year survival rate of 97.5 versus 89.8%. There was, however, no statistically relevant difference between those treated with tamoxifen and those treated with chemotherapy. Also, systemic treatment, when subjected to a Cox regression analysis, was a more important predictor than young age or positive hormonal receptor status (52).

■ ADJUVANT THERAPY

After definitive local therapy is completed, it is important to plan for adjuvant systemic therapy. The use of chemotherapy, hormonal therapy, or both has had a significant effect on the management and treatment of breast malignancies. It has been demonstrated that all women with node-positive disease and a significant percentage of node-negative women with tumors that are hormone receptor–negative or >1 cm in size benefit from chemotherapy. The choice of agents to be used for chemotherapy and hormonal therapy should be guided by the patient's age, concomitant medical issues, positive or negative axillary lymph node involvement, and the status of the hormone receptors.

CHEMOTHERAPY

Historical Perspective

Studies in the 1960s to 1970s evaluated whether single-agent chemotherapy after local therapy had any benefit

TABLE 24-3	**TEN-YEAR DISEASE-FREE SURVIVAL ESTIMATES WITH LOCOREGIONAL THERAPY ALONE***

	TUMOR SIZE					
No. of Positive Nodes	*<1 cm*	*1-2 cm*	*2-3 cm*	*3-4 cm*	*4-5 cm*	*>5 cm*
0	90	81	75	69	63	56
1-3	60	56	50	47	42	37
4-6	46	42	38	35	31	27
6-9	36	32	29	26	21	18
≥10	22	19	17	16	14	13

*Values in the body of this table are percentages.
Reproduced, with permission, from Loprinzi CL, Thome SD. Understanding the utility of adjuvant systematic therapy for primary breast cancer. J Clin Oncol 2001;19:972-979.

TABLE 24-4

ESTIMATED 10-YEAR DISEASE-FREE SURVIVAL PERCENTAGES FOR ESTROGEN RECEPTOR–POSITIVE WOMEN

No. of Positive Nodes	TUMOR SIZE																	
	<1 cm			1-2 cm			2-3 cm			3-4 cm			4-5 cm			>5 cm		
	Ø	T	T and AC	Ø	T	T and AC	Ø	T	T and AC	Ø	T	T and AC	Ø	T	T and AC	Ø	T	T and AC
Women ≤50 years																		
0	90	92	94	81	85	89	75	81	86	69	76	82	63	71	78	56	65	73
1-3	60	68	76	56	65	73	50	60	69	47	57	67	42	53	63	37	48	59
4-6	46	56	66	42	53	63	38	49	59	35	46	57	31	42	53	27	38	50
6-9	36	47	58	32	43	54	29	40	52	26	37	49	21	32	44	18	28	40
≥10	22	33	45	19	30	42	17	27	39	16	26	38	14	24	36	13	23	34
Women >50 years																		
0	90	92	93	81	85	87	75	81	83	69	76	79	63	71	74	56	65	69
1-3	60	68	72	56	65	69	50	60	64	47	57	62	42	53	57	37	48	53
4-6	46	56	61	42	53	57	38	49	54	35	46	51	31	42	47	27	38	44
6-9	36	47	52	32	43	48	29	40	46	26	37	42	21	32	37	18	28	34
≥10	22	33	38	19	30	35	17	27	33	16	26	32	14	24	29	13	23	28

AC, standard primary adjuvant chemotherapy such as doxorubicin/cyclophosphamide; Ø, no systemic adjuvant therapy; T, tamoxifen.

Reproduced, with permission, from Loprinzi CL, Thome SD. Understanding the utility of adjuvant systematic therapy for primary breast cancer. J Clin Oncol 2001;19:972-979.

TABLE 24-5 | **ESTIMATED 10-YEAR DISEASE-FREE SURVIVAL PERCENTAGES FOR ESTROGEN RECEPTOR–NEGATIVE WOMEN**

TUMOR SIZE

No. of Positive Nodes	<1 cm			1-2 cm			2-3 cm			3-4 cm			4-5 cm			>5 cm		
	Ø	AC	AC and P*	Ø	AC	AC and P	Ø	AC	AC and P	Ø	AC	AC and P	Ø	AC	AC and P	Ø	AC	AC and P
Women ≤50 years																		
0	90	93	95	81	87	90	75	83	87	69	79	84	63	74	80	56	69	76
1-3	60	72	78	56	69	76	50	64	72	47	62	70	42	57	66	37	53	62
4-6	46	61	69	42	57	66	38	54	63	35	51	61	31	47	57	27	44	54
6-9	36	52	61	32	48	58	29	46	56	26	43	53	21	37	48	18	34	45
≥10	22	38	49	19	35	46	17	33	44	16	32	43	14	29	40	13	28	39
Women >50 years																		
0	90	92	94	81	85	88	75	79	84	69	74	80	63	69	76	56	63	71
1-3	60	67	74	56	63	71	50	58	66	47	55	64	42	50	60	37	46	56
4-6	46	54	63	42	50	60	38	46	57	35	44	54	31	40	50	27	36	47
6-9	36	45	55	32	41	51	29	38	48	26	35	46	21	29	40	18	26	37
≥10	22	30	41	19	27	38	17	25	36	16	24	35	14	21	32	13	20	31

*Paclitaxel.

Reproduced, with permission, from Loprinzi CL, Thome SD. Understanding the utility of adjuvant systematic therapy for primary breast cancer. J Clin Oncol 2001;19:972-979.

compared with observation alone. The single agents studied included cyclophosphamide and melphalan, and most reports documented that single agents have little or no effect on DFS. Subsequently the focus shifted to polychemotherapy, with most trials evaluating variations of the three-drug regimen of cyclophosphamide, methotrexate, and 5-FU (CMF) or anthracycline-containing regimens (53,54).

While these polychemotherapy regimens clearly showed a greater benefit in DFS, it was often unclear to clinicians which regimens were superior and which were equivalent. The Oxford Overview published in 1998 helped to provide clarity to this issue by reviewing data from about 18,000 women in 47 trials that compared polychemotherapy or no chemotherapy, about 6000 women in 11 trials that compared longer versus shorter polychemotherapy, and about 6000 women in 11 trials of anthracycline-containing regimes versus CMF (55). The final interpretation revealed that adjuvant polychemotherapy for patients under 50 years of age resulted in an absolute improvement in 10-year survival of 7 to 11%, whereas the overall 10-year survival benefit was 2 to 3% for patients from 50 to 69 years of age.

The review compared trials including the Milan trial, which revealed that treatment of node-positive patients with CMF for 12 courses versus no therapy resulted in an OS of 47 versus 22%. The NSABP B-15 trial then documented that Adriamycin (doxorubicin) plus cyclophosphamide (AC) for four courses was equivalent to CMF for six courses, with a 10-year OS of 56% in each group. SWOG 8897 then examined FAC for six courses versus CMF for six courses in 2700 high-risk node-negative patients; the result in terms of 5-year OS was 92 versus 90%, respectively. The NCIC trial then compared cyclophosphamide, epirubicin, and 5-fluorouracil (CEF) for six courses with CMF for six courses in 710 node-positive patients and noted that the 5-year OS was 77 versus 70%, respectively.

The Role of Anthracyclines

The 1998 Oxford Overview further demonstrated that anthracycline-containing regimens were superior to CMF. There was noted to be a statistically significant 12% reduction in risk of recurrence for anthracycline-containing regimens. Also there was a 2.7% decrease in mortality and a 3.2% decrease in relapse. The information gained from this important systematic analysis began a shift toward administration of anthracycline-based regimens for adjuvant therapy of breast cancer.

Official recommendations have been made based on the above data; these were presented at the National

Premedications 30 Min Prior to Chemotherapy

Ondansetron 8 mg PO
Lorazepam 1 mg PO
Dexamethasone 20 mg in 50 mL NS IVPB

Chemotherapy

5-Fluorouracil 500 mg/m^2 in 50 mL NS IVPB on days 1 and 4
Doxorubicin 50 mg/m^2 in NS IV continuous infusion through a central venous catherer over 72 h (days 1-3)
Cyclophosphamide 500 mg/m^2 in 100 mL NS IVPB (if total dose $<$1 g) or in 250 mL NS IVPB (if total dose $\geq$1 g) on day 1

Cycles are repeated every 21 days

FIGURE 24-3. FAC regimen: 5-fluorouracil, Adriamycin (doxorubicin), cyclophosphamide.

Institute of Health Consensus Development Conference in 2000 and suggested that anthracycline be included as a part of breast cancer adjuvant therapy. Several studies have investigated the role of *HER-2/neu* in the positive response to anthracyclines. Both the CALGB-8082 and NASBP-11 studies have shown a benefit in DFS in those patients who overexpressed *HER-2/neu* and received anthracycline therapy (56,57).

Currently the standard-of-care anthracycline regimen at the University of Texas MD Anderson Cancer Center (MDACC) is the use of FAC (Fig. 24-3).

Evaluation of this regimen began in 1974; for 1107 women with node-positive disease, the results were favorable, with a 10-year DFS of 72% for patients with one to three positive nodes, a 55% DFS for patients with four to ten positive nodes, and a 36% DFS for those with more than 10 nodes. One of the more severe toxicities of doxorubicin is congestive heart failure; however, since according to the MDACC regimen this drug is given over 72 h via an infusion pump, there is only a 1% risk of cardiac dysfunction (58,59).

Epirubicin in place of doxorubicin has been evaluated with 5-FU and cyclophosphamide (FEC). Six cycles of FEC have been shown to be similar, in terms of safety and efficacy, to FAC (60). One of the benefits touted for epirubicin is that it causes less cardiac toxicity than doxorubicin. However, when a prolonged infusion of doxorubicin is given, the risk of cardiac dysfunction is minimal. No published studies have directly compared FEC with FAC.

For patients with *HER-2/neu*-positive tumors, trastuzumab is establishing its place in the neoadjuvant and adjuvant settings. It has proven efficacy in the treatment of metastatic *HER-2/neu*-expressing tumors and that efficacy is being seen in earlier stages of disease (see section Other Systemic Therapy Topics, later). To this end, the question has been raised regarding the need for anthracyclines in these patients. BCIRG 006 aims to compare non-trastuzumab based adjuvant therapy to trastuzumab-based regimens with and without an anthracycline. The regimens in this trial are adriamycin 60 mg/m^2 plus cyclophophomide 600 mg/m^2 every 21 days for 4 cycles followed by docetaxel 100 mg/m^2 every 21 days for 4 cycles (AC→T) or AC for four cycles followed by docetaxel 100 mg/m^2 for four cycles plus trastuzumab weekly during chemotherapy then every 21 days for a total of 1 year of trastuzumab (AC→TH) or docetaxel 75 mg/m^2 plus carboplatin (AUC 6) for six cycles plus trastuzumab weekly during chemotherapy then every 21 days for a total of 1 year (TCH). In the most recent third planned analysis with median follow-up of 65 months presented at San Antonio Breast Cancer Symposium (SABCS) 2009, BCIRG 006 demonstrates superiority in disease-free survival and overall survival with the AC→TH and TCH regimens. The AC→TH regimen appears to have a slight advantage over TCH with an absolute reduction in recurrence of 11% (AC→TH hazard ratio 0.64, 95% confidence interval (CI) 0.53-0.78; TCH hazard ratio 0.75, 95% confidence interval 0.63-0.90), thereby maintaining a role for anthracyclines in the adjuvant setting for all breast cancer patients, including those with *HER-2/neu*-positive tumors (61). Additonally, there is no validated test to predict sensitivity to anthracyclines, and combination regimens which include anthracyclines remain the standard for adjuvant therapy in early breast cancer.

Taxanes

The role of taxanes for breast cancer treatment was first investigated in metastatic disease. Paclitaxel and docetaxel in randomized controlled trials were shown to improve response rates, duration of response, and OS (62,63). It was these positive results of taxanes in the metastatic setting that prompted their investigation in the treatment of early breast cancer. Several major studies have contributed to the current use of taxanes in the adjuvant setting. CALGB 9344, NSABP B-28, MDACC 94-002, and CALGB 9741 studied paclitaxel, while BCIRG 001 investigated docetaxel.

The CALGB 9344 Intergroup trial was a randomized controlled trial that enrolled 3121 node-positive breast cancer patients. Based on randomization, patients received doxorubicin at either 60, 75, or 90 mg/m^2, with cyclophosphamide at a fixed dose of 600 mg/m^2, every

3 weeks for four courses. This was followed by further randomization, with patients receiving either paclitaxel 175 mg/m^2 every 3 weeks for four courses or no further therapy. In addition, all hormone receptor–positive tumors were treated with tamoxifen 20 mg a day for 5 years. Data analysis supported the conclusion that an escalated dose of doxorubicin beyond 60 mg/m^2 did not provide any significant further benefit. The DFS at 69 months for the paclitaxel arm was 70%, as compared with 65% for the control arm ($p = .001$), and OS at 69 months was 80 versus 77% ($p = .01$), respectively (64). These data led to the approval of paclitaxel by the FDA for the treatment of lymph node–positive disease.

NSABP B-28 enrolled 3060 patients with resected breast cancer and positive lymph nodes on pathology. Every 3 weeks, these patients received Adriamycin (doxorubicin) (60 mg/m^2) and cyclophosphamide (600 mg/m^2) (AC) for a total of four courses. Then they received four additional courses of paclitaxel (T) at 225 mg/m^2 every 3 weeks versus no further therapy. Patients with hormone receptor–positive tumors were treated with tamoxifen for 5 years. The 5-year analysis for DFS was 76% for those in the arm providing AC followed by T and 72% for those in the arm providing AC alone ($p = .008$) (65). However, the 5-year OS was 85% in each group. Thus, this study demonstrated a slight improvement in DFS and no improvement in OS. Grade 3 + paclitaxel toxicities occurred in 50% of the patients treated; the most predominant toxicities noted were neurosensory symptoms (14%), arthralgia/myalgia (11%), and neuromotor manifestations (7%).

MDACC 94-002 was a smaller prospectively conducted study at MDACC. A total of 524 patients were evaluated with early breast cancer; 350 of these were enrolled in an adjuvant setting and 174 in the neoadjuvant setting. In this study, patients were randomized to receive paclitaxel every 3 weeks for four courses or FAC for four courses. Those in the neoadjuvant group then underwent surgery followed by FAC for four courses, radiation therapy, and tamoxifen if they were 50 years of age or above and ER-positive (Figs. 24-4 and 24-5).

In the neoadjuvant setting, the complete response (CR) was 24% for the FAC-alone arm versus 27% for the paclitaxel-FAC arm. For all patients treated, the 4-year DFS was 83% for the FAC-alone arm and 86% for the paclitaxel-FAC arm; however, this was not statistically significant ($p = .09$). The overall hazard ratio adjusted for prognostic factors for paclitaxel followed by FAC as compared to FAC alone was 0.66 (66). Thus this study indicated that the addition of paclitaxel to FAC produced a trend toward risk reduction, although it

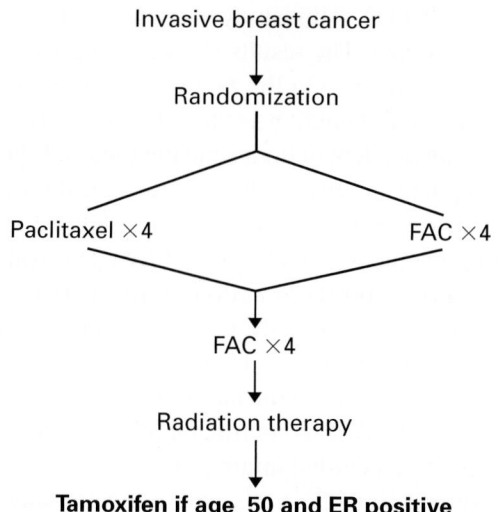

Invasive breast cancer

↓

Randomization

Paclitaxel ×4   FAC ×4

FAC ×4

↓

Radiation therapy

↓

Tamoxifen if age 50 and ER positive

FIGURE 24-4. Overall schema of MDACC 94-002 study. *(Reproduced, with permission, from Buzdar AU, Singletary SE, Valero V, et al. Evaluation of paclitaxel in adjuvant chemotherapy for patients with operable breast cancer: preliminary data of a prospective randomized trial. Clin Cancer Res 2002 May;8[5]:1073-1079.)*

was not statistically significant. Also of note is the fact that patients with ER-positive disease had a similar degree of clinical benefit with paclitaxel when compared with those with ER-negative disease.

The use of docetaxel was evaluated in a large phase III study. The BCIRG 001 study compared TAC (docetaxel plus AC) versus FAC for the adjuvant treatment of

Anaphylactic Medications

Prior to administering paclitaxel ensure that these medications are readily available: epinephrine (1:1000) .5 mL IV, diphenhydramine 25 mg IV, hydrocortisone 100 mg IV

Premedications

Dexamathasone 20 mg PO 12 and 6 h prior to paclitaxel
Dexamathasone 20 mg in 50 mL NS IVPB 30 min prior to course #1
Cimetidine 300 mg in 50 mL NS IVPB 30 min prior
Diphenhydramine 50 mg in 50 mL NS IVPB 30 min prior

Chemotherapy

Paclitaxel 250 mg/m² IV as 24-h continuous infusion

Repeat every 21 days times 4 courses

↓

FAC every 21 days times 4 courses (see Fig. 24-3)

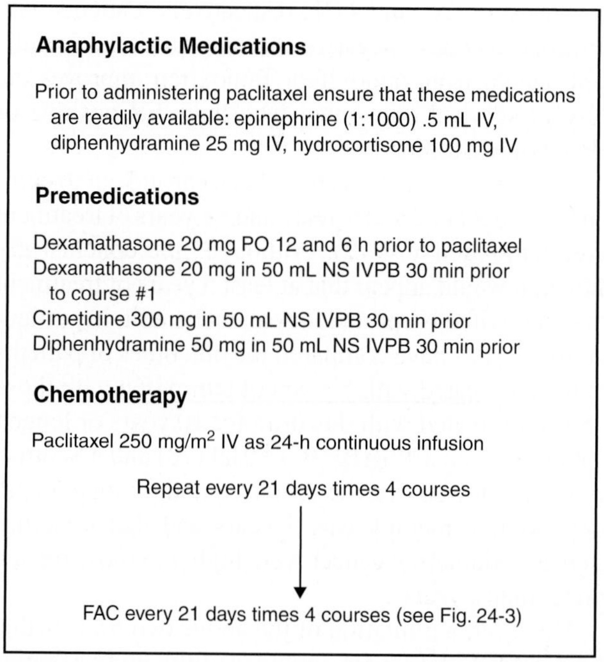

FIGURE 24-5. MDACC 94-002 regimen: paclitaxel every 3 weeks for four courses followed by FAC for four courses.

node-positive breast cancer patients. A total of 1491 women were randomized to receive docetaxel, Adriamycin (doxorubicin), and cyclophosphamide (TAC) at respective doses of 75/50/500 mg/m² every 3 weeks or FAC at respective doses of 500/50/500 mg/m² every 3 weeks. Each chemotherapy regimen was given for a total of six cycles. Patients with ER-positive disease were to be treated with tamoxifen for 5 years. The most common hematologic toxicities experienced in the TAC arm were neutropenia, both febrile and nonfebrile (65 and 24% respectively), amenorrhea (51%), and asthenia (11.2%). Both first analysis at 33 months and second interim analysis data at 55 months have shown significant improvement in DFS in favor of TAC (67,68). At 4 years, the DFS for the TAC arm was 80 versus 71% for the FAC arm; at 5 years, the DFS was 75 versus 68%. At 33 months, the relative risk of relapse was 0.68 (p = .001), which demonstrated a 32% reduction in risk of recurrence. When this was stratified by ER status, the ER-negative women had a relative risk of relapse of 0.62 (p = .005) and the ER-positive women had a relative risk of relapse of 0.68 (p = .02). Further stratification was based on level of nodal involvement of 1 to 3, 4 to 9, and ≥10 nodes. This analysis revealed that the benefit from TAC was greatest for those with 1 to 3 nodes, less but still present for those with 4 to 9 nodes, and not present for those with more than 10 nodes. On analysis of OS, there was a non–statistically significant trend toward improved OS for the TAC arm. These data showed that regimens with docetaxel could reduce the risk of recurrence of breast cancer in the adjuvant setting compared to the standard FAC regimen. However, with the higher rates of myelosuppression and febrile neutropenia seen with TAC, the use of this regimen requires extensive supportive care including utilization of granulocyte colony-stimulating growth factor.

ENDOCRINE THERAPY

The correlation between the endocrine system and breast cancer was first recognized more than 100 years ago. Surgical adrenalectomy was studied some 55 years ago and found to be an effective method for second-line endocrine therapy. However, the true understanding of the biological mechanisms that cause estrogen to stimulate the growth of hormone receptor–positive tumors is more recent. This knowledge has enabled the development of multiple therapies. Many of these therapies have varying mechanisms of action, but all have the common goal of decreasing estrogen availability for hormone receptor–positive malignancies.

Monotherapy

In the late 1970s, tamoxifen was shown to be an effective agent for the treatment of metastatic breast cancer. This form of treatment was especially well received, since data from trials showed that patients experienced fewer side effects than they did with traditional chemotherapy. It was tamoxifen's proven efficacy in the metastatic setting that first enabled it to be studied for adjuvant use.

Tamoxifen was the first drug to be used as an endocrine treatment for early breast cancer. An early placebo-controlled trial of tamoxifen as adjuvant therapy for early breast cancer, NATO, showed that 2 years of tamoxifen treatment reduced treatment failure at 21 months compared with control (14.2 versus 20.5%, respectively) (69). Since then, tamoxifen's efficacy in the adjuvant treatment of primary breast cancer has been demonstrated repeatedly.

Since tamoxifen was made available over 25 years ago, a large number of trials have been undertaken to investigate its efficacy and tolerability in the treatment of primary breast cancer. Although some individual trials are too small to justify firm conclusions, a meta-analysis has increased confidence in the effectiveness of tamoxifen in improving DFS and OS.

Several key trials have made considerable contributions. The most important of these is the National Surgical Adjuvant Breast and Bowel Project (NSABP) B-14 trial, which is a placebo-controlled trial involving 2644 node-negative, ER-positive patients receiving either placebo or tamoxifen (20 mg daily) following primary treatment (70). The update of this trial (at 5-year treatment) showed a significant improvement in DFS ($p < .0001$) and OS ($p < .01$), decreased local recurrence ($p < .00001$), and lower contralateral breast recurrence rates ($p < .0001$) with tamoxifen compared with placebo.

The Stockholm trial included 1344 postmenopausal patients with node-negative breast cancer who received either tamoxifen (40 mg daily for 2 or 5 years) or no adjuvant therapy. Median follow-up was 7 years. Results showed a significant increase in DFS in the tamoxifen group versus the control group ($p < .01$). There were also fewer deaths ($p = .02$) and improved survival ($p = .11$) in the group treated with tamoxifen compared with the control group, although this did not reach significance for survival (71). As reported in the NSABP B-14 trial, the beneficial effects observed with tamoxifen were restricted to the ER-positive subgroup.

The Scottish trial investigated the rate of relapse in patients taking 5 years of tamoxifen treatment compared with control (72). This study included 1312 patients <80 years of age. The results showed a highly significant delay in relapse in the tamoxifen arm versus the control arm. This benefit was maintained in terms of OS and was independent of nodal and menopausal status. A further update of this study (the median duration of tamoxifen treatment was 60 months) showed significant improvements in recurrence-free survival with tamoxifen ($p = .0001$) in node-negative patients compared with controls, with the greatest benefit seen in the postmenopausal patients. There was a trend toward improved OS in favor of the tamoxifen group, and there was also a reduction in contralateral breast cancer and incidence of myocardial infarction.

An overview of 55 trials with adjuvant tamoxifen for 1, 2, or 5 years versus no treatment in patients with primary breast cancer showed that tamoxifen treatment produced highly significant benefits in terms of both recurrence of first events and mortality (proportional reductions in recurrence were 18, 25, and 41%; and proportional reductions in death rate were 10, 15, and 22% for 1, 2, and 5 years of tamoxifen treatment, respectively; $p < .00001$ for each) (73). These benefits were found to occur almost exclusively in the hormone receptor–positive population (proportional reductions in recurrence were 21, 28, and 50%; proportional reductions in death rate were 14, 18, and 28% for 1, 2, and 5 years of tamoxifen treatment, respectively; $p < .00001$ for each). Furthermore, tamoxifen treatment for 1, 2, and 5 years reduced the incidence of contralateral breast cancer by 13, 26, and 47%, respectively. Patients with hormone receptor–negative disease derive no significant benefit from tamoxifen. Tamoxifen improves the 10-year survival of women who have ER-positive or ER-unknown tumors.

Further investigations have been carried out to compare the effect of 2 and 5 years and >5 years of treatment with tamoxifen (74-77). Although not conclusively shown, it would appear that at least 5 years of treatment with tamoxifen is optimal for patient benefit. In particular, three trials have compared the outcomes of patients who were treated with 5 years of tamoxifen with those who were treated with this drug for 10 years or longer. Data from both a NSABP B-14 trial (78) and a Scottish trial (79) showed that the preferred and optimal length of tamoxifen therapy was 5 years and that toxicities such as endometrial cancer were higher in those treated longer than 5 years.

However, a limitation of the above two trials is that the NSABP B-14 trial included only node-negative patients, and most of the patients in the Scottish trial also had node-negative disease. Thus a third trial sponsored by Eastern Cooperative Oncology Group (ECOG) (80), which enrolled women with only node-positive disease, demonstrated in an initial report that therapy with tamoxifen for more than 5 years could lengthen relapse-free survival (RFS) and possibly OS for women with node-positive disease that is ER-positive. Further clarification of optimal treatment duration with tamoxifen is also currently being investigated in two ongoing adjuvant trials (ATTOM [Adjuvant Tamoxifen Treatment Offers More] and ATLAS [Adjuvant Tamoxifen—Longer Against Shorter]). Both trials are aiming to recruit 20,000 women. The ATTOM trial, which is a Cancer Research Campaign (CRC) trial, is investigating women who have already been taking tamoxifen for at least 2 years. Eligible patients will be randomized to either discontinuation of treatment or continuation of treatment for a further 3 years (81). The ATLAS trial also aims to recruit women already taking tamoxifen, and eligible patients will be randomized to tamoxifen for 5 years or to discontinuation of therapy (82).

With Chemotherapy

The addition of chemotherapy in intermediate- or high-risk groups is recommended (83). The Early Breast Cancer Trialists' Collaborative Group (EBCTCG) overviews in 1990 showed that chemotherapy in combination with tamoxifen demonstrated a beneficial effect in premenopausal women. More recently, the results of the 1998 EBCTCG overview (73) showed that the benefits of chemotherapy combined with tamoxifen in patients with ER-positive disease was irrespective of age or menopausal status. Furthermore, the benefits of chemotherapy in terms of contralateral breast cancer and improved survival were also irrespective of age or menopausal status.

It was not until fairly recently that the appropriate sequence of chemotherapy and hormonal therapy was definitively documented. One difficulty was that evidence had existed in experimental systems that tamoxifen could antagonize the cytotoxic effects of particular chemotherapeutic agents.

In 2002 the results of two prospective studies were presented. One study (84) enrolled 1477 patients. Patients were divided among three groups, with 361 receiving tamoxifen alone, 566 receiving CAF chemotherapy followed by tamoxifen, and 550 receiving concomitant CAF and tamoxifen. Patients were followed up for a median of 8.5 years. The estimated DFS was 67% in the sequential treatment group compared with 62% in the concurrent treatment group. Risk of recurrence was decreased by 18% in the sequential administration group.

In a second study (85), chemotherapy consisted of epirubicin and cyclophosphamide (EC) with, once again, sequential or concomitant administration of tamoxifen. A total of 485 patients were enrolled; 242 received sequential administration and 243 were treated with concomitant tamoxifen. Length of follow-up ranged from 15 to more than 70 months. While there was no significant difference in DFS, there was a trend toward improved DFS in the sequential tamoxifen treatment group.

Aromatase Inhibitors

First-Line

Although tamoxifen has proven efficacy for the treatment of hormone-positive breast cancer both alone and in combination with chemotherapy, its usefulness is in part curtailed by its partial estrogen agonist activity. The documented negative secondary effects of tamoxifen include an increased incidence of endometrial cancer, uterine sarcoma, and thromboembolic disease. Thus there has been great interest in exploring other avenues of endocrine therapy.

In women whose ovarian function has ceased, the primary remaining estrogen source is the conversion of adrenal androgens to estrogens in peripheral tissues by the cytochrome P-450 enzyme aromatase. Aromatase inhibitors act by reducing the availability of estrogen by inhibiting the aromatase enzyme (86) and are indicated for the treatment of breast cancer in postmenopausal women, whose ovarian function has ceased. The first-generation aromatase inhibitor (AI) aminoglutethimide became available approximately 25 years ago (87). Although efficacious, aminoglutethimide was unable to rival tamoxifen owing to its excessive toxicity compared with tamoxifen and its lack of selectivity for the aromatase enzyme, creating the need for concomitant corticosteroid supplementation. Formestane, an effective second-generation AI, became available in 1993. Formestane has fewer side effects than aminoglutethimide (88); however, formestane is not available in the United States.

Newer-generation selective AIs—including anastrozole, letrozole, fadrozole, and exemestane—are now commercially available for the treatment of metastatic breast cancer, although fadrozole can be obtained only in Japan. Anastrozole is indicated for use as either first- or second-line therapy for locally advanced and metastatic breast cancer, as is letrozole. Exemestane is indicated only for second-line use after the failure of other hormonal agents. In addition, anastrozole is also indicated for use in the adjuvant setting in early hormone receptor–positive breast cancer in postmenopausal women.

Based on the antitumor activity of the third-generation AIs in the setting of metastatic disease, these drugs have been assessed in the adjuvant setting. The ATAC (Arimidex [anastrozole], Tamoxifen, Alone, or in Combination) trial was a randomized, double-blind, multicenter study involving 9366 postmenopausal women with invasive operable breast cancer who had completed primary therapy and were eligible for adjuvant treatment. A total of 83.7% of tumors were hormone receptor–positive, 8.2% of tumors were hormone receptor–negative, and 8.1% of tumors were hormone receptor–unknown; the mean age of patients was 64 years, and 34% were node-positive. Patients received either anastrozole alone (1 mg), tamoxifen alone (20 mg), or a combination of the two. The primary objectives of the trial were to evaluate DFS and safety/tolerability. Secondary endpoints were time to recurrence (TTR; defined similarly to DFS but censoring non–breast cancer deaths prior to recurrence) and incidence of new

contralateral primary breast tumors. The first results of the ATAC trial became available in December 2001. These showed that anastrozole was superior to tamoxifen for the treatment of postmenopausal women with primary breast cancer, demonstrating improved efficacy and a more favorable tolerability profile (89).

The first analysis of the ATAC trial was planned to occur when there were 1056 events, including recurrence or death from any cause, and it was actually carried out when 1079 events were recorded, at a median follow-up of 33.3 months. A subsequent updated analysis of the efficacy data was based on a median follow-up of 47 months and a total of 1373 events (90), while the updated analysis of safety data was performed after an additional 7 months of follow-up (37 months) from the first safety analysis at 30 months (Figs. 24-6 and 24-7; Tables 24-6 and 24-7) (91).

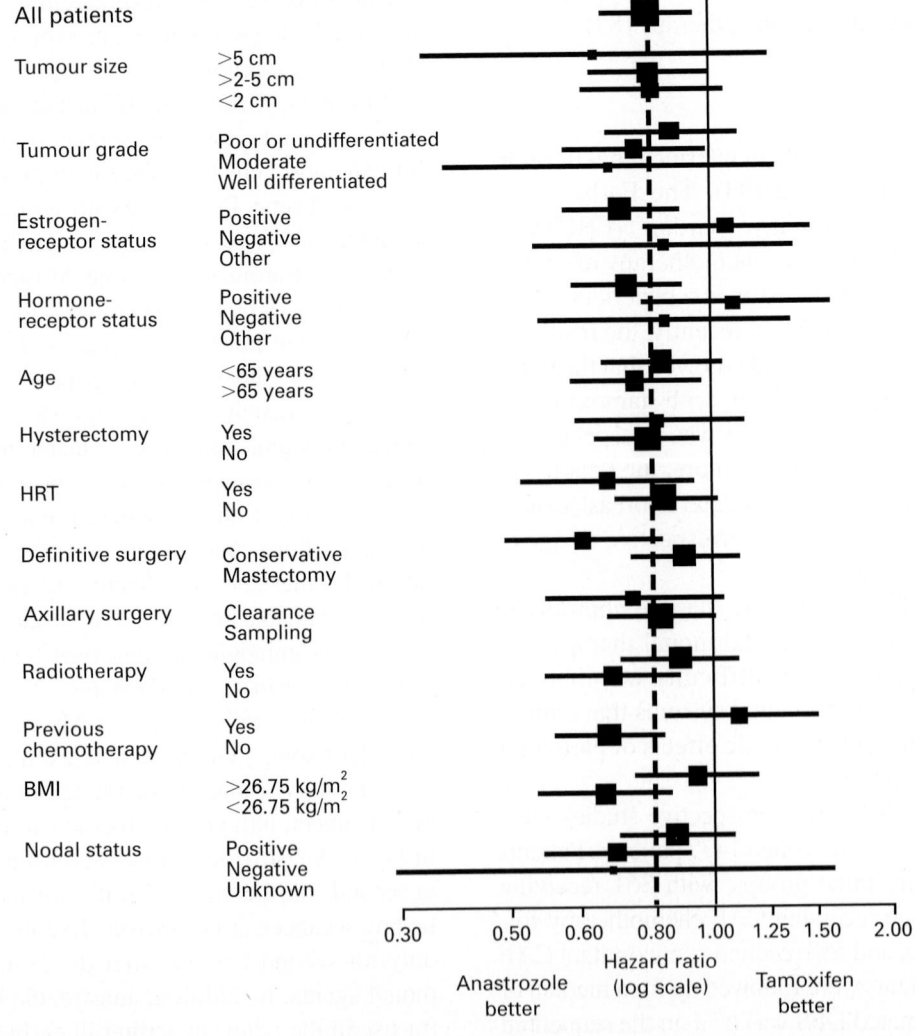

FIGURE 24-6. Subgroup analysis of time to recurrence for tamoxifen versus anastrozole. *(Reproduced, with permission, from Baum M, Budzar AU, Cuzick J, et al. Anastrozole alone or in combination with tamoxifen versus tamoxifen alone for adjuvant treatment of postmenopausal women with early breast cancer: first results of the ATAC randomised trial. Lancet 2002 June 22;359[9324]:2131-2139.)*

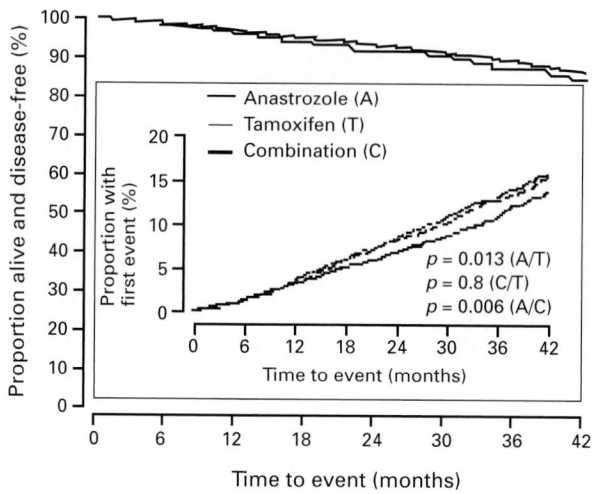

FIGURE 24-7. Kaplan-Meier curves for disease-free survival in the intention-to-treat population. Insert shows data as related to probability of first event. *(Reproduced, with permission, from Baum M, Budzar AU, Cuzick J, et al. Anastrozole alone or in combination with tamoxifen versus tamoxifen alone for adjuvant treatment of postmenopausal women with early breast cancer: first results of the ATAC randomised trial. Lancet 2002 June 22;359[9324]:2131-2139.)*

At the first analysis, anastrozole was found to be superior to tamoxifen for the primary endpoint of DFS and the secondary endpoint of contralateral breast cancer, while the combination was not significantly different from tamoxifen alone for any efficacy endpoints. DFS was significantly longer in the anastrozole group compared with both the tamoxifen and the combination groups. Due to the lack of superiority over tamoxifen alone in either efficacy or safety, follow-up of the combination arm was discontinued after the first analysis.

At 3 years, the DFS estimates were 89.4, 87.4, and 87.2% for anastrozole, tamoxifen, and the combination,

TABLE 24-6	UPDATED EFFICACY RESULTS BASED ON A MEDIAN FOLLOW-UP OF 47 MONTHS		
	AN (N = 3125)	*TAM* (N = 3116)	*AN + TAM* (N = 3125)
First event	413	472	488
Locoregional	84	101	107
Distant	195	222	246
CL (invasive)	20	35	30
CL (DCIS)	5	5	5
Deaths before recurrent	109	109	100

AN, anastrozole; BC, breast cancer; CL, contralateral breast cancer; DCIS, ductal carcinoma in situ; TAM, tamoxifen.
Reproduced, with permission, from Buzdar AU, Obot ATG. The ATAC (Arimidex, Tamoxifen, Alone or in Combination) trial in postmenopausal women with early stage breast cancer: Updated efficacy results based on a median follow-up of 47 months. Breast Cancer Res Treat 2003;77:295.

respectively. In the hormone receptor–positive population, DFS was also significantly longer for those treated with anastrozole compared with those receiving tamoxifen or the combination. Anastrozole was significantly superior to tamoxifen for time to recurrence. Time to recurrence was also significantly longer for those treated with anastrozole compared with tamoxifen in the hormone receptor–positive population. There was a significant reduction in contralateral breast cancers as a first event in the anastrozole group (0.5%; 14 of 3125 patients) versus the tamoxifen group (1.1%; 33 of 3116 patients): the odds were reduced by 58%, which equated to a 58% reduction in risk of developing contralateral breast cancer for women in the anastrozole group compared with women in the tamoxifen group.

Following the first analysis, it was decided that the combination arm should be discontinued, since it showed no benefit over tamoxifen monotherapy in terms of either efficacy or tolerability. At the updated efficacy analysis in the overall and hormone receptor–positive population, DFS remained significantly longer in the anastrozole arm versus the tamoxifen arm of the trial. Time to recurrence was significantly longer for the anastrozole group versus the tamoxifen group in the overall population, with a larger benefit seen in the hormone receptor–positive population. A reduction in the incidence of contralateral breast cancers remained in favor of anastrozole, with statistical significance in the hormone receptor–positive population. DFS estimates at 4 years were 86.9 and 84.5% for anastrozole and tamoxifen, respectively, with an absolute difference of 2.4% (90).

In terms of tolerability, anastrozole was associated with significantly fewer withdrawals from treatment than tamoxifen (anastrozole versus tamoxifen, 21.9 versus 26.0%, $p = .0002$), and significantly fewer withdrawals due to adverse events (anastrozole versus tamoxifen, 7.8 versus 11.1%, $p < .0001$). For the updated safety analysis, the corresponding figures were 24.1 versus 28.3% for anastrozole versus tamoxifen, respectively, and 8.8 versus 12.2% for anastrozole versus tamoxifen, respectively, which demonstrates that the benefit in favor of anastrozole was maintained with longer follow-up. Anastrozole showed a lower incidence compared with tamoxifen for hot flashes, vaginal discharge, and vaginal bleeding ($p < .0001$ for each), ischemic cerebrovascular events and thromboembolic events ($p = .0006$ for each), including deep venous thrombosis ($p = .02$), and for endometrial cancer ($p = .02$). Tamoxifen showed a lower incidence compared with anastrozole for musculoskeletal disorders (including myalgias and arthralgias) and fractures ($p < .0001$ for both). The tolerability results at the updated analysis showed no major difference from those seen at the first analysis (91).

TABLE 24-7 | **OCCURRENCE OF ADVERSE EVENTS FOR TAMOXIFEN VERSUS ANASTRAZOLE**

	Anastrozole (N = 3092)	*Tamoxifen* (N = 3094)	*Combination* (N = 3097)	*p (A versus T)*
Hot flushes	1060 (34.3%)	1229 (39.7%)	1243 (40.1%)	<.0001
Nausea and vomiting	324 (10.5%)	315 (10.2%)	363 (11.7%)	.7
Fatigue/tiredness	483 (15.6%)	466 (15.1%)	435 (14.0%)	.5
Mood disturbances	480 (15.5%)	469 (15.2%)	482 (15.6%)	.7
Musculoskeletal disorders	860 (27.8%)	660 (21.3%)	685 (22.1%)	<.0001
Vaginal bleeding	138 (4.5%)	253 (8.2%)	238 (7.7%)	<.0001
Vaginal discharge	86 (2.8%)	354 (11.4%)	357 (11.5%)	<.0001
Endometrial cancer	3 (0.1%)	13 (0.5%)	6 (0.3%)	.02
Fractures	183 (5.9%)	115 (3.7%)	142 (4.6%)	<.0001
Hip	11 (0.4%)	13 (0.4%)	10 (0.3%)	ND
Spine	23 (0.7%)	10 (0.3%)	14 (0.5%)	ND
Wrist/colles	36 (1.2%)	25 (0.8%)	27 (0.9%)	ND
Ischemic cardiovascular disease	76 (2.5%)	9 (1.9%)	68 (2.2%)	.14
Ischemic cardiovascular event	31 (1.0%)	65 (2.1%)	51 (1.6%)	.0006
Any venous thromboembolic events	64 (2.1%)	109 (3.5%)	124 (4.0%)	.0006
Deep venous thromboembolic events PE	32 (1.0%)	54 (1.7%)	63 (2.0%)	.02
Cataracts	107 (3.5%)	116 (3.7%)	105 (3.4%)	.6

A, anastrozole; ND, no data; PE, pulmonary embolism; T, tamoxifen.

Reproduced, with permission, from Baum M, Budzar AU, Cuzick J, et al. Anastrozole alone or in combination with tamoxifen versus tamoxifen alone for adjuvant treatment of postmenopausal women with early breast cancer: first results of the ATAC randomised trial. Lancet 2002;359:2131-2139.

An investigation of the first-generation aromatase inhibitor aminoglutethimide was done by the Austrian Breast and Colorectal Cancer Study Group Trial 6 (92), which recruited 2021 hormone receptor–positive, lymph node–negative or –positive postmenopausal patients, randomly assigned patients to receive either tamoxifen monotherapy (40 mg/day for 2 years and 20 mg/day for the subsequent 3 years) and in combination (40 mg/day for 2 years and 20 mg/day for the subsequent 3 years) with aminoglutethimide (500 mg/day for 2 years). Results showed that after a median follow-up of 5.3 years, there were no differences between the two groups for DFS (aminoglutethimide plus tamoxifen versus tamoxifen, 83.6 versus 83.7%, p = .89) and for OS (aminoglutethimide plus tamoxifen versus tamoxifen, 91.4 versus 91.2%, p = .74). Significantly more patients in the combination group failed to complete treatment because of side effects (aminoglutethimide plus tamoxifen versus tamoxifen, 13.7 versus 5.2%, p = .0001). Thus the authors conclude that the combination of aminoglutethimide with tamoxifen versus tamoxifen alone does not improve clinical outcome in postmenopausal women with hormone receptor–positive, lymph node–negative or –positive tumors. Although this trial does not include an aminoglutethimide monotherapy arm, the profile of results seen in the tamoxifen monotherapy and combination arms are similar to those seen in the ATAC trial for the tamoxifen and combination arms.

A meta-analysis published in 2010 reviewed the use of AIs versus tamoxifen in postmenopausal women with ER-positive tumors. This quantitative review compared AIs as initial monotherapy to tamoxifen monotherapy, or as a hormone switch after 2 to 3 years of tamoxifen for a total of 5 years. The conclusion was that AI therapy was associated with a lower rate of recurrence when used as an initial monotherapy or after 2 to 3 years of tamoxifen when compared to tamoxifen monotherapy (Fig. 24-8) (93).

Following Tamoxifen

Recent publications have now brought about significant discussion regarding the use of aromatase inhibitors after tamoxifen in the adjuvant setting. It is postulated that tamoxifen might stop being effective because breast cancer cells develop resistance to tamoxifen, dependence on tamoxifen, or great sensitivity to circulating estrogen.

MA-17 (94) was a phase III randomized, double-blind study of adjuvant letrozole 2.5 mg a day versus placebo in women with primary breast cancer after completing 5 years of tamoxifen therapy. To study efficacy, 2575 women received letrozole 2.5 mg a day versus 2582 women who received placebo for a total of 5 years. In order to be eligible, patients needed to be postmenopausal, have a history of estrogen-dependent tumors, have completed 4.5 to 6 years of tamoxifen, and

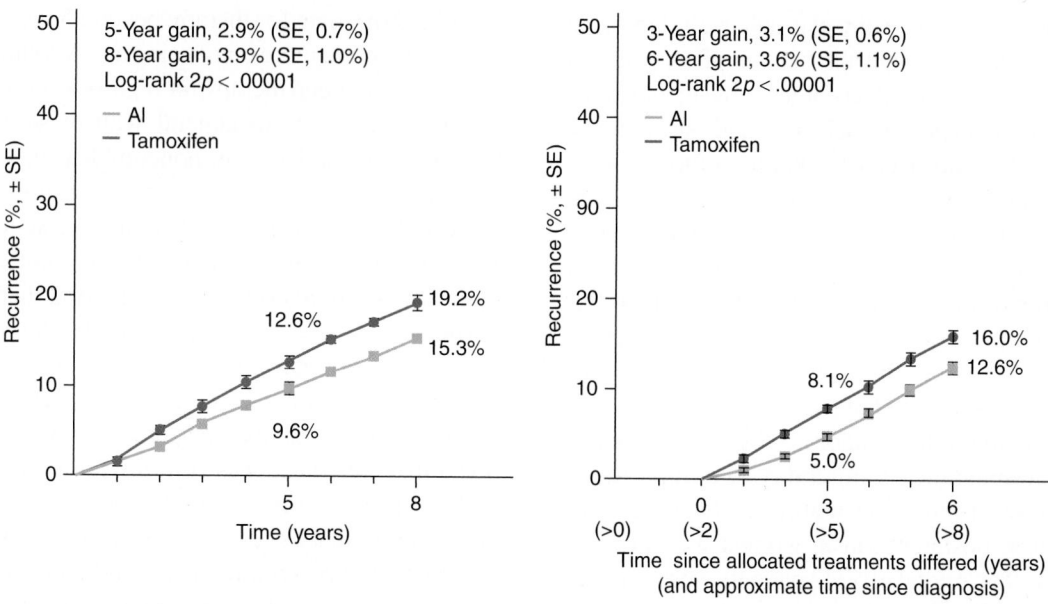

FIGURE 24-8. Life-table curves for recurrence after 5 years aromatase inhibitor (AI) therapy versus tamoxifen (left) and after 2 to 3 years of tamoxifen followed by 2 to 3 years of AI versus tamoxifen (right). *(Reproduced, with permission, from Dowsett M, Cuzick J, Ingle J, et al. Meta-analysis of breast cancer outcomes in adjuvant trials of aromatase inhibitors versus tamoxifen. J Clin Oncol 2010 January 20;28[3]509-518.)*

have no evidence of recurrence. The primary endpoint was defined as DFS. Interim analysis was prospectively planned at 171 and 342 events, with a stopping boundary of $p = .00079$. Median duration of follow-up was 2.4 years. The 4-year DFS rate was 93% in the letrozole arm versus 87% in the placebo arm ($p = .00008$). Letrozole lowered the risk of recurrence by 43% versus

placebo (Table 24-8). A more recent analysis of this trial involved a subset of patients who became menopausal during treatment. As presented at SABCS 2009, ER-positive premenopausal breast cancer patients appear to benefit from extended AI therapy after they become menopausal and this benefit extended to up to 6 years after tamoxifen therapy (95). Thus, letrozole has

TABLE 24-8	RECURRENCE OF PRIMARY CANCERS AND NEW CONTRALATERAL BREAST CANCERS IN LETROZOLE GROUP VERSUS PLACEBO GROUP	
Variable	*Letrozole Group* *(N = 2575)*	*Placebo Group* *(N = 2582)*
Recurrence*	61 (2.4%)	106 (4.1%)
Local, ipsilateral breast only	6	19
Local, ipsilateral chest wall only	2	7
Regional nodes only	6	4
Distant site or sites[†]	47	76
Bone marrow	4	4
Lungs	9	14
Bone	29	44
Pleural effusion	0	8
Liver	14	13
Central nervous system	0	2
Other	11	18
New primary tumor in the contralateral breast only	14 (0.5%)	26 (1.0%)
Total with recurrence or new contralateral breast cancer	75	132

Reproduced, with permission, from Goss PE, Ingle JN, Martino S, et al. A randomized trial of letrozole in postmenopausal women after five years of tamoxifen therapy for early-stage breast cancer. N Engl J Med 2003;349:1793-1802.

been shown to be the first treatment to achieve a significant DFS in the extended adjuvant setting after adjuvant tamoxifen. Common side effects of letrozole included hot flashes, arthritis, joint pain, muscle pain, and osteoporosis.

The Big 1-98 trial was designed to compare letrozole with tamoxifen in postmenopausal hormone-positive women and was later amended to include two sequential strategies using letrozole either before or after tamoxifen for a total of 5 years. The results of this study are that upfront AI reduces the risk of recurrence and disease-free survival better than upfront tamoxifen and better than either switching strategy (96,97).

Another double-blind randomized trial investigated the use of exemestane 25 mg a day to complete the 5 years of adjuvant endocrine treatment after 2 to 3 years of tamoxifen in postmenopausal women with primary breast cancer (98). A total of 4742 patients were enrolled with 2362 assigned to switch to exemestane and 2380 to continue to receive tamoxifen. Median follow-up was 30.6 months. The unadjusted hazard ratio was 0.68 ($p < .001$) for exemestane as compared to the tamoxifen group, and the absolute benefit in DFS was 4.7% (Fig. 24-9). OS was not statistically different between the two groups. Analysis of adverse events demonstrated that there was a lower incidence of thromboembolic events among women who were switched to exemestane, and, as expected, there was a slight nonsignificant increase in osteoporosis and related fractures for the exemestane group. Thus, exemestane therapy following 2 to 3 years of tamoxifen did significantly improve DFS.

The above data for therapy beyond 5 years of tamoxifen is becoming more convincing and AIs should be considered as extended therapy for high-risk postmenopausal patients. Outcomes in general with these antiestrogen therapies are hindered by noncompliance, with reports indicating 20 to 50% nonadherence rates. This is the same difficulty faced in other disease states, and the presence of a cancer diagnosis does not necessarily command optimal compliance with oral therapy. Many barriers influence compliance including medication cost, access to mail-order pharmacies, and a lack of understanding of the benefits of such medicine. A population-based study performed in British Columbia noted that adherence was still difficult even when these oral agents are given free of charge in a country with a national formulary system. Patients who are on oral medication should be seen regularly and compliance should be reinforced as highly important as shown in multiple studies even when drug cost is excluded as a barrier (99).

Ovarian Ablation and Suppression

The use of oophorectomy or ovarian irradiation to cause ovarian ablation has been documented to be an efficacious method for treating early-stage disease in premenopausal patients. The 1996 meta-analysis by the EBCTCG demonstrated that for women below age 50 there was a distinct advantage in OS and DFS when they were treated with ovarian ablation compared with those who received no adjuvant therapy. In addition, the outcomes for these

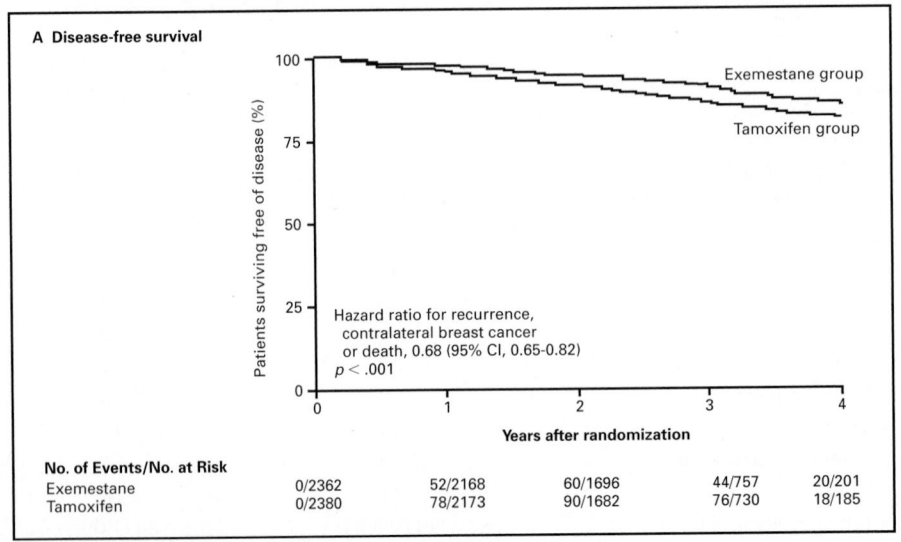

FIGURE 24-9. Kaplan-Meier estimates of disease-free survival for exemestane group as compared with tamoxifen group. An additional 6 patients in the exemestane group and 4 patients in the tamoxifen group had a recurrence or a second primary cancer in the contralateral breast or died more than 4 years after randomization. *(Reproduced, with permission, from Coombes RC, Hall E, Gibson LJ, et al. A randomized trial of exemestane after two to three years of tamoxifen therapy in postmenopausal women with primary breast cancer. N Engl J Med 2004 March 11;350[11]:1081-1092.)*

patients were similar to those who received the CMF regimen. However, the permanent creation of premature menopause is not without complications. Thus multiple studies are now investigating the outcome of inducing reversible ovarian ablation or ovarian suppression.

LH-RH Agonists

Monotherapy

The most currently studied luteinizing hormone–releasing hormone (LH-RH) agonist is goserelin acetate, or Zoladex. The Zoladex Early Breast Cancer Research Association (ZEBRA) trial (100) is the largest adjuvant trial to investigate goserelin acetate in the adjuvant treatment of women with early breast cancer. A total of 1640 premenopausal or perimenopausal women who were less than 50 years old were enrolled. All patients were systemic treatment–naive and had node-positive stage II disease. Patients received either goserelin 3.6 mg every 28 days for 2 years or CMF (cyclophosphamide, methotrexate, 5-flurouracil) for six cycles. Patients were followed up for a median of 6 years. Data was stratified for ER status. DFS was noted to be equivalent to CMF for the ER-positive group. Conversely, goserelin was inferior to CMF for DFS in the ER-negative group. Treatment with goserelin resulted in an insignificant trend toward longer survival.

Amenorrhea was noted to occur with a higher incidence in the goserelin group, with 95% at 24 weeks in the goserelin group versus 65% in the CMF group. However, while amennorhea occurred early in the goserelin group, it was reversible. In the CMF group, the amenorrhea continued at 3 years for the majority of women, likely resulting in irreversible ovarian ablation. The most notable other side effects for goserelin were vaginal dryness and hot flashes, which were noted to cease after completion of therapy.

With Tamoxifen

In 1990 the Austrian Breast Cancer Study Group (ABCSG) ac05 trial (101) was established to compare outcomes for women treated with CMF for six cycles versus goserelin 3.6 mg every 28 days plus tamoxifen 20 mg a day for 5 years. The patients enrolled were all premenopausal but varied in their hormonal and nodal status. Median follow-up was for 5 years. DFS was significantly better for the goserelin-plus-tamoxifen arm as compared with the CMF arm for patients with hormone receptor–positive disease, with a risk ratio of 1.35 (CMF: goserelin + tamoxifen), $p = .04$. OS was not statistically significantly different between the two groups. The side effects of goserelin were similar to those seen in the ZEBRA trial, with hot flashes being the most common.

The results of INT0142 (102) were presented at the 2003 meeting of the American Society of Clinical Oncology (ASCO). This was a prospective randomized trial planned to assess DSF, OS, TTR, and quality of life for adjuvant tamoxifen alone versus tamoxifen plus ovarian ablation. Over a 3-year time course, 345 women were enrolled with tumors less than or equal to 3 cm, negative nodes, and positive ER and/or PR status. Patients were treated with either tamoxifen 20 mg a day for 5 years or tamoxifen for 5 years plus ovarian ablation. Methods for ovarian ablation included LH-RH analogs (goserelin or leuprolide acetate), oophorectomy, or ovarian radiation. The trial was designed to accrue 1684 patients, but it accrued slowly and was closed before reaching this target. Survival analyses were under-powered, but DFS was notably similar, with 87% in the tamoxifen arm and 89% in the arm providing tamoxifen plus ovarian ablation. However, menopausal symptoms as measured by questionnaire were significantly worse in the ovarian ablation arm.

After Chemotherapy

The ZIPP (Zoladex in Premenopausal Patients) analysis (103) involved a combination of data from randomized trials carried out by four international collaborative groups. Patients were all premenopausal and were treated with surgery followed by chemotherapy ± radiation therapy followed by randomization to an endocrine therapy. The most common chemotherapy regimen used was CMF. The four endocrine therapy groups were goserelin 3.6 mg every 28 days for 2 years, tamoxifen 20 mg a day for 5 years, combination of goserelin and tamoxifen, and the control group of no endocrine treatment. Analysis of the data revealed that there was a distinctly significant benefit for the goserelin in decreasing the risk of recurrence and increasing OS. This benefit was noted regardless of which chemotherapy regimen was given and whether tamoxifen was given.

At the ASCO 2003 meeting a trial was presented that investigated whether ovarian suppression added benefit to chemotherapy. This study included 926 women who were treated with adjuvant chemotherapy after surgery (104). Patients were then randomized to ovarian irradiation versus triptorelin or goserelin versus no further therapy. Hormone-positive tumors were present in 76% of the patients and axillary nodal involvement in 90%. Ten-year DFS was 49% in the chemotherapy-alone arm and 48% in the arm providing chemotherapy plus ovarian suppression. The respective 10-year OS results were 68 versus 65%. Thus there is no apparent benefit from ovarian suppression after chemotherapy. This is independent of age, hormone receptor status, or method of ovarian suppression.

In the end, although there are promising data from the use of goserelin as monotherapy for adjuvant therapy of hormone receptor–positive disease, there is no convincing randomized trial that shows a clear benefit beyond what is achieved by tamoxifen or anastrazole. In addition, the data from studies combining goserelin with tamoxifen or chemotherapy are conflicting. Data from multiple studies support using tamoxifen for the premenopausal patient and considering anastrazole for the postmenopausal hormone receptor–positive patient. However, the recent results from the MA-17 trial now provides evidence for the use of tamoxifen followed by letrozole. In addition, data from multiple trials including the NSABP B-23 (105) do not support the use of endocrine agents such as tamoxifen in the estrogen receptor–negative patient.

BISPHOSPHONATES

Bisphosphonates have an established role in metastatic breast cancer as they have proven efficacy in reducing skeletal-related events in patients with bone metastases. In a high percentage of patients even at early stage, there are tumor cells which are detectable in peripheral blood and are thought to seek sites for quiescence. The highest reservoir of these cells is in bone. Newer data suggest that zoledronic acid, specifically, possesses antitumor activity due to regulation of molecular pathways involved in adhesion, invasion, and angiogenesis. This has prompted rapid research in the adjuvant setting using zoledronic acid as demonstrated in the Austrian Breast and Colorectal Cancer Study Group trial 12 (ABCSG-12). This trial reported that the addition of zoledronic acid to adjuvant endocrine therapy prolongs disease-free survival compared to endocrine therapy alone (106). The United States initiated a similar trial known as Z-FAST, the Zometa-Femara Adjuvant Synergy Trial, and Europe led the ZO-FAST trial of the same name, both of which concurred with the results of ABCSG-12 (107,108).

Other trials are now under way evaluating bisphosphonates in the adjuvant setting for early and locally advanced breast cancer. NSABP B34 is testing oral clodronate versus placebo for 3 years. The largest study to complete enrollment to date is the AZURE trial comparing zoledronic acid versus placebo and has completed enrollment of 3360 patients. Results are expected in the near future.

■ NEOADJUVANT THERAPY

CHEMOTHERAPY

The concept of giving chemotherapy in the preoperative setting was first evaluated more than 30 years ago for the treatment of locally advanced and inoperable breast cancer. There are multiple possible benefits. One is the ability to downstage a tumor, which would result in making an unresectable tumor operable or enable breast-conserving surgery or segmental mastectomies to be offered to a greater number of patients with operable breast cancer. In addition, there are biological advantages, such as the ability to assess response or resistance to chemotherapy early, delivering the chemotherapy prior to surgical alterations to the vasculature, and using molecular profiling in conjunction with pathologic response to predict outcomes for patients.

In 1978, a study was published that addressed whether there was a benefit for those with inoperable breast cancer who were treated with neoadjuvant chemotherapy. A total of 110 patients were enrolled and were treated with doxorubicin and vincristine. CR was seen in 16% and PR in 55% of patients. All patients also received standard radiation therapy. The 36-month survival data were 53% for the study group and 41% for the historical controls. The positive results of this study led to other trials (109).

In 1983, MDACC reported on 52 patients with locally advanced breast cancer who were treated with three cycles of neoadjuvant anthracycline-based chemotherapy followed by local therapy, and then further adjuvant treatment for 2 years. This resulted in a 40% DFS at 5 years (110).

Outcomes from neoadjuvant chemotherapy have also been compared directly with adjuvant chemotherapy. One such study enrolled a total of 272 patients. All patients had tumors greater than 3 cm that were considered operable. Patients were randomized to either the traditional treatment arm with surgery followed by chemotherapy or the neoadjuvant arm with neoadjuvant therapy preceding surgery. This trial did show an increased OS that was statistically significant for the neoadjuvant therapy arm; however, more patients were enrolled in this neoadjuvant group than in the traditional treatment arm (111).

The NASBP B-18 trial was the largest to date to investigate neoadjuvant chemotherapy. A total of 1523 patients with T1 to T3 and N0 to N1 disease were randomized to receive preoperative Adriamycin (doxorubicin) and cytoxan (AC) versus postoperative AC for four cycles (112). In addition to using traditional response criteria, patients who had a CR also underwent tissue analysis for a pathologic complete response (pCR). It was found that tumor size and nodal status were independent clinical predictors of response, and 36% of patients achieved a CR. Lumpectomy was initially proposed for only 3% of women with tumor sizes >5 cm; however, there was a 175% increase in lumpectomies performed in the neoadjuvant treatment group. Final comparison of the two groups revealed no difference in DFS or OS at 5 years. This was true for all groups including those with tumors larger than 5 cm.

Another trial investigated downstaging of axillary nodal metastases after primary chemotherapy (113). A total of 152 patients with invasive T1 to T3 tumors and axillary nodal metastases were enrolled. All patients underwent neoadjuvant chemotherapy followed by lumpectomy or mastectomy, axillary lymph node dissection, and irradiation. Patients were treated with three or four monthly courses of FAC or 5-fluorouracil, cyclophosphamide, and methotrexate or thiotepa. A pCR was achieved for the axillary nodes in 23% of the patients and 13.2% of the primary tumors. An initial tumor size of less than 3 cm was associated with a pCR of the primary tumor. From Cox regression analysis it was shown that one of the parameters associated with poor distant disease survival was persistent nodal involvement after neoadjuvant therapy. Thus it was concluded that the response of the axillary nodes to neoadjuvant chemotherapy was a better predictor than the response of the primary tumor.

Epirubicin-based therapy given in either the preoperative or the postoperative setting was evaluated by the European Organization for Research and Treatment of Cancer (EORTC) group in a phase III trial. The primary outcomes addressed by this trial included OS and RFS as well as rates of breast-conserving therapy (114). Nearly 700 patients were enrolled with T1c to T4b, N0 to N1, and M0 disease. All patients were treated with four cycles of FEC either preoperatively or postoperatively. Patients were followed up for a median of 56 months and there was no significant difference in OS, RFS. However, as previously noted by other trials, more patients could be given breast-conserving treatment.

A 2002 paper addressed the question of the efficacy of neoadjuvant docetaxel with anthracycline-based treatment with a secondary goal of addressing the effectiveness of the use of docetaxel for patients who had failed anthracyline therapy (115). Patients with tumors more than 3 cm in size or T3, T4, or N2 disease were treated with four cycles of cyclophosphamide, vincristine, Adriamycin (doxorubicin), and prednisolone (CVAP). Patients who achieved a CR or PR were then treated with either four cycles of CVAP or four cycles of

docetaxel. Patients who were nonresponders were treated with four cycles of docetaxel. Those who achieved a CR or PR with initial CVAP and who then received docetaxel achieved significantly higher CR, PR, and pCR rates. In addition, the use of docetaxel for anthracycline-resistant tumors also resulted in improved clinical responses.

Paclitaxel was also evaluated in the preoperative setting for locally advanced breast cancer. Patients who had stage IIB to III disease were eligible for this phase I/II (116). Treatment strategy included twice-weekly paclitaxel at a dose of 30 mg/m^2 for 8 to 10 weeks and then concurrent radiation with a total of 45 Gy. Patients then all underwent modified radical mastectomy. Postoperative treatment was based on response to preoperative therapy. Those who had shown good response went on to receive doxorubicin and paclitaxel, whereas those with a poor preoperative response were treated with doxorubicin and cyclophosphamide. The overall clinical response rate for the preoperative therapy was 91%. The total pathologic response rate was 34%, with 16% CRs. Thus a combined neoadjuvant therapy approach with concurrent radiation treatment was shown to be an effective approach for locally advanced breast cancer.

A phase III randomized trial (117) at MDACC was performed to evaluate the effect of a dose-dense approach to weekly paclitaxel as compared with standard every-3-week paclitaxel. MDACC, which had previously investigated paclitaxel every 3 weeks in the adjuvant setting followed by FAC, has also studied the use of weekly paclitaxel followed by FAC as neoadjuvant systemic therapy. This study accrued 258 patients with operable breast cancer with T1 to T3, N0 to N1, M0 disease; they were randomized to receive either weekly paclitaxel or the standard every-3-week paclitaxel regimen. The endpoints were to address whether different schedules or dose densities of paclitaxel improved the pCR rates. The patients on the weekly paclitaxel regimen who were N0 received 80 mg/m^2 per week for 12 weeks, whereas N1 patients received 150 mg/m^2 per week for 3 weeks followed by a 1-week break for a total of four cycles, or 12 weeks. The standard paclitaxel dose was 225 mg/m^2 every 3 weeks for four cycles. All patients then received four cycles of FAC after paclitaxel, and this was followed by locoregional therapy. Data presented at the ASCO 2002 meeting documented that weekly paclitaxel provided a statistically significant benefit in improvement of pCR rates as compared to every-3-week paclitaxel. For N1 patients, the pCR was 28% with weekly paclitaxel as compared to 13.7% with every-3-week paclitaxel (Table 24-9).

TABLE 24-9	PATHOLOGIC COMPLETE REMISSION RATES IN WEEKLY VERSUS EVERY-3-WEEK NEOADJUVANT PACLITAXEL			
	NODE-POSITIVE		NODE-NEGATIVE	
	Weekly	*Every 3 Weeks*	*Weekly*	*Every 3 Weeks*
pCR	28%	13.7%	29.4%	13.4%

pCR, pathologic complete response.
Data from Green MC, Budzar AU, Smith T et al. Weekly paclitaxel followed by FAC as primary systemic chemotherapy of operable breast cancer improves pathologic complete remission rates when compared to every 3-week paclitaxel therapy followed by FAC-final results of a preospective phase III randomized trial. J Clin Oncol Sep 1;23(25):5983-5992, 2005.

In patients with *HER-2/neu* positive breast cancer, neoadjuvant therapy includes utilization of trastuzumab. In most instances, trastuzumab is combined with the taxane portion of systemic therapy, given the increased risk of cardiac toxicity when combined with anthracyclines. Nonetheless, a trial from MD Anderson recently demonstrated the safe employment of trastuzumab and epirubicin (118). Also, data supports that the initiation of trastuzumab concomitant with taxane-based chemotherapy rather than sequentially results in significant improvement in DFS with a 4.4% absolute risk reduction in the number of events at 5 years (119).

Thus, in general, neoadjuvant therapy with either anthracycline- or taxane-containing regimens has been shown in multiple trials to result in an increase in the number of women who are able to undergo breast-conserving surgery. Studies have also shown that the use of neoadjuvant therapy, especially with taxanes, can lead to pCRs as well as clinical responses. These responses have been well-correlated to disease-free and overall survival making response to preoperative chemotherapy a novel prognostic factor in the treatment of early and locally advanced breast cancer. At this time the majority of neoadjuvant studies have not yet shown an increase in OS for patients treated with this approach. Preoperative chemotherapy is especially clinically warranted for those with tumors greater than 3 cm and for axillary node disease. More studies are also planned to address quality-of-life issues for patients treated with this modality.

ENDOCRINE THERAPY

The concept of neoadjuvant hormonal therapy is also being evaluated currently. Most studies have investigated the potential of using this approach for patients with locally advanced disease rather than early-stage disease. It is a treatment option for women with tumors expressing the estrogen receptor or progesterone receptor or both, and for patients with low histologic grade tumors.

In 1981, tamoxifen therapy was investigated in postmenopausal advanced breast cancer with locally advanced noninflammatory inoperable T3 to T4 disease (120). Patients were treated with neoadjuvant tamoxifen 10 to 20 mg twice a day for a minimum of 6 weeks. A total of 17% of patients had an objective response after 6 weeks of treatment; with continued therapy a total of 30% of patients achieved a response. The outcome of this study revealed that while response rates were lower than those for chemotherapy, endocrine therapy is a safe and at least moderately effective treatment.

A decade later, a pilot study was done that investigated chemotherapy versus endocrine therapy for patients with locally advanced breast cancer. A total of 60 patients were randomized to receive endocrine therapy or chemotherapy (121). The endocrine therapy used was goserelin, an LH-RH analog, for premenopausal women and 4-hydroxyandrostenedione for postmenopausal women. Complete clinical response of the primary tumor was noted in 27% of the patients treated with chemotherapy. However, no patients in the endocrine therapy group had a complete clinical response, although 10% had PRs. The conclusion of the study was that response rates were significantly better with chemotherapy but that overall outcomes such as DFS were similar over a 65-week follow-up interval.

In 2000, MDACC published a study that addressed the use of neoadjuvant tamoxifen in multimodality treatment for the care of patients who were above 75 years of age or frail and had locally advanced breast cancer (122). All 47 patients studied were treated with tamoxifen for 3 to 6 months, then surgery, followed by radiation therapy, followed by adjuvant tamoxifen for 5 years. Both stage II and stage III patients were enrolled, with respective percentages of 22 and 78%. After 6 months of treatment, a response rate of 47% was noted. Median follow-up was 40 months, and 49% of patients remained disease-free during this time. The estimated 5-year progression-free survival (PFS) and OS rates were 83 and 59%. Thus tamoxifen was shown to be a good option for patients who, because of age or comorbidities, would not be ideal candidates for chemotherapy.

A phase III trial investigated the use of the AI letrozole as a neoadjuvant endocrine therapy for postmenopausal patients with c-*erb* B-1– and/or c-*erb* B-2 (*HER-2/neu*)–positive, ER-positive breast cancer (123). Letrozole was studied, since it is known that c-*erb* B-1/-2–positive tumors are likely more resistant to tamoxifen. Treatment included either tamoxifen 20 mg daily or letrozole 2.5 mg daily for a total of 4 months. For the letrozole arm, patients had a 60% overall response rate, with 48% undergoing breast-conserving therapy, whereas the tamoxifen group had inferior responses, with a 41% response rate and a 36% rate of breast-conserving surgery. Thus it appears that for this subgroup of ER-positive tumors, the use of an AI is more potent than the use of tamoxifen.

A 2003 ASCO abstract detailed the results of a trial that investigated the use of third-generation AIs alone or in combination with tamoxifen for versus tamoxifen alone. Patients enrolled were all postmenopausal and had either ER- or PR-positive breast cancers with T2,N1, T3,N0-1, and T4,N0 disease (124). Patients were treated with anastrazole 1 mg daily, tamoxifen 20 mg daily, or tamoxifen plus anastrazole for 3 months. The clinical overall response rates were superior in the anastrazole arm, with 70 versus 44% in the tamoxifen arm and 49% in the combined-treatment arm. Breast-conserving therapy was able to be performed in 42% of the anastrazole group, 28% in the tamoxifen group, and 30% in the combined-treatment group. Anastrazole was shown to be more effective than tamoxifen or combined treatment for postmenopausal patients with ER- or PR-positive breast cancer. Although clinical responses are observed with preoperative endocrine therapy, pCRs occur in less than 5% of patients. The proliferative index marker Ki67 is being studied as a predictor of long-term response after therapy in this setting (125,126).

At this time, neoadjuvant hormonal therapy based on trial results seems to be best suited to women who have locally advanced breast cancer who are otherwise thought to be not suitable for neoadjuvant chemotherapy or whose tumors are noted to be low-grade with expression of the estrogen or progesterone receptors. However, at this time the standard neoadjuvant approach for node-positive or locally advanced breast cancer remains chemotherapy.

■ OTHER SYSTEMIC THERAPY TOPICS

DOSE DENSITY

One method of increasing response rate to chemotherapy that has been investigated is the concept of dose density. This term represents the administration of chemotherapeutic agents with a shortened interval between treatments, based on the knowledge that a given dose always kills a particular fraction of cancer cells. Thus it has been proposed that more frequent administration of cytotoxic therapy would be more efficacious than dose escalation for minimizing tumor burden. To this effect several recently published trials have explored the outcomes from dose-density regimens.

CALGB 9741 (127,128) explored the possible superiority of dose-dense over conventional scheduling of adjuvant chemotherapy for node-positive breast cancer. Endpoints to be evaluated were OS, DFS, and toxicities. A total of 2005 patients with T0 to T3, N1-2, M0 disease were enrolled. They were then randomly assigned to receive one of four treatment regimens. There were two each of sequential and concurrent treatment arms. Patients in the first group received sequential treatment with doxorubicin (60 mg/m^2) for four doses every 3 weeks followed by four doses of paclitaxel (175 mg/m^2) every 3 weeks followed by cyclophosphamide (600 mg/m^2) for four doses every 3 weeks. The second sequential treatment group received the same regimen as above but with dosing modifications, so that the dosing frequency for all chemotherapeutic agents was decreased from every 3 weeks to every 2 weeks; in addition, all patients received granulocyte colony-stimulating factor (G-CSF) for days 3 to 10 of each cycle. The third treatment group received chemotherapy with concurrent doxorubicin (60 mg/m^2) and cyclophosphamide (600 mg/m^2) for four doses every 3 weeks followed by paclitaxel (175 mg/m^2) for four doses every 3 weeks. The fourth treatment group received similar concurrent chemotherapy as group three, but with the dosing frequency once again increased to every 2 weeks plus G-CSF for days 3 to 10 of each cycle.

Median follow-up for CALGB 9741 was 36 months. Dose-dense treatment did improve DFS to 82% (every 2 weeks) versus 75% (every 3 weeks), with $p = .01$. OS was also improved with 92% (every 2 weeks) versus 90% (every 3 weeks), with $p = .013$. However, there was no difference between OS or DFS between the sequential and concurrent schedules. In terms of toxicities, the highest neutropenia rates were noted in groups one and three (23 and 43%) as compared to groups two and four (3 and 9%). The decreased rates of neutropenia can be attributed to the fact that groups two and four received growth factor support. In addition there was a significant increase in red blood cell transfusions (13%) for group four, which received concurrent every-2-week therapy (Figs. 24-10 through 24-12, Table 24-10).

Thus this study was able to document that dose density does improve clinical outcome. However, sequential chemotherapy appears to be as effective as concurrent chemotherapy at this time.

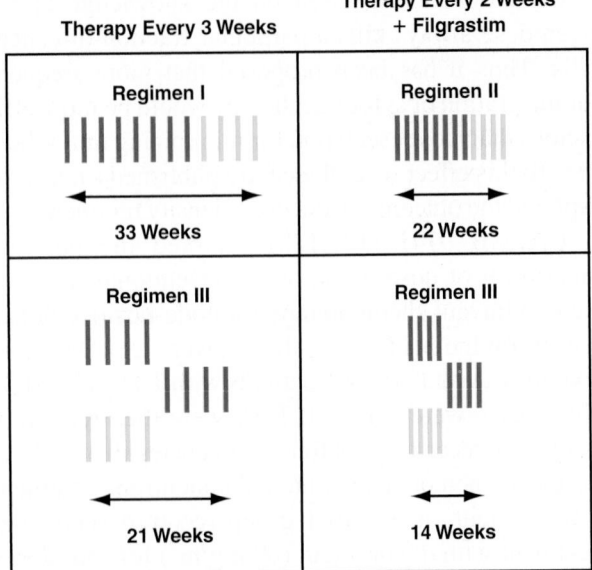

Doxorubicin 60 mg/m² IV

Cyclophosphamide 600 mg/m² IV

Paclitaxel 175 mg² IV over 3 h

Regimen 1: A×4→T×4→C×4 every 3 weeks
Regimen 2: A×4→T×4→C×4 every 2 weeks with G-CSF
Regimen 3: AC×4→T×4 every 3 weeks
Regimen 4: AC×4→T×4 every 2 weeks with G-CSF

A = Doxorubicin 60 mg/m²
T = Paclitaxel 175 mg/m² over 3 h
C = Cyclophosphamide 600 mg/m²

FIGURE 24-10. Treatment regimens for CALGB 9741. (*Reproduced, with permission, from Citron ML, Berry DA, Cirrincione C, et al. Randomized trial of dose-dense versus conventionally scheduled and sequential versus concurrent combination chemotherapy as postoperative adjuvant treatment of node-positive primary breast cancer: first report of Intergroup Trial C9741/ Cancer and Leukemia Group B Trial 9741. J Clin Oncol 2003 April 15;21[8]:1431-1439.*)

A smaller study (129) evaluated dose-dense anthracycline-based therapy in combination with cyclophosphamide with and without 5-FU. A total of 52 patients were enrolled who had either node-positive, ER-negative disease, *HER-2/neu*–positive disease, or four or more positive lymph nodes. Patients were treated with doxorubicin on a weekly basis of 20 mg/m² per week and 5-FU at 300 mg/m² per week, both given intravenously, for 24 weeks. Cyclophosphamide was then administered at 60 mg/m² per day orally for 24 weeks. In the last 22 patients, 5-FU was omitted mainly because of symptomatic hand-foot syndrome,

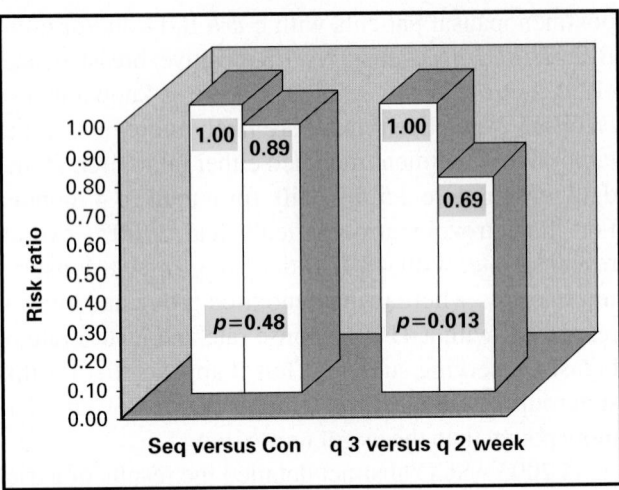

FIGURE 24-11. Disease-free survival of patients on CALGB 9741. (*Reproduced, with permission, from Citron M, Berry D, Cirrincione C, et al. Superiority of dose-dense over conventional scheduling and equivalence of sequential vs. combination adjuvant chemotherapy for node-positive breast cancer [CALGB 9741, INT C9741]. Breast Cancer Res Treat 76 [Suppl. 1], S32 [abst 15]. 2002.*)

and the doxorubicin dose was increased to 24 mg/m² per week for 20 weeks, such that both groups of patients received the same total dose of doxorubicin. All patients also received G-CSF on each day of therapy except for the days when intravenous chemotherapy was given. Also all hormone-positive patients were treated with tamoxifen for 5 years. The observed DFS was 85% at 5 years; this was contrasted to the 62 and

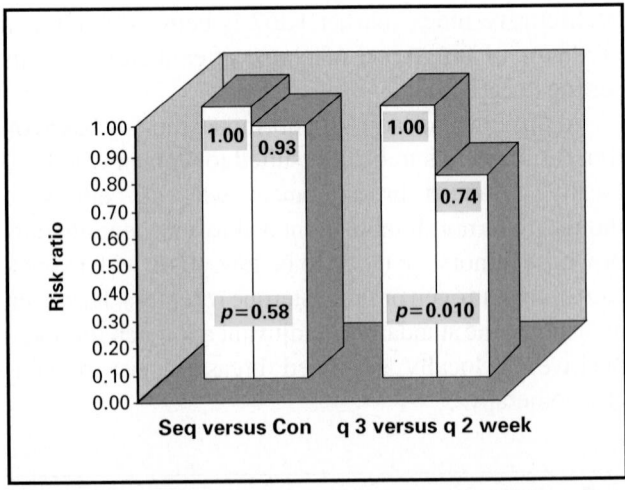

FIGURE 24-12. Overall survival of patients on CALGB 9741. (*Reproduced, with permission, from van der Hage JA, van de Velde CJ, Julien JP, et al. Preoperative chemotherapy in primary operable breast cancer: results from the European Organization for Research and Treatment of Cancer trial 10902. J Clin Oncol 2001 November 15;19[22]:4224-4237.*)

TABLE 24-10 | **ADVERSE EFFECTS DURING TREATMENT ON CALGB 9741**

| | TREATMENT ARMS | | | | | | | |
| | ARM 1 $(A \to T \to C\ q\ 3\ weeks)$ | | ARM 2 $(A \to T \to C\ q\ 2\ weeks)$ | | ARM 3 $(AC \to T\ q\ 3\ weeks)$ | | ARM 4 $(AC \to T\ q\ 2\ weeks)$ | |
Complication, Patients, and Cycles	N	%	N	%	N	%	N	%
Total no. of patients	103	100	101	100	104	100	104	100
Total no. of cycles	1209	100	1143	100	818	100	803	100
Patients with any delay	40	39	45	45	41	39	32	31
Cycles delayed	81	7	80	7	68	8	44	6
Patients transfused (RBCs)	0	0	3	3	4	4	13	3
Cycles transfused	0	0	10	1	5	1	22	13
Patients hospitalized for febrile neutropenia	3	3	2	2	6	6	2	2
Cycles hospitalized for febrile neutropenia	3	1	5	1	7	1	2	1

A, doxorubicin; AC, doxorubicin, cyclophosphamide; C, cyclophosphamide; RBCs, red blood cells; T, paclitaxel.
Reproduced, with permission, from Citron ML, Berry DA, Cirrincione C, et al. Randomized trial of dose-dense versus conventionally scheduled and sequential versus concurrent combination chemotherapy as postoperative adjuvant treatment of node-positive primary breast cancer: first report of Intergroup Trial C9741/Cancer and Leukemia Group B Trial 9741. J Clin Oncol 2003 April 15;21(8):1431-1439.

65% DFS at 5 years seen in the NSABP studies using a traditional regimen of doxorubicin 60 mg/m^2 and cyclophosphamide 600 mg/m^2 given every 3 weeks. Hospitalization was required for 6% of patients for febrile neutropenia. Notably it was reported that one patient subsequently died from acute leukemia with a translocation that was thought to be secondary to anthracycline-related exposure. Thus it was concluded that dose-dense anthracycline in combination with GCSF produced encouraging results, with a seemingly higher response rate as compared to traditional every-3-week dosing. However, this dose-dense approach seemed to limit the ability of patients to receive the concomitant 5-FU because of increased side effects, such as hand-foot syndrome.

In addition, as previously described above under "Taxanes," a phase III randomized trial (117) at MDACC has documented that weekly paclitaxel is superior in achieving pCR for both node-positive and node-negative patients (Table 24-9).

At this time there are multiple ongoing trials evaluating the pCR, DFS, and OS for those patients treated with a dose-dense chemotherapy as compared with standard-regimen chemotherapy. While it makes biological sense that those treated with the dose-dense chemotherapy regimen should have an improved clinical outcome, one always needs to evaluate how large this benefit is, especially in relation to the side effects. The side effects noted in the above trials included the increased transfusion requirement in the concurrent every-2-week therapy arm for the CALGB trial as well

as an elevated incidence of hand-foot syndrome for those treated with dose-dense anthracyline-based chemotherapy. However, the benefit for the paclitaxel weekly arm in the MDACC trial was significant, without any notable increase in side effects.

TRASTUZUMAB

Trastuzumab is a high-affinity humanized monoclonal antibody that recognizes the c-*erb* B-2 (or *HER-2/neu*) receptor and is a targeted therapeutic for tumors that overexpress this growth factor receptor. Trastuzumab has been evaluated extensively in the *HER-2/neu*–overexpressing metastatic setting and has been shown to be effective as a single agent both before (130) and after chemotherapy (131) and in combination (132) with multiple agents. One notable side effect has been a high rate of cardiotoxicity, particularly when trastuzumab is combined with anthracyline-based chemotherapy, which is due in part to overlapping toxicities in combination with trastuzumab's long half-life of up to 32 days. (Please refer to detailed information in Chap. 25.)

Therefore trastuzumab is an accepted and standard therapy for metastatic breast cancer that overexpresses *HER-2/neu*. However, the safety and efficacy of trastuzumab-based therapy is not yet firmly established for earlier-stage breast cancer. There is currently a great deal of interest in resolving this issue. To this effect a pilot study (133) was conducted that enrolled 40 women with stage II or III *HER-2/neu*–over-expressing breast cancer (2+ or 3+ by IHC). All patients then received preoperative trastuzumab based on the established dosing parameters used in the metastatic setting, with a 4-mg/kg loading dose for 1 week followed by a maintenance dose of 2 mg/kg for 11 weeks. Trastuzumab was given in combination with paclitaxel 175 mg/m^2 every 3 weeks for four cycles. Patients then underwent definitive breast surgery. Following surgery they all were treated with standard doses of Adriamycin (doxorubicin) and cyclophosphamide (AC) therapy for four cycles. Preoperative therapy with paclitaxel and trastuzumab achieved a clinical response in 75%, with a pCR in 18% of the women enrolled. It was shown that women with *HER-2/neu* IHC 3+ disease were more likely to respond than those with 2+ disease. Four patients did develop grade 2 cardiotoxicity with asymptomatic declines in the left ventricular ejection fraction. Also of note, *HER-2/neu* extracellular domains were measured both before and after preoperative therapy and were noted to decline in 24% of the patients. Thus preoperative therapy with combined trastuzumab and paclitaxel was shown to be effective in the treatment of stages II and III breast cancers with *HER-2/neu* overexpression.

Currently, ongoing studies at MDACC are also seeking to address the use of trastuzumab both in neoadjuvant and adjuvant therapy. MDACC ID 99-146 is evaluating the addition of trastuzumab to standard chemotherapy with paclitaxel and FEC in the neoadjuvant setting for T2 to T3 and N0 to N1 operable breast cancers that overexpress *HER-2/neu*. In addition, a multicenter phase III study is ongoing to investigate doxorubicin and cyclophosphamide followed by docetaxel plus or minus trastuzumab with docetaxel plus a platinum salt plus trastuzumab for the treatment of node-positive and high- risk node-negative cancers that overexpress *HER-2/neu*. Trastuzumab continues to show promise for the treatement of *HER-2/neu* overexpressing breast cancers in multiple treatment settings and continues to generate interest for clinical trials.

ONCO*TYPE* DX

Recently, efforts have been made to identify a multigene assay that can help quantify a patient's risk of breast cancer recurrence (134). Onco*type* DX is a commercially available, validated laboratory test performed on a tumor specimen that analyzes 21 various genes associated with receptor expression, proliferation, invasion, and other factors. Calculations based on the expression of these 21 genes result in a recurrence score which relays the likelihood of breast cancer recurrence in the first 10 years after diagnosis (135). These studies found that those patients with a low recurrence score derive

little benefit from chemotherapy while those with a high recurrence score are likely to benefit more from chemotherapy. For women with an intermediate recurrence score, the benefit of chemotherapy was uncertain (Fig. 24-13). In order to elucidate the benefit of systemic cytotoxic therapy for this middle group, ECOG has designed a trial known at TAILORx, the Trial Assigning Individualized Options for Treatment (Rx). This study, which plans to enroll 10,000 patients, will randomly assign node-negative, Her2/neu-negative, estrogen- and/or progesterone-positive women with early breast cancer with a mid-range recurrence score to either treatment with hormonal therapy or chemotherapy followed by hormonal therapy. Disease-free survival, recurrence-free interval, and overall survival will be compared in these large cohorts.

More data is emerging that perhaps analysis of 21 genes is no better than immunohistochemical analysis of receptor status and Ki-67 percentage. At the 2009 San Antonio Breast Cancer Symposium, a prognostic score based upon staining of ER, PR, Her2/neu, and Ki-67, known collectively as IHC4, correlated with the prognostic information provided by the Onco*type* DX score (136). This relevant comparison may scale back the elaborate, costly, and time-consuming testing that currently accompanies the evaluation of early stage breast cancer. This observation regarding IHC4, however, is based upon a single institution report and merits confirmation and validation.

The use of a genomic-derived recurrence score helps predict recurrences in patients with node-negative, hormone receptor-positive early breast cancer. However, the details regarding which assay will emerge the most useful, innovative, and cost-effective remain to be seen. What is also up in the air is how to manage middle range risk patients in terms of adjuvant therapy. As of now, intermediate risk patients should be counseled regarding the uncertainty of their benefit with chemotherapy and encouraged to enroll on clinical trials.

■ MD ANDERSON CANCER CENTER MANAGEMENT STRATEGIES

EARLY-STAGE BREAST CANCER (STAGES I AND II)

At MD Anderson, every effort is made to integrate clinical information with pathologic staging, and molecular characteristics to optimize treatment efficacy and whenever possible, perform breast-conserving surgery (Fig. 24-14). Early-stage tumors comprise those that are neither fixed to the chest wall nor inflammatory. Stage I breast cancer includes primary malignancies that are ≤ 2 cm in greatest

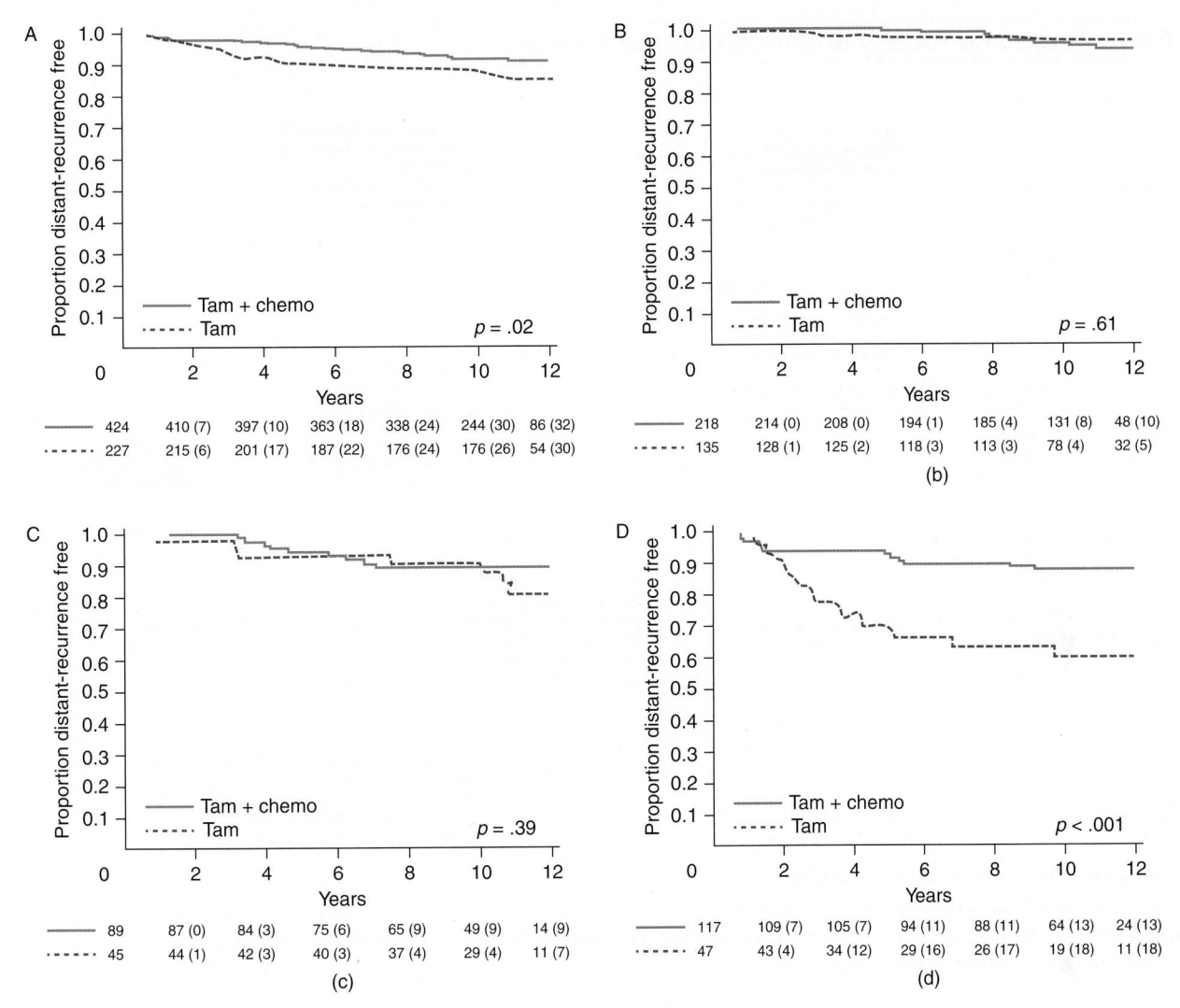

FIGURE 24-13. Kaplan-Meier curves for recurrence after treatment with tamoxifen (Tam) alone versus tamoxifen plus chemotherapy (Tam + chemo). (A) All patients; (B) low-risk recurrence score (RS) <18; (C) intermediate risk (RS = 18-30); (D) high risk (RS ≥ 31). *(Reproduced, with permission, from Paik S, Tang G, Shak S, et al. Gene expression and benefit of chemotherapy in women with node-negative, estrogen receptor-positive breast cancer. J Clin Oncol 2006 August 10;24[23]:3726-3734.)*

dimension and do not involve the lymph nodes and microinvasive tumors that are ≤ 0.1 cm in greatest dimension. Stage II breast cancer encompasses primary tumors of 2 to 5 cm that can involve ipsilateral axillary lymph nodes and tumors >5 cm without lymph node involvement. All patients at MDACC undergo receptor testing for hormone receptor status for ER and PR status. In addition, patients are also tested for *HER-2/neu* status by IHC, and 2/3+ results are confirmed by FISH.

STAGE I

Breast-Conserving Therapy

Breast-conserving surgery (BCS) or segmental resection has revolutionized patient care for breast cancer over the last two decades. Women today are

able to preserve their breasts without a negative effect on their survival. Breast-conserving therapy involves the surgical removal of tumor followed by radiation therapy to the breast. Multiple studies have shown that patients with stage I breast cancer who are treated with breast-conserving surgery have DFS and OS rates similar to those of patients who are treated with modified radical mastectomies (137).

There are only a few true absolute contraindications to BCS, including persistently positive resection margins, multicentric disease, diffuse malignant-appearing microcalcifications, a history of prior radiation to the breast or mantle region (for Hodgkin disease), and pregnancy, although it might be possible to perform BCS in the third trimester. Relative contraindications include a history of connective tissue disease suggesting that radiation would

Early-stage and locally advanced breast cancer

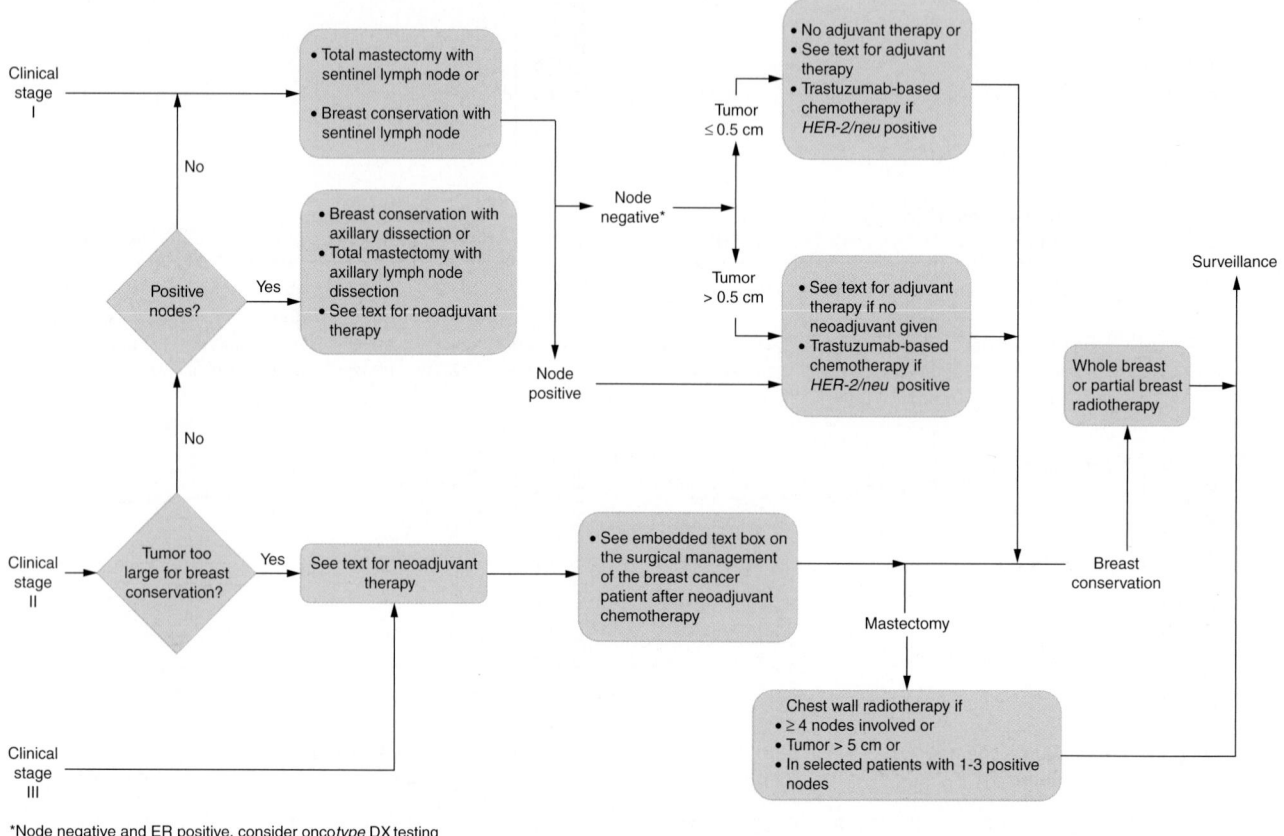

*Node negative and ER positive, consider oncotype DX testing

FIGURE 24-14. MDACC algorithm for management of early stage and locally advanced breast cancer. *(Adapted with permission from the MD Anderson Invasive Breast Cancer algorithm.)*

be poorly tolerated, centrally located tumors involving the nipple-areolar complex, and a large tumor in a small breast that might lead to a poor cosmetic result. At MDACC, while the final decision about whether to offer BCS is left to the discretion of our surgical colleagues, most patients who do not meet one of the absolute or relative contraindications are offered this surgical approach.

Risk Factors for Ipsilateral Recurrence With Breast-Conserving Surgery

The risk of ipsilateral tumor recurrence has been reported to range from 0.5 to 2.0% per year. These risk factors include age <35 years, an extensive intraductal component, major lymphocytic stromal reaction, peritumoral invasion, positive margins of resection, and presence of tumor necrosis.

Axillary Lymph Node Dissection

There is still significant controversy regarding the role of axillary lymph node dissection in the patient with

clinically negative axillary nodes. Sentinel lymph node biopsy is currently the standard of care at MDACC. Previous studies have shown that the sensitivity and specificity of sentinel node biopsy could be increased by using both vital blue dye and lymphoscintigraphy. It has been noted that the sensitivity can be up to 97% when blue dye and technetium-99m sulfur colloid are paired (138).

Currently, there are trials ongoing at multiple centers evaluating the use of axillary lymph node dissection when the sentinel lymph node is negative. There are also ongoing trials at MDACC and elsewhere exploring the role of axillary lymph node dissection for patients with a positive sentinel lymph node but clinically negative nodal status and T1 or T2 disease.

Radiation Therapy after Breast-Conserving Surgery

Patients with node-negative disease are treated at MDACC to achieve a total dose of 5000 cGy with an approximate dose of 200 cGy/day on a schedule of 5 days per week for a total of 5 weeks. Of note, there have been two recently published randomized clinical trials that attempted to address the question of whether a boost to the tumor bed is needed. One such study evaluated 5000 patients treated with BCS. Patients were treated with a 16-Gy boost to the tumor bed following the standard of 50 Gy of radiation. The median follow-up for patients was 5.1 years, and the 5-year rates of local relapse were 7.3 (no boost) versus 4.3% (with boost), $p \le .001$ (139). At MDACC, a boost of radiation to the tumor bed is standard. Regional nodal irradiation is no longer used for negative axillary lymph nodes. Radiation is usually begun after chemotherapy is completed, but it can be given concomitantly with hormone-based therapy.

Adjuvant Therapy

Estrogen and Progesterone Receptor–Negative Tumors Chemotherapy

Based on data detailed under the section Overall Benefits of Adjuvant Therapy, above, both pre- and post-menopausal women are offered chemotherapy at MDACC. However, we do not routinely give chemotherapy to node-negative breast tumors that are estrogen-receptor positive and/or progesterone-receptor positive and Her2/neu negative. For these patients, we are currently incorporating the use of the Onco*type DX* test for an estimation of the risk of recurrence (see section Other Systemic Therapy Topics). Patients with a low recurrence score are recommended for adjuvant endocrine therapy, patients with a high recurrence score are counseled for chemotherapy followed by endocrine therapy, and patients with a mid-range recurrence score offered a choice of either therapy or randomization via the ongoing TAILORx trial. Our current standard chemotherapy is FAC for node-negative disease, and its use is based on data that were published over 20 years ago (140).

Chemotherapy is usually initiated approximately 4 weeks after surgery, although studies have shown that delaying chemotherapy up to 8 to 10 weeks does not seem to have a negative effect on development of metastasis or survival. Prior to beginning chemotherapy, our patients undergo the insertion of a subclavian catheter.

FAC or FEC, using epirubicin 100 mg/m^2, is given for a total of six cycles every 3 weeks by nurses in our ambulatory treatment centers. Chemotherapy is administered if the absolute neutrophil count (ANC) ≥ 1500/mm^3 and platelets $\ge 100,000$/mm^3. A complete blood count with differential is checked prior to each chemotherapy cycle and also weekly after the first cycle. Growth factor support is not used routinely and is given only

for the indications detailed in the current ASCO guidelines (141).

Estrogen and/or Progesterone Receptor–Positive Tumors

Endocrine Therapy

Our standard approach, based on previously described information (see page 647) is to treat receptor-positive stage I disease utilizing a hormonal treatment regimen. MDACC's cutoff for tumor hormone receptor positivity is 5%. Based on the ATAC trial data discussed previously, tamoxifen is given to premenopausal women, whereas postmenopausal women receive either anastrazole or tamoxifen; however, anastrazole is our preferred agent. Both are taken for a total of 5 years. The recent data from the MA-17 trial concerning letrozole for 5 years after completion of tamoxifen is also discussed with our postmenopausal patients, as are the data on exemestane following 2 to 3 years of tamoxifen to complete the 5 years of endocrine therapy. However, for early stage I patients, the potential side effects from letrozole or exemestane should be very carefully weighed against the potential benefits. Endocrine therapies are begun after completion of chemotherapy but can be given concomitantly with radiation therapy (Table 24-11).

STAGE II

Surgery

As in the case of stage I disease, multiple studies of stage II patients treated with either breast-conserving therapy and modified radical mastectomy have documented similar long-term outcomes. Patients with tumors of >4 to 5 cm are often not considered to be ideal candidates for BCS, often because of the potential for residual tumor and poor cosmetic result.

TABLE 24-11	ADJUVANT ENDOCRINE TREATMENT REGIMENS COMMONLY USED AT THE MD ANDERSON CANCER CENTER*	
Premenopausal	*Postmenopausal*
Tamoxifen 20 PO daily for 5 years	Anastrazole 1 mg PO daily for 5 years or Tamoxifen 20 mg PO daily for 5 years

*Based on recent MA-17 data in postmenopausal women, to complete the 5 years of adjuvant hormonal therapy, the use of letrozole 2.5 mg daily for 5 years should be considered after completion of tamoxifen or exemestane 25 mg daily should be considered after 2 to 3 years of tamoxifen.

Radiation Therapy

After Breast-Conserving Therapy

Radiation of the breast after this form of surgery is similar in terms of area treated and dose given to the treatment of stage I patients. Regional nodal irradiation to negative axillary lymph nodes is no longer routinely given. Some groups do recommend irradiation of the supraclavicular fossa or internal mammary chain for those with positive lymph nodes.

After Mastectomy

Postmastectomy irradiation should be considered for patients with positive postmastectomy margins, primary tumors >5 cm, or ≥4 positive lymph nodes. ASCO clinical care guidelines do recommend routine use of postmastectomy radiation for women with stage III or T3 disease or those with ≥4 positive lymph nodes (142). As yet there are no clear guidelines for patients with T1 or T2 disease and one to three positive lymph nodes. At this time an intergroup randomized trial is investigating this issue. Patients in this trial will receive standard chemotherapy and be randomized to receive postmastectomy radiation to the chest wall, internal mammary lymph nodes, and the supraclavicular lymph nodes.

According to current recommendations the dose to be delivered ranges from 4500 to 5000 cGy. Electron boosts to doses of 6000 cGy can be considered if there is gross residual disease or there are positive margins. At this time treatment of the axilla, even for those who have multiple positive lymph nodes in the absence of gross residual disease, is not routinely recommended.

Neoadjuvant Therapy

At MDACC, neoadjuvant therapy is typically given to patients with positive axillary nodal involvement. These MDACC guidelines are based on information previously discussed under the sections Neoadjuvant Therapy and Dose Density.

Neoadjuvant therapy combines preoperative taxane therapy with FAC adjuvant chemotherapy. Our neoadjuvant taxane of choice is paclitaxel, which is given on a weekly basis based on the data of Green et al. (117), previously described.

Central intravenous access is also obtained. Patients are then treated with paclitaxel on a weekly basis for 12 weeks. This is followed by surgical intervention and then completion of chemotherapy with FAC every 3 weeks for four cycles.

Clinical response is documented by serial examinations. If there is evidence of a level of response that could possibly lead to a pCR of the tumor, a marker is placed in the breast to identify the primary tumor site. This is done to guide resection, so that if a pCR has occurred, the "scar" tissue from the prior tumor can be resected.

This approach of using neoadjuvant therapy allows one to document therapeutic response to taxanes prior to surgical intervention and also allows some patients who otherwise would not be eligible for BCS to undergo this type of surgery.

Adjuvant Therapy

Chemotherapy

Patients who do not meet the criteria for neoadjuvant therapy are treated with adjuvant chemotherapy in a fashion similar to those with stage I breast cancer. FAC chemotherapy is given every 3 weeks for a total of six courses (Fig. 24-3).

Endocrine Therapy

Whether patients are treated with neoadjuvant or adjuvant therapy, those with hormone receptor–positive tumors are treated with hormone-based therapy in a similar fashion to those with stage I breast cancer (Table 24-11).

LOCALLY ADVANCED BREAST CANCER (STAGE III)

Unfortunately approximately 20 to 25% of women do present with locally advanced cancer. These patients usually have easily palpable tumors with large breast masses and/or axillary nodal disease. Inflammatory breast cancer is also included in locally advanced disease and represents 1 to 3% of diagnosed breast cancers. Patients with this very aggressive form of breast cancer can present without a discrete mass and only erythema and edema.

One challenging issue about this group of patients is the heterogeneous nature of their disease, with multiple different subgroups including tumors >5 cm, those with extensive regional lymph node involvement, direct involvement of the skin or chest wall, tumors that have no metastases but are still considered inoperable, and inflammatory breast cancer. The majority of locally advanced patients will have involved lymph nodes at time of diagnosis and approximately 50% will have

Commentary: Surgical Management of the Breast Cancer Patient After Neoadjuvant Chemotherapy

Neoadjuvant chemotherapy has traditionally been administered in cases of inoperable or locally advanced disease to facilitate local-regional treatment with surgery and radiation. The success of this approach, in addition to the known benefits of adjuvant chemotherapy, has led to the increasing use of neoadjuvant therapy for the treatment of patients with operable breast cancer. A well-recognized role of neoadjuvant chemotherapy is the ability to improve surgical options for patients by downsizing tumors and increasing the chances for breast conservation. The success of this approach depends on the involvement of a multidisciplinary team.

Patients should have imaging of the breast and regional nodal basins at presentation with biopsy of any suspicious lesions. This helps to define the extent of disease and outline the potential treatment options. Response to therapy should be assessed at defined intervals during the treatment. Patients with significant clinical tumor reduction after the first or second chemotherapy cycle and those who start with a primary tumor less than 2 cm in size undergo sonography and placement of metallic markers to facilitate subsequent localization of the tumor under ultrasound or mammographic guidance and to facilitate specimen radiography. At the conclusion of preoperative chemotherapy, these patients undergo repeat breast imaging to determine the options for local treatment. It is preferable that the residual tumor size after preoperative chemotherapy is less than 4 cm, but the size of the tumor in relation to the size of the breast is a major consideration. Patients who have extensive microcalcifications on mammography, multicentric disease on physical examination or mammography, or persistent skin edema on physical examination are not considered to be candidates for breast conservation therapy.

The MD Anderson Cancer Center published our institutional experience with breast conservation after preoperative chemotherapy in patients with locally advanced breast cancer and those with large primary tumors. The 5-year rates of ipsilateral breast tumor recurrence-free and local-regional

recurrence-free survival were 95% and 91%, respectively. Factors that correlated with ipsilateral breast tumor recurrence and local-regional recurrence were clinical N2 or N3 disease, pathologic residual tumor size >2 cm, a multifocal pattern of residual disease, and lymphovascular space invasion. A prognostic scoring index utilizing these factors has been proposed to assist clinicians in counseling their patients regarding the use of breast conservation therapy after chemotherapy.

The use of axillary lymph node dissection (ALND) has been standard practice for management of the axilla following neoadjuvant chemotherapy. As the use of sentinel lymph node dissection (SLND) has gained acceptance in early-stage breast cancer and has been shown to reduce the need for ALND in node-negative patients, surgeons have begun to utilize this procedure following chemotherapy. It has been our practice to perform SLND following chemotherapy in patients who present with N0 disease. We have recently reported that SLN identification rates and false-negative rates are similar between patients undergoing surgery first and those who undergo neoadjuvant chemotherapy followed by surgery. Overall there were fewer positive SLNs in the neoadjuvant chemotherapy group confirming previous reports that chemotherapy eradicates disease in the regional nodal basins. After adjusting for clinical stage there were no differences in local-regional recurrences, disease-free or overall survival between the groups. SLN surgery after chemotherapy is as accurate for axillary staging as SLN surgery prior to chemotherapy. Chemotherapy eradicates disease in the breast and regional lymph nodes and utilizing SLN surgery after chemotherapy results in fewer positive SLNs and decreases unnecessary axillary dissections. Based on the available data, SLND appears to be feasible in N0 patients but is not yet proven accurate in women with node-positive disease at presentation, a group that should continue to undergo ALND following chemotherapy.

Kelly K. Hunt

four or more lymph nodes involved. DFS rates are also variable. The most common cause of treatment failure is distant metastases, usually occurring within 2 years of diagnosis.

The significant importance of a multimodality approach cannot be stressed enough. Previously women with locally advanced disease were classified as being inoperable. It was known that patients who were treated with a single modality of therapy with surgery or radiation had 5-year survival rates of less than 20%. Chemotherapy was first introduced into the treatment algorithm for this subset of breast cancer patients in the

1970s (143). It was noted by the Early Breast Cancer Collaborative Group review (55) that there was a modest benefit in survival for those treated with postoperative chemotherapy. It was the high risk of developing metastatic disease faced by these patients that led to the use of neoadjuvant therapy as part of a multimodality approach.

Neoadjuvant-Based Therapy

This form of therapy offers many important benefits, including direct in vivo measurement of sensitivity of tumor cells to chemotherapy, which allows for early discontinuation of ineffective therapy. Also, treatment prior to surgical intervention allows the delivery of the chemotherapy through an intact vasculature and therefore possibly decreases the probability of developing resistant tumor cells.

As with node-positive stage II breast cancer, these patients are treated with a taxane-based neoadjuvant approach at MDACC, as described above. Paclitaxel is given on a weekly basis for 12 weeks. This is followed by chemotherapy with FAC every 3 weeks for cycles, followed by surgery and potentially two more cycles of FAC (Fig. 24-15).

Clinical response is documented by serial physical examinations, mammograms, and ultrasounds of the breast and nodal regions. If there is evidence of a level of response that could possibly lead to a pCR of the tumor, a radioopaque marker is placed in the breast. On average, the range of responses with neoadjuvant therapy regimens is variable, with clinical complete responses of 10 to 60% and an average overall clinical response of 75% (144). Of note, only approximately 30 to 50% of clinical CRs are confirmed to be complete

pCRs. It is known that neoadjuvant therapy can also convert clinically positive axillary lymph nodes to negative ones in approximately 33% of breast cancer patients. In addition, it has been demonstrated that the tumor's effect on the axillary lymph nodes, rather than the response of the primary tumor itself, may be more important in predicting long-term patient outcomes (145).

Surgery

The historical surgical procedure for locally advanced disease is mastectomy. However, overall, clinical trials using neoadjuvant chemotherapy have noted that 50% or more of women with locally advanced breast cancer can be treated with BCS after neoadjuvant therapy (146). One concern that still remains is that the women who need to be staged downward with preoperative chemotherapy in order to be eligible for segmental mastectomy have a higher local failure rate (147). This can be improved in part through accurate localization of the tumor using a radioopaque clip, so that the appropriate area of tumor involvement can be resected even if a complete or near-complete response is achieved with neoadjuvant therapy.

The role of sentinel lymph node biopsy in locally advanced breast cancer has not been formally established. One concern is that the lymphatics might undergo fibrosis after neoadjuvant chemotherapy. This, in turn, might make the mapping procedure prone to high false-negative rates.

Radiation Therapy

Multiple nonrandomized trials have tried to address the issue of postsurgical radiation for locally advanced breast cancer. Most have shown decreased local recurrence rates for those patients treated with both surgery and radiation, including patients who had achieved a pCR with neoadjuvant chemotherapy. One randomized trial performed by ECOG (148) assigned women to neoadjuvant chemohormonal therapy followed by surgery alone or surgery plus radiation therapy. Interestingly, even with 9 years of follow-up, there was no significant benefit in terms of time to relapse or OS for those in the treatment arm, which included radiation therapy. However, a benefit was noted with radiation in terms of a decreased locoregional failure rate.

Thus, at this time, radiation treatment guidelines recommend that patients with a pathologic response in the primary tumor and axillary lymph nodes, whether they undergo lumpectomy or mastectomy, should receive radiation to the breast and/or chest wall and/or internal mammary lymph nodes to a total dose of 5000 to 6000 cGy.

Paclitaxel Weekly Times 12 Courses

Anaphylactic Medications

Prior to administering paclitaxel have epinephrine (1:1000) .5 mL IV, diphenhydramine 25 mg IV, and hydrocortisone 100 mg IV immediately available

Premedications

Dexamathasone 10 mg in 50 mL NS IVPB 30 min prior to course #1
Cimetidine 300 mg in 50 mL NS IVPB 30 min prior
Diphenhydramine 50 mg in 50 mL NS IVPB 30 min prior

Chemotherapy

Paclitaxel 80 mg/m^2 IV in 250 mL NS IVPB (if total dose is <300 mg) or in 500 mL NS IVPB (if total dose ≥300 mg) over 1 h every week

Repeat every week times 12 courses

↓

FAC every 21 days times 4 courses (see Fig. 24-3)

↓

Surgery

FIGURE 24-15. MDACC neoadjuvant chemotherapy with weekly paclitaxel followed by FAC.

Patients who achieve a PR in the primary tumor and have residual comprehensive radiation should have radiation in a comprehensive fashion, including the axillary field.

Adjuvant Therapy

Endocrine Therapy

As in the case of stage I and stage II disease, our standard approach is based in part on results of the ATAC trial. Premenopausal women are treated with tamoxifen. For postmenopausal women, either anastrazole or tamoxifen can be given, but anastrazole is the drug of choice at our institution. Both are taken for a total of 5 years. For women treated with tamoxifen who are postmenopausal, letrozole is considered following tamoxifen, based on the results of the MA-17 trial. In addition, the data on the use of exemestane after 2 to 3 years of tamoxifen to complete the 5 years of endocrine therapy is also discussed with our postmenopausal patients. Endocrine therapies are begun after completion of chemotherapy but can be given concomitantly with radiation therapy (Table 24-11).

Prognosis

Clinical endpoints have been shown to improve with neoadjuvant therapy involving a combined-modality approach. Patients who are treated with a multimodality treatment approach can achieve long-term survival upward of 50%, whereas those who do not respond to neoadjuvant therapy have poorer outcomes. It has been shown that of those women who fail to respond to neoadjuvant anthracycline-based therapy, only 30% remain free of distant disease (149).

■ CONCLUSION

Treatment for breast cancer patients has evolved from single-agent therapies to more contemporary combinations. Combined-modality approaches with refinement in local therapies (surgery, irradiation) have resulted in progressive improvement in survival in this disease. This is reflected in a single-center series of breast cancer patients treated from diagnosis at our institution from the 1940s to the present (Fig. 24-16).

Over the past six decades there have been significant advances in the care of early-stage, locally advanced breast cancer. Between 1991 and 2005, the rate of death from breast cancer decreased by 37% in the United States (1). The use of optimal stage- and hormone receptor–specific therapy is of utmost importance,

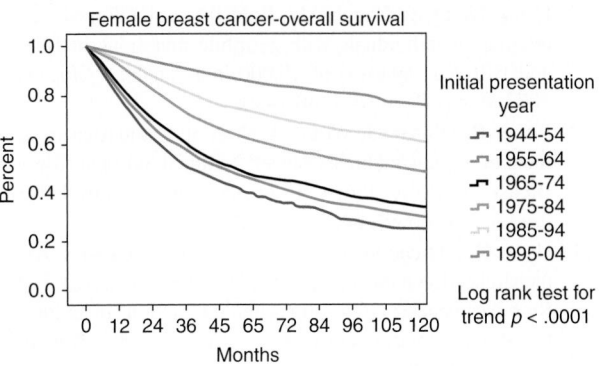

FIGURE 24-16. Survival of breast cancer patients treated at MD Anderson Cancer Center by decades.

since through doing so we can significantly affect the risk of recurrence and death from breast cancer and thus our patients' lives. As outcomes have been improved through the addition of neoadjuvant therapy, taxanes, and hormonal therapies, so shall current and future investigation shape the care of breast cancer patients, especially investigations of the use of targeted therapeutic approaches.

References

1. Jemal A, Siegel R, Ward E, et al. Cancer statistics, 2009. *CA: A Cancer J Clinicians* 2009 July;59(4):225-249.
2. Chu KC, Tarone RE, Kessler LG, et al. Recent trends in U.S. breast cancer incidence, survival, and mortality rates. *J Natl Cancer Inst* 1996;88(21):1571-1579.
3. Li CI, Daling JR, Malone KE. Incidence of invasive breast cancer by hormone receptor status from 1992 to 1998. *J Clin Oncol* 2003 January 1;21(1):28-34.
4. Willett WC, Rockhill B, Hankinson SE, Hunter DJ, Colditz GA. Epidemiology and nongenetic causes of breast cancer. In: Harris JR, Lippman ME, Morrow M, Osborne CK, (eds): *Diseases of the Breast.* 2nd ed. Philadelphia: Lippincott Williams & Wilkins; 2000:175-220.
5. Chevarley F, White E. Recent trends in breast cancer mortality among white and black US women. *Am J Public Health* 1997 May;87(5):775-781.
6. Gail MH, Brinton LA, Byar DP, et al. Projecting individualized probabilities of developing breast cancer for white females who are being examined annually. *J Natl Cancer Inst* 1989;81(24):1879-1886.
7. Claus EB, Risch N, Thompson WD. Genetic analysis of breast cancer in the cancer and steroid hormone study. *Am J Hum Genet* 1991 February;48(2):232-242.
8. Collaborative Group on Hormonal Factors in Breast Cancer. Familial breast cancer: Collaborative reanalysis of individual data from 52 epidemiological studies including 58,209 women with breast cancer and 101,986 women without the disease. *Lancet* 2001 October 27;358(9291):1389-1399.

9. Frank TS, Deffenbaugh AM, Reid JE, et al. Clinical characteristics of individuals with germline mutations in BRCA1 and BRCA2: Analysis of 10,000 individuals. *J Clin Oncol* 2002 March 15;20(6): 1480-1490.

10. Fisher B, Dignam J, Wolmark N, et al. Tamoxifen in treatment of intraductal breast cancer: National Surgical Adjuvant Breast and Bowel Project B-24 randomised controlled trial. *Lancet* 1999;353(9169):1993-2000.

11. Hsieh CC, Trichopoulos D, Katsouyanni K, Yuasa S. Age at menarche, age at menopause, height and obesity as risk factors for breast cancer: Associations and interactions in an international case-control study. *Int J Cancer* 1990 November 15;46(5):796-800.

12. Layde PM, Webster LA, Baughman AL, et al. The independent associations of parity, age at first full term pregnancy, and duration of breastfeeding with the risk of breast cancer. Cancer and Steroid Hormone Study Group. *J Clin Epidemiol* 1989;42(10):963-973.

13. Brinton LA, Schairer C, Hoover RN, Fraumeni JF, Jr. Menstrual factors and risk of breast cancer. *Cancer Investigation* 1988;6(3):245-254.

14. Bruzzi P, Negri E, La Vecchia C, et al. Short term increase in risk of breast cancer after full term pregnancy. *Brit Med J* 1988 October 29;297(6656):1096-1098.

15. Hankinson SE, Colditz GA, Manson JE, et al. A prospective study of oral contraceptive use and risk of breast cancer (Nurses' Health Study, United States). *Cancer Causes Control* 1997 January;8(1):65-72.

16. Marchbanks PA, McDonald JA, Wilson HG, et al. Oral contraceptives and the risk of breast cancer. *N Engl J Med* 2002 June 27;346(26):2025-2032.

17. Collaborative Group on Hormonal Factors in Breast Cancer. Breast cancer and hormonal contraceptives: Collaborative reanalysis of individual data on 53, 297 women with breast cancer and 100, 239 women without breast cancer from 54 epidemiological studies. *Lancet* 1996 June 22;347(9017): 1713-1727.

18. Rossouw JE, Anderson GL, Prentice RL, et al. Risks and benefits of estrogen plus progestin in healthy postmenopausal women: Principal results From the Women's Health Initiative randomized controlled trial. *J Am Med Assoc* 2002 July 17;288(3):321-333.

19. American Joint Committee on Cancer. In: Greene FL (ed). *AJCC Cancer Staging Manual.* 6th ed. 2002:223-240.

20. Singletary SE, Allred C, Ashley P, et al. Revision of the American Joint Committee on Cancer staging system for breast cancer. *J Clin Oncol* 2002 September 1;20(17): 3628-3636.

21. Elston CW, Ellis IO. Pathological prognostic factors in breast cancer I. The value of histological grade in breast cancer: Experience from a large study with long-term follow-up. *Histopathology* 1991 November;19(5):403-410.

22. Woodward WA, Strom EA, Tucker SL et al. Changes to the 2003 American Joint Commission on Cancer staging for breast cancer dramatically affect stage-specific survival. *J Clin Oncol* 2003 September 1;21(17):3244-3248.

23. Gasparini G, Pozza F, Harris AL. Evaluating the potential usefulness of new prognostic and predictive indicators in node-negative breast cancer patients. *J Natl Cancer Inst* 1993 Aug 4;85(15):1206-1219.

24. Hayes DF, Trock B, Harris AL. Assessing the clinical impact of prognostic factors: When is "statistically significant" clinically useful? *Breast Cancer Res Treat* 1998;52(1-3):305-319.

25. Rosen PP, Groshen S, Kinne DW, et al. Factors influencing prognosis in node-negative breast carcinoma: Analysis of 767 T1N0M0/T2N0M0 patients with long-term follow-up. *J Clin Oncol* 1993;11(11):2090-2100.

26. Fitzgibbons PL, Page DL, Weaver D, et al. Prognostic factors in breast cancer. College of American Pathologists Consensus Statement 1999. *Arch Pathol Lab Med* 2000 July;124(7): 966-978.

27. Weiss RB, Woolf SH, Demakos E, et al. Natural history of more than 20 years of node-positive primary breast carcinoma treated with cyclophosphamide, methotrexate, and flurorouracil-based adjuvant chemotherapy: A study by the Cancer and Leukemia Group B. *J Clin Oncol* 2003 May 1;21(9):1825-35.

28. Early Breast Cancer Trialists' Collaborative Group. Systemic treatment of early breast cancer by hormonal, cytotoxic, or immune therapy. 133 randomised trials involving 31,000 recurrences and 24,000 deaths among 75,000 women. Early Breast Cancer Trialists' Collaborative Group. *Lancet* 1992 Jan 11;339(8785):71-85.

29. Nemoto T, Vana J, Bedwani RN, Baker HW, McGregor FH, Murphy GP. Management and survival of female breast cancer: Results of a national survey by the American College of Surgeons. *Cancer* 1980 June 15;45(12):2917-2924.

30. Allred DC, Harvey JM, Berardo M, et al. Prognostic and predictive factors in breast cancer by immunohistochemical analysis. *Modern Pathology* 1998 February;11(2):155-168.

31. Malmström P, Bendahl PO, Boiesen P, et al. S-phase fraction and urokinase plasminogen activator are better markers for distant recurrences than Nottingham Prognostic Index and histologic grade in a prospective study of premenopausal lymph node-negative breast cancer. *J Clin Oncol* 2001 April 1;19(7):2010-2019.

32. Rudolph P, Alm P, Heidebrecht HJ, et al. Immunologic proliferation marker Ki-S2 as prognostic indicator for lymph node-negative breast cancer. *J Natl Cancer Inst* 1999 February 3;91(3):271-278.

33. Paik S, Bryant J, Tan-Chiu E et al. Real-world performance of HER2 testing–National Surgical Adjuvant Breast and Bowel Project experience. *J Natl Cancer Inst* 2002 June 5;94(11):852-854.

34. Roche PC, Suman VJ, Jenkins RB, et al. Concordance between local and central laboratory HER2 testing in the breast intergroup trial N9831. *J Natl Cancer Inst* 2002 June 5;94(11):855-857.

35. Mass RD, Press MF, Anderson S, et al. Evaluation of clinical outcomes according to HER2 detection by fluorescence in situ hybridization in women with metastatic breast cancer treated with trastuzumab. *Clin Breast Cancer* 2005 Aug;6(3): 240-246.

36. Perez EA, Roche PC, Jenkins RB, et al. HER2 testing in patients with breast cancer: Poor correlation between weak positivity by immunohistochemistry and gene amplification by fluorescence in situ hybridization. *Mayo Clin Proc* 2002 February;77(2):148-154.

37. Tandon AK, Clark GM, Chamness GC, et al. HER-2/neu oncogene protein and prognosis in breast cancer. *J Clin Oncol* 1989;7(8):1120-1128.

38. Allred DC, Clark GM, Tandon AK, et al. HER-2/neu in node-negative breast cancer: Prognostic significance of over-expression influenced by the presence of in situ carcinoma. *J Clin Oncol* 1992;10(4):599-605.

39. De Placido S, Carlomagno C, De Laurentiis M, et al. c-erbB2 expression predicts tamoxifen efficacy in breast cancer patients. *Breast Cancer Res Treat* 1998;52(1-3):55-64.

40. Knoop AS, Bentzen SM, Nielsen MM, et al. Value of epidermal growth factor receptor, HER2, p53, and steroid receptors in predicting the efficacy of tamoxifen in high-risk postmenopausal breast cancer patients. *J Clin Oncol* 2001 July 15;19(14):3376-3384.

41. Berry DA, Muss HB, Thor AD, et al. HER-2/neu and p53 expression versus tamoxifen resistance in estrogen receptor-positive, node-positive breast cancer. *J Clin Oncol* 2000 October 15;18(20):3471-3479.

42. Keyomarsi K, Tucker SL, Buchholz TA, et al. Cyclin E and survival in patients with breast cancer. *N Engl J Med* 2002 November 14;347(20):1566-1575.

43. Rosen PP, Lesser ML, Arroyo CD, et al. p53 in node-negative breast carcinoma: An immunohistochemical study of epidemiologic risk factors, histologic features, and prognosis. *J Clin Oncol* 1995;13(4):821-830.

44. Elledge RM, Fuqua SA, Clark GM, et al. Prognostic significance of p53 gene alterations in node-negative breast cancer. *Breast Cancer Res Treat* 1993;26(3):225-235.

45. Weidner N, Folkman J, Pozza F, et al. Tumor angiogenesis: A new significant and independent prognostic indicator in early-stage breast carcinoma. *J Natl Cancer Inst* 1992 December 16;84(24):1875-1887.

46. Eppenberger U, Kueng W, Schlaeppi JM H, et al. Markers of tumor angiogenesis and proteolysis independently define high- and low-risk subsets of node-negative breast cancer patients. *J Clin Oncol* 1998 September;16(9):3129-3236.

47. Linderholm B, Grankvist K, Wilking N, et al. Correlation of vascular endothelial growth factor content with recurrences, survival, and first relapse site in primary node-positive breast carcinoma after adjuvant treatment. *J Clin Oncol* 2000 April;18(7):1423-1431.

48. Ferrandina G, Scambia G, Bardelli F, et al. Relationship between cathepsin-D content and disease-free survival in node-negative breast cancer patients: A meta-analysis. *Brit J Cancer* 1997;76(5):661-666.

49. van de Vijver MJ, He YD, van't Veer LJ, et al. A gene-expression signature as a predictor of survival in breast cancer. *N Engl J Med* 2002 December 19;347(25):1999-2009.

50. Ayers M, Symmans WF, Stec J, et al. Gene expression profiles predict complete pathologic response to neoadjuvant paclitaxel and fluorouracil, doxorubicin, and cyclophophamide chemotherapy in breast cancer. *J Clin Oncol* 2004 June 15;22(12):2284-2293.

51. Loprinzi CL, ThomÈ SD. Understanding the utility of adjuvant systemic therapy for primary breast cancer. *J Clin Oncol* 2001 February 15;19(4):972-979.

52. Buchholz TA, Tucker SL, Erwin J, et al. Impact of systemic treatment on local control for patients with lymph node-negative breast cancer treated with breast-conservation therapy. *J Clin Oncol* 2001 April 15;19(8):2240-2246.

53. Nissen-Meyer R, Kjellgren K, Mansson B. Preliminary report from the Scandinavian adjuvant chemotherapy study group. *Cancer Chemother Rep* 1971 December;55(5):561-566.

54. Fisher B, Ravdin RG, Ausman RK, et al. Surgical adjuvant chemotherapy in cancer of the breast: Results of a decade of cooperative investigation. *Annals Surg* 1968 September; 168(3):337-356.

55. Early Breast Cancer Trialists' Collaborative Group. Polychemotherapy for early breast cancer: An overview of the randomised trials. *Lancet* 1998 September 19;352(9132): 930-942.

56. Paik S, Bryant J, Tan-Chiu E, et al. HER2 and choice of adjuvant chemotherapy for invasive breast cancer: National Surgical Adjuvant Breast and Bowel Project Protocol B-15. *J Natl Cancer Inst* 2000 December 20;92(24):1991-1998.

57. Thor AD, Berry DA, Budman DR, et al. erbB-2, p53, and efficacy of adjuvant therapy in lymph node- positive breast cancer. *J Natl Cancer Inst* 1998 September 16;90(18): 1346-1360.

58. Buzdar AU, Hortobagyi GN, Singletary SE, et al. Impact of FAC-adjuvant therapy on mortality of early breast cancer: Long-term results of the M.D. Anderson Cancer Center Studies. In: Salmon SE, (ed). *Adjuvant Therapy of Cancer VIII*. Philadelphia: Lippincott-Raven; 1997:93-100.

59. Buzdar AU, Marcus C, Smith TL, et al. Early and delayed clinical cardiotoxicity of doxorubicin. *Cancer* 1985;55(12): 2761-2765.

60. Levine MN, Bramwell VH, Pritchard KI, et al. Randomized trial of intensive cyclophosphamide, epirubicin, and fluorouracil chemotherapy compared with cyclophosphamide, methotrexate, and fluorouracil in premenopausal women with node-positive breast cancer. National Cancer Institute of Canada Clinical Trials Group. *J Clin Oncol* 1998 August;16(8):2651-2658.

61. Slamon D, Eiermann W, Robert N, et al. Phase III Randomized Trial comparing doxorubicin and cyclophosphamide Followed by docetaxel (ACT) with doxorubicin and cyclophosphamide followed by docetaxel and trastuzumab (AC→TH) with docetaxel, carboplatin and trastuzumab (TCH) in Her2neu positive early breast cancer patients: BCIRG 006 Study. 32nd Annual San Antonio Breast Cancer Symposium 2009. Ref Type: Abstract

62. Nabholtz JM, Senn HJ, Bezwoda WR, et al. Prospective randomized trial of docetaxel versus mitomycin plus vinblastine in patients with metastatic breast cancer progressing despite previous anthracycline-containing chemotherapy. 304 Study Group. *J Clin Oncol* 1999 May;17(5):1413-1424.

63. Bishop JF, Dewar J, Toner GC, et al. Initial paclitaxel improves outcome compared with CMFP combination chemotherapy as front-line therapy in untreated metastatic breast cancer. *J Clin Oncol* 1999 August;17(8):2355-2364.

64. Henderson IC, Berry DA, Demetri GD, et al. Improved outcomes from adding sequential paclitaxel but not from escalating doxorubicin dose in an adjuvant chemotherapy regimen for patients with node-positive primary breast cancer. *J Clin Oncol* 2003 March 15;21(6):976-983.

65. Mamounas EP, Bryant J, Lembersky BC, et al. Paclitaxel after doxorubicin plus cyclophosphamide as adjuvant chemotherapy for node-positive breast cancer: Results from NSABP B-28. *J Clin Oncol* 2005 June 1;23(16):3686-3696.

66. Buzdar AU, Singletary SE, Valero V, et al. Evaluation of paclitaxel in adjuvant chemotherapy for patients with operable breast cancer: Preliminary data of a prospective randomized trial. *Clin Cancer Res* 2002 May;8(5):1073-1079.

67. Nabholtz JM, Pienkowski T, Mackey J, et al. Phase III trial comparing TAC (docetaxel, doxorubicin, cyclophosphamide) with FAC (5-fluorouracil, doxorubicin, cyclophosphamide) in the adjuvant treatment of node positive breast cancer (BC) patients: Interim analysis of the BCIRG 001 study. *Proc Am Soc Clin Oncol* 2002;21:36a. Ref Type: Abstract

68. Martin M, Pienkowski T, Mackey J, et al. Adjuvant docetaxel for node-positive breast cancer. *N Engl J Med* 2005 June 2;352(22):2302-2313.

69. Nolvadex Adjuvant Trial Organization. Controlled trial of tamoxifen as adjuvant agent in management of early breast cancer. Interim analysis at four years. *Lancet* 1983 February 5;1(8319):257-261.

70. Fisher B, Costantino J, Redmond C, et al. A randomized clinical trial evaluating tamoxifen in the treatment of patients with node-negative breast cancer who have estrogen-receptor-positive tumors. *N Engl J Med* 1989;320(8):479-484.

71. Rutqvist LE, Cedermark B, Glas U, et al. Randomized trial of adjuvant tamoxifen in node negative postmenopausal breast cancer. Stockholm Breast Cancer Study Group. *Acta Oncologica* 1992;31(2):265-270.

72. Stewart HJ. The Scottish trial of adjuvant tamoxifen in node-negative breast cancer. Scottish Cancer Trials Breast Group. *J Natl Cancer Inst* Monographs 1992;(11):117-120.

73. Early Breast Cancer Trialists' Collaborative Group. Tamoxifen for early breast cancer: An overview of the randomised trials. *Lancet* 1998 May 16;351(9114):1451-167.

74. Current Trials working Party of the Cancer Research Campaign Breast Cancer Trials Group. Preliminary results from the cancer research campaign trial evaluating tamoxifen duration in women aged fifty years or older with breast cancer. *J Natl Cancer Inst* 1996 December 18;88(24):1834-1839.

75. Fisher B, Dignam J, Bryant J, et al. Five versus more than five years of tamoxifen therapy for breast cancer patients with negative lymph nodes and estrogen receptor- positive tumors. *J Natl Cancer Inst* 1996 November 6;88(21):1529-1542.

76. Breast Cancer Trials Committee. Adjuvant tamoxifen in the management of operable breast cancer: The Scottish Trial. *Lancet* 1987 July 25;2(8552):171-175.

77. Swedish Breast Cancer Cooperative Group. Randomized trial of two versus five years of adjuvant tamoxifen for postmenopausal early stage breast cancer. Swedish Breast Cancer Cooperative Group. *J Natl Cancer Inst* 1996 November 6;88(21):1543-1549.

78. Fisher B, Dignam J, Bryant J, et al. Five versus more than five years of tamoxifen for lymph node-negative breast cancer: Updated findings from the National Surgical Adjuvant Breast and Bowel Project B-14 randomized trial. *J Natl Cancer Inst* 2001 May 2;93(9):684-690.

79. Stewart HJ, Forrest AP, Everington D, et al. Randomised comparison of 5 years of adjuvant tamoxifen with continuous therapy for operable breast cancer. The Scottish Cancer Trials Breast Group. *Brit J Cancer* 1996;74(2):297-299.

80. Tormey DC, Gray R, Falkson HC. Postchemotherapy adjuvant tamoxifen therapy beyond five years in patients with lymph node-positive breast cancer. Eastern Cooperative Oncology Group. *J Natl Cancer Inst* 1996;88(24):1828-1833.

81. Earl H, Gray R, Kerr D, et al. The optimal duration of adjuvant tamoxifen treatment for breast cancer remains uncertain: Randomize into aTTom. *Clin Oncol* (Royal College of Radiology) 1997;9(3):141-143.

82. Bryant J, Fisher B, Dignam J. Duration of adjuvant tamoxifen therapy. *J Natl Cancer Inst* Monographs 2001;(30):56-61.

83. Goldhirsch A, Glick JH, Gelber RD, et al. Meeting highlights: International Consensus Panel on the Treatment of Primary Breast Cancer. *J Natl Cancer Inst* 1998 November 4;90(21):1601-1608.

84. Albain KS, Barlow WE, Ravdin PM, et al. Adjuvant chemotherapy and timing of tamoxifen in postmenopausal patients with endocrine-responsive, node-positive breast cancer: A phase 3, open-label, randomised controlled trial. *Lancet* 2009 December 19;374(9707):2055-2063.

85. Pico C, Martin M, Jara C, et al. Epirubicin-cyclophosphamide (EC) chemotherpy plus tamoxifen (T) administered concurrent (Con) versus sequential (Sec): Randomized phase III trial in postmenopausal node-positive breast cancer (BC) patients. *Proc Am Soc Clin Oncol* 2002. Ref Type: Abstract

86. Brodie AM, Njar VC. Aromatase inhibitors and breast cancer. *Semin Oncol* 1996 August;23(4 Suppl 9):10-20.

87. Wells SA, Jr., Santen RJ, Lipton A, et al. Medical adrenalectomy with aminoglutethimide: Clinical studies in postmenopausal patients with metastatic breast carcinoma. *Annals Surg* 1978 May;187(5):475-484.

88. Goss PE, Powles TJ, Dowsett M, et al. Treatment of advanced postmenopausal breast cancer with an aromatase inhibitor, 4-hydroxyandrostenedione: Phase II report. *Cancer Res* 1986 September;46(9):4823-4826.

89. Baum M, Budzar AU, Cuzick J, et al. Anastrozole alone or in combination with tamoxifen versus tamoxifen alone for adjuvant treatment of postmenopausal women with early breast cancer: First results of the ATAC randomised trial. *Lancet* 2002 June 22;359(9324):2131-2139.

90. Buzdar AU. Data from the Arimidex, tamoxifen, alone or in combination (ATAC) trial: Implications for use of aromatase inhibitors in 2003. *Clin Cancer Res* 2004 January 1;10 (1 Pt 2):355S-361S.

91. Sainsbury R, ATAC Trialists' Group. Beneficial side-effect profile of anastrozole compared with tamoxifen by additional 7 months of exposure data: A safety update from the "Arimidex", Tamoxifen, Alone or in Combination (ATAC) trial. *Breast Cancer ResTreat* 2002;76(Suppl 1):156S (abst 633). Ref Type: Abstract.

92. Schmid M, Jakesz R, Samonigg H, et al. Randomized trial of tamoxifen versus tamoxifen plus aminoglutethimide as adjuvant treatment in postmenopausal breast cancer patients with hormone receptor-positive disease: Austrian breast and colorectal cancer study group trial 6. *J Clin Oncol* 2003 March 15;21(6):984-990.

93. Dowsett M, Cuzick J, Ingle J, et al. Meta-analysis of breast cancer outcomes in adjuvant trials of aromatase inhibitors versus tamoxifen. *J Clin Oncol* 2010 January 20;28(3) 509-518.

94. Goss PE, Ingle JN, Martino S, et al. A randomized trial of letrozole in postmenopausal women after five years of tamoxifen therapy for early-stage breast cancer. *N Engl J Med* 2003 November 6;349(19):1793-1802.

95. Goss PE, Ingle JN, Martino S, et al. Outcomes of women who were premenopausal at diagnosis of early stage breast cancer in the NCIC CTG MA17 Trial. 32nd Annual San Antonio Breast Cancer Symposium 2009. Ref Type: Abstract.

96. Breast International Group (BIG) 1-98 Collaborative Group; Thurlimann B, Keshaviah A, Coates AS, et al. A comparison of letrozole and tamoxifen in postmenopausal women with early breast cancer. *N Engl J Med* 2005 December 29;353(26): 2747-2757.

97. BIG 1-98 Collaborative Group; Mouridsen H, Giobbie-Hurder A, Goldhirsch A, et al. Letrozole therapy alone or in sequence with tamoxifen in women with breast cancer. *N Engl J Med* 2009 August 20;361(8):766-776.

98. Coombes RC, Hall E, Gibson LJ, et al. A randomized trial of exemestane after two to three years of tamoxifen therapy in postmenopausal women with primary breast cancer. *N Engl J Med* 2004 March 11;350(11):1081-1092.

99. Chan A, Speers C, O'Reilly S, et al. Adherence of adjuvant hormonal therapies in post-menopausal hormone receptor positive (HR+) early stage breast cancer: A Population Based Study from British Columbia. 32nd Annual San Antonio Breast Cancer Symposium 2009. Ref Type: Abstract

100. Jonat W, Kaufmann M, Sauerbrei W, et al. Goserelin versus cyclophosphamide, methotrexate, and fluorouracil as adjuvant therapy in premenopausal patients with node-positive breast cancer: The Zoladex Early Breast Cancer Research Association Study. *J Clin Oncol* 2002 December 15;20(24): 4628-4635.

101. Jakesz R, Hausmaninger H, Kubista E, et al. Randomized adjuvant trial of tamoxifen and goserelin versus cyclophosphamide, methotrexate, and fluorouracil: Evidence for the superiority of treatment with endocrine blockade in premenopausal patients with hormone-responsive breast cancer–Austrian Breast and Colorectal Cancer Study Group Trial 5. *J Clin Oncol* 2002 December 15;20(24):4621-4627.

102. Robert NJ, Wang M, Cella D, et al. Phase III comparison of tamoxifen versus tamoxifen with ovarian ablation in premenopausal women with axillary node-negative receptor-positive breast cancer <3 cm. *Proc Am Soc Clin Oncol* 2003;22:5 (abst 16). Ref Type: Abstract.

103. Baum M, Hackshaw A, Houghton J, et al. Adjuvant goserelin in pre-menopausal patients with early breast cancer: Results from the ZIPP study. *Eur J Cancer* 2006 May;42(7):895-904.

104. Arriagada R, LÍ MG, Spielmann M, et al. Randomized trial of adjuvant ovarian suppression in 926 premenopausal patients with early breast cancer treated with adjuvant chemotherapy. *Annals Oncol* 2005 March;16(3):389-396.

105. Fisher B, Anderson S, Tan-Chiu E, et al. Tamoxifen and chemotherapy for axillary node-negative, estrogen receptor-negative breast cancer: Findings from National Surgical Adjuvant Breast and Bowel Project B-23. *J Clin Oncol* 2001 February 15;19(4):931-942.

106. Gnant M, Mlineritsch B, Schippinger W, et al. Endocrine therapy plus zoledronic acid in premenopausal breast cancer. *N Engl J Med* 2009 February 12;360(7):679-691.

107. Brufsky A, Bundred N, Coleman R, et al. Integrated analysis of zoledronic acid for prevention of aromatase inhibitor-associated bone loss in postmenopausal women with early breast cancer receiving adjuvant letrozole. *Oncologist* 2008 May;13(5):503-514.

108. Bundred NJ, Campbell ID, Davidson N, et al. Effective inhibition of aromatase inhibitor-associated bone loss by zoledronic acid in postmenopausal women with early breast cancer receiving adjuvant letrozole: ZO-FAST Study results. *Cancer* 2008 March 1;112(5):1001-1010.

109. De Lena M, Zucali R, Viganotti G, et al. Combined chemotherapy-radiotherapy approach in locally advanced (T3b-T4) breast cancer. *Cancer Chemother Pharmacol* 1978; 1(1):53-59.

110. Hortobagyi GN, Spanos W, Montague ED, et al. Treatment of locoregionally advanced breast cancer with surgery, radiotherapy, and combination chemoimmunotherapy. *Int J Radiat Oncol, Biol, Phys* 1983 May;9(5):643-650.

111. Mauriac L, Durand M, Avril A, et al. Effects of primary chemotherapy in conservative treatment of breast cancer patients with operable tumors larger than 3 cm. Results of a randomized trial in a single centre. *Annals Oncol* 1991 May;2(5):347-354.

112. Fisher B, Brown A, Mamounas E, et al. Effect of preoperative chemotherapy on local-regional disease in women with operable breast cancer: Findings from National Surgical Adjuvant Breast and Bowel Project B-18. *J Clin Oncol* 1997 Jul;15(7):2483-2493.

113. Rouzier R, Extra JM, Klijanienko J, et al. Incidence and prognostic significance of complete axillary downstaging after primary chemotherapy in breast cancer patients with T1 to T3 tumors and cytologically proven axillary metastatic lymph nodes. *J Clin Oncol* 2002 March 1;20(5):1304-1310.

114. van der Hage JA, van de Velde CJ, Julien JP, et al. Preoperative chemotherapy in primary operable breast cancer: Results from the European Organization for Research and Treatment of Cancer trial 10902. *J Clin Oncol* 2001 November 15;19(22):4224-4237.

115. Smith IC, Heys SD, Hutcheon AW, et al. Neoadjuvant chemotherapy in breast cancer: Significantly enhanced response with docetaxel. *J Clin Oncol* 2002 March 15;20(6):1456-1466.

116. Formenti SC, Volm M, Skinner KA, et al. Preoperative twice-weekly paclitaxel with concurrent radiation therapy followed by surgery and postoperative doxorubicin-based chemotherapy in locally advanced breast cancer: A phase I/II trial. *J Clin Oncol* 2003 March 1;21(5):864-870.

117. Green MC, Buzdar AU, Smith T, et al. Weekly paclitaxel improves pathologic complete remission in operable breast cancer when compared with paclitaxel once every 3 weeks. *J Clin Oncol* 2005 September 1;23(25):5983-5992.

118. Buzdar AU, Valero V, Ibrahim NK, et al. Neoadjuvant therapy with paclitaxel followed by 5-fluorouracil, epirubicin, and cyclophosphamide chemotherapy and concurrent trastuzumab in human epidermal growth factor receptor 2-positive operable breast cancer: An update of the initial randomized study population and data of additional patients treated with the same regimen. *Clin Cancer Res* 2007 January 1;13(1):228-233.

119. Perez EA, Suman VJ, Davidson NE, et al. Results of Chemotherapy Alone, with Sequential or Concurrent Addition of 52 Weeks of Trastuzumab in the NCCTG N9831 HER2-Positive Adjuvant Breast Cancer Trial. 32nd Annual San Antonio Breast Cancer Symposium 2009. Ref Type: Abstract

120. Veronesi A, Frustaci S, Tirelli U, et al. Tamoxifen therapy in postmenopausal advanced breast cancer: Efficacy at the primary tumor site in 46 evaluable patients. *Tumori* 1981 May-Jun;67(3):235-238.

121. Gazet JC, Ford HT, Coombes RC. Randomised trial of chemotherapy versus endocrine therapy in patients presenting with locally advanced breast cancer (a pilot study). *Brit J Cancer* 1991 February;63(2):279-282.

122. Hoff PM, Valero V, Buzdar AU, et al. Combined modality treatment of locally advanced breast carcinoma in elderly patients or patients with severe comorbid conditions using tamoxifen as the primary therapy. *Cancer* 2000 May 1;88(9):2054-2060.

123. Ellis MJ, Coop A, Singh B, et al. Letrozole is more effective neoadjuvant endocrine therapy than tamoxifen for ErbB-1- and/or ErbB-2-positive, estrogen receptor-positive primary breast cancer: Evidence from a phase III randomized trial. *J Clin Oncol* 2001 September 15;19(18):3808-3816.

124. Semiglazov V, Ivanov V, Ziltzova EK, et al. Anastrozole vs tamoxifen vs combined anastrozole and tamoxifen as neoadjuvant endocrine therapy of postmenopausal breast cancer patients. *Proc Am Soc Clin Oncol* 2003;22:880. Ref type: Abstract.

125. Dowsett M, Smith IE, Ebbs SR, et al. Short-term changes in Ki-67 during neoadjuvant treatment of primary breast cancer with anastrozole or tamoxifen alone or combined correlate with recurrence-free survival. *Clin Cancer Res* 2005 January 15;11(2 Pt 2):951S-958S.

126. Dowsett M, Smith IE, Ebbs SR, et al. Prognostic value of Ki67 expression after short-term presurgical endocrine therapy for primary breast cancer. *J Natl Cancer Inst* 2007 January 17;99(2):167-170.

127. Citron M, Berry D, Cirrincione C, et al. Superiority of dose-dense over conventional scheduling and equivalence of sequential vs. combination adjuvant chemotherapy for node-positive breast cancer (CALGB 9741, INT C9741). *Breast Cancer Res Treat* 2002;76(Suppl. 1):32S; (abst 15). Ref Type: Abstract.

128. Citron ML, Berry DA, Cirrincione C, et al. Randomized trial of dose-dense versus conventionally scheduled and sequential versus concurrent combination chemotherapy as postoperative adjuvant treatment of node-positive primary breast cancer: First report of Intergroup Trial C9741/Cancer and Leukemia Group B Trial 9741. *J Clin Oncol* 2003 April 15;21(8):1431-1439.

129. Ellis GK, Livingston RB, Gralow JR, et al. Dose-dense anthracycline-based chemotherapy for node-positive breast cancer. *J Clin Oncol* 2002 September 1;20(17):3637-3643.

130. Vogel CL, Cobleigh MA, Tripathy D, et al. Efficacy and safety of trastuzumab as a single agent in first-line treatment of HER2-overexpressing metastatic breast cancer. *J Clin Oncol* 2002 February 1;20(3):719-726.

131. Cobleigh MA, Vogel CL, Tripathy D, et al. Multinational study of the efficacy and safety of humanized anti-HER2 monoclonal antibody in women who have HER2-overexpressing metastatic breast cancer that has progressed after chemotherapy for metastatic disease. *J Clin Oncol* 1999 September;17(9):2639-2648.

132. Slamon DJ, Leyland-Jones B, Shak S, et al. Use of chemotherapy plus a monoclonal antibody against HER2 for metastatic breast cancer that overexpresses HER2. *N Engl J Med* 2001 March 15;344(11):783-792.

133. Burstein HJ, Harris LN, Gelman R, et al. Preoperative therapy with trastuzumab and paclitaxel followed by sequential adjuvant doxorubicin/cyclophosphamide for HER2 overexpressing stage II or III breast cancer: A pilot study. *J Clin Oncol* 2003 January 1;21(1):46-53.

134. Paik S, Shak S, Tang G, et al. A multigene assay to predict recurrence of tamoxifen-treated, node-negative breast cancer. *N Engl J Med* 2004 December 30;351(27):2817-2826.

135. Paik S, Tang G, Shak S, et al. Gene expression and benefit of chemotherapy in women with node-negative, estrogen receptor-positive breast cancer. *J Clin Oncol* 2006 August 10;24(23):3726-3734.

136. Cuzick J, Dowsett M, Wale C, et al. Prognostic value of a combined ER, PgR, Ki67, HER2 immunohistochemical (IHC4) score and comparison with the GHI recurrence score–results from TransATAC. 32nd Annual San Antonio Breast Cancer Symposium 2009. Ref Type: Abstract.

137. Fisher B, Anderson S, Bryant J, et al. Twenty-year follow-up of a randomized trial comparing total mastectomy, lumpectomy, and lumpectomy plus irradiation for the treatment of invasive breast cancer. *N Engl J Med* 2002 October 17;347(16):1233-1241.

138. Derossis AM, Fey J, Yeung H, et al. A trend analysis of the relative value of blue dye and isotope localization in 2,000 consecutive cases of sentinel node biopsy for breast cancer. *J Am Coll Surg* 2001 November;193(5):473-478.

139. Bartelink H, Horiot JC, Poortmans P, et al. Recurrence rates after treatment of breast cancer with standard radiotherapy with or without additional radiation. *N Engl J Med* 2001 November 8;345(19):1378-1387.

140. Hortobagyi GN, Gutterman JU, Blumenschein GR, et al. Combination chemoimmunotherapy of metastatic breast cancer with 5-fluorouracil, adriamycin, cyclophosphamide, and BCG. *Cancer* 1979 April;43(4):1225-1233.

141. Ozer H, Armitage JO, Bennett CL, et al. 2000 update of recommendations for the use of hematopoietic colony-stimulating factors: Evidence-based, clinical practice guidelines. American Society of Clinical Oncology Growth Factors Expert Panel. *J Clin Oncol* 2000 October 15;18(20):3558-3585.

142. Recht A, Edge SB, Solin LJ, et al. Postmastectomy radiotherapy: clinical practice guidelines of the American Society of Clinical Oncology. *J Clin Oncol* 2001 March 1;19(5):1539-1569.

143. Gröhn P, Heinonen E, Klefstrom P, et al. Adjuvant postoperative radiotherapy, chemotherapy, and immunotherapy in stage III breast cancer. *Cancer* 1984 August 15;54(4):670-674.

144. Chollet P, Charrier S, Brain E, et al. Clinical and pathological response to primary chemotherapy in operable breast cancer. *Eur J Cancer* 1997 May;33(6):862-866.

145. McCready DR, Hortobagyi GN, Kau SW, et al. The Prognostic significance of lymph node metastases after preoperative chemotherapy for locally advanced breast cancer. *Arch Surg* 1989 Jan;124(1):21-25.

146. Veronesi U, Bonadonna G, Zurrida S, et al. Conservation surgery after primary chemotherapy in large carcinomas of the breast. *Annals Surg* 1995;222(5):612-618.

147. Rouzier R, Extra JM, Carton M, et al. Primary chemotherapy for operable breast cancer: Incidence and prognostic significance of ipsilateral breast tumor recurrence after breast-conserving surgery. *J Clin Oncol* 2001 September 15;19(18):3828-3835.

148. Olson JE, Neuberg D, Pandya KJ, et al. The role of radiotherapy in the management of operable locally advanced breast carcinoma: results of a randomized trial by the Eastern Cooperative Oncology Group. *Cancer* 1997 March 15;79(6):1138-1149.

149. Huang E, McNeese MD, Strom EA, et al. Locoregional treatment outcomes for inoperable anthracycline-resistant breast cancer. *Int J Radiat Oncol, Biol, Phys* 2002 August 1;53(5):1225-1233.

METASTATIC BREAST CANCER

Mariana Chavez-MacGregor
Vicente Valero

Breast cancer is a significant cause of morbidity and mortality among women. In the United States, it is the most common malignancy among women. It is estimated that approximately 194,280 new cases of invasive breast cancer will have occurred in the United States in 2009 (1). Although lung cancer has surpassed breast cancer as the leading cause of cancer death among women, nearly 40,200 deaths are expected to occur from breast cancer alone in 2009 (1).

Since the 1970s, advances in primary and adjuvant systemic therapies have substantially improved both survival and quality of life in patients with newly diagnosed, early, and locally advanced breast cancer. In spite of these advances, approximately 10 to 60% of patients with initial localized breast cancer will suffer a systemic relapse. Furthermore, metastatic disease is diagnosed at the time of presentation in 3 to 6% of patients, but can be as high as 10 to 12% depending on the series (1,2). Bone is the most common site of first distant relapse; other common sites of metastases include lymph nodes, lung, liver, and less frequently brain. The 5-year survival rate for localized breast cancer is 97%, but for women with metastatic disease, this rate is only 17 to 28% (1,2). As is true with cancer in general, the clinical course for patients with metastatic breast cancer varies from patient to patient, but as a group, patients with metastatic breast cancer (MBC) have a median survival of 23 months (3). Patients with bone-only disease tend to live longer than patients with visceral involvement. Untreated patients with MBC will have a median overall survival time of 9 to 12 months. With chemotherapy, the mean survival time is 21 months for patients with visceral disease, and is as long as 60 months for patients with bone-only disease. Survival and response to therapy are affected by several factors, including estrogen receptor (ER), progesterone receptor (PR), and HER2/neu receptor status; performance status; site of disease; number of disease sites; and duration of disease-free interval.

The therapeutic objectives and approach to patients with advanced breast cancer is distinct from that of those patients with early-stage disease. Treatment for MBC is triaged to endocrine therapy, biological therapy, or chemotherapy, depending on the hormonal and HER-2/neu receptor status of the tumor and the severity of the symptoms and site and extent of disease. Systemic treatment prolongs survival, provides palliation of symptoms, and enhances quality of life, but in general terms is not considered curative; therefore, a discussion regarding goals of care is imperative between the patient and treating oncologist. Cure in MBC is rare; less than 2% of patients with chemotherapy-naïve MBC may remain disease-free after anthracycline-containing therapy. It is possible to prolong the median survival of patients with MBC as much as 18 to 36 months. In a review of the survival of patients with recurrent breast cancer, Giordano et al. found that the prognosis for patients with recurrent breast cancer improved between 1974 and 2000, with a 1% reduction in risk for each succeeding year (4). This occurred for several reasons, including more effective therapies, staging migration, and trial design. In recent years, several new agents have contributed to the improvements in overall survival. In the same review, other factors associated with improved survival after breast cancer recurrence included smaller initial tumor size, lower stage of disease at the time of initial diagnosis, fewer lymph nodes involved, longer disease-free interval, estrogen receptor-positive tumors, and nonvisceral dominant site of disease recurrence.

This chapter reviews standard care for patients with MBC and discusses some unique approaches used at The University of Texas MD Anderson Cancer Center (MDACC).

■ DIAGNOSTIC WORKUP

Once metastatic disease is suspected, careful evaluation of the primary disease history, current symptoms, and existing comorbid diseases is essential. The history of the primary disease should include a review of the initial presentation, stage of disease, histology, hormone-receptor and HER2/neu status, nuclear grade, and treatment modalities employed. Knowledge of the initial tumor type may yield clues about the sites of disease as well as its biology. For instance, infiltrating ductal carcinoma most commonly involve the lungs, pleura, liver, and brain, whereas infiltrating lobular carcinoma may metastasize to unusual sites such as the bone marrow, meninges, peritoneum, and retroperitoneal structures, such as the ureters (5). Other ancillary information, such as DNA ploidy and S-phase fraction, have been studied in primary breast cancer, but the influence of these factors on metastatic disease progression is unclear. However, among patients who develop extraosseous metastatic disease, those with highly aneuploid tumors at initial presentation have significantly shorter survival times than do patients with diploid tumors at initial presentation (6).

If possible, it should be strongly considered to perform a biopsy of the metastatic or recurrence site to confirm the histologic type, as well as estrogen- and progesterone-receptor and HER2/neu status, as there is some evidence of significant discordance in the receptor status between the time of diagnosis of the primary tumor and the time of diagnosis of metastasis (7,8). Pathologic confirmation is also essential in patients suspected of clinical metastases if the clinical course is not apparent. Such relapse scenarios include single-lesion metastasis, unusual metastatic sites, and long disease-free interval (DFI). Autopsy data from a 1993 series showed that second primary nonmammary malignancies, most commonly of the female genital and gastrointestinal systems, occurred in 11% of patients with breast cancer at a mean interval of nearly 7 years after diagnosis of primary breast cancer (9). Furthermore, half of these occurred in the first 4 years following diagnosis. In this series, a nonmammary primary tumor was the cause of death in 54% of patients, whereas breast cancer was the cause of death in 29%. The length of the disease-free interval and menopausal status should also be ascertained.

A comprehensive physical examination is essential. Evaluation of the soft tissues includes a careful survey of all the lymph-node basins of the upper torso, with documentation of the size and location of enlarged nodes and assessment of the chest wall, surgical scar, and all breast tissue. A complete neurologic examination in combination of a good history can determine the need for specific diagnostic imaging. Ascites caused by peritoneal metastasis is less common but not rare and should be evaluated.

A basic laboratory evaluation includes a complete blood count with differential, liver and renal function tests, and serum calcium determination. In addition, CA 15.3 and CA 27-29 are potentially helpful in monitoring response to therapy. The CA 15.3 test is a combination of two monoclonal antibodies bearing two reactive determinants directed against DF3 and MAM-6 antigens expressed on mammary epithelial cells (10,11). CA 15.3 and CA 27-29, which are more sensitive than CEA, are elevated in 70 to 85% of patients with metastases, but they lack sensitivity and specificity for breast cancer progression. Therefore their prognostic significance remains indeterminate (10). CEA is elevated in 40 to 50% of patients with metastatic disease (11,12). Current recommendations from the American Society of Clinical Oncology establish that CA27.29, CA 15-3, or CEA can be used in conjunction with diagnostic imaging, history, and physical examination for monitoring patients with metastatic disease during active therapy; however data are insufficient to recommend use of CA 15-3, CA 27.29, or CEA alone for monitoring response to treatment (13). It is important to mention that in the absence of readily measurable disease, an increasing level of any of these markers may be used to indicate treatment failure. Caution should be used when interpreting tumor marker levels during the first 4 to 12 weeks of a new therapy, since spurious early rises may occur (10,13). The measurement of circulating tumor cells (CTC) has recently been studied in patients with MBC. Several studies showed that high levels of CTCs are correlated with poor survival in MBC and with response to treatment (14-16). However based on current recommendations, the measurement of CTCs should not be used to make the diagnosis of breast cancer or to influence any treatment decisions. Similarly, the use of the recently FDA (Food and Drug Administration)-cleared test for CTC (CellSearch Assay) in patients with MBC cannot be recommended until further validation confirms the clinical value of the test. An intergroup trial is underway to determine the implication of changing treatment based on the CTC level (13).

A chest radiograph is usually sufficient to assess, but in most cases we perform a baseline evaluation that also includes a computed tomography (CT). In addition to liver parenchymal involvement, metastases to peri-portal nodes with compression of the biliary tree or hepatic/portal vessels may also occur. These metastases are detected by CT or ultrasonography, but occasionally magnetic resonance imaging (MRI) of the abdomen may be indicated (17). The presence of bone metastases should be evaluated and in general, we recommend a bone scan. Only 30 to 60% of patients with true-positive bone scans have increased levels of alkaline phosphatase (18,19), and conversely, only 20% of patients with elevated levels of alkaline phosphatase are disease-free (19). If the bone scan shows areas of abnormal uptake, plain radiographs of the affected sites are necessary to confirm metastatic disease and exclude a benign etiology. Impending fractures in the weight-bearing bones, such as the femur, and an unstable spine must be ruled out. The preferred test for spinal evaluation for metastases is MRI. Radiographic evaluations of the brain, leptomeninges, and spinal cord have low yield unless the patient is symptomatic or has abnormal neurologic findings (17). Current guidelines discourage the use of PET/CT except in those situations where other staging studies are equivocal or suspicious (17).

TREATMENT

GENERAL CONSIDERATIONS

The decision whether to use chemotherapy or biological or hormonal therapy for the initial treatment of MBC should be guided by several factors including hormone receptor and HER2/neu status, the presence of symptomatic visceral disease or life-threatening disease (Fig. 25-1). Patients with moderately symptomatic visceral disease or life-threatening disease should be considered for treatment with systemic chemotherapy regardless of hormone receptor status because systemic therapy offers faster palliation of symptoms for most patients. Among women who do not have life-threatening or symptomatic visceral disease, those whose tumors are negative for ER and PR should be also considered for systemic chemotherapy. Those whose tumors are positive for ER or PR should be treated with hormonal therapy. Since the discovery of the importance of HER2/neu gene amplification in breast cancer and the development of anti-HER2/neu therapy with trastuzumab (Herceptin), those patients with tumors positive for HER2/neu overexpression by immunohistochemistry (IHC 3+) or gene amplification by fluorescent in situ hybridization (FISH) should be treated with trastuzumab in combination with chemotherapy as this provides a significant survival advantage.

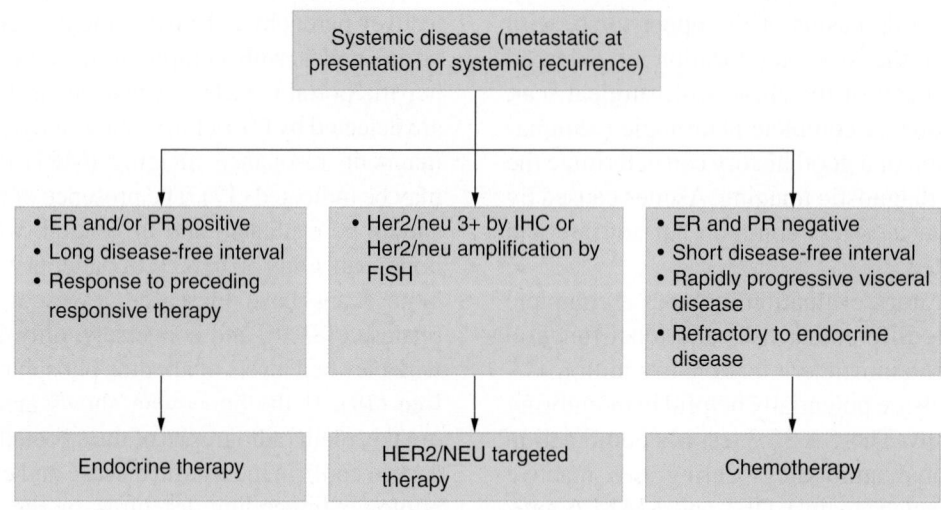

FIGURE 25-1.   Algorithm for treatement selection in patients with metastatic breast cancer.

Multiple agents are active against hormone-responsive tumors. Endocrine therapy tends to be associated with fewer side effects and helps to maintain quality of life for many patients. If the tumor does not respond to endocrine therapy or becomes unresponsive to hormonal therapy, systemic chemotherapy should be initiated.

As previously mentioned, as a general rule, there is no cure for MBC. However, few studies have shown prolonged remissions in patients who receive systemic chemotherapy. A review of patients with anthracycline-naive MBC treated at MDACC showed that among individuals who have a complete remission after anthracycline-containing therapy, 17% (3% of the overall population) will remain free of disease for more than 10 years (5). In patients who have received no prior chemotherapy in the setting of metastasis, objective response rates of 25 to 55% have been observed in multicenter randomized trials. In women with advanced disease, chemotherapy was shown to improve survival, however there are no phase III trials evaluating the use of chemotherapy versus best supportive care in patients with untreated or refractory MBC.

Currently, the primary goals of chemotherapy for MBC should be palliation of symptoms attributable to cancer and prolongation of life. It is the physician's duty to balance the benefits of therapy with possible toxic effects and to fully discuss therapeutic options with patients. The patient's multiple previous therapies, decline in performance status, comorbid conditions, and organ function should be taken into consideration in the treatment decision. In the setting of metastatic disease, as in the adjuvant setting, high-dose chemotherapy with

stem cell transplantation remains investigational. The treatment algorithm of patients with metastatic breast cancer at the MDACC is illustrated in Fig. 25-2; for details, please refer to the Endocrine Therapy, Chemotherapy, and Targeted Therapy sections of this chapter.

■ ENDOCRINE THERAPY

Endocrine therapy has dramatically improved outcomes in patients with hormone receptor–positive breast cancer; it can result in significant palliation of symptoms and improvement in quality of life as well as overall survival in patients with hormone receptor–positive MBC. Manipulation of the endocrine system as a treatment for metastatic breast cancer was introduced in 1896, when Beatson demonstrated objective regression of breast cancer after oophorectomy. Now a number of endocrine therapies are used in patients with hormone-sensitive MBC; most of these therapies are directed at reducing the synthesis of estrogen or blocking estrogen receptors in hormone-dependent tumors.

The presence of ER or PR in breast tumors is predictive of a higher likelihood of response to endocrine therapy (20,21). Patients who have tumors that are both ER-positive and PR-positive will have a 50 to 70% probability of receiving clinical benefit from endocrine therapy. Patients with either ER-positive or PR-positive tumors will have about a 30% probability of receiving clinical benefit from endocrine therapy. Quantitative PR levels have been shown to correlate significantly and independently with increased response to tamoxifen, longer time to treatment failure (TTF), and also

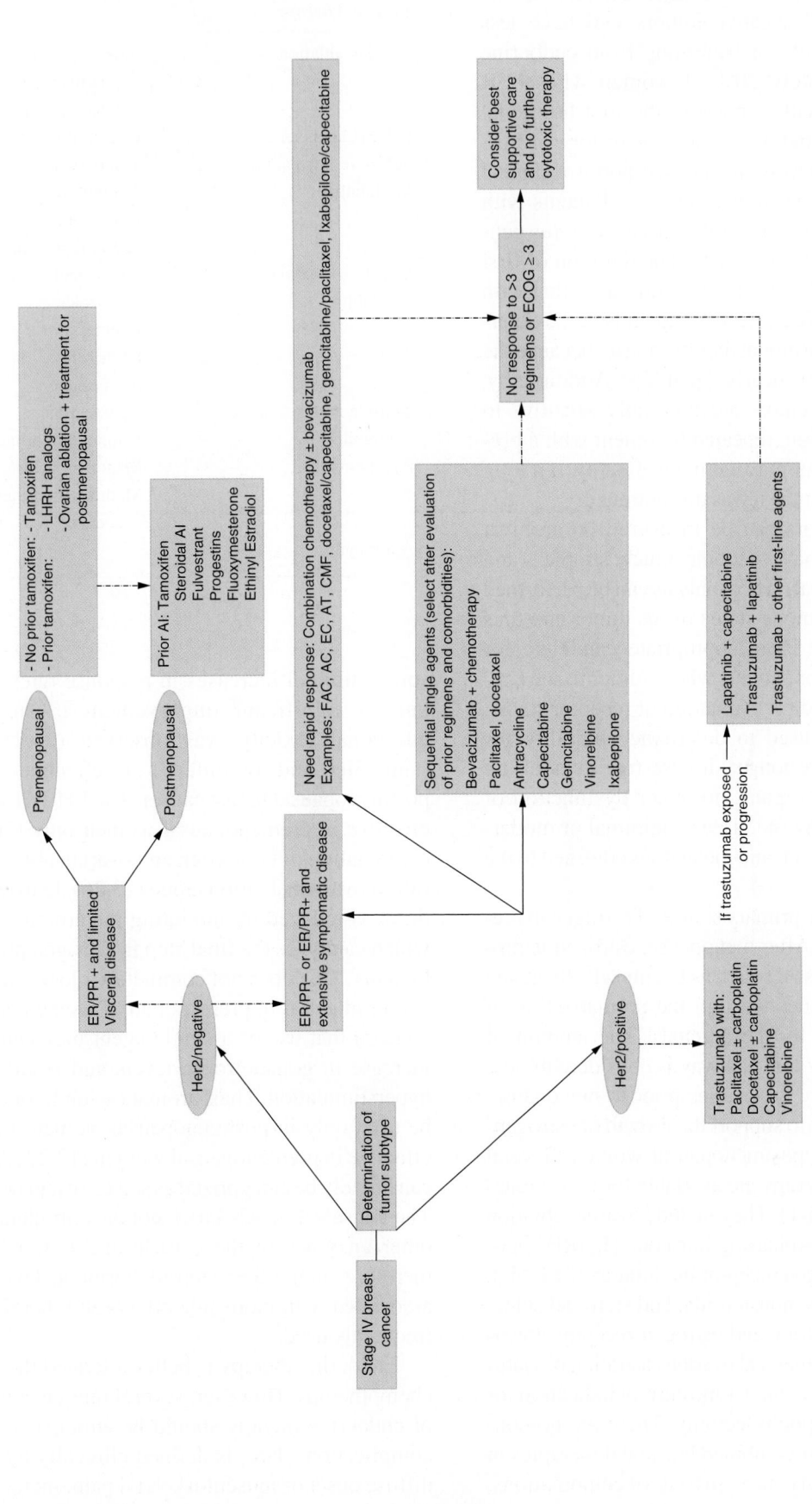

FIGURE 25-2. Treatment of metastatic breast cancer.

longer overall survival (OS) times in patients with ER-positive tumors (22). On the other hand, those with ER-negative and PR-negative tumors will have less than a 10% probability of benefiting from endocrine therapy. Approximately 30% of women whose ER status is unknown will respond to the first hormonal manipulation. Of patients with a prior history of hormonal response, 30 to 50% will have a response or clinical benefit from another hormonal regimen. Patients with low-volume disease and better performance status generally have higher response rates. The duration of first response is usually 9 to 12 months, similar to that with chemotherapy. The side-effect profile aids in the determination of which hormonal therapy to use, because the efficacy of all agents is nearly equal (23). Additionally, for patients whose tumors are unusually sensitive to hormonal manipulation, repeated treatment with a previously effective agent may again be effective if a long interval has elapsed since it was discontinued.

Hormone receptors can be measured on archival tissue. The assays have become much simpler, and immunohystochemical (IHC) analysis can be performed to determine the hormone status of the tumor and thus whether that patient is an appropriate candidate for endocrine therapy. For patients whose tumor tissue cannot be easily accessed for evaluation of receptor status, the clinical criteria used to determine eligibility for endocrine therapy are longer disease-free interval, no involvement of vital organs, no major dysfunction of the organs involved by the disease, minimal or moderate visceral involvement, and metastases confined to the soft tissue or bone.

The ovaries are the primary source of estrogen in premenopausal women. After menopause, estrogen is produced in peripheral tissues such as fat, muscle, liver, and the breast tumor tissues through the aromatization of androgens produced by the adrenals. The amount of estrogen produced by this pathway is considerably less than that produced by the ovaries prior to menopause, but it is still sufficient to support the growth of estrogen-dependent tumors in postmenopausal women. Several types of endocrine therapy are available for use in managing MBC (Table 25-1). They include ovarian ablation (luteinizing hormone-releasing hormone [LHRH] agonists), selective estrogen receptor modulators [SERMs], progestins, androgens, nonsteroidal and steroidal selective aromatase inhibitors, and estrogen receptor down-regulators. Currently, medical ovarian castration obviates surgery as a first choice; there is no current indication for adrenalectomy or hypophysectomy. There are no conclusive data to support combined hormonal therapies in postmenopausal breast cancer. In trials of combinations,

TABLE 25-1	TYPES OF ENDOCRINE THERAPY FOR METASTATIC BREAST CANCER
Type of Therapy	
Ovarian ablation	Surgery, radiation therapy, pharmacologic interventions
LH-RH agonists	Groserelin acetate
Selective estrogen receptor Modulators	Tamoxifen
	Toremifene
	Raloxifene
	Arzoxifene hydrochloride
Selective aromatase inhibitors	Anastrozole
	Letrozole
	Exemestane
	Fadrozole
	Formestane
Nonselective aromatase inhibitors	Testolactone
	Aminoglutethimide
Progestins	Megestrol acetate
	Medroxyprogesterone acetate
Androgens	

some minimal increases in response rates were seen, but no significant improvement in survival, and additional toxicity was observed (24,25). SERMs (tamoxifen and toremifene) are effective in pre- and postmenopausal breast cancer. The LH-RH agonists are effective in premenopausal women only (26), and the combination of tamoxifen and ovarian ablation is superior to ovarian ablation alone (23,26). Estrogen biosynthesis is reduced by inhibiting the aromatase enzyme, which catalyzes the final step in estrogen production in humans. This does not completely block ovarian estrogen production in premenopausal women, and there is concern that use of a single agent may cause a reflex increase in gonadotropin levels and result in ovarian hyperstimulation. Thus, aromatase inhibitors (AIs) must be used only in postmenopausal women; they are not effective in premenopausal women (17,27-29). The AIs can broadly be categorized as selective and nonselective. The nonselective AIs block not only aromatase but also other enzymes in the cytochrome P-450 family and therefore alter other steroid hormone levels and are associated with more side effects and therefore are not frequently used.

Endocrine therapy is better tolerated than cytotoxic chemotherapy. However, several unique complications of endocrine therapy should be anticipated. One such complication, flare, is defined clinically by an abrupt, diffuse onset of musculoskeletal pain, increased size of skin lesions, or erythema surrounding the skin lesion within the first month of endocrine therapy. There is no published evidence that tumor growth rates increase during this period. The most serious manifestation of flare is hypercalcemia, which can be seen with several hormonal therapies except AIs and surgical castration. Hypercalcemia usually occurs in patients with bone metastases and manifests itself within the first 2 weeks after treatment. The underlying mechanism is the predominating early agonist effect of hormonal agents. Low doses of prednisone (10-30 mg/day) may abrogate the initial flare of bone pain. The patient should be instructed about the possibility of flare and should undergo monitoring of serum calcium level within the first 2 weeks of treatment. If hypercalcemia develops, the calcium level should be controlled and treatment continued provided that it is lower than 14 mg/dL.

Many side effects of endocrine therapy, such as hot flashes and mood disturbances, are related to estrogen deprivation and are common to tamoxifen and AIs, reflecting the mechanism of action of these drugs (30). Tamoxifen has estrogenic effects that are beneficial in some tissues; it lowers serum cholesterol levels and protects against bone loss and cardiovascular disease, but is also associated with potentially life-threatening side effects, such as endometrial cancer and thromboembolic disease (30,31). AIs lack estrogenic activity, therefore they are not associated with these serious adverse events, and in general are associated with a lower incidence of gynecologic symptoms and hot flashes when compared to tamoxifen. However, they are associated with musculoskeletal side effects, such as arthralgias, myalgias, and bone loss. Other side effects, including abnormalities of the lipid metabolism and the cardiovascular system are still debatable according to some authors (30,32). All hormonal regimens except the AIs may cause weight gain. This side effect is most common with progestins, which can cause both a true increase in weight, from their anabolic effect, and fluid retention, secondary to their glucocorticoid effect. Progestins are the drugs most likely to cause thromboembolism; tamoxifen is the next most likely drug to cause this complication. Both drugs have been reported to prolong prothrombin time in patients who are also receiving warfarin (33).

The preferred agent for endocrine therapy depends on the menopausal status of the patient. In premenopausal women, tamoxifen is recommended as the initial therapy, although ovarian suppression with an LH-RH agonist alone or plus tamoxifen can also be used. In patients that are within 1 year of antiestrogen exposure, the preferred second-line therapy is surgical oophorectomy or an LHRH agonist with endocrine therapy (17). In postmenopausal women who are antiestrogen naïve or who are more than 1 year from previous antiestrogen therapy, an aromatase inhibitor is recommended as initial first-line therapy but tamoxifen can also be used. AIs appear to have superior outcome compared with tamoxifen, but differences are modest (34,35). The use of anastrozole or letrozole, both aromatase inhibitors, as initial therapy in postmenopausal women with ER-positive tumors results in increased response rates, longer control of disease, and fewer side effects than tamoxifen therapy (36). Patients who respond to initial therapy have a higher probability of response to second and third endocrine therapies. There is a partial lack of cross-resistance between steroidal and nonsteroidal aromatase inhibitors; thus, these agents may provide palliation of disease if used sequentially in patients with hormone receptor–positive tumors. Many patients with hormone-responsive breast cancer benefit from the sequential use of endocrine therapies at the time of disease progression. In patients that respond to endocrine therapy with either shrinkage of the tumor or long-term disease stabilization should receive additional endocrine therapy at the time of disease progression (17).

Fulvestrant is an ER antagonist that downregulates ER and has no agonist effects. It was compared with tamoxifen in a large randomized, multicenter trial involving 587 postmenopausal women with advanced or metastatic breast cancer who had not previously been treated with endocrine therapy. Patients were given either fulvestrant 250 mg IM monthly or tamoxifen 20 mg PO daily. At a median follow-up of 14.5 months, there was no significant difference between fulvestrant and tamoxifen in TTP (median 6.8 versus 8.3 months, respectively) (37). Fulvestrant also appears to be, at least as effective as anastrozole in patients whose disease progressed on tamoxifen (38,39). Furthermore, the clinical benefit rates of examestane and fulvestrant observed in a phase III trial of postmenopausal women with hormone receptor–positive breast cancer who experienced disease progression on prior nonsteroidal-AIs were comparable (32.2 versus 31.5%) (40). The CONFIRM trial (N = 736) compared the use of fulvestrant at different doses (250 mg and 500 mg) in postmenopausal women with advanced disease recurring or progressing after prior endocrine therapy. Response rates observed were similar in both groups (13.8 versus 14.6%) but TTP was significantly longer for the patients that received 500 mg (HR 0.80; 95% CI 0.68-0.94) (41).

After second-line endocrine therapy, little high level evidence exists to assist selecting the optimal sequence of endocrine therapy. There are many available hormonal

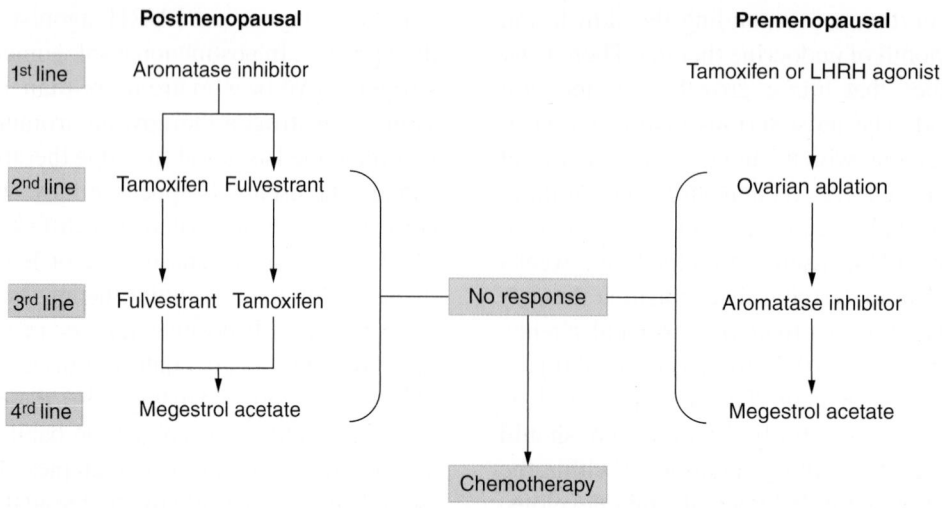

Postmenopausal

1st line   Aromatase inhibitor

2nd line   Tamoxifen   Fulvestrant

3rd line   Fulvestrant   Tamoxifen

4th line   Megestrol acetate

No response

Chemotherapy

Premenopausal

Tamoxifen or LHRH agonist

Ovarian ablation

Aromatase inhibitor

Megestrol acetate

FIGURE 25-3. Endocrine therapy algorithm for patients with hormone-receptor positive metastatic breast cancer.

agents; progestins, for example are synthetic derivates of progesterone that have a progesterone-agonist effect. Progestins such as megestrol acetate and medroxyprogesterone acetate are effective in treating MBC but their exact mechanism of action is unknown. They have antiestrogenic properties and may result in interruption of the pituitary-ovarian axis. Androgens have been also evaluated and used in patients with MBC who have been treated with multiple endocrine agents and still have hormone-dependent disease. Recent data suggest that the use of estrogen can be beneficial for patients with AI-resistant breast cancer (42). In a phase II study, 66 patients with AI-resistant MBC were randomized to receive 6 versus 30 mg of estradiol. The clinical benefit rates were 25% on the 30 mg arm and 29% on the 6 mg arm. The authors concluded that 6 mg of estradiol was as effective as the 30 mg arm with greater safety, and that this regimen could be a palliative therapeutic strategy for patients with MBC that have progressed to other endocrine therapies (42). The treatment algorithm used for treating patients with hormone-receptor MBC at MDACC is illustrated in this chapter (Fig. 25-3).

■ **CHEMOTHERAPY**

Unlike hormonal receptors and endocrine therapy, no predictive test for a response to chemotherapy has been sufficiently validated to use in a standard clinical setting. For patients with MBC that have not been previously treated with chemotherapy, the benefit ratio is in the order of 30 to 75%. Some of the predictors of response

to chemotherapy include disease-free interval, sites of disease, organ function, and performance status among others (43,44) (Table 25-2). Distinct molecular markers have been evaluated as potential predictive factors for chemotherapy in general, or for specific agents. Data are mixed for ER receptor status and response to chemotherapy. There is some suggestion that patients with ER-positive tumors are less likely to respond to chemotherapy than those with ER-negative tumors (45). Other markers of cellular proliferation—such as flow cytometry evaluation of the fractions of cells in S phase, determination of radiolabeled thymidine uptake, and IHC staining for the proliferation antigen Ki67—have all been associated with higher chemotherapy response rates (46,47). However, none of these markers is sufficiently accurate to form the basis of a decision to treat or withhold therapy. A number of gene products are under active investigation as chemotherapy response markers. These include p170-glycoprotein (gp170), a

TABLE 25-2	CLINICAL PREDICTORS OF IMPROVED RESPONSE TO CHEMOTHERAPY FOR METASTATIC BREAST CANCER

- Low tumor burden
- Normal organ function
- Good performance status
- No recent weight loss
- No prior chemotherapy or radiation therapy
- Soft-tissue metastases
- Premenopausal status
- Prolonged disease-free interval after adjuvant chemotherapy

drug efflux pump that mediates multidrug resistance (MDR), and p53. It is not yet clear what roles gp170 and p53 have in defining chemotherapy treatment in MBC.

SELECTION OF AGENTS/REGIMEN

In deciding which cytotoxic regimen to use in the setting of negative ER/PR and HER2/neu status, or in patients that have progressed to endocrine therapy, considerations should be given to the patient's previous therapies, organ function, and comorbid conditions. Typically, chemotherapy within the conventional range of doses is associated with higher response rates than is "low-dose chemotherapy." As in the setting of adjuvant therapy, high-dose chemotherapy with peripheral/ bone marrow stem cell transplantation remains investigational.

The choice between sequential single agents and combination chemotherapy is also controversial. The principle of nonoverlapping mechanisms of resistance and toxicities has been the basis of combination chemotherapy. Curability with combination therapy in lymphoma, leukemia, and testicular cancer had been proof of this concept. Multiple randomized trials involving single-agent versus multiple-agent regimens in MBC have generally demonstrated that combination chemotherapy has improved response rates and TTP, but OS remains little altered or unchanged. Fossati et al. (48), in a systematic review that included 31,510 patients, estimated that the proportional reduction in overall mortality for combinations versus single-agent regimens is only 18%, translating to an absolute benefit in survival of 9% at 1 year, 5% at 2 years, and only 3% after 5 years. More toxicity was associated with combination therapy. In two randomized trials of combination versus single-agent therapy in MBC, formal quality-of-life analyses favored the single-agent arms even though response rates were slightly lower (49,50).

More recently, a Cochrane review (51) including 28 trials and 5707 patients with MBC that were randomly assigned to receive single-agent or combination chemotherapy found that combination therapy was associated with a higher response rate (OR 1.28; 95% CI 1.15-1.42), longer time to progression (HR 0.78; 95% CI 0.73-0.83), and longer OS (HR 0.88; 95% CI 0.83-0.94) than single-agent therapy. It is important to mention that most trials including in the Cochrane review did not specifically investigate the combination versus the sequential use of the single agents, and very few studies reported the rate of "crossover" to an additional therapy following progression in the monotherapy arm. Therefore, the studies included evaluated the value of the use of two agents versus a single agent and do not address whether a combination or a sequential monotherapy strategy should be pursued.

Two well-conducted phase III clinical trials (52,53) demonstrated that median OS is improved by approximately 3 months with a combination regimen using a taxane in patients previously treated with anthracyclines. Both studies showed that response rates and TTP were improved in the combination arm at the expense of greater toxicity. Unfortunately, very few patients in the single-agent arm crossed over to receive the additional drug, making difficult to apply the conclusions to clinical practice. Other clinical trials (54-59) evaluated a variety of combination regimens and included in its design the use of sequential agents. Results suggest that the efficacy of the combined and sequential therapy is similar, with greater toxicity seen in the combination arm.

We believe that in the absence of strong evidence to guide the decision, both combination and single-agent chemotherapy are reasonable options as first-line systemic treatment. However at MDACC, in agreement with different oncological societies (60), we believe that single-agent therapy should be used preferably, in the absence of rapid clinical progression, life-threatening visceral metastases, or the need for rapid symptom or disease control. Ultimately the choice of the use of sequential versus combination chemotherapy should involve an open discussion and will depend on the careful evaluation of risks and benefits for individual patients.

DURATION OF CHEMOTHERAPY

The optimal duration of chemotherapy for MBC remains somewhat controversial. Several studies have compared continuous (maintenance) chemotherapy with intermittent therapy as treatment of MBC. Several studies found that continuous therapy was associated with a longer time to relapse (61-65) but worse side effects (64). None of the individual studies comparing continuous and intermittent therapy showed prolongation of life with continuous therapy. However, a recent meta-analysis of these data showed a statistically significant improvement in survival for patients receiving chemotherapy for a longer versus a shorter time (65). Some regimens, such as anthracycline-containing treatments, have inherent dose-limiting toxic effects that prohibit prolonged use. Other agents, such as trastuzumab, capecitabine, and, possibly, low-dose taxanes given weekly lend themselves to indefinite continued therapy. In an unplanned interim analysis, the recently presented Italian MANTA trial found no progression-free or overall survival benefits for maintenance treatment with paclitaxel (175 mg/m^2 every 3 weeks for

8 cycles) after first-line chemotherapy for MBC with an anthracycline/taxane-containing regimen (6-8 cycles) (66). Many trials are designed to treat patients until they have progression of disease or for 2 to 3 cycles after maximum benefits are seen. Currently, there is no single right answer regarding treatment duration except that the right choice is the one that provides the most benefit for the individual patient. Open communication between the patient and clinician is essential to determine the correct length of treatment. The usual practice at MDACC is to treat patients with MBC with continuous chemotherapy, at least until a third-line regimen comes into play and/or ECOG performance status is ≥3 in patients with MBC.

SINGLE-AGENT CHEMOTHERAPY

Anthracyclines

The introduction of anthracyclines (doxorubicin and epirubicin) in the 1970s represented a significant advance in the treatment of advanced breast cancer. In patients with MBC, response rates to single-agent doxorubicin (25-75 mg/m^2 every 3 weeks) range from 25 to 60% and are heavily influenced by patient characteristics such as prior chemotherapy exposure, performance status, and extent and sites of disease (67-71). At MDACC, doxorubicin-containing regimens have historically been the initial treatment of choice for patients with MBC who previously received non-anthracycline-containing chemotherapy. Patients who received anthracyclines and had a prolonged disease-free interval before the development of metastatic disease occasionally benefit from repeat administration of doxorubicin. However, given the increasing number of active agents available to treat MBC, repeat management with anthracyclines should be reserved for patients in whom other treatments have failed.

Epirubicin is a doxorubicin analog that has been shown to have similar efficacy and somewhat less toxicity than doxorubicin at equimolar doses (72). The mean elimination half-life of epirubicin and its circulating metabolite epirubicinol are shorter than the half-lives of doxorubicin and doxorubicinol, respectively (73). It has been suggested that the pharmacologic kinetic characteristics of doxorubicin and epirubicin are responsible for their different toxicity profiles. Although not designed to perform a head-to-head comparison, results from a randomized trial suggested that epirubicin may be as efficacious as doxorubicin (74). This trial compared the use of different anthracyclines in combination (FAC versus FEC) at equimolar doses; both regimens were found to be equally effective in terms of response rate,

TTP, and survival. The FEC regimen was associated with less gastrointestinal, hematologic, and cardiac toxicity. It is important to mention that the optimal dose of epirubicin is unknown. Indirect evidence suggests that 75 mg/m^2 of epirubicin is superior with respect to response rate and survival compared with combination regimens that include epirubicin at a 50 mg/m^2 dose (75).

Efforts to improve the safety profile of doxorubicin while preserving efficacy have resulted in liposomal formulations of doxorubicin. To date, three liposomal anthracycline formulations have been developed: liposomal daunorubicin (DaunoXome); liposomal doxorubicin (Myocet); and pegylated liposomal doxorubicin (Doxil), the latter being the more studied and used formulation in MBC. Response rates with these products appear comparable to those seen in other multicenter trials using conventional single-agent doxorubicin (76,77). In a phase III clinical trial, O'Brien and colleagues compared the efficacy and safety of pegylated liposomal doxorubicin with those of conventional doxorubicin as first-line therapy in patients with MBC (78). A total of 509 women received 1-h infusion of pegylated liposomal doxorubicin (50 mg/m^2 once every 4 weeks), or conventional doxorubicin (60 mg/m^2 once every 3 weeks). The median PFS and OS were similar in both treatment groups (6.9 versus 7.8 months and 20.1 versus 22.0 months, respectively). The incidence of alopecia, myelosuppression, and nausea and vomiting were lower in patients treated with pegylated liposomal doxorubicin than in patients treated with conventional doxorubicin. Perhaps most notably, pegylated liposomal doxorubicin was associated with a significantly lower incidence of cardiotoxicity, even at higher cumulative doses ($p < .001$) (78). Probably the most important dose-limiting toxicity of pegylated liposomal doxorubicin is palmar-plantar erythrodysesthesia which is both dose- and duration-related. The polyethylene glycol coating results in preferential concentration of the drug in the skin, and that explains why small amounts of the drug can leak from capillaries in the palms and soles, resulting in redness, tenderness, and peeling of the skin that can be uncomfortable and even painful. As with all liposomal drug delivery systems, there is a low incidence of hypersensitivity reactions. The non-pegylated liposomal doxorubicin formulation has been approved in Europe and Canada for the treatment of MBC in combination with cyclophosphamide, but has not yet been approved by the FDA for use in the United States (77).

Taxanes

The taxanes, paclitaxel (Taxol), docetaxel (Taxotere), and the nanoparticle albumin-bound paclitaxel (Abraxane), are among of the most active classes of cytotoxic drugs available today for the treatment of breast cancer. They rival the anthracyclines in terms of response rates and positive impact on time to progression. Response rates with paclitaxel range from 21 to 62%. In early studies, some patients were heavily pretreated with prior anthracyclines, and paclitaxel doses and administration schedules were variable. Because the definition of anthracycline resistance varies from study to study, it is important to recognize the criteria for determining resistance in reviewing and comparing these data. Different definitions of resistance can lead to large differences in response rates and other measures of efficacy. Taxanes are frequently used as first-line chemotherapy for MBC patients that are naïve to treatment or also in those previously treated with anthracyclines or in whom anthracyclines are contraindicated. In anthracycline-resistant breast cancer, response rates of 48% were reported when paclitaxel was administered as a 96-hour continuous infusion (79). The NSAPB B-26 (80) trial compared paclitaxel given over 24 or 3 h in patients with MBC. OS was similar among groups but the response rates in the longer infusion arm were higher (51 versus 40%; $p = .02$). More cases of grade 4 neutropenia were also seen among the patients that received 24 h infusion (80).

Single-agent paclitaxel has been directly compared with mitomycin C and with CMFP (cyclophosphamide/methotrexate/fluorouracil/prednisone). Response rates and TTP were superior with paclitaxel compared with mitomycin C (81). The response rate, TTP, and OS were similar when paclitaxel was compared with CMFP (49). The CMFP trial included untreated patients only, whereas the mitomycin C trial included heavily pretreated patients. Two trials have directly compared doxorubicin and paclitaxel, utilizing different dosing and administration schedules. In the Intergroup E1193 study (57), similar response rates and TTF were demonstrated with doxorubicin administered at 60 mg/m^2 and paclitaxel at 175 mg/m^2 over 24 h. Therefore it appears that paclitaxel may be as effective as doxorubicin when it is administered as a single agent. The dose and administration schedule may influence the response to paclitaxel.

Paclitaxel-induced myelosuppression is schedule-related, with shorter infusions producing less myeloid toxicity and less mucositis (82). However, shorter infusions are associated with higher rates of myalgia and neurotoxicity. In the palliative setting, individualization of treatment should include a thorough assessment of all potential risks and benefits as certain patients may be better candidates for different doses or schedules due to the improved side-effect profiles. The use of weekly paclitaxel has recently become very popular due to the improvement in the toxicity profile and the ability to deliver a more dose-intensive regimen. Phase II studies investigating this administration schedule have found the maximum tolerated dose (MTD) to be quite high, depending on the schedule of administration. When given weekly on a continuous basis, the MTD is 80 to 100 mg/m^2/week (83). Approximately 240 to 270 mg/m^2 of paclitaxel can be delivered over a 3-week period with a weekly schedule, which is greater than that given as a single dose every 3 weeks (175-250 mg/m^2). The dose can be increased if patients receive paclitaxel every week for 3 weeks, followed by 1 week of rest. This "3 weeks on, 1 week off" approach allows patients to receive up to 250 mg/m^2 consistently for long periods of time. Weekly paclitaxel causes less myeloid toxicity, but more nerve toxicity. At these doses, fluid retention, fatigue, and peripheral neuropathy become dose-limiting. In the setting of MBC most clinicians administer paclitaxel 80 mg/m^2/week continuously; at MDACC we frequently use a "3 weeks on, 1 week off" schedule.

Docetaxel is a semisynthetic taxane; it has several preclinical, pharmacokinetic, biological, and clinical differences in comparison to paclitaxel. It has demonstrated a 37 to 57% response rate in patients with anthracycline-resistant tumors and was initially FDA-approved for this indication (84). In patients who had received paclitaxel previously, docetaxel administration was associated with response rates of 18 to 21%, demonstrating a lack of cross-resistance between these two agents (85). Compared with mitomycin plus vinblastine, docetaxel has demonstrated superiority in terms of response rate, TTP, and OS (30 versus 11.6%, $p < .0001$; 19 versus 11 weeks, $p = .001$; and 11.4 versus 8.7 months, $p = .0097$, respectively) (86). Methotrexate plus fluorouracil is also inferior to docetaxel in terms of response rate and time to progression (42 versus 21%, $p < .001$; 6.3 versus 3 months, $p = .001$, respectively) (56). The Food and Drug Administration-approved dose of docetaxel is 100 mg/m^2, every 3 weeks. At this dose, hematologic toxicity is the greatest and the rates of neutropenia are similar to those seen when paclitaxel is given every 3 weeks. The approved dose of docetaxel has been associated with the greatest response rates when used as frontline therapy in patients with MBC. In a large clinical trial 527 patients were randomized to receive docetaxel 60, 75, or 100 mg/m^2 every 3 weeks. A relationship between increasing dose of docetaxel and increased tumor response was observed, but toxicities were also related to increasing doses (87). Docetaxel every 3 weeks at doses between 100 and 75 mg/m^2 are appropriate choices as first-line therapy for

MBC. Compared to every-3-week paclitaxel, docetaxel 100 mg/m^2 was associated with longer TTP (HR 1.64; 94% CI 1.33-2.02) and improved OS (HR 1.64; 95% CI 1.33-2.02), but also greater incidence of treatment-related toxicities (88). Although interpreting this data is important to remember that paclitaxel has greater activity when given on a weekly schedule, yet it is not clear whether docetaxel or paclitaxel provide superior outcomes when each agent is administered at its optimal dose and schedule.

Several studies have investigated weekly administration of docetaxel. The MTD was found to be 43 mg/m^2/week when given weekly for 6 weeks every 8 weeks, but a dose of 36 mg/m^2/week was recommended for phase II studies (89). In a clinical trial using a dose of 40 mg/m^2 a response rate of 41% was seen with 28% of the patients developing grade-3 toxicities (90). Most patients are able to tolerate docetaxel 30 to 35 mg/m^2/week only when it is administered either weekly for 3 weeks every 4 weeks or weekly for 6 weeks every 8 weeks continuously. Dose-limiting fatigue and asthenia are associated with weekly administration. Moderate nail changes and fatigue are commonly seen with weekly paclitaxel and docetaxel; excessive tearing due to partial or complete canalicular stenosis is seen with weekly docetaxel. However, diarrhea, stomatitis, and neutropenia and its complications are uncommon with weekly taxane administration. Fluid retention is seen in patients that receive a docetaxel cumulative dose greater than 300 mg/m^2. Premedication with steroids greatly reduces the magnitude of fluid retention; the optimal doses and schedules for steroid administration are not well established. At MDACC we routinely prescribe dexamethasone 4 mg PO bid for 3 days beginning the day before chemotherapy administration.

ABI-007 is a nanoparticle albumin-bound paclitaxel (Abraxane) that has been investigated in the treatment of MBC. In different comparisons it has proven to be better or at least as effective as the other taxanes (91,92), with the advantage that does not require cremophor for solubility and therefore is associated with less hypersensitivity reactions. In a phase III study, 454 patients were randomly assigned to 3-week cycles of ABI-007 260 mg/m^2 or paclitaxel 175 mg/m^2. ABI-007 demonstrated significantly higher response rates compared with paclitaxel (33 versus 19%, p = .001) and longer TTP (23.0 versus 16.9 weeks, p = .006). Grade-3 sensory neuropathy was more common in the ABI-007 arm, the incidence of grade-4 neutropenia was significantly lower for ABI-007, but rate of febrile neutropenia was similar in both groups (92). Recently a phase II-four arm study was published comparing the use of albumin-bound

paclitaxel (300 mg/m^2 every 3 weeks, 100 mg/m^2 weekly, or 150 mg/m^2 weekly) and docetaxel (100 mg/m^2 every 3 weeks). The weekly dose of 150 mg/m^2 of albumin-bound paclitaxel demonstrated longer PFS than docetaxel (12.9 versus 7.5 months, p = .006), but no difference in PFS or response rates were seen when comparing docetaxel and the 3-week schedule of albumin-bound paclitaxel. Grade-3 or -4 fatigue, neutropenia, and febrile neutropenia were less frequent in all albumin-bound paclitaxel arms, but the frequency and grade of peripheral neuropathy were similar in all groups (91).

The use of weekly (100 mg/m^2), every 3 week (300 mg/m^2), or every 28 days (150 mg/m^2 on day 1,8, and 15) albumin-bound paclitaxel was compared to every 3-week docetaxel in a clinical trial that included 300 patients with MBC (93). Results from an interim analysis showed greater response rates with the weekly or the every 28-day schedule with less cases of neutropenia in all the albumin-bound paclitaxel groups when compared to docetaxel (93). Currently, investigations are ongoing to define the optimal dose and schedule. At MD Anderson the albumin-bound paclitaxel is frequently used as first- or second-line therapy administered in a weekly schedule.

Antimetabolites

Capecitabine

Capecitabine (Xeloda) is an oral fluoropyrimidine that was approved by the FDA in April 1998 as single-agent therapy for the treatment of MBC in patients resistant to anthracyclines and taxanes. In September 2001, capecitabine was approved for use in combination with docetaxel in MBC patients previously treated with an anthracycline. Capecitabine is a systemic prodrug of 5'-deoxy-5-fluorouridine (5'-FUdR) that is activated by a three-step conversion process in the liver and tumor tissues to the active form, fluorouracil. This provides more directed cytotoxicity and leads to less direct fluorouracil release into the bowel, potentially reducing the incidence of diarrhea. Capecitabine is well absorbed and not altered by the small bowel's mucosa. Clinically, its activity mimics that of continuous-infusion fluorouracil.

The first phase II study of capecitabine in breast cancer involved 162 patients who were previously treated with paclitaxel for metastatic disease (94). The majority of patients had also received previous anthracycline therapy. Those who had previously received a taxane, an anthracycline, or both were designated as either having failed or having resistant disease. Capecitabine was administered at 2500 mg/m^2/day in two divided doses for 14 days, followed by 1 week of rest. Twenty-seven (20%) of the 135 women with measurable disease demonstrated complete (N = 3) or partial (N = 24) responses. Median duration of response was 8.1 months, and the median survival time was 12.8 months. Blum and colleagues reported results of a randomized phase II study with a similar design (95). In this trial, all patients had failed treatment or had disease that was refractory to two or three previous chemotherapy regimens. The overall response rate was 26%. Among patients who were pretreated with paclitaxel and docetaxel, the objective response rates seen were 27 and 20%, respectively. In a phase II trial, O'Shaughnessy and colleagues randomized patients to receive CMF or capecitabine in the frontline setting (96). The overall response rate was 30% for capecitabine and 16% for CMF; median TTP was similar between the two groups. Similar levels of nausea, vomiting, and stomatitis were observed for both groups, whereas more cases of grade-3 or -4 diarrhea (8%), fatigue (5%), and hand-foot syndrome (15%) were seen in patients treated with capecitabine. In a randomized phase II trial comparing capecitabine with paclitaxel (175 mg/m^2), patients whose disease was unresponsive or resistant to anthracycline therapy appeared to respond better to capecitabine (response rate 36%) than to paclitaxel (response rate 26%) (97). However, the confidence intervals and the size and design of the study do not preclude that this difference was due to chance alone. TTP and overall survival were similar between the two groups.

The previously mentioned studies demonstrated that capecitabine is an active agent in the treatment of MBC and that significant response rates can be achieved in women previously treated with an anthracycline and a taxane. The FDA-approved dose and schedule are 2500 mg/m^2/day given orally in two divided doses for 14 days, followed by 1 week of rest. However, retrospective studies suggest that a slightly lower starting dose (2000 mg/m^2/day) is better tolerated, with preserved efficacy. There is evidence that capecitabine as first-line therapy for MBC results in response rates between 30 and 58% and is a reasonable option for many patients. At MD Anderson it is often used as first-line therapy for patients who were previously treated with anthracylines or taxanes in the adjuvant or neoadjuvant setting. Capecitabine is a well-tolerated agent suitable for use in the outpatient setting. The most frequently reported clinical adverse events experienced by patients treated with capecitabine include hand-foot syndrome, diarrhea, and nausea. Alopecia was very rare. The majority of treatment-related events are classified as grade 1 or 2. Myelosuppression and blood chemistry abnormalities are relatively rare, with grade-3 or -4 hyperbilirubinemia occurring in >5% of patients.

Gemcitabine

In April 2004, gemcitabine (Gemzar), a nucleoside analog, was approved by the FDA for the first-line treatment of MBC in the United States. In patients with MBC, single-agent response rates have ranged from 14 to 37% (98-100). These were small trials, and the disparate results may be due to dosing differences. Generally, chemotherapy-naive patients are able to tolerate doses of 1000 to 1250 mg/m^2/week on days 1, 8, and 15 every 28 days; however, omitting the day-15 dose or reducing the dose in subsequent cycles of chemotherapy may improve the patient's ability to tolerate therapy beyond initial cycles. Pretreated patients may require dose reductions in order to decrease the risk of thrombocytopenia. In a phase II study, Charmichael et al. (100) studied the efficacy and tolerability of gemcitabine (800 mg/m^2) administered as once a week for 3 weeks followed by a 1-week rest every 4 weeks. The overall response rate was 25.0%, median survival was 11.5 months. Grade-3 and -4 neutropenia occurred in 23.3 and 7.0% of patients, respectively. Flu-like symptoms which were mild, transient, and treatable with acetominophen were reported in 6.8% of patients.

Gemcitabine has been investigated in many different doublet and triplet combination regimens; it is a promising agent for its efficacy as a single drug, but also due to its ability to readily combine with paclitaxel, vinorelbine, docetaxel, or cisplatin/carboplatin as first- or second-line therapy. At present, gemcitabine is appropriate treatment strategy for patients with MBC that have failed to standard regimens.

Other agents

Vinorelbine

Vinorelbine (Navelbine) is a semisynthetic vinca alkaloid that interferes with microtubule assembly and it is an important active agent in the treatment of MBC. Phase II trials investigating its efficacy in pretreated MBC patients have demonstrated response rates ranging from 25 to 47% (101-103). Response rates to vinorelbine as first-line therapy range from 35 to 53%, and as second-line therapy estimated response rates are close to 20 to 30% (104,105). Vinorelbine may have a role in therapy after patients have been exposed to anthracyclines and taxanes. Dose-intensive vinorelbine with filgrastim support has shown to produce 25% response rates in patients previously exposed to paclitaxel (103). Zelek and colleagues found a 25% response rate with weekly vinorelbine (25 mg/m^2) in patients whose disease had progressed following anthracycline and taxane therapy (105). The primary side effects seen with the use of vinorelbine are neutropenia, pain with infusion, flu-like symptoms, and gastrointestinal symptoms such as nausea or constipation. Vinorelbine is appropriate as third-line (or later) therapy for patients with MBC.

Ixabepilone

Ixabepilone (Ixempra) is an epothilone B analog that binds to microtubules and causes microtubule stabilization and mitotic arrest. It was approved in October 2007 by the FDA (alone or in combination with capecitabine) for the treatment of patients with MBC resistant to treatment with an anthracycline and a taxane, or whose cancer is taxane resistant and for whom further anthracycline therapy is contraindicated. As a single agent, is also indicated for patients with tumors that are resistant or refractory to capecitabine.

Ixabepilone monotherapy was evaluated in a single arm trial of 126 who had previously received an anthracycline, a taxane and capecitabine (106). Ixabepilone was administered at a dose of 40 mg/m^2 every 3 weeks, the objective response rate was 11.5%, the median response duration was 5.7 months and the median OS was 8.6 months. Grade-3 or -4 neutropenia was seen in 54% of patients and grade-3 or -4 peripheral neuropathy was seen in 14%; this neuropathy was generally reversible to grade 1 or better with cessation of therapy. Other commonly observed toxicities included anemia, fatigue, myalgias, arthralgias, nausea, vomiting, stomatitis, diarrhea, and decrease in blood counts (106). Thomas et al. (107) studied the effect of ixabepilone (50 or 40 mg/m^2 every 3 weeks) among MBC patients who had experienced disease progression while receiving or within 4 months of taxane therapy. The response rate was 12% and among responders the median response duration was 10.4 months. Forty-one percent of the patients achieved stable disease. Median time to progression was 2.2 months and median survival was 7.9 months. When used as first-line therapy in patients with MBC that received anthracyline-based chemotherapy in the adjuvant setting, response rates of 41.5% have been reported, with median duration of response of 8.2 months and median survival of 22 months (108).

Different doses and schedules of ixabepilone have been evaluated, Denduluri et al., in a small trial with taxane-naïve patients, used ixabepilone at 6 mg/m^2 on days 1 to 5 every 3 weeks (109). Fifty-seven percent of

patients had partial responses, and median time to progression and duration of response were 5.5 and 5.6 months, respectively. Minimal hematologic toxicity and no grade-3 sensory neuropathy were noted. Currently, several trials are evaluating the use of ixabepilone alone or in combination with different subgroups of patients with MBC, it is a promising drug and at MDACC we frequently use it in patients who have received anthracyclines, taxanes, and capecitabine.

COMBINATION CHEMOTHERAPY

Anthracycline-Based Combination Regimens

Doxorubicin-containing combinations have been reported to result in overall response rates ranging from 50 to 80% with observed response duration of 8 to 15 months. Median survival with doxorubicin–alkylating agent combinations was 17 to 25 months. Although doxorubicin-containing regimens are more efficacious in the metastatic setting than are non-doxorubicin-containing combinations, sometimes anthracycline-based combinations are not used because of the side effects associated with such regimens. Almost all patients treated with doxorubicin develop alopecia and some degree of nausea and vomiting. Additionally, approximately 2 to 4% of patients develop congestive heart failure (with bolus administration up to a cumulative lifetime dose of 450 mg/m^2). Extravasation may cause severe skin and subcutaneous damage.

As was discussed previously, the issue of whether combination chemotherapy is superior to single-agent chemotherapy in the treatment for MBC continues to be debated. For patients with rapidly progressing disease, treatment regimens most likely to produce an objective tumor response are highly desirable; therefore there is still an important role for the use of combination chemotherapy. For many years FAC (500/50/500 mg/m^2) was the standard regimen for patients with MBC treated at MDACC. With this regimen, chemotherapy is given for 6 to 8 cycles or until progression of disease, with objective responses rates of 50 to 80%. Several randomized clinical trials have compared different anthracycline-based chemotherapy regimens in patients with MBC. Nabholtz et al. (110,111), compared the use of docetaxel/doxorubicin/cyclophosphamide (TAC 75/50/500 mg/m^2) to FAC as first-line therapy for MBC (N = 484). The objective response rate with TAC was 55%, compared with 44% with FAC ($p = .02$) (HR 1.5; 95% CI 1.1-2.2). However, there was no significant difference in TTP or OS between treatment arms. Febrile neutropenia occurred more frequently in those receiving TAC (29 versus 5%) but similar rates of infection were seen.

Carmichael et al. reported the results of a clinical trial comparing epirubicin and cyclophosphamide (EC) with epirubicin and paclitaxel (EP) in patients with MBC (112). A total of 705 patients received up to 6 cycles of therapy. The objective response rate was higher in patients receiving EP (67%) than in those receiving EC (56%). However, the TTP and OS were similar between treatment arms. Doxorubicin and cyclophosphamide (AC) were compared to doxorubicin and docetaxel (AT) in 429 patients with MBC (113). At significantly improved TTP (37.9 versus 31.9 weeks, $p = 0.014$) and overall response rate (59 versus 47%, $p = .008$) compared with AC, but there was no difference in OS. AT represents a valid option for the treatment of MBC. Biganzoli et al. reported the results of a randomized trial comparing doxorubicin and paclitaxel to AC in 275 patients with MBC (114). The overall response rate was higher for patients receiving AP (58%) than in those given AC (54%), but this difference did not reach statistical significance. TTF and OS were different between the treatment arms.

Anthracycline-taxane combinations have been compared with classic anthracycline combinations in several phase III trials in patients with MBC. Data suggest a modest benefit with the taxane-anthracycline combinations in terms of response rates but no difference in TTP or OS. In one trial that compared doxorubicin and paclitaxel with FAC (115), the taxane combination found to have improved response rates ($p = .032$), TTP ($p = .034$) and OS ($p = .013$). One of the problems associated with this trial is that only 25% of patients in the FAC arm received a taxane as second-line treatment. Thus, patients treated initially with doxorubicin and paclitaxel received two of the most effective single agents in the treatment of breast cancer, whereas the vast majority of patients initially treated with FAC were denied treatment with a taxane. The question whether the differences in outcome in patients treated with FAC may be compensated by the addition of a taxane as a second-line therapy remains to be established.

Non-Anthracycline-Based Combination Regimens

As single agents, the platinum salts (primarily cisplatin and carboplatin) have had limited use in the treatment of MBC. Typically, platinum compounds have been reserved for third-line therapy or beyond. Objective responses in this setting have generally been reported in fewer than 10% of patients (116). In the limited number of clinical trials in which cisplatin or carboplatin was administered as first-line chemotherapy for MBC, objective responses were reported in up to 50% of patients (116). Nevertheless, the availability of many active chemotherapeutic regimens and the significant toxicities associated with the platinum salts resulted in their use being reserved largely for the salvage setting. With the introduction of newer cytotoxic agents and preclinical data demonstrating synergy between some of these agents and platinum salts, there is renewed interest in incorporating the platinum compounds into regimens for MBC.

A heterogeneous mix of phase II clinical trials has been reported with the combination of paclitaxel and cisplatin. In the trials in which this combination was administered as first-line therapy for MBC, overall response rates have ranged from 50 to 90%. Clinical trials evaluating this combination as second- or third-line therapy have reported response rates of 30 to 50% (116). These results suggest that the combination of cisplatin and paclitaxel produces response rates higher than those expected with paclitaxel alone. Perez et al. reported the results of a clinical trial combining paclitaxel (200 mg/m^2) with carboplatin (AUC 6 every 3 weeks) as first-line treatment of MBC (117). In 53 patients, an overall response rate of 62% was observed, including a CR rate of 16%. The median time to disease progression was 7.3 months, with a 1-year survival estimate of 72%. Grade-3 peripheral neuropathy was seen in 16% of patients. A similarly designed trial combining paclitaxel (175 mg/m^2) and carboplatin (AUC 6) administered every 3 weeks was reported by Fountzilas et al. on behalf of the Hellenic Cooperative Oncology Group (118). In 37 patients, an objective response rate of 43% (14% CR) was observed, with 27% of patients experiencing grade-3 or -4 leukopenia. Prophylactic granulocyte colony-stimulating factor (G-CSF) was administered in this study. The objective response rate was higher among patients who had received prior adjuvant therapy (76 versus 45%). One phase II study examined the combination of a platinum compound and docetaxel (119). Thirty-six women who had previously been treated with chemotherapy for MBC were treated with docetaxel 75 mg/m^2 as a 1-h infusion followed by carboplatin AUC 6, cycling every 21 days. The overall response rate was 61%. The median duration of response was 8 months and the median TTP was 10 months. Toxicities were manageable.

Combinations with vinorelbine also have been investigated. A trial of single-agent doxorubicin compared to doxorubicin plus vinorelbine failed to demonstrate a superior response rate with the combination (120). Despite the disappointing results seen in this study, vinorelbine has been successfully combined with taxanes. Although there are no phase III trials to confirm that these combinations are better than either single agent, different phase II studies combining vinorelbine and paclitaxel in MBC have been reported (121). The overall response rates with first-line vinorelbine/paclitaxel range from 49 to 60%. Similarly, the overall response rates for second-line vinorelbine/paclitaxel and vinorelbine/docetaxel range from 46 to 56% and 37 and 59%, respectively. The primary toxicities associated with vinorelbine/taxane combinations were myelosuppression and mild neurotoxicity (121).

Gemcitabine in Combination With Other Agents

Gemcitabine is unique in its mechanism of action and toxicity profile, allowing it to be combined with many other chemotherapeutic agents potentially without the need for dose reduction. The activity of the cisplatin/gemcitabine combination in MBC had been explored with promising results. In one trial patients who had previously received treatment with an anthracycline and/or taxane received cisplatin (30 mg/m^2) plus gemcitabine (750 or 1000 mg/m^2) on days 1, 8, and 15 of 21-day cycles. An objective response rate of 50% was reported, with 10% of patients attaining a CR. The most common toxicities associated with this combination have been peripheral neuropathy, nausea/vomiting, and hematologic toxicities (neutropenia, thrombocytopenia, and anemia) (122). Recently, two parallel phase II studies were published (123). One-hundred and thirty-six patients with MBC were included. Patients were divided in two cohorts according to prior treatments (heavily pretreated and not heavily pretreated), they received cisplatin 25 mg/m^2 on days 1 through 4 and gemcitabine 1000 mg/m^2 on days 2 and 8 of a 21-day cycle. The heavily pretreated group received GCSF support. The response rate for both the heavily and minimally pretreated cohorts was 26%, and the median durations of response were 5.3 and 5.9 months, respectively. The most common grades-3 or -4 toxicities were thrombocytopenia (71%), neutropenia (66%), and anemia (38%) (123). In a phase III study, the combination of gemcitabine (1250 mg/m^2 day 1and 8) and paclitaxel (175 mg/m^2 day 1) was associated with an improvement in response rate and TTP compared with paclitaxel alone (39.3 versus 25.6%, and 5.4 versus 3.5 months respectively) in first-line therapy for MBC (124). Median OS was significantly improved in the combination arm (18.5 versus 15.8 months, HR 0.77, 95% CI 0.62-0.95). The safety profile included significantly more frequent grade-4 hematologic toxicity in the combination arm. It should be noted that most patients randomized to paclitaxel alone did not receive subsequent gemcitabine.

Several published phase II clinical trials have investigated salvage therapy with docetaxel/gemcitabine combinations in MBC (125-127). Drug doses and schedules varied between individual clinical trials. These trials included heavily pretreated patients; the objective response rates ranged from 36 to 79%, with up to 14% of patients attaining a CR. Grade-3 or -4 neutropenia was reported in 29 to 92% of patients. Grade-3 or -4 thrombocytopenia occurred in up to 21% of patients. Grade-3 or -4 nonhematologic toxicity occurred in >10% of patients, including asthenia, alopecia, and fatigue. Recently the results of an European phase III trial where no difference between gemcitabine-docetaxel (1000 mg/m^2 days 1 and 8 and 75 mg/m^2 day 1) and capecitabine-docetaxel (1250 mg/m^2 bid days 1-14 and 75 mg/m^2 day 1) were published (128). No differences in PFS, OS, or response rates were seen, however the toxicity profile for the gemcitabine-docataxel combination was better.

Gemcitabine-anthracycline combinations have been evaluated using both doxorubicin and epirubicin showing significant antitumor activity and a manageable toxicity profile. A phase III trial comparing gemcitabine/epirubicin/paclitaxel (GET) to FEC as first-line treatment of MBC did not show any statistically significant differences in response rate (63.2 versus 51.2%, $p = .093$) or time to progression (9.0 versus 9.1 months) between the two arms (129). Grade-3 and -4 toxicities were more frequently in the GET arm, and they were certainly very high for a regimen that is administered with a palliative intent.

Capecitabine Combination Regimens

In September 2001, the FDA-approved capecitabine in combination with docetaxel for patients with MBC previously treated with an anthracycline. This was based on the results of a multinational phase III trial that randomly assigned 511 anthracycline-refractory patients to receive docetaxel 100 mg/m^2 or capecitabine 1250 mg/m^2 twice daily for 14 days plus docetaxel 75 mg/m^2 IV every 3 weeks (53). The response rates for the single-agent and combination regimens were 30 and 42% ($p = .006$) respectively, and TTP was 4.2 and 6.1 months ($p = .0001$). Of note, the OS was significantly superior with the combination (HR 0.775; 95% CI, 0.63-0.94). This is one of the few randomized clinical trials that reported a survival benefit of one treatment over the other, but the design of the trial does not confirm that the combination is better than the sequential administration of single-agent docetaxel followed by capecitabine or vice versa. Grade-3 treatment–related adverse events were more common in the combination therapy group

(71 versus 49%, respectively), grade-4 treatment–related adverse events were slightly lower with the combination therapy (25 versus 31%). Overall, the incidence of treatment–related adverse events was similar between the two groups (98 versus 94%). Patients receiving the combination therapy experienced a higher incidence of gastrointestinal side effects and hand-foot syndrome.

Capecitabine in combination with ixabepilone has been approved for the management of MBC in patients that are considered to have disease that is resistant or has progresses to anthracyclines and taxanes. The clinical trial that led to the approval of this combination randomized 752 patients to receive ixabepilone (40 mg/m^2 IV every 3 weeks) plus capecitabine (2000 mg/m^2 on days 1 through 14 of a 21-day cycle), or capecitabine alone (2500 mg/m^2 on the same day schedule) (130). Patients had previously received an anthracycline and a taxane, had evidence of disease progression or resistance, or, in the case of the anthracycline, received a minimum required cumulative dose. Patients receiving the combination had a 25% reduction in the estimated risk of disease progression (HR 0.75; 95% CI 0.64-0.88). Median PFS (5.8 versus 4.2 months) and response rates (35 versus 14%) were also higher in the combination arm. Grade 3/4 treatment-related sensory neuropathy, fatigue, and neutropenia were more frequent with combination therapy, as was the rate of death as a result of toxicity (3 versus 1%). Patients with liver dysfunction were at higher risk of complications and therefore should not be treated with this regimen. This combination despite its toxicity represents a good alternative for patients with resistant disease that have been previously treated with anthracyclines and taxanes in whom a fast response is needed.

■ TARGETED THERAPIES

HER2/NEU-TARGETED THERAPIES

Trastuzumab

The HER2/neu protein, a receptor tyrosine kinase, is overexpressed in 25 to 30% of human breast cancers and plays an important role in tumor development and progression. Patients with tumors that overexpress HER2/neu have a more aggressive disease than those whose tumors do not (131-133). HER2/neu status has been implicated as a prognostic factor independent of systemic therapy, but several investigators have also suggested that it may be a predictive factor for resistance to certain types of systemic therapy or benefit from it. However, the results of preclinical and clinical

studies have been mixed. Some studies have suggested that HER2/neu amplification is associated with resistance to endocrine therapy (134-138). The relationship between HER2-neu overexpression and hormone-receptor status is not clearly defined. The Trans-ATAC study (139) showed that approximately 10% of hormone-positive tumors also overexpress HER2-neu; results suggest that the benefit from tamoxifen was smaller in this group of patients. Similarly, a subgroup analysis of the BIG 1-98 study (140) revealed that among patients with hormone-receptor positive disease, those with HER2-neu overexpression have worse prognosis. These observations are likely secondary to a crosstalk between HER2-neu and hormone receptors that could induce resistance to endocrine treatment. Results of several studies have suggested that patients whose tumors overexpress HER2/neu are less likely to benefit from adjuvant non-doxorubicin-containing regimens, suggesting further that these patients seem to benefit from the addition of an anthracycline (141,142). Trastuzumab (Herceptin) is a murine-human chimeric monoclonat antibody targeted against the HER2/neu protein. Trastuzumab has been evaluated in two pivotal multinational trials in women with HER2/neu overexpressed MBC. In one trial, trastuzumab (4 mg/kg loading dose, then 2 mg/kg weekly) was evaluated as a single agent in 222 heavily pretreated women with MBC (143). Nine of 213 treated patients (4%) achieved a CR and 37 (17%) achieved a PR. Median duration of response was 9.1 months; for all treated patients, the median TTP was 3.1 months and the median OS was 13 months. The most clinically significant adverse event was cardiac dysfunction, which occurred in 10 patients (4.7%), 9 of whom had received prior anthracycline therapy. This trial demonstrated that trastuzumab can induce durable objective responses and is associated with an acceptable toxicity profile. The second pivotal trial evaluated the use of chemotherapy with or without trastuzumab in 469 patients who had not received prior chemotherapy for metastatic disease (144). Women who had received anthracycline in the adjuvant setting received paclitaxel 175 mg/m^2 every 3 weeks. All of the other patients received doxorubicin 60 mg/m^2 or epirubicin 75 mg/m^2 plus cyclophosphamide 600 mg/m^2 every 3 weeks. Trastuzumab 2 mg/kg (after a 4-mg/kg loading dose) was administered weekly until disease progression. The combination of chemotherapy plus trastuzumab resulted in a significantly higher objective response rate than chemotherapy alone (50 versus 32%). Women in the chemotherapy plus trastuzumab arm also had a significantly longer TTP and OS than those treated with chemotherapy alone. Symptomatic or asymptomatic cardiac dysfunction was seen in 27% of women treated with concurrent anthracycline/cyclophosphamide and trastuzumab. On the basis of the results of this trial, the FDA approved the combination of paclitaxel and trastuzumab for use as first-line therapy for HER2/neu overexpressed MBC.

Given the success of the trastuzumab and paclitaxel combination, this agent has been combined with others known to have activity against breast cancer (145). The combination of trastuzumab and vinorelbine has been studied in a phase II trial in which 40 women with HER2/neu–positive MBC were treated with weekly vinorelbine (25 mg/m^2) and trastuzumab (146). The overall response rate was 75%. Approximately 50% of the patients in this trial had received at least one prior regimen in the metastatic setting and still responded to this combination. TTP and OS were longer in women receiving treatment as first-line therapy than in those who had received prior chemotherapy for metastatic disease. This regimen was generally well tolerated. To further evaluate it, a multicenter phase III study comparing trastuzumab/vinorelbine to trastuzumab/taxane (TRAVIOTA study) randomized 81 patients to receive trastuzumab with weekly vinorelbine or weekly taxane therapy (paclitaxel or docetaxel at the investigator's choice) (147). Response rates were 51 and 40% for the vinorelbine/trastuzumab arm and the taxane/trastuzumab arm, respectively. The median time to disease progression was 8.5 and 6.0 months for the vinorelbine- and taxane-based arms, respectively ($p = .09$). Treatment with either regimen generally was well tolerated, yielding comparable toxicity. Another trial led by MDACC compared vinorelbine alone to vinorelbine/trastuzumab in patients with disease progression on a taxane/trastuzumab regimen and final results are awaited.

Trastuzumab has also been safely combined with other agents. The trastuzumab/gemcitabine combination provides response rates of 30 to 44% in heavily pretreated patients (145,148,149). There is an ongoing a phase III study evaluating gemcitabine/trastuzumab versus gemcitabine alone in HER2/neu–positive patients who progressed on a prior trastuzumab-containing regimen. This study is designed to examine the clinical benefit of continuous trastuzumab therapy after disease progression. For patients that had filed anthracylines, taxanes, and vinorelbine, the combination of capecitabine (1250 mg/m^2 divided bid for 14 days) and trastuzumab has shown to be very effective (150,151). In different trials, the response rates seen were between 20 and 45% with clinical benefit rates that ranged from 70 to 85%. The safety profile of the combination was favorable and predictable, with a low incidence of grade 3/4 adverse events. The most common adverse events were pain, hand-foot syndrome, and gastrointestinal toxicities. These trials support the use of the combination of capecitabine and trastuzumab in heavily pretreated MBC patients with tumors that have Her2-neu overexpression (150,151).

The combination of trastuzumab and docetaxel has a high level of activity and an acceptable toxicity profile (152,153). When the use of docetaxel (100 mg/m^2 every 3 weeks) with or without trastuzumab (4 mg/kg loading dose followed by 2 mg/kg weekly) was evaluated, the combination arm was significantly superior to docetaxel alone in terms of overall response rate (61 versus 34%; $p = .0002$), OS (31.2 versus 22.7 months; $p = .0325$), TTP (11.7 versus 6.1 months; $p = .0001$) and duration of response (11.7 versus 5.7 months; $p = .009$) (154). There was little difference in the number and severity of adverse events between the arms. Results from a small single-institution phase II trial of 30 patients, treated with weekly docetaxel and trastuzumab as first- or second-line therapy, demonstrated a response rate of 63%, with a median TTP of 9 months (152). Another trial using trastuzumab (4 mg/kg load followed by a weekly dose of 2 mg/kg) and docetaxel (35 mg/m^2/week for 6 weeks) showed an overall response rate of 50% with a median time to progression of 12.4 months and median survival of 22.1 months (155).

A number of trials evaluating triplet combinations have also been published or are ongoing (145,156). A phase III clinical trial evaluated the combination of trastuzumab/paclitaxel/carboplatin (TPC) (trastuzumab 4 mg/kg loading dose followed by 2 mg/kg weekly, paclitaxel 175 mg/m^2 and carboplatin AUC 6 every 21 days) and compared it with TP in 196 patients with MBC. The combination arm had statistically significant improved response rates and PFS. Both treatments were well tolerated but more cases of grade-4 neutropenia were seen in the combination arm (157). When evaluating the combination of docetaxel (75 mg/m2) and trastuzumab (loading dose 4 mg/kg followed by 2 mg/kg weekly) in combination with either cisplatin (75 mg/m^2) or carboplatin (AUC 6) every 21 days. High response rates were seen (79% for the patients who received cisplatin and 58% for those receiving carboplatin). Median times to progression were 9.9 and 12.7 months, respectively (158). Without any doubt, the use of trastuzumab in the metastatic setting has changed HER2-positive status from a marker of poor prognosis to one of better overall outcome, and ongoing studies should expand further treatment options for patients with HER2-positive MBC.

Trastuzumab-DM1 (TDM1) is the first HER2-antibody drug conjugate drug that combines trastuzumab with a linked antimicrotubule drug, maytansine (DM1). The potential advantage of this immunoconjugate agent is that the antibody targets DM1 specifically into tumor tissues. Phase I study conducted in heavily pretreated patients with HER2-overexpression showed clinical activity. A recent preliminary report of phase II study in 112 patients with HER2 overexpression who had failed to trastuzumab, lapatinib, or both showed a promising activity with a response rate of 25% and clinical benefit of 34% (159). Phase III studies evaluating the activity of TDM1 versus therapy with lapatinib-capecitabine for second-line therapy of patients with metastatic HER2-positive breast cancer and docetaxel plus trastuzumab versus single-agent TDM-1 as first-line therapy for MBC are ongoing. The use of TDM1 is investigational and is used only in the setting of a clinical trial.

Lapatinib

Lapatinib (Tykerb) is a selective, reversible dual EGFR-HER2 inhibitor. Phase II trials of single-agent lapatinib have shown modest clinical benefit in patients with HER2-positive breast cancer (160-162). Lapatinib in combination with capecitabine was approved by the FDA on March 2007, for the treatment of patients with advanced or HER2-overexpressing MBC previously treated with an anthracycline, a taxane, and trastuzumab. The trial that led to the approval of the combination showed that patients treated with lapatinib and capecitabine had a significant increase in PFS compared to capecitabine alone (163). The study was closed prematurely because the first interim analysis showed that the addition of lapatinib was associated with a 51% reduction in the risk of disease progression. The median TTP for patients treated with lapatinib plus capecitabine compared with capecitabine plus placebo were 8.4 versus 4.4 months, respectively (HR 0.49; 95% CI 0.34-0.71). In a recent phase II study of patients with HER2-positive breast cancer and brain metastasis treated with lapatinib, 6% of patients had an objective response, defined as ≥50% volumetric reduction of the brain metastasis (164). Other patients treated with lapatinib and capecitabine had a 20% CNS objective response and 40% experienced a 20% volumetric reduction in their CNS lesions.

Preclinical studies showed a synergistic interaction between trastuzumab and lapatinib in HER2-overexpressing breast cancer cell lines and tumor xenografts (165). Preliminary results of a randomized phase III trial combining lapatinib with trastuzumab compared with lapatinib alone in heavily pretreated HER2-positive MBC (N = 296) demonstrated synergy and improved the response rates as well as PFS. Despite a high crossover rate, there was a significant improvement in OS in patients that received lapatinib and trastuzumab combination (HR 0.71; 95% CI 0.54-0.93) (166).

Lapatinib has also been combined with hormonal agents. In a preclinical model, lapatinib restored tamoxifen sensitivity in tamoxifen-resistant breast cancer (167). The EGF3008, a phase III study combining letrozole plus lapatinib versus letrozole, demonstrated a 29% reduction in risk of disease progression ($p = .019$), and an improvement in median PFS (3 High response 8.2 months) in the combination arm (168). A detailed description of the trials evaluating the use of lapatinib (160-162) as single agent and in combination (163,166, 168,169) is shown in Table 25-3.

VASCULAR ENDOTHELIAL GROWTH FACTOR (VEGF)-TARGETED THERAPIES

Bevacizumab

Bevacizumab (Avastin), a monoclonal antibody against all VEGF-A isoforms. This monoclonal antibody has single-agent response rates of 9% in patients with refractory MBC. In a randomized phase III trial comparing the efficacy and safety of capecitabine with or without bevacizumab in patients previously treated with an anthracycline and a taxane, the addition of bevacizumab produced a significant increase in response rates but not in PFS or OS (170).

The trial that resulted in FDA approval (February, 2008) of bevacizumab for the treatment of MBC was the ECOG 2100 trial. Six-hundred and eighty patients with previously untreated locally recurrent or MBC received weekly paclitaxel (90 mg/m^2 on days 1, 8, and 15) with or without bevacizumab (10 mg/kg on days 1 and 15) in 4-week cycles until progression (171). The overall response rate (29.9 versus 13.8%, $p = .0001$) and the PFS were significantly better with combination therapy (11.4 versus 6.11 months; HR 0.51; 95% CI 0.43-0.62). The benefit of bevacizumab was observed, regardless of age, number of metastatic sites, previous adjuvant taxane use, disease-free interval after adjuvant therapy, and hormone receptor status.

Based on the ECOG 2100 trial, the combination of bevacizumb and paclitaxel was approved for first-line therapy of patients with MBC. Several phase III studies using bevacizumab combined with different

TABLE 25-3 | **PHASE II AND III TRIALS OF LAPATINIB FOR TREATMENT OF METASTATIC BREAST CANCER**

Trial	N	Patient Population	Lapatinib Dose (mg/day) Combination dose	Response PR (%)	CR (%)	CB (%)	Patient Outcome
LAPATINIB SINGLE AGENT							
Blackwell (159) Phase II	78	HER2 (+) Trastuzumab refractory	1250–1500	5.1	0	9	TTP was 15.3 weeks, and PFS 15.3 weeks (range 9.7–16.3). Adverse events included skin rash (47%), diarrhea (46%), and nausea (31%).
Burstein (160) Phase II	229	Anthracycline, taxane, capecitabine refractory	1500	4	0		No response rate observed in HER2 (−). Independent review assessment of median TTP and PFS were similar in HER2 (+) and HER2 (−) (9.1 weeks and 7.6 weeks, respectively). Adverse events: diarrhea (54%), skin rash (30%), nausea (24%).
Gomez (161) Phase II	138	HER2 (+) First line	1500 qday 500 twice daily	24	0	31	Median TTP was 7.9 weeks; median duration of response was 28.4 weeks. Similar responses with both doses. Adverse events: diarrhea, rash, pruritus, and nausea.
LAPATINIB IN COMBINATION							
Geyer (162) Phase III	324	HER2 (+) Anthracycline, taxane, capecitabine, and trastuzumab refractory	Lapatinib 1250 + capecitabine 2000 mg/m²/day versus capecitabine 2500 mg/m²/day	35 23	1 0	44 29	The median TTP for the combination arm was 8.4 versus 4.4 months (HR 0.49 [0.34–0.71]). Most common AE were gastrointestinal toxicity. Diarrhea 60 versus 39%, nausea 44 versus 42%, and vomiting 26 versus 24%. All more common in combination arm.

(Continued)

Study	N	Patients	Treatment				Comments
Di Leo (168) Phase III	579	HER2 (−) or HER2-untested	Lapatinib 1500+ paclitaxel 17 5 mg/m² q3wk versus paclitaxel+ placebo	30	5	40.5	There were no significant differences in TTP, EFS, or OS between treatment arms. In 86 patients (15%) with HER2 (+) treatment with paclitaxol + lapatinib resulted in statistically significant improvements in TTP, EFS, ORR, and CB.
Johnston (167) Phase III	1286	HR (+), HER2 (−) or HR (+), HER2 (+)	Lapatinib 1500 + letrozole 2.5 mg daily versus letrozole + placebo	23	2	32 48	HR (+)/HER2 (−): no significant treatment benefit on PFS (HR 0.90; 95% CI 0.77–1.05) Subgroup analysis of patients HER2 (−) and lower expression of ER had significant improvement in median PFS (13.6 versus 6.6 months, HR = 0.65, 95% CI 0.47–0.9) when are treated with combination treatment. HR (+)/HER2 (+). The PFS was 8.2 versus 3 months for lapatinib arm. Significant improvement in CB rate for the combination arm.
						29	
Blackwell (165) Phase III	296	HER2 (+) Anthracycline, taxane, capecitabine, trastuzumab refractory	Lapatinib 1000 + trastuzumab 2 mg/kg qwk versus lapatinib 1500	10.3 6.9		24.7 12.4	PFS in the combination arm was 12.0 versus 8.0 months (HR 0.73;95% CI 0.57–0.93), OS was also improved 14.0 versus 9.5 months (HR 0.74; 95% CI 0.57–0.97).

699

chemotherapy agents have been reported. A detailed description of the results of such trials is shown. (Table 25-4). Mature data from four studies (171-174) demonstrated an increment in the PFS when bevacizumab is added to chemotherapy, but final results of three of those trials are awaited.

■ OTHER AGENTS

Bisphosphonates are analogs of pyrophosphates that bind to hydroxyapatite crystals and inhibit bone resorption by osteoclasts. They are widely used for the treatment of osteoporosis and to prevent both skeletal complications in patients with bone metastases and the bone loss associated with cancer treatment. In vitro, bisphosphonates have antiangiogenic effect, reduce cell proliferation, and induce apoptosis of tumor cell lines, reflecting either a direct antitumor effect or an indirect effect by decreasing the local release of bone-derived growth factors and through the inhibition of tumor-induced osteolysis (175,176).

Bisphosphonate treatment is a very important palliative strategy in patients with MBC to the bone, especially in patients with lytic lesions and expected survival of more than 3 months (17). Clinical trials have shown that the use of pamidronate or zoledronic acid are associated with fewer skeletal-related events, pathologic fractures, and less need for radiation therapy and surgery to treat bone pain (177-186), with even some suggesting that zoledronic acid is superior (185). In the United States, pamidronate 90 mg IV over 2 h or zoledronic acid 4 mg IV over 15 min is recommended. They should be given on 3 to 5 week intervals in conjunction with antineoplastic therapy and should be accompanied by calcium and vitamin D supplementation. During bisphosphonate treatment monitoring of renal function is needed. Physicians should also be aware of the risk of developing osteonecrosis of the jaw, a rare but serious complication associated to bisphosphonate therapy. Current clinical trial results support the use of bisphosphonates for 2 years, but there are limited long-term safety data.

Clinical trials using clodronate have suggested a decrease in the incidence of bone metastases as well as a survival benefit. Diel et al. (187) in an open-label, non-placebo-controlled study which included 302 patients with evidence of tumor cells in the bone marrow observed a reduction in the incidence and number of bone and visceral metastases ($p = .003$) that conferred a survival advantage ($p = .001$) in patients that received bisphosphonate therapy (187). After follow-up was

extended to 53 months, the OS and the reduction in bone metastases benefit were maintained but weakened; however, the effect of clodronate on visceral metastases was no longer statistically different between the two groups. Other trials in the adjuvant setting have failed to show a decrease in the risk of developing metastatic disease in patients treated with clodronate (188,189).

Several studies are exploring whether zoledronic acid can decrease the presence of disseminated tumor cells in the bone marrow, decrease the incidence of metastases, and improve survival. Lin et al. (190) showed that the use of zoledronic acid in patients with known bone marrow micrometastasis decreases the number of disseminated tumor cells at 1 and 2 years (190). The ABCSG-12 trial is a phase III 2×2 trial (N = 1803) that demonstrated that the addition of zoledronic acid to adjuvant endocrine therapy prolongs DFS, contralateral breast cancer, distant metastases, and local-regional recurrence (191). This results suggest that maybe bisphosphonates can be a treatment that could prevent the development of metastatic disease.

Denosumab is a fully human monoclonal antibody that targets RANK ligand, a protein that acts as the primary signal to promote bone removal. Denosumab is being studied in the treatment of osteoporosis, treatment-induced bone loss, and bone metastases. Recently, the results of a large (N = 2033) randomized-placebo-controlled clinical trial evaluating the use of denosumab (120 mg subcutaneously) versus zoledronic acid (4 mg IV) in patients with MBC and bone metastases were presented. Denosumab was superior to zoledronic acid in delaying or preventing skeletal-related events, and delayed or prevented hypercalcemia, radiation to bone and bone pain, suggesting that monthly denosumab is a viable option for the management of bone metastases.

■ INVESTIGATIONAL THERAPY

Despite our advances, the prognosis for many women with breast cancer is still poor. With the availability of new discoveries and new drugs, the treatment for MBC will continue to evolve and change in the near future. Investigational therapies for MBC include new molecules and agents with novel mechanisms of action.

In breast cancer, EGFR plays a major role in promoting cell proliferation and malignant growth. Multiple studies evaluating the use of tyrosine kinase (TK) inhibitors in MBC are currently ongoing. Phase II studies of gefitinib (Iressa) used as a single agent or in combination with chemotherapy or hormonotherapy have been

TABLE
25-4

PHASE III CLINICAL TRIALS EVALUATING THE USE OF BEVACIZUMAB IN PATIENTS WITH MBC

Trial Name	Number of Patients	Patient Population	Bevacizumab dose	Combination Therapy	Benefit in Anti-VEGF therapy	Endpoint (PFS)	Study Primary Results
AVF2119 (170)	462	Second-line	15 mg/kg q3wk	Capecitabine 2500 mg/m^2/day from day 1 to day 14	No	4.2 versus 4.0 months. HR 0.98	Combination increased response rate (9.1 versus 19.8%, $p = .001$), but not PFS. No differences in the incidence of diarrhea, hand-foot syndrome, and serious bleeding between treatment groups.
ECOG1200 (171)	722	Frontline	10 mg/kg q2wk	Paclitaxel 90 mg/m^2 days 1, 8, 15	Yes	11.8 versus 5.9 months HR 0.60, $p < .001$	Increased response rate in combination arm (36.9 versus 21.2%). No differences in OS between two groups (median 26.7 versus 25.5 months) Significantly more cases of grade-3 or -4 hypertension, proteinuria, headache, and cerebrovascular ischemia in the combination arm.
AVADO (173)	736	Frontline	7.5 mg/kg q3wk 15 mg/kg q3wk	Docetaxel 100 mg/m^2 q3wk	Yes	7.5 mg/kg dose: HR 0.80 (95% CI 0.65–1.00) 15 mg/kg dose: HR 0.67 (95% CI 0.54–0.83)	Response rate was 46.1% for placebo, 55.2% for 7.5 mg/kg dose and 64.1% for 15 mg/kg dose. No OS differences.
RIBBON1 (174)	1237	Frontline	15 mg/kg q3wk	Capecitabine, taxanes, anthracycline	Yes	Capecitabine HR 0.66 (95% CI 0.56–0.84) Taxanes and anthracyclines HR 0.66 (95% CI 0.52–0.79)	Response rates in capecitabine were 23.45 versus 35.4% favouring bevacizumab. In the combines taxanes and anthracycline group, 37.9 versus 53.1% also favouring bevacizumab. No OS differences.
RIBBON2 (172)	684	Second-line	15 mg/kg or 10 mg/kg	Paclitaxel, docetaxel, gemcitabine, capecitabine, vinorelbine	Yes	7.2 versus 5.1 months HR 0.78 (95% CI 0.64–0.93)	Response rate was increased in those receiving bevacizumab (39.5 versus 29.6%). Interim analysis for OS shows no differences. Grade-3 adverse events 35.2% in bevacizumab and 22.6% in placebo.

completed. Single-agent gefitinib showed minimal clinical benefit and no improvement in response rates or TTF were seen when it was used in combination. More recently, an exploratory analysis of two randomized phase II trials comparing anastrozole or tamoxifen plus gefitinib versus single-agent anastrozole or tamoxifen plus placebo were published (192). In both trials, among endocrine-naïve patients, gefitinib was associated to improved PFS when combined with hormonal therapy compared to anastrozole or tamoxifen alone. Erlotinib (Tarceva) is a small molecule that reversibly inhibits the EGFR TK and prevents receptor autophosphorylation. Combinations of erlotinib with drugs known to be active in breast cancer have also been conducted. In a dose-escalation study of capecitabine, docetaxel, and erlotinib in patients with MBC, the overall response rate was 67% (193). The regimen was generally well tolerated; manageable skin and gastrointestinal problems were the most common treatment–related adverse effects.

Multikinase inhibitors that inhibit VEGF receptors are undergoing active research. Sunitinib malate (Sutent) is an oral TK inhibitor that targets several receptor TKs, including VEGFR-1,-2, and -3. In a phase II trial in patients with MBC previously treated with anthracyclines and taxanes (N = 64), sunitinib was associated with a clinical benefit rate of 16% (194). In a phase II randomized study, 46 patients with HER2-negative MBC were randomized to receive paclitaxel (90 mg/m^2 weekly), bevacizumab (10 mg/kg every 2 weeks), and sunitinib (25 mg daily for 21 days) as first-line chemotherapy (195). High rates of dose modification and treatment discontinuation due to toxic effects were seen, leading to closure of the study. In previously treated MBC patients, sunitinib (37.5 mg PO daily dose) was compared to capecitabine (N = 482), no differences in PFS or OS were seen and, in general, capecitabine was better tolerated (196).

Sorafenib (Nexavar) has been evaluated in patients with MBC refractory to anthracyclines and taxanes. Results from the SOLTI-0701 trial, evaluating the combination of sorafenib (400 mg PO bid) and capecitabine (1000 mg/m^2 days 1-14 from a 21-day cycle) versus capecitabine and placebo in HER2-negative MBC, were recently presented (197). Similar response rates were seen (38.3 versus 30.7%), but improved PFS (6.4 versus 4.1 months, $p < .001$) was observed in the group treated with sorafenib and capecitabine. The combination treatment was associated with 45% rate of grade-3 hand and foot syndrome. The TIES program evaluated the combination of sorafenib and paclitaxel versus paclitaxel and placebo in the frontline setting. TTP and overall response rate, but not PFS, were improved in the active combination arm, with also increased cases of grade-3 toxicities and an imbalance in the number of deaths due to unusual causes in the paclitaxel and sorafenib group (198). Other VGEF-TK inhibitors such as vandetanib (Zactima), valatinib, and axitinib are currently being tested in phase II clinical trials.

Active research is ongoing evaluating insulin-like growth factor inhibitors (CP-751, 856, AMG 479, IMC-A12) as well as RAS/MEK/ERK (tipifarnib) and PI3K/AKT/mTOR pathway inhibitors. Three mTOR antagonists (sirolimus, temsirolimus, and everolimus) are being studied for breast cancer treatment as all have shown activity against breast cancer in preclinical studies (199,200). In a phase II study in previously treated patients with locally advanced or MBC, the use of temsirolimus (Toricel) was associated with a clinical benefit of 13.8% (201). Preliminary results of a phase III study including more than 1200 postmenopausal patients with estrogen receptor-positive MBC suitable for first-line therapy was published (202). Patients were randomized to letrozole with or without temsirolimus. The trial was terminated early after interim analysis demonstrated a complete lack of additional benefit for the combination. Probably the agents that have produced the most important results in recent times are the PARP inhibitors. Poly (ADP-ribose) polymerase 1 (PARP-1) is a critical enzyme of cell proliferation and DNA repair. PARP-1 and -2 are fundamental in the repair of single-stranded DNA breaks (203). A preliminary analysis of a randomized phase II study of BSI-201 in combination with gemcitabine plus carboplatin showed higher objective response rates and increased PFS and OS in patients with MBC and triple receptor negative tumors (204). The promising efficacy and low toxicity results have prompted the initiation of a phase III study. Several phase II studies using other PARP inhibitors (ABT-888, AGO14699, and MK4827) are under way.

■ LOCAL THERAPY

Recent retrospective studies suggest that there is a potential survival benefit from complete excision of the tumor in selected patients with MBC. Substantial selection biases exist in all of those reports that are likely to confound the study results (205-209). No clinical trials have evaluated such question, and debate exists among some groups. According to the most recent guidelines, patients with MBC and an intact primary should be treated based on systemic therapy as has been discussed earlier in this chapter. Consideration for surgery for palliation is indicated in women with impending complications that may compromise quality of life such as skin ulceration, bleeding, fungation, and pain (17). Surgery in such cases should be performed only if complete local tumor clearance can be achieved and if other sites of disease are not immediately threatening the patient's life. Frequently, such surgery requires the collaboration between the breast surgeon and the reconstructive surgeon to provide optimal cancer control and wound closure. Alternatively, radiation therapy may be considered as an option to surgery.

■ SUMMARY

Breast cancer is by far the most common malignancy in women in the western world and MBC is largely incurable. The median survival of women with MBC is in the range of 2 years. The concept of MBC has changed with the realization that breast cancer is a conglomerate of several molecularly defined subtypes, each with a distinct prognosis, clinical course, and sensitivity to existing therapeutics. Treatment for MBC has dramatically evolved, incorporating new hormonal therapies, cytotoxic agents, and monoclonal agents. Refinements of chemotherapy with different combinations of newer agents along with modulating agents and growth-factor support have allowed for further advancement in the treatment of MBC. Despite great enthusiasm for targeted therapy, these agents have exhibited modest activity when used as single agents in unselected patients. The development of new drugs in oncology faces multiple challenges. We need a better understanding of the molecular biology of signaling pathways and the discovery of new biomarkers to help us better select the patients that will benefit from specific treatments. Our main objective should be the improvement of survival and quality of life of our patients.

References

1. American Cancer Society. *Breast Cancer Facts and Figures 2007-2008*. Atlanta, GA: American Cancer Society; 2009.
2. SEER Cancer Statistics Review 1975-2006., National Cancer Institute, DC-CPS, Surveillance Research Program, Cancer Staistics Branch, Released May 2009. Available at: http://www.seer.cancer.gov.
3. Dawood S, Broglio K, Gonzalez-Angulo AM, et al. Trends in survival over the past two decades among white and black patients with newly diagnosed stage IV breast cancer. *J Clin Oncol* 2008;26:4891-4898.
4. Giordano SH, Buzdar AU, Smith TL, et al. Is breast cancer survival improving? *Cancer* 2004;100:44-52.
5. Jain S, Fisher C, Smith P, et al. Patterns of metastatic breast cancer in relation to histological type. *Eur J Cancer* 1993;29A:2155-2157.
6. De Lena M, Romero A, Rabinovich M, et al. Metastatic pattern and DNA ploidy in stage IV breast cancer at initial diagnosis. Relation to response and survival. *Am J Clin Oncol* 1993;16:245-249.
7. Amir E, Ooi WS, Simmons C, et al. Discordance between receptor status in primary and metastatic breast cancer: an exploratory study of bone and bone marrow biopsies. *Clin Oncol (R Coll Radiol)* 2008;20:763-768.
8. Broom RJ, Tang PA, Simmons C, et al. Changes in estrogen receptor, progesterone receptor and Her-2/neu status with time: discordance rates between primary and metastatic breast cancer. *Anticancer Res* 2009;29:1557-1562.
9. Mamounas EP, Perez-Mesa C, Penetrante RB, et al. Patterns of occurrence of second primary non-mammary malignancies in breast cancer patients: Results from 1382 consecutive autopsies. *Surg Oncol* 1993;2:175-185.
10. Saad A, Abraham J. Role of tumor markers and circulating tumors cells in the management of breast cancer. *Oncology (Williston Park)* 2008;22:726-731; discussion 734, 739, 743-744.
11. Tondini C, Hayes DF, Gelman R, et al. Comparison of CA15-3 and carcinoembryonic antigen in monitoring the clinical course of patients with metastatic breast cancer. *Cancer Res* 1988;48:4107-4112.
12. Tormey DC, Waalkes TP. Clinical correlation between CEA and breast cancer. *Cancer* 1978;42:1507-1511.
13. Harris L, Fritsche H, Mennel R, et al. American Society of Clinical Oncology 2007 update of recommendations for the use of tumor markers in breast cancer. *J Clin Oncol* 2007;25:5287-5312.
14. Cristofanilli M, Budd GT, Ellis MJ, et al. Circulating tumor cells, disease progression, and survival in metastatic breast cancer. *N Engl J Med* 2004;351:781-791.
15. Cristofanilli M, Reuben J, Uhr J. Circulating tumor cells in breast cancer: fiction or reality? *J Clin Oncol* 2008;26:3656-3657; author reply 3657-3658.
16. Hayes DF, Cristofanilli M, Budd GT, et al. Circulating tumor cells at each follow-up time point during therapy of metastatic breast cancer patients predict progression-free and overall survival. *Clin Cancer Res* 2006;12:4218-4224.
17. NCCN Clinical Practice Guidelines in Oncology. Breast Cancer V.I.2009, National Comprehensive Cancer Network.
18. Khansur T, Haick A, Patel B, et al. Evaluation of bone scan as a screening work-up in primary and local-regional recurrence of breast cancer. *Am J Clin Oncol* 1987;10:167-170.
19. White DR, Maloney JJ, 3rd, Muss HB, et al. Serum alkaline phosphatase determination. Value in the staging of advanced breast cancer. *JAMA* 1979;242:1147-1149.
20. Allegra JC, Lippman ME. Estrogen receptor status and the disease-free interval in breast cancer. *Recent Results Cancer Res* 1980;71:20-25.
21. Allegra JC, Lippman ME, Thompson EB, et al. Estrogen receptor status: an important variable in predicting response to endocrine therapy in metastatic breast cancer. *Eur J Cancer*, 1980;16:323-331.

22. Ravdin PM, Green S, Dorr TM, et al. Prognostic significance of progesterone receptor levels in estrogen receptor-positive patients with metastatic breast cancer treated with tamoxifen: Results of a prospective Southwest Oncology Group study. *J Clin Oncol* 1992;10:1284-1291.

23. Buzdar AU. Current status of endocrine treatment of carcinoma of the breast. *Semin Surg Oncol* 1990;6:77-82.

24. Ingle JN, Ahmann DL, Green SJ, et al. Randomized clinical trial of megestrol acetate versus tamoxifen in paramenopausal or castrated women with advanced breast cancer. *Am J Clin Oncol* 1982;5:155-160.

25. Smith IE, Harris AL, Stuart-Harris R, et al. Combination treatment with tamoxifen and aminoglutethimide in advanced breast cancer. *Br Med J (Clin Res Ed)* 1983;286:1615-1616.

26. Saphner T, Troxel AB, Tormey DC, et al. Phase II study of goserelin for patients with postmenopausal metastatic breast cancer. *J Clin Oncol* 1993;11:1529-1535.

27. Come SE, Buzdar AU, Ingle JN, et al. Endocrine and targeted manipulation of breast cancer: summary statement for the Sixth Cambridge Conference. *Cancer* 2008;112:673-678.

28. Goss PE, Gwyn KM. Current perspectives on aromatase inhibitors in breast cancer. *J Clin Oncol* 1994;12:2460-2470.

29. Klijn JG, Blamey RW, Boccardo F, et al. Combined tamoxifen and luteinizing hormone-releasing hormone (LHRH) agonist versus LHRH agonist alone in premenopausal advanced breast cancer: a meta-analysis of four randomized trials. *J Clin Oncol* 2001;19:343-353.

30. Perez EA. Safety profiles of tamoxifen and the aromatase inhibitors in adjuvant therapy of hormone-responsive early breast cancer. *Ann Oncol* 2007; 18 (Suppl 8):viii26-35.

31. Cella D, Fallowfield LJ. Recognition and management of treatment-related side effects for breast cancer patients receiving adjuvant endocrine therapy. *Breast Cancer Res Treat* 2008;107:167-180.

32. Mouridsen HT. Incidence and management of side effects associated with aromatase inhibitors in the adjuvant treatment of breast cancer in postmenopausal women. *Curr Med Res Opin* 2006;22:1609-1621.

33. Lundgren S, Kvinnsland S, Utaaker E, et al. Effect of oral high-dose progestins on the disposition of antipyrine, digitoxin, and warfarin in patients with advanced breast cancer. *Cancer Chemother Pharmacol* 1986;18:270-275.

34. Bonneterre J, Thurlimann B, Robertson JF, et al. Anastrozole versus tamoxifen as first-line therapy for advanced breast cancer in 668 postmenopausal women: results of the Tamoxifen or Arimidex Randomized Group Efficacy and Tolerability study. *J Clin Oncol* 2000;18:3748-3757.

35. Nabholtz JM, Buzdar A, Pollak M, et al. Anastrozole is superior to tamoxifen as first-line therapy for advanced breast cancer in postmenopausal women: results of a North American multicenter randomized trial. Arimidex Study Group. *J Clin Oncol* 2000;18:3758-3767.

36. Mouridsen H, Gershanovich M, Sun Y, et al. Phase III study of letrozole versus tamoxifen as first-line therapy of advanced breast cancer in postmenopausal women: Analysis of survival and update of efficacy from the International *Letrozole Breast Cancer Group J Clin Oncol* 2003;21:2101-2109.

37. Howell A, Robertson JF, Abram P, et al. Comparison of fulvestrant versus tamoxifen for the treatment of advanced breast cancer in postmenopausal women previously untreated with endocrine therapy: a multinational, double-blind, randomized trial. *J Clin Oncol* 2004; 22:1605-1613.

38. Osborne CK, Pippen J, Jones SE, et al. Double-blind, randomized trial comparing the efficacy and tolerability of fulvestrant versus anastrozole in postmenopausal women with advanced breast cancer progressing on prior endocrine therapy: results of a North American trial. *J Clin Oncol* 2002; 20:3386-3395.

39. Robertson JF, Osborne CK, Howell A, et al. Fulvestrant versus anastrozole for the treatment of advanced breast carcinoma in postmenopausal women: a prospective combined analysis of two multicenter trials. *Cancer* 2003;98:229-238.

40. Chia S, Gradishar W, Mauriac L, et al. Double-blind, randomized placebo controlled trial of fulvestrant compared with exemestane after prior nonsteroidal aromatase inhibitor therapy in postmenopausal women with hormone receptor-positive, advanced breast cancer: results from EFECT. *J Clin Oncol* 2008; 26:1664-1670.

41. Di Leo A JG, Petruzelka L, Torres R et al. CONFIRM: a phase III, randomized, parallel-group trial comparing fulvestrant 250 mg vs fulvestrant 500 mg in postmenopausal women with estrogen receptor-positive advanced breast cancer. *Cancer Research* 2009;69(24):491s.

42. Ellis MJ DF, Kommareddy A, Jamalabadi-Majidi S, et al. A randomized phase 2 trial of low dose (6 mg daily) versus high dose (30 mg daily) estradiol for patients with estrogen receptor positive aromatase inhibitor resistant advanced breast cancer. In: Proceedings of the 31st San Antonio Breast Cancer Symposium, 2008.

43. Hortobagyi GN, Smith TL, Legha SS, et al. Multivariate analysis of prognostic factors in metastatic breast cancer. *J Clin Oncol* 1983;1:776-786.

44. Swenerton KD, Legha SS, Smith T, et al. Prognostic factors in metastatic breast cancer treated with combination chemotherapy. *Cancer Res* 1979;39:1552-1562.

45. Kiang DT. Correlation between estrogen-receptor proteins and response to chemotherapy in patients with breast cancer. *Cancer Treat Rep* 1984;68:577-579.

46. Amadori D, Volpi A, Maltoni R, et al. Cell proliferation as a predictor of response to chemotherapy in metastatic breast cancer: a prospective study. *Breast Cancer Res Treat* 1997;43:7-14.

47. Krajewski S, Blomqvist C, Franssila K, et al. Reduced expression of proapoptotic gene BAX is associated with poor response rates to combination chemotherapy and shorter survival in women with metastatic breast adenocarcinoma. *Cancer Res* 1995;55:4471-4478.

48. Fossati R, Confalonieri C, Torri V, et al. Cytotoxic and hormonal treatment for metastatic breast cancer: a systematic review of published randomized trials involving 31,510 women. *J Clin Oncol* 1998;16:3439-3460.

49. Bishop JF, Dewar J, Toner GC, et al. Initial paclitaxel improves outcome compared with CMFP combination chemotherapy as front-line therapy in untreated metastatic breast cancer. *J Clin Oncol* 1999;17:2355-2364.

50. Joensuu H, Holli K, Heikkinen M, et al. Combination chemotherapy versus single-agent therapy as first- and second-line treatment in metastatic breast cancer: a prospective randomized trial. *J Clin Oncol* 1998;16:3720-3730.

51. Carrick S, Parker S, Wilcken N, et al. Single agent versus combination chemotherapy for metastatic breast cancer. Cochrane Database Syst Rev: CD003372, 2005.

52. Albain KS, Nag SM, Calderillo-Ruiz G, et al. Gemcitabine plus paclitaxel versus paclitaxel monotherapy in patients with metastatic breast cancer and prior anthracycline treatment. *J Clin Oncol* 2008;26:3950-3957.

53. O'Shaughnessy J, Miles D, Vukelja S, et al. Superior survival with capecitabine plus docetaxel combination therapy in anthracycline-pretreated patients with advanced breast cancer: phase III trial results. *J Clin Oncol* 2002;20:2812-2823.

54. Alba E, Martin M, Ramos M, et al. Multicenter randomized trial comparing sequential with concomitant administration of doxorubicin and docetaxel as first-line treatment of metastatic breast cancer: A Spanish Breast Cancer Research Group (GEICAM-9903) phase III study. *J Clin Oncol* 2004; 22:2587-2593.

55. Conte PF, Guarneri V, Bruzzi P, et al. Concomitant versus sequential administration of epirubicin and paclitaxel as first-line therapy in metastatic breast carcinoma: results for the Gruppo Oncologico Nord Ovest randomized trial. *Cancer* 2004;101:704-712.

56. Sjostrom J, Blomqvist C, Mouridsen H, et al. Docetaxel compared with sequential methotrexate and 5-fluorouracil in patients with advanced breast cancer after anthracycline failure: a randomised phase III study with crossover on progression by the Scandinavian Breast Group. *Eur J Cancer* 1999;35: 1194-1201.

57. Sledge GW, Neuberg D, Bernardo P, et al. Phase III trial of doxorubicin, paclitaxel, and the combination of doxorubicin and paclitaxel as front-line chemotherapy for metastatic breast cancer: An intergroup trial (E1193). *J Clin Oncol* 2003; 21:588-592.

58. Soto C, Torrecillas L, Reyes S. Capecitabine (X) and taxanes in patients with anthracyline-pretreated metastatic breast cancer (MBC): Sequential vs. combined therapy results from a MOSG randomized phase III trial. Proceedings from the American Society of Clinical Oncology Annual Meeting. 2006;24:570.

59. Tomova A, Brodowicz T, Tzekova V, et al. Concomitant docetaxel plus gemcitabineversus sequential docetaxel followed by gemcitabine. Proceedings from the American Society of Clinical Oncology Annual Meeting. 2008;26(s15):1106.

60. Cardoso F, Bedard PL, Winer EP, et al. International guidelines for management of metastatic breast cancer: combination vs sequential single-agent chemotherapy. *J Natl Cancer Inst* 2009;101:1174-1181.

61. Coates A, Gebski V, Bishop JF, et al. Improving the quality of life during chemotherapy for advanced breast cancer. A comparison of intermittent and continuous treatment strategies. *N Engl J Med* 1987;317:1490-1495.

62. Ejlertsen B, Pfeiffer P, Pedersen D, et al. Decreased efficacy of cyclophosphamide, epirubicin and 5-fluorouracil in metastatic breast cancer when reducing treatment duration from 18 to 6 months. *Eur J Cancer* 1993;29A:527-531.

63. Falkson G, Gelman RS, Pandya KJ, et al. Eastern Cooperative Oncology Group randomized trials of observation versus maintenance therapy for patients with metastatic breast cancer in complete remission following induction treatment. *J Clin Oncol* 1998;16:1669-1676.

64. Muss HB, Case LD, Richards F, 2nd, et al. Interrupted versus continuous chemotherapy in patients with metastatic breast cancer. The Piedmont Oncology Association. *N Engl J Med* 1991;325:1342-1348.

65. Stockler M, Wilcken N, Coates A. Chemotherapy for metastatic breast cancer–when is enough enough? *Eur J Cancer* 1997; 33:2147-2148.

66. Gennari A, Conte P, Nanni O, et al. Multicenter randomized trial of paclitaxel (P) for maintenance chemotherapy (CT) versus control in metastatic breast cancer (MBC) patients achieving a response or stable disease to first-line CT including anthracyclines and paclitaxel: Final results from the Italian MANTA study. Proceedings from the American Society of Clinical Oncology Annual Meeting. 2005; 23(s16) (abstract 522).

67. Weiss RB. The anthracyclines: will we ever find a better doxorubicin? *Semin Oncol* 1992;19:670-686.

68. Hoogstraten B, George SL, Samal B, et al. Combination chemotherapy and adriamycin in patients with advanced breast cancer. A Southwest Oncology Group study. *Cancer* 1976;38:13-20.

69. Jain KK, Casper ES, Geller NL, et al. A prospective randomized comparison of epirubicin and doxorubicin in patients with advanced breast cancer. *J Clin Oncol* 1985;3:818-826.

70. Lawton PA, Spittle MF, Ostrowski MJ, et al. A comparison of doxorubicin, epirubicin and mitozantrone as single agents in advanced breast carcinoma. *Clin Oncol (R Coll Radiol)* 1993;5:80-84.

71. Van Oosterom AT, Mouridsen HT, Wildiers J, et al. Carminomycin versus doxorubicin in advanced breast cancer, a randomized phase II study of the E.O.R.T.C. Breast Cancer Cooperative Group. *Eur J Cancer Clin Oncol* 1986;22:601-605.

72. Camaggi CM, Strocchi E, Carisi P, et al. Epirubicin metabolism and pharmacokinetics after conventional- and high-dose intravenous administration: A cross-over study. *Cancer Chemother Pharmacol* 1993;32:301-309.

73. Plosker GL, Faulds D. Epirubicin. A review of its pharmacodynamic and pharmacokinetic properties, and therapeutic use in cancer chemotherapy. *Drugs* 1993;45:788-856.

74. A prospective randomized phase III trial comparing combination chemotherapy with cyclophosphamide, fluorouracil, and either doxorubicin or epirubicin. French Epirubicin Study Group. *J Clin Oncol* 1988;6:679-688.

75. A prospective randomized trial comparing epirubicin monochemotherapy to two fluorouracil, cyclophosphamide, and epirubicin regimens differing in epirubicin dose in advanced breast cancer patients. The French Epirubicin Study Group. *J Clin Oncol* 1991;9:305-312.

76. Minisini AM, Andreetta C, Fasola G, et al. Pegylated liposomal doxorubicin in elderly patients with metastatic breast cancer. *Expert Rev Anticancer Ther* 2008;8:331-342.

77. Rivera E. Liposomal anthracyclines in metastatic breast cancer: clinical update. *Oncologist* 2003; 8 (Suppl 2):3-9.

78. O'Brien ME, Wigler N, Inbar M, et al. Reduced cardiotoxicity and comparable efficacy in a phase III trial of pegylated liposomal doxorubicin HCl (CAELYX/Doxil) versus conventional doxorubicin for first-line treatment of metastatic breast cancer. *Ann Oncol* 2004;15:440-449.

79. Wilson WH, Berg SL, Bryant G, et al. Paclitaxel in doxorubicin-refractory or mitoxantrone-refractory breast cancer: a phase I/II trial of 96-hour infusion. *J Clin Oncol* 1994;12:1621-1629.

80. Mamounas EP, Brown A, Smith R, et al. Effect of taxol duration of infusion in advanced breast cancer (ABC): Results from NSABP B-26 trial comparin 3- to 24-h infusion of high dose taxol. Proceedings from the American Society of Clinical Oncology Annual Meeting. 1998;21 (abstract 137).

81. Dieras V, Marty M, Tubiana N, et al. Phase II randomized study of paclitaxel versus mitomycin in advanced breast cancer. *Semin Oncol* 1995;22:33-39.

82. Eisenhauer EA, Vermorken JB. The taxoids. Comparative clinical pharmacology and therapeutic potential. *Drugs* 1998; 55:5-30.

83. Seidman AD, Hudis CA, Albanell J, et al. Dose-dense therapy with weekly 1-hour paclitaxel infusions in the treatment of metastatic breast cancer. *J Clin Oncol* 1998;16:3353-3361.

84. Ravdin PM, Burris HA, 3rd, Cook G, et al. Phase II trial of docetaxel in advanced anthracycline-resistant or anthracenedione-resistant breast cancer. *J Clin Oncol* 1995;13:2879-2885.

85. Valero V, Jones SE, Von Hoff DD, et al. A phase II study of docetaxel in patients with paclitaxel-resistant metastatic breast cancer. *J Clin Oncol* 1998;16:3362-3368.

86. Nabholtz JM, Senn HJ, Bezwoda WR, et al. Prospective randomized trial of docetaxel versus mitomycin plus vinblastine in patients with metastatic breast cancer progressing despite previous anthracycline-containing chemotherapy. 304 Study Group. *J Clin Oncol* 1999;17:1413-1424.

87. Harvey V, Mouridsen H, Semiglazov V, et al. Phase III trial comparing three doses of docetaxel for second-line treatment of advanced breast cancer. *J Clin Oncol* 2006;24:4963-4970.

88. Jones SE, Erban J, Overmoyer B, et al. Randomized phase III study of docetaxel compared with paclitaxel in metastatic breast cancer. *J Clin Oncol* 2005;23:5542-5551.

89. Hainsworth JD, Burris HA, 3rd, Erland JB, et al. Phase I trial of docetaxel administered by weekly infusion in patients with advanced refractory cancer. *J Clin Oncol* 1998;16: 2164-2168.

90. Burstein HJ, Manola J, Younger J, et al. Docetaxel administered on a weekly basis for metastatic breast cancer. *J Clin Oncol* 2000;18:1212-1219.

91. Gradishar WJ, Krasnojon D, Cheporov S, et al. Significantly longer progression-free survival with nab-paclitaxel compared with docetaxel as first-line therapy for metastatic breast cancer. *J Clin Oncol* 2009;27:3611-3619.

92. Gradishar WJ, Tjulandin S, Davidson N, et al. Phase III trial of nanoparticle albumin-bound paclitaxel compared with polyethylated castor oil-based paclitaxel in women with breast cancer. *J Clin Oncol* 2005;23:7794-7803.

93. Gradishar W, Krasnojon D, Cheporov S, et al. A randomized phase 2 trial of qw or q3w ABI-007 (ABX) vs. q3W solvent-based docetaxel (TXT) as first-line therapy in metastatic breast cancer (MBC). Presented at the San Antonio Breast Cancer Symposium. *Breast Cancer Res Treat* 2006; 100 (suppl 1).

94. Blum JL, Jones SE, Buzdar AU, et al. Multicenter phase II study of capecitabine in paclitaxel-refractory metastatic breast cancer. *J Clin Oncol* 1999;17:485-493.

95. Blum JL, Dieras V, Lo Russo PM, et al. Multicenter, phase II study of capecitabine in taxane-pretreated metastatic breast carcinoma patients. *Cancer* 2001;92:1759-1768.

96. Oshaughnessy JA, Blum J, Moiseyenko V, et al. Randomized, open-label, phase II trial of oral capecitabine (Xeloda) vs. a reference arm of intravenous CMF (cyclophosphamide, methotrexate and 5-fluorouracil) as first-line therapy for advanced/metastatic breast cancer. *Ann Oncol* 2001;12: 1247-1254.

97. Talbot DC, Moiseyenko V, Van Belle S, et al. Randomised, phase II trial comparing oral capecitabine (Xeloda) with paclitaxel in patients with metastatic/advanced breast cancer

pretreated with anthracyclines. *Br J Cancer* 2002;86: 1367-1372.

98. Blackstein M, Vogel CL, Ambinder R, et al. Gemcitabine as first-line therapy in patients with metastatic breast cancer: a phase II trial. *Oncology* 2002;62:2-8.

99. Possinger K, Kaufmann M, Coleman R, et al. Phase II study of gemcitabine as first-line chemotherapy in patients with advanced or metastatic breast cancer. *Anticancer Drugs* 1999; 10:155-162.

100. Carmichael J, Possinger K, Phillip P, et al. Advanced breast cancer: a phase II trial with gemcitabine. *J Clin Oncol* 1995; 13:2731-2736.

101. Canobbio L, Boccardo F, Pastorino G, et al. Phase-II study of Navelbine in advanced breast cancer. *Semin Oncol* 1989; 16:33-36.

102. Jones S, Winer E, Vogel C, et al. Randomized comparison of vinorelbine and melphalan in anthracycline-refractory advanced breast cancer. *J Clin Oncol* 1995;13:2567-2574.

103. Livingston RB, Ellis GK, Gralow JR, et al. Dose-intensive vinorelbine with concurrent granulocyte colony-stimulating factor support in paclitaxel-refractory metastatic breast cancer. *J Clin Oncol* 1997;15:1395-1400.

104. Weber BL, Vogel C, Jones S, et al. Intravenous vinorelbine as first-line and second-line therapy in advanced breast cancer. *J Clin Oncol* 1995;13:2722-2730.

105. Zelek L, Barthier S, Riofrio M, et al. Weekly vinorelbine is an effective palliative regimen after failure with anthracyclines and taxanes in metastatic breast carcinoma. *Cancer* 2001; 92:2267-2272.

106. Perez EA, Lerzo G, Pivot X, et al. Efficacy and safety of ixabepilone (BMS-247550) in a phase II study of patients with advanced breast cancer resistant to an anthracycline, a taxane, and capecitabine. *J Clin Oncol* 2007;25:3407-3414.

107. Thomas E, Tabernero J, Fornier M, et al. Phase II clinical trial of ixabepilone (BMS-247550), an epothilone B analog, in patients with taxane-resistant metastatic breast cancer. *J Clin Oncol* 2007;25:3399-3406.

108. Roche H, Yelle L, Cognetti F, et al. Phase II clinical trial of ixabepilone (BMS-247550), an epothilone B analog, as first-line therapy in patients with metastatic breast cancer previously treated with anthracycline chemotherapy. *J Clin Oncol* 2007;25:3415-3420.

109. Denduluri N, Low JA, Lee JJ, et al. Phase II trial of ixabepilone, an epothilone B analog, in patients with metastatic breast cancer previously untreated with taxanes. *J Clin Oncol* 2007;25:3421-3427.

110. Nabholtz J, Paterson A, Dirix L, et al. A phase III randomized trial comparing docetaxel (T), doxorubicin (A) and cyclophosphamide (C) (TAC) to FAC as first line chemotherapy (CT) for patients (Pts) with metastatic breast cancer (MBC). *Proc Am Soc Clin Oncol* 2001;20 (abstract 83).

111. Mackey J, Paterson A, Dirix L, et al. Final results of the phase III randomized trial comparing docetaxel (T), doxorubicin (A) and cyclophosphamide (C) to FAC as first line chemotherapy (CT) for patients (pts) with metastatic breast cancer (MBC). *Proc Am Soc Clin Oncol* 2002;21 (abstract 137).

112. Carmichael J. UKCCCR trial of epirubicin and cyclophosphamide (EC) vs. epirubicin and taxol (ET) in the first line treatment of women with metastatic breast cancer (MBC). *Proc Am Soc Clin Oncol* 2001;20 (abstract 84).

113. Nabholtz JM, Falkson C, Campos D, et al. Docetaxel and doxorubicin compared with doxorubicin and cyclophosphamide as first-line chemotherapy for metastatic breast cancer: results of a randomized, multicenter, phase III trial. *J Clin Oncol* 2003;21:968-975.

114. Biganzoli L, Cufer T, Bruning P, et al. Doxorubicin and paclitaxel versus doxorubicin and cyclophosphamide as first-line chemotherapy in metastatic breast cancer: the European Organization for Research and Treatment of Cancer 10961 Multicenter Phase III Trial. *J Clin Oncol* 2002;20: 3114-3121.

115. Jassem J, Pienkowski T, Pluzanska A, et al. Doxorubicin and paclitaxel versus fluorouracil, doxorubicin, and cyclophosphamide as first-line therapy for women with metastatic breast cancer: final results of a randomized phase III multicenter trial. *J Clin Oncol* 2001;19:1707-1715.

116. Martin M. Platinum compounds in the treatment of advanced breast cancer. *Clin Breast Cancer* 2001;2:190-208; discussion 209.

117. Perez EA, Hillman DW, Stella PJ, et al. A phase II study of paclitaxel plus carboplatin as first-line chemotherapy for women with metastatic breast carcinoma. *Cancer* 2000;88: 124-131.

118. Fountzilas G, Athanassiadis A, Kalogera-Fountzila A, et al. Paclitaxel by 3-h infusion and carboplatin in anthracycline-resistant advanced breast cancer. A phase II study conducted by the Hellenic Cooperative Oncology Group. *Eur J Cancer* 1997;33:1893-1895.

119. Mavroudis D, Alexopoulos A, Malamos N, et al. Salvage treatment of metastatic breast cancer with docetaxel and carboplatin. A multicenter phase II trial. *Oncology* 2003;64: 207-212.

120. Norris B, Pritchard KI, James K, et al. Phase III comparative study of vinorelbine combined with doxorubicin versus doxorubicin alone in disseminated metastatic/recurrent breast cancer: National Cancer Institute of Canada Clinical Trials Group Study MA8. *J Clin Oncol* 2000;18:2385-2394.

121. Domenech GH, Vogel CL. A review of vinorelbine in the treatment of breast cancer. *Clin Breast Cancer* 2001;2:113-128.

122. Nagourney RA, Link JS, Blitzer JB, et al. Gemcitabine plus cisplatin repeating doublet therapy in previously treated, relapsed breast cancer patients. *J Clin Oncol* 2000;18:2245-2249.

123. Chew HK, Doroshow JH, Frankel P, et al. Phase II studies of gemcitabine and cisplatin in heavily and minimally pretreated metastatic breast cancer. *J Clin Oncol* 2009;27:2163-2169.

124. Albain S, Nag S, Calderillo-Ruiz G, et al. Global phase III study of gemcitabine plus paclitaxel (GT) vs. paclitaxel (T) as frontline therapy for metastatic breast cancer (MBC): first report of overall survival. 2004 ASCO Annual Meeting Proceedings. *J Clin Oncol*, 2004;22 (14S): 510.

125. Fountzilas G, Nicolaides C, Bafaloukos D, et al. Docetaxel and gemcitabine in anthracycline-resistant advanced breast cancer: a Hellenic Cooperative Oncology Group Phase II study. *Cancer Invest* 2000;18:503-509.

126. Kornek GV, Haider K, Kwasny W, et al. Treatment of advanced breast cancer with docetaxel and gemcitabine with and without human granulocyte colony-stimulating factor. *Clin Cancer Res* 2002;8:1051-1056.

127. Laufman LR, Spiridonidis CH, Pritchard J, et al. Monthly docetaxel and weekly gemcitabine in metastatic breast cancer: a phase II trial. *Ann Oncol* 2001;12:1259-1264.

128. Chan S, Romieu G, Huober J, et al. Phase III study of gemcitabine plus docetaxel compared with capecitabine plus docetaxel for anthracycline-pretreated patients with metastatic breast cancer. *J Clin Oncol* 2009;27:1753-1760.

129. Zielinski C, Beslija S, Mrsic-Krmpotic Z, et al. Gemcitabine, epirubicin, and paclitaxel versus fluorouracil, epirubicin, and cyclophosphamide as first-line chemotherapy in metastatic breast cancer: a Central European Cooperative Oncology Group International, multicenter, prospective, randomized phase III trial. *J Clin Oncol* 2005;23:1401-1408.

130. Thomas ES, Gomez HL, Li RK, et al. Ixabepilone plus capecitabine for metastatic breast cancer progressing after anthracycline and taxane treatment. *J Clin Oncol* 2007;25: 5210-5217.

131. Hynes NE: Amplification and overexpression of the erbB-2 gene in human tumors: its involvement in tumor development, significance as a prognostic factor, and potential as a target for cancer therapy. *Semin Cancer Biol* 1993;4:19-26.

132. Slamon DJ, Clark GM, Wong SG, et al. Human breast cancer: correlation of relapse and survival with amplification of the HER-2/neu oncogene. *Science* 1987;235:177-182.

133. Slamon DJ, Godolphin W, Jones LA, et al: Studies of the HER-2/neu proto-oncogene in human breast and ovarian cancer. *Science* 1989;244:707-712.

134. Carlomagno C, Perrone F, Gallo C, et al. c-erb B2 overexpression decreases the benefit of adjuvant tamoxifen in early-stage breast cancer without axillary lymph node metastases. *J Clin Oncol* 1996;14:2702-2708.

135. Elledge RM, Green S, Ciocca D, et al. HER-2 expression and response to tamoxifen in estrogen receptor-positive breast cancer: a Southwest Oncology Group Study. *Clin Cancer Res* 1998;4:7-12.

136. Leitzel K, Teramoto Y, Konrad K, et al. Elevated serum c-erbB-2 antigen levels and decreased response to hormone therapy of breast cancer. *J Clin Oncol* 1995;13:1129-1135.

137. Pietras RJ, Arboleda J, Reese DM, et al: HER-2 tyrosine kinase pathway targets estrogen receptor and promotes hormone-independent growth in human breast cancer cells. *Oncogene* 1995;10:2435-2446.

138. Yamauchi H, O'Neill A, Gelman R, et al. Prediction of response to antiestrogen therapy in advanced breast cancer patients by pretreatment circulating levels of extracellular domain of the HER-2/c-neu protein. *J Clin Oncol* 1997;15: 2518-2525.

139. Howell A, Cuzick J, Baum M, et al. Results of the ATAC (Arimidex, tamoxifen, alone or in combination) trial after completion of 5 years' adjuvant treatment for breast cancer. *Lancet* 2005;365:60-62.

140. Rasmussen BB, Regan MM, Lykkesfeldt AE, et al. Adjuvant letrozole versus tamoxifen according to centrally-assessed ERBB2 status for postmenopausal women with endocrine-responsive early breast cancer: supplementary results from the BIG 1-98 randomised trial. *Lancet Oncol* 2008;9:23-28.

141. Muss HB, Thor AD, Berry DA, et al. c-erbB-2 expression and response to adjuvant therapy in women with node-positive early breast cancer. *N Engl J Med* 1994;330:1260-1266.

142. Paik S, Bryant J, Park C, et al. erbB-2 and response to doxorubicin in patients with axillary lymph node-positive, hormone receptor-negative breast cancer. *J Natl Cancer Inst* 1998;90: 1361-1370.

143. Cobleigh MA, Vogel CL, Tripathy D, et al. Multinational study of the efficacy and safety of humanized anti-HER2 monoclonal antibody in women who have HER2-overexpressing metastatic breast cancer that has progressed after chemotherapy for metastatic disease. *J Clin Oncol* 1999;17: 2639-2648.

144. Slamon DJ, Leyland-Jones B, Shak S, et al. Use of chemotherapy plus a monoclonal antibody against HER2 for metastatic breast cancer that overexpresses HER2. *N Engl J Med* 2001;344:783-792.

145. Pegram MD, Lopez A, Konecny G, et al. Trastuzumab and chemotherapeutics: drug interactions and synergies. *Semin Oncol* 2000;27:21-25; discussion 92-100.

146. Burstein HJ, Kuter I, Campos SM, et al. Clinical activity of trastuzumab and vinorelbine in women with HER2-overexpressing metastatic breast cancer. *J Clin Oncol* 2001;19: 2722-2730.

147. Burstein HJ, Keshaviah A, Baron AD, et al. Trastuzumab plus vinorelbine or taxane chemotherapy for HER2-overexpressing metastatic breast cancer: the trastuzumab and vinorelbine or taxane study. *Cancer* 2007;110:965-972.

148. Yardley DA, Burris HA, 3rd, Hanson S, et al. Weekly gemcitabine and trastuzumab in the treatment of patients with HER2-overexpressing metastatic breast cancer. *Clin Breast Cancer* 2009;9:178-183.

149. O'Shaughnessy JA, Vukelja S, Marsland T, et al. Phase II study of trastuzumab plus gemcitabine in chemotherapy-pretreated patients with metastatic breast cancer. *Clin Breast Cancer* 2004;5:142-147.

150. Bartsch R, Wenzel C, Altorjai G, et al. Capecitabine and trastuzumab in heavily pretreated metastatic breast cancer. *J Clin Oncol* 2007; 25:3853-3858.

151. Schaller G, Fuchs I, Gonsch T, et al. Phase II study of capecitabine plus trastuzumab in human epidermal growth factor receptor 2 overexpressing metastatic breast cancer pretreated with anthracyclines or taxanes. *J Clin Oncol* 2007; 25:3246-3250.

152. Esteva FJ, Valero V, Booser D, et al. Phase II study of weekly docetaxel and trastuzumab for patients with HER-2-overexpressing metastatic breast cancer. *J Clin Oncol* 2002; 20:1800-1808.

153. Montemurro F, Choa G, Faggiuolo R, et al. Safety and activity of docetaxel and trastuzumab in HER2 overexpressing metastatic breast cancer: a pilot phase II study. *Am J Clin Oncol* 2003;26:95-97.

154. Marty M, Cognetti F, Maraninchi D, et al. Randomized phase II trial of the efficacy and safety of trastuzumab combined with docetaxel in patients with human epidermal growth factor receptor 2-positive metastatic breast cancer administered as first-line treatment: the M77001 study group. *J Clin Oncol* 2005;23:4265-4274.

155. Tedesco KL, Thor AD, Johnson DH, et al. Docetaxel combined with trastuzumab is an active regimen in HER-2 3+ overexpressing and fluorescent in situ hybridization-positive metastatic breast cancer: a multi-institutional phase II trial. *J Clin Oncol* 2004; 22:1071-1077.

156. Jackisch C. HER-2-positive metastatic breast cancer: optimizing trastuzumab-based therapy. *Oncologist* 2006;11 (Suppl 1):34-41.

157. Robert N, Leyland-Jones B, Asmar L, et al. Randomized phase III study of trastuzumab, paclitaxel, and carboplatin compared with trastuzumab and paclitaxel in women with HER-2-overexpressing metastatic breast cancer. *J Clin Oncol* 2006;24:2786-2792.

158. Pegram MD, Pienkowski T, Northfelt DW, et al. Results of two open-label, multicenter phase II studies of docetaxel, platinum salts, and trastuzumab in HER2-positive advanced breast cancer. *J Natl Cancer Inst* 2004;96:759-769.

159. Vogel C, Burris H, Limentani S, et al. A phase II study of trastuzumab-DM1, a HER2 antibody conjugate, in patients with HER2 metastatic breast cancer: Final Results. *J Clin Oncol* 2009;27: 15s (abstract 1017).

160. Blackwell KL, Pegram MD, Tan-Chiu E, et al. Single-agent lapatinib for HER2-overexpressing advanced or metastatic breast cancer that progressed on first- or second-line trastuzumab-containing regimens. *Ann Oncol* 2009;20: 1026-1031.

161. Burstein HJ, Storniolo AM, Franco S, et al. A phase II study of lapatinib monotherapy in chemotherapy-refractory HER2-positive and HER2-negative advanced or metastatic breast cancer. *Ann Oncol* 2008;19:1068-1074.

162. Gomez HL, Doval DC, Chavez MA, et al. Efficacy and safety of lapatinib as first-line therapy for ErbB2-amplified locally advanced or metastatic breast cancer. *J Clin Oncol* 2008;26:2999-3005.

163. Geyer CE, Forster J, Lindquist D, et al. Lapatinib plus capecitabine for HER2-positive advanced breast cancer. *N Engl J Med* 2006; 355:2733-2743.

164. Lin NU, Dieras V, Paul D, et al. Multicenter phase II study of lapatinib in patients with brain metastases from HER2-positive breast cancer. *Clin Cancer Res* 2009;15: 1452-1459.

165. Konecny GE, Pegram MD, Venkatesan N, et al. Activity of the dual kinase inhibitor lapatinib (GW572016) against HER-2-overexpressing and trastuzumab-treated breast cancer cells. *Cancer Res* 2006;66:1630-1639.

166. Blackwell K, Burstein H, Sledge G, et al. Updated survival analysis of a randomized study of lapatinib alone or in combination with trastuzumab in women with HER2-Positive metastatic breast cancer progressing on trastuzumab therapy. *Cancer Research* 2009;69(24):499s.

167. Chu I, Blackwell K, Chen S, et al. The dual ErbB1/ErbB2 inhibitor, lapatinib (GW572016), cooperates with tamoxifen to inhibit both cell proliferation- and estrogen-dependent gene expression in antiestrogen-resistant breast cancer. *Cancer Res* 2005;65:18-25.

168. Johnston S, Pegram M, Press M, et al. Lapatinib combined with letrozole vs. letrozole alone for front line postmenopausal hormone receptor positive metastatic breast cancer: first results from the EGF30008 trial. *Breast Cancer Res Treat* 2008;102 (suppl; abstract 46).

169. Di Leo A, Gomez HL, Aziz Z, et al. Phase III, double-blind, randomized study comparing lapatinib plus paclitaxel with placebo plus paclitaxel as first-line treatment for metastatic breast cancer. *J Clin Oncol* 2008;26:5544-5552.

170. Miller KD, Chap LI, Holmes FA, et al. Randomized phase III trial of capecitabine compared with bevacizumab plus capecitabine in patients with previously treated metastatic breast cancer. *J Clin Oncol* 2005;23:792-799.

171. Miller K, Wang M, Gralow J, et al. Paclitaxel plus bevacizumab versus paclitaxel alone for metastatic breast cancer. *N Engl J Med* 2007;357:2666-2676.

172. Brufsky A BI, Smirnov V, Hurvitz S, et al. RIBBON-2: A randomized, double-blind, placebo-controlled, phase III trial evaluating the efficacy and safety of bevacizumab in combination with chemotherapy for second-line treatment of HER2-negative metastatic breast cancer. *Cancer Research* 2009;69(24):495s.

173. Miles DW CA, Romieu G, Dirix LY et al. Final overall svival (OS) results from the randomised, double-blind, placebo-controlled, phase III AVADO study of bevacizumab (BV) plus docetaxel (D) compared with placebo (PL) plus D for the first-line treatment of locally recurrent (LR) or metastatic breast cancer (mBC). *Cancer Research* 2009;69(24):495s.

174. Robert N, Dieras V, Glaspy J, et al. RIBBON-1: randomized, double-blind, placebo-controlled, phase III trial of chemotherapy with or without bevacizumab (B) for first-line treatment of HER2-negative locally recurrent or metastatic breast cancer (MBC). *J Clin Oncol* 2009;27:15s (suppl; abstract 1005).

175. Clezardin P. The antitumor potential of bisphosphonates. *Semin Oncol* 2002;29:33-42.

176. Green JR, Clezardin P. Mechanisms of bisphosphonate effects on osteoclasts, tumor cell growth, and metastasis. *Am J Clin Oncol* 2002;25:3S-9S.

177. Ali SM, Esteva FJ, Hortobagyi G, et al. Safety and efficacy of bisphosphonates beyond 24 months in cancer patients. *J Clin Oncol* 2001;19:3434-3437.

178. Berenson JR, Rosen LS, Howell A, et al. Zoledronic acid reduces skeletal-related events in patients with osteolytic metastases. *Cancer* 2001;91:1191-1200.

179. Gordon MN, King DL, Diamond DM, et al. Correlation between cognitive deficits and Abeta deposits in transgenic APP+PS1 mice. *Neurobiol Aging* 2001;22:377-385.

180. Harbour JW, Brantley MA, Jr., Hollingsworth H, et al. Association between posterior uveal melanoma and iris freckles, iris naevi, and choroidal naevi. *Br J Ophthalmol* 2004;88:36-38.

181. Hortobagyi GN, Theriault RL, Lipton A, et al. Long-term prevention of skeletal complications of metastatic breast cancer with pamidronate. Protocol 19 Aredia Breast Cancer Study Group. *J Clin Oncol* 1998;16:2038-2044.

182. Hortobagyi GN, Theriault RL, Porter L, et al. Efficacy of pamidronate in reducing skeletal complications in patients with breast cancer and lytic bone metastases. Protocol 19 Aredia Breast Cancer Study Group. *N Engl J Med* 1996; 335:1785-1791.

183. Lewis JL, Marley SB, Ojo M, et al. Opposing effects of PI3 kinase pathway activation on human myeloid and erythroid progenitor cell proliferation and differentiation in vitro. *Exp Hematol* 2004;32:36-44.

184. Rosen LS, Gordon D, Kaminski M, et al. Zoledronic acid versus pamidronate in the treatment of skeletal metastases in patients with breast cancer or osteolytic lesions of multiple myeloma: a phase III, double-blind, comparative trial. *Cancer J* 2001;7:377-387.

185. Rosen LS, Gordon DH, Dugan W, Jr., et al. Zoledronic acid is superior to pamidronate for the treatment of bone metastases in breast carcinoma patients with at least one osteolytic lesion. *Cancer* 2004;100:36-43.

186. Theriault RL, Lipton A, Hortobagyi GN, et al. Pamidronate reduces skeletal morbidity in women with advanced breast cancer and lytic bone lesions: a randomized, placebo-controlled trial. Protocol 18 Aredia Breast Cancer Study Group. *J Clin Oncol* 1999;17:846-854.

187. Diel IJ, Solomayer EF, Costa SD, et al. Reduction in new metastases in breast cancer with adjuvant clodronate treatment. *N Engl J Med* 1998;339:357-363.

188. Saarto T, Blomqvist C, Virkkunen P, et al. Adjuvant clodronate treatment does not reduce the frequency of skeletal metastases in node-positive breast cancer patients: 5-year results of a randomized controlled trial. *J Clin Oncol* 2001; 19:10-17.

189. Powles T, Paterson S, Kanis JA, et al. Randomized, placebo-controlled trial of clodronate in patients with primary operable breast cancer. *J Clin Oncol* 2002;20:3219-3224.

190. Lin AY, Park JW, Scott J, et al. Zoledronic acid as adjuvant therapy for women with early stage breast cancer and disseminated tumor cells in bone marrow. *Proc Am Soc Clin Oncol* 2008;26 (abstract 559).

191. Gnant M, Mlineritsch B, Schippinger W, et al. Endocrine therapy plus zoledronic acid in premenopausal breast cancer. *N Engl J Med* 2009;360:679-691.

192. Cristofanilli M, Schiff R, Valero V. Exploratory subset analysis according to prior endocrine treatment of two randomized phase II trials comparing gefitinib with placebo in combination with tamoxifen or anastrozole in hormone receptor-positive metastatic breast cancer. *J Clin Oncol* 2009; 27:15s (abstract 1014).

193. Twelves C, Trigo J, Jones R, et al. Erlotinib in combination with capecitabine and docetaxel in patients with metastatic breast cancer: a dose-escalation study. *Eur J Cancer* 2008; 44:419-426.

194. Burstein H, Elias A, Rugo H, et al. Phase II study of sunitinib malate, an oral multitargeted tyrosine kinase inhibitor, in patients with metastatic breast cancer previously treated with an anthracycline and taxane. *J Clin Oncol* 2008;26: 1810-1816.

195. Mayer E, Kozloff M, Qamar R, et al. SABRE-B: A randomized phase II trial evaluating the safety and efficacy of combining sunitinib with paclitaxel and bevacizumab as first-line treatment for HER2-negative metastatic breast cancer: final results. *Breast Cancer Res Treat* 2008;102 (abstract 3126).

196. Barrios C, Liu M-C, Lee S, et al. Phase III randomized trial of sunitinib (SU) vs. capecitabine (C) in patients (Pts) with previously treated HER2-negative advanced breast cancer (ABC). *Cancer Research* 2009;69(24):497s.

197. Baselga J, Roché H, Costa F, et al. SOLTI-0701: A multinational double-blind, randomized phase 2b study evaluating the efficacy and safety of sorafenib compared to placebo when administered in combination with capecitabine in patients with locally advanced or metastatic breast cancer (BC). *Cancer Research* 2009;69(24):497.

198. Gradishar W, Kaklamani V, Prasad Sahoo T, et al. Double-blind, randomized, placebo-controlled, phase 2b study evaluating the efficacy and safety of sorafenib (SOR) in combination with paclitaxel (PAC) as a first-line therapy in patients (pts) with locally recurrent or metastatic breast cancer (BC). *Cancer Research* 2009;69(24):496s.

199. Meric-Bernstam F, Gonzalez-Angulo A. Targeting the mTOR signaling network for cancer therapy. *J Clin Oncol* 2009; 27:2278-2287.

200. Lane H, Wood J, McSheehi P, et al. mTOR inhibitor RAD001 (everolimus) has antiangiogenic/vascular properties distinct from a VEGFR tyrosine kinase inhibitor. *Clin Cancer Res* 2009;15:1612-1622.

201. Chan S, Scheulen M, Johnston S, et al. Phase II study of temsirolimus (CCI-779), a novel inhibitor of mTOR, in heavily pretreated patients with locally advanced or metastatic breast cancer. *J Clin Oncol* 2006;23:5314-5322.

202. Chow L, Jassem J, Baselga J, et al. Phase III study of temsirolimus with letrozole or letrozole alone in postmenopausal women with locally advanced or metastatic breast cancer. *Breast Cancer Res Treat* 2006;97 (abstract 6091).

203. Schreiber V, Dantzer F, Ame JC, et al. Poly(ADP-ribose): novel functions for an old molecule. *Nat Rev Mol Cell Biol* 2006;7:517-528.

204. O'Shaughnessy J, Osborne C, Pippen J, et al. Efficacy of BSI-201, a poly (ADP-ribose) polymerase-1 (PARP1) inhibitor, in combination with gemcitabine/carboplatin in patients with metastatic triple negative cancer: results of a randomized phase II trial. *J Clin Oncol* 2009;27:18s (abstract 3).

205. Babiera GV, Rao R, Feng L, et al. Effect of primary tumor extirpation in breast cancer patients who present with stage IV disease and an intact primary tumor. *Ann Surg Oncol* 2006;13:776-782.

206. Khan SA, Stewart AK, Morrow M. Does aggressive local therapy improve survival in metastatic breast cancer? *Surgery* 2002;132:620-626; discussion 626-627.

207. Morrow M, Goldstein L. Surgery of the primary tumor in metastatic breast cancer: closing the barn door after the horse has bolted? *J Clin Oncol* 2006;24:2694-2696.

208. Rao R, Feng L, Kuerer HM, et al. Timing of surgical intervention for the intact primary in stage IV breast cancer patients. *Ann Surg Oncol* 2008;15:1696-1702.

209. Rapiti E, Verkooijen HM, Vlastos G, et al. Complete excision of primary breast tumor improves survival of patients with metastatic breast cancer at diagnosis. *J Clin Oncol* 2006;24:2743-2749.

INFLAMMATORY BREAST CANCER

Windy Marie Dean-Colomb
Massimo Cristofanilli

Inflammatory breast carcinoma (IBC) represents a rare but very aggressive subtype of breast cancer. It is a clinicopathologic entity that is characterized by distinct skin changes suggestive of infection or inflammation, usually of fairly abrupt onset and rapid progression. The breast often appears red, swollen, and inflamed, hence the term *inflammatory breast cancer*. Since IBC has historically been a clinical diagnosis, its true incidence has been hard to quantify based in large part on a lack of consensus about a case definition for IBC. Acknowledging variations in the case definitions for IBC in population-based registries, it is estimated that IBC accounts for almost 2% of all breast cancer cases here in the United States (1).

Because of its unique appearance, IBC has often been confused with locally advanced breast cancer (LABC). However, emerging epidemiologic and molecular evidence indicates that IBC is not a part of the spectrum of LABC, but is in fact a separate entity (2). Furthermore, a distinction must be made between primary IBC, which is the simultaneous development of inflammatory skin changes and carcinoma in a previously healthy breast, and secondary IBC, which is the development of inflammatory changes in a breast known to have had a prior malignancy; the outcomes from these two diseases are quite different. Patients with primary IBC usually have a relatively short duration of symptoms prior to diagnosis, usually less than 3 months. Patients that have had symptoms for more than 3 months are a more heterogeneous group and include patients with previous non-IBC that develop a new primary tumor or recurrence with clinical characteristics of IBC.

■ EPIDEMIOLOGY

INCIDENCE

Worldwide, the incidence of IBC appears to be higher than in the United States, ranging from 2.1% in Turkey to as high as 50% in Tunisia (3). In fact, much of the information about IBC was initially derived from studies in Tunisia where about half of the breast cancer cases were attributed to IBC (4). More recent and updated data from Tunisia and other North African Countries now suggest a lower incidence using the criteria of the American Joint Commission for Cancer (AJCC) (5). Data from the National Cancer Institute's Surveillance, Epidemiology, and End Results (SEER) program demonstrate that while there has been a steady decline in non-IBC in general in the United States, the incidence of

IBC has been on the rise over the last three decades. From 1973 to 2002, IBC has increased at an annual rate ranging from 1.23 to 4.35% per year, depending on the specific database analyzed and the case definition (1,3,6).

MORTALITY

IBC is an aggressive and usually lethal form of breast cancer. Women diagnosed with IBC have statistically significantly poorer survival than women with either LABC or non-T4 breast cancer ($p < 0.001$), with a median overall survival (OS) of 2.9 years (1,11). Additionally, although IBC accounted for only 2.5% of all breast cancer cases in the period 1988 to 2000, it led to 7% of all breast cancer–specific deaths during that timeframe (1).

As with non-IBC, overall mortality rates for IBC have been declining. A modest trend for improved survival (8.4 months) was noted from 1988 to 1999 in a study reported by Hance et al. (1) This trend toward improved survival is supported by retrospective data from the University of Texas, MD Anderson Cancer Center (MDACC). We reviewed the outcomes of 635 patients with locally advanced breast cancer, including IBC, with a median follow-up of 90 months. The 2-year OS rates of a historical control group of 178 patients treated with anthracycline-based protocols compared with patients treated on a paclitaxel-containing regimen were 71 and 74%, respectively. This suggested a marginal, but not statistically significant, difference in favor of the paclitaxel-containing regimen (7). The trend in decreasing mortality from IBC may also be related to increasing awareness of IBC, resulting in earlier diagnosis, and the use of more effective multimodality treatments.

However, mortality rates from IBC continue to be higher for African-American women with median survival for African-American women at 2.0 versus 2.9 years for their Caucasian counterparts ($p < .001$) (1). The early age at diagnosis and poor survival outcomes observed in African-American patients with IBC suggests that there are also race- or ethnicity-related biologic determinants of this disease.

EPIDEMIOLOGIC FACTORS

Despite limited epidemiologic data regarding IBC, several important epidemiologic factors have been associated with IBC. First, there is a higher incidence of IBC in African Americans compared to other ethnic groups, with African Americans having at least a 50% higher incidence than whites (3.1 versus 2.2 per 100,000 woman-years, $p < .001$) (1). Second, age of onset also varies according to race or ethnicity with African Americans having a younger age at onset (median 55.2 versus 58.1 years) and a poorer prognosis when compared with Caucasians. Of note, Hispanic women have the youngest mean age of onset of the disease (median 50.5 years) (8).

IBC appears to develop at a younger age (median 57 years) compared with non-IBC (61.9 years). There are also differences between genders and age of onset with men usually diagnosed 10 years later than women (median 66.5 versus 57 years, $p < .001$) (3). Geographic variations for IBC have also been noted. Using the SEER program registries from 1992 to 2002, rates ranged from 2.064 per 100,000 woman-years in Jose-Monterey up to 3.042 cases per 100,000 in Los Angeles (3). Tumor-specific factors include a higher tumor grade, an equal proportion of estrogen receptor–positive and –negative tumors and an increased incidence of IBC over time, which is in contrast to the decrease observed in non-IBC (1).

■ RISK FACTORS

Identifying risk factors associated with the development of IBC has been challenging. However, when studies involving IBC are combined with studies involving rapidly developing breast cancer, which includes some cases of IBC, several interesting findings emerge (Table 26-1).

FAMILY HISTORY

While clearly established risk factors have been associated with the development of non-IBC, this is not the case with IBC, which is much less frequent and not consistently defined. For example, while family history, menopausal status, and age at menarche are important risk factors for non-IBC, they have not been consistently established as risk factor for the development of IBC. In a study analyzing 68 patients with IBC and

TABLE 26-1	RISK FACTORS ASSOCIATED WITH THE DEVELOPMENT OF INFLAMMATORY BREAST CANCER

- Early age at first birth
- Pregnancy/lactation
- Increased body mass index
- Blood type A
- Rural residency

143 patients with non-IBC seen at MDACC, 13% of IBC patients reported a positive family history of breast cancer, compared with 8% of non-IBC patients; this was not statistically significant (9). However, in a Pakistani study, 20% of patients with IBC reported a positive family history of breast cancer, compared to 5% in the non-IBC group, which was statistically significant (10).

REPRODUCTIVE HISTORY

Although IBC is diagnosed at a younger age than non-IBC, there does not appear to be a consistent association between IBC and premenopausal status. Of the patients evaluated at MDACC, 49% of IBC patients were premenopausal compared to 39% of non-IBC patients (9). But again, in the Pakistani study, no significant difference in menopausal status was noted (10). Thus, larger studies will be required to establish relationships between IBC and menopausal status.

Early age at first birth has also been associated with the development of IBC. Women with aggressive breast cancer, including IBC, are more likely to have their first child before the age of 20 when compared to patients with non-aggressive breast cancer (3). In a study of Tunisian patients with IBC as defined by the *Poussée Évolutive* (PEV) System described later in the chapter, 14 out of 15 premenopausal women diagnosed with IBC had their first births at the age of 18 or earlier (11). These data are weakly supported by our study, in which the lowest median age at first birth was seen among the IBC patients, although this was not statistically significant (9).

Many studies have also reported an association of IBC with pregnancy and/or lactation. Although not observed in the MDACC cohort, several other studies from Tunisia and the United States have supported this association. IBC accounts for approximately 21 to 26% of breast cancer cases in patients that developed breast cancer during or after pregnancy (11-13) No association between oral contraceptive use and development of IBC has been found (9).

BODY MASS INDEX, BLOOD TYPE, AND GEOGRAPHIC LOCATION

Body mass index (BMI) and the risk of developing IBC has also been studied. Usually, a high BMI is associated with an increased risk of postmenopausal non-IBC. We were among the first to evaluate the association between IBC and high BMI. In our initial study, a case-comparison between patients with IBC and non-IBC, patients with IBC were heavier (median weight 77.6 kg) than those with non-IBC (70.0 kg) or those having no history of breast cancer (68.0 kg) (9). Additionally, after adjusting for other factors, women with the highest BMI (>26 kg/m^2) had an increased risk for development of IBC when compared to those with non-IBC (odds ratio 2.54). This was irrespective of menopausal status, age at menarche, or family history of breast cancer.

We also evaluated whether obesity and menopausal status had an impact on IBC survival in a cohort of 177 female IBC patients seen from 1974 to 1993 at MDACC. After adjusting for axillary lymph node involvement and chemotherapy protocol, a modifying effect of menopausal status at diagnosis was noted on the association between obesity and IBC survival ($p = .02$) (14). Relative to postmenopausal women, premenopausal women had significantly worse survival (HR = 1.51). After stratifying by menopausal status, premenopausal obese women had non-significantly better survival than their leaner premenopausal counterparts (HR = 0.63) while postmenopausal obese women had significantly worse survival than their leaner counterparts (HR = 1.86). These findings suggest that factors associated with larger body size at diagnosis may contribute to shorter IBC survival among postmenopausal women but not premenopausal women, who were found to have poorer survival regardless of body size.

Finally, we retrospectively evaluated the association and prognostic value of BMI at the time of initial diagnosis in 602 patients with LABC, which included a subset with IBC (18%). Obese patients were more commonly associated with a diagnosis of IBC compared with overweight and normal or underweight groups ($p = 0.01$) (15). Additionally, patients with LABC who were obese or overweight had a significantly worse overall survival (OS) and relapse-free survival (RFS), and a higher incidence of visceral recurrence compared with normal/underweight patients. In a multivariable model, BMI remained significantly associated with both OS and RFS for the entire cohort. The interactions between BMI and LABC subsets and between BMI and menopausal status were not statistically significant.

Other factors that have been associated with the development of IBC include blood type and area of residence. A higher proportion of Tunisian patients with IBC have blood type A. Additionally, a larger proportion of them live in rural locations (11). Smoking and alcohol use were not associated with a risk of developing IBC (9).

IMMUNOLOGIC FACTORS

Given its rapid progression and its clinicopathologic appearance, there have been efforts to identify immunologic factors that may be important in the development of IBC. Delayed hypersensitivity studies have shown that IBC is not due to immune deficiency (16). However, in Tunisian patients, a hyperimmune response has been noted in patients with rapidly progressive breast cancer (17).

Additionally, 81% of tumors from patients with PEV3 (ie, clinicopathologic IBC) in Tunisia, were positive for a variant of the mouse mammary tumor virus (MMTV). The percentage of patients with breast cancer in Tunisia who were MMTV-positive were two-fold higher than those here in the United States (74 versus 36%) (18). While these data are alarming, these results are from cases diagnosed in the late 1970s, when the incidence of IBC in this population was reported to be as high as 55% (4,11). More recent studies have shown that, as the incidence of IBC had declined in this population, so has the prevalence of MMTV-positive cancer cases (19). The relationship between MMTV and IBC is currently being investigated here in the United States.

■ PATHOLOGICAL ASPECTS OF INFLAMMATORY BREAST CANCER

The cancer we currently define as primary IBC was first described in 1814 by Sir Charles Bell who noted a condition where "a purple color on the skin over the tumor accompanied by shooting pains is a very unpropitious beginning" (20). However, the term "Inflammatory Carcinoma of the Breast" (ie, IBC) was not coined until 1924 when Lee and Tannenbaum noted that "as the disease progresses, the skin becomes deep red or reddish-purple, and to the touch is brawny and infiltrated (21).

Despite the very early clinical identification of IBC, the clinical case definition of this disease has continued to be debated. Since 1924, several definitions for IBC have emerged. Over time, the definition of IBC has evolved with the eventual proposal of three subtypes of IBC: (1) clinicopathologically apparent IBC, (2) clinically apparent IBC, and (3) pathologic (ie, occult) IBC. Of note, two population-based studies using this classification for IBC show that patients with "occult IBC" have a better OS than patients with clinically apparent IBC (22,23).

MACROSCOPIC PATHOLOGY

The classic criterion for diagnosis of IBC established by Haagensen in 1971 included diffuse erythema and edema involving more than two-thirds of the breast, tenderness, induration, warmth, enlargement, and a diffuse tumor revealed on palpation (24). Indeed, the gross pathology of IBC tends to correspond with its clinical characteristics. One of the commonly described changes associated with IBC is erythema. The extent of the erythema can vary from merely a flush of pink to red to bronze. Comparison with the contralateral, unaffected breast is therefore important to clearly identify the erythema (Fig. 26-1A-B). The erythema may also be associated with a sensation of heat in the affected breast.

Subsequently, the breast begins to enlarge rapidly, sometimes increasing in size two- to three-fold in a period of a few weeks. The thickening of the skin is usually significant and can measure up to 1 cm. The increased size of the breast is the result of edema caused by obstruction of the lymphatic channels. The edema is associated with exaggerated hair follicle pits, causing a characteristic orange peel (*peau d'orange*) appearance to the skin.

In African and African-American women, where erythema may be more difficult to distinguish, *peau d'orange* changes may be easier to identify (Fig. 26-1C).

It is important to mention that the rapid rate of progression, along with the diffuse erythema of more than one-third of the skin overlying the breast, should be used as criteria to distinguish IBC from neglected locally advanced breast cancer with skin involvement. These gross skin changes associated with IBC become less prominent following neoadjuvant chemotherapy.

MICROSCOPIC PATHOLOGY

In conjunction with the clinical features associated with IBC, several histopathological features have also been identified. Histologically, IBC does not correspond to any specific breast carcinoma subtype. IBC tumors are generally characterized by higher-grade, ductal-type breast tumors with significant angiolymphatic invasion (25). In 1887, Thomas Bryant observed that the marked swelling of the breast and inflammatory signs were probably related to tumor invasion of the dermal lymphatics causing obstruction (Fig. 26-1D) (26). In fact

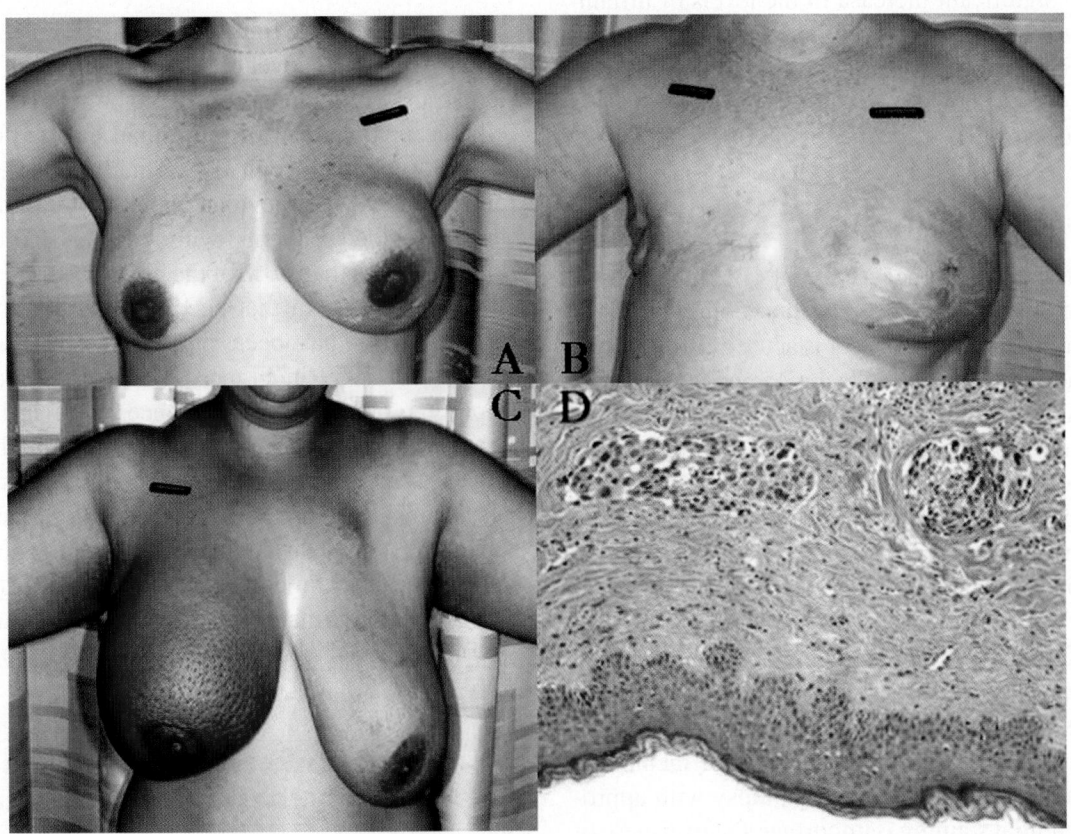

FIGURE 26-1. Clincal appearance of inflammatory breast cancer. **A.** Erythema and enlargement noted when compared to normal breast; **B.** Diffuse erythema of the left breast in a woman with prior history of right breast cancer. **C.** Peau d'orange appearance of the skin of the right breast. **D.** Photomicrograph of breast biopsy from a woman with inflammatory breast cancer showing normal appearing epidermis (bottom of figure) with tumor cells infiltrating the lymphatic channels of the dermis.

dermal lymphatic invasion (DLI) was considered to offer "pathologic proof" of IBC (27). However, in 1974, Saltzstein described a form of IBC he identified as "clinically occult inflammatory carcinoma of the breast" in which DLI was pathologically present, but there was no clinical signs of IBC (28). Nonetheless, although the presence of DLI is the histological hallmark of IBC and responsible for the clinical inflammatory signs of IBC invasion, it is not required for diagnosis.

The metastatic potential of IBC has been attributed to DLI and the molecular basis for DLI has been evaluated in several studies. E-cadherin overexpression appears to contribute to the development of this condition. E-cadherin in normally thought to be a tumor suppressor protein, with its loss associated with disease progression in most malignancies. However, in IBC, overexpression of E-cadherin has been shown to be necessary for tumor emboli formation by enhancing tumor cell-cell contact (29).

Its rapid onset, progression, and name, all suggest an inflammatory process as part of the underlying cause of IBC. However, infiltration of the affected breast tissue by inflammatory cells is rare. Moreover, there is no significant increase in the levels of inflammatory cytokines produced by the tumor cells. In fact, similar mRNA expression levels for the more common inflammatory cytokines were noted in both IBC and non-IBC tumors (30).

DIFFERENTIAL DIAGNOSIS

The aggressive and lethal nature of IBC calls for its early and accurate diagnosis. The most common misdiagnosis for inflammatory cancer is acute mastitis (AM). This condition occurs during lactation and is characterized by acute inflammation of the breast, with swelling, redness, and breast pain. Mastitis usually resolves in several days, but if left untreated, mastitis may become a breast abscess requiring surgical drainage. Thus, the acute nature, along with the clinical scenario and other constitutional symptoms, should help in distinguishing IBC from mastitis. Other infectious entities that can mimic IBC include erysipelas, which is usually caused by group A streptococcus.

Various other cancers can also mimic IBC, including LABC, sarcoma, inflammatory metastatic melanoma and lymphoma. In these instances, biopsy with appropriate differential staining is important. Paget disease of the nipple can also mimic IBC, but generally develops more slowly and is usually associated with destruction of the nipple. Radiation dermatitis, in its acute phase, may also appear to be IBC, however, desquamation of the skin usually occurs with resolution of skin changes in 2 to 3 weeks.

■ STAGING OF INFLAMMATORY BREAST CANCER

TUMOR-NODE-METASTASES (TNM) SYSTEM

In the United States, the most widely used case definition for IBC is that of the AJCC which states that "inflammatory carcinoma is a clinicopathologic entity characterized by diffuse erythema and edema of the breast (*peau d'orange*), often without an underlying mass. These clinical findings should involve the majority of the breast. Involvement of the dermal lymphatics alone does not indicate inflammatory carcinoma in the absence of clinical findings" (31). Based upon this definition, IBC is designated as a T4d tumor in TNM classification (32). Thus patients with IBC will have at least stage IIIB disease (Table 26-2).

POUSSÉE ÉVOLUTIVE (PEV) SYSTEM

While the AJCC definition of IBC is clinically appropriate, it does not cover the entire spectrum of IBC since it restricts the diagnosis of IBC to only those cases with clinical involvement of more than half the breast and does not include occult IBC. This limited definition is problematic since previous population-based registries have included patients with occult IBC or tumors involving less than 50% of the breast (1,8,33).

Thus, a system that encompasses the entire spectrum of IBC has been proposed. This system was devised in 1959 in France in an effort to describe a rapidly progressive breast cancer with inflammatory features (Table 26-2). Using this French PEV breast cancer classification, PEV2 (inflammatory signs involving less than half the breast) and PEV3 (inflammatory signs involving more than half the breast) would coincide with IBC here in the United States. When utilizing this classification, approximately 50% of the breast cancer cases in Tunisia have been attributed to IBC (11,34).

■ MOLECULAR DETERMINANTS OF INFLAMMATORY BREAST CANCER

Notwithstanding the obstacles noted in making a clinical diagnosis of IBC, our knowledge of the molecular basis of IBC has expanded tremendously in the past several decades. Development of in vivo and in vitro

TABLE 26-2 | CLASSIFICATION SYSTEMS USED IN THE DIAGNOSIS OF INFLAMMATORY BREAST CANCER

A. *POUSSÉE ÉVOLUTIVE* (PEV) CLASSIFICATION

Tumor Classification	Definition
T4	Any size tumor growing into the chest wall or affecting the skin
T4a	Extension of tumor to the chest wall
T4b	Edema (including peau d'orange), ulceration of the skin or satellite skin nodules confined to the same breast
T4c	Both 4a and 4b
T4d	Inflammatory breast carcinoma

B. *POUSSÉE ÉVOLUTIVE* (PEV) CLASSIFICATION

PEV Classification	Clinical Presentation
PEV-0	A tumor without recent increase in volume and without inflammatory signs
PEV-1	A tumor showing marked increase in volume during the previous 2 months but without inflammatory signs
PEV-2	A tumor in which breast tissue, particularly the skin, is affected by subacute inflammation and edema involving less than half of the breast surface
PEV-3*	A tumor with actue and subacute inflammation and edema involving more than half of the breast surface

TNM, tumor, nodes, metastasis.
*PEV-3 is equivalent to T4d AJCC classification for IBC.

models of IBC has also allowed for molecular profiling. This has led to the identification of two IBC signatures (30,35-38). While IBC shares some of the molecular characteristics associated with breast cancer in general, some very distinct differences have been noted. For example, as would be expected in highly aggressive tumors, IBC tumors are usually of higher grade (10). Additionally, IBC tumors are more likely to be estrogen receptor–negative when compared to non-IBC tumors (66 versus 36%) (39). Furthermore, overexpression of c-erB1/ ErbB1/EGFR and c-erB2/ErbB2/Her2-neu has been noted, with 42 to 57% of IBC tumors noted to be Her2-positive (40,41).

Not surprisingly, IBC is a very vascular tumor with overexpression of lymphangiogenic factors such as VEGF and Flt-4 (29,42). Additionally, a significantly higher intratumoral microvessel density has been reported in IBC tumors when compared to non-IBC tumors (43). Furthermore, increased expression of E-cadherin and non-sialylated mucin-1 (MUC1) have also been identified in IBC tumors. In one study, 100% of IBC tumors were positive for E-cadherin compared to 68% in non-IBC tumors (44). In another study using a xenograft model, a 10- to 20-fold increased expression of E-cadherin and MUC-1 was noted and thought to contribute to the passive dissemination of tumor

emboli in IBC (45). Dual overexpression of these two proteins in IBC is thought to play a role in the aggressive, invasive nature of this disease (46,47).

Studies evaluating p53 overexpression in IBC have also yielded interesting findings. In a study performed at MDACC evaluating 48 patients with IBC, p53 overexpression was noted in 58% of IBC tumors (48). In this study, patients who had p53 overexpression were found to have lower 5-year progression-free survival (PFS) rates (35 versus 55%; $p = .3$) and 5-year OS rates (44 versus 54%; $p = .4$). This is supported by another study in which p53 overexpression was also associated with a poorer prognosis, with an 8.6-fold increased risk of death in patients with IBC (49).

Other studies have described increased chromosomal instability in patients with IBC and resulted in the identification of two distinct genotypes of IBC (36). RhoC GTPase, a novel transforming oncogene in human mammary epithelial cells that partially mimic the inflammatory breast cancer phenotype has been shown to be overexpressed in IBC tumors more frequently than in non-IBC tumors (91 versus 38%) (50). The overexpression of RhoC GTPase has been associated with increased mRNA expression of cyclin D1, VEGF, fibronectin, and caveolin-2, proteins which are important in tumor invasion (50,51). It is believed that the

TABLE 26-3 | **SUMMARY OF POTENTIAL BIOLOGICAL TARGETS IN THE TREATMENT OF INFLAMMATORY BREAST CANCER**

Category	Molecular Marker	Agents
Oncogenes (40,41,51,100)	Her-2/neu	mAbs, TKIs
	EGFR	TKIs
	RhoC GTPase	FTIs
Tumor suppressor genes (10,48,49,101)	p53	Gene therapy, p53-stabilizing agents
	PTEN	Proteasome inhibitors, PI3K-inhibitors
Angiogenesis modulators (29,44,45,47)	Tie-2	Tie-2 kinase inhibitor
	VEGF	Angiogenesis inhibitors
	Flt-1/Flk-1	TKIs, mAbs
	E-cadherin	E-cadherin inhibitors
	MUC-1	MUC-1 inhibitors, PIAS
	RhoC GTPase	FTIs

FTIs, farnesyltransferase inhibitors; mAbs, monoclonal antibodies; MUC1, mucin-1; PIAS, protein inhibitor of activated signal transducer and activator of transcription; PI3K, phosphatidylinositol-3-kinase; TKIs, tyrosine kinases inhibitors; VEGF, vascular endothelial growth factor.

overexpression of RhoC GTPase, combined with the loss of WISP3/WINT-1, another tumor suppressor gene, is largely responsible for the aggressive phenotype of IBC (52). The expanded knowledge gained from these studies about the biological basis of IBC has resulted in several potential molecular targets for directed therapy (Table 26-3).

■ EVOLVING ROLE OF IMAGING MODALITIES IN INFLAMMATORY BREAST CANCER

Although IBC is a clinicopathologic entity, the use of modern imaging modalities has played a key role in the diagnosis and staging of this disease. In fact, multimodality imaging comprised of mammography, sonography, and magnetic resonance imaging is considered the minimal imaging needed to diagnose IBC, and to adequately stage it.

MAMMOGRAPHY

Mammographic findings in patients with IBC can be quite subtle, with the mammogram often read as "negative." In fact, in a retrospective analysis of various imaging modalities in the diagnosis of IBC, mammography was found to be the least sensitive and effective method, detecting only 43% of primary breast parenchymal lesions (53). The most common sign of IBC noted on mammogram is skin thickening (Fig. 26-2) (54). Although it is usually always present in patients with IBC, it is often missed on mammograms based on low

levels of suspicion. Diagnosis is often not made without comparison to the contralateral breast.

The most variable mammographic finding in patients with IBC is that of a visible mass. While often not visible on mammograms, a palpable mass has been reported in 82% of cases of IBC, calling into question the clinical diagnoses in those patients (see criteria for clinical diagnosis of IBC) (55). The lack of a visible mass on mammogram has been attributed to the increased density of the breast in patients with IBC, which often obscures the underlying mass. Calcifications are also less common in patients with IBC and typically only become apparent after therapy, when there has been a decrease in breast density (55). Furthermore, in some instances, the only mammographic finding of IBC may be that of axillary lymphadenopathy. This finding is often useful in distinguishing IBC from other breast abnormalities such as postradiation change.

In our retrospective study evaluating the mammographic findings of 26 women with IBC, 92% of them had skin thickening, 81% had diffusely increased breast tissue density, 62% had trabecular thickening, 58% had axillary lymphadenopathy, 50% had architectural distortion or focal asymmetric density, and 38% had nipple retraction.

ULTRASOUND

Information regarding the role of ultrasound in the diagnosis of IBC is limited. As with non-IBC, ultrasound is very useful in localizing sites for biopsy in patients with masses. In a series evaluating 142 women with histologically proven IBC, in contrast to mammography,

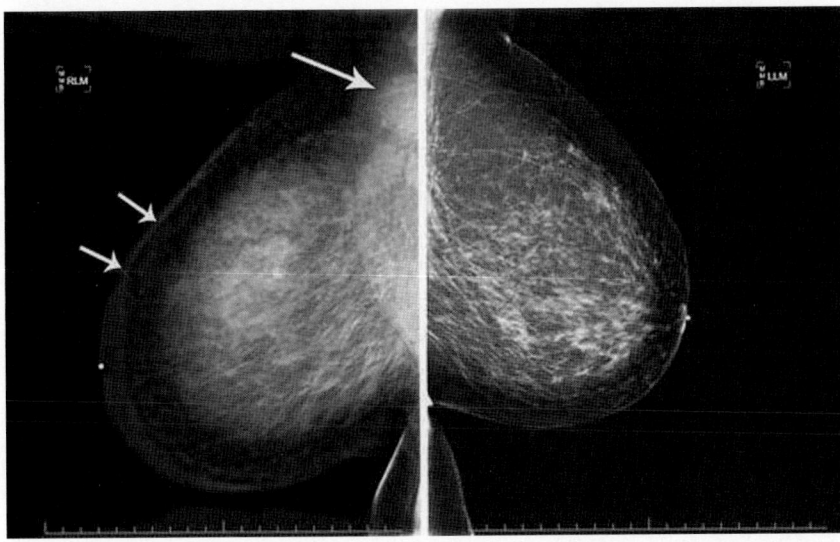

FIGURE 26-2. Bilateral mediolateral oblique mammograms in a 54-year-old female show global skin and trabecular thickening (short arrows) of the right breast with associated right axillary adenopathy (long arrow). No visible primary breast parenchymal lesion is noted in the right breast. *(Reproduced, with permission, from Yang WT, Le-Petross HT, Macapinlac H, et al. Inflammatory breast cancer: PET/CT, MRI, mammography, and sonography findings. Breast Cancer Res Treat 2008;109:417-426.)*

ultrasound was able to detect an additional 24 masses (18%) obscured by edema, when compared to mammogram alone (56). The greatest benefit of ultrasound may be its potential to provide comprehensive evaluation of the nodal stations and pectoral muscle invasion. In this same series, ultrasound was able to detect axillary lym-

phadenopathy in the majority (73%) of these patients and pectoral muscle invasion in 10%. These findings have been confirmed in our series, in which sonography found a parenchymal breast lesion and skin thickening in 95% of patients and regional axillary nodal disease in 93% of cases (Fig. 26-3) (54).

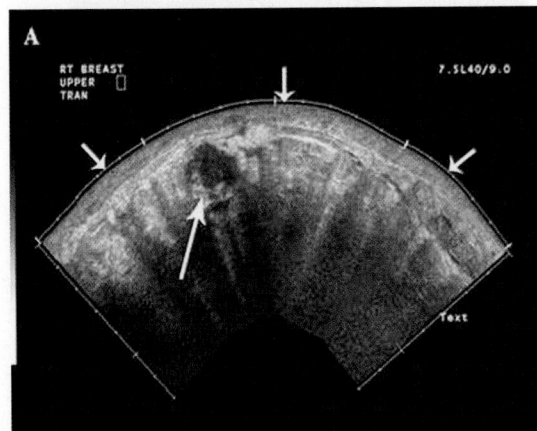

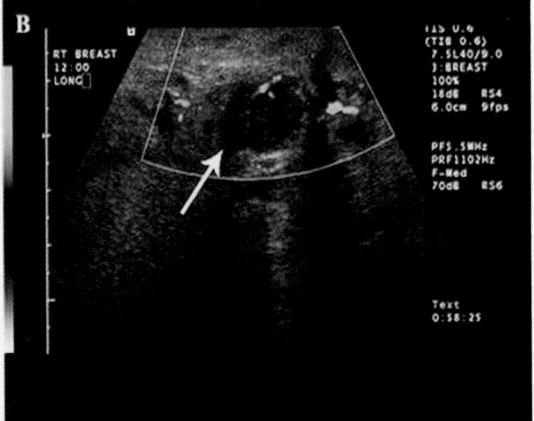

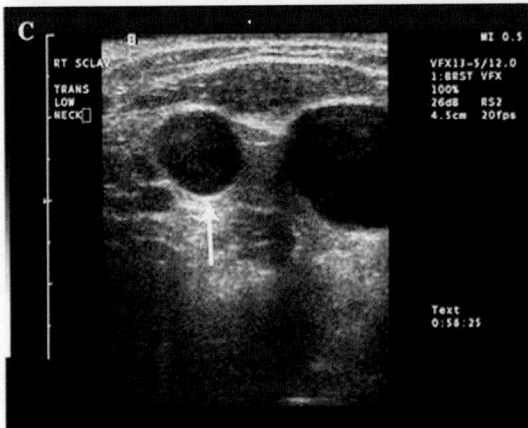

FIGURE 26-3. Ultrasound images of the right breast from patient described in Fig. 26-2. **(A)** Extended-field-of-view ultrasound of the right breast in the patient of Fig. 26-2 showing marked diffuse skin thickening and subcutaneous edema (short arrows) and a focal solid hypoechoic mass (long arrow) representing primary breast parenchymal lesion. **(B)** Transverse ultrasound with power Doppler imaging of the primary mass in the right breast shows marked internal hypervascularity. **(C)** Transverse ultrasound of the right supraclavicular region shows a solid hypoechoic node that showed metastatic carcinoma on biopsy. *(Reproduced, with permission, from Yang WT, Le-Petross HT, Macapinlac H, et al. Inflammatory breast cancer: PET/CT, MRI, mammography, and sonography findings. Breast Cancer Res Treat 2008;109:417-426.)*

MAGNETIC RESONANCE IMAGING

The use of magnetic resonance imaging (MRI) in the diagnosis of breast cancer has steadily increased over the past several decades based on its superior sensitivity and lack of ionizing radiation. However, only a few studies have evaluated its use in the diagnosis of IBC. Nevertheless, it is clear that MRI plays an important role in the diagnosis of IBC, with 90-100% of patients noted to have skin thickening on MRI and 75% of patients also having axillary lymphadenopathy (53,54,

57,58). A discreet mass could also be seen in up to 38% of the cases (57,59). Thus, MRI is considered by some to be the imaging modality of choice in the diagnosis of IBC (Fig. 26-4).

MRI use in differentiating between AM and IBC has also been evaluated. For the most part, the MRI findings with AM and IBC were very similar with edema and skin thickening noted in both (59,60). However, in a recent study evaluating 90 patients (48 with IBC and 42 with AM), MRIs of the breast were able to statistically

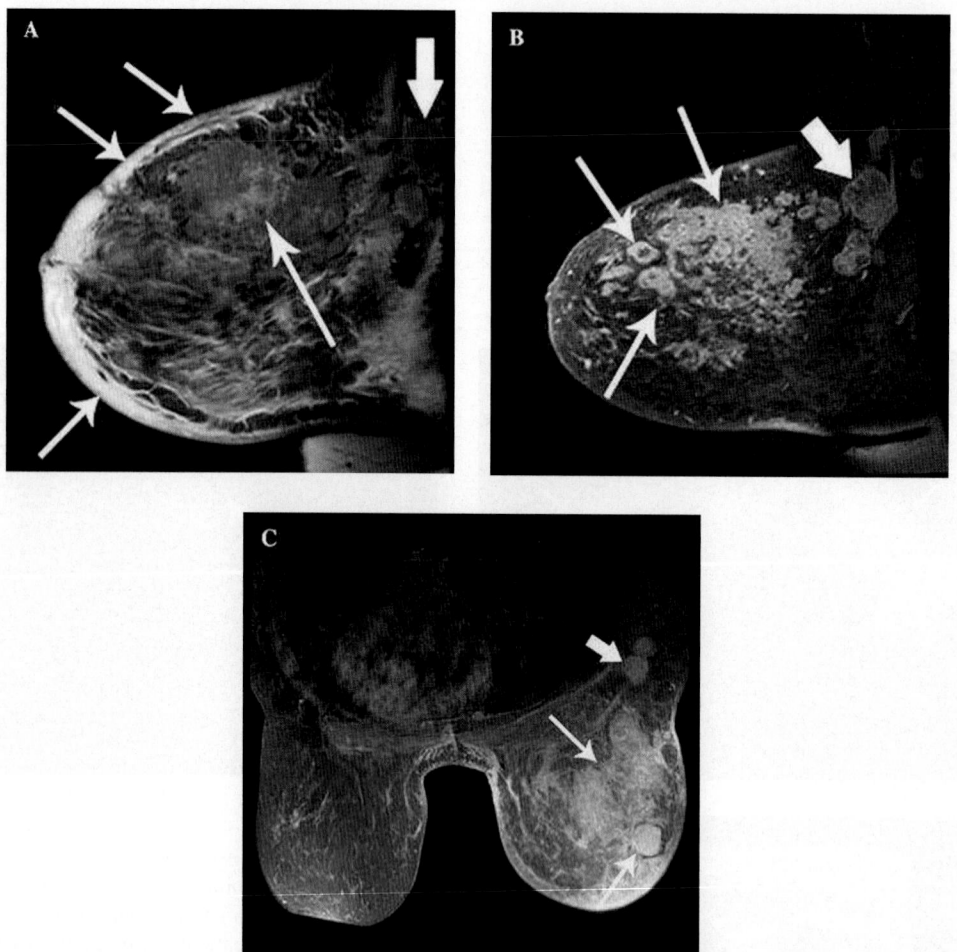

FIGURE 26-4. (A) Sagittal T2-weighted fast spin-echo image with fat suppression shows a dominant heterogeneous mass in the superior right breast (long arrow), global skin and subcutaneous edema (medium arrows), and right axillary adenopathy (broad arrow). (B) Sagittal fat suppressed 3D spoiled gradient-recalled-echo sequence with parallel imaging at 2 min post-contrast administration demonstrates multiple rim enhancing tumor masses (arrows) in the right breast and malignant-appearing necrotic right axillary lymph nodes (broad arrow). (C) Delayed axial fat suppressed contrast-enhanced 3D fast spoiled gradient-recalled echo MR image reveals multiple heterogeneously enhancing masses in the central and lateral right breast (arrows), and right axillary adenopathy (broad arrow). *(Reproduced, with permission, from Yang WT, Le-Petross HT, Macapinlac H, et al. Inflammatory breast cancer: PET/CT, MRI, mammography, and sonography findings. Breast Cancer Res Treat 2008;109:417-426.)*

detect more T2-hypodense masses, infiltration of pectoralis major muscle, and pectoralis edema (60). Additionally, MRI has been shown to be useful in follow-up of AM by evaluating success of antibiotic treatment and diagnosis of coexisting or confounding inflammatory carcinoma (59).

Breast MRI has also been used to monitor response to therapy with correlation with pathologic size ranging from 0.75 to 0.89 (61,62). Several studies have shown that pathologic complete response (pCR) was the strongest prognostic factor for IBC and in a recent study by Chen et al., the accuracy of complete clinical response on MRI to predict pCR was 69% (11 of 16), with a sensitivity of 58% (7 of 12), specificity of 92% (11 of 12), and a false-negative rate of 21% (5 of 24) (63). These results suggest that interpretation of and future treatment decisions based upon MRI findings should be done with extreme caution, especially in cases where no discrete mass was identified, since cases with no identifiable discrete mass accounted for 80% of the false-negative cases (4 of 5).

COMPUTERIZED TOMOGRAPHY

The utility of helical **computerized tomography** (CT) which provides high-resolution thin cuts has also been investigated in the diagnosis of IBC. In a study by Mogavero et al., as with MRI, skin thickening was found in 100% of the patients with IBC (Fig. 26-5). However, unlike mammography, axillary lymphadenopathy was

found in 82% of patients and distant metastases noted in 64% of patients (64). Helical CT has also been evaluated for its ability to monitor response to therapy in patients with IBC. When compared to clinical examination and mammography, breast helical CT was found to be very useful in the quantitative assessment of response to neoadjuvant chemotherapy and preoperative determination of residual tumor volume in patients with round opacities (correlation coefficients of 0.97) (65). However, it was not as reliable for tumors with diffuse, scattered or multinodular opacities (correlation coefficient 0.60). Thus some have been cautious about the role of helical CT in determining the extent of residual disease following neoadjuvant chemotherapy (66).

POSITRON EMISSION TOMOGRAPHY

The data regarding the role of **positron emission tomography** (PET) in the diagnosis of IBC is very limited. In one study that evaluated PET in seven patients with IBC, skin enhancement was noted in 100% of the patients, with axillary lymphadenopathy in 85%, and skeletal metastases in 14% (Fig. 26-6). Postchemotherapy PET scans performed in four patients showed response in the primary tumor, axillary lymph nodes, and skeletal metastases (67). Given that 20 to 35% of patients with IBC have distant metastases at the time of diagnosis, PET, and increasingly PET/CT may have a useful role in staging.

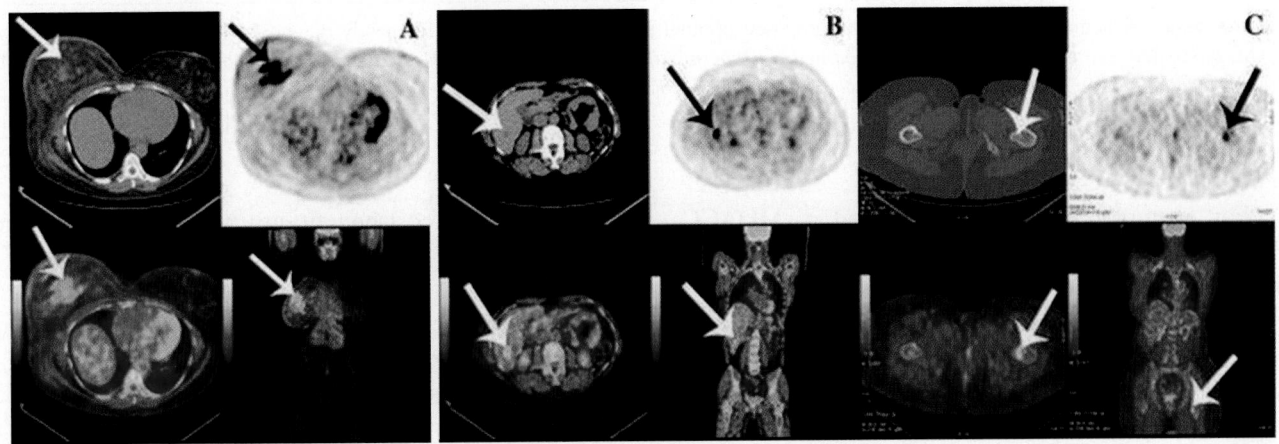

FIGURE 26-5. **(A)** PET/CT shows multicentric hypermetabolism in the right breast (arrow) associated with hypermetabolic diffuse skin thickening. **(B)** PET/CT shows a solitary focal hypermetabolic focus in the right lobe of the liver (arrows) that showed a maximum SUV of 5.7. Corresponding CT of the liver shows a focal hypoechoic mass with indistinct margins. **(C)** PET/CT shows a solitary focal hypermetabolic focus in the left proximal femur (arrows) that showed a maximum SUV of 7.7. Corresponding CT of the proximal femur shows this area of hypermetabolism to be within the marrow (whole body bone imaging was negative in this patient). *(Reproduced, with permission, from Yang WT, Le-Petross HT, Macapinlac H, et al. Inflammatory breast cancer: PET/CT, MRI, mammography, and sonography findings. Breast Cancer Res Treat 2008;109:417-426.)*

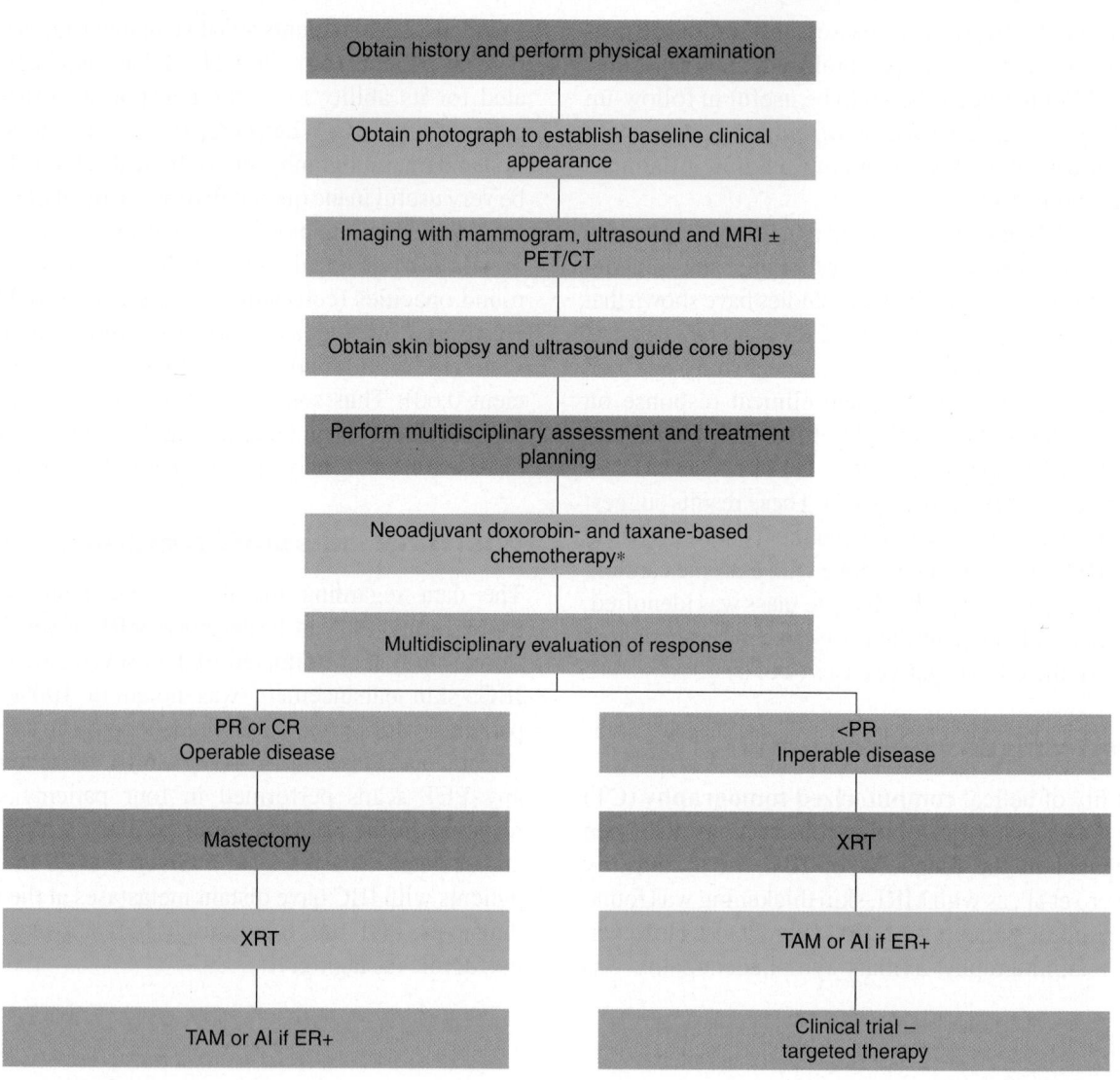

FIGURE 26-6. Schematic representation of the proposed optimal sequence of treatment for newly diagnosed IBC. XRT, radiotherapy; TAM, tamoxifen; AI, aromatase inhibitor. *(Modified, with permission, from Cristofanilli M, Buzdar AU, Hortobagyi GN: Update on the management of inflammatory breast cancer. Oncologist 8:141-8, 2003.)*

For example, in studies performed at MDACC, PET/CT was able to identify patients with distant metastases at diagnosis. In one study in which PET/CT was performed on 24 patients with IBC, 63% of patients were noted to have multicentric disease, 88% noted to have regional nodal disease, and 38% found to have distant metastases (53,54,58,68). In more recent studies, up to 98% of patients were found to have parenchymal breast lesions on PET/CT (54,58,68). Additionally, when PET/CT was used in initial staging of IBC, 17% more cases of distant metastases were identified in patients who were not previously known to have metastases (68). However, further studies are needed to

determine the cost-benefit utility of this diagnostic modality.

■ THE MULTIDISCIPLINARY TREATMENT OF INFLAMMATORY BREAST CANCER

There have been significant advances in the care of the IBC patients over the last 40 years. While once considered a uniformly fatal disease, with fewer than 5% of patients alive at 5 years, the introduction of primary system chemotherapy in combination with other treatment modalities has drastically altered the survival outcomes compared to locoregional treatments alone.

SURGERY

Historically, surgery was the primary modality for IBC, but it yielded poor results. In fact, the inadequacy of surgery to provide local control or increase survival was first noted in the 1920s when Lee and Tannenbaum observed an "almost immediate recurrence following radical surgery" for IBC, thus making them "certain of the inefficiency of surgery in this disease" (21). In a review article evaluating the efficacy of surgery in the treatment of IBC from 1924 to 1981, a median survival of 19.8 months was noted, with a 5-year OS less than 5% (69). Upfront surgery for IBC also provides poor local control with a local recurrence rate around 50% (21,70-72). As it became apparent that nearly all the patients with IBC died despite surgery, this treatment was abandoned. Thus, by the 1950s, the only indication for surgery was to establish a diagnosis with biopsy.

However, as multimodality treatment became the standard of care for patients with IBC, the role of surgery expanded (69). In a study examining the treatment of 485 patients with IBC, there was an increase in the use of mastectomy from 11 to 69%, with a concurrent decrease in the number of patients having no surgery from 67 to 22% (73). During this time the sequencing of surgery also changed with mastectomy occurring following neoadjuvant chemotherapy.

A more recent study of 178 women with IBC treated with neoadjuvant chemotherapy showed that the addition of mastectomy to combination chemotherapy plus radiotherapy improved local control in patients with IBC. Furthermore, the addition of mastectomy to chemotherapy plus radiotherapy improved distant disease-free survival (DFS) and OS in patients with a clinical complete response (CR) or partial response (PR) to induction chemotherapy (74). Patients are now considered candidates for a modified radical mastectomy when there has been complete resolution of inflammatory skin changes.

RADIOTHERAPY

Since initial studies indicated that IBC was not a disease amendable to surgical intervention, studies evaluating the benefit of radiation in local control emerged with radiotherapy alone being the treatment of choice (33). Although treatment with radiotherapy yielded better overall responses with 50% local control, which was the best rate reported at the time, survival was still poor with less than 5% of patients alive by 5 years (75). Even in more recent studies evaluating radiotherapy alone in the treatment of IBC, local control remains a problem. For example, in a 1980 study in which 62 patients with localized clinical IBC were treated with radiotherapy to the breast and draining lymphatics, 69% of the patients developed local and regional recurrence (76).

To improve these results, studies using different radiotherapy regimens were investigated. A team from MDACC was the first to use hyperfractionated radiotherapy in the treatment of IBC. Locoregional recurrence was decreased from 47% in patients with once-daily radiation therapy to 27% with twice-daily administration.

Other studies have shown improved survival with radiotherapy especially with the use of dose escalation. For example, at MDACC, in a study evaluating 115 nonmetastatic patients with IBC from 1977 to 1993 treated with curative intent, twice-daily postmastectomy radiation to a total dose of 66 Gy, resulted in significant improvements in rates of locoregional control ($p = 0.03$) and OS ($p = .03$), and a trend toward better DFS ($p = .06$) (77).

NEOADJUVANT CHEMOTHERAPY

Despite the ability of radiation therapy to provide some improvement in locoregional control, the development of distant metastatic disease has remained a challenge, and for many years, no standard chemotherapeutic regimen existed for IBC. The rarity and poor overall prognosis associated with IBC often resulted in these patients being excluded from most clinical trials. As a result, most patients with IBC were previously treated with regimens intended for those with non-IBC cancer. More recently, clinical trials of chemotherapy specifically designed for patients with IBC have been conducted. Importantly, based upon emerging data showing that response to neoadjuvant chemotherapy had prognostic significance, studies were designed using neoadjuvant chemotherapy in the treatment of IBC. For example, in a study evaluating 372 patients with LABC treated with a doxorubicin-containing regimen showed that neoadjuvant chemotherapy was able to completely clear the breast and axillary lymph nodes of invasive tumor before surgery. Furthermore, patients with LABC who have a pCR in the breast and axillary nodes have a significantly improved DFS rate (78). Therefore, treatment with doxorubicin-containing regimens in the

TABLE 26-4

SUMMARY OF CLINICAL RESPONSES IN FIVE CONSECUTIVE CLINICAL TRIALS CONDUCTED AT MDACC FOR PATIENTS WITH INFLAMMATORY BREAST CANCER (81-83,86)

Clinical Response	Protocol A N (%)	Protocol B N (%)	Protocol E N (%)	Protocol C N (%)	Protocol D N (%)
CR	6 (15)	3 (13)	3 (7)	9 (13)	3 (7)
PR	26 (65)	10 (44)	25 (58)	45 (63)	31 (70)
MR	6 (15)	8 (35)	11 (26)	13 (18)	0 (0)
SD	1 (3)	0 (0)	0 (0)	2 (3)	1 (2)
PD	1 (3)	2 (9)	0 (0)	1 (1)	6 (14)
N/A	0 (0)	0 (0)	4 (9)	2 (3)	3 (7)
Total	40 (100)	23 (100)	43 (100)	72 (100)	44 (100)

N/A, not applicable; PD, progressive disease.

neoadjuvant setting became the standard for treatment of IBC.

The largest experience to date on the systemic management of IBC comes from MDACC. From 1974 to 2001, we treated 242 IBC patients on clinical trials designed solely for this disease (Table 26-4). These trials established the need for neoadjuvant chemotherapy to improve DFS and OS in patients with IBC. Additionally, they showed that response to neoadjuvant chemotherapy was a surrogate marker of long-term outcome in patients with IBC. In a retrospective study examining 489 patients (7.5% with IBC) that received an anthracycline-based chemotherapy as their primary mode of treatment, patients with IBC were found to have lower RFS rates and a greater hazard of death than patients with clinical stage I/II/IIIA disease. Additionally, patients with IBC who failed to achieve CR with primary systemic chemotherapy also had decreased OS (79). Thus, not only did neoadjuvant chemotherapy become a mainstay in the treatment of IBC, but trials to identify the chemotherapeutic regimen that yielded the best pathological response were also begun.

Anthracyclines

Four consecutive protocols took place at MDACC between 1974 and 1993 (80-83). The first protocol evaluated the use of 5-fluorouracil, doxorubicin, and cyclophosphamide (FAC) as induction/neoadjuvant therapy, followed by radiation and further chemotherapy with FAC or cyclophosphamide, methotrexate, and 5-FU (CMF). A second protocol investigated the same induction regimen followed by mastectomy, adjuvant FAC, and radiation, while a third protocol investigated the addition of vincristine and prednisone to FAC (FACVP). Finally, a fourth study gave IBC patients induction

chemotherapy with FACVP and surgery followed by FACVP for those who had a CR after induction with FACVP. Patients who achieved a PR with a clinical reduction in tumor size of more than 50% received postoperative treatment with FACVP plus methotrexate and vinblastine (MV); those who achieved a minimal response (MR) of a 25 to 50% decrease in tumor size were treated postoperatively with MV alone.

The ORR for all four trials was 72%, with a 12% clinical CR rate. There were no significant differences in DFS or OS between the four protocols. Of note, the use of surgery did not alter the risk of local recurrence for those with poorly responsive disease. Results from the fourth protocol showed that the vincristine and prednisone and methotrexate and vinblastine had no effect on DFS or OS. Importantly, the rarity of IBC resulted in modest sample sizes for all four trials. Nevertheless, for all 178 patients treated on these protocols, the DFS ranged from 32% at 5 years to 28% at 15 years, with a median survival of 37 months.

A 20-year follow-up regarding these initial 178 patients reported by Ueno et al. showed among those patients with recurrence, 20% of patients had local failure, 39% systemic failure, and 9% CNS recurrence (83). Initial response to induction chemotherapy was found to be an important prognostic factor. DFS at 15 years was 44% in patients who had a CR to induction chemotherapy, 31% in those who had a partial response (PR), and 7% in those who had less than a PR. There was no improvement in OS or DFS among patients who underwent alternate chemotherapy (MV) compared with those who did not. Using surgery and radiotherapy as opposed to radiotherapy alone as local therapy did not have an impact on the DFS or OS rate.

These long-term follow-up data showed that with a combined-modality approach, a significant fraction of patients (28%) remained free of disease beyond 15 years compared to 5% following single-modality treatments. These findings have helped to establish combined-modality treatment (anthracycline-based neoadjuvant chemotherapy, then mastectomy, then adjuvant chemotherapy and radiotherapy) as the standard of care for treatment of inflammatory breast carcinoma.

Taxanes

The importance of achieving a pCR following neoadjuvant chemotherapy has been observed in patients with IBC as it has been for those with non-IBC. In a study of 175 patients with IBC that were treated with neoadjuvant chemotherapy, 61 were found to have residual disease in the axillary lymph nodes. These patients were noted to have a lower 5-year RFS (82.5 versus 37.1%) and OS (78.6 versus 25.4%) when compared to patients who attained a pCR. Thus, the significance of a pCR to induction chemotherapy as an important prognosticator of survival has led to the investigation of novel chemotherapeutic regimens that might increase pCR rates.

In 1994, a fifth protocol opened at MDACC, which evaluated the use of paclitaxel in the treatment of IBC. A total of 44 patients were enrolled. All patients were treated with FAC for induction and adjuvant chemotherapy. Paclitaxel was given preoperatively to those patients who achieved only a minimal response or stable disease after receiving FAC and it was delivered to all patients in the adjuvant setting. The treatment course consisted of neoadjuvant chemotherapy, mastectomy, adjuvant chemotherapy, and radiation therapy. While this approach was promising with higher objective response rates compared with the four prior trials (81 versus 72%) and better OS rates (46 versus 37 months), the results were not statistically significant (84).

Thus a sixth trial involving 18 IBC patients was begun, which was designed to determine the effect of FAC plus high-dose weekly paclitaxel as induction chemotherapy. Postoperative therapy then consisted of cyclophosphamide, etoposide, and cisplatin (CVP). This treatment was followed by bone marrow mobilization, high-dose chemotherapy with cyclophosphamide, carmustine (BCNU), and thiotepa, and subsequent peripheral blood stem cell support. Analysis of the data showed that 31% of patients achieved a clinical CR and 72% of patients proceeded to mastectomy (84).

More recently, a retrospective study evaluated the outcomes of 240 patients with IBC treated on these six MDACC protocols. Patients were stratified on the basis of whether they had received paclitaxel as part of either their induction or adjuvant chemotherapy. There was a trend toward an increased objective response rate (ORR) for the paclitaxel regimens (79%) compared with anthracycline-based therapy (72%) and increased 3-year OS rates (71 versus 53%, respectively). While, statistical significance was not reached in the general analysis, subset analysis of the ER-negative group of patients did reveal a significantly higher 3-year OS (54 versus 32 months, $p = .03$) and PFS (27 versus 18 months, $p = .04$). Additionally, a significantly higher pCR rate was noted with the addition of paclitaxel compared with treatment using FAC alone (25 versus 10%, $p = .012$) (85).

These results established the addition of paclitaxel to anthracycline-based therapy in the treatment of patients with ER-negative IBC. Furthermore, these results indicate that anthracyclines and taxanes are the most effective chemotherapeutic agents in the treatment of IBC, thus securing their use in the frontline setting.

MULTIMODALITY TREATMENT

As outcomes in patients with IBC began to improve following the introduction of primary systemic chemotherapy, combining this treatment with local therapies such as radiation therapy and surgery became more common. One of the first studies evaluating multimodality treatment of IBC was performed at MDACC. Thirty-two patients with inflammatory breast cancer were treated with a combined modality approach consisting of FAC, followed by radiation therapy and compared with 32 patients with inflammatory breast cancer treated with irradiation without systemic therapy at our institution in the past. After a median follow-up of 62 months (range 42-76 months), 11 patients in combined modality group and 3 patients in the irradiation group were free of disease. Overall median disease-free interval was 22.8 months for the combined modality group and 9 months for the irradiation group, with a median survival of 30.1 months and 18 months, respectively. In subgroup analysis, this treatment was effective in prolonging the disease-free interval and survival of patients greater than or equal to 50 years of age, with an estimated 45% of the patients surviving free of disease beyond 42 months. However, in patients <50 years old, although an improved disease-free interval was still noted, survival of this subgroup was not significantly improved (86).

To reexamine the benefit of surgery in IBC, Fleming et al. performed a retrospective analysis of 178 patients that had received multimodality treatment between 1974 and 1993. They found that the addition of mastectomy to combination chemotherapy plus radiotherapy improved local control, distant DFS and OS in IBC patients with a clinical complete or partial response to induction chemotherapy (74). These studies laid the foundation for the multimodality treatment for IBC (87).

As improved responses to chemotherapy in combination with local therapies were noted, questions regarding the best sequencing of these modalities emerged. Thus, studies were performed combining chemotherapy with radiation, with the addition of surgery, depending on response to chemotherapy. The efficacy of neoadjuvant chemotherapy was shown in a study that retrospectively examined 179 patients with nonmetastatic IBC treated with curative intent. Patients who received multimodality treatment with neoadjuvant chemotherapy, surgery, and radiation had a higher 5-year DFS (40%), when compared to patients who received only definitive radiation (6%), surgery with radiation (24%), or chemotherapy with radiation (6%) (88). Similar results were seen at 10 years and this improvement has been confirmed by other studies.

The use of high-dose chemotherapy (HDCT) supported by stem cell transplantation (SCT) as a component of multimodality therapy regimens has also been assessed. Several small phase II trials have shown a survival benefits for patients with IBC treated with HDCT with SCT. These trials generally reported 3 to 4 year OS rates of 52 to 89% and DFS rates of 45 to 65%, which were favorable compared to historical survival data with standard-dose chemotherapy (89-92). However, in the absence of definitive, prospective, randomized trials, the use of HDCT remains controversial.

■ MOLECULAR TARGETS OF INFLAMMATORY BREAST CANCER

With the identification of molecular determinants of IBCs, focus then turned to the introduction of novel biologic therapies to the primary systemic chemotherapy. The identification of Her2 overexpression in IBC soon led to the incorporation of trastuzumab, a humanized monoclonal antibody against Her2, to anthracycline/taxane-based chemotherapy regimes. To date, at least four prospective trials have added trastuzumab to primary systemic therapy in the treatment of IBC. In a study by Hurley et al., 48 patients with Her2-positive LABC (including IBC) were treated with docetaxel, cisplatin, and trastuzumab, followed by surgery, adjuvant chemotherapy, and radiation. An OS rate of 100% was noted in those who attained a pCR, compared to 76 to 83% for those who had residual disease (93).

In another study by of 22 patients with LABC, 9 of whom had IBC, treated with docetaxel and tratuzumab,

a complete response rate of 40% was observed (94). Other studies have yielded similar results, with pCR rates of 18 to 39% (95,96). Taken together, these studies showed that the addition of trastuzumab contributed to higher rates of pCR in patients with Her2-positive IBC. Encouraging results have also been obtained with lapatinib, a dual-action Her1 and Her2 tyrosine kinase inhibitor, in Her2-positive IBC. The combination of lapatinib and paclitaxel in 21 patients with Her2-positive IBC resulted in a 95% clinical response rate (97). These results are currently undergoing prospective validation.

Several other novel agents have been or are currently being studied in the treatment of IBC. The identification of increased expression of VEGF has led to the investigation of angiogenesis as a therapeutic target. Bevacizumab, a VEGF inhibitor, has been evaluated in combination with primary system chemotherapy in IBC. Thus far, results have been disappointing, but other multitargeted tyrosine kinase inhibitors of angiogenesis such as pazopanib are now being investigated (98).

The discovery that low-affinity insulin-like growth-binding protein (LIBC/WINT1) and RhoC GTPase, which are part of the Ras pathway, are respectively absent and overexpressed in IBC, leading to their evaluation as potential targets in the treatment of IBC (51). It has been shown that farnesyl transferase inhibitors (FTIs), which inhibit RhoC proteins, decrease angiogenesis, and therefore RhoC-targeted therapy merits further investigation in the treatment of IBC (99).

■ CURRENT THERAPEUTIC STRATEGIES AT MD ANDERSON CANCER CENTER

Multimodality therapy for IBC is of utmost importance with neoadjuvant chemotherapy acting as the backbone. Anthracyclines and taxanes are the cytotoxic agents of choice for the management of IBC. Our standard of care is the use of an anthracycline-containing regimen (FAC) followed by a taxane (paclitaxel or docetaxel). For paclitaxel, the data suggest that a weekly schedule may be more beneficial, with achievement of a higher pCR rates. Patients are deemed to have a poor prognosis if extensive residual disease is present after induction chemotherapy.

Locoregional treatment after neoadjuvant chemotherapy consists of radiation therapy with or without surgical intervention. After resolution of the characteristic skin changes associated with IBC, most patients are considered to be appropriate candidates for a modified radical mastectomy and subsequent radiation treatment.

Radiation therapy alone is an adequate method of locoregional treatment for patients who have not achieved sufficient debulking. Increased complete pathologic response rates are currently being evaluated by combining chemotherapy with biologically directed agents. Our recommended schema for multimodality treatment of IBC is presented in Fig. 26-6.

■ CONCLUSION

IBC is an aggressive and often lethal form of breast cancer. Thus, early and accurate diagnosis is essential. Although IBC is a clinicopathologic entity, imaging modalities such as mammography, ultrasound, MRI, CT, and PET/ CT have been useful in diagnosing and staging this disease. While primary systemic chemotherapy with anthracycline- and taxane-based regimens are the mainstay of therapy, a multidisciplinary approach using adjuvant chemotherapy, radiation, and/or surgery is of critical importance. This multidisciplinary approach to the treatment of IBC has resulted in significant increases in survival over the past four decades, with OS up from less than 5 to 44% at 15 years in patients who achieve a pCR. As our knowledge of the biological basis of IBC continues to expand, one would expect further improvement in survival as targeted therapies are added to these regimens.

References

1. Hance KW, Anderson WF, Devesa SS, et al. Trends in inflammatory breast carcinoma incidence and survival: the surveillance, epidemiology, and end results program at the National Cancer Institute. *J Natl Cancer Inst* 2005;97:966-975.
2. Anderson WF, Chu KC, Chang S. Inflammatory breast carcinoma and noninflammatory locally advanced breast carcinoma: distinct clinicopathologic entities? *J Clin Oncol* 2003; 21:2254-2259.
3. Anderson WF, Schairer C, Chen BE, et al. Epidemiology of inflammatory breast cancer (IBC). *Breast Dis* 2005;22:9-23.
4. Tabbane F, Muenz L, Jaziri M, et al. Clinical and prognostic features of a rapidly progressing breast cancer in Tunisia. *Cancer* 1977;40:376-382.
5. Boussen H, Bouzaiene H, Ben Hassouna J, et al. Inflammatory breast cancer in Tunisia: reassessment of incidence and clinicopathological features. *Semin Oncol* 2008;35:17-24.
6. Chang S, Parker SL, Pham T, et al. Inflammatory breast carcinoma incidence and survival: the surveillance, epidemiology, and end results program of the National Cancer Institute, 1975-1992. *Cancer* 1998;82:2366-2372.
7. Cristofanilli M, Buzdar AU, Hortobagyi GN. Update on the management of inflammatory breast cancer. *Oncologist* 2003; 8:141-148.
8. Wingo PA, Jamison PM, Young JL, et al. Population-based statistics for women diagnosed with inflammatory breast cancer (United States). *Cancer Causes Control* 2004;15: 321-328.
9. Chang S, Buzdar AU, Hursting SD. Inflammatory breast cancer and body mass index. *J Clin Oncol* 1998;16:3731-3735.
10. Aziz SA, Pervez S, Khan S, et al. Case control study of prognostic markers and disease outcome in inflammatory carcinoma breast: a unique clinical experience. *Breast J* 2001; 7:398-404.
11. Mourali N, Muenz LR, Tabbane F, et al. Epidemiologic features of rapidly progressing breast cancer in Tunisia. *Cancer* 1980;46:2741-2746.
12. Bonnier P, Romain S, Dilhuydy JM, et al. Influence of pregnancy on the outcome of breast cancer: a case-control study. Societe Francaise de Senologie et de Pathologie Mammaire Study Group. *Int J Cancer* 1997;72:720-727.
13. Chiedozi LC. Rapidly progressing breast cancer in Nigeria. *Eur J Surg Oncol* 1987;13:505-509.
14. Chang S, Alderfer JR, Asmar L, et al. Inflammatory breast cancer survival: the role of obesity and menopausal status at diagnosis. *Breast Cancer Res Treat* 2000;64:157-163.
15. Dawood S, Broglio K, Gonzalez-Angulo AM, et al. Prognostic value of body mass index in locally advanced breast cancer. *Clin Cancer Res* 2008;14:1718-1725.
16. Levine PH, Mourali N, Tabbane F, et al. Studies on the role of cellular immunity and genetics in the etiology of rapidly progressing breast cancer in Tunisia. *Int J Cancer* 1981;27: 611-615.
17. Mourali N, Levine PH, Tabanne F, et al. Rapidly progressing breast cancer (poussee evolutive) in Tunisia: studies on delayed hypersensitivity. *Int J Cancer* 1978;22:1-3.
18. Levine PH, Pogo BG, Klouj A, et al. Increasing evidence for a human breast carcinoma virus with geographic differences. *Cancer* 2004;101:721-726.
19. Hachana M, Trimeche M, Ziadi S, et al. Prevalence and characteristics of the MMTV-like associated breast carcinomas in Tunisia. *Cancer Lett* 2008;271:222-230.
20. Bell C. *A System of Operative Surgery founded on the Basis of Anatomy*. 2nd ed. Hartford, CT: Hale & Homser;1816.
21. Lee BJ, Tannenbaum N. Inflammatory Carcinoma of the breat: a report of twenty-eight cases from the breast clinic of Memorial Hospital. *Surg Gynecol Obstet* 1924;39:580-595.
22. Amparo RS, Angel CD, Ana LH, et al. Inflammatory breast carcinoma: pathological or clinical entity? *Breast Cancer Res Treat* 2000;64:269-273.
23. Lucas FV, Perez-Mesa C. Inflammatory carcinoma of the breast. *Cancer* 1978;41:1595-1605.
24. Haagensen CD. *Inflammatory Carcinoma*. 2nd ed. Philadelphia, PA: WB Saunders;1971.
25. Wu M, Merajver SD. Molecular biology of inflammatory breast cancer: applications to diagnosis, prognosis, and therapy. *Breast Dis* 2005;22:25-34.
26. Bryant T. Disease of the breast. New York, Wood's Medical and Surgical Monographs, 1889.
27. Taylor GW, Metzler A. Inflammatory carcinoma of the breast. *Am J Cancer* 1938;33:33-49,
28. Saltzstein SL. Clinically occult inflammatory carcinoma of the breast. *Cancer* 1974;34:382-388.
29. Colpaert CG, Vermeulen PB, Benoy I, et al. Inflammatory breast cancer shows angiogenesis with high endothelial proliferation rate and strong E-cadherin expression. *Br J Cancer* 2003;88:718-725.

30. Bieche I, Lerebours F, Tozlu S, et al. Molecular profiling of inflammatory breast cancer: identification of a poor-prognosis gene expression signature. *Clin Cancer Res* 2004;10:6789-6795.

31. Greene FL, Page DL, Fleming ID, et al. *AJCC Cancer Staging Handbook*. 6th ed. New York, NY: Springer;2002.

32. Singletary SE, Allred C, Ashley P, et al. Revision of the American Joint Committee on Cancer staging system for breast cancer. *J Clin Oncol* 2002;20:3628-3636.

33. Levine PH, Steinhorn SC, Ries LG, et al. Inflammatory breast cancer: the experience of the surveillance, epidemiology, and end results (SEER) program. *J Natl Cancer Inst* 1985;74:291-297.

34. Costa J, Webber BL, Levine PH, et al. Histopathological features of rapidly progressing breast carcinoma in Tunisia: a study of 94 cases. *Int J Cancer* 1982;30:35-37.

35. Bertucci F, Finetti P, Rougemont J, et al. Gene expression profiling identifies molecular subtypes of inflammatory breast cancer. *Cancer Res* 2005;65:2170-2178.

36. Lerebours F, Bertheau P, Bieche I, et al. Two prognostic groups of inflammatory breast cancer have distinct genotypes. *Clin Cancer Res* 2003;9:4184-4189.

37. Van den Eynden GG, Van der Auwera I, Van Laere S, et al. Validation of a tissue microarray to study differential protein expression in inflammatory and non-inflammatory breast cancer. *Breast Cancer Res Treat* 2004;85:13-22.

38. Van Laere S, Van der Auwera I, Van den Eynden GG, et al. Distinct molecular signature of inflammatory breast cancer by cDNA microarray analysis. *Breast Cancer Res Treat* 2005;93:237-246.

39. Paradiso A, Tommasi S, Brandi M, et al. Cell kinetics and hormonal receptor status in inflammatory breast carcinoma. Comparison with locally advanced disease. *Cancer* 1989;64:1922-1927.

40. Parton M, Dowsett M, Ashley S, et al. High incidence of HER-2 positivity in inflammatory breast cancer. *Breast* 2004;13:97-103.

41. Turpin E, Bieche I, Bertheau P, et al. Increased incidence of ERBB2 overexpression and TP53 mutation in inflammatory breast cancer. *Oncogene* 2002;21:7593-7597.

42. Van der Auwera I, Van Laere SJ, Van den Eynden GG, et al. Increased angiogenesis and lymphangiogenesis in inflammatory versus noninflammatory breast cancer by real-time reverse transcriptase-PCR gene expression quantification. *Clin Cancer Res* 2004;10:7965-7971.

43. McCarthy NJ, Yang X, Linnoila IR, et al. Microvessel density, expression of estrogen receptor alpha, MIB-1, p53, and c-erbB-2 in inflammatory breast cancer. *Clin Cancer Res* 2002;8:3857-3862.

44. Kleer CG, van Golen KL, Braun T, et al. Persistent E-cadherin expression in inflammatory breast cancer. *Mod Pathol* 2001;14:458-464.

45. Alpaugh ML, Tomlinson JS, Shao ZM, et al. A novel human xenograft model of inflammatory breast cancer. *Cancer Res* 1999;59:5079-5084.

46. Alpaugh ML, Tomlinson JS, Kasraeian S, et al. Cooperative role of E-cadherin and sialyl-Lewis X/A-deficient MUC1 in the passive dissemination of tumor emboli in inflammatory breast carcinoma. *Oncogene* 2002;21:3631-3643.

47. Tomlinson JS, Alpaugh ML, Barsky SH. An intact overexpressed E-cadherin/alpha,beta-catenin axis characterizes the lymphovascular emboli of inflammatory breast carcinoma. *Cancer Res* 2001;61:5231-5241.

48. Gonzalez-Angulo AM, Sneige N, Buzdar AU, et al. p53 expression as a prognostic marker in inflammatory breast cancer. *Clin Cancer Res* 2004;10:6215-6221.

49. Riou G, Le MG, Travagli JP, et al. Poor prognosis of p53 gene mutation and nuclear overexpression of p53 protein in inflammatory breast carcinoma. *J Natl Cancer Inst* 1993;85:1765-1767.

50. van Golen KL, Bao LW, Pan Q, et al. Mitogen activated protein kinase pathway is involved in RhoC GTPase induced motility, invasion and angiogenesis in inflammatory breast cancer. *Clin Exp Metastasis* 2002;19:301-311.

51. van Golen KL, Wu ZF, Qiao XT, et al. RhoC GTPase, a novel transforming oncogene for human mammary epithelial cells that partially recapitulates the inflammatory breast cancer phenotype. *Cancer Res* 2000;60:5832-5838.

52. Kleer CG, Zhang Y, Pan Q, et al. WISP3 is a novel tumor suppressor gene of inflammatory breast cancer. *Oncogene* 2002;21:3172-3180.

53. Chow CK. Imaging in inflammatory breast carcinoma. *Breast Dis* 2005;22:45-54.

54. Yang WT, Le-Petross HT, Macapinlac H, et al. Inflammatory breast cancer: PET/CT, MRI, mammography, and sonography findings. *Breast Cancer Res Treat* 2008;109:417-426.

55. Dershaw DD, Osborne M. Imaging techniques in breast cancer. *Semin Surg Oncol* 1989;5:82-93.

56. Gunhan-Bilgen I, Ustun EE, Memis A. Inflammatory breast carcinoma: mammographic, ultrasonographic, clinical, and pathologic findings in 142 cases. *Radiology* 2002;223:829-838.

57. Lee KW, Chung SY, Yang I, et al. Inflammatory breast cancer: imaging findings. *Clin Imaging* 2005;29:22-25.

58. Le-Petross CH, Bidaut L, Yang WT. Evolving role of imaging modalities in inflammatory breast cancer. *Semin Oncol* 2008;35:51-63.

59. Rieber A, Tomczak RJ, Mergo PJ, et al. MRI of the breast in the differential diagnosis of mastitis versus inflammatory carcinoma and follow-up. *J Comput Assist Tomogr* 1997;21:128-132.

60. Renz DM, Baltzer PA, Bottcher J, et al. Inflammatory breast carcinoma in magnetic resonance imaging: a comparison with locally advanced breast cancer. *Acad Radiol* 2008;15:209-221.

61. Kuhl CK. High-risk screening: multi-modality surveillance of women at high risk for breast cancer (proven or suspected carriers of a breast cancer susceptibility gene). *J Exp Clin Cancer Res* 2002;21:103-106.

62. Rieber A, Brambs HJ, Gabelmann A, et al. Breast MRI for monitoring response of primary breast cancer to neo-adjuvant chemotherapy. *Eur Radiol* 2002;12:1711-1719.

63. Chen JH, Mehta RS, Nalcioglu O, et al. Inflammatory breast cancer after neoadjuvant chemotherapy: can magnetic resonance imaging precisely diagnose the final pathological response? *Ann Surg Oncol* 2008;15:3609-3613.

64. Mogavero GT, Fishman EK, Kuhlman JE. Inflammatory breast cancer: CT evaluation. *Clin Imaging* 1992;16:183-186.

65. Moyses B, Haegele P, Rodier JF, et al. Assessment of response by breast helical computed tomography to neoadjuvant chemotherapy in large inflammatory breast cancer. *Clin Breast Cancer* 2002;2:304-310.

66. Akashi-Tanaka S, Fukutomi T, Watanabe T, et al. Accuracy of contrast-enhanced computed tomography in the prediction of residual breast cancer after neoadjuvant chemotherapy. *Int J Cancer* 2001;96:66-73.

67. Baslaim MM, Bakheet SM, Bakheet R, et al. 18-Fluorodeoxyglucose-positron emission tomography in inflammatory breast cancer. *World J Surg* 2003;27:1099-1104.

68. Carkaci S, Macapinlac HA, Cristofanilli M, et al. Retrospective study of 18F-FDG PET/CT in the diagnosis of inflammatory breast cancer: preliminary data. *J Nucl Med* 2009;50:231-238.

69. Kell MR, Morrow M. Surgical aspects of inflammatory breast cancer. *Breast Dis* 2005;22:67-73.

70. Barber KW, Jr., Dockerty MB, Clagett OT. Inflammatory carcinoma of the breast. *Surg Gynecol Obstet* 1961;112:406-410.

71. Bozzetti F, Saccozzi R, De Lena M, et al. Inflammatory cancer of the breast: analysis of 114 cases. *J Surg Oncol* 1981;18:355-361.

72. Haagensen CD, Stout AP. Carcinoma of the breast. III. Results of treatment, 1935-1942. *Ann Surg* 1951;134:151-172.

73. Panades M, Olivotto IA, Speers CH, et al. Evolving treatment strategies for inflammatory breast cancer: a population-based survival analysis. *J Clin Oncol* 2005;23:1941-1950.

74. Fleming RY, Asmar L, Buzdar AU, et al. Effectiveness of mastectomy by response to induction chemotherapy for control in inflammatory breast carcinoma. *Ann Surg Oncol* 1997;4:452-461.

75. Barker JL, Nelson AJ, Montague ED. Inflammatory carcinoma of the breast. *Radiology* 1976;121:173-176.

76. Chu AM, Wood WC, Doucette JA. Inflammatory breast carcinoma treated by radical radiotherapy. *Cancer* 1980;45:2730-2737.

77. Liao Z, Strom EA, Buzdar AU, et al. Locoregional irradiation for inflammatory breast cancer: effectiveness of dose escalation in decreasing recurrence. *Int J Radiat Oncol Biol Phys* 2000;47:1191-1200.

78. Kuerer HM, Newman LA, Smith TL, et al. Clinical course of breast cancer patients with complete pathologic primary tumor and axillary lymph node response to doxorubicin-based neoadjuvant chemotherapy. *J Clin Oncol* 1999;17:460-469.

79. Dawood S, Broglio K, Gong Y, et al. Prognostic significance of HER-2 status in women with inflammatory breast cancer. *Cancer* 2008;112:1905-1911.

80. Buzdar AU, Singletary SE, Booser DJ, et al. Combined modality treatment of stage III and inflammatory breast cancer. M.D. Anderson Cancer Center experience. *Surg Oncol Clin N Am* 1995;4:715-734.

81. Koh EH, Buzdar AU, Ames FC, et al. Inflammatory carcinoma of the breast: results of a combined-modality approach– M.D. Anderson Cancer Center experience. *Cancer Chemother Pharmacol* 1990;27:94-100.

82. Singletary SE, Ames FC, Buzdar AU. Management of inflammatory breast cancer. *World J Surg* 1994;18:87-92.

83. Ueno NT, Buzdar AU, Singletary SE, et al. Combined-modality treatment of inflammatory breast carcinoma: twenty years of experience at M. D. Anderson Cancer Center. *Cancer Chemother Pharmacol* 1997;40:321-329.

84. Cristofanilli M, Buzdar AU, Sneige N, et al. Paclitaxel in the multimodality treatment for inflammatory breast carcinoma. *Cancer* 2001;92:1775-1782.

85. Cristofanilli M, Gonzalez-Angulo AM, Buzdar AU, et al. Paclitaxel improves the prognosis in estrogen receptor negative inflammatory breast cancer: the M. D. Anderson Cancer Center experience. *Clin Breast Cancer* 2004;4:415-419.

86. Buzdar AU, Montague ED, Barker JL, et al. Management of inflammatory carcinoma of breast with combined modality approach - an update. *Cancer* 1981;47:2537-2542.

87. Hagelberg RS, Jolly PC, Anderson RP. Role of surgery in the treatment of inflammatory breast carcinoma. *Am J Surg* 1984;148:125-131.

88. Perez CA, Fields JN, Fracasso PM, et al. Management of locally advanced carcinoma of the breast. II. Inflammatory carcinoma. *Cancer* 1994;74:466-476.

89. Arun B, Slack R, Gehan E, et al. Survival after autologous hematopoietic stem cell transplantation for patients with inflammatory breast carcinoma. *Cancer* 1999;85:93-99.

90. Cagnoni PJ, Nieto Y, Shpall EJ, et al. High-dose chemotherapy with autologous hematopoietic progenitor-cell support as part of combined modality therapy in patients with inflammatory breast cancer. *J Clin Oncol* 1998;16:1661-1668.

91. Chevallier B, Roche H, Olivier JP, et al. Inflammatory breast cancer. Pilot study of intensive induction chemotherapy (FEC-HD) results in a high histologic response rate. *Am J Clin Oncol* 1993;16:223-228.

92. Dazzi C, Cariello A, Rosti G, et al. Neoadjuvant high dose chemotherapy plus peripheral blood progenitor cells in inflammatory breast cancer: a multicenter phase II pilot study. *Haematologica* 2001;86:523-529.

93. Hurley J, Doliny P, Reis I, et al. Docetaxel, cisplatin, and trastuzumab as primary systemic therapy for human epidermal growth factor receptor 2-positive locally advanced breast cancer. *J Clin Oncol* 2006;24:1831-1838.

94. Van Pelt AE, Mohsin S, Elledge RM, et al. Neoadjuvant trastuzumab and docetaxel in breast cancer: preliminary results. *Clin Breast Cancer* 2003;4:348-353.

95. Burstein HJ, Harris LN, Gelman R, et al. Preoperative therapy with trastuzumab and paclitaxel followed by sequential adjuvant doxorubicin/cyclophosphamide for HER2 overexpressing stage II or III breast cancer: a pilot study. *J Clin Oncol* 2003;21:46-53.

96. Limentani SA, Brufsky AM, Erban JK, et al. Phase II study of neoadjuvant docetaxel, vinorelbine, and trastuzumab followed by surgery and adjuvant doxorubicin plus cyclophosphamide in women with human epidermal growth factor receptor 2-overexpressing locally advanced breast cancer. *J Clin Oncol* 2007;25:1232-1238.

97. Cristofanilli M, Boussen H, Baselga Jea. A phase II combination study of lapatinib and paclitaxel as a neoadjuvant therapy in patients with newly diagnosed inflammatory breast cancer (IBC). *Breast Cancer Res Treat* 2006;100:5S (abstract 1).

98. Sonpavde G. Lapatinib plus capecitabine in breast cancer. *N Engl J Med* 2007;356:1471;author reply1471-1472.

99. End DW. Farnesyl protein transferase inhibitors and other therapies targeting the Ras signal transduction pathway. *Invest New Drugs* 1999;17:241-258.

SPECIAL SITUATIONS IN BREAST CANCER

Rachel L. Theriault
Karin M.E. Hahn

■ BREAST CANCER DURING PREGNANCY

EPIDEMIOLOGY

Although cancer of the breast is one of the most common cancers diagnosed during pregnancy, it is a rare event, with 1 in 3000 to 3 in 10,000 deliveries being to women who were diagnosed with breast cancer while pregnant (1). The majority of data on this unique group of breast cancer patients are derived from retrospective case-control studies as well as case series and reports. Complicating the interpretation of the literature on breast cancer diagnosed during pregnancy is that this is often combined with pregnancy diagnosed in the year following delivery. Breast cancer diagnosed during pregnancy and the 12 months following delivery is referred to as pregnancy-associated breast cancer (PABC). It has been estimated that 0.2 to 3.8% of all breast cancers coincide with pregnancy or lactation (2). Given that increasing age is a risk factor for breast cancer, it has been postulated that the incidence of breast cancer during pregnancy may increase as more women delay childbearing (1).

DIAGNOSIS

A pregnant woman with breast cancer usually presents with a mass in her breast. However, the physiologic changes in a pregnant woman's breast, physician familiarity with PABC, as well as patient age, socioeconomic, cultural, and psychosocial factors are all thought to contribute to the delays in diagnosis that have been documented in older studies of pregnant and lactating women. These delays may be among the factors contributing to the later stage of diagnosis that has been documented in a number of case-control studies (1).

Biopsy

Although the majority of breast biopsies performed in pregnant women will demonstrate benign pathology, a breast mass that persists for 2 to 4 weeks should be further investigated. Any clinically suspicious breast mass should be biopsied for a definitive diagnosis whether a patient is pregnant or not. Even though a number of small studies have shown the accuracy of fine-needle

aspiration (FNA) in the diagnosis of PABC, a core or excisional biopsy of the breast lesion is necessary to make a diagnosis of invasion (3).

Two large surgical series of pregnant patients who had general anesthesia for a variety of underlying medical problems failed to demonstrate an increase in the risk of congenital malformations as compared with pregnant women who did not undergo surgery (4,5). One of these series suggested that there may be an increased risk of spontaneous abortion with surgery in the first and second trimesters, especially after gynecologic procedures (4). The other surgical series found an increased incidence of very low and low-birth-weight infants among pregnant women, particularly in the first and second trimesters (5). The authors suggest that the underlying illness precipitating the surgery in pregnant women may have played a role in the incidence of very low and low-birth-weight infants.

Ultimately, the least invasive and most technically accurate method(s) available should be utilized to determine the nature of a breast mass in a pregnant woman.

Diagnostic Imaging

Few studies have addressed the effectiveness of mammography or ultrasound in the diagnosis of breast cancer in a pregnant or lactating woman. However, Yang et al. performed a retrospective survey of 23 pregnant breast cancer patients treated at The MD Anderson Cancer Center (MDACC) (6). They found that breast cancer diagnosed during pregnancy was mammographically evident in 18 of the 20 patients with preoperative mammograms despite dense parenchymal background. They also found that breast ultrasound (US), when performed (N = 20), demonstrated all masses and provided information regarding response to neoadjuvant chemotherapy (N = 12). Mammography can be performed safely with the use of abdominal shielding and may provide important information particularly regarding calcifications which may not be seen on US. Clearly, ultrasound of the breast and nodal basins is safe during pregnancy and may be helpful in the initial evaluation and staging of a breast mass.

Magnetic resonance imaging (MRI) is currently not considered part of the standard evaluation of a nonpregnant breast cancer patient and thus is not considered in the evaluation of the pregnant woman with a breast mass. In addition, the safety of gadolinium during pregnancy has not been established (7).

PATHOLOGIC FEATURES OF BREAST CANCER DURING PREGNANCY

Although a number of studies have examined the pathologic features of breast cancer diagnosed during delivery or in the year following delivery, differences in study populations, sample size, and study design make it difficult to make comparisons between pregnant and nonpregnant patients when matched for age. An MDACC case series by Middleton et al. examined the tumor characteristics of a cohort of breast cancer patients treated with chemotherapy while they were pregnant (8). They found that pregnant women tended to present with advanced-stage disease and had tumors with poor histologic and prognostic features, including a high nuclear grade as well as estrogen and progesterone receptor negativity. As seen in Fig. 27-1, the tumors of pregnant breast cancer patients are often poorly differentiated. Middleton et al. felt that the characteristics of these tumors were similar to those reported in young, nonpregnant women with breast cancer, making age at breast cancer diagnosis more likely than pregnancy to determine the biologic characteristics of the tumor.

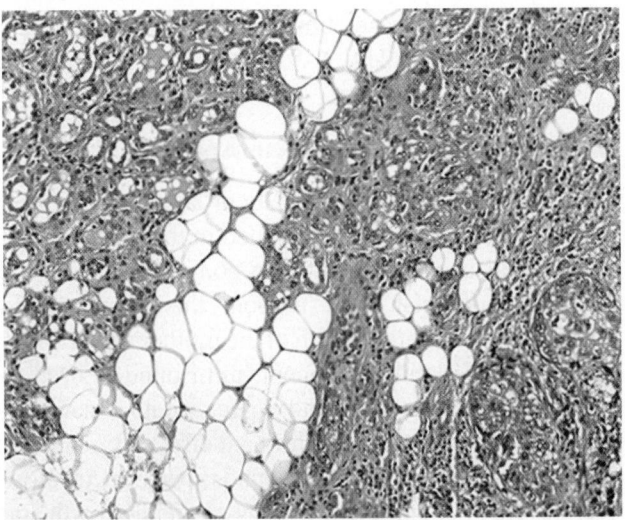

FIGURE 27-1. Right: hematoxylin and eosin-stained specimen of high-grade invasive and in situ ductal carcinoma (original magnification 100×). Pregnancy changes are seen in nonneoplastic acini in the upper left-hand corner. (*Courtesy of Lavinia Middleton, MD, Department of Pathology, The University of Texas MD Anderson Cancer Center.*)

Staging

The tumor-node-metastasis (TNM) system should be used to stage both pregnant and nonpregnant breast cancer patients. Given that stage of diagnosis may have significant psychosocial implications, particularly if a pregnant breast cancer patient presents with metastatic disease, accurate staging is important.

After a thorough clinical examination of the breast and lymph node–bearing regions, local imaging of the breast with mammography and ultrasound can be helpful earlier. Given that women with PABC often present with advanced-stage disease, metastatic disease, especially to lungs, liver, and bone, should also be ruled out. Chest radiography with abdominal shielding is not contraindicated in the pregnant patient, even though the utility of these radiographs in the third trimester is limited by the compression of the lower lung parenchyma by the gravid uterus. Abdominal ultrasound can be used to evaluate the liver for metastases, but it may be less accurate if the woman has developed fatty infiltration of the liver during pregnancy. Computed tomography (CT) of the abdomen and pelvis is not usually performed during pregnancy because of the risk of fetal exposure to radiation (7). MRI can be used when further evaluation of visceral organs is required, although radiologists may not recommend it during the first trimester, when there is an increased incidence of spontaneous abortion independent of MRI exposure. MRI should be performed without gadolinium-based intravenous contrast medium because its safety in pregnant women has not been established (7).

Given that a higher stage of disease increases the likelihood of bone metastases, pregnant women with later-stage disease should be evaluated to rule these out. Bone scans are difficult to perform in the pregnant patient because of the recommendation that there be adequate hydration and an indwelling Foley catheter for 8 h to prevent urinary retention of radioactivity (9). If there is clinical or radiographic suspicion of bone metastases, a screening MRI of the thoracic and lumbosacral spine without contrast can be used provided the patient has no complaints suggestive of bony metastases outside the spine.

TREATMENT OF BREAST CANCER DURING PREGNANCY

The goal of treatment in both pregnant and nonpregnant patients is the same: the control of local and systemic disease. Although the treatment strategies for pregnant and nonpregnant patients are similar, the impact of the treatment on the fetus and the outcome of the pregnancy should be considered in the pregnant breast cancer patient.

Surgery and Radiation Therapy

As previously discussed, surgery can be performed in the pregnant breast cancer patient with minimal risk to the developing fetus (4,5). In most reports of pregnant breast cancer patients, the majority of women underwent modified radical mastectomy with axillary lymph node dissection, possibly reflecting treatment practice during that time period, later stage of diagnosis, and/or concerns over the need for radiation if breast-conserving surgery is performed (10,11). In general, breast radiation is contraindicated during pregnancy because of the risk of radiation exposure to the fetus (10).

Breast-conserving surgery can be an option for a pregnant woman who presents in the third trimester or whose advanced stage at presentation warrants the use of neoadjuvant chemotherapy prior to surgery, such that surgery could be performed either later in pregnancy or even postpartum.

Although sentinel lymph node biopsy is often performed in nonpregnant breast cancer patients who are clinically node-negative, the use of this procedure in pregnant breast cancer patients has not been systematically evaluated as an alternative to axillary dissection. It has been estimated that fetal exposure to radiation would be very low using the technetium-99m localization method for sentinel lymph node biopsy (11). However, there are no studies on the safety of isosulfan blue dye for sentinel lymph node biopsy in pregnant women and there have even been reports of anaphylaxis when this dye has been used in nonpregnant women (11).

The indications for systemic therapy in a pregnant breast cancer patient are similar to those in the nonpregnant patient. However, information on the effects of antineoplastic drugs administered during pregnancy has been derived from case reports, case series, and collected reviews. In a review of 289 pregnant cancer patients treated with chemotherapy for a variety of malignancies, the 17% incidence of fetal malformations with first-trimester exposure dropped to 1.3% with exposure in the second and third trimesters (12).

Chemotherapy

The only published prospective cohort of pregnant breast cancer patients treated with systemic chemotherapy during the second and third trimesters of pregnancy did not report any congenital malformations, stillbirths, or spontaneous abortions (13). The 57 women in this prospective series were treated with FAC chemotherapy (5-fluorouracil, 500 mg/m^2 intravenously [IV] on days 1 and 4; doxorubicin 50 mg/m^2 IV continuous infusion over 72 h; and cyclophosphamide 500 mg/m^2 IV on day 1; every 21 days if blood counts have recovered) for a median of four cycles while pregnant. At MDACC, pregnant women with breast cancer continue to be treated with FAC chemotherapy during their second and third trimesters of pregnancy.

There are case reports on the use of taxanes during pregnancy for women with breast or ovarian cancer (14-17). Although these reports did not describe any detrimental effects to the children, given the scarcity of the evidence, the routine use of taxanes in pregnant breast cancer patients cannot be recommended. For our node-positive patients, taxanes are given after delivery.

Hormonal Therapy

The routine use of tamoxifen in pregnant breast cancer patients is not recommended, given limited clinical data on safety in humans and the availability of animal data suggesting that it could be teratogenic (18).

Other Agents

Methotrexate is not recommended for the treatment of pregnant breast cancer patients because it is an abortifacient and can cause severe fetal malformations when given in the first trimester (12,19). Oligohydramnios has been reported in pregnant breast cancer patients treated with single-agent trastuzumab as well as trastuzumab and vinorelbine (20,21).

MONITORING THE PREGNANCY

The pregnant breast cancer patient should be closely monitored by a team highly skilled in the management of maternal and fetal health. In conjunction with the medical oncologist and surgeon, this team should assess and monitor the health of the mother and fetus.

Prior to initiating treatment, ultrasound is used to determine gestational age and expected date of delivery, because both will have a significant effect on treatment planning. In our practice, ultrasound is performed before every cycle of chemotherapy to assess fetal growth and development. Amniocentesis may be recommended by the maternal/fetal health team if the fetus is thought to be at higher than average risk for karyotype abnormalities or if there are abnormalities detected by ultrasound that should be investigated further. Although not part of the routine evaluation, amniocentesis may be necessary to assess fetal lung maturity, particularly if early induction of labor is being considered.

Timing of delivery should be optimized with relation to the systemic treatment of the breast cancer, occurring approximately 3 weeks after the last dose of anthracycline-based chemotherapy, to minimize the effects of cytopenias (13).

LONG-TERM IMPLICATIONS FOR THE OFFSPRING

MDACC has reported that out of 40 children born to mothers who underwent chemotherapy for breast cancer in the second and/or third trimesters, the majority of children were healthy and had no developmental delays, with the exception of one child born with Down syndrome (13). However, longer follow-up of these children will be needed to evaluate possible late side effects such as impaired cardiac function and fertility. Another study by Aviles et al. described similar outcomes for a cohort of 84 children born to mothers who received chemotherapy for hematologic malignancies while pregnant (22). They also evaluated 81 of these children for cardiac toxicity, using clinical evaluation and echocardiography, every 5 years after birth until 29 years of age. There was no evidence of cardiac dysfunction among the children ranging in age from 9.3 to 29.5 years (mean 17.1 years) (23).

PREGNANCY TERMINATION

A number of case series do not appear to support the previously held belief that pregnancy termination improved the survival of pregnant breast cancer patients (1). A pregnant woman with breast cancer must be fully aware of the evidence, or lack thereof, regarding pregnancy termination and survival. In situations of known or suspected fetal teratogenesis or if maternal health is in jeopardy, pregnancy termination may be an appropriate medical recommendation.

■ PREGNANCY AFTER A DIAGNOSIS OF BREAST CANCER

EPIDEMIOLOGY

Of the 247,782 women in the Surveillance Epidemiology End Results (SEER) database diagnosed with breast cancer between 2002 and 2006, a total of 4708 (1.9%) were 20 to 34 years of age and 26,017 (10.5%) were 35 to 44 years of age (24).

According to the National Center for Health Statistics, the average age of first-time mothers increased from 21.4 years in 1970 to 25 years in 2006 (25). From 1970 to 2006 the proportion of first births to women aged 35 years and older increased by almost eight times. In 2006, about 1 out of 12 first births were to women aged 35 years and older compared with 1 out of 100 in 1970.

Therefore, younger women diagnosed with breast cancer may not have had children at the time of their breast cancer diagnosis and may seek to do so after their breast cancer treatment is completed. Of course, breast cancer patients who have had children before their diagnosis may wish to have additional children after treatment.

CHEMOTHERAPY-RELATED AMENORRHEA

Chemotherapy-related amenorrhea (CRA) is variably defined as cessation of menstruation of 3 to 12 months in women who have been exposed to chemotherapy (26). The definition of the interval from the beginning of chemotherapy to menstruation cessation is also variable (interval defined from starting treatment, during treatment, or after completion of treatment). The incidence of CRA varies with age, cytotoxic agent used, and cumulative cytotoxic dose (26). Taxanes may result in a higher rate of CRA in the first year but have not been shown to cause a longer duration of CRA; this effect is primarily seen in older women, and when age is controlled for, adding a taxane appears to have little to no effect on subsequent risk of CRA (27). Adjuvant endocrine therapy with tamoxifen has been associated with decreased likelihood of monthly bleeding 1 year following chemotherapy, but this effect became statistically nonsignificant by 3 years (28).

There are studies such as Southwest Oncology Group (SWOG) S0230 that examine whether ovarian suppression during chemotherapy will improve preservation of fertility among premenopausal women (29,30). S0230 is an ongoing randomized phase III trial comparing goserelin with no goserelin in preventing early menopause in premenopausal women undergoing chemotherapy for stage I, II, or III hormone receptor–negative breast cancer.

IMPACT OF PREGNANCY AFTER BREAST CANCER

A number of reviews have concluded that pregnancy after a diagnosis of breast cancer does not worsen survival (31-33). In a retrospective case-control study by

Mueller et al., data from three SEER populations were linked to vital records data to identify women under the age of 45 at diagnosis who had a live birth ≥10 months after diagnosis. When these women were matched to nonpregnant women with a history of breast cancer, women who became pregnant after a diagnosis of breast cancer had a decreased risk of dying as compared with women who did not become pregnant (34). The improved survival noted in this and other studies may reflect a "healthy-mother effect," whereby women who become pregnant after a diagnosis of breast cancer may have already been at decreased risk of recurrence.

Women who are considering pregnancy after a diagnosis of breast cancer should understand that most data come from retrospective case-control studies in different populations and with different data-collection techniques. Women with a history of breast cancer must be aware of their personal risk of recurrence and should weigh this against their desire to have a child. Although it has been suggested that women should wait 2 years after their breast cancer diagnosis before becoming pregnant, there are no data suggesting that a pregnancy in the first 2 years increases the risk of recurrence; rather, data indicate that this is the period of increased recurrence regardless of pregnancy (35).

■ MALE BREAST CANCER

EPIDEMIOLOGY

It was estimated that 1910 new cases of breast cancer would be diagnosed in men in the United States in 2009 and that 440 men would die of the disease (36). A large population-based study done by Giordano et al. suggest that the incidence of male breast carcinoma is increasing, albeit at a slower rate than that of women and that the median age of diagnosis is slightly older than that of women, 67 versus 62 years, respectively (37). Giordano et al. had previously published a systematic review of the literature on male breast cancer from 1942 to 2000 (38). This review listed a number of possible risk factors for development of breast cancer in men, including testicular abnormalities, infertility, Klinefelter syndrome, positive family history, benign breast conditions, radiation exposure, increasing age, obesity, and Jewish ancestry. Gynecomastia does not appear to be more frequent among men with breast cancer than in the general male population.

Although mutations in the *BRCA1* gene have been described among men with breast cancer, *BRCA1* does not appear to be associated with an increased risk of breast cancer in men (39). However, men with germline

mutations in the *BRCA2* gene appear to be at increased risk (40). Given the prevalence of *BRCA2* mutations in male breast cancer patients, genetic counseling and testing should be considered (41).

DIAGNOSIS AND STAGING

Men with breast cancer are more likely to have a delay in diagnosis when compared to women, and this delay is thought to be one of the reasons men appear to present with later-stage disease, including larger tumors and more frequent lymph node involvement (37,38). The most common presenting signs and symptoms in men with breast cancer are, in order of decreasing frequency, breast mass, nipple retraction, local pain, nipple ulceration, nipple bleeding, and nipple discharge (38).

To help differentiate between gynecomastia and malignancy, mammography can be useful (38), as depicted in Fig. 27-2. A biopsy should be performed of any suspicious mass. If breast cancer is diagnosed, the male breast cancer patient should undergo staging evaluations appropriate for the given tumor stage, based on the TNM staging system.

PATHOLOGIC FEATURES OF MALE BREAST CANCER

As in women with breast cancer, increasing tumor size, lymph node involvement (including increasing numbers of positive lymph nodes), and higher histologic grade are poor prognostic features (38). In men with breast cancer, the majority of cases are invasive ductal carcinoma with invasive lobular carcinomas being rarely diagnosed (37). Breast cancers in men are also significantly more likely than those in women to be ER/PR positive: approximately 90% express the estrogen receptor and 81% express the progesterone receptor (41).

TREATMENT OF MALE BREAST CANCER

Overall prognosis for men with breast cancer is similar to that of women with similar stage disease (37) and the goals of treatment are the same: to control local and systemic disease.

Local Therapy

For the local therapy of male breast cancer that has not metastasized, a modified radical mastectomy is the current recommendation, as this has been shown to be equivalent to a radical mastectomy in this unique group of cancer patients (38). Given the limited amount of

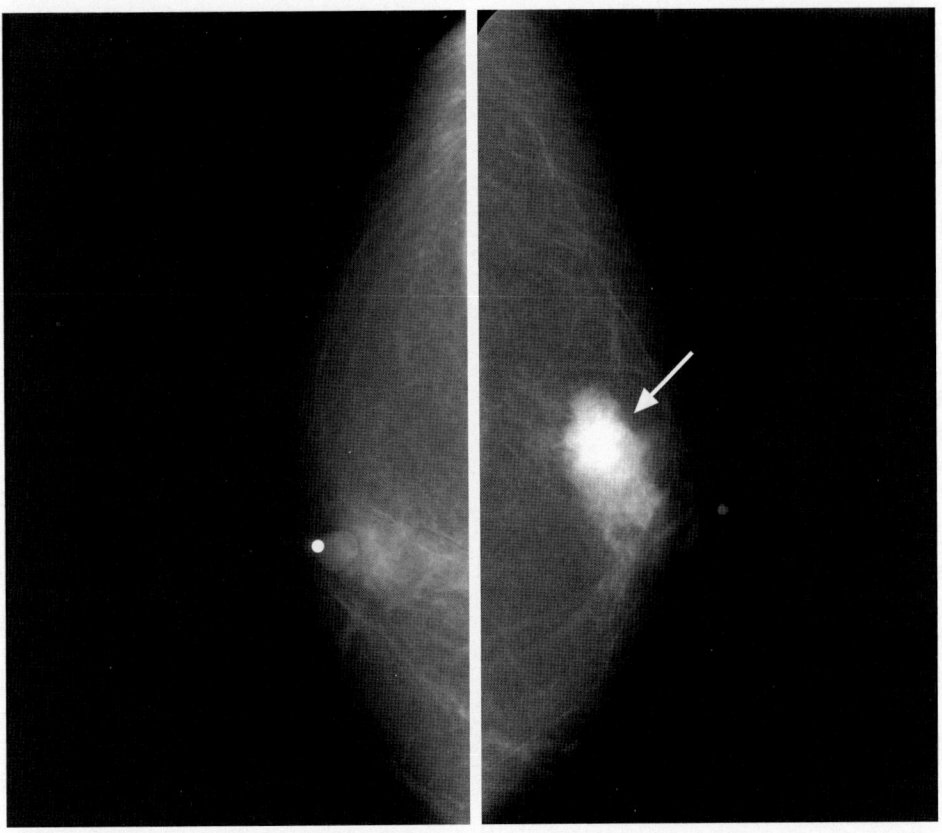

FIGURE 27-2. Bilateral mammograms of a 69-year-old man with a 2-month history of a palpable left breast mass. This abnormality (*arrow*), on biopsy, was consistent with low-grade invasive ductal carcinoma.

breast tissue and the often more advanced stage of disease at presentation, breast conservation is usually not an option. To assess the extent of regional disease, an axillary lymph node dissection or, if appropriate, a sentinel lymph node biopsy are also considered part of standard of care (38,42).

Based on the retrospective data available, Giordano et al. conclude that radiation therapy appears to decrease the risk of local recurrence but does not improve overall survival (38).

Adjuvant Systemic Therapy

No randomized clinical trials have evaluated the efficacy of adjuvant treatment for men with breast cancer. Based on retrospective analyses, men who received adjuvant tamoxifen had improved survival over those who received no hormonal therapy (43-46). It is currently recommended that all men with hormone receptor–positive breast cancer be treated with adjuvant tamoxifen for 5 years (41). The role of aromatase inhibitors in the adjuvant setting requires further investigation because the limited published data have reflected their use for metastatic breast cancer (47,48).

Although prospective data are limited, retrospective reviews suggest that adjuvant chemotherapy may be of benefit for men at higher risk of recurrence (38,41).

Therapy for Metastatic Disease

Given the high proportion of hormone-sensitive tumors among men with breast cancer, a variety of hormonal therapies have been used for the treatment of metastatic disease (41). In men with metastatic breast cancer, Jaiyesimi et al. reported response rates to a variety of hormonal therapies: 75% for androgens, 57% for antiandrogens, 50% for steroids, 32% for estrogens, 50% for progestins, 40% for aminoglutethimide, and 49% for tamoxifen (49). Tamoxifen has been recommended as first-line hormonal therapy because of its limited toxicity and established efficacy in men (41). The role of aromatase inhibitors in metastatic disease is not yet clear, though some case reports with disease response exist (47,48). A phase II SWOG trial investigating anastrozole and goserelin for the treatment of male patients with hormone receptor–positive metastatic or recurrent breast cancer closed in 2007 because of a lack of enrollment (30).

In men with hormone receptor–negative disease or who fail hormonal therapy, systemic chemotherapy may offer significant palliation for metastatic disease. Jaiyesimi et al. reported an overall response rate of 40% for the use of chemotherapeutic agents or regimens such as FAC in men with metastatic breast cancer (49). Systematic evaluation of the newer chemotherapeutic agents such as the taxanes in this unique breast cancer population is lacking.

■ THE RISKS AND BENEFITS OF HORMONE REPLACEMENT THERAPY

Over the past 20 years, a number of case-control studies, meta-analyses, and systematic reviews have attempted to determine whether exposure to hormone replacement therapy (HRT), consisting of either estrogen or estrogen and progesterone, posed a risk for the development of breast cancer. Some of these studies suggested that HRT may be a risk factor for the development of breast cancer, but that HRT may be beneficial in the primary prevention of cardiac disease.

The combined estrogen and progesterone arm of the Women's Health Initiative (WHI), a large randomized clinical trial designed to evaluate the role of HRT in the primary prevention of coronary artery disease, demonstrated an increased risk of breast cancer and ischemic stroke without any decrease in cardiovascular events (50). Combined HRT failed to improve cognitive function and health-related quality of life, although there was an improvement in vasomotor symptoms (51,52). Although there may have been an increase in ovarian cancer incidence, colon cancer incidence appeared to be reduced in women on combined HRT (53). There was an improvement in bone mineral density as well as a decreased risk of fracture in women on combined HRT (54). Given the information obtained from the WHI, the decision to recommend combined HRT in a postmenopausal woman for either the vasomotor symptoms of menopause or bone health must be made carefully by weighing the risks and benefits for that individual.

The estrogen-only arm of the WHI closed for a lack of improvement in cardiovascular health among those treated with estrogen (55). Although there was a non–statistically significant decrease in breast cancer among those women randomized to the estrogen arm, the decision to recommend estrogen alone as HRT for a postmenopausal woman must be made carefully by weighing the risks and benefits for that individual.

A Cochrane review, last updated in 2008, evaluated the effect of long-term HRT by reviewing 19 trials involving 41,904 women (56). It found that continuous combined HRT significantly increased the risk of breast cancer, among other conditions. In contrast, continuous estrogen-only HRT did not significantly increase the risk of breast cancer. The significant benefits of HRT were a decreased incidence of fractures and of colon cancer. This review concluded that HRT is not indicated for the routine management of chronic disease at this time and more evidence is needed regarding its safety.

HORMONE REPLACEMENT THERAPY IN BREAST CANCER SURVIVORS

The majority of studies of HRT use in breast cancer survivors were conducted before the results of the WHI were available. For example, a cohort of 319 breast cancer survivors from the MDACC was evaluated for use of estrogen replacement therapy (ERT). Among the 39 who were randomly assigned to ERT, there did not appear to be an increased risk of breast cancer events when compared to controls (57). In the limited number of cohort and case-control studies examining the use of HRT in breast cancer survivors, an increased risk of breast cancer recurrence was not demonstrated (58-60). However, such studies cannot possibly control for biases in the selection of breast cancer survivors who are offered HRT.

The first published, randomized trial evaluating the safety of HRT in breast cancer survivors was the HABITS (Hormone replacement after breast cancer-Is it safe?) trial (61). This study was a randomized, non–placebo-controlled, noninferiority trial which evaluated the risk of a new breast cancer in women with a history of breast cancer if they subsequently received HRT. Of the planned recruitment of 1300, 447 women were randomized, 221 women received HRT, and 221 women acted as controls. This study was terminated early after the results of the WHI trials became available. With a median of 4 years of follow-up, the hazard ratio (HR) for the development of a new breast cancer in women receiving HRT in the HABITS trial was 2.4 (95% CI, 1.3-4.2). The cumulative incidences of breast cancer at 5 years were 22.2% in the HRT arm and 8% in the control arm. Thus, there was a statistically significant increased risk of a new breast cancer in survivors on HRT. By the end of follow-up, six women in the HRT arm had died of breast cancer and six were alive with distant metastases. In the control arm, five women had died of breast cancer and four had metastatic breast cancer ($p = .51$).

Given the results of the HABITS trial and the WHI data regarding the risks and benefits of HRT in women without a history of breast cancer, one must carefully consider the use of estrogen and progestin or estrogen alone in postmenopausal breast cancer survivors. Among postmenopausal women without a history of breast cancer, HRT appears most beneficial for the treatment of vasomotor symptoms and the prevention of bone loss and fracture. In women with a history of breast cancer, it may be best to pursue other pharmacologic therapies for bone health and/or vasomotor symptoms before prescribing HRT.

◼ DUCTAL CARCINOMA IN SITU

EPIDEMIOLOGY

Ductal carcinoma in situ (DCIS), also called intraductal carcinoma, is a noninvasive breast cancer whose age-adjusted incidence between 1973 and 1992 rose from 2.3 to 15.8 per 100,000 women (62). The increase in incidence is likely secondary to screening mammography. The most common presentation of DCIS is an abnormal mammogram demonstrating clustered microcalcifications (63).

PATHOLOGIC FEATURES

DCIS traditionally has been classified primarily on the basis of architectural pattern (solid, papillary, micropapillary, or cribriform), even though such a classification system may have limitations (63). Nuclear grade (low, intermediate, or high) and the presence or absence of comedonecrosis have also used to classify DCIS (64). Morrow and Harris (63) concluded that most studies have shown that comedo or high-grade DCIS was more frequently estrogen and progesterone receptor–negative and HER-2/neu–positive as compared with noncomedo or low-grade lesions.

Although an axillary or sentinel lymph node biopsy is not the standard of care for all women presenting with DCIS, a small proportion have axillary lymph node involvement. For example, a National Cancer Data Base review of almost 11,000 women with DCIS who had a lymph node dissection between 1985 and 1991 found that 3.6% had axillary metastases (65).

DCIS is classified as having microinvasion if the invasive component is 0.1 cm or less in greatest dimension (66). If there are multiple foci of microinvasion, the size of the largest area is used to classify the microinvasion. The clinical significance of microinvasion is controversial and the incidence of axillary involvement with women who have a diagnosis of DCIS with microinvasion is said to range from 0 to 20% (63).

TREATMENT

▨ Local Therapy

The options for the surgical management of DCIS range from excision alone to mastectomy. In 98 to 99% of women with DCIS alone, mastectomy is a curative treatment (63). Given that it is unclear which DCIS lesions will progress to invasive disease and over what time frame, mastectomy may be considered to be an aggressive approach. There are, however, no randomized trials comparing DCIS treated by mastectomy to segmental mastectomy followed by radiation.

Although the routine use of axillary dissection or sentinel lymph node biopsy is not recommended for women with DCIS, nodal evaluation may be appropriate for those tumors that are more likely to harbor microinvasive disease, that is, large (>3 cm) tumors, which frequently have a high nuclear grade and are of the comedo subtype (67,68). In addition, sentinel lymph node biopsy may be discussed as an option for those undergoing a simple mastectomy for DCIS. If microinvasive or invasive disease is subsequently found in the mastectomy tissue, the opportunity for a sentinel lymph node biopsy is lost because the tumor bed is no longer in place.

The National Surgical Adjuvant Breast and Bowel Project (NSABP) B-17 study compared lumpectomy to lumpectomy with radiation for women with primarily small-volume DCIS (≤2 cm) and negative resection margins. Through 8 years of follow-up, the use of radiation therapy significantly reduced the incidence of noninvasive breast cancer from 13.4 to 8.2% and that of invasive disease from 13.4 to 3.9% (69). In 8 years of follow-up for NSABP B-17, only moderate-to-marked and absent-to-slight comedo necrosis was found to be an independent high- and low-risk predictor for ipsilateral breast tumor recurrence, respectively (70).

In a European trial that included women with DCIS up to 5 cm in size at the time of excision, women were randomly assigned to no further treatment or radiation (71). With a median follow-up of 10.5 years, the 10-year local recurrence-free rate was 74% in the group treated with excision alone compared with 85% in the women treated by excision and radiation ($p < .0001$; HR, 0.53; 95% CI, 0.4-0.7). The HRs for DCIS and invasive local recurrence were 0.52 (95% CI, 0.34-0.77) and 0.58 (95% CI, 0.39-0.86), respectively. In multivariate analysis, factors significantly associated with an increased local recurrence risk in this study were young age, symptomatic detection of DCIS, intermediate or poorly differentiated DCIS, cribriform or solid growth pattern, involved or close margins, and treatment by local excision alone. The effect of radiation therapy was homogeneous across all assessed risk factors.

The need for radiation therapy in women with low-volume, good-prognosis DCIS was to have been evaluated in a randomized trial conducted by the Radiation Therapy Oncology Group (RTOG). Unfortunately, this study which randomized women with good prognosis DCIS to radiation ± tamoxifen to observation ± tamoxifen was closed due to slow accrual (72). A recent Cochrane review has confirmed the benefit of adding radiation therapy to breast conserving surgery in the treatment of all patients with DCIS (73).

Systemic Therapy

The only approved therapy in the United States for the systemic treatment of DCIS is tamoxifen. In the NSABP B-24 study, 1804 women with small-volume DCIS (most ≤2 cm), including some with positive margins, who had undergone a lumpectomy and radiation therapy, were randomly assigned to either placebo or tamoxifen 20 mg by mouth daily for 5 years (74). There was a statistically significant absolute risk reduction of 5.2% in all breast cancer events (invasive and noninvasive combined) in women who received tamoxifen. This risk reduction is mainly the result of a decrease in ipsilateral invasive disease and contralateral noninvasive disease. The risk of the development of breast cancer at regional or distant sites was not significantly reduced among tamoxifen users. The most serious but rare side effects of tamoxifen were deep venous thrombosis (1%), nonfatal pulmonary embolism (0.2%), and uterine cancer (approximately 0.1%).

Subsequent analysis of available tumor tissue from women who participated in NSABP B-24 was performed to determine if response to tamoxifen was influenced by estrogen-receptor (ER) status (75). Although tamoxifen was beneficial among women with ER-positive DCIS, the number of women with ER-negative DCIS was small in this subanalysis so the investigators concluded that the benefit of tamoxifen was unclear in this group of women. At MDACC, tamoxifen is recommended for women with ER-positive DCIS but not those with ER-negative DCIS. The benefit of tamoxifen in women with ER-negative but PR-positive DCIS is unclear.

Anastrozole is an aromatase inhibitor currently approved for the treatment of adjuvant and metastatic breast cancer. In clinical trials such as NSABP-B35, anastrozole is currently being compared to tamoxifen in postmenopausal women with hormone-sensitive

DCIS who have undergone lumpectomy and radiation therapy (76). Until the results of these clinical trials are available, anastrozole should not be used for the treatment of DCIS because the risk/benefit ratio is unknown.

In the Study of Tamoxifen and Raloxifene (STAR) trial, a breast cancer prevention trial, Vogel et al. demonstrated that raloxifene, a selective estrogen receptor modulator (SERM), was as effective as tamoxifen in reducing the risk of invasive breast cancer in post-menopausal women (77). The women in the STAR trial had to have at least a 5-year predicted breast cancer risk of 1.66% based on the Gail model, but none had DCIS. In the STAR trial, raloxifene was as effective as tamoxifen in reducing the risk of invasive breast cancer and had a lower risk of thromboembolic events and cataracts. There was, however, a non–statistically significant higher risk of noninvasive breast cancer among those who received raloxifene.

■ HIGH-DOSE CHEMOTHERAPY WITH TRANSPLANTATION

In an attempt to decrease the risk of death for women with early-stage, poor-prognosis, or metastatic breast cancer, the effectiveness of more aggressive chemotherapeutic regimens including high-dose chemotherapy (HDC) with either bone marrow or stem cell support has been and continues to be investigated.

Data have shown a dose-response relationship in the action of chemotherapeutic drugs against cancer (78). Response to chemotherapy is also associated with the dose intensity of the drugs received (79). Through the use of autologous bone marrow or peripheral blood stem cells, chemotherapy can be delivered at higher doses than could otherwise be used.

Initial animal studies and nonrandomized trials in patients with advanced breast cancer were encouraging (80-82). Not surprisingly, these nonrandomized trials have been criticized for design weaknesses, including participant selection bias (83).

As a result, randomized trials have been and continue to be conducted to determine the possible benefit of HDC in women with either poor-prognosis, early-stage breast cancer, or metastatic disease.

POOR-PROGNOSIS, EARLY-STAGE BREAST CANCER

A number of randomized clinical trials have been conducted to determine whether there is a role for HDC with autologous bone marrow or stem cell transplant in women with poor-prognosis, early-stage breast cancer. The women included in these trials were defined as poor prognosis by having multiple axillary lymph nodes involved with tumor.

The Cochrane Breast Cancer Group performed a systematic review of the available literature on HDC in poor-prognosis breast cancer and identified 13 randomized controlled trials that met their criteria for inclusion (84). This analysis included 5064 women with a median age of 43 to 47 years, but ranging in age from 22 to 66 years. These women were defined as having poor-prognosis breast cancer by having multiple positive axillary lymph nodes and no evidence of distant metastases.

The majority of the studies in this systematic review included women who had been enrolled immediately after a full or partial mastectomy and axillary lymph node dissection. In two trials, however, some or all of the women were randomized to HDC or conventional therapy based on response to preoperative chemotherapy. In the 13 studies in this systematic review, there was substantial variation in the chemotherapy regimens used. However, in most of the trials, both arms received the same initial chemotherapy regimen, though the women randomized to the high-dose chemotherapy were also given GCSF. The control arms then went on to receive no further treatment, continuation of the initial chemotherapy or another standard chemotherapy regimen or other alternative regimens. The experimental arm went on to receive one or two cycles of high-dose chemotherapy followed by autologous peripheral blood progenitor cell transplantation and/or bone marrow transplantation.

The Cochrane Breast Cancer Group concluded that among the studies they analyzed, there was statistically significant evidence of increased event-free survival for women in the high-dose group at 3 and 4 years follow-up. However, this significance was decreasing at 5-year follow-up and was not evident in the one trial with 6-year follow-up. There was also no evidence of overall survival benefit; rather, the HDC arm showed evidence of harm with increased numbers of treatment-related deaths and adverse events.

Although this meta-analysis was updated in 2006, more mature data are still awaited from several of the trials. Nevertheless, they concluded in this update that there is insufficient evidence to support the use, outside of a clinical trial, of high-dose chemotherapy with autologous bone marrow or peripheral stem cell transplant for women with early-stage, poor-prognosis breast cancer.

A subgroup analyses of the Dutch Intergroup study showed statistically significant improved event-free survival for women with lower *HER-2/neu* expression, as well as younger age and lower histologic grade (85) Data from the West German Study Group suggest that younger women with large, higher-grade tumors benefit most from high-dose treatment. These subgroup analyses were unplanned although they do point to areas of interest for further study (86).

In conclusion, on the basis of the studies published thus far, HDC with autologous bone marrow or stem cell support has not yet shown an improvement in overall survival in women with early-stage, poor-prognosis breast cancer. However, not all studies have completed their follow-up and there may be subsets of high-risk patients who are more likely to benefit to HDC. However, at MDACC breast cancer patients with high-risk disease are offered HDC only in the setting of a clinical trial.

METASTATIC BREAST CANCER

The Cochrane Breast Cancer Group has systematically reviewed the use of HDC with autologous bone marrow or peripheral blood stem cell transplant versus conventional chemotherapy for women with metastatic breast cancer (87). Based on their search strategy and their selection, they identified six randomized controlled trials to include in their systematic review.

In this six-study analysis, a total of 438 women were randomized to receive HDC with autologous transplant and 413 were randomized to receive conventional therapy. No statistically significant difference in overall survival was seen between the two groups at 1, 3, and 5 years, even though at both 1 and 5 years, there was a statistically significant difference in event-free survival, favoring the HDC group. Of note, only one of the trials followed up all women for 5 years. The Cochrane Breast Cancer Group concluded that there was insufficient evidence to support the routine use of HDC with autologous transplant for women with metastatic breast cancer. However, further follow-up of ongoing studies as well as analysis of those subgroups who may benefit most from HDC is warranted.

■ RISK-REDUCTION STRATEGIES FOR *BRCA1* AND *BRCA2* CARRIERS

Although a family history of breast cancer, especially in a first-degree relative, has been identified as a risk factor for the development of breast cancer, most women with breast cancer do not have a significant family history (88-90). It is believed that approximately 5 to 10% of breast cancer cases are due to the inheritance of rare, highly penetrant germline mutations, particularly in the *BRCA1* and *BRCA2* genes (91,92). Women with mutations in one of these two genes can have a cumulative lifetime risk of invasive breast cancer (up to age 70 years) of 55 to 85% and a risk of invasive epithelial ovarian cancer of 15 to 65% (93,94).

CHEMOPREVENTION

The benefit of tamoxifen for risk reduction among women with mutations in either the *BRCA1* or *BRCA2* gene is unclear. A subgroup analysis of the 288 patients in the P1 breast cancer prevention trial who developed breast cancer examined whether tamoxifen decreased the risk of breast cancer among those subsequently found to have *BRCA1* or *BRCA2* mutations (95). Of the 288 tested, 19 (6.6%) had inherited disease-predisposing *BRCA1* or *BRCA2* mutations. Of the eight with *BRCA1* mutations, five received tamoxifen and three received placebo (risk ratio, 1.67; 95% CI, 0.32-10.7). Of the 11 with *BRCA2* mutations, 3 received tamoxifen and 8 received placebo (risk ratio, 0.38; 95% CI, 0.06-1.56). Thus in this small subset of patients, the use of tamoxifen in women ≥35 years of age did not reduce the risk of breast cancer among healthy *BRCA1* carriers. Other retrospective analyses examining the efficacy of tamoxifen for reducing the risk of contralateral breast cancer in women with invasive breast cancer who carry mutations in the *BRCA1* and *BRCA2* genes have demonstrating conflicting results (96,97).

While the NSABP STAR P-2 trial demonstrated that raloxifene was as effective as tamoxifen in reducing the risk of invasive breast cancer in women at increased risk for breast cancer (defined as a Gail score of >1.66%) (77), the effectiveness of raloxifene in women with either *BRCA1* or *BRCA2* mutations is unknown. For women with known *BRCA1* or *BRCA2* mutations, the most effective class of endocrine agent, the optimal duration of its use and the age at which to begin chemoprevention have not yet been demonstrated (98). Patients with a known mutation in the *BRCA1* or *BRCA2* gene, a unique population at risk for the development of breast cancer, should be encouraged to participate in clinical trials evaluating the efficacy of chemopreventative agents for breast cancer.

PROPHYLACTIC MASTECTOMIES

A woman with a mutation in either *BRCA1* or *BRCA2* gene should be counseled regarding the potential role of prophylactic mastectomy in reducing her future risk of developing breast cancer. The two groups of women who are usually candidates for this procedure are those with a genetic predisposition for breast cancer due to a known germline mutation in *BRCA1* or *BRCA2* or those with a known mutation as well as a personal history of unilateral invasive breast cancer.

Both types of prophylactic mastectomies, subcutaneous or total, are likely to leave behind a small amount of residual breast tissue, making this a risk-reduction strategy that is not 100% effective in preventing subsequent breast cancer.

Hartmann et al. examined the effectiveness of prophylactic mastectomies among women at increased risk of breast cancer (99,100). Initially, they examined its efficacy in 214 women thought to be at high risk of breast cancer based on family history alone (99). After a median follow-up of 14 years, the incidence of breast cancer in the women who underwent prophylactic mastectomies as compared to their sisters who had not was 1.4 and 39%, respectively. The investigators then genotyped 176 of the women who had prophylactic mastectomies and they found that 26 had germline mutations (100). Of these 26 women who had a prophylactic mastectomy, none developed breast cancer over a median follow-up of 13 years, although 6 incidental breast cancers were found at the time of prophylactic mastectomy.

Meijers-Heijboer et al. prospectively followed 139 women with germline *BRCA1* or *BRCA2* gene mutations (101). After a mean follow-up of 2.9 years, no breast cancers were observed in the 76 women who underwent prophylactic mastectomy. Eight breast cancers were detected in the 63 women without mastectomies under regular surveillance after a mean follow-up of 3.0 years.

In the PROSE study group, Rebbeck et al. prospectively followed 483 women with *BRCA1* or *BRCA2* gene mutations (102). 105 women underwent bilateral prophylactic mastectomy and 378 did not have the procedure, serving as matched controls. With a mean follow-up of 6.1 years, 2 cases of breast cancer were diagnosed in the 105 who underwent surgery and 184 cases were diagnosed in the control group.

A 2004 Cochrane review of a number of observational studies concluded that bilateral prophylactic mastectomies were effective at reducing both the incidence of and death from breast cancer, but that prospective, ideally randomized studies were needed. There was insufficient evidence that contralateral prophylactic mastectomy improves survival in breast cancer survivors although the risk of contralateral breast cancer was reduced (103).

At MDACC, a woman with a known mutation in either the *BRCA1* or *BRCA2* gene are counseled by our genetic counselors and our breast surgeons as to the potential breast cancer risk reduction by bilateral prophylactic mastectomies or bilateral mastectomies in those who already have a diagnosis of breast cancer.

PROPHYLACTIC BILATERAL OOPHORECTOMIES

In addition to decreasing the risk of gynecologic cancer among women with a known mutation in either the *BRCA1* or *BRCA2* gene, prophylactic bilateral salpingo-oophorectomy (BSO) may also decrease the risk of developing breast cancer (104,105). One prospective study of 170 women ≥35 years of age with either a *BRCA1* or *BRCA2* mutation that chose to undergo either surveillance or prophylactic BSO found that those who underwent a BSO had a decreased risk of breast cancer and *BRCA*-related gynecologic malignancies (104). With a median follow-up of 24.2 months, breast cancer and peritoneal cancer were diagnosed in 3 and 1, respectively, of the 98 women who chose prophylactic BSO. Of the 72 women who chose surveillance, breast cancer was diagnosed in 8 women, ovarian cancer in 4, and peritoneal cancer in 1. Although a prophylactic BSO may significantly decrease the risk of ovarian cancer among women carrying a germline mutation in *BRCA1* or *BRCA2*, there is still a small risk of developing peritoneal cancer.

In a large, multicenter prospective study, 1079 women 30 years of age and older with ovaries in situ and a deleterious *BRCA1* or *BRCA2* mutation were enrolled at one of 11 centers from November 1, 1994 to December 1, 2004 (105). Women self-selected prophylactic BSO or observation. Follow-up information through November 30, 2005, was collected by questionnaire and medical record review. During the 3-year follow-up, prophylactic BSO was associated with an 85% reduction in *BRCA1*-associated gynecologic cancer risk (HR, 0.15; 95% CI, 0.04-0.56) and a 72% reduction in *BRCA2*-associated breast cancer risk (HR, 0.28; 95% CI, 0.08-0.92). While protection against *BRCA1*-associated breast cancer and *BRCA2*-associated gynecologic cancer was suggested, neither effect reached statistical significance. They concluded that the protection provided by prophylactic BSO against breast and gynecologic cancers might differ between carriers of *BRCA1* and *BRCA2* mutations. Further studies evaluating the efficacy of risk-reduction strategies in *BRCA* mutation carriers should stratify by the specific gene mutated.

Our patients with germline mutations in either *BRCA1* or *BRCA2* are counseled by qualified professionals on the possible reduction in ovarian cancer risk through the use of bilateral prophylactic salpingo-oophorectomy. Prophylactic BSO may also decrease breast cancer risk in patients with known mutations in *BRCA1*. However, fertility is clearly impaired by this risk-reduction strategy. Also, the premenopausal patient with a known mutation in *BRCA1* or *BRCA2* who is considering a prophylactic BSO should be counseled regarding the physiologic changes that may be associated with premature menopause, including bone loss and psychosocial changes, such as changes in mood and sexual function.

References

1. Gwyn K, Theriault R. Breast cancer during pregnancy. *Oncology* 2001;15:39-46.
2. Wallack MK, Wolf Jr JA, Bedwinek J, et al. Gestational carcinoma of the female breast. *Curr Probl Cancer* 1983;7:1-58.
3. Gupta RK. The diagnostic impact of aspiration cytodiagnosis of breast masses in association with pregnancy and lactation with an emphasis on clinical decision making. *Breast J* 1997; 3:131-134.
4. Duncan PG, Pope WDB, Cohen MM, et al. Fetal risk of anesthesia and surgery during pregnancy. *Anesthesiology* 1986;64: 790-794.
5. Mazze RI, Kallen B. Reproduction outcome after anesthesia and operation during pregnancy: A registry study of 5405 cases. *Am J Obstet Gynecol* 1989;161:1178-1185.
6. Yang WT, Dryden MJ, Gwyn K, et al. Imaging of breast cancer diagnosed and treated with chemotherapy during pregnancy. *Radiology* 2006;239:52-60
7. Chen MM, Coakley FV, Kaimal A, et al. Guidelines for computed tomography and magnetic resonance imaging use during pregnancy. *Ostet Gynecol* 2008;112:333-339
8. Middleton LP, Amin M, Gwyn K, et al. Breast carcinoma in pregnant women: Assessment of clinicopathologic and immunohistochemical features. *Cancer* 2003;98:1055-1060.
9. Baker J, Ali A, Groch MW, et al. Bone scanning in pregnant patients with breast carcinoma. *Clin Nucl Med* 1987;12:519-524.
10. Mazonakis M, Vaveris H, Damilakis J, et al. Radiation dose to conceptus resulting from tangential breast radiation. *Int J Radiat Biol Phys* 2003;55:386-391.
11. Keleher AJ, Theriault RL, Gwyn KM, et al. Multidisciplinary management of breast cancer concurrent with pregnancy. *J Am Coll Surg* 2001;194:54-64.
12. Doll DC, Ringenberg S, Yarbro JW. Antineoplastic agents and pregnancy. *Semin Oncol* 1989;16:337-346.
13. Hahn KM, Johnson PH, Gordon N, et al. Treatment of pregnant breast cancer patients and outcomes of children exposed to chemotherapy in utero. *Cancer* 2006;107:1219-1226.
14. De Santis M, Lucchese A, DeCarolis S, et al. Metastatic breast cancer in pregnancy: First case of chemotherapy with docetaxel. *Eur J Cancer Care* 2000;9:235-237.
15. Sood AK, Shahin MS, Sorosky JI. Paclitaxel chemotherapy for ovarian carcinoma during pregnancy. *Gynecol Oncol* 2001; 83:599-600.
16. Mendez LE, Mueller A, Salom E, et al. Paclitaxel and carboplatin chemotherapy administered during pregnancy for advanced ovarian cancer. *Obstet Gynecol* 2003;102:1200-1202.

17. Gonzalez-Angulo, AM, Walters RS, Carpenter RJ, et al. Paclitaxel chemotherapy in a pregnant patient with bilateral breast cancer. *Clin Breast Cancer* 2004;5:317-319.

18. Ignuchi T, Hirokawa M, Takasugi N. Occurrence of genital tract abnormalities and bladder hernia in female rats exposed neonatally to tamoxifen. *Toxicology* 1986;42:1-11.

19. Ebert U, Loffler H, Kirch W. Cytotoxic therapy and pregnancy. *Pharmacol Ther* 1997;74:207-220.

20. Watson WJ. Herceptin (trastuzumab) therapy during pregnancy: Association with reversible anhydramnios. *Obstet Gynecol*. 2005;10:642-643.

21. Fanale MA, Uyei AR, Theriault RL, et al. Treatment of metastatic breast cancer with trastuzumab and vinorelbine during pregnancy. *Clin Breast Cancer* 2005;6:354-356.

22. Avilés A, Neri N. Hematological malignancies and pregnancy: A final report of 84 children who received chemotherapy in utero. *Clin Lymphoma* 2001;2:173-177.

23. Avilés A, Neri N, Nambo MJ. Long-term evaluation of cardiac function in children who received anthracyclines during pregnancy. *Ann Oncol* 2006;17:286-288.

24. www.seer.cancer.gov

25. www.cdc.gov

26. Bines J, Oleske DM, Cobleigh MA. Ovarian function in premenopausal women treated with adjuvant chemotherapy for breast cancer. *J Clin Oncol* 1996;14:1718-1729.

27. Han HS, Ro J, Lee KS, et al. Analysis of chemotherapy-induced amenorrhea rates by three different anthracycline and taxane containing regimens for early breast cancer. *Breast Cancer Res Treat* 2009;115:335-342.

28. Petrek JA, Naughton MJ, Case LD, et al. Incidence, time course and determinants of menstrual bleeding after breast cancer treatment: A prospective study. *J Clin Oncol* 2006;24:1045-1051.

29. Maltaris T, Weigel M, Mueller A, et al. Cancer and fertility preservation: Fertility preservation in breast cancer patients. *Breast Cancer Res* 2008;10:206-216.

30. www.swog.org

31. Upponi SS, Ahmad F, Whitaker IS, et al. Pregnancy after breast cancer. *Eur J Cancer* 2003;39:736-741.

32. Surbone A, Petrek JA. Childbearing issues in breast cancer survivors. *Cancer* 1997;79:1271-1278.

33. Morrow PK, Theriault RL. Pregnancy after the diagnosis of breast cancer. *Clin Breast Cancer* 2006;7:173-175.

34. Mueller BA, Simon MS, Deapen D, et al. Childbearing and survival after breast carcinoma in young women. *Cancer* 2003;98:1131-1140.

35. Early Breast Cancer Trialists' Collaborative Group (EBCTCG). Effects of chemotherapy and hormonal therapy for early breast cancer on recurrence and 15-year survival: An overview of the randomised trials. *Lancet* 2005;365:1687-1717.

36. Jemal A, Seigel R, Ward E, et al. Cancer statistics, 2009. *CA Cancer J Clin* 2009;59:225-249.

37. Giordano SH, Cohen D, Buzdar AU, et al. Breast carcinoma in men: A population-based study. *Cancer* 2004;101:51-57.

38. Giordano SH, Buzdar AU, Hortobagyi GN. Breast cancer in men. *Ann Intern Med* 2002;137:678-687.

39. Stuewing JP, Brody LC, Erdos MR, et al. Detection of eight *BRCA1* mutations in 10 breast/ovarian cancer families, including 1 family with male breast cancer. *Am J Hum Genet* 1995;57:1-7.

40. Wooster R, Neuhausen SL, Mangion J, et al. Localization of a breast cancer susceptibility gene, *BRCA2*, to chromosome 13q12–13. *Science* 1994;265:2088-2090.

41. Giordano SH. A review of the diagnosis and management of male breast cancer. *Oncologist* 2005;10:471-479.

42. Boughey JC, Bedrosian I, Meric-Bernstam F, et al. Comparative analysis of sentinel lymph node operation in male and female breast cancer patients. *J Am Coll Surg* 2006;203:475-480.

43. Goss PE, Reid C, Pintilie M, et al. Male breast carcinoma: A review of 229 patients who presented to the Princess Margaret Hospital during 40 years: 1955–1996. *Cancer* 1999;85:629-639.

44. Ribeiro GG, Swindell R, Harris M, et al. A review of the management of the male breast carcinoma based upon an analysis of 420 treated cases. *Breast* 1996;5:141-146.

45. Ribeiro G, Swindell R. Adjuvant tamoxifen for male breast cancer MBC. *Br J Cancer* 1992;65:252-254.

46. Giordano SH, Perkins GH, Broglio K, et al. Adjuvant systemic therapy for male breast cancer. *Cancer* 2005;104:2359-2364.

47. Giordano SH, Valero V, Buzdar AU, et al. Efficacy of anastrozole in male breast cancer. *Am J Clin Oncol* 2002;25:235-237.

48. Giordano SH, Hortobagyi GN. Leuprolide acetate plus aromatase inhibition for male breast cancer. *J Clin Oncol* 2006;24:e42-e43.

49. Jaiyesimi IA, Buzdar AU, Sahin AA, et al. Carcinoma of the male breast. *Ann Intern Med* 1992;117:771-777.

50. Writing Group for the Women's Health Initiative Investigators. Risks and benefits of estrogen plus progestin in healthy postmenopausal women: Principal results from the Women's Health Initiative Randomized Controlled Trial. *JAMA* 2002;288:321-333.

51. Hays J, Ockene JK, Brunner RL, et al. Effects of estrogen plus progestin on health-related quality of life. *N Engl J Med* 2003;348:1839-1854.

52. Rapp SR, Espeland MA, Shumaker SA, et al. Effect of estrogen plus progestin on global cognitive function in post-menopausal women: The Women's Health Initiative Memory Study: Randomized controlled trial. *JAMA* 2003;289:2663-2672.

53. Anderson GL, Judd HL, Kaunitz AM, et al. Effects of estrogen plus progestin on gynecologic cancers and associated diagnostic procedures: The Women's Health Initiative randomized trial. *JAMA* 2003;290:1739-1748.

54. Cauley JA, Robbins J, Chen Z, et al. Effects of estrogen plus progestin on risk of fracture and bone mineral density: The Women's Health Initiative randomized trial. *JAMA* 2003;290:1729-1738.

55. The Women's Health Initiative Steering Committee. Effects of conjugated equine estrogen in postmenopausal women with hysterectomy: The Women's Health Initiative Randomized Controlled Trial. *JAMA* 2004;291:1701-1712.

56. Farquhar C, Marjoribanks J, Lethaby A, et al. Long term hormone therapy for perimenopausal and postmenopausal women. *Cochrane Database Syst Rev* 2009;(2):CD004143.

57. Vassilopoulou-Sellin R, Asmar L, Hortobagyi GN, et al. Estrogen replacement therapy after localized breast cancer: Clinical outcome of 319 women followed prospectively. *J Clin Oncol* 1999;17:1482-1487.

58. O'Meara ES, Rossing MA, Daling JR, et al. Hormone replacement therapy after a diagnosis of breast cancer in relation to recurrence and mortality. *J Natl Cancer Inst* 2001;93:754-761.

59. Decker DA, Pettinga JE, VanderVelde N, et al. Estrogen replacement therapy in breast cancer survivors: A matched-controlled series. *Menopause* 2003;10:277-285.

60. Di Saia PJ, Brewster WR, Ziogras A, et al. Breast cancer survival and hormone replacement therapy. *Am J Clin Oncol* 2000;23:541-545.

61. Holmberg L, Iverson OE, Rudenstam CM, et al. Increased risk of recurrence after hormone replacement therapy in breast cancer survivors. *J Natl Cancer Inst* 2008;100:475-482.

62. Ernster VL, Barclay J, Kerlikowske K, et al. Incidence of and treatment for ductal carcinoma in situ of the breast. *JAMA* 1996;275:913-918.

63. Morrow M, Harris JR. Ductal carcinoma in situ. In Harris JR, Lippmann ME, Morrow M, Osborne CK (eds). *Diseases of the Breast*. Philadelphia: Lippincott, Williams, and Wilkins, 2010;349-362.

64. Burstein HJ, Polyak K, Wong JS, et al. Ductal carcinoma in situ of the breast. *N Engl J Med* 2004;350:1430-1441.

65. Winchester DP, Menck HR, Osteen RT, et al. Treatment trends for ductal carcinoma in situ of the breast. *Ann Surg Oncol* 1995;2:207-213.

66. American Joint Committee on Cancer. Greene FL, Page DL, Fleming ID, et al. (eds): *AJCC Cancer Staging Manual*, 6th ed. New York: Springer; 2002:233-240.

67. Sakorafas GH, Farley DR. Optimal management of ductal carcinoma in situ of the breast. *Surg Oncol* 2003;12:221-240.

68. Cox CE, Nguyen K, Gray RJ, et al. Importance of lymphatic mapping in ductal carcinoma in situ (DCIS): Why map DCIS? *Am Surg* 2001;67:513-519.

69. Fisher B, Dignam J, Wolmark N, et al. Lumpectomy and radiation therapy for the treatment of intraductal breast cancer: Findings from National Surgical Adjuvant Breast and Bowel Project B-17. *J Clin Oncol* 1998;16:441-452.

70. Fisher ER, Dignam J, Tan-Chiu E, et al. Pathologic findings from the National Surgical Adjuvant Breast Project (NSABP). Eight-year Update Protocol B-17. *Cancer* 1999; 86:429-438.

71. EORTC Breast Cancer Cooperative Group; EORTC Radiotherapy Group, Bijker N, Meijnen P, Peterse JL, et al. Breast-conserving treatment with or without radiotherapy in ductal carcinoma-in-situ: Ten-year results of European Organisation for Research and Treatment of Cancer randomized phase III trial 10853-a study by the EORTC Breast Cancer Cooperative Group and EORTC Radiotherapy Group. *J Clin Oncol* 2006;24:3381-3387.

72. www.rtog.org

73. Goodwin A, Parker S, Ghersi D, et al. Post-operative radiotherapy for ductal carcinoma in situ of the breast. *Cochrane Database Syst Rev* 2009;(4):CD000563.

74. Fisher B, Dignam J, Wolmark N, et al. Tamoxifen in treatment of intraductal breast cancer: National Surgical Adjuvant Breast and Bowel Project B-24 randomised controlled trial. *Lancet* 1999;353:1993-2000.

75. Allred DC, Bryant J, Land S, et al. Estrogen receptor expression as a predictive marker of the effectiveness of tamoxifen in the treatment of DCIS: Findings from NSABP Protocol B-24. *Breast Cancer Res Treat* 2002;76(Suppl 1): S36 (abstract 30).

76. Julian TB, Land SR, Wolmark N. NSABP B-35: A Clinical Trial to Compare Anastrozole and Tamoxifen for Postmenopausal Patients With Ductal Carcinoma in Situ Undergoing Lumpectomy With Radiation Therapy. *Breast Diseases: A Year Book Quarterly* 2003;14:121-122.

77. Vogel VG, Costantino JP, Wickerham DL, et al. Effects of tamoxifen vs. raloxifene on the risk of developing invasive breast cancer and other disease outcomes: The NSABP Study of Tamoxifen and Raloxifene (STAR) P-2 trial. *JAMA* 2006; 295:2727-2741.

78. Frei E III, Canellos GP. Dose: A critical factor in cancer chemotherapy. *Am J Med* 1980;69:585-594.

79. Hryniuk W, Bush H. The importance of dose intensity in chemotherapy of metastatic breast cancer. *J Clin Oncol* 1984;2:1281-1288.

80. Antman K, Ayash L, Elias A, et al. A phase II study of high-dose cyclophosphamide, thiotepa, and carboplatinum with autologous marrow support in women with measurable advanced breast cancer responding to standard-dose therapy. *J Clin Oncol* 1992;10:102-110.

81. Peters WP, Shpall EJ, Jones RB, et al. High-dose combination alkylating agents with bone marrow support as initial treatment for metastatic breast cancer. *J Clin Oncol* 1988; 6:1368-1376.

82. Williams SF, Gilewski T, Mick R, et al. High-dose consolidation therapy with autologous stem-cell rescue in stage IV breast cancer: A follow-up report. *J Clin Oncol* 1992;10: 1743-1747.

83. Eddy DM. High-dose chemotherapy with autologous bone marrow transplantation for the treatment of metastatic breast cancer. *J Clin Oncol* 1992;10:657-670.

84. Farquhar C, Majoribanks J, Basser R, et al. High dose chemotherapy and autologous bone marrow or stem cell transplantation versus conventional chemotherapy for women with early prognosis breast cancer. *Cochrane Database Syst Rev* 2005;3:CD003149.

85. Rodenhuis S, Bontenbal M, Beex LVAM, et al. High-dose chemotherapy with hematopoietic stem-cell rescue for high-risk breast cancer. *N Engl J Med* 2003;349:7-16.

86. Gluz O, Nitz UA, Harbeck N, et al. Triple negative high-risk breast cancer derives particular benefit from dose-intensification of adjuvant chemotherapy: Results of WSG AM-01 trial. *Ann Oncol* 2008;19:861-870.

87. Farquhar C, Basser R, Hetrick S, et al. High dose chemotherapy and autologous bone marrow or stem cell transplantation versus conventional chemotherapy for women with metastatic breast cancer. *Cochrane Database Syst Rev* 2005;3:CD003142.

88. Adami, H-O, Hansen J, Jung B, et al. Characteristics of familial breast cancer in Sweden. *Cancer* 1981;48:1688-1695.

89. Bain C, Speizer FE, Rosner B, et al. Family history of breast cancer as a risk indicator for the disease. *Am J Epidemiol* 1980;111:301-308.

90. Lubin JH, Burns PE, Blot WJ, et al. Risk factors for breast cancer in women in northern Alberta, Canada, as related to age at diagnosis. *J Natl Cancer Inst* 1982;68:211-217.

91. Easton DF, Bishop DT, Ford DE, et al. Genetic linkage analysis in familial breast and ovarian cancer: Results from 214 families. *Am J Hum Genet* 1993;52:678-701.

92. Wooster R, Bignell G, Lancaster J, et al. Identification of breast cancer susceptibility gene BRCA2. *Nature* 1995;378: 789-92.

93. Ford D, Easton DF, Stratton M, et al. Genetic heterogeneity and penetrance analysis of the BRCA1 and BRCA2 genes in breast cancer families. *Am J Hum Genet* 1998;62:676-689.

94. Struewing JP, Hartge P, Wacholder S, et al. The risk of cancer associated with specific mutations of *BRCA1* and *BRCA2* among Ashkenazi Jews. *N Engl J Med* 1997;336:1401-1408.

95. King M-C, Wieand S, Hale K, et al. Tamoxifen and breast cancer incidence among women with inherited mutations in *BRCA1* and *BRCA2*. *JAMA* 2001;286:2251-2256.

96. Narod SA, Brunet J-S, Ghadirian P, et al. Tamoxifen and risk of contralateral breast cancer in *BRCA1* and *BRCA2* mutation carriers: A case-control study. *Lancet* 2000;356:1876-1881.

97. Li CI, Malone KE, Weiss NS, et al. Tamoxifen therapy for primary breast cancer and risk of contralateral breast cancer. *J Natl Cancer Inst* 2001;93:1008-1013.

98. Pichert G, Bolliger B, Buser K, et al. Evidence-based management options for women at increased breast/ovarian risk. *Ann Oncol* 2003;14:9-19.

99. Hartmann LC, Schaid DJ, Woods JE, et al. Efficacy of bilateral prophylactic mastectomy in women with a family history of breast cancer. *N Engl J Med* 1999;340:77-84.

100. Hartmann LC, Sellers TA, Schaid DJ, et al. Efficacy of bilateral prophylactic mastectomy in *BRCA1* and *BRCA2* gene mutation carriers. *J Natl Cancer Inst* 2001;93:1633-1637.

101. Meijers-Heijboer H, van Geel B, van Putten WLJ, et al. Breast cancer after prophylactic bilateral mastectomy in women with a *BRCA1* or *BRCA2*. *N Engl J Med* 2001;345:159-164.

102. Rebbeck TR, Freibel T, Lynch HT, et al. Bilateral prophylactic mastectomy reduces breast cancer risk in *BRCA1* and *BRCA2* mutation carriers: The PROSE study group. *J Clin Oncol* 2004;22:1055-1062.

103. Lostumbo L, Carbine N, Wallace J, et al. Prophylactic mastectomy for the prevention of breast cancer. *Cochrane Database Syst Rev* 2004;4:CD002748.

104. Kauff ND, Satagopan JM, Robson ME, et al. Risk-reducing salpingo-oophorectomy in women with a *BRCA1* or *BRCA2* mutation. *N Engl J Med* 2002;346:1609-1615.

105. Kauff ND, Domchek SM, Friebel TM, et al. Risk-reducing salpingo-oophorectomy for the prevention of BRCA1- and BRCA2-associated breast and gynecologic cancer: A multicenter, prospective study. *J Clin Oncol* 2008;26:1331-1337.

Gynecologic Malignancies

OVARIAN CANCER

Bryan T. Hennessy
Grace K. Suh
Maurie Markman

■ EPIDEMIOLOGY

Epithelial ovarian cancer is the commonest cancer of the female genital tract. It is the sixth most common cancer in the United States. The incidence is 33 cases per 100,000 women aged ≥50 years; the lifetime risk of a woman in the United States developing ovarian cancer is approximately 1 in 70 (1.7%) (1). 90% of ovarian cancers are epithelial in origin, accounting for 21,650 women diagnosed with ovarian cancer in 2008. It is the fifth leading cause of cancer death in women, accounting for 4% of all new cancer diagnoses and 5% of all cancer deaths. It is estimated that ovarian cancer will result in 15,520 deaths in 2008 in the United States (2).

Ovarian cancer is more common in industrialized nations, with the highest rate among women in Scandinavian countries (21 cases per 100,000 in Sweden). The lifetime risk of developing ovarian cancer is highest in Sweden (1.73%), followed by the United States (1.53%), United Kingdom (1.25%), South Europe (1.11%), South America (0.87%), India (0.75%), and Japan (0.47%) (3). In most parts of Europe and North America, the incidence of ovarian cancer was constant during the decades prior to the 1990s (4). Ovarian cancer is also more common among white women than among African-American or Asian-American women in the United States (2), although the differences are narrowing (4,5). Among white women, ovarian cancer incidence rates were reported to have declined from 1973 to 1981, increased from 1981 to 1991, and then reversed again to decline significantly from 1991 to 1997 (5). Trends between 1992 and 1998 revealed a significant decline in incidence rates of 1.4% per year for all races combined, as well as significant annual declines in white and Hispanic women (6).

This cancer is predominantly a cancer of the perimenopausal and the postmenopausal period, with 80 to 90% of cases occurring after the age of 40. The incidence is higher in older women, and the median age at diagnosis is about 62 years (7). Hereditary ovarian cancers generally occur about 10 years earlier (8). Data from the Gilda Radner Foundation Registry suggest the occurrence of anticipation (9). The majority of ovarian cancer occurs sporadically in population, and only about 5 to 10% is familial (10).

MORTALITY

Ovarian cancer accounts for more than half of the deaths from cancer that occur in women between 55 and 74 years of age, while only approximately one-quarter of ovarian cancer deaths occur in women between 35 and 54 years of age. Prognosis among women with ovarian cancer is dependent on the stage of disease at the time of diagnosis. Statistics reported during the period 1989 to 1996 estimate that the 5-year survival rate among women with localized disease was 94.6%, compared with 79.0% for women with regional disease and 28.2% for women with distant-stage disease at the time of diagnosis (5). Relative survival rates for ovarian cancer have improved substantially in the past several decades in the United States, with approximately half (50.4%) of women diagnosed with ovarian cancer between 1989 and 1996 surviving 5 years (5). Survival among white women with ovarian cancer in the United States is reportedly better than survival among black women (50.1 versus 47.5%), regardless of age or disease stage at the time of diagnosis (5,11). By contrast, Asian and Hispanic women reportedly present with a more favorable stage at diagnosis and have better 5-year survival rates than do white women (12).

ETIOLOGY

The etiology of ovarian cancer is not fully understood. Numerous studies have attempted to demonstrate possible links between environmental, dietary, reproductive, endocrine, viral, and hereditary factors and the risk of developing ovarian cancer. So far, the strongest risk factor for ovarian cancer is a familial pattern, reported in about 7% of women with the disease (13).

Distinct genetic patterns influence the etiology of ovarian cancer. Some 5 to 10% of ovarian cancers are familial, with the highest risk noted among women with ≥2 first-degree relatives with ovarian cancer (14,15). Women with *BRCA1* (chromosome 17) mutations are at a substantially higher risk of ovarian cancer than are women in the general population (15). A smaller proportion of cases of familial ovarian cancer are associated with mutations in *BRCA2* (chromosome 13) or mismatch repair genes related to hereditary nonpolyposis colorectal cancer syndrome (14,15).

Certain risk factors for ovarian cancer, such as nulliparity, may be more strongly associated with familial than with spontaneous ovarian cancer (16). Schildkraut et al. (17) have reported that increased ovulatory cycles were associated with *p53* overexpression in ovarian tumors, although others did not support this (18). Mutations of *p53* are found more frequently in nonmucinous tumors, especially serous types, and may represent the accumulation of spontaneous DNA replication errors during normal epithelial cell proliferation associated with ovulation. Overexpression of *p53* in borderline lesions, although uncommon, is associated with metastatic disease (19). Histologic differences in the patterns of *p53* mutations may influence the association of ovarian cancer with ovulation-related risk factors such as parity, use of the oral contraceptive pill, and lactation. In addition to *p53*, the inactivation of the tumor suppressor gene *PTEN* is commonly found in endometrioid and clear cell tumors (20). In addition to tumor suppressor genes, oncogenes also have been shown to be overexpressed or mutated in association with ovarian cancer. For example, the overexpression of *HER-2/neu* in ovarian tissue is predictive of a poorer response to therapy and poorer survival in ovarian cancer patients (21).

Two reported risk factors for ovarian cancer have been consistently shown to reduce the risk for this cancer: the use of oral contraceptives (22,23) and increasing number of pregnancies. Other risk factors have also been studied: asbestos-talc powder absorption through the vagina or cervix, increased dietary galactose consumption, and low serum levels of galactose-l-phosphatase uridyltransferase, increased fat consumption, menstrual history, age at first pregnancy, infertility, and hormone replacement therapy (24-28). None, however, has shown a consistent and significant effect on ovarian cancer risk (25,26). No association has been found between ovarian cancer and the use of coffee, alcohol, or tobacco (25). By far the strongest correlation found is between risk reduction and decreased ovulation; this has been explained to a certain extent by two theories: the excess gonadotropin secretion theory of Cramer and Welch (29) and the incessant ovulation theory of Fathalla (30).

■ SCREENING

The most crucial prognostic factor in ovarian cancer is the stage of disease (31,32). The main purpose of a screening test is thus to increase survival by allowing diagnosis at a more localized and curable stage. Many screening techniques are currently available. However, although there are enough reliable data to suggest that screening can detect cancer in asymptomatic women, there is still no proof that detection leads to an improvement in length and quality of life.

AVAILABLE SCREENING TECHNIQUES

Physical Examination

Pelvic examination is of limited value in screening asymptomatic women for ovarian cancer. Its sensitivity and specificity in the detection of adnexal masses have not been well documented. Although sensitivity increases with the size of the mass, this is of little use, since the disease has already disseminated in two thirds of patients whose disease is palpable (32). Some studies, however, suggest that a pelvic examination by a highly skilled examiner may reveal early-stage ovarian cancer. Unfortunately, this procedure detects only 1 ovarian cancer in 10,000 asymptomatic women (32).

Cancer Antigen 125

Cancer antigen 125 (CA 125) is a high-molecular-weight antigenic determinant on a glycoprotein shed into the bloodstream by malignant cells derived from coelomic epithelium. It has been used for a very long time in postsurgical surveillance but has recently also been studied as a screening tool. Over 85% of ovarian cancers (half of which are confined to the ovary) have a CA 125 level higher than 35 U/mL. A single CA 125 level that exceeds this may mean a positive test for ovarian cancer. Unfortunately, 6% of normal women have a CA 125 exceeding this level thus significantly impairing the sensitivity of this marker in screening for ovarian cancer (33). Nevertheless, elevated serum CA 125 levels have been associated with an increased incidence of ovarian cancer in a prospective cohort study (34). About 9320 postmenopausal women underwent an initial screen and then an average of 2.8 yearly screens with the CA 125 assay and were followed for an average of 6.8 years. Forty-nine cancers were identified. A serum CA 125 concentration of at least 30 U/mL was associated with a relative risk of 35.9 (95% confidence interval [CI] 18.3-70.4) during the first year after the screen and a relative risk of 14.3 (95% CI 8.5-24.4) during the 5 years after the screen. At a CA 125 concentration of 100 U/mL, the relative risks were 204.8 and 74.5, respectively. Women with CA 125 levels below 30 U/mL had risks of 0.13 and 0.54, respectively. At a reference level of 35 U/mL, the sensitivity of CA 125 as a marker of clinically diagnosed ovarian cancer ranges from 61 to 96%: 25 to 75% for stage I and 67 to 100% for stage II. The reported specificity is 98.6 to 99.2% (35). In about one third of women who eventually develop cancer, CA 125 levels rise above 35 U/mL 18 months before the disease is clinically detected (36).

Levels of CA 125 are also increased in patients with endometrial, pancreatic, and other cancers. They may also be increased in patients with some benign conditions—including early pregnancy, endometriosis, uterine leiomyoma, and benign ovarian cysts—in pelvic inflammatory disease (PID) (33). The serum level of CA 125 fluctuates during the menstrual cycle (37). Consequently, screening with CA 125 in premenopausal women has been little studied.

Transvaginal Sonography

Transvaginal sonography (TVS) is considered safe, time-efficient, and acceptable to patients for screening of ovarian cancer. In diagnosing ovarian cancer, the morphology and size of the mass are the most important factors. Uniform hypoechogenic or entirely cystic patterns are usually of no concern, as opposed to complex or solid patterns (38,39). Also important to consider is that cyclic changes in ovary size during the menstrual cycle can give an abnormal TVS; therefore an abnormal TVS must always be repeated.

Three trials involving a total of 66,620 screened women have been completed. In total, 545 operations were prompted and 45 cancers detected, 34 of which were invasive. Approximately 78% of the cancers were stage I. Van Nagell et al. reported the trial with the highest predictive value. From among more than 14,000 patients, the positive predictive value of an abnormal TVS screening was 9.3%, indicating that approximately 11 patients had benign ovaries removed for every malignant tumor detected (40-42). Another major limitation of transvaginal screening was the inability to detect primary peritoneal cancer or ovarian malignancy in which the ovarian size is normal.

Combination of Screening Strategies

One promising strategy may be the combination of ultrasound screening and serum CA 125 examination. Data collected from early screening trials have revealed that postmenopausal women from the general population with an elevated CA 125 level but normal ovarian morphology on ultrasound had a cumulative risk of 0.15%, which was similar to the general risk of 0.22% (43). On the other hand, women with elevated CA 125 and an abnormal ovarian morphology had a cumulative risk of 24%, translated to a relative risk of 327 (44). Jacobs et al. (45) reported a series of 22,000 women whose ovarian morphology was evaluated only if the CA 125 was greater than 30 μg/mL. The control group was observed, while the screened group underwent combined-modality screening every year. Results of the prevalence screen suggest a sensitivity of 85% at 1 year follow-up and 58% at 2 years. The end specificity was 99.6%. The results of this study were positive for a trend toward better median survival in the screened group (72.9 versus 41.8 months in the others), although this was not statistically significant. The positive predictive value of the screen was 21%. The criticism, however, was that the outcome for women with ovarian cancer in the control group was unexpectedly poor.

New Modalities

Because of the limitations of either TVS or CA 125 alone, and even the combination, there is an ongoing search for more accurate screening tools. Radiologically, color Doppler and magnetic resonance imaging (MRI) have been studied. New markers are also under investigation, most notably HE4, the M-CSF serum marker and the LPA plasma tumor marker (46,47). Although the screening of women in the general population is still considered nonstandard, the possible benefits of screening women with hereditary ovarian cancer syndromes results in an increasing number of women being encouraged to undergo screening both within trial settings and outside of them. At the University of Texas MD Anderson Cancer Center (MDACC), we encourage women at high risk to undergo genetic counseling and to enroll in a screening program.

■ BIOLOGY, IMMUNOLOGY, TUMOR MARKERS, ETIOLOGY, AND PATHOGENESIS

Although the different subtypes of EOC possess unique molecular aberrations (Table 28-1) and transcriptional signatures, their morphologic features resemble the specialized epithelia of the reproductive tract that derive from the mullerian ducts and recent studies suggest that they may all arise from a single OSE precursor cell with the specific path of differentiation regulated by embryonic pathways involving *HOX* genes (48,49). *HOX* genes are not normally expressed in OSE. However, expression of *HOXA9, HOXA10,* and *HOXA11* in tumorigenic mouse OSE-derived cells induces these cells to differentiate along distinct mullerian lineages, giving rise to tumors that exhibit morphologic features that are characteristic of serous, endometrioid, and mucinous ovarian tumors, respectively (Table 28-2). *HOXA7* has been found to control the degree of differentiation and grade of ovarian tumors. Since sex steroids regulate HOX expression throughout the menstrual cycle, it is plausible that prolonged exposure of OSE cells to these hormones in the adult female contributes to inappropriate HOX activation, perhaps in the context of epithelial inclusion cysts and excessive autocrine/paracrine stimulation leading to proliferation and genomic instability.

Genomic mutations are felt to play a key role in the pathogenesis of multiple forms of cancer. High prevalence

TABLE 28-1 | CURRENT CONCEPTS REGARDING THE ORIGINS AND MOLECULAR PATHOLOGY OF EPITHELIAL OVARIAN CANCER

Histology	*Precursor*	*Molecular Features*
Low-grade serous carcinoma	Cystadenoma-borderline tumor-carcinoma sequence	Mutations in K-RAS and/or b-RAF
High-grade serous carcinoma	"De novo" in epithelial inclusion cysts	p53 mutation and BRCA1 dysfunction (usually promoter methylation) PIK3CA† amplification (25-40%)
Low-grade endometrioid carcinoma	Endometriosis and endometrial-like hyperplasia*	Mutations in CTNNB1 (B-catenin gene) and PTEN with microsatellite instability
High-grade endometrioid carcinoma	Epithelial inclusion glands/cysts	p53 mutation and BRCA1 dysfunction (usually promoter methylation) PIK3CA mutation
Mucinous carcinoma	Cystadenoma-borderline tumor-carcinoma sequence	Mutations in K-RAS; ?p53 mutation associated with transition from borderline tumor to carcinoma
Clear cell carcinoma	?endometriosis	?PTEN mutation/loss of heterozygosity PIK3CA mutation

*Endometriosis and adjacent low-grade endometrioid carcinoma share common genetic events such as loss of heterozygosity at the same loci involving the same allele (eg, PTEN). In contrast, high-grade and poorly differentiated endometrioid carcinomas are similar to high-grade serous carcinomas.
†PIK3CA is the gene at chromosome 3q26 which specifically encodes the p110α subunit of the phosphatidylinositol-3-kinase (PI3K) protein.

TABLE 28-2	IMPORTANT ROLE FOR THE HOMEOBOX GENES HOXA7, A9, A10, AND A11 IN THE MORPHOLOGIC HETEROGENEITY OF EPITHELIAL OVARIAN CANCERS AND THEIR ASSUMPTION OF MÜLLERIAN-LIKE FEATURES (48)		
Homeobox (HOX) Gene	*Normally Expressed in**	*Epithelial Ovarian Cancer Expression*	*Stable Expression in TransforMed Mouse OSE Cells Induces Formation of*
*HOX*A9	Fallopian tubes, endometrium, endocervix	Serous, endometrioid, mucinous	Cystic, papillary tumors resembling serous carcinomas
*HOX*A10	Endometrium, endocervix	Mucinous, endometrioid	Glandular tumors resembling endometrioid carcinomas
*HOX*A11	Endocervix, lower uterine segment	Mucinous	Tumors resembling mucinous carcinomas

*Little or no staining for HOX proteins is present in normal human ovarian surface epithelial cells.

somatic (non-germline) mutations (>5%) have been found in only a limited number of genes in EOC, occur like *HOX* gene changes in a histologic subtype- and grade-specific fashion, and identify genes whose functional perturbation likely plays a key role in ovarian carcinogenesis. These genes include *TP53*, *CTNNB1*, *PTEN* (all inactivated), *KRAS*, *PIK3CA*, and *AKT1* (all activated) (50). Hereditary (germline) *BRCA1/2* mutation-related EOCs tend to occur at an earlier age than sporadic tumors and are more commonly high-grade serous tumors with p53 dysfunction (51).

Like many solid tumors, EOCs frequently have a high degree of chromosomal instability (gene copy number amplifications and deletions), and both total and regional instability are associated with tumor grade and altered patient outcomes (50). Although such aberrant areas of DNA frequently carry multiple genes, it is presently thought that only a limited number of genes are "key drivers" of the process; these "key drivers" are thought to be the most critical markers and potential treatment targets. Since inhibition of protein function is generally believed to be more achievable than restoration of function, most studies focus on areas of chromosomal gain (amplicons) for identification of novel potential therapy targets. Candidate "drivers" at areas of copy number gain that have been identified to date in ovarian tumors include *RAB25* at 1q22, ecotropic viral integration site-1 (*EVI1*), protein kinase C iota (*PKCi*), *SnoN*, *BCL6*, the initiation factor *EIF5A2* and *PIK3CA* at 3q26.2, *MYC* and *PVT1* at 8q24.2, remodeling and spacing factor 1 (rsf-1, *HBXAP*) and *PAK1* at 11q13, *HER2/neu* at 17q12, *AKT2* at 19q13.2, and *ZNF217*, *BTAK* (Aurora Kinase), *BRK,* and *EEF1A2* at 20q13.2 (50,52). Some of these genes are targetable with novel agents that are currently undergoing preclinical or early clinical assessment. In addition, rearrangements, epigenetic changes and imprinting also affect cellular function

and identify potentially important markers and therapy targets in EOC (52).

In one model of ovarian carcinogenesis (48,52), EOCs are divided into two categories designated type I and type II tumors that correspond to two main pathways of tumorigenesis. Type I tumors arise in a stepwise manner from borderline tumors and include low-grade serous carcinomas, mucinous, endometrioid, and clear cell carcinomas. Type II tumors arise de novo and include high-grade serous carcinoma, malignant mixed mesodermal tumors, and undifferentiated carcinomas. Type II tumors are characterized by frequent *TP53* mutations, by marked genomic instability and by *BRCA* gene mutations in some cases. This model of carcinogenesis reconciles the relationship of borderline tumors to invasive carcinoma and provides a morphological and molecular framework for studies aimed at elucidating EOC pathogenesis.

STEROID HORMONES

Many ovarian cancers have histologic characteristics of classic endocrine-responsive tissues. This alone suggests a role for hormones in the etiology and progression of such cancers. Estrogen receptors and progesterone receptors are expressed in approximately 50% of all ovarian cancers (53). There are, however, conflicting data on the relationship of the estrogen receptor to the prognosis of the cancer. Many have demonstrated that estrogen receptor status is not an independent prognostic factor. In contrast, the expression of progesterone receptor has been shown to be associated with a positive prognosis (54). There is also controversy as to the role of estrogens and progesterone in the pathogenesis of ovarian cancer. Recently, there has been a greater interest in the activity of aromatase in the ovary. This is an enzyme that catalyzes the conversion of androgens to estrone.

Aromatase activity has been demonstrated in the majority of ovarian cancers and has been localized to the stromal cells while benign ovarian tumors do not demonstrate aromatase activity. Intratumoral aromatase is more common in serous than in mucinous carcinomas (55).

GROWTH FACTORS AND CYTOKINES

Several cytokines and growth factors have been studied in ovarian carcinogenesis. For instance, levels of interleukin-10 (IL-10) and interleukin-6 (IL-6) are particularly elevated in ovarian cancer ascites (56,57). Preliminary studies have shown that on one hand, endogenously produced IL-6 can protect tumor cells from natural killer cell–mediated killing (57), while, on the other hand, high levels of IL-10 may play a role in immune responsiveness and the promotion of tumor growth (56-59).

Epidermal growth factor (EGF) receptors have been detected in a high percentage of ovarian cancer specimens, and overexpression of the receptor has been correlated with poor prognosis. The effects of tumor growth factor beta (TGF-β), which is closely related to EGF, are mediated through the EGF receptor, and TGF-β has been shown to inhibit the growth of normal surface epithelium and some ovarian cancer cell lines. Furthermore, fibroblast growth factor (FGF) was shown in one study to be mitogenic in one of four ovarian cancer cell lines (60). Receptors for two other factors, c-erb-2 and c-fms, have been identified, and increased levels of their oncogenes have been correlated with poor prognosis in ovarian cancer (61-66).

However, although *HER-2/neu* is overexpressed in about 30% of ovarian malignancies, it is infrequently amplified at the oncogene level and has thus not emerged as a promising clinical target in ovarian cancer.

TUMOR SUPPRESSOR GENES

The loss of normal *p53* function, due to mutation with deletion of the normal *p53* gene, is often associated with a malignant phenotype. The *p53* gene is located on chromosome 17p and has been seen to be mutated in 30 to 50% of ovarian cancers, more commonly in high-grade tumors (67,68). *MDR-1* is specifically stimulated by mutant *p53* and repressed by wild-type *p53* leading to increased drug resistance and a growth advantage in cells that express a mutated *p53* gene (69).

Tumor necrosis factor alpha (TNF-α), levels of which are also increased in ascites, has been shown to upregulate *p53* mRNA expression and to induce apoptosis in an ovarian cancer cell line (70). TNF-α also was recently found to follow a distinct pathway in inducing apoptosis (71). Upregulation by TNF-alpha of the mutated oncogene *p53* could induce proliferation of ovarian cancer cells, whereas its upregulation of wild-type *p53* would induce apoptosis (72,73).

■ PROGNOSTIC FACTORS

Prognostic factors are tumor-related characteristics that determine the biologic behavior and risk of death from the disease; their predictive value may change during the course of treatment and thereafter. Stage is a dominant prognostic factor in ovarian cancer. The main prognostic factors in early-stage ovarian cancer (stages I-IIA) are International Federation of Gynecology and Obstetrics (FIGO) stage, histologic grade, histologic type, and patient's age (74,75). Ovarian cancer is discovered early in fewer than 30% of patients; in such cases, the 5-year survival is good, ranging from 51 to 98% (74,76,77). Unfortunately, however, the histologic grading of ovarian tumors is based on subjective criteria and varies widely between and among observers (78-80).

CANCER ANTIGEN 125

The prognostic value of the preoperative CA 125 level in epithelial ovarian cancer is debatable (81,82). Most aggressive tumors are not necessarily those with the highest CA 125 levels. Although such levels are seen in the most poorly differentiated tumors, there is no big difference in the percentages of patients with low-grade and high-grade tumors who have elevated CA 125 levels (83,84). This suggests that the absolute level of CA 125 does not relate to the volume of ovarian tumor; furthermore, the expression of CA 125 in tissue shows no association with tumor grade, DNA ploidy, or S-phase fraction (85).

DNA PLOIDY ANALYSIS

DNA ploidy, which is the expression of a cell's nuclear DNA content, is an independent prognostic factor (86). Aneuploidy increases with age, stage, histology other than serous and mucinous, and degree of atypia and in the presence of *Pseudomyxoma peritonei*. In patients with invasive cancer, most tumors are aneuploid; most borderline tumors are diploid. To establish an individual tumor's ploidy, at least two biopsies from the solid tumor are required. S-phase fraction is currently not a reliable prognostic factor (87). Among stage I (early ovarian cancer) patients, diploid tumors are associated with an extremely good survival independent of adjuvant treatment. The 5-year disease-free survival for patients with diploid tumors is 90%, versus 64% for those with aneuploid tumors (88,89).

Factors associated with a poor prognosis in advanced ovarian cancer (stage III or IV) fall into two subgroups (as determined by multivariate analysis in clinical trials):

1. *Variables prior to systemic treatment predictive of survival:* Residual tumor >1 cm diameter, FIGO stage IV, poorer performance status, older age, undifferentiated tumor, presence of ascites, 20 or more sites of disease, clear cell or mucinous histology, aneuploid and polyploid tumors, clonogenic growth in vitro, and treatment center (90,91).
2. *Variables at the time of relapse predictive of time to progression:* Less than 180 days from last chemotherapy, poorer performance status, mucinous histology, larger number of sites of disease, best previous response to chemotherapy versus progression, serum CA 125 levels (92).

Low-risk patients with invasive advanced carcinomas are below age 40; have tumors that are euploid, of stage III, serous and/or endometrioid in type, and grade 1; they have no residual tumors. High-risk patients are above age 70; have tumors that are aneuploid, of stage IV, clear cell and/or unclassified in type, and grade III; they have bulky disease (87).

RESIDUAL DISEASE

Postoperative residual tumor volume may simply reflect the natural biology and history of the disease. Tumors that are more advanced are more difficult to resect and therefore associated with larger residual disease. Therefore, how advanced the tumor was before debulking may be more important than how much disease was left behind (93). Other features—such as the type of chemotherapy, the intrinsic chemosensitivity of the tumor, and the presence of other biological variables—may be as important as or even more important than the extent of the surgery (94-99). Indeed, Heintz et al. found that factors influencing the ability to perform optimal cytoreductive surgery were the same as those influencing disease-free and overall survival (95).

The literature on second-look surgery in ovarian cancer covers its diagnostic, prognostic, and therapeutic aspects. The earlier assumption that a negative second-look surgery is associated with excellent survival is evidently not true (100,101), since it is now quite clear that at least 30 to 50% of patients with no pathologic

evidence of disease will experience a relapse (101-103). Furthermore, patients with grade 3 tumors or grossly visible disease at completion of initial surgery also are at high risk. The question then remains whether additional treatment will affect outcome in these high-risk patients (survival difference) (92,102,103).

Some investigators have attempted to quantify the impact of pretreatment prognostic factors on survival and to construct a prognostic index (PI) from these factors. Five pretreatment characteristics so far used in calculating the PI are performance status, FIGO stage, residual tumor size, tumor grade, and presence of ascites (98,104,105). Prognostic factors under study that have produced promising results include *p53* immunostaining of epithelial ovarian cancers. It has been shown that those individuals whose tumors express excessive amounts of mutated *p53* experience shorter overall survival. However, those same studies failed to show that *p53* expression is an independent prognostic factor (99).

■ PATHOLOGY

The ovarian stroma and epithelium are of the same mesodermal origin (52). The epithelium lining the ovary and the peritoneum is similar to the coelomic epithelium that gives rise to the fallopian tube, uterus, cervix, and müllerian duct and from which approximately 75% of all primary ovarian neoplasms arise (Fig. 28-1). "Epithelial" ovarian tumors contain varying amounts and activities of the gonadal mesenchyme and are all potentially hormone-producing. They are classified

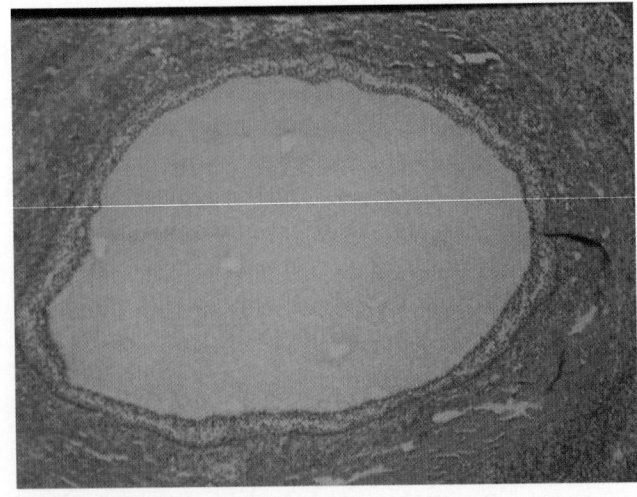

FIGURE 28-1. Histology of normal ovarian tissue.

according to cell type and behavior as benign, border-line malignant or of low malignant potential, or malignant. Criteria for the diagnosis of borderline malignant tumors are as follows:

1. Epithelial proliferation with papillary formation and pseudostratification
2. Nuclear atypia and increased mitotic activity
3. Absence of true stromal invasion

Some 20 to 25% of borderline malignant tumors have truly spread beyond the ovary, although rare examples of microinvasion have been reported; the prognosis of these tumors is determined by the nature of metastatic implants.

The major cell types of epithelial tumors are serous, mucinous, endometrioid, clear cell, transitional, and undifferentiated. The importance of distinguishing among different epithelial subtypes lies in their different biological behaviors, likelihood of spread, and consequent variation in prognosis and treatment. For the invasive epithelial carcinomas, however, the current consensus is that histologic type has limited prognostic significance in comparison with clinical stage, extent of residual disease, and histologic grade.

SEROUS TUMORS (FIGS. 28-2, 28-3)

Serous tumors represent 50% of epithelial ovarian tumors. Of these, 10% are borderline malignant serous tumors and 50% occur before the age of 40. The 5-year survival is 80 to 90%. Malignant calcified psammoma bodies are found in 80% of serous carcinomas (see Fig. 28-3).

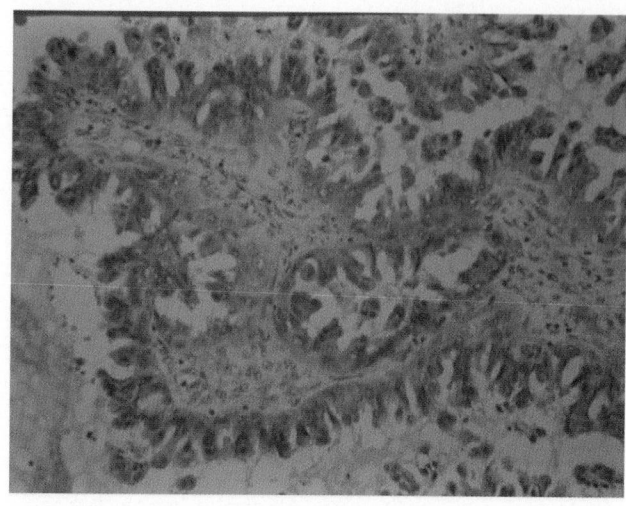

FIGURE 28-3. Histology of serous adenocarinoma.

MUCINOUS TUMORS (FIG. 28-4)

Mucinous tumors make up 8 to 10% of epithelial ovarian tumors. These tumors may reach enormous size, filling the entire abdominal cavity (Fig. 28-5). The tumors are bilateral in 8 to 10% of cases, and the mucinous lesions are intraovarian in 95 to 98% of cases. Pseudomyxoma peritonei is most commonly secondary to an ovarian mucinous carcinoma (Fig. 28-6).

ENDOMETRIOID TUMORS

Overall, 6 to 8% of epithelial ovarian tumors resemble endometrial adenocarcinoma, and both types occur

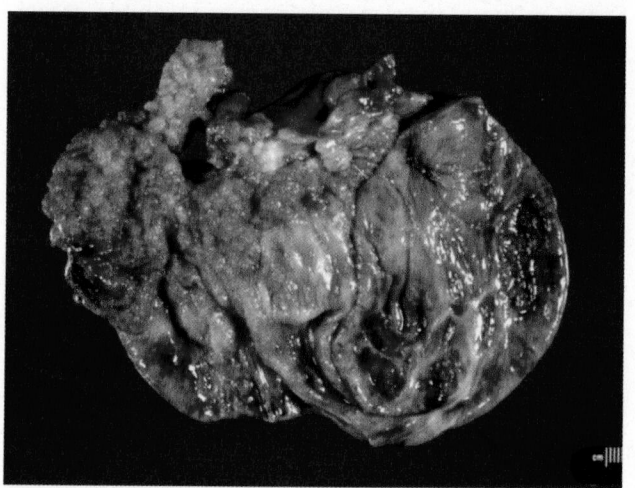

FIGURE 28-2. Gross specimen of serous adenocarcinoma of the ovary.

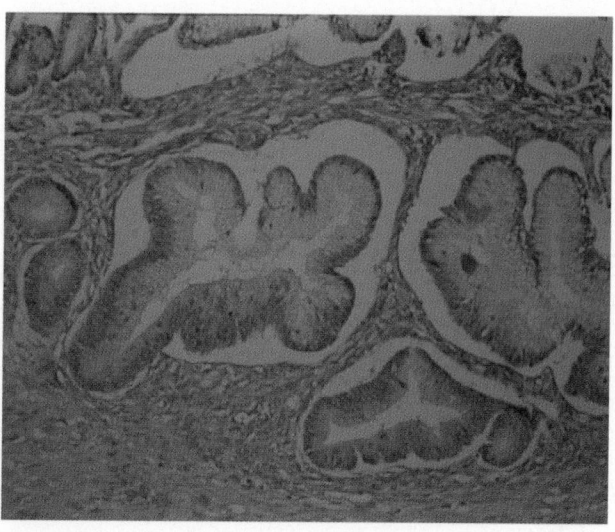

FIGURE 28-4. Histology of mucinous adenocarcinoma.

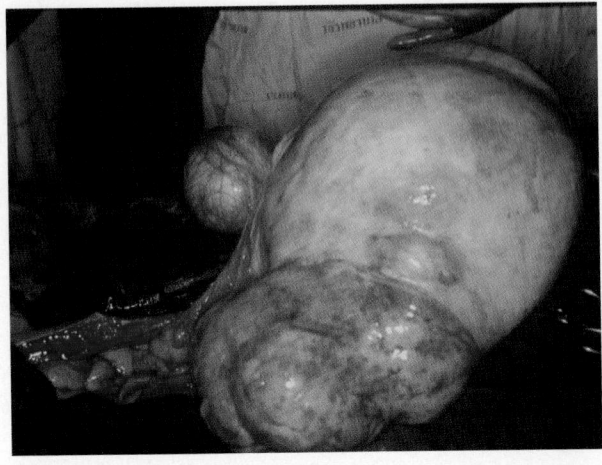

FIGURE 28-5. Operative removal of mucinous ovarian tumor.

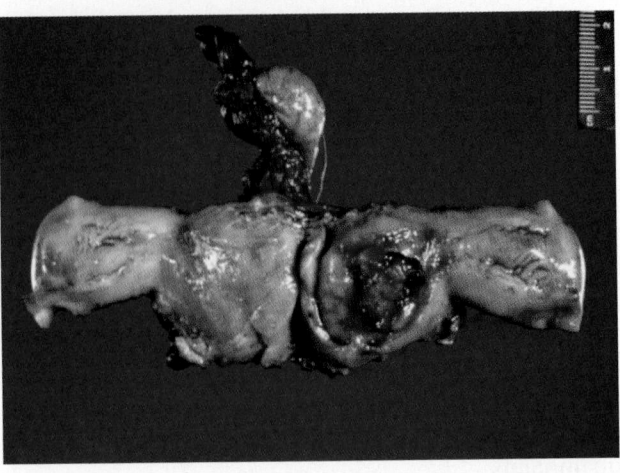

FIGURE 28-7. Gross specimen of clear cell carcinoma of the ovary.

simultaneously as synchronous primary tumors in 30% of cases. Identification of multifocal disease is important because patients with disease metastatic from the uterus to the ovaries have a 5-year survival rate of 30 to 40%. Those with synchronous multifocal disease have a 5-year survival rate of 75 to 80%. Concurrent endometriosis is present in 10% of cases. The malignant potential of endometriosis is very low, although a transition from benign to malignant epithelium may be seen.

Adenocarcinoma with benign-appearing squamous metaplasia has an excellent prognosis. Conversely, mixed adenosquamous carcinoma (malignant glandular and squamous epithelial) has a very poor one.

CLEAR CELL CARCINOMAS (FIGS. 28-7, 28-8)

Clear cell carcinomas occur in 5% of cases and may also be associated with endometriosis or endometrial cancer. Often the clear cell type coexists with other cell types. It is sometimes associated with hypercalcemia or hyperpyrexia. These tumors may have a worse prognosis than others.

BRENNER TUMORS

Brenner tumors can be malignant, borderline, or benign; they are very rare.

TRANSITIONAL CELL TUMORS

Some primary ovarian carcinomas resemble transitional cell carcinoma of the urinary bladder without a recognizable Brenner tumor. Ovarian carcinomas that are more than 50% transitional cell tumors are more sensitive to chemotherapy and have a more favorable prognosis (106).

UNDIFFERENTIATED CARCINOMAS

Undifferentiated carcinomas make up 17% of epithelial ovarian tumors; the prognosis for patients with these tumors is poor.

PRIMARY PERITONEAL CARCINOMA

Primary peritoneal carcinoma is characterized by carcinomatosis with peritoneal epithelium as the primary

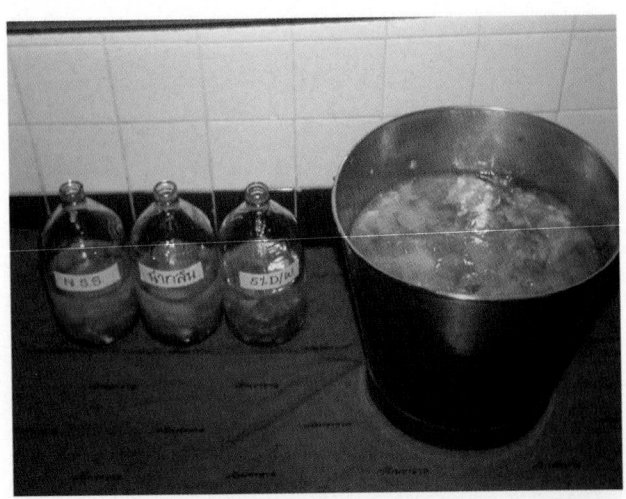

FIGURE 28-6. Copious mucinous material removed from peritoneal cavity from mucinous ovarian tumor.

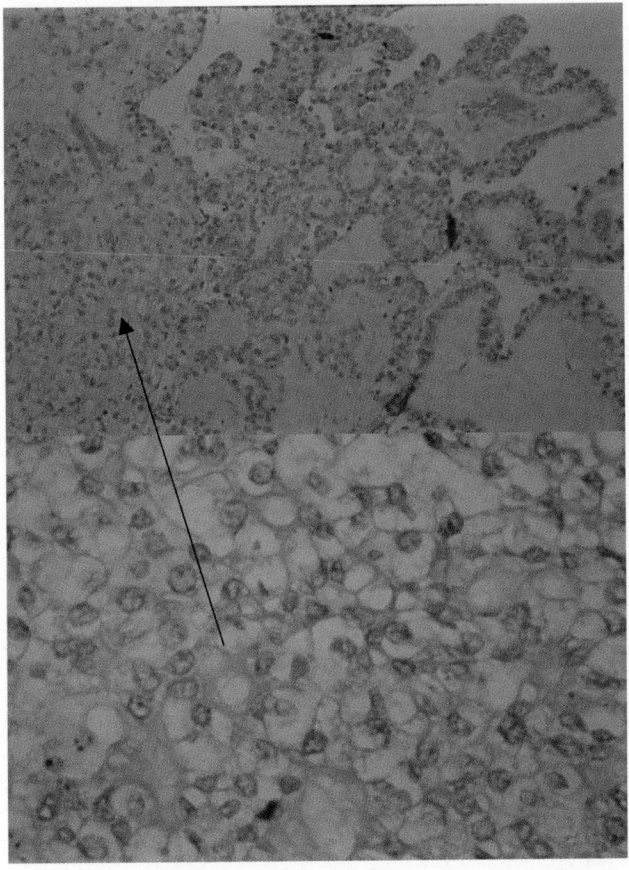

FIGURE 28-8. Histology of clear cell carcinoma of the ovary.

source. The ovaries are not involved with tumor, or only their surfaces may be involved. Women with such tumors may have a remote history of oophorectomy.

HISTOLOGIC GRADING

Two histologic grading systems are in common use. The pattern system considers the general microscopic appearance of a lesion. Lesions range from grade 1 (well differentiated) to grade 2 (moderately differentiated and predominantly glandular) to grade 3 (poorly differentiated and predominantly solid). Broder grading system classifies lesions from grade 1 to 4, depending on the lesions' cytologic and nuclear characteristics. This system assumes grade 4 to be an undifferentiated lesion. Pathologists usually use a combination of both systems. The value of grade as an independent prognostic variable has not been fully clarified. A number of reports state that tumor grade may be of value in early-stage ovarian cancer but that its value falls off in patients with advanced-stage disease.

■ STAGING

Accurate staging is critical to the success of surgery and adjuvant therapy. The staging of ovarian cancer is based on the gross and pathologic findings of the initial surgical evaluation. The FIGO classification uses the sites and extent of the disease, including capsule rupture and ascites, to categorize ovarian cancer into four stages. This is summarized in Table 28-3. Procedures required to confirm staging are described later in the chapter.

■ DIAGNOSIS

Objective signs of ovarian carcinoma are nonspecific and include a pelvic mass, ascites, pleural effusion, and occasionally supraclavicular lymphadenopathy. Patients with ovarian cancer may occasionally present with various types of paraneoplastic conditions, such as humorally mediated hypercalcemia (clear cell, small cell), cerebellar degeneration (associated with antibodies to Purkinje cells), the sudden appearance of seborrheic keratosis (a sign of Leser-Trelat syndrome), or chronic intravascular coagulation (Trousseau syndrome). Preoperative evaluation should include a barium enema, an abdominal/pelvic computed tomography (CT), blood chemistries, chest x-ray, and CA 125 measurement. If symptoms of obstruction are present, an upper gastrointestinal (GI) series may be indicated. Mammograms may be helpful in ruling out metastatic breast cancer. Ascitic or pleural fluid should be tapped and examined.

■ MANAGEMENT

SURGERY

A full staging laparotomy with the following steps should be performed as far as possible as follows:

- Midline vertical incision
- Evacuation and cytologic analysis of ascites
- Peritoneal washings of pelvis and paracolic gutters
- Inspection and palpation of all peritoneal (intraperitoneal and retroperitoneal) surfaces, including the subdiaphragmatic areas
- Frozen section of ovarian mass (unilateral or bilateral) followed by bilateral salpingo-oophorectomy of carcinoma
- Omentectomy with optimal bulk reduction of remaining tumor masses

TABLE 28-3 | STAGING

FIGO		TNM
0	Primary tumor cannot be assessed	TX
	No evidence of primary tumor	T0
I	Tumor confined to ovaries	T1
IA	Tumor limited to one ovary, capsule intact	T1a
	No tumor on ovarian surface	
	No malignant cells in the ascites or peritoneal washings	
IB	Tumor limited to both ovaries, capsules intact	T1b
	No tumor on ovarian surface	
	No malignant cells in the ascites or peritoneal washings	
IC	Tumor limited to one or both ovaries, with any of the following capsules ruptured, tumor on ovarian surface, positive malignant cells in the ascites, or positive peritoneal washings	T1c
II	Tumor involves one or both ovaries with pelvic extension	T2
IIA	Extension and/or implants in uterus and/or tubes	T2a
	No malignant cells in the ascites or peritoneal washings	
IIB	Extension to other pelvic organ	T2b
	No malignant cells in the ascites or peritoneal washings	
IIC	IIA/B with any of the following:	T2c
	Capsule ruptured, tumor on ovarian surface, positive malignant cells in the ascites, or positive peritoneal washings	
III	Tumor involves one or both ovaries with microscopically confirmed peritoneal metastasis outside the pelvis and/or regional lymph node metastasis	T3
IIIA	Microscopic peritoneal metastases beyond the pelvis	T3a
IIIB	Macroscopic peritoneal metastases beyond the pelvis 2 cm or less in greatest dimension	T3b
IIIC	Peritoneal metastases beyond pelvis more than 2 cm in greatest dimension and/or regional lymph node metastasis	T3c
IV	Distant metastases beyond the peritoneal cavity	M1

NOTE: Liver capsule metastasis is T3/stage III, liver parenchymal metastasis M1/stage IV. Pleural effusion must have positive cytology.

- Relief of intestinal obstruction by resection or colostomy
- If disease limited to ovaries, multiple biopsies including the paracolonic gutters, cul-de-sac, lateral pelvic walls, vesicouterine reflection, subdiaphragmatic sites, and intraabdominal areas
- Ipsilateral and paraaortic lymph node sampling if conservative therapy is planned

A unilateral salpingo-oophorectomy without hysterectomy may be considered for those patients with low-risk early-stage disease who wish to maintain fertility (107). Repeat surgery for staging may be indicated in patients who have been inadequately staged and in whom this will provide further information affecting treatment. After surgery is completed, the patient's histologic grade, stage, and residual disease should be characterized.

FIGO staging criteria, whose prognostic value is well established, are used to stage these tumors. According to FIGO, stage I has a 5-year survival rate of 80 to 90%; stage II has a 5-year survival rate of 40 to 60%; stage III has a 5-year survival rate of 10 to 15%; and stage IV has a 5-year survival rate of less than 5%. Differences in survival among patients with the same FIGO stage of disease may indicate incomplete staging. This may limit stage as a prognostic factor. Frequently unrecognized sites of disease include the pelvic lymph nodes, cul-de-sac peritoneum, paraaortic nodes, omentum, and diaphragm.

When comprehensive staging is performed, a substantial number of patients initially believed to have disease confined to the pelvis will be staged upward. Young et al. (108) initially reported on a group of 100 patients, 62 of whom agreed to be restaged after being referred for treatment of stage I or II cancer. Approximately one third (31%) of these patients were staged upward, with the final stage in most becoming stage III. Soper et al. (109) undertook a comparable study and reported similar results. The benefit of cytoreductive surgery is most clear at the time of diagnosis and initial surgery for ovarian cancer. There are no prospective randomized trials comparing patients with optimal versus suboptimal cytoreduction, but accumulated retrospective data shows a strong correlation between the volume of residual tumor and survival (110).

The earliest data to support maximal cytoreduction came from Griffith et al. in 1975, when he published a retrospective study demonstrating improved survival in women with advanced-stage disease who had no residual disease after primary surgery (111). His data indicated, however, that there was no improvement in survival if there were residual tumor deposits greater than 1.5 cm in size. These findings have been confirmed by at least two Gynecologic Oncology Group (GOG) studies comprising more than 500 patients demonstrating improved pathologic response, survival, disease-free interval, and complete clinical response in patients with no residual nodules greater than 1.0 cm in size (111,112). These data have also been confirmed by many single-institution trials. The rationale for cytoreductive surgery is based on kinetic as well as retrospective studies, which have shown that patients with small-volume residual disease following initial surgery respond better to subsequent chemotherapy and survive longer.

Optimal surgical cytoreduction can be performed with acceptable morbidity in a large proportion of those patients with advanced-stage ovarian cancer (113-117). If one cannot cytoreduce the tumor burden to less than 1 to 2 cm of residual disease, no significant survival benefit is realized. The role of surgical cytoreduction in stage IV disease is somewhat more controversial than it is in stage III disease, since these patients have parenchymal liver disease or extraperitoneal disease. However, over the past decade, emerging data suggest a survival advantage for those patients who can be optimally cytoreduced, a likelihood that is smaller than in patients with stage III disease (118-121). Together, these studies suggest that survival in patients with advanced bulky ovarian carcinoma is influenced by many factors other than the surgeon's technical ability to cytoreduce tumor bulk. Instead, tumor biology probably plays an important but undefined role in the natural history of the disease.

Cytoreductive surgery in properly selected patients probably helps palliate intestinal obstruction and abdominal discomfort. However, there are no prospective randomized studies to prove the survival benefit of cytoreductive surgery (122). Nevertheless, in the absence of a prospective randomized trial, the standard practice remains cytoreductive surgery when it can be accomplished with acceptable morbidity. The importance of secondary cytoreduction following chemotherapy, however, remains controversial, since there is no evidence to suggest that second-look laparotomy prolongs survival (123,124).

Secondary Cytoreduction

Second-Look Surgery

The information obtained at a second look is primarily prognostic. However, information from a negative second look is of limited clinical benefit: in 30 to 50% of patients who obtain a surgically confirmed complete response (CR), disease will recur (112,123). Nevertheless, one randomized study reports that patients with recurrent or progressive ovarian cancer who had optimal (<2 cm) secondary cytoreduction survived longer (mean, 27.1 months) than those who had unsuccessful surgery (mean, 9 months) (125).

Interval Cytoreduction

Two phase III trials have reached opposing conclusions regarding any favourable effect of interval cytoreduction after several cycles of chemotherapy in a patient who has already undergone an initial attempt at cytoreduction (126,127). Different patient cohorts, type of chemotherapy, intent of primary surgery, and use of maintenance therapy might have contributed to this disagreement.

Secondary Cytoreduction for Recurrent Disease

The benefits of secondary cytoreduction for recurrent disease are also unclear, although accumulating data suggest that, in certain circumstances, this may be of significant survival benefit. Eisenkop et al. published a large series of patients with recurrent ovarian cancer undergoing cytoreduction for recurrent disease (128). There were 106 patients who had enjoyed a complete clinical response to initial therapy. These patients had a disease-free interval of at least 6 months prior to recurrence. Sixty percent underwent reexploration and debulking, and 82% were rendered disease-free at that time. The authors evaluated factors that might be predictive of surgical outcome (optimal debulking) as well as those that might be indicative of survival. Predictors of complete cytoreduction included (1) size of recurrent tumor less than 10 cm, (2) the use of chemotherapy before cytoreduction, and (3) good Karnofsky performance status.

The following influenced survival: (1) disease-free interval (DFI) after primary treatment (DFI 6-12 months, with a median survival of 25 months, versus DFI 13-36 months, with a median survival of 44.4 months versus DFI more than 36 months, with a median survival of 56.8 months); (2) completeness of surgical cytoreduction, no residual (median survival, 44 months) versus macroscopic disease (median survival, 19.3 months); and (3) the use of salvage chemotherapy.

A study from MDACC looked at a similar group of patients who also had a disease-free interval of at least 6 months, with similar results (129). These investigators noted that there was significantly improved survival in women who underwent optimal cytoreduction of tumor to less than 2 cm (19.5 versus 8.3 months). Others have published similar findings, all noting that the duration of prior clinical response is important in terms of survival and chances of optimal cytoreduction (125). These data underscore the need for all patients with ovarian cancer to be followed by a gynecologic oncologist. This allows complex decisions to be made correctly with regard to surgical or medical therapy.

■ TREATMENT OF PRIMARY DISEASE

CHEMOTHERAPY

Limited Disease

The Royal Marsden Study reviewed 194 patients with stage I epithelial ovarian cancer who had received no adjuvant treatment but were under regular follow-up with physical examination, CA 125, and CT scan. At a median follow-up of 54 months, 5-year disease-free survival of patients with stage IA disease was 87%; stage IB, 65%; and stage IC disease, 62%. Five-year overall survival for stage IA patients was 93.7%; stage IB, 92%; and stage IC, 84%. It was observed that factors associated with an increased risk of relapse in multivariate analyses included extraovarian spread, grade 3 histology/ poorly differentiated, rupture of capsule, dense adhesions, clear cell histology, extracystic tumor, and positive peritoneal washing (130).

The first trial in the United States was in patients with good prognosis and early stage 1A or 1B. A total of 92 patients were randomized to either melphalan or no treatment. Their 5-year disease-free survival was 91 versus 98%, respectively, while 5-year overall survival was 94 versus 98%. The authors concluded that patients with early good prognoses do not require adjuvant treatment (77). The second trial involved 141 patients with stages I and II disease and poorly differentiated

histology. They were given melphalan versus intraperitoneal chronic phosphate (P-32). The 5-year disease-free survival was 80% for both arms (77). The 5-year overall survival at 81% (melphalan arm) versus 78% (P-32) was not statistically significant. It was concluded, after multivariate analysis showed clear cell tumor and histologic grading to be related to outcome, that the preferred adjuvant treatment was P-32 for high-risk patients.

The Gruppo Interregionale Collaborativo in Ginecologia Oncologica (GICOG) then had two randomized trials comparing adjuvant cisplatin (CDDP) versus no treatment and CDDP versus P-32. In total, there were 271 patients with stage I ovarian cancer after radical surgery. In the first trial, patients were randomized to receiving CDDP versus no adjuvant treatment. The 5-year disease-free survival was 65% in the control arm and 83% in the CDDP arm; the 5-year overall survival was 82% in the control arm and 88% in the CDDP arm. The second trial randomized 161 patients to CDDP versus P-32. The 5-year disease-free survival was 65% in the P-32 arm and 85% in the CDDP arm ($p = .008$); the 5-year overall survival was 79% in the P-32 arm and 81% in the CDDP arm ($p = .354$). Both trials were criticized as containing too few patients, thus resulting in low statistical power, and the dose of CDDP was considered to be suboptimal (131).

At the same time, a Norwegian trial randomized patients to CDDP versus P-32 or whole abdominal radiotherapy (WAR) as adjuvant treatment (N = 347). Patients with early epithelial ovarian cancer (EOC) were accrued (a few FIGO stage III patients were included) from 1982 to 1988. CDDP was given at 50 mg/m^2 every 3 weeks for six cycles (N = 169), P-32 or WAR (N = 171, WAR, N = 28), or WAR and abdominal pelvic radiotherapy (RT). Anteroposterior (AP) fields received 2200 cGy in 20 patients and 11 patients were given 2200 cGy to the pelvis. The 5-year disease-free survival for patients who received P-32 was 81%, while it was 75% for those who received CDDP ($p = .57$ NS). The 5-year overall survival (OS) for P-32 was 83%; and for CDDP, it was 81% ($p = .6$ NS). It was concluded that CDDP should be standard of treatment in view of its lower toxicity compared to P-32 (132).

The GOG 95 trial studied stages IC and II and poorly differentiated stages IA and IB. The 205 evaluable patients were randomized to intraperitoneal P-32 (N = 98) versus cyclophosphamide (1000 mg/m^2 every 21 days for three cycles) and cisplatin 100 mg/m^2 (CP) every 21 days for three cycles) (N = 107). The 5-year disease-free survival for P-32 was 66%, while it was 77% ($p = .08$) for CP, with a 31% reduction in time to progression. The 5-year overall survival for P-32 was 76%; for CP, it was 84% (not significant). It was concluded that although there were no statistical differences between two groups, CP was preferred standard treatment because of a better progression-free interval (133). The largest international randomized trials, the ACTION and ICON trials, in early ovarian cancer were reported in 2003 (134). Between November 1990 and January 2000, a total of 925 patients who had had surgery for early-stage ovarian cancer were randomly assigned to receive platinum-based adjuvant chemotherapy (N = 465) or observation (N = 460) until chemotherapy was indicated. When the ACTION (Adjuvant Chemotherapy in Ovarian Neoplasms) trial was analyzed alone, the overall survival was not significant and the recurrence-free survival advantage was limited to suboptimally debulked patients (135). However, when all the patients in the ICON (International Collaborative Ovarian Neoplasm) trial and ACTION trials were combined, the overall survival at 5 years was 82% in the chemotherapy arm and 74% in the observation arm. Recurrence-free survival at 5 years was also better in the adjuvant chemotherapy arm than it was in the observation arm. Both of these results were significant. In conclusion, it is the consensus that patients with early-stage ovarian cancer can also benefit from adjuvant chemotherapy.

More recently, one clinical trial involving patients with limited disease was completed. The goal was to determine whether six cycles of carboplatin and paclitaxel would significantly lower the rate of cancer recurrence, compared to three cycles of the same agents following surgical staging operations on patients with stage IA grade 3, stage IB grade 3, stage IC, and completely resected stage II ovarian epithelial cancer. A secondary objective was to compare the toxicities of the two treatments. Following surgical staging laparotomy, TAH (Total Abdominal Hysterectomy), and BSO (Bilateral Salpingo-Oophorectomy), 321 patients were randomized to either three or six cycles of paclitaxel 175 mg/m^2 infused over 3 h followed by carboplatin 7.5 AUC (area under the curve) infused over 30 min. Cycles were repeated every 21 days. A total of 70% of these patients had stage I disease. In the standard three-cycle arm, the estimated probability of cancer recurring within 5 years was 27%, compared to 19% in the six-cycle arm. The risk of recurrence was 33% lower for patients treated with six cycles of chemotherapy, with a relative hazard of 0.672. If the treatment comparison includes the patients considered ineligible due to incomplete surgical staging, then the recurrence rate was 24% less on the six-cycle regimen, with a relative hazard of 0.762. It was concluded that the addition of three cycles of

carboplatin and paclitaxel over the standard three cycles did not significantly alter the rate of cancer recurrence in patients with early-stage ovarian epithelial carcinoma. In addition, six cycles caused significantly more toxicity than three cycles (136).

Advanced Disease

Before the 1990s, patients with advanced ovarian cancer had little to look forward to after cytoreductive surgery. There were few studies to suggest that—apart from whole-abdominal radiotherapy—adjuvant therapy made any difference in disease-free and overall survival. Until the 1990s, chemotherapy had been largely based on alkylating agents such as melphalan and cyclophosphamide. Adjuvant chemotherapy with such agents was less than satisfactory. With the development of cisplatin came the first hopes that adjuvant chemotherapy could make a difference in patients' prognosis. Then carboplatin was developed and found to be better tolerated. Soon, it became clear that platinum-containing chemotherapies were superior to nonplatinum-containing regimens.

In 1991, the Advanced Ovarian Cancer Trialist Group (AOCTG) published a meta-analysis considering the role of platinum and the relative merits of single-agent and combination chemotherapy in the treatment of advanced ovarian cancer. This represented a quantitative overview of updated individual patient data from 8139 patients in 45 available randomized trials (137). There were three conclusions. First, the results suggested that, in terms of survival, immediate platinum-based treatment was better than any nonplatinum regimen, with the overall relative risk at 0.93. Second, platinum in combination was better than single-agent platinum when used at the same dose, with an overall relative risk of 0.85. Finally, cisplatin and carboplatin were equally effective, with an overall relative risk of 1.05. A similar conclusion came from two large North American trials: a trial by the Southwest Oncology Group (342 patients with stage III or IV disease randomized to receive cisplatin and cyclophosphamide versus carboplatin plus cyclophosphamide [138]) and a trial by the National Cancer Institute of Canada (139). None of these failed trials demonstrated a significant difference in overall survival, though the carboplatin regimen was found to have a better therapeutic index and to produce a better quality of life.

In contrast, a French trial involving 144 patients with stage III or IV disease who received either cisplatin or carboplatin had very different results (140). The pathologic complete remission and overall response rates were significantly higher in the cisplatin arm than in the carboplatin arm (33 versus 15% and 73 versus 47%, respectively). The median survival time was 27.9 months for the cisplatin arm and 20.6 months for the carboplatin arm. The actual delivered dose intensity of the drugs in the two arms was not reported.

In 1992, another systematic overview of 54 randomized clinical trials testing a variety of chemotherapeutic approaches in advanced ovarian carcinoma was reported. Prolonged follow-up data are available for most patients, and individual patient data were made available for all patients; analysis was made on the basis of "intention to treat." This report concentrated on two comparisons: (1) platinum alone versus platinum in combination, apparently showing a long-term survival advantage for the combination; and (2) carboplatin versus cisplatin, showing no obvious survival differences. It was striking that no single study to date has been large enough to detect the modest survival differences expected from current therapy (141).

As a result of these studies, the ICON group in Europe decided to look at single-agent carboplatin, the least toxic of all chemotherapies, compared to the combination containing carboplatin. ICON II compared the combination of cyclophosphamide, doxorubicin, and cisplatin (CAP) with single-agent carboplatin in women with ovarian cancer requiring chemotherapy. A total of 1526 patients were entered from 132 centers in nine European countries. The overall survival curves showed no evidence of a difference between CAP and carboplatin, with a hazard ratio of 1.00. The results indicate a median survival of 33 months and a 2-year survival of 60% for both groups. It was concluded that in view of the greater toxicities of CAP compared to carboplatin, single-agent carboplatin was the appropriate standard of treatment for women with advanced ovarian cancer (142). Meanwhile, in the United States, paclitaxel, extracted from the Pacific yew tree, was discovered by the drug screen of the National Cancer Institute (NCI) in the forests of South America. The success of paclitaxel in recurrent ovarian cancer prompted efforts to look into paclitaxel as a component of frontline therapy. Two large phase III trials were published; these formed the basis for our current standard of care. The first of these was GOG protocol 111, which randomized patients with large-volume advanced disease to cyclophosphamide plus cisplatin or paclitaxel plus cisplatin. This study showed superiority for the paclitaxel-and-cisplatin regimen compared with cyclophosphamide and cisplatin in regard to five parameters: (1) response rate, (2) clinical CR rate, (3) percentage of patients grossly disease-free at second-look

laparotomy, (4) progression-free survival (PFS), and (5) overall survival (143). Approximately $1\frac{1}{2}$ years after the publication of this trial, a confirmatory study from a European-Canadian consortium called OV-10 was presented (144). This study also randomized patients to either cyclophosphamide and cisplatin or paclitaxel and cisplatin. The population here comprised women with stage IIB through IV disease and included both small- and large-volume patients. The combination of paclitaxel and platinum proved to be superior to the cyclophosphamide and platinum combination with regard to response rate, clinical CR rate, PFS (progression-free survival), and overall survival. The numbers also closely reproduced the numbers seen with GOG protocol 111.

That led to the conclusion, in the middle to latter 1990s, that the standard of care in ovarian carcinoma was paclitaxel plus a platinum compound, although the preferred dosing schedule of each agent was not totally clear at that time.

Now that a possibly superior regimen had been found, the question of carboplatin versus cisplatin arose: whether carboplatin could be substituted for cisplatin in order to improve the regimen from the standpoint of both toxicity and ease of administration. Two large trials were done, a German trial and a GOG trial in the United States. The German trial, presented in 1998, randomized 798 patients with advanced ovarian cancer to either paclitaxel and cisplatin or paclitaxel and carboplatin (145). The results showed equivalence between the two regimens with regard to response rate, clinical CR rate, PFS (progression-free survival), and overall survival. The large number of patients in this study, 798, made it possible to conclude that the regimens were equivalent.

Confirmation came from GOG protocol 158, a study that focused on patients with stage III optimal or minimal residual disease. Patients were again randomized to either paclitaxel and cisplatin or paclitaxel and carboplatin. The results showed equivalence between the two regimens with regard to pathologic CR rate and PFS. The study continues to be followed for purposes of survival analysis when enough events have occurred (146). As a result of these two large trials, it was concluded that cisplatin and carboplatin were equivalent in combination with paclitaxel and that it would be not only feasible but also easier to treat these patients with paclitaxel plus carboplatin as opposed to other regimens.

The results of OV 10 and GOG 111 led to another ICON trial. ICON III aimed to compare the safety and efficacy of paclitaxel plus carboplatin with a control of cisplatin, doxorubicin, and cyclophosphamide (CAP) or carboplatin alone. Between 1995 and 1998, a total of 2074 patients from 130 centers in eight European countries were accrued. Women were randomly assigned paclitaxel plus carboplatin or control, the control (CAP or single-agent carboplatin) being chosen by the patient and clinician before randomization. At a median follow-up of 51 months, the survival curves showed no evidence of a difference in overall survival between paclitaxel plus carboplatin and control, the hazard ratio being 0.98. The median overall survival was 36.1 months on paclitaxel plus carboplatin and 35.4 months on control. Median PFS was 17.3 months on paclitaxel plus carboplatin and 16.1 months on control. When this trial was interpreted, it was concluded that single-agent carboplatin and CAP are as effective as paclitaxel plus carboplatin as first-line treatment for women requiring chemotherapy for ovarian cancer. The favorable toxicity profile of single-agent carboplatin suggests that this drug is a reasonable option as first-line chemotherapy for ovarian cancer (147).

Alternative Chemotherapeutic Agents

Docetaxel (Taxotere) is a semisynthetic compound structurally related to paclitaxel. The toxicity of docetaxel is in many ways similar to that of paclitaxel. However, prolonged treatment with docetaxel increases skin toxicity and produces significant edema. A very recent trial by the Europeans concluded that docetaxel could be an alternative to paclitaxel. A total of 1077 patients with FIGO stage IC to IV EOC (epithelial ovarian cancer) were randomized to receive either paclitaxel and carboplatin or docetaxel with carboplatin; the median follow-up in surviving patients was 21 months. Median PFS and overall survival (at 18 months) for patients treated with docetaxel and carboplatin was 15.1 months and 73.5% and for paclitaxel and carboplatin was 15.4 months and 76.6%, respectively. The main on-treatment toxicity differences between the two arms were neurotoxicity (more common with the paclitaxel combination) and myelosuppression (more common with the docetaxel combination). Statistically significantly less neurotoxicity following the docetaxel combination appeared to be still evident at 10 months postrandomization. Global quality-of-life parameters were comparable in both arms. However, there were significantly less arthralgic/myalgic symptoms during treatment with the docetaxel combination at 33.0% compared with paclitaxel combination at 48.0%, as well as less weakness in legs or arms with the docetaxel combination at 33.9%, whereas the combination with paclitaxel had a 47.7% occurrence. The authors concluded that

the docetaxel combination appears to be a viable alternative to the paclitaxel combination as first-line chemotherapy in EOC because of an improved therapeutic index while maintaining similar efficacy (148).

Back in North America, the search for better frontline chemotherapy continued. Of interest was the combination of a third agent, creating sequential or combination triplets. In the first trial, GOG 132, patients with large-volume advanced disease were randomized to either single-agent cisplatin; single-agent paclitaxel; or a combination of paclitaxel and cisplatin. In terms of survival, there were no significant differences among these three arms (149). That prompted a further look to determine why the combination did not prove to be superior. What soon became apparent was the fact that in this particular study, if there was any residual disease at the conclusion of frontline therapy, patients immediately received the other agent. Effectively, therefore, instead of studying single-agent therapy versus combination chemotherapy, sequential single-agents versus combination chemotherapy was being tested. This may have affected the results.

Nevertheless, this trial formed the basis for some novel ways of incorporating a third agent into frontline therapy. The agents that GOG focused on were those that had demonstrated the ability to get responses in paclitaxel- and platinum-resistant disease. There are four such drugs, oral etoposide, topotecan, liposomal doxorubicin, and gemcitabine. Oral etoposide, unfortunately, when combined with paclitaxel and carboplatin, induces acute leukemia in a small percentage of patients but one that is high enough to raise concerns. So the focus instead was on topotecan, doxorubicin, and gemcitabine introduced as new agents in frontline therapy.

This has resulted in GOG protocol 182/ICON V. The control arm is paclitaxel plus carboplatin for eight cycles. The experimental arms include two triplet regimens. Regimen II is paclitaxel, carboplatin, and gemcitabine given on each of eight cycles. Regimen V is paclitaxel, carboplatin, and doxorubicin, with the doxorubicin given on cycles 1, 3, 5, and 7. There are also two sequential doublet regimens: (1) regimen III, gemcitabine and carboplatin, followed by paclitaxel and carboplatin, and (2) regimen IV, topotecan and carboplatin, followed by paclitaxel and carboplatin. However, in this now completed phase III trial, investigators have reported no improvement for any arm in comparison with the control arm (150).

Additional Combination Chemotherapy

Researchers also looked at the addition of anthracycline to make concurrent triplets. It was accepted that either cyclophosphamide (750 mg/m^2) plus cisplatin (75 mg/m^2) every 3 weeks or cyclophosphamide (500 mg/m^2) plus doxorubicin (50 mg/m^2) plus cisplatin (50 mg/m^2) every 3 weeks (CAP) is acceptable standard therapy. However, four prospective randomized trials comparing cisplatin and cyclophosphamide with the CAP regimen failed to show statistically significant differences in overall survival (151-153). The largest of the above trials was that of the Italian Cooperative Gynecologic Oncology Group (GICOG), which randomized 529 patients to receive CAP, cisplatin/cyclophosphamide, or single-agent cisplatin (151). No statistical difference was seen in overall survival (minimum follow-up 5 years) among the three groups. Meta-analysis of the above four trials (154) revealed a 6-year survival advantage of 7% in patients receiving the doxorubicin-containing regimen, but it remains unclear whether the benefit was a result of doxorubicin or the greater dose intensity reached by adding it. There was also a very large German trial with 1281 patients comparing paclitaxel, epirubicin, and carboplatin with paclitaxel and carboplatin. As presented at the American Society of Clinical Oncology meetings, there were no significant differences in response, PFS, or overall survival even though a meta-analysis 10 years ago suggested that adding an anthracycline might be of benefit. As a result, it does not appear that the addition of either doxorubicin or epirubicin to frontline therapy is beneficial (155).

Neoadjuvant chemotherapy

The preliminary results of a large phase III trial (EORTC55971) showed that neoadjuvant chemotherapy followed by debulking surgery produces similar outcomes to primary debulking followed by chemotherapy in stages IIIC and IV disease (156).

Consolidation Therapy

The high risk of recurrent disease after treatment of advanced-stage epithelial ovarian cancer has prompted an intensive search for therapeutic strategies that can be given after standard-of-care therapy to improve patient outcomes. More than 12 phase III trials have been undertaken in this setting, including extension of frontline agents, administration of short duration non-cross resistant chemotherapy, high-dose chemotherapy, whole-abdominal or intraperitoneal radiotherapy, immunotherapy, vaccine therapy, biologic therapy, and single-agent paclitaxel; however, none have shown a survival advantage against various controls (usually no treatment) (51,157). The single-agent paclitaxel strategy has been assessed in two phase III trials giving paclitaxel for 6 or 12 months.

Only S9701/GOG178, a phase III trial that administered paclitaxel intravenously for 12 months (versus 3 months) after an initial response to first-line chemotherapy showed improved progression-free survival.

Intraperitoneal Chemotherapy

The intraperitoneal administration of cisplatin as primary chemotherapy for debulked epithelial ovarian cancer results in a 20 to 30% improvement in both progression-free and overall survival times by comparison with intravenous delivery (158-162). However, the randomized trials have been criticized (162) and intraperitoneal chemotherapy has not been universally accepted for at least three reasons: toxic effects, intraperitoneal treatment delivery issues (eg, technical experience with catheter placement and management), and complications (eg, intraperitoneal adhesions, infections) (163). In response to concerns about underuse, a National Cancer Institute clinical announcement made on January 5, 2006, encouraged oncologists to use intraperitoneal cisplatin after optimum cytoreduction in patients with epithelial ovarian cancer. However, for intraperitoneal therapy to become widely accepted, an ambulatory regimen needs to be established with acceptable toxic effects that preserve the survival advantage (164). The Gynecology Oncology Group is also planning a phase III trial that will test whether intraperitoneal chemotherapy is associated with survival benefits by comparison with intravenous chemotherapy when the targeted agent bevacizumab is added to the treatment regimen. Finally, early data suggest that hyperthermic intraperitoneal chemotherapy is promising, but this treatment is still highly investigational (165).

Dose Intensity

The relationship between the dose of chemotherapy and response and/or survival has been investigated extensively. There have now been seven randomized trials of dose intensity in the treatment of ovarian cancer, and two more with intraperitoneal chemotherapy. Clinically, it is possible for a dose intensity of two- to threefold with cytokine support and five to ten times with stem cell support for cancer treatment.

Cisplatin

The landmark meta-analysis was that of a collection of 60 studies where there seemed to be a correlation between the dose intensity of the chemotherapy and response in ovarian cancer. However, the dose intensity studied translated into a difference of 18 mg/m^2 compared to 36 mg/m^2 (166), a range well below the dose of

50 to 75 mg/m^2 that is conventionally used in patients. A similar meta-analysis in 1993 came to the same conclusion for cisplatin up to 75 mg/m^2, but again suffered the same handicap of not being able to support dose intensity beyond 75 mg/m^2 (167).

■■■ Uncontrolled Trials

Evidence from nonrandomized trials initially led to the observation that higher doses or alternative administration of IP cisplatin resulted in responses in patients who were initially resistant to cisplatin (168). However, a closer look revealed that many of those who were deemed to have responded to reinduction cisplatin had actually responded originally to platinum, but they merely had a shorter relapse interval than the conventional 6 months.

■■■ Randomized Trials

Seven randomized trials have been performed (169-175). These are summarized in Table 28-4.

Overall, they seem to conclude that by doubling the dose of platinum, it increased toxicity without providing further therapeutic gain. Five of the seven studies showed no difference in response rate or survival. The other randomized trials showed advantages in dose-intensity regimen. The large Scottish trial also showed a difference in survival but included in its population optimally debulked patients with stage IC to IV disease.

However, a separate analysis by the Scottish investigators of patients with advanced ovarian cancer still showed a difference favoring the high-dose arm with respect to PFS and overall survival. Patients on the high-dose arm received the same number of treatment cycles as those in the low-dose arm; as a result, the total dose of cisplatin was 67% higher (174). The Hong Kong trial included stage III to IV patients who showed improved survival with high-dose regimens, but the patient population was small and staging criteria were not uniform (175). Further, the multiple chemotherapy-related toxicities in ovarian cancer preclude marked increases in dose intensity for prolonged periods.

Paclitaxel

Studies in dose intensification with paclitaxel also began with preclinical studies that seem to suggest a dose-response relationship. However, it soon became apparent that the duration of the infusion was more important than the absolute dose of the paclitaxel (176). In vitro studies have demonstrated that prolonged exposure to paclitaxel increased the cytotoxicity in many different tumor lines to a greater extent than that observed by merely increasing the dose. This, in addition to the fact that this drug exhibits nonlinear pharmacokinetics with saturable parameters of distribution and elimination, meant that increasing the dose would not result in a proportional increase in maximum plasma concentration or

TABLE 28-4	DOSE-INTENSITY TRIALS IN OVARIAN CANCER			
Trials	*N*	*Platinum Dose*	*Response Rate*	*Overall Survival*
No difference				
GOG (McGuire 1995) (169)	458	CDDP 16.7 mg/m^2/week	65	21
		CDDP 33.3 mg/m^2/week	59	24
GICOG (Columbo 1993) (170)	306	CDDP 25 mg/m^2/week	61	33
		CDDP 50 mg/m^2/week	66	36
GONO (Conte 1996) (171)	145	CDDP 12.5 mg/m^2/week	61	24
		CDDP 25 mg/m^2/week	58	29
London GOG (Ehrlich 1983) (172)	241	CBDA AUC 6 q 28	57	HR: 0.91
		CBDA AUC 12 q 28	63	
Austrian trial (Dittrich 1996) (173)	253	CDDP 25 mg/m^2/week	42	38
		CDDP 25 mg/m^2/week+ CBDA 75 mg/m^2/week	39	42
Difference				
Scottish trial (Kaye 1996) (174)	159	CDDP 16.7 mg/m^2/week	34	27% at 4 years
		CDDP 33.3 mg/m^2/week	61	32% at 4 years
Hong Kong trial (Ngam 1989) (175)	50	CDDP 15-20 mg/m^2/week	30	30% at 3 years
		CDDP 30-40 mg/m^2/week	55	60% at 3 years

AUC, area under the curve; CBDA, carboplatin; HR, hazard ratio; N, number of patients; OS, overall survival; RR, response rate.
Reproduced, with permission, from Vasey P, Kaye SB, Thigpen JT. Importance of dose intensity in ovarian cancer. In: Gershenson D, McGuire W (eds). Ovarian Cancer: Controversies in Management. New York: Churchill Livingstone; 2002;169-194.

drug exposure. Nevertheless, dose intensity studies were performed, but only with the coadministration of growth factors (177,178).

A meta-analysis of phase II studies comprising a total of 191 patients showed that for the majority of patients who were considered platinum-resistant, an increased dose of paclitaxel did not correlate with an improved response rate (177). A randomized study of more than 300 patients was positive, in that a higher 250 mg/m^2 q21 dose of paclitaxel was associated with a 36% response rate, while a lower dose of 175 mg/m^2 q21 led to a lower response rate of 27%. Both regimens administered the chemotherapy over 24 h. There was no overall difference in the PFS or overall survival. However, the higher dose was associated with higher toxicities (178).

Studies indicate that there is no evidence that dose intensity is crucial in the chemotherapeutic responses of ovarian carcinoma. And, in fact, there is no evidence that going above a cisplatin dose of 75 mg/m^2, carboplatin AUC 5, or a dose of 350 to 500 mg/m^2, or paclitaxel 175 mg/m^2 shows any additional advantage.

■ FOLLOW-UP AND TREATMENT OF RECURRENT DISEASE

Most patients with ovarian cancer will have disease that either persists or recurs following primary treatment. These patients would need retreatment. EOC is not just a single entity. There is a widely variable spectrum of behavior. The extent and the virulence of the primary tumor often dictate not only the subsequent natural history of the cancer but also the likelihood of relapse and interval of ensuing events.

Regular follow-up with tumor marker can detect disease recurrence (179,180). In women with previously treated ovarian cancer that is in clinical remission, the National Comprehensive Cancer Network has recommended assessment of serum CA125 concentration at every follow-up visit if this concentration was raised at initial diagnosis. After documentation of CA125 increase in such women, the median time to a clinical relapse of ovarian cancer is 2 to 6 months. There is, however, controversy over the benefit of early treatment versus treatment later. The results of a large study showed no survival benefit from early treatment on the basis of a raised serum CA125 concentration alone, and therefore questioned the value of routine measurement of CA125 in the follow-up of patients with epithelial ovarian cancer (181). Some authors also suggest that smaller tumors are more often responsive to treatment (182),

but this does not eliminate the lead-time bias. It is also argued that larger tumors have an inferior primary response and grow rapidly. Recurrent ovarian cancer is a mortal disease; but—in absence of data showing that treatment improves quality of life—this does not justify haste in treating patients. In fact, it is the concern of many clinicians that early treatment may lead to immediate symptoms.

One of the problems with recurrent ovarian cancer is the lack of a truly effective salvage therapy. Approximately 50% of ovarian carcinomas are intrinsically resistant to conventional chemotherapy. The other problem is the uniformity of prognostic factors by which one can predict the behavior of recurrent disease. Observations over the past 10 years have perhaps allowed clinicians to cast light on this issue. The first observation is the interval from primary treatment to time of recurrence. This has now come to be known as the treatment interval or platinum interval, as most patients would have received platinum in the primary treatment. The treatment-free interval has been widely accepted to be 6 months based on the better response to chemotherapy in a salvage setting (183). The natural history of the disease after relapse is characterized by the eventual development of a broad cross-resistance to various treatments. Patients who relapse within 6 months of a CR have only a 10 to 20% chance of responding to platinum retreatment, whereas those with treatment-free intervals of 21 months or longer have a 90% response rate (165). In general, drug resistance may result from alterations in host-drug metabolism, from the spread of tumor cells to sites poorly accessible to chemotherapy, and/or from biochemical changes at the cellular or subcellular level.

TREATMENT OF LESS RESISTANT DISEASE

After identifying patients who seem to belong to the less resistant group, one can then embark on the treatment. As mentioned, patients who had a treatment-free interval of more than 6 months have a very good chance of response to repeat platinum treatment. On average, about 25, 33, and 60% of patients respond to salvage platinum therapy if the interval is 6 to 12 months, 12 to 24 months, and greater than 24 months, respectively. One choice would be to use carboplatin as a single agent for its equivalence in efficacy (137) and favorable toxicities compared with cisplatin (183). Prospective trials and retrospective analyses of patients who have received paclitaxel and platinum therapy as first-line treatment have recently been published. In the two small prospective trials, response was seen in 87 to 91% of the patients.

However, the number of patients treated was small, in total only 43 (184,185). In the retrospective studies, activity ranging from 70 to 84% was observed (186,187). Unfortunately, the lack of quality-of-life correlations for these makes it difficult, in looking at overall benefit, to interpret the trials.

Two phase III trials (188,189) have shown that combination platinum-based chemotherapy with paclitaxel or gemcitabine improves progression-free survival compared with single-agent platinum or conventional platinum-based chemotherapy in women with recurrent platinum-sensitive disease. A phase III study (CALYPSO) showed that a pegylated liposomal doxorubicin and carboplatin combination was better than was paclitaxel with carboplatin in terms of progression-free survival in relapsed platinum-sensitive cancer (190). By contrast, nonplatinum topotecan combinations do not provide a survival advantage over topotecan alone in relapsed disease (191).

As long as patients continue to respond to platinum and have a more than a 6-month interval between each treatment, it seems reasonable to continue treatment with platinum, either as a single agent or in a combination regimen. As mentioned, the likelihood of patients responding to nonplatinum-based therapy is also greater if the treatment-free interval is greater (182). Using paclitaxel as single-agent therapy, a total of 110 patients with advanced ovarian cancer received doses ranging from 100 to 250 mg/m^2 infused over 24 h every 3 weeks. Overall, in 20 to 37% of patients, tumors regressed partially; in 7 patients, regression was complete. Responses were 40 to 50% in platinum sensitive tumors (182). In patients with relapsed ovarian cancer, the overall response rates on treatment with topotecan ranged from 19 to 33% in those who had platinum-sensitive tumors, while 48% of patients achieved stable disease (192-194).

TREATMENT OF MORE RESISTANT DISEASE

The GOG refers to this group of patients as platinum-refractory. These patients also exhibit a poorer prognosis to other nonplatinum agents.

Paclitaxel

In three phase II trials, a total of 110 patients with advanced ovarian cancer received paclitaxel as single-agent therapy in doses ranging from 100 to 250 mg/m^2 infused over 24 h every 3 weeks. Overall, tumors regressed partially in 20 to 37% of patients; in 7 patients, regression was complete. Responses were seen in 24 to 30% of platinum-resistant tumors. At least 2 patients with platinum-resistant disease achieved a CR. The median duration of response was 6 months. The overall median survival was 11 months (17 months in patients with platinum-sensitive tumors and 9 months in those with platinum-resistant tumors) (195-198). The major toxic effect was granulocytopenia. Trimble et al. found that 22% of patients who had undergone multiple prior regimens had objective responses to this regimen (4% CR, 18% PR [partial response]) and that the median survival was 9 months (199).

Topotecan

Topotecan, a semisynthetic camptothecin derivative, has shown activity in both preclinical and phase I studies. Compared to paclitaxel in patients with refractory ovarian cancer, it was found to produce a response rate of 20%, compared to the 13% in patients who received paclitaxel (200). This resulted in its approval for use by the FDA. In patients with relapsed platinum-resistant ovarian cancer, the overall response rates on treatment with topotecan ranged from 5 to 18%. The proportion of these patients who achieved stable disease was 17% (201). In phase III studies, topotecan was shown to have an efficacy equal to both paclitaxel and liposomal doxorubicin as second-line therapy in patients with relapsed ovarian cancer.

Liposomal Doxorubicin

A pegylated liposomal formulation of doxorubicin was first tested in patients with platinum-refractory disease; the resulting response rate was approximately 26% (202). Compared to topotecan or paclitaxel in phase III settings in two separate trials, liposomal doxorubicin was associated with lower toxicities but with equivalent efficacy (203,204). Based on the data from Gordon et al., the drug was FDA-approved for use in ovarian cancer.

Gemcitabine

Gemcitabine is a primary antimetabolite that closely resembles cytarabine. In patients with platinum-refractory disease, single-agent gemcitabine produced responses ranging from 14 (205) to 19% (206). Gemcitabine has been frequently studied in combination with cisplatin. The response rates ranged from 40 to 70% (207-209). However, the small number of patients treated as well as their heterogeneity disallows any further conclusion. Furthermore, it is difficult to justify the use of combination chemotherapy in patients without evidence that responses correlated with improvements in quality of life.

Etoposide

This topoisomerase II inhibitor has the advantage of being administered as an oral agent. In patients with platinum-refractory disease who were given 100-mg doses of etoposide orally for 14 days every 21 days, the response rate was about 26% (210). Lower doses of etoposide, at 50 mg/d, produced less reported response, typically 10 to 20% (211,212).

Docetaxel

In four phase II trials in patients with extensively platinum-pretreated ovarian cancer, docetaxel 100 mg/m^2 administered as a 1-h infusion every 3 weeks showed promising activity (213-216). Among 155 patients whose disease was judged most refractory (ie, in whom the platinum-free interval was less than 4 months), the overall response rate was 28% (217). In addition, there is evidence that docetaxel is active in paclitaxel-resistant disease; this has been observed in both the preclinical and clinical settings in ovarian cancer (218). In a small study conducted at MDACC, an overall response rate of 23% was seen in such patients (1 patient had a CR, 6 had a PR, and 9 had stable disease (219). Median overall survival was 9.5 months.

Other Chemotherapeutic Agents

CPT-11, also a topoisomerase II inhibitor, produced an objective response rate of between 14 and 21% (220). Oxaliplatin was tried in patients with platinum-refractory ovarian cancer and was found to produce a response of 17% as compared with topotecan (221). Vinorelbine, a vinca alkaloid, has shown activity in patients with ovarian cancer, with a response rate of 21% in a small phase II study (222). Capecitabine, an oral pro-drug of 5 fluorouracil, has also been tried in patients; it is associated with a response of 22 to 40% in small studies (223,224). Epirubicin has also been tried in patients, with a range of responses varying from 90 to 27% (225, 226). Altretamine is associated with maximum response rates of 10 to 15% in platinum-refractory patients. It has been considered by many to be an unsatisfactory treatment because it has toxicities that are potentially detrimental to the patient's quality of life, and also because of its schedule for dosing (227-231).

The evidence available does not support firm conclusions about the preferred chemotherapy regimen for recurrent ovarian cancer. Randomized trials that compare new drugs with current standard treatments are needed. A summary of treatment for ovarian cancer at MDACC is seen in Fig. 28-9.

■ HIGH-DOSE CHEMOTHERAPY WITH STEM CELL SUPPORT

The initial trials used autologous bone marrow transplant (ABMT) rescue in heavily treated patients who were treated with single agents followed by transplantation. Subsequently, combinations of high-dose alkylating agents and platinum compounds were evaluated. The overall responses were in the region of 70 to 80%. Although this was considered promisingly high, these responses are brief and associated with high toxicities. It is also often difficult to interpret the results because the patient population is often too heterogeneous (232). There are two settings in which high-dose chemotherapy has been considered in ovarian cancer: (1) at first remission of patients with disease who have a high risk for relapse and (2) in the patients who have recurrent disease.

The major obstacle is that giving high-dose chemotherapy in a single course produces a dose-dependent antitumor effect; this, in turn, can induce a high but not durable response rate in patients with advanced disease (233,234). A single intensification course is inadequate because of the low-growth fraction of tumor cells, which comprises a significant number of clonogenic tumor cells and is unaffected by most chemotherapeutic agents. Since dose intensity is important in achieving responses in ovarian cancer, a viable alternative to ABMT is to administer repeated courses of dose-intensified therapy with peripheral blood stem cell (PBSC) support (235-237).

There have been many studies of high-dose chemotherapy with autologous support in the treatment of patients with refractory ovarian cancer. This is outlined in Table 28-5. Although the number of patients in each treatment regimen is small, the results have been consistent in that the responses in heavily pretreated patients have been high at 70 to 82%. However, the progression-free interval has been uniformly short, with no clear impact on overall survival (238).

The longest response durations have been in patients with platinum-sensitive disease and in those with minimal residual disease at the time of the therapy. The inability to eradicate all tumors with high-dose chemotherapy is likely due to the drug resistance that is prevalent in ovarian cancer. The majority of studies suggest that high-dose chemotherapy with autologous stem cell support will be most effective in producing high response rates and improved long-term survival in patients with minimal residual disease and in tumors that are still relatively sensitive to cytotoxic chemotherapy.

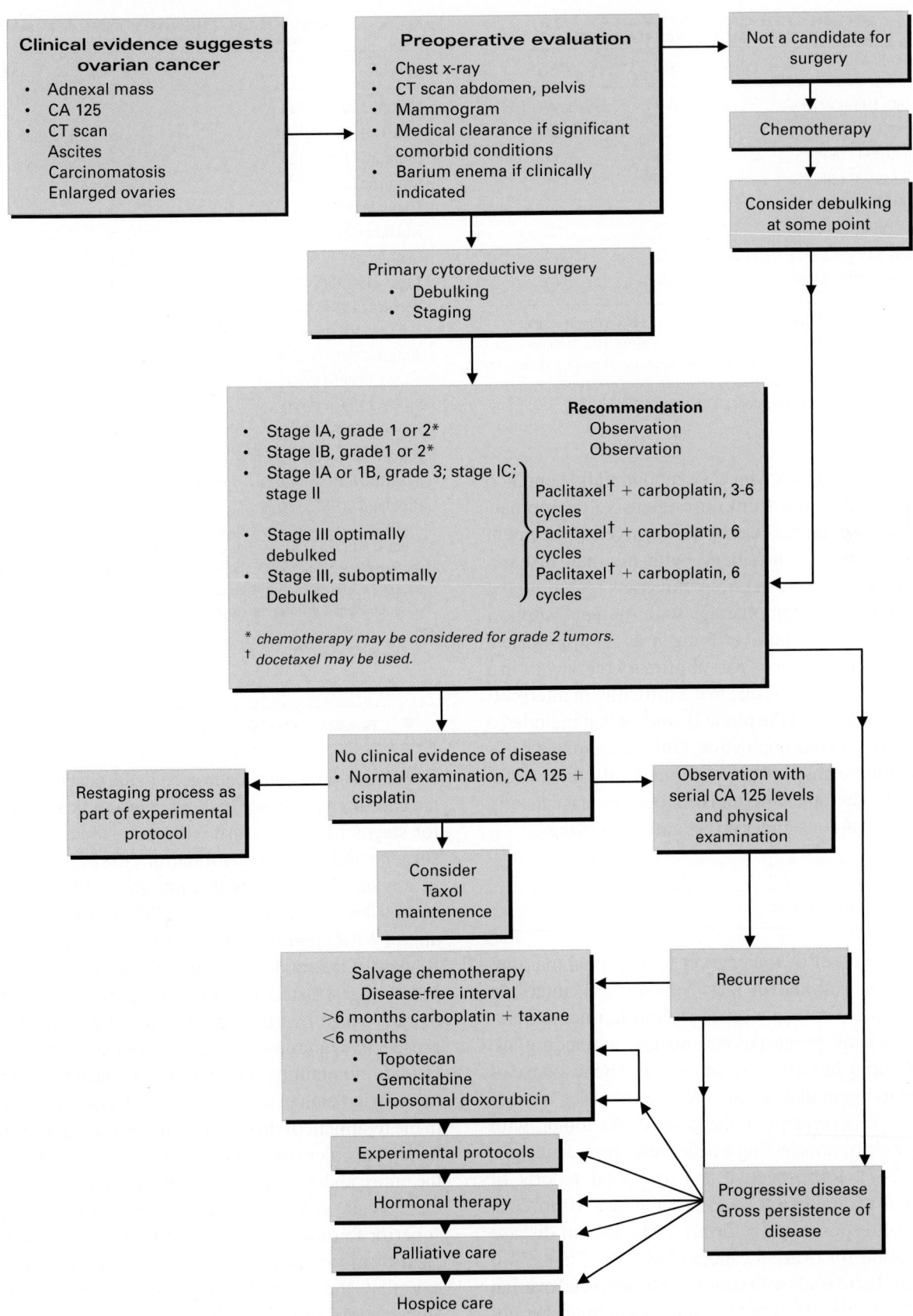

FIGURE 28-9. Summary of treatment of ovarian cancer.

TABLE 28-5	HIGH-DOSE CHEMOTHERAPY FOR ADVANCED OVARIAN CANCER		
Trial	**sN**	**RR**	**PFS**
Dauplat (1989) (239)	14	NA	33% 3-year PFS
Mulder (1989) (240)	11	55	15
Broun (1994) (241)	8	63	6
Shpall (1990) (242)	8	75	6
Stiff (1995) (243)	30	89	7
Viens (1990) (244)	12	75	5
Fennelly (1994) (245)	27	78	NA
Fennelly (1995) (246)	13	100	NA

NA, not available; PFS, progression-free survival; RR, response rate.
Adapted, with permission, from Swenerton K, Muss HB, Robinson EG. Salvage chemotherapy for refractory disease in ovarian cancer. In: Gershenson D, McGuire W (eds). *Ovarian cancer controversies in management*. Churchill Livingstone; 2002:169-194.

It is clear that patients who have suboptimally debulked disease benefit little from dose-intensive chemotherapy, while dose-intense therapy with stem cell replacement is most promising in patients with minimal disease. However, the conclusion from clinicians regarding the use of high-dose chemotherapy with stem cell support is that there is no data verifying it as an appropriate form of therapy either as part of primary therapy or in a salvage therapy. This is due to the difficulty in interpreting the data from all the phase II studies that included a very heterogeneous population. Only randomized trials will be able to answer this question. Untill then, high-dose chemotherapy with stem cell replacement can only be given to patients under investigational settings.

■ HORMONES

The sensitivity of ovarian cancer to hormonal manipulations is a well-known fact. Nevertheless, there are several reports of responses to various hormonal treatments such as progestational agents, antiandrogens, gonadotropin agonists, and tamoxifen. The response of hormonal manipulation in advanced ovarian cancer seems to be dependent on the grade of the tumor, with lower grade tumors having a better response to manipulation (247). Retrospective and anecdotal reports of hormonal manipulation seem to suggest a 10 to 20% chance of response and a further 10 to 20% of disease stabilization for ovarian cancer (248-250). Table 28-6 shows the list of trials with tamoxifen in advanced ovarian cancer (251-267). The use of aromatase inhibitors has not been completely evaluated for advanced ovarian cancer. A trial has just recently started at MDACC looking into the treatment of epithelial ovarian cancer with letrozole.

TABLE 28-6	TAMOXIFEN THERAPY FOR ADVANCED OVARIAN CANCER	
Trials	**OR (%)**	**SD (%)**
Hatch (1991) (251)	17	38
Marth (1997) (252)	6	77
Landoni (1985) (253)	0	35
Osborne (1988) (254)	2	9
Gennatas (1996) (255)	6	NS
Rolski (1991) (256)	6	47
Quinn (1987) (257)	23	30
Jager (1995) (258)	0	6
Weiner (1987) (259)	10	19
Van der Velden (1995) (260)	13	38
Ahlgren (1993) (261)	17	62
Shirey (1985) (262)	0	83
Slevin (1986) (263)	0	5
Pagel (1983) (264)	38	57
Hamerlynck (1985) (265)	6	11
Schwartz (1982) (266)	8	31
Rowland (1985) (267)	0	NS

NS, not significant; OR, overall survival; SD, stable disease.
Data from Perez-Gracia JL, Carrasco EM. Tamoxifen therapy for ovarian cancer in the adjuvant and advanced settings: systematic review of the literature and implications for future research. *Gynecol Oncol* 2002;84(2):201-209.

■ RADIATION THERAPY

Radiation therapy has been used in the past to treat ovarian carcinoma in two situations: (1) as adjuvant therapy for stages I to III disease without residual tumor after surgery and (2) as consolidation after chemotherapy in advanced disease with minimal residual tumor at second-look laparotomy (268). Whole abdominal radiation (WAR) and IP isotopes were used in this setting. Review of the randomized and nonrandomized data for WAR suggest that it can help prolong disease-free survival in early-stage ovarian cancer (269). Unfortunately, no prospective randomized trial has compared WAR with a cisplatin-containing regimen. The metastatic pattern of the ovarian cancer and the normal tissue bed involved in the treatment of this disease makes effective radiation therapy problematic. The limitation is in the dosage, as the entire abdomen must be considered at risk. To date, there is no proof that adjuvant radiation therapy is superior to other treatment modalities. However, it is clear from two studies of consolidation radiation therapy that the related complications are significant. Hoskins et al. evaluated patients with stage III or IV disease and found a 10-year OS of 4% (270). Whelan et al. evaluated 105 patients and found no survival advantage and an increased risk (8.6%) of complications (bowel obstruction) (271). Overall, the complication rate of radiation therapy as consolidation treatment is considerable and the effect on survival unremarkable. With the understanding of and greater use of chemotherapeutic agents in ovarian cancer, the role of radiation therapy in this disease has diminished in prominence.

The use of P-32 is really of only historic importance. However, three trials in the past did not show any benefit, despite greater toxicities (272-274). Although, retrospectively, the cure rate of patients with early-stage disease completely resected in combination with P-32 appears to be comparable to that of patients who were treated with WAR, there has been no direct prospective comparison. Two trials by the GOG and the NCIC-CTG have compared the use of P-32, melphalan, and WAR. There was no advantage of any treatment. Like WAR, radioisotopic P-32 in ovarian cancer has diminished in use and importance due to the greater understanding of chemotherapy and improvements in preventing the toxicities of systemic chemotherapy.

■ BORDERLINE TUMORS

Borderline malignant tumors represent approximately 4 to 14% of all ovarian tumors. Compared to obviously malignant neoplasms, these borderline tumors tend to affect a younger population. They constitute 15% of all EOC. Nearly 75% of these are stage I at the time of diagnosis. Onset tends to be earlier, the mean age of onset being 40 years, approximately 10 to 20 years younger than the women with frankly malignant tumors (275). The borderline tumors share the same risk factors (276). The cause of death has been determined to be benign complications of disease (eg, small bowel obstruction), complications of therapy, and only rarely malignant transformation.

The mainstay of treatment is primary surgical staging and cytoreduction in the same manner as malignant tumors. However, the survival is far better. In a large review, stage I patients had a 99% chance of being alive at 7 years; stage II and III patients had a 92% survival rate at 7 years. In this review, more patients perished from the complications of treatment than from disease progression (277). Another study observed that 146 patients with stage I disease showed 100% disease-free survival after a median follow-up of 42.4 months (278). Because of the excellent survival of patients with stage I disease, it is suggested that young patients with disease limited to one ovary should potentially be subjected to limited surgery so as to preserve fertility (275,279). This can be considered only after intraoperative inspection

of the contralateral ovary to exclude involvement. All other patients should receive optimal cytoreduction with full surgical staging.

Postoperatively, optimally cytoreduced patients in all stages of disease should receive only expectant treatment without adjuvant chemotherapy provided that the metastases are also borderline tumors histologically. There have been no prospective studies suggesting a benefit of adjuvant therapy. A retrospective review of four studies of adjuvant therapy in patients with borderline tumor looked at treatment with external beam radiation; IP gold therapy; P-32; treatment with thiotepa; and treatment with cisplatin. It revealed that there was no significant difference between any of these treatments (280). Another observational review of patients treated with adjuvant radiation showed no impact of adjuvant therapy (281). Many other retrospective reviews have also concluded that patients do not benefit from adjuvant chemotherapy (277,282-285). A very small percentage of patients may still require chemotherapy should they fail surgery. These are patients in whom the histologic specimens reveal invasive implants on the peritoneal surfaces or omentum and those who develop a rapid recurrence of IP disease after surgery. They should be treated as for invasive ovarian cancer.

For patients with slow recurrence of the disease, especially after a long disease-free interval, it is widely practiced to repeat optimal cytoreduction and postoperative observation, leaving chemotherapy for only the seemingly rapidly progressing tumors. Follow-up of patients with no evidence of disease is as those of malignant EOC, but less frequent intervals are appropriate. If the contralateral ovary has been retained, it should be followed by transvaginal ultrasonography at least on an annual basis.

■ GERM CELL TUMORS

This group of ovarian tumors consists of a variety of histologically different entities that are all derived from the primitive germ cells of the embryonic gonad. Malignant germ cell tumors represent a relatively small proportion of all ovarian tumors. Prior to advances in chemotherapy, the prognosis for these aggressive tumors was poor. Over the past decade, however, new chemotherapeutic regimes have made germ cell tumors among the most highly curable cancers. The highest incidence of germ cell tumor occurs in the second and the third decades of life. These tumors are frequently diagnosed by the discovery of a palpable abdominal mass in a young woman who complains of abdominal pain. The following, in order of frequency, are the symptoms of germ cell tumors (286): acute abdominal pain, chronic abdominal pain, asymptomatic abdominal mass, abnormal vaginal bleeding, abdominal distention. The classification of germ cell tumors of the ovary is important for prognostication and for treatment with chemotherapy. Germ cell tumors are classified as below (287):

- Germ cell tumors
- Dysgerminoma
- Nondysgerminoma (embryonal cancer)
- Embryonal differentiation
- Mixed
- Mature
- Immature
- Extraembryonal differentiation
- Choriocarcinoma
- Endodermal sinus tumor (yolk sac tumor) (Fig. 28-10)
- Extraembryonal carcinoma

Germ cell tumors are staged in the same way as epithelial ovarian cancer. Dysgerminoma is the equivalent of seminoma in testicular cancer. It is exquisitely sensitive to chemotherapy and radiotherapy. The cure rate is high irrespective of the stage of the neoplasm. The other histologies are really equivalent to nonseminomas in testicular cancer. The aggressiveness of the disease is dependent on the type, the most aggressive being endodermal sinus and choriocarcinoma. With chemotherapy, these tumors are also highly curable (286, 288-292). Because chemotherapy can cure the majority of patients even with advanced disease, conservative surgery is standard for germ cell tumors at all stages. By conservative surgery is meant full laparotomy with

careful examination and detailed biopsies of all suspicious areas and with limited cytoreduction, thereby avoiding major morbidity. However, if any bulky disease is found during laparotomy, it should be removed as completely as is reasonably possible. Patients who have had complete surgical staging and adjuvant chemotherapy almost always remain disease-free regardless of stage (288), while those who had bulky residual disease have a lower cure rate. It is therefore important that all visible tumors should be removed as completely as possible. Nonetheless, with the aim of preserving fertility, the uterus and contralateral ovary should be left intact if they are normal. Only then can the patient be considered adequately staged and a proper prognosis arrived at. Wedge biopsy of a normal ovary is not recommended, as it defeats the purpose of conservative therapy by causing possible infertility. Patients who received conservative surgery with the preservation of one ovary may retain acceptable fertility rates despite adjuvant treatment with chemotherapy. There have also been no reports of any adverse obstetric outcome or long-term unfavorable sequelae in the offspring (286,293-296).

Second-look surgery is of no proven benefit except in a minority of patients whose tumor was not completely resected at the initial surgical procedure and who had teratomatous elements in their primary tumor. Surgical resection of residual masses detected by clinical examination or by radiographic procedures may be beneficial, as such masses may contain mature teratoma or residual tumor (286,297-299).

For patients who are considered for either nondysgerminoma or dysgerminoma who did not have a full staging yet have seemingly localized disease (stages I-II) after minimal surgery, there is debate as to the optimal adjuvant management. All nonpatients with dysgerminoma should receive adjuvant chemotherapy. For these patients, some authors recommend obtaining a CT scan of the abdomen and pelvis and a determination of the hCG and AFP (alpha-fetal protein). Assuming that all these tests are normal, it may be possible just to observe these patients without providing adjuvant therapy. The patients, however, must be aware that the rate of recurrence of seemingly localized disease without full staging is 15 to 25% (300). Should the cancers recur, however, the cure rate remains high (290,291).

DYSGERMINOMA

Patients with stage IA disease may be observed after surgery. A small portion of these patients may experience recurrence, but they can be treated successfully at the time of recurrence, with a high rate of cure (286). This applies to patients who have been completely staged.

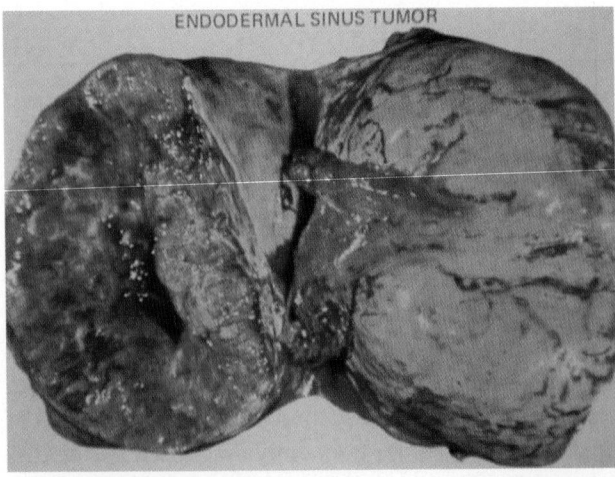

FIGURE 28-10. Gross specimen of endodermal sinus tumor of the ovary.

Incompletely staged patients with presumed stage IA disease and those with higher-stage disease should receive adjuvant chemotherapy treatment. For any stage beyond stage IA, chemotherapy should be given. Radiotherapy for early stages is probably as effective as an adjuvant treatment, but concerns over ovarian failure make radiotherapy undesirable for patients with an intact ovary. However, for patients with a contraindication to chemotherapy, radiotherapy remains an effective option.

Dysgerminoma is extremely sensitive to chemotherapy, and such treatment cures the majority of patients even with advanced disease. The recommended chemotherapy regime is etoposide 100 mg/m^2 per day for 5 days with cisplatin 20 mg/m^2 per day for 5 days, with or without bleomycin at 10 U/day for days 1, 8, and 15 (EP [etoposide + cisplatin] or BEP [bleomycin + etoposide + cisplatin]; various schedules of bleomycin are utilized). When there is bulky residual disease, it is common to give three to four courses of combination BEP chemotherapy. As BEP chemotherapy is associated with a lower relapse rate and shorter treatment time (288), it is preferred to the older regimen of vincristine, dactinomycin, and cyclophosphamide (VAC) (289) given in an adjuvant setting. Other tested chemotherapy regimens include combinations of ifosfamide and doxorubicin; vinblastine, ifosfamide, and cisplatin; and cyclophosphamide, doxorubicin, and cisplatin. All patients who do not respond to standard therapy are candidates for clinical trials. All patients should have their levels of lactate dehydrogenase (LDH) and human chorionic gonadotropin (β-hCG) measured so as to monitor the treatment. All patients treated with chemotherapy may be followed up with medical history, physical examination, and tumor markers (LDH, β-hCG) every 1 to 2 months for year 1, every 2 months for year 2, every 3 months for year 3, every 4 months for year 4, every 6 months for year 5, and once a year subsequently. Although tumor markers are important, radiologic imaging is also pertinent, especially for patients whose tumor markers were not raised at diagnosis. CT scans should be performed as clinically indicated.

Patients who did not receive chemotherapy should be followed up more closely. Some 90% of relapses in patients treated with chemotherapy usually occur within the first 2 years after primary diagnosis. At relapse, these patients can be successfully treated (286).

NONDYSGERMINOMA

With chemotherapy, these tumors are also highly curable, even with advanced disease. Patients with stage IA grade 1 immature teratoma or mature teratoma have a very good prognosis and should be only observed after

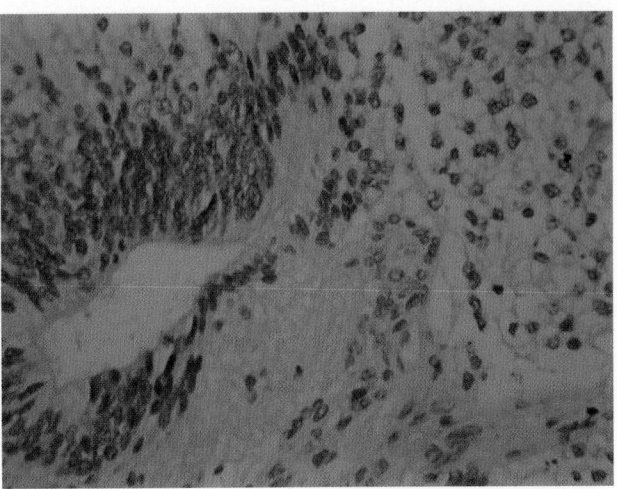

FIGURE 28-11. Histology of immature teratoma of the ovary.

primary conservative surgery. Patients with stage I grade 2 immature teratoma also have a very good prognosis (Fig. 28-11). It is controversial whether adjuvant chemotherapy adds any further overall survival benefit in this subgroup of patients. All other patients with higher-stage and higher-grade tumors should receive postoperative adjuvant chemotherapy. The recommended chemotherapy regimen is as dysgerminoma. Potential salvage treatments include an ifosfamide combination or high-dose chemotherapy and autologous bone marrow rescue. Although the role of secondary cytoreductive surgery for patients with recurrent or progressive ovarian germ cell tumors remains controversial, it may have some benefit for a select group of patients, particularly those with immature teratoma. After a maximal effort at surgical cytoreduction, chemotherapy should be considered. All patients who do not respond to standard therapy are candidates for clinical trials.

Measurements of LDH, AFP, and β-hCG should be made in all patients in order to monitor treatment. All patients treated with chemotherapy should be followed up with medical history, physical examination, and appropriate tumor markers as for dysgerminoma. Patients who did not receive chemotherapy should be followed up more closely. Relapses usually occur within the first 2 years after diagnosis.

■ THE FUTURE

Advances in our understanding of pathogenesis have identified novel potential targets for therapy (Table 28-7) (49, 301-309). Several of these targets have been implicated in chemotherapy resistance (eg, PI3K/AKT and

TABLE 28-7 | PROMISING NOVEL THERAPY TARGETS THAT ARE CURRENTLY BEING EXPLORED IN WOMEN WITH EPITHELIAL OVARIAN CANCER (EOC)

Target	Drug Examples	Most Advanced Clinical Trial Phase	FDA Approval	References
CA125	Abagovomab	Phase III	No	301
DNA methylation	Azacitidine	Phase II	Yes	302
E1A gene transfer	tgDCC-E1 adenovirus	Phase I/II	No	303
Endothelin receptors	ZD4054	Phase II	No	49
Folate receptor alpha	Farletuzumab	Phase II	Orphan drug designation	ClinicalTrials.gov
LPA signaling	Preclinical	Preclinical	–	49
Mitotic motor protein kinesin spindle protein (KSP)	Ispinesib	Phase II	No	ClinicalTrials.gov
Mucin	Pemtumomab	Phase III	No	304
PARP	AZD2281 BSI201 ABT888	Phase II	No	305,306
PI3K/AKT signaling pathway	SF1126 XL147 BEZ235 Perifosine	Phase I/II	No	49
PKC iota signaling	Preclinical	Preclinical	Preclinical	49
RAS/MEK signaling pathway	AZD6244	Phase II	No	49
Liposomal siRNA gene targeting, eg, EPHA2	Liposomal siRNA	Phase I	No	307
SRC signaling	Dasatinib AZD0530	Phase II	No	49
Telomerase	GRN163L	Phase I	No	ClinicalTrials.gov
VEGF signaling pathway	Bevacizumab Sunitinib Vandetanib AEE788 Aflibercept Cediranib DMXAA IMC-1121B Pazopanib Sorafenib SU6668 Vatalanib	Phase I-III	Yes: Bevacizumab Sunitinib Vandetanib	308,309

DNA, deoxyribonucleic acid; LPA, lysophosphatidic acid; MEK, mitogen-activated protein kinase (MAPK); PARP, poly ADP-ribose polymerase; PI3K, phosphatidylinositol-3-kinase; PKC, protein kinase C; siRNA, small interfering ribonucleic acid; VEGF, vascular endothelial growth factor.

SRC signalling, DNA methylation), and results of preclinical experiments suggest that combination of the appropriate inhibitors with cytotoxic drugs can overcome chemoresistance in models of epithelial ovarian cancer. Aberrant kinase signaling plays a key part in the pathogenesis and chemoresistance of many epithelial ovarian cancers. Further, several of the potential therapy targets shown in Table 28-7 are aberrant at the genomic level, and the corresponding targeted therapies might thus show most striking antitumour efficacy in cancers that express the aberrant target. For example, trials are assessing drugs that inhibit RAS signalling in the treatment of borderline and low-grade epithelial ovarian cancers because of the frequency of activation of *KRAS* by mutations in these tumours. Similarly, PI3K/AKT pathway inhibitors might have substantial antitumour activity in cancers that harbour amplification or mutations in the *PIK3CA* oncogene or mutations in *PTEN*. Hence, with targeted therapies, rigorous correlative studies should be designed in association with clinical trials to validate predictive and pharmacodynamic biomarkers of efficacy that are identified in preclinical studies. Inability to assess potential targets in tumour tissue, inappropriate study designs, and poor attention to an appropriate clinical setting for novel therapy assessment are all likely to contribute to the frequent failure in clinical trials of drugs that seem promising in preclinical and early clinical assessment.

VEGF and its receptors are essential for angiogenesis in epithelial ovarian cancer. Furthermore, VEGF is an important autocrine growth factor in this disease. Thus, several agents and strategies to target VEGF signaling have been developed (see Table 28-7) (308). Bevacizumab, the first drug approved by the US Food and Drug Administration to target angiogenesis, is a humanised monoclonal anti-VEGF antibody. In preclinical models of epithelial ovarian cancer, monoclonal VEGF antibody eliminates ascites, extends survival of mice, and, in combination with cytotoxic drugs, reduces tumour burden compared with either agent alone (308). Bevacizumab has shown promising antitumour activity alone and in combination with cytotoxic chemotherapy in phase II trials in women with relapsed disease (309). Bevacizumab and cediranib are currently in phase III development.

■ CONCLUSION

A plateau has been reached regarding the benefits associated with intravenous administration of cytotoxic chemotherapy in epithelial ovarian cancer. However, advances in screening, novel targeted therapies, and widespread use of practical intraperitoneal drug delivery techniques will probably improve patient outcomes. Although the list of genomic aberrations in this disease is daunting, a systems approach and the integration of therapies targeting multiple component genes of important genetic aberrations has potential in treatment and in the potentiation of chemotherapy efficacy. Such efforts will be aided by the continuing comprehensive molecular characterisation of epithelial ovarian cancer by The

Cancer Genome Atlas (TCGA). The optimum route of administration for novel therapies and how best to schedule these therapies with cytotoxic chemotherapy has to be defined. Our responsibility to patients demands that we develop a new framework to make more efficient progress toward improved management of this devastating disease.

References

1. Garcia M, Jemal A, Ward EM, et al. *Global Cancer Facts and Figures 2007*. Atlanta, GA: American Cancer Society; 2007.
2. Jemal A, Thomas A, Murray T, Thun M. Cancer Statistics, 2002. *CA Cancer J Clin* 2002;52(1):23-47.
3. World Health Organization. *World Health Statistics Annuals, 1987-1992*. Geneva: World Health Organization; 1987-1992.
4. Coleman MP, Esteve J, Damiecki P, et al. *Trends in Cancer Incidence and Mortality*. Vol 121. Lyon, France: IARC Scientific Publications; 1993;477-498.
5. Ries LAG, Wingo PA, Miller DS, et al. The annual report to the nation on the status of cancer, 1973-1997, with a special section on colorectal cancer. *Cancer* 2000;88:2398-2424.
6. Howe HL, Wingo PA, Thun MJ, et al. Annual report to the nation on the status of cancer, 1973-1998, featuring cancers with recent increasing trends. *J Natl Cancer Inst* 2001;93:824-842.
7. Yancik R. Ovarian cancer. Age contrasts in incidence, histology, disease stage at diagnosis, and mortality (review). *Cancer* 1993;71(2 suppl):517-523.
8. Boyd J, Rubin SC. Hereditary ovarian cancer: Molecular genetics and clinical implications (review). *Gynecol Oncol* 1997;64:196-206.
9. Goldberg JM, Piver MS, Jishi MF, Blumenson L. Age at onset of ovarian cancer in women with a strong family history of ovarian cancer. *Gynecol Oncol* 1997;66:3-9.
10. Hartge P, Whittemore AS, Itnyre J, et al. Rates and risks of ovarian cancer in subgroups of white women in the United States. *Obstet Gynecol* 1994;84:760-764.
11. Harlow BL, Cramer DW, Bell DA, Welch WR. Perineal exposure to talc and ovarian cancer risk. *Obstet Gynecol* 1992; 80:19-26.
12. Parham G, Phillips JL, Hicks ML, et al. The National Cancer Data Base report on malignant epithelial ovarian carcinoma in African-American women. *Cancer* 1997;80:816-826.
13. Schildkraut JM, Thompson WD. Familial ovarian cancer: A population-based case control study. *Am J Epidemiol* 1988; 128:456-466.
14. Wooster R, Neuhausen SL, Mangion J, et al. Localization of a breast cancer susceptibility gene, BRCA2, to chromosome 13q12-13. *Science* 1994;265:2088-2090.
15. Struewing JP, Hartge P, Wacholder S, et al. The risk of cancer associated with specific mutations of BRCA1 and BRCA2 among Ashkenazi Jews. *N Engl J Med* 1997;336:1401-1408.
16. Vachon CM, Mink PJ, Janney CA, et al. Association of parity and ovarian cancer risk by family history of breast or ovarian cancer in a population-based study of postmenopausal women. *Epidemiology* 2002;13:66-71.
17. Schildkraut JM, Bastos E, Berchuck A. Relationship between lifetime ovulatory cycles and overexpression of mutant p53 in epithelial ovarian cancer. *J Natl Cancer Inst* 1997;89:932-938.

18. Webb PM, Green A, Cummings MC, et al. Relationship between number of ovulatory cycles and accumulation of mutant p53 in epithelial ovarian cancer. *J Natl Cancer Inst* 1998;90:1729-1734.

19. Berchuck A, Kohler MF, Hopkins MP, et al. Overexpression of p53 is not a feature of benign and early-stage borderline epithelial ovarian tumors. *Gynecol Oncol* 1994;52:232-236.

20. Sato N, Tsunoda H, Nishida M, et al. Loss of heterozygosity on 10q23.3 and mutation of the tumor suppressor gene PTEN in benign endometrial cyst of the ovary: Possible sequence progression from benign endometrial cyst to endometrioid carcinoma and clear cell carcinoma of the ovary. *Cancer Res* 2000;60:7052-7056.

21. Berchuck A, Kamel A, Whitaker R, et al. Overexpression of HER-2/neu is associated with poor survival in advanced epithelial ovarian cancer. *Cancer Res* 1990;50:4087-4091.

22. Whittemore AS, Harris R, Huyre J. Characteristics relating to ovarian cancer risk: Collaborative analysis of twelve US case-control studies. II. Invasive epithelial ovarian cancers in white women. *Am J Epidemiol* 1992;136:1184-1203.

23. Haukinson SE, Colditz GA, Hunter DJ, et al. A quantitative assessment of oral contraceptive use and risk of ovarian cancer. *Obstet Gynecol* 1992;80:708-714.

24. Cramer DW, Welch WR, Scully RE, et al. Ovarian cancer and talc: A case control study. *Cancer* 1982;50:372-376.

25. Whittemore AS, Wu ML, Paffenbarger RS, et al. Personal and environmental characteristics related to epithelial ovarian cancer: II. Exposure to talcum powder, tobacco, alcohol and coffee. *Am J Epidemiol* 1988;128:1228-1240.

26. Cramer DW, Willet WC, Bell DA, et al. Galactose consumption and metabolism in relation to the risk of ovarian cancer. *Lancet* 1989;2:66-71.

27. Piver MS, Mattlin C. A case-control study of milk-drinking and ovary cancer risk. *Am J Epidemiol* 1990;132:871-876.

28. Cramer DW, Welch WR, Hutchison GB, et al. Dietary animal fat in relation to ovarian cancer risk. *Obstet Gynecol* 1984;63:833-838.

29. Cramer DW, Welch WR. Determinants of ovarian cancer risk. II. Inferences regarding pathogenesis. *J Natl Cancer Inst.* 1983;71(4):717-721.

30. Fathalla MF. Incessant ovulation. A factor in ovarian neoplasia. *Lancet* 1971;2:163.

31. Annual report on the results of treatment in gynecological cancer: Twenty-first volume: Statements of results obtained in patients treated in 1982 to 1986, inclusive 3- and 5-year survival up to 1990. *Int J Gynaecol Obstet* 1991;36(suppl):238-277.

32. DiSaia P, Creasman W. *Clinical Gynecologic Oncology,* 6th ed. St. Louis: Mosby; 2002.

33. Jacobs F, Bast RC Jr. The CA-125 tumor associated antigen: A review of the literature. *Hum Reprod* 1989;4:1-12.

34. Jacobs IJ, Skates S, Davies AP, et al. Risk of diagnosis of ovarian cancer after raised serum CA 125 concentration: A prospective cohort study. *BMJ* 1996;313(7069):1355-1358.

35. Carlson KJ, Skates SJ, Singer DE. Screening for ovarian cancer. *Ann Intern Med* 1994;121:124-132.

36. Zurawski VR Jr, Orgaseter H, Andersen A, et al. Elevated serum CA 125 levels prior to diagnosis of ovarian neoplasia: Relevance for early detection of ovarian cancer. *Int J Cancer* 1988;42:677-680.

37. Pittaway DE, Fayez JA. Serum CA-125 antigen levels increase during menses. *Am J Obstet Gynecol* 1987;56:75-76.

38. van Nagell JJ, Higgins R, Donaldson E, et al. Transvaginal sonography as a screening method for ovarian cancer: A report of the first 1000 screened. *Cancer* 1990;65:573-577.

39. Grauberg S, Wikland M, Jansson I. Microscopic characterization of ovarian tumors and the relation to the histological diagnosis: Criteria to be used for ultrasound evaluation. *Gynecol Oncol* 1989;35:139-144.

40. van Nagell JR Jr, DePriest PD, Reedy MB, et al. The efficacy of transvaginal sonographic screening in asymptomatic women at risk for ovarian cancer. *Gynecol Oncol* 2000;77(3):350-356.

41. Bourne TH, Campbell S, Reynolds KM, et al. Screening for early familial ovarian cancer with transvaginal ultrasonography and colour blood flow imaging. *BMJ* 1993;306(6884):1025-1029.

42. Sato S, Yokoyama Y, Sakamoto T, et al. Usefulness of mass screening for ovarian carcinoma using transvaginal ultrasonography. *Cancer* 2000;89(3):582-588.

43. Menon U, Talaat A, Jeyarajah AR, et al. Ultrasound assessment of ovarian cancer risk in postmenopausal women with CA 125 elevation. *Br J Cancer* 1999;80(10):1644-1647.

44. Menon U, Talaat A, Rosenthal AN, et al. Performance of ultrasound as a second line test to serum CA 125 in ovarian cancer screening. *Br J Obstet Gynaecol* 2000;107(2):165-169.

45. Jacobs IJ, Skates SJ, MacDonald N, et al. Screening for ovarian cancer: A pilot randomized controlled trial. *Lancet* 1999;353(9160):1207-1210.

46. Hellstrom I, Raycraft J, Hayden-Ledbetter M, et al. The HE4 (WFDC2) protein is a biomarker for ovarian carcinoma. *Cancer Res* 2003;63:3695-3700.

47. Xu Y, Shen Z, Wiper DW, et al. Lysophosphatidic acid as a potential biomarker for ovarian and other gynecologic cancers. *JAMA* 1998;280(8):719-723.

48. Shih IeM, Kurman RJ. Ovarian tumorigenesis: A proposed model based on morphological and molecular genetic analysis. *Am J Pathol* 2004;164:1511-1518.

49. Cheng W, Liu J, Yoshida H, et al. Lineage infidelity of epithelial ovarian cancers is controlled by HOX genes that specify regional identity in the reproductive tract. *Nat Med* 2005;11:531-537.

50. Hennessy BT, Mills GB. Ovarian cancer: Homeobox genes, autocrine/paracrine growth, and kinase signaling. *Int J Biochem Cell Biol* 2006;38:1450-1456.

51. Shaw PA, Zweemer RP, McLaughlin J, et al. Characteristics of genetically determined ovarian cancer [abstract]. *Mod Pathol* 1999;12:124A.

52. Hennessy BT, Coleman RL, Markman M. Ovarian cancer. *Lancet* 2009;374(9698):1371-1382.

53. Geisinger KR, Kute TE, Pettenati MJ, et al. Characterization of a human ovarian carcinoma cell line with estrogen and progesterone receptors, *Cancer* 1989;63:280-288.

54. Slotman BJ, Nauta JJ, Rao BR. Survival of patients with ovarian cancer. Apart from stage and grade, tumor progesterone receptor content is a prognostic indicator. *Cancer* 1990;66(4):740-744.

55. Seidman JD, Russell P, Kurman R. Surface epithelial tumors of the ovary. In: Kurman RJ (ed): *Blaustein's Pathology of the Female Genital Tract*. New York: Springer; 2002.

56. Gotlieb WH, Abrams JS, Watson JM, et al. Presence of IL-10 in the ascites of patients with ovarian and other intra-abdominal cancers. *Cytokine* 1992;4:385-390.

57. Ray A, Tatter SB, Santhanam V, et al. Regulation of expression of IL-6. Molecular and clinical studies. *Ann NY Acad Sci* 1989;557:353-361.

58. Bogdan C, Vodovotz Y, Nathan C. Macrophage deactivation by IL-10. *J Exp Med* 1991;174:1549-1555.

59. de Waal Malefyt R, Abrams J, et al. IL-10 inhibits cytokine synthesis by human monocytes. *J Exp Med* 1991;174:1209-1226.

60. Berek JS, Martinez-Maza O, Hamilton T, et al. Molecular and biological factors in the pathogenesis of ovarian cancer. *Semin Oncol* 1993;4(suppl):S3-S16.

61. Berchuck A, Bast RC Jr, Kohler M. Oncogenes in ovarian cancer. *Hematol Oncol Clin North Am* 1992;6:813-827.

62. Kommoss F, Bauknecht T, Birmelin G, et al. Oncogene and growth factor expression in ovarian cancer. *Acta Obstet Gynecol Scand* 1992;155(suppl):19-24.

63. Lichtenstein A, Berenson J, Gera JF, et al. Resistance of human ovarian cancer cells to tumor necrosis factor and lymphokine-activated killer cells: Correlation with expression of HER-2/neu oncogenes. *Cancer Res* 1990;50:7364-7370.

64. Berchuck A, Marks JR, Bast RC Jr. Expression of the epidermal growth factor receptor, HER-2/neu, and P53 in ovarian cancer. In: Sharp F, Mason WP, Creasman W (ed): *Ovarian Cancer 2: Biology, Diagnosis, and Management.* London: Chapman and Hall; 1992:53-59.

65. Slamon DJ, Goddphin W, Jones LA, et al. Studies of HER-2/neu proto-oncogene in human breast and ovarian cancer. *Science* 1989;244:707-712.

66. Berchuck A, Kamel A, Whitaker R, et al. Overexpression of HER-2/neu is associated with poor survival in advanced epithelial ovarian cancer. *Cancer Res* 1990;50:4087-4091.

67. Marks JR, Davidoff AM, Kerus BJ, et al. Overexpression and mutation of P53 in epithelial ovarian cancer. *Cancer Res* 1991;51:2979-2984.

68. Mazars R, Pujol P, Mandelonde T, et al. P53 mutations in ovarian cancer: A late event? *Oncogene* 1991;6:1685-1690.

69. Chin KV, Veda K, Pastan I, et al. Modulation of activity of the promoter of the human MDR I gene by ras and P53. *Science* 1992;255:459-462.

70. Gotheb WH, Watson JM, Rezai AR, et al. Cytokine-induced modulation of tumor suppressor gene expression in ovarian cancer cells: Up-regulation of P53 gene expression and induction of apoptosis by tumor necrosis factor-alpha. *Am J Obstet Gynecol* 1994;4:1121-1128.

71. Wong GHW, Goeddel DV. Fas antigen and P55 TNF receptor signal apoptosis through distinct pathways. *J Immunol* 1994;52:1751-1755.

72. Wu S, Boyer CM, Whitaker RS, et al. Tumor necrosis factor alpha as an autocrine and paracrine growth factor for ovarian cancer: Monokine induction of tumor cell proliferation and tumor necrosis factor alpha expression. *Cancer Res* 1993;53:1939-1944.

73. Naylor MS, Stamp GW, Foulkes WD, Eccles D, et al. Tumor necrosis factor and its receptors in human ovarian cancer: Potential role in disease progression. *J Clin Invest* 1993;91:2194-2206.

74. Sigurdsson K, Alm P, Gullberg B. Prognostic factors in malignant epithelial ovarian tumors. *Gynecol Oncol* 1983;15:370-380.

75. Dembo AJ, Davy M, Stenwig AE, et al. Prognostic factors in patients with stage I epithelial ovarian cancer. *Obstet Gynecol* 1990;75:263-273.

76. Petterson F, Coppleson M, Creasman W, et al. *Annual Report on the Result of Treatment in Gynecological Cancer.* Stockholm: International Federation of Gynecology and Obstetrics; 1988;110-151.

77. Young RC, Walton LA, Ellenberg SS, et al. Adjuvant therapy in stage I and stage II epithelial ovarian cancer. Results of two prospective randomized trials. *N Engl J Med* 1990;322(15):1021-1027.

78. Hernandez E, Bhagavan BS, Pamiley TH, et al. Interobserver variability in the interpretation of epithelial ovarian cancer. *Gynecol Oncol* 1984;17:117-123.

79. Baak JPA, Langley FA, Talerman A, et al. Interpathologist and intrapathologist disagreement in ovarian tumor grading and typing. *Anal Quant Cytol Histol* 1986;8:354-357.

80. Cramer SF, Roth LM, Ulbright TM, et al. Evaluation of the reproducibility of the WHO classification of common ovarian cancers. *Arch Pathol Lab Med* 1987;111:819-829.

81. Cruickshank DJ, Paul J, Lewis CR, et al. An independent evaluation of the potential clinical usefulness of proposed CA-125 indices previously shown to be of prognostic significance in epithelial ovarian cancer. *Br J Cancer* 1992;65(4):597-600.

82. Mobus V, Kreinberg R, Crowbuch G, et al. Evaluation of CA 125 as prognostic and predictive factor in ovarian cancer. *J Tumour Marker Oncol* 1988;3:251-258.

83. Tholander B, Taube A, Lindgren A, et al. Pretreatment serum levels of CA125, CEA, tissue polypeptide antigen, and placental alkaline phosphatase in patients with ovarian carcinoma: Influence of histological type, grade of differentiation, and clinical stage of disease. *Gynecol Oncol* 1990;39:26-33.

84. Zanaboni F, Vergadoro F, Presti M, et al. Tumour antigen CA 125 as a tumor marker of ovarian epithelial carcinoma. *Gynecol Oncol* 1987;28:61-67.

85. Tholander B, Lindgren A, Taube A, et al. Immunohistochemical detection of CA 125 and CEA in ovarian tumors in relation to corresponding preoperative S levels. *Int J Gynecol* 1992;2:263-270.

86. Kaern J, Tropé CG, Kristensen GB, et al. Evaluation of deoxyribonucleic acid ploidy and S-phase fraction as prognostic parameters in advanced epithelial ovarian carcinoma: a prospective study. *Am J Obstet Gynecol.* 1994;170(2):479-487.

87. Berek JS, Martinez-Maza O, Hamilton T, et al. Molecular and biological factors in the pathogenesis of ovarian cancer. *Ann Oncol* 1993;4(suppl 4):3-16.

88. Chambers JT, Merino MJ, Kohory EI, et al. Borderline ovarian tumors. *Am J Obstet Gynecol* 1988;59:1088-1094.

89. Klemi PJ, Jaensuu H, Kilholma P, et al. Clinical significance of abnormal nuclear DNA content in serous ovarian tumors. *Cancer* 1988;62:2005-2010.

90. Alberts DS, Dahlberg S, Green SJ, et al. Analysis of patient age as an independent prognostic factor for survival in a phase I study of cisplatin-cyclophosphamide vs carboplatin-cyclophosphamide in stage III (suboptimal) and IV ovarian cancer: A SWOG study. *Cancer* 1993;71:2(suppl):618-627.

91. deSouza PL, Friedlander ML. Prognostic factors in ovarian cancer. *Hematol Oncol Clin North Am* 1992;6:4:761-781.

92. Hoskins PJ, O'Reilly SE, Swenerton KD. The "failure free interval" defines the likelihood to resistance to carboplatin in patients with advanced epithelial ovarian cancer previously treated with cisplatin: Relevance to therapy and new drug testing. *Int J Gynecol Cancer* 1991;1(5):205-208.

93. Omura GA, Brady MF, Homesley HD, et al. Long-term follow up and prognostic factor analysis in advanced ovarian carcinoma: The GOG experience. *J Clin Oncol* 1991;9(7):1138-1150.

94. Levin L, Lund B, Heintz AP. Advanced ovarian cancer. An overview of multivariate analysis of prognostic variables with special reference to the role of cytoreductive surgery. *Ann Oncol* 1993;(4):23-29.

95. Heintz APM. Surgery in advanced ovarian carcinoma. Is there proof to show the benefit? *Eur J Surg Oncol* 1988;14: 91-99.

96. Gershenson DM, Copeland LJ, Wharton JT, et al. Prognosis of surgically determined complete responders in advanced ovarian cancer. *Cancer* 1985;55:1129-1135.

97. Bertelsen E, Hansen MK, Pedersen PH, et al. The prognostic and therapeutic value of second look laparotomy in advanced ovarian cancer. *Br J Obstet Gynaecol* 1988;95:1231-1236.

98. van Houwelingen JC, Ten Bokkel Huinink WW, van der Burg MEL, et al. Predictability of the survival of patients with advanced ovarian cancer. *J Clin Oncol* 1989;7:769-773.

99. Hartmann LC, Podratz KC, Keeney GL, et al. Prognostic significance of P53 immunostaining in epithelial ovarian carcinoma. *J Clin Oncol* 1994;12:64-69.

100. Ozols RF: Ovarian cancer: Part II. Treatment. *Curr Probl Cancer* 1992;16:63-126.

101. Hunter RW, Alexander NDE, Stouter WA, et al. Metaanalysis of surgery in advanced ovarian carcinoma: Is maximum cytoreductive surgery an independent determinant of prognosis? *Am J Obstet Gynecol* 1992;166(2):504-511.

102. Goodman HM, Harlow BL, Sheets EE, et al. The role of cytoreductive surgery in the management of stage IV epithelial ovarian carcinoma. *Gynecol Oncol* 1992;46:367-371.

103. Potter ME, Hatch KD, Soong SJ, et al. Second look laparotomy and salvage therapy: A research modality only? *Gynecol Oncol* 1992;44:39.

104. Lund B, Williamson P, van Houwelingen HC, et al. Comparison of the predictive power of different prognostic indices for survival in patients with advanced ovarian cancer. *Cancer Res* 1990;50:4626-4629.

105. Morgan MA, Noumoff IS, King S, et al. A formula for predicting the risk of a positive second look laparotomy in epithelial ovarian cancer: Implications for a randomized trial. *Obstet Gynecol* 1992;80:944-948.

106. Silva EG, Robey-Cafferty SS, Smith TL, et al. Ovarian carcinomas with transitional cell carcinoma pattern. *Am J Clin Pathol* 1990;93:457.

107. Allan DG, Baak J, Belpomme D, et al. Advanced epithelial ovarian cancer: 1993 consensus statements. *Ann Oncol* 1993; 4(suppl 4):83-89.

108. Young RH, Decker DG, Wharton JT, et al. Staging laparotomy in early ovarian cancer. *JAMA* 1983;250:3072-3076.

109. Soper JT, Johnson P, Johnson V, et al. Comprehensive restaging laparotomy in women with apparent early ovarian carcinoma. *Obstet Gynecol* 1992;80:949-953.

110. Mutch DG. Surgical management of ovarian cancer. A Review. *Semin Oncol* 2002;29(1 suppl 1):3-8.

111. Griffiths CT. Surgical resection of tumor bulk in the primary treatment of ovarian carcinoma. *Natl Cancer Inst Monogr* 1975;42:101-104.

112. Hoskins WH, Bundy BN, Thigpen JT, et al. The influence of cytoreductive surgery on recurrence-free interval and survival in small-volume stage III epithelial ovarian cancer: A Gynecologic Oncology Group study. *Gynecol Oncol* 1992; 47:159-166.

113. Young RH, Clement PB, Skully RD. The ovary. In: Sternberg SS, Antonioli DA, Carter D, et al. (eds): *Diagnostic Surgical Pathology,* 2nd ed. New York: Raven Press; 1994; 2195-2210.

114. Smith JP, Day TG Jr. Review of ovarian cancer at the University of Texas Systems Cancer Center, M.D. Anderson Hospital and Tumor Institute. *Am J Obstet Gynecol* 1979; 135:984-993.

115. Wharton J, Edwards CL. Cytoreductive surgery for common epithelial tumours of the ovary. *Clin Obstet Gynaecol* 1983; 10:235-244.

116. Piver MS, Lele SB, Marchetti DL, et al. The impact of aggressive debulking surgery and cisplatin-based chemotherapy on progression-free survival in stage III and IV ovarian carcinoma. *J Clin Oncol* 1988;6:983-989.

117. Eisenkop SM, Spirtos NM, Montag TW, et al. The impact of subspecialty training on the management of advanced ovarian cancer. *Gynecol Oncol* 1992;47:203-209.

118. Curtin JP, Malik R, Venkatraman ES, et al. Stage IV ovarian cancer: Impact of surgical debulking. *Gynecol Oncol* 1991; 41:101-110.

119. Liu PC, Benjamin I, Morgan MA, et al. Effect of surgical debulking on survival in stage IV ovarian cancer. *Gynecol Oncol* 1997;64:4-8.

120. Munkarah AR, Hallum AV III, Morris M, et al. Prognostic significance of residual disease in patients with stage IV epithelial ovarian cancer. *Gynecol Oncol* 1997;4:13-17.

121. Bristow RE, Montz FJ, Lagasse LD, et al. Survival impact of surgical cytoreduction in stage IV epithelial ovarian cancer. *Gynecol Oncol* 1999;72:278-287.

122. Ozols, RF. Treatment of ovarian cancer: Current status. *Semin Oncol* 1994;21(suppl 2):1-9.

123. Potter M, Partridge E, Hatch K, et al. Primary surgical therapy of ovarian cancer: How much and when? *Gynecol Oncol* 1991;40:195-200.

124. Friedman JB, Weiss NS. Second thoughts about second look laparotomy in advanced ovarian cancer. *N Engl J Med* 1990; 322:1079-1082.

125. Segna RA, Dottino PR, Mandeli JP, et al. Secondary cytoreduction for ovarian cancer following cisplatin therapy. *J Clin Oncol* 1993;11:434-439.

126. van der Burg MEL, van Lent M, Buyse M, et al. The effect of debulking surgery after induction chemotherapy on the prognosis in advanced epithelial ovarian cancer. *N Engl J Med* 1995;332:629-634.

127. Rose PG, Nerenstone S, Brady M, et al. A phase III randomized study of interval secondary cytoreduction in patients with advanced stage ovarian carcinoma with suboptimal residual disease: A Gynecologic Oncology Group study. *Proc Am Soc Clin Oncol* 2002;21:201A (abstract 802).

128. Eisenkop SM, Friedman RL, Spirtos NM. The role of secondary cytoreductive surgery in the treatment of patients with recurrent epithelial ovarian carcinoma. *Cancer* 2000;88: 144-153.

129. Morris M, Gershenson DM, Wharton JT, et al. Secondary cytoreductive surgery for recurrent epithelial ovarian cancer. *Gynecol Oncol* 1989;34:334-338.

130. Ahmed FY, Wiltshaw E, A'Hern RP, et al. Natural history and prognosis of untreated stage I epithelial ovarian carcinoma. *J Clin Oncol* 1996;14(11):2968-2975.

131. Bolis G, Colombo N, Pecorelli S, et al. Adjuvant treatment for early epithelial ovarian cancer: Results of two randomised clinical trials comparing cisplatin to no further treatment or chromic phosphate (32P). GICOG: Gruppo Interregionale Collaborativo in Ginecologia Oncologica. *Ann Oncol* 1995; 6(9):887-893.

132. Vergote IB, Vergote-De Vos LN, Abeler VM. Randomized trial comparing cisplatin with radioactive phosphorus or whole-abdomen irradiation as adjuvant treatment of ovarian cancer. *Cancer* 1992;69(3):741-749.

133. Young RC, Brady MF, Nieberg RM, et al. Randomized Clinical Trial of Adjuvant Treatment of Women with Early (Figo-I-IIA High Risk) Ovarian Cancer—GOG #95. *Proc Am Soc Clin Oncol* 1999;18:358a(abstract 1376).

134. Trimbos JB, Parmar M, Vergote I, et al. International Collaborative Ovarian Neoplasm trial 1 and Adjuvant Chemotherapy in Ovarian Neoplasm trial: Two parallel randomized phase III trials of adjuvant chemotherapy in patients with early-stage ovarian carcinoma. *J Natl Cancer Inst* 2003;95(2): 105-112.

135. Trimbos JB, Vergote I, Bolis G, et al. Impact of adjuvant chemotherapy and surgical staging in early-stage ovarian carcinoma: European Organisation for Research and Treatment of Cancer–Adjuvant ChemoTherapy in Ovarian Neoplasm trial. *J Natl Cancer Inst* 2003;95(2):113-125.

136. Bell J, Brady MF, Young RC, et al. Randomized phase III trial of three versus six cycles of adjuvant carboplatin and paclitaxel in early stage epithelial ovarian carcinoma: a Gynecologic Oncology Group study. *Gynecol Oncol*. 2006; 102(3):432-439.

137. Advanced Ovarian Cancer Trialist Group: Chemotherapy in advanced ovarian cancer: An overview of randomized clinical trials. *Br Med J* 1991;303:884-893.

138. Alberts DS, Green S, Hanningan EV, et al. Improved therapeutic index of carboplatin plus cyclophosphamide vs. cisplatin plus cyclophosphamide: Final report by the Southwest Oncology Group of a phase III randomized trial in stages III and IV ovarian cancer. *J Clin Oncol* 1992;10:706-717.

139. Swenerton K, Jeffrey J, Stuart G, et al. Cisplatin-cyclophosphamide vs carboplatin-cyclophosphamide in advanced ovarian cancer: A randomized phase III study of National Cancer Institute of Canada Clinical Trial Group. *J Clin Oncol* 1992; 10:718-726.

140. Belpomme D, Bugat R, Rives M, et al. Carboplatin vs cisplatin in association with cyclophosphamide and doxorubicin as first line therapy in stage III-IV ovarian carcinoma: Results of an ARTAC phase III trial (abstr). *Proc Am Soc Clin Oncol* 1992;11:227.

141. Williams CJ, Stewart L, Parmar M, et al. Metaanalysis of the role of platinum compounds in advanced ovarian carcinoma. The Advanced Ovarian Cancer Trialists Group. *Semin Oncol* 1992;19(1 suppl 2):120-128.

142. ICON collaborators. ICON2: Randomised trial of single-agent carboplatin against three-drug combination of CAP (cyclophosphamide, doxorubicin, and cisplatin) in women with ovarian cancer. ICON collaborators. International Collaborative Ovarian Neoplasm Study. *Lancet* 1998;352(9140): 1571-1576.

143. McGuire WP, Hoskins WJ, Brady MF, et al. Cyclophosphamide and cisplatin compared with paclitaxel and cisplatin in patients with stage III and stage IV ovarian cancer. *N Engl J Med* 1996;334(1):1-6.

144. Piccart MJ, Bertelsen K, James K, et al. Randomized intergroup trial of cisplatin-paclitaxel versus cisplatin-cyclophosphamide in women with advanced epithelial ovarian cancer: Three-year results. *J Natl Cancer Inst* 2000;92(9):699-708.

145. du Bois A, Lück HJ, Meier W, et al. A randomized clinical trial of cisplatin/paclitaxel versus carboplatin/paclitaxel as first-line treatment of ovarian cancer. *J Natl Cancer Inst*. 2003;95(17):1320-1329.

146. Ozols RF, Bundy BN, Fowler J, et al. Randomized phase III study of cisplatin (CIS)/paclitaxel (PAC) versus carboplatin (CARBO)/PAC in optimal stage III epithelial ovarian cancer (OC): A Gynecologic Oncology Group trial (GOG 158). *Proc Am Soc Clin Oncol* 1999;18:A-1373(abstract 356a).

147. ICON collaborators. Paclitaxel plus carboplatin versus standard chemotherapy with single-agent carboplatin or cyclophosphamide, doxorubicin, and cisplatin in women with ovarian cancer: The ICON3 randomised trial. International Collaborative Ovarian Neoplasm Study. *Lancet* 2002; 360 (9332): 505-515.

148. Vasey PA, Jayson GC, Gordon A, et al. Phase III randomized trial of docetaxel-carboplatin versus paclitaxel-carboplatin as first-line chemotherapy for ovarian carcinoma. *J Natl Cancer Inst* 2004;96:1682-1691.

149. Muggia FM, Braly PS, Brady MF, et al. Phase III randomized study of cisplatin versus paclitaxel versus cisplatin and paclitaxel in patients with suboptimal stage III or IV ovarian cancer: A Gynecologic Oncology Group study. *J Clin Oncol* 2000; 18(1):106-115.

150. Bookman M, for the Gynecologic Cancer Intergroup. GOG182-ICON5: 5-arm phase III randomized trial of paclitaxel and carboplatin versus combinations with gemcitabine, pegylated liposomal doxorubicin or topotecan in patients with advanced-stage epithelial ovarian or primary peritoneal carcinoma. *J Clin Oncol* 2006;24(18S):256s (abstract 5002).

151. GICOG. Randomized comparison of cisplatin with cyclophosphamide/cisplatin and with cyclophosphamide/doxorubicin/cisplatin in advanced ovarian cancer. *Lancet* 1989;2:353-359.

152. Bertelsen K, Jakobsen A, Andersen JE, et al. A randomized study of cyclophosphamide and cisplatinum with or without doxorubicin in advanced ovarian carcinoma. *Gynecol Oncol* 1987;28:161-169.

153. Conte PF, Bruzzon M, Chiara S, et al. A randomized trial comparing cisplatin plus cyclophosphamide vs cisplatin, doxorubicin, and cyclophosphamide in advanced ovarian cancer. *J Clin Oncol* 1986;4:965-971.

154. Ovarian Cancer Metaanalysis Project. Cyclophosphamide + cisplatin vs cyclophosphamide, doxorubicin, and cisplatin chemotherapy of ovarian carcinoma: A metaanalysis. *J Clin Oncol* 1991;9:166-167.

155. du Bois A, Weber B, Pfisterer J, et al. Epirubicin/paclitaxel (TEC) vs paclitaxel/carboplatin (TC) in first line treatment of ovarian cancer FIGO stages IIb-IV. Interim results of an AGO-GINECO intergroup phase III trial. *Proc Am Soc Clin Oncol* 2001;20:202a(abstract 805).

156. Bessette AR, Benedetti-Panici PL, Boman K, et al. Randomised trial comparing primary debulking surgery (PDS) with neoadjuvant chemotherapy (NACT) followed by interval debulking (IDS) in stage IIIC-IV ovarian, fallopian tube and peritoneal cancer. IGCS Biennial Meeting Proceedings; Bangkok, Oct 25-28, 2008.

157. Markman M, Liu PY, Wilczynski S, et al. Phase III randomized trial of 12 versus 3 months of maintenance paclitaxel in patients with advanced ovarian cancer after CR to platinum and paclitaxel-based chemotherapy: A Southwest Oncology Group and Gynecologic Oncology Group trial. *J Clin Oncol* 2003;21(13):2460-2465.

158. Armstrong DK, Bundy B, Wenzel L, et al. Intraperitoneal cisplatin and paclitaxel in ovarian cancer. *N Engl J Med* 2006;354:34-43.

159. Alberts DS, Liu PY, Hannigan EV, et al. Intraperitoneal cisplatin plus intravenous cyclophosphamide versus intravenous cisplatin plus intravenous cyclophosphamide for stage III ovarian cancer. *N Engl J Med* 1996;335:1950-1955.

160. Markman M, Bundy BN, Alberts DS, et al. Phase III trial of standard-dose intravenous cisplatin plus paclitaxel versus moderately high-dose carboplatin followed by intravenous paclitaxel and intraperitoneal cisplatin in small-volume stage III ovarian carcinoma: an intergroup study of the Gynecologic Oncology Group, Southwestern Oncology Group, and Eastern Cooperative Oncology Group. *J Clin Oncol* 2001; 19:1001-1007.

161. Hess LM, Ham-Hutchins M, Herzog TJ, et al. A meta-analysis of the efficacy of intraperitoneal cisplatin for the front-line treatment of ovarian cancer. *Int J Gynecol Cancer* 2007;17: 561-570.

162. Elit L, Oliver TK, Covens A, et al. Intraperitoneal chemotherapy in the first-line treatment of women with stage III epithelial ovarian cancer: A systematic review with metaanalyses. *Cancer* 2007;109:692-702.

163. Gore M, du Bois A, Vergote I. Intraperitoneal chemotherapy in ovarian cancer remains experimental. *J Clin Oncol* 2006; 24:4528-4530.

164. Markman M, Walker JL. Intraperitoneal chemotherapy of ovarian cancer: A review, with a focus on practical aspects of treatment. *J Clin Oncol* 2006;24:988-994.

165. Markman M. Hyperthermic intraperitoneal chemotherapy in the management of ovarian cancer: A critical need for an evidencebased evaluation. *Gynecol Oncol* 2009;113:4-5.

166. Levin L, Hryniuk W. Dose intensity analysis of chemotherapy regimens in ovarian carcinoma. *J Clin Oncol* 1987;5(5): 756-767.

167. Levin L, Simon R, Hryniuk W. Importance of multiagent chemotherapy regimens in ovarian carcinoma: Dose intensity analysis. *J Natl Cancer Inst* 1993;85(21):1732-1742.

168. Ozols RF, Ostchega Y, Curt G, Young RC. High-dose carboplatin in refractory ovarian cancer patients. *Clin Oncol* 1987; 5(2):197-201.

169. McGuire WP, Hoskins WJ, Brady MF, et al. Assessment of dose-intensive therapy in suboptimally debulked ovarian cancer: A Gynecologic Oncology Group study. *J Clin Oncol* 1995;13(7):1589-1599.

170. Columbo N, Pittelli MR, Parma G. Cisplatin (P) dose intensity in advanced ovarian cancer (AOC): A randomized study of conventional dose (DC) vs dose-intense (DO) cisplatin monochemotherapy. *Proc Am Soc Clin Oncol* 1993;12:255.

171. Conte P, Bruzzone M, Carnino F, et al. High-dose versus low-dose cisplatin in combination with cyclophosphamide and epidoxorubicin in suboptimal ovarian cancer: A randomized study of the Gruppo Oncologico Nord-Ovest. *J Clin Oncol* 1996;14(2):351-356.

172. Ehrlich CE, Einhorn L, Stehman FB, et al. treatment of advanced epithelial ovarian cancer using cisplatin, Adriamycin and cytoxan—The Indiana University experience. *Clin Obstet Gynecol* 1983;10:325-335.

173. Dittrich C, Obermair A, Kurz C, et al. Prospective randomized trial of cisplatin/carboplatin versus conventional cisplatin/ cyclophosphomide in epithelial ovarian cancer: First results of the impact of platinum dose intensity on patient outcome. *Proc Am Soc Clin Oncol* 1996;15:279.

174. Kaye SB, Paul J, Cassidy J. Mature results of a randomized trial of two doses of cisplatin for the treatment of ovarian cancer. Scottish Gynecology Cancer Trials Group. *J Clin Oncol* 1996;14(7):2113-2119.

175. Ngam HY, Choo YC, Cheung M, et al. A randomized trial of high dose vs low dose cisplatin combined with cyclophosphamide in the treatment of advanced ovarian cancer. *Chemotherapy* 1989;35:221-227.

176. Eisenhauer EA, ten Bokkel Huinink WW. European-Canadian randomized trial of paclitaxel in relapsed ovarian cancer: High-dose versus low-dose and long versus short infusion. *J Clin Oncol* 1994;12(12):2654-2666.

177. EK Rowinsky, MK Mackey, SN Goodman. Metaanalysis of paclitaxel (P) dose-response and dose intensity (DI) in recurrent or refractory ovarian cancer (OC) (abstr). *Proc Am Soc Clin Oncol* 1996;15:284.

178. Omura GA, Brady MF, Look KY, et al. Phase III Trial of paclitaxel at two dose levels, the higher dose accompanied by filgrastim at two dose levels in platinum-pretreated epithelial ovarian cancer: An Intergroup Study. *J Clin Oncol* 2003; 21(15):2843-2848.

179. Guppy AE, Rustin GJ. CA125 response: Can it replace the traditional response criteria in ovarian cancer? *Oncologist* 2002;7(5):437-443.

180. van der Burg ME, Lammes FB, Verweij J. The role of CA 125 in the early diagnosis of progressive disease in ovarian cancer. *Ann Oncol* 1990;1(4):301-302.

181. Rustin GJ, van der Burg ME. On behalf of MRC and EORTC collaborators. A randomized trial in ovarian cancer (OC) of early treatment of relapse based on CA125 level alone versus delayed treatment based on conventional clinical indicators (MRC OV05/EORTC 55955 trials). *J Clin Oncol* 2009; 27(suppl):1 (abstract).

182. Neijt JP. New therapy for ovarian cancer. *N Engl J Med* 1996;334(1):50-51.

183. Swenerton K, Muss HB, Robinson EG. Salvage chemotherapy for refractory disease in ovarian cancer. In: Gershenson D, McGuire W (eds): *Ovarian Cancer: Controversies in Management*. Churchill Livingstone; 2002;169-194.

184. Balbi G, Di Prisco L, Musone R. Second-line with paclitaxel and carboplatin for recurrent disease following first paclitaxel and platinum compounds in ovarian carcinoma. *Eur J Gynaecol Oncol* 2002;23(4):347-349.

185. Rose PG, Fusco N, Fluellen L, et al. Second-line therapy with paclitaxel and carboplatin for recurrent disease following first-line therapy with paclitaxel and platinum in ovarian or peritoneal carcinoma. *J Clin Oncol* 1998;16(4):1494-1497.

186. Dizon DS, Hensley ML, Poynor EA, et al. Retrospective analysis of carboplatin and paclitaxel as initial second-line therapy for recurrent epithelial ovarian carcinoma: Application toward a dynamic disease state model of ovarian cancer. *J Clin Oncol* 2002;20(5):1238-1247.

187. Gronlund B, Hogdall C, Hansen HH, et al. Results of reinduction therapy with paclitaxel and carboplatin in recurrent epithelial ovarian cancer. *Gynecol Oncol* 2001;83(1):128-134.

188. Parmar MK, Ledermann JA, Colombo N, et al. Paclitaxel plus platinum-based chemotherapy versus conventional platinum-based chemotherapy in women with relapsed ovarian cancer: The ICON4/AGO-OVAR-2.2 trial. *Lancet* 2003;361(9375): 2099-2106.

189. Pfisterer J, Plante M, Vergote I, et al. Gemcitabine plus carboplatin compared with carboplatin in patients with platinumsensitive recurrent ovarian cancer: An intergroup trial of the AGO-OVAR, the NCIC CTG, and the EORTC GCG. *J Clin Oncol* 2006;24:4699-4707.

190. Pujade-Lauraine E, Mahner S, Kaern J, et al. A randomized, phase III study of carboplatin and pegylated liposomal doxorubicin versus carboplatin and paclitaxel in relapsed platinum-sensitive ovarian cancer (OC): CALYPSO study of the Gynecologic Cancer Intergroup (GCIG). *J Clin Oncol* 2009;27(suppl):LBA5509 (abstract).

191. Sehouli J, Stengel D, Oskay-Oezcelik G, et al. Nonplatinum topotecan combinations versus topotecan alone for recurrent ovarian cancer: Results of a phase III study of the North-Eastern German Society of Gynecological Oncology Ovarian Cancer Study Group. *J Clin Oncol* 2008;26:3176-3182.

192. Swisher EM, Mutch DG, Rader JS, et al. Topotecan in platinum- and paclitaxel-resistant ovarian cancer. *Gynecol Oncol* 1997; 66(3):480-486.

193. Bookman MA, Malmstrom H, Bolis G, et al. Topotecan for the treatment of advanced epithelial ovarian cancer: An open-label phase II study in patients treated after prior chemotherapy that contained cisplatin or carboplatin and paclitaxel. *J Clin Oncol* 1998;16(10):3345-3352.

194. McGuire WP, Blessing JA, Bookman MA, et al. Topotecan has substantial antitumor activity as first-line salvage therapy in platinum-sensitive epithelial ovarian carcinoma: A Gynecologic Oncology Group study. *J Clin Oncol* 2000;18(5): 1062-1067.

195. McGuire WP, Rowinsky EK, Rosenshein NB, et al. Taxol: A unique antineoplastic agent with significant activity in advanced ovarian epithelial neoplasms. *Ann Intern Med* 1989;111(4): 273-279.

196. Thigpen JT, Blessing JA, Ball H, et al. Phase II trial of paclitaxel in patients with progressive ovarian carcinoma after platinum-based chemotherapy: A Gynecologic Oncology Group study. *J Clin Oncol* 1994;12(9):1748-1753.

197. Einzig AI, Wiernik PH, Sasloff J, et al. Phase II study and long-term follow-up of patients treated with Taxol for advanced ovarian adenocarcinoma. *J Clin Oncol* 1992;10(11):1748-1753.

198. McGuire WP. Paclitaxel in the treatment of ovarian cancer. In: *American Society of Clinical Oncology Educational Book.* Dallas, TX: American Society of Clinical Oncology; 1994;204-213 (abstract 3014).

199. Trimble EL, Adams JD, Vena D, et al. Paclitaxel for platinum-refractory ovarian cancer: Results from the first 1,000 patients registered to National Cancer Institute Treatment Referral Center 9103. *J Clin Oncol* 1993;11(12):2405-2410.

200. ten Bokkel Huinink W, Gore M, Carmichael J, et al. Topotecan versus paclitaxel for the treatment of recurrent epithelial ovarian cancer. *J Clin Oncol* 1997;15:2183-2193.

201. Kudelka AP, Tresukosol D, Edwards CL. Phase II study of intravenous topotecan as a 5-day infusion for refractory epithelial ovarian carcinoma. *J Clin Oncol* 1996;14(5): 1552-1557.

202. Muggia FM, Hainsworth JD, Jeffers S. Phase II study of liposomal doxorubicin in refractory ovarian cancer: Antitumor activity and toxicity modification by liposomal encapsulation. *J Clin Oncol* 1997;15(3):987-993.

203. Gordon AN, Fleagle JT, Guthrie D, et al. Recurrent epithelial ovarian carcinoma: A randomized phase III study of pegylated liposomal doxorubicin versus topotecan. *J Clin Oncol* 2001;19(14):3312-3322.

204. O'Byrne KJ, Bliss P, Graham JD, et al. A phase III study of Doxil/Caelyx versus paclitaxel in platinum-treated, taxane-naive relapsed ovarian cancer. *Proc Am Soc Clin Oncol* 2002; 21:203a (abstract 808).

205. Friedlander M, Millward MJ, Bell D, et al. A phase II study of gemcitabine in platinum pre-treated patients with advanced epithelial ovarian cancer. *Ann Oncol* 1998;9(12):1343-1345.

206. Lund B, Hansen OP, Neijt JP, et al. Phase II study of gemcitabine in previously platinum-treated ovarian cancer patients. *Anticancer Drugs* 1995;6(suppl 6):61-62.

207. Nagourney RA, Brewer CA, Radecki S, et al. Phase II trial of gemcitabine plus cisplatin repeating doublet therapy in previously treated, relapsed ovarian cancer patients. *Gynecol Oncol* 2003;88(1):35-39.

208. Rose PG, Mossbruger K, Fusco N, et al. Gemcitabine reverses cisplatin resistance: Demonstration of activity in platinum- and multidrug-resistant ovarian and peritoneal carcinoma. *Gynecol Oncol* 2003;88(1):17-21.

209. Nogue M, Cirera L, Arcusa A, et al. Phase II study of gemcitabine and cisplatin in chemonaive patients with advanced epithelial ovarian cancer. *Anticancer Drugs* 2002;13(8): 839-845.

210. Hoskins PJ, Swenerton KD. Oral etoposide is active against platinum resistant ovarian cancer. *J Clin Oncol* 1994;12:60-63.

211. Markman M, Hakes T, Reichman B, et al. Phase 2 trial of chronic low-dose oral etoposide as salvage therapy of platinum-refractory ovarian cancer. *J Cancer Res Clin Oncol* 1992; 119(1):55-57.

212. de Wit R, van der Burg ME, van den Gaast A, et al. Phase II study of prolonged oral etoposide in patients with ovarian cancer refractory to or relapsing within 12 months after platinum-containing chemotherapy. *Ann Oncol* 1994;5(7):656-657.

213. Piccart MJ, Gore M, Ten Bokkel Huinink W, et al. Docetaxel: An active new drug for treatment of advanced epithelial ovarian cancer. *J Natl Cancer Inst* 1995;87(9):676-681.

214. Aapro M, Bruno R. Early clinical studies with docetaxel. Docetaxel Investigators Group. *Eur J Cancer* 1995;31A (suppl 4):S7-S10.

215. Francis P, Schneider J, Hann L, et al. Phase II trial of docetaxel in patients with platinum-refractory advanced ovarian cancer. *J Clin Oncol* 1994;12(11):2301-2308.

216. Kavanagh JJ, Kudelka AP, de Leon CG, et al. Phase II study of docetaxel in patients with epithelial ovarian carcinoma refractory to platinum. *Clin Cancer Res* 1996;2(5):837-842.

217. Kaye SB, Piccart M, Aapro M, et al. Phase II trials of docetaxel (Taxotere) in advanced ovarian cancer—An updated overview. *Eur J Cancer* 1997;33(13):2167-2170.

218. Untch M, Untch A, Sevin BU, et al. Comparison of paclitaxel and docetaxel (Taxotere) in gynecologic and breast cancer cell lines with the ATP-cell viability assay. *Anticancer Drugs* 1994;5(1):24-30.

219. Verschraegen CF, Sittisomwong T, Kudelka AP, et al. Docetaxel for patients with paclitaxel-resistant Müllerian carcinoma. *J Clin Oncol* 2000;18(14):2733-2739.

220. Bodurka DC, Levenback C, Wolf JK, et al. Phase II trial of irinotecan in patients with metastatic epithelial ovarian cancer or peritoneal cancer. *J Clin Oncol* 2003;21(2):291-297.

221. Vermorken J, Gore M, Perren T, et al. Multicenter randomized phase II study of oxaliplatin (OXA) or topotecan (TOPO) in platinum-pretreated epithelial ovarian cancer (EOC) patients. *Proc Am Soc Clin Oncol* 2001;20:212a (abstract 847).

222. Sorensen P, Hoyer M, Jakobsen A, et al. Phase II study of vinorelbine in the treatment of platinum-resistant ovarian carcinoma. *Gynecol Oncol* 2001;81(1):58-62.

223. Boehmer Ch, Jaeger W. Capecitabine in treatment of platinum-resistant recurrent ovarian cancer. *Anticancer Res* 2002;22(1A):439-443.

224. Vasey PA, McMahon L, Paul J, et al. A phase II trial of capecitabine (Xeloda) in relapsed ovarian cancer. *Ann Oncol* 2000;11(suppl 4):84a.

225. Coleman R, Towlson K, Wiltshaw E. Epirubicin for pretreated advanced ovarian cancer. *Eur J Cancer* 1990;26(7):850-851.

226. Pelaez I, Lacave AJ, Palacio I, et al. Phase II trial of epirubicin at standard dose in relapsed ovarian cancer. *Eur J Cancer* 1996;32A(5):899-900.

227. Rosen GF, Lurain JR, Newton M. Hexamethylmelamine in ovarian cancer after failure of cisplatin-based multiple-agent chemotherapy. *Gynecol Oncol* 1987;27(2):173-179.

228. Stehman FB, Ehrlich CE, Callangan MF. Failure of hexamethylmelamine as salvage therapy in ovarian epithelial adenocarcinoma resistant to combination chemotherapy. *Gynecol Oncol* 1984;17(2):189-195.

229. Manetta A, MacNeill C, Lyter JA, et al. Hexamethylmelamine as a single second-line agent in ovarian cancer. *Gynecol Oncol* 1990;36(1):93-96.

230. Vergote I, Himmelmann A, Frankendal B, et al. Hexamethylmelamine as second-line therapy in platin-resistant ovarian cancer. *Gynecol Oncol* 1992;47(3):282-286.

231. Moore DH, Valea F, Crumpler LS, et al. Hexamethylmelamine/altretamine as second-line therapy for epithelial ovarian carcinoma. *Gynecol Oncol* 1993;51(1):109-112.

232. Vasey P, Kaye SB, Thigpen JT. Importance of dose intensity in ovarian cancer. In: Gershenson D, McGuire W (eds): *Ovarian Cancer: Controversies in Management.* New York: Churchill Livingstone; 2002:139-167.

233. Cure H, Legros M, Fleury J, et al. High-dose chemotherapy and autologous bone marrow transplantation in advanced epithelial ovarian cancer. *Bone Marrow Transplant* 1992;10(suppl 2):50.

234. Menichella G, Pierelli L, Foddai ML, et al. Autologous blood stem cell harvesting and transplantation in patients with advanced ovarian cancer. *Br J Haematol* 1991;79(3):444-450.

235. Herrmann F, Brugger W, Kanz L, et al. In vivo biology and therapeutic potential of hematopoietic growth factors and circulating progenitor cells. *Semin Oncol* 1992;19:422-431.

236. Korbling M, Juttner C, Henon P, et al. Autologous blood stem cell vs bone marrow transplant. *Bone Marrow Transplant* 1992;10(suppl 10):144-148.

237. Shea TC, Mason JR, Storniolo AM, et al. Sequential cycles of high dose carboplatin administered with recombinant human granulocyte-macrophage colony-stimulating factor and repeated infusions of autologous peripheral blood progenitor cells: A novel and effective method for delivering multiple courses of dose-intensive therapy. *J Clin Oncol* 1992; 10:464-473.

238. Shpall EJ, Jones RB, Bearman SI, et al. Future strategies for the treatment of advanced epithelial ovarian cancer using high-dose chemotherapy and autologous bone marrow support. *Gynecol Oncol* 1994;54(3):357-361.

239. Dauplat J, Legros M, Condat P, et al. High-dose melphalan and autologous bone marrow support for treatment of ovarian cancer with positive second-look operation. *Gynecol Oncol* 1989;34:294-298.

240. Mulder PO, Willemse PH, Aalders JG, et al. High-dose chemotherapy with autologous bone marrow transplantation in patients with refractory ovarian cancer. *Eur J Cancer Clin Oncol* 1989;25(4):645-649.

241. Broun ER, Belinson JL, Berek JS, et al. Salvage therapy for recurrent and refractory ovarian cancer with high-dose chemotherapy and autologous bone marrow support: A Gynecologic Oncology Group pilot study. *Gynecol Oncol* 1994;54(2):142-146.

242. Shpall EJ, Pearson-Clarke D, Soper JT, et al. High dose alkylating agent chemotherapy with ABMT in patients with stage III/IV epithelial ovarian cancer. *Gynecol Oncol* 1990; 38:386-391.

243. Stiff P, Bayer R, Camarda M, et al. A phase II trial of high-dose mitoxantrone, carboplatin, and cyclophosphamide with autologous bone marrow rescue for recurrent epithelial ovarian carcinoma: Analysis of risk factors for clinical outcome. *Gynecol Oncol* 1995;57(3):278-285.

244. Viens P, Maraniuch D, Legros M, et al. High dose melphalan and autologous marrow rescue in advanced epithelial ovarian carcinomas: A retrospective analysis of 35 patients treated in France. *Bone Marrow Transplant* 1009;5:227-233.

245. Fennelly D, Wasserheit C, Schneider J, et al. Simultaneous dose escalation and schedule intensification of carboplatin-based chemotherapy using peripheral blood progenitor cells and filgrastim: A phase I trial. *Cancer Res* 1994;54(23):6137-6142.

246. Fennelly D, Schneider J, Spriggs D, et al. Dose escalation of paclitaxel with high-dose cyclophosphamide, with analysis of progenitor-cell mobilization and hematologic support of advanced ovarian cancer patients receiving rapidly sequenced high-dose carboplatin/cyclophosphamide courses. *J Clin Oncol* 1995;13(5):1160-1166.

247. Rendina GM, Donadio C, Giovannini M, et al. Steroid receptors and progestinic therapy in ovarian endometrioid carcinoma. *Eur J Gynaecol Oncol* 1982;3(3):241-246.

248. Kavanagh JJ, Roberts W, Townsend P, et al. Leuprolide acetate in the treatment of refractory or persistent epithelial ovarian cancer. *J Clin Oncol* 1989;7:115-118.

249. Ahlgren JD, Ellison NM, Gottlieb RJ, et al. Hormonal palliation of chemoresistant ovarian cancer: Three consecutive phase II trials of the Mid-Atlantic Oncology Program. *J Clin Oncol* 1993;11:1957-1968.

250. Sevelda P, Vavra N, Fitz R, et al. Goserelin alpha GnRH analogue as third-line therapy of refractory ovarian cancer. *Int J Gynecol Cancer* 1992;2:160-162.

251. Hatch KD, Beecham JB, Blessing JA, Creasman WT. Responsiveness of patients with advanced ovarian carcinoma to tamoxifen. A Gynecologic Oncology Group study of second-line therapy in 105 patients. *Cancer.* 1991;68(2):269-271.

252. Marth C, Sorheim N, Kaern J, Trope C. Tamoxifen in the treatment of recurrent ovarian carcinoma. *Int J Gynecol Cancer* 1997;7:256-261.

253. Landoni F, Epis A, Gorga G, et al. Hormonal treatment in advanced epithelial ovarian cancer. In: Panutti F (ed): *Antiestrogens in Oncology: Past, Present and Prospects.* Amsterdam: Excerpta Medica; 1985.

254. Osborne RJ, Malik S, Slevin ML, et al. Tamoxifen in refractory ovarian cancer: The use of a loading dose. *Br J Cancer* 1988;57:115.

255. Gennatas C, Dardoufas C, Karvouni H, et al. Phase II trial of tamoxifen in patients with advanced epithelial ovarian cancer. *Proc Am Soc Clin Oncol* 1996;15.

256. Rolski J, Pawlicki M. Evaluation of efficacy and toxicity of tamoxifen in patients with advanced chemotherapy resistant ovarian cancer. *Ginekol Pol* 1998;69:586-589.

257. Quinn MA. Hormonal therapy of ovarian cancer. In: F Sharp F, Soutter WP (eds): *Ovarian Cancer: The Way Ahead.* London: Royal College of Obstetricians and Gynaecologists; 1987: 383-393.

258. Jager W, Sauerbrei W, Beck E, et al. A randomized comparison of triptorelin and tamoxifen as treatment of progressive ovarian cancer. *Anticancer Res* 1995;15:2639-2642.

259. Weiner SA, Alberts DS, Surwitt EA, et al. Tamoxifen therapy in recurrent epithelial ovarian carcinoma. *Gynecol Oncol* 1987;27:208-213.

260. Van Der Velden J, Gitsch G, Wain GV, et al. Tamoxifen in patients with advanced epithelial ovarian cancer. *Int J Gynecol Cancer* 1995;5(4):301-305.

261. Ahlgren JD, Ellison NM, Gottlieb RJ, et al. Hormonal palliation of chemoresistant ovarian cancer: Three consecutive phase II trials of the Mid-Atlantic Oncology Program. *J Clin Oncol* 1993;11:1957-1968.

262. Shirey DR, Kavanagh JJ, Gershenshon DM, et al. Tamoxifen therapy of epithelial ovarian cancer. *Obstet Gynecol* 1985; 66:575-578.

263. Slevin ML, Harvey VJ, Osborne RJ, et al. A phase II study of tamoxifen in ovarian cancer. *Eur J Cancer Clin Oncol* 1986; 22:309-312.

264. Pagel J, Rose C, Thorpe S, et al. Treatment of advanced ovarian carcinoma with tamoxifen: A phase II trial. *Proc 2nd Eur Conf Clin Oncol* 1983:42.

265. Hamerlynck JV, Vermorken JB, Van der Burgh ME. Tamoxifen therapy in advanced ovarian cancer: A phase II study. *Proc Am Soc Clin Oncol* 1985;4:115.

266. Schwartz PE, Keating G, MacLusky N, et al. Tamoxifen therapy for advanced ovarian cancer. *Obstet Gynecol* 1982; 59:583-588.

267. Rowland K, Bonomi P, Wilbanks G, et al. Hormone receptors in ovarian carcinoma. *Proc Am Soc Clin Oncol* 1985;4:117.

268. Bertlesen K, Jacobsen A. Radiotherapy for gynecologic cancers. *Curr Opin Oncol* 1993;5:885-894.

269. Smith JP, Rutledge FN, Delclos L, et al. Postoperative treatment of early cancer of the ovary: A random trial between postoperative irradiation and chemotherapy. *J Natl Cancer Inst* 1975;42:149-153.

270. Hoskins PJ, O'Reilly SE, Swenerton KD, et al. Ten-year outcome of patients with advanced epithelial ovarian carcinoma treated with cisplatin-based multimodality therapy. *J Clin Oncol* 1992;10:1561-1568.

271. Whelan TJ, Dembo AJ, Bush RS, et al. Complications of whole abdominal and pelvic radiotherapy following chemotherapy for advanced ovarian cancer. *Int J Radiat Oncol Biol Phys* 1992;22:853-858.

272. Soper JT, Berchuck A, Dopdge R, et al. Adjuvant therapy with intraperitoneal chronic phosphate (P-32) in women with early ovarian carcinoma after comprehensive surgical staging. *Obstet Gynecol* 1992;79:993-997.

273. Spanos WJ, Day T, Abner A, et al. Complications in the use of intra-abdominal P-32 for ovarian carcinoma. *Gynecol Oncol* 1992;45:243-247.

274. Vergotte IB, DeVos LN, Abeler VM, et al. Randomized trial comparing cisplatin with radioactive phosphorus or whole-abdomen irradiation as adjuvant treatment of ovarian cancer. *Cancer* 1992;63:741-749.

275. Barnhill D, Heller P, Brzozowski P, et al. Epithelial ovarian carcinoma of low malignant potential. Obstet Gynecol. 1985; 65(1):53-59.

276. Goldman TL, Chalas E, Chumas J, et al. Management of borderline tumors of the ovary. *South Med J* 1993;86(4): 423-425.

277. Kurman RJ, Trimble CL. The behavior of serous tumors of low malignant potential: Are they ever malignant? *Int J Gynecol Pathol* 1993;12(2):120-127.

278. Barnhill DR, Kurman RJ, Brady MF, et al. Preliminary analysis of the behavior of stage I ovarian serous tumors of low malignant potential: A Gynecologic Oncology Group study. *J Clin Oncol* 1995;13(11):2752-2756.

279. Chambers JT, Merino MJ, Kohorn EI, et al. Borderline ovarian tumors. *Am J Obstet Gynecol* 1988;159(5):1088-1094.

280. Zanetta G, Rota S, Chiari S, et al. Behavior of borderline tumors with particular interest to persistence, recurrence, and progression to invasive carcinoma: A prospective study. *J Clin Oncol* 2001;19(10):2658-2664.

281. Tropé C, Kaern J, Vergote IB, et al. Are borderline tumors of the ovary overtreated both surgically and systemically? A review of four prospective randomized trials including 253 patients with borderline tumors. *Gynecol Oncol* 1993; 51(2): 236-243.

282. Nikrui N. Survey of clinical behavior of patients with borderline epithelial tumors of the ovary. *Gynecol Oncol* 1981;12(1): 107-119.

283. Kliman L, Rome RM, Fortune DW. Low malignant potential tumors of the ovary: A study of 76 cases. *Obstet Gynecol* 1986;68(3):338-344.

284. Kaern J, Tropé CG, Abeler VM. A retrospective study of 370 borderline tumors of the ovary treated at the Norwegian Radium Hospital from 1970 to 1982. A review of clinico-pathologic features and treatment modalities. *Cancer* 1993; 71(5):1810-1820.

285. Gershenson DM, Silva EG, Tortolero-Luna G, et al. Serous borderline tumors of the ovary with noninvasive peritoneal implants. *Cancer* 1998;83(10):2157-2163.

286. DiSaia P, Creasman W. Germ cell, stromal and other ovarian tumors. In: *Clinical Gynecologic Oncology,* 6th ed. St. Louis, MO: Mosby; 2002;351-378.

287. Scully RE. Tumors of the ovary and maldeveloped gonads, fallopian tubes and broad ligaments. In: Young RH, Clements PB (eds): *Atlas of Tumor Pathology,* third series. Washington, DC: Armed Forces Institute of Pathology; 1996;27.

288. Williams S, Blessing JA, Liao SY, et al. Adjuvant therapy of ovarian germ cell tumors with cisplatin, etoposide, and bleomycin: A trial of the Gynecologic Oncology Group. *J Clin Oncol* 1994;12(4):701-706.

289. Slayton RE, Park RC, Silverberg SG, et al. Vincristine, dactinomycin, and cyclophosphamide in the treatment of malignant germ cell tumors of the ovary. A Gynecologic Oncology Group Study (a final report). *Cancer* 1985;56(2): 243-248.

290. Gershenson DM, Morris M, Cangir A, et al. Treatment of malignant germ cell tumors of the ovary with bleomycin, etoposide, and cisplatin. *J Clin Oncol* 1990;8(4):715-720.

291. Williams SD, Blessing JA, Hatch KD, Homesley HD. Chemotherapy of advanced dysgerminoma: Trials of the Gynecologic Oncology Group. *J Clin Oncol* 1991;9(11):1950-1955.

292. Williams SD, Blessing JA, Moore DH, et al. Cisplatin, vinblastine, and bleomycin in advanced and recurrent ovarian germ-cell tumors. A trial of the Gynecologic Oncology Group. *Ann Intern Med* 1989;111(1):22-27.

293. Wu PC, Huang RL, Lang JH, et al. Treatment of malignant ovarian germ cell tumors with preservation of fertility: A report of 28 cases. *Gynecol Oncol* 1991;40(1):2-6.

294. Zanetta G, Bonazzi C, Cantu M, et al. Survival and reproductive function after treatment of malignant germ cell ovarian tumors. *J Clin Oncol* 2001 15;19(4):1015-1020.

295. Casey AC, Bhodauria S, Shapter A, et al. Dysgerminoma: The role of conservative surgery. *Gynecol Oncol* 1996;63(3): 352-357.

296. Ezzat A, Raja M, Bakri Y, et al. Malignant ovarian germ cell tumours—A survival and prognostic analysis. *Acta Oncol* 1999;38(4):455-460.

297. Gershenson DM. The obsolescence of second-look laparotomy in the management of malignant ovarian germ cell tumors. *Gynecol Oncol* 1994;52(3):283-285.

298. William SD, Blessing JA, DiSaia PJ, et al. Second look -laparotomy in ovarian germ cell tumors: The gynecologic oncology group experience. *Gynecol Oncol* 1994;52(3):287-291.

299. Culine S, Lhomme C, Michel G, et al. Is there a role for second-look laparotomy in the management of malignant germ cell tumors of the ovary? Experience at Institut Gustave Roussy. *J Surg Oncol* 1996;62(1):40-45.

300. Thomas GM, Dembo AJ, Hacker NF, et al. Current therapy for dysgerminoma of the ovary. *Obstet Gynecol* 1987;70(2): 268-275.

301. Berek J, Taylor P, McGuire W, et al. Oregovomab maintenance monoimmunotherapy does not improve outcomes in advanced ovarian cancer. *J Clin Oncol* 2009;27:418-425.

302. Bast RC, Iyer RB, Hu W, et al. A phase IIa study of a sequential regimen using azacitidine to reverse platinum resistance to carboplatin in patients with platinum resistant or refractory epithelial ovarian cancer. *J Clin Oncol* 2008; 26:3500.

303. Breidenbach M, Rein DT, Everts M, et al. Mesothelin-mediated targeting of adenoviral vectors for ovarian cancer gene therapy. *Gene Ther* 2005;12:187-193.

304. Nicholson S, Gooden CS, Hird V, et al. Radioimmunotherapy after chemotherapy compared to chemotherapy alone in the treatment of advanced ovarian cancer: A matched analysis. *Oncol Rep* 1998;5:223-226.

305. Fong PC, Boss DS, Carden CP, et al. AZD2281 (KU-0059436), a PARP (poly ADP-ribose polymerase) inhibitor with single agent anticancer activity in patients with BRCA defi cient ovarian cancer: Results from a phase I study. *J Clin Oncol* 2008;26:5510.

306. Fong PC, Boss DS, Yap TA, et al. Inhibition of poly(ADP-ribose) polymerase in tumors from *BRCA* mutation carriers. *N Engl J Med* 2009;361:123-134.

307. Merritt WM, Lin YG, Spannuth WA, et al. Effect of interleukin-8 gene silencing with liposome-encapsulated small interfering RNA on ovarian cancer cell growth. *J Natl Cancer Inst* 2008;100:359-372.

308. Collinson FJ, Hall GD, Perren TJ, Jayson GC. Development of antiangiogenic agents for ovarian cancer. *Expert Rev Anticancer Ther* 2008;8:21-32.

309. Burger RA, Sill MW, Monk BJ, et al. Phase II trial of bevacizumab in persistent or recurrent epithelial ovarian cancer or primary peritoneal cancer: A Gynecologic Oncology Group Study. *J Clin Oncol* 2007;25:5165-5171.

TUMORS OF THE UTERINE CORPUS

Grace K. Suh
Bryan T. Hennessy
Maurie Markman

■ EPITHELIAL UTERINE TUMORS 787

■ NONEPITHELIAL UTERINE TUMORS 811

■ EPITHELIAL UTERINE TUMORS

EPIDEMIOLOGY

Cancer of the lining of the uterine corpus, endometrial cancer (EC), is the most common gynecologic malignancy in the United States. Adenocarcinoma of the endometrium, the most common histologic subtype, ranks fourth in cancer prevalence after breast, lung, and colorectal. Endometrial adenocarcinoma will account for approximately 7500 deaths this year and is the eighth leading cause of death from malignancy in women (1).

Endometrial cancer is primarily a disease of postmenopausal women. Ninety percent of cases are diagnosed in women over the age of 50 with a median age of diagnoses at 61. About 20 to 25% of women diagnosed are premenopausal with fewer than 5% under the age of 40 (2).

RISK FACTORS

Both genotypic and phenotypic risk factors are noted in the development of EC. There are two types of EC as well as a hereditary of genetic variant. Type I tumors are the most common, accounting for about 75% of endometrial cancers, and are associated with chronic exposure to exogenous or endogenous estrogen. These tumors arise on a background of benign endometrial hyperplasia and progress to carcinomas, have minimal myometrial invasion, and usually have more favorable prognoses (3). Type II disease represents approximately 10 to 20% of cases and generally consists of high-grade tumors with myometrial invasion. These neoplasms are associated with less differentiated cell type and have worse prognosis than type I. Type II disease is not associated with hormone exposure. Finally, genetic disease can represent the remainder of up to 10% of cases with Lynch II syndrome or hereditary nonpolyposis colorectal cancer (HNPCC) being the most common. Endometrial cancer is the most common cancer associated with HNPCC with 40 to 60% lifetime risk of developing the disease (4) (Table 29-1).

Unopposed Estrogen

The association between chronic exposure to estrogen replacement therapy and EC is well-established, and both the duration and dose of estrogen affect the risk.

The relative risk of developing EC for women taking estrogen replacement therapy is two to six times the risk for control groups (5-7). This risk remains elevated for more than 5 years after the drug is discontinued. Adding progestins to estrogen replacement therapy has a protective effect and reduces the relative risk of EC to 0.8 (5). The duration of progestin use and its use over the course of the cycle also seem significant. Use of progestin for at least 10 days per cycle is associated with a relative risk of 1.07 per 5 years of use (6), whereas continuous use of progestin reduces that risk to 0.2 (7).

Tamoxifen

Tamoxifen, a selective estrogen receptor modulator, is used as chemoprevention of breast cancer and increase the risk of endometrial cancer by threefold. Tamoxifen acts by blocking the binding of estrogen to estrogen receptors but also has a weak agonist effect on the endometrium. Its estrogenic effects lead to a significant increase in the risk of developing endometrial cancer, with an overall increase in relative risk of 1.9 to 7.5 and an absolute annual risk of about 2 per 1000 patients (8-12).

A Swedish study evaluated the incidence of endometrial cancers among 4914 women with history of early invasive breast cancers with a median follow-up of 9 years. In this trial, women with invasive breast cancer were randomly allocated to receive either 2 years of adjuvant tamoxifen (40 mg daily) or no adjuvant

TABLE 29-1	CHARACTERISTIC FEATURES OF TYPES I AND II UTERINE CANCER	
Features	*Type I*	*Type II*
Estrogenic status–related	Estrogen-related	Not estrogen-related
Menstrual history	Anovulatory	No association
Fertility	Reduced or infertile	No association
Age at diagnosis	Younger, perimenopause	Late postmenopause
Ovarian or exogenous estrogen	Yes	No association
Hormone replacement therapy	Yes	No association
Endometrial status	Hyperplastic	Atrophic
Personal history		
Obesity	Often associated	No association
Diabetes mellitus	Often associated	No association
Duration of symptoms	Long	Short
Pathology		
Histology	Endometrioid, mucinous, villoglandular	Nonendometrioid: clear cell carcinoma or serous carcinoma
Staging and grading	Low stage, low grade	High grade, advanced stage
Clinical course and prognosis	Slow progressive, favorable prognosis	Aggressive behavior, unfavorable prognosis
Hormone receptor expression	High	Low

endocrine therapy. Secondary cancer incidence was obtained retrospectively. This study reported a nearly sixfold increase in endometrial cancers in the tamoxifen-treated group (12).

Subsequently, the National Surgical Adjuvant Breast and Bowel Project (NSABP) reported analysis on 2843 patients with node-negative, estrogen receptor–positive, invasive breast cancer randomly assigned to placebo or tamoxifen (20 mg/day) and on further 1220 tamoxifen-treated patients registered subsequently in NSABP B-14. The annual hazard rate through all follow-up was 0.2 per 1000 cases in the placebo group and 1.6 per 1000 in the tamoxifen-treated group. The relative risk of endometrial cancer for the tamoxifen-treated group was 7.5. The mean duration of treatment was 35 months, and 36% of endometrial cancers developed by 2 years following initiation of tamoxifen. Of note, however, the 5-year cumulative hazard ratio for death in the randomized tamoxifen group was 38% less than that in the placebo group, indicating an overall benefit from tamoxifen treatment in terms of breast cancer recurrence (9).

In light of the elevated risk of developing endometrial cancer, the benefit of adjuvant tamoxifen for early-stage breast cancer has been questioned. However, in women with estrogen receptor–positive breast cancer, adjuvant tamoxifen reduces the annual risk of recurrence by 39% and annual odds of death by 31% (13). Although tamoxifen may increase the risk of developing EC, its proven benefits in preventing or controlling recurrences of breast cancer and occurrence of cancer in the contralateral breast must be weighed against this risk, and patients must be counseled accordingly.

There is no formal guideline on screening women on tamoxifen for endometrial cancer. At MD Anderson, we educate patients about the signs and symptoms that would warrant further evaluation such as abnormal bleeding, spotting, or discharge. There have been cost-effectiveness analyses of screening asymptomatic, high-risk patients, including those on tamoxifen (14). However, we do not recommend the routine use of screening trans-vaginal ultrasonography, endometrial biopsy, or serum studies.

Obesity

Obesity is a well-established risk factor for development of endometrial cancer. Women who are obese have higher levels of endogenous estrogen because of the conversion of androstenedione into estrone and the aromatization of androgens to estradiol which occurs in the peripheral adipose tissue. In Western societies where obesity is more prevalent, the number of type I endometrial cancer cases attributed to excess body weight is increasing, and in different studies, obesity has been associated with a two- to fivefold increase in endometrial risk (15-17). Several studies have shown an increase in risk only among obese women with a BMI of ≥ 30 kg/m^2 (16).

Obesity increases the risk of endometrial cancer in both post- and premenopausal women. A study at the MD Anderson and elsewhere found that the majority of women diagnosed with endometrial cancer at a young age were obese (18,19). Although there is a strong association between obesity and endometrial cancer, preventative strategies are not currently recommended. A study conducted at MD Anderson found that endometrial cancer risk in obese women had to be 13 times greater than the general population risk before oral contraceptive pills were a cost-effective intervention (20).

Endometrial Hyperplasia

Women with histologic diagnoses of endometrial hyperplasia often present with postmenopausal bleeding or menometrorrhagia (Fig. 29-1 and 29-2). The risk factors associated with the development of endometrial hyperplasia, mainly obesity and unopposed estrogen, are similar to those associated with endometrial cancer (21). The World Health Organization defines endometrial hyperplasia based on two characteristics: (1) Simple or complex glandular/stromal architectural pattern. (2) The presence or absence of nuclear atypia. The presence of nuclear atypia correlates highest with the risk of developing malignancy. In this spectrum, those with simple hyperplasia without atypia are least likely to develop endometrial carcinoma, while women with complex hyperplasia with atypia are most likely to develop carcinoma. In a long-term follow-up study conducted by Kurman et al., endometrial carcinoma occurred in simple, complex, simple atypical, and complex atypical hyperplasia in 1, 3, 8, and 29% of cases, respectively (22). A report from one meta-analysis showing a wider range of risk of cancer progression based on four prospective follow-up studies is summarized in Table 29-2 (23).

Because of their resemblance to each other, distinguishing between endometrial hyperplasia and well-differentiated endometrioid adenocarcinoma can be challenging (23). A recent study by the Gynecologic Oncology Group (GOG-0167) addressed the reproducibility of classifying endometrial lesions based on the WHO classification. In this prospective study, there was only 38% concordance in cases of endometrial hyperplasia with atypia between the referring institution's

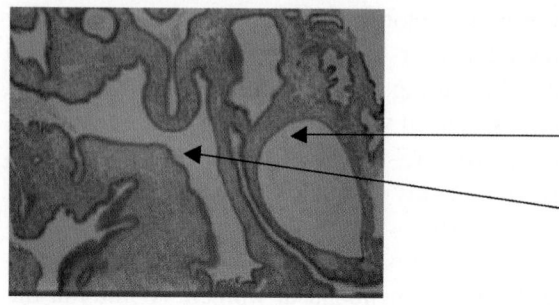

Increased glandular components with dilated lumen giving Swiss-cheese appearance

FIGURE 29-1. Simple cystic hyperplasia. The ratio of endometrial glands to stroma is increased and the glands are dilated, giving a Swiss-cheese appearance. The single-layer cuboidal or flattened epithelial lining of the glands shows no atypia.

pathologist and a majority of study panel consisting of three expert pathologists. The severity of the lesions was both underestimated and overestimated as the remaining specimens were classified as adenocarcinoma in 29% of cases, normal cycling endometrium in 7%, and nonatypical hyperplasia in 18%. Furthermore, between the three pathologists in the expert panel, unanimous agreement for any diagnosis was reached in only 40% of cases, demonstrating the variability and difficulty in classifying endometrial lesions. The authors site a number of factors that may have contributed to the variability, including small sample size and quality of specimen fixation (24).

DIAGNOSIS AND SCREENING

Screening

Except patients with HNPCC, there is insufficient evidence to support screening for endometrial cancer in the general population, even those with risk factors such as tamoxifen use, history of unopposed estrogen, obesity, diabetes, or hypertension. The American Cancer Society currently recommends that all women be informed about the risks and symptoms of endometrial cancer at menopause. Women should alert their physicians of any unexpected bleeding or spotting (25).

The optimal interval for screening members of women affected by HNPCC continues to be under debate. However, the value of screening this high-risk

population of women is well established. The American Cancer Society recommends yearly screening with endometrial biopsy beginning at age 35 for women who are known to carry HNPCC-associated mutations, those who have a family member known to carry this mutation, or women from families with an autosomal dominant predisposition to colon cancer in the absence of genetic testing for HNPCC (25).

In a recent Finnish study, the effect of screening was evaluated among 175 mutation carriers. The authors of this study compared transvaginal ultrasound to intrauterine biopsy as the method of detection and concluded that EC surveillance in HNPCC seems more effective with endometrial biopsies than with TVUS alone (26). A subsequent study evaluated the long-term effectiveness of surveillance over a 10-year follow-up period. For women, intrauterine biopsy and transvaginal ultrasonography were offered beginning at the age of 35 years. Surveillance of the 103 women at risk detected 19 cases (18%) of EC, with affected individuals having a median age of 49 years. Surveillance visits in this study were recommended at 2- to 3-year intervals (27).

Diagnosis

Dilation and Curettage

Until recently, the traditional means of diagnosing an endometrial lesion was fractional dilation and curettage, but this technique has largely been replaced by

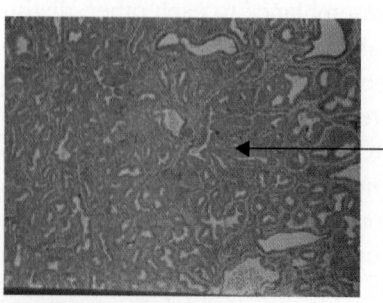

Proliferation of endometrial glands giving proportion of gland: stroma ratio >1, However, intervening stroma is still evidenced.

FIGURE 29-2. Adenomatous hyperplasia. Endometrial gland proliferation is out of proportion to the stromal component. However, the lack of morphologic atypia and the presence of intervening stroma between the glands distinguish adenomatous hyperplasia from atypical endometrial hyperplasia and endometrial cancer, respectively.

TABLE 29-2	RISK OF PROGRESSION FROM ENDOMETRIAL HYPERPLASIA TO ENDOMETRIAL CANCER		
Hyperplastic Type	*No. of Cases*	*Risk of Progression (%)*	*Mean Risk (%)*
Simple hyperplasia	164	0-10	4.3
Complex hyperplasia	193	3-22	16.1*
Simple hyperplasia with atypia	27	7.8	7.4*
Complex hyperplasia with atypia	151	29-100	47.0

*Complex hyperplasia architecture carries a higher risk of progressing to carcinoma than does atypical simple hyperplasia.

endometrial biopsy, which can be performed on an outpatient basis and under hysteroscopic guidance in difficult cases. Results from endometrial biopsy with a small-caliber Pipelle suction curette performed in the office correlate well with results from curettage specimens. However, biopsy methods involve random, "blind" selection of tissue for pathologic examination and thus may miss focal lesions. Hysteroscopy, on the other hand, has the potential benefit of increased sensitivity but carries additional expense as well as the risk of peritoneal dissemination of EC cells (28).

HISTOPATHOLOGY

Endometrioid Carcinoma

Endometrioid carcinoma contributes 75 to 80% of EC cases and is the most common subtype. There is a spectrum of differentiation from well differentiated to undifferentiated. Well-differentiated tumors are composed of glands resembling normal endometrial tissue (Fig. 29-3). In less differentiated tumors, glandular formations are less evident or are replaced with solid areas. The percentage of tumor consisting of these nonsquamous or nonmorular solid areas is the criterion for grading. Notably, the presence of nuclear atypia that does not correlate with the architectural features should lead to a one-step upgrade of the tumor.

Endometrioid Carcinoma With Squamous Differentiation

Generally 15 to 25% of endometrioid carcinomas have a squamous component. This subtype of tumor was previously called "adenoacanthoma" if the coexisting squamous portion was benign or "adenosquamous carcinoma" if both parts were malignant. The name "endometrioid carcinoma with squamous differentiation" is now recommended, because the degree of squamous

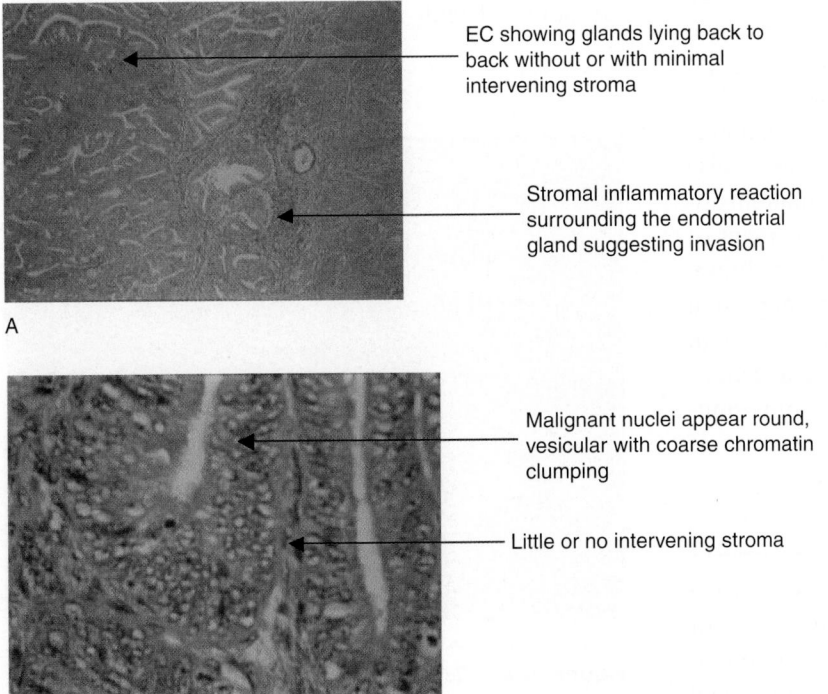

A

EC showing glands lying back to back without or with minimal intervening stroma

Stromal inflammatory reaction surrounding the endometrial gland suggesting invasion

Malignant nuclei appear round, vesicular with coarse chromatin clumping

Little or no intervening stroma

B

FIGURE 29-3. **A.** Endometrial cancer with superficial myometrial invasion. The stromal inflammatory reaction surrounding the endometrial gland can aid in the diagnosis in some equivocal cases. **B.** High-power magnification shows malignant nuclei in the endometrial glands.

differentiation generally reflects that of the glandular component, which in turn predicts the clinical behavior of the tumor.

Villoglandular Adenocarcinoma

Villoglandular adenocarcinoma is considered a well-differentiated variant of endometrioid carcinoma. The significance of being able to recognize this tumor is the ability to distinguish it from papillary serous carcinoma, which behaves more aggressively.

Secretory Carcinoma

A rare variant of endometrioid carcinoma, secretory carcinoma is more common among women in early menopause. Its appearance is characterized by the presence of well-differentiated glands with minimal nuclear atypia and prominent intracytoplasmic vacuoles that resemble normal secretory endometrium. These cytoplasmic vacuoles contain glycogen rather than mucin (as in mucinous tumors). It is also important to distinguish secretory carcinoma, which has a good prognosis, from the more aggressive clear cell carcinoma; the clue to the differential diagnoses is that secretory carcinoma has more uniform architectural and cytologic features, but clear cell carcinoma displays a histologic spectrum that can include clear cell, tubulocystic, papillary, or solid patterns with much more nuclear atypia.

Mucinous Carcinoma

Mucinous carcinomas constitute about 5% of ECs. The histologic features of mucinous carcinoma resemble those of mucinous tumors of the cervix or ovary. At least 50% of the tumor should consist of intracytoplasmic mucinous lesions for it to be considered a mucinous carcinoma. Both the site of tumor (uterine versus cervix) and its cellular origin (as determined by immunohistochemistry) may influence the surgical management of the disease. Histologic features indicative of an endometrial origin are the presence of a transition from normal or hyperplastic endometrial tissue to tumor, stromal foam cells, areas of squamous differentiation, and areas of typical endometrioid tumor. The presence of perinuclear vimentin on immunohistochemical staining is characteristic of EC but not of cervical cancer.

Papillary Serous Carcinoma

Papillary serous carcinomas are highly aggressive tumors that should be distinguished from other types of uterine carcinoma, particularly the histologically similar villoglandular type. Papillary serous carcinomas tend to occur in older women, usually present in advanced stages, and represent 1 to 5% of cases. Deep myometrial invasion, extensive lymphovascular space invasion, and extrauterine spread are common. Intraperitoneal involvement is often observed even when the primary lesion is localized. The histologic features of papillary serous carcinoma resemble those of ovarian or tubal carcinoma. Papillary fronds usually have broader cores than in villoglandular tumors. Cytologic atypia is so prominent that papillary serous carcinomas should always be graded as poorly-differentiated tumors.

Clear Cell Carcinoma

Another aggressive form of uterine carcinoma, clear cell carcinoma, represents 5 to 10% of EC cases and should always be considered a high-grade tumor. Clear cell carcinoma tends to occur in older women. Morphologically, it resembles clear cell carcinoma arising from other sites (eg, vagina, cervix, ovary), but clear cell carcinoma of the uterine corpus, unlike that of the vagina or cervix, is not associated with intrauterine exposure to diethylstilbestrol. The microscopic appearance varies and can include solid clear cell features, prominent glycogen content, and a glandular, tubulocystic, or papillary pattern. The cells have abundant clear or eosinophilic cytoplasm, sometimes containing periodic acid-Schiff-positive hyaline globules (Fig. 29-4). The nuclei show marked atypia with frequent mitotic figures. The characteristic "hobnail" appearance is seen as cells with scanty cytoplasm and nuclei protruding into the lumen of the gland. At least half of the clear cell carcinomas are admixed with uterine papillary serous carcinoma

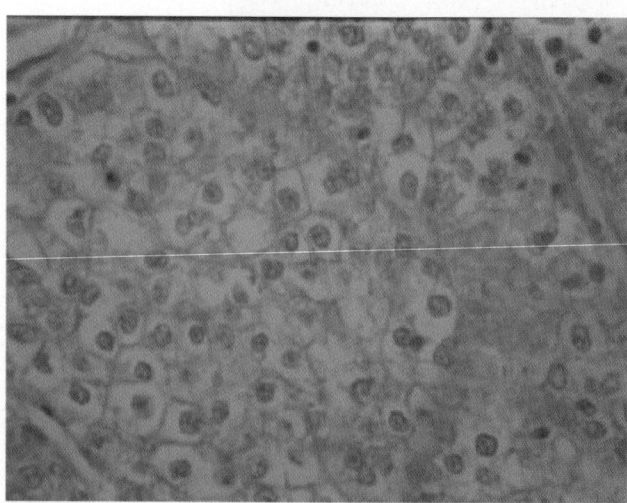

FIGURE 29-4. Clear cell carcinoma. A more aggressive type of endometrial cancer than the usual endometrioid carcinoma. The clear cytoplasmic content is glycogen rather than mucin.

(UPSC); this has contributed to ideas that the poor prognosis associated with clear cell carcinoma is due to the presence of UPSC.

Squamous Cell Carcinoma

Squamous cell carcinoma, another rare tumor of the endometrium, has a grave prognosis. Histologically, its uterine origin is confirmed by the absence of histologic connection to cervical squamous epithelium and the absence of existing cervical squamous cell carcinoma. Squamous cell carcinoma of the uterus often presents with cervical stenosis, chronic inflammation, and pyometra at diagnosis.

Mixed Cell Type

As the name implies, mixed cell ECs contain more than one type of tumor. The proportion of the minor component should exceed 10% for a tumor to be designated a mixed cell type.

SURGICAL METHODS

FIGO Staging

In 1988, the International Federation of Gynecology and Obstetrics (FIGO) committee established a surgical staging system for EC (FIGO1988) (Table 29-3A). Tumor stages based on this system have been shown to

TABLE 29-3A | THE 1988 FIGO STAGING SYSTEM

Stages	Characteristics
I	Tumor limited to uterus
IA	Confined to endometrium
IB	Invades ≤1/2 the myometrial depth*
IC	Invades >1/2 the myometrial depth*
II	Cervical extension
IIA	Involves endocervical gland only
IIB	Invades cervical stroma
III	Pelvic structures or intra-abdominal lymph node involvement
IIIA	Invades serosa or adnexa, or is peritoneal cytology–positive
IIIB	Vaginal metastasis
IIIC	Pelvic or para-aortic lymph node metastasis
IV	Other organ involvement
IVA	Invades bladder or rectal mucosa
IVB	Distant metastasis including inguinal lymph node involvement

*Ideally, width (depth) of myometrial invasion should be measured and recorded with the depth (thickness) of the entire myometrium.

TABLE 29-3B | 2009 FIGO SURGICAL STAGING FOR ENDOMETRIAL CARCINOMA

Stage I*	Tumor confined to the corpus uteri
Stage IA*	No or less than half myometrial invasion
Stage IB*	Invasion equal to or more than one-half the myometrium
Stage II*	Tumor invades cervical stroma, but does not extend beyond the uterus†
Stage III*	Local and/or parametrial involvement‡
Stage IIIA*	Tumor invades serosa and/or adnexae‡
Stage IIIB*	Vaginal and/or parametrial involvement‡
Stage IIIC*	Metastases to pelvic and/or para-aortic lymph nodes‡
Stage IIIC1*	Positive pelvic nodes
Stage IIIC2	Positive para-aortic lymph nodes with or without positive pelvic lymph nodes
Stage IV*	Tumor invasion of bladder and/or bowel mucosa, and/or distant metastases
Stage IVA*	Tumor invasion of bladder and/or bowel mucosa
Stage IVB*	Distant metastases, including intra-abdominal metastases and/or inguinal lymph nodes

FIGO, International Federation of Gynecology and Obstetrics.
*Either G1, G2, or G3.
†Endocervical glandular involvement only should be considered as stage I and no longer as stage II.
‡Positive cytology has to be reported separately without changing stage.
(Reprinted from the International Journal of Gynecology & Obstetrics, Pellecino S.; Vol. 105, Issue 2. Revised FIGO Staging for Carcinoma of the Vulva, Cervix, and Endometrium, Copyright 2009, with permission from Elsevier.)

correlate with survival (Table 29-4 and Fig. 29-5) (29). In 2009, this staging system was updated to incorporate four major changes (FIGO 2009, Table 29-3B): (1) Previous stages IA and IB have been combined as stage IA in the new staging system. Stage IB now represents invasion at or into the outer one-half of the myometrium. Stage 1C has been removed. (2) Involvement of the endocervical gland of the cervix is considered stage IA, and stage II no longer has subgroups A and B. (3) Previous stage IIIC has been subdivided into IIIC1 (positive pelvic nodes) and IIIC2 (indicates positive para-aortic lymph nodes with or without positive pelvic nodes). (4) Peritoneal cytology is no longer a factor in FIGO staging.

The 2009 FIGO staging system reflects outcome analysis of over 43,000 EC patients who have been surgically staged according to the 1988 FIGO staging system. Hence, the substages more accurately reflect their respective prognoses. However, most of the landmark studies and treatment recommendations, including those of the National Comprehensive Cancer Network, are based on FIGO 1988. Hence, we will primarily use

TABLE 29-4 | **SURVIVAL BY FIGO SURGICAL STAGE IN 5694 CASES OF CARCINOMA OF THE CORPUS UTERI IN 1999-2001**

			OVERALL SURVIVAL RATE (%) AT:					
Stage	No. of Patients	Mean Age (Years)	1 Year	2 Years	3 Years	4 Years	5 Years	Hazards Ratio* (95% CI)
Ia	1054	59.0	98.2	96.6	95.3	93.7	90.8	Reference
Ib	2833	62.1	98.7	96.6	94.6	92.5	91.1	0.9 (0.7-1.2)
Ic	1426	62.2	97.5	93.7	89.7	87.2	85.4	1.4 (1.1-1.8)
IIa	430	63.8	95.2	93.2	89.0	86.0	83.3	1.8 (1.3-2.5)
IIb	543	63.8	93.5	85.3	80.3	76.7	74.2	2.8 (2.1-3.7)
IIIa	612	63.0	89.0	79.9	73.3	69.4	66.2	4.4 (3.4-5.8)
IIIb	80	67.0	73.5	61.6	56.7	52.7	49.9	7.3(4.8-10.9)
IIIc	356	61.6	89.9	74.5	66.3	61.5	57.3	6.2 (4.7-8.2)
IVa	49	64.5	63.4	46.7	34.4	29.1	25.5	14.0 (9.2-21.2)
IVb	206	63.9	59.5	37.0	29.0	22.3	20.1	16.1 (12.2-21.3)

*Hazards ratio and 95% confidence interval (CI) obtained from a Cox model adjusted for age and country.
(Reprinted from the International Journal of Gynecology & Obstetrics, Creasman WT, Odicino F, Maisonneuve P, et al. Vol. 95, Suppl[1]. Carcinoma of the Corpus Uteri, Copyright 2006, with permission from Elsevier.)

this older staging system in this chapter. FIGO 2009 is beginning to be adopted and utilized in clinical trials and other studies; therefore, we expect the new staging system to be incorporated into future management recommendations.

Surgical Staging

Surgical staging should be applied in all stages (stages I-IV) of uterine cancer provided that the patient is medically stable to undergo surgery. Although the role of cytoreductive surgery for stage IV patients has been questioned (30), the current recommendation is

for all patients, even those with stage IV disease, to undergo surgical debulking (31,32).

The basic procedures to be used in surgical staging are outlined in Table 29-5; however, the details can vary depending on the patient's condition, institutional practices, and the surgeon's preference. At MD Anderson, we pay special attention to tumor size, location, and depth of invasion; cervical and extrauterine involvement should be assessed by opening and inspecting the uterus in the operating room. Surgical pathologists can aid in describing these features by gross or frozen section analysis (Fig. 29-6).

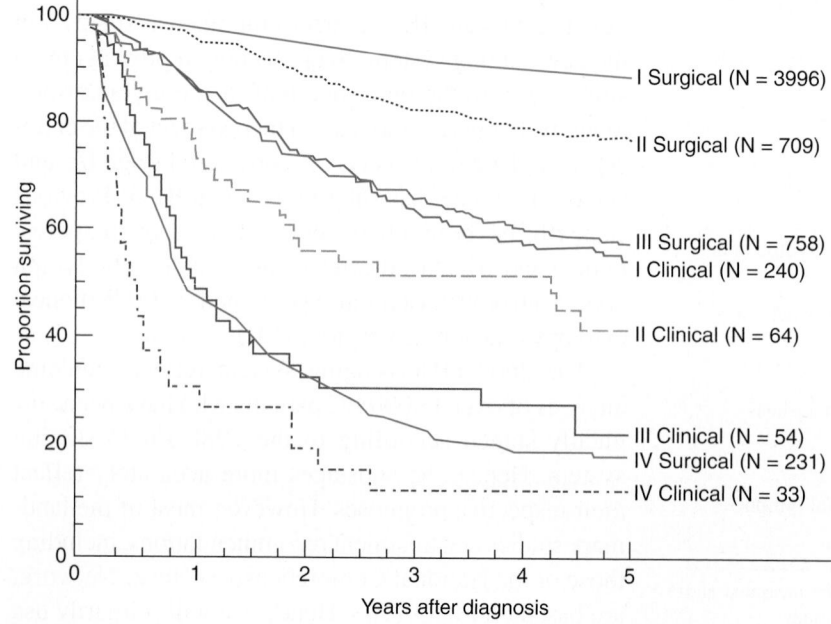

FIGURE 29-5. Five-year survival rates for 6085 patients with carcinoma of the corpus uteri according to mode of staging (clinical versus surgical). *(Reproduced, with permission, from Creasman WT, Odicino F, Maisonneuve P, et al. Carcinoma of the corpus uteri. FIGO 6th Annual Report on the Results of Treatment in Gynecological Cancer. Int J Gynaecol Obstet 2006;95 Suppl 1:S105-43.)*

TABLE 29-5	STEPS TO BE TAKEN TO OBTAIN CORRECT SURGICAL STAGING OF ENDOMETRIAL CANCER ACCORDING TO THE FIGO SYSTEM
Steps	*Remarks*
Adequate abdominal incision	Vertical incision is preferred as it yields better exposure and access to the operative field than transverse incision
Abdominal and pelvic exploration	To evaluate any extrauterine spread, biopsy area suspicious for tumor
Abdominal total hysterectomy and bilateral salpingo-oophorectomy	Inspect for uterine serosal involvement, tumor characteristics, and extension (see details given in the text)
Pelvic and para-aortic lymph node sampling	Details given in the text
Omental biopsy or infracolic omentectomy	Required in cases suspected of or having histologic evidence of extrauterine spread, such as papillary serous carcinoma, malignant mixed müllerian tumor, squamous cell carcinoma
Appendectomy	Optional

The involvement of infiltrative lesions, particularly the depth of invasion, may well be more extensive than is evident at gross examination; thus gross findings should not be considered definitive in evaluating the depth of myometrial involvement. Several studies have shown the accuracy of gross inspection (as compared with histopathologic examination) to range from 85 to 91% (33-36), a range similar to that of frozen section analysis (87-95%) (33,37,38).

Several preoperative histologic findings and intraoperative pathologic findings correlate with an increased risk of nodal involvement. Specific indications for retroperitoneal node sampling are as follows: grade 3 endometrioid tumor; aggressive tumors such as clear cell, serous, or squamous carcinoma; invasion of more than half of the myometrium; extension to the cervical isthmus; tumor size >2 cm; and the presence of extrauterine disease (39,40). The para-aortic nodes should be sampled when pelvic nodes are grossly involved or when macroscopic adnexal disease or deep myometrial invasion is evident. However, in about one-third of cases, para-aortic nodes can be involved even in the absence of pelvic node disease (40), so the judgment as to whether to remove the para-arotic nodes should be based on other risk factors as well.

In the process of lymph node resection, mere palpation of the fatty tissue of node-bearing areas is inadequate for the evaluation of node status, because only about half of metastatic nodes are enlarged (41) and fewer than 30% can be identified as abnormal on palpation (40,42). Aside from its value in predicting prognosis, adequate lymph node sampling can improve survival independently of tumor grade or depth of invasion or use of postoperative adjuvant radiation therapy (43). Thus, some clinicians advocate extensive node sampling or lymphadenectomy for surgical staging in EC (44).

Laparoscopic Methods

Since the early 1990s, the Gynecologic Oncology Group (GOG) has been evaluating minimally invasive surgical approaches to staging women with endometrial cancer. Numerous studies have compared laparoscopy with laparotomy with respect to surgical complications, perioperative morbidity, length of hospital stay, the incidence of subcutaneous metastases, and patients' quality of life

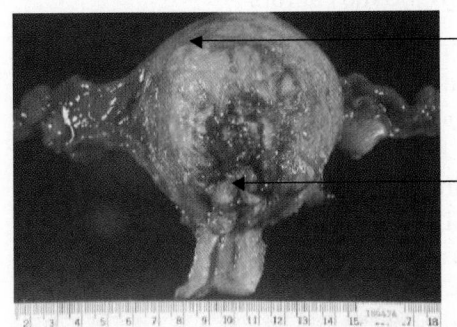

A. Depth of myometrial invasion should be carefully evaluated, more than half in this case

B. Tumor filled up uterine cavity and invaded down to lower uterine segment

FIGURE 29-6. A uterus and bilateral adnexae showing endometrial cancer filling the endometrial cavity, with deep invasion of the myometrium near the uterine serosa at the right cornual area and extension to the lower uterine segment. The ovaries are usually removed with the uterus because they are the main estrogen-producing organs as well as being a possible site of metastasis.

(QOL) and have attempted to define the indications where laparoscopic methods would be most appropriate. Although laparoscopic surgery takes longer to perform, it is associated with fewer intra- and postoperative complications than laparotomy. Laparoscopic surgery requires less pain medication and shorter hospital stays. Lymphadenectomy can be performed safely by laparoscopy and yields adequate numbers of nodes (45,46). Several long-term follow-ups have shown no significant differences in recurrence or disease-free survival rates between patients treated by laparoscopy and those treated by traditional laparotomy (47,48). A complication specific to the laparoscopic procedure has been recurrent at the portal site owing to dissemination of tumor cells (49,50).

In two recent reports by the GOG, laparoscopic surgical methods were compared to conventional laparotomy. The GOG LAP-2 study is the largest randomized trial ever performed in endometrial cancer. In this phase III prospective, multi-institutional, randomized study, 2616 patients with stage I to IIA uterine cancer were assigned to laparoscopy (N = 1696) or laparotomy (N = 920). Study endpoints were morbidity and mortality at 6 weeks, length of hospitalization, failure to complete laparoscopy, site of recurrence, and recurrence-free survival. Consistent with previous studies, laparoscopy required longer operative time but led to fewer postoperative adverse events and shorter hospitalization. The rate of intraoperative complications was similar. One unexpected outcome was that as many as 26% of patients in the laparoscopy arm were converted to laparotomy. Laparoscopic failure was associated with increasing age and body mass index (51).

In a companion report, patients undergoing surgical staging via laparoscopy versus laparotomy were assessed with QOL measures. The study's objective was to compare the QOL of patients with endometrial cancer undergoing surgical staging via laparoscopy versus laparotomy. Although patients in the laparoscopy arm had overall better QOL measures at 6 weeks postsurgery, except for better body image in the laparoscopy arm, no difference was detected between the two arms at 6 months (52).

The decision to perform open or minimally invasive surgery depends on patient preference, the skill and experience of the surgeon, the availability of the equipment, the size of the uterus, the parity of the patient, and the patients' medical condition.

PROGNOSTIC FACTORS

Seventy-five to 80% of patients with EC present with postmenopausal vaginal bleeding. Because symptoms

TABLE 29-6	PROGNOSTIC FACTORS IN ENDOMETRIAL CANCER	
Uterine Factors	*Extrauterine Factors*	*Clinical and Genetic Factors*
Histologic subtype	Lymph node metastasis	Age
Tumor grade	Peritoneal fluid cytologic findings	Hormone receptor status
Lymphovascular space invasion	Histologic cell type	Ploidy
Myometrial invasion		Microsatellite instability
Cervical extension		Oncogenic influence
Adnexal metastasis		

occur at early stages, for most patients with EC, prognosis is favorable with 5-year survival above 70 to 90%. However, despite no change in the incidence of endometrial cancer, there has been an increase in mortality over the past two decades. A study published in 2008 suggests that this increase may be attributed to an increased rate of advanced-stage cancers and high-risk histologies (53). Thus, it is important to identify high-risk patients and tailor treatment based on various prognostic factors, including clinical, pathologic, and genetic characteristics (Table 29-6).

Endometrial cancer is a surgically staged disease. However, the role of pelvic and para-aortic lymphadenectomy in determining prognosis has not been demonstrated in a randomized trial. Several landmark studies in the 1980s identified inadequacies of clinical staging, and based on these studies, FIGO incorporated many of the prognostic factors into the current staging process (39,40,54). Identifying additional markers for prognosis remains an active area of research.

Uterine Prognostic Factors

Prognostic factors can be broadly grouped into uterine, extrauterine, and other clinical and genetic features. A recent report concluded that high-risk uterine factors such as grade 3 tumor, deep myometrial invasion, and cervical extension may be more significant determinants of survival in endometrial cancer than extrauterine features such as pelvic-node status. At MD Anderson, we consider these factors in addition to surgical stage in determining treatment (55).

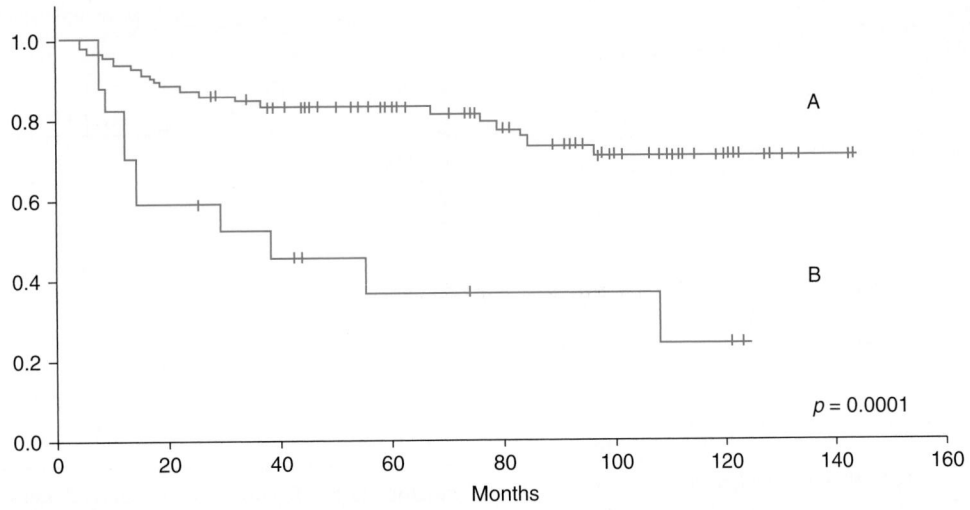

FIGURE 29-7. Tumor histology and survival. **A.** Estimated overall survival rate for patients with adenocarcinoma, including typical adenoacanthoma and adenosquamous carcinoma, was approximately 80%. **B.** Overall survival for those with other histologic types, including papillary serous and clear cell carcinoma, was about 35%. *(Reproduced, with permission, from Steiner E, Eicher O, Sagemuller J, et al. Multivariate independent prognostic factors in endometrial carcinoma: a clinicopathologic study in 181 patients: 10 years experience at the Department of Obstetrics and Gynecology of the Mainz University. Int J Gynecol Cancer 2003;13:197-203.)*

Histologic Subtype

Papillary serous carcinoma, clear cell carcinoma, and squamous cell carcinoma are associated with worse prognosis than endometrioid carcinoma; these subtypes should always be considered high-grade tumors (Fig. 29-7).

Tumor Grade

Tumor grade correlates well with myometrial invasion, pelvic and para-aortic node involvement, and recurrence (39,40) (Table 29-7, Fig. 29-8).

The current FIGO guidelines recommend that histologic grade be determined in terms of both architectural pattern (proportion of tumor with glandular arrangement) and nuclear features (pleomorphism and size of the nucleoli). In adenocarcinoma, the architectural grade is defined by the proportion of solid area; nuclear atypia

that is inappropriate for architectural grade raises the grade by one point. Adenocarcinomas with squamous differentiation are graded according to the nuclear grade of the glandular component. In serous adenocarcinomas, clear cell adenocarcinomas, and squamous cell carcinomas, nuclear grading takes precedence.

Some authors have suggested that architectural arrangement is superior to nuclear grade for predicting survival because of the tediousness and lack of reproducibility of nuclear grading (56). Subdivision of architectural grade based on the extent of nuclear atypia does not improve predictability. Because grading based on nuclear pleomorphism does not provide better prognostic information than that resulting from architectural grading, Zaino et al., from the GOG, do not advocate use of nuclear grading in routine surgical pathology practice (56). Recently, some authors proposed using a two-tier instead of a three-tier nuclear grading system

TABLE 29-7	PATHOLOGIC FEATURES OF ENDOMETRIAL CARCINOMA GRADES AND THEIR ASSOCIATION WITH DEPTH OF MYOMETRIAL INVASION				
		PERCENT OF PATIENTS WITH EACH DEPTH OF MYOMETRIUM INVASION			
Grade	*Pathologic Features*	*Endometrial Only*	*Superficial*	*Middle*	*Deep*
1	5% or less of nonsquamous solid area	24	53	12	10
2	6-50% of nonsquamous solid area	11	45	24	20
3	>50% of nonsquamous solid area	7	35	16	42

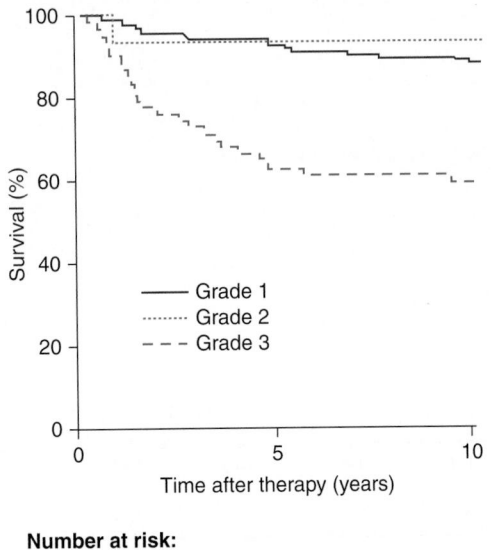

Number at risk:

Grade 1:	164	132	88
Grade 2:	25	20	12
Grade 3:	64	37	22

FIGURE 29-8. Tumor grade and survival in endometrial cancer. Use of the two-tiered grading system is favored because of less interobserver variability and similar outcome for patients with grade 1 or 2 tumors. (N = 243). *(Reproduced, with permission, from Scholten AN, Creutzberg CL, Noordijk EM, Smit VT. Long-term outcome in endometrial carcinoma favors a two- instead of a three-tiered grading system. Int J Radiat Oncol Biol Phys 2002; 52:1067-74.)*

for EC owing to lower interobserver variability and better correlation with long-term clinical outcome for the two-tier system (57,58) (see Fig. 29-8).

Lymphovascular Space Invasion

Lymphovascular space invasion, an independent risk factor for recurrence, is present in about 15% of EC cases (59-62). Multivariate analyses have shown angioinvasion, depth of myometrial invasion, and DNA ploidy to be associated with survival in EC regardless of disease stage. Angioinvasion, independently of tumor grade or depth of myometrial invasion, is also associated with risk of pelvic and para-aortic node involvement and thus should lead to surgical nodal assessment or empiric radiation in patients with unstaged disease (40,63).

Myometrial Invasion

The depth of myometrial invasion is associated with degree of tumor differentiation, angioinvasion, lymph node involvement, extrauterine spread, recurrence, and overall survival (Fig. 29-9).

Whether the depth of invasion should be judged in terms of thirds or halves of the total myometrial depth has been controversial. In the 1988 FIGO staging

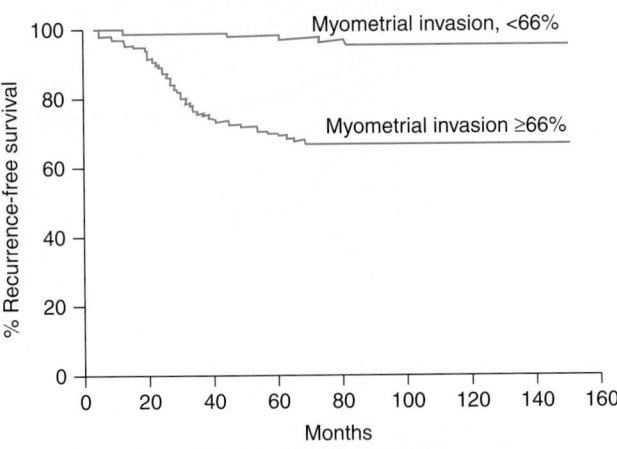

FIGURE 29-9. Recurrence-free survival rates for 282 patients with stage I endometrial cancer were significantly reduced when the depth of myometrial invasion exceeded two-thirds of the total thickness of the myometrium (p < .001). *(Reproduced, with permission, from Mariani A, Webb MJ, Keeney GL, et al. Surgical stage I endometrial cancer: predictors of distant failure and death. Gynecol Oncol 2002;87:274-80.)*

system, invasion to less than half the depth of the myometrium is considered stage IB disease and invasion to more than half is considered stage IC; however, much of the data on prognostic factors have grouped myometrial invasion by thirds rather than by halves (64,65). A report by Alektiar et al. involving 251 patients with stage IB EC revealed no significant differences in locoregional control, disease-free survival, and overall survival rates between patients with tumor invading more than one-third but less than one-half the myometrial depth and those with tumor invading less than half the myometrial depth (66). These findings seem to support the FIGO staging system. Other authors have proposed that neither the depth of myometrial invasion nor the ratio of tumor thickness to myometrium is as important as the margin between the tumor and the uterine serosa (65,67). Invasion of adenocarcinoma in areas of preexisting adenomyosis is another topic of interest (68,69). Patients with EC in which myometrial involvement is limited to areas of adenomyosis have better 5-year survival rates than those with truly invading EC at similar depth. Some histologic features that distinguish these two conditions are listed in Table 29-8.

Cervical Stromal Invasion

Tumors that involve the cervix have a worse prognosis than those limited to the fundus, as such tumors are associated with increased risk of extrauterine disease, lymph node involvement, and recurrence (40,65,70) (Fig. 29-10).

TABLE 29-8	HISTOLOGIC FEATURES DISTINGUISHING TRUE MYOMETRIAL INVASION FROM MYOMETRIAL INVOLVEMENT BY ADENOMYOSIS	
Tumor Involvement in Adenomyosis	***Tumor Invasion Into Myometrium***
Lesion has distinct border	Lesion has irregular or shaggy outline
Residual benign gland or basalis-type stroma	Minimal or absent normal endometrial tissue
Tissue commonly surrounded by myofibroblastic stroma	Malignant tissue surrounded by desmoplastic stroma
Associated with other areas of adenomyosis	No adenomyosis

Cervical stromal invasion confers a poor prognosis in EC and should be distinguished from involvement of the lower uterine segment, which occurs in up to 50% of cases of stage I EC (71). Involvement of the lower segment has been considered important in that the risk of recurrence would be greater if adjuvant radiation therapy were not given (72). However, multivariate analyses have shown that lower uterine involvement does not independently affect survival or recurrence in the absence of other accompanying risk factors (71).

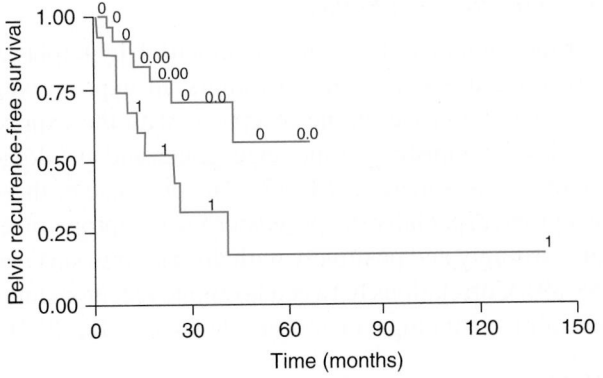

FIGURE 29-10. Correlation of cervical involvement and pelvic recurrence in endometrial cancer. The 3-year actuarial pelvic recurrence rate of patients with cervical involvement (1) was 67%, as compared with 33% in patients without cervical involvement (0) (*p* = .01) (N = 43). (*Reproduced, with permission, from Mundt AJ, McBride R, Rotmensch J, et al. Significant pelvic recurrence in high-risk pathologic stage I-IV endometrial carcinoma patients after adjuvant chemotherapy alone: implications for adjuvant radiation therapy. Int J Radiat Oncol Biol Phys 2001;50:1145-53.*)

Uterine Size

Uterine size is not considered an independent prognostic factor.

Extrauterine Prognostic Factors

Adnexal Metastasis

Adnexal metastasis correlates strongly with metastatic involvement of pelvic and para-aortic nodes; in one study, 32% of patients with adnexal involvement had positive pelvic nodes, as compared with 8% of those without adnexal disease (40). However, the alternative possibility of simultaneous ovarian and endometrial primaries must be ruled out as the surgical management and prognosis is vastly different.

Lymph Node Metastasis

Up to 11% of patients with clinical stage I or II disease have lymph node involvement (40). The risk of para-aortic node involvement increases if the pelvic nodes are positive for tumor. A recent multivariate analysis found that lymph node metastasis was not an important independent prognostic factor, but that it correlated with the depth of myometrial invasion, which significantly influences survival (73). Aside from depth of myometrial invasion, the presence of tumor metastases to lymph nodes is also associated with other risk factors (Table 29-9). Para-aortic spread may occur via tubo-ovarian vessels. Among these patients (25-30%), para-aortic nodal involvement in the absence of significant myometrial invasion does not portend worse prognosis.

Peritoneal Fluid Cytology

Positive findings on peritoneal cytology are often associated with other unfavorable prognostic factors, such as deep myometrial invasion, cervical extension, and extrauterine spread. UPSCs in particular demonstrate a high rate of positive washings. Even in clinical stage I disease that is confined to the uterus, cytologic findings have been positive in as many as 16 to 17% of cases (74,75). Recurrence rates in this circumstance have been high, especially in combination with high-grade tumors or papillary serous cell type (74,76). However, others have found no significant relationship between positive peritoneal cytology (in the absence of other factors associated with poor prognosis) and recurrence, disease-free survival, or 5-year survival rates (75,77-79). In at least two studies, the 5-year survival rates for patients with cytologically positive disease but no other risk factors have been higher than 90% (75) (Fig. 29-11).

The current FIGO staging system does not incorporate peritoneal washings, as the evidence for its prognostic value is weak.

TABLE 29-9	ASSOCIATION OF LYMPH NODE METASTASIS WITH OTHER PROGNOSTIC FACTORS IN ENDOMETRIAL CARCINOMA	
Risk Factors	Percent of Patients With Positive Pelvic Nodes	Percent of Patients With Positive Para-aortic Nodes
Histology		
Endometrioid carcinoma	9	5
Others	9	18
Tumor grade		
Grade 1	3	2
Grade 2	9	5
Grade 3	18	11
Depth of myometrial invasion		
None	1	1
Superficial	5	3
Middle	6	1
Deep	25	17
Tumor site		
Fundus	8	4
Isthmus or cervix	16	14
Lymphovascular space invasion		
Absent	7	9
Present	27	19
Peritoneal cytologic findings		
Negative	7	4
Positive	25	19
Extrauterine metastasis		
Absent	7	4
Present	51	23

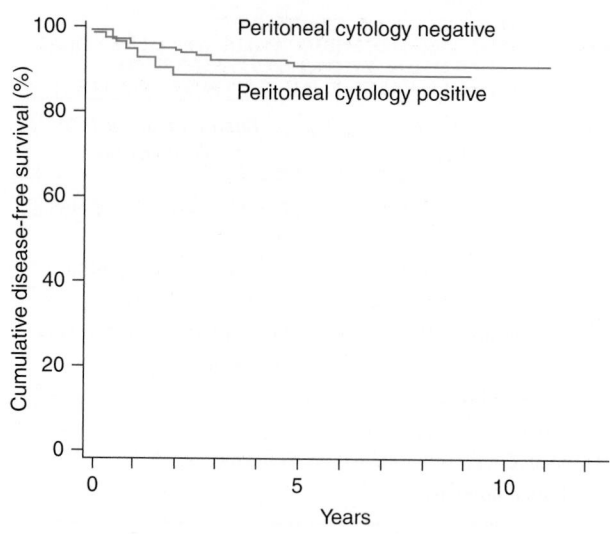

FIGURE 29-11. Five-year survival rates for patients with endometrial cancer confined to the uterus with positive findings on peritoneal cytology (91%) were not different from those with cytonegative findings (95%) (N = 280). *(Reproduced, with permission, from Kasamatsu T, Onda T, Katsumata N, et al. Prognostic significance of positive peritoneal cytology in endometrial carcinoma confined to the uterus. Br J Cancer 2003;88:245-50.)*

higher-grade (grade 3) disease, and advanced-stage disease compared to those <45 years old. Evaluation of patients with endometrioid tumors revealed a similar pattern of deeper myometrial invasion and higher tumor grade as age increased (85). Other studies have shown that the risks of locoregional relapse and death among patients older than 60 years were twice as high as the risks among those aged 60 years or younger (80,81).

Hormone Receptor Status

Normal endometrial tissue, endometrial hyperplasia, and low-grade endometrioid tumors all express both estrogen and progesterone receptors, with the expression level diminishing as the stage, grade, and histologic aggressiveness increase (86,87). The presence of these receptors, especially the progesterone receptor, correlates strongly and positively with disease-free survival (88,89). Correlations between hormone receptor status and clinicopathologic factors are shown in Table 29-10.

Ploidy

DNA ploidy in endometrial tumors is associated with the degree of differentiation and the clinical course of disease. Tumors that are less differentiated tend to have higher proportions of aneuploid cells. Tumor ploidy and proliferative index have also been linked to other prognostic factors, such as extrauterine spread and recurrence (90-92).

Other Clinical and Genetic Prognostic Factors

Age

Generally studies have shown outcomes for women with EC are more favorable among younger patients (80-84). There is higher incidence of deep myometrial invasion and high-grade tumors among older patients (84). For instance, a recent retrospective report showed that patients <45 years old were statistically more likely to have endometrioid histology, grade I tumors, and stage IA disease while women over age 65 were significantly more likely to have papillary serous histology, grade 3 tumors, and stage IC. A subset analysis of patients >75 years of age showed an increase in the percentage of patients with aggressive papillary serous histology,

TABLE 29-10	ASSOCIATIONS BETWEEN CYTOPLASMIC HORMONE RECEPTOR STATUS AND CLINICOPATHOLOGIC FACTORS			
	PERCENT ESTROGEN RECEPTOR-POSITIVE		PERCENT PROGESTERONE RECEPTOR-POSITIVE	
Clinicopathologic Characteristics	*Liao Study*	*Creasman Study*	*Liao Study*	*Creasman Study*
Clinical stage				
I	94	72 IA, 71 IB	92	72 IA, 61 IB
II	72	60	72	72
III/IV	50	–	44	–
Histologic cell type				
Adenocarcinoma	81	75	79	76
Adenoacanthoma	78	71	86	86
Adenosquamous	50	71	33	78
Papillary serous	–	53	–	27
Clear cell	–	60	–	29
Histologic grade				
1	94	82	92	82
2	72	72	72	60
3	50	46	44	59
Menopausal status				
Premenopausal	86	–	86	–
Postmenopausal	77	–	75	–

Microsatellite Instability

Microsatellite instability, previously known as replication error repair, has been found in 9 to 45% of cases of EC (93-95). Its presence correlates well with atypical hyperplasia associated with cancer but not with hyperplasia in the absence of cancer (95). Sherman postulated that microsatellite instability might be acquired during the process of malignant transformation (96).

Tumor Oncogenes

Several oncogene mutations have been reported to be associated with EC (97). Mutations in *ras* (98,99) have been found in 10 to 46% of ECs. Although *ras* mutations can be present in hyperplasia, more often the mutations are associated with degree of atypical hyperplasia and cancer (96). With regard to *PTEN* (100,101), because most ECs contain clusters of *PTEN*-negative glands, detection of individual *PTEN*-negative glands has been proposed as an early sign of endometrial carcinogenesis (100). *PTEN*-negative glands have been found in 40 to 83% of endometrioid carcinomas (96,100), and up to 86% coexist with microsatellite instability. Mutations in *p53* have been found in approximately 20% of ECs (90). Most endometrioid carcinomas that harbor *p53* mutations are large, high-grade tumors with dedifferentiation (96).

In conclusion, these prognostic factors correlate with clinical course of disease, recurrence, and risk of death. However, the relative importance of each factor is not always clear because of interrelations and interdependence among them. Results of a multivariate analysis by Zaino and colleagues of factors affecting survival in stages I and II EC are summarized in Table 29-11 (101).

THERAPEUTIC OPTIONS FOLLOWING SURGICAL STAGING

Surgery

At MD Anderson, we stratify patients according to features of the disease and prognostic factors described above. The risk group helps guide the choice adjuvant treatment. The consideration of grade is especially relevant in stage I disease where the depth of myometrial invasion along with tumor grade determines risk category and recommendation for adjuvant treatment (Table 29-12).

There is lack of evidence on the benefit of adjuvant therapy in patients with uterine-confined disease. Grade 1 or 2 tumors without demonstrable myometrial invasion (stages IA and IB, FIGO 1988) are associated with excellent prognosis with 5-year survival

| TABLE | ASSOCIATIONS BETWEEN PATHOLOGIC PROGNOSTIC FACTORS AND RELATIVE |
| 29-11 | RISK AND SURVIVAL RATES |

| | | RELATIVE RISK OF SURGICAL STAGE I–II TUMORS[†] | | |
Prognostic Factors	*5-Year Survival Rate (%)*	*Grade 1*	*Grade 2*	*Grade 3*
Histologic cell type				
Clear cell	67.7	5.1	3.5	2.5
Mucinous	100	—	—	—
Serous	55	2.2	3.1	4.4
Endometrioid	82.1	1.0	1.3	1.8
Endometrioid with squamous differentiation	89.4	1.2	1.0	0.8
Villoglandular	91.2	0.01	0.5*	41.9*
Myometrial invasion				
Endometrial only	92.9		1	
Superficial	87.6		0.5	
Middle	84.5		3.3	
Deep	62.6		4.6	
Lymphovascular space invasion				
No	85.8		—	
Yes	60.9		1.4	
Grade				
1	91.1		—	
2	82		—	
3	66.4		—	
Peritoneal washings				
Negative	85.3		—	
Positive	56		—	

*p < .05.
[†]Typical endometrioid grade 1 as the reference for all cell types.

approaching 90% and are at low risk of recurrence after surgery. Other factors such as invasion of the myometrium, cervix, or lower uterus, positive findings on peritoneal cytology, and extrauterine extension indicate more advanced disease and a higher risk of recurrence.

In a series of studies by Mariani et al., deep myometrial invasion was the strongest predictor of relapse in patients with surgical stage 1 endometrial cancer (64,102-104).

Radiation Therapy

Radiation Therapy in the Adjuvant Setting

At MD Anderson, we tailor postoperative adjuvant therapy based on the results of the surgical staging procedure. Depending on the perceived risks of recurrence in the vagina or in the regional lymph nodes, radiation may be delivered using intravaginal brachytherapy alone, external beam radiation alone, or a combination of the two. Intravaginal radiation may be accomplished as an inpatient using low dose-rate techniques or, more commonly, as an outpatient using fractionated high dose-rate intravaginal brachytherapy. External

TABLE	RISK OF ENDOMETRIAL CANCER
29-12	RECURRENCE FOR STAGE I
	ENDOMETRIAL CANCERS

Risk	*Stage*	*Grade*
Low	IA	1,2
Risk of recurrence 2-4%	IIA	1,2
Intermediate	IA	3
	IB	3
	IC	1,2
High	IC	3
Risk of recurrence 21-23%		

beam irradiation usually focuses on the vagina, paravaginal tissues, and regional lymph nodes in the pelvis or pelvic and aortic regions.

The radiation oncologists at MD Anderson consider two main groups of patients for whom radiation therapy can be considered in the postoperative setting: (1) selected high intermediate-risk stage I or II disease, or (2) patients with more advanced disease (eg, stage IIIC) that still has a high likelihood of being locoregionally confined. Most patients with low risk, FIGO 2009 stage IA, grade 1 to 2 disease probably do not benefit from adjuvant therapy, and radiation is generally not recommended for this group of patients. However, there is fairly broad consensus that most patients who have FIGO 2009 stage III to IV disease are at high risk of recurrence and need some form of adjuvant therapy.

A number of trials have addressed the question of radiotherapy in early-stage endometrial cancers. Patients in *low-risk* groups do not derive benefit from adjuvant radiotherapy (105). For *intermediate-risk* patients, adjuvant radiation therapy reduces the incidence of pelvic recurrence without prolonging overall survival (Fig. 29-12) (81,106,107). *Vaginal irradiation alone* is adequate for preventing pelvic recurrence in patients who are at risk of only isolated vaginal recurrence (eg, those with low-risk stage I disease). Vaginal irradiation has a higher therapeutic ratio than whole-pelvis radiation because it produces fewer long-term sequelae (65,108,109). The rate of recurrence after vaginal irradiation is low in women with negative or unknown lymph node status (108,110-112). Patients in *high-risk* groups in whom disease is limited to the uterus would probably require adjuvant *whole-pelvis external pelvic radiation*; the addition of *brachytherapy* for such patients does not seem to improve the results. One study showed that the addition of brachytherapy to external irradiation did not affect 5-year pelvic disease control or disease-free survival rates in patients with stage I or II disease (108).

Two large, randomized controlled trials compared external beam radiotherapy following surgery to no adjuvant therapy in stage I endometrial cancer. GOG-99 randomized 392 surgically staged patients to external beam radiation (50.4 Gy) or no treatment (control) (106). The study was included "intermediate-risk" endometrial cancers; patients with any degree of myometrial invasion, adenocarcinoma of any grade, with stages IB, IC, and occult stage II disease. The 2-year pelvic recurrence rate was 3% in the radiation arm versus 12% in the control arm (relative hazard: 0.42; p = .007). In subgroup analysis, the treatment difference was particularly evident among the high intermediate-risk

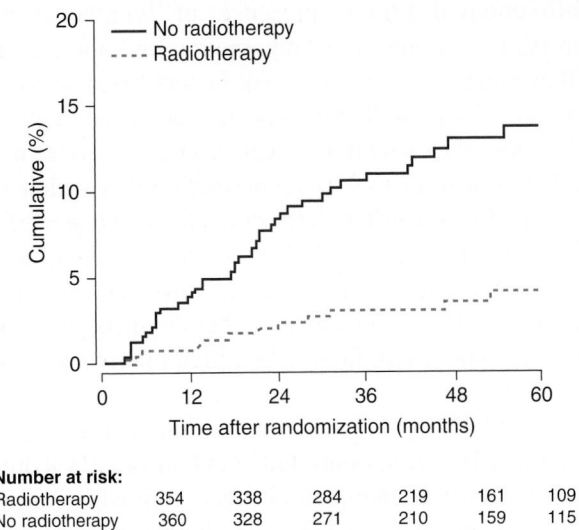

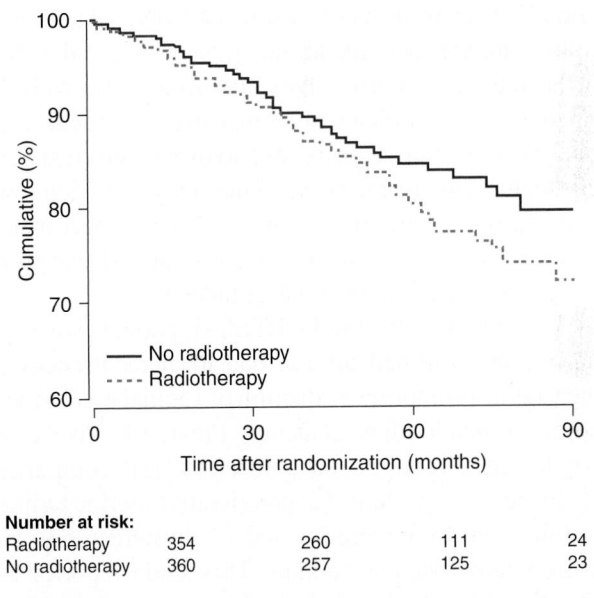

FIGURE 29-12. Pelvic radiotherapy in stage I endometrial cancer. The PORTEC Study Group multicenter randomized trial of 715 patients with stage I endometrial cancer of any type (excluding grade 3 tumors or those with >50% myometrial invasion) showed that pelvic radiotherapy reduced locoregional relapse rates (4 versus 14%, top panel) but did not affect 5-year overall survival rates (81% radiotherapy versus 85% observation, bottom panel). (*Reproduced, with permission, from Creutzberg CL, van Putten WL, Koper PC, et al. Surgery and postoperative radiotherapy versus surgery alone for patients with stage-1 endometrial carcinoma: multicentre randomised trial. PORTEC Study Group. Post Operative Radiation Therapy in Endometrial Carcinoma. Lancet 2000;355:1404-11.*)

subgroup (2-year cumulative incidence rate 6 versus 26% in radiation versus no radiation arms; relative hazard ratio, 0.42). High intermediate-risk subgroup was defined as those with (1) moderate to poorly differentiated tumor, presence of lymphovascular invasion, and outer third myometrial invasion; (2) age 50 or greater with any two risk factors listed above; or (3) age of at least 70 with any risk factor listed above. However, the estimated 4-year survival was 92% in the radiation arm versus 92% for the control arm, which was not significantly different (hazard ratio = 0.86; p = .557). The authors concluded that adjunctive radiation in early-stage intermediate-risk endometrial carcinoma decreases the risk of recurrence, but should be limited to patients whose risk factors fit a high intermediate-risk definition.

The PORTEC-1 (Post Operative Radiation Therapy in Endometrial Carcinoma) study randomized 714 women with early-stage endometrial cancer following surgical staging to either external beam radiotherapy (46 Gy) or no adjuvant treatment (81). At 5 years, local recurrence was significantly lower for patients in the experimental arm (4%) versus the control arm (14%) (81). At 10-year follow-up, the local recurrence rates were similar; 5% in the radiotherapy arm versus 14% in control arm (107). There was no significant difference in distant recurrence rates at either 5 or 10 years, and no overall survival benefit seen at either time points. This study excluded low- and high-risk patients and was primarily performed to evaluate patients in the intermediate-risk category (stage IB, grades 2, 3; stage IC, grades 1, 2).

In both GOG-99 and PORTEC-1, patients with initial uterine-confined disease had local recurrences in the vagina, prompting evaluation of vaginal brachytherapy as a possible adjuvant therapy. Previously, Piver et al. conducted a randomized controlled trial comparing (1) hysterectomy alone, (2) preoperative uterine radium followed by hysterectomy, and (3) hysterectomy and postoperative vaginal radium. This study reported no significant local control rates, disease-free survival, or overall survival at a follow-up of 10 years (109).

More recently, Alektiar et al. compared intravaginal brachytherapy to external beam pelvic radiotherapy in the adjuvant setting. Three hundred eighty-two patients with stage IB to IIB endometrial carcinoma were treated with simple hysterectomy followed by vaginal brachytherapy alone (range, 6-21 Gy). The study is limited in that this was a single-arm, single-institution study. Furthermore, only 20% of the patients had complete surgical staging. However, this study concluded that intracavitary vaginal brachytherapy alone provided adequate tumor control with limited morbidity (113).

PORTEC-2 addresses the question of adjuvant pelvic radiation versus vaginal brachytherapy alone for patients with uterine-confined disease following surgical staging (114). Final results of this study are pending. Preliminary

reports suggest excellent vaginal and pelvic control with both approaches with less short- and long-term toxicity from vaginal brachytherapy, suggesting that vaginal cuff irradiation may be the more effective treatment for the subsets of patients included in that trial.

Some evidence suggests that patients with uterine-confined disease but with high-intermediate risk (stage 1C, grade 3, FIGO 1988) benefit in overall survival from adjuvant radiotherapy. A retrospective analysis of over 21,000 women with stage I disease from the Surveillance, Epidemiology, and End Results (SEER) program of the US National Cancer Institute found that adjuvant pelvic radiotherapy led to improved overall survival in patients with stage IC disease (115). Other meta-analyses also showed improved overall survival with pelvic radiotherapy for patients with high-risk patients (116,117).

At MD Anderson, adjuvant therapy is recommended for all patients with extrauterine disease. We are currently investigating the role of chemotherapy in advanced endometrial cancers, whether in combination with radiotherapy or chemotherapy alone. The current recommendations for adjuvant therapy from the 2010 version of the National Comprehensive Cancer Network's Clinical Practice Guidelines for completely surgically staged patients is summarized in Table 29-13 (118).

Radiation Therapy for Recurrent Disease

At MD Anderson, radiation therapy plays an important role in the treatment of locally recurrent disease. Patients who have local recurrence and have not received prior radiation often can be cured with radiation therapy alone. Five-year survival rates for patients with locoregional recurrence treated with radiation range from 30 to 50% (119,120). Creutzberg et al. reported on survival of intermediate-risk, early-stage patients entered in the PORTEC trial (121). For patients who did not receive adjuvant radiation, 5-year survival after vaginal relapse was 65%. However, possibly because of earlier detection of the relapses and the exclusion of grade 3 disease, the survival rates may be higher than previously reported. At MD Anderson, Jhingran et al. led a retrospective study of 91 patients treated with radiation for vaginal recurrence following definitive surgery for endometrial carcinoma (122). Radiation in this setting provided excellent local control of isolated vaginal recurrences, particularly using the combination of external beam pelvic radiation and brachytherapy. However, perhaps due to the inclusion of grade 3 disease, distant metastases frequently develop despite local disease control, contributing to a 5-year overall survival rate of <50%, much lower than that shown in the Creutzberg study.

TABLE 29-13 | **THE 2010 PRACTICE GUIDELINES OF THE NATIONAL COMPREHENSIVE CANCER NETWORK FOR THE ADJUVANT TREATMENT OF ENDOMETRIAL CANCER FOLLOWING SURGICAL STAGING BASED ON UPDATED 2009 FIGO STAGING. ALL RECOMMENDATIONS CATEGORY 2A UNLESS OTHERWISE INDICATED**

STAGE	ADVERSE RISK FACTORS*	HISTOLOGICAL GRADE		
		G1	**G2**	**G3**
IA (<50% myometrial invasion)	Not present	Observe	Observe or Vaginal brachytherapy	Observe or Vaginal brachytherapy
	Present	Observe or Vaginal brachytherapy	Observe or Vaginal brachytherapy and/or pelvic RT (category 2B for pelvic RT)	Observe or Vaginal brachytherapy and/or Pelvic RT
IB (≥50% myometrial invasion)	Not present	Observe or Vaginal brachytherapy	Observe or Vaginal brachytherapy	Observe or Vaginal brachytherapy and/or Pelvic RT
	Present	Observe or Vaginal brachytherapy and/or Pelvic RT	Observe or Vaginal brachytherapy and/or Pelvic RT	Observe or Pelvic RT and/or Vaginal brachytherapy ± chemotherapy (category 2B for chemotherapy)
II		Vaginal brachytherapy and/or Pelvic RT	Pelvic RT +Vaginal brachytherapy	Pelvic RT + Vaginal brachytherapy ± chemotherapy (category 2B for chemotherapy)
IIIA		Chemotherapy ± RT or Tumor-directed RT ± chemotherapy or Pelvic RT ± vaginal brachytherapy	Chemotherapy ± RT or Tumor-directed RT ± chemotherapy or Pelvic RT ± vaginal brachytherapy	Chemotherapy ± RT or Tumor-directed RT ± chemotherapy or Pelvic RT ± vaginal brachytherapy
IIIB		Chemotherapy and/or tumor-directed RT	Chemotherapy and/or tumor-directed RT	Chemotherapy and/or tumor-directed RT
IIIC (IIIC1 pelvic node positive) (IIIC2 para-aortic node positive ± pelvic node positive)		Chemotherapy and/or tumor-directed RT	Chemotherapy and/or tumor-directed RT	Chemotherapy and/or tumor-directed RT
IVA, IVB (Debulked and with no gross residual disease or microscopic abdominal disease)		Chemotherapy ± RT	Chemotherapy ± RT	Chemotherapy ± RT

*Adverse risk factors include: age, positive lymphovascular invasion, tumor size, lower uterine (cervical/ glandular) involvement.
RT, radiation therapy

Our current recommendation is for patients to receive adjuvant radiation and not to reserve this option as salvage therapy.

Chemotherapy in Advanced or Recurrent Disease

At MD Anderson, we consider all patients with advanced or recurrent endometrial cancer for systemic therapy. Our approach is based on extensive clinical trial data. Numerous phase II trials have shown single-agent activity with response rates above 20% using platinum compounds, taxanes, and anthracyclines in patients with advanced or recurrent endometrial cancer (123). In addition, several randomized trials have compared combination treatments to single-agent activity in patients with FIGO stage III, stage IV, and recurrent disease.

Doxorubicin has been the most extensively studied cytotoxic agent for the treatment of advanced and recurrent disease. As a single agent, the response rate is reported to be 22 to 27% (124,125). Two trials, European Organization for Research and Treatment of Cancer (EORTC)-55872 and GOG-107, have compared combination therapies of doxorubicin with cisplatin to single-agent doxorubicin in the advanced or recurrent disease setting (125,126). In both studies, doxorubicin was more effective when used in combination with cisplatin (overall response rate 43 versus 17% in EORTC-55872; 42 versus 25% in GOG-107). However, there was only a modest effect on overall survival; 9 versus 7 months in the EORTC study, and 9.2 versus 9 months in the GOG study. Toxicity, primarily hematologic, was significantly higher in the combination arms for both studies (125,126).

There have been a number of trials using three-drug combination with doxorubicin. Burke et al. reported a high overall response rate (45%) in a prospective study of the three-drug combination cisplatin, doxorubicin, and cyclophosphamide (127). However, the significant toxicity and brief median response duration were thought to limit the clinical application of this combination. A pegylated liposomal form of doxorubicin was studied for recurrent or persistent EC on the basis of expected benefits in improved pharmacologic effect and reduced toxicity (128). Although the antitumor activity of this formulation was demonstrated to be only about 9%, its lesser toxicity compared with that of traditional doxorubicin could merit further study in combination drug regimens.

One prospective, phase III trial compared the combination of doxorubicin plus cisplatin to doxorubicin, cisplatin, and paclitaxel (129). Two hundred seventy-three women patients, either with chemonaïve stage III, stage IV, or recurrent disease, were randomized to receive doxorubicin 60 mg/m^2 and cisplatin 50 mg/m^2 (AP), or doxorubicin 45 mg/ m^{2}and cisplatin 50 mg/m^2 (day 1), followed by paclitaxel 160 mg/m^2 (day 2) with filgrastim support (TAP). Both regimens were repeated every 3 weeks to a maximum of seven cycles. Results were significantly favorable for the three-drug combination with objective response (57 versus 34%; $p < .01$), PFS (median, 8.3 versus 5.3 months; $p < .01$), and OS (median, 15.3 versus 12.3 months; $p = .037$). Of note, neurologic toxicity was greater for those in the TAP arm compared to AP, with 12 versus 1% grade 3 and 27 versus 4% grade 2 peripheral neuropathy.

Paclitaxel has also been extensively studied for EC. Response rates for paclitaxel in a phase II GOG trial have been as high as 35.7% for chemonaïve patients and 27.3% for patients who had previously been given chemotherapy (130,131). Given the high response rates shown in phase 2 studies of single-agent paclitaxel, there have been a number of attempts to improve response rates by combining paclitaxel with other drugs (129,132). GOG-163 was a randomized trial comparing doxorubicin and cisplatin to doxorubicin with 24-h paclitaxel with granulocyte colony-stimulating factor (G-CSF) in patients with stages III and IV or recurrent EC. There was no difference in response rate, progression-free survival, or overall survival (132). In a subsequent randomized study (GOG-177), both experimental arms contained cisplatin: doxorubicin and cisplatin compared to doxorubicin and cisplatin with paclitaxel and G-CSF. In this study, the three-drug combination led to an improvement in response rate (overall response rate 57% in three-drug arm compared to 34% in control). Median progression-free survival and overall survival were also improved with the addition of paclitaxel to doxorubicin and cisplatin (median PFS 8.3 versus 5.3 months [$p < .01$] and median overall survival 15.3 versus 12.3 months [$p = .037$]). However, patients who received the three-drug combination experienced greater toxicity, particularly neurologic (132).

Carboplatin, another drug studied for advanced or recurrent EC, can be given in outpatient settings and produces manageable myelosuppression. Response rates have ranged from 28 to 33% (133-135), with median response durations of 2.7 to 4.0 months (133,134), an interval comparable to the 4.8 months obtained with cisplatin, doxorubicin, and cyclophosphamide (127). Outcome in another study by Burke and others was excellent, with approximately 44% of patients surviving disease-free for more than 2 years (133).

Chemotherapy trials for EC are summarized in Table 29-14.

TABLE | **DRUGS USED IN THE TREATMENT OF PERSISTENT, RECURRENT, OR ADVANCED**
29-14 | **ENDOMETRIAL CANCER**

Drug Regimen	First Author and Year of Study (Reference)	No. of Patients	Prior Chemotherapy	Dose	Overall Response Rate (%)
Carboplatin	Burke, 1993 (133)	33	No	360-450 mg/m^2	33
	Long, 1988 (135)	26	No	300-400 mg/m^2	28
	Green, 1990 (134)	23	No	400 mg/m^2	30
Ifosfamide + mesna	Sutton, 1994 (323)	52	Yes	1.2 g/m^2 (ifosfamide)	15
Dox versus dox + cisplatin	Thigpen, 1993 (125)	223	Yes and no	60 mg/m^2 ± 50 mg/m^2	27 versus 45 (S)
Dox + cisplatin	Deppe, 1994 (324)	19	Yes	50 mg/m^2 + 50 mg/m^2	36
Dox versus dox + cyclophosphamide	Thigpen, 1994 (124)	276	Yes and no	60 mg/m^2 ± 500 mg/m^2	22 versus 30 (NS)
Dox + cisplatin versus dox + paclitaxel	Fleming, 2004 (132)	314	Yes and no	60 mg/m^2 + 50 mg/m^2 versus 50 mg/m^2 + 150 mg/m^2 G-CSF used in both arms	NS
Dox + cisplatin + cyclophosphamide	Burke, 1991 (127)	87	Yes and no	50 mg/m^2 + 50 mg/m^2 + 500 mg/m^2	45
Liposomal dox	Muggia, 2002 (128)	32	Yes	50 mg/m^2	9.5
Escalated paclitaxel + fixed-dose cisplatin + dox	Fleming, 2001 (325)	80	No	90-250 mg/m^2 + 60 mg/m^2 45 mg/m^2	46
Paclitaxel	Ball, 1996 (130)	30	No	250 mg/m^2	35.7
	Lincoln, 2003 (131)	44	Yes	110-200 mg/m^2	27.3
Topotecan	Miller, 2002 (326)	22	Yes	0.5-1.5 mg/m^2	9
Cisplatin + epirubicin + cyclophosphamide	Gaducci, 1999 (327)	19	Yes and no	50 mg/m^2 + 60 mg/m^2 + 600 mg/m^2	43.7
Dox + cisplatin versus dox + cisplatin + paclitaxel	Fleming, 2004 (132)	266	Yes and no	60 mg/m^2 + 50 mg/m^2 versus 45 mg/m^2 + 50 mg/m^2 + 160 mg/m^2	NS

Dox, doxorubicin; G-CSF, granulocyte colony-stimulating factor; NS, not significant; S, significant.

Adjuvant Chemotherapy for Early-Stage Disease

To date, evidence supporting the use of adjuvant systemic therapy in early-stage, high-risk disease is limited. The first adjuvant trial was GOG-34, published in 1990, comparing whole-pelvis radiation versus radiation plus doxorubicin in high-risk stages I and II patients. Following TAH-BSO, lymph node dissection, and peritoneal cytology, 224 patients underwent adjuvant pelvic external radiotherapy. They were then randomized to observation or doxorubicin 45 mg/m^2 after completion of radiotherapy. Results showed no significant difference in the recurrence or overall survival between the two treatment arms. However, because of the small sample size, protocol violations, and the number of patients lost to follow-up, the authors of this study were unable to conclude definitively whether the use of doxorubicin as adjuvant therapy had an effect on recurrence, progression, and survival of the endometrial cancer study population (136).

At MD Anderson, Stringer et al. undertook a prospective study in early-stage (stage 1 and occult stage 2) patients considered high risk for recurrence (grade 2 tumor with middle- or outer-third myometrial invasion, grade 3 tumor with any myometrial invasion, grade 2 or 3 tumor with documented extrauterine disease and no macroscopic residual disease following the initial surgical procedure, or a high-risk histologic subtype, including papillary serous, adenosquamous, or clear cell tumors with any myometrial invasion). Patients were treated with the combination regimen of cyclophosphamide, doxorubicin, and cisplatin (500/50/50 mg/m^2) every 4 weeks for six cycles based on efficacy seen in the recurrent setting. The resulting 2-year progression-free survival rate and overall survival rate were 79% and 83%, respectively. Toxicity, primarily hematologic, was moderate (137). These results are comparable to those of GOG-34 (136).

The Japanese GOG (JGOG-2033) designed a multicenter randomized phase III trial to address the relative efficacy of combination chemotherapy cyclophosphamide 333 mg/m^2, doxorubicin 40 mg/m^2, and cisplatin 50 mg/m^2 (CAP) every 4 weeks for three or more cycles in patients with stage IC to IIIC and ≥50% myometrial invasion. All patients underwent TAH-BSO ± lymphadenectomy. They were then randomized to pelvic XRT or chemotherapy with CAP. At 5 years, there was no difference in progression-free survival or overall survival between the two groups. Although subgroup analysis of high- to intermediate-risk patients (stage IC in patients >70 years old or grade 3 histology or stage II or IIIA patients with positive cytology) did show significantly improved progression-free (84 versus 66%, log-rank test $p = .024$; hazard ratio, 0.44) and overall survival (90 versus 74%, log-rank test $p = .006$; hazard ratio, 0.24), this analysis is limited (138).

The Nordic Society of Gynecologic Oncology (NSGO) in collaboration with the EORTC presented early reports of a randomized phase III study in patients with surgical stage I, II, IIIA, or IIIC with high-risk features. Following surgery, patients received pelvic XRT with or without vaginal brachytherapy, then were randomized to observation versus chemotherapy given before or after XRT. Regimens included combinations of (1) cisplatin and doxorubicin or epirubicin, (2) paclitaxel, epirubicin, and carboplatin, or (3) paclitaxel and carboplatin. There were several limitations of this study, including high rate of attrition in the chemotherapy arm with 27% of patients not completing planned therapy, early termination due to slow accrual, and lower dose of XRT (44 Gy versus standard 45-50 Gy). There was a significant improvement in PFS in the XRT + chemotherapy arm (hazard ratio 0.58 in favor of RT + CT [95% confidence interval, 0.34-0.99; $p = 0.046$]). This translates to an estimated 7% absolute difference in 5-year PFS from 75% (95% CI, 67-82 %) to 82% (95% CI, 73-88 %). However, there was no significant difference in overall survival (139).

Trials Comparing Chemotherapy Versus Radiation

In GOG-122, patients with FIGO stages III and IV disease of any histology were treated with either whole-abdomen irradiation or chemotherapy as adjuvant treatment (140). Of 396 evaluable patients, 202 were randomized to receive adjuvant whole-abdominal irradiation (30 Gy) and a pelvic boost (15 Gy), and 194 were received cisplatin (50 mg/m^2) plus doxorubicin (60 mg/m^2) every 3 weeks for seven cycles, followed by one cycle of cisplatin. At a median follow-up time of 74 months, the hazard ratio for progression adjusted for stage was 0.71 favoring chemotherapy (95% CI, 0.55-0.91; $p < .01$). Adjuvant chemotherapy significantly improved both progression-free and overall survival compared with radiation alone. However, treatment-related toxicities were greater in the chemotherapy arm with fewer than two-thirds of patients completing all eight cycles. In addition, there were significantly more incidences of hematologic and cardiac toxicities. Therefore, we recommend the use of growth factor support and monitoring of left ventricular function for patients receiving cisplatin and doxorubicin-based adjuvant therapy.

Hormonal Therapy

Although hormonal agents have been used for the treatment of EC, they have not had a dramatic impact on overall survival. Furthermore, reports are conflicting on their benefit. For example, in a 2002 meta-analysis of six randomized controlled trials, Martin-Hirsch et al. reported that adjuvant progestin therapy was of no benefit in the treatment of EC and might even have adversely affected survival because of intercurrent deaths from cardiovascular accident, thromboembolism, and cardiac failure (141). Progestin treatment may have a more suitable role in the recurrent disease setting.

Progestin has long been used in the treatment of EC. The drug was originally given parenterally and later as an oral formulation. A dose-response study of oral medroxyprogesterone acetate found that higher doses (1000 mg/day) yielded higher serum concentrations but were not more beneficial than lower doses (200 mg/day) (142,143). The response of EC to progestin correlates directly with and is predictive of the degree of tumor differentiation, which is linked to hormone receptor status, particularly progesterone receptor levels (143). A wide range of response rates have been reported, with responses lasting 16 to 287 months and survival times lasting 18 to 33 months. These wide ranges reflect variations in recruitment criteria as well as methods in the evaluation of response. In one GOG study that was limited to patients with advanced or recurrent disease, the response rate was only 18%, with median progression-free survival time of only 4 months and median overall survival time of only 10.5 months (143).

High-dose megestrol has also been evaluated in the treatment of advanced or recurrent ED. Patients enrolled in this study had not received prior cytotoxic or hormonal therapy, had either failed to respond, or had been considered incurable with local therapy. Response rate of patients with grade 1 or 2 lesions (37%) was significantly higher (*p* = .02) than that of patients with more poorly differentiated tumors (8%). Four of the responses lasted longer than 18 months (142). The authors concluded that although high-dose megestrol is active in treatment of advanced or recurrent EC, there was no advantage over lower-dose progestins but with greater side effects.

Tamoxifen has also been used to treat advanced or recurrent EC. When bound to cytoplasmic endoplasmic reticulum, tamoxifen stimulates the production and expression of progesterone receptors (144); theoretically, therefore, tamoxifen should potentiate the efficacy of progestins. However, no clinically significant improvements have been demonstrated by using tamoxifen and progestins together (145-147). At doses of 20 to 40 mg/day, tamoxifen given for EC produces response rates of 0 to 53% (148,149). Despite this wide range, a dose-response effect may have been present in some cases, as the highest dose used (40 mg/day) yielded the highest response rate (53%) (148).

Preclinical data suggest that gonadotropin-releasing hormone analogs can inhibit the growth and enhance the apoptosis of EC cells. In the few trials conducted using this drug to treat advanced, metastatic, or recurrent EC, response rates have varied from 0 to 35% (99,150,151). Gallagher et al. showed a relatively high response rate of 35%, despite the fact that 82% of their patients had had prior treatment with progestin. The duration of response was also prolonged, ranging from 7 to 20 months (152). However, this study included only 12 patients. A later report by Asbury et al. of a similar study conducted by the GOG with 40 patients showed a response rate of only 11%, with median overall survival time of only 7.3 months (153). The recommendation from that study was that further study of goserelin acetate alone was not justified but that this drug might be more effective in combination with other drugs.

Another agent being evaluated for the treatment of EC is anastrozole, a nonsteroidal aromatase inhibitor that acts by blocking the peripheral conversion of adrenal androstenedione to estrone. In a phase II study conducted of anastrozole for 23 patients with recurrent EC, the GOG found only two cases of partial response and two cases of stable disease (154). None of the patients who had responded to previous hormonal therapy responded to anastrozole. Note that most patients also tended to have poorly differentiated tumors, which might have influenced the results.

Selective estrogen-receptor modulators oppose the actions of estrogen on the breast and endometrium but exert an estrogen-agonist effect on bones and on lipid profiles. Burke, et al. as well as others reported findings from phases I and II trials of arzoxifene for refractory, metastatic, or recurrent EC (155,156). Clinical response rates were significant at 25 to 31%, and disease progression was stabilized in a substantial proportion of women studied. To date, there have not been any phase III trials of arzoxifene (157).

Surgery for Relapsed Disease

At MD Anderson, we evaluate all patients who have experienced an isolated central pelvic recurrence after radiotherapy for radical pelvic surgery or pelvic exenteration; these procedures remain the only potentially curative options that offer the possibility of long-term survival. However, given the high incidence of major postoperative complications such as urinary/intestinal tract fistulas, pelvic abscesses, septicemia, pulmonary emboli, and cerebrovascular accidents, we consider only selected patients with isolated central recurrences for this treatment (31,158-160).

CONSERVATIVE TREATMENT

At MD Anderson, we rarely undertake a conservative, nonsurgical approach to EC, but for younger patients wishing to preserve their fertility, several options may be explored (161). Currently, no treatment recommendations or guidelines exist for nonsurgical management of EC. However, for women with early-stage disease, fertility-sparing hormonal treatment has been explored (162-164). The use of progestins has been shown to have efficacy in women with low-grade tumors (165). However, it should be noted that even among responders to progestins, a 50% recurrence rate is observed (164).

Other conservative surgical option is the omission of a bilateral salpingo-oophorectomy (BSO) in young women with EC (166,167). This strategy offers the potential for future oocyte retrieval and avoids the adverse consequences of estrogen deprivation (ie, hot-flashes, vaginal atrophy, cardiovascular disease, and osteoporosis). However, this strategy risks missing occult ovarian metastases (168) and coexisting synchronous ovarian primary tumors (166,168-170). There is also a risk of hormonal stimulation of residual microscopic endometrial cancer foci.

TREATMENT AFTER INCOMPLETE STAGING

EC patients are incompletely staged when the patient undergoes total abdominal hysterectomy and bilateral salpingo-oophorectomy without adequate lymph node dissection. There have been two published randomized clinical trials in patient who had incomplete staging (81,110). In Aalders et al. 540 stage I EC patients received TAH-BSO and adjuvant radiation to the vaginal vault. These patients were then randomized to receive external beam radiation to the pelvis/pelvic lymph nodes or observation. At 3- and 10-year follow-ups, the patient who received additional pelvic radiation had fewer local recurrences but also had more distant metastasis. Thus, there was no effect of external beam pelvic radiation on overall survival. Based on subset analyses, the authors concluded that only patients with grade 3, poorly differentiated tumors, which infiltrate more than half the myometrial thickness, might benefit from additional external radiotherapy (110).

In a more recent study, investigators in the PORTEC-1 trial reported similar results in a randomized trial with stage IB, grades 2 and 3, and stage IC, grades 1 and 2 patients who underwent TAH-BSO without lymph node assessment. There was a significant reduction in locoregional recurrence in patients who received pelvic RT but no effect on overall survival (81). The National Comprehensive Cancer Network Clinical Practice Guidelines for adjuvant treatment of cases in which surgical staging is incomplete is shown in Figure 29-13.

POSTOPERATIVE SURVEILLANCE

There are no prospective studies to guide frequency of postoperative follow-up. At MD Anderson, we recommend follow-up visits to include a routine physical examination with pelvic examination along with examination of abdomen, peripheral lymph nodes, and lungs every 3 to 6 months for the first 2 years, followed by an examination every 6 months to 1 year.(171-174).

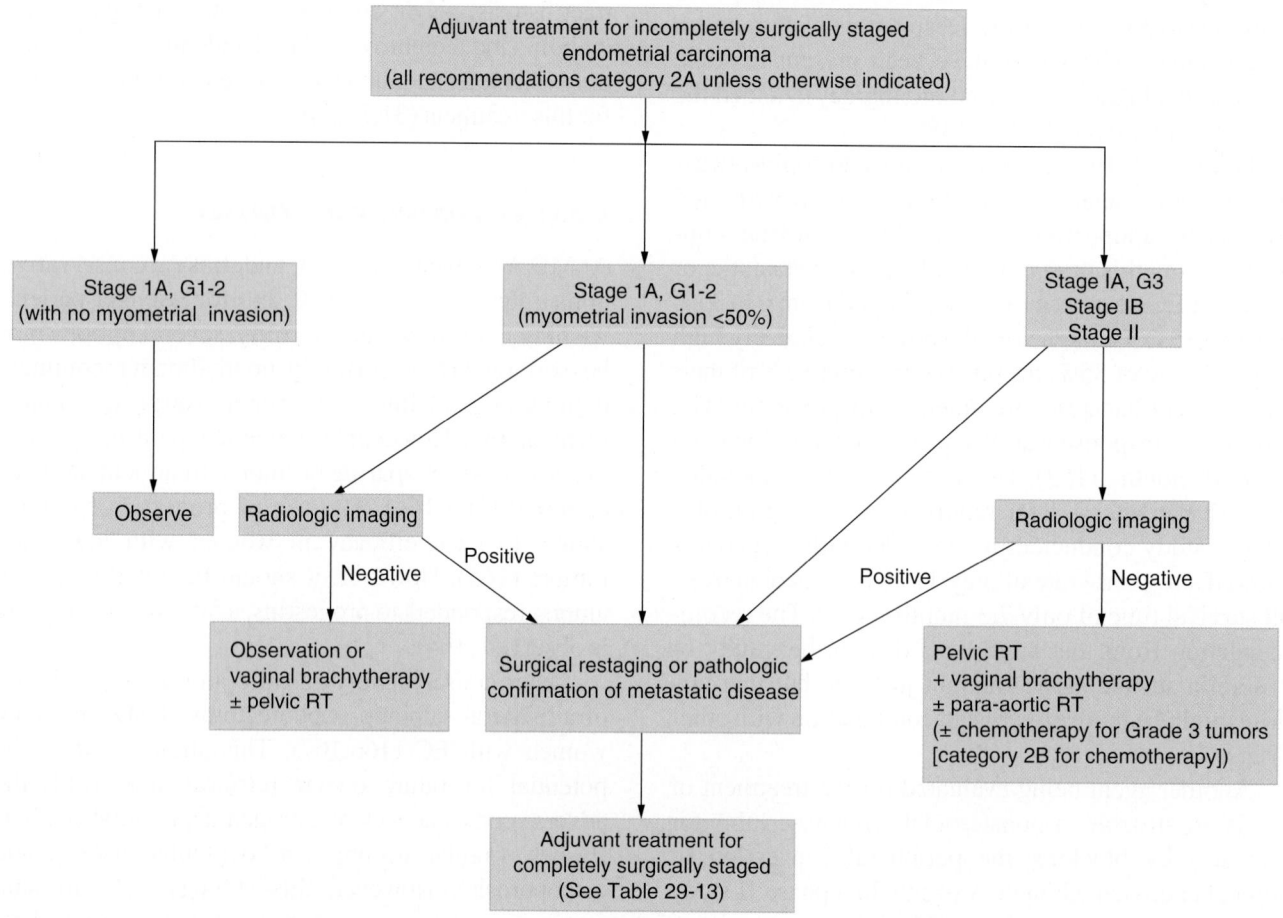

FIGURE 29-13. Treatment guideline for incompletely staged endometrial cancer, based on 2009 FIGO staging. *(Reproduced, with permission, from National Comprehensive Cancer Network. (NCCN) Clinical Practice Guidelines in Oncology. 2010 [Available from: http://www. nccn.org])*

The cost-effectiveness of regular Pap smears for uterine cancer surveillance is questionable, as only a few recurrences are detected through an abnormal Pap test. We recommend vaginal cytology every 6 months for 2 years, then annually. Chest x-rays should be obtained annually for the first 2 years after diagnosis, as recurrences are most likely to appear during that period.

Serum CA 125 level measurements are optional, although we perform them on a routine basis. In patients with elevated serum CA 125 levels at diagnosis, they can be used as a marker for recurrent disease. In one study, among patients with advanced EC who initially had high CA 125 levels, 26 to 58% showed elevated CA 125 levels at recurrence (175). The use of serial CA 125 assays is most beneficial in diagnosing recurrence in a high-risk population, although there have been no studies to show that their use improves survival. False elevations may occur following radiation therapy.

USE OF HORMONE REPLACEMENT THERAPY AFTER TREATMENT OF ENDOMETRIAL CANCER

The use of estrogen replacement therapy in women who have been treated for endometrial cancer is controversial. Most of the evidence regarding the effects of hormone replacement therapy in women with previously treated EC comes from retrospective studies. (176-179) In one study, Chapman et al. found no significant difference in disease-free survival rates between women who used estrogen replacement therapy and those who did not (176). However, in this study, the group that used estrogen had earlier-stage disease with less depth of invasion compared to the control group. A subsequent cohort study by Suriano et al., who matched cases for tumor status and treatment, also found lower recurrence rates and longer disease-free survival among women who used estrogen (179). Notably, 49% of patients in the estrogen replacement group in that study were also given progestin, which might have influenced the apparent improvement in outcome.

In a study reported in 2006, the GOG conducted a double-blind, randomized phase III trial to evaluate the safety of estrogen replacement therapy following treatment for endometrial cancer (GOG-137) (180). One thousand, two hundred and thirty-six women with a history of stage I or occult stage II endometrial cancer were enrolled within 20 weeks following surgery. All enrolled patients had an indication for treatment with estrogen replacement therapy, including hot flashes, vaginal atrophy, increased risk of cardiovascular disease, or an increased risk of osteoporosis and were randomized to receive estrogen replacement or placebo for 3 years following surgery. This study closed early when the results of the Women's Health Initiative (WHI) study showed increased overall risks in the estrogen and progestin arm (181). Based on the results of the WHI study, GOG-137 closed prematurely, and the study was left with insufficient power to detect a difference in patients with intermediate- or high-risk early endometrial cancers. The results of this study are inconclusive. However, the authors noted that in the low-risk population, the absolute recurrence rate (2.1%) was low. The relative risk of recurrence/death in the estrogen replacement therapy group was 1.27 compared with the placebo group (80% CI, 0.916-1.77).

At MD Anderson, we approach the use of estrogen replacement therapy on an individual basis. Overall risk of disease recurrence in low-risk patients is low, even in the setting of exogenous estrogen replacement. Therefore, estrogen replacement therapy may be considered for this population. If adjuvant therapy is given following surgery, we recommend a 6- to 12-month waiting period prior to initiation of hormone replacement therapy.

■ NONEPITHELIAL UTERINE TUMORS

Uterine sarcoma is uncommon, accounting for only 2 to 6% of all tumors arising from the uterine corpus (182-184). Most uterine sarcomas originate from mesodermal tissue, although some are derived from specialized müllerian mesenchyme, such as endometrial stroma, and a few originate from nonspecific or nonmüllerian mesenchyme (eg, smooth or skeletal muscle, vessels, or lymphoid tissue). The three most common types of uterine sarcoma are leiomyosarcoma, endometrial stromal sarcoma (ESS), and carcinosarcoma, also referred to as malignant mixed müllerian tumor (MMMT); leiomyosarcomas and carcinosarcomas represent about two-thirds of all uterine sarcomas (183). Uterine sarcomas are generally aggressive with overall mortality approaching 90% (185).

Previously, the 1988 FIGO criteria for endometrial carcinoma have been used to stage uterine sarcomas. Recently, a new FIGO classification and staging system designed for uterine sarcomas has been devised (186,187). This staging system includes three new classifications for staging, including leiomyosarcoma, ESS, and adenosarcoma (Table 29-15). Note that carcinosarcoma is still staged according to the FIGO staging for endometrial carcinoma.

| TABLE 29-15 | FIGO STAGING FOR UTERINE SARCOMAS |

(1) LEIOMYOSARCOMAS AND ENDOMETRIAL STROMAL SARCOMAS*

Stage	Definition
I	Tumor limited to uterus
IA	≤5 cm
IB	≥5 cm
II	Tumor extends beyond the uterus, within the pelvis
IIA	Adnexal involvement
IIB	Involvement of other pelvic tissues
III	Tumor invades abdominal tissues (not just protruding into the abdomen)
IIIA	One site
IIIB	More than one site
IIIC	Metastasis to pelvic and/or para-aortic lymph nodes
IV	
IVA	Tumor invades bladder and/or rectum
IVB	Distant metastasis

(2) ADENOSARCOMAS

Stage	Definition
I	Tumor limited to uterus
IA	Tumor limited to endometrium/endocervix with no myometrial invasion
IB	Less than or equal to half myometrial invasion
IC	More than half myometrial invasion
II	Tumor extends beyond the uterus, within the pelvis
IIA	Adnexal involvement
IIB	Involvement of other pelvic tissues
III	Tumor invades abdominal tissues (not just protruding into the abdomen)
IIIA	One site
IIIB	More than one site
IIIC	Metastasis to pelvic and/or para-aortic lymph nodes
IV	
IVA	Tumor invades bladder and/or rectum
IVB	Distant metastasis

(3) CARCINOSARCOMAS

Carcinosarcomas should be staged as carcinomas of the endometrium.

FIGO, International Federation of Gynecology and Obstetrics.
*Note: Simultaneous endometrial stromal sarcomas of the uterine corpus and ovary/pelvis in association with ovarian/pelvic endometriosis should be classified as independent primary tumors.
Reprinted from the International Journal of Gynecology & Obstetrics; Vol. 106, Issue 3. Corrigendum to "FIGO staging for uterine sarcomas," Copyright 2009, with permission from Elsevier.

EPIDEMIOLOGY

Each type of sarcoma tends to appear in a different age group. Leiomyosarcoma and ESS usually affect women in their early 50s; carcinosarcomas usually appear in older women aged 60 or above (188-190). Adenosarcomas have been reported in women 14 to 84 years old; the median age at appearance is between 51 and 57 years (59,191,192).

Although uterine sarcoma differs somewhat from EC in its clinical and pathologic characteristics, some risk factors—such as hypertension, diabetes mellitus, and obesity—are common to both. Previous history of pelvic irradiation has been associated with uterine sarcoma, occurring in 2 to 29% of patients so exposed at an interval ranging from 2 to 20 years (193,194). Although the link between estrogen and EC is well established, no such clear relationship is evident for estrogen and uterine sarcoma. Nevertheless, an association between tamoxifen use and uterine sarcoma has been reported (195-201). This association was confirmed in the P-1 trial of the NSABP and a study by Bergman et al., both of which showed increased numbers of adenocarcinomas and uterine sarcomas among women taking tamoxifen, and sarcomas constituting about 10% of total malignancies in these cases (202,203).

HISTOPATHOLOGY

Leiomyosarcoma

Leiomyosarcomas represent only 1.3% of uterine malignancies; however, in six studies of uterine sarcomas, leiomyosarcoma constituted 33 to 42% (mean 34%) of the 321 sarcomas studied (183,188,204-207). Gross features of leiomyosarcoma (Fig. 29-14) are typified by variegation at the cut surface (unlike the whorl-like surface typical of a benign leiomyoma).

Cells are spindle-shaped and arranged in fascicles with eosinophilic cytoplasm. The nuclei are usually elongated with rounded ends, appearing hyperchromatic with coarse chromatin and prominent nucleoli. The most important criterion for the diagnosis of leiomyosarcoma is a high mitotic rate generally exceeding 15 mitotic figures per 10 high-power fields. Other features such as extrauterine extension, large size, and infiltrating border, necrosis, and atypical mitotic figures can also aid in the diagnosis (187).

Other variants of leiomyosarcoma include myxoid and epithelioid leiomyosarcoma. In myxoid leiomyosarcoma, tumor cellularity is low, cells are separated by myxoid material, and the tumor cells are still characterized by nuclei atypia and high mitotic index (187,208,209).

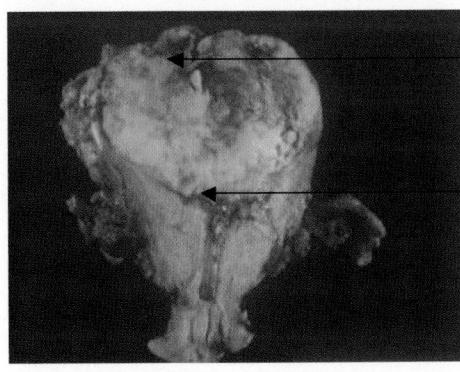

Tumor mass located in the myometrium invading through the uterine serosa

The endoterium was compressed but showed no gross involvement

FIGURE 29-14. Gross appearance of a leiomyosarcoma in the upper uterus. The cut surface shows a grayish-tan tumor with hemorrhage and necrosis, without the whorl-like appearance typical of benign leiomyoma. The mass clearly involves most of the myometrium but not the endometrium.

The tumor cells in epithelioid leiomyosarcoma, in contrast, exhibit epithelioid features distinct from the usual characteristics of leiomyosarcoma (210).

Smooth Muscle Tumor of Uncertain Malignant Potential

Uterine smooth muscle tumors with histologic features of necrosis, nuclear atypia, or mitoses but do not meet all diagnostic criteria for leiomyosarcoma fall into the category of smooth muscle tumor of uncertain malignant potential (STUMP) (187,211). STUMPs are a group of smooth muscle tumors for which a diagnosis of sarcoma cannot be made because of their uncertain malignant characteristics. Most of these tumors are associated with favorable prognosis and only follow-up of the patients is recommended (212). In a recent study of 41 cases of STUMP conducted at MD Anderson, the recurrence rate was 7%. One of the three recurrences was a leiomyosarcoma; the others were STUMP (213).

Endometrial Stromal Sarcoma

ESS accounts for about 23% of all uterine sarcomas (183,188,190,204,206,207). ESSs originate from endometrial stromal cells that invade the myometrium. Low- and high-grade variants differ in their clinical behavior. Gross features of a low-grade ESS presenting as multiple small lobulated tumor masses in the myometrium are shown in Fig. 29-15A.

In fresh specimens, tumor invading the lymphovascular spaces can sometimes be compressed out of the vascular lumen, giving a vermiform appearance. Tumor cells resemble endometrial stromal cells during the proliferative phase of the menstrual cycle and are monotonous and of uniform shape and size (214). The presence of spiral arteriole-like vessels is a characteristic finding of ESS, as is the propensity of the tumor cells to invade the lymphovascular spaces (Fig. 29-15B).

In high-grade ESS, the tumor cells tend to be larger, with more vesicular nuclei, coarse clumps of chromatin, and more prominent nucleoli (215). Mitotic counts are usually low in low-grade ESS, and this is the principal criterion for distinguishing between the low- and high-grade forms (215). However, numerous mitotic figures can be present in otherwise typical low-grade tumors, and high-grade tumors can have only a few mitotic figures (216,217). Flow cytometry with DNA ploidy seems to be associated more with the behavior of the tumor than with mitotic count (218). In the 2002 classification of ESS by the World Health Organization, high-grade tumors are considered as pleomorphic or undifferentiated sarcoma rather than as a type of ESS because of their distinctive and aggressive clinical behavior.

Carcinosarcoma

Carcinosarcomas or malignant mixed müllerian tumors (MMMTs) account for less than 5% of malignant neoplasms of the uterus but approximately 37% of all uterine sarcomas (183,188,190,204,206,207). Four theories have been proposed about the histologic origin of carcinosarcomas: *collision theory* suggests that the carcinomatous and sarcomatous components are two independent neoplasms; *composition theory* considers the sarcoma component to be a pseudosarcomatous reaction to the carcinoma; *combination theory* suggests that both components arise from a common stem cell; and *conversion theory* suggests that the sarcomatous component is derived from the carcinoma during the evolution of the tumor (219,220). In recent years, clinical, histopathologic, immunohistochemical, ultrastructural, tissue culture, and molecular evidence has supported the combination or conversion theories; that is, carcinosarcomas are metaplastic carcinomas. These important findings are useful in that they will lead to proper treatment for carcinosarcomas as a high-grade carcinoma rather than a

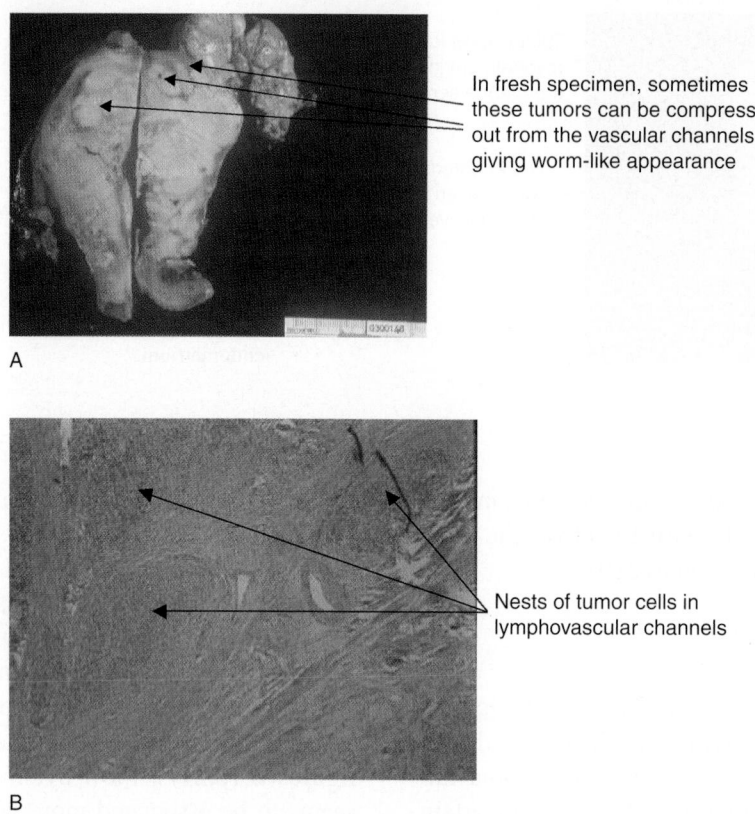

In fresh specimen, sometimes
these tumors can be compressed
out from the vascular channels
giving worm-like appearance

Nests of tumor cells in
lymphovascular channels

FIGURE 29-15. **A.** Gross appearance of an endometrial stromal sarcoma infiltrating most of the myometrium. The lobulated appearance corresponds with the presence of tumor in the lymphovascular spaces, as verified on microscopy in panel B. **B.** Endometrial stromal sarcoma cells with invasion of the intralymphatic spaces.

sarcoma. Nevertheless, if carcinosarcomas truly represent two tumors in "collision" (a sarcoma and a carcinoma), the prognosis would be better than that of a metaplastic carcinoma at a similar stage (221).

The gross appearance of a polypoid carcinosarcoma mass protruding into the endometrial cavity is shown in Fig. 29-16. Although not pathognomonic of carcinosarcoma, this feature in a postmenopausal woman should alert the clinician to the possibility of carcinosarcoma.

Histologically, carcinosarcomas consist of two components—malignant epithelial and mesenchymal tissue. The two most common types of EC are the endometrioid and serous types (222-224). In homologous MMMT, the sarcomatous component can be tissue that is normally found in the uterus; ESS or leiomyosarcoma are common. The so-called heterologous type of MMMT consists of tissue that does not normally appear in the uterus; rhabdomyosarcoma and chondrosarcoma are two common types. Homologous and heterologous MMMTs occur at approximately the same frequency (224).

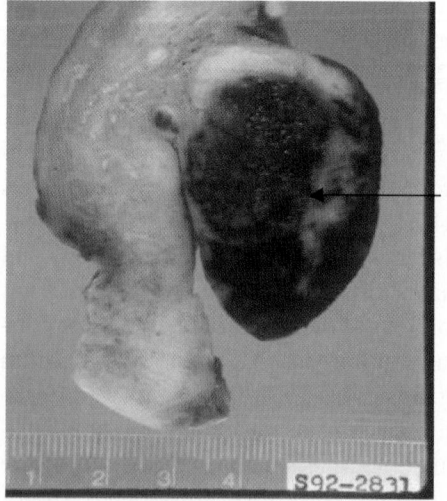

Polypoid mass
protruding into the
endometrial

FIGURE 29-16. Gross appearance of a fleshy hemorrhagic polypoid MMMT protruding into the endometrial cavity in a hemiuterus specimen. Such tumors, which typically present with vaginal bleeding, must be distinguished from submucous myoma. Several endometrial tissue biopsies are sometimes needed for diagnosis because of the necrotic and hemorrhagic nature of this tumor.

Adenosarcoma

Adenosarcomas have two tissue components; the mesenchymal tissue is malignant and the epithelial part is benign. The epithelial component commonly resembles a proliferative or inactive endometrial gland, often appearing as cleft-like spaces dispersed throughout the proliferative stroma in a phyllode pattern. Slight atypia may be present (190). The mesenchymal stromal component is usually homologous tissue such as stromal sarcoma, fibrosarcoma, or leiomyosarcoma (191,225). The pattern of stromal cell hypercellularity surrounding the glands is characteristic, and the stromal cells show variable atypia and mitosis (59). Adenosarcomas with extensive stromal sarcoma proliferation are called *adenosarcoma with sarcoma overgrowth* if the sarcomatous component constitutes more than 25% of the tumor (59,191). This subtype should be recognized, because its prognosis is worse than that of a typical adenosarcoma and more similar to that of carcinosarcoma (226).

CLINICAL PRESENTATION

Vaginal bleeding is the most common presenting symptom of uterine sarcomas. Another common presenting symptom in ESS, carcinosarcoma, and adenosarcoma is the appearance of a prolapsed polypoid mass through the cervical os. Other symptoms such as back pain, urinary retention or hematuria, gastrointestinal symptoms, or weight loss may indicate an invading or metastasizing tumor (227-229).

Patients with carcinosarcoma most commonly present with uterine enlargement and vaginal bleeding. Carcinosarcomas are large polypoid masses and may be seen prolapsing through the cervical os. Although not diagnostic, serum CA125 levels are elevated (230,231). Up to one-third of cases present with extrauterine spread (224).

Patients with ESS often present with uterine bleeding and pelvic pain, but up to 25% of women may be asymptomatic. Up to one-third of patients may have extrauterine pelvic extension, most often affecting the ovary (187,217).

Women with leiomyosarcomas may present with signs and symptoms similar to benign leiomyomas. Patients can exhibit abnormal vaginal bleeding (56%), palpable pelvic mass (54%), and/or pelvic pain (22%). On rare instances, women may present with signs of ruptured tumors such as hemoperitoneum (187).

Adenosarcomas are rare and can present with similar symptoms of vaginal bleeding. Some patients also experience pelvic pain, abdominal mass, or vaginal discharge.

Adenosarcomas rarely have extrauterine extension to the ovary, pelvis, or abdominal cavity (187,191).

DIAGNOSIS

Uterine sarcomas are most commonly diagnosed following myomectomy or hysterectomy, and the diagnosis is based on histologic examination. Data regarding diagnostic accuracy of serum markers, biopsy, or imaging are limited.

Endometrial sampling can either be performed via a simple endometrial aspiration or dilation and curettage. Both techniques are used for the detection of epithelial uterine tumors, but since uterine sarcomas typically originate in the deep muscular myometrial layer of the uterus, these tumors may be less accessible by standard endometrial sampling techniques.

Endometrial sampling will yield the correct diagnosis in some patients whose tumors arise from the endometrium (eg, ESS or carcinosarcoma), but can miss between 20 and 75% of uterine sarcomas, particularly leiomyosarcomas, which are generally found in the myometrium (232,233). A retrospective analysis of endometrial sampling (endometrial biopsy or curettage) for uterine sarcoma reported that while invasive neoplasm was identified in 86% of patients with uterine sarcomas, a correct histologic diagnosis was made in 64% of cases (232).

Methods utilizing pulsed Doppler ultrasonography to preoperatively distinguish between a benign leiomyoma and uterine sarcoma are reported (234). Although useful for detecting extrauterine disease, imaging studies such as CT and MRI are not specific for diagnosing sarcomas (235).

In summary, the diagnostic accuracy of serum markers, biopsy, imaging, or their combination are limited in uterine sarcomas. Endometrial biopsy may lead to an accurate diagnosis in some but not all patients, and a negative biopsy does not rule out the disease. Thus, additional diagnostic procedures must be performed if the suspicion of cancer remains high.

PROGNOSIS AND CLINICAL COURSE

Many prognostic factors affect outcome in uterine sarcoma, but the most important is the clinical stage at presentation (205,206,236-239). Disease stage directly affects disease-free and overall survival rates (183,206,239,240).

Leiomyosarcomas are aggressive tumors with recurrence rate of 50 to 70% even at early stages (184). The overall 5-year survival rate ranges from 15 to 25%, and the 5-year survival rate for patients with stages I and II is 40 to 70% (241,242). There has been no consensus on prognostic indicators for leiomyosarcoma. Previous studies have reported mitotic index, cellular atypia, vascular invasion, and tumor size to correlate with survival.

Endometrial stromal sarcomas are indolent tumors (243). Generally, patients with ESS have favorable prognoses; however, recurrence can appear late after primary diagnosis and treatment, even in stage I disease (217,244). FIGO stage, depth of myometrial invasion, tumor grade, positive margins, and patient characteristics such as age, race, and menopausal have been reported to be prognostic factors (188,245-247). Mitotic activity and cytologic atypia were found to be important by some (188,241,248) but not by others (214,217). Extrauterine and nodal disease is prevalent in ESS.

Adenosarcoma is considered a low-grade malignant tumour (59,191,192). Prognosis for patients with adenosarcoma is more favorable than those with carcinosarcoma (191). Distant metastases have been reported in 5% of cases (249). The recurrence rate is approximately 23%, with about one-third of recurrences occurring more than 5 years after initial treatment (59,191). Extrauterine spread at diagnosis, deep infiltrating tumors, sarcomatous overgrowth, and tumor cell necrosis have been associated with increased risk of recurrence (59,241,247,250).

TREATMENT

Surgery

Surgery remains the mainstay of treatment for uterine sarcoma, regardless of histologic type. However, there is some controversy regarding the need for oophorectomy and/or lymph node dissection for each subtype of uterine sarcoma. In general, hysterectomy including oophorectomy with or without lymph node dissection is the treatment of choice.

Oophorectomy for early-stage leiomyosarcomas, particularly in premenopausal women, is controversial, as the incidence of adnexal metastases is low (184). In one study, multivariate analysis showed that oophorectomy for leiomyosarcoma was associated with significantly worse disease-specific survival. Furthermore, case-control investigations implied that ovarian preservation does not adversely affect survival (251). In another study, ovarian metastases were found in about 10% of all cases, despite most having been detected at an early stage (183). Hence, the choice of oophorectomy for the treatment of early-stage leiomyosarcoma should be judged on an individual basis.

The need for lymph node dissection is also controversial. Leiomyosarcoma has substantially lower risk of nodal involvement than clinical stage I or stage II EC with other risk factors. A GOG study of early-stage

sarcoma found that nodal metastases were present in only 3.5% of leiomyosarcoma cases, and the pelvic nodes were twice as likely to be involved than the para-aortic nodes (184). However, the patients in this series underwent lymph node sampling rather than intended dissection, so the reported incidence may be falsely low. Goff et al. found lymph node involvement in about 27% of leiomyosarcoma cases, but only in those cases that involved recurrent or disseminated intraperitoneal disease (227). Two more recent studies identified lymph node metastases in 7 to 11% of patients who underwent lymph node dissection (251,252). In the series by Kapp et al., the 5-year disease-specific survival rate was 26% in patients who had positive lymph nodes compared with 64% in those who had negative nodes (252).

For recovery from ESS, treatment is largely surgical, and hysterectomy with bilateral salpingo-oophorectomy is recommended. ESS is often sensitive to hormones, and patients with in-tact ovaries may be at a higher risk for recurrence (253-256). However, there is no consensus on the absolute need for oophorectomy in early-stage ESS. In a study by Li et al., bilateral salpingo-oophorectomy did not appear to affect time to recurrence or overall survival in patients with stage I ESS (254). In a recent report of 384 women with low-grade ESS, lymph node metastasis and ovarian preservation were not significant prognostic factors for survival in this study. Lymph node metastasis was found in 7% of patients (255). In two smaller series, only two of the nine patients with ESS who had undergone lymph node sampling were found to have lymph node metastases (227,248). The choice of lymph node dissection for ESS should be individualized.

Carcinosarcoma is an aggressive type of uterine sarcoma, and surgical management of carcinosarcoma includes total abdominal hysterectomy with bilateral salpingo-oophorectomy and pelvic and aortic lymph node dissection (257-260). Peritoneal cytology, omentectomy, and peritoneal biopsies are also recommended (257,261-264). Approximately 20 to 60% of patients will have more advanced disease during surgical staging (182,184,265). A recent study reported that in patients with stages I to III uterine carcinosarcomas, 5-year overall survival, disease-free survival, and median survival were significantly improved for patients receiving lymph node dissection compared to those who did not (266). Currently, there are no data regarding the role of cytoreduction in women with advanced carcinosarcoma.

In the absence of strong data on the optimal surgical management of patients with uterine adenosarcoma, we recommend hysterectomy with bilateral salpingo-oophorectomy.

Radiation Therapy

No standard recommendation exists regarding the role of adjuvant radiation for uterine sarcoma. Many studies have reported benefit in locoregional control without a significant impact on survival (206,223,236,267-269). Only a few studies have shown that adjuvant radiation therapy decreases not only locoregional recurrence and is beneficial in terms of 5-year disease-free and overall survival (239,240,270,271).

There are several issues in interpreting these studies. First, many previously-published studies are non-randomized and retrospective. Because of the small number of cases, the different histologic subtypes of uterine sarcoma have been grouped together, further limiting the interpretation of results. There may be differences in radiosensitivity among sarcoma subtypes. Furthermore, there is a propensity for patients with more advanced disease to receive adjuvant radiotherapy, possibly leading to selection bias.

Recently, the EORTC reported on the results of a phase III randomized trial evaluating the role of postoperative radiation in stages I and II uterine sarcomas. The study spanned 13 years and accrued 224 patients with all uterine sarcoma subtypes. All patients were required to have undergone a TAH, BSO, and pelvic cytology. Nodal sampling was optional. Patients were randomized to either observation or pelvic radiation, 51 Gy in 28 fractions over 5 weeks following primary surgery. Results showed a reduction in local relapse for patients with carcinosarcoma and ESS but not patients with leiomyosarcoma. There was no difference in either progression-free survival or overall survival for any subtype (272).

Chemotherapy

Even in the absence of intraperitoneal or lymph node disease, uterine sarcoma has a high rate of distant metastases. Furthermore, recurrence rate is high even for early-stage disease, up to 50 to 70% for carcinosarcoma and leiomyosarcoma in one GOG study (184). The high metastatic potential of uterine sarcoma may necessitate the use of systemic adjuvant treatment such as chemotherapy. Unfortunately, the rarity of this disease along with the heterogeneity in uterine sarcoma subtypes have limited interpretation from randomized controlled trials. Response to systemic therapy is dependent on histologic subtype.

Leiomyosarcoma

Numerous single agents have been used to treat leiomyosarcoma; we recommend doxorubicin and ifosfamide, as these are the most active of these agents for the treatment of advanced uterine leiomyosarcomas. In one GOG study of 28 patients with leiomyosarcoma, the response rate to doxorubicin given every 3 weeks was 25% (273). A subsequent GOG study of liposomal doxorubicin reported overall response rate of 16%, not better than historical comparison to the parent compound (274). Ifosfamide showed more moderate activity, with response rates of about 17% (275,276); paclitaxel showed only limited activity, with a response rate of only 9% (277); and intravenous etoposide led to a response rate of 11% (278), but prolonged oral treatment with the same drug yielded a response rate of only 6.9% (279). Another more recent GOG study of intravenous etoposide showed no response (280). Cisplatin had only limited activity against leiomyosarcoma, producing overall response rates of only 3 to 5% in phase II trials as first- and second-line treatment for advanced or recurrent disease (281,282). Other drugs used in single-agent therapy such as mitoxantrone (283), diaziquone (284), amonafide (285), topotecan (280), and trimetrexate (286) have little activity against leiomyosarcoma (Table 29-16).

Combination chemotherapy for leiomyosarcoma improves response rates. In one phase II trial, the GOG demonstrated an overall response rate to a combination of doxorubicin and dacarbazine of 30% (273); however, another randomized phase III study of doxorubicin and cyclophosphamide showed a response rate of 19%, equal to that of single-agent doxorubicin in this study. In 1996, the same group demonstrated an overall response rate of 18% with a combination of dacarbazine, etoposide, and hydroxyurea (287). A combination of ifosfamide and doxorubicin yielded an overall response rate of 30.3% in advanced, previously untreated leiomyosarcoma (288). More recently, a combination of mitomycin C, doxorubicin, and cisplatin produced an overall response rate of 23% (289); however, this moderate activity was associated with severe pulmonary toxicity, leading to a low therapeutic index. The combination of gemcitabine plus docetaxel in patients with previously treated and untreated leiomyosarcoma led to a response rate of 53% while limiting toxicity (290). Examples of these combination chemotherapies are shown in Table 29-17.

Endometrial Stromal Sarcoma

Because of its rarity and because low-grade ESS usually responds well to hormonal therapy, ESS has not been well studied in chemotherapeutic trials. A GOG study demonstrated an overall response rate of 33.3% among 21 patients given ifosfamide for recurrent or metastatic ESS; none of these patients had been previously treated (291). Information from other studies is limited by small numbers of patients, but the drugs

TABLE
29-16 | **DRUGS USED IN SINGLE-AGENT THERAPY FOR LEIOMYOSARCOMA**

Drug	First Author and Year of Study (Reference)	No. of Patients	Prior Chemotherapy	Drug Dose	Overall Response Rate (%)
Doxorubicin	Omura, 1983 (273)	28	No	60 mg/m^2 q 3 weeks	25
Liposomal Doxorubicin	Sutton, 2005 (274)	35	No	50 mg/m^2 q 4 weeks	16
Ifosfamide	Sutton, 1990(276),* 1992 (275)*	35	No	$1.5 \text{ mg/m}^2 \times 5$ days q 4 weeks	17
Paclitaxel	Sutton, 1999 (277)	33	Yes	175 mg/m^2 q 3 weeks	9
Etoposide	Thigpen, 1996 (280)*	28	No	$100 \text{ mg/m}^2 \times 3$ days q 3 weeks	0
Cisplatin	Thigpen, 1986 (282)*	33	No	50 mg/m^2 q 3 weeks	3
	Thigpen, 1991 (281)*	19	No	50 mg/m^2 q 3 weeks	5
Topotecan	Miller, 2000 (328)	36	Yes	$1.5 \text{ mg/m}^2 \times 5$ days q 3 weeks	11
Trimetrexate	Smith, 2002 (286)*	28	Yes	5 mg/m^2 orally $\times 7$ days q 2 weeks	4.3

*Indicates phase II study.

studied to date have included carboplatin and paclitaxel in an accelerated regimen (292) and oral etoposide (293). Recently, a cisplatin-based chemotherapy regimen was tested in a study of uterine sarcoma in which about 10% of the cases were ESS (294). Despite a relatively high response rate of 54%, the regimen was too toxic to be clinically useful.

Carcinosarcoma

Of the drugs studied as single-agent therapy for carcinosarcoma, three seem to have clear-cut activity: cisplatin (281,295,296), ifosfamide (given with mesna) (297-300), and paclitaxel (301). Of these three drugs, ifosfamide is the most active, producing response rates of approximately 30% regardless of whether or not patients had been treated previously (299,300). One GOG study found that 18% of patients with prior chemotherapy exposure responded to cisplatin (296), nearly the same as the 19% response rate in a repeat trial with previously untreated patients (281). An MD Anderson study in which cisplatin was given at higher doses (75-100 mg/m^2) increased the response rate to 42%, but that study was not a randomized trial and included only a few patients (295). Doxorubicin has inconsistent response rates in the treatment of carcinosarcoma. A study of high-dose doxorubicin conducted at MD Anderson showed no response. Other drugs such as etoposide and mitoxantrone have shown only minimal activity and thus have not been developed further for clinical application (281,302). Findings from

single-agent chemotherapy studies for carcinosarcoma are summarized in Table 29-18.

A combination chemotherapeutic treatment for carcinosarcoma has not had an impressive impact on survival; therefore, we do not routinely recommend this approach. A study of cyclophosphamide, vincristine, doxorubicin, and dacarbazine showed a response rate of only 23% (303). Another study found that adding dacarbazine to doxorubicin insignificantly raised the response rate, from 16.3 to 24.2%, at the cost of higher hematologic and gastrointestinal toxicity (273). However, from this study, the combination therapy was found to be more beneficial (relative to single-agent therapy), particularly in heterologous malignant mixed müllerian tumors, than in other sarcomas. In a phase III randomized comparison of chemonaïve uterine sarcoma, the GOG found that adding cyclophosphamide to doxorubicin did not extend the progression-free interval or improve survival (304). In another study, the same group found that a combination of hydroxyurea, dacarbazine, and etoposide was moderately active, with a response rate of 15.7% (305). A more recent phase II trial by the EORTC involved 41 patients with primary or recurrent carcinosarcoma being treated with a combination of cisplatin, doxorubicin, and ifosfamide. The overall response rate was an impressive 56%, but unfortunately this regimen was associated with severe hematologic and renal toxicity. The authors of this study concluded that cytoreduction and a less toxic platinum-based regimen would be more beneficial for carcinosarcomas (306).

TABLE
29-17

DRUG COMBINATIONS USED TO TREAT UTERINE SARCOMAS

Type of Tumor	Drug Regimen	First Author and Year of Study (Reference)	No. of Patients	Intent	Results
Carcinosarcoma	Dox vs dox + dacarbazine	Omura, 1983 (273)	72	Pall	OR 10 vs 23%
Malignant mixed müllerian tumor	Dox vs dox + cyclophos	Muss, 1985 (304)	20	Pall	OR 25% for both, no benefit of combined Rx
	Dox + cisplatin + ifosfamide	Van Rijswijk, 2003 (306)	41	Pall	OR 56%
	Cyclophos + vincr + dox + dacarbazine	Piver, 1982 (303)	26	Pall	OR 23%
	Eto + hydroxyurea + dacarbazine	Currie, 1996 (287)	32	Pall	OR 15.7%
	Eto + cisplatin + dox	Resnik, 1995 (329)	23	Adj	92% 2-year overall survival
	Epirubicin + cisplatin	Manolitsas, 2001 (330)	38	Adj	74% alive at median follow-up 55 months
	Ifosfamide vs ifosfamide + cisplatin	Sutton, 2000 (298)	194	Pall	36 vs 54%, median PFS 4 vs 6 months ($p < .05$)
	Ifosfamide vs ifosfamide + paclitaxel	Homesley, 2007 (307)	88	Pall	OR 29 vs 45%
Leiomyosarcoma	Dox vs dox + dacarbazine	Omura, 1983 (273)	48	Pall	OR 25 vs 30%
	Dox vs dox + cisplatin	Muss, 1985 (304)	23	Pall	OR 13% for both
	Dox + ifosfamide	Sutton, 1996 (288)	33	Pall	OR 30.3%
	Eto+ hydroxyurea + dacarbazine	Currie, 1996 (287)	39	Pall	OR 18.4%
	Mitomycin C + dox + cisplatin	Edmonson, 2002 (331)	23	Pall	OR 23%
	Gemcitabine + docetaxel	Hensley, 2002 (290)	34	Adj	OR 53%
Sarcoma, not otherwise specified	Dox vs dox + dacarbazine	Omura, 1983 (273)	26	Pall	OR 18 vs 20%
	Dox vs dox + cisplatin	Muss, 1985 (304)	9	Pall	OR 22% for both
	Dox vs no adjuvant therapy	Omura, 1985 (332)	156	Adj	Median overall survival 73 vs 55 months (NS)

Adj, adjuvant; dox, doxorubicin; eto, etoposide; NS, not significant; OR, overall response rate; Pall, palliative; PFS, progression-free survival; SVR, survival rate; Vincr, vincristine; vs, versus.

TABLE
29-18
DRUGS USED IN SINGLE-AGENT THERAPY FOR CARCINOSARCOMA (MIXED MULLERIAN TUMOR) TUMOR

Drug Tested	First Author and Year of Study (Reference)	No. of Patients	Prior Chemotherapy*	Dose	Overall Response Rate (%)
Ifosfamide	Sutton, 1989 (300)[†]	28	Yes	1.2-1.5 g/m^2	32.2
	Sutton, 1990 (299)[†]	26	No	1.5 g/m^2	30.7
Cisplatin	Gershenson, 1987 (295)[†]	12	Yes	75-100 mg/m^2	42
	Thigpen, 1986 (282)[†]	28	Yes	50 mg/m^2	18
	Thigpen, 1991 (281)[†]	63	No	50 mg/m^2	19
Doxorubicin	Gershenson, 1987 (333)	9	Yes and no	50-90 mg/m^2	0
	Omura, 1985 (332)	41	Yes and no	60 mg/m^2	10
Paclitaxel	Curtin, 2001 (301)[†]	33	Yes	170 mg/m^2	21.2
Etoposide	Slayton, 1987 (302)[†]	31	Yes	100 mg/m^2	6
Mitoxantrone	Muss, 1990 (283)	17	Yes and no	12 mg/m^2	0

*Yes and no indicates that some patients had had previous chemotherapy and others had not.
[†]Indicates a phase II study.

A large randomized trial comparing ifosfamide with or without cisplatin for carcinosarcoma found that the combination regimen slightly improved the overall response rate and prolonged the median progression-free interval, but there was no improvement in overall survival (298). More recently, the GOG conducted a phase III trial of ifosfamide with or without paclitaxel in advanced uterine carcinosarcoma. There was an improvement in overall response rate with the addition of paclitaxel to ifosfamide (45% for the combination versus 29% in single-agent ifosfamide). Both median progression-free survival and overall survival were improved (PFS 3.6 versus 5.8 months and OS 8.4 versus 13.5 months, for ifosfamide and ifosfamide and paclitaxel groups, respectively) (307). Examples of these combination chemotherapy regimens are shown in Table 29-18.

Adenosarcoma

Only a few reports have described cases in which adenosarcoma was successfully treated with chemotherapeutic drugs such as liposomal doxorubicin (192). Krivak and colleagues reported adjuvant chemotherapeutic treatment of nine patients with residual or recurrent adenosarcoma with sarcomatous overgrowth. The drugs used were cisplatin and ifosfamide; doxorubicin; and cisplatin and doxorubicin. The progression-free interval for four patients ranged from 7 to 22 months; all patients had died of recurrent or progressive disease by 39 months (226).

In summary, until clear-cut, evidence-based data can be found to support the use of combination chemotherapy regimens for uterine sarcoma, we do not recommend such treatments due to their cost, toxicity, and lack of proven benefit to survival.

Hormonal Treatment

A significant percentage of endometrial stromal sarcomas, leiomyosarcomas, and carcinosarcomas express estrogen receptors. The discovery that estrogen and progesterone receptors are present on over half of all uterine sarcomas has led to the use of hormonal agents as adjuvant therapy, especially for ESS, which has higher rate of hormone receptor expression (308).

Most studies of hormonal agents have focused on treatment outcomes of patients with ESS who had received progestin therapy (309). Isolated cases have been reported in which metastatic or recurrent ESS responded to hormonal agents such as medroxyprogesterone acetate (310,311). Recurrent ESSs have been reported to regress or stabilize using progestin treatment (312,313). Furthermore, progestin therapy in adjuvant setting may prevent recurrences (253). Side effects of long-term high-dose progestin therapy are weight gain, severe depression, and thromboembolic complications (314).

ESS tumor shrinkage following preoperative treatment with gonadotropin-releasing hormone analogs has been reported (315,316). There have been also reports of using aromatase inhibitors such as aminoglutethimide and letrozole for the treatment of ESS (256,317). For recurrent ESS, aromatase inhibitors may have better efficacy in the recurrent disease setting (318,319). Tamoxifen is contraindicated in the treatment of ESS due to its stimulatory effect on the endometrial stromal cells (317,319-321).

Data on the use of other types of hormonal therapy and the other subtypes of uterine sarcoma are more limited.

Summary of diagnosis and management of uterine cancer is shown in Fig. 29-17.

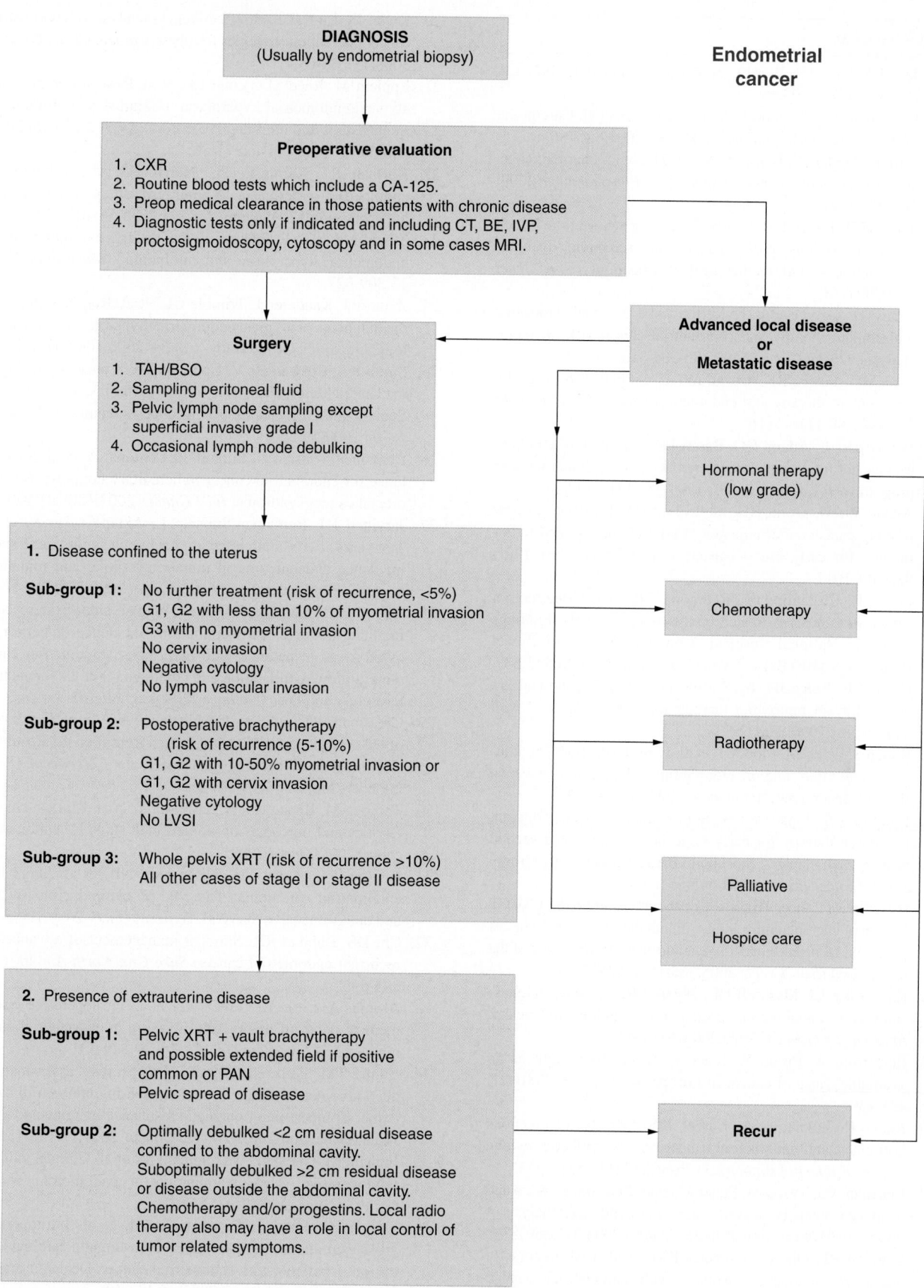

FIGURE 29-17. Uterine algorithm.

References

1. Jemal A, Siegel R, Ward E, et al. Cancer statistics, 2008. *CA Cancer J Clin* 2008;58:71-96.

2. Creasman WT, Odicino F, Maisonneuve P, et al. Carcinoma of the corpus uteri. *J Epidemiol Biostat* 2001;6:47-86.

3. Barrena Medel NI, Bansal S, Miller DS, et al. Pharmacotherapy of endometrial cancer. *Expert Opin Pharmacother* 2009; 10:1939-1951.

4. Lynch HT, Lynch PM, Lanspa SJ, et al. Review of the Lynch syndrome: History, molecular genetics, screening, differential diagnosis, and medicolegal ramifications. *Clin Genet* 2009;76:1-18.

5. Grady D, Gebretsadik T, Kerlikowske K, et al. Hormone replacement therapy and endometrial cancer risk: A meta-analysis. *Obstet Gynecol* 1995;85:304-313.

6. Pike MC, Peters RK, Cozen W, et al. Estrogen-progestin replacement therapy and endometrial cancer. *J Natl Cancer Inst* 1997;89:1110-1116.

7. Weiderpass E, Adami HO, Baron JA, et al. Risk of endometrial cancer following estrogen replacement with and without progestins. *J Natl Cancer Inst* 1999;91:1131-1137.

8. Andersson M, Storm HH, Mouridsen HT. Incidence of new primary cancers after adjuvant tamoxifen therapy and radiotherapy for early breast cancer. *J Natl Cancer Inst* 1991; 83:1013-1017.

9. Fisher B, Costantino JP, Redmond CK, et al. Endometrial cancer in tamoxifen-treated breast cancer patients: Findings from the National Surgical Adjuvant Breast and Bowel Project (NSABP) B-14. *J Natl Cancer Inst* 1994;86:527-537.

10. Curtis RE, Boice JD, Jr., Shriner DA, et al. Second cancers after adjuvant tamoxifen therapy for breast cancer. *J Natl Cancer Inst* 1996;88:832-834.

11. Ryden S, Ferno M, Moller T, et al. Long-term effects of adjuvant tamoxifen and/or radiotherapy. The South Sweden Breast Cancer Trial. *Acta Oncol* 1992;31:271-274.

12. Rutqvist LE, Johansson H, Signomklao T, et al. Adjuvant tamoxifen therapy for early stage breast cancer and second primary malignancies. Stockholm Breast Cancer Study Group. *J Natl Cancer Inst* 1995;87:645-651.

13. Early Breast Cancer Trialists' Collaborative Group (EBCTCG). Effects of chemotherapy and hormonal therapy for early breast cancer on recurrence and 15-year survival: An overview of the randomised trials. *Lancet* 2005;365:1687-1717.

14. Havrilesky LJ, Maxwell GL, Myers ER. Cost-effectiveness analysis of annual screening strategies for endometrial cancer. *Am J Obstet Gynecol* 2009;200:640 e1-e8.

15. Bergstrom A, Pisani P, Tenet V, et al. Overweight as an avoidable cause of cancer in Europe. *Int J Cancer* 2001;91: 421-430.

16. Kaaks R, Lukanova A, Kurzer MS. Obesity, endogenous hormones, and endometrial cancer risk: A synthetic review. *Cancer Epidemiol Biomarkers Prev* 2002;11:1531-1543.

17. Renehan AG, Tyson M, Egger M, et al. Body-mass index and incidence of cancer: A systematic review and meta-analysis of prospective observational studies. *Lancet* 2008;371:569-578.

18. Soliman PT, Oh JC, Schmeler KM, et al. Risk factors for young premenopausal women with endometrial cancer. *Obstet Gynecol* 2005;105:575-580.

19. Thomas CC, Wingo PA, Dolan MS, et al. Endometrial cancer risk among younger, overweight women. *Obstet Gynecol* 2009; 114:22-27.

20. Kwon JS, Lu KH. Cost-effectiveness analysis of endometrial cancer prevention strategies for obese women. *Obstet Gynecol* 2008;112:56-63.

21. Epplein M, Reed SD, Voigt LF, et al. Risk of complex and atypical endometrial hyperplasia in relation to anthropometric measures and reproductive history. *Am J Epidemiol* 2008; 168:563-570; discussion 71-76.

22. Kurman RJ, Kaminski PF, Norris HJ. The behavior of endometrial hyperplasia. A long-term study of "untreated" hyperplasia in 170 patients. *Cancer* 1985;56:403-412.

23. Silverberg SG. Problems in the differential diagnosis of endometrial hyperplasia and carcinoma. *Mod Pathol* 2000; 13:309-327.

24. Zaino RJ, Kauderer J, Trimble CL, et al. Reproducibility of the diagnosis of atypical endometrial hyperplasia: A Gynecologic Oncology Group study. *Cancer* 2006;106:804-811.

25. Smith RA, Cokkinides V, Brawley OW. Cancer screening in the United States, 2009: A review of current American Cancer Society guidelines and issues in cancer screening. *CA Cancer J Clin* 2009;59:27-41.

26. Renkonen-Sinisalo L, Butzow R, Leminen A, et al. Surveillance for endometrial cancer in hereditary nonpolyposis colorectal cancer syndrome. *Int J Cancer* 2007;120:821-824.

27. Jarvinen HJ, Renkonen-Sinisalo L, Aktan-Collan K, et al. Ten years after mutation testing for Lynch syndrome: Cancer incidence and outcome in mutation-positive and mutation-negative family members. *J Clin Oncol* 2009;27:4793-4797.

28. Obermair A, Geramou M, Gucer F, et al. Does hysteroscopy facilitate tumor cell dissemination? Incidence of peritoneal cytology from patients with early stage endometrial carcinoma following dilatation and curettage (D & C) versus hysteroscopy and D & C. *Cancer* 2000;88:139-143.

29. Creasman WT, Odicino F, Maisonneuve P, et al. Carcinoma of the corpus uteri. FIGO 6th Annual Report on the Results of Treatment in Gynecological Cancer. *Int J Gynaecol Obstet* 2006;95(Suppl 1):S105-S143.

30. Tanioka M, Katsumata N, Sasajima Y, et al. Clinical characteristics and outcomes of women with stage IV endometrial cancer. *Med Oncol* 2009.

31. Bristow RE, Zerbe MJ, Rosenshein NB, et al. Stage IVB endometrial carcinoma: The role of cytoreductive surgery and determinants of survival. *Gynecol Oncol* 2000;78:85-91.

32. Chi DS, Barakat RR. Surgical management of advanced or recurrent endometrial cancer. *Surg Clin North Am* 2001;81: 885-896.

33. Altintas A, Cosar E, Vardar MA, et al. Intraoperative assessment of depth of myometrial invasion in endometrial carcinoma. *Eur J Gynaecol Oncol* 1999;20:329-331.

34. Cunha TM, Felix A, Cabral I. Preoperative assessment of deep myometrial and cervical invasion in endometrial carcinoma: Comparison of magnetic resonance imaging and gross visual inspection. *Int J Gynecol Cancer* 2001;11:130-136.

35. Franchi M, Ghezzi F, Melpignano M, et al. Clinical value of intraoperative gross examination in endometrial cancer. *Gynecol Oncol* 2000;76:357-361.

36. Vorgias G, Hintipas E, Katsoulis M, et al. Intraoperative gross examination of myometrial invasion and cervical infiltration in patients with endometrial cancer: Decision-making accuracy. *Gynecol Oncol* 2002;85:483-486.

37. Fanning J, Tsukada Y, Piver MS. Intraoperative frozen section diagnosis of depth of myometrial invasion in endometrial adenocarcinoma. *Gynecol Oncol* 1990;37:47-50.

38. Kayikcioglu F, Pata O, Cengiz S, et al. Accuracy of frozen section diagnosis in borderline ovarian malignancy. *Gynecol Obstet Invest* 2000;49:187-189.

39. Boronow RC, Morrow CP, Creasman WT, et al. Surgical staging in endometrial cancer: Clinical-pathologic findings of a prospective study. *Obstet Gynecol* 1984;63:825-832.

40. Creasman WT, Morrow CP, Bundy BN, et al. Surgical patho-logic spread patterns of endometrial cancer. A Gynecologic Oncology Group study. *Cancer* 1987;60:2035-2041.

41. Girardi F, Petru E, Heydarfadai M, et al. Pelvic lymphadenec-tomy in the surgical treatment of endometrial cancer. *Gynecol Oncol* 1993;49:177-180.

42. Chuang L, Burke TW, Tornos C, et al. Staging laparotomy for endometrial carcinoma: Assessment of retroperitoneal lymph nodes. *Gynecol Oncol* 1995;58:189-193.

43. Kilgore LC, Partridge EE, Alvarez RD, et al. Adenocarci-noma of the endometrium: Survival comparisons of patients with and without pelvic node sampling. *Gynecol Oncol* 1995;56:29-33.

44. Orr JW, Jr., Orr PF, Taylor PT. Surgical staging endometrial cancer. *Clin Obstet Gynecol* 1996;39:656-668.

45. Holub Z, Jabor A, Sprongl L, et al. Clinical outcome, inflam-matory response and tissue trauma in total laparoscopic hys-terectomy: Comparison to laparoscopically-assisted vaginal hysterectomy. *Ceska Gynekol* 2002;67:315-320.

46. Lee YS. Early experience with laparoscopic pelvic lym-phadenectomy in women with gynecologic malignancy. *J Am Assoc Gynecol Laparosc* 1999;6:59-63.

47. Holub Z, Jabor A, Bartos P, et al. Laparoscopic surgery for endometrial cancer: Long-term results of a multicentric study. *Eur J Gynaecol Oncol* 2002;23:305-310.

48. Magrina JF, Mutone NF, Weaver AL, et al. Laparoscopic lymphadenectomy and vaginal or laparoscopic hysterectomy with bilateral salpingo-oophorectomy for endometrial cancer: Morbidity and survival. *Am J Obstet Gynecol* 1999;181:376-381.

49. Muntz HG, Goff BA, Madsen BL, et al. Port-site recurrence after laparoscopic surgery for endometrial carcinoma. *Obstet Gynecol* 1999;93:807-809.

50. Wang PH, Yen MS, Yuan CC, et al. Port site metastasis after laparoscopic-assisted vaginal hysterectomy for endometrial cancer: Possible mechanisms and prevention. *Gynecol Oncol* 1997;66:151-155.

51. Walker JL, Piedmonte MR, Spirtos NM, et al. Laparoscopy compared with laparotomy for comprehensive surgical stag-ing of uterine cancer: Gynecologic Oncology Group study LAP2. *J Clin Oncol* 2009;27:5331-5336.

52. Kornblith AB, Huang HQ, Walker JL, et al. Quality of life of patients with endometrial cancer undergoing laparoscopic International Federation of Gynecology and Obstetrics stag-ing compared with laparotomy: A Gynecologic Oncology Group study. *J Clin Oncol* 2009;27:5337-5342.

53. Ueda SM, Kapp DS, Cheung MK, et al. Trends in demo-graphic and clinical characteristics in women diagnosed with corpus cancer and their potential impact on the increasing number of deaths. *Am J Obstet Gynecol* 2008;198:218 e1-e6.

54. Cowles TA, Magrina JF, Masterson BJ, et al. Comparison of clinical and surgical-staging in patients with endometrial car-cinoma. *Obstet Gynecol* 1985;66:413-416.

55. Kwon JS, Qiu F, Saskin R, et al. Are uterine risk factors more important than nodal status in predicting survival in endome-trial cancer? *Obstet Gynecol* 2009;114:736-743.

56. Zaino RJ, Silverberg SG, Norris HJ, et al. The prognostic value of nuclear versus architectural grading in endometrial adenocarcinoma: A Gynecologic Oncology Group study. *Int J Gynecol Pathol* 1994;13:29-36.

57. Lax SF, Kurman RJ, Pizer ES, et al. A binary architectural grading system for uterine endometrial endometrioid carci-noma has superior reproducibility compared with FIGO grading and identifies subsets of advance-stage tumors with favorable and unfavorable prognosis. *Am J Surg Pathol* 2000;24:1201-1208.

58. Scholten AN, Creutzberg CL, Noordijk EM, et al. Long-term outcome in endometrial carcinoma favors a two- instead of a three-tiered grading system. *Int J Radiat Oncol Biol Phys* 2002;52:1067-1074.

59. Kaku T, Silverberg SG, Major FJ, et al. Adenosarcoma of the uterus: A Gynecologic Oncology Group clinicopathologic study of 31 cases. *Int J Gynecol Pathol* 1992;11:75-88.

60. Ambros RA, Kurman RJ. Identification of patients with stage I uterine endometrioid adenocarcinoma at high risk of recur-rence by DNA ploidy, myometrial invasion, and vascular invasion. *Gynecol Oncol* 1992;45:235-239.

61. Hanson MB, van Nagell JR, Jr., Powell DE, et al. The prog-nostic significance of lymph-vascular space invasion in stage I endometrial cancer. *Cancer* 1985;55:1753-1757.

62. Sivridis E, Buckley CH, Fox H. The prognostic significance of lymphatic vascular space invasion in endometrial adeno-carcinoma. *Br J Obstet Gynaecol* 1987;94:991-994.

63. Cohn DE, Horowitz NS, Mutch DG, et al. Should the presence of lymphvascular space involvement be used to assign patients to adjuvant therapy following hysterectomy for unstaged endometrial cancer? *Gynecol Oncol* 2002;87:243-246.

64. Mariani A, Webb MJ, Keeney GL, et al. Surgical stage I endometrial cancer: Predictors of distant failure and death. *Gynecol Oncol* 2002;87:274-280.

65. Morrow CP, Bundy BN, Kurman RJ, et al. Relationship between surgical-pathological risk factors and outcome in clin-ical stage I and II carcinoma of the endometrium: A Gyneco-logic Oncology Group study. *Gynecol Oncol* 1991;40:55-65.

66. Alektiar KM, McKee A, Lin O, et al. The significance of the amount of myometrial invasion in patients with stage IB endometrial carcinoma. *Cancer* 2002;95:316-321.

67. Kaku T, Tsuruchi N, Tsukamoto N, et al. Reassessment of myometrial invasion in endometrial carcinoma. *Obstet Gynecol* 1994;84:979-982.

68. Hall JB, Young RH, Nelson JH, Jr. The prognostic signifi-cance of adenomyosis in endometrial carcinoma. *Gynecol Oncol* 1984;17:32-40.

69. Jacques SM, Lawrence WD. Endometrial adenocarcinoma with variable-level myometrial involvement limited to ade-nomyosis: A clinicopathologic study of 23 cases. *Gynecol Oncol* 1990;37:401-407.

70. DiSaia PJ, Creasman WT, Boronow RC, et al. Risk factors and recurrent patterns in stage I endometrial cancer. *Am J Obstet Gynecol* 1985;151:1009-1015.

71. Phelan C, Montag AG, Rotmensch J, et al. Outcome and management of pathological stage I endometrial carcinoma patients with involvement of the lower uterine segment. *Gynecol Oncol* 2001;83:513-517.

72. Mayr NA, Wen BC, Benda JA, et al. Postoperative radiation therapy in clinical stage I endometrial cancer: Corpus, cervi-cal, and lower uterine segment involvement–patterns of fail-ure. *Radiology* 1995;196:323-328.

73. Steiner E, Eicher O, Sagemuller J, et al. Multivariate independent prognostic factors in endometrial carcinoma: A clinicopathologic study in 181 patients: 10 years experience at the Department of Obstetrics and Gynecology of the Mainz University. *Int J Gynecol Cancer* 2003;13:197-203.

74. Creasman WT, Disaia PJ, Blessing J, et al. Prognostic significance of peritoneal cytology in patients with endometrial cancer and preliminary data concerning therapy with intraperitoneal radiopharmaceuticals. *Am J Obstet Gynecol* 1981;141: 921-929.

75. Kasamatsu T, Onda T, Katsumata N, et al. Prognostic significance of positive peritoneal cytology in endometrial carcinoma confined to the uterus. *Br J Cancer* 2003;88:245-250.

76. Kodama S, Kase H, Tanaka K, et al. Multivariate analysis of prognostic factors in patients with endometrial cancer. *Int J Gynaecol Obstet* 1996;53:23-30.

77. Kadar N, Homesley HD, Malfetano JH. Positive peritoneal cytology is an adverse factor in endometrial carcinoma only if there is other evidence of extrauterine disease. *Gynecol Oncol* 1992;46:145-149.

78. Lurain JR, Rice BL, Rademaker AW, et al. Prognostic factors associated with recurrence in clinical stage I adenocarcinoma of the endometrium. *Obstet Gynecol* 1991;78:63-69.

79. Lurain JR, Rumsey NK, Schink JC, et al. Prognostic significance of positive peritoneal cytology in clinical stage I adenocarcinoma of the endometrium. *Obstet Gynecol* 1989;74:175-179.

80. Alektiar KM, Venkatraman E, Abu-Rustum N, et al. Is endometrial carcinoma intrinsically more aggressive in elderly patients? *Cancer* 2003;98:2368-2377.

81. Creutzberg CL, van Putten WL, Koper PC, et al. Surgery and postoperative radiotherapy versus surgery alone for patients with stage-1 endometrial carcinoma: Multicentre randomised trial. PORTEC Study Group. Post Operative Radiation Therapy in Endometrial Carcinoma. *Lancet* 2000;355:1404-1411.

82. Jolly S, Vargas CE, Kumar T, et al. The impact of age on long-term outcome in patients with endometrial cancer treated with postoperative radiation. *Gynecol Oncol* 2006;103:87-93.

83. Lee NK, Cheung MK, Shin JY, et al. Prognostic factors for uterine cancer in reproductive-aged women. *Obstet Gynecol* 2007;109:655-662.

84. Mundt AJ, Waggoner S, Yamada D, et al. Age as a prognostic factor for recurrence in patients with endometrial carcinoma. *Gynecol Oncol* 2000;79:79-85.

85. Lachance JA, Everett EN, Greer B, et al. The effect of age on clinical/pathologic features, surgical morbidity, and outcome in patients with endometrial cancer. *Gynecol Oncol* 2006;101: 470-475.

86. Creasman WT. Endometrial cancer: Incidence, prognostic factors, diagnosis, and treatment. *Semin Oncol* 1997;24: S1-140-S1-150.

87. Nyholm HC, Nielsen AL, Lyndrup J, et al. Biochemical and immunohistochemical estrogen and progesterone receptors in adenomatous hyperplasia and endometrial carcinoma: Correlations with stage and other clinicopathologic features. *Am J Obstet Gynecol* 1992;167:1334-1342.

88. Liao BS, Twiggs LB, Leung BS, et al. Cytoplasmic estrogen and progesterone receptors as prognostic parameters in primary endometrial carcinoma. *Obstet Gynecol* 1986;67: 463-467.

89. Creasman WT, Soper JT, McCarty KS, Jr., et al. Influence of cytoplasmic steroid receptor content on prognosis of early stage endometrial carcinoma. *Am J Obstet Gynecol* 1985; 151:922-932.

90. Homesley HD, Zaino R. Endometrial cancer: Prognostic factors. *Semin Oncol* 1994;21:71-78.

91. Susini T, Rapi S, Massi D, et al. Preoperative evaluation of tumor ploidy in endometrial carcinoma: An accurate tool to identify patients at risk for extrauterine disease and recurrence. *Cancer* 1999;86:1005-1012.

92. Zaino RJ, Davis AT, Ohlsson-Wilhelm BM, et al. DNA content is an independent prognostic indicator in endometrial adenocarcinoma. A Gynecologic Oncology Group study. *Int J Gynecol Pathol* 1998;17:312-319.

93. Gurin CC, Federici MG, Kang L, et al. Causes and consequences of microsatellite instability in endometrial carcinoma. *Cancer Res* 1999;59:462-466.

94. MacDonald ND, Salvesen HB, Ryan A, et al. Frequency and prognostic impact of microsatellite instability in a large population-based study of endometrial carcinomas. *Cancer Res* 2000;60:1750-1752.

95. Mutter GL, Boynton KA, Faquin WC, et al. Allelotype mapping of unstable microsatellites establishes direct lineage continuity between endometrial precancers and cancer. *Cancer Res* 1996;56:4483-4486.

96. Sherman ME. Theories of endometrial carcinogenesis: A multidisciplinary approach. *Mod Pathol* 2000;13:295-308.

97. Emons G, Fleckenstein G, Hinney B, et al. Hormonal interactions in endometrial cancer. *Endocr Relat Cancer* 2000;7: 227-242.

98. Berchuck A, Boyd J. Molecular basis of endometrial cancer. *Cancer* 1995;76:2034-2040.

99. Jeyarajah AR, Gallagher CJ, Blake PR, et al. Long-term follow-up of gonadotrophin-releasing hormone analog treatment for recurrent endometrial cancer. *Gynecol Oncol* 1996; 63:47-52.

100. Mutter GL. Histopathology of genetically defined endometrial precancers. *Int J Gynecol Pathol* 2000;19:301-309.

101. Zaino RJ, Kurman RJ, Diana KL, et al. Pathologic models to predict outcome for women with endometrial adenocarcinoma: The importance of the distinction between surgical stage and clinical stage—a Gynecologic Oncology Group study. *Cancer* 1996;77:1115-1121.

102. Mariani A, Dowdy SC, Keeney GL, et al. Predictors of vaginal relapse in stage I endometrial cancer. *Gynecol Oncol* 2005; 97:820-827.

103. Mariani A, Webb MJ, Keeney GL, et al. Predictors of lymphatic failure in endometrial cancer. *Gynecol Oncol* 2002; 84:437-442.

104. Mariani A, Webb MJ, Keeney GL, et al. Hematogenous dissemination in corpus cancer. *Gynecol Oncol* 2001;80:233-238.

105. Lukka H, Chambers A, Fyles A, et al. Adjuvant radiotherapy in women with stage I endometrial cancer: A systematic review. *Gynecol Oncol* 2006;102:361-368.

106. Keys HM, Roberts JA, Brunetto VL, et al. A phase III trial of surgery with or without adjunctive external pelvic radiation therapy in intermediate risk endometrial adenocarcinoma: A Gynecologic Oncology Group study. *Gynecol Oncol* 2004;92: 744-751.

107. Scholten AN, van Putten WL, Beerman H, et al. Postoperative radiotherapy for stage 1 endometrial carcinoma: Long-term outcome of the randomized PORTEC trial with central pathology review. *Int J Radiat Oncol Biol Phys* 2005;63:834-838.

108. Greven KM, Lanciano RM, Herbert SH, et al. Analysis of complications in patients with endometrial carcinoma receiving adjuvant irradiation. *Int J Radiat Oncol Biol Phys* 1991; 21:919-923.

109. Piver MS, Yazigi R, Blumenson L, et al. A prospective trail comparing hysterectomy, hysterectomy plus vaginal radium, and uterine radium plus hysterectomy in stage I endometrial carcinoma. *Obstet Gynecol* 1979;54:85-89.

110. Aalders J, Abeler V, Kolstad P, et al. Postoperative external irradiation and prognostic parameters in stage I endometrial carcinoma: Clinical and histopathologic study of 540 patients. *Obstet Gynecol* 1980;56:419-427.

111. Eltabbakh GH, Piver MS, Hempling RE, et al. Excellent long-term survival and absence of vaginal recurrences in 332 patients with low-risk stage I endometrial adenocarcinoma treated with hysterectomy and vaginal brachytherapy without formal staging lymph node sampling: Report of a prospective trial. *Int J Radiat Oncol Biol Phys* 1997;38:373-380.

112. Fanning J. Long-term survival of intermediate risk endometrial cancer (stage IG3, IC, II) treated with full lymphadenectomy and brachytherapy without teletherapy. *Gynecol Oncol* 2001;82:371-374.

113. Alektiar KM, Venkatraman E, Chi DS, et al. Intravaginal brachytherapy alone for intermediate-risk endometrial cancer. *Int J Radiat Oncol Biol Phys* 2005;62:111-117.

114. Nout RA, Putter, H., Jürgenliemk-Schulz IM, et al. Vaginal brachytherapy versus external beam pelvic radiotherapy for high-intermediate risk endometrial cancer: Results of the randomized PORTEC-2 trial [abstract]. *J Clin Oncol* 2008;26: LBA5503.

115. Lee CM, Szabo A, Shrieve DC, et al. Frequency and effect of adjuvant radiation therapy among women with stage I endometrial adenocarcinoma. *JAMA* 2006;295:389-397.

116. Johnson N, Cornes P. Survival and recurrent disease after postoperative radiotherapy for early endometrial cancer: Systematic review and meta-analysis. *BJOG* 2007;114:1313-1320.

117. Kong A, Johnson N, Cornes P, et al. Adjuvant radiotherapy for stage I endometrial cancer. *Cochrane Database Syst Rev* 2007:CD003916.

118. National Comprehensive Cancer Network. NCCN Guidelines Version 1.2011 Endometrial Carcinoma. http://www.nccn.org. Accessed 12-1-10.

119. Kuten A, Grigsby PW, Perez CA, et al. Results of radiotherapy in recurrent endometrial carcinoma: A retrospective analysis of 51 patients. *Int J Radiat Oncol Biol Phys* 1989;17:29-34.

120. Sears JD, Greven KM, Hoen HM, et al. Prognostic factors and treatment outcome for patients with locally recurrent endometrial cancer. *Cancer* 1994;74:1303-1308.

121. Creutzberg CL, van Putten WL, Koper PC, et al. Survival after relapse in patients with endometrial cancer: Results from a randomized trial. *Gynecol Oncol* 2003;89:201-209.

122. Jhingran A, Burke TW, Eifel PJ. Definitive radiotherapy for patients with isolated vaginal recurrence of endometrial carcinoma after hysterectomy. *Int J Radiat Oncol Biol Phys* 2003;56:1366-1372.

123. Humber CE, Tierney JF, Symonds RP, et al. Chemotherapy for advanced, recurrent or metastatic endometrial cancer: A systematic review of Cochrane collaboration. *Ann Oncol* 2007;18:409-420.

124. Thigpen JT, Blessing JA, DiSaia PJ, et al. A randomized comparison of doxorubicin alone versus doxorubicin plus cyclophosphamide in the management of advanced or recurrent endometrial carcinoma: A Gynecologic Oncology Group study. *J Clin Oncol* 1994;12:1408-1414.

125. Thigpen JT, Brady MF, Homesley HD, et al. Phase III trial of doxorubicin with or without cisplatin in advanced endometrial carcinoma: A Gynecologic Oncology Group study. *J Clin Oncol* 2004;22:3902-3908.

126. Aapro MS, van Wijk FH, Bolis G, et al. Doxorubicin versus doxorubicin and cisplatin in endometrial carcinoma: Definitive results of a randomised study (55872) by the EORTC Gynaecological Cancer Group. *Ann Oncol* 2003;14:441-448.

127. Burke TW, Stringer CA, Morris M, et al. Prospective treatment of advanced or recurrent endometrial carcinoma with cisplatin, doxorubicin, and cyclophosphamide. *Gynecol Oncol* 1991;40:264-267.

128. Muggia FM, Blessing JA, Sorosky J, et al. Phase II trial of the pegylated liposomal doxorubicin in previously treated metastatic endometrial cancer: A Gynecologic Oncology Group study. *J Clin Oncol* 2002;20:2360-2364.

129. Fleming GF, Brunetto VL, Cella D, et al. Phase III trial of doxorubicin plus cisplatin with or without paclitaxel plus filgrastim in advanced endometrial carcinoma: A Gynecologic Oncology Group study. *J Clin Oncol* 2004;22:2159-2166.

130. Ball HG, Blessing JA, Lentz SS, et al. A phase II trial of paclitaxel in patients with advanced or recurrent adenocarcinoma of the endometrium: A Gynecologic Oncology Group study. *Gynecol Oncol* 1996;62:278-281.

131. Lincoln S, Blessing JA, Lee RB, et al. Activity of paclitaxel as second-line chemotherapy in endometrial carcinoma: A Gynecologic Oncology Group study. *Gynecol Oncol* 2003;88: 277-281.

132. Fleming GF, Filiaci VL, Bentley RC, et al. Phase III randomized trial of doxorubicin + cisplatin versus doxorubicin + 24-h paclitaxel + filgrastim in endometrial carcinoma: A Gynecologic Oncology Group study. *Ann Oncol* 2004;15:1173-1178.

133. Burke TW, Munkarah A, Kavanagh JJ, et al. Treatment of advanced or recurrent endometrial carcinoma with single-agent carboplatin. *Gynecol Oncol* 1993;51:397-400.

134. Green JB, 3rd, Green S, Alberts DS, et al. Carboplatin therapy in advanced endometrial cancer. *Obstet Gynecol* 1990;75:696-700.

135. Long HJ, Pfeifle DM, Wieand HS, et al. Phase II evaluation of carboplatin in advanced endometrial carcinoma. *J Natl Cancer Inst* 1988;80:276-278.

136. Morrow CP, Bundy BN, Homesley HD, et al. Doxorubicin as an adjuvant following surgery and radiation therapy in patients with high-risk endometrial carcinoma, stage I and occult stage II: A Gynecologic Oncology Group study. *Gynecol Oncol* 1990;36:166-171.

137. Stringer CA, Gershenson DM, Burke TW, et al. Adjuvant chemotherapy with cisplatin, doxorubicin, and cyclophosphamide (PAC) for early-stage high-risk endometrial cancer: A preliminary analysis. *Gynecol Oncol* 1990;38:305-308.

138. Susumu N, Sagae S, Udagawa Y, et al. Randomized phase III trial of pelvic radiotherapy versus cisplatin-based combined chemotherapy in patients with intermediate- and high-risk endometrial cancer: A Japanese Gynecologic Oncology Group study. *Gynecol Oncol* 2008;108:226-233.

139. Hogberg T, Rosenberg P, Kristensen G, et al. A randomized phase-III study on adjuvant treatment with radiation (RT) ± chemotherapy (CT) in early-stage high-risk endometrial cancer (NSGO-EC-9501/EORTC 55991). ASCO Annual Meeting Proceedings Part I 2007. *J Clin Oncol* 2007;25:5503.

140 Randall ME, Filiaci VL, Muss H, et al. Randomized phase III trial of whole-abdominal irradiation versus doxorubicin and cisplatin chemotherapy in advanced endometrial carcinoma: A Gynecologic Oncology Group study. *J Clin Oncol* 2006; 24:36-44.

141. Martin-Hirsch PL, Lilford RJ, Jarvis GJ. Adjuvant progestagen therapy for the treatment of endometrial cancer: Review and meta-analyses of published randomised controlled trials. *Eur J Obstet Gynecol Reprod Biol* 1996;65:201-207.

142. Lentz SS, Brady MF, Major FJ, et al. High-dose megestrol acetate in advanced or recurrent endometrial carcinoma: A Gynecologic Oncology Group study. *J Clin Oncol* 1996;14: 357-361.

143. Thigpen JT, Brady MF, Alvarez RD, et al. Oral medroxyprogesterone acetate in the treatment of advanced or recurrent endometrial carcinoma: A dose-response study by the Gynecologic Oncology Group. *J Clin Oncol* 1999;17:1736-1744.

144. Vishnevsky AS, Tsyrlina EV, Sofroniy DF, et al. Criteria of endometrial carcinoma sensitivity to hormone therapy: Pathogenetic type of the disease and the tumor reaction to tamoxifen. *Eur J Gynaecol Oncol* 1993;14:139-143.

145. Kline RC, Freedman RS, Jones LA, et al. Treatment of recurrent or metastatic poorly differentiated adenocarcinoma of the endometrium with tamoxifen and medroxyprogesterone acetate. *Cancer Treat Rep* 1987;71:327-328.

146. Moore TD, Phillips PH, Nerenstone SR, et al. Systemic treatment of advanced and recurrent endometrial carcinoma: Current status and future directions. *J Clin Oncol* 1991;9:1071-1088.

147. Pandya KJ, Yeap BY, Weiner LM, et al. Megestrol and tamoxifen in patients with advanced endometrial cancer: An Eastern Cooperative Oncology Group Study (E4882). *Am J Clin Oncol* 2001;24:43-46.

148. Bonte J, Ide P, Billiet G, et al. Tamoxifen as a possible chemotherapeutic agent in endometrial adenocarcinoma. *Gynecol Oncol* 1981;11:140-161.

149. Slavik M, Petty WM, Blessing JA, et al. Phase II clinical study of tamoxifen in advanced endometrial adenocarcinoma: A Gynecologic Oncology Group study. *Cancer Treat Rep* 1984;68:809-811.

150. Covens A, Thomas G, Shaw P, et al. A phase II study of leuprolide in advanced/recurrent endometrial cancer. *Gynecol Oncol* 1997;64:126-129.

151. Markman M, Kennedy A, Webster K, et al. Leuprolide in the treatment of endometrial cancer. *Gynecol Oncol* 1997; 66:542.

152. Gallagher CJ, Oliver RT, Oram DH, et al. A new treatment for endometrial cancer with gonadotrophin releasing-hormone analogue. *Br J Obstet Gynaecol* 1991;98:1037-1041.

153. Asbury RF, Brunetto VL, Lee RB, et al. Goserelin acetate as treatment for recurrent endometrial carcinoma: A Gynecologic Oncology Group study. *Am J Clin Oncol* 2002;25: 557-560.

154. Rose PG, Brunetto VL, VanLe L, et al. A phase II trial of anastrozole in advanced recurrent or persistent endometrial carcinoma: A Gynecologic Oncology Group study. *Gynecol Oncol* 2000;78:212-216.

155. Burke TW, Walker CL. Arzoxifene as therapy for endometrial cancer. *Gynecol Oncol* 2003;90:S40-S46.

156. McMeekin DS, Gordon A, Fowler J, et al. A phase II trial of arzoxifene, a selective estrogen response modulator, in patients with recurrent or advanced endometrial cancer. *Gynecol Oncol* 2003;90:64-69.

157. Decruze SB, Green JA. Hormone therapy in advanced and recurrent endometrial cancer: a systematic review. *International Journal of Gynecological Cancer* 2007;(17)5:964-978.

158. Barakat RR, Goldman NA, Patel DA, et al. Pelvic exenteration for recurrent endometrial cancer. *Gynecol Oncol* 1999; 75:99-102.

159. Morris M, Alvarez RD, Kinney WK, et al. Treatment of recurrent adenocarcinoma of the endometrium with pelvic exenteration. *Gynecol Oncol* 1996;60:288-291.

160. Scarabelli C, Campagnutta E, Giorda G, et al. Maximal cytoreductive surgery as a reasonable therapeutic alternative for recurrent endometrial carcinoma. *Gynecol Oncol* 1998;70:90-93.

161. Zivanovic O, Carter J, Kauff ND, et al. A review of the challenges faced in the conservative treatment of young women with endometrial carcinoma and risk of ovarian cancer. *Gynecol Oncol* 2009;115:504-509.

162. Gotlieb WH, Beiner ME, Shalmon B, et al. Outcome of fertility-sparing treatment with progestins in young patients with endometrial cancer. *Obstet Gynecol* 2003;102:718-725.

163. Kim YB, Holschneider CH, Ghosh K, et al. Progestin alone as primary treatment of endometrial carcinoma in premenopausal women. Report of seven cases and review of the literature. *Cancer* 1997;79:320-327.

164. Ushijima K, Yahata H, Yoshikawa H, et al. Multicenter phase II study of fertility-sparing treatment with medroxyprogesterone acetate for endometrial carcinoma and atypical hyperplasia in young women. *J Clin Oncol* 2007;25:2798-2803.

165. Ramirez PT, Frumovitz M, Bodurka DC, et al. Hormonal therapy for the management of grade 1 endometrial adenocarcinoma: A literature review. *Gynecol Oncol* 2004;95:133-138.

166. Lee TS, Jung JY, Kim JW, et al. Feasibility of ovarian preservation in patients with early stage endometrial carcinoma. *Gynecol Oncol* 2007;104:52-57.

167. Wright JD, Buck AM, Shah M, et al. Safety of ovarian preservation in premenopausal women with endometrial cancer. *J Clin Oncol* 2009;27:1214-1219.

168. Walsh C, Holschneider C, Hoang Y, et al. Coexisting ovarian malignancy in young women with endometrial cancer. *Obstet Gynecol* 2005;106:693-699.

169. Gitsch G, Hanzal E, Jensen D, et al. Endometrial cancer in premenopausal women 45 years and younger. *Obstet Gynecol* 1995;85:504-508.

170. Shamshirsaz AA, Withiam-Leitch M, Odunsi K, et al. Young patients with endometrial carcinoma selected for conservative treatment: A need for vigilance for synchronous ovarian carcinomas, case report and literature review. *Gynecol Oncol* 2007;104:757-760.

171. Berchuck A. Biomarkers in the endometrium. *J Cell Biochem Suppl* 1995;23:174-178.

172. Podczaski E, Kaminski P, Gurski K, et al. Detection and patterns of treatment failure in 300 consecutive cases of "early" endometrial cancer after primary surgery. *Gynecol Oncol* 1992; 47:323-327.

173. Reddoch JM, Burke TW, Morris M, et al. Surveillance for recurrent endometrial carcinoma: Development of a follow-up scheme. *Gynecol Oncol* 1995;59:221-225.

174. Shumsky AG, Stuart GC, Brasher PM, et al. An evaluation of routine follow-up of patients treated for endometrial carcinoma. *Gynecol Oncol* 1994;55:229-233.

175. Rose PG, Sommers RM, Reale FR, et al. Serial serum CA 125 measurements for evaluation of recurrence in patients with endometrial carcinoma. *Obstet Gynecol* 1994;84:12-16.

176. Chapman JA, DiSaia PJ, Osann K, et al. Estrogen replacement in surgical stage I and II endometrial cancer survivors. *Am J Obstet Gynecol* 1996;175:1195-1200.

177. Creasman WT, Henderson D, Hinshaw W, et al. Estrogen replacement therapy in the patient treated for endometrial cancer. *Obstet Gynecol* 1986;67:326-330.

178. Lee RB, Burke TW, Park RC. Estrogen replacement therapy following treatment for stage I endometrial carcinoma. *Gynecol Oncol* 1990;36:189-191.

179. Suriano KA, McHale M, McLaren CE, et al. Estrogen replacement therapy in endometrial cancer patients: A matched control study. *Obstet Gynecol* 2001;97:555-560.

180. Barakat RR, Bundy BN, Spirtos NM, et al. Randomized double-blind trial of estrogen replacement therapy versus placebo in stage I or II endometrial cancer: A Gynecologic Oncology Group study. *J Clin Oncol* 2006;24:587-592.

181. Rossouw JE, Anderson GL, Prentice RL, et al. Risks and benefits of estrogen plus progestin in healthy postmenopausal women: Principal results from the Women's Health Initiative randomized controlled trial. *JAMA* 2002;288:321-333.

182. Amant F, Coosemans A, Debiec-Rychter M, et al. Clinical management of uterine sarcomas. *Lancet Oncol* 2009;10:1188-1198.

183. Gonzalez-Bosquet E, Martinez-Palones JM, Gonzalez-Bosquet J, et al. Uterine sarcoma: A clinicopathological study of 93 cases. *Eur J Gynaecol Oncol* 1997;18:192-195.

184. Major FJ, Blessing JA, Silverberg SG, et al. Prognostic factors in early-stage uterine sarcoma. A Gynecologic Oncology Group study. *Cancer* 1993;71:1702-1709.

185. Doss LL, Llorens AS, Henriquez EM. Carcinosarcoma of the uterus: A 40-year experience from the state of Missouri. *Gynecol Oncol* 1984;18:43-53.

186. Prat J. FIGO staging for uterine sarcomas. *Int J Gynaecol Obstet* 2009;104:177-178.

187. D'Angelo E, Prat J. Uterine sarcomas: A review. *Gynecol Oncol* 2010;116:131-139.

188. Bodner K, Bodner-Adler B, Obermair A, et al. Prognostic parameters in endometrial stromal sarcoma: A clinicopathologic study in 31 patients. *Gynecol Oncol* 2001;81:160-165.

189. Olah KS, Dunn JA, Gee H. Leiomyosarcomas have a poorer prognosis than mixed mesodermal tumours when adjusting for known prognostic factors: The result of a retrospective study of 423 cases of uterine sarcoma. *Br J Obstet Gynaecol* 1992;99:590-594.

190. Piura B, Rabinovich A, Yanai-Inbar I, et al. Uterine sarcoma in the south of Israel: Study of 36 cases. *J Surg Oncol* 1997;64:55-62.

191. Clement PB, Scully RE. Mullerian adenosarcoma of the uterus: A clinicopathologic analysis of 100 cases with a review of the literature. *Hum Pathol* 1990;21:363-381.

192. Verschraegen CF, Vasuratna A, Edwards C, et al. Clinicopathologic analysis of mullerian adenosarcoma: The M.D. Anderson Cancer Center experience. *Oncol Rep* 1998;5: 939-944.

193. Meredith RF, Eisert DR, Kaka Z, et al. An excess of uterine sarcomas after pelvic irradiation. *Cancer* 1986;58: 2003-2007.

194. Sutton G, Kavanagh J, Wolfson A, et al. Corpus: Mesenchymal Tumors. In: Barakat RR, Markman M, Randall ME, (eds). *Principles and Practice of Gynecologic Oncology, 5th ed.* Baltimore, MD: Lippincott Williams & Wilkins; 2009:733-762.

195. Arici DS, Aker H, Yildiz E, et al. Mullerian adenosarcoma of the uterus associated with tamoxifen therapy. *Arch Gynecol Obstet* 2000;264:105-107.

196. Beer TW, Buchanan R, Buckley CH. Uterine stromal sarcoma following tamoxifen treatment. *J Clin Pathol* 1995;48:596.

197. Bouchardy C, Verkooijen HM, Fioretta G, et al. Increased risk of malignant mullerian tumor of the uterus among women with breast cancer treated by tamoxifen. *J Clin Oncol* 2002;20:4403.

198. Eddy GL, Mazur MT. Endolymphatic stromal myosis associated with tamoxifen use. *Gynecol Oncol* 1997;64:262-264.

199. Gillett D. Leiomyosarcoma of the uterus in a woman taking adjuvant tamoxifen therapy. *Med J Aust* 1995;163:160-161.

200. Pang LC. Endometrial stromal sarcoma with sex cord-like differentiation associated with tamoxifen therapy. *South Med J* 1998;91:592-594.

201. Wickerham DL, Fisher B, Wolmark N, et al. Association of tamoxifen and uterine sarcoma. *J Clin Oncol* 2002;20: 2758-2760.

202. Bergman L, Beelen ML, Gallee MP, et al. Risk and prognosis of endometrial cancer after tamoxifen for breast cancer. Comprehensive Cancer Centres' ALERT Group. Assessment of Liver and Endometrial cancer Risk following Tamoxifen. *Lancet* 2000;356:881-887.

203. Fisher B, Costantino JP, Wickerham DL, et al. Tamoxifen for prevention of breast cancer: Report of the National Surgical Adjuvant Breast and Bowel Project P-1 Study. *J Natl Cancer Inst* 1998;90:1371-1388.

204. Amant F, Dreyer L, Makin J, et al. Uterine sarcomas in South African black women: A clinicopathologic study with ethnic considerations. *Eur J Gynaecol Oncol* 2001;22:194-200.

205. El Husseiny G, Al Bareedy N, Mourad WA, et al. Prognostic factors and treatment modalities in uterine sarcoma. *Am J Clin Oncol* 2002;25:256-260.

206. Jereczek B, Jassem J, Kobierska A. Sarcoma of the uterus. A clinical study of 42 patients. *Arch Gynecol Obstet* 1996;258: 171-180.

207. Tinkler SD, Cowie VJ. Uterine sarcomas: A review of the Edinburgh experience from 1974 to 1992. *Br J Radiol* 1993; 66:998-1001.

208. Kunzel KE, Mills NZ, Muderspach LI, et al. Myxoid leiomyosarcoma of the uterus. *Gynecol Oncol* 1993;48: 277-280.

209. Schneider D, Halperin R, Segal M, et al. Myxoid leiomyosarcoma of the uterus with unusual malignant histologic pattern– a case report. *Gynecol Oncol* 1995;59:156-158.

210. Clement PB. The pathology of uterine smooth muscle tumors and mixed endometrial stromal-smooth muscle tumors: A selective review with emphasis on recent advances. *Int J Gynecol Pathol* 2000;19:39-55.

211. Bell SW, Kempson RL, Hendrickson MR. Problematic uterine smooth muscle neoplasms. A clinicopathologic study of 213 cases. *Am J Surg Pathol* 1994;18:535-558.

212. Ip PP, Cheung AN, Clement PB. Uterine smooth muscle tumors of uncertain malignant potential (STUMP): A clinicopathologic analysis of 16 cases. *Am J Surg Pathol* 2009;33:992-1005.

213. Guntupalli SR, Ramirez PT, Anderson ML, et al. Uterine smooth muscle tumor of uncertain malignant potential: A retrospective analysis. *Gynecol Oncol* 2009;113:324-326.

214. Evans HL. Endometrial stromal sarcoma and poorly differentiated endometrial sarcoma. *Cancer* 1982;50:2170-2182.

215. Zaloudek C, Hendrickson MR. *Mesenchymal Tumor of the Uterus*, 5th ed. New York: Springer-Verlag; 2002.

216. Berchuck A, Rubin SC, Hoskins WJ, et al. Treatment of endometrial stromal tumors. *Gynecol Oncol* 1990;36:60-65.

217. Chang KL, Crabtree GS, Lim-Tan SK, et al. Primary uterine endometrial stromal neoplasms. A clinicopathologic study of 117 cases. *Am J Surg Pathol* 1990;14:415-438.

218. August CZ, Bauer KD, Lurain J, et al. Neoplasms of endometrial stroma: Histopathologic and flow cytometric analysis with clinical correlation. *Hum Pathol* 1989;20:232-237.

219. McCluggage WG. Uterine carcinosarcomas (malignant mixed Mullerian tumors) are metaplastic carcinomas. *Int J Gynecol Cancer* 2002;12:687-690.

220. McCluggage WG. Malignant biphasic uterine tumours: Carcinosarcomas or metaplastic carcinomas? *J Clin Pathol* 2002;55:321-325.

221. Lam KY, Khoo US, Cheung A. Collision of endometrioid carcinoma and stromal sarcoma of the uterus: A report of two cases. *Int J Gynecol Pathol* 1999;18:77-81.

222. Larson B, Silfversward C, Nilsson B, et al. Prognostic factors in uterine leiomyosarcoma. A clinical and histopathological study of 143 cases. The Radiumhemmet series 1936-1981. *Acta Oncol* 1990;29:185-191.

223. Nielsen SN, Podratz KC, Scheithauer BW, et al. Clinico-pathologic analysis of uterine malignant mixed mullerian tumors. *Gynecol Oncol* 1989;34:372-378.

224. Silverberg SG, Major FJ, Blessing JA, et al. Carcinosarcoma (malignant mixed mesodermal tumor) of the uterus. A Gynecologic Oncology Group pathologic study of 203 cases. *Int J Gynecol Pathol* 1990;9:1-19.

225. Fehmian C, Jones J, Kress Y, et al. Adenosarcoma of the uterus with extensive smooth muscle differentiation: Ultra-structural study and review of the literature. *Ultrastruct Pathol* 1997;21:73-79.

226. Krivak TC, Seidman JD, McBroom JW, et al. Uterine adenosarcoma with sarcomatous overgrowth versus uterine carcinosarcoma: Comparison of treatment and survival. *Gynecol Oncol* 2001;83:89-94.

227. Goff BA, Rice LW, Fleischhacker D, et al. Uterine leiomyosarcoma and endometrial stromal sarcoma: Lymph node metastases and sites of recurrence. *Gynecol Oncol* 1993;50:105-109.

228. Iwasa Y, Haga H, Konishi I, et al. Prognostic factors in uterine carcinosarcoma: A clinicopathologic study of 25 patients. *Cancer* 1998;82:512-519.

229. Larson B, Silfversward C, Nilsson B, et al. Endometrial stromal sarcoma of the uterus. A clinical and histopathological study. The Radiumhemmet series 1936-1981. *Eur J Obstet Gynecol Reprod Biol* 1990;35:239-249.

230. Hoskins PJ, Le N. Preoperative tumor markers at diagnosis in women with malignant mixed mullerian tumors/carcinosarcoma of the uterus. *Int J Gynecol Cancer* 2008;18:1200-1201.

231. Huang GS, Chiu LG, Gebb JS, et al. Serum CA125 predicts extrauterine disease and survival in uterine carcinosarcoma. *Gynecol Oncol* 2007;107:513-517.

232. Bansal N, Herzog TJ, Burke W, et al. The utility of preoperative endometrial sampling for the detection of uterine sarcomas. *Gynecol Oncol* 2008;110:43-48.

233. Sagae S, Yamashita K, Ishioka S, et al. Preoperative diagnosis and treatment results in 106 patients with uterine sarcoma in Hokkaido, Japan. *Oncology* 2004;67:33-39.

234. Hata K, Hata T, Maruyama R, et al. Uterine sarcoma: Can it be differentiated from uterine leiomyoma with Doppler ultrasonography? A preliminary report. *Ultrasound Obstet Gynecol* 1997;9:101-104.

235. Rha SE, Byun JY, Jung SE, et al. CT and MRI of uterine sarcomas and their mimickers. *AJR Am J Roentgenol* 2003;181:1369-1374.

236. Kahanpaa KV, Wahlstrom T, Grohn P, et al. Sarcomas of the uterus: A clinicopathologic study of 119 patients. *Obstet Gynecol* 1986;67:417-424.

237. Peters WA, 3rd, Kumar NB, Fleming WP, et al. Prognostic features of sarcomas and mixed tumors of the endometrium. *Obstet Gynecol* 1984;63:550-556.

238. Wolfson AH, Wolfson DJ, Sittler SY, et al. A multivariate analysis of clinicopathologic factors for predicting outcome in uterine sarcomas. *Gynecol Oncol* 1994;52:56-62.

239. Soumarova R, Horova H, Seneklova Z, et al. Treatment of uterine sarcoma. A survey of 49 patients. *Arch Gynecol Obstet* 2002;266:92-95.

240. Knocke TH, Kucera H, Dorfler D, et al. Results of postoperative radiotherapy in the treatment of sarcoma of the corpus uteri. *Cancer* 1998;83:1972-1979.

241. Abeler VM, Royne O, Thoresen S, et al. Uterine sarcomas in Norway. A histopathological and prognostic survey of a total population from 1970 to 2000 including 419 patients. *Histopathology* 2009;54:355-364.

242. D'Angelo E, Spagnoli LG, Prat J. Comparative clinicopathologic and immunohistochemical analysis of uterine sarcomas diagnosed using the World Health Organization classification system. *Hum Pathol* 2009;40:1571-1585.

243. Dionigi A, Oliva E, Clement PB, et al. Endometrial stromal nodules and endometrial stromal tumors with limited infiltration: A clinicopathologic study of 50 cases. *Am J Surg Pathol* 2002;26:567-581.

244. Thomas MB, Keeney GL, Podratz KC, et al. Endometrial stromal sarcoma: Treatment and patterns of recurrence. *Int J Gynecol Cancer* 2009;19:253-256.

245. Chan JK, Kawar NM, Shin JY, et al. Endometrial stromal sarcoma: A population-based analysis. *Br J Cancer* 2008;99:1210-1215.

246. Haberal A, Kayikcioglu F, Boran N, et al. Endometrial stromal sarcoma of the uterus: Analysis of 25 patients. *Eur J Obstet Gynecol Reprod Biol* 2003;109:209-213.

247. Nordal RR, Kristensen GB, Kaern J, et al. The prognostic significance of surgery, tumor size, malignancy grade, menopausal status, and DNA ploidy in endometrial stromal sarcoma. *Gynecol Oncol* 1996;62:254-259.

248. Gadducci A, Sartori E, Landoni F, et al. Endometrial stromal sarcoma: Analysis of treatment failures and survival. *Gynecol Oncol* 1996;63:247-253.

249. Moinfar F, Azodi M, Tavassoli FA. Uterine sarcomas. *Pathology* 2007;39:55-71.

250. Seidman JD, Wasserman CS, Aye LM, et al. Cluster of uterine mullerian adenosarcoma in the Washington, DC metropolitan area with high incidence of sarcomatous overgrowth. *Am J Surg Pathol* 1999;23:809-814.

251. Giuntoli RL, 2nd, Metzinger DS, DiMarco CS, et al. Retrospective review of 208 patients with leiomyosarcoma of the uterus: Prognostic indicators, surgical management, and adjuvant therapy. *Gynecol Oncol* 2003;89:460-469.

252. Kapp DS, Shin JY, Chan JK. Prognostic factors and survival in 1396 patients with uterine leiomyosarcomas: Emphasis on impact of lymphadenectomy and oophorectomy. *Cancer* 2008;112:820-830.

253. Chu MC, Mor G, Lim C, et al. Low-grade endometrial stromal sarcoma: Hormonal aspects. *Gynecol Oncol* 2003;90:170-176.

254. Li AJ, Giuntoli RL, 2nd, Drake R, et al. Ovarian preservation in stage I low-grade endometrial stromal sarcomas. *Obstet Gynecol* 2005;106:1304-1308.

255. Shah JP, Bryant CS, Kumar S, et al. Lymphadenectomy and ovarian preservation in low-grade endometrial stromal sarcoma. *Obstet Gynecol* 2008;112:1102-1108.

256. Spano JP, Soria JC, Kambouchner M, et al. Long-term survival of patients given hormonal therapy for metastatic endometrial stromal sarcoma. *Med Oncol* 2003;20:87-93.

257. Gadducci A, Cosio S, Romanini A, et al. The management of patients with uterine sarcoma: A debated clinical challenge. *Crit Rev Oncol Hematol* 2008;65:129-142.

258. Callister M, Ramondetta LM, Jhingran A, et al. Malignant mixed Mullerian tumors of the uterus: Analysis of patterns of failure, prognostic factors, and treatment outcome. *Int J Radiat Oncol Biol Phys* 2004;58:786-796.

259. Livi L, Paiar F, Shah N, et al. Uterine sarcoma: Twenty-seven years of experience. *Int J Radiat Oncol Biol Phys* 2003; 57:1366-1373.

260. Villena-Heinsen C, Diesing D, Fischer D, et al. Carcinosarcomas—a retrospective analysis of 21 patients. *Anticancer Res* 2006;26:4817-4823.

261. Ali S, Wells M. Mixed Mullerian tumors of the uterine corpus: A review. *Int J Gynecol Cancer* 1993;3:1-11.

262. Morice P, Rodriguez A, Rey A, et al. Prognostic value of initial surgical procedure for patients with uterine sarcoma: Analysis of 123 patients. *Eur J Gynaecol Oncol* 2003;24: 237-240.

263. Sartori E, Bazzurini L, Gadducci A, et al. Carcinosarcoma of the uterus: A clinicopathological multicenter CTF study. *Gynecol Oncol* 1997;67:70-75.

264. Vaccarello L, Curtin JP. Presentation and management of carcinosarcoma of the uterus. *Oncology (Williston Park)* 1992; 6:45-49; discussion 53-54, 59.

265. Yamada SD, Burger RA, Brewster WR, et al. Pathologic variables and adjuvant therapy as predictors of recurrence and survival for patients with surgically evaluated carcinosarcoma of the uterus. *Cancer* 2000;88:2782-2786.

266. Nemani D, Mitra N, Guo M, et al. Assessing the effects of lymphadenectomy and radiation therapy in patients with uterine carcinosarcoma: A SEER analysis. *Gynecol Oncol* 2008; 111:82-88.

267. Echt G, Jepson J, Steel J, et al. Treatment of uterine sarcomas. *Cancer* 1990;66:35-39.

268. Salazar OM, Bonfiglio TA, Patten SF, et al. Uterine sarcomas: Analysis of failures with special emphasis on the use of adjuvant radiation therapy. *Cancer* 1978;42:1161-1170.

269. Sorbe B. Radiotherapy and/or chemotherapy as adjuvant treatment of uterine sarcomas. *Gynecol Oncol* 1985;20:281-289.

270. Le T. Adjuvant pelvic radiotherapy for uterine carcinosarcoma in a high risk population. *Eur J Surg Oncol* 2001;27: 282-285.

271. Moskovic E, MacSweeney E, Law M, et al. Survival, patterns of spread and prognostic factors in uterine sarcoma: A study of 76 patients. *Br J Radiol* 1993;66:1009-1015.

272. Reed NS, Mangioni C, Malmstrom H, et al. Phase III randomised study to evaluate the role of adjuvant pelvic radiotherapy in the treatment of uterine sarcomas stages I and II: An European Organisation for Research and Treatment of Cancer Gynaecological Cancer Group Study (protocol 55874). *Eur J Cancer* 2008;44:808-818.

273. Omura GA, Major FJ, Blessing JA, et al. A randomized study of adriamycin with and without dimethyl triazenoimidazole carboxamide in advanced uterine sarcomas. *Cancer* 1983; 52:626-632.

274. Sutton G, Blessing J, Hanjani P, et al. Phase II evaluation of liposomal doxorubicin (Doxil) in recurrent or advanced leiomyosarcoma of the uterus: A Gynecologic Oncology Group study. *Gynecol Oncol* 2005;96:749-752.

275. Sutton GP, Blessing JA, Barrett RJ, et al. Phase II trial of ifosfamide and mesna in leiomyosarcoma of the uterus: A Gynecologic Oncology Group study. *Am J Obstet Gynecol* 1992;166:556-559.

276. Sutton GP, Blessing JA, Photopulos G, et al. Gynecologic Oncology Group experience with ifosfamide. *Semin Oncol* 1990;17:6-10.

277. Sutton G, Blessing JA, Ball H. Phase II trial of paclitaxel in leiomyosarcoma of the uterus: A Gynecologic Oncology Group study. *Gynecol Oncol* 1999;74:346-349.

278. Slayton RE, Blessing JA, Angel C, et al. Phase II trial of etoposide in the management of advanced and recurrent leiomyosarcoma of the uterus: A Gynecologic Oncology Group study. *Cancer Treat Rep* 1987;71:1303-1304.

279. Rose PG, Blessing JA, Soper JT, et al. Prolonged oral etoposide in recurrent or advanced leiomyosarcoma of the uterus: A Gynecologic Oncology Group study. *Gynecol Oncol* 1998; 70:267-271.

280. Thigpen T, Blessing JA, Yordan E, et al. Phase II trial of etoposide in leiomyosarcoma of the uterus: A Gynecologic Oncology Group study. *Gynecol Oncol* 1996;63:120-122.

281. Thigpen JT, Blessing JA, Beecham J, et al. Phase II trial of cisplatin as first-line chemotherapy in patients with advanced or recurrent uterine sarcomas: A Gynecologic Oncology Group study. *J Clin Oncol* 1991;9:1962-1966.

282. Thigpen JT, Blessing JA, Wilbanks GD. Cisplatin as second-line chemotherapy in the treatment of advanced or recurrent leiomyosarcoma of the uterus. A phase II trial of the Gynecologic Oncology Group. *Am J Clin Oncol* 1986;9:18-20.

283. Muss HB, Bundy BN, Adcock L, et al. Mitoxantrone in the treatment of advanced uterine sarcoma. A phase II trial of the Gynecologic Oncology Group. *Am J Clin Oncol* 1990; 13:32-34.

284. Slayton RE, Blessing JA, Clarke-Pearson D. A phase II trial of diaziquone (AZQ) in mixed mesodermal sarcomas of the uterus. A Gynecologic Oncology Group study. *Invest New Drugs* 1991;9:93-94.

285. Asbury R, Blessing JA, Smith DM, et al. Aminothiadiazole in the treatment of advanced leiomyosarcoma of the uterine corpus. A Gynecologic Oncology Group study. *Am J Clin Oncol* 1995;18:397-399.

286. Smith HO, Blessing JA, Vaccarello L. Trimetrexate in the treatment of recurrent or advanced leiomyosarcoma of the uterus: A phase II study of the Gynecologic Oncology Group. *Gynecol Oncol* 2002;84:140-144.

287. Currie J, Blessing JA, Muss HB, et al. Combination chemotherapy with hydroxyurea, dacarbazine (DTIC), and etoposide in the treatment of uterine leiomyosarcoma: A Gynecologic Oncology Group study. *Gynecol Oncol* 1996;61:27-30.

288. Sutton G, Blessing JA, Malfetano JH. Ifosfamide and doxorubicin in the treatment of advanced leiomyosarcomas of the uterus: A Gynecologic Oncology Group study. *Gynecol Oncol* 1996;62:226-229.

289. Edmonson JH, Marks RS, Buckner JC, et al. Contrast of response to dacarbazine, mitomycin, doxorubicin, and cisplatin (DMAP) plus GM-CSF between patients with advanced malignant gastrointestinal stromal tumors and patients with other advanced leiomyosarcomas. *Cancer Invest* 2002;20:605-612.

290. Hensley ML, Maki R, Venkatraman E, et al. Gemcitabine and docetaxel in patients with unresectable leiomyosarcoma: Results of a phase II trial. *J Clin Oncol* 2002;20:2824-2831.

291. Sutton G, Blessing JA, Park R, et al. Ifosfamide treatment of recurrent or metastatic endometrial stromal sarcomas previously unexposed to chemotherapy: A study of the Gynecologic Oncology Group. *Obstet Gynecol* 1996;87:747-750.

292. Szlosarek PW, Lofts FJ, Pettengell R, et al. Effective treatment of a patient with a high-grade endometrial stromal sarcoma with an accelerated regimen of carboplatin and paclitaxel. *Anticancer Drugs* 2000;11:275-278.

293. Lin YC, Kudelka AP, Tresukosol D, et al. Prolonged stabilization of progressive endometrial stromal sarcoma with prolonged oral etoposide therapy. *Gynecol Oncol* 1995;58:262-265.

294. Pautier P, Genestie C, Fizazi K, et al. Cisplatin-based chemotherapy regimen (DECAV) for uterine sarcomas. *Int J Gynecol Cancer* 2002;12:749-754.

295. Gershenson DM, Kavanagh JJ, Copeland LJ, et al. Cisplatin therapy for disseminated mixed mesodermal sarcoma of the uterus. *J Clin Oncol* 1987;5:618-621.

296. Thigpen JT, Blessing JA, Orr JW, Jr., et al. Phase II trial of cisplatin in the treatment of patients with advanced or recurrent mixed mesodermal sarcomas of the uterus: A Gynecologic Oncology Group study. *Cancer Treat Rep* 1986;70:271-274.

297. Kushner DM, Webster KD, Belinson JL, et al. Safety and efficacy of adjuvant single-agent ifosfamide in uterine sarcoma. *Gynecol Oncol* 2000;78:221-227.

298. Sutton G, Brunetto VL, Kilgore L, et al. A phase III trial of ifosfamide with or without cisplatin in carcinosarcoma of the uterus: A Gynecologic Oncology Group study. *Gynecol Oncol* 2000;79:147-153.

299. Sutton GP, Blessing JA, Photopulos G, et al. Early phase II Gynecologic Oncology Group experience with ifosfamide/mesna in gynecologic malignancies. *Cancer Chemother Pharmacol* 1990;26(Suppl):S55-S58.

300. Sutton GP, Blessing JA, Rosenshein N, et al. Phase II trial of ifosfamide and mesna in mixed mesodermal tumors of the uterus (a Gynecologic Oncology Group study). *Am J Obstet Gynecol* 1989;161:309-312.

301. Curtin JP, Blessing JA, Soper JT, et al. Paclitaxel in the treatment of carcinosarcoma of the uterus: A Gynecologic Oncology Group study. *Gynecol Oncol* 2001;83:268-270.

302. Slayton RE, Blessing JA, DiSaia PJ, et al. Phase II trial of etoposide in the management of advanced or recurrent mixed mesodermal sarcomas of the uterus: A Gynecologic Oncology Group study. *Cancer Treat Rep* 1987;71:661-662.

303. Piver MS, DeEulis TG, Lele SB, et al. Cyclophosphamide, vincristine, adriamycin, and dimethyl-triazeno imidazole carboxamide (CYVADIC) for sarcomas of the female genital tract. *Gynecol Oncol* 1982;14:319-323.

304. Muss HB, Bundy B, DiSaia PJ, et al. Treatment of recurrent or advanced uterine sarcoma. A randomized trial of doxorubicin versus doxorubicin and cyclophosphamide (a phase III trial of the Gynecologic Oncology Group). *Cancer* 1985;55:1648-1653.

305. Currie JL, Blessing JA, McGehee R, et al. Phase II trial of hydroxyurea, dacarbazine (DTIC), and etoposide (VP-16) in mixed mesodermal tumors of the uterus: A Gynecologic Oncology Group study. *Gynecol Oncol* 1996;61:94-96.

306. van Rijswijk RE, Vermorken JB, Reed N, et al. Cisplatin, doxorubicin and ifosfamide in carcinosarcoma of the female genital tract. A phase II study of the European Organization for Research and Treatment of Cancer Gynaecological Cancer Group (EORTC 55923). *Eur J Cancer* 2003;39:481-487.

307. Homesley HD, Filiaci V, Markman M, et al. Phase III trial of ifosfamide with or without paclitaxel in advanced uterine carcinosarcoma: A Gynecologic Oncology Group study. *J Clin Oncol* 2007;25:526-531.

308. Sutton GP, Stehman FB, Michael H, et al. Estrogen and progesterone receptors in uterine sarcomas. *Obstet Gynecol* 1986;68:709-714.

309. Reich O, Regauer S. Hormonal therapy of endometrial stromal sarcoma. *Curr Opin Oncol* 2007;19:347-352.

310. Mansi JL, Ramachandra S, Wiltshaw E, et al. Endometrial stromal sarcomas. *Gynecol Oncol* 1990;36:113-118.

311. O'Brien AA, O'Briain DS, Daly PA. Aggressive endometrial stromal sarcoma responding to medroxyprogesterone following failure of tamoxifen and combination chemotherapy. Case report. *Br J Obstet Gynaecol* 1985;92:862-866.

312. Gadducci A, Cosio S, Genazzani AR. Use of estrogen antagonists and aromatase inhibitors in breast cancer and hormonally sensitive tumors of the uterine body. *Curr Opin Investig Drugs* 2004;5:1031-1044.

313. Geas FL, Tewari DS, Rutgers JK, et al. Surgical cytoreduction and hormone therapy of an advanced endometrial stromal sarcoma of the ovary. *Obstet Gynecol* 2004;103:1051-1054.

314. Jordan VC. Medroxyprogesterone acetate and metastases: Of mice and (wo)men. *J Natl Cancer Inst* 2005;97:619-621.

315. Burke C, Hickey K. Treatment of endometrial stromal sarcoma with a gonadotropin-releasing hormone analogue. *Obstet Gynecol* 2004;104:1182-1184.

316. Mesia AF, Demopoulos RI. Effects of leuprolide acetate on low-grade endometrial stromal sarcoma. *Am J Obstet Gynecol* 2000;182:1140-1141.

317. Leunen M, Breugelmans M, De Sutter P, et al. Low-grade endometrial stromal sarcoma treated with the aromatase inhibitor letrozole. *Gynecol Oncol* 2004;95:769-771.

318. Maluf FC, Sabbatini P, Schwartz L, et al. Endometrial stromal sarcoma: Objective response to letrozole. *Gynecol Oncol* 2001;82:384-388.

319. Pink D, Lindner T, Mrozek A, et al. Harm or benefit of hormonal treatment in metastatic low-grade endometrial stromal sarcoma: Single center experience with 10 cases and review of the literature. *Gynecol Oncol* 2006;101:464-469.

320. Reich O, Regauer S. Is tamoxifen an option for patients with endometrial stromal sarcoma? *Gynecol Oncol* 2005;96:561; author reply.

321. Reich O, Regauer S. Estrogen replacement therapy and tamoxifen are contraindicated in patients with endometrial stromal sarcoma. *Gynecol Oncol* 2006;102:413-414; author reply 4.

322. Mundt AJ, McBride R, Rotmensch J, et al. Significant pelvic recurrence in high-risk pathologic stage I-IV endometrial carcinoma patients after adjuvant chemotherapy alone: Implications for adjuvant radiation therapy. *Int J Radiat Oncol Biol Phys* 2001;50:1145-1153.

323. Sutton GP, Blessing JA, Homesley HD, et al. Phase II study of ifosfamide and mesna in refractory adenocarcinoma of the endometrium. A Gynecologic Oncology Group study. *Cancer* 1994;73:1453-1455.

324. Deppe G, Malviya VK, Malone JM, et al. Treatment of recurrent and metastatic endometrial carcinoma with cisplatin and doxorubicin. *Eur J Gynaecol Oncol* 1994;15:263-266.

325. Fleming GF, Fowler JM, Waggoner SE, et al. Phase I trial of escalating doses of paclitaxel combined with fixed doses of cisplatin and doxorubicin in advanced endometrial cancer and other gynecologic malignancies: A Gynecologic Oncology Group study. *J Clin Oncol* 2001;19:1021-1029.

326. Miller DS, Blessing JA, Lentz SS, et al. A phase II trial of topotecan in patients with advanced, persistent, or recurrent endometrial carcinoma: A Gynecologic Oncology Group study. *Gynecol Oncol* 2002;87:247-251.

327. Gadducci A, Romanini A, Cosio S, et al. Combination of cisplatin, epirubicin, and cyclophosphamide (PEC regimen) in advanced or recurrent endometrial cancer: A retrospective clinical study. *Anticancer Res* 1999;19:2253-2256.

328. Miller DS, Blessing JA, Kilgore LC, et al. Phase II trial of topotecan in patients with advanced, persistent, or recurrent uterine leiomyosarcomas: A Gynecologic Oncology Group study. *Am J Clin Oncol* 2000;23:355-357.

329. Resnik E, Chambers SK, Carcangiu ML, et al. A phase II study of etoposide, cisplatin, and doxorubicin chemotherapy in mixed mullerian tumors (MMT) of the uterus. *Gynecol Oncol* 1995;56:370-375.

330. Manolitsas TP, Wain GV, Williams KE, et al. Multimodality therapy for patients with clinical stage I and II malignant mixed Mullerian tumors of the uterus. *Cancer* 2001;91:1437-1443.

331. Edmonson JH, Blessing JA, Cosin JA, et al. Phase II study of mitomycin, doxorubicin, and cisplatin in the treatment of advanced uterine leiomyosarcoma: A Gynecologic Oncology Group study. *Gynecol Oncol* 2002;85:507-510.

332. Omura GA, Blessing JA, Major F, et al. A randomized clinical trial of adjuvant adriamycin in uterine sarcomas: A Gynecologic Oncology Group study. *J Clin Oncol* 1985;3:1240-1245.

333. Gershenson DM, Kavanagh JJ, Copeland LJ, et al. High-dose doxorubicin infusion therapy for disseminated mixed mesodermal sarcoma of the uterus. *Cancer* 1987;59:1264-1267.

334. Pecorelli S, Denny L, Ngan H, et al. Revised FIGO staging for carcinoma of the vulva, cervix, and endometrium. *International Journal of Gynecology and Obstetrics* 2009;S105:103-104.

TUMORS OF THE UTERINE CERVIX

Pedro T. Ramirez
Maria Jimena Lange
John J. Kavanagh
Alexandria T. Phan
Siriwan Tangjitgamol

■ **EPIDEMIOLOGY**

DEMOGRAPHICS

Cancer of the cervix is the third most common gynecologic malignancy in the United States. In 2009, a total of 11,270 new cases of cervical cancer and 4070 deaths were estimated (1). The incidence of this disease has decreased steadily over the past several decades. However, cervical cancer remains one of the most common cancers in women worldwide with approximately 490,000 new cases diagnosed each year and 275,000 related deaths (2). The areas with the highest incidence are Latin America, sub-Saharan Africa, and southern and southeastern Asia, while the areas with the lowest incidence are Western Europe, North America, the Middle East, and China (3). The incidence also varies by race and socioeconomic status, as it is higher in African Americans and Hispanics than in whites in the general population. Women in the lowest socioeconomic groups have the highest incidence of cervical cancer, due at least in part to inadequate screening. Generally, as Papanicolaou (Pap) screening has become more prevalent, preinvasive lesions of the cervix have been detected far more frequently than invasive cancer.

Squamous cell carcinoma (SCC) of the cervix may occur at any age from the second decade of life onward. The mean age at diagnosis is approximately 51 years, with the number of cases evenly divided between patients at 30 to 39 and 60 to 69 years of age (4). This represents a combination of earlier onset of sexual activity (ie, earlier acquisition of human papillomavirus [HPV] infection) and active Pap screening programs in the United States, which detect cancerous and precancerous lesions earlier in life. There has been an increase in the incidence of adenocarcinoma of the cervix compared with that of SCC over the past 2 decades (5), particularly among women below the age of 35 years (6,7). Adenocarcinoma (ACA) now makes up 15 to 25% of all invasive cervical cancers. This does not appear to be due to a relative decrease in SCC incidence caused by effective screening practices but rather an absolute increase in the incidence of adenocarcinoma and adenocarcinoma in situ (AIS) in younger women. Some have also hypothesized that this is due to an increase in oral contraceptive use, changes in the prevalence of HPV infection, or an increase in the reports of cervical cancer with this histology (8,9).

ETIOLOGY AND RISK FACTORS

Epidemiologic studies have been examined for many possible explanations of the development of cervical cancer. Age at first intercourse, number of sexual partners, high parity, cigarette smoking, race, low socioeconomic status, and so on have been shown to be associated with an increased risk of cervical cancer (8,10,11). However, most of these factors have not been shown to be independent risk factors but rather are associated with sexual behavior and HPV infection, the latter of which is known to be the most important risk factor (12). Some may be cofactors with other risk factors; for example, socioeconomic status is related to the pattern of sexual activity, and limited access to Pap screening

TABLE 30-1	RISK FACTORS FOR CERVICAL CANCER	
Gynecologic Factor	*Male Factor*	*Others*
Human papillomavirus	History of penile cancer	Immunodeficiency
Number of sexual partners	Cervical cancer in ex-wife	Smoking
Age at first intercourse	Multiple sexual partners	Genetic predisposition
Multiparity		Nutrient deficiency
Sexually transmitted disease		
Oral contraception		

may also contribute to increased risk. Risk factors for cervical cancer are listed in Table 30-1.

Human Papillomavirus

To understand the current methods for cervical screening, a basic understanding of the nature of cervical abnormalities is essential. Human papillomavirus is the critical factor for the development of preinvasive and invasive cervical lesions. An estimated 75% of the US population is infected with the virus. More than 5.5 million incident cases are reported annually, the majority of which occur in persons aged 15 to 24 (13,14). HPV is a small, non-enveloped double-stranded DNA virus predominantly transmitted through sexual intercourse. The most consistent risk factors for acquiring HPV are number of sexual partners, age of first sexual intercourse, and a partner infected with HPV.

There are over 100 genotypes of HPV, of which at least 40 genotypes are known to infect the anogenital tract (15). These subtypes are further classified into "high-risk" HPV (HR-HPV) and "low-risk" HPV (LR-HPV) depending on their oncogenic potential for cervical cancer and its precursors. LR-HPV genotypes include HPV6 and 11, and typically cause benign anogenital warts, though they may occasionally be associated with neoplastic cervical changes (16). Invasive lesions, on the other hand, are much more commonly caused by HR-HPV including, in order of frequency, types 16, 18, 45, 31, 33, 52, 58, and 35. While the majority of premalignant and invasive disease can be directly attributed to types 16 or 18, HPV DNA from any genotype is detectable in greater than 99% of all cervical cancer specimens (16).

Immunodeficiency Status

Many studies have reported an increased risk of HPV infection and preinvasive and invasive cervical cancer in women who have low immunity, such as those with human immunodeficiency virus (HIV) infection (17-19) or who have undergone renal transplantation (20). Women with immunodeficiency syndromes have a higher prevalence of squamous intraepithelial lesion when compared with normal women (20 versus 4-5% [relative risk, 3.2-5.7]) (21,22). Rapid progression of cervical intraepithelial neoplasia to cancer has also been observed in this patient group. Cervical cancer is one of the criteria used to define women with HIV infection as having acquired immunodeficiency syndrome (AIDS).

Number of Sexual Partners

The number of sexual partners is one of the important risk factors for both preinvasive and invasive cervical cancer. Many studies have found an increased relative risk of cervical cancer in women who had more than six sexual partners (23,24). This is related to a higher risk of acquiring HPV infection. In a study limited to women with HPV infection, however, the risk of cervical cancer was not increased with an increased number of partners (25). These two factors, the number of sexual partners and HPV infection, are also significant independent predictors of regression. In one multivariate analysis study, women with five or fewer lifetime sexual partners had a higher rate of regression of untreated CIN2 and CIN3 than did women with more than five partners (26).

Age at First Intercourse

Women who have intercourse early in life are more prone to develop cervical cancer. This increase in risk has been proposed because the process of transformation of columnar epithelium to squamous epithelium is active and is vulnerable to carcinogenic agents during early adolescence. However, these women frequently have other associated risk factors, such as multiple sexual partners and HPV infection. When these factors are controlled, as in studies of women with HPV infection, this factor appears not to impose an increased risk of cervical cancer (27).

Contraception

Many studies have produced controversial results on the effect of oral contraception (OC) on cervical cancer risk. In a recent systematic review by Smith et al. (28) in

women with HPV infection in 28 eligible studies—after controlling for the confounding effect of other factors such as number of sexual partners, smoking, and use of barrier contraception—the risk of cervical cancer increased according to the duration of OC use (relative risk of 0.9, 1.3, and 2.5 in women who used OC for <5 years, 5-10 years, and >10 years, respectively). This increased risk was found in both preinvasive and invasive cancer and both in cancer with squamous and adenocarcinoma histology. Other studies also found the association between OC use and certain types of invasive adenocarcinoma—for example, well-differentiated villoglandular adenocarcinoma and adenosquamous carcinoma. However, this association between ACA and OC disappeared after adjustment for HPV infection and number of sexual partners except in cases of AIS, in which the association remained (29). In comparison, use of both barrier contraception and spermicidal agents has been found to decrease the risk of cervical cancer (30,31).

Smoking

The carcinogenic effect of smoking is due to various chemicals, such as the nicotine derivative cotinine and tobacco-specific nitrosamines (32). Local immune mechanisms are also affected, including reductions in the number of Langerhans cells and other markers of immune function (33). Whether smoking as a risk factor for cervical cancer is independent of HPV, infection remains a controversial issue. In one case-control study, smoking appeared to be a genuine risk factor for cervical intraepithelial neoplasia independent of other sexual risk factors (34). Another study in patients with high-grade intraepithelial lesions (HSILs) found that smoking was associated with CIN2 and CIN3 (odds ratio, 2.6) in a dose-dependent manner even after adjusting for HPV infection (35). However, others have evaluated the role of smoking as a cofactor of progression from HPV infection to cancer in a pooled analysis of 10 previously published case-control studies of cofactors of HPV in the etiology of cervical cancer (36). They found that smoking increased the risk of cervical cancer in HPV-positive women, but they did not find an association between smoking and HPV infection in those who did not have cervical cancer.

Male Factors

Women with cervical cancer frequently report a history of having a male partner who has multiple other female partners, a history of condyloma infection, a history of intercourse with prostitutes, or an ex-wife or former partner with cervical cancer (37,38). Approximately 50% of these men are found to have subclinical HPV infection in the urethra or external genitalia as revealed via colposcopic examination (39).

Other less important factors—including parity, sexually transmitted diseases such as *Chlamydia,* and deficiency of nutrients (eg, vitamin A, vitamin C, folate)—have also been reported to be associated with cervical cancer. However, the body of evidence regarding these factors is not solid. Some are associated with HPV infection, while others are still controversial and are therefore not discussed here in detail.

■ HISTOPATHOLOGY

ANATOMY AND HISTOLOGY

The cervix is the region of the uterus from the isthmus to its vaginal termination. It is generally divided into the ectocervix and endocervix. Centrally located within the ectocervix is the external cervical os. Proximal to the external os is the elliptical endocervical canal, which terminates at the internal cervical os. Here, the cervix joins the uterine isthmus. The ectocervix is visible on examination; histologically, it is lined with stratified nonkeratinizing squamous epithelium continuous with the vaginal vault. The endocervix is lined with a single layer of columnar mucus-secreting epithelium that often enfolds into the underlying stroma, producing crypts or endocervical glands (Fig. 30-1).

The point at which the squamous and glandular epithelia meet is the *squamocolumnar junction.* Although its original position is at the cervical os, the location of this abrupt transformation is variable, and it undergoes continuous change during a woman's reproductive years, partly influenced by the lower vaginal pH

after puberty. In this process, the columnar epithelium undergoes a metaplastic change or differentiation of subcolumnar reserve cells to the more resilient squamous epithelium. The area of squamous epithelium between the original and new squamocolumnar junction is called the *transformation zone,* which is the area at which most preinvasive and invasive lesions arise (Figs. 30-2 and 30-3).

SQUAMOUS CELL TUMORS AND PRECURSORS

Squamous Intraepithelial Lesions

Cervical SCCs are believed to develop from precursor or preinvasive lesions, which have been classified in a variety of ways but are generally based on the degree of disruption of epithelial differentiation. The oldest such system is the *dysplasia–carcinoma in situ (CIS) system,* with mild dysplasia at one end and severe dysplasia/CIS at the other. Another is the *CIN classification,* with mild dysplasia, termed CIN1, and CIS, termed CIN3. The Bethesda System for reporting cervical/vaginal cytologic abnormalities categorizes squamous abnormalities as LSIL, encompassing HPV infection and CIN1; HSIL, encompassing CIN2 and CIN3; and SCC. These systems are compared in Table 30-2 (40).

Generally a lesion originates at the squamocolumnar junction in the transformation zone. The spectrum of morphologic changes is found in association with cervical HPV infection. The histopathology of CIN1 is indistinguishable from that of condyloma infection with viral cytopathic effects; they are considered to be in the same Bethesda category. Mild nuclear abnormalities are present throughout, with mitotic figures limited to the basal third. In CIN2, maturation is present in the upper third of the epithelium, while the mitotic figures are seen in the basal two-thirds, with some abnormal

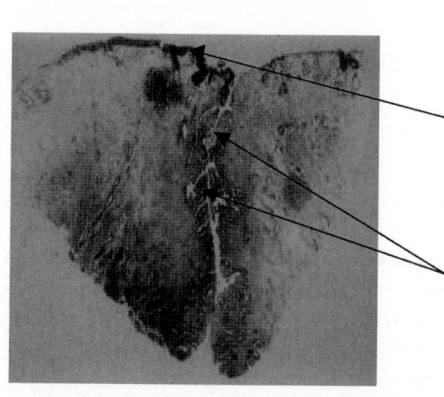

Squamous epithelium covering ectocervix

Along the endocervical canal lined by columnar epithelium

FIGURE 30-1. Giant section of the cervix shows the ectocervix in continuation with the endocervix.

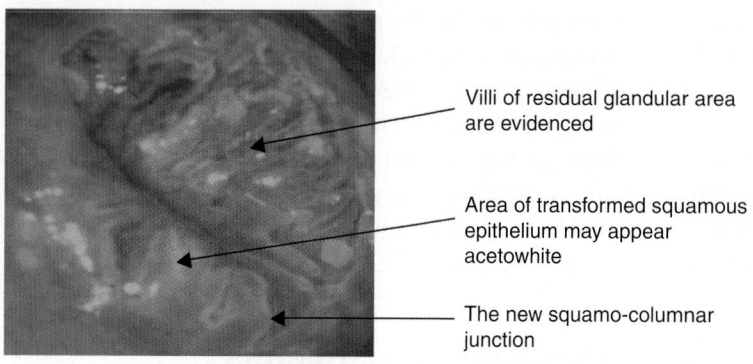

Villi of residual glandular area are evidenced

Area of transformed squamous epithelium may appear acetowhite

The new squamo-columnar junction

FIGURE 30-2. Colpophotograph of the cervix showing active transformation zone. The squamocolumnar junction, or "transformation zone" of the cervix, changes continually during a woman's reproductive life.

forms. These changes correlate strongly but not invariably with low- and intermediate-risk HPV. The next point in the spectrum, CIN3, consists of alterations of the cells throughout the epithelium with no surface maturation, presumably signifying immortalization of these cells by high-risk HPV types. The atypical cells show changes in the nucleocytoplasmic ratio; variations in nuclear size (anisokaryosis); loss of polarity; more mitotic figures, including abnormal mitoses; and hyperchromasia. These features have been associated with aneuploid cell populations. The cellular changes on Pap smears corresponding with this histologic spectrum are illustrated in Fig. 30-4.

Microinvasive Carcinoma

Microinvasion has been defined variably depending on the recommendations of the International Federation of Gynecology and Obstetrics (FIGO) ("preclinical invasive carcinoma diagnosed microscopically only," depth of lesion, ≤5 mm; width, ≤7 mm) or Society of Gynecologic Oncology (depth of invasion, ≤3 mm with no lymphovascular space invasion [LVSI] or confluent pattern) (41,42). The depth of stromal invasion is measured from the base of the epithelium, either squamous or glandular, to the deepest point of invasion. Microinvasion can be diagnosed only with a conization specimen containing the entire lesion, having uninvolved margins, and having a sufficient number of sections examined by the pathologist (43).

The pathologic features of microinvasive SCC include an invasive tongue of malignant cells penetrating through the basement membrane and a desmoplastic response in the adjacent stroma. The histology of

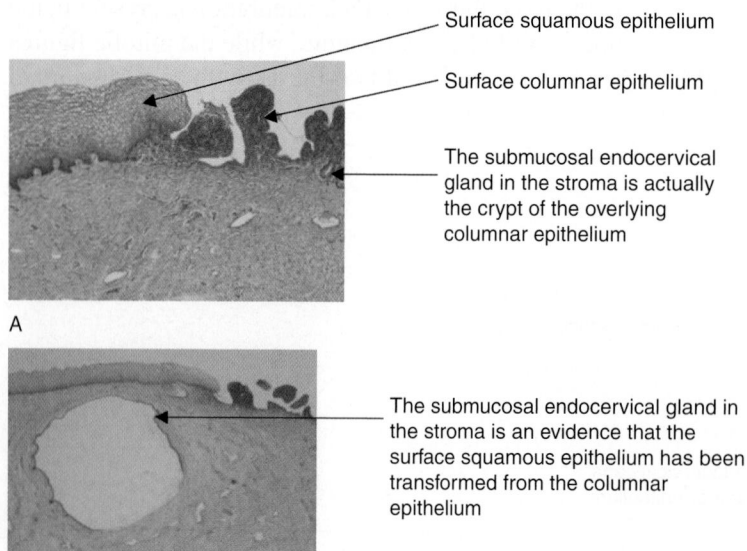

Surface squamous epithelium

Surface columnar epithelium

The submucosal endocervical gland in the stroma is actually the crypt of the overlying columnar epithelium

A

The submucosal endocervical gland in the stroma is an evidence that the surface squamous epithelium has been transformed from the columnar epithelium

B

FIGURE 30-3. **A.** Histology of the cervical squamocolumnar junction in the transformation zone. **B.** The endocervical gland in the stroma with overlying surface squamous epithelium in the transformation zone.

TABLE 30-2	CLASSIFICATION OF HPV-ASSOCIATED INTRAEPITHELIAL LESIONS OF THE CERVIX AND CYTOLOGIC CLASSIFICATION

COMPARISON OF CLASSIFICATION SYSTEMS

HPV Risk Category	Dysplasia/CIN	Pap System	Bethesda System
—	Normal	Class I	Normal
Low risk	Inflammation	Class II	LSIL
Low risk	Inflammation	Class II	LSIL
Low and high risk	Inflammation	Class II	LSIL
Low and high risk	Mild dysplasia/CIN1	Class III	LSIL
High risk	Moderate dysplasia/CIN2	Class III	HSIL
High risk	Severe dysplasia/CIS/CIN3	Class IV	HSIL
	Cancer	Class V	Cancer

CIN, cervical intraepithelial neoplasia; CIS, carcinoma in situ; HPV, human papillomavirus; HSIL, high-grade squamous intraepithelial lesion; LSIL, low-grade squamous intraepithelial lesion.

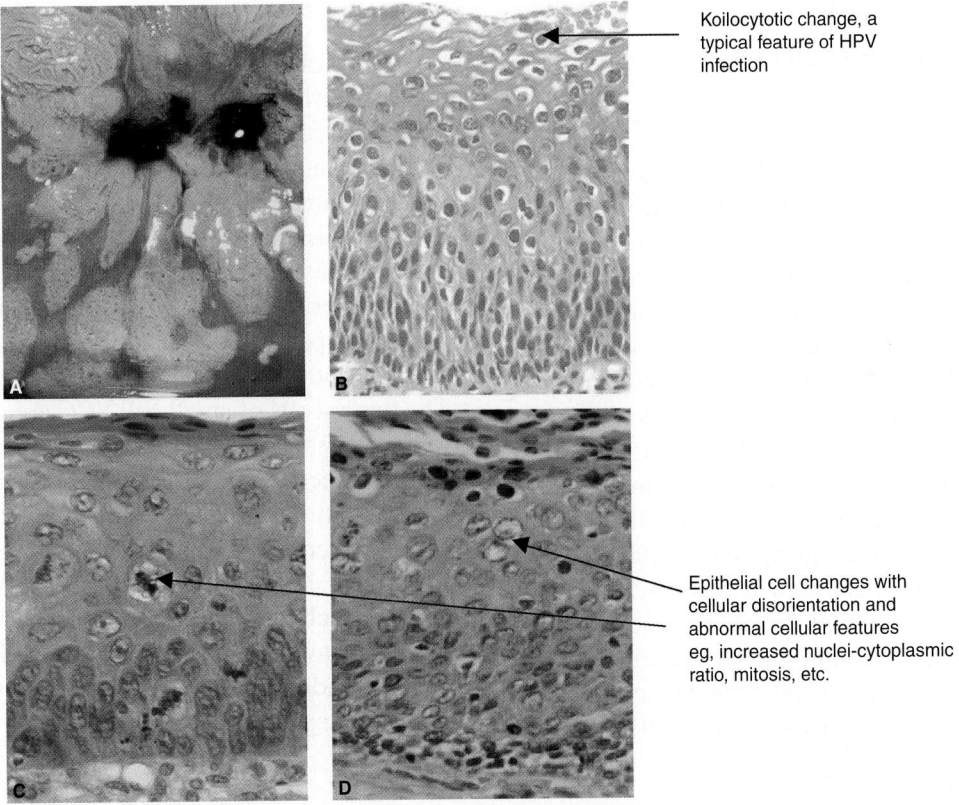

Koilocytotic change, a typical feature of HPV infection

Epithelial cell changes with cellular disorientation and abnormal cellular features eg, increased nuclei-cytoplasmic ratio, mitosis, etc.

FIGURE 30-4. **A.** Colpophotograph illustrating a low-grade cervical intraepithelial neoplasia (CIN) in the transformation zone. **B, C,** and **D.** Histopathology of cervical intraepithelial neoplasia (CIN I, II, and III, respectively) (H&E stain; ×400 magnification).

invasive foci is usually better differentiated than that of the nearby SIL (Figs. 30-5 and 30-6).

In the presence of an intense inflammatory response, which may obscure the basement membrane or desmoplastic reaction, the additional features that aid in recognizing invasion are scalloping or marginal irregularities of the epithelial-stromal interface and duplication or folding of neoplastic epithelium.

Clinicians should read the pathologic report carefully and clarify the extent of the lesion with the pathologist, because invasive lesions less than 3 mm in depth may be treated with a conservative approach, while

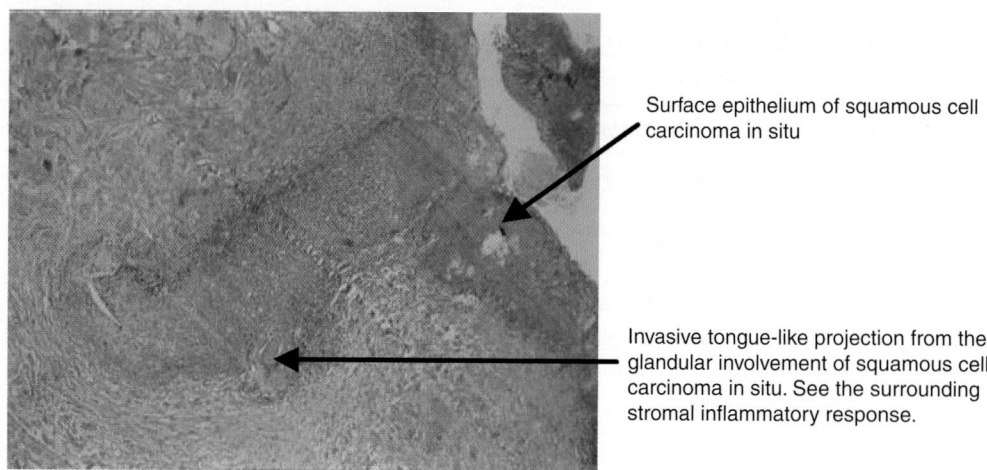

Surface epithelium of squamous cell carcinoma in situ

Invasive tongue-like projection from the glandular involvement of squamous cell carcinoma in situ. See the surrounding stromal inflammatory response.

FIGURE 30-5. Microinvasive squamous cell carcinoma (H&E stain, ×100).

deeper lesions or lesions with LVSI may require more radical therapy (44).

<hr/>

Invasive Squamous Cell Carcinoma

The gross features of SCC vary from focal elevated, to granular, to ulcerated areas. As the disease becomes more advanced, lesions may have an exophytic polypoid or papillary appearance. An endophytic lesion can result in an enlarged nodular and indurate cervix underneath the intact epithelium. The cervix may also grow to a considerable size and shape ("barrel-shaped cervix").

In 2003, the World Health Organization (WHO) divided SCC into eight subtypes: keratinizing, nonkeratinizing, basaloid, verrucous, warty, papillary, lymphoepithelioma-like, and squamotransitional cell. The histopathology of SCC is shown in Figs. 30-7 and 30-8.

The small cell nonkeratinizing SCC is not included in the WHO classification of the two-tiered system to avoid confusion with small cell neuroendocrine carcinoma; however, some still include small cell tumors as

a subtype of SCC. Large cell squamous carcinomas appear as irregular sheets of angulated to round cells with sharp cell borders and intercellular bridges, coarse chromatin nuclei, and prominent nucleoli. Also, necrosis is common. For the designation of keratinizing SCC, at least one well-formed keratin pearl should be present. This keratin pearl is not cytoplasmic keratinaceous material, which can be found in both cell types; rather, it appears as a cluster of squamous cells arranged in a concentric nest that have undergone keratinization. The tumor cells of small cell SCC are small and basaloid in shape, with uniform hyperchromatic nuclei showing necrosis and mitotic activity. Focal squamous differentiation without keratin pearl formation may also be seen. This subtype should be differentiated from small cell undifferentiated neuroendocrine carcinoma, which has a poorer prognosis. This classification may have prognostic significance in patients who undergo radiation therapy (45) but not in those who undergo surgery (46).

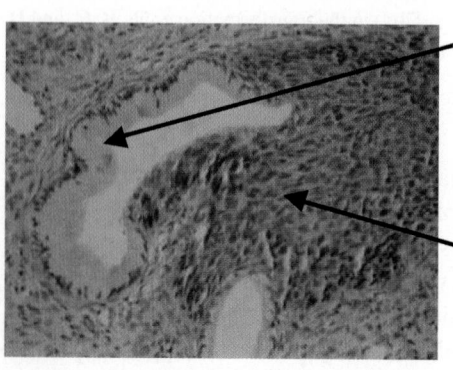

A portion of the endocervical gland showing residual columnar epithelial lining

Squamous cell carcinoma in situ involving the endocervical gland

FIGURE 30-6. Squamous cell carcinoma in situ with glandular involvement (H&E stain, ×400). This should not be interpreted as invasive carcinoma.

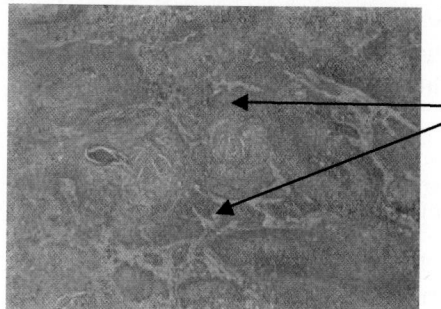

Invasive squamous cell carcinoma appears sheets of tumor tissue invading into the cervical stroma

FIGURE 30-7. Invasive squamous cell carcinoma (H&E stain, ×10).

A modification of the Broder grading system according to the histologic features of skin tumors is commonly used to grade SCC (47). However, this histologic grading and other features of keratinization—including nuclear pleomorphism, the mitotic rate, the pattern of invasion at the stromal interface, and inflammatory cell infiltrates—do not correlate with prognosis (48).

Variants of Squamous Cell Carcinoma

Verrucous Carcinoma

Verrucous carcinoma is a rare lesion that usually presents as a large sessile lesion resembling a condyloma (49). Histologically, it is characterized by both an exophytic and endophytic growth pattern. The tumor appears as well-differentiated squamous epithelium expanding into the underlying stroma via blunt invasion with intense inflammatory stromal reaction. It can be differentiated from a large exophytic condyloma; in that it lacks the more delicate architecture of condyloma. The finger-like or angulated invasive epithelial tongues of marked nuclear atypia seen in well-differentiated SCC are not found in verrucous carcinoma. The diagnosis may be difficult without multiple biopsies or hysterectomy. Local excision is not usually possible, and extension into the adjacent pelvic tissues may occur.

Metastasis to lymph nodes (LNs) is very rare, although the recurrence rates have been as high as 50% (49). Very few cases with aggressive behavior or metastasis have been reported after radiation therapy (49).

Warty Carcinoma

Warty carcinoma is also a rare variant of SCC with pronounced koilocytic changes. It is less aggressive than conventional SCC and associated with HPV types found in cases of LSIL (50).

Papillary Squamous Cell Carcinoma

Papillary SCC has been described as an exophytic papillary tumor with fibrovascular cores lined by squamous cells that resembles HSIL but is devoid of significant koilocytic changes (51,52). However, it has been reported to be positive for HPV-16 (52). Papillary SCC tends to metastasize and recur late; its treatment appears to be the same as that of ordinary SCC at an equivalent clinical stage (51).

Transitional Cell Carcinoma

Transitional cell carcinoma of the cervix resembles papillary transitional cell tumors of the urinary tract (53).

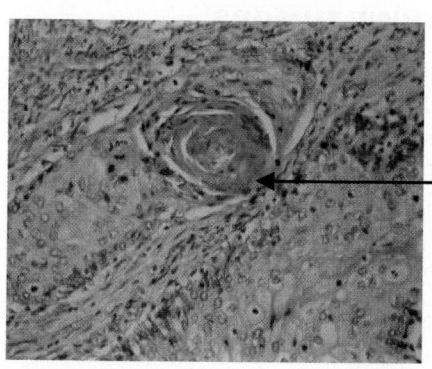

Focal area of keratin pearl demonstrated in the sheet of neoplastic epithelium

FIGURE 30-8. High-power magnification (×40) of epithelial sheets of squamous cell carcinoma.

This tumor should be distinguished from the more common benign papillary lesions of the cervix because it is an aggressive malignant tumor that often presents at an advanced clinical stage and frequently recurs and metastasizes. Some tumors may have intermediate features between those of squamous papillary and transitional cell carcinoma, hence presenting another entity, *papillary squamotransitional cell carcinoma* (54).

Spindle Cell (Sarcomatoid) Squamous Carcinoma

Spindle cell squamous carcinoma is not included in the new WHO classification, but its distinctive features merit attention. It is a rare form of squamous carcinoma composed of large spindle sarcomatoid cells, which are transformed from and frequently seen to emerge with squamous carcinoma (55,56). Immunohistochemistry has demonstrated coexpression of cytokeratin and vimentin in these tumor cells (56). It has an aggressive clinical course (55,56). However, a few early-stage cases have been reported to be cured with primary treatment, while patients with advanced disease at presentation or recurrence died of the disease (56).

GLANDULAR TUMORS AND PRECURSORS

The WHO has classified cervical into adenocarcinoma eight categories: (1) adenocarcinoma in situ, (2) early invasive adenocarcinoma, (3) adenocarcinoma not otherwise specified, (4) mucinous adenocarcinoma (including endocervical, intestinal, minimal deviation ACA or adenoma malignum, and villoglandular adenocarcinoma), (5) endometrioid adenocarcinoma, (6) clear cell adenocarcinoma, (7) serous adenocarcinoma, and (8) mesonephric adenocarcinoma.

Adenocarcinoma in Situ

AIS is an intraepithelial glandular neoplasm that occurs in women at a younger age than invasive adenocarcinoma (57,58). It is a precursor of and often coexists with invasive disease and is associated with HPV-18 and, less often, HPV-16 (59). Typically, AIS involves the transformation zone, may spread 3 cm upward into the endocervical canal (60), and may be associated with a squamous precursor, usually CIN3. The principal morphologic features are cytologic malignant glandular epithelium with stratification, atypia, mitotic activity, and frequent apoptosis without stromal invasion. The cellular changes may be found focally in the glands and may have features of endocervical, endometrial, intestinal, or mixed cell types. The distinction between AIS and nonneoplastic glandular epithelium may at times be difficult; some authors have coined terms such as

glandular dysplasia and *glandular atypia* for these lesser changes. Diagnoses of glandular dysplasia should always be met with skepticism and a request for further clarification.

Early Invasive or Microinvasive Adenocarcinoma

Although the concept of microinvasive adenocarcinoma has not been universally accepted, recent studies suggest that lesions with invasion <5 mm in depth behave similarly to so-called microinvasive squamous carcinomas and may be amenable to conservative therapy (61). The depth of invasion should be measured from the surface rather than the basement membrane at the site of origin, and the term tumor *thickness* should be used instead of *depth*.

Adenocarcinoma

Various subtypes of adenocarcinoma have been noted due to their differentiation, as their respective names imply, such as mucinous adenocarcinoma, which can have endocervical or intestinal goblet cell features and the appearance of endometrioid, clear cell, serous, or mesonephric types. Adenoma malignum is usually an extremely benign-appearing cancer that is often diagnosed late and thus has a clinically poor prognosis. Clear cell adenocarcinomas may or may not be associated with diethylstilbestrol exposure in utero, but they have no known association with HPV (62). These tumors are found at two age peaks: 26 and 71 years; they are also associated with an unfavorable outcome (63). Serous adenocarcinoma is rare, with a histology identical to its ovarian counterpart, and it carries a similarly bad prognosis. Mesonephric carcinomas, such as clear cell carcinomas, are variants that are not associated with papillomaviruses but are derived from mesonephric rests in Gartner duct, so they are most commonly found in the deep lateral portions of the cervical walls (64) (Fig. 30-9).

UNCOMMON CARCINOMAS AND NEUROENDOCRINE TUMORS

The WHO has classified cervical carcinomas into five categories: (1) adenosquamous carcinoma (including glassy cell carcinoma), (2) adenoid cystic carcinoma, (3) adenoid basal cell carcinoma, (4) neuroendocrine tumors, and (5) undifferentiated carcinoma.

Adenosquamous Carcinoma

Gompel and Silverberg (65) defined this tumor, which has both squamous and glandular features as evidenced

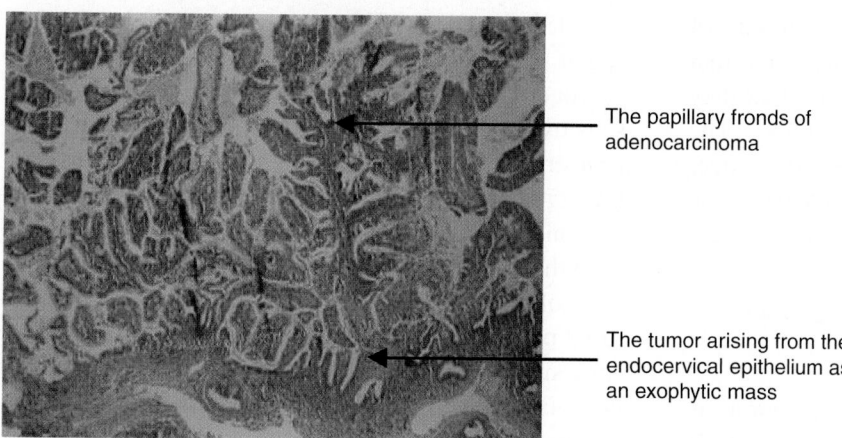

The papillary fronds of adenocarcinoma

The tumor arising from the endocervical epithelium as an exophytic mass

FIGURE 30-9. Endocervical papillary adeno-carcinoma (H&E stain, ×10).

via hematoxylin and eosin (H&E) staining. Some have included tumors with other histologic features—such as typical squamous carcinoma staining for mucin (mucoepidermoid carcinoma), collision tumors of separate SCC and ACA, and endometrioid carcinoma with squamous differentiation—in this group. In a study by dos Reis et al. (66), the authors evaluated whether histology (adenocarcinoma versus adenosquamous carcinoma) is an independent prognostic indicator in patients with stage IB1 cervical cancer after radical hysterectomy. The authors found no evidence that histologic subtype affects outcome; however, the median time to recurrence was shorter in patients with adenosquamous carcinoma.

Glassy Cell Carcinoma

Glassy cell carcinoma is a rare, aggressive form of adenosquamous carcinoma that rarely responds to radiation therapy (67) but may respond to chemotherapy (68). It appears as a sheet of pleomorphic cells with distinct cellular borders, abundant ground-glass cytoplasm, prominent nucleoli, and a high mitotic rate; it is often infiltrated with eosinophils and plasma cells.

Adenoid Basal Carcinoma Versus Adenoid Cystic Carcinoma

Both adenoid basal carcinoma and adenoid cystic carcinoma occur more often in older patients and contain the glandular and basaloid squamous components that arise from reserve cells (69). However, accurate pathologic distinction is necessary due to their different clinical behavior: adenoid basal carcinoma has a good prognosis, while adenoid cystic carcinoma has a poor one (69,70). Adenoid basal carcinoma, which has not been reported to metastasize, is usually small and occurs in association with squamous dysplasia, CIS, and early invasive

carcinoma; this has not been seen in patients with adenoid cystic carcinoma (70).

Neuroendocrine Tumors

Neuroendocrine tumors include carcinoid, atypical carcinoid, and large and small cell neuroendocrine carcinoma. Carcinoid tumors have the characteristic organoid appearance of those at other sites: nuclear atypia, necrosis, and mitotic activity (>5 to 10 per high-power field) are the criteria used to differentiate between typical and atypical carcinoids (71). Small cell carcinoma accounts for 1 to 6% of all cervical carcinomas and is notorious for its aggressive behavior, with a 5-year survival rate of only 14 to 39% (72-74). Its histologic features are similar to those of its counterpart in the lung. Large cell neuroendocrine carcinoma is rare, with abundant cytoplasm and large nuclei and nucleoli. It frequently has focal ACA differentiation and should be distinguished from ACA and other undifferentiated tumors. It has a poor prognosis, similar to that of the small cell type (75).

Undifferentiated Carcinoma

Undifferentiated carcinoma shows no specific differentiation and should be distinguished from poorly differentiated SCC, adenocarcinoma, glassy cell carcinoma, and large cell neuroendocrine carcinoma.

■ SCREENING

The concept that invasive cervical cancer develops from its precursor or dysplastic lesions was first introduced in the early twentieth century. In the 1960s, based on clinical studies and supporting laboratory data, Richart and Barron (76) proposed that dysplastic lesions were preinvasive lesions that preceded the development of invasive cancer in the cervix. They also suggested that those lesions formed a biological continuum that they called cervical intraepithelial neoplasia (CIN). The presence of a preinvasive stage at which cervical cancer can be diagnosed and treated makes it the ideal disease for the effectiveness of screening and prevention.

PAP SMEAR AND BETHESDA SYSTEM

Pap Smear

The Pap smear is the result of the observation by Dr. George Papanicolaou in 1924 that cancer cells derived from the uterine cervix could be detected on vaginal smears (77). Since then, cytologic screening using the Pap smear has been the standard of gynecologic care around the world and led to a significant reduction in the incidence of invasive cervical cancer as well as its mortality. Specifically, the cervical cancer rate has dropped 70 to 90% in well-screened populations. In developing countries, the limited access to screening programs continues to be a major contributor to the high mortality rates of cervical cancer.

AIS as well as ACA may be detected by the Pap smear. However, the Pap smear has been less effective at reducing the incidence of ACA because it may be less sensitive and is more prone to sampling and interpretation errors when compared with the squamous cell type (78). In women with HIV infection, the Pap smear was initially not considered to be reliable, so all women with this infection were recommended to undergo routine colposcopy. However, after much initial fear about rapid progression, it appears that patients with precursor lesions do not experience rapid progression to cervical cancer (79,80). Regular screening with appropriate treatment of preinvasive lesions is vital in this patient group to prevent cervical cancer.

Guidelines for screening have been put forth by both the American Cancer Society (1) and American College of Obstetricians and Gynecologists (81) and are summarized in Table 30-3.

Since the Pap smear was initially developed, there have been several changes in nomenclature and interpretation to make the results more clinically relevant. At present, the Bethesda System is being used worldwide for cytologic diagnosis (see Table 30-2).

TABLE 30-3	THE AMERICAN COLLEGE OF OBSTETRICIANS AND GYNECOLOGISTS RECOMMENDATIONS FOR CERVICAL CYTOLOGY SCREENING*
Initial Screening	*Age 21 Years*
Frequency	Low-risk women • <30 years → every 2 years[†][*] • ≥30 year → after three consecutive negative annual smears → extend interval to 3 years* • Cytology with HPV screening is appropriate for women ≥30 years if negative → not more frequently than every 3 years High-risk women[‡] • Require more frequent screening • HIV women → twice in the first year after diagnosis, then annually • History of CIN2/CIN3, posttreatment follow-up → annually until at least three consecutive negative smears
Following hysterectomy	• No prior history of CIN2/CIN3 and had hysterectomy for benign condition → discontinue • History of CIN2/CIN3, after three consecutive satisfactory negative smears following treatment before hysterectomy → discontinue
Discontinuation[§]	Reasonable to stop screening at age 65 or 70 among women who have three or more negative cytology results in a row and no abnormal test results in the past 10 years. If discontinued, risk factors should be assessed during annual examination

CIN, cervical intraepithelial neoplasia.
*According to the American College of Obstetricians and Gynecologists, liquid-based and conventional methods of cervical cytology are acceptable.
[†]The American Cancer Society recommends that women <30 years of age undergo screening annually with conventional methods and every 2 years with a liquid-based method.
[‡]High-risk women are those who have history of CIN2/CIN3, are immunocompromised, are positive for HIV, and have had diethylstilbestrol exposure in utero.
[§]The American Cancer Society recommends discontinuation of the test in low-risk women >70 years of age. The US Preventive Services task force sets the upper age limit at 65 years. The exceptions are women who are sexually active and have had multiple partners and those who have a history of abnormal cytology.
Data from American College of Obstetricians and Gynecologists (81).

Bethesda System

The Bethesda System is another procedure used for the cytologic diagnosis of cervical cancer. It was developed in 1988, last updated in 2001, and is now used widely (82). The Bethesda System report is divided into three sections:

1. *Specimen adequacy*
   Satisfactory for evaluation
   Unsatisfactory for evaluation

2. *General categorization* (*optional*)
   Negative for intraepithelial lesion or malignancy
   Epithelial cell abnormality
   Other

3. *Interpretation/result*
   Negative for intraepithelial lesion or malignancy
       Organism
       Other nonneoplastic findings (optional to report; list not comprehensive)
           Reactive cellular changes associated with (descriptive findings)
           Glandular cells status posthysterectomy
           Atrophy
   Epithelial cell abnormalities
       Squamous cell
           Atypical squamous cells (ASCs); ASC-US, and ASC-H
           LSIL
           HSIL
       Glandular cell (specify endocervical, endometrial, or not otherwise specified)
           Atypical glandular cells (AGCs)
           Atypical glandular cells, favor neoplastic
           Endocervical AIS
   ACA
       Other (list not comprehensive)
           Endometrial cells in a woman ≥40 years of age
           Automated review and ancillary testing (include as appropriate)
       Educational notes and suggestions (optional)

Note the following:

1. ASC: Some cells were seen that cannot be called normal but do not meet the requirements to call them precancerous. The abnormal cells may be caused by an infection, irritation, or intercourse or may be precancerous.

   a. Atypical squamous cell of undetermined significance (ASC-US).
   b. ASC cannot exclude HSIL (ASC-H).

2. SIL: Changes were seen in the cells that may show precancerous signs. SIL can be low or high grade.
   a. LSIL: Early, mild changes in the size or shape of cells were seen.
   b. HSIL: Moderate or severe cell changes are seen. HSIL changes on a Pap smear suggest an increased risk of "precancer" when compared with LSIL changes.

3. AGC: Cell changes were seen that represent an abnormality that must be evaluated more closely. The type of evaluation depends on patient age and other factors.

Examples of cytologic feature of HPV and cervical intraepithelial neoplasia are shown in Fig. 30-10.

LIQUID-BASED CERVICAL CYTOLOGY

With the Pap smear, a considerable number of patients still have false-positive and false-negative results due to either sampling or diagnostic errors. The reported sensitivity of the Pap smear in a meta-analysis of the procedure was only approximately 50% (83). The false-negative rate was reported to be as high as 15 to 30% for HSIL (83-85) and 50% for invasive cancer (86,87). The errors may be due to uneven cellular distribution, as the thick cell layers on the surface of the slides render the conditions for diagnosis less than optimal. Mucus, blood, and inflammatory debris may make interpretation even more difficult.

Recently, the liquid-based cervical cytology system, or ThinPrep, and a automated computerized system evolved to improve the rate of detection of abnormal cells by eliminating the troublesome factors described above. Many studies reported relatively higher sensitivity than the conventional method (88-91). These two systems have been used more widely since their approval by the US Food and Drug Administration (FDA) in 1996. The American College of Obstetricians and Gynecologists has announced the committee opinion and stated that liquid-based cervical cytology and conventional methods are both acceptable for screening, depending on the patient's history and risk, cost of the test, and possible false-positive and false-negative results.

AUTOMATED SYSTEMS: PAPNET AND AUTOCYTEPREP

PAPNET and AutoCytePrep are the commonly used automated computerized screening systems, both of which increase the rate of abnormal cytologic detection. The PAPNET system is equipped with neural

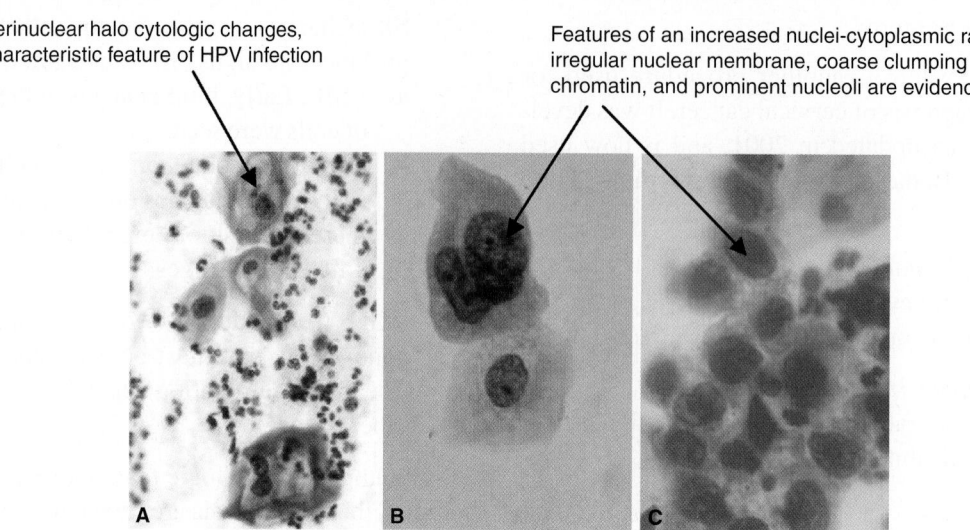

Perinuclear halo cytologic changes, characteristic feature of HPV infection

Features of an increased nuclei-cytoplasmic ratio, irregular nuclear membrane, coarse clumping chromatin, and prominent nucleoli are evidenced

FIGURE 30-10. Cytologic changes associated with cervical intraepithelial neoplasia (CIN), including CIN1 with koilocytotic feature of HPV infection **A.** ×600 magnification, CIN2 **B.** ×1000 magnification, and CIN3 **C.** ×1000 magnification.

network programming, which can detect cancer cells that are missed by visual cytologic diagnosis (92). In a study of HSIL or invasive cancer with normal findings of an ordinary Pap smear, rescreening of the slides using PAPNET yielded an abnormality in up to 95% of the cases (93).

The AutoCytePrep system uses a high-speed video microscope and image-interpretation software program to image, analyze, and classify cells on Pap smear slides. Its sensitivity in detecting lesions at a grade higher than LSIL is better than that of conventional microscopic examination (98 versus 89%) (94). Also, the false-negative rate was significantly reduced from 15.7 to 10.5%.

Despite the improved sensitivity of these tests when compared with conventional Pap smears, the New Technology Task Force of the George Papanicolaou Society of Cytopathology published the results of a survey on the value of automation in cytology showing that most laboratories do not regard automation as essential for cervicovaginal cytology due to the added expense (95). The American College of Obstetricians and Gynecologists has previously stated that these technologies do not represent the current standard of care in cervical cancer screening.

TESTING FOR HUMAN PAPILLOMAVIRUS

HPV, particularly the high-risk type, is an important etiologic factor for cervical cancer. This has led to the clinical application of HPV testing as a screening method alone or together with the Pap smear in cases of ASC or LSIL lesions in order to predict cancer risk—and such testing may result in subsequent management modifications. The period in which an LSIL progresses to invasive cancer is approximately 12 to 13 years (96); therefore women who have a normal Pap smear and do not have a high-risk HPV infection can be followed up for a longer interval (97).

HPV testing can be achieved through detection of HPV DNA using various techniques, such as the polymerase chain reaction, in situ hybridization, and Hybrid Capture. Hybrid Capture II is a commercially available HPV test designed to detect 18 different types of HPV. The test detects HPV in terms of high- and low-risk groups, but it cannot specify the type. In one study, the sensitivity of HPV testing for detection of a histologically proven HSIL was 100%, which was significantly higher than that of conventional (68.1%) and liquid-based cytology (87.8%) (98). The specificities of HPV testing were 85.6% in scrapes treated for liquid-based cytology and 87.3% in smears examined by conventional cytology. The specificities were slightly increased to 88.4 and 90.1% from the liquid-based and conventional cytology, respectively, when testing was reserved for women above the age of 30 years.

OTHER SCREENING METHODS

There are several other methods of cervical cancer screening. These include *chemiluminescent speculoscopy,* which uses a chemical substance that can illuminate more of the acetowhite than normal tissue, making the lesion easily visible with a speculoscope at a magnification of ×4 to ×6 (99). The other methods are *Fourier transform infrared spectrophotometry* and use of the *optoelectronic device,* both of which are based on differential molecular infrared energy absorption in conjunction with the illumination of visible infrared signals and electrical measurement of the decay curves at various points from the cervical tissues, respectively (100,101). Fourier transform infrared spectrophotometry has higher sensitivity and specificity, with lower false-negative and false-positive rates, than the standard Pap smear (100). Use of the optoelectronic *device* in combination with the Pap smear has also resulted in a significant improvement in the sensitivity of cervical screening (101). A fourth method, *electrical current flow impedance,* is based on the differential impedance patterns of normal and abnormal cervical epithelium to electrical frequency (102). Finally, *fluorescence spectroscopy* discriminates normal and precancerous tissues of the cervix that have a heterogeneous molecular and cellular composition of fluorophores. This technique uses a fiberoptic probe that is placed on the cervix, obtaining a spectrum of different fluorescence wavelengths that are translated by the computerized system (103). Mitchell et al. (104) found better receiver operating characteristic curve performance with fluorescence spectroscopy than with standard Pap smear screening and worse performance than with screening colposcopy, cervicography, HPV testing, and cervicoscopy. Although these tests are noninvasive and produce results rapidly, the clinical implication of some of these tests for large population–based screening must await further studies.

■ NATURAL HISTORY

Knowledge of the natural history of cervical cancer is important for optimal management of its precursor lesions. It is crucial to realize that not all lesions begin as condyloma or CIN1. Cervical cancer may present at any point in the spectrum, depending on the associated HPV type and other host factors. The rates of progression are also by no means uniform, even with the same HPV type, which is a potential predictor of a lesion's behavior; this means that it is still difficult to predict the outcome in an individual patient. These findings underscore the fact that the risk of cancer is conferred only in part by the HPV type and depends on other carcinogens as well as genetic alterations that bring about the evolution of a precancerous lesion.

Most mild and moderate dysplasias will regress. One historical cohort study reported on the course of cervical dysplasia in 17,000 women with an abnormal Pap smear who were followed or cared for conservatively (105). Only 2.1% of the women with mild dysplasia and 16.3% of those with moderate dysplasia had progression to severe dysplasia or worse. The rate of progression at any severity was highest in the first 2 years and increased constantly at a rate of 1% per year up to 10 years. At 10 years, more than half of the women with mild or moderate dysplasia did not experience progression to a more severe lesion. Predictably, lesions in which the whole epithelial thickness has evolved completely (CIN3) constitute the greatest risk to progression to cervical cancer. Many longitudinal studies of untreated patients with squamous CIS have documented progression to invasive disease in a significant number of cases when followed up sufficiently. The studies of CIS that have been reported on this finding are summarized in Table 30-4 (106-110).

HPV infection is present and has been identified in more than 95% of cervical cancer cases (111). However, the molecular events that drive CIS to invasion and therefore establish the diagnosis of cancer are not well known. Recent information suggests that the viral load may increase the risk for subsequent cancer development (112).

The natural history of growth of a cervical lesion is believed to progress through a state of microscopic invasion into the stroma and radial growth on the surface. Ultimately, a mass is formed, which, in general, grows locally to invade first the deeper stroma and later the

TABLE 30-4	PROGRESSION RATE OF SQUAMOUS CARCINOMA IN SITU TO INVASIVE CANCER WITHOUT TREATMENT		
Study, Year (Ref)	*Number of Patients*	*Median Follow-Up (Months)*	*Invasive Disease (%)*
Holowaty (105), 1999	507	4-24	1.4
Peterson (106), 1956	127	108	33.0
Koss (107), 1963	67	39	13.0
Clemmensen (108), 1971	67	99	40.0
Luthra (109), 1987	43	24	32.0
Saito (110), 1999	45	26	58.0

paracervical and parametrial tissues. If left untreated, the disease will expand through these tissues to involve the lateral pelvic side wall and nearby viscera, such as the urinary bladder and rectum. Cancer arising from the cervix has been reported to involve the uterine corpus in 10 to 30% of cases and rare with the ovaries; 0.5% for SCC and 1.6% for adenocarcinoma (113).

Lateral spread of cervical cancer is the rule, although up to 17% of patients with early-stage cervical cancer have been found to have lymphatic metastatic disease (114). As a primary group, the pelvic nodes are most commonly involved. It is very uncommon to find isolated para-aortic lymphatic disease in the absence of metastatic pelvic disease (115). However, the node group at greatest risk is variable and dependent on the tumor size and location.

Hematogenous spread of disease is generally found with late presentation and most commonly involves bone, the lungs, or other intra-abdominal viscera (116). Variant cell types, such as neuroendocrine and glassy cell carcinoma, may be associated with distant disease in the absence of local involvement.

CLINICAL PRESENTATION

SYMPTOMS

The clinical signs and symptoms of patients with cervical cancer vary depending on the stage and characteristic features of their lesions. Patients with early-stage disease may not have any abnormal symptoms; rather, their lesions may be discovered incidentally on a Pap smear. In patients with gross lesions, the most common presenting symptom is vaginal bleeding, which may have a characteristic pattern of mucous bloody discharge, postcoital bleeding, and/or intermenstrual, intermittent, or continuous vaginal bloody discharge. Vaginal bleeding is often found with exophytic cervical lesions. Tumor necrosis with superimposed infection may cause a mucopurulent bloody discharge with a foul smell due to anaerobic organisms. The symptoms in patients with more advanced disease include leg swelling due to compression of the venous or lymphatic system, pain due to nerve or bone involvement, and other urinary or bowel symptoms due to cancer invasion, such as hematuria or hematochezia.

SIGNS AND CLINICAL FEATURES OF LESIONS

The characteristic features of cervical lesions may be those of endophytic lesions, such as an ulcer or infiltrative lesion. These may not be visible but are palpable, with

abnormal consistency. Alternatively, the lesions may be exophytic. Important parameters to evaluate include the size of the cervix as well as involvement of vagina, parametrium, and pelvic side wall. Any palpable rectal involvement should be documented. Attention should be directed to the possible distant sites of metastasis, such as the supraclavicular and inguinal regions, especially in cases involving an advanced primary lesion.

FIGO STAGING

Cervical cancer is currently staged clinically using the FIGO system (41). Routine evaluation includes physical examination, pelvic and rectal examination, and pathologic review of cervical or cone biopsy specimens. Basic imaging studies such as chest x-ray, intravenous pyelography, cystoscopy, and proctoscopy are allowed in order to classify the disease into four stages, as shown in Table 30-5.

DIAGNOSTIC IMAGING

The reason that FIGO does not include special imaging studies such as CT scan, MRI, or PET scan in the standard clinical staging system is to allow every institution throughout the world to acquire basic information for staging in a similar manner. However, many important prognostic factors, including those most important for cervical cancer (eg, lymphnode [LN] status and subclinical distant metastasis), may not be identified with the basic imagings (117). Lymphangiography, computed tomography (CT), and magnetic resonance imaging (MRI) have long been used in the clinical management of cervical cancer. One meta-analysis comparing CT and MRI found that these tests have similarly modest sensitivity and specificity in determining the LN status of patients with cervical cancer (118). However, another recent systematic review of these two imaging studies in the staging of cervical carcinoma reported that the sensitivity of MRI was better than that of CT in detecting invasion and metastasis to the parametrium (74 versus 55%), LNs (60 versus 43%), urinary bladder (75 versus 64%), and rectum (71 versus 45%) (119). The difference was significant for parametrial and LN invasion but not for urinary bladder and rectal invasion.

Whole-body positron emission tomography (PET) is a new imaging technique that uses the glucose analog of (18F) fluoro-2-deoxy-D-glucose to detect malignant tumors based on their functional increased glycolytic activity. PET has an advantage over lymphangiography,

TABLE
30-5 | **FIGO STAGING OF CERVICAL CARCINOMA**

Stage I	Confined to cervix
Stage IA	Microscopic lesion; stromal invasion ≤ 5 mm in depth, ≤ 7 mm in width
Stage IA1	≤ 3 mm in depth, ≤ 7 mm in width
Stage IA2	Stromal invasion > 3 mm and ≤ 5 mm in depth, ≤ 7 mm in width
Stage IB	Preclinical lesion greater than stage 1A or clinically visible (all gross lesions, even those with superficial invasion, are stage IB cancers)
Stage IB1	Size ≤ 4 cm
Stage IB2	Size > 4 cm
Stage II	Lesions extend beyond the cervix but not onto the pelvic side wall
Stage IIA	IIA1
	Involves upper two-thirds of vagina, no obvious parametrial involvement, visible lesion ≤ 4 cm in greatest dimension
	IIA2
	Involves upper two-thirds of vagina, no obvious parametrial involvement, visible lesion > 4 cm in greatest dimension
Stage IIB	Obvious parametrial involvement
Stage III	Extension to pelvic side wall or hydronephrosis or nonfunctioning kidney* or involves lower third of the vagina
Stage IIIA	Involves lower one-third of vagina, no extension onto the pelvic side wall
Stage IIIB	Extension onto the pelvic side wall or hydronephrosis or nonfunctioning kidney
Stage IV	Beyond the true pelvis or involvement of the mucosa of the bladder or rectum[†]
Stage IVA	Involves urinary bladder or rectal mucosa
Stage IVB	Spread to distant organs.

*All cases of hydronephrosis or nonfunctioning kidney should be included unless they are known to be due to another cause.
[†]Bullous edema of the urinary bladder or rectal mucosa does not permit a case to be designated as stage IV disease.

CT, and MRI in that it can detect abnormal tissues even when they are of normal size or structural appearance. In cervical cancer, the role of PET has evolved, with many published reports describing its role in the evaluation of patients with newly diagnosed disease, in devising a plan of treatment, or as a prognostic study and in the follow-up period to detect recurrences. Many studies have shown that the sensitivity of PET is higher than that of CT and MRI in determining the LN status and detecting extrapelvic sites of metastasis (120-124), locally advanced or recurrent cervical cancer who underwent PET scanning (125). The sensitivity of PET, CT, and MRI in this study was the same (93%) for primary, residual, and local recurrent cancer. However, PET was significantly superior in detecting most sites of metastases except for the liver, for which its diagnostic value was similar.

In patients who had undergone radiation therapy, the LN status as determined by PET is a significant prognostic factor for progression-free survival (PFS) (126,127). One retrospective study of 101 patients with stage IAIVB cervical cancer who underwent CT and PET prior to radiation therapy or concurrent chemoradiation found a 2-year PFS rate of 64% with disease-negative LNs on both CT and PET scans, 18% with

disease-negative LNs on CT scans but disease-positive LNS on PET scans, and 14% with disease-positive LNs on both CT and PET scans (126). Another similar study evaluating 47 patients with stage IIIB cervical cancer who underwent concurrent chemoradiation demonstrated that the LN status according to pretreatment PET evaluation was a significant predictor of survival (127). The survival rate decreased as the level of LN involvement went from the pelvic nodes to the para-aortic and supraclavicular nodes.

For surveillance after treatment, information on local pelvic recurrence is sometimes difficult to obtain via physical examination due to reactive tissue changes after surgery or radiation therapy, especially if the recurrence does not appear as a discrete mass but rather as an infiltrating tissue. In metastatic LNs or other sites of metastasis, CT and MRI have a limited role if the lesions do not increase in size (126). PET has been found to be superior to CT in the detection of recurrences, with a sensitivity and specificity of approximately 90 to 100% (127-131).

Reduction in a tumor's metabolic activity, which reflects tumor response, is also of prognostic significance. CT and MRI have a limited role in follow-up evaluation of abnormal LNs regardless of whether tumors persist or recur if they do not increase in size. In a multivariate analysis of patients with cervical cancer who underwent PET scan before and after radiation therapy, Grigsby et al. (126) showed that posttreatment PET findings were the most significant prognostic factors for survival. The 2-year PFS rate was 86% in patients with disease-negative PET findings and 40% in those with persistent lesions after treatment.

■ PROGNOSTIC FACTORS

STAGE IA

Three potential areas of concern in considering microinvasion are *tumor depth, confluence of growth pattern,* and *LVSI.* The depth of stromal invasion correlates with the risk of pelvic LN metastases and progression-free interval. In their review, Raspagliesi et al. (132) found many studies reporting that in the case of tumors with a depth of invasion <1, 1 to 3, and >3 mm, the risk of LN involvement was 0 to 1.6%, 0 to 5.3%, and 1.3 to 13.8%, respectively; the risk of parametrial invasion was 0%, 0 to 2.3%, and 0 to 3.3%, respectively.

A confluent growth pattern is defined as the presence of anatomizing tongues of epithelium with pushing borders or a lesion front of >1 mm (133). Despite a report emphasizing the prognostic importance of confluent patterns of invasion, some have found this growth pattern in association with depth of invasion and this, by itself, is not considered an independent factor once the depth of invasion is controlled (134).

The incidence of LVSI in microinvasive carcinoma (MIC) varies widely from many studies, ranging from 19 to 57% (135-137). LVSI is another area of controversy in defining the MIC; whether it is an independent prognostic factor in lesions ≤3 mm in depth remains an area of debate (135). In a review by Ostor (136), 50% of the tumors with LN metastasis or recurrence were associated with LVSI, compared with only 18 and 14% of the patients with negative nodes and no recurrences, respectively. In patients with stage IA1 cervical cancer, the incidence of LN involvement increased from 0.3% without LVSI to 2.6% with LVSI (138); a recurrence rate of 3.1% was reported in the presence of LVSI (139). In patients with stage IA2 disease, the tumor recurrence rate was significantly increased in patients with positive LVSI from 3.2 to 9.7% in one study (140) and to 15.7% in another (139). Also, the 5-year survival rate in patients with LVSI decreased from 98 to 89% (140). In a study by Milam et al. (141), the authors aimed to determine the association between findings on review of preoperative biopsy specimens and the risk of lymph node

involvement (LNI) at radical hysterectomy in patients with early-stage (stage IA-IB1) cervical cancer. In that study, the authors found that twelve patients (14.8%) had LNI at radical hysterectomy. Stage, grade, and histologic subtype were not associated with LNI. LVSI and depth of invasion >4 mm were both significantly associated with LNI (25.6 versus 4.8%, $p = .01$, and 25.0 versus 4.5%, $p = .01$, respectively). LVSI with >4 mm invasion was 6.6 times more likely to have LNI at the time of radical hysterectomy (RR = 6.6; 95% confidence interval, 2.1-21.9). The authors concluded that patients with preoperative LVSI are at higher risk for LNI at radical hysterectomy and should be counseled regarding potential implications for management.

STAGE IB-IIA

▬▬▬ Lymph Node Status

The incidence of LN metastasis in patients with stage IB1 and IB2 cervical cancer has been reported to be as high as 15 to 20% and 30 to 50%, respectively (142,143). LN involvement is the most important prognostic factor for survival, as the 5-year survival rate has been reported to be 85 to 95% and 40 to 60% in patients with stage IB disease with negative and positive nodes, respectively (143,144).

▬▬▬ Parametrial Invasion

Parametrial involvement is noted in up to 31% of patients with stage IB1 and 63% of patients with stage IB2 (142). The 5-year survival rate in patients whose disease had parametrial involvement was reported to decrease to 62%, compared with 86% in those without parametrial invasion (145). Parametrial invasion is related to the grade of the tumor, depth of stromal invasion, and presence of LVSI (146). In their study, described above, Benedetti-Panici et al. (142) also reported that the most important predictor of parametrial invasion was the presence of LVSI, which was directly related to the size of the tumor and depth of stromal invasion. A recent study by Frumovitz et al. (147) evaluated the incidence of parametrial involvement and the factors associated with parametrial spread in women with early-stage cervical cancer. In that study, the authors sought to also identify a cohort of patients at low risk for parametrial spread who may benefit from less radical surgery. Three hundred fifty patients met the inclusion criteria. Overall, 27 women (7.7%) had parametrial involvement. The majority of specimens with parametrial involvement (52%) had tumor spread through direct microscopic extension. Patients with parametrial involvement were more likely to have a primary tumor size larger than 2 cm (larger than 2 cm: 14%, smaller than 2 cm: 4%, $p = .001$), higher histologic grade (grade 3: 12%, grades 1 and 2: 3%, $p = .01$), lymphovascular space invasion (positive: 12%, negative: 3%, $p = .002$), and metastasis to the pelvic lymph nodes (positive: 31%, negative: 4%, $p < .001$). One hundred twenty-five women (36%) had squamous, adenocarcinoma, or adenosquamous lesions, all grades, with primary tumor size 2 cm or smaller and no lymphovascular space invasion. In this group of patients, there was no pathologic evidence of parametrial involvement.

Depth of Stromal Invasion

Increased depth of invasion is significantly correlated with nodal spread, recurrence, and poor survival (148). Together with LVSI, depth of invasion is considered the intermediate risk factor necessitating postoperative adjuvant radiation therapy to reduce local recurrence (149).

Size of Tumor

Tumor size is an important prognostic factor for recurrence and survival. The recurrence rate for cervical tumors >6, 4 to 6, 2 to <4, and 1 to <2 cm was found to be 67, 58, 38, and 31%, respectively. The 5-year survival rate in patients with a tumor <2, >2, and >4 cm in size was approximately 90, 60, and 40%, respectively (150).

Surgical Margins

Free space between a tumor and outer cervicoparacervical tissue border of <3 mm is considered a close margin (151). This finding is related to LVSI and is an important risk factor for parametrial and LN involvement (151-153). However, close tumor margin as an isolated finding without the other related risk factors appears to have no impact on prognosis (151). A distance from the tumor to the vaginal margin of <5 mm is regarded as close. A 5-year survival rate of only 28% has been reported in patients with a close vaginal margin, compared with 81% in those with a more distant vaginal margin (154).

Lymphovascular Space Invasion

The significance of LVSI as a prognostic factor in stage IB-IIA tumors is still an issue of debate. Delgado et al. (155) reported an incidence of LN metastasis as high as 25% in the presence of LVSI, compared with only 8% without LVSI. The 3-year disease-free interval rate was 77.0% in those with positive LVSI and 88.9% in those with negative LVSI. However, when adjusted according to size and extent of tumor or depth of parametrial invasion, the prognosis in patients with or without LVSI appeared not to differ.

Tumor Histology

Neuroendocrine and glassy cell carcinoma are generally accepted as being more aggressive than common SCC. The results of studies of adenocarcinoma (ACA) are controversial regarding whether it is worse than SCC. However, unlike the case with SCC, the grade of ACA appears to be an important prognostic factor for determining the risk of metastasis to LNs, recurrence rate, and survival. Patients with grade 1 tumors have longer survival duration than those with grade 2 or 3 tumors do, with a 5-year survival rate of 80, 69, and 41%, respectively (156-158).

■ VACCINATIONS

The inverse relationship between host immune response and HPV infection and preinvasive and invasive cervical lesions has been well recognized. Because HPVs are responsible for the majority of cervical cancer cases, a vaccine that stimulates the host immune response which can subsequently reduce the incidence of cancer-related HPV may be advantageous. Many preclinical and a few clinical trials have been performed in an attempt to prevent this infection or to treat the preinvasive lesion.

PREVENTIVE SETTING

Koutsky et al. (159) conducted a double-blinded randomized study in 2392 women at risk for infection who received three doses of a placebo or HPV-16–like particle vaccine (40 µg/dose). After a median follow-up duration of 17.4 months from administration of the last dose, the incidence of HPV-16 infection was significantly lower in the study group (3.8% in the placebo group, 0.0% in the vaccinated group; $p < .001$). In their review of the vaccines for cervical cancer, Crum and Rivera (160) found that many questions have yet to be answered and resolved. These include vaccine safety, the multiplicity of the cancer-associated HPVs, the inconsistency in assembly in different strains, the lack of cross-protection between different HPV types, and the lack of data on other HPV strains associated with cancer risk, such as HPV-45, which, together with HPV-16 and -18, is the important causative agent for aggressive adenocarcinoma (ACA) and neuroendocrine tumors (NEC). Another major issue is the timing in prevention, specifically whether vaccination at the time of infection or soon after would effectively prevent an HPV infection.

Two HPV vaccines are currently on the market: Gardasil and Cervarix. Both vaccines protect against two of the HPV types (HPV-16 and HPV-18) that can cause cervical cancer, and some other genital cancers; Gardasil also protects against two of the HPV types (HPV-6 and HPV-11) that cause genital warts. These two vaccines have been shown to have nearly 100% efficacy in preventing development of cervical cancer for the HPV strains that they are targeted. Gardasil is given by injection and requires three doses; the first injection is followed by a second and third dose 2 and 6 months later, respectively. Cervarix is also given by injection and requires three doses, although the schedule is slightly different than with Gardasil; the first injection is followed by a second and third dose 1 and 6 months later, respectively. In the United States, Gardasil is recommended for all girls and women who are between ages 9 and 26 years. Cervarix is recommended for girls and women of any age.

THERAPEUTIC SETTING

Usually, expression of the oncoproteins E6 and E7 is due to covalent integration of a virus into the host genome. These oncoproteins are necessary for tumor maintenance, so any vaccine or therapeutic intervention that stimulates the host immune response against these oncoproteins may reverse or delay the growth of existing tumors transformed by them. In their review, Gissman et al. (161) reported that vaccines for cervical cancer, consisting of either a recombinant vaccine virus or peptides derived from E6 and E7, can stimulate both humoral and cytotoxic T-lymphocyte responses. A randomized controlled trial of a DNA vaccine in 150 women with high-grade SIL (HSIL) showed a higher regression rate in the treated group than in the placebo group, 44 versus 25% ($p = .12$) (162). The difference in regression rate was significant only to women <25 years of age, 70 versus 30% ($p = .007$).

■ TUMOR MARKERS

SQUAMOUS CELL CARCINOMA ANTIGEN

Measurement of SCC antigen has been used clinically as a prognostic factor in patients undergoing either radiation therapy or surgery (163-166). One study reported the prognostic role of SCC antigen in predicting tumor response in patients who had been treated with radiation; >70% decrease of SCC antigen was significantly correlated with complete tumor response (163). Others found that normalization of antigen level after treatment

was also significantly associated with higher 2-year recurrence-free survival (164). In patients undergoing surgical treatment, preoperative serum SCC antigen was found in one study to be associated with recurrence-free and overall survival ($p = 0.003$ and 0.0078), independent of other factors such as tumor size, pelvic nodal status, cervical stroma infiltration, parametrial spread, and tumor grading (165). Another study, by Takeda et al., demonstrated that preoperative serum levels of SCC antigen as well as serum CA 125 were significantly related to the FIGO stage, tumor diameter, depth of cervical stromal invasion, LVSI, and lymph node metastasis (166).

The other clinical use of SCC antigen is in the detection of early recurrence in SCC of the cervix (167-169). In a study of Micke et al., 71% of patients with recurrent disease had a significant increase of SCC serum levels before clinical manifestation of relapse (167). The lead time ranged between 1 and 16 months (median: 3.1 months). A study by Hung et al. including 50 patients with recurrent cervical cancer demonstrated abnormal value of serum SCC antigen or tissue polypeptide-specific antigen prior to clinical recurrence in 27 and 30 patients, respectively (168). The combination of SCC antigen and tissue polypeptide-specific, provided lead-time detection in 42 cases. Esajas et al. evaluated 225 patients with a history of cervical cancer and demonstrated that the sensitivity of SCC antigen in detecting recurrence was 74% (26 of 35 patients); only 14% had this elevation as the first measured clinical indicator (169). However, the early detection of recurrence did not contribute to better survival. Median survival after recurrence in patients with an elevated serum SCC antigen at recurrence was worse than that of patients with normal serum values, 9 months (range 2-112 months) and 20 months (range 4-96 months) respectively. Other authors found that the median lead time of SCC antigen elevation prior to clinical detection was 7.8 months (170). However, the authors concluded that SCC monitoring is not cost-effective because most recurrences to distant spread were not amenable to curative treatment; that is, detection did not alter clinical management and offered no advantage over clinical examination in detecting local recurrence.

■ TREATMENTS

TREATMENT OF ABNORMAL PAP SMEARS

In a conference sponsored by the American Society for Colposcopy and Cervical Pathology held in September 2001, participants from many organizations, federal agencies, and national and international health organizations came up with a consensus on guidelines for the treatment of SILs, which is summarized below (171).

Atypical Squamous Cells

Treatment of ASC depends on the subcategory based on the Pap smear: undetermined significance (ASC-US) or cannot exclude HSIL (ASC-H).

1. ASC-US: The risk of co-HSIL lesions is only 5 to 17%, and patients with these lesions can be cared for with "triage" methods: follow-up of Pap smears at 4- to 6-month intervals, immediate colposcopy, or DNA testing for high-risk types of HPV. HPV DNA typing is recommended if the cytology is obtained with a liquid-based method. This can be achieved via the polymerase chain reaction, which can verify the specific type of HPV, or Hybrid Capture II, which can indicate only the risk group of HPV infection.

   However, immunosuppressed and postmenopausal women may require special management, as the former group has a greater risk of high-risk types of HPV infection and HSIL, while the latter appears to have a lower risk of HSIL than premenopausal women do. All immunosuppressed patients should be referred for colposcopy immediately. Postmenopausal women may be given intravaginal estrogen followed by a repeat cervical cytology test at 1 week after treatment.

2. ASC-H: Because the risk of co-HSIL lesions in this group of patients is high, ranging from 24 to 94%, these patients should be referred for immediate colposcopic evaluation.

Low-Grade Squamous Intraepithelial Lesion

Approximately 15 to 30% of women with a cytologic diagnosis of LSIL have a high-grade lesion detected after colposcopy-directed biopsy; colposcopy is recommended as the next step in the management of these lesions. Further management depends on the result of the colposcopic examination or presence of any identified lesions. In women who have a satisfactory colposcopic examination with an identified lesion, biopsy analysis with or without endocervical sampling is recommended. Endocervical sampling is obtained only if a lesion is seen at the transformation zone. In cases with an unsatisfactory colposcopic examination, either biosy analysis of the lesion or endocervical sampling is done. Women with negative results can undergo follow-up with repeat cytologic testing at 6 and 12 months or

HPV testing at 12 months and managed according to those results.

High-Grade Squamous Intraepithelial Lesion

Because women with a cytologic diagnosis of HSIL have an approximately 70 to 75% chance of having biopsy confirmation of HSIL and a 1 to 2% chance of having invasive cervical cancer, colposcopy with endocervical assessment is recommended for disease management in these women. If the colposcopy does not reveal a lesion or biopsy analysis does not show LSIL, all cytologic and histologic results should be reviewed and a diagnostic excisional procedure should be performed.

Atypical Glandular Cells

The presence of AGCs is associated with a greater risk of cervical neoplasia than that of ASCs or LSIL. Women in this group have an incidence of CIN, AIS, and invasive carcinoma detected via tissue biopsy as high as 9 to 54%, 0 to 8%, and <1 to 9%, respectively. The 2001 Bethesda System classifies glandular cell abnormalities less severe than adenocarcinoma into three categories:

1. AGCs, either endocervical, endometrial, or not otherwise specified: high-grade lesions, including CIN2, CIN3, AIS, and invasive cancer, have been found in 9 to 41% of women in this group.
2. AGCs, either endocervical or glandular cells "favor neoplasia": HSIL, AIS, or invasive cancer has been found in 27 to 96% of women in this group.
3. Endocervical AIS: The cytologic interpretation of AIS is associated with a very high risk of either AIS (48-69%) or invasive cervical adenocarcinoma (38%).

The management of all subcategories of AGCs is colposcopy with endocervical sampling except in women older than 35 years or with AGCs specified with atypical endometrial cells, which should also be evaluated with endometrial sampling. If the lesion identified via tissue diagnosis is less than invasive disease, women with AGCs that "favor neoplasia" or endocervical AIS should undergo a diagnostic excisional procedure. Cold-knife conization is more appropiate than electrical loop excision in women with AGCs or AIS due to better assessment of higher and multiple disconnected lesions. Repeat cervical cytologic testing is unacceptable, and assessment of HPV DNA testing is not recommended due to insufficient supporting data.

TREATMENT OF CERVICAL INTRAEPITHELIAL NEOPLASIA

Eradication of precursor lesions is mandatory as an effective approach to the prevention of cervical cancer. Options for the management of CIN have varied owing to several factors. One factor is the poor reproducibility of histologic diagnosis of CIN due to a high level of intraobserver and interobserver variability in many studies and by the National Cancer Institute's ASCUS/LSIL Triage Study (172). Another factor is the wide variation in the natural history of CIN. In patients with CIN1, more than half of the lesions have spontaneous regression, and the rate of progression to CIN2 and CIN3 or cancer is very low. In comparison, in patients with CIN2 and CIN3, approximately 30 to 40% have spontaneous regression if the lesion goes untreated, and more than half have progression to CIS or invasive cancer. This led to management guidelines for management of biopsy-confirmed CIN as summarized by the American Society for Colposcopy and Cervical Pathology, described below (173).

CIN1

Women who have a satisfactory colposcopy can undergo follow-up without immediate treatment and have a repeat Pap smear at 6 and 12 months, HPV testing at 12 months, or a combination of repeat cytology and colposcopy at 12 months. However, they can also undergo treatment with ablative methods such as cryotherapy, laser vaporization, or electrocautery, or they can undergo lesion excision as deemed necessary by the physician. Endocervical sampling should be performed prior to ablative treatment. In the recurrence setting after ablative methods, use of excisional modalities is the better option. If the colposcopy is unsatisfactory, a diagnostic excisional procedure such as cold-knife conization should be performed. However, follow-up is acceptable in pregnant women, those who are immunosuppressed, and adolescents.

CIN2, CIN3

The type of treatment of CIN depends on the severity of the lesion, degree of suspicion for invasive cancer, experience of the clinician, available resources, and patient preference.

Both excision and ablation are acceptable for women with CIN2 or CIN3 documented after a satisfactory colposcopy and in whom invasive cervical cancer has been ruled out. However, diagnostic excisional procedures are recommended for women with these lesions and an unsatisfactory colposcopy or in the recurrent setting. Excision or conization has an advantage over the ablative procedures in that the resected tissue can be examined pathologically. It can be achieved with either a cold knife, laser surgery, or a loop electrosurgical excision procedure (LEEP), the last of which has become more popular in recent years due to its greater convenience, shorter operative times, less blood loss, and better cervical visualization after treatment when compared with the other methods.

Hysterectomy is unacceptable as primary therapy due to its risk of morbidity compared with excisional or ablative procedures. Nevertheless, the procedure is acceptable for recurrent or persistent CIN2 or CIN3.

TREATMENT OF INVASIVE CERVICAL CARCINOMA

Type of Treatment

Treatment of invasive cervical cancer depends on many factors: disease stage, patient age, performance status, fertility of the patient, and skill and resources of the care providers. Generally, four major types of treatment are implemented as described below.

Surgery
Conization
Radical trachelectomy (RT)
Hysterectomy

In 1974, Piver et al. (174) categorized hysterectomy into five classes according to the extent of tissue resection.

Class I

Simple hysterectomy is removal of the uterus along with the cervix in an extrafascial manner without incision into the cervical or uterine tissue.

Class II

Modified radical hysterectomy is removal of the uterus with part of the paracervical and parametrial tissue in the lateral aspect of the cervix after dissecting the ureters away. Half of the cardinal ligament (lateral aspect), the uterosacral ligament (posterior aspect), and one-third of the upper vagina are all removed. This is usually performed in cases of stage IA2 or persistent or local recurrent cervical cancer after radiation therapy.

Class III

Radical hysterectomy is removal of the uterus in a manner similar to that of class II hysterectomy, but the tissue structure is removed to a greater extent, generally close to the pelvic side wall laterally and sacrum posteriorly; the upper half of the vagina is also removed. Conventionally, this class of hysterectomy is done for cases of stage IB-IIA disease. However, it can be performed for persistent or recurrent cervical cancer after primary radiation therapy as an alternative procedure to exenteration in highly selected patients. These include patients with stage IB-IIA disease at primary diagnosis, no clinical parametrial involvement, and a tumor diameter of ≤4 cm at the time of recurrence.

Class IV

Extended radical hysterectomy is complete removal of cervix, uterus, parametrial tissue, cardinal, and uterosacral ligaments. In addition, the ureter is completely dissected from the vesicouterine ligament, and the superior vesical artery is sacrificed. This is a possible procedure for central locoregional recurrence.

Class V

Partial exenteration is partial excision of the involved organs. In addition to the above procedures, this encompasses the removal of the distal ureter and urinary bladder. This procedure is performed in cases of central recurrence.

A more recent classification has been introduced by Querleu and Morrow (175):

Type A: Minimum Resection of Paracervix

This resection is an extrafascial hysterectomy, in which the position of the ureters is determined by palpation or direct vision (after opening of the ureteral tunnels) without freeing the ureters from their beds. The paracervix is transected medial to the ureter, but lateral to the cervix. The uterosacral and vesicouterine ligaments are not transected at a distance from the uterus. Vaginal resection is generally at a minimum, routinely less than 10 mm, without removal of the vaginal part of the paracervix (paracolpos).

Type B: Transection of Paracervix at the Ureter

Partial resection of the uterosacral and vesicouterine ligaments is a standard part of this category. The ureter is unroofed and rolled laterally, permitting transection of the paracervix at the level of the ureteral tunnel. The caudal (posterior, deep) neural component of the paracervix caudal to the deep uterine vein is not resected. At least 10 mm of the vagina from the cervix or tumour is resected.

Type C: Transection of Paracervix at Junction With Internal Iliac Vascular System

This type is transection of the uterosacral ligament at the rectum and vesicouterine ligament at the bladder. The ureter is mobilized completely. Fifteen to twenty mm of vagina from the tumour or cervix and the corresponding paracolpos is resected routinely, depending on vaginal and paracervical extent and on surgeon choice.

Type D: Laterally Extended Resection

This group of rare operations feature additional ultraradical procedures, mostly indicated at the time of pelvic exenteration. Type D1 is resection of the entire paracervix at the pelvic sidewall along with the hypogastric vessels, exposing the roots of the sciatic nerve. There is total resection of the vessels of the lateral part of the paracervix; these vessels (ie, inferior gluteal, internal pudendal, and obturator vessels) arise from the internal iliac system. Type D2 is D1 plus resection of the entire paracervix with the hypogastric vessels and adjacent fascial or muscular structures.

▨▨ Radiation Therapy

Pelvic Irradiation
Extended-Field Para-aortic Irradiation

▨▨ Chemotherapy

Until recently, the role of chemotherapy was limited to the management of advanced-stage cervical cancer with systemic dissemination and recurrent cervical cancer, which are not amenable to other treatment modalities. Recently, its role was expanded for locally advanced disease in concurrence with radiation therapy.

▨▨ Combination Treatment

Concurrent Chemoradiation
Neoadjuvant Chemotherapy Prior to Radiation Therapy
Neoadjuvant Chemotherapy Prior to Surgery
Adjuvant Radiation Therapy After Surgery
Adjuvant Simple Hysterectomy After Radiation Therapy

TREATMENT BY STAGE OF DISEASE

▨▨ Stage IA1

Stage IA1 cervical cancer should be diagnosed using a conization specimen, because small tissue biopsy study may not be accurate enough to rule out other areas of a more extensive lesion. The treatment depends on the need for fertility preservation.

Conization

Conization is a cone-shaped resection of a portion of cervix either as a diagnostic procedure in cases in which invasive cancer cannot be ruled out via biopsy or as a therapeutic procedure.

In cases with clear margins in the cone biopsy specimen, there is a place for conservative management in a select group of patients who wish to preserve fertility. These women should undergo regular long-term surveillance in a colposcopy clinic. If either the internal margin or postconization endocervical curettage contains dysplasia or carcinoma, the risk of residual invasion is high: 22% for a positive internal margin and 33% with positive of both internal margin and endocervical curettage (176). Therefore these women must undergo repeat conization before definitive treatment planning. This second cone biopsy may be appropriate "definitive treatment" in young women who wish to preserve their fertility if the margins in the second biopsy specimen are clear and there is no evidence of invasion. Even in those for whom a hysterectomy is proposed, a second cone biopsy analysis may be required before hysterectomy to avoid inappropriate treatment of an occult invasive lesion.

Simple Hysterectomy

Simple hysterectomy may be performed in women with stage IA1 cervical cancer in whom preservation of fertility function is not required. However in patients with LVSI, a modified radical hysterectomy may be the procedure of choice.

Stage IA2

Because the incidence of LN involvement in patients with this stage cervical cancer is as high as 7% with a recurrence rate of 3 to 5%, they should be treated with a radical hysterectomy with pelvic LN dissection and conservative treatment, as conization or simple hysterectomy is not appropiate. The other conservative approach that has been reported to have a successful outcome is radical trachelectomy with extraperitoneal or laparoscopic pelvic lymphadenectomy, in which the body of uterus is preserved for fertility function (177).

Individualization of therapy based on findings from extensive pathologic review of an adequate cone biopsy specimen is important for treatment planning. In patients with inoperable stage IA disease, radiation therapy with only intracavitary implants is an option that has been shown to have excellent results (178).

Stage IB1

In early-stage (stage IA-IB1) cervical cancer, surgery and radiation therapy yield comparable overall 5-year survival rates ranging from 80 to 90% (179). These two methods have both advantages and disadvantages, including side effects, and may be appropriate for different individuals. Surgery has many advantages over radiation therapy: shorter treatment time, preservation of ovarian and vaginal function, and increased accuracy compared with clinical staging in evaluating primary lesions and intraperitoneal and retroperitoneal spread (including to LNs), treatment of other associated pelvic pathologies in the same setting, and fewer long-term complications. The advantages of radiation therapy over surgery are that it can be employed for disease at any stage and all patients, including those with medical disease or contraindications to surgery.

Radical Hysterectomy and Pelvic Irradiation With or Without Para-aortic Lymph Node Dissection

Traditionally, surgery for stage IB disease consists of radical hysterectomy performed in conjunction with pelvic lymphadenectomy. Lately, many authors have recommended class II hysterectomy rather than conventional class III hysterectomy in stages IB and IIA disease with a tumor size <2 cm owing to fewer complications from the former and no difference in the 5-year survival (180-182) (Figs. 30-11 and 30-12).

In patients with negative nodes and high-risk local findings, the Gynecologic Oncology Group (GOG) randomized 137 patients with stage IB cervical cancer treated with radical hysterectomy and pelvic lymphadenectomy who had at least two of the following risk factors: more than one-third stromal invasion, capillary lymphatic space involvement, and a large clinical tumor diameter to have postoperative radiation therapy compared to 140 patients to receive no further treatment (183). The risk of recurrence was significantly reduced to 15.3% in the radiation group versus 27.9% in group that received no further treatment ($p = .008$). The 2-year recurrence-free survival was also higher among the patients receiving radiation compared with those without treatment, 88 versus 79%; however, this benefit was obtained at the cost of an increasing rate of complications, 6 versus 2.1%, respectively.

In those with LN-positive disease, pelvic irradiation certainly reduces the risk of recurrence, but with no improvement in overall survival (184-186). The survival

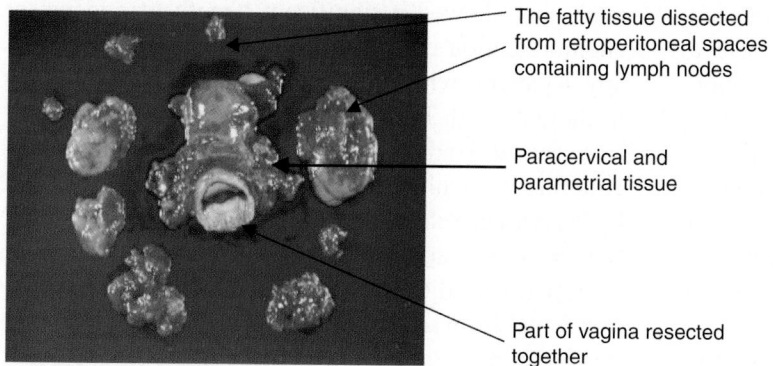

The fatty tissue dissected from retroperitoneal spaces containing lymph nodes

Paracervical and parametrial tissue

Part of vagina resected together

FIGURE 30-11. Gross specimen from a radical hysterectomy with lymph nodes dissected.

benefit of pelvic irradiation was later demonstrated in a study by the Southwest Oncology Group (187), which indicated that concurrent chemoradiation was superior to radiation therapy alone in patients with stage IA2-IIA disease who had positive LNs or parametrial involvement or a positive surgical margin (3-year survival rate, 87 versus 77%) (206). In a recent presentation at the 2004 Society of Gynecologic Oncology meeting by Im et al. (188), the benefit of adding chemotherapy to radiation therapy postoperatively in patients in this study (SWOG 8797) appeared to be limited to those with tumors >2 cm, >2 positive nodes, and parametrial extension.

Sentinel Lymph Node Mapping

Cervical cancer commonly spreads through the lymphatic system in a stepwise pattern from the cervical stroma and serosal lymphatics to paracervical pelvic groups and further distant groups of the common iliac and para-aortic area (189). LN dissection is a crucial part of surgical procedure, together with radical hysterectomy, for the treatment of early-stage cervical cancer. Owing to the relatively low rate of LN involvement in

early-stage disease and the risk of radical lymphadenectomy, which may outweigh the benefit, a procedure of sentinel node (SN) mapping for cervical cancer has been evolved. The concept of the SN was first clinically developed by Cabanas in association with penile carcinoma (190). It is based on the principle that if the SN or the first node receiving drainage from tumor is negative, more extensive lymphadenectomy may be exempted to avoid the morbidity of the procedure.

Generally, the techniques used to map SNs involve identification of the lymphatic duct by injecting of isosulfan blue dye or lymphoscintigraphy, using gamma probe detection of technetium 99m–labeled colloid, which is injected into the cervix. This can be done either before or during the operation. More than 10 studies of SN mapping for cervical cancer have been published; in these instances the investigators used either blue dye, lymphoscintigraphy, or both with varying degrees of success. The first study was reported in 1999 by Etch et al., with a detection rate of only approximately 15% with the blue-dye technique (191). Later studies reported that the detection rate from blue dye ranged from 40 to 100%. Many factors have contributed to the varying

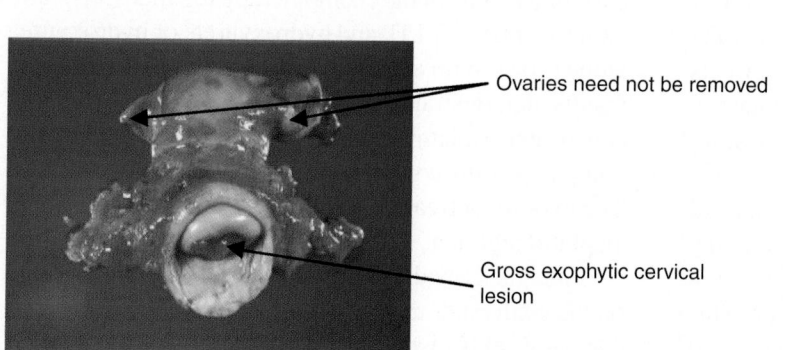

Ovaries need not be removed

Gross exophytic cervical lesion

FIGURE 30-12. A radical hysterectomy specimen with a portion of upper vagina. Note that the ovaries need not be removed unless indicated by the associated pathology.

degrees of success, such as the amount of dye injected (191); difficult and unreliable visual detection of dye uptake, which is a fast transition; or the size of tumor, where the larger tumors are less likely to be detected by the dye because of more congested nodes and lymphatic channels invaded by tumor and inflammatory debris. The detection rate of lymphoscintigraphy ranges from 76 to 93%. With the combination of two techniques, using both blue dye and lymphoscintigraphy, the rate of detection increased to 87 to 100% (192-203).

The success rate of detection depends partly on the learning curve experience of the performer. This is evidenced by the study of Plante et al., which was the largest study on SN mapping in cervical cancer to date (N = 70). The authors clearly demonstrated the importance of the learning curve to the success of the procedure. The rate of detection in the last 15 cases was significantly improved over that of the first 55 cases, 51 versus 93% (203).

At present, the procedure is still considered only on a trial basis, with an apparent benefit. However, a few issues remain unresolved, particularly in the pathologic aspect, such as the lack of consensus among the pathologists as to the management of the sentinel lymph node with the number of frozen sections and whether the evaluation of molecular marker should be included. It is questionable whether a single micrometastatic focus in the SN implies poor prognosis and increased mortality. The clinical relevance of micrometastatic disease and treatment has not been appreciated even in breast cancer, where the concept of SN mapping has long been applied (204). Although early information on SN biopsy in breast cancer suggested no adverse outcome for patients with micrometastases (205), this remains to be proven. The issue becomes even more pertinent if molecular marker techniques are applied, which could certainly identify a greater number of metastases.

Concurrent Chemoradiation

The synergistic effect of chemotherapy and radiation therapy reduces the tumor hypoxic fraction, synchronizes cell cycles, inhibits cellular repair, and recruits non-proliferating cells into cell cycles. These effects account for the improved treatment efficacy obtained with concurrent chemoradiation as opposed to irradiation alone.

In 1999, the US National Cancer Institute announced its support of concurrent cisplatin-based chemotherapy and radiation therapy in women who require radiation therapy for the management of cervical cancer. This was based on data from five randomized controlled trials that showed a significant benefit of concurrent chemoradiation either as postoperative adjuvant therapy in patients with high-risk factors or primary therapy in patients with locally advanced cervical cancer. All five trials utilized concurrent cisplatin either alone or in combination with 5-fluorouracil (5-FU) or 5-FU and hydroxyurea. Peters et al. (187), in the GOG trial 109/SWOG 8797, applied concurrent chemoradiation as postoperative adjuvant therapy in patients with risk factors found from radical hysterectomy in stage IA2-IIA; this report has been described in the section on adjuvant radiation therapy above. Keys et al. (206), in the GOG trial 123, compared chemoradiation and radiation with adjuvant hysterectomy in both groups as the definitive treatment in patients with stage IB2 disease. Significant improvement of 3-year survival was found in the chemoradiation group, 83 versus 74%. Pathologic examination of the hysterectomy specimens demonstrated a significant decrease in persistent disease with chemoradiation.

Three other studies comprised patients with more advanced disease (207-209). The Radiation Therapy Oncology Group trial 9001 (RTOG) by Morris et al. randomized stage IB-IVA patients to concurrent chemoradiation with cisplatin and 5-FU versus extended-field radiation (207). Chemoradiation was superior, with an increased in overall survival of 73%, compared with 58% for radiation alone. Acute toxicity was more common with chemoradiation, but the rates of late complications (>60 days posttreatment) were similar. Another GOG trial (GOG 85) in stage IIB-IVA cervical cancer by Whitney et al. compared the efficacy of a chemotherapy regimen in the concurrent chemoradiation setting (209). The result showed superiority of cisplatin and 5-FU over hydroxyurea; survival at a median follow-up of 8.7 years was 55 versus 43%. Leukopenia occurred less often in the group receiving cisplatin and 5-FU than in those receiving hydroxyurea. Another GOG investigation (GOG 120), by Rose et al. studied the optimal chemoradiation regimen by randomizing patients with stage IIB-IVA disease to receive radiation therapy concurrent with one of the chemotherapy regimens: cisplatin alone; cisplatin, 5-FU, and hydroxyurea; or hydroxyurea alone (208). With a median follow-up of 35 months, the results demonstrated superior survival rates for both concurrent cisplatin regimens (66 and 64%, respectively) compared with concurrent hydroxyurea alone (39%). The toxicity of treatment was least with the single-agent cisplatin regimen.

Later the Canadian National Cancer Institute reported on the sixth randomized controlled trial comparing concurrent weekly cisplatin and irradiation with irradiation alone (210). However, their study failed to show a significant benefit of the concurrent treatment. However, the 3- and 5-year survival slightly favored the chemoradiation group, 69 versus 66% and 62 versus 58%, respectively ($p = .42$). These seemingly different outcomes compared with the five mentioned studies may be due to a variety of factors. The patients in this trial were staged only by CT and some positive LNs may have gone undetected. This would have lessened the overall response, especially to local radiation therapy. Also, patients in the chemoradiation arm had significant anemia, which would impair the effect of treatment.

A summary of these six trials is presented in Table 30-6. Green et al. (211) conducted a systematic review of 19 randomized controlled trials of concurrent chemoradiation for cervical cancer (12 platinum-based and 7 non–platinum-based trials) in a large number of

patients. They showed a significant improvement in overall and progression-free survival and decreased local and distant recurrences (Table 30-7). Acute toxic effects, consisting of leukopenia and gastrointestinal problems, were more common in the chemoradiation group. However, these effects were brief and medically manageable.

Focusing on toxicity, Kirwan et al. (212) extensively reviewed 19 randomized trials of concurrent chemoradiation in 1766 patients with available data regarding acute and late toxic effects. The toxicity criteria were based on the combined criteria for irradiation (Radiation Therapy Oncology Group/Acute Radiation Morbidity Scoring Criteria) and chemotherapy (National Cancer Institute/Common Toxicity Criteria and WHO). Overall, acute toxic effects were more common in the concurrent chemoradiation group (odds ratio, 1.5 and

TABLE 30-6 | SIX RANDOMIZED CONTROL TRIALS OF CONCURRENT CHEMORADIATION FOR CERVICAL CANCER

Study (Protocol)	Setting	N	Rx	Outcome*	Remarks
Keys (206), 1999 (GOG 123)	IB2	369	1. RT + weekly C 2. RT (followed by TAH in both groups)	RR of progression and death, 0.51 and 0.54 in CRT arm	Higher severe hematologic and GIT toxicity in CRT arm (21 versus 4% and 14 versus 5%)
Peters (187), 2000 (SWOG 8797/ GOG 109)	PO IA2-IIA with risk factors	243	1. RT + CF 2. RT alone	4-year PFS and SVR, 80 and 81% in group 1 4-year PFS and SVR, 63 and 71% in group 2	ACA had similar outcomes as SCC in CRT arm ACA did worse in RT arm
Whitney (209), 1999 (GOG 85)	IIB-IVA	368	1. RT + CF 2. RT + HU	RR of progression and death, 0.79 and 0.74 of group 1 compared to group 2 (21 and 26% decreased risk of progression and death)	Severe leukopenia more common in HU arm (24 versus 4%)
Morris (207), 1999 (RTOG 9001)	IB-IVA	388	1. RT + CF 2. RT + extended field radiation	5-year OS and DFS, 73 and 67% 5-year OS and DFS, 58 and 40%	Higher reversible hematologic side effects in CRT arm
Rose (208), 1999 (GOG 120)	IIB-IVA	526	1. RT + weekly C 2. RT + CF + HU 3. RT + HU	2-year PFS, 67 and 64% in groups 1 and 2 and 47% in group 3 RR of death, 0.61 and 0.58 in groups 1 and 2 compared with group 3	Group 1 least toxic
Pearcey (210), 2002 (NCIC)	IB-IVA	253	1. RT + weekly C 2. RT alone	3-year SVR, 69 versus 66% 5-year SVR, 62 versus 58%	No statistically significant difference

ACA, adenocarcinoma; C, cisplatin; CF, cisplatin plus 5-fluorouracil; CRT, concurrent chemoradiation; DFS, disease-free survival; GIT, gastrointestinal tract; GOG, Gynecologic Oncology Group; HU, hydroxyurea; OS, overall survival; PFS, progression-free survival; PO, postoperative; RR, relative risk; RT, radiation therapy; SCC, squamous cell carcinoma; SVR, survival rate; SWOG, Southwest Oncology Group; vs, versus.
*There was a significant difference in all outcomes between the study and control groups except in the study by Pearcey et al.

TABLE 30-7	META-ANALYSIS OF RANDOMIZED CONTROLLED TRIALS OF CONCURRENT CHEMORADIATION		
Clinical Outcome	No. of Trials for Analysis	No. of Patients	Benefit
Overall survival	11	2865	HR 0.71 (95% CI 0.63-0.81) 29% reduction risk of death 12% absolute improvement of SVR (42-52%)
Progression-free survival	13	3611	HR 0.61 (95% CI 0.55-0.68) 13% absolute improvement of PFS (47-63%)
Local recurrence	12	3186	OR 0.61 (95% CI 0.51-0.73)
Distant recurrence	12	3186	OR 0.57 (95% CI 0.46-0.77)

CI, confidence interval; HR, hazard ratio; OR, overall response; PFS, progression-free survival; SVR, survival rate.

2.4 in grades 1 to 2 and grades 3 to 4 toxicity, respectively). The most striking toxicity was hematologic (odds ratio, 5.5 and 31.5 in grades 1 to 2 and grades 3 to 4 toxicity, respectively). Regarding late toxicity, no statistically significant differences in long-term effects were found. Overall, bowel complications from irradiation accounted for most of the nonhematologic toxic effects.

Other drugs have also been studied in concurrent chemoradiation, but with less satisfactory outcomes compared with cisplatin. For example, mitomycin produced significant late gastrointestinal toxic effects in a retrospective study at the rate of 21.8% in a concurrent setting and thus was not incorporated in the prospective study (213). Also, fluorouracil was studied in a prospective trial by Thomas et al. (214), but no benefit was seen. Another drug of interest is carboplatin, because it is less neurotoxic, nephrotoxic, and emetogenic than cisplatin and requires no hydration. However, there have been no controlled trials showing that the efficacy of carboplatin is comparable with that of cisplatin. Only a few phase I and II studies of carboplatin have been performed. Examples of these studies are listed in Table 30-8 (215-218).

Radical Trachelectomy

RT is resection of the cervix together with paracervical and parametrial tissue, with retention of the corpus

TABLE 30-8	STUDIES OF CONCURRENT CARBOPLATIN AND RADIATION THERAPY			
	Duenas-Gonzalez (215), 2003	Higgins (216), 2003	Muderspach (217), 1997	Corn (218), 1998
Number of patients	24	31	22	15
Stage and disease	IIIB	IB1-IVA	IIA-IIIB	IB2-IIIB, recurrence
Characteristics	PAN not evaluated	Negative PAN	32% positive LN (3 PAN, 4 PN)	(no prior chemotherapy) 20% positive LN
Carboplatin dose	100-150 mg/m² weekly	AUC 2, weekly	30-50 mg/m² twice a week	60 or 90 mg/m² weekly
Toxicity	50% toxicity at 150 mg/m² 33% leukopenia at 133 mg/m²	Unusual	No grade 4 toxicity Most common toxicity was anemia	Mild and transient (no grade 3-4 toxicity)
Response	OR 75% (18 CR, 4 SD, 2 PD)	OR 90% (28 CR, 1SD, 2 PD)	OR 96% (19 CR, 2 PR, 1 SD)	OR 87% (7 CR, 6 PR, 2 SD or PD)
Remark	Recommend dose, 133 mg/m²	—	Extended-field RT given in three patients with positive PAN	Extended-field RT given in three patients with positive LN

AUC, area under curve; CR, complete response; LN, lymph node; OR, overall response; PAN, para-aortic lymph node; PD, progressive disease; PN, pelvic lymph node; RT, radiation therapy; SD, stable disease.

uteri. The procedure is indicated in reproductive-age women with disease stage IA1 (with LVSI), IA2, or IB1 who wish to preserve fertility (219-222). The following are the tumor characteristics appropriate for RT: *tumor size* should be <2 cm. An increase in tumor size is usually accompanied by extension to the upper endocervix or parametrium, with an increased possibility of LN metastasis and recurrence (223). The considerable exception is a large exophytic mass with a narrow base (224), described by Covens as mushroom-shaped (225). In another series by Schlaerth et al. (224) in which 5 of 10 cases were ACA and 1 of 10 was adenosquamous carcinoma, the authors reported success of treatment with no recurrence and that 2 of 4 pregnant patients had ACA. Hence, they did not regard ACA as a contraindication to RT as long as conization revealed free margins, a negative endocervical curettage, and no LVSI. *Negative lymph nodes* should be confirmed by frozen section before beginning the RT procedure. There is *no endocervical involvement* and all surgical margins should be free, as revealed by frozen section. The superior endocervical margin should be at least 5 to 8 mm (225), otherwise more endocervix is removed. Preferably, the procedure should leave a cervical length of at least 1 cm for fertility function (224). The presence of LVSI was also considered as a risk factor for recurrence. Both recurrences in the series of Dargent had evidence of LVSI. However, Covens et al. did not regard this as a contraindication unless accompanied by other poor prognostic factors (219).

Many studies have reported on preservation of fertility function and cancer recurrence after RT. The rate of pregnancy loss is high due to the possibility of cervical incompetence from a shorter cervical length, increased subclinical or chorioamnionitis from the cerclage, or absence of the cervical mucus plug barrier. Covens summarized data from four large published articles comprising 237 women who underwent RT (225). Tumor size was less than 2 cm in 89%, with SCC histology of 65%. Presence of LVSI was noted in 30%. At the median follow-up of 37 months, the recurrence rate was 3%. Among 92 women who attempted conception, pregnancies were achieved in 102 events, with 65 live births.

Diaz et al. compared the oncologic outcomes of women who underwent a fertility-sparing radical trachelectomy (RT) to those who underwent a radical hysterectomy (RH) for stage IB1 cervical carcinoma (226). Forty stage IB1 patients underwent an RT and 110 patients underwent an RH. There were no statistical differences between the two groups for the following prognostic variables: histology, median number of lymph nodes removed, node-positive rate, lymph-vascular space

involvement (LVSI), or deep stromal invasion (DSI). The median follow-up for the entire group was 44 months. The 5-year RFS rate was 96% (for the RT group compared to 86% for the RH group (p-value not significant). On multivariate analysis in this group of stage IB1 lesions, tumor size <2 cm was not an independent predictor of outcome, but both LVSI and DSI retained independent predictive value ($p = .033$ and $.005$, respectively). The authors concluded that for selected patients with stage IB1 cervical cancer, fertility-sparing radical trachelectomy appears to have a similar oncologic outcome to radical hysterectomy. LVSI and DSI appear to be more valuable predictors of outcome than tumor diameter in this subgroup of patients.

More recently, Ramirez et al. (227) showed that robotic radical trachelectomy and bilateral pelvic lymphadenectomy is feasible and safe and should be considered for patients desiring fertility-sparing surgery. This option offers patients the benefits of minimally invasive surgery to patients who wish to preserve their fertility.

Stage IB2-IIA

The risk of metastasis to LNs and the parametrium in patients with stage IB2 cervical cancer is much higher than that in patients with stage IB1 disease (30-50% versus 15-25%), and the subsequent 5-year survival rate is lower (60-70% versus 80-90%). Until recently, women with cancer at these stages underwent radical hysterectomy or received radiation therapy alone. However, with the decreased survival, other treatments have been developed with variable success. These are discussed below.

Concurrent Chemoradiation

The concurrent chemoradiation treatment is considered a standard practice in these stages of disease. This has been previously discussed and will not be explored further.

Radiation Treatment

Generally, radiation therapy for cervical cancer consists of a combination of external whole pelvic irradiation (ERT) and intracavitary irradiation (ICRT). The aim is to eradicate cancer in the primary site, paracervical tissue, and regional pelvic LNs (228). ERT is given initially to decrease the bulk of the tumor, providing a better geometric anatomy and allowing optimal dose delivery in ICRT. ERT also covers the pelvic tissue up to the side wall. A course of 40 to 45 Gy of ERT is given over approximately 4 to 5 weeks, with the use of anteroposterior and posteroanterior beams or additional left-and right-lateral beams (to minimize the dose delivered to the small bowel). The extent of the irradiated fields encompasses the level of the midpubis or 3 to 4 cm below the cervical or vaginal lesions inferiorly, L5 to S1 level to cover the area of common iliac nodes superiorly (or up to L4 to L5 if para-aortic nodes are at high risk), and at least 1 cm lateral to bony pelvic margins. ICRT is employed by means of uterine tandem and vaginal ovoid to provide a high radiation dose to the cervical tumor after it is partially shrunken by ERT. This application of ICRT has been proven by many authors to reduce the rate of local failure and to improve the survival rate compared with ERT alone: 78 versus 53% for local control (229) and 43 to 87% versus 21.0 to 60.5% for survival (229-231). Low-dose-rate brachytherapy has long been used (232), but immobilization and hospitalization of patients and exposure of medical personnel to radiation have been by-products of the increasing popularity of the high-dose-rate technique in the recent years (233,234). It remains difficult to compare the superiority of the two methods due to poor methodology in reporting complications and loss of a large number of patients to follow-up in most studies (235). In a study of approximately 2000 patients, Lorvidhaya et al. (236) reported similar survival and complications at each disease stage in patients undergoing high- and low-dose-rate brachytherapy. Conventional high-dose radiation therapy for bulky tumors may result in a high rate of complications, such as rectovaginal fistula, vesicovaginal fistula, stricture ureter, and vaginal necrosis and stenosis. Recently, intensity-modulated radiation therapy (IMRT) has emerged as a new treatment with fewer complications than conventional radiation therapy. It is performed via computerized optimized modulation to generate the dose distribution, so it provides a highly conformal dose to tumors of almost any shape and is more advantageous than conventional three-dimensional radiation therapy, which is generally limited to lesions with convex volumes (237). The therapeutic ratio is improved in that IMRT allows selective normal tissue dose reduction and concomitant integrated boost dose to the tumor. With this increased dose delivered to the tumor, subsequent improved local control has been reported in many studies (238-240). One study by Low et al. (239) demonstrated an advantage with external beam intensity-modulated conformal dose distributions over ICRT in treating cervical cancer in that it covered the point-A isodose surface and reduced the dose delivered to the bladder and rectum, while ICRT showed extensive underdosed regions in the target area. The flexibility of IMRT, which enables customized dose

distributions, clearly reduces acute and potentially late treatment-related toxic effects in the urinary bladder, rectum, and small bowel in addition to improving local control, especially of locally advanced disease. However, one study found that IMRT is likely to increase the risk of a second cancer from 1.00 to 1.75% compared with conventional radiation therapy in patients who survive for 10 years (241). This was explained by the fact that IMRT involves more fields, although at lower doses, so a larger volume of normal tissue is exposed to radiation. Last, the number of patients in each study was limited, so more prospective trials are necessary to better evaluate IMRT before a definite conclusion for the advantage of the procedure can be drawn.

Regarding prognostic factors for patients who receive radiation therapy, *tumor size* has long been known to be an important factor affecting the result of radiation therapy. Principally, radiation therapy destroys tumor tissue through the formation of oxygen-free radicals. Large tumors are usually hypoxic and are considered radioresistant, with subsequent poor local tumor control and decreased survival (242). Anemia, which results in tissue hypoxia, is also considered a negative factor for prognosis. The mean weekly nadir hemoglobin and, less likely, hemoglobin level at the time of presentation are correlated with local control, disease-free survival, and overall survival; the rate of 5-year survival or greater was 74, 52, and 45 when the mean weekly nadir hemoglobin levels were ≥120, 110 to 119, and <110 g/L, respectively (243). An attempt to keep the hemoglobin level above 12 g/dL using erythropoietin has been evaluated in a study by the GOG. However, this study was closed prior to an accrual completion due to an increase in venous thrombosis in the patients receiving erythropoietin. *The duration of radiation therapy* is another important prognostic factor; the rate of local tumor control is decreased by 0.7 to 1.0% (244,245) and survival is decreased by 0.6% (245) for each day of treatment delay.

Extended-Field Radiation Therapy (Prophylactic Para-aortic Irradiation)

As the incidence of para-aortic node involvement in stages IB, IIB, and IIIB disease is approximately 7, 17, and 29%, respectively, this area might be a site of treatment failure if only conventional pelvic irradiation is used. An attempt to include this field in the treatment of locally advanced cervical cancer has evolved.

A prospective randomized trial by the Radiation Therapy Oncology Group first published in 1990 (246) and updated in 1995 (247) demonstrated a significantly improved 10-year overall survival rate when prophylactic extended-field irradiation was added to standard locoregional pelvic irradiation in patients with high-risk stage IB or IIA (≥4 cm) or stage IIB cervical cancer who had no evidence of para-aortic node metastasis (55% for pelvic plus para-aortic irradiation versus 44% for pelvic irradiation only). However, the disease-free survival and locoregional failure rates were similar. These findings were attributed to a lower incidence of distant failure in complete responders and better response to salvage treatment in the complete responders who later experienced local treatment failure. As expected, the toxicity and death rates were higher in the extended-irradiation arm, although not significantly.

Radiation Therapy Followed by Adjuvant Simple Hysterectomy

The efficacy of radiation therapy alone is less than optimum for large, bulky cervical tumors due to an inadequate or poor dose distribution with standard intracavitary irradiation, which results in a high local failure rate and poor survival. Many studies have reported a benefit of postirradiation hysterectomy in patients with a tumor larger than 6 cm (248,249). However, its effect on survival was not clearly demonstrated, with similar or higher morbidity rate from complications (248,249). In our institution, Thoms et al. (250) reported retrospective data on the treatment of bulky endocervical stage IB-IIB cervical carcinoma over a 23-year period. The benefit in pelvic control and survival from the addition of adjuvant hysterectomy appeared to be limited to a subset of patients with stage IIB disease who had disease-negative lymph-angiograms, tumors ≥8 cm in size, and a good response to external irradiation (64 versus 45%). Other studies could not demonstrate a benefit of surgery after irradiation when compared with irradiation alone (251,252). The GOG recently reported the results of a randomized controlled trial with 256 eligible patients with exophytic or barrel-shaped tumors measuring ≥4 cm (253). There was no significant difference in the 5-year survival of patients by treatment regimen; relative risk of the combined-treatment group to the radiation-only group was 0.89 (90% confidence interval [CI], 0.65-1.21; $p = .26$). The 5-year progression-free survival was significantly increased in the combined-treatment group, 62 versus 53% ($p = .09$). The frequency of any reported adverse effect was higher for the hysterectomy group (63 versus 56%) but severe adverse effects from the gastrointestinal or genitourinary tract exclusively were similar in both groups (10%).

Findings from hysterectomy specimens clearly affect overall survival, as 92% of patients with disease-negative specimens survived 5 years, compared with 71% of patients with disease-positive specimens (254).

Neoadjuvant Chemotherapy

The role of neoadjuvant chemotherapy for cervical cancer has evolved to two settings: prior to radiation therapy and prior to surgery. Cisplatin has been the main drug used in all neoadjuvant chemotherapy regimens in most trials.

Prior to Radiation Therapy

Theoretically, chemotherapy prior to radiation therapy may decrease tumor size, treat micrometastases outside the radiation field, and be less toxic compared to concurrent administration with radiation therapy. However, patients who receive prior chemotherapy have unavoidable toxic effects and cannot tolerate the subsequent radiation therapy well.

Neoadjuvant chemotherapy followed by radiation therapy has been studied in patients with stage IB2, IIA, and IIB disease. However, randomized controlled trials of neoadjuvant chemotherapy prior to irradiation have not demonstrated a definite benefit when compared with irradiation alone, with a similar (255-259) or worse outcome in the neoadjuvant groups (260,261). This has led most clinicians to abandon the use of neoadjuvant chemotherapy followed by radiation therapy. This finding was recently confirmed in a systematic review by Tierney et al. (262), who found a 2- and 3-year survival odd ratio in neoadjuvant and control groups of 1.09 (95% CI, 0.83-1.45) and 0.96 (95% CI, 0.73-1.25), respectively. A larger multicenter collaboration group reconducted the meta-analysis by reviewing the individual patient data in all randomized studies (263). The authors found a highly significant level of statistical heterogeneity in treatment provided. Thus, they separately analyzed the outcomes to the treatment characteristics by grouping the trials by cycle length and cisplatin dose. The beneficial effects of neoadjuvant chemotherapy on survival and other endpoints were demonstrated in certain subgroups with short cycles of treatment and at a certain minimum dose of cisplatin. The reviewers explained that the short cycle and dose intensity would limit the accelerated regrowth of tumors after their size was reduced by the chemotherapy. The benefit on survival is shown in Table 30-9.

TABLE 30-9	META-ANALYSIS OF RANDOMIZED CONTROLLED TRIALS OF NEOADJUVANT CHEMOTHERAPY PRIOR TO RADIATION THERAPY			
Trial Grouping Characteristics	*No. of Trials*	*No. of Events/ Patients*	*HR (95% CI), p Value*	*Remarks*
Chemotherapy cycles				
>14 days	11	639/1214	1.25 (1.07-1.46), .005	25% increased risk of death
≤14 days	7	445/860	0.83 (0.69-1.00), .046	17% decreased risk of death and improved 5-year SVR from 45 to 52%
Cisplatin dose/week				
<25 mg/m^2	7	413/845	1.35 (1.11-1.64), .002	35% increased risk of death
≥25 mg/m^2	11	671/1229	0.91 (0.78-1.05), .200	9% decreased risk of death and improved 5-year SVR from 45 to 48%

CI, confidence interval; HR, hazard ratio; SVR, survival rate.

Data from the Neoadjuvant Chemotherapy for Locally Advanced Cervical Cancer Meta-Analysis Collaboration. Neoadjuvent chemotherapy for locally advanced cervical cancer: a systematic review and meta-analysis of individual patient data from 21 randomised trials. Eur J Cancer 2003;39:2470-2486.

Prior to Surgery

When neoadjuvant chemotherapy is administered prior to surgery, it reduces the tumor's size, rendering it more operable, reduces some of the risk factors necessitating postoperative adjuvant therapy, and controls systemic micrometastasis.

One study by Sardi et al. (264) showed a benefit of neoadjuvant chemotherapy prior to surgery. The authors conducted their trial in patients with stage IB2 cervical cancer with a long-term follow-up duration of 7 years. They found a significant decrease in pathologic risk factors, such as parametrial involvement, LVSI, and nodal metastasis in the neoadjuvant group, which had a higher overall survival rate than did the group not receiving neoadjuvant chemotherapy (80 versus 61%).

A review by the Neoadjuvant Chemotherapy for Locally Advanced Cervical Cancer Meta-Analysis Collaboration group discovered seven randomized controlled trials available for analysis, comprising 872 patients (263). The overall analysis and analysis of each individual trial showed significant improvement of all outcomes: hazard ratio of 0.65 for survival with 14% absolute improvement in 5-year survival rate (50 to 64%); hazard ratio of 0.68 for DFS with 13% absolute improvement of DFS (45 to 58%); and hazard ratio of 0.63 for metastasis-free survival, with 15% absolute improvement in metastasis-free survival (45 to 60%). However, many confounding factors were inherent and unavoidable in this systematic analysis: these factors were that a number of patients, ranging from 28 to 90% in each trial, also received postoperative adjuvant radiation therapy or triple-modality treatment compared with radiation therapy, the route of cisplatin administration

(intra-arterial in one trial), and different stages of disease in patients recruited to each trial. Until a large, well-designed, randomized controlled trial is conducted, neoadjuvant chemotherapy prior to surgery cannot be recommended as the standard of care.

Stage IIB-IVA

Patients with advanced lesions in this stage range usually receive concurrent radiation therapy and chemotherapy, as described in the concurrent chemoradiation section above. However, the optimal drug regimen, optimal radiation therapy technique, and role of surgery in selected cases continue to be subjects of controversy.

Stage IVB

In patients with stage IVB cervical cancer, which implies systemic disease, treatment is palliative rather than curative. Radiation therapy has a role for local primary disease to alleviate symptoms such as bleeding and pain. In patients who have distant metastases, symptoms such as bone pain can be relieved with high-dose radiation.

The use of many chemotherapeutic agents has been reported for stage IVB cervical cancer, with, however, only a modest response. This is based on the fact that most of these studies were conducted in patients with advanced disease with many poor prognostic factors or recurrent disease that had been treated with surgery, radiation therapy, or even chemotherapy. These prior treatments certainly subjected the patients to less than optimal conditions, such as poor vascular supply and bone marrow reserve, leading to lower chemotherapeutic response. In his review of the role of chemotherapy in the management of cervical carcinoma, Thigpen (265) reported on almost 60 agents in various studies in SCC but found that only 21 agents were active, with a response rate of >15%. Among these drugs, cisplatin and ifosfamide are the most active single agents. Cisplatin administered in different doses, schedules, and settings as primary or salvage therapy yielded response rates ranging from 17 to 50%. Examples of single-agent chemotherapy for cervical cancer are shown in Table 30-10 (266-289).

Ifosfamide as a primary drug treatment after radiation therapy yielded response rates of 16 to 40% in phase II trials (269,271). However, in patients with prior radiation therapy and chemotherapy, the response rates were reported to be only partial, ranging from 11 to 31% (269,270).

Only a few phase II studies have reported on the efficacy of carboplatin, with response rates of 15 to 28% (286,287). No controlled trials have found the efficacy of carboplatin to be definitely comparable with that of cisplatin.

TABLE 30-10 | SINGLE DRUGS USED IN THE TREATMENT OF PERSISTENT, RECURRENT, OR ADVANCED CERVICAL CANCER

Drug Regimen	Study	No. of Patients	Prior CT	Dose	Response Rate (%)
Cisplatin	Thigpen (266), 1981	22	No	50 mg/m^2 q3weeks	50
		12	Yes		17
	Bonomi (267), 1985	150	No	50 mg/m^2 q3weeks	21
		166	No	100 mg/m^2 q3weeks	31
		128	No	20 mg/m^2 days 1-5 q3weeks	25
	Thigpen (268), 1989	164	No	50 mg/m^2 q3weeks	17
		156	No	50 mg/m^2 q3weeks (24-h infusion)	18
Ifosfamide	Coleman (269), 1986	41	Yes or no	1.5 g/m^2 days 1-5	31 (prior CT), 40 (no prior CT)
	Sutton (270), 1989	27	Yes	1.2-1.5 g/m^2 days 1-5	11
	Sutton (271), 1993	51	No	1.5 g/m^2 days 1-5	16
	Sutton (272), 1993 (non-SCC)	40	Yes	1.2-1.5 g/m^2 days 1-5	15
Paclitaxel	McGuire (273), 1996	22	No	170 mg/m^2 or 135 mg/m^2 with prior RT	17
	Kudelka (274), 1997	32	No	250 mg/m^2 with G-CSF	25
	Curtin (275), 2001 (non-SCC)	42	Yes	135 or 170 mg/m^2 q3weeks	31
Gemcitabine	Fukuoka (276), 1996	23	No	800 mg/m^2 × 3 weeks	9
	Schilder (277), 2000	25	Yes	800 mg/m^2 × 3 weeks	8
Vinorelbine	Morris (278), 1998	33	No	30 mg/m^2 weekly	18
	Lhomme (279), 2000	41	No	30 mg/m^2 weekly	17
Topotecan	Muderspach (280), 2001	43	No	1.5 mg/m^2 days 1-5	19
	Bookman (281), 2000	40	Yes	1.5 g/m^2 days 1-5	13
Irinotecan	Verschraegen (282), 1997	42	Yes	125 mg/m^2 weekly	21
	Irvin (283), 1998	14	Yes	125 mg/m^2 weekly	0
	Look (284), 1998	49	No	125 mg/m^2 weekly	13
	Lhomme (285), 1999	51	No	350 mg/m^2 q3weeks	16
Carboplatin	McGuire (286), 1989	?	No	400 mg/m^2 (340 mg/m^2 with prior RT	15
	Arseneau (287), 1986	39	No	400 mg/m^2 (340 mg/m^2 with prior RT)	28
Oxiliplatin	Fracasso (288), 2003	22	Yes*	130 mg/m^2 q3weeks	8
Oral etoposide	Rose (289), 2003 (non-SCC)	42	Yes	40-60 mg/m^2/day	12

CT, chemotherapy; G-CSF, granulocyte colony-stimulating factor; RT, radiation therapy; SCC, squamous cell carcinoma.
*Prior treatment with cisplatin or carboplatin was allowed.

The role of chemotherapy for adenocarcinoma has been less well studied than that for squamous cancers. Only cisplatin, paclitaxel, and ifosfamide have shown a response rate >15% (266,272,275).

Although combination chemotherapy appears to produce higher response rates than single drug, it does not seem to yield a significant benefit in overall survival. Examples of combination chemotherapy for cervical cancer are shown in Table 30-11 (290-307).

In caring for patients with recurrent or advanced cervical cancer, aside from the response and benefit, their accompanying toxic effects, cost benefit, and ethical issues should be considered. Zanetta et al. (308) conducted a multivariate analysis regarding the prognostic factors that predict treatment response and survival in 140 patients with metastatic or recurrent cervical SCC. Only the performance status and interval from irradiation (>1 year) were significant in

TABLE 30-11 | DRUG COMBINATIONS USED IN THE TREATMENT OF PERSISTENT, RECURRENT, AND ADVANCED CERVICAL CANCER

Drug Regimen	Study	N	Prior CT	Dose	Response Rate (%)
P+I	Filtenborg (290), 1993	31	No	P 50 mg/m^2 + I 1.5 g/m^2 days 1-3 + carbo 200 mg/m^2 day 1	64
	Omura (291), 1997	438	No	P 50 mg/m2 ± I 5 g/m^2	18 (P) vs 31 (P+I)
P+I ± B	Bloss (292), 2002	287	No	P 50 mg/m^2 + I 5 g/m^2 vs P + I + B 30 U	32 (two drugs) vs 31 (three drugs)
P+CPT-11	Chitapanarux (293), 2003	30	No	P 60 mg/m^2 q 4 weeks + CPT-11 60 mg/m^2 weekly	67
	Sugiyama (294), 2000	21	No	P 60 mg/m^2 day 1 q 4 weeks + CPT-11 60 mg/m^2 weekly	59
Platinum + 5-FU	Ghaemmaghami (295), 2003	8	No	P 50 mg/m^2 or carbo 300 mg/m^2 + 5-FU 1 g/m^2 days 1-4	30
P+Topo	Fiorica (296), 2002	32	No	P 50 mg/m^2 day 1 + topo 0.75 mg/m^2 days 1-3 q3weeks	28
	Long (297), 2004	148	NA	P 50 mg/m^2 ± topo 0.75 mg/m^2 days 1-3 q3weeks	13 (P) vs 26 (P+Topo)
P+NVB	Gebbia (298), 2002	42	No	P 80 mg/m^2 day 1 + NVB 25 mg/m^2 days 1, 8 q3weeks	48
	Pignata (299), 1999	50	No	P 80 mg/m^2 day 1 + NVB 25 mg/m^2 days 1, 8 q3weeks	64
P+pacl	Rose (300), 1999	41	No	P 75 mg/m^2 + pacl 135-170 mg/m^2	46
	Moore (301), 2001	NA	No	P 50 mg/m^2 ± pacl 135 mg/m^2	19 (P) vs 36 (P + pacl)
P+I+pacl	Dimopoulos (302), 2002	57	No	I 1.5 g/m^2 days 1-3 + pacl 175 mg/m^2 day 1 + P 50 mg/m^2 day 2	46
	Zanetta (303), 1999	45	No	I 1.5 g/m^2 + pacl 175 mg/m^2 + P 50-75 mg/m^2	67
P+Gem	Burnett (304), 2000	17	No	P 50 mg/m^2 day 1 + Gem 1.25 g/m^2 days 1 and 8	41
	Duenas-Gonzalez (305), 2001	11	NA	Weekly P 33 mg/m^2 + gemc 100 mg/m^2	36
Carboplatin + lip. doxo	Verschraegen (306), 2001	29	No	Carbo AUC 5 + lip doxo 40 mg/m^2 q4weeks	38
P+Mito	Wagenaar (307), 2001	42	No	P 50 mg/m^2 + Mito 6 mg/m^2	42

B, bleomycin; carbo, carboplatin; CPT-11, irenotecan; CT, chemotherapy; 5-FU, 5-fluorouracil; Gem, gemcitabine; I, ifosfamide; lip doxo, liposomal doxorubicin; Mito, mitomycin C; NVB, vinorelbine; P, cisplatin; pacl, paclitaxel; Topo, topotecan; vs, versus.

predicting response to treatment, whereas the interval from first diagnosis, site of tumor, and response to treatment were significant in predicting survival. Notably, none of the chemotherapeutic combinations significantly improved survival despite their four-fold increase in cost over that of single-drug regimens. These prognostic factors may be part of clinical decision making regarding whether to treat disease further.

Monk and colleagues (309) published the most recent phase III trial from the Gynecologic Oncology Group evaluating the toxicity and efficacy of cisplatin (Cis) doublet combinations in advanced and recurrent cervical carcinoma. Patients were randomly assigned to paclitaxel 135 mg/m(2) over 24 h plus Cis 50 mg/m^2 day 2 every 3 weeks (PC, reference arm); vinorelbine 30 mg/m^2 days 1 and 8 plus Cis 50 mg/m^2 day 1 every 3 weeks (VC); gemcitabine 1000 mg/m^2 day 1 and 8 plus Cis 50 mg/m^2 day 1 every 3 weeks (GC); or topotecan 0.75 mg/m^2 days 1, 2, and 3 plus Cis 50 mg/m^2 day 1 every 3 weeks (TC). Survival was the primary end point with a 33% improvement relative to PC considered important (85% power, alpha = 5%). Quality-of-life data were prospectively collected. A total of 513 patients were enrolled when a planned interim analysis recommended early closure for futility. The experimental-to-PC hazard ratios of death were 1.15 (95% CI, 0.79-1.67) for VC, 1.32 (95% CI, 0.91 to 1.92) for GC, and 1.26 (95% CI, 0.86-1.82) for TC. The hazard ratios for progression-free survival (PFS) were 1.36 (95% CI, 0.97-1.90) for VC, 1.39 (95% CI, 0.99-1.96) for GC, and 1.27 (95% CI, 0.90-1.78) for TC. Response rates (RRs) for PC, VC, GC, and TC were 29.1%, 25.9%, 22.3%, and 23.4%, respectively. The arms were comparable with respect to toxicity except for leucopenia, neutropenia, infection, and alopecia. The authors concluded that none of the regimens studied were superior to paclitaxel and cisplatin combination in terms of overall survival (OS). However, the trend in RR, PFS, and OS favored paclitaxel and cisplatin.

In conclusion, a variety of therapies for cervical cancer have been developed and dictated by the stage of the disease. Therapies for cervical cancer at each stage are summarized in Table 30-12.

TABLE 30-12 | SUMMARY OF TREATMENT BY STAGE

Stage	Surgery	Radiation Therapy
0 (CIS)	Ablative or excisional conization	Brachytherapy
IA1	Conization or simple hysterectomy	Brachytherapy
IA2	Modified radical hysterectomy with pelvic lymphadenectomy or radical trachelectomy with pelvic lymphadenectomy*	Brachytherapy ± pelvic RT
IB-IIA (≤ 4 cm)	Radical hysterectomy with pelvic lymphadenectomy +/– para-aortic sampling Radical trachelectomy with pelvic lymphadenectomy in select patients with lesions ≤2cm	Pelvic RT brachytherapy as primary therapy or as adjuvant postoperative therapy[†]
IB2 or IIA (> 4 cm)	Radical hysterectomy with pelvic lymphadenectomy +/– para-aortic sampling or neoadjuvant chemotherapy followed by radical hysterectomy[‡]	Concurrent chemoradiation therapy brachytherapy (± adjuvant simple hysterectomy) as primary therapy or adjuvant postoperative therapy[‡]
IIB-IVA	Optional imaging study ± retroperitoneal lymph node sampling (or FNA)	
	– or + pelvic node/– para-aortic node ⟶	Concurrent chemoradiation therapy + brachytherapy
	+ pelvic node/+ para-aortic node/– scalene node ⟶	Concurrent chemoradiation therapy + brachytherapy + extended-field RT to para-aortic area
	+ pelvic node/+ para-aortic node/scalene node ⟶	Systemic chemotherapy ± individualized RT
IVB	Palliative chemotherapy or radiation therapy depending on site of disease	

CIS, carcinoma in situ; FNA, fine-needle aspiration; LVSI, lymphovascular space invasion; RT, radiation therapy.

*Pelvic lymphadenectomy may be achieved with an extraperitoneal approach.

[†]Postoperative adjuvant radiation therapy with pelvic RT ± brachytherapy in cases of negative nodes with deep stromal invasion or LVSI or with concurrent chemoradiation in cases of positive pelvic nodes, a positive surgical margin, or a positive parametrium (+ brachytherapy if a positive vaginal margin).

[‡]Considered under a clinical trial.

INVASIVE CANCER DISCOVERED IN SIMPLE HYSTERECTOMY SPECIMENS

Not uncommonly, invasive cervical cancer may be incidentally discovered in simple hysterectomy specimens. One of the most common reasons for this catastrophic event is the negligence of preoperative Pap smears or lack of further investigation in cases with an abnormal Pap smear. The prognosis for women who fall into this category is poor due to their lack of a uterus and cervix for adequate radiation-dose delivery; deterred vascular supply to the area, which will consequently hinder radiation therapy and chemotherapy efficacy; and possible systemic spread of tumor cells due to operative manipulation (310,311). Treatment options for such patients include simple follow-up, pelvic irradiation, radical parametrectomy, upper vaginectomy, and pelvic LN dissection. Choosing the treatment depends mainly on the disease stage and pathologic risk factors, such as tumor size, depth of stromal invasion, presence of a tumor at the surgical margin, LVSI, performance status, and ability of the radiation or gynecologic oncologist in the institution. One study found that radical parametrectomy may obviate radiation therapy in patients who are unlikely to have a residual tumor, with satisfactory 5-year survival of 96% (312).

In patients with stage IA1 cervical cancer, the recurrence rate varies from 1 to 3%, depending on the presence or absence of LVSI, which carries a risk of spread to LNs of 0.6% and 2.6%, respectively. These patients can be observed in the absence of LVSI or undergo an optional LN dissection via an extraperitoneal approach in the presence of LVSI, which would help with a decision for further management.

The incidence of LN involvement in patients with stage IA2 cervical cancer without LVSI is approximately 5.8 to 7.8%, whereas the recurrence rate is 3 to 5%. The incidences are higher with the presence of LVSI; 16.0% of LN involvement and 15.7% recurrence rate. The incidence of LN involvement in patients with stage IB disease is higher, ranging from 15 to 50% (160), so that further management is mandatory.

■ POSTTREATMENT SURVEILLANCE

Conventionally, patients with cervical cancer are followed up at different intervals after treatment to detect any recurrences. However, the value of this practice is questionable. Many authors have found that this surveillance has a limited role in the detection of recurrence (313-316); in particular, one study found a detection rate of recurrence of 32% (313). Most recurrences

are recognized when the disease presents with clinical symptoms rather than signs or objective manifestations (87 versus 9%). Moreover, the survival benefit in clinical findings of routine surveillance is not increased over that in patients who are found to have recurrence with presenting symptoms or referred by a primary care physician (313,314). Generally, the surveillance includes the patient's history of any abnormal symptoms, a physical examination, and a simple laboratory examination, such as a Pap smear and chest x-ray.

The clinical value of detecting recurrences with Pap smears is questionable. The sensitivity of the test in this setting is only 2 to13% (313). Studies at our institution have reported a low recurrence detection rate with Pap smears. Specifically, a study of patients with stage IB cervical cancer who underwent surgery reported an abnormal Pap smear in only 1 of 27 recurrence cases (316). However, Pap smear is a simple, inexpensive means of surveillance, and it remains a standard of surveillance.

Because lung is the most common site of distant metastasis of recurrent cervical cancer, a chest x-ray is often recommended at least yearly. This may aid in the detection of asymptomatic pulmonary recurrences. Some authors have not agreed though, and they do not recommend routine chest x-rays for surveillance (317). In their study, Barter et al. reported the incidence of pulmonary recurrence of cervical cancer to be 3.6% (317). Chest x-rays detected such a recurrence in about 38% of patients with no presenting symptoms. However, the survival in this group of asymptomatic patients was not different from that in patients who had clinical symptoms.

Other investigations may be justified by suspicious clinical findings. Some abnormal signs and symptoms may be due to treatment complications or recurrence and cannot be differentiated via a simple physical examination. For example, leg swelling may be due to LN dissection, radiation therapy, venous thromboembolism, or pelvic recurrence with a lymphatic obstruction. These different diagnoses necessitate further evaluation for appropriate management.

Some of the imaging studies used to detect recurrences are discussed above, in the section on diagnostic imaging. However, these tests—such as CT scan, MRI, or PET scan—are not routinely recommended, and it remains to be proven whether early detection of recurrences will improve survival.

In conclusion, posttreatment surveillance guidelines recommended by the National Comprehensive Cancer Network group for surveillance of cervical cancer are interval history, physical examination, and Pap testing every 3-6 months in the first two years, every 6 months in the third to fifth years, and then annually. Annual chest x-ray, testing for CBC, BUN, and creatinine every 6 months, and PET-CT scan are considered optional as clinically indicated (318).

■ **HORMONE REPLACEMENT THERAPY**

Generally, cervical cancer is not a contraindication for hormone replacement therapy. However, a randomized controlled trial by the Women's Health Initiative found that hormone replacement therapy increases the risk of cardiovascular disease (both arterial and venous), stroke, pulmonary embolism, cancer in general, and breast cancer in particular (319). The only FDA-approved indication for estrogen-based hormone replacement therapy that has remained unchanged is for relieving moderate to severe vasomotor symptoms associated with menopause. The use of topical forms of estrogen or nonestrogen products for other menopausal symptoms should be considered (320). Thus, hormone replacement therapy should be administered only after meticulous consideration, and patients should be counseled carefully regarding the risks associated with hormone replacement therapy before any such therapy is begun.

■ **RECURRENT CERVICAL CANCER**

It is generally accepted that any lesions detected within 6 months after treatment should be considered persistent. The diagnosis of recurrence is usually made after 6 months. If a lesion is noted within 3 months after radiation therapy, no treatment is recommended due to the ongoing effects of irradiation at this time period.

Choosing the type of therapy for recurrent cervical cancer depends on many factors: site of recurrence, previous therapy, and performance status of the patients.

LOCOREGIONAL

A study of patients with stage IB cervical cancer who underwent treatment primarily with surgery reported a recurrence rate of approximately 11%; half of the recurrences occurred within 1 year, and most appeared within 2 years (321). Approximately 60% of the recurrences were in the pelvis or vulva, while 37% were outside the pelvis. The overall survival rates in these patients with local recurrence ranged from 6 to 74% (321-325). Recurrence limited to the central pelvis carries a better prognosis than does recurrence involving the pelvic side wall. The size of the recurrence is also important, as one study found that the 10-year survival rate in patients with nonpalpable lesions and lesions <3 cm is 77 and 48%, respectively, while patients with lesions >3 cm did not experience long-term survival (323).

In patients whose primary treatment is surgery or radiation therapy and whose recurrent disease is limited to the pelvis, radical surgery, such as extended radical hysterectomy or pelvic exenteration, has a specific role in selected patients. Maneo et al. reported a series of 34 patients who underwent radical hysterectomy for persistent or recurrent cervical cancer after primary radiotherapy (325). Although major complications occurred in 44%, the same figures of 44% were alive without evidence of disease at a median survival of 81 months (range 33-192). Actuarial 5-year survival rate for the whole group was 49%. Patients with FIGO stage IB-IIA at primary diagnosis, no clinical parametrial involvement, and small (≤4 cm) tumor diameter at the time of recurrence carried a better prognosis. Larson et al. also suggested that these patients should have no evidence of pelvic side wall or extrapelvic disease and have a good performance status, and can withstand major surgery (321). However, a recent study by Hockel (326) reported good results of laterally extended endopelvic resection in patients with recurrent cervical carcinomas involving the side wall of an irradiated pelvis. The 5-year survival rate was as high as 49% in the whole group and 46% in patients considered only for palliation with the use of current treatment options. Most patients without evidence of disease at least 1 year after the procedure had a good quality of life.

DISTANT

Distant recurrence with or without associated locoregional lesions denotes systemic disease and carries a poor prognosis and minimal chance of a cure. Chemotherapy has a specific role in this setting. The details of chemotherapy have been previously discussed.

In cases with an isolated metastatic lesion in any distant organ, resection of the metastasis may have a role in selected cases. In patients who experience bony metastases from or pain due to metastatic lesions, focal short-term, high-dose radiation therapy may alleviate these symptoms.

Treatment guidelines for cervical cancer are shown in Fig. 30-13.

Clinical presentation   Initial evaluation   Primary treatment

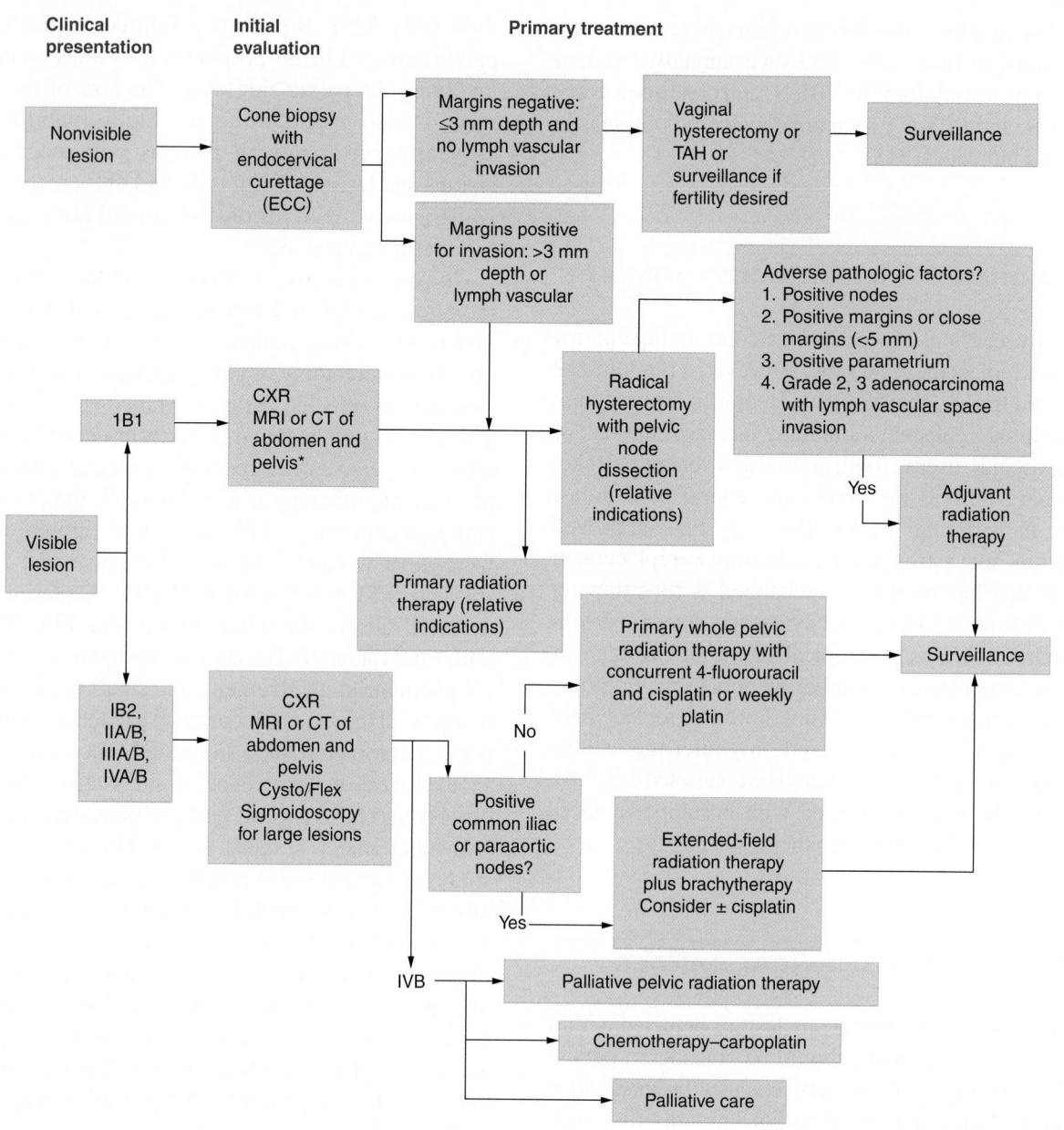

FIGURE 30-13. Cervical cancer algorithm and treatment guidelines for cervical cancer. (*Adapted from the Memorial-Sloan Kettering Cancer Center & MD Anderson Cancer Center Handbook of Gynecologic Oncology.*)

■ ACKNOWLEDGMENT

We thank Dr. Muriel Camarillo for her contribution to this work.

References

1. American Cancer Society. Cancer statistics *2009*. American Cancer Society; 2009. www.cancer.org.
2. Parkin DM, Bray F, Ferlay J, et al. Global cancer statistics 2002. *CA Cancer J Clin.* 2005;55:74-108.
3. Herrero R, Brinton LA, Hartge P, et al. Determinants of the geographic variation of invasive cervical cancer in Costa Rica. *Bull Pan Am Health Org* 1993;27:15-25.
4. Hacker NF. Cervical cancer. In: Berek JS, Hacker NF (eds): *Practical Gynecologic Oncology,* 3rd ed. Philadelphia, PA: Lippincott Williams & Wilkins; 2000:345-406.
5. Zaino RJ. Glandular lesions of the uterine cervix. *Mod Pathol* 2000;13:261-274.
6. Vizcaino AP, Moreno V, Bosch FX, et al. International trends in the incidence of cervical cancer: I. Adenocarcinoma and adenosquamous cell carcinomas. *Int J Cancer* 1998;75:536-545.

7. Kjaer SK, Brinton LA. Adenocarcinomas of the uterine cervix: The epidemiology of an increasing problem. *Epidemiol Rev* 1993;15:486-498.

8. Herrero R, Brinton LA, Reeves WC. Sexual behavior, venereal diseases, hygiene practices, and invasive cervical cancer in a high-risk population. *Cancer* 1990;65:380-386.

9. Ursin G, Peters RK, Henderson BE, et al. Oral contraceptive use and adenocarcinoma of cervix. *Lancet* 1994;344:1390-1394.

10. Clarke EA, Morgan RW, Newman AM. Smoking as a risk factor in cancer of the cervix: Additional evidence from a case-control study. *Am J Epidemiol* 1982;115:59-66.

11. Brinton LA, Hamman RF, Huggins GR. Sexual and reproductive risk factors for invasive cervical cancer. *J Natl Cancer Inst* 1987;79:23-30.

12. Palefski JM, Holly EA. Molecular virology and epidemiology of human papillomavirus and cervical cancer. *Cancer Epidemiol Biomarkers Prev* 1995;4:415-428.

13. Kjaer SK, Chackerian B, van den Brule AJ, et al. High-risk human papillomavirus is sexually transmitted: Evidence from a follow-up study of virgins starting sexual activity (intercourse). *Cancer Epidemiol Biomarkers Prev* 2001;10:101-106.

14. Schiffman M, Castle PE. Human papillomavirus: Epidemiology and public health. *Arch Pathol Lab Med* 2003;127:930-934.

15. Munoz N, Bosch FX, de Sanjose S, et al. Epidemiologic classification of human papillomavirus types associated with cervical cancer. *N Engl J Med* 2003;348:518-527.

16. Castellsague X, Diaz M, de Sanjose S, et al. Worldwide human papillomavirus etiology of cervical adenocarcinoma and its cofactors: Implications for screening and prevention. *J Natl Cancer Inst* 2006;98:303-315.

17. Chiasson MA, Ellerbrock TV, Bush TJ, et al. Increased prevalence of vulvovaginal condyloma and vulvar intraepithelial neoplasia in women infected with the human immunodeficiency virus. *Obstet Gynecol* 1997;89:690-694.

18. Sun XW, Kuhn L, Ellerbrock TV, et al. Human papillomavirus infection in women infected with the human immunodeficiency virus. *N Engl J Med* 1997;337:1343-1349.

19. Ferenczy A, Coutlee F, Franco E, Hankins C. Human papillomavirus and HIV coinfection and the risk of neoplasias of the lower genital tract: A review of recent developments. *CMAJ* 2003;169:431-434.

20. Halpert R, Fruchter RG, Sedlis A, et al. Human papillomavirus and lower genital neoplasia in renal transplant patients. *Obstet Gynecol* 1986;68:251-258.

21. Ellerbrock TV, Chiasson MA, Bush TJ, et al. Incidence of cervical squamous intraepithelial lesions in HIV-infected women. *JAMA* 2000;283:1031-1037.

22. Wright TC Jr, Ellerbrock TV, Chiasson MA, et al. Cervical intraepithelial neoplasia in women infected with human immunodeficiency virus: Prevalence, risk factors, and validity of Papanicolaou smears. New York Cervical Disease Study. *Obstet Gynecol* 1994;84:591-597.

23. Munoz N, Bosch FX, de Sanjose S, et al. Risk factors for cervical intraepithelial neoplasia grade III/carcinoma in situ in Spain and Colombia. *Cancer Epidemiol Biomarkers Prev* 1993;2:423-431.

24. Becker TM, Wheeler CM, McGough NS, et al. Cigarette smoking and other risk factors for cervical dysplasia in southwestern Hispanic and non-Hispanic white women. *Cancer Epidemiol Biomarkers Prev* 1994;3:113-119.

25. Schiffman MH, Bauer HM, Hoover RN, et al. Epidemiologic evidence showing that human papillomavirus infection causes most cervical intraepithelial neoplasia. *Natl Cancer Inst* 1993;85:958-964.

26. Chan JK, Monk BJ, Brewer C, et al. HPV infection and number of lifetime sexual partners are strong predictors for "natural" regression of CIN 2 and 3. *Br J Cancer* 2003;89:1062-1066.

27. Bosch FX, Munoz N, de Sanjose S, et al. Risk factors for cervical cancer in Colombia and Spain. *Int J Cancer* 1992;52:750-758.

28. Smith JS, Green J, Berrington de Gonzalez A, et al. Cervical cancer and use of hormonal contraceptives: A systematic review. *Lancet* 2003;361:1159-1167.

29. Lacey JV Jr, Brinton LA, Abbas FM, et al. Oral contraceptives risk factors for cervical adenocarcinomas and squamous cell carcinomas. *Cancer Epidemiol Biomarkers Prev* 1999;8:1079-1085.

30. Jones CJ, Brinton LA, Hamman RF, et al. Risk factors for in situ cervical cancer: Results from a case-control study. *Cancer Res* 1990;50:3657-3662.

31. Parazzini F, Negri E, La Vecchia C, Fedele L. Barrier methods of contraception and the risk of cervical neoplasia. *Contraception* 1989;40:519-530.

32. Hellberg D, Nilsson S, Haley NJ, et al. Smoking and cervical intraepithelial neoplasia: Nicotine and cotinine in serum and cervical mucus in smokers and nonsmokers. *Am J Obstet Gynecol* 1988;158:910-913.

33. Poppe WA, Ide PS, Drijkoningen MP, et al. Tobacco smoking impairs the local immunosurveillance in the uterine cervix. An immunohistochemical study. *Gynecol Obstet Invest* 1995;39:34-38.

34. Hellberg D, Valentin J, Nilsson S. Smoking and cervical intraepithelial neoplasia. An association independent of sexual and other risk factors? *Acta Obstet Gynecol Scand* 1986;65:625-631.

35. Kjellberg L, Hallmans G, Ahren AM, et al. Smoking, diet, pregnancy and oral contraceptive use as risk factors for cervical intra-epithelial neoplasia in relation to human papillomavirus infection. *Br J Cancer* 2000;82:1332-1338.

36. Plummer M, Herrero R, Franceschi S, et al. IARC Multi-centre Cervical Cancer Study Group. Smoking and cervical cancer: Pooled analysis of the IARC multi-centric case-control study. *Cancer Causes Control* 2003;14:805-814.

37. Agarwal SS, Sehgal A, Sardana S, et al. Role of male behavior in cervical carcinogenesis among women with one lifetime sexual partner. *Cancer* 1993;72:1666-1669.

38. Kjaer SK, de Villiers EM, Dahl C, et al. Case-control study of risk factors for cervical neoplasia in Denmark. I: Role of the "male factor" in women with one lifetime sexual partner. *Int J Cancer* 1991;48:39-44.

39. Barrasso R. HPV-related genital lesions in men. *IARC Sci Publ* 1992;119:85-92.

40. IARC. Tumours of the uterine cervix. In: Tavassoli FA, Devilee P (eds): *Pathology and Genetics of Tumours of the Breast and Female Genital Organs. World Health Organization Classification of Tumours.* Lyon, France: International Agency for Research on Cancer; 2003:259-290.

41. Pecorelli S. Revised FIGO staging for carcinoma of the vulva, cervix, and endometrium. *Int J Gynecol Obstet* 2009:105:103-104.

42. Sevin B. Carcinoma of the cervix uteri. In: Jones HI, Burke T, Creasman W, et al. (eds): *SGO Handbook: Staging of Gynecologic Malignancies.* Chicago, IL: Society of Gynecologic Oncologists; 1994:15-22.

43. Silverberg SG, Ioffe OB. Pathology of cervical cancer. *Cancer J* 2003;9:335-347.

44. Creasman WT. New gynecologic cancer staging. *Gynecol Oncol* 1995;58:157-158.

45. Randall ME, Constable WC, et al. Results of the radiotherapeutic management of carcinoma of the cervix with emphasis on the influence of histologic classification. *Cancer* 1988;62:48-53.

46. Zaino RJ, Ward S, Delgado G, et al. Histopathologic predictors of the behavior of surgically treated stage IB squamous cell carcinoma of the cervix. A Gynecologic Oncology Group study. *Cancer* 1992;69:1750-1758.

47. Robert ME, Fu YS. Squamous cell carcinoma of the uterine cervix—A review with emphasis on prognostic factors and unusual variants. *Semin Diagn Pathol* 1990;7:173-189.

48. Jennings RH, Barclay DL. Verrucous carcinoma of the cervix. *Cancer* 1972;30:430-434.

49. Tiltman AJ, Nel CP. Verrucous carcinoma of the uterine cervix. Case reports. *S Afr Med J* 1982;62:490-492.

50. Cho NH, Joo HJ, Ahn HJ, et al. Detection of human papillomavirus in warty carcinoma of the uterine cervix: Comparison of immunohistochemistry, in situ hybridization and in situ polymerase chain reaction methods. *Pathol Res Pract* 1998;194:713-720.

51. Randall ME, Andersen WA, Mills SE, et al. Papillary squamous cell carcinoma of the uterine cervix: A clinicopathologic study of nine cases. *Int J Gynecol Pathol* 1986;5:1-10.

52. Brinck U, Jakob C, Bau O, et al. Papillary squamous cell carcinoma of the uterine cervix: Report of three cases and a review of its classification. *Int J Gynecol Pathol* 2000;19:231-235.

53. Albores-Saavedra J, Young RH. Transitional cell neoplasms (carcinomas and inverted papillomas) of the uterine cervix: A report of five cases. *Am J Surg Pathol* 1995;19:1138-1145.

54. Koenig C, Turnicky RP, Kankam CF, et al. Papillary squamotransitional cell carcinoma of the cervix: A report of 32 cases. *Am J Surg Pathol* 1997;21:915-921.

55. Steeper TA, Piscioli F, Rosai J. Squamous cell carcinoma with sarcoma-like stroma of the female genital tract. Clinicopathologic study of four cases. *Cancer* 1983;52:890-898.

56. Brown J, Broaddus R, Koeller M, et al. Sarcomatoid carcinoma of the cervix. *Gynecol Oncol* 2003;90:23-28.

57. Schwartz SM, Weiss NS. Increased incidence of adenocarcinoma of the cervix in young women in the United States. *Am J Epidemiol* 1986;124:1045-1047.

58. Lee KR, Flynn CE. Early invasive adenocarcinoma of the cervix. *Cancer* 2000;89:1048-1055.

59. Tase T, Okagaki T, Clark BA, et al. Human papillomavirus DNA in adenocarcinoma in situ, microinvasive adenocarcinoma of the uterine cervix, and coexisting cervical squamous intraepithelial neoplasia. *Int J Gynecol Pathol* 1989;8:8-17.

60. Bertrand M, Lickrish GM, Colgan TJ. The anatomic distribution of cervical adenocarcinoma in situ: Implications for treatment. *Am J Obstet Gynecol* 1987;157:21-25.

61. Ostor A, Ome R, Quinn M. Microinvasive adenocarcinoma of the cervix: A clinicopathological study of 77 women. *Obstet Gynecol* 1997;89:88-93.

62. Pirog EC, Kleter B, Olgac S, et al. Prevalence of human papillomavirus DNA in different histological subtypes of cervical adenocarcinoma. *Am J Pathol* 2000;157:1055-1062.

63. Hanselaar A, van Loosbroek M, Schuurbiers O, et al. Clear cell adenocarcinoma of the vagina and cervix: An update of the central Netherlands registry showing twin age incidence peaks. *Cancer* 1997;79:2229-2236.

64. Clement PB, Young RH, Keh P, et al. Malignant mesonephric neoplasms of the uterine cervix. A report of eight cases, including four with a malignant spindle cell component. *Am J Surg Pathol* 1995;19:1158-1171.

65. Gompel C, Silverberg S. *Pathology in Gynecology and Obstetrics,* 4th ed. Philadelphia, PA: Lippincott; 1994.

66. dos Reis R, Frumovitz M, Milam MR, et al. Adenosquamous carcinoma versus adenocarcinoma in early-stage cervical cancer patients undergoing radical hysterectomy: An outcomes analysis. *Gynecol Oncol* 2007;107:458-463.

67. Pak HY, Yokota SB, Paladugu RR, et al. Glassy cell carcinoma of the cervix. Cytologic and clinicopathologic analysis. *Cancer* 1983;52:307-312.

68. Mikami M, Ezawa S, Sakaiya N, et al. Response of glassy-cell carcinoma of the cervix to cisplatin, epirubicin, and mitomycin C. *Lancet* 2000;355:1159-1160.

69. Grayson W, Taylor LF, Cooper K. Adenoid cystic and adenoid basal carcinoma of the uterine cervix: Comparative morphologic, mucin, and immunohistochemical profile of two rare neoplasms of putative "reserve cell" origin. *Am J Surg Pathol* 1999;23:448-458.

70. Brainard JA, Hart WR. Adenoid basal epitheliomas of the uterine cervix: A reevaluation of distinctive cervical basaloid lesions currently classified as adenoid basal carcinoma and adenoid basal hyperplasia. *Am J Surg Pathol* 1998;22:965-975.

71. Albores-Saavedra J, Gersell D, Gilks CB, et al. Terminology of endocrine tumors of the uterine cervix. Results of a workshop sponsored by the College of American Pathologists and the National Cancer Institute. *Arch Pathol Lab Med* 1997;121:34-39.

72. Abeler VM, Holm R, Nesland JM, et al. Small cell carcinoma of the cervix. A clinicopathologic study of 26 patients. *Cancer* 1994;73:672-677.

73. Bermudez A, Vighi S, Garcia A, et al. Neuroendocrine cervical carcinoma: A diagnostic and therapeutic challenge. *Gynecol Oncol* 2001;82:32-39.

74. Straughn JM Jr, Richter HE, Conner MG, et al. Predictors of outcome in small cell carcinoma of the cervix—A case series. *Gynecol Oncol* 2001;83:216-220.

75. Gilks CB, Young RH, Gersell DJ, et al. Large cell neuroendocrine [corrected] carcinoma of the uterine cervix: A clinicopathologic study of 12 cases. *Am J Surg Pathol* 1997;21:905-914.

76. Richart RM, Barron BA. A follow-up study of patients with cervical dysplasia. *Am J Obstet Gynecol* 1969;105:386-393.

77. Papanicolaou GN, Traut HF. The diagnostic value of vaginal smears in carcinoma of the uterus. *Am J Obstet Gynecol* 1941;42:193-206.

78. Crum CP, Nuovo G, Lee KR. The cervix. In: Sternberg S (ed): *Diagnostic Surgical Pathology,* 3rd ed. Philadelphia, PA: Lippincott Williams & Wilkins; 1999:2155-2202.

79. Korn AP, Autry M, DeRemer PA, et al. Sensitivity of the Papanicolaou smear in human immunodeficiency virus-infected women. *Obstet Gynecol* 1994;83:401-404.

80. Adachi A, Fleming I, Burk RD. Women with human immun-odeficiency virus infection and abnormal Papanicolaou smears: A prospective study of colposcopy and clinical outcome. *Obstet Gynecol* 1993;81:372-377.

81. American College of Obstetricians and Gynecologists. Cervical cytology screening. ACOG practice bulletin No. 109. Washington, DC: *Obstet Gynecol* 2009 Dec;114(6): 1409-1420.

82. Solomon D, Davey D, Kurman R, et al. Forum Group Members; Bethesda 2001 Workshop. The 2001 Bethesda System: Terminology for reporting results of cervical cytology. *JAMA* 2002;287:2114-2119.

83. Fahey MT, Irwig L, Macaskill P. Meta-analysis of Pap test accuracy. *Am J Epidemiol* 1995;141:680-689.

84. Koss LG, Sherman M, Cohen M, et al. Significant reduction in the rate of false negative cervical smears with neural network-based technology (PAPNET testing system). *Human Pathol* 1997;28:1196-1203.

85. Wilkinson EJ. Pap smears and screening for cervical neoplasia. *Clin Obstet Gynecol* 1990;33:817-825.

86. Kristensen GB, Skyggebjerg KD, Holund B, et al. Analysis of cervical smears obtained within three years of the diagnosis of invasive cervical cancer. *Acta Cytol* 1991;35: 47-50.

87. Sherman ME, Kelly D. High-grade squamous intraepithelial lesions and invasive carcinoma following the report of three negative Papanicolaou smears: Screening failures or rapid progression? *Mod Pathol* 1992;5:337-342.

88. Hutchinson ML, Zahniser DJ, Sherman ME, et al. Utility of liquid-based cytology for cervical carcinoma screening: Results of a population-based study conducted in a region of Costa Rica with a high incidence of cervical carcinoma. *Cancer* 1999;87:48-55.

89. Ferenczy A, Robitaille CS, Franco F, et al. Conventional cervical cytology vs. ThinPrep smears. *Acta Cytol* 1996;40: 1136-1142.

90. Vassilakos P, Schwartz D, de Marval F, et al. Biopsy-based comparison of liquid-based, thin-layer preparations to conventional Pap smears. *J Reprod Med* 2000;45:11-16.

91. Minge L, Fleming M, VanGeem T, et al. AutoCyte Prep system vs. conventional cervical cytology. Comparison based on 2,156 cases. *J Reprod Med* 2000;45:179-184.

92. Boon ME, Kok LP. Neural network processing can provide means to catch errors that slip through human screening of Pap smears. *Diagn Cytopathol* 1993;9:411-416.

93. Sherman ME, Mango LJ, Kelly D, et al. PAPNET analysis of reportedly negative smears preceding the diagnosis of a high-grade squamous intraepithelial lesion or carcinoma. *Mod Pathol* 1994;7:578-581.

94. Bishop JW, Kaufman RH, Taylor DA. Multicenter comparison of manual and automated screening of AutoCyte gynecologic preparations. *Acta Cytol* 1999;43:34-38.

95. Masood S, Cajulis RS, Cibas ES, et al. Automation in cytology: A survey conducted by the New Technology Task Force, Papanicolaou Society of Cytopathology. *Diagn Cytopathol* 1998;18:47-54.

96. Gustafsson L, Adami HO. Natural history of cervical neoplasia: Consistent results obtained by an identification technique. *Br J Cancer* 1989;60:132-141.

97. Meijer CJ, Helmerhorst TJ, Rozendaal L, et al. HPV typing and testing in gynaecological pathology: Has the time come? *Histopathology* 1998;33:83-86.

98. Clavel C, Masure M, Bory JP, et al. Human papillomavirus testing in primary screening for the detection of high-grade cervical lesions: A study of 7932 women. *Br J Cancer* 2001; 84:1616-1623.

99. Mann W, Lonky N, Massad S, et al. Papanicolaou smear screening augmented by a magnified chemiluminescent exam. *Int J Gynaecol Obstet* 1993;43:289-296.

100. Fung Kee Fung M, Senterman M, Eid P, et al. Comparison of Fourier-transform infrared spectroscopic screening of exfoliated cervical cells with standard Papanicolaou screening. *Gynecol Oncol* 1997;66:10-15.

101. Singer A, Coppleson M, Canfell K, et al. A real time opto-electronic device as an adjunct to the Pap smear for cervical screening: A multicenter evaluation. *Int J Gynecol Cancer* 2003;13:804-811.

102. Brown BH, Tidy JA, Boston K, et al. Relation between tissue structure and imposed electrical current flow in cervical neoplasia. *Lancet* 2000;355:892-895.

103. Ramanujam N, Mitchell MF, Mahadevan A, et al. Fluorescence spectroscopy: A diagnostic tool for cervical intraepithelial neoplasia (CIN). *Gynecol Oncol* 1994;52:31-38.

104. Mitchell MF, Cantor SB, Ramanujam N, et al. Fluorescence spectroscopy for diagnosis of squamous intraepithelial lesions of the cervix. *Obstet Gynecol* 1999;93:462-470.

105. Holowaty P, Miller AB, Rohan T, To T. The natural history of dysplasia of the uterine cervix. *J Natl Cancer Inst* 1999; 91:252-258.

106. Peterson O. Spontaneous course of cervical precancerous conditions. *Am J Obstet Gynecol* 1956;72:1063-1067.

107. Koss L, Stewart F, Foote F. Some histological aspects of behavior of epidermoid carcinoma in situ and related lesions of the uterine cervix. *Cancer* 1963;16:1160.

108. Clemmensen J, Poulsen H. *Report of the Ministry of the Interior*. Copenhagen: Ministry of the Interior; 1971.

109. Luthra UK, Prabhakar AK, Seth P, et al. Natural history of precancerous and early cancerous lesions of the uterine cervix. *Acta Cytol* 1987;31:226-234.

110. Saito J, Fukuda T, Hoshaiai H, et al. High-risk types of human papillomavirus associated with the progression of cervical dysplasia to carcinoma. *J Obstet Gynaecol Res* 1999; 25:281-286.

111. Walboomers JM, Jacobs MV, Manos MM, et al. Human papillomavirus is a necessary cause of invasive cervical cancer worldwide. *J Pathol* 1999;189:12-19.

112. Josefsson A, Magnusson P, Yliato N, et al. Viral load of human papilloma virus 16 as a determinant for development of cervical carcinoma in situ: A nested case-control study. *Lancet* 2000;355:2189-2193.

113. Sutton GP, Bundy BN, Delgado G, et al. Ovarian metastases in stage IB carcinoma of the cervix: A Gynecologic Oncology Group study. *Am J Obstet Gynecol* 1992;166(1 pt 1): 50-53.

114. Hopkins MP, Morley GW. A comparison of adenocarcinoma and squamous cell carcinoma of the cervix. *Obstet Gynecol* 1991;77:912-917.

115. Sakuragi N, Satoh C, Takeda N, et al. Incidence and distribution pattern of pelvic and para-aortic lymph node metastasis in patients with stages IB, IIa, and IIB cervical carcinoma treated with radical hysterectomy. *Cancer* 1999;85:1547-1554.

116. Carlson V, Delclos L, Fletcher G. Distant metastases in squamous cell carcinoma of the uterine cervix. *Radiology* 1967; 88:961-965.

117. Stehman FB, Bundy BN, DiSaia PJ, et al. Carcinoma of the cervix treated with radiation therapy: A multi-variate analysis of prognostic variables in the Gynecologic Oncology Group. *Cancer* 1991;67:2776-2785.

118. Scheidler J, Hricak H, Yu KK, et al. Radiological evaluation of lymph node metastases in patients with cervical cancer. A meta-analysis. *JAMA* 1997;278:1096-1101.

119. Bipat S, Glas AS, van der Velden J, et al. Computed tomography and magnetic resonance imaging in staging of uterine cervical carcinoma: A systematic review. *Gynecol Oncol* 2003;91:59-66.

120. Rose PG, Adler LP, Rodriguez M, et al. Positron emission tomography for evaluating para-aortic nodal metastasis in locally advanced cervical cancer before surgical staging: A surgicopathologic study. *J Clin Oncol* 1999;17:41-45.

121. Grigsby PW, Siegel BA, Dehdashti F. Lymph node staging by positron emission tomography in patients with carcinoma of the cervix. *J Clin Oncol* 2001;19:3745-3749.

122. Narayan K, Hicks RJ, Jobling T, et al. A comparison of MRI and PET scanning in surgically staged loco-regionally advanced cervical cancer: Potential impact on treatment. *Int J Gynecol Cancer* 2001;11:263-271.

123. Belhocine T, Thille A, Fridman V, et al. Contribution of whole-body 18FDG PET imaging in the management of cervical cancer. *Gynecol Oncol* 2002;87:90-97.

124. Sugawara Y, Eisbruch A, Kosuda S, et al. Evaluation of FDG PET in patients with cervical cancer. *J Nucl Med* 1999;40:1125-1131.

125. Yen TC, Ng KK, Ma SY, et al. Value of dual-phase 2-fluoro-2-deoxy-d-glucose positron emission tomography in cervical cancer. *J Clin Oncol* 2003;21:3651-3658.

126. Grigsby PW, Siegel BA, Dehdashti F, et al. Posttherapy surveillance monitoring of cervical cancer by FDG-PET. *Int J Radiat Oncol Biol Phys* 2003;55:907-913.

127. Singh AK, Grigsby PW, Dehdashti F, et al. FDG–PET lymph node staging and survival of patients with FIGO stage IIIb cervical carcinoma. *Int J Radiat Oncol Biol Phys* 2003;56:489-493.

128. Havrilesky LJ, Wong TZ, Secord AA, et al. The role of PET scanning in the detection of recurrent cervical cancer. *Gynecol Oncol* 2003;90:186-190.

129. Nakamoto Y, Eisbruch A, Achtyes ED, et al. Prognostic value of positron emission tomography using F-18-fluorodeoxyglucose in patients with cervical cancer undergoing radiotherapy. *Gynecol Oncol* 2002;84:289-295.

130. Sun SS, Chen TC, Yen RF, et al. Value of whole body 18F-fluoro-2-deoxyglucose positron emission tomography in the evaluation of recurrent cervical cancer. *Anticancer Res* 2001;21:2957-2961.

131. Park DH, Kim KH, Park SY, et al. Diagnosis of recurrent uterine cervical cancer: Computed tomography versus positron emission tomography. *Korean J Radiol* 2000;1:51-55.

132. Raspagliesi F, Ditto A, Solima E, et al. Microinvasive squamous cell cervical carcinoma. *Crit Rev Oncol Hematol* 2003;48:251-261.

133. Savage EW. Microinvasive carcinoma of the cervix. *Am J Obstet Gynecol* 1972;113:708.

134. Hasumi K, Sakamoto A, Sugano H. Microinvasive carcinoma of the uterine cervix. *Cancer* 1980;45:928.

135. Van Nagell Jr, Greenwell N, Powell DF. Microinvasive carcinoma of the cervix. *Am J Obstet Gynecol* 1983;145:981.

136. Ostor AG. Studies on 200 cases of early squamous cell carcinoma of the cervix. *Int J Gynecol Pathol* 1993;12:193-207.

137. Roche WD, Norris HJ. Microinvasive carcinoma of the cervix: The significance of lymphatic invasion and confluent patterns of growth. *Cancer* 1975;36:180.

138. Ostor AG. Pandora's box or Ariadne's thread? Definition and prognostic significance of microinvasion in the uterine cervix. *Squamous Lesions Pathol Annu* 1995;30(pt 2):103-136.

139. Copeland LJ, Silva EG, Gershenson DM, et al. Superficially invasive squamous cell carcinoma of the cervix. *Gynecol Oncol* 1992;45:307-312.

140. Benedet JL, Anderson GH. Stage IA carcinoma of the cervix revisited. *Obstet Gynecol* 1996;87:1052-1959.

141. Milam MR, Frumovitz M, dos Reis R, et al. Preoperative lymph-vascular space invasion is associated with nodal metastases in women with early-stage cervical cancer. *Gynecol Oncol* 2007;106:12-15.

142. Benedetti-Panici P, Maneschi F, D'Andrea G, et al. Early cervical carcinoma: The natural history of lymph node involvement redefined on the basis of thorough parametrectomy and giant section study. *Cancer* 2000;88:2267-2274.

143. Landoni F, Maneo A, Colombo A, et al. Randomised study of radical surgery versus radiotherapy for stage Ib-IIa cervical cancer. *Lancet* 1997;350:535-540.

144. Moore DH, Stehman FB. What is the appropriate management of early stage cervical cancer (International Federation of Gynecology and Obstetrics stages I and IIA), surgical assessment of lymph nodes, and role of therapeutic resection of lymph nodes involved with cancer? *Natl Cancer Inst Monogr* 1996;43-46.

145. Burghardt E, Baltzer J, Tulusan AH, et al. Results of surgical treatment of 1028 cervical cancers studied with volume-try. *Cancer* 1992;70:648-655.

146. Covens A, Rosen B, Murphy J, et al. How important is removal of the parametrium at surgery for carcinoma of the cervix? *Gynecol Oncol* 2002;84:145-149.

147. Frumovitz M, Sun CC, Schmeler KM, et al. Parametrial involvement in radical hysterectomy specimens for women with early-stage cervical cancer. *Obstet Gynecol* 2009;114:93-99.

148. Boyce J, Fruchter RG, Nicastri AD, et al. Prognostic factors in stage I carcinoma of the cervix. *Gynecol Oncol* 1981;12:154-165.

149. Sedlis A, Bundy BN, Rotman MZ, et al. A randomized trial of pelvic radiation therapy versus no further therapy in selected patients with stage IB carcinoma of the cervix after radical hysterectomy and pelvic lymphadenectomy: A Gynecologic Oncology Group Study. *Gynecol Oncol* 1999;73:177-183.

150. Alvarez RD, Potter ME, Soong SJ, et al. Rationale for using pathologic tumor dimensions and nodal status to subclassify surgically treated stage IB cervical cancer patients. *Gynecol Oncol* 1991;43:108-112.

151. Okada M, Kigawa J, Minagawa Y, et al. Indication and efficacy of radiation therapy following radical surgery in patients with stage IB to IIB cervical cancer. *Gynecol Oncol* 1998;70(1):61-64.

152. Rotman M, John M, Boyce J. Prognostic factors in cervical carcinoma: Implications in staging and management. *Cancer* 1981;48(2 suppl):560-567.

153. Inoue T. Prognostic significance of the depth of invasion relating to nodal metastases, parametrial extension, and cell types. A study of 628 cases with stage IB, IIA, and IIB cervical carcinoma. *Cancer* 1984;54:3035-3042.

154. Averette HE, Nguyen HN, Donato DM, et al. Radical hysterectomy for invasive cervical cancer. A 25-year prospective experience with the Miami technique. *Cancer* 1993;71 (4 suppl):1422-1437.

155. Delgado G, Bundy B, Zaino R, et al. Prospective surgical-pathological study of disease-free interval in patients with stage IB squamous cell carcinoma of the cervix: A Gynecologic Oncology Group study. *Gynecol Oncol* 1990;38:352-357.

156. Hopkins MP, Schmidt RW, Roberts JA, et al. The prognosis and treatment of stage I adenocarcinoma of the cervix. *Obstet Gynecol* 1988;72:915-921.

157. Hopkins MP, Schmidt RW, Roberts JA, et al. Gland cell carcinoma (adenocarcinoma) of the cervix. *Obstet Gynecol* 1988; 72:789-795.

158. Hopkins MP, Morley GW. A comparison of adenocarcinoma and squamous cell carcinoma of the cervix. *Obstet Gynecol* 1991;77:912-917.

159. Koutsky LA, Ault KA, Wheeler CM, et al. Proof of Principle Study Investigators. A controlled trial of a human papillomavirus type 16 vaccine. *N Engl J Med* 2002;347:1645-1651.

160. Crum CP, Rivera MN. Vaccines for cervical cancer. *Cancer J* 2003;9:368-376.

161. Gissmann L, Osen W, Muller M, et al. Therapeutic vaccines for inducing antitumor immunity against human papillomavirus type human papillomaviruses. *Intervirology* 2001;44: 167-175.

162. Garcia F, Petry KU, Muderspach L, et al. ZYC101a for treatment of high-grade cervical intraepithelial neoplasia: A randomized controlled trial. *Obstet Gynecol* 2004;103:317-326.

163. Ohno T, Nakayama Y, Nakamoto S, et al. Measurement of serum squamous cell carcinoma antigen levels as a predictor of radiation response in patients with carcinoma of the uterine cervix. *Cancer* 2003;97:3114-3120.

164. Ohara K, Tanaka Y, Tsunoda H, et al. Assessment of cervical cancer radioresponse by serum squamous cell carcinoma antigen and magnetic resonance imaging. *Obstet Gynecol* 2002;100:781-787.

165. Strauss HG, Laban C, Lautenschlager C, et al. SCC antigen in the serum as an independent prognostic factor in operable squamous cell carcinoma of the cervix. *Eur J Cancer* 2002; 38:1987-1991.

166. Takeda M, Sakuragi N, Okamoto K, et al. Preoperative serum SCC, CA125, and CA19-9 levels and lymph node status in squamous cell carcinoma of the uterine cervix. *Acta Obstet Gynecol Scand* 2002;81:451-457.

167. Micke O, Prott FJ, Schafer U, et al. The impact of squamous cell carcinoma (SCC) antigen in the follow-up after radiotherapy in patients with cervical cancer. *Anticancer Res* 2000;20:5113-5115.

168. Hung YC, Shiau YC, Chang WC, et al. Early predicting recurrent cervical cancer with combination of tissue polypeptide specific antigen (TPS) and squamous cell carcinoma antigen (SCC). *Neoplasma* 2002;49:415-417.

169. Esajas MD, Duk JM, de Bruijn HW, et al. Clinical value of routine serum squamous cell carcinoma antigen in follow-up of patients with early-stage cervical cancer. *J Clin Oncol* 2001;19:3960-3966.

170. Chan YM, Ng TY, Ngan HY, et al. Monitoring of serum squamous cell carcinoma antigen levels in invasive cervical cancer: Is it cost-effective? *Gynecol Oncol* 2002;84:7-11.

171. Wright TC Jr, Cox JT, Massad LS, et al. 2001 Consensus Guidelines for the management of women with cervical cytological abnormalities. *JAMA* 2002;287:2120-2129.

172. Stoler MH, Schiffman M. Atypical squamous cells of undetermined significance—Low-grade Squamous Intraepithelial Lesion Triage Study (ALTS) group. Interobserver reproducibility of cervical cytologic and histologic interpretations: Realistic estimates from the ASCUS-LSIL Triage Study. *JAMA* 2001;285:1500-1505.

173. Wright TC Jr, Cox JT, Massad LS, et al. American Society for Colposcopy and Cervical Pathology. 2001 consensus guidelines for the management of women with cervical intraepithelial neoplasia. *Am J Obstet Gynecol* 2003;189: 295-304.

174. Piver MS, Rutledge F, Smith JP. Five classes of extended hysterectomy for women with cervical cancer. *Obstet Gynecol* 1974;44:265-272.

175. Querleu D. and Morrow CP. Classification of radical hysterectomy. *Lancet Oncol* 2008;9:297-303.

176. Roman LD, Felix JC, Muderspach LI, et al. Risk of residual invasive disease in women with microinvasive squamous cancer in a conization specimen. *Obstet Gynecol* 1997;90: 759-764.

177. Dargent D, Martin X, Sacchetoni A, et al. Laparoscopic vaginal radical trachelectomy: A treatment to preserve the fertility of cervical carcinoma patients. *Cancer* 2000;88: 1877-1882.

178. Grigsby PW, Perez CA. Radiotherapy alone for medically inoperable carcinoma of the cervix: Stage IA and carcinoma in situ. *Int J Radiat Oncol Biol Phys* 1991;21:375-378.

179. Roddick JW Jr, Greenelaw RH. Treatment of cervical cancer. A randomized study of operation and radiation. *Am J Obstet Gynecol* 1971;109:754-764.

180. Magrina JF, Goodrich MA, Lidner TK, et al. Modified radical hysterectomy in the treatment of early squamous cervical cancer. *Gynecol Oncol* 1999;72:183-186.

181. Kinney WK, Hodge DO, Egorshin EV, et al. Identification of a low-risk subset of patients with stage IB invasive squamous cancer of the cervix possibly suited to less radical surgical treatment. *Gynecol Oncol* 1995;57:3-6.

182. Landoni F, Maneo A, Cormio G, et al. Class II versus class III radical hysterectomy in stage IB-IIA cervical cancer: A prospective randomized study. *Gynecol Oncol* 2001;80:3-12.

183. Sedlis A, Bundy BN, Rotman MZ, et al. A randomized trial of pelvic radiation therapy versus no further therapy in selected patients with stage IB carcinoma of the cervix after radical hysterectomy and pelvic lymphadenectomy: A Gynecologic Oncology Group Study. *Gynecol Oncol* 1999; 73:177-183.

184. Soisson AP, Soper JT, Clarke-Pearson DL, et al. Adjuvant radiotherapy following radical hysterectomy for patients with stage IB and IIA cervical cancer. *Gynecol Oncol* 1990;37: 390-395.

185. Morrow CP. Panel report. Is pelvic radiation beneficial in the post operative management of stage IB squamous cell carcinoma of the cervix with pelvic node metastasis treated by radical hysterectomy and pelvic lymphadenectomy? *Gynecol Oncol* 1980;10:105-110.

186. Kinney WK, Alvarez RD, Reid GC, et al. Value of adjuvant whole-pelvis irradiation after Wertheim hysterectomy for early-stage squamous carcinoma of the cervix with pelvic nodal metastasis: A matched-control study. *Gynecol Oncol* 1989;34:258-262.

187. Peters WA III, Liu PY, Barrett RJ, et al. Cisplatin and 5-fluorouracil plus radiation therapy are superior to radiation therapy as adjunctive in high-risk early stage carcinoma of the cervix after radical hysterectomy and pelvic lymphadenectomy: Report of a phase III intergroup study. *J Clin Oncol* 2000;18:1606-1613.

188. Monk BJ, Wang J, Im S, et al. Rethinking the use of radiation and chemotherapy after radical hysterectomy: a clinical-pathologic analysis of a Gynecologic Oncology Group/Southwest Oncology Group/Radiation Therapy Oncology Group trial. *Gynecol Oncol* 2005;96(3):721-728.

189. Plentl AA, Friedman EA. Lymphatic system of the female genitalia. The morphologic basis of oncologic diagnosis and therapy. *Major Probl Obstet Gynecol* 1971;2:1-223.

190. Cabanas R. An approach for the treatment of penile carcinoma. *Cancer* 1977;39:456-466.

191. Echt ML, Finan MA, Hoffman MS, et al. Detection of sentinel lymph nodes with lymphazurin in cervical, uterine, and vulvar malignancies. *South Med J* 1999;92:204-208.

192. Malur S, Krause N, Kohler C, et al. Sentinel lymph node detection in patients with cervical cancer. *Gynecol Oncol* 2001;80:254-257.

193. O'Boyle JD, Coleman RL, Bernstein SG, et al. Intraoperative lymphatic mapping in cervix cancer patients undergoing radical hysterectomy: A pilot study. *Gynecol Oncol* 2000;79:238-243.

194. Verheijen RH, Pijpers R, van Diest PJ, et al. Sentinel node detection in cervical cancer. *Obstet Gynecol* 2000;96:135-138.

195. Dargent D, Martin X, Mathevet P. Laparoscopic assessment of the sentinel lymph node in early stage cervical cancer. *Gynecol Oncol* 2000;79:411-415.

196. Chung YA, Kim SH, Sohn HS, et al. Usefulness of lymphoscintigraphy and intraoperative gamma probe detection in the identification of sentinel nodes in cervical cancer. *Eur J Nucl Med Mol Imaging* 2003;30:1014-1017.

197. Barranger E, Grahek D, Cortez A, et al. Laparoscopic sentinel lymph node procedure using a combination of patent blue and radioisotope in women with cervical carcinoma. *Cancer* 2003;97:3003-3009.

198. Lantzsch T, Wolters M, Grimm J, et al. Sentinel node procedure in Ib cervical cancer: A preliminary series. *Br J Cancer* 2001;85:791-794.

199. van Dam PA, Hauspy J, Vanderheyden T, et al. Intraoperative sentinel node identification with technectium-99m-labeled nanocolloid in patients with cancer of the uterine cervix: A feasibility study. *Int J Gynecol Cancer* 2003;13: 182-186.

200. Levenback C, Coleman RL, Burke TW, et al. Lymphatic mapping and sentinel node identification in patients with cervix cancer undergoing radical hysterectomy and pelvic lymphadenectomy. *J Clin Oncol* 2002;20:688-693.

201. Lambaudie E, Collinet P, Narducci F, et al. Laparoscopic identification of sentinel lymph nodes in early stage cervical cancer: Prospective study using a combination of patent blue dye injection and technetium radiocolloid injection. *Gynecol Oncol* 2003;89:84-87.

202. Rhim CC, Park JS, Bae SN, et al. Sentinel node biopsy as an indicator for pelvic nodes dissection in early stage cervical cancer. *J Korean Med Sci* 2002;17: 507-511.

203. Plante M, Renaud MC, Tetu B, et al. Laparoscopic sentinel node mapping in early-stage cervical cancer. *Gynecol Oncol* 2003;91:494-503.

204. Noguchi M. Therapeutic relevance of breast cancer micrometastases in sentinel lymph nodes. *Br J Surg* 2002;89: 1505-1515.

205. Weaver DL. Sentinel lymph nodes and breast carcinoma: Which micrometastases are clinically significant? *Am J Surg Pathol* 2003;27:842-845

206. Keys HM, Bundy BN, Stehman FB, et al. Cisplatin, radiation, and adjuvant hysterectomy compared with radiation and adjuvant hysterectomy for bulky stage IB cervical carcinoma. *N Engl J Med* 1999;340:1154-1161.

207. Morris M, Eifel PJ, Lu J, et al. Pelvic radiation with concurrent chemotherapy versus pelvic and para-aortic radiation for high-risk cervical cancer: A randomized Radiation Therapy Oncology Group clinical trial. *N Engl J Med* 1999;340: 1137-1143.

208. Rose PG, Bundy BN, Watkins EB, et al. Concurrent cisplatin-based chemoradiation improves progression free and overall survival in advanced cervical cancer: Results of a randomized Gynecologic Oncology Group study. *N Engl J Med* 1999;340:1144-1153.

209. Whitney CW, Sause W, Bundy BN, et al. A randomized comparison of fluorouracil plus cisplatin versus hydroxyurea as an adjunct to radiation therapy in stages IIB-IVA carcinoma of the cervix with negative para-aortic lymph nodes. A Gynecologic Oncology Group and Southwest Oncology Group study. *J Clin Oncol* 1999;17:1339-1348.

210. Pearcey R, Brundage M, Drouin P, et al. Phase III trial comparing radical radiotherapy with and without cisplatin chemotherapy in patients with advanced squamous cell cancer of the cervix. *J Clin Oncol* 2002;20:966-972.

211. Green JA, Kirwan JM, Tierney JF, et al. Survival and recurrence after concomitant chemotherapy and radiotherapy for cancer of the uterine cervix: A systematic review and meta-analysis. *Lancet* 2001;358:781-786.

212. Kirwan JM, Symonds P, Green JA, et al. A systematic review of acute and late toxicity of concomitant chemoradiation for cervical cancer. *Radiother Oncol* 2003;68:217-226.

213. Thomas G, Dembo A, Fyles A, et al. Concurrent chemoradiation in advanced cervical cancer. *Gynecol Oncol* 1990;38: 446-451.

214. Thomas G, Dembo A, Ackerman I, et al. A randomized trial of standard versus partially hyperfractionated radiation with or without concurrent 5-fluorouracil in locally advanced cervical cancer. *Gynecol Oncol* 1998;69:137-145.

215. Duenas-Gonzalez A, Cetina L, Sanchez B, et al. A phase I study of carboplatin concurrent with radiation in FIGO stage IIIB cervix uteri carcinoma. *Int J Radiat Oncol Biol Phys* 2003;56:1361-1365.

216. Higgins RV, Naumann WR, Hall JB, et al. Concurrent carboplatin with pelvic radiation therapy in the primary treatment of cervix cancer. *Gynecol Oncol* 2003;89:499-503.

217. Muderspach LI, Curtin JP, Roman LD, et al. Carboplatin as a radiation sensitizer in locally advanced cervical cancer: A pilot study. *Gynecol Oncol* 1997;65:336-342.

218. Corn BW, Micaily B, Dunton CJ, et al. Concomitant irradiation and dose-escalating carboplatin for locally advanced carcinoma of the uterine cervix: An updated report. *Am J Clin Oncol* 1998;21:31-35.

219. Covens A, Shaw P, Murphy J, et al. Is radical trachelectomy a sage alternative to radical hysterectomy for patients with Stage IA-B carcinoma of the cervix? *Cancer* 1999;86: 2273-2279.

220. Roy M, Plante M. Radical vaginal trachelectomy for invasive cervical cancer. *J Gynecol Obstet Biol Reprod* 2000;29: 279-281.

221. Dargent D. Radical trachelectomy: An operation that preserves the fertility of young women with invasive cervical cancer. *Bull Acad Natl Med* 2001;185:1295-1304.

222. Shepherd JH, Mould T, Oram DH. Radical trachelectomy in early stage carcinoma of the cervix: Outcome as judged by recurrence and fertility rates. *BJOG* 2001;108:882-885.

223. Burnett AF, Roman LD, O'Meara AT, et al. Radical vaginal trachelectomy and pelvic lymphadenectomy for preservation of fertility in early cervical carcinoma. *Gynecol Oncol* 2003; 88:419-423.

224. Schlaerth JB, Spirtos NM, Schlaerth AC. Radical trachelectomy and pelvic lymphadenectomy with uterine preservation in the treatment of cervical cancer. *Am J Obstet Gynecol* 2003; 188:29-34.

225. Covens A. Preserving fertility in early cervical CA with radical trachelectomy. *Contemp OB/Gyn* 2003;48:46-66.

226. Diaz JP, Sonoda Y, Leitao MM, et al. Oncologic outcome of fertility-sparing radical trachelectomy versus radical hysterectomy for stage IB1 cervical carcinoma. *Gynecol Oncol* 2008;111:255-260.

227. Ramirez PT, Schmeler KM, Malpica A, et al. Safety and feasibility of robotic radical trachelectomy in patients with early-stage cervical cancer. *Gynecol Oncol* 2009 (in Press).

228. Eifel PJ. Radiation therapy. In: Berek JS, Hacker NF (eds): *Practical Gynecologic Oncology,* 3rd ed. Philadelphia, PA: Lippincott Williams & Wilkins; 2000:117-158.

229. Coia L, Won M, Lanciano R, et al. The Patterns of Care Outcome Study for cancer of the uterine cervix: Results of the Second National Practice Survey. *Cancer* 1990;66:2451-2456.

230. Komaki R, Brickner TJ, Hanlon AL, et al. Long-term results of treatment of cervical carcinoma in the United States in 1973, 1978, and 1983: Patterns of Care Study (PCS). *Int J Radiat Oncol Biol Phys* 1995;31:973-982.

231. Logsdon MD, Eifel PJ. FIGO IIIB squamous cell carcinoma of the cervix: An analysis of prognostic factors emphasizing the balance between external beam and intracavitary radiation therapy. *Int J Radiat Oncol Biol Phys* 1999;43:763-775.

232. Eifel PJ, Moughan J, Owen J, et al. Patterns of radiotherapy practice for patients with squamous carcinoma of the uterine cervix: Patterns of Care study. *Int J Radiat Oncol Biol Phys* 1999;43:351-358.

233. Patel FD, Sharma SC, Negi PS, et al. Low dose rate vs. high dose rate brachytherapy in the treatment of carcinoma of the uterine cervix: A clinical trial. *Int J Radiat Oncol Biol Phys* 1994;28:335-341.

234. Hareyama M, Sakata K, Oouchi A, et al. High-dose-rate versus low-dose-rate intracavitary therapy for carcinoma of the uterine cervix: A randomized trial. *Cancer* 2002;94: 117-124.

235. Petereit DG, Sarkaria JN, Potter DM, et al. High-dose-rate versus low-dose-rate brachytherapy in the treatment of cervical cancer: Analysis of tumor recurrence—The University of Wisconsin experience. *Int J Radiat Oncol Biol Phys* 1999;45: 1267-1274.

236. Lorvidhaya V, Tonusin A, Changwiwit W, et al. High-dose-rate afterloading brachytherapy in carcinoma of the cervix: An experience of 1992 patients. *Int J Radiat Oncol Biol Phys* 2000;46:1185-1191.

237. Heron DE, Gerszten K, Selvaraj RN, et al. Conventional 3D conformal versus intensity-modulated radiotherapy for the adjuvant treatment of gynecologic malignancies: A comparative dosimetric study of dose-volume histograms small star, filled. *Gynecol Oncol* 2003;91:39-45.

238. Mundt AJ, Lujan AE, Rotmensch J, et al. Intensity-modulated whole pelvic radiotherapy in women with gynecologic malignancies. *Int J Radiat Oncol Biol Phys* 2002;52:1330-1337.

239. Low DA, Grigsby PW, Dempsey JF, et al. Applicator-guided intensity-modulated radiation therapy. *Int J Radiat Oncol Biol Phys* 2002;52:1400-1406.

240. Kavanagh BD, Schefter TE, Wu Q, et al. Clinical application of intensity-modulated radiotherapy for locally advanced cervical cancer. *Semin Radiat Oncol* 2002;12:260-271.

241. Hall EJ, Wuu CS. Radiation-induced second cancers: The impact of 3D-CRT and IMRT. *Int J Radiat Oncol Biol Phys* 2003;56:83-88.

242. Knocke TH, Weitmann HD, Feldmann HJ, et al. Intratumoral PO_2-measurements as predictive assay in the treatment of carcinoma of the uterine cervix. *Radiother Oncol* 1999;53:99-104.

243. Grogan M, Thomas GM, Melamed I, et al. The importance of hemoglobin levels during radiotherapy for carcinoma of the cervix. *Cancer* 1999;86:1528-1536.

244. Fyles A, Keane TJ, Barton M, Simm J. The effect of treatment duration in the local control of cervix cancer. *Radiother Oncol* 1992;25:273-279.

245. Petereit DG, Sarkaria JN, Chappell R, et al. The adverse effect of treatment prolongation in cervical carcinoma. *Int J Radiat Oncol Biol Phys* 1995;32:1301-1307.

246. Rotman M, Choi K, Guse C, et al. Prophylactic irradiation of the para-aortic lymph node chain in stage IIB and bulky stage IB carcinoma of the cervix, initial treatment results of RTOG 7920. *Int J Radiat Oncol Biol Phys* 1990;19:513-521.

247. Rotman M, Pajak TF, Choi K, et al. Prophylactic extended-field irradiation of para-aortic lymph nodes in stages IIB and bulky IB and IIA cervical carcinomas. Ten-year treatment results of RTOG 79-20. *JAMA* 1995;274:387-393.

248. Gallion HH, van Nagell JR Jr, Donaldson ES, et al. Combined radiation therapy and extrafascial hysterectomy in the treatment of stage IB barrel-shaped cervical cancer. *Cancer* 1985;56:262-265.

249. Weems DH, Mendenhall WM, Bova FJ, et al. Carcinoma of the intact uterine cervix, stage IB–IIA–B, greater than or equal to 6 cm in diameter: Irradiation alone vs preoperative irradiation and surgery. *Int J Radiat Oncol Biol Phys* 1985; 11:1911-1914.

250. Thoms WW Jr, Eifel PJ, Smith TL, et al. Bulky endocervical carcinoma: A 23-year experience. *Int J Radiat Oncol Biol Phys* 1992;23:491-499.

251. Rotman M, John MJ, Moon SH, et al. Limitations of adjunctive surgery in carcinoma of the cervix. *Int J Radiat Oncol Biol Phys* 1979;5:327-332.

252. Perez CA, Camel HM, Kao MS, et al. Randomized study of preoperative radiation and surgery or irradiation alone in the treatment of stage IB and IIA carcinoma of the uterine cervix: Preliminary analysis of failures and complications. *Cancer* 1980;45:2759-2768.

253. Keys HM, Bundy BN, Stehman FB, et al. Gynecologic Oncology Group. Radiation therapy with and without extra-fascial hysterectomy for bulky stage IB cervical carcinoma: A randomized trial of the Gynecologic Oncology Group. *Gynecol Oncol* 2003;89:343-353.

254. Maruyama Y, van Nagell JR, Powell D, et al. Predictive value of specimen histology after preoperative radiotherapy in the treatment of bulky/barrel carcinoma of the cervix. *Am J Clin Oncol* 1992;15:150-156.

255. Tobias J, Buxton EJ, Blackledge G, et al. Neoadjuvant bleomycin, ifosfamide and cisplatin in cervical cancer. *Cancer Chemother Pharmacol* 1990;26(suppl):S59-S62.

256. Kumar L, Kaushal R, Nandy B, et al. Chemotherapy followed by radiotherapy versus radiotherapy alone in locally advanced cervical cancer: A randomized study. *Gynecol Oncol* 1994; 301-315.

257. Leborgne F, Leborgne JH, Doldaân R, et al. Induction chemotherapy and radiotherapy of advanced cancer of the cervix: A pilot study and phase III randomized trial. *Int J Radiat Oncol Biol Phys* 1997;37:343-350.

258. Sundfor K, Tropeâ CG, Hoègberg T, et al. Radiotherapy and neoadjuvant chemotherapy for cervical carcinoma. A randomized multicenter study of sequential cisplatin and 5-fluorouracil and radiotherapy in advanced cervical carcinoma stage 3B and 4A. *Cancer* 1996;77:2371-2378.

259. Chiara S, Bruzzone M, Merlini L, et al. Randomized study comparing chemotherapy plus radiotherapy versus radiotherapy alone in FIGO stage IIB±III cervical carcinoma. *Am J Clin Oncol* 1994;17:294-297.

260. Souhami L, Gil RA, Allan SE, et al. A randomized trial of chemotherapy followed by pelvic radiation therapy in stage IIIB carcinoma of the cervix. *J Clin Oncol* 1991;9:970-977.

261. Tattersall MHN, Lorvidhaya V, Vootiprux V, et al. Randomized trial of epirubicin and cisplatin chemotherapy followed by pelvic radiation in locally advanced cervical cancer. *J Clin Oncol* 1995;13:444-451.

262. Tierney JF, Stewart LA, Parmar MK. Can the published data tell us about the effectiveness of neoadjuvant chemotherapy for locally advanced cancer of the uterine cervix? *Eur J Cancer* 1999;35:406-409.

263. Neoadjuvant Chemotherapy for Locally Advanced Cervical Cancer Meta-Analysis Collaboration. Neoadjuvant chemotherapy for locally advanced cervical cancer: A systematic review and meta-analysis of individual patient data from 21 randomised trials. *Eur J Cancer* 2003;39:2470-2486.

264. Sardi JE, Giaroli A, Sananes C, et al. Long-term follow-up of the first randomized trial using neoadjuvant chemotherapy in stage Ib squamous carcinoma of the cervix: The final results. *Gynecol Oncol* 1997;67:61-69.

265. Thigpen T. The role of chemotherapy in the management of carcinoma of the cervix. *Cancer J* 2003;9:425-432.

266. Thigpen T, Shingleton H, Homesley H, et al. Cis-platinum in treatment of advanced or recurrent squamous cell carcinoma of the cervix: A phase II study of the Gynecologic Oncology Group. *Cancer* 1981;48:899-903.

267. Bonomi P, Blessing JA, Stehman FB, et al. Randomized trial of three cisplatin dose schedules in squamous-cell carcinoma of the cervix: A Gynecologic Oncology Group study. *J Clin Oncol* 1985;3:1079-1085.

268. Thigpen JT, Blessing JA, DiSaia PJ, et al. A randomized comparison of a rapid versus prolonged (24 hr) infusion of cisplatin in therapy of squamous cell carcinoma of the uterine cervix: A Gynecologic Oncology Group study. *Gynecol Oncol* 1989;32:198-202.

269. Coleman RE, Harper PG, Gallagher C, et al. A phase II study of ifosfamide in advanced and relapsed carcinoma of the cervix. *Cancer Chemother Pharmacol* 1986;18:280-283.

270. Sutton GP, Blessing JA, Adcock L, et al. Phase II study of ifosfamide and mesna in patients with previously-treated carcinoma of the cervix. A Gynecologic Oncology Group study. *Invest New Drugs* 1989;7:341-343.

271. Sutton GP, Blessing JA, DiSaia PJ, McGuire WP. Phase II study of ifosfamide and mesna in nonsquamous carcinoma of the cervix: A Gynecologic Oncology Group study. *Gynecol Oncol* 1993;49:48-50.

272. Sutton GP, Blessing JA, McGuire WP, et al. Phase II trial of ifosfamide and mesna in patients with advanced or recurrent squamous carcinoma of the cervix who had never received chemotherapy: A Gynecologic Oncology Group study. *Am J Obstet Gynecol* 1993;168(3 pt 1):805-807.

273. McGuire WP, Blessing JA, Moore D, et al. Paclitaxel has moderate activity in squamous cervix cancer. A Gynecologic Oncology Group study. *J Clin Oncol* 1996;14:792-795.

274. Kudelka AP, Winn R, Edwards CL, et al. An update of a phase II study of paclitaxel in advanced or recurrent squamous cell cancer of the cervix. *Anticancer Drugs* 1997;8: 657-661.

275. Curtin JP, Blessing JA, Webster KD, et al. Paclitaxel, an active agent in nonsquamous carcinomas of the uterine cervix: A Gynecologic Oncology Group study. *J Clin Oncol* 2001;19: 1275-1278.

276. Fukuoka M, Noda K, Hasegawa K, et al. An early phase II study of gemcitabine hydrochloride (LY 188011). Gemcitabine Cooperative Study Group for Early Phase II (abstract). *Gan To Kagaku Ryoho* 1996;23(13):1813-1824.

277. Schilder RJ, Blessing JA, Morgan M, et al. Evaluation of gemcitabine in patients with squamous cell carcinoma of the cervix: A phase II study of the gynecologic oncology group. *Gynecol Oncol* 2000;76:204-207.

278. Morris M, Brader KR, Levenback C, et al. Phase II study of vinorelbine in advanced and recurrent squamous cell carcinoma of the cervix. *J Clin Oncol* 1998;16:1094-1098.

279. Lhomme C, Vermorken JB, Mickiewicz E, et al. Phase II trial of vinorelbine in patients with advanced and/or recurrent cervical carcinoma: An EORTC Gynaecological Cancer Cooperative Group study. *Eur J Cancer* 2000;36:194-199.

280. Muderspach LI, Blessing JA, Levenback C, et al. A phase II study of topotecan in patients with squamous cell carcinoma of the cervix: A Gynecologic Oncology Group study. *Gynecol Oncol* 2001;81:213-215.

281. Bookman MA, Blessing JA, Hanjani P, et al. Topotecan in squamous cell carcinoma of the cervix: A phase II study of the Gynecologic Oncology Group. *Gynecol Oncol* 2000;77: 446-449.

282. Verschraegen CF, Levy T, Kudelka AP, et al. Phase II study of irinotecan in prior chemotherapy-treated squamous cell carcinoma of the cervix. *J Clin Oncol* 1997;15:625-631.

283. Irvin WP, Price FV, Bailey H, et al. A phase II study of irinotecan (CPT-11) in patients with advanced squamous cell carcinoma of the cervix. *Cancer* 1998;82:328-333.

284. Look KY, Blessing JA, Levenback C, et al. A phase II trial of CPT-11 in recurrent squamous carcinoma of the cervix: A Gynecologic Oncology Group study. *Gynecol Oncol* 1998;70: 334-338.

285. Lhomme C, Fumoleau P, Fargeot P, et al. Results of a European Organization for Research and Treatment of Cancer/Early Clinical Studies Group phase II trial of first-line irinotecan in patients with advanced or recurrent squamous cell carcinoma of the cervix. *J Clin Oncol* 1999;17:3136-3142.

286. McGuire WP III, Arseneau J, Blessing JA, et al. A randomized comparative trial of carboplatin and iproplatin in advanced squamous carcinoma of the uterine cervix: A Gynecologic Oncology Group study. *J Clin Oncol* 1989;7:1462-1468.

287. Arseneau J, Blessing JA, Stehman FB, et al. A phase II study of carboplatin in advanced squamous cell carcinoma of the cervix: A Gynecologic Oncology Group study. *Invest New Drugs* 1986;4:187-191.

288. Fracasso PM, Blessing JA, Wolf J, et al. Phase II evaluation of oxaliplatin in previously treated squamous cell carcinoma of the cervix: A Gynecologic Oncology Group study. *Gynecol Oncol* 2003;90:177-180.

289. Rose PG, Blessing JA, Buller RE, et al. Prolonged oral etoposide in recurrent or advanced non-squamous cell carcinoma of the cervix: A Gynecologic Oncology Group study. *Gynecol Oncol* 2003;89:267-270.

290. Filtenborg TA, Hansen HH, Aage Engelholm S, et al. A phase II study of ifosfamide, carboplatin and cisplatin in advanced and recurrent squamous cell carcinoma of the uterine cervix. *Ann Oncol* 1993;4:485-488.

291. Omura GA, Blessing JA, Vaccarello L, et al. Randomized trial of cisplatin versus cisplatin plus mitolactol versus cisplatin plus ifosfamide in advanced squamous carcinoma of the cervix: A Gynecologic Oncology Group study. *J Clin Oncol* 1997;15:165-171.

292. Bloss JD, Blessing JA, Behrens BC, et al. Randomized trial of cisplatin and ifosfamide with or without bleomycin in squamous carcinoma of the cervix: A Gynecologic Oncology Group study. *J Clin Oncol* 2002;20:1832-1837.

293. Chitapanarux I, Tonusin A, Sukthomya V, et al. Phase II clinical study of irinotecan and cisplatin as first-line chemotherapy in metastatic or recurrent cervical cancer. *Gynecol Oncol* 2003;89:402-407.

294. Sugiyama T, Yakushiji M, Noda K, et al. Phase II study of irinotecan and cisplatin as first-line chemotherapy in advanced or recurrent cervical cancer. *Oncology* 2000;58:31-37.

295. Ghaemmaghami F, Behtash N, Yarandi F, et al. First-line chemotherapy with 5-FU and platinum for advanced and recurrent cancer of the cervix: A phase II study. *J Obstet Gynaecol* 2003;23:422-425.

296. Fiorica J, Holloway R, Ndubisi B, et al. Phase II trial of topotecan and cisplatin in persistent or recurrent squamous and nonsquamous carcinomas of the cervix. *Gynecol Oncol* 2002;85:89-94.

297. Long HJ 3rd, Bundy BN, Grendys EC Jr et al. Randomized phase III trial of cisplatin with or without topotecan in carcinoma of the uterine cervix: a Gynecologic Oncology Group Study. *J Clin Oncol* 2005;23(21):4626-4633.

298. Gebbia V, Caruso M, Testa A, et al. Vinorelbine and cisplatin for the treatment of recurrent and/or metastatic carcinoma of the uterine cervix. *Oncology* 2002;63:31-37.

299. Pignata S, Silvestro G, Ferrari E, et al. Phase II study of cisplatin and vinorelbine as first-line chemotherapy in patients with carcinoma of the uterine cervix. *J Clin Oncol* 1999;17:756-760.

300. Rose PG, Blessing JA, Gershenson DM, et al. Paclitaxel and cisplatin as first-line therapy in recurrent or advanced squamous cell carcinoma of the cervix: A Gynecologic Oncology Group study. *J Clin Oncol* 1999;17:2676-2680.

301. Moore DH, McQuellon RP, Blessing JA, et al. A randomized phase III study of cisplatin versus cisplatin plus paclitaxel in stage IVB, recurrent or persistent squamous cell carcinoma of the cervix: A Gynecologic Oncology Group Study (abstract). *Proc Amer Soc Clin Oncol* 2001;20:20a.

302. Dimopoulos MA, Papadimitriou CA, Sarris K, et al. Combination of ifosfamide, paclitaxel, and cisplatin for the treatment of metastatic and recurrent carcinoma of the uterine cervix: A phase II study of the Hellenic Cooperative Oncology Group. *Gynecol Oncol* 2002;85:476-482.

303. Zanetta G, Fei F, Parma G, et al. Paclitaxel, ifosfamide and cisplatin (TIP) chemotherapy for recurrent or persistent squamous-cell cervical cancer. *Ann Oncol* 1999;10:1171-1174.

304. Burnett AF, Roman LD, Garcia AA, et al. A phase II study of gemcitabine and cisplatin in patients with advanced, persistent, or recurrent squamous cell carcinoma of the cervix. *Gynecol Oncol* 2000;76:63-66.

305. Duenas-Gonzalez A, Hinojosa-Garcia LM, Lopez-Graniel C, et al. Weekly cisplatin/low-dose gemcitabine combination for advanced and recurrent cervical carcinoma. *Am J Clin Oncol* 2001;24:201-203.

306. Verschraegen CF, Kavanagh JJ, Loyer E, et al. Community Clinical Oncology Program. Phase II study of carboplatin and liposomal doxorubicin in patients with recurrent squamous cell carcinoma of the cervix. *Cancer* 2001;92:2327-2333.

307. Wagenaar HC, Pecorelli S, Mangioni C, et al. Phase II study of mitomycin-C and cisplatin in disseminated, squamous cell carcinoma of the uterine cervix. A European Organization for Research and Treatment of Cancer (EORTC) Gynecological Cancer Group study. *Eur J Cancer* 2001;37:1624-1628.

308. Zanetta G, Torri W, Bocciolone L, et al. Factors predicting response to chemotherapy and survival in patients with metastatic or recurrent squamous cell cervical carcinoma: A multivariate analysis. *Gynecol Oncol* 1995;58:58-63.

309. Monk BJ, Sill MW, McMeekin DS, et al. Phase III trial of four cisplatin-containing doublet combinations in stage IVB, recurrent, or persistent cervical carcinoma: A Gynecologic Oncology Group study. *J Clin Oncol* 2009;27:4649-4655

310. Heller PB, Barnhill DR, Mayer AR, et al. Cervical carcinoma found incidentally in a uterus removed for benign indications. *Obstet Gynecol* 1986;67:187-190.

311. Hopkins MP, Peters WA III, Andersen W, et al. Invasive cervical cancer treated initially by standard hysterectomy. *Gynecol Oncol* 1990;36:7-12.

312. Leath CA, Straughn JM, Bhoola SM, et al. The role of radical parametrectomy in the treatment of occult cervical carcinoma after extrafascial hysterectomy. *Gynecol Oncol* 2004;92:215-219.

313. Duyn A, Van Eijkeren M, Kenter G, et al. Recurrent cervical cancer: Detection and prognosis. *Acta Obstet Gynecol Scand* 2002;81:759-763.

314. Gerdin E, Cnattingius S, Johnson P, et al. Prognostic factors and relapse patterns in early-stage cervical carcinoma after brachytherapy and radical hysterectomy. *Gynecol Oncol* 1994;53:314-319.

315. Look KY, Rocereto TF. Relapse patterns in FIGO stage IB carcinoma of the cervix. *Gynecol Oncol* 1990;38:114-120.

316. Larson DM, Copeland LJ, Malone JM Jr, et al. Diagnosis of recurrent cervical carcinoma after radical hysterectomy. *Obstet Gynecol* 1988;71:6-9.

317. Barter JF, Soong SJ, Hatch KD, et al. Diagnosis and treatment of pulmonary metastases from cervical carcinoma. *Gynecol Oncol* 1990;38:347-351.

318. National Comprehensive Cancer Network. NCCN Clinical Practice Guidelines for Cervical Cancer, Version 1.2011. http.//www.nccn.org/professionals/physician_gls/pdf/cervical.pdf. Accessed 2/15/2011.

319. Writing Group for the Women's Health Initiative Investigators. Risks and benefits of estrogen plus progestin in healthy postmenopausal women: Principal results from the Women's Health Initiative randomized controlled trial. *JAMA* 2002;288:321-333.

320. Stephenson J. FDA orders estrogen safety warnings: Agency offers guidance for HRT use. *JAMA* 2003;289:537-538.

321. Larson DM, Copeland LJ, Stringer CA, et al. Recurrent cervical carcinoma after radical hysterectomy. *Gynecol Oncol* 1988;30:381-387.

322. Webb MJ, Symmonds RE. Site of recurrence of cervical cancer after radical hysterectomy. *Am J Obstet Gynecol* 1980;138 (7 pt 1): 813-817.

323. Ito H, Shigematsu N, Kawada T, et al. Radiotherapy for centrally recurrent cervical cancer of the vaginal stump following hysterectomy. *Gynecol Oncol* 1997;67:154-161.

324. Jobsen JJ, Leer JW, Cleton FJ, et al. Treatment of locoregional recurrence of carcinoma of the cervix by radiotherapy after primary surgery. *Gynecol Oncol* 1989;33:368-371.

325. Maneo A, Landoni F, Cormio G, et al. Concurrent carboplatin/5-fluorouracil and radiotherapy for recurrent cervical carcinoma. *Ann Oncol* 1999;10:803-807.

326. Hockel M. Laterally extended endopelvic resection. Novel surgical treatment of locally recurrent cervical carcinoma involving the pelvic sidewall. *Gynecol Oncol* 2003;91: 369-377.

GESTATIONAL TROPHOBLASTIC TUMORS

Maurie Markman
John J. Kavanagh

Gestational trophoblastic tumors (GTTs) comprise a wide spectrum of neoplastic disorders that arise from placental trophoblastic tissue after abnormal fertilization (Fig. 31-1). In the United States, GTTs account for fewer than 1% of all gynecologic malignancies. Their importance as an oncologic entity stems from the fact that they can often be cured with appropriate treatment, usually with the preservation of reasonable fertility

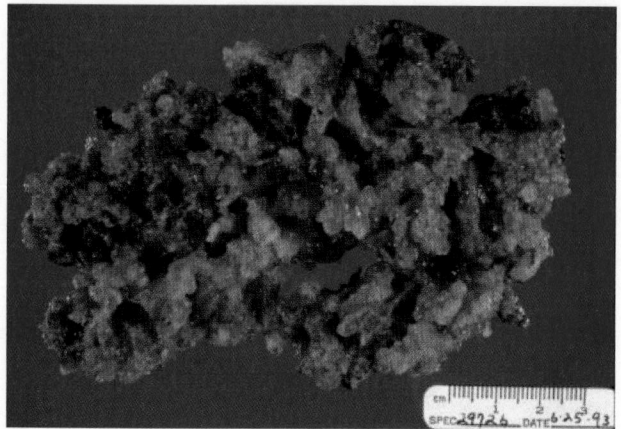

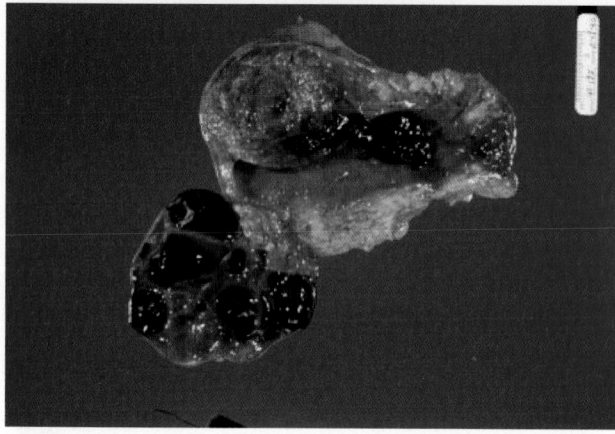

FIGURE 31-1. Gross specimen of two complete molar pregnancies. Note the absence of fetal tissue, which is replaced by abundant trophoblastic tissue.

The hydatidiform mole is the most common type of GTT. It is essentially a benign condition with variable potential for malignant transformation. Most molar pregnancies resolve spontaneously after uterine evacuation, with no further event or adverse outcome. At any time during or after gestation, however, approximately 10 to 20% undergo malignant transformation to invasive nonmetastatic or metastatic trophoblastic disease. Nearly two-thirds of these lesions develop into persistent nonmetastatic gestational trophoblastic disease, while the remaining one-third develop distant metastases (3,4). In the 1950s, a woman with choriocarcinoma had a less than 5% chance of survival. With improved understanding of the natural history and prognostic factors of this disease and the development of a reliable tumor marker for diagnosis (the beta subunit of human chorionic gonadotropin, or β-hCG) as well as effective chemotherapy for treatment, even advanced metastatic gestational trophoblastic disease is associated with a cure rate of greater than 90% (5).

■ EPIDEMIOLOGY

In the United States, GTTs develop in approximately 1 in 1000 to 2000 pregnancies (6-8). Overall, approximately 80% of GTTs are hydatidiform moles, 15% are invasive moles, and 5% are choriocarcinomas. Choriocarcinoma is associated with an antecedent mole in 50% of the cases, a history of abortion in 25%, term delivery in 20%, and ectopic pregnancy in 5% (9).

Molar pregnancies are reported in approximately 3000 patients per year, and malignant transformation occurs in 6 to 19% of these cases (3,10). About 1 in 40 molar pregnancies is complete, and complete molar pregnancies occur 1 in 15,000 abortions, and 1 in 150,000 normal pregnancies. The estimated incidence of twin pregnancy consisting of a molar pregnancy and a normal fetus is 1 per 22,000 to 100,000 pregnancies (11).

True estimates of the incidence of molar pregnancy are difficult to obtain owing to the vast variation in presentation and management of normal and abnormal pregnancies around the world. Early observations suggest a 5- to 15-fold higher incidence in the East and Southeast Asian countries than in the United States. The incidence has been reported to be as high as 1 in 120 pregnancies in East Asia (12). Native Alaskans have been found to have an incidence three- to fourfold that of white women (13), and a Hawaiian study demonstrated lower GTT rates in white and native Hawaiians

with no adverse outcome. Even advanced-stage disease is potentially highly curable. Patients are classified into different prognostic groups on the basis of factors such as tumor histologic subtype, extent of disease, human gonadotropin titer, duration of disease, nature of the antecedent pregnancy, and extent of prior treatment. All patients should receive individualized management after careful prognostication under the care of a multidisciplinary team.

GTTs are classified into two distinct groups: benign and malignant trophoblastic disease (1). Benign disease consists of a complete and partial hydatidiform mole or an invasive mole. Malignant disease comprises nonmetastatic and metastatic gestational trophoblastic disease. A hydatidiform mole is confined to the uterine cavity. Invasive moles and placental site tumors are locally invasive but rarely metastatic. Both tumors are rare, but they can be distinguished histologically (2). Choriocarcinomas are highly malignant and tend to metastasize extensively.

than in Filipino and Japanese populations (14). Another study showed that American Indian women had a higher incidence than other predominant ethnic groups in New Mexico (15). In the United Arab Emirates, women born in the Persian Gulf region had a higher GTT incidence than women of Arab or Asian origin (16). However, not all available data have confirmed the importance of ethnic background. For example, the observation that Malaysian, Indian, and Chinese populations in Kuala Lumpur have similar incidences of molar disease implies a lesser role for cultural or racial differences in the etiology of GTT (17).

This inconsistent relationship between GTT incidence and geographic region, culture, and socioeconomic status suggests that diet and nutrition may contribute to the etiology, although nothing further can be concluded. Parazinni and colleagues reported that low beta-carotene consumption was associated with GTT (18). No strong association between cigarette smoking and GTT has been found (19).

Women above age 40 have as much as a fivefold greater risk of molar pregnancy (20), whereas those younger than 20 years have a 1.5- to 2-fold relative risk (7,20,21). Younger women seem to have a better disease-free survival rate than older women (14). Women with a history of previous hydatidiform mole have a 10-fold greater risk for a second molar pregnancy (20) and a more than 1000-fold greater risk of choriocarcinoma than do women with normal pregnancies. The New England Trophoblastic Disease Center demonstrated the increased risk of subsequent molar pregnancy to be 1% (22).

Women of lower socioeconomic status seem to have a 10-fold greater rate of molar pregnancy than their more affluent counterparts. This trend is apparent not just in the East Asia but also in the Middle East and in the United States. In the Philippines, women of lower socioeconomic standing have a rate of molar disease 10 times higher than that of affluent populations (23).

Likewise, Bertini reported a higher incidence of GTT among Israeli women of poorer Middle Eastern and African heritage than among those of European descent (24). Moreover, as the standard of living improved for Israeli women of Middle Eastern origin, the incidence of GTT declined. In the Western Hemisphere, the rate of molar pregnancy is 10 times higher in Mexicans than in other North Americans.

The ABO blood groups of parents appear to be related to the development of choriocarcinoma. There is a particular risk for women in blood group A whose male partner is blood group O (25). Thus far, studies of human leukocyte antigen (HLA) have been inconclusive in clarifying the significant association between the ABO blood group and GTT.

■ PATHOLOGY

Based on these morphologic and cytogenetic features, Szulman and Surti divided hydatidiform moles into two unique syndromes: complete (classic) and partial (Table 31-1) (26,27).

COMPLETE MOLES (SEE FIG. 31-1)

Molar pregnancy is characterized by the lack of a fetus, trophoblastic hyperplasia, edematous chorionic villi, and a loss of normal villous blood vessels. A complete mole is usually detected during the second trimester and identified by total hydatidiform enlargement of the villi, which are enveloped by hyperplastic and atypical trophoblasts (28). There is a notable absence of any embryonic or amniotic remnant. Approximately 20% of complete moles give rise to persistent trophoblastic disease (29).

PARTIAL MOLES (FIG. 31-2)

Partial moles, in contrast to complete moles, are typically accompanied by an identifiable embryo or amniotic membranes. These moles are described as partial because the hydatidiform changes in the villi tend to be focal. The hydropic villi are usually irregularly scalloped and have stromal hyperplastic inclusions (27).

The villous capillaries appear to be functional because they possess the same proportion of nucleated fetal erythrocytes as the embryo. In partial moles, hydatidiform change occurs at a slower rate, and the proportion of relatively normal villi appears to correlate with fetal survival rate.

TABLE 31-1	FEATURES OF COMPLETE AND PARTIAL HYDATIDIFORM MOLES	
	Complete	*Partial*
Fetal or embryonic tissue	Absent	Present
Hydatidiform swelling of chorionic villi	Diffuse	Focal
Trophoblastic hyperplasia	Diffuse	Focal
Trophoblastic stromal inclusions	Absent	Present
Genetic parentage	Paternal	Biparental
Karyotype	46XX; 46XY	69XXY; 69XYY
Persistent β-hCG elevation	20%	0.5%

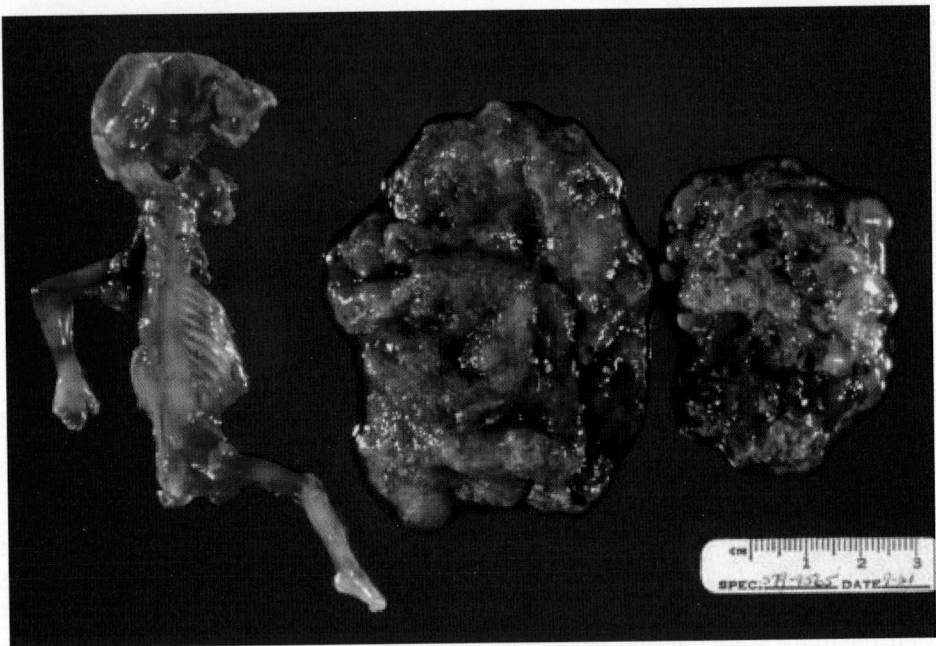

FIGURE 31-2. Partial molar pregnancy removed along with partially formed fetal tissue.

Maturation of mesenchymal elements is only minimally delayed in partial moles, and there is a paucity of fibroblast karyorrhexis. Approximately 2% of partial moles undergo malignant degeneration. Because of this sporadic malignant potential, follow-up and treatment of patients with partial moles are the same as for patients with complete moles.

INVASIVE MOLES

Locally invasive moles have the same histologic features as complete moles; in addition, they are characterized by myometrial invasion without involvement of intervening endometrial stroma (30). Invasive moles are typically diagnosed approximately 6 months after molar evacuation. They tend to invade locally, causing hemorrhage and necrosis. Rarely, uterine perforation results. Hematogenous metastasis may occur, often to the lungs. Occasionally, metastatic deposits display hydropic villi rather than the sheets of anaplastic cells that typify metastatic choriocarcinoma.

PLACENTAL-SITE TUMORS

Placental site tumors are rare. They are derived from intermediate trophoblast cells of the placenta, which are identified by their secretion of placental lactogen and small amounts of β-hCG (31). Occasionally, after a complete hydatidiform mole is removed, an unusual complication develops, characterized by proliferation of intermediate trophoblast-forming nodules in the endometrium and myometrium (32). The nodules are usually numerous and appear microscopically as cells with oval nuclei having an abundant eosinophilic cytoplasm. No chorionic villi are seen. These tumors usually present as nodules confined to the endometrium and myometrium.

CHORIOCARCINOMAS

Choriocarcinomas have a unique histology distinct from that of moles (11). The tumor is grossly red and granular and exhibits extensive necrosis and hemorrhage. On microscopic examination, the neoplasm is composed of a disordered array of syncytiotrophoblastic and cytotrophoblastic elements, frequent mitoses, and multinucleated giant cells. Vascular invasion occurs early, with resultant metastases to the lungs, vagina, brain, kidneys, liver, and gastrointestinal tract.

Malignant gestational trophoblastic tumors tend to occur after evacuation of a mole. These GTTs exhibit the histologic features of either hydatidiform moles or choriocarcinomas. On the other hand, persistent GTTs after a nonmolar pregnancy almost always have the histologic pattern of choriocarcinoma. Choriocarcinoma is characterized by sheets of anaplastic syncytiotrophoblasts and cytotrophoblasts with no preserved chorionic villous structures. Placental-site trophoblastic tumor is an uncommon form of GTT that predominantly consists of intermediate trophoblasts and a few syncytial elements.

■ PATHOGENESIS

Pathologic characteristics alone generally do not allow adequate discrimination of molar pregnancies. With the advent of cytogenetic techniques, such as chromosomal banding and restriction fragment length polymorphism (RFLP) analysis of DNA, unique chromosomal patterns of molar pregnancies were discovered (33,34), allowing complete and partial moles to be distinguished from one another (26,35).

CELL BIOLOGY (FIG. 31-3)

Normal fertilization results from the union of a single sperm and an egg, followed by rapid cellular division and the creation of an embryo. Early embryonic differentiation gives rise to trophoblasts, specialized epithelial cells responsible for developing the placenta and the villi. GTTs arise from abnormal unions of sperm with

the ovum, resulting in distinct pathologic characteristics. This is a remarkable event involving activated transcription factors, cytokines, hormone secretion, cell-adhesion molecules, and immunologic activity (36).

A complete mole is now known to contain nuclear chromosomes of all-paternal origin and cytoplasmic chromosomes of maternal origin. This occurs when a sperm fertilizes an empty ovum and this subsequently divides or two sperm unite with an ovum that is devoid of genetic material. Both methods result in a diploid complete mole. A partial mole, on the other hand, is the abnormal union of two sperms with one ovum with intact chromosomes, resulting in a triploid karyotype.

As first reported by Kajii and Ohama on the basis of chromosomal banding studies, complete moles contain only paternal chromosomes (33). Yamashita and colleagues confirmed this finding by showing that when paternal heterozygotes for the HLA locus give rise to a mole, the HLA expression of the molar tissue is

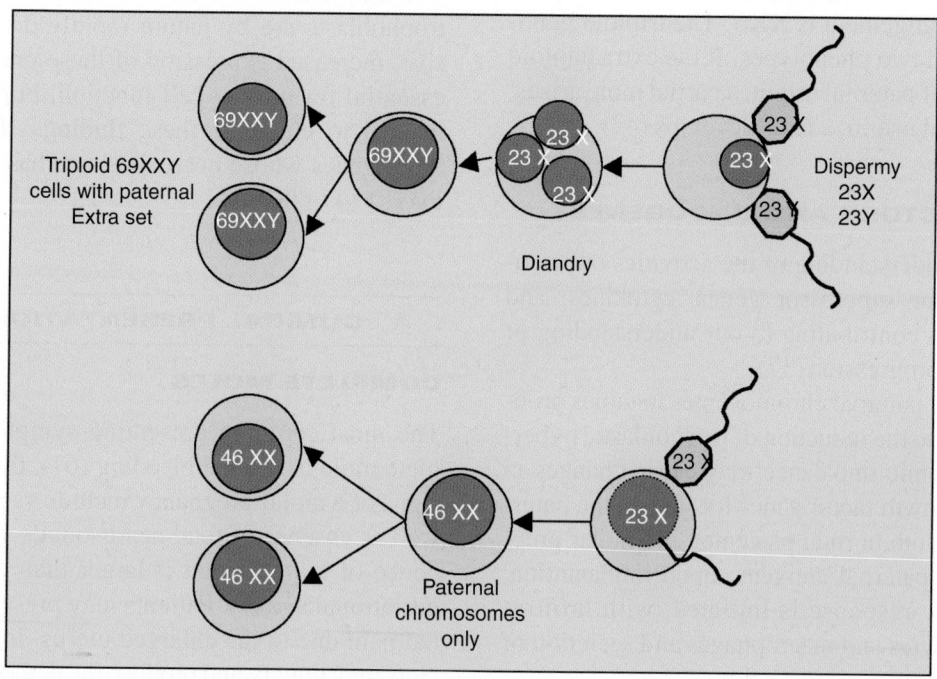

FIGURE 31-3. Schematic diagram of the pathogenesis of molar pregnancies. A partial mole, on the other hand, is the abnormal union of two sperms with one ovum with intact chromosomes, resulting in a triploid karyotype. The classic partial mole has a triploid karyotype (69 chromosomes), and both paternal and maternal chromosomes are present. The most common sex chromosome arrangement is XXY. The triploid genotype can result in two phenotypes. If the extra haploid chromosome is of paternal origin, a partial mole arises; if it is of maternal origin, a fetus develops. A complete mole is now known to contain nuclear chromosomes of all-paternal origin and cytoplasmic chromosomes of maternal origin. This occurs when a sperm fertilizes an empty ovum and then divides, or when two sperms unite with an ovum that is devoid of genetic material. Both methods result in a diploid complete mole. Approximately 85 to 92% of complete moles have a 46XX karyotype, which results from fertilization of an egg by a haploid sperm (23X) that undergoes duplication to create a diploid set of chromosomes. Some 4 to 15% of complete moles have a 46XY karyotype, which results from dispermy, the fertilization of an empty ovum by two spermatozoa, 23X and 23Y.

homozygous (37). Approximately 85 to 92% of complete moles have a 46XX karyotype (33,38), which results from fertilization of an egg by a haploid sperm (23X) that undergoes duplication to create a diploid set of chromosomes. Why maternal DNA is lost is uncertain; it may involve extrusion of maternal chromosomes or fertilization of an empty egg. Regardless of the mechanism, the finding of maternal mitochondrial DNA suggests that the mole resulted from an abnormal fertilization event (39).

Approximately 4 to 15% of complete moles have a 46XY karyotype (40,41) which results from dispermy, or the fertilization of an empty ovum by two spermatozoa, 23X and 23Y. There is no strong evidence that dispermic or Y chromosome–containing moles have greater malignant potential than the monospermic 46XX karyotype (39). Fisher and colleagues (41) also found that nearly 5% of complete moles are heterozygous 46XX. A 46YY mole has not been reported because the X chromosome is probably required for survival.

The classic partial mole has a triploid karyotype (69 chromosomes), and both paternal and maternal chromosomes are present (36). The most common sex chromosome arrangement is XXY. The triploid genotype can result in two phenotypes. If the extra haploid chromosome is of paternal origin, a partial mole arises; if it is of maternal origin, a fetus develops (42).

GROWTH FACTORS AND ONCOGENES

Our improved understanding of the activities of proto-oncogenes, tumor suppressor genes, cytokines, and growth factors is contributing to our understanding of GTT and tumor progression (37).

The excess of paternal chromosomes in moles probably contributes to the induction of trophoblastic hyperplasia. The genomic imbalance may cause changes in expression of growth factor genes located on the paternal allele (39). Both normal placentas and molar pregnancies contain paternal antigens; upon implantation, an immunologic response is initiated, with infiltration of lymphocytes and macrophages and secretion of cytokines (36).

The growth of choriocarcinomas may be related to the abundant expression of epidermal growth factor (EGF) receptor. Macrophage-derived cytokines—interleukin-1 (IL-1-α, IL-1-β) and tumor necrosis factor—can suppress cell growth and increase the expression of EGF receptor in choriocarcinoma cell lines, thus acting as paracrine mediators of cell growth (43).

The contribution of several oncogenes to the malignant transformation of GTT has also been examined.

TABLE 31-2	GENES THAT HAVE BEEN IMPLICATED IN GESTATIONAL TROPHOBLASTIC DISEASE
p53	
p21[WAF1/CIP1]	
Mdm2	
Rb (retinoblastoma)	
C-myc7q21–q31	
C-erbB2	
C-fms	
bcl-2	
Telomerase	

Growth regulation in the trophoblast has been found to be associated with expression of the transcription factor Mash-2 (44). Cheung et al. have demonstrated increased expression of c-fms RNA in complete moles compared with that in normal placentas (45). In choriocarcinoma, increased expression of oncogenes has been observed, and progression of some tumors has been associated with inactivation of tumor suppressor genes (46). The significance of these findings is uncertain. Because trophoblasts are by nature rapidly dividing and invasive, increased expression of these oncogenes may be essential for normal cell function. Further studies are needed to elucidate these findings. Table 31-2 lists other genes whose overexpression has been implicated in GTT (47-60).

■ CLINICAL PRESENTATION

COMPLETE MOLES

The most common presenting symptom of the complete mole is vaginal bleeding (61), though the classic signs of a molar pregnancy include vaginal bleeding as well as absence of fetal heart sounds and physical evidence of a uterus that is larger than expected for the gestational age (9). Patients may present with abdominal pain due to the enlarged uterus. Intrauterine blood clots may liquefy and produce the pathognomonic prune juice–like vaginal discharge. Because of the recurrent bleeding, patients may also present with iron deficiency beyond that expected for a normal pregnancy. Symptoms of anemia are noted in approximately 50% of patients at the time of diagnosis (9). Theca-luteal cysts, caused by beta–human chorionic gonadotropin (β-hCG)-induced hyperstimulation of both ovaries in about 50% of patients, may result in a sensation of pelvic pressure or fullness. Usually, these cysts regress spontaneously after uterine evacuation, although their rupture or tension can cause acute abdominal symptoms occasionally requiring surgery (9).

Some 20 to 30% of patients present with early toxemia, thought to be precipitated by the release of large amounts of vasoactive substances from necrotic trophoblastic tissue; there is a possibility of toxemic convulsions, but this is fortunately a rare event (22). Ten percent of patients present with hyperemesis gravidarum, and 7% with hyperthyroidism, presumably due to the structural similarities of β-hCG to thyroid-stimulating hormone (62-64). Thyroid storm has been reported. Other rare presentations include respiratory distress, disseminated intravascular coagulation, and microangiopathic hemolytic anemia (9).

PARTIAL MOLES

Unlike complete moles, partial moles do not usually present with an enlarged uterus. Fewer than 10% of patients with partial moles present in this manner. Notably, however, an intact fetus can coexist with a partial mole, although this occurs in fewer than 1 in 100,000 pregnancies. Patients with partial moles typically do not have the hormonal symptoms experienced by patients with complete moles, and toxemia occurs only rarely. Goldstein and Berkowitz reviewed the cases of 81 patients with partial moles and found that none had prominent theca-luteal cysts, hyperthyroidism, or respiratory insufficiency and only one had toxemia (64). In general, patients with partial moles present with the signs and symptoms of a missed or incomplete abortion, and the diagnosis of a partial mole is made only after histologic review of curettage specimens.

MALIGNANT GESTATIONAL TROPHOBLASTIC TUMORS

Patients treated surgically for molar pregnancy should be monitored closely for any signs and symptoms of malignant transformation. Signs, symptoms, and serum evaluation constitute the monitoring system. Details of this are outlined under the section Future Childbearing, later. Fifty percent of all malignant GTTs follow molar pregnancy, while 25% follow normal pregnancy and the remaining 25% follow ectopic pregnancy or abortion (65). Persistent invasive nonmetastatic GTT usually presents with recurrence of symptoms or signs such as irregular vaginal bleeding, theca-luteal cysts, asymmetric uterine enlargement, or persistently elevated serum β-hCG levels. The tumor may even perforate the myometrium,

causing intraperitoneal bleeding, or into uterine vessels, causing vaginal hemorrhage. Patients can also present with sepsis and abdominal pain, as the uterine tumor presents a nidus for infection. Placental site tumors present in the same manner as invasive moles tend to be confined to the uterus, and produce small amounts of β-hCG relative for their size.

Metastatic GTT occurs in as many as 19% of patients who have undergone molar evacuation (9). Metastatic GTTs most often arise from choriocarcinoma. Molar pregnancy is the most common antecedent of choriocarcinoma, but this tumor may also occur after normal pregnancy, ectopic pregnancy, or abortion. These highly vascular tumors, which tend to metastasize extensively, may cause spontaneous hemorrhage at the metastatic foci causing symptoms. The metastases are sometimes histologically identical to molar disease, but the vast majority are choriocarcinomas. Metastatic spread is hematogenous. Because of its extensive vascular network, metastatic GTT often produces local spontaneous bleeding. Common metastatic sites of GTT as reported by the New England Trophoblastic Disease Center are summarized in Table 31-3.

Pulmonary metastases are quite common, occurring in 80% of patients with metastatic disease (61), and result when trophoblastic tissue enters the circulation via uterine venous sinuses. Most often this happens spontaneously, but it may also occur after molar evacuation. Because choriocarcinoma is a vascular tumor, hemoptysis is a frequent symptom of lung involvement. Other symptoms include chest pain, dyspnea, and cough.

Pulmonary hypertension and pleural effusions may also develop. An asymptomatic lesion on a chest x-ray or computed tomography (CT) scan may be the only sign of pulmonary involvement (66). Radiologic features may be subtle and include alveolar, nodular, and

TABLE 31-3	COMMON METASTATIC SITES IN ORDER OF FREQUENCY	
Lungs	80%
Vagina	30%
Pelvis	20%
Brain	10%
Liver	10%
Bowel, kidney, spleen	<5%
Other	<5%
Serum*	<5%

*Persistent hCG after hysterectomy.
Data from Berkowitz RS, Goldstein DP. Pathogenesis of gestational trophoblastic neoplasms. Pathol Annu 1981;11:391–411.

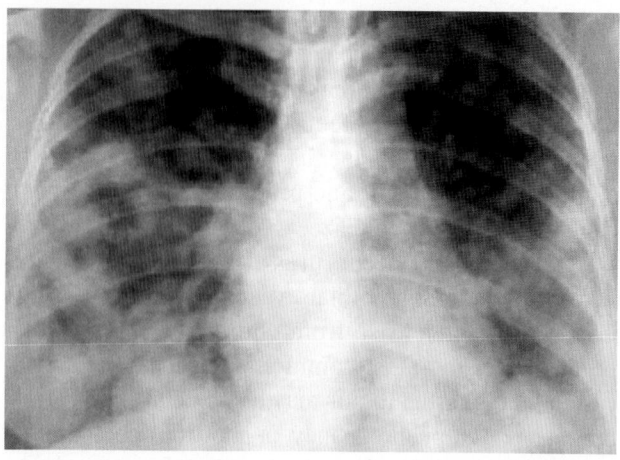

FIGURE 31-4. Chest x-ray and chest CT scan of a patient with metastatic choriocarcinoma. In this case, the patient had refused further treatment and died of the disease.

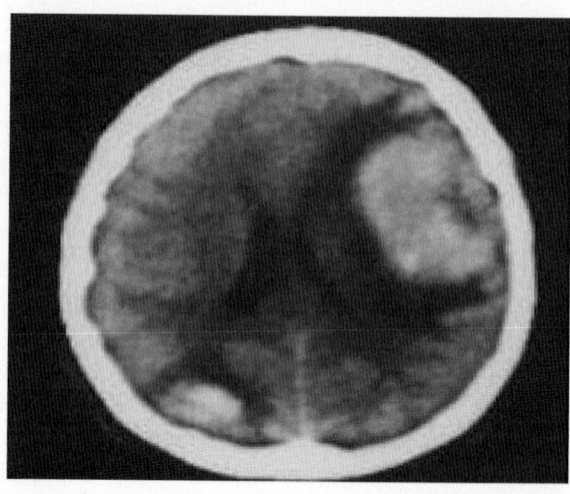

FIGURE 31-5. MRI scan of patient with metastatic choriocarcinoma.

miliary patterns (67). Pulmonary metastases (Fig. 31-4) can be extensive and can cause respiratory failure and death.

Patients may experience right-upper-quadrant pain when hepatic metastases stretch Glisson capsule. Gastrointestinal lesions can result in severe hemorrhage or in perforation with peritonitis, either of which requires emergency intervention. Vaginal examination may reveal bluish metastatic deposits; biopsy of these and other metastatic sites is contraindicated because severe uncontrolled bleeding may occur.

Central nervous system (CNS) involvement from metastatic GTT suggests widespread disease. CNS metastases are clinically evident in 7 to 28% of patients with metastatic choriocarcinoma (61, 68-70). Bakri and colleagues reported that 17% of patients with metastatic GTT in their study had metastases to the brain (71). The presenting neurologic symptoms included headache, hemiparesis, vomiting, dizziness, coma, grand mal seizure, visual disturbances, aphasia, and slurred speech. Cerebral metastases tend to respond favorably to both radiotherapy and chemotherapy (Fig. 31-5).

■ DIAGNOSIS

RADIOLOGIC IMAGING

Radiographic studies are needed to confirm a diagnosis of GTT. Ultrasonography is a reliable and sensitive technique for the confirmation of complete molar pregnancy. It is therefore the first modality of radiographic imaging used when GTT is considered. The ultrasound

may reveal the classic "snowstorm" appearance, which is due to the numerous chorionic villi exhibiting diffuse hydatidiform swelling (72-74) (see Fig. 31-5; Figs. 31-6 and 31-7).

Because 70 to 80% of patients with metastatic GTT have lung involvement, a chest x-ray should be performed in all patients (9,61) (see Fig. 31-4). As 97 to 100% of patients with CNS disease from choriocarcinoma have concomitant pulmonary metastases, a CNS work-up is not routinely warranted for asymptomatic patients with a normal chest x-ray (75).

An abnormal chest x-ray associated with a β-hCG level that plateaus or rises during treatment is an indication for a more thorough evaluation for metastatic disease. CT scans of the brain, abdomen, and pelvis should be performed to evaluate other likely sites of metastatic spread.

At the University of Texas MD Anderson Cancer Center (MDACC), magnetic resonance imaging (MRI) is the preferred modality for localized disease. MRI can be considered the most promising imaging modality to delineate the invasiveness of local disease as well as the tumor's vascularity (Fig. 31-8) (76).

LABORATORY TESTS

The complete blood count usually reveals anemia and thrombocytopenia, clotting times may be prolonged, and consumption of coagulation factors may be unusually high in patients with disseminated intravascular coagulation. Hepatic or renal impairment is sometimes noted but is rare. Thyroid function studies are mandated in patients with a clinical history or physical examination findings suggestive of hyperthyroidism.

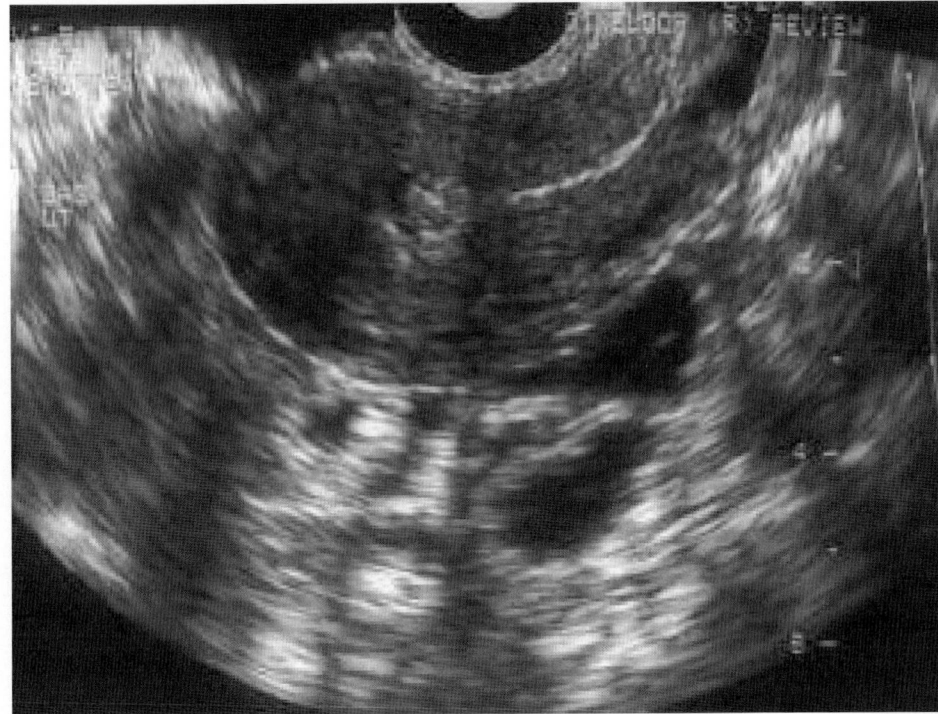

FIGURE 31-6. Ultrasound of a gestational trophoblastic tumor.

Chorionic gonadotropin is glycoprotein hormone secreted by the syncytiotrophoblast: it is essential to maintaining normal function of the corpus luteum during pregnancy (70). This hormone has an alpha subunit identical to the alpha subunit of the pituitary hormones and a beta subunit (β-hCG) that confers the hormone's unique biological activity. The hormone becomes detectable 8 days after ovulation; its level doubles every 2 to 4 days, reaching its peak at 10 to 12 weeks of gestation. After that, the β-hCG level declines steadily. All trophoblastic tumors secrete β-hCG; thus its level serves as an excellent marker for tumor activity in the nonpregnant patient (77-80). The urine pregnancy test is not considered adequate for detecting GTTs, although it is sometimes used to confirm a positive blood test.

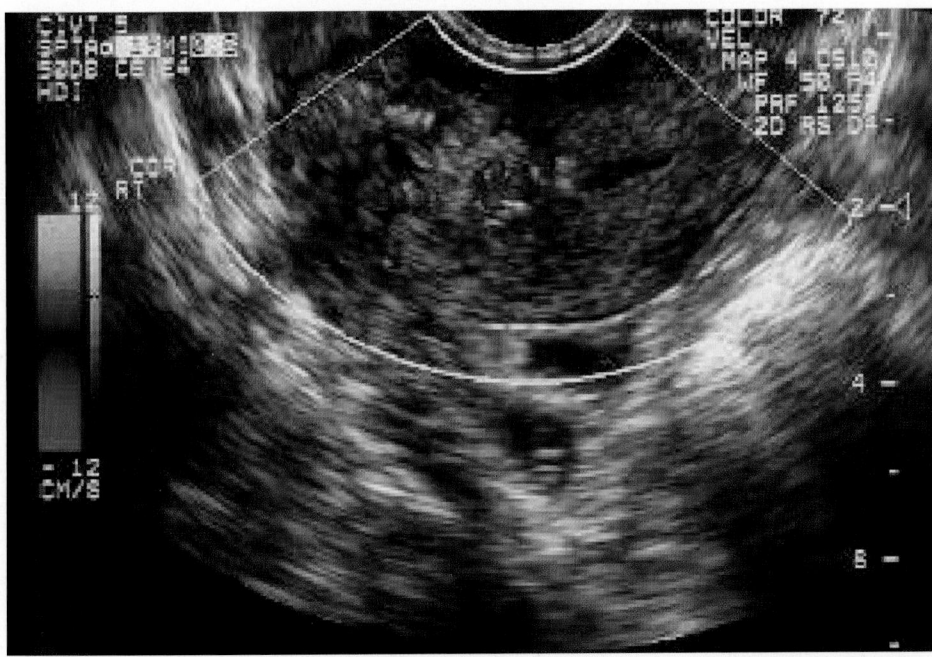

FIGURE 31-7. Doppler ultrasound of a gestational trophoblastic tumor.

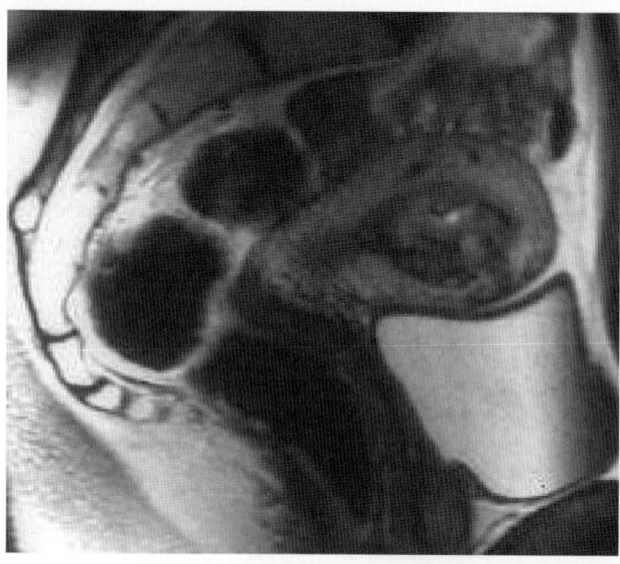

FIGURE 31-8. MRI scan of a gestational trophoblastic tumor.

Monitoring of the serial β-hCG levels is mandatory during therapy for GTTs to ensure adequate treatment. The level of β-hCG can be considered approximately proportional to the tumor burden and inversely proportional to therapeutic outcome. The 10 to 20% of patients with hydatidiform mole who are not cured by local therapy or do not achieve a spontaneous remission can be identified by a rising or plateaued β-hCG titer on serial determinations after evacuation of a mole. These patients may have persistent trophoblastic disease and therefore require additional therapy.

At one time, the ratio of β-hCG in serum to that in cerebrospinal fluid (CSF) was used to detect brain metastases in GTT. A serum:CSF β-hCG ratio of less than 60:1 is considered a positive predictor for brain metastases (75). Bagshawe and Harland reported that 29 of 33 of their patients who had CT-documented GTT brain involvement also had a positive serum:CSF β-hCG ratio (81). With the availability of MRI, this test is rarely used. CA125 may also have a role as a marker for GTT. In at least one study of patients with hydatidiform mole, the CA-125 level was elevated; more significant was the association of the degree of CA-125 elevation with the development of persistent GTT (80).

■ **PHANTOM hCG SYNDROME**

Phantom hCG or phantom choriocarcinoma syndrome is also called pseudohypergonadotropinemia. It refers to persistent mild elevation of hCG when no true hCG or trophoblastic tissue is present. This may result in the patient being treated further by her physician during the follow-up period either after primary surgery for molar pregnancy or chemotherapy for metastatic disease. It is mentioned here because clinicians may encounter this problem during the follow-up period and should rule out this syndrome before deciding to label a patient as having persistent disease.

hCG is a glycoprotein whose two subunits, alpha and beta, are held together by charge and hydrophobic interactions. Over 40 different professional laboratory tests are available for assaying the level of serum hCG. Most of these work through the multiantibody "sandwich assay," using the labeled-enzyme or chemoimmunoassay (RIA) method developed in the 1950s. The mechanism by which heterophilic antibodies cause false-positive results relates to the nature of this immunometric assay. One antibody, commonly a mouse monoclonal immunoglobulin (IgG), immobilizes hCG by binding one site on the molecule; a second antibody, commonly a polyclonal antibody labeled with an enzyme or chemiluminescent agent, marks the first antibody. Heterophilic antibodies usually bind the assay of IgG at sites common to humans and other species. They are bivalent and therefore link the capture and tracer antibodies, mimicking hCG immunoactivity. Binding of human antibodies to mouse IgG is the most common form of interference. The positivity of this test, however, is not correlated with positivity in the urine. Therefore a simple urine hCG test can support or refute a phantom hCG test result. If both the urine test and the serum test results are positive, searching for occult disease is prudent. If the urine test is negative, assuming that no clear radiologic sites of disease are identified, different assay systems can then be used to confirm the first serum result (82). It is recommended that the serum be tested by a reference laboratory in these cases.

Phantom hCG reemphasizes the clinical dilemma that arises when patient care is based primarily on laboratory data. It is the clinician's responsibility to interpret test results with caution. Unfortunately, the prevalence of false-positive hCG results is not known. In one series of healthy individuals, it has been found to be 3.4% (83).

■ **STAGING AND PROGNOSIS**

There are many staging and prognosticating systems in GTT. All are attempts to define prognostic groups that can direct a rational therapeutic strategy aiming at the highest possible cure rate. For patients with nonmetastatic disease, the staging system of the International Federation of Gynecology and Obstetrics (FIGO) is used (Table 31-4). For patients with metastatic disease, the

TABLE 31-4	FIGO STAGING OF GESTATIONAL TROPHOBLASTIC TUMORS

Stage I: GTT confined to the uterus

Stage IA	Disease confined to the uterus with no risk factors
Stage IB	Disease confined to the uterus with one risk factor
Stage IC	Disease confined to the uterus with two risk factors

Stage II: GTT extends outside the uterus but is limited to the genital structures (ovary, tube, vagina, broad ligament)

Stage IIA	Disease involving genital structures without risk factors
Stage IIB	Disease extends outside the uterus but is limited to the genital structures with one risk factor
Stage IIC	Disease extents outside of the uterus but is limited to the genital structures with two risk factors

Stage III: GTT extends to the lungs with or without known genital tract involvement

Stage IIIA	Disease extends to the lungs with or without known genital tract involvement and no risk factors
Stage IIIB	Disease extends to the lungs with or without known genital tract involvement with one risk factor
Stage IIIC	Disease extends to the lungs with or without known genital tract involvement with two risk factors

Stage IV: All other metastatic sites

Stage IVA	All other metastatic sites without risk factors
Stage IVB	All other metastatic sites with one risk factor
Stage IVC	All other metastatic sites with two risk factors

risk stratification is defined by FIGO 2000 criteria, which were adapted from the World Health Organization (WHO) scoring system, shown in Table 31-5 (84).

■ MANAGEMENT

A large proportion of women who have been treated for a GTT retain reasonable fertility with no long-term sequelae in the offspring. Each patient is considered individually and treated by a multidisciplinary team. Figure 31-9 succinctly outlines the general diagnostic and therapeutic approaches used at MDACC.

MOLAR PREGNANCY

Hydatidiform mole is 100% curable. The treatment is mainly surgical (85,86), but optimal management is dependent on the desire to preserve reproductive capability. All patients are evaluated for any medical condition

TABLE 31-5	FIGO 2000 PROGNOSTIC SCORING FOR GESTATIONAL TROPHOBLASTIC DISEASE

FIGO (WHO) Risk Factor Scoring With FIGO Staging	*0*	*1*	*2*	*4*
Age (year)	<40	≥40		
Antecedent pregnancy	Hydatidiform mole	Abortion	Term	
Interval months from index pregnancy	<4	4-6	7-12	>12
Pretreatment in hCG mIU/ml	$<10^3$	10^3-10^4	10^4-10^5	$>10^5$
Largest tumor size including uterus	3-4 cm	≥5 cm		
Site of metastases including uterus		Spleen, kidney	Gastrointestinal tract	Brain, liver
Number of metastases identified	0	1-4	5-8	>8
Previous failed chemotherapy			Single drug	Two or more drugs

Low risk ≤6, High risk ≥7.

This combination of the modified WHO risk factor scoring system with the FIGO Cancer Staging and Nomenclature Committee in September 2000 and ratified in June 2002 with the FIGO announcement.

Source: Kohorn, E.I. (2001), The new FIGO 2000 staging and risk factor scoring system for gestational trophoblastic disease: Description and critical assessment. *International Journal of Gynecological Cancer*, 11:73-77. doi: 10.1046/j.1525-1438.2001.011001073.x.

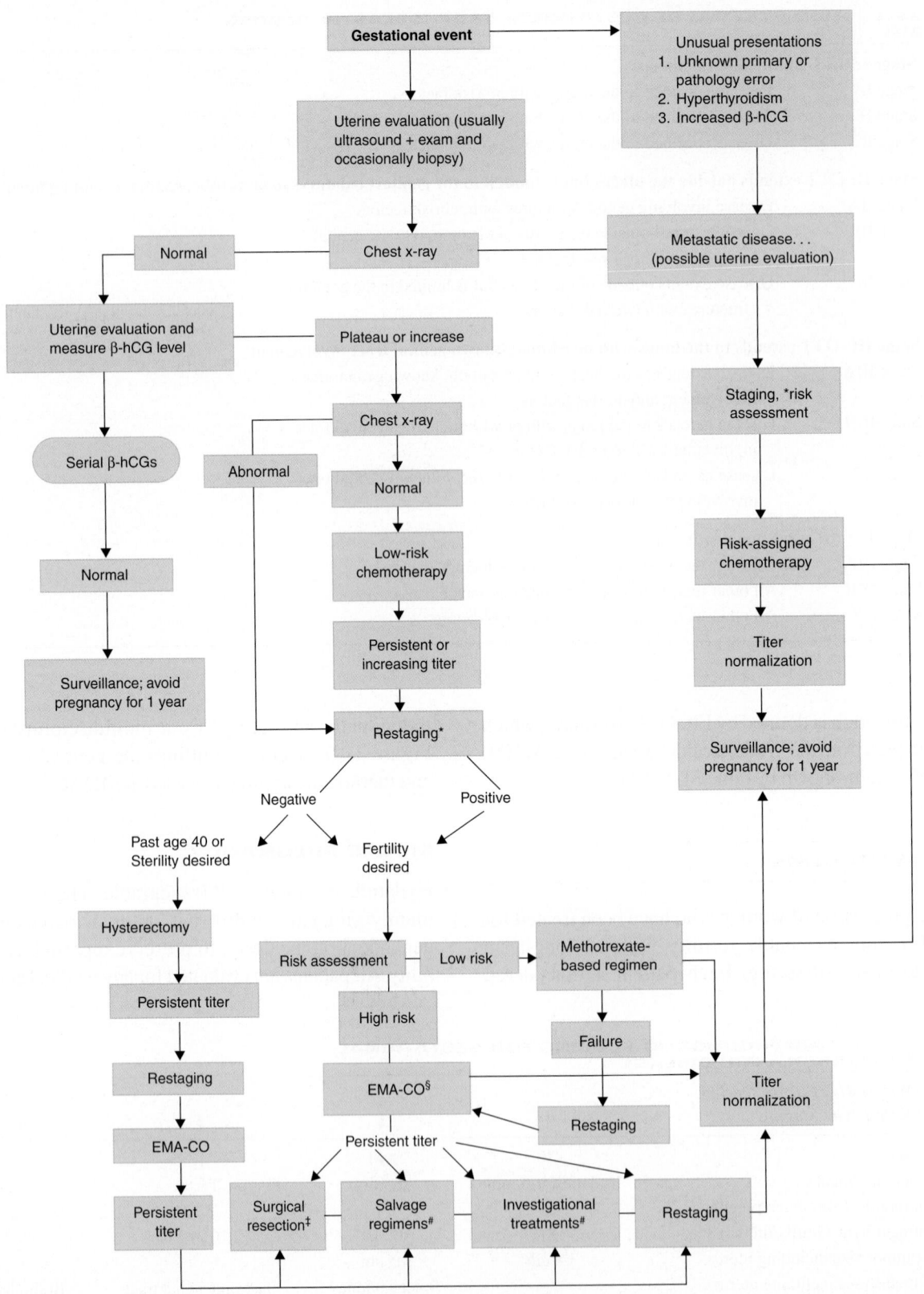

FIGURE 31-9. Management algorithm for gestational trophoblastic disease. β-hCG, beta–human chorionic gonadotropin; EMA-CO, etoposide/methotrexate/Adriamycin (dactinomycin)/cyclophosphamide/vincristine. *Includes radiologic evaluation of brain, liver, kidney, and lungs (MRI of brain preferred). †β-hCG titers every month for 1 year, then every 4 months for 1 year, and then every 12 months for 2 years. ‡Of prior or suspected disease sites, including uterus. #No other active sites on radiologic restaging. §No prior EMA-CO.

secondary to the mole and treated appropriately before surgery. If a patient has completed her family and does not wish to retain the ability to conceive, a hysterectomy is performed with the mole in situ. In younger patients who wish to retain reproductive ability, the ovaries are preserved even if theca-luteal cysts are present. These patients should be counseled with regard to the possibility of another molar pregnancy and of malignant transformation (65).

Primary Treatment

Should the decision be made to retain the uterus, treatment comprises suction and curettage (85). Depending on the trophoblastic elements, the amount of bleeding can vary widely. Oxytocin is often infused immediately prior to surgery to limit the volume of blood lost, although caution is necessary in patients with medical complications because of the concerns with hyponatremia and fluid overload associated with the infusion (87). Specimens from surgery are sent for pathologic evaluation.

Postsurgical Care

After primary surgical treatment, all patients undergo weekly serum β-hCG tests until the level returns to normal on three consecutive assays (ie, three consecutive weeks). Three consecutive normal β-hCG levels define complete remission.

Urine pregnancy tests alone are considered inadequate for monitoring. The level of β-hCG typically normalizes within 8 weeks, but this may take up to 14 to 16 weeks in 20% of patients. Once the β-hCG level has normalized, it should be checked monthly for 12 months, every 4 months for the following year, and then yearly for 2 years. Eighty percent of patients need no further treatment (3,4,32). The other 20%, who will go on to develop a malignant sequelae, will be treated as appropriate for their status as either low- or high-risk patients as defined by the FIGO 2000 criteria (see Table 31-5). They would no longer be considered as having molar pregnancies but as malignant GTTs. These patients are identified through the following events:

- Rising β-hCG level for 2 weeks measured over three separate intervals
- Tissue diagnosis of choriocarcinoma
- Failure to reach normal serum titers of β-hCG
- Evidence of metastatic disease
- Elevation of β-hCG level after a normal result
- Postevacuation bleeding not due to retained tissues

Patients who receive treatment for molar pregnancy are encouraged to use effective contraception with hormonal or barrier methods during the entire interval of β-hCG follow-up. Intrauterine devices are not used because of the potential for uterine perforation. At MDACC, patients are advised to avoid pregnancy for at least 1 year. Subsequent pregnancy is discussed later under the section Future Childbearing.

Prophylactic Chemotherapy

Administration of prophylactic adjuvant chemotherapy after molar evacuation still cannot be considered routine. Although a short course of dactinomycin and methotrexate after molar evacuation has reduced the incidence of persistent or recurrent disease in patients at high risk, the same benefit has not been proven for patients at low risk. In 1965, a prospective study was conducted of the use of chemotherapy at the time of molar evacuation (88). Of the three schedules evaluated, the one comprising dactinomycin, given intravenously for 5 days starting 3 days prior to molar evacuation, was found to be optimal in effectiveness and toxicity. Goldstein randomized 200 patients to receive the same regimen or observation at the time of molar evacuation (89). He found no cases of metastatic trophoblastic disease in the treated group, while there were four cases among those who did not receive treatment. Nevertheless, the disease remained treatable at progression, indicating that prophylactic chemotherapy yielded no overall survival benefit.

Kim et al., in their study of 71 patients, found that adjuvant chemotherapy significantly reduced the incidence of persistent molar disease in high-risk patients from 47 to 14% (90). Among low-risk patients, however, more courses of adjuvant chemotherapy were required to produce a complete response in the group receiving chemotherapy compared to those who had not had adjuvant chemotherapy. This implied that the chemotherapy may have induced tumor resistance (90). The only role for adjuvant chemotherapy, therefore, seems to be in patients whose ability to be compliant in follow-up is doubtful.

A small minority of patients who have undergone removal of a complete hydatidiform mole may develop the unusual complication of intermediate trophoblastic disease (35). They usually present with vaginal bleeding and a slightly elevated β-hCG titer. Examination of the uterus may reveal multiple nodules involving the endometrium and myometrium. Surgical intervention is warranted as progressive disease tends to develop, and the disease does not readily respond to chemotherapy.

PLACENTAL-SITE TUMOR

Originally known as trophoblastic pseudotumor, these tumors have been retermed placental-site trophoblastic tumor to better reflect their malignant potential. These tumors present with metastases in about 10% of cases (91) and an additional 10% of patients develop metastases during the follow-up interval (65). Hysterectomy is the preferred treatment for nonmetastatic disease, which is highly curable. A small number of patients, however, require chemotherapy and/or radiation. These patients are usually those who present with metastatic disease or recurrent disease not amenable to surgery. Combination chemotherapy regimens with etoposide, methotrexate, actinomycin, cyclophosphamide, and Oncovin (vincristine) (EMA-CO) and combination chemotherapy with etoposide, methotrexate, actinomycin, and cisplatin (EMA-EP) are the most useful (92-94). For patients whose tumors do not respond, radiation can be useful for palliation. Unfortunately, this rare tumor rarely produces β-hCG, so the serum β-hCG level is typically not helpful in diagnosis, treatment, or follow-up (95). Some patients who have had surgery may require immediate chemotherapy, typically those with any of the following risk factors: metastatic disease, time from antecedent pregnancy greater than 2 years, or tumor mitotic index greater than 5 mitoses per 10 high-power fields. The chemotherapy of choice is EMA-EP (96).

MALIGNANT GESTATIONAL TROPHOBLASTIC TUMOR

For malignant GTTs, the treatment depends on the cell type, stage, level of serum β-hCG, duration of the disease, specific sites of metastases, and extent of prior treatment.

Nonmetastatic Tumors

For patients who do not wish to preserve fertility, hysterectomy is the treatment of choice. Prophylactic single-agent chemotherapy may be considered but is not routine. The rationale behind chemotherapy is to reduce the likelihood of disseminating viable tumor cells at surgery and during the immediate postoperative period as well as to eliminate any occult metastases. Notably, however, the benefit of such practice is controversial on the basis of clinical trial data. For patients wishing to retain fertility, chemotherapy is offered as primary treatment for low-risk disease. The first choice at MDACC is a combination of methotrexate and folinic acid. Other chemotherapy regimens are listed in Table 31-6.

Persistent elevation or increase in titer of β-hCG mandates restaging. If the tumor is still limited to the uterus and the patient is older than 40 years and/or has no wish to retain fertility, hysterectomy is offered. If the patient prefers to retain fertility and belongs to the low-risk category, she can be treated with other combination chemotherapy. Despite a high rate of resistance to first-line chemotherapy, a cure rate of almost 100% is achieved with combination chemotherapy. In the rare instances of tumor resistance to combination chemotherapy in a patient who wishes to retain fertility, localized resection should be offered after careful evaluation by perioperative MRI, ultrasonography, and/or arteriography.

Metastatic Tumors

More than 50 years ago, metastatic gestational trophoblastic disease was not curable. Since that time, treatments have improved such that the cure rate of these tumors now exceeds 90% (5). This success is the result of a combination of factors:

- The discovery that these tumors are chemosensitive
- Our ability to diagnose and monitor therapy by using β-hCG levels
- Identification of prognostic factors

TABLE 31-6	CHEMOTHERAPY REGIMES FOR LOW-RISK* GESTATIONAL TROPHOBLASTIC DISEASE	
Drug	*Administration*	*Cycle*†
Methotrexate and folinic acid	1 mg/kg (up to 70 mg) IM or IV days 1, 3, 5, 7 0.1 mg/kg IM or IV days 2, 4, 6, 8	14 days
Methotrexate	0.4 mg/kg IM or IV daily for 5 days	14 days
Methotrexate	30 to 50 mg/m² IM	7 days
Dactinomycin	10 µg/kg (max 0.5 mg) IV daily for 5 days	14 days
Dactinomycin	1.25 mg/m²	14 days

*Therapy based on WHO risk criteria in Table 31-5.
†Withhold treatment for marrow recovery if necessary.

- Use of combination therapy
- Referral of these patients to specialized centers for treatment

Low-Risk Disease

Patients with metastatic low-risk disease as determined by the WHO prognostic scoring system have a high potential for cure with chemotherapy alone (89). The first choice at MDACC is a combination of methotrexate and folinic acid. This combination induces remission in 90% of patients with low-risk disease, with little short- or long-term toxicity (95-97). Other regimens that are used at MDACC are listed in Table 31-6. In patients for whom single-agent therapy with methotrexate or dactinomycin fails to achieve remission, cure can still be attained with other regimens. Approximately 40% of patients fall into this category (95).

Patients in whom treatment does not produce a complete response may have undetected metastatic disease. Mutch et al. reported that at least 40% of patients with a negative chest radiograph result will have a positive chest CT scan and may be at higher risk of resistance to single-agent therapy (66).

Patients should be treated for two to three courses after attaining serologic remission (ie, normal β-hCG level). The very rare patient who does not attain serologic remission, or in whom β-hCG level raises after reaching a normal value, is restaged and stratified again according to the findings of the second restaging. At this time, it is prudent to check with the laboratory to make sure that the rising β-hCG level is not a result of phantom hCG syndrome. In the event of confirmed persistent GTT, either experimental therapy or salvage chemotherapy is given. Salvage chemotherapy is discussed in the section below.

High-Risk Disease

High-risk disease is not likely to be cured by single-agent chemotherapy and patients with high-risk disease are at the highest risk of treatment failure. These patients should be treated with combination chemotherapy (5). The most widely employed regimen includes MAC (methotrexate, dactinomycin, and cyclophosphamide or chlorambucil, EMA-CO) (Table 31-7) (98).

The MAC combination has produced cure rates ranging from 63 to 80% (99-102). In intermediate- to high-risk GTT, MAC is most effective when used as initial chemotherapy (65% survival), rather than second-line treatment (39% survival) following failed single-agent therapy (100).

An older regimen, CHAMOCA (cyclophosphamide, hydroxyurea, actinomycin D [dactinomycin], methotrexate with leucovorin rescue, Oncovin [vincristine], cyclophosphamide, and Adriamycin [doxorubicin]), has been associated with a remission rate of 82% (98) in a Gynecologic Oncology Group trial published in 1989; however, CHAMOCA was inferior to MAC in terms of toxicity and efficacy (103).

TABLE 31-7	CHEMOTHERAPY REGIMES FOR INTERMEDIATE- AND HIGH-RISK* GESTATIONAL TROPHOBLASTIC DISEASE	
Drug Regimen		*Administration*
EMA-CO[†] (preferred regimen)		
Course I (EMA)		
Day 1	Etoposide	100 mg/m^2 IV over 30 min
	Methotrexate	100 mg/m^2 IV bolus
	Methotrexate[‡]	200 mg/m^2 IV as 12-h continuous infusion
	Dactinomycin	0.5 mg IV bolus
Day 2	Etoposide	100 mg/m^2 IV over 30 min
	Folinic acid	15 mg IV/IM/PO every 6 h for four doses, beginning 24 h after start of methotrexate
	Dactinomycin	0.5 mg IV bolus
Course II (CO)		
Day 8	Cyclophosphamide	600 mg/m^2 IV over 30 min
	Vincristine	1 mg/m^2 (up to 2 mg) IV bolus

*Therapy based on the WHO risk criteria (see Table 31-5).
[†]Repeat each regimen in sequence every 14 days as toxicity permits.
[‡]In case of CNS metastases, the dose of infused methotrexate is increased to 1000 mg/m^2 IV over 12 h after alkalinization of the urine. Increase the number of folinic acid doses to eight given every 6 h. This regimen is called "high-dose methotrexate EMA-CO."

Etoposide became known early on as an effective agent against trophoblastic disease; this led to development of the EMA-CO regimen by Bagshawe. He reported a survival rate of 83% in patients with high-risk choriocarcinoma (104). Berkowitz et al. (102) and Bower et al. (105) separately corroborated the high degree of effectiveness of this regimen. To date, many different groups have confirmed its efficacy (106,107). At MDACC, EMA-CO is therefore the preferred regimen for high-risk GTT. It is generally well tolerated, with no life-threatening toxic effects. Although originally developed for high-risk disease, it is also the regime of choice for intermediate-risk disease at MDACC. Toxic effects include alopecia, and mild anemia, neutropenia, and stomatitis. Reproductive function is preserved in 75% of patients. In patients with significant tumor volume, extreme care is taken to look out for complications of rapid tumor necrosis, which may lead to hemorrhage. Twenty-five percent of patients with high-risk disease do not attain complete remission. If this occurs, salvage chemotherapy is administered.

Metastases Requiring Special Care

Pulmonary Metastases

Pulmonary metastases can be extensive and may cause respiratory failure and death (108). Some factors that may predict early death from respiratory compromise include cyanosis, pulmonary hypertension, anemia, tachycardia, extensive lung opacification, and a high WHO prognostic score (109). Bakri et al. studied 75 patients with pulmonary metastases and found that factors such as dyspnea, anemia, clinical pulmonary hypertension, cyanosis, more than 50% lung opacification, mediastinal involvement, and bilateral pleural effusion were associated with poorer outcome (110). Patients with extensive lung opacification (particularly when associated with anemia), pulmonary hypertension, or cyanosis were at risk for respiratory failure. In such patients with extensive pulmonary metastases, reduced doses of initial chemotherapy have been suggested to abate the risk of respiratory failure, although this strategy does not seem to protect completely against pulmonary failure and death (109-111).

CNS Choriocarcinoma

Like pulmonary metastases, CNS metastases pose a significant threat to patients with GTT. Although clinically apparent in only 7 to 28% of patients with choriocarcinoma (68-70,81), CNS involvement is found in as many as 40% of patients on postmortem examination (112). Multimodality therapy for this group of patients seems to be the optimal treatment. Weed and Hammond reported a survival rate of 50% disease-free intervals of 12 to 120 months in patients with CNS involvement by choriocarcinoma who received multimodality therapy (113).

Athanassiou et al. reported that 8.8% of their 782 patients had CNS metastases (75). The overall survival rate of patients who had CNS metastases at the outset was 80%, while the overall survival of patients who developed CNS metastases after initial diagnosis and treatment was only 25%. The authors concluded that the outcome was likely improved by CNS prophylaxis. Ayhan et al. reached the same conclusions in 1996 (114). Around the same time, Evans et al. reported 42 patients with CNS metastases. They also concluded that patients who developed CNS metastases during active treatment had a poorer survival than those who had brain metastases at the beginning (115). Gillespie et al. reported 69 patients with lung metastases who might have had CNS metastases at the outset and concluded that, without evidence of CNS metastases, CNS prophylaxis is not required (116). We support his conclusion.

Yordan et al. reported a retrospective analysis of 70 cases of GTT involving the CNS (117). Of the 70 patients, half died before therapy was initiated. Of the remaining patients, 24% of those given chemotherapy alone survived, and 50% of patients given concurrent chemotherapy plus whole-brain irradiation achieved long-term remission. In the chemotherapy-plus-radiation group, none of the deaths was attributed to CNS disease. For patients with CNS metastases at presentation, we advocate aggressive treatment with combination chemotherapy after stabilizing the brain metastases. The need for primary treatment of the brain prior to chemotherapy is related to the high chance of tumor hemorrhage, which may further compromise a patient's long-term outcome. Primary treatment should be either surgical resection for solitary metastasis or radiotherapy. Surgical decompression should be considered for patients who have symptoms of raised intracranial pressure (118,119).

A slightly higher dose of radiation given at 3000 cGy seemed to yield a better overall cure rate compared to less than 2500 cGy. Yordan et al. therefore concluded that at the time of diagnosis of CNS disease, irradiation of the brain with 3000 cGy given over 10 fractions should be initiated simultaneously with the start of chemotherapy. Schechter et al. also showed that patients who received a total dose of greater than 2200 cGy achieved a 91% local control rate, while those who received less than 2200 cGY achieved a lower control rate of 24% (120).

PATIENTS IN FIRST REMISSION

Patients who are in first remission and are thought to have a high risk of recurrence are observed closely with serum β-hCG levels and posttherapy baseline radiologic imaging. For a patient who has had lung metastases, a repeat high-resolution CT scan at the end of chemotherapy serves as a baseline for follow-up. Many patients who have had lung metastases have residual nodules in the lung field on CT scans or chest x-ray, signifying fibrous scar tissue. For a patient who has had brain metastases, an MRI of the head would be obtained. Likewise, for a patient who has had liver metastases, a CT scan of the liver would be obtained. If the uterus is in place and was a site of previous disease, consideration is also given to baseline MRI of the uterus. The rationale is that modest increases in the β-hCG level, signifying relapse, may be accompanied by subtle changes in "sterile" lesions noted on earlier images. This finding raises the issue of surgical resection of a chemotherapy-resistant site. If the imaging obtained after chemotherapy reveals suspicious nodules or masses and the β-hCG level is normal, a baseline positron emission tomography (PET) scan is sometimes obtained to serve as a baseline. If the β-hCG level rises during follow-up, this PET scan would be helpful in identifying active disease.

SALVAGE THERAPY

Approximately one-quarter of patients with high-risk metastatic disease do not achieve complete remission when treated with EMA-CO. These patients require salvage therapy. Unfortunately, a standard salvage regimen has not yet been defined for these patients. The essential strategy is identification of chemotherapy-resistant sites for possible surgical resection and salvage chemotherapy. Patients who are not amenable to surgery would require platinum-containing chemotherapy regimens (5,121,122).

In the past, numerous regimens have been administered at MDACC, including combinations of cisplatin, etoposide, vinca alkaloids, and bleomycin. Because of their significant nephrotoxicity, cisplatin-containing regimens are withheld as primary therapy. In salvage therapy, cisplatin serves as a very effective element of combination regimes. Cisplatin in combination with vincristine and methotrexate achieved a 33% response rate as salvage therapy (123). At MDACC, Gordon et al. reported a sustained remission rate of 20% in 10 patients treated with cisplatin, vinblastine, and bleomycin (PVB) (124). The dose-intensive regimen EMA-EP utilizing cisplatin (100 mg/m^2) and etoposide (200 mg/m^2) in combination with EMA has also been tested with favorable results (125), as has the PEBA regimen (cisplatin, etoposide, bleomycin, Adriamycin) in China (126). Ninety-six percent of patients whose disease was refractory to EMA-CO achieve complete remission. Seventy-three percent had a sustained complete response that lasted at least 1 year. In a small study, ifosfamide alone and in combination with etoposide and cisplatin (VIP) showed promise as an effective salvage drug in GTT (127). Lotz et al. treated five women who had refractory GTT with high-dose ifosfamide, carboplatin, and etoposide (ICE) (128). Only one of these women attained a durable complete response (68+ months). The risks and benefits of high-dose chemotherapy in the treatment of GTT are still under investigation. Combinations of bleomycin and ifosfamide have also been used with efficacy (127,129,130).

■ COEXISTING GESTATIONAL TROPHOBLASTIC TUMORS AND NORMAL PREGNANCY

GTTs have been known to coexist, although, very rarely, with normal intrauterine pregnancy (131). This entity has been described in the context of both spontaneous and in vitro fertilization (IVF) gestations. GTTs in such cases have been either molar pregnancy or malignant neoplasm. The estimated incidence of twin pregnancies consisting of a molar pregnancy and a normal fetus is 1 per 22,000 to 100,000 pregnancies (65). This incidence may increase with the increase in the number of pregnancies involving assisted fertility. A patient with this rare condition poses a therapeutic dilemma. At MDACC, all such patients go through thoughtful and careful evaluation which judges the threat of the disease to the mother and child. This is especially so in patients with paraneoplastic endocrine and hematologic emergencies. In many cases, the actual diagnosis can be made only after a therapeutic abortion. The decision on any therapy is made only after consultation with the patient, a perinatologist, and a gynecologic oncologist. This is especially true in the rare case of metastatic malignant GTT with normal pregnancy.

■ FUTURE CHILDBEARING

Women who have undergone effective treatment for molar pregnancy have a risk of future molar pregnancy of 1 to 2%. Strict contraception is required during the surveillance period because pregnancy would obviate the usefulness of β-hCG as a tumor marker. Patients are advised to use effective hormonal or barrier contraception. Intrauterine devices are not employed as contraception for patients with intact uteri in view of concerns over uterine perforation. In general, once a 12-month surveillance establishes disease-free status, conception is acceptable, although these women are always at high risk for future molar disease and will require close observation during future pregnancies (132). Standard chemotherapy seems to have minimal impact on patients' subsequent ability to reproduce, and most patients are able to carry a pregnancy to term successfully, with a live birth (133). These women seem to have no increase in adverse events such as first- or second-trimester abortions or stillbirths, prematurity, or need for cesarean section. Similarly, their offsprings have no increased risk of anomalies. Nevertheless, patients at MDACC are monitored closely throughout any subsequent pregnancy, especially in the first trimester. A pelvic ultrasound examination should be performed during any subsequent pregnancies to confirm that gestation is normal (116). Patients who have difficulty with conception are considered for fertility treatment, although these patients are at increased risk of repeat molar pregnancy. These patients will be advised accordingly and presented with options for implantation with fertilized donor oocytes.

■ CONCLUSION

Gestational trophoblastic tumors (GTTs) comprise a wide spectrum of neoplastic disorders that arise from placental trophoblastic tissue after abnormal fertilization. Patients are classified into different prognostic groups on the basis of factors such as tumor histologic subtype, extent of disease, human gonadotropin titer, duration of disease, nature of the antecedent pregnancy, and extent of prior treatment. The probability of cure depends on the group designated. All patients should receive individualized management after careful prognostication under the care of a multidisciplinary team. GTT patients are followed long term with regular laboratory tests of complete blood count and β-hCG. Patients are counseled regarding the higher risk of leukemia in patients treated with combination chemotherapy with etoposide. GTT survivors are also followed up with management of any psychosocial problems that may be associated with GTTs and their treatment.

References

1. World Health Organization Scientific Group. *Gestational Trophoblastic Disease. Technical Report Series No 692.* Geneva: World Health Organization; 1983.
2. Shih LM, Mazur M, Kurman RJ. Gestational Trophoblastic disease and related lesions. In: Kurman RJ (ed): *Blaustein's Pathology of the Female Genital Tract.* New York: Springer; 2002;1193-1247.
3. Lurain JR, Brewer JI, Torok EE, et al. Natural history of hydatidiform mole after primary evacuation. *Am J Obstet Gynecol* 1983;145:591-595.
4. Miller JM, Surwit EA, Hammond CB. Choriocarcinoma following term pregnancy. *Obstet Gynecol* 1979;53:207-212.
5. Lurain JR. Advances in management of high-risk gestational trophoblastic tumors. *J Reprod Med* 2002;47(6):451-459.
6. Goldstein DP. Worldwide controversies in gestational trophoblastic neoplasms. *Int J Gynaecol Obstet* 1977;15:207-215.
7. Hayashi K, Bracken MB, Freeman DH, et al. Hydatidiform mole in the United States (1970-1977): A statistical and theoretical analysis. *Am J Epidemiol* 1982;115:67-77.
8. Buckley JD. The epidemiology of molar pregnancy and choriocarcinoma. *Clin Obstet Gynecol* 1984;27:153-159.
9. Page RD, Kudelka AP, Freedman RS, et al. Gestational trophoblastic tumors. In: Pazdur R (ed): *Medical Oncology, A Comprehensive Review.* Huntington: PRR; 1995:377-391.
10. Bagshawe KD, Golding PR, Off AM. Choriocarcinoma after hydatidiform mole: Studies related to the effectiveness of follow-up practice after hydatidiform mole. *BMJ* 1969;2:733-737.
11. Mazur MT, Kurman RJ. Choriocarcinoma and placental site trophoblastic tumor. In: Szulman AE, Buchsbaum HJ (eds): *Gestational Trophoblastic Disease.* New York: Springer-Verlag; 1987;45-68.
12. Wei PY, Ouyang PC. Trophoblastic diseases in Taiwan. *Am J Obstet Gynecol* 1963;85:844-849.
13. Martin PM. High frequency of hydatidiform mole in native Alaskans. *Int J Gynaecol Obstet* 1978;15:395-396.
14. Matsuura J, Chui D, Jacobs PA, et al. Complete hydatidiform mole in Hawaii: An epidemiological study. *Genet Epidemiol* 1984;1(3):271-284.
15. Smith HO, Hilgers RD, Bedrick EJ, et al. Ethnic differences at risk for gestational trophoblastic disease in New Mexico: A 25-year population based study. *Am J Obstet Gynecol* 2003;188(2):357-366.
16. Graham IH, Fajardo AM. The incidence and morphology of hydatidiform mole in Abu Dhabi, United Arab Emirates. *Br J Obstet Gynaecol* 1988;95:391-392.
17. Joint project for the study of choriocarcinoma and hydatidiform mole in Asia. Geographic variation in the occurrence of hydatidiform mole and choriocarcinoma. *Ann N Y Acad Sci* 1959;80:174-196.
18. Parazinni F, LaVecchia C, Mangili G, et al. Dietary factors and risk of trophoblastic disease. *Am J Obstet Gynecol* 1988;158:93.
19. Berkowitz RS, Cramer DW, Bernstein MR, et al. Risk factors for complete molar pregnancy from a case-control study. *Am J Obstet Gynecol* 1985;152:1016-1020.
20. Bagshawe KD, Dent J, Webb J. Hydatidiform mole in England and Wales, 1973—1983. *Lancet* 1986;11:673-677.

21. Teoh ES, Dagwood MY, Ratnam SS. Epidemiology of hyda-tidiform mole in Singapore. *Am J Obstet Gynecol* 1971;110: 415-420.

22. Berkowitz RS, Bernstein MR, Laborde O, et al. Subsequent pregnancy experience with gestational trophoblastic disease: New England Trophoblastic Disease Center, 1965-1992. *J Re-prod Med* 1994;39:228-232.

23. Acosta-Sison H. Statistical study of chorioepithelioma in the Philippine General Hospital. *Am J Obstet Gynecol* 1949; 58:125.

24. Bertini B. Epidemiology of hydatidiform mole in Israel: A study based on 113 patients. *Int J Gynaecol Obstet* 1973;11:55.

25. Bagshawe KD, Rawlings G, Pike MC, et al. The ABO group in trophoblastic neoplasia. *Lancet* 1971;1:553-555.

26. Szulman AE, Surti U. The syndromes of hydatidiform mole: I. Cytogenic and morphologic correlations. *Am J Obstet Gynecol* 1978;131:665-671.

27. Szulman AE, Surti U. The syndromes of hydatidiform mole: II. Morphologic evolution of the complete and partial mole. *Am J Obstet Gynecol* 1978;132:20-27.

28. Driscoll SG. Trophoblastic growths: Morphologic aspects and taxonomy. *J Reprod Med* 1981;26(4):181-191.

29. Morrow CP. Postmolar trophoblastic disease: Diagnosis, man-agement, and prognosis. *Clin Obstet Gynecol* 1984;27:211-220.

30. Lurain JR, Brewer JI. Invasive mole. *Semin Oncol* 1982; 9:174-180.

31. Kurman RJ, Main CS, Chen HC. Intermediate trophoblast: A distinctive form of trophoblast with specific morphological, biochemical, and functional features. *Placenta* 1984;5:349-370.

32. Silva EG, Tomos C, Lage J, et al. Multiple nodules of inter-mediate trophoblast following hydatidiform moles. *Int J Gynecol Pathol* 1993;12:324-332.

33. Kajii T, Ohama K. Androgenetic origin of hydatidiform mole. *Nature* 1977;268:633-655.

34. Lawler S, Fisher RA, Dent J. A prospective genetic study of complete and partial hydatidiform moles. *Am J Obstet Gynecol* 1991;164:1270-1277.

35. Jacobs PA, Wilson CM, Sprenkle JA, et al. Mechanisms of ori-gin of complete hydatidiform moles. *Nature* 1980;286:714-716.

36. Cross JC, Werb Z, Fisher SJ. Implantation and the placenta: Key pieces of the development puzzle. *Science* 1994;266: 1508-1518.

37. Yamashita K, Wake N, Araki T, et al. Human lymphocyte antigen expression in hydatidiform mole: Androgenesis fol-lowing fertilization by a haploid sperm. *Am J Obstet Gynecol* 1979;135:597-600.

38. Wake N, Fujino T, Hoshi S, et al. The propensity to malignancy of dispermic heterozygous mole. *Placenta* 1987;8:319-326.

39. Wallace DC, Surti U, Adams CW, et al. Complete moles have paternal chromosomes but maternal mitochondrial DNA. *Hum Genet* 1982;61:145-147.

40. Ohama K, Kajii T, Okamoto E, et al. Dispermic origin of XY hydatidiform moles. *Nature* 1981;292:551-552.

41. Fisher RA, Povey S, Jeffries AJ, et al. Frequency of heterozy-gous complete hydatidiform moles, estimated by locus-specific minisatellite and Y chromosome-specific probes. *Hum Genet* 1989;82:259-263.

42. McFadden DE, Kalousek DK. Two different phenotypes of fetuses with chromosomal triploidy: Correlation with parental origin of the extra haploid set. *Am J Med Genet* 1991; 38:535-538.

43. Steller MA, Mok SC, Yeh J. Effects of cytokines on epider-mal growth factor receptor expression by malignant tro-phoblast cells in vitro. *J Reprod Med* 1994;39:209-216.

44. Guillemot F, Nagy A, Auerbach A, et al. Essential role of Mash2 in extraembryonic development. *Nature* 1994;371: 333-336.

45. Cheung AN, Srivastava G, Pittaluga S, et al. Expression of c-myc and c-fins oncogenes in hydatidiform mole and nor-mal human placenta. *J Clin Pathol* 1993;46:204-207.

46. Sarkar S, Kacinski BM, Kohorn EI, et al. Demonstration of myc and ras oncogene expression by hybridization in situ in hydatidiform mole and in the BeWo choriocarcinoma cell line. *Am J Obstet Gynecol* 1986;154:390-393.

47. Li HW, Tsao SW, Cheung AN. Current understandings of the molecular genetics of gestational trophoblastic diseases. *Placenta* 2002;23(1):20-31.

48. Cameron B, Gown AM, Tamini HK. Expression of c-erb B2 oncogene product in persistent gestational trophoblastic dis-ease. *Am J Obstet Gynecol* 1994;170:1616-1621.

49. Park JS, Namkoong SE, Lee HY, et al. Expression and ampli-fication of cellular oncogenes in human developing placenta and neoplastic trophoblastic disease. *Asia Oceania J Obstet Gynaecol* 1992;18:57-64.

50. Cheung ANY, Srivastava G, Chung LP, et al. Expression of the p53 gene in trophoblastic cells in hydatidiform moles and normal human placentas. *J Reprod Med* 1994;39:223-227.

51. Lee YS. p53 expression in gestational trophoblastic disease. *Int J Gynecol Pathol* 1995;14:119-124.

52. Cheville JC, Robinson A, Benda JA. p53 expression in pla-centas with hydropic change and hydatidiform moles. *Mod Pathol* 1996;9:392-396.

53. Fulop V, Mok SC, Genest DR et al. p53, p21, Rb and mdm2 oncoproteins: Expression in normal placenta, partial and complete mole, and choriocarcinoma. *J Reprod Med* 1998; 43:119-127.

54. Fulop V, Mok SC, Genest DR, et al. c-myc, c-erbB-2, c-fms and bcl-2 oncoproteins: Expression in normal placenta, par-tial and complete mole, and choriocarcinoma. *J Reprod Med* 1998;43:101-110.

55. Cheung ANY, Shen DH, Khoo US, et al. p21WAF1/CIP1 expression in gestational trophoblastic disease: Correlation with clinicopathological parameters, and Ki67 and p53 gene expression. *J Clin Pathol* 1998;51:159-162.

56. Nishi H, Yahata N, Ohyashiki K, et al. Comparison of telom-erase activity in normal chorionic villi to trophoblastic dis-eases. *Int J Oncol* 1998;12:81-85.

57. Cheung ANY, Shen DH, Khoo US, et al. Immunohistochem-ical and mutational analysis of p53 tumour suppressor gene in gestational trophoblastic disease—correlation with mdm2, proliferation index and clinicopathological parameters. *Int J Gynecol Cancer* 1999;9:123-130.

58. Cheung ANY, Zhang DK, Liu Y, et al. Telomerase activity in gestational trophoblastic disease. *J Clin Pathol* 1999;52: 588-592.

59. Bae SN, Kim SJ. Telomerase activity in complete hydatidi-form mole. *Am J Obstet Gynecol* 1999;180:328-333.

60. Halperin R, Peller S, Sandbank J, et al. Expression of the p53 gene and apoptosis in gestational trophoblastic disease. *Plac-enta* 2000;21:58-62.

61. Berkowitz RS, Goldstein DP. Pathogenesis of gestational tro-phoblastic neoplasms. *Pathol Annu* 1981;11:391-411.

62. Yuen BH, Carron W, Benedet JL, et al. Plasma beta-subunit human chorionic gonadotropin assay in molar pregnancy and choriocarcinoma. *Am J Obstet Gynecol* 1977;127:711-712.

63. Amir SM, Osathanondh R, Berkowitz RS, et al. Human chorionic gonadotropin and thyroid function in patients with hydatidiform mole. *Am J Obstet Gynecol* 1984;150:723.

64. Goldstein DP, Berkowitz RS. Current management of complete and partial molar pregnancy. *J Reprod Med* 1994;39:139-146.

65. DiSaia PJ, Creasman WT, eds. Gestational trophoblastic neoplasia. In: *Clinical Gynecologic Oncology*. St. Louis: Mosby; 2002:185-210.

66. Mutch D, Soper JT, Baker ME, et al. Role of computed axial tomography of the chest in staging patients with nonmetastatic gestational trophoblastic disease. *Obstet Gynecol* 1986;68:348-352.

67. Kumar J, Ilancheran A, Ratnam SS. Pulmonary metastases in gestational trophoblastic disease: A review of 97 cases. *Br J Obstet Gynaecol* 1988;95:70-74.

68. Bagshawe KD. Risk and prognostic factors in trophoblastic neoplasia. *Cancer* 1976;38:1373-1385.

69. Park WW, Lees JC. Choriocarcinoma: A general review with analysis of 516 cases. *Arch Pathol* 1950;49:73-104 and 205-224.

70. Stilp TJ, Bucy PC, Brewer JI. Cure of metastatic choriocarcinoma of the brain. *JAMA* 1972;221:276-279.

71. Bakri Y, Berkowitz RS, Goldstein DP, et al. Brain metastases of gestational trophoblastic tumor. *J Reprod Med* 1994;39:179-183.

72. Palmer JR, Schorge JO, Goldstein DP, et al. Recent advances in gestational trophoblastic disease. *J Reprod Med* 2000;45(9):692-700.

73. Benson CB, Genest DR, Bernstein MR, et al. Sonographic appearance of first trimester complete hydatidiform moles. *Ultrasound Obstet Gynecol* 2000;16(2):188-191.

74. Dobkin GR, Berkowitz RS, Goldstein DP, et al. Duplex ultrasonography for persistent gestational trophoblastic tumor. *J Reprod Med* 1991;36(1):14-16.

75. Athanassiou A, Begent RHL, Newlands ES, et al. Central nervous system metastases of choriocarcinoma: Twenty-three years' experience at Charing Cross Hospital. *Cancer* 1983;52:1728-1735.

76. Ha HK, Jung JK, Jee MK, et al. Gestational trophoblastic tumors of the uterus: MR imaging—pathologic correlation. *Gynecol Oncol* 1995;57(3):340-350.

77. Pastorfide GB, Goldstein DP, Kosasa TS. The use of a radio-immunoassay specific for human chorionic gonadotropin in patients with molar pregnancy and gestational trophoblastic disease. *Am J Obstet Gynecol* 1974;120:1025-1028.

78. Vaitukaitis JL, Braunstein GD, Ross GT. A radioimmuno-assay which specifically measures human chorionic gonadotropin in the presence of human luteinizing hormone. *Am J Obstet Gynecol* 1972;113:751-758.

79. Kenimer JG, Hershman JM, Higgins HP. The thyrotropin in hydatidiform moles is human chorionic gonadotropin. *J Clin Endocrinol Metab* 1975;40:482-491.

80. Koonongs PP, Schalerth JB. CA125: A marker for persistent gestational trophoblastic disease? *Gynecol Oncol* 1993;49:240-242.

81. Bagshawe KD, Harland J. Immunodiagnosis and monitoring of gonadotropin-producing metastases in the central nervous system. *Cancer* 1976;39:112-118.

82. Rotmensch S, Cole LA. False diagnosis and needless therapy of presumed malignant disease in women with false-positive human chorionic gonadotropin concentrations. *Lancet* 2000; 355(9205):712-715. Erratum in *Lancet* 2000; 356(9229):600.

83. Ward G, McKinnon L, Badrick T, et al. Heterophilic antibodies remain a problem for the immunoassay laboratory. *Am J Clin Pathol* 1997;108:417-421.

84. Kohorn EI, Goldstein DP, Hancock BW, et al. Combining the staging system of the International Federation of Gynecology and Obstetrics with the scoring system of the World Health Organization for trophoblastic neoplasia. Report of the Working Committee of the International Society for the Study of Trophoblastic Disease and the International Gynecologic Cancer Society. *Int J Gynecol Cancer* 2000;(10):84-88.

85. Hammond CB, Weed JC, Jr., Currie JL. The role of operation in the current therapy of gestational neoplastic disease. *Am J Obstet Gynecol* 1980;136:844-858.

86. Hancock BW, Tidy JA. Current management of molar pregnancy. *J Reprod Med* 2002;47(5):347-354.

87. Soper JT. Surgical therapy for gestational trophoblastic disease. *J Reprod Med* 1994;39:168-174.

88. Goldstein DP. Prevention of gestational trophoblastic disease by use of actinomycin D in molar pregnancies. *Obstet Gynecol* 1974;43:475-479.

89. Goldstein DP. Prophylactic chemotherapy of molar pregnancy. *Obstet Gynecol* 1971;38:817-822.

90. Kim DS, Hyung M, Kyung TK, et al. Effects of prophylactic chemotherapy for persistent trophoblastic disease in patients with complete hydatidiform mole. *Obstet Gynecol* 1986;67:690-694.

91. Larsen LG, Theilade K, Skibsted L, et al. Malignant placental site trophoblastic tumor. A case report and a review of the literature. *APMIS* 1991;23(Suppl):138-145.

92. Newlands ES, Bower M, Fisher RA, et al. Management of placental site trophoblastic tumors. *J Reprod Med* 1998;43(1):53-59.

93. Swisher E, Drescher C. Metastatic placental site trophoblastic tumor: Long-term remission in a patient treated with EMA/CO chemotherapy. *Gynecol Oncol* 1998;68(1):62-65.

94. Newlands ES, Mulholland PJ, Holden L, et al. Etoposide and cisplatin/etoposide, methotrexate, and actinomycin D (EMA) chemotherapy for patients with high-risk gestational trophoblastic tumors refractory to EMA/cyclophosphamide and vincristine chemotherapy and patients presenting with metastatic placental site trophoblastic tumors. *J Clin Oncol* 2000;18(4):854-859.

95. Berkowitz RS, Goldstein DP, Bernstein MR. Ten years' experience with methotrexate and folinic acid as primary therapy for gestational trophoblastic disease. *Gynecol Oncol* 1986;23:111-118.

96. Feltmate CM, Genest DR, Wise L, et al. Placental site trophoblastic tumor: A 17-year experience at the New England Trophoblastic Disease Center. *Gynecol Oncol* 2001;82(3):415-419.

97. Gleeson NC, Finan MA, Fiorica JV, et al. Nonmetastatic gestational trophoblastic disease: Weekly methotrexate compared with 8-day methotrexate-folinic acid. *Eur J Gynaecol Oncol* 14:461-465.

98. Jones WB. Management of low-risk metastatic gestational trophoblastic disease. *J Reprod Med* 1981;26:213-217.

99. Hammond CB, Borchert LG, Tyrey L, et al. Treatment of metastatic trophoblastic disease: Good and poor prognosis. *J Obstet Gynecol* 1973;115:451-457.

100. Lurain JR, Brewer JI. Treatment of high-risk gestational trophoblastic disease with methotrexate, actinomycin D, and cyclophosphamide chemotherapy. *Obstet Gynecol* 1985;65: 830-836.

101. Gordon AN, Gershenson DM, Copeland LJ, et al. High-risk metastatic gestational trophoblastic disease. *Obstet Gynecol* 1985;65:550-556.

102. Berkowitz RS, Goldstein DP, Bernstein MR. Modified triple chemotherapy in the management of high-risk metastatic gestational trophoblastic tumors. *Gynecol Oncol* 1984;19: 173-181.

103. Curry SL, Blessing JA, Disaia PJ, et al. A prospective randomized comparison of methotrexate, actinomycin D, and chlorambucil (MAC) versus modified Bagshawe regimen in "poor-prognosis" gestational trophoblastic disease. *Obstet Gynecol* 1989;73:357-362.

104. Bagshawe KD. Treatment of high-risk choriocarcinoma. *J Reprod Med* 1984;29:813-820.

105. Bower M, Newlands ES, Holden L, et al. EMA/CO for high-risk gestational trophoblastic tumors: Results from a cohort of 272 patients. *J Clin Oncol* 1997;15(7):2636-2643. Erratum in *J Clin Oncol* 1997;15(9):3168.

106. Quinn M, Murray J, Friedlander M, et al. EMACO in high risk gestational trophoblast disease—The Australian experience. Gestational Trophoblast Subcommittee, Clinical Oncological Society of Australia. *Aust N Z J Obstet Gynaecol* 1994;34(1):90-92.

107. Soper JT, Evans AC, Clarke-Pearson DL, et al. Alternating weekly chemotherapy with etoposide-methotrexate-dactinomycin/cyclophosphamide-vincristine for high-risk gestational trophoblastic disease. *Obstet Gynecol* 1994; 83(1):113-117.

108. DuBeshter B, Berkowitz RS, Goldstein DP, et al. Analysis of treatment failure in high-risk metastatic gestational trophoblastic disease. *Gynecol Oncol* 1988;29(2):199-207.

109. Kelly MP, Rustin GJS, Ivory C, et al. Respiratory failure due to choriocarcinoma: A study of 103 dyspneic patients. *Gynecol Oncol* 1990;38:149-154.

110. Bakri YN, Berkowitz RS, Khan J, et al. Pulmonary metastases of gestational trophoblastic tumor: Risk factors for early respiratory failure. *J Reprod Med* 1994;38:175-178.

111. Rustin GJS, Bagshawe KD. Gestational trophoblastic tumours. *CRC Crit Rev Oncol Haematol* 1985;3:103.

112. Gilbert HA, Kagan AR. Incidence, detection, and evaluation without histologic confirmation. In: Weiss L (ed): *Fundamental Aspects of Metastases*. Amsterdam: North Holland; 1976; 385-405.

113. Weed JC, Hammond CB. Cerebral metastatic choriocarcinoma: Intensive therapy and prognosis. *Obstet Gynecol* 1980; 55:89-94.

114. Ayhan A, Tuncer ZS, Tanir M, et al. Central nervous system involvement in gestational trophoblastic neoplasia. *Acta Obstet Gynecol Scand* 1996;75(6):548-550.

115. Evans AC, Jr., Soper JT, Clarke-Pearson DL, et al. Gestational trophoblastic disease metastatic to the central nervous system. *Gynecol Oncol* 1995;59(2):226-230.

116. Gillespie AM, Siddiqui N, Coleman RE, et al. Gestational trophoblastic disease: Does central nervous system chemoprophylaxis have a role? *Br J Cancer* 1999;79(7-8): 1270-1272.

117. Yordan EL, Jr., Schlaerth JB, Gaddis O, et al. Radiation therapy in the management of gestational choriocarcinoma metastatic to the central nervous system. *Obstet Gynecol* 1987;69: 627-630.

118. Ishizuka T, Tomoda Y, Kaseki S, et al. Intracranial metastasis of choriocarcinoma. A clinicopathologic study. *Cancer* 1983;52(10):1896-1903.

119. Kobayashi T, Kida Y, Yoshida J, et al. Brain metastasis of choriocarcinoma. *Surg Neurol* 1982;17(6):395-403.

120. Schechter NR, Mychalczak B, Jones W, et al. Prognosis of patients treated with whole-brain radiation therapy for metastatic gestational trophoblastic disease. *Gynecol Oncol* 1998; 68(2):183-192.

121. Hartenbach EM, Saltzman AK, Carter JR, et al. A novel strategy using G-CSF to support EMA/CO for high-risk gestational trophoblastic disease. *Gynecol Oncol* 1995;56(1): 105-108.

122. Soper JT, Evans AC, Rodriguez G, et al. Etoposide-platin combination therapy for chemorefractory gestational trophoblastic disease. *Gynecol Oncol* 1995;56(3):421-424.

123. Newlands ES. New chemotherapeutic agents in the management of gestational trophoblastic disease. *Semin Oncol* 1982; 9(2):239-243.

124. Gordon AN, Kavanagh JJ, Gershenson DM, et al. Cisplatin, vincristine, and bleomycin combination therapy in resistant gestational trophoblastic disease. *Cancer* 1986;58: 1407-1410.

125. Surwit EA, Childers JM. High-risk metastatic gestational trophoblastic disease: A new dose-intensive, multiagent chemotherapeutic regimen. *J Reprod Med* 1991;36:45-48.

126. Li-Pai C, Shu-Mo C, Jian-Xuan F, et al. PEBA regimen (cisplatin, etoposide, bleomycin, and Adriamycin) in the treatment of drug-resistant choriocarcinoma. *Gynecol Oncol* 1995;56:231-234.

127. Sutton GP, Soper JT, Blessing JA, et al. Ifosfamide alone and in combination in the treatment of refractory malignant gestational trophoblastic disease. *Am J Obstet Gynecol* 1992; 167:489-495.

128. Lotz JP, Andre T, Donsimoni R, et al. High dose chemotherapy with ifosfamide, carboplatin, and etoposide combined with autologous bone marrow transplantation for the treatment of poor-prognosis germ cell tumors and metastatic trophoblastic disease in adults. *Cancer* 1995;75:874-885.

129. Garris PD, Gallup DG, Melton K. Long-term remission of previously resistant choriocarcinoma with a combination of etoposide, ifosfamide, and cisplatin. *Gynecol Oncol* 1995; 57(2):254-256.

130. Piamsomboon S, Kudelka AP, Termrungruanglert W. Remission of refractory gestational trophoblastic disease in the brain with ifosfamide, carboplatin, and etoposide (ICE): First report and review of literature. *Eur J Gynaecol Oncol* 1997;18(6):453-456.

131. Steigrad SJ, Cheung AP, Osborn RA. Choriocarcinoma coexistent with an intact pregnancy: Case report and review of the literature. *J Obstet Gynaecol Res* 1999;25(3):197-203.

132. Walden PAM, Bagshawe KD. Pregnancies after chemotherapy for gestational trophoblastic tumors. *Lancet* 1979;2(8154):1241.

133. Garner EI, Lipson E, Bernstein MR, et al. Subsequent pregnancy experience in patients with molar pregnancy and gestational trophoblastic tumor. *J Reprod Med* 2002;47(5):380-386.

Genitourinary Carcinomas

RENAL CELL CARCINOMA

Eric Jonasch
Surena F. Matin
Lance C. Pagliaro
Christopher G. Wood
Nizar M. Tannir

■ INCIDENCE AND DIAGNOSIS

The American Cancer Society predicts that there will be over 56,000 new cases of renal neoplasms in the coming year in the United States and that 13,000 patients will die as a consequence of disease progression (1). Renal cell carcinoma (RCC) is the most common histology found in kidney tumors, with clear cell (conventional) RCC being the most common histologic subtype (Fig. 32-1). Non–clear cell subtypes include chromophobe, papillary, oncocytoma, collecting duct carcinoma (CDC), and unclassified RCC.

The incidence of RCC has been increasing over the last several decades. This increase in incidence is partly attributed to the increased use of better-quality abdominal imaging in patients who present with either unrelated or nonspecific complaints. As a consequence, one would predict an increase in the earlier detection of RCC, in earlier stages, and better outcomes associated with definitive therapy. Several reports have examined large epidemiologic databases to determine whether other causative factors may explain the increased incidence of RCC (1,2). Chow and colleagues (2) examined the database of the National Cancer Institute's Surveillance, Epidemiology, and End Results (SEER) Program looking at patients who were diagnosed with kidney cancer from 1975 through 1995. This database reflects approximately 10% of the US population. They noted an increasing incidence of RCC in men and women regardless of race and also that the increases were greatest for localized tumors, but there was an increased incidence of more advanced and unstaged tumors as well. These data are corroborated in

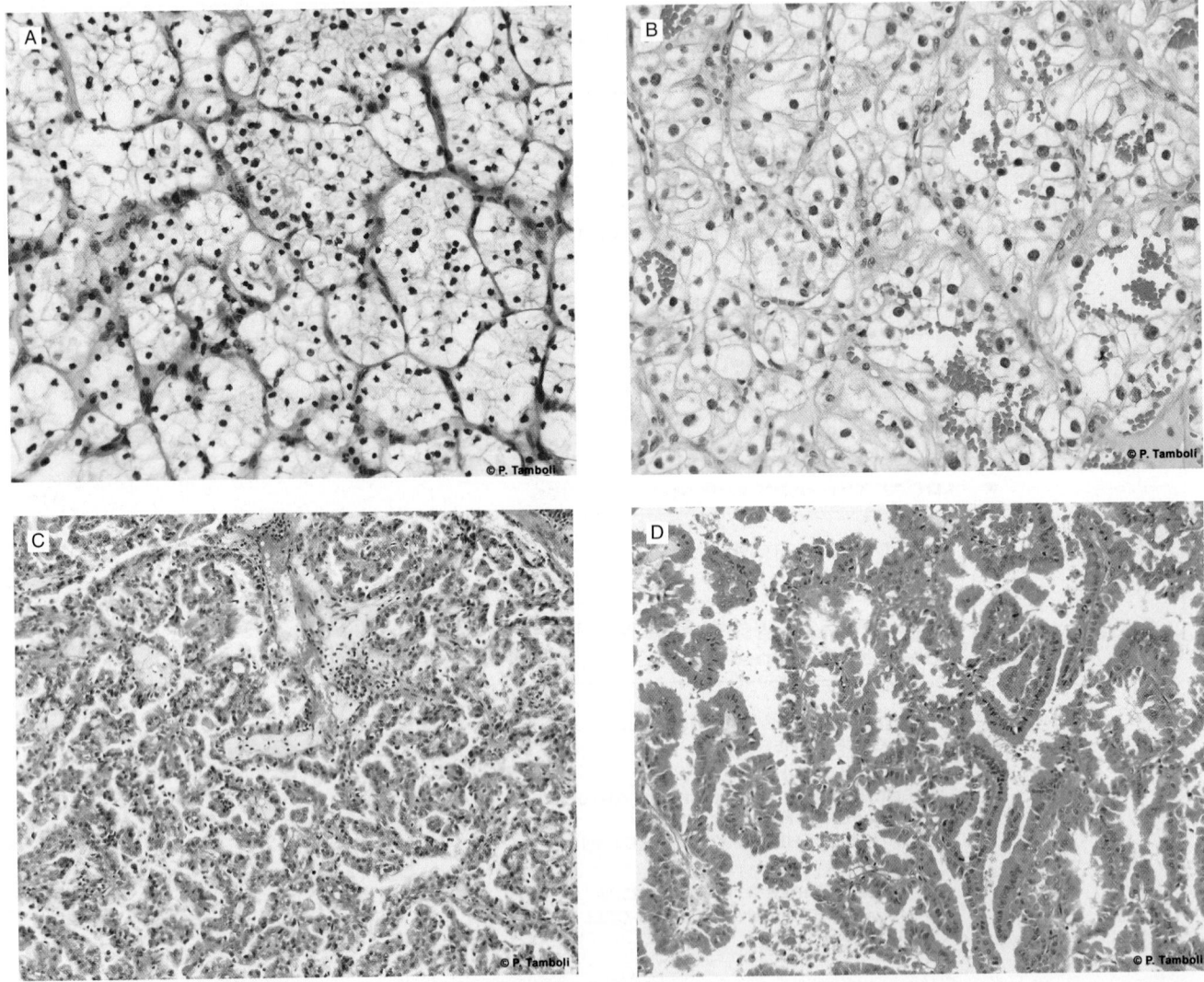

FIGURE 32-1.   Photomicrographs of clear cell (conventional) RCC with low-grade **A.** and high-grade **B.** nuclear features. Photomicrographs of a type 1 papillary RCC **C.** showing papillae lined by short cuboidal cells, and type 2 papillary RCC **D.** showing papillae lined by tall columnar cells, with eosinophilic cytoplasm and high grade nuclear features. (*Reprinted with permission from Pheroze Tamboli, MD.*)

other studies and suggest that there has been an increase in the prevalence of RCC across both gender and racial lines and that, despite the earlier detection, there has not been an improvement in disease-specific mortality rates.

■ STAGING, EPIDEMIOLOGY, AND RISK FACTORS

The American Joint Commission on Cancer staging schema for renal cell carcinoma was updated in 2010. Major staging categories are as follows: Stage 1: T1 tumors, which are less than 7 centimeters (cm) in maximum diameter and are confined to the kidney. Stage 2: T2 tumors that exceed 7 cm in diameter but are confined to the kidney. Stage 3: T3 tumors, which demonstrate extracapsular invasion, renal or inferior vena caval invasion. Stage 3 also includes tumors with regional node positivity. Stage 4: Extension of the primary tumor into the adrenal gland or beyond gerota's fascia, or distant metastases (3).

It has been well documented that there are racial differences in the incidence of RCC. Both the incidence and mortality of RCC are increasing in African Americans faster than in whites. The biology of RCC in African Americans appears more virulent and less responsive to conventional therapies. This may reflect differences in access to health care or dietary influences. It may also reflect a difference in the incidence of comorbidities, such as hypertension or diabetes that are associated with an increased risk of RCC (see below).

The link between germline genetic mutations and the development of RCC is well established and applies to a small but biologically important subset of RCC cases (4). While these genetic alterations certainly play an important role in the biology of RCC in both familial and sporadic cases, there are also some environmental factors that contribute to the risk of developing a renal neoplasm. Smoking has long been linked to an increase in the risk of developing RCC, in addition to its association with multiple other malignancies (5). As is the case with other malignancies, cessation of smoking can be associated with a diminution in the risk of developing RCC. Interestingly, this diminution in risk appears to be slower and requires a significantly longer time frame to reach baseline than that seen with other malignancies, such as lung cancer.

Obesity or increased body mass index (BMI) has also been linked to increased risk of developing RCC. Several studies have demonstrated a higher incidence of obesity or increased BMI in patients with RCC, suggesting an epidemiologic linkage (6). As is the case in most retrospective epidemiologic studies, these observations are confounded by other associated variables, including diet, occupational history, and smoking. In a report by Kamat et al., obese patients were not more likely to present with advanced-stage tumors; overall, they had a more favorable prognosis following surgery than did patients with a lower BMI (6).

Several studies have pointed to an increase in the risk of developing RCC in association with the diagnosis of diabetes mellitus or hypertension (7,8). Some of the therapies employed for the treatment of hypertension, such as diuretic therapy (9), have been associated with an increased risk of developing RCC. Given the retrospective nature of these studies, it remains unclear whether it is the underlying medical condition or its treatment that increases the risk of developing RCC. Some insight may be forthcoming from a study published in the *New England Journal of Medicine* (7), which demonstrated that successful treatment of hypertension lowered the risk of developing RCC.

Dietary factors have been linked to the development of RCC. These include a high-fat or high-protein diet or the ingestion of significant quantities of fried foods (10). Increased alcohol consumption and increased consumption of red meat have also been identified as risk factors (11). A study published by Yuan et al. suggested that increased intake of cruciferous vegetables may decrease the risk of developing RCC (12).

■ PROGNOSTIC FACTORS, PATHOLOGY, AND MOLECULAR MARKERS

The natural history is variable, depending on tumor genetic factors, the general medical condition of the patient, and host factors such as angiogenesis and immune response. Patients who undergo nephrectomy for localized disease remain at risk of recurrence for many years and require appropriate counseling and surveillance.

The traditional measures of performance status (PS), tumor stage, and tumor grade each demonstrate good correlation with clinical outcome (13). Integration of these parameters and other clinical prognostic variables allows the classification of patients into groups with statistically significant differences in survival. There are a variety of clinical, pathologic, and molecular features that have been proposed and studied as prognostic factors (Table 32-1) (14,15). A better understanding of the tumor biology and its putative biomarkers is needed to develop better predictive models (16), and ultimately more effective treatment, of this heterogeneous disease.

TABLE
32-1   **PROGNOSTIC FACTORS IN ADVANCED RENAL CELL CARCINOMA**

Patient- or Treatment-Related Factors	Laboratory Studies	Tumor-Related Factors	Molecular Markers
Performance status	Lactate dehydrogenase	Site and/or no of metastatic sites	VHL mutation or hypermethylation
Age, gender, race	Alkaline phosphatase	Disease-free interval	Carbonic anhydrase IX expression
Symptoms: weight loss, fatigue, pain, appetite, fever	Calcium	Metastasis-free interval	Phospho-extracellular signal-regulated kinase (pERK)
Overweight	Albumin	Tumor burden	Cytoplasmic mTOR staining
Prior nephrectomy	Liver dysfunction	Histologic type	PTEN deletion
Prior therapy	Anemia	Sarcomatoid dedifferentiation	p53 overexpression
	Thrombocytosis	Ploidy	MMP-2 and MMP-9 overexpression

CLINICAL PROGNOSTIC VARIABLES

Investigators at MSKCC identified five prognostic factors for survival in patients with metastatic RCC. The adverse features were low PS (Karnofsky <80%), high LDH (>1.5 times normal), anemia, hypercalcemia (corrected serum calcium >10 mg/dL), and absence of prior nephrectomy (17). In a cohort of 670 patients with median survival duration of 10 months, 22% of patients had 3 or more risk factors (poor-risk), 53% had 1 or 2 (intermediate-risk), and 25% had none (favorable-risk). The median survival for each group was 4.9 months, 10 months, and 20 months, respectively, with significant differences also seen in 1-, 2-, and 3-year survival.

The MSKCC system based on these five parameters gives reproducible results and can greatly facilitate the design and interpretation of clinical trials by allowing appropriate comparisons between similar groups of patients. After cytoreductive nephrectomy became standard of care, time from initial diagnosis of RCC to initiation of systemic therapy of less than 1 year replaced nephrectomy status as a risk factor in the updated MSKCC prognostic model. Non–clear-cell histology has been associated with lower probability of response to systemic therapy (18,19). In an attempt to improve on the MSKCC clinical prognostic model, we investigated the role of cytokines and angiogenic factors (CAF) in serum of patients treated with interferon-alpha, and found elevated baseline levels of interleukin-5, interleukin-6, interleukin-12p40 and VEGFA (vascular endothelial growth factor A) to be independent risk factors associated with inferior survival. Incorporating the CAF model with the MSKCC clinical model improved the concordance index for predicting overall survival (OS). Patients having 3 or more of the 4 CAF or MSKCC poor-risk group had a median OS of 9 months, compared with 32 months median OS for patients with 2 or

less of these risk factors (20). Similar efforts have been made to develop serum and plasma-based prognostic and predictive biomarkers in individuals who received antiangiogenic therapy (21).

PATHOLOGY AND MOLECULAR MARKERS

There are several major histological subtypes in RCC, including clear cell, papillary, and chromophobe variants (see Fig. 32-1). Historically, patients with non–clear-cell RCC variants do poorly once they develop metastatic disease, mainly due to the dearth of effective systemic therapy.

The VHL gene product regulates the hypoxia-induced pathway and is commonly mutated in clear-cell RCC (22). The hypoxia-induced pathway leads to the activation of survival genes that mediate glucose transport, proliferation, angiogenesis, and pH regulation, and is also implicated in the other tumor types. In a study of 187 patients undergoing nephrectomy for clear-cell RCC in Japan, mutation or hypermethylation of the VHL gene was found in 58% of tumors, and was associated with significantly improved disease-free and cancer-specific survival in patients with organ-confined tumors (N = 134), but not in those with stage IV disease at the time of nephrectomy (N = 53) (23). VHL abnormalities probably occur early in the development of clear-cell RCC, potentially identifying the subset of patients who respond well to surgery.

Loss of VHL allows accumulation of HIF-1α protein, activation of the HIF-1 complex, and HIF-1-induced expression of genes including VEGF and carbonic anhydrases (24). Carbonic anhydrase IX (CA IX), a hypoxia-inducible enzyme that controls cellular pH, is highly expressed in RCC but absent in most normal tissues. A study of CA IX expression in 321 clear-cell

RCC nephrectomy specimens showed expression in 94%, most of which were highly positive (>90% of cells) (25). Expression was lower in metastases than in primary tumors. Low or absent CA IX was an independent predictor of death from cancer in patients who had metastases at the time of nephrectomy (N = 140), but not for those with organ-confined, that is, curable, disease.

Studies are currently underway to determine whether CA IX expression can be used to predict responses to systemic therapy such as IL-2. Progress in the characterization of this and other molecular markers may also reveal new opportunities for targeted therapy. Putative molecular markers hold promise for application in the prediction of response to therapy, but none are yet valid enough for routine clinical application (15).

■ CONTROL OF THE PRIMARY TUMOR

CYTOREDUCTIVE NEPHRECTOMY

The role of initial cytoreductive radical nephrectomy as part of a multidisciplinary treatment approach for patients with metastatic RCC has remained a subject of much controversy in the urologic literature. At issue is the question of whether surgical control of the primary can be performed safely and also provide benefit in patient outcome. Prior to the completion and publication of two large phase III trials, the evidence regarding efficacy for this treatment paradigm consisted of single-institution series (26,27).

The EORTC Genitourinary Group trial 30947 was a prospective randomized trial that included 85 patients with metastatic RCC randomized to either interferon-alpha 2b (IFNα) or nephrectomy followed by IFNα (28). The study demonstrated no difference in overall response (complete plus partial) to IFNα between the two groups (surgery 19% versus control 12%, p = .38), but the surgery group had improved median survival (17 versus 7 months, p = .03) and time to progression (5 versus 3 months, p = .04).

The Southwest Oncology Group (SWOG) trial 8949 also examined the role of cytoreductive nephrectomy in 241 patients with metastatic RCC treated with IFNα (29). Ninety-eight percent of the patients who underwent surgery were able to receive IFNα. The mean time from surgery to initiation of systemic therapy was 19.9 days, with three responses seen in each group, and an overall survival difference favoring patients who underwent cytoreductive nephrectomy (median 11.1 versus 8.1 months, p = .012). Of note, there were more patients

with impaired PS (SWOG score = 1) in the control arm (58.1 versus 45.0%, p = .04). Because the groups were not balanced for PS, the investigators performed a proportional-hazards analysis and found no significant interaction between treatment group and PS. Furthermore, there was a survival advantage favoring surgery for both PS subgroups (6.9 versus 4.8 months for PS 1; 17.4 versus 11.7 months for PS 0).

One of the important issues that has come to light is the wholesale application of cytoreductive nephrectomy to patients regardless of their suitability for this procedure. In the larger US study, patients with a SWOG PS of 1 (Zubrod ≥1) who underwent cytoreductive nephrectomy demonstrated a clinically insignificant benefit, with median overall survival increased from approximately 4.9 months for those without nephrectomy to 6.9 months with the procedure (29). Based on these data, many urologic oncologists are now performing cytoreductive nephrectomies on selected patients with metastatic RCC, particularly those with good PS, absence of sarcomatoid histology, and without central nervous system or bone metastases.

Further complicating the debate surrounding the role of cytoreductive nephrectomy is the emergence of targeted molecular therapy as the standard of care in the treatment of metastatic renal cell carcinoma. These agents, which target specific molecular pathways important in tumor growth, angiogenesis, and metastatic progression, have produced unprecedented tumor response rates, as well as improvements in progression-free, and overall survival (30-34). As such, some have questioned the need for cytoreductive nephrectomy, citing primarily anecdotal evidence that we are now seeing significant antitumor responses both in metastatic sites as well as in the primary tumor, in those patients treated with their primary in situ. The CARMENA trial was initiated in France in 2009 to address this question, and randomizes patients between upfront cytoreductive nephrectomy followed by sunitinib versus sunitinib alone. Proponents of continuing the practice of cytoreductive nephrectomy as part of a multidisciplinary approach in the treatment of patients with advanced disease cite that complete responses to targeted therapy are rare to non-existent, that a resistant phenotype will eventually emerge, and that significant primary tumor downstaging or tumor volume reduction is not a common phenomenon with the current generation of targeted agents as evidence to continue the practice of cytoreductive nephrectomy and metastasectomy. Furthermore, in the clinical trials performed to verify the activity of these agents, the vast majority of patients had prior nephrectomy, thus demonstrating the significant activity of these agents largely in the context of patients with their primary tumor removed.

Other investigators have initiated studies to investigate the importance of timing of cytoreductive nephrectomy in patients who receive molecularly targeted agents. The concept of presurgical therapy, whereby patients receive a defined course of therapy with targeted agents prior to cytoreductive nephrectomy has shown promise in a phase II clinical trial (35). The purported benefit of this management approach is that surgery will be reserved only for patients demonstrating a response to therapy, thus sparing highly morbid surgery in patients who are not destined to respond to systemic therapy. In addition, there is the real possibility of primary tumor downstaging as a consequence of presurgical therapy, thus potentially reducing the morbidity of cytoreductive surgery. This concept is currently being investigated in a phase III trial design by the EORTC.

■ SYSTEMIC THERAPY

The integration of systemic therapy and surgical management is one of the key challenges in RCC treatment. Figure 32-2 summarizes an algorithm that outlines how to approach an individual with RCC. The decision to surgically resect the primary tumor or metastatic disease and the choice of systemic therapy requires a multidisciplinary approach. Input from surgical colleagues and from the patient with regards to their expectations and acceptance of treatment related toxicity is essential for proper patient management.

IMMUNOTHERAPY

Clear-cell RCC is considered an immunogenic tumor. This is based on the observation of up to a 4% spontaneous regression rate in metastatic lesions (34), the presence of tumor infiltrating lymphocytes in tumor specimens, and well-documented responses to therapies presumed to act via stimulation of the immune system. The following discussion of immunotherapy apply mainly to patients with clear-cell RCC, as very little data exist supporting the use of immunotherapy in variant histology RCC.

The genes for IL-2 and IFNα 2a and 2b were cloned in 1983 and 1981, respectively. A number of studies were performed testing these agents in RCC, and due to the absence of other effective therapies, the modest benefit seen in RCC was a welcome change. High-dose

intravenous bolus IL-2 was FDA-approved in 1992 based on a compilation of 255 patients from a number of phase II trials, with results demonstrating a response rate of 15% and a durable complete response rate of 5% (37).

Two randomized studies assessing the effect of IFNα therapy on survival were published in 1999 (38,39). The Medical Research Council Renal Cancer Collaborators reported on 335 patients randomized to IFNα or medroxyprogesterone acetate, demonstrating a median survival advantage of 2.5 months for the IFN group (37). Similar results were found by Pyrhonen et al. in a smaller study, with a 7-month survival improvement for patients treated with IFN plus vinblastine versus those treated with vinblastine alone (38). Despite these findings, IFN was never FDA approved for RCC in the USA. Efforts to improve on these results involved the combination of IL-2, IFNα, and 5-fluorouracil (5-FU) (40-42). Early enthusiasm for combination therapy was dampened as more rigorous testing demonstrated response rates for the combination therapies that were no higher than those of cytokine monotherapy (40).

With the advent of molecularly targeted agents, IFN has fallen out of favor as a frontline agent. High-dose IL-2 is still considered a frontline therapy option for patients with grade 2 or 3 clear-cell RCC who are younger than 70, have an excellent performance status, and exhibit no significant cardiac or pulmonary comorbidities. A retrospective analysis suggests that the presence of retroperitoneal adenopathy at the time of cytoreductive nephrectomy is a negative predictor for outcome (43). Additionally, the use of high-dose IL-2 in patients who were previously treated with anti-VEGF agents was associated with a substantially higher rate of cardiac toxicity and lack of response among 23 patients treated, compared to historic controls (44).

A number of vaccines strategies have been tested in RCC. Unfortunately, the published studies fail to demonstrate convincing or consistent efficacy for any of these strategies. In particular, autologous dendritic cells (45) or allogeneic dendritic cells (46) failed to demonstrate a strong clinical signal in published trials.

Nonmyeloablative transplantation has the potential for harnessing a potent graft-versus-tumor effect, but with lower toxicity from the conditioning regimen. This approach demonstrated promise in a National Cancer Institute study (47). An analysis of studies published by other centers shows an aggregate response rate of approximately 30%, with treatment-related mortality averaging 20% (48,49). In addition to the mortality risk, long-term consequences of graft-versus-host disease and other morbidities are associated with transplantation.

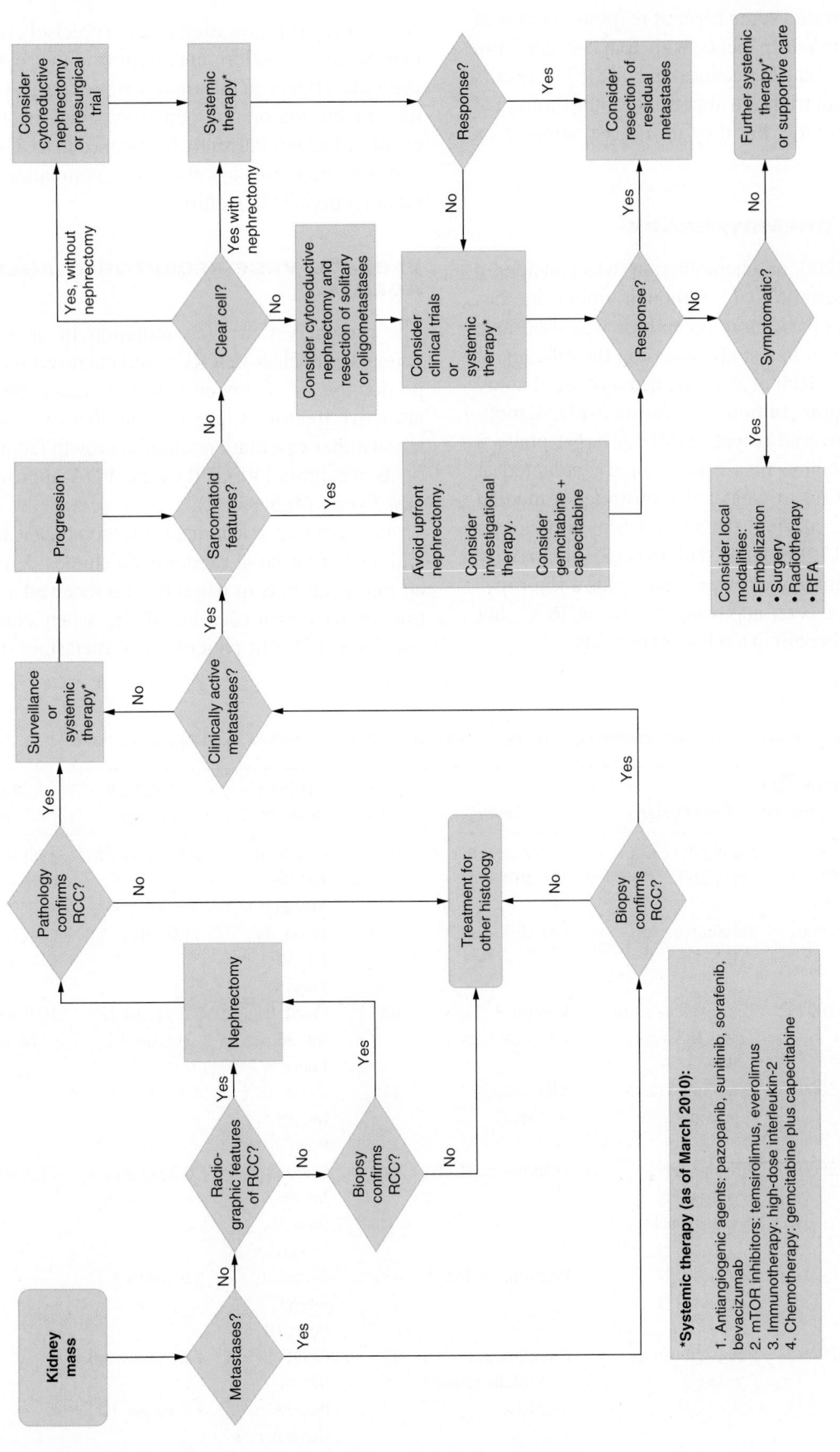

FIGURE 32-2. Management algorithm for patients diagnosed with a renal mass.

A study by Ueno et al. from MD Anderson Cancer Center demonstrated some form of response occurred in 7 of 14 evaluable patients with RCC; death from transplant-related causes occurred in 5 (48). The results of these transplant trials are important for the biological insights they provide, but they do not yet support its routine use.

CYTOTOXIC CHEMOTHERAPY

Until the year 2000, no chemotherapy was considered effective in metastatic RCC. Although vinblastine has been used in the past, more recently it was used as a comparator control in a study assessing the efficacy of IFN therapy (38). Rini et al. published a phase II study of gemcitabine plus continuous infusion 5-FU, demonstrating a 17% overall response (50). A larger phase 2 study of gemcitabine plus capecitabine conducted at MD Anderson Cancer Center demonstrated a median progression-free survival (PFS) of 4.6 months and a median OS of 17.9 months, with manageable toxicity (51). The combination of gemcitabine plus a fluoropyrimidine has not been approved for use in RCC, but clearly provides benefit in a subset of patients.

MOLECULARLY TARGETED AGENTS

A major effort is now underway to precisely target aberrant cellular function, and achieve either cytostatic or cytocidal effects on the tumor cells, or target vulnerabilities in the tumor microenvironment. The two major classes of agents currently being used in RCC are VEGF pathway blocking agents, and mammalian target of rapamycin (mTOR) inhibitors.

VEGF- OR VEGF-RECEPTOR-TARGETED AGENTS

The presence of a *VHL* mutation in up to 80% of patients with clear-cell RCC and the resultant increased production of angiogenic factors make this axis an attractive treatment target. A number of agents which target either vascular endothelial growth factor (VEGF) or its receptors (VEGFR) were FDA approved in the past 5 years (Table 32-2).

Bevacizumab is a humanized recombinant anti-VEGF antibody. Two large randomized studies demonstrated an improved PFS in patients who received a combination of bevacizumab plus IFNa, when compared to interferon IFNa in patients with metastatic RCC who

TABLE 32-2 | PHASE III STUDIES OF APPROVED MOLECULARLY TARGETED AGENTS IN RCC

Agent	Year FDA Approved	Trial Design	Setting	N	MSKCC Risk (%)*	MedPFS (mos)	Med OS (mos)
Sorafenib	2005	Sorafenib versus placebo	Cytokine failures ccRCC	903	Good: 50 Int.: 49 Missing: 1	5.5 versus 2.8	19.3 versus 15.9 (NS)
Sunitinib	2006	Sunitinib versus IFN	Frontline ccRCC	750	Good: 34 Int: 59 Poor: 7	11.0 versus 5.0	26.4 versus 21.8 (p =.051)
Temsirolimus	2007	Temsi versus temsi plus IFN versus IFN	Frontline Any histology	626	Good: 0 Int: 26 Poor: 74	5.5 versus 4.7 versus 3.1	10.9 versus 8.4 versus 7.3
Everolimus	2009	Everolimus versus placebo	TKI failures ccRCC	416	Good: 28.5 Int: 56.5 Poor: 15	4.9 versus 1.9	NA
Bevacizumab	2009	Bev plus IFN versus IFN plus placebo	Frontline ccRCC	649	Good: 28 Int: 56 Poor: 9 Unknown: 8	10.2 versus 5.4	23.3 versus 21.8
		Bev plus IFN versus IFN	Frontline ccRCC	732	Good: 26 Int: 64 Poor: 10	8.5 versus 5.2	
Pazopanib	2009	Pazopanib versus placebo	Frontline and cytokine failures ccRCC	435	Good: 39 Int: 54 Poor: 3 Unknown: 3	11.1 versus 2.8 7.4 versus 4.2	

*MSKCC criteria in Everolimus study for second line therapy.

had not received prior systemic therapy (52,53). The AVOREN study showed a median PFS of 10.2 months in bevacizumab plus IFN-treated patients, compared with a median PFS of 5.4 months for IFN-treated patients. The Cancer and Leukemia Group B (CALGB) 90206 study showed a median PFS of 8.5 months for the combination arm versus 5.2 months for IFN monotherapy. Of note, the OS for both studies was numerically superior in the bevacizumab-containing arm, but did not reach statistical significance. Bevacizumab plus IFN was FDA approved for advanced RCC in 2009.

Sorafenib is an orally bioavailable small molecule inhibitor of VEGFR, platelet-derived growth factor (PDGFR), and Raf, and was FDA approved in 2005 for the treatment of advanced RCC. In a randomized phase 3 trial, sorafenib showed a doubling of median PFS to 5.5 months, compared to placebo in patients who had failed one prior therapy, the majority having received prior cytokines (30). A phase II frontline study comparing sorafenib to IFN showed equivalent median PFS of 5.7 months, (54) and for this reason sorafenib has fallen out of favor in the frontline setting.

Sunitinib malate is an oral inhibitor of VEGFR and PDGFR. When it was first tested in the cytokine refractory population, a time to progression (TTP) of 8.7 months was achieved (55), earning it provisional FDA approval in early 2006. A follow-up phase III trial randomizing patients between sunitinib and IFN showed a median PFS of 11.0 months for sunitinib versus 5.0 months for IFN (33). Median overall survival of sunitinib treated patients was 26.4 months, versus a surprising 21.8 months for the interferon-treated group ($p = .051$), likely due to crossover to molecularly targeted agents (56). When a subgroup analysis was performed of the individuals who did not receive any subsequent therapy, it was found that those who received sunitinib alone had a median OS of 28 months, versus 14 months for the IFN-only group.

Pazopanib is an oral small molecule with a lower IC50 for VEGFR when compared to sorafenib and sunitinib (57). A randomized, phase III trial compared pazopanib to placebo in a mixed population of cytokine treated and previously untreated patients, and demonstrated an overall PFS of 9.2 versus 4.2 months; HR 0.46; 95% CI 0.34, 0.62; $p < .0000001$ (58). Pazopanib was FDA approved in 2009 for the treatment of advanced RCC.

MAMMALIAN TARGET OF RAPAMYCIN INHIBITORS

Temsirolimus is an intravenous sirolimus ester, which was tested in an intermediate- and poor-risk patient population, after phase II data had suggested that this was the subgroup of patients most likely to benefit from temsirolimus (59). This frontline phase III trial randomized patients among temsirolimus, temsirolimus plus IFN, versus IFN monotherapy. The median OS in the temsirolimus arm was 10.9 months, versus 8.4 months for the combination arm and 7.3 months for IFN monotherapy (32). Temsirolimus obtained FDA approval in 2007.

Everolimus is an orally bioavailable sirolimus ester, which was evaluated in patients who had progressed on sorafenib, sunitinib, or both. This phase 3 trial randomized patients between everolimus 10 mg by mouth daily versus placebo in a 2:1 fashion. Median PFS was 4.0 months for everolimus versus 1.9 months for placebo (60). Everolimus obtained FDA approval in 2009 for the treatment of patients who had progressed on sorafenib or sunitinib.

SIDE EFFECT PROFILES

The major side effects of the targeted agents are summarized in Table 32-3. Blockade of VEGF receptors or depletion of the VEGF ligand causes class effects, which include hypertension, fatigue, proteinuria, and a slightly increased risk of bleeding and thromboembolic events. All of the anti-VEGF agents will cause these side effects to varying degrees. Sorafenib, sunitinib, and pazopanib are also inhibitors of PDGF, Flt3, and a number of other receptor tyrosine kinases (RTKs), and will as a result induce hand-foot-syndrome, diarrhea, and dysgeusia. Sunitinib appears to be particularly prone to inducing hypothyroidism (61) and, in some cases, cardiomyopathy with decreased ejection fraction (EF) (62,63). Emerging data suggest that scrupulous control of blood pressure in patients on sunitinib will decrease cardiac stress and resultant cardiac failure.

Other side effects include wound dehiscence, and increased thromboembolic events. Perioperative complications in patients pretreated with antiangiogenic agents were reported in both prospective and retrospective studies published by the UTMDACC. In the prospective study (35), perioperative wound healing complications in patients who received 8 weeks of bevacizumab therapy were increased when compared to a set of matched controls. The retrospective study, which looked at 44 individuals who received either sorafenib, sunitinib, or bevacizumab preoperatively, did not detect a significant elevation of any perioperative events (64).

The mTOR inhibitors demonstrate several unique side effects, including hyperglycemia, hypertriglyceridemia, and noninfectious pneumonitis. On the other hand, these agents do not appear to induce hypertension, or hand foot syndrome.

TABLE
32-3 SIDE EFFECT SUMMARY OF MOLECULARLY TARGETED AGENTS

Agent	Sorafenib	Sunitinib	Bevacizumab	Pazopanib	Temsirolimus	Everolimus
Hypertension	XX	XX	XX	X		
Fatigue	XX	XX	X	X	X	X
Hand-foot syndrome	XX	XX		X		
Diarrhea	XX	XX		X	X	X
Dysgeusia	X	XX		X		
Mouth sores	X	X			X	X
Cardiac toxicity	X	XX	X	X		
Pulmonary toxicity					XX	XX
Hepatotoxicity				XX		
Hypertriglyceridemia					XX	XX
Rash	XX	XX			XX	XX
Hyperglycemia				X	XX	XX
Hypothyroidism	X	XX	?	?		
Proteinuria	X	X	XX	X		
Cytopenias	X	XX		X	X	X
Renal insufficiency	X	X	X	X	X	X

X, XX, and XXX: Low, Intermediate, and High Incidence

AGENT SELECTION AND SIDE EFFECT MANAGEMENT

A number of different factors come into play when choosing the best agent for patients with mRCC. Clearly, evidence-based criteria for usage are vital, but as seen in Table 32-4, there are several agents available for a particular treatment stage. For example, if we are dealing with a patient who has undergone nephrectomy, has good-risk characteristics, and is younger than 70 years, we can reasonably choose among high-dose interleukin-2, sunitinib, bevacizumab plus IFN or pazopanib. We need to take into consideration the patient's tolerance for

TABLE
32-4 DOSE REDUCTION ALGORITHM USED IN PIVOTAL TRIALS OF APPROVED TARGETED AGENTS*

Agent	Standard Dose	Dose Reduction Schema
Sorafenib	400 mg PO bid	Dose level -1: 400 mg PO daily
		Dose level -2: 400 mg PO every other day
		Alternate[†]: Dose reduction to 600 mg PO daily.
Sunitinib	50 mg PO daily 4 weeks on, followed by 2 weeks off	Dose level -1: 37.5 mg PO daily
		Dose level -2: 25 mg PO daily
		Alternate[†]: Schedule change to 50 mg PO 14 days on and 7 days off
Temsirolimus	25 mg IV weekly	Dose level -1: 20 mg IV weekly
		Dose level -2: 15 mg IV weekly
Everolimus	10 mg PO daily	Standard: Dose level -1: 5 mg PO daily
Bevacizumab	Bevacizumab 10 mg/kg IV every 14 days	IFN: Dose level -1 6MU SQ TIW
Plus IFN	IFN 9 Million Units (MU) subcutaneously (SQ) TIW	Dose level -2: 3MU SQ TIW
		Bevacizumab: for proteinuria: If greater than 2 g/dL hold until below 500 mg/dL
Pazopanib	800 mg PO daily	600 mg/day (Dose level -1); 400 mg/day (Dose level -2)

*Once patients are on therapy, there are several ways to mitigate side effects. The package inserts of each agent outline the standard algorithm for dose reduction. This table summarizes the standard dose reduction algorithms used in clinical trials of these agents.
[†]Not prospectively validated, but used empirically with good effect.

TABLE
32-5

MANAGEMENT RECOMMENDATIONS FOR COMMONLY EXPERIENCED TOXICITIES

Side Effect	*Preventative Measures*	*Supportive Care Measures*		
Diarrhea	In patients with prior history of diarrhea on agent, consider loperamide once daily in AM.	Loperamide 1-2 tabs post diarrhea	Diphenoxylate plus atropine	1 scoop psyllium with 1 oz water daily
Hand-foot syndrome	Heavy emollients applied to hands and feet bid and prn	As in preventive measures, plus urea-based callus creams		
Fatigue	Regular physical activity	Consider modafenil or methylphenidate	Check thyroid function	Short naps Regular exercise Regularized diet
Hypertension		Maintain BP below 140/90 using: 1. Ca channel blockers (Norvasc ok but not diltiazem) 2. Angiotensin-converting enzyme inhibitors 3. Beta blockers		
Hypothyroidism		Levothyroxine		
Dysgeusia	Salt and soda mouthwash four times a day	Avoidance of hot and spicy foods Salt and soda mouthwash	Carafate	
Mouth sores	Salt and soda mouthwash four times a day	Xylocaine-based mouthwash		
Hyperglycemia	Scrupulous glycemic control	Scrupulous glycemic control		
Rash (sorafenib)		Dose adjustment Aveeno baths		
Rash (temsirolimus and everolimus)		Topical steroids		

specific side effects. Table 32-5 provides a summary of some of the most common side effects seen with these agents. A review of these side effects may aid in treatment choice for specific patients. Some may have occupational considerations that make hand-foot syndrome a particular problem. Others may have cardiac comorbidities that make an agent like sunitinib, with a known effect on cardiac output in a subset of patients, less favorable.

Once patients are on therapy, there are several ways to mitigate side effects. The package inserts of each agent outline the standard algorithm for dose reduction. Table 32-4 summarizes the standard dose reduction algorithms used in clinical trials of these agents.

In addition to these maneuvers, a change in schedule may be beneficial for some patients. As the development of side effects will generally occur after a discrete period of time, it is sometimes possible to incorporate breaks in therapy that minimize normal tissue toxicity and maximize the amount of drug taken over a specific time period. Examples of such schedule changes include administering sunitinib for 14 days followed by a 7-day break. The same number of capsules is taken over a 6-week period, but with potentially less toxicity. These types of schedule changes have not been prospectively validated to show equivalent efficacy, but can be considered when the alternative is a dose reduction of the agent being used.

Symptom control is essential for patients receiving molecularly targeted agents. Table 32-5 outlines supportive care maneuvers that can mitigate or prevent specific side effects. It is essential that the patient and the health care team maintain an ongoing dialogue during each cycle of therapy to ensure that patients proactively and appropriately manage these toxicities. Successful side effect management will translate into higher drug compliance, and a greater probability of achieving a successful outcome.

NON-CLEAR-CELL RENAL CELL CARCINOMA

The large majority of studies performed to date excluded non–clear-cell RCC. The exception was the phase III temsirolimus study, where 20% of the 626 patients had **non–clear-cell** histology. A post-hoc analysis of papillary RCC showed outcomes similar to clear-cell RCC after treatment with temsirolimus (65). A 52-patient trial evaluating erlotinib in papillary RCC showed a response rate of 11%, and an overall survival of 27 months (66). A retrospective review of sunitinib and sorafenib use in non–clear-cell RCC suggested reasonable efficacy (67), but preliminary data from an ongoing study at UTMDACC contradict these findings (68). Unfortunately choosing the right agent for this relatively heterogeneous group of patients is hampered by a lack of studies, and relatively small patient numbers to gain experience from. In the absence of clinical trials, an mTOR inhibitor is a reasonable first step for patients with papillary RCC. Other histologies are even more difficult to select agents due to very small numbers and poor understanding of their underlying biology. Clinical trials are the preferred route for these patients. An ongoing prospective phase II trial at UTMDACC is evaluating the efficacy of sunitinib in patients with **non–clear-cell** histology.

SARCOMATOID RENAL CELL CARCINOMA

Approximately 5% of all patients with RCC will demonstrate sarcomatoid dedifferentiation in their tumors (69). Varying percentages of sarcomatoid involvement can be seen, and in cases where there is a predominance of sarcomatoid cells, it is difficult to determine the underlying histological background. In these extreme cases, epithelial tumor markers are still present on the tumor cells, distinguishing these tumors from frank sarcomas.

Presence of sarcomatoid features in the tumor portends a poor prognosis (70). In a retrospective review at UTMDACC, the median survival for patients with all stages of sarcomatoid RCC was 9 months (71). Use of a fluoropyrimidine-containing regimen at some point in the disease course was associated with better outcome. Several reports were published in the past decade describing the use of a variety of agents, including the combination of gemcitabine plus doxorubicin, which may provide short-term control in some patients (72). A retrospective analysis of an empirical regimen consisting of the combination of gemcitabine, capecitabine plus bevacizumab in 28 patients with mRCC, several of whom having poor-risk characteristics, including 8 with sarcomatoid features, showed a median PFS of 5.9 months and a median OS of 10.4 months. These observations formed the basis of a prospective ongoing study at UTMDACC using this three-drug combination in patients with sarcomatoid histology.

COLLECTING DUCT CARCINOMA

Tumors arising from the collecting duct epithelium are located in the medulla or center portion of the kidney, in contrast to RCC tumors, which arise from tubules in the cortex (73). The diagnosis of collecting duct carcinoma (CDC) is based on both clinical and histologic features. Sarcomatoid dedifferentiation is not uncommon, and patterns of metastasis are similar to those of a high-grade, rapidly progressive RCC. There is no established effective systemic therapy for metastatic CDC, although marginal benefit is occasionally seen with IFNα or chemotherapy regimens developed for transitional cell carcinoma (70,74).

MEDULLARY CARCINOMA

Renal medullary carcinoma is a rare and virulent malignancy, afflicting patients with sickle cell hemoglobinopathies, usually sickle cell trait, sickle thalassemia, or hemoglobin SC disease (75). It arises from the caliceal epithelium and can be morphologically distinguished from RCC and CDC. Some investigators have suggested that it is a dedifferentiated form of transitional cell carcinoma. Other kidney disorders associated with sickle cell hemoglobinopathies include unilateral hematuria, papillary necrosis, nephrotic syndrome, renal infarction, inability to concentrate urine, and pyelonephritis. These associated conditions may contribute to the development of renal medullary carcinoma. The majority of cases reported have a highly aggressive clinical course, presenting with metastatic disease and with survival averaging only 3 months. It is refractory to most forms of systemic therapy (76), with some responses to M-VAC reported and also observed at our institution.

A recent case series from UTMDACC evaluated the impact of using antiangiogenic agents to treat patients with medullary RCC (34). Longer OS was seen in patients with medullary RCC who were treated with a bevacizumab-containing regimen. Validation of this finding will require a prospective study, a difficult undertaking in this extremely rare disease entity.

XP11.2 TRANSLOCATION CARCINOMA

Xp11.2 translocation carcinoma is a rare disease entity that is proportionally more common in children, but can occur in young adults (77). The specific chromosomal translocation t(X;1)(p11.2;q21.2 results in the fusion of a novel gene designated PRCC at 1q21.2 to the TFE3 gene at Xp11.2 (78). Histologically, these tumors may resemble clear-cell RCC or show mixed clear and papillary features. These histological findings in a young adult should prompt further histological and molecular characterization of the tumor. Staining for TFE3 permits relatively specific identification of this disease entity (79). In a case series of 28 adult patients, a strong female predominance was observed, and 14 patients presented with metastatic disease (77). Response to standard immunotherapy or chemotherapy is poor, and patients have a relatively short overall survival. A retrospective review of 15 adult patients (12 females; median age 40 years) with translocation carcinoma who were treated with targeted therapy at four centers in the United States showed an overall response rate (ORR) of 20%, with median PFS of 7.1 months and median OS of 14.3 months (80). A French study reported on 21 patients with adult translocation carcinoma treated with anti-VEGF agents or mTOR inhibitors. The authors reported objective responses, PFS, and OS results in the range of those previously reported for clear-cell RCC (81).

PRIMITIVE NEUROECTODERMAL TUMOR OF THE KIDNEY

Neuroectodermal tumors are most familiar as Ewing sarcoma in children, but are also seen, rarely, in adults and in peripheral organs (82). A small cell tumor of the kidney may be described on the basis of this morphology as adult Wilms tumor, adult Ewing sarcoma, or primitive neuroectodermal tumor (PNET). The immunohistochemical detection of CD99 antigen (mic-2) establishes the diagnosis of PNET; in this instance, there is no meaningful distinction between the terms *Ewing sarcoma* and *PNET*. The treatment algorithms developed for pediatric/skeletal Ewing sarcoma involve combined chemotherapy, radiotherapy, and surgical excision and are not well suited for PNET of the kidney. In case reports, patients with metastatic PNET have received drugs for Ewing sarcoma or soft tissue sarcomas (eg, vincristine, ifosfamide, actinomycin D, and doxorubicin) and frequently have partial responses, but without long-term tumor control and with reported survival of less than 5 years. At UTMDACC, we have recently used a dose-dense regimen developed for small cell carcinoma of the urinary tract consisting of etoposide and cisplatin, alternating with doxorubicin and ifosfamide, given every 3 weeks. Additional patients and follow-up are needed to determine whether this approach merits further study in metastatic PNET of the kidney or as adjuvant therapy.

■ LOCAL THERAPY FOR METASTASES

Local therapy decisions in metastatic RCC frequently and significantly affect the clinical course beyond the mere palliation of symptoms. Metastasectomy is appropriate in selected patients depending on the number and sites of metastases, presence of symptoms or threatening location, and other coexisting risk factors (80). Solitary lesions in the brain, spine, chest, or extremities are usually amenable to surgical control; however, systemic therapy should be considered for early recurrences (<1 year from nephrectomy), with surgical consolidation in the event of a response. Late recurrences have an excellent prognosis with metastasectomy alone, and systemic therapy can be deferred in most of these cases. The histologic subtype is not predictive of disease velocity, which must be determined empirically. Exceptions are high-grade or sarcomatoid tumors, which metastasize quickly, with median time to progression of only 2 months; these are usually poor candidates for surgery (71,84).

METASTASECTOMY

RCC metastases in the thorax are often amenable to resection. Pulmonary parenchymal metastases can usually be resected with negative margins, whereas lymph node and pleural disease tends to be more diffuse. A solitary pulmonary parenchymal recurrence more than 1 year from diagnosis is an indication for surgery in selected patients, but patients with additional disease are better managed initially with systemic therapy. Patients who achieve partial response and have residual masses in the chest should be considered for surgical consolidation and, whenever possible, rendered disease-free.

Aggressive management of vertebral metastases in RCC can be rewarding. Lytic metastases to the vertebrae are common, often associated with a soft tissue component or epidural extension, and have a high potential for spinal cord compression. Responses to conventional radiotherapy in this location are suboptimal and of limited benefit. Vertebrectomy with internal reconstruction is the preferred approach at MD Anderson Cancer Center and should be performed by an experienced team. Postoperative radiotherapy to the spine should be considered when residual disease is suspected.

In some circumstances, sterotactic radiosurgery with any of a number of currently available systems may forestall surgery, and can be considered in cases where there is no imminent threat of neurologic compromise.

Lesions in the humerus or femur associated with fracture or loss of cortical integrity are best controlled with en bloc resection, hemiarthroplasty, and postoperative radiation. Smaller lesions can be initially controlled with radiation or placement of an intramedullary nail.

■ ADJUVANT THERAPY FOR NONMETASTATIC PATIENTS

Currently, no effective adjuvant therapy exists for patients who undergo nephrectomy for locally advanced RCC. Risk stratification for this patient population is determined by a variety of factors implicated in RCC tumor biology, including tumor stage, Fuhrman grade, and PS (85). Ideally, an effective adjuvant therapy should be relatively nontoxic, demonstrate some efficacy in the metastatic setting, and be easily administered in the outpatient setting. Currently, proven effective adjuvant therapy for RCC does not exist. Results are anticipated from several other ongoing adjuvant trials, which may redefine the role of adjuvant therapy in RCC.

Immunotherapy was a logical choice as an adjuvant strategy in RCC, since IL-2 and IFNα had demonstrated some efficacy in the metastatic setting. Unfortunately, even the limited benefits of immunotherapy for metastatic disease have not been realized in the adjuvant setting (87-89). To date, no trial utilizing adjuvant immunotherapy has demonstrated a survival benefit, and there has been significant toxicity, thus further dampening enthusiasm for this approach.

Vaccine strategies have also been explored as potential adjuvant therapies for RCC. Initial studies in tumor vaccination for RCC examined the role of whole-tumor cell lysates harvested from radical nephrectomy specimens at the time of surgery (86,90). Jocham et al. performed a randomized study involving 558 patients at 55 institutions (86). Before surgery, all patients were centrally randomized to receive autologous renal tumor cell vaccine or no adjuvant treatment. A total of 379 patients were assessable for the intention-to-treat analysis. At 5-year and 70-month follow-up, the hazard ratios for tumor progression were 1.58 (95% confidence interval

1.05-2.37) and 1.59 (1.07-2.36), respectively, in favor of the vaccine group (p = .0204, log-rank test). Another vaccine strategy that has been applied in a variety of solid tumors including RCC is the heat-shock protein 96 vaccine. Heat-shock proteins are intra-cellular molecular chaperones that bind peptide fragments, which represent the antigenic complement of the cell. These proteins, with their associated peptides, can be highly purified from excised surgical specimens and utilized for vaccine preparation. A multicenter phase III study of adjuvant heat-shock protein 96 vaccines for patients with RCC at high risk of relapse following nephrectomy was reported and no PFS advantage was seen in those who received vaccine (91). The ongoing Rencarex trial is assessing the efficacy of a monoclonal chimeric antibody (cG250) against CAIX, a cell surface molecule overexpressed in VHL-mutated tumors. Patients received cG250 IV once weekly for 24 weeks, or a placebo injection. This trial accrued 864 patients, and final results are expected by 2013.

Several clinical trials evaluating the role of adjuvant antiangiogenic therapy are currently enrolling patients. These include the ASSURE trial, led by Eastern Cooperative Oncology Group, which randomizes patients between 1 year of sunitinib, sorafenib, or placebo. A large, placebo-controlled, phase 3 British trial is evaluating the efficacy of 1 year of sorafenib versus 3 years of sorafenib. Other similar trials are also recruiting patients.

■ SUCCESSFUL STRATEGIES: CASE EXAMPLES

Treatment strategies must be individualized according to the extent of disease, prior treatment, and level of illness. Disease that is unresectable and refractory to systemic therapy should receive a symptom-directed approach, whereas patients with good PS and minimal pretreatment can be managed aggressively with both local and systemic modalities.

CASE EXAMPLE 1: SEQUENTIAL-TARGETED THERAPY

A 51-year-old man developed gross hematuria, and was found to have a 6 cm renal mass. He underwent nephrectomy, revealing a grade 3-4 clear-cell RCC. Six months later, follow-up scans showed new multifocal bilateral pulmonary nodules. He was placed on a clinical trial of sorafenib therapy, and demonstrated progression after 2 months, with 29% growth of his lesions. He was then placed on sunitinib therapy, and showed progression with 3 months. He was then placed on gemcitabine and capecitabine, and progressed after 8 weeks. He was experiencing worsening night sweats, weight loss, and fatigue. He now had enlarging pulmonary nodules, and had developed multiple intra-abdominal metastatic deposits. He was then switched over to temsirolimus, and showed a rapid resolution of constitutional symptoms, and regression of all sites of disease. After a year of temsirolimus therapy, he showed asymptomatic slight disease progression, and bevacizumab 10 mg/kg IV every 14 days was added to temsirolimus. He remained stable for another 9 months, at which point he was placed on a clinical trial.

Comment: At this point we still do not know how to match therapy to disease phenotype. The key for positive patient outcome is to move from one therapy to another when clinically appropriate and to maintain the patient's performance status, to make a therapy switch feasible. Despite the aggressive course of his disease at the outset, he has been alive for over 3 years.

CASE EXAMPLE 2: EFFICACY OF GEMCITABINE AND CAPECITABINE IN IMMUNOTHERAPY AND TARGETED-THERAPY REFRACTORY PATIENTS

A 51-year-old man underwent cytoreductive nephrectomy for clear-cell RCC metastatic to lungs and intrathoracic lymph nodes. He started high-dose IL-2 2 months later, and showed progression after two cycles of therapy with new liver and lung metastases. He was then started on bevacizumab plus erlotinib, and showed further progression of disease, and the interval development of hypercalcemia. He was then started on gemcitabine and capecitabine combination therapy, and showed a rapid improvement of clinical and radiographic findings. He achieved a CR 18 months later (Fig. 32-3), and was kept on maintenance capecitabine for 3 months, and has been off all therapy for the past $2^{1}/_{2}$ years.

Comment: The combination of gemcitabine and a fluoropyrimidine has been shown to provide benefit in prospective trials (50,51). Here is a further example of two principles: (1) Careful sequencing of therapy may lead to a regimen that is effective in a specific patient and (2) Gemcitabine and capecitabine provide non-overlapping efficacy to immunotherapy and targeted therapy, and should be considered in patients refractory to these agents.

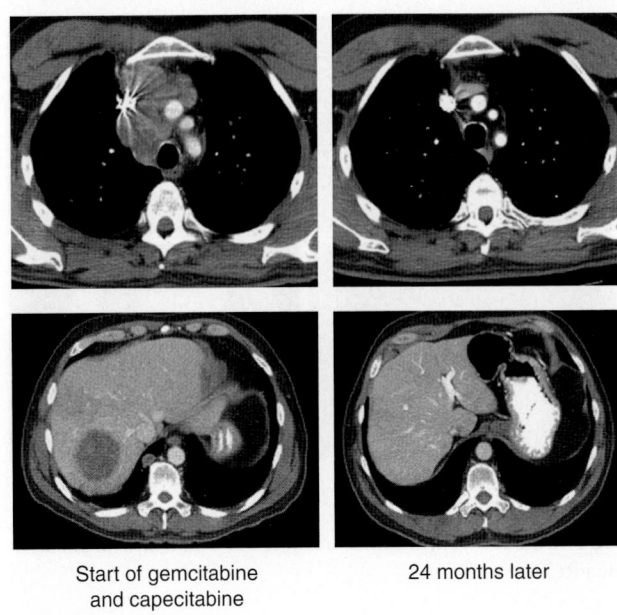

Start of gemcitabine and capecitabine   24 months later

FIGURE 32-3.   Response to gemcitabine and capecitabine in an immunotherapy and antiangiogenic therapy refractory patient.

CASE EXAMPLE 3: RAPAMYCIN ANALOGUES IN NON-CLEAR-CELL HISTOLOGY

A 67-year-old woman presented with anemia, a right renal mass and possible pulmonary metastases. She underwent right cytoreductive nephrectomy for a 14-cm unclassified T4 N0 MX RCC. Three months post-op, she developed progression in the renal fossa, liver, right chest wall, lungs and presented to UTMDACC. She received sunitinib on a phase 2 protocol, and experienced grade 3 LFT elevations, worsening PS, worsening anemia and had progressive disease (PD) at the 6-week restaging visit. Temsirolimus was started at 20 mg IVPB weekly. After six infusions, she noted improvement in her symptoms, and restaging showed dramatic tumor regression at all sites of disease (Fig. 32-4). She developed asymptomatic pneumonitis, but continued therapy with temsirolimus for approximately 13 months until she developed PD. She did not receive further therapy and died of PD 22 months after initial diagnosis of stage IV RCC.

Comment: Unclassified RCC does not have a standard therapy associated with it, due to the fact that most recent phase III studies included only patients with clear cell histology. The exception is the randomized phase III study of temsirolimus, where 20% had non–clear-cell histology. A post-hoc review of these patients suggests that temsirolimus may be effective in patients with **non–clear-cell** histology (65).

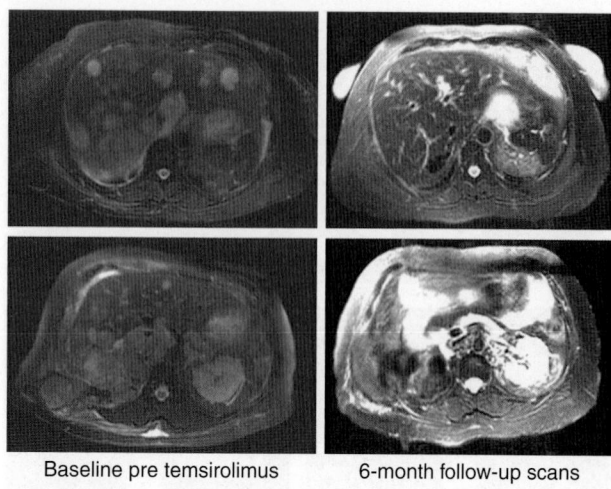

Baseline pre temsirolimus   6-month follow-up scans

FIGURE 32-4. Temsirolimus treatment in a patient with unclassified RCC.

CASE EXAMPLE 4: METASTASECTOMY IN A PATIENT WITH INDOLENT DISEASE

A 55-year-old man presented with an 8-cm left kidney tumor and clear-cell histology. He was observed after radical nephrectomy and developed bilateral pulmonary nodules after 15 months. Wedge resections were performed, of which two contained metastatic RCC. There was no evidence of disease postoperatively, and he was followed. He had a second pulmonary recurrence 9 years later but was asymptomatic. He was kept on observation, demonstrating gradual progression in the lungs and a new adrenal metastasis. At last follow-up he was 13 years postnephrectomy and remained asymptomatic.

Comment: Patients with metastatic RCC can be safely observed when they are asymptomatic and have no threatening sites of disease, thereby avoiding unnecessary surgery or premature administration of systemic therapy.

CASE EXAMPLE 5: BRAIN METASTASES

A 64-year-old man underwent a right partial nephrectomy for a cystic renal cell carcinoma. Two years later he developed mediastinal, and pulmonary metastases with biopsy consistent with metastatic RCC. On workup for a clinical trial, he was found to have a solitary, asymptomatic temporal lobe brain metastasis. He underwent stereotactic radiosurgery, and was started on sorafenib therapy. Seventeen months later, a second brain metastasis was found, and also treated with stereotactic

radiosurgery. Two months later several new brain lesions were found and he received whole brain radiation therapy. Subsequent to his whole brain radiation he has not experienced any further progression in his brain. His mediastinal adenopathy progressed after 6 months, and he was switched to sunitinib therapy. His systemic disease remained stable on sunitinib therapy for 2 years, upon which he demonstrated progression and had his systemic therapy further modified. He is still alive after 4 years.

Comment: Stereotactic radiosurgery is appropriate for patients with solitary or oligometastatic lesions, which are less than 2 cm in size. For multiple brain metastases, whole brain radiation therapy is a reasonable approach, and can achieve CNS control in a subset of individuals. In this case, sequential systemic therapy provided benefit and the patient has been alive for over 4 years.

CASE EXAMPLE 6: MANAGEMENT OF BONE METASTASES

A 42-year-old man was found to have an 8.2-cm renal mass after complaining of worsening bone pain. He underwent nephrectomy, confirming a grade 3 clear-cell RCC, and workup of his bone pain revealed multifocal metastatic disease, including a lesion on the T7 vertebral body. He underwent radical nephrectomy, and upon recovery received stereotactic radiosurgery to his T7 lesion and T11 lesions. He also received conventional radiation to his L5-S1 spine and to his right femur. He was placed on an experimental study of zolendronic acid, gamma interferon, and thalidomide, and demonstrated minimal progression after 4 months. He was continued on zolendronic acid alone, and did not experience substantial further progression for close to a year, when he developed a left iliac lesion, which was treated with external beam radiation. Nine months later, a scapular lesion was radiated, and he was then started off study on bevacizumab and erlotinib. He remained stable on this combination, plus zolendronic acid, for close to 9 months, at which point further local interventions were needed.

Comment: Bone metastases are a particularly difficult issue for patients with RCC, and may demonstrate an attenuated response to most commonly used systemic therapies. An integration of radiation, surgery, thermal ablation (radiofrequency ablation, cryoablation), and embolization can provide relief and improved quality of life. Zolendronic acid is undoubtedly also of value in RCC (92), and should be administered to patients with bone metastases.

References

1. Jemal A, Siegel R, Ward E, et al. Cancer statistics, 2009. *CA Cancer J Clin* 2009;59:225-249.

2. Chow WH, Devesa SS, Warren JL, et al. Rising incidence of renal cell cancer in the United States. *JAMA* 1999;281: 1628-1631.

3. Kidney. In: Edge SB, Byrd DR, Compton CC, et al., eds.: AJCC Cancer Staging Manual. 7th ed. New York, NY: Springer, 2010, pp. 479-489.

4. Linehan WM, Walther MM, Zbar B. The genetic basis of cancer of the kidney. *J Urol* 2003;170:2163-2172.

5. Parker AS, Cerhan JR, Janney CA, et al. Smoking cessation and renal cell carcinoma. *Ann Epidemiol* 2003;13:245-251.

6. Kamat AM, Shock RP, Naya Y, et al. Prognostic value of body mass index in patients undergoing nephrectomy for localized renal tumors. *Urology* 2004;63:46-50.

7. Chow WH, Gridley G, Fraumeni JF Jr, et al. Obesity, hypertension, and the risk of kidney cancer in men. *N Engl J Med* 2000;343:1305-1311.

8. Grossman E, Messerli FH, Boyko V, et al. Is there an association between hypertension and cancer mortality? *Am J Med* 2002;112:479-486.

9. Grossman E, Messerli FH. Diuretics and renal cell carcinoma–What is the risk/benefit ration? *Kidney Int* 1999;56: 1603-1604.

10. Lindblad P, Wolk A, Bergstrom R, et al. Diet and risk of renal cell cancer: A population-based case-control study. *Cancer Epidemiol Biomarkers Prev* 1997;6:215-223.

11. Parker AS, Cerhan JR, Lynch CF, et al. Gender, alcohol consumption, and renal cell carcinoma. *Am J Epidemiol* 2002; 155:455-462.

12. Yuan JM, Gago-Dominguez M, Castelao JE, et al. Cruciferous vegetables in relation to renal cell carcinoma. *Int J Cancer* 1998;77:211-216.

13. Zisman A, Pantuck AJ, Dorey F, et al. Improved prognostication of renal cell carcinoma using an integrated staging system. *J Clin Oncol* 2001;19:1649-1657.

14. Bukowski RM. Prognostic factors for survival in metastatic renal cell carcinoma: Update 2008. *Cancer* 2009;115:2273-2281.

15. Eichelberg C, Junker K, Ljungberg B, et al. Diagnostic and prognostic molecular markers for renal cell carcinoma: A critical appraisal of the current state of research and clinical applicability. *Eur Urol* 2009;55:851-863.

16. Isbarn H, Karakiewicz PI. Predicting cancer-control outcomes in patients with renal cell carcinoma. *Curr Opin Urol* 2009; 19:247-257.

17. Motzer RJ, Mazumdar M, Bacik J, et al. Survival and prognostic stratification of 670 patients with advanced renal cell carcinoma. *J Clin Oncol* 1999;17:2530-2540.

18. Motzer RJ, Bacik J, Mariani T, et al. Treatment outcome and survival associated with metastatic renal cell carcinoma of **non–clear-cell** histology. *J Clin Oncol* 2002;20:2376-2381.

19. Tannir NM, Cohen L, Wang X, et al. Improved tolerability and quality of life with maintained efficacy using twice-daily low-dose interferon-alpha-2b: Results of a randomized phase II trial of low-dose versus intermediate-dose interferon-alpha-2b in patients with metastatic renal cell carcinoma. *Cancer* 2006; 107:2254-2261.

20. Montero AJ, Diaz-Montero CM, Millikan RE, et al. Cytokines and angiogenic factors in patients with metastatic renal cell carcinoma treated with interferon-alpha: Association of pretreatment serum levels with survival. *Ann Oncol* 2009;20: 1682-1687.

21. Zurita AJ, Jonasch E, Wu HK, et al. Circulating biomarkers for vascular endothelial growth factor inhibitors in renal cell carcinoma. *Cancer* 2009;115:2346-2354.

22. Shuin T, Kondo K, Torigoe S, et al. Frequent somatic mutations and loss of heterozygosity of the von Hippel-Lindau tumor suppressor gene in primary human renal cell carcinomas. *Cancer Res* 1994;54:2852-2855.

23. Yao M, Yoshida M, Kishida T, et al. VHL Tumor suppressor gene alterations associated with good prognosis in sporadic clear-cell renal carcinoma. *J Natl Cancer Inst* 2002;94: 1569-1575.

24. Ashida S, Nishimori I, Tanimura M, et al. Effects of von Hippel-Lindau gene mutation and methylation status on expression of transmembrane carbonic anhydrases in renal cell carcinoma. *J Cancer Res Clin Oncol* 2002;128:561-568.

25. Bui M, Seligson D, Han K, et al. Carbonic anhydrase IX is an independent predictor of survival in advanced renal clear cell carcinoma: Implications for prognosis and therapy. *Clinical Cancer Research* 2003;9:802-811.

26. Levy DA, Swanson DA, Slaton JW, et al. Timely delivery of biological therapy after cytoreductive nephrectomy in carefully selected patients with metastatic renal cell carcinoma. *J Urol* 1998;159:1168-1173.

27. Wood CG, Huber N, Madsen L, et al. Clinical variables that predict survival following cytoreductive nephrectomy for metastatic renal cell carcinoma. *J Urol* 2001;165(5):184A.

28. Mickisch GH, Garin A, van Poppel H, et al. Radical nephrectomy plus interferon-alfa-based immunotherapy compared with interferon alfa alone in metastatic renal-cell carcinoma: A randomised trial. *Lancet* 2001;358:966-970.

29. Flanigan RC, Salmon SE, Blumenstein BA, et al. Nephrectomy followed by interferon alfa-2b compared with interferon alfa-2b alone for metastatic renal-cell cancer. *N Engl J Med* 2001;345:1655-1659.

30. Escudier B, Eisen T, Stadler WM, et al. Sorafenib in advanced clear-cell renal-cell carcinoma. *N Engl J Med* 2007; 356:125-134.

31. Escudier B, Pluzanska A, Koralewski P, et al. Bevacizumab plus interferon alfa-2a for treatment of metastatic renal cell carcinoma: A randomised, double-blind phase III trial. *Lancet* 2007;370:2103-2111.

32. Hudes G, Carducci M, Tomczak P, et al. Temsirolimus, interferon alfa, or both for advanced renal-cell carcinoma. *N Engl J Med* 2007;356:2271-2281.

33. Motzer RJ, Hutson TE, Tomczak P, et al. Sunitinib versus interferon alfa in metastatic renal-cell carcinoma. *N Engl J Med* 2007;356:115-124.

34. Johnson ED, Tannir NM, Logothetis CJ, et al. Survival benefit in bevacizumab based therapy in sickle cell trait patients diagnosed with renal medullary carcinoma. In: American Society of Clinical Oncology Genitourinary Cancers Symposium, 2009; Orlando, FL. (Abstract 335). 2009, 335.

35. JonaAch E, Wood CG, Matin SF, et al. Phase II presurgical feasibility study of bevacizumab in untreated patients with metastatic renal cell carcinoma. *J Clin Oncol* 2009;27(25): 4076-4081.

36. Freed SZ, Halperin JP, Gordon M. Idiopathic regression of metastases from renal cell carcinoma. *J Urol* 1977;118:538-542.

37. Fyfe G, Fisher RI, Rosenberg SA, et al. Results of treatment of 255 patients with metastatic renal cell carcinoma who received high-dose recombinant interleukin-2 therapy. *J Clin Oncol* 1995;13:688-696.

38. Pyrhonen S, Salminen E, Ruutu M, et al. Prospective randomized trial of interferon alfa-2a plus vinblastine versus vinblastine alone in patients with advanced renal cell cancer. *J Clin Oncol* 1999;17:2859-2867.

39. Interferon-alpha and survival in metastatic renal carcinoma: Early results of a randomised controlled trial. Medical Research Council Renal Cancer Collaborators. *Lancet* 1999;353:14-17.

40. Negrier S, Caty A, Lesimple T, et al. Treatment of patients with metastatic renal carcinoma with a combination of subcutaneous interleukin-2 and interferon alfa with or without fluorouracil. *J Clin Oncol* 2000;18:4009-4015.

41. Atzpodien J, Lopez Hanninen E, Kirchner H, et al. Multiinstitutional home-therapy trial of recombinant human interleukin-2 and interferon alfa-2 in progressive metastatic renal cell carcinoma. *J Clin Oncol* 1995;13:497-501.

42. Ellerhorst JA, Sella A, Amato RJ, et al. Phase II trial of 5-flurorouracil, interferon-alpha and continuous infusion interleukin-2 for patients with metastatic renal cell carcinoma. *Cancer* 1997; 80:2128-2132.

43. Pantuck AJ, Zisman A, Dorey F, et al. Renal cell carcinoma with retroperitoneal lymph nodes. Impact on survival and benefits of immunotherapy. *Cancer* 2003;97:2995-3002.

44. Cho DC, Puzanov I, Regan MM, et al. Retrospective analysis of the safety and efficacy of interleukin-2 after prior VEGF-targeted therapy in patients with advanced renal cell carcinoma. *J Immunother* 2009;32:181-185.

45. Marten A, Flieger D, Renoth S, et al. Therapeutic vaccination against metastatic renal cell carcinoma by autologous dendritic cells: Preclinical results and outcome of a first clinical phase I/II trial. *Cancer Immunol Immunother* 2002;51:637-644.

46. Avigan DE, Vasir B, George DJ, et al. Phase I/II study of vaccination with electrofused allogeneic dendritic cells/autologous tumor-derived cells in patients with stage IV renal cell carcinoma. *J Immunother* 2007;30:749-761.

47. Childs R, Chernoff A, Contentin N, et al. Regression of metastatic renal-cell carcinoma after nonmyeloablative allogeneic peripheral-blood stem-cell transplantation. *N Engl J Med* 2000;343:750-758.

48. Ueno NT, Cheng YC, Rondon G, et al. Rapid induction of complete donor chimerism by the use of a reduced-intensity conditioning regimen composed of fludarabine and melphalan in allogeneic stem cell transplantation for metastatic solid tumors. *Blood* 2003;102:3829-3836.

49. Rini BI, Zimmerman T, Stadler WM, et al. Allogeneic stem-cell transplantation of renal cell cancer after nonmyeloablative chemotherapy: Feasibility, engraftment, and clinical results. *J Clin Oncol* 2002;20:2017-2024.

50. Rini BI, Vogelzang NJ, Dumas MC, et al. Phase II trial of weekly intravenous gemcitabine with continuous infusion fluorouracil in patients with metastatic renal cell cancer. *J Clin Oncol* 2000;18:2419-2426.

51. Tannir NM, Thall PF, Ng CS, et al. A phase II trial of gemcitabine plus capecitabine for metastatic renal cell cancer previously treated with immunotherapy and targeted agents. *J Urol* 2008;180:867-872; discussion 872.

52. Escudier B, Koralewski P, Pluzanska A, et al and investigators, o. b. o. t. A. A randomized, controlled, double-blind phase III study (AVOREN) of bevacizumab/interferon-α2a vs placebo/interferon- α2a as first-line therapy in metastatic renal cell carcinoma. *J Clin Oncol* 2007;25:3.

53. Rini BI, Halabi S, Rosenberg JE, et al. Bevacizumab plus interferon alfa compared with interferon alfa monotherapy in patients with metastatic renal cell carcinoma: CALGB 90206. *J Clin Oncol* 2008;26:5422-5428.

54. Escudier B, Szczylik C, Hutson TE, et al. Randomized phase II trial of first-line treatment with sorafenib versus interferon Alfa-2a in patients with metastatic renal cell carcinoma. *J Clin Oncol* 2009;27:1280-1289.

55. Motzer RJ, Michaelson MD, Redman BG, et al. Activity of SU11248, a multitargeted inhibitor of vascular endothelial growth factor receptor and platelet-derived growth factor receptor, in patients with metastatic renal cell carcinoma. *J Clin Oncol* 2006;24:16-24.

56. Motzer RJ, Hutson TE, Tomczak P, et al. A. Overall survival and updated results for sunitinib compared with interferon alfa in patients with metastatic renal cell carcinoma. *J Clin Oncol* 2009;27:3584-3590.

57. Harris PA, Boloor A, Cheung M, et al. Discovery of 5-[[4-[(2,3-dimethyl-2H-indazol-6-yl)methylamino]-2-pyrimidinyl]amino]-2-m ethyl-benzenesulfonamide (Pazopanib), a novel and potent vascular endothelial growth factor receptor inhibitor. *J Med Chem* 2008;51:4632-4640.

58. Sternberg CN, Davis ID, Mardiak J, et al. Pazopanib in locally advanced or metastatic renal cell carcinoma: results of a randomized phase III trial. *J Clin Oncol* 2010;28: 1061-1068.

59. Atkins MB, Hidalgo M, Stadler WM, et al. Randomized phase II study of multiple dose levels of CCI-779, a novel mammalian target of rapamycin kinase inhibitor, in patients with advanced refractory renal cell carcinoma. *J Clin Oncol* 2004; 22:909-918.

60. Motzer RJ, Escudier B, Oudard S, et al. Efficacy of everolimus in advanced renal cell carcinoma: A double-blind, randomised, placebo-controlled phase III trial. *Lancet* 2008;372:449-456.

61. Rini BI, Tamaskar I, Shaheen P, et al. Hypothyroidism in patients with metastatic renal cell carcinoma treated with sunitinib. *J Natl Cancer Inst* 2007;99:81-83.

62. Schmidinger M, Zielinski CC, Vogl UM, et al. Cardiac toxicity of sunitinib and sorafenib in patients with metastatic renal cell carcinoma. *J Clin Oncol* 2008;26:5204-5212.

63. Khakoo AY, Kassiotis CM, Tannir N, et al. Heart failure associated with sunitinib malate: A multitargeted receptor tyrosine kinase inhibitor. *Cancer* 2008;112:2500-2508.

64. Margulis V, Matin SF, Tannir N, et al. Surgical morbidity associated with administration of targeted molecular therapies before cytoreductive nephrectomy or resection of locally recurrent renal cell carcinoma. *J Urol* 2008;180:94-98.

65. Dutcher JP, de Souza P, McDermott D, et al. Effect of temsirolimus versus interferon-alpha on outcome of patients with advanced renal cell carcinoma of different tumor histologies. *Med Oncol,* 2009;26:202-209.

66. Gordon MS, Hussey M, Nagle RB, et al. Phase II Study of Erlotinib in Patients With Locally Advanced or Metastatic Papillary Histology Renal Cell Cancer: SWOG S0317. *J Clin Oncol* 2009;27(34):5788-5793.

67. Choueiri TK, Plantade A, Elson P, et al. Efficacy of sunitinib and sorafenib in metastatic papillary and chromophobe renal cell carcinoma. *J Clin Oncol* 2008;26:127-131.

68. Plimack ER, Jonasch E, Bekele BN, et al. Sunitinib in non-clear cell renal cell carcinoma (ncc-RCC): A phase II study. *J Clin Oncol* 2008; 26 (May 20 suppl): (Abstract 5112).

69. Cheville JC, Lohse CM, Zincke H, et al. Sarcomatoid renal cell carcinoma: An examination of underlying histologic subtype and an analysis of associations with patient outcome. *Am J Surg Pathol* 2004;28:435-441.

70. Cheville JC, Lohse CM, Zincke H, et al. Comparisons of outcome and prognostic features among histologic subtypes of renal cell carcinoma. *Am J Surg Pathol* 2003;27:612-624.

71. Mian BM, Bhadkamkar N, Slaton JW, et al. Prognostic factors and survival of patients with sarcomatoid renal cell carcinoma. *J Urol* 2002;167:65-70.

72. Nanus DM, Garino A, Milowsky MI, et al. Active chemotherapy for sarcomatoid and rapidly progressing renal cell carcinoma. *Cancer* 2004;101:1545-1551.

73. Peyromaure M, Thiounn N, Scotte F, et al. Collecting duct carcinoma of the kidney: A clinicopathological study of 9 cases. *J Urol* 2003;170:1138-1140.

74. Gollob JA, Upton MP, DeWolf WC, et al. Long-term remission in a patient with metastatic collecting duct carcinoma treated with taxol/carboplatin and surgery. *Urology* 2001; 58:1058.

75. Davis CJ Jr, Mostofi FK, Sesterhenn IA. Renal medullary carcinoma. The seventh sickle cell nephropathy. *Am J Surg Pathol* 1995;19:1-11.

76. Avery RA, Harris JE, Davis CJ Jr, et al. Renal medullary carcinoma: Clinical and therapeutic aspects of a newly described tumor. *Cancer* 1996;78:128-132.

77. Argani P, Olgac S, Tickoo SK, et al. Xp11 translocation renal cell carcinoma in adults: Expanded clinical, pathologic, and genetic spectrum. *Am J Surg Pathol* 2007;31:1149-1160.

78. Sidhar SK, Clark J, Gill S, et al. The t(X;1)(p11.2;q21.2) translocation in papillary renal cell carcinoma fuses a novel gene PRCC to the TFE3 transcription factor gene. *Hum Mol Genet* 1996;5:1333-1338.

79. Argani P, Lal P, Hutchinson B, et al. Aberrant nuclear immunoreactivity for TFE3 in neoplasms with TFE3 gene fusions: A sensitive and specific immunohistochemical assay. *Am J Surg Pathol* 2003;27:750-761.

80. Choueiri TK, Lim ZD, Hirsch MS, et al. Vascular endothelial growth factor-targeted therapy for the treatment of adult metastatic Xp11.2 translocation renal cell carcinoma. *Cancer* 2010;116(22):5219-5225.

81. Malouf G, Camparo P, Oudard S, et al. Targeted agents in metastatic Xp11 Translocation/TFE3 gene fusion renal cell carcinoma (RCC): A report from the Juvenile RCC Network. In: ECCO Berlin, 2009: O-7104.

82. Kennedy JG, Eustace S, Caulfield R, et al. Extraskeletal Ewing's sarcoma: A case report and review of the literature. *Spine* (Phila PA 1976) 2000;25:1996-1999.

83. Daliani DD, Tannir NM, Papandreou CN, et al. Prospective assessment of systemic therapy followed by surgical removal of metastases in selected patients with renal cell carcinoma. *BJU Int* 2009;104:456-460.

84. Leibovich BC, Han KR, Bui MH, et al. Scoring algorithm to predict survival after nephrectomy and immunotherapy in patients with metastatic renal cell carcinoma: A stratification tool for prospective clinical trials. *Cancer* 2003;98: 2566-2575.

85. Kattan MW, Reuter V, Motzer RJ, et al. A postoperative prognostic nomogram for renal cell carcinoma. *J Urol* 2001;166: 63-67.

86. Jocham D, Richter A, Hoffmann L, et al. Adjuvant autologous renal tumour cell vaccine and risk of tumour progression in patients with renal-cell carcinoma after radical nephrectomy: phase III, randomised controlled trial. *Lancet* 2004;363:594-599.

87. Messing EM, Manola J, Wilding G, et al. Phase III study of interferon alfa-NL as adjuvant treatment for resectable renal cell carcinoma: An Eastern Cooperative Oncology Group/ Intergroup trial. *J Clin Oncol* 2003;21:1214-1222.

88. Pizzocaro G, Piva L, Colavita M, et al. Interferon adjuvant to radical nephrectomy in Robson stages II and III renal cell carcinoma: A multicentric randomized study. *J Clin Oncol* 2001; 19:425-431.

89. Clark JI, Atkins MB, Urba WJ, et al. Adjuvant high-dose bolus interleukin-2 for patients with high-risk renal cell carcinoma: A cytokine working group randomized trial. *J Clin Oncol* 2003;21:3133-3140.

90. Repmann R, Goldschmidt AJ, Richter A. Adjuvant therapy of renal cell carcinoma patients with an autologous tumor cell lysate vaccine: A 5-year follow-up analysis. *Anticancer Res* 2003;23:969-974.

91. Wood C, Srivastava P, Bukowski R, et al. An adjuvant autologous therapeutic vaccine (HSPPC-96; vitespen) versus observation alone for patients at high risk of recurrence after nephrectomy for renal cell carcinoma: A multicentre, open-label, randomised phase III trial. *Lancet* 2008;372:145-154.

92. Lipton A, Zheng M, Seaman J. Zoledronic acid delays the onset of skeletal-related events and progression of skeletal disease in patients with advanced renal cell carcinoma. *Cancer* 2003;98:962-969.

BLADDER CANCER

Arlene Siefker-Radtke
Colin P.N. Dinney
Bogdan A. Czerniak
Randall E. Millikan
Commentary: David J. McConkey

■ OVERVIEW

The urinary tract conveys urine from the confluence of urinary tubules in the renal papillae to the outside world. This entire path is lined by a specialized epithelial surface known as the urothelium, which is composed primarily of transitional cells, and extends from the renal pelvis through the ureters, bladder, and urethra. In males, it also lines the terminal prostatic ducts and prostatic urethra. While tumors arising from the urothelium can involve any organ along this path, about 90% of these cancers arise in the urinary bladder.

■ EPIDEMIOLOGY

Urothelial cancer is the fifth most common cancer diagnosis in the United States and is strikingly related to cigarette smoking. In 2009, about 74,500 new cases were expected, with about 71,000 arising in the bladder.

Altogether, these cases account for just over 15,000 deaths (1). These incidence figures are somewhat misleading, however, since it is an historical anomaly that only in the bladder are histologically bland hyperplastic lesions counted as cancers. In other sites, such lesions would be counted as benign or at most premalignant, and thus the incidence figures include many patients with lesions that do not meet the conventional definition of malignancy. (Imagine what the incidence figures for colon cancer would be if every patient with a polyp was counted as a case of colon cancer!) Many such lesions recur but few progress to true malignancy, and thus it is critically important to separate risk models that are designed to predict recurrence from those that predict progression, which is far more biologically significant. Because of this anomaly of classification, the literature on "risk of bladder cancer," both for incidence and recurrence must be interpreted very carefully.

In contrast to most other carcinomas, the majority of patients with urothelial cancer (even after excluding the low-grade papillary "cancers") have early-stage, potentially curable disease at presentation. Only about 20% of patients present with disease that invades into the muscle wall. Fewer than 5% of patients present with locally advanced (ie, clinically extravesical) disease, and another 5% or so present with clinically apparent metastatic disease. Once clinically metastatic, urothelial cancer is remarkably aggressive, exhibiting a natural history reminiscent of small cell carcinoma of the lungs: untreated, the survival is measured in weeks; it is markedly chemosensitive; responses are typically short-lived; the brain is a typical "sanctuary" site of relapse after response to initial therapy; and cure of patients with distant metastases, while well documented, remains anecdotal.

The ready accessibility of urine, and the fact that the urothelium itself can be accessed via minimally invasive cystoscopy, makes urothelial cancer an important context for understanding the processes of carcinogenesis and clonal evolution, and an important platform for the development of human gene therapy.

The current state of the art is rather sobering:

- Careful patient selection has made it possible for some patients to have organ preservation, but this strategy clearly results in some patients dying unnecessarily.
- While the combination of chemotherapy and surgery does improve the cure fraction for patients with locally advanced disease, a disturbing fraction (30-40% even at referral centers) of patients with invasive disease but no detectable involvement beyond the bladder at the time of diagnosis still succumb to the disease.

- There have been no substantive advances in systemic treatment since the introduction of M-VAC in the early 1980s, and indeed, reported outcomes for patients with metastatic urothelial cancer are getting worse as marginally effective systemic therapies (such as gemcitabine and carboplatin) are now widely used.
- To date, there are no biologic insights that have been widely applied to improve detection, prognostic stratification, treatment selection, or therapy development.

To say the field is ripe for an advance is egregious understatement.

■ CLASSICAL EPIDEMIOLOGY

Malignant transformation of the urothelium parallels observations with other epithelial tumors (2), in that it is distinctly uncommon before age 40 and has a peak incidence in the seventh decade. The male:female ratio is about 3:1, reflecting, in part, differences in exposure to smoking and industrial toxins. Malignant transformation is the result of a multistep process in which multiple genes are implicated. The appearance of clinical cancer typically follows carcinogenic exposure by decades. Fluid intake is inversely associated with risk (3), supporting the concept that contact time of excreted carcinogens with the urothelial surface contributes to carcinogenesis.

There is a striking correlation of urothelial cancer incidence with exposure to certain environmental toxins. About half of all cases are related to smoking. Industrial exposures, especially to petrochemicals, account for another 10 to 15%. Many occupations with "chemical" exposures have been linked to an excess risk of urothelial cancer. An association with aniline dye exposure was noted more than a century ago, and many aromatic amines (prototypically beta-naphthyl amine) have now been shown to be potent urothelial carcinogens. Cigarette smoke is rich in both aromatic amines and the highly reactive bladder toxin acrolein. Another source of acrolein, which is strongly linked to urothelial carcinogenesis, is the metabolism of cyclophosphamide and ifosfamide. In one report (4), prolonged exposure to oral cyclophosphamide (as was a common intervention for some forms of cancer and for autoimmune disease in the 1970s) increased the risk of bladder cancer by a factor of nine. Also noteworthy are exposures to the analgesic phenacetin and to the plant-toxin–related "Balkan Nephropathy" in which the risk of upper tract tumors is increased (5).

As is generally true for epithelial carcinogenesis, chronic irritation and inflammation have also been associated with malignant transformation. This is seen prototypically in settings such as staghorn calculus and other cases of chronic urolithiasis, chronic bladder catheterization (a particularly distressing complication of spinal cord injury [6] or congenital malformations) and classically, chronic schistosomiasis in the Middle East. Urothelial cancers that arise in the context of chronic irritation typically show squamous differentiation.

MOLECULAR EPIDEMIOLOGY

Assessment of genomic variations, as well as functional assessment of certain metabolic pathways, is now routinely integrated with classical aspects of cancer risk assessment. As might have been anticipated from the classical epidemiologic studies of environmental exposures, it has now been confirmed that polymorphisms of various genes involved in xenobiotic metabolism are correlated with the risk of developing bladder cancer. However, these pathways are complex, and the impact of genetic changes is of course context-dependent. A classic example of this is provided by *N*-acetyltransferase 2 (*NAT-2*)–mediated *N*-acetylation, which constitutes a detoxification step for some carcinogens, but can be an activation step for others (7,8). A meta-analysis (9) suggests a possible role for some of these variants in risk of bladder cancer and clearly demonstrates an interaction with smoking status, as would be expected on the hypothesis that these genes are important for the response to smoking-induced DNA damage (10).

Telomere length, which also contributes to the maintenance of genetic integrity, may also be relevant to urothelial carcinogenesis since patients with bladder cancer have been found to have shortened telomeres or telomerase abnormalities (11,12).

■ TUMOR BIOLOGY

CARCINOGENESIS

Chromosomal instability is a hallmark of invasive urothelial cancer (13). Overexpression of the serine/threonine kinase Aurora A (also known as STK15/BTAK) is associated with chromosomal instability and aggressive behavior in many cancers, and has been reported to correlate with bladder cancer progression (14). A subsequent tissue microarray (TMA) study (15) in 246 patients with Ta/T1 tumors demonstrated that Aurora A overexpression was associated with recurrence. Even though some investigators have not found Aurora A expression to be correlated with outcome (16),

it is very clear that gene amplification and protein overexpression is a common and early event in urothelial carcinogenesis and leads to chromosomal instability (17). More recently, quantitation of Aurora A copy number in urine sediment (18) was shown to be a promising biomarker for urothelial cancer detection.

There are also markers that appear to be able to identify the least aggressive end of the biologic spectrum. In the previously cited TMA study (15), preservation of E-cadherin expression (a classic manifestation of the "epithelial phenotype") was associated with low risk of recurrence. Two studies (19,20) have shown that the ratio of E-cadherin to matrix metalloproteinase-9, a surrogate for the "epithelial to mesenchymal transformation," is inversely correlated with outcome. Recently, an immunohistochemical phenotype was described which reliably identified a subset of patients with low-grade papillary lesions that to not recur (21). This phenotype, consisting of strong expression of fibroblast growth factor receptor 3, in combination with a low proliferative index, and superficial expression of cytokeratin-20, has not yet been validated in a larger population, but clearly this is a potential example of the sort of "molecular diagnostics" that are desperately needed to better inform clinical management.

Since the bladder is readily accessible, and most patients present before life-threatening progression is apparent, bladder cancer is well suited for studying the details of the molecular pathogenesis of transformation, invasion, and metastasis. Molecular genetics investigations have revealed that numerous loci are lost, and have confirmed that clonal expansion is an early event; that is, morphologically normal urothelium in bladders harboring urothelial tumors is genetically altered, and multifocal disease generally represents multifocal expansion of a preexisting clonal lesion (22). Thus the classical notion of "field carcinogenesis" is amply confirmed by these molecular genetic studies. These studies demonstrate that early carcinogenesis involves relatively few key loci that provide the fertile context for more generalized chromosomal instability that is apparent in grossly established invasive tumors.

Loss of the retinoblastoma gene (*Rb*), or indeed any inactivation of Rb function, is clearly associated with an adverse prognosis (23).

The *p53* gene is also frequently mutated in urothelial cancer (24) and appears to interact with *Rb* (25). In surgical series, abnormal p53 immunostaining (which in the context of bladder cancer is in fact highly correlated with nonfunctional mutation) correlates strongly with an adverse prognosis. In a recent confirmatory study (26) of 272 patients (92 pT1 and 180 pT2) with long-term follow-up, there were 34 cancer-specific deaths. The Kaplan-Meier estimate of long-term cause-specific survival was 82% for patients with wild-type immunostaining, and 48% for those with altered p53 immunophenotype. In a multivariate analysis of cause-specific survival considering age, gender, number of lymph nodes removed, lymphovascular invasion (LVI), concomitant carcinoma in situ (CIS) and p53 status, only LVI was significant in the final model. Thus it appears that p53 status is a potentially powerful tool for discriminating risk among patients with cT1 cancers. Prospective validation of this predictive power and especially prospective trials of management strategies for cT1 disease that are informed by p53 status are needed.

In our own series of locally advanced patients treated with chemotherapy (27), we found no relation of p53 expression and survival, strongly suggesting that p53 status is indeed related to chemosensitivity. This issue is being prospectively addressed in a national trial in which patients with an abnormal phenotype for p53 protein are offered adjuvant chemotherapy.

NOVEL THERAPEUTIC TARGETS

Epidermal growth factor (EGF), and transforming growth factor-alpha, an important physiologic ligand for EGF receptor, are known to be present in significant amounts in urine. Likewise, EGF receptors (EGFR) have been detected on urothelial cells. Overexpression of EGFR in superficial bladder cancers was one of the first phenotypic features to identify patients with an increased likelihood of progression to invasive cancer. Interestingly, however, overexpression of EGFR in the context of invasive cancers has no independent prognostic value, presumably because it is nearly universal among patients with threatening, muscle-invasive cancers. As with many other epithelial cancers, blocking growth signals mediated by EGFR is an antitumor strategy under investigation (28). A small randomized trial of EGFR blockade as a consolidative strategy after best response to frontline multiagent chemotherapy has completed accrual. The results are expected soon.

At least 40% of clinically aggressive urothelial cancers overexpress the *HER-2* gene product which is a receptor in the EGF family and is known to modulate EGFR signaling, an effect likely mediated by formation of receptor heterodimers. A multi-institutional phase II clinical trial of chemotherapy (gemcitabine, carboplatin, and paclitaxel) with the HER-2 blocking antibody trastuzumab has been reported (29). This trial was notable for prospective evaluation of 109 registered patients for Her-2 status. The investigators found that 49% showed 2+ or 3+ staining by IHC; 14% were positive for gene amplification by FISH, and 12% showed elevated serum levels of Her-2 protein. Only 21 patients of the 109 were positive by two tests and only 3 patients by all three criteria. Overall, 57 of 109 (52%) were "positive" by any criterion, and 44 of those were treated with the regimen containing trastuzumab. The treated population included 3 patients with PS >1 and 24 with visceral metastases. There were three treatment-related deaths (7%), and the median survival was 14 months. These results are well within expectation for chemotherapy alone (see below), and thus the role (if any) for Her-2–directed therapy in urothelial cancer remains to be defined.

Induction of angiogenesis has emerged as a fundamental property of tumor cells, and markers of an "angiogenic phenotype" such as VEGF expression have been found to correlate with outcome in many cancers. In urothelial cancer, EGF signaling is associated with significant upregulation of proangiogenic factors, including interleukin-8, basic fibroblast growth factor and VEGF. In addition, high expression of VEGF is a powerful predictor of treatment failure among locally advanced patients treated with chemotherapy and surgery (30). A preclinical study (31) of sunitinib and cisplatin in a mouse model suggested some activity for sunitinib as a single agent and synergistic activity for the combination. A human phase II study of single-agent sunitinib as salvage therapy has been reported in abstract form (32). In a trial of 31 patients with intact performance status and 25 of 31 with visceral disease, only one partial response was observed and the median survival was 7 months, strongly suggesting that this agent will not be useful as a single agent in an unselected population.

Numerous other agents and other potential therapeutic targets are being identified. Youssef et al. has provided a recent review (33).

HISTOLOGY

In the United States, approximately 90% of all urothelial malignancies are within the histologic spectrum of transitional cell carcinoma (TCC), which, in our view, merges without obvious demarcation with the "sarcomatoid" and "small cell" variants at the extreme of dedifferentiation. Most of the remainder exhibit squamous histology (especially prominent in the more distal urethra) or glandular differentiation (ie, adenocarcinoma). The finding of adenocarcinoma apart from the context of bladder exstrophy or a urachal tumor (see below) should prompt consideration of metastatic disease from some other primary site, since bona fide primary adeno-carcinomas originating from the urothelium are distinctly uncommon.

As noted above, primarily hyperplastic lesions, biologically akin to polyps in the GI tract, account for a large portion of incident cases. In 1999, the World Health Organization put forward a new classification of noninvasive papillary urothelial tumors in recognition of the fact that the malignant potential of these lesions varies widely (34). The WHO terminology for these lesions, which together account for more than half of all new cases of urothelial neoplasia is:

Papillary urothelial neoplasm of low malignant potential (PUNLMP). This lesion is characterized by orderly progression of morphology within the urothelium and no cellular atypia. Recurrence is seen in about 25% of cases, but progression is rare.

Noninvasive papillary urothelial carcinoma, low-grade. This lesion shows some architectural variation and mild atypia. Such lesions commonly recur (in 50% or more of cases) but progression is seen in only 5 to 10%. It is classified by the WHO as a borderline tumor.

Noninvasive papillary urothelial carcinoma, high-grade. This lesion shows predominantly disorganized architecture and moderate to marked cytological atypia. Such lesions do not invade below the basement membrane, but they have substantial biologic potential, with progression to invasive, potentially life-threatening disease in up to 65% of cases. These are classified by the WHO as malignant. Note that in the WHO system grades are collapsed to a two-tier system of low grade and high grade. In general, this would map to the older three-tier system as grade 1 = low grade, and grades 2 and 3 = high grade.

In contrast to these papillary cancers, some urothelial cancers exhibit dysplasia and chromosomal instability early on and constitute a "second pathway" of carcinogenesis (35-37), and most of the cases with lethal potential are in this class (Figs. 33-1 and 33-2). In contrast to the classic "mulberry" appearance, the non-papillary lesions have a grossly flat or infiltrative appearance at cystoscopy. In older literature such cancers have been known as *flat*, *sessile*, *solid*, or *tentacular*. Currently, the preferred nomenclature is simply "nonpapillary" although "flat" persists in the AJCC Cancer Staging Manual, 7th edition. These morphologic differences were noted long before an understanding of the genetic changes associated with cancer was appreciated. As expected for such distinct phenotypes, the characteristic genetic lesions have been found to be distinct.

In addition to papillary and nonpapillary variants, a *micropapillary* pattern is increasingly recognized (38-41). The term micropapillary originally came from the recognition of morphologic resemblance to an aggressive variant of ovarian cancer. Indeed, this general histologic pattern has been reported in many epithelial malignancies, and invariably identifies a more aggressive subset, as was first reported for bladder cancer in 1994. Thus, the biologic potential of urothelial neoplasia extends from relatively nonthreatening in papillary lesions, to potentially life-threatening in nonpapillary lesions, to remarkably aggressive micropapillary lesions, all of which are recognizable as "transitional cell" cancer.

Depending on the series, about 30% (or more) of muscle-invasive urothelial cancers are found to have focal areas of squamous or glandular morphology when examined in detail. It is not clear that such "mixed" tumors have a different prognosis than "pure" TCC, and we do not consider this a meaningful subset at MD Anderson. Certainly, tumors with only focal areas of squamous or glandular differentiation do not exhibit the distinctive natural history of pure squamous cancers or pure adenocarcinomas. Primary nonepithelial cancers (eg, sarcomas, lymphomas, and melanomas) are exceedingly uncommon in the bladder. When they do occur, they do not appear to have a distinctive natural history or clinical management from what would be expected of similar tumors arising in more typical sites.

Urothelial cancers can dedifferentiate to include spindled ("sarcomatoid") and small cell variants. In these cases, the clinical expression of the overall disease process is dominated by the aggressive component, even if most of the primary cancer is well within the typical morphologic spectrum of TCC.

Small cell carcinoma of the urothelium is a remarkably aggressive malignancy and exhibits a similar propensity for spread to the brain as does small cell carcinoma arising in other sites. Even in the setting of clinically localized disease, the prognosis with local therapy alone remains poor, reflecting the early development of micrometastases. We strongly favor management of patients with cT2 or lower disease that is based on neoadjuvant chemotherapy, followed by surgical consolidation (42). In our hands this provides about 50 to 60% cure. Patients with locally advanced disease have a high incidence (8 of 16 in our series) of relapse in the brain, and thus we feel these patients are candidates for prophylactic cranial irradiation. Patients with metastatic disease at presentation continue to have nearly a 100% response rate, with a 100% relapse rate and a median survival of only 11 months.

Cancers arising in a urachal remnant, while not strictly "bladder cancers" in the sense of this chapter,

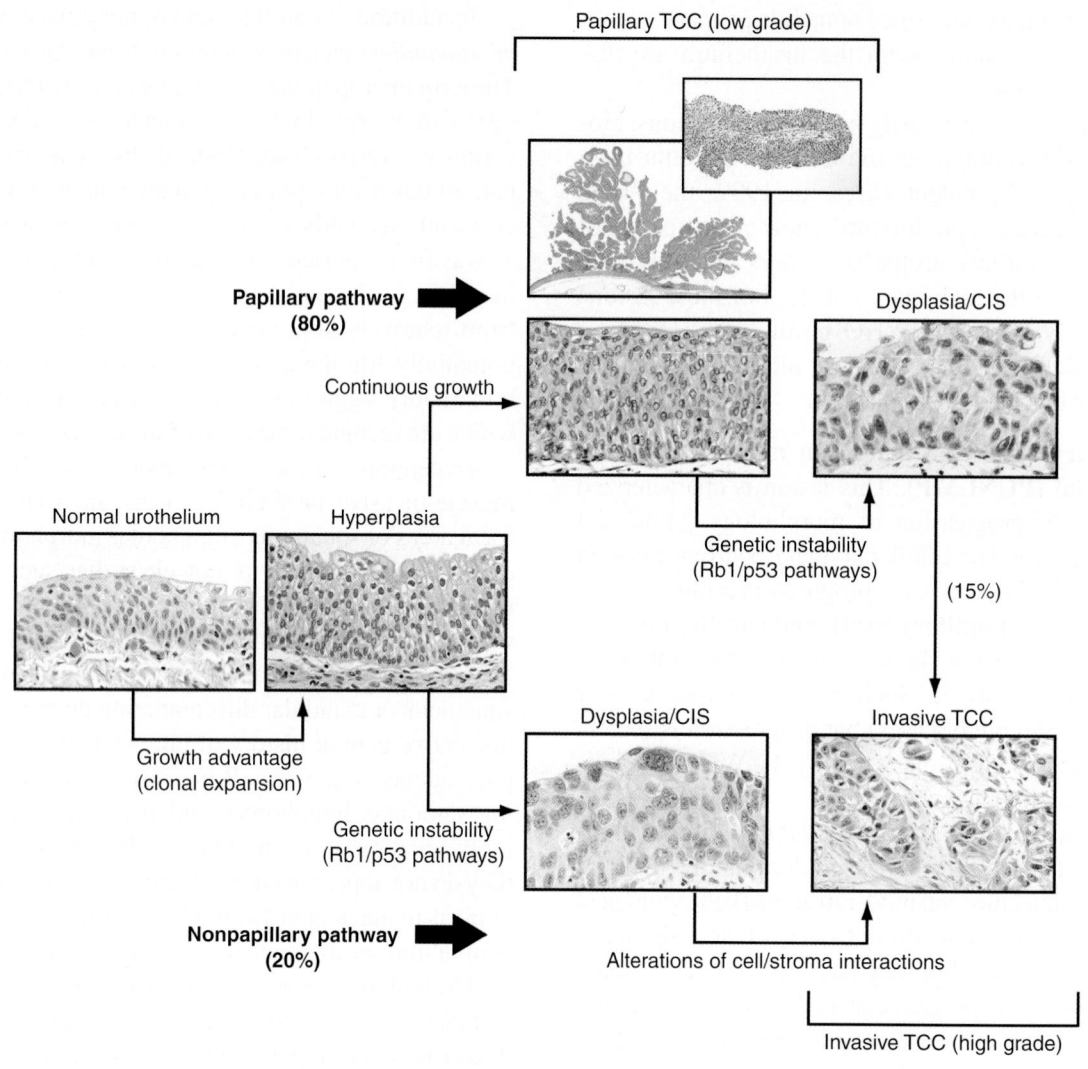

FIGURE 33-1.   Histomorphologic classification of transitional cell carcinoma.

merit a comment. These cancers typically involve the dome of the bladder, and histologically are enteric-type adenocarcinomas. They are thought to reflect malignant transformation of an enteric epithelial rest within the urachal remnant, producing a cancer readily recognized as a mucinous adenocarcinoma (43). The Memorial Sloan-Kettering experience in 50 patients was recently published (44,45) and demonstrated long-term survival in 26 of 28 patients (93%) with pathologically localized disease, in 9 of 13 (69%) patients with extension through the bladder or urachal cavity, and in none of 9 patients with peritoneal involvement initially. Similarly, the Mayo Clinic experience (46,47) in 49 patients demonstrated apparent cure in the majority of patients with confined disease and relapse in the majority with nonconfined disease, the latter group having a median

survival of only 16 months. All investigators have emphasized the importance of an attempt at margin-negative, en bloc resection if at all possible.

Urachal cancers have a tendency to recur locally, often with peritoneal carcinomatosis, and the typical metastatic sites are (about equally) lungs and liver. Although dramatic responses are infrequent, the use of modern combination regimens with activity in enteric adenocarcinoma is associated with about a 40% objective response rate. Thus, in essentially every clinical respect, urachal cancer behaves like colon cancer and, based on the available data, should be treated accordingly. Median survival from the recognition of metastases was 24 months in our retrospective series of 26 patients with metastatic disease, although some patients with grossly metastatic disease have been long-term

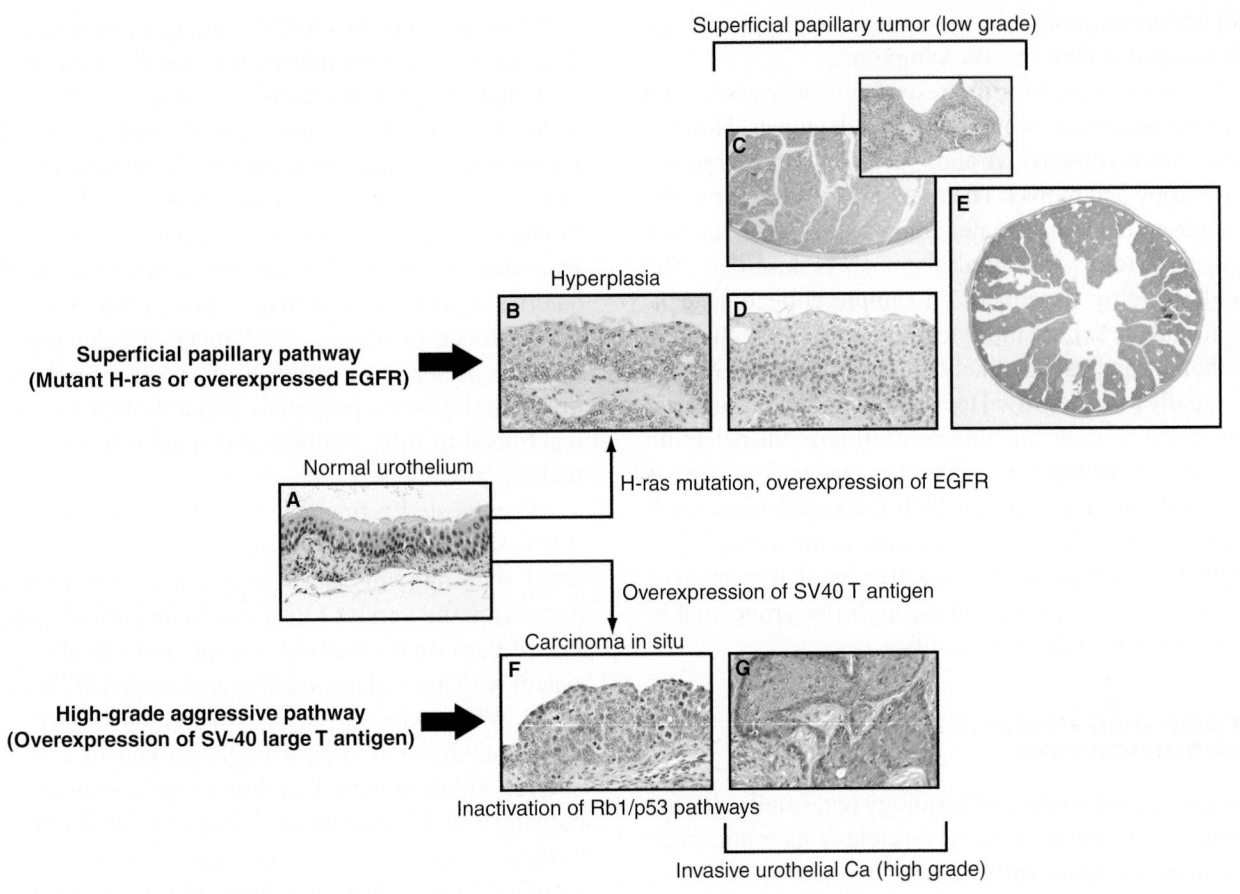

Superficial papillary tumor (low grade)

Hyperplasia

**Superficial papillary pathway
(Mutant H-ras or overexpressed EGFR)**

Normal urothelium

H-ras mutation, overexpression of EGFR

Overexpression of SV40 T antigen

Carcinoma in situ

**High-grade aggressive pathway
(Overexpression of SV-40 large T antigen)**

Inactivation of Rb1/p53 pathways

Invasive urothelial Ca (high grade)

FIGURE 33-2. Characteristic genetic lesions in transitional cell carcinoma carcinogenesis. EGFR, epidermal growth factor receptor.

survivors (48). This experience led us to open a prospective phase II study of 5-fluorouracil, leucovorin, cisplatin, and gemcitabine. Results from this recently completed trial are expected soon.

■ DIAGNOSIS, STAGING, AND PROGNOSIS

PRESENTATION

About 80% of patients present with hematuria, usually painless. The "typical patient" is a smoker in his late 60s. Such patients frequently suffer from pulmonary disease and cardiovascular disease, magnifying the morbidity of both chemotherapy and surgery. They are also at high risk for other smoking-related malignancies. A high percentage of patients have diminished renal function as a result of hypertension and obstructive nephropathy. Thus, the use of nephrotoxic chemotherapy is especially challenging in this population. Hospitalization and meticulous attention to detail are typically required in order to safely deliver multiple cycles of cisplatin or ifosfamide-based therapy.

Irritative voiding symptoms, including frequency, dysuria, and dribbling, are important points in the medical history, since the presence of irritative symptoms raises the possibility of extensive carcinoma in situ or large, infiltrative tumors that may be far more extensive than is revealed by the initial cystoscopy. Obstructive symptoms (nocturia, double voiding, overflow incontinence, low anterior abdominal pain) are often encountered from tumors of the bladder neck or prostatic urethra. Tumors in these locations are far less likely to be anatomically confined (ie, curable with surgery) than are similarly muscle-invasive bladder cancers that are well away from these areas where the detrusor muscle is discontinuous.

In evaluating patients presenting with hematuria, it is mandatory to evaluate the upper urinary tracts. Even if a bladder tumor is confirmed on initial cystoscopy, excretory urography is still appropriate, since synchronous or metachronous tumors of the upper tracts typically are not associated with specific symptoms.

Recently, several urine tests for cancer-associated antigens have been promulgated for diagnosis. None of these tests is yet sensitive and specific enough to replace cystoscopy and biopsy. The role of these tests for widespread screening is also not defined. Likewise, the role of urine cytology in initial diagnosis is unsettled. The yield is highly dependent on sample collection technique and the skill of the cytopathologist. As with many epithelial cancers, it is likely that DNA-based tests will eventually be widely used to find pathognomonic genetic alterations in urine, and thus revolutionize the detection and clinical follow-up of bladder cancer. The role of some form of surveillance in high-risk populations (such as petrochemical workers) remains controversial. The relatively low positive and negative predictive value of cytology, even when applied to a high-risk group, makes such screening difficult to justify.

STAGE AND PROGNOSTIC CLASSIFICATION

Excepting the extremes of histology (eg, small cell), the dominant prognostic clinical variable is anatomic stage at diagnosis. Classically, this is defined by depth of invasion. The currently used staging system is summarized in Fig. 33-3. This system is of course historically rooted in pathologic findings related to cystectomy specimens. As a result, it is not well suited for *clinical* staging. For example, the distinction between deep muscle invasion (T2b) and more superficial muscle invasion (T2a) cannot be reliably made by cystoscopic biopsy, and indeed the differentiation of muscle fibers in the lamina propria from muscularis propria (ie, the distinction between deep cT1 and cT2) is often problematic. As with most solid tumors, one must be extraordinarily careful regarding staging information, especially when comparing surgical and radiotherapy series, which necessarily rely on very different primary information.

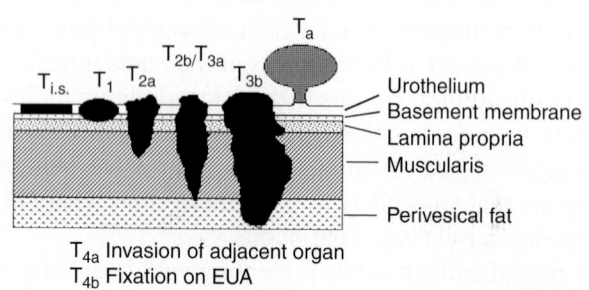

FIGURE 33-3. Current scheme for tumor (T) staging of urothelial cancer. EUA, examination under anesthesia.

Unfortunately the AJCC staging system does not account for available information about tumor biology. Although "staging" has come to be understood as "prognostic assessment" for most cancers, urologic oncology lags behind in laying aside the historical notion of stage as essentially an anatomic concept. As noted above, the biology of papillary cancers is fundamentally different from that of nonpapillary cancers. Other biologic characteristics such as location of tumor within the bladder, the presence or absence of lymphovascular invasion, and the presence or absence of specific markers are known to influence prognosis, and thus there is a significant need to fully evaluate and standardize how such features are reported.

A suggested refinement to the currently dominant AJCC system relates to the subdivision of cT1. Several ways of doing this have been suggested, including measuring the depth of invasion (with a break point at 1.5 mm), or on the basis of whether muscle fibers consistent with muscularis *mucosa* are invaded (T1b) or not (T1a). While many subspecialty pathologists have found such a subdivision to be strongly prognostic (49), it is not yet widely reported, and there are questions about both intra- and interobserver variability (50,51). We tend to think of the commonly reported "extensive involvement" of lamina propria as a useful way of identifying higher-risk cT1 disease. What is clear is that there is significant variability of prognosis among patients with cT1 disease, and better ways of refining this group remains a worthy goal for clinical investigators.

Although there is no official system for *clinical* staging, there are several important factors that largely define prognosis that can be reasonably well assessed by clinical evaluation:

- The presence or absence of muscle invasion (ie, T1 versus ≥T2). This is fairly reliably established by transurethral resection (TUR), especially if the surgeon provides deep enough samples that contain muscularis propria.
- The presence or absence of a definable mass (ie, assessable in three dimensions) by *examination under anesthesia* (EUA) following a "complete" TUR. This is the clinical definition of cT3b disease and is of critical prognostic importance. The role of cross-sectional imaging criteria for cT3b disease is controversial. We do not believe that routinely available studies can make this distinction reliably at the present time. The EUA is an essential component of the evaluation of a patient with muscle-invasive bladder cancer (52) and is most informative when it is done following drainage of the bladder once the

TUR has been completed. A proper EUA provides important staging information complementing data obtained by imaging modalities such as CT scan or MRI. The presence of induration indicates deep muscle invasion, while the palpation of a discreet, mobile three-dimensional mass implies gross invasion into extravesical tissue and carries a significant risk (30-40%) of occult lymph node metastasis. At EUA, it is possible to identify masses extending directly into the prostate in men or into the vagina in women. These findings are also associated with a high risk of occult lymph node metastasis. The finding of a mass by EUA, which extends and is fixed to the pelvic sidewall (ie, cT4b), indicates an unresectable cancer. These patients have a similar prognosis to those with overt distant metastases.

- The presence or absence of nodal disease, as assessed clinically by CT or MRI imaging of the pelvis. Patients with radiographically detectable adenopathy should have a biopsy prior to surgery. If positive, primary chemotherapy is appropriate, since distant recurrence dominates the clinical course in these patients. That being said, we certainly advocate surgical consolidation with cystectomy and pelvic node dissection in patients with no clinical evidence of disease after chemotherapy.

- The presence or absence of lymphovascular invasion (LVI) on the TUR biopsy specimen is also a powerful prognostic feature. While it must be admitted that TUR samples are often difficult to assess secondary to crush and cautery artifact, the unequivocal finding of tumor cells in vascular spaces identifies a group of patients with a high risk of occult nodal involvement. In fact, LVI is associated with a risk of pN+ status of about 35%, comparable to the risk associated with a large cT3b tumor. (It should be noted that tumors in the dome are difficult both to completely resect by TUR and are also more difficult to evaluate by EUA, and thus clinical staging is even less reliable in this subset.)

Other clinical factors that routinely "stay in the model" when investigators construct Cox proportional hazard models for the prognosis of urothelial cancer patients treated with cystectomy are age, gender (females consistently do worse), and time from diagnosis to definitive therapy.

In addition to the routinely available pathologic and clinical features that are related to outcome, many new methods of molecular characterization are being investigated as prognostic and predictive markers. Many studies (using either germ-line or tumor-derived material) have investigated genomic, transciptomic or proteomic profiles. A recent review (53) confirms that it is relatively easy to outperform AJCC stage groupings, but there is not as yet a consensus about which genes (or gene products) are most important, and certainly none of the molecular techniques have come into routine clinical practice.

From a medical oncology perspective, the most important issue is how to recognize which patients will benefit from the addition of systemic chemotherapy to definitive surgery. The current management guidelines for bladder cancer as promulgated by the NCCN (54) suggest the use of neoadjuvant chemotherapy for patients with cT2 disease. In our view, this is a wonderful example of how "evidence-based medicine" can pave the way for uncritical and even irrational management guidelines.

In evaluating this recommendation, it should first be noted that cT2 cancers could easily be pT0 (ie, no residual disease in cystectomy specimen following initial TUR), pTis, pTa, pT1, pT2a, pT2b, or pT3a without constituting a clinical staging error. However, it is abundantly clear that the burden of residual disease (ie, the burden of disease found at cystectomy) after TUR is strongly related to the risk of disease relapse and death. In a series of 208 patients, Isbarn (55) recently demonstrated that those with residual invasive disease (ie, pT1 and pT2) were cured about 70% of the time, while all 55 of those with no residual invasive disease (pTa, pTis, or pT0) were cured.

To further highlight the enormous heterogeneity of patients with cT2 cancers, consider that we know of many features that have a dramatic influence on prognosis:

1. Cancers arising at the bladder neck are notoriously difficult to adequately stage, monitor, and have a higher rate of occult nodal involvement.

2. Cancers presenting with hydronephrosis from tumors in the region of the ureterovessical junctions have a very high rate of pT3b extension, occult nodal involvement, and inferior outcome. This was first reported in the 1980s and has been amply confirmed. In a recent study of 241 patients with cT2 disease treated by cystectomy (56), the 5-year cause-specific survival (a very good surrogate for cure) was 63% for those without this feature versus 12% for those with hydronephrosis. This remained prognostically significant after accounting for pathologic stage. Similar results were obtained by Bartsch et al. (57) who observed 68 versus 30%, again remaining significant after accounting for pathologic stage.

3. As noted above, cancers exhibiting micropapillary, sarcomatoid, and small cell histology have a much

more aggressive biology and inferior "stage-for-stage" outcome with cystectomy.

4. Large nonpapillary tumors (cut points range from 3-5 cm) that are muscle invasive over a broad front are much worse (ie, much more likely to be upstaged at cystectomy) than those with focal muscle invasion.

5. Cancers showing lymphovascular invasion, especially when appreciated in the TUR specimen, are associated with about a 30% rate of occult nodal involvement (58).

6. Cancers with an abnormal immunophenotype for *p53* and *Rb* gene products have a decreased probability of cure with cystectomy, and the prognosis is especially unfavorable when both are altered. In a large study of patients with cT2 disease, the cure rate for patients with both genes showing wild type expression was 80%, while only 20% with both genes altered were cured (23). All were stage cT2, all operated on by the same surgeon, and a flip from 80% cured to 80% dead by IHC status!

7. Cancers with prominent neovascularity in the tumor (ie, microvessel density as revealed by CD34 staining or other methods) or strong expression of VEGF are consistently associated with a higher risk of recurrent disease after cystectomy (59).

8. Cancers with an "invasive phenotype" characterized, for example, by high expression of matrix metalloprotease-9 and/or low expression of E-cadherin, are consistently associated with an increased risk of recurrent and metastatic disease.

9. In addition to these tumor characteristics, it is now well established that circulating levels of tumor markers are independent predictors of outcome. This has been demonstrated for hCG, CA19-9, and CA 125 (60-62).

It is apparent that on the basis of information that can be gathered preoperatively, it is possible to very substantially refine the clinical risk of a patient with cT2 bladder cancer. Recently, Vickers et al. (63) have provided a compelling numerical analysis of just how powerful the application of a multivariate model to decision making can be, and how this consistently outperforms the simple-minded notion that all patients with cT2 cancer should get chemotherapy.

In addition to these clinical features that can be ascertained preoperatively, there are of course surgical factors that impact outcome. For example, we know that outcome is dependent on the experience of both the surgeon and the center where surgery is performed (64,65), and that cure is consistently related to extent of pelvic node dissection (66), and of course,

patients with involved surgical margins nearly always relapse.

■ CLINICAL MANAGEMENT

MANAGEMENT OF SUPERFICIAL DISEASE (cTa, cTi.s.)

The management of low-grade papillary disease is by TUR, and since these lesions recur but rarely progress, there is generally no thought of cystectomy except in the rare case that the bladder surface is a carpet of lesions. In such a case, just as with overwhelming colon polyposis, radical surgery prior to progression to more threatening disease is appropriate.

High-grade noninvasive cancers present a difficult dilemma for the urologist, who must balance the risk of recurrent, invasive disease (which occurs despite therapy and surveillance in at least 20% of patients), with the risk of overtreating patients not destined to have a threatening cancer. As noted above, there is currently much interest in finding markers that will stratify the risk of progression and allow optimized management. The presence of CIS increases the probability of both recurrence and progression. Typically, patients with either high-grade Ta disease or CIS (or both) are now treated with both TUR and BCG.

Intravesical BCG was introduced in 1976, and since the first controlled trial establishing the efficacy of BCG was reported by Lamm et al. in 1980 (67), it has had a remarkable impact on the clinical management of bladder cancer. Although standard criteria for therapy are still evolving, BCG has been shown in randomized trials to be superior to intravesical chemotherapy and TUR alone and will delay recurrence and progression, decreasing the need for immediate cystectomy. It is important to note that complete responses to BCG are required for significant alteration of the natural history of the disease (68). Partial responses should prompt referral for experimental therapy or consideration of early cystectomy. Especially in the context of any invasive component, BCG therapy will be associated with progression to potentially life-threatening disease in a substantial fraction and thus, persistent treatment with BCG in the context of less than complete response is a major cause of potentially avoidable mortality from bladder cancer. In our experience, Urologists are likely to emphasize the advantages of avoiding cystectomy, but place less emphasis on the dangers of progression to the point that a cystectomy will no longer be curative. The decision to delay cystectomy in the face of less than an initial complete response to BCG is responsible for many deaths from disease that was not caught early enough, despite close surveillance (69).

The other feature of BCG therapy of particular interest from a medical oncology perspective (because it relates to assessment of the need for perioperative systemic therapy) is the increasing incidence of cancers in the distal ureter and prostatic urethra. In each case, these lesions are a challenge for cystoscopic surveillance, and particularly for ureteral lesions, minimal progression can be associated with a sharply rising risk of life-threatening disease. BCG therapy can clear the bladder proper, while urothelial carcinogenesis and progression continue just millimeters away. Patients treated with BCG (especially those with CIS) who have negative cystoscopy but positive cytology are at very substantial risk of having such disease, and it is often fatal if definitive management is delayed (70).

MANAGEMENT OF MINIMALLY INVASIVE DISEASE (cT1)

Patients with cancers that are invasive into the lamina propria (cT1) are at high risk of developing muscle-invasive disease. In general, patients with an invasive or high-grade component recognized on the initial TUR should have a re-excision approximately 4 weeks later (71). A second TUR provides another opportunity to sample muscle and thus more definitively establish the status of muscle invasion, which is a key prognostic feature. In addition, the re-resection establishes which patients have persistent disease vs. those who do not. Those with persistent disease have a prognosis similar to cT2 patients and should be informed of the risk associated with bladder preserving therapy. Conversely, a complete TUR, as demonstrated by a negative re-resection, may be adequate therapy for many patients with cT1 disease, especially if there is no CIS present, and noninvolved muscle has been sampled. In this context, it is especially important to have a highly sensitive test for CIS Although not yet standard, there is substantial interest in looking at tissue fluorescence to enhance conventional cystoscopy (72). In the United States, most patients with cT1 disease receive BCG, and the caveats about BCG use as noted above apply even more strongly to this group. It is also important to recognize that tumors that overlie the ureteral orifices or involve the bladder neck are sometimes difficult to confirm as only T1 lesions and require a lower threshold for definitive surgery.

Men with a positive cytology and no obvious tumor within the bladder should undergo transurethral biopsy of the prostate at 5 and 7 o'clock at the verumontanum in addition to random bladder biopsies. Prostate

recurrence is detected in approximately 10 to 15% of patients within 5 years of treatment of their bladder tumor and in 20 to 40% by 10 years.

At MD Anderson, patients with persistent T1 disease despite resection and intravesical therapy are generally cautioned against second-line therapy and guided toward radical cystectomy. Esrig et al. have provided a useful perspective on this situation (73).

MANAGEMENT OF CLINICALLY LOCALIZED, MUSCLE-INVASIVE DISEASE (cT2)

In the United States, cystectomy is the standard therapy for muscle-invasive bladder cancer. In older surgical series, cystectomy was curative in about half of these patients. More contemporary series typically report cure in the range of 80%, but this is on the basis of *pathologic stage*. Thus, while it is true that in experienced centers 80 to 85% of patients undergoing cystectomy for cancers that are found to be pathologically confined to the muscular wall of the bladder (ie, pT2b or less, N0) will be cured, it is not absolutely clear that the old figure of about 50% cure for *clinical stage* T2 patients is now obsolete, although modern series do seem better (74). At the very least, the finding of muscle invasion signals a potentially life-threatening problem; in fact, this seems to constitute an oncologic urgency. In a study of 214 patients treated with cystectomy at the University of Michigan (75), a cut point of 93 days from recognition of muscle invasion to surgery was associated with statistically inferior cause-specific and overall survival. Specifically, about 60% of patients with timely surgery were long-term survivors versus about 40% of those with delay, even though there was no clinical or pathologic stage migration!

In view of available knowledge of prognostic features reviewed above, it is clearly inappropriate in the current era to speak of "muscle-invasive" bladder cancer as though it were a single disease state with a well-defined prognosis and a single best management. We know that there are many patients with cT2 bladder cancer with such a favorable prognosis that no available systemic therapy would be expected to improve outcome over that achieved with radical cystectomy and template pelvic node dissection (76). Likewise, we know that some patients at high risk will benefit from currently available chemotherapy in addition to surgery. The challenge for clinicians, and especially for clinical investigators, is to better define those at each end of this spectrum and then continue to work on subdivision of the remaining patients where we currently do not know how to define the role of systemic chemotherapy. This issue of identifying the appropriate patients for systemic chemotherapy is the single most important question related to bladder cancer from a medical oncology perspective. There is no longer any question that perioperative chemotherapy can improve outcome for some patients; likewise, it is all too obvious that it can do much harm. Thus, as always, the central question for the medical oncologist is: How are we to balance risk and benefit for each patient?

Based on our understanding of the impact of currently available therapy, it is our sense that patients with a 70% chance or more of cure should not be offered chemotherapy as it currently exists. Conversely, when the probability of surgical cure falls to about 40% or less, then it seems clear that chemotherapy should be offered. In between these extremes, the decision is a highly personal issue of risk abatement versus burden of therapy. As a practical implementation of this intuitive sense that 40% cure probability is about the right threshold for chemotherapy plus surgery, we offer chemotherapy to patients with any of the following: direct invasion of the prostate or vagina (ie, cT4a disease), a three-dimensional mass on EUA (ie, cT3b disease), lymphovascular invasion on TUR material, bladder neck involvement, and hydronephrosis or an excessive delay (ie, >4 months) between the finding of muscle-invasive disease and definitive management. We look forward to implementing more refined prognostic tools in our own practice.

PRIMARY RADIOTHERAPY

In our view, radiotherapy is inferior to surgery as a local modality for bladder cancer. Available data (77) clearly demonstrate that long-term control can be achieved in about 40% of patients with small primary tumors amenable to complete resection, not associated with CIS, not arising at the bladder neck or UVJ, and without hydronephrosis. This is precisely the subset that have about an 80% cure with surgery, and to claim that the available results are "comparable" to surgical series is not justified (78). Clearly some patients could decide that the risks are acceptable and rationally choose radiotherapy, but this must not be presented as an option associated with a comparable outcome to surgery.

MANAGEMENT OF LOCALLY ADVANCED, RESECTABLE DISEASE (HIGH-RISK cT2, cT3, cT4a)

Tumors that are clinically beyond the bladder wall (ie, those which are identified clinically by a definable three-dimensional mass at EUA *after* TUR of intravesical

tumor) carry a much worse prognosis with cystectomy alone, with most authorities citing a figure of about 35% as the reasonable range for the surgical cure rate in this group. Many patients with cT2 and high-risk features have a similar chance for surgical cure. Patients with prostatic stromal involvement (from the bladder, *not* from TCC of prostatic ducts), or extension into the vaginal wall (ie, anatomic clinical stage cT4a), have a surgical cure rate in the range of 5 to 20%. Collectively, these groups have what we term "locally advanced but resectable" disease, and at MDACC they are treated primarily with chemotherapy, followed by surgical consolidation as appropriate. While this is a patient cohort with truly threatening disease, it is also true that this is the population for whom combined application of best systemic therapy and best surgical therapy has the greatest patient benefit. In the MD Anderson experience (79), the benchmark outcome in this cohort is cure in about 60% of patients (by intent to treat), with about 40% having no residual invasive cancer in the resected specimen following chemotherapy (so-called "p-zero" status), which we and others have noted to be a reliable indicator of long-term disease-free survival.

Since the publication of the SWOG trial (80) of cystectomy with or without neoadjuvant M-VAC, many (including the NCCN guidelines) have advocated that this is the standard of care for patients with cT2 cancers. Clearly we feel this is an unrefined interpretation of the data, and would urge that some notion of probability of recurrence be the guide.

A recent retrospective multicenter study (81) of 583 patients with pT4 disease (all obviously deemed resectable on clinical grounds) found cause-specific survival of about 30%. Univariate analysis confirmed female gender, lymphovascular invasion, nodal involvement, positive surgical margins, and pT4b substage to be associated with inferior outcome. None of these patients received neoadjuvant therapy. Some did receive adjuvant therapy, but it was not obvious that chemotherapy improved outcome in this cohort.

MANAGEMENT OF LOCALLY ADVANCED, UNRESECTABLE DISEASE (cT4b, cN+)

This group has a dismal prognosis. In our experience, patients presenting with large tumors that are clinically fixed to the rectum, pelvic sidewall, or pubic symphysis actually have a worse prognosis than patients with extrapelvic nodes or lung-only metastases. These patients are considered unresectable, and are treated with chemotherapy initially, and then reassessed for the possibility of surgical consolidation in light of the quality of response and their fitness for surgery postchemotherapy (82).

Investigators from Memorial Sloan-Kettering (83) have published their experience with this strategy. Forty-one patients presenting with initially unresectable disease were treated primarily with chemotherapy, but with the intention of intervening surgically in those patients with a high-quality response to systemic therapy. After chemotherapy, 29 of 41 (71%) were explored, and 24 were able to have cystectomy. At a minimum of 4 years of follow-up, none of the 12 patients without initial response to chemotherapy (and therefore not explored) were alive, while all but one of the 10 patients who were pT0, N0 after chemotherapy were alive. These data confirm that response to systemic therapy is the dominant prognostic feature, and that surgical consolidation is both feasible and associated with long-term survival in selected patients. This experience also confirmed that patients with significant residual disease after chemotherapy did not benefit from surgery, and that overall the prognosis is still poor, with only 9 of 41 patients surviving. Still, 22% survival among initially unresectable bladder cancer patients is much better than what could be expected of any single modality.

Radiotherapy has not been useful as a single modality with these large cancers. As with surgery, there probably is a role for radiotherapy in the "consolidation" of patients who show an excellent response to primary chemotherapy. It is worth emphasizing that sensitivity to chemotherapy and radiotherapy do tend to be parallel in the context of urothelial cancer. We have never seen a chemorefractory cancer respond to radiation, and we have seen some excellent long-term results from use of radiotherapy to consolidate an initially unresectable mass after an excellent response to combination chemotherapy.

MANAGEMENT OF DISTANTLY METASTATIC DISEASE

Bladder cancer typically spreads first to regional nodes, then disseminates with about equal frequency to the lungs, liver, and bone. Late in the course, subcutaneous and brain metastases are common. Brain involvement is especially likely in patients who have elevated serum levels of beta-hCG.

Even with strictly palliative goals in mind, most patients with metastatic bladder cancer should be treated with multicomponent chemotherapy, pitched at their level of physiologic tolerance. Metastatic urothelial cancer remains a clinical situation in which toxic side effects are typically encountered if chemotherapy is given in a way that has any chance of substantially altering the natural history of the disease. Unfortunately, "kinder, gentler" therapy is likely to be of little benefit. Metastatic urothelial cancer is a very aggressive malignancy, with an untreated natural history from the time it causes symptoms to death on the order of 3 to 4 months. Quality of life is essentially completely dependent on the efficacy of therapy. Even extraordinarily toxic regimens can be truly palliative in light of how rapidly (and morbidly) the disease progresses.

Since the mid-1980s, the use of cisplatin-based combination chemotherapy has been standard. In the modern era with a bit of lead time bias compared to practice in the early 1980s, such treatment results in median survival of about 16 months, with few survivors beyond 3 years. This is the benchmark where therapy has plateaued for more than a decade.

Of course, some patients with distantly metastatic disease still have disease restricted to one (or a few) anatomic areas, and one might imagine that local therapy would have a role in such a setting. However, in contrast to the situation with renal cell carcinoma for example, surgery is almost never an appropriate initial intervention for metastatic urothelial cancer. Almost always, the disease is not really localized, and one finds rapid progression in the postoperative setting. Thus, even in cases of anatomically threatening lesions such as threatened cord compression, we generally advocate primary chemotherapy to get the disease under some control that will then permit safe surgical intervention. Nonetheless, it is only natural to ask if there is a role for surgical consolidation after a good response to chemotherapy for (highly) selected patients with metastatic urothelial cancer. The MD Anderson experience with this strategy has been published in the setting of retroperitoneal lymph node metastases (82) and in a very small, select subset of patients with visceral metastases (84). Selection criteria for this approach have not yet matured. In the absence of more data, we have adopted the following guidelines. For patients with pelvic or retroperitoneal nodal involvement (below the renal vessels) we typically offer an extended node dissection to patients with a complete radiographic response to initial chemotherapy. Since judging the "completeness" of response in a lymph node is problematic, we include in our working definition a negative biopsy for any node that is large enough for CT-guided biopsy. For patients with visceral involvement, we typically treat to maximum response and observe. Only when patients progress in the initially involved area (with no progression elsewhere) and then go on to have a significant response to a second course of chemotherapy do we consider surgical removal of residual metastatic disease.

Just as with patients with germ cell cancers, failure of markers to normalize is nearly an absolute contraindication to surgical consolidation.

The exception to this is the rare patient with a long interval from initial management to the onset of resectable, oligometastatic visceral disease. In this setting we typically give two cycles of systemic therapy and then excise the lesions. Note that in our view surgery without some chemotherapy is essentially never appropriate as these cancers have a high propensity of seeding surgical wounds. Even in the face of cord compression, chemotherapy followed by surgery is usually the preferred management.

Patients relapsing after cystectomy essentially always have systemic disease, but a substantial fraction have clinically detectable involvement confined to local and/ or regional nodes. We know that some of these patients will have an excellent response to chemotherapy and with surgical consolidation will be long-term survivors. Thus, while it has not been rigorously shown to produce a better overall outcome, surveillance by periodic CT is usually performed. Relapse is stereotypically circumscribed between 9 and 18 months, by which time about 85% of those destined to relapse will have done so, and this is when we advocate surveillance.

In our experience, CIS of the distal ureter is the pathological feature most closely associated with upper tract recurrence (85). In fact, 15% of those with postcystectomy tumor within the distal intramural ureter developed an upper tract recurrence. Intraoperative ureteral margin status by itself was of little consequence. Patients with TCC involving the prostatic urethra also had a higher incidence of upper tract recurrence following cystectomy, in keeping with the field-change hypothesis of urothelial carcinogenesis. Upper tract surveillance of these patients can be accomplished with urine cytology and upper tract imaging. Traditionally, the intravenous pyelogram (IVP) was the primary imaging tool for surveillance of the upper tract because it provides visualization of filling defects and can detect obstruction. More recently, CT urography has been found to be a more sensitive surveillance tool following cystectomy because not only can it identify local and distant recurrences but early upper tract recurrences as well.

■ SYSTEMIC THERAPY FOR UROTHELIAL CANCER

Currently, *combination therapy is standard* in the treatment of metastatic TCC. The development of methotrexate, vinblastine, Adriamycin, and cisplatin

(M-VAC) at Sloan-Kettering (86) was an important achievement. Subsequent landmark trials have confirmed that M-VAC is superior to single-agent cisplatin (87), the combination of cyclophosphamide, doxorubicin, and cisplatin (88), the combination of 5-fluorouracil, interferon-alpha, and cisplatin (89), and the combination of docetaxel and cisplatin (90). In fact, there are at least nine randomized trials involving M-VAC, and to date, the only challenger to even suggest improved clinical outcome was a trial of a dose-dense variant of M-VAC given with G-CSF support versus "classic" M-VAC (91). The dose-dense version was associated with markedly less mucositis, and the cycles are only 14 days (compared to 28 in the classic schedule) and thus this variant has supplanted the original. With overall response rates in the 50 to 60% range and up to 30% clinical CR rate, there is no doubt that dose-dense M-VAC provides meaningful palliation for most patients and can significantly change the natural history of the disease for a few.

Nonetheless, for most oncologists, M-VAC has overstayed its welcome. Despite having been the standard of care for 20 years, it is nearly completely abandoned because of significant toxicity and the availability of regimens of similar efficacy that are slightly less toxic. While we freely acknowledge the considerable shortcomings of M-VAC, it is distressing to us to see phase II studies of newer doublets consistently show survival results inferior to the well-established benchmark established by M-VAC and to see widespread use of these regimens. While one might argue that this is acceptable in the metastatic setting, where a shorter overall survival might be associated with "more good days" if one uses a less toxic treatment, we see no rationale for the widespread use of inferior regimens in the setting of perioperative therapy for locally advanced disease. In that context, improvement of cure fraction has been demonstrated for M-VAC, but not established for other regimens. Thus, in the absence of a clinical trial, the dose-dense version of M-VAC is the standard frontline therapy at MD Anderson when chemotherapy is given with curative intent.

In the setting of metastatic disease, for which the goals are clearly palliative, the doublet of gemcitabine and cisplatin (Gem/Cis) has become a standard option. Gem/Cis was compared to M-VAC in a large international phase III trial (92). The doublet was shown to be similar with respect to median survival and was associated with significantly less mucositis and neutropenic fever. Gem/Cis did cause more thrombocytopenia however. As expected for two regimens with comparable efficacy, quality-of-life measures were not different between the two treatments, despite the favorable treatment-related side-effect profile of Gem/Cis. In our view this is not a surprising finding, but rather reinforces the notion that the burden of morbidity in patients with metastatic bladder cancer is far more likely to be due to the disease, rather than secondary to the treatment. Metastatic urothelial cancer is a very bad disease.

Gemcitabine, the taxanes, and ifosfamide all have activity in urothelial cancer, and there have been many new doublets and triplets investigated over the past 10 years. From this experience, it is clear that all regimens substituting carboplatin for cisplatin show inferior results (the triplet of gemcitabine, paclitaxel, and carboplatin may be an exception).

Urothelial cancer is a disease of the elderly. The lifetime accumulation of risk factors predisposing patients to bladder cancer often lead to other comorbid conditions such as coronary artery disease and chronic obstructive pulmonary disease. These diseases, in addition to other conditions found in an aging population such as diabetes and hypertension, often contribute to poor renal function, or a performance status unable to tolerate aggressive cisplatin- or ifosfamide-based therapy.

Ureteral obstruction is also a frequent factor contributing to diminished renal function, and nephrostomy tubes are an indispensable tool in the treatment of advanced bladder cancer. Nephrostomy tubes are much to be preferred over ureteral stents in patients undergoing chemotherapy for locally advanced bladder cancer. This is so because chemotherapy often engenders periods of neutropenia that can lead to chronic infection associated with foreign bodies. Nephrostomies are much more easily changed out than stents. Furthermore, stents are far more irritating and likely to bleed during periods of thrombocytopenia. It is not uncommon to have stents clog from bleeding, and this is much less problematic with nephrostomies. Finally, nephrostomies will reliably decompress the kidneys, even if the cancer grows, while stents can be collapsed by tumor, and even by desmoplastic reaction to therapy.

Relatively effective chemotherapy for patients with impaired renal function is now fairly easy to come by. Vinblastine, gemcitabine, taxanes, and doxorubicin can all be given safely in the context of renal insufficiency. At the present time, we favor a triplet of gemcitabine (900 mg/m^2 given over 90 min), paclitaxel (100 mg/m^2), and doxorubicin (30 mg/m^2) repeated every 14 days for patients with poor renal function. This regimen is reliably deliverable and has useful clinical activity.

■ FUTURE PROSPECTS

The ready availability of the bladder surface makes bladder cancer an ideal clinical model for the development of gene therapy. Investigators at MDACC have reported that adenoviral-mediated gene expression (in this case of interferon-alpha 2b) within the bladder can be achieved using the detergent Syn3 (93). A phase I trial has been completed, and further work with this and other intravesical gene transfer therapies is ongoing.

The efficacy of BCG strongly suggests that immune recognition and reaction to bladder cancer antigens is a clinical strategy that could be further developed. Moreover, tumor-infiltrating CD8 expressing T cells are predictive of survival in patients with urothelial carcinoma (94). In addition, the tumor antigen NY-ESO-1 occurs in approximately 30 to 40% of muscle-invasive tumors, and CD8 expressing T cells can recognize the NY-ESO-1 antigen (95). A clinical trial (96) based on NY-ESO-1 vaccine was conducted in patients with urothelial cancer whose tumors expressed the NY-ESO-1 antigen and who received vaccination in the adjuvant setting. Six patients were enrolled on this exploratory study and all developed antigen-specific immune responses, consisting of antibody or CD8 or CD4 T-cell responses specific for NY-ESO-1. This work, and other approaches based on specific antigens, clearly shows enough promise that we can expect further advances in the near term.

In a complementary approach, some investigators are pursuing modulation of immune-cell signaling. The best-characterized inhibitory cell signaling system consists of the interactions between the cytotoxic lymphocyte antigen-4 (CTLA-4) and the B7 family of membrane proteins. Anti-CTLA-4 antibody, developed as a therapeutic agent with an aim to overcome the inhibitory B7-CTLA-4 signal to downregulate T cells, has shown promise for the immunologic treatment of cancer. To date, over 3000 patients with different tumor types (including melanoma, renal cell carcinoma, ovarian carcinoma, pancreatic cancer, and prostate cancer) have been treated with anti-CTLA-4. Although clinical responses have been limited to a small subset (approximately 10% of patients), there is ongoing research to understand the biologic basis for the effect. Clearly, a trial of NY-ESO-1 vaccine in combination with anti-CTLA-4 antibody for patients with metastatic urothelial cancer is of substantial interest.

Finally, there is much reason to think that soon we will see significantly refined prognostic models that will allow substantial refinement of how we apply currently available therapies (97). This could result in better outcomes for many patients even without the appearance of new treatments.

Commentary: Molecular Markers for Risk Stratification and Personalized Therapy in Urothelial Tumors

As aptly outlined in the accompanying chapter, urothelial cancer poses significant scientific and public health challenges. On the one hand, most urothelial cancers are low-grade papillary lesions that recur at high frequency. While they are not life threatening, these "tumors" are the most expensive cancers to manage, and it is not yet possible for clinicians to distinguish the ones that will become lethal from the ones that will not. On the other hand, muscle-invasive urothelial tumors often progress rapidly and are often fatal. Although a significant subset of these tumors responds well to cisplatin-based chemotherapy, another large fraction does not, and many of the tumors that initially respond to therapy become resistant. It is at present impossible to distinguish these tumors from one another, and no real progress has been made in targeting resistant tumors over the last 20 years, presumably because we do not understand the biological basis of resistance. Finally, urothelial cancers actually comprise an even more heterogeneous group of different tumor phenotypes (TCC, squamous tumors, micropapillary tumors, small cell cancer, etc), and it is not clear at present whether they should all be considered one disease or several.

Although funding for basic research on urothelial cancer has been modest, enormous progress has been made in defining the genetic and biological mechanisms that influence urothelial cancer susceptibility and disease progression, and with the emergence of new technical advances (including whole genome SNP, micro RNA, and mRNA expression profiling and "next generation" sequencing), we expect that even more dramatic breakthroughs are forthcoming within the next 5 years. We expect that this information will prove to be critical in addressing the existing challenges described earlier. Specifically, we expect that advances in whole genome molecular biology will help to resolve current questions about which non-invasive tumors will progress to become life threatening, which therapies will be most active in cisplatin-refractory muscle-invasive and metastatic disease, how the various histologic subsets of urothelial cancer are related to one another, and how the biology of each subset relates to vulnerability to certain agents. These new developments will lead to a "personalized medicine" approach to the management of urothelial cancers that should dramatically improve patient outcomes and require the authors of this chapter to drastically revise their contribution for the next edition of this volume.

David J. McConkey

References

1. Jemal A, Siegel R, Ward E, et al. Cancer statistics, 2009. *CA Cancer J Clin* 2009;59:225-249.
2. Wu X, Ros MM, Gu J, et al. Epidemiology and genetic susceptibility to bladder cancer. *BJU Int* 2008;102:1207-1215.
3. Michaud DS, Spiegelman D, Clinton SK, et al. Fluid intake and the risk of bladder cancer in men. *N Engl J Med* 1999; 340:1390-1397.
4. Levine LA, Richie JP. Urological complications of cyclophosphamide. *J Urol* 1989;141:1063-1069.
5. Ross RK, Paganini-Hill A, Landolph J, et al. Analgesics, cigarette smoking, and other risk factors for cancer of the renal pelvis and ureter. *Cancer Res* 1989;49:1045-1048.
6. Groah SL, Weitzenkamp MS, Lammertse DP, et al. Excess risk of bladder cancer in spinal cord injury: Evidence for an association between indwelling catheter use and bladder cancer. *Arch Phys Med Rehabil* 2002;83:346-351.
7. Taylor JA, Umbach DM, Stephens E, et al. The role of N-acetylation polymorphisms in smoking-associated bladder cancer: Evidence of a gene-gene-exposure three-way interaction. *Cancer Res* 1998;58:3603-3610.
8. Reszka E, Wasowicz W. Genetic polymorphism of N-acetyltransferase and glutathione S-transferase related to neoplasm of genitourinary system. *Neoplasma* 2002;49:209-216.
9. Wang M, Gu D, Zhang Z et al. XPD polymorphisms, cigarette smoking, and bladder cancer risk: A meta-analysis. *J Toxicol Environ Health Part A* 2009;72:698-705.
10. Stern MC, Lin J, Figueroa JD, et al. Polymorphisms in DNA repair genes, smoking and bladder cancer risk: Findings from the International Consortium of Bladder Cancer. *Cancer Res* 2009;69:6857-6864.
11. Wu X, Amos CI, Zhu Y, et al. Telomere dysfunction: A potential cancer predisposition factor. *J Natl Cancer Inst* 2003; 95:1211-1218.
12. McGrath M, Wong JY, Michaud D, et al. Telomere length, cigarette smoking, and bladder cancer risk in men and women. *Cancer Epidemiol Biomarkers Prev* 2007;16:815-819.
13. Yamamoto Y, Matsuyama H, Kawauchi S, et al. Biological characteristics in bladder cancer depend on the type of genetic instability. *Clin Cancer Res* 2006;12:2752-2758.
14. Sen S, Zhou H, Zhang R-D, et al. Amplification/overexpression of a mitotic kinase gene in human bladder cancer. *J Natl Cancer Inst* 2002;94:1320-1329.

15. Mhawech-Fauceglia P, Fischer G, Beck A, et al. Raf1, Aurora-A/STK15 and E-cadherin biomarkers expression in patients with pTa/pT1 urothelial bladder carcinoma: A retrospective TMA study of 246 patients with long-term follow-up. *Eur J Surg Oncol* 2006;32:439-444.

16. Bruyere F, Corcoran NM, Berdjis N, et al. Arora kinase B is an independent protective factor in superficial bladder tumours with a dysfunctional G1 checkpoint. *BJU International* 2008; 102:247-252.

17. Comperat E, Bieche I, Dargere D, et al. Gene expression study of Aurora-A reveals implication during bladder carcinogenesis and increasing values in invasive urothelial cancer. *Urology* 2008;72:873-877.

18. Park H-S, Park WS, Bondaruk J, et al. Quantitation of Aurora A gene copy number in urine sediments and bladder cancer detection. *J Natl Cancer Inst* 2008;100:1401-1411.

19. Imao T, Koshida K, Endo Y, et al. Dominant role of E-cadherin in the progression of bladder cancer. *J Urol* 1999;161:692-698.

20. Inoue K, Slaton JW, Karashima T, et al. The prognostic value of angiogenesis factor expression for predicting recurrence and metastasis of bladder cancer following neoadjuvant chemotherapy and radical cystectomy. *Clin Cancer Res* 2000; 6:4866-4873.

21. Barbisan F, Santinelli A, Mazzucchelli R, et al. Strong immunohistochemical expression of fibroblast growth factor receptor 3, superficial staining pattern of cytokeratin 20, and low proliferative activity define those papillary urothelial neoplasms of low malignant potential that do not recur. *Cancer* 2008;112:636-644.

22. Majewski T, Lee S, Jeong J, et al. Understanding the development of human bladder cancer by using a whole-organ genomic mapping strategy. *Lab Invest* 2008;88:694-721.

23. Cote RJ, Dunn MD, Chatterjee SJ, et al. Elevated and absent pRb expression is associated with bladder cancer progression and has cooperative effects with p53. *Cancer Res* 1998;58: 1090-1094.

24. Esrig D, Elmajian D, Groshen S, et al. Accumulation of nuclear p53 and tumor progression in bladder cancer. *N Engl J Med* 1994;331:1259-1264.

25. Sarkar S, Julicher KP, Burger MS, et al. Different combinations of genetic/epigenetic alterations inactivate the p53 and pRb pathways in invasive human bladder cancers. *Cancer Res* 2000;60:3862-3871.

26. Shariat SF, Lotan Y, Karakiewicz PI, et al. p53 Predictive value for pT1-2 N0 disease at radical cystectomy. *J Urol* 2009;182:907-913.

27. Millikan RE, Dinney C, Swanson D, et al. Final Report of a Randomized Trial of Cystectomy Plus Adjuvant M-VAC vs. Cystectomy With Both Pre-and Post-Operative M-VAC. *J Clin Oncol* 2001;19:4005-4013.

28. Mendelsohn J, Dinney CP. The Willet F. Whitmore, Jr., Lectureship: Blockade of epidermal growth factor receptors as anticancer therapy. *J Urol* 2001;165:1152-1157.

29. Hussain MH, MacVicar GR, Petrylak DP, et al. Trastuzumab, paclitaxel, carboplatin, and gemcitabine in advanced human epidermal growth factor receptor-2/neu-positive urothelial carcinoma: Results of a multicenter phase II National Cancer Institute trial. *J Clin Oncol* 2007;25:2218-2224. [Erratum appears in *J Clin Oncol* 2008;26: 3295.]

30. Slaton JW, Millikan R, Inoue K, et al. Correlation of metastasis related gene expression and relapse-free survival in patients with locally advanced bladder cancer treated with cystectomy and chemotherapy. *J Urol* 2004;171:570-574.

31. Sonpavde G, Jian W, Liu H, et al. Sunitinib malate is active against human urothelial carcinoma and enhances the activity of cisplatin in a preclinical model. *Urologic Oncol* 2009;27: 391-399.

32. Milowsky SR, Gerst S, Tickoo N, et al. A phase II study of sunitinib on a continuous dosing schedule in patients (pts) with relapsed or refractory urothelial carcinoma (UC). *J Clin Oncol* 2008;72:252s (suppl abstr 5072).

33. Youssef RF, Mitra AP, Bartsch G Jr., et al. Molecular targets and targeted therapies in bladder cancer management. *World J Urol* 2009;27:9-20.

34. Epstein JI, Amin MB, Reuter VR, et al. The Bladder Consensus Conference Committee. The World Health Organization/International Society of Urologic Pathology consensus classification of urothelial (transitional cell) neoplasms of the urinary bladder. *Am J Surg Pathol* 1998;22:1435-1448.

35. Dinney CP, McConkey DJ, Millikan RE, et al. Focus on bladder cancer. *Cancer Cell* 2004;6:111-116.

36. Mitra AP, Datar RH, Cote RJ. Molecular pathways in invasive bladder cancer: New insights into mechanisms, progression and target identification. *J Clin Oncol* 2006;24:5552-5564.

37. Spiess PE, Czerniak B. Dual-track pathway of bladder carcinogenesis: Practical implications. *Archiv Pathol Lab Med* 2006;130:844-852.

38. Amin MB, Ro JY, el-Sharkawy T, et al. Micropapillary variant of transitional cell carcinoma of the urinary bladder. Histologic pattern resembling ovarian papillary serous carcinoma. *Am J Surg Pathol* 1994;18:1224-1232

39. Ohtsuki Y, Kuroda N, Umeoka T, et al. KL-6 is another useful marker in assessing a micropapillary pattern in carcinomas of the breast and urinary bladder, but not the colon. *Medical Molec Morphol* 2009;42:123-127.

40. Sangoi AR, Higgins JP, Rouse RV, et al. Immunohistochemical comparison of MUC1, CA125, and Her2Neu in invasive micropapillary carcinoma of the urinary tract and typical invasive urothelial carcinoma with retraction artifact. *Mod Pathol* 2009;22:660-667.

41. Kamat AM, Dinney CP, Gee JR, et al. Micropapillary bladder cancer: A review of the University of Texas MD Anderson Cancer Center experience with 100 consecutive patients. *Cancer* 2007;110:62-67.

42. Siefker-Radtke AO, Kamat AM, Grossman HB, et al. Phase II clinical trial of neoadjuvant alternating doublet chemotherapy with ifosfamide/doxorubicin and etoposide/cisplatin in small-cell urothelial cancer. *J Clin Oncol* 2009;27:2592-2597.

43. Siefker-Radtke A. Urachal carcinoma: Surgical and chemotherapeutic options. *Expert Rev Anticancer Ther* 2006;6: 1715-1721.

44. Herr HW, Bochner BH, Sharp D, et al. Urachal carcinoma: Contemporary surgical outcomes. *J Urol* 2007;178:74-78.

45. Gopalan A, Sharp DS, Fine SW, et al. Urachal carcinoma: A clinicopathologic analysis of 24 cases with outcome correlation. *Am J Surg Path* 2009;33:659-668.

46. Molina JR, Quevedo JF, Furth AF, et al. Predictors of survival from urachal cancer: A Mayo Clinic study of 49 cases. *Cancer* 2007;10:2434-2440.

47. Ashley RA, Inman BA, Sebo TJ, et al. Urachal carcinoma: Clinicopathologic features and long-term outcomes of an aggressive malignancy. *Cancer* 2006;107:712-720.

48. Siefker-Radtke AO, Gee J, Shen Y, et al. Multimodality management of urachal carcinoma: The M.D. Anderson Cancer Center experience. *J Urol* 2003;169:1295-1298.

49. Mhawech-Fauceglia P, Fischer G, Alvarez V Jr., et al. Predicting outcome in minimally invasive (T1a and T1b) urothelial bladder carcinoma using a panel of biomarkers: A high throughput tissue microarray analysis. *BJU Int* 2007;100: 1182-1187.

50. Platz CE, Cohen MB, Jones MP, et al. Is microstaging of early invasive cancer of the urinary bladder possible or useful? *Mod Pathol* 1996;9:1035.

51. Engel P, Anagnostaki L, Braendstrup O. The muscularis mucosae of the human urinary bladder. Implications for tumor staging or biopsies. *Scand J Urol Nephrol* 1992;26:249.

52. Wijkstrom H, Norming U, Lagerkvist M, et al. Evaluation of clinical staging before cystectomy in transitional cell bladder carcinoma: A long-term follow-up of 276 consecutive patients. *Br J Urol* 1998;81:686-691.

53. Shariat SF, Karakiewicz PI, Gody G, et al. Use of nomograms for predictions of outcome in patients with advanced bladder cancer. *Ther Adv Urol* 2009;1:13-26.

54. Galsky MD, Herr HW, Bajorin DF. Integration of chemotherapy and surgery for bladder cancer. *J Natl Compr Canc Netw* 2005;3:45-51.

55. Isbarn H, Karakiewica PI, Shariat SF, et al. Residual pathological stage at radical cystectomy significantly impacts outcomes for initial T2N0 bladder cancer. *J Urol* 2009;182:459-465.

56. Resorlua B, Baltacia S, Resorluc M, et al. Prognostic significance of hydronephrosis in bladder cancer treated by radical cystectomy. *Urol Int* 2009;83:285-288.

57. Bartsch GC, Kuefer R, Gschwend JE, et al. Hydronephrosis as a prognostic marker in bladder cacner in a cystectomy-only series. *Eur Urol* 2007;51:690-697.

58. Quek ML, Stein JP, Nichols PW, et al. Prognostic significance of lymphovascular invasion of bladder cancer treated with radical cystectomy. *J Urol* 2005;174:103-106.

59. Goddard JC, Sutton CD, Furness PN, et al. Microvessel density at presentation predicts subsequent muscle invasion in superficial bladder cancer. *Clin Cancer Res* 2003;9:2583-2586.

60. Margel D, Tal R, Neuman A, et al. Prediction of extravesical disease by preoperative serum markers in patients with clinically organ confined invasive bladder cancer. *J Urol* 2006;175: 1253-1258.

61. Margel D, Tal R, Baniel J. Serum tumor markers may predict overall and disease-specific survival in patients with clinically organ-confined invasive bladder cancer. *J Urol* 2007;178: 2297-2233.

62. Pectasides D, Bafaloucos D, Antoniou F, et al. TPA, TATI, CEA, AFP, beta-HCG, PSA, SCC, and CA 19-9 for monitoring transitional cell carcinoma of the bladder. *Am J Clin Oncol* 1996;19:271-277.

63. Vickers AJ, Cronin AM, Kattan MW, et al. Clinical benefits of a multivariate prediction model for bladder cancer. *Cancer* 2009;115:5460-5469.

64. Herr HW. Extent of surgery and pathology evaluation has an impact on bladder cancer outcomes after radical cystectomy. *Urology* 2003;61(1):105-108.

65. Elting LS, Pettaway C, Bekele BN, et al. Correlation between annual volume of cystectomy, professional staffing, and outcomes: A statewide, population-based study. *Cancer* 2005; 104:975-984.

66. Herr HW, Faulkner JR, Grossman HB, et al. Pathologic evaluation of radical cystectomy specimens: A cooperative group report. *Cancer* 2004;100:2470-2475.

67. Lamm DL, Thor DE, Harris SC, et al. Bacillus Calmette-Guérin immunotherapy of superficial bladder cancer. *J Urol* 1980;124:38-40.

68. Lerner SP, Tangen CM, Sucharew H, et al. Failure to achieve a complete response to induction BCG therapy is associated with increased risk of disease worsening and death in patients with high risk non-muscle invasive bladder cancer. *Urol Oncol* 2009;27:155-159.

69. Herr HW, Sogani P. Does early cystectomy improve the survival of patients with high risk superficial bladder tumors? *J Urol* 2001;168:1296-1299.

70. Cookson MS, Herr HW, Zhang ZF, et al. The treated natural history of high risk superficial bladder cancer: 15-year outcome. *J Urol* 1997;158:62-67.

71. Herr HW. The value of a second transurethral resection in evaluating patients with bladder tumors. *J Urol* 1999;162(1):74-76.

72. Fradet Y, Grossman H, Gomella L, et al. A comparison of hexaminolevulinate fluorescence cystoscopy and white light cystoscopy for the detection of carcinoma in situ in patients with bladder cancer: A phase III, multicenter study. *J Urol* 2007;178:68-73.

73. Esrig D, Freeman JA, Stein JP, et al. Early cystectomy for clinical stage T1 transitional cell carcinoma of the bladder. *Semin Urol Oncol* 1997;15:154-160.

74. Madersbacher S, Hochreiter W, Burkhard F, et al. Radical cystectomy for bladder cancer today—a homogeneous series without neoadjuvant therapy. *J Clin Oncol* 2003;21:690.

75. Lee CT, Madii R, Daignault S, et al. Cystectomy delay more than 3 months from initial bladder cancer diagnosis results in decreased disease specific and overall survival. *J Urol* 2006; 175:1262-1267.

76. Herr HW. Extent of pelvic lymph node dissection during radical cystectomy: Where and Why! *Eur Urol* 2009;57:212-213.

77. Shipley WU, Zietman AL, Kaufman DS, et al. Selective bladder preservation by trimodality therapy for patients with muscularis propria-invasive bladder cancer and who are cystectomy candidates—the Massachusetts General Hospital and Radiation Therapy Oncology Group experiences. *Semin Radiat Oncol* 2005;15:36-41.

78. Logothetis CJ. Organ preservation in bladder carcinoma: A matter of selection. *J Clin Oncol* 1991;9:1525-1526.

79. Millikan R, Dinney C, Swanson D, et al. Integrated therapy for locally advanced bladder cancer: Final report of a randomized trial of cystectomy plus adjuvant M-VAC versus cystectomy with both preoperative and postoperative M-VAC. *J Clin Oncol* 2001;19:4005-4013.

80. Grossman HB, Natale RB, Tangen CM, et al. Neoadjuvant chemotherapy plus cystectomy compared with cystectomy alone for locally advanced bladder cancer. *N Engl J Med* 2003; 349:859-866.

81. Tilki D, Svatek RS, Karakiewicz PI, et al. Characteristics and outcomes of patients with pT4 urothelial carcinoma at radical cystectomy: A retrospective international study of 583 patients. *J Urol* 2010;183:87-93.

82. Sweeney P, Millikan R, Donat M, et al. Is there a therapeutic role for post-chemotherapy retroperitoneal lymph node dissection in metastatic transitional cell carcinoma of the bladder? *J Urol* 2003;169:2113-2117.

83. Donat SM, Herr HW, Bajorin DF, et al. Methotrexate, vinblastine, doxorubicin and cisplatin chemotherapy and cystectomy for unresectable bladder cancer. *J Urol* 1996;156:368-371.

84. Siefker-Radtke AO, Walsh GL, Pisters LL, et al. Is there a role for surgery in the management of metastatic urothelial cancer? The M.D. Anderson experience. *J Urol* 2004;171:145-148.

85. Kenworthy P, Tanguay S, Dinney CP. The risk of upper tract recurrence following cystectomy in patients with transitional cell carcinoma involving the distal ureter. *J Urol* 1996;155:501-503.

86. Sternberg CN, Yagoda A, Scher HI, et al. Preliminary results of M-VAC (methotrexate, vinblastine, doxorubicin and cisplatin) for transitional cell carcinoma of the urothelium. *J Urol* 1985;133:403-407.

87. Loehrer PJ Sr, Einhorn LH, Elson PJ, et al. A randomized comparison of cisplatin alone or in combination with methotrexate, vinblastine, and doxorubicin in patients with metastatic urothelial carcinoma: A cooperative group study. *J Clin Oncol* 1992;10:1066-1073.

88. Logothetis CJ, Dexeus FH, Finn L, et al. A prospective randomized trial comparing MVAC and CISCA chemotherapy for patients with metastatic urothelial tumors. *J Clin Oncol* 1990;8:1050-1055.

89. Siefker-Radtke AO, Millikan RE, Tu SM, et al. Phase III trial of fluorouracil, interferon alpha-2b, and cisplatin versus methotrexate, vinblastine, doxorubicin, and cisplatin in metastatic or unresectable urothelial cancer. *J Clin Oncol* 2002; 20:1361-1367.

90. Bamias A, Aravantinos G, Deliveliotis C, et al. Docetaxel and cisplatin with granulocyte colony-stimulating factor (G-CSF) versus MVAC with G-CSF in advanced urothelial carcinoma: A multicenter, randomized, phase III study from the Hellenic Cooperative Oncology Group. *J Clin Oncol* 2004; 22:220-228.

91. Sternberg CN, de Mulder PH, Schornagel JH, et al. Randomized phase III trial of high-dose-intensity methotrexate, vinblastine, doxorubicin, and cisplatin (MVAC) chemotherapy and recombinant human granulocyte colony-stimulating factor versus classic MVAC in advanced urothelial tract tumors: European Organization for Research and Treatment of Cancer Protocol no. 30924. *J Clin Oncol* 2001;19:2638-2646.

92. von der Maase H, Hansen SW, Roberts JT, et al. Gemcitabine and cisplatin versus methotrexate, vinblastine, doxorubicin, and cisplatin in advanced or metastatic bladder cancer: Results of a large, randomized, multinational, multi-center, phase III study. *J Clin Oncol* 2000;18:3068-3077.

93. Nagabhushan TL, Maneval DC, Benedict WF, et al. Enhancement of intravesical delivery with Syn3 potentiates interferon-alpha2b gene therapy for superficial bladder cancer. *Cytokine Growth Factor Rev* 2007;18:389-94.

94. Sharma P, Shen Y, Wen S, et al. CD8 tumor-infiltrating lymphocytes are predictive of survival in muscle-invasive urothelial carcinoma. *Proc Natl Acad Sci USA* 2007;104:3967-3972.

95. Sharma P, Gnjatic S, Jungbluth A, et al. Frequency of NY-ESO-1 and LAGE-1 expression in bladder cancer and evidence of a new NY-ESO-1 T-cell epitope in a patient with bladder cancer. *Cancer Immun* 2003;3:19.

96. Sharma P, Bajorin D, Jungbluth A, et al. Immune responses detected in urothelial carcinoma patients after vaccination with NY-ESO-1 protein plus BCG and GM-CSF. *J Immunol* 2008; 31:849-857.

97. Shariat SF, Chade DC, Karakiewicz PI et al. Combination of multiple molecular markers can improve prognostication in patients with locally advanced and lymph node positive bladder cancer. *J Urol* 2010;183:68-75.

PROSTATE CANCER

Paul Corn
Christopher Logothetis

Over the past decade, insight into the biological basis of prostate cancer development and progression has influenced our approach to treating patients with the disease. While research efforts have historically focused on the prostate cancer epithelial cell, there is growing evidence that interactions between the host tissue microenvironment and the cancer epithelial cell are critical for tumorigenesis. For example, prostate cancer epithelial cells preferentially metastasize to bone by acquiring osteomimetic properties that usurp normal bone homeostasis maintained by osteoblasts, osteoclasts, endothelial cells, and other bone stromal elements. Understanding

the bidirectional cancer cell-host interaction now dominates prostate cancer research. The knowledge gained from this effort has led to novel treatment strategies that target the bone microenvironment (eg, with antiangiogenesis inhibitors) in addition to the epithelial cell (eg, with chemotherapy).

Prostate cancers have recognizable clinical features that allow anticipation of their clinical behavior. Fortunately, the progression from localized, androgen-dependent disease to castration-resistant disease with bone-forming metastases occurs in only a minority of patients. To conceptualize the clinical heterogeneity displayed along this continuum, we assign patients to different prostate cancer "clinical states" to help structure treatment recommendations and therapy development. The goal of our research program at MD Anderson is to more reliably predict prostate cancer progression and apply therapy to only those patients who need it. This strategy will favorably improve the outcome of selected patients threatened by their disease while avoiding unnecessary morbidity to the majority who are not.

EPIDEMIOLOGY AND CLINICAL FEATURES

Prostate cancer is a major health care challenge in the United States (1). It is the second most common cancer in men (behind skin cancer) and the second leading cause of cancer death (behind lung cancer). In 2009, it is estimated that 192,280 men will be newly diagnosed with prostate cancer and 27,360 men will die from prostate cancer. There are a number of unique clinical features of prostate cancer that distinguish it from other solid tumor types:

1. Despite the high prevalence of prostate cancer, the majority of patients diagnosed with the disease eventually die from other causes. This is in striking contrast to lung cancer, where the majority of patients diagnosed with the disease die from it.
2. Cancer of the prostate often has a prolonged natural history. This is evidenced by a high incidence of occult malignancy in autopsy series of men who die from non–prostate cancer causes and in clinically normal prostates of men undergoing cysto-prostatectomy for bladder cancer. Therefore, over the course of a normal lifetime, most men will develop "clinically occult" prostate cancer that will never produce symptoms, require treatment, or cause death.
3. The incidence of detected carcinoma increases with age.
4. Androgens are a major driving force in normal prostate development and are implicated in tumorigenesis.
5. Prostate cancer is typically multifocal, commonly presenting as synchronous carcinomas arising in multiple locations, and the malignant potential is determined by the sum of the primary and secondary grades (Gleason score). Thus, biologic heterogeneity is an inherent property of each tumor.
6. Clinical prostate cancer is more prevalent in Western than Eastern societies, although incidence rates increase for men from China and Japan who immigrate to the United States. This observation implicates environmental factors (diet, lifestyle, etc) in prostate cancer development.
7. Prostate cancers have a predictable rate and pattern of progression, with bone-forming metastases dominating the clinical progression in the majority of patients with advanced disease. This observation supports the view that the bone-epithelial interaction is central to the progression of prostate cancer.

AGING

It has long been recognized that prostate cancer is a disease of the elderly, and epidemiologic data demonstrate that rates of prostate cancer incidence and mortality increase with age (2,3). While prostate-specific antigen (PSA) screening has led to an earlier average age at diagnosis, mortality is still largely seen in patients 70 years of age or older. As the longevity of populations increases worldwide, the burden of prostate cancer creates a significant health care challenge. This has generated a sense of urgency among physicians to refine our ability to predict cancer virulence and apply therapy to those patients who need it.

ENDOCRINE

Androgens are central to the normal growth, differentiation, and function of the prostate gland, although the role of androgen-receptor (AR) signaling in prostate carcinogenesis and progression has not been fully elucidated. Even in the clinically castrate state (serum testosterone <50 ng/mL), there is growing evidence that prostate cancer cells continue to rely on AR signaling for proliferation (4). Potential mechanisms accounting for this include intratumoral amplification of the androgen receptor, mutations of the androgen receptor, changes in levels of androgen receptor cofactors, ligand-independent activation of the androgen receptor, upregulation of enzymes involved in androgen synthesis, and conversion of testosterone to dihydrotestosterone (DHT). Thus, during prostate cancer progression there is a gradual shift from endocrine sources of androgens (ie, from the testes and adrenal glands) to paracrine/autocrine/intracrine sources (Fig. 34-1). All these events can occur in the setting of a low serum testosterone.

Although we lack experimental data and supporting clinical evidence, other hormones that may be implicated in prostate cancer progression include insulin-like growth factor-1 (IGF-1), leptin, prolactin, and bombesin (5,6).

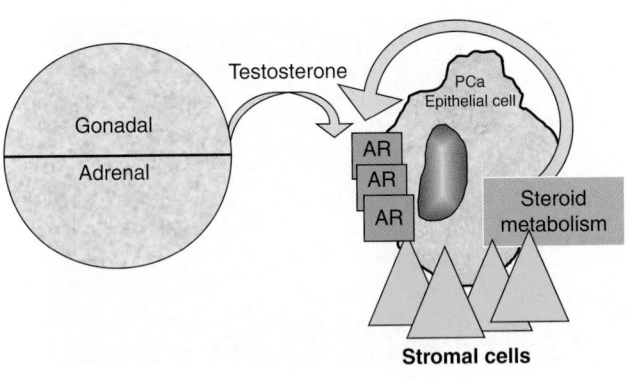

FIGURE 34-1. Androgen sources switch from endocrine to paracrine/autocrine during disease progression.

DIET AND OBESITY

Several lines of clinical and experimental evidence support a central role for diet, caloric intake, and obesity in the development of prostate cancer with lethal potential. Obesity, defined as body mass index (BMI) above 30, is manifested by overgrowth of white adipose tissue (WAT). Recently, obesity has been associated with progression of a number of different cancer types, including prostate cancer (7). For example, obese patients with prostate cancer are more likely to develop a recurrence following radical prostatectomy or radiation therapy for localized disease (8-10). The mechanism for the association between obesity and prostate cancer progression is poorly understood. Current models suggest that predetermined genetic traits associated with both obesity and cancers are influenced by lifestyle components such as diet and physical activity. However, epidemiological studies show that cancer can be accelerated in obese patients irrespective of their lifestyle. Thus, it has been proposed that WAT itself may have a direct effect on cancer progression.

One hypothesis is that WAT acts as a potent endocrine organ that secretes numerous soluble growth and inflammatory factors (such as leptin, adiponectin, insulin-like growth factor (IGF-1), and hepatocyte growth factor [HGF]) that stimulate tumor growth (11,12). In support of this, abdominal adiposity causes a metabolic syndrome characterized by insulin resistance and hyperinsulinemia (13). Previous research efforts have focused on measuring adipokine levels to explain a functional link between obesity and cancer. Results, however, have been inconsistent, suggesting alternate mechanisms account for the association between obesity and cancer. Ongoing clinical trials will test many of these hypotheses (eg, by targeting the IGF-1 signaling axis as a therapy strategy).

RACE AND ETHNICITY

African Americans have a higher frequency of death from prostate cancer compared to Caucasian and Hispanic Americans. This has variably been attributed to differences in steroid metabolism, genetics, environmental effects, or social factors. There is a reduced incidence of prostate cancer among Chinese and Japanese Americans, but their incidence is higher than that reported in native Chinese or Japanese persons. Of interest is the fact that northern European males have a higher frequency of prostate cancer than males from southern Europe. A similar finding has been reported in the United States, suggesting that the incidence of prostate cancer is inversely related to sun exposure. These findings have epidemiologically linked prostate cancer to vitamin D metabolism.

GENETIC PREDISPOSITION

As with breast and colon cancer, familial clustering of prostate cancer has been reported. Unlike with breast and colon cancer, however, specific genetic lesions have not been identified to merit the routine use of genetic screening for prostate cancer. The search for "prostate cancer genes" has identified candidate genetic events implicated in tumorigenesis, but these findings have been more useful in understanding the underlying etiology of prostate cancer than in screening. For example, a major hereditary prostate cancer susceptibility locus resides at 1q24, though the responsible gene(s) remains under investigation (14,15). More recently, men carrying *BRCA1/BRCA2* mutations have been shown to be at increased risk of developing prostate cancer (16,17). However, it has not been established that familial cases of prostate cancer are more virulent than nonfamilial cases; so it is unclear how this information will influence management decisions for individual patients.

■ RELEVANT HISTOMORPHOLOGY OF PROSTATE CANCER

Most epithelial cancers arise from the prostatic acinus, with fewer than 10% having a pure ductal origin (this is the opposite of the pattern seen in cancers of the pancreas and breast, where ductal cancers are far more common than those arising in the acinar portion of the secretory unit). The majority show glandular differentiation (ie, adenocarcinoma) (Fig. 34-2A). Importantly, mucin is essentially never seen in prostate

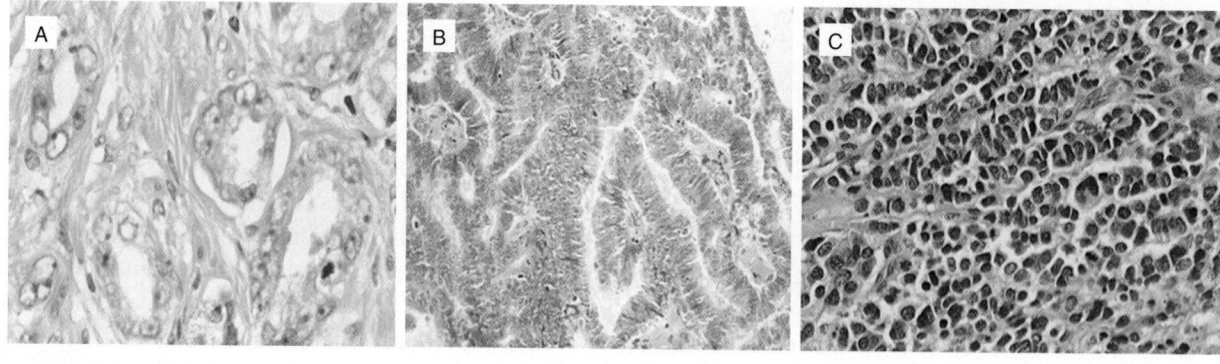

FIGURE 34-2. **A.** Architecture of prostate adenocarcinoma. **B.** Architecture of prostate ductal carcinoma. **C.** Architecture of prostate small cell carcinoma.

cancer. Historically, numerous grading systems have been devised, using all of the typical morphologic criteria by which pathologists can sometimes infer biologic potential. While more than 20 systems have been put forward, prostate cancers are now almost universally graded according to the system of Gleason.

GLEASON GRADING SYSTEM

The Gleason system is unique among pathologic grading systems because it is a composite classification based on a combination of architectural and cellular features often considered in the grading of other epithelial cancers. As originally described, the Gleason system includes two components:

(1) There are five patterns, or grades, ranging from normal architecture to arrays of cells without any glandular organization at all. At our institution, because unequivocal criteria for malignancy already correspond to Gleason grade 2 and the Gleason grade 1 category is rarely reported, prostate cancers are assigned Gleason grades ranging from 2 through 5. (2) The Gleason score is obtained by assigning one Gleason grade to the most dominant (ie, "primary") pattern, and another to the next most common (ie, "secondary") pattern. By convention, such data are expressed as a sum, with the primary pattern listed first. Thus the Gleason score can range from 2 (ie, 1 + 1) to 10 (5 + 5). At MD Anderson, these scores range from 4 to 10, reflecting our decision not to assign a Gleason grade of 1.

A major advantage of the Gleason grading system is its reproducibility and ability to distinguish different cancer phenotypes that influence clinical management. The system is most useful for tumors falling at one the extremes (eg, Gleason 6 or less versus Gleason 8-10). However, a major disadvantage of the system is that it

does not provide a refined view of Gleason 7 tumors, the most commonly reported type. Gleason 7 cancers (ie, 3 + 4 or 4 + 3) represent a very clinically heterogeneous group with variable biologic potential and clinical outcome (18). Despite efforts to improve stratification of Gleason 7 tumors, it is clear the Gleason system is inherently limited by light microscopic methodology to evaluate morphology. Thus, most investigators are now looking to incorporate molecular characterization of tumors into the current grading system.

ASSESSMENT OF PROSTATE BIOPSIES

Gleason grading is a validated system to prognosticate untreated prostate cancers sampled at initial diagnosis. However, the common practice of applying Gleason grading to treat cancers may be misleading. At MD Anderson, for example, pathology reports of specimens obtained after hormone ablation typically indicate "hormonal treatment effect" rather than a Gleason grade per se. Thus, Gleason scores from serial biopsies obtained pre- and posttherapy from the same patient should be interpreted with careful regard to treatment effects. To address this problem, our group has recently proposed a novel "posttherapy" histologic classification to introduce uniformity in analysis of treated tissue specimens (19). If prospectively validated, this system should prove useful in prognosticating preoperatively treated prostate cancers.

An additional confounding variable is tissue sampling. We recognize that there is intratumoral heterogeneity of grade within individual prostates. Thus, it logically follows that the extent and areas of sampling will affect the accuracy of grading and staging. The development of techniques to obtain prostate tissue samples with ultrasound guidance and limited patient morbidity has had a major effect on stage and grade assignment. We increasingly find that the completeness of tissue sampling as measured by the number and distribution of transrectal biopsies greatly influences the adequacy of tumor staging and grading. Biopsy algorithms have been developed to ensure adequate number and distribution of the biopsies (20).

ASSESSMENT OF THE PROSTATECTOMY SPECIMEN

Many of the challenges attributed to the sampling error that occur with needle biopsies can be overcome with proper handling of the prostate following surgery. Assigning a primary and secondary Gleason score is straightforward in a properly processed specimen. This requires great attention to detail in assessing whether the cancer has invaded beyond the prostate capsule (extracapsular) or beyond the margin of resection (margin-positive). Effective communication between the surgeon and pathologist is essential to properly identify the extent and site of surgical margin involvement. As the therapeutic benefit of postoperative radiation therapy is better appreciated, the importance of these aspects has proportionally increased.

Many studies have sought to refine the diagnostic classification of prostate cancer through molecular methods. Unfortunately, no consensus yet exists about the usefulness of molecular phenotypic (or genotypic) characterization in prostate cancer. Using immunohistochemistry, we do know that expression of specific proteins in human specimens has been linked to the clinical course of the disease. For example, loss of functional protein tyrosine phosphatase (PTEN), mutations in p53, and increased expression of BCL-2 are some of the widely reported gain- and loss-of-function changes that have been correlated with prostate cancer progression and mechanistically lined to castration-resistant growth (21,22). Despite this link to biology and correlation with clinical outcome, the methods provide insufficient additional clinical information to justify their routine use.

PROSTATE CANCER VARIANTS

It is apparent that prostate cancer is a heterogeneous disease, and morphologic variants of the cancer may account for some of the heterogeneity (23). The two most prominent morphologic subtypes seen at MD Anderson are ductal and small cell/anaplastic variants.

DUCTAL CANCERS

The ductal variant of prostate cancer in its pure form is unusual. More often, ductal and acinar components are mixed and the relative contribution of the ductal variant to the clinical phenotype of the cancer is unclear. Our impression of the behavior of ductal cancers of the prostate is based on those tumors that are either dominant or pure ductal in origin (Fig. 34-2B). The clinical features that lead us to suspect its presence include the lack of proportional rises in serum PSA concentrations with invasion of the base of the bladder (occasionally mistaken for urothelial cancer), soft tissue distribution of metastases, or lytic bone metastases. For localized disease, patients with pure ductal adenocarcinoma have a better clinical outcome after radical prostatectomy than patients with mixed ductal adenocarcinoma (24). However, metastatic cancers are more aggressive and demonstrate a higher probability of developing visceral metastases than pure acinar adenocarcinomas. We regard endometrioid features as ductal elements of a high-grade acinar adenocarcinoma and have interpreted this to indicate that ductal elements are implicated in prostate cancer progression. However, given the difficulty of establishing objective criteria for the presence of ductal carcinoma as a component of cancer, we are not certain of the frequency of the event.

Small Cell/Anaplastic Cancers

Small cell carcinoma of the prostate is clinically distinguishable from prostate adenocarcinoma in predictable ways. It is castration-resistant, highly metastatic, produces little or no PSA, and causes lytic rather than blastic bone metastases. In addition, in comparison to adenocarcinoma, small cell prostate cancer more frequently metastasizes to lymph nodes and visceral organs (eg, liver or lungs). It can arise de novo or more commonly as a delayed manifestation of progression in patients with a history of high-grade (Gleason 9 and 10) adenocarcinomas following therapy (hormone ablation, radiation therapy, or chemotherapy). The classic clinical presentation is a patient with a precipitously enlarging prostate associated with obstructive symptoms and very little (to no) PSA production. Interestingly, the evolution to a neuroendocrine phenotype is often associated with expression of carcinoembryonic antigen (CEA). For many patients, the CEA will be a much more useful monitoring tool than PSA.

In our experience, small cell carcinomas are also frequently detected in metastatic sites. Our approach is to biopsy sites with unusual features (lytic as opposed to blastic metastases or soft tissue metastases), particularly in those patients whose PSA concentration is judged to be lower than would be expected for the volume of cancer. Requests are made to pathology to analyze the tissue for neuroendocrine markers (chromogranin, synaptophysin, etc). Although standard criteria for establishing a diagnosis have not emerged, most of these cancers will show "salt and pepper" chromatin, express synaptophysin and chromogranin, and display a high nuclear:cytoplasm ratio (Fig. 34-2C). However, the diagnosis of small cell does not require proof of neuroendocrine differentiation. For this reason, we have recently added the term "anaplastic" to our nomenclature to describe tumors presenting clinically as "neuroendocrine-like" but lacking neuroendocrine markers. Until more precise genotype-phenotype associations are elucidated, we recognize that tumors displaying the clinical phenotype described above may display heterogeneity with respect to neuroendocrine differentiation. Small cell/anaplastic carcinomas are highly responsive to etoposide and cisplatin-based chemotherapy but are generally incurable (25).

Rare prostate cancers can take on a squamous appearance, and these cancers are typically much more aggressive and much less amenable to therapy than are typical adenocarcinomas. Cancers displaying intrinsic squamous features are to be distinguished from the squamous appearance often seen in the setting of androgen deprivation and radiation therapy, in which context such features do not imply a poor prognosis. Other rare epithelial cancers include Paneth cell tumors, prostate carcinoids, and sarcomatoid cancers. In general, these cancers are considered unresponsive to androgen ablation and, if localized, are managed with surgery. Clinical decisions are based largely on experience from anecdotal observations.

CANDIDATE PREMALIGNANT LESIONS

Prostatic Intraepithelial Neoplasia

The search for premalignant lesions of the prostate has resulted in the identification of two candidate morphologic lesions (26). The first and most promising premalignant lesion is prostatic intraepithelial neoplasia (PIN). Grades I and II PIN are observed but have not been reliably associated with cancer, nor have they been linked with confidence to prostate cancer development or progression. Thus the reporting of grades I and II PIN has fallen into disfavor at MD Anderson and at most leading institutions. Grade III PIN has been linked to the presence of cancer in many studies, but it does not justify a therapeutic intervention (eg, prostatectomy). Rather, its presence leads to the recommendation of a more thorough biopsy to search for coexistent cancer and/or a repeat biopsy within 6 to 12 months. Grade III

PIN is frequently linked to the presence of established cancer in other regions of the prostate, and as a consequence it rarely serves as a useful early predictive marker. Therein lies the difficulty of performing prevention studies targeting PIN. Most MD Anderson clinicians share the view that a report of multifocal PIN III is nearly identical to a report of low-grade prostate cancer, but with the important caveat that there is insufficient evidence to justify routine intervention (surgery or radiation).

The second potential premalignant lesion is proliferative inflammatory atrophy (PIA) (27). Histologically, these lesions are characterized by inflammatory infiltrates associated with atrophic epithelium. Compared with normal epithelium, there is an increased fraction of proliferating epithelial cells within PIAs. These lesions are thought to provide a mechanistic link between chronic infection and/or inflammation and the predisposition to develop prostate cancer. However, in contrast to PINs, adenocarcinomas rarely arise from PIAs, and PIAs are often observed in prostate biopsies that have no evidence of cancer. Thus, it remains unclear if PIAs are truly precursor lesions for prostate cancer. Ongoing studies seek to address this.

STAGING

It is difficult to precisely assess the extent of prostate cancer on clinical criteria alone. The major benchmark of local extent that influences treatment—organ confined versus non–organ confined—is essentially impossible to distinguish by rectal examination and is not easily appreciated by any imaging modality. Furthermore, PSA levels do not accurately inform about extraprostatic extension of disease. Thus it is common to employ an array of modalities, including transrectal ultrasound, CT, conventional MRI, MRI with an endorectal receiver coil, complex biopsy strategies designed to sample the seminal vesicles and extraprostatic space, and even pelvic lymph node sampling, to determine disease extent. Clearly, each of these modalities offers a different level of sensitivity for detecting lesions and can vary markedly in efficacy. In the final analysis the concept of clinical stage is meaningless without proper context. One must ask, "What is the clinical stage by a particular set of diagnostic tests?"

THE CASE FOR PROSATE CANCER SCREENING

With the advent of PSA screening, there has been a dramatic increase in the number of younger men detected with localized disease. Along with improved outcomes for local therapy (surgery or radiation), it logically follows that PSA screening has contributed to the improved survival rates for men diagnosed with localized prostate cancer. However, the benefits of PSA screening remain controversial for clinicians and a source of confusion for patients. For clinicians, there has been a conspicuous lack of level 1 evidence supporting the use of PSA screening. The recent publication of two large randomized screening trials (with >250,000 patients) has not helped clarify the issue, since one trial did not show a survival benefit (The PLCO [Prostate, Lung, Colorectal, and Ovarian] Cancer Screening Trial in the United States) while the other one did (the European Randomized Study of Screening for Prostate Cancer [ERSPC] trial in Europe) (28,29). While confounding factors to each study limit a definitive conclusion about PSA screening, the enormous expense and time required may discourage future PSA screening trials. Nonetheless, both trials are ongoing, and it is possible that future interim analyses and statistical modeling may provide further evidence for the role of PSA screening.

In our practice, we recommend annual PSA and digital rectal examination (DRE) for all healthy males starting at age 50 or age 40 for those at high risk (eg, those men with a family history or African Americans). Early inclusion of the patient in the decision-making process is essential to optimize patient care given the ambiguities regarding the cost-effectiveness and clinical value of widespread screening for prostate cancer. The rationale for routine screening that justifies routine application is outlined in Table 34-1.

THE CASE FOR CHEMOPREVENTION

Given the high prevalence of prostate cancer and the significant burden of therapy for patients, their families, and society at large, there is great interest in preventing the disease altogether and/or preventing lethal progression of the disease. Inhibitors of 5α-reductase enzymes

TABLE 34-1	RATIONALE FOR PROSTATE CANCER SCREENING

- Reduction in prostate cancer mortality coincides with the introduction of routine PSA screening.
- Patients whose cancers are detected with PSA screening have early-stage disease.
- Long-term disease-free survival is linked to treatment of early-stage disease.
- Randomized trials demonstrate a survival advantage for early surgical intervention for early-stage disease.

(types 1 and 2 enzymes convert testosterone to DHT, the predominant and more potent agonist of androgen-receptor signaling in prostate tissues) have demonstrated potential in this regard. Two randomized, placebo-controlled clinical trials utilizing finasteride (a type II inhibitor) and dutasteride (a type I/II inhibitor) have demonstrated a reduction in prostate cancer in healthy men who had no evidence for prostate cancer at enrollment but did have risk for developing disease (based on age and PSA) (30-32). A third clinical trial is evaluating the ability of dutasteride to prevent prostate cancer progression in patients with low-grade, low-risk, localized prostate cancer at study entry (REDEEM: Reduction by Dutasteride of Clinical Progression Events in Expectant Management Trial). While we have not adapted chemoprevention as standard of care, we are encouraging patients with low-risk prostate cancer to participate in preoperative trials that offer short duration 5α-reductase inhibition prior to radical prostatectomy. Our goal is to elucidate molecular signatures that: (1) predict response (or resistance) to 5α-reductase inhibition, (2) characterize therapy-specific effects on epithelial-stromal compartments, and (3) refine existing risk stratification schemas.

■ PATIENT MANAGEMENT BY DISEASE STATE

CLINICALLY LOCALIZED DISEASE AT PRESENTATION

As a result of widespread screening of men by PSA and DRE, the majority of patients are seen with clinically localized disease at diagnosis. Unfortunately, it is not always obvious how to match the individual patient with the most appropriate management. In an abstract sense, patients with clinically localized prostate cancer fall into one of four theoretical categories:

- *Those not destined to have any clinical manifestations of their disease.* These patients are actually harmed by any intervention, including further surveillance.
- *Those destined to have a clinical manifestation of cancer but will not die of it.* These patients might benefit from definitive therapy (such as prostatectomy or radiation), but would likely benefit equally from less morbid intervention (eg, minimally invasive surgery).
- *Those destined to have life-threatening disease for whom definitive therapy will be curative.* Patients who can be cured, or for whom there will be a substantial alteration of the natural history of their disease,

constitute the group that will unequivocally benefit from definitive local therapy.

- *Those destined to have life-threatening disease for whom the opportunity to cure by means of local therapy either never existed or passed.* For these patients, however, control of the primary tumor could still be an important component of an overall treatment strategy that considers the probability of local versus distant progression, comorbidity, and other factors.

The common practice of urologists and radiation therapists is to assume that nearly every patient falls into the third category, and thus they recommend definitive therapy for the vast majority of newly diagnosed cases of localized prostate cancer. Unfortunately, available evidence suggests that fewer than half of patients are in category 3, so it is not surprising that understanding the role of definitive therapy in eliminating prostate cancer morbidity and mortality has been both difficult and controversial. In fact, these issues underscore the fact that overtreatment of "clinically insignificant" prostate cancers certainly occurs. The significant cost and morbidity associated with local treatment also adds to the difficulty of managing these patients (whether the patient ultimately benefited from the therapy or not).

A number of successful efforts to improve prognostication of patients with localized disease have been made. The large prostatectomy experience at Johns Hopkins has provided valuable insights that have been remarkably influential in directing clinical decision making. The Hopkins investigators initially published a predictive model relating the rate of finding disease that is not confined to the prostate (by assessing the surgical specimen) as a function of three readily available preoperative clinical parameters: PSA, Gleason score from the core biopsy, and the clinical stage based on DRE (33,34). The correlation of these features with pathologically organ-confined disease, summarized in the famous "Partin tables," provided sobering evidence that commonly encountered subsets of patients had a surprisingly high risk of disease that was not confined to the prostate. Of course, not all patients with pathologically organ-confined disease relapse, and not all patients with pathologically organ-confined cancers are cured. Thus the importance of this particular surrogate outcome was uncertain and remains so. Nevertheless, the effect of the Partin tables on clinical practice has been profound. They have driven the application of prostatectomy to patients with smaller and smaller volumes of cancer. It is very clear that although more patients are remaining free of disease after prostatectomy, this comes paradoxically at the cost of operating on many patients who may not have needed surgery or not

operating on many patients who would have benefited from good local control even if the surgery were not curative.

Additional models have been developed to predict outcomes following radical prostatectomy or radiation therapy. Based on the work of D'Amico, a combination of pretherapy PSA, Gleason score, and clinical stage can be used to stratify patients into low (T1-T2a and Gleason score 2-6 and PSA<10 ng/mL), intermediate (T2b-T2c or Gleason score 7 or PSA 10-20 ng/mL), high (T3a or Gleason score 8-10 or PSA >20 ng/mL), and locally advanced (T3b-T4) groups that predict risk for both biochemical recurrence and survival following definitive local therapy (radical prostatectomy or radiation) (35-37). Similarly, Kattan et al. have developed postoperative nomograms for predicting prostate cancer recurrence after radical prostatectomy (38,39). These tools help not only guide recommendations for individual patients, but also stratify patients for clinical trials. For example, low-risk patients can be directed toward "active surveillance" trials while high-risk patients can be direct toward adjuvant/neoadjuvant trials. The rationale for the use of predictive nomograms is outlined in Table 34-2.

Despite the efforts detailed above, tumors with identical morphology and clinicopathologic characteristics often display biologic heterogeneity (ie, some low-risk tumors rapidly progress while some high-risk tumors are relatively indolent). Thus, more refined models are needed. Investigational approaches to improve risk stratification include assessing suspicious nodes or small-volume extracapsular extension by MRI or PET, staging biopsies of seminal vesicles and extraprostatic tissue, and incorporating molecular signatures. Within our group, a significant effort is under way to relate the expression of genes that may affect apoptotic threshold, invasion, angiogenesis, and AR signaling to biologic potential and ultimately clinical outcome of localized tumors. These data suggest that both loss of tumor suppressor pathways (eg, p53) and gain of oncogene/antiapoptotic pathways (eg, BCL-2) contribute to prostate

TABLE 34-2	RATIONALE FOR USE OF PREDICTIVE NOMOGRAMS

- Gleason grade, clinical stage, and initial PSA are predictive of surgical stage, risk of subsequent relapse, and risk of cancer-specific mortality.
- Improving the ability to predict outcome will inform both physicians and patients about the risk/benefits of local therapy.
- Fewer patients will undergo unnecessary or futile surgery.

cancer progression. In addition to these and other "epithelial" events, the importance of the host-epithelial interaction in prostate cancer progression has been supported by evidence that pathways involved in paracrine regulation of normal stromal-epithelial interactions have also been implicated in prostate cancer progression (40-42). For example, sonic hedgehog and src kinase signaling pathways are involved in normal bone development, but their aberrant activation contributes to tumor progression. Clinical trials targeting sonic hedgehog and src kinase are ongoing.

THERAPY

Localized Low-Stage Prostate Cancer

In patients with localized low-stage disease (generally including low- and intermediate-risk groups based on D'Amico et al.), the options offered include active surveillance, surgery, radiation, or presurgical clinical trials. Educating the patient about his/her treatment options is critical to make the best decision for each individual. Patients who are undecided or request more information about treatments and side effects are seen in our multidisciplinary clinic.

Critical evaluation of the relative merits of different therapies for localized low-stage prostate cancer is difficult. This is because patients in this category have a >80% chance of 10-year progression-free survival following local therapy (43-45). Prostate cancer has a long natural history, and 10-year data for patients with low-risk prostate cancer remain immature with respect to cause-specific and disease-free survival. The contribution of delayed hormonal therapy and the appreciation that not all patients with a delayed PSA recurrence after local therapy are threatened by their disease have made comparisons between different treatment modalities difficult. As a consequence, the modification of older therapies or the application of new ones (such as brachytherapy, cryoablation, or proton beam therapy) is often judged by their complication profile and the rate of PSA-free survival with a relatively short follow-up. While seemingly logical, interpreting potential benefit from "new and improved" therapies is challenged by the impact of "stage migration" on outcomes. Stage migration refers to fact that as a consequence of awareness and PSA screening, younger patients with lower-stage cancer are diagnosed with increasing frequency. This trend of earlier therapy in younger patients with earlier-stage disease likely has an effect on the analysis of therapy efficacy and morbidity for low-stage cancer. Therefore the practice of deriving conclusions from the comparison of nonrandomized study groups in low-stage prostate cancer is a dubious exercise.

In fact, in localized, low-stage prostate cancer, the principal therapeutic dilemma is whether to intervene at all. Increasingly, many investigators are recognizing that not all patients diagnosed with prostate cancer by histologic criteria have a disease that has lethal potential (46). Hence many clinicians have explored a strategy of observation followed by delayed therapy if required. This strategy has historically been called "watchful waiting" but in recent years we have adapted the term "active surveillance." This is because the definition of watchful waiting is ambiguous and includes the practice of not following or evaluating patients after diagnosis until they present with a prostate cancer associated symptom(s). In contrast, active surveillance implies regular follow-ups with PSA, DRE, and repeat biopsies as indicated to inform the need for local therapy. Active surveillance acknowledges the reality that many patients with prostate cancer survive despite diagnosis and therapy, as opposed to a benefit directly from the intervention. At MD Anderson, the rationale for offering active surveillance is the idea that carefully monitored patients will require therapy with curative intent only if accompanied by objective evidence that their cancer has become life threatening. In this way, patients with truly indolent disease can be spared the morbidities of local therapy, while patients who show progression over time to potentially lethal disease will preserve the opportunity for curative therapy.

Active Surveillance With Deferred Treatment

Two categories of patients with low-stage disease are generally considered for active surveillance: (1) men who have a higher probability of dying from a comorbid illness (such as coronary artery disease) than from prostate cancer, (2) men whose cancer poses some risk for lethality but choose active surveillance because of concerns about consequences of therapy (eg, impotence and/or incontinence). The rationale for active surveillance is outlined in Table 34-3.

TABLE 34-3 | RATIONALE FOR ACTIVE SURVEILLANCE

- A significant portion of newly diagnosed patients will not develop clinical progression.
- Complications of local therapy exceed benefits in some patients.
- Close monitoring of selected patients with serial PSA measurements, DREs, and biopsies may avoid or delay initiation of potentially morbid or unnecessary therapy.

There are two central challenges of the active surveillance strategy. The first is that we do not yet have a validated method to anticipate progression of the disease to avoid "closing the window" on curative therapy. The second is that we lack methods to ensure reliable selection of all patients in whom the disease will be unlikely to spread while excluding all patients who will have lethal progression of the disease despite its initial morphologic appearance as being low-stage. Thus this strategy, while supported by compelling logic, must be regarded as unproven. This is particularly true for those patients with a life expectancy of 15 years or more. As a patient's life span shortens due to comorbid conditions, the unproven nature of this strategy has less predicted impact on outcome. Thus, outside of a clinical trial, active surveillance in our practice is routinely reserved for patients with low-stage disease and an expected survival of less than 10 years due to comorbidities.

Active surveillance for category 1 patients is not codified and follow-up strategies (such as annual PSA checks) are designed by mutual agreement between the physician and patient. Select elderly patients whose cancer diagnosis was precipitated by an ill-advised PSA screening test may choose no further follow-up. In contrast, active surveillance for category 2 patients involves close observation with quarterly PSA checks and annual prostate biopsies. Often these patients elect to undergo local therapy as the physical and emotional burden of close observation becomes more obvious. Despite the intensity of follow-up, the ability to anticipate progression of disease based on true biologic evidence as opposed to apparent progression caused by the randomness of the biopsies remains a major problem. These problems will be clarified with prospective studies accruing at several institutions.

Treatment of Low-Stage Disease With Available Therapy

Although there is much debate about the relative merits of radiation therapy and surgery for patients with localized low-stage prostate cancer, the inescapable conclusion is that both treatment groups have an excellent survival and the principal issues influencing choice are related to therapy-associated morbidity. Interestingly, competition between radiation therapy and surgery has resulted in the reduction in morbidity to both therapies. The morbidity of radiation therapy—while retaining its effectiveness—has been greatly reduced, as has morbidity related to improvements in surgical techniques. Thus for low-stage prostate cancer, the principal therapeutic recommendation is to treat those patients who

TABLE 34-4	RATIONALE FOR SELECTION OF LOCAL TREATMENT MODALITY

- There are no clinical trials showing a therapeutic advantage of surgery over radiation therapy for localized disease.
- Either approach is associated with some risk of significant morbidity (initial impotence rates are higher with surgery).
- There is a reduction in impotence rates over time with radiation.
- Surgery provides better assessment of risk for future relapse by allowing molecular-pathologic analysis of the radical prostatectomy specimen.
- Radiation is ideally suited for patients who are physically unfit for surgery or those who have disease extending beyond the bounds of traditional surgical fields.
- Surgery improves symptom-free and overall survival in patients with localized disease.

have a >15-year expected life expectancy. The primary recommendation is surgery or radiation therapy, with a bias toward surgery for those patients with an expected longevity of >20 years, and a bias toward radiation therapy for those patients with an expected longevity of 15 or fewer years (Table 34-4).

Preoperative Trials for Low-Stage Disease

Preoperative trials facilitate the development of novel therapies and treatment strategies in prostate cancer by providing proof of "target engagement" by the drug(s) and modulation of the tumor phenotype in a therapeutically favorable manner (47). The principal goal of a preoperative clinical trial is to identify short-term molecular and pathologic tissue surrogates that establish target engagement and modulation of key signaling pathways by the drug(s). Because surgery is performed before cytoreduction or significant changes in the tumor phenotype are expected (as opposed to neoadjuvant trials), preoperative trials provide only limited inferences about the therapeutic potential of the drug(s) being tested. However, data from preoperative trials help identify the most promising therapeutic candidates worthy of further study. Preoperative studies of low-stage prostate cancer seek to identify molecular markers that characterize response to therapy and predict tumor biology.

High-Risk and Locally Advanced Prostate Cancer

As a general principle of oncology, high-risk and locally advanced tumors (based on the D'Amico risk stratification groups) are best treated with a combination of systemic therapy and aggressive local therapy.

This strategy addresses occult disseminated disease while preventing local complications of the primary tumor. Despite the widely recognized poor outcomes for patients with seminal vesicle and/or regional node involvement, the application of optimum local control with systemic therapy has only recently become accepted (48,49).

Current multimodal therapies include radiation plus hormones and neoadjuvant therapy plus surgery. It is now well established that the addition of hormones to radiation therapy is superior to radiation therapy or hormones alone for patients with high-risk and locally advanced tumors (50). The duration and sequence of the combination are important in maximizing therapy benefit from the combination. Several lines of evidence suggest that initiating the androgen ablation 2 months prior to the radiation therapy is more effective than combined therapy from the outset or sequential therapy with radiation followed by androgen ablation. The available data demonstrate an increase in survival with a 3-year period of androgen ablation. However, the optimal duration of androgen ablation in the context of locally advanced prostate cancer treated with radiation remains an area of investigation.

It also appears that improved local control represents another strategy to improve overall survival in patients with T3 N0 M0 tumors. Randomized controlled trials have demonstrated that adjuvant radiation therapy following radical prostatectomy for T3 N0 M0 tumors significantly reduces the risk of metastases and improves overall survival (51). These data support the hypothesis that untreated residual disease at the primary site can act as a source for metastatic progression.

Preoperative Trials in High-Risk and Locally Advanced Prostate Cancer

At MD Anderson we recognize two different categories of patients with high-risk or locally advanced disease: (1) those whom we believe can be effectively treated with hormones and radiation therapy, and (2) those whom we believe will not be effectively treated with this approach because of the extent of their disease, adverse histologic features of the tumor, or the relative youth and expected long survival of the patient. Patients in the second category are candidates for a novel preoperative therapy given prior to prostatectomy. The rationale for preoperative therapy in this setting is based on progress made in other cancer types and is described as follows: (1) in high-risk and locally advanced disease, the posttherapy pathology specimen will inform both prognosis and future treatment

decisions and (2) controlling the primary tumor is an essential part of an integrated strategy for patients with high-risk and locally advanced disease (although this strategy is not always curative) (52). At MD Anderson, we are using preoperative trial designs with increasing frequency to develop novel agents (eg, angiogenesis inhibitors) in prostate cancer. Analysis of the prostatectomy specimen permits detailed analysis of molecular (eg, apoptosis) and pathologic surrogates for therapy benefit (eg, achievement of P0). We believe the preoperative model will significantly enhance our ability to identify the most promising agents worthy of development in a time-efficient manner.

Castration-Resistant Locally Advanced Prostate Cancer

In order to determine whether a patient's prostate cancer is castration-resistant, serum testosterone levels should be analyzed concurrently with other measures. Castration-resistant prostate cancer (CRPC) should only be considered in patients whose serum testosterone is <50 ng/dL (53). It must be appreciated, however, that CRPC is an "umbrella" term that encompasses a spectrum of disease states ranging from rising PSA alone to rising PSA associated with osseous and/or soft tissue metastases (54). Furthermore, patients receiving combined androgen blockade are typically screened for an antiandrogen withdrawal response before being considered castration-resistant. Patients with CRPC and PSA-only recurrence will be discussed below.

For patients with castration-resistant locally advanced prostate cancer, clinical progression presents significant clinical symptoms (pain, hematuria, bladder outlet, and bowel obstruction), but optimal management remains a difficult therapeutic problem. The critical decision is whether or not to offer consolidative therapy. For patients without metastatic disease, we offer neoadjuvant chemotherapy followed by surgery for consolidation. If not used as primary therapy, salvage radiation therapy is another rational strategy, particularly for patients who are not candidates for salvage surgery.

For patients with both castration-resistant locally advanced and metastatic disease, these approaches are more controversial. Nonetheless, we recognize that these patients experience significant morbidity from local tumor progression that is comparable to patients without metastases. Thus for select candidates, we still offer consolidative therapy. As an example, consider the case of a patient who presented with metastatic prostate cancer at diagnosis and was successfully treated with androgen

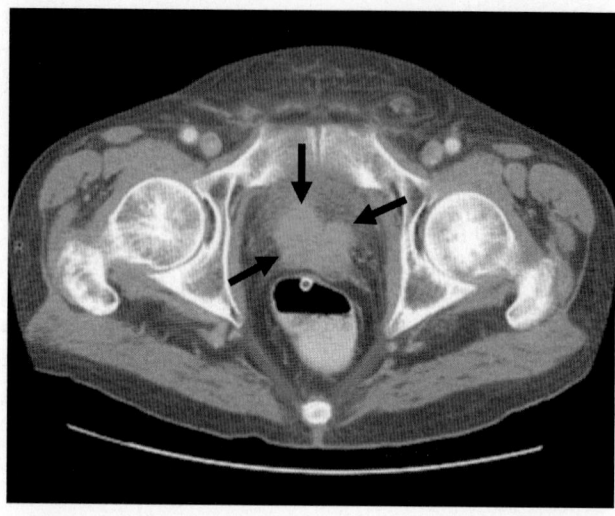

FIGURE 34-3. Recurrent prostate cancer invading the base of the bladder.

ablation for 10 years. He then developed castration-resistant progression and presented with invasion of his primary tumor into the bladder (Fig. 34-3). To relieve painful voiding symptoms attributed to the bladder invasion, induction chemotherapy followed by salvage cystoprostatectomy was performed. At 3 years follow-up, the patient continued to have evidence of active metastases but was free of cancer-associated local symptoms. While this patient benefited longer than most, striking relief of intractable symptoms is common using this approach. The clinical rationale to apply chemotherapy followed by salvage surgery is summarized in Table 34-5.

Rising Prostate-Specific Antigen After Definitive Local Therapy

The utility of PSA measurements is greatest in monitoring cancer progression and effects of therapy in patients with radiographic evidence of disease. In contrast, the significance of PSA in patients without detectable

TABLE 34-5	RATIONALE FOR SALVAGE SURGERY

- Patients can avoid significant morbidity associated with local progression.
- Improved local control may contribute to longer overall survival.
- Patients who develop a delayed local relapse after treatment with primary radiation therapy may still have surgically curable disease.

disease is less clear. Although available evidence suggests that patients with a measurable PSA following prostatectomy will eventually develop a recurrence given sufficient time, these recurrences are not uniformly fatal. Furthermore, in patients treated with radiation therapy, interpretation of PSA posttherapy is very different than in patients treated with surgery.

Significance of Prostate-Specific Antigen Following Prostatectomy

The serum PSA concentration should be undetectable using standard commercial assays within 6 weeks of prostatectomy. Persistent PSA following surgery usually indicates persistent cancer secondary to inadequate surgery, persistent cancer despite adequate surgery, or the presence of occult metastases. The experience from Johns Hopkins suggests that, given sufficient time, patients with early PSA recurrence (<2 years) or short PSA doubling time (<10 months) will develop metastatic disease within 15 years of surgery (55-57). In contrast, patients with late PSA recurrence or a longer PSA doubling time are more likely to have a recurrence confined to the prostatic fossa. Patients who have a striking discordance between the predicted behavior of the cancer (eg, low-stage) and early elevations of postoperative serum PSA may have had inadequate surgery and are considered for adjuvant radiation therapy. In patients who undergo nerve-sparing prostatectomy, consideration must also be given to the possibility that normal prostate gland left behind at surgery is producing PSA.

Significance of Prostate-Specific Antigen Following Radiation Therapy

In contrast to surgery, serum PSA concentrations are not expected to become undetectable following curative therapy. In addition, the phenomenon of a PSA "bounce" is well described following radiation of the primary tumor (58). The PSA bounce is a modest, self-limited rise in PSA concentration without evidence of cancer progression. It typically occurs within the first 18 months following completion of radiation and can last for as long as 3 months before reaching a plateau and then declining. PSA bounces are attributed to radiation-induced inflammation, although no definitive etiology exists. The central clinical dilemma with PSA bounces is that their presence can only be determined with confidence in retrospect. Thus, clinicians need to be aware of this phenomenon and show restraint in introducing therapy to patients displaying delayed PSA elevation after radiation without evidence for metastases.

Management of the Patient With Prostate-Specific Antigen-Only Recurrence

As the incidence of men diagnosed and treated for localized prostate cancer increases, so does the incidence of men presenting with PSA-only recurrent disease (in other words, no radiographic evidence for metastases). This scenario poses a therapeutic dilemma for physicians and considerable anxiety for patients. As experience with this disease state matures, it is becoming clear that PSA-only recurrences do not uniformly portend morbidity/mortality from the disease. Our general approach is to offer hormone ablative therapy (commonly using an intermittent strategy) during the androgen-dependent phase of the disease (59). Notably, we never use chemotherapy for PSA-only recurrences that occur in the setting of CRPC. Instead, we advocate placing these patients on clinical trials testing novel compounds.

METASTATIC CANCER

Metastatic Androgen-Dependent Disease

For patients with visible disease in the bone and/or lymph nodes, the standard approach is continuous androgen ablation. In a recent randomized clinical trial completed at our institution, the addition of chemotherapy to androgen ablation did not delay the time to development of castrate-resistant progression (60). Thus, we no longer incorporate chemotherapy into our management of patients with metastatic androgen-dependent disease. The clinical rationale for the use of androgen ablation is summarized in Table 34-6.

Castration-Resistant Progression

Second-Line Hormonal Therapies

Although not as well established as in breast cancer, second-line hormonal therapies are useful in men with castration-resistant prostate cancer. The principal reasons why these therapies work include (1) a lack of predictable cross-resistance between different antiandrogens that block androgen receptor activation, and (2) extragonadal sources of testosterone (eg, produced in the adrenal gland or within the tumor) not blocked by standard castration are excellent targets for inhibition. With respect to (2), drugs that inhibit enzymes involved in androgen synthesis have proven useful as second-line therapies. For example, there is considerable research interest in blocking CYP17, a key enzyme in androgen biosynthesis in the adrenal glands and tumor tissue (61). Ketoconazole is an antifungal with weak and nonspecific CYP17 inhibitory properties that has been around for

TABLE 34-6 | CLINICAL RATIONALE FOR ANDROGEN ABLATION

1. Androgen ablation enhances local therapy.
   - Concurrent androgen ablation and radiation therapy increases survival in selected patients.
   - Early use of androgen ablation in patients noted to be node-positive following radical prostatectomy increases overall survival.
2. Timing of androgen ablation.
   - The decision to introduce androgen ablation among patients with a rising PSA following local therapy should be based on assessment of risk for recurrence and cancer-associated mortality.
   - Androgen ablation therapy reduces the duration of time patients experience symptomatic progression.
   - Symptoms are reliably relieved and should be initiated in the presence of symptomatic progression.
3. Types of androgen ablation.
   - Surgical castration and LHRH agonists or antagonists are considered to be equally effective.
   - Combined androgen ablation is not convincingly superior to serial use of an LHRH agonist followed by an antiandrogen upon progression. However, antiandrogen therapy should precede the use of an LHRH agonist in the setting of threatening disease in order to avoid a "surge."
4. Secondary hormonal therapy
   - Experimental and clinical data demonstrate that most prostate cancers growing in a castrate environment still rely on androgen signaling for continued growth.
5. Management of complications associated with androgen ablation.
   - Patients on sustained androgen ablation should be monitored for bone complications and considered for bisphosphonate therapy to reduce the risk of osteopenia.
   - Supplementation with calcium (500 mg) and vitamin D (400 IU) is recommended.
   - Antidepressants should be considered for androgen ablation–associated depression.

decades. However, poor tolerance prevents its broad use. Novel CYP17 inhibitors are currently being developed. Abiraterone, a potent irreversible oral inhibitor of CYP17, has demonstrated promising activity in phase II studies for patients with CRPC in terms of both PSA response, palliation of symptoms, and radiographic responses (62). This drug is active in both chemotherapy-naïve and docetaxel-treated CRPC patients. Phase III randomized, placebo-controlled trials are under way to establish an indication for this drug in both disease states.

Diethylstilbestrol (DES) has demonstrated consistent responses in patients with well-documented castration-resistant progression. The responses occur in all clinical presentations, but most experienced clinicians believe patients with less threatening disease are more likely to respond. We have all observed occasional remarkable responses in patients with castration-resistant prostate cancer, even when all other strategies have failed. The major complications attributed to DES are cardiovascular and include increased risk of stroke, thrombosis, and ischemic heart disease. Parenteral estrogens are being studied as an alternative to this approach. The parenteral use of DES also has the theoretical advantage of avoiding initial hepatic metabolism to which the thrombotic complications have been attributed.

Thus in our practice, an example of one approach to a patient with asymptomatic castration-resistant prostate cancer (who has progressed through luteinizing hormone-releasing hormone [LHRH] agonist therapy and first-line antiandrogen therapy) would be to offer a second antiandrogen + Avodart (to block intratumoral DHT production). Upon progression, the antiandrogen and Avodart would be discontinued and DES prescribed. If DES fails, we then try to offer patients clinical trials with novel agents. With each of these scenarios, we continue with LHRH agonist therapy to maintain castrate levels of testosterone in the systemic circulation. For patients who continue to progress and/or develop (or are anticipated to develop) cancer-associated symptoms, we move to chemotherapy.

Chemotherapy

Prostate cancer has now entered the realm of the other adult common solid tumors in that chemotherapy is routinely applied to patients with castration-resistant locally advanced and/or metastatic disease. For more than a decade, patients have been treated with docetaxel-based regimens. However, while these therapies improve quality of life, prolongation in survival is modest and therapy-related toxicities are common. Faced with these challenges, the approach at MD Anderson has been to delay cytotoxic therapy until second-line hormonal (or experimental) options have been explored. Of course, patients with rapidly progressive disease-causing (or expecting to cause) symptoms are offered chemotherapy sooner rather than later, particularly when additional hormonal manipulations are predicted to fail. The rationale for the use of chemotherapy is outlined in Table 34-7.

Given the limitations of docetaxel-based chemotherapy, there has been a global research initiative to improve on it, principally by combining docetaxel with other agents. These efforts have met with little success

TABLE 34-7	RATIONALE FOR THE USE OF CHEMOTHERAPY

- Chemotherapy palliates and/or prevents symptoms associated with progression of disease.
- Docetaxel-based regimens result in modest improvements in survival in patients with metastatic castration-resistant cancer.
- Other active agents in prostate cancer (eg, mitoxantrone) can be used as second-line therapy.

until recently, when insights about basic prostate cancer biology encouraged rational integration of novel "targeted" agents that inhibit critical growth-promoting pathways. A guiding principle derived from translational research has been the discovery that growth signaling pathways involved in normal prostate gland or bone development frequently become dysregulated in prostate cancer (63). These pathways present novel targets for small molecule therapeutics that inhibit host-epithelial interactions in the tumor microenvironment (64). Thus, several randomized phase III trials are currently under way comparing docetaxel to combinations of docetaxel plus bevacizumab (a vascular endothelial growth factor inhibitor), dasatinib (a src-kinase inhibitor), or atrasentan (an endothelin receptor antagonist).

These trials seek to build on our experience with bone-targeting radiopharmaceuticals. The merits of targeting the bone microenvironment have been established by the use of strontium 89 as a single agent or in combination with cytotoxic therapy (65,66) (Table 34-8). Emerging data support the view that targeting bone will prolong overall patient survival, even in those with advanced-stage disease. While we continue to research the potential benefits of bone-targeting radiopharmaceuticals, our hope is that the novel agents described above will more specifically inhibit the bone-epithelial interaction with less toxicity.

TABLE 34-8	RATIONALE FOR BONE-TARGETED THERAPY

- Osseous metastases are the preferred site of castration-resistant progression.
- Osseous metastases significantly contribute to the morbidity and mortality of prostate cancer.
- Bone-targeting radiopharmaceuticals prolong symptom-free survival in patients with castration-resistant progression and skeletal metastases.

Optimizing Therapy Benefit Using Different Cytotoxic Agents

The gold standard for the FDA (U.S. Food and Drug Administration) approval of chemotherapy agents in patients with castration-resistant metastatic prostate cancer is evidence for prolongation of patient survival. Thus, oncologists who practice "evidence-based" medicine have routinely offered docetaxel-based chemotherapy regimens as first-line therapy since 2004, when data from two randomized phase III trials showed a median improvement in survival of approximately 2 months when compared to mitoxantrone chemotherapy alone (67,68). While the prolongation in survival was statistically significant, the relatively short duration of benefit has continued to raise questions about the clinical significance of docetaxel-based chemotherapy compared to other active cytotoxic agents, especially in light of docetaxel toxicity.

In reality, while the drug approval process (with overall survival as the primary endpoint) remains indispensable for drug development, it does not consistently guide therapy decisions routinely used in caring for patients with castration-resistant metastatic disease. There are two principal reasons for this. First, the goal to effectively palliate symptoms arguably influences the clinical decision to offer chemotherapy as much as the evidence for a small survival benefit. Second, physicians typically switch cytotoxic therapies if clinical benefit is not observed. Again, this decision is gauged as much by the quality of the response and the number of active agents available in the salvage setting rather than evidence-based guidelines on how to optimize survival. Reflecting this, multiple chemotherapy regimens with modest activity are routinely applied in a sequential manner to patients who have failed docetaxel-based chemotherapy. However, there is no standard chemotherapy in the second- or third-line setting and we do not have randomized comparisons testing whether the sequential application of therapy prolongs survival.

Here at MDACC, we have sought to investigate these challenges by using a novel clinical trial design referred to as "adaptive." Adaptive trial design refers to a clinical trial methodology that allows design modifications to be made after patients have enrolled on study. For example, interim safety and efficacy data may be used in real time to modify treatment arms for responding versus nonresponding patients. We recently published a study of 150 chemonaïve patients with castration-resistant prostate cancer who were randomly assigned to one of four chemotherapy regimens (cyclophosphamide, vincristine, and dexamethasone [CVD]; ketoconazole plus doxorubicin alternating with vinblastine plus estramustine [KA/VE]; weekly paclitaxel, estramustine, and carboplatin [TEC]; paclitaxel, estramustine, and etoposide [TEE]) (69). Patients were evaluated every 8 weeks to assess response and adverse events. Patients who responded continued with the same treatment while those who did not were randomly assigned to one of the other three treatments. Response was assessed by considering tumor-specific symptoms, tumor regression, and PSA changes. Treatment was continued until two consecutive courses induced a response or until patients were given two different regimens that failed to induce a response. Thus, during the trial, successful treatments were "selected for" while unsuccessful treatments were "selected against."

Notably, median survival was 22 months, and the estimated 3-year survival was 26%. These data compare favorably to median and 3-year survival rates reported in the landmark docetaxel trials (~17-19 months median survival and ~17% 3-year survival) and suggest a survival benefit to second-line chemotherapy. Overall success was achieved in 35 patients with the initial treatment (4 treated with CVD, 7 with KA/VE, 14 with TEC, and 10 with TEE) and in 9 more patients using a second-line regimen (ie, two with CVD, five with KA/VE, and two with TEC). TEC produced the greatest number and proportion of successful courses of treatment, and TEC followed by KA/VE was the most promising two-stage sequential strategy. This trial illustrates the strength of the adaptive trial design in: (1) identifying the most promising therapies in castration-resistant prostate cancer and (2) optimizing the application of different therapies in sequence so as to minimize cross-resistance. We are currently using the adaptive trial design to test multiple novel therapies that target the epithelial-host microenvironment.

Immune-Based Therapies

Historically, there has been a long-standing interest in stimulating a patient's immune system as a therapy strategy for prostate cancer. Despite enthusiasm for this paradigm, studies have consistently demonstrated no clinical benefit. Recently, however, several new strategies have emerged that reveal the potential of immunotherapy in treating prostate cancer. Two randomized, placebo-controlled phase III trials demonstrated an overall survival benefit for men with castration-resistant prostate cancer treated with sipuleucel-T, an immunotherapy agent that stimulates T-cell immunity to prostatic acid phosphatase (an antigen expressed on the vast majority of prostate cancer cells but not in nonprostate tissue) (70). Another immunotherapy agent is GVAX, a cellular vaccine product that uses exogenous tumor cells that secrete GM-CSF to induce a host antitumor response. GVAX has shown promising activity in phase II studies and is currently being compared in phase III trials to docetaxel (71). Finally, ipilimumab is a humanized anti-CTLA-4 antibody that promotes stimulation of T-cell responses and has elicited PSA responses in phase I/II trials (71). Further development of these agents (and others) could dramatically change the way we treat prostate cancer in the coming decade.

Management of Metastases

Avoiding neurologic and bone marrow complications for patients with prostate cancer and skeletal metastases is a major challenge. Close monitoring of patients and use of palliative radiation therapy is important to avoid base-of-skull syndrome, spinal cord compression, or fractures. While bisphosphonates appear to reduce some bone-related events, they do not convincingly benefit patients clinically and it is not clear that they inhibit tumor progression per se. Thus, our practice is to offer bisphosphonate therapy to reduce osteoporosis associated with androgen deprivation rather than as a cancer-related therapy.

■ FUTURE DIRECTIONS

The majority of patients with advanced prostate cancer demonstrate a predictable clinical pattern of progression. Elucidation of the biologic events responsible for invasion, castration-resistant progression, and bone metastases is already influencing therapy discovery in an unprecedented manner. Along with the integration of improved predictive and prognostic markers, we believe it is realistic to expect individualized treatment algorithms for prostate cancer patients in the very near future. The application of biologically based, rational therapy is the foundation of our mission at MD Anderson to cure prostate cancer. Recent progress has created a strong sense of hope that we are well on our way to achieving this goal.

References

1. Jemal A, Siegel R, Ward E, et al. Cancer statistics, 2009. *CA Cancer J Clin* 2009 Jul;59(4):225-249.

2. Gann PH. Risk factors for prostate cancer. *Rev Urol* 2002;4(Suppl 5):S3-S10.

3. Patel AR, Klein EA. Risk factors for prostate cancer. *Nat Clin Pract Urol* 2009 Feb;6(2):87-95.

4. Scher HI, Sawyers CL. Biology of progressive, castration-resistant prostate cancer: Directed therapies targeting the androgen-receptor signaling axis. *J Clin Oncol* 2005 Nov 10; 23(32):8253-8261.

5. Rowlands MA, Gunnell D, Harris R, et al. Circulating insulin-like growth factor peptides and prostate cancer risk: A systematic review and meta-analysis. *Int J Cancer* 2009 May 15; 124(10):2416-2429.

6. Ben-Jonathan N, Liby K, McFarland M, et al. Prolactin as an autocrine/paracrine growth factor in human cancer. *Trends Endocrinol Metab* 2002 Aug;13(6):245-250.

7. Calle EE, Rodriguez C, Walker-Thurmond K, et al. Overweight, obesity, and mortality from cancer in a prospectively studied cohort of U.S. adults. *N Engl J Med* 2003 Apr 24; 348(17):1625-1638.

8. Freedland SJ, Aronson WJ, Kane CJ, et al. Impact of obesity on biochemical control after radical prostatectomy for clinically localized prostate cancer: A report by the Shared Equal Access Regional Cancer Hospital database study group. *J Clin Oncol* 2004 Feb 1;22(3):446-453.

9. Freedland SJ, Isaacs WB, Mangold LA, et al. Stronger association between obesity and biochemical progression after radical prostatectomy among men treated in the last 10 years. *Clin Cancer Res* 2005 Apr 15;11(8):2883-2888.

10. Strom SS, Wang X, Pettaway CA, et al. Obesity, weight gain, and risk of biochemical failure among prostate cancer patients following prostatectomy. *Clin Cancer Res* 2005 Oct 1;11(19 Pt 1): 6889-6894.

11. Baillargeon J, Rose DP. Obesity, adipokines, and prostate cancer (review). *Int J Oncol* 2006 Mar;28(3):737-745.

12. Buschemeyer WC, III, Freedland SJ. Obesity and prostate cancer: Epidemiology and clinical implications. *Eur Urol* 2007 Aug;52(2):331-343.

13. Barnard RJ. Prostate cancer prevention by nutritional means to alleviate metabolic syndrome. *Am J Clin Nutr* 2007 Sep;86(3): S889-S893.

14. Smith JR, Freije D, Carpten JD, et al. Major susceptibility locus for prostate cancer on chromosome 1 suggested by a genome-wide search. *Science* 1996 Nov 22;274(5291):1371-1374.

15. Xu J, Gillanders EM, Isaacs SD, et al. Genome-wide scan for prostate cancer susceptibility genes in the Johns Hopkins hereditary prostate cancer families. *Prostate* 2003 Dec 1; 57(4):320-325.

16. Ford D, Easton DF, Bishop DT, et al. Risks of cancer in BRCA1-mutation carriers. Breast Cancer Linkage Consortium. *Lancet* 1994 Mar 19;343(8899):692-695.

17. Gayther SA, de Foy KA, Harrington P, et al. The frequency of germ-line mutations in the breast cancer predisposition genes BRCA1 and BRCA2 in familial prostate cancer. The Cancer Research Campaign/British Prostate Group United Kingdom Familial Prostate Cancer Study Collaborators. *Cancer Res* 2000 Aug 15;60(16):4513-4518.

18. Stark JR, Perner S, Stampfer MJ, et al. Gleason score and lethal prostate cancer: Does 3 + 4 = 4 + 3? *J Clin Oncol* 2009 Jul 20;27(21):3459-3464.

19. Efstathiou E, Abrahams NA, Tibbs RF, et al. Morphologic characterization of preoperatively treated prostate cancer: Toward a post-therapy histologic classification. *Eur Urol* 2009 Oct 17.

20. Srigley JR, Humphrey PA, Amin MB, et al. Protocol for the examination of specimens from patients with carcinoma of the prostate gland. *Arch Pathol Lab Med* 2009 Oct;133(10): 1568-1576.

21. McDonnell TJ, Navone NM, Troncoso P, et al. Expression of bcl-2 oncoprotein and p53 protein accumulation in bone marrow metastases of androgen independent prostate cancer. *J Urol* 1997 Feb;157(2):569-574.

22. Assikis VJ, Do KA, Wen S, et al. Clinical and biomarker correlates of androgen-independent, locally aggressive prostate cancer with limited metastatic potential. *Clin Cancer Res* 2004 Oct 15;10(20):6770-6778.

23. Grignon DJ. Unusual subtypes of prostate cancer. *Mod Pathol* 2004 Mar;17(3):316-327.

24. Tu SM, Lopez A, Leibovici D, et al. Ductal adenocarcinoma of the prostate: Clinical features and implications after local therapy. *Cancer* 2009 Jul 1;115(13):2872-2880.

25. Papandreou CN, Daliani DD, Thall PF, et al. Results of a phase II study with doxorubicin, etoposide, and cisplatin in patients with fully characterized small-cell carcinoma of the prostate. *J Clin Oncol* 2002 Jul 15;20(14):3072-3080.

26. Epstein JI. Precursor lesions to prostatic adenocarcinoma. *Virchows Arch* 2009 Jan;454(1):1-16.

27. De Marzo AM, Platz EA, Sutcliffe S, et al. Inflammation in prostate carcinogenesis. *Nat Rev Cancer* 2007 Apr;7(4):256-269.

28. Andriole GL, Crawford ED, Grubb RL, III, et al. Mortality results from a randomized prostate-cancer screening trial. *N Engl J Med* 2009 Mar 26;360(13):1310-1319.

29. Schroder FH, Hugosson J, Roobol MJ, et al. Screening and prostate-cancer mortality in a randomized European study. *N Engl J Med* 2009 Mar 26;360(13):1320-1328.

30. Thompson IM, Goodman PJ, Tangen CM, et al. The influence of finasteride on the development of prostate cancer. *N Engl J Med* 2003 Jul 17;349(3):215-224.

31. Andriole GL, Roehrborn C, Schulman C, et al. Effect of dutasteride on the detection of prostate cancer in men with benign prostatic hyperplasia. *Urology* 2004 Sep;64(3):537-541.

32. Andriole GL. Overview of pivotal studies for prostate cancer risk reduction, past and present. *Urology* 2009 May;73(Suppl 5):S36-S43.

33. Partin AW, Kattan MW, Subong EN, et al. Combination of prostate-specific antigen, clinical stage, and Gleason score to predict pathological stage of localized prostate cancer. A multi-institutional update. *JAMA* 1997 May 14;277(18):1445-1451.

34. Makarov DV, Trock BJ, Humphreys EB, et al. Updated nomogram to predict pathologic stage of prostate cancer given prostate-specific antigen level, clinical stage, and biopsy Gleason score (Partin tables) based on cases from 2000 to 2005. *Urology* 2007 Jun;69(6):1095-1101.

35. D'Amico AV, Whittington R, Malkowicz SB, et al. Biochemical outcome after radical prostatectomy, external beam radiation therapy, or interstitial radiation therapy for clinically localized prostate cancer. *JAMA* 1998 Sep 16;280(11):969-974.

36. D'Amico AV, Moul JW, Carroll PR, et al. Surrogate end point for prostate cancer-specific mortality after radical prostatectomy or radiation therapy. *J Natl Cancer Inst* 2003 Sep 17;95(18):1376-1383.

37. Hernandez DJ, Nielsen ME, Han M, et al. Contemporary evaluation of the D'Amico risk classification of prostate cancer. *Urology* 2007 Nov;70(5):931-935.

38. Kattan MW, Wheeler TM, Scardino PT. Postoperative nomogram for disease recurrence after radical prostatectomy for prostate cancer. *J Clin Oncol* 1999 May;17(5):1499-1507.

39. Graefen M, Karakiewicz PI, Cagiannos I, et al. Validation study of the accuracy of a postoperative nomogram for recurrence after radical prostatectomy for localized prostate cancer. *J Clin Oncol* 2002 Feb 15;20(4):951-956.

40. Sanchez P, Hernandez AM, Stecca B, et al. Inhibition of prostate cancer proliferation by interference with SONIC HEDGEHOG-GLI1 signaling. *Proc Natl Acad Sci U S A* 2004 Aug 24;101(34):12561-12566.

41. Zunich SM, Douglas T, Valdovinos M, et al. Paracrine sonic hedgehog signalling by prostate cancer cells induces osteoblast differentiation. *Mol Cancer* 2009;8:12.

42. Park SI, Zhang J, Phillips KA, et al. Targeting SRC family kinases inhibits growth and lymph node metastases of prostate cancer in an orthotopic nude mouse model. *Cancer Res* 2008 May 1;68(9):3323-3333.

43. Holmberg L, Bill-Axelson A, Helgesen F, et al. A randomized trial comparing radical prostatectomy with watchful waiting in early prostate cancer. *N Engl J Med* 2002 Sep 12;347(11):781-789.

44. Bill-Axelson A, Holmberg L, Ruutu M, et al. Radical prostatectomy versus watchful waiting in early prostate cancer. *N Engl J Med* 2005 May 12;352(19):1977-1984.

45. D'Amico AV, Moul J, Carroll PR, et al. Cancer-specific mortality after surgery or radiation for patients with clinically localized prostate cancer managed during the prostate-specific antigen era. *J Clin Oncol* 2003 Jun 1;21(11):2163-2172.

46. Johansson JE, Holmberg L, Johansson S, et al. Fifteen-year survival in prostate cancer. A prospective, population-based study in Sweden. *JAMA* 1997 Feb 12;277(6):467-471.

47. Efstathiou E, Kim J, Logothetis CJ. Informative clinical investigation: A demanding taskmaster. *J Clin Oncol* 2009 Oct 20;27(30):4937-4938.

48. Messing EM, Manola J, Sarosdy M, et al. Immediate hormonal therapy compared with observation after radical prostatectomy and pelvic lymphadenectomy in men with node-positive prostate cancer. *N Engl J Med* 1999 Dec 9;341(24):1781-1788.

49. Miyamoto H, Messing EM. Early versus late hormonal therapy for prostate cancer. *Curr Urol Rep* 2004 Jun;5(3):188-196.

50. Bolla M, Collette L. pT3N0M0 prostate cancer: A plea for adjuvant radiation. *Nat Rev Urol* 2009 Aug;6(8):410-412.

51. Thompson IM, Tangen CM, Paradelo J, et al. Adjuvant radiotherapy for pathological T3N0M0 prostate cancer significantly reduces risk of metastases and improves survival: Long-term followup of a randomized clinical trial. *J Urol* 2009 Mar;181(3):956-962.

52. Pettaway CA, Pisters LL, Troncoso P, et al. Neoadjuvant chemotherapy and hormonal therapy followed by radical prostatectomy: Feasibility and preliminary results. *J Clin Oncol* 2000 Mar;18(5):1050-1057.

53. Scher HI, Halabi S, Tannock I, et al. Design and end points of clinical trials for patients with progressive prostate cancer and castrate levels of testosterone: Recommendations of the Prostate Cancer Clinical Trials Working Group. *J Clin Oncol* 2008 Mar 1;26(7):1148-1159.

54. Scher HI, Heller G. Clinical states in prostate cancer: Toward a dynamic model of disease progression. *Urology* 2000 Mar;55(3):323-327.

55. Pound CR, Partin AW, Eisenberger MA, et al. Natural history of progression after PSA elevation following radical prostatectomy. *JAMA* 1999 May 5;281(17):1591-1597.

56. Han M, Partin AW, Pound CR, et al. Long-term biochemical disease-free and cancer-specific survival following anatomic radical retropubic prostatectomy. The 15-year Johns Hopkins experience. *Urol Clin North Am* 2001 Aug;28(3):555-565.

57. Cannon GM, Jr., Walsh PC, Partin AW, et al. Prostate-specific antigen doubling time in the identification of patients at risk for progression after treatment and biochemical recurrence for prostate cancer. *Urology* 2003 Dec 29; 62(Suppl 1):2-8.

58. Rosser CJ, Kuban DA, Levy LB, et al. Prostate specific antigen bounce phenomenon after external beam radiation for clinically localized prostate cancer. *J Urol* 2002 Nov;168(5): 2001-2005.

59. Bhandari MS, Crook J, Hussain M. Should intermittent androgen deprivation be used in routine clinical practice? *J Clin Oncol* 2005 Nov 10;23(32):8212-8218.

60. Millikan RE, Wen S, Pagliaro LC, et al. Phase III trial of androgen ablation with or without three cycles of systemic chemotherapy for advanced prostate cancer. *J Clin Oncol* 2008 Dec 20;26(36):5936-5942.

61. Reid AH, Attard G, Barrie E, et al. CYP17 inhibition as a hormonal strategy for prostate cancer. *Nat Clin Pract Urol* 2008 Nov;5(11):610-620.

62. Attard G, Reid AH, A'Hern R, et al. Selective inhibition of CYP17 with abiraterone acetate is highly active in the treatment of castration-resistant prostate cancer. *J Clin Oncol* 2009 Aug 10;27(23):3742-3748.

63. Logothetis CJ, Lin SH. Osteoblasts in prostate cancer metastasis to bone. *Nat Rev Cancer* 2005 Jan;5(1):21-28.

64. Cher ML, Towler DA, Rafii S, et al. Cancer interaction with the bone microenvironment: A workshop of the National Institutes of Health Tumor Microenvironment Study Section. *Am J Pathol* 2006 May;168(5):1405-1412.

65. Tu SM, Lin SH, Logothetis C. Re: A randomized, placebo-controlled trial of zoledronic acid in patients with hormone-refractory metastatic prostate carcinoma. *J Natl Cancer Inst* 2003 Aug 6;95(15):1174-1175.

66. Tu SM, Lin SH. Current trials using bone-targeting agents in prostate cancer. *Cancer J* 2008 Jan;14(1):35-39.

67. Tannock IF, de WR, Berry WR, et al. Docetaxel plus prednisone or mitoxantrone plus prednisone for advanced prostate cancer. *N Engl J Med* 2004 Oct 7;351(15):1502-1512.

68. Petrylak DP, Tangen CM, Hussain MH, et al. Docetaxel and estramustine compared with mitoxantrone and prednisone for advanced refractory prostate cancer. *N Engl J Med* 2004 Oct 7; 351(15):1513-1520.

69. Thall PF, Logothetis C, Pagliaro LC, et al. Adaptive therapy for androgen-independent prostate cancer: A randomized selection trial of four regimens. *J Natl Cancer Inst* 2007 Nov 7; 99(21):1613-1622.

70. Higano CS, Schellhammer PF, Small EJ, et al. Integrated data from 2 randomized, double-blind, placebo-controlled, phase 3 trials of active cellular immunotherapy with sipuleucel-T in advanced prostate cancer. *Cancer* 2009 Aug 15;115(16): 3670-3679.

71. Harzstark AL, Ryan CJ. Novel therapeutic strategies in development for prostate cancer. *Expert Opin Investig Drugs* 2008 Jan;17(1):13-22.

CHAPTER
35

PENILE CANCER

Lance C. Pagliaro

■ INCIDENCE AND ETIOLOGY

INCIDENCE IN UNITED STATES

Penile cancer is a disease of older men, with an abrupt increase in incidence in the sixth decade of life and a peak around 80 years of age (1). In two studies, the mean age was 58 years and 55 years (2,3). The tumor is not unusual in younger men; in one large series, 22% of patients were younger than 40 years and 7% were younger than 30 years (2). The Surveillance, Epidemiology, and End Results (SEER) database reveals no racial difference in incidence of penile cancer between African American and Caucasian men in the United States (incidence for Caucasian men, 0.8 of 100,000; for African American men, 0.7 of 100,000) (3,4). In 2009 there were an estimated 1400 new cases in the United States (3).

EPIDEMIOLOGY—DEVELOPING COUNTRIES

Penile carcinoma accounts for 0.4% to 0.6% of all malignant neoplasms among men in the United States and Europe, but it may represent up to 10% of malignant neoplasms in men in some Asian, African, and South American countries (4). However, reports suggest that the incidence of penile cancer is decreasing in many countries, including Finland, the United States, India, and other Asian countries (4-7). The reasons are unclear but may be related in part to increased attention to personal hygiene.

INCIDENCE AND SIGNIFICANCE WORLDWIDE

Among uncircumcised tribes of Africa and within uncircumcised Asian cultures, penile cancer may amount to 10 to 20% of all male malignant neoplasms (8,9). The annual number of new cases per year worldwide is approximately 26,000 (10). Squamous cell carcinoma is the most common histologic subtype, accounting for over 95% of cases (Table 35-1) (11,12).

TABLE 35-1	HISTOPATHOLOGY SUBTYPES OF PENILE CANCER
Squamous cell carcinoma	
Adenocarcinoma	
Lymphoma	
Melanoma	
Kaposi sarcoma	
Leiomyosarcoma	

■ CAUSES OF PENILE CANCER

LACK OF CIRCUMCISION

The incidence of carcinoma of the penis varies according to circumcision practice, hygienic standard, phimosis, number of sexual partners, human papilloma virus (HPV) infection, exposure to tobacco products, and other factors (13-15). Neonatal circumcision has been well established as a prophylactic measure that removes most of the risk of penile carcinoma because it eliminates the closed preputial environment where penile carcinoma most commonly develops.

The chronic irritative effects of smegma, a byproduct of bacterial action on desquamated cells that are within the preputial sac, have been proposed as an etiologic agent in penile cancer. Poor hygiene can lead to buildup of smegma beneath the preputial foreskin, with resulting inflammation. Healing by fibrosis leads to phimosis of the preputial skin, which tends to perpetuate the cycle. Phimosis is found in 25 to 75% of patients with penile carcinoma described in most large series. Reddy et al. (16) studied the foreskins of 26 men undergoing circumcision because of phimosis and found epithelial atypia in one-third of the specimens. Definitive evidence that human smegma itself is a carcinogen, however, has not been established (8).

Carcinoma of the penis is rare among the Jewish population, for whom neonatal circumcision is a universal practice (9). Data from most large series show that penile cancer is rare among neonatally circumcised individuals but more frequent when circumcision is delayed until puberty (2,22,23). Adult circumcision appears to offer little or no protection from subsequent development of the disease (17). These data suggest that the critical period of exposure to certain etiologic agents may have already occurred at puberty and certainly by adulthood, rendering later circumcision relatively ineffective as a prophylactic tool for penile cancer.

HUMAN PAPILLOMAVIRUS

Although human papillomavirus (HPV) is not a reportable sexually transmitted disease, a current estimate puts the number of new infections at 500,000 to 1 million annually in the United States (17). The terms *genital condyloma, venereal warts, genital warts,* and *genital HPV infection* all refer to a sexually transmitted disease caused by HPV. Factors associated with higher rates of infection with HPV include: presence of foreskin, increasing numbers of sexual partners, lack of condom use, and smoking (18). The overall prevalence of HPV in females was found to be 26.8% among US females aged 14 to 59 years and highest among women aged 20 to 24 years (44.8%) (19). HPV is recognized as the principal etiologic agent in cervical dysplasia and cervical cancer (20-22).

On histologic examination, the koilocyte—a cell characterized by an empty cavity surrounding an atypical nucleus—is pathognomonic for HPV infection (Fig. 35-1) (23). DNA hybridization techniques have been used to identify and classify HPV infections, and some 60 genotypes of HPV virus have been identified that involve the genital tract (13). Virus types 6, 11, and 42 to 44 are associated with gross condylomata and low-grade dysplasia. Types 16, 18, 31, 33, 35, and 39 have a higher association with malignant disease (14).

In men, condylomata have been associated with squamous cell carcinoma of the penis (18-20). Malignant transformation of condylomata to squamous cell carcinoma has been reported (24-26). Condylomata acuminata located in the perianal, scrotal, and oral areas have also demonstrated malignant degeneration (24,25). An increased incidence of penile intraepithelial neoplasia has been found in the male partners of women with cervical intraepithelial neoplasia (27,28).

More than 25 types of HPV infect genital sites. HPV types 6 and 11 are most commonly associated with nondysplastic lesions such as genital warts, but these are also noted in nonmetastatic verrucous carcinomas. In contrast, HPV types 16, 18, 31, and 33 are associated with in situ and invasive carcinomas (29). HPV-16 appears to be the most frequently detected type in primary carcinomas and has also been detected in metastatic lesions (29-32). Thus, preventive strategies are

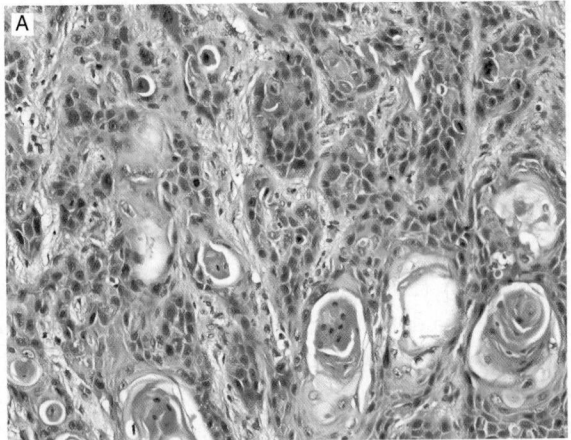

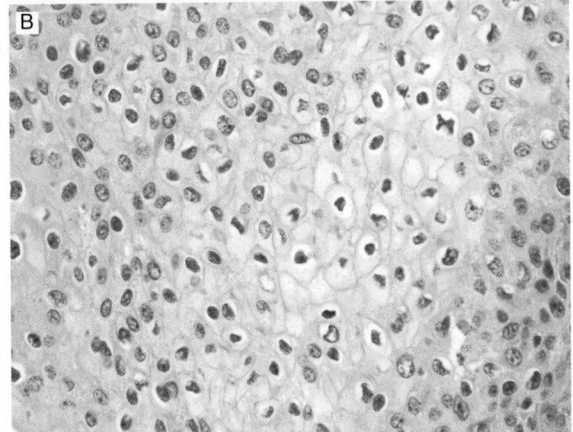

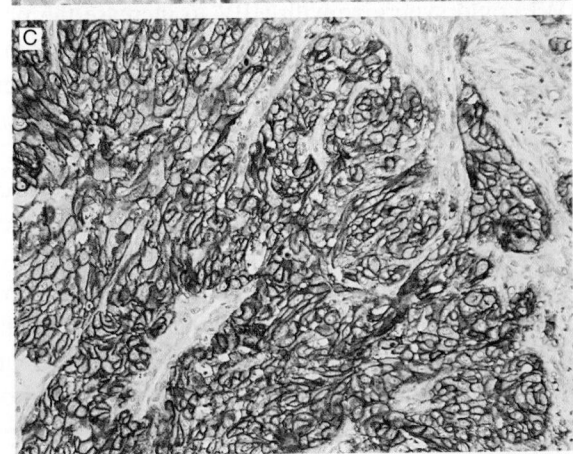

FIGURE 35-1. **(A)** Moderately differentiated keratinizing squamous cell carcinoma, **(B)** human papilloma virus related changes, including koilocytosis, and **(C)** immunohistochemical stain for epidermal growth factor receptor. *(Reprinted with permission from Pheroze Tamboli, MD.)*

relevant, and two prophylactic HPV vaccines are available (HPV 16/18 vaccine Cervarix [GlaxoSmithKline] and the quadrivalent HPV 16/18/6/11 vaccine Gardasil [Sanofi Pasteur, Merck Sharpe &Dome]) (10). The efficacy of preventing HPV infection among HPV negative women has been demonstrated (33,34). The safety and immunogenicity of the vaccines has also been established among adolescent boys, but efficacy in prevention of HPV infection in such populations awaits the results of ongoing studies (13,48). Currently, the vaccines are not approved for use in young men.

Although HPV infection is probably an important factor in the development of penile cancer, its presence is not invariable (31-63% of patients with penile carcinoma test positive) (29), indicating that additional factors may be involved in the development of the disease or its subtypes. Rubin et al. (35) performed a sensitive polymerase chain reaction assay on penile cancer specimens from the United States and Paraguay. Overall, 42% of penile carcinomas were HPV positive. Only 34.9% and 33.3% of keratinizing and verrucous carcinomas, respectively, were positive, whereas 80% and 100% of basaloid and warty tumor subtypes, respectively, exhibited HPV DNA.

HUMAN IMMUNODEFICIENCY VIRUS

Human immunodeficiency virus (HIV) infection may predispose affected patients to rapid development of squamous carcinoma from preexisting condyloma infection (36). Poblet et al. (37) reported on two cases of coexisting HIV-1 and HPV infection and postulated that HIV-1 could synergize with HPV to increase the progression of HPV penile lesions into penile carcinoma. Whereas there is evidence supporting this effect in cervical and anal neoplasia, definitive proof for penile cancer awaits further study (38).

In the patient with acquired immunodeficiency syndrome (AIDS), the underlying immune deficiency predisposes the host to Kaposi sarcoma by a factor of 7000 (39). The first case of HIV-related epidemic Kaposi sarcoma was reported in 1981 and the first with penile involvement in 1986 (40). Subsequently, Kaposi sarcoma of the penis has become a relatively common lesion in patients with AIDS.

Kaposi sarcoma of the penis is now probably the second most common malignant neoplasm of the penis after squamous cell carcinoma. Penile involvement is more common in the gay male population than in others with AIDS.

OTHER INFECTIOUS AGENTS

Several reports suggest a strong relationship between infection with human herpesvirus 8, also known as Kaposi sarcoma–related herpesvirus, and the development of Kaposi sarcoma lesions in patients with HIV infection (41,42). Some studies have found epidemic Kaposi sarcoma in patients who are HIV negative,

which suggests that certain sexual practices and a separate sexually transmitted agent may be responsible for this form of the disease (39,43). Recently human herpesvirus 8 has been isolated from penile Kaposi lesions in patients who were HIV negative supporting the notion that this may be sexually transmitted (44).

■ MOLECULAR FEATURES

OVERIEW OF MOLECULAR FEATURES

Human papillomavirus infection has been implicated as an etiologic factor in squamous cell carcinoma of the penis, as noted above, but the correlation of HPV with prognostic variables is still unclear. The high-risk types HPV 16 and 18 occur in 60 to 75% of in situ and invasive tumors, whereas the low-risk types 6 and 11 are associated with condylomata acuminata and Buschke-Lowenstein tumors (an advanced condylomatous lesion without malignant change) (29,32). The viral genes *E6* and *E7* are overexpressed in HPV transformed cells, and they are known to interact with Rb/E2F and p53 tumor suppressor pathways. These molecular events play a critical role in the development of cervical cancer (45), and a similar mechanism probably exists in at least some cases of penile cancer (12). A study comparing survival of patients with HPV positive penile cancer with HPV negative found a 5-year disease-specific survival of 92% and 78%, respectively, suggesting a survival advantage in patients who are HPV DNA positive (46). An analogous association of HPV with favorable outcome has been observed in patients with squamous cell carcinoma of the head and neck (47).

The tumor suppressor gene *p53* is commonly mutated in human solid tumors, where the abnormal protein accumulates and can be detected by positive immunostaining. In penile cancer, p53 immunostaining is an independent predictor of lymph node metastasis (48-50). In a study by Lopes et al., 34 of 82 (41.5%) primary tumor samples showed nuclear accumulation of p53. The p53 positive cases had a lower overall survival and higher incidence of lymph node metastasis (50). Martins et al. studied 50 patients of which 14 had clinically positive lymph nodes. After penectomy, tumors were stained for p53 and proliferating cell nuclear antigen (PCNA), and these results were compared with stage, grade, nodal status, and cause of death. Overexpression of p53 was associated with pT stage, grade, nodal metastasis, and cause-specific survival. PCNA was associated with nodal metastasis, but not survival (48). Presently, standardization of methodologies for assessment of gene expression, and the lack of large tissue banks with well annotated clinical data for validation studies hamper efforts to rigorously evaluate the potential utility of such biomarkers.

Matrix metalloproteinases and cellular adhesion molecules have been studied in penile cancer. Campos et al. (51) measured MMP-2 and MMP-9 expression and found that MMP-9 was an independent risk factor for disease recurrence. In the same study, low E-cadherin was associated with a greater risk of lymph node metastasis. A Chinese study (49) found that 45% of tumors had low E-cadherin, and that it was associated with shorter cause-specific survival. These alterations have been found in both HPV-positive and -negative penile tumors (10).

EPIDERMAL GROWTH FACTOR RECEPTOR

The epidermal growth factor receptor (EGFR) is overexpressed in a variety of human solid tumors, including squamous cell carcinomas (61). The published data on EGFR in penile cancer are limited to two studies. Borgermann et al. (52) recently reported the results of immunostain for EGFR on samples of tumor tissue from 44 patients, of which 40 tumors (90.9%) showed positive EGFR expression. The patients included 3 with distant metastases and 20 with pathologically proven lymph node metastasis. Nineteen patients were pathologically lymph node negative. Twenty-four patients died, and there was no statistical association of EGFR expression with mortality. In a series from MD Anderson Cancer Center (53), tumor tissue from 13 patients was immunostained and all were EGFR positive (Fig. 35-1*C*). Six of the samples were from primary tumors and 7 were from metastases. The data from these two studies suggest that EGFR overexpression is common in both metastatic and nonmetastatic penile cancer. EGFR negative cases are few or absent, so it is not likely to have relevance as a prognostic factor. The high frequency of expression, however, suggests that it may be a useful target for therapy (53), as it has been successfully targeted in squamous cell carcinoma of the head and neck (47).

■ PATTERN OF METASTASIS

ANATOMY OF LYMPHATIC DRAINAGE

Penile cancers have a predictable pattern of local, regional, and systemic spread. The earliest route of dissemination from the penis is metastasis to the regional femoral and iliac nodes. The lymphatics of the prepuce form a connecting network that joins with the lymphatics from the skin of the shaft. These tributaries drain into the superficial inguinal nodes, that is nodes that are external to the fascia lata. The lymphatics of the glans join the lymphatics draining the corporal bodies, and they form a collar of connecting channels at the base of the penis that drain by way of the superficial lymph nodes. The superficial nodes drain to the deep inguinal nodes (those deep to the fascia lata). From there, drainage is to the pelvic nodes (external iliac, internal iliac, and obturator). Penile lymphangiographic studies demonstrate a consistent pattern of drainage that proceeds from superficial inguinal to deep inguinal to pelvic node sites without evidence of preferential ipsilateral drainage (54,55). Multiple cross-connections exist at all levels of drainage, so that penile lymphatic drainage is bilateral to both inguinal areas. Some tumors metastasize directly to deep inguinal lymph nodes, but skip metastases to pelvic lymph nodes are unusual (56).

FREQUENCY OF METASTASES—PROGNOSTIC FACTORS

Tumor grade, lymphovascular invasion, and perineural invasion appear to be the most important pathologic prognostic factors for nodal spread and mortality (56). Other frequently cited risk factors are pT stage, tumor thickness, anatomical site (proximal versus distal), pathologic subtype, urethral invasion, and positive margins of resection.

Vascular invasion (embolism) by tumor cells has significant prognostic importance. Four studies have assessed its presence or absence, and it was an important predictor of nodal metastasis in all the reports (57-60). The pathologist should specifically comment on the presence or absence of vascular invasion in the surgical specimen. Lopes et al. (58) studied the prognostic value of lymphatic invasion in 146 patients with penile cancer. In a univariate analysis, clinical nodal stage, tumor thickness, lymphatic and venous embolization, and urethral infiltration were all associated with lymph node metastasis. However, subsequent to multivariate analysis, only venous and lymphatic invasion remained significant predictors for positive lymph nodes. Data from the MD Anderson Cancer Center revealed that vascular invasion was absent in all patients with T1 tumors (60). These patients were also lymph node negative at surgery. In contrast, patients with stage pT2 primary tumors exhibited nodal metastasis in 75% of cases (15 of 20) when vascular invasion was present but in only 25% of cases (3 of 12) when it was absent.

Perineural invasion was recently found to be present in 36% of cases analyzed in a multi-institutional data set of 134 patients, and was also a strong predictor of lymph node metastasis (61).

Several authors have evaluated the risk of nodal metastasis for pT1 lesions according to tumor grade. Among 73 patients with pT1, grade 1 or grade 2 primary tumors, metastasis occurred in only 5 patients (7%). Among 3 series reporting specifically on the T1 grade 2 subset the risk of metastases in 24 initially node-negative patients was 9 (38%). However, 5 patients in this subset also exhibited either lymphatic or venous invasion. Ficarra et al. (62) developed the first penile cancer nomogram utilizing data from 175 patients. Based on tumor thickness and growth pattern, patients with T1 grade 2 tumors exhibited rates of metastasis between 5 and 20%. Thus grade 2 tumors represent a heterogeneous group where the histologic criteria used to describe grade 2 and the presence or absence of other poor prognostic features ultimately determines prognosis (56). In this regard the European Association of Urology (EAU) Guidelines assigned patients with T1 grade 2 tumors to the intermediate risk category where the risk of lymph node metastasis is greater than 16% (low risk) and less than 68% (high-risk group) (63).

DISTANT METASTASIS AND MORTALITY

Metastatic penile cancer is characterized by a relentlessly progressive course, causing death for the majority of untreated patients within 2 years (15,64,65). Metastatic enlargement of the regional nodes eventually leads to skin necrosis, chronic infection, and death from sepsis, hemorrhage secondary to erosion into the femoral vessels, and failure to thrive.

Clinically detectable distant metastatic lesions to the lung, liver, bone, or brain are uncommon and are reported to occur in 1 to 10% of cases in most large series (3,23,33). Such metastases usually occur late in the course of the disease after the local lesion has been treated. Distant metastases in the absence of regional node metastases are unusual.

■ EVALUATION OF THE PATIENT

STAGING SYSTEM

The American Joint Committee on Cancer (AJCC) seventh edition TNM staging system for penile cancer (Table 35-2) differs from the sixth edition in that pT1 tumors are stratified as to whether there is high-grade histology or lymphovascular invasion (pT1b) (66). Considering pathologic nodal factors further, the seventh edition distinguishes patients with a single positive node (N1) from those with multiple or bilateral nodes (N2) and further recognizes the ominous prognosis

TABLE 35-2	DEFINITIONS OF TNM

Primary Tumor (T)

TX	Primary tumor cannot be assessed
T0	No evidence of primary tumor
Tis	Carcinoma in situ
Ta	Noninvasive verrucous carcinoma
T1a	Tumor invades subepithelial connective tissue without lymph vascular invasion and is not poorly differentiated (ie, grade 3-4)
T1b	Tumor invades subepithelial connective tissue and exhibits lymph vascular invasion or is poorly differentiated
T2	Tumor invades corpus spongiosum or cavernosum
T3	Tumor invades urethra
T4	Tumor invades other adjacent structures

Regional Lymph Nodes (N)

Clinical Stage Definition

cNX	Regional lymph nodes cannot be assessed
cN0	No palpable or visibly enlarged inguinal lymph nodes
cN1	Palpable mobile unilateral inguinal lymph node
cN2	Palpable mobile multiple or bilateral inguinal lymph nodes
cN3	Palpable fixed inguinal nodal mass or pelvic lymphadenopathy unilateral or bilateral

Pathologic Stage Definition

pNX	Regional lymph nodes cannot be assessed
pN0	No regional lymph node metastasis
pN1	Metastasis in a single inguinal lymph node
pN2	Metastasis in multiple or bilateral inguinal lymph nodes
pN3	Extranodal extension of lymph node metastasis or pelvic lymph nodes(s) unilateral or bilateral

Distant Metastasis (M)

M0	No distant metastasis
M1	Distant metastasis*

*Lymph node metastasis outside the true pelvis in addition to visceral or bone sites.

Used with the permission of the American Joint Committee on Cancer (AJCC), Chicago, Illinois. The original source for this material is the AJCC Cancer Staging Manual, Seventh Edition (2010) published by Springer Science and Business Media LLC, www.springer.com.

(5-18% 5-year survival) associated with extranodal extension of cancer (67-69).

LIMITATIONS OF THE STAGING SYSTEM

A study from the Netherlands Cancer Institute evaluated the practical and prognostic value of the sixth edition TNM classification for penile carcinoma (Table 35-3) (70). The current T2 category combines tumors that invade either the corpus spongiosum or corpora cavernosa (66). The 5-year disease-specific survival for tumors invading the corpus spongiosum in the Dutch series was 77.7%, and for tumors invading the corpora

TABLE
35-3 | STAGE GROUPING FOR PENILE
CANCER

Stage 0	Tis	N0	M0
	Ta	N0	M0
Stage I	T1a	N0	M0
Stage II	T1b	N0	M0
	T2	N0	M0
	T3	N0	M0
Stage IIIa	T1-3	N1	M0
Stage IIIb	T1-3	N2	M0
Stage IV	T4	Any N	M0
	Any T	N3	M0
	Any T	Any N	M1

Used with the permission of the American Joint Committee on Cancer (AJCC), Chicago, Illinois. The original source for this material is the AJCC Cancer Staging Manual, Seventh Edition (2010) published by Springer Science and Business Media LLC, www.springer.com.

cavernosa was 52.6%, suggesting that the capacity of a tumor to penetrate the tunica albuginea covering the corpora cavernosa is a more invasive characteristic. The Dutch investigators also suggested that the T3 category appears to be obsolete, since a distally located tumor that invades the urethra can still be treated with good prognosis; they proposed that invasion of the corpora cavernosa should be designated T3 (71).

The Dutch study did not find a significant difference in 5-year disease-specific survival between the N1 and N2 category (70.2 and 58.3%, respectively; $p = .18$), and the authors proposed designating all unilateral inguinal (mobile) lymph node metastases as N1, bilateral inguinal (mobile) lymph nodes as N2, and any fixed groin mass as N3 (70). They also noted the difficulty of distinguishing superficial from deep inguinal lymph nodes, which is not always possible to do either clinically or on histopathologic analysis of a surgical specimen. The seventh edition TNM does not distinguish superficial from deep inguinal lymph nodes and does recognize the prognostic significance of a fixed groin mass as N3. The N2 category, however, still includes ≥ 2 unilateral, mobile lymph nodes, where the prognosis with 2 to 3 nodes is probably better than with more than 3 nodes involved (71).

Thus, the current TNM classification, while it is an improvement over the previous version, still necessitates caution with respect to prognosis in the assessment of deep inguinal lymph nodes (as to whether they are truly inguinal or pelvic lymph nodes) and in considering laterality as well as the number of inguinal lymph nodes involved. Also, bulky inguinal lymph nodes that are mobile and suspected of having extranodal extension based on imaging are still classified as N1 or N2; such cases would be pN3 upon histopathologic confirmation of extranodal involvement. Patients with clinical N1 or N2 and suspicion of extranodal extension should be regarded as being at higher risk. The new TNM version awaits validation with contemporary data.

EVALUATION OF PALPABLE LYMPH NODES

Palpable inguinal lymph nodes are found at presentation in 28 to 64% of patients with penile cancer, but not all of these represent metastatic tumor. Lymphadenopathy is caused by metastasis in 47 to 85% of cases, and the remainder is secondary to inflammation (72). Approximately 25% of patients with palpable lymph nodes will have bilateral metastases. Careful note should be made of the uni- or bilateral location of palpable adenopathy, diameter, number in each inguinal area, mobile or fixed, relationship to other structures (eg, skin) with respect to infiltration or perforation, and presence of leg or scrotal edema.

Persistent adenopathy after treatment of the primary lesion and 4 to 6 weeks of antibiotic therapy is most often the consequence of metastatic disease. Similarly, the development of new adenopathy during follow-up is much more likely to be due to tumor than inflammatory response. Historically a course of antibiotics was recommended for patients with suspicious nodes to potentially discern metastasis from cancer (69). However, several authors have raised the issue that this causes a significant delay and could impact survival especially among patients who are likely to be truly positive by virtue of the stage/grade of the primary tumor (73). An alternative approach for such patients is to perform fine-needle aspiration cytology of palpable nodes either at the time of or immediately after treatment of the primary tumor. In the case of a positive result, definite therapy can be planned without a 4-to 6-week delay.

Saisorn et al. (74) recently reported a 93% sensitivity and a 91% specificity in 16 patients with palpable adenopathy (mean size 1.47 cm) undergoing fine-needle aspirate (FNA) prior to lymphadenectomy. The recommendation for FNA among patients with palpable nodes was also recently incorporated in the EAU Penile Cancer Guidelines.

STAGING GROIN DISSECTION

While treatment of the primary tumor and a period of antibiotics may be useful to help sterilize the inguinal region, this practice is no longer advocated as a tool to select patients for that either should or should not undergo lymphadenectomy. One alternative to immediate lymphadenectomy for all patients has been to observe patients with normal findings on inguinal examination. Lymphadenectomy is subsequently reserved for those patients who develop palpable lymph nodes. The reluctance to advocate automatic ilioinguinal lymphadenectomy in all patients with penile cancer stems from the substantial morbidity the procedure can produce. Early complications of phlebitis, pulmonary embolism, wound infection, flap necrosis, and permanent and disabling lymphedema of the scrotum and lower limbs were frequent after both inguinal and ilioinguinal node dissections (57,65,75,76). Postoperative complications have been reduced by improved preoperative and postoperative care and advances in surgical technique (77). The mortality of complete inguinal lymph node dissection is about 3% (72).

Several studies have analyzed the survival of men undergoing early versus delayed lymphadenectomy according to pathologic evaluation of nodal status. McDougal et al. (76) reported a series of 23 patients with invasive primary lesions and nonpalpable nodes; 9 patients were treated with immediate adjunctive lymph node dissection (6 were positive), and 14 were treated with surveillance and delayed lymph node dissection. The 5-year survival in the node-positive immediate adjunctive lymphadenectomy group was 83% (5 of 6 patients), whereas in the surveillance group, the 5-year survival was 36% (5 of 14 patients). A third subset in this series had palpable nodes at presentation and had immediate *therapeutic lymph node dissection*, with 10 of 15 patients (66%) surviving 5 years (76). The best results were from immediate adjunctive lymph node dissection (83%), with the next best from immediate therapeutic lymphadenectomy (66%). The worst results were from the surveillance and delayed lymphadenectomy group (36%), in whom dissection was delayed until palpable nodes developed. The interval of opportunity for cure in this third group appears to have been lost.

Similarly, Fraley et al. (57) reported that immediate adjunctive lymphadenectomy resulted in a 5-year disease-free survival in 6 of 8 node-positive patients (75%) compared with 1 of 12 patients (8%) who had been followed up and then treated by delayed lymphadenectomy when nodal enlargement occurred. Six other patients in that series also presented with unresectable adenopathy after initial surveillance, and all died of disease. Although only two of six immediate lymphadenectomy patients had more than two positive nodes, all the patients treated by delayed lymph node dissection had three or more positive nodes.

A series from MD Anderson Cancer Center compared 5-year disease-free survival of 14 patients undergoing early lymphadenectomy for clinically suspicious and histologically node-positive disease with that of 8 patients who were followed up and later underwent lymphadenectomy when clinical nodal enlargement was undisputed (78). The primary tumors were of similar stage. The 5-year disease-free survival was 57% for early lymphadenectomy compared with 13% for delayed node dissection. Of note, the number of involved nodes in the immediate lymphadenectomy group (median, 2) was half that of the delayed lymphadenectomy group (median, 4), and no patient with more than two positive nodes survived more than 5 years.

Data from these and other studies suggest that a policy of immediate adjunctive or early lymphadenectomy gives greater assurance that surgical intervention will occur when tumor volume is small (55,67,71,73,77). For patients at highest risk of lymph node metastases based on features in the primary tumor, surgical staging can be performed by complete, bilateral inguinal lymph node dissection, which may also be curative in cases of small volume metastases. Moreover, experience has suggested that lymphadenectomy in the setting of microscopic disease may be less likely to produce complications than node dissection in the presence of bulky nodal metastases (57,79,80). This is presumably due to the reduced amount of lymphatic tissue removed, preservation of venous drainage, and blood supply compromised, which affect the viability of skin flaps and lymphatic flow.

In patients with nonpalpable inguinal lymph nodes, if ultrasound-guided FNA is tumor negative, dynamic sentinel lymph nodes biopsy (DSLNB) can be performed if the equipment and expertise are available (72). In patients at intermediate risk of inguinal lymph node metastases, sentinel lymph node biopsy or modified (limited) inguinal lymph node dissection may be performed if DSLNB is not feasible (95).

CT IMAGING

Patients with clinically palpable lymph nodes should undergo imaging to define the extent of disease. Historically, lymphangiography was used as an adjunct to physical examination in the identification of microscopic inguinal and pelvic nodal metastases and to direct needle biopsy (81). The technical difficulty of the procedure, combined with the availability of CT scanning and magnetic resonance imaging (MRI) has made lymphangiography obsolete in staging of this disease. Both CT and MRI scanning techniques depend primarily on lymph node enlargement for detection of metastases, but are unable to define the internal architecture of normal-sized nodes. Because CT and MRI have similar accuracy in detecting lymphadenopathy in other cancers, CT has often been the imaging modality chosen in penile cancer to examine the inguinal and pelvic areas as well as to rule out more distant metastases (see Fig. 35-2).

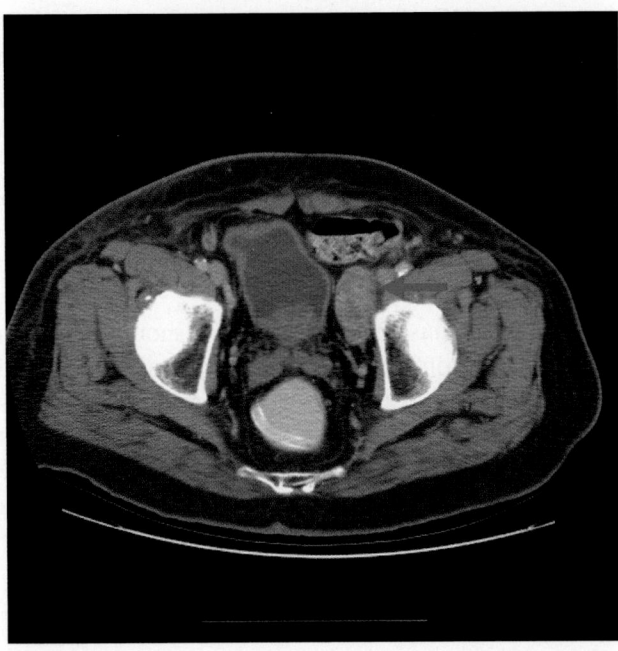

FIGURE 35–2. CT scan showing bulky metastasis in left external iliac lymph node.

CT scanning facilitates the examination of the inguinal region in obese patients or in those who have had prior inguinal surgery, for whom the physical examination may be unreliable. In addition, in patients with known inguinal metastases, CT-guided biopsy of enlarged pelvic nodes may provide important information for consideration of neoadjuvant chemotherapeutic strategies. Otherwise, the addition of CT imaging does not appear to improve the sensitivity or specificity of lymph node detection when compared to physical examination in patients with a normal inguinal examination (72).

POSITRON EMISSION TOMOGRAPHY (PET) IMAGING

Recently, squamous carcinoma was shown to take up the radiopharmaceutical ^{18}F-FDG and be amenable to detection utilizing PET/CT scanning. Scher et al. (82) evaluated PET/CT among 13 patients with penile cancer. Five of thirteen patients had metastatic disease and PET/CT detected four of five patients (80% sensitivity). There may be a role for PET/CT in the detection of lymph node disease in penile cancer; however, this promising initial report requires validation among larger data sets (Fig. 35-3).

■ TREATMENT

LOCAL CONTROL

Surgery

Surgical amputation of the primary tumor remains the oncologic gold standard for rapid definitive treatment of the penile primary tumor; local recurrence rates range from 0 to 8% (76,83,84). Amputation is often necessary for bulky stage T2-T4 tumors, but it has been shown to decrease sexual quality of life (85). It is generally accepted that patients with penile primary tumors exhibiting favorable histologic features (stages Tis, Ta, T1; grade 1 and grade 2 tumors) are at a lower risk for metastases. These patients are also best suited for *organ-sparing* or *glans-sparing* procedures (63). The goal of treatment is to preserve glans sensation where possible or at least to maximize penile shaft length. Such approaches include topical treatments (fluorouracil or imiquimod cream for Tis only), radiotherapy, Mohs surgery, limited excision strategies (eg, circumcision), and laser ablation (63,86-88).

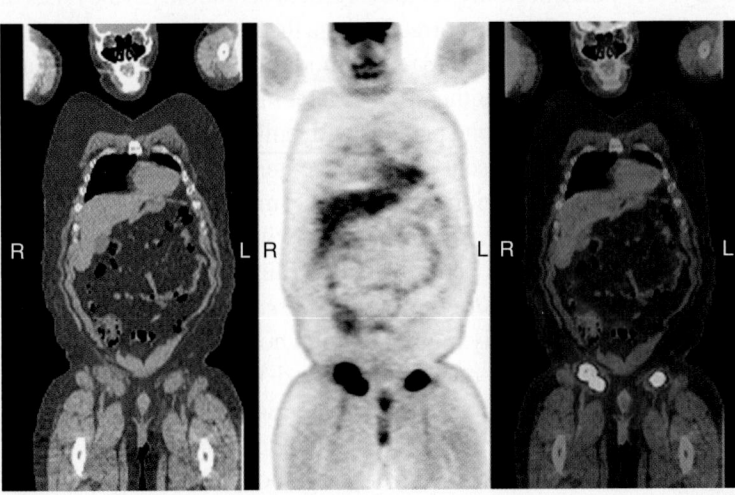
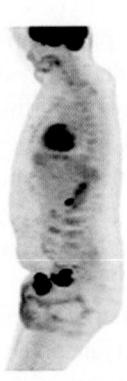

FIGURE 35–3. CT and PET images of bilateral inguinal and left external iliac lymph node metastases.

Laser Ablation

Laser ablation is feasible and may achieve results equivalent to those of surgery, especially when it is performed in well-selected patients in conjunction with frozen-section biopsies. In addition, laser ablation has been associated with high rates of resumption of sexual activity (75%) and overall satisfaction (78%) (89). Until additional long-term studies become available, however, laser ablation should be performed with the understanding that local recurrences may develop and that close surveillance and patient self-examination are necessary for early detection. Although well-selected patients who develop small recurrent lesions may be candidates for repeated laser ablation, recurrences are best treated with wide local excision or partial amputation.

Radiotherapy

Radiotherapy as primary treatment to the primary tumor has significant curative potential, and may permit relative preservation of penile form and function. If local control is not achieved, salvage surgery may still be curative, and therefore in a subset of men with penile cancer radiation as an initial strategy is reasonable. Both external beam radiotherapy and interstitial brachytherapy are currently utilized in treating the primary penile tumor. Circumcision must be performed before radiotherapy to expose the lesion, to allow resolution of any surface infection, and to prevent maceration and preputial edema (87).

External beam radiotherapy has several advantages as it is widely available, delivers a homogeneous dose, and does not require the same expertise with respect to technical skills required for delivery of brachytherapy. In a recent review, Crook et al. (87) describe contemporary doses and fractions as ranging from 60 Gy in 25 fractions delivered over 5 weeks to 74 Gy in 37 fractions over 7.5 weeks. This contrasts with lower doses of 50 to 55 Gy cited in older series (105,106). Five-year local control rates among patients treated using a variety of techniques ranged from 44 to 69.7% with penile preservation rates of 50 to 65%. These results show that the ability of primary external beam radiotherapy to control the primary tumor was inferior to traditional surgical techniques. Further local control in most cases of radiation treatment failure was achieved by partial or total penectomy. Cause-specific survival ranged from 58 to 86% depending on primary tumor stage, and lymph node status.

The benefits of avoiding a mutilating surgical procedure are obvious, and although sexual function is generally reported to be preserved, the sideeffects of radiation of sexual quality of life have not been studied with validated

instruments (87). In addition, patients and physicians must carefully consider the unique acute and long-term side effects of radiation therapy to the penis. Radiation therapy is usually administered for a period of 3 to 6 weeks and is followed by several months of morbidity. This may pose a formidable burden in elderly patients. By contrast, partial penectomy offers a prompt and effective treatment, with relatively few side effects limiting activity in the postoperative period.

Finally, it must be accepted that should radiation therapy fail, prompt penectomy must be done to avoid jeopardizing survival. Careful long-term follow-up is essential to detect postradiation recurrence, and it must be recognized that recurrence may develop relatively late. In one series, 7 of 11 recurrences (63%) were detected after 2 years, and 2 recurrences (18%) were detected after 5 years (90).

PENECTOMY

Partial or total penectomy should be considered in patients exhibiting adverse features that defy adequate control by organ preservation strategies. These include tumors of size 4 cm or more, grade 3 lesions, and those invading deeply into the glans urethra or corpora cavernosa (91-93).

THERAPEUTIC LYMPH NODE DISSECTION

The biology of penile cancer is such that it exhibits a prolonged locoregional phase before distant dissemination. Lymphadenectomy alone can be curative and should be incorporated into the treatment planning for most patients. However, due to the morbidity of traditional lymphadenectomy, especially among those patients with clinically negative groins, contemporary controversial issues include: (1) The selection of patients for lymphadenectomy versus careful observation; (2) the types of procedures to correctly stage the inguinal region with low morbidity; and (3) multimodality strategies (eg, neoadjuvant chemotherapy, see later in the chapter) to improve survival among patients with bulky inguinal metastases.

The presence and the extent of metastasis to the inguinal region are the most important prognostic factors for survival in patients with squamous cell carcinoma of the penis. This was illustrated in the preceding section on *Staging Groin Dissection*, in which prophylactic or early inguinal lymph node dissection led to better survival rates that delayed lymph node dissection. The survival rates for therapeutic lymph node dissection in patients with established regional lymph node metastases are variable, averaging about 60% (range, 0-86%)

(57,67-69,83,94,95). This variability in survival rates is directly attributable to the extent of nodal metastasis. Patients with pN1 or pN2 with a minimal number of lymph nodes involved have an average 5-year survival of 77%, compared with only 25% when a greater degree of nodal involvement was present. In one study (68), the 5-year survival of patients with extranodal involvement was only 6% (1 of 17 patients). The combined results of several small series suggest an average 5-year survival of 15% when pelvic lymph nodes are present.

Taken together, these data suggest that the pathologic criteria that predict long-term survival (ie, 80% 5-year survival rate) after attempted curative surgical resection of inguinal metastases are: (1) minimal nodal disease (up to two involved nodes in most series); (2) unilateral involvement; (3) no evidence of extranodal extension of cancer; and (4) absence of pelvic nodal metastases.

CHEMOTHERAPY FOR STAGE IIIB/IV PENILE CARCINOMA

The first candidate drugs for the treatment of penile carcinoma were identified on the basis of their antitumor activity in squamous cell carcinomas arising in other sites. These included cisplatin, vincristine, methotrexate, fluorouracil, mitomycin, and bleomycin. Responses to single-agent bleomycin were reported in 1969 (96) and to methotrexate, in 1972 (97). Cisplatin and cisplatin-based combinations were studied in the 1980s (98). In a multicenter study conducted by the Southwest Oncology Group (SWOG), 26 patients with metastatic penile cancer received single-agent cisplatin at a dosage of 50 mg/m^2 on days 1 and 8 of each 28-day cycle (99). Only four patients (15%) experienced responses that persisted for 1 to 3 months.

The combination of bleomycin, methotrexate, and cisplatin was studied in phase II clinical trials. In a single-institution study conducted at MD Anderson Cancer Center (100), 30 patients with squamous cell carcinoma of the urinary tract, including 21 men with metastatic penile carcinoma, received bleomycin at a dosage of 50 mg/m^2 on days 2 to 6, cisplatin at 20 mg/m^2 on days 2 to 6, and methotrexate at 200 mg/m^2 with

leucovorin rescue on days 1, 15, and 22 of each 28-day cycle. There were 12 responses (55%) in the group with penile carcinoma, and the median duration of response was 4.7 months for the entire study. A second phase II study was conducted by the Southwest Oncology Group, in which patients received bleomycin at a dosage of 10 units/m^2 on days 1 and 8, methotrexate at 25 mg/m^2 on days 1 and 8, and cisplatin 75 mg/m^2 on day 1 of each 21-day cycle (101). Among 40 evaluable patients there were 5 complete and 8 partial responses for an overall response rate of 32.5%, which exceeded the predetermined target rate of 30%. The median response duration was 16 weeks, and the estimated median survival time was 28 weeks. The toxicity of the regimen was considerable, however, with 5 treatment-related deaths. Nine additional patients withdrew from treatment because of toxicity. The most common toxic effects were gastrointestinal and hematologic, and the treatment-related deaths were due to bleomycin lung toxicity, other pulmonary causes, and infection.

The use of bleomycin in the treatment of men with penile cancer was associated with an unacceptable level of toxicity. Bleomycin is associated with potentially fatal pulmonary toxicity, in which there is a greater risk in patients older than 50 years (102). The median age of men with penile cancer is 55 to 58 years, so bleomycin is a poor choice of drug for this group. Single-agent methotrexate had a 61.5% response rate in a small series (98), but was also associated with life-threatening toxicity, and the high response rate was never confirmed or supported by the results of combination regimens that contained methotrexate (101). The median survival with these treatments in patients with advanced metastatic penile cancer was only 4 to 5 months.

Other cisplatin-based combinations demonstrated response rates of 25 to 50% (Table 35-4) (103-105). A regimen would be of interest if it has an overall response rate greater than 30% with acceptable toxicity. The study of irinotecan/cisplatin (102) conducted by EORTC was a prospective study with 26 evaluable patients, but was interpreted as a negative result by the authors because the response rate had an 80% confidence interval (18.8-45.1%) extending well below

TABLE 35-4	CISPLATIN-BASED CHEMOTHERAPY REGIMENS WITHOUT BLEOMYCIN		
Regimen	Overall Response Rate	Treatment-Related Deaths	Median Overall Survival, (Months)
Fluorouracil, cisplatin (103)	25%	0/8	11.5
Irinotecan, cisplatin (104)	31%	0/28	4.7
Paclitaxel, ifosfamide, cisplatin (105)	50%	0/30	17.1

TABLE 35-5	TAXANE-BASED CHEMOTHERAPY REGIMENS FOR PENILE CANCER	
Regimen	**Dose**	**Schedule**
Paclitaxel	175 mg/m^2	Day 1 over 3 hours
Ifosfamide	1200 mg/m^2	Days 1-3
Cisplatin	25 mg/m^2	Days 1-3
Cycle every 3 weeks (105)		
Paclitaxel	120 mg/m^2	Day 1
Cisplatin	50 mg/m^2	Days 1 and 2
Fluorouracil	1000 mg/m^2/day	Days 3-5
Cycle every 3 weeks (106)		

30%. The study of paclitaxel, ifosfamide, and cisplatin (105) was a neoadjuvant study, as discussed below, in which all patients had stage III or IV penile cancer, but with metastases limited to the inguinal and pelvic lymph nodes. This difference in patient eligibility may have influenced the response rate and overall survival in relation to previous studies. Nevertheless, the response rate of 50% and safety profile of this regimen compare favorably to the historical experience with other drug combinations, and those containing bleomycin in particular. Further study of taxanes for the treatment of metastatic penile cancer is warranted, and a prospective study of docetaxel, fluorouracil, and cisplatin is currently ongoing in Europe (Table 35-5). (106).

MULTIMODALITY THERAPY

Neoadjuvant Chemotherapy

As discussed in the preceding section on *Therapeutic Lymph Node Dissection*, the 5-year overall and disease-free survival rates with surgery alone are as high as 80% for unilateral, superficial inguinal lymph node involvement with no more than two nodes (stage N1 or limited N2), only 10 to 20% for stages N2 and N3 (multiple, bilateral, or pelvic lymph nodes involved), and less than 10% in the presence of extranodal extension. Nearly all recurrences are detected within 2 years of surgery, and an aggressive, multimodality approach to the treatment of high-risk patients could result in better overall survival.

In 1988, a team of Italian investigators reported their experience with adjuvant or preoperative (neoadjuvant) bleomycin, vincristine, and methotrexate for patients with penile carcinoma and metastases confined to the inguinal lymph nodes (107). Five patients with fixed inguinal nodes received weekly bleomycin (30 mg intramuscularly), vincristine (1 mg intravenously), and methotrexate (30 mg orally). Three of those five patients had a sufficient tumor response that they could undergo surgical consolidation, and they were reported to be alive and disease-free at 20, 27, and 72 months after surgery. The other two patients experienced less than partial responses, did not undergo surgery, and survived less than 12 months. This study, although small, demonstrated that perioperative chemotherapy for locally advanced penile carcinoma was feasible.

A group from the Netherlands reported on their retrospective analysis of 20 patients who had received preoperative chemotherapy to downstage unresectable disease (108). Seventeen patients had had bulky lymph node metastases (Tx, N3), and the other three had had advanced primary tumors (T3-4, N0-1). The most commonly used regimens in the Dutch series, which spanned a 34-year period, were: bleomycin, methotrexate, and cisplatin (N = 10); bleomycin, vincristine, and methotrexate (N = 5); and single-agent bleomycin (N = 3). Severe toxicity had occurred in four patients, including three treatment-related deaths. Twelve patients had experienced an objective tumor response; nine of the twelve had undergone surgery, and eight had achieved long-term disease-free survival. Two patients had had no residual tumor in the surgical specimen.

A retrospective study (109) from MD Anderson Cancer Center reported a series of 10 patients who had received neoadjuvant chemotherapy. The reported experience spanned a 15-year period at one institution and was limited to patients who had undergone aggressive lymph node dissections after having experienced a response or stable disease after chemotherapy. The regimens given preoperatively had been bleomycin, methotrexate, and cisplatin (N = 3); paclitaxel and carboplatin (N = 2); and paclitaxel, ifosfamide, and cisplatin (N = 5). Four patients had had complete responses and one had had a partial response to chemotherapy. Three patients had experienced a pathologic complete response in the lymph nodes, all of whom had received paclitaxel, ifosfamide, and cisplatin, and all had had biopsy-confirmed metastases prior to chemotherapy. Four patients had experienced long-term disease-free survival.

A prospective study of neoadjuvant paclitaxel, ifosfamide, and cisplatin was recently completed at MD Anderson Cancer Center (105). In this single-institution study, 30 patients with TX N2 (or N3) M0 penile cancer received 4 courses of chemotherapy prior to a planned complete bilateral inguinal lymph node dissection and uni- or bilateral pelvic lymph node dissection. Twenty-two patients completed the neoadjuvant chemotherapy and surgery. Fifteen patients (50%) experienced a partial or complete responses to chemotherapy, and three patients (10%) had a pathologic complete response

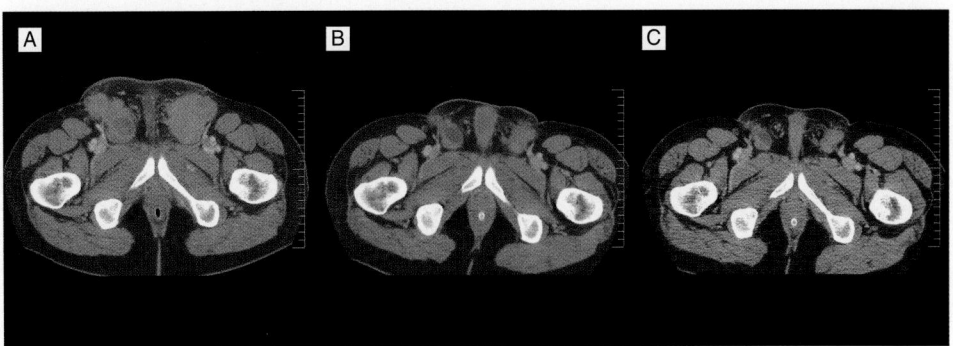

FIGURE 35–4. A patient with bilateral bulky superficial and deep inguinal lymph node metastases, shown (**A**) at baseline, (**B**) after 2 courses and (**C**) 4 courses of paclitaxel, ifosfamide, and cisplatin chemotherapy. Bilateral inguinal and pelvic lymph node dissections revealed no viable tumor, ie, a pathologic complete response.

in the lymph nodes (Fig. 35-4). Response to chemotherapy, absence of bilateral residual tumor, and absence of extranodal extension on histopathology were all associated with a higher rate of overall and progression-free survival that was statistically significant (Fig. 35-5).

Adjuvant Chemotherapy

In the Italian study of adjuvant or neoadjuvant bleomycin, vincristine, and methotrexate, there were 12 patients who had received chemotherapy after inguinal lymphadenectomy, and 11 of them were free of relapse at their last follow-up (107). These data were inconclusive due to the absence of measurable disease, small number of patients, and single-arm design of the study, although it did demonstrate safety and feasibility of the approach.

A German retrospective study involved 13 patients treated over a 7-year period who had received bleomycin, methotrexate, and cisplatin for metastatic or locally advanced penile carcinoma (110). Eight of the patients had received chemotherapy as adjuvant treatment for radically resected local or nodal disease. Only three of the eight patients had survived; four had died of tumor progression, and one died of treatment-related toxicity.

A randomized clinical trial of adjuvant chemotherapy would not be feasible due to the low frequency of penile carcinoma and the large number of patients necessary to power such a trial. The development of neoadjuvant chemotherapy as standard treatment appears to be more achievable, and has advantages of downstaging to facilitate surgery, better tolerance of chemotherapy in the preoperative setting, and earlier exposure of micrometastases to the chemotherapy agents.

Tumor response can be detected in the neoadjuvant setting, and the histopathologic findings of post-chemotherapy surgery provide and early indicator of

effect. In cases where patients have undergone surgery without neoadjuvant chemotherapy and are found to have multiple or pelvic lymph nodes involved, or extranodal extension, then a regimen such as paclitaxel, ifosfamide, and cisplatin can be administered as adjuvant the basis of extrapolation from the neoadjuvant data.

Radiotherapy Combined With Surgery or Chemotherapy

Studies of radiotherapy in penile carcinoma have included penis-sparing treatment for small (T1-2, <4 cm) primary tumors (111), treatment of lymph node metastases (112), postoperative radiotherapy (113), and chemoradiotherapy (114). There are no published randomized trials of multimodality treatment in penile cancer, as there are in squamous cell carcinomas from other sites. Comparison of radiotherapy with surgical lymphadenectomy has been studied in women with cancer of the vulva, a disease site that has natural history and nodal drainage similar to those of the penis. In this setting, Hyde et al. (115) reported that node debulking was equally effective as full groin dissection when followed by adjuvant radiotherapy (50-54 Gy) to the groin. Moreover, Parthasarathy et al. (116) found that when node dissection removed fewer than 12 nodes, even patients with a single positive node showed improved disease-free survival when they received adjuvant postoperative radiotherapy. These results suggest a role for postoperative adjuvant radiotherapy for regional nodal metastases in penile cancer.

For bulky inguinal nodes at presentation the Gynecologic Oncology Study Group performed a phase II study to assess the efficacy of preoperative chemoradiation prior to inguinal lymphadenectomy among patients with bulky N2/N3 inguinal nodes from vulvar

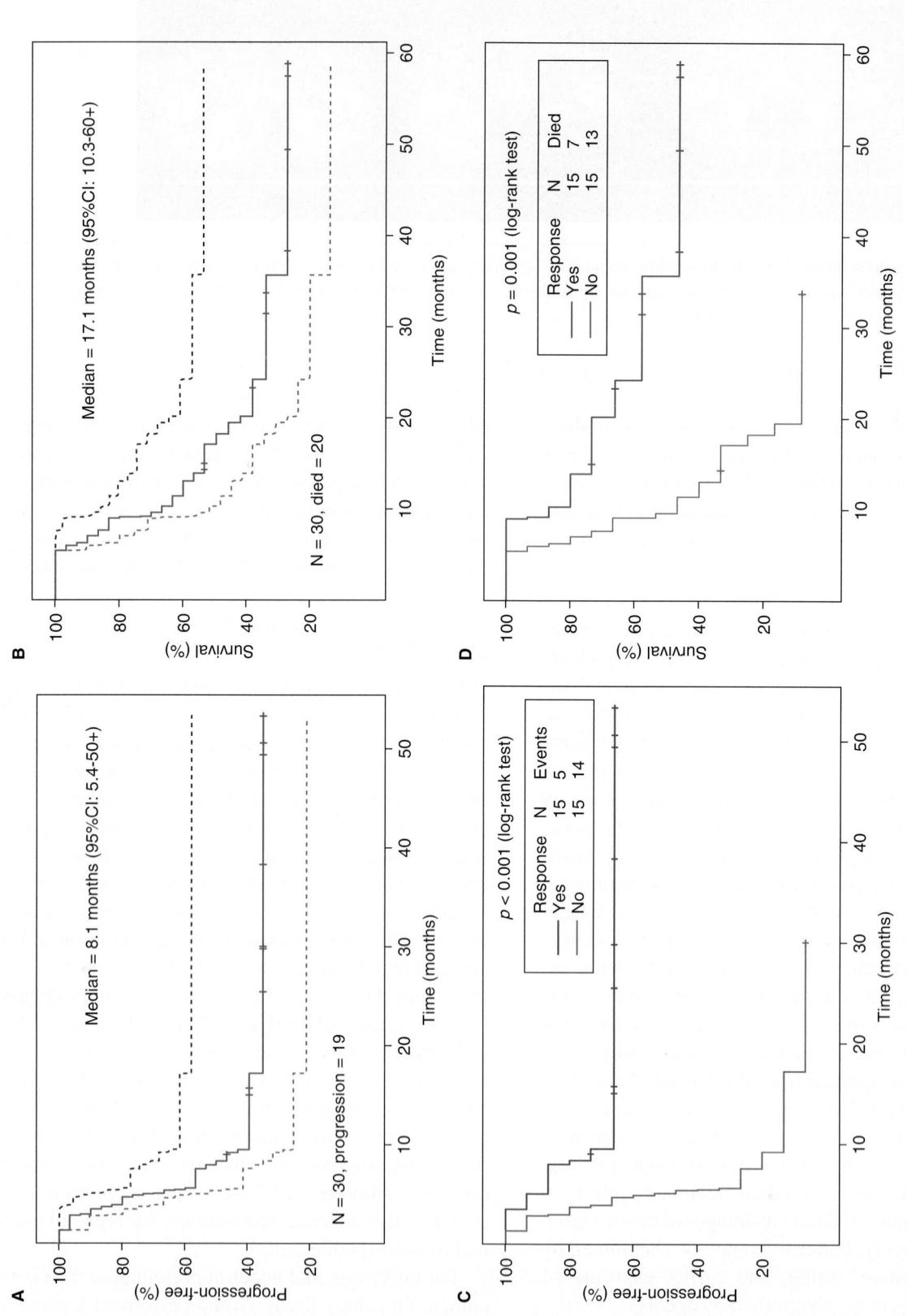

FIGURE 35-5. Kaplan-Meier plots (with 95% CIs as dotted lines) of (**A**) time to progression of disease, (**B**) overall survival; patients are grouped by response for (**C**) time to progression and (**D**) overall survival. Treatment consisted of neoadjuvant paclitaxel, ifosfamide, and cisplatin. (*Reproduced, with permission, from Pagliaro LC, Williams DL, Daliani D, et al. Neoadjuvant Paclitaxel, Ifosfamide, and Cisplatin Chemotherapy for Metastatic Penile Cancer: A Phase II Study. J Clin Oncol 2010;28(24):3851-7. Copyright 2010 American Society of Clinical Oncology. All rights reserved.*)

squamous cancer (117). Forty-two patients received split course chemoradiation consisting of cisplatin (50 mg/m^2) and fluorouracil (1000 mg/m^2) combined with 47.60 Gy to the primary tumor and inguinal nodes. Thirty-seven of 38 patients taken to surgery had an inguinal dissection and in 15 (40.5%) no tumor was found. Thirty-six of 37 patients (97%) had no inguinal recurrence. Only twelve patients (31%) remained alive without evidence of disease at 78 months follow-up as death due to other causes (N = 7) and distant metastases (N = 9) occurred. Thus preoperative chemoradiation in this prospective study improved resectability and local control among patients with bulky inguinal metastases.

In light of these lessons from squamous cell carcinoma in analogous sites, radiotherapy may also have a role in the treatment of penile cancer when inguinal adenopathy is initially unresectable (Fig. 35-6). Although primary radiotherapy in these circumstances will be palliative at best, chemoradiotherapy (114) or initial chemotherapy alone may render disease resectable. In the latter case, postoperative groin and/or pelvic radiotherapy can be offered, depending on the amount of residual disease after chemotherapy.

■ PREVENTION

NEONATAL CIRCUMCISION

With respect to penile cancer, neonatal circumcision and good hygiene to prevent phimosis represent the most important prevention strategies (Fig. 35-7). Although circumcision can nearly eliminate risk of the disease, especially where facilities for daily hygiene may be lacking, it may not be as important in countries where good hygiene is practiced. Frisch et al. (6) reported a falling incidence of penile cancer (from 1.15 of 100,000 men to 0.82 of 100,000 men) in the Danish population, which has a circumcision rate of only 1.6%. They attributed this trend to improved hygiene because the percent of homes having a bath facility increased from 35% in the 1940s to 90% in the 1990s. The recommendation of neonatal circumcision as a health-promoting measure remains controversial, and the procedure is usually performed or not performed according to cultural preferences.

HPV VACCINE

HPV vaccination could play a role in the future with respect to preventing transmission of HPV between males and females and thereby decreasing the risk of penile cancer. There is evidence that HPV vaccines are safe and immunogenic in men 10 to 15 years old (10).

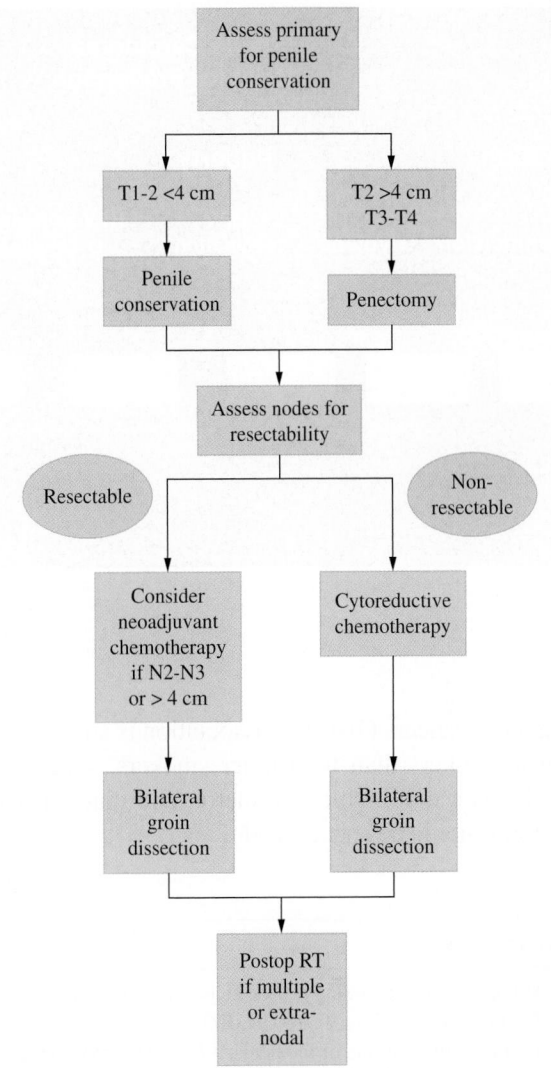

FIGURE 35-6. Treatment algorithm for penile cancer with bulky or unresectable regional lymph node metastases. *(Reproduced, with permission, from Chen MF, Chen WC, Wu CT, et al: Contemporary management of penile cancer including surgery and adjuvant radiotherapy: an experience in Taiwan. World J Urol 2004;22:60-6.)*

The efficacy for prevention of HPV-associated penile lesions is, however, unknown (118).

CONDOM USE

Condom use is effective in preventing the spread of sexually transmitted infections, including HPV. This may have consequences for viral persistence and the natural history of genital lesions, but it is unknown whether it would decrease the risk of penile cancer (10).

TOBACCO CESSATION

The precise role of tobacco in penile carcinogenesis has not been defined. There is an association between tobacco use and penile, as well as other HPV-associated

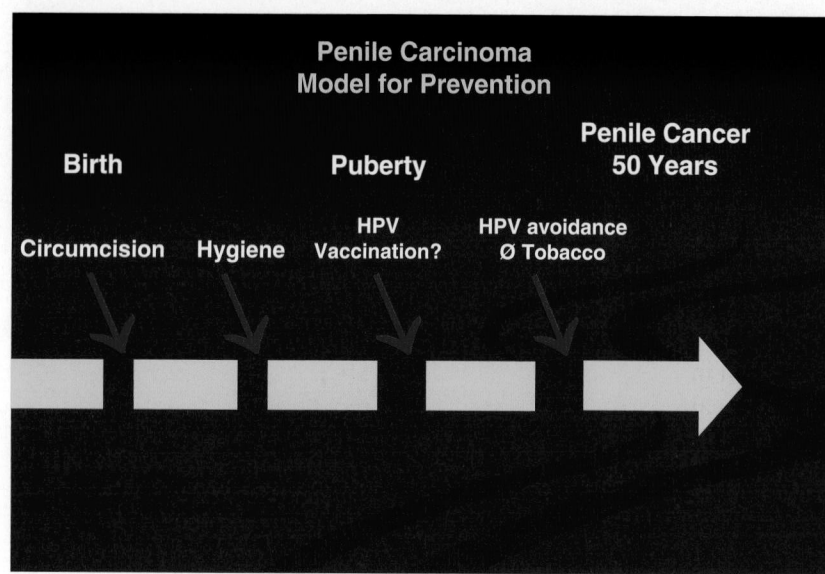

FIGURE 35–7.   Prevention model based on the pathogenesis of penile cancer. *(Reprinted, with permission, from Curtis A. Pettaway, MD)*

anogenital cancers (10). The association is stronger for current smokers than for former smokers, suggesting that this is a modifiable risk factor, and that smoking cessation should be encouraged.

References

1. Persky L. Epidemiology of cancer of the penis. Recent Results. *Cancer Res* 1977;60:97-109.
2. Dean A. Epithelioma of the penis. *J Urol* 1935;33:252-283.
3. Jemal A, Siegel R, Ward E, et al. Cancer statistics, 2009. *CA Cancer J Clin* 2009;59:225-249.
4. Vatanasapt V, Martin N, Sriplung H, et al. Cancer incidence in Thailand, 1988-1991. *Cancer Epidemiol Biomarkers Prev* 1995;4:475-483
5. Maiche AG. Epidemiological aspects of cancer of the penis in Finland. *Eur J Cancer Prev* 1992;1:153-158.
6. Frisch M, Friis S, Kjaer SK, et al. Falling incidence of penis cancer in an uncircumcised population (Denmark 1943-90). *BMJ* 1995;311:1471.
7. Yeole BB, Jussawalla DJ. Descriptive epidemiology of the cancers of male genital organs in greater Bombay. *Indian J Cancer* 1997;34:30-39.
8. Reddy DG, Baruah IK. Carcinogenic action of human smegma. *Arch Pathol* 1963;75:414-420.
9. Licklider S. Jewish penile carcinoma. *J Urol* 1961;86:98.
10. Bleeker MC, Heideman DA, Snijders PJ, et al. Penile cancer: Epidemiology, pathogenesis and prevention. *World J Urol* 2009;27:141-150.
11. Cubilla AL, Reuter V, Velazquez E, et al. Histologic classification of penile carcinoma and its relation to outcome in 61 patients with primary resection. *Int J Surg Pathol* 2001; 9:111-120.
12. Muneer A, Kayes O, Ahmed HU, et al. Molecular prognostic factors in penile cancer. *World J Urol* 2009;27:161-167.
13. Nielson CM, Flores R, Harris RB, et al. Human papillomavirus prevalence and type distribution in male anogenital sites and semen. *Cancer Epidemiol Biomarkers Prev* 2007; 16:1107-1114.
14. Smotkin D. Virology of human papillomavirus. *Clin Obstet Gynecol* 1989;32:117-126.
15. Beggs JH, Spratt JS, Jr.. Epidermoid carcinoma of the penis. *J Urol* 1964;91:166-172.
16. Reddy CR, Devendranath V, Pratap S. Carcinoma of penis— Role of phimosis. *Urology* 1984;24:85-88.
17. Stone KM. Epidemiologic aspects of genital HPV infection. *Clin Obstet Gynecol* 1989;32:112-116.
18. Giuliano AR, Lazcano E, Villa LL, et al. Circumcision and sexual behavior: Factors independently associated with human papillomavirus detection among men in the HIM study. *Int J Cancer* 2009;124:1251-1257.
19. Dunne EF, Unger ER, Sternberg M, et al. Prevalence of HPV infection among females in the United States. *JAMA* 2007; 297:813-819.
20. Lancaster WD, Castellano C, Santos C, et al. Human papillomavirus deoxyribonucleic acid in cervical carcinoma from primary and metastatic sites. *Am J Obstet Gynecol* 1986;154: 115-119.
21. Alani RM, Munger K. Human papillomaviruses and associated malignancies. *J Clin Oncol* 1998;16:330-337.
22. Gross G, Pfister H. Role of human papillomavirus in penile cancer, penile intraepithelial squamous cell neoplasias and in genital warts. *Med Microbiol Immunol* 2004;193:35-44.
23. Schneider V. Microscopic diagnosis of HPV infection. *Clin Obstet Gynecol* 1989;32:148-156.
24. Boxer RJ, Skinner DG. Condylomata acuminata and squamous cell carcinoma. *Urology* 1977;9:72-78.
25. Coetzee T. Condyloma acuminatum: A precancerous condition? *S Afr J Surg* 1977;15:75-80.
26. Malek RS, Goellner JR, Smith TF, et al. Human papillomavirus infection and intraepithelial, in situ, and invasive carcinoma of penis. *Urology* 1993;42:159-170.

27. Barrasso R, De Brux J, Croissant O, et al. High prevalence of papillomavirus-associated penile intraepithelial neoplasia in sexual partners of women with cervical intraepithelial neoplasia. *N Engl J Med* 1987;317:916-923.

28. Iversen T, Tretli S, Johansen A, et al. Squamous cell carcinoma of the penis and of the cervix, vulva and vagina in spouses: Is there any relationship? An epidemiological study from Norway, 1960-92. *Br J Cancer* 1997;76:658-660.

29. Wiener JS, Walther PJ. The association of oncogenic human papillomaviruses with urologic malignancy. The controversies and clinical implications. *Surg Oncol Clin N Am* 1995; 4:257-276.

30. Varma VA, Sanchez-Lanier M, Unger ER, et al. Association of human papillomavirus with penile carcinoma: A study using polymerase chain reaction and in situ hybridization. *Hum Pathol* 1991;22:908-913.

31. Iwasawa A, Kumamoto Y, Fujinaga K. Detection of human papillomavirus deoxyribonucleic acid in penile carcinoma by polymerase chain reaction and in situ hybridization. *J Urol* 1993;149:59-63.

32. Heideman DA, Waterboer T, Pawlita M, et al. Human papillomavirus-16 is the predominant type etiologically involved in penile squamous cell carcinoma. *J Clin Oncol* 2007;25: 4550-4556.

33. Harper DM, Franco EL, Wheeler C, et al. Efficacy of a bivalent L1 virus-like particle vaccine in prevention of infection with human papillomavirus types 16 and 18 in young women: A randomised controlled trial. *Lancet* 2004;364: 1757-1765.

34. Villa LL, Costa RL, Petta CA, et al. Prophylactic quadrivalent human papillomavirus (types 6, 11, 16, and 18) L1 virus-like particle vaccine in young women: a randomised double-blind placebo-controlled multicentre phase II efficacy trial. *Lancet Oncol* 2005;6:271-278.

35. Rubin MA, Kleter B, Zhou M, et al. Detection and typing of human papillomavirus DNA in penile carcinoma: Evidence for multiple independent pathways of penile carcinogenesis. *Am J Pathol* 2001;159:1211-1218.

36. Sanders CJ. Condylomata acuminata of the penis progressing rapidly to invasive squamous cell carcinoma. *Genitourin Med* 1997;73:402-403.

37. Poblet E, Alfaro L, Fernander-Segoviano P, et al. Human papillomavirus-associated penile squamous cell carcinoma in HIV-positive patients. *Am J Surg Pathol* 1999;23:1119-1123.

38. Northfelt DW. Cervical and anal neoplasia and HPV infection in persons with HIV infection. *Oncology* (Williston Park) 1994;8:33-37; discussion 38-40.

39. Miles SA. Pathogenesis of HIV-related Kaposi's sarcoma. *Curr Opin Oncol* 1994;6:497-502.

40. Seftel AD, Sadick NS, Waldbaum RS. Kaposi's sarcoma of the penis in a patient with the acquired immune deficiency syndrome. *J Urol* 1986;136:673-675.

41. Jaffe HW, Pellett PE. Human herpesvirus 8 and Kaposi's sarcoma—Some answers, more questions. *N Engl J Med* 1999;340:1912-1913.

42. Sitas F, Carrara H, Beral V, et al. Antibodies against human herpesvirus 8 in black South African patients with cancer. *N Engl J Med* 1999;340:1863-1871.

43. Chitale SV, Peat D, Meaden JD, et al. Kaposi's sarcoma of the glans penis in an HIV negative patient. *Int Urol Nephrol* 2002;34:251-253.

44. Morelli L, Pusiol T, Piscioli F, et al. Herpesvirus 8-associated penile Kaposi's sarcoma in an HIV-negative patient: First report of a solitary lesion. *Am J Dermatopathol* 2003;25:28-31.

45. Snijders PJ, Steenbergen RD, Heideman DA, et al. HPV-mediated cervical carcinogenesis: Concepts and clinical implications. *J Pathol* 2006;208:152-164.

46. Lont AP, Kroon BK, Horenblas S, et al. Presence of high-risk human papillomavirus DNA in penile carcinoma predicts favorable outcome in survival. *Int J Cancer* 2006;119:1078-1081.

47. Kies MS, Holsinger FC, Lee JJ, et al. Induction chemotherapy and cetuximab for locally advanced squamous cell carcinoma of the head and neck: Results from a phase II prospective trial. *J Clin Oncol* 2010;28:8-14.

48. Martins AC, Faria SM, Cologna AJ, et al. Immunoexpression of p53 protein and proliferating cell nuclear antigen in penile carcinoma. *J Urol* 2002;167:89-92; discussion 92-93.

49. Zhu Y, Zhou XY, Yao XD, et al. The prognostic significance of p53, Ki-67, epithelial cadherin and matrix metalloproteinase-9 in penile squamous cell carcinoma treated with surgery. *BJU Int* 2007;100:204-208.

50. Lopes A, Bezerra AL, Pinto CA, et al. p53 as a new prognostic factor for lymph node metastasis in penile carcinoma: Analysis of 82 patients treated with amputation and bilateral lymphadenectomy. *J Urol* 2002;168:81-86.

51. Campos RS, Lopes A, Guimaraes GC, et al. E-cadherin, MMP-2, and MMP-9 as prognostic markers in penile cancer: Analysis of 125 patients. *Urology* 2006;67:797-802.

52. Borgermann C, Schmitz KJ, Sommer S, et al. Characterization of the EGF receptor status in penile cancer: Retrospective analysis of the course of the disease in 45 patients. *Urologe A* 2009;48:1483-1489.

53. Pagliaro L, Osai W, Tamboli P, et al. Epidermal growth factor receptor expression in and targeted therapy for metastatic squamous cell carcinoma of the penis. ASCO Annual Meeting Proceedings Part I 2007. *J Clin Oncol* 2007;25:14045.

54. Cabanas RM. An approach for the treatment of penile carcinoma. *Cancer* 1977;39:456-466.

55. Cabanas RM. Anatomy and biopsy of sentinel lymph nodes. *Urol Clin North Am* 1992;19:267-276.

56. Cubilla AL. The role of pathologic prognostic factors in squamous cell carcinoma of the penis. *World J Urol* 2009; 27:169-177.

57. Fraley EE, Zhang G, Manivel C, et al. The role of ilioinguinal lymphadenectomy and significance of histological differentiation in treatment of carcinoma of the penis. *J Urol* 1989; 142:1478-1482.

58. Lopes A, Hidalgo GS, Kowalski LP, et al. Prognostic factors in carcinoma of the penis: multivariate analysis of 145 patients treated with amputation and lymphadenectomy. *J Urol* 1996; 156:1637-1642.

59. Heyns CF, van Vollenhoven P, Steenkamp JW, et al. Carcinoma of the penis–appraisal of a modified tumour-staging system. *Br J Urol* 1997;80:307-312.

60. Slaton JW, Morgenstern N, Levy DA, et al. Tumor stage, vascular invasion and the percentage of poorly differentiated cancer: Independent prognosticators for inguinal lymph node metastasis in penile squamous cancer. *J Urol* 2001;165:1138-1142.

61. Velazquez EF, Ayala G, Liu H, et al. Histologic grade and perineural invasion are more important than tumor thickness as predictor of nodal metastasis in penile squamous cell carcinoma invading 5 to 10 mm. *Am J Surg Pathol* 2008;32:974-979.

62. Ficarra V, Zattoni F, Artibani W, et al. Nomogram predictive of pathological inguinal lymph node involvement in patients with squamous cell carcinoma of the penis. *J Urol* 2006; 175:1700-1704; discussion 1704-1705.

63. Solsona E, Algaba F, Horenblas S, et al. EAU Guidelines on Penile Cancer. *Eur Urol* 2004; 46:1-8.

64. Derrick FC, Jr., Lynch KM, Jr., Kretkowski RC, et al. Epidermoid carcinoma of the penis: Computer analysis of 87 cases. *J Urol* 1973;110:303-305.

65. Skinner DG, Leadbetter WF, Kelley SB. The surgical management of squamous cell carcinoma of the penis. *J Urol* 1972;107:273-277.

66. Edge S, Byrd DR, Compton CC, et al. *AJCC Cancer Staging Manual*, 7th ed. New York: Springer; 2010.

67. Lont AP, Kroon BK, Gallee MP, et al. Pelvic lymph node dissection for penile carcinoma: Extent of inguinal lymph node involvement as an indicator for pelvic lymph node involvement and survival. *J Urol* 2007;177:947-952; discussion 952.

68. Ravi R. Correlation between the extent of nodal involvement and survival following groin dissection for carcinoma of the penis. *Br J Urol* 1993;72:817-819.

69. Srinivas V, Morse MJ, Herr HW, et al. Penile cancer: Relation of extent of nodal metastasis to survival. *J Urol* 1987;137: 880-882.

70. Leijte JA, Gallee M, Antonini N, et al. Evaluation of current TNM classification of penile carcinoma. *J Urol* 2008;180: 933-938; discussion 938.

71. Leijte JA, Horenblas S. Shortcomings of the current TNM classification for penile carcinoma: Time for a change? *World J Urol* 2009;27:151-154.

72. Mendoza-Valdes A, Heyns CF, Pompeo ACL. Diagnosis and staging of penile cancer. In: Pompeo A, Heyns CF, Abrams P, eds. *Penile Cancer*. Montreal, Quebec, Canada: Societe Internationale d'Urologie; 2007:71-99.

73. Kroon BK, Horenblas S, Lont AP, et al. Patients with penile carcinoma benefit from immediate resection of clinically occult lymph node metastases. *J Urol* 2005;173:816-819.

74. Saisorn I, Lawrentschuk N, Leewansangtong S, et al. Fine-needle aspiration cytology predicts inguinal lymph node metastasis without antibiotic pretreatment in penile carcinoma. *BJU Int* 2006;97:1225-1228.

75. Johnson DE, Lo RK. Complications of groin dissection in penile cancer. Experience with 101 lymphadenectomies. *Urology* 1984;24:312-314.

76. McDougal WS, Kirchner FK, Jr., Edwards RH, et al. Treatment of carcinoma of the penis: The case for primary lymphadenectomy. *J Urol* 1986;136:38-41.

77. Bevan-Thomas R, Slaton JW, Pettaway CA. Contemporary morbidity from lymphadenectomy for penile squamous cell carcinoma: The M.D. Anderson Cancer Center Experience. *J Urol* 2002;167:1638-1642.

78. Johnson DE, Lo RK. Management of regional lymph nodes in penile carcinoma. Five-year results following therapeutic groin dissections. *Urology* 1984; 24:308-311.

79. Ornellas AA, Seixas AL, Marota A, et al. Surgical treatment of invasive squamous cell carcinoma of the penis: Retrospective analysis of 350 cases. *J Urol* 1994;151:1244-1249.

80. Coblentz TR, Theodorescu D. Morbidity of modified prophylactic inguinal lymphadenectomy for squamous cell carcinoma of the penis. *J Urol* 2002;168:1386-1389.

81. Vapnek JM, Hricak H, Carroll PR. Recent advances in imaging studies for staging of penile and urethral carcinoma. *Urol Clin North Am* 1992;19:257-266.

82. Scher B, Seitz M, Reiser M, et al. 18F-FDG PET/CT for staging of penile cancer. *J Nucl Med* 2005;46:1460-1465.

83. de Kernion JB, Tynberg P, Persky L, et al. Proceedings: Carcinoma of the penis. *Cancer* 1973;32:1256-1262.

84. Horenblas S, van Tinteren H, Delemarre JF, et al. Squamous cell carcinoma of the penis. II. Treatment of the primary tumor. *J Urol* 1992;147:1533-1538.

85. Opjordsmoen S, Fossa SD. Quality of life in patients treated for penile cancer. A follow-up study. *Br J Urol* 1994;74: 652-657.

86. Sanchez-Ortiz RF, Pettaway CA. Natural history, management, and surveillance of recurrent squamous cell penile carcinoma: A risk-based approach. *Urol Clin North Am* 2003; 30:853-867.

87. Crook J, Ma C, Grimard L. Radiation therapy in the management of the primary penile tumor: An update. *World J Urol* 2009;27:189-196.

88. Minhas S, Kayes O, Hegarty P, et al. What surgical resection margins are required to achieve oncological control in men with primary penile cancer? *BJU Int* 2005;96:1040-1043.

89. Windahl T, Skeppner E, Andersson SO, et al. Sexual function and satisfaction in men after laser treatment for penile carcinoma. *J Urol* 2004;172:648-651.

90. Mazeron JJ, Langlois D, Lobo PA, et al. Interstitial radiation therapy for carcinoma of the penis using iridium 192 wires: The Henri Mondor experience (1970-1979). *Int J Radiat Oncol Biol Phys* 1984;10:1891-1895.

91. Mohs FE, Snow SN, Larson PO. Mohs micrographic surgery for penile tumors. *Urol Clin North Am* 1992;19:291-304.

92. Gotsadze D, Matveev B, Zak B, et al. Is conservative organ-sparing treatment of penile carcinoma justified? *Eur Urol* 2000;38:306-312.

93. Kiltie AE, Elwell C, Close HJ, et al. Iridium-192 implantation for node-negative carcinoma of the penis: the Cookridge Hospital experience. *Clin Oncol (R Coll Radiol)* 2000;12:25-31.

94. Fossa SD, Hall KS, Johannessen NB, et al. Cancer of the penis. Experience at the Norwegian Radium Hospital 1974-1985. *Eur Urol* 1987;13:372-377.

95. Horenblas S, van Tinteren H. Squamous cell carcinoma of the penis. IV. Prognostic factors of survival: Analysis of tumor, nodes and metastasis classification system. *J Urol* 1994;151: 1239-1243.

96. Ichikawa T, Nakano I, Hirokawa I. Bleomycin treatment of the tumors of penis and scrotum. *J Urol* 1969;102:699-707.

97. Mills EE. Intermittent intravenous methotrexate in the treatment of advanced epidermoid carcinoma. *S Afr Med J* 1972; 46:398-401.

98. Ahmed T, Sklaroff R, Yagoda A. Sequential trials of methotrexate, cisplatin and bleomycin for penile cancer. *J Urol* 1984;132:465-468.

99. Gagliano RG, Blumenstein BA, Crawford ED, et al. cis-Diamminedichloroplatinum in the treatment of advanced epidermoid carcinoma of the penis: A Southwest Oncology Group Study. *J Urol* 1989;141:66-67.

100. Corral DA, Sella A, Pettaway CA, et al. Combination chemotherapy for metastatic or locally advanced genitourinary squamous cell carcinoma: A phase II study of methotrexate, cisplatin and bleomycin. *J Urol* 1998;160:1770-1774.

101. Haas GP, Blumenstein BA, Gagliano RG, et al. Cisplatin, methotrexate and bleomycin for the treatment of carcinoma of the penis: A Southwest Oncology Group study. *J Urol* 1999;161:1823-1825.

102. Yagoda A, Mukherji B, Young C, et al. Bleomycin, an antitumor antibiotic. Clinical experience in 274 patients. *Ann Intern Med* 1972;77:861-870.

103. Shammas FV, Ous S, Fossa SD. Cisplatin and 5-fluorouracil in advanced cancer of the penis. *J Urol* 1992;147:630-632.

104. Theodore C, Skoneczna I, Bodrogi I, et al. A phase II multicentre study of irinotecan (CPT 11) in combination with cisplatin (CDDP) in metastatic or locally advanced penile carcinoma (EORTC PROTOCOL 30992). *Ann Oncol* 2008;19:1304-1307.

105. Pagliaro LC, Williams DL, Daliani D, et al. Neoadjuvant paclitaxel, ifosfamide, and cisplatin chemotherapy for metastatic penile cancer: A phase II study. *J Clin Oncol* 2010;28: 3851-3857.

106. Pizzocaro G, Nicolai N, Milani A. Taxanes in combination with cisplatin and fluorouracil for advanced penile cancer: Preliminary results. *Eur Urol* 2009;55:546-551.

107. Pizzocaro G, Piva L. Adjuvant and neoadjuvant vincristine, bleomycin, and methotrexate for inguinal metastases from squamous cell carcinoma of the penis. *Acta Oncol* 1988; 27:823-824.

108. Leijte JA, Kerst JM, Bais E, et al. Neoadjuvant chemotherapy in advanced penile carcinoma. *Eur Urol* 2007;52:488-494.

109. Bermejo C, Busby JE, Spiess PE, et al. Neoadjuvant chemotherapy followed by aggressive surgical consolidation for metastatic penile squamous cell carcinoma. *J Urol* 2007; 177:1335-1338.

110. Hakenberg OW, Nippgen JB, Froehner M, et al. Cisplatin, methotrexate and bleomycin for treating advanced penile carcinoma. *BJU Int* 2006;98:1225-1227.

111. Rozan R, Albuisson E, Giraud B, et al. Interstitial brachytherapy for penile carcinoma: A multicentric survey (259 patients). *Radiother Oncol* 1995;36:83-93.

112. Horenblas S, van Tinteren H, Delemarre JF, et al. Squamous cell carcinoma of the penis. III. Treatment of regional lymph nodes. *J Urol* 1993;149:492-497.

113. Chen MF, Chen WC, Wu CT, et al. Contemporary management of penile cancer including surgery and adjuvant radiotherapy: An experience in Taiwan. *World J Urol* 2004;22:60-66.

114. Modig H, Duchek M, Sjodin JG. Carcinoma of the penis. Treatment by surgery or combined bleomycin and radiation therapy. *Acta Oncol* 1993;32:653-655.

115. Hyde SE, Valmadre S, Hacker NF, et al. Squamous cell carcinoma of the vulva with bulky positive groin nodes-nodal debulking versus full groin dissection prior to radiation therapy. *Int J Gynecol Cancer* 2007;17:154-158.

116. Parthasarathy A, Cheung MK, Osann K, et al. The benefit of adjuvant radiation therapy in single-node-positive squamous cell vulvar carcinoma. *Gynecol Oncol* 2006;103: 1095-1099.

117. Montana GS, Thomas GM, Moore DH, et al. Preoperative chemo-radiation for carcinoma of the vulva with N2/N3 nodes: A gynecologic oncology group study. *Int J Radiat Oncol Biol Phys* 2000;48:1007-1013.

118. Garnett GP. Role of herd immunity in determining the effect of vaccines against sexually transmitted disease. *J Infect Dis* 2005;191 (Suppl 1):97S-106S.

CHAPTER
36

GERM CELL TUMORS

Heather D. Brooks
Lance C. Pagliaro
Zita Dubauskas Lim
Louis L. Pisters
Nizar M. Tannir

■ INTRODUCTION

Germ cell tumors (GCTs), the majority arising from the testicle, are a highly curable group of cancers primarily seen in young men. This group of patients should present a special consideration for oncologists, as appropriate management in the frontline setting can lead to many years of life recovered, making GCT the paradigm of the curable solid tumors. This chapter will primarily discuss GCTs arising in the testicle, dividing this category into seminoma versus nonseminoma germ cell tumors (NSGCTs). Then, the rare entity of extragonadal GCTs, which can arise in the mediastinum, retroperitoneum, or pineal body, will be described.

■ OVERVIEW OF GERM CELL TUMORS

EPIDEMIOLOGY

GCTs are the most common cancer in young men. Roughly 8400 new cases were being diagnosed in the United States in 2009, representing only a fraction of new genitourinary cancers which are estimated to be over 280,000 (1). Highlighting the high curability of this cancer, GCTs only claimed approximately 380 lives in 2009 (1) and carry a 5-year overall survival (OS) rate of greater than 90% (2,3). GCTs have a bimodal age distribution, with most men diagnosed between ages 15 and 25. There is a second peak of diagnosis around age 60, which largely represents seminoma histology and a lower mortality risk. Lifetime risk for the development of GCTs is approximately 0.5% or 1 in 200 (4).

Worldwide, GCTs are six times more common in developed countries, with the largest incidence reported in Denmark and Switzerland and the lowest in Japan, Finland, and Israel (4). In the United States, the overall incidence of GCTs appears to be gradually increasing. The incidence has specifically increased among African Americans, with the greatest increase in seminoma histology. This does not appear to be related to screening or earlier diagnosis. Caucasian men, although still representing the group most likely to be diagnosed, are more likely to be identified at an earlier stage than in the past (5,6).

RISK FACTORS

Cryptorchidism is one of the major identifiable risk factors for the development of GCTs, although representing only about 10% of cases. When present, cryptorchidism imparts a relative risk between 2.5 and

17.1 (7,8). This increased risk includes the contralateral testicle, even if descended normally or via orchiopexy. It is unclear if orchiopexy reduces the lifetime risk of GCTs, although data showing increased incidence even in the contralateral testicle supports the theory that the etiology of GCTs lie in abnormal gonadal development rather than anatomic malposition (9,10). Men with a prior history of GCTs also have an increased risk of GCTs in the contralateral testicle, suggesting a genetic predisposition, although men with a family history of GCTs account for only 1.5% of patients with new diagnosis (11). A personal history of GCT carries an increased lifetime risk of secondary cancers, irrespective of histologic type (12).

TUMOR BIOLOGY

The most common genetic abnormality in GCTs is an isochromosome of the short arm of chromosome 12, which has been identified in approximately 80% of GCT (13). This abnormality can be found in all histologic subtypes, including intratubular germ cell neoplasia (ITGCN) (14,15). Other chromosomal anomalies have also been identified. Overexpression of *c-kit* is seen in seminoma (16). Of note, p53 is rarely altered in GCTs, a fact that may be related to the qualitatively different results seen with chemotherapy and radiation when applied to GCTs compared to other solid tumors (17). Recently, Korkola et al. (18) identified a gene expression signature which may improve prediction of prognosis in GCTs.

Carcinoma in situ (CIS), or ITGCN, has been identified as the precursor lesion in most GCTs. It is histologically described as atypical germ cells in the seminiferous tubules. Such changes are found adjacent to most invasive GCTs, with the notable exception of spermatocytic seminoma. The ITGCN cells express numerous proto-oncogenic proteins that play a role in tumorigenesis, including the receptor tyrosine kinase CD-117 or *c-kit*, a protein normally involved in germ cell migration and early differentiation (19,20).

TUMOR HISTOLOGY

The main histologies encountered in GCTs are seminoma, embryonal carcinoma, endodermal sinus tumor (EST, also known as yolk sac tumor), choriocarcinoma, and teratoma. The latter can be further classified as mature, immature, or teratoma with malignant transformation. It is very common to see more than one histologic subtype within a tumor. Importantly, the clinical course can be largely inferred from the histology. GCTs which show exclusively the seminoma histology constitute pure seminomas, while those containing any other histologic pattern are classified as NSGCT, even if the dominant histologic pattern is seminoma. Thus, the term *seminoma* is used in two very different senses: as a histologic pattern and as a main subdivision of GCT. The biology and clinical expression are dominated by the nonseminoma component, and thus the presence of any histologic component other than seminoma places the tumor in the category of NSGCT.

CLINICAL PRESENTATION

Most patients with GCTs present with painless testicular swelling or a nodule. In some cases, testicular swelling can be accompanied by pain secondary to bleeding or infarction within the tumor. In the presence of pain or a history of injury, an appropriate differential diagnosis would include testicular torsion, epididymitis, orchitis, hydrocele, spermatocele, and hematoma. *It is extremely important that regardless of pain or other associated symptoms, all scrotal masses should be approached as if they were malignant.* In patients who present with gynecomastia, especially bilateral, GCTs should be considered (21). Other symptoms can include fever, weight loss, back pain, and hemoptysis (most often seen in patients presenting with high-volume disease).

DIAGNOSIS

The importance of early diagnosis cannot be stressed enough because the extent of disease at presentation predicts overall prognosis. Increased awareness of the occurrence of GCTs in young men is important for both general practitioners and the general public. Radiographic evaluation of a suspected primary should include high resolution, trans-scrotal ultrasonography with color Doppler of both testicles, and any suspicious lesion should be definitively evaluated with radical orchiectomy.

Trans-scrotal biopsy is contraindicated in the diagnostic workup of a suspected testicular neoplasm, as this procedure can disrupt regional lymphatics, potentially altering the otherwise predictable nodal spread. Since the diagnosis of GCTs is rarely in question, the preferred diagnostic and therapeutic procedure for a testicular mass is radical inguinal orchiectomy. If a tissue diagnosis is felt to be necessary prior to orchiectomy, an open biopsy should be performed via an inguinal incision to allow for proper examination and tissue sampling with minimal risk of inguinal or scrotal contamination.

TUMOR MARKERS

Serum markers, specifically human chorionic gonadotropin (hCG), alpha-fetoprotein (AFP), and lactate dehydrogenase (LDH), have unique diagnostic and prognostic significance in GCTs. These markers enable the clinician to infer clinical behavior, monitor therapy, decide when to apply surgical consolidation, and detect residual or recurrent disease.

Elevated in pregnancy, hCG is not normally detectable in males except in the setting of GCTs. With a half-life of 18 to 36 hours, hCG can also be markedly elevated in gestational trophoblastic disease, and rarely detectable in epithelial cancers (22). It is composed of two subunits, α and β, which exist in multiple isoforms. The α subunit is highly homologous to the α subunit of thyroid-stimulating hormone (TSH), follicle-stimulating hormone (FSH), and luteinizing hormone (LH) which leads to "cross-talk" between these hormones and hCG. For this reason, hCG assays measure the β subunit. This "cross-talk" can be clinically significant in high-volume disease accompanied by high levels of hCG, where hCG binds to the TSH receptor. Prophylactic use of β-blockers is often needed for symptom management and relief of clinical hyperthyroidism (23). *Extreme elevation of hCG in males should be considered pathognomonic for GCTs, and, in selected cases of threatening disease, justifies initiation of therapy even before tissue confirmation.*

AFP is normally produced by the fetal yolk sac and also exists in multiple isoforms. It is elevated in GCT cells derived from the embryological yolk sac, including endodermal sinus tumor and embryonal carcinoma. It has also been found to be elevated in other neoplasms such as hepatocellular carcinoma, pancreatic, gastric, and lung cancer, and has a half-life of approximately 5 days (24). In general, any presence of AFP in the setting of GCTs implies that the histology is not that of a pure seminoma (25).

LDH is expressed normally by multiple tissues including muscle, liver, brain, and kidney and is elevated in many diseases, malignant and otherwise. It is also found in multiple isoforms, and although elevation of LDH is a nonspecific marker for GCTs, LDH-1 is most specific for GCTs. To date, there is no established routine use for the fractionation of LDH and precise measurement of LDH-1, although total LDH can be used to estimate the prognosis as it relates to the volume of disease, or to detect recurrent disease (26).

ANATOMIC PROGRESSION

GCTs follow a distinct pattern of spread and metastasis. The lymphatic drainage from the testicle reflects embryologic origin, and thus the right testicle drains to the interaortocaval lymph nodes and the left testicle drains to the left para-aortic lymph nodes. These initial nodes of spread are termed the "landing zone." Epididymal lymphatics drain via the external iliac chain and scrotal lymphatics via the pelvic chain; therefore, locally advanced disease (involving the epididymis and scrotum) can present with involvement of these nodal basins. Distant metastasis involves the lungs principally, followed by the liver, brain, and bones.

STAGING

Table 36-1 shows the most recent American Joint Commission on Cancer (AJCC) TNM staging of testicular cancer (27). This system is based on the anatomic characteristics of the tumor, the presence of elevated tumor markers, and the presence of distant disease. These well-defined risk factors are used to place patients in risk stratification groups. In general, stage I disease is confined to the testes, stage II disease is confined to the retroperitoneum with markers in the good prognosis range, and stage III disease includes nodes that extend beyond the retroperitoneum, extranodal metastases, and elevation of tumor markers to the intermediate- or poor-prognosis range.

CONSIDERATION OF FERTILITY PRESERVATION

Of particular importance in GCTs is the preservation of fertility. Both the diagnosis and treatment of GCTs can affect fertility negatively, potentially decreasing a man's ability to conceive indefinitely. It is recommended that, if clinically feasible, the patient be counseled about and offered the opportunity to pursue sperm banking before starting chemotherapy. It is not recommended to delay chemotherapy in symptomatic poor-risk patients, as poor physical condition often makes sperm donation difficult or even impossible (28).

■ TESTICULAR SEMINOMA

HISTOLOGY

Under microscopic visualization, classic seminoma has a "fried-egg" appearance defined as a monotonous proliferation of large, rounded cells arranged in sheets or cords with large centralized nuclei and nucleoli. These tumors can be difficult to distinguish from lymphoma if there is a background of lymphocytic infiltration. Further confirmation (ie, negativity for lymphocyte

markers such as common leukocyte antigen) is often required. Although not specific, seminomas stain positive for placental alkaline phosphatase (PLAP) and are routinely negative for AFP and hCG. Figure 36-1 shows the histological appearance of classic seminoma.

On pathologic examination of the testis, seminoma tends to be a semisolid tumor that readily oozes onto the gross examination table. This makes the presence of malignant cells on the surface of the spermatic cord and at the margins of resection a ubiquitous finding. Thus, the clinician must be careful not to be unduly influenced by reports of "margin positivity" and "involvement of the spermatic cord" in the pathology report (29). Figure 36-2 shows the typical gross appearance of seminoma.

Even in the presence of significant metastatic disease, it is not uncommon to find only a scar in the testicle. This phenomenon is known as "burned-out" seminoma and is not a prominent feature of NSGCTs, except choriocarcinoma. The biological basis for this spontaneous regression of the primary is not known. Seminomas are typically associated with a significant inflammatory infiltration, and they characteristically leave a dense desmoplastic residual mass after treatment often making them difficult to resect.

CLINICAL FEATURES

Pure seminoma is the most common GCT of the testicle, accounting for approximately 50% of GCTs. By definition, seminomas have no evidence of a nonseminoma component and do not produce AFP, but may have modest elevation of β-hCG. Spermatocytic seminomas, a rare variant comprising only 10% of seminomas, are not associated with ITGCN. These tumors typically occur in men over 50 years old, in stage I disease, and have a low metastatic rate. This subtype portends an excellent prognosis with resection alone (± radiotherapy) (30). Seminomas tend to spread via lymphatics initially, with late hematogenous spread, and are more likely to spread locally, as evidenced by positive margins and involvement of the spermatic cord on histology. The most common hematogenous spread is to the lungs, and metastatic seminomas rarely metastasize to the brain. Remarkably, very bulky tumors rapidly respond, with dramatic loss of tumor bulk, but tumor lysis syndrome is never encountered.

PROGNOSIS

The International Germ Cell Cancer Collaborative Group (IGCCCG) established a standard risk classification for both seminomas and NSGCTs. Patients

TABLE 36-1 | **GERM CELL TUMOR: THE NEW AJCC TNM STAGING OF TESTICULAR CANCER**

PRIMARY TUMOR (T)

The extent of primary tumor is usually classified after radical orchiectomy, and for this reason a pathologic stage is assigned.

pTX   Primary tumor cannot be assessed

pT0   No evidence of primary tumor (eg, histologic scar in testis)

pTis   Intratubular germ cell neoplasia (carcinoma in situ)

pT1   Tumor limited to the testis and epididymis without vascular/lymphatic invasion; tumor may invade into the tunica albuginea but not the tunica vaginalis

pT2   Tumor limited to the testis and epididymis with vascular/lymphatic invasion, or tumor extending through the tunica albuginea with involvement of the tunica vaginalis

pT3   Tumor invades the spermatic cord with or without vascular/lymphatic invasion

pT4   Tumor invades the scrotum with or without vascular/lymphatic invasion

REGIONAL LYMPH NODES (N)

CLINICAL

NX   Regional lymph nodes cannot be assessed

N0   No regional lymph node metastasis

N1   Metastasis with a lymph node mass ≤2 cm in greatest dimension or multiple lymph nodes, none >2 cm in greatest dimension

N2   Metastasis with a lymph node mass >2 cm but not >5 cm in greatest dimension; or multiple lymph nodes, any one mass >2 cm but not >5 cm in greatest dimension

N3   Metastasis with a lymph node mass >5 cm in greatest dimension

PATHOLOGIC (PN)

pNX   Regional lymph nodes cannot be assessed

pN0   No regional lymph node metastasis

pN1   Metastasis with a lymph node mass ≤2 cm in greatest dimension and ≤5 nodes positive, none >2 cm in greatest dimension

pN2   Metastasis with a lymph node mass >2 cm but not >5 cm in greatest dimension; or >5 nodes positive, none >5 cm; or evidence of extranodal extension of tumor

pN3   Metastasis with a lymph node mass >5 cm in greatest dimension

DISTANT METASTASIS (M)

M0   No distant metastasis

M1   Distant metastasis

M1a   Nonregional nodal or pulmonary metastasis

M1b   Distant metastasis other than to nonregional lymph nodes and lungs

SERUM TUMOR MARKERS (S)

SX   Marker studies not available or not performed

S0   Marker study levels within normal limits

S1   LDH <1.5 × **N AND**

     hCG (mIU/mL) <5000 **AND**

     AFP (ng/mL) <1000

S2   LDH >1.5-10 × **N OR**

     hCG (mIU/mL) 5000-50,000 **OR**

     AFP (ng/mL) 1000-10,000

S3   LDH >10 × **N OR**

     hCG (mIU/mL) >50,000 **OR**

     AFP (ng/mL >10,000

N indicates the upper limit of normal for the LDH assay.

(Continued)

TABLE 36-1	GERM CELL TUMOR: THE NEW AJCC TNM STAGING OF TESTICULAR CANCER (*Continued*)

STAGE GROUPING

Stage 0	pTis	N0	M0	S0
Stage I	pT1-4	N0	M0	SX
Stage IA	pT1	N0	M0	S0
Stage IB	pT2	N0	M0	S0
	pT3	N0	M0	S0
	pT4	N0	M0	S0
Stage IS	Any pT/Tx	N0	M0	S1-3
Stage II	Any pT/Tx	N1-3	M0	SX
Stage IIA	Any pT/Tx	N1	M0	S0
	Any pT/Tx	N1	M0	S1
Stage IIB	Any pT/Tx	N2	M0	S0
	Any pT/Tx	N2	M0	S1
Stage IIC	Any pT/Tx	N3	M0	S0
	Any pT/Tx	N3	M0	S1
Stage III	Any pT/Tx	Any N	M1	SX
Stage IIIA	Any pT/Tx	Any N	M1a	S0
	Any pT/Tx	Any N	M1a	S1
Stage IIIB	Any pT/Tx	N1-3	M0	S2
	Any pT/Tx	Any N	M1a	S2
Stage IIIC	Any pT/Tx	N1-3	M0	S3
	Any pT/Tx	Any N	M1a	S3
	Any pT/Tx	Any N	M1b	Any S

Reproduced, with permission, from Edge SB, Byrd DR, Compton CC, eds. AJCC Cancer Staging Manual, 7th edition. New York, Springer, 2010, pp. 475-77.

with seminoma are divided into either good- or intermediate-risk categories, with no definable poor-risk category. The one characteristic that predicted patient prognosis was the presence or absence of nonpulmonary visceral metastases. Interestingly, prechemotherapy tumor markers did not influence prognosis (unlike in NSGCTs to be discussed later). The prognostic categories from this research are outlined in Table 36-2. Ninety percent of patients with seminoma fell into the good-prognosis category and had 5-year OS of 86%. Patients with seminoma in the intermediate-prognosis category had a 5-year OS of 72% (2).

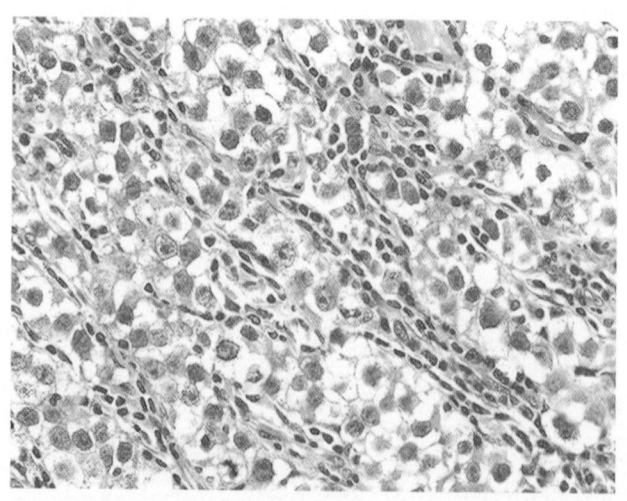

FIGURE 36-1. Histological appearance of classic seminoma.

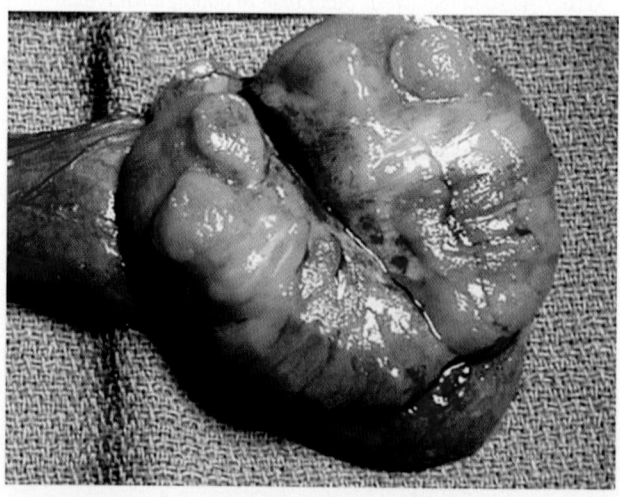

FIGURE 36-2. Gross appearance of seminoma.

TABLE 36-2	IGCCCG CLASSIFICATION PROGNOSTIC RISK STRATIFICATION (2)	
Seminoma	**Nonseminoma**	
GOOD RISK		
Any primary site and No nonpulmonary visceral metastases and Normal AFP, any hCG, any LDH	Testis/retroperitoneal primary and No nonpulmonary visceral metastases and AFP <1000 ng/mL hCG <5000 mIU/mL LDH <1.5 × ULN	
82% 5-year PFS; 86% 5-year OS	**86% 5-year PFS; 90% 5-year OS**	
INTERMEDIATE RISK		
Any primary site and Nonpulmonary visceral metastases and Normal AFP, any hCG, any LDH	Testis/retroperitoneal primary and No nonpulmonary visceral metastases and AFP 1000-10,000 ng/mL hCG 5000-50,000 mIU/mL LDH 1.5-10 × ULN	
67% 5-year PFS; 72% 5-year OS	**75% 5-year PFS; 80% 5-year OS**	
POOR RISK		
— — — —	Mediastinal primary or Nonpulmonary visceral metastases or AFP >10,000 ng/mL hCG >50,000 mIU/mL LDH >10 × ULN	
—	**41% 5-year PFS; 48% 5-year OS**	

MANAGEMENT OF CLINICAL STAGE I SEMINOMA

Clinical stage I seminoma patients, representing 70% of patients at diagnosis, generally have disease confined to the testicle with no evidence of nodal or distant metastasis. Most patients will be cured by radical orchiectomy alone, but between 12 and 32% will recur without further treatment. Defining the patients who are at high risk for recurrent disease could avoid unnecessary intervention and exposure to treatment risks.

Active Surveillance

With the majority of patients cured postsurgery, active surveillance remains a reasonable option for the motivated and reliable patient. The benefits of surveillance include avoidance of unnecessary treatment and risk in patients who can have disease control regained at the first sign of recurrence. Warde et al. reported data on 638 patients managed with surveillance with a median follow-up of 7 years. Patients with a primary tumor less than 4 cm and without invasion of rete testis had 5-year risk of relapse of 12%. Patients with both risk factors had risk of recurrence of 32%, while one of the two risk factors portends a 16% risk of relapse (31). Because of excellent outcomes of patients later treated for recurrent disease, active surveillance is still considered a reasonable option in patients with both risk factors.

Radiotherapy

Delivery of 20 Gy to the para-aortics alone is a standard management strategy for clinical stage I seminoma. The radiation field to the para-aortics is defined as a 10-cm-wide field between T12 and L5. This current standard is based on data from two trials. The first, by Jones et al., randomly assigned patients to either 20 Gy in 10 fractions over 2 weeks or 30 Gy in 15 fractions over 3 weeks. Patients receiving the 30-Gy dose reported more symptoms at 4 weeks (no difference at 12 weeks), with no evidence for decreased relapse rate at median follow-up of 61 months (32). Fossa et al. reported their experience with 478 patients with stage I disease randomly assigned to receive radiation to both the para-aortic and ipsilateral iliac fields versus the para-aortic field alone. Those treated with reduced fields had 3-year survival of 99.3% versus 100% with the extended field. This minimal loss of treatment efficacy was accompanied by a reduction in both gastrointestinal side effects and infertility risk. A determination of the risk of secondary malignancies was not yet assessable, but it is presumed to be reduced in the face of the decreased size of radiation portals (33).

Chemotherapy

Recently, data have been reported from a randomized comparison of single-agent carboplatin dose based on AUC 7 versus radiotherapy for the adjuvant treatment of clinical stage I seminoma (34). Median follow-up was 4 years, and the relapse-free survival was similar in both groups, 96.7% and 97.7%, respectively, showing non-inferiority of the one-cycle, single-agent carboplatin strategy. This treatment approach is a valuable option for patients who cannot tolerate or have contraindications to radiation therapy. There are no data currently comparing

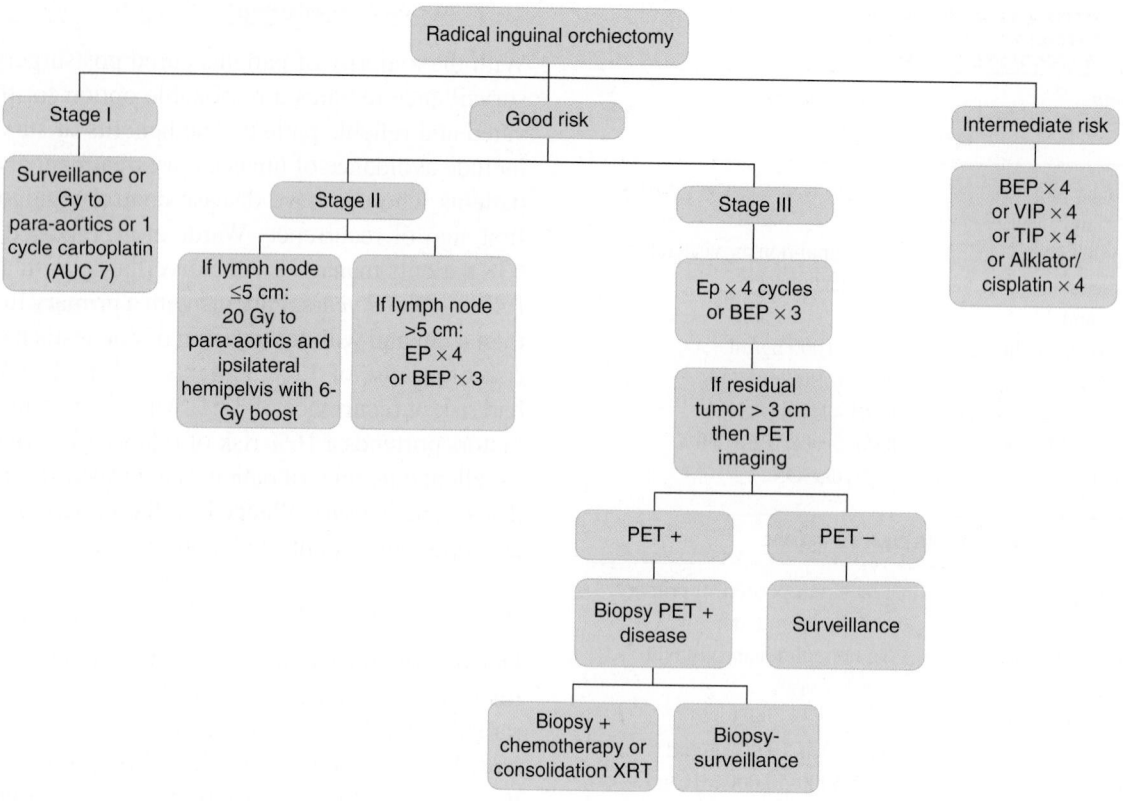

FIGURE 36-3. Management of testicular cancer (seminoma).

the long-term safety of this strategy or sufficient evidence to comment on any risk of secondary malignancy. Figure 36-3 outlines our approach to therapy for stage I seminoma.

MANAGEMENT OF NONBULKY, GOOD-RISK SEMINOMA (STAGES IIA/IIB)

Patients with stage II seminoma are often divided into nonbulky versus bulky disease for treatment discussion. In general, nonbulky disease is defined as nodes less than 5 cm in the CT or MRI. The primary mode of therapy for patients in this category is radiotherapy unless the patient has contraindication or is unable to tolerate radiation treatment.

Radiotherapy

It is no longer recommended that stages IIA and IIB seminoma patients receive high-dose radiation (30-35 Gy), mediastinal radiation, or left supraclavicular radiation. The current recommendation is for radiotherapy to a dose of 20 Gy to the para-aortic and ipsilateral iliac nodal fields with a 6-Gy boost to the para-aortic lymph nodes (35). Occasionally, radiographic evidence for residual disease

is present postradiotherapy, but if the abnormality is less than 3 cm, observation is recommended.

Alternatives to Radiotherapy

There is a subset of patients who will not be able to receive radiation therapy for various reasons. These reasons may include patient refusal, inflammatory bowel disease, horseshoe or pelvic kidney, and history of abdominal surgery. In this setting, systemic chemotherapy could be offered. In a series published by Xiao et al. (36), good-prognosis seminoma patients were included in the analysis and were treated with four cycles of etoposide and cisplatin (EP). Although this does not represent the standard of care for stages IIA and IIB seminoma, it is a reasonable alternative for patients who absolutely cannot receive radiation therapy.

MANAGEMENT OF ADVANCED, GOOD-RISK SEMINOMA (STAGES IIC/III)

This treatment group includes stage II patients with bulky lymphadenopathy (>5 cm) and stage III patients with good-risk disease. In this group of patients, the risk of recurrence remains high despite local therapy and therefore the primary treatment recommendation is systemic chemotherapy. It is also in this category of patients that the role of positron emission tomography (PET) scan may be introduced in its limited role for GCTs.

Chemotherapy

The recommended systemic chemotherapy regimen for patients with good-risk advanced seminoma (stages IIC or IIIA) is three cycles of bleomycin, etoposide, and cisplatin (BEP). The evidence for use of three cycles of BEP versus four cycles was presented by de Wit et al. (37,38). These investigators showed that three cycles of BEP is equivalent to four cycles, with 2-year progression-free survival (PFS) of 90.4% and 89.4%, respectively (39). Alternatively, patients who are unable or refuse to receive bleomycin or are older than 50 years can be successfully treated with four cycles of EP.

Residual Disease After Chemotherapy and the Role of PET

After completion of chemotherapy, restaging CT scans are performed. If a patient is found to have no residual disease or residual disease measuring less than 3 cm in size with normal tumor markers, active surveillance should be pursued. Postchemotherapy, residual disease measuring greater than 3 cm can be further evaluated by PET imaging. Evidence for the role of PET imaging in the setting of residual disease greater than 3 cm was presented by De Santis et al. (40). In this evaluation of 33 patients with follow-up time of 23 months, the positive predictive value of FDG PET was 100%, with a specificity and sensitivity of 100% and 89%, respectively, for the identification of residual disease in lesions more than 3 cm. Although encouraging, the role of PET imaging in this setting is being reexamined, because several false-positive cases from our institution have been recently identified.

PET-Negative Disease Postchemotherapy

If there is no evidence of avid uptake on PET, the patient enters the active surveillance strategy. If the patient is unable to have PET imaging, surgical biopsy or consolidative radiation therapy can be considered for those patients with residual disease measuring greater than 3 cm.

PET-Positive Disease Postchemotherapy

At MD Anderson, a positive PET scan requires a confirmatory biopsy. If residual disease is confirmed, several options can be considered. First, salvage radiation therapy

to the residual mass can be offered, but this does not provide long-term control. Second, the patient can be offered salvage chemotherapy. Finally, the patient may undergo high-dose chemotherapy with autologous stem cell transplantation. See Figure 36-3 for the algorithm of our management strategy.

MANAGEMENT OF ADVANCED, INTERMEDIATE-RISK SEMINOMA

Patients with advanced, intermediate-risk seminoma have nonpulmonary visceral metastasis. The most common sites of disease are the liver and bone. These rare patients are offered systemic chemotherapy upon presentation (see figure 36-3). The chemotherapy regimens commonly used are four cycles of BEP, four cycles of etoposide, ifosfamide, cisplatin (VIP), or four cycles of paclitaxel, ifosfamide, cisplatin (TIP) (41).

CASE 36-1: Seminoma Presenting With Renal Insufficiency

A 37-year-old man had a left inguinal orchiectomy for classic seminoma. Laboratory data at presentation to MDACC revealed serum creatinine of 1.8 mg/dL, calcium 12.7 mg/dL, Hgb 10.5 g/dL, hCG 113 mIU/mL, Alk phos 194 IU/L, and LDH 1773 IU/L (ULN 618). A CT scan of abdomen and pelvis revealed a large retroperitoneal mass with marked left hydronephrosis (Fig 36-4A). The patient received initially one cycle of cyclophosphamide and carboplatinum. Repeat laboratory data revealed serum creatinine of 1.1 mg/dL, calcium 8.2 mg/dL, LDH 483 IU/L, and undetectable hCG. He subsequently received three full cycles of EP with excellent response. Repeat imaging shown in Fig 36-4B revealed marked improvement in the size of the mass (from 14-7 cm). Postchemotherapy PET imaging showed the residual mass to be metabolically inactive.

Comment: A patient with advanced seminoma presenting with hydronephrosis and renal insufficiency may receive induction chemotherapy with cyclophosphamide and carboplatinum rather than placing nephrostomy tubes to allow administration of BEP or EP in the first cycle. The patient can subsequently receive standard therapy after normalization of renal function.

SALVAGE THERAPY FOR REFRACTORY/RECURRENT SEMINOMA

The primary treatment of recurrent seminoma is salvage chemotherapy. For patients with lung metastasis (good-risk category), the standard of care is administration of either three cycles of BEP or four cycles of EP. In

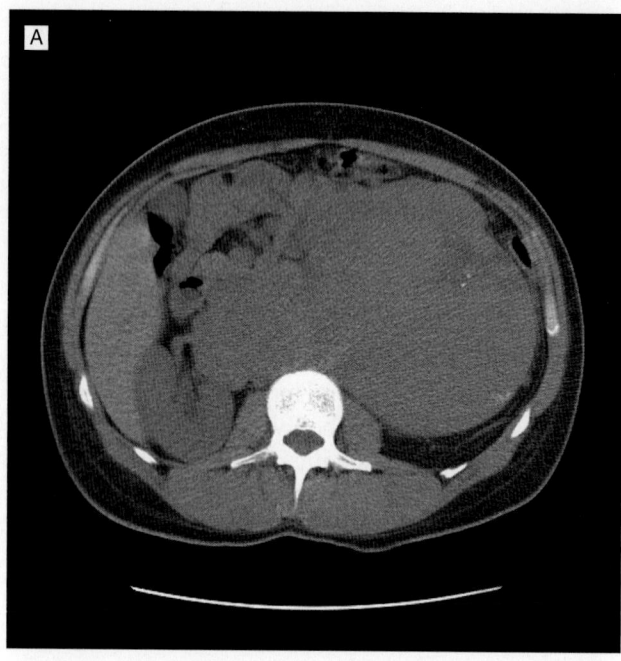

FIGURE 36-4A. Baseline imaging from case 36-1 showing a large left retroperitoneal mass with left hydronephosis.

patients with bone or liver metastasis (intermediate-risk category), salvage chemotherapy is pursued with either four cycles of BEP, TIP, or VIP. Bleomycin should be avoided in men older than 50 years.

Clinical signs of refractory disease should be approached with an aggressive change of strategy,

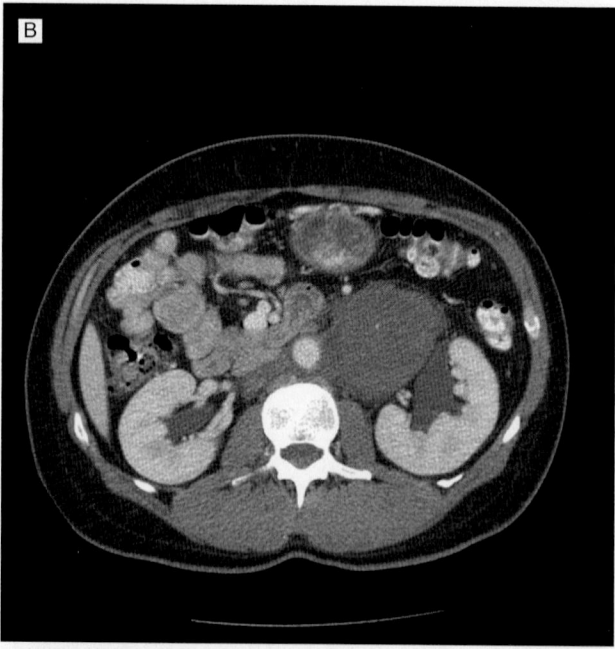

FIGURE 36-4B. Repeat imaging from patient in case 36-1 showing marked improvement in mass after 3 cycles of chemotherapy.

including the option of high-dose chemotherapy and stem cell transplantation. Usually reserved for BEP failures and recurrent disease, the role of stem cell transplantation in refractory/recurrent advanced seminoma was addressed by Einhorn et al. (42). Nineteen percent of a series of 184 patients were patients with metastatic testicular seminoma. At a median follow-up of 48 months, 26 of 35 seminoma patients treated were in complete remission. Patients in this category should be considered for referral to transplant centers if possible.

■ NONSEMINOMATOUS GERM CELL TUMORS

HISTOLOGY

Embryonal Carcinoma

Embryonal carcinoma is the second most common pure presentation of GCT. It is rarely seen at the extremes of age, most commonly presenting in the 20- to 30-year age group and presents with metastasis in one-third of cases. Microscopically, embryonal carcinoma cells are the most undifferentiated of the GCT types and are characterized by microscopically varied cells with indistinct borders and scant cytoplasm, giving the appearance of overlapping nuclei. Tumor cells can be seen in sheets or arranged as papillary or tubular structures with a high mitotic rate. There is a propensity for vascular invasion. Phenotypic characterization can reveal positivity for cytokeratin, CD30, PLAP, AFP, and hCG. Modest elevations of both AFP and hCG are typical, but importantly, pure embryonal cancers can be marker-negative in the serum. Figure 36-5 shows the typical histologic appearance of embryonal carcinoma.

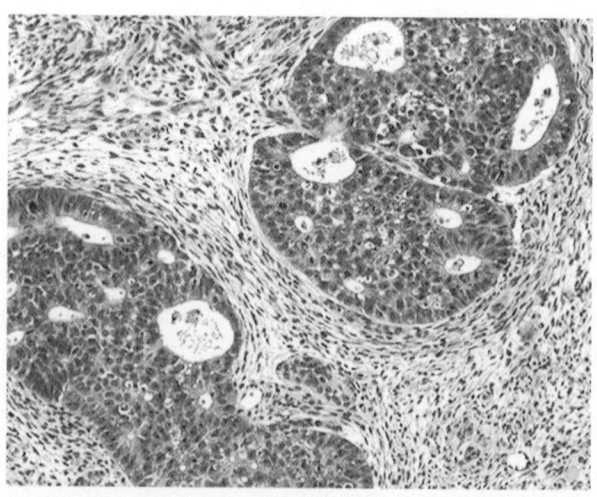

FIGURE 36-5. Histological appearance of embryonal carcinoma.

Endodermal Sinus Tumors (or Yolk Sac Tumors)

Pure yolk sac tumors are extremely rare in the adult patient but account for the majority of childhood GCTs. In adults, endodermal sinus tumor (EST) or yolk sac elements are commonly seen as a component of mixed NSGCTs. Microscopically, EST can manifest as macrocystic, papillary, solid, or a glandular/alveolar pattern with perivascular arrangements of epithelial cells known as glomeruloid or Schiller-Duval bodies. High AFP levels generally reflect an EST component, and serum levels of AFP are important prognostically in the classification of good-, intermediate-, and poor-risk metastatic NSGCTs. Figure 36-6 shows the typical histological appearance of an EST carcinoma.

Choriocarcinoma

Also rare in the pure form in the adult population, choriocarcinoma frequently presents as a component of NSGCTs. Choriocarcinomas comprise both syncytiotrophoblasts and cytotrophoblasts, typically arranged in sheets or nests. Choriocarcinomas generally make copious amounts of hCG, and the level of this marker is also an indication of prognosis in metastatic NSGCTs. Half of choriocarcinomas are PLAP positive. Choriocarcinoma elements tend to dominate the clinical course and frequently metastasize to the brain. Figure 36-7 shows the typical histological appearance of choriocarcinoma.

Teratoma

Teratomas possess somatic cells from at least two germ cell layers (ectoderm, endoderm, and mesoderm).

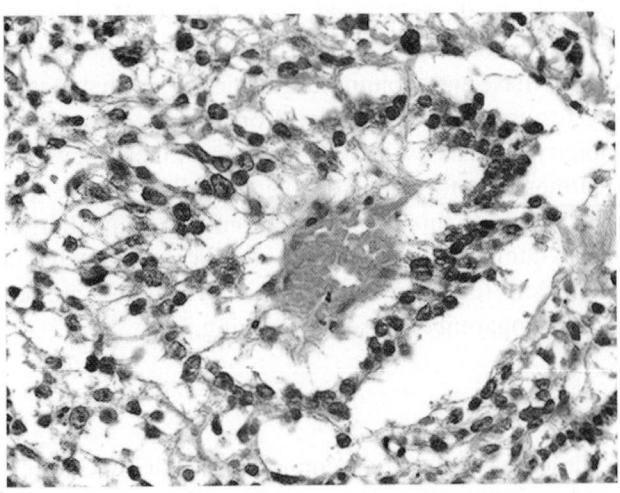

FIGURE 36-6. Histological appearance of EST carcinoma.

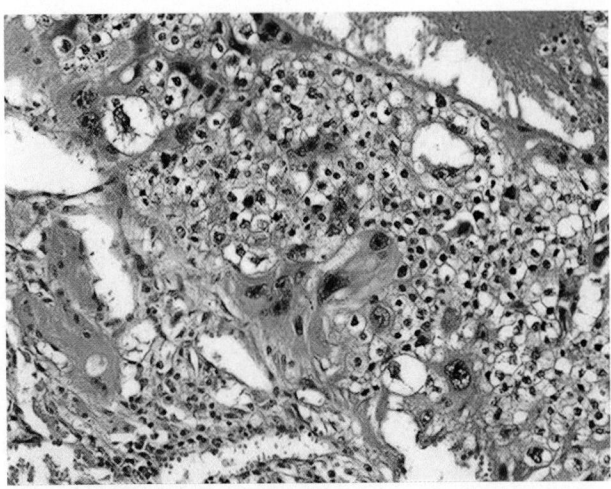

FIGURE 36-7. Histological appearance of choriocarcinoma.

Variable degrees of differentiation allow for the subclassification of mature and immature forms. Mature teratoma consists of terminally differentiated tissues and can form cystic structures. Although histologically bland, this low-grade malignancy can grow to a threatening dimension and become unresectable. Only about 2 to 3% of all GCTs show mature teratoma as the only histologic component, but teratoma is commonly present as an element of a mixed GCT. Immature teratoma is less differentiated and displays a correspondingly more aggressive biology. One of the unfortunate manifestations is the development of non-GCT within the teratoma. Known as teratoma with malignant transformation, this entity typically displays the biology of whatever histology develops and can range from leukemias to sarcomas to carcinomas. In general, such a transformation belies a poor prognosis (43). Figures 36-8 and 36-9 represent the typical histological and gross appearance of teratoma, respectively.

CLINICAL FEATURES

As described previously, approximately half of testicular GCTs show histologic elements other than seminoma or produce serum elevation of AFP indicating nonseminoma. These cancers are collectively known as mixed GCTs or NSGCTs, and they form a group of histologically and clinically diverse cancers (44). NSGCTs are more likely to spread hematogenously with increased risk of distant metastasis when compared to seminomas. Because of the unique and heterogeneous nature of NSGCTs, there are several clinical presentations which warrant further discussion, because of their significance to patient care and prognosis.

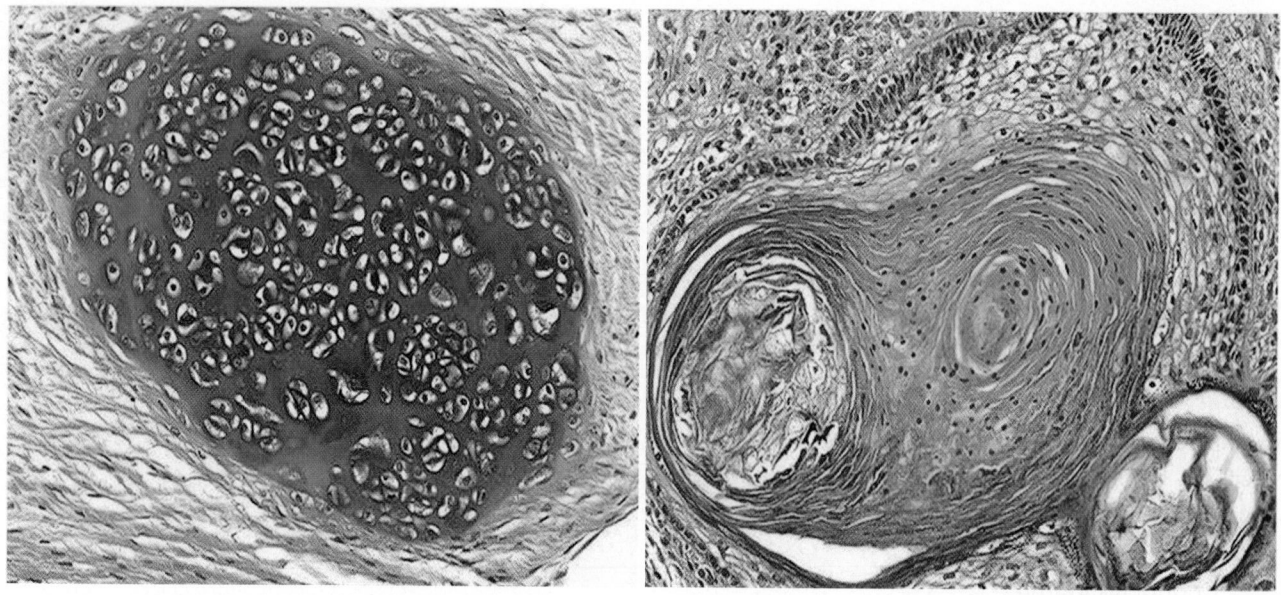

FIGURE 36-8. Histological appearance of teratoma.

Growing Teratoma Syndrome

Residual teratoma is a low-grade, slow-growing malignancy that can be fatal by inexorable growth. This can take 10 or even 20 years to become threatening and thus can be missed without dedicated lifelong follow-up of patients with NSGCTs. One of the most remarkable and clinically important features of teratomas is that they are often "pushing," and rarely invasive. Thus at surgery, even very large masses are sometimes removed far more easily than would be expected on the basis of the preoperative imaging. It is important to consult a center where sufficient surgical experience is available before concluding that a residual teratoma is "unresectable" (45).

Choriocarcinoma Syndrome

As the name implies, this is seen in the setting of high-volume NSGCT that shows predominantly choriocarcinoma histology and is associated with very high (typically about 1,000,000 U/L) levels of β-hCG. This syndrome is characterized by prominent constitutional symptoms that represent the effects of both a bulky cancer, and secondary hyperthyroidism caused by cross-reaction of hCG with TSH receptors. Typically, patients are rapidly losing weight, tachycardic, anxious, diaphoretic, and have tender, swollen breasts from secondary hyperprolactinemia. In addition, most patients have high-volume lung metastases with impending respiratory compromise from the burden of pulmonary metastasis. This is a medical emergency, and treatment should not be delayed for histologic confirmation, since this is a pathognomonic constellation in a young man. Metastatic choriocarcinoma has a propensity for brain metastasis, although they are not always apparent on baseline imaging.

PROGNOSIS

As described above with seminoma, the IGCCCG developed a prognostic staging system for NSGCTs with non-pulmonary visceral metastasis found as a major factor in

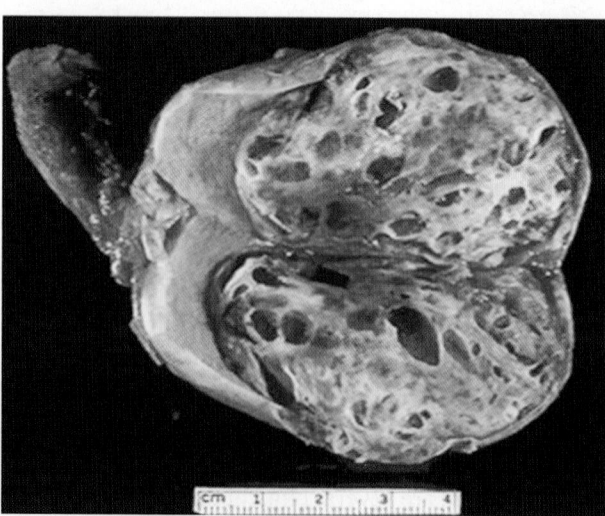

FIGURE 36-9. Gross appearance of teratoma.

prognosis. Unlike seminoma, prechemotherapy tumor markers were identified as significant in the prognosis of these patients. The prognostic categories are outlined in Table 36-2. In general, patients with mediastinal primary, nonpulmonary visceral metastasis and "poor markers" as defined in the figure are considered to have poor prognosis and have a 5-year OS of 48%. Patients with testis or retroperitoneal primary, no nonpulmonary visceral metastasis are placed in the good prognosis category based on tumor marker levels as described in the figure. Good-prognosis patients have a 5-year OS of 92%. All others are placed in the intermediate-risk group and have a 5-year OS of 80% (2). Van Dijk et al. (3) updated the 5-year OS data for NSGCTs in a pooled meta-analysis. The authors reported 5-year OS of 94% for good-prognosis, 83% for intermediate-prognosis, and 71% for poor prognosis. This illustrates the improving survival rates in the high-risk group.

MANAGEMENT OF CLINICAL STAGE I NSGCT

In general, clinical stage I NSGCT includes patients with normal markers postorchiectomy and no evidence of disease outside the resected testis, epididymis, or cord. As with seminoma, radical inguinal orchiectomy is the initial therapy for early-stage NSGCT. Appropriate surgery will cure approximately 70% of clinical stage I patients. The two identified risk factors in these patients include percentage of embryonal histology and lymphovascular invasion (LVI), with LVI the most predictive (46). Patients are considered low-risk for recurrence postorchiectomy, if there is less than 50% embryonal component in the tumor and no evidence of LVI. The role of percentage of embryonal component is debatable. In fact, European guidelines utilize only absence of LVI for determination of "low-risk" for recommendation of observation (47).

Observation

Observation is a reasonable strategy for the reliable, low-risk patient, which in practice can be those with absence of LVI. The active surveillance schedule as outlined by the National Comprehensive Cancer Network (NCCN) Clinical Practice Guidelines in Oncology recommends that patients should have a physical examination, chest radiography, and tumor marker measurements every month during the first year, every 2 months during the second year, and every third month during the third year. Abdominal and pelvic CT is recommended approximately every 3 months during the first year and every 4 months for years 2 and 3 (48).

Retroperitoneal Lymph Node Dissection

Retroperitoneal lymph node dissection (RPLND) is a surgical removal of the "landing zone" lymph nodes. An accurate staging strategy, its role in primary prevention of recurrence in stage I NSGCT patients is controversial. Morbidity of RPLND includes sympathetic nerve damage that may lead to failure of ejaculation and infertility; however, use of a modified surgical template is a nerve-sparing approach that can preserve the sympathetic nerves and may facilitate antegrade ejaculation in 90% or more patients. Stephenson et al. (49) reported that RPLND in clinical stage I patients yielded a 4-year progression-free probability of 96% and is an option for therapy in this patient population. Higher failure rates have been reported for patients with high-risk clinical stage I NSGCT. Patients who do not undergo prophylactic RPLND must undergo periodic CT scanning of the abdomen to rule out growing teratoma in the retroperitoneum.

Chemotherapy

In the past, adjuvant chemotherapy for stage I NSGCT patients with high risk of recurrence consisted of two cycles of BEP. Recently, two randomized trials evaluated the impact of one cycle of BEP. Albers et al. (50) compared RPLND to one cycle of BEP in 382 patients with a median follow-up of 4.7 years. The 2-year recurrence-free survival was 99.46% in the chemotherapy group and 91.87% in the RPLND group, suggesting an advantage of one cycle of BEP chemotherapy, although this finding did not reach statistical significance. Tandstad et al. (51), in the SWENOTECA study, confirmed these findings in 745 patients who were prospectively randomized based on the presence of LVI. These investigators reported that one cycle of BEP reduced the risk of recurrence by 90% in patients with or without LVI. Our algorithm for management of non-seminoma testicular cancer is shown in Figure 36-10.

MANAGEMENT OF GOOD-RISK CLINICAL STAGES IIA AND IIB NSGCT

Patients with tumor marker negative, stages IIA or IIB NSGCTs present a unique clinical situation. At our institution, these patients are divided into groups by CT evidence of disease greater than or less than 3 cm. If patients have negative tumor markers with a retroperitoneal mass less than 3 cm after orchiectomy, surgical biopsy is pursued. If negative, then observation is a reasonable alternative for the reliable patient. Patients with larger than 3 cm disease, positive tumor markers, or positive biopsy are treated with primary chemotherapy with BEP for three cycles. As discussed, several groups have reported long-term follow-up data confirming the

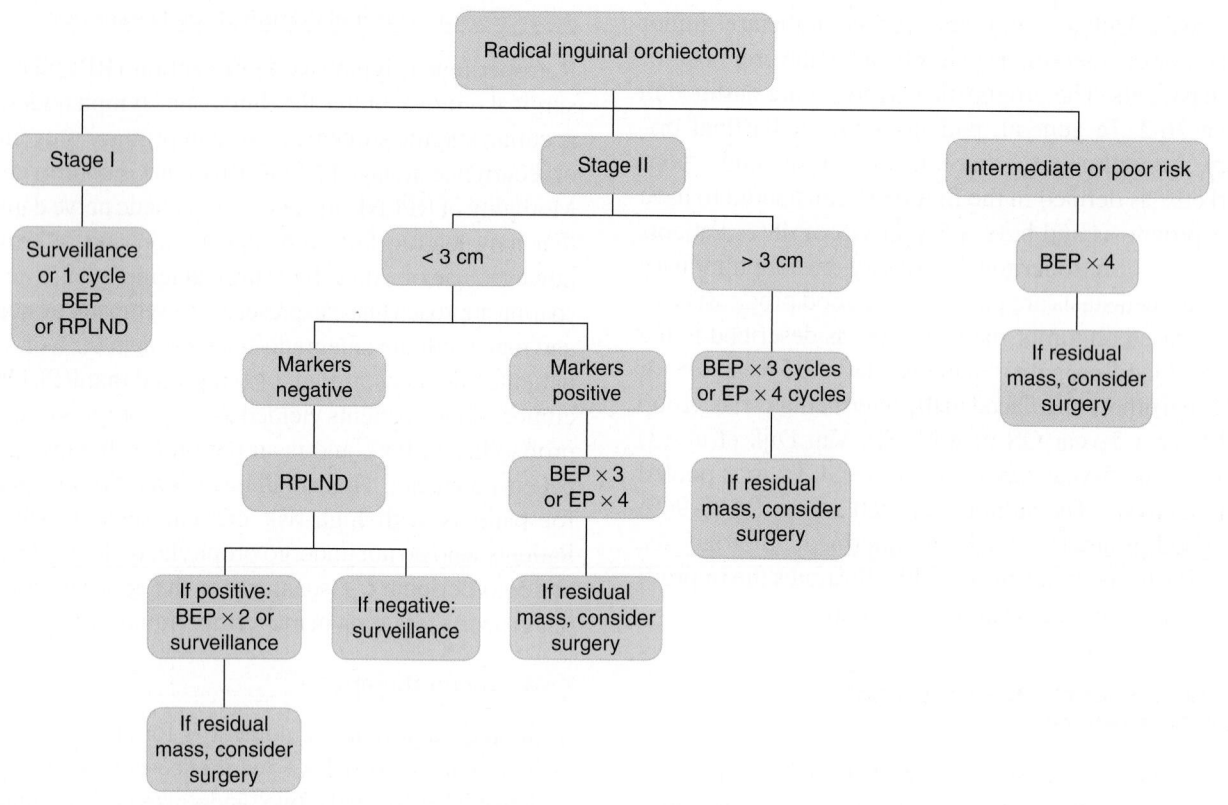

FIGURE 36-10. Management of testicular cancer (nonseminoma).

equivalence of three cycles when compared to four cycles of BEP (37,38). As previously recommended, four cycles of EP is also a reasonable alternative in patients who refuse or have a contraindication to receive bleomycin (39). If residual tumor is detected on follow-up staging, surgical resection is recommended.

MANAGEMENT OF GOOD-RISK STAGES IIC AND III NSGCT

Patients with bulky retroperitoneal disease of greater than 5 cm or pulmonary metastasis, with relatively low serum markers constitute those with advanced disease, but still with favorable prognosis. These patients may be either stage IIC or IIIA according to the AJCC criteria and are considered together in this discussion. The primary mode of treatment in this patient population is systemic chemotherapy. This may be administered before or after radical orchiectomy as long as surgical resection of the primary is performed after completion of therapy. Once again, three cycles of BEP chemotherapy is considered standard of care and four cycles of EP considered a reasonable alternative for patients with a contraindication to receive bleomycin. Resection of residual disease present on restaging should be performed (37-39).

Pathology of the resected tumor after salvage chemotherapy is different than after primary chemotherapy.

Following primary chemotherapy, viable GCT, fibrosis, or teratoma are found in approximately 20%, 40%, and 40% of pathological specimens, respectively, compared to 50%, 10%, and 40% following salvage chemotherapy, respectively. Patients with greater than 10% viable GCT in the residual pathology specimen after primary chemotherapy should receive additional two cycles of platinum-based chemotherapy (Figure 36-10).

MANAGEMENT OF INTERMEDIATE- AND POOR-RISK ADVANCED-STAGES IIIB AND IIIC NSGCT

Patients with advanced NSGCTs who present with intermediate- or poor-risk features are managed with systemic chemotherapy consisting of four cycles of BEP. This may be given prior to radical orchiectomy. For advanced-, intermediate- or poor-risk patients with a contraindication to receive bleomycin, VIP, or TIP is recommended (52). These patients should also be considered for participation in clinical trials.

MANAGEMENT OF RECURRENT AND REFRACTORY NSGCT

Several chemotherapy regimens with clinical activity in the salvage setting have been reported, and these include VIP, TIP, VeIP (vinblastine, ifosfamide, cisplatin), IPO (irinotecan, paclitaxel, oxaliplatin), or gemcitabine/oxaliplatin. In general, many patients respond and some are even cured with salvage chemotherapy and surgical consolidation, especially those with a small or moderate volume of disease. There has been some suggestion that rotation of chemotherapy regimens may offer some benefit. We are currently evaluating our own experience with this treatment strategy.

The strategy most supported by recent data is the role of high-dose induction chemotherapy with stem cell transplantation. Einhorn et al. (42) retrospectively reviewed 184 patients (149 patients with advanced NSGCT) with a median follow-up of 48 months. Ninety of the 149 patients with NSGCT treated with high-dose chemotherapy and subsequent autologous stem cell transplantation were disease free at follow-up. The authors suggest that use of this aggressive treatment as second-line therapy is distinctly advantageous when compared to patients who receive this treatment in the third-line setting. Based on this study and despite the absence of a randomized trial, patients with recurrent or refractory advanced-stage NSGCT may be considered for this aggressive, yet effective, treatment strategy.

CASE 36-2: BEP/TIP Failure

A 24-year-old man presented with lower back pain, anorexia, night sweats, and weight loss. Imaging studies revealed extensive retroperitoneal lymphadenopathy, a right testicular mass, and bilateral lung nodules. Tumor markers were hCG 33,261, AFP 4.1, and LDH 1847. A fine-needle aspiration of the retroperitoneal mass revealed embryonal carcinoma. BEP chemotherapy was initiated. The kinetics of decline of serum hCG levels are shown below for the first three out of four planned cycles:

- s/p cycle 1: 1507
- s/p cycle 2: 279
- s/p cycle 3: 323

Salvage chemotherapy is commenced after the third cycle of BEP. The patient received four cycles of TIP, with decrease in adenopathy and decline of serum hCG to undetectable. The patient was then referred for RPLND and right radical orchiectomy. Pathology revealed no viable tumor. Two months postoperatively, serum hCG rose to 161. He received one cycle of irinotecan, paclitaxel, and oxaliplatin with tumor marker normalization. He then underwent tandem peripheral blood stem cell transplantation (SCT) with high-dose ICE. He remains disease free 3.5 years later.

Comments: For symptomatic patients with intermediate- or poor-risk GCTs, chemotherapy can be initiated before orchiectomy. Rising tumor markers during BEP chemotherapy signal BEP failure and dictate change of therapy. The best results are achieved with high-dose chemotherapy and SCT.

SPECIAL CONSIDERATIONS

Pitfalls in Tumor Marker Elevation

Mild elevation of β-hCG (usually <20) may occur secondary to hypogonadism or marijuana use, and therefore, should not always be attributed to residual or recurrent tumor. Modest elevation of AFP may be present with residual teratoma and will normalize following surgical resection, but may also be constitutionally elevated or indicate presence of liver disease. Additionally, elevated tumor markers may indicate unidentified CNS disease or residual primary testicular tumor.

CASE 36-3: The Challenge of Managing Intercurrent Illness

A 35-year-old heavy smoker and marijuana user man underwent a left orchiectomy for a 3.5-cm mixed NSGCT and presented 2 months later to MDACC with left groin pain and left thigh numbness. Tumor markers were AFP 6575, hCG 1059, and LDH 2441. CT scans revealed bilateral lung nodules, a large (14.7 cm) retroperitoneal mass, left hydronephrosis, and multiple other enlarged abdominal and pelvic lymph nodes. During the first BEP chemotherapy cycle, he suffered an inferior myocardial infarction (MI) secondary to an occluding atherosclerotic plaque in the right coronary artery. After coronary stenting and optimal medical therapy, the patient was able to complete four cycles of BEP on schedule and at full dose, without delay or significant complications, except for moderate peripheral neuropathy. His tumor markers declined as follows:

- s/p cycle 1   AFP = 3853 hCG = 34.7
- s/p cycle 2   AFP = 542 hCG = 5.2
- s/p cycle 3   AFP = 88.1 hCG = 4.6
- s/p cycle 4   AFP = 42 hCG = 4.7

The patient received intramuscular testosterone injection for low serum testosterone level, and 3 weeks later serum hCG was <1.0. Six months after his MI, the patient had resection of the large left retroperitoneal mass, the left kidney and left adrenal gland, RPLND, and segmental resection of the left psoas muscle. Pathology of the specimen revealed 98% necrosis and only two microscopic foci of residual viable EST in transition to adenocarcinoma. The patient has been recurrence free for 3 years.

Comments: This case illustrates three points. The first is the importance of pursuing chemotherapy while managing an intercurrent illness. The second point is to remember that there are causes of elevated tumor markers other than tumor. The third point is that we do not treat foci of MTT.

Role of Desperation Surgery

There are patients with NSGCTs who have rising tumor markers, despite optimal systemic therapy. In these instances, surgery to resect all visible disease, a term we

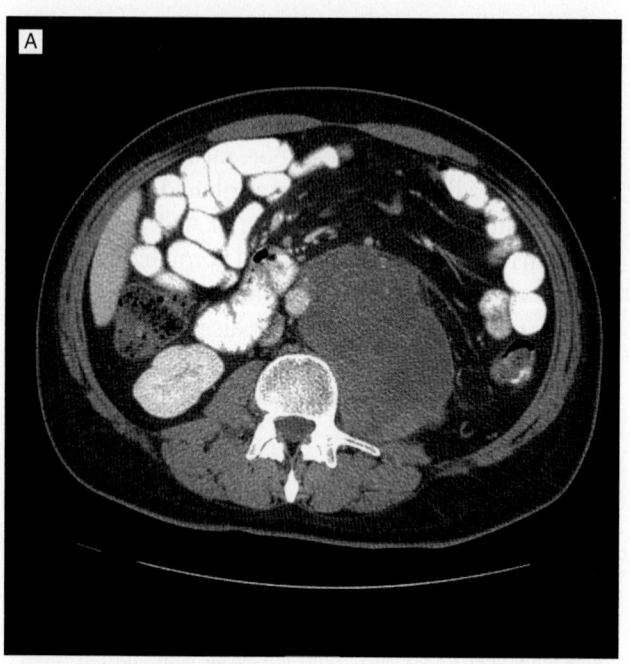

FIGURE 36-11A. Baseline imaging of patient described in case 36-4 with large retroperitoneal mass.

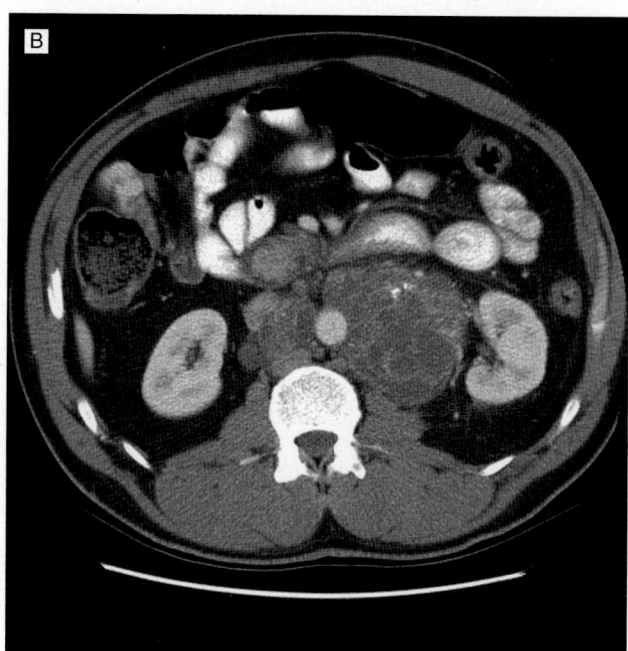

FIGURE 36-11B. Repeat imaging of patient in case 36-4 after six cycles of EP.

coin "desperation surgery" could be considered. It is estimated that up to 20% of patients who fit these criteria may be cured with surgical resection. Patients with isolated retroperitoneal lymph node disease, AFP-only elevation, and who undergo a complete resection of residual disease have the most favorable outcome. Referral to a center with high surgical expertise in this setting is recommended, as potentially large en bloc

resections may be required to achieve the desired outcome of complete resection.

Treatment of Late Relapse

Late relapse is defined as disease recurrence after 24 months from primary BEP chemotherapy. Teratoma and yolk sac are the most common histologies in this

---

CASE 36-4: Desperation Surgery

A 46-year-old man presented with back pain and was found to have an 11-cm retroperitoneal mass, biopsy of which revealed high-grade GCT (Figure 36-11A). He underwent a left radical orchiectomy for a 2.8-cm mixed GCT (99% seminoma, 1% teratoma). Postoperatively, serum AFP was greater than 10,000. He received six cycles of EP, followed by one cycle of VeIP but never achieved tumor marker normalization (Figure 36-11B). At presentation to MDACC, his serum AFP was 604. The patient received multiple additional cycles of rotating salvage chemotherapy, including actinomycin-D, cyclophosphamide, and etoposide (ACE); TIP, cisplatinum, vincristine, methotrexate, and bleomycin (POMB); doxorubicin, paclitaxel, and gemcitabine (ATG); and cisplatinum, cyclophosphamide, and doxorubicin (CisCa) (Figure 36-11C). The patient developed renal insufficiency, recalcitrant anemia,

and grade 3 peripheral neuropathy, and had transient normalization of serum tumor markers while awaiting surgical resection. At the time of surgery, serum AFP was 46.9. The patient underwent RPLND with excision of retroperitoneal masses, left radical nephrectomy, and excision of retrocrural lymph node masses. Pathology demonstrated metastatic mixed GCT, including areas of EST, mature teratoma, and focal areas suspicious for embryonal carcinoma and choriocarcinoma. He remains disease free past 5 years from the time of his salvage surgery.

  Comments: Four cycles of BEP and not EP is the standard for patients with intermediate- and poor-risk NSGCT. In rare cases, where the tumor markers do not normalize, even after exhausting all chemotherapeutic options, patients may be salvaged surgically. Patients who have primarily AFP elevation and EST or teratoma benefit the most from such an approach.

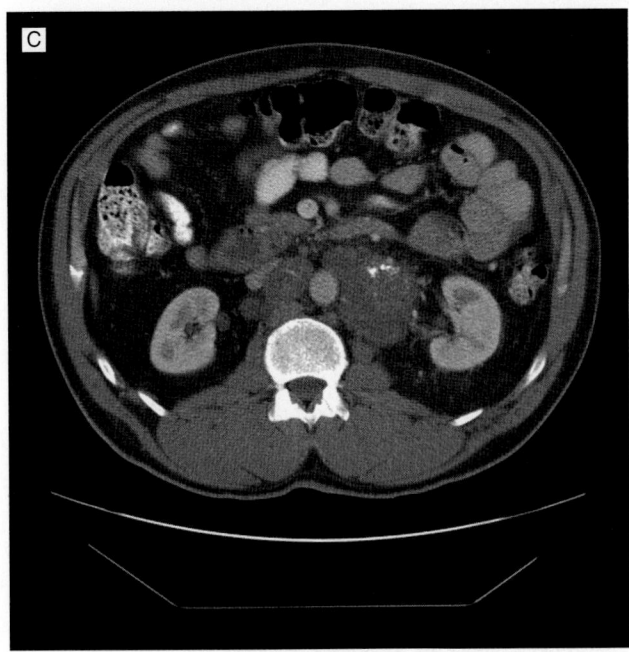

FIGURE 36-11C. Imaging of patient from case 36-4 showing residual disease despite multiple lines of salvage chemotherapy prior to desperation surgery.

setting, with pure teratoma conferring a better prognosis. Surgery is the preferred initial treatment in these cases, if the tumor is felt to be completely resectable.

Late Complications of Therapy

Although rare, there are specific complications associated with treatment of GCTs, which are especially important in this patient population, as curability may lead to a normal life expectancy. Secondary leukemias occur in fewer than 0.5% patients and are associated with use of etoposide. Bleomycin toxicity can appear early and is most associated with dose greater than 200 IU. Patients may also have increased risk of vascular side effects, including Raynaud syndrome and hypertension. Up to 25% of patients may develop the metabolic syndrome. Additional complications include renal insufficiency, chronic peripheral neuropathy, chronic electrolyte abnormalities, and neuropsychiatric abnormalities.

■ EXTRAGONADAL GERM CELL TUMORS

Patients with seminomas arising in the mediastinum have similar prognosis to patients with testicular seminomas and are treated with four cycles of EP at our institution, if they do not have nonpulmonary visceral metastasis. Nonseminomatous extragonadal GCTs represent a distinct subset of GCTs and carry a poorer prognosis than primary testicular NSGCTs. The most common origin is the mediastinum, but they can also arise in the retroperitoneum or pineal region. Rare cases involve the vagina, prostate, liver, and orbit.

Mediastinal EGCTs appear as large anterior masses on radiographs. This subset is characterized by prominence of EST and teratoma histology, compared to primary testicular GCTs (53). Initial diagnosis may be aided by elevations of AFP or hCG. Klinefelter syndrome is associated with increased risk of primary nonseminomatous mediastinal GCTs (54). Additional associations include acute megakaryoblastic leukemia, acute myeloid leukemia, myelodysplastic syndrome, and malignant histiocytosis. Some of these cases represent malignant transformation of immature teratoma elements.

Nonseminomatous GCTs are classified as high-risk GCTs (2), and data suggest that long-term survival is as low as 20% (55-57). The aggressive nature of this entity is coupled by the surgical difficulty of resection of residual disease after therapy. Early diagnosis and aggressive resection of mediastinal NSGCTs may improve the outcome. At our institution, the treatment strategy for this rare entity includes presurgical chemotherapy to optimum response and then consolidation surgery.

CASE 36-5: GST With Occult Primary

A 29-year-old man presented with weight loss and left supraclavicular lymphadenopathy (see Figure 36-12), but had a negative testicular examination and ultrasound. Imaging studies confirmed a 5-cm left supraclavicular lymph node and showed a small left pleural effusion. A biopsy of the supraclavicular lymph node demonstrated poorly differentiated adenocarcinoma. Embryonal carcinoma could not be excluded. Immunostains for PLAP and Ki-1 were positive but were negative for AFP and inconclusive for hCG. Laboratory evaluation revealed azoospermia but normal serum chemistries and tumor markers. The patient was treated with three cycles of BEP and achieved a complete remission and is now disease free for 5 years without surgical consolidation (Figure 36-12B).

Comments: The case of unknown primary carcinoma in a young man, even if tumor markers are negative, should raise the diagnosis of GCT and should be treated as such. Surgical consolidation is not always necessary, when a clinical complete response is achieved with chemotherapy.

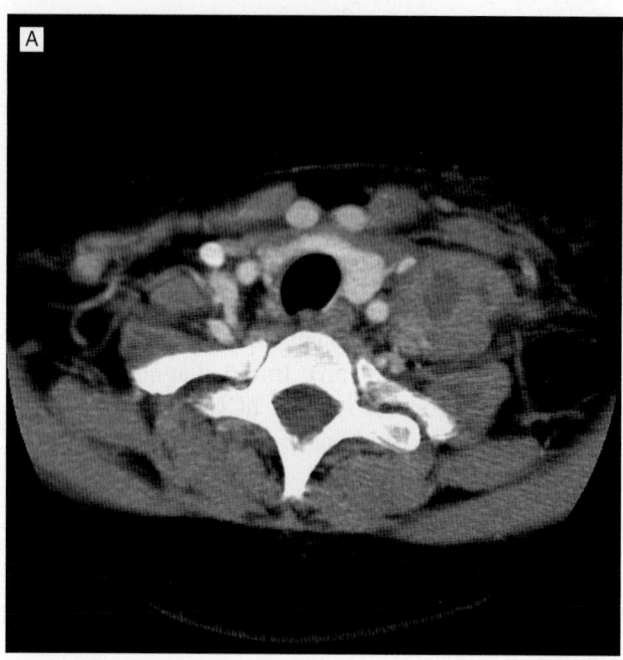

FIGURE 36-12A. Baseline imaging of patient described in Case 36-5 showing bulky left supraclavicular adenopathy..

■ CONCLUSION

GCTs represent the paradigm of curable solid tumors. Optimal management of these patients requires a multidisciplinary approach, integrating chemotherapy and surgery, to achieve the highest cure rates. Patients who

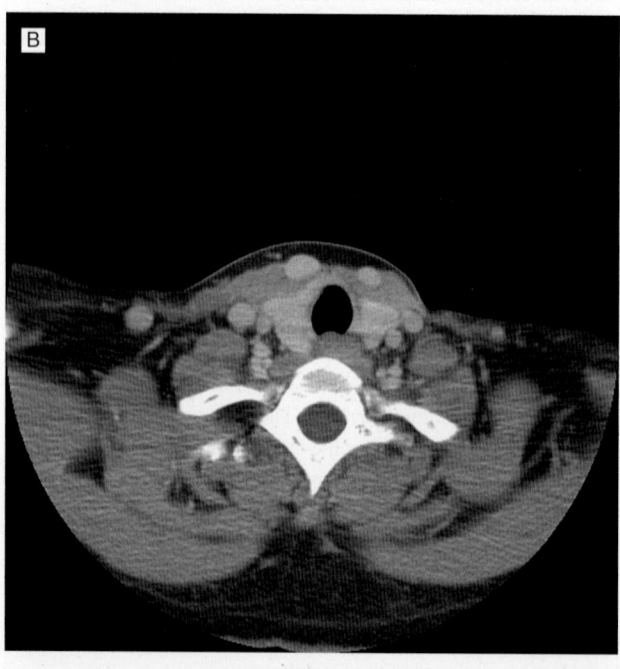

FIGURE 36-12B. Imaging after three cycles of chemotherapy.

pose a unique diagnostic or therapeutic challenge should be considered for early referral to a large tertiary care center.

REFERENCES

1. American Cancer Society. *Cancer Facts and Figures 2009.* Atlanta: American Cancer Society; 2009.
2. International Germ Cell Cancer Collaborative Group. International germ cell consensus classification: A prognostic factor-based staging system for metastatic germ cell cancers. *J Clin Onc* 1997;15:594-603.
3. Van Dijk MR, Steyerberg EW, Habbema DF. Survival of non-seminomatous germ cell cancer patients according to the IGC-CCG classification: An update based on meta-analysis. *Eur J Cancer* 2006;42:820-826.
4. Bray F, Ferlay J, Devesa SS, et al. Interpreting the international trends in testicular seminoma and nonseminoma incidence. *Nat Clin Pract Urol* 2006;3:532-543.
5. McGlynn KA, Devesa SS, Graubard BI, et al. Increasing incidence of testicular germ cell tumors among black men in the United States. *JCO* 2005;23:5757-5761.
6. McGlynn KA, Devesa SS, Sigurdson AJ, et al. Trends in the incidence of testicular germ cell tumors in the United States. *Cancer* 2003;97:63-70.
7. Dieckmann KP, Picjlmeier U. Clinical epidemiology of testicular germ cell tumors. *World J Urol* 2004;22:2-14.
8. Hanna N, Timmerman R, Foster R, et al. Testis cancer. In: Kufe D, Pollock R, Weichselbaum R, et al (eds): *Cancer Medicine.* Hamilton, Ontario: BC Decker; 2003:1747-1768.
9. Moller H, Cortes D, Engholm G, et al. Risk of testicular cancer with cryptorchidism and with testicular biopsy: Cohort study. *Br J Med* 1998;317:729-730.
10. Giwercman A, Brunn E, Frimodt-Moller C, et al. Prevalence of carcinoma in situ and other histopathologic abnormalities in testes of men with cryptorchidism. *J Urol* 1989;142:998-1001.
11. Dieckmann KP, Pichlmeier U. The prevalence of familial testicular cancer: An analysis of two patient populations and a review of the literature. *Cancer* 1997;80:1954-1960.
12. Travis LB, Curtis RE, Storm H, et al. Risk of second malignant neoplasms among long-term survivors of testicular cancer. *J Natl Cancer Inst* 1997;89:1429-1439.
13. Bosl GJ, Ilson DH, Rodriguez E, et al. Clinical relevance of the i(12p) marker chromosome in germ cell tumors. *J Natl Cancer Inst* 1994;86:349-355.
14. Atkin NB, Baker MC. Specific chromosome change i(12p) in testicular tumors. *Lancet* 1982;2:1349.
15. Rodriguez E, Matthew S, Reuter V, et al. Cytogenetic analysis of 124 prospectively ascertained germ cell tumors. *Cancer Res* 1992;52:2285-2291.
16. Sumersgill G, Goker H, Weber-Hall S, et al. Molecular cytogenetic analysis of adult testicular germ cell tumors and identification of regions of consensus copy number change. *Br J Cancer* 1998;77:305-313.
17. Kersemaekers A-MF, Mayer F, Molier M, et al. Role of p53 and MDM2 in treatment response of human germ cell tumors. *J Clin Oncol* 2002;20:1551-1561.
18. Korkola JE, Houldsworth J, Feldman DR, et al. Identification and validation of a gene expression signature that predicts outcome in adult men with germ cell tumors. *J Clin Oncol* 2009; 27:5240-5247.

19. Horie K, Fujita J, Takakura H, et al. The expression of c-kit protein in human adult and fetal tissues. *Hum Reprod* 1993; 8:1955-1962.

20. Hoei-Hanseni CE, Rajpert-De Meytsi E, Daugaard G, et al. Carcinoma in situ testis, the progenitor of testicular germ cell tumours: A clinical review. *Ann Oncol* 2005;16:863-868.

21. Braunstein GD. Gynecomastia. *N Engl J Med* 2007;357: 1229-1237.

22. Wehmann RE, Nisula BC. Metabolic and renal clearance rates of purified human chorionic gonadotropin. *J Clin Invest* 1981; 68:184-194.

23. Giralt SA, Dexeus F, Amato R, et al. Hyperthyroidism in men with germ cell tumors and high levels of beta-human chorionic gonadotropin. *Cancer* 1992;69:1286-1290.

24. Light PA. Tumour markers in testicular cancer. *J R Soc Med* 1985;78(Suppl 6):19-24.

25. Yuasa T, Yoshiki T, Ogawa O, et al. Detection of alpha-fetoprotein mRNA in seminoma. *J Androl* 1999;20:336-340.

26. Mencel PJ, Motzer RJ, Mazumdar M, et al. Advanced seminoma: Treatment results, survival, and prognostic factors in 142 patients. *J Clin Oncol* 1994;12:120-126.

27. Edge SB, Byrd DR, Compton CC, et al. *AJCC Cancer Staging Manual*, 6th ed. New York, Springer, 2009.

28. Jeruss JS, Woodruff TK. Preservation of fertility in patients with cancer. *N Engl J Med* 2009;360:902-911.

29. Nazeer T, Ro JY, Kee KH, et al. Spermatic cord contamination in testicular cancer. *Mod Pathol* 1996;9:762-766.

30. Chung PWM, Bayley AJS, Sweet J, et al. Spermatocytic seminoma: A review. *Eur Urol* 2004;45:495-498.

31. Warde P, Specht L, Horwich A, et al. Prognostic factors for relapse in stage I seminoma managed by surveillance: A pooled analysis. *J Clin Oncol* 2002;20:4448-4452.

32. Jones WG, Fossa SD, Mead GM, et al. Randomized trial of 30 versus 20 Gy in the adjuvant treatment of stage I testicular seminoma: A report on Medical Research Council Trial TE18, European Organisation for the Research and Treatment of Cancer Trial 30942. *J Clin Oncol* 2005;23:1200-1208.

33. Fosså SD, Horwich A, Russell JM, et al. Optimal planning target volume for stage I testicular seminoma: A Medical Research Council randomized trial. Medical Research Council Testicular Tumor Working Group. *J Clin Oncol* 1999; 17:1146.

34. Oliver RTD, Mason MD, Mead GM, et al. Radiotherapy versus single-dose carboplatin in adjuvant treatment of stage I seminoma: A randomized trial. *Lancet* 2005;366:293-300.

35. Classen J, Schmidberger H, Meisner C, et al. Radiotherapy for stages IIA/B testicular seminoma: Final report of a prospective multicenter clinical trial. *J Clin Oncol* 2003;21:1101-1106.

36. Xiao H, Mazumdar M, Bajorin D, et al. Long-term follow-up of patients with good-risk germ cell tumors treated with etoposide and cisplatin. *J Clin Oncol* 1997;15:2553-2558.

37. Saxman SB, Finch D, Gonin R, et al. Long-term follow-up of a phase III study of three versus four cycles of bleomycin, etoposide, and cisplatin in favorable-prognosis germ-cell tumors: The Indiana University Experience. *J Clin Oncol* 1998;16:702-706.

38. de Wit R, Roberts JT, Wilkinson PM, et al. Equivalence of three or four cycles of bleomycin, etoposide, and cisplatin chemotherapy and of a 3- or 5-day schedule in good-prognosis germ cell cancer: A randomized study of the European Organization for Research and Treatment of Cancer Genitourinary Tract Cancer Cooperative Group and the Medical Research Council. *J Clin Oncol* 2001;19:1629-1640.

39. Kondagunta GV, Bacik J, Bajorin D, et al. Etoposide and cisplatin chemotherapy for metastatic good-risk germ cell tumors. *J Clin Oncol* 2005;23:9290-9294.

40. De Santis M, Bokemeyer C, Becherer A, et al. Predictive Impact of 2-[18]Fluoro-2-Deoxy-D-Glucose positron emission tomography for residual postchemotherapy masses in patients with bulky seminoma. *J Clin Oncol* 2001;19:3740-3744.

41. Vuky J, Tickoo SK, Sheinfeld J, et al. Salvage chemotherapy for patients with advanced pure seminoma. *J Clin Oncol* 2002;20:297-301.

42. Einhorn LH, Williams SD, Chamness A, et al. High-dose chemotherapy and stem-cell rescue for metastatic germ-cell tumors. *N Engl J Med* 2007;357:340-348.

43. Spiess PE, Pisters LL, Liu P, et al. Malignant transformation of testicular teratoma: A chemoresistant phenotype. *Urol Oncol* 2008;26:595-599.

44. Bosl GJ, Geller N, Cirrincione C, et al. Interrelationships of histopathology and other clinical variables in patients with germ cell tumors of the testis. *Cancer* 1983;51:2121-2125.

45. Logothetis CJ, Samuels ML, Trindade A, et al. The growing teratoma syndrome. *Cancer* 1982;50:1629-1635.

46. Albers P, Siener R, Kliesch S, et al. Risk factors for relapse in clinical stage I nonseminomatous testicular germ cell tumors: Results of the German Testicular Cancer Study Group Trial. *J Clin Oncol* 2003;21:1505-1512.

47. Krege S, Beyer J, Souchon R, et al. European consensus conference on diagnosis and treatment of germ cell cancer: A report of the Second Meeting of the European Germ Cell Cancer Consensus group (EGCCCG): Part 1. *Eur Urol* 2008;53: 478-496.

48. Motzer RJ, Bolger GB, Boston B, et al. Testicular cancer: Clinical practice guidelines in oncology. *J Natl Compr Canc Netw* 2006;4:1038-1058.

49. Stephenson AJ, Bosl GJ, Motzer RJ, et al. Retroperitoneal lymph node dissection for nonseminomatous germ cell testicular cancer: Impact of patient selection factors on outcome. *J Clin Oncol* 2005;23:2781-2788.

50. Albers P, Siener R, Krege S, et al. Randomized phase III trial comparing retroperitoneal lymph node dissection with once course of bleomycin and etoposide plus cisplatin chemotherapy in the adjuvant treatment of clinical stage I nonseminomatous testicular germ cell tumors: AUO Trial AH 01/94 by the German Testicular Cancer Study Group. *J Clin Oncol* 2008; 26:2966-2972.

51. Tandstad T, Dahl O, Cohn-Cedermark G, et al. Risk-adapted treatment in clinical stage I nonseminomatous germ cell testicular cancer: The SWENOTECA Management Program. *J Clin Oncol* 2009;27:2122-2128.

52. Hinton S, Catalano PJ, Einhorn LH, et al. Cisplatin, etoposide and either bleomycin or ifosfamide in the treatment of disseminated germ cell tumors: Final analysis of an intergroup trial. *Cancer* 2003;97:1869-1875.

53. Moran CA, Suster S. Primary germ cell tumors of the mediastinum: I. Analysis of 322 cases with special emphasis on teratomatous lesions and a proposal for histopathologic classification and clinical staging. *Cancer* 1997;80:681-690.

54. Nichols CR, Heerema NA, Palmer C, et al. Klinefelter's syndrome associated with mediastinal germ cell neoplasms. *J Clin Oncol* 1987;5:1290-1294.

55. Logothetis CJ, Samuels ML, Selig DE, et al. Chemotherapy of extragonadal germ cell tumors. *J Clin Oncol* 1985;3: 316-325.

56. Toner GC, Geller NL, Lin SY, et al. Extragonadal and poor risk nonseminomatous germ cell tumors. Survival and prognostic features. *Cancer* 1991;67:2049-2057.

57. Moran CA, Suster S, Koss MN. Primary germ cell tumors of the mediastinum: III. Yolk sac tumor, embryonal carcinoma, choriocarcinoma, and combined nonteratomatous germ cell tumors of the mediastinum—a clinicopathologic and immunohistochemical study of 64 cases. *Cancer* 1997;80: 699-707.

Miscellaneous Tumors

TUMORS OF THE CENTRAL NERVOUS SYSTEM

Nicole A. Shonka
Sigmund H. Hsu
W.K. Alfred Yung
Commentary: Anita Mahajan, Sujit Prabhu

■ OVERVIEW

Brain tumors are a heterogeneous group of lesions that range from benign, slow-growing tumors found only incidentally on autopsy to malignant, rapidly growing tumors that cause death within months. The most common intracranial tumors are brain metastases from systemic cancer, estimated to be up to 200,000 per year in the United States, based on a 10 to 15% incidence (1,2), whereas the expected number of all new cancer diagnoses in 2009 was 1.48 million (3). In comparison, the incidence of primary brain tumors in 2009 was an estimated 22,070 new cases (3). Because of the heterogeneous histology and often refractory nature of these tumors, their management is complex, ideally requiring a multidisciplinary team and individualized treatment. Diagnosis is made on the basis of histology, so an accurate characterization of the lesion's pathology is crucial, often necessitating confirmation at a specialized cancer center. Optimal outcomes involve the coordination of neurosurgery, radiation oncology, and neuro-oncology, although low-grade tumors may not require initial therapy other than observation following optimal surgical resection. Despite advances in neurosurgical techniques, radiation therapy, and chemotherapy, the prognosis for patients with high-grade gliomas such as glioblastoma (GB), the most common form of glioma, remains dismal. For patients with GB, median survival is approximately 1 year. A review of eight consecutive phase II chemotherapy trials for recurrent GB demonstrated only a 6% response rate (complete response [CR] and partial response [PR]), with a 6-month progression-free survival (PFS) of 15% and a 1-year overall survival of 21% (4). It is, therefore, important to consider patients with high-grade gliomas for entry into clinical trials at all stages of disease, since new therapies target patients from initial diagnosis with presurgical protocols to salvage therapy at relapse. This chapter aims to provide basic principles that can be used for diagnosing and treating patients with brain tumors. Areas that present special challenges for the treating physician are highlighted, along with an introduction to the underlying molecular mechanisms of gliomagenesis.

■ CLASSIFICATION AND INCIDENCE

Brain tumors are either primary tumors that arise de novo or secondary brain metastases, the latter being far more common. The most common brain metastases result from lung cancer, followed by breast, melanoma, renal, and colorectal cancers (5). Most patients with brain metastases die from progression of their systemic cancer, although, because of improvements in systemic therapy, brain metastases are seen more frequently and have produced escalating morbidity and mortality (1). On a more hopeful note, advances in treating brain metastasis with surgery and radiotherapy have improved overall survival when the patient's systemic disease is controlled.

Primary brain tumors are classified by the World Health Organization (WHO) grading system (Table 37-1), which is based on the histologic pattern of cell differentiation in the tumor. Tumor grade is inversely correlated with prognosis. The most common primary brain tumors are gliomas (all glial tumors), followed by meningiomas, nerve sheath tumors, and pituitary tumors (6).

■ EPIDEMIOLOGY

BRAIN METASTASES

As previously mentioned, brain metastases occur far more commonly than primary brain tumors. Nearly any type of primary cancer can metastasize to the brain, including the hematologic malignancies (7).

The most common brain metastasis originates from lung cancer, which represents the second most common

TABLE 37-1	WORLD HEALTH ORGANIZATION (WHO) CLASSIFICATION OF TUMORS OF THE CENTRAL NERVOUS SYSTEM
WHO grade I	
Pilocytic astrocytoma	Meningioma
Myxopapillary ependymoma	Craniopharyngioma
Subependymoma	
WHO grade II	
Diffuse astrocytoma	Ependymoma
Pleomorphic	Pineocytoma
xanthoastrocytoma	Atypical meningioma
Oligodendroglioma	
Oligoastrocytoma	
WHO grade III	
Anaplastic astrocytoma	Anaplastic oligoastrocytoma
Anaplastic oligodendroglioma	Anaplastic ependymoma
Anaplastic (malignant)	
meningioma	
WHO grade IV	
Glioblastoma	Pineoblastoma
Gliosarcoma	Medulloblastoma

systemic cancer in men and women and the cancer responsible for the greatest mortality (3). The next most common pathology to metastasize to the brain is breast cancer, followed by melanoma, renal cancer, and colorectal cancer (5), although melanoma is the tumor most likely to metastasize to the brain. Based on autopsy findings, 40 to 60% of patients with melanoma develop brain metastases (8). Most brain metastases, particularly melanoma, present with multiple lesions (9), although when renal cancer metastasizes to the brain, it often results in a single lesion. Overall, however, the pattern of distribution of metastases in the brain varies depending on the primary cancer (10).

The incidence of brain metastases appears to be rising, which may be a consequence of increasingly sensitive imaging modalities such as magnetic resonance imaging (MRI), combined with the prolonged survival of patients with metastatic disease. The development of brain metastases usually occurs in the context of systemic relapse, although relapses can be isolated to the central nervous system (CNS). The impermeability of the blood–brain barrier (BBB), which often limits chemotherapy penetration into the CNS, may be the culprit in circumstances of isolated brain relapse.

PRIMARY BRAIN TUMORS

Gliomas are the most frequently occurring primary brain tumors and include astrocytomas, oligodendrogliomas (OD), and ependymomas. Combined, these histologies

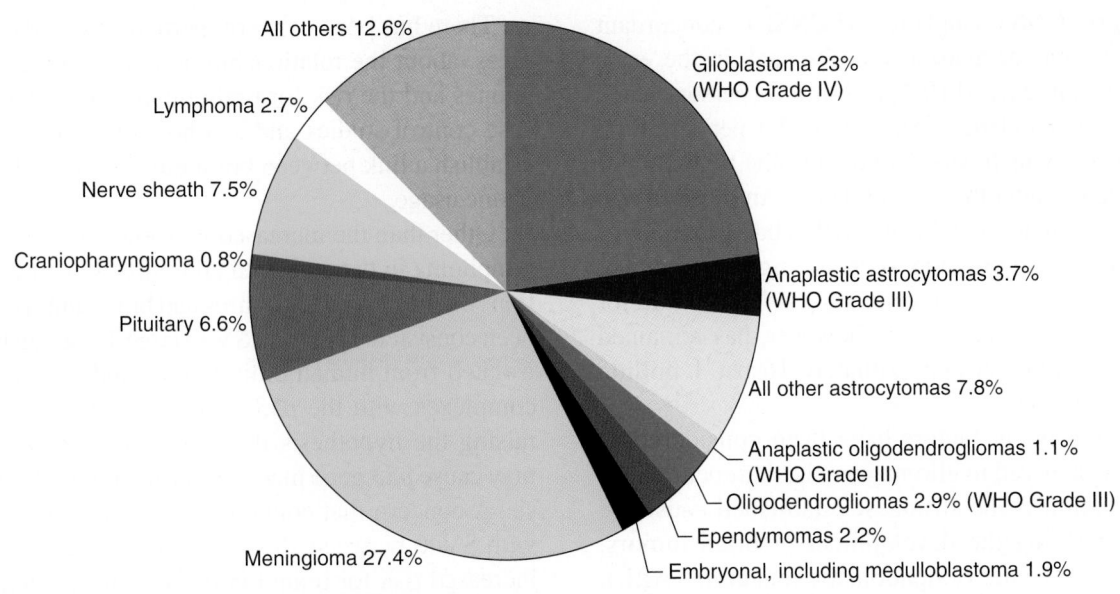

FIGURE 37-1. Distribution of all primary brain and central nervous system tumors by histology, CBTRUS 1995 to 1999 (N = 37,788).

account for approximately 40% of all primary brain tumors and over 80% of all malignant CNS tumors (6). The next most common tumor is meningioma (32%), followed by nerve sheath tumor (9%) and pituitary tumor (8%) (6). The most recent data from the Central Brain Tumor Registry of the United States report an incidence of all primary benign and malignant CNS tumors of 16.5 cases per 100,000 person-years and a prevalence rate of 130.8 per 100,000 (6).

The incidence of primary brain tumors differs by age, with the incidence for all tumors peaking between the ages of 75 and 84 years. Although this is also the peak incidence of gliomas, low-grade glioma is more likely to occur in patients younger than 35 years. Unfortunately, after age 35, a diagnosis of GB is much more common and accounts for more than half of all gliomas. In addition to the disparities of age, gender differences are seen in the incidence of primary brain tumors. The incidence of malignant brain tumors per 100,000 person-years in males is 7.7, compared with 5.4 for females. In contrast, meningioma is more common in females, with an incidence ratio of 2.85:1 (6) (Figs. 37-1 and 37-2).

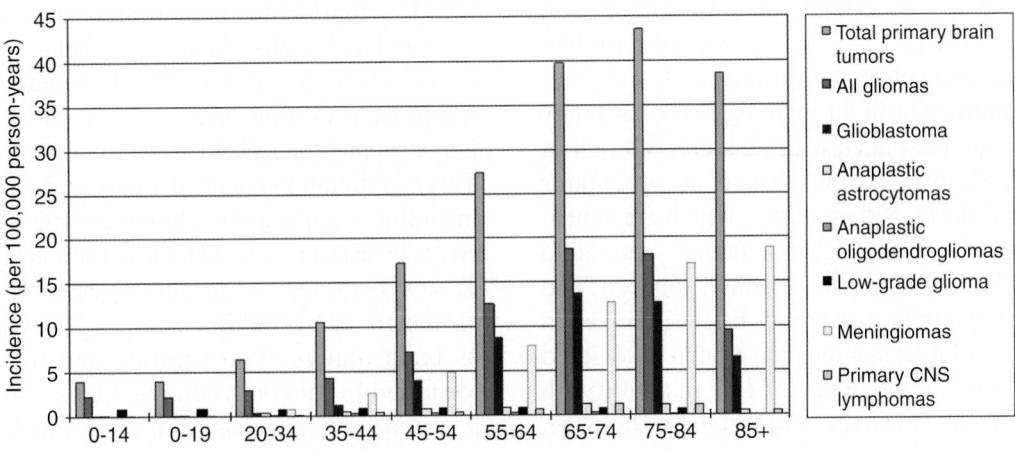

FIGURE 37-2. Age-specific incidence of primary brain and central nervous system tumors by selected histologies, CBTRUS 1995 to 1999.

Primary CNS lymphoma (PCNSL), concordant with AIDS, has decreased since its peak in the early 1990s, when it reached 10.2 per 1 million person-years. By 1998, the incidence decreased to 5.1 per 1 million person-years, which was attributed to the treatment of HIV in males under the age of 60 (11). An escalation in PCNSL is seen not only in HIV/AIDS but also in iatrogenic immunosuppression such as organ transplant, autoimmune disease, and cancer (12-14). The rate for persons over 60 years of age, however, has remained stable since 1994, at approximately 16 per 1 million person-years (11).

Although many factors have been considered as putatively involved in gliomagenesis, therapeutic ionizing radiation is the strongest established causative agent underlying the development of brain tumors. Children with acute lymphoblastic leukemia (ALL), following prophylactic cranial irradiation, have a 27-fold increased risk of brain tumors (15). Increased risk of brain tumors has been seen following therapeutic irradiation for pituitary tumors, even with the low doses of radiation previously used to treat scalp ringworm, which has specifically increased the risk of developing nerve sheath tumors, meningiomas, and gliomas (16). Fortunately, diagnostic radiation does not appear to be strongly associated with the development of gliomas (17).

While brain tumors have been linked to chemical exposure, no specific agent has been identified with a link to brain tumors that can be validated with an exposure-disease correlation. Despite the fact that pesticides have been shown to cause tumors in experimental animal models and there is an association between the use of pesticides and the development of tumors, no consistent link has been proven for the occurrence of cancer in agricultural workers (18). Positive correlations, but not causation, have been drawn between the occurrence of brain tumors and occupations involving exposure to synthetic rubber, vinyl chloride, and petroleum refining (19). Whereas smoking is implicated in an increased risk for many cancers, it is not associated with an increased risk of brain tumors, despite the fact that tobacco contains nitrosamines (20,21). *Nitrosamines*, which are neuro-carcinogens in animals, are highly ubiquitous, and found in cured foods, auto interiors, alcohol, tobacco, and cosmetics. Exposure to cured foods has been linked to meningioma, and nitrosamines have been associated with glioma with a relative risk of 1.48 in adults with a high intake of cured meat (22). No correlation between alcohol intake or cosmetic use and brain tumors has been found (17,21).

There has been concern, particularly in the popular press, about the relationship between exposure to cell phones and the risk for brain tumors. Thus far, several case control studies and a cohort study have failed to establish a link between brain tumors and cellular telephone usage.

Other than the increased incidence of primary CNS lymphoma in patients with HIV infection, any associations between viral exposures and brain tumors have not been consistent (20). The SV40 large T antigen has been isolated from human brain tumors and is able to form complexes with the *p53* tumor suppressor gene (23), raising the hypothesis that expression of this antigen may cause *p53* gene inactivation and favor gliomagenesis. A concern that contamination of the polio vaccine with SV40 between 1955 and 1963 would result in an increased risk for brain tumors was invalidated by two case control studies (24,25). A protective effect of allergies (asthma, eczema, and hay fever) was noted in a meta-analysis of over 3000 patients, with a relative risk of glioma incidence of 0.61 (26), supporting a role for immune modulation in brain tumorigenesis. A retrospective case-control series demonstrated a decreased incidence of glioma in patients who reported histories of chickenpox, shingles, HSV, and EBV (27), and as a surrogate for exposure to infections in early life, birth order was recently correlated with increased risk for the development of glioma in adulthood. With each one-unit increase in birth order, there was a 13% decreased absolute risk for glioma (28).

Relatively few brain tumors are attributable to heredity; studies have cited from 2 to 4% (29,30). Brain tumors can arise as a component of familial tumor syndromes, such as neurofibromatosis type 1 (NF1), resulting in glioma and optic nerve glioma. NF1 is caused by a mutation of the *NF-1* gene and is also associated with leukemia and pheochromocytoma. Neurofibromatosis type II is marked by a mutation of the *NF-2* gene and is associated with bilateral vestibular schwannomas, meningioma, and glioma. The Li-Fraumeni syndrome results from an autosomal dominant mutation of the *p53* tumor suppressor gene, located on chromosome 17p (31). This *p53* mutation results in many types of malignancy, including glioma and medulloblastoma, as well as sarcoma, breast cancer, leukemia, and adrenocortical cancer. Turcot syndrome is an autosomal dominant disease characterized by multiple polyps of the GI tract as well as brain tumors. Two separate mutations have been identified in Turcot syndrome. One involves the *APC* gene (adenomatous polyposis coli), which is associated with medulloblastoma. A second mutation of the *hMLH1* DNA mismatch repair gene is associated with GB (32).

■ BIOLOGY AND MOLECULAR GENETICS

Increasingly, the focus of understanding various cancers resides in a clear view of underlying molecular biologic mechanisms and signaling pathways. Delineating such mechanisms is confounded by the tremendous molecular and histologic heterogeneity from tumor to tumor. Glial tumors can have areas composed both of low- and high-grade tissue. Additionally, most tumors have multiple genetic mutations that can affect growth factor signaling, cell cycle events, apoptosis, cell survival pathways, and DNA repair mechanisms.

Newer drugs target specific extracellular receptors or block intracellular signal transduction systems. Owing to their specificity, these drugs often lack the side effects commonly associated with standard cytotoxic chemotherapy. If the therapeutic target is crucial for the cancer cell's continued viability, the drug can be especially effective. An example is the use of imatinib for chronic myelogenous leukemia (33,34). If the target is heterogeneous or is not critical for continued cell survival, the benefits can be more modest, such as the use of gefitinib in lung cancer (35). Technologic advances in the development of transgenic mice, cDNA microarrays, and protein analysis approaches make possible a highly sophisticated and powerful molecular analysis of brain tumors. Molecular characterization of brain tumors using cDNA microarray technology has identified specific genetic profiles that are directly correlated with tumor grading and prognosis (36,37). Ultimately, tumors will be identified on the basis of their underlying molecular makeup and individual treatments will be targeted to these specific diseases rather than to broad categories such as glioma.

GLIAL TUMORS

Malignant glial tumors often exhibit significant histologic heterogeneity, which is reflected at the molecular level. One proposed explanation for this diversity is that an underlying genetic instability results in a progressive accumulation of mutations and leads to an increasingly malignant phenotype. Some believe that cancer originates when progenitor cell populations become active in different locations in the body. The adult brain is one such organ that has a population of stem cells that could become targets for neoplastic transformation (38). Glial tumors have known mutations in critical cellular pathways, including cell cycle regulation, proliferation, cellular metabolism, cell death, and survival. Separate mutations may have

an equivalent phenotypic effect if they are involved in the same signaling pathway. Intracellular signaling pathways are complicated; they interact at multiple levels and can directly affect gene transcription, post-transcription processing, protein modification and transport, and protein-protein interactions.

Several growth factor pathways have been identified in glioma growth. The epidermal growth factor (EGF) pathway is overexpressed in GB (39). It is estimated that the EGF receptor (EGFR) is amplified in 30 to 50% of GB (40,41). An alternate mutation in the external domain generates a truncated receptor, the EGFRvIII mutant, which is constitutively activated in gliomas (42). Growth factors such as EGF and platelet-derived growth factor (PDGF) activate multiple signal transduction pathways that lead to cell survival and proliferation. EGFR can activate the PI3Kinase pathway, which is frequently mutated in glioma. When the PI3Kinase pathway is activated, the activation of *AKT* (protein kinase B) is triggered, in turn activating multiple prosurvival pathways such as NFkB, forkhead, and glycolysis (43). The activation of the PI3Kinase pathway has been associated with the reduced survival of glioma patients (44). Growth factors can also stimulate the *ras* pathway, which initiates a signal cascade through *Raf/MEK/Erk,* and also promotes cell survival and tumorigenesis (45).

The deletion of *MMAC/PTEN* is a key mutation in GB (46). PTEN has phosphatase activity that inhibits the PI3Kinase pathway. The deletion of *MMAC/PTEN* leads to *AKT* pathway activation. One effector of the AKT signal involves mTOR. mTOR inhibitors are being investigated in clinical trials for GB. The importance of these pathways has been shown in transgenic mouse-modeling studies; these have produced primary brain tumors that mimic many of the characteristics of human primary brain tumors (47,48) as well as allowing direct mapping of mutated pathways found in human tumor samples.

A commonly mutated gene in gliomas is *p53,* a transcription factor that, among other signals, is activated in response to DNA damage in an attempt to control the cell cycle. The activation of *p53* can result either in apoptosis or cell cycle arrest and initiation of DNA repair mechanisms (49). The functions of *p53* are complex and have been studied for many years. Initially, *p53* was thought to act mainly through *p21, BAX, GADD45,* and *MDM2.* Sequencing and scanning the promoter and enhancer regions of more than 2500 human genes has identified 300 genes that are putatively directly regulated by *p53* (50). An alternate mechanism that decreases *p53* pathway activity involves MDM2 protein, which binds to *p53* and inactivates it. Amplification of

MDM2, seen in 10% of GB that lack the mutant form of *p53*, decreases the activity of *p53* (51). The abrogation of *p53* activity would be expected to increase proliferation and mutations, leading to genetic instability, the prodrome of tumorigenesis.

The cell cycle represents stages of development via cell division that are necessary for cell replication, including DNA synthesis and the duplication of chromosomes (S phase), mitosis (M phase), and the intervals in between these events: cellular quiescence and differentiation (G0 phase), cell preparation and signaling to commit the cell to division (G1 phase), and cellular checks to DNA replication prior to cell division (G2 phase). Cell cycle regulation is a key target of carcinogenesis. The transition from each phase to the next phase is characterized by checkpoints. These cell cycle checkpoints are affected by multiple proteins, acting either as accelerators or inhibitors of cell regulation. Important molecules in this process include *p53, p21,* and *MDM2,* which can both inhibit and accelerate the degradation of *p53*. Another cell cycle regulation pathway important for glial tumors involves the retinoblastoma (*RB*) gene. When the *RB* gene is phosphorylated, the E2F transcription factor is released and activates cellular proliferation. The regulation of *RB* activity is complex and involves multiple cyclins (cyclin D), cyclin-dependent kinases (CDK4/6), and cyclin-dependant kinase inhibitors (p16), whose activities continue to be investigated (52). Tests are being done using gene therapy to take advantage of the *RB* mutation to allow replication of a mutated adenovirus, and to generate an oncolytic effect (53).

Apoptosis is genetically programmed cell death, an important process in embryogenesis, normal tissue turnover, ischemia, and degenerative disorders. Antiapoptotic proteins such as bcl-2 and proapoptotic proteins such as myc and bax are important regulators of this pathway. Apoptosis can be activated through binding of the fas/apo-1 receptor (CD95) by the fas ligand (tumor necrosis factor), which in turn activates caspases via proteolytic cleavage and ends in cell death. It is suspected that alterations in the regulation of apoptosis and response to apoptosis signals may be in part responsible for the resistance of glial tumors to chemotherapy.

The production of enzymes that repair the effects of chemotherapy is another mechanism of the resistance of cancer cells. O6-methylguanine-DNA methyltransferase (MGMT) is expressed by glial tumors and removes the DNA adduct produced by nitrosourea compounds. Hypermethylation of the promoter region of the *MGMT* gene, which inactivates *MGMT* gene transcription, has been associated with response to alkylating agents and increased survival in glioma patients (51,52). The mechanism of gene inactivation by hypermethylation

can target other cellular pathways, including those involving DNA repair, cell cycle regulation, apoptosis, and tumor suppressor genes (54).

One of the hallmarks of glial tumors is their propensity to invade neighboring brain tissue, generally within 1 to 2 cm of the original tumor mass. Glial tumor cells can generate an extracellular matrix (ECM) that promotes migration through the production of tenascin, vitronectin, and fibronectin. Glial tumor cells can also express receptors for integrin, CD44 (a transmembrane glycoprotein), RHAMM (a hyaluronan-binding protein that regulates ras signaling), the ECM proteoglycan versican, and the neural cell adhesion molecule (NCAM). Glial tumors also secrete matrix metalloproteinases (MMPs) that degrade the adjacent ECM and facilitate invasion (54). Downregulation of MMP-2 activity by the *PTEN* gene has been shown to reduce invasion in glial tumor cell lines (55). These various molecules will hopefully be able to offer viable targets that will be instrumental in producing efficacious glioma therapies.

The molecular and cytogenetic characterization of brain tumors has suggested two models that can explain the development of GB. One model, resting on the multihit hypothesis, attributes the development of GB to a stepwise accumulation of mutations beginning in low-grade astrocytoma and progressing to high-grade astrocytoma. This process is marked by the presence of mutated *p53*. In this model, progression from a normal astrocyte to a low-grade astrocytoma is marked by *p53* mutation (>65%) and PDGF-A or PDGFR-alpha overexpression (60%). Progression from low-grade astrocytoma to anaplastic astrocytoma (AA) involves loss of heterozygosity (55) at 19q (50%) and alterations in the RB pathway (25%). Progression from AA to GB is marked by LOH at 10q/mutation of PTEN (5%), loss of expression of DCC (which induces apoptosis by a mechanism requiring receptor proteolysis (50%)), and amplification of PDGFR-alpha (<10%). A separate model has been proposed for primary de novo GB, which is characterized by the lack of *p53* mutation, by EGFR amplification (40%) or overexpression (60%), MDM2 amplification (<10%) or overexpression (50%), *p16* deletion (30-40%), LOH at 10p and 10q/PTEN mutation (30%), and *RB* alterations (56,57). These models are descriptive more than they are mechanistic and do not adequately take into account the genetic or histologic heterogeneity that is found within a single tumor. The persistence of glioma is likely due to multiple mechanisms combining to generate a common tumor phenotype (40).

Tumor tissue studies suggest that a patient's response to chemotherapy might be correlated with his or her cytogenetic profile. Patients with anaplastic oligodendroglioma (AOD) are generally considered to be more chemosensitive than those with other anaplastic gliomas. However, not all AODs respond to standard alkylating agent chemotherapy. The allelic loss of chromosomes 1p and 19q has been linked to the response of oligodendroglioma (OD) and AOD to chemotherapy and radiation therapy, and the presence of intact 1p and 19q has been correlated with both lack of response and decreased survival (58-62).

MENINGIOMAS

A mutation in the *NF2* gene, on chromosome 22q12, has been closely associated with meningiomas. Germline mutations of this gene result in neurofibromatosis type 2, an autosomal dominant disorder that can manifest as multiple meningiomas, schwannomas, gliomas, and intracranial calcifications (63). Mutations of the *NF2* gene have also been detected in as many as 60% of sporadic meningiomas (64). Merlin, the product of the *NF2* gene, functions as a tumor suppressor gene. Merlin is a member of a family of cytoskeleton-associated proteins linked to receptor tyrosine kinase activity and ECM interactions (65). Merlin has also been reported to stabilize *p53* by inhibiting *MDM2*-mediated degradation of *p53* (66).

Cytogenetic alterations have similarly been described in higher-grade meningiomas. Atypical meningioma has been associated with chromosomal losses of 1p, 6q, 10q, 14q, and 18q and gains of 1q, 9q, 12q, 15q, 17q, and 20q. Malignant meningioma has been associated with these changes as well as losses of *9p,* rare mutations of *p53* and *PTEN,* and rare deletions of *CDKN2A* (67).

Several oncogenes and growth factor receptors have been identified in meningiomas. The oncogenes include *c-myc, n-myc, IGF-I,* and *IGF-II.* The growth factor receptors include EGF, interferon-alpha (INFα), PDGF-β, progesterone, somatostatin, and androgens (68). Meningiomas are sometimes associated with significant edema, which is unusual for a slow-growing tumor. This edema has been linked to the direct production of vascular endothelial growth factor (VEGF) by the tumor (69). EGF and basic fibroblast growth factor (bFGF) can induce VEGF secretion by meningioma cells, whereas the corticosteroid dexamethasone decreases VEGF secretion (70) and is often prescribed for patients with edema-causing brain tumors.

BRAIN METASTASES

The development of brain metastases is an intricate sequential process (71). In addition to proliferating, tumor cells must migrate and enter the systemic circulation, survive, be transported through the blood to the brain, adhere to and extravasate through the endothelium, invade the brain parenchyma, and proliferate, which requires the recruitment of a secondary blood supply. Failure at any of these steps will halt the metastatic process (72-74). Each of these steps requires complex interactions between the tumor cell and its changing microenvironment. The location of tumor metastases is not random and involves the interface between the tumor cell and tissue in a process that has been characterized as the "seed and soil" hypothesis, described by Stephen Paget more than 100 years ago (75-77). The primary tumor is regarded as biologically and molecularly heterogeneous, subject to a biological imperative favoring the selection of tumor cells that can survive the arduous process required for metastasis, that is, the "seed." Experimentally, metastases arising from the same primary tumor can have different clonal origins and be traced back to different single cells (78). The local environment of the tumor cell greatly affects its success in proliferating and recruiting an adequate blood supply through angiogenesis, that is, the "soil." The properties that allow success in producing tumor metastases are unrelated to the proliferative capacity of the cells at the primary site. In clinical practice, this is seen when distant metastases develop in the context of good local response of the tumor to treatment (79). The discovery of unique molecules expressed on endothelial cells that allow preferential targeting of tumor cells may also contribute to conditions that facilitate tumor metastases (80,81).

An understanding of the biological processes of brain metastases and the role of the BBB provides potential targets for intervention to improve treatment. There are multiple complex regulators of cell adhesion, including molecules such as integrins, cadherins, selectins, and heparin sulfate proteoglycans (79). Additionally, integrins can recruit intracellular signaling molecules such as focal adhesion kinase and src, which can lead to a cascade of cellular signaling that affects cell cycle control and proliferation (82,83). Integrins also play a part in regulating angiogenesis and tumor invasion (84). Other molecules that mediate invasion include the MMP family, serine proteases, and heparinase. The MMPs are proenzymes that degrade the ECM and basement membrane, promoting tumor invasion. The gelatinases (MMP-2 and MMP-9) are thought to have especially important roles in brain tumor invasion (85). Heparinase is an enzyme that degrades heparin sulfate chains, which are important components of the basement membrane (86), and heparinase activity has been detected in melanoma cells derived from brain metastasis (87). Tumor cells must generate their own blood supply if they are to grow successfully and remain viable. The regulation of such angiogenesis is influenced both by activators and inhibitors, which can be expressed either by tumor cells or other cells in the tumor's microenvironment. Important activators of angiogenesis include VEGF, angiopoietin, hypoxia-inducible transcription factor (HIF), cyclooxygenase 2 (COX-2), PDGF, integrins, MMPs, and others. Important inhibitors of angiogenesis include angiostatin, endostatin, tissue inhibitors of matrix metalloproteinases (TIMPs), interferons, and platelet factor 4 (88). Upregulation of activators or downregulation of inhibitors favor angiogenesis. As tumors grow, they begin to produce increasing numbers of angiogenic molecules that can participate in metastasis (88). Because a multitude of pathways are involved in tumor growth and invasion, it is likely that if one pathway is inhibited, cells may escape through alternate pathways.

The BBB is formed by tight junctions and non-fenestrated endothelial cells. The brain lacks lymphatic drainage and depends on the BBB to filter and block the entrance of macromolecules and invasion by micro-organisms (89). Effective drug delivery through the BBB to tumor cells is a significant obstacle to chemotherapy, both for brain metastases and primary brain tumors. The blockade to charged hydrophilic molecules created by the BBB is passive, but it is also augmented by active transport from P-glycoprotein, which is expressed at high levels in the brain's endothelium (90). The P-glycoprotein family of transporters actively exports drugs such as anthracyclines, Vinca alkaloids, taxanes, and etoposide (91). The integrity of the BBB also depends on dynamic interactions between endothelial cells with astrocytes and oligodendrocytes (76,92).

The BBB can be breached by circulating cancer cells, a process that has been duplicated experimentally by direct carotid artery injection of tumor cell lines into nude mice (93). The selected tumor cells migrate across the BBB without degrading its permeability and proliferate. Once the tumor reaches a size that requires recruitment of new vessels, the BBB is disrupted, which allows imaging of brain tumors with contrast agents. In experimental models, brain metastases smaller than 0.25 mm in diameter are associated with an intact BBB, whereas larger tumors demonstrate BBB permeability (76). Despite the presence of the BBB, studies of drug levels in brain tumors from systemic delivery administered before surgery demonstrate pharmacologically relevant concentrations of drugs (94,95). Decreasing amounts of drug reach the tumor periphery and adjacent brain in animals, and comparatively lower drug levels are achieved in brain tumors compared to levels

in subcutaneously implanted tumors (96). Measurements of drug levels in cerebrospinal fluid are not accurate indicators of tissue drug levels in tumor metastases and should not be assumed to predict activity (97).

■ CLINICAL PRESENTATION, DIAGNOSIS, AND PATHOLOGY

CLINICAL PRESENTATION (FIGS. 37-3 TO 37-10)

Brain tumors are usually diagnosed on presentation with symptoms such as seizure, headache, or focal neurologic deficits. High-grade malignant tumors typically present with headache, which reflects elevated intracranial pressure, and focal neurologic signs, such as weakness or aphasia. Low-grade glial tumors often come to attention with seizure, while other slow-growing tumors, such as meningioma, may be clinically silent and incidentally detected during imaging for an unrelated problem. Contrast-enhanced MRI is the diagnostic standard for brain tumor imaging. In addition to its superior sensitivity, MRI provides more detailed anatomic as well as physiologic information that can contribute to a differential diagnosis. While contrast-enhanced CT is able to detect high-grade lesions that cause BBB breakdown, low-grade lesions may be detectable only on MRI, using sequences sensitive for edema and tissue changes (98). However, even in the case of known systemic primary

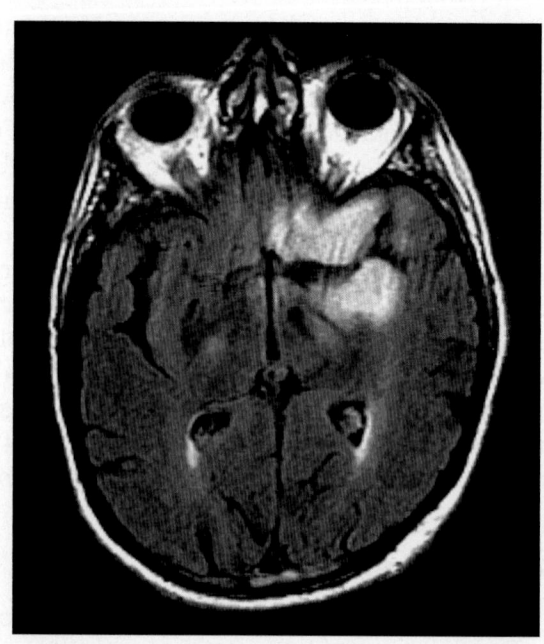

FIGURE 37-3. Low-grade glioma.

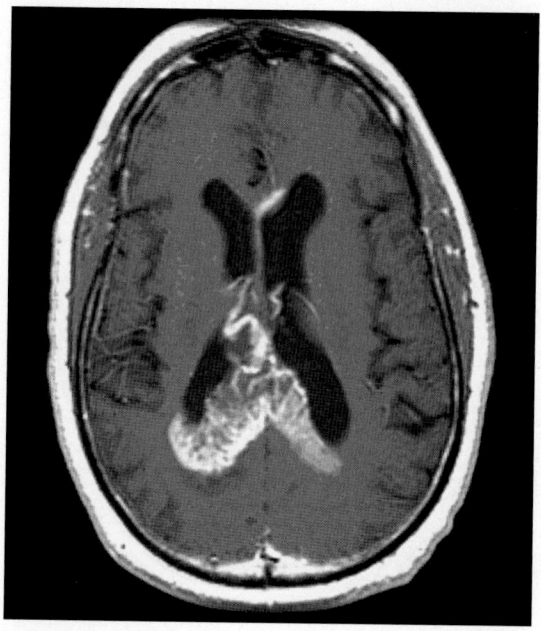

FIGURE 37-4. Glioblastoma.

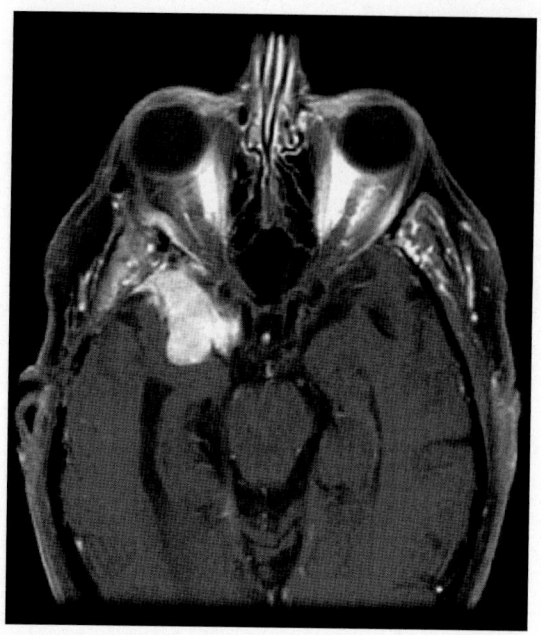

FIGURE 37-6. Meningioma.

cancer, contrast-enhanced CT may miss small foci of metastatic disease that are visible on MRI.

The brain tumor imaging characteristics seen in MRI are helpful in making a diagnosis. However, confirmation of the diagnosis with pathology is necessary in nearly all cases. Noncancerous brain lesions that

have been mistaken for malignancy include infection, demyelinating disease, vascular malformations, and stroke. A particular variant of a demyelinating disease with large focal tumor-like lesions is known for resembling a malignant brain tumor (99). Unfortunately, some of these lesions have been irradiated, under the

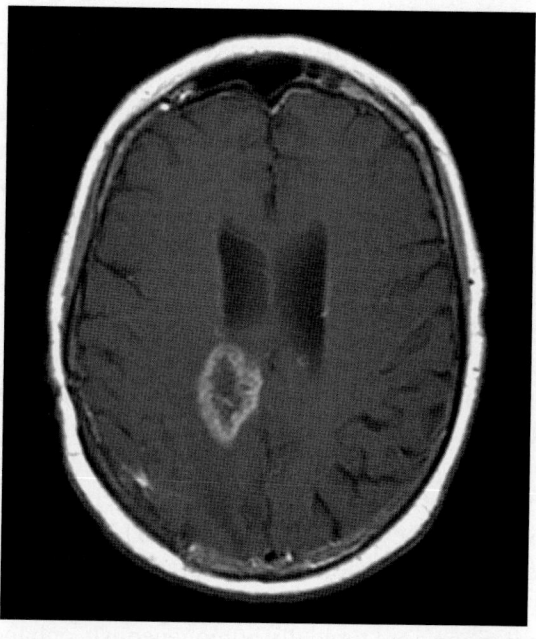

FIGURE 37-5. Radiation necrosis.

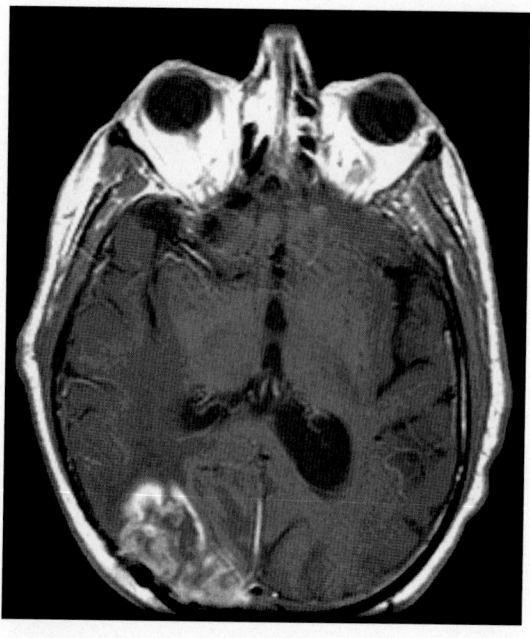

FIGURE 37-7. Malignant meningioma.

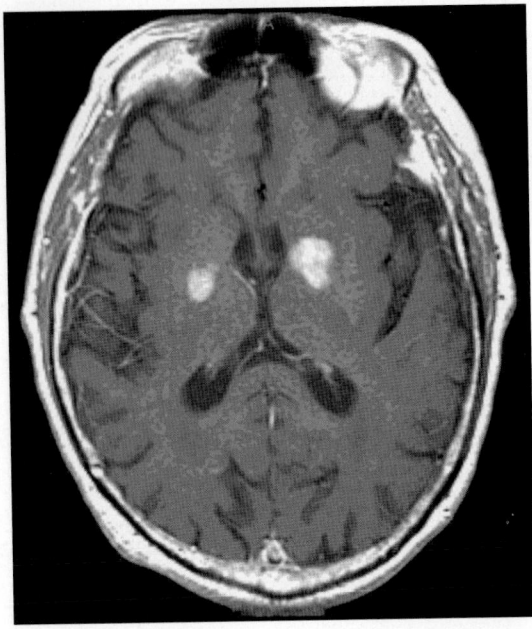

FIGURE 37-8. Central nervous system lymphoma.

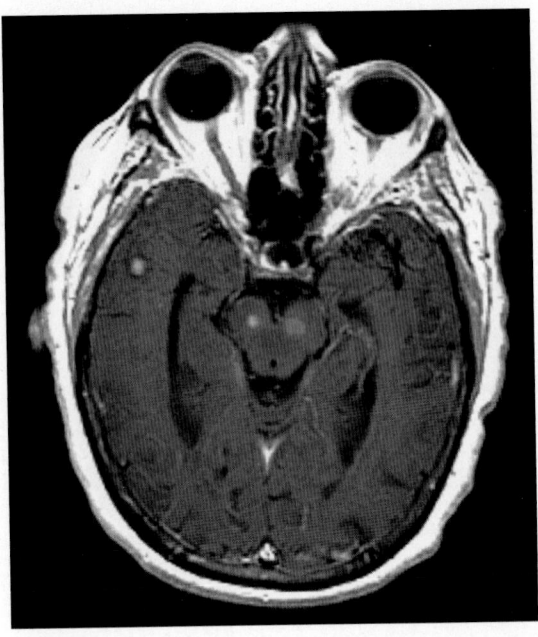

FIGURE 37-10. Multiple brain metastases, breast.

presumptive diagnosis of GB, which only increases the severity of the demyelination (100). Conversely, patients with primary brain tumors are sometimes initially diagnosed with stroke or demyelinating disease. Further complicating the picture are patients who have brain tumor in addition to stroke, which is far more prevalent with increasing age. Patients with systemic cancer, often in remission, or a stable condition, can present with brain lesions that are suspected to be brain metastases but turn out to be a second primary brain tumor. These types of cases often benefit from an interpretation by a specialized neuroradiologist who has been provided with a relevant patient history. A history of immunosuppression and multiple subcortical enhancing lesions may prompt the suspicion of a primary CNS lymphoma or infection with toxoplasmosis. In this case, further workup with brain thallium single photon emission computed tomography (SPECT) scanning or fluorodeoxyglucose–positron emission tomography (FDG-PET) imaging may serve to distinguish between these two possibilities.

There are several classic radiographic appearances of brain tumors that suggest malignancy. An irregular enhancing lesion with extensive edema following white matter pathways indicates a malignant glioma. Non-contrast-enhancing lesions with increased diffuse signals on FLAIR (fluid attenuated inversion recovery) imaging suggest a low-grade astrocytoma. As a general rule for glial tumors, the presence of contrast enhancement suggests a high-grade malignancy. WHO grade IV tumors nearly always enhance, as opposed to grade II tumors, which are nonenhancing. Two notable exceptions to this guideline include pilocytic astrocytoma (WHO grade I) and pleomorphic xanthoastrocytoma (WHO grade II), which typically have an enhancing nodule and associated cyst. Meningiomas are typically homogeneously enhancing dural-based lesions, associated with calcification. The

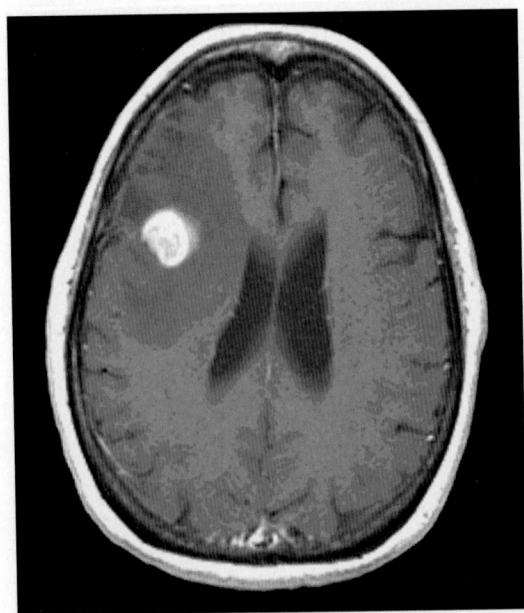

FIGURE 37-9. Single brain metastasis, lung adenocarcinoma.

appearance of multiple enhancing subcortical lesions with a homogeneous enhancement suggests primary CNS lymphoma. However, the same lesions, if associated with a known primary malignancy, may indicate brain metastases.

DIAGNOSIS

The discovery of a brain lesion should prompt referral to a neurosurgeon for consideration of biopsy or resection. The management of brain tumors is crucially dependent on definitive pathology for diagnosis. Our institution insists on reviewing patient diagnostic slides prior to rendering a treatment recommendation, and it is not uncommon for our neuropathologists to disagree with the diagnosis provided by the referring physician. A referral to a specialized neuropathologist may be necessary for diagnosis of uncommon or rare tumors and also in cases where there is only limited biopsy tissue available. Biopsies must be of adequate quality and be representative of the overall tumor to allow accurate diagnosis. Primary brain glial tumors are graded according to the most malignant portion of the tumor. A brain lesion that is predominantly grade III astrocytoma but has a few regions that meet the criteria for grade IV astrocytoma (GB) is graded as a GB. The tumor grade may be underestimated if the most malignant portion of the tumor is not sampled. Typically the most malignant region corresponds to an area of contrast enhancement. In the case of a non-contrast-enhancing tumor, the biopsy may be guided by MR spectroscopy or PET imaging (101). Clinically, this issue is critical in assessing a purported grade II astrocytoma in a patient who, because of his or her age, is more likely to have a grade III astrocytoma. With the former diagnosis, the patient might be followed by observation, whereas for the latter, the patient would require maximal resection, radiation therapy, and chemotherapy.

If a patient is suspected of having primary CNS lymphoma, the use of corticosteroids should be avoided. Primary CNS lymphoma can be quite sensitive to steroids during initial presentation, and the preoperative use of even small doses of corticosteroids can lead to a nondiagnostic biopsy. These patients usually require repeat biopsy after steroid discontinuation. Patients may also present with deep central lesions involving the brainstem or thalamus. These cases may require referral to a specialized neurosurgical center to evaluate whether open biopsy, resection, or stereotactic-guided biopsy is appropriate. In these cases close coordination with a department of neuropathology will be critical in obtaining adequate tissue for diagnosis.

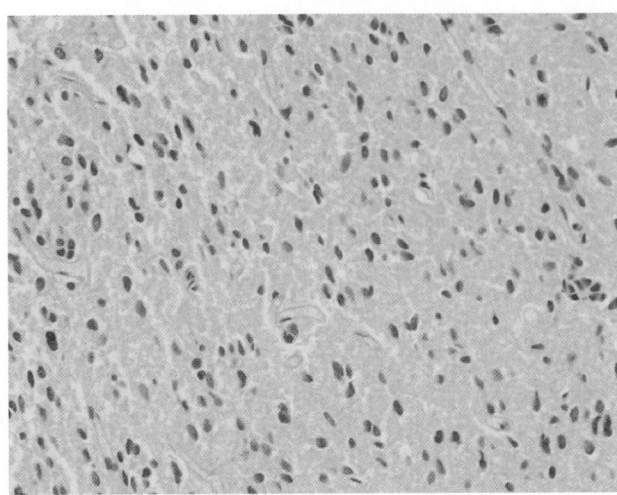

FIGURE 37-11. Low-grade astrocytoma, WHO grade II (×200). (*Courtesy of Dr. Gregory N. Fuller.*)

PATHOLOGY

Diffuse astrocytomas are characterized by well-differentiated astrocytes—either fibrillary, gemistocytic, or rarely protoplasmic—with mildly increased cellularity. The cellular morphology of the tumor cells may differ within the same tumor sample and show great variability between tumors. Necrosis and microvascular proliferation are absent. Rare mitotic figures may occur and nuclear atypia may be present, but not sufficiently to characterize the tumor as AA. The typical MIB-1 labeling index is less than 4% (Figs. 37-11 and 37-12).

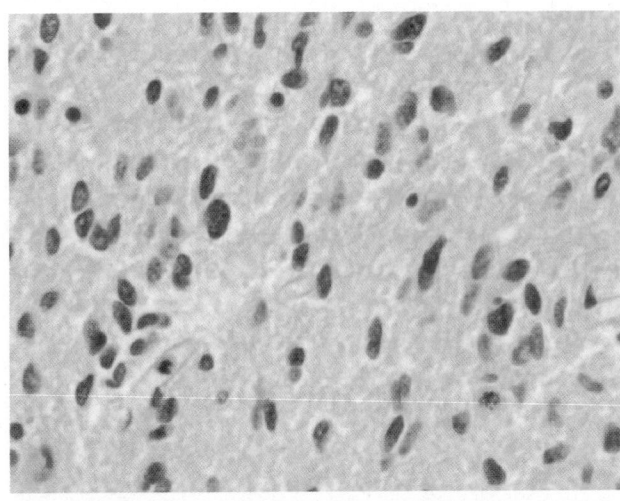

FIGURE 37-12. Low-grade astrocytoma, WHO grade II (×400). (*Courtesy of Dr. Gregory N. Fuller.*)

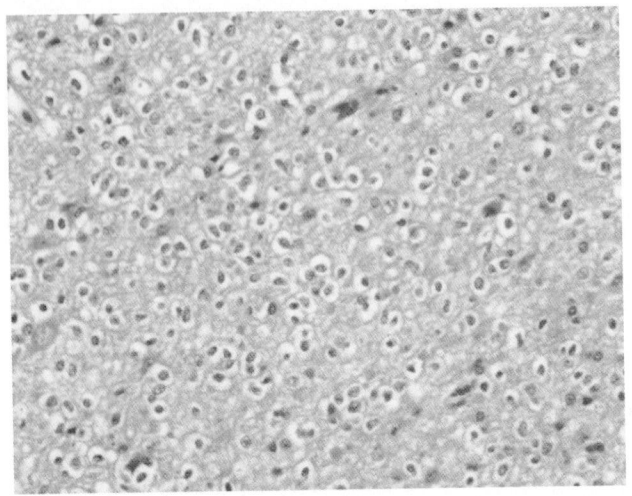

FIGURE 37-13. Oligodendroglioma, WHO grade II (×200).

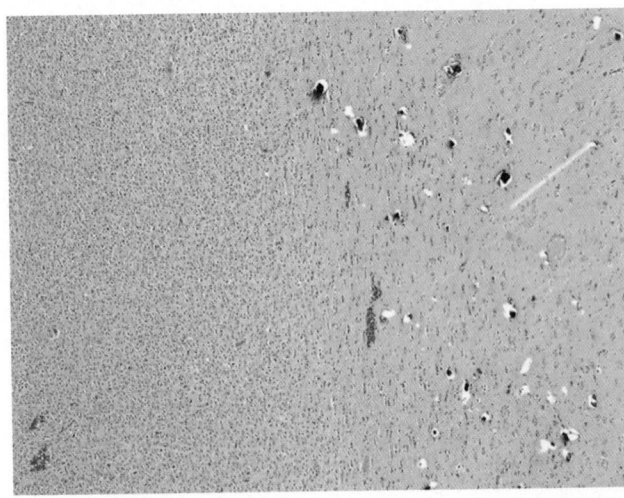

FIGURE 37-15. Anaplastic oligodendroglioma, WHO grade III (×40).

ODs are characterized by moderately cellular tumor cells with rounded, homogenous nuclei, giving a "fried egg" artifactual appearance which is referred to as "classical OD." A recent RTOG trial found that 80% of tumors with classic oligodendroglial morphology were associated with 1p 19q deletion, compared with only 13% of 1p and 19q deletions seen in nonclassical ODs (102). Microcalcifications, microcyst formation, extracellular mucin deposition, and a dense network of branching capillaries are other oligodendrogliomal features. Nuclear atypia may be seen, but significant mitotic activity or microvascular proliferation is suggestive of an anaplastic tumor. The MIB-1 index is typically less than 5% (Figs. 37-13 and 37-14).

AODs are characterized by oligodendroglial cells, with signs of increased cellularity, nuclear atypia, and mitotic activity. Cellular pleomorphism may be present, with formation of multi-nucleated giant cells or spindle cells. Gliofibrillary oligodendrocytes and minigemistocytes are common. Although microvascular proliferation and necrosis may be present, their presence does not change the diagnosis to GB. There is currently no designation for a WHO grade IV OD. The MIB-1 ratio is usually greater than 5% (Figs. 37-15 to 37-17).

AA is characterized by diffusely infiltrating astrocytes with increased cellularity, nuclear atypia, and mitotic activity. They are more cellular than low-grade

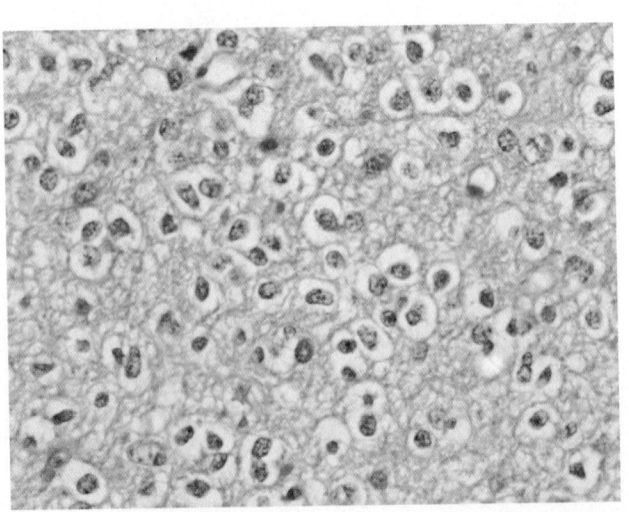

FIGURE 37-14. Oligodendroglioma, WHO grade II (×400).

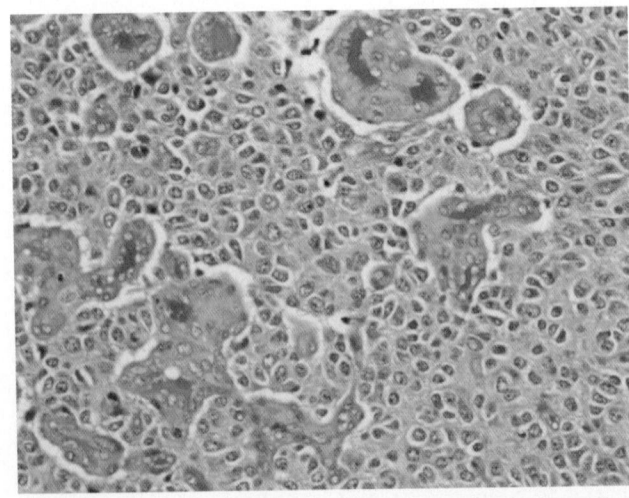

FIGURE 37-16. Anaplastic oligodendroglioma, WHO grade III (×200).

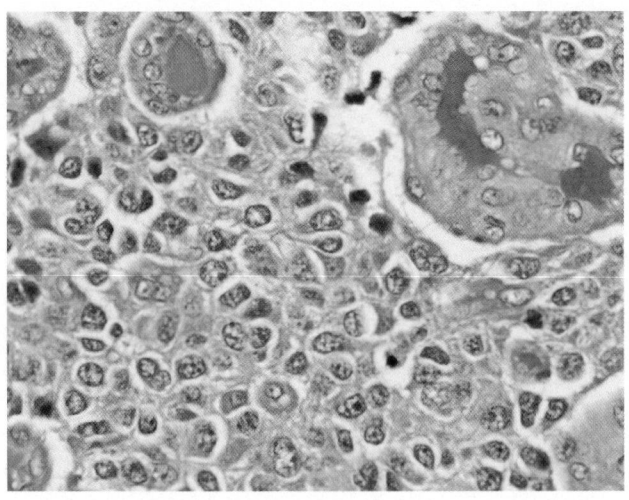

FIGURE 37-17. Anaplastic oligodendroglioma, WHO grade III (×400).

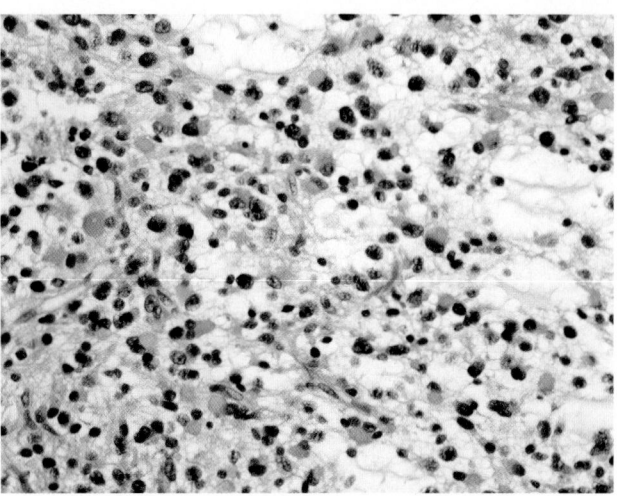

FIGURE 37-19. Anaplastic astrocytoma, WHO grade III (×200).

astrocytomas, and the nuclear atypia include formation of nuclear inclusions, multinucleated cells, and abnormal mitoses. Microvascular proliferation is absent; if present, it would upgrade the tumor to GB. Previous classifications distinguished the presence of necrosis as a hallmark of GB. Currently, microvascular proliferation is a sufficient criterion, so an AA with necrosis is as valid a characterization as GB without necrosis. The typical MIB-1 labeling index ranges from 5 to 10% and can occasionally overlap with index values for low-grade astrocytoma and GB (Figs. 37-18 and 37-19).

GB and GB multiforme are synonymous; "multiforme" was dropped from the title in the 2007 World Health Organization (WHO) classification book. GB is an anaplastic cellular tumor with marked nuclear atypia and mitotic activity, often with marked regional heterogeneity and cellular polymorphism. The presence of either microvascular proliferation or necrosis differentiates this lesion from AA. Other features associated with GB include formation of epithelial "adenoid" structures, multinucleated giant cells, granular cells, lipidized cells, perivascular lymphocytes, and metaplasia. GB is associated with a high proliferative rate, and MIB-1 labeling typically ranges from 15 to 20% (Figs. 37-20 to 37-22).

Meningiomas can have a wide range of appearances and are subtyped according to their appearance. Most

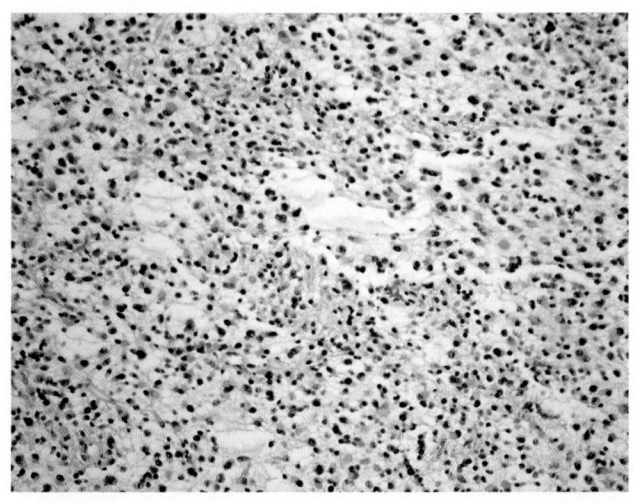

FIGURE 37-18. Anaplastic astrocytoma, WHO grade III (×100).

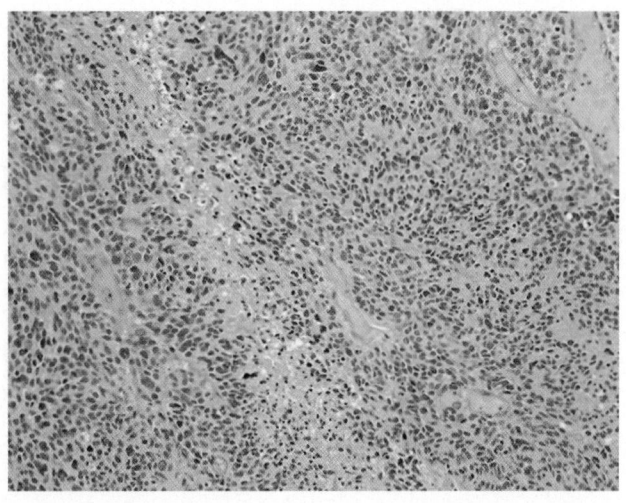

FIGURE 37-20. Glioblastoma, WHO grade IV (×100).

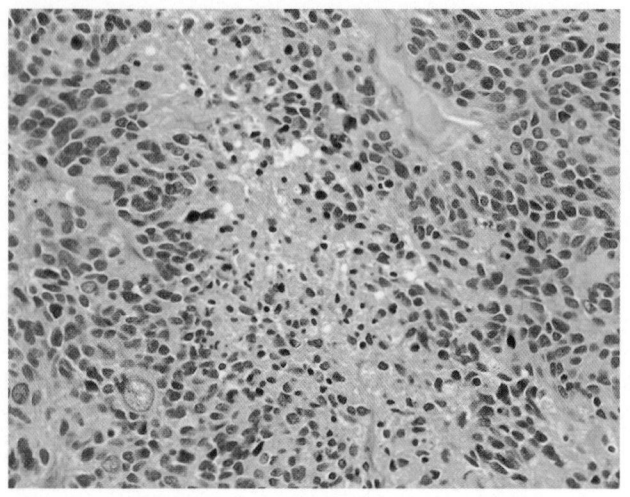

FIGURE 37-21. Glioblastoma, WHO grade IV (×200).

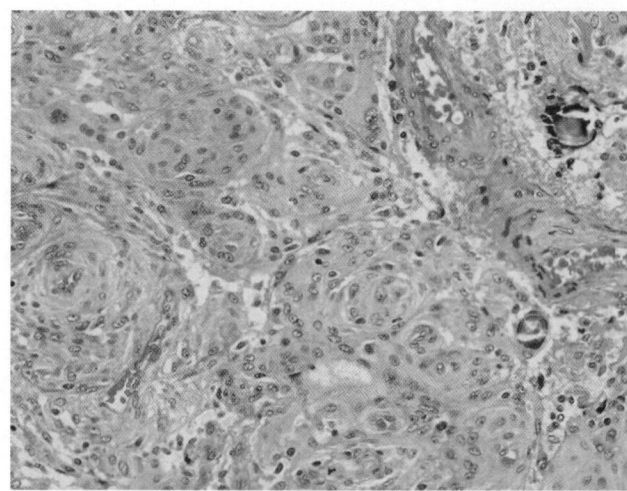

FIGURE 37-23. Meningioma (×100).

meningiomas are grade I. The transitional variant has numerous concentric "onionbulb" structures. The psammomatous variant has calcified psammoma bodies. Pleomorphic nuclei and occasional mitoses are allowed, although four or more mitoses per 10 high-power fields would qualify in diagnosing atypical meningioma, grade II. Increased cellularity, high nuclear-to-cytoplasmic ratio, prominent nucleoli, and foci of necrosis will also upgrade these to a grade II. Anaplastic meningiomas, grade III, have more than 20 mitoses per 10 high-power fields, or obviously malignant cytology resembling carcinoma, melanoma, or high-grade sarcoma (103) (Figs. 37-23 and 37-24).

■ TREATMENT AND PROGNOSIS

LOW-GRADE GLIOMA

Diffuse astrocytomas are disseminated, infiltrative low-grade brain tumors. Their peak incidence is in the third decade, followed by the second decade. Ten percent of diffuse astrocytomas occur in patients younger than 20 years of age and 30% in patients older than 45. Overall, these low-grade tumors represent 4% of glial tumors (6). Although these tumors are considered benign compared with malignant astrocytoma, they are still lethal. The median survival time of patients with

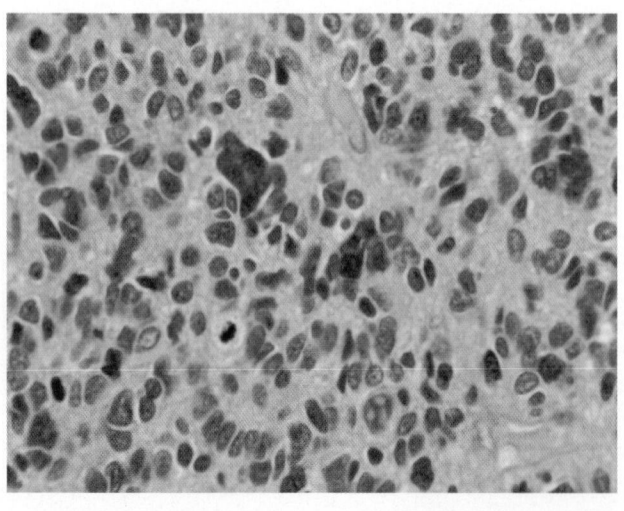

FIGURE 37-22. Glioblastoma, WHO grade IV (×400).

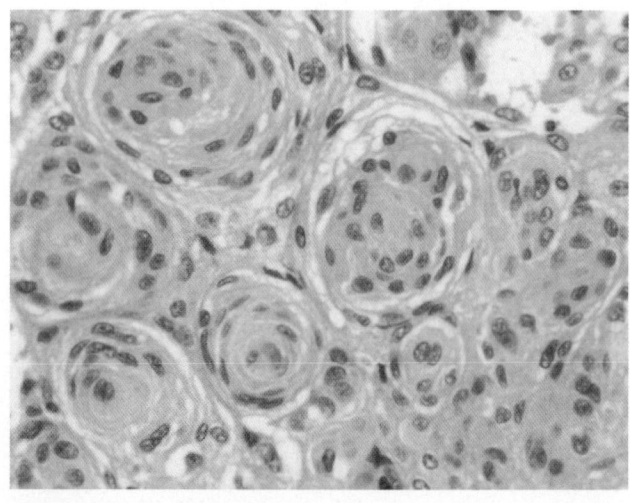

FIGURE 37-24. Meningioma (×200).

diffuse astrocytoma is between 5 and 8 years (104). Variation in length of survival depends on patient age, performance status at diagnosis, and total versus partial tumor resection (105-107).

OD is a diffusely infiltrative, well-differentiated tumor composed of oligodendrocytes. These tumors comprise 3 to 4% of all primary brain tumors and approximately 7% of glial tumors, with an incidence of 0.3 per 100,000 per year. The peak incidence is from the ages of 30 to 50. Children can be affected and represent approximately 6% of all patients with OD. Tumors with pure OD differentiation behave more indolently than astrocytomas. ODs appear to be more sensitive to both chemotherapy and radiation therapy than astrocytomas, and the benefit from these therapies is more pronounced and durable. Median survival ranges from 4 to 12 years, and both OD and oligoastrocytoma (OA) have been included in the reported data (104).

OA is a mixed tumor composed of cells that resemble both OD and diffuse astrocytoma. Based on only a few cytogenetic studies, these tumors are thought to be of monoclonal origin (108). Clinically, these tumors present in a similar fashion to other low-grade glial tumors, which are best imaged with MRI and have imaging characteristics that indicate a diffuse, nonenhancing tumor. There has been no demonstration of a better prognosis with an increased proportion of the OD component. Treatment is similar to that for other low-grade glial tumors. Median survival ranges from 3 to 6 years. In general, these mixed tumors behave more aggressively than pure ODs but are possibly less malignant than pure astrocytomas (109).

CLINICAL MANAGEMENT

Once a diagnosis of low-grade glioma is suspected, it is typical to probe this diagnosis with biopsy or resection so as to differentiate between a low-grade glioma and a nonenhancing anaplastic glioma (Tables 37-2 and 37-3).

In cases where gross total resection or a major resection is possible without significant morbidity,

TABLE 37-2	INITIAL BRAIN TUMOR WORKUP
Contrast-enhanced MRI or MR spectroscopy may be helpful to diagnose nonenhancing tumors
Referral to neurosurgery for resection versus biopsy for tissue diagnosis
Confirmation of pathology with second opinion
Postoperative MRI taken within 3 days of surgery

MRI, magnetic resonance imaging.

TABLE 37-3	EVALUATION BY TUMOR TYPE
Astrocytoma, oligodendroglioma, anaplastic astrocytoma Anaplastic oligodendroglioma, glioblastoma
MRI brain (with and without contrast)
MRI spine (with and without contrast) only if patient is symptomatic
Primary CNS lymphoma
MRI brain and spine (with and without contrast)
Lumbar puncture
Ophthalmology evaluation including slit-lamp examination
CT chest/abdomen/pelvis

CNS, central nervous system; CT, computed tomography; MRI, magnetic resonance imaging.

neuro-oncologists generally recommend a complete resection, which may obviate the need for irradiation and decrease the risk of malignant transformation from residual tumor cells. It has been shown in multiple retrospective series that a total resection of nonenhancing tumor improves survival (104), and a volumetric analysis of the preoperative tumor in addition to analysis of postoperative residual tumor showed a correlation with time to recurrence and the likelihood of malignant transformation (110). There are several low-grade tumors—such as pilocytic astrocytoma, ependymoma and subependymoma, pleomorphic xanthoastrocytoma, ganglioglioma, and dysembryoplastic neuroepithelial tumor—that may be definitively treated by complete surgical resection alone. These patients may benefit from treatment at a specialized neurosurgic center that treats a large volume of brain tumors (Table 37-4 and Fig. 37-25).

TABLE 37-4	MANAGEMENT OF LOW-GRADE GLIOMAS
Confirmation of diagnosis with biopsy is preferred, although observation is acceptable with close follow-up.
Option for complete resection should be considered.
Options after diagnosis include observation (especially if patient is at high risk for treatment morbidity) or treatment (especially if patient is symptomatic).
Radiation therapy is the current standard of treatment (focal brain irradiation to 54 Gy), although the role of chemotherapy is being investigated.
Formal serial neuropsychologic testing is helpful in assessing cognitive function.
Consider use of psychostimulants to improve cognitive function and quality of life.
Consider biopsy/resection of progressive tumor to confirm diagnosis and consider same salvage regimens as for malignant glioma.

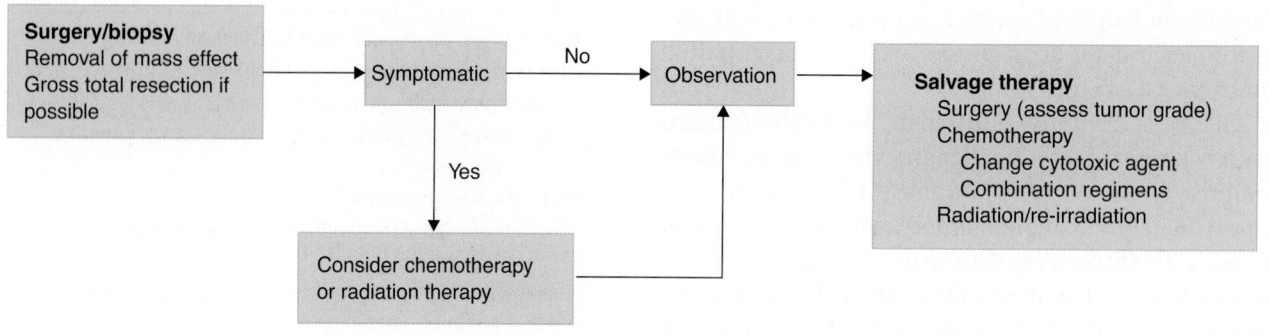

FIGURE 37-25. Treatment algorithm for low-grade glioma.

In cases where a complete resection is not recommended, therapeutic options range from observation to treatment with focal brain irradiation. Older studies of low-grade astrocytomas suggested that radiation improved survival. The 5-year survival rates ranged from 49 to 68% for irradiated tumors compared with 32% for nonirradiated tumors (111). The EORTC 22845 trial randomized patients to either upfront radiotherapy (54 Gy in 6 weeks) or delayed radiation therapy at progression. The patients were randomized and stratified to control for institution, tumor pathology, and amount of resection. One-hundred and fifty-seven patients were assigned to each group, and PFS was 5.3 years in the early radiation group and 3.4 years in the control group. Overall survival, however, was 7.4 years in the upfront radiation group versus 7.2 years in the control group (112). No data was collected on quality of life. The use of this data as a guide suggests that it is acceptable to delay radiation therapy until there are signs of tumor progression, especially for asymptomatic patients or patients who have had a complete tumor resection.

Patients with low-grade glioma should be carefully assessed to determine whether their symptoms are caused by the tumor. Formal neuropsychologic testing may reveal cognitive deficits that are not apparent in the simple mental status screening used for dementia. In addition, these tests can be repeated to detect subtle cognitive decline, which may lead to a decision to alter a prescribed therapy. Patients who are symptomatic from their tumor from seizures, altered mental status due to tumor bulk or location, or who have other focal neurologic signs would be expected to improve with treatment of the tumor. Although there are concerns about the long-term effects of brain irradiation, radiation therapy is the current treatment standard (113). The

dose of radiotherapy currently used by the Radiation Therapy Oncology Group (RTOG) for low-grade glioma is 54 Gy to localized treatment fields as defined by the tumor's appearance on T2-weighted MRI and including a 2-cm margin. A large European trial involving 379 patients with low-grade glioma did not demonstrate a benefit for higher radiation dose when comparing 45 Gy with 59.4 Gy (114). A second prospective study that randomized 203 patients with low-grade glioma to radiation therapy with either 50.4 or 64.8 Gy found a slightly lower survival (64 versus 72% at 5 years) and higher incidence of radiation necrosis in the group receiving the higher dose of 64.8 Gy (115).

Much less is known about the usefulness of chemotherapy for low-grade tumors. A small study of patients with incompletely resected tumors randomized to radiotherapy alone or radiotherapy with CCNU (lomustine) demonstrated a median survival time of 4.5 years with no difference between the two treatment arms (116). A RTOG trial (RTOG 98-02) that randomized patients with low-grade glioma and a high risk of recurrence (age ≥40 or subtotal resection/biopsy) to either radiation therapy alone or radiation therapy followed by six cycles of procarbazine, CCNU, and vincristine (PCV) was closed to accrual in 2002 and continues with follow-up. The usefulness of chemotherapy as an initial treatment for patients with low-grade gliomas is unproven (117). The rationale for using chemotherapy as an alternative to radiation therapy for these patients is that although radiation therapy has a proven record of treatment response, it does not improve survival and may be associated with the significant long-term side effect of cognitive decline. It is hoped that chemotherapy will delay the need for radiation therapy without reducing treatment efficacy or survival (118). Several limited studies have demonstrated an encouraging radiographic response by low-grade gliomas (primarily ODs but also astrocytomas) after treatment with temozolomide and PCV (62,119-123). Patients who have residual tumor and would be at a high risk of cognitive side effects from radiation therapy may benefit from this strategy; however, there are no results from prospective randomized studies to recommend it. Patients with OD or OA may be more attractive candidates for applying this strategy as they tend to have higher response rates to chemotherapy than patients with astrocytoma. The cytogenetic analysis of the tumor sample for LOH at 1p and 19q may predict patients who might benefit from this strategy.

The etiology of cognitive decline in primary brain tumor patients is multifactorial. The causes include direct tumor effects from invasion and destruction as well as side effects from radiation therapy, chemotherapy, and anticonvulsants (113). We have found the use of psychostimulants such as methylphenidate to be helpful in improving cognitive function, mood, and fatigue (124).

■ MALIGNANT GLIOMAS—GRADES III AND IV

The survival of patients who have primary malignant brain tumors is unsatisfactory; it is particularly dismal for those with WHO grade IV tumors. The National Cancer Institute Surveillance, Epidemiology, and End Results (SEER) program reported a 32% 5-year survival from 1992 to 1998. These data include survival statistics for both WHO grade III and grade IV tumors (125). The median survival of patients with GB, the most common primary glioma, has remained at approximately 12 months in recent clinical trials (126-128).

ANAPLASTIC OLIGODENDROGLIOMA

AODs comprise between 20 and 50% of all oligodendroglial tumors, approximately 5% of anaplastic tumors, and between 20 and 50% of all oligodendroglial tumors. The peak incidence is between ages 40 and 50. The clinical presentation of these tumors is similar to that of other anaplastic tumors, with focal neurologic signs, seizures, or symptoms of increased intracranial pressure. These lesions, which are usually contrast-enhancing, can show calcification on CT scans as well as cystic structures, necrosis, and hemorrhage. The standard therapy for AOD does not significantly differ from that used for other anaplastic gliomas (WHO grade III). Initial therapy is surgery, with the goal of gross total resection, followed by radiation therapy. AOD is more responsive to chemotherapy than AA. Adjuvant chemotherapy is recommended, and although PCV is the most studied regimen, temozolomide is usually favored for its more tolerable toxicity profile.

Increasing evidence has shown that codeletion of 1p and 19q portends a more favorable prognosis for patients with both ODs and AODs, although its usefulness as a predictive marker for treatment response has not yet been validated. In the RTOG 9402 study, both classical oligodendroglial morphology and 1p 19q deletion remained significantly associated with PFS and OS in both treatment arms (102). This finding was supported by the EORTC 26951 as well, and increased survival of both AOD and anaplastic oligoastrocytoma (AOA) with 1p/19q codeletion has been noted regardless of the treatment given: radiation alone or radiation with chemotherapy (129). Further study is ongoing from the RTOG/NCCTG/EORTC trial to determine if chemotherapy (PCV or Temozolomide) can replace radiation and maintain this survival benefit.

Despite initially high response rates, these tumors usually recur. Many centers, including MD Anderson, are treating codeleted AOD and AOA with Temozolomide initially and utilizing radiation later for progressive disease. Median survival for AOD treated with surgery, irradiation, and chemotherapy ranges from 3 to 5 years, although some patients survive past 10 years (109,130). Recurrent tumors are treated with salvage regimens similar to those used for AA and GB (Tables 37-5 and 37-6).

ANAPLASTIC ASTROCYTOMA

AAs are diffusely infiltrating with nuclear atypia and anaplasia as well as marked proliferation, features that distinguish them from low-grade astrocytomas. The highest incidence of this tumor is in the fourth decade, followed by the third decade, with nearly equal incidence rates in the second, fifth, and sixth decades. These tumors account for approximately 7.5% of all glial tumors (6).

Patients with AA can present with seizures but are more likely to show signs of increased intracranial pressure and focal neurologic deficits. Some patients have a history of prior low-grade astrocytoma. Brain imaging shows diffuse hypointense tumor on CT scans and T1-weighted MRI. There is usually more mass effect and edema compared with low-grade astrocytomas and contrast enhancement is typical. However, since these tumors can occasionally be nonenhancing, neuroimaging alone is not sufficient to distinguish

TABLE 37-5	MANAGEMENT OF MALIGNANT GLIOMAS

Consider clinical trials at all stages, especially up front, adjuvant, and at relapse (especially at first or second recurrence).

Multidisciplinary approach is necessary for optimal outcome:
- Neurosurgery
- Neuro-oncology
- Radiation therapy
- Psychiatry
- Neuropsychology
- Rehabilitation
- Social work

Maximal resection when possible.

Standard conformal radiation therapy—chemoradiation (temozolomide) for glioblastoma.

Adjuvant chemotherapy for both anaplastic glioma (temozolomide or nitrosourea regimens) and glioblastoma (temozolomide).

Avoid use of anticonvulsants that induce cytochrome P-450 3A4 metabolism when possible (Table 30-7).

Progressive disease
- Consider clinical trials.
- Consider surgical resection at relapse (especially to rule out radiation necrosis).
- Salvage chemotherapy agents include single-agent and combination regimens incorporating temozolomide, nitrosoureas, retinoic acid, irinotecan, and platinum agents.
- Consider stereotactic radiotherapy.

TABLE 37-6	CHEMOTHERAPY REGIMENS FOR GLIOMAS

Temozolomide
75 mg/m^2/day PO days 1-42 during radiotherapy
200 mg/m^2/day PO days 1-5 (patients with no prior chemotherapy)
or
150 mg/m^2/day PO days 1-5 (patients with prior chemotherapy)

Temozolomide and CRA (repeat every 28 days) 200 mg/m^2/day PO days 1-5 (patients with no prior chemotherapy)
or
150 mg/m^2/day PO days 1-5 (patients with prior chemotherapy)
with
13–*cis*-retinoic acid 100 mg/m^2/days 1-21

Temozolomide and irinotecan
Temozolomide 150 mg/m^2/day PO days 1-5 (patients with prior chemotherapy)
with
Irinotecan 200 mg/m^2/day IV days 1 and 14
or
Irinotecan 450 mg/m^2/day IV days 1 and 14 (if the patient is on a cytochrome P-450–inducing anticonvulsant)

Irinotecan (repeat every 3 weeks)
$300\text{-}350 \text{ mg/m}^2$/day IV day 1
or
$700\text{-}750 \text{ mg/m}^2$/day IV day 1 (if patient receiving cytochrome P-450–inducing anticonvulsant)

PCV (repeat every 6 weeks)
Procarbazine
60 mg/m^2/day PO days 8-21
Lomustine
110 mg/m^2/day PO day 1
Vincristine
1.4 mg/m^2/day IV days 8 and 29 (maximum dose = 2 mg)

Carmustine (repeat every 6 weeks)
80 mg/m^2/day IV days 1-3

6-Thioguanine and carmustine (repeat every 6 weeks)
6-Thioguanine
$80\text{-}100 \text{ mg/m}^2$ PO every 6 h for 12 doses followed by carmustine
80 mg/m^2/day IV days 1-3

TPCH (repeat every 6 weeks)
6-Thioguanine
$80\text{-}100 \text{ mg/m}^2$ PO every 6 h for 12 doses, days 1-4
Procarbazine
70 mg/m^2 PO every 6 h for 6 doses, days 4-6
Lomustine
130 mg/m^2 PO 6 h after third procarbazine dose on day 5
Hydroxyurea
600 mg/m^2 PO every 6 h for 11 doses, days 5-8
except at time of lomustine dosing

CRA (repeat every 28 days)
13–*cis*-retinoic acid
100 mg/m^2/day PO in two divided doses, days 1-21

these lesions from low-grade astrocytomas. The median survival for patients with anaplastic astrocytoma ranges from 3 to 5 years; an increased survival is seen when chemotherapy is used in addition to radiotherapy. Optimal initial management begins with surgery with the goal of gross total resection, both to provide adequate tissue for accurate analysis of pathology and to improve survival. Following surgery, limited-field radiation therapy to a target dose of 60 Gy is commonly recommended. The target radiation field typically includes the contrast-enhancing region of the tumor as well as the surrounding edema or nonenhancing tumor plus a 2-cm margin. This size of this field is often reduced after a 46-Gy dose has been applied to the contrast-enhancing lesion alone plus a 2-cm margin. Chemotherapy has been used during irradiation in an effort to improve radiation sensitivity and efficacy. Hydroxyurea and bromodeoxyuridine have been used safely, but there is no randomized trial demonstrating benefit with this strategy compared to chemotherapy following standard radiation. Clinical trials using alternate radiation schemes of hyperfractionation or accelerated fractionation have not demonstrated an increased survival benefit over conventional fractionated conformal radiation therapy (130,131). Adjuvant chemotherapy following radiation therapy increases time to progression and survival. Standard agents include combination therapy composed of procarbazine/lomustine/vincristine (PCV) or another nitrosourea-based regimen of 6-thioguanine/bischloroethylnitrosourea (6TG +BCNU) (see Table 37-6). Temozolomide is the newest alkylating agent to show activity against anaplastic astrocytoma and GB (126,132). Delivered via an oral route, it is better tolerated by patients than PCV combination.

Patients with recurrent anaplastic astrocytoma should be considered for clinical trials. Surgical resection should also be considered to provide a palliative benefit, relieve mass effect, allow dose reduction of steroids, and confirm histology. The recurrent tumor may actually have progressed to GB from AA, and such patients are often eligible for a wider array of clinical trials than are available for recurrent AA. Recent clinical trials have used temolozomide in combination with agents such as IFNα, *cis*-retinoic acid, metalloproteinase inhibitors, carmustine, irinotecan, and thalidomide (133-135). Other agents that have been used for recurrent AA include tamoxifen, carboplatin, etoposide, irinotecan, and combination chemotherapy. Stereotactic radiosurgery for recurrent tumors can also provide benefit if recurrence is local and if it can be targeted to limit dosage to the often previously irradiated tissue (Fig. 37-26).

GLIOBLASTOMA

GB is the most common and most malignant glial tumor of the brain and comprises approximately 50% of all glial tumors, with an incidence of approximately 2 to 3 per 100,000 per year (6). GBs are characterized by poorly differentiated astrocytes with cellular polymorphism, nuclear atypia, microvascular proliferation, and necrosis. The peak incidence is in the fifth decade, followed by the sixth and fourth decades. GB is rare in children and young adults (6,136). Clinically, these tumors often present with signs of increased intracranial pressure such as headache. They also present with focal neurologic symptoms such as hemiparesis and aphasia, often with a short history of symptoms. Seizures are common. Imaging with CT or MRI usually reveals a contrast-enhancing lesion with irregular borders, frequently with a necrotic center. Vasogenic edema and nonenhancing tumor often surround the area of contrast enhancement, which is best seen on T2-weighted or FLAIR imaging on MRI. GBs commonly spread through white matter tracts across the corpus callosum, internal capsule, and optic radiations. Multifocal lesions are possible. If these multiple lesions truly arise independently as opposed to spreading diffusely through tracts that are not visualized by imaging or pathology, they may have a polyclonal origin. GB is extremely lethal. Despite extensive clinical research, the rate of survival has not changed greatly during the last 20 years. Median survival is 9 to 14 months with a 5-year survival rate of approximately 3% (4). Prognostic factors include age and KPS (Karnofsky Performance Scale). Surgical resection

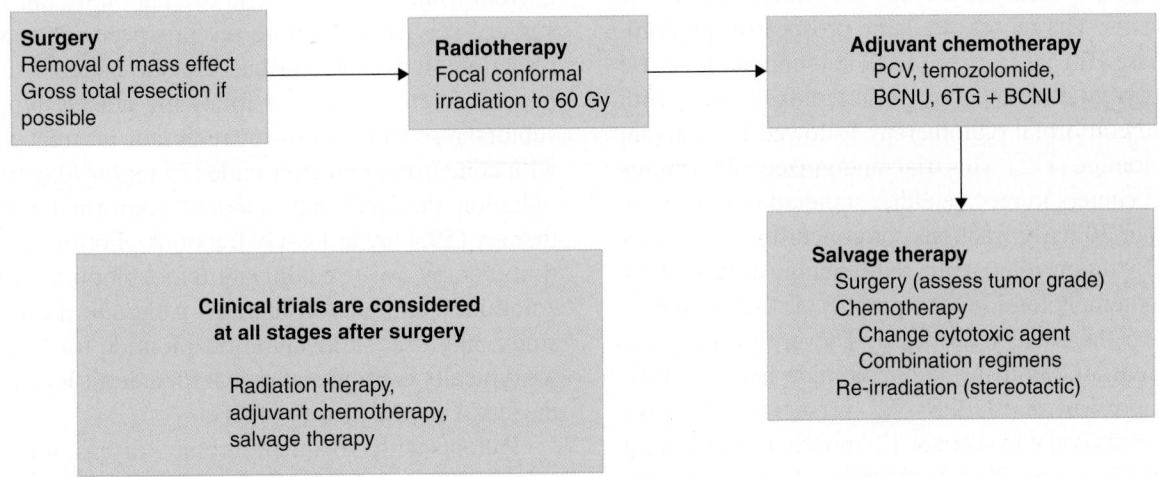

FIGURE 37-26. Treatment algorithm for anaplastic astrocytoma.

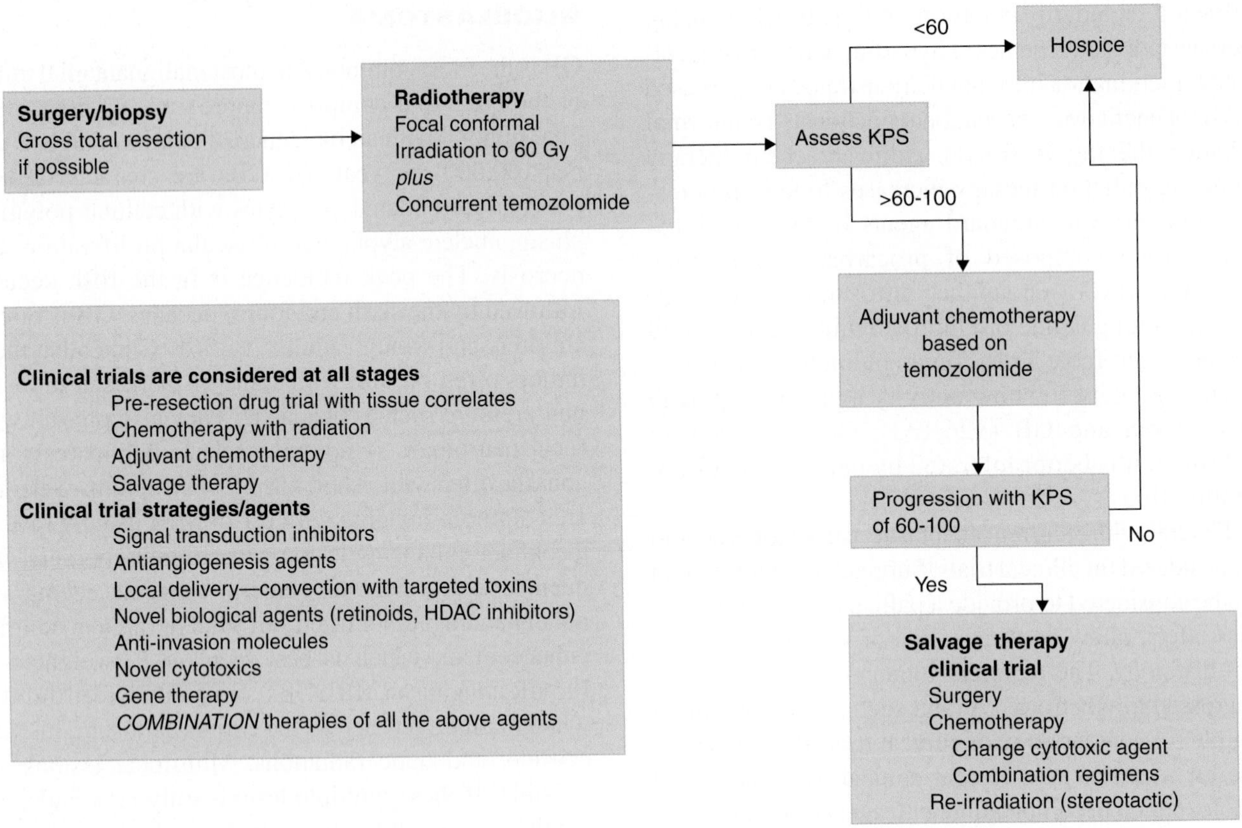

FIGURE 37-27. Treatment algorithm for glioblastoma.

has shown some benefit, especially gross total resection (of enhancing tumor) or when 90% or more of the tumor is removed (137). There are also intriguing data indicating that the volume of residual GB tumor may correlate with subsequent response to chemotherapy, with a higher likelihood of response if the residual tumor volume is less than 10 cm^3 (138) (Fig. 37-27).

The current standard therapy for GB changed in the last 5 years. The report of a large prospective randomized phase III trial from the EORTC supported the use of concurrent chemotherapy with temozolomide, with standard conformal radiotherapy followed by adjuvant temozolomide (112). This trial randomized 573 patients from 85 centers to receive either standard radiotherapy (60 Gy in 30 daily fractions) or concurrent temozolomide (75 mg/m^2/day) with radiotherapy followed by adjuvant temozolomide for 6 months (150-200 mg/m^2/day for 5 days every 28 days). The group receiving concurrent and adjuvant temozolomide had a significant improvement in PFS (7.2 versus 5.0 months), median survival (15 versus 12 months), and 2-year survival (26 versus 8%). Both groups had similar age, KPS, and surgical resection rates. Previously, although

investigators had suspected that adjuvant chemotherapy could be of benefit, no phase III trials supported this strategy.

Our center continues to strongly recommend patient participation in clinical trials, which enroll patients from initial resection to radiation therapy and salvage therapy at relapse. If the patient is not enrolled in an upfront trial, we recommend evaluation by our neurosurgery service to explore the prospect of gross total resection. It is not unusual for our patients to have repeat resection of tumor following outside biopsy or subtotal resection. Following resection, we treat patients with concurrent temozolomide (75 mg/m^2/day through radiation therapy) and standard conformal radiation therapy (59.4 Gy in 1.8-Gy fractions). Following radiation therapy, we use adjuvant temozolomide or temozolomide combination therapy. Although the EORTC study only used adjuvant temozolomide for 6 months, we typically continue treatment for at least 1 year, given the lethal natural history of GB.

Patients with GB and progressive disease are offered salvage therapy if their KPS is adequate. We consider options including resection of tumor, chemotherapy, and stereotactic radiation therapy. Some novel neurosurgical clinical trials have offered local therapy with gene therapy using *p53*, although this was limited by lack of dispersion of the therapy into surrounding tissues (139). An IL-13–conjugated *Pseudomonas* exotoxin has been studied using convection-enhanced delivery to lead to higher tissue concentration with larger volumes of distribution in phase I (140,141). Another ongoing trial uses a conditionally replication-competent adenovirus (Delta-24-RGD) injected into the resection cavity for recurrent malignant gliomas.

One advantage of re-resection of progressive disease is to confirm pathology and specifically to determine whether the progressive enhancement on MRI represents tumor or radiation necrosis. MRI dynamic contrast imaging, MR spectroscopy, FDG-PET scanning, and brain SPECT thallium imaging sometimes help to distinguish between these two possibilities. However, all of these modalities have limited sensitivity and specificity, and sometimes the pathology reveals both treatment-related necrosis and foci of active tumor. Patients with pathology-confirmed radiation necrosis are often treated with steroids and antiplatelet agents or anticoagulation, whose putative value is based on anecdotal case reports (142). Hyperbaric oxygen therapy has also been reported to produce a radiologic response (143,144). More recently, bevacizumab, a monoclonal antibody targeted against the vascular endothelial growth factor (VEGF) has been utilized to treat radiation necrosis with promising results (145,146).

Chemotherapy for recurrent disease typically produces response rates that are less than 10% and a 6-month PFS of 15% (4). Response rates that include stable disease and complete or partial responses are 40% at best, but as the 6-month progression-free survival value indicates, these responses are not durable. It is hypothesized that the multiple mutations and alterations in GB and the heterogeneity of the tumor cell population may partially explain the striking resistance of these tumors to therapy. Younger patients respond best to chemotherapy, although responses to alkylating agents can be seen in patients older than 60 years of age. Long-term survivors of GB (over 5 years) have typically had gross total resection, radiation therapy to a dose of 60 Gy, and chemotherapy, generally with temozolomide or a nitrosourea or other alkylating agent.

Salvage agents used for malignant glioma are identical to those used for recurrent AA (see Table 37-6). After treatment failure with temozolomide and nitrosourea-based therapy (PCV, 6TG, and BCNU), switching to a biologic agent such as high-dose *cis*-retinoic acid may be

helpful, especially as it does not cause myelosuppression (147). Most recently, bevacizumab has been approved by the FDA for progressive disease following prior therapy, based on two trials. One study showed a 6-month PFS of 42% and overall survival of 8.7 months in patients receiving bevacizumab alone (148). Another study showed a 19.6% response rate with median duration of 3.9 months. PFS at 6 months was 29%, and 6 month survival was 57%. Additionally, 50% of patients experienced decreased cerebral edema, 58% were able to decrease their corticosteroid dependency, and 52% had improvement in their neurologic symptoms (149)

Other active agents include irinotecan (150), carboplatin, and etoposide (151). Other agents targeting angiogenesis have also been studied, although the use of interferon, thalidomide, epidermal growth factor–receptor tyrosine kinase antagonists, and integrin receptor antagonists is not yet standard. In general, many of these targeted therapies demonstrated only limited activity as single agents and efforts are under way to combine them with cytotoxic therapy (152,153). Other cellular pathways being investigated with small-molecule inhibitors include the *ras* pathway with farnesyl-transferase inhibitors and the PI3Kinase pathway with *mTOR* inhibitors. Other novel approaches to malignant brain tumor therapy include use of oncolytic adenovirus, vaccine and dendritic cell immunotherapy, and histone deacetylase inhibitors (see Fig. 37-27).

An important reaction has been discovered from the interaction between anticonvulsants that induce the hepatic cytochrome P-450 3A4 enzyme and other chemotherapy agents also metabolized by this same enzyme. Pharmacokinetic studies of patients with malignant glioma on single-agent irinotecan and sirolimus found significantly lower levels of active drug in patients on enzyme-inducing anticonvulsant drugs (EIAEDs) (154,155). In a phase I trial of irinotecan administered every 3 weeks, the recommended dose for patients not on enzyme-inducing agents was 350 mg/m^2, whereas the dose for patients on enzyme-inducing agents was 750 mg/m^2. Based on pharmacologic data, our patients on EIAEDs receiving irinotecan every 2 weeks are given 340 mg/m^2, and patients not taking EIAEDs receive 125 mg/m^2 (148). We recommend that brain tumor patients on chemotherapy avoid use of anticonvulsants that induce the expression of the P-450 3A4 enzyme whenever possible (see Table 37-7).

SEIZURE CONTROL

The management of seizures in brain tumor patients is important in order to improve patient functioning and

TABLE 37-7	CYTOCHROME P-450 3A4–INDUCING AGENTS (ANTICONVULSANTS IN RED)
Carbamazepine	Phenytoin
Dexamethasone	Primidone
Ethosuximide	Progesterone
Glucocorticoids	Rifabutin
Griseofulvin	Rifampin
Nafcillin	Rofecoxib (mild)
Nelfinavir	St. John's wort
Nevirapine	Sulfadimidine
Oxcarbazepine	Sulfinpyrazone
Phenobarbital	Troglitazone
Phenylbutazone	

quality of life. A degeneration of seizure control in brain tumor patients may indicate tumor progression and worsening edema. However, it may also indicate a systemic infection or a drug interaction leading to decreased anticonvulsant drug levels. In the case of tumor progression, a reduction in the amount of brain edema through the use of high-potency corticosteroids (dexamethasone) may be sufficient to prevent further seizures. However, often a second anticonvulsant is necessary. It should also be noted that dexamethasone is a hepatic P-450 3A4–inducing agent. We often see a reduction in serum levels of phenytoin or carbamazepine (also enzyme inducers) when the dose of dexamethasone is increased. Similarly, patients can become symptomatic with toxic levels of anticonvulsants in the middle of a dexamethasone taper. It is important to follow serum anticonvulsant levels when using agents metabolized by the cytochrome P-450 system. Anticonvulsants that are highly protein-bound can demonstrate significant changes in levels of circulating free drug without significantly changing the total serum level. It is useful to check serum-free phenytoin or valproic acid levels when patients taking these agents have seizures or show signs of toxicity. Unfortunately, despite the numerous choices of anticonvulsants, it can be quite difficult to control seizures in brain tumor patients. Of the newer generation of anticonvulsants, we have had success using levetiracetam (Keppra), which is easily titrated without significant drug interactions, and topiramate (Topamax), which is one of the few anticonvulsants associated with weight loss and not weight gain. Phenobarbital and clonazepam can also be useful in resistant cases. Short-term use of lorazepam (Ativan) can be helpful to bridge changes in anticonvulsant regimens. Ultimately, if the tumor is successfully treated, the resulting reduction in mass effect and edema will improve seizure control.

It is critical to provide effective supportive care to brain tumor patients to improve their functional status, as well as quality of life for themselves and their caregivers. Unfortunately, this care is typically very labor-intensive and often beyond the means of patients and their families to provide. We involve social work and case management early in the treatment of brain tumor patients. They can provide interventions that may prevent a later breakdown in care. The incidence of depression is high among this population and should be treated early. The causes of depression are typically multifactorial and may include direct effects of the tumor, side effects of chemotherapy and radiation therapy, and side effects of steroids in addition to issues associated with a loss of independence and a diagnosis of cancer. We suggest referral to psychiatry to optimally address these issues. A related concern is the impact of fatigue in this population. A common side effect of brain radiation therapy is somnolence and fatigue. We advocate use of psychostimulants such as methylphenidate to treat both fatigue and cognitive side effects (124). Although there are theoretical concerns that the use of stimulants in this population may exacerbate seizures, we have not observed this in practice.

Brain tumor patients often require high doses of steroids to manage edema, and they experience both acute and chronic toxicity from their administration. Acutely, the steroids may induce hyperglycemia requiring an insulin sliding scale. Patients often become agitated, irritable, suffer extreme mood swings, and even become psychotic when taking steroids. Low-dose standing neuroleptics can be effective in treating these side effects. Clinicians should aim to taper steroid use to the lowest doses necessary. Patients typically tolerate initial steroid weaning but often experience fatigue or worsening of neurologic function as dexamethasone doses fall below 4 mg daily. This can be ameliorated somewhat by providing an extremely slow steroid taper and only lowering doses every week to 2 weeks by increments of 1 mg or even 0.5 mg. The use of psychostimulants can help treat the inevitable fatigue patients experience as they taper the steroid dose. There is no effective treatment for steroid myopathy other than tapering off steroids and prescribing physical therapy and rehabilitation as early as possible.

MENINGIOMA

Meningiomas comprise 32.1% of all primary brain tumors, with a rate of 5.35 per 100,000 person-years.

The incidence of meningioma rises with age, and the median age at diagnosis is 64 (6). The tumor is often discovered incidentally without any symptoms. Clinically, these tumors typically present with headache, cognitive or personality changes, persistent focal neurologic deficits, and sometimes seizure. The main treatment for these tumors is surgical resection, with the goal of complete resection when possible, accounting for relative risks and benefits depending on the patient's age and condition (156). Options for residual tumor include observation and radiation therapy, which can incorporate stereotactic delivery to minimize effects to local tissue (157-159).

Chemotherapy for meningioma has been used for patients who have progressive disease after resection and radiotherapy; it is sometimes used adjuvantly following radiotherapy when pathology indicates malignant meningioma. In general, response rates have been disappointing in small case series. Chemotherapy agents that have been used include hydroxyurea (160,161), IFNα (162,163), and liposomal doxorubicin (164). Results using temozolomide have been discouraging, with no responders (165). As there are no established treatments after surgery and radiation have been exhausted, and response to chemotherapy has been disappointing, the use of targeted agents is being explored. The epidermal growth factor receptor (EGFR) is frequently overexpressed in meningiomas. Clinical trials using small-molecule signal transduction inhibitors such as erlotinib, gefitinib, and imatinib are still being explored, but have not yet shown significant efficacy (166,167).

PRIMARY CNS LYMPHOMA

In contrast to most other brain tumors, chemotherapy is the initial treatment of choice for CNS lymphoma. The incorporation of high-dose methotrexate (>1 g/m^2) has resulted in a significantly greater response and improved survival compared to previous regimens that used a CHOP regimen prior to whole-brain radiation therapy. Although 64% of patients in one study responded to CHOP prior to radiation therapy, their median survival was 9.6 months, but it was 20.7 months for those who were able to complete the entire regimen (168). The report by DeAngelis, incorporating methotrexate (1 g/m^2), followed by whole-brain irradiation and two cycles of high-dose cytarabine (ara-C) (3 g/m^2), demonstrated a median survival of 42.5 months (169). This strategy is the basis for current CNS lymphoma protocols that have increased the dose of methotrexate and incorporated agents that more easily cross the BBB, such as procarbazine. A follow-up clinical trial incorporating

methotrexate at 3.5 g/m^2 with procarbazine and vincristine, followed by whole-brain irradiation and cytarabine demonstrated a median survival of 60 months (170). The improvement in patient survival has also brought to attention the significant rates of cognitive decline and radiation-induced dementia, especially in patients above age 60 (171,172). Current approaches to therapy of CNS lymphoma are investigating whether radiation therapy can be avoided or delayed in the hope of reducing rates of cognitive decline and dementia without adversely affecting survival. Preliminary results from a trial using single-agent methotrexate at 8 g/m^2 every 2 weeks demonstrated a PFS of 12.8 months. Median survival had not been reached at 22.8+ months (173). Many clinicians at our center are cautiously delaying radiation therapy until relapse and continuing to use high-dose–based methotrexate regimens. In hopes of improving the results of the single-agent methotrexate study (173), some regimens continue to incorporate procarbazine. Other agents that may be active in this setting include temozolomide and rituximab.

Patients with recurrent disease may respond to methotrexate a second time. Other regimens that have been used include PCV (174), high-dose cytarabine (171), temozolomide (175), rituximab (176), and the combination of temozolomide and rituximab (177).

BRAIN METASTASIS

To achieve optimal results, the treatment of brain metastasis involves taking into account the interaction between oncology, neurosurgery, and radiation therapy. Depending on the setting of relapse, patient survival may depend more on local tumor control in the brain or on systemic control for progressive metastasis. Advances in local brain tumor control with surgery and radiosurgery will not improve patient survival if the patient ultimately succumbs to progressive systemic disease or continues to develop new brain metastasis. Overall, the median survival of patients with brain metastases is 3 to 6 months (178). Local therapy and systemic chemotherapy will need further development to improve patient survival.

The options for therapy include surgical resection, whole-brain irradiation, stereotactic radiosurgery if the target is smaller than 3 cm, and systemic chemotherapy. The advantage of surgical resection is that mass effect can be immediately ameliorated and removal of the tumor decreases edema. Surgical resection also provides pathologic confirmation of diagnosis. Surgery can be considered for large lesions that are not amenable to stereotactic radiosurgery. The drawback of surgery is the need for an invasive procedure that requires general anesthesia, especially in a patient who has additional sites of metastatic disease and who has an elevated medical risk for surgical complications.

Whole-brain radiation therapy (30 Gy in 10 fractions) is the standard therapy for brain metastasis, with an established body of literature supporting its use for multiple metastases. Whole-brain irradiation has the ability to eradicate micrometastatic disease to delay recurrence (178,179) and is often used in conjunction with surgical resection or radiosurgery. It is tolerated fairly well and can be very effective for radiosensitive tumors such as metastases from small cell lung cancer or germ cell tumors. However, whole-brain irradiation can be associated with cognitive loss and leukoencephalomalacia.

There is increasing evidence that radiosurgery can effectively achieve local control of a brain metastasis that is smaller than 3 cm. This modality is also less invasive than surgical resection and does not require the patient to undergo general anesthesia. The disadvantage of radiosurgery is that mass effect is not relieved and, in the short term, tumor edema may increase. There are no prospective randomized studies comparing radiosurgery to surgery. Retrospective comparative studies that match similar patient selection criteria have reached opposite conclusions (180,181).

We frequently treat patients at our institution with surgery if their lesions are greater than 3 cm and they are symptomatic. If the patient's medical condition makes a surgical procedure too risky, the patient may receive whole-brain radiation therapy. Patients who have lesions smaller than 3 cm can receive radiosurgery if they are asymptomatic or their lesion is in a deep region that is not amenable to resection. However, patients with symptoms resulting from their lesions more frequently receive surgery to remove mass effect as long as their medical condition permits. There is also debate over the role of whole-brain irradiation following surgery or radiosurgery to single lesions.

CHEMOTHERAPY FOR BRAIN METASTASIS

Several small clinical trials and case reports in the literature support the concept that systemic chemotherapy demonstrates activity in treating brain metastases. Chemosensitive tumor types include breast cancer, small cell lung cancer, and germ cell tumors. The primary consideration in choosing a given regimen of chemotherapy is to use agents with known activity in a given tumor type (182). A confounding problem in brain tumor chemotherapy is the use of corticosteroids, which are often necessary to control cerebral edema, but can reestablish disrupted BBB function, which may impair delivery of chemotherapy (183). A review of treatment with systemic chemotherapy of brain metastases from small cell lung cancer pooled data from five clinical trials. A 66% response rate was demonstrated (184). Unfortunately, this response is not often durable when chemotherapy is used as a single modality, even in cases of complete response.

In many trials, the response rate of brain metastases has been comparable to the response rates of the systemic disease. Patients who have had prior chemotherapy usually respond at lower rates. A small trial of first-line chemotherapy for brain metastases from non–small cell lung cancer demonstrated a response rate of 45%, with an equal number of minor responses and stable disease. The median time to response was 10 weeks and the median duration of response was 25 weeks. However, although the median survival was 33 weeks for the group, it was only 48 weeks for the responders (185). A trial of patients who had failed prior radiotherapy utilizing a multidrug regimen composed of 6-thioguanine, procarbazine, dibromodulcitol, lomustine, 5-flourouracil, and hydroxyurea demonstrated an overall (complete and partial responses and stable disease) response rate of 60% for breast cancer, 52% for non–small cell lung cancer (NSCLC), and 66% for small cell lung cancer (SCLC). The disease-free period of survival for these patients was 27 weeks for breast cancer, 21 weeks for non–small cell lung cancer, and 133 weeks for small cell lung cancer (186). Temozolomide resulted in a modest response and disease control) in 41% of a small group of patients in one study of NSCLC patients. Overall median survival was 6.6 months (187). A case report demonstrated a response of brain metastases to capecitabine following failure of whole-brain irradiation, hormonal therapy, and systemic chemotherapy that included 5-fluorouracil (188).

After demonstrating single-agent activity, the next step is to investigate combination therapy. A trial using a combination of cyclophosphamide, 5-fluorouracil, methotrexate, vincristine, and prednisone for treatment of breast cancer in patients who had not received prior chemotherapy demonstrated a greater than 50% response rate, although the median duration of response was only 7 months (189) Another study of patients with recurrent NSCLC investigated the combination of cisplatin, ifosfamide, and irinotecan in 121 patients. Thirty of these patients had brain metastases and had a 50% response rate without the use of radiotherapy (190). Other strategies for devising combination therapy have used novel biological agents combined with traditional cytotoxic agents. Temozolomide on a daily low-dose schedule combined with thalidomide was given to patients with metastatic melanoma in a small phase I trial. Five major responses were reported using a temozolomide daily dosing schedule of 75 mg/m^2/day, with a median duration of 6 months and median survival of 12.3 months (191). Patients with brain metastases were excluded from the trial because of concern of overlapping neurotoxicity from thalidomide; however, a case report from the same institution demonstrated a complete response of metastatic melanoma to brain and leptomeninges treated with temozolomide combined with thalidomide (192).

Chemotherapy produces a high response rate for brain metastases arising from germ cell tumors. A regimen of etoposide, methotrexate, dactinomycin, vincristine, cyclophosphamide, and cisplatin for gestational choriocarcinoma induced a 72% durable response rate (193). In a study of brain metastases from germinoma, 8 of 10 patients had a complete response to a combination regimen of cisplatin, vincristine, methotrexate, bleomycin, etoposide, dactinomycin, and cyclophosphamide (194).

Considering the widespread prevalence of brain metastases, relatively few clinical trials have addressed this issue. Most clinical trials of investigational agents for solid tumors explicitly exclude patients with brain metastases. Compounding this omission is their common inclusion into studies of a heterogeneous group of patients with mixed tumor types and differing prior exposure to chemotherapy. Patients might also be expected to be more resistant to treatment with chemotherapeutic agents if they have failed radiotherapy. If chemotherapy is given during and after radiotherapy, it may be difficult to separate efficacy due to radiotherapy and efficacy due to chemotherapy. These factors combined make it difficult to compare treatment regimens and meaningfully interpret studies (195). One approach to this problem is to stratify patients according to pretreatment factors. These can be analyzed to determine factors that have prognostic value. The RTOG analyzed a database of 1200 patients using differing radiation fractionation schemes or radiosensitizers for brain metastasis treatment. First, a univariate analysis was performed, which considered 18 pretreatment factors, including age, tumor

histology, control of systemic tumor, neurologic status, KPS, location of lesions, and three treatment-related variables, such as radiation dose. A recursive partitioning analysis (RPA) was performed to rank the significance of these factors. The study grouped patients into 3 classes. Class 1 patients had a KPS ≥70, age <65, a controlled primary tumor site, and no extracranial metastases. Class 3 patients had a KPS <70, and class 2 patients were all others. The median survival was 7.1 months for class 1, 4.2 months for class 2, and only 2.3 months for class 3 patients (178). The validity of this database was verified by a second RPA on a trial of 445 patients randomized to an accelerated hyperfractionation group or to an accelerated fractionation group. Class 1 patients had a median survival of 6.2 months, compared with 7.1 months for the database as a whole, and a 1-year survival of 29%, compared with 32% for the database (179). The use of RPA allows the most important pretreatment prognostic factors to be identified and provides a historic database against which to compare future studies.

Bioimmunotherapy is being assessed for the treatment of patients with malignant melanoma and a few responses have been demonstrated in a setting of brain metastases. A retrospective review at the National Cancer Institute of high-dose IL-2 in 36 patients with evaluable brain metastases found 2 patients with a regression of their brain lesions, a response that reflected the systemic response. The overall response rate for patients with previously untreated brain metastases demonstrated only a 5.6% response rate, compared with 19.8% for patients without brain metastases. The patients with brain metastases did not exhibit excess toxicity compared to the overall group (196). A study of interferon-alpha with IL-2 following chemotherapy with cisplatin, dacarbazine, and carmustine included 15 patients with brain metastases. Seven (47%) of these patients had a partial response, with a median time to progression of 6 months and a median survival of 6.5 months (197).

The use of chemotherapy for brain metastases is faced with great challenges. The most important imperative is to discover new agents that can overcome the resistance of tumor cells to standard chemotherapy agents, whether through selection by prior pretreatment or inherent chemoresistance of tumor cell clones that metastasize from a primary site. Because most patients with brain metastases succumb to progressive systemic disease, improvement of local control in the brain will likely have a limited effect on survival. Conversely, development of agents that are effective in establishing durable tumor control, both systemically and in the brain, will improve survival, as in the unique case of germ cell tumors. If patients with a good performance status who have brain metastases are excluded from clinical trials of novel agents, it will be difficult to accurately determine the possible effectiveness of these agents against CNS disease. The use of RPA may help to identify patients who might benefit from chemotherapy as well as to design clinical trials that take into account specific tumor histology and prior exposure to chemotherapy. Improvement in patient survival will result from improved local control of CNS disease if the primary disease site remains dormant, illustrating the need for a multimodality approach to the treatment of the patient with brain metastases.

Commentary: The Role of Radiation Therapy for Brain Tumors

Radiation therapy is used to enhance local control and overall survival as a sole modality or in combination with surgery and/or chemotherapy for many benign and malignant central nervous system (CNS) tumors.

Radiotherapy is prescribed in the unit of Gray which measures the energy absorbed in a material (J/kg). Typically, radiation treatments are fractionated in 1.8 to 2 Gy per day. The prescribed dose of radiation depends on the inherent radiosensitivity of the lesion and the risk to the normal tissues that are in or close to the radiotherapy volumes. For example, CNS leukemia is treated with 18 to 24 Gy in 10 to 12 fractions; whereas, glioblastoma requires 60 Gy delivered in 30 fractions. The risk of cataract formation increases after a total dose of only 2 Gy, but brain necrosis typically will not occur below a dose of 60 Gy.

A variety of different radiotherapy techniques and modalities are available for treatment of the CNS. All of current treatment techniques—three-dimensional conformal radiotherapy (3DCRT), intensity-modulated radiotherapy (IMRT), stereotactic radiosurgery (SRS), proton therapy, and intensity-modulated proton therapy (IMPT)—use three-dimensional algorithms which calculate dose distributions in all planes and display dose in the axial, coronal, and sagittal views. The tumor and normal tissues are delineated using the planning CT scan and any other imaging modality such as MRI or PET that may facilitate this process. The tumor delineation involves determination of the gross tumor volume (GTV) which represents the macroscopic visible tumor, the clinical target volume (CTV) which is GTV with a margin that incorporates areas of possible microscopic extension, and planning target volume (PTV) that gives an additional margin for day-to-day setup differences.

The basic form of 3D planning is 3DCRT. These plans use conformal fields from different angles optimized to the individual patient's needs. Any radiotherapy modality, that is, photons, electrons, or protons, can be used for 3DCRT.

SRS and fractionated stereotactic radiotherapy (FSRT) are techniques that use stereotactic position using an external fiducial system to immobilize and position patients allowing submillimeter precision for radiotherapy treatments. A large single fraction of radiation is given with SRS; whereas, FSRT uses multiple fractions of repeated doses of radiation with a noninvasive stereotactic frame. SRS is typically used for noninfiltrating tumors that are less than 3 cm and away from critical structures such as the optic chiasm. FSRT may be used for a tumor that is close to a critical structure where the highest precision for delivery is required.

IMRT is typically used with photon beams with a few centers now using it with proton beams (IMPT). Intensity modulation can also be implemented with the stereotactic approach which may allow an increase in precision of delivery and conformality. IMRT plans use multiple beams optimized for the tumor location and patient. For each beam the multileaf collimation varies during the dose delivery to modulate the dose from that beam to "paint" dose to allow improved conformality and reduction in normal tissue doses.

Proton radiotherapy is a modality that is becoming more available worldwide and allows treatment of larger deeper tumors without an exit dose, thereby reducing the volume of normal tissue receiving low to moderate doses which could result in a reduction in acute and late toxicities. Proton radiotherapy may be a useful technology in young patients with curable tumors.

The results of radiotherapy vary according to the type of tumor that is being treated. Benign tumors such as meningiomas or acoustic schwannomas have control rates of as high as 90%, whereas malignant tumors such as glioblastoma have lower durable control rates

Anita Mahajan

Commentary: Surgical Management of Primary Brain Tumors

The primary goal in the surgical management of primary brain tumors like gliomas is a maximum safe resection. The decision to resect or not to resect should be made after close collaboration between the neurosurgeons, neuro-oncologists, and radiation oncologists. The surgeon must consider a number of critical factors prior to making the decision to operate: these include age, neurologic status, location and size of the tumor, number and extent of recurrences, and whether the patient would be suitable for adjuvant treatments including radiation and chemotherapy. In both low-grade (LGG) and high-grade gliomas (HGG) compared with patients having lesser degrees of resection, those undergoing gross total resections have a better neurologic outcome on long-term follow-up without added perioperative morbidity or mortality. Recent surgical series in LGG have shown maximum safe resection if the tumor is an independent predictor of both progression-free and overall survival of patients. Lacroix et al. described 416 consecutive glioblastoma patients, and demonstrated that radical resection of the main tumor mass (≥98% by volumetric analysis) was an independent variable which significantly prolonged patient survival (137). The median survival for these patients was 13.4 months compared with 8.8 months for patients who had lesser resections ($p < .0001$). The study relied on a prospective computerized measurement of the volume of the tumors, with the extent of resection expressed as a percentage of the preoperative volume. Overall the results showed that a 90% resection did not result in a statistically significant prolongation of survival and the greatest benefit was noted when the extent of resection reached 98% or greater. These data are particularly important because of their precision and their avoidance of subjective terms such as "gross total" or "subtotal" to describe degree of resection.

Beyond extending survival, several other benefits can result from more radical resections of gliomas in our experience. These include: (1) a diagnostic advantage in terms of better sampling of tumors and better tissue quality acquired for immunohistochemical and other analysis; (2) a symptomatic advantage through relief of mass effect, leading to improved performance status and enhanced tolerance to radiotherapy; (3) an oncologic advantage by reducing the number of neoplastic cells by almost two logs; and (4) a research advantage by harvesting ample tissue material for molecular analysis and fingerprinting, with the eventual identification of novel and specific molecular targets that will form the basis of the therapies of the future.

Several technological adjuncts to surgery are available to aid in localizing the brain mass, in identifying zones of brain function, and in aiding the surgeon to maintain proper orientation in reference to the mass and to its surrounding anatomic structures. Of these, intraoperative ultrasound is an inexpensive, readily accessible surgical tool that allows localization of the mass in real time and aids in the assessment of the completeness of tumor resection. Most gliomas and metastases are hyperechoic with respect to normal brain and thus can be localized easily with the ultrasound probe. It is, indeed, almost inconceivable to perform such procedures without intraoperative ultrasound.

Frameless stereotactic systems have provided significant assistance on many levels, including adequate placement and sizing of the bone flap, identification of the surface margins, and localization of the mass and the navigational direction of the dissection around or into the mass. The obvious drawback of these systems is their inability to provide a true assessment of residual tumor, because of brain shifts that occur necessarily during surgery. Experience with these systems and correlation of the image-derived data with the ultrasound data and with what is visible in the operative field are necessary for safe use of these techniques in obtaining maximum tumor resection.

Neurophysiologic techniques are employed primarily when the tumor is in or adjacent to eloquent brain. The most commonly used techniques for cortical mapping include somatosensory evoked potentials and direct cortical stimulation. For motor and sensory localization, the patient is usually (although not invariably) under general anesthesia; for speech localization, however, an awake craniotomy is necessary. The introduction of these techniques to surgery for malignant gliomas has made it possible to perform larger resections with an increased margin of safety.

Recently, intraoperative MRI has been introduced in a few centers. This technique identifies residual tumor more accurately than any other method. Its main drawback, however, is substantial in that it includes an expensive and sometimes cumbersome piece of equipment. Early systems had low field strength, and as such were less sensitive and provided more indistinct images than the current generation of such equipment.

Existing data concerning the benefits of surgical resection suggest a survival advantage in patients with gliomas who undergo a complete resection of the tumor mass. Careful preoperative planning should allow for the gross total resection of most gliomas. Until convincing data to the contrary are presented, the goal of a neurooncologic operation should be a complete resection of the tumor mass.

Sujit Prabhu

References

1. Posner JB, Chernik NL. Intracranial metastases from systemic cancer. *Adv Neurol* 1978;19:579-592.

2. Schouten LJ, Rutten J, Huveneers HA, et al. Incidence of brain metastases in a cohort of patients with carcinoma of the breast, colon, kidney, and lung and melanoma. *Cancer* 2002; 94(10):2698-2705.

3. American Cancer Society Cancer Facts and Figures 2009. Surveillance Research. 2009 ed: American Cancer Society, 2009.

4. Wong ET, Hess KR, Gleason MJ, et al. Outcomes and prognostic factors in recurrent glioma patients enrolled onto phase II clinical trials. *J Clin Oncol* 1999;17(8):2572-2578.

5. Sawaya R, Bindal, RK, Lang, FF. Metastatic brain tumors. In: Kaye AH, Laws ER (eds): *Brain Tumors*. London: Churchill Livingstone; 2001.

6. CBTRUS. Statistical Report: Primary Brain Tumors in the United States 2000-2004. Central Brain Tumor Registry of the United States, 2008.

7. Tremont-Lukats IW, Bobustuc G, Lagos GK, et al. Brain metastasis from prostate carcinoma: The M. D. Anderson Cancer Center experience. *Cancer* 2003;98(2):363-368.

8. Patel JK, Didolkar MS, Pickren JW, et al. Metastatic pattern of malignant melanoma. A study of 216 autopsy cases. *Am J Surg* 1978;135(6):807-810.

9. Lang F, Wildrick DM, Sawaya R. Metastatic brain tumors. In: Hazuka MB (ed): *Neuro-Oncology: The Essentials*. New York: Thieme; 2000:329-337.

10. Delattre JY, Krol G, Thaler HT, et al. Distribution of brain metastases. *Arch Neurol* 1988;45(7):741-744.

11. Kadan-Lottick NS, Skluzacek MC, Gurney JG. Decreasing incidence rates of primary central nervous system lymphoma. *Cancer* 2002;95(1):193-202.

12. Cote TR, Manns A, Hardy CR, et al. Epidemiology of brain lymphoma among people with or without acquired immunodeficiency syndrome. AIDS/Cancer Study Group. *J Natl Cancer Inst* 1996;88(10):675-679.

13. Tomlinson FH, Kurtin PJ, Suman VJ, et al. Primary intracerebral malignant lymphoma: A clinicopathological study of 89 patients. *J Neurosurg* 1995;82(4):558-566.

14. DeAngelis LM, Wong E, Rosenblum M, et al. Epstein-Barr virus in acquired immune deficiency syndrome (AIDS) and non-AIDS primary central nervous system lymphoma. *Cancer* 1992;70(6):1607-1611.

15. Nygaard R, Garwicz S, Haldorsen T, et al. Second malignant neoplasms in patients treated for childhood leukemia. A population-based cohort study from the Nordic countries. The Nordic Society of Pediatric Oncology and Hematology (NOPHO). *Acta Paediatr Scand* 1991;80(12):1220-1228.

16. Wrensch M, Bondy ML, Wiencke J, et al. Environmental risk factors for primary malignant brain tumors: A review. *J Neurooncol* 1993;17(1):47-64.

17. Preston-Martin S, Mack W. Neoplasms of the nervous system. *Cancer Epidemiology and Prevention*. New York: Oxford University Press; 1996:1231-1281.

18. Bohnen NI, Kurland LT. Brain tumor and exposure to pesticides in humans: A review of the epidemiologic data. *J Neurol Sci* 1995;132(2):110-121.

19. Wrensch M, Minn Y, Chew T, et al. Epidemiology of primary brain tumors: Current concepts and review of the literature. *Neuro Oncol* 2002;4(4):278-299.

20. Wrensch M, Minn, Y, Bondy, ML. Epidemiology. In: Bernstein M, Berger MS, (eds): *Neuro-Oncology: The Essentials*. New York: Thieme; 2000:2-17.

21. Hurley SF, McNeil JJ, Donnan GA, et al. Tobacco smoking and alcohol consumption as risk factors for glioma: A case-control study in Melbourne, Australia. *J Epidemiol Community Health* 1996;50(4):442-446.

22. Huncharek M, Kupelnick B, Wheeler L. Dietary cured meat and the risk of adult glioma: A meta-analysis of nine observational studies. *J Environ Pathol Toxicol Oncol* 2003;22(2): 129-137.

23. Martini F, De Mattei M, Iaccheri L, et al. Human brain tumors and simian virus 40. *J Natl Cancer Inst* 1995;87(17):1331.

24. Rollison DE, Helzlsouer KJ, Alberg AJ, et al. Serum antibodies to JC virus, BK virus, simian virus 40, and the risk of incident adult astrocytic brain tumors. *Cancer Epidemiol Biomarkers Prev* 2003;12(5):460-463.

25. Strickler HD, Rosenberg PS, Devesa SS, et al. Contamination of poliovirus vaccines with simian virus 40 (1955-1963) and subsequent cancer rates. *JAMA* 1998;279(4):292-295.

26. Linos E, Raine T, Alonso A, et al. Atopy and risk of brain tumors: A meta-analysis. *J Natl Cancer Inst* 2007;99(20): 1544-1550.

27. Scheurer ME, El-Zein R, Thompson PA, et al. Long-term anti-inflammatory and antihistamine medication use and adult glioma risk. *Cancer Epidemiol Biomarkers Prev* 2008; 17(5):1277-1281.

28. Amirian E, Scheurer ME, Bondy ML. The association between birth order, sibship size, and glioma development in adulthood. *Int J Cancer* 2009;126(11):2752-2756.

29. Narod SA, Stiller C, Lenoir GM. An estimate of the heritable fraction of childhood cancer. *Br J Cancer* 1991;63(6): 993-999.

30. Bondy ML, Lustbader ED, Buffler PA, et al. Genetic epidemiology of childhood brain tumors. *Genet Epidemiol* 1991;8(4): 253-267.

31. Malkin D, Li FP, Strong LC, et al. Germ line p53 mutations in a familial syndrome of breast cancer, sarcomas, and other neoplasms. *Science* 1990;250(4985):1233-1238.

32. Hamilton SR, Liu B, Parsons RE, et al. The molecular basis of Turcot's syndrome. *N Engl J Med* 1995;332(13):839-847.

33. Kantarjian H, Sawyers C, Hochhaus A, et al. Hematologic and cytogenetic responses to imatinib mesylate in chronic myelogenous leukemia. *N Engl J Med* 2002;346(9):645-652.

34. O'Brien SG, Guilhot F, Larson RA, et al. Imatinib compared with interferon and low-dose cytarabine for newly diagnosed chronic-phase chronic myeloid leukemia. *N Engl J Med* 2003; 348(11):994-1004.

35. Cohen MH, Williams GA, Sridhara R, et al. FDA drug approval summary: Gefitinib (ZD1839) (Iressa) tablets. *Oncologist* 2003;8(4):303-306.

36. Nutt CL, Mani DR, Betensky RA, et al. Gene expression-based classification of malignant gliomas correlates better with survival than histological classification. *Cancer Res* 2003;63(7):1602-1607.

37. Fuller GN, Hess KR, Rhee CH, et al. Molecular classification of human diffuse gliomas by multidimensional scaling analysis of gene expression profiles parallels morphology-based classification, correlates with survival, and reveals clinically-relevant novel glioma subsets. *Brain Pathol* 2002; 12(1):108-116.

38. Reynolds BA, Weiss S. Generation of neurons and astrocytes from isolated cells of the adult mammalian central nervous system. *Science* 1992;255(5052):1707-1710.

39. Libermann TA, Nusbaum HR, Razon N, et al. Amplification, enhanced expression and possible rearrangement of EGF receptor gene in primary human brain tumours of glial origin. *Nature* 1985;313(5998):144-147.

40. Louis DN, Gusella JF. A tiger behind many doors: Multiple genetic pathways to malignant glioma. *Trends Genet* 1995; 11(10):412-415.

41. Wong AJ, Bigner SH, Bigner DD, et al. Increased expression of the epidermal growth factor receptor gene in malignant gliomas is invariably associated with gene amplification. *Proc Natl Acad Sci USA* 1987;84(19):6899-6903.

42. Wong AJ, Ruppert JM, Bigner SH, et al. Structural alterations of the epidermal growth factor receptor gene in human gliomas. *Proc Natl Acad Sci USA* 1992;89(7):2965-2969.

43. Choe G, Horvath S, Cloughesy TF, et al. Analysis of the phosphatidylinositol 3'-kinase signaling pathway in glioblastoma patients in vivo. *Cancer Res* 2003;63(11):2742-2746.

44. Chakravarti A, Zhai G, Suzuki Y, et al. The prognostic significance of phosphatidylinositol 3-kinase pathway activation in human gliomas. *J Clin Oncol* 2004;22(10):1926-1933.

45. Guha A, Feldkamp MM, Lau N, et al. Proliferation of human malignant astrocytomas is dependent on Ras activation. *Oncogene* 1997;15(23):2755-2765.

46. Steck PA, Lin H, Langford LA, et al. Functional and molecular analyses of 10q deletions in human gliomas. *Genes Chromosomes Cancer* 1999;24(2):135-143.

47. Holland EC, Celestino J, Dai C, et al. Combined activation of Ras and Akt in neural progenitors induces glioblastoma formation in mice. *Nat Genet* 2000;25(1):55-57.

48. Ding H, Shannon P, Lau N, et al. Oligodendrogliomas result from the expression of an activated mutant epidermal growth factor receptor in a RAS transgenic mouse astrocytoma model. *Cancer Res* 2003;63(5):1106-1113.

49. Levine AJ. p53, the cellular gatekeeper for growth and division. *Cell* 1997;88(3):323-331.

50. Hoh J, Jin S, Parrado T, et al. The p53MH algorithm and its application in detecting p53-responsive genes. *Proc Natl Acad Sci USA* 2002;99(13):8467-8472.

51. Reifenberger G, Liu L, Ichimura K, et al. Amplification and overexpression of the MDM2 gene in a subset of human malignant gliomas without p53 mutations. *Cancer Res* 1993; 53(12):2736-2739.

52. Maher EA, Furnari FB, Bachoo RM, et al. Malignant glioma: Genetics and biology of a grave matter. *Genes Dev* 2001; 15(11):1311-1333.

53. Fueyo J, Alemany R, Gomez-Manzano C, et al. Preclinical characterization of the antiglioma activity of a tropism-enhanced adenovirus targeted to the retinoblastoma pathway. *J Natl Cancer Inst* 2003;95(9):652-660.

54. Esteller M. CpG island hypermethylation and tumor suppressor genes: A booming present, a brighter future. *Oncogene* 2002;21(35):5427-5440.

55. Suh CO, Loh JJ, Kim GE, et al. Primary malignant lymphomas of the central nervous system: radiotherapy results in 12 cases. *Yonsei Med J* 1989;30(1):54-64.

56. Kleihues P, Ohgaki H. Primary and secondary glioblastomas: From concept to clinical diagnosis. *Neuro Oncol* 1999;1(1): 44-51.

57. Watanabe K, Tachibana O, Sata K, et al. Overexpression of the EGF receptor and p53 mutations are mutually exclusive in the evolution of primary and secondary glioblastomas. *Brain Pathol* 1996;6(3):217-223; discussion 23-24.

58. Cairncross JG, Ueki K, Zlatescu MC, et al. Specific genetic predictors of chemotherapeutic response and survival in patients with anaplastic oligodendrogliomas. *J Natl Cancer Inst* 1998;90(19):1473-1479.

59. Jenkins RB, Curran W, Scott CB, et al. Pilot evaluation of 1p and 19q deletions in anaplastic oligodendrogliomas collected by a national cooperative cancer treatment group. *Am J Clin Oncol* 2001;24(5):506-508.

60. Ino Y, Betensky RA, Zlatescu MC, et al. Molecular subtypes of anaplastic oligodendroglioma: Implications for patient management at diagnosis. *Clin Cancer Res* 2001; 7(4):839-845.

61. Smith JS, Perry A, Borell TJ, et al. Alterations of chromosome arms 1p and 19q as predictors of survival in oligodendrogliomas, astrocytomas, and mixed oligoastrocytomas. *J Clin Oncol* 2000;18(3):636-645.

62. Hoang-Xuan K, Capelle L, Kujas M, et al. Temozolomide as initial treatment for adults with low-grade oligodendrogliomas or oligoastrocytomas and correlation with chromosome 1p deletions. *J Clin Oncol* 2004;22(15):3133-3138.

63. Louis D, Stemmer-Rachamimov AO, Wiestler OD. Neurofibromatosis type 2. In: Kleihues P, Cavenee WK (eds): *Pathology and Genetics of Tumors of the Nervous System.* Lyon, France: IARC Press; 2000:219-222.

64. Lee JH, Sundaram V, Stein DJ, et al. Reduced expression of schwannomin/merlin in human sporadic meningiomas. *Neurosurgery* 1997;40(3):578-587.

65. Xiao GH, Chernoff J, Testa JR. NF2: The wizardry of merlin. *Genes Chromosomes Cancer* 2003;38(4):389-399.

66. Kim H, Kwak NJ, Lee JY, et al. Merlin neutralizes the inhibitory effect of Mdm2 on p53. *J Biol Chem* 2004;279(9): 7812-7818.

67. Louis D, Scheithauer B, Budka H. Meningiomas. In: Kleihues P, Cavenee, WK (eds): *Pathology and Genetics of Tumors of the Nervous System.* Lyon, France: IARC Press; 2000: 176-184.

68. Mcdermott M, Quinones-Hinosa A, Fuller GN. Meningiomas. In: Levin V (ed): *Cancer in the Nervous System.* New York: Oxford University Press; 2000;269-299.

69. Kalkanis SN, Carroll RS, Zhang J, et al. Correlation of vascular endothelial growth factor messenger RNA expression with peritumoral vasogenic cerebral edema in meningiomas. *J Neurosurg* 1996;85(6):1095-1101.

70. Tsai JC, Hsiao YY, Teng LJ, et al. Regulation of vascular endothelial growth factor secretion in human meningioma cells. *J Formos Med Assoc* 1999;98(2):111-117.

71. Fidler I. The biology of brain metastasis. In: Sawaya R (ed): *Intracranial Metastases: Current Management Strategies.* Malden: Blackwell Futura; 2004: 35-54.

72. Price JE, Aukerman SL, Fidler IJ. Evidence that the process of murine melanoma metastasis is sequential and selective and contains stochastic elements. *Cancer Res* 1986;46(10): 5172-5178.

73. Posner J. *Neurologic Complications of Cancer. Contemporary Neurology Series. Philadelphia*, PA: FA Davis; 1995;77-110.

74. Fidler IJ. Host and tumour factors in cancer metastasis. *Eur J Clin Invest* 1990;20(5):481-486.

75. Kendal WS, Lagerwaard FJ, Agboola O. Characterization of the frequency distribution for human hematogenous metastases: evidence for clustering and a power variance function. *Clin Exp Metastasis* 2000;18(3):219-229.

76. Fidler IJ, Yano S, Zhang RD, et al. The seed and soil hypothesis: Vascularisation and brain metastases. *Lancet Oncol* 2002;3(1):53-57.

77. Marchetti D, Li J, Shen R. Astrocytes contribute to the brain-metastatic specificity of melanoma cells by producing heparanase. *Cancer Res* 2000;60(17):4767-4770.

78. Fidler IJ, Kripke ML. Metastasis results from preexisting variant cells within a malignant tumor. *Science* 1977;197(4306): 893-895.

79. Puduvalli VK. Brain metastases: Biology and the role of the brain microenvironment. *Curr Oncol Rep* 2001;3(6):467-475.

80. Pasqualini R, Ruoslahti E. Organ targeting in vivo using phage display peptide libraries. *Nature* 1996;380(6572): 364-366.

81. Pasqualini R, Arap W, McDonald DM. Probing the structural and molecular diversity of tumor vasculature. *Trends Mol Med* 2002;8(12):563-571.

82. Felding-Habermann B, O'Toole TE, Smith JW et al.. Integrin activation controls metastasis in human breast cancer. *Proc Natl Acad Sci USA* 2001;98(4):1853-1858.

83. Cary LA, Han DC, Guan JL. Integrin-mediated signal transduction pathways. *Histol Histopathol* 1999;14(3):1001-1009.

84. Jin H, Varner J. Integrins: Roles in cancer development and as treatment targets. *Br J Cancer 2004*;90(3):561-565.

85. Stamenkovic I. Matrix metalloproteinases in tumor invasion and metastasis. *Semin Cancer Biol* 2000;10(6):415-433.

86. Marchetti D, Nicolson GL. Human heparanase: A molecular determinant of brain metastasis. *Adv Enzyme Regul* 2001;41: 343-359.

87. Borsig L, Wong R, Feramisco J, et al. Heparin and cancer revisited: mechanistic connections involving platelets, P-selectin, carcinoma mucins, and tumor metastasis. *Proc Natl Acad Sci USA* 2001;98(6):3352-3357.

88. Carmeliet P, Jain RK. Angiogenesis in cancer and other diseases. *Nature* 2000;407(6801):249-257.

89. Drewes LR. What is the blood-brain barrier? A molecular perspective. Cerebral vascular biology. *Adv Exp Med Biol* 1999;474:111-122.

90. Bendayan R, Lee G, Bendayan M. Functional expression and localization of P-glycoprotein at the blood brain barrier. *Microsc Res Tech* 2002;57(5):365-380.

91. Gottesman MM, Fojo T, Bates SE. Multidrug resistance in cancer: role of ATP-dependent transporters. *Nat Rev Cancer* 2002;2(1):48-58.

92. Abbott NJ. Astrocyte-endothelial interactions and blood-brain barrier permeability. *J Anat* 2002;200(6):629-638.

93. Schackert G, Fidler IJ. Site-specific metastasis of mouse melanomas and a fibrosarcoma in the brain or meninges of syngeneic animals. *Cancer Res* 1988;48(12):3478-3484.

94. Savaraj N, Lu K, Feun LG, et al. Intracerebral penetration and tissue distribution of 2,5-diaziridinyl 3,6-bis(carboethoxyamino) 1,4-benzoquinone (AZQ, NSC-182986). *J Neurooncol* 1983; 1(1):15-19.

95. Stewart DJ, Leavens M, Maor M, et al. Human central nervous system distribution of cis-diamminedichloroplatinum and use as a radiosensitizer in malignant brain tumors. *Cancer Res* 1982;42(6):2474-2479.

96. Stewart PA, Hayakawa K, Farrell CL. Quantitation of blood-brain barrier ultrastructure. *Microsc Res Tech* 1994;27(6): 516-527.

97. Stewart DJ, Lu K, Benjamin RS, et al. Concentration of vinblastine in human intracerebral tumor and other tissues. *J Neurooncol* 1983;1(2):139-144.

98. Graif M, Bydder GM, Steiner RE, et al. Contrast-enhanced MR imaging of malignant brain tumors. *AJNR Am J Neuroradiol* 1985;6(6):855-862.

99. Kepes JJ. Large focal tumor-like demyelinating lesions of the brain: Intermediate entity between multiple sclerosis and acute disseminated encephalomyelitis? A study of 31 patients. *Ann Neurol* 1993;33(1):18-27.

100. Peterson K, Rosenblum MK, Powers JM, et al. Effect of brain irradiation on demyelinating lesions. *Neurology* 1993; 43(10):2105-2112.

101. Herminghaus S, Dierks T, Pilatus U et al. Determination of histopathological tumor grade in neuroepithelial brain tumors by using spectral pattern analysis of in vivo spectroscopic data. *J Neurosurg* 2003;98(1):74-81.

102. Giannini C, Burger PC, Berkey BA, et al. Anaplastic oligodendroglial tumors: Refining the correlation among histopathology, 1p 19q deletion and clinical outcome in Intergroup Radiation Therapy Oncology Group Trial 9402. *Brain Pathol* 2008; 18(3):360-369.

103. World Health Organization Classification of Tumours. In: Louis D, Ohgaki, H, Wiestler OD, Cavenee, WK, (eds): *WHO Classification of Tumours of the Central Nervous System*, 4th ed. Lyon: International Agency for Research on Cancer; 2007:164-172.

104. Shaw E. Management of low-grade gliomas in adults. In: Prados M (ed): *Brain Cancer*. Hamilton, Ontario: BC Decker; 2002:279-302.

105. Westergaard L, Gjerris F, Klinken L. Prognostic parameters in benign astrocytomas. *Acta Neurochir* (Wien) 1993; 123(1-2):1-7.

106. Philippon JH, Clemenceau SH, Fauchon FH, et al. Supratentorial low-grade astrocytomas in adults. *Neurosurgery* 1993;32(4):554-559.

107. Piepmeier J, Christopher S, Spencer D, et al. Variations in the natural history and survival of patients with supratentorial low-grade astrocytomas. *Neurosurgery* 1996;38(5):872-878; discussion 878-879.

108. Kraus JA, Koopmann J, Kaskel P, et al. Shared allelic losses on chromosomes 1p and 19q suggest a common origin of oligodendroglioma and oligoastrocytoma. *J Neuropathol Exp Neurol* 1995;54(1):91-95.

109. Berger M, Leibel, S, Bruner, J. Primary cerebral tumors. In: Levin V (ed). *Cancer in the Nervous System*. Oxford, UK: Oxford University Press; 2002:75-157.

110. Berger MS, Deliganis AV, Dobbins J, et al. The effect of extent of resection on recurrence in patients with low grade cerebral hemisphere gliomas. *Cancer* 1994;74(6):1784-1791.

111. Shaw EG, Daumas-Duport C, Scheithauer BW, et al. Radiation therapy in the management of low-grade supratentorial astrocytomas. *J Neurosurg* 1989;70(6):853-861.

112. Stupp R, Mason WP, van den Bent MJ et al. Radiotherapy plus concomitant and adjuvant temozolomide for glioblastoma. *N Engl J Med* 2005;352(10):987-996.

113. Taphoorn MJ. Neurocognitive sequelae in the treatment of low-grade gliomas. *Semin Oncol* 2003;30(6 Suppl 19):45-48.

114. Karim AB, Maat B, Hatlevoll R, et al. A randomized trial on dose-response in radiation therapy of low-grade cerebral glioma: European Organization for Research and Treatment of Cancer (EORTC) Study 22844. *Int J Radiat Oncol Biol Phys* 1996;36(3):549-556.

115. Shaw E, Arusell R, Scheithauer B et al. Prospective randomized trial of low- versus high-dose radiation therapy in adults with supratentorial low-grade glioma: Initial report of a North Central Cancer Treatment Group/Radiation Therapy Oncology Group/Eastern Cooperative Oncology Group study. *J Clin Oncol* 2002;20(9):2267-2276.

116. Eyre HJ, Crowley JJ, Townsend JJ et al. A randomized trial of radiotherapy versus radiotherapy plus CCNU for incompletely resected low-grade gliomas: A Southwest Oncology Group study. *J Neurosurg* 1993;78(6):909-914.

117. Stupp R, Baumert BG. Promises and controversies in the management of low-grade glioma. *Ann Oncol* 2003;14(12): 1695-1696.

118. van den Bent M. Can chemotherapy replace radiotherapy in low-grade gliomas? Time for randomized studies. *Semin Oncol* 2003;30:39-44.

119. Buckner JC, Gesme D, Jr., O'Fallon JR, et al. Phase II trial of procarbazine, lomustine, and vincristine as initial therapy for patients with low-grade oligodendroglioma or oligoastrocytoma: Efficacy and associations with chromosomal abnormalities. *J Clin Oncol* 2003;21(2):251-255.

120. Diabira S, Rousselet MC, Gamelin E, et al. PCV chemotherapy for oligodendroglioma: Response analyzed on T2 weighted-MRI. *J Neurooncol* 2001;55(1):45-50.

121. Pace A, Vidiri A, Galie E, et al. Temozolomide chemotherapy for progressive low-grade glioma: Clinical benefits and radiological response. *Ann Oncol* 2003;14(12):1722-1726.

122. Sanson M, Cartalat-Carel S, Taillibert S et al. Initial chemotherapy in gliomatosis cerebri. *Neurology* 2004;63(2): 270-275.

123. Quinn JA, Reardon DA, Friedman AH et al. Phase II trial of temozolomide in patients with progressive low-grade glioma. *J Clin Oncol* 2003;21(4):646-651.

124. Meyers CA, Weitzner MA, Valentine AD, et al. Methylphenidate therapy improves cognition, mood, and function of brain tumor patients. *J Clin Oncol* 1998;16(7):2522-2527.

125. Horner M, Ries LAG, Krapcho M, et al. *SEER Cancer Statistics Review, 1975-2006*, 11th ed. National Cancer Institute; 2008.

126. Yung WK, Albright RE, Olson J, et al. A phase II study of temozolomide vs. procarbazine in patients with glioblastoma multiforme at first relapse. *Br J Cancer* 2000;83(5):588-593.

127. Brada M, Hoang-Xuan K, Rampling R, et al. Multicenter phase II trial of temozolomide in patients with glioblastoma multiforme at first relapse. *Ann Oncol* 2001;12(2): 259-266.

128. Prados MD, Larson DA, Lamborn K, et al. Radiation therapy and hydroxyurea followed by the combination of 6-thioguanine and BCNU for the treatment of primary malignant brain tumors. *Int J Radiat Oncol Biol Phys* 1998;40(1):57-63.

129. van den Bent MJ, Carpentier AF, Brandes AA, et al. Adjuvant procarbazine, lomustine, and vincristine improves progression-free survival but not overall survival in newly diagnosed anaplastic oligodendrogliomas and oligoastrocytomas: A randomized European Organisation for Research and Treatment of Cancer phase III trial. *J Clin Oncol* 2006; 24(18):2715-2722.

130. Levin VA, Yung WK, Bruner J, et al. Phase II study of accelerated fractionation radiation therapy with carboplatin followed by PCV chemotherapy for the treatment of anaplastic gliomas. *Int J Radiat Oncol Biol Phys* 2002;53(1):58-66.

131. Prados MD, Wara WM, Sneed PK, et al. Phase III trial of accelerated hyperfractionation with or without difluoromethylornithine (DFMO) versus standard fractionated radiotherapy with or without DFMO for newly diagnosed patients with glioblastoma multiforme. *Int J Radiat Oncol Biol Phys* 2001; 49(1):71-77.

132. Yung WK, Prados MD, Yaya-Tur R, et al. Multicenter phase II trial of temozolomide in patients with anaplastic astrocytoma or anaplastic oligoastrocytoma at first relapse. Temodal Brain Tumor Group. *J Clin Oncol* 1999;17(9): 2762-2771.

133. Jaeckle KA, Hess KR, Yung WK, et al. Phase II evaluation of temozolomide and 13-cis-retinoic acid for the treatment of recurrent and progressive malignant glioma: A North American Brain Tumor Consortium study. *J Clin Oncol* 2003;21(12): 2305-2311.

134. Groves MD, Puduvalli VK, Hess KR, et al. Phase II trial of temozolomide plus the matrix metalloproteinase inhibitor, marimastat, in recurrent and progressive glioblastoma multiforme. *J Clin Oncol* 2002;20(5):1383-1388.

135. Gilbert M. Phase I/II study of combination temozolomide (TMZ) and irinotecan (CPT-11) for recurrent malignant gliomas: A North American Brain Tumor Consortium (NABTC) study. *Proc Am Soc Clin Oncol* 2003;22(103): (Abstract 410).

136. Dohrmann GJ, Farwell JR, Flannery JT. Glioblastoma multiforme in children. *J Neurosurg* 1976;44(4):442-448.

137. Lacroix M, Abi-Said D, Fourney DR, et al. A multivariate analysis of 416 patients with glioblastoma multiforme: Prognosis, extent of resection, and survival. *J Neurosurg* 2001; 95(2):190-198.

138. Keles GE, Lamborn KR, Chang SM, et al. Volume of residual disease as a predictor of outcome in adult patients with recurrent supratentorial glioblastomas multiforme who are undergoing chemotherapy. *J Neurosurg* 2004;100(1):41-46.

139. Lang FF, Bruner JM, Fuller GN, et al. Phase I trial of adenovirus-mediated p53 gene therapy for recurrent glioma: Biological and clinical results. *J Clin Oncol* 2003;21(13): 2508-2518.

140. Kunwar S. Convection enhanced delivery of IL13-PE38QQR for treatment of recurrent malignant glioma: Presentation of interim findings from ongoing phase 1 studies. *Acta Neurochir Suppl* 2003;88:105-111.

141. Kunwar S, Prados MD, Chang SM, et al. Direct intracerebral delivery of cintredekin besudotox (IL13-PE38QQR) in recurrent malignant glioma: A report by the Cintredekin Besudotox Intraparenchymal Study Group. *J Clin Oncol* 2007;25(7): 837-844.

142. Glantz MJ, Burger PC, Friedman AH, et al. Treatment of radiation-induced nervous system injury with heparin and warfarin. *Neurology* 1994;44(11):2020-2027.

143. Kohshi K, Imada H, Nomoto S, et al. Successful treatment of radiation-induced brain necrosis by hyperbaric oxygen therapy. *J Neurol Sci* 2003;209(1-2):115-117.

144. Chuba PJ, Aronin P, Bhambhani K, et al. Hyperbaric oxygen therapy for radiation-induced brain injury in children. *Cancer* 1997;80(10):2005-2012.

145. Gonzalez J, Kumar AJ, Conrad CA, et al. Effect of bevacizumab on radiation necrosis of the brain. *Int J Radiat Oncol Biol Phys* 2007;67(2):323-326.

146. Torcuator R, Zuniga R, Mohan YS, et al. Initial experience with bevacizumab treatment for biopsy confirmed cerebral radiation necrosis. *J Neurooncol* 2009;94(1):63-68.

147. Yung WK, Kyritsis AP, Gleason MJ, et al. Treatment of recurrent malignant gliomas with high-dose 13-cis-retinoic acid. *Clin Cancer Res* 1996;2(12):1931-1935.

148. Vredenburgh JJ, Desjardins A, Herndon JE, II, et al. Phase II trial of bevacizumab and irinotecan in recurrent malignant glioma. *Clin Cancer Res* 2007;13(4):1253-1259.

149. Kreisl TN, Kim L, Moore K, et al. Phase II trial of single-agent bevacizumab followed by bevacizumab plus irinotecan at tumor progression in recurrent glioblastoma. *J Clin Oncol* 2009;27(5):740-745.

150. Reardon DA, Friedman HS, Powell JB, Jr., et al. Irinotecan: Promising activity in the treatment of malignant glioma. *Oncology* 2003;17(5 suppl 5):9-14.

151. Franceschi E, Cavallo G, Scopece L et al. Phase II trial of carboplatin and etoposide for patients with recurrent high-grade glioma. *Br J Cancer* 2004;91(6):1038-1044.

152. Reardon DA. A phase I/II trial of PTK787/ZK 222584 (PTK/ZK): A novel oral angiogenesis inhibitor in combination with either temozolomide or lomustine for patients with recurrent glioblastoma multiforme (GBM). ASCO Annual Meeting Proceedings. *J Clin Oncol* 2004;22(suppl 14S):1513.

153. Conrad C, Friedman, H, Reardon, D. A Phase I/II trial of single-agnet PTK 787/ZK 222584 (PTK/ZK) a novel oral angiogenesis inhibitor in patients with recurent glioblastoma multiforme (GBM). ASCO Annual Meeting Proceedings. *J Clin Oncol* 2004;22(suppl 14S):1512.

154. Prados MD, Yung WK, Jaeckle KA, et al. Phase 1 trial of irinotecan (CPT-11) in patients with recurrent malignant glioma: A North American Brain Tumor Consortium study. *Neuro Oncol* 2004;6(1):44-54.

155. Chang SM, Kuhn J, Wen P, et al. Phase I/pharmacokinetic study of CCI-779 in patients with recurrent malignant glioma on enzyme-inducing antiepileptic drugs. *Invest New Drugs* 2004;22(4):427-435.

156. Mcdermott M, Quinones-Hinosa A, Bollen AW. Meningiomas. In: Prados M (ed): *Brain Cancer*. Hamilton, Ontario: BC Decker; 2002:333-364.

157. Goldsmith BJ, Wara WM, Wilson CB, et al. Postoperative irradiation for subtotally resected meningiomas. A retrospective analysis of 140 patients treated from 1967 to 1990. *J Neurosurg* 1994;80(2):195-201.

158. Hakim R, Alexander E III, Loeffler JS, et al. Results of linear accelerator-based radiosurgery for intracranial meningiomas. *Neurosurgery* 1998;42(3):446-453; discussion 453-454.

159. Ojemann SG, Sneed PK, Larson DA, et al. Radiosurgery for malignant meningioma: Results in 22 patients. *J Neurosurg* 2000;93 (suppl 3): 62-67.

160. Newton HB, Slivka MA, Stevens C. Hydroxyurea chemotherapy for unresectable or residual meningioma. *J Neurooncol* 2000;49(2):165-170.

161. Mason WP, Gentili F, Macdonald DR, et al. Stabilization of disease progression by hydroxyurea in patients with recurrent or unresectable meningioma. *J Neurosurg* 2002;97(2):341-346.

162. Kaba SE, DeMonte F, Bruner JM, et al. The treatment of recurrent unresectable and malignant meningiomas with interferon alpha-2B. *Neurosurgery* 1997;40(2):271-275.

163. Kyritsis AP. Chemotherapy for meningiomas. *J Neurooncol* 1996;29(3):269-272.

164. Travitzky M, Libson E, Nemirovsky I, et al. Doxil-induced regression of pleuro-pulmonary metastases in a patient with malignant meningioma. *Anticancer Drugs* 2003;14(3):247-250.

165. Chamberlain MC, Tsao-Wei DD, Groshen S. Temozolomide for treatment-resistant recurrent meningioma. *Neurology* 2004;62(7):1210-1212.

166. Gupta V, Samuleson CG, Su S, et al. Nelfinavir potentiation of imatinib cytotoxicity in meningioma cells via survivin inhibition. *Neurosurg Focus* 2007;23(4):E9.

167. Norden AD, Raizer JJ, Abrey LE, et al. Phase II trials of erlotinib or gefitinib in patients with recurrent meningioma. *J Neurooncol* 2010;96(2):211-217.

168. O'Neill BP, Wang CH, O'Fallon JR, et al. Primary central nervous system non-Hodgkin's lymphoma (PCNSL): Survival advantages with combined initial therapy? A final report of the North Central Cancer Treatment Group (NCCTG) Study 86-72-52. *Int J Radiat Oncol Biol Phys* 1999;43(3):559-563.

169. DeAngelis LM, Yahalom J, Thaler HT, et al. Combined modality therapy for primary CNS lymphoma. *J Clin Oncol* 1992;10(4):635-643.

170. Abrey LE, Yahalom J, DeAngelis LM. Treatment for primary CNS lymphoma: The next step. *J Clin Oncol* 2000;18(17): 3144-3150.

171. Abrey LE, DeAngelis LM, Yahalom J. Long-term survival in primary CNS lymphoma. *J Clin Oncol* 1998;16(3):859-863.

172. Harder H, Holtel H, Bromberg JE, et al. Cognitive status and quality of life after treatment for primary CNS lymphoma. *Neurology* 2004;62(4):544-7.

173. Batchelor T, Carson K, O'Neill A et al. Treatment of primary CNS lymphoma with methotrexate and deferred radiotherapy: A report of NABTT 96-07. *J Clin Oncol* 2003;21(6): 1044-1049.

174. Herrlinger U, Brugger W, Bamberg M, et al. PCV salvage chemotherapy for recurrent primary CNS lymphoma. *Neurology* 2000;54(8):1707-1708.

175. Lerro KA, Lacy J. Case report: A patient with primary CNS lymphoma treated with temozolomide to complete response. *J Neurooncol* 2002;59(2):165-168.

176. Pels H, Schulz H, Schlegel U, et al. Treatment of CNS lymphoma with the anti-CD20 antibody rituximab: Experience with two cases and review of the literature. *Onkologie* 2003; 26(4):351-354.

177. Enting RH, Demopoulos A, DeAngelis LM, et al. Salvage therapy for primary CNS lymphoma with a combination of rituximab and temozolomide. *Neurology* 2004;63(5):901-903.

178. Gaspar L, Scott C, Rotman M, et al. Recursive partitioning analysis (RPA) of prognostic factors in three Radiation Therapy Oncology Group (RTOG) brain metastases trials. *Int J Radiat Oncol Biol Phys* 1997;37(4):745-751.

179. Gaspar LE, Scott C, Murray K, et al. Validation of the RTOG recursive partitioning analysis (RPA) classification for brain metastases. *Int J Radiat Oncol Biol Phys* 2000; 47(4):1001-1006.

180. Bindal AK, Bindal RK, Hess KR, et al. Surgery versus radiosurgery in the treatment of brain metastasis. *J Neurosurg* 1996;84(5):748-754.

181. Auchter RM, Lamond JP, Alexander E, et al. A multiinstitutional outcome and prognostic factor analysis of radiosurgery for resectable single brain metastasis. *Int J Radiat Oncol Biol Phys* 1996;35(1):27-35.

182. Yung W, Kunschner, LJ, Sawaya, R. Intracranial metastases. In: Levin V (ed): *Cancer in the Nervous System*, 2nd ed. Oxford: Oxford University Press; 2002:321-340.

183. Nakagawa H, Groothuis DR, Owens ES, et al. Dexamethasone effects on [125I]albumin distribution in experimental RG-2 gliomas and adjacent brain. *J Cereb Blood Flow Metab* 1987;7(6):687-701.

184. Grossi F, Scolaro T, Tixi L, et al. The role of systemic chemotherapy in the treatment of brain metastases from small-cell lung cancer. *Crit Rev Oncol Hematol* 2001;37(1):61-67.

185. Bernardo G, Cuzzoni Q, Strada MR, et al. First-line chemotherapy with vinorelbine, gemcitabine, and carboplatin in the treatment of brain metastases from non-small-cell lung cancer: A phase II study. *Cancer Invest* 2002;20(3):293-302.

186. Kaba SE, Kyritsis AP, Hess K, et al. TPDC-FuHu chemotherapy for the treatment of recurrent metastatic brain tumors. *J Clin Oncol* 1997;15(3):1063-1070.

187. Abrey LE, Christodoulou C. Temozolomide for treating brain metastases. *Semin Oncol* 2001;28(4 suppl 13):34-42.

188. Wang ML, Yung WK, Royce ME, et al. Capecitabine for 5-fluorouracil-resistant brain metastases from breast cancer. *Am J Clin Oncol* 2001;24(4):421-424.

189. Rosner D, Nemoto T, Lane WW. Chemotherapy induces regression of brain metastases in breast carcinoma. *Cancer* 1986;58(4):832-839.

190. Fujita A, Fukuoka S, Takabatake H, et al. Combination chemotherapy of cisplatin, ifosfamide, and irinotecan with rhG-CSF support in patients with brain metastases from non-small cell lung cancer. *Oncology* 2000;59(4):291-295.

191. Hwu WJ, Krown SE, Panageas KS, et al. Temozolomide plus thalidomide in patients with advanced melanoma: Results of a dose-finding trial. *J Clin Oncol* 2002;20(11):2610-2615.

192. Hwu WJ, Raizer J, Panageas KS, et al. Treatment of metastatic melanoma in the brain with temozolomide and thalidomide. *Lancet Oncol* 2001;2(10):634-635.

193. Rustin GJ, Newlands ES, Begent RH, et al. Weekly alternating etoposide, methotrexate, and actinomycin/vincristine and cyclophosphamide chemotherapy for the treatment of CNS metastases of choriocarcinoma. *J Clin Oncol* 1989;7(7):900-903.

194. Rustin GJ, Newlands ES, Bagshawe KD, et al. Successful management of metastatic and primary germ cell tumors in the brain. *Cancer* 1986;57(11):2108-2113.

195. Gilbert M: Brain metastases: Still an 'orphan' disease? *Curr Oncol Rep* 2001;3(6):463-466.

196. Guirguis LM, Yang JC, White DE, et al. Safety and efficacy of high-dose interleukin-2 therapy in patients with brain metastases. *J Immunother* 2002;25(1):82-87.

197. Richards JM, Gale D, Mehta N, et al. Combination of chemotherapy with interleukin-2 and interferon alfa for the treatment of metastatic melanoma. *J Clin Oncol* 1999;17(2):651-657.

CHAPTER
38

ENDOCRINE MALIGNANCIES

Naifa Lamki Busaidy
Mouhammed Amir Habra
Rena Vassilopoulou-Sellin

■ DIFFERENTIATED THYROID CARCINOMA

INTRODUCTION

Carcinoma of the thyroid gland is the most common endocrine malignancy, accounting for 1.6% of all new malignant disease (1). It has a prevalence rate of 335,000, and approximately 37,200 new cases of thyroid carcinoma were diagnosed in the United States in 2009 alone (1,2). Despite the generally good prognosis of thyroid carcinoma, 5 to 10% of patients will die of the disease (3,4). Differentiated thyroid carcinomas, those that derive from the follicular epithelial cells (papillary and follicular), account for 94% of these malignancies; 5% are medullary thyroid cancers, a neuroendocrine tumor derived from C cells in the thyroid gland; and the remaining 1% are anaplastic thyroid carcinoma.

Papillary carcinoma is the most common type of thyroid carcinoma, except that in regions where there is an iodine insufficiency, the follicular type is more common. Follicular thyroid carcinoma occurs in older people, with peak incidence in the fifth decade of life. Follicular thyroid malignancies have a worse prognosis than papillary tumors, especially in patients with fixed/invasive lesions. In one report from the Surveillance, Epidemiology, and Endocrine Points database, of approximately 15,700 patients in the United States, overall survival rates corrected for age and sex were 98% for papillary, 92% for follicular, 80% for medullary, and 13% for anaplastic carcinoma (5). Worse prognoses are associated with increasing age at diagnosis and metastatic disease at presentation.

Women are affected twice as often as men, although the latter gender dies of cancer twice as often as women (1). Although the median age of diagnosis is 45 years, thyroid carcinoma does affect children. In our institution, fewer than 10% of all patients with thyroid cancer were diagnosed before 20 years of age (6).

DIAGNOSTIC EVALUATION OF THE SOLITARY THYROID NODULE

The most common presentation of a patient with thyroid carcinoma is the presence of a solitary thyroid nodule found either on physical examination or discovered as an incidental nodule on imaging studies performed for other purposes. Cytologic examination of a fine-needle aspirate of a nodule more than 1cm in diameter is the most appropriate first diagnostic procedure. Papillary, medullary, and anaplastic carcinomas can be readily diagnosed by fine-needle aspiration (FNA), but distinguishing benign from malignant follicular lesions proves more difficult. Histologic examination showing capsular or vascular invasion is necessary to classify a lesion as malignant. Because follicular adenoma and carcinoma cannot be differentiated cytologically, they are grouped as "indeterminate or suspicious follicular neoplasms." The false-positive and false-negative rates for all nodules categorized as malignant or benign, respectively, is less than 5% (7). The rate of carcinoma for suspicious follicular neoplasms is about 20%. The incidence of malignancy increases with larger nodule size, male sex, and increasing age. Fifteen to 25% of the time, the FNA will yield "inadequate diagnostic material," and this necessitates repeat aspiration. The availability of ultrasound guidance has increased the diagnostic yield.

The majority (85-95%) of thyroid nodules are benign. Radionuclide scans usually show malignant lesions as hypofunctioning or "cold," although 85% of "cold" nodules are still benign (Fig. 38-1). Radionuclide scanning is no longer advocated in the initial evaluation of thyroid nodules unless the thyroid-stimulating hormone (TSH) concentration is suppressed; in this situation, a radioiodine scan is done to assess for a functioning ("hot") adenoma. The algorithm for evaluating the patient with a thyroid nodule is outlined in Table 38-1 (8).

DIFFERENTIATED THYROID CARCINOMA

Etiology

External low-dose radiation therapy to the head and neck during infancy and childhood, used frequently from the 1940s to the 1960s to treat a variety of benign diseases, has been shown to predispose to thyroid cancer, specifically of the papillary type. The average time duration between irradiation and recognition of the tumor is 10 years but may be longer than 30 years (9).

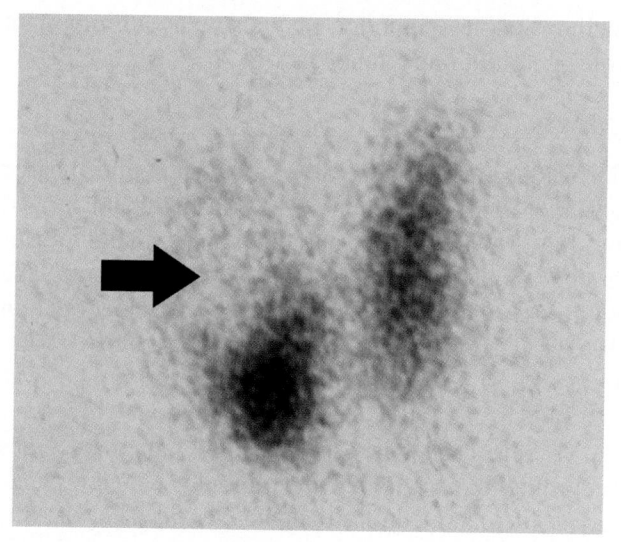

FIGURE 38-1. Thyroid scan showing a "cold" nodule in the right superior pole of the thyroid.

Patients exposed to head or neck irradiation experience an increased frequency of benign tumors, but malignancy occurs in up to 30% of cases. Treatment of malignant diseases with higher radiation doses (>2000 cGy), especially at a young age, also has been associated with an increased risk of both benign and malignant neoplasms of the thyroid. Exposure to external sources of radiation after the Chernobyl nuclear accident led to a 3- to 75-fold increase in the incidence of papillary thyroid carcinoma in fallout regions, especially in younger children.

Except for reports of radiation-induced thyroid cancer, there is little information about the etiology of this malignancy. Prolonged TSH stimulation has been implicated as a potential risk factor; however, patients with primary hypothyroidism do not exhibit increased frequency of thyroid carcinoma. Thyroid-stimulatory immunoglobulins present in patients with Graves

T A B L E 38-1	EVALUATION OF THE THYROID NODULE

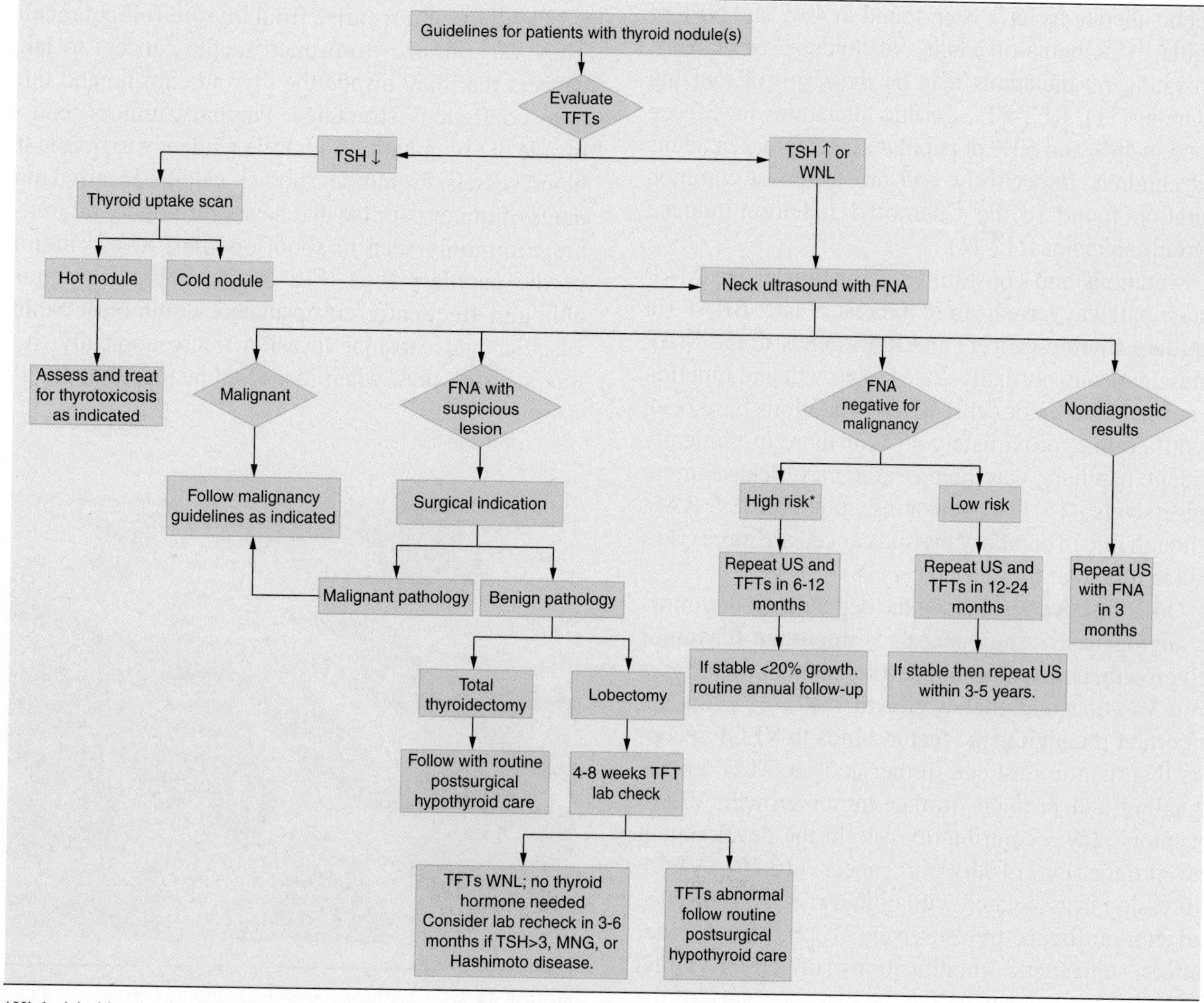

Guidelines for patients with thyroid nodule(s)

Evaluate TFTs

TSH ↓ — TSH ↑ or WNL

Thyroid uptake scan

Hot nodule — Cold nodule → Neck ultrasound with FNA

Assess and treat for thyrotoxicosis as indicated

Malignant → Follow malignancy guidelines as indicated ← Malignant pathology

FNA with suspicious lesion → Surgical indication → Benign pathology

FNA negative for malignancy → High risk* → Repeat US and TFTs in 6-12 months → If stable <20% growth, routine annual follow-up

Low risk → Repeat US and TFTs in 12-24 months → If stable then repeat US within 3-5 years.

Nondiagnostic results → Repeat US with FNA in 3 months

Total thyroidectomy → Follow with routine postsurgical hypothyroid care

Lobectomy → 4-8 weeks TFT lab check

TFTs WNL; no thyroid hormone needed Consider lab recheck in 3-6 months if TSH>3, MNG, or Hashimoto disease.

TFTs abnormal follow routine postsurgical hypothyroid care

*High risk: history of radiation exposure to the head and neck or family history of thyroid cancer.

disease have also been implicated, and associations between thyroid cancer and Hashimoto thyroiditis, Graves disease, and multinodular goiter have been reported. However, any causative relationship between these diseases remains poorly documented.

There are a few uncommon familial syndromes associated with differentiated thyroid carcinomas: familial adenomatous polyposis (also known as Gardner syndrome) and Cowden disease, which is characterized by inherited multiple hamartomas. Familial cases have been reported in 5% of all patients with papillary thyroid carcinoma and may portend a more aggressive disease course.

Understanding the follicular cell tumorigenesis pathways is key to the development of clinical trials testing novel therapies to treat thyroid cancer. Mutations in either BRAF, RAS, or RET/PTC rearrangements are present in most differentiated thyroid cancers (10). Chromosomal rearrangement of the gene encoding the transmembrane tyrosine kinase receptors *ret* and *trk* have been implicated as an early step in the development of these tumors. These genetic alterations have been found in 40% and 60% of papillary carcinomas in adults and children, respectively. Activating *ret* mutations may be the result of ionizing radiation (11). RET-PTC genetic alterations have been found in 40% and 60% of papillary carcinomas in adults and children, respectively, and are the most common mutation found in the Chernobyl radiation-induced thyroid carcinomas (12-14).

Mutations and constitutive activation of the MAP kinase pathway have been of interest of late. BRAF (in papillary thyroid cancer) and RAS genes in the MAP kinase pathway normally code for growth and function in normal and tumor cells. BRAF mutations have been identified in approximately 45% or more of clinically evident papillary carcinomas and may behave more aggressively (15-17). Activating mutations of RAS, although rare in papillary thyroid cancer, are more common in follicular thyroid cancer (18).

Other discoveries include the dependence of tumors on angiogenesis. Angiogenesis is important for tumor cell growth, promotion, and development of metastases (19). Vascular endothelial growth factor (VEGF), an important proangiogenic factor, binds to VEGF receptors that then in turn can further activate MAP-kinase signaling and promote further tumor growth. VEGF receptors play a contributory role in the development and progression of thyroid cancer (10,20). VEGF expression is associated with higher risk of recurrence and shorter disease-free survival (21,22). Like in other tumors, epigenetic modifications of chromosomal DNA and histones, including the promoter gene of the sodium-iodine symporter, may also play an important role in promotion of tumor growth.

Pathology

Thyroid cancer is generally subdivided into a large group of well-differentiated neoplasms characterized by slow growth and high curability and a small group of highly anaplastic tumors with a bleak outlook. The pathologic classification proposed by Woolner et al. in 1961 was adopted by the American Thyroid Association with a few modifications, and in 1974, it was accepted by the World Health Organization.

Thyroid cancer is classified into four main types according to morphology and biologic behavior: papillary, follicular, medullary, and anaplastic. This classification scheme has an advantage over systems based purely on histologic patterns in that it relates morphology to methods of treatment and prognosis. Primary lymphoma of the thyroid, metastases from other primary sites, and other uncommon thyroid tumors are also encountered, though rarely.

Papillary tumors arise from thyroid follicular cells. They vary in size from microscopic cancers to large cancers that may invade the thyroid capsule and infiltrate contiguous structures. Papillary tumors tend to invade the lymphatics with little tendency to invade the blood vessels. Psammoma bodies, calcified scarred remnants of tumor papillae that have presumably infarcted, are commonly seen in about one-half of carcinomas of the papillary type (Fig. 38-2). Follicular tumors, although frequently encapsulated, commonly exhibit vascular and capsular invasion microscopically; it is this invasion that, when identified histopathologically,

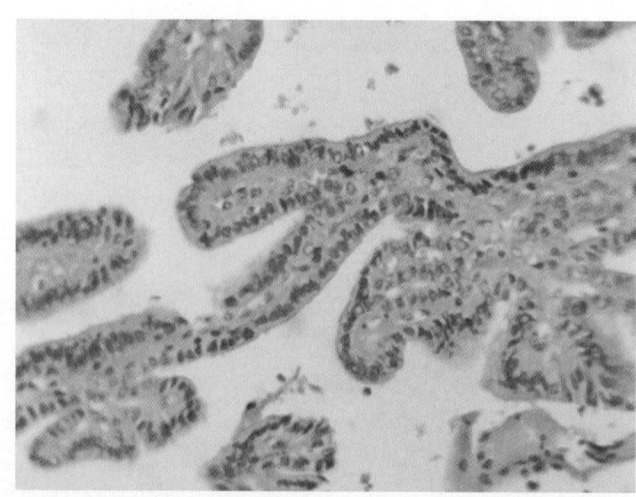

FIGURE 38-2. Classic histology for papillary thyroid carcinoma.

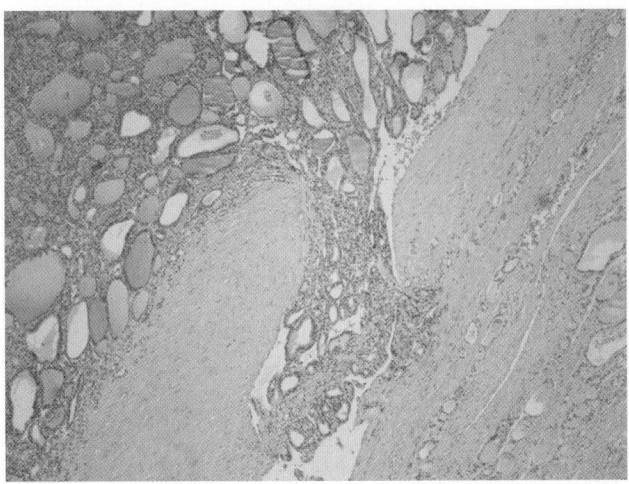

FIGURE 38-3. Histology of follicular carcinoma at the site at which the cancer invades the capsule of the nodule. Capsular and vascular invasion of nodules in a lesion that contains cells with the features of follicular neoplasm is follicular carcinoma by definition.

distinguishes benign neoplasms from malignant follicular neoplasms (Fig. 38-3). Cytology alone cannot be used to diagnose follicular carcinoma. Hurthle-cell carcinomas, neoplasms formed from granular, eosinophilic cells with numerous mitochondria, are considered a type of follicular cancer.

Many tumors have both papillary and follicular elements histologically; they are called follicular variants of papillary carcinoma and are classified as papillary lesions because their clinical behavior is typically indistinguishable from that of pure papillary cancers (Fig. 38-4). Occasionally, both papillary and follicular

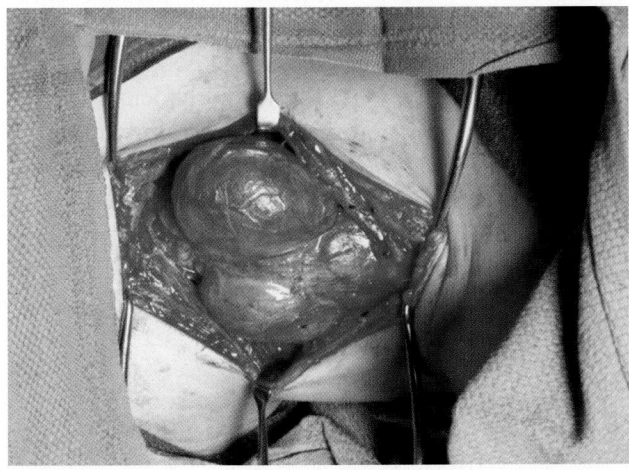

FIGURE 38-4. Intraoperative thyroid gland containing large foci of follicular variant of papillary thyroid carcinoma as seen on postoperative pathology.

tumors occur as small lesions surrounded by a dense fibrotic reaction; they are called occult sclerosing lesions and may be associated with lymph-node metastases. Tall-cell variants, columnar-cell variants, and the Hurthle-cell variant are histologic subtypes that may portend a worse prognosis.

Staging

Many clinicopathologic staging systems exist for differentiated thyroid carcinomas (23-27). The TNM (tumor, node, metastasis) method might be most useful for prediction of disease-free survival and is generally used in our institution (28). Tumor size and presence of extrathyroidal invasion carry prognostic importance and therefore should be reported by pathologists on every case. Anaplastic thyroid carcinoma by convention is always stage IV (Table 38-2*A* and *B*).

Therapy

Surgical Management

Total thyroidectomy is the preferred initial surgical procedure for most patients with differentiated thyroid carcinoma at our institution. Arguments for total thyroidectomy rather than lobectomy are that: (1) papillary foci are seen in bilateral lobes in 60 to 85% of patients (29) and (2) 5 to 10% of recurrences of papillary thyroid carcinoma after a unilateral lobectomy arise in the contralateral lobe (30). Whether the disease seen in the contralateral lobe is caused by tumor growth de novo or contralateral metastases is the subject of debate. Of the 1685 low-risk patients reviewed in a retrospective analysis of outcomes of patients with papillary carcinoma at the Mayo Clinic, the recurrence rate at 20 years after total thyroidectomy was 8 versus 22% after unilateral lobectomy, although there was no difference in cause-specific mortality rates (31). Other retrospective studies support these findings of lower recurrence and show only minimal improvement in survival (26,32,33). A third reason that lends support to a total thyroidectomy as the preferred surgical procedure is that treatment with radioiodine and the specificity of serum thyroglobulin (Tg) concentrations as a tumor marker become most efficacious after as much thyroid tissue removed as possible.

Some institutions still advocate unilateral surgery due to the lack of survival benefit with more extensive surgery and the apparent lower risk of hypoparathyroidism and recurrent laryngeal nerve injury (34); these latter two complications of thyroidectomy occur in 1% or less of total thyroidectomies when done by an experienced surgeon.

TABLE
38-2A **STAGING OF THYROID CARCINOMA**

Primary Tumor (T)

Note: all categories may be subdivided into (a) solitary tumor and (b) multifocal tumor (the largest determines the classification).

TX	Primary tumor cannot be assessed
T0	No evidence of primary tumor
T1	Tumor 2 cm or less in greatest dimension limited to the thyroid
T2	Tumor more than 2 cm but not more than 4 cm in greatest dimension limited to the thyroid
T3	Tumor more than 4 cm in greatest dimension limited to the thyroid or any tumor with minimal extrathyroid extension (eg, extension to sternothyroid muscle or perithyroid soft tissues)
T4a	Tumor of any size extending beyond the thyroid capsule to invade subcutaneous soft tissues, larynx, trachea, esophagus, or recurrent laryngeal nerve
T4b	Tumor invades prevertebral fascia or encases carotid artery or mediastinal vessels

All anaplastic carcinomas are considered T4 tumors

T4a	Intrathyroidal anaplastic carcinoma—surgically resectable
T4b	Extrathyroidal anaplastic carcinoma—surgically unresectable

Regional Lymph Nodes (N)

Regional lymph nodes are those of the central compartment as well as lateral cervical and upper mediastinal lymph nodes.

NX	Regional lymph nodes cannot be assessed
N0	No regional lymph node metastasis
N1	Regional lymph node metastasis
N1a	Metastasis to level VI (pretracheal, paratracheal, and prelaryngeal/Delphian lymph nodes)
N1b	Metastasis to unilateral, bilateral, or contralateral cervical or superior mediastinal lymph nodes

Distant Metastasis (M)

MX	Distant metastasis cannot be assessed
M0	No distant metastasis
M1	Distant metastasis

Reproduced, with permission, from Edge SB, Byrd DR, Compton CC, eds. AJCC Cancer Staging Manual, 7th edition. New York, Springer, 2010, pp. 87-88.

Many consensus guidelines state that a total thyroidectomy is indicated if the primary tumor is >1 cm, if there is extrathyroidal invasion, or if metastases are present. Patients with a history of head and neck irradiation should have the above preferred surgery as they are at higher risk for multicentric disease and the subsequent higher recurrence risk that follows. For patients whose primary tumor is <1 cm, a unilateral lobectomy may be sufficient (5).

For patients with a cytologically suspicious follicular neoplasm, a unilateral lobectomy and isthmusectomy is the initial procedure of choice. If a malignant follicular lesion is confirmed on histopathology, then a completion thyroidectomy is warranted to allow for treatment with radioiodine therapy. Direct invasion of the strap muscles and trachea may occur and compromise resectability.

Microscopic regional nodal metastases are present in 80% of patients with papillary carcinoma. Only 35% of patients will have grossly detectable nodal (cervical or mediastinal) metastases (35). The presence of lymph node metastases increases risk for disease recurrence; however, unlike other malignancies, it is only a minor risk factor for mortality. Nodal metastases represent an uncommon finding in follicular carcinoma, but when present may indicate decreased survival.

It thus follows that neck dissection should be performed on patients with identifiable nodal disease, as their presence impacts recurrence. Preoperative ultrasound of the entire neck (not just of the thyroid) is indicated to help identify the presence of nodal metastases and help the surgeon to perform a more focused operation in the hope that doing so will decrease both recurrence and complication rates. This modality is routinely done at our institution.

Calcium and phosphorus levels should be monitored postoperatively due to the distinct possibility of hypoparathyroidism due to either vascular damage intraoperatively or inadvertent removal.

Postoperative Iodine-131 Therapy (Radioactive Iodine Treatment)

Iodine 131 (^{131}I) has been advocated as adjuvant therapy for thyroid carcinoma; iodine is preferentially taken up and trapped by the thyroid follicular cells and malignant counterparts. ^{131}I destroys cells of follicular origin by

TABLE 38-2B	STAGE GROUPING FOR THYROID CARCINOMA

Separate stage groupings are recommended for papillary or follicular, medullary, and anaplastic (undifferentiated) carcinomas.

PAPILLARY OR FOLLICULAR (<45 YEARS)

Stage I	Any T	Any N	M0
Stage II	Any T	Any N	M1

PAPILLARY OR FOLLICULAR (≥45 YEARS)

Stage I	T1	N0	M0
Stage II	T2	N0	M0
Stage III	T3	N0	M0
	T1/T2/T3	N1a	M0
Stage IVA	T4a	N0/N1a	M0
	T1/T2/T3/T4a	N1b	M0
Stage IVB	T4b	Any N	M0
Stage IVC	Any T	Any M	M1

MEDULLARY CARCINOMA

Stage I	T1	N0	M0
Stage II	T2	N0	M0
Stage III	T3	N0	M0
	T1/T2/T3	N1a	M0
Stage IVA	T4a	N0/N1a	M0
	T1/T2/T3/T4a	N1b	M0
Stage IVB	T4b	Any N	M0
Stage IVC	Any T	Any N	M1

ANAPLASTIC CARCINOMA

All anaplastic carcinomas are stage IV.

Stage IVA	T4a	Any N	M0
Stage IVB	T4b	Any N	M0
Stage IVC	Any T	Any N	M1

Reproduced, with permission, from Edge SB, Byrd DR, Compton CC, eds. AJCC Cancer Staging Manual, 7th edition. New York, Springer, 2010, pp. 87-88.

first becoming concentrated in the cell where beta rays are released and the high-energy electrons spewed induce radiation cytotoxicity; simultaneously, gamma rays are released that allow for detection of the emission by a camera. Postoperative examination with radioiodine scanning, therefore, allows the identification of residual regional or distant foci of disease and radioiodine can be used therapeutically to ablate such tumor deposits.

The rationale for using ^{131}I as adjuvant therapy are that: (1) destroys any residual microscopic foci of disease, (2) increases specificity of subsequent ^{131}I scanning for detection of recurrent or metastatic disease by elimination of uptake by residual normal tissue, and

(3) improves the value of measurements of serum Tg as a serum marker; hence, any elevation in Tg would be representative of recurrent or metastatic disease and not residual normal thyroid tissue (5). Combined retrospective data suggest that radioiodine ablation reduces long-term, disease-specific mortality in patients with primary tumors 1cm in diameter or larger, those with multicentric disease, or in whom there is evidence of soft-tissue invasion at presentation (2,26,36,37).

More recent data have shown that some low-risk patients may not benefit from radioiodine, however (38). Patients with known residual disease, be it nodal disease or distant metastatic disease postoperatively, do have prolonged disease-free survival postoperation with radioiodine treatment. Radioactive iodine (RAI) treatment is not recommended for solitary primary tumors <1 cm in size unless high-risk features or metastatic disease are present.

The efficacy of radioiodine is dependent on tumor characteristics, patient preparation, sites of disease, and radioiodine activity (35). Uptake of iodine by follicular cells (malignant and benign) is stimulated by TSH and is suppressed by increased iodide stores. For maximum uptake of radioiodine, thyroid hormone concentrations should be dropped sufficiently to allow the TSH rise to >25 mU/L. Postoperative hypothyroidism develops after 4 weeks. To help alleviate symptoms of hypothyroidism for the first 2 weeks, liothyronine (T3) may be administered at 25 μg two times per day. Lower doses are given to elderly patients and patients with coronary artery disease. Two weeks prior to radioiodine scanning, the T3 is stopped and patients should avoid foods with high iodine content for these 2 weeks as well. Administration of "cold" (nonradioactive) iodine, such as that found in contrast material routinely used for computed tomography (CT) imaging and various invasive procedures, should be avoided for at least 3 months prior to a radioactive iodine scan. This "cold" iodine will interfere with the therapeutic radioactive iodine and may make the radioiodine scans falsely "negative" in these instances. Urinary concentrations of iodine can be checked to assess total body iodine content prior to scanning and treating a patient with [131]I. Using 2 to 5 mCi of either ^{123}I or ^{131}I, a radioiodine scan for localization of uptake prior to ablation (pretreatment scan) is recommended. Twenty-four to 96 h after dosing, whole-body scans and spot images of the neck are performed using a gamma camera. After the thyroidectomy, most patients will demonstrate uptake of radioiodine in the thyroid bed (presumably normal residual tissue) less than 5%. An uptake of more than 5% on a whole-body scan indicates excessive thyroid tissue remaining and may warrant further surgical resection. If extensive locoregional disease is seen, additional surgery should be considered. Once the decision is made to treat the patient with radioactive iodine, an empiric dose of radioactive iodine treatment is generally chosen for patients: 30 to 100 mCi for adjuvant ablation, approximately 150 mCi for nodal disease, and 200 mCi or more for metastatic disease outside the lungs. More strict-dosing calculations using elaborate dosimetric techniques can be computed; however, these are not routinely used clinically at present.

A posttreatment scan is performed to assess for further uptake of radioactive iodine that was not previously seen on the pretreatment scan (ie, regional or distant metastases). The posttreatment scan is a more sensitive technique to detect metastatic disease, as the ability to demonstrate radioactive iodine-avid lesions is directly proportional to amount of radioactive iodine given (Fig. 38-5).

Treatment with radioiodine is usually done in a hospital setting to adhere to radiation safety issues. In most institutions and for most cases of thyroid cancer, treatment with radioactive iodine is now done as an outpatient with appropriate radiation safety precautions.

Short-term complications, though rare, include radiation thyroiditis, neck edema, sialoadenitis, and tumor hemorrhage. These occur more often in the presence of bulky disease. Long-term complications, which increase with cumulative doses, include xerostomia, nasolacrimal duct obstruction (39,40); pulmonary fibrosis (if pulmonary metastasis is present and treated at high doses); and secondary malignant diseases, such as acute myelogenous leukemia. It has been suggested by some small studies that patients treated with ^{131}I may be at a small but increased risk for other secondary malignancies such as bladder cancer, salivary gland tumors, colon cancer, and female breast carcinomas. However, a recent meta-analysis found that the relative risk of any secondary primary malignancy was 1.19 (95% CI, 1.04-1.36) relative to thyroid cancer survivors not treated with radioactive iodine and that those treated with RAI were at 2.5 times increased risk of developing leukemia (41). There was no increased risk of bladder, breast, central nervous system, colorectal, digestive tract, stomach, pancreas, kidney, lung, or melanoma skin cancers. In other studies, oligospermia and transient ovarian failure have also been described, but there is no definite dose relation.

There are no reports of congenital abnormalities in children conceived after radioactive iodine treatment; however, most physicians would recommend that women not conceive for at least 6 months after treatment. Radioactive iodine should not be given to pregnant

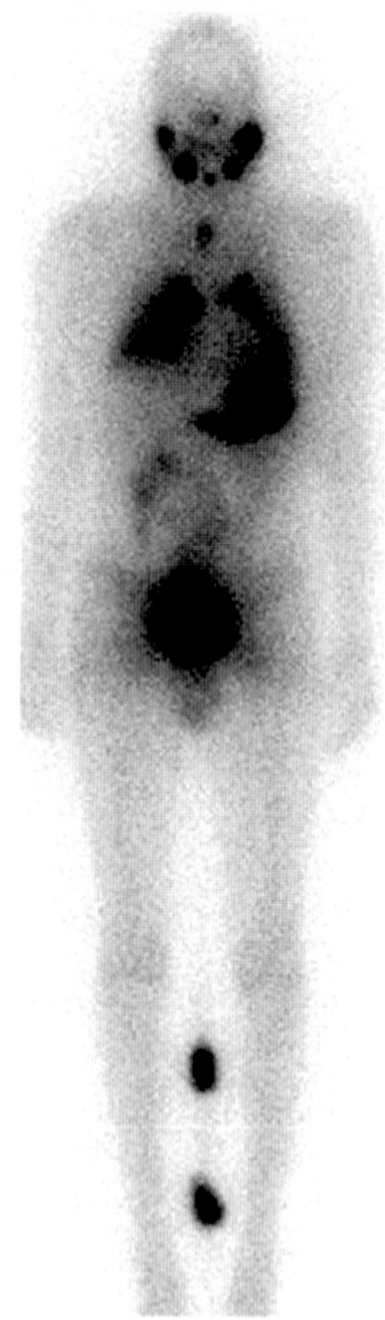

FIGURE 38-5.   Whole-body scan with iodine 138 showing multiple metastatic deposits in the neck and lungs, with physiologic uptake in the salivary gland, stomach, intestines, and bladder.

women due to the potential teratogenic effects for the fetus's growth and thyroid development; all women of childbearing age must have a negative pregnancy test prior to treatment.

Thyroid Hormone Therapy

Patients are placed on thyroid hormone therapy after receiving radioactive ablation for 2 reasons. The first and foremost reason is that it corrects the iatrogenic hypothyroidism and avoids all subsequent long-term complications. Secondly, it minimizes potential TSH-stimulated growth of thyroid cancer cells. TSH suppressive therapy has been shown to increase disease-free survival two- to threefold, especially in high-risk patients. Oversuppression of TSH can present morbid consequences. Some of the complications of thyroid hormone suppression are osteopenia, atrial fibrillation, and possible cardiac hypertrophy. Enough thyroid hormone should be given to suppress TSH to 0.1 to 0.5 mU/L. In patients at higher risk of recurrence, TSH should be suppressed to less than 0.1 mU/L.

External Beam Radiotherapy

External beam radiotherapy (EBRT) has a role in the treatment of papillary thyroid carcinoma. Although it is controversial, two retrospective studies have shown that it may be an effective adjuvant therapy to prevent local-regional recurrence in patients 45 years of age and older with locally invasive papillary carcinoma (42,43). Ten-year local relapse-free rates (93 versus 78%) and disease-specific survival rates (100 versus 95%) were significantly improved in a subgroup of 155 patients with papillary histology and presumed microscopic disease (disease within 2-mm margin resections, tumor-shaved off structures) treated with EBRT (42). Patients younger than 45 years are generally not treated with EBRT both because of their better prognosis and the possible late side effects of therapy, including secondary malignancies.

Doses in the range of 40 to 50 Gy may aid in local-regional control in patients with papillary thyroid carcinoma who are over 45 years of age and have incomplete resection near the aerodigestive tract and/or those with gross extrathyroidal invasion and presumed microscopic residual disease. A multidisciplinary approach and discussion with the surgeon, radiation oncologist, and endocrinologist of risks and benefits should ensue.

Long-Term Follow-up

Imaging

After the patient has had a total thyroidectomy followed by radioiodine ablation, the patient needs lifelong monitoring using both clinical and radiographic data. It is recommended that patients have a follow-up radioiodine scan 6 to 12 months after initial radioiodine ablation. The predictive value for 10-year disease-free survival is approximately 90% with one negative scan post ablation (44). Recombinant human TSH (rhTSH) may be used in this follow-up scan at the clinician's discretion

(a discussion of rhTSH follows). Scanning beyond this first follow-up needs to be individualized and is no longer routine for all thyroid cancer patients. Ultrasonography (U/S) of the neck (thyroid bed and cervical neck compartments) is used more in the pre- and postoperative follow-up of these patients today. It can be used to accurately diagnose and identify lesions in the neck as small as 3 mm. Although it can aid in distinguishing benign lesions from malignant lesions, FNA (U/S-guided) is most helpful to definitively prove recurrent cancer. Routine use of U/S in the 3- to 12-month monitoring of patients with extrathyroidal invasion or local-regional nodal metastases is advocated in many consensus guidelines (8,45,46). As many as half the patients with findings of recurrence on U/S may have no uptake on radioiodine scanning or may have an undetectable serum Tg.

Other imaging techniques that can be used in individual cases of thyroid cancer follow-up include CT scan of the neck and chest, chest radiographs, fluorodeoxyglucose positron emission tomography (FDG-PET or PET) and magnetic resonance imaging (MRI). MRI and CT scan of the neck play important roles in the detection of recurrent disease; they are not as sensitive as U/S but are much less operator-dependent. Chest radiographs may show macronodular pulmonary metastases that do not routinely take up iodine; however, they are less sensitive for micronodular metastases. CT scan of the chest may be more helpful in these situations. FDG-PET imaging is approved for the follow-up of thyroid cancer patients who have a Tg greater than 10 and have negative radioiodine imaging. PET imaging is sensitive in detecting metastatic disease; however, it is not specific for thyroid cancer, and caution should be exercised when searching for recurrent disease. PET imaging is, therefore, not useful in the routine follow-up of patients with thyroid cancer, but may play a role in the less common radioiodine-negative, Tg-positive disease (Figs. 38-6 and 38-7). The latest technology in detection of recurrent thyroid cancer is PET/CT. This imaging technique takes advantage of both CT image technology and a PET image and fuses the two making for more accurate localization and detection of both function (PET) and anatomy (CT).

Fluorodeoxyglucose positron emission tomography (FDG-PET or PET)-CT imaging is an increasingly more useful tool in the detection of radioiodine-negative thyroglobulin-positive thyroid cancer (47,48).

Thyroid carcinomas with little to no iodine activity tend to have higher glucose metabolism and positive FDG-PET scans and vice versa (47,49,50). This tends to be representative of tumor dedifferentiation (51).

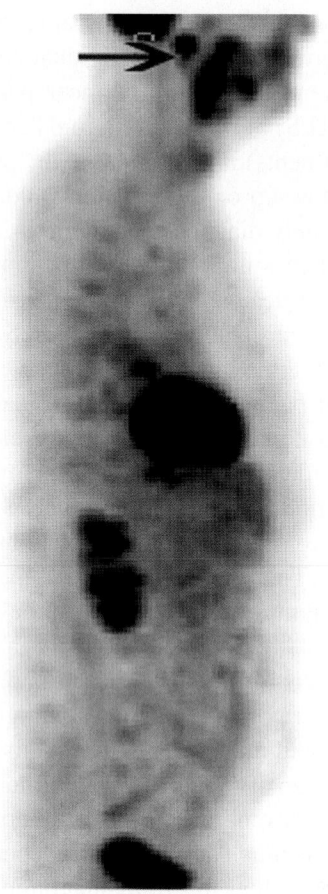

FIGURE 38-6. PET scan showing posterior pharyngeal metastatic papillary thyroid carcinoma. Thyroglobulin was 35 and radioiodine whole-body scan was negative for disease.

¹⁸FDG-PET can aid in both localization of the recurrent tumor (49,52) and also aids in prognostication (52,53). FDG-PET is not sensitive enough to detect subcentimeter metastases, as are common in metastatic papillary thyroid carcinoma and should be used in conjunction with CT chest imaging. Patients with larger volumes of FDG-avid disease or higher SUVs are less likely to respond to radioiodine and have a higher mortality over a 3-year follow-up compared with the patients with no FDG uptake (54,55).

¹⁸FDG-PET has been approved for reimbursement for the follow-up of thyroid cancer patients who have a Tg greater than 10 ng/mL and have negative radioiodine imaging. ¹⁸FDG-PET CTs are also used in those patients whose cancers are very poorly differentiated and make no Tg.

TSH stimulates ¹⁸FDG uptake by differentiated thyroid carcinoma (56), suggesting that PET scans may be more sensitive after TSH stimulation with rhTSH or withdrawal (56-58). One study recently evaluated the incremental value of rhTSH stimulated PET-CT and

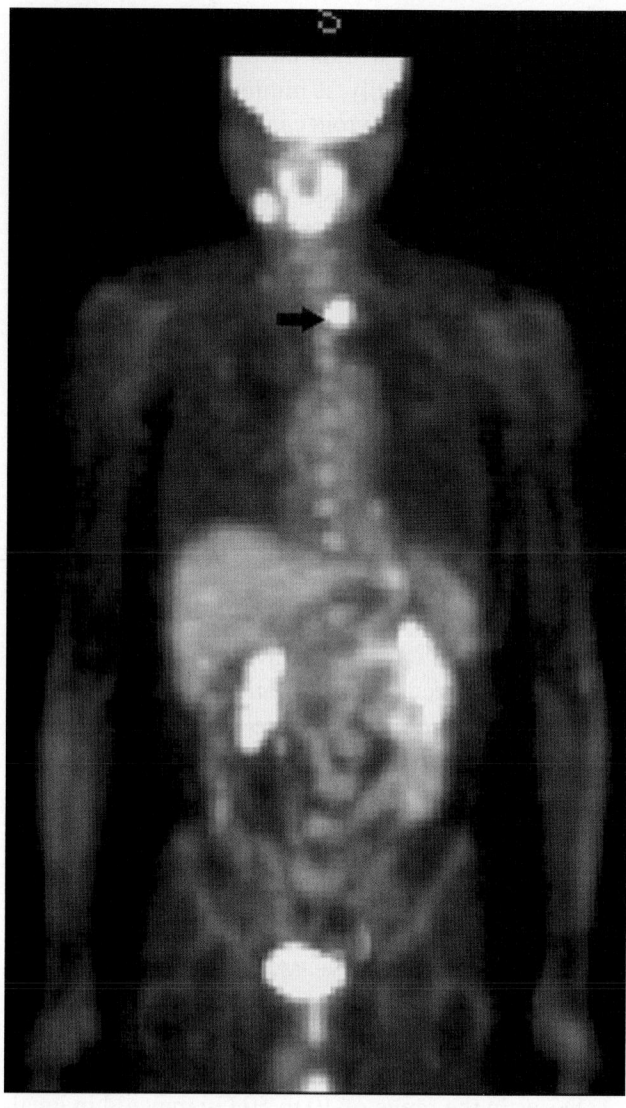

FIGURE 38-7. PET scan illustrating incidentally discovered papillary thyroid carcinoma during staging workup for lymphoma.

found while rhTSH stimulated PET-CT identifies more total FDG-avid lesions, it changed treatment planning only 6% of the time (59).

Eleven to 25% of cases will have imaging that is convincingly positive (false positive) but intra- and postoperative pathology is not consistent with thyroid carcinoma but rather confirms benign disease such as scar. Malignant nature of the disease should be confirmed prior to further therapy (59,60-62).

Monitoring Serum Thyroglobulin

Tg is a protein synthesized only by the thyroid follicular cells (both benign and differentiated malignant tissue) and, therefore, is a good biochemical test to assess the presence of residual, recurrent or metastatic disease.

After total thyroidectomy and ablation, the Tg should be undetectable. The nadir should be reached within 3 months posttreatment but may take as long as 1 to 2 years. Tg should always be measured and recorded in the context of the TSH value because Tg production is dependent on TSH secretion. The sensitivity of Tg measurements to detect cancer is increased to 85 to 95% during thyroid hormone withdrawal with its subsequent elevated TSH levels and is approximately 50% during TSH-suppressive therapy (63). When the tumor has dedifferentiated and no longer secretes the Tg protein, Tg levels will be falsely low and cannot be relied upon.

Autoantibodies to Tg can falsely lower the reported Tg concentrations in immunometric assays as the antibodies interfere with the assay's ability to bind to Tg. Tg antibodies are present in approximately 25% of patients with thyroid cancer and the presence of antibodies after total thyroidectomy and postradioactive ablation may be indicative of the presence of cancer (64). It can take years for Tg antibodies to disappear even in the absence of disease. Sensitive methods to detect Tg mRNA are being developed and, if proven to be valid and useful, may circumvent the above mentioned problem. It is also important that the assay used for Tg measurement be repeated in the same laboratory to avoid erroneous misinterpretations of interassay variability (64,65).

Recombinant Human TSH

Thyrotropin alfa, an rhTSH, may be used in lieu of standard thyroid hormone withdrawal to increase thyrotropin concentrations, as needed for adequate stimulation of both radioiodine uptake for scanning and serum Tg concentrations. The use of rhTSH is of particular benefit in the patient in whom endogenous TSH levels cannot rise due to hypopituitarism or in whom the clinician prefers to avoid prolonged hypothyroidism and its resultant complications due to concurrent medical problems. Studies have shown that the accuracy of diagnostic radioiodine scanning and Tg measurement to detect residual thyroid tissue or carcinoma after two injections of thyrotropin alfa is almost as efficacious as thyroid hormone withdrawal. In general, patients who are at lower risk of recurrence (stage I/II TNM) may be eligible for rhTSH-stimulated Tg measurement and scanning on their first follow-up scan. If there is evidence of abnormal uptake on this scan currently, the patient would have to be withdrawn from thyroid hormone to be treated with radioiodine ablation. An ongoing randomized multicenter trial will answer the question of whether rhTSH can be used for treatment with radioiodine as efficaciously as withdrawal in patients with evidence of radioiodine uptake.

Metastatic Disease

Gross nodal disease should be resected at the time of initial surgery or later at recurrence; this has been shown to increase relapse-free survival. Microscopic nodal metastases occur in up to 80% of cases at diagnosis, and their presence is associated with a high rate of recurrence. Resection of gross nodal disease and RAI treatment (approximately 150 mCi) should be performed for nodal metastases.

Distant metastases are evident in fewer than 1% of patients at the time of presentation. The most common sites of metastasis, in decreasing order of frequency, are the lungs, bones, and other soft tissues (Figs. 38-8A, 38-8B, and 38-9). Older patients have a higher risk for distant metastases. The clinical course and prognosis of patients who have received head and neck irradiation predating the cancer is similar to that of random cases, even though the former group may present with more extensive disease.

Pulmonary metastases in differentiated thyroid carcinoma are often classified radiographically as either "micronodular" or "macronodular" disease. Micronodular metastases present a miliary, diffusely reticular pattern predominating in the lower lung fields and tend to concentrate radioiodine diffusely; this is the pattern of metastasis seen most often in children (Fig. 38-10) (6). Macronodular (coarse) metastases with nodular masses of unequal size (varying between 0.5 and 3.0 cm) occur more frequently overall. Radioiodine incorporation is heterogeneous but often not present. The transition from micro- to macronodular metastasis may occur during the course of the disease.

In a review of 101 patients with differentiated thyroid carcinoma and pulmonary metastases, Samaan et al. (66) analyzed potential prognostic factors and the efficacy of RAI treatment over time. Uptake of RAI by lung metastases conferred a favorable prognosis, especially in patients with negative radiological findings. The probability of RAI uptake was related to the degree of differentiation of the primary tumor. Pulmonary metastases were least common in patients with papillary carcinoma and most common in those with Hurthle-cell carcinoma. Patients younger than 40 years had a better prognosis than those older than 40. Patients with radioactive iodine uptake in pulmonary metastases have a 5-year survival rate of 60% compared with 30% in patients with no uptake in their lungs on RAI scanning. Radioiodine treatments in the range of 150 to 175 mCi are used to treat pulmonary metastases; higher doses are avoided to decrease the rare possibility of pulmonary fibrosis.

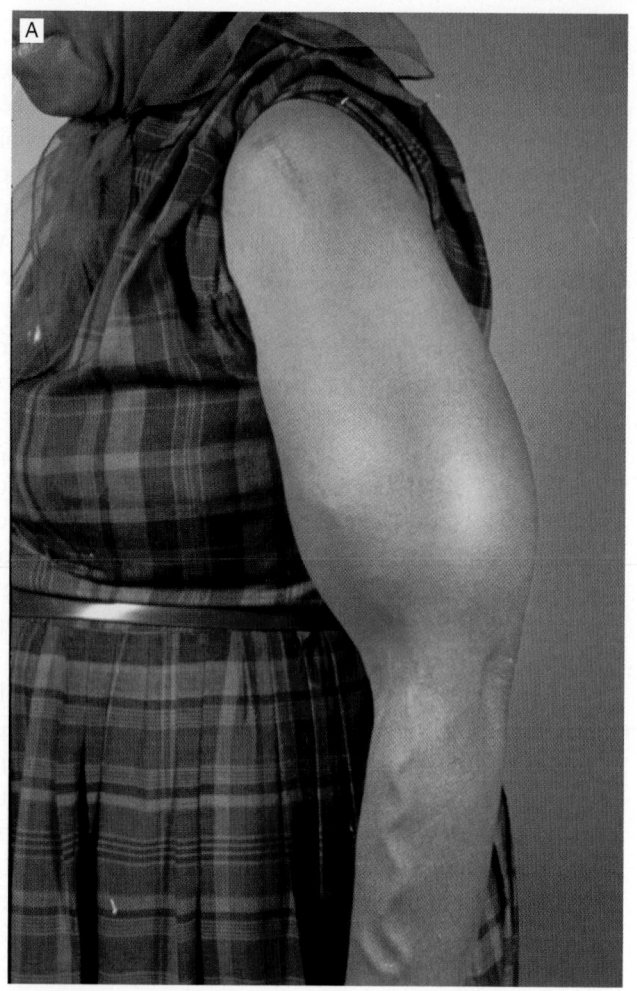

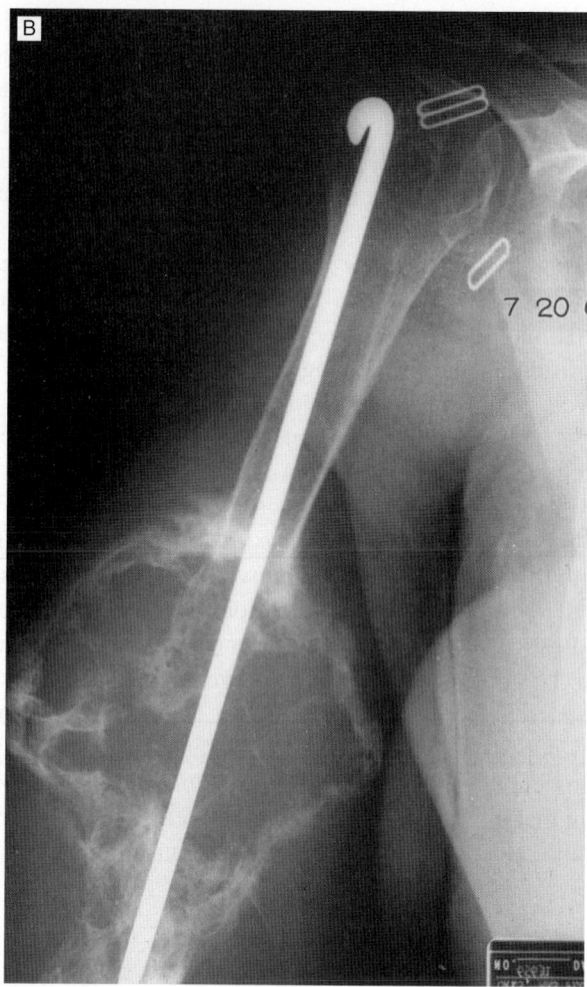

FIGURE 38-8.   **A.** A woman with metastatic follicular thyroid carcinoma to left humerus. **B.** Radiograph of metastatic follicular thyroid carcinoma to left humerus in the same patient.

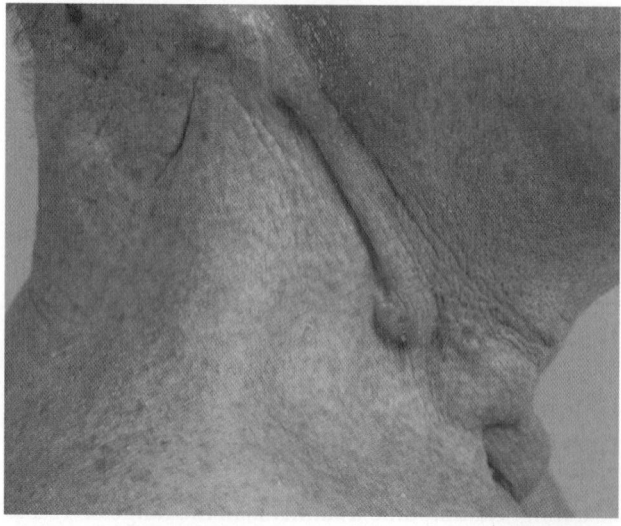

FIGURE 38-9.   Patient with multiple metastatic deposits of papillary thyroid carcinoma to the skin.

Median survival duration of patients with one or more brain metastases improves significantly from 4 to 22 months with surgical resection (67). Bone lesions tend to concentrate RAI as well as pulmonary metastases. Complete resolution is achieved in fewer than 10% of these cases. Follicular thyroid carcinoma tends to spread to bone (producing osteolytic lesions) and lungs more readily than papillary carcinoma and may respond better to ^{131}I treatment. Symptoms from painful bone lesions or spinal-cord–compressing lesions may be relieved by surgical treatment. EBRT has also been used successfully to render bone lesions pain free. In follicular thyroid carcinoma, where the lesions are highly vascular, arterial embolization has been used anecdotally with successful reduction in pain at our institution. Intravenous bisphosphonates (pamidronate or zoledronic acid) are prescribed for painful bony metastases with some success as well.

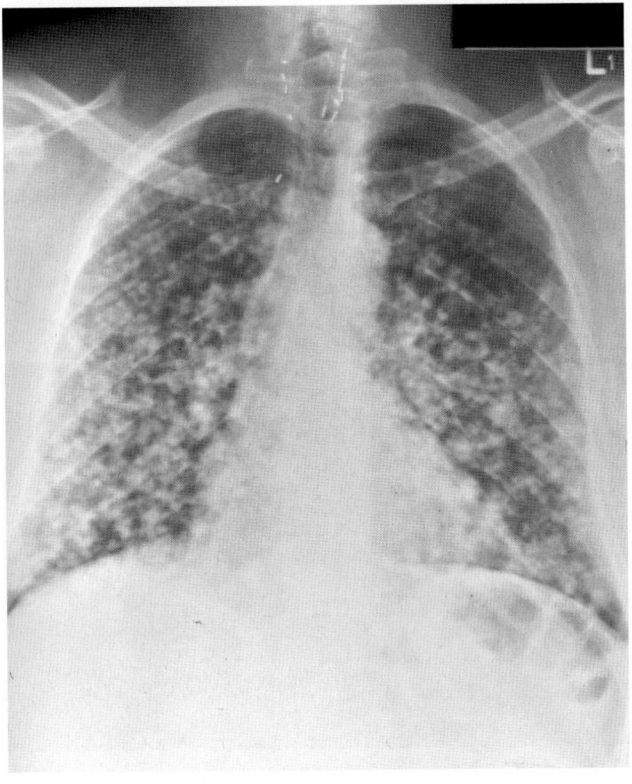

FIGURE 38-10. Chest radiograph showing classic miliary pattern of metastatic papillary thyroid carcinoma in the lungs.

[131]I treatment follows surgical resection of distant metastatic disease if the tumor takes up radioactive iodine. This represents a setting (especially with Central Nervous System lesions) where we are increasingly using rhTSH for treatment of thyroid cancer in order to avoid the potential complications, such as edema, inherent to the prolonged hypothyroid state.

In general, doses of 200 mCi are used for the treatment of distant metastatic disease. This dose may then be repeated 6 to 12 months later. [131]I treatment should be used judiciously to avoid red marrow toxicity and pulmonary fibrosis.

EBRT may prove useful in patients with unresectable, grossly locally invasive or metastatic disease to the neck. This may also aid to control compressive symptomatology from residual/recurrent disease.

Systemic chemotherapy is used in certain cases of widespread disease, although available regimens have not been well studied and are not very effective to date. Doxorubicin is associated with a response rate of up to 40% for progressive differentiated cancers that do not respond to radioactive iodine. The recommended dosage is 60 to 75 mg/m every 3 weeks. Combination therapies are also used but data are limited because of the small number of patients in reported series.

Systemic Therapy for Metastatic Thyroid Cancer

Approximately 15 to 20% of patients will recur locoregionally or have distant metastases. Although it is the most effective medical treatment for differentiated thyroid carcinoma, only about 50 to 80% of primary tumors and their metastases take up radioactive iodine (66,68-71). Five percent of patients will succumb to their disease.

Because metastatic differentiated thyroid cancer can be stable and quiescent for many years, only patients with progressive or symptomatic disease should be treated with systemic treatments. Clinical trials should be considered first-line therapy for those patients that do not take up radioactive iodine. If a clinical trial is not available or patient is not suitable for one, then off-label use of sorafenib or cytotoxic chemotherapy should be considered (45).

Cytotoxic chemotherapies have been used in various combinations with response rates of 25 to 38%, mostly partial responses. Doxorubicin, cis- and carboplatin, epirubicin, and taxol have all been used as single agent or in various combinations (72-76). Response rates appear to be short lived and with high toxicity. Cytotoxic chemotherapies are reserved for patients who can not enter clinical trial or tyrosine kinase inhibitors.

With the knowledge that many differentiated thyroid cancers have oncogenic mutations in the MAP-kinase pathway, the dependence of these tumors on angiogenesis and the development of biologic agents that inhibit these pathways, tyrosine kinase, and other antiangiogenic inhibitors have been studied in various phase II trials. Although many of these agents have a partial response rate similar to cytotoxic chemotherapy, their have higher stable disease rates, more durable response rates, and less toxicity.

There were two small phase II trials evaluating sorafenib in differentiated thyroid carcinoma showing a partial response rate around 20 to 27% and a large majority developing stable disease rate (60%). Sorafenib is FDA approved for renal cancer and is, therefore, available for off-label use for patients who can not enroll in a clinical trial. We recently reviewed our off-label experience with sorafenib and found similar response rates to the phase II trials, and progression-free survival was prolonged from 4 months predrug to 19 months afterdrug treatment (77).

Other agents have been evaluated in clinical trials and most are being further analyzed and appear promising, including motesanib, axitinib, lenalidomide, sunitinib, and pazopanib (78-82).

In summary, for asymptomatic stable disease, thyroid hormone suppression and close observation is warranted. For progressive or symptomatic disease, consideration should be given to putting a patient on clinical trials or tyrosine kinase inhibitors (8,45). Cytotoxic chemotherapies should be reserved for patients who are felt inappropriate or ineligible for above.

Differentiated Thyroid Carcinoma in Children

Thyroid cancer infrequently affects children; at our institution, fewer than 10% of all patients diagnosed with thyroid cancer were under the age of 20. Little data, therefore, exist regarding the optimal treatment in this population. Children with thyroid cancer generally have a good prognosis despite the initial extent of disease. In our review of outcomes of differentiated thyroid carcinoma in children, we found that 25% of patients diagnosed in childhood had recurrences, and 6% died of their disease. Three percent of patients died of late complications of external beam radiotherapy, including tracheal necrosis and cervical sarcomas. Two patients treated with radioactive iodine and surgery died of breast carcinoma at young ages (83).

Cervical node involvement is more common in children than adults. Up to 10% of children and adolescents may have lung involvement at the time of diagnosis (84). Regardless of the extent of disease, however, children with thyroid carcinoma live for many years posttreatment.

In view of the high incidence of recurrence, multifocality, local-regional spread, and extracervical metastases, total thyroidectomy with nodal dissection and adjuvant radioiodine therapy is recommended for children with thyroid cancer. Lifelong surveillance, however, is of the utmost importance.

For the few children with metastatic differentiated thyroid carcinoma that does not take up radioactive iodine, these patients should be referred to a referral center with pediatric endocrine neoplasia expertise. Pediatric endocrinologists at our institution are currently researching treatment options for these rare cases (85,86).

■ MEDULLARY THYROID CARCINOMA

INTRODUCTION

Medullary thyroid carcinomas (MTC) represent 5% of all thyroid neoplasms. About 80% of patients with MTC have a sporadic form of the disease, and the remaining 20% inherit MTC as an autosomal dominant trait as part of the distinct clinical syndromes of multiple endocrine

neoplasia (MEN) type 2A, type 2B, or familial MTC. In MEN 2A, MTC occurs in association with pheochromocytoma and multigland parathyroid tumors; MTC is usually the first manifested disease of the three aforementioned components of this syndrome. In MEN 2B, MTC occurs in association with pheochromocytoma and mucosal neuromas (Fig. 38-11A and B) or neurofibromas and marfanoid habitus.

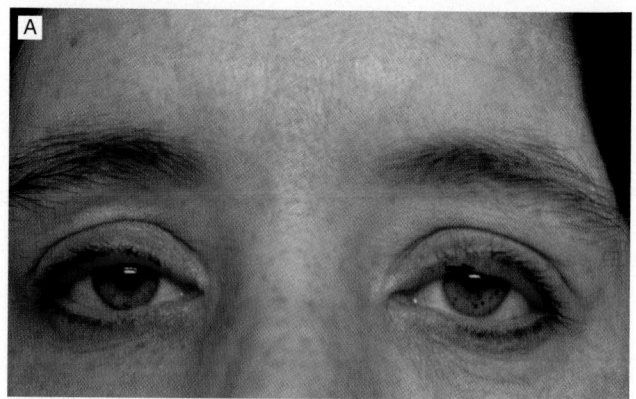

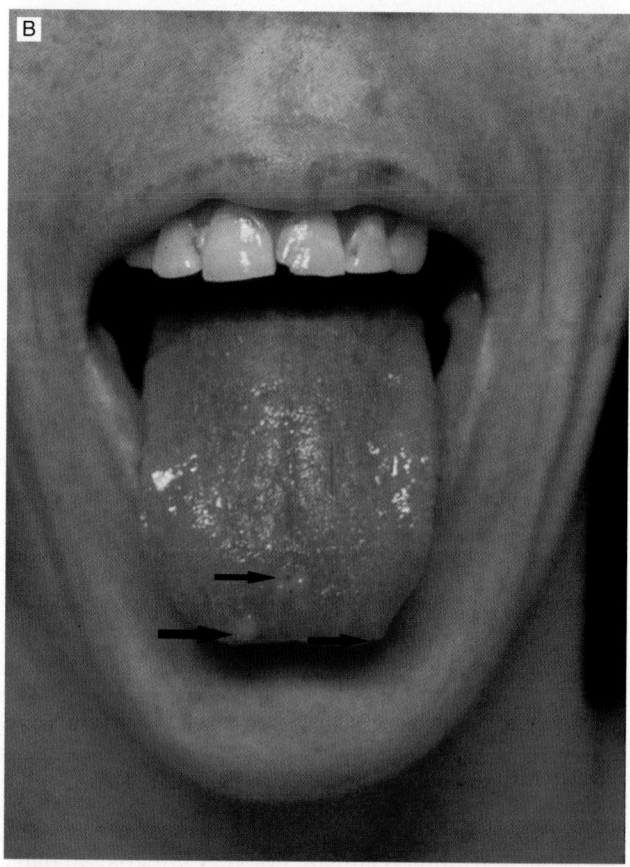

FIGURE 38-11. **A.** Patient with MEN 2B, with typical thickening of the palpebrum. Note also the ganglioneuroma on the left superior eyelid. **B.** Multiple ganglioneuromas on the tongue of a patient with MEN 2B.

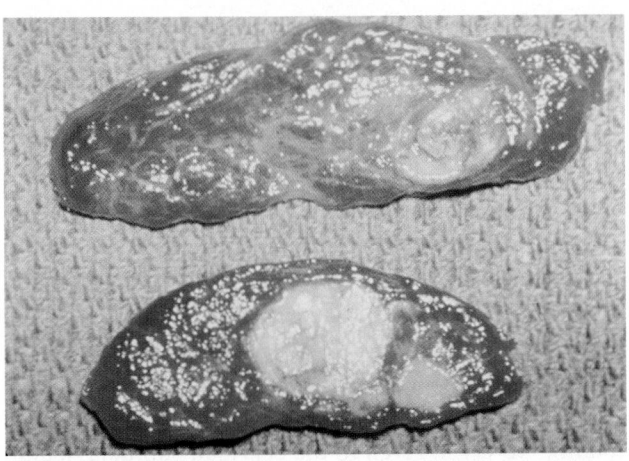

FIGURE 38-12. Gross specimen of thyroid gland containing medullary thyroid carcinoma.

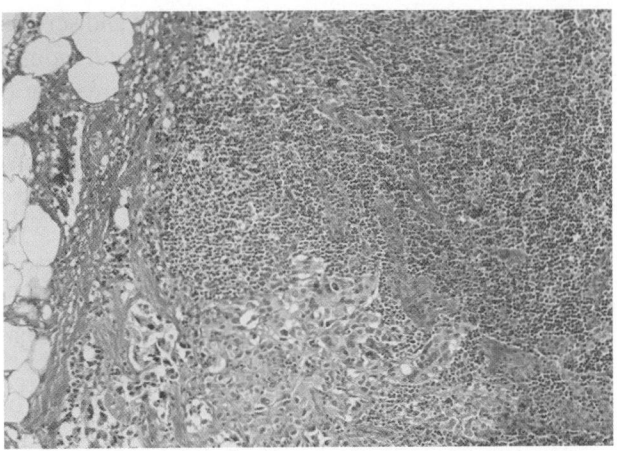

FIGURE 38-13. Hematoxylin and eosin staining of areas of lymph node containing metastasis from medullary thyroid carcinoma.

MTC is derived from C cells (or calcitonin-secreting cells) that are of neural crest origin. MTC arises primarily in the upper two-thirds of the gland where the C cells are normally found (Fig. 38-12). C cells secret a 32-amino-acid peptide called calcitonin, which serves as a useful biochemical marker in patients with this cancer. MTC occurs as a solid mass or a cluster of C-cell hyperplasia interspersed between normal-appearing thyroid follicles. These can be visualized with calcitonin immunostaining, which shows variable amounts of fibrosis and deposits of amyloid in 60 to 80% of tumors. Even the smallest visible tumors can be associated with metastases.

The most common clinical presentation of sporadic medullary thyroid cancer is a solitary thyroid mass found incidentally during routine examination. Routine measurement of serum calcitonin concentrations is not recommended for the assessment of a thyroid nodule as the results may be misleading and it is not cost-effective (87-90); there are other etiologies of elevated calcitonin levels that may make the level difficult to interpret. Most patients with sporadic MTC present in the fifth or sixth decade of life with a male:female ratio of 1.4:1. Metastases to cervical and mediastinal lymph nodes are found in about 50% of the patients at the time of initial presentation (Fig. 38-13). Distant metastases to the lungs, liver, bones, and adrenal glands most commonly occur late in the course of the disease (Fig. 38-14).

Secretory diarrhea, often severe, is the most prominent hormone-mediated clinical features of medullary carcinoma. Facial flushing is also a symptom commonly seen with hormone overproduction. Rarely, ectopic production of adrenocorticotropin hormone (ACTH) and/or corticotropin-releasing hormone (CRH) may cause paraneoplastic Cushing syndrome.

INHERITED MEDULLARY THYROID CANCER

In kindreds with inherited MTC, prospective family screening is essential due to the 90 to 95% penetrance of the disease (91-93). MTC, in these cases, is usually present by the third decade of life. Inherited syndromes of MTC are all transmitted in an autosomal dominant form. The mutation is detected in the tyrosine kinase proto-oncogene RET and can be identified in 98% of affected family members with appropriate screening (91,93-95). There is a 2 to 5% false-negative rate in patients known to have inherited medullary carcinoma (93). Six percent of patients with sporadic MTC carry a germline RET mutation (96). Genetic testing should, thus, be offered to all patients with newly diagnosed apparent sporadic disease. MEN 2B patients tend to

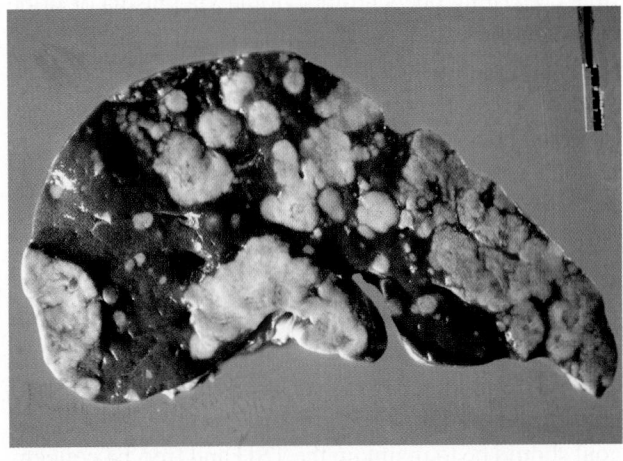

FIGURE 38-14. Gross specimen of liver containing metastatic lesions of medullary thyroid carcinoma.

exhibit more locally aggressive MTC (97), and screening with RET testing is recommended at age 6 months or prior; for familial MTC and MEN 2A screening is recommended by 5 years of age (45,46,93,98).

Analysis of the RET gene should include the most common sites of mutation, initially exons 10 and 11, and if no mutation is found, testing should proceed with exons 13 to 16 (93,98).Appropriate genetic counseling must be a part of the initial evaluation, including the possibilities of errors in testing, the potential for discrimination, and changes that may occur in quality of life.

Five- and 10-year disease-specific survival rates of about 95% and 75%, respectively, for patients under 40 years contrasts with rates of 65% and 50%, respectively, for those older than 40 years (99). Better outlooks seem to bias patients with inherited disease even after correction for younger age at diagnosis.

THERAPY

Surgery

In MTC there is a high propensity for bilateral disease in both the sporadic and familial forms and, therefore, the usual treatment is total thyroidectomy with central neck compartment dissection in all patients. In unilateral sporadic disease, if the primary tumor is greater than 1 cm or central compartment disease is present, strong consideration should be given to ipsilateral modified radical neck or mediastinal dissections, or both. Bilateral neck dissections are usually performed in many institutions, including our own, to patients with inherited disease (46,93,98,100). Radical neck dissections are not favored as they cause major disfigurement without improving prognosis; rather, a function-preserving approach is preferred.

Patients should have a preoperative evaluation for possible coexisting pheochromocytoma via plasma or urine metanephrines and catecholamines and hyperparathyroidism via serum calcium testing. If the pheochromocytoma is present, appropriate control of catecholamine hypersecretion should precede thyroid surgery.

Hormone Replacement

Patients should be placed on thyroid hormone replacement therapy postoperatively. TSH has not been implicated in the growth or recurrence of MTC (as neuroendocrine C cells are the cell of origin); therefore, unlike differentiated thyroid carcinoma, there is no role for thyroid hormone suppression therapy; hence, the goal should be to maintain the TSH and free T4 concentrations within normal levels. There is also no role of radioactive iodine therapy in the treatment of MTC and,

therefore, thyroid hormone replacement may be started immediately after surgery.

External Beam Radiotherapy

External beam radiotherapy (EBRT) should be considered for patients who are at high risk for local-regional recurrence. The relapse-free rate at 10 years was 86% for patients with microscopic residual disease, extraglandular invasion, or lymph node metastases after optimal surgical excision who were treated with EBRT compared with 52% for those not given adjuvant radiation therapy in one study (101). In general, in MTC, 20 fractions totaling 40 Gy is given to the cervical, supraclavicular, and upper mediastinal lymph nodes over 4 weeks; subsequent booster doses of 10 Gy are then given to the thyroid bed, especially if there was gross residual disease (102). EBRT can also be given to treat painful skeletal metastases.

MONITORING AND FOLLOW-UP

Biochemical testing with serum calcitonin and carcinoembryonic antigen (CEA) is used in the routine follow-up of patients with MTC. Two to 3 months postoperatively, these markers should be within the normal ranges (a nadir of 6 months has been reported). Sensitive detection of residual disease may be done by measuring calcitonin after calcium or pentagastrin stimulation tests when these tumor markers are within normal range. Patients with palpable recurrent/residual disease, in general, will have stimulated calcitonin levels of at least 10 pg/mL; the exception being those tumors that are dedifferentiated and no longer secrete calcitonin (these tumors usually secrete CEA). Values of serum calcitonin greater than 100 pg/mL are indicative of residual neck disease or distant metastases, and these patients should be aggressively assessed clinically and radiographically. Because of MTC's propensity for neck, mediastinal, and liver metastasis, diagnostic imaging should include U/S of the neck, CT of the chest, and MRI of the liver. Routine use of PET, metaiodobenzylguanidine (MIBG), and bone scans is not recommended. The liver should be the organ of highest suspect for distant metastases for basal calcitonin levels greater than 1000 pg/mL and no obvious neck disease. Occasionally, venous catheterization is necessary to localize distant metastases.

Postoperative hypercalcitoninemia in one study was associated with 5- and 10-year survival rates of 90% and 86%, respectively (103); in other studies high clinical recurrence rates are reported. Outcomes of hypercalcitoninemia in these patients correlate with their initial presentation of disease. Although there is a lack of long-term outcome studies, few reports indicate normalization of calcitonin levels after surgical resection for nodal recurrences. The clinical significance of this remains to be elucidated.

PROPHYLACTIC SURGERY FOR KINDREDS WITH RET MUTATIONS

Carriers of a familial RET mutation are recommended to have prophylactic thyroidectomy; this is an area of much controversy. The controversy lies in the age at which this should occur. The specifically mutated codon on the RET gene correlates with the MEN 2 variant and subsequently with the aggressiveness of MTC (93,98,104). The latest consensus guidelines suggest risk stratification based on these four known levels of aggressiveness (ATA levels A-D) of the known codon mutation (98). MEN 2B patients and patients with codons known to have the highest risk (ATA level D) and most aggressive form of MTC are recommended to have prophylactic thyroidectomy as soon as possible and within the first year of life. It has been recommended that patients classified as level B or C and considered at high risk for MTC should have prophylactic thyroidectomy by age 5 years or delayed if stringent criteria are met. Most felt that a level VI compartmental dissection should be performed. For patients with level A risk, surgery can be delayed beyond age 5 if stringent criteria are met and good follow-up is adhered to. It was also emphasized that because of the high risk of complications in children and the difficulty in managing hypoparathyroidism, these surgeries, especially in children, should be done by surgeons with expertise in MEN disease and prophylactic thyroidectomies.

Metastatic Disease

Almost all familial forms of MTC have a germline-activating mutation in the RET tyrosine kinase. Sporadic disease can have similar mutations of the C cells. Similar to differentiated thyroid carcinoma, these tumors tend to be dependent on angiogenesis as well. Clinical trials thus far have focused on VEGF inhibitors or RET and c-MET inhibition.

Patients with stable and asymptomatic metastatic disease may not need any therapy. Once the disease is progressive or symptomatic (including difficult to control diarrhea), treatment is recommended. Similar to metastatic differentiated thyroid carcinoma, treatment of individual metastatic sites causing symptoms or problems can be addressed individually (bone, spine and brain - see Differentiated Thyroid Carcinoma section).

Otherwise, clinical trials are considered first line in patients with symptomatic or progressive disease, since cytotoxic chemotherapy even in combination is limited at best (45).

Motesanib diphosphonate, a VEGF inhibitor, was recently studied in a phase II study evaluating progressive metastatic MTC and it was found that of 91 patients enrolled 2% had a partial response and 47% had stable disease for 24 weeks (105). Vandetanib, an oral tyrosine kinase inhibitor that inhibits VEGFR, RET, and EGFR, was recently studied in a phase II study. Seventeen percent of patients had a partial response and an additional 33% developed stable disease for 24 weeks or more (106).

Sorafenib and sunitinib, both oral small molecule tyrosine kinase inhibitors with VEGF inhibition and some raf (sorafenib) and ret (sunitinib) inhibition, are undergoing studies in medullary thyroid cancer. Both appear promising with significant stable disease development in patients with progressive cancer. Both drugs are FDA approved for the treatment of metastatic renal cell carcinoma and so are available for off-label use for patients who can not get into a clinical trial.

■ ANAPLASTIC THYROID CARCINOMA

INTRODUCTION

Anaplastic thyroid carcinoma is a locally and systemically aggressive undifferentiated tumor derived from follicular cells. In fact, it has the poorest prognosis of all thyroid carcinomas, with a disease-specific mortality rate approaching 100% (107-110). More than 90% of patients with this disease are over the age of 50 years, and a male:female ratio of 2:3 exists.

In sharp contrast with differentiated thyroid carcinomas, anaplastic thyroid carcinoma confers a dismal prognosis. Median survival duration after diagnosis ranges from 4 to 12 months with a long-term survival of more than 5 years considered rare. Better survival rates are seen only in those patients with well-localized anaplastic tumors. Favorable prognostic features seem to be unilateral tumors, tumor size less than 5 cm, no invasion of adjacent tissue, and absence of nodal involvement or distant metastases.

PATHOLOGY

Anaplastic thyroid carcinoma most commonly presents as the rapid growth of a thyroid mass, frequently in a preexisting goiter. A history of a long-standing thyroid enlargement is noted in about 80% of the patients. FNA

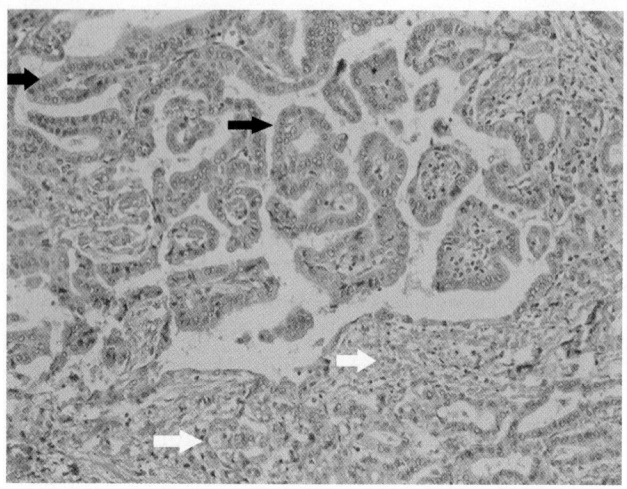

FIGURE 38-15. Hematoxylin and eosin staining of thyroid illustrating papillary thyroid carcinoma (*black arrows*) in transition to anaplastic thyroid carcinoma (*white arrows*).

or surgical biopsy can usually establish the diagnosis. In 50% of cases, this disease arises from preexisting well-differentiated thyroid carcinoma (Fig. 38-15). The presence of argyrophilic cytoplasmic granules distinguishes tumor of follicular origin from that of parafollicular origin and thus can differentiate anaplastic follicular thyroid lesions from undifferentiated variants of MTC. Tg, normally synthesized in the follicular epithelium of the thyroid, is present in well-differentiated papillary and follicular carcinomas and infrequently in anaplastic carcinomas. The absence of Tg immunoreactivity in anaplastic carcinomas does not exclude follicular epithelial origin, because undifferentiated carcinoma cells may have lost the ability to synthesize this glycoprotein. EGFR was overexpressed in 58% of anaplastic thyroid carcinomas compared to the more well-differentiated thyroid carcinoma components in the same patient (111). In a separate study, although PI3 kinase mutations were found only in 14% of specimens, PI3 kinase gain of copy number was found in 39% (112). This information may help guide clinical trials in the near future.

THERAPY

Treatment is generally palliative in nature as anaplastic thyroid carcinoma is rarely cured and almost always fatal. Death occurs from upper airway obstruction and suffocation in half the patients and complications of therapy or distant metastases in the others. For resectable lesions (no extracervical disease) in anaplastic carcinoma, surgical excision with wide margins of adjacent soft tissue on the side of the tumor is appropriate followed

by adjuvant radiotherapy. Prolonged survival of 75 to 80% at 2 years has been reported for the 20% of patients whose tumor is confined to the neck and grossly resectable when treated by complete surgical resection followed by adjuvant radiotherapy and chemotherapy (107,110). Total thyroidectomy and radical neck dissection result in an increased complication rate and are not likely to increase survival time in patients in whom disease cannot be completely resected (107,110,113,114). Hyperfractionated radiotherapy and radiosensitizing doxorubicin may increase local response rate. Paclitaxel has shown promise of late in newly diagnosed patients and may provide benefit (76,108). Radiotherapy and chemotherapy are important alternative approaches, but further evaluation is needed to optimize their effectiveness. Clinical trials are under way, including cytotoxic chemotherapy and combretastatin. Other trials are currently in phase I that may seem promising for anaplastic thyroid carcinoma. Biologic response modifiers aimed at restoring dedifferentiated functions of thyroid tissue in combination with chemotherapy may also be of some benefit in the future, but they are still under investigation at present.

■ PHEOCHROMOCYTOMA

INTRODUCTION

Pheochromocytoma is a chromaffin-cell neoplasm that can arise as an adrenal (adrenal medulla) or extra-adrenal tumor. Extra-adrenal pheochromocytoma is also referred to as paraganglioma. Pheochromocytoma is an infrequent but potentially curable cause of secondary hypertension. If undiagnosed or improperly treated, it can lead to life-threatening complications that can be avoided by considering pheochromocytoma early in the differential diagnosis of symptomatic hypertension, which presents with headache, palpitations, or sweating.

These tumors are most often benign; in general, 10% are thought to be malignant, 10% extra-adrenal, and 10% bilateral (most often in the setting of familial syndromes) (Fig. 38-16). This classic teaching has been challenged in the past few years with data estimating that close to 25% of all pheochromocytomas/paragangliomas are associated with underlying germ line mutations of various genes (RET, VHL, SDHD, and SDHB) (115). Even more, some genetic mutations such as succinate dehydrogenase B (SDHB) are associated with high rate of malignant pheochromocytomas/paragangliomas approaching 30 to 40% of SDHB gene carriers while only 3% of SDHD mutations are reported to have malignant paraganglioma (116,117).

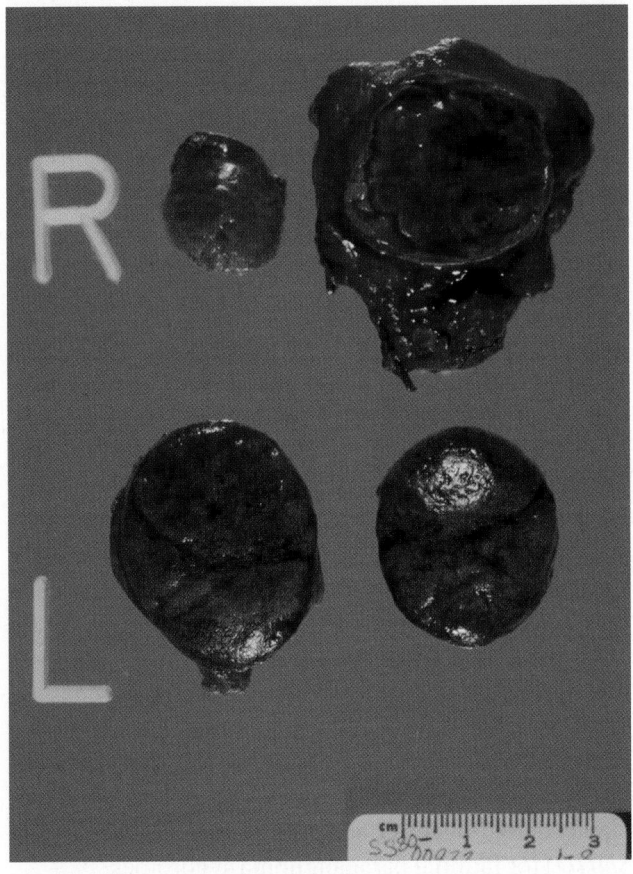

FIGURE 38-16. Bilateral pheochromocytoma in multiple endocrine neoplasia 2A.

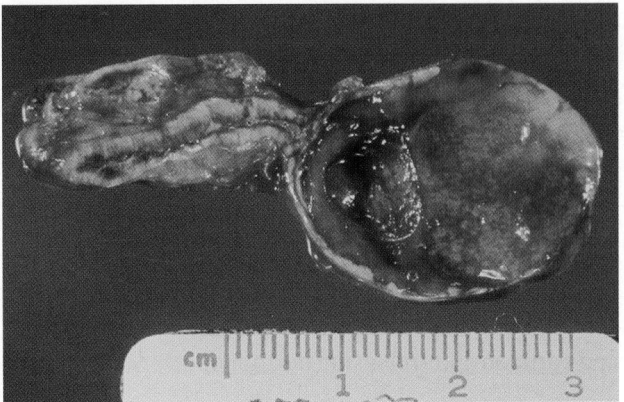

FIGURE 38-17. Adrenal gland with pheochromocytoma.

The incidence of reported pheochromocytomas depends on the screening method chosen. In the general population, the incidence rate has been estimated at 0.95 per 100,000 person-years (118), whereas on autopsy series, the incidence rate was reported as 0.05% (one tumor per 2031 autopsies) (119). In one study, sporadic cases accounted for 84% of the patients and hereditary cases for the other 16% (120). Tumor is located in the adrenal gland in 81% of cases (Fig. 38-17) and is extra-adrenal (Fig. 38-18) in 19% (121), with a slight female predominance (53.6% females and 46.4% males) (122). It is believed that extra-adrenal pheochromocytomas are more likely to be malignant than adrenal tumors and they carry a poorer prognosis especially if measured more than 5 cm (123).

CLINICAL FEATURES

The clinical presentation of pheochromocytoma is variable, ranging from asymptomatic to catastrophic sudden death. Hypertension is commonly reported with pheochromocytoma and has been reported to be

paroxysmal in 48% of patients and persistent in 39%; 13% of patients were normotensive. Rarely, hypotension may occur with tumors that secrete mainly epinephrine. The symptomatic triad (headaches, palpitations, and sweating attacks) has a specificity of 93.8% and a sensitivity of 90.9% in the diagnosis of pheochromocytoma. The presence of the above symptoms in hypertensive patients justifies systematic assays of blood or urinary catecholamines; in their absence, the probability of pheochromocytoma is less than 1 in 1000 (124). Patients may have characteristic "spells" of paroxysmal headaches, pallor or flushing, hypertension, and diaphoresis that may persist anywhere from a few minutes to several hours. Attacks may be provoked by body position, straining, exercise, emotional stress, or voiding. Orthostatic hypotension in the presence of hypertension may be an additional clue to a diagnosis of

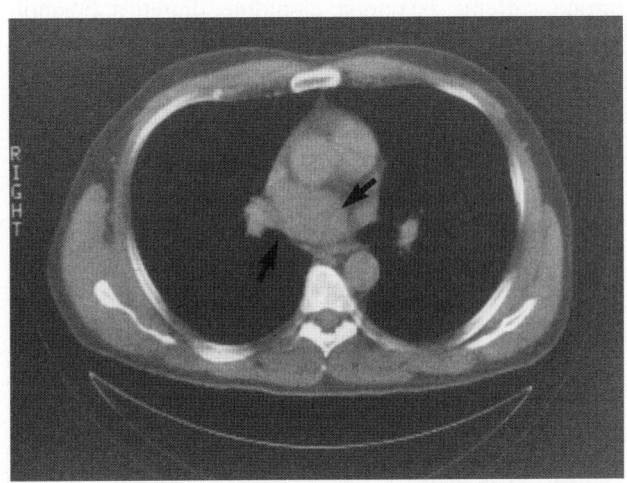

FIGURE 38-18. CT of the chest showing extra-adrenal pheochromocytoma in the pericardium (*arrows*).

pheochromocytoma; this may be due to the intravascular volume depletion associated with vasoconstriction. Patients may have impaired glucose tolerance from the suppressive effects of catecholamines on insulin secretion. Patients also may have constipation, cholelithiasis, or abdominal distention from the inhibitory effects of catecholamines on gut motility.

Rarely, pheochromocytoma can lead to the ectopic production of vasoactive intestinal polypeptide (VIP), growth hormone–releasing factor, adrenocorticotropin, and corticotropin-releasing hormone.

DIAGNOSIS

Laboratory Findings

There is ongoing discussion as to the optimal screening test for pheochromocytomas. Biochemical testing is indicated in the presence of (1) features or family history suggestive of syndromes associated with pheochromocytoma, including MEN 2A, MEN 2B, von Hippel-Lindau (VHL) disease, familial paraganglioma syndromes, and neurofibromatosis 1 (NF-1); (2) clinical features of symptomatic pheochromocytoma (headache, diaphoresis, or palpitations), especially in the presence of hypertension; (3) adrenal incidentalomas; and (4) a hypertensive crisis at the time of delivery or induction of anesthesia (Table 38-3).

It is important to have chemical confirmation of pheochromocytoma before attempting costly localization procedures. At our institution, plasma-free metanephrines and 24-hour urine fractionated metanephrines are the two most commonly used laboratory tests to diagnose pheochromocytoma. Results must be interpreted with caution because several medications (eg, monoamine oxidase inhibitors, amphetamines, bromocriptine, buspirone, caffeine, levodopa, clonidine, diuretics, ethanol, nicotine, theophylline, tricyclic antidepressants, vasodilators, methyldopa, and labetalol) may affect the results. In a multicenter study, plasma-free metanephrines were superior to plasma catecholamines in the diagnosis of pheochromocytoma (125). In hereditary pheochromocytoma, plasma-free metanephrines (with an upper reference limit of 0.9 nmol/L) had a sensitivity and specificity of 97 and 96%, respectively; whereas in sporadic tumors, sensitivity and specificity were 99 and 82%, respectively.

In the same study, urinary fractionated metanephrines (with upper reference limit of 2.4 μmol/day for women and 4.2 μmol/day for men) had a sensitivity and specificity of 96 and 82% in hereditary tumors, respectively, and 97 and 45% in sporadic tumors, respectively.

Chromogranin A (CgA) is an acidic protein that is stored and released with catecholamines. It is nonspecific and widely distributed in neuroendocrine cells, particularly in chromaffin adrenal medullary cells. There is a significant concordance between CgA levels and ^{131}I MIBG imaging data (126). Elevated levels of serum CgA are not specific for the diagnosis of pheochromocytoma and may be of less benefit in patients with impaired renal function.

Genetic Testing

Pheochromocytoma is thought to be hereditary in about 10 to 16% of cases, although this may be an underestimate as more recent studies put this close to 25% (115). Multiple familial syndromes are associated with the development of pheochromocytoma, including MEN 2A and 2B, familial paraganglioma syndromes, NF-1, and VHL disease. Routine genetic testing in apparently sporadic pheochromocytomas is not widely practiced in the United States, but in the presence of any of the aforementioned syndromes or a family history suggestive of familial pheochromocytoma, multiple genes are now available in selected laboratories and should be analyzed. These include *RET* for MEN 2, *VHL* for VHL disease, *NF-1* for neurofibromatosis, and, recently, succinate dehydrogenase subunits B and D (*SDHB* and *SDHD*) for familial paraganglioma syndromes.

Other syndromes include Carney triad (paraganglioma, gastric stromal tumor, and pulmonary chondroma) and Carney-Stratakis syndrome (paraganglioma and gastric stromal tumors) (127). Genetic counseling is imperative prior to and after any familial testing and should include an explanation of the pros and cons of testing, some of which are the possibility of errors in the test, genetic discrimination, and potential quality-of-life changes.

Imaging

Ninety-five percent of pheochromocytomas are intra-abdominal, and the majority of these are localized to the adrenal gland. When a pheochromocytoma is suspected on clinical and laboratory grounds, CT or MRI of the abdomen and pelvis can be performed as an initial step for tumor localization. If an adrenal mass is not seen, attention should be directed to the paraspinous region and urinary bladder; even less commonly, extra-adrenal tumors may be located in the head and neck region. Pheochromocytoma has a characteristic hyperintense appearance on T2-weighted MRI scans; however, not all pheochromocytomas have this imaging characteristic, and pheochromocytoma cannot be excluded on the basis of a lack of high-signal intensity on T2-weighted MRI scans.

TABLE 38-3 | ALGORITHM FOR CLINICAL APPROACH AND MANAGEMENT OF PHEOCHROMOCYTOMA

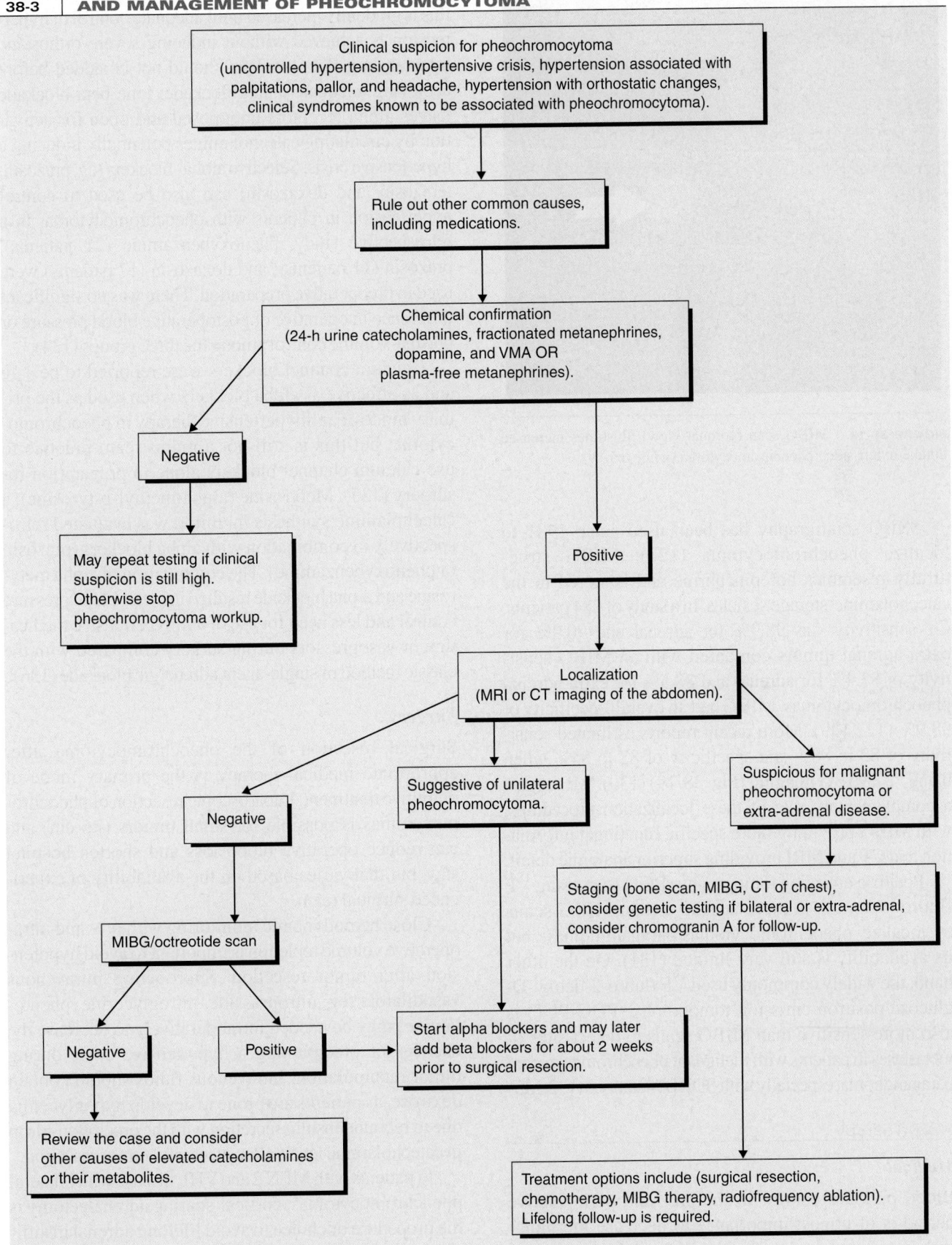

CT, computed tomography; MIBG, metaiodenzylguanidine; MRI, magnetic resonance imaging; VMA, vanillylmandelic acid.

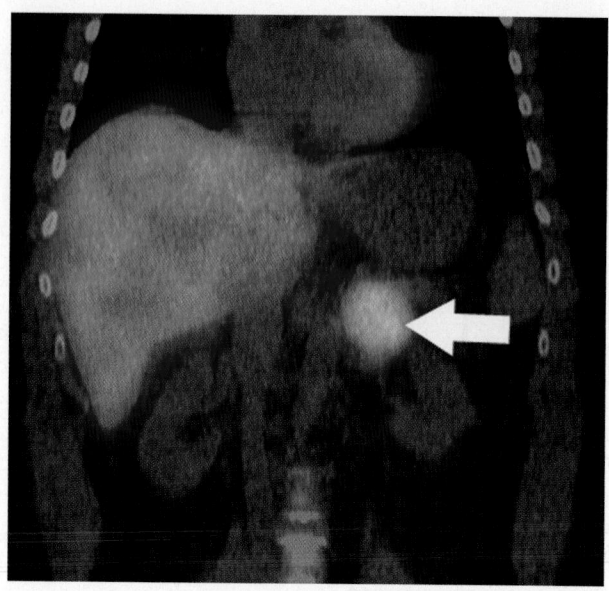

FIGURE 38-19. MIBG scan (coronal view) illustrates increased uptake in left-sided pheochromocytoma (*white arrow*).

MIBG scintigraphy has been used since 1981 to localize pheochromocytoma (128). MIBG structurally resembles norepinephrine and is stored in the catecholamine-storage vesicles. In a study of 284 patients, CT sensitivity was 98.9% for adrenal and 90.9% for extra-adrenal tumors compared with an MIBG sensitivity of 87.4% for adrenal and 88.5% for extra-adrenal pheochromocytomas. MIBG had an overall specificity of 98.9% (122,129). More recent reports estimated sensitivity of 82 to 88% and specificity of 82 to 84% when using ^{123}I MIBG imaging (Fig. 38-19) (130). We suggest a complementary role of these localization procedures, with MIBG providing more specific functional information and CT and MRI providing superior anatomic detail.

Positron emission tomography (PET) scan using ^{18}F fluorodopamine is more sensitive than MIBG scans to localize pheochromocytomas/paragangliomas, but its availability is still very limited (131). On the other hand, the widely commonly used ^{18}F fluoro-2-deoxy-D-glucose positron emission tomography (FDG-PET) is also more sensitive than MIBG scans to detect sites of metastases in patients with malignant pheochromocytoma/paraganglioma, especially with SDHB mutations (132,133).

Therapy

Medical

Blood pressure control in the pre- and perioperative period is of utmost importance to decrease morbidity and mortality associated with a potential hypertensive crisis at the time of surgical resection. Patients are usually given a long-acting alpha blocker (phenoxybenzamine)

starting at 10 mg twice a day (2 weeks before surgery); this is gradually increased until adequate control of hypertension is achieved without inducing severe orthostatic hypotension. Beta blockers should not be added before achieving adequate alpha blockade; lone beta blockade leaves alpha receptors unopposed and open for activation by circulating catecholamines potentially inducing a hypertensive crisis. Selective alpha₁ blockers (eg, prazosin, terazosin, and doxazosin) can also be used to control hypertension in patients with pheochromocytoma. In a retrospective study, phenoxybenzamine (21 patients), prazosin (11 patients), and doxazosin (17 patients) were used in preoperative preparation. There was no significant difference in operative or postoperative blood pressure or plasma-volume control among the three groups (134).

Calcium channel blockers were reported to be safe and as effective as alpha blockers when used as the primary mode of antihypertensive therapy in pheochromocytoma, but this is still not a mainstream practice to use calcium channel blockers alone in preparation for surgery (135). Metyrosine (alpha-methyl-p-tyrosine), a catecholamine synthesis inhibitor, was evaluated retrospectively in combination with alpha blockers (prazosin or phenoxybenzamine). The combination of alpha metyrosine and alpha blockade resulted in better blood pressure control and less need for use of antihypertensive medication or vasopressors during surgery compared with the classic method of single-agent adrenergic blockade (136).

Surgery

Surgical resection of the pheochromocytoma after appropriate medical therapy is the primary mode of definitive treatment. Laparoscopic resection of pheochromocytomas is possible for small tumors (<6 cm) and can reduce operative blood loss and shorten hospital stay, but that varies based on the availability of experienced surgical team.

Close hemodynamic monitoring with pre- and intraoperative volume repletion is important to avoid hypotension after tumor resection. Short-acting intravenous vasodilators (eg, nitroprusside, nitroglycerine, phentolamine) may be needed intraoperatively to decrease the chances of precipitating a hypertensive crisis during tumor manipulation. Intravenous fluids should contain dextrose, as patients are prone to develop hypoglycemia due to rebound insulin secretion with the precipitous drop in catecholamine levels after successful tumor resection.

In patients with MEN 2 and VHL disease with bilateral pheochromocytomas, cortical-sparing adrenalectomy is the procedure of choice to avoid lifelong adrenal insufficiency, but patients still require long-term follow-up, as recurrence may develop many years after operation and some may still develop adrenal insufficiency (137).

■ MALIGNANT PHEOCHROMOCYTOMA

INTRODUCTION

The exact prevalence of malignant pheochromocytoma is not well known. Pheochromocytoma has been reported to recur at intervals from 5 to 13 years following initial resection of a benign-appearing tumor (138); thus, after seemingly successful resection of benign tumor, life-long follow-up is mandated in these patients (120). The malignancy rate is estimated to be 9.9 to 14% of all pheochromocytomas (122,138). The presence of familial syndromes (MEN 2 and VHL) is associated with bilateral pheochromocytomas, though these are rarely malignant (121,139). The axial skeleton is the most common site of metastases (Fig. 38-20), followed by the liver, lymph nodes, lungs, and peritoneum. Familial paraganglioma syndromes are associated with succinate dehydrogenase (SDH) complex mutations. In particular, SDHB mutations are associated with increased risk of malignant pheochromocytomas and paragangliomas approaching 40% (117,140).

DIAGNOSIS

As in the case of many endocrine tumors, in the absence of clinically evident metastases or recurrences, there are no reliable histological features that can distinguish benign from malignant pheochromocytoma. Various markers have been proposed to differentiate benign from malignant pheochromocytomas. These include chromogranin A (CgA), secretogranin II–derived peptide EM66, neuron-specific enolase (NSE), and neuropeptide Y (NPY) (141-143). In most studies these markers have been shown to be higher in malignant

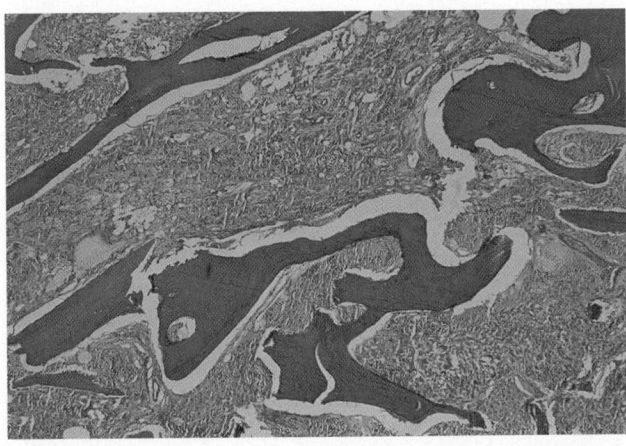

FIGURE 38-20. Histopathologic picture of metastatic pheochromocytoma to a rib.

pheochromocytomas as compared to benign ones. Loss of inhibin/activin beta B subunit expression in pheochromocytomas may be used as an indicator of malignant potential (144). Ki-67 staining combined with histological features may also predict malignant potential of pheochromocytomas (145). The zinc-finger transcription factor SNAIL and its target gene (TWIST) are also thought to be involved in the malignant transformation of pheochromocytomas (146,147).

THERAPY

In the few selected cases of malignant pheochromocytoma with limited disease, surgery can be attempted in conjunction with other therapeutic measures. The role of debulking surgery is more controversial in cases where total resection is deemed impossible.

^{131}I MIBG therapy has been suggested as a useful palliative adjunct in selected patients with malignant pheochromocytoma (148).

Radiolabeled somatostatin analogue (DOTATOC) was studied in patients with surgically incurable paragangliomas and pheochromocytomas. While the treatment was well tolerated, it only led to few partial responses while most patients had stable or progressive disease (149). Streptozocin-based regimens were used in metastatic pheochromocytoma with variable results ranging from no response to partial response (150,151).

Combination chemotherapy of cyclophosphamide (750 mg/m^2 body-surface area on day 1), vincristine (1.4 mg/m^2 on day 1), and dacarbazine (600 mg/m^2 on days 1 and 2) every 21 days (CVD regimen) achieved complete and partial responses in 57% of patients, while 79% of patients had a complete or partial response biochemically. All responding patients had objective improvement in performance status and blood pressure (152). Subsequent update of this series as well as other recent retrospective review did not find survival benefit in patients treated with CVD especially for women or having malignant pheochromocytoma of adrenal origin though it helped improving symptoms associated with catecholamine excess (153,154). At MD Anderson the most commonly used regimen for metastatic pheochromocytoma is CVAD (cyclophosphamide, vincristine, Adriamycin [doxorubicin], and dacarbazine).

While initial reports using multityrosine kinase inhibitor (sunitinib) suggested partial short-term responses in a very small number of reported patients, the long-term efficacy and validation of these findings is still lacking (155-157). Similarly, the use of mammalian target of rapamycin inhibitor (everolimus) was reported in four patients with malignant paraganglioma but did not lead to significant results (158).

Fractionated EBRT is mainly used for symptomatic relief of bony metastases. It can lead to short-lived reduction in catecholamine production and reduced need for analgesics (159). Radiofrequency ablation (RFA) has been attempted in a very limited number of patients with metastatic pheochromocytoma and proposed as a potential treatment modality (160-162).

PROGNOSIS

In a series of 86 patients with 85 benign and 10 malignant pheochromocytomas, the 5-year survival rate for malignant pheochromocytomas was reported at 20%, and all patients with malignant pheochromocytomas died within 10 years (121).

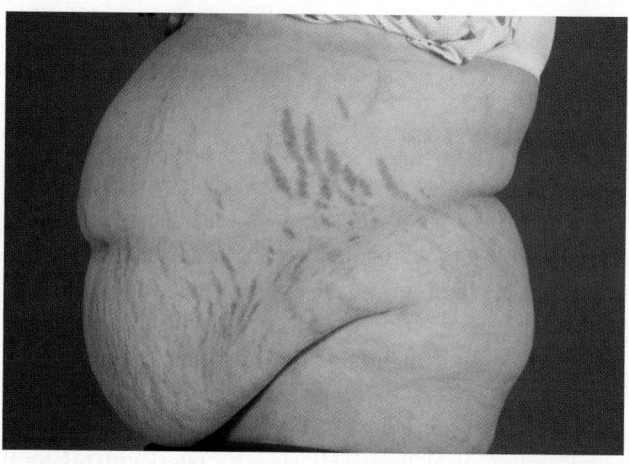

FIGURE 38-21.　Purple striae on the abdomen associated with Cushing syndrome.

■ ADRENOCORTICAL CARCINOMA

INTRODUCTION

Adrenocortical carcinoma (ACC) is a rare malignancy with significant morbidity and mortality. The increasing use of body imaging techniques (eg, US, CT, and MRI) has led to the discovery of silent adrenal tumors that may have malignant potential. The earlier identification of ACC by such detection methods facilitates earlier intervention and may translate into improved survival rates.

The incidence of ACC is approximately two cases per million populations per year. It can occur at any age with reported bimodal age incidence in the first and fourth decades of life with near equal sex distribution. Hormonally functional tumors are found in 34 to 62% of ACC cases (163,164), with variable clinical signs and symptoms based on the predominantly produced hormone. The various syndromes seen with functioning adrenal

cancers are presented in Table 38-4 (see Fig. 38-20; Figs. 38-21 and 38-22).

Adrenocortical tumors may also present as nonfunctioning tumors, with nonspecific symptoms of abdominal discomfort or pain, indigestion, or site-specific symptoms based on the location of the metastatic disease (Figs. 38-23 and 38-24).

PATHOGENESIS

ACC is considered a monoclonal disease in contrast to benign adrenal adenomas. ACC may present in the setting of inherited cancer syndromes. Li-Fraumeni syndrome, one such example, is a constellation of diseases that all have a *p53* germline mutation in common; this raises the possibility that loss of *p53* tumor suppressor activity can lead to the development of ACC (165). The

TABLE 38-4	CLINICAL SYNDROMES ASSOCIATED WITH FUNCTIONAL ADRENOCORTICAL CARCINOMA	
Clinical Syndrome	*Suggestive Clinical Features*	*Suggested Laboratory Workup*
Cushing syndrome	Obesity, moon face, purple striae, cervical fat pads, easy bruising, myopathy, hypertension, diabetes mellitus	Plasma electrolytes, plasma glucose, ACTH, cortisol, 24-h urine-free cortisol
Virilizing syndrome	Hirsutism, clitoromegaly, temporal balding, increased muscle mass, amenorrhea, male precocious puberty, advanced bone age in children.	DHEA sulfate, testosterone, 17-OH progesterone
Feminizing syndrome	Gynecomastia, loss of libido	Estradiol, prolactin, testosterone
Hyperaldosteronism	Hypertension, hypokalemia	Plasma renin activity, plasma aldosterone concentration, plasma electrolytes, 18-OH corticosterone
Mixed syndromes		

ACTH, adrenocorticotropic hormone; DHEA, dehydroepiandrosterone.

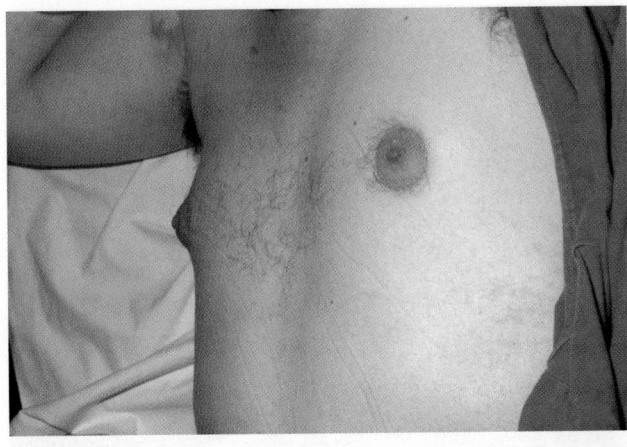

FIGURE 38-22. Gynecomastia associated with feminizing adrenocortical carcinoma.

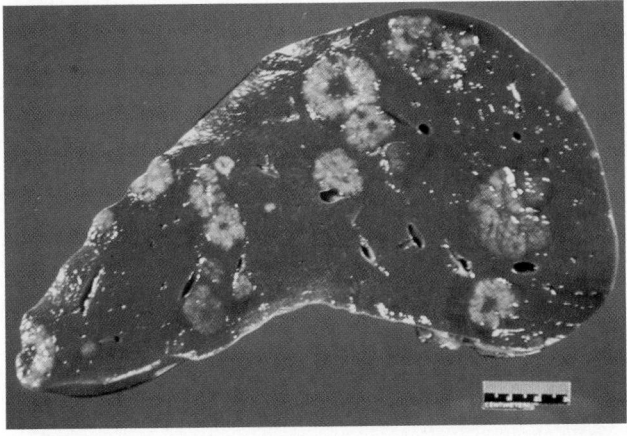

FIGURE 38-23. Liver metastases from adrenocortical carcinoma.

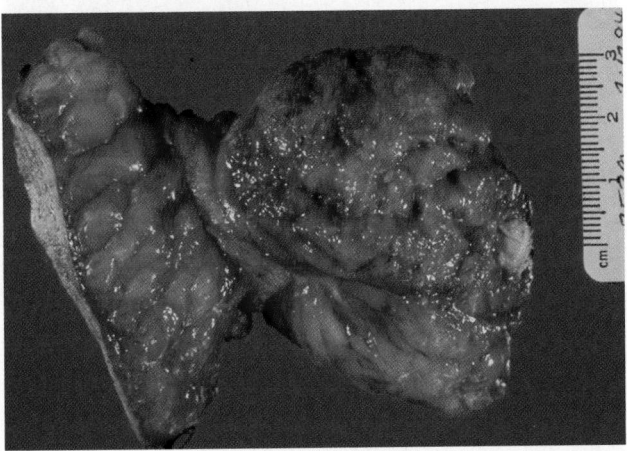

FIGURE 38-24. Adrenocortical carcinoma invading the abdominal wall.

Beckwith-Wiedemann syndrome (BWS) is characterized by somatic overgrowth and a predisposition to tumors, including ACC. BWS results from mutations or epimutations affecting imprinted genes on chromosome 11p15.5 (166). ACC can be rarely seen in patients with multiple endocrine neoplasia type 1 (mutation of menin gene on 11q13).

DIAGNOSIS

Laboratory Findings

In patients found to have an adrenal mass, it is necessary to obtain a complete blood count and serum chemistries. Hormonal evaluation could include random plasma renin activity, plasma aldosterone concentration, ACTH, serum cortisol, and 24-h urine-free cortisol and plasma-free metanephrines. Total testosterone, dehydroepiandrosterone sulfate (DHEAS), and estradiol can be obtained if there is a clinical suspicion of increased sex-hormone secretion (ie, virilizing or feminizing features).

Radiologic Findings

The expanding use of body imaging methods has led to the increasing discovery of adrenal masses. Radiologic studies play a critical role in detecting adrenal masses and characterizing malignant potential. Numerous imaging modalities—including CT, MRI, US, and nuclear medicine imaging—can be used to evaluate the adrenal gland.

Benign adrenal adenomas are usually smaller than the malignant variety and have higher lipid content, giving them characteristic features on imaging. CT scanning with thin cuts targeted to the adrenal gland is a useful tool for both the detection and characterization of adrenal masses. A nonenhanced examination should initially be performed, followed by a contrast-enhanced study if necessary (Figs. 38-25 and 38-26).

Benign adenomas usually have low attenuation on nonenhanced CT scans; using a threshold of 10 Hounsfield units (HU), the sensitivity of nonenhanced CT for characterizing adrenal adenomas was 79%, with a specificity of 96% (167). Almost 30% of adenomas do not contain sufficient lipid to have low attenuation at CT. On the other hand, benign adenomas enhance rapidly with intravenous contrast media and wash out rapidly. More than 50% washout between the dynamic phase of contrast enhancement and the 10-min delayed images is highly diagnostic of benign adenoma and confirms the finding on the low attenuation on nonenhanced CT scan.

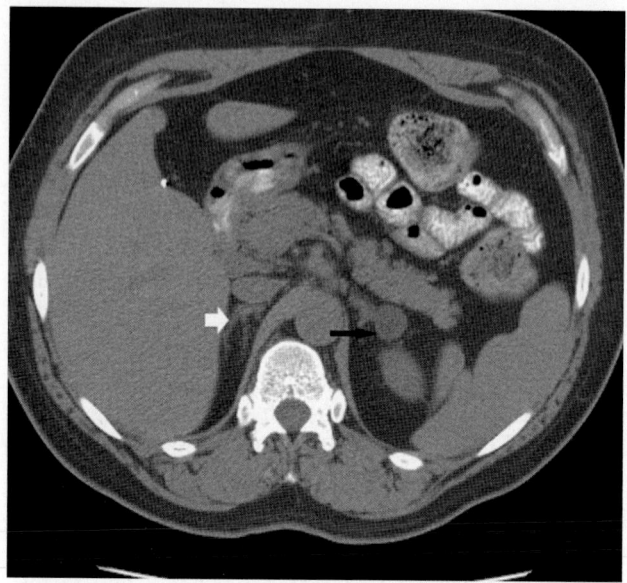

FIGURE 38-25. CT scan of the abdomen showing a left adrenal mass (*black arrow*) with low attenuation (<10 Hounsfield units) on precontrast images, compatible with benign adenoma.

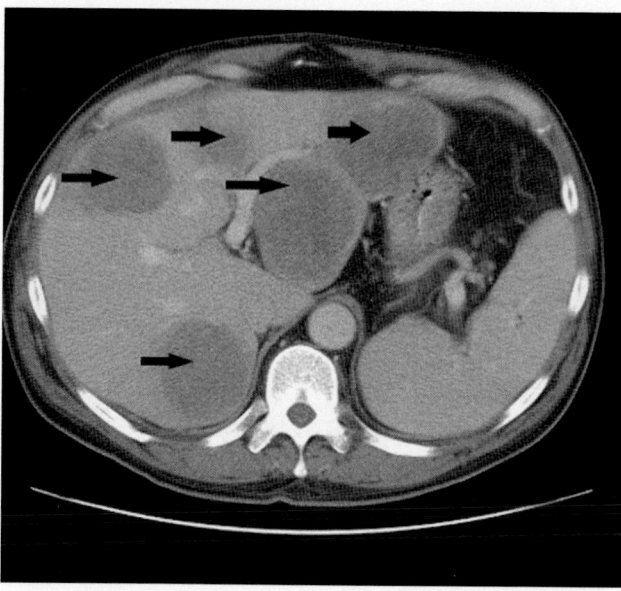

FIGURE 38-27. CT of the abdomen showing hepatic metastases from adrenocortical carcinoma (*black arrows*).

Larger adrenal lesions have a greater likelihood of being malignant; an increase in the size of the lesion is a useful indicator of malignancy, as adenomas in general tend to grow slowly and often do not change in size over time. An adrenal tumor diameter of 5 cm identifies ACC with a sensitivity of 93% and a specificity of 64% (168). Other radiologic features suggestive of malignancy include heterogeneity, irregular shape, irregular margins, or hemorrhage (Figs. 38-27 and 38-28). Although these findings are helpful in differentiating a benign from a malignant adrenal mass, they are not specific.

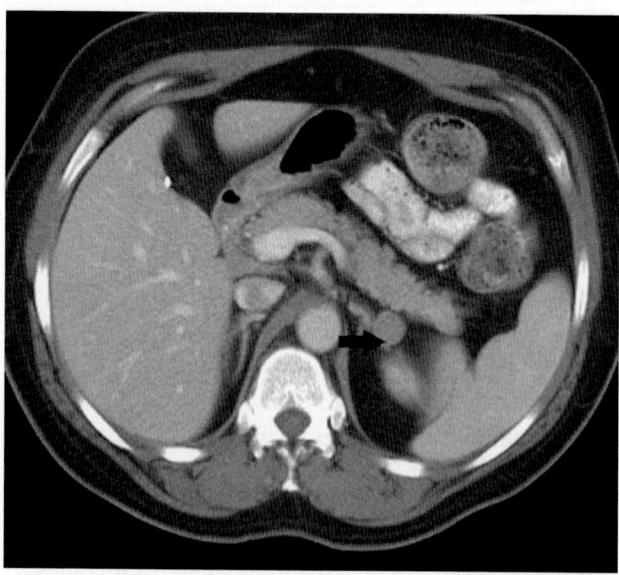

FIGURE 38-26. Postcontrast CT scan images showing enhancement of the left adrenal mass (*black arrow*), but these images still have lower attenuation than those of the normal right adrenal gland.

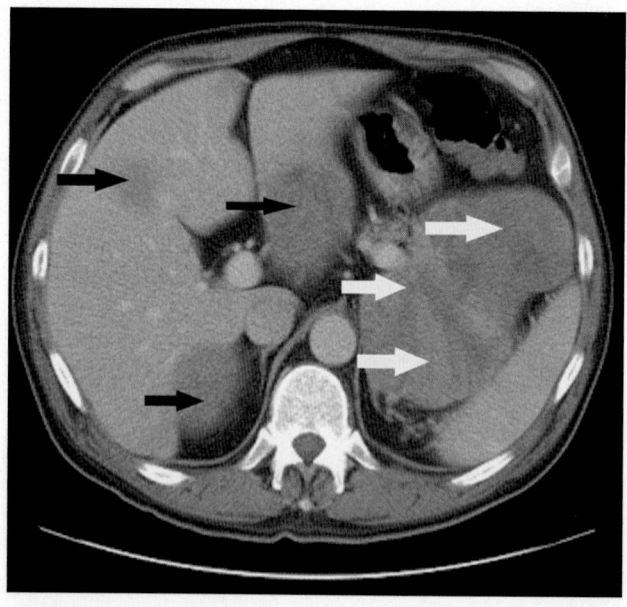

FIGURE 38-28. Left-sided adrenocortical carcinoma (*white arrows*) with liver metastases (*black arrows*).

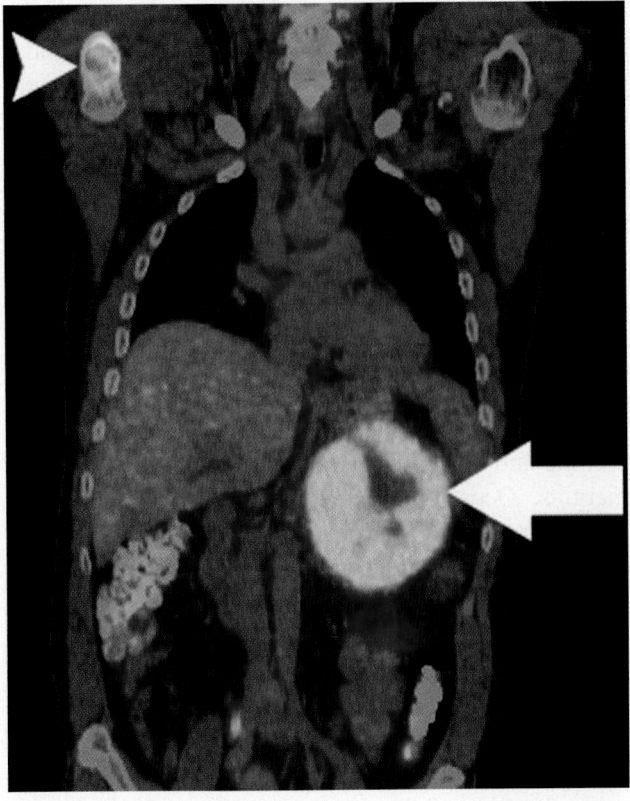

FIGURE 38-29. FDG-PET scan (coronal view) showing FDG-avid left adrenal mass (*white arrow*) with bony metastases (*arrowhead*).

When results of CT examinations are equivocal, MRI is another good study of choice for characterizing adrenal lesions. Tissues with higher lipid content (benign adenomas) show loss of signal intensity (ie, appear darker) on out-of-phase images on chemical-shift MRI. MRI with T2-weighted imaging is also a useful modality when the adrenal gland is being evaluated because in addition to the heterogeneous characteristics of ACC due to hemorrhage or tumor necrosis typically seen on other radiographic studies, malignant adrenal masses usually have higher signal intensity with this modality than benign adrenal adenomas in addition to the heterogeneity of ACC because of hemorrhage or tumor necrosis as well as intravascular extension.

PET shows promise in differentiating benign from malignant masses (Fig. 38-29). In small series studies, FDG-PET had 100% sensitivity and 80 to 100% specificity for differentiating malignant masses versus benign adrenal masses (169,170).

Although FDG-PET scans seem to be a sensitive tool for detecting malignant tissue, the false-positive results and the lack for cost-effective analysis make it premature to recommend the routine use of this modality in patients with adrenal cancer.

Fine-Needle Aspiration

Adrenal incidentalomas are relatively common, whereas occult metastatic cancers only rarely present as isolated asymptomatic adrenal masses. An adrenal mass may also represent pheochromocytoma, and performing FNA may therefore precipitate a hypertensive crisis. For these reasons, the routine FNA of asymptomatic adrenal masses is not indicated unless a patient has a known primary malignant tumor with possible metastases to the adrenal gland (ie, small cell lung cancer). In this instance, FNA may be considered if the result seems to affect the management plan. In a study of 1639 patients found to have cancer, the adrenal gland was involved at diagnosis in 95 patients (5.8%), and only one patient had ACC. In four patients (0.2%), the disease was limited to the adrenal gland at presentation, with tumor size ≥6 cm (171).

The cytological features of ACCs vary from well-differentiated tumor resembling adrenal adenomas to poorly differentiated carcinoma. Hypercellularity, necrotic debris, nuclear pleomorphism, mitotic figures, and prominent nucleoli are the most noticeable features on FNA with necrosis and/or mitosis seen in all studied cases (172).

PATHOLOGY

Adrenal tumor size has been suggested as a predictor of malignancy. ACCs are usually large (>5-6 cm), whereas benign adenomas are usually small (<5 cm); however, there is remarkable overlap, and tumor size cannot be used as a sole pathologic criterion for predicting malignancy (173).

ACCs, especially the nonfunctioning tumors, are often large at diagnosis. They are commonly encapsulated and lobulated and can be solid or cystic, with areas of necrosis and hemorrhage evident on gross sections.

Microscopically, it can be hard to differentiate ACC from benign adenomas based on histologic features alone. ACC is described as polygonal cells arranged in sheets, nests, trabeculae, or ribbons and at times contains anaplastic features. Cells are usually eosinophilic, in contrast to the clear cells of normal adrenals or benign adenomas, although clear cells can be found in some ACCs. Increased mitotic figures and vascular and capsular invasion are other signs that suggest a diagnosis of ACC. Weiss proposed a scoring system consisting of nine criteria to aid in the diagnosis of adrenal cancer (174). The criteria were later modified and include (1) mitotic rate greater than five mitoses per 50 high-power fields in the most active areas of the tumor, (2) atypical mitoses, (3) venous invasion, (4) clear cells comprising

25% or less of the tumor, (5) tumor necrosis, (6) nuclear grade III or IV tumor (Fuhrman method), (7) diffuse (solid) architecture in more than one-third of the tumor, (8) invasion of sinusoidal structures, and (9) capsular invasion. The presence of three or more of these nine features is highly suggestive of ACC. Despite this system, there are still borderline cases in which a systematic approach is needed to make a definitive diagnosis.

Recent data suggested that Ki-67 immunohistochemistry staining combined with overexpression of insulin-like growth factor-2 (IGF-2) carried high sensitivity and specificity to differentiate adrenal adenomas from carcinomas (175).

ACC usually spreads early by direct invasion, lymphatic invasion, or hematogenous spread. Liver, lungs, bones, and regional lymph nodes are the main sites for metastases.

Table 38-5 summarizes the staging system used at MD Anderson (176); it is modified from the earlier accepted system proposed by MacFarlane in 1958 (177). Recent study validated the earlier reports that stage IV ACC should be limited to patients with distant metastases while the presence of local invasion, venous tumor thrombus, or local lymphadenopathy define stage III disease (178).

THERAPY

Surgery

At our institution, adrenalectomy is performed for adrenal masses that are either functional or have suspicious radiologic features. For benign-appearing nonfunctional tumors, surgery is considered if the tumor is ≥4 cm and the patient is a good surgical candidate (168); however, the National Institutes of Health (NIH) consensus guidelines for adrenal nonfunctional incidentalomas currently state that all tumors greater than 6 cm should be surgically resected, whereas surgical decisions should be individualized for tumors between 4 and 6 cm (179).

Complete surgical resection is the mainstay of therapy for ACC and offers the best chance for prolonged disease-free survival (176). Subcostal transabdominal or thoracoabdominal incision is the preferred approach at our institution; if ACC is suspected, laparoscopic adrenalectomy is not recommended, as it can result in early locoregional recurrence through tumor spillage and seeding and decreases the ability to achieve tumor-free margins. Occasionally, en bloc resection sacrificing adjacent organs is performed with the aim of complete resection of tumor and invaded structures. Tumor encasement of the celiac axis, aorta, or proximal superior mesenteric artery (SMA) may make tumor unresectable. The presence of tumor thrombus in the inferior vena cava (IVC), or renal vein, or tumor invasion of the pancreas, spleen, or kidney is not a contraindication for complete resection in selected patients. Although there is limited evidence of benefit from resection of the primary tumor in the presence of metastatic disease, there might still be a role for resection of primary tumor and all visible metastases in an otherwise young, healthy patient, especially in cases of functioning tumors (176).

In corticosteroid-producing ACC, preoperative blockade of steroid production using agents such as ketoconazole or metyrapone may reduce postoperative morbidity. In these cases, the contralateral adrenal gland is usually atrophic and the patients require peri- and postoperative corticosteroid replacement. This

TABLE 38-5	**STAGING OF ADRENOCORTICAL CARCINOMA**	
Stage	*MacFarlane (177)*	*Lee et al. (176)*
I	T1 (≤5 cm), N0, M0	T1 (≤5 cm), N0, M0
II	T2 (>5 cm), N0, M0	T2 (>5 cm), N0, M0
III	T3 (local invasion without involvement of adjacent organs) or mobile positive lymph nodes, M0	T3/T4 (local invasion as shown by histological evidence of adjacent organ invasion, direct tumor extension to IVC, or tumor thrombus within IVC (or renal vein), and/or N1 (positive regional lymph nodes), M0
IV	T4 (invasion of adjacent organs) or fixed positive lymph nodes or M1 (distant metastases)	T1-4, N0-1, M1 (distant metastases)

IVC, inferior vena cava.

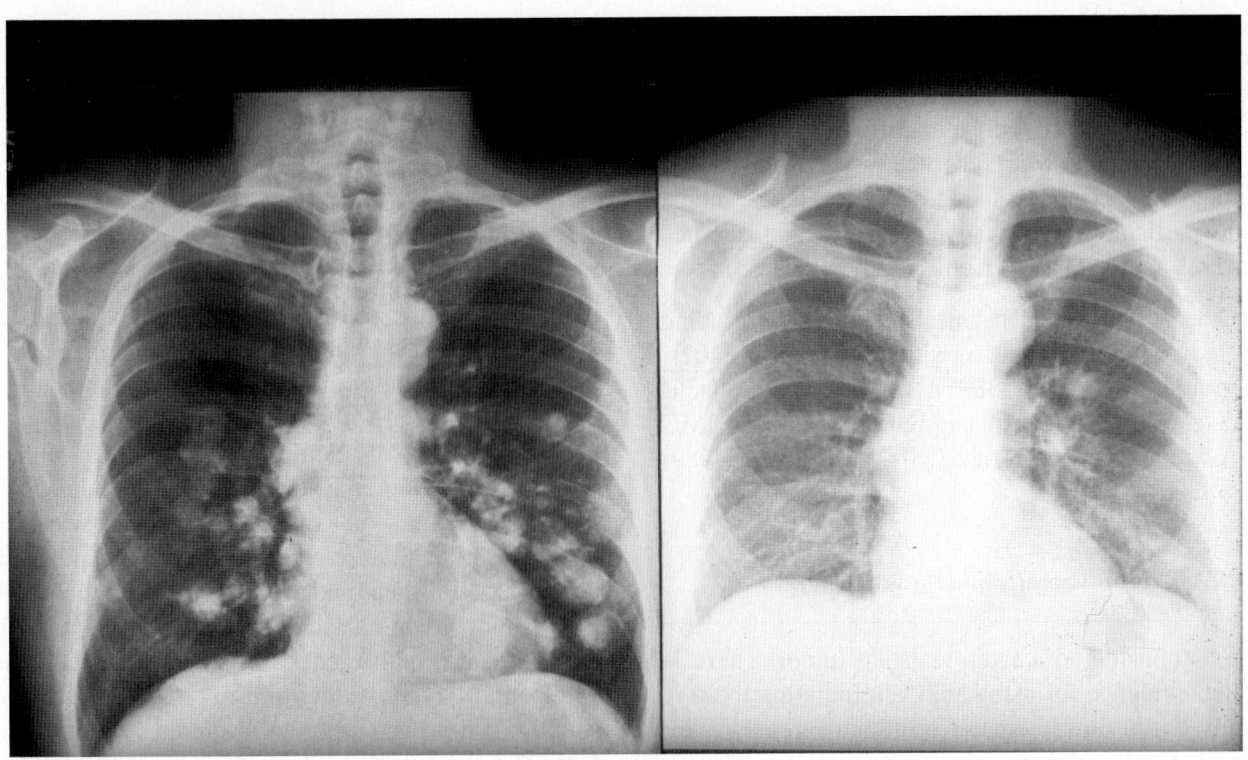

FIGURE 38-30.   Resolution of adrenocortical carcinoma metastases with mitotane therapy (before mitotane on the left and after mitotane on the right).

relative adrenal insufficiency may last for months after successful resection.

Chemotherapy

In 1949, it was found that oral administration of insecticide (DDD, or Rothane) to dogs induced selective necrosis of zona fasciculata and zona reticularis of the adrenal cortex. Mitotane (o,p′-DDD) has been used to treat ACC since 1960.

Until now, o,p′-DDD has been considered an efficacious agent in treating patients with cancer, especially when its plasma levels exceed 14 mg/L (180,181) (Fig. 38-30).

Mitotane blocks adrenal 11β hydroxylase and cholesterol side-chain cleavage, alters zona fasciculata mitochondrial morphology, and destroys the adrenal cortex. Treatment starts with 1 g twice daily and increases to 9 to 10 g/day, depending on plasma levels (target 14-20 mg/L) and tolerability. Patients receiving mitotane should receive glucocorticosteroid replacement. Mitotane increases corticosteroid-binding globulin and enhances steroids clearance, which explains the increased corticosteroid requirements during mitotane therapy. Steroid replacement can be potentially guided by ACTH monitoring for two reasons: to ensure adequate replacement and to probably suppress endogenous ACTH production in a

manner similar to thyroxine-suppression therapy in differentiated thyroid cancer. Mitotane is mainly used for inoperable and metastatic disease. Recent retrospective review suggested potential benefit of adjuvant mitotane use, but this has not been universally accepted yet. Adjuvant mitotane can be used in selected patients who have high risk of recurrence based on surgical and pathological findings (182,183).

The combination of mitotane with etoposide, doxorubicin, and cisplatin (EDP) is mainly based on limited literature showing evidence of response approaching 50% (184). Streptozocin with mitotane: The initial report about this combination reported three patients with ACC. Two patients had neoadjuvant therapy and later had surgical resection, and one patient had metastatic disease and showed regression of lymph node and lung metastases lasting more than 6 years (185). A later phase II study enrolled 40 ACC patients and the patients were given intravenous streptozocin with mitotane showing improved overall survival. Overall response rate was about 36% and the overall 5-year survival was 32% (186).

Currently, an international phase III study (FIRM-ACT) is the first ever conducted mainly in Europe randomizing ACC patient to either EDP-mitotane or streptozocin-mitotane with a focus on overall survival and quality of life, time to progression, response rate, and response duration.

A recent review compared different regimens in 57 ACC patients who received first-line systemic chemotherapy in our institution. There was no advantage of any particular regimen and no significant difference in overall survival between different subgroups(187).

- Other agents are under clinical investigation, including *gossypol* (NCT00848016), gefitinib (NCT00215202), sunitinib (NCT00453895), sorafenib with paclitaxel (NCT00786110), and IGF-1R inhibitors IMC A-12 (NCT00810537) and OSI-906 (NCT00924989) (188-199).

Radiation Therapy and Radiofrequency Ablation

ACC is considered a radio-resistant tumor. There is limited evidence for using adjuvant radiation therapy mainly based on retrospective literature review with proposed reduced local recurrence rate in high-risk patients but no clear effect on survival or distant metastases (200,201). At MD Anderson, radiation treatment is used as a palliative measure in selected patients with metastatic ACC. Percutaneous image-guided radiofrequency ablation has been attempted in the treatment of unresectable primary or metastatic ACC. The procedure was effective for the short-term local control of small adrenal tumors, especially for tumors less than 5 cm (202); however, further data are needed to examine its long-term efficacy and its effect on survival.

PROGNOSIS

Adrenal cancer remains a tumor with high morbidity and mortality. Long-term survival is possible in these patients if complete resection with tumor-free margins can be achieved (176). Survival is inversely correlated with disease stage at diagnosis.

High mitotic figures, but not DNA aneuploidy, have been associated with reduced survival and hence proposed as a prognostic factor. Younger age may portend a better prognosis, as children, when adjusted for stage; seem to have improved outcomes compared with adults (203). At our institution, the 5-year survival rate improved from 30% in 1983 to 60% in 2001, which is likely secondary to the improvement in supportive measures (163,204). Recent data suggested that aberrant microRNA expression (miR-195, miR-483-5p) is

associated with poor prognosis in ACC, but these data have not been validated in other studies yet (205).

■ PARATHYROID CARCINOMA

INTRODUCTION

Parathyroid carcinoma is the least-common endocrine malignancy, with a prevalence of 0.005% of all cancers (206) and 5.73 per 10 million (207). It is a rare cause of primary hyperparathyroidism, accounting for 0.4 to 5% of all cases.

The etiology of parathyroid carcinoma remains obscure. Radiation exposure has been implicated in a number of reports of carcinoma occurring within an adenoma, hyperplastic gland or even normal glands; however, overall, head and neck irradiation does not seem to be as significant a factor in malignant parathyroid disease, as it is in the genesis of parathyroid adenomas and benign hyperparathyroidism (208). Parathyroid carcinoma has been reported in families with isolated familial hyperparathyroidism, in patients with MEN types 1 and 2A, and hereditary hyperparathyroidism jaw tumor syndrome. Thus, it may be prudent to screen the relatives of certain patients with parathyroid carcinoma for hypercalcemia to improve the chance of early diagnosis of parathyroid disease. Parathyroid carcinoma has also been described in patients with chronic renal failure and dialysis, raising the possibility of malignant transformation of benign hyperplastic parathyroid glands.

CLINICAL PRESENTATION

Patients with parathyroid carcinoma tend to be approximately a decade younger than patients with benign hyperparathyroidism. The disease occurs with similar frequency in both sexes. Most patients with malignant disease are symptomatic and have moderate to severe hypercalcemia (serum calcium >12); although patients with parathyroid carcinoma can present anywhere along the calcemic spectrum, including asymptomatic and mild hypercalcemia. Parathyroid hormone levels are generally five times normal. Rare cases of nonfunctioning parathyroid carcinoma have been described; their clinical course is similar to that in patients with functioning tumors.

Unlike patients with benign disease, patients with parathyroid carcinoma are more likely to have a palpable mass in the neck. Manifestations of hypercalcemia in peripheral target organs, such as kidneys or bone, are no longer considered characteristic of benign hyperparathyroidism, but are somewhat common in patients with functioning parathyroid cancer. This is probably related to the generally more severe hypercalcemia at presentation in the malignant disease.

DIAGNOSIS

The diagnosis of parathyroid carcinoma in the absence of regional or distant metastases is a challenging issue. Differentiating benign adenoma from a malignant parathyroid carcinoma can be difficult based on pathology alone. Palpable neck masses, high calcium values (>13.5 mg/dL), and high intact parathyroid hormone (iPTH) values raise the suspicion of this disease (209,210). Gross invasion and adherence at the time of surgery, recurrences, or the classic histopathologic criteria are available as other clues to assist in diagnosis.

PATHOLOGY

Pathologic criteria may not definitively differentiate parathyroid carcinoma from the more common adenoma. The classic histopathologic criteria initially described by Schantz and Castleman (211) are still used today. These include the presence of a trabecular or lobular pattern, mitotic figures, thick fibrous bands, and capsular or blood vessel invasion. Although cytologic evidence of mitoses is generally necessary to confirm malignancy, mitotic activity alone is an unreliable indicator of such malignancy. The likelihood of malignancy increases the more aforementioned histologic features present in the tumor. DNA aneuploidy determined by flow cytometry is a valuable adjunct marker in the diagnosis of malignancy and is associated with a poor prognosis (212,213). Aneuploid parathyroid carcinomas are likely to show more malignant behavior than those with a diploid DNA pattern. It should be pointed out; however, that DNA aneuploidy may be found in some benign lesions. Therefore, this feature should be interpreted with caution (214). Immunohistochemical staining for various markers, including tumor suppressor genes, retinoblastoma, p53, cyclin D1, and others, may, perhaps in the future, help differentiate benign from malignant parathyroid disease (215,216). Other important distinguishing features include metastases and gross or histologic evidence of tumor infiltration into the surrounding tissues (including macroscopic adherence or vocal cord paralysis).

On occasion, some highly differentiated tumors without distinct nuclear atypia or classic histopathologic criteria are initially considered to be adenomas but are later reclassified when recurrence or metastases appear. On the other hand, a few parathyroid tumors may be classified as malignant because of their atypia, but neither metastasis nor relapse develops. One view is that the only reliable microscopic findings of malignancy are invasion of surrounding structures or metastasis. Thus, the ultimate diagnosis of parathyroid carcinoma can be made with confidence only after recurrence or metastatic spread occurs. Local invasion (micro- or macroscopically) of adjacent structures may be present at initial operation. This malignancy rarely metastasizes to lymph nodes. The thyroid gland is the most common site of involvement, but any of the following may be involved: recurrent laryngeal nerve, strap muscles, esophagus, and trachea. Distant metastases to the lungs, bone, and liver can be present at initial presentation or may develop later in the disease. Parathyroid carcinomas are most often located originating from the inferior parathyroid glands (217); rarely are they found in the mediastinum. To improve the accuracy of diagnosis of malignant parathyroid disease, pathologic specimens of suspected cases should be reviewed by experienced pathologists.

STAGING

There are no accepted staging criteria for parathyroid carcinoma. The standard TNM staging system cannot be applied to this disease for two reasons. First, parathyroid carcinoma is not a disease that frequently metastasizes to lymph nodes; second, tumor size does not seem to play a role in prognosis (206). No current staging system can be used to determine prognosis of this rare disease.

THERAPY

Preoperative suspicion and intraoperative identification of malignancy and appropriate initial surgery are critical in the therapy for parathyroid carcinoma. Comprehensive resection of the tumor along with the ipsilateral lobe of the thyroid and abnormal or involved adjacent tissues (the so-called "en bloc" resection) is indicated. This may improve survival and decrease recurrence (130,218,219). Ideally these tumors should be identified and removed by experienced parathyroid surgeons. A gray, dark, husky, gross appearance on intraoperative examination may be one clue to performing the more comprehensive resection required of malignant parathyroid disease. Every effort should be made to maintain the integrity of the capsule to prevent seeding of tumor, as this will contribute to recurrence. Because this tumor does not typically metastasize to lymph nodes, routine lymph node dissection is not indicated unless involved by tumor (206). For recurrences, a wide excision of locally recurrent tumor and an aggressive surgical resection of metastases whenever possible are recommended. Although these repeat operations are not always curative, they usually offer palliation of the marked hypercalcemia (the cause of true morbidity in these patients) for a considerable although variable period.

Chemotherapeutic agents, as of yet, do not seem to be efficacious in this disease.

The role of radiation therapy has been the subject of much debate in this malignancy. Select patients treated in the Princess Margaret Hospital and our institution have benefited from radiotherapy (102,217,220). Radiotherapy seems to effectively decrease local relapse rate in patients at high risk for recurrence. Radiotherapy has not become the standard of care in patients with parathyroid carcinoma because it is difficult to prove its efficacy with such small numbers of patients being treated in reported series. There is a potential benefit of adjuvant radiation therapy after initial surgery as seen in six patients in whom only one patient recurred (217). Radiation therapy should be considered in select patients at high risk of local relapse (those with gross or local invasion or tumor spillage intraoperatively) or those left with gross disease.

Morbidity and mortality are generally caused by the effects of unremitting hypercalcemia rather than tumor growth. Medical treatments, especially in patients with unresectable disease, such as intravenous fluids, diuretics, calcitonin, plicamycin (Mithracin), and bisphosphonates offer only temporary and palliative control of hypercalcemia. However, therapies such as calcimimetic agents that focus on decreasing parathyroid hormone secretion may better prevent complications and improve survival in patients with no curable disease (221). Because of the variable clinical course of this disease, it is important to individualize therapeutic strategies. Nevertheless, surgical resection where possible remains the most effective treatment for both local and metastatic disease.

Parathyroid carcinoma is a slow-growing but tenacious malignancy, and the hypercalcemia it engenders may have catastrophic consequences. Recurrences usually appear regionally within the neck and occur anywhere from 1 to 20 years post initial diagnosis. Therefore, regular lifetime surveillance of serum calcium and parathyroid hormone (PTH) levels is essential because of protracted and unpredictable course of malignant parathyroid disease. The 5-year survival rate of this disease has improved over the years to approximately 85%, and the 10-year survival rate is approximately 70 to 77% (217,220). Death usually results from hypercalcemia and its associated complications.

Because of its rarity and unpredictable clinical course, an individualized, multidisciplinary approach to caring for the patient with parathyroid carcinoma that involves the endocrinologist, surgeon, oncologist, and radiotherapist offers the best chance for cure.

References

1. Jemal A, Siegel R, Ward E, et al. Cancer statistics, 2009. *CA Cancer J Clin*. 2009;59(4):225-249.
2. Taylor T, Specker B, Robbins J, et al. Outcome after treatment of high-risk papillary and non-Hurthle-cell follicular thyroid carcinoma. *Ann Intern Med* 1998;129(8):622-627.
3. Robbins J, Merino MJ, Boice JD, Jr., et al. Thyroid cancer: A lethal endocrine neoplasm. *Ann Intern Med* 1991;115(2):133-147.
4. Gilliland FD, Hunt WC, Morris DM, et al. Prognostic factors for thyroid carcinoma. A population-based study of 15,698 cases from the Surveillance, Epidemiology and End Results (SEER) program 1973-1991. *Cancer* 1997;79(3):564-573.
5. Sherman SI. Thyroid carcinoma. *Lancet* 2003;361(9356):501-511.
6. Vassilopoulou-Sellin R. Long-term outcome of children with papillary thyroid cancer. *Surgery* 2001;129(6):769.
7. Gharib H, Goellner JR. Fine-needle aspiration biopsy of the thyroid: An appraisal. *Ann Intern Med* 1993;118(4):282-289.
8. Cooper DS, Doherty GM, Haugen BR, et al. Revised American Thyroid Association management guidelines for patients with thyroid nodules and differentiated thyroid cancer. *Thyroid* 2009;19(11):1167-1214.
9. DeGroot L, Paloyan E. Thyroid carcinoma and radiation. A Chicago endemic. *JAMA* 1973;225(5):487-491.
10. Fagin JA. How thyroid tumors start and why it matters: Kinase mutants as targets for solid cancer pharmacotherapy. *J Endocrinol* 2004;183(2):249-256.
11. Bounacer A, Wicker R, Caillou B, et al. High prevalence of activating ret proto-oncogene rearrangements, in thyroid tumors from patients who had received external radiation. *Oncogene* 1997;15(11):1263-1273.
12. Jhiang SM. The RET proto-oncogene in human cancers. *Oncogene* 2000;19(49):5590-5597.
13. Jhiang SM, Sagartz JE, Tong Q, et al. Targeted expression of the ret/PTC1 oncogene induces papillary thyroid carcinomas. *Endocrinology* 1996;137(1):375-378.
14. Zafon C, Obiols G, Castellvi J, et al. Clinical significance of RET/PTC and p53 protein expression in sporadic papillary thyroid carcinoma. *Histopathology* 2007;50(2):225-231.
15. Ugolini C, Giannini R, Lupi C, et al. Presence of BRAF V600E in very early stages of papillary thyroid carcinoma. *Thyroid* 2007;17(5):381-388.
16. Kim TY, Kim WB, Rhee YS, et al. The BRAF mutation is useful for prediction of clinical recurrence in low-risk patients with conventional papillary thyroid carcinoma. *Clin Endocrinol (Oxf)* 2006;65(3):364-368.
17. Xing M, Westra WH, Tufano RP, et al. BRAF mutation predicts a poorer clinical prognosis for papillary thyroid cancer. *J Clin Endocrinol Metab* 2005;90(12):6373-6379.

18. Fagin JA. Molecular Pathogenesis of Tumors of Thyroid Follicular Cells. In: Fagin JA, ed. *Thyroid Cancer*. Boston: Kluwer, 1998.

19. Carmeliet P. Mechanisms of angiogenesis and arteriogenesis. *Nat Med* 2000;6(4):389-395.

20. Laird AD, Cherrington JM. Small molecule tyrosine kinase inhibitors: Clinical development of anticancer agents. *Expert Opin Investig Drugs* 2003;12(1):51-64.

21. Lennard CM, Patel A, Wilson J, et al. Intensity of vascular endothelial growth factor expression is associated with increased risk of recurrence and decreased disease-free survival in papillary thyroid cancer. *Surgery* 2001;129(5):552-558.

22. Klein M, Vignaud JM, Hennequin V, et al. Increased expression of the vascular endothelial growth factor is a pejorative prognosis marker in papillary thyroid carcinoma. *J Clin Endocrinol Metab* 2001;86(2):656-658.

23. Hay ID, Grant CS, Taylor WF, et al. Ipsilateral lobectomy versus bilateral lobar resection in papillary thyroid carcinoma: A retrospective analysis of surgical outcome using a novel prognostic scoring system. *Surgery* 1987;102(6):1088-1095.

24. Cady B, Rossi R. An expanded view of risk-group definition in differentiated thyroid carcinoma. *Surgery* 1988;104(6): 947-953.

25. Byar DP, Green SB, Dor P, et al. A prognostic index for thyroid carcinoma. A study of the E.O.R.T.C. Thyroid Cancer Cooperative Group. *Eur J Cancer* 1979;15(8):1033-1041.

26. Mazzaferri EL, Jhiang SM. Long-term impact of initial surgical and medical therapy on papillary and follicular thyroid cancer. *Am J Med* 1994;97(5):418-428.

27. Sherman SI, Brierley JD, Sperling M, et al. Prospective multicenter study of thyrois carcinoma treatment: Initial analysis of staging and outcome. National Thyroid Cancer Treatment Cooperative Study Registry Group. *Cancer* 1998; 83(5):1012-1021.

28. Sherman SI. Toward a standard clinicopathologic staging approach for differentiated thyroid carcinoma. *Semin Surg Oncol* 1999;16(1):12-15.

29. Katoh R, Sasaki J, Kurihara H, et al. Multiple thyroid involvement (intraglandular metastasis) in papillary thyroid carcinoma. A clinicopathologic study of 105 consecutive patients. *Cancer* 1992;70(6):1585-1590.

30. Silverberg SG, Hutter RV, Foote FW, Jr. Fatal carcinoma of the thyroid: Histology, metastases, and causes of death. *Cancer* 1970;25(4):792-802.

31. Hay ID, Grant CS, Bergstralh EJ, et al. Unilateral total lobectomy: Is it sufficient surgical treatment for patients with AMES low-risk papillary thyroid carcinoma? *Surgery* 1998;124(6): 958-964; discussion 964-966.

32. Samaan NA, Schultz PN, Hickey RC, et al. The results of various modalities of treatment of well differentiated thyroid carcinomas: A retrospective review of 1599 patients. *J Clin Endocrinol Metab* 1992;75(3):714-720.

33. DeGroot LJ, Kaplan EL, Straus FH, et al. Does the method of management of papillary thyroid carcinoma make a difference in outcome? *World J Surg* 1994;18(1):123-130.

34. Cady B. Papillary carcinoma of the thyroid gland: Treatment based on risk group definition. *Surg Oncol Clin N Am* 1998;7(4):633-644.

35. Sherman SI, Gillenwater A. Neoplasms of the thyroid. In: Bast RJ, Kufe D, Pollock R, (eds): *Cancer Medicine*. Hamilton: B.C. Decker, 2000;1105-1114.

36. DeGroot LJ, Kaplan EL, McCormick M, et al. Natural history, treatment, and course of papillary thyroid carcinoma. *J Clin Endocrinol Metab* 1990;71(2):414-424.

37. Wong JB, Kaplan MM, Meyer KB, et al. Ablative radioactive iodine therapy for apparently localized thyroid carcinoma. A decision analytic perspective. *Endocrinol Metab Clin North Am* 1990;19(3):741-760.

38. Jonklaas J, Sarlis NJ, Litofsky D, et al. Outcomes of patients with differentiated thyroid carcinoma following initial therapy. *Thyroid* 2006;16(12):1229-1242.

39. Shepler TR, Sherman SI, Faustina MM, et al. Nasolacrimal duct obstruction associated with radioactive iodine therapy for thyroid carcinoma. *J Ophthal Plast Reconstr Surg* 2003 Nov;19(6):479-781.

40. Kloos RT, Duvuuri V, Jhiang SM, et al. Nasolacrimal drainage system obstruction from radioactive iodine therapy for thyroid carcinoma. *J Clin Endocrinol Metab* 2002; 87(12):5817-5820.

41. Sawka AM, Thabane L, Parlea L, et al. Second primary malignancy risk after radioactive iodine treatment for thyroid cancer: A systematic review and meta-analysis. *Thyroid* 2009; 19(5):451-457.

42. Tsang RW, Brierley JD, Simpson WJ, et al. The effects of surgery, radioiodine, and external radiation therapy on the clinical outcome of patients with differentiated thyroid carcinoma. *Cancer* 1998;82(2):375-388.

43. Farahati J, Reiners C, Stuschke M, et al. Differentiated thyroid cancer. Impact of adjuvant external radiotherapy in patients with perithyroidal tumor infiltration (stage pT4). *Cancer* 1996;77(1):172-180.

44. Grigsby PW, Baglan K, Siegel BA. Surveillance of patients to detect recurrent thyroid carcinoma. *Cancer* 1999;85(4): 945-951.

45. Sherman S. Thyroid Carcinoma: Practice Guidelines in Oncology v.1.2009. *J Natl Compreh Network* 2009; cited: available at www.nccn.org.

46. AACE/AAES medical/surgical guidelines for clinical practice: Management of thyroid carcinoma. American Association of Clinical Endocrinologists. American College of Endocrinology. *Endocr Pract* 2001;7(3):202-220.

47. Hooft L, Hoekstra OS, Deville W, et al. Diagnostic accuracy of 18F-fluorodeoxyglucose positron emission tomography in the follow-up of papillary or follicular thyroid cancer. *J Clin Endocrinol Metab* 2001;86(8):3779-3786.

48. Khan N, Oriuchi N, Higuchi T, et al. PET in the follow-up of differentiated thyroid cancer. *Br J Radiol* 2003;76(910): 690-695.

49. Chung JK, So Y, Lee JS, et al. Value of FDG PET in papillary thyroid carcinoma with negative 131I whole-body scan. *J Nucl Med* 1999;40(6):986-992.

50. Alnafisi NS, Driedger AA, Coates G, et al. FDG PET of recurrent or metastatic 131I-negative papillary thyroid carcinoma. *J Nucl Med* 2000;41(6):1010-1015.

51. Feine U, Lietzenmayer R, Hanke JP, et al. Fluorine-18-FDG and iodine-131-iodide uptake in thyroid cancer. *J Nucl Med* 1996;37(9):1468-1472.

52. Wang W, Macapinlac H, Larson SM, et al. [18F]-2-fluoro-2-deoxy-D-glucose positron emission tomography localizes residual thyroid cancer in patients with negative diagnostic (131)I whole body scans and elevated serum thyroglobulin levels. *J Clin Endocrinol Metab* 1999;84(7):2291-2302.

53. Robbins RJ, Wan Q, Grewal RK, et al. Real-time prognosis for metastatic thyroid carcinoma based on 2-[18F)fluoro-2-deoxy-D-glucose-positron emission tomography scanning. *J Clin Endocrinol Metab* 2006;91(2):498-505.

54. Wang W, Larson SM, Tuttle RM, et al. Resistance of [18f]-fluorodeoxyglucose-avid metastatic thyroid cancer lesions to treatment with high-dose radioactive iodine. *Thyroid* 2001; 11(12):1169-1175.

55. Wang W, Larson SM, Fazzari M, et al. Prognostic value of [18F]fluorodeoxyglucose positron emission tomographic scanning in patients with thyroid cancer. *J Clin Endocrinol Metab* 2000;85(3):1107-1113.

56. Petrich T, Borner AR, Otto D, et al. Influence of rhTSH on [(18)F]fluorodeoxyglucose uptake by differentiated thyroid carcinoma. *Eur J Nucl Med Mol Imaging* 2002;29(5): 641-647.

57. Moog F, Linke R, Manthey N, et al. Influence of thyroid-stimulating hormone levels on uptake of FDG in recurrent and metastatic differentiated thyroid carcinoma. *J Nucl Med* 2000;41(12):1989-1995.

58. Chin BB, Patel P, Cohade C, et al. Recombinant human thyrotropin stimulation of fluoro-D-glucose positron emission tomography uptake in well-differentiated thyroid carcinoma. *J Clin Endocrinol Metab* 2004;89(1):91-95.

59. Leboulleux S, Schroeder PR, Busaidy NL, et al. Assessment of the incremental value of recombinant thyrotropin stimulation before 2-[18F]-Fluoro-2-deoxy-D-glucose positron emission tomography/computed tomography imaging to localize residual differentiated thyroid cancer. *J Clin Endocrinol Metab* 2009;94(4):1310-1316.

60. Schluter B, Bohuslavizki KH, Beyer W, et al. Impact of FDG PET on patients with differentiated thyroid cancer who present with elevated thyroglobulin and negative 131I scan. *J Nucl Med* 2001;42(1):71-76.

61. Helal BO, Merlet P, Toubert ME, et al. Clinical impact of (18)F-FDG PET in thyroid carcinoma patients with elevated thyroglobulin levels and negative (131)I scanning results after therapy. *J Nucl Med* 2001;42(10):1464-1469.

62. Zimmer LA, McCook B, Meltzer C, et al. Combined positron emission tomography/computed tomography imaging of recurrent thyroid cancer. *Otolaryngol Head Neck Surg* 2003; 128(2):178-184.

63. Haugen BR, Pacini F, Reiners C, et al. A comparison of recombinant human thyrotropin and thyroid hormone withdrawal for the detection of thyroid remnant or cancer. *J Clin Endocrinol Metab* 1999;84(11):3877-3885.

64. Spencer CA, Bergoglio LM, Kazarosyan M, et al. Clinical impact of thyroglobulin (Tg) and Tg autoantibody method differences on the management of patients with differentiated thyroid carcinomas. *J Clin Endocrinol Metab* 2005;90(10): 5566-5575.

65. Spencer CA, Lopresti JS. Measuring thyroglobulin and thyroglobulin autoantibody in patients with differentiated thyroid cancer. *Nat Clin Pract Endocrinol Metab* 2008;4(4): 223-233.

66. Samaan NA, Schultz PN, Haynie TP, et al. Pulmonary metastasis of differentiated thyroid carcinoma: Treatment results in 101 patients. *J Clin Endocrinol Metab* 1985;60(2):376-380.

67. Chiu AC, Delpassand ES, Sherman SI. Prognosis and treatment of brain metastases in thyroid carcinoma. *J Clin Endocrinol Metab* 1997;82(11):3637-3642.

68. Franceschi M, Kusic Z, Franceschi D, et al. Thyroglobulin determination, neck ultrasonography and iodine-131 whole-body scintigraphy in differentiated thyroid carcinoma. *J Nucl Med* 1996;37(3):446-451.

69. Simpson WJ, Panzarella T, Carruthers JS, et al. Papillary and follicular thyroid cancer: Impact of treatment in 1578 patients. *Int J Radiat Oncol Biol Phys* 1988;14(6): 1063-1075.

70. Ruegemer JJ, Hay ID, Bergstralh EJ, et al. Distant metastases in differentiated thyroid carcinoma: A multivariate analysis of prognostic variables. *J Clin Endocrinol Metab* 1988;67(3): 501-508.

71. Schlumberger M, Challeton C, De Vathaire F, et al. Radioactive iodine treatment and external radiotherapy for lung and bone metastases from thyroid carcinoma. *J Nucl Med* 1996; 37(4):598-605.

72. Santini F, Bottici V, Elisei R, et al. Cytotoxic effects of carboplatinum and epirubicin in the setting of an elevated serum thyrotropin for advanced poorly differentiated thyroid cancer. *J Clin Endocrinol Metab* 2002;87(9):4160-4165.

73. Haugen BR. Management of the patient with progressive radioiodine non-responsive disease. *Semin Surg Oncol* 1999; 16(1):34-41.

74. Gottlieb JA, Hill CS, Jr. Chemotherapy of thyroid cancer with Adriamycin. Experience with 30 patients. *N Engl J Med* 1974;290(4):193-197.

75. Gottlieb JA, Hill CS, Jr., Ibanez ML, et al. Chemotherapy of thyroid cancer. An evaluation of experience with 37 patients. *Cancer* 1972;30(3):848-853.

76. Ain KB, Egorin MJ, DeSimone PA. Treatment of anaplastic thyroid carcinoma with paclitaxel: Phase 2 trial using ninety-six-hour infusion. Collaborative Anaplastic Thyroid Cancer Health Intervention Trials (CATCHIT) Group. *Thyroid* 2000;10(7):587-594.

77. Cabanillas M. Treatment with tyrosine kinase inhibitors for patients with differentiated thyroid cancer: The M.D. Anderson Cancer Center experience. *J Clin Oncol* 2009;27(Suppl S15; abstract 6060).

78. Sherman SI, Wirth LJ, Droz JP, et al. Motesanib diphosphate in progressive differentiated thyroid cancer. *N Engl J Med* 2008;359(1):31-42.

79. Cohen EE, Rosen LS, Vokes EE, et al. Axitinib is an active treatment for all histologic subtypes of advanced thyroid cancer: Results from a phase II study. *J Clin Oncol* 2008; 26(29):4708-4713.

80. Ain K, al. E. Phase II study of lenalidomide in distantly metastatic, rapidly progressive, and radioiodine-unresponsive thyroid carcinomas: Preliminary results. *J Clin Oncol* 2008; 26(May 20 Suppl 6027).

81. Cohen E. Phase 2 study of sunitinib in refractory thyroid cancer. *J Clin Oncol* 2008;26:6025.

82. Bible KC. Phase II trial of pazopanib in progressive, metastatic, iodine-insensitive differentiated thyroid cancers. *J Clin Oncol* 2009;27(15sL;3521).

83. Vassilopoulou-Sellin R, Goepfert H, Raney B, et al. Differentiated thyroid cancer in children and adolescents: Clinical outcome and mortality after long-term follow-up. *Head Neck* 1998;20(6):549-555.

84. Vassilopoulou-Sellin R, Klein MJ, Smith TH, et al. Pulmonary metastases in children and young adults with differentiated thyroid cancer. *Cancer* 1993;71(4):1348-1352.

85. Waguespack SG, Sherman SI, Williams MD, et al. The successful use of sorafenib to treat pediatric papillary thyroid carcinoma. *Thyroid* 2009;19(4):407-412.

86. Ying AK, Huh W, Bottomley S, et al. Thyroid cancer in young adults. *Semin Oncol* 2009;36(3):258-274.

87. Horvit PK, Gagel RF. The goitrous patient with an elevated serum calcitonin–what to do? *J Clin Endocrinol Metab* 1997;82(2):335-337.

88. Hahm JR, Lee MS, Min YK, et al. Routine measurement of serum calcitonin is useful for early detection of medullary thyroid carcinoma in patients with nodular thyroid diseases. *Thyroid* 2001;11(1):73-80.

89. Bennedbaek FN, Perrild H, Hegedus L. Diagnosis and treatment of the solitary thyroid nodule. Results of a European Survey. *Clin Endocrinol (Oxf)* 1999;50(3):357-363.

90. Redding AH, Levine SN, Fowler MR. Normal preoperative calcitonin levels do not always exclude medullary thyroid carcinoma in patients with large palpable thyroid masses. *Thyroid* 2000;10(10):919-922.

91. Gagel RF, Cote GJ. *Pathogenesis of Medullary Thyroid Carcinoma*. Boston: Kluwer Academic Publishers, 1998 Thyroid Cancer.

92. Ponder BA, Ponder MA, Coffey R, et al. Risk estimation and screening in families of patients with medullary thyroid carcinoma. *Lancet* 1988;1(8582):397-401.

93. Brandi ML, Gagel RF, Angeli A, et al. Guidelines for diagnosis and therapy of MEN type 1 and type 2. *J Clin Endocrinol Metab* 2001;86(12):5658-5671.

94. Niccoli-Sire P, Murat A, Rohmer V, et al. Familial medullary thyroid carcinoma with noncysteine ret mutations: Phenotype-genotype relationship in a large series of patients. *J Clin Endocrinol Metab* 2001;86(8):3746-3753.

95. Hansford JR, Mulligan LM. Multiple endocrine neoplasia type 2 and RET: From neoplasia to neurogenesis. *J Med Genet* 2000;37(11):817-827.

96. Wohllk N, Cote GJ, Bugalho MM, et al. Relevance of RET proto-oncogene mutations in sporadic medullary thyroid carcinoma. *J Clin Endocrinol Metab* 1996;81(10):3740-3745.

97. O'Riordain DS, O'Brien T, Weaver AL, et al. Medullary thyroid carcinoma in multiple endocrine neoplasia types 2A and 2B. *Surgery* 1994;116(6):1017-1023.

98. Kloos RT, Eng C, Evans DB, et al. Medullary thyroid cancer: Management guidelines of the American Thyroid Association. *Thyroid* 2009;19(6):565-612.

99. Saad MF, Ordonez NG, Rashid RK, et al. Medullary carcinoma of the thyroid. A study of the clinical features and prognostic factors in 161 patients. *Medicine (Baltimore)* 1984;63(6):319-342.

100. Hyer SL, Vini L, A'Hern R, et al. Medullary thyroid cancer: Multivariate analysis of prognostic factors influencing survival. *Eur J Surg Oncol* 2000;26(7):686-690.

101. Brierley J, Tsang R, Simpson WJ, et al. Medullary thyroid cancer: Analyses of survival and prognostic factors and the role of radiation therapy in local control. *Thyroid* 1996;6(4):305-310.

102. Chow E, Tsang RW, Brierley JD, et al. Parathyroid carcinoma–the Princess Margaret Hospital experience. *Int J Radiat Oncol Biol Phys* 1998;41(3):569-572.

103. van Heerden JA, Grant CS, Gharib H, et al. Long-term course of patients with persistent hypercalcitoninemia after apparent curative primary surgery for medullary thyroid carcinoma. *Ann Surg* 1990;212(4):395-400; discussion 400-401.

104. Waguespack SG. A perspective from pediatric endocrinology on the hereditary medullary thyroid carcinoma syndromes. *Thyroid* 2009;19(6):543-546.

105. Schlumberger MJ, Elisei R, Bastholt L, et al. Phase II study of safety and efficacy of motesanib in patients with progressive or symptomatic, advanced or metastatic medullary thyroid cancer. *J Clin Oncol* 2009;27(23):3794-3801.

106. Wells SA, Jr., Gosnell JE, Gagel RF, et al. Vandetanib for the treatment of patients with locally advanced or metastatic hereditary medullary thyroid cancer. *J Clin Oncol* 28(5):767-772.

107. Pierie JP, Muzikansky A, Gaz RD, et al. The effect of surgery and radiotherapy on outcome of anaplastic thyroid carcinoma. *Ann Surg Oncol* 2002;9(1):57-64.

108. Xu G, Pan J, Martin C, et al. Angiogenesis inhibition in the in vivo antineoplastic effect of manumycin and paclitaxel against anaplastic thyroid carcinoma. *J Clin Endocrinol Metab* 2001;86(4):1769-1777.

109. McIver B, Hay ID, Giuffrida DF, et al. Anaplastic thyroid carcinoma: A 50-year experience at a single institution. *Surgery* 2001;130(6):1028-1034.

110. Haigh PI, Ituarte PH, Wu HS, et al. Completely resected anaplastic thyroid carcinoma combined with adjuvant chemotherapy and irradiation is associated with prolonged survival. *Cancer* 2001;91(12):2335-2342.

111. Elliott DD, Sherman SI, Busaidy NL, et al. Growth factor receptors expression in anaplastic thyroid carcinoma: Potential markers for therapeutic stratification. *Hum Pathol* 2008;39(1):15-20.

112. Santarpia L, El-Naggar AK, Cote GJ, et al. Phosphatidylinositol 3-kinase/akt and ras/raf-mitogen-activated protein kinase pathway mutations in anaplastic thyroid cancer. *J Clin Endocrinol Metab* 2008;93(1):278-284.

113. Venkatesh YS, Ordonez NG, Schultz PN, et al. Anaplastic carcinoma of the thyroid. A clinicopathologic study of 121 cases. *Cancer* 1990;66(2):321-330.

114. Junor EJ, Paul J, Reed NS. Anaplastic thyroid carcinoma: 91 patients treated by surgery and radiotherapy. *Eur J Surg Oncol* 1992;18(2):83-88.

115. Neumann HP, Bausch B, McWhinney SR, et al. Germ-line mutations in nonsyndromic pheochromocytoma. *N Engl J Med* 2002;346(19):1459-1466.

116. Neumann HP, Pawlu C, Peczkowska M, et al. Distinct clinical features of paraganglioma syndromes associated with SDHB and SDHD gene mutations. *JAMA* 2004;292(8):943-951.

117. Burnichon N, Rohmer V, Amar L, et al. The succinate dehydrogenase genetic testing in a large prospective series of patients with paragangliomas. *J Clin Endocrinol Metab* 2009;94(8):2817-2827.

118. Beard CM, Sheps SG, Kurland LT, et al. Occurrence of pheochromocytoma in Rochester, Minnesota, 1950 through 1979. *Mayo Clin Proc* 1983;58(12):802-804.

119. McNeil AR, Blok BH, Koelmeyer TD, et al. Phaeochromocytomas discovered during coronial autopsies in Sydney, Melbourne and Auckland. *Aust N Z J Med* 2000;30(6):648-652.

120. Goldstein RE, O'Neill JA, Jr., Holcomb GW, III, et al. Clinical experience over 48 years with pheochromocytoma. *Ann Surg* 1999;229(6):755-764; discussion 764-766.

121. John H, Ziegler WH, Hauri D, et al. Pheochromocytomas: Can malignant potential be predicted? *Urology* 1999;53(4):679-683.

122. Mannelli M, Ianni L, Cilotti A, et al. Pheochromocytoma in Italy: A multicentric retrospective study. *Eur J Endocrinol* 1999;141(6):619-624.

123. O'Riordain DS, Young WF, Jr., Grant CS, et al. Clinical spectrum and outcome of functional extraadrenal paraganglioma. *World J Surg* 1996;20(7):916-921; discussion 922.

124. Plouin PF, Degoulet P, Tugaye A, et al. (Screening for phaeochromocytoma: In which hypertensive patients? A semiological study of 2585 patients, including 11 with phaeochromocytoma [author's transl]). *Nouv Presse Med* 1981;10(11):869-872.

125. Lenders JW, Pacak K, Walther MM, et al. Biochemical diagnosis of pheochromocytoma: Which test is best? *JAMA* 2002;287(11):1427-1434.

126. d'Herbomez M, Gouze V, Huglo D, et al. Chromogranin A assay and (131)I-MIBG scintigraphy for diagnosis and follow-up of pheochromocytoma. *J Nucl Med* 2001;42(7):993-997.

127. Stratakis CA, Carney JA. The triad of paragangliomas, gastric stromal tumours and pulmonary chondromas (Carney triad), and the dyad of paragangliomas and gastric stromal sarcomas (Carney-Stratakis syndrome): Molecular genetics and clinical implications. *J Intern Med* 2009;266(1):43-52.

128. Sisson JC, Frager MS, Valk TW, et al. Scintigraphic localization of pheochromocytoma. *N Engl J Med* 1981;305(1):12-17.

129. Shapiro B, Copp JE, Sisson JC, et al. Iodine-131 metaiodobenzylguanidine for the locating of suspected pheochromocytoma: Experience in 400 cases. *J Nucl Med* 1985;26(6):576-585.

130. Wiseman SM, Rigual NR, Hicks WL, Jr., et al. Parathyroid carcinoma: A multicenter review of clinicopathologic features and treatment outcomes. *Ear Nose Throat J* 2004;83(7):491-494.

131. Ilias I, Chen CC, Carrasquillo JA, et al. Comparison of 6-18F-fluorodopamine PET with 123I-metaiodobenzylguanidine and 111in-pentetreotide scintigraphy in localization of nonmetastatic and metastatic pheochromocytoma. *J Nucl Med* 2008;49(10):1613-1619.

132. Takano A, Oriuchi N, Tsushima Y, et al. Detection of metastatic lesions from malignant pheochromocytoma and paraganglioma with diffusion-weighted magnetic resonance imaging: Comparison with 18F-FDG positron emission tomography and 123I-MIBG scintigraphy. *Ann Nucl Med* 2008;22(5):395-401.

133. Timmers HJ, Chen CC, Carrasquillo JA, et al. Comparison of 18F-Fluoro-L-DOPA, 18F-Fluoro-Deoxyglucose, and 18F-Fluorodopamine PET and 123I-MIBG Scintigraphy in the Localization of Pheochromocytoma and Paraganglioma. *J Clin Endocrinol Metab* 2009;94(12):4757-4767.

134. Kocak S, Aydintug S, Canakci N. Alpha blockade in preoperative preparation of patients with pheochromocytomas. *Int Surg* 2002;87(3):191-194.

135. Ulchaker JC, Goldfarb DA, Bravo EL, et al. Successful outcomes in pheochromocytoma surgery in the modern era. *J Urol* 1999;161(3):764-767.

136. Steinsapir J, Carr AA, Prisant LM, et al. Metyrosine and pheochromocytoma. *Arch Intern Med* 1997;157(8):901-906.

137. Lee JE, Curley SA, Gagel RF, et al. Cortical-sparing adrenalectomy for patients with bilateral pheochromocytoma. *Surgery* 1996;120(6):1064-1070; discussion 1070-1071.

138. van Heerden JA, Roland CF, Carney JA, et al. Long-term evaluation following resection of apparently benign pheochromocytoma(s)/paraganglioma(s). *World J Surg* 1990;14(3):325-329.

139. Kebebew E, Duh QY. Benign and malignant pheochromocytoma: Diagnosis, treatment, and follow-Up. *Surg Oncol Clin N Am* 1998;7(4):765-789.

140. Gimenez-Roqueplo AP, Favier J, Rustin P, et al. Mutations in the SDHB gene are associated with extra-adrenal and/or malignant phaeochromocytomas. *Cancer Res* 2003;63(17):5615-5621.

141. Rao F, Keiser HR, O'Connor DT. Malignant pheochromocytoma. Chromaffin granule transmitters and response to treatment. *Hypertension* 2000;36(6):1045-1052.

142. Yon L, Guillemot J, Montero-Hadjadje M, et al. Identification of the secretogranin II-derived peptide EM66 in pheochromocytomas as a potential marker for discriminating benign versus malignant tumors. *J Clin Endocrinol Metab* 2003;88(6):2579-2585.

143. Grouzmann E, Gicquel C, Plouin PF, et al. Neuropeptide Y and neuron-specific enolase levels in benign and malignant pheochromocytomas. *Cancer* 1990;66(8):1833-1835.

144. Salmenkivi K, Arola J, Voutilainen R, et al. Inhibin/activin betaB-subunit expression in pheochromocytomas favors benign diagnosis. *J Clin Endocrinol Metab* 2001;86(5):2231-2235.

145. Kimura N, Watanabe T, Noshiro T, et al. Histological grading of adrenal and extra-adrenal pheochromocytomas and relationship to prognosis: A clinicopathological analysis of 116 adrenal pheochromocytomas and 30 extra-adrenal sympathetic paragangliomas including 38 malignant tumors. *Endocr Pathol* 2005;16(1):23-32.

146. Hayry V, Salmenkivi K, Arola J, et al. High frequency of SNAIL-expressing cells confirms and predicts metastatic potential of phaeochromocytoma. *Endocr Relat Cancer* 2009;16(4):1211-1218.

147. Waldmann J, Slater EP, Langer P, et al. Expression of the transcription factor snail and its target gene twist are associated with malignancy in pheochromocytomas. *Ann Surg Oncol* 2009;16(7):1997-2005.

148. Loh KC, Fitzgerald PA, Matthay KK, et al. The treatment of malignant pheochromocytoma with iodine-131 metaiodobenzylguanidine (131I-MIBG): A comprehensive review of 116 reported patients. *J Endocrinol Invest* 1997;20(11):648-658.

149. Forrer F, Riedweg I, Maecke HR, et al. Radiolabeled DOTA-TOC in patients with advanced paraganglioma and pheochromocytoma. *Q J Nucl Med Mol Imaging* 2008;52(4):334-340.

150. Hamilton BP, Cheikh IE, Rivera LE. Attempted treatment of inoperable pheochromocytoma with streptozocin. *Arch Intern Med* 1977;137(6):762-765.

151. Feldman JM. Treatment of metastatic pheochromocytoma with streptozocin. *Arch Intern Med* 1983;143(9):1799-1800.

152. Averbuch SD, Steakley CS, Young RC, et al. Malignant pheochromocytoma: Effective treatment with a combination of cyclophosphamide, vincristine, and dacarbazine. *Ann Intern Med* 1988;109(4):267-273.

153. Huang H, Abraham J, Hung E, et al. Treatment of malignant pheochromocytoma/paraganglioma with cyclophosphamide, vincristine, and dacarbazine: Recommendation from a 22-year follow-up of 18 patients. *Cancer* 2008;113(8):2020-2028.

154. Nomura K, Kimura H, Shimizu S, et al. Survival of patients with metastatic malignant pheochromocytoma and efficacy of combined cyclophosphamide, vincristine, and dacarbazine chemotherapy. *J Clin Endocrinol Metab* 2009;94(8):2850-2856.

155. Jimenez C, Cabanillas ME, Santarpia L, et al. Use of the tyrosine kinase inhibitor sunitinib in a patient with von Hippel-Lindau disease: Targeting angiogenic factors in pheochromocytoma and other von Hippel-Lindau disease-related tumors. *J Clin Endocrinol Metab* 2009;94(2):386-391.

156. Joshua AM, Ezzat S, Asa SL, et al. Rationale and evidence for sunitinib in the treatment of malignant paraganglioma/pheochromocytoma. *J Clin Endocrinol Metab* 2009; 94(1):5-9.

157. Park KS, Lee JL, Ahn H, et al. Sunitinib, a novel therapy for anthracycline- and cisplatin-refractory malignant pheochromocytoma. *Jpn J Clin Oncol* 2009;39(5):327-331.

158. Druce MR, Kaltsas GA, Fraenkel M, et al. Novel and evolving therapies in the treatment of malignant phaeochromocytoma: Experience with the mTOR inhibitor everolimus (RAD001). *Horm Metab Res* 2009;41(9):697-702.

159. Edstrom Elder E, Hjelm Skog AL, Hoog A, et al. The management of benign and malignant pheochromocytoma and abdominal paraganglioma. *Eur J Surg Oncol* 2003;29(3): 278-283.

160. Pacak K, Fojo T, Goldstein DS, et al. Radiofrequency ablation: A novel approach for treatment of metastatic pheochromocytoma. *J Natl Cancer Inst* 2001;93(8):648-649.

161. Ohkawa S, Hirokawa S, Masaki T, et al. Examination of percutaneous microwave coagulation and radiofrequency ablation therapy for metastatic liver cancer. *Gan To Kagaku Ryoho* 2002;29(12):2149-2151.

162. Venkatesan AM, Locklin J, Lai EW, et al. Radiofrequency ablation of metastatic pheochromocytoma. *J Vasc Interv Radiol* 2009;20(11):1483-1490.

163. Vassilopoulou-Sellin R, Schultz PN. Adrenocortical carcinoma. Clinical outcome at the end of the 20th century. *Cancer* 2001;92(5):1113-1121.

164. Ng L, Libertino JM. Adrenocortical carcinoma: Diagnosis, evaluation and treatment. *J Urol* 2003;169(1):5-11.

165. Reincke M, Karl M, Travis WH, et al. p53 mutations in human adrenocortical neoplasms: Immunohistochemical and molecular studies. *J Clin Endocrinol Metab* 1994;78(3):790-794.

166. Henry I, Jeanpierre M, Couillin P, et al. Molecular definition of the 11p15.5 region involved in Beckwith-Wiedemann syndrome and probably in predisposition to adrenocortical carcinoma. *Hum Genet* 1989;81(3):273-277.

167. Lee MJ, Hahn PF, Papanicolaou N, et al. Benign and malignant adrenal masses: CT distinction with attenuation coefficients, size, and observer analysis. *Radiology* 1991;179(2):415-418.

168. Dackiw AP, Lee JE, Gagel RF, et al. Adrenal cortical carcinoma. *World J Surg* 2001;25(7):914-926.

169. Boland GW, Goldberg MA, Lee MJ, et al. Indeterminate adrenal mass in patients with cancer: Evaluation at PET with 2-[F-18]-fluoro-2-deoxy-D-glucose. *Radiology* 1995;194(1): 131-134.

170. Erasmus JJ, Patz EF, Jr., McAdams HP, et al. Evaluation of adrenal masses in patients with bronchogenic carcinoma using 18F-fluorodeoxyglucose positron emission tomography. *AJR Am J Roentgenol* 1997;168(5):1357-1360.

171. Lee JE, Evans DB, Hickey RC, et al. Unknown primary cancer presenting as an adrenal mass: Frequency and implications for diagnostic evaluation of adrenal incidentalomas. *Surgery* 1998;124(6):1115-1122.

172. Ren R, Guo M, Sneige N, et al. Fine-needle aspiration of adrenal cortical carcinoma: Cytologic spectrum and diagnostic challenges. *Am J Clin Pathol* 2006;126(3):389-398.

173. Barnett CC, Jr., Varma DG, El-Naggar AK, et al. Limitations of size as a criterion in the evaluation of adrenal tumors. *Surgery* 2000;128(6):973-982; discussion 982-983.

174. Weiss LM. Comparative histologic study of 43 metastasizing and nonmetastasizing adrenocortical tumors. *Am J Surg Pathol* 1984;8(3):163-169.

175. Soon PS, Gill AJ, Benn DE, et al. Microarray gene expression and immunohistochemistry analyses of adrenocortical tumors identify IGF2 and Ki-67 as useful in differentiating carcinomas from adenomas. *Endocr Relat Cancer* 2009; 16(2):573-583.

176. Lee JE, Berger DH, el-Naggar AK, et al. Surgical management, DNA content, and patient survival in adrenal cortical carcinoma. *Surgery* 1995;118(6):1090-1098.

177. MacFarlane DA. Cancer of the adrenal cortex; the natural history, prognosis and treatment in a study of fifty-five cases. *Ann R Coll Surg Engl* 1958;23(3):155-186.

178. Fassnacht M, Johanssen S, Quinkler M, et al. Limited prognostic value of the 2004 International Union Against Cancer staging classification for adrenocortical carcinoma: Proposal for a Revised TNM Classification. *Cancer* 2009;115(2): 243-250.

179. Grumbach MM, Biller BM, Braunstein GD, et al. Management of the clinically inapparent adrenal mass ("incidentaloma"). *Ann Intern Med* 2003;138(5):424-429.

180. Baudin E, Pellegriti G, Bonnay M, et al. Impact of monitoring plasma 1,1-dichlorodiphenildichloroethane (o,p'DDD) levels on the treatment of patients with adrenocortical carcinoma. *Cancer* 2001;92(6):1385-1392.

181. van Slooten H, Moolenaar AJ, van Seters AP, et al. The treatment of adrenocortical carcinoma with o,p'-DDD: Prognostic implications of serum level monitoring. *Eur J Cancer Clin Oncol* 1984;20(1):47-53.

182. Terzolo M, Angeli A, Fassnacht M, et al. Adjuvant mitotane treatment for adrenocortical carcinoma. *N Engl J Med* 2007; 356(23):2372-2380.

183. Lee JE. Adjuvant mitotane in adrenocortical carcinoma. *N Engl J Med* 2007;357(12):1258; author reply 1259.

184. Berruti A, Terzolo M, Pia A, et al. Mitotane associated with etoposide, doxorubicin, and cisplatin in the treatment of advanced adrenocortical carcinoma. Italian Group for the Study of Adrenal Cancer. *Cancer* 1998;83(10): 2194-2200.

185. Eriksson B, Oberg K, Curstedt T, et al. Treatment of hormone-producing adrenocortical cancer with o,p'DDD and streptozocin. *Cancer* 1987;59(8):1398-1403.

186. Khan TS, Imam H, Juhlin C, et al. Streptozocin and o,p'DDD in the treatment of adrenocortical cancer patients: Long-term survival in its adjuvant use. *Ann Oncol* 2000;11(10): 1281-1287.

187. Fareau GG, Lopez A, Stava C, et al. Systemic chemotherapy for adrenocortical carcinoma: Comparative responses to conventional first-line therapies. *Anticancer Drugs* 2008;19(6): 637-644.

188. Cuellar A, Ramirez J. Further studies on the mechanism of action of gossypol on mitochondrial membrane. *Int J Biochem* 1993;25(8):1149-1155.

189. Le Blanc M, Russo J, Kudelka AP, et al. An in vitro study of inhibitory activity of gossypol, a cottonseed extract, in human carcinoma cell lines. *Pharmacol Res* 2002;46(6): 551-555.

190. Cuellar A, Diaz-Sanchez V, Ramirez J. Cholesterol side-chain cleavage and 11 beta-hydroxylation are inhibited by gossypol in adrenal cortex mitochondria. *J Steroid Biochem Mol Biol* 1990;37(4):581-585.

191. Wu YW, Chik CL, Knazek RA. An in vitro and in vivo study of antitumor effects of gossypol on human SW-13 adrenocortical carcinoma. *Cancer Res* 1989;49(14):3754-3758.

192. Flack MR, Pyle RG, Mullen NM, et al. Oral gossypol in the treatment of metastatic adrenal cancer. *J Clin Endocrinol Metab* 1993;76(4):1019-1024.

193. Bates SE, Shieh CY, Mickley LA, et al. Mitotane enhances cytotoxicity of chemotherapy in cell lines expressing a multidrug resistance gene (mdr-1/P-glycoprotein) which is also expressed by adrenocortical carcinomas. *J Clin Endocrinol Metab* 1991;73(1):18-29.

194. Bates S, Kang M, Meadows B, et al. A Phase I study of infusional vinblastine in combination with the P-glycoprotein antagonist PSC 833 (valspodar). *Cancer* 2001;92(6):1577-1590.

195. Abraham J, Bakke S, Rutt A, et al. A phase II trial of combination chemotherapy and surgical resection for the treatment of metastatic adrenocortical carcinoma: Continuous infusion doxorubicin, vincristine, and etoposide with daily mitotane as a P-glycoprotein antagonist. *Cancer* 2002;94(9):2333-2343.

196. Quinkler M, Hahner S, Wortmann S, et al. Treatment of advanced adrenocortical carcinoma with erlotinib plus gemcitabine. *J Clin Endocrinol Metab* 2008;93(6):2057-2062.

197. Lee JO, Lee KW, Kim CJ, et al. Metastatic adrenocortical carcinoma treated with sunitinib: A case report. *Jpn J Clin Oncol* 2009;39(3):183-185.

198. Almeida MQ, Fragoso MC, Lotfi CF, et al. Expression of insulin-like growth factor-II and its receptor in pediatric and adult adrenocortical tumors. *J Clin Endocrinol Metab* 2008;93(9):3524-3531.

199. Barlaskar FM, Spalding AC, Heaton JH, et al. Preclinical targeting of the type I insulin-like growth factor receptor in adrenocortical carcinoma. *J Clin Endocrinol Metab* 2009;94(1):204-212.

200. Markoe AM, Serber W, Micaily B, et al. Radiation therapy for adjunctive treatment of adrenal cortical carcinoma. *Am J Clin Oncol* 1991;14(2):170-174.

201. Polat B, Fassnacht M, Pfreundner L, et al. Radiotherapy in adrenocortical carcinoma. *Cancer* 2009;115(13):2816-2823.

202. Wood BJ, Abraham J, Hvizda JL, et al. Radiofrequency ablation of adrenal tumors and adrenocortical carcinoma metastases. *Cancer* 2003;97(3):554-560.

203. Mendonca BB, Lucon AM, Menezes CA, et al. Clinical, hormonal and pathological findings in a comparative study of adrenocortical neoplasms in childhood and adulthood. *J Urol* 1995;154(6):2004-2009.

204. Nader S, Hickey RC, Sellin RV, et al. Adrenal cortical carcinoma. A study of 77 cases. *Cancer* 1983;52(4):707-711.

205. Soon PS, Tacon LJ, Gill AJ, et al. miR-195 and miR-483-5p Identified as Predictors of Poor Prognosis in Adrenocortical Cancer. *Clin Cancer Res* 2009;15(24):7684-7692.

206. Hundahl SA, Fleming ID, Fremgen AM, et al. Two hundred eighty-six cases of parathyroid carcinoma treated in the U.S. between 1985-1995: A National Cancer Data Base Report. The American College of Surgeons Commission on Cancer and the American Cancer Society. *Cancer* 1999;86(3):538-544.

207. Ain KB, Lee C, Williams KD. Phase II trial of thalidomide for therapy of radioiodine-unresponsive and rapidly progressive thyroid carcinomas. *Thyroid* 2007;17(7):663-670.

208. Cohn K, Silverman M, Corrado J, et al. Parathyroid carcinoma: The Lahey Clinic experience. *Surgery* 1985;98(6):1095-1100.

209. Shane E, Bilezikian JP. Parathyroid carcinoma: A review of 62 patients. *Endocr Rev* 1982;3(2):218-226.

210. Shane E. Clinical review 122: Parathyroid carcinoma. *J Clin Endocrinol Metab* 2001;86(2):485-493.

211. Schantz A, Castleman B. Parathyroid carcinoma. A study of 70 cases. *Cancer* 1973;31(3):600-605.

212. Obara T, Fujimoto Y, Hirayama A, et al. Flow cytometric DNA analysis of parathyroid tumors with special reference to its diagnostic and prognostic value in parathyroid carcinoma. *Cancer* 1990;65(8):1789-1793.

213. Obara T, Fujimoto Y, Kanaji Y, et al. Flow cytometric DNA analysis of parathyroid tumors. Implication of aneuploidy for pathologic and biologic classification. *Cancer* 1990;66(7):1555-1562.

214. Joensuu H, Klemi PJ. DNA aneuploidy in adenomas of endocrine organs. *Am J Pathol* 1988;132(1):145-151.

215. Westin G, Bjorklund P, Akerstrom G. Molecular genetics of parathyroid disease. *World J Surg* 2009;33(11):2224-2233.

216. Woodard GE, Lin L, Zhang JH, et al. Parafibromin, product of the hyperparathyroidism-jaw tumor syndrome gene HRPT2, regulates cyclin D1/PRAD1 expression. *Oncogene* 2005;24(7):1272-1276.

217. Busaidy NL, Jimenez C, Habra MA, et al. Parathyroid carcinoma: A 22-year experience. *Head Neck* 2004;26(8):716-726.

218. Koea JB, Shaw JH. Parathyroid cancer: Biology and management. *Surg Oncol* 1999;8(3):155-165.

219. Shortell CK, Andrus CH, Phillips CE, Jr., et al. Carcinoma of the parathyroid gland: A 30-year experience. *Surgery* 1991;110(4):704-708.

220. Anderson BJ, Samaan NA, Vassilopoulou-Sellin R, et al. Parathyroid carcinoma: Features and difficulties in diagnosis and management. *Surgery* 1983;94(6):906-915.

221. Collins MT, Skarulis MC, Bilezikian JP, et al. Treatment of hypercalcemia secondary to parathyroid carcinoma with a novel calcimimetic agent. *J Clin Endocrinol Metab* 1998;83(4):1083-1088.

MALIGNANT MELANOMA

Kevin B. Kim
Michael A. Davies
Ronald P. Rapini
Patrick Hwu
Agop Y. Bedikian

■ EPIDEMIOLOGY

In the United States, malignant melanoma is the fifth most prevalent cancer among men and the sixth most common in women, and the incidence has been increasing every year over the last several decades (1). The median age at diagnosis for melanoma is 59 years, and approximately 21% of the patients are under 45 years of age at the time of diagnosis (2). In women in the 25 to 29-year age group, melanoma is the most common cancer. In women between 30 and 34 years of age, it is the second most common type of malignancy, breast cancer being the most common (3). Between 2002 and 2006, the age-adjusted incidence for cutaneous malignant melanoma was 19.6 per 100,000 males and females per year in the United States (2). The high rate of malignant melanoma in the United States is surpassed only in Australia, New Zealand, Norway, and Israel. Although the incidence of melanoma in the United States rose dramatically from the 1970s through the 2000s, this trend appears to be slowing for those born after 1945 (2,4). The cause for the slowing trend is multifaceted, including reduced exposure to ultraviolet rays, widespread use of sunscreen, and improvements in community-based education and screening.

■ RISK FACTORS

Malignant melanoma is mostly curable if identified at an early stage. Therefore understanding the host and environmental factors that predispose individuals to an increased risk is of paramount importance. Those individuals at increased risk of developing melanoma benefit from regular screening examinations and education regarding the warning signs of melanoma.

Exposure to ultraviolet light is the most significant cause of the development of skin melanoma (5,6), as suggested by the fact that the increase in incidence of cutaneous melanoma is associated with the increasing distance from the poles (7-10) and that freckles and nevi, the risk factors for the development of melanoma, are induced by exposure to sunlight (11-13). In addition, severe sunburns during adolescence years and the use of tanning beds have been linked to an increased risk of cutaneous melanoma (5,14).

The color of the skin is related to the risk of developing cutaneous melanoma. The age-adjusted incidence rates of malignant melanoma are lower in ethnic groups with darker skin colors. For instance, the incidence rates among white, Hispanic, and black populations are 28.9, 4.6, and 1.1 per 100,000 men, respectively, and 18.7, 4.7, and 1.0 per 100,000 women, respectively (2). In addition, people whose skin tends to burn easily with sun exposure have a higher risk of melanoma (15-17). Likewise, lighter hair color or red hair and blue eye color are associated with a greater risk of developing melanoma (relative risks of 1.5-2.4 fold) (18).

Although commonly acquired nevi typically appear after the first year of life and are benign in and of themselves, several studies have demonstrated that higher numbers of nevi are directly related to an increased risk of developing melanoma. Swerdlow et al. demonstrated a relative risk of 12.1 in patients with 50 or more nevi (19). Similarly, studies by Weiss et al. demonstrated a relative risk of 14.9 in patients with more than 50 benign nevi (20).

Irregular borders, contour, and color characterize dysplastic or atypical nevi. In contrast to benign nevi, the dysplastic nevi tend to appear in the second decade of life and continue developing throughout adulthood. These nevi can occur sporadically or can be inherited in a familial pattern; this has been given several names, including "the B-K mole syndrome," "familial atypical mole and melanoma syndrome," and the "dysplastic nevus syndrome." The familial syndrome is characterized by the occurrence of melanoma in at least one first- or second-degree relative; the presence of a large number of acquired nevi, some of which are atypical; and nevi that demonstrate specific histologic features. The risk of eventually developing melanoma is 184-fold greater for theses patients than for the general population (21). Studies have demonstrated that the occurrence of malignant melanoma is significantly greater in patients with atypical nevi but who do not meet the criteria for the familial syndrome. Tucker et al. demonstrated a twofold increase in the risk of developing melanoma in patients with even just one atypical nevus. The risk increased to 12-fold in patients with at least 10 dysplastic nevi (22).

Congenital nevi present at birth are divided into groups according to size: small (<1.5 cm), medium (1.5-20 cm), and large (>20 cm). Only patients with large nevi have been shown to be at increased risk of developing melanoma (19, 23-27).

Patients with a history of prior cutaneous melanoma are also at increased risk of developing a second primary melanoma (28). The lifetime risk of developing a second primary melanoma is estimated to be 3 to 6% (29).

■ CLINICAL-PATHOLOGIC SUBTYPES

MAJOR SUBTYPES

Melanoma is a malignancy of melanocytes which arise from the neural crest and migrate to the epidermis although it can migrate to uveal tract, meninges, and ectodermal mucosal. As a consequence, melanomas are most commonly found in the epidermal skin layer, and less frequently in the eyes, oral, nasal, rectal, and vaginal mucosal surface. There are four major clinical-pathologic subtypes of cutaneous melanoma: superficial spreading melanoma, nodular melanoma, lentigo maligna melanoma, and acral lentiginous melanoma. Distinctions among these subtypes are based primarily on histology and anatomic site.

Superficial Spreading Melanoma

Superficial spreading melanoma is the most common subtype of malignant melanoma, comprising approximately 70% of cases (30) (Figs. 39-1 through 39-4). These lesions can occur anywhere on sun-protected skin and often occur on the upper back in both sexes and the lower extremities in women. The lesions demonstrate irregular and asymmetrical borders. Their size is typically greater than 6 to 8 mm, with notable color variegation. These lesions are often confused with traumatized nevi, commonly acquired nevi, and seborrheic keratoses.

Nodular Melanoma

The second most common melanoma subtype, nodular melanoma, accounts for between 15 and 30% of

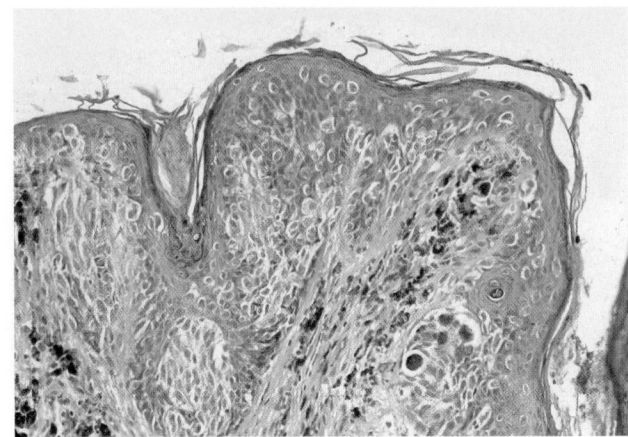

FIGURE 39-2. Superficial spreading melanoma. Note the variegated color and irregular border.

cases (30). Unlike the other three major subtypes, nodular melanoma lacks a preceding radial growth phase. Thus, these melanomas are characterized by rapid growth over weeks to months. The lesions, which typically occur on the trunk or legs, appear as raised dark brown to black nodules. Ulceration and bleeding are common. For this reason amelanotic variants may mimic squamous or basal cell carcinomas.

Lentigo Maligna Melanoma

Lentigo maligna melanoma accounts for 4 to 15% of cutaneous melanomas (31). This subtype typically appears on the head, neck, and arms (Fig. 39-5). Like other skin cancers, lentigo maligna melanoma is linked

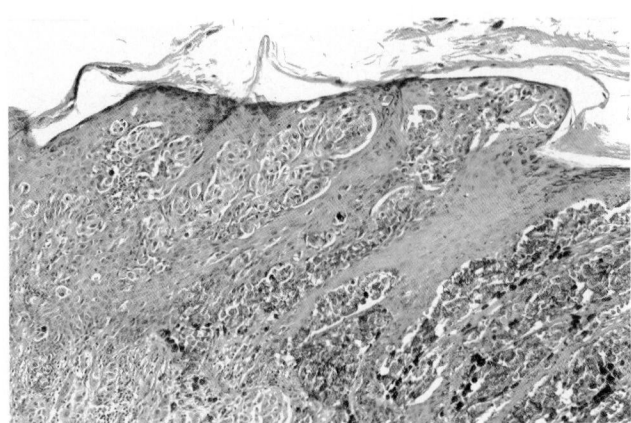

FIGURE 39-1. Melanoma pathology (superficial spreading melanoma). Atypical pagetoid melanocytes are seen within the epidermis, invading the dermis.

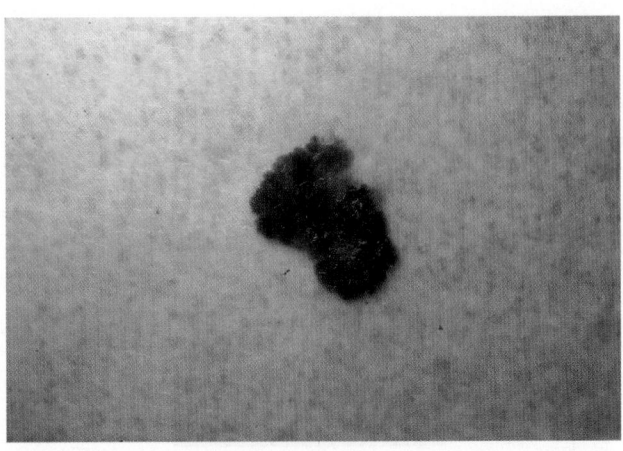

FIGURE 39-3. Melanoma of the trunk with notched borders and variegated blue, black, and brown pigmentation.

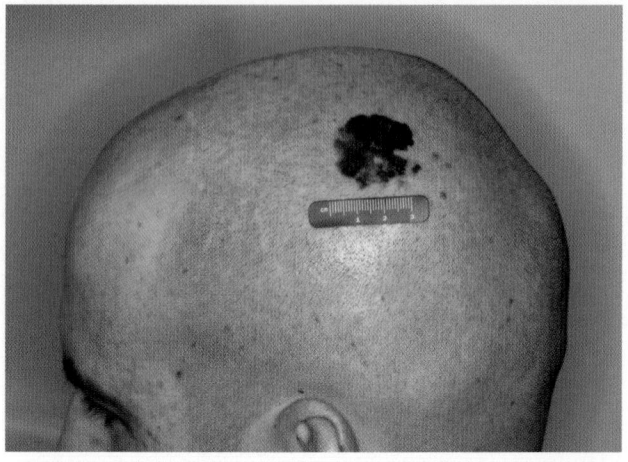

FIGURE 39-4. This melanoma of the scalp did not become apparent until the patient developed alopecia from chemotherapy for another primary cancer.

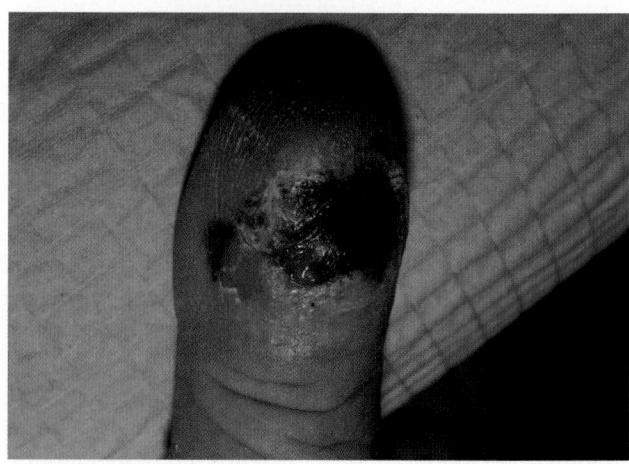

FIGURE 39-6. Acral lentiginous melanoma of the toe.

to cumulative sun exposure. The precursor lesion, lentigo maligna, may be present for up to two decades and grow to sizes greater than 3 cm in diameter before being transformed into lentigo maligna melanoma. Clinically, these lesions appear as flat tan to brown macules with areas that appear hypopigmented. Approximately 5 to 8% of them will transform to invasive melanoma; clinically, this is often heralded by the development of a nodule within the flat precursor lesion (31).

Acral Lentiginous Melanoma

Acral lentiginous melanoma is the least common subtype of cutaneous malignant melanoma, accounting for 2 to 8% of cases in Caucasians (32). However, among

African Americans, Asians, and Hispanics, this subtype accounts for 29 to 72% of cases (32). Typically occurring on the palms or soles or beneath the nail plate, these melanoma tend to be large and irregularly pigmented (Figs. 39-6 and 39-7). The presence of pigmentation in the proximal or lateral nail fold (Hutchinson sign) is diagnostic of subungual melanoma. These lesions may be mistaken for pyogenic granuloma, subungual hematoma, or a bacterial or fungal infection.

LESS COMMON SUBTYPES

Amelanotic melanomas lack the typical pigment expected to be present in most melanomas (Fig. 39-8). These lesions are notorious for resembling other lesions,

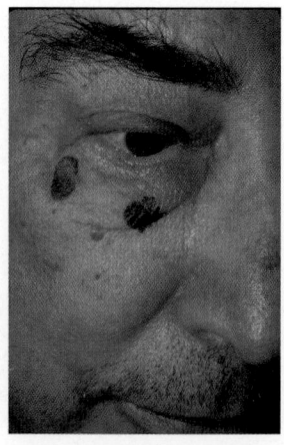

FIGURE 39-5. Melanoma of the face. Lentigo maligna (melanoma in situ) of the eyelid. The lateral lesion was a seborrheic keratosis.

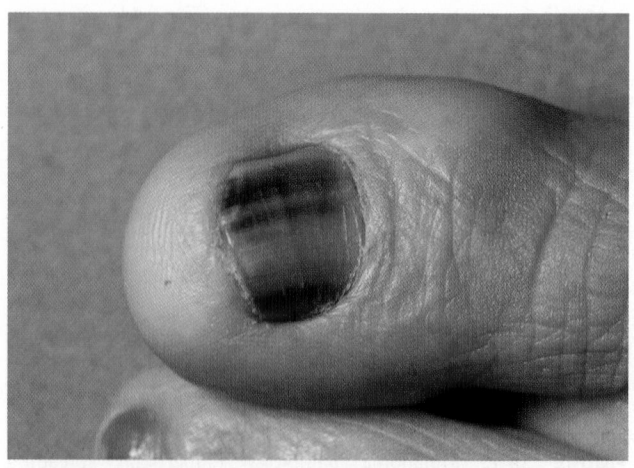

FIGURE 39-7. Acral lentiginous melanoma of the subungual surface.

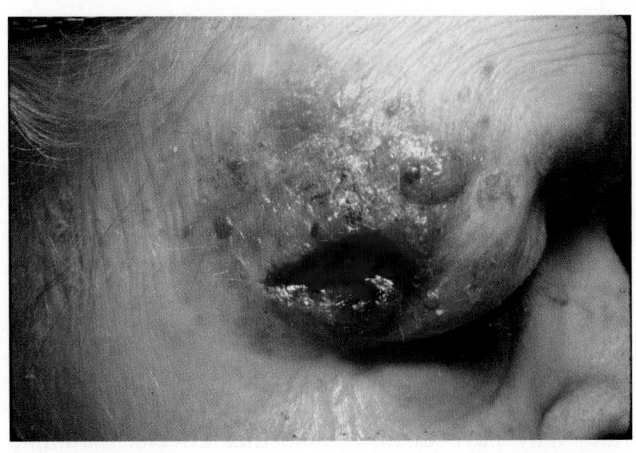

FIGURE 39-8. An amelanotic melanoma that was initially thought to be a basal cell carcinoma.

such as inflammatory conditions, basal cell carcinoma, and pyogenic granuloma. The pathologist frequently has to perform immunostaining for antigens such as S-100, HMB-45, or MART-1 to make the diagnosis.

Desmoplastic melanoma is a rare subtype that is locally aggressive and tends to have a high rate of local reoccurrence. This subtype has a male predominance (2:1) and typically develops on the sun-exposed area of the head and neck in the elderly. Most are deeply invasive at the time of diagnosis (>5 mm) and tend to invade perineurally, which may cause the patient significant discomfort (33). The lesion may appear as a nodule or pigmented macule with or without an associated nodule. Frequently desmoplastic melanomas develop in association with lentigo maligna.

Mucosal melanomas can arise in the head and neck, anus, genital tract, respiratory tract, or the gastrointestinal tract (34). Like acral lentiginous melanoma, mucosal melanoma is more frequently diagnosed in darker skin populations. This melanoma subtype tends to present at an advanced stage with a very aggressive natural history. Patients with mucosal melanomas tend to have a poor prognosis, likely due to the delayed diagnosis in many cases and possibly due to the aggressiveness of its survival mechanism.

Uveal melanomas are tumors that arise from melanocytes of the uveal tract of the eye, which includes the iris, ciliary body, and the choroid. Uveal melanomas are quite rare, with a prevalence of 4 to 7 individuals per million, but they are one of the most common primary tumors of the eye (35). Tumors are often discovered in asymptomatic patients on routine eye examinations, but patients may also present with visual disturbances, including visual loss, flashing lights, or visual field defects (36). Uveal melanoma has a distinct pattern of spread, with an absence of spread to regional lymph nodes, but frequent and often exclusive metastatic involvement of the liver. Patients with metastatic disease generally succumb within a few months, as these tumors are highly resistant to therapy.

■ GENETIC BASIS OF MELANOMA

While some malignancies are caused by infectious agents, the predominant mechanism underlying most cancers is alteration of DNA that predisposes to oncogenic transformation and progression. A number of genetic events have been identified in melanoma, including both germline changes that predispose individuals to melanoma and somatic changes that contribute to the development and progression of the tumors. In addition to providing information about the processes that may be critical to the pathogenesis of this disease, these genetic events somewhat reflect the different subtypes of melanoma, and present possible therapeutic opportunities.

GERMLINE MUTATIONS

CDKN2A

Approximately 10% of melanomas are familial, defined as occurring in families with at least three affected individuals (37). The most common genetic alteration observed in this subset of melanomas is loss of the *CDKN2A* locus on chromosome 9. The *CDKN2A* locus encodes two different proteins due to alternative splicing mechanisms, p16^{INK4A} and p14^{ARF}. Deletion or inactivating mutations of this locus are identified in up to 40% of melanoma-prone families (37). P16 regulates cell cycle progression by inhibiting the complex of CDK4/CDK6 and cyclin D. Loss of P16 function activates the CDK4/6—cyclin D complex—which results in hyperphosphorylation of the RB protein and promotes progression from the G1 phase of the cell cycle into the S phase. The importance of this mechanism is supported by the additional finding of rare germline mutations of *CDK4* in familial melanoma (37). The mutations in *CDK4* affect the residues that interact with p16, blocking this interaction from occurring, and thus functionally recapitulate loss of p16. The second protein encoded by the *CDKN2A* locus, p14, also functions as a regulator of cell cycle progression but through a different mechanism. P14 sequesters and inactivates MDM2, which is a ubiquitin ligase that normally targets p53 for proteasome-mediated degradation (37). Loss of p14 function therefore results in increased degradation of p53 and thus loss of cell cycle regulation and the apoptotic response after various genotoxic events, such as DNA damage. The frequent loss of p14 may explain the comparative low frequency (≤15%) of *p53* mutations in melanoma compared with other cancers (38). The contributory role of altered responses to DNA damage to melanoma development is also suggested by the identification of polymorphisms in DNA repair genes that confer an increased risk of melanoma (39).

MC1R

In addition to cell cycle regulation, polymorphisms in genes involved in melanin synthesis have also been associated with an increased risk of melanoma. Epidemiologic studies have previously implicated a number of factors related to pigmentation in association with melanoma, including fair skin, red or blonde hair, freckling, and poor tanning (40). Genetic studies have identified several variants in the *MC1R* gene, which encodes the melanocortin-1 receptor (MC1R), as conferring an increased risk of melanoma, and these variants are specifically associated with the red hair-fair skin–freckled phenotype (37). Activation of MC1R triggers a signaling cascade that results in the increased expression of several genes involved in melanin synthesis, including microphthalmia transcription factor (MITF), tyrosinase (TYR), and tyrosinase-related proteins 1 and 2 (TYRP1 and TYRP2, respectively). Several of the polymorphisms in *MC1R* that confer an increased risk of melanoma have been demonstrated to reduce the activation of this signaling following stimulation of the receptor, presumably resulting in compromised melanin production. Additional validation of the importance of this biochemical pathway is provided by the identification of polymorphisms in both the *TYR* and *TYRP1* loci that confer an increased risk of melanoma (37).

SOMATIC MUTATIONS

BRAF and NRAS

There is now evidence that the overwhelming majority of melanomas have acquired somatic mutations that result in hyperactivation of protein kinase signaling pathways. The most common somatic mutations in melanoma are point mutations in the *BRAF* gene (38,41). BRAF is a serine-threonine kinase that is part of the RAS-RAF-MAPK signaling cascade. This pathway has been implicated in promoting cancer cell growth and survival in many different tumor types,

most commonly by activation of growth factor receptors that are upstream of the pathway, or by activating mutations of *RAS* family members (42). Studies in both cell lines and tumors have identified point mutations in *BRAF* in approximately 50% of melanomas (38). Almost 90% of the detected mutations result in a single nucleotide change, the V600E mutation. The V600E mutation alters the structure of the BRAF protein so that it is constitutively active, and results in growth factor-independent activation of the RAS-RAF-MAPK signaling pathway (42). There is some evidence to support the idea that the non-V600 mutations in *BRAF*, although rare, may have distinct molecular effects, including dependence upon other signaling pathways (43). While the prevalence of *BRAF* mutations is quite high in melanomas, there are several lines of evidence demonstrating that this change alone cannot fully explain the aggressive nature of this disease. In preclinical models, including experiments using human melanocytes, genetically engineered mice, and zebrafish, expression of the mutated form of the BRAF protein was able to change the growth property of melanocytes, but failed to result in malignant lesions without additional genetic events (44-46). Clinically, the requirement of other genetic events is supported by the fact that *BRAF* mutations have a similar prevalence in benign nevi, which have virtually no malignant potential, compared with invasive melanomas (47,48).

Activating mutations of *NRAS* are detected in approximately 20% of cutaneous melanomas (38). Similar to mutations in BRAF, the mutant forms of the NRAS protein result in constitutive activation of the RAS-RAF-MAPK signaling pathway. In contrast to *BRAF* mutations, *NRAS* mutations are very rare in common nevi, but they have been detected in the more rare congenital nevi (49). Mutant NRAS is a potent inducer of transformation in preclinical models. This functional difference from mutant BRAF may be due to activation of additional signaling pathways by mutant NRAS, as has been observed with mutations of other RAS isoforms (50). One pathway that has been of particular interest is the PI3K-AKT pathway.

The PI3K-AKT Pathway

The PI3K-AKT pathway is affected by mutations more frequently than any other pathway in cancer, and it has been shown to promote tumor proliferation, survival, anchorage-independence, invasion, and other oncogenic properties (51). The most common PI3K-AKT pathway mutations detected in melanoma are deletions and inactivating mutations of PTEN, a lipid phosphatase that inhibits the pathway (52). Loss of PTEN has been detected in up to 30% of melanomas, and results in increased activation of AKT. Activating mutations have also been identified at a low prevalence (<5%) in *PIK3CA*, which encodes the catalytic subunit of PI3K, and in *AKT* (53,54).

The pattern of the mutations in *BRAF*, *NRAS*, and *PTEN* indicates that concurrent activation of multiple signaling pathways is common in melanoma. *NRAS* mutations are mutually exclusive with both *BRAF* and *PTEN* mutations (55,56). In contrast, *PTEN* mutations frequently occur in tumors with concurrent *BRAF* mutations, suggesting that these two events may functionally be equivalent to the activation of multiple pathways achieved by *NRAS* mutations. The complementation of *BRAF* and *PTEN* mutations is supported by transgenic mouse models. Transgenic mice engineered to express the V600E mutant form of BRAF developed melanocyte hyperplasia, but no invasive lesions. However, crossing these mice with a strain in which PTEN expression was abrogated in the melanocytes resulted in frankly invasive and metastatic melanomas (44). While these experiments demonstrate the potential synergy of *BRAF* mutations and activation of the PI3K-AKT pathway, additional studies have demonstrated that AKT hyperactivation is present is a subset of BRAF-mutant melanomas, but not all (57).

Subtype-Specific Mutations: *c-KIT*

While mutations of *BRAF* and *NRAS* are frequent events in melanoma, additional research has demonstrated that the prevalence of these mutations varies in the different melanoma subtypes. For example, although *BRAF* mutations are detected in approximately 60% of cutaneous melanomas arising in areas with intermittent sun exposure, much lower rates are detected in acral lentiginous (AL) (20%), mucosal (MM) (3%), and uveal (0%) melanomas (58). Interestingly, cutaneous melanomas with evidence of chronic sun damage (CSD) also have a lower incidence of *BRAF* mutations (5%). *NRAS* mutations are also seen with relatively low frequency (0-10%) in these subtypes. Analysis of DNA copy number changes in a diverse set of melanomas showed that the subtypes were each characterized by alterations in different chromosomal regions, supporting the idea that the molecular pathogenesis of these tumors may be quite different (58).

The identification of frequent amplifications in chromosomal region 4q12 in the AL, MM, and CSD melanomas led to detailed investigation of the genes in this region, which included several potential therapeutic targets. These studies found that these subtypes had frequent focal amplification of the *c-KIT* gene (59). C-KIT is a transmembrane receptor tyrosine kinase that is mutated in approximately 80% of gastrointestinal stromal tumors (GIST) (60). Subsequent studies demonstrated that similar mutations of *c-KIT* also occur in the AL, MM, and CSD melanomas. Overall, amplification and/or mutations of *c-KIT* were detected in 20 to 40% of the tumors in these subtypes, while virtually none were detected in cutaneous melanomas without cutaneous sun damage (59,61). Mutant forms of the c-KIT protein have been demonstrated to activate the RAS-RAF-MAPK, the PI3K-AKT, and other signaling pathways in melanoma cells (62).

SOMATIC AMPLIFICATIONS

In addition to *c-KIT*, amplifications in other genes in pathways previously implicated in melanoma have been identified. The *MITF* gene, which is downstream of MC1R and which regulates the transcription of several key genes involved in melanin synthesis, is amplified in 10 to 20% of melanomas (63). Amplifications of the *MITF* gene appear to be specific for melanoma, and overexpression of MITF was able to cooperate with the V600E BRAF to transform melanocytes. Point mutations in *MITF* have also been reported in some metastatic melanomas (64).

Amplification of *CCND1* has also been reported in melanomas, particularly in the acral subtype (44%) (65). Expression of cyclin D1, the protein encoded by *CCND1*, is also increased by activation of the RAS-RAF-MAPK pathway, which occurs with both *BRAF* and *NRAS* mutations. Cyclin D1 interacts with CDK4 and CDK6 to phosphorylate RB and promote S-phase cell cycle entry. As noted previously, germline mutations that activate *CDK4* have been reported in some familial melanomas, and somatic amplifications of the gene have also been identified (58). In addition, p16 is a critical negative regulator of the cyclin D1—CDK4/6 complex—which thus is activated by loss of the *CDKN2A* locus. Thus, multiple genetic events detected in melanoma may theoretically promote cyclin D1 expression and function, which recently have been shown to contribute to therapeutic resistance by melanoma cells (66).

GENOMIC CHANGES OF UVEAL MELAOMA

Uveal melanomas appear to be molecularly distinct from the other melanoma subtypes. Genetic alterations in *BRAF*, *NRAS*, and *c-KIT* have not been detected in these tumors (67). Recently, point mutations in *GNαQ*, a G-protein coupled receptor, were identified in approximately 50% of uveal melanoma tumors and cell lines (68). These mutations were not detected in cutaneous or mucosal melanomas. Although it is likely that these mutations may activate additional pathways, initial studies demonstrated that the mutant form of the GNαQ protein that was observed in the tumors causes activation of the RAS-RAF-MAPK signaling pathway (68). Additional functional studies are ongoing to further characterize this mutation, as well as to screen for mutations in other similar genes. Uveal melanomas are also characterized by frequent events affecting whole chromosomes, including monosomy of chromosome 3 and gain of chromosome 8q (67).

■ PATTERN OF SPREAD OF MALIGNANT MELANOMA

Despite the differences in the appearance of the four subtypes of cutaneous melanoma, they have similar patterns of metastatic spread, and all have ability to metastasize to virtually any organ or tissue (69,70). Cutaneous and mucosal melanomas tend to spread to regional lymph nodes through the lymphatic channels at an early stage of progression. Regional lymph nodes are the first site of recurrence in 50 to 60% of patients (71). Distant skin, subcutaneous tissues, or lymph nodes are the most common sites of distant metastases, and they account for nearly 42 to 59% of all sites of recurrences (71). Spread to distal visceral organs occurs through invasion of local capillaries at the later stage of progression. However, approximately 25% of all patients whose disease ultimately relapses have distant visceral metastases as the initial sites of recurrence (72-74). The most common sites of visceral metastases are the lung, liver, brain, bone, and gastrointestinal tract (71) (Fig. 39-9).

Uveal melanomas may involve the iris, ciliary body, or, most frequently, the choroids. Localized disease is often treated with local excision, photocoagulation, external-beam radiotherapy, or enucleation (75). The uveal tract is poor in lymphatics; therefore metastasis is typically hematogenous in origin. The pattern of spread of uveal melanoma is significantly different from that of cutaneous melanoma (Fig. 39-10). The rates of metastasis to the liver and to the brain differ significantly in patients with skin and uveal melanoma. By far, the liver is the most common site of metastasis for uveal melanoma (76). In our review, over 95% of the patients had liver metastasis. About half of the patients had the

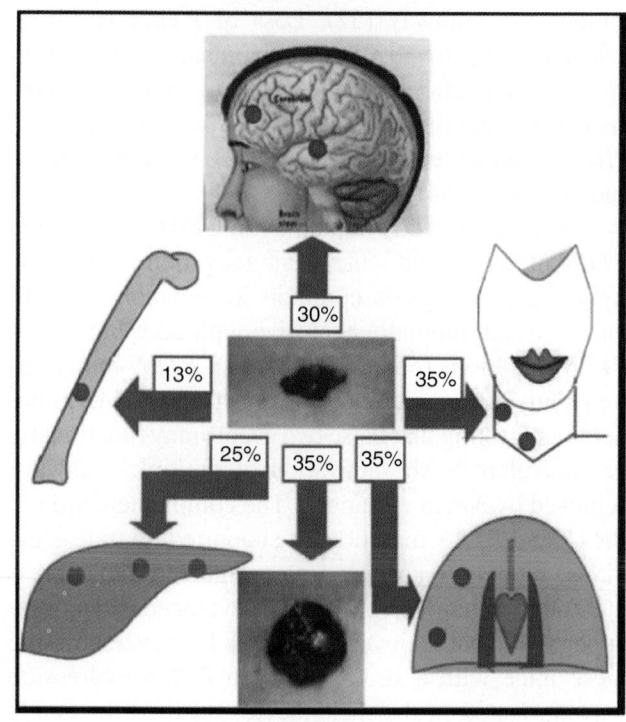

FIGURE 39-9. Pattern of systemic spread of cutaneous melanoma.

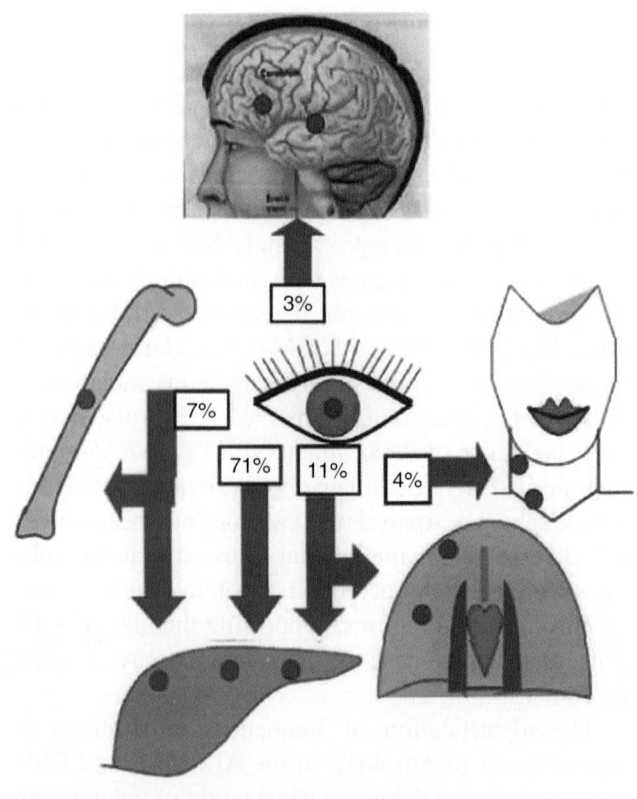

FIGURE 39-10. Pattern of systemic spread of uveal melanoma.

disease confined in the liver; another third have liver and other organ involvement (see Fig. 39-10). Brain involvement with metastasis, which occurs in 20 to 40% of patients with metastatic skin melanoma, occurred in less than 3% patients with uveal melanoma. In contrast to patients with cutaneous melanoma, none of the patients with uveal melanoma had tumor spread to the regional lymph nodes. Four percent of patients had metastasis to distant lymph node basins, most commonly in the abdomen. The median time from diagnosis of primary uveal melanoma to discovery of metastatic disease was 36 months. The median of survival from date of detection of metastatic disease was 8 months.

■ STAGING

The American Joint Committee on Cancer (AJCC) staging system for cutaneous melanoma has recently been revised to more accurately reflect variables of prognostic significance. Revisions in the tumor microstaging, nodal staging, and metastasis staging were published in 2009 (77) and have replaced the prior staging system in the sixth edition of the *AJCC Staging Manual* (78) (Tables 39-1 and 39-2).

Tumor staging (T) in the old systems was based on both the Clark level and Breslow thickness. The new staging system focuses on melanoma thickness,

TABLE 39-1	2009 AMERICAN JOINT COMMITTEE ON CANCER STAGING SYSTEM FOR MELANOMA	
T Classification	**Thickness (mm)**	**Ulceration Status/Mitoses**
T1s	NA	NA
T1	≤1.00	a: without ulceration and mitosis <1/mm^2 b: with ulceration or mitoses ≥1/mm^2 (or Clark level IV or V only if mitotic rate cannot be determined)
T2	1.01–2.00	a: without ulceration b: with ulceration
T3	2.01–4.00	a: without ulceration b: with ulceration
T4	>4.00	a: without ulceration b: with ulceration
N Classification	**No. of Metastatic Nodes**	**Nodal Metastatic Burden**
N0	0	NA
N1	1	a: micrometastasis* b: macrometastasis†
N2	2–3	a: micrometastasis* b: macrometastasis† c: in-transit met(s)/satellite(s) without metastatic lymph nodes
N3	4 + metastatic nodes, or matted lymph nodes, or in-transit met(s)/satellite(s) with metastatic node(s)	
M Classification	**Site**	**Serum LDH**
M0	No distant metastases	NA
M1a	Distant skin, subcutaneous or nodal met(s)	Normal
M1b	Lung met(s)	Normal
M1c	All other visceral met(s)	Normal
	Any distant met(s)	Elevated

LDH, lactate dehydrogenase; mets, metastases; NA, not applicable.

*Micrometastases are diagnosed after sentinel lymph node biopsy.

†Macrometastases are defined as clinically detectable lymph node metastases confirmed pathologically (or by finding of gross [not microscopic] extracapsular extension).

Reproduced, with permission, from Balch CM, et al., Final version of 2009 AJCC melanoma staging and classification. J Clin Oncol, 2009. 27(36): p. 6199-206.

TABLE 39-2 · AJCC STAGE GROUPINGS FOR CUTANEOUS MELANOMA

	CLINICAL STAGING*					PATHOLOGIC STAGING†		
	T	*N*	*M*			*T*	*N*	*M*
0	Tis	N0	M0		0	Tis	N0	M0
IA	T1a	N0	M0		IA	T1a	N0	M0
IB	T1b	N0	M0		IB	T1b	N0	M0
	T2a	N0	M0			T2a	N0	M0
IIA	T2b	N0	M0		IIA	T2b	N0	M0
	T3a	N0	M0			T3a	N0	M0
IIB	T3b	N0	M0		IIB	T3b	N0	M0
	T4a	N0	M0			T4a	N0	M0
IIC	T4b	N0	M0		IIC	T4b	N0	M0
III	any T	N> N0	M0		IIIA	T1-4a	N1a	M0
						T1-4a	N2a	M0
					IIIB	T1-4b	N1a	M0
						T1-4b	N2a	M0
						T1-4a	N1b	M0
						T1-4a	N2b	M0
						T1-4a	N2c	M0
					IIIC	T1-4b	N1b	M0
						T1-4b	N2b	M0
						T1-4b	N2c	M0
						any T	N3	M0
IV	any T	any N	M1		IV	any T	any N	M1

*Clinical staging includes microstaging of the primary melanoma and clinical/radiologic evaluation for metastases. By convention, it should be used after complete excision of the primary melanoma with clinical assessment for regional and distant metastases.

†Pathologic staging includes microstaging of the primary melanoma and pathologic information about the regional lymph nodes after partial (ie, sentinel node biopsy) or complete lymphadenectomy. Pathologic stage 0 or stage IA patients are the exception; they do not require pathologic evaluation of their lymph nodes.

Reproduced, with permission, from Balch CM, et al., Final version of 2009 AJCC melanoma staging and classification. J Clin Oncol, 2009. 27(36): p. 6199-206.

ulceration, and mitosis of the primary melanoma lesions, three strong predictors of outcome as determined by Cox regression analysis (77). Clark level of invasion and mitotic rates (per mm^2) are used in further staging only of T1 tumors (<1 mm) because they are independent predictors of outcome in that subgroup.

The major revision to nodal staging (N) places an emphasis on the number of involved lymph nodes. Cox regression analysis has demonstrated that the number, not the size, of metastatic lymph nodes was the strongest predictor of outcome (77). N1, N2, and N3 include patients with one involved lymph node, two or three involved lymph nodes, and four or more involved lymph nodes, respectively. The next most important predictor of outcome is the tumor burden within the involved lymph nodes (77). N groups are further characterized as having microscopic metastases or macroscopic metastases that are clinically or radiographically

apparent and confirmed pathologically. Both satellite lesions and in-transit metastases involve the lymphatics and portend a poor prognosis. These were grouped separately in the old staging system but are now grouped together as N2c disease in the revised AJCC staging system. The presence of satellite lesions or in-transit metastases in patients with nodal metastasis represents N3 disease. Finally, in patients with lymph node metastasis, ulceration of the primary tumor was the feature that independently predicted an adverse outcome among patients with stage III disease. In the revised AJCC staging system, all stage III patients whose primary tumor is ulcerated are staged upward by one substage.

In patients with metastasis, the metastases (M) staging has been broken down into three subgroups (M1a, M1b, and M1c) in the revised AJCC staging system. The subgroups reflect the site of metastasis and whether or not lactate dehydrogenase (LDH) is elevated.

■ SURGICAL THERAPY FOR LOCALIZED MELANOMA

In the early 1900s, Handley described the existence of a satellite lesion as far as 3 to 5 cm from the primary melanoma lesion (30) (Fig. 39-11). For that reason, for much of the twentieth century, surgeons typically resected melanomas with 5-cm margins. Data to support more conservative resection margins have come from the World Health Organization Melanoma Programme Trial and the Intergroup Trial as well as many studies conducted in the 1970s and 1980s. Today, surgeons in the United States generally follow the guidelines proposed during the 1997 World Health Organization (WHO) Melanoma Programme meeting (79). These guidelines recommend more conservative surgical margins that are based on tumor thickness. Lesions more than 2-mm thick require a 2-cm margin, those less than 2-mm thick require a 1-cm margin, and excision of melanoma in situ requires a 0.5-cm margin (79). Fig. 39-12 depicts the scheme for the management of primary melanoma.

MOHS SURGERY

The role of Mohs micrographic surgery in the management of cutaneous malignant melanoma remains controversial. Findings from one study in 1997 support the efficacy of the Mohs technique for the treatment of melanoma versus wide local excision (80). Furthermore, the local recurrence rate was lower in the Mohs group than for the group that underwent conventional surgery (81). The margins required to remove the tumor

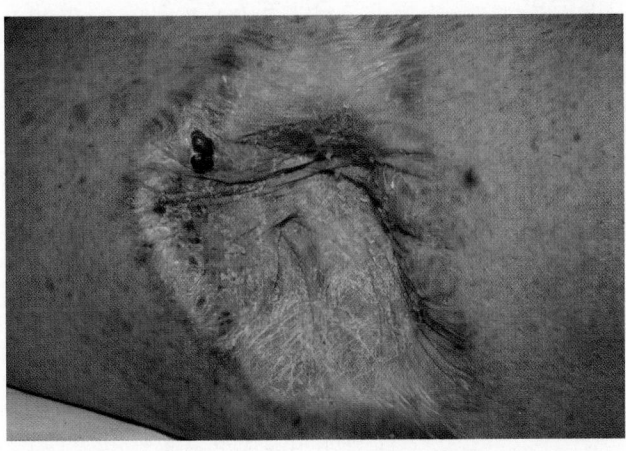

FIGURE 39-11. Metastatic melanoma appearing within and around a graft site.

averaged 6 mm in 83% of the cases (81). At present, Mohs surgery is not widely used in the management of melanoma. It is labor intensive, time intensive, and costly. Furthermore, no randomized prospective studies have been conducted comparing this technique to conventional surgery. Results of such a study would, of course, be dependent on the experience of the Mohs surgeon. Finally, cutting part of the tumor in an attempt to obtain a strict margin is a risk that is not deemed acceptable by most surgeons. Others have advocated its use in areas where tissue conservation is desired, such as on the face.

ELECTIVE LYMPH NODE DISSECTION

As in the case of other tumors, lymph node metastasis remains the most important predictor of survival in patients with malignant melanoma (82,83). Studies have shown that the number of lymph nodes bearing cancer, rather than their size, is the most important prognostic feature in this disease (84). The 10-year survivals for patients with one, two to four, or five or more lymph nodes involved with melanoma are approximately 40, 26, and 15%, respectively (84). Therefore many believe that elective lymph node dissection (ELND) is important not only for staging but also for potential cure through removal of disseminated tumor foci. Indeed, many studies have shown a survival advantage for patients who undergo ELND as part of staging compared with those who wait until the development of clinically evident metastases (85-87). However, the WHO trial concluded that ELND offered no survival benefit over delayed lymph node dissection (88).

SENTINEL LYMPH NODE BIOPSY

ELND carries risks of morbidity. These include lymphedema, nerve damage, and wound complications. To circumvent these problems, intraoperative lymphatic mapping and sentinel lymph node (SLN) biopsy have now become the standard of care in most institutions for staging the lymphatic basin. The indication for SLN is the presence of primary melanoma without clinical, radiographic, or histologic evidence of distant metastases. At present, there is still disagreement as to when to perform SLN biopsy. Many surgeons feel that this procedure is appropriate for melanomas at least 0.75-mm thick, whereas others would argue that it should be employed only for lesions at least 1-mm thick.

Morton et al. have published one of the first clinical studies demonstrating the efficacy of SLN biopsy (89). In this study they identified the SLN(s) in 82% of

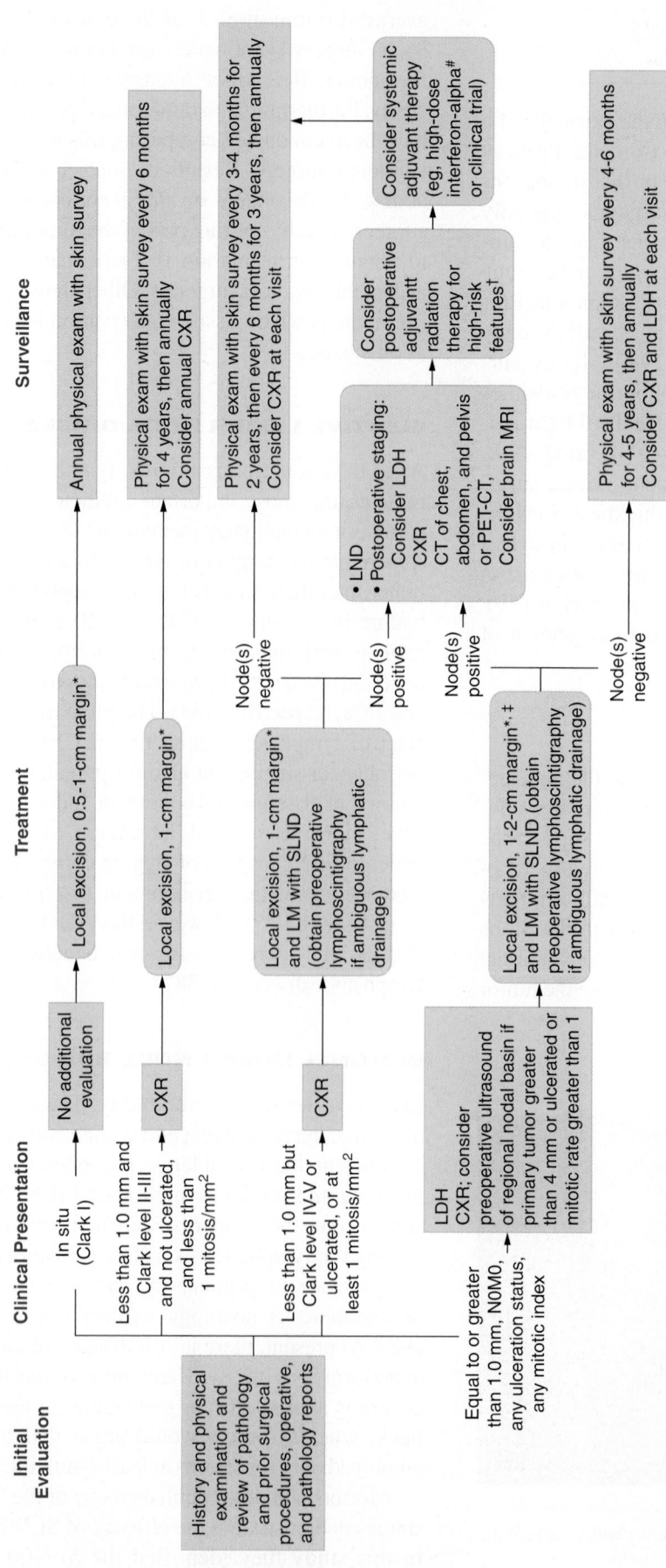

FIGURE 39-12. Management of primary melanoma.

LM, lymphatic mapping and sentinel lymph node biopsy; LMD, leptomeningeal disease; LND, lymph node dissection; SLND, selective lymph node dissection based on results of sentinel lymph node evaluation.

*Consider function and cosmesis

†High-risk features include: Extracapsular extension, Greater than or equal to 4 nodes involved, Greater than or equal to 3 cm, or Regional nodal or soft tissue recurrence.

‡Consider postoperative adjuvant radiation therapy for pure desmoplastic and neurotropic histology.

#See references in Adjuvant Interferon-Alpha section.

NOTE: Consider clinical trials as treatment options for eligible patients

Adapted with permission from The University of Texas MD Anderson Cancer Center.

lymphatic basins. Metastases were present in approximately 18% of the SLNs identified (89). This correlates well with prior studies indicating metastases in 12 to 15% of SLNs (90,91). Combinations of blue dye and radiocolloid-guided lymphatic mapping are accurate in determining the SLN. This accuracy is reduced, however, in patients who have previously had surgical disruption of their tumor site. This is most problematic if the primary site was resected with large margins or a rotational flap was used for closure. For this reason, it is preferred that SLN biopsies occur at the time of excision. It is a standard of practice to evaluate histologic features and immunohistochemical staining for S-100, HMB-45, and MART-1 in the SLNs to diagnose the nodal micrometastases. The presence of cells with tyrosinase with S-100, MART-1, or MAGE-3 mRNA detected by RT-PCR does not seem to correlate with the risk of recurrence in the absence of positive histology or immunohistochemical staining (92). If there is histopathologic or immunohistochemical evidence of metastasis in the SLN, it is standard to proceed with lymphadenectomy. Although ELND and SLN biopsies may not increase survival in patients with regional lymph node involvement, they clearly provide accurate staging information, which may help guide the clinician's decision as to whether or not to offer adjuvant therapy.

■ ADJUVANT THERAPY FOR PATIENTS WITH HIGH RISK FOR MELANOMA RECURRENCE

The risk of melanoma recurrence and death is closely related to Breslow thickness, presence of ulceration of the primary tumor, and the number of regional lymph nodes involved. Surgery can be curative in more than 90% of low-risk patients with stage I disease (Breslow thickness <2 mm, without ulceration) and 70% of intermediate-risk patients with stage IIA disease (Breslow thickness 2-4 mm) at presentation (see Fig. 39-12). In contrast, patients with stage IIB or C disease (Breslow thickness >4 mm) have a 5-year survival of about 30 to 50% despite complete surgical excision. The survival rates decrease to 30% at 5 years with local-regional recurrences and to less than 5% with systemic metastasis. Adjuvant therapies are prescribed following surgery to patients at high risk for tumor recurrence, with the hope that such treatments might be most successful in patients with micrometastasis. Patients with clinically detectable metastatic melanoma have a median survival of 7 to 9 months.

A number of modalities of treatments have been tested to reduce the risk of recurrence in high-risk patients through eradication of occult micrometastases. Chemotherapy, nonspecific immune response modifiers, hormonal agents, and lymphokines have been tried. Unfortunately, despite the promising results from pilot studies, none of these therapies, except a high-dose interferon-alpha, has proved consistently to be beneficial in prospectively randomized clinical trials when compared with observation or placebo.

Chemotherapy outcomes in adjuvant settings have been reviewed (93), and the following general conclusions were reached. First, dacarbazine (DTIC), a cytotoxic drug approved by the US Food and Drug Administration (FDA) specifically for the treatment of metastatic melanoma, has been found to be of no significant benefit. The Central Oncology Group (COG) and the Southwest Oncology Group (SWOG) studies were relatively large. In the COG trial (94) after surgery for regional lymph node metastasis, 174 patients were prospectively randomized to observation or treatment with dacarbazine for four courses. At a median follow-up of 2.5 years, the control group had superior relapse-free survival (RFS) and overall survival (OS) compared with the dacarbazine-treated group. In the SWOG study (95), after resection of the primary tumor, 123 patients were randomized to either carmustine, hydroxyurea, and dacarbazine for 1 year or observation. At the 6-year point, the two groups had similar OS durations.

Immunotherapy trials in melanoma began over four decades ago based on the observation of tumor regression with the administration of bacillus Calmette-Guérin (BCG) (96). Several pilot studies with BCG gave encouraging results in patients with stage I to III melanoma who were rendered free of disease by surgery. One of the large studies was conducted by the Eastern Cooperative Oncology Group (ECOG) (97) in which 474 patients with stage I-III disease were randomized to receive immunotherapy with Tice strain BCG (18 months) or observation after curative surgery. No significant benefit in RFS or OS was observed with BCG. Similarly, compared with observation, no improvement over observation was seen with methyl-lomustine (CCNU), BCG, or BCG plus allogeneic cultured melanoma cells in a study conducted by the National Cancer Institute (98). ECOG evaluated the role of adjuvant BCG and dacarbazine in Trial E1673 (99). After surgery, 652 patients with stage I-III melanoma were randomly assigned to one of three study groups: (1) treatment with immunotherapy with BCG, (2) dacarbazine plus BCG, or (3) observation. There were no significant differences in RFS or OS among the treatment groups compared with the control arm.

In a trial conducted by WHO (100) in patients with advanced primary or stage III melanoma, 761 patients were prospectively randomized to one of four groups: (1) 185 patients to surgery alone; (2) 192 to surgery plus dacarbazine at 200 mg/m² per day × 5 days every 4 weeks; (3) 203 to surgery plus BCG; and (4) 181 to surgery plus dacarbazine and BCG. Veronisi reported in 1982 that over 70% of these patients experienced tumor recurrence. There was no significant difference in RFS and OS among the four groups.

Levamisole trials in melanoma were initiated after the discovery of its immunomodulating activity. Two adjuvant trials with levamisole, one conducted by the European Organization for Research on the Treatment of Cancer (EORTC) comparing dacarbazine (250 mg/m² per day × 5 days monthly for 6 months), levamisole, or placebo (101) and the second by Spitler comparing levamisole with placebo (102) found no benefit with regard to RFS and OS compared with observation. However, a Phase III study conducted by the National Cancer Institute of Canada compared the roles of BCG and levamisole with observation (103). Following complete resection, 543 patients with poor-prognosis melanoma were randomly assigned to four treatment groups: (1) levamisole for 3 years, (2) BCG for 3 years, (3) BCG alternating with levamisole for 3 years, and (4) observation (103). At a median follow-up of 8.5 years, a trend in favor of levamisole was observed in OS and RFS ($p = .08$ and .09, respectively).

Melanoma vaccines—including whole cell, cell lysates or shed antigen vaccines as well as ganglioside vaccines—have been evaluated in intermediate- and high-risk patients with melanoma. These vaccines were reported to result in significantly prolonged survival when administered as a surgical adjuvant compared with historical controls. However, the initial promising results could not be confirmed with these agents when used alone or in combination in the few prospectively randomized adjuvant studies designed to compare them with placebo or observation in stages III and IV in the postoperative settings.

Vaccinia melanoma oncolysates (VMO) resulted in significant improvement in survival relative to historical controls in the pilot clinical trial. In the subsequent randomized clinical trial using a VMO derived from four melanoma cell lines infected with vaccinia virus, 215 patients with stage III melanoma were randomized to VMO or vaccinia alone. There was no evidence of RFS or OS benefit (104). In another trial, 700 patients with high-risk (66% with clinically detectable regional lymph node metastasis) melanoma, after definitive surgery, were prospectively randomized either to therapy with VMO for 2 years or to observation. At a median follow-up of 8 years, statistically significant prolongation of RFS or OS was not observed (105).

Allogeneic melanoma vaccine (Melacine) was evaluated by the SWOG in patients with stage II melanoma. Six hundred patients with intermediate-thickness (1.5-4.0 mm or Clark level IV) melanoma and without clinical or histologic evidence of lymph node metastasis were randomly assigned after surgery to treatment with Melacine for 2 years or to observation. After follow-up of 5.6 years, no improvement in RFS or OS with adjuvant vaccine was found (106).

GM2 ganglioside vaccine induced antibody responses in a study conducted by Livingston et al. They postulated that T cells infiltrating melanoma lesions recognized specific tumor antigens located on the surface of melanoma cells. The presence of IgM antibody against GM2 ganglioside was associated with prolonged survival in patients with melanoma (107). In a randomized Phase III trial, 122 patients who had undergone resection of regional node metastases were assigned to receive either GM2/BCG vaccine or BCG alone (108). The patients with no pretreatment anti-GM2 antibodies who had IgM antibody production in response to administration of GM2/BCG had improvement in RFS and OS, but only the improvement in RFS was statistically significant ($p = .02$).

A large Phase III EORTC 18961 trial of ganglioside GM2-KLH21 vaccination treatment versus observation in 1314 patients with stage II (T3-T4N0M0) melanoma was stopped early by the Independent Data Monitoring Committee because of inferior survival in the vaccine treatment arm (109).

Allogeneic cancer vaccine (Canvaxin) developed from three melanoma cell lines was used in two clinical trials. In a large, randomized trial, 1166 patients with stage III melanoma after lymphadenectomy were randomly allocated to receive Canvaxin plus BCG or placebo plus BCG after surgery. The trial was closed prematurely on the advice of the Independent Data Monitoring Committee because of safety concerns. The patients who received Canvaxin treatment had shorter survival than did controls. The 5-year survivals were 59% for those who received Canvaxin and 68% for control patients (110). A similar result was observed in another adjuvant trial of Canvaxin with a similar clinical design in patients with stage IV disease rendered free of disease surgically.

INTERFERON-ALPHA THERAPY

Interferon-alpha (IFNα) induces immune modulation and tumor regression in patients with metastatic melanoma. The antiviral and immunomodulatory properties of IFN could stimulate host rejection of tumor cells and induction of MHC antigens. The IFNs may inhibit angiogenesis and may have direct growth-inhibitory effects. A series of clinical trials were initiated to examine the role of IFN in the treatment and prevention of melanoma. The significant toxicity and cost associated with the higher-dose schedules and the marginal antitumor efficacy of IFN have been important factors in the decision to adopt different-dose schedules as standard in Europe and the United States. In western Europe, the low-dose chronic (1-5 years) IFN administration schedule was preferred by the European Medicine Evaluation Agency as standard over the high-dose IFN schedule for 1 year approved by the FDA in the United States. The outcomes of the adjuvant clinical trials with IFN have been inconsistent. A brief summary of a few selected trials is presented below.

The data from high-dose IFN adjuvant trials in patients with lymph node metastasis at high risk for melanoma recurrence quite often showed an improvement in RFS. However, the only clinical trial that showed significant OS benefit with IFN compared with observation was that of the ECOG study E1684 (111). In that study, patients with thick primary melanoma (>4 mm Breslow thickness) or lymph node metastases treated with high-dose IFN after surgical resection of the primary tumor and complete lymph node dissection had a median RFS that was prolonged by about 9 months, and their 5-year RFS rate was increased to 37%, compared with 26% for the control group. The corresponding improvements in OS were about 1 year for median survival and a 9% improvement in 5-year survival. These results led the FDA in 1996 to recommend the approval of this IFN regimen as standard therapy for patients with high-risk melanoma. However, an updated analysis by Kirkwood et al. indicated that, at median follow-up of 12.6 years, there was no significant survival benefit with IFN (112).

Confirmatory Intergroup Trial E1690, a three-arm trial comparing the IFN high-dose IV/SC regimen or low-dose subcutaneous regimen for 2 years with observation, showed no OS benefit (113). It confirmed the RFS advantage of the high-dose therapy observed in the prior trial. The observation group of this trial did significantly better than the E1684 trial group. One possible cause for this finding was the crossover effect made possible by the FDA's approval of IFN during the life of the trial. Other randomized trials of adjuvant IFN in high-risk patients employed lower doses; differing doses, durations, and routes of administration showed no significant survival benefit.

In the E1694 clinical trial, 1 year of high-dose IFN was compared with 2 years of GMK, a ganglioside vaccine (114). In this study, the patients who received IFN arm had significantly better RFS and OS than those who received GMK vaccine. It is still uncertain whether the difference in efficacy is related to a possible negative effect of GMK vaccine or the superiority of IFN.

Thus, although data from high-dose IFN clinical trials consistently demonstrated RFS benefit when IFN was given as surgical adjuvant to patients with thick primary melanoma or regional lymph node involvement after lymphadenectomy, its impact on OS has been less clear. Quantitative meta-analysis based on published data was performed to determine the effect of IFN on RFS and OS (115). A subgroup analysis by dose of IFNα was performed. Endpoints evaluated were RFS and OS. A subgroup analysis by dose of IFNα was performed. It was concluded that adjuvant IFNα produced clear reductions in recurrence of high-risk melanoma, with some evidence of an effect of dose of IFNα, but it was unclear whether this translated into a worthwhile survival benefit or not.

Because benefit from IFN therapy cannot be demonstrated while adjuvant therapy is being administered, an attempt was made to identify patients who are likely to benefit from this therapy early in the treatment by measuring the serum levels of autoantibodies in response to IFN treatments. Since most immunotherapies that confer survival benefit in patients with advanced melanoma induce an appearance of autoimmunity, a study was conducted to correlate induction of immune response as determined by increased production of serum levels of autoantibodies, including antithyroid, antinuclear, anti-DNA, antiplatelet, and anti–islet-cell antibodies, in response to IFN therapy with prolonged survival. Although autoantibody production in response to IFN therapy in a subpopulation of melanoma patients receiving IFN therapy has been confirmed (116), the prognostic implication of this finding in terms of long-term survival remains debatable.

Eggermont et al. reported on EORTC 18991 trial with adjuvant PEGylated IFNα-2b (PEG-IFNα-2b) versus observation in patients with stage III melanoma (117). A total of 1256 patients with stage III melanoma were randomly assigned after full lymphadenectomy to receive either observation (N = 629) or PEG-IFNα-2b (N = 627): induction 6 g/kg/week for 8 weeks and then maintenance 3 g/kg/week for an intended total duration of 5 years. The patients whose metastatic melanoma was discovered by SLN biopsy rather than as a clinically palpable node (N2/3) benefited the most from PEG-IFNα-2b. Patients with N1 disease who were randomized to PEG-IFNα-2b had improved recurrence-free and distant metastasis-free survival and a nonsignificant improvement in OS compared with patients with N2 disease, with more extensive lymph node metastases.

A trial comparing the efficacy of high-dose IFNα-2b to IL-2–based biochemotherapy is currently under way nationally. In this SWOG study, patients with stage III melanoma are prospectively randomized following surgery to receive either high-dose IFN administered for 1 year or three courses of biochemotherapy including cisplatin, vinblastine, dacarbazine, IFN, and IL-2 over a 9-week period. The effects of these treatments on RFS and OS will be compared. A similar study was recently reported from our institution (118). One hundred and thirty-eight patients were enrolled: 71 in the biochemotherapy group, 34 in the high-dose IFN subgroup, and 33 in the intermediate-dose IFN subgroup. No significant differences in median RFS or OS between the high-dose IFN and the intermediate-dose IFN subgroups were observed. With a median follow-up of 49.3 months, neither the biochemotherapy group nor the IFN group had reached median RFS or OS, and there were no significant differences in estimated median RFS or OS ($p = .86$ and 0.45, respectively) between the two groups. Biochemotherapy is not more effective than IFN.

IFN therapy remains the standard of care for adjuvant therapy of patients with melanoma at high risk for tumor recurrence (stage II with at least 4-mm thick primary melanoma or stage III with regional lymph node metastases). It is associated with considerable but generally manageable toxicity. Side effects include flu-like symptoms (fever, fatigue, and nausea), depression, neutropenia, and reversible hepatotoxicity. Despite these problems, over 60% of patients are able to complete a year of therapy without serious toxicity. Contraindications to high-dose IFNα-2b adjuvant therapy include recent history of myocardial infarction or arrhythmias, preexisting liver or central nervous system disorders, and overall debility. The importance of dose and schedule in the use of IFN is still under investigation.

Recently, the Hellenic Collaborative Oncology Group reported the equivalency of 1 month of induction interferon-alpha to 1 year of interferon-alpha therapy (119). However, the results of this study have not been widely accepted because the assumption in the study design that a difference in the median RFS rates of less than 15% at 3 years is clinically equivalent is controversial, and this study was underpowered to detect a clinically significant difference in OS rate. The clinical utility of 1 month of induction therapy of high-dose interferon-alpha without 11 months of the maintenance therapy in an adjuvant setting in patients with high risk

for melanoma recurrence will be determined in an ongoing large Phase III study (ECOG 1697) which compares the survival durations of patients receiving 4 weeks of induction IFNα therapy with those of patients receiving no treatment. Table 39-3 lists the randomized studies of adjuvant interferon therapy in patients with high risk for melanoma recurrence.

■ MANAGEMENT OF METASTATIC DISEASE

It is estimated that between 2 and 5% of patients will present with metastatic disease. On the whole, survival time for patients with metastasis ranges from 6 to 9 months with long-term survival of less than 10%. In these patients, the site of metastasis is of prognostic value. Patients with skin, subcutaneous, and distant lymph node metastases have a better prognosis than those with lung or liver and bone metastases. The development of brain metastasis has a significant negative impact on prognosis (survival of 3-4 months). The number of metastatic sites is also predictive of patient outcome. In those patients with a single metastatic focus to the brain, lungs, gastrointestinal tract, skin, or subcutaneous tissue following a long disease-free interval after treatment of local/regional disease, surgical excision may render the patient disease-free. Such patients have respectable 2-year survival rates. Unfortunately, patients who are not candidates for surgical intervention are left with few medical treatment options. These options include single-agent chemotherapy, combination chemotherapy, biotherapy, biochemotherapy, radiation therapy, and vaccines. Because metastatic melanomas of skin and mucosal primaries generally respond to systemic chemotherapy and immunotherapy better than metastatic melanomas of uveal origin, their management is described separately. Fig. 39-13 depicts the scheme for the management of recurrent, regional, and/or distant melanoma metastases. Table 39-4 lists the results of the recently completed Phase III clinical trials in patients with metastatic melanoma of cutaneous priamy conducted since the year 2000.

METASTATIC SKIN/MUCOSAL MELANOMA

Cytotoxic Therapy

Single-Agent Chemotherapy

Dacarbazine remains the most commonly used FDA-approved single agent in malignant melanoma. Dacarbazine has a response rate of about 15%; however,

TABLE 39-3 | ADJUVANT INTERFERON THERAPY OF PATIENTS AT HIGH RISK FOR MELANOMA RECURRENCE

Trial, Year of Publication	Eligibility	No. of Pts.	Interferon	Control	Outcome*
WHO Melanoma 16, Cascinelli et al., 2001 (120)	Regional lymph node metastases	424	IFNα-2a 3 MU SC 3 × per week for 3 years	Observation	No significant RFS or OS benefit
SWOG 8642, Meykens et al., 1995 (121)	T ≥1.5 mm or regional lymph node metastases	284	IFNγ 0.2 mg SC 3 × per week for 1 year	Observation	No significant RFS or OS benefit
NCCTG, Creagan et al., 1995 (122)	T >1.69 mm or regional lymph node metastases	262	IFNα-2a 20 MU/m^2 IM 3 × per week for 3 months	Observation	No significant RFS or OS benefit
ECOG 1684, Kirkwood et al., 1996 (111)	T >4.0 mm or regional lymph node metastases	287	IFNα-2b 20 MU/m^2/ day IV × 5 q7days for 4 weeks, then 10 MU/m^2 SC 3 × per week for 11 months	Observation	IFN has significant RFS or OS benefit
French Multicenter Trial, Grob et al., 1998 (123)	T >1.5 mm and no clinically detectable regional lymph nodes	489	IFNα-2a 3 MU/m^2 SC 3 × per week for 18 months	Observation	Significant RFS but no OS benefit
Austrian Malignant Melanoma Co-op. Group, Pehamberger et al., 1998 (124)	T ≥1.5 mm and no regional/distant metastases	311	IFNα-2a 3 MU SC daily for 3 weeks, then 3 × per week for 12 months	Observation	Significant RFS but no OS benefit
ECOG 1690, Kirkwood et al., 2000 (113)	T >4.0 mm or regional lymph node metastases	642	IFNα-2b 20 MU/m^2/ day IV × 5 q7days for for 4 weeks, then 10 MU/m^2 SC 3 × per week × 11 months versus 3 MU SC 3 × per week for 2 years	Observation	No significant RFS or OS benefit
ECOG 1694, Kirkwood et al., 2001 (114)	T > 4.0 mm or regional lymph node metastases	880	IFNα-2b 20 MU/m^2/ day IV × 5 q7days for 4 weeks, then 10 MU/m^2 SC 3 × per week for 11 months	G$_{M2}$ ganglioside vaccine	IFN has significant DFS and OS benefit
EORTC 18952, Eggermont et al., 2005 (125)	T ≥4.0 mm or regional lymph node metastases	1388	IFNα-2b 10 MU/day × 5 q7days × 4 weeks, 5 MU SC 3 × per week for 23 months versus 10 MU/day × 5 q7days for 4 weeks, 10 MU SC 3 × per week for 11 months	Observation	Significant RFS but no OS benefit with low-dose IFN versus control
EORTC 18871, Kleeberg et al., 2004 (126)	T >3 mm or regional lymph node metastases	830	IFNα-2b 1 MU 3 × per week for 1 year	IFNγ 0.2 mg SC 3 × per week for 1 year	No significant RFS or OS benefit
UKCCCR study, Hancock et al., 2004 (127)	T ≥4.0 mm or regional lymph node metastases	674	IFNα-2a 3 MU SC 3 × per week for 2 years	Observation	No significant RFS or OS benefit

*OS, overall survival; RFS, relapse-free survival.

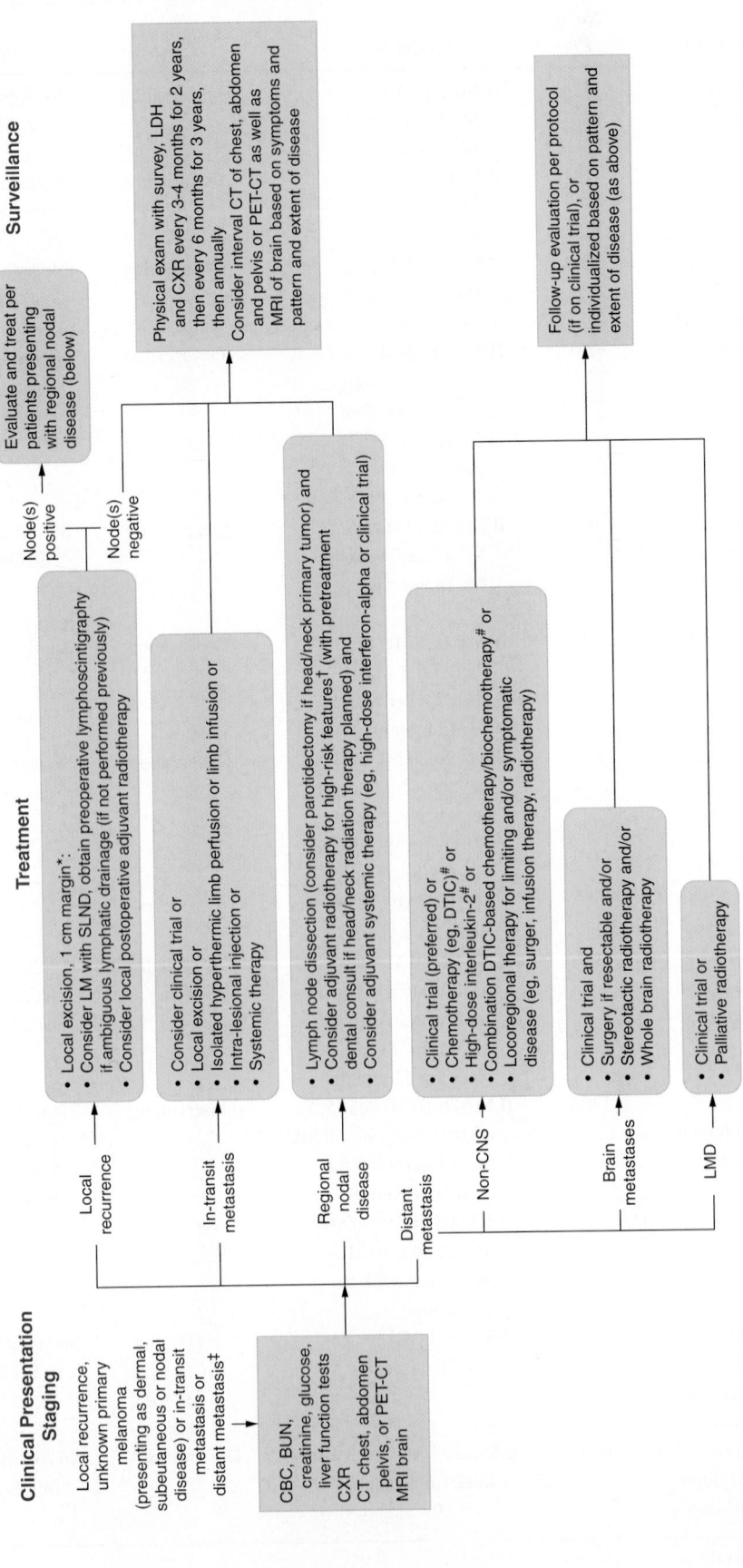

FIGURE 39-13. Management of recurrent, regional, and/or distant melanoma metastases.

*Consider function and cosmesis

†High-risk features include: Extracapsular extension, Greater than or equal to 3 cm, Greater than or equal to 4 nodes, Recurrent regional nodal or soft tissue recurrence.

‡Note: If patient presents with clinically suspicious lymph node or nodule, or history of melanoma, consider FNA to establish the diagnosis prior to excision to facilitate definitive treatment planning.

#See references in Chemotherapy, Biochemotherapy, and Targeted Therapy section.

NOTE: Consider clinical trials as treatment options for eligible patients.

Adapted with permission from The University of Texas MD Anderson Cancer Center.

1094

TABLE 39-4 | RECENTLY COMPLETED PHASE III CLINICAL TRIALS WITH NEW DRUGS IN METASTATIC MELANOMA OF CUTANEOUS PRIMARY

Author, Year	Therapy	N	Chemonaive/ Prior Therapy	ORR (%)	Median OS*	Result
Avril et al., 2004 (203)	Fotemustine versus dacarbazine	229 221	Chemonaive	15.2 7.2	7.3 5.6	Not significant
Bedikian et al., 2006 (134)	Dacarbazine versus dacarbazine + oblimersen	385 386	Chemonaive	7.5 13.5	9.0 7.8	Not significant
Ribas et al., 2008 (204)	Tremelimumab versus Temozolomide or dacarbazine	328 327	Chemonaive	9 10	11.8 10.7	Not significant
O'Day et al., 2009 (205)	Paclitaxel + elesclemol versus paclitaxel	225 226	Chemonaive	7.4 4.4	10.6 11.3	Not significant
Hauschild et al., 2009 (187)	Carboplatin/paclitaxel versus Carboplatin/paclitaxel/ sorafenib	134 134	Second-line	11 12	42 weeks 42 weeks	Not significant
Eisen et al., 2009 (206)	Lenalidomide versus placebo	152 154	Prior chemo	5.3 5.8	5.9 7.4	Not significant
Glaspy et al., 2009 (207)	Lenalidomide 25 mg versus Lenalidomide 5 mg	148 146	Prior chemo	5.5 4.4	6.8 7.2	Not significant
Flaherty et al., 2009 (188)	Carboplatin/Paclitaxel versus Carboplatin/Paclitaxel/ Sorafenib	390 384	Chemonaive	16 18	11.4 10.7	Not significant

ORR, overall response rate; OS, overall survival.

*In months unless stated otherwise.

complete responses (CRs) are rare and the response duration is short (4-6 months) (128-132). In large Phase III melanoma clinical trials that included dacarbazine as the control arm, the response rate to dacarbazine was only 8 to 12% (129,130). Side effects include nausea and mild marrow suppression; rare cases of hepatic veno-occlusive disease have also been reported (133). The dacarbazine response rate is lower when RECIST criteria are used to assess tumor response (134).

Temozolomide (TMZ), a dacarbazine analogue, has several properties that are advantageous compared with dacarbazine. TMZ has high oral bioavailability, does not require metabolic conversion to an active metabolite, and readily crosses the blood–brain barrier making it the preferred drug for the management of brain metastasis. Phase III trials comparing dacarbazine and TMZ reported comparable response rates and survivals (135,136).

Cisplatin has been shown to have modest activity in melanoma, with a response rate of approximately 15% (137). Higher doses of cisplatin have resulted in response rates and require coadministration with amifostine (138). Carboplatin has been used as a substitute for cisplatin in combination with paclitaxel in several recent trials with equal efficacy.

Nitrosoureas, which include carmustine and CCNU, have response rates that range from 13 to 18% (137). Several Phase II studies completed in Europe showed that the nitrosourea fotemustine has a superior response rate as single-agent with an average response rate of 20% (139-142). Fotemustine also demonstrated significant efficacy in brain metastasis (average response rate 21%) (140).

Other agents with single-agent efficacy in melanoma include the vinca alkaloids (vindesine and vinblastine) (143,144) and the taxanes (paclitaxel and docetaxel), (145-147) with response rates of 16 to 17%.

Combination Chemotherapy

The principle of combining drugs that have single-agent efficacy to achieve additive or synergistic effects has been extensively studied in metastatic melanoma.

The CVD regimen (cisplatin, vinblastine, and dacarbazine) and the Dartmouth regimen (cisplatin, dacarbazine, carmustine, and tamoxifen) were initially reported to be superior to dacarbazine with response rates of 35 to 45% (148,149). Unfortunately, Phase III prospectively randomized clinical trials have failed to confirm the superiority of multidrug chemotherapy regimens over dacarbazine alone (129,130).

■ Cytokines and Immunotherapy

High-Dose Interleukin-2

Melanoma is an immunogenic tumor, capable of being recognized and destroyed by immune cells including cytotoxic T cells. Antigens have been cloned from melanoma cells that are capable of being recognized by T cells. In addition, dramatic responses can be seen in some patients treated with immune therapies, including cytokines, immunomodulating antibodies, and T cells. Infusion of interleukin-2 (IL-2), a natural protein produced by T cells, has a 10 to 20% response rate in patients with metastatic melanoma. Complete responses (CRs) are seen in approximately half of the responding patients, and these are highly durable with long-term disease-free intervals in over 50% of patients with CRs (Fig. 39-14) (150). Because of this potential for long-term survival, albeit in a minority of patients, IL-2 is considered a standard frontline therapy for metastatic melanoma. Current studies are aimed at identifying the host and tumor characteristics at the molecular level that will predict responses and in combining IL-2 with other agents to increase the number of long-term survivors.

High-dose IL-2 therapy has a significant number of toxicities, including hypotension, capillary leak syndrome resulting in pulmonary edema, and transient renal toxicity. Therefore, safe administration requires adequate prescreening of patients to ensure adequate cardiac and pulmonary function as well as significant training and experience of the health care team. As with interferon, clinical response to IL-2 is associated with autoimmunity. The development of hypothyroidism or vitiligo, an autoimmune destruction of melanocytes following IL-2 therapy, has been correlated with clinical response (151,152).

In patients with metastatic, nonvisceral disease, response rates from IL-2 are particularly high, and have been reported to be as high as 50% for patients with cutaneous- or subcutaneous-only metastases (153). Therefore, high-dose IL-2 may be considered as a first-line therapeutic (154). However, Phase II studies by other groups failed to replicate this response rate (155). Currently, a randomized multicenter study comparing high-dose IL-2 with vaccine and IL-2 only will help to shed light on whether the combination is beneficial (156). Initial results of this study demonstrated an increased response rate and progression-free survival in patients receiving the combination.

Interferon-Alpha

IFNs exhibit antiviral, immunomodulatory, and growth-inhibitory properties and have a definite, though limited efficacy against metastatic melanoma with an overall response rate of 7 to 23% (157-160). Despite the modest response rate, durable responses have been observed in patients with low-volume and soft-tissue disease. However, interferon-alpha is rarely used as a single agent in patients with metastatic melanoma.

Biochemotherapy

On the basis of clinical observations about lack of cross-resistance between chemotherapy and biotherapy with IL-2 and the possibility of synergy between these

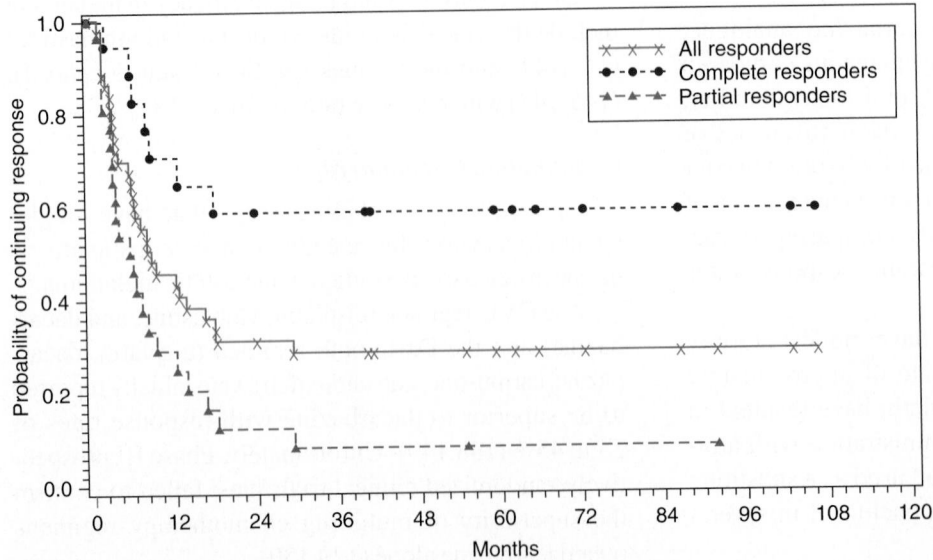

FIGURE 39-14. Responses are durable following treatment with high-dose IL-2 treatment.

TABLE 39-5	PHASE III TRIALS OF BIOCHEMOTHERAPY				
Author, Year	*Regimens*	*N*	*Response (CR + PR)*	*Median Survival*
Rosenberg et al.,	CDT/IL-2, IFN	50	44% (6+38)	10.7 months
1999 (161)	versus CDT	52	27% (8+19)	15.8 months
Eton et al.,	CVD/IL-2, IFN	91	48% (6+42)	11.8 months
2002 (162)	versus CVD	92	25% (1+24)	9.5 months
Ridolfi et al.,	CD/IL-2, IFN	87	25% (3+22)	11 months
2002 (163)	versus CD	89	20% (3+17)	9.5 months
Keilholz et al.,	CD/IL-2, IFN	182	20.8%	9.0 months
2005 (171)	versus CD/INF	181	22.8%	9.0 months
Atkins et al.,	CVD/IL-2, IFN	200	19.5%	9.0 months
2008 (164)	versus CVD	195	13.8%	8.7 months

CVD, cisplatin, vinblastine, dacarbazine; IFN, interferon ; CR, complete response; TTP, time to progression.

treatments, different combinations of chemotherapy with IL-2 and IFN, namely biochemotherapy, have been investigated. Cisplatin, vinblastine, and dacarbazine in combination with interleukin-2 and interferon-alpha have been evaluated with a variety of schedules. Multiple randomized studies have been performed comparing combination chemotherapy with biochemotherapy (Table 39-5) (161-165). While the majority of studies have shown no differences in median survival between patients treated with biochemotherapy and those receiving combination chemotherapy, long-term survival is seen in some patients treated with biochemotherapy. Bedikian et al. recently reported that 10-year survival of patients with metastatic melanoma treated with biochemotherapy was 12.5% (166,167). For this reason, it is still reasonable to utilize biochemotherapy as a frontline regimen, especially in patients with rapidly progressive disease. In addition, response rates are consistently higher in patients treated with biochemotherapy compared with combination chemotherapy. Therefore, in some patients with aggressive locoregional disease that is borderline resectable, neoadjuvant therapy with biochemotherapy may increase the likelihood that the disease could be rendered surgically resectable.

Although the majority of trials have been performed in patients with metastatic melanoma from a primary cutaneous lesion, response rates are likely similar for patients with mucosal melanoma primaries (168-170).

Anti-CTLA-4 Antibody

The immune system has evolved a number of regulatory mechanisms to prevent autoimmune tissue damage. One of these is the CTLA-4 molecule, which is expressed on T cells following activation (Fig. 39-15). CTLA-4

binds strongly to the costimulatory molecules CD80 and CD86 (B7-1 and B7-2) on antigen presenting cells, thereby preventing the binding of these molecules to CD28, which is required for full T-cell activation. Thus, the CTLA-4 molecule acts as a "braking" mechanism to decrease function of activated T cells. Antibodies blocking CTLA-4 thus release this braking mechanism, allowing increased activation of T cells. Anti-CTLA-4 therapy has been evaluated in multiple trials in patients with advanced melanoma. Overall response rates are approximately 15% (Table 39-6) (172-174). Importantly, though, some patients receiving this agent have had long-term disease-free survival. Further follow-up will be required to determine how this compares with standard high-dose IL-2 in the ability to induce long-term survival in a subset of patients. In addition, because anti-CTLA-4 has an immune-mediated mechanism of

- Blocks CTLA-4, an inhibitory receptor on T cells.
- CTLA-4 is only expressed on the surface of T cells after stimulation with antigen.

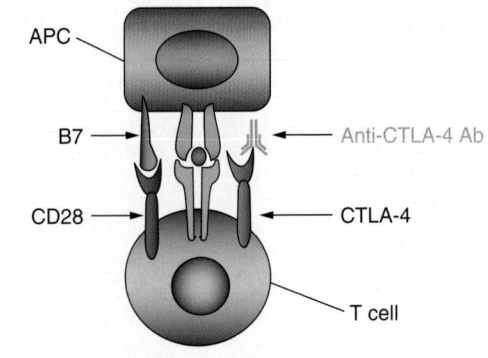

FIGURE 39-15. Anti-CTLA-4: Mechanism of action.

TABLE 39-6 | **CLINICAL RESPONSES TO ANTI-CTLA-4 THERAPY**

Author, Year	N	CR	PR	Total Response	Treatment
Attia et al., 2005 (175)	56	2 (3.5%)	5 (9%)	7 (12.5%)	MDX-010 (3 mg/kg, then 3 mg/kg or 1 mg/kg q3weeks) + gp100 vaccine
Ribas et al., 2005 (174)	29	2 (7%)	2 (7%)	4 (14%)	CP-675,206 (0.01-15 mg/kg)

CR, complete response; PR, partial response.

action, delayed, durable clinical responses have been observed in some patients, highlighting a possible need for unique criteria to measure response rates using this class of agents.

Because anti-CTLA-4 strongly stimulates activated T cells throughout the body, autoimmune adverse reactions are frequently seen, including hypophysitis (inflammation of the pituitary gland), rash, diarrhea, and hepatitis. Skin and colonic biopsies demonstrate immune infiltration, thereby suggesting the mechanism of toxicity in the release of CTLA-4 regulation on the surface of immune effector cells. As with the general autoimmunity seen with interferon therapy and the vitiligo seen with IL-2 treatment, the development of autoimmunity appears to be linked to clinical response in patients receiving anti-CTLA-4 (Table 39-7) (175). The severity of autoimmune toxicities can range from mild to life-threatening. Severe diarrhea or hepatitis may require treatment with steroids. Diarrhea not responsive to steroids may require administration of anti-TNF agents.

Adoptive T-cell Therapy

The infusion of antigen-specific T cells, often cultured and expanded in the laboratory, termed adoptive T-cell therapy (ACT), has been shown to be successful in treating a number of diseases including CMV infection posttransplant (176,177), EBV-induced lymphoproliferative disease posttransplant (178), EBV-induced nasopharyngeal cancer (179), leukemias treated with donor lymphocyte infusions (180), and melanoma

(180,181). The most successful T-cell therapies for metastatic melanoma have been reported following treatment with tumor infiltrating lymphocytes (TILs). In a subset of melanoma metastases, tumor-specific T cells can be isolated and expanded from the tumor itself, and reinfused into the patient (Fig. 39-16). Response rates have been higher with this approach if the infusion is performed following lymphodepleting chemotherapy, which may enhance the treatment effect by increasing homeostatic proliferation of antigen-specific T cells (ie, making "space" in the lymphoid compartment prior to infusion) or through the elimination of regulatory T cells. Response rates for patients receiving lymphodepleting chemotherapy followed by TIL infusion and high dose IL-2 have been reported to be approximately 50% (181) and perhaps even higher if whole-body radiation and stem cell transfer are included (182). With the addition of 2 or 12 Gy of total-body irradiation, response rates increased to 52% and 72%, respectively.

▬ Targeted Therapy

BRAF Inhibition

Since the initial report of the frequent occurrence of *BRAF* mutations in melanomas (41), a number of drugs that target mutated *BRAF* kinase have been investigated. Despite the early debate regarding the role of *BRAF* mutations in the development and progression of melanoma cells, there has been a great interest in these *BRAF* inhibitors among oncologists and researchers.

Sorafenib is a small-molecule inhibitor of multiple kinases, including C-RAF, B-RAF, vascular endothelial growth factor receptor 2 (VEGFR-2), VEGFR-3, platelet-derived growth factor receptor (PDGRF), FLT-3, and C-KIT (183). Sorafenib was shown to downregulate the MAPK signaling in melanomas in preclinical study (184). Unfortunately, a Phase II study of sorafenib showed a lack of clinical activity as a single agent (185). However, a Phase I/II study of sorafenib in combination with carboplatin and paclitaxel had an overall response rate of 31% among 35 patients with metastatic melanoma,

TABLE 39-7 | **CORRELATION OF AUTOIMMUNITY WITH RESPONSE TO ANTI-CTLA-4 THERAPY (175)**

Grade III/IV Autoimmune Toxicity	N	CR + PR	
Yes	14	5 (36%)	
No	42	2 (5%)	$p = .008$

CR, complete response; PR, partial response.

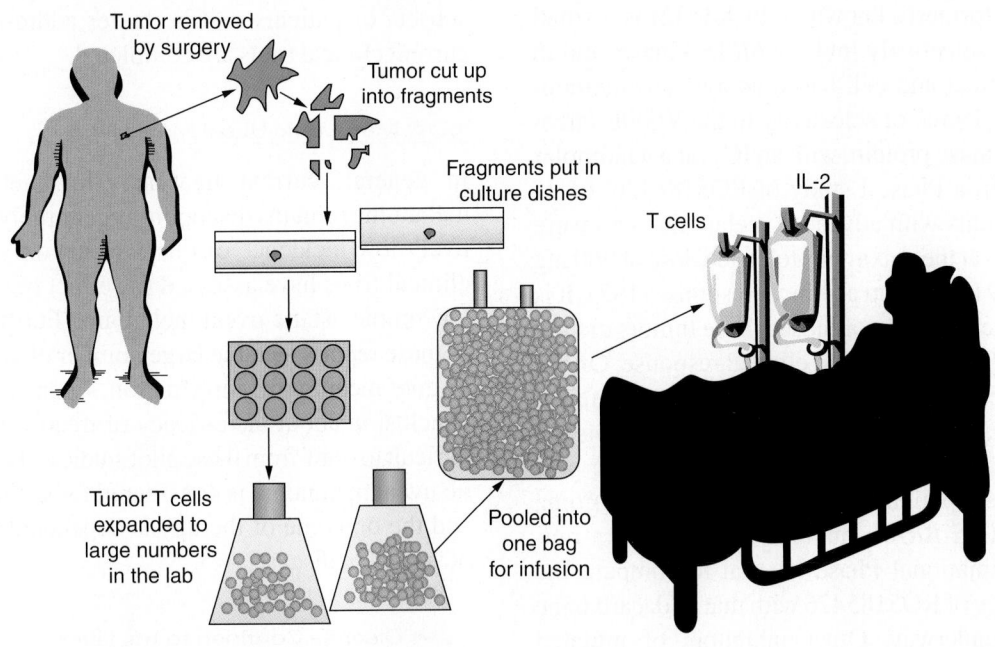

FIGURE 39-16. A schema diagram of adoptive cell therapy (ACT) with antigen-specific T cells.

and nearly 85% of the patients had either a clinical response or disease stabilization (186). Contrary to an initial expectation, the correlation between the clinical benefit and the presence of *BRAF* mutation was not apparent. On the basis of the encouraging results of the clinical study, two large randomized double-blind Phase III studies were conducted to evaluate the survival advantage of combining carboplatin and paclitaxel with sorafenib in patients with metastatic melanoma (187,188). The first study to be reported was a multinational study, which randomized 270 previously treated patients with unresectable stage III or IV melanoma to receive either the combination of carboplatin, paclitaxel, and sorafenib, or the combination of carboplatin, paclitaxel, and placebo (187). This study failed to show the progression-free survival (PFS) advantage of the three-drug combination over the two-drug combination, which was the primary endpoint. The median PFS durations were 17.4 weeks and 17.9 weeks in the sorafenib-containing combination regimen and placebo combination groups, respectively. The median OS durations, the secondary objective, were also equivalent in both groups. The second Phase III study had the same randomized design between the two groups, but only chemonaïve patients were enrolled (188). Between the two groups, there were no statistical differences in response rates (16 versus 18%), the median progression-free survival durations (4.4 months versus 4.9 months), and the

median overall survival durations (11.4 months versus 10.7 months). It appears that the addition of sorafenib to the combination of carboplatin and paclitaxel does not have any efficacy advantage over the cytotoxic combination only.

Sorafenib has also been combined with dacarbazine or temozolomide in separate Phase II studies, which showed encouraging results of the clinical efficacies of the combination approach. In a double-blind, placebo-controlled, randomized Phase II study, the combination of dacarbazine and sorafenib had superior response rate and PFS rate at day 180 over dacarbazine alone among 101 chemonaïve patients (189). In another Phase II study, nearly the two-thirds of the 47 patients who had not previously received temozolomide and who had not had brain metastases had either a clinical response or disease stabilization with the combination of sorafenib and temozolomide (190). However, these combination regimens have not been accepted as standard therapy because randomized Phase III studies of these combinations have not been conducted.

One of the possible reasons that sorafenib does not improve OS in patients with metastatic melanoma when it is combined with carboplatin and paclitaxel is its property to inhibit multiple kinase proteins and the fact that a higher dose to sufficiently inhibit the MAPK pathway cannot be achieved due to adverse events resulting from its effect on other nonspecific kinases.

RO5185426 (formerly known as PLX4032) is a small molecule that selectively inhibits *BRAF* kinase, and in vitro biochemical and cell-based assays have demonstrated a high degree of selectivity to the V600E oncogenic B-Raf kinase protein, with an IC_{50} at a nanomolar range (191). In a Phase I study of RO5185426, of 27 evaluable patients with advanced melanoma who were treated at doses at the maximum-tolerated dose of 960 mg twice daily, 19 (70%) had a clinical response (192). It is striking to note that none of those whose tumors did not harbor a *BRAF* mutation had a clinical response. On the basis of the very promising result of the first-in-human Phase I study, a large Phase II study is underway to evaluate the clinical efficacy of RO5185426 in previously treated patients with metastatic melanoma harboring V600E *BRAF* mutation. In addition, a randomized multinational Phase III trial to compare the clinical efficacy of RO5185426 with that of dacarbazine is currently underway. Other inhibitors of mutated *BRAF* kinase protein, including RAF265, XL281, and GSK2118436, are being evaluated in Phase I or II studies.

c-KIT Inhibition

Imatinib is a small molecule that inhibits a number of protein tyrosine kinases, including the Bcr-Abl fusion protein, C-ABL, abl-related gene (ARG), PDGFR-α, PDGFR-β, and the c-KIT tyrosine kinase receptor (193-195). Although c-KIT is frequently expressed in melanoma cells (196), imatinib had a minimal clinical efficacy among 62 patients in three Phase II trials combined (197-199).

However, enthusiasm for imatinib and other c-KIT inhibitors, such as dasatinib or nilotinib, resurfaced when Curtin et al. reported oncogenic mutation and/or copy number increases of c-KIT in 39%, 36%, and 28% of mucosal, acral lentiginous melanoma, and melanomas on chronically sun-damaged skin, respectively, while c-KIT mutation is rare in melanomas on skin without chronic sun damage, which are the most common form of melanoma (59). A number of case reports have since described the dramatic clinical response observed with imatinib treatment in patients with c-KIT mutations (200,201). Currently, several Phase II clinical trials are testing the clinical efficacy of c-KIT–inhibiting small molecules (eg, imatinib, dasatinib, and nilotinib) in patients with c-KIT mutation or gene amplification. In a Phase II study of imatinib in patients with c-KIT mutation, preliminary analyses showed that three of seven treated patients had a clinical response (202). The c-KIT mutations as a relevant target for therapy in these

subsets of patients will be better addressed when the current clinical trials are completed.

Metastatic Uveal Melanoma

In general, current treatment for metastatic uveal melanoma remains disappointing. Largely due to a relatively low incidence of this disease, only a handful of clinical trials have assessed the effect of systemic therapy on metastatic uveal melanoma. Furthermore, most of these reports lack the large number of patients needed to give meaningful information. Therefore a clear-cut conclusion about the efficacy of treatment regimens is difficult to draw from these pilot studies. Overall, metastatic uveal melanoma is considered to be chemoresistant, and the outcome of therapy is dependent on the extent of spread of disease.

Disease Confined to the Liver

In selected cases of solitary metastasis, surgical excision and radiofrequency thermal ablation have been reported to yield long-lasting control of local disease. In view of the fact that in most patients with metastatic uveal melanoma the disease is multifocal even if the metastatic disease is confined to one organ, only a small subset of patients are candidates for management with such modalities of therapy.

Hepatic Arterial Infusion

The purpose of hepatic arterial infusion is to expose the liver to high doses of chemotherapy in order to achieve maximal tumor shrinkage. Fotemustine (208), carboplatin (209), and cisplatin (76,210) have been used in small clinical trials with limited success. Likewise, hepatic arterial infusion of cytokines, such as interferon-alpha or interleukin-2, failed to induce tumor regression in patients with uveal melanoma metastatic to the liver (211,212).

Transhepatic Arterial Chemoembolization

Embolization is the process of injecting a foreign substance such as starch particles or Ivalon into the tumor to transiently stop the blood flow, thus depriving the tumor of needed oxygen and nutrients and eventually causing the cancer cells to die (213). Chemoembolization include administration of anticancer drugs, such as cisplatin or BCNU together with an embolizing agent. Chemoembolization of hepatic metastasis from uveal melanoma was first reported by our group in an earlier publication (213). Cisplatin was used as the chemotherapy drug of choice. About half of the treated patients responded to chemoembolization as the first-line therapy for metastatic uveal melanoma confined to the liver. The median survival of the patients was 12 months. Response to chemoembolization was associated with statistically significant longer survival (median 14.5 months) compared with the nonresponders (5 months) (213). About a third of the patients responded if they were previously treated with systemic therapy. The addition of other cytotoxic drugs such as IA vinblastine or IV dacarbazine did not significantly affect the outcome of therapy (76). The adverse side effects of the procedure included nausea, vomiting, abdominal discomfort, fever, and paralytic ileus. There was transient elevation of the liver enzymes. Other investigators have had mixed success with chemoembolization using cisplatin (214,215) or BCNU (216). To improve the outcome of their patients with metastatic uveal melanoma, Sato et al. added immunotherapy with granulocyte-macrophage colony-stimulating factor (GM-CSF, Leukine, Immunex Corp., Seattle, WA) to embolization of liver metastasis (217). Of the 34 patients treated, 30% had a partial response. The median survival was 14.5 months. Responses at sites outside the liver were seen in a few of the patients with extrahepatic metastasis.

Isolated Hepatic Perfusion

The basis of this treatment is to expose the liver containing metastatic melanoma to high doses of chemotherapy in order to achieve maximal tumor shrinkage. It requires complete isolation of the liver from the systemic circulation so that the body is not exposed to the high dose of drugs administered directly to the liver. There have been a number of clinical trials utilizing this technique with melphalan infusion with or without tumor necrosis factor (TNF), and the results among patients with unresectable hepatic metastases from uveal primary melanoma were encouraging in these early studies (218,219).

Multiorgan Metastasis

Systemic therapy of metastatic uveal melanoma was recently reviewed (220). Anticancer drugs such as dacarbazine alone or together with combination chemotherapy have been shown to be ineffective. The CVD and Dartmouth regimens have resulted in responses in less than 10% of the patients. The most commonly used multidrug regimen, BOLD-IFN (bleomycin + oncovin + [lomustine CCNU] + dacarbazine + IFN), is of marginal efficacy, with an average response rate of about 11% (221-223). Biotherapy has had limited evaluation for efficacy against metastatic uveal melanoma, and the available medical literature suggests it has only marginal efficacy.

Immunotherapy alone or with combination chemotherapy have been shown to be ineffective. Interleukin-2-based biochemotherapy has been found to have marginal efficacy against metastatic uveal melanoma. Dorval et al. conducted a Phase II trial with IL-2 in 27 patients with metastatic melanoma (224). He administered IL-2 at 18 to 20 million units/m^2/day as a 5-day continuous IV infusion over 2 weeks as induction therapy, and after 4 weeks dacarbazine at 800 mg/m^2 was given with IL-2 every 3 weeks as maintenance. He observed six objective tumor responses, including two complete responses. All the responses occurred among the 20 patients with skin melanoma. All seven patients with uveal melanoma had disease progression during IL-2 therapy. Proebstle et al. treated 22 poor-risk patients with metastatic melanoma, including eight patients with uveal primary (225). The treatment included dacarbazine, cisplatin, IFNα, and high-dose IL-2. Five patients had partial response, including a patient with metastatic uveal melanoma. We reviewed the result of therapy of previously untreated patients with metastatic uveal melanoma. Fourteen patients were treated with CVD (cisplatin, vinblastine, dacarbazine), CVD-IFN, and CVD-IFN-IL-2 protocols. One patient had partial response. Four patients had stable disease. The median time to progression and the survival were 3.2 and 8.5 months, respectively.

In view of the chemoresistance of uveal melanoma cells to cytotoxic drugs, ATP-based tumor cell ex vivo chemosensitivity assays were used to examine the sensitivity of uveal melanoma cells separated from enucleated eyes of uveal melanoma patients to anticancer agents alone and in combination (226,227). Significant activity was observed with gemcitabin, treosulfan, cytosine arabinoside, paclitaxel, and mitoxantrone. The combinations of treosulfan with gemcitabine and with cytosine arabinoside were active in over 70% of the tumor specimens tested. On the basis of these results, clinical trials using the treosulfan-gemcitabine combination were initiated to evaluate clinical activity in patients with metastatic uveal melanoma (228-232). Unfortunately, the initial results of these studies indicate only marginal efficacy against uveal melanoma.

During the past few years, molecular marker studies have identified genetic and molecular pathways that may play a role in the development of liver metastases in patients with uveal melanoma and the pathways that melanoma cells use for proliferation, metastasis, and survival (233-235). Therapies targeting these pathways and mutations are being developed that carry the potential for better outcomes for patients with metastatic uveal melanoma.

References

1. Jemal A, Siegel R, Ward E, et al. Cancer statistics, 2009. *CA Cancer J Clin* Jul-Aug 2009;59(4):225-249.

2. Horner MJ, Ries LAG, Krapcho M et al. SEER Cancer Statistics Review, 1975-2006, National Cancer Institute, http://seer.cancer.gov/csr/1975_2006/, based on November 2008 SEER data submission, posted to the SEER web site, 2009.

3. Brochez L, Naeyaert JM. Understanding the trends in melanoma incidence and mortality: Where do we stand? *Eur J Dermatol* Jan-Feb 2000;10(1):71-75; quiz 76.

4. Dennis LK, White E, Lee JA. Recent cohort trends in malignant melanoma by anatomic site in the United States. *Cancer Causes Control* Mar 1993;4(2):93-100.

5. Elwood JM, Jopson J. Melanoma and sun exposure: An overview of published studies. *Int J Cancer* Oct 9 1997;73(2):198-203.

6. Longstreth J. Cutaneous malignant melanoma and ultraviolet radiation: A review. *Cancer Metastasis Rev* Dec 1988;7(4):321-333.

7. Swerdlow AJ. Incidence of malignant melanoma of the skin in England and Wales and its relationship to sunshine. *Br Med J* Nov 24 1979;2(6201):1324-1327.

8. Magnus K. Incidence of malignant melanoma of the skin in Norway, 1955-1970. Variations in time and space and solar radiation. *Cancer* Nov 1973;32(5):1275-1286.

9. Eklund G, Malec E. Sunlight and incidence of cutaneous malignant melanoma. Effect of latitude and domicile in Sweden. *Scand J Plast Reconstr Surg* 1978;12(3):231-241.

10. Elwood JM, Lee JA, Walter SD, et al. Relationship of melanoma and other skin cancer mortality to latitude and ultraviolet radiation in the United States and Canada. *Int J Epidemiol* Dec 1974;3(4):325-332.

11. Richard MA, Grob JJ, Gouvernet J, et al. Role of sun exposure on nevus. First study in age-sex phenotype-controlled populations. *Arch Dermatol* Oct 1993;129(10):1280-1285.

12. Garbe C, Buttner P, Weiss J, et al. Associated factors in the prevalence of more than 50 common melanocytic nevi, atypical melanocytic nevi, and actinic lentigines: Multicenter case-control study of the Central Malignant Melanoma Registry of the German Dermatological Society. *J Invest Dermatol* May 1994;102(5):700-705.

13. Slade J, Marghoob AA, Salopek TG et al. Atypical mole syndrome: Risk factor for cutaneous malignant melanoma and implications for management. *J Am Acad Dermatol* Mar 1995;32(3):479-494.

14. Tsao H, Sober AJ. Ultraviolet radiation and malignant melanoma. *Clin Dermatol* Jan-Feb 1998;16(1):67-73.

15. MacKie RM, Aitchison T. Severe sunburn and subsequent risk of primary cutaneous malignant melanoma in scotland. *Br J Cancer* Dec 1982;46(6):955-960.

16. Weinstock MA. Assessment of sun sensitivity by questionnaire: Validity of items and formulation of a prediction rule. *J Clin Epidemiol* May 1992;45(5):547-552.

17. Beral V, Evans S, Shaw H, et al. Cutaneous factors related to the risk of malignant melanoma. *Br J Dermatol* Aug 1983;109(2):165-172.

18. Bliss JM, Ford D, Swerdlow AJ, et al. Risk of cutaneous melanoma associated with pigmentation characteristics and freckling: Systematic overview of 10 case-control studies. The International Melanoma Analysis Group (IMAGE). *Int J Cancer* Aug 9 1995;62(4):367-376.

19. Swerdlow AJ, English JS, Qiao Z. The risk of melanoma in patients with congenital nevi: A cohort study. *J Am Acad Dermatol* Apr 1995;32(4):595-599.

20. Weiss J, Bertz J, Jung EG. Malignant melanoma in southern Germany: Different predictive value of risk factors for melanoma subtypes. *Dermatologica* 1991;183(2):109-113.

21. Greene MH, Clark WH, Jr., Tucker MA, et al. High risk of malignant melanoma in melanoma-prone families with dysplastic nevi. *Ann Intern Med* Apr 1985;102(4):458-465.

22. Tucker MA, Halpern A, Holly EA, et al. Clinically recognized dysplastic nevi. A central risk factor for cutaneous melanoma. *JAMA* May 14 1997;277(18):1439-1444.

23. Rhodes AR. Melanocytic precursors of cutaneous melanoma. Estimated risks and guidelines for management. *Med Clin North Am* Jan 1986;70(1):3-37.

24. Sahin S, Levin L, Kopf AW, et al. Risk of melanoma in medium-sized congenital melanocytic nevi: A follow-up study. *J Am Acad Dermatol* Sep 1998;39(3):428-433.

25. Ruiz-Maldonado R, Tamayo L, Laterza AM, et al. Giant pigmented nevi: Clinical, histopathologic, and therapeutic considerations. *J Pediatr* Jun 1992;120(6):906-911.

26. Quaba AA, Wallace AF. The incidence of malignant melanoma (0 to 15 years of age) arising in "large" congenital nevocellular nevi. *Plast Reconstr Surg* Aug 1986;78(2):174-181.

27. Marghoob AA, Schoenbach SP, Kopf AW, et al. Large congenital melanocytic nevi and the risk for the development of malignant melanoma. A prospective study. *Arch Dermatol* Feb 1996;132(2):170-175.

28. Goggins WB, Tsao H. A population-based analysis of risk factors for a second primary cutaneous melanoma among melanoma survivors. *Cancer* Feb 1 2003;97(3):639-643.

29. Giles G, Staples M, McCredie M, et al. Multiple primary melanomas: An analysis of cancer registry data from Victoria and New South Wales. *Melanoma Res* Dec 1995;5(6):433-438.

30. Langley RG, Sober AJ. Clinical recognition of melanoma and its precursors. *Hematol Oncol Clin North Am* Aug 1998;12(4):699-715, v.

31. Weinstock MA, Sober AJ. The risk of progression of lentigo maligna to lentigo maligna melanoma. *Br J Dermatol* Mar 1987;116(3):303-310.

32. Reintgen DS, McCarty KM Jr., Cox E, et al. Malignant melanoma in black American and white American populations. A comparative review. *JAMA* Oct 15 1982;248(15):1856-1859.

33. Jain S, Allen PW. Desmoplastic malignant melanoma and its variants. A study of 45 cases. *Am J Surg Pathol* May 1989;13(5):358-373.

34. Cooper PH, Mills SE, Allen MS Jr. Malignant melanoma of the anus: Report of 12 patients and analysis of 255 additional cases. *Dis Colon Rectum* Oct 1982;25(7):693-703.

35. Harbour JW. Molecular Prognostic Testing and Individualized Patient Care in Uveal Melanoma. *Am J Ophthalmol* 2009;148(6):823-829.e821.

36. Shields CL, Shields JA. Ocular melanoma: Relatively rare but requiring respect. *Clin Dermatol* 2009;27(1):122-133.

37. Meyle KD, Guldberg P. Genetic risk factors for melanoma. *Hum Genet* Oct 2009;126(4):499-510.

38. Hocker T, Tsao H. Ultraviolet radiation and melanoma: A systematic review and analysis of reported sequence variants. *Hum Mutat* Jun 2007;28(6):578-588.

39. Mocellin S, Verdi D, Nitti D. DNA repair gene polymorphisms and risk of cutaneous melanoma: A systematic review and meta-analysis. *Carcinogenesis* Oct 1 2009;30(10):1735-1743.

40. Miller AJ, Mihm MC Jr. Melanoma. *N Engl J Med* Jul 6 2006;355(1):51-65.

41. Davies H, Bignell GR, Cox C, et al. Mutations of the BRAF gene in human cancer. *Nature* Jun 27 2002;417(6892):949-954.

42. Dhomen N, Marais R. New insight into BRAF mutations in cancer. *Curr Opin Genet Devel* 2007;17(1):31-39.

43. Smalley KS, Xiao M, Villanueva J, et al. CRAF inhibition induces apoptosis in melanoma cells with non-V600E BRAF mutations. *Oncogene* Jan 8 2009;28(1):85-94.

44. Dankort D, Curley DP, Cartlidge RA, et al. Braf(V600E) cooperates with Pten loss to induce metastatic melanoma. *Nat Genet* May 2009;41(5):544-552.

45. Michaloglou C, Vredeveld LC, Soengas MS, et al. BRAFE600-associated senescence-like cell cycle arrest of human naevi. *Nature* Aug 4 2005;436(7051):720-724.

46. Patton EE, Widlund HR, Kutok JL, et al. BRAF mutations are sufficient to promote nevi formation and cooperate with p53 in the genesis of melanoma. *Curr Biol* Feb 8 2005;15(3):249-254.

47. Pollock PM, Harper UL, Hansen KS, et al. High frequency of BRAF mutations in nevi. *Nat Genet* Jan 2003;33(1):19-20.

48. Yazdi AS, Palmedo G, Flaig MJ, et al. Mutations of the BRAF gene in benign and malignant melanocytic lesions. *J Invest Dermatol* Nov 2003;121(5):1160-1162.

49. Bauer J, Curtin JA, Pinkel D, et al. Congenital melanocytic nevi frequently harbor NRAS mutations but no BRAF mutations. *J Invest Dermatol* Jan 2007;127(1):179-182.

50. Giehl K. Oncogenic Ras in tumor progression and metastasis. *Biol Chem* 2005;386(3):193-205.

51. Hennessy BT, Smith DL, Ram PT, et al. Exploiting the PI3K/AKT pathway for cancer drug discovery. *Nat Rev Drug Discov* Dec 2005;4(12):988-1004.

52. Wu H, Goel V, Haluska FG. PTEN signaling pathways in melanoma. *Oncogene* May 19 2003;22(20):3113-3122.

53. Davies MA, Stemke-Hale K, Tellez C, et al. A novel AKT3 mutation in melanoma tumours and cell lines. *Br J Cancer* Oct 21 2008;99(8):1265-1268.

54. Omholt K, Krockel D, Ringborg U et al. Mutations of PIK3CA are rare in cutaneous melanoma. *Melanoma Res* Apr 2006;16(2):197-200.

55. Goel VK, Lazar AJ, Warneke CL et al. Examination of mutations in BRAF, NRAS, and PTEN in primary cutaneous melanoma. *J Invest Dermatol* Jan 2006;126(1):154-160.

56. Tsao H, Goel V, Wu H et al. Genetic interaction between NRAS and BRAF mutations and PTEN//MMAC1 inactivation in melanoma. *J Investig Dermatol* 2004;122(2):337-341.

57. Davies MA, Stemke-Hale K, Lin E, et al. Integrated molecular and clinical analysis of AKT activation in metastatic melanoma. *Clin Cancer Res* Dec 15 2009;15(24):7538-7546.

58. Curtin JA, Fridlyand J, Kageshita T, et al. Distinct sets of genetic alterations in melanoma. *N Engl J Med* Nov 17 2005;353(20):2135-2147.

59. Curtin JA, Busam K, Pinkel D et al. Somatic activation of KIT in distinct subtypes of melanoma. *J Clin Oncol* Sep 10 2006;24(26):4340-4346.

60. Hirota S, Isozaki K, Moriyama Y, et al. Gain-of-function mutations of c-kit in human gastrointestinal stromal tumors. *Science* Jan 23 1998;279(5350):577-580.

61. Beadling C, Jacobson-Dunlop E, Hodi FS, et al. KIT gene mutations and copy number in melanoma subtypes. *Clin Cancer Res* Nov 1 2008;14(21):6821-6828.

62. Jiang X, Zhou J, Yuen NK, et al. Imatinib targeting of KIT-mutant oncoprotein in melanoma. *Clin Cancer Res* Dec 1 2008;14(23):7726-7732.

63. Garraway LA, Widlund HR, Rubin MA, et al. Integrative genomic analyses identify MITF as a lineage survival oncogene amplified in malignant melanoma. *Nature* 2005;436(7047):117-122.

64. Cronin JC, Wunderlich J, Loftus SK, et al. Frequent mutations in the MITF pathway in melanoma. *Pigment Cell Melanoma Res* 2009;22(4):435-444.

65. Sauter ER, Yeo U-C, von Stemm A, et al. Cyclin D1 is a candidate oncogene in cutaneous melanoma. *Cancer Res* June 1 2002;62(11):3200-3206.

66. Smalley KSM, Lioni M, Palma MD, et al. Increased cyclin D1 expression can mediate BRAF inhibitor resistance in BRAFV600E-mutated melanomas. *Mol Cancer Ther*; 7(9):2876-2883.

67. Landreville S, Agapova OA, Harbour JW. Emerging insights into the molecular pathogenesis of uveal melanoma. *Future Oncol* Oct 2008;4(5):629-636.

68. Van Raamsdonk CD, Bezrookove V, Green G, et al. Frequent somatic mutations of GNAQ in uveal melanoma and blue naevi. *Nature* 2009;457(7229):599-602.

69. Patel JK, Didolkar MS, Pickren JW, et al. Metastatic pattern of malignant melanoma. A study of 216 autopsy cases. *Am J Surg* Jun 1978;135(6):807-810.

70. Lee YT. Malignant melanoma: Pattern of metastasis. *CA Cancer J Clin* May-Jun 1980;30(3):137-142.

71. Hwu WJ, Balch CM, Houghton AN. Diagnosis of stage IV disease. In: Balch CM, Houghton AN, Sober AJ et al. (eds): *Cutaneous Melanoma*, 4th ed. St. Louis, MO: Quality Medical Publishing, Inc.; 2003:525.

72. Balch CM, Soong SJ, Murad TM, et al. A multifactorial analysis of melanoma. IV. Prognostic factors in 200 melanoma patients with distant metastases (stage III). *J Clin Oncol* Feb 1983;1(2):126-134.

73. McCarthy WH, Shaw HM, Thompson JF, et al. Time and frequency of recurrence of cutaneous stage I malignant melanoma with guidelines for follow-up study. *Surg Gynecol Obstet* Jun 1988;166(6):497-502.

74. Nambisan RN, Alexiou G, Reese PA, Karakousis CP. Early metastatic patterns and survival in malignant melanoma. *J Surg Oncol* Apr 1987;34(4):248-252.

75. Hungerford J. Uveal melanoma. *Eur J Cancer* 1993;29A(10):1365-1368.

76. Bedikian AY, Legha SS, Mavligit G, et al. Treatment of uveal melanoma metastatic to the liver: A review of the M. D. Anderson Cancer Center experience and prognostic factors. *Cancer* Nov 1 1995;76(9):1665-1670.

77. Balch CM, Gershenwald JE, Soong SJ, et al. Final version of 2009 AJCC melanoma staging and classification. *J Clin Oncol* Dec 20 2009;27(36):6199-6206.

78. Balch CM, Buzaid AC, Soong SJ, et al. Final version of the American Joint Committee on Cancer staging system for cutaneous melanoma. *J Clin Oncol* Aug 15 2001;19(16): 3635-3648.

79. Ross MI, Balch CM. Surgical treatment of primary melanoma. In: Balch CM, Houghton AN, Sober AJ, Soong SJ (eds). *Cutaneous Melanoma,* 3rd ed. St. Louis, MO: Quality Medical Publishing; 1998:141-153.

80. Zitelli JA, Brown C, Hanusa BH. Mohs micrographic surgery for the treatment of primary cutaneous melanoma. *J Am Acad Dermatol* Aug 1997;37(2 Pt 1):236-245.

81. Zitelli JA, Brown CD, Hanusa BH. Surgical margins for excision of primary cutaneous melanoma. *J Am Acad Dermatol* Sep 1997;37(3 Pt 1):422-429.

82. Coit DG, Rogatko A, Brennan MF. Prognostic factors in patients with melanoma metastatic to axillary or inguinal lymph nodes. A multivariate analysis. *Ann Surg* Nov 1991; 214(5):627-636.

83. Morton DL, Wanek L, Nizze JA, et al. Improved long-term survival after lymphadenectomy of melanoma metastatic to regional nodes. Analysis of prognostic factors in 1134 patients from the John Wayne Cancer Clinic. *Ann Surg* Oct 1991; 214(4):491-499; discussion 499-501.

84. Buzaid AC, Tinoco LA, Jendiroba D, et al. Prognostic value of size of lymph node metastases in patients with cutaneous melanoma. *J Clin Oncol* Sep 1995;13(9):2361-2368.

85. Drepper H, Kohler CO, Bastian B, et al. Benefit of elective lymph node dissection in subgroups of melanoma patients. Results of a multicenter study of 3616 patients. *Cancer* Aug 1 1993;72(3):741-749.

86. Coates AS, Ingvar CI, Petersen-Schaefer K, et al. Elective lymph node dissection in patients with primary melanoma of the trunk and limbs treated at the Sydney Melanoma unit from 1960 to 1991. *J Am Coll Surg* Apr 1995;180(4): 402-409.

87. Slingluff CL Jr., Stidham KR, Ricci WM, et al. Surgical management of regional lymph nodes in patients with melanoma. Experience with 4682 patients. *Ann Surg* Feb 1994;219(2):120-130.

88. Veronesi U, Adamus J, Bandiera DC, et al. Delayed regional lymph node dissection in stage I melanoma of the skin of the lower extremities. *Cancer* Jun 1 1982;49(11):2420-2430.

89. Morton DL, Wen DR, Wong JH, et al. Technical details of intraoperative lymphatic mapping for early stage melanoma. *Arch Surg* Apr 1992;127(4):392-399.

90. Krag DN, Weaver DL, Alex JC, et al. Surgical resection and radiolocalization of the sentinel lymph node in breast cancer using a gamma probe. *Surg Oncol* Dec 1993;2(6):335-339; discussion 340.

91. Albertini JJ, Cruse CW, Rapaport D, et al. Intraoperative radio-lympho-scintigraphy improves sentinel lymph node identification for patients with melanoma. *Ann Surg* Feb 1996;223(2):217-224.

92. McMasters KM, Ross MI, Reintgen DS, et al. Final results of the Sunbelt Melanoma Trial. *J Clin Oncol* 2008;26 (May 20 suppl): (Abstract 9003).

93. Bedikian AY, Legha SS. Adjuvant chemotherapy for malignant melanoma. In: Kirkwood JM (ed): *Molecular Diagnosis and Treatment of Melanoma.* New York: Marcel Dekker; 1998:195-216.

94. Hill GJ, 2nd, Moss SE, Golomb FM, et al. DTIC and combination therapy for melanoma: III. DTIC (NSC 45388) Surgical Adjuvant Study COG PROTOCOL 7040. *Cancer* Jun 1 1981;47(11):2556-2562.

95. Tranum BL, Dixon D, Quagliana J, et al. Lack of benefit of adjunctive chemotherapy in stage I malignant melanoma: A Southwest Oncology Group Study. *Cancer Treat Rep* Jun 1987;71(6):643-644.

96. Morton D, Eilber FR, Malmgren RA et al. Immunological factors which influence response to immunotherapy in malignant melanoma. *Surgery* Jul 1970;68(1):158-163; discussion 163-154.

97. Cunningham TJ, Schoenfeld D, Nathanson L. A controlled ECOG study of adjuvant therapy with BCG or BCG plus DTIC in patients with stage I and II malignant melanoma. In: Terry WD, Rosenberg SA (eds): *Immunotherapy of Human Cancer.* New York: Excerpta Medica; 1982:271-277.

98. Terry WD, Hodges RJ, Rosenberg SA. Treatment of stage I and II malignant melanoma with adjuvant immunotherapy or chemotherapy: Preliminary analysis of a prospective randomized trial. In: Terry WD, Rosenberg SA (eds): *Immmunotherapy of Human Cancer.* New York: Excerpta Media; 1982:251-257.

99. Cunningham TJ, Schoenfeld DL, Nathanson L. A controlled ECOG study of adjuvant therapy in patients with stage I & II malaignant melanoma. In: Jones SE, Salmon SE (eds): *Adjuvant Therapy of Cancer IV.* New York: Grune & Stratton; 1984:507-577.

100. Veronesi U, Adamus J, Aubert C, et al. A randomized trial of adjuvant chemotherapy and immunotherapy in cutaneous melanoma. *N Engl J Med* Oct 7 1982;307(15):913-916.

101. Czarnetzki BM, Macher E, Behrendt H, et al. Current status of melanoma chemotherapy and immunotherapy. *Recent Results Cancer Res* 1982;80:264-268.

102. Spitler LE. A randomized trial of levamisole versus placebo as adjuvant therapy in malignant melanoma. *J Clin Oncol* May 1991;9(5):736-740.

103. Quirt IC, Shelley WE, Pater JL, et al. Improved survival in patients with poor-prognosis malignant melanoma treated with adjuvant levamisole: A phase III study by the National Cancer Institute of Canada Clinical Trials Group. *J Clin Oncol* May 1991;9(5):729-735.

104. Wallack MK, Sivanandham M, Balch CM, et al. A phase III randomized, double-blind multiinstitutional trial of vaccinia melanoma oncolysate-active specific immunotherapy for patients with stage II melanoma. *Cancer* Jan 1 1995;75(1): 34-42.

105. Hersey P, Coates AS, McCarthy WH, et al. Adjuvant immunotherapy of patients with high-risk melanoma using vaccinia viral lysates of melanoma: Results of a randomized trial. *J Clin Oncol* Oct 15 2002;20(20):4181-4190.

106. Sondak VK, Liu PY, Tuthill RJ, et al. Adjuvant immunotherapy of resected, intermediate-thickness, node-negative melanoma with an allogeneic tumor vaccine: Overall results of a randomized trial of the Southwest Oncology Group. *J Clin Oncol* Apr 15 2002;20(8):2058-2066.

107. Livingston PO, Natoli EJ, Calves MJ, et al. Vaccines containing purified GM2 ganglioside elicit GM2 antibodies in melanoma patients. *Proc Natl Acad Sci USA* May 1987; 84(9):2911-2915.

108. Livingston PO, Wong GY, Adluri S, et al. Improved survival in stage III melanoma patients with GM2 antibodies: A randomized trial of adjuvant vaccination with GM2 ganglioside. *J Clin Oncol* May 1994;12(5):1036-1044.

109. Eggermont AM, Suciu S, Ruka W, et al. EORTC 18961: Post-operative adjuvant ganglioside GM2-KLH21 vaccination treatment vs observation in stage II (T3-T4N0M0) melanoma: 2nd interim analysis led to an early disclosure of the results. *J Clin Oncol* 26((May 20 suppl)): (Abstract 9004).

110. Eggermont AM. Immunotherapy: Vaccine trials in melanoma—time for reflection. *Nat Rev Clin Oncol* May 2009;6(5):256-258.

111. Kirkwood JM, Strawderman MH, Ernstoff MS et al. Interferon alfa-2b adjuvant therapy of high-risk resected cutaneous melanoma: The Eastern Cooperative Oncology Group Trial EST 1684. *J Clin Oncol* Jan 1996;14(1):7-17.

112. Kirkwood JM, Manola J, Ibrahim J, et al. A pooled analysis of eastern cooperative oncology group and intergroup trials of adjuvant high-dose interferon for melanoma. *Clin Cancer Res* Mar 1 2004;10(5):1670-1677.

113. Kirkwood JM, Ibrahim JG, Sondak VK, et al. High- and low-dose interferon alfa-2b in high-risk melanoma: First analysis of intergroup trial E1690/S9111/C9190. *J Clin Oncol* Jun 2000;18(12):2444-2458.

114. Kirkwood JM, Ibrahim JG, Sosman JA, et al. High-dose interferon alfa-2b significantly prolongs relapse-free and overall survival compared with the GM2-KLH/QS-21 vaccine in patients with resected stage IIB-III melanoma: Results of intergroup trial E1694/S9512/C509801. *J Clin Oncol* May 1 2001;19(9):2370-2380.

115. Wheatley K, Ives N, Hancock B, et al. Does adjuvant interferon-alpha for high-risk melanoma provide a worthwhile benefit? A meta-analysis of the randomised trials. *Cancer Treat Rev* Aug 2003;29(4):241-252.

116. Gogas H, Ioannovich J, Dafni U, et al. Prognostic significance of autoimmunity during treatment of melanoma with interferon. *N Engl J Med* Feb 16 2006;354(7):709-718.

117. Eggermont AM, Suciu S, Santinami M, et al. Adjuvant therapy with pegylated interferon alfa-2b versus observation alone in resected stage III melanoma: Final results of EORTC 18991, a randomised phase III trial. *Lancet* Jul 12 2008; 372(9633):117-126.

118. Kim KB, Legha SS, Gonzalez R, et al. A randomized phase III trial of biochemotherapy versus interferon-alpha-2b for adjuvant therapy in patients at high risk for melanoma recurrence. *Melanoma Res* Feb 2009;19(1):42-49.

119. Pectasides D, Dafni U, Bafaloukos D, et al. Randomized phase III study of 1 month versus 1 year of adjuvant high-dose interferon alfa-2b in patients with resected high-risk melanoma. *J Clin Oncol* Feb 20 2009;27(6):939-944.

120. Cascinelli N, Belli F, MacKie RM, et al. Effect of long-term adjuvant therapy with interferon alpha-2a in patients with regional node metastases from cutaneous melanoma: A randomised trial. *Lancet* Sep 15 2001;358(9285):866-869.

121. Meyskens FL Jr., Kopecky KJ, Taylor CW, et al. Randomized trial of adjuvant human interferon gamma versus observation in high-risk cutaneous melanoma: A Southwest Oncology Group study. *J Natl Cancer Inst* Nov 15 1995;87(22): 1710-1713.

122. Creagan ET, Dalton RJ, Ahmann DL, et al. Randomized, surgical adjuvant clinical trial of recombinant interferon alfa-2a in selected patients with malignant melanoma. *J Clin Oncol* Nov 1995;13(11):2776-2783.

123. Grob JJ, Dreno B, de la Salmoniere P, et al. Randomised trial of interferon alpha-2a as adjuvant therapy in resected primary melanoma thicker than 1.5 mm without clinically detectable node metastases. French Cooperative Group on Melanoma. *Lancet* Jun 27 1998;351(9120):1905-1910.

124. Pehamberger H, Soyer HP, Steiner A, et al. Adjuvant interferon alfa-2a treatment in resected primary stage II cutaneous melanoma. Austrian Malignant Melanoma Cooperative Group. *J Clin Oncol* Apr 1998;16(4):1425-1429.

125. Eggermont AM, Suciu S, MacKie R, et al. Post-surgery adjuvant therapy with intermediate doses of interferon alfa 2b versus observation in patients with stage IIb/III melanoma (EORTC 18952): Randomised controlled trial. *Lancet* Oct 1 2005;366(9492):1189-1196.

126. Kleeberg UR, Suciu S, Brocker EB, et al. Final results of the EORTC 18871/DKG 80-1 randomised phase III trial. rIFN-alpha2b versus rIFN-gamma versus ISCADOR M versus observation after surgery in melanoma patients with either high-risk primary (thickness >3 mm) or regional lymph node metastasis. *Eur J Cancer* Feb 2004;40(3):390-402.

127. Hancock BW, Wheatley K, Harris S, et al. Adjuvant interferon in high-risk melanoma: The AIM HIGH Study–United Kingdom Coordinating Committee on Cancer Research randomized study of adjuvant low-dose extended-duration interferon Alfa-2a in high-risk resected malignant melanoma. *J Clin Oncol* Jan 1 2004;22(1):53-61.

128. Carbone PP, Costello W. Eastern Cooperative Oncology Group studies with DTIC (NSC-45388). *Cancer Treat Rep.* Feb 1976;60(2):193-198.

129. Buzaid AC, Legha SS, Winn R. Cisplatin, vinblastine, and dacarbazine versus dacarbazine alone in metastatic melanoma: Preliminary results of a phase III Cancer Community Oncology Program (CCOP) trial. Paper presented at: American Society of Clinical Oncology1993; Orlando, FL.

130. Chapman PB, Einhorn LH, Meyers ML, et al. Phase III multicenter randomized trial of the Dartmouth regimen versus dacarbazine in patients with metastatic melanoma. *J Clin Oncol* Sep 1999;17(9):2745-2751.

131. Costanza ME, Nathanson L, Schoenfeld D, et al. Results with methyl-CCNU and DTIC in metastatic melanoma. *Cancer* Sep 1977;40(3):1010-1015.

132. Hill GJ, 2nd, Krementz ET, Hill HZ. Dimethyl triazeno imidazole carboxamide and combination therapy for melanoma. IV. Late results after complete response to chemotherapy (Central Oncology Group protocols 7130, 7131, and 7131A). *Cancer* Mar 15 1984;53(6):1299-1305.

133. McClay E, Lusch CJ, Mastrangelo MJ. Allergy-induced hepatic toxicity associated with dacarbazine. *Cancer Treat Rep* Feb 1987;71(2):219-220.

134. Bedikian AY, Millward M, Pehamberger H, et al. Bcl-2 antisense (oblimersen sodium) plus dacarbazine in patients with advanced melanoma: The Oblimersen Melanoma Study Group. *J Clin Oncol* Oct 10 2006;24(29):4738-4745.

135. Middleton MR, Grob JJ, Aaronson N, et al. Randomized phase III study of temozolomide versus dacarbazine in the treatment of patients with advanced metastatic malignant melanoma. *J Clin Oncol* Jan 2000;18(1):158-166.

136. Patel PM, Suciu S, Mortier L, et al. Extended schedule, escalated dose temozolomide versus dacarbazine in stage IV malignant melanoma: Final results of the randomised phase III study EORTC 18032. Paper presented at: 33rd European Society of Medical Oncology (ESMO) Congress2008; Stockholm.

137. Atkins MB. The treatment of metastatic melanoma with chemotherapy and biologics. *Curr Opin Oncol* Mar 1997; 9(2):205-213.

138. Glover D, Glick JH, Weiler C et al. WR-2721 and high-dose cisplatin: An active combination in the treatment of metastatic melanoma. *J Clin Oncol* Apr 1987;5(4):574-578.

139. Calabresi F, Aapro M, Becquart D, et al. Multicenter phase II trial of the single agent fotemustine in patients with advanced malignant melanoma. *Ann Oncol* May 1991;2(5):377-378.

140. Jacquillat C, Khayat D, Banzet P, et al. Final report of the French multicenter phase II study of the nitrosourea fotemustine in 153 evaluable patients with disseminated malignant melanoma including patients with cerebral metastases. *Cancer* Nov 1 1990;66(9):1873-1878.

141. Kleeberg UR, Engel E, Israels P, et al. Palliative therapy of melanoma patients with fotemustine. Inverse relationship between tumour load and treatment effectiveness. A multi-centre phase II trial of the EORTC-Melanoma Cooperative Group (MCG). *Melanoma Res* Jun 1995;5(3):195-200.

142. Schallreuter KU, Wenzel E, Brassow FW, et al. Positive phase II study in the treatment of advanced malignant melanoma with fotemustine. *Cancer Chemother Pharmacol* 1991;29(1):85-87.

143. Bajetta E, Del Vecchio M, Bernard-Marty C, et al. Metastatic melanoma: Chemotherapy. *Semin Oncol* Oct 2002;29(5):427-445.

144. Quagliana JM, Stephens RL, Baker LH, et al. Vindesine in patients with metastatic malignant melanoma: A Southwest Oncology Group study. *J Clin Oncol* Apr 1984;2(4):316-319.

145. Einzig AI, Hochster H, Wiernik PH, et al. A phase II study of taxol in patients with malignant melanoma. *Invest New Drugs* Feb 1991;9(1):59-64.

146. Bedikian AY, Weiss GR, Legha SS, et al. Phase II trial of docetaxel in patients with advanced cutaneous malignant melanoma previously untreated with chemotherapy. *J Clin Oncol* Dec 1995;13(12):2895-2899.

147. Einzig AI, Schuchter LM, Recio A, et al. Phase II trial of docetaxel (Taxotere) in patients with metastatic melanoma previously untreated with cytotoxic chemotherapy. *Med Oncol* Jun 1996;13(2):111-117.

148. Legha SS, Ring S, Papadopoulos N, et al. A prospective evaluation of a triple-drug regimen containing cisplatin, vinblastine, and dacarbazine (CVD) for metastatic melanoma. *Cancer* Nov 15 1989;64(10):2024-2029.

149. McClay EF, Mastrangelo MJ, Berd D, et al. Effective combination chemo/hormonal therapy for malignant melanoma: Experience with three consecutive trials. *Int J Cancer* Feb 20 1992;50(4):553-556.

150. Atkins MB, Lotze MT, Dutcher JP, et al. High-dose recombinant interleukin 2 therapy for patients with metastatic melanoma: Analysis of 270 patients treated between 1985 and 1993. *J Clin Oncol* Jul 1999;17(7):2105-2116.

151. Phan GQ, Attia P, Steinberg SM, et al. Factors associated with response to high-dose interleukin-2 in patients with metastatic melanoma. *J Clin Oncol* Aug 1 2001;19(15):3477-3482.

152. Rosenberg SA, White DE. Vitiligo in patients with melanoma: Normal tissue antigens can be targets for cancer immunotherapy. *J Immunother Emphasis Tumor Immunol* Jan 1996;19(1):81-84.

153. Chang E, Rosenberg SA. Patients with melanoma metastases at cutaneous and subcutaneous sites are highly susceptible to interleukin-2-based therapy. *J Immunother* Jan-Feb 2001;24(1):88-90.

154. Rosenberg SA, Yang JC, Schwartzentruber DJ, et al. Immunologic and therapeutic evaluation of a synthetic peptide vaccine for the treatment of patients with metastatic melanoma. *Nat Med* Mar 1998;4(3):321-327.

155. Sosman JA, Carrillo C, Urba WJ, et al. Three phase II cytokine working group trials of gp100 (210M) peptide plus high-dose interleukin-2 in patients with HLA-A2-positive advanced melanoma. *J Clin Oncol* May 10 2008;26(14):2292-2298.

156. Schwartzentruber DJ, Lawson D, Richards J, et al. A phase III multi-institutional randomized study of immunization with the gp100:209-217(210M) peptide followed by high-dose IL-2 compared with high-dose IL-2 alone in patients with metastatic melanoma. *J Clin Oncol* 2009;27(18s (suppl): (Abstract CRA9011).

157. Creagan ET, Ahmann DL, Green SJ, et al. Phase II study of recombinant leukocyte A interferon (rIFN-alpha A) in disseminated malignant melanoma. *Cancer* Dec 15 1984;54(12):2844-2849.

158. Dorval T, Palangie T, Jouve M, et al. Clinical phase II trial of recombinant DNA interferon (interferon alpha 2b) in patients with metastatic malignant melanoma. *Cancer* Jul 15 1986;58(2):215-218.

159. Legha SS, Papadopoulos NE, Plager C, et al. Clinical evaluation of recombinant interferon alfa-2a (Roferon-A) in metastatic melanoma using two different schedules. *J Clin Oncol* Aug 1987;5(8):1240-1246.

160. Sertoli MR, Bernengo MG, Ardizzoni A, et al. Phase II trial of recombinant alpha-2b interferon in the treatment of metastatic skin melanoma. *Oncology* 1989;46(2):96-98.

161. Rosenberg SA, Yang JC, Schwartzentruber DJ, et al. Prospective randomized trial of the treatment of patients with metastatic melanoma using chemotherapy with cisplatin, dacarbazine, and tamoxifen alone or in combination with interleukin-2 and interferon alfa-2b. *J Clin Oncol* Mar 1999;17(3):968-975.

162. Eton O, Legha SS, Bedikian AY, et al. Sequential biochemotherapy versus chemotherapy for metastatic melanoma: Results from a phase III randomized trial. *J Clin Oncol* Apr 15 2002;20(8):2045-2052.

163. Ridolfi R, Chiarion-Sileni V, Guida M, et al. Cisplatin, dacarbazine with or without subcutaneous interleukin-2, and interferon alpha-2b in advanced melanoma outpatients: Results from an Italian multicenter phase III randomized clinical trial. *J Clin Oncol* Mar 15 2002;20(6):1600-1607.

164. Atkins MB, Hsu J, Lee S, et al. Phase III trial comparing concurrent biochemotherapy with cisplatin, vinblastine, dacarbazine, interleukin-2, and interferon alfa-2b with cisplatin, vinblastine, and dacarbazine alone in patients with metastatic malignant melanoma (E3695): A trial coordinated by the Eastern Cooperative Oncology Group. *J Clin Oncol* Dec 10 2008;26(35):5748-5754.

165. Ives NJ, Stowe RL, Lorigan P, et al. Chemotherapy compared with biochemotherapy for the treatment of metastatic melanoma: A meta-analysis of 18 trials involving 2,621 patients. *J Clin Oncol* Dec 1 2007;25(34):5426-5434.

166. Bedikian AY, Johnson MM, Warneke CL, et al. Prognostic factors that determine the long-term survival of patients with unresectable metastatic melanoma. *Cancer Invest* Jul 2008;26(6):624-633.

167. Bedikian AY, Johnson MM, Warneke CL, et al. Systemic therapy for unresectable metastatic melanoma: Impact of biochemotherapy on long-term survival. *J Immunotoxicol* Apr 2008;5(2):201-207.

168. Kim KB, Sanguino AM, Hodges C, et al. Biochemotherapy in patients with metastatic anorectal mucosal melanoma. *Cancer* Apr 1 2004;100(7):1478-1483.

169. Harting MS, Kim KB. Biochemotherapy in patients with advanced vulvovaginal mucosal melanoma. *Melanoma Res* Dec 2004;14(6):517-520.

170. Bartell HL, Bedikian AY, Papadopoulos NE, et al. Biochemotherapy in patients with advanced head and neck mucosal melanoma. *Head Neck* Dec 2008;30(12):1592-1598.

171. Keilholz U, Punt CJ, Gore M, et al. Dacarbazine, cisplatin, and interferon-alfa-2b with or without interleukin-2 in metastatic melanoma: A randomized phase III trial (18951) of the European Organisation for Research and Treatment of Cancer Melanoma Group. *J Clin Oncol* Sep 20 2005; 23(27):6747-6755.

172. Weber J. Overcoming immunologic tolerance to melanoma: Targeting CTLA-4 with ipilimumab (MDX-010). *Oncologist* 2008;13 (suppl 4):16-25.

173. Phan GQ, Yang JC, Sherry RM, et al. Cancer regression and autoimmunity induced by cytotoxic T lymphocyte-associated antigen 4 blockade in patients with metastatic melanoma. *Proc Natl Acad Sci USA* Jul 8 2003;100(14): 8372-8377.

174. Ribas A, Camacho LH, Lopez-Berestein G, et al. Antitumor activity in melanoma and anti-self responses in a phase I trial with the anti-cytotoxic T lymphocyte-associated antigen 4 monoclonal antibody CP-675,206. *J Clin Oncol* Dec 10 2005;23(35):8968-8977.

175. Attia P, Phan GQ, Maker AV, et al. Autoimmunity correlates with tumor regression in patients with metastatic melanoma treated with anti-cytotoxic T-lymphocyte antigen-4. *J Clin Oncol* Sep 1 2005;23(25):6043-6053.

176. Riddell SR, Greenberg PD. T cell therapy of human CMV and EBV infection in immunocompromised hosts. *Rev Med Virol* Sep 1997;7(3):181-192.

177. Rooney CM, Aguilar LK, Huls MH, et al. Adoptive immunotherapy of EBV-associated malignancies with EBV-specific cytotoxic T-cell lines. *Curr Top Microbiol Immunol* 2001;258:221-229.

178. Straathof KC, Bollard CM, Popat U, et al. Treatment of nasopharyngeal carcinoma with Epstein-Barr virus—specific T lymphocytes. *Blood* Mar 1 2005;105(5):1898-1904.

179. Luznik L, Fuchs EJ. Donor lymphocyte infusions to treat hematologic malignancies in relapse after allogeneic blood or marrow transplantation. *Cancer Control* Mar-Apr 2002;9(2): 123-137.

180. Dudley ME, Wunderlich JR, Robbins PF, et al. Cancer regression and autoimmunity in patients after clonal repopulation with antitumor lymphocytes. *Science* Oct 25 2002; 298(5594):850-854.

181. Dudley ME, Wunderlich JR, Yang JC, et al. Adoptive cell transfer therapy following non-myeloablative but lymphodepleting chemotherapy for the treatment of patients with refractory metastatic melanoma. *J Clin Oncol* Apr 1 2005; 23(10):2346-2357.

182. Dudley ME, Yang JC, Sherry R, et al. Adoptive cell therapy for patients with metastatic melanoma: Evaluation of intensive myeloablative chemoradiation preparative regimens. *J Clin Oncol* Nov 10 2008;26(32):5233-5239.

183. Strumberg D. Preclinical and clinical development of the oral multikinase inhibitor sorafenib in cancer treatment. *Drugs Today (Barc)* Dec 2005;41(12):773-784.

184. Panka DJ, Wang W, Atkins MB, et al. The Raf inhibitor BAY 43-9006 (Sorafenib) induces caspase-independent apoptosis in melanoma cells. *Cancer Res* Feb 1 2006;66(3):1611-1619.

185. Eisen T, Ahmad T, Flaherty KT, et al. Sorafenib in advanced melanoma: A Phase II randomised discontinuation trial analysis. *Br J Cancer* Sep 4 2006;95(5):581-586.

186. Flaherty KT, Schiller J, Schuchter LM, et al. A phase I trial of the oral, multikinase inhibitor sorafenib in combination with carboplatin and paclitaxel. *Clin Cancer Res* Aug 1 2008; 14(15):4836-4842.

187. Hauschild A, Agarwala SS, Trefzer U, et al. Results of a phase III, randomized, placebo-controlled study of sorafenib in combination with carboplatin and paclitaxel as second-line treatment in patients with unresectable stage III or stage IV melanoma. *J Clin Oncol* Jun 10 2009;27(17):2823-2830.

188. Flaherty KF, investigators EC-r. E2603: A randomized phase III trial comparing sorafenib, carboplatin & paclitaxel to carboplatin & paclitaxel in metastatic melanoma. Paper presented at: Perspectives in Melanoma XIII; October 10, 2009; Baltimore, MA.

189. McDermott DF, Sosman JA, Gonzalez R, et al. Double-blind randomized phase II study of the combination of sorafenib and dacarbazine in patients with advanced melanoma: A report from the 11715 Study Group. *J Clin Oncol* May 1 2008;26(13):2178-2185.

190. Amaravadi RK, Schuchter LM, McDermott DF, et al. Phase II Trial of Temozolomide and Sorafenib in Advanced Melanoma Patients with or without Brain Metastases. *Clin Cancer Res* Dec 15 2009;15(24):7711-7718.

191. Sala E, Mologni L, Truffa S et al. BRAF silencing by short hairpin RNA or chemical blockade by PLX4032 leads to different responses in melanoma and thyroid carcinoma cells. *Mol Cancer Res* May 2008;6(5):751-759.

192. Chapman P, Puzanov I, Sosman J, et al. Early efficacy signal demonstrated in advanced melanoma in a phase I trial of the oncogenic BRAF-selective inhibitor PLX4032. *Eur J Cancer* 2009;7(3 suppl):5 (Abstract 6BA).

193. Druker BJ, Lydon NB. Lessons learned from the development of an abl tyrosine kinase inhibitor for chronic myelogenous leukemia. *J clin invest* Jan 2000;105(1):3-7.

194. Okuda K, Weisberg E, Gilliland DG, et al. ARG tyrosine kinase activity is inhibited by STI571. *Blood* Apr 15 2001; 97(8):2440-2448.

195. Schindler T, Bornmann W, Pellicena P, et al. Structural mechanism for STI-571 inhibition of abelson tyrosine kinase. *Science* Sep 15 2000;289(5486):1938-1942.

196. Shen SS, Zhang PS, Eton O, et al. Analysis of protein tyrosine kinase expression in melanocytic lesions by tissue array. *J Cutan Pathol* Oct 2003;30(9):539-547.

197. Wyman K, Atkins MB, Prieto V, et al. Multicenter Phase II trial of high-dose imatinib mesylate in metastatic melanoma: Significant toxicity with no clinical efficacy. *Cancer* May 1 2006;106(9):2005-2011.

198. Kim KB, Eton O, Davis DW, et al. Phase II trial of imatinib mesylate in patients with metastatic melanoma. *Br J Cancer* Sep 2 2008;99(5):734-740.

199. Ugurel S, Hildenbrand R, Zimpfer A, et al. Lack of clinical efficacy of imatinib in metastatic melanoma. *Br J Cancer* Apr 25 2005;92(8):1398-1405.

200. Hodi FS, Friedlander P, Corless CL, et al. Major response to imatinib mesylate in KIT-mutated melanoma. *J Clin Oncol* Apr 20 2008;26(12):2046-2051.

201. Lutzky J, Bauer J, Bastian BC. Dose-dependent, complete response to imatinib of a metastatic mucosal melanoma with a K642E KIT mutation. *Pigment Cell Melanoma Res* Aug 2008;21(4):492-493.

202. Carvajal RD, Chapman PB, Wolchok JD, et al. A phase II study of imatinib mesylate (IM) for patients with advanced melanoma harboring somatic alterations of KIT. *J Clin Oncol* 2009;27(15s suppl):(Abstract 9001).

203. Avril MF, Aamdal S, Grob JJ, et al. Fotemustine compared with dacarbazine in patients with disseminated malignant melanoma: A phase III study. *J Clin Oncol* Mar 15 2004; 22(6):1118-1125.

204. Ribas A, Hauschild A, Kefford R, et al. Phase III, open-label, randomized, comparative study of tremelimumab (CP-675,206) and chemotherapy (temozolomide [TMZ] or dacarbazine [DTIC]) in patients with advanced melanoma. *J Clin Oncol*. 2008;26 (suppl):(Abstract LBA9011).

205. O'Day S. A Randomized, Double-blind, Phase 3 Trial of elesclomol in combination with paclitaxel versus paclitaxel alone for treatment of patients with stage IV metastatic melanoma (SYMMETRY). Updated Results presentation. Paper presented at: Perspectives in Melanoma XIII; October 10, 2009; Baltimore, MA.

206. Eisen T, Trefzer U, Hamilton A, et al. Results of a multicenter, randomized, double-blind phase 2/3 study of lenalidomide in the treatment of pretreated relapsed or refractory metastatic malignant melanoma. *Cancer* Jan 1;116(1):146-154.

207. Glaspy J, Atkins MB, Richards JM, et al. Results of a multicenter, randomized, double-blind, dose-evaluating phase 2/3 study of lenalidomide in the treatment of metastatic malignant melanoma. *Cancer* Nov 15 2009;115(22):5228-5236.

208. Becker JC, Terheyden P, Kampgen E, et al. Treatment of disseminated ocular melanoma with sequential fotemustine, interferon alpha, and interleukin 2. *Br J Cancer* Oct 7 2002; 87(8):840-845.

209. Cantore M, Fiorentini G, Aitini E, et al. Intra-arterial hepatic carboplatin-based chemotherapy for ocular melanoma metastatic to the liver. Report of a phase II study. *Tumori* Feb 28 1994;80(1):37-39.

210. Agarwala SS, Panikkar R, Kirkwood JM. Phase I/II randomized trial of intrahepatic arterial infusion chemotherapy with cisplatin and chemoembolization with cisplatin and polyvinyl sponge in patients with ocular melanoma metastatic to the liver. *Melanoma Res* Jun 2004;14(3):217-222.

211. Bedikian AY, Mavligit G, Carrasco CH, et al. Phase I evaluation of hepatic arterial infusion of interferon alfa-2b in patients with liver cancer. *Reg Cancer Treat* 1996;9:17-20.

212. Keilholz U, Scheibenbogen C, Brado M, et al. Regional adoptive immunotherapy with interleukin-2 and lymphokine-activated killer (LAK) cells for liver metastases. *Eur J Cancer* 1994;30A(1):103-105.

213. Mavligit GM, Charnsangavej C, Carrasco CH, et al. Regression of ocular melanoma metastatic to the liver after hepatic arterial chemoembolization with cisplatin and polyvinyl sponge. *JAMA* Aug 19 1988;260(7):974-976.

214. Feun LG, Reddy KR, Yrizarry JM, et al. A phase I study of chemoembolization with cisplatin and lipiodol for primary and metastatic liver cancer. *Am J Clin Oncol* Oct 1994;17(5): 405-410.

215. Sato T, Nathan FE, Berd D, et al. Lack of effect from chemoembolization for liver metastasis from uveal melanoma. Paper presented at: Proc Am Soc Clin Oncol 1995; Los Angeles, CA.

216. Patel K, Sullivan K, Berd D, et al. Chemoembolization of the hepatic artery with BCNU for metastatic uveal melanoma: Results of a phase II study. *Melanoma Res* Aug 2005;15(4): 297-304.

217. Sato T, Eschelman DJ, Gonsalves CF, et al. Immunoembolization of malignant liver tumors, including uveal melanoma, using granulocyte-macrophage colony-stimulating factor. *J Clin Oncol* Nov 20 2008;26(33):5436-5442.

218. Alexander HR, Jr., Libutti SK, Pingpank JF, et al. Hyperthermic isolated hepatic perfusion using melphalan for patients with ocular melanoma metastatic to liver. *Clin Cancer Res* Dec 15 2003;9(17):6343-6349.

219. Noter SL, Rothbarth J, Pijl ME, et al. Isolated hepatic perfusion with high-dose melphalan for the treatment of uveal melanoma metastases confined to the liver. *Melanoma Res* Feb 2004;14(1):67-72.

220. Bedikian AY. Metastatic uveal melanoma therapy: Current options. *Int Ophthalmol Clin* Winter 2006;46(1):151-166.

221. Nathan FE, Berd D, Sato T, et al. BOLD+interferon in the treatment of metastatic uveal melanoma: First report of active systemic therapy. *J Exp Clin Cancer Res* Jun 1997;16(2): 201-208.

222. Pyrhonen S, Hahka-Kemppinen M, Muhonen T, et al. Chemoimmunotherapy with bleomycin, vincristine, lomustine, dacarbazine (BOLD), and human leukocyte interferon for metastatic uveal melanoma. *Cancer* Dec 1 2002;95(11): 2366-2372.

223. Kivela T, Suciu S, Hansson J, et al. Bleomycin, vincristine, lomustine and dacarbazine (BOLD) in combination with recombinant interferon alpha-2b for metastatic uveal melanoma. *Eur J Cancer* May 2003;39(8):1115-1120.

224. Dorval T, Fridman WH, Mathiot C, et al. Interleukin-2 therapy for metastatic uveal melanoma. *Eur J Cancer* 1992; 28A(12):2087.

225. Proebstle TM, Scheibenbogen C, Sterry W, et al. A phase II study of dacarbazine, cisplatin, interferon-alpha and high-dose interleukin-2 in 'poor-risk' metastatic melanoma. *Eur J Cancer* Aug 1996;32A(9):1530-1533.

226. Myatt N, Cree IA, Kurbacher CM, et al. The ex vivo chemosensitivity profile of choroidal melanoma. *Anticancer Drugs* Sep 1997;8(8):756-762.

227. Neale MH, Myatt N, Cree IA, et al. Combination chemotherapy for choroidal melanoma: Ex vivo sensitivity to treosulfan with gemcitabine or cytosine arabinoside. *Br J Cancer* Mar 1999;79(9-10):1487-1493.

228. Corrie PG, Shaw J, Spanswick VJ, et al. Phase I trial combining gemcitabine and treosulfan in advanced cutaneous and uveal melanoma patients. *Br J Cancer* Jun 6 2005;92(11): 1997-2003.

229. Keilholz U, Schuster R, Schmittel A, et al. A clinical phase I trial of gemcitabine and treosulfan in uveal melanoma and other solid tumours. *Eur J Cancer* Sep 2004;40(14): 2047-2052.

230. Pfohler C, Cree IA, Ugurel S, et al. Treosulfan and gemcitabine in metastatic uveal melanoma patients: Results of a multicenter feasibility study. *Anticancer Drugs* Jun 2003;14(5):337-340.

231. Schmittel A, Schuster R, Bechrakis NE, et al. A two-cohort phase II clinical trial of gemcitabine plus treosulfan in patients with metastatic uveal melanoma. *Melanoma Res* Oct 2005;15(5):447-451.

232. Schmittel A, Schmidt-Hieber M, Martus P, et al. A randomized phase II trial of gemcitabine plus treosulfan versus treosulfan alone in patients with metastatic uveal melanoma. *Ann Oncol* Dec 2006;17(12):1826-1829.

233. Onken MD, Worley LA, Long MD, et al. Oncogenic mutations in GNAQ occur early in uveal melanoma. *Invest Ophthalmol Vis Sci* Dec 2008;49(12):5230-5234.

234. Bakalian S, Marshall JC, Logan P, et al. Molecular pathways mediating liver metastasis in patients with uveal melanoma. *Clin Cancer Res* Feb 15 2008;14(4):951-956.

235. Petrausch U, Martus P, Tonnies H, et al. Significance of gene expression analysis in uveal melanoma in comparison to standard risk factors for risk assessment of subsequent metastases. *Eye (Lond)* Aug 2008;22(8):997-1007.

SOFT TISSUE AND BONE SARCOMAS

Anthony Conley
Min S. Park
Jonathan C. Trent
Shreyaskumar Patel

■ INCIDENCE

Sarcomas are an extremely rare and heterogeneous group of tumors that arise from mesenchymal tissues. According to the estimates of the American Cancer Society, approximately 1.4 million people were estimated to be diagnosed with cancer in the year 2009, with only 13,230 cases representing sarcomas (1); 10,660 of these represented new soft tissue sarcomas and 2570 bone sarcomas diagnosed in 2009, with 3820 and 1470 deaths, respectively, resulting from these tumors (1).

■ EPIDEMIOLOGY AND PATHOGENESIS

The etiology and pathogenesis of sarcomas, like most cancers, is not well understood. Multiple environmental factors have been associated with the development of soft tissue and bone sarcomas. Many studies have shown that patients who have received radiation therapy for prior cancers have an increased risk of developing soft tissue sarcomas near or within the field of radiation (2-7). In one series, patients developed sarcoma between 3 and 23 years after radiation therapy (5). The average time for development is between 10 and 13 years (2, 4-6). Postirradiation sarcomas have been reported to occur most commonly in patients who received radiation for breast cancer, Hodgkin and non-Hodgkin lymphoma, and cervical cancer. These have also been reported in patients who received radiation for other benign and malignant conditions (2,3). Postirradiation sarcomas comprise a variety of histologic types, including malignant fibrous histiocytoma, osteosarcoma, fibrosarcoma, malignant peripheral nerve sheath tumor, and angiosarcoma (3,5,6). Most postirradiation sarcomas are high-grade lesions, which may be less responsive to chemotherapy than their de novo counterparts and are associated with a poorer prognosis (2-7).

Exposure to various chemicals and environmental toxins—such as asbestos, phenyl herbicides, chlorophenols (wood preservatives), dioxins (Agent Orange), and hexachlorobenzene (pesticide)—has been linked to the development of sarcoma (8-15). Arsenic, vinyl chloride, and Thorotrast have also been associated with the occurrence of sarcomas (15-18). Tamoxifen, which is used to treat and to prevent breast cancer, has been implicated in the etiology uterine sarcomas (19).

Trauma and foreign bodies have also been associated with sarcoma development. There are reports of sarcomas developing after recent trauma (20,21), although a causal relationship is unclear; the trauma is likely responsible for bringing the tumor to medical attention. Chronic inflammation has been associated with sarcoma development and may be a risk factor (15). Lymphangiosarcoma can occur in the setting of chronic lymphedema and is known as Stewart-Treves syndrome (22). Sarcomas have also been associated with viral infections; the best-known examples are herpesvirus 8 (HHV-8), HIV-1, and Kaposi sarcoma (15,16). Other viral infections have been suggested, but no epidemiologic data have been found to establish a true causal relationship (15).

Molecular and genetic alterations have been shown to be responsible for the development of soft tissue sarcomas and bone sarcomas. Though most of these genetic aberrations are sporadic in origin, some of the known mutations are inherited. One of the most notable of these is the Li-Fraumeni syndrome (23). First described in 1969 in four families with an autosomal dominant pattern of soft tissue sarcoma, breast cancer, and other cancers in children and young adults, subsequent studies found that the syndrome includes osteosarcoma, brain tumors, acute leukemia, adrenocortical carcinoma, and germ cell tumors (15,23). Li-Fraumeni syndrome is associated with a germline mutation of the

p53 tumor suppressor gene, which is located on chromosome 17p13 (24). Inherited retinoblastoma is also associated with the development of sarcomas, both osteosarcoma and soft tissue sarcoma (15). The inciting event appears to be a germline mutation in the *rb-1* tumor suppressor gene, which leads to the development of a sarcoma (15,18). Neurofibromatosis-1 (von Recklinghausen disease) is a single-gene disorder inherited in an autosomal dominant pattern (25). The *nf-1* gene is located on chromosome 17 and codes for a protein called neurofibromin, which is involved in the regulation of Ras oncoproteins (18,25,26). Neurofibromatosis-1 is associated with an increased risk of development of sarcoma in a preexisting neurofibroma, resulting in a malignant peripheral nerve sheath tumor (18, 25-27). Sarcomas have been associated with other cancer family syndromes, including basal cell nevus syndrome, Werner syndrome, familial adenomatous polyposis, and Gardner syndrome (15,28).

Many sarcomas are known to have characteristic cytogenetic abnormalities (Table 40-1) such as translocations, amplifications, and partial loss of specific chromosomes.

Because many of these are relatively tumor-specific, it has been postulated that molecular therapies could be developed for each of them (26,29). Imatinib (Gleevec) in the treatment of gastrointestinal stromal tumors (GISTs) is one example of a successful targeted therapy. Many of these specific abnormalities can also be useful in the diagnosis of certain histologic subtypes (26,30). Molecular testing of tumors is becoming more useful in the diagnosis and treatment of soft tissue sarcomas. For example, the t(x;18) translocation is a specific marker for synovial sarcomas. The transcript formed from this translocation (SYT-SSX) can be detected using polymerase chain reaction (PCR) testing. Coindre et al. evaluated over 200 cases of synovial sarcoma and classified these into three groups: (1) those in which the diagnosis of synovial sarcoma was certain; (2) those in which the diagnosis of synovial sarcoma was probable; and (3) those in which the diagnosis of synovial sarcoma was possible but where it was not the first on the list. After evaluation all the specimens underwent PCR examination for the SYT-SSX transcript. Tumors in the first category did not need molecular evaluation, as 84.5% of these tumors were positive for the transcript. In the second category, where the diagnosis of synovial sarcoma was probable, these tumors were found to have the SYT-SSX transcript 74.4% of the time. However, for the third category, where the diagnosis of synovial sarcoma was possible but not the first in the differential, 24.3% tumors were positive for the transcript, which

TABLE 40-1	CYTOGENETIC TRANSLOCATION AND OTHER ABNORMALITIES IN SARCOMA	
Tumor	*Cytogenetic Abnormality*	*Gene Product*
Alveolar rhabdomyosarcoma	t(2;13)(q35;q14)	PAX3-FOXO1A
	t(1;13)(p36;q14)	PAX7-FOXO1A
Alveolar soft tissue sarcoma	t(X;17)(p11.2;q25)	ASPL-TFE3
Clear cell sarcoma	t(12;22)(q13;q12)	EWSR1-ATF1
	t(2;22)(q32;q12)	EWSR1-CREB1
Congenital fibrosarcoma	t(12;15)(p13;q25)	ETV6-NTRK3
Dermatofibrosarcoma protuberans	t(17;22)(q22;q13)	COL1A1-PDGFB
Desmoplastic small round cell tumor	t(11;22)(p13;q12)	EWSR1-WR1
Endometrial stromal sarcoma	t(7;17)(p15;q11)	JAZF1-SUZ12
Ewing sarcoma	t(11;22)(q24;q12)	EWSR1-FLI1
	t(21;22)(q22;q12)	EWSR1-ERG
	t(7;22)(p22;q12)	EWSR1-ETV1
	t(17;22)(q21;q12)	EWSR1-ETV4
	t(2;22)(q33;q12)	EWSR1-FEV
Gastrointestinal stromal tumor	Activating mutations	KIT, PDGFR
	Loss of 14q	
	LOH of 22q	
	Loss of 1p	
Inflammatory myofibroblastic tumor	t(1;2)(q22-23;p23)	TPM3-ALK
	t(2;19)(p23;p13.1)	TPM4-ALK
Lipoma	12q abnormalities	Amplified 12q
Malignant peripheral nerve sheath tumor	Deletion of NF1	
Myxoid chondrosarcoma	t(9;22)(q22-31;q11-12)	EWSR1-NR4A3
	t(9;17)(q22;q11)	TAF15-NR4A3
	t(9;15)(q22;q21)	TCF12-NR4A3
Myxoid liposarcoma	t(12;16)(q13;p11)	FUS-DDIT3
	t(12;22)(q13;q12)	EWSR1-DDIT3
Synovial sarcoma	t(X;18)(p11;q11)	SS18-SSX1
		SS18-SSX2
		SS18-SSX4
Uterine leiomyosarcoma	t(12,14)(q7-)	

aided in the diagnosis of synovial sarcoma (31). These data suggest that molecular genetics may also be a useful adjunct in the diagnosis of some sarcomas.

■ SOFT TISSUE SARCOMA

Soft tissues are the nonepithelial extraskeletal tissues of the body that support, connect, and surround other discrete anatomic structures. These tissues include fibrous, adipose, and vascular structures as well as muscles and tendons and represent more than 50% of body weight. Soft tissues are derived embryologically primarily from the mesoderm, making tumors from these tissues mesenchymal in origin. Soft tissue sarcomas represent approximately 0.6% of all adult cancers and tend to occur more frequently in men (1). These cancers are

also more common in older adults, but this is somewhat dependent on tumor type as well (32).

Soft tissue sarcomas are an extremely heterogeneous group and are classified based on their resemblance to normal tissues rather than the tissue of origin. When the spindle or round cell tumor is very poorly differentiated, it can be almost impossible to classify it despite immunohistochemical techniques and electron microscopy. Each tumor type has a varying degree of aggressiveness and ability to metastasize, depending on the histologic grade.

CLINICAL PRESENTATION

Soft tissue sarcomas can occur in any anatomic region of the body because of the ubiquitous nature of connective tissue. The majority of soft tissue sarcomas arise from the extremities (60%), more commonly in the lower extremities. They can also develop in the trunk (30%) and the head and neck region (10%). The most common symptom reported is that of a soft tissue mass or swelling. Pain is reported by only about one-third of patients with soft tissue sarcoma at presentation (33). Therefore, because of the lack of symptoms, there is often a delay in the diagnosis (34). Many times these tumors are mistaken for other benign tumors, such as hematomas or lipomas. In the case of retroperitoneal and intra-abdominal sarcomas, delay in diagnosis is likely due to the fact that tumors can grow extensively in this area without causing any symptoms.

EVALUATION

As with any suspected illness or disease, evaluation should start with a thorough history and physical examination. This can give some indication as to how long the symptoms have been present and can help guide further study, including imaging and biopsy.

The imaging modalities recommended for the evaluation of sarcomas depend on the site of disease. A plain film of the involved area is a good initial imaging modality. For soft tissue tumors of the extremities as well as the head and neck, magnetic resonance imaging (MRI) is preferred. By using contrast-enhanced T1- and T2-weighted images, MRI studies can distinguish between tumor, fat, vessels, bone, and other surrounding structures (34-36). Soft tissue sarcomas of the pelvis may also be better visualized with MRI studies. Soft tissue sarcomas found in the retroperitoneum and abdomen are generally best evaluated by computed tomography (CT). Though still considered investigational, positron emission tomography (PET) has become increasingly utilized in the diagnosis and management of sarcomas. PET imaging can distinguish histologic grade to a degree based on tumor standardized uptake values (SUV) (37). It can be used to monitor neurofibromatosis type I (NF1) patients for malignant transformation of neurofibromas (38). For both soft tissue sarcomas and bone sarcomas, PET imaging has a predictive role in determining response to chemotherapy and targeted agents, such as imatinib, but also has prognostic value for outcome (39-43). Arteriograms and other invasive studies are almost never required to evaluate soft tissue sarcomas.

A biopsy should be performed for any soft tissue mass if it is symptomatic, enlarging, is greater than 5 cm, and has persisted for more than 4 to 6 weeks. The method of biopsy chosen depends on the least invasive technique available to make a definitive diagnosis of both histology and grade of the tumor. Most often a core-needle biopsy is sufficient to provide enough tissue for definitive diagnosis; however, open biopsy may still need to be performed in cases where more tissue is needed to evaluate the histology (44,45). If an open biopsy is performed, the biopsy site should be removed at the time of definitive surgical resection, as there are reports of tumor recurrences within the needle tract after percutaneous biopsy (46). An excisional biopsy may be used for small or superficial lesions; however, careful examination of margins and planning of the orientation of the resection should always be performed. Fine-needle aspiration can also be a useful tool in diagnosis, assuming that an experienced sarcoma cytopathologist is available (47-49); however, core biopsies are preferred for the diagnosis of sarcoma.

Once the diagnosis of sarcoma is established, screening for metastatic disease is required. The most common site of metastatic disease in sarcoma is the lungs; however in abdominal and retroperitoneal sarcomas, the liver is also a common site. Therefore staging workup should include chest x-ray but may also include chest CT, depending on the size, grade, and location of the primary tumor. Patients with low-grade or intermediate-/high-grade tumors less than 5 cm in diameter need only a chest x-ray during staging; those with high-grade tumors greater than 5 cm in diameter need a chest CT at diagnosis for staging (50). Patients with abdominal or retroperitoneal soft tissue sarcomas should also undergo CT scanning of the abdomen and pelvis, with appropriate imaging of the liver and peritoneal space, to evaluate for metastatic disease.

PATHOLOGY

Malignancies are classified according to histologic grade, which is determined by assessment of several features: (1) degree of cellularity, (2) cellular pleomorphism or anaplasia, (3) mitotic activity, (4) degree of necrosis, and (5) expansive or infiltrative and invasive growth (51). Sarcomas are classified primarily according to their tissue appearance, histologic grade, and sometimes the cell of origin. This can be quite difficult, as approximately 70 different histologic types of soft tissue sarcoma are recognized (Table 40-2).

Pathologists often separate sarcomas into three histologic grades. Grade 1 (low-grade) describes tumors that are well differentiated, grade 2 describes tumors with an intermediate differentiation, and grade 3 (high-grade) describes tumors with a poorly differentiated histology. Biological aggressiveness can be predicted based on histologic grade, and this spectrum

| TABLE 40-2 | SOFT TISSUE SARCOMAS—HISTOLOGIC DIAGNOSIS |

Sarcomas of adipose tissue
  Liposarcoma
    Atypical lipomatous tumor
    Myxoid liposarcoma
    Cellular myxoid liposarcoma
    Round cell liposarcoma
    Dedifferentiated liposarcoma
    Pleomorphic liposarcoma
Sarcomas of peripheral nervous tissue
  Malignant peripheral nerve sheath tumor
    (Malignant schwannoma, neurofibrosarcoma,
      neurogenic sarcoma)
Sarcomas of smooth muscle
  Leiomyosarcoma
Sarcomas of fibrous tissue
  Desmoid fibromatosis
  Dermatofibrosarcoma protuberans
  Low-grade fibromyxoid sarcoma
  Fibrosarcoma
  Malignant fibrous histiocytoma (MFH)
Sarcomas of blood vessels and lymphatics
  Epithelioid hemangioendothelioma
  Hemangiopericytoma
  Angiosarcoma/lymphangiosarcoma
Sarcomas of skeletal muscle
  Embryonal rhabdomyosarcoma
  Alveolar rhabdomyosarcoma
  Pleomorphic rhabdomyosarcoma
Sarcomas of unknown origin
  Synovial sarcoma
    Monophasic
    Biphasic
  Alveolar soft tissue sarcoma
  Epithelioid sarcoma
  Unclassified sarcoma
  Extraskeletal osteosarcoma
  Extraskeletal chondrosarcoma
  Extraskeletal Ewing sarcoma (PNET)
Soft tissue tumors of melanocytic tissue
  Melanoma of soft tissue or clear cell sarcoma

varies among the histologic subtypes of sarcoma (Fig. 40-1) (52,53).

STAGING AND PROGNOSIS

The staging system of the American Joint Committee on Cancer (AJCC) is one of the most often used systems for soft tissue sarcomas (Table 40-3) (54).

All soft tissue sarcoma subtypes are included except Kaposi sarcoma, dermatofibrosarcoma protuberans, infantile fibrosarcoma, and angiosarcoma.

This system is designed to classify tumors of the extremities, trunk, head and neck, and retroperitoneum, but it was not designed for evaluation of sarcomas of the gastrointestinal (GI) tract. This system has its limitations because anatomic site and certain histologic subtypes (eg, small cell histologies), which are known to influence outcome, are not taken into account (55,56).

Several clinicopathologic factors are important for treatment planning and prognosis assessment. These form the basis for the AJCC classification system and include tumor grade, size of the primary tumor, depth of invasion, and extent of disease (52,53,57). Patients at highest risk for local recurrence or distant metastases would be those with a high-grade lesion, a primary tumor >5 cm, and deep tumor location (52,53,56,57). Whether local recurrence of soft tissue sarcomas affects overall survival is unclear, though a multivariate analysis in at least one study conducted by a large single institution found local recurrence at presentation to be an adverse prognostic factor for disease-specific-survival (58,59). In addition, adverse prognostic factors for local recurrence differ from those that predict distant metastasis and tumor-related mortality (52).

TREATMENT

Evaluation for the treatment of sarcoma requires a multidisciplinary approach with experienced medical, surgical, and radiation oncologists, pathologists, and radiologists, working together to develop the best plan of action. Treatment depends on tumor type, location, and extent of disease. The primary endpoint of any sarcoma therapy is to eradicate all gross and microscopic evidence of disease with aggressive multimodality treatment. In patients in whom this endpoint is achievable, the therapeutic intent is cure; where this is not achievable, the objective is palliation of existing or potential symptoms and perhaps extension of life.

Treatment of Local Disease

Surgery

For local disease, surgical resection is the mainstay of treatment. Sarcomas tend to expand and compress tissue planes, which produce a pseudocapsule comprising normal tissue interlaced with tumor tissue. When surgical resection does not include the plane of tissue adjacent to the pseudocapsule, the local recurrence rates are between 33 and 66% (60-64). Wide local excision with a margin of normal tissue surrounding the tumor is associated with lower local recurrence rates of approximately 10 to 30% (63-65). The ideal surgical margins

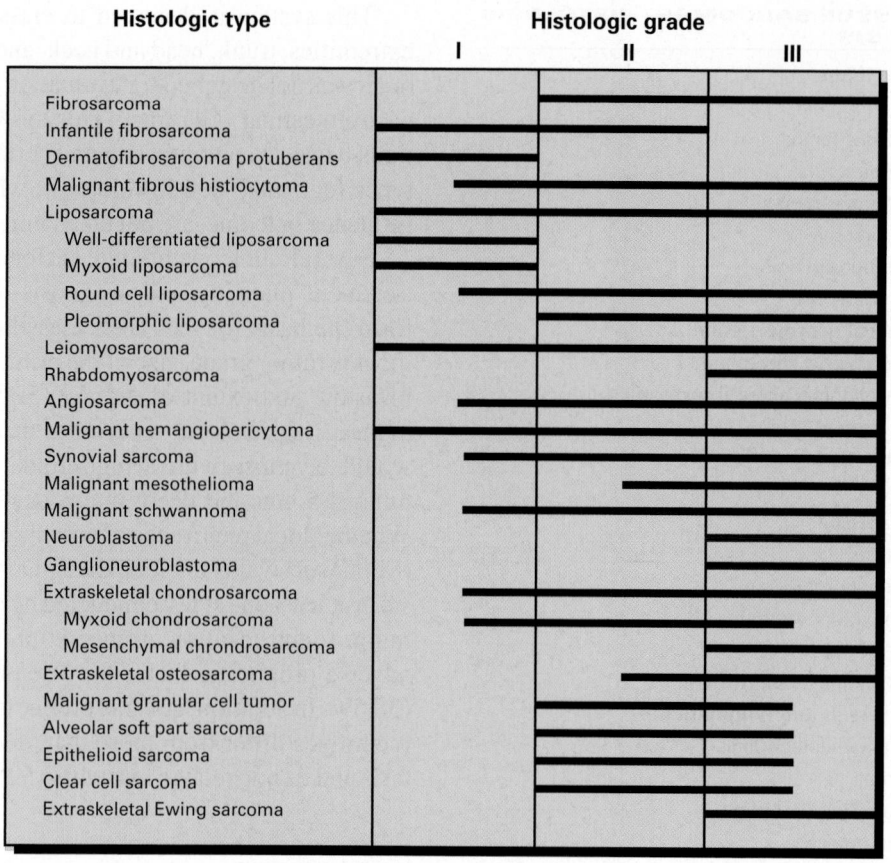

FIGURE 40-1. Spectrum of grades observed among histologic subtypes of soft tissue sarcoma. (*Reproduced, with permission, from Weiss S, Goldblum J: Enzinger and Weiss's Soft Tissue Tumors, 4th ed. St. Louis: Mosby, 2001.*)

should be 2 to 3 cm without tumor involvement; however, this can vary depending on feasibility. If positive margins are confirmed by pathology, re-excision to obtain negative margins is important when feasible. Pre- or postoperative radiation therapy can be a very useful adjunct to wide local excision and has been shown to improve local control in tumors at high risk for local recurrence.

Adult sarcomas have a less than 4% prevalence of lymph node metastases (66-68). For this reason routine regional lymph node dissection is often not required. However, patients with synovial sarcoma, clear cell sarcoma, rhabdomyosarcoma, angiosarcoma, and epithelioid sarcomas have a higher incidence of lymph node metastases and should be evaluated closely for lymphadenopathy; if found, this should be treated appropriately (66,67).

Because of better surgical techniques and a multimodality approach to the care of patients, a decrease in radical resection of extremity tumors, such as amputation or compartment resection, has resulted with a corresponding rise in limb-sparing procedures combining wide

local resection with pre- or postoperative chemotherapy and radiotherapy (69,70). Approximately 90% patients with localized sarcomas of the extremities can safely undergo limb-sparing procedures to preserve limb function and adequately maintain local control (70,71). A study conducted at the National Cancer Institute (NCI) showed no survival advantage to amputation over limb-sparing surgery with postoperative radiation; thus, amputation should be utilized as a last resort (72). However, there are contraindications to limb-sparing surgery, for example extensive or circumferential involvement of the extremity, or involvement of major vessels and/or nerves within the tumor which could critically compromise function (73).

Isolated limb perfusion with or without regional hyperthermia has been studied in patients with soft tissue sarcoma of the extremities and is still under investigation as a treatment modality (74-77). Both modalities have been studied in resectable and unresectable disease settings. European studies of isolated limb perfusion with a combination of recombinant TNF-α-1A and melphalan resulted in its European approval for patients

TABLE 40-3	STAGING—FROM THE AMERICAN JOINT COMMITTEE ON CANCER

PRIMARY TUMOR (T)

TX	Primary tumor cannot be assessed
T0	No evidence of primary tumor
T1	Tumor ≤5 cm in greatest dimension
T1a*	Superficial tumor
T1b*	Deep tumor
T2	Tumor >5 cm in greatest dimension
T2a	Superficial tumor
T2b	Deep tumor

REGIONAL LYMPH NODES (N)

NX	Regional lymph nodes cannot be assessed
N0	No regional lymph node metastasis
N1[†]	Regional lymph node metastasis

DISTANT METASTASIS (M)

M0	No distant metastasis
M1	Distant metastasis

HISTOLOGIC GRADE (G)

GX	Grade cannot be assessed
G1	Well differentiated
G2	Moderately differentiated
G3	Poorly differentiated

ANATOMIC STAGE/PROGNOSTIC GROUPS

Stage IA	T1a, T1b	N0	M0	G1, GX
Stage IB	T2a, T2b			
Stage IIA	T1a, T1b	N0	M0	G2, G3
Stage IIB	T2a, T2b			G2
Stage III	T2a, T2b	N0	M0	G3
	Any T	N1		Any G
Stage IV	Any T	Any N	M1	Any G

*Superficial tumors are located exclusively above the superficial fascia without invasion of the fascia; deep tumors are located either exclusively beneath the superficial fascia, superficial to the fascia with invasion of or through the fascia, or both superficial yet beneath the fascia.

†Note: Presence of positive nodes (N1) in M0 tumors is considered Stage III.

Used with the permission of the American Joint Committee on Cancer (AJCC), Chicago, Illinois. The original source for this material is the AJCC Cancer Staging Manual, 7th ed. Springer Science and Business Media LLC; 2010, www.springer.com.

with high-grade extremity soft tissue sarcoma. A phase III trial, the European Organization for the Research and Treatment of Cancer 62961 (EORTC-62961), comparing regional hyperthermia with systemic chemotherapy (etoposide, ifosfamide, and Adriamycin) versus chemotherapy alone revealed improvement of overall response rate and survival in the combination group for patients with extremity involvement (78). While the data for both therapies are compelling, these modalities are still under investigation and should, therefore, only be performed at an experienced sarcoma center. We currently do not employ isolated limb perfusion or regional hyperthermia as options in our multimodality approach in the treatment of soft tissue sarcomas.

The same principles of surgical resection for soft tissue sarcomas of extremities are applied to soft tissue sarcomas in other parts of the body. However, many times these lesions are located in areas that are not amenable to "radical" resection. This makes it even more important to incorporate radiation and/or chemotherapy in a sequence deemed appropriate by a multidisciplinary group with experience and expertise in these areas. Unfortunately, even with the multimodality approach, local recurrences are common in head and neck and retroperitoneal sarcomas.

Radiation

Although radiation is not effective for the treatment of gross disease, it has been a useful adjunct to surgery in the treatment of microscopic local disease and for palliation of symptoms. In the past, soft tissue sarcomas were thought to be relatively resistant to radiation for several reasons. Tumors treated with radiation regress slowly, low-energy radiation beams initially used in treatment of these tumors were less effective than the beams currently available, and previous clinical experience demonstrating resistance was based in large part on studies where radiation was the sole therapy used (79). Now, however, both experimental and clinical studies have shown that radiation is an effective adjuvant treatment modality for soft tissue sarcomas (79,80). In patients with sarcomas arising from certain anatomic locations, there are limitations on the amount of radiation that may be delivered to the tumor or tumor bed due to the proximity to vital normal tissues. These locations include the abdomen, paraspinal region, lungs, and mediastinum. Some of these limitations are being overcome with better planning (intensity-modulated radiation therapy [IMRT]) or the use of heavier particles, for example proton beam radiation, which limits the scatter to surrounding normal tissues and therefore minimizes toxicity while delivering a full therapeutic dose to the target volume.

Radiation therapy is occasionally used as the sole treatment modality for palliation for some patients with soft tissue sarcomas. These patients are often those who have unresectable disease or who are not appropriate candidates for surgery and/or chemotherapy. There have been reports of 5-year survival rates ranging from 25 to 40% with radiation therapy alone, and of local control rates of approximately 30%, depending on the primary tumor's size and biology (80-82).

Radiation therapy is commonly used in the pre- or postoperative adjuvant setting. Studies comparing pre- and postoperative radiation therapy found that wound complications were twice as common with preoperative as opposed to postoperative radiation. Larger field sizes and higher doses were required with postoperative radiation and grade 2 or greater fibrosis or edema was more common in patients receiving this treatment (83-85). Because there are pros and cons about the timing of radiation therapy, this topic remains controversial; appropriate discussion between radiation oncologists, medical oncologists, and surgeons is required in planning the treatment of each patient (86,87).

Preoperative radiation has several advantages over postoperative radiation, including smaller radiation portals, easier surgical resection from vital structures, conversion to a limb-sparing procedure, reduction of the extent of the surgical procedure, and lower radiation doses, which can be utilized because there are theoretically fewer radioresistant hypoxic cells within the tumor and surgical removal can supplement the boost (83, 88-90). However, preoperative radiotherapy may lead to difficulty in assessing pathologic responses to preoperative chemotherapy and may also contribute to delayed wound healing. Several studies have shown improved local control rates with preoperative radiation, especially with larger tumors that were initially considered unresectable (64,72,91-93). The modality of choice is external beam radiotherapy (EBRT), and a dose of 50 Gy or more is often required to obtain local control. At these dose levels, the entire circumference of the extremity must not be irradiated in order to avoid lymphedema (64,72,93). A period of 4 to 6 weeks is needed following preoperative radiation to prevent wound complications. Following the surgical resection, close or positive margins could be treated with a radiation boost if feasible. Brachytherapy (BRT), EBRT, or intraoperative radiotherapy (IORT) can be used by experienced clinicians in appropriate situations (Fig. 40-2) (94,95).

As compared to preoperative radiation therapy, there is more literature regarding the use of postoperative radiation. In patients with high-grade soft tissue sarcomas of the extremities with positive microscopic margins (<1 mm from the inked margin, despite all efforts at achieving negative margins),

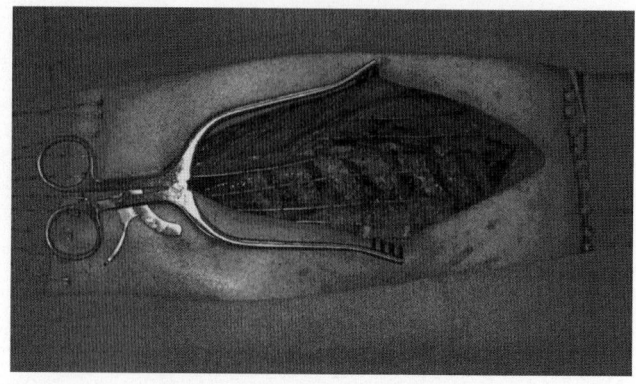

FIGURE 40-2. Brachytherapy wires used intraoperatively. (*Courtesy of Dr. Matthew Ballo, Department of Radiation Oncology, The University of Texas MD Anderson Cancer Center.*)

adjuvant radiation can improve 5-year local control rate compared to the no-RT group (74 versus 56% and *p* = .01, respectively) (96,97). Adjuvant BRT has been shown in a prospective study to improve 5-year local control rates compared to patients randomized to the BRT group (82 versus 69% and *p* = .04, respectively) except for low-grade tumors where EBRT is preferred (63). IMRT has also been shown to provide a great 5-year local control rate of 94% in high-risk patients following limb-sparing surgery with negative or positive margins (98).

The interval of time between surgery and initiation of radiation therapy is a controversial but legitimate concern. The most recent soft tissue sarcoma guidelines issued by the National Comprehensive Cancer Network (NCCN) suggest the interval to be no longer than 6 weeks (94). The primary concern is whether delayed adjuvant radiation therapy may contribute to local failure. The University of Texas MD Anderson Cancer Center (MDACC) investigators have conducted a retrospective review of 799 patients with soft tissue sarcoma treated with postoperative radiation therapy between 1960 and 2000 (99). Using local recurrence as the primary endpoint, the overall local control rate at 10 and 15 years was 79 and 78%, respectively. The interval between surgery and radiation therapy ranged from 6 to 490 days and the median interval was 34 days. Although a trend toward decreased 10-year local control rate was noted for patients initiating radiotherapy more than 30 days from surgery, the difference was not statistically significant. Although this is a retrospective analysis with the potential for bias, this large series suggest that justifiable treatment delays may not adversely affect local control rates;

however, long treatment delays should be avoided if possible.

Chemotherapy

Some soft tissue sarcomas are more sensitive to chemotherapy than others. Small cell sarcomas, synovial sarcomas, angiosarcomas, uterine leiomyosarcomas (LMS), and myxoid liposarcomas are sensitive to conventional chemotherapy. Aside from small cell sarcomas, synovial sarcomas are among the most responsive to chemotherapy, particularly to ifosfamide-based regimens (100-103). Evidence also suggests that myxoid liposarcomas are very responsive to doxorubicin-based regimens (104,105). Extraskeletal osteosarcomas, chondrosarcomas, and Ewing sarcomas are treated in a similar fashion as soft tissue sarcomas. In our experience at MDACC, extraskeletal osteosarcomas are not as responsive to chemotherapy as osseous osteosarcomas and do not respond to cisplatin or high-dose methotrexate unlike their skeletal counterparts. (106). GISTs (discussed further on), alveolar soft part sarcomas, clear cell sarcomas, and hemangiopericytomas, on the other hand, are resistant to standard chemotherapy and therefore should not be treated with standard therapies, as the toxicities and risks clearly outweigh any benefit.

The two most active agents in the treatment of soft tissue sarcoma are doxorubicin and ifosfamide. Unfortunately very few other known active agents are currently available. Studies have shown that both doxorubicin and ifosfamide also exhibit a positive dose-response curve (Fig. 40-3) (107,108). Doxorubicin is most active at doses of ≥75 mg/m^2, with single-agent response rates of approximately 20 to 35%. When given by a 48- to 96-h continuous infusion, it is less cardiotoxic (107). Ifosfamide has been shown to produce single-agent response rates similar to those of single-agent doxorubicin when used at doses of 10 g/m^2 or higher (108). Ifosfamide has also been shown to have greater efficacy when administered as a 2- to 3-h infusion as opposed to a 24-h infusion (108-111). Dacarbazine (DTIC) has activity as a single agent, with response rates of 10 to 15%. The three-drug regimen MAID (mesna, Adriamycin [doxorubicin], ifosfamide, dacarbazine) has been studied and has shown response rates varying from 25 to 47% (112,113). When the MAID regimen was studied at MDACC, significant toxicities related to the addition of DTIC were seen (114). The combination of doxorubicin (75 or 90 mg/m^2) and ifosfamide at 10 g/m^2 without DTIC was then evaluated in two pilot studies at MDACC in patients with soft tissue sarcomas; objective response rates of 66% (95% confidence interval [CI], 46-82%) were seen. This regimen is most often used in the clinic at MDACC in patients who are otherwise healthy, ≤65 years of age, and with high-risk tumors (115). Because of these encouraging results, this regimen was further studied and thrombopoietin was added for platelet support. The results showed a 75% response rate (95 CI, 59-71%; complete response [CR] 12%) in patients with primary tumors of the extremities and a 68% response rate (95% CI, 56-80%; CR 12%) in patients with primary disease at any site (116). The breakdown of response rates according to histology from this study was as follows: malignant fibrous histiocytoma (MFH) 69%, synovial sarcoma 88%, unclassified sarcomas 60%, non-GI–leiomyosarcomas 50%, liposarcomas 56%, angiosarcomas 83%, neurogenic sarcomas 40%; other miscellaneous histologies demonstrated objective response rates of 45% (116). These data show that sensitivity to chemotherapy depends on the histologic type of sarcoma and points to the importance of proper histologic diagnosis in determining prognosis.

Other agents have been studied in soft tissue sarcomas. Often, these are used after failure of doxorubicin and ifosfamide. Response rates in patients whose disease failed doxorubicin-based therapy and then received high-dose ifosfamide, as a single agent, was 29% for soft tissue sarcomas (108). The response rate (RR) was higher (30-40%) for the bolus schedule; therefore, high-dose ifosfamide as a single agent with doses of 14 g/m^2 is sometimes used as a salvage regimen at MDACC.

Gemcitabine alone but, more commonly, in combination with docetaxel is frequently used for the

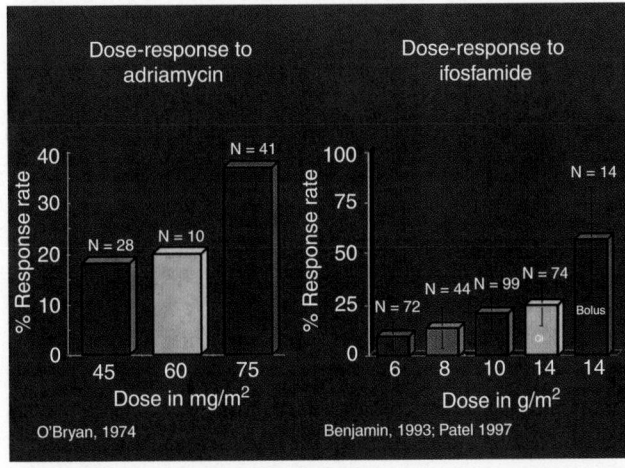

FIGURE 40-3. Doxorubicin and ifosfamide dose-response curves.

treatment of advanced, recurrent, or metastatic disease once patients fail doxorubicin- and ifosfamide-based therapy or in patients who may not tolerate intensive chemotherapy. A two-arm phase II study using gemcitabine as a single agent was performed using doses of $1g/m^2$ on a weekly schedule (117). A response rate of 18% (95% CI, 7-29%) was seen even though many patients had received prior chemotherapies. The median duration of response was 3.5 months, ranging from 2 to 13 months. Four patients with leiomyosarcomas (LMS) of non-GI origin achieved a partial response, which suggests that there may be selective activity in this subset of patients. Studies by the GI medical oncology group at MDACC demonstrated benefit with prolonged infusions of gemcitabine at $10 mg/m^2/min$ or a "fixed-dose rate" (118,119). Soon after, a study evaluated gemcitabine given at $900 mg/m^2$ on days 1 and 8 and docetaxel $100 mg/m^2$ on day 8, after gemcitabine, repeated every 21 days in patients with unresectable LMS of gynecologic origin (120). The results showed that 3 of 34 patients achieved CR and 15 achieved a partial response, for an overall response rate of 53% (95% CI, 35-70%). To address the additive/synergistic effect of docetaxel to gemcitabine, a randomized phase II study was designed and conducted by SARC. Patients were randomized to receive gemcitabine (fixed dose rate of $10 mg/m^2/min$ at $1200 mg/m^2$ days 1 and 8, every 21 days) or gemcitabine-docetaxel (gemcitabine dose was fixed-dose rate $900 mg/m^2$ days 1 and 8, and docetaxel $100 mg/m^2$ on day 8, of a 21-day cycle) (121). The investigators used the Response Evaluation Criteria in Solid Tumors (RECIST) criteria to measure their primary endpoint, tumor response (complete or partial response, or stable disease for duration greater than 24 weeks). Utilizing a bayesian adaptive design to incorporate response data and toxicity data, the schema randomized more patients to the gemcitabine-docetaxel arm compared to the gemcitabine arm due to the better response rates and acceptable toxicity (60 and 40% patients, respectively). The response rate for the gemcitabine-docetaxel arm and gemcitabine arm was 16 and 8%, respectively. Furthermore, an improvement in median progression-free survival (PFS) (6.2 versus 3.0 months) and overall survival (17.9 versus 11.5 months) was noted in the gemcitabine-docetaxel arm compared to the gemcitabine arm. The primary grade 3/4 toxicity from the combination arm was thrombocytopenia (40%). Interestingly, the two histologies most responsive to the gemcitabine-docetaxel arm were LMS and high-grade undifferentiated pleomorphic sarcomas (HGUPS).

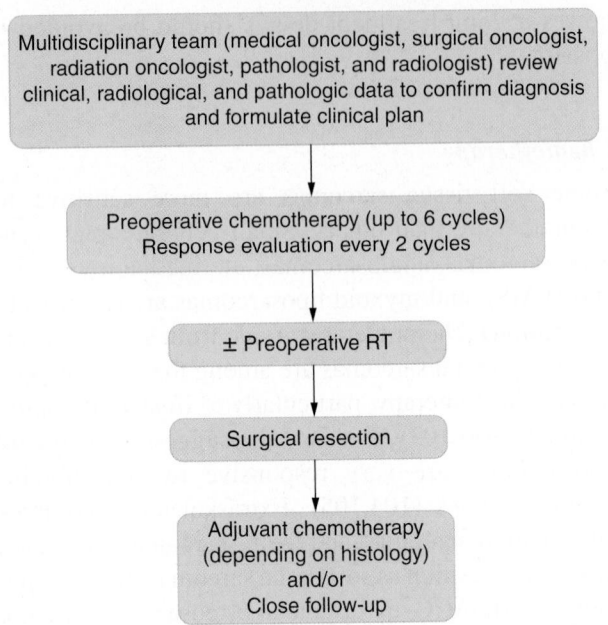

FIGURE 40-4.   Treatment approach for patients with stage III soft tissue sarcomas.

Adjuvant/Neoadjuvant chemotherapy

The goals of chemotherapy in the treatment of high-risk local disease are to eradicate micrometastasis, decrease risk of local recurrence, and downsize tumors to facilitate either limb-sparing procedures for extremity tumors or resection for tumors initially deemed unresectable. For all patients with small cell sarcomas (eg, rhabdomyosarcoma, Ewing sarcoma/primitive neuroectodermal tumor [PNET]) of any size, systemic chemotherapy is considered standard of care (Fig. 40-4). At MDACC, preoperative chemotherapy is preferred in patients with high-risk (>5 cm or high-grade) tumors.

Postoperative chemotherapy and its benefits have been debated over the last couple of decades. The majority of randomized trials conducted, mainly in the 1970s and 80s, were very small and were therefore underpowered to evaluate clinically significant improvements in disease-free and overall survival. Many of these studies also used suboptimal doses of chemotherapy and included patients with a variety of tumor histologies and grades, making evaluation of these studies difficult in terms of the current knowledge of chemotherapy dose and prognostic factors. The Sarcoma Meta-Analysis Collaboration (SMAC) undertook a quantitative intention-to-treat meta-analysis of all 14 randomized trials of adjuvant chemotherapy from the 1970s and 80s to answer some of the questions regarding benefit of doxorubicin-based chemotherapy in patients with localized, resectable soft tissue sarcomas. This meta-analysis showed a significant improvement for local and distant recurrence-free survival and for overall survival in patients with extremity sarcomas; however, the survival advantage for the entire group failed to achieve statistical significance (116). Recently, a Canadian group reviewed the published trials from the SMAC meta-analysis and factored in four more trials into the analysis (122). The additional trials consisted of doxorubicin-ifosfamide combinations, not previously represented in the original SMAC meta-analysis. The addition of these four trials increased the total number of trials to 18, and the total number of patients included in the analysis was 1953. As with the previous analysis, the results of this updated meta-analysis detected favorable odds-ratios (OR) of local recurrence and distant recurrence for chemotherapy. Although the absolute risk reduction (ARR) in distant recurrence with adjuvant doxorubicin-based chemotherapy for all studies was 9% (95% CI, 5-14%, $p = .000$), the ARR with adjuvant doxorubicin-ifosfamide chemotherapy was 10% (95% CI, 1-19%; $p = .03$) (122). By pooling all the data, the numbers needed to treat (NNT) to prevent distant recurrence was 12. Although a survival benefit was not noted with single-agent doxorubicin, a statistically significant survival advantage was observed with the doxorubicin-ifosfamide combination. The OR for overall survival with the doxorubicin-ifosfamide cohort was 0.56 (95% CI, 0.36-0.85; $p = .01$). Combining all trials in the meta-analysis, the NNT to prevent 1 death was 17. Although the obvious limitation to this study is the use of published results rather than review of actual patient files, it does provide more evidence to suggest that, for certain patients with localized soft tissue sarcomas and high-risk features, adjuvant chemotherapy is beneficial. Therefore, the common practice at our institution regarding adjuvant chemotherapy is to offer treatment with doxorubicin (75 mg/m^2, continuous intravenous infusion over 72 h) in combination with ifosfamide (total bolus dose of 10 g/m^2 over 4 or 5 days) to healthy patients with intact organ function who have high-risk disease (tumor size >5 cm, high-grade histology, and deep soft tissue involvement). If toxicity becomes concerning or excessive, patients are usually treated in the hospital rather than in the outpatient setting.

Locally Recurrent Disease

During the evaluation of the patient with locally recurrent disease, an attempt is made to determine possible reasons for treatment failure and whether this is truly recurrent disease versus a new primary tumor. Workup is conducted to evaluate the primary tumor as well to look for metastatic disease. Surgical, chemotherapeutic, and radiation options for treatment depend on the management of the initial tumor and are sometimes limited; however, patients with local recurrence can be potentially cured of their disease. Surgery, radiation, and chemotherapy should be considered as outlined above.

Metastasectomy

Patients with obvious metastatic disease to multiple organ systems are generally incurable and considered appropriate for palliative systemic therapy, as described above. The subset of patients with lung-only metastatic disease, especially with a greater than 12-month disease-free interval, have a favorable biology and prognosis and should be considered for resection if feasible. This approach results in 3- to 5-year survival of up to 20%. Chemotherapy is the mainstay of therapy for patients with metastatic disease although surgical resection of residual disease to render patients free of gross disease is often pursued. The sequencing of chemotherapy is similar to that of isolated local disease. In a study done at MDACC, patients with metastatic disease showed a 57% response rate to doxorubicin (75-90 mg/m^2) and ifosfamide (10 g/m^2) (116). If patients fail this regimen, the choice of treatment may depend on the histology of the tumor and/or the performance status of the patient. High-dose ifosfamide as described above is an acceptable salvage therapy for most soft tissue sarcoma subtypes. For patients with compromised renal function, declining performance status, or LMS histology, gemcitabine in combination with docetaxel is a possibility. Most other therapies would be best utilized in the context of a clinical trial. There are times when surgery and/or radiation may also be used for palliation of symptoms. These cases are very selective and should be discussed in a multimodality planning conference, as the risks and benefits of such therapies must be weighed carefully.

GASTROINTESTINAL STROMAL TUMORS

GISTs are the most common mesenchymal tumors of the GI tract (123). Until recently, they were often designated smooth muscle tumors of the GI tract—specifically, GI leiomyosarcoma, leiomyoblastoma, leiomyosarcoma, and leiomyomas. Investigators discovered that GISTs express the KIT (CD-117) receptor tyrosine kinase and possibly originate from the interstitial cell of Cajal (or a closely related cell), the intestinal pacemaker cell responsible for peristalsis (124). These tumors most commonly arise in the stomach (60-70%), small intestine (20-30%), colon and rectum (5%), and esophagus (<5%), although they can arise anywhere in the GI tract or omentum/peritoneum (extra-GI GIST). The liver, peritoneum, and abdominal wall are the most common sites of metastatic disease; however, there are reports of associated central nervous system (CNS), lymph node, lung, and bone metastasis (125). The incidence of GIST is equal in men and women; it generally peaks between the fourth and sixth decades of life, and patients are more commonly Caucasian. Presenting symptoms often represent the site of tumor origin, but they may be vague, including abdominal pain, anorexia, weight loss, and dyspepsia.

Traditional chemotherapy or radiotherapy has historically not been effective in the treatment of GIST. As early as 1975, Gottlieb et al. at MDACC observed that leiomyosarcomas arising from the GI tract did not respond to doxorubicin-based chemotherapy, as leiomyosarcomas that arose from other organ systems did (126). Other agents have been studied in GISTs, also with disappointing results. A phase II study of gemcitabine in patients with metastatic GI leiomyosarcoma found no objective responses in 17 patients treated (117). Prior to the availability of imatinib, we published a phase II trial of temozolomide in patients with GIST in which there were no objective responses (127).

Since the last edition of this book, treatment guidelines for GIST have changed. Imatinib mesylate, which has now been extensively studied, selectively inhibits BCR-ABL, KIT, and PDGFR tyrosine kinases (128,129). GISTs occur due to gain-of-function mutations in the KIT gene (130). The first case report of imatinib use for GIST described a patient with widely metastatic, chemotherapy-resistant disease who, after several weeks of therapy, had a durable major objective clinical response for more than 18 months (131). Early clinical trial results were also encouraging. A single-arm phase I study conducted by the EORTC and the B2222 phase II trial, a study of two-dose schedules for imatinib, noted objective response rates of 69 and 53.7%, respectively (132,133). An update to the B2222 trial revealed an ORR of 68% and, at median follow-up of 71 months, no difference in time to progression (TTP) was noted between treatment arms, though the 5-year survival rate for both arms was about 50% (134). These trial results led to the implementation of two phase III trials (EORTC 62005 and SWOG S0033), which were designed to compare imatinib at two-dose

levels (400 mg/day versus 800 mg/day) (135,136). In both studies, the higher-dose arm (800 mg/day) failed to show a statistically significant difference in response or overall survival (OS) as compared to the once-daily dosing schedule. A subsequent meta-analysis of both trials did, in fact, show a slight increase in PFS at the higher dose compared to the lower dose (137). As with metastatic GIST, imatinib has shown efficacy in the adjuvant setting (138). These studies have demonstrated that the sensitivity of GIST to imatinib is, in part, a function of the KIT genotype. GIST with KIT exon 11 mutations, which are generally deletions, are most responsive to imatinib as compared with tumors expressing mutations in KIT exon 9 or in wild-type KIT-expressing GIST (139). Before imatinib, KIT exon 11 mutation expressing GIST carried a worse prognosis than patients with no KIT mutation (140). So the presence of the mutation portends an aggressive clinical course, while the actual site of mutation is of predictive significance. The most common site of KIT mutation is in exon 11. Patients with this mutation have a significantly higher response rate, PFS, and OS with imatinib compared to those with exon 9 mutation (139,141). Of equal importance is that the primary cause of secondary resistance to imatinib is the development of new mutations within the KIT gene (142,143). These new mutations generally occur within exon 13 and exon 17 of the KIT gene (Fig. 40-5). Sunitinib, a multikinase inhibitor, appears to have activity in patients with secondary KIT

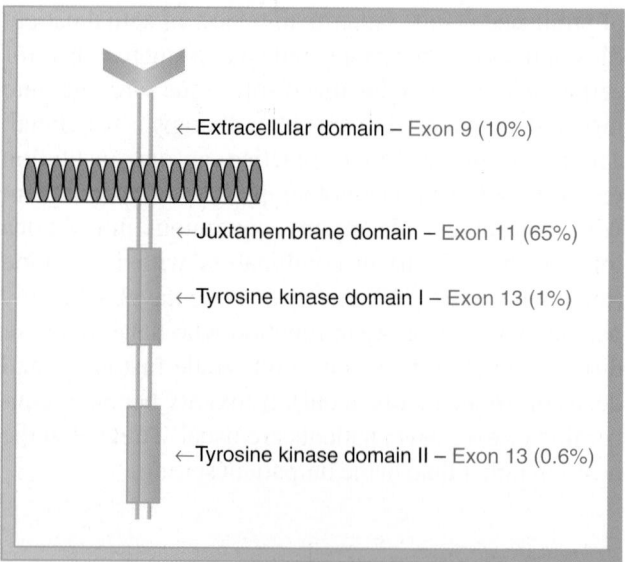

FIGURE 40-5. The KIT receptor tyrosine kinase with mutation sites observed in GISTs which are tested at MDACC.

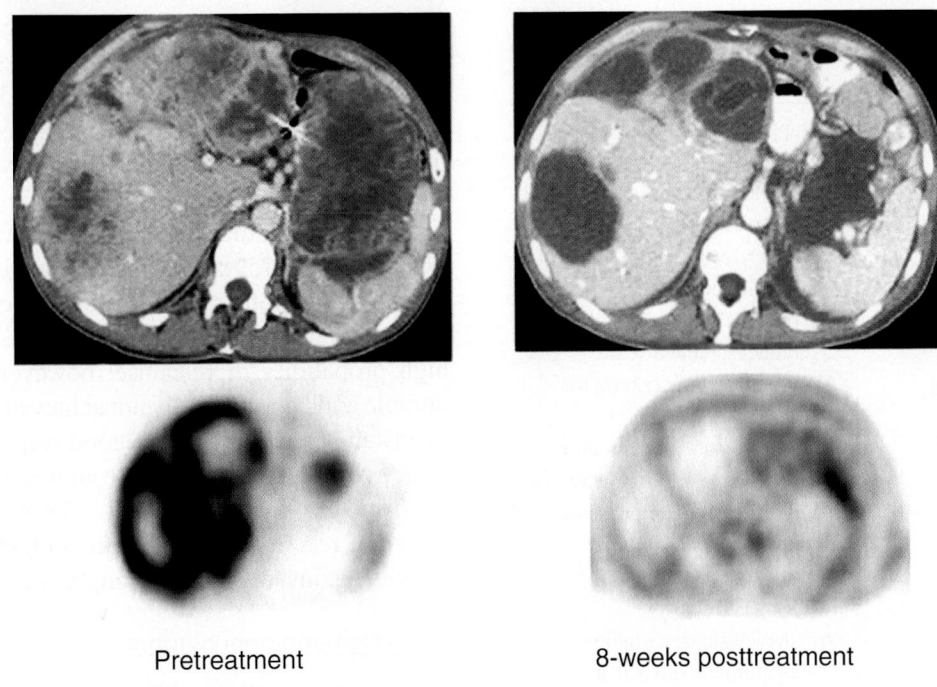

Pretreatment   8-weeks posttreatment

FIGURE 40-6. Gastrointestinal stromal tumor response to Gleevec therapy, CT, and PET imaging. (*Courtesy of Dr. Haesun Choi, Department of Diagnostic Radiology, The University of Texas MD Anderson Cancer Center.*)

mutations (144,145). Other KIT inhibitors such dasatinib and nilotinib are still under investigation for the treatment of imatinib-refractory GIST.

Assessment of imatinib plasma levels may be useful when patients develop progression of disease while on imatinib. Data from B2222 and a retrospective review conducted at MDACC suggest that imatinib levels greater than 1100 ng/mL usually correspond with a better outcome (146,147). Because patients with GIST commonly have a history of surgery involving portions of the GI tract, it is possible to surmise that drug absorption may be altered. Other factors that may affect imatinib plasma levels include drugs that alter hepatic metabolism, serum albumin levels, and noncompliance. Studies are in development to prospectively study the use of imatinib plasma testing in guiding treatment decisions.

The role of radiographic imaging for response assessment has also changed since the last edition of this book. Though the standard measurement of response is by CT scan, PET is increasingly being utilized for treatment decisions. PET was initially noted to show treatment response at an earlier time point compared to standard CT imaging (39). Clinicians at MDACC have demonstrated that certain molecular events, such as apoptosis, occur early on and may partially explain the rationale behind early PET response related to

imatinib (148). Our institution also demonstrated that RECIST criteria may underestimate early tumor response seen in GIST. In fact, patients who respond to imatinib clinically may show a decrease in tumor size and/or a decrease in tumor radiodensity by CT radiography (Fig. 40-6). Further analysis of patients treated with imatinib at MDACC revealed that, when tumor density is taken into account, sensitivity of CT imaging is comparable to PET response (149-151). These data culminated in the development of the Choi criteria of response assessment (Table 40-4). These response criteria have been evaluated in a prospective setting, but the results have yet to be published. It is our experience that decisions to discontinue therapy should not be based solely on CT radiography or PET imaging, but instead the patient's overall clinical condition should also be taken into consideration.

In summary, the frontline therapy for patients with newly diagnosed, metastatic GIST is imatinib at 400 mg daily. Imatinib should be continued indefinitely or until progression, as defined by Choi criteria. CT imaging is used to assess response initially at 2 months and then at 3-month intervals for at least the first 2 years. At the time of progression, we check the plasma imatinib level and, if tolerable, we increase the dose of imatinib to a total of 800 mg daily. If or when this strategy fails, we switch to sunitinib. For patients with isolated or

TABLE 40-4 | CHOI RESPONSE CRITERIA

Response	Response Definition
Complete response (CR)	Disappearance of all disease
	No new lesions
Partial response (PR)	A decrease in size of >10% *or* a decrease in CT density (HU) >15%
	No new lesions
	No obvious progression of nonmeasurable disease
Stable disease (SD)	Does not meet the criteria for CR, PR, or PD
	No symptomatic deterioration attributed to tumor progression
Progression of disease (PD)	An increase in unidimensional tumor size of >10% *and* does not meet criteria for PR by CT density
	Any new lesions, including new tumor nodules in a previous cystic tumor

resectable metastatic disease, surgery and/or hepatic artery embolization or radiofrequency ablation is offered if feasible. For resectable GIST patients with high-risk features, such as a high mitotic count and/or large tumor size, adjuvant imatinib for at least 1 year should be administered to increase recurrence-free survival. The duration of imatinib use, in the adjuvant setting, beyond 1 year is still under investigation.

SPECIFIC SOFT TISSUE SARCOMAS

Angiosarcomas

Angiosarcomas represent a rare subset (2%) of soft tissue sarcomas with a vascular origin, the endothelial cell (152-154). This disease generally affects people over the age of 50 years and has a male predominance. This heterogeneous disease is generally visible on the scalp and face of elderly men but can also be found on the breast, extremities, pelvis, and trunk. The etiology is also varied; exposure to vinyl chloride and previous radiation represent the root cause for some but not all cases (17,155). Chronic lymphedema has been implicated in Stewart-Treves syndrome, in which women previously treated for breast cancer with radical mastectomy develop chronic lymphedema leading to the development of lymphangiosarcoma (156). Diagnosis is often based on the patient's history, visual inspection,

but, ultimately, confirmed by pathologic examination. By immunohistochemistry, these tumors generally stain for factor VIII–related antigen, CD 34 antigen, and vimentin (157). The initial site of disease and presentation of metastasis at diagnosis greatly influence survival (158). When these lesions are amenable to surgical resection, 5-year disease-specific survival (DSS) can be as high as 60% (159). In terms of systemic treatment, conventional chemotherapy with anthracycline/ifosfamide and gemcitabine/docetaxel combinations provides a very high probability of response; however, these are not durable and cure is usually not achieved in patients with metastatic disease despite a good response. Paclitaxel, an active drug for unresectable angiosarcoma, has been confirmed by several studies (153,160,161). However, there are recent reports of antiangiogenic agents with activity against unresectable angiosarcoma (162,163).

Hemangiopericytoma

Hemangiopericytoma and solitary fibrous tumor (HPC/SFT) are closely related rare soft tissue sarcomas which are thought to arise from fibroblasts (164). HPCs/SFTs primarily affect adults aged 20 to 70 and are found in virtually at any body site (165). HPCs/SFTs are classically characterized by a presence of "staghorn" thick-walled vessels, sheaths of spindle-cells, and CD34 positivity, but in reality these histopathologic features vary greatly. Complete surgical resection is an effective primary therapy for a majority of HPC/SFT, resulting in cure. Approximately 15 to 20% of HPC/SFT patients, however, display a more aggressive behavior and develop local and/or distant metastases (166,167). Repeat surgical resections, whenever possible, should be attempted. For unresectable or metastatic disease, systemic chemotherapy, radiation therapy, and/or stereotactic radiosurgery are utilized (168,169). The efficacy of conventional systemic chemotherapy in advanced HPC/SFT is very limited and therefore not recommended for routine use.

Recently, a MDACC retrospective study of 14 patients with unresectable, locally recurrent, or metastatic HPC/SFT who received temozolomide and bevacizumab has found this combination therapy to be a potentially more effective regimen than doxorubicin-based therapy (170). All patients were treated with temozolomide 150 mg/m^2 orally on days 1 to 7 and 15 to 21 and bevacizumab 5 mg/kg intravenously on days 8 and 22 on a 28-day cycle. Overall response rate, using the Choi criteria, showed 79% PR and 14% SD. The median PFS was 8.6 months. Currently, at MDACC the temozolomide and bevacizumab combination therapy is our treatment of choice for advanced HPC/SFT.

The exact mechanisms by which temozolomide and bevacizumab exert their action on HPC/SFT are not clear, but antiangiogenic pathways, especially that involving the vascular endothelial growth factor (VEGF) pathway, are implicated. Additional case reports of HPC/SFT achieving disease control on anti-VEGFR agents including sorafenib, sunitinib, and pazopanib also support this hypothesis (163,171-173). Future studies will need to better determine the utility of these agents in HPC/SFT.

Myxoid Liposarcoma

Liposarcomas represent the second most common soft tissue sarcoma in the United States. There are several histologic subtypes of liposarcoma with unique clinical and biological features. Myxoid liposarcoma represents the most common variant of liposarcoma. Other subsets include well-differentiated, dedifferentiated, and pleomorphic subtypes. Myxoid liposarcoma derives its name from the appearance of its myxoid matrix in addition to its unique plexiform capillary network and signet-ring lipoblasts (104,174,175). Myxoid liposarcomas often occur in the third through fifth decade of life. These tumors generally develop in the extremities with the thigh representing the most common location. Though this disease is regarded a low-grade tumor, local recurrence and distant metastasis occur in about 30% of patients. One single-institution study of 214 patients with myxoid liposarcoma found that local recurrence occurred by a median time of 24 months from diagnosis (176). Interestingly, for patients who developed distant metastatic disease, the median time from diagnosis to distant metastasis was 20 months. Sites of metastasis include the lungs and soft tissue regions such as the axilla, retroperitoneum, the pleural lining, and even the pericardium. A rare variant of myxoid liposarcoma, round cell liposarcoma, is considered to be a more malignant variant of a spectrum of this disease. One study observed an increase in round cell percentage as a correlate to metastasis and poor survival compared with myxoid liposarcomas containing less round cell predominance (175). Though most cases contain a diploid karyotype, a common chromosomal abnormality is the t(12;16), *FUS-CHOP* (177,178). The product of this arrangement is thought to contribute to the oncogenesis, resulting in myxoid liposarcoma (179). Treatment options for this disease depend on the location and size of the lesion. Whereas surgery and radiation are more feasible for extremity locations, retroperitoneal involvement is less amenable to surgery for curative intent. As with other soft tissue sarcomas, large size and depth of invasion are considered high-risk features that warrant treatment with chemotherapy. Importantly, myxoid liposarcoma is considered a chemosensitive disease. Reports from MDACC using doxorubicin-based chemotherapy yield response rates of 44%. Trabectedin (also known as ecteinascidin 743 [ET-743]), a unique alkylating agent derived from the marine tunicate, *Ecteinascidia turbinata*, has been shown in various trials to have higher activity in myxoid liposarcoma (180-183). Aside from binding to the minor groove of DNA and forming covalent adducts, this agent is thought to promote differentiation of myxoid liposarcoma lipoblasts. This agent is approved for use by European Medicines Evaluation Agency (EMEA) in Europe but remains investigational in the United States.

FOLLOW-UP MANAGEMENT

The major goals of follow-up surveillance and management should be early identification of potentially curable recurrences, identification of treatment-related complications, and patient reassurance. Much of the surveillance of patients treated for soft tissue sarcomas is based on known prognostic factors, outcomes in individual subsets of patients, and patterns of tumor recurrence. These patterns vary depending on the anatomic site of the primary tumor; it is also important to realize that lymph node metastases occur extremely rarely in soft tissue sarcomas (<5%). Patients with extremity and superficial trunk primaries often have distant lung metastasis rather than local or regional recurrences, whereas patients whose primary is located in the retroperitoneum, head and neck, or visceral organs tend to have higher incidences of local rather than distant metastasis.

For patients with low-risk T1 primaries of the extremities (or other sites) who have undergone treatment with curative intent and are free of any gross evidence of disease, follow-up should include a history and physical, cross-sectional imaging to encompass the tumor bed to evaluate for local recurrence, and routine chest x-rays for surveillance of metastatic disease (50). Imaging of the primary tumor site should be done with the modality best for that particular site. For tumors of the head and neck and extremities, MRI imaging is appropriate; for tumors of the chest cavity, abdomen, and retroperitoneum, CT scans are appropriate (50). Ultrasound technology can be a useful tool in imaging primary tumor sites of the extremity and superficial trunk when in the hands of an experienced ultrasonographer, but this is extremely operator-dependent and requires expertise, experience, and consistency (50).

The routine use of chest CT for evaluation of metastatic disease in soft tissue sarcomas has been studied and found not to be cost-effective; further, when it was used, the group that underwent both CT and chest x-ray was found to have a lower (65%) 5-year metastases-free survival than the group followed with chest x-ray alone (90%) (184). The interval and length of time to follow these patients depends on the clinician to some degree. The NCCN guidelines recommend follow-up with annual scanning of the primary site for at least 5 years; however, often these patients are seen every 3 to 4 months in the immediate postoperative period for the first 2 years, then every 4 to 6 months for the next 2 years, and yearly thereafter (50,185).

Patients with high-risk T2 (>5 cm) soft tissue sarcomas are at a greater risk for distant lung metastases than those with low-risk tumors. In patients with high-risk tumors who have undergone treatment with curative intent and are free of any gross evidence of disease, follow-up should include a history and physical, cross-sectional imaging to encompass the tumor bed to evaluate for local recurrence, and routine chest x-rays for surveillance of metastatic disease (50). These patients are followed in the same manner as low-risk patients, with follow-up visits with the above studies every 3 months for the first 1 to 2 years, then visits every 4 months for the next 1 to 2 years, followed by visits every 6 months for 1 to 2 years, and yearly visits thereafter (50). As for local recurrence surveillance, the cross-sectional imaging is omitted after 5 years, as most local recurrences appear within 5 years of initial treatment (50). There is a fair amount of variability in the frequency of visits based on the clinician's suspicion for the possibility of metastatic or locally recurrent disease, as well as patient preference.

■ BONE SARCOMA

Bone sarcomas are rare tumors. In 2009, an estimated 2570 new cases of bone sarcomas were diagnosed in the United States and 1470 deaths were attributed to this group of diseases (1). Bone tumors account for approximately 9% of all childhood cancers and comprise approximately 15% of all cancer deaths for patients below 20 years of age (1). The most common malignant tumor of bone is osteosarcoma, which accounts for approximately 20 to 45% of all bone tumors. Chondrosarcoma is second most common, accounting for approximately 20%, and the Ewing sarcoma/PNET family of tumors accounts for 11% of malignant bone tumors. The incidence of osteosarcoma is slightly higher in men than in women whereas chondrosarcoma has an equal distribution between genders. The Ewing sarcoma/PNET family of tumors also has a slightly greater predilection for men (186). This class of tumors tends to occur more frequently in children and adolescents (187,188), whereas osteosarcoma has a biphasic pattern of incidence that peaks in adolescents with the growth of long bones, and in the elderly with tumors arising in association with Paget disease or previously radiated tissues (189,190). Chondrosarcomas are usually seen in patients after the fifth decade of life, but they can also occur in younger patients, where the tumors tend to be of a higher-grade malignancy. Dedifferentiated chondrosarcomas, however, tend to occur in patients over the age of 60 years (191).

CLINICAL PRESENTATION

The clinical presentation of any bone tumor depends on its location. Virtually any bone in the body may be affected by a sarcoma (Table 40-5).

TABLE 40-5 | **FEATURES OF COMMON BONE TUMORS**

Type	Frequency (%)	Age Distribution (year)	Gender	Common Sites	Radiologic Features	Pathologic Features
Osteosarcoma	45	10-20	M > F	Metaphysis	Sunburst calcifications	Spindle cells, osteoid matrix
MFH	8	20-80	M > F	Long bones	Radiolucent with ill-defined margins	Pleomorphic spindle cells, NO osteoid
Chondrosarcoma	22	20-80	M > F	Pelvis/shoulder girdles	Lobulated appearance	Lobules, chondroid matrix
Ewing/PNET	15	10-20	F > M	Diaphyses	Lytic with soft tissue component	Small round blue cells

MFH, malignant fibrous histiocytoma; PNET, primitive neuroectodermal tumor.

Most osteosarcomas arise in the metaphyseal region of long bones, specifically the distal femur, proximal tibia, and proximal humerus. Approximately 55% of osteosarcomas occur around the knee joint. Chondrosarcomas can also arise in any bone of the body; however, they generally occur in the pelvis and other flat bones (192). Ewing sarcoma/PNET tumors tend to occur in the diaphyseal portion of the long bones and in flat bones of the body—for example, the pelvis and scapula.

The most common presenting symptom is pain and swelling or a mass. This pain is often described as initially insidious and transient, gradually becoming progressively more severe and unremitting. Swelling can also occur; it is usually localized and can be associated with warmth and erythema. Patients can have decreased range of motion and increased pain with movement or weight bearing in the affected extremity. Patients who have pelvic tumors may have neurologic impairment and severe pain, typically because these tumors are often not recognized until late in the disease course. In the case of Ewing sarcoma, patients often present with night sweats and fevers.

EVALUATION

As with all patients, evaluation of those with sarcoma should begin with a careful history, physical examination, and routine laboratory tests, followed by imaging tailored to the given complaint. The imaging of any bone tumor should begin with a plain film of the involved area. Such an x-ray image is often helpful in the diagnosis of bone sarcomas; for example, osteosarcoma often has a "sunburst" appearance of calcification on x-ray imaging, which is virtually diagnostic (Fig. 40-7).

The amount of calcification associated with osteosarcoma depends on the histologic subtype, for example, osteoblastic osteosarcoma usually has very dense calcification whereas telangiectatic osteosarcoma is primarily lytic. Chondrosarcoma also has a distinct appearance on x-ray imaging, with destruction of the bone and endosteal scalloping of the bony cortex and a chondroid matrix, which appears lobulated (see Fig. 40-7). Ewing sarcoma has a typical "onion skin" appearance on x-ray imaging (see Fig. 40-7). Other initial imaging should include a CT scan and/or MRI of the primary lesion to further evaluate involvement of the neurovascular

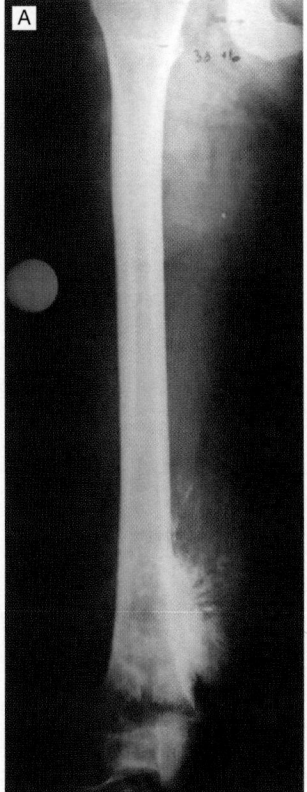
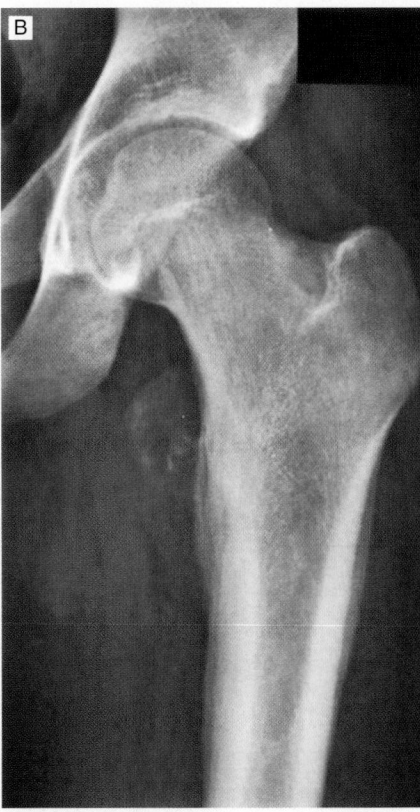
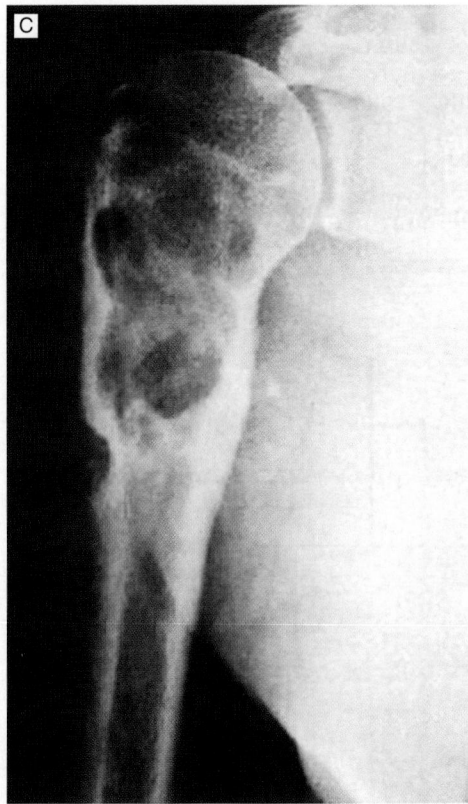

FIGURE 40-7. X-ray imaging of osteosarcoma, Ewing sarcoma, and chondrosarcoma. **A.** The typical "sunburst" appearance of osteosarcoma. **B.** The "onionskin" appearance often seen in Ewing sarcoma. **C.** The lobulated appearance of chondrosarcoma.

structures, surrounding soft tissues, and adjacent joints and to better evaluate any associated soft tissue mass. MRI may be useful to evaluate soft tissue masses associated with extremity and pelvic tumors; CT tends to be more useful in defining the cortical/bony details of involvement. These scans are often used together in the workup of bone sarcomas as complementary tests. Plain x-rays and CT scans are usually adequate for the evaluation of tumors arising from the thoracic skeleton.

As with soft tissue sarcomas, biopsy of bone sarcomas is critical to the diagnosis, and careful planning is essential. When patients are diagnosed with bone sarcoma or the diagnosis is suspected, it is important to have a multidisciplinary team approach with physicians who are experienced in the treatment of bone sarcomas. The biopsy method chosen should be the least invasive required to make the diagnosis. Most often, however, a core-needle biopsy is performed, as this tends to suffice. An open biopsy should be performed only when core-needle biopsy does not provide enough material for a conclusive diagnosis (193). When surgery is ultimately performed, care should be taken that the biopsy site is also completely resected. The pathologist should be provided not only with the specimen but also with the patient's x-ray images, as these can help make the diagnosis (194).

Once the diagnosis has been established, a chest x-ray, CT scan of the chest, and bone scan should be performed to evaluate for metastatic disease. As with soft tissue sarcomas, the most common site of metastasis from bone sarcoma is the lungs; therefore a chest x-ray and CT chest are warranted. A bone scan should be included in the workup for metastatic disease in patients with bone sarcoma to evaluate for distant bone metastases or skip metastases. For patients with Ewing sarcoma, an MRI of the spine should be performed because there is a risk of bone marrow metastases in these patients. The usefulness of PET is still under investigation. PET imaging is frequently used in pretreatment assessments for patients with osteosarcoma. At least one study has shown that a 25 to 50% reduction in SUV following 1 week of neoadjuvant chemotherapy is often found in patients who have >90% tumor necrosis on pathologic evaluation (195). Further studies are needed to confirm these results.

PATHOLOGY

As with soft tissue sarcomas, there are many histologic subsets of bone sarcoma. Osteosarcoma can be broken down into two major categories: conventional osteosarcoma and variant osteosarcoma (Fig. 40-8).

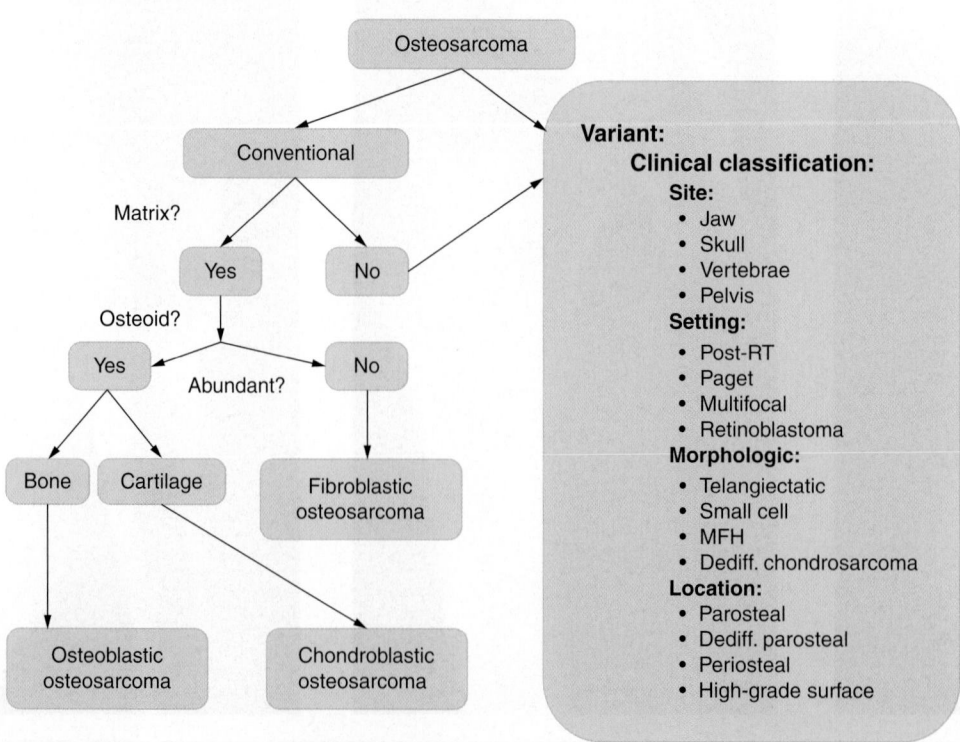

FIGURE 40-8.   Flowchart of osteosarcoma: pathologic diagnosis rationale.

Conventional osteosarcoma comprises approximately 60 to 75% of all osteosarcomas, while the 11 variants comprise the other 35 to 40% (196). Conventional osteosarcoma includes osteoblastic osteosarcoma, chondroblastic osteosarcoma, and fibroblastic osteosarcoma. These classifications are made based on the histologic features of the tumor, such as the amount of matrix present within the tumor and whether bone or cartilage is predominant. The classification of the osteosarcoma variants relies more on the clinical correlation, such as the site of disease (ie, jaw, skull, or pelvis); the setting in which the disease presents (ie, postradiation, Paget disease, multifocal, and retinoblastoma); and the morphology, such as telangiectatic, small cell, malignant fibrous histiocytoma of bone, dedifferentiated chondrosarcoma, and surface lesions such as parosteal, periosteal, and high-grade surface osteosarcoma.

MFH of bone is similar to that of soft tissue histologically and often appears to constitute the high-grade component of dedifferentiated chondrosarcoma. MFH is also sometimes seen as a component of fibroblastic osteosarcomas, the only difference between the two being the presence or absence of osteoid. MFH is thought to be part of a spectrum of osteosarcoma where the spindle cells do not produce osteoid visible by light microscopy; however, it may become possible to visualize these at some time in the future, especially postchemotherapy in responding tumors.

Chondrosarcoma is a malignant tumor of bone characterized by malignant cartilaginous proliferation. These tumors produce chondroid matrix and can arise from benign processes such as enchondroma. Chondrosarcoma is characterized by the permeation of cartilage into the bone marrow. This process is virtually pathognomonic for chondrosarcoma when other possibilities, such as chondroblastic osteosarcoma and fracture callus formation, have been excluded. It should be noted that chondroblastic osteosarcoma and chondrosarcoma are two completely separate entities with different prognoses and treatments. Dedifferentiated chondrosarcoma is a unique subset of chondrosarcomas, where the overriding component of MFH or osteosarcoma dictates therapeutic strategy, as opposed to the low-grade chondrosarcoma.

Ewing sarcoma is a completely separate histology and is grouped with the PNETs because of its similarities in histology, immunohistochemical staining, and molecular genetics. This family of tumors includes Ewing tumors of bone, extraosseous Ewing sarcoma, PNETs, and Askin tumors (PNET of the chest wall). These tumors are often referred to as "small round blue cell tumors" because, under the microscope, the cells contain scanty cytoplasm and round to oval nuclei with fine chromatin that are tightly packed together.

An important part of the pathologic review of bone tumors is the grading of the tumors by the pathologist. Bone sarcomas are classified as either high- or low-grade lesions, similar to the three-tier grading system of soft tissue sarcomas. Grading is an important factor that helps to determine the overall "stage" and prognosis.

STAGING AND PROGNOSIS

The staging of bone sarcomas is an area of debate. There are two widely accepted staging systems: the AJCC and the Musculoskeletal Tumor Society staging systems (197,198). In a comparison of these systems, there was no significant difference between them and neither had any notable advantage (199). At MDACC, instead of routinely using a staging system, we prefer to emphasize prognostic factors—for example, size of the primary, location and extent of bone involvement, soft tissue involvement, histologic grade, and presence or absence of distant metastases. The prognosis of patients with bone sarcomas largely depends on the specific histology, grade, location, and presence of metastatic disease. The most important predictive factor relating to prognosis and survival of patients with bone sarcoma is the percent of tumor necrosis achieved with preoperative chemotherapy.

TREATMENT

The treatment of bone sarcomas is best accomplished by a multidisciplinary team comprising medical oncologists, surgical oncologists, pathologists, and radiation oncologists working together to provide comprehensive care. The treatment required depends on the tumor type, location, and extent of disease. As with soft tissue sarcomas, the primary endpoint of therapy is to eradicate all gross and microscopic evidence of disease with multimodality treatment whenever possible.

Osteosarcoma

Osteosarcoma is the prototype of most other bone sarcomas. Chemotherapy is the mainstay of treatment for osteosarcoma which is a systemic disease, because most patients have micrometastatic disease at presentation. That is why there is a <20% long-term survival in patients who are treated with surgery alone (200). Patients who receive surgery alone as treatment for localized osteosarcoma tend to have pulmonary metastasis within months of surgery. Aggressive combination chemotherapy with adjuvant surgery for local control

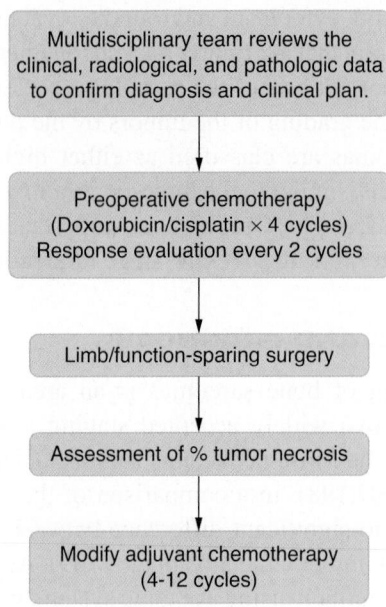

FIGURE 40-9. Treatment approach for patients with osteosarcoma/malignant fibrous histiocytoma/dedifferentiated chondrosarcoma.

can offer "cure" rates of close to 70% in patients with localized, conventional osteosarcoma of an extremity (200). With the use of preoperative chemotherapy, the majority of patients can undergo limb-sparing procedures, which offer increased function and a better quality of life.

At MDACC, patients with conventional high-grade osteosarcoma of an extremity receive treatment consisting of preoperative chemotherapy followed by limb-sparing surgery, followed by postoperative chemotherapy (Fig. 40-9).

The postoperative therapy chosen is based on the knowledge of the percent necrosis found in the pathologic specimen after surgery. The most active agents for the treatment of osteosarcoma are cisplatin, doxorubicin (Adriamycin), ifosfamide, and high-dose methotrexate (108,109,201-204). Intra-arterial administration of cisplatin (120 mg/m^2) in combination with doxorubicin (90 mg/m^2 continuous infusion over 96 h) given preoperatively has been studied by investigators at MDACC (200). This regimen is given every 3 weeks for a total of four cycles prior to surgery. Tumor is continually reassessed prior to each two cycles of therapy. Despite the utility of imaging as a determinant of response to treatment, the percentage of tumor necrosis is the single most important predictor of long-term disease-free and overall survival (205). Generally, patients with ≥90% tumor necrosis after preoperative chemotherapy have a

5-year continuous disease-free survival of approximately 80% (200). The 5-year continuous disease-free survival of patients with <90% tumor necrosis after preoperative chemotherapy with doxorubicin and cisplatin depended on their postoperative chemotherapy. If the same doxorubicin-based regimen was continued, it was 13%, compared to 34% with the addition of high-dose methotrexate and 67% with the addition of high-dose methotrexate and ifosfamide (200). For patients who achieve ≥90% tumor necrosis with four cycles of doxorubicin and cisplatin preoperatively, we recommend four additional cycles of doxorubicin (75 mg/m^2) combined with ifosfamide (10 g/m^2). For those with <90% tumor necrosis after preoperative doxorubicin and cisplatin, we favor six cycles of high-dose ifosfamide and six cycles of high-dose methotrexate given sequentially.

Memorial Sloan Kettering Cancer Center randomized patients to receive the T10 regimen (high-dose methotrexate, bleomycin, cyclophosphamide, dactinomycin) preoperatively, followed by doxorubicin and cisplatin postoperatively, or patients received a more intense regimen of two cycles of doxorubicin or cisplatin in addition to the T10 chemotherapy (T12 protocol) followed by doxorubicin or cisplatin postoperatively (206). The 5-year event-free survival was similar in both groups, at 78 and 73%, respectively. Researchers in Italy performed a series of studies in which they used high-dose methotrexate with one of three combinations (cisplatin and ifosfamide, cisplatin and doxorubicin, or doxorubicin and ifosfamide) (207). Each of the four chemotherapeutic agents was used as a single agent in the postoperative setting. A total of 121 patients with primary osteosarcoma of an extremity were evaluated; the resulting data showed that the limb-salvage rate was 97% and that 32% of patients achieved total tumor necrosis. With a median follow-up of 36 months, 76% of patients remained without recurrence. The projected 3-year continuous disease-free survival was 75%, and the overall survival was 91%. Several other studies with similar combinations support the use of doxorubicin, cisplatin, ifosfamide, and high-dose methotrexate in the pre- and postoperative treatment of osteosarcoma (208-211).

Patients with high-grade osteosarcomas of other sites are treated in a similar fashion; however, their overall outcome appears to be worse than that of patients with extremity tumors. This may be due in part to poor sensitivity to the chemotherapy agents and also to difficulties in achieving a negative surgical margin of resection owing to anatomic constraints. Patients with low-grade and variant osteosarcomas—such as well-differentiated intramedullary osteosarcoma or parosteal osteosarcoma and jaw osteosarcoma, typically arising in the mandible, which have a lower tendency to produce distant metastases—are treated with surgical resection with negative margins alone without routine use of adjuvant chemotherapy. If surgical resection with negative margins cannot be achieved in osteosarcoma of the jaw, preoperative chemotherapy should be considered. Patients with intermediate-grade periosteal osteosarcoma should also receive preoperative chemotherapy.

MFH of bone is treated according to the same basic principles as conventional osteosarcoma. Patients are given preoperative chemotherapy, followed by surgical resection, followed by postoperative chemotherapy, which is based on the knowledge of the response to preoperative chemotherapy or percent tumor necrosis. Studies performed at MDACC showed that with preoperative chemotherapy with doxorubicin and cisplatin, approximately 50% of the patients with localized MFH of bone had percent tumor necrosis of ≥90% (212). The median survival was 23 months for all patients who received this preoperative regimen, with the patients who achieved ≥90% having a median survival of 66 months and those with <90% necrosis a median survival of 20 months. The European Osteosarcoma Intergroup had similar results in studies using doxorubicin and cisplatin pre- and postoperatively, with 5-year PFS and overall survival of 56 and 59%, respectively (213).

With regard to rare histologic variants of osteosarcoma—such as small cell osteosarcoma, unclassified sarcoma, or dedifferentiated osteosarcoma—it should be noted that while these are treated in the same fashion as described, they have a worse prognosis than the histologies as discussed above. Patients with these tumors are better treated on investigational protocols that evaluate more intensive regimens or standard regimens in combination with biological agents to improve efficacy.

Metastatic and Recurrent Disease

Most often, osteosarcoma metastasizes to the lungs; however, osteosarcoma can also metastasize to almost any bone in the body. Rarely are lymph node metastases seen; when they are, it is usually later in the disease process, after or in conjunction with other metastasis. Patients who have resectable pulmonary metastases are treated with curative intent with primary chemotherapy, as described above, followed by surgical resection of all lesions either at the same time or in staged operations. These patients have a 15 to 30% chance of long-term disease-free survival and potential cure, depending on the biology of the disease. Patients with bone metastasis have a poorer prognosis, with therapy usually directed at palliation and prolongation of life as the primary outcomes.

Patients with metastasis or recurrence later are approached in a similar way as those with metastasis at the time of diagnosis; however, options for chemotherapy may be somewhat limited.

Chondrosarcoma

Chondrosarcoma is refractory to most of the chemotherapeutic agents used for the treatment of bone sarcomas. Most patients with chondrosarcoma are treated primarily with surgical resection regardless of the grade of the tumor. The exceptions to this rule are mesenchymal chondrosarcoma and dedifferentiated chondrosarcoma. Dedifferentiated chondrosarcoma is associated with low-grade chondrosarcoma, with foci of high-grade sarcoma that resemble osteosarcoma of MFH of bone and are often thought of as variants of osteosarcoma (214,215). These tumors can respond to chemotherapy and are treated in the same manner as conventional osteosarcomas (216). Mesenchymal chondrosarcoma is a very rare variant that presents in the jaw, spinal column, and ribs with lytic lesions on x-ray. The histology consists of a biomorphic appearance of benign to low-grade cartilaginous components with poorly differentiated small cell components (217). Mesenchymal chondrosarcomas do respond to chemotherapy; they are treated in a similar fashion as Ewing sarcoma, discussed below.

Ewing Sarcoma

Like osteosarcoma, Ewing sarcoma and the PNET family of tumors are treated primarily with chemotherapy prior to surgery, because patients with localized disease most likely have occult metastasis at the time of diagnosis. These tumors are extremely responsive to the following chemotherapeutic agents: doxorubicin, actinomycin D, ifosfamide, cyclophosphamide, vincristine, and etoposide. The most commonly used combinations are vincristine, Adriamycin (doxorubicin), and cyclophosphamide (VAC); ifosfamide and etoposide (IE); and vincristine, Adriamycin, and ifosfamide (VAI). Multiple trials have shown that with these combinations of chemotherapy, survival rates greater than 50% can be achieved (218-221). At MDACC, we usually give vincristine (up to 2 mg) with doxorubicin (75-90 mg/m^2) and ifosfamide (10 g/m^2) as our preoperative chemotherapy regimen. This is followed by surgical resection, if possible, or radiation therapy. Ewing

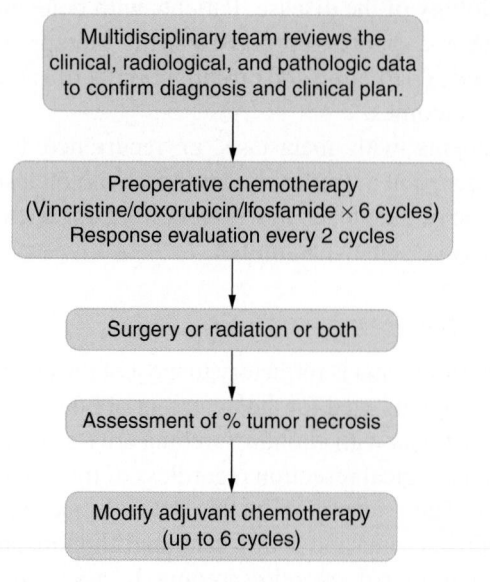

FIGURE 40-10. Treatment approach for patients with Ewing sarcoma/PNET and mesenchymal chondrosarcoma.

sarcoma is very radiosensitive; often, when surgical resection is not an option or positive margins remain, consolidative radiation therapy is used. There are studies that show good survival results in patients who have consolidative radiation therapy when needed (222). After definitive resection, tumor necrosis is assessed and postoperative therapy modified as needed (Fig. 40-10).

Metastatic/Recurrent Disease

Metastatic or recurrent Ewing sarcoma is treated in a similar manner as metastatic or recurrent disease in osteosarcoma. Patients who have metastatic disease in their lungs at the time of presentation are treated as outlined above, with curative intent. Those patients with recurrent or metastatic disease after primary therapy are treated on the basis of their disease-free interval. If there is a long interval (>12 months), a retrial of previous chemotherapeutic regimens preferably at higher dose intensity (eg, high-dose ifosfamide) is reasonable. For patients with a shorter interval between therapy and recurrence or metastasis, investigational therapies are appropriate. Of recent interest, the insulin-like growth factor-1 receptor (IGF-1R) is a tyrosine kinase receptor expressed on the cell surface of Ewing sarcoma cells. As with GIST, ubiquitous activation of this tyrosine kinase receptor is thought to play a key role in the pathogenesis of Ewing sarcoma (186,223). At least two

antibodies to IGF-1R have been reported to have antitumor activity against Ewing sarcoma (224,225). Further studies will be necessary to determine when and how this potential therapy may be incorporated into our current methods of treatment for Ewing sarcoma.

FOLLOW-UP MANAGEMENT

Similar to other treatable and potentially curable malignancies, long-term follow-up is essential. It is important to follow patients frequently with good-quality chest x-rays to evaluate for pulmonary metastasis and plain films of the primary tumor area to evaluate for local recurrence and to determine the condition of any prosthesis that may be in place. Patients are followed at MDACC with x-rays and physical examination every 3 months for the first 2 years, every 4 months for the next 2 years, every 6 months for the next 2 years, and then yearly thereafter. There are also occasional side effects from chemotherapy that are seen later after treatment. Anthracycline-induced cardiomyopathy is rare, the incidence varying with the cumulative dose and the duration of infusion. Nephrotoxicity due to ifosfamide can present within weeks to months after chemotherapy, especially when patients are simultaneously taking nonsteroidal anti-inflammatory drugs (NSAIDs) or other nephrotoxic agents. Sensory neuropathy due to cisplatin is often seen in patients who receive more than a 300 mg/m^2 cumulative dose; while this tends to be self-limited, it can take several months to years after chemotherapy before it resolves. The incidence of secondary malignancies such as leukemia is low; however, this is a real possibility and clinicians should be aware of it.

RARE BONE TUMORS

Some mention should be made of tumors that, while rare, are occasionally seen. Chordoma is a tumor that arises from the remnants of the primitive notochord. While biologically indolent, it can be locally aggressive, with a tendency to occur at either end of the spinal canal. Chordomas occur more frequently in men and tend to affect younger adults. Patients present with symptoms related to location. Sacrococcygeal chordomas tend to cause pelvic pain by extrinsic compression of surrounding structures and can result in impaired bowel and bladder function. Distal neuropathies may occur in this setting as well. Chordomas that occupy the superior portion of the spinal canal tend to present with localized pain, cranial nerve deficits, and radiculopathies. These tumors rarely metastasize.

An MDACC retrospective review of 37 patients with spinal or sacrococcygeal chordoma treated with surgery identified seven patients (19%) who developed metastatic disease. The sites of metastasis included the lungs, liver, and other areas of the spine (226). Treatment of these tumors is primarily surgical when feasible. Recently, adjuvant proton beam therapy has been noted to provide excellent local control compared to conventional photon therapy, especially for patients with chordomas located at the base of skull (227). Unresectable chordomas are treated with radiation therapy, as chemotherapy is of little value for chordoma unless dedifferentiation is seen. In the last decade, several studies have noted the expression of platelet-derived growth factor receptor-beta (PDGFR-β) expression (228). Casali et al. have reported on the limited role of imatinib mesylate, a PDGFR inhibitor, for the treatment of chordoma (228,229). Preliminary evidence points to the ability of imatinib to at least induce durable stable disease of 6 months; however, completion of this and other studies will be needed to appropriately conclude on the activity of imatinib for treatment of chordoma. There are cases when the chordoma undergo dedifferentiation, resulting in a highly metastatic phenotype (230). Few cases have been reported regarding treatment for dedifferentiated chordoma, though at least one MDACC report shows significant activity of high-dose ifosfamide and CyVADIC (cyclophosphamide, vincristine, doxorubicin, dacarbazine, and cisplatin) (231). Unfortunately, the prognosis is still poor.

Another rare tumor is giant cell tumor of the bone. These tumors have an uncertain cell of origin. They are characterized by osteoclast-like giant cells that are usually surrounded by oval mononuclear cells. There is a female predominance reported in the literature. These tumors tend to involve the epiphyses of long bones and usually result in pain, swelling, and decreased range of motion. Giant cell tumors appear as lytic, eccentrically located lesions in the epiphyses of a long bone on x-ray imaging. While this rare bone tumor has benign histologic features, local recurrence does occur frequently, and a small subset of these patients develop distant metastatic disease, primarily to the lungs. The primary treatment consists of surgical intervention, usually intralesional curettage and cementation. When the primary location precludes surgical resection due to morbidity, or patients develop distant metastatic disease, systemic therapy becomes the treatment of choice. These are vascular tumors and, therefore, antiangiogenic therapy may be beneficial. At MDACC, we treat patients with interferon alpha-2b therapy with either 3 million units subcutaneously every day for 6 to 12 months or 10 million units subcutaneously every Monday, Wednesday, and Friday for 6 to 12 months (232). Clinicians must be aware that these tumors respond gradually and can even grow initially on treatment. Often, responses are not fully appreciated until interferon therapy has been completed. Preliminary data suggest activity of denosumab, an antibody to the RANK ligand which inhibits osteoclastic function, increases calcification with improvement in pain in patients with recurrent or metastatic GCT (233).

References

1. Jemal A, Siegel R, Ward E, et al. Cancer statistics, 2009. *CA Cancer J Clin* 2009;59(4):225-249.
2. Mark RJ, Poen J, Tran LM, et al. Postirradiation sarcomas. A single-institution study and review of the literature. *Cancer* 1994;73(10):2653-2662.
3. Brady MS, Gaynor JJ, Brennan MF. Radiation-associated sarcoma of bone and soft tissue. *Arch Surg* 1992;127(12):1379-1385.
4. Pitcher ME, Davidson TI, Fisher C, et al. Post irradiation sarcoma of soft tissue and bone. *Eur J Surg Oncol* 1994;20(1):53-56.
5. Wiklund TA, Blomqvist CP, Raty J, et al. Postirradiation sarcoma. Analysis of a nationwide cancer registry material. *Cancer* 1991;68(3):524-531.
6. Laskin WB, Silverman TA, Enzinger FM. Postradiation soft tissue sarcomas. An analysis of 53 cases. *Cancer* 1988;62(11):2330-2340.
7. Robinson E, Neugut AI, Wylie P. Clinical aspects of postirradiation sarcomas. *J Natl Cancer Inst* 1988;80(4):233-240.
8. Kogevinas M, Kauppinen T, Winkelmann R, et al. Soft tissue sarcoma and non-Hodgkin's lymphoma in workers exposed to phenoxy herbicides, chlorophenols, and dioxins: Two nested case-control studies. *Epidemiology* 1995;6(4):396-402.
9. Grimalt JO, Sunyer J, Moreno V, et al. Risk excess of soft-tissue sarcoma and thyroid cancer in a community exposed to airborne organochlorinated compound mixtures with a high hexachlorobenzene content. *Int J Cancer* 1994;56(2):200-203.
10. Smith JG, Christophers AJ. Phenoxy herbicides and chlorophenols: A case control study on soft tissue sarcoma and malignant lymphoma. *Br J Cancer* 1992;65(3):442-448.
11. Johnson CC, Feingold M, Tilley B. A meta-analysis of exposure to phenoxy acid herbicides and chlorophenols in relation to risk of soft tissue sarcoma. *Int Arch Occup Environ Health* 1990;62(7):513-520.
12. Wingren G, Fredrikson M, Brage HN, et al. Soft tissue sarcoma and occupational exposures. *Cancer* 1990;66(4):806-811.
13. Eriksson M, Hardell L, Adami HO. Exposure to dioxins as a risk factor for soft tissue sarcoma: A population-based case-control study. *J Natl Cancer Inst* 1990;82(6):486-490.
14. Hardell L, Eriksson M. The association between soft tissue sarcomas and exposure to phenoxyacetic acids. A new case-referent study. *Cancer* 1988;62(3):652-656.
15. Zahm SH, Fraumeni JF, Jr. The epidemiology of soft tissue sarcoma. *Semin Oncol* 1997;24(5):504-514.

16. Froehner M, Wirth MP. Etiologic factors in soft tissue sarcomas. *Onkologie* 2001;24(2):139-142.

17. Marion MJ, Boivin-Angele S. Vinyl chloride-specific mutations in humans and animals. *IARC Sci Publ* 1999;(150):315-324.

18. Helman LJ, Meltzer P. Mechanisms of sarcoma development. *Nat Rev Cancer* 2003;3(9):685-694.

19. Wickerham DL, Fisher B, Wolmark N, et al. Association of tamoxifen and uterine sarcoma. *J Clin Oncol* 2002;20(11):2758-2760.

20. Raney RB, Jr. Localized sarcoma of the chest wall. *Med Pediatr Oncol* 1984;12(2):116-118.

21. Joss R, Ganz R, Ryssel HJ, et al. Posttraumatic soft tissue sarcoma: A case study of a malignant fibrous histiocytoma of the elbow joint which appeared six and a half years after a severe injury. *Schweiz Med Wochenschr* 1980;110(52):2021-2024.

22. Stewart FW, Treves N. Classics in oncology: Lymphangiosarcoma in postmastectomy lymphedema: A report of six cases in elephantiasis chirurgica. *CA Cancer J Clin* 1981;31(5):284-299.

23. Li FP, Fraumeni JF, Jr. Soft-tissue sarcomas, breast cancer, and other neoplasms. A familial syndrome? *Ann Intern Med* 1969;71(4):747-752.

24. Malkin D, Li FP, Strong LC, et al. Germ line p53 mutations in a familial syndrome of breast cancer, sarcomas, and other neoplasms. *Science* 1990;250(4985):1233-1238.

25. Goldberg Y, Dibbern K, Klein J, et al. Neurofibromatosis type 1—an update and review for the primary pediatrician. *Clin Pediatr (Phila)* 1996;35(11):545-561.

26. Tuveson DA, Fletcher JA. Signal transduction pathways in sarcoma as targets for therapeutic intervention. *Curr Opin Oncol* 2001;13(4):249-255.

27. Neville H, Corpron C, Blakely ML, et al. Pediatric neurofibrosarcoma. *J Pediatr Surg* 2003;38(3):343-346; discussion 343-346.

28. Lynch HT, Deters CA, Hogg D, et al. Familial sarcoma: Challenging pedigrees. *Cancer* 2003;98(9):1947-1957.

29. Mackall CL, Meltzer PS, Helman LJ. Focus on sarcomas. *Cancer Cell* 2002;2(3):175-178.

30. Sandberg AA, Bridge JA. Updates on the cytogenetics and molecular genetics of bone and soft tissue tumors: Osteosarcoma and related tumors. *Cancer Genet Cytogenet* 2003;145(1):1-30.

31. Coindre JM, Pelmus M, Hostein I, et al. Should molecular testing be required for diagnosing synovial sarcoma? A prospective study of 204 cases. *Cancer* 2003;98(12):2700-2707.

32. Weiss S, Goldblum J. *Enzinger and Weiss's Soft Tissue Tumors*, 4th ed. St. Louis: Mosby; 2001.

33. Mann GB, Lewis JJ, Brennan MF. Adult soft tissue sarcoma. *Aust N Z J Surg* 1999;69(5):336-343.

34. Lawrence W, Jr., Donegan WL, Natarajan N, et al. Adult soft tissue sarcomas. A pattern of care survey of the American College of Surgeons. *Ann Surg* 1987;205(4):349-359.

35. Hanna SL, Fletcher BD. MR imaging of malignant soft-tissue tumors. *Magn Reson Imaging Clin N Am* 1995;3(4):629-650.

36. Chang AE, Matory YL, Dwyer AJ, et al. Magnetic resonance imaging versus computed tomography in the evaluation of soft tissue tumors of the extremities. *Ann Surg* 1987;205(4):340-348.

37. Folpe AL, Lyles RH, Sprouse JT, et al. (F-18) fluorodeoxyglucose positron emission tomography as a predictor of pathologic grade and other prognostic variables in bone and soft tissue sarcoma. *Clin Cancer Res* 2000;6(4):1279-1287.

38. Ferner RE, Golding JF, Smith M, et al. [18F]2-fluoro-2-deoxy-D-glucose positron emission tomography (FDG PET) as a diagnostic tool for neurofibromatosis 1 (NF1) associated malignant peripheral nerve sheath tumours (MPNSTs): A long-term clinical study. *Ann Oncol* 2008;19(2):390-394.

39. Van den Abbeele AD, Badawi RD. Use of positron emission tomography in oncology and its potential role to assess response to imatinib mesylate therapy in gastrointestinal stromal tumors (GISTs). *Eur J Cancer* 2002;38(Suppl 5):S60-S65.

40. Schuetze SM, Rubin BP, Vernon C, et al. Use of positron emission tomography in localized extremity soft tissue sarcoma treated with neoadjuvant chemotherapy. *Cancer* 2005;103(2):339-348.

41. Evilevitch V, Weber WA, Tap WD, et al. Reduction of glucose metabolic activity is more accurate than change in size at predicting histopathologic response to neoadjuvant therapy in high-grade soft-tissue sarcomas. *Clin Cancer Res* 2008;14(3):715-720.

42. Schwarzbach MH, Hinz U, Dimitrakopoulou-Strauss A, et al. Prognostic significance of preoperative (18-F) fluorodeoxyglucose (FDG) positron emission tomography (PET) imaging in patients with resectable soft tissue sarcomas. *Ann Surg* 2005;241(2):286-294.

43. Eary JF, O'Sullivan F, O'Sullivan J, et al. Spatial heterogeneity in sarcoma 18F-FDG uptake as a predictor of patient outcome. *J Nucl Med* 2008;49(12):1973-1979.

44. Skrzynski MC, Biermann JS, Montag A, et al. Diagnostic accuracy and charge-savings of outpatient core needle biopsy compared with open biopsy of musculoskeletal tumors. *J Bone Joint Surg Am* 1996;78(5):644-649.

45. Heslin MJ, Lewis JJ, Woodruff JM, et al. Core needle biopsy for diagnosis of extremity soft tissue sarcoma. *Ann Surg Oncol* 1997;4(5):425-431.

46. Schwartz HS, Spengler DM. Needle tract recurrences after closed biopsy for sarcoma: Three cases and review of the literature. *Ann Surg Oncol* 1997;4(3):228-236.

47. Kilpatrick SE, Cappellari JO, Bos GD, et al. Is fine-needle aspiration biopsy a practical alternative to open biopsy for the primary diagnosis of sarcoma? Experience with 140 patients. *Am J Clin Pathol* 2001;115(1):59-68.

48. Ward WG, Savage P, Boles CA, et al. Fine-needle aspiration biopsy of sarcomas and related tumors. *Cancer Control* 2001;8(3):232-238.

49. Palmer HE, Mukunyadzi P, Culbreth W, et al. Subgrouping and grading of soft-tissue sarcomas by fine-needle aspiration cytology: A histopathologic correlation study. *Diagn Cytopathol* 2001;24(5):307-316.

50. Patel SR, Zagars GK, Pisters PW. The follow-up of adult soft-tissue sarcomas. *Semin Oncol* 2003;30(3):413-416.

51. Broders AC, Hargrave R, Meyerding HW. Pathologic features of soft tissue fibrosarcoma with special reference to the grading of its malignancy. *Surg Gynecol Obstet* 1939;69:pp.267-280.

52. Pisters PW, Leung DH, Woodruff J, et al. Analysis of prognostic factors in 1,041 patients with localized soft tissue sarcomas of the extremities. *J Clin Oncol* 1996;14(5):1679-1689.

53. Coindre JM, Terrier P, Bui NB, et al. Prognostic factors in adult patients with locally controlled soft tissue sarcoma. A study of 546 patients from the French Federation of Cancer Centers Sarcoma Group. *J Clin Oncol* 1996;14(3):869-877.

54. Green FL, Page D.L, Fleming I.D., et al. *Soft Tissue Sarcoma. AJCC Cancer Staging Handbook*, 6th ed. Philadelphia: Lippincott-Raven, 2002;221-228.

55. Kattan MW, Leung DH, Brennan MF. Postoperative nomogram for 12-year sarcoma-specific death. *J Clin Oncol* 2002; 20(3):791-796.

56. Stojadinovic A, Yeh A, Brennan MF. Completely resected recurrent soft tissue sarcoma: Primary anatomic site governs outcomes. *J Am Coll Surg* 2002;194(4):436-447.

57. Gaynor JJ, Tan CC, Casper ES, et al. Refinement of clinicopathologic staging for localized soft tissue sarcoma of the extremity: A study of 423 adults. *J Clin Oncol* 1992;10(8): 1317-1329.

58. Lewis JJ, Leung D, Heslin M, et al. Association of local recurrence with subsequent survival in extremity soft tissue sarcoma. *J Clin Oncol* 1997;15(2):646-652.

59. Weitz J, Antonescu CR, Brennan MF. Localized extremity soft tissue sarcoma: Improved knowledge with unchanged survival over time. *J Clin Oncol* 2003;21(14):2719-2725.

60. Bowden L, Booher RJ. The principles and technique of resection of soft parts for sarcoma. *Surgery* 1958;44(6):963-977.

61. Cantin J, McNeer GP, Chu FC, et al. The problem of local recurrence after treatment of soft tissue sarcoma. *Ann Surg* 1968;168(1):47-53.

62. Gerner RE, Moore GE, Pickren JW. Soft tissue sarcomas. *Ann Surg* 1975;181(6):803-808.

63. Pisters PW, Harrison LB, Leung DH, et al. Long-term results of a prospective randomized trial of adjuvant brachytherapy in soft tissue sarcoma. *J Clin Oncol* 1996;14(3):859-868.

64. Yang JC, Chang AE, Baker AR, et al. Randomized prospective study of the benefit of adjuvant radiation therapy in the treatment of soft tissue sarcomas of the extremity. *J Clin Oncol* 1998;16(1):197-203.

65. Karakousis CP, Proimakis C, Walsh DL. Primary soft tissue sarcoma of the extremities in adults. *Br J Surg* 1995;82(9): 1208-1212.

66. Fong Y, Coit DG, Woodruff JM, et al. Lymph node metastasis from soft tissue sarcoma in adults. Analysis of data from a prospective database of 1772 sarcoma patients. *Ann Surg* 1993;217(1):72-77.

67. Weingrad DN, Rosenberg SA. Early lymphatic spread of osteogenic and soft-tissue sarcomas. *Surgery* 1978;84(2): 231-240.

68. Behranwala KA, A'Hern R, Omar AM, et al. Prognosis of lymph node metastasis in soft tissue sarcoma. *Ann Surg Oncol* 2004;11(7):714-719.

69. Rosenberg SA, Tepper J, Glatstein E, et al. Prospective randomized evaluation of adjuvant chemotherapy in adults with soft tissue sarcomas of the extremities. *Cancer* 1983;52(3): 424-434.

70. Williard WC, Collin C, Casper ES, et al. The changing role of amputation for soft tissue sarcoma of the extremity in adults. *Surg Gynecol Obstet* 1992;175(5):389-396.

71. Johnstone PA, Wexler LH, Venzon DJ, et al. Sarcomas of the hand and foot: Analysis of local control and functional result with combined modality therapy in extremity preservation. *Int J Radiat Oncol Biol Phys* 1994;29(4):735-745.

72. Rosenberg SA, Tepper J, Glatstein E, et al. The treatment of soft-tissue sarcomas of the extremities: Prospective randomized evaluations of (1) limb-sparing surgery plus radiation therapy compared with amputation and (2) the role of adjuvant chemotherapy. *Ann Surg* 1982;196(3):305-315.

73. Yang JC, Rosenberg SA. Surgery for adult patients with soft tissue sarcomas. *Semin Oncol* 1989;16(4):289-296.

74. Eggermont AM, Schraffordt Koops H, Lienard D, et al. Isolated limb perfusion with high-dose tumor necrosis factor-alpha in combination with interferon-gamma and melphalan for nonresectable extremity soft tissue sarcomas: A multicenter trial. *J Clin Oncol* 1996;14(10):2653-2665.

75. Yang JC, Fraker DL, Thom AK, et al. Isolation perfusion with tumor necrosis factor-alpha, interferon-gamma, and hyperthermia in the treatment of localized and metastatic cancer. *Recent Results Cancer Res* 1995;138:161-166.

76. Lienard D, Ewalenko P, Delmotte JJ, et al. High-dose recombinant tumor necrosis factor alpha in combination with interferon gamma and melphalan in isolation perfusion of the limbs for melanoma and sarcoma. *J Clin Oncol* 1992;10(1): 52-60.

77. Issels RD. Regional hyperthermia in high-risk soft tissue sarcomas. *Curr Opin Oncol* 2008;20(4):438-443.

78. Issels RD, Lindner LH, Wust P, et al. Regional hyperthermia (RHT) improves response and survival when combined with systemic chemotherapy in the management of locally advanced, high grade soft tissue sarcomas (STS) of the extremities, the body wall and the abdomen: A phase III randomised pros. *J Clin Oncol* 2007;25(Suppl 18). Abstract 10009.

79. Suit H, Spiro I. Radiation as a therapeutic modality in sarcomas of the soft tissue. *Hematol Oncol Clin North Am* 1995;9(4):733-746.

80. Tepper JE, Suit HD. Radiation therapy alone for sarcoma of soft tissue. *Cancer* 1985;56(3):475-479.

81. Pickering DG, Stewart JS, Rampling R, et al. Fast neutron therapy for soft tissue sarcoma. *Int J Radiat Oncol Biol Phys* 1987;13(10):1489-1495.

82. Slater JD, McNeese MD, Peters LJ. Radiation therapy for unresectable soft tissue sarcomas. *Int J Radiat Oncol Biol Phys* 1986;12(10):1729-1734.

83. O'Sullivan B, Davis AM, Turcotte R, et al. Preoperative versus postoperative radiotherapy in soft-tissue sarcoma of the limbs: A randomised trial. *Lancet* 2002;359(9325):2235-2241.

84. O'Sullivan B, Davis, A. A randomized phase III trial of preoperative compared to postoperative radiotherapy in extremity soft tissue sarcoma. *Proc. ASTRO* 2001:151.

85. Wayne JD, Langstein H., Pollack A, et al. Preoperative radiotherapy for extremity soft tissue sarcoma (STS): Site-specific wound complication rates and the impact of reconstructive surgery. *Proc Am Soc Clin Oncol* 2000:558a.

86. Robinson MH, Keus RB, Shasha D, et al. Is pre-operative radiotherapy superior to postoperative radiotherapy in the treatment of soft tissue sarcoma? *Eur J Cancer* 1998;34(9): 1309-1316.

87. Zagars GK, Ballo MT, Pisters PW, et al. Preoperative vs. postoperative radiation therapy for soft tissue sarcoma: A retrospective comparative evaluation of disease outcome. *Int J Radiat Oncol Biol Phys* 2003;56(2):482-488.

88. Suit HD, Mankin HJ, Wood WC, et al. Preoperative, intraoperative, and postoperative radiation in the treatment of primary soft tissue sarcoma. *Cancer* 1985;55(11):2659-2667.

89. Nielsen OS, Cummings B, O'Sullivan B, et al. Preoperative and postoperative irradiation of soft tissue sarcomas: Effect of radiation field size. *Int J Radiat Oncol Biol Phys* 1991; 21(6):1595-1599.

90. Stinson SF, DeLaney TF, Greenberg J, et al. Acute and long-term effects on limb function of combined modality limb sparing therapy for extremity soft tissue sarcoma. *Int J Radiat Oncol Biol Phys* 1991;21(6):1493-1499.

91. Pollack A, Zagars GK, Goswitz MS, et al. Preoperative vs. postoperative radiotherapy in the treatment of soft tissue sarcomas: A matter of presentation. *Int J Radiat Oncol Biol Phys* 1998;42(3):563-572.

92. Suit HD, Mankin HJ, Wood WC, et al. Treatment of the patient with stage M0 soft tissue sarcoma. *J Clin Oncol* 1988; 6(5):854-862.

93. Fein DA, Lee WR, Lanciano RM, et al. Management of extremity soft tissue sarcomas with limb-sparing surgery and postoperative irradiation: Do total dose, overall treatment time, and the surgery-radiotherapy interval impact on local control? *Int J Radiat Oncol Biol Phys* 1995;32(4):969-976.

94. Thomas J, Ferme C, Noordijk EM, et al. Results of the EORTC-GELA H9 randomized trials: The H9-F trial (comparing 3 radiation dose levels) and H9-U trial (comparing 3 chemotherapy schemes) in patients with favorable or unfavorable early stage Hodgkin's lymphoma (HL). *Haematologica* 2007;92:27-27.

95. Sadoski C, Suit HD, Rosenberg A, et al. Preoperative radiation, surgical margins, and local control of extremity sarcomas of soft tissues. *J Surg Oncol* 1993;52(4):223-230.

96. Alektiar KM, Velasco J, Zelefsky MJ, et al. Adjuvant radiotherapy for margin-positive high-grade soft tissue sarcoma of the extremity. *Int J Radiat Oncol Biol Phys* 2000;48(4): 1051-1058.

97. Cahlon O, Spierer M, Brennan MF, et al. Long-term outcomes in extremity soft tissue sarcoma after a pathologically negative re-resection and without radiotherapy. *Cancer* 2008;112(12):2774-2779.

98. Alektiar KM, Brennan MF, Healey JH, et al. Impact of intensity-modulated radiation therapy on local control in primary soft-tissue sarcoma of the extremity. *J Clin Oncol* 2008;26(20):3440-3444.

99. Ballo MT, Zagars GK, Cormier JN, et al. Interval between surgery and radiotherapy: Effect on local control of soft tissue sarcoma. *Int J Radiat Oncol Biol Phys* 2004;58(5): 1461-1467.

100. Rosen G, Forscher C, Lowenbraun S, et al. Synovial sarcoma. Uniform response of metastases to high dose ifosfamide. *Cancer* 1994;73(10):2506-2511.

101. Tascilar M, Loos WJ, Seynaeve C, et al. The pharmacologic basis of ifosfamide use in adult patients with advanced soft tissue sarcomas. *Oncologist* 2007;12(11):1351-1360.

102. Spurrell EL, Fisher C, Thomas JM, et al. Prognostic factors in advanced synovial sarcoma: An analysis of 104 patients treated at the Royal Marsden Hospital. *Ann Oncol* 2005; 16(3):437-444.

103. Sleijfer S, Ouali M, van Glabbeke M, et al. Prognostic and predictive factors for outcome to first-line ifosfamide-containing chemotherapy for adult patients with advanced soft tissue sarcomas: An exploratory, retrospective analysis on large series from the European Organization for Research and Treatment of Cancer-Soft Tissue and Bone

Sarcoma Group (EORTC-STBSG). *Eur J Cancer* 2010; 46(1):72-83.

104. Patel SR, Burgess MA, Plager C, et al. Myxoid liposarcoma. Experience with chemotherapy. *Cancer* 1994;74(4): 1265-1269.

105. Jones RL, Fisher C, Al-Muderis O, et al. Differential sensitivity of liposarcoma subtypes to chemotherapy. *Eur J Cancer* 2005;41(18):2853-2860.

106. Ahmad SA, Patel SR, Ballo MT, et al. Extraosseous osteosarcoma: Response to treatment and long-term outcome. *J Clin Oncol* 2002;20(2):521-527.

107. O'Bryan RM, Baker LH, Gottlieb JE, et al. Dose response evaluation of Adriamycin in human neoplasia. *Cancer* 1977; 39(5):1940-1948.

108. Patel SR, Vadhan-Raj S, Papadopolous N, et al. High-dose ifosfamide in bone and soft tissue sarcomas: Results of phase II and pilot studies–dose-response and schedule dependence. *J Clin Oncol* 1997;15(6):2378-2384.

109. Patel SR, Benjamin RS. Ifosfamide in sarcomas: Is it a schedule-dependent drug? *Cancer Invest* 1996;14(3):290-291.

110. Benjamin RS, Legha SS, Patel SR, et al. Single-agent ifosfamide studies in sarcomas of soft tissue and bone: The M.D. Anderson experience. *Cancer Chemother Pharmacol* 1993; 31(Suppl 2):S174-S179.

111. Antman KH, Ryan L, Elias A, et al. Response to ifosfamide and mesna: 124 previously treated patients with metastatic or unresectable sarcoma. *J Clin Oncol* 1989;7(1):126-131.

112. Bramwell V, Quirt I, Warr D, et al. Combination chemotherapy with doxorubicin, dacarbazine, and ifosfamide in advanced adult soft tissue sarcoma. Canadian Sarcoma Group–National Cancer Institute of Canada Clinical Trials Group. *J Natl Cancer Inst* 1989;81(19):1496-1499.

113. Elias A, Ryan L, Sulkes A, et al. Response to mesna, doxorubicin, ifosfamide, and dacarbazine in 108 patients with metastatic or unresectable sarcoma and no prior chemotherapy. *J Clin Oncol* 1989;7(9):1208-1216.

114. Vadhan-Raj S, Patel S, Burgess MA, et al. Phase II Trial of Adriamycin (A), ifosfamide (I), mesna (M) uroprotection, dacarbazine (D)(MAID) with PIXY321 (GM-CSF/IL-3 fusion protein) of G-CSF in patients (PTS) with soft tissue sarcoma (STS). *Proc Am Soc Clin Oncol* 1996:525.

115. Patel SR, Vadhan-Raj S, Burgess MA, et al. Results of two consecutive trials of dose-intensive chemotherapy with doxorubicin and ifosfamide in patients with sarcomas. *Am J Clin Oncol* 1998;21(3):317-321.

116. Patel SR. *Dose Intensive Chemotherapy for Soft Tissue Sarcoma*. Alexandria: Lippincott Williams & Wilkins, 2000, American Society of Clinical Oncology Educational Booklet.

117. Patel SR, Gandhi V, Jenkins J, et al. Phase II clinical investigation of gemcitabine in advanced soft tissue sarcomas and window evaluation of dose rate on gemcitabine triphosphate accumulation. *J Clin Oncol* 2001;19(15):3483-3489.

118. Touroutoglou N, Gravel D, Raber MN, et al. Clinical results of a pharmacodynamically-based strategy for higher dosing of gemcitabine in patients with solid tumors. *Ann Oncol* 1998;9(9):1003-1008.

119. Tempero M, Plunkett W, Ruiz Van Haperen V, et al. Randomized phase II comparison of dose-intense gemcitabine: Thirty-minute infusion and fixed dose rate infusion in patients with pancreatic adenocarcinoma. *J Clin Oncol* 2003;21(18): 3402-3408.

120. Hensley ML, Maki R, Venkatraman E, et al. Gemcitabine and docetaxel in patients with unresectable leiomyosarcoma: Results of a phase II trial. *J Clin Oncol* 2002;20(12):2824-2831.

121. Maki RG, Wathen JK, Patel SR, et al. Randomized phase II study of gemcitabine and docetaxel compared with gemcitabine alone in patients with metastatic soft tissue sarcomas: Results of sarcoma alliance for research through collaboration study 002 [corrected]. *J Clin Oncol* 2007;25(19):2755-2763.

122. Pervaiz N, Colterjohn N, Farrokhyar F, et al. A systematic meta-analysis of randomized controlled trials of adjuvant chemotherapy for localized resectable soft-tissue sarcoma. *Cancer* 2008;113(3):573-581.

123. Fletcher CD, Berman JJ, Corless C, et al. Diagnosis of gastrointestinal stromal tumors: A consensus approach. *Hum Pathol* 2002;33(5):459-465.

124. Kindblom LG, Remotti HE, Aldenborg F, et al. Gastrointestinal pacemaker cell tumor (GIPACT): Gastrointestinal stromal tumors show phenotypic characteristics of the interstitial cells of Cajal. *Am J Pathol* 1998;152(5):1259-1269.

125. DeMatteo RP, Lewis JJ, Leung D, et al. Two hundred gastrointestinal stromal tumors: Recurrence patterns and prognostic factors for survival. *Ann Surg* 2000;231(1):51-58.

126. Gottlieb J, Baker, L., O'Bryan, R., et al. Adriamycin (NSC-123-127) used alone and in combination for soft tissue and bony sarcomas. *Cancer Chemother Rep* 1974;6:271-282.

127. Trent JC, Beach J, Burgess MA, et al. A two-arm phase II study of temozolomide in patients with advanced gastrointestinal stromal tumors and other soft tissue sarcomas. *Cancer* 2003;98(12):2693-2699.

128. Buchdunger E, Cioffi CL, Law N, et al. Abl protein-tyrosine kinase inhibitor STI571 inhibits in vitro signal transduction mediated by c-kit and platelet-derived growth factor receptors. *J Pharmacol Exp Ther* 2000;295(1):139-145.

129. Savage DG, Antman KH. Imatinib mesylate–a new oral targeted therapy. *N Engl J Med* 2002;346(9):683-693.

130. Hirota S, Isozaki K, Moriyama Y, et al. Gain-of-function mutations of c-kit in human gastrointestinal stromal tumors. *Science* 1998;279(5350):577-580.

131. Joensuu H, Roberts PJ, Sarlomo-Rikala M, et al. Effect of the tyrosine kinase inhibitor STI571 in a patient with a metastatic gastrointestinal stromal tumor. *N Engl J Med* 2001;344(14):1052-1056.

132. van Oosterom AT, Judson I, Verweij J, et al. Safety and efficacy of imatinib (STI571) in metastatic gastrointestinal stromal tumours: A phase I study. *Lancet* 2001;358(9291):1421-1423.

133. Demetri GD, von Mehren M, Blanke CD, et al. Efficacy and safety of imatinib mesylate in advanced gastrointestinal stromal tumors. *N Engl J Med* 2002;347(7):472-480.

134. Blanke CD, Demetri GD, von Mehren M, et al. Long-term results from a randomized phase II trial of standard-versus higher-dose imatinib mesylate for patients with unresectable or metastatic gastrointestinal stromal tumors expressing KIT. *J Clin Oncol* 2008;26(4):620-625.

135. Verweij J, Casali PG, Zalcberg J, et al. Progression-free survival in gastrointestinal stromal tumours with high-dose imatinib: Randomised trial. *Lancet* 2004;364(9440):1127-1134.

136. Blanke CD, Rankin C, Demetri GD, et al. Phase III randomized, intergroup trial assessing imatinib mesylate at two dose levels in patients with unresectable or metastatic gastrointestinal stromal tumors expressing the kit receptor tyrosine kinase: S0033. *J Clin Oncol* 2008;26(4):626-632.

137. Van Glabbeke M, Owzar K., Rankin C, et al. Comparison of two doses of imatinib for the treatment of unresectable or metastatic gastrointestinal stromal tumors (GIST): A meta-analysis based on 1,640 patients (pts). *J Clin Oncol* (Annual Meeting Abstracts) 2007;25(S18):10004.

138. Dematteo RP, Ballman KV, Antonescu CR, et al. Adjuvant imatinib mesylate after resection of localised, primary gastrointestinal stromal tumour: A randomised, double-blind, placebo-controlled trial. *Lancet* 2009;373(9669):1097-1104.

139. Heinrich MC, Corless CL, Demetri GD, et al. Kinase mutations and imatinib response in patients with metastatic gastrointestinal stromal tumor. *J Clin Oncol* 2003;21(23):4342-4349.

140. Taniguchi M, Nishida T, Hirota S, et al. Effect of c-kit mutation on prognosis of gastrointestinal stromal tumors. *Cancer Res* 1999;59(17):4297-4300.

141. Heinrich MC, Owzar K, Corless CL, et al. Correlation of kinase genotype and clinical outcome in the North American Intergroup Phase III Trial of imatinib mesylate for treatment of advanced gastrointestinal stromal tumor: CALGB 150105 Study by Cancer and Leukemia Group B and Southwest Oncology Group. *J Clin Oncol* 2008;26(33):5360-5367.

142. Chen LL, Trent JC, Wu EF, et al. A missense mutation in KIT kinase domain 1 correlates with imatinib resistance in gastrointestinal stromal tumors. *Cancer Res* 2004;64(17):5913-5919.

143. Antonescu CR, Besmer P, Guo T, et al. Acquired resistance to imatinib in gastrointestinal stromal tumor occurs through secondary gene mutation. *Clin Cancer Res* 2005;11(11):4182-4190.

144. Demetri GD, van Oosterom AT, Garrett CR, et al. Efficacy and safety of sunitinib in patients with advanced gastrointestinal stromal tumour after failure of imatinib: A randomised controlled trial. *Lancet* 2006;368(9544):1329-1338.

145. Heinrich MC, Maki RG, Corless CL, et al. Primary and secondary kinase genotypes correlate with the biological and clinical activity of sunitinib in imatinib-resistant gastrointestinal stromal tumor. *J Clin Oncol* 2008;26(33):5352-5359.

146. Demetri GD, Wang Y, Wehrle E, et al. Imatinib plasma levels are correlated with clinical benefit in patients with unresectable/metastatic gastrointestinal stromal tumors. *J Clin Oncol* 2009;27(19):3141-3147.

147. Nolden LK, Shum L, Dumont A, et al. Steady-state plasma imatinib levels in 142 GIST patients. Connective Tissue Oncology Society, Miami, 2009.

148. McAuliffe JC, Hunt KK, Lazar AJ, et al. A randomized, phase II study of preoperative plus postoperative imatinib in GIST: Evidence of rapid radiographic response and temporal induction of tumor cell apoptosis. *Ann Surg Oncol* 2009;16(4):910-919.

149. Choi H, Charnsangavej C, de Castro Faria S, et al. CT evaluation of the response of gastrointestinal stromal tumors after imatinib mesylate treatment: A quantitative analysis correlated with FDG PET findings. *AJR Am J Roentgenol* 2004;183(6):1619-1628.

150. Choi H, Charnsangavej C, Faria SC, et al. Correlation of computed tomography and positron emission tomography in patients with metastatic gastrointestinal stromal tumor treated at a single institution with imatinib mesylate: Proposal of new computed tomography response criteria. *J Clin Oncol* 2007;25(13):1753-1759.

151. Benjamin RS, Choi H, Macapinlac HA, et al. We should desist using RECIST, at least in GIST. *J Clin Oncol* 2007; 25(13):1760-1764.

152. Holden CA, Spittle MF, Jones EW. Angiosarcoma of the face and scalp, prognosis and treatment. *Cancer* 1987;59(5): 1046-1057.

153. Fata F, O'Reilly E, Ilson D, et al. Paclitaxel in the treatment of patients with angiosarcoma of the scalp or face. *Cancer* 1999;86(10):2034-2037.

154. Orchard GE, Zelger B, Jones EW, et al. An immunocyto-chemical assessment of 19 cases of cutaneous angiosarcoma. *Histopathology* 1996;28(3):235-240.

155. Scow JS, Reynolds CA, Degnim AC, et al. Primary and secondary angiosarcoma of the breast: The Mayo Clinic experience. *J Surg Oncol* 2010 Apr 1;101(5):401-407.

156. Stewart FW, Treves N. Lymphangiosarcoma in postmastectomy lymphedema; A report of six cases in elephantiasis chirurgica. *Cancer* 1948;1(1):64-81.

157. Meis-Kindblom JM, Kindblom LG. Angiosarcoma of soft tissue: A study of 80 cases. *Am J Surg Pathol* 1998;22(6): 683-697.

158. Fayette J, Martin E, Piperno-Neumann S, et al. Angiosarcomas, a heterogeneous group of sarcomas with specific behavior depending on primary site: A retrospective study of 161 cases. *Ann Oncol* 2007;18(12):2030-2036.

159. Abraham JA, Hornicek FJ, Kaufman AM, et al. Treatment and outcome of 82 patients with angiosarcoma. *Ann Surg Oncol* 2007;14(6):1953-1967.

160. Casper ES, Waltzman RJ, Schwartz GK, et al. Phase II trial of paclitaxel in patients with soft-tissue sarcoma. *Cancer Invest* 1998;16(7):442-446.

161. Penel N, Bui BN, Bay JO, et al. Phase II trial of weekly paclitaxel for unresectable angiosarcoma: The ANGIOTAX Study. *J Clin Oncol* 2008;26(32):5269-5274.

162. Agulnik M, Okuno SH, Von Mehren M, et al. An open-label multicenter phase II study of bevacizumab for the treatment of angiosarcoma. *Journal of Clinical Oncology*, Orlando, FL, 2009.

163. Maki RG, D'Adamo DR, Keohan ML, et al. Phase II study of sorafenib in patients with metastatic or recurrent sarcomas. *J Clin Oncol* 2009;27(19):3133-3140.

164. Fletcher CD. The evolving classification of soft tissue tumours: An update based on the new WHO classification. *Histopathology* 2006;48(1):3-12.

165. Park MS, Araujo DM. New insights into the hemangiopericytoma/solitary fibrous tumor spectrum of tumors. *Curr Opin Oncol* 2009;21(4):327-331.

166. Spitz FR, Bouvet M, Pisters PW, et al. Hemangiopericytoma: A 20-year single-institution experience. *Ann Surg Oncol* 1998;5(4):350-355.

167. Espat NJ, Lewis JJ, Leung D, et al. Conventional hemangiopericytoma: Modern analysis of outcome. *Cancer* 2002; 95(8):1746-1751.

168. Galanis E, Buckner JC, Scheithauer BW, et al. Management of recurrent meningeal hemangiopericytoma. *Cancer* 1998; 82(10):1915-1920.

169. Soyuer S, Chang EL, Selek U, et al. Intracranial meningeal hemangiopericytoma: The role of radiotherapy: Report of 29 cases and review of the literature. *Cancer* 2004;100(7): 1491-1497.

170. Park MS, Lazar AJ, Trent JC, et al. Combination therapy with temozolomide and bevacizumab in the treatment of hemangiopericytoma/solitary fibrous tumor: An updated analysis. 14th Connective Tissue Oncologic Society Annual Meeting, London, UK, November 13-15, 2008.

171. Casali PG, Stacchiotti S, Palassini E, et al. Evaluation of the antitumor activity of sunitinib malate (SM) in solitary fibrous tumor (SFT). *J Clin Oncol* 27:15s, 2009 (suppl; abstr 10571).

172. George S, Merriam P, Maki RG, et al. Multicenter phase II trial of sunitinib in the treatment of nongastrointestinal stromal tumor sarcomas. *J Clin Oncol* 2009;27(19):3154-3160.

173. Sleijfer S, Ray-Coquard I, Papai Z, et al. Pazopanib, a multi-kinase angiogenesis inhibitor, in patients with relapsed or refractory advanced soft tissue sarcoma: A phase II study from the European organisation for research and treatment of cancer-soft tissue and bone sarcoma group (EORTC study 62043). *J Clin Oncol* 2009;27(19):3126-3132.

174. Dei Tos AP. Lipomatous tumours. *Curr Diagn Pathol* 2001; 7:8-16.

175. Kilpatrick SE, Doyon J, Choong PF, et al. The clinicopathologic spectrum of myxoid and round cell liposarcoma. A study of 95 cases. *Cancer* 1996;77(8):1450-1458.

176. Fiore M, Grosso F, Lo Vullo S, et al. Myxoid/round cell and pleomorphic liposarcomas: Prognostic factors and survival in a series of patients treated at a single institution. *Cancer* 2007;109(12):2522-2531.

177. Forni C, Minuzzo M, Virdis E, et al. Trabectedin (ET-743) promotes differentiation in myxoid liposarcoma tumors. *Mol Cancer Ther* 2009;8(2):449-457.

178. Perez-Losada J, Pintado B, Gutierrez-Adan A, et al. The chimeric FUS/TLS-CHOP fusion protein specifically induces liposarcomas in transgenic mice. *Oncogene* 2000;19(20): 2413-2422.

179. Riggi N, Cironi L, Provero P, et al. Expression of the FUS-CHOP fusion protein in primary mesenchymal progenitor cells gives rise to a model of myxoid liposarcoma. *Cancer Res* 2006;66(14):7016-7023.

180. Le Cesne A, Blay JY, Judson I, et al. Phase II study of ET-743 in advanced soft tissue sarcomas: A European Organisation for the Research and Treatment of Cancer (EORTC) soft tissue and bone sarcoma group trial. *J Clin Oncol* 2005; 23(3): 576-584.

181. Garcia-Carbonero R, Supko JG, Manola J, et al. Phase II and pharmacokinetic study of ecteinascidin 743 in patients with progressive sarcomas of soft tissues refractory to chemotherapy. *J Clin Oncol* 2004;22(8):1480-1490.

182. Grosso F, Jones RL, Demetri GD, et al. Efficacy of trabectedin (ecteinascidin-743) in advanced pretreated myxoid liposarcomas: A retrospective study. *Lancet Oncol* 2007;8(7):595-602.

183. Demetri GD, Chawla SP, von Mehren M, et al. Efficacy and safety of trabectedin in patients with advanced or metastatic liposarcoma or leiomyosarcoma after failure of prior anthracyclines and ifosfamide: Results of a randomized phase II study of two different schedules. *J Clin Oncol* 2009;27(25): 4188-4196.

184. Fleming JB, Cantor SB, Varma DG, et al. Utility of chest computed tomography for staging in patients with T1 extremity soft tissue sarcomas. *Cancer* 2001;92(4):863-868.

185. Demetri GD, Delaney T. NCCN: Sarcoma. *Cancer Control* 2001;8(6 Suppl 2):94-101.

186. Ludwig JA. Ewing sarcoma: Historical perspectives, current state-of-the-art, and opportunities for targeted therapy in the future. *Curr Opin Oncol* 2008;20(4):412-418.

187. Paulussen M, Ahrens S, Craft AW, et al. Ewing's tumors with primary lung metastases: Survival analysis of 114 (European Intergroup) Cooperative Ewing's Sarcoma Studies patients. *J Clin Oncol* 1998;16(9):3044-3052.

188. Cotterill SJ, Ahrens S, Paulussen M, et al. Prognostic factors in Ewing's tumor of bone: Analysis of 975 patients from the European Intergroup Cooperative Ewing's Sarcoma Study Group. *J Clin Oncol* 2000;18(17):3108-3114.

189. Dahlin DC, Coventry MB. Osteogenic sarcoma. A study of six hundred cases. *J Bone Joint Surg Am* 1967;49(1):101-110.

190. Wick MR, Siegal GP, Unni KK, et al. Sarcomas of bone complicating osteitis deformans (Paget's disease): Fifty years' experience. *Am J Surg Pathol* 1981;5(1):47-59.

191. Dickey ID, Rose PS, Fuchs B, et al. Dedifferentiated chondrosarcoma: The role of chemotherapy with updated outcomes. *J Bone Joint Surg Am* 2004;86-A(11):2412-2418.

192. Evans HL, Ayala AG, Romsdahl MM. Prognostic factors in chondrosarcoma of bone: A clinicopathologic analysis with emphasis on histologic grading. *Cancer* 1977;40(2):818-831.

193. Ayala AG, Raymond AK, Ro JY, et al. Needle biopsy of primary bone lesions. M.D. Anderson experience. *Pathol Annu* 1989;24(Pt 1):219-251.

194. Raymond AK, Simms W, Ayala AG. Osteosarcoma. Specimen management following primary chemotherapy. *Hematol Oncol Clin North Am* 1995;9(4):841-867.

195. Brenner W, Bohuslavizki KH, Eary JF. PET imaging of osteosarcoma. *J Nucl Med* 2003;44(6):930-942.

196. Bone cancer. NCCN Clinical Practice Guidelines in Oncology, 2010.

197. Enneking WF, Spanier SS, Goodman MA. A system for the surgical staging of musculoskeletal sarcoma. *Clin Orthop Relat Res* 1980;(153):106-120.

198. Green FL, Page DL, Fleming ID, et al. *Bone. AJCC Cancer Staging Handbook*, 6th ed. New York: Springer-Verlag, 2002;213-319.

199. Heck RK, Jr., Stacy GS, Flaherty MJ, et al. A comparison study of staging systems for bone sarcomas. *Clin Orthop Relat Res* 2003 Oct;(415):64-71.

200. Jaffe N, Patel SR, Benjamin RS. Chemotherapy in osteosarcoma. Basis for application and antagonism to implementation; early controversies surrounding its implementation. *Hematol Oncol Clin North Am* 1995;9(4):825-840.

201. Petrilli S, Penna V, Lopes A, et al. IIB osteosarcoma. Current management, local control, and survival statistics–São Paulo, Brazil. *Clin Orthop Relat Res* 1991 Sep;(270):60-66.

202. Cortes EP, Holland JF, Glidewell O. Osteogenic sarcoma studies by the Cancer and Leukemia Group B. *Natl Cancer Inst Monogr* 1981 Apr;(56):207-209.

203. Antman KH, Montella D, Rosenbaum C, et al. Phase II trial of ifosfamide with mesna in previously treated metastatic sarcoma. *Cancer Treat Rep* 1985;69(5):499-504.

204. Jaffe N. Recent advances in the chemotherapy of metastatic osteogenic sarcoma. *Cancer* 1972;30(6):1627-1631.

205. Raymond AK, Chawla SP, Carrasco CH, et al. Osteosarcoma chemotherapy effect: A prognostic factor. *Semin Diagn Pathol* 1987;4(3):212-236.

206. Meyers PA, Heller G, Healey J, et al. Chemotherapy for nonmetastatic osteogenic sarcoma: The Memorial Sloan-Kettering experience. *J Clin Oncol* 1992;10(1):5-15.

207. Bacci G, Ferrari S, Mercuri M, et al. Neoadjuvant chemotherapy for extremity osteosarcoma–preliminary results of the Rizzoli's 4th study. *Acta Oncol* 1998;37(1):41-48.

208. Goorin AM, Schwartzentruber DJ, Devidas M, et al. Presurgical chemotherapy compared with immediate surgery and adjuvant chemotherapy for nonmetastatic osteosarcoma: Pediatric Oncology Group Study POG-8651. *J Clin Oncol* 2003;21(8):1574-1580.

209. Souhami RL, Craft AW, Van der Eijken JW, et al. Randomised trial of two regimens of chemotherapy in operable osteosarcoma: A study of the European Osteosarcoma Intergroup. *Lancet* 1997;350(9082):911-917.

210. Benjamin RS, Patel SR, Armen T. et al. The value of ifosfamide in the postoperative neoadjuvant chemotherapy for osteosarcoma. *Proc Am Soc Clin Oncol* 1995;14:516 (abstr 1690).

211. Link MP, Goorin AM, Miser AW, et al. The effect of adjuvant chemotherapy on relapse-free survival in patients with osteosarcoma of the extremity. *N Engl J Med* 1986;314(25):1600-1606.

212. Patel SR, Armen T, Carrasco CH, et al. Primary chemotherapy in malignant fibrous histiocytoma of bone. In: Banzet P, Holland J, Khayat D. (eds): *U.T.M.D. Anderson Cancer Center Experience*. Houston, TX: MDACC, 1994;577-580.

213. Bramwell VH, Steward WP, Nooij M, et al. Neoadjuvant chemotherapy with doxorubicin and cisplatin in malignant fibrous histiocytoma of bone: A European Osteosarcoma Intergroup study. *J Clin Oncol* 1999;17(10):3260-3269.

214. Dahlin DC, Beabout JW. Dedifferentiation of low-grade chondrosarcomas. *Cancer* 1971;28(2):461-466.

215. Frassica FJ, Unni KK, Beabout JW, et al. Dedifferentiated chondrosarcoma. A report of the clinicopathological features and treatment of seventy-eight cases. *J Bone Joint Surg Am* 1986;68(8):1197-1205.

216. Benjamin RS, Chu P, Patel SR, et al. *De-differentiated Chondrosarcoma: A Treatable Disease*. American Association of Cancer Research, 1995.

217. Nakashima Y, Unni KK, Shives TC, et al. Mesenchymal chondrosarcoma of bone and soft tissue. A review of 111 cases. *Cancer* 1986;57(12):2444-2453.

218. Paulussen M, Ahrens S, Dunst J, et al. Localized Ewing tumor of bone: Final results of the cooperative Ewing's Sarcoma Study CESS 86. *J Clin Oncol* 2001;19(6):1818-1829.

219. Burgert EO, Jr., Nesbit ME, Garnsey LA, et al. Multimodal therapy for the management of nonpelvic, localized Ewing's sarcoma of bone: Intergroup study IESS-II. *J Clin Oncol* 1990;8(9):1514-1524.

220. Rosito P, Mancini AF, Rondelli R, et al. Italian Cooperative Study for the treatment of children and young adults with localized Ewing sarcoma of bone: A preliminary report of 6 years of experience. *Cancer* 1999;86(3):421-428.

221. Craft A, Cotterill S, Malcolm A, et al. Ifosfamide-containing chemotherapy in Ewing's sarcoma: The Second United Kingdom Children's Cancer Study Group and the Medical Research Council Ewing's Tumor Study. *J Clin Oncol* 1998;16(11):3628-3633.

222. Dunst J, Schuck A. Role of radiotherapy in Ewing tumors. *Pediatr Blood Cancer* 2004;42(5):465-470.

223. Toretsky JA, Kalebic T, Blakesley V, et al. The insulin-like growth factor-I receptor is required for EWS/FLI-1 transformation of fibroblasts. *J Biol Chem* 1997;272(49):30822-30827.

224. Patel S, Pappo A, Crowley J, et al. A SARC global collaborative phase II trial of R1507, a recombinant human monoclonal antibody to the insulin-like growth factor-1 receptor (IGF1R) in patients with recurrent or refractory sarcomas. *J Clin Oncol* 2009;27(Suppl S15; abstr 10503), 27(Suppl S15; abstr 10503).

225. Olmos D, Postel-Vinay S, Molife LR, et al. Safety, pharmacokinetics, and preliminary activity of the anti-IGF-1R antibody figitumumab (CP-751,871) in patients with sarcoma and Ewing's sarcoma: A phase 1 expansion cohort study. *Lancet Oncol* 2009;11(2):129-135.

226. McPherson CM, Suki D, McCutcheon IE, et al. Metastatic disease from spinal chordoma: A 10-year experience. *J Neurosurg Spine* 2006;5(4):277-280.

227. Amichetti M, Cianchetti M, Amelio D, et al. Proton therapy in chordoma of the base of the skull: A systematic review. *Neurosurg Rev* 2009;32(4):403-416.

228. Casali PG, Messina A, Stacchiotti S, et al. Imatinib mesylate in chordoma. *Cancer* 2004;101(9):2086-2097.

229. Stacchiotti S, Ferrari S, Ferraresi V, et al. Imatinib mesylate in advanced chordoma: A multicenter phase II study. *J Clin Oncol* 2007;25(Suppl S18; abstr 10003).

230. Meis JM, Raymond AK, Evans HL, et al. "Dedifferentiated" chordoma. A clinicopathologic and immunohistochemical study of three cases. *Am J Surg Pathol* 1987;11(7):516-525.

231. Fleming GF, Heimann PS, Stephens JK, et al. Dedifferentiated chordoma. Response to aggressive chemotherapy in two cases. *Cancer* 1993;72(3):714-718.

232. Benjamin RS, Patel SR, Gutterman JU, et al. Interferon alpha-2b as anti-angiogenesis therapy of giant cell tumor of bone: Implications for the study of newer angiogenesis-inhibitors. *Proc Am Soc Clin Oncol* 1999;548a.

233. Thomas D, Henshaw R, Skubitz K, et al. Denosumab in patients with giant-cell tumour of bone: An open-label, phase 2 study. *Lancet Oncol* 2010;11(3):275-280.

CHAPTER
41

THE AIDS-RELATED CANCERS

Adan Rios
Fredrick B. Hagemeister

■ THE CHANGING INCIDENCE OF MALIGNANCIES

The relationship between malignancies and AIDS began changing in 1996 (1,2) when the highly active antiretroviral (HAART) therapy regimens were introduced in the industrial nations. Thanks to the United Nations efforts and to general programs of economic support and philanthropy, HAART has also been successfully introduced into a significant number of developing nations. Africa, the main epicenter of the pandemic, has been the exception, due to the sheer magnitude of the African epidemic. Significant political and social turmoil has hampered the efficiency of these efforts in Africa. (3). Prior to 1996, epidemiologists noted that specific malignancies afflicted patients with AIDS, and that the risk of development of a malignancy was directly proportional to the degree of immunodeficiency of the infected host. Before the development of HAART, patients with AIDS could be separated into two groups: patients who would have an opportunistic infection as their first manifestation of AIDS (60%) and those who would have a malignancy as the mode of presentation (40%) (4).

Of those with an AIDS-related malignancy, up to 90% would have Kaposi sarcoma (KS) and the rest had non-Hodgkin lymphomas (NHL), including primary central nervous system lymphoma (PCNSL) and systemic diffuse large B-cell lymphoma (DLBCL). While there was, and continues to be, an increase in HPV-related invasive cervical cancers, particularly in women with high-grade uterine cervical dysplasias, recent findings of a lack of a clear association between the occurrence of cervical cancer and the degree of HIV-related immunosuppression has created questions about the validity of including cervical cancer among the AIDS-defining or associated malignancies (5). Epithelial dysplasia and squamous cell carcinomas of the anal canal, rectum, and oral cavity are also observed in men infected by HIV (human immunodeficiency virus). After the introduction of HAART, these previously obvious relationships between AIDS and AIDS-related malignancies have been significantly challenged. This has been most clearly observed with HIV-related Burkitt lymphoma, a NHL initially associated with the AIDS-induced immunosuppression. Investigators studying the incidence of HIV-related Burkitt lymphoma before and after introduction of HAART have found that although the improvement in immunity due to the administration of HAART has been associated with significant reductions in KS, PCNSL, and systemic DLBCL, the same is not true with Burkitt lymphoma, once considered a typical AIDS-defining malignancy (6). As in the case with invasive cervical cancer, the incidence of Burkitt lymphoma has remained stable between the pre-HAART and the post-HAART eras, thereby increasing its proportional frequency. In addition to these observations, there has been in the post-HAART era an increase in Hodgkin lymphoma (Epstein-Barr virus related), lung cancer, and non-melanoma skin cancer, which carries significant etiologic implications related to the complex relationship between immunity, aging, chronic antigenic stimulation, and viral oncogenesis. Overall, the excess risk of a malignancy in HIV disease has been observed, before and after HAART introduction, mostly in cancers with an established or suspected infectious cause (7).

In this chapter, we first discuss HIV and its effect on the immune system. We then concentrate on the discussion of those malignancies associated to the AIDS immunosuppression. We also include a discussion of other malignancies such as Burkitt lymphoma and HPV-related cancers, which although not directly associated with the HIV-induced immunosuppression do occur with a high enough incidence in HIV-infected patients to merit study.

■ HIV DISEASE

HISTORICAL SIGNIFICANCE OF THE VIRUS

The AIDS epidemic came into the medical world in 1980 with the publication in the CDC MMWR (Center for Diseases Control and Prevention Morbidity and Mortality Weekly Report) of a series of cases of patients afflicted by de novo opportunistic infections, mostly *Pneumocystis jiroveci* (formerly known as *P carinii*) pneumonia and CMV (cytomegalovirus) infections. This first report was important since these conditions usually occurred in patients with an established immunodeficiency status (8). It was soon followed by another one in which KS, an infrequent malignancy, was reported in 26 homosexual men, thought to be previously immunologically healthy (9). As the numbers of similar cases exponentially increased throughout the United States and Europe, reports of other parts of the world helped to confirm that a new pandemic with an epicenter in sub-Saharan Africa had occurred (10). This exponential increase in the number of reported cases with similar clinical presentations gave way to the designation of a new syndrome, the acquired immunodeficiency syndrome, or AIDS (11). Today, more than 25 years after those initial reports, much is known and much is still to be learned about the cause of the syndrome, the HIV virus, and its associated complications, including opportunistic infections and malignancies (12).

HIV disease is caused by the infection of a human subject with a retrovirus, HIV. HIV is transmitted only through blood or unprotected sexual contact, causing a progressive destruction of the immune system followed by a high occurrence of opportunistic infections and malignancies. When either an opportunistic infection or a specific type of malignancy occurs, it signals a significant degree of impairment of the immune system function. The occurrence or association of opportunistic infections and a status of immune suppression was a well-established phenomenon in the medical literature and clinical practice. The relationship between immune surveillance dysfunction and development of malignancies had been described to some degree in the medical literature (13). It was not until the early 1970s, with the initiation of kidney transplantation programs in Canada, that an increased incidence of malignancies in patients treated with an immunosuppressant, azathioprine, was formally described (14). Subsequent to those reports it became clear that pharmacologically immune-suppressed patients had increases of several folds of magnitude in certain types of cancers and opportunistic infections. Typically these patients had either KS or lymphoproliferative malignancies, although other types of malignancies were also reported. In a sense, these patients had a chemically induced AIDS whereas HIV patients have a biologically induced AIDS. No discussion of AIDS-related malignancies can occur without a review of what is known about HIV virus, the cause of AIDS, and the status of the HIV pandemic.

ORIGIN OF THE DISEASE

With the discovery of the HIV in 1983 (15), much of the mystery surrounding AIDS was dispelled. Today, it is known that AIDS is caused in humans by a retrovirus, more specifically a lentivirus (Latin, lentus, slow, + virus), endemic in African monkeys, which entered the human population as a result of a cross-species transmission or zoonosis (16,17). There are two types of HIV virus that have infected humans: HIV-1 and HIV-2. HIV-1 originated from chimpanzees infected by a retrovirus, the SIVcpz (the chimpanzee simian immunodeficiency virus) and HIV-2 from sooty mangabeys monkeys, also endemically infected by a retrovirus, the SIVsm. The SIVcpz is itself the product of recombination in chimpanzees of two retroviruses of monkeys predated by chimpanzees: the SIVrcm and the SIVgsn (the red capped mangabeys, *Cerocebus torquatus*, and the great spot-nosed monkeys, *Ceropithecus nictitans*, respectively). These viruses do not cause any disease in their natural hosts and were named simian immunodeficiency viruses or SIV after their genetic and structural similarities with HIV. Each one is then subclassified in groups and clades based on phylogenetic criteria: HIV-1 having three groups, M, N, and O with the predominant group M comprising 11 clades A to K and HIV-2 with six clades, A to F. In both HIV-1 and HIV-2, there is evidence of recombination among clades giving origin to genetically complex viral quasispecies. The transmission from animals to humans occurs when endemically SIVcpz infected chimpanzees enter in contact with humans as a result of hunting and butchering or through contact with infected animals used as domestic pets, as is the case of the sooty mangabeys monkeys (18).

HIV-2 is endemic in coastal West Africa and HIV-1 in west equatorial Africa (19). While HIV-2 has been for the most part contained to Africa, several HIV-1 clades from the group M have been responsible for the vast majority of worldwide infections. In the western world, HIV-1 B is responsible for over 90% of infections, while in Africa types A, G, and D and in Asia the types A and the circulating recombinant forms CRF-001 and CRF-002 can be found (20). The disease is diagnosed by detecting the presence of anti-HIV antibodies in the serum by an ELISA (enzyme linked immunoadsorbent assay) test. The initial result can be corroborated with a second ELISA test or by a Western blot blood test. The amount of actively replicating virus in the host can be measured by quantitative PCR (polymerase chain reaction) or via signal amplification techniques such as branch-DNA HIV viral load (21,22).

STATUS OF THE PANDEMIC AND ITS EFFECTS ON THE IMMUNE SYSTEM

HIV disease and its consequence, AIDS, are responsible for a human tragedy of incalculable proportions. It is estimated that since the beginning of the pandemic there have been over 16 million deaths, more than 50 million persons have been infected (including those who have died), and the rate of new infections is estimated to be 15,000 new infections per day. Most of these new infections occur in developing nations affecting a significant number of women and children. The two most frequent modes of HIV transmission are unprotected sex and the use of intravenous drugs. While the main epicenter of the pandemic continues to be sub-Saharan Africa, there are new epicenters in the former Soviet Union, China, India, and Latin-America. In the United States, minority groups such as Hispanics and African Americans as well as younger generations of gay men continued to be disproportionately affected by HIV (23).

HIV is an enveloped diploid RNA virus, meaning that each viral particle contains two RNA ribbons each with its genetic material and an armamentarium of enzymes essential for the virus to go through its natural life cycle. These viral components and elements are within a viral particle with a membrane composed of HLA groups and other surface membrane proteins as well as the viral protein gp120 in a trimer form (24). Among the enzymes packaged within the viral particle are reverse transcriptase, integrase, and proteases, all essential for survival of the virus. Once the virus enters a susceptible host, through sex or blood, the viral envelope spikes composed of the viral protein gp120 trimers bind to receptors (CD4) and coreceptors (CCR-5) of cells of the immune system, entering the cells through a process of membrane fusion. The content of the viral particle is released into the cytoplasm of the infected cell. The viral RNA is transcribed into DNA which is then integrated at random into the genomic material of the infected cell. From there, through a complex process of transcription activators and as a direct result of the natural frequent cycles of cell replication of the immune system, the virus with the participation of its enzymatic machinery generates new viral particles. These new viral particles are released through a process of budding and lysis continuing to infect new susceptible cells. This complex process occurs at an unusually fast pace (25). Recent findings have shown that the initial process of HIV infection is characterized in simian models of AIDS and in man by a rapid destruction of the memory cells of the gut-associated tissue, GALT (gut-associated lymphoid tissue). This process occurs in a matter of days to few weeks in the animal models and in several weeks in man. GALT harbors the majority of body lymphocytes in comparison to the 2 to 5% of lymphocytes located in the peripheral circulation (26,27).

The result of destruction of GALT, together with the aberrant activation of B cells and inhibition of the immune system function by HIV viral gene products such as the vif protein induce a severe immune dysfunction and depletion (28). The vif protein inhibits the *APOBEC3* gene family, implicated in the control of HIV infection including the production of neutralizing antibodies. Once HIV is integrated into the genome of the susceptible cells, there is a process of destruction by attrition of the immune system, which in the absence of effective inhibition of viral replication, leads to a progressive status of immunodeficiency, with the development of opportunistic infections and tumors characteristic of AIDS. This process of early senescence of the immune system is implicated in changes at a molecular level resulting in the loss of control of oncogenic viruses and molecular changes associated with the malignant transformations observed in AIDS.

■ AIDS-DEFINING MALIGNANCIES

KAPOSI SARCOMA

Epidemiology

At the beginnings of the AIDS pandemic, KS was a disease not entirely unknown to the medical world. It was initially described by Dr. Moritz Kaposi in 1872 (29) as

an indolent dermatological disease characterized by the appearance of purplish nodules or plaques, particularly in the lower extremities of older men of Eastern Europe, Mediterranean, or Jewish descent (classical KS). Canadian investigators first noted in the 1970s that it occurred in patients who had undergone renal transplants and were exposed to immunosuppressant regimens, particularly azathioprine (transplant or iatrogenic KS) (30). These observations included the first reports of remission of the disease when immunosuppressant regimens were temporarily discontinued, suggesting a relationship between immunodeficiency and the malignancies. In this same group of patients, investigators also noted a high incidence of NHL. Previously in the 1960s, British investigators had reported the appearance of an aggressive lymphadenopathic form of KS geographically confined to equatorial Africa (African KS) (31). This form of KS occurred in younger patients and was characterized by aggressive involvement of lymph nodes and the appearance of nodules and plaques that rapidly progressed to severe ulcerations of the lower extremities. These reports were considered to be almost a medical curiosity, and it was not until a report, published in the CDC Morbidity and Mortality Weekly Report of 26 gay men with KS, that the disease became and still is one of the hallmarks of the AIDS epidemic (epidemic or AIDS-related KS) (9). In contrast to the known characteristics of KS in patients with the classical form, in patients with AIDS, the KS lesions appeared with an aggressive pattern of distribution which included the trunk, arms, and face in addition to the lower extremities. In the absence of effective antiretroviral therapies, many patients died of a combination of tumor progression and associated opportunistic infections as terminal events. Despite the advent of HAART (highly active antiretroviral therapy) in 1996, KS continues to be the most prevalent cancer among HIV-infected patients, although the use of HAART has significantly changed the incidence of the disease. From 1990 to 1995 the incidence of KS in the United States was 1838.9 cases per 100,000 person-years in contrast to 334.6 cases per 100,000 person-years from 1996 to 2002. In the United States and in Europe, AIDS-related KS has been almost exclusively diagnosed in homosexual men, suggesting that the prevalence of the disease may vary among different categories of AIDS patients. However, in Africa, where the human herpes virus-8 (HHV-8) or KSHV (KS herpesvirus) is endemic, the male-to-female ratio of AIDS-related KS in some African countries is 2:1, almost the same ratio observed in transplant- or iatrogenic-related KS. Thus, in the presence of profound immune suppression such as the exogenous immunosuppression in transplant patients or HIV infection in AIDS patients, factors that made the disease more prevalent in males than in females prior to the AIDS pandemic appear to be of little relevance (32). What is clear is that the incidence of AIDS-related KS is related to the degree of the immune suppression of the infected hosts, with most afflicted patients having CD4+ cell counts of 200 CD4+ cells/μL or less.

The Viral Etiology of Kaposi Sarcoma

The etiologic agent of all forms of KS is HHV-8, also called KSHV (33). Early in the pandemic, several other viruses or agents were implicated as the cause of AIDS-related KS, including cytomegalovirus (CMV). In 1994, sequences of a new herpes-like virus were isolated from the lesions of an AIDS-KS patient using a subtractive PCR technique called representative differential analysis. This technique allowed the preferential amplification of DNA sequences present in the affected tissue and absent in normal tissue from the same individual. Investigators found that sequences isolated with this technique from KS lesions were homologous but not identical to other known herspesvirues and thus were named HHV-8, since it became the eighth known herpes virus (34). Not all patients infected with HHV-8 developed KS; however, viral DNA and seroconversion can be detected in patients prior to the development of KS, confirming the role of HHV-8 as the cause of KS and the relationship of its pathogenesis to immunosuppression in addition to other cofactors.

HHV-8 belongs to the gamma-herpesvirus subfamily, to the subgroup gamma-2 or rhadinovirus (from the Latin term rhadino, referring to the tendency of the viral genome to break apart when it is isolated) and is the first human virus of this subfamily identified. As with many other infectious diseases, the detection of the infection relies on the presence of antibodies against viral antigens using immunofluorescence assays (IFAs) based on the use of B lymphocytes as the antigen source or ELISA with recombinant immunogenic proteins or peptides of HHV-8 (35,36). The seroprevalence of the infection mirrors the distribution of AIDS-related KS, with the highest infection rates in Central African countries (80%) to 25 to 50% among homosexual men in the western world and an intermediate level in the Mediterranean regions. Of epidemiological interest, the adult general population of blood donors in North America and Europe has an HHV-8 seroprevalence ranging from 0 to 8%. This seroprevalence of HHV-8 is also closely related to the geographic incidence of KS, with the highest HHV-8 infection rate in geographic areas where classic or endemic forms of KS are more common. In addition to being the etiologic agent of AIDS-related KS, HHV-8 has been associated with two other lymphoproliferative disorders: primary effusion lymphoma (PEL, a subset of body cavity–based lymphomas [BCBL] [Fig. 41-1], which were subsequently called PELs) and multicentric Castleman disease (33).

Pathogenesis of KS

In addition to its own unique viral genes, HHV-8 incorporates into its genome a significant number of host genes such as cyclin-D and growth factor IL-6 (37). These genes, many of which are directly involved in control of the replication and survival of the host cells, become involved in the replication, survival, and transformation of the infected tumor cells. Genes such as the viral K1 gene kaposin and viral G protein–coupled receptor (vGPCR) have transformation potential. Others deregulate cell growth and lead to transformation including viral IL-6, viral IL-10, viral cc-class chemokines, and viral FLICE-inhibitory protein (vFLIP) (38). The expression of the different key genes in transformation, increased replication, survival of the tumor cells, immunosuppression, and modulation of immune surveillance is related to the latency and lytic cycles of HHV-8. During the latency-phase, genes such as *LANA-1* (latency-associated nuclear antigen), in addition to the maintenance of latency of the viral infection, inactivate p53, inhibiting apoptosis. Also, during the latency phase, a viral cyclin prevents cell-cycle arrest by cyclin-dependent kinases, pRB and vFLIP, avoiding the activation of the Fas death receptor pathway. During the HHV-8 lytic phase, homologues of genes involved in replication promote the replication and proliferation of tumor cells. Such genes include the K1 kaposin gene, a Bcl-2 homologue, a viral G protein–coupled receptor gene (vGPCRP), a viral homologue of interleukin (IL-6), and viral macrophages and interferon regulatory factors (39). Some of these genes also have immune suppression functions such as the inhibition by vFLIP of cytotoxicity of T cells against HHV-8 infected cells and the inhibition of HHV-8 class 2 major histocompatibility complex (MHC)–mediated T-cell activation by K1 (40). Finally, other viral proteins such as K3 and K5 downregulate the presentation of MHC class 1 molecules on the cell surface (41).

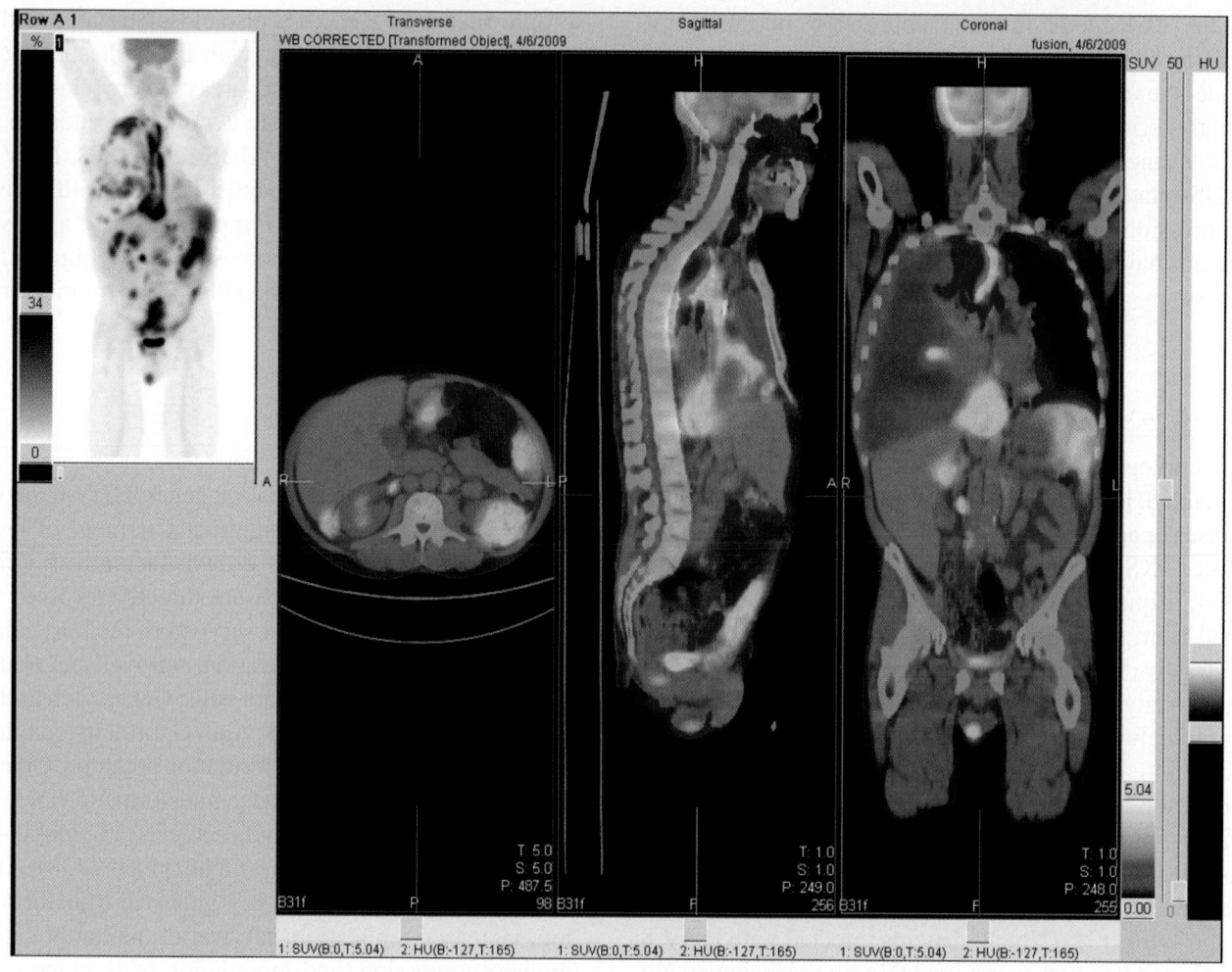

FIGURE 41-1.   Scan in a patient with PEL (primary effusion lymphoma) showing multiple sites of increased FDG activity and a large right pleural effusion.

Pathology of KS

Typically, the histology of KS is characterized by the abundance of spindle cells in a matrix of neovascular formation and a rich background of mononuclear inflammatory cells and collagen. The vascular spaces are dilated and contain extravasated erythrocytes. The histological findings correlate with the clinical findings. Involvement of the reticular dermis, reflected by patchy lesions and the involvement of all the layers of the skin, clinically presents as nodular or plaque lesions that can coalesce, interfering with the lymphatic circulation and are histologically and clinically associated with surrounding subcutaneous edema (42). The spindle KS cells are rich in endothelial Factor VIII as demonstrated by the use of immunohistochemistry techniques (43). Recent microarray studies have recognized the origin of the KS cell to be virally transformed lymphatic endothelial cells (44). Spindle cells derived from KS lesions express a variety of

angiogenic/inflammatory cytokines and growth factors, including VEGF, basic fibroblast growth factor (bFGF), interleukin-1 (IL-1), and IL-6, among others (45). In addition KS cells overexpress receptors for multiple cytokines suggesting that they grow through autocrine or paracrine mechanisms (46). They also proliferate in response to IL-1, IFNγ, IL-6, and tumor necrosis factor (TNF), abundantly present in the serum of patients with poorly controlled HIV infection, and MMPs (matrix metalloproteinases), enzymes involved in the destruction of extracellular matrix proteins required for angiogenesis and metastasis (47,48). In AIDS-related KS Tat (the trans-activator of transcription protein) is a costimulator of the KS spindle and endothelial cell replication, promoting an increase in the concentrations of bFGF. This in turn upregulates the integrins $\alpha_5\beta_1$ and $\alpha_v\beta_3$, receptors for fibronectin and vitronectin, which are highly expressed in AIDS-KS (49).

Clinical Features of KS

Most patients with AIDS-related KS will have the initial presentation of their disease with CD4+ cell counts of 200 CD4+ cells/μL of blood with increased severity in the number and aggressiveness of the lesions in those who are more severely immunosuppressed. There are periods of exacerbation alternated with periods of quiescence related to the oscillations of the immune status of the patient. Finally, extensive reviews of the medical literature seem to indicate that the tumor never or exceptionally invades the central nervous system. This is of great biological interest as many other human malignant tumors are characterized as they progress by the invasion of the central nervous system (50,56).

Most patients with AIDS-related KS will have the appearance of purplish lesions located either in the lower extremities or the trunk as the initial physical manifestation of the disease (51). The distribution of the lesions in the skin often follows the Langer's folds of the skin. The occurrence of lesions in acral regions of the body such as the tip of the nose is common. The evolution of the skin lesions correlates directly with the status of the patient's immune system. In the pre-HAART era, severe involvement of the skin of the face by typical, raised purplish lesions was frequent.

With progression of the disease, there is frequent involvement of the gastrointestinal tract. Lesions of the palate and gums are often the first ones to be noted (52), and diarrhea and occasional bleeding can be manifestations of involvement of the gastrointestinal tract by KS (52). In the case of disease involvement of the lower extremities, progressive edema with nodular and plaque lesions that coalesce can cause significant discomfort

and pain. Prior to the introduction of HAART in 1996, this was one of the most frequent and serious complications of the disease, since cases of "elephantiasis" secondary to the progression of the disease were extremely difficult to manage and treat (53). This type of presentation was the cause of significant morbidity and even mortality. Advanced cases of AIDS-related KS often involve ulceration of some lesions particularly when located in the lower extremities (53). Lymph node involvement is frequent and there are occasions in which there is only generalized involvement of lymph nodes requiring a biopsy for confirmation of the diagnosis. In advanced cases, lung involvement is frequent and usually manifested by bilateral basilar infiltrates mixed with a nodular appearance (54). However, even in the cases of severe involvement of the lungs and the mucosa of the gastrointestinal tract, the occurrence of severe hemoptysis or gastrointestinal bleeding is infrequent. During the early years of the epidemic, there were a significant number of patients who in the absence of HIV treatment had involvement of vital organs such as the liver and heart with large masses of Kaposi sarcoma. These patients often died from a combination of progression of their KS tumors and associated opportunistic infections (55,56).

Staging and Prognostic Factors of KS

The staging of AIDS-related KS is complicated by the fact that the tumor usually occurs as multiple skin lesions and the usual TNM system used in other solid tumors is not easily applicable. A new system based on the work of Chachoua and colleagues was proposed in 1989 by the AIDS Clinical Trial Group (ACTG) (57) (Table 41-1). This staging system takes into account the

TABLE 41-1 | TIS STAGING SYSTEM FOR AIDS-RELATED KAPOSI SARCOMA AND RISK STATUS

Characteristics	GOOD RISK (0) *All of the Following*	POOR RISK (1) *Any of the Following*
Tumor (T)	Tumor confined to skin and lymph nodes and/or minimal oral disease*	Tumor-associated edema or ulceration; extensive oral KS; gastrointestinal KS; KS in other nonnodal viscera
Immune system (I)	CD4 cells ≥150/mm^3	CD4 cells <150/mm^3
Systemic illness (S)	No history of opportunistic infection or thrush; no B symptoms[†]; performance status ≥70 (Karnofsky)	History of opportunistic infection and/or thrush; B symptoms; performance status <70 (Karnofsky); other HIV-related illness (eg, neurologic disease, lymphoma)

KS, Kaposi sarcoma.
*Minimal oral disease defined as nonnodular KS confined to the palate.
[†]B symptoms: fever, drenching night sweats, and/or >10% involuntary weight loss.
Reproduced, with permission, from Levine AM, Tulpule A. Clinical aspects and management of AIDS-related Kaposi's sarcoma. Eur J Cancer 2001;37:1288-1295.

extent of tumor involvement, the immune status as measured by the level of CD4+ cell count, and the presence or absence of any systemic illness (B symptoms). In addition to a complete physical examination, it includes a complete blood count, serum chemistries, HIV viral load, a panendoscopy of the gastrointestinal tract, CT of the abdomen and pelvis, and when indicated, based on signs and symptoms, the performance of bronchoscopy for those cases where pulmonary involvement by KS is suspected(58). When in doubt, biopsies of skin or lymph nodes should be performed to confirm the diagnosis or rule out entities which may be similar in presentation such as bacillary angiomatosis or pyoderma gangrenosum (59). After the advent of HAART, the extent of disease and the presence of HIV-systemic symptoms became the most important prognostic factors. Pulmonary involvement by KS carries a particular poor prognosis. Correlations with the levels of HIV viral load, and the status of HHV-8 infection are under study in relationship to their impact on survival (60).

Therapy of KS

Highly Active Antiretroviral Therapy

The initiation of HAART brought with it a dramatic and significant decrease in the incidence of AIDS-related KS (61). HAART consists of the administration of a combination of agents with anti-HIV activity, including inhibitors of HIV reverse transcriptase and HIV protease inhibitors. Inhibitors of the HIV reverse transcriptase can in turn consist of nucleoside analogue inhibitors of HIV reverse transcriptase (NRTI) and nonnucleoside analogue inhibitors of HIV reverse transcriptase (NNRTI). HAART usually includes two NRTIs and one HIV protease inhibitor or two NRTIs and one NNRTI. The consensus of experts in the field about which anti-HIV drugs should be used frontline as components of HAART therapy is periodically published in *Guidelines for the Use of Antiretroviral Agents in HIV-1 Infected Adults and Adolescents* by the Department of Human and Health Services (DHHS). These Guidelines are frequently updated and are available online by visiting the DHHS web site (62). For those patients in whom KS is part of the initial diagnosis of AIDS, HAART therapy should be started irrespective of the extent of the disease. For most patients with minimal, asymptomatic tumor burden, the initiation of HAART for HIV treatment constitutes frontline therapy of their AIDS-related KS. This approach can control KS lesions for long periods of time (often more than 1 year) and in many instances results in complete disappearance of the KS lesions (63).

Patients with extensive disease or visceral involvement can receive systemic chemotherapy in addition to HAART.

Radiation Therapy for KS

The use of radiotherapy in the management and treatment of AIDS-related KS lesions has become more effective due to HAART and effective systemic chemotherapeutic regimens (64). It can be useful for treatment of minimal local disease and in cases where the use of systemic treatment other than HAART is not absolutely indicated. It can also be used as an adjunct treatment modality for patients where the administration of chemotherapy leads to incomplete results enhancing the beneficial effects of the systemic treatment. Depending on the general condition of the patient and the size of the lesions to be treated, doses range from the administration of a single fraction to fractionated doses over periods of 2 to 4 weeks. For the treatment of single lesions and for patients who are more frail, a frequently used strategy includes the administration of a single 800-cGy dose. In selected cases, radiotherapy can be used for cosmetic reasons, although this should be done carefully to avoid secondary side effects such as postradiation cataracts in the case of periorbital lesions (64). For larger lesions or when the therapeutic intent is cosmetic, fractionated doses between 200 and 4000 cGy are effective and carry less risk (65). For patients receiving systemic therapy, radiotherapy can be an adjuvant for the treatment of complicated single lesions, particularly when they are bleeding, ulcerated, painful or when there is complication by the lesion of the well-being of the patient. Such is the case of patients with disseminated disease receiving systemic treatment and in whom oral lesions due to local pain or size may affect the ingestion of food.

Local Therapy Other Than Radiotherapy for KS

The local treatment of KS lesions with other modalities than radiotherapy is indicated when the burden of disease is minimal, for cosmetic reasons and/or palliative purposes (local ulcerated lesions, painful oral lesions). Prior to the development of HAART and effective systemic chemotherapy for AIDS-related KS, local therapies were an important component of the treatment for these patients. Techniques such as cryotherapy, laser photocoagulation, intralesional injections of chemotherapeutic agents, and application of alitretinoin topical gel were used with varied success and risks of complications. Better results could be achieved when the lesions were small and located in areas where the side effects of the treatment were not subject to anatomical complications (66,67). For example, the injection of oral cavity lesions with chemotherapy can often be accompanied by severe pain and ulceration of the treated lesions. Patients can develop difficulties in eating and this could have an adverse impact in their overall well-being (68). In general, the physical destruction of lesions is accompanied by a rate of success of 60 to 80%, depending on the size of the lesions and the frequency of the treatments. All these modalities of local therapies produce local scarring. During the early years of the pandemic in the absence of better treatments, they were useful therapeutic interventions. The use of surgery may be appropriate in selected cases such as large skin lesions or when there are complications (bleeding or obstruction of a hollow viscus).

In the modern era, the use of local therapies such as cryo and laser therapies may have a role for patients with few and small lesions. Other treatments such as intralesional injection of chemotherapeutic agents and application of alitretinoin gel (69) have been replaced by a more sophisticated use of radiotherapy techniques, HAART, and systemic chemotherapy.

Immunomodulators in Therapy of KS

Since the demonstration of the activity of interferon-alpha (IFNα) in hairy cell leukemia and renal cell cancer in 1984 (70), there was an impetus to use the same doses of interferon in patients with AIDS-related KS. However, the relatively low doses of interferon-alpha which were highly effective against hairy cell leukemia and had demonstrable activity against renal cell carcinoma were ineffective against AIDS-related KS (71). Known reported results of a dose-response study that unequivocally demonstrated the therapeutic effect of interferon-alpha in KS when used at doses of 20 to 30 MU/m^2. The interferon-alpha was administered daily for several weeks (at least a month) followed by a less intense schedule of administration (three times a week for at least 6 months) (72). Other investigators confirmed that the response was not related to the type of interferon-alpha used. Both recombinant and lymphoblastoid forms of interferon-alpha produced the same results (73). A different situation was observed with interferon-gamma. Under the angiogenic stimuli of interferon-gamma, KS have the capacity to replicate resulting in a deleterious impact on patients treated with this agent in pilot studies (74). As a result of these interferon trials, recombinant IFNs α-2a (Roferon-A) and α-2b (Intron-A) were approved for the systemic treatment of patients with AIDS-related KS. Response rates in these early trials were in the range of 25 to 30%. Subsequent expanded use of these agents revealed their true activity to be in the range of 15 to 20%.

Interferon has various modes of action in the treatment of KS. It can block the synthesis of viral proteins and the budding of viral particles from infected cells in addition to other complex pleiotropic effects (75). Interferon has other potent immunomodulatory effects as well as antiproliferative activity resulting in an antitumoral response, but its actions are also accompanied by significant systemic side effects including tiredness, fatigue, anorexia, hepatotoxicity, and severe myelosuppression. These side effects occur more frequently in patients with severe immunosuppression, as measured by counts of less than 200 CD4+ cells/μL of blood, and in patients with previous opportunistic infections or in those already exposed to chemotherapy. Therefore, in an attempt to capitalize on the effectiveness of interferon-alpha as monotherapy, investigators combined reduced doses of interferon with the antiretroviral agents zidovudine and didanosine. Although patients had responses to this approach, the side effects were not ameliorated with reductions in the doses of interferon (76). In addition, the combination of interferon with these myelosuppressive agents caused an increase in the frequency of neutropenia and immunosuppression in these patients. Other attempts to reduce interferon side effects have included studies that incorporated the use of pegylated interferon (77). However, the side effects of this drug observed in therapy of patients treated for hepatitis C makes it unlikely that toxicities in these trials will be any different from those noted in previous studies with interferon-alpha. With the development of HAART and the use of more effective systemic chemotherapy regimens in the treatment of AIDS-related KS, the interest in the use of interferon-alpha in the treatment of AIDS-related KS has declined.

Chemotherapy for KS

Indications for the use of systemic chemotherapy in AIDS-related KS have been the same prior to and after the introduction of HAART: extensive skin, mucocutaneous and/or visceral involvement by tumor. Often, in patients who require systemic chemotherapy, local radiotherapy is used to treat local complications in addition to the systemic disease. Since the introduction of HAART, there has been a dramatic change in the use of chemotherapeutic agents with activity against AIDS-related KS. This has resulted in better and more durable responses with increased tolerability and durability, than those observed prior to HAART.

Before the discovery of antiretrovirals, a variety of chemotherapeutic agents had modest to significant activity as monotherapy for KS. This was, more evident when used in patients with relatively good immunological status and low tumor burden. These agents included etoposide, vinblastine, vincristine, bleomycin, doxorubicin, vinorelbine, and epirubicin (78-84). These drugs induced responses in 40 to 69% of patients. Most of these studies were not randomized trials, and for the most part, performed in very heterogeneous groups of patients. In part this was due to the inherent difficulties associated with the need to treat a large number of patients during the early years of the AIDS pandemic. With the introduction of antiretroviral therapy in the early 1990s, combination chemotherapy became the standard of treatment for AIDS-related KS. The most frequently used and established regimen was the combination of doxorubicin (Adriamycin), bleomycin, and vincristine (ABV). Standard doses of ABV included doxorubicin 20 mg/m^2, bleomycin 10 U/m^2, and vincristine in maximum doses of 1 to 2 mg. ABV became the standard of treatment with an accepted response rate of 60%, with complications and tolerance depending on the performance status and general condition of the patient (85). Antiretroviral and other supportive therapies with growth factors (GM-CSF and G-CSF) paired with vigorous prophylaxis of opportunistic infections reduced the treatment's risks for these patients. The ABV regimen complications were the expected ones with systemic chemotherapy and included alopecia and myelosuppression in addition to the potential for cardiac toxicity by doxorubicin.

The recognition of ABV as an effective treatment of AIDS-related KS was followed by the introduction of agents which today are considered the standard of care for AIDS-related KS, including liposomal encapsulated anthracyclines (doxorubicin or Doxil and daunorubicin or Daunoxome) (86) and taxanes (paclitaxel) (87). Paclitaxel promotes apoptosis and downregulates Bcl-2 protein expression in KS cells in vitro and in KS-like lesions in mice. In addition, it has an important antimitotic effect associated with its capacity for the disruption of tubulin activity during mitosis (88).

The current treatment of AIDS-related KS is based on the combination of an anthracycline (liposomal doxorubicin, 20 mg/m^2 or liposomal daunorubicin, 40 mg/m^2 but *not both* together) with paclitaxel 25 mg/m^2 with or without bleomycin or vincristine. Escalation of the dose of liposomal doxorubicin is not recommended due to the production of a syndrome of desquamation of the skin of the palm of soles and feet known as palmar-plantar erythrodysesthesia (89). In contrast, the dose of liposomal-encapsulated daunorubicin can be increased to up to 60 mg/m^2 or even higher for patients who tolerate the lower doses (90). Since liposomal doxorubicin is encapsulated in a pegylated pseudoliposome, its half-life is longer than liposomal daunorubicin which is encapsulated in a true liposome, allowing for dose escalation if necessary. This is of particular relevance in patients with advanced disease or significant pulmonary involvement and for whom prompt control and achievement of a quick therapeutic response is of great importance (Fig. 41-2).

Future Therapies for KS

Despite the described efficiency of HAART and of systemic and local treatments for AIDS-related KS, only patients with early disease and relatively good performance status consistently achieve durable remissions. For the rest of patients with advanced disease, only significant palliation and stabilization of disease can be achieved with the current regimen of treatments. For these reasons efforts are underway to develop new therapies based on the knowledge of the physiopathology of the disease. For example, since angiogenesis is an important component of AIDS-related KS, agents such as thalidomide and anti-VEGF agents such as bevacizumab are of great interest in the therapy of this disease. Metalloprotease inhibitors are also of great interest and active clinical trials are in progress. Viruses associated with the production of malignancies tend to constitutively activate the NF-κB pathway and thus agents that can inhibit this pathway may be of some value (91). Clinical trials with agents such as bortezomib, an agent with activity against multiple myeloma, a drug that putatively inhibits the NF-κB pathway, may also be useful in treatment of AIDS-related KS (92). There is also great interest in the inhibition of signaling cell receptors implicated in the stimulation of angiogenesis such as platelet-derived growth factor receptor (PDGF-R) and C-kit receptor by agents such as imatinib, an orally administered tyrosine kinase inhibitor, approved by the FDA for treatment of chronic myeloid leukemia (CML) and gastrointestinal stromal tumor (GIST) (93).

Finally, there is significant interest in the development of therapies against the latent phase of HHV-8, the most common form of HHV-8 in KS cells, since this viral illness cannot be treated with standard antiherpetic drugs such as foscarnet and cidofovir (94). This area of research has led to potential development of a possible vaccine against HHV-8. Despite all these new and better potential therapeutic developments, the significant impact of HAART in the incidence of AIDS-related KS cannot

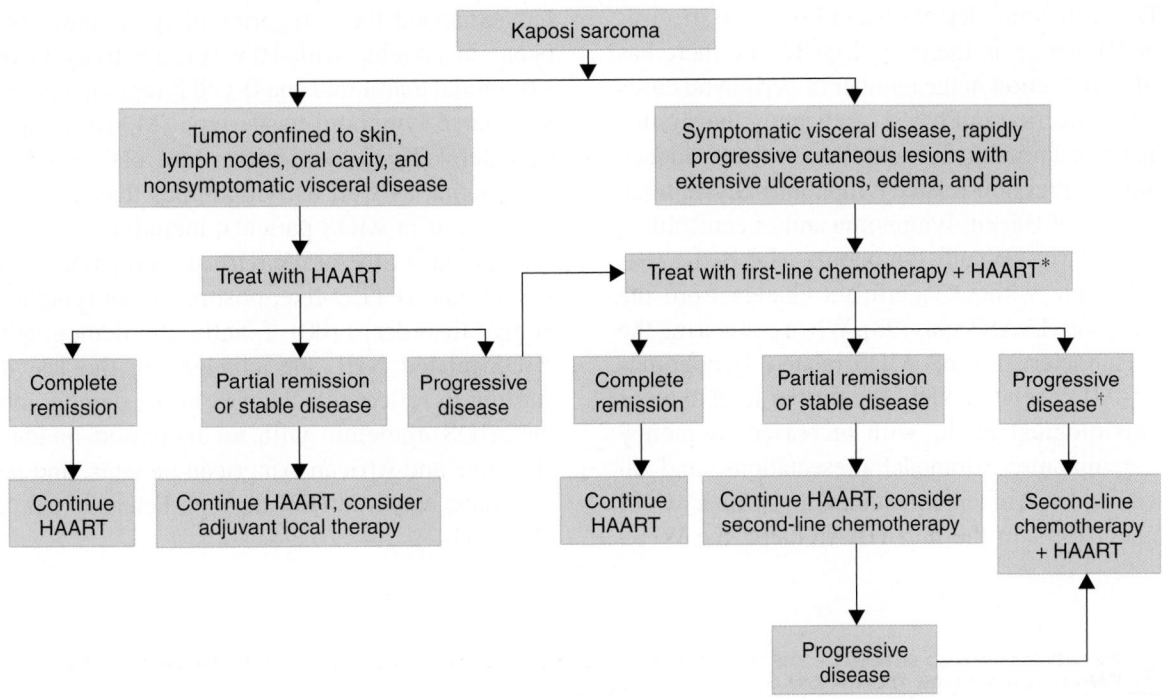

FIGURE 41-2. Algorithm for the management of AIDS-related Kaposi sarcoma. *Monthly evaluation of Kaposi sarcoma clinical response and estimation of CD4+ cell count and HIV-RNA levels. [†]HAART regimen should be changed in the case of immunovirologic failure. HAART, highly active antiretroviral therapy. *(Reproduced, with permission, from Catellan AM, et al. Recent advances in the treatment of AIDS-related Kaposi sarcoma. Am J Clin Dermatol 2002;3[7]:451-462.)*

be overemphasized. The development of more potent and less toxic HAART regimes and the acceptance of earlier therapeutic intervention against HIV seem to be the main paths to the control of the epidemic of AIDS-related KS.

AIDS-RELATED NON-HODGKIN LYMPHOMA: SYSTEMIC NHL

Epidemiology

Soon after the AIDS pandemic began, it became clear that NHL was second to KS, the most frequent malignancy associated with AIDS. It was also clear that both KS and NHL were occurring with an incidence that had an almost linear relationship to the degree of the patient's immunodeficiency status (95). In 1985, high- or intermediate-grade B-cell NHLs were considered part of the spectrum of AIDS-related malignancies (96). Eighty percent of AIDS-related NHLs are systemic (peripheral) lymphomas, involving nodal or extranodal sites, with 15 to 20% originating in the primary central nervous system (PCNSL). A small proportion, less than 3%, of the systemic AIDS-related NHL patients have primary

effusion lymphomas (PEL), also known as "body cavity" lymphomas. In general, the risk of AIDS-related NHL in patients with HIV appears to be highest in those who have poor immune function with average CD4+ cell counts of 150 CD4+ cells/μL of blood (96).

As with other immunodeficiency-associated malignancies, a viral relationship is implicated in the development of the disease. EBV (Epstein-Barr virus) appears to contribute to the development of most of these tumors, although HHV-8 is specifically associated with the development of PEL (97). This influence of EBV in the development of AIDS-related NHL may be the reason why there is no relationship between the risk of development of AIDS-related NHL and specific modes of HIV transmission. In the pre-HAART era, the incidence of AIDS-related NHL was 60 to 200 times higher than in a matched HIV seronegative population; the relative risk was even higher for PCNSL. Age, nadir of CD4+ cell count, and the absence of anti-HIV therapy were three critical factors that predicted for the development of AIDS-related NHL. In the pre-HAART era, 80% of these NHLs, including 60% of systemic cases and 20% of PCNSL, were immunoblastic variants associated with CD4+ cell count depletion and Epstein-Barr virus infection. However, in the post-HAART era, there has been a 30% reduction in the number of peripheral cases and a 70% reduction in PCNSL, indicating the significant impact of immune reconstitution in the incidence of immunosuppression-related lymphomas. In contrast, the incidence of Burkitt lymphoma and of centroblastic diffuse large B-cell lymphoma (DLBCL) has remained stable without significant change from the pre- to the post-HAART eras (98). When comparing the clinical characteristics of AIDS-related lymphomas with non–AIDS-related NHL, the former tend to be of higher histological grade, with increased frequency of "B" symptoms, extranodal presentations, and an increased incidence of leptomeningeal and primary CNS involvement (99). In the post-HAART era, the WHO has expanded the categories of lymphomas that can occur in patients with HIV seropositivity to include extranodal marginal zone B-cell lymphoma of mucosa-associated lymphoid tissue type (MALT lymphoma), peripheral T-cell lymphoma, and classical Hodgkin lymphoma, as well as lymphomas that more specifically occur in AIDS patients, including plasmablastic lymphomas of the oral cavity and polymorphic B-cell lymphomas (PTLD-like, posttransplant lymphoproliferative disorder) (100). Finally, the demographics of AIDS-related NHL has changed in the last decade starting to reflect the changes in the demographics of the AIDS epidemic with an increased incidence in Hispanic and African-American patients, and patients who have acquired HIV through heterosexual contact (Table 41-2).

TABLE 41-2	DEMOGRAPHIC PROFILE OF 369 PATIENTS WITH AIDS-RELATED LYMPHOMA OVER DIFFERENT TIME INTERVALS					
	1982-1986 (%)	*1987-1990 (%)*	*1991-1994 (%)*	*1995-1998 (%)*	*Total (%)*	*p value*
No of patients	44	88	132	105	369	
Median age (years)	40	36	38	39	38	0.18
Sex						0.25
Female	0 (0)	2 (2)	6 (5)	7 (7)	15 (4)	
Male	44 (100)	86 (98)	126 (95)	98 (93)	354 (96)	
Race						0.001
Caucasian	33 (75)	50 (57)	64 (48)	42 (40)	189 (51)	*
Hispanic	7 (16)	26 (33)	51 (39)	58 (55)	145 (39)	†
Black	4 (9)	4 (5)	17 (13)	5 (5)	30 (8)	
Asian	0 (0)	5 (6)	0 (0)	0 (0)	5 (1)	
Risk						0.039
MSM	37 (84)	67 (76)	105 (80)	69 (66)	278 (75)	‡
IDU ± MSM	3 (7)	7 (8)	4 (3)	3 (3)	17 (5)	
Hetero	2 (5)	4 (5)	13 (10)	19 (18)	38 (10)	#
Transfusion	0	3 (3)	1 (0.5)	4 (4)	8 (2)	
Unknown	2 (5)	7 (8)	9 (7)	10 (10)	28 (8)	
KPS						0.0008
>80%	14 (32)	28 (32)	75 (57)	45 (43)	162 (44)	
<80%	30 (68)	60 (68)	57 (43)	60 (57)	207 (56)	
Prior OI§	14 (32)	40 (45)	58 (44)	53 (50)	165 (45)	0.22
Prior KS§	2 (5)	13 (15)	11 (8)	14 (13)	40 (11)	0.20
Median CD4¶	177	113	54	53	66	0.0006
Range	0-1703	2-1927	0-710	0-700	0-1927	

Hetero, heterosexual risk factor for HIV; IDU, injection drug use; KPS, Karnofsky performance status; KS, Kaposi sarcoma; MSM, men who have sex with men; OI = opportunistic infection.

*p value, .0007, comparing Caucasian versus all other races.

†p value = <.0001, comparing Hispanics versus all other races.

‡p value = .045, comparing MSM with all other HIV-risk groups.

#p value = .011, comparing heterosexual transmission with all other HIV-risk groups.

§Patients without a diagnosis of OI or KS prior to development of lymphoma presented with lymphoma as the first AIDS-defining condition.

¶CD4 cell count at time of diagnosis of AIDS-related lymphoma.

Reproduced, with permission, from Levine AM, Seneviratne L, Espina BM, et al. Evolving characteristics of AIDS-related lymphoma. Blood 2000;96(13): 4084-4090.

Pathogenesis of AIDS-Related NHLs

In many respects, the development of NHLs in patients with HIV seropositivity is similar to the pathogenesis of malignancies associated with other immunodeficiency disorders, including congenital or posttransplant immunodeficiency (102). In such conditions, most of the malignancies consist of NHL and KS. In the case of HIV, the immunodeficiency together with other cofactors, including oncogenic viruses, chronic antigenic stimulation, and cytokine overproduction, are responsible for the development of AIDS-related NHL malignancies. In contrast to AIDS-associated KS, where investigators have clearly demonstrated the presence of the HHV-8 sequences in the DNA of the malignant cells, no one has yet found HIV sequences in the biopsies or tumor cells of AIDS-related NHLs (103), although polymerase chain reaction analysis has revealed the presence of HIV in infiltrating T cells. Most recently, the roles of immunodeficiency and cofactors such as the EBV virus in the development of AIDS-related NHL has have been better defined. For patients with severe HIV immunodeficiency, the oncogenic nature of both, EBV and HHV-8 are responsible for the malignant transformation of DLBCL the immunoblastic subtype, PCNSL, plasmablastic lymphoma of the oral cavity and PEL. Often PEL is the result of coinfection with HHV-8 and EBV. These lymphomas are the result of active oncogenic viruses released from control by an effective immune surveillance.

The role of EBV is central to the pathogenesis of both types of AIDS-related non-Hodgkin lymphomas, those that are truly related to immunodeficiency and those that occur in the presence of a reconstituted immune system, such as centroblastic DLBCL and Burkitt lymphoma. The presence of the EBV genome is very high in immunodeficiency-associated AIDS-related NHLs, although it can only be detected in around 60% of the centroblastic DLBCL and 30% of Burkitt lymphoma, suggesting that some other factor or additional common latent or chronic viral infections may be involved in the development of these tumors. In contrast, the EBV genome is found in almost 100% of pre-HAART AIDS-associated NHLs. It is present in almost 100% of PCNSL and in 90% of PEL, both of which have significantly decreased in incidence since the advent of HAART (104). In EBV infected cells the EBV virus is for the most part in a state of latency with brief periods of lytic activity. The malignant transformation of B cells occurs in the latent phase, requiring multiple molecular events (105). EBV contributes to the cellular transformation process through the expression of genes with oncogenic activity such as LMP-1, LMP-2, and EBNA-1 and 2. There is also expression of small EBV-encoded, nonpolyadenylated nuclear RNAs (EBERs) all of which are participants in the oncogenic transformation phenomenon. These proteins can rescue cells that otherwise would have followed a path toward apoptosis by mimicking cell receptors such as CD40 and BCR (B-cell receptor). For example, LMP-1 (latent membrane protein-1) is capable of replacing the function of CD40 in germinal B-cells which otherwise would follow an apoptotic fate.

The Impact of HAART on Distribution of AIDS-Related NHL

In the post-HAART era there has been a significant decline in the incidence of non-Hodgkin lymphomas associated with immunodeficiency. In contrast, the incidence of both centroblastic DLBCL and Burkitt lymphoma appears to be similar pre and post introduction of HAART. Factors influencing the pathogenesis of these diseases may include an increase in regulatory cells of the immune system, associated with recovery of the immune status of the host and the effects of chronic antigenic stimulation by HIV with a resultant overproduction of cytokines. Regardless, the existence of more than one pathogenic mechanism for the occurrence of AIDS-related NHLs can be inferred from the variety of genetic abnormalities displayed by the malignant cells (106). The number and type of these genetic abnormalities vary according to the anatomic site and tumor histology. They include: *c-myc* rearrangement, *bcl-6* gene rearrangement, *ras* gene mutations, and *p53* mutations/deletions (107).

Pathology of Systemic NHLs

The hallmark of AIDS-related NHL is high-grade histology, regardless of the histological subtype, including diffuse large cell, immunoblastic, or small noncleaved cell lymphomas, including Burkitt and Burkitt-like lymphoma. The cells of PEL express CD45, activation-associated antigens such as HLA-DR, CD30, CD38, CD71, epithelial membrane antigen, and CD 138/ syndecan-1. The PEL cells often lack B-cell antigens and c-myc gene rearrangements and mutations and uniformly contain HHV-8 and frequently also contain EBV (108,109). Other hematological neoplasms, including low-grade B-cell lymphomas and lymphocytic leukemia, multiple myeloma/plasmacytomas, T-cell neoplasms, and various acute myeloid leukemias and myeloproliferative disorders have been reported in patients with AIDS and

HIV infection. However, there is no evidence to suggest that the incidence of these neoplasms has increased in parallel with the AIDS epidemic (110-113).

Clinical Features of Systemic NHLs

Patients with AIDS-related NHLs usually present with advanced stages of the disease and B-symptoms including fever, loss of weight, and enlarged lymph nodes or masses. It is estimated that over 60% of the patients will present with stage III or IV disease. The most frequent extranodal sites of involvement are the bone marrow, the CNS parenchyma and meninges, the lungs, and the spleen. Patients with PEL typically present with ascites or a pleural effusion and less frequently with a pericardial effusion. Masses are typically absent in the presentation of PEL although occasionally a mass may accompany the development of the effusion (114,115) (see Fig. 41-1).

The staging of patients with AIDS-related NHL is similar to the staging of non-HIV patients with NHL, and should be reported according to the Ann Arbor Staging System (Table 41-3). The International Prognostic Index has been validated in pre-HAART studies, although there has been significant changes in treatment outcomes since the initiation of HAART (117). Complete blood count, beta-2-microglobulin, lactic dehydrogenase, and complete blood chemistries should be performed, and a radiologic staging should include an MRI of the brain and a PET-CT scan. This is particularly

TABLE 41-3	ANN ARBOR STAGING CLASSIFICATION FOR HODGKIN LYMPHOMA (116)
Stage	**Characteristics**
I	Involvement of a single lymph node region (I) or a single extralymphatic organ or site (IE).
II	Involvement of two or more lymph node regions on the same side of the diaphragm (II) or localized involvement of an extralymphatic organ or site (IIE).
III	Involvement of lymph node regions on both sides of diaphragm (III) or localized involvement of an extralymphatic organ or site (IIIE) or spleen (IIIS) or both (IIISE).
IV	Diffuse or disseminated involvement of one or more extralymphatic organs with or without associated lymph node involvement. The organ(s) involved should be identified by a symbol: A, asymptomatic; B, fever, sweats, weight loss >10% of body weight.

Data from Carbone PP, Kaplan HS, Mushoff K, et al. Report of the Committee on Hodgkin's Disease Staging. Cancer Res 1971;31:1860-1861.

relevant since patients who have high-grade tumors and are in remission after two courses of treatment will tend to remain in remission for the duration of induction therapy. In addition, all patients should have a bone marrow aspiration and biopsy and a diagnostic lumbar puncture if there is bone marrow involvement or the tumor is of Burkitt type. Finally, all patients should be screened for hepatitis B, since rituximab has become an important component of the anti-lymphoma regimens. The exacerbation of untreated active hepatitis B can be prevented by screening the patients for hepatitis BsAg, and hepatitis B core antibody. Those patients seropositive for hepatitis BsAg or who have a history of hepatitis B with a positive antigen should be concurrently treated for hepatitis B prior to the administration of rituximab. Less is known regarding therapy for those with only positive core antibody. In these cases, measurement of HBV DNA and of the presence or absence of anti-HBs are important in guiding the decision to intervene (118).

Before HAART, the presence of an opportunistic infection, less than 100 CD4+ cells/μL of blood, bone marrow involvement, and increased age predicted for a poor survival. This was complicated by the fact that patients were often suboptimally treated, due to the poor tolerance to standard doses of chemotherapy (119). After HAART, only two factors predict for poor survival: a CD4+ cell count of less than 100 CD4+ cells/μL and high-intermediate IPI (international prognostic index) scores (120).

Therapy for AIDS-Related Systemic NHL

Prior to HAART, a series of regimens were developed all of which had in common reduced doses of chemotherapy. After 1996, it became clear that patients on HAART can receive standard doses of chemotherapy. The outcomes of treatment in the presence of HAART are more related to the subtype of lymphoma and specific treatment administered for the lymphoma than to the degree of immunodeficiency of the patient (Table 41-4). Vigorous strategies of prevention of infections by the administration of prophylactic antibiotics, aggressive use of growth factors (G-CSF and Peg-G-CSF), and the use of rituximab in cases where indicated have significantly improved the outcomes for these patients (Table 41-5). Although investigators were originally concerned that rituximab might compromise the immune status of patients with CD20 positive B-cell lymphomas who received this drug, studies have since demonstrated that rituximab can safely be used for patients with 50 CD4+ cells/μL of blood or more. (121)

Today, regimens commonly used to treat patients with AIDS-related DLBCL, including CHOP or R-CHOP,

TABLE
41-4

SUMMARY OF SELECTED HRL TRIALS

Chemo Regimen	N	Median CD4 Cell Count at Enrollment (/μL)	CR (%)	ORR (%)	HAART	OI (%)	OS	Year (ref.)
Modified m-BACOD vs	98	100	41	69	NR	22	35 weeks	1997 (119)
m-BACOD+GM-CSF	94	107	52	78	NR	23		
MTX/LV	29	132	46	77	AZT	NR	12 months	1997 (122)
CHOP-HAART vs	24	190	50	NR	Yes	18	62% at 8.5 months	2001 (123)
CHOP	80	146	36					
G-CSF+CHOP-R vs	95	133 total	58	NR	NR	NR	Median F/U	2003 (124)
G-CSF+CHOP	47		50				26 weeks	
Infusional CDE	62	NR	48	74	NR	NR	2.7 years	2002 (125)
G-CSF+CDE-R	30	132	86	90	Yes	7	80% at 2 years	2002 (126)
EPOCH	39	198	74	87	Held during chemotherapy	*	60% at 53 months	2003 (127)

AZT, azidothymidine; CR, complete response; HAART, highly active antiretroviral therapy; NR, not reported; OI, opportunistic infection; ORR, overall response rate; OS, overall survival; vs, versus.
*0% during chemotherapy, 9% after.

TABLE
41-5

SUGGESTED SUPPORTIVE CARE FOR THE PATIENT WITH HIV INFECTION AND LYMPHOMA OR OTHER MALIGNANCIES

Indication	Drug(s)
Primary infection prophylaxis	
Pneumocystis carinii, Toxoplasma	Trimethoprim-sulfamethoxazole 1 DS daily
Oral and/or esophageal candidiasis	Fluconazole 100 mg daily
MAI complex (CD4 <50 cells/μL)	Azithromycin 1200 mg weekly
Secondary infection prophylaxis	
Herpes simplex infections	Acylovir 400 mg bid or 200 mg tid
Cytomegalovirus infection	Ganciclovir 1 g tid
Mycobacterium avium complex	Clarithromycin 500 mg bid plus ethambutol 15 mg/kg daily, with or without rifabutin 300 mg daily
Toxoplasma gondii	Sulfadiazine 1-1.5 g q6h, pyrimethamine 25-75 mg daily Leucovorin 10-25 mg daily-qid
Cryptococcus neoformans	Fluconazole 200 mg daily
Salmonella bacteremia	Ciprofloxacin 500 mg bid
Hematopoietic growth factors	
For selected patients in whom the risk of febrile neutropenia ≥40%	G-CSF 5 μg/kg or GM-CSF 250 μg/m² SC daily beginning after completion of chemotherapy and continuing until neutrophil recovery
Antiretroviral agents	
Selecting patients for therapy	Follow NIH guidelines (62)
Role of therapy in controlling malignancy	
Kaposi sarcoma	Essential
Lymphoma	Unknown
Other tumors	Unknown
May be used with myelosuppressive drugs	Didanosine, zalcitabine
Avoid with myelosuppressive drugs/regimens	Zidovudine
Avoid with neurotoxic drugs/regimens	Didanosine, zalcitabine, stavudine
May alter the metabolism of cytotoxic drugs metabolized by cytochrome P-450 enzymes	All protease inhibitors and nonnucleoside RTIs

bid, two times daily; G-CSF, granulocyte colony-stimulating factor; GM-CSF, granulocyte-macrophage colony-stimulating factor; NIH, National Institute of Health; tid, three times daily; qid, four times daily; RTIs, reverse transcriptase inhibitors; SC, subcutaneous.
Reproduced, with permission, from Sparano JA. Clinical aspects and management of AIDS-related lymphoma. Eur J Cancer 2001;37(10):1296-1305.

R-CDE, and dose-adjusted EPOCH or dose-adjusted EPOCH -R. Progression-free survival rates at 2 years for these different schemas of treatment are approximately 70% for R-CHOP and R-CDE, while for dose-adjusted EPOCH-R it is closer to 90% (129). In the case of Burkitt lymphoma, CHOP or similar regimens are not recommended since the response to these regimens is poor. Burkitt lymphoma should be treated with R-HyperCVAD (130,131) or R-CODOX-M/IVAC (132). Either protocol can achieve remissions of more than 92% and a 2-year overall survival rate of 49% (Figs. 41-3 and 41-4). Recent data have suggested that dose-adjusted EPOCH-R also has excellent activity against Burkitt lymphoma establishing this regimen as a potential new standard of care. This regimen consists of a 4-day infusion of etoposide (50 mg/m^2/day), vincristine (0.4 mg/m^2/day), and doxorubicin (10 mg/m^2/day) admixed in the same solution, along with prednisone, at a dose of 60 mg/m^2/day orally on days 1 to 5. Cyclophosphamide is given with an adjusted-dose based upon CD4 cell count at initiation of therapy, and given by bolus on day 5 (187 mg/m^2 for patients with CD4 cells <100/μL) and 375 mg/m^2 for patients with CD4 cells over 100/μL of blood. Rituximab is given at a standard doses of 375 mg/m^2. Filgrastin is given SC starting on day 6 until absolute neutrophil count is 5000/μL (past nadir). Cyclophosphamide 187 mg is increased or decreased from previous course dose if the neutrophil count nadir is over 500 ANC or less than 500 ANC, respectively (133). Only cyclophosphamide is dose-adjusted for hematologic

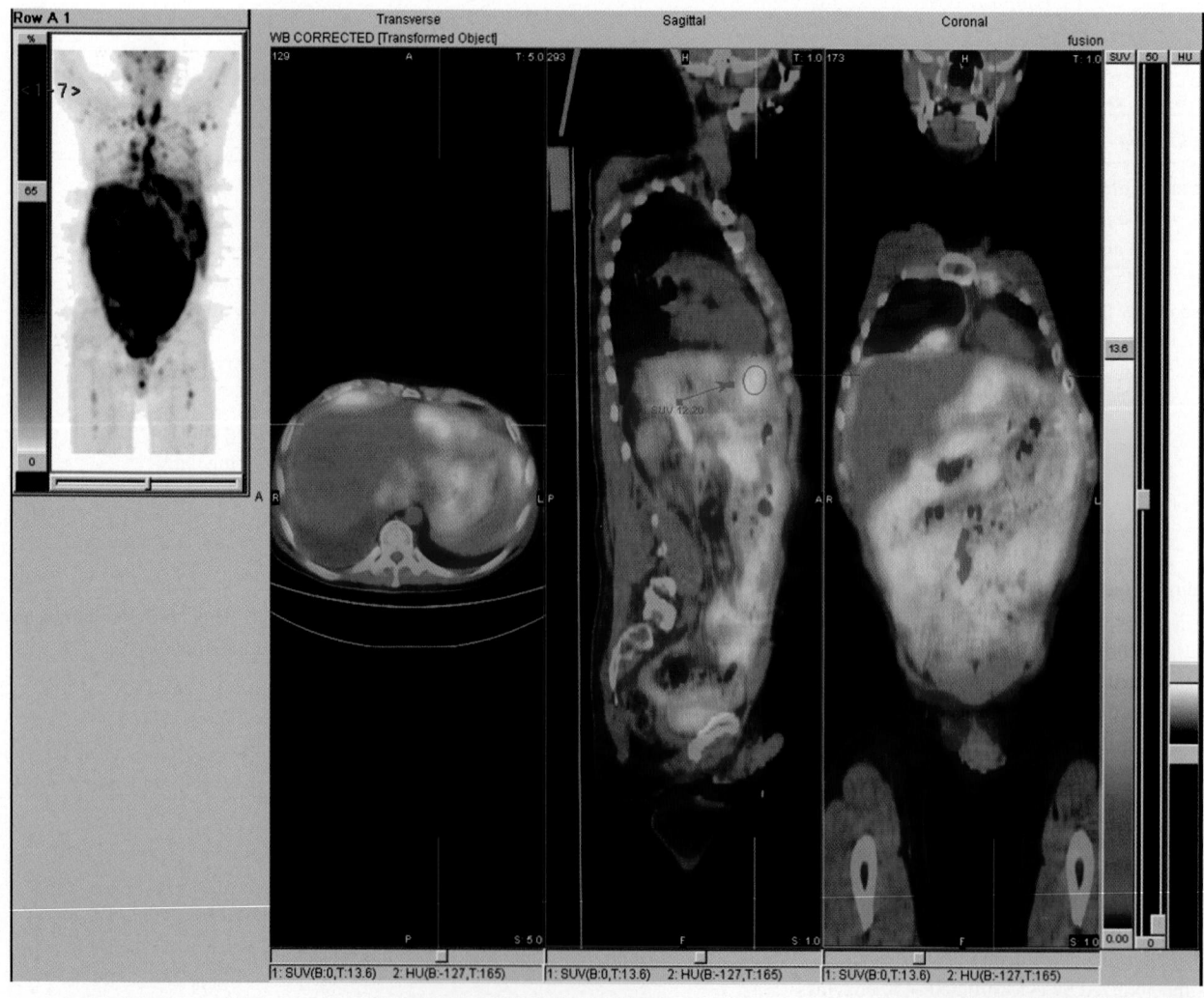

FIGURE 41-3. CT PET scan in a 51-year-old HIV-positive patient demonstrating extensive involvement by Burkitt lymphoma of the chest, abdomen, and pelvis.

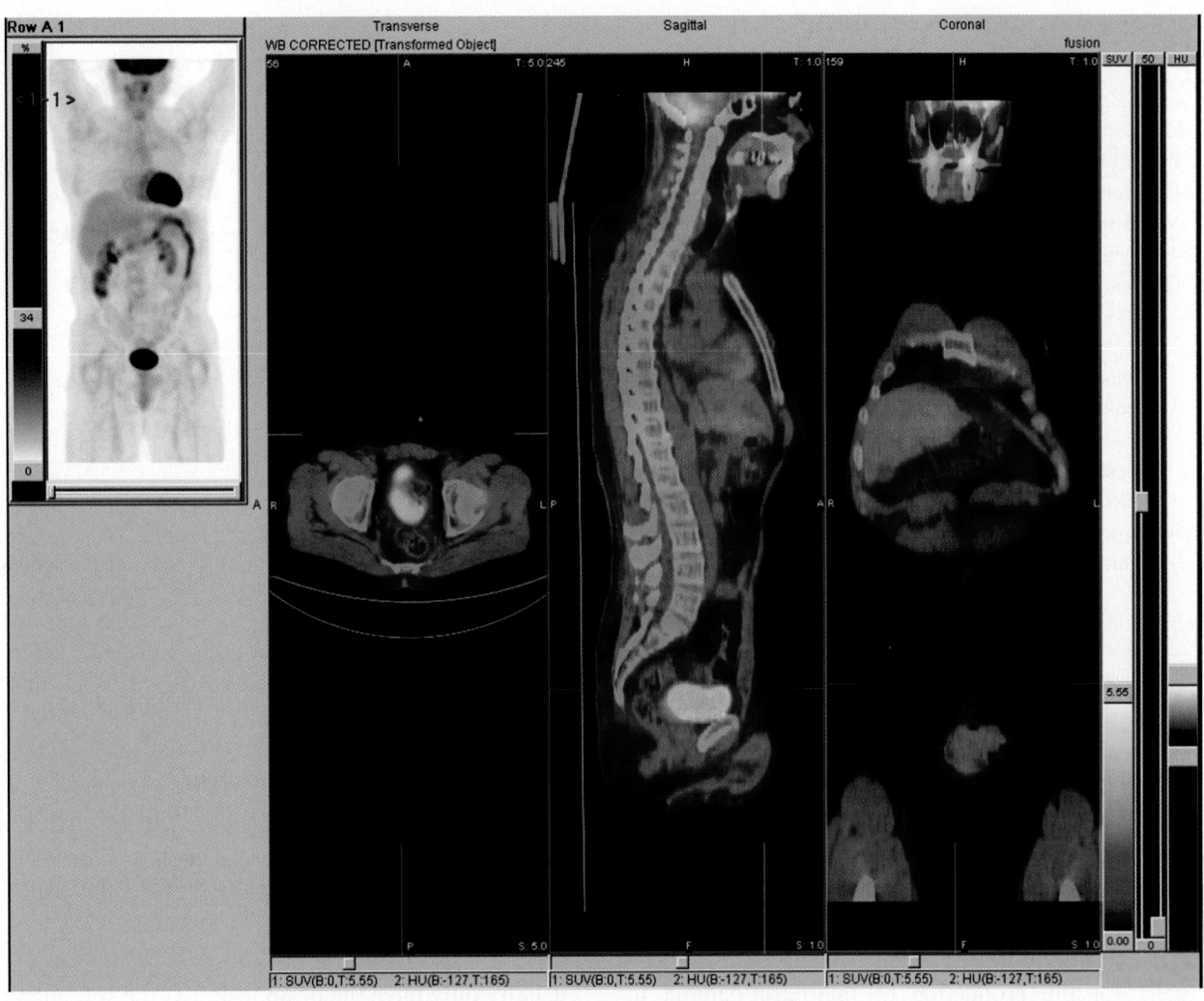

FIGURE 41-4. Same patient as in Fig. 41-3. The CT PET scan after 4 courses of hyperCVAD-ARA-C-methotrexate reveals a dramatic improvement with no residual hypermetabolic activity. The patient went on to complete 8 courses of treatment with hyperCVAD. He remains in complete remission of the Burkitt lymphoma 4 years after treatment and on HAART.

toxicity (Table 41-6). For patients with relapsed or refractory lymphoma R-ICE or ESHAP can be of value. Patients with disease responsive to salvage therapy can be considered for high-dose chemotherapy and autologous stem-cell transplant or experimental therapies (134).

AIDS-RELATED NHL: PRIMARY CNS LYMPHOMA

Epidemiology and Pathogenesis

Primary CNS lymphoma (PCNSL) became an AIDS-defining malignancy in 1983 (135). During the early years of the epidemic, the occurrence of PCNSL was related to the severity of the immunosuppression in patients with HIV. Initially described in 1929 as a sarcoma (136), PCNSL accounts for up to 15% of NHLs in

HIV-infected patients compared to only 1% of NHLs in the general population. In the pre-HAART era, typical patients with PCNSL were men of a younger age (median age: 40 years) than their immunocompetent counterparts, with CD4+ cell counts of less than 50 CD4+ cells/μL of blood. The impact of HAART on the incidence of PCNSL can be seen in its significant decrease after 1996 (from 313.2 per 100,000 person-years to 77.4 per 100,000 person-years) (5). The development of PCNSL is directly related to the immunodeficiency induced by HIV and its effect on the activity of EBV. Since EBV does not replicate in CNS tissue, infected B-cells most likely reach the CNS in increased numbers as a direct result of the progression of the HIV infection. As the immunological control of EBV by the host immune system declines there is a loss of capacity by specific

TABLE
41-6   **DOSE-ADJUSTED EPOCH**[¶]

Drug	Dose	Route	Treatment Days
Infused agents*			
Etoposide	50 mg/m^2/day	CIV	1,2,3,4 (96 h)
Doxorubicin	10 mg/m^2/day	CIV	1,2,3,4 (96 h)
Vincristine[†]	0.4 mg/m^2/day	CIV	1,2,3,4 (96 h)
Bolus agents			
Cyclophosphamide (cycle 1)			
CD4+ cells ≥100/mm^3	375 mg/m^2/day	IV	5
CD4+ cells <100/mm^3	187 mg/m^2/day	IV	5
Cyclophosphamide dose- adjustment (after cycle 1)[‡]			
nadir ANC >500/μL	↑187 mg above previous cycle	NA	NA
nadir ANC <500/μL or platelets <25000/μL	↓187 mg below previous cycle	NA	NA
Prednisone	60 mg/m^2/day	PO	1,2,3,4,5
Filgrastim	5 μg/kg/day	SC	6→ANC >5000/μL (past nadir)
Next cycle[#]			Day 21

ANC, absolute neutrophil count; NA, not applicable.

*Etoposide, doxorubicin, and vincristine can be admixed in the same solution. Etoposide, doxorubicin, and vincristine are never dose-adjusted for hematologic toxicity.

[†]Vincristine dose should never be routinely capped.

[‡]Dose based on previous cycle absolute neutrophil count (ANC) nadir (CBC BIW); maximum cyclophosphamide dose 750 mg/m^2.

[#]Begin day 21 if ANC ≥1000/μL and platelets ≥50 000/μL.

[¶]Data are for cycle 1 except where noted in "cyclophosphamide dose-adjustment."

Reproduced, with permission, from Little RF, Pittaluga S, Grant N, et al. Highly effective treatment of acquired immunodeficiency syndrome-related lymphoma with dose-adjusted EPOCH: impact of antiretroviral therapy suspension and tumor biology. Blood 2003;101(12):4653-4659.

T cells for the production of interferon-gamma in response to EBV peptides with increased expression of EBNA-2, LMPs, and EBERs, a pattern of EBV latency known as latency type III (138). This is the pattern seen when EBV transforms primary B cells in vitro. The expression of type III latency upregulates genes involved in transformation, including *Bcl-2* and *IRF-7*, and inactivation of the *p53* and *Rb* tumor suppressor gene products (139).

Clinical Presentation and Diagnosis

Patients with AIDS and PCNSL usually present with a florid acute organic brain syndrome, in contrast to immunocompetent patients, in whom neurological deterioration can be slow and progressive. Headaches, seizures, and focal neurological signs and symptoms are common. Personality changes are frequent and nausea and vomiting are indications of increased intracranial pressure. Rarely the patient will become comatose. When this occurs, it is usually an indication of an acute intracranial catastrophe such as intra-tumoral hemorrhage.

Patients who present with a primary lesion in the brain and no history of previous systemic lymphoma usually only have the brain lesion as the sole manifestation of their disease. As with other CNS oncological disorders, radiological diagnostic methods paired with the analysis of the cerebrospinal fluid are the cornerstones of the diagnosis of PCNSL. The use of MRI is preferred to CT scan due to its capacity to detect smaller lesions. Whenever MRI is not available the use of CT scan is acceptable as it can allow the detection of larger lesions (≥1 cm) and provide information about the safety of performing a lumbar puncture (140). Prior to and after the introduction of HAART, the most important differential diagnosis of PCNSL has been cerebral toxoplasmosis, still the most frequent cause of cerebral infection and masses in severely HIV-immunosuppressed patients (141). In both instances, PCNSL and cerebral toxoplasmosis, multiple lesions can occur and also have enhancing ring lesions. The distinction between the two can sometimes be difficult. In such cases, a positive serology for toxoplasmosis can be helpful if titers are >1:256. If the serology for toxoplasmosis is negative, the presence of EBV DNA by polymerase chain reaction in the cerebral spinal fluid and a positive SPECT-thallium scan of the brain have high specificity for diagnosis of the PCNSL (142,143). More recently, flow cytometry examination of the CSF has been used to detect occult disease (144).

During the early years of the AIDS pandemic, one of the more difficult subjects encountered by physicians treating patients with advanced HIV disease and cerebral lesions was the performance of invasive procedures in patients afflicted by an infectious process of which very little was known and much was feared. These difficulties resulted in the development of a series of practices that were borne out of necessity rather than of the use of rational approaches to the management and treatment of these patients. While at the time some of these practices were useful, today there is little room for their continuation, including the routine empirical treatment of brain lesions

with antitoxoplasmosis therapy and gauging the diagnosis of the patient based on the clinical response to the antitoxoplasmosis treatment. This is a practice which today should be completely avoided. It causes unnecessary delays in diagnosis and complicates the patient's management as there are potential side effects associated with a treatment for an illness the patient may not have. Therefore, unless there is an absolute contraindication, the standard of care for a patient with a brain lesion and AIDS is the performance of a stereotactic biopsy of the brain. This is of particular relevance for patients with a negative serology for toxoplasmosis. Patients who present with a primary lesion in the brain and no history of systemic lymphoma usually only have the brain lesion as the sole manifestation of their disease (Fig. 41-5).

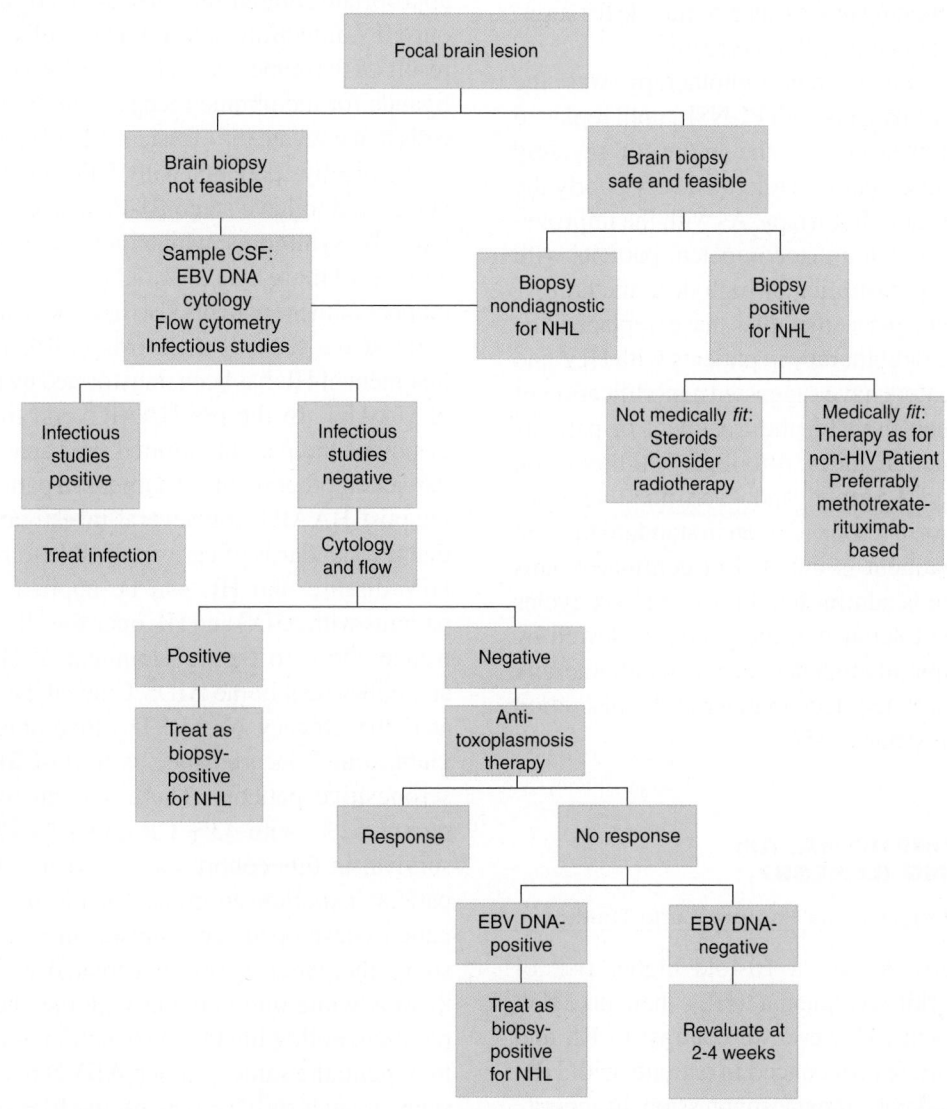

FIGURE 41-5. Evaluation of brain lesions in patients with HIV disease. CSF, cerebrospinal fluid; EBV, Epstein-Barr virus; RT, radiotherapy. *(Reproduced, with permission, from Sparano JA. Clinical aspects and management of AIDS-related lymphoma. Eur J Cancer 2001;37(10): 1296-1305.)*

Treatment of PCNSL

In addition to a significant impact in the incidence of AIDS-related PCNSL, HAART is the first step in the treatment of these patients. There is a clear correlation between the immune status of the patient and prognosis. The use of steroids and anticonvulsants is of debate among some investigators concerned with the potential of steroids to confound the histological diagnosis. However, a few days of steroids (4-5) can be of great clinical benefit to the patient particularly when there is an obvious mass effect, whereas high doses of steroids for 2 weeks would not be advisable. The same situation applies to anticonvulsive therapy which when administered for few days can allow the stabilization of the neurological condition of the patient by controlling the risk of focal or grand mal seizures. Since even solitary lesions of PCNSL tend to infiltrate the surrounding tissues, there is no role for surgical resection in the treatment of this disease.

Pre-HAART, whole brain radiotherapy was the standard of care for patients with PCNSL, until replaced by best comfort measures as the brains of severely immunocompromised patients tolerated very poorly the antitumoral doses of radiotherapy. As with the improvement in the treatment immunocompetent patients with PCNSL by the administration of high-dose methotrexate and rituximab, these therapies have replaced the administration of radiotherapy in patients with HIV and PCNSL. Investigators have suggested a modification of a standard regimen used for the treatment of patients without HIV which includes: rituximab 500 mg/m^2 on day 1; methotrexate 3.5 gm/m^2 and vincristine 1.4 mg/m^2 on day 2. Leucovorin rescue is given in standard fashion and HAART treatment is initiated or continued. This modified regimen is administered for five to six cycles depending on the tolerance of the patient followed by four courses of monthly maintenance with radiotherapy administered in a stereotactic manner at the discretion of the treating physician (145).

HODGKIN LYMPHOMA: AN AIDS-DEFINING ILLNESS?

Epidemiology, Clinical Features, and Therapy

HIV-infected persons have a 10-fold higher risk of developing Hodgkin lymphoma (HL) than do HIV-seronegative persons. However, in contrast to KS and NHL, the risk is more pronounced in patients with HIV who only have moderate immunosuppression. In general, patients with HIV disease have a higher incidence of unfavorable histologies, including mixed cellularity and lymphocyte depletion subtypes of HL, when compared to those without HIV infection. Interestingly, instead of observing a decrease in HL in patients in the post-HAART era (146), as with certain NHL subtypes, investigators have noted an increase in the incidence of HL in HIV patients. This observation has made the relationship between immunodeficiency and HL uncertain. Despite its inclusion by the WHO as an AIDS-defining malignancy, HL is not considered by most experts as a true AIDS-associated disease. From the pathogenetic point of view, EBV is often associated with HIV-related HL, in the range of 80 to 100%. The Reed-Sternberg cells of HIV-related HL express the EBV-encoded latent membrane protein1 (LMP-1), known to have oncogenic properties (147). In the post-HAART era, it has been postulated that an increase in CD4+ cells as a result of antiretroviral therapy fosters the development of the appropriate cellular milieu seen in HL in patients without HIV infection. These CD4+ cells, generated as a result of immune reconstitution by HAART, produce ligands for membrane receptors in the Reed-Sternberg cells that activate the classical NF-κB pathway (148).

Clinically, patients with HIV and HL tend to be young and to have stage III-IV disease at presentation, with "B" symptoms, which include fever, night sweats, and loss of more than 10% of body weight. A significant number of these patients also have bone marrow involvement at the time of diagnosis (149). Fortunately, the treatment of HL has been transformed by the introduction of HAART. In the pre-HAART era, the immunodeficiency of the patients limited the capacity to use standard chemotherapeutic regimens in patients with HL. In the post-HAART era, several investigators have found that the standards of care applicable to patients without HIV disease and HL can be applied successfully to patients with AIDS and HL once the HIV disease is controlled. Prior to the development of HAART, Levine and colleagues in the AIDS Clinical Trial Group evaluated the efficacy of ABVD (doxorubicin, bleomycin, vinblastine, dacarbazine) with G-CSF in 21 HIV-seropositive patients. There was an overall response rate of 62%, with 43% CR and 19% PR. The median survival in this cohort was 1.5 years. Almost half the patients experienced grade 4 neutropenia, and 29% of patients developed opportunistic infections (150). In this study, the patients were not treated with antiretroviral therapy while on treatment with the chemotherapeutic regimen. Following the introduction of HAART during treatment, the same regimen ABVD resulted in a retrospective analysis of 68 patients in a 91% complete remission rate and a median time to relapse of over 36 months (151). Spina and colleagues used the Stanford V regimen, administering only short-term chemotherapy

(12 weeks) with adjuvant radiotherapy. Of 59 patients who received this therapy, 69% completed the treatment without dose reduction or delays in the administration of the chemotherapy. Eighty-one percent of the patients achieved a complete remission, and with a median follow-up of 17 months, 33 out of 59 (56%) patients were alive and free of disease (152). High-dose chemotherapy and autologous stem cell transplantation is currently being explored for those patients who have disease progression while on treatment or relapse after remission induction. Thus, because of HAART, Hodgkin lymphoma patients with HIV can be treated with standard of care options, similar to those used for Hodgkin lymphoma patients who do not have HIV.

■ OTHER MALIGNANCIES AFFECTING HIV-INFECTING PATIENTS

CERVICAL NEOPLASMS

Epidemiology

In the early 1980s, reports appeared in the medical literature signaling an increased association between HIV infection and cervical intraepithelial neoplasia in HIV infected women. These reports initially attracted considerable attention. It was not until 1993, following an intense debate that cervical cancer was officially added to the WHO recommendations as an AIDS-related malignancy (153). Women with HIV disease have a higher incidence of infection with multiple types of oncogenic HPV and have a higher incidence of dysplastic changes of the cervix than do women without HIV disease, events that can culminate in the development of cervical cancer (154) (Table 41-7). Presently, no obvious association between the level of CD4+ cell count and cervical cancer has been established and the statistical correlations between the association of HIV and HPV-induced cervical cancer remain moderately strong at best. There has also been no significant decline in the incidence of HPV-related malignancies after HAART, a

decline observed for KS, NHL, and PCNSL, all of which are accepted as being AIDS-related malignancies.

There may be inherent reasons of why HPV, the etiologic agent of cervical cancer, causes this disease regardless of the immune status of the infected host (155). HPV infects the basal keratinocytes of the stratified epithelium and its replication is closely coupled to the process of keratinocyte differentiation in the infected squamous epithelium. From an initial low-copy number episome in the basal keratinocytes, there is a dramatic increase in the concentrations of proteins E1 and E2 by the time the keratinocytes differentiate and enter the stratum spinosum layer of the epithelium. In addition, for oncogenic strains of HPV such as 16, 18, and 31, there is also an increase in the increased expression of E6 and E7, which have a high oncogenic capacity manifested by the functional inactivation of p53 and Rb (156,157). Regardless, this is a slow process, and it takes several years for an HPV-induced cervical lesion to transform into cancer. Hence, the uncertainty of relationship between HIV and cervical cancer as an AIDS-related malignancy.

Epidemiologically, the increased incidence of infections by oncogenic HPV types in patients with HIV in contrast to non–HIV-infected women highlights the importance of mandatory cervical screening of HIV infected women. This is so despite the controversies regarding the exact relationship between HIV, HPV, and cervical cancer. Despite this recommendation, recent studies have shown that HIV-infected women are not being offered cervical screening, even though older women without HIV for whom the relevance of the screening may not be considered as important are routinely screened are routinely screened, for whom the relevance of the screening may not be considered as important. Clearly, educational efforts are necessary as the number of HIV-infected woman increases in the United States and elsewhere (158).

Cervical Cytology and Screening

Papanicolaou tests in HIV-infected women have a high prevalence of cytologic abnormalities, ranging from 20 to 40%. Even those women with negative Pap smears will, over the course of 3 to 5 years, develop cytological abnormalities at a higher rate than will HIV-negative women (159). There is also evidence that there is a higher rate of progression to cervical cancer following the longevity induced by HAART. Therefore, it is imperative that patients with HIV infection be screened appropriately with Pap smears, colposcopy and biopsy when needed for the early detection of cervical cancer.

TABLE 41-7	TRADITIONAL FACTORS FOR CERVICAL CANCER RISK
History of more than six sexual partners	
Cigarette smoking	
Early age of first intercourse	
History of sexually transmitted disease	
Immunosuppression	
Human papillomavirus	

Data from Stier E. Cervical neoplasia and the HIV-infected patient. Hematol Oncol Clin North Am 2003;17:873-887.

Pap smears read as "atypical squamous cells, cannot exclude a high-grade squamous intraepithelial lesion," (HGSIL), atypical glandular cells of undetermined significance, low-grade squamous intraepithelial lesion (LGSIL). HGSIL, adenocarcinoma, and squamous carcinoma must be evaluated with colposcopic examination (see Fig. 41-4). Current US Public Health Service (USPHS) and Infectious Diseases Society of America (IDSA) (160) guidelines recommend Pap smears every 6 months during the first year after HIV diagnosis; if

both tests are normal, annual screening is suggested (Fig. 41-6).

Treatment for Cervical Cancer

The American Society for Colposcopy and Cervical Cytopathology recommend close observation for CIN grade 1 lesions, the reason being that they rarely progress and often go away on their own.

The treatment of invasive cervical cancer is the same as for HIV seronegative women. It involves the

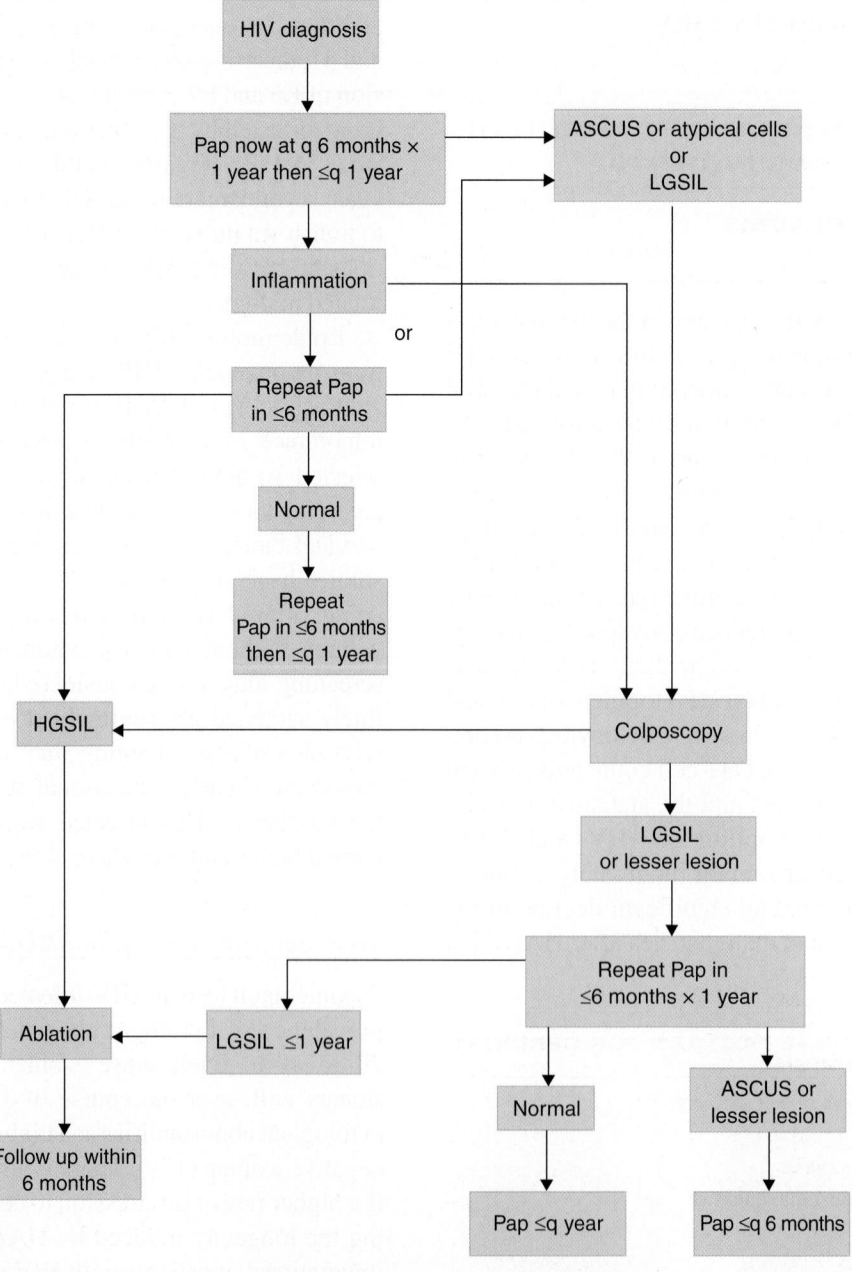

FIGURE 41-6. Screening/treatment algorithm for cervical cancer. ASCUS, atypical squamous cells of undetermined significance; LGSIL, low-grade squamous intraepithelial lesion; HGSIL, high-grade squamous intraepithelial lesion.

use of surgery in early stages and a combination of surgery and chemo-radiotherapy in intermediate stages. For CIN type II the preferred mode of treatment is LEEP (loop electrosurgical excision procedure). Cryotherapy and laser surgery can also be used although these methods are usually reserved for larger lesions. Chemotherapy alone is used for more advanced cases (161). The immune status of the patient can influence the response to treatment.

One of the most important advances against HPV-induced cervical cancer has been the development of preventive HPV vaccines. Papillomaviruses comprise a family of hundreds of different viruses. Cervical cancer is primarily caused by HPV types 16, 18, and 31, and by at least a dozen of other "high-risk" types that infect the genital mucosa. (162) The structure of the HPV virus consists of a capsid made of two structural proteins, L1 and L2. L1 is a major structural protein and L2 a minor one. The capsid contains the double-stranded viral DNA associated with cellular nucleosomal proteins. Two-thirds of the viral genome is composed of the early proteins E1 to E7, approximately one-third codes for the structural proteins L1 and L2, and the remainder contains the elements necessary for viral DNA replication and transcription. The expression of L1 or L2 in yeast systems or cells is accompanied by the assembly of the proteins into viral-like particles (VLP). These particles display a remarkable structural and antigenic similitude to HPV virions and can induce the production of high titers of neutralizing antibodies. Two versions of L1-only HPV viral-like particle vaccines are available for immunization of humans against HPV. Gardasil (Merck, Sharp, and Dohme) has viral-like particles of HPV subtypes 16 and 18 (oncogenic subtypes) and 6 and 11 (the causes of genital warts). Cervarix (GlaxoSmith-Kline) contains viral-like particles of HPV 16 and 18. They both are administered intramuscularly, and have demonstrated almost 100% protection in clinical trials prior to their approval by the FDA. They should be used prior to the initiation of sexual activity and neither have demonstrated therapeutic efficacy in the treatment of preexisting infections. Future work is aimed at increasing the immunogenicity of the viral-like particles by adding L2 to the vaccine component and by expanding the number of HPV oncogenic subtypes available for vaccination (163).

ANORECTAL CARCINOMA

The infection of the anogenital tract in men with oncogenic strains of HPV has the same consequences as in

TABLE 41-8	RISK FACTORS FOR AIDS-ASSOCIATED ANAL CARCINOMA
HIV seropositivity	
Low CD4 cell count	
Persistent HPV infection	
High-risk HPV genotypes	
Multiple HPV genotypes	
History of anal intercourse	
Cigarette smoking	
Immunosuppression	

HPV, Human papillomavirus.
Data from Martin F, Bowers M. Anal intraepithelial neoplasia in HIV-positive people. Sex Transm Inf 2001;77:327-331.

women. Just as it had happened in women, the incidence of the disease has not decreased with the introduction of HAART but rather increased as patients live longer and the biological characteristics unique to the HPV oncogenic transformation are expressed over time (Table 41-8). The incidence of anal cancer has increased from 19.0 per 100,000 person-years in the pre-HAART era (1992-1995) to 48.3 persons per 100,000 person-years in the immediate post-HAART period (1996-1999) to 78.2 per 100,000 person-years more recently (2000-2003, $p < .001$) (165).

The same subtypes of HPV and the same pathogenic mechanisms involved in the oncogenic activity of HPV in women apply to men. The screening and treatment of CIN II and III is of greatest relevance in these patient populations. Now that we have a better understanding of the oncogenic potential of HPV, there has been a greater understanding of the need for anal screening of both men and women with HIV disease (166) (Fig. 41-7). The treatment of high-grade squamous intraepithelial lesions includes the use of local therapies such as podophyllotoxin, liquid nitrogen, and laser surgery (Fig. 41-8). Just as investigators have recommended that women undergo screening with Pap smears every 6 months the first year following diagnosis and yearly thereafter, the same recommendations apply to men with HIV infection and anal HPV-related lesions. Invasive lesions are treated as in the general population. The standards of care are the use of chemoradiotherapy followed by salvage surgery when there is no response or relapse after initial treatment (166).

OTHER MALIGNANCIES

Patients with HIV can develop other malignancies not necessarily associated to their HIV condition. Lung cancer continues to steadily increase in its incidence in

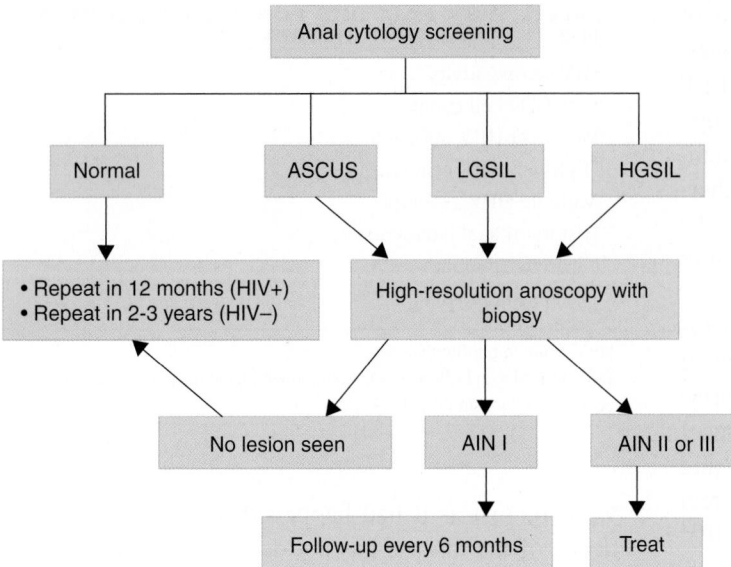

FIGURE 41-7. Protocol for screening anal intraepithelial neoplasia (AIN). ASCUS = atypical squamous cells of indeterminate significance; HGSIL = high-grade squamous intraepithelial lesion; LGSIL = low-grade squamous intraepithelial lesion. *(Reproduced, with permission, from Chin-Hong PV, Palefsky JM. Natural history and clinical management of anal human papillomavirus disease in men and women infected with human immunodeficiency virus. Clin Infect Dis. 2002 Nov 1;35(9):1127-34.)*

this population. In general smoking is one of the most important negative factors predicting for poor survival in HIV patients even in the presence of HAART. In general, patients with HIV who develop malignant tumors often do so at an earlier age, tend to have atypical presentations, and frequently their tumors follow a very aggressive course.

■ **IMMUNE RECONSTITUTION INFLAMMATORY SYNDROME (IRIS)**

In patients with advanced HIV disease (fewer than 100 CD4+ cells/μL of blood) the initiation of antiretroviral therapy (ART) can be accompanied by a paradoxical worsening of established infections or appearance of new ones. This phenomenon is most frequent with patients who have tuberculosis or cryptococcal disease as their opportunistic infection but can happen with any other type of infection. This syndrome is known as the Immune Reconstitution Inflammatory Syndrome or IRIS. The management of IRIS consists of the administration of the indicated specific therapies and of a short course of steroids for one to two weeks with a rapid taper. The recommended dose of prednisone is 1-2 mg/Kg. Antiretroviral therapy should only be interrupted in severe cases as most patients respond to the use of steroid or anti-inflammatory agents depending on the severity of the IRIS. Since the management of patients with AIDS related malignancies involves a multi-disciplinary team and given the importance of the use of ART in the management of patients with AIDS and malignancies, treating oncologists must be familiar with this condition as to avoid unnecessary delays or interruptions in the ART of their patients. (168)

■ **MD ANDERSON CANCER CENTER AND THE AIDS PANDEMIC**

When the AIDS pandemic first began in the early 1980s there was much that was unknown about this illness. That unknown created a fear that gripped the soul and minds not only of the public, but also of the general medical community. Most of the initial cases of AIDS were initially reported from east and west coast centers. Houston, an international port of entry into the United States, quickly became one of the epicenters of the AIDS pandemic, occupying the fourth place among cities with the highest in the number of cases of AIDS in the United States for several years. Since many of the early cases of AIDS initially presented with malignancies and opportunistic infections, the Department of Epidemiology, under the leadership of Peter W. Mansell and its Director, Guy Newell, took a leading role in studying methods for prevention of AIDS and public education efforts. With the collaboration of R. Palmer Beasley, Dean of the UT Health Science Center School of Public Health, this group thoroughly mapped the AIDS epidemic in the State of Texas. The Department of Immunology and Biological Therapy, under the direction of Evan Hersh and the collaboration of immunologists and virologists, including James M. Reuben and Blaine F. Hollinger, became a departmental leader in the treatment of the malignant complications of AIDS, the understanding of the associated immunological abnormalities and of the carcinogenic potential of AIDS. Their scientific, clinical, and public health work was recognized with one of the first ATEU (AIDS Treatment Evaluation Units) Grants awarded

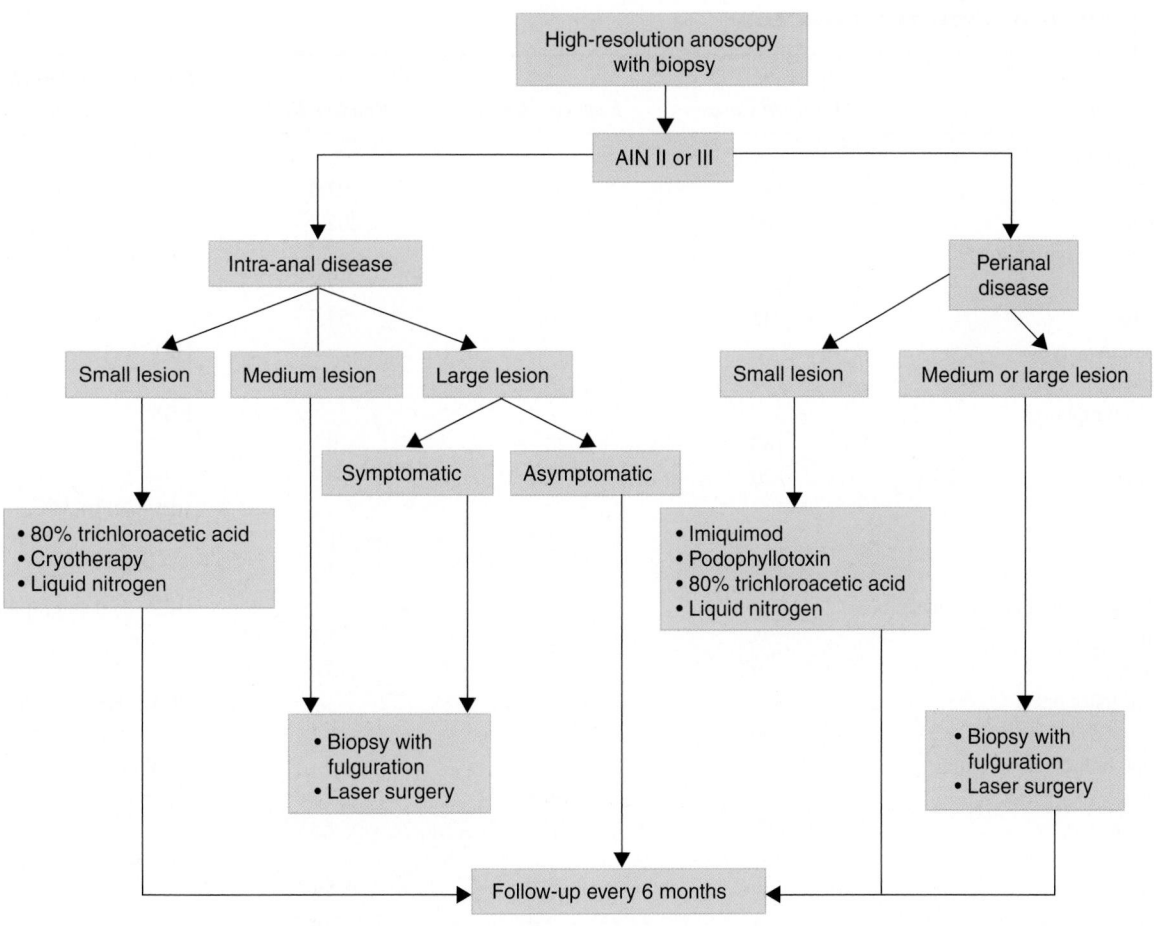

FIGURE 41-8. Treatment of anal intraepithelial neoplasia (AIN) II and III. Imiquimod and podophyllotoxin have not been approved by the US Food and Drug Administration for this indication. *(Reproduced, with permission, from Chin-Hong PV, Palefsky JM. Natural history and clinical management of anal human papillomavirus disease in men and women infected with human immunodeficiency virus. Clin Infect Dis. 2002 Nov 1;35(9):1127-34.)*

for basic science and clinical research in AIDS in the nation. This work led to the creation of the Institute for Immunological Disorders under the direction of Peter W. Mansell and Adan Rios. While the Institute was ahead of its time, it opened the doors for a humane treatment of AIDS patients, contributing to the development of new therapies and strategies for research of the disease, and provided Houston and the surrounding areas with a base of knowledge that was instrumental in the development of the community strategies subsequently developed for the management and treatment of AIDS in the State of Texas. This work that ranged from epidemiological studies to the treatment of AIDS-related malignancies has extended to current times with the pioneer work done at the institution in the treatment of Burkitt lymphoma in HIV patients, using what is considered today a standard strategy for treatment of AIDS-related malignancies: the use of HAART in combination with the best known strategy for the treatment of the malignancy.

AIDS is a pandemic and the work of the world scientific and medical community has provided in a relatively short period of time multiple advances in the management and treatment of this disease and its related complications. At MD Anderson Cancer Center, the current approach for all of these AIDS and HIV associated malignancies is to provide the best known therapy for each of these cancers, while supporting the patient with modern HAART treatment and prophylaxis against infectious and other complications of the underlying disease.

■ CONCLUSIONS

The complexities of the AIDS pandemic are captured in the history of the AIDS-related malignancies (Table 41-9). However, despite this, the introduction of effective anti-HIV therapy or HAART in 1996 has brought a profound change in the overall management of cancer in HIV

TABLE | **AIDS-ASSOCIATED CANCERS***
41-9

Cancer Type	Observed Cases	Expected Cases	Relative Risk	Etiologic or Contributing Factors
Kaposi sarcoma				KSHV
Men	5583	57.3	97.5[†]	
Women	200	1.0	202.7[†]	
Non-Hodgkin lymphoma				EBV and KSHV
Men	2434	65	37.4	
Women	342	6.3	54.6	
Cervical, invasive				HPV
Women	133	14.7	9.1	
Hodgkin lymphoma				EBV
Men	160	20	8	
Women	20	3.1	6.4	
Tongue				HPV and EBV
Men	17	9.3	1.8	
Women	5	0.7	7.1	
Rectal, rectosigmoidal, and anal				HPV (anal carcinoma)
Men	75	22.7	3.3	
Women	9	3.0	3.0	
Liver (primary only)				HCV,[‡] HBV, alcohol
Men	36	7.1	5.1	
Tracheal, bronchial, and lung				Smoking[#]
Men	217	66.1	3.3	
Women	50	6.7	7.5	
Brain and CNS				EBV for CNS lymphoma
Men	42	13.4	3.1	
Women	7	2.0	3.4	
Skin, excluding KS				HPV[§] and ultraviolet-light exposure
Men	133	6.4	20.8	
Women	8	1.1	7.5	
Melanoma, skin				
Men	24	17.3	1.4	
Testicular				
Men	38	25.6	1.5	
Colon				
Men	32	38.2	0.8	
Women	5	6.3	0.8	
Prostate				
Men	37	53.7	0.7	
Breast				
Women	47	59.9	0.8	
Ovarian				
Women	6	7.8	0.8	

CNS, central nervous system; EBV, Epstein-Barr virus; HBV, hepatitis B virus; HCV, hepatitis C virus; HPV, human papillomavirus; KSHV, Kaposi' sarcoma–associated herpesvirus.

*Data are based on the observed number of cases in HIV-positive individuals (men and women aged 15-69 years), expected cases based on the incidence in a nonimmunocompromised population in New York State (NYS), relative risk and etiologic factors. Data from the AIDS/Cancer Matched Cohort NYS, 1981-1991.

[†]Relative risk for Kaposi sarcoma (KS) is lower than in other studies, probably because the background population in NYS is enriched with population groups (eg, Italians, Greeks, and Jews) that have an increased risk for classic KS.

[‡]HCV contributes to increased incidence of liver cancer, particularly in HIV-infected men with hemophilia, and in intravenous drug users.

[#]The increase in lung cancer might be confounded by the fact that HIV-infected individuals have been reported to smoke more cigarettes per day than HIV-negative individuals.

[§]In Africa, HPV and ultraviolet-light exposure have been implicated in the high incidence of conjunctival squamous carcinoma, and HPV is also implicated as the cause of skin cancers seen after an organ transplant. Misdiagnosis of KS might also contribute to increased risk of skin cancer.

Reprinted by permission from MacMillan Magazines Ltd: Nature Reviews Cancer. Boshoff C, Weiss R. AIDS-related malignancies. Nature 2002;2:373–382.

patients. This profound change is a common theme in the diagnosis and therapy of all malignancies in this population. One of the most important predictors of good outcomes in the therapy of cancer of AIDS in HIV-infected patients is the administration of HAART (169). The common goals for treatment of patients with AIDS and cancer should be to treat the HIV with HAART and the cancer with the same standards of oncological care that exists for patients without HIV disease, along with the vigorous prophylaxis of opportunistic infections and supportive therapy including growth factors and appropriate nutritional and emotional support.

References

1. Ho DD, Avidan U, Neumann AU, et al.: Rapid turnover of plasma virions and CD4 lymphocytes in HIV-1 infection. Nature 373:123-126, 1995.
2. Hogg RS, Heath KV, Yip B, et al.: Improved survival among HIV-infected individuals following initiation of anti-retroviral therapy. JAMA 279:450-454, 1998.
3. Veneman A: Point of view: Child survival in Africa– Seven signs of hope. UNICEF Press Centre May 28 2008. Available at: http://www.unicef.org/childsurvival/index_44202. html. Accessed 15 Jan 2011.
4. Sepkowitz KA: AIDS—The first 20 years. N Engl J Med 344:1764-1772, 2001.
5. Biggar RJ, Anil K, Chaturvedi AK, et al.: AIDS-related cancer and severity of immunosuppression in persons with AIDS. J Natl Cancer Inst 99:962-972, 2007.
6. Palmieri C, Treibel T, Large O, et al.: AIDS-related non-Hodgkin's lymphoma in the first decade of highly active antiretroviral therapy. Q J Med 99:811-826, 2006.
7. Stebbing J, Duru O, and Bower M: Non-AIDS-defining cancers. Curr Opin Infect Dis 22:7-10, 2009.
8. CDC: Pneumocystis pneumonia—Los Angeles MMWR Morb Mortal Wkly Rep 30:250-2, 1981.
9. CDC: Kaposi's sarcoma and pneumocystis pneumonia among homosexual men—New York City and California MMWR Morb Mortal Wkly Rep 30:305, 1981.
10. Morison L: The global epidemiology of HIV/AIDS. Br Med Bull 58:7-18, 2001.
11. Gottlieb MS: AIDS—Past and future. N Engl J Med 344:1788-1791, 2001.
12. Hammer SM: Management of newly diagnosed HIV infection. N Engl J Med 353:1701-1710, 2005.
13. Stiehm ER, Chin TW, Hass A, et al.: Infectious complications of the primary immunodeficiencies. Clin Immunol Immunopathol 40:69-86, 1986.
14. Farge D, Lebbé C, Marjanovic Z, et al.: Human herpes virus-8 and other risk factors for Kaposi's sarcoma in kidney transplant recipients1. Groupe Cooperatif de Transplantation d'Ile de France (GCIF). Transplantation 67: 1236-42, 1999.
15. Barré-Sinoussi F, Chermann JC, Rey F, et al.: Isolation of a T-lymphotropic retrovirus from a patient at risk for acquired immune deficiency syndrome (AIDS). Science 220:868-71, 1983.
16. Hahn BH, Shaw GM, De Cock KM, et al.: AIDS as a zoonosis: Scientific and public health implications. Science 287:607-614, 2000.
17. Gao F, Bailes E, Robertson DL, et al.: Origin of HIV-1 in the chimpanzee pan troglodytes troglodytes. Nature 397: 436-441, 1999.
18. Chen Z, Telfer P, Gettie A, et al.: Genetic characterization of new West African simian immunodeficiency virus SIVsm: Geographic clustering of household-derived SIV strains with human immunodeficiency virus tupe 2 subtypes and genetically diverse viruses from a single feral sooty mangabey troop. J Virol 70:3617-3627, 1996.
19. De Cock KM, Adjorlolo G, Ekpini E, et al.: Epidemiology and transmission of HIV-2: Why there is no HIV-2 pandemic. JAMA 1270:2083-2086, 1993.
20. Kahn P: Do clades matter for HIV vaccines? IAVI Report 7:May- August, 2003.
21. Constantine NT, Saville RD, Dax EM: Retroviral testing and quality assurance. Essentials for laboratory diagnosis. Halifax: MedMira Laboratories, 2005.
22. WHO/UNAIDS: The importance of simple/rapid assays in HIV testing. Wkly Epidemiol Rec 73:321-328, 1998.
23. WHO/UNAIDS: AIDS Epidemic Update – November 2009. Available at: http://data.unaids.org/pub/Report/2009/JC1700_Epi_Update_2009_en.pdf. Accessed 15 Jan 2011.
24. Kieny MP: Structure and regulation of the human AIDS virus. J Acquir Immune Defic Syndr 3:395, 1990.
25. Greene WC: The molecular biology of human immunodeficiency virus type 1 infection. N Engl J Med 324:308, 1991.
26. Veazey RS, Lackner AA: Getting to the guts of HIV pathogenesis. J Exp Med 200:697-700, 2004.
27. Veazey RS, DeMaria M, Chalifoux LV, et al.: Gastrointestinal tract as a major site of CD4+ T cell depletion and viral replication in SIV infection. Science 280:427-431, 1998.
28. Santiago ML, Montano M., Benitez R, et al.: Apobec3 encodes Rfv3, a gene influencing neutralizing antibody control of retrovirus infection. Science 321:1343-1346, 2008.
29. Kaposi M: Idiopathisches multiples Pigmentsarkom der Haut. Arch Dermatol Syph 4:265-73, 1872.
30. Ivabnoski N, Popov Z, Kolevski P, et al.: Cancer after kidney transplantation and immunosuppression. Ann Urol (Paris) 34:336-9, 2000.
31. Dedicoat M and Newton R: Review of the distribution of Kaposi's sarcoma-associated herpesvirus(KSHV) in Africa in relation to the incidence of Kaposi's sarcoma. Br J Cancer 88:1-3, 2003.
32. Simonart T: Role of environmental factors in the pathogenesis of classic and African-endemic Kaposi sarcoma. Cancer Lett 244:1-7, 2006.
33. Gessain A: Human herpesvirus 8 (HHV-8): Clinical and epidemiological aspects and clonality of associated tumors. Bull Acad Natl Med 192:1189-1204, 2008. discussion 1204-6.
34. Chang Y, Cesarman E, Pessin MS, et al.: Identification of herpesvirus-like DNA sequences in AIDS-associated Kaposi's sarcoma. Science 266:1865-1869, 1994.
35. Cannon MJ, Dollard SC, Smith KD, et al.: Blood-borne and sexual transmission of human herpesvirus 8 in women with or at risk for Human Immunodeficiency Virus infection. N Engl J Med 344:637, 2001.
36. Pauk J, Huang ML, Brodie JS, et al.: Mucosal shedding of Human Herpesvirus 8 in men. N Engl J Med 343:1369, 2000.

37. Moore PS, Boshoff C, Weiss RA, et al.: Molecular mimicry of human cytokine and cytokine response pathways genes by KSHV. Science 274:1739-1744, 1996a.

38. Nicholas J: Human herpesvirus 8-encoded proteins with potential roles in virus-associated neoplasia. Front Biosci 12:265-81, 2007.

39. Long E, Ilie M, Hoffman V, et al.: LANA-1, Bcl-2, Mcl-1 and HIF-1 alpha protein expression in HIV-associated Kaposi sarcoma. Virchows Arch 455:159-70, 2009.

40. Djerbi M, Screpanti V, Catrina AL, et al.: The inhibitor of death-receptor signaling, FLICE-inhibitory protein defines a new class of tumor progression factors. J Exp Med 190:1025, 1999.

41. Lee BS, Alvarez X, Ishido S, et al.: Inhibition of intracellular transport of B cell antigen receptor complexes by Kaposi's sarcoma-associated herpesvirus K1. J Exp Med 192:11-22, 2000.

42. Grayson W, Pantanowitz L: Histological variants of Kaposi sarcoma. Diag Pathol 3:31, 2008.

43. Hashimot H, Müller H, Falk S, et al.: Histogenesis of Kaposi's sarcoma associated with AIDS: A histologic, immunohistochemical and enzyme histochemical study. Pathol Res Pract 182:658-68, 1987.

44. Wang HW, Trotter MWB, Lagos D, et al.: Kaposi sarcoma herpesvirus-induced cellular reprogramming contributes to the lymphatic endothelial gene expression in Kaposi sarcoma. Nat. Genet 36:687, 2004.

45. Samaniego F, Pati S, Karp JE, et al.: Human herpesvirus 8 K1-associated nuclear factor-kappa B-dependent promoter activity: Role in Kaposi's sarcoma inflammation? J Natl Cancer Inst Monograph Dec:15-23, 2000.

46. Stürzl M, Roth WK, Brockmeyer NH, et al.: Expression of platelet-derived growth factor and its receptor in AIDS-related Kaposi sarcoma in vivo suggests paracrine and autocrine mechanisms of tumor maintenance. Proc Natl Acad Sci USA 89:704-50, 1992.

47. Hazenberg MD, Otto SA, van Benthem BH, et al.: Persistent immune activation in HIV-1 infection is associated with progression to AIDS. AIDS 17:1881-1888, 2003.

48. Pantanowitz L, Dezube BH, Hernandez-Barrantes S, et al.: Matrix metalloproteinases in the progression and regression of Kaposi's sarcoma. J Cutan Pathol 33:793-8, 2006.

49. Aoki Y, Tosato G: Interactions between HIV-1 Tat and KSHV. Curr Top Microbiol Immunol 312:309-26, 2007.

50. Dezube BJ: Clinical presentation and natural history of AIDS-related Kaposi's sarcoma. Hematol Oncol Clin North Am 5:1023-9, 1996.

51. Kalpidis CD, Lysitsa SN, Lombardi T, et al.: Gingival involvement in a case series of patients with acquired immunodeficiency syndrome-related Kaposi sarcoma. J Periodontol 77:523-33, 2006.

52. Parente F, Cernuschi M, Orlando G, et al.: Kaposi's sarcoma and AIDS: Frequency of gastrointestinal involvement and its effect on survival. A prospective study in a heterogeneous population. Scand J Gastroenterol 10:1007-12, 1991.

53. Allen PJ, Gillespie DL, Redfield RR, et al.: Lower extremity lymphedema caused by acquired immune deficiency syndrome-related Kaposi's sarcoma: Case report and review of the literature. J Vasc Surg 2:178-81, 1995.

54. Kaplan LD, Hopewell PC, Jaffe H, et al.: Kaposi's sarcoma involving the lung in patients with the acquired immunodeficiency syndrome. J Acquir Immune Defic Syndr 1:23, 1988.

55. Ioachim HL, Adsay V, Giancotti FR, et al.: Kaposi's sarcoma of internal organs. A multiparameter study of 86 cases. Cancer 75:1376-85, 1995.

56. Bahat E, Akman S, Karpozoglu G, et al.: Visceral Kaposi's sarcoma with intracranial metastasis: A rare complication of renal transplantation. Pediatr Transplant 6:505-8, 2002.

57. Chachoua A, Krigel R, Lafleur F, et al.: Prognostic factors and staging classification of patients with epidemic Kaposi's sarcoma. J Clin Oncol 7:774-780, 1989.

58. Levina AM, Tulpule A. Clinical aspects and management of AIDS-related Kaposi's sarcoma. Eur J Cancer 2001;37:1288-1295.

59. Kayaselçuk F, Ceken I, Bircan S, et al.: Bacillary angiomatosis of the scalp in a human immunodeficiency virus-negative patient. J Eur Acad Dermatol Venereol 6:612-4, 2002.

60. Cattelan AM, Calabró ML, Gasperini P, et al.: Acquired immunodeficiency syndrome-related Kaposi's sarcoma regression after highly active antiretroviral therapy: Biologic correlates of clinical outcome. J Natl Cancer Inst Monograph 28:44-9, 2001.

61. Biggar RJ: AIDS-related cancers in the era of highly active antiretroviral therapy. Oncology Williston Park 4:439-448, 2001, discussion 448-9.

62 Panel on Antiretroviral Guidelines for Adults and Adolescents. Guidelines for the use of antiretroviral agents in HIV-1-infected adults and adolescents. Department of Health and Human Services. December 1, 2009; 1-161. Available at: http://www.aidsinfo.nih.gov/ContentFiles/AdultandAdolescentGL.pdf. Accessed 15 Jan 2011.

63. Cattelan AM, Calabró ML, De Rossia A, et al.: Long-term clinical outcome of AIDS-related Kaposi's sarcoma during highly active antiretroviral therapy. Int J Oncol 3:779-85, 2005.

64. Becker G, Bottke D: Radiotherapy in the management of Kaposi's sarcoma. Onkologie 7:329-33, 2006.

65. Stelzer KJ, Griffin TW: A randomized prospective trial of radiation therapy for AIDS-associated Kaposi's sarcoma. Int J Radiat Oncol Biol Phys 27:1057, 1993.

66. Krown SE, Myskowski PL, Paredes J: Kaposi's sarcoma. Med Clin North Am 76:235-252, 1992.

67. Pluda JM, Broder S, Yarchoan R: Therapy of AIDS and AIDS-related tumors. Cancer Chemother Biol Response Modif 12:395-429, 1991.

68. Epstein JB: Treatment of oral Kaposi sarcoma with intralesional vinblastine. Cancer 71:1722-5, 1993.

69. Walmsley S, Northfelt DW, Melosky B, et al.: Treatment of AIDS-related cutaneous Kaposi's sarcoma with topical alitretinoin (9-cis retinoic) gel. J Acquir Immunodef Syndr 22:235-246, 1999.

70. Quesada JR, Reuben J, Manning JT, et al.: Alpha interferon for induction of remission in hairy-cell leukemia. N Engl J Med 310:15-8, 1984.

71. Rios A. Personal observation.

72. Krown SE: The role of interferon in the therapy of epidemic Kaposi's sarcoma. Semin Oncol 14(2 Suppl 3):27-33, 1987.

73. Rios A, Mansell PW, Newell GR, et al.: Treatment of acquired immunodeficiency syndrome-related Kaposi's sarcoma with lymphoblastoid interferon. J Clin Oncol 4:506-12, 1985.

74. Fiorelli V, Barillari G, Toschi E, et al.: IFN-gamma induces endothelial cells to proliferate and to invade the extracellular matrix in response to the HIV-1 Tat protein: Implications for AIDS-Kaposi's sarcoma pathogenesis. J Immunol 162:1165-70, 1999.

75. Battistini AJ: Interferon regulatory factors in hematopoietic cell differentiation and immune regulation. Interferon Cytokine Res 12:765-80, 2009.

76. Stadler R, Bratzke B, Schaart F, et al.: Long-term combined rIFN-alpha-2a and zidovudine therapy for HIV-associated Kaposi's sarcoma: Clinical consequences and side effects. J Invest Dermatol Dec(6 Suppl):170S-175S, 1990.

77. Angel JB, Greaves W, Long J, et al.: Virologic and immunologic activity of PegIntron in HIV disease. AIDS 23:2431-8, 2009.

78. Bakker PJM, Danner SA, Lange JMA, et al.: Etoposide for epidemic Kaposi's sarcoma: A phase II study. Eur J Cancer Clin Oncol 24:1047, 1988.

79. Volberding PA, Abrams DI, Conant M, et al.: Vinblastine therapy for Kaposi's sarcoma in the acquired immunodeficiency syndrome. Ann Intern Med 103:335, 1985.

80. Mintzer DM, Real FX, Jovino L, et al.: Treatment of Kaposi's sarcoma and thrombocytopenia with vincristine in patients with acquired immunodeficiency syndrome. Ann Intern Med 102:200, 1985.

81. Caumes E, Guermonprez G, Katlama C, et al.: AIDS-associated mucocutaneous Kaposi's sarcoma treated with bleomycin. AIDS 6:1483, 1992.

82. Fischl MA, Krown SE, O'Boyle KP, et al.: Weekly doxorubicin in the treatment of patients with AIDS-related Kaposi's sarcoma. J Acquir Immune Defic Syndr 6:259, 1993.

83. Nasti G, Errante D, Talamini R, et al.: Vinorelbine is an effective and safe drug for AIDS-related Kaposi's sarcoma: Results of a phase II study. J Clin Oncol 18:1550, 2000.

84. Shepherd FA, Burkes RL, Paul KE, et al.: A phase II study of epirubicin in the treatment of poor-risk Kaposi's sarcoma and AIDS. AIDS 5:305, 1991.

85. Gill PS, Mitsuyasu RT, Montgomery T, et al.: AIDS Clinical Trials Group Study 094: A phase I/II trial of ABV chemotherapy with zidovudine and recombinant human GM-CSF in AIDS-related Kaposi's sarcoma. Cancer J Sci Am 5:278-83, 1997.

86. Krown SE, Northfelt DW, Osoba D, et al.: Use of liposomal anthracyclines in Kaposi's sarcoma. Semin Oncol 6(Suppl 13):36, 2004.

87. Welles L, Saville MW, Lietzau J, et al.: Phase II trial with dose titration of paclitaxel for the therapy of human immunodeficiency virus-associated Kaposi's sarcoma. J Clin Oncol 16:1112, 1998.

88. Belotti D, Vergani V, Drudis T, et al.: The microtubule-affecting drug paclitaxel has antiangiogenic activity. Clin Cancer Res 2:1843, 1996.

89. Uziely B, Jeffers S, Isaacson R, et al.: Liposomal doxorubicin: Antitumor activity and unique toxicities during two complementary phase I studies. J Clin Oncol 13:1777, 1995.

90. Petre CE, Dittmer DP: Liposomal daunorubicin as treatment for Kaposi's sarcoma. Int J Nanomedicine 2:277-88, 2007.

91. Martellotta F, Berretta M, Vaccher E, et al.: AIDS-related Kaposi's sarcoma: State of the art and therapeutic strategies. Curr HIV Res 6:634-8, 2009.

92. Clinical Trial Verified by National Cancer Institute (NCI): Pilot study bortezomib in treating patients with relapsed or refractory AIDS-related Kaposi sarcoma. Available at: http://www.cancer.gov/search/ViewClinicalTrials.aspx?cdrid=659554&protocolsearchid=7440516&version=patient. Accessed 15 Jan 2011.

93. Koon HB, Bubley GJ, Pantanowitz L, et al.: Imatinib-induced regression of AIDS-related Kaposi's sarcoma. J Clin Oncol 23:982-9, 2005.

94. Little RF, Merced-Galindez F, Staskus K, et al.: A pilot study of cidofovir in patients with Kaposi sarcoma. J Infect Dis 187:149, 2003.

95. Scadden DT: AIDS-related malignancies. Ann Rev Med 54:285-303, 2003.

96. Lym ST, Levine AM: Recent advances in acquired immunodeficiency syndrome (AIDS)-related lymphoma. CA Cancer J Clin 55:229-241, 2005.

97. Carbone A, Cesarman E, Spina M, et al.: HIV-associated lymphomas and gamma-herpesviruses. Blood 113:1213-24, 2009.

98. National Cancer Institute sponsored study of classifications of non-Hodgkin's lymphomas: Summary and description of a working formulation for clinical usage. The Non-Hodgkin's Lymphoma Pathologic Classification Project. Cancer 49:2112-2135, 1982.

99. Barclay LR, Buskin SE, Kahle EM, et al.: Clinical and immunologic profile of AIDS-related lymphoma in the era of highly active antiretroviral therapy. Clin Lymphoma Myeloma 4:272-9, 2007.

100. Jaffe ES, Harris NL, Stein H, et al.: World Health Organization Classification of Tumors: Pathology & Genetics: Tumors of Haematopoietic and Lymphoid Tissues. Lyon: IARC Press; 2001.

101. Levine AM: Acquired immunodeficiency-syndrome related lymphoma. Blood 80:8–20, 1992.

102. Vajdic CM, van Leeuwen MT: What types of cancers are associated with immune suppression in HIV? Lessons from solid organ transplant recipients. Curr Opin HIV/AIDS 1:35-41, 2009.

103. Pelicci P, Knowles DM, Arlin ZA, et al.: Multiple monoclonal B cell expansions and c-myc oncogene rearrangements in acquired immune deficiency syndrome-related lymphoproliferative disorders. J Exp Med 164:2049–2076, 1986.

104. Carbone A, Gloghini A: AIDS-related lymphomas: From pathogenesis to pathology. Br J Haematol 130:662-670, 2005.

105. Angeletti PC, Luwen Z, Wood C: The viral etiology of AIDS-associated malignancies. Adv Pharmacol 56:509-557, 2008.

106. Vaghefi P, Martin A, Prévot S, et al.: Genomic imbalances in AIDS-related lymphomas: Relation with tumoral Epstein-Barr virus status. AIDS 20:2285-91, 2006.

107. Gaidano G, Pastore C, Lanza C, et al.: Molecular pathology of AIDS-related lymphomas. Biologic aspects and clinicopathologic heterogeneity. Ann Hematol 69:281-290, 1994.

108. Knowles DM: Molecular pathology of acquired immunodeficiency syndrome-related non-Hodgkin's lymphoma. Semin Diagn Pathol 1:67-82, 1997.

109. Voelkerding KV, Sandhaus LM, Kim HC, et al.: Plasma cell malignancy in the acquired immune deficiency syndrome. Am J Clin Pathol 92:222–228, 1989.

110. Levine AM, Sadeghi S, Espina B, et al.: Characteristics of indolent non-Hodgkin lymphoma in patients with type 1 human immunodeficiency virus infection. Cancer 94:1500–1506, 2002.

111. Goldstein J, Becker N, Delrowe J, et al.: Cutaneous T-cell lymphoma in a patient infected with human immunodeficiency virus type 1. Use of radiation therapy. Cancer 66:1130-1132, 1990.

112. Tsimberidou AM, Medina J, Cortes J, et al.: Chronic myeloid leukemia in a patient with acquired immune deficiency syndrome: Complete cytogenetic response with imatinib mesylate: Report of a case and review of the literature. Leuk Res 6:657-60, 2004.

113. Ziegler JL, Beckstead JA, Volberding PA, et al.: Non-Hodgkin's lymphoma in 90 homosexual men. Relation to generalized lymphadenopathy and the acquired immunodeficiency syndrome. N Engl J Med 311:565–570, 1984.

114. Kaplan LD, Abrams DI, Feigal E, et al.: AIDS-associated non-Hodgkin's lymphoma in San Francisco. JAMA 261: 719–724, 1989.

115. Ikebe T., Amemiya Y., Saburi M., Ando T., Kohno K., Ogata M., Hiramatusu K., Kadota J. Rare primary effusion lymphoma associated with HHV-8 in Japan Intern Med 2010; 49(13):1303-6.

116. Carbone PP., Kaplan H.S., Mushoff K et al. Report of the Committee on Hodgkin's Disease Staging. Cancer Res 1971;31:1860-1861.

117. Rossi G, Donisi A, Casari S, et al.: The International Prognostic Index can be used as a guide to treatment decisions regarding patients with human immunodeficiency virus-related systemic non-Hodgkin lymphoma. Cancer 86:2391-2397, 1999.

118. Francisci D, Falcinelli F, Schiaroli E, et al.: Management of hepatitis B virus reactivation in patients with hematological malignancies treated with chemotherapy. Infection 38:58-61, 2010.

119. Kaplan LD, Straus DJ, Testa MA, et al.: Low-dose compared with standard-dose m-BACOD chemotherapy for non-Hodgkin's lymphoma associated with human immunodeficiency virus infection. National Institute of Allergy and Infectious Diseases AIDS Clinical Trials Group. N Engl J Med 336:1641-1648, 1997.

120. Bower M., Gazzard B., Mandallia S., Newson-Davis T., Thirwell C., Dhillon T., Young A.M., Powles T., Gaya A., Nelsor S.J. A prognostic index for systemic AIDS-related non-Hodgkin lymphoma treated in the era of highly active antiretroviral therapy. Ann Intern Med 2005 Aug 16;143(4):265-73.

121. Levine A. HIV associated lymphoma Blood 115(15):2986. (2010)

122. Tosi P, Gherlinzoni F, Mazza P., et al. 3′-Azido-3′-deoxythymidine plus methotrexate as a novel antineoplastic combination in the treatment of human immunodeficiency virus-related non-Hodgkin's lymphomas. Blood 1997;89:419-425.

123. Vaccher E, Spina M, di gennaro G, et al. Concomitant cyclophosphamide, doxorubicin, vincristine, and prednisone chemotherapy plus highly active antiretroviral therapy in patients with human immunodeficiency virus-related, non-Hodgkin lymphoma. Cancer 2001;91(1):155-163.

124. Kaplan LD, Scadden DT. No benefit from rituximab in a randomized phase III trial of CHOP with or without rituximab for patients with HIV-associated non-Hodgkin's lymphoma: AIDS malignancies consortium study 010. Proc Am Soc Clin Oncol 2003; abstr 2268).

125. Sparano JA, Weller E., Nazeer T., et al. Phase II trial of infusional cyclophosphamide, doxorubicin, and etoposide in patients with poor-prognosis, intermediate-grade non-Hodgkin lymphoma: An Eastern Cooperative Oncology Group trial (E3493). Blood 2002;100(5):1634-1640.

126. Tirelli U, SpinaM., Jaeger U., et al. Infusional CDE with rituximab for the treatment of human immunodeficiency virus-associated non-Hodgkin's lymphoma: Preliminary results of a phase 1/II study. Recent Results Cancer Res 2002;159: 149-153.

127. Little RF, Pittaluga S, Grant N. et al. highly effective treatment of acquired immunodeficiency syndrome-related lymphoma with dose-adjusted EPOCH: Impact of antiretroviral therapy suspension and tumor biology. Blood 2003;101(12): 4653-4659.

128. Sparano JA,. Clinical aspects and management of AIDS-related lymphoma. Eur J cancer 2001;37(10):1296-1305.

129. Antinori A, Cingolani A., Alba L. et al. Better response to chemotherapy and prolonged survival in AIDS-related lymphomas responding to highly active antiretroviral therapy. AIDS 2001;15:1483-1491.

130. Levine AM: Management of AIDS-related lymphoma. Curr Opin Oncol 20:522-528, 2008.

131. Cortes J, Thomas D, Rios A, et al.: Hyperfractionated cyclophosphamide, vincristine, doxorubicin, and dexamethasone and highly active antiretroviral therapy for patients with acquired immunodeficiency syndrome-related Burkitt lymphoma/ leukemia. Cancer 94:1492-1499, 2002.

132. Wang ES, Straus DJ, Teruya-Feldstein J, et al.: Intensive chemotherapy with cyclophosphamide, doxorubicin, high dose methotrexate/ifosfamide, etoposide, and high-dose cytarabine (CODOX-M/IVAC) for human immunodeficiency virus associated Burkitt lymphoma. Cancer 98:1196-1205, 2003.

133. Dunleavy K, Healy Bird BR, Pittaluga S, et al.: Efficacy and toxicity of dose-adjusted EPOCH-rituximab in adults with newly diagnosed Burkitt lymphoma. J Clin Oncol 18S(June suppl):8035, 2007.

134. Krishnan A, Molina A, Zaia J, et al.: Durable remissions with autologous stem cell transplantation for high risk HIV associated lymphomas. Blood 105:874-878, 2004.

135. CDC: Revision of the CDC surveillance case definition for acquired immunodeficiency syndrome. MMWR 36:1-15S, 1987.

137. Bailey P: Intracranial sarcomatous tumors of leptomeningeal origin. Arch Surg 18:1359-1402, 1929.

138. Ivers LC, Kim AY, Sax PE. Predictive value of polymerase chain reaction of cerebrospinal fluid for detection of Epstein-Barr virus to establish the diagnosis of HIV-related primary central nervous system lymphoma. Clin. Infect. Dis.2004; 38(11):1629-1632.

139. Pagano JS, Epstein-Barr virus: The first human tumor virus and its role in cancer. Proc Assoc AM Physicians 111:573-580, 1999.

140. Antinori A, Ammassari A, De Luca A, et al.: Diagnosis of AIDS-related focal brain lesions: A decision-making analysis based on clinical and neuroradiologic characteristics combined with polymerase chain reaction assays in CSF. Neurology 48:687, 1997.

141. Wong SY, Israeliski DM, Remington JS: AIDS-associated toxoplasmosis, in Sande MA, Volberding PA, (eds): The Medical Management of AIDS, 4th ed. Philadelphia: WB Saunders, 1995; p 460.

142. Lorberboym M, Wallach F, Estok L, et al.: Thallium-201 retention in focal intracranial lesions for differential diagnosis of primary lymphoma and nonmalignant lesions in AIDS patients. J Nucl Med 39:1366-1369, 1998.

143. Corcoran C., Rebe K., van de Plas H., Myer L., Hardie D.R. The predictive value of cerebrospinal fluid Epstein-Barr viral load as a marker of primary central nervous system lymphoma in HIV-infected persons. Journal of Clinical Virology 42(2008) p 433-436.

144. Broomberg JEC, Breems DA, Kran J, et al.: CSF flow cytometry greatly improves diagnostic accuracy in CNS hematologic malignancies. Neurology 68:1674-1679, 2007.

145. Shah GD, Yahalom J, Correa DD, et al.: Combined immunochemotherapy with reduced whole-brain radiotherapy for newly diagnosed primary CNS lymphoma. J Clin Oncol 25:4730-5, 2007.

146. Carbone A, Gloghini A, Serraino D, et al.: HIV-associated Hodgkin lymphoma. Curr Opin HIV/AIDS 4:3-10, 2009.

147. Carbone A, Gloghini A, Dotti G: EBV-associated lymphproliferative disorders: Classification and treatment. Oncologist 13:577-585, 2008.

148. Vaccher E, Spina M, Tirelli U: Clinical aspects and management of Hodgkin's disease and other tumours in HIV-infected individuals. Eur J Cancer 37:1306–1315, 2001.

149. Hessol NA, Katz MH, Liu JU, et al.: Increased incidence of Hodgkin's disease in homosexual men with HIV infection. Ann Intern Med 117:309–311, 1992.

150. Levine AM, Li P, Cheung T, et al.: Chemotherapy consisting of doxorubicin, bleomycin, vinblastine, and dacarbazine with granulocyte-colony-stimulating factor in HIV-infected patients with newly diagnosed Hodgkin's disease: A prospective, multi-institutional AIDS clinical trials group study (ACTG 149). J AIDS 15:444–450, 2000.

151. Berenguer J, Miralles P, Ribera JM, et al.: Characteristics and outcome of AIDS-related Hodgkin's lymphoma before and after the introduction of highly active antiretroviral therapy. J Acquire Immune Defic Syndr 47:422-428, 2008.

152. Spina M, Gabarre J, Rossi G, et al. Stanford V regimen and concomitant HAART in 59 patients with Hodgkin's disease and HIV infection. Blood 2002;100:1984-1988.

153. Massad LS, Evans CT, Wilson TE, et al.: Knowledge of cervical cancer prevention and human papillomavirus among women with HIV. Gynecol Oncol [Epub January 27, 2010].

154. Stier E. Cervical neoplasia and the HIV-infected patient. Hematol Oncol Clin North Am 2003;17:873-887.

155. Chow LT, Brooker TR: Papillomavirus DNA replication. Intervirology 37:150-158, 1994.

156. Munger K, Phelps WC, Bubb V, et al.: The E6 and E7 genes of the human papillomavirus type 16 together are necessary and sufficient for transformation of primary human keratinocytes. J Virol 63:4417-4421, 1989.

157. Ellerbrock TV, Chiasson MA, Bush TJ, et al.: Incidence of cervical squamous intraepithelial lesions in HIV-infected women. JAMA 282:1031–1037, 2000.

158. US Preventive Services Task Force. Screening for cervical cancer. In: AHRQ Publication No. 03–515A, January 2003. Rockville, MD: Agency for Healthcare Research and Quality; 2003.

159. Palefsky J: Human papillomavirus-related disease in people with HIV. Curr Opin HIV AIDS Jan 4(1);52-6, 2009.

160. Chaturvedi AK, Madeleine MM, Biggar RJ, et al.: Risk of human Papillomavirus-associated cancers among persons with AIDS. J Natl Cancer Inst 101:1120-1130, 2009.

161. NCCN Clinical Practice Guidelines in Oncology: Cervical cancer version 1.2010. Natl Comp Cancer Network, 2010. Available at: http://www.nccn.org/professionals/ physician_gls/ PDF/cervical.pdf. Accessed 15 Jan 2015.

162. zur Hausen.H. 2002. Papillomaviruses and cancer: from basic studies to clinical application. Nature Rev, cancer 2:342-350.

163. Campo MS, Roden RBS. Papillomavirus prophylactic vaccines: Established successes, new approaches. J Virol 84:1214-1220, 2010.

164. Martin F., Bowers M. Anal intraepithelial neoplasia in HIV-positive people. Sex Transm Inf 2001;77:327-331.

165. Chin-Hong PV, Palefsky JM: Natural history and clinical management of anal human papillomavirus disease in men and women infected with human immunodeficiency virus. HIV/AIDS 35:1127–1134, 2002.

166. NCCN Clinical Practice Guidelines in Oncology: Anal cancer version 1.2011. Natl Comp Cancer Network, 2010. Available at: http://www.nccn.org/professionals/physician_gls/PDF/anal.pdf. Accessed 15 Jan 2011.

167. Boshoff C., Weiss R. AIDS-related malignancies. Nature 2002;2:373-382.

168. French MA: Immune Reconstitution syndrome: A reappraisal. Clinical Infectious Diseases. 2009; 48:101-7.

169. Valencia Ortega ME: AIDS-related malignancies-A new approach. AIDS Rev 10:125-7, 2008.

170. Catellan AM, Trevenzoli M, Aversa SML, et al. Recent advances in the treatment of AIDS-related Kaposi sarcoma. Am J Clin Dermatol 2002;3(7):451-462.

CARCINOMA OF UNKNOWN PRIMARY

Gauri R. Varadhachary

Carcinomas of unknown primary, with their heterogeneous presentations, pose a major problem for oncologists; depending on the extent of evaluation, they comprise 3 to 10% of all tumors diagnosed (1-3). A working definition for carcinoma of unknown primary (CUP) is biopsy-proven metastatic cancer with no identifiable primary source by history, physical examination, chest radiography, complete blood count, chemistry, computed tomography (CT) of the chest, abdomen and pelvis, prostate-specific antigen (PSA) in men, and mammography in women. The natural history of disease for CUP is diverse and is dependent on multiple variables such

as, age, number of metastatic sites, dominant area of disease, and histology (2,4,5). It is this considerable heterogeneity that has presented a challenge to the systematic study of CUP. Depending on histologic features, sites of disease, and performance status, a small but significant minority of patients will be long-term survivors (4,6).

This chapter discusses the evaluation of patients with CUP and optimal therapeutic strategies in the era of sophisticated diagnostics. The differing natural histories in CUP, depending on both the sites of disease and histology, are also discussed. Studies show that in this population, a search for the primary tumor beyond "routine" evaluation is unrewarding in >90% of cases (2,3,7). This fact has caused much consternation for both patients and physicians. The foundation for cancer treatment traditionally relies on identification of the tumor origin, thereby allowing treatment to be chosen based on the known natural history as well as specific therapies which have been proven effective for the cancer; this is becoming even more important with the rapid emergence of targeted therapies. Without knowledge of the primary site, the oncologist is often hesitant to recommend therapy especially given the disease heterogeneity. Although most patients with metastatic CUP have tumors that respond poorly to current treatments and will consequently have a poor prognosis, it has become evident over the last two decades that subsets of patients with CUP have a favorable prognosis and respond to chemotherapy or can be successfully treated with regional therapy alone. The current era of sophisticated diagnostics and introduction of targeted therapies has been particularly important in the CUP setting, since this cancer diagnosis is the epitome of personalized therapy.

■ EPIDEMIOLOGY

The incidence of CUP is difficult to determine because many patients are given other diagnoses, and CUP is therefore underreported (6). It was estimated that 31,490 new cases of cancer of "other and unspecified primary sites" were diagnosed in 2009, representing more than 2% of all cancers (8). Based on studies explicitly designed to evaluate CUP, the true incidence is thought to be much higher, closer to 6% of all new cancers (9). CUP seems to affect men and women equally and recent large series show a median age at presentation between 59 and 66 years (1,5,10).

A minority of patients (10%) with CUP have a history of an antecedent cancer (11). In autopsies performed before the advent of CT, the occult primary tumor was identified in 60 to 80% of cases. In one autopsy series, the two most commonly identified primary sites were the pancreas (20%) and lungs (18%) (12). Given the current high-quality CT imaging and PET scans, it is unclear whether these cancer profiles are still the majority. The poor prognosis for patients with these malignancies reflects the overall poor prognosis for those with CUPs as a group. Although breast and prostate cancers represent the most common cancers in women and men, these usually account for only 2% of the primary sites identified in patients with CUP (13).

■ BIOLOGY AND CHROMOSOMAL ABERRATIONS

CUPs, despite their heterogeneity, are a clinically unique oncologic entity; as such, they share many common features that set them apart from other malignancies. The central unifying clinical feature of CUP is the absence of a detectable primary tumor. Previous studies have shown that even after an autopsy, the primary site will not be identified in 20 to 40% of cases and that number is likely much lower with significant improvements in imaging (14). At present, it is not known why primary carcinomas exhibit this unique biological behavior. One current hypothesis is that the acquisition of a "metastatic phenotype" is an early event in CUPs, soon after oncogenesis, thus enabling cells to metastasize early, before the development of a clinically detectable tumor (15-17). It has also been hypothesized that the primary tumors may regress or involute before the metastases become clinically evident, attributed to a host immunologic response. A third hypothesis is that the primary tumor is exposed to antiangiogenic factors locally, whereas the metastases acquire the angiogenic phenotype after a period of dormancy (18).

Several studies have demonstrated a specific nonrandom pattern of chromosomal aberrations that seems to be unique to CUPs. These data suggest that some of these genetic changes may be the underlying cause of the metastatic phenotype. CUP is characterized by greater genetic instability, with massive genomic alterations, when compared with other distant metastases. In a study by Pantou and colleagues (19), cytogenetic profiling of tumors from 20 patients with CUP was performed, revealing an average of 11 chromosomal changes per case. Of the three histologic subtypes in this study, adenocarcinomas had not only the highest number of cytogenetic changes (16 versus 3) but also involvement of distinct sites (4q31, 6q15, 10q25, and 13q22) when compared with carcinomas or undifferentiated malignancies. The latter group was distinguished by the involvement of changes at 11q22. Overall, the most commonly rearranged chromosomal regions were 1q21, 3p13, 6q21-23, 7q22, 11p15-12, and 11q14-24. The number of cytogenetic alterations was found to be prognostically relevant. Median survival was significantly greater for patients with five or fewer cytogenetic changes compared with those with more than five changes (3 versus 18 months, $p = .003$) (19). An older study of 12 CUP cell lines also demonstrated a preponderance of chromosome 1 abnormalities. These changes were observed on both the long arm (eg, 1p deletion, isochromosome 1p, and translocations with a 1p breakpoint) and on the short arm (1q21), suggesting the importance of chromosome 1 in the biology of CUPs (16). Chromosome 1p aberrations are also commonly associated with advanced malignancies (20).

Chromosome 12 abnormalities have also been shown in CUP. This is of particular interest because one of the observed alterations, isochromosome 12p (i12p), is present in as many as 80% of germ cell tumors. Motzer and colleagues (21,22) reported that 30% of patient tumors in their series had either i12p or 12q deletions. The presence of either of these two cytogenetic abnormalities was found to be predictive of a complete response to cisplatin-based chemotherapy (75 versus 17%, $p = .002$) (21,22).

The tumor suppressor gene *p53* is commonly mutated in human cancers, especially in advanced malignancies. Paradoxically, this does not seem to be true in CUP. Bar-Eli and colleagues (15) found *p53* mutations to be less frequent than expected (26%) in CUP after evaluating 15 biopsy specimens and 8 cell lines (15). However, work by other researchers evaluating immunohistochemical studies of *p53* in CUP has found this protein to be highly expressed in 70% of the tumors examined (23,24). Nevertheless, *p53* expression has not been found to have prognostic relevance. Molecular studies have also demonstrated the overexpression of other oncogenes, such as c-*myc*, *ras*, *bcl-2*, and *Her2/neu*, in CUPs, but none have been found to have any correlation with either survival or response to chemotherapy (23,25).

■ NATURAL HISTORY AND CLINICAL PRESENTATION

The clinical course of patients with CUP varies widely. Consequently, median survival in large retrospective studies has ranged from 11 weeks to 11 months (1,5,26). In the University of Texas MD Anderson Cancer Center database, the 5-year overall survival (OS) rate was only 11%. Although survival is poor as a whole, there are certain prognostic variables that correlate with longer survival, including disease limited to one organ site, involvement of lymph nodes only, and histologic diagnoses of squamous or neuroendocrine carcinoma. Variables suggestive of a poor prognosis include male sex, histologic diagnosis of adenocarcinoma, and metastatic involvement of the liver, lungs, bone, pleura, or brain (Table 42-1) (5,10).

By performing multivariate analyses on a consecutive series of 1000 patients with CUP with classification and regression tree (CART) analysis, Hess and colleagues (5) were able to more closely study the interactions between

TABLE 42-1 | FAVORABLE-VERSUS POOR-PROGNOSIS CARCINOMA OF UNKNOWN PRIMARY

Favorable	*Poor Prognosis*
Extragonadal germ cell syndrome	Liver metastases (non-neuroendocrine)
Isolated single small metastasis	Pleural and/or lung metastases
Papillary peritoneal adenocarcinoma (women)	Adrenal metastases
Isolated axillary adenocarcinoma (women)	Multiple brain metastases
Cervical adenopathy (squamous cell)	
Isolated inguinal adenopathy	
Neuroendocrine histology	

different clinical variables and how this influenced survival (Fig. 42-1).

Patients with CUP present with symptoms and signs similar to those of patients with advanced malignancies of known origin. In one review, the most common symptoms at presentation of CUP were general deterioration (73%), digestive symptoms (58%), liver enlargement (58%), abdominal pain (56%), respiratory symptoms (45%), ascites (26%), and node enlargement (16%) (27). Most patients with CUP present with multiple metastases, with three or more organs involved (10). Moreover, CUPs are also distinguished from other solid tumors by an unusual metastatic pattern, with a relatively high number of metastases found in the skin, kidneys, heart, and adrenal gland (12,28). In patients with a dominant (or single) site of metastasis, the most common reported sites were liver (25%), bone (22%), lungs (20%), lymph nodes (15%), pleural space (10%), and brain (5%) (10).

■ DIAGNOSTIC EVALUATION

Much has been written about the proper approach to the diagnostic evaluation of CUPs. In the past, minimalist diagnostic strategies had been advocated, limiting the scope of initial evaluations to differentiate only between treatable and untreatable disease (29). Others have supported a more aggressive approach, wherein a complete assessment of the extent of the disease and detection of the primary tumor site are attempted. In our experience, a more pragmatic approach is better. Extensive evaluation

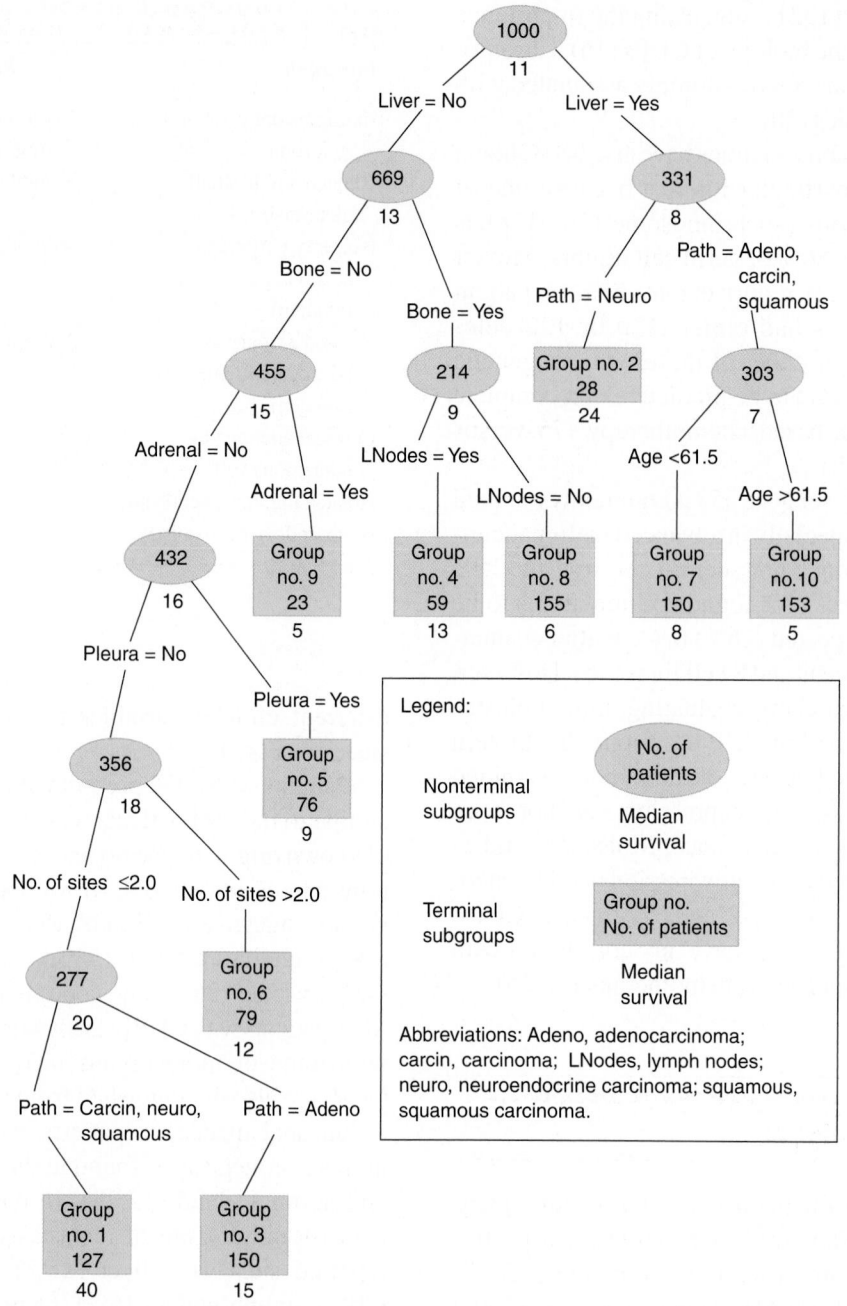

FIGURE 42-1. Classification and regression tree (CART) analysis of 1000 consecutive patients with CUP (default tree). (*Reproduced, with permission, from Hess KR, Abbruzzese MC, Lenzi R, et al. Classification and regression tree analysis of 1000 consecutive patients with unknown primary carcinoma. Clin Cancer Res 1999;5[11]:3403–3410.*)

of all patients presenting with metastases of CUP is an expensive and wasteful extreme that does not benefit patients. In one study, the average cost of evaluating a patient with CUP was $17,973 (and much higher in this day and age) (30). In that study, mean survival was 8.1 months, representative of the natural history of CUPs, with only 18% of patients surviving 1 year.

However, a strictly minimalist approach may result in the oversight of treatable and potentially curable neoplasms.

An important determinant of the appropriate extent of evaluation for a given patient with an unknown primary is whether the data obtained by a diagnostic test will influence treatment decisions. If a treatable or potentially curable cancer is strongly suspected (eg, a germ cell tumor or lymphoma), further investigation should proceed until a precise clinical diagnosis can be made, provided that therapy is not unreasonably delayed. Clinical data support the observation that patients who have CUPs that are later proved to have originated from a particular site have an overall prognosis similar to that of patients who present with a known primary tumor (31). The recommended general approach at the present time is thus one of a directed evaluation based on clinical presentation and pathologic findings; predictions of tumor origin from molecular profiling techniques may ultimately also play a role in narrowing the scope of evaluation.

PHYSICAL EXAMINATION AND LABORATORY TESTS INCLUDING SERUM TUMOR MARKERS

In each case, a thorough medical history should be obtained and a physical examination, including a digital prostate examination in men and a breast and pelvic examination in women, should be performed. Determination of the patient's performance status, nutrition, and the presence or absence of concomitant medical illnesses and malignancy-related complications (eg, paraneoplastic syndromes, painful metastases, or spinal cord compression) that may affect patient care that is required.

Laboratory tests should include routine biochemical and hematologic surveys. The role of tumor markers in the evaluation of patients with CUP is unclear. Most tumor markers are nonspecific and are not useful for identifying a primary site or for prognostic purposes. Adenocarcinoma markers (eg, carcinoembryonic antigen [CEA], cancer antigen 125 [CA 125], CA 15-3, and CA 19-9) are often elevated in patients with CUP and cannot be reliably used to identify a specific primary site or to predict either overall survival or the exact burden of metastatic disease (32). Serum tumor markers may play an important role in helping to evaluate patients for responses to therapy, although levels are not always predictive of response to chemotherapy (33).

Their selective use in a directed approach is more helpful than ordering a large battery of tumor markers on all patients who present with CUP (34). Men who present with metastatic adenocarcinoma should have PSA and prostatic acid phosphatase levels measured, especially in the presence of bony metastases. In all men with undifferentiated (or poorly differentiated) carcinoma, beta-human chorionic gonadotropin and alpha-fetoprotein levels should be measured, especially if the clinical presentation suggests an extragonadal germ cell

tumor (34). In patients with hepatic tumors, alpha-fetoprotein levels should also be measured if there are risk factors or pathologic characteristics that suggest a possibility of primary hepatocellular carcinoma.

DIAGNOSTIC IMAGING AND INVASIVE STUDIES

Initial radiographic studies should include CT of the chest, abdomen, and pelvis. CT scanning of the abdomen or pelvis in CUP has been shown to detect the primary site in 30 to 35% of patients with an initial metastatic site presentation (35,36). Not surprisingly, the tumors most often identified on CT scans are those that arise from the pancreas, kidneys, hepatobiliary tract, and ovary. Imaging or endoscopy of the upper and lower gastrointestinal (GI) tract is indicated for patients with abdominal complaints, ascites, liver metastases, or other findings in the initial workup that are suggestive of a possible GI primary tumor.

All women with CUP and adenocarcinoma should undergo mammography. In cases of suspicious findings on a breast examination and negative mammography findings, patients should have breast sonography and a biopsy as indicated. Because both the sensitivity (23-29%) and specificity (71-73%) of mammography in detecting an occult carcinoma are low, breast magnetic resonance imaging (MRI) has been evaluated as an alternative. In the setting of isolated axillary adenopathy, MRI is very sensitive in detecting occult primary breast cancers (>75%) and should be performed in women with isolated axillary adenopathy and negative mammography findings (37-40). Women with adenocarcinoma presenting with metastatic sites other than cervical or axillary adenopathy that are compatible with breast cancer (ie, bone, liver, or lungs) may also undergo breast MRI if the mammography findings are negative (41).

Patients with upper or midcervical adenopathy with a squamous cell carcinoma on pathology should undergo a thorough head and neck evaluation, including panendoscopy (ie, laryngoscopy, bronchoscopy, and esophagoscopy) with random biopsies. Ipsilateral or (more often) bilateral tonsillectomy has also been recommended as part of the staging process, because this has been shown to identify an occult primary lesion deep in the tonsillar crypts in up to 30% of patients with this presentation of CUP (42). CT of the head and neck region is routinely done as part of the initial workup. In addition, the utility of 18-fluorodeoxyglucose positron emission tomography (FDG-PET) has been well documented in patients with squamous carcinoma and cervical adenopathy; small prospective and retrospective studies suggest that a primary head and neck tumor is identified in 25 to 30% of these patients (43-45). A recent retrospective review found that the primary tumor site was identified in 44% of these patients undergoing PET-CT fusion scans (46), and this modality appears to be emerging as a superior alternative to either PET or CT alone.

Lower cervical or supraclavicular adenopathy suggests a primary tumor arising from below the clavicle. Patients with a pathologic diagnosis of adenocarcinoma or papillary carcinoma in the neck or chest region should be evaluated for thyroid carcinoma. Patients with inguinal lymphadenopathy may have a detectable primary site in the perineal or anorectal area, and anoscopy and colposcopy should be performed (2,47). Evaluation by an urologist may reveal a primary carcinoma of the distal urinary tract.

The role of PET imaging in patients with CUP other than those presenting with cervical adenopathy remains unproven. Data from small retrospective studies evaluating PET for diagnosis in CUP suggest a primary tumor detection rate of approximately 20% (48-50). Even after combined PET-CT, the primary site remains undetermined in a small percentage of patients (43,51-53). In one retrospective study by Alberini and colleagues, the primary site remained unknown after complete imaging in 20% of patients (54). As the PET-CT imaging modality is becoming more readily available, its utility and cost-effectiveness should be studied in larger, well-designed trials.

Finally, another nuclear imaging technology, ^{111}In-pentetreotide scanning, may also prove to be of use in helping to identify the primary site of occult neuroendocrine tumors (55).

HISTOPATHOLOGIC EVALUATION INCLUDING IMMUNOHISTOCHEMICAL STUDIES AND CYTOGENETICS

All pathologic material obtained at biopsy from a patient with CUP should be evaluated by an experienced pathologist who is familiar with the special diagnostic problems of CUPs. The pathologist should also be informed of the patient's pertinent history and clinical findings so that he or she can recommend further analysis on the basis of this information. Adenocarcinoma is the most common histologic diagnosis by light microscopy (approximately 55%). Another 30% of patients will have either undifferentiated or poorly differentiated carcinoma (PDC) or adenocarcinoma (PDAC). The remainder will have one of a variety of carcinomas that include squamous cell carcinomas (6%) and

| TABLE 42-2 | MAJOR HISTOLOGIES IN CARCINOMA OF UNKNOWN PRIMARY |

Histology	Proportion (%)
Well to moderately differentiated adenocarcinoma	55
Poorly differentiated adenocarcinoma Poorly differentiated carcinoma	30
Squamous	6
Neuroendocrine	4
Undifferentiated malignancy	5

neuroendocrine tumors (4%), as well as malignancies that upon more detailed study are determined to be sarcomas, lymphomas, germ cell tumors, melanomas, or unclassifiable undifferentiated malignant neoplasms (Table 42-2) (3,5).

Adequacy of tissue is essential, especially in cases where the pathologist has to make a diagnosis on deep fine-needle aspirations and there is insufficient tissue for immunohistochemical staining. The diagnosis of a poorly differentiated neoplasm implies that the pathologist is unable to classify it into any of the general neoplastic categories (carcinoma, lymphoma, melanoma, or sarcoma). Subsequent evaluation of this group of poorly differentiated lesions by means of special immunohistochemical techniques is warranted, because some of these patients will have tumors that are potentially curable and very responsive to treatment. Many immunohistochemical reagents are at the disposal of the pathologist, making the histologic classification of the tumor easier (Table 42-3).

Especially useful are the antibodies to common leukocyte antigens present in lymphoma and the antibodies to PSA present in most prostate cancers (56,57). Other useful immunohistochemical markers include cytokeratin (CK) 7, CK20, and TTF-1. TTF-1 is a nuclear transcription factor that is normally expressed in lung and thyroid tissues and in their neoplasms. Staining for TTF-1 is frequently positive in lung cancer, especially in adenocarcinomas (60-75%) and small cell lung cancers (66-87%); however, it is inconsistently expressed in squamous cell carcinoma (58-61). Among the various monoclonal antibodies against various cytokeratins, CK7 and CK20 can help differentiate between different solid tumors. For instance, CK7 is more commonly associated with pulmonary or gynecologic malignancies, whereas CK20 is frequently seen in gastrointestinal adenocarcinomas. The CK7+/CK20– immunophenotype, in conjunction with TTF-1 staining, is suggestive

TABLE 42-3	**COMMONLY UTILIZED IMMUNOPEROXIDASE STAINS TO ASSIST IN THE DIFFERENTIAL DIAGNOSIS OF POORLY DIFFERENTIATED NEOPLASMS**
Stain	*Likely Primary Site*
Estrogen/progesterone receptor, gross cystic disease fluid protein-15 (GCDFP-15), low-molecular-weight cytokeratin (CK)	Breast cancer
Thyroid transcription factor (TTF-1), CK7, CK20, surfactant protein A precursor (SP-A1)	Lung cancer
Prostate-specific antigen (PSA), epithelial membrane antigen (EMA), alpha-methylacyl CoA racemase/P504S (AMACR/P504S)	Prostate cancer
Leukocyte common antigen (LCA), CD3, CD4, CD5, CD20, CD45	Lymphoma
Vimentin, desmin[†], factor VIII[‡]	Sarcoma
Chromogranin/synaptophysin, neuron-specific enolase, cytokeratin	Neuroendocrine tumor
EMA, β-hCG, αFP, placental alkaline phosphatase (PLAP)	Germ cell tumor
CK7, CK20*, uroplakin III	Urothelial malignancies
S100, vimentin, HMB-45, neuron-specific enolase	Melanoma
CK7, CK20*, CDX-2, carcinoembryonic antigen (CEA)	Colorectal cancer

*Whereas a CK7+/CK20– staining pattern is typical of lung neoplasms, CK7–/CK20+ is suggestive of a colorectal primary. Dual CK7+/CK20+, however, is suggestive of urothelial primary.
[†]Positive in desmoid tumors, rhabdomyosarcomas, and leiomyosarcomas.
[‡]Positive in angiosarcomas.

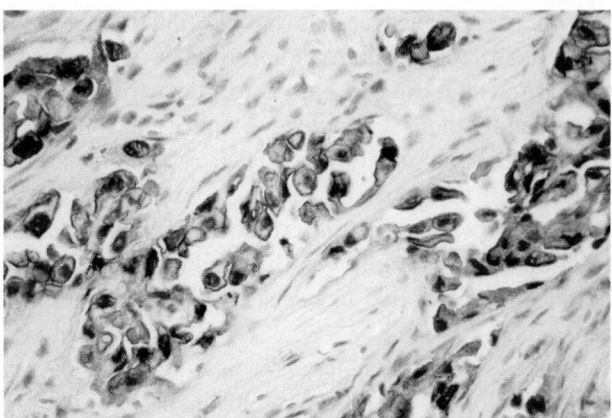
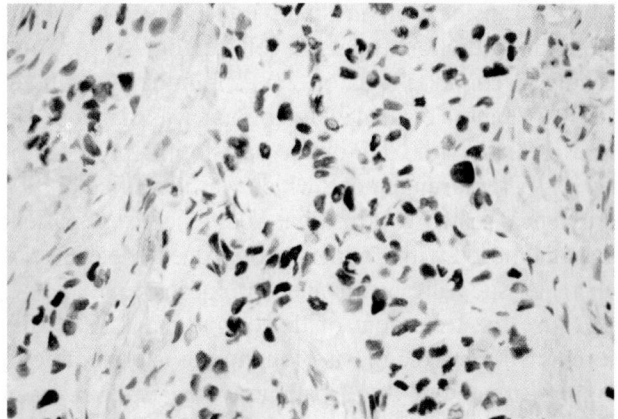
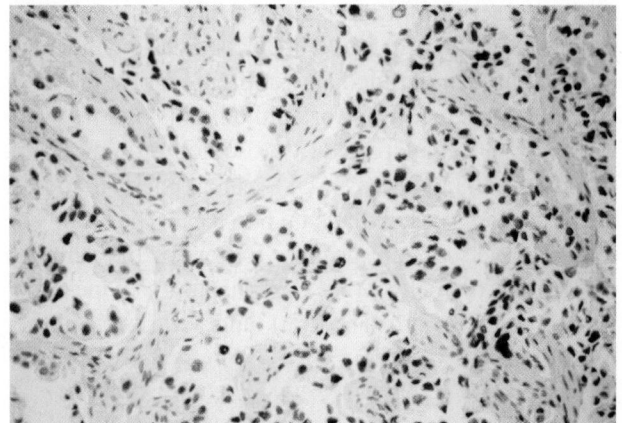

FIGURE 42-2. Immunohistochemical stains performed on the biopsy specimen from a patient with primary metastatic adenocarcinoma to a supraclavicular lymph node. Immunoperoxidase stains were positive for CK-7 (**A**) and TTF-1 (**B**) but negative for CK-20 (**C**), thus suggestive of metastatic non–small cell lung cancer. (*Courtesy of Dr. Nelson Ordoñez, Department of Pathology MDACC.*)

of a lung primary and is a highly sensitive and specific method for differentiating primary pulmonary adenocarcinomas from metastatic extrapulmonary adenocarcinomas (Fig. 42-2) (62-64). By contrast, the CK7–/CK20+ immunophenotype is suggestive of a colorectal primary site. CK7+ and CK20+ dual staining suggest a malignancy of urothelial origin (65).

Hep par 1 is an antigen whose expression is confined to benign and malignant hepatocytes and aids in the diagnosis of hepatocellular carcinoma in patients with CUP presenting with liver lesions. In women, depending on the pathology and pattern of metastasis, estrogen receptor (ER) and progesterone receptor (PR) staining is done to look for a breast primary. Another marker for a breast primary is gross cystic disease fluid protein 15 (GCDFP-15), which is present in 62 to 72% of breast cancers.

Dennis and colleagues (66) have identified other novel molecular markers using a bioinformatics approach. All publicly available gene expression data from various adenocarcinomas were pooled together and four novel proteins not previously recognized as tumor markers were found to be significantly upregulated. This was confirmed by reverse transcription–polymerase chain reaction. One example was lipophilin B, which was found to be restricted to breast, ovarian, and prostate cancers.

The use of cytogenetic analysis in the diagnosis of CUPs is limited. Specific chromosomal abnormalities have been identified in several types of lymphoma (8; 14 translocation in small non–cleaved-cell non-Hodgkin lymphoma), germ cell tumors (i12p), and Ewing sarcoma (t11; 22 or t21; 22). In the cytogenetic study by Pantou et al. (19), lymphoma was diagnosed in four patients with CUP on the basis of the presence of IgH/Alk-1 rearrangement, which was identified by fluorescence in situ hybridization. Additionally, one patient was diagnosed with Ewing sarcoma due to detection of characteristic rearrangement of chromosomes 11 and 22. Because the treatment of these malignancies is different, a correct diagnosis of the tumor is preferable to empiric treatment of all patients with cisplatin-based chemotherapy.

In our series of 1380 patients with suspected CUP, primary tumors were found in 27.5% by using the diagnostic approach outlined above. In this series, the most common sites of origin for epithelial histologies were lungs (15%), pancreas (13%), colon/rectum (6%), kidneys (5%), and breast (4%). Melanomas, sarcomas, and lymphomas each made up 6 to 8% of the total. The remaining cases were primary tumors of the stomach (4%), ovary (3%), liver (3%), esophagus (3%), mesothelial tissue (2%), prostate (2%), and a variety of other histologies (19%) (13).

MOLECULAR PROFILING OF CARCINOMA OF UNKNOWN PRIMARY

Over the past decade, there has been considerable progress in the development of platforms using gene expression profiling to identify the tissue of origin of CUP. Initial studies evaluated gene expression profiles of primary and metastatic tumors of known origin to identify tumor-specific patterns; when applied to test sets, the predictive accuracy for tissue site ranged from 78 to 85% (67,68). These studies served as proof of principle but are somewhat less feasible in routine clinical practice due to requirement of frozen tissue blocks for RNA recovery and array preparation. More recent promising platforms permit evaluation of mRNA expression from formalin-fixed, paraffin-embedded tissue (69-72).

One of these assays (69) uses 10 mRNA markers via quantitative reverse transcriptase polymerase chain reaction (qRT-PCR), to identify the tissue of origin for lung, colon, breast, ovary, prostate, and pancreas tumors. In the initial validation study, the accuracy of the prediction ranged from 73 to 77%. In a follow-up study employing this method to analyze specimens from 120 clinical tissue specimens (71), the assay was technically feasible in 87% of samples and predicted a diagnosis in 61%, yielding an overall rate of diagnosis of 53%. It is likely that the diagnostic rate could be improved further with the addition of more genes to be analyzed. Another assay (72) uses a 495-gene microarray to predict tissue of origin among 48 tumor types; in an initial validation study, 83% of known samples were classified correctly.

Monzon and colleagues evaluated another assay with the aim of their blinded study, which was to validate a predefined 1550-gene expression profile (73). The group processed 547 frozen specimens representing 15 tissues of origin using oligonucleotide microarrays. Half of the specimens were metastatic tumors, with the remainder being poorly differentiated and undifferentiated primary cancers chosen to resemble those that present as a clinical challenge. The study found overall sensitivity of 87.8% (95% CI, 84.7-90.4%) and overall specificity of 99.4% (95% CI, 98.3-99.9%). Performance within the subgroup of metastatic tumors (N = 258) was found to be slightly lower than that of the poorly differentiated and undifferentiated primary tumor subgroup, 84.5 and 90.7%, respectively ($p = .04$). Differences between individual (4) laboratories were not statistically significant (73).

Validation of molecular profiling assay predictions for patients with true CUP is inherently difficult because the primary site is never identified for most patients; however, one study (71) employed clinical correlation with therapeutic response and immunohistochemical staining. In this study, the assay agreed with immunohistochemical staining in the few cases where immunohistochemistry results were specific enough to make a diagnosis. Clinically, patients predicted by the assay to have a colon cancer profile responded better to colon-specific chemotherapy regimens. Future efforts to further correlate molecular profiling with clinical treatment outcome will be illustrative. At the present time, the most valuable, feasible, and economic approach to utilizing molecular profiling in relation to other diagnostic testing, including immunohistochemistry, remains to be determined.

■ MANAGEMENT OF SPECIFIC CLINICOPATHOLOGIC SUBGROUPS

CUP PRESENTING AS BRAIN METASTASES (WITHOUT ANY EXTRACRANIAL DISEASE)

It is estimated that brain metastases occur in 20 to 40% of patients with cancer. In as many as 15% of these, the primary site remains unknown (74). The important factor in treating patients with brain lesions is to distinguish patients with metastatic disease from those with primary brain tumors. Once this distinction has been made, patients with single metastatic lesions should be considered for surgery and those with multiple lesions should receive radiotherapy. In a recent small prospective study, patients with CUP who had single brain metastases treated with gross total resection and subsequent whole-brain radiotherapy (WBRT) had a median survival of 13 months. Patients with CUP who had multiple brain metastases and who underwent either WBRT alone or gross resection of symptomatic lesions followed by adjuvant WBRT had a median survival of only 6 to 8 months (75). After treatment, patients should be monitored for recurrence or the appearance of the primary site, which in most cases is the lungs (75,76).

CUP PRESENTING AS METASTATIC CERVICAL ADENOPATHY

In this subgroup, patients present with high to midcervical or supraclavicular adenopathy; on histopathology, these tumors are squamous cell or PDCs. For squamous cell carcinoma, the primary site is eventually identified during follow-up in approximately 20% of patients, with the tonsil being the most common site, followed by the pyriform sinus and base of the tongue (77-79).

Adenocarcinoma is much less common and is generally from either metastatic nonpapillary thyroid carcinoma or advanced malignant disease from a distant site (gastrointestinal, lung, or breast carcinoma presenting as a metastatic supraclavicular node). Of all malignancies of the head and neck, only 5 to 10% are classified as unknown primary after imaging and panendoscopy (78). The prognosis for patients with cervical CUP overall is better than that for other CUP clinical subgroups, but even within this group, significant heterogeneity exists. Yalin et al. (80), in a retrospective study of 107 patients with cervical CUP (62% PDC, 24% squamous carcinoma, and 14% adenocarcinoma), reported a 5-year OS rate of 35.5% (80). In a recent retrospective study by Issing et al. (77), 5- and 10-year OS rates were 42.7 and 30.6%, respectively. The prognosis is significantly worse in the presence of any of the following: adenocarcinoma, level III/IV lymphadenopathy, multiple lymph nodes, and bulky disease.

Patients with supraclavicular adenopathy have a far worse prognosis than those with adenopathy in other lymph node–bearing areas. Carcinoma affecting supraclavicular lymph nodes on the right most commonly arises from occult primary tumors of the lungs and breast. When disease affects the lymph nodes on the left side, spread from intra-abdominal malignancies by way of the thoracic duct (Virchow node) is an additional possibility.

The management of patients with cervical CUP has become increasingly controversial, primarily because of the question of postoperative radiation therapy. The notion of adjuvant irradiation of all potential mucosal sites has been questioned because of the absence of any demonstrated survival benefit in randomized studies. To date, postoperative radiation therapy in cervical CUP significantly improves locoregional control, but this does not translate into improved OS (81). This being said, combined-modality therapy (surgery and radiation therapy) is better than either modality alone (81,82). Most patients with only cervical or supraclavicular involvement should have regional therapy consisting of surgery, postoperative radiation therapy, and close follow-up. Patients who undergo an excisional biopsy for diagnosis usually do not need additional surgery if no gross disease is left behind, only a single lymph node measuring less than 6 cm is involved, and no extracapsular extension is noted on pathologic review. If any of these features are present, a neck dissection is indicated. Additionally, for patients with squamous cell carcinoma, unilateral tonsillectomy ipsilateral to the presenting neck mass is commonly advocated as part of the surgical treatment, because occult tonsillar carcinomas are usually found in 18 to 39% of patients who undergo tonsillectomy (78,79). Identification of the primary site would thereby reduce morbidity by limiting the field of radiation and would improve surveillance.

In patients with N1 or N2a disease (squamous cell), it is unclear whether postoperative radiation improves local control, because studies have been contradictory (2,83). In this case, close surveillance would also be an acceptable option after surgery. All other patients should receive postoperative radiation to the bilateral neck covering all potential occult primary sites (ie, nasopharynx, oropharynx, and hypopharynx). The 3-year survival rate after radical neck dissection and/or radical neck irradiation ranges from 35 to 60%. Within this group, patients with N1 disease have a better prognosis; patients with N3 disease, regardless of the local treatment modality used (surgery, radiotherapy, or both), fail to achieve complete remission in 65% of cases.

Although the role of chemotherapy in patients with cervical CUP remains poorly defined, extrapolation of phase II/III data in head and neck cancer indicates a role in patients with advanced nodal disease (N3). A recent large meta-analysis of more than 10,000 patients in 63 trials with head and neck squamous cell carcinoma demonstrated a small but significant absolute survival benefit of 4% at 5 years for chemotherapy (84). Intensive concurrent chemoradiotherapy in unresectable squamous cell head and neck cancers with cisplatin/ 5-fluorouracil–based regimens has resulted in improved complete response rates, locoregional control, and preservation of organ function, albeit at the cost of significant toxicities. Taxanes have also been shown to be efficacious in this setting, either as single agents or in combination with cisplatin. In patients with N3 cervical CUP, there is a role for both chemotherapy and radiation therapy. Currently, insufficient data exist to know whether concurrent chemoradiation is superior to sequential chemotherapy followed by radiation in this group of patients with unresectable tumors (85).

WOMEN WITH CUP AND ISOLATED AXILLARY ADENOPATHY

Women who present with adenocarcinoma in the axillary lymph nodes compose another subset with a more favorable prognosis. These patients are often managed as women with stage II breast cancer. Isolated axillary adenopathy is an uncommon presentation of breast cancer, accounting for only 1 to 3 of every 1000 diagnosed breast cancers. Mammography and ultrasound should be performed, and biopsies should be performed on any identified lesions. If mammography findings are normal, additional imaging of the breast with MRI is indicated because of its greater ability to detect small primary breast tumors (70-95% sensitivity) (37-40). MRI has a very low false-negative rate. Of approximately 40 women reported in the literature with isolated axillary adenocarcinoma and negative breast MRI findings, only 4 were found to have breast cancer at surgery or during follow-up (39,86).

Modified radical mastectomy has been traditionally recommended in women with isolated axillary adenocarcinoma, even when physical examination and mammography studies fail to identify a primary breast cancer. A report by Ellerbroek et al. (87) documented actuarial disease-free survival rates of 71% at 5 years and 65% at 10 years (87). Survival rates were higher in patients who received systemic chemotherapy plus radiation therapy. Local control was also enhanced by irradiating the affected breast and axilla. Foroudi and Tiver (88) also reported similar results in a small retrospective study of 20 women with axillary metastases who had received local therapy to the axilla (excisional biopsy, axillary dissection, or radiation). Recurrence-free survival was significantly longer for patients who had local therapy to the breast (either radiotherapy or mastectomy) than for those who did not (182 versus 7 months; $p = .003$). Interestingly, this was true despite the fact that a greater proportion of patients in the latter group received systemic therapy with tamoxifen and/or chemotherapy (88).

The present recommended management of women with CUP of the axilla includes axillary dissection, axillary radiotherapy for those at high risk of local recurrence (eg, extracapsular invasion or more than four positive lymph nodes), and appropriate systemic therapy for breast cancer, depending on age and menopausal status. In cases where breast MRI findings are negative, neither mastectomy nor breast irradiation is recommended (89). If the breast MRI is positive or suspicious, radiation to the breast is usually recommended. The prognosis is not as favorable in men who present with axillary adenopathy only (90).

This management paradigm may change as molecular profiling complements pathology as a diagnostic tool in this subset of patients. All women with axillary adenopathy may not have occult breast cancer. Profiling for tissue of origin can help with treatment decisions especially if the immunohistochemistry does not correlate with breast cancer and ER, PR, and Her-2 status is negative.

CUP PRESENTING AS ISOLATED INGUINAL ADENOPATHY

A few patients with CUP present with inguinal adenopathy. Undifferentiated (anaplastic) carcinoma is identified in at least half of these cases (6). Some of these anaplastic "carcinomas" appear to be melanomas with no obvious primary skin lesion. The remaining patients have squamous cell carcinomas arising from the skin, genitourinary tract, anus, or pelvis. A detailed investigation for primary lesions in these areas is important, because curative therapy is available for carcinomas of the anus, vulva, vagina, and cervix even with spread to regional lymph nodes. In patients with carcinomas and PDCs confined to the groin nodes, where no primary site was identified, a superficial groin dissection should be performed with or without radiation therapy (11). Bimodality therapy with surgery and radiation may increase the risk of significant lymph edema and requires careful planning. Chemotherapy, before definitive therapy and in the context of a clinical trial, may be offered to patients with bulky locoregional adenopathy and is not an uncommon practice in the clinic.

CUP AND ISOLATED PLEURAL EFFUSIONS

Most patients with isolated pleural effusions have adenocarcinomas, which may sometimes be difficult to differentiate from mesotheliomas. Newer immunohistochemical markers (eg, calretinin, CK 5/6, and WT1) that are more sensitive in differentiating epithelioid malignant mesothelioma from pulmonary adenocarcinoma can assist in the diagnosis (91). Additional IHC markers including TTF-1, CK 7/20, and breast markers should routinely be done as first and second tier diagnostics to aid in treatment. If the effusion reaccumulates quickly, pleurodesis may be attempted to slow the rate of fluid reaccumulation or as done more often nowadays, pleural catheter with daily aspirations is preferred (this can be removed after chemotherapy response noted and the flow decreases). Chemotherapy is initiated in most patients based on their IHC profile and taxane + carboplatin versus gemcitabine + cisplatin are commonly used doublets.

CUP PRESENTING AS MALIGNANT ASCITES

Patients with malignant ascites usually belong to one of two subsets, each with a very different natural history of disease. The first group consists of patients with mucin-producing adenocarcinoma, who may present with ascitic fluid that contains signet-ring cells. These patients often have multiple peritoneal implants with the primary site most likely being the GI tract (ie, stomach, small bowel, appendix, colon, or pancreaticobiliary). Given the current armamentarium of drugs available for treatment of metastatic colon cancer and the improved survival, it is important to consider those combinations for patients with IHC suggestive of colon profile (CK20+, CK7–, and CDX-2+). The second subset is composed of women patients with primary serous papillary peritoneal carcinomatosis. This disease is often also associated with pelvic adenopathy or masses. These patients may have elevated CA 125 levels but do not have detectable ovarian cancer. Some investigators consider these patients to have true unknown primary ovarian tumors or primary serous carcinomas of the peritoneum (92,93).

Disease management should be the same as for women with ovarian carcinoma. A prolonged median survival of 13 months, with 25% of patients having a progression-free survival lasting more than 2 years, was reported for paclitaxel/carboplatin-based chemotherapy in patients with peritoneal carcinomatosis. In this study, a high overall response rate (ORR) and number of complete responses were reported for this subgroup of patients with CUP (68.4 and 20%, respectively) (94).

CUP PRESENTING AS ISOLATED BONY METASTASES

When bone metastases are detected, men should be evaluated for prostate cancer and women for breast cancer given that they may be candidates for hormonal therapy which is relatively simple compared to cytotoxic therapies. Other cancer profiles include lung, cholangiocarcinoma, renal, and rarely melanoma. Patients with a single bony metastasis may be candidates for surgery and/or radiation and then monitored. Patients with multiple sites disease and good performance status and whose tumors progress after radiation therapy should be offered a trial of chemotherapy. Many experimental agents are currently available in ongoing clinical trials. Therapy with bone-seeking radioisotopes (eg, strontium 89) may be useful in the treatment of disseminated painful bone metastases (95). Bisphosphonates are routinely used as in other malignancies, such as multiple myeloma, breast cancer, and prostate cancer and are used in CUP patients as well (89).

CUP PRESENTING AS HEPATIC METASTASES

Patients with hepatic metastases constitute 30 to 40% of people with CUPs; they compose a clinical subgroup with a relatively poor prognosis, with reported median OS between 49 days and 7 months (96,97). The most important diagnostic considerations in this class are to distinguish primary liver and biliary tumors (hepatocellular carcinoma and cholangiocarcinoma) from cancers that have metastasized to the liver and to identify patients with neoplasms of a more indolent nature (eg, neuroendocrine tumors). A careful pathologic review with IHC of liver biopsy specimens is therefore essential. The two most common histologies in primary CUP of the liver are adenocarcinoma (55%) and undifferentiated carcinoma (30%). The recommended initial therapy for unresectable disease is systemic chemotherapy. In one large retrospective study, the benefit of chemotherapy was most pronounced in patients with adenocarcinoma, significantly prolonging survival by 5 months compared with no chemotherapy ($p < .0001$) (97). Hepatic intra-arterial therapy is also an option for some patients, and surgery may be considered an option for those with resectable disease.

NEUROENDOCRINE TUMORS OF UNKNOWN PRIMARY SITE

Neuroendocrine tumors compose about 4% of all CUPs and commonly present with diffuse liver or bone metastases. Histologically, neuroendocrine tumors can be well differentiated or low grade, with features that are typical of carcinoid or islet cell tumors exhibiting a more indolent behavior. Management of these tumors should be similar to established guidelines for metastatic low-grade neuroendocrine tumors from a known primary site. In patients with limited disease, surgical resection or chemoembolization may be appropriate. If not amenable to local therapy, then a trial of chemotherapy or targeted therapy may be considered (anti–vascular endothelial growth factor [anti-VEGF] agents, mammalian target of rapamycin [mTOR] inhibitors are currently in trial). Cisplatin-based chemotherapy in well-differentiated neuroendocrine tumors has typically yielded low response rates (6).

A second group involves high-grade neuroendocrine tumors that may present as poorly differentiated carcinoma by light microscopy but have neuroendocrine features revealed by immunohistochemistry (ie, neuron-specific enolase, chromogranin A, and synaptophysin-positive) (83). These high-grade neuroendocrine tumors act aggressively and are treated like small cell lung carcinoma with etoposide + platinum or irinotecan + platinum combinations, with high reported response rates (98,99). A combination of paclitaxel, carboplatin, and oral etoposide has also been reported as an active regimen for patients with high-grade neuroendocrine tumors of unknown primary site (6,100).

CUP AND EXTRAGONADAL GERM CELL SYNDROME

As a group, patients who have undifferentiated carcinoma or PDC are younger than 50 years and present with rapidly growing midline tumors involving the lymph nodes, mediastinum, or retroperitoneum; their tumors have been found to be very responsive to chemotherapy, particularly to platinum-containing regimens. It is believed that these patients have poorly differentiated

extragonadal germ cell tumors. They have response rates to chemotherapy of 35 to 50%, and those who achieve a complete response often enjoy a durable remission. In a prospective study by Hainsworth and colleagues (99) of 220 patients with PDC or PDAC treated between 1978 and 1989 with cisplatin-based chemotherapy regimens, approximately half of the patients had a predominant tumor location in the mediastinum, retroperitoneum, or peripheral lymph nodes. The ORR was 63%, with 26% complete responses and an actuarial 10-year disease-free survival rate of 16%.

However, this was not found to be true by Lenzi and colleagues (4), who retrospectively reviewed the clinical outcomes of 337 patients with PDC/PDAC. No prolonged survival was observed in this cohort of patients, and no significant survival advantage resulted from cisplatin-based chemotherapy. Moreover, elevated serum levels of alpha-fetoprotein or beta-human chorionic gonadotropin, contrary to other reports in the literature, were not found to be predictive of an improved median OS. This discrepancy may have resulted from several confounding factors.

First, older studies of extragonadal germ cell syndrome included patients with PDCs who in actuality did not have CUP but had other highly treatable malignancies (4). In a study by Hainsworth et al. (99), of the 36 long-term survivors, 20% were subsequently found to have either lymphoma (5), testicular cancer (1), or leiomyosarcoma (1). Conversely, in the study by Lenzi, patients in whom the primary site was identified were excluded from the analysis. Most of these patients were found to have highly treatable malignancies, such as lymphoma (6%), breast cancer (8%), ovarian cancer (3%), germ cell tumors (2%), and prostate cancer (1%). Exclusion of these patients would significantly reduce response and median survival rates.

Second, even among patients with PDC/PDAC of unknown primary, significant heterogeneity exists. In the study by Lenzi, CART analysis on 337 patients revealed different groups with widely discrepant survival times. The group with the longest median OS (40 months) included patients with PDC, lymph node involvement, and only one or two metastatic sites. By contrast, patients with non–lymph node metastases had a very poor prognosis, with a median OS of only 7 months (4).

CUP AND SINGLE SITES DISCOVERED INCIDENTALLY ON RESECTION

CUPs are notorious for unusual, isolated presentations. Such lesions may appear on the skin, in single isolated lymph nodes removed during surgery for benign unrelated conditions, and at other, even more unusual sites. Patients should be examined for primary tumors and other sites of metastasis, as described earlier. If no primary tumor and no additional sites of metastasis are found, complete removal of the lesion must be ensured; this often requires additional excision with wider margins (if skin or subcutaneous). The patient may then be monitored without therapy and in selected cases are candidates for radiation. Many such patients may enjoy prolonged survival. Patients with isolated skin lesions may have an undifferentiated primary integumentary tumor with a potential for cure after adequate local surgical treatment.

CUP AND DISSEMINATED VISCERAL DISEASE

Developing a strategy to care for patients with CUP and disseminated visceral metastases has proven exceedingly difficult. As noted previously, some subsets of patients in this category have disease that is responsive to therapy (eg, those with features of germ cell tumors and their equivalents, women with papillary abdominal carcinomatosis, and patients with neuroendocrine tumors). Such patients should be treated aggressively with platinum-based chemotherapy regimens and may have ORRs as high as 50% and complete response rates ranging from 20 to 35% (101,102).

■ CHEMOTHERAPEUTIC STRATEGIES FOR CUP

Data from chemotherapy trials enrolling patients with CUPs have historically been difficult to interpret. Many early studies were done before the era of controlled clinical trials, and the methods used in interpreting the results of these studies have been questioned. Additionally, combination regimens using newer chemotherapeutic agents have consistently demonstrated greater benefit than did older single-agent therapies. Several difficulties arise when survival and response rates reported in different chemotherapy trials are compared. For example, histologic criteria for patient selection often varied from study to study. Moreover, in older studies, immunohistochemical methods were not used to evaluate pathologic specimens. Despite these difficulties, no study has firmly established any chemotherapy regimen as the "gold standard" in CUP. The median survival in most studies, regardless of regimen, has ranged between 5 and 13 months, with response rates of

less than 30% and without a significant improvement in survival (Table 42-4).

Nevertheless, patients with certain clinical subtypes (eg, peritoneal carcinomatosis and lymph node–predominant disease) do benefit from chemotherapy. Historically, cisplatin-based combination chemotherapy regimens were frequently used to treat patients with CUP. Response rates in the literature range from 12 to 26% and median survival from 5 to 7 months. Combining paclitaxel with carboplatin has modestly improved both survival and response rates. In patients with widespread metastases and poor performance status, however, systemic chemotherapy is unlikely to be beneficial, and only supportive therapy is usually indicated.

In a phase II study by Hainsworth and colleagues (100), patients with CUP (N = 55) received paclitaxel (200 mg/m^2 day 1), carboplatin (AUC = 6 day 1), and oral etoposide (50 mg alternating with 100 mg days 1-10) every 21 days. Most were previously untreated, with only four having received prior chemotherapy. Most patients had moderately to well-differentiated adenocarcinoma (55%) or PDC/PDAC (38%), with squamous (2%) and neuroendocrine (5%) histologies being less prevalent. The dominant sites of disease were lymph nodes (25%), liver (16%), and lungs (16%). Approximately 24% of patients in the study had multiple sites of disease, with 42% of patients having more than two metastatic sites. Response rates were equivalent in all histologic subgroups, with a reported ORR of 47% and a median OS of 13.4 months. This regimen was well tolerated, with myelosuppression being the most common grade 3/4 toxicity. No treatment-related deaths were reported.

Briasoulis and colleagues (94) found equivalent response rates and median OS in CUP with carboplatin (AUC = 6) and paclitaxel (200 mg/m^2) without oral etoposide. In this phase II trial, patients (N = 77) were given a maximum of eight cycles of chemotherapy. Additionally, granulocyte colony–stimulating factor was administered on days 5 to 12. The proportions of differing histologic subtypes were comparable to those in the Hainsworth study: adenocarcinoma (61%), undifferentiated (35%), and squamous (4%). Three distinct clinical subsets were present in this study: peritoneal carcinomatosis (25%, mostly women); visceral and/or bony metastases (43%); and predominant nodal and/or pleural disease (30%). The reported ORR, median response duration, and median OS were 38.7%, 6 months, and 13 months, respectively. Although response rates were equivalent for adenocarcinoma and undifferentiated carcinoma, significant differences were seen among the three clinical subsets: liver/bone or disseminated

TABLE 42-4 | **SELECTED PHASE II STUDIES IN CARCINOMA OF UNKNOWN PRIMARY**

						OVERALL SURVIVAL		
Reference	*N*	*Chemotherapy Regimen*	*Two or More Metastatic Sites (%)*	*ORR (%)*	*Median TTP (Months)*	*Median (Months)*	*1 year (%)*	*2 years (%)*
Assersohn et al. (108)	45	5-FU versus	44	11.6	4.1	6.6	28	NR
	43	5-FU+ Mi		20	3.6	4.7	21	NR
Culine et al. (109)	82	AC→EP, alt q14d + GCSF	68	39	NR	10		
McDonald et al. (110)	31	Mi/P/CI 5-FU	52	27	3.4	7.7	28	
Greco et al. (111)	120	Gem/Cb/Pac	65	25	NR	9	42	23
Saghatchian et al. (112)	33	PDC/PDAC: EP × 2→BI	57	40	8.1	9.4	NR	28
	18	Adeno: P/CI-5FU/ IFNα	44	44	8.6	16.1	NR	39
Hainsworth et al. (107)	39	Gem	NR	33	5	NR		
Dowell et al. (113)	17	Pac + 5FU/ leucovorin versus	59	19	NR	8.4		
	17	CbE	65	19		6.5		
Briasoulis et al. (94)	77	Cb + Pac	22% with 3 or more	38.7	6	13		
Greco et al. (103)	23	DP versus	73	26	NR	8	42	
	40	DCb	68	22		8	29	
Culine et al. (104)	20	HDCT + Auto SCT versus	80	42	NR	11		
	40	AC alt with EP	75	39		8		
Falkson et al. (114)	43	Mi/Epi/P versus	53	50	4.5*	9.4*		
	41	Mi	44	17	2.0	5.4		
Warner et al. (115)	33	Cb + E (PO)	91	23	NR	5.6	NR	
Hainsworth et al. (100)	55	Pac/Cb/E (PO)	67	47	NR	13.4	58	NR
Hainsworth et al. (99)	220	BEvP ± Doxo; after 1985: BEP	74	63	NR			10-year survival: 16%
Van der Gaast et al. (116)	34	BEP × 4→EP × 2	53	53	NR	NR		
Eagen et al. (117)	28	MiA→CAM versus	NR	14	NR	5.5	19	8
	27	MiAP→CAM		26		4.6	12	0

5FU, 5-flurouracil; A, doxorubicin; Adeno, adenocarcinoma; alt, alternating; AutoSCT, autologous stem cell transplant; B, bleomycin; C, cyclophosphamide; Cb, carboplatin; CI, continuous infusion; D, docetaxel; Doxo, doxorubicin; E, etoposide; Epi, epirubicin; Gem, gemcitabine; GCSF, Graulocyte colony stimulating factor; HDCT, high-dose chemotherapy; I, ifosfamide; IFN, interferon; M, methotrexate; Mi, mitomycin; Neuro, neuroendocrine; NR, not reported; P, cisplatin; Pac, paclitaxel; PDC/PDAC, poorly differentiated carcinoma/adenocarcinoma; Undif, undifferentiated malignancy; v, vinblastine.
*Statistically significant difference $p = .05$.

metastases (ORR, 15.1%; median OS, 10 months), nodal/pleural disease (ORR, 47.8%; median OS, 13 months), and peritoneal (ORR, 68.4% [75% for women]; median OS, 15 months), $p = .01$. Three patients with nodal-predominant disease had durable responses lasting longer than 2 years. Grade 3/4 neutropenia was only 4%, with two reported septic deaths.

The results of docetaxel in combination with carboplatin in one small phase II study appear to be inferior to those of paclitaxel/carboplatin in the above-mentioned trials. The ORR was 22%, the median OS was 8 months, and the 1-year OS rate was 29%. Differences in sites of disease and histology among these three studies may account for the discrepancy. Severe grade 3/4 myelosuppression was more frequent with docetaxel (50%) than with paclitaxel, with two reported septic deaths (103).

High-dose chemotherapy followed by autologous stem cell transplant has not been found to play any role in CUP. In a phase II study, patients (N = 60) were randomized to receive either high-dose chemotherapy followed by autologous stem cell rescue or conventional chemotherapy with doxorubicin at 50 mg/m^2 and cyclophosphamide at 1000 mg/m^2 alternating with etoposide at 300 mg/m^2 and cisplatin at 100 mg/m^2 on the basis of clinical features. Patients in the high-dose arm (N = 12) were younger than 61 years, with good performance status, PDAC or PDC, and no evidence of brain or bone marrow involvement. ORRs (42 versus 39%) and median OS (11 versus 8 months) in the two arms were equivalent (104).

Patients with undifferentiated or PDCs not fitting into the extragonadal germ cell or neuroendocrine clinical subgroups have traditionally been given a trial of a cisplatin-based regimen (47). Patients with squamous cell carcinomas who require chemotherapy are also often treated effectively using a cisplatin-based regimen. Investigators have discussed the merits of a combination of 5-fluorouracil and cisplatin in squamous cell carcinomas of the head and neck in addition to taxane-based chemotherapy (105,106).

The role of salvage chemotherapy in CUP is poorly defined. Gemcitabine is the only agent that has been shown to have modest activity as second-line therapy in patients with previously treated CUP. In a phase II study by Hainsworth and colleagues (107), gemcitabine was administered weekly at 1000 mg/m^2 (on days 1, 8, and 15 of a 28-day cycle). All patients (N = 39) received two cycles and were then evaluated for response. Chemotherapy was continued for a maximum of six cycles for either an objective response or stable disease. Approximately 90% of patients had failed a prior regimen containing platinum and a taxane. Most patients had either adenocarcinoma (59%) or PDC/PDAC (31%). Median time to progression was 5 months. Gemcitabine was well tolerated, with 92% of patients receiving two or more cycles. The most common grades 3 to 4 toxicities were fatigue/weakness and mucositis/esophagitis.

Hainsworth et al. reported on a combination-targeted therapy trial of bevacizumab and erlotinib in 51 patients; 25% of whom were chemotherapy naïve with advanced bone or liver metastases and 75% had been treated with one or two chemotherapy regimens. Responses were noted in 4 patients (8%), and 30 patients (59%) experienced stable disease or a minor response. The median overall survival duration was 8.9 months, with 42% of patients alive at 1 year.

These combination therapy trials have been a significant contribution in the post 5-flurouracil and cisplatin era of second-generation chemotherapeutic agents. They have certainly served their function in allowing the access to several broad-spectrum chemotherapies in CUP patients and helped us understand the responses to these therapies. Although evaluation of empiric regimens was the preferred approach in the past, with the emergence of modern molecular diagnostic trials that help define CUP subtypes, our focus needs to shift from empiric combinations to more tailored regimens. Further, as therapies for known cancers improve and become more selective based on evolving predictive markers, the newer therapeutic approaches should be evaluated in the appropriate CUP subtypes as well.

SUMMARY AND FUTURE TRENDS

All CUP patients should undergo a directed diagnostic evaluation for the primary tumor and a detailed pathologic evaluation of the metastatic specimen. A subset of patients defined by clinicopathologic criteria and considered to have favorable prognosis benefit significantly from selective and or aggressive treatments. For most patients who present with advanced disseminated CUP, the prognosis remains poor, and no unique combination therapy of established efficacy is available. We have moved away from the paradigm of one treatment fits all to a more focused approach that integrates clinical presentation, pathologic evaluation, and the evolving diagnostic tool of molecular profiling. Our current focus is to study the impact of molecular profiling studies on CUP patients' outcomes. Although there are some obstacles to progress including tumor heterogeneity, challenging study designs including validation trials for profiling assays and adequate tissue availability for research studies, it is important to pursue an individualized approach to CUP patients.

ACKNOWLEDGMENT

The authors would like to thank Carolyn Morrison for her assistance with editing this chapter.

References

1. van de Wouw AJ, Janssen-Heijnen ML, Coebergh JW, et al. Epidemiology of unknown primary tumours; incidence and population-based survival of 1285 patients in Southeast Netherlands, 1984-1992. *Eur J Cancer* 2002;38(3):409-413.

2. Hainsworth JD, Greco FA. Treatment of patients with cancer of an unknown primary site. *N Engl J Med* 1993;329(4): 257-263.

3. Greco FA, Burris HA, III, Erland JB, et al. Carcinoma of unknown primary site. *Cancer* 2000;89(12):2655-2660.

4. Lenzi R, Hess KR, Abbruzzese MC, et al. Poorly differentiated carcinoma and poorly differentiated adenocarcinoma of unknown origin: Favorable subsets of patients with unknown-primary carcinoma? *J Clin Oncol* 1997;15(5):2056-2066.

5. Hess KR, Abbruzzese MC, Lenzi R, et al. Classification and regression tree analysis of 1000 consecutive patients with unknown primary carcinoma. *Clin Cancer Res* 1999;5(11): 3403-3410.

6. Greco FA, Hainsworth JD. Cancer of unknown primary site. In: DeVita VT (ed): *Cancer: Principles and Practice of Oncology.* Philadelphia: Lippincott, Williams & Wilkins; 2001:2537-2560.

7. Raber MN, Abbruzzese JL, Frost P. Unknown primary tumors. *Curr Opin Oncol* 1992;4(1):3-9.

8. Jemal A, Siegel R, Ward E, et al. Cancer statistics, 2009. *CA Cancer J Clin* 2009;59:225-249.

9. Saad ED, Abbruzzese JL. Prognostic stratification in CUP: A role for assessing the value of conventional-dose and high-dose chemotherapy for unknown primary carcinoma. *Crit Rev Oncol Hematol* 2002;41(2):205-211.

10. Abbruzzese JL, Abbruzzese MC, Hess KR, et al. Unknown primary carcinoma: Natural history and prognostic factors in 657 consecutive patients. *J Clin Oncol* 1994;12(6):1272-1280.

11. Casciato DA, Tabbarah HJ. Metastases of unknown origin. In: Haskell CM (ed): *Cancer Treatment.* Philadelphia: Saunders; 1990:1128.

12. Nystrom JS, Weiner JM, Heffelfinger-Juttner J, et al. Metastatic and histologic presentations in unknown primary cancer. *Semin Oncol* 1977;4(1):53-58.

13. Abbruzzese JL, Abbruzzese MC, Lenzi R, et al. Analysis of a diagnostic strategy for patients with suspected tumors of unknown origin. *J Clin Oncol* 1995;13(8):2094-2103.

14. Daugaard G. Unknown primary tumours. *Cancer Treat Rev* 1994;20(2):119-147.

15. Bar-Eli M, Abbruzzese JL, Lee-Jackson D, et al. *p53* gene mutation spectrum in human unknown primary tumors. *Anticancer Res* 1993;13(5A):1619-1623.

16. Bell CW, Pathak S, Frost P. Unknown primary tumors: Establishment of cell lines, identification of chromosomal abnormalities, and implications for a second type of tumor progression. *Cancer Res* 1989;49(15):4311-4315.

17. van de Wouw AJ, Jansen RL, Speel EJ, et al. The unknown biology of the unknown primary tumour: A literature review. *Ann Oncol* 2003;14(2):191-196.

18. Naresh KN. Do metastatic tumours from an unknown primary reflect angiogenic incompetence of the tumour at the primary site? A hypothesis. *Med Hypoth* 2002;59(3):357-360.

19. Pantou D, Tsarouha H, Papadopoulou A, et al. Cytogenetic profile of unknown primary tumors: Clues for their pathogenesis and clinical management. *Neoplasia* 2003;5(1):23-31.

20. Atkin NB. Chromosome 1 aberrations in cancer. *Cancer Genet Cytogenet* 1986;21(4):279-285.

21. Motzer RJ, Rodriguez E, Reuter VE, et al. Molecular and cytogenetic studies in the diagnosis of patients with poorly differentiated carcinomas of unknown primary site. *J Clin Oncol* 1995;13(1):274-282.

22. Motzer RJ, Rodriguez E, Reuter VE, et al. Genetic analysis as an aid in diagnosis for patients with midline carcinomas of uncertain histologies. *J Natl Cancer Inst* 1991;83(5): 341-346.

23. Pavlidis N, Briassoulis E, Bai M, et al. The expression of *cmyc, ras,* and c-erbB-2 in patients with carcinoma of unknown primary. *Proc Am Soc Clin Oncol* 1994;13:(abstr 1374).

24. Soong R, Robbins PD, Dix BR, et al. Concordance between p53 protein overexpression and gene mutation in a large series of common human carcinomas. *Hum Pathol* 1996; 27(10): 1050-1055.

25. Hainsworth JD, Lennington WJ, Greco FA. Overexpression of Her-2 in patients with poorly differentiated carcinoma or poorly differentiated adenocarcinoma of unknown primary site. *J Clin Oncol* 2000;18(3):632-635.

26. Culine S, Gazagne L, Ychou M, et al. Carcinoma of unknown primary site. Apropos of 100 patients treated at the Montpellier regional center of cancer prevention. *Rev Med Interne* 1998;19(10):713-719.

27. Mayordomo JI, Guerra JM, Guijarro C, et al. Neoplasms of unknown primary site: A clinicopathological study of autopsied patients. *Tumori* 1993;79(5):321-324.

28. Le Chevalier T, Cvitkovic E, Caille P, et al. Early metastatic cancer of unknown primary origin at presentation. A clinical study of 302 consecutive autopsied patients. *Arch Intern Med* 1988;148(9):2035-2039.

29. Stewart JF, Tattersall MH, Woods RL, et al. Unknown primary adenocarcinoma: Incidence of overinvestigation and natural history. *Br Med J* 1979;1(6177):1530-1533.

30. Schapira DV, Jaret AR. Cost of diagnosis and survival of patients with unknown primary cancer. *Proc Am Soc Clin Oncol* 1994;13:(abstr 481).

31. Horning SJ, Carrier EK, Rouse RV, et al. Lymphomas presenting as histologically unclassified neoplasms: Characteristics and response to treatment. *J Clin Oncol* 1989;7(9): 1281-1287.

32. Milovic M, Popov I, Jelic S. Tumor markers in metastatic disease from cancer of unknown primary origin. *Med Sci Monit* 2002;8(2):MT25-MT30.

33. Bates SE. Clinical applications of serum tumor markers. *Ann Intern Med* 1991;115(8):623-638.

34. Abbruzzese JL, Raber MN, Frost P. The role of CA-125 in patients with unknown primary tumors. *Proc Am Soc Clin Oncol* 1991;10:(abstr 39).

35. McMillan JH, Levine E, Stephens RH. Computed tomography in the evaluation of metastatic adenocarcinoma from an unknown primary site. A retrospective study. *Radiology* 1982; 143(1):143-146.

36. Karsell PR, Sheedy PF, O'Connell MJ. Computed tomography in search of cancer of unknown origin. *JAMA* 1982; 248(3):340-343.

37. Bedrosian I, Mick R, Orel SG, et al. Changes in the surgical management of patients with breast carcinoma based on preoperative magnetic resonance imaging. *Cancer* 2003;98(3): 468-473.

38. Podo F, Sardanelli F, Canese R, et al. The Italian multi-centre project on evaluation of MRI and other imaging modalities in early detection of breast cancer in subjects at high genetic risk. *J Exp Clin Cancer Res* 2002;21(Suppl 3): 115-124.

39. Schelfout K, Kersschot E, Van Goethem M, et al. Breast MR imaging in a patient with unilateral axillary lymphadenopathy and unknown primary malignancy. *Eur Radiol* 2003;13(9): 2128-2132.

40. Henry-Tillman RS, Harms SE, Westbrook KC, et al. Role of breast magnetic resonance imaging in determining breast as a source of unknown metastatic lymphadenopathy. *Am J Surg* 1999;178(6):496-500.

41. Schorn C, Fischer U, Luftner-Nagel S, et al. MRI of the breast in patients with metastatic disease of unknown primary. *Eur Radiol* 1999;9(3):470-473.

42. Koch WM, Bhatti N, Williams MF, et al. Oncologic rationale for bilateral tonsillectomy in head and neck squamous cell carcinoma of unknown primary source. *Otolaryngol Head Neck Surg* 2001;124:331-333.

43. Lassen U, Daugaard G, Eigtved A, et al. 18F-FDG whole body positron emission tomography (PET) in patients with unknown primary tumours (UPT). *Eur J Cancer* 1999;35(7): 1076-1082.

44. Regelink G, Brouwer J, de Bree R, et al. Detection of unknown primary tumours and distant metastases in patients with cervical metastases: Value of FDG-PET versus conventional modalities. *Eur J Nucl Med Mol Imaging* 2002;29: 1024-1030.

45. Rusthoven KE, Koshy M, Paulino AC. The role of fluorodeoxyglucose positron emission tomography in cervical lymph node metastases from an unknown primary tumor. *Cancer* 2004;101:2641-2649.

46. Waltonen JD, Ozer E, Hall NC, et al. Metastatic carcinoma of the neck of unknown primary origin. *Arch Otolaryngol Head Neck Surg* 2009;135:1024-1029.

47. Hainsworth JD, Greco FA. Poorly differentiated carcinoma and poorly differentiated adenocarcinoma of unknown primary tumor site. *Semin Oncol* 1993;20(3):279-286.

48. Kolesnikov-Gauthier H, Levy E, Merlet P, et al. FDG PET in patients with cancer of an unknown primary. *Nucl Med Commun* 2005;26:1059-1066.

49. Pelosi E, Pennone M, Deandreis D, et al. Role of whole body positron emission tomography/computed tomography scan with 18F-fluorodeoxyglucose in patients with biopsy proven tumor metastases from unknown primary site. *Q J Nucl Med Mol Imaging* 2006;50:15-22.

50. Nanni C, Rubello D, Castellucci P, et al. Role of 18F-FDG PET-CT imaging for the detection of an unknown primary tumour: Preliminary results in 21 patients. *Eur J Nucl Med Mol Imaging* 2005;32:589-592.

51. Mantaka P, Baum RP, Hertel A, et al. PET with 2-[F-18]-fluoro-2-deoxy-D-glucose (FDG) in patients with cancer of unknown primary (CUP): Influence on patients' diagnostic and therapeutic management. *Cancer Biother Radiopharm* 2003;18(1):47-58.

52. Johansen J, Eigtved A, Buchwald C, et al. Implication of 18F-fluoro-2-deoxy-D-glucose positron emission tomography on management of carcinoma of unknown primary in the head and neck: A Danish cohort study. *Laryngoscope* 2002; 112(11):2009-2014.

53. Delgado-Bolton RC, Fernandez-Perez C, Gonzalez-Mate A, et al. Meta-analysis of the performance of 18F-FDG PET in primary tumor detection in unknown primary tumors. *J Nucl Med* 2003; 44(8):1301-1314.

54. Alberini JL, Belhocine T, Hustinx R, et al. Whole-body positron emission tomography using fluorodeoxyglucose in patients with metastases of unknown primary tumours (CUP syndrome). *Nucl Med Commun* 2003;24(10):1081-1086.

55. Lenzi R, Kim EE, Raber MN, et al. Detection of primary breast cancer presenting as metastatic carcinoma of unknown primary origin by ^{111}In-pentetreotide scan. *Ann Oncol* 1998; 9(2):213-216.

56. Warnke RA, Gatter KC, Falini B, et al. Diagnosis of human lymphoma with monoclonal antileukocyte antibodies. *N Engl J Med* 1983;309(21):1275-1281.

57. Allhoff EP, Proppe KH, Chapman CM, et al. Evaluation of prostate specific acid phosphatase and prostate specific antigen in identification of prostatic cancer. *J Urol* 1983;129(2): 315-318.

58. Tan D, Li Q, Deeb G, et al. Thyroid transcription factor-1 expression prevalence and its clinical implications in non-small cell lung cancer: A high-throughput tissue microarray and immunohistochemistry study. *Hum Pathol* 2003;34(6): 597-604.

59. Kaufmann O, Dietel M. Thyroid transcription factor-1 is the superior immunohistochemical marker for pulmonary adenocarcinomas and large cell carcinomas compared to surfactant proteins A and B. *Histopathology* 2000;36(1): 8-16.

60. Fujita J, Ohtsuki Y, Bandoh S, et al. Expression of thyroid transcription factor-1 in 16 human lung cancer cell lines. *Lung Cancer* 2003;39(1):31-36.

61. Wu M, Wang B, Gil J, et al. p63 and TTF-1 immunostaining. A useful marker panel for distinguishing small cell carcinoma of lung from poorly differentiated squamous cell carcinoma of lung. *Am J Clin Pathol* 2003;119(5): 696-702.

62. Ng WK, Chow JC, Ng PK. Thyroid transcription factor-1 is highly sensitive and specific in differentiating metastatic pulmonary from extrapulmonary adenocarcinoma in effusion fluid cytology specimens. *Cancer* 2002;96(1): 43-48.

63. Chhieng DC, Cangiarella JF, Zakowski MF, et al. Use of thyroid transcription factor 1, PE-10, and cytokeratins 7 and 20 in discriminating between primary lung carcinomas and meta-static lesions in fine-needle aspiration biopsy specimens. *Cancer* 2001;93(5):330-336.

64. Reis-Filho JS, Carrilho C, Valenti C, et al. Is TTF1 a good immunohistochemical marker to distinguish primary from metastatic lung adenocarcinomas? *Pathol Res Pract* 2000; 196(12):835-840.

65. Rubin BP, Skarin AT, Pisick E, et al. Use of cytokeratins 7 and 20 in determining the origin of metastatic carcinoma of unknown primary, with special emphasis on lung cancer. *Eur J Cancer Prev* 2001;10(1):77-82.

66. Dennis JL, Vass JK, Wit EC, et al. Identification from public data of molecular markers of adenocarcinoma characteristic of the site of origin. *Cancer Res* 2002;62(21): 5999-6005.

67. Ramaswamy S, Tamayo P, Rifkin R, et al. Multiclass cancer diagnosis using tumor gene expression signatures. *Proc Natl Acad Sci U S A* 2001;98:15149-15154.

68. Su AI, Welsh JB, Sapinoso LM, et al. Molecular classification of human carcinomas by use of gene expression signatures. *Cancer Res* 2001;61:7388-7393.

69. Talantov D, Baden J, Jatkoe T, et al. A quantitative reverse transcriptase-polymerase chain reaction assay to identify metastatic carcinoma tissue of origin. *J Mol Diagn* 2006;8: 320-329.

70. Tothill RW, Kowalczyk A, Rischin D, et al. An expression-based site of origin diagnostic method designed for clinical application to cancer of unknown origin. *Cancer Res* 2005; 65,4031-4040.

71. Varadhachary GR, Talantov D, Raber MN, et al. Molecular profiling of carcinoma of unknown primary and correlation with clinical evaluation. *J Clin Oncol* 2008b;26: 4442-4448.

72. Horlings HM, van Laar RK, Kerst JM, et al. Gene expression profiling to identify the histogenetic origin of metastatic adenocarcinomas of unknown primary. *J Clin Oncol* 2008;26: 4435-4441.

73. Monzon FA, Lyons-Weiler M, Buturovic LJ, et al. Multicenter validation of a 1,550-gene expression profile for identification of tumor tissue of origin. *J Clin Oncol* 2009;27(15): 2503-2508.

74. Soffietti R, Ruda R, Mutani R. Management of brain metastases. *J Neurol* 2002;249(10):1357-1369.

75. Ruda R, Borgognone M, Benech F, et al. Brain metastases from unknown primary tumour: A prospective study. *J Neurol* 2001;248(5):394-398.

76. Srodon M, Westra WH. Immunohistochemical staining for thyroid transcription factor-1: A helpful aid in discerning primary site of tumor origin in patients with brain metastases. *Hum Pathol* 2002;33(6):642-645.

77. Issing WJ, Taleban B, Tauber S. Diagnosis and management of carcinoma of unknown primary in the head and neck. *Eur Arch Otorhinolaryngol* 2003;260:436-443.

78. Randall DA, Johnstone PA, Foss RD, et al. Tonsillectomy in diagnosis of the unknown primary tumor of the head and neck. *Otolaryngol Head Neck Surg* 2000;122(1):52-55.

79. Kazak I, Haisch A, Jovanovic S. Bilateral synchronous tonsillar carcinoma in cervical cancer of unknown primary site (CUPS). *Eur Arch Otorhinolaryngol* 2003;260:436-443.

80. Yalin Y, Pingzhang T, Smith GI, et al. Management and outcome of cervical lymph node metastases of unknown primary sites: A retrospective study. *Br J Oral Maxillofac Surg* 2002; 40(6):484-487.

81. Iganej S, Kagan R, Anderson P, et al. Metastatic squamous cell carcinoma of the neck from an unknown primary: Management options and patterns of relapse. *Head Neck* 2002; 24(3):236-246.

82. Zuur CL, van Velthuysen ML, Schornagel JH, et al. Diagnosis and treatment of isolated neck metastases of adenocarcinomas. *Eur J Surg Oncol* 2002;28(2):147-152.

83. Garrow GC, Greco FA, Hainsworth JD. Poorly differentiated neuroendocrine carcinoma of unknown primary tumor site. *Semin Oncol* 1993;20(3):287-291.

84. Pignon JP, Bourhis J, Domenge C, et al. Chemotherapy added to locoregional treatment for head and neck squamous-cell carcinoma: Three meta-analyses of updated individual data. MACH-NC Collaborative Group. Meta-Analysis of Chemotherapy on Head and Neck Cancer. *Lancet* 2000; 355(9208):949-955.

85. Posner MR, Glisson B, Frenette G, et al. Multicenter phase I–II trial of docetaxel, cisplatin, and fluorouracil induction chemotherapy for patients with locally advanced squamous cell cancer of the head and neck. *J Clin Oncol* 2001;19(4):1096-1104.

86. Olson JA, Jr., Morris EA, Van Zee KJ, et al. Magnetic resonance imaging facilitates breast conservation for occult breast cancer. *Ann Surg Oncol* 2000;7(6):411-415.

87. Ellerbroek N, Holmes F, Singletary E, et al. Treatment of patients with isolated axillary nodal metastases from an occult primary carcinoma consistent with breast origin. *Cancer* 1990;66(7):1461-1467.

88. Foroudi F, Tiver KW. Occult breast carcinoma presenting as axillary metastases. *Int J Radiat Oncol Biol Phys* 2000;47(1): 143-147.

89. Bugat R, Bataillard A, Lesimple T, et al. Standards, options and recommendations for the management of patient with carcinoma of unknown primary site. *Bull Cancer* 2002;89(10): 869-875.

90. Jackson B, Scott-Conner C, Moulder J. Axillary metastasis from occult breast carcinoma: Diagnosis and management. *Am Surg* 1995;61(5):431-434.

91. Ordonez NG. The immunohistochemical diagnosis of mesothelioma: A comparative study of epithelioid mesothelioma and lung adenocarcinoma. *Am J Surg Pathol* 2003;27(8): 1031-1051.

92. Gershenson DM, Silva EG. *Serous* ovarian tumors of low malignant potential with peritoneal implants. *Cancer* 1990; 65(3):578-585.

93. Strnad CM, Grosh WW, Baxter J, et al. Peritoneal carcinomatosis of unknown primary site in women. A distinctive subset of adenocarcinoma. *Ann Intern Med* 1989;111(3):213-217.

94. Briasoulis E, Kalofonos H, Bafaloukos D, et al. Carboplatin plus paclitaxel in unknown primary carcinoma: A phase II Hellenic Cooperative Oncology Group Study. *J Clin Oncol* 2000;18(17):3101-3107.

95. Porter AT, McEwan AJ, Powe JE, et al. Results of a randomized phase-III trial to evaluate the efficacy of strontium-89 adjuvant to local field external beam irradiation in the management of endocrine resistant metastatic prostate cancer. *Int J Radiat Oncol Biol Phys* 1993;25(5):805-813.

96. Hogan BA, Thornton FJ, Brannigan M, et al. Hepatic metastases from an unknown primary neoplasm (UPN): Survival, prognostic indicators and value of extensive investigations. *Clin Radiol* 2002;57(12):1073-1077.

97. Ayoub JP, Hess KR, Abbruzzese MC, et al. Unknown primary tumors metastatic to liver. *J Clin Oncol* 1998;16(6): 2105-2112.

98. Greco FA, Johnson DH, Hainsworth JD. Etoposide/cisplatin-based chemotherapy for patients with metastatic poorly differentiated carcinoma of unknown primary site. *Semin Oncol* 1992;19(6 Suppl 13):14-18.

99. Hainsworth JD, Johnson DH, Greco FA. Cisplatin-based combination chemotherapy in the treatment of poorly differentiated carcinoma and poorly differentiated adenocarcinoma of unknown primary site: Results of a 12-year experience. *J Clin Oncol* 1992;10(6):912-922.

100. Hainsworth JD, Erland JB, Kalman LA, et al. Carcinoma of unknown primary site: Treatment with 1-hour paclitaxel, carboplatin, and extended-schedule etoposide. *J Clin Oncol* 1997; 15(6):2385-2393.

101. Greco FA, Vaughn WK, Hainsworth JD. Advanced poorly differentiated carcinoma of unknown primary site: Recognition of a treatable syndrome. *Ann Intern Med* 1986;104(4): 547-553.

102. Richardson RL, Schoumacher RA, Fer MF, et al. The unrecognized extragonadal germ cell cancer syndrome. *Ann Intern Med* 1981;94(2):181-186.

103. Greco FA, Erland JB, Morrissey LH, et al. Carcinoma of unknown primary site: Phase II trials with docetaxel plus cisplatin or carboplatin. *Ann Oncol* 2000;11(2):211-215.

104. Culine S, Fabbro M, Ychou M, et al. Chemotherapy in carcinomas of unknown primary site: A high-dose intensity policy. *Ann Oncol* 1999;10(5):569-575.

105. Jeremic B, Zivic DJ, Matovic M, et al. Cisplatin and 5-fluorouracil as induction chemotherapy followed by radiation therapy in metastatic squamous cell carcinoma of an unknown primary tumor localized to the neck. A phase II study. *J Chemother* 1993;5(4):262-265.

106. Glisson BS, Murphy BA, Frenette G, et al. Phase II trial of docetaxel and cisplatin combination chemotherapy in patients with squamous cell carcinoma of the head and neck. *J Clin Oncol* 2002;20(6):1593-1599.

107. Hainsworth JD, Burris HA III, Calvert SW, et al. Gemcitabine in the second-line therapy of patients with carcinoma of unknown primary site: A phase II trial of the Minnie Pearl Cancer Research Network. *Cancer Invest* 2001;19(4):335-339.

108. Assersohn L, Norman AR, Cunningham D, et al. A randomised study of protracted venous infusion of 5-fluorouracil (5-FU) with or without bolus mitomycin C (MMC) in patients with carcinoma of unknown primary. *Eur J Cancer* 2003;39(8): 1121-1128.

109. Culine S, Fabbro M, Ychou M, et al. Alternative bimonthly cycles of doxorubicin, cyclophosphamide, and etoposide, cisplatin with hematopoietic growth factor support in patients with carcinoma of unknown primary site. *Cancer* 2002;94(3): 840-846.

110. McDonald AG, Nicolson MC, Samuel LM, et al. A phase II study of mitomycin C, cisplatin and continuous infusion 5-fluorouracil (MCF) in the treatment of patients with carcinoma of unknown primary site. *Br J Cancer* 2002;86(8): 1238-1242.

111. Greco FA, Burris HA III, Litchy S, et al. Gemcitabine, carboplatin, and paclitaxel for patients with carcinoma of unknown primary site: A Minnie Pearl Cancer Research Network study. *J Clin Oncol* 2002;20(6):1651-1656.

112. Saghatchian M, Fizazi K, Borel C, et al. Carcinoma of an unknown primary site: A chemotherapy strategy based on histological differentiation–Results of a prospective study. *Ann Oncol* 2001;12(4):535-540.

113. Dowell JE, Garrett AM, Shyr Y, et al. A randomized phase II trial in patients with carcinoma of an unknown primary site. *Cancer* 2001;91(3):592-597.

114. Falkson CI, Cohen GL. Mitomycin C, epirubicin and cisplatin versus mitomycin C alone as therapy for carcinoma of unknown primary origin. *Oncology* 1998;55(2):116-121.

115. Warner E, Goel R, Chang J, et al. A multicentre phase II study of carboplatin and prolonged oral etoposide in the treatment of cancer of unknown primary site (CUPS). *Br J Cancer* 1998;77(12):2376-2380.

116. van der Gaast, Verweij J, Henzen-Logmans SC, et al. Carcinoma of unknown primary: Identification of a treatable subset? *Ann Oncol* 1990;1(2):119-122.

117. Eagan RT, Therneau TM, Rubin J, et al. Lack of value for cisplatin added to mitomycin-doxorubicin combination chemotherapy for carcinoma of unknown primary site. A randomized trial. *Am J Clin Oncol* 1987;10(1):82-85.

PART
XI

Supportive Care

INFECTION IN THE NEUTROPENIC PATIENT

Kenneth V.I. Rolston

Infection is the most common complication associated with neutropenia (1). Bacterial infections occur early, whereas most fungal and some viral infections are more common in patients with persistent neutropenia (2). The spectrum of infection is influenced by several factors, including the nature and intensity of chemotherapy, antimicrobial prophylaxis, and the use of catheters and other medical devices (3,4). Febrile neutropenic patients are a heterogeneous group. Risk prediction rules have been developed that can reliably identify a "low-risk" subset among febrile neutropenic patients (5,6). The administration of prompt broad-spectrum parenteral antibiotic therapy to a neutropenic patient who becomes febrile is the accepted standard of care (7). Oral and parenteral outpatient regimens represent new options in the management of "low-risk" febrile neutropenic patients (8). Antimicrobial prophylaxis is useful for preventing infections in high-risk patients. Hematopoetic growth factors and granulocyte transfusions are useful in refractory infections. All these issues are discussed in this chapter, with an emphasis on strategies that have been developed at the University of Texas MD Anderson Cancer Center.

■ DEFINITIONS

Fever is defined as a single temperature $\geq 38.3°C$ (101°F). Some neutropenic patients may be unable to mount an adequate inflammatory response and may be afebrile or even hypothermic when infected. Neutropenia is defined as an absolute neutrophil count (ANC) of $\leq 500/mm^3$, although the risk of infection begins to increase as the ANC falls below $1000/mm^3$ (7,9).

■ SPECTRUM OF INFECTION

The epidemiology of bacterial infections in neutropenic cancer patients undergoes periodic changes, and it is important to conduct epidemiologic surveys in order to detect these changes in a timely manner (Fig. 43-1). Currently, in approximately 50% of febrile neutropenic patients no clinical site of infection (eg, cellulitis, pneumonia) is identified, and all microbiological cultures are negative (Fig. 43-2). These are referred to as episodes of unexplained fever and probably represent low-grade or undetectable infection (2). The most common sites of infection include the respiratory tract, urinary tract, bloodstream, gastrointestinal tract, and skin/skin structure infections (Fig. 43-3) (4).

Gram-positive organisms are the most frequent cause of bloodstream infections in neutropenic patients (3,10). Bloodstream infections however, account for only 20 to 35% of documented infections. Infections at most other sites are caused more often by gram-negative bacilli and are frequently polymicrobial (see Fig. 43-4) (11). The most common fungal organisms causing infections in neutropenic patients are *Candida* and *Aspergillus* species, although the spectrum of opportunistic fungal pathogens keeps expanding (12). Certain subsets among neutropenic patients (hematopoetic stem cell transplant

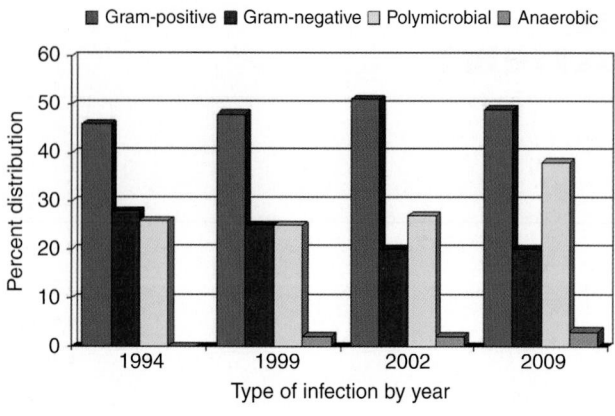

FIGURE 43-1. Changing epidemiology of bacterial infections in patients with cancer* (1994-2009).

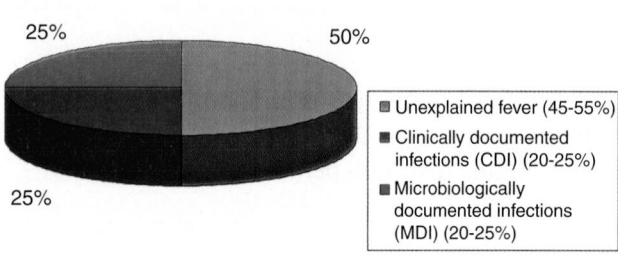

FIGURE 43-2. Nature of febrile episodes in neutropenic patients.

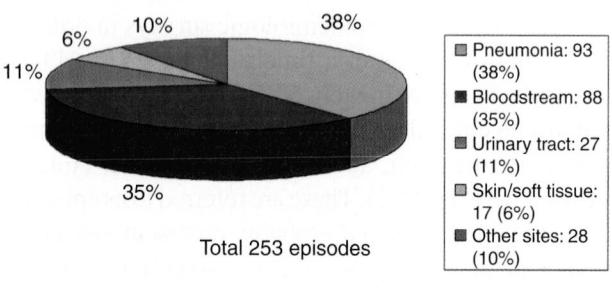

FIGURE 43-3. Breakdown of microbiologically documented infections in neutropenic patients.

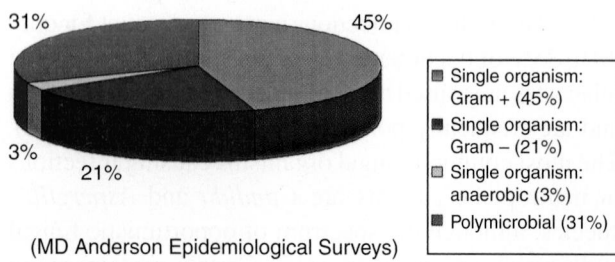

(MD Anderson Epidemiological Surveys)

FIGURE 43-4. Overall spectrum of bacterial infections in neutropenic cancer patients.

TABLE 43-1	ORGANISMS FREQUENTLY ISOLATED FROM NEUTROPENIC PATIENTS
Gram-Positive Bacteria	**Fungi**
Coagulase-negative staphylococci	*Candida* species
Staphylococcus aureus (including MRSA)	*Aspergillus* species
Enterococcus species (including VRE)	*Fusarium* species
Viridans streptococci	Zygomycetes
Corynebacterium species	*Trichosporon beigelii*
Bacillus species	*Scedosporium* species
Micrococcus species	
Stomatococcus mucilaginosus	
Gram-Negative Bacteria	**Viruses**
*Escherichia coli**	Herpes simplex virus I and II
*Pseudomonas aeruginosa**	Varicella-zoster virus
Klebsiella species*	Cytomegalovirus
Enterobacter species	Epstein-Barr virus
Citrobacter species	Human herpesvirus 6
*Stenotrophomonas maltophilia**	Respiratory syncytial virus
Acinetobacter species*	Influenza A and B
Serratia species	Parainfluenza viruses Adenovirus

*These organisms exhibit multiple mechanisms of resistance.

recipients and patients with hematologic malignancies) are at increased risk of developing viral infections, predominantly those caused by the herpes groups of viruses (herpes simplex virus [HSV], varicella-zoster virus [VZV], cytomegalovirus [CMV], Epstein-Barr virus [EBV], human herpesvirus 6 [HHV-6]) and the community respiratory viruses (RSV, influenza A and B, parainfluenza) (13). Table 43-1 lists the common pathogens causing infection in neutropenic patients.

■ INITIAL EVALUATION

A detailed history and a thorough physical examination are of paramount importance. Useful bits of information include the nature and intensity of antineoplastic therapy, travel history or environmental exposure, the use and nature of antimicrobial prophylaxis, history and nature of previous infection and/or surgical procedures, and drug allergies. A careful and systematic search for infected sites—including the oropharynx, upper and lower gastrointestinal tracts, skin (including scalp), perianal and genital regions, lungs, skin, nail beds, vascular access and biopsy sites—is mandatory. Blood cultures should be performed in all patients from a peripheral site and through each lumen of multilumen catheters. Any drainage site should also be cultured and appropriate stains (Gram, acid-fast, fungal, viral) should be performed. Stool cultures are recommended only for patients with diarrhea, and in these cases assays for *Clostridium difficile* toxin should also be performed. Urine cultures should be performed in symptomatic patients and those with urinary catheters in place. Testing of cerebrospinal fluid and joint fluid should be performed only in patients suspected to have central nervous system infection or septic arthritis. In institutions where resistant organisms such as methicillin-resistant *S aureus* (MRSA), vancomycin-resistant enterococci (VRE), or *Stenotrophomonas maltophilia* are common, surveillance cultures to detect colonization with these organisms for purposes of infection control are indicated.

A baseline chest radiograph, although not considered mandatory, might provide useful information in some patients. Repeat studies should be obtained only if respiratory symptoms develop. Significant infiltrates may not develop in patients with pneumonia and severe neutropenia. All cutaneous lesions should be biopsied and sent for appropriate stains and cultures. All patients should have a complete blood count, liver and renal function tests, and a serum electrolyte panel at baseline with repeat studies every 3 to 4 days to screen for side effects (Table 43-2).

■ RISK ASSESSMENT

As our understanding of the clinical syndrome of febrile neutropenia has evolved, it has become evident that not all febrile neutropenic patients have the same risk for developing serious infection and/or complications during a neutropenic episode. It has now become possible to accurately predict different risk groups at the time of clinical presentation (8). The purpose of risk assessment is to stratify this heterogeneous population into meaningful subgroups based on clinical outcomes.

The initial observations made by Bodey and colleagues indicated that the risk and severity of infection were greatest in patients with severe neutropenia ($\leq 100/mm^3$) that lasted for 2 weeks or more (9). Several clinical trials conducted at MD Anderson also demonstrated significantly better response rates in patients with

TABLE 43-2	INITIAL EVALUATION OF THE FEBRILE NEUTROPENIC PATIENT

Detailed history

Comprehensive physical examination (search for potential sites of infection (skin, nail, oropharynx, gastrointestinal and respiratory tracts, perianal and genital regions, vascular access and biopsy sites)

Blood cultures × 2 (for bacterial and fungal organisms), peripheral blood, and each catheter lumen

Chest radiograph: baseline and with symptoms

Urine cultures: symptoms or catheter in place

Cerebrospinal fluid, joint fluid: local infection suspected

Diarrheal stools: cultures, ova/parasites, *C difficile* toxin assays

Cutaneous lesions: biopsy, stain, and culture

CBC, LFTs, RFTs, electrolyte panel: at baseline and every 3-4 days, as necessary

Surveillance cultures: for infection control purposes only (MRSA, VRE)

Drainage sites: stain and culture (bacteremia, AFB, fungi, viruses)

AFB, acid-fast bacilli; LFT, liver function test; MRSA, methicillin-resistant *S aureus*; RFT, renal function test; VRE, vancomycin-resistant enterococci.

neutrophil recovery compared to those with persistent neutropenia (14). This was confirmed in a study from the National Cancer Institute (15). Patients with ≤ 7 days of neutropenia had a response rate to initial antibiotic therapy of 95%, with a 6.6 % rate of recurrent fever, compared to a response rate of only 32% and a 38% rate of recurrent fever in patients with ≥ 15 days of neutropenia. At greatest risk are patients with hematologic malignancies, particularly acute leukemia, and recipients of allogeneic hematopoietic stem cell transplants (HSCT), since the duration of severe neutropenia is likely to exceed 14 days in many of these patients. Various other factors—including damage to natural barriers (skin, mucosal surfaces), the presence of vascular access and other medical devices, and the general medical and nutritional status of the patient—have an impact on the risk and nature of infections in neutropenia patients.

Risk assessment can be performed using simple clinical criteria initially developed at MD Anderson and subsequently adopted by the National Cancer Institute (NCI) and the European Organization for the Research and Treatment of Cancer (EORTC) (16-18). These are outlined in Table 43-3 and include evidence of hemodynamic stability and lack of medical comorbidity. Two statistically derived risk prediction rules

TABLE 43-3 | CLINICAL CRITERIA FOR RISK ASSESSMENT AND PARADIGM FOR RISK-BASED THERAPY FOR FEBRILE NEUTROPENIC PATIENTS

Risk Group	Clinical Criteria	Treatment Options
Low risk	Solid tumor (breast, sarcoma, etc) on conventional chemotherapy; clinically/hemodynamically stable at onset of febrile episode; minimal medical comorbidity; short-lived neutropenia (≤7 days); favorable compliance profile	Outpatient therapy → parenteral, sequential (IV → PO), or oral
Moderate risk	Solid tumor; high-dose chemotherapy (±) autologous PBSCT; clinically stable with minimal comorbidity; moderate duration of neutropenia (7-14 days); early response to initial antibiotic therapy	Hospital-based parenteral antibiotic therapy followed by early discharge on parenteral or oral antibiotics
High risk	Hematologic malignancy, allogeneic SCT, substantial comorbidity, clinical and/or hemodynamic instability; prolonged neutropenia (>14 days); slow response to initial therapy	Hospital-based parenteral antibiotics, close follow-up, appropriate modifications of initial regimen

TABLE 43-4A | RISK-GROUPING IN FEBRILE NEUTROPENIC PATIENTS BASED ON THE TALCOTT SYSTEM

Risk Group	Characteristics	Percent Morbidity/ Mortality
Group 1 (high risk)	Hospitalized at onset of fever: hematologic malignancy and/or BMT/HSCT	35/13
Group 2 (high risk)	Outpatient at onset of fever: substantial concurrent comorbidity	40/12
Group 3 (moderate to high risk)	Outpatient at onset of fever: no comorbidity but unresponsive/ progressive tumors	25/18
Group 4 (low risk)	Outpatient at onset of fever: mainly solid tumor, clinically/ hemodynamically stable, no comorbidity, responsive tumors	3/0

BMT, bone marrow transplantation; HSCT, hematopoietic stem cell transplantation.

Data from Talcott JA, Siegel RD, Finberg R, et al. Risk assessment in cancer patients with fever and neutropenia. A prospective, two-center validation of a prediction rule. J Clin Oncol 1992; 10:316–322.

Talcott JA, Finbert R, Mayer RJ, et al. The medical course of cancer patients with fever and neutropenia. Arch Intern Med 1988;148:2501–2568.

TABLE 43-4B | THE MASCC RISK-INDEX FOR IDENTIFICATION OF LOW-RISK FEBRILE NEUTROPENIC PATIENTS

Clinical Features	Score
Burden of illness*	
No symptoms	5
Mild symptoms	5
No hypotension	5
No chronic obstructive pulmonary disease	4
Solid tumor or no previous fungal infection	4
No dehydration	3
Moderate symptoms	3
Outpatient at fever onset	3
Age <60 years	2

MASCC, Multinational Association of Supportive Care in Cancer.

*Choose only one; maximum theoretical score is 26. A score ≥21 denotes low risk for severe complications or mortality.

Reproduced, with permission, from Klastersky J, Paesmans M, Rubenstein E, et al. The MASCC Risk Index: A multinational scoring system to predict low-risk febrile neutropenic cancer patients. J Clin Oncol 2000;18: 3038–3051.

have also been developed and validated (5,6,19). Details of these two prediction rules are outlined in Tables 43-4A and B. Most low-risk patients have solid tumors that are being treated in the outpatient setting with conventional chemotherapy. They have minimal comorbidity and have short-lived (≤7 days) neutropenia. Regardless of which method is used for risk assessment, some patients will be misclassified, making close observation and monitoring of all neutropenic patients being treated for fever a necessity.

■ EMPIRIC ANTIBIOTIC THERAPY

All febrile neutropenic patients need to be treated with empiric broad-spectrum antibiotic therapy based on local epidemiologic and susceptibility/resistance patterns (7).

TABLE 43-5A	COMMONLY USED OUTPATIENT ANTIBIOTIC REGIMENS FOR LOW-RISK FEBRILE NEUTROPENIC PATIENTS

Parenteral regimens

    Aztreonam + clindamycin (or ampicillin/sulbactam)

    Ciprofloxacin + clindamycin (or ampicillin/sulbactam)

    Ceftriaxone (±) amikacin

    Ceftazidime

    Cefepime

    Ertapenem

Oral regimens

    Ciprofloxacin + amoxicillin/clavulanate

    Ciprofloxacin + clindamycin or a macrolide

    Moxifloxacin or levofloxacin+*

*Only pilot data for these agents as monotherapy are currently available (20,23).

It has become customary to treat low-risk patients with oral or parenteral antibiotic regimens without admitting them to the hospital (8). Most oral regimens are quinolone-based combinations, although newer broad-spectrum quinolones are being evaluated for monotherapy (16-18,20). Several parenteral regimens are also available for low-risk patients who might have some mucositis or whose chemotherapy-induced emesis is not under full control. Commonly used outpatient regimens are listed in Tables 43-5A and B, which also outline the advantages and disadvantages of outpatient antibiotic therapy.

Patients who do not fall into the low-risk subset should receive parenteral, broad-spectrum antibiotics in the hospital so that they can be closely monitored for response, development of adverse events, or other complications. Two types of antibiotic regimens are used for empiric therapy in such patients: (1) combination regimens and (2) single-agent (monotherapy) regimens. Although a large number of prospective randomized trials have shown that monotherapy is as effective as combination therapy, some clinicians are still hesitant to prescribe monotherapy, particularly to high-risk patients with documented infections due to organisms such as *P aeruginosa*. This debate continues to rage and might never be settled by a definitive study, because it would take a single study of several thousand such high-risk patients to demonstrate a meaningful difference.

Since a large number of clinical trials of empiric therapy in febrile neutropenic patients have been considered at MD Anderson over the past three decades, we took a closer look at the outcomes of patients with bacteremic infection enrolled in these studies (14). In the 909 episodes studied, extensive tissue infection significantly compromised response to initial therapy (38 versus 74%), ultimate outcome of infection (73 versus 94%), median time to defervescence (5.3 versus 2.5 days), and survival. Other poor prognostic factors were shock and bacteremia caused by *Pseudomonas* or *Clostridium* species or a pathogen resistant to the initial antibiotic(s) (Fig. 43-5). Although the mortality rate was not significantly increased when patients with gram-negative bacteremia initially received monotherapy, this strategy increased the duration of therapy by 25%. It might be prudent to administer combination regimens initially to patients who have extensive tissue involvement or the other factors listed above and monotherapy to those who present with fever, hemodynamic stability, and no documented site of infection.

TABLE 43-5B	ADVANTAGES AND DISADVANTAGES OF OUTPATIENT ANTIBIOTIC THERAPY

Advantages

    Economic advantage (reduced costs)

    Enhanced quality of life (both for patient and caregivers)

    Reduced nosocomial infection rate

    More appropriate utilization of health care resources (material and personnel)

Disadvantages

    Potential for adverse events in an unmonitored setting

    Potential for poor compliance or noncompliance

    Need for adequate infrastructure to manage patients at home or in the clinic

    False sense of security

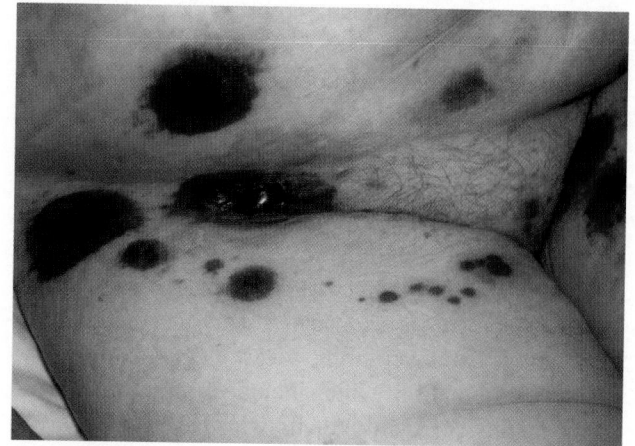

FIGURE 43-5. Typical cutaneous lesions (ecthyma gangrenosum) associated with *P aeruginosa* bacteremia.

TABLE 43-6	OPTIONS FOR EMPIRIC ANTIBIOTIC THERAPY IN HIGH-RISK FEBRILE NEUTROPENIC PATIENTS*†

Combination regimens (without glycopeptide)
   Aminoglycoside + piperacillin/tazobactam
   Aminoglycoside + cefepime (ceftazidime)
   Aminoglycoside + imipenem or meropenem (doripenem)

Combination regimens (with glycopeptide)‡
   Vancomycin + piperacillin/tazobactam
   Vancomycin + cefepime (ceftazidime)
   Vancomycin + imipenem or meropenem
   Vancomycin + aztreonam (±) aminoglycoside
   Vancomycin + ciprofloxacin (±) aminoglycoside

Single agents (monotherapy)
   Cefepime
   Imipenem
   Meropenem
   Doripenem
   Piperacillin/tazobactam

*Amikacin (used most often), tobramycin, or gentamicin.
†Choice of specific agent(s) depends on local susceptibility/resistance patterns.
‡In some settings, linezolid or daptomycin may be used instead of vancomycin.

The various choices for combination therapy and monotherapy are listed in Table 43-6. Specific agents should be chosen based on local epidemiologic trends and susceptibility/resistance patterns. Periodic surveillance studies should be conducted in order to detect epidemiologic shifts and changes in susceptibility patterns (including the emergence of multidrug-resistant organisms) in a timely manner (21,22).

When opting for combination therapy, a decision regarding the initial administration of a glycopeptide (vancomycin) must be made. If a glycopeptide is not deemed necessary, combination therapy usually consists of an aminoglycoside (eg, amikacin) with an extended spectrum cephalosporin (cefepime), and antipseudomonal penicillin (piperacillin ± tazobactam), or a carbapenem (imipenem, meropenem). Doripenem may be slightly more potent in vitro against *P aeruginosa* than other carbapenems, but has not been clinically evaluated in this setting. Ertapenem should not be used for empiric monotherapy since its activity against *P aeruginosa* and *Acinetobacter* species is suboptimal. When vancomycin is deemed necessary, any of the agents listed above can be combined with it (±), an aminoglycoside. Combinations which include a quinolone should only be considered in patients who have not received quinolone prophylaxis (Fig. 43-6).

Some antibiotic combinations are synergistic against both gram-positive and gram-negative pathogens and may be associated with better response rates. Combination therapy may also be associated with less emergence of resistant organisms, although data regarding this issue are conflicting. The major disadvantages are increased toxicity, drug–drug interactions, and cost.

Agents recommended for monotherapy include cefepime, imipenem, and meropenem. Recent studies have also indicated a potential role for piperacillin/tazobactam as monotherapy for febrile neutropenic patients. The quinolones are not currently recommended for use as single agents, although the potential of newer quinolones (moxifloxacin) for monotherapy in low-risk patients is being evaluated (20,23). Aminoglycosides should not be used as single agents in neutropenic patients under any circumstances (24).

■ SUBSEQUENT TREATMENT INCLUDING MODIFICATIONS AND DURATION OF THERAPY

Defervescence in febrile neutropenic patients does not happen overnight. It is customary to allow approximately 72 h to ascertain whether the initial regimen is effective or not. If fever persists unabated after 3 days, the patient should be reassessed. If initial cultures are negative and there has been no clinical deterioration, the same regimen can be continued for an additional 3 to 4 days, since a substantial proportion of patients will defervescence by day 7. The initial regimen should be changed if there are signs of progressive infection or if microbiological cultures dictate the need for a change. The most frequent modifications include:

1. A specific gram-positive agent (vancomycin, linezolid, daptomycin, quinupristin-dalfopristin) for organisms such as MRSA, methicillin-resistant *Staphylococcus epidermidis* (MRSE), VRE, or other resistant gram-positive pathogens.

2. Additional gram-negative coverage (an agent belonging to a different class than the original regimens) particularly in some documented infections (*P aeruginosa, Stenotrophomonas maltophilia, Acinetobacter* species, *Enterobacter* species, etc).

3. Additional anaerobic coverage, particularly if an abdominal, pelvic, or perianal site of infection has been documented.

4. When fever persists beyond 5 to 7 days in the absence of a documented pathogen, empiric antifungal therapy should be initiated. Empiric antifungal therapy should be considered sooner in patients with hematologic malignancies, those with a focus

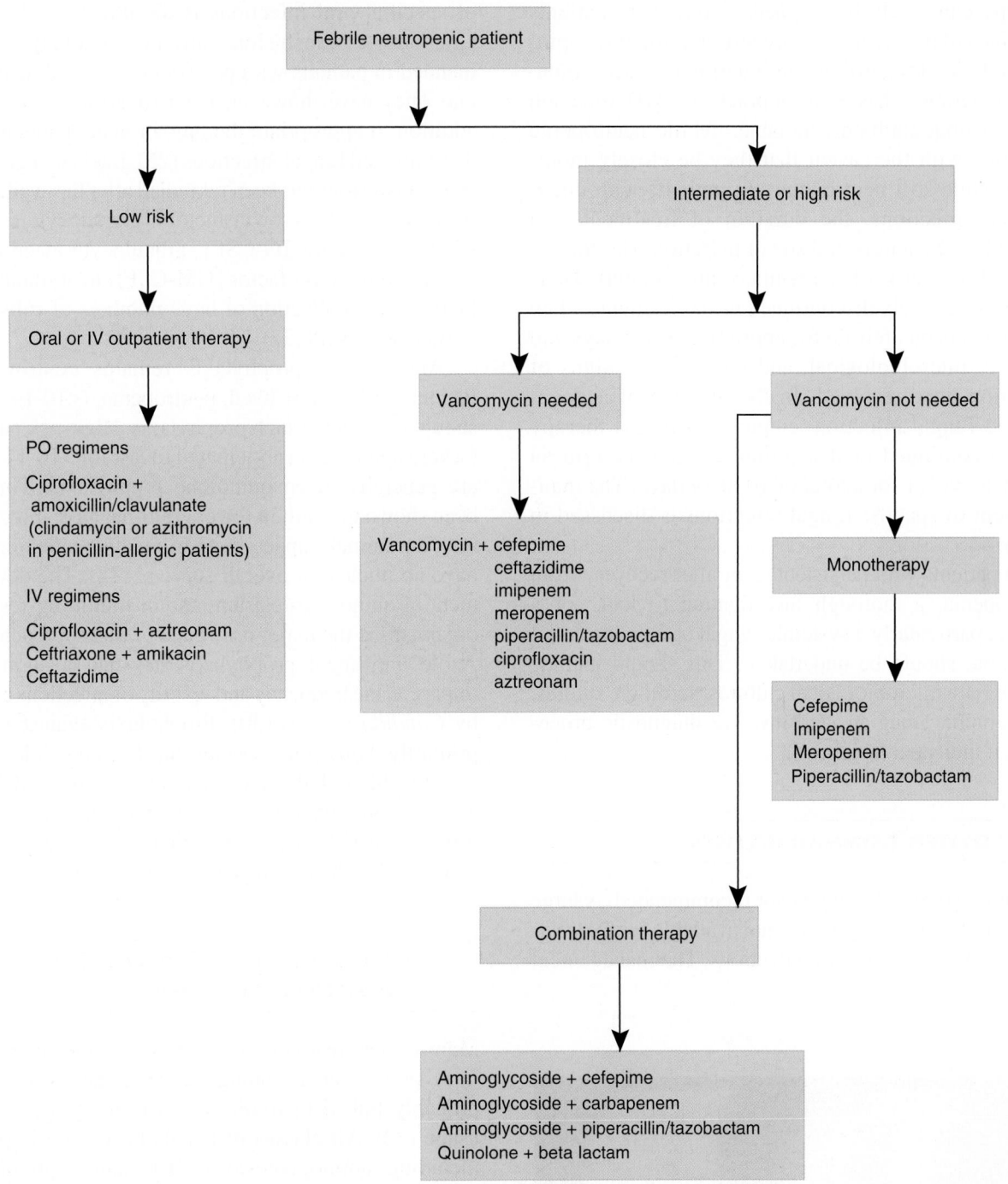

FIGURE 43-6. Algorithm for the management of febrile neutropenic patients.

of infection in the lungs or paranasal sinuses, and those with a previously documented fungal infection or fungal colonization at multiple sites.

The duration of therapy depends on several factors, including:

1. The nature of the febrile episode (ie, unexplained fever versus documented infection)

2. The nature of the infection, if documented (bacteremia, urinary tract infection [UTI], pneumonia, perirectal infection, enterocolitis, etc)

3. Recovery from neutropenia

In patients who did not have a documented infection, have been afebrile for approximately 48 h, and have an ANC that has risen above 500/mm^3, antibiotic therapy can safely be stopped by day 7. In patients who have defervesced but are still neutropenic, opinion is divided regarding continuation or discontinuation of therapy. It has been our practice at MD Anderson to discontinue antibiotics in stable, afebrile, neutropenic patients, with the caveat that they be closely monitored while still neutropenic. In patients with documented infections, the duration of treatment will depend on the nature and site of infections (ie, shorter for UTI, longer for bacteremia or pneumonia). Therapy may be safely discontinued in such patients when they have been afebrile for approximately 4 days and clinical, microbiological, and radiographic signs of infection have resolved. In the absence of a documented fungal infection, empiric antifungal therapy is also continued or discontinued using the criteria listed above, or for a total of 10 to 14 days. The management of specific fungal infections is discussed in Chap. 44.

In patients with persistent fever after recovery from neutropenia, a thorough investigation to look for a source, particularly a systemic fungal or mycobacterial infection, should be undertaken. This should include appropriate microbiological cultures, serologic studies, radiographic imaging, and invasive diagnostic procedures if indicated (Fig. 43-7).

◼ OTHER CONSIDERATIONS

Empiric antiviral therapy is not recommended. A large number of antiviral agents are not available for the treatment of documented viral infections. The management

of specific viral infections is discussed in Chap. 44. Granulocyte transfusions are not routinely recommended in patients with persistent fever and neutropenia. They have, however, been found to be useful in addition to appropriate therapy, in many patients with disseminated fungal infections (25). Interest in granulocyte transfusions has been rekindled after the availability of hematopoietic growth factors (granulocyte colony-stimulating factor [G-CSF], granulocyte-macrophage colony-stimulating factor [GM-CSF]) to stimulate and facilitate the collection of large numbers of cells from normal donors (26,27).

Antibacterial prophylaxis remains controversial. Patients with short-lived neutropenia (<10-14 days) should not receive such prophylaxis. High-risk patients (severe neutropenia anticipated to last for >10-14 days) are generally given quinolone prophylaxis. This has been shown to result in fewer gram-negative infections, have a minimal impact on gram-positive infection, and have no impact on overall survival (28). The development of quinolone-resistant and/or multidrug-resistant organisms is the major drawback of this approach (29). Azole antifungal prophylaxis has had a significant impact on the frequency and severity of infections caused by *Candida* species (30). Prophylaxis against molds, primarily *Aspergillus* species, has been much less successful, although the development of agents with better activity against many molds (voriconazole, posaconazole) is promising (31). Increased voriconazole usage has been associated with infrequency of zygomycosis.

◼ ANTIMICROBIAL STEWARDSHIP & INFECTION CONTROL

Many cancer treatment centers have reported increasing rates of resistance among bacterial pathogens, most probably linked to frequent and prolonged antibiotic usage (32). All classes of agents have been impacted including aminoglycosides, B-lactams, quinolones, and glycopeptides (33). Some organisms (*P aeruginosa, Stenotrophomonas maltophilia, Acinetobacter* species, *Klebsilla* species, *Enterobacter* species, *Escherichia coli*) acquire several mechanisms of resistance and become multi drug-resistant (34). The number of novel agents in the development pipeline is rather limited, and judicious use of currently available agents (antimicrobial stewardship) to prevent the emergence of resistant organisms, along with strict adherence to infection control practices in order to limit the spread of resistant organisms, have become vital strategies in the overall management of infections in cancer patients.

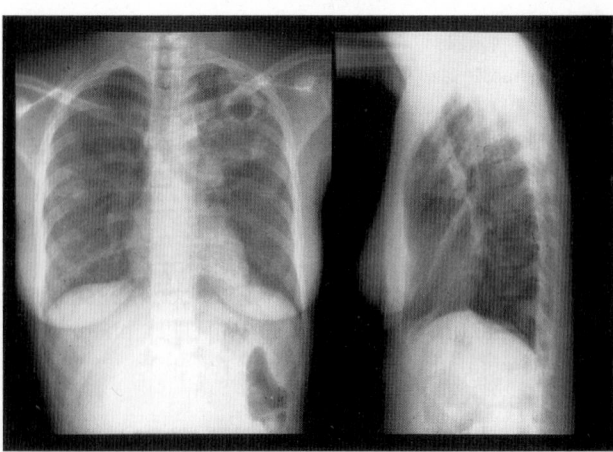

FIGURE 43-7. Cavitary pulmonary lesion located in the left upper lobe and caused by *Mycobacterium tuberculosis.*

TABLE 43-7	ANTIMICROBIAL STEWARDSHIP STRATEGIES

- Baseline data/infrastructure
  Determine local epidemiology and resistance patterns
  Know institutional formulary and prescribing habits
  Develop multidisciplinary antimicrobial stewardship team (MAST)
- Recommendations for antimicrobial usage
  Limit antimicrobial prophylaxis
  Encourage targeted/specific therapy
  Consider formulary restrictions or preauthorization of selective agents
  Create institutional guidelines and pathways
  Consider antimicrobial heterogeneity
  Consider deescalation (streamlining) of empiric regiment
  Practice dose optimization
  Optimize duration of therapy
- Other strategies
  Prospective audits of antimicrobial usage with feedback to prescribers
  Monitor susceptibility/resistant data after starting stewardship program
  Educational activities (grand rounds, in services meetings)
- Strict adherence to infection control policies

Several methods for reducing problems associated with emerging resistance have been suggested (see Table 43-7) and are summarized in the joint guidelines published by the Infectious Diseases Society of America and the Society for Healthcare Epidemiology of America (35). These have been implemented with some success at several cancer centers (36,37). Collecting baseline local data before embarking on a stewardship program is important as institutional/regional differences do exist. These data include local epidemiology, susceptibility/resistance patterns, hospital formulary, and prescribing habits of physicians. Armed with these data a multidisciplinary antibiotic stewardship team (MAST) can implement the strategies for judicious antimicrobial outlined in Table 43-7.

■ SUMMARY

The management of febrile neutropenic patients has evolved considerably over the past two decades. The spectrum of infection in such patients undergoes periodic changes that must be anticipated and monitored so that prophylactic/therapeutic strategies can be changed in a timely manner. The recognition of a low-risk subset has simplified management, that is, oral outpatient

therapy of such patients. Conversely, the numbers of high-risk patients has actually increased as a result of widespread use of intensive chemotherapy and/or peripheral blood stem cell transplantation, producing severe and prolonged myelosuppression. These patients still need prompt and sophisticated management in a hospital-based setting. Accurate and rapid diagnostic techniques must be developed, particularly for fungal infections. The prevention and treatment of many fungal and viral infections remains suboptimal. These issues will continue to challenge us for years to come.

References

1. Bodey GP. Infection in cancer patients: A continuing association. *Am J Med* 1986;81 (Suppl 1A):11-26.
2. Rolston KVI, Bodey GP. Infections in patients with cancer. In: Holland JF, Frei E (eds): *Cancer Medicine,* 6th ed. Montreal: BC Decker; 2003:2633-2658.
3. Wisplinghoff H, Seifert H, Wenzel RP, et al. Current trends in the epidemiology of nosocomial bloodstream infections in patients with hematological malignancies and solid neoplasms in hospitals in the United States. *Clin Infect Dis* 2003;36:1103-1110.
4. Yadegarynia D, Rolston KV, Tarrand J, et al. Current spectrum of bacterial infections in patient with hematological malignancies (HM) and solid tumors (st). 40th Annual Meeting of Infectious Diseases Society of America. Chicago, IL. Oct. 24-27, 2002 (abstr 139).
5. Talcott JA, Siegel RD, Finberg R, et al. Risk assessment in cancer patients with fever and neutropenia. A prospective, two-center validation of a prediction rule. *J Clin Oncol* 1992;10:316-322.
6. Klastersky J, Paesmans M, Rubenstein E, et al. The MASCC Risk Index: A multinational scoring system to predict low-risk febrile neutropenic cancer patients. *J Clin Oncol* 2000;18:3038-3051.
7. Hughes WT, Armstrong D, Bodey GP, et al. 2002 guidelines for the use of antimicrobial agents in neutropenic patients with cancer. *Clin Infect Dis* 2002;34:730-751.
8. Rolston K. New trends in patient management: Risk-based therapy for febrile patients with neutropenia. *Clin Infect Dis* 1999;29:515-521.
9. Bodey GP, Buckley M, Sathe YS, et al. Quantitative relationships between circulating leukocytes and infection in patients with acute leukemia. *Ann Intern Med* 1966;64:328-340.
10. Zinner SH. Changing epidemiology of infections in patients with neutropenia and cancer: Emphasis on gram-positive and resistant bacteria. *Clin Infect Dis* 1999;3:490-494.
11. Yadegarynia D, Tarrand J, Raad I, et al. Current spectrum of bacterial infections in cancer patients. *Clin Infect Dis* 2003;37:1144-1145.
12. Anaissie EJ, Bodey GP, Rinaldi MG. Emerging fungal pathogens. *Eur J Clin Microbiol Infect Dis* 1989;8:323-330.
13. Whimbey E, Englund JA, Couch RB. Community respiratory virus infections in immunocompromised patients with cancer. *Am J Med* 1997;102:10-18.
14. Elting LS, Rubenstein EB, Rolston K, et al. Time to clinical response: An outcome of antibiotic therapy of febrile neutropenia with implications for quality and cost of care. *J Clin Oncol* 2000;18:3699-3706.

15. Rubin M, Hathorn JW, Pizzo PA. Controversies in the management of febrile neutropenic cancer patients. *Cancer Invest* 1988;6:167-184.

16. Rubenstein EB, Rolston K, Benjamin RS, et al. Outpatient treatment of febrile episodes in low risk neutropenic cancer patients. *Cancer* 1993;71:3640-3646.

17. Freifeld A, Marchigiani D, Walsh T, et al. A double-blind comparison of empirical oral and intravenous antibiotic therapy for low-risk febrile patients with neutropenia during cancer chemotherapy. *N Engl J Med* 1999;341:305-311.

18. Kern KV, Cometta A, De Bock R, et al. Oral versus intravenous empirical antimicrobial therapy for fever in patients with granulocytopenia who are receiving cancer chemotherapy. *N Engl J Med* 1999;341:312-318.

19. Talcott JA, Finbert R, Mayer RJ, et al. The medical course of cancer patients with fever and neutropenia. *Arch Intern Med* 1988;148:2501-2568.

20. Chamilos G, Bamias A, Efstathiou E, et al. Outpatient treatment of low-risk neutropenic fever in cancer patients using oral moxifloxacin. *Cancer* 2005;103:2629-2635.

21. Jacobson K, Rolston K, Elting L, et al. Susceptibility surveillance among gram-negative bacilli at a cancer center. *Chemotherapy* 1999;45:325-334.

22. Rolston KVI, Kontoyiannis DP, Raad II, et al. Susceptibility surveillance among gram-negative bacilli at a comprehensive cancer center. 103rd General Meeting American Society of Microbiology. Washington, DC, May 18-22; 2003 (abstr 2362).

23. Rolston KVI, Frisbee-Hume SE, Patel S, Manzullo EF, Benjamin RS. Oral moxifloxacin for outpatient treatment of low-risk, febrile neutropenic patients. *Support Care Cancer* 2010;18:89-94.

24. Bodey GP. Synergy: Should it determine antibiotic selection in neutropenic patients (editorial). *Arch Intern Med* 1985;145:1964-1966.

25. Dignani MC, Anaissie EJ, Hester JP, et al. Treatment of neutropenia-related fungal infections with granulocyte colony-stimulating factor-elicited white blood cell transfusions: A pilot study. *Leukemia* 1997;82:362-363.

26. Jendiroba DB, Lichtiger B, Anaissie E, et al. Evaluation and comparison of three mobilization methods for the collection of granulocytes. *Transfusion* 1998;38:722-728.

27. Hubel K, Dale DC, Engert A, et al. Current status of granulocyte (neutrophil) transfusion therapy for infectious diseases. *J Infect Dis* 2001;183:321-328.

28. Engels EA, Lau J, Barza M. Efficacy of quinolone prophylaxis in neutropenic cancer patients: A meta-analysis. *J Clin Oncol* 1998;16:1179-1187.

29. Rolston KVI. Commentary: Chemoprophylaxis and bacterial resistance in neutropenic patients. *Infect Dis Clin Pract* 1998;7:202-204.

30. Marr KA, Seidel K, Slavin MA, et al. Prolonged fluconazole prophylaxis is associated with persistent protection against candidiasis-related death in allogeneic marrow transplant recipients: Long-term follow-up of a randomized, placebo-controlled trial. *Blood* 2003;96:2055-2061.

31. Johnson LB, Kauffman CA. Voriconazole: A new triazole antifungal agent. *Clin Infect Dis* 2003;36:630-637.

32. Rolston KVI. Challenges in the treatment of infections caused by gram-positive and gram-negative bacteria in patients with cancer and neutropenia. *Clin Infect Dis* 2005;40:246S-252S.

33. Boucher HW, Talbot GH, Bradley JS, et al. Bad Bugs, No Drugs: No ESKAPE! An Update from the Infectious Diseases Society of America. *Clin Infect Dis* 2009;48:1-12.

34. Talbot GH, Bradley J, Edward JE Jr, et al. Bad bugs need drugs: An update on the development pipeline from the Antimicrobial Availability Task Force of the Infectious Diseases Society of America. *Clin Infect Dis* 2006;42:657-668.

35. Dellit TH, Owens RC, McGowan JE, et al. Infectious Diseases Society of America and the Society for Heathcare Epidemiology of America Guidelines for developing an institutional program to enhance antimicrobial stewardship. *Clin Infect Dis* 2007;44:159-177.

36. Paskovaty A, Pflomm JM, Myke N, et al. A multidisciplinary approach to antimicrobial stewardship: Evolution into the 21st century. *Int J Anticrob Agents* 2005;25:1-10.

37. Adachi J, Perego C, Vigil K, et al. Antibiotic stewardship initiative in the intensive care unit (ICU): Evidence from a quality improvement project supporting the development of a multidisciplinary antimicrobial stewardship team (MAST). [abstr 08-059] In: *Programs and Abstracts of the Multinationals Association for Supportive Care in Cancer (MNASCC/ISOO) 2008 International Symposium*. Multinational Association for Supportive Care in Cancer (MASCC): Houston, Texas, 26-28, June 2008.

FUNGAL AND VIRAL INFECTIONS IN CANCER PATIENTS

Bruno P. Granwehr
Roy F. Chemaly
Dimitrios P. Kontoyiannis
Commentary: Jeffrey J. Tarrand

Fungal and viral infections have emerged as a significant cause of morbidity and mortality in cancer patients. Modern management of infections in cancer requires knowledge of the epidemiology, pathogenesis, treatment, and prevention of such infections. Fungal infections range from nosocomial infections with *Candida* species to endemic fungi acquired outside the hospital, such as *Histoplasma capsulatum*. Opportunistic fungi, especially molds, have emerged as a leading cause of death in patients with leukemia or hematopoietic stem cell transplant (HSCT) (1). Viral infections such as varicella-zoster virus (VZV), herpes simplex virus (HSV), or cytomegalovirus (CMV) have been associated with disease and treatment for multiple myeloma and chronic lymphocytic leukemia (CLL) (2-4). Respiratory viruses, such as respiratory syncytial virus (RSV), adenovirus, and influenza, are increasingly recognized as significant pathogens in cancer patients, particularly as molecular diagnostic methods improve. In addition, viruses such as novel influenza H1N1, West Nile virus, bocaviruses, and noroviruses have emerged as newly recognized pathogens in cancer patients.

■ FUNGAL INFECTIONS

Fungal infections remain a challenge for oncology patients. Exposure to fungi is common, with exposure typically occurring in the environment. Cancer patients are susceptible not only to new infection with endemic fungi (such as *H capsulatum*), but also to reactivation of latent infections. Opportunistic molds, such as *Fusarium* species, *Scedosporium* species, and Zygomycetes cause devastating disease in hematologic patients. Cases of nosocomial infection due to molds are reported in the setting of hospital construction, leading to routine air sampling and filtration. In contrast, *Candida* species are a common component of the patient's and/or health care workers' endogenous microbial flora. Manifestations of infection may not present until the patient receives chemotherapy or undergoes HSCT.

RISK FACTORS

Severe neutropenia, particularly prolonged, has long been associated with invasive fungal infections. Chemotherapy resulting in prolonged and severe CD4 lymphocytopenia can also result in infections similar to those seen in untreated HIV/AIDS patients, such as cryptococcosis and reactivation of endemic fungi, including histoplasmosis and coccidioidomycosis. In addition, conditioning regimens for stem cell transplant and immunosuppressives to treat and/or prevent graft-versus-host disease (GVHD) result in deficient cell-mediated immunity increasing risk for invasive fungal infection (4-6). Disruption of mucocutaneous barriers predisposes to invasive candidal infection, exemplified by catheter-related bloodstream infections caused by *Candida* species (7). Aside from catheter infection, damage from radiation, GVHD, and mucositis are risk factors for invasive infection (8).

Finally, another aspect of importance is the change in flora that takes place with broad-spectrum antibacterial and antifungal therapy. The latter may result in suppression of normal bacterial flora and candidal overgrowth in the oropharynx and gastrointestinal tract. Antifungal therapy or prophylaxis may result in breakthrough infection with non-*Candida albicans* species, such as *Candida krusei* (resistant to fluconazole) (9). Aside from non-*C albicans* species, prophylaxis with nonmold active antifungals (eg, fluconazole) may predispose to infection with molds, such as aspergillosis.

CANDIDIASIS

Candidiasis remains the most common invasive fungal infection in cancer patients. Modern medical care is increasingly complex, involving frequent antimicrobial and device utilization that alter patient flora and disrupt the mucocutaneous barrier. *Candida* species commonly arise from the patient's endogenous flora, but rare hospital-acquired cases have been reported due to contaminated equipment, solutions, and hospital personnel. The range of manifestations of candidiasis is from local infection of the skin or oral mucosa to candidemia and widely disseminated infection.

Superficial Candidiasis

Oral Infection

Thrush is the most common superficial candidal infection among cancer patients, typically those with cancers involving the head and neck undergoing chemoradiation (10). Oropharyngeal candidiasis is characterized by whitish plaques on the buccal mucosa, palate, or tongue (Fig. 44-1) that may be painful if removed, exposing the erythematous base. Oral thrush may also be a manifestation of esophagitis (10). The diagnosis is commonly made clinically, but is confirmed by finding yeast and pseudohyphae on scraping and/or culture. Therapy may initially begin with clotrimazole troches or nystatin suspension and then, depending on severity, proceed to oral fluconazole (11).

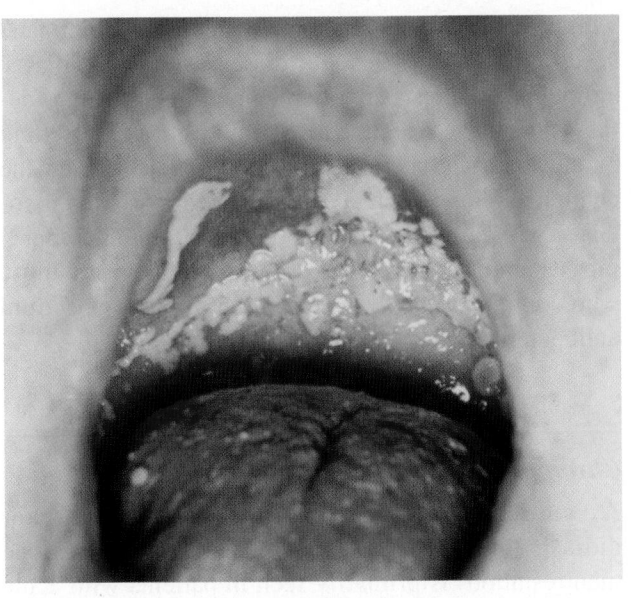

FIGURE 44-1. Typical appearance of oropharyngeal candidiasis on palatal and buccal mucosa.

Esophagitis

Esophageal candidiasis may cause dysphagia, retrosternal pain, and odynophagia in cancer patients (12). Serious complications of this infection can occur, including chronic esophageal strictures, bronchoesophageal fistulas, and mediastinitis (12). Candidal *esophagitis* can occur in conjunction with CMV or HSV esophagitis. Esophagoscopy with biopsy and culture are necessary to confirm the diagnosis of candidal esophagitis (12). Unfortunately, thrombocytopenia often makes esophagoscopy challenging so empiric therapy is often used. Esophageal candidiasis requires systemic therapy, typically utilizing fluconazole as initial therapy (11). Caspofungin or other echinocandins may be used if fluconazole fails or is not well tolerated, but it is available only as an intravenous preparation (11). Itraconazole, voriconazole, posaconazole, or amphotericin B formulations are rarely indicated for these infections (11).

Urinary Tract Infection

Cancer patients, as with many other hospitalized patients, may develop primary infections of the urinary tract in the setting of urinary obstruction and particularly urinary catheters (13). Differentiating between colonization and infection is challenging in the presence of urinary catheters. Urinalysis may be normal and high organism counts are not sufficient to confirm infection (13). Demonstration of urine candidal casts is rare but diagnostic (13). Aside from cystitis, fungus ball

formation and necrotizing papillitis may occur secondary to migration of *Candida* species to the renal pelvis via the ureter. In febrile neutropenic patients, candiduria should be carefully considered as a harbinger of disseminated candidiasis. Recent guidelines recommend treatment with fluconazole, with amphotericin B formulations used for resistant *Candida* species (11). Of note, echinocandins fail to penetrate the urinary tract, so should not be used in this setting. Amphotericin B bladder wash is generally not a useful modality, although may be rarely used for fluconazole-resistant organisms in circumstances where there is concern of nephrotoxicity with systemic amphotericin B (11). Relapse of infection will, however, be likely unless the urinary catheter is removed.

Candidemia

Neutropenia, presence of colonization of oropharynx and other sites, steroid use, presence of central venous catheters, and persistent fever in the setting of broad-spectrum antibacterial therapy suggest the diagnosis of candidemia (14). A recent study from a multicenter database demonstrated that *C albicans* now represents a minority of candidemia infections (45.6%) (15). In that study, candidemia resulted in an overall 12-week crude mortality of 35.2%, with highest mortality rate associated with *C krusei* (52.9%) and lowest with *Candida parapsilosis* (23.7%) (15). *C parapsilosis* candidemia was associated with central venous catheters (16). Patients with *C parapsilosis*, including nononcology patients from a multicenter database, were less likely to be neutropenic and immunosuppressed, perhaps explaining the lower mortality rate (15). *C krusei* was associated with prior antifungal use, hematologic malignancy (including stem cell transplant), neutropenia, and steroid use. These host factors associated with infection suggest why *C krusei* exhibits the highest mortality rate of species causing candidemia (52.9%) (15).

Disseminated Candidiasis

Disseminated candidiasis is difficult to differentiate from other disseminated fungal and bacterial infections. Persistent fever in the setting of antibacterial therapy and liver dysfunction may suggest consideration of disseminated candidiasis (15). Patients are chronically ill with prior or concomitant bacterial infection, but can rarely exhibit signs of septic shock, more commonly exhibited by children (17).

In cancer patients, disseminated candidiasis typically originates from the gastrointestinal tract or central venous catheters. Dissemination affects multiple organs,

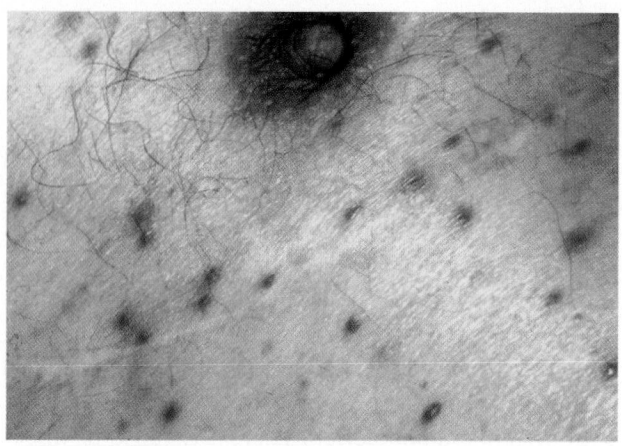

FIGURE 44-2. Widespread nodular skin lesions in a patient with disseminated candidiasis.

such as the kidneys, heart, gastrointestinal tract, lungs, liver, spleen, and skin (18). *Candida tropicalis* is more likely to cause the characteristic skin lesions associated with disseminated candidiasis and occasionally causes a syndrome of skin lesions and painful myositis (19,20). Skin lesions have been described in about 10 to 25% of patients (20,21). Lesions may appear as clusters of pustules, larger nodules, and may even develop necrotic centers similar to ecthyma gangrenosum (22). Common presentation is nontender, firm, nonblanching, raised nodules that are pink to red in color (Fig. 44-2).

Eye lesions may occur, manifested by a complaint of blurred vision or ocular pain (20). Frequency of involvement is as low as 3% to as high as 78%, rarely noted in neutropenic patients presumably secondary to less prominent inflammatory reaction (20). This is suggested by single or multiple, whitish, fluffy exudates with indistinct margins.

Diagnosis

The diagnosis of disseminated candidiasis may be difficult to establish because culture of the organism from sputum, urine, and feces may be positive in patients without infection. On the other hand, 40% of patients with widespread infection demonstrated at autopsy examination had multiple negative blood cultures (18,20). The use of lysis centrifugation, the BacT-Alert system (which monitors CO_2 production), and the BACTEC system with infrared detection have improved yield blood cultures (20). In addition, molecular methodologies including polymerase chain reaction (PCR), antimannan antibodies, and β-glucan testing are utilized. The β-glucan test detects this component of the cell wall present in many fungal pathogens. Sensitivity and specificity are over 90% for disseminated candidiasis, although serial tests are often helpful in ensuring accuracy since false-negative tests may result in the setting of elevated triglycerides or bilirubin (20). Given the challenge of appropriate diagnosis and morbidity associated with failure to treat the severely immunocompromised, empiric therapy is commonly given for those who continue to be ill in the setting of broad-spectrum antibacterial therapy.

▨ Other Candidal Infections

Chronic Disseminated Candidiasis

A syndrome known as chronic disseminated candidiasis (CDC) (hepatosplenic candidiasis the classic manifestation) is primarily seen in patients with acute leukemia (23). In contrast to many patients, they fail to improve symptomatically from neutropenic fever despite recovery of neutrophils. They may exhibit anorexia, progressive debilitation, and weight loss with hepatosplenomegaly. Pain in the right upper quadrant may be associated with highly elevated alkaline phosphatase with other liver enzymes less elevated. CT, MRI, or ultrasound may demonstrate multiple small lesions (Fig. 44-3). Unfortunately, this disease may persist for months despite adequate therapy and may result in delayed administration of chemotherapy. Diagnosis is made by culture in only 50% of biopsy specimens, but can also be confirmed by visualizing hyphae on biopsy. This syndrome is much less frequent in the last 20 years due to routine use of fluconazole and other antifungal prophylaxis.

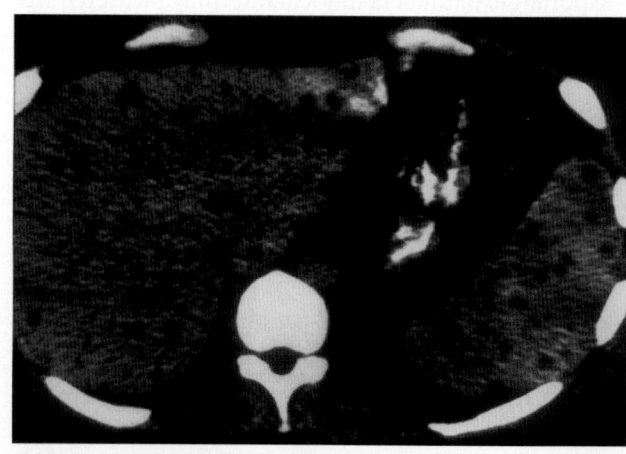

FIGURE 44-3. CT scan showing multiple lesions in liver and spleen of patient with chronic disseminated candidiasis.

Pneumonia

The isolation of *Candida* species from sputum and bronchoalveolar lavage has a low positive predictive value for pneumonia, based on an autopsy study of cancer patients (24). The lung may, however, be a site of disseminated infection, but primary Candidal pneumonia is rare, particularly with routine use of fluconazole and other antifungal prophylaxis in many centers. Potential mechanisms of primary pneumonia include aspiration of oral secretions. Histopathologic evidence of infection is confirmatory, but is difficult to obtain with the at-risk population that is often thrombocytopenic. Radiographs may be difficult to distinguish from other invasive fungal infections, with nodular opacities, cavitary lesions, ground-glass opacities, and consolidation (25). For high-risk patients with positive sputum or BAL cultures and progressive pulmonary disease with infiltrates on broad-spectrum antibacterial therapy, empiric antifungal therapy is prudent.

Meningitis

Meningitis and brain abscesses rarely occur in the setting of disseminated candidiasis, particularly when central venous catheters, ventricular shunts, or other devices may be present (26). With intact immune responses, symptoms may be difficult to differentiate from bacterial meningitis. In contrast, if the immune response is diminished, then symptoms may be absent, unless a mass is present. In addition, cerebrospinal fluid (CSF) may show increased protein and decreased glucose, also making it difficult to differentiate from bacterial meningitis (27). Direct visualization of *Candida* species is unusual, but cultures may demonstrate *Candida* species (27). As with pneumonia and chronic disseminated candidiasis, this is an uncommon entity in the setting of fluconazole and other antifungal therapy and prophylaxis.

Therapy

Therapy for candidiasis includes three classes of medications: azoles (eg, voriconazole), echinocandins (eg, caspofungin), and the polyenes (eg, amphotericin B). Dosing regimens, major toxicities, and general considerations are shown in Tables 44-1 through 44-3. Appropriate therapy is necessary since the mortality rate for candidemia ranges from 24% for *C parapsilosis* to as high as 53% for *C krusei* (15). *Candida glabrata* exhibits decreased susceptibility to fluconazole (14). Mortality, however, is not significantly different from *C albicans* candidemia (14). *C krusei*, inherently resistant to fluconazole, is increasingly isolated in institutions where fluconazole is commonly used for prophylaxis (16). *C lusitaniae*, more commonly seen in patients with stem cell transplant or neutropenia, is of concern due to amphotericin B resistance (28).

Recently published guidelines suggest that echinocandins be utilized as first-line therapy in neutropenic patients with candidemia, with lipid formulations of amphotericin B as second-line therapy (11). Species-specific recommendations, however, are provided, given inherent differences in resistance. The guidelines emphasize that if a therapeutic approach is resulting in

TABLE 44-1	DOSAGE REGIMENS FOR SERIOUS FUNGAL INFECTIONS		
Drug	**Loading Dose**	**Daily Dose**	**Route**
D-AMB	—	1-1.5 mg/kg	IV only
Lipid AMB	—	3-5 mg/kg	IV only
Fluconazole	800 mg	400-800 mg	IV, PO
Itraconazole IV	200 mg bid × 2 days	200 mg	IV
Itraconazole solution	200 mg bid × 2 days	200 mg	PO
Itraconazole capsules	200 mg tid × 3 days	200 mg bid	PO
Voriconazole IV	6 mg/kg q12h × 2 doses	4 mg/kg q12h	IV
Voriconazole tablets	—	200 mg q12h (>40 kg)	PO
		100 mg q12h (<40 kg)	
Posaconazole solution	—	200 mg q6h	PO
Caspofungin	70 mg × 1 dose	50 mg	IV
Micafungin	—	150 mg	IV
Anidulafungin	200 mg × 1 dose	100 mg	IV

D-AMB, deoxycholate amphotericin B; IV, intravenous; PO, per os (oral).

TABLE 44-2 MAJOR TOXICITIES OF ANTIFUNGAL AGENTS

Agent	Toxicities
Amphotericin B	Infusion-related (headache, chills, hypotension, etc); nephrotoxicity; hypo K, hypo/Mg; anemia
Fluconazole	Nausea, vomiting; headache; hepatotoxicity (rare); drug interactions
Itraconazole	Nausea, vomiting; headache; hepatotoxicity (rare); pulmonary edema; drug interactions
Voriconazole	Visual; rash; nausea, vomiting; headache; hepatotoxicity; drug interactions
Posaconazole	Nausea, vomiting; headache; hepatotoxicity (rare); drug interactions
Echinocandins (eg, caspofungin)	Fever; nausea; flushing; rash; some drug interactions; phlebitis

clinical improvement, then current therapy can be continued. For *C glabrata*, an echinocandin or lipid formulation of amphotericin B is recommended (11). For infection with *C parapsilosis*, an azole or lipid formulation of amphotericin B is recommended. For *C krusei*, fluconazole is contraindicated due to innate resistance (11). For neutropenic patients with invasive candidiasis (but not candidemia), lipid formulations of amphotericin B, echinocandins, or voriconazole are recommended (11). In candidemia and invasive candidiasis, fluconazole may be used in patients who have no prior exposure to azoles and are not critically ill (11). If fluconazole is used, the initial recommended dose is 12 mg/kg/day. The guidelines recommend the use of lipid formulations of amphotericin B, rather than deoxycholate amphotericin B (D-AMB), in order to avoid nephrotoxicity (11).

Caspofungin was the first Food and Drug Administration (FDA)–approved echinocandin, showing broad-spectrum activity against *Candida* species In comparison to D-AMB in a study of invasive candidiasis (80% of which was candidemia), caspofungin showed similar outcomes with fewer adverse events (29). Of note, however, few patients were neutropenic in this study. The three currently available echinocandins, caspofungin, micafungin, and anidulafungin, are comparable in their efficacies, although only one study in nononcologic candidemia patients directly compared micafungin and caspofungin and showed equivalent outcomes (30).

TABLE 44-3 THERAPEUTIC OPTIONS FOR DISSEMINATED AND MAJOR ORGAN CANDIDIASIS

Regimen	Advantages	Disadvantages
Deoxycholate amphotericin B (D-AMB)	Broad-spectrum activity.	Acute and chronic toxicities, minimally effective in patients with neutropenia and with chronic disseminated candidiasis, IV preparations only.
Lipid formulations of AMB	Broad-spectrum activity, reduced nephrotoxicity. Higher doses can be administered.	Prospective randomized trial showed no advantage in efficacy over AMB deoxycholate despite higher doses. More expensive. IV preparations only.
Fluconazole	Oral and intravenous preparation. As effective as AMB in randomized trials of nonneutropenic. Minimal toxicity. More effective for chronic disseminated candidiasis. Little experience in neutropenic patients, but appears to be as effective as AMB.	Variable activity against *C glabrata*, inactive against *C krusei*. Some drug-drug interactions.
Echinocandins (eg, caspofungin)	Broad-spectrum activity. Minimal toxicity. In randomized trials, as active as amphotericin B and fluconazole. Limited experience in neutropenic patients.	No oral preparation.
Flucytosine	Synergistic with AMB and fluconazole. Combination of flucytosine and AMB may be superior to AMB alone for chronic disseminated candidiasis and *C tropicalis* infection.	No IV preparation. Causes myelosuppression. Often need monitoring of serum concentrations. Emergence of resistance if used alone.

CDC is challenging to treat. Response is slow, requiring weeks for radiologic response, and duration of 2 to 6 months of therapy is typical (23). Fluconazole has traditionally been used for treatment, even in patients who failed treatment with D-AMB. Given the lack of significant experience with echinocandins, fluconazole should still be considered the preferred drug for CDC, particularly for stable patients. Residual lesions in the liver and spleen may not represent persistent infection, but rather scarring.

The management of catheter-related bloodstream infections is controversial. Debate exists with respect to need for catheter removal. Patients with indwelling intravascular catheters typically require them for chemotherapy and/or supportive care. The removal of surgically implanted catheters is particularly difficult, given thrombocytopenia is often present in this patient population and also the high costs of placement. Studies suggest a role for catheter removal, particularly if it is clear that the catheter is the source or in the setting of persistent candidemia without other source. Removal of the catheter may improve response rates and reduce duration of candidemia (7,29). Infection with *C parapsilosis*, in particular, is associated with persistent candidemia without catheter removal (31). In vitro studies have suggested that caspofungin and lipid formulations of AMB were more active against *Candida* species growing in the biofilms that characteristically form on catheters, compared to various azoles (32).

In brief, *Candida* causes a wide spectrum of syndromes from superficial oral candidiasis to candidemia in cancer patients. The therapeutic approach should take into consideration host risk factors, medication interactions, antifungal toxicities, and comorbidities when selecting a particular agent.

ASPERGILLOSIS

One of the most common and important invasive fungal infections is aspergillosis. *Aspergillus* species are the most common invasive mold infections in cancer patients (33). *Aspergillus fumigatus* is the species most commonly associated with infection, although *Aspergillus terreus* and *Aspergillus flavus*, more resistant *Aspergillus* species, are becoming increasingly common (33,34). Infections are typically acquired by spore inhalation, but construction in hospitals and surrounding areas have been associated with infection (34,35). The most important risk factor is prolonged neutropenia (33). In stem cell transplant patients, risk-reported risk factors for increased mortality include poor baseline pulmonary status, high doses of steroids (≥2 mg/kg/day), disseminated

aspergillosis, proved invasive aspergillosis, increased bilirubin, increased creatinine, HLA-mismatched stem cells, and invasive aspergillosis occurring 40 or more days after transplant (36). *Aspergillus* species are angioinvasive, causing thrombosis and infarction (37). Similar to Zygomycetes, they can also erode through fascial planes, cartilage, and even bone (37).

Pulmonary Infection

The most common syndrome associated with aspergillosis is pneumonia. Because of the angioinvasive nature of the infection, symptoms suggesting pulmonary involvement are pulmonary embolism, pleuritic chest pain, fever, hemoptysis, and friction rub are occasionally encountered (34). Initial chest x-ray may initially be unremarkable with fever proceeding in the setting of broad-spectrum antibacterials (34).

Radiologic findings are variable, with wedge-shaped infarcts, necrotizing bronchopneumonia, lobar consolidation, or diffuse infiltrates noted (34). If suspicion is high for infection, CT scan of the thorax is essential, potentially demonstrating a halo sign (area of low attenuation surrounding a nodular infiltrate), an important early sign that disappears in 75% of cases within the first week (34) (Fig. 44-4). Analysis of radiologic studies from a clinical trial suggested that patients with the halo sign had an improved response to treatment and also improved mortality compared to those who did not exhibit the halo sign (38). Cavitation occurs as the infection progresses, with lesions often increasing in size until neutrophil recovery occurs.

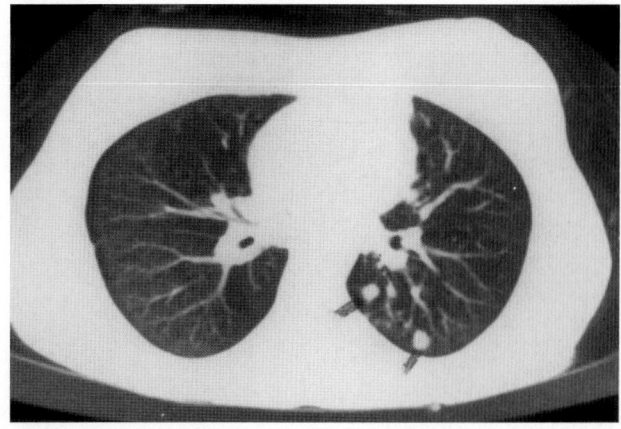

FIGURE 44-4. CT scan showing nodular lesions in lung of patient on high-dose adrenal corticosteroid therapy who developed sudden onset of pleuritic chest pain and a pleural friction rub due to pulmonary aspergillosis. The chest roentgenogram was normal.

Differentiation from other molds like mucormycosis can be difficult. A recent study suggested that CT of the thorax with greater than 10 nodules and pleural effusion are more often seen in pulmonary mucormycosis rather than invasive pulmonary aspergillosis (39).

Sinusitis

Immunocompromised patients may exhibit acute sinusitis as a component of invasive diseases, occurring in 15 to 20% of neutropenic patients (37). Fever, headache, cough, epistaxis, and sinus discharge are signs and symptoms that are nonspecific symptoms suggestive of fungal sinusitis (37). On examination, necrotic lesions may be seen in the nose or palate (Fig. 44-5), with accurate diagnosis improved by examination and confirmed by biopsy by experienced otolaryngologists (40,41). Imaging of the sinuses by CT or MRI scan may show opacification of the sinuses and/or bony destruction. Mortality may be as high as 20% in leukemia patients in remission to 100% for those with invasive sinusitis who have refractory leukemia or undergoing HSCT (42).

Skin Infection

Aspergillosis as part of dissemination is discussed below, although primary cutaneous infection occurs with direct inoculation. These infections are rarely associated with central venous access device (43). Mechanism of spread is presumed to be via inoculation during catheter insertion or possibly dressing changes or application. Initially lesions may appear as erythematous plaques, then progressing to necrotic ulcers with black eschars (43).

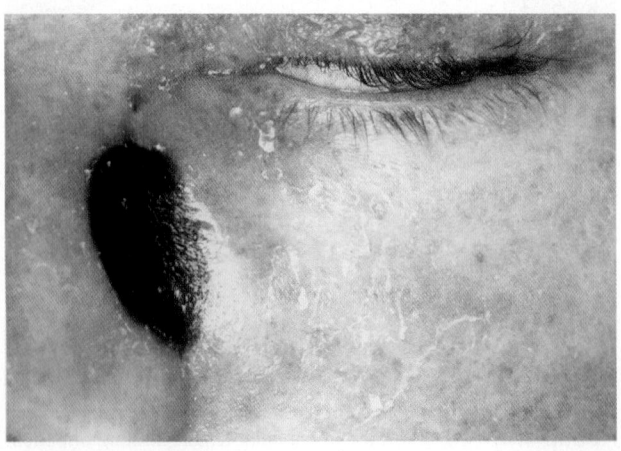

FIGURE 44-5. Black eschar on bridge of nose in a patient with *Aspergillus* sinusitis.

A flavus is the most common cause of cutaneous invasive aspergillosis.

Disseminated Infection

Given the angioinvasive nature of aspergillosis, hematogenous dissemination occurs in approximately 20% of patients with active hematologic malignancy or HSCT (44). Common sites of dissemination include the central nervous system, gastrointestinal tract, and skin. Central nervous system (CNS) involvement may be evidenced by cerebral infarction causing symptoms ranging from focal neurologic deficits to coma (45). Gastrointestinal involvement is apparent in 40 to 50% of cases, affecting the esophagus and large bowel (46). Perforation or massive hemorrhage may occur in this setting. Skin infection may also occur, evolving from erythematous plaques to ulcers that ultimately may be covered by black eschar (47). Given the broad differential diagnosis of skin lesions in this patient population, skin biopsy is critical.

Diagnosis

A continuing challenge in management of aspergillosis is early and reliable diagnosis (34). Tissue biopsies from infected tissue may reveal invading hyphae. Paradoxically, cultures of the biopsy specimens fail to grow the fungus in over 50% of cases. Similarly, blood cultures will rarely (except in the case of *A terreus*) demonstrate the organism, in contrast to fusariosis (48). Unfortunately, *Aspergillus* species fail to grow well from sputum or bronchoscopy, with only 30% of biopsy-proven aspergillosis cases having sputum cultures (49). Because of these challenges of diagnosis, patients commonly receive antifungal therapy based on presumed, rather than proven infection.

In order to increase the likelihood of detection of aspergillosis, various nonculture-based tests have been developed. Available tests detect circulating antigens or immune complexes. Galactomannan and 1,3-β-D-glucan are the most commonly used tests. A sandwich enzyme-linked immunosorbent assay used to detect the polysaccharide cell wall component of *Aspergillus* species can be detected in the serum of infected patients (34). Sensitivity ranges from 67 to 100% and specificity from 86 to 99%, but the test has been studied primarily in hematologic malignancy patients with profound neutropenia. The positive predictive value of this test is poor in solid tumor and other cancer patients (34).

1,3-β-D-glucan is an integral component of the cell wall of several yeasts and fungi (34). Sensitivity ranges from 67 to 100% and specificity from 84 to 100%, but false positives are noted, due to cirrhosis, hemodialysis

TABLE 44-4	PRINCIPLES OF THERAPY OF ASPERGILLOSIS

Early, aggressive treatment with high doses of voriconazole or a lipid formulation of deoxycholate amphotericin B (D-AMB)

Rapid tapering of dose of adrenal corticosteroids if possible

Consideration for G-CSF-primed granulocyte transfusions in selected cases

Long-term antifungal therapy, which should be individualized based on response

Debridement of necrotic tissue of localized disease (onychomycosis, sinusitis, abscess)

patients, and some chemotherapeutic agents (34). PCR tools are in development that are anticipated to play a significant role in early detection, but will require significant standardization, optimization, and validation.

Therapy

Early diagnosis of aspergillosis utilizing the various available tools has allowed for earlier treatment, but challenges continue in assessing the impact of various treatments, given categorization of infection as proven, probable, or possible (41). Table 44-4 describes various principles for management of aspergillosis. Persistence of neutropenia is a host factor that is critical in determining the outcome of infection, regardless of therapy. In fact, in a study of acute myeloid leukemia (AML) patients, mortality was 90% in those patients who failed to recover from neutropenia (50).

Voriconazole is currently recommended as first-line therapy of invasive pulmonary aspergillosis (42). A randomized trial comparing voriconazole to D-AMB for patients with definite or probable aspergillosis showed decreased mortality in the voriconazole group (71 versus 58%) (51). Both oral and intravenous formulations are available, with decreased nephrotoxicity compared to amphotericin B. Voriconazole does, however, cause visual disturbances, hallucinations, and liver dysfunction in a subset of patients.

Posaconazole, the newest azole, is available only as an oral solution. Posaconazole was recently compared to high-dose liposomal amphotericin B ± caspofungin in a retrospective single institution study (52). Posaconazole was associated with increased response to therapy and decreased mortality compared to Liposomal amphotericin B (L-AMB) ± caspofungin (52). In addition, nephrotoxicity and change in liver function tests were more likely in the L-AMB– containing regimens. Posaconazole has been approved for salvage treatment

with the major challenge being poor absorption related to issues from diarrhea to proton pump inhibitor therapy to mucositis (33,42). A reference laboratory demonstrated that 84% of serum samples were subtherapeutic or had undetectable posaconazole levels (53).

Lipid formulations of amphotericin B are now recommended in lieu of amphotericin B deoxycholate, given the decreased risk of nephrotoxicity. In a randomized study of early treatment of aspergillosis, in neutropenic patients, doses of 10 mg/kg/day were compared with 3 mg/kg/day with comparable outcomes (46% high dose versus 50% low dose), but the higher dose resulted in greater toxicity (32 versus 20%) (42). As salvage therapy for those who failed D-AMB or could not tolerate it, the efficacy rate was 40 to 60% (54). Tissue distribution may differ with respect to different lipid formulations, but no data are available to suggest superiority of one formulation over the other (54,55).

Echinocandins are the newest class of antifungal agents that inhibit the synthesis of 1,3-β-D-glucan, an essential component of the fungal cell wall. The echinocandin with the greatest experience is caspofungin. A disadvantage of echinocandins is that they are available only as an intravenous preparation (42). In a noncomparative trial of 90 patients with definite or probable aspergillosis who had failed other therapy, a complete or partial response occurred in 45% (56). Responses were observed in 50% of patients with pulmonary infection but in only 26% of those with neutropenia. Micafungin, another echinocandin, has also been studied for prophylaxis, but compared only against fluconazole with only a trend toward reduction in infections (42).

Treatment of aspergillosis is challenging, particularly in the setting of prolonged neutropenia. This has led to the use of combination therapy and various sequences of therapy (57). Previous studies have demonstrated responses from synergy to antagonism for the combination of itraconazole and amphotericin B (57). Other combinations have included amphotericin B formulations with mold-active azoles, echinocandins, 5-fluorocytosine, and rifampin with variable in vivo and in vitro results (42,57). Limited data suggest a potential role for caspofungin in combination with voriconazole (58) and liposomal amphotericin B (59). Given the tissue distribution of lipid formulations of amphotericin B, combinations that include this agent as well as combinations of others need to be studied carefully to optimize the sequence and timing of various combinations of agents in various settings (34). Antifungal agents utilized for prophylaxis against aspergillosis in high-risk patients have included posaconazole, itraconazole, voriconazole, aerosolized or nebulized formulations of amphotericin B, and micafungin (33,42). Posaconazole is the only agent currently approved for the indication of prevention of invasive aspergillosis in patients with acute leukemia and high-risk stem cell transplant recipients, but significant expense and absorption limit the utility of this agent (60).

Surgery may play a role in selected circumstances where patients are failing to adequately respond completely to therapy or if there may be a risk for pulmonary hemorrhage. In a study of pediatric invasive aspergillosis, the only factor in a multivariate model associated with improved mortality was surgery after diagnosis (61). The role of surgery in adults, however, is unclear. A small retrospective study suggested a benefit for patients with limited disease without prolonged neutropenia (62). There may also be a potential benefit for those patients with residual lesions that may then pose a risk for late hemorrhage or sources of reactivation (63). Surgical intervention early in those at high risk for pulmonary hemorrhage (62) or late for those with residual lesions may reduce mortality (63).

CRYPTOCOCCOSIS

Cryptococci are encapsulated yeasts that have a worldwide distribution, with a dramatic increase in incidence corresponding with the HIV/AIDS (64). *Cryptococcus neoformans* is the most common pathogen, found in the pigeon excretions, with infection acquired by inhalation into the lungs. HIV/AIDS patients had the highest incidence of infection prior to the initiation of highly active antiretroviral therapy (64). Factors associated with cryptococcosis in cancer patients include lymphopenia, chemotherapy, and steroid use less than 1 month prior to diagnosis (65). Those at particular risk include those with lymphoma or CLL. Risk in patients with hematologic malignancy is low because of widespread use of fluconazole and other agents for antifungal prophylaxis.

Pneumonia

Given inhalation as the mechanism of entry, the lung typically serves as the primary site of infection. Despite this fact, fewer than 40% of patients present with symptoms suggestive of pneumonia (66). Symptoms may, however, include chest pain, fever, or dyspnea. Chest radiographic findings may include single or multiple nodules, airspace consolidation, reticular patterns, ground-glass opacities, cavitary lesions, and occasionally pleural effusions with all findings unilateral or bilateral (67). Cryptococcal pneumonia can rapidly progress, resulting

in higher mortality in cancer patients. For susceptible patients, finding of this organism in a patient with chest radiography and symptoms consistent with infection is sufficient indication for therapy. In a series from a cancer center, fine-needle aspiration, bronchoalveolar lavage, and open lung biopsy had a yield of over 90% on culture (65). If serum cryptococcal antigen is positive in patients with confirmed pulmonary infection, this is suggestive of extrapulmonary disease.

Central Nervous System Infection

Many series showed a predominance of central nervous system (CNS) infection in cancer patients, primarily with meningoencephalitis, but rarely with meningitis alone or with cryptococcoma (68). Depending on degree of immunosuppression, patients may exhibit an indolent course with initial symptoms of fever and headache. As the disease progresses, symptoms may include nausea, vomiting, dizziness, somnolence, irritability, confusion, photophobia, or obtundation. Absence of nuchal rigidity (a finding exhibited in only 15% of patients) does not rule out infection (68). In patients with CNS disease, findings include elevated opening pressure, decreased glucose, and high protein concentration. Leukocyte count may also be elevated, with lymphocyte predominance (65). Available diagnostic tests include India ink, serum cryptococcal antigen, and culture. India ink detects 50% of infections, whereas serum cryptococcal antigen is positive in 90% of CSF and 70% of blood in patients with CNS infection. False positives may occur with cross-reactivity reported with *Trichosporon beigelii* and *Capnocytophaga canimorsus* (69,70).

Disseminated Infection

Multiple organs, including the liver, prostate, eyes, skin, and bone may serve as sites of dissemination. Serum cryptococcal antigen has greater than 90% sensitivity and specificity for invasive cryptococcal disease (71). Skin lesions, present in only approximately 10% of patients, tend to be painless and located on the face, neck, and scalp (66). The lesions may appear as papules, plaques, ulcerations, acneiform, lesions, or even draining sinuses. With wide use of antifungal prophylaxis, skin, soft tissue, and osteoarticular lesions appear to be less common (72).

Therapy

Treatment of cryptococcal disease depends largely on site of infection. D-AMB combined with flucytosine is the traditional approach of choice for severe pulmonary cryptococcosis and CNS disease in non-HIV–infected immunocompromised patients as induction therapy (71). Flucytosine is available only as an oral preparation with myelosuppressive toxicity (see Tables 44-1 and 44-2). The recommended dose is D-AMB 0.7 to 1.0 mg/kg/day plus flucytosine 100 mg/kg/day for 2 weeks, as induction therapy, consolidation with fluconazole 400 to 800 mg daily for 8 weeks, and then 200 mg daily maintenance therapy for 6 to 12 months (71). In mild-to-moderate cases of pulmonary disease, fluconazole 400 mg daily alone may be given for 6 to 12 months (71). Of note, synergy has been noted between some antifungal agents and calcineurin inhibitors, associated with improved outcomes for solid-organ transplant patients (73), potentially of relevance in HSCT patients although not established.

Management of cryptococcal meningitis requires monitoring of CSF pressure and appropriate measures if elevated pressures are noted to prevent complications and reduce mortality (71). Complications of elevated intracranial pressures (>200 mmH$_2$O) include papilledema, hearing loss, vision loss, severe headache, and cognitive impairment (74). Therefore, management is aggressive, including daily lumbar puncture or, if necessary, ventricular shunt placement (71). Timely intervention is necessary to prevent irreversible neurologic complications or death.

FUSARIOSIS

Humans are exposed to various *Fusarium* species found in the air and soil. Syndromes include superficial (cutaneous, keratitis, onychomycosis), locally invasive, and disseminated infection. The most common species that causes human disease is *Fusarium solani* (approximately 50% of cases), but others include *Fusarium moniliforme*, *Fusarium oxysporum*, and *Fusarium dimerum* (75). Entry points for infection by *Fusarium* spores are typically skin, onychomycosis, and respiratory tract (75). Systemic infections occur primarily in severely immunocompromised patients, particularly HSCT and acute leukemia patients, accounting for up to 70% of cases in this population (75). Risk factors for disease and poor outcome are persistent neutropenia and steroid therapy (75).

Infection may be manifested simply by persistent fever in the setting of broad-spectrum antibacterial therapy. In immunocompromised hosts, however, signs of specific organ disease may quickly occur. Given the predilection for angioinvasion, this organism may cause thrombosis and infarction. In addition, multiple organisms can be affected, including the skin, sinuses, lungs, eyes (endophthalmitis), liver, spleen, and brain.

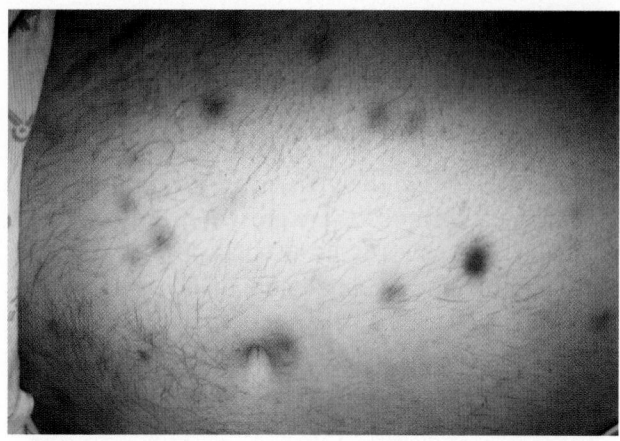

FIGURE 44-6. Skin lesions in a patient with disseminated fusariosis.

Sinus-based infections may produce retroorbital pain, headache, or erythema. Pulmonary infection may result in signs and symptoms suggestive of pulmonary embolism.

Sinus infection and pneumonia occur in 80% of patients and blood cultures are positive in 50 to 70% of cases (76). In neutropenic patients, dissemination occurs 75% of the time. Disseminated fusariosis is commonly associated with multiple skin lesions (77). Skin lesions may appear as red or gray macules, pustules, or classically papules with central necrosis or eschar (Fig. 44-6). Lesions may also appear to be different types of lesions at different stages of evolution (77). Myalgias or subcutaneous lesions are also noted in disseminated fusariosis. In non-neutropenic patients with less severe immunocompromise, infection may be relatively localized, with paronychia, erythematous nodules, hemorrhagic bullae, or trauma-associated tender, necrotic lesions (76).

Therapy

The significance of in vitro susceptibility results is unclear, with conflicting reports of species-specific susceptibility to amphotericin B in some series (75), whereas others do not demonstrate such an association. Azoles, particularly voriconazole and posaconazole, exhibit variable in vitro activity against different *Fusarium* species (76). Posaconazole and voriconazole have both been used as salvage therapy after initial monotherapy with high-dose lipid formulations of amphotericin B have failed (76). Combination therapy has been used with anecdotal success, but definitive evidence of effectiveness is lacking. In neutropenic patients, however, neutrophil recovery is the critical component improving outcomes (78).

TRICHOSPORONOSIS

Trichosporon asahi (*beigelii*) and *Blastoschizomyces capitatus*, related yeast, are present in soil and fresh water (79). These yeasts are associated with syndromes including meningitis, pneumonia, and osteomyelitis (80). The geographic distribution of *Trichosporon* and *Blastoschizomyces* infections is predominantly the United States and Europe, respectively (81). Patients who are most susceptible are those with hematologic malignancies, including acute leukemia and HSCT recipients (79). Fungemia is present in over 70% of cases (82). A recent study suggested a shift from predominance of disseminated infection to catheter-related fungemia (70% of cases) perhaps associated with routine azole prophylaxis (82).

Disseminated trichosporonosis may present with fever with potential organs infected, including kidneys, lungs, and heart. Manifestations of trichosporonosis depend on organ affected, with hematuria and proteinuria occurring in those with renal involvement. In those with disseminated infection, pulmonary involvement occurs in up to 60% of patients, although less common in a recent series (79). Hypoxia may occur in the setting of relatively minimal findings on chest radiography and scant hemoptysis may also be noted (83). Hepatosplenic *Trichosporon* infection can have a similar appearance to chronic disseminated candidiasis (83). In approximately 30% of patients with disseminated infection, skin lesions appear, initially beginning as red papular or nodulapapular lesions that subsequently may ulcerate (47). The mortality rate in the setting of disseminated trichosporonosis ranges from 50 to 80% (79,82).

Up to 70% of *B capitatus* infections consist of fungemia with a recent study showing almost 50% disseminated infection in patients with hematologic malignancy (82). Liver involvement may appear similar to trichosporonosis and invasive candidiasis (82). Meningitis or brain abscess have also been reported with *B capitatus* infection.

Therapy

A key issue to keep in mind is the lack of effectiveness of echinocandins in treatment of trichosporonosis as evidenced by high minimum inhibitory concentrations (MICs) combined with reports of breakthrough infection (82). Data are limited on the optimal agent, as there are only few in vitro and clinical data (82). Combination therapy has been anecdotally successful, with animal studies suggesting a potential role for AMB combined with an azole for disseminated infection (84). *B capitatus* infection is rare with experience primarily with amphotericin B. Current recommendation is treatment with 5 mg/kg of a lipid-based formulation of amphotericin B (82).

MUCORMYCOSIS

Mucormycosis is an infection caused by molds of the order *Mucorales* present in the environment, acquired by inhalation of spores (85). These molds, similar to *Aspergillus* species, are angioinvasive, causing thrombosis and infarction. Macrophages and neutrophils are key components of the immune response to mucormycosis. Patients with acute leukemia, diabetic ketoacidosis, iron overload, HSCT recipients, and those treated with adrenal corticosteroids (86). Syndromes include rhinocerebral, pulmonary, gastrointestinal, and cutaneous (86). Patients with hematologic malignancy tend to have pulmonary or disseminated disease, whereas those with diabetes have predominantly sinus involvement (85).

Overall mortality is 44%, but cancer patients with definite or probably mucormycosis have a mortality rate of 71% (87). Patients with neutropenia are more likely to have disseminated disease, which has a mortality over 90% (86).

Therapy

Amphotericin B, more recently in lipid formulations, has been the most commonly used approach to treatment for mucormycosis (85,88). High doses of amphotericin B (5-10 mg/kg/day) can be provided with lipid formulations (88). Other modalities that have been used include hyperbaric oxygen, iron-chelating agents (deferasirox), surgical intervention, immunomodulatory therapy with granulocyte-macrophage colony-stimulating factor (GM-CSF) or interferon gamma (INFγ), and granulocyte transfusions (88). The addition of posaconazole typically occurs in transition to oral therapy, but rarely may be used as a frontline agent, if there is a contraindication to amphotericin B formulations and/or relatively mild, localized disease that has been surgically resected (88). In addition to monotherapy with amphotericin B formulations, various combinations of antifungals, including echinocandins, are given with any or all of the above modalities (88).

ENDEMIC FUNGI

The list of common endemic fungi that may infect cancer patients in North America includes *Coccidioides immitis* and *H capsulatum* (89). The distribution of these organisms is determined by climate and geography. These may infect patients without severe immunosuppression and may manifest as lung lesions that may even be confused with malignancy, such as lung cancer, or as disseminated disease (89). In patients with hematologic malignancies with cellular immunity impaired by the disease process or by treatments including steroids (eg, CLL), these infections may represent reactivation of latent infection (89,90).

Histoplasmosis

Presentation of histoplasmosis is with pulmonary lesions in solid tumor patients, but is predominantly with disseminated disease in hematologic malignancy patients (89). In the United States, histoplasmosis is most common in the Ohio and Mississippi River valleys. Hepatosplenomegaly and mucocutaneous ulcerations, particularly in the oral cavity, may be present (90). Histoplasmosis is identified by culture from infected tissues, including respiratory samples and rarely the bloodstream on culture (90). Histoplasmosis antigen testing can be used to detect evidence of histoplasmosis in urine (91). Recent guidelines suggest utilizing liposomal AMB (3-5 mg/kg/day) for severe pulmonary or disseminated disease, followed by itraconazole (200 mg twice daily for 2 days then 200 mg daily) (92). For most infections requiring treatment, therapy is provided for 6 to 9 months (92). Severely immunocompromised patients may require even more prolonged therapy. Successful therapy with voriconazole has been used for histoplasmosis (93).

Coccidioidomycosis

C immitis is reported to cause fever, hypoxemia, and diffuse pulmonary infiltrates in immunocompromised patients (90). In the United States, coccidioidomycosis is endemic to west Texas, central California, southern New Mexico, and southern Arizona. Disseminated infection may involve the skin and bone (90). In patients with hematologic malignancy, serologic tests may be negative. As in most cases, specimens from the lung, CSF, or other tissue provide the best approach for diagnosis (94). Current guidelines recommend therapy for severe pulmonary or severe disseminated infection should begin with an amphotericin B formulation, D-AMB (0.7-1.0 mg/kg/day) or liposomal amphotericin B (3-5 mg/kg/day). For meningitis, guidelines recommend fluconazole (400-800 mg/day), possibly combined with intrathecal amphotericin B (94). After completing

initial aggressive therapy according to syndrome on presentation, fluconazole (400 mg/day) or itraconazole (400 mg/day) are continued for at least a year for most cases and indefinitely for immunocompromised patients (94). Lifelong therapies with fluconazole or voriconazole, which penetrate the CNS, are recommended for those with meningitis (90).

ADJUVANT THERAPY FOR FUNGAL INFECTIONS

White Blood Cell Transfusions

Recovery of neutropenia is essential to recovery from invasive fungal infection. Almost five decades ago, transfusions of leukocytes were first utilized to assist neutropenic patients in recovery. Some studies have suggested that this approach could be effective in management of invasive fungal infection, but doubts remain (95). Issues include the challenge of the dose of cells and the length of time during which they remain active (96). Administration of granulocyte colony-stimulating factor (G-CSF) has allowed healthy volunteers to provide adequate numbers of cells (96). The effectiveness of this approach may be as a bridge to recovery of bone marrow. Finally, clinical issues with granulocyte transfusions include an initial worsening of respiratory symptoms, although skin and soft tissue infections appear to improve.

Cytokines

Proinflammatory cytokines, exemplified by IFNγ, tumor necrosis factor alpha (TNFα), and interleukin 2 (IL-2), are produced by Th1 lymphocytes, activating effector immune cells (97). Treatment with IFNγ, sometimes in combination with GM-CSF, has been used to stimulate immune response to fungal infections (97). IFNγ enhances hyphal damage to fungal pathogens by neutrophils and monocytes (98). IL-2, used for treatment of melanoma, is considered to be too toxic for patients with fungal infection (97). The duration and depth of neutropenia can be decreased by use of colony-stimulating factors, including G-CSF (filgrastim) and GM-CSF (sargramostim, molgramostim). GM-CSF may be of particular use because it not only increases number of granulocytes, but improves function of macrophages and granulocytes (97). Case reports and case series have suggested potential benefit of several of these adjunct therapies, although data are not adequate to make firm recommendations for use of these immunomodulators (97,99).

■ VIRAL INFECTIONS

Viral infections are an important cause of morbidity and mortality in cancer patients. Although morbidity and mortality are greater for patients with hematologic malignancy, viral infections, such as norovirus or influenza virus, can increase length of hospital stay and delay chemotherapy, radiation, or surgery in a broad patient population. The most common viral infections are respiratory viral infections, including adenovirus, influenza, parainfluenza, respiratory syncytial virus, rhinovirus, and human metapneumovirus. DNA viruses, such as herpes simplex, varicella, and cytomegalovirus, are well known to cause serious infections in patients with hematologic malignancy, resulting in intense monitoring and prophylaxis directed against such infections. Hematopoietic stem cell transplant patients are at particular risk for severe viral infections. Nonmyeloablative regimens have, however, resulted in stratification of risks of infection posttransplant. Modern tools of diagnosis can quickly identify infection, but treatment options are limited for many viral infections. The following sections will provide an overview of viral infections in cancer patients. Special focus will be placed on those with hematologic malignancy and transplant patients since this population is uniquely susceptible to infection.

HUMAN HERPESVIRUSES

Human herpesviruses are among the most common causes of viral infections in immunocompetent as well as in immunocompromised patients. Morbidity and mortality from these viruses are high among immunosuppressed patients. Herpesviruses are double-stranded DNA viruses. The herpesvirus group has eight members, six of which are important pathogens in immunosuppressed patients (ie, patients with hematologic malignancies and solid-organ or stem cell transplant recipients). This group of pathogens includes herpes simplex virus (HSV) 1 and 2, varicella-zoster virus (VZV), cytomegalovirus (CMV), Epstein-Barr virus (EBV), and human herpesvirus 6 (HHV-6).

Herpesviruses establish a latent phase after primary infection. The reactivation of these DNA viruses can be triggered by several stimuli; this is perhaps best recognized in the recurrent blisters and ulcers associated with HSV. The likelihood of reactivation of these viruses is increased during profound T-cell immunosuppression, as host defenses against these viruses are dependent on virus-specific helper and cytotoxic T lymphocytes (CTLs). Over the past decade substantial improvements have been made in the techniques used to detect these infections, such as real-time PCR (RT-PCR), as well as the development of effective antiviral agents and the use of different strategies for prophylaxis and treatment. Currently available drugs with activity against herpesviruses are acyclovir (with its prodrug valacyclovir), penciclovir (with the prodrug famciclovir), ganciclovir (GCV) (with its prodrug valganciclovir), cidofovir, and foscarnet. All these antiviral agents except foscarnet are nucleoside analogs that require phosphorylation by viral or cellular enzymes to become activated (Table 44-5).

TABLE 44-5	ANTIVIRAL COMPOUNDS		
Antiviral	*Dosage*	*Mechanism of Action*	*Active Against*
Acyclovir	5-10 mg/kg IV every 8 h	Inhibits DNA polymerase	HSV, VZV
Famciclovir	500 mg PO every 8 h	Inhibits DNA polymerase	HSV, VZV
Valacyclovir	0.5-1 g every 8-12 h	Inhibits DNA polymerase	HSV, VZV
Ganciclovir	5 mg/kg every 12 h	Inhibits DNA polymerase	CMV
Foscarnet	60 mg/kg IV every 8 h	Inhibits DNA polymerase	CMV, HSV, VZV, HHV-6
Cidofovir*	5 mg/kg IV once a week	Inhibits DNA polymerase	CMV, ADV, HSV, VZV, BK
Ribavirin	PO or aerosolized	Inhibits viral replication	HCV, RSV
Oseltamivir	75 mg PO every 12 h	Neuraminidase inhibitor	Influenza A and B
Zanamivir	2 inhalations every 12 h (IV formulation available, clinical trial)	Neuraminidase inhibitor	Influenza A and B

*Licensed for CMV retinitis.
ADV, adenovirus; CMV, cytomegalovirus; HCV, hepatitis C virus; HSV, herpes simplex viruses; IV, intravenous; PO, oral; RSV, respiratory syncytial virus; VZV, varicella-zoster virus.

HERPES SIMPLEX VIRUSES

Among the most common causes of mucocutaneous lesions in immunocompromised patients are HSV types 1 and 2 (100). Approximately 70 to 80% of seropositive patients undergoing induction chemotherapy for leukemia or conditioning for bone marrow transplant (BMT) will experience HSV reactivation, usually in early stages, when immunosuppression is most intense (101,102). HSV reactivation may cause severe disease during neutropenia. Patients with a CD4 count less than 50 who received purine analogs or alemtuzumab are at highest risk of reactivation (103). Oropharyngeal and esophageal disease is usually but not exclusively caused by HSV-1. The clinical manifestations of oropharyngeal HSV disease can range from gingivitis to stomatitis and cheilitis. HSV esophagitis may occur from local spread. Clinical presentation ranges from fever, malaise, myalgias, dysphagia, and bleeding to severe oral pain and odynophagia. Pneumonitis occurs rarely and requires a pulmonary biopsy for diagnosis. It is acquired from aspiration of infected oropharyngeal secretions. A recent retrospective study from our center of solid tumor patients with HSV lower respiratory tract infection, underlying breast cancer and APACHE II score greater than 15 were associated with increased mortality (104). HSV disease may progress and disseminate to the skin, gastrointestinal tract, liver (causing necrotizing hepatitis), and brain (causing meningoencephalitis). HSV-2 disease is more likely to cause genital and anal disease.

Diagnosis

The diagnosis of HSV infection can be made by isolating the virus in culture or by performing a biopsy showing the characteristic inclusions by immunohistochemistry. Direct detection methods of the virus in clinical specimens are generally not as sensitive as culture methods but offer the advantage of a rapid diagnosis. Direct or indirect immunofluorescence can be used to detect HSV-1, HSV-2, and VZV from specimens of cutaneous lesions.

Prophylaxis

Antiviral prophylaxis should be strongly considered in HSV-seropositive patients at risk for reactivation during intensive chemotherapy for acute leukemia and during early stages of HSCT (102,105). Oral acyclovir and valacyclovir are the agents of choice for prophylaxis. If patients are receiving IV foscarnet or ganciclovir for treatment of another viral infection, then they do not need to continue acyclovir prophylaxis (106). Guidelines suggest that continuing prophylaxis for over a year post-HSCT significantly reduces reactivation, with a finding that this may even decrease the risk of acyclovir-resistant HSV (103,106,107).

Therapy

The available antiviral agents for the treatment of HSV disease include acyclovir, valacyclovir, famciclovir, foscarnet, and cidofovir (see Table 44-5; Table 44-6) (106). The bioavailability of oral valacyclovir and famciclovir is three to five times superior to that of oral acyclovir. All of these drugs are dependent on the virus-encoded thymidine kinase for their intracellular phosphorylation for activity.

Established HSV disease can be treated either orally or intravenously. The most commonly used drug is acyclovir. Immunosuppressed patients with disseminated or severe HSV disease should be treated with intravenous

TABLE 44-6	COMMON AND SERIOUS TOXICITIES OF ANTIVIRALS
Acyclovir	Transient renal insufficiency (IV), nausea, vomiting, agitation, confusion, TTP (rare)
Famciclovir	Headache, somnolence, nausea, diarrhea
Valacyclovir	Headache, nausea, vomiting, TTP (rare)
Ganciclovir	Anemia, neutropenia (more common), thrombocytopenia, fever, phlebitis, anorexia
Foscarnet	Nephrotoxicity (major toxicity), electrolyte disturbances (hypocalcemia, hypophosphatemia, hyperphosphatemia, hypomagnesemia, hypokalemia), diarrhea, nausea, vomiting
Cidofovir	Headache, rash, severe nephrotoxicity, metabolic acidosis, decreased intraocular pressure, neutropenia
Ribavirin	Fatigue, headache, nausea, rash, pruritus, conjunctivitis (inhalation, health care workers administering ribavirin), hemolytic anemia (cardiac and pulmonary events have occurred), worsening respiratory status including death (inhalation)
Oseltamivir	Insomnia, vertigo, nausea, vomiting (most common), bronchitis
Zanamivir	Headache, nausea, diarrhea, cough, bronchospasm, decline in lung function (some fatal outcomes)

IV, intravenous; TTP, thrombotic thrombocytopenic purpura.

acyclovir (5-10 mg/kg every 8 h). Otherwise, an oral regimen can be used for milder HSV disease (famciclovir, 500 mg three times a day, or valacyclovir, 1 g three times a day). Foscarnet and cidofovir can be used for resistant disease, but are only available in intravenous formulations (106).

VARICELLA-ZOSTER VIRUS

VZV reactivation occurs primarily in elderly individuals, seropositive organ transplant and HSCT recipients, patients with cancer, and those with AIDS. Disseminated VZV infection can be life-threatening in HSCT recipients and patients receiving intensive corticosteroid therapy.

VZV can be transmitted from person to person, and this can become problematic in a hospital or clinic setting. To prevent nosocomial transmission, immunocompromised patients with cutaneous lesions suspicious of VZV eruption and those with disseminated zoster should be placed under contact and respiratory isolation. In addition, it is recommended that the family members, caregivers, and visitors of patients scheduled to undergo transplant be vaccinated against VZV, preferably at least 4 weeks prior to conditioning for transplant (103,106).

The clinical manifestations of VZV infection are primary varicella infection or chickenpox and herpes zoster. VZV infections are less common but usually more severe. The clinical presentation includes low-grade fever, malaise, and a vesicular rash that evolves to scabs. Constitutional symptoms usually develop after the onset of rash and include pruritus, anorexia, and listlessness. Primary VZV infection or chickenpox occurs mainly in children under 10 years of age. Children with acute leukemia who develop primary VZV infection are at particularly high risk for VZV pneumonia, which may occur in up to one-third of patients, with a mortality rate of about 10% (108).

Reactivation of latent VZV or herpes zoster is frequently observed among cancer patients, mainly patients with leukemia or lymphoma, as well as in HSCT recipients. Visceral herpes zoster may follow cutaneous dissemination in immunocompromised patients and can result in pneumonia, encephalitis, retinal necrosis, hepatitis, and small bowel disease. Cutaneous VZV eruption can be complicated by secondary bacterial infections, thrombocytopenia, and vasculitis (Fig. 44-7).

Diagnosis

The diagnosis of VZV reactivation in a single dermatomal distribution can usually be made on a clinical

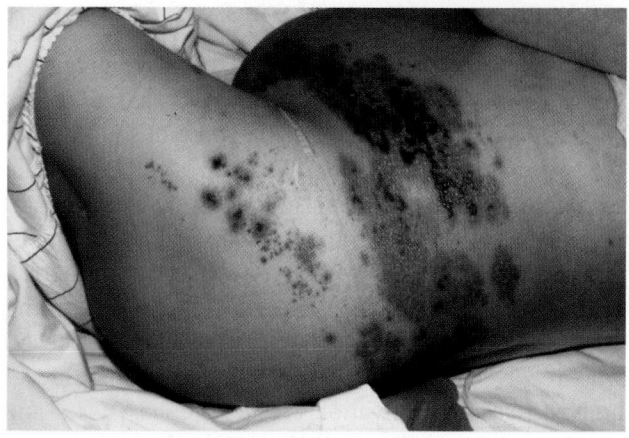

FIGURE 44-7. Hemorrhagic vesicular lesions of herpes zoster.

basis alone. On the other hand, immunocompromised patients usually develop multidermatomal or disseminated cutaneous disease, which can make the clinical diagnosis less certain on visual inspection alone. The diagnosis can be established within hours by the direct method of immunofluorescent staining on material collected from a skin lesion or from a skin biopsy. Viral culture should also be performed. In some cases, a biopsy is required to establish the diagnosis, because other diseases can mimic VZV, such as streptococcal impetigo and various noninfectious bullous diseases.

Therapy

The treatment of choice for chickenpox or VZV in immunocompromised patients is high-dose intravenous acyclovir (10 mg/kg every 8 h) (see Tables 44-5 and 44-6). Early initiation of acyclovir is paramount because it may reduce progression to end-organ disease and usually prevents death in patients with reactivated disease. Therapy can be changed to an oral agent once clinical improvement has occurred, such as resolution of fever or healing/crusting of lesions. The options for an oral regimen for treatment of localized herpes zoster among patients with mild immunosuppression include acyclovir, valacyclovir, and famciclovir (109).

Prevention of Infection

Immunosuppressed patients with negative VZV titers and no history of chickenpox should be offered varicella-zoster immune globulin after being in close contact with individuals with either chickenpox or herpes zoster. Close contact includes prolonged face-to-face contact, a household or playmate contact, or exposure to a roommate in a shared hospital room. Varicella-zoster immune globulin, if available, should be administered within 96 h of exposure to be most effective in preventing infection (103).

Active immunization with a live attenuated varicella vaccine using the live Oka strain (Merck) has been shown to be immunogenic, effective, and safe in children with leukemia (110,111). Immunocompromised persons should avoid contact with individuals who developed a rash after receiving varicella vaccine. No precaution is required if a rash has not developed (103,106). Two inactivated varicella vaccines studied in HSCT patients resulted in decreased incidence and severity of zoster, but are not currently available (103).

CYTOMEGALOVIRUS

Evidence of prior cytomegalovirus (CMV) infection is present in approximately 85% of the US population (103). Therefore, reactivation of latent CMV infection is the primary concern in the hematologic malignancy and HSCT patient populations (103,106). Reactivation can manifest as viremia alone, a mononucleosis-like syndrome with lymphadenopathy, or more severe disease with end-organ damage. Other symptoms of CMV reactivation include fever, lymphadenopathy, splenomegaly, lymphocytosis, and polyradiculopathy. Manifestations of end-organ disease include retinitis, encephalitis, and hepatitis, but pneumonitis and gastrointestinal disease are most common and life-threatening (103).

The most common sites of CMV infection in the gastrointestinal tract are the esophagus and colon. The hallmarks of CMV colitis are abdominal pain and diarrhea. CMV esophagitis is associated with pain and dysphagia. On upper gastrointestinal endoscopy, ulcerations can be seen in the esophagus and a biopsy must be obtained to rule out other infectious etiologies, such as HSV or candidal esophagitis. As with esophagitis, the diagnosis of colitis requires biopsy. In a retrospective study at our institution, 72% of patients diagnosed with gastrointestinal (GI) CMV disease had hematologic malignancy, 25% had AIDS, and overall CMV-attributable mortality rate was 42% (112). Independent predictors of mortality were disseminated CMV and AIDS (112).

CMV pneumonitis is associated with a mortality rate of 80 to 100% in high-risk leukemia and HSCT patients (103). Pneumonitis typically presents with severe dyspnea, hypoxia, and interstitial disease on chest radiograph. Similar to gastrointestinal disease, finding of CMV from bronchoscopy specimens without accompanying pathology is of unclear significance. Thrombocytopenia

present in most leukemia and HSCT patients often prevents acquisition of a biopsy specimen that can accurately confirm diagnosis of CMV pneumonitis. A study of autopsy-proven CMV pneumonia in HSCT and hematologic malignancy patients showed that incidence decreased over the time of the study (from 1990-2004) (113). In addition, complete remission and prolonged lymphopenia (over 3 months) were associated with CMV pneumonia in this population (113). On the other hand, in a recent study we found an increasing incidence of CMV pneumonia in lymphoma patients, with attributable mortality of 30% (114). Over 90% of pneumonia cases were diagnosed in non-Hodgkin lymphoma patients (114). Approximately 90% had received chemotherapy and corticosteroids (114).

▨ Risk Factors

HSCT and hematologic malignancy patients are at highest risk for CMV infection and reactivation. In leukemia patients, those at highest risk include patients who have received purine analogs (eg, fludarabine) and T-cell depleting monoclonal antibodies (eg, alemtuzumab) (103). Reactivation can occur in almost 5% of those receiving purine analogs and in 15 to 66% of those receiving alemtuzumab, with the highest-risk period for the latter group being in the first 1 to 3 months after therapy (103). Reactivation in the setting of alemtuzumab therapy was, however, significantly reduced (0 versus 35% in the control arm) with prophylaxis utilizing valganciclovir 450 mg orally twice per day when compared to 500 mg daily valacyclovir (115).

In HSCT patients, the highest-risk group is the CMV-seropositive recipient, regardless of donor status followed by the seronegative recipient with seropositive donor (103). Nonmyeloablative regimens for HSCT patients have resulted in decreased risk of CMV reactivation, although cases have occurred later after transplant (116,117). The period of highest risk is in the first 100 days after transplant, although prophylaxis and preemptive strategies have resulted in CMV infections of the day 100 after transplant (117). Risk factors for late disease in HSCT patients include GVHD, CMV reactivation before day 100 posttransplant, steroid use, low CD4 count (<50), use of unmatched stem cells, cord blood, T-cell depleted stem cells, and receipt of allograft-negative donors in CMV-positive recipients (106,118). CMV can also be transmitted to HSCT recipients from seropositive donors and from blood products (103). The utilization of CMV-seronegative blood for transfusions and leukoreduction of blood products has resulted in significantly reduced CMV infection (103).

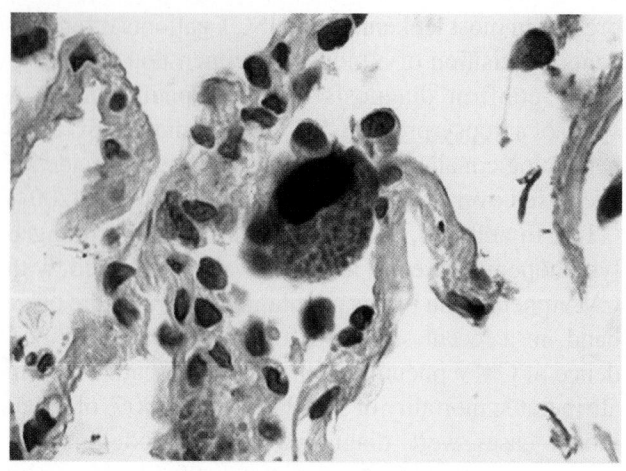

FIGURE 44-8. Typical cytomegalovirus inclusions in the lung parenchyma of a lymphoma patient with pneumonia.

Diagnosis

Diagnosis of CMV depends on the site of infection. For detection of disseminated infection or reactivation, the three types of tests available and recommended for diagnosis of CMV include pp65 testing, detection of DNA, and detection of RNA (106). Serologic testing is not useful, except for donor selection for transplant, since CMV antibodies demonstrate evidence of prior exposure, rather than active infection. For detection of end-organ disease such as liver and lungs, the recommended approach is biopsy with detection of viral inclusions on histopathology or by immunohistochemistry (Fig. 44-8), that has greater sensitivity. If available, in situ PCR and nucleic acid hybridization are also useful diagnostic tools for biopsy samples.

Antigen detection is by immunofluorescence, quantitating leukocytes that are positive for CMV pp65 in a cytospin preparation of 2×10^5 peripheral blood leukocytes (119). The test can be completed within a few hours and can be used to monitor the response to treatment. This test, however, is labor intensive and requires an adequate number of leukocytes (106). The latter is of particular concern in hematologic malignancy and HSCT patients.

Detection of CMV DNA is a widely available test in transplant centers, utilizing quantitative RT-PCR for CMV DNA detection (103,106,120). These tests, although not standardized between institutions, are more sensitive and timely than CMV pp65 antigen. Institutional thresholds are typically defined in order to establish risk strata (120). Samples may be obtained of whole blood or plasma, contributing to variability unless institutional standards are established (121).

Finally, nucleic-acid sequence-based amplification (NASBA) is a rapid and sensitive test that is used to detect CMV RNA, although it is rarely used at transplant centers (120). The messenger RNA (mRNA) sequence detected is late protein pp67. The utility of this tool continues to be investigated.

Therapy

Antiviral agents are used for prevention and treatment of CMV infection. Available agents are described in Tables 44-5 and 44-6. Strategies for utilization of these agents include treatment of established disease, preemptive therapy, and prophylaxis (103). The latter two strategies focus on disease prevention in high-risk HSCT patients. Preemptive strategies involve regular surveillance of CMV pp65 antigen, CMV DNA, or rarely pp67 mRNA, triggering treatment after established thresholds are exceeded (103). Prophylaxis utilizes antivirals to prevent onset of infection (120). At MD Anderson Cancer Center, prophylaxis with ganciclovir or foscarnet is used for high-risk HSCT patients, whereas preemptive therapy is used in low-risk HSCT patients.

Ganciclovir functions as a competitive inhibitor of viral DNA polymerase, requiring phosphorylation in the infected cell followed by dephosphorylation by cellular kinases (103). Its major side effect is myelosuppression, limiting its use as a prophylactic agent and requiring frequent blood count monitoring (103). Dosing for treatment is 5 mg/kg intravenously every 12 h (103). Valganciclovir, a prodrug of ganciclovir available in capsule form, is significantly better absorbed than its prodrug ganciclovir in oral form (103). A common induction dose is 900 mg twice daily by mouth.

An alternative agent, foscarnet, functions as a noncompetitive inhibitor of the pyrophosphate-binding site of CMV DNA polymerase, which does not require phosphorylation to become active (103). Foscarnet is typically used when resistance to ganciclovir is suspected or bone marrow suppression is excessive with ganciclovir. It is also useful in patients with delayed engraftment (120). Foscarnet has been reported to clear antigenemia faster, but without change in side effects or mortality (103). Side effects of foscarnet include nephrotoxicity, azotemia, and electrolyte abnormalities. Foscarnet is a useful agent that has broad activity against all herpesviruses, but requires aggressive monitoring of renal function and electrolytes to prevent long-term sequelae.

Cidofovir, a nucleotide analog, has been approved for treatment of CMV retinitis in HIV patients. It works as a competitive inhibitor of the CMV DNA polymerase. Its role in treatment or prophylaxis of CMV in immunocompromised patients, however, is limited due to nephrotoxicity. The long half-life makes once-weekly administration possible, but also results in lasting impact of adverse effects (120). Modalities used to reduce risk of nephrotoxicity include use of hydration and probenecid. Although the target of cidofovir is the same as ganciclovir, cidofovir can be attempted, although some experts suggest resistance testing (106). Finally, a novel agent inhibiting the UL97 protein kinase inhibitor, maribavir, showed promise for prophylaxis in a phase II study of an allogeneic HSCT cohort (122), but failed to affirm the findings in a subsequent multicenter study (unpublished data).

HUMAN HERPESVIRUS 6

Human herpesvirus 6 (HHV-6) is a beta herpesvirus with two variant groups (A and B). Primary infection with HHV-6 is very common in children. Exanthem subitum, the most common cause of fever and hospitalization of infants younger than 1 year, is caused by HHV-6 subtype B (106,123). In addition to fever, children present with mild upper respiratory symptoms and a classic diffuse maculopapular exanthem. It is unclear whether HHV-6 subtype A causes any primary infection. In immunosuppressed individuals, typically AIDS patients and transplant recipients, HHV-6 may cause opportunistic viral infections. As this infection is very common early in life, positive titers are found in more than 95% of adults. In immunosuppressed individuals, especially HSCT recipients, this virus occasionally may cause interstitial pneumonia, fever, encephalitis, hepatitis, and delayed engraftment (106). Up to 40 to 60% of HSCT patients may demonstrate viremia by PCR, but the significance of this finding is unclear, so routine surveillance is not currently recommended (106,123).

Therapy

Both ganciclovir and foscarnet are used to treat HHV-6 infections, but this is based on in vitro studies only, since clinical experience is minimal. Both ganciclovir and foscarnet have been reported to be effective against HHV-6 meningoencephalitis after HSCT in a small number of patients (124). Also, an epidemiologic study showed lower HHV-6 DNA levels in patients who received high-dose acyclovir, and these patients were less likely to experience delayed marrow engraftment (125).

EPSTEIN-BARR VIRUS

Epstein-Barr virus (EBV) infection is very common in the adult population. EBV is the cause of infectious mononucleosis and has also been linked to several geographically defined cancers. EBV-associated post-transplant lymphoproliferative disorder (PTLD) is an important cause of morbidity and mortality in HSCT and solid-organ transplant recipients. PTLD is reported in 0.45 to 29% of HSCT patients, depending on the source of hematopoietic cells (cord blood higher risk), manipulation of those cells, and immunosuppressive regimen (126). Although variable in incidence, PTLD can be fulminant and lethal. The disease is essentially the result of suppression of cytotoxic T-cell function. The first step in the management of PTLD is to reduce the dose of any immunosuppressive therapy if possible. Another therapeutic approach using the anti-CD20 monoclonal antibody (rituximab) has been tested for therapy of EBV-induced PTLD. It has been successful for the treatment or prevention of PTLD in solid-organ transplant and HSCT-recipients as well as those with proven EBV lymphomas (127,128). Another approach is utilization of EBV-cytotoxic T lymphocytes (EBV-CTLs), typically derived from EBV-positive stem cell donors or from third-party donors (126). In a recent report, EBV-CTLs were effective in prophylaxis of PTLD, with no cases reported in the treated cohort (129). The same group also showed an almost 85% response rate in patients with biopsy-proven or probable PTLD (129). There is no apparent role for antivirals in treatment of EBV-associated PTLD. Treatment with rituximab and EBV-targeted CTLs has resulted in over 85% survival, compared with less than 20% before these modalities were available (126).

■ COMMUNITY RESPIRATORY VIRAL INFECTIONS

Infections caused by community respiratory viruses (CRV) were not considered to be a significant problem for cancer patients until the early 1990s. Since then it has been recognized that they represent a threat to patients undergoing chemotherapy for acute leukemia and to HSCT recipients, especially recipients of allogeneic transplants (130). Early surveys indicated that about 30% of respiratory illnesses occurring during the winter and spring among these patient populations were due to CRVs. Recent studies have reported CRVs as the cause of as few as 5% to as many as 48% of respiratory infections (130). Although many patients acquire only upper respiratory infections (URIs), some develop pneumonias, which may be fatal. In a retrospective study conducted at our institution, progression from URI to pneumonia was noted in 35% of HSCT and hematologic malignancy patients (130). Many of these pneumonias may be due to bacterial or fungal pathogens and not attributed to the virus. For example, it has been recognized for many years that influenza can predispose to bacterial pneumonia. Epidemics of CRV have occurred on leukemia and transplant units, where the virus may be transmitted by patients, visitors, and hospital personnel. Clinics may serve as important starting point for epidemics. Also, epidemics may occur among these susceptible patients in the absence of a recognized epidemic in the community. An additional problem is that these immunocompromised patients may have very prolonged viral shedding (in some cases 100 days) after resolution of symptoms (131). Shedding of influenza virus continued in a small study despite antiviral therapy, halting only when lymphopenia resolved (132).

The most commonly reported viruses causing infection are influenza A and B (predominantly influenza A), respiratory syncytial virus (RSV), and parainfluenza virus (almost entirely type 3). Rhinoviruses are the most common cause of community respiratory illnesses but are identified infrequently in most surveys of cancer patients, suggesting that they are underdiagnosed. It is uncertain whether these viruses can cause pneumonia. Influenza, RSV, and parainfluenza types 1 and 2 occur during the winter and spring, whereas parainfluenza 3 infection occurs throughout the year. Some patients may be infected by multiple viruses simultaneously or have multiple episodes of the same viral infection separated by only a few weeks. There is considerable variability in the relative frequency of the three major viruses in different geographical areas and in different years, most likely reflecting the relative prevalence of the infections within the community.

Recently discovered community respiratory viral infections include bocaviruses, human metapneumovirus (hMPV), and new coronaviruses (103,106,133,134). Bocaviruses are recently described as parvoviruses that are associated with symptoms ranging from rhinorrhea and cough to fever with wheezing and hypoxia (134-136). Disseminated bocavirus infection has been reported in HSCT patients, but the clinical significance of this virus in the rest of the cancer population remains an area of investigation (136). A nested PCR-based study of samples sent to a referral laboratory in the United Kingdom, however, demonstrated that this virus was third in prevalence

behind RSV and adenovirus (135). New coronaviruses NL63, HKU1, as well as established strains OC43 and 229E are detected in cancer patients, although typically with other pathogens (134). A study of coronavirus and rhinovirus infection in HSCT patients showed high incidence in the first 100 days after transplant, but rare lower respiratory tract infection (133). The significance of these viruses remains an area of investigation.

Human metapneumovirus is a recently discovered paramyxovirus similar to RSV that was first described in children (137), but has now been described in immunocompetent and immunocompromised adults (134,138). Fatal cases in HSCT patients were reported from Seattle, but surveys of HSCT patients from Latin America and New York City demonstrate approximately a 3% incidence and a low mortality rate (139-141). Cough and fever were common and shedding was prolonged (140).

The recent influenza season witnessed the emergence of a pandemic strain of influenza, the 2009 novel H1N1 influenza A virus (142). Fever was seen in 83 to 100%, cough in 75 to 89%, shortness of breath in 56%, and nausea or vomiting in 33% of cases (143). The pandemic H1N1 influenza virus attacks younger populations than seasonal influenza, although case-fatality rate remained highest among those over 50 for this novel strain (143,144). Obesity and pregnancy also increase mortality (143). Oseltamivir resistance is rarely reported to date (145). No published data are currently available regarding the impact of novel H1N1 influenza virus infection in cancer patients.

PREDISPOSING FACTORS

Several important predisposing factors for these infections have been identified in HSCT recipients and patients with hematologic malignancies. These include age >65 years, severe neutropenia, severe lymphopenia, allogeneic transplantation, transplant conditioning regimen, graft-versus-host disease (GVHD), and adrenal corticosteroid therapy (130,134,146). HSCT recipients are at greatest risk within the first 100 days post-transplant, although nonmyeloablative transplant has resulted in an increase in disease occurring after this initial period (146). Failure to provide therapy for RSV and age over 65 years were risk factors for RSV pneumonia (130). Aerosolized ribavirin reduced the likelihood of developing pneumonia in leukemia patients who presented with URI (147). Development of influenza pneumonia was associated with lymphopenia ($\leq$200 cells/mL) (130).

PNEUMONIA

There is great variability in the frequency of pneumonia in different studies, ranging from 15 to over 70%, but most surveys have reported only small patient populations. Data on incidence and mortality rate associated with human metapneumovirus, bocavirus, rhinoviruses, and coronaviruses in cancer patients are currently under investigation (134). Fatality rates from pneumonia vary widely in different reports, but most include only small numbers of cases. In our institution, mortality in hematologic malignancy was 15%, although reports in HSCT patients range as high as 50 to 70% (130). The same factors that predispose for pneumonia may predispose for death.

Diagnosis

The diagnosis of CRV infection is established from nasopharyngeal wash, sputum, swab, or bronchoalveolar lavage specimens (130). Rapid antigen detection tests are available for influenza and RSV, whereas tissue cell cultures are used for detecting parainfluenza and rhinoviruses. Modern tools for diagnosis include available multiplex PCR platforms that are capable of detecting up to 17 respiratory viruses simultaneously with improved sensitivity compared to cell culture or direct fluorescent-antibody (134).

Therapy

Therapy for these infections has been limited (see Tables 44-5 and 44-6). At present, there is no demonstrably effective therapy for parainfluenza infection. Currently available agents for influenza include the adamantanes, amantadine, and rimantadine, useful for seasonal H1N1 influenza virus infection, but otherwise not recommended for treatment of serious influenza infection. Neuraminidase inhibitors, inhaled zanamivir and oral oseltamivir, are the only currently recommended antivirals against influenza (148). A study in leukemia patients showed mortality reduced from 38 to 0% in the patients treated with neuraminidase inhibitors (148). In the pandemic 2009 H1N1 influenza A outbreak, early therapy was shown to be critical in improving mortality in cancer patients (unpublished data). Viral resistance to these agents developed in some patients during therapy, particularly among those with lymphopenia who may shed the viruses for weeks to months (132). Among

high-risk patients, administration of oseltamivir during the URI reduces the risk of progression to pneumonia (149). If patients are unable to inhale zanamivir or tolerate oral oseltamivir, intravenous zanamivir or peramivir are also neuraminidase inhibitors that are available via clinical trials or for emergency use authorization from the FDA (144).

Ribavirin is available for the therapy of RSV infection (Fig. 44-9). Ribavirin is administered by aerosolization 2 to 3 h every 8 h or continuously over 18 h, requiring the patient to be confined in a tent (147). In leukemia patients, lack of aerosolized ribavirin and high APACHE II scores were independent predictors of developing pneumonia in this population (147). Ribavirin may also be combined with immunoglobulin therapy (134). Initially, intravenous gamma globulins have been used (134). Palivizumab, a humanized monoclonal antibody directed against the F glycoprotein of RSV, is currently available and approved for prophylaxis of RSV infection in high-risk pediatric patients (150). Most patients with RSV pneumonia are being treated with combination therapy, but the limited numbers of patients and lack of clinical trial data reported make interpretation of results difficult.

HEPATITIS VIRUSES

Hepatitis B

Hepatitis B (HBV) and C (HCV) infections are common in many countries. There is a global epidemic of HBV infections affecting more than 350 million people worldwide. Chronic HBV or HCV infections lead to progressive liver disease, cirrhosis, and hepatocellular cancer. Hepatitis can be a serious problem in cancer patients for various reasons. Chemotherapy-induced immunosuppression may lead to reactivation and fulminant infection in patients with chronic HBV infection. Furthermore, the presence of hepatitis may require substantial delays in the administration of antineoplastic therapy. In HSCT patients, reactivation is more likely in those who have received high-dose steroids, fludarabine, rituximab, or alemtuzumab (106).

Therapy

Although clinical experience is limited, lamivudine may potentially suppress HBV reactivation secondary to chemotherapy in patients with chronic HBV infection (positive HBV DNA and/or positive HBs Ag). It may also be beneficial for preventing reactivation in patients who have recovered from prior infection (positive hepatitis B core antibody with or without HBs Ab).

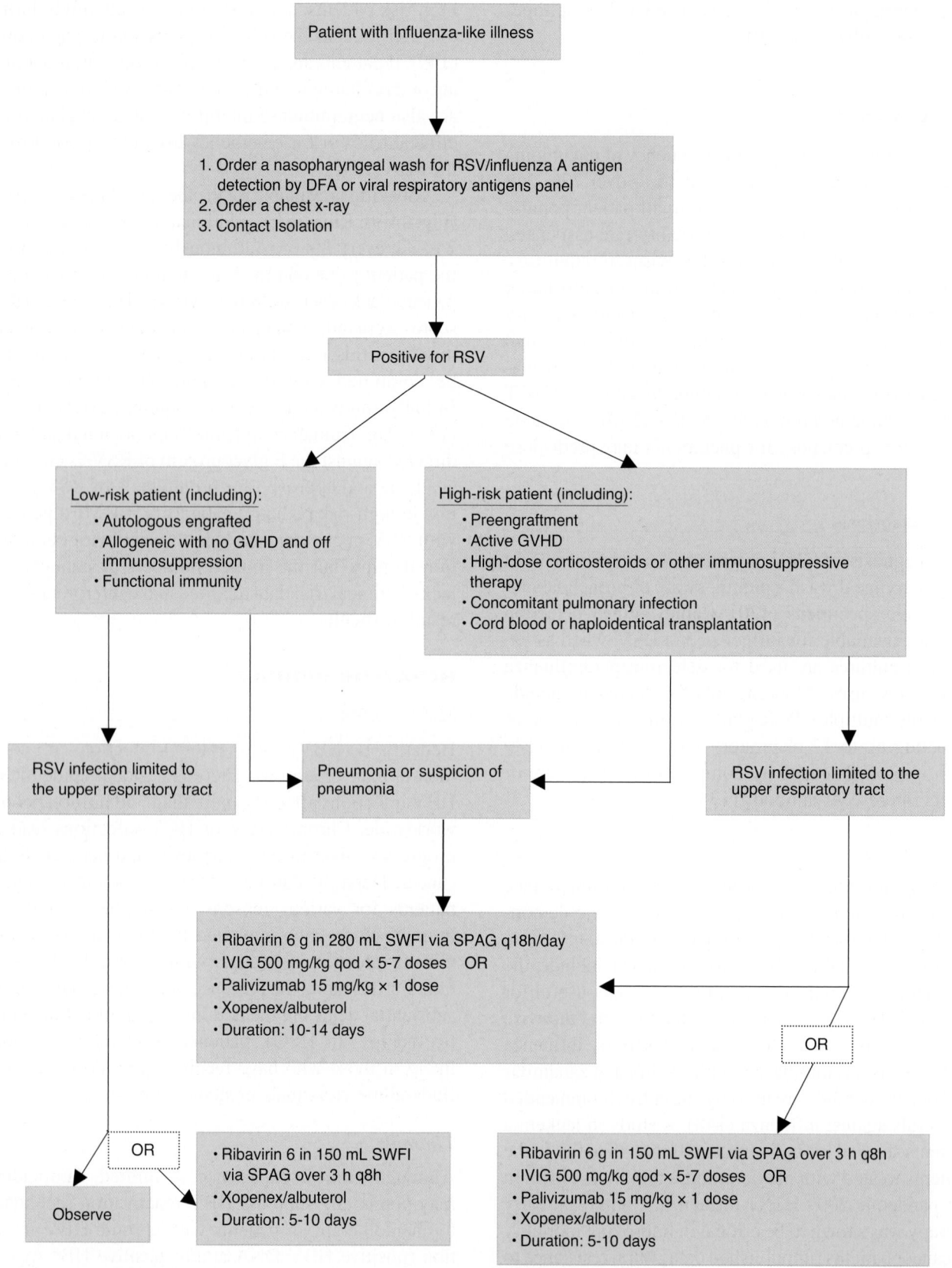

FIGURE 44-9.   Management of RSV infection after hematopoietic stem cell transplantation. GVHD, graft-versus-host disease; RSV, respiratory syncytial virus. *(Adapted with permission from The University of Texas MD Anderson Cancer Center.)*

Determining screening markers of chronic HBV infection or past exposure is important in immunosuppressed patients for determining the need for treatment of chronic infection or prophylaxis against acute reactivation (151,152). Interferon alpha (INFα), lamivudine, and adefovir are antiviral agents with efficacy against HBV that can be used for prevention or treatment of HBV infection in seropositive patients undergoing chemotherapy for cancer or in HSCT recipients. Additional studies are needed to assess the usefulness of these agents to prevent HBV-associated complications in HSCT recipients. At this time, lamivudine continues to be the preferred agent for prevention of reactivation in high-risk patients (106). Preexposure vaccination of persons at risk using recombinant HBV vaccines offers protection against HBV infection (106). Postexposure prophylaxis includes the administration of HBV vaccine and HBV immunoglobulins (106).

Hepatitis C

Hepatitis C is the most common chronic blood-borne infection. In the United States, 4 million individuals (1.6% of the population) have been infected (153). It is the leading indication for liver transplantation. HCV transmission occurs primarily through exposure to infected blood. It can be acquired from intravenous drug abuse, blood transfusion before 1992, solid-organ transplantation from infected donors, unsafe medical practices, occupational exposure to infected blood, birth to an infected mother, sexual contact with an infected person, and possibly via intranasal cocaine use.

Several studies suggest an association between HCV infection and several B-cell lymphoproliferative disorders. Furthermore, epidemiologic studies from Italy, Japan, and California found a high prevalence of HCV among patients with non-Hodgkin lymphoma (154,155). Treatment of these lymphomas with chemotherapy can be complicated by viral reactivation and immune reconstitution hepatitis, which is more commonly encountered in cases of infection with HBV. In high-prevalence areas, screening for the virus should be performed when lymphoma is diagnosed. Antibody testing should be the first test used to assess exposure to HCV, but in cases of persistent liver disease with immunocompromised status that may prevent adequate response, HCV RNA testing should be undertaken (153). Patients who are seropositive for HCV should be tested for HCV RNA to determine if virus is circulating and to determine likelihood of response to currently available therapies (153). The combination of pegylated INFα plus ribavirin produces sustained virologic responses in HCV infection in approximately 50% of genotype 1 infections and 80% of other genotypes (153). Treatment is uniformly recommended for HCV-infected HSCT recipients, although timing should be at least 2 years after transplant with no evidence of GVHD and off immunosuppression (106). At present, no active or passive immunizations are available for HCV.

ADENOVIRUS

Adenoviruses are a common cause of self-limited respiratory and gastrointestinal infections in normal individuals. Transmission occurs by aerosolized droplets or the oral-fecal route. Adenovirus infections have been recognized in patients undergoing intensive chemotherapy for hematologic and occasionally other malignancies, but they are especially prevalent among HSCT recipients. The frequency of infection among HSCT recipients has varied from 3 to 21%, and it is more prevalent among children than adults (156,157). There is no seasonal variation, and the onset of infection from time of transplantation can be quite variable, although the median interval is about 50 days. The virus may persist for prolonged periods in normal individuals; hence, some infections in cancer patients represent reactivation.

Important risk factors have been identified for adenovirus infection, including childhood, allogeneic transplantation, GVHD, total-body irradiation (in children), T-cell depleting conditioning regimens, adrenal corticosteroid therapy, and lymphopenia (156,158). Use of antibody-positive donors may also be a predisposing factor for infection. About 50% of adenoviral infections occur in patients with other concomitant infections.

Immunocompromised patients may have asymptomatic infection, single-organ disease, or disseminated disease (159). The most common disease is gastroenteritis presenting as fever and diarrhea, which may become bloody. Infections of the respiratory tract may vary from mild URI to severe pneumonitis with respiratory failure. Adenovirus may cause nephritis, and as many as 50% of patients with positive urine cultures develop hemorrhagic cystitis. Hepatitis may lead to liver failure and death. Other types of infection include encephalitis, pancreatitis, and disseminated infection with multiple organ failure.

Diagnosis

The virus may be identified from nasopharyngeal washings, throat swabs, lower respiratory specimens, urine, stool, blood, and infected tissues. The diagnosis can be established by culture or more rapidly by the use of commercially available tests for antigen detection. Positive cultures are most often obtained from stool or urine specimens. PCR is a useful diagnostic tool, and the amount of DNA load detected can discriminate between nonfatal disease and fatal disseminated disease (160). Persistent, high load adenoviremia has been linked to progressive disease in pediatric HSCT patients (161).The histopathologic findings in tissue biopsies are pathognomonic for adenovirus infection.

Outcome

The mortality rate from symptomatic infection is about 25%, but it is 60 to 75% in patients with definite disseminated disease (156). Death is mainly due to pneumonitis, hepatitis, or multiorgan failure. Many patients who die have other concomitant infections. There is no established therapy for these infections. In one series of 45 patients, cidofovir produced successful results in 69% and was as effective in asymptomatic patients as in those with definite disease (162). Lipid esters of cidofovir have been developed to improve bioavailability and reduce toxicity associated with this compound (161). Other approaches to treatment include ribavirin and immunotherapy. The latter involves utilizing adenovirus-specific cytotoxic T lymphocyte infusions from donors (161,163).

■ PARVOVIRUS B19 INFECTION

Parvovirus B19 causes erythema infectiosum in children. It has been associated with aplastic crises in diseases in which the life span or production of red blood cells is reduced (164). Anti-B19 IgG has been found to be more prevalent among cancer patients undergoing chemotherapy than among the general population. In this study, 63% of the seropositive cancer patients had unexplained anemia (165). Prolonged erythroid aplasia in childhood acute lymphocytic leukemia was associated with detection B19 DNA in the bone marrow. Several CLL patients have developed severe parvovirus B19 infection, manifested by a flu-like illness followed by anemia caused by pure red cell aplasia in the bone marrow. The infection may be followed by an incapacitating polyarthritis. Intravenous immunoglobulin is a treatment available for infection, but with significant risk of relapse (166). A recent concern is the potential risk posed for infection or reactivation with parvovirus B19 for patients on dasatinib (a tyrosine kinase inhibitor) (167).

■ BK (POLYOMA) VIRUS INFECTION

Polyoma hominis, or BK virus, infects 80% of the general population without causing clinical manifestations. It persists in the genitourinary tract (168) and is a major cause of hemorrhagic cystitis among HSCT recipients. About 50% of these patients have persistent viruria, and half of these develop hemorrhagic cystitis. Risk is higher in allogeneic HSCT recipients (169). Patients with hemorrhagic cystitis have higher viral loads in the urine, as detected by PCR (106). The disease may vary from asymptomatic microscopic hematuria to severe dysuria, frequency, and passage of clots, which may cause outflow obstruction and renal failure. Patients who develop this disease >100 days posttransplantation are more likely to survive. Symptomatic therapy includes red blood cell and platelet transfusions, saline bladder irrigations, and cauterization. Intravesical cidofovir, bladder irrigations with GM-CSF, and IV cidofovir have been reported to be of benefit in hemorrhagic cystitis (169), although no specific therapy is currently recommended.

■ PROGRESSIVE MULTIFOCAL LEUKOENCEPHALOPATHY

Progressive multifocal leukoencephalopathy (PML) is a demyelinating disease of the brain caused by the JC virus, a polyomavirus which is related to BK virus (170). The disease results from reactivation of latent infection. About 80% of normal adults demonstrate JC virus antibodies by middle age. PML was first described in patients with CLL and Hodgkin disease. Subsequent reports centered on HIV patients, who currently account for 80% of new PML cases (170). Symptoms include visual disturbances, speech defects, and mental deterioration leading to dementia and coma. The mortality rate is 80% at 1 year and the mean time from diagnosis to death is 4 months. A recent association has been reported with steroid use, fludarabine, cyclophosphamide, methotrexate, mycophenolate, and, more recently, monoclonal antibodies, including rituximab (170,171). Therapeutic choices are limited, with the individual and combination therapy attempted with cytarabine, cidofovir, IL-2, IFNα, immunoglobulin, zidovudine, ganciclovir, donor lymphocyte infusion, and, if possible, discontinuation of GVHD prophylaxis (172). No consistently effective therapy is available.

Commentary: Role of the Microbiology Laboratory in the Diagnosis of Infectious Diseases in Cancer Patients

Laboratories need to make specific adaptations to provide adequate microbiological diagnosis in cancer patients. Detection of molds and reactivation of endogenous virus infection is particularly problematic. *Aspergillus* galactomannan detection is plagued with false positives; however, periodic "endotoxin stripping" procedures for all plastic containers as well as lines and a quick-freeze-thaw of the sample prior to extraction will reduce intrinsic test variability. Similarly, the pan-fungal β-glucan assay has high variability and shows cross-reactivities with penicillins. Quantitative blood culturing detects yeast well, but rarely detects invasive aspergillosis. PCR assays for *Aspergillus* species offer the potential for definitive results; however limited sensitivity has confined this testing to a research setting. Separate molecular tests would be required, of course, for detection of Zygomycetes, *Scedosporium*, *Fusarium*, and other molds. Culture is insensitive and slow, yet has utility. In our center the simple expedient of 37°C incubation of fungal cultures has doubled the recovery of *Aspergillus* species and resulted in a sixfold improvement in the yield of Zygomycetes from tissue. In clinical specimens molds appear to die rapidly at room temperature; transport of samples for fungal culture at 37°C should yield further improvements. The introduction of molecular assays will eventually revolutionize virology diagnostics; however, a few caveats remain. An RSV molecular assay will occasionally find RSV in asymptomatic patients—similar to current DFA and culture methods. It seems likely that the molecular assays will eventually need quantitative thresholds for interpretation as do many other assays in microbiology. It is reasonable therefore to ask whether these molecular thresholds are, at the level of decision making, likely to be substantially different from current 48-h culture method for respiratory viruses. Influenza provides a cautionary example as well—we now have concern for H5N1 (avian influenza), H3N2, H1N1 seasonal, and the H1N1 2009 variant—all important—but we appear to have more tests chasing fewer dollars. Substantial progress has been made in converting open-system (homebrew) molecular assays to closed-system automatable assays, with major benefits in quality control and decreased in interlaboratory variation; however, the costs are high and the platforms remain inflexible. The cost-effectiveness of fully implementing a molecular approach must be carefully evaluated at each institution and will require close collaboration between microbiology, infectious diseases, and other services.

Jeffrey J. Tarrand

References

1. Bodey GP. Fungal infections complicating acute leukemia. *J Chronic Dis* 1966;19(6):667-687.
2. Egerer G, Hensel M, Ho AD. Infectious complications in chronic lymphoid malignancy. *Curr Treat Options Oncol* 2001;2(3):237-244.
3. Dearden C. Disease-specific complications of chronic lymphocytic leukemia. Hematology/the Education Program of the American Society of Hematology American Society of Hematology 2008:450-456.
4. Nucci M, Anaissie E. Infections in patients with multiple myeloma in the era of high-dose therapy and novel agents. *Clin Infect Dis* 2009;49(8):1211-1225.
5. Nucci M, Anaissie E. Fungal infections in hematopoietic stem cell transplantation and solid-organ transplantation—focus on aspergillosis. *Clin Chest Med* 2009;30(2):295-306, vii.
6. Wolff D, Roessler V, Steiner B, et al. Treatment of steroid-resistant acute graft-versus-host disease with daclizumab and etanercept. *Bone Marrow Transplant* 2005;35(10):1003-1010.
7. Raad I, Hanna H, Boktour M, et al. Management of central venous catheters in patients with cancer and candidemia. *Clin Infect Dis* 2004;38(8):1119-1127.
8. Lehrnbecher T, Koehl U, Wittekindt B, et al. Changes in host defence induced by malignancies and antineoplastic treatment: Implication for immunotherapeutic strategies. *Lancet Oncol* 2008;9(3):269-278.
9. Wingard JR, Merz WG, Rinaldi MG, et al. Increase in *Candida krusei* infection among patients with bone marrow transplantation and neutropenia treated prophylactically with fluconazole. *N Engl J Med* 1991;325(18):1274-1277.
10. Samonis G, Skordilis P, Maraki S, et al. Oropharyngeal candidiasis as a marker for esophageal candidiasis in patients with cancer. *Clin Infect Dis* 1998;27(2):283-286.
11. Pappas PG, Kauffman CA, Andes D, et al. Clinical practice guidelines for the management of candidiasis: 2009 update by the Infectious Diseases Society of America. *Clin Infect Dis* 2009;48(5):503-535.
12. Roseff SA, Sugar AM. Oral and esophageal candidiasis. In: Bodey GP (ed): *Candidiasis: Pathogenesis, Diagnosis, and Treatment*, 2nd ed. New York: Raven Press; 1993:185-203.
13. Kauffman CA. Candiduria. *Clin Infect Dis* 2005;41(Suppl 6): S371-S376.
14. Klevay MJ, Horn DL, Neofytos D, et al. Initial treatment and outcome of *Candida glabrata* versus *Candida albicans* bloodstream infection. *Diagn Microbiol Infect Dis* 2009;64(2): 152-157.
15. Horn DL, Neofytos D, Anaissie EJ, et al. Epidemiology and outcomes of candidemia in 2019 patients: Data from the prospective antifungal therapy alliance registry. *Clin Infect Dis* 2009;48(12):1695-1703.
16. Hachem R, Hanna H, Kontoyiannis D, et al. The changing epidemiology of invasive candidiasis: *Candida glabrata* and *Candida krusei* as the leading causes of candidemia in hematologic malignancy. *Cancer* 2008;112(11):2493-2499.

17. Krupova Y, Sejnova D, Dzatkova J, et al. Prospective study on fungemia in children with cancer: Analysis of 35 cases and comparison with 130 fungemias in adults. *Support Care Cancer* 2000;8(5):427-430.

18. Maksymiuk AW, Thongprasert S, Hopfer R, et al. Systemic candidiasis in cancer patients. *Am J Med* 1984;77(4D):20-27.

19. Kontoyiannis DP, Vaziri I, Hanna HA, et al. Risk factors for *Candida tropicalis* fungemia in patients with cancer. *Clin Infect Dis* 2001;33(10):1676-1681.

20. Dignani MC, Solomkin, JS, Anaissie EJ. Candida. In: Anaissie EJ, McGinnis MR, Pfaller MA, (ed): *Clinical Mycology*, 2nd ed. China: Churchill-Livingstone, Elsevier; 2009:197-229.

21. Bodey GP, Luna M. Skin lesions associated with disseminated candidiasis. *JAMA* 1974;229(11):1466-1468.

22. Bae GY, Lee HW, Chang SE, et al. Clinicopathologic review of 19 patients with systemic candidiasis with skin lesions. *Int J Dermatol* 2005;44(7):550-555.

23. Kontoyiannis DP, Luna MA, Samuels BI, et al. Hepatosplenic candidiasis. A manifestation of chronic disseminated candidiasis. *Infect Dis Clin North Am* 2000;14(3):721-739.

24. Kontoyiannis DP, Reddy BT, Torres HA, et al. Pulmonary candidiasis in patients with cancer: An autopsy study. *Clin Infect Dis* 2002;34(3):400-403.

25. Franquet T, Muller NL, Lee KS, et al. Pulmonary candidiasis after hematopoietic stem cell transplantation: Thin-section CT findings. *Radiology* 2005;236(1):332-337.

26. Chen S, Slavin M, Nguyen Q, et al. Active surveillance for candidemia, Australia. *Emerg Infect Dis* 2006;12(10):1508-1516.

27. van Hal SJ, Stark D, Harkness J, et al. *Candida dubliniensis* meningitis as delayed sequela of treated *C. dubliniensis* fungemia. *Emerg Infect Dis* 2008;14(2):327-329.

28. Atkinson BJ, Lewis RE, Kontoyiannis DP. *Candida lusitaniae* fungemia in cancer patients: Risk factors for amphotericin B failure and outcome. *Med Mycol* 2008;46(6):541-546.

29. Mora-Duarte J, Betts R, Rotstein C, et al. Comparison of caspofungin and amphotericin B for invasive candidiasis. *N Engl J Med* 2002;347(25):2020-2029.

30. Pappas PG, Rotstein CM, Betts RF, et al. Micafungin versus caspofungin for treatment of candidemia and other forms of invasive candidiasis. *Clin Infect Dis* 2007;45(7):883-893.

31. Girmenia C, Martino P, De Bernardis F, et al. Rising incidence of *Candida parapsilosis* fungemia in patients with hematologic malignancies: Clinical aspects, predisposing factors, and differential pathogenicity of the causative strains. *Clin Infect Dis* 1996;23(3):506-514.

32. Kuhn DM, George T, Chandra J, et al. Antifungal susceptibility of *Candida* biofilms: Unique efficacy of amphotericin B lipid formulations and echinocandins. *Antimicrob Agents Chemother* 2002;46(6):1773-1780.

33. Leventakos K, Lewis RE, Kontoyiannis DP. Fungal infections in leukemia patients: How do we prevent and treat them? *Clin Infect Dis* Feb 1 2010;50(3):405-415.

34. Kontoyiannis DP, Bodey GP. Invasive aspergillosis in 2002: An update. *Eur J Clin Microbiol Infect Dis* 2002;21(3):161-172.

35. Vonberg RP, Gastmeier P. Nosocomial aspergillosis in outbreak settings. *J Hosp Infect* 2006;63(3):246-254.

36. Upton A, Kirby KA, Carpenter P, et al. Invasive aspergillosis following hematopoietic cell transplantation: Outcomes and prognostic factors associated with mortality. *Clin Infect Dis* 2007;44(4):531-540.

37. Bodey GP, Vartivarian S. Aspergillosis. *Eur J Clin Microbiol Infect Dis* 1989;8(5):413-437.

38. Greene RE, Schlamm HT, Oestmann JW, et al. Imaging findings in acute invasive pulmonary aspergillosis: Clinical significance of the halo sign. *Clin Infect Dis* 2007;44(3):373-379.

39. Chamilos G, Marom EM, Lewis RE, et al. Predictors of pulmonary zygomycosis versus invasive pulmonary aspergillosis in patients with cancer. *Clin Infect Dis* 2005;41(1):60-66.

40. de Carpentier JP, Ramamurthy L, Denning DW, et al. An algorithmic approach to *Aspergillus* sinusitis. *J Laryngol Otol* 1994;108(4):314-318.

41. De Pauw B, Walsh TJ, Donnelly JP, et al. Revised definitions of invasive fungal disease from the European Organization for Research and Treatment of Cancer/Invasive Fungal Infections Cooperative Group and the National Institute of Allergy and Infectious Diseases Mycoses Study Group (EORTC/MSG) Consensus Group. *Clin Infect Dis* 2008;46(12):1813-1821.

42. Walsh TJ, Anaissie EJ, Denning DW, et al. Treatment of aspergillosis: Clinical practice guidelines of the Infectious Diseases Society of America. *Clin Infect Dis* 2008;46(3):327-360.

43. Allo MD, Miller J, Townsend T, et al. Primary cutaneous aspergillosis associated with Hickman intravenous catheters. *N Engl J Med* 1987;317(18):1105-1108.

44. Patterson TF, Kirkpatrick WR, White M, et al. Invasive aspergillosis. Disease spectrum, treatment practices, and outcomes. I3 *Aspergillus* Study Group. *Medicine* 2000;79(4):250-260.

45. Pagano L, Ricci P, Montillo M, et al. Localization of aspergillosis to the central nervous system among patients with acute leukemia: Report of 14 cases. Gruppo Italiano Malattie Ematologiche dell'Adulto Infection Program. *Clin Infect Dis* 1996;23(3):628-630.

46. Young RC, Bennett JE, Vogel CL, et al. Aspergillosis. The spectrum of the disease in 98 patients. *Medicine* 1970;49(2):147-173.

47. Mays SR, Bogle MA, Bodey GP. Cutaneous fungal infections in the oncology patient: Recognition and management. *Am J ClinDermatol* 2006;7(1):31-43.

48. Kontoyiannis DP, Sumoza D, Tarrand J, et al. Significance of aspergillemia in patients with cancer: A 10-year study. *Clin Infect Dis* 2000;31(1):188-189.

49. Tarrand JJ, Lichterfeld M, Warraich I, et al. Diagnosis of invasive septate mold infections. A correlation of microbiological culture and histologic or cytologic examination. *Am J Clin Pathol* 2003;119(6):854-858.

50. Pagano L, Caira M, Candoni A, et al. Invasive aspergillosis in patients with acute myeloid leukemia: SEIFEM-2008 registry study. *Haematologica* 2010;95(4):644-650.

51. Herbrecht R, Denning DW, Patterson TF, et al. Voriconazole versus amphotericin B for primary therapy of invasive aspergillosis. *N Engl J Med* 2002;347(6):408-415.

52. Raad, II, Hanna HA, Boktour M, et al. Novel antifungal agents as salvage therapy for invasive aspergillosis in patients with hematologic malignancies: Posaconazole compared with high-dose lipid formulations of amphotericin B alone or in combination with caspofungin. *Leukemia* 2008;22(3):496-503.

53. Thompson GR, 3rd, Rinaldi MG, Pennick G, et al. Posaconazole therapeutic drug monitoring: A reference laboratory experience. *Antimicrobial Agents Chemoth* 2009;53(5):2223-2224.

54. Arikan S, Rex JH. Lipid-based antifungal agents: Current status. *Curr Pharma Des* 2001;7(5):393-415.

55. Wingard JR. Lipid formulations of amphotericins: Are you a lumper or a splitter? *Clin Infect Dis* 2002;35(7):891-895.

56. Keating G, Figgitt D. Caspofungin: A review of its use in oesophageal candidiasis, invasive candidiasis and invasive aspergillosis. *Drugs* 2003;63(20):2235-2263.

57. Steinbach WJ, Stevens DA, Denning DW. Combination and sequential antifungal therapy for invasive aspergillosis: Review of published in vitro and in vivo interactions and 6281 clinical cases from 1966 to 2001. *Clin Infect Dis* 2003;37(Suppl 3): S188-S224.

58. Singh N, Limaye AP, Forrest G, et al. Combination of voriconazole and caspofungin as primary therapy for invasive aspergillosis in solid organ transplant recipients: A prospective, multicenter, observational study. *Transplantation* 2006;81(3): 320-326.

59. Kontoyiannis DP, Hachem R, Lewis RE, et al. Efficacy and toxicity of caspofungin in combination with liposomal amphotericin B as primary or salvage treatment of invasive aspergillosis in patients with hematologic malignancies. *Cancer* 2003; 98(2):292-299.

60. Chandrasekar P. Prophylaxis against *Aspergillus* is not perfect: Problems and perils in stem cell transplantation. *Med Mycol* 2009;47(Suppl 1):S349-S354.

61. Burgos A, Zaoutis TE, Dvorak CC, et al. Pediatric invasive aspergillosis: A multicenter retrospective analysis of 139 contemporary cases. *Pediatrics* 2008;121(5):e1286-e1294.

62. Salerno CT, Ouyang DW, Pederson TS, et al. Surgical therapy for pulmonary aspergillosis in immunocompromised patients. *Ann Thorac Surg* 1998;65(5):1415-1419.

63. Yeghen T, Kibbler CC, Prentice HG, et al. Management of invasive pulmonary aspergillosis in hematology patients: A review of 87 consecutive cases at a single institution. *Clin Infect Dis* 2000;31(4):859-868.

64. Mirza SA, Phelan M, Rimland D, et al. The changing epidemiology of cryptococcosis: An update from population-based active surveillance in 2 large metropolitan areas, 1992-2000. *Clin Infect Dis* 2003;36(6):789-794.

65. Kontoyiannis DP, Peitsch WK, Reddy BT, et al. Cryptococcosis in patients with cancer. *Clin Infect Dis* 2001;32(11): E145-E150.

66. Pappas PG, Perfect JR, Cloud GA, et al. Cryptococcosis in human immunodeficiency virus-negative patients in the era of effective azole therapy. *Clin Infect Dis* 2001;33(5): 690-699.

67. Chang WC, Tzao C, Hsu HH, et al. Pulmonary cryptococcosis: Comparison of clinical and radiographic characteristics in immunocompetent and immunocompromised patients. *Chest* 2006;129(2):333-340.

68. Gupta SK, Sarosi GA. Cryptococcal meningitis. *Curr Opin Infect Dis* 2002;4:503-511.

69. Westerink MA, Amsterdam D, Petell RJ, et al. Septicemia due to DF-2. Cause of a false-positive cryptococcal latex agglutination result. *Am J Med* 1987;83(1):155-158.

70. Campbell CK, Payne AL, Teall AJ, et al. Cryptococcal latex antigen test positive in patient with *Trichosporon beigelii* infection. *Lancet* 1985;2(8445):43-44.

71. Saag MS, Graybill RJ, Larsen RA, et al. Practice guidelines for the management of cryptococcal disease. Infectious Diseases Society of America. *Clin Infect Dis* 2000;30(4):710-718.

72. Sun HY, Wagener MM, Singh N. Cryptococcosis in solid-organ, hematopoietic stem cell, and tissue transplant recipients: Evidence-based evolving trends. *Clin Infect Dis* 2009;48(11): 1566-1576.

73. Kontoyiannis DP, Lewis RE, Alexander BD, et al. Calcineurin inhibitor agents interact synergistically with antifungal agents in vitro against *Cryptococcus neoformans* isolates: Correlation with outcome in solid organ transplant recipients with cryptococcosis. *Antimicrobial Agents Chemother* 2008; 52(2):735-738.

74. Graybill JR, Sobel J, Saag M, et al. Diagnosis and management of increased intracranial pressure in patients with AIDS and cryptococcal meningitis. The NIAID Mycoses Study Group and AIDS Cooperative Treatment Groups. *Clin Infect Dis* 2000;30(1):47-54.

75. Nucci M, Anaissie E. *Fusarium* infections in immunocompromised patients. *Clin Microbiol Rev* 2007;20(4):695-704.

76. Lionakis MS, Kontoyiannis DP. *Fusarium* infections in critically ill patients. *Semin Respir Crit Care Med* 2004;25(2): 159-169.

77. Bodey GP, Boktour M, Mays S, et al. Skin lesions associated with *Fusarium* infection. *J Am Acad Dermatol* 2002;47(5): 659-666.

78. Kontoyiannis DP, Bodey GP, Hanna H, et al. Outcome determinants of fusariosis in a tertiary care cancer center: The impact of neutrophil recovery. *Leuk Lymphoma* 2004;45(1): 139-141.

79. Kontoyiannis DP, Torres HA, Chagua M, et al. Trichosporonosis in a tertiary care cancer center: Risk factors, changing spectrum and determinants of outcome. *Scand J Infect Dis* 2004;36(8):564-569.

80. Groll AH, Walsh TJ. Uncommon opportunistic fungi: New nosocomial threats. *Clin Microbiol Infect* 2001;7 (Suppl 2): 8-24.

81. Walsh TJ. Trichosporonosis. *Infect Dis Clin North Am* 1989;3(1):43-52.

82. Girmenia C, Pagano L, Martino B, et al. Invasive infections caused by *Trichosporon* species and *Geotrichum capitatum* in patients with hematological malignancies: A retrospective multicenter study from Italy and review of the literature. *J Clin Microbiol* 2005;43(4):1818-1828.

83. Walsh TJ, Melcher GP, Lee JW, et al. Infections due to *Trichosporon* species: New concepts in mycology, pathogenesis, diagnosis and treatment. *Curr Top Med Mycol* 1993;5: 79-113.

84. Anaissie EJ, Hachem R, Karyotakis NC, et al. Comparative efficacies of amphotericin B, triazoles, and combination of both as experimental therapy for murine trichosporonosis. *Antimicrob Agents Chemotherapy* 1994;38(11):2541-2544.

85. Roden MM, Zaoutis TE, Buchanan WL, et al. Epidemiology and outcome of zygomycosis: A review of 929 reported cases. *Clin Infect Dis* 2005;41(5):634-653.

86. Spellberg B, Edwards J, Jr., Ibrahim A. Novel perspectives on mucormycosis: Pathophysiology, presentation, and management. *Clin Microbiol Rev* 2005;18(3):556-569.

87. Kontoyiannis DP, Wessel VC, Bodey GP, et al. Zygomycosis in the 1990s in a tertiary-care cancer center. *Clin Infect Dis* 2000;30(6):851-856.

88. Spellberg B, Walsh TJ, Kontoyiannis DP, et al. Recent advances in the management of mucormycosis: From bench to bedside. *Clin Infect Dis* 2009;48(12):1743-1751.

89. Torres HA, Rivero GA, Kontoyiannis DP. Endemic mycoses in a cancer hospital. *Medicine* 2002;81(3):201-212.

90. Kauffman CA. Endemic mycoses in patients with hematologic malignancies. *Semin Respir Infect* 2002;17(2):106-112.

91. Freifeld AG, Wheat LJ, Kaul DR. Histoplasmosis in solid organ transplant recipients: Early diagnosis and treatment. *Curr Opin Organ Transplant* 2009;14(6):601-605.

92. Wheat LJ, Freifeld AG, Kleiman MB, et al. Clinical practice guidelines for the management of patients with histoplasmosis: 2007 update by the Infectious Diseases Society of America. *Clin Infect Dis* 2007;45(7):807-825.

93. Freifeld A, Proia L, Andes D, et al. Voriconazole use for endemic fungal infections. *Antimicrob Agents Chemother* 2009;53(4):1648-1651.

94. Galgiani JN, Ampel NM, Blair JE, et al. Coccidioidomycosis. *Clin Infect Dis* 2005;41(9):1217-1223.

95. Strauss RG. Clinical perspectives of granulocyte transfusions: Efficacy to date. *J Clin Apher* 1995;10(3):114-118.

96. Drewniak A, Kuijpers TW. Granulocyte transfusion therapy: Randomization after all? *Haematologica* 2009;94(12):1644-1648.

97. Safdar A. Strategies to enhance immune function in hematopoietic transplantation recipients who have fungal infections. *Bone Marrow Transplant* 2006;38(5):327-337.

98. Gaviria JM, van Burik JA, Dale DC, et al. Comparison of interferon-gamma, granulocyte colony-stimulating factor, and granulocyte-macrophage colony-stimulating factor for priming leukocyte-mediated hyphal damage of opportunistic fungal pathogens. *J Infect Dis* 1999;179(4):1038-1041.

99. Bodey GP, Anaissie E, Gutterman J, et al. Role of granulocyte-macrophage colony-stimulating factor as adjuvant treatment in neutropenic patients with bacterial and fungal infection. *Eur J Clin Microbiol Infect Dis* 1994;13(Suppl 2):S18-S22.

100. Bustamante CI, Wade JC. Herpes simplex virus infection in the immunocompromised cancer patient. *J Clin Oncol* 1991;9(10):1903-1915.

101. Meyers JD, Flournoy N, Thomas ED. Infection with herpes simplex virus and cell-mediated immunity after marrow transplant. *J Infect Dis* 1980;142(3):338-346.

102. Saral R, Ambinder RF, Burns WH, et al. Acyclovir prophylaxis against herpes simplex virus infection in patients with leukemia. A randomized, double-blind, placebo-controlled study. *Ann Intern Med* 1983;99(6):773-776.

103. Angarone M, Ison MG. Prevention and early treatment of opportunistic viral infections in patients with leukemia and allogeneic stem cell transplantation recipients. *J Natl Compr Canc Netw* 2008;6(2):191-201.

104. Aisenberg GM, Torres HA, Tarrand J, et al. Herpes simplex virus lower respiratory tract infection in patients with solid tumors. *Cancer* 2009;115(1):199-206.

105. Wade JC, Newton B, Flournoy N, et al. Oral acyclovir for prevention of herpes simplex virus reactivation after marrow transplantation. *Ann Intern Med* 1984;100(6):823-828.

106. Zaia J, Baden L, Boeckh MJ, et al. Viral disease prevention after hematopoietic cell transplantation. *Bone Marrow Transplant* 2009;44(8):471-482.

107. Erard V, Wald A, Corey L, et al. Use of long-term suppressive acyclovir after hematopoietic stem-cell transplantation: Impact on herpes simplex virus (HSV) disease and drug-resistant HSV disease. *J Infect Dis* 2007;196(2):266-270.

108. Feldman S, Lott L. Varicella in children with cancer: Impact of antiviral therapy and prophylaxis. *Pediatrics* 1987;80(4):465-472.

109. Tyring S, Barbarash RA, Nahlik JE, et al. Famciclovir for the treatment of acute herpes zoster: Effects on acute disease and postherpetic neuralgia. A randomized, double-blind, placebo-controlled trial. Collaborative Famciclovir Herpes Zoster Study Group. *Ann Intern Med* 1995;123(2):89-96.

110. Gershon AA, Steinberg SP. Persistence of immunity to varicella in children with leukemia immunized with live attenuated varicella vaccine. *N Engl J Med* 1989;320(14):892-897.

111. Hardy I, Gershon AA, Steinberg SP, et al. The incidence of zoster after immunization with live attenuated varicella vaccine. A study in children with leukemia. Varicella Vaccine Collaborative Study Group. *N Engl J Med* 1991;325(22):1545-1550.

112. Torres HA, Kontoyiannis DP, Bodey GP, et al. Gastrointestinal cytomegalovirus disease in patients with cancer: A two decade experience in a tertiary care cancer center. *Eur J Cancer* 2005;41(15):2268-2279.

113. Torres HA, Aguilera E, Safdar A, et al. Fatal cytomegalovirus pneumonia in patients with haematological malignancies: An autopsy-based case-control study. *Clin Microbiol Infect* 2008;14(12):1160-1166.

114. Chemaly RF, Torres HA, Hachem RY, et al. Cytomegalovirus pneumonia in patients with lymphoma. *Cancer* 2005;104(6):1213-1220.

115. O'Brien S, Ravandi F, Riehl T, et al. Valganciclovir prevents cytomegalovirus reactivation in patients receiving alemtuzumab-based therapy. *Blood* 2008;111(4):1816-1819.

116. Junghanss C, Boeckh M, Carter RA, et al. Incidence and outcome of cytomegalovirus infections following nonmyeloablative compared with myeloablative allogeneic stem cell transplantation, a matched control study. *Blood* 2002;99(6):1978-1985.

117. Nakamae H, Kirby KA, Sandmaier BM, et al. Effect of conditioning regimen intensity on CMV infection in allogeneic hematopoietic cell transplantation. *Biol Blood Marrow Transplant* 2009;15(6):694-703.

118. Fries BC, Riddell SR, Kim HW, et al. Cytomegalovirus disease before hematopoietic cell transplantation as a risk for complications after transplantation. *Biol Blood Marrow Transplant* 2005;11(2):136-148.

119. van der Bij W, Schirm J, Torensma R, et al. Comparison between viremia and antigenemia for detection of cytomegalovirus in blood. *J Clin Microbiol* 1988;26(12):2531-2535.

120. Boeckh M, Ljungman P. How we treat cytomegalovirus in hematopoietic cell transplant recipients. *Blood* 2009;113(23):5711-5719.

121. Gerna G, Furione M, Baldanti F, et al. Quantitation of human cytomegalovirus DNA in bone marrow transplant recipients. *Br J Haematol* 1995;91(3):674-683.

122. Winston DJ, Young JA, Pullarkat V, et al. Maribavir prophylaxis for prevention of cytomegalovirus infection in allogeneic stem cell transplant recipients: A multicenter, randomized, double-blind, placebo-controlled, dose-ranging study. *Blood* 2008;111(11):5403-5410.

123. Wade JC. Viral infections in patients with hematological malignancies. Hematology/the Education Program of the American Society of Hematology American Society of Hematology 2006:368-374.

124. Wang FZ, Dahl H, Linde A, et al. Lymphotropic herpesviruses in allogeneic bone marrow transplantation. *Blood* 1996;88(9):3615-3620.

125. Wang FZ, Linde A, Hagglund H, et al. Human herpesvirus 6 DNA in cerebrospinal fluid specimens from allogeneic bone marrow transplant patients: Does it have clinical significance? *Clin Infect Dis* 1999;28(3):562-568.

126. Styczynski J, Einsele H, Gil L, Ljungman P. Outcome of treatment of Epstein-Barr virus-related post-transplant lymphoproliferative disorder in hematopoietic stem cell recipients: A comprehensive review of reported cases. *Transpl Infect Dis* 2009;11(5):383-392.

127. Milpied N, Vasseur B, Parquet N, et al. Humanized anti-CD20 monoclonal antibody (rituximab) in post transplant B-lymphoproliferative disorder: A retrospective analysis on 32 patients. *Ann Oncol* 2000;11(Suppl 1):113-116.

128. van Esser JW, Niesters HG, van der Holt B, et al. Prevention of Epstein-Barr virus-lymphoproliferative disease by molecular monitoring and preemptive rituximab in high-risk patients after allogeneic stem cell transplantation. *Blood* 2002;99(12):4364-4369.

129. Heslop HE, Slobod KS, Pule MA, et al. Long term outcome of EBV specific T-cell infusions to prevent or treat EBV-related lymphoproliferative disease in transplant recipients. *Blood* 2010;115(5):925-935.

130. Chemaly RF, Ghosh S, Bodey GP, et al. Respiratory viral infections in adults with hematologic malignancies and human stem cell transplantation recipients: A retrospective study at a major cancer center. *Medicine* 2006;85(5):278-287.

131. Couch RB, Englund JA, Whimbey E. Respiratory viral infections in immunocompetent and immunocompromised persons. *Am J Med* 1997;102(3A):2-9; discussion 25-26.

132. Gooskens J, Jonges M, Claas EC, et al. Prolonged influenza virus infection during lymphocytopenia and frequent detection of drug-resistant viruses. *J Infect Dis* 2009;199(10):1435-1441.

133. Milano F, Campbell AP, Guthrie KA, et al. Human rhinovirus and coronavirus detection among allogeneic hematopoietic stem cell transplantation recipients. *Blood* 2010;115(10):2088-2094.

134. Boeckh M. The challenge of respiratory virus infections in hematopoietic cell transplant recipients. *Br J Haematol* 2008;143(4):455-467.

135. Manning A, Russell V, Eastick K, et al. Epidemiological profile and clinical associations of human bocavirus and other human parvoviruses. *J Infect Dis* 2006;194(9):1283-1290.

136. Schenk T, Strahm B, Kontny U, et al. Disseminated bocavirus infection after stem cell transplant. *Emerg Infect Dis* 2007;13(9):1425-1427.

137. van den Hoogen BG, de Jong JC, Groen J, et al. A newly discovered human pneumovirus isolated from young children with respiratory tract disease. *Nat Med* 2001;7(6):719-724.

138. Walsh EE, Peterson DR, Falsey AR. Human metapneumovirus infections in adults: Another piece of the puzzle. *Arch Intern Med* 2008;168(22):2489-2496.

139. Englund JA, Boeckh M, Kuypers J, et al. Brief communication: Fatal human metapneumovirus infection in stem-cell transplant recipients. *Ann Intern Med* 2006;144(5):344-349.

140. Kamboj M, Gerbin M, Huang CK, et al. Clinical characterization of human metapneumovirus infection among patients with cancer. *J Infect* 2008;57(6):464-471.

141. Oliveira R, Machado A, Tateno A, et al. Frequency of human metapneumovirus infection in hematopoietic SCT recipients during 3 consecutive years. *Bone Marrow Transplant* 2008;42(4):265-269.

142. Centers for Disease Control and Prevention (CDC). Swine influenza A (H1N1) infection in two children—Southern California, March-April 2009. *MMWR Morb Mortal Wkly Rep* 2009;58(15):400-402.

143. Louie JK, Acosta M, Winter K, et al. Factors associated with death or hospitalization due to pandemic 2009 influenza A(H1N1) infection in California. *JAMA* 2009;302(17):1896-1902.

144. Casper C, Englund J, Boeckh M. How we treat influenza in patients with hematologic malignancies. *Blood* 2010;115(7):1331-1342.

145. Centers for Disease Control and Prevention (CDC). Oseltamivir-resistant 2009 pandemic influenza A (H1N1) virus infection in two summer campers receiving prophylaxis—North Carolina, 2009. *MMWR Morb Mortal Wkly Rep* 2009;58(35):969-972.

146. Schiffer JT, Kirby K, Sandmaier B, et al. Timing and severity of community acquired respiratory virus infections after myeloablative versus non-myeloablative hematopoietic stem cell transplantation. *Haematologica* 2009;94(8):1101-1108.

147. Torres HA, Aguilera EA, Mattiuzzi GN, et al. Characteristics and outcome of respiratory syncytial virus infection in patients with leukemia. *Haematologica* 2007;92(9):1216-1223.

148. Chemaly RF, Torres HA, Aguilera EA, et al. Neuraminidase inhibitors improve outcome of patients with leukemia and influenza: An observational study. *Clin Infect Dis* 2007;44(7):964-967.

149. Kaiser L, Wat C, Mills T, et al. Impact of oseltamivir treatment on influenza-related lower respiratory tract complications and hospitalizations. *Arch Intern Med* 2003;163(14):1667-1672.

150. Georgescu G, Chemaly RF. Palivizumab: Where to from here? *Expert Opin Biol Ther* 2009;9(1):139-147.

151. Simpson ND, Simpson PW, Ahmed AM, et al. Prophylaxis against chemotherapy-induced reactivation of hepatitis B virus infection with Lamivudine. *J Clin Gastroenterol* 2003;37(1):68-71.

152. Picardi M, Selleri C, De Rosa G, et al. Lamivudine treatment for chronic replicative hepatitis B virus infection after allogeneic bone marrow transplantation. *Bone Marrow Transplant* 1998;21(12):1267-1269.

153. Ghany MG, Strader DB, Thomas DL, et al. Diagnosis, management, and treatment of hepatitis C: An update. *Hepatology* 2009;49(4):1335-1374.

154. Zuckerman E, Zuckerman T, Levine AM, et al. Hepatitis C virus infection in patients with B-cell non-Hodgkin lymphoma. *Ann Intern Med* 1997;127(6):423-428.

155. Izumi T, Sasaki R, Tsunoda S, et al. B cell malignancy and hepatitis C virus infection. *Leukemia* 1997;11(Suppl 3):516-518.

156. La Rosa AM, Champlin RE, Mirza N, et al. Adenovirus infections in adult recipients of blood and marrow transplants. *Clin Infect Dis* 2001;32(6):871-876.

157. Baldwin A, Kingman H, Darville M, et al. Outcome and clinical course of 100 patients with adenovirus infection following bone marrow transplantation. *Bone Marrow Transplant* 2000;26(12):1333-1338.

158. Chakrabarti S, Mautner V, Osman H, et al. Adenovirus infections following allogeneic stem cell transplantation: Incidence and outcome in relation to graft manipulation, immunosuppression, and immune recovery. *Blood* 2002;100(5):1619-1627.

159. Kojaoghlanian T, Flomenberg P, Horwitz MS. The impact of adenovirus infection on the immunocompromised host. *Rev Med Virol* 2003;13(3):155-171.

160. Schilham MW, Claas EC, van Zaane W, et al. High levels of adenovirus DNA in serum correlate with fatal outcome of adenovirus infection in children after allogeneic stem-cell transplantation. *Clin Infect Dis* 2002;35(5):526-532.

161. Ison MG. Adenovirus infections in transplant recipients. *Clin Infect Dis* 2006;43(3):331-339.

162. Ljungman P, Ribaud P, Eyrich M, et al. Cidofovir for adenovirus infections after allogeneic hematopoietic stem cell transplantation: A survey by the Infectious Diseases Working Party of the European Group for Blood and Marrow Transplantation. *Bone Marrow Transplant* 2003;31(6):481-486.

163. Feuchtinger T, Matthes-Martin S, Richard C, et al. Safe adoptive transfer of virus-specific T-cell immunity for the treatment of systemic adenovirus infection after allogeneic stem cell transplantation. *Br J Haematol* 2006;134(1):64-76.

164. Chisaka H, Morita E, Yaegashi N, et al. Parvovirus B19 and the pathogenesis of anaemia. *Rev Med Virol* 2003;13(6):347-359.

165. Kuo SH, Lin LI, Chang CJ, et al. Increased risk of parvovirus B19 infection in young adult cancer patients receiving multiple courses of chemotherapy. *J Clin Microbiol* 2002;40(11):3909-3912.

166. Eid AJ, Brown RA, Patel R, et al. Parvovirus B19 infection after transplantation: A review of 98 cases. *Clin Infect Dis* 2006;43(1):40-48.

167. Torres HA, Chemaly RF. Viral infection or reactivation in patients during treatment with dasatinib: A call for screening? *Leuk Lymphoma* 2007;48(12):2308-2309.

168. Reploeg MD, Storch GA, Clifford DB. Bk virus: A clinical review. *Clin Infect Dis* 2001;33(2):191-202.

169. Cesaro S, Hirsch HH, Faraci M, et al. Cidofovir for BK virus-associated hemorrhagic cystitis: A retrospective study. *Clin Infect Dis* 2009;49(2):233-240.

170. Carson KR, Focosi D, Major EO, et al. Monoclonal antibody-associated progressive multifocal leucoencephalopathy in patients treated with rituximab, natalizumab, and efalizumab: A review from the Research on Adverse Drug Events and Reports (RADAR) Project. *Lancet Oncol* 2009;10(8):816-824.

171. Garcia-Suarez J, de Miguel D, Krsnik I, et al. Changes in the natural history of progressive multifocal leukoencephalopathy in HIV-negative lymphoproliferative disorders: Impact of novel therapies. *Am J Hematol* 2005;80(4):271-281.

172. Pelosini M, Focosi D, Rita F, et al. Progressive multifocal leukoencephalopathy: Report of three cases in HIV-negative hematological patients and review of literature. *Ann Hematol* 2008;87(5):405-412.

ENDOCRINE AND METABOLIC COMPLICATIONS OF CANCER THERAPY

Mouhammed Amir Habra
Naifa Lamki Busaidy
Sai-Ching Jim Yeung
Rena Vassilopoulou-Sellin

In the past two decades, cancer research has rapidly advanced, spurred by the development of high throughput technology and the maturation of genomic and proteomic research methods. These advances have resulted in treatments that have substantial effects on the outcomes of certain cancers. The continuous development of new antineoplastic agents adds increasing challenges to practicing physicians.

Current cancer treatments include surgery, radiation, cytotoxic chemotherapy, hormonal therapy, bioimmunotherapy, and targeted therapy. Adverse effects of antineoplastic agents on the endocrine system are caused by several different mechanisms and can range from a subtle laboratory abnormality with limited clinical significance to a clinical syndrome with significant morbidity. Antineoplastic agents in general can be cytotoxic to endocrine cells and result in glandular dysfunction. Antineoplastic agents can also interfere with the synthesis or postsynthesis processing of hormones at different levels (ie, transcription, translation, or posttranslation). An agent may inhibit or induce secretion of a hormone by interacting with receptors, perturbating intracellular second messenger metabolism or may affect hormone delivery by changing carrier protein levels in serum or by competing for binding on the carrier protein. Finally, antineoplastic agents can interact with signal transduction pathway to inhibit or enhance hormonal action in the end organs.

In this chapter, we summarize the major and common endocrine complications of cancer therapy and discuss screening and surveillance of these complications in cancer patients and survivors.

■ METABOLIC DISORDERS

GLUCOSE METABOLISM

Diabetes Mellitus

Serum glucose is under continuous complex regulation. Many processes can affect glucose levels, including gut absorption, cellular uptake, gluconeogenesis, and glycogenolysis. Multiple hormones also play important roles in overall glucose homeostasis, including insulin, glucagon, growth hormone (GH), cortisol, somatostatin, and incretins.

Glucocorticoids are frequently used with many chemotherapy protocols and can have profound effects on glucose levels by increasing insulin resistance. Glucocorticoids can unmask preexisting prediabetic states by precipitating overt diabetes or make diabetes more difficult to control. The severity may range from

asymptomatic hyperglycemia to nonketotic hyperosmolar coma. Most patients taking glucocorticoids with elevated glucose may require insulin therapy to achieve blood glucose control, especially when given high-dose steroids. Long-acting and intermediate-acting insulin formulations are more effective at controlling glucose levels when they are combined with meal time rapid-acting or short-acting insulins than are regimens that use short-acting insulin alone on the basis of sliding scales. Currently, there are no evidence-based specific guidelines for the management of steroid-induced diabetes mellitus in cancer patients. Recent concerns about promotion of malignancy by the mitogenic effect of insulin (1,2) and especially insulin analogues (3) which cross-activate IGF-1 receptors (4) but conflicting clinical study results about glargine and cancer (5,6) have brought attention to the gap in knowledge about the proper diabetic management strategy for cancer patients and survivors to maximize their survival.

Temsirolimus, L-asparaginase, streptozocin, and interferon-alpha (IFNα) are other antineoplastic agents that have been associated with impaired glucose homeostasis or frank diabetes mellitus.

Temsirolimus is an inhibitor of mTOR. It may cause secondary diabetes in 10 to 30% of renal cell carcinoma patients (7,8). The mechanism by which temsirolimus leads to diabetes may be similar to that of tacrolimus which decreases glucose-stimulated insulin release in the pancreatic islets by reducing ATP production and glycolysis (9).

L-**asparaginase** is an enzyme derived from *Escherichia coli* or *Erwinia* species that inhibits protein synthesis by depleting L-asparagine. This drug is mainly used in the treatment of hematologic malignancies. Pegaspargase is formed by the linking of monomethoxy-polyethylene glycol to *E coli* asparaginase to decrease immunogenicity. Pegylated *E coli* asparaginase has been reported to have a similar risk of hyperglycemia compared with native asparaginase; in one study, the risk was about 5% in children with acute lymphoblastic leukemia treated with either agent (10).

The exact mechanism of hyperglycemia is not known, although it has been postulated that inhibition of insulin, insulin receptor synthesis, or both may be the cause, leading to a combined insulin deficiency and resistance syndrome. Pancreatitis, which might occur with L-asparaginase therapy, is another possible mechanism for hyperglycemia through islet cell destruction.

Hyperglycemia and glycosuria without ketonemia occurs in 1 to 14% of patients treated with L-asparaginase, an effect that is reversible upon discontinuation of the drug (11-13). Insulin therapy is frequently required.

One potential complication is hypoglycemia after cessation of L-asparaginase, thus, close monitoring of blood glucose is recommended. Diabetic ketoacidosis has been reported during L-asparaginase therapy (13,14). Long-term insulin therapy may not be needed in all cases of L-asparaginase–induced diabetes mellitus.

Streptozocin is an *N*-nitrosourea derivative of glucosamide that is primarily used to treat malignant islet cell tumors and other neuroendocrine tumors. Pancreatic β cells exposed to streptozocin develop long-lasting impairment to the production and release of insulin, although other cell functions are better preserved. Streptozocin's effect on islet cells is species-specific and dose-related; rat islet cells appear to be more susceptible to the cytotoxic effects of streptozocin than do human islet cells. Most of streptozocin's effects are reversible upon discontinuation of the drug. Although the reported incidence of glucose intolerance varies from 6 to 60%, most cases are mild to moderate in severity (15-17).

Interferon-alpha: Use of recombinant IFNα-2a and -2b to treat malignancies has been associated with the development of hyperglycemia in patients without diabetes and deterioration of glycemic control in diabetics. Although the incidence of IFNα-induced diabetes mellitus in patients with cancer is unclear, the incidence of diabetes mellitus is about 0.7% among patients who have received high-dose IFNα for chronic active hepatitis C (18). Diabetic ketoacidosis has been reported in a variety of conditions treated with IFNα-2 (19,20). The exact mechanism of IFNα-induced diabetes is not well known. IFNα acts as an immunomodulatory agent, inducing autoantibody production and the development of autoimmune disease in susceptible patients, but in a study of 58 patients who received IFNα for treatment of chronic, active hepatitis C, neither islet cell antibodies nor type I diabetes mellitus developed during IFNα therapy, though hemoglobin-A1c levels increased in two patients (21). IFNs may also directly inhibit preproinsulin synthesis in islet β cells and thus contribute to insulin deficiency (22). Ironically some reports postulated that IFNα may preserve residual β-cell function in newly diagnosed type I diabetes (23). Insulin resistance is thought to contribute to diabetes mellitus in patients with hepatitis, and IFNα therapy may improve insulin sensitivity.

Glucosuria

Some antineoplastic drugs (eg, ifosfamide and mercaptopurine) cause a proximal tubular defect and lower the renal threshold for glucosuria without affecting glucose metabolism. 2-Mercaptoethane sulfonate sodium (MESNA) is often used with ifosfamide to decrease the incidence of hemorrhagic cystitis and has been reported to give a false-positive reaction for urinary ketones.

LIPID DISORDERS

Lipid disorders are seldom evaluated in the process of active anticancer therapy as patients are often encouraged to maintain a positive metabolic balance via liberal oral intake. Investigation or treatment of mild lipid abnormalities is often overlooked because the focus is on maintaining a positive caloric balance during cancer treatment. Some lipid disorders may be short-lived without clear clinical consequences, but some may be of clinical importance and need to be detected and treated. In general, triglyceride levels higher than 1000 mg/dL increase the rate of complications, including pancreatitis and visual impairment, and need to be treated urgently.

Hypertriglyceridemia

IFNs may induce hypertriglyceridemia by increasing hepatic and peripheral fatty acid production and suppressing hepatic triglyceride lipase. Elevation of serum triglyceride levels to more than 1000 mg/dL can occur. In one case, a controlled diet and gemfibrozil had therapeutic effects despite continued IFNα therapy (24).

All-trans retinoic acid (tretinoin) and other retinoic acid derivatives have been used in the treatment of several malignancies including head and neck cancer and acute promyelocytic leukemia. They are well known to induce hypertriglyceridemia with elevated very-low-density lipoprotein (VLDL) (25-29) and hypercholesterolemia associated with increased low-density lipoproteins (LDL). Cerebrovascular accidents and pancreatitis have been described in association with retinoid-induced hypertriglyceridemia.

Bexarotene is a synthetic retinoid X receptor (RXR)-selective retinoid used in the treatment of cutaneous T-cell lymphoma. Hypertriglyceridemia is the most frequent drug-related adverse effect and occurred in 79% of patients (30,31). Hypertriglyceridemia is considered a dose-limiting toxicity, with three reported cases of pancreatitis during phase II/III trials. These three patients were taking 300 mg/m^2 or more of oral bexarotene per day and had triglyceride levels higher than 1300 mg/dL (31). Retinoid-induced hyperlipidemia has been successfully treated with fibrates or fish oil.

Hypercholesterolemia

Dose-related hypercholesterolemia has been described in patients with adrenocortical carcinoma treated with mitotane (32); inhibition of cholesterol oxidase is the likely mechanism. Patients with adrenocortical carcinoma usually have a poor prognosis, making mild to moderate elevation of cholesterol of less clinical importance, but in long-term (5-10 year) survivors, continued mitotane therapy can lead to early development of atherosclerotic disease. In long-term survivors, the benefits of treating mitotane-induced lipid abnormalities have not been established.

Hypercholesterolemia is the second most common side effect of bexarotene and has been reported in 48% of treated patients (31). The long-term significance of this drug-induced hypercholesterolemia is unclear; however, atorvastatin has been successfully used in patients at our institution.

Serum cholesterol and low-density lipoprotein cholesterol were increased in 41% of patients with germ cell tumors treated with cisplatin-containing chemotherapy regimens; the long-term significance of this is also not clear (33).

WATER AND ELECTROLYTES DISORDERS

Serum osmolality is tightly regulated, primarily by the interaction of the hypothalamic osmoreceptors that regulate secretion of antidiuretic hormone from cells in the paraventricular and supraoptic nuclei, the hypothalamic thirst center, and the kidneys. The disruption of any of the above mentioned regulators may lead to a disturbance in free water clearance and subsequent abnormalities in serum sodium levels.

Syndrome of Inappropriate Antidiuretic Hormone Secretion and Hyponatremia

Hyponatremia is a relatively common electrolyte abnormality in patients with cancer. The syndrome of inappropriate antidiuretic hormone (SIADH) secretion is one of the most common underlying causes for hyponatremia in this patient population. This syndrome is characterized by hyponatremia, low serum osmolality, and an inappropriately high urine osmolality with elevated urine sodium in the absence of diuretics use, heart failure, cirrhosis, adrenal insufficiency, or hypothyroidism. In patients with cancer, SIADH may be caused by ectopic antidiuretic hormone (ADH) production by a variety of tumors. This is most commonly seen in patients with small cell lung cancer (SCLC). Other tumors

are rarely described in association with SIADH and include malignant thymoma, oral squamous cell carcinoma, prostate carcinoma, and pancreatic carcinoma. Chemotherapy-induced lysis of ADH-containing cancer cells may lead to more severe hyponatremia at the time of chemotherapy induction.

Other factors that may increase ADH secretion include nausea, pain, narcotics, nicotine, and antineoplastic agents such as high-dose intravenous cyclophosphamide, vincristine, vinblastine, and cisplatin.

SIADH is a diagnosis of exclusion after ruling out hypovolemia, adrenal insufficiency, hypothyroidism, renal insufficiency, congestive heart failure, cirrhosis, and rarely, cerebral salt-wasting syndrome.

In cases of hyponatremia secondary to SIADH, urine osmolality is higher than plasma osmolality, and urine sodium is determined by sodium intake. Urine sodium is usually higher than 40 mEq/L in patients with SIADH. Fluid restriction (usually 700-1200 mL of free water a day), increasing salt intake, and occasionally loop diuretics are usually attempted first in most cases of SIADH when the patient is asymptomatic or having mild symptoms. In the presence of severe symptoms (seizures or obtundation), hypertonic saline infusions might be needed with close and frequent monitoring of sodium levels to avoid rapid correction and possible central pontine myelinolysis. Demeclocycline (600-1200 mg/day) can be used in few cases in which hyponatremia do not respond to more conservative treatments. Vasopressin receptor (V2) antagonists are still being evaluated in clinical trials, but carry the potential of being a more specific therapy for cases of SIADH.

Diabetes Insipidus and Hypernatremia

Central diabetes insipidus can happen after brain surgery and occasionally in cases of tumors invading the neurohypophysis or disrupting the pituitary stalk. These cases are often recognized by a clinical presentation of polyuria, polydipsia in patients who have undergone recent brain or pituitary surgery or who have known tumors near the sella or the hypothalamus. These cases are usually treated with 1-desamino-8-delta-arginine vasopressin (DDAVP) (subcutaneously, intranasally, or orally) to control the symptoms and correct the hypernatremia.

Nephrogenic diabetes insipidus (DI) can occur in patients with cancer. Multiple antineoplastic agents have been described in association with this syndrome. Ifosfamide is well known to induce renal tubular damage at the level of the proximal renal tubules and to a lesser extent, the distal renal tubules, where it has been found to induce nephrogenic DI. Streptozocin has also been reported to cause nephrogenic DI.

Another common cause of hypernatremia in patients with cancer is the failure to deliver enough free water, especially when patients are on parenteral or tube feeding regimens or are too debilitated to obtain water for themselves.

■ DISORDERS OF BONE AND MINERAL METABOLISM

OSTEOPOROSIS

Normal bone remodeling requires a delicate balance between bone formation by osteoblasts and bone resorption by osteoclasts. Antineoplastic therapy may affect this balance by increasing the activity of osteoclasts (eg, interleukin-2) and sometimes by having direct toxic effects on osteoblast function. Hormones and cytokines (ie, ACTH, PTH, PTH-related peptide and interleukin-1) can also affect the overall bone turnover rate. Malnutrition and poor calcium and vitamin D intake may be major factors affecting bone turnover in patients with cancer.

Antineolastic agents have been implicated in chemotherapy-associated osteoporosis. Prolonged therapy with oral methotrexate for acute lymphoblastic leukemia (ALL) has led to distal extremity pain, severe osteoporosis, and associated fractures with significant improvement after cessation of methotrexate therapy (34).

Other agents reported to reduce bone density include cisplatin and carboplatin.

In addition, many chemotherapy protocols include corticosteroids, which decrease bone density and increase the risk of fractures. Hypogonadism resulting from chemotherapy, hormonal therapy, or radiation therapy will also add to the reduced bone density in patients with cancer.

Patients who have undergone bone marrow transplantation have been reported to have low bone mass. The reduced bone density is likely to be secondary to the long-term side effects of bone marrow radiation, chemotherapy, corticosteroids, and hypogonadism. Aromatase inhibitors, including anastrozole and letrozole, have been shown to decrease bone density and increase the rate of fractures in postmenopausal women. This is in sharp contrast to the positive effect on bone (both bone mineral density and fracture rates) seen with the alternative adjuvant hormonal treatment of breast cancer with tamoxifen, a selective estrogen receptor modulator (SERMs) (Fig. 45-1). In the Arimidex,

Tamoxifen Alone or in Combination (ATAC) trial, 9366 postmenopausal women with invasive operable breast cancer who had completed primary therapy were randomly assigned to receive anastrozole, tamoxifen, or both. The anastrozole group had significantly more fractures of all kinds than did the tamoxifen alone group (35). Patients treated with aromatase inhibitors should undergo bone mineral density prior to treatment with aromatase inhibitors and followed up annually thereafter. A bisphosphonate should be added to the treatment regimen if the patient's bone density is within the osteopenic or osteoporotic range pretreatment or if a decline in bone mineral density is seen during follow-up.

Osteoblasts and osteoclasts are controlled and under the influence of many hormonal and signaling pathways including tyrosine kinase receptors for the platelet-derived growth factor (PDGF-R alpha and beta) and c-Abl. The activation of the PDGF pathway increases bone mineral density in ovariectomized rats and accelerates fracture healing (36,37). The absence of c-Abl is associated with impaired osteoblast maturation leading to an osteoporosis phenotype (37).

Multikinase inhibitors such as sorafenib, sunitninb, and imatinib amongst others can inhibit many of the pathways that are common to the pathways that affect the normal bone remodeling. Not much is known about the tyrosine kinase inhibitors' clinical effects on bone. Imatinib has been the best studied and will be discussed here.

After 2 to 4 years of treatment with imatinib in patients with chronic myelogenous leukemia (CML), a significant increase of the trabecular bone volume in the iliac crest has been shown (38). Preosteoblast cells exposed to imatinib causes suppression of PDGF-induced PI3 kinase/Akt activation with upregulation of genes associated with osteoblast differentiation and bone formation.

Patients with gastrointestinal stromal tumors (GIST) and CML treated with imatinib may develop mild to moderate hypophosphatemia (phosphate < 2.5 mg/dL) soon after initiation of imatinib (<2 weeks) in a dose-dependent manner.(39). This may be accompanied with decreased levels of serum calcium, and secondary hyperparathyroidism with phosphaturia, normal 25-hydroxyvitamin D3, and elevated calcitriol (39). Increased markers of bone formation (osteocalcin and procollagen type 1 N-terminal propeptide) (40), but not markers of bone resorption has also been described. Although exact mechanisms are not clear, hypocalcemia may be due to inhibition of c-FMS in osteoclasts and perhaps other tyrosine kinase receptor–mediated mechanisms. Other,

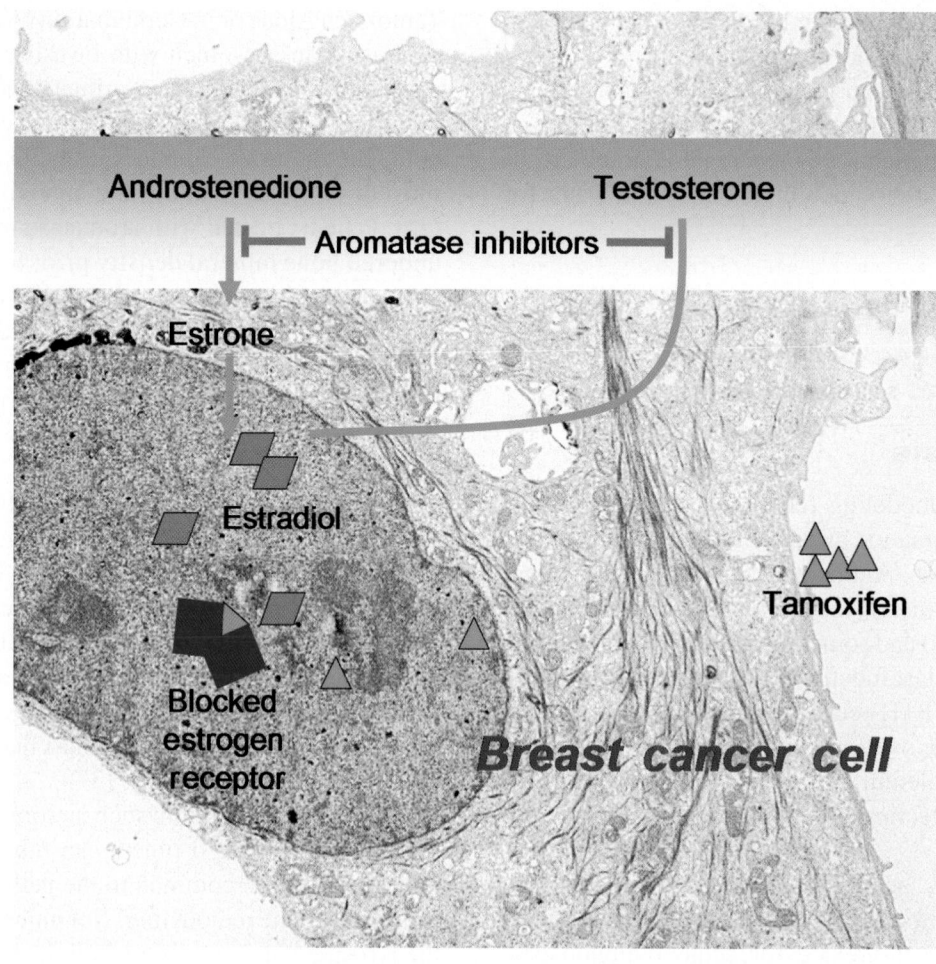

FIGURE 45-1. Mechanism of action of selective estrogen receptor modulators (SERMs) and aromatase inhibitors.

perhaps simultaneous mechanisms to explain these metabolic bone and mineral abnormalities include: an increase in bone formation (inhibition of PDGF-R and Abl receptor in osteoblasts) with subsequent sequestration of calcium and phosphate to the skeleton causing a compensatory increase in the secretion of PTH and decreased renal phosphate absorption leading to hypophosphatemia (38). More simplistic mechanisms including decreased absorption and increased clearance may also explain the reason for hypocalcemia.

While imatinib may improve bone mineral density and may help to prevent fractures, the opposing effects on electrolytes such as phosphate and calcium may be associated with muscular weakness and osteoporosis. The long-term effects of imatinib on skeletal health are unknown. Appropriate monitoring in these patients is warranted. More studies are needed for imatinib and other tyrosine kinase inhibitors effects on bone and mineral metabolism.

OSTEOMALACIA AND RICKETS

Osteomalacia results when normal mineralization of the organic bone matrix fails. In children, the abnormal mineralization and maturation of the growth plate at the epiphysis is called rickets. Nutritional deficiency (especially vitamin D) and renal wasting of phosphorus leading to hypocalcemia or hypophosphatemia are among the common causes of osteomalacia. Other contributing factors include drugs such as anticonvulsants or aluminum and systemic acidosis. Antineoplastic agents can also cause or worsen osteomalacia. Ifosfamide-induced tubular damage leads to renal phosphate wasting, hypophosphatemia, and rickets. Estramustine has also been used in prostrate cancer metastatic to bone and leads to hypocalcemia, hypophosphatemia, secondary hyperparathyroidism, and osteomalacia with normal vitamin D levels. Tumor-induced osteomalacia (TIO) is a rare form of hypophosphatemic rickets that is characterized by phosphaturia and hypophosphatemia. TIO has been reported mainly with benign tumors (especially hemangiopericytoma), but it has also been reported in a variety of malignant tumors (usually of mesenchymal origin). Fibroblast growth factor 23 (FGF-23) is secreted from these tumors and causes hyperphosphaturia with subsequent hypophosphatemia. Surgical removal of the tumor corrects the hyperphosphaturic abnormality and subsequently, the hypophosphatemia and the bone mineralization defect. Radiolabeled octreotide has been reported to detect some of these tumors, and octreotide therapy has been used to treat these tumors with varying results (41,42).

HYPERCALCEMIA

Calcium homeostasis is normally maintained by the interplay of parathyroid hormone (PTH), calcitonin, phosphorus, and vitamin D metabolites on several target organs, including bones, parathyroid glands, intestines, and kidneys. In patients with cancer, multiple factors can affect this delicate balance, including nutritional status, medications, tumor secretion of cytokines, hormones, or other humoral factors.

Hypercalcemia occurs in 5 to 10% of all patients with advanced cancer, and severe hypercalcemia (calcium level >12 mg/dL) is seen in about 0.5% of all patients with cancer (43). Renal cell carcinoma, non–small cell lung carcinoma, breast carcinoma, leukemia, non-Hodgkin lymphoma, and multiple myeloma are among the most common malignancies associated with hypercalcemia. Retinoic acid derivatives have been reported to induce hypercalcemia during the treatment of acute promyelocytic leukemia (44). Similarly, bexarotene has been reported to cause hypercalcemia in initial studies (45).

Hyperparathyroidism occurs 2.5 to 3 times more often in patients treated with low-dose (2-7.5 Gy) external radiation to the head and neck area than it does in the age-matched control population. Hyperparathyroidism after high-dose irradiation is uncommon. Radiation exposure from radioactive iodine treatment has also been reported in association with hyperparathyroidism.

HYPOCALCEMIA

Many factors can increase patients' risk of hypocalcemia. These include the patient's nutritional status, the antineoplastic agents used, and the type of surgical procedures performed (ie, neck dissection). Cytotoxic chemotherapy can result in tumor lysis syndrome and its resultant hypocalcemia; this is more commonly seen in the treatment of hematologic malignancies.

Hyperphosphatemia, hyperkalemia, hypocalcemia, and hyperuricemia can occur after induction chemotherapy; it is of vital importance to preempt this and prevent the complications of tumor lysis by hydration, alkaline diuresis, inhibition of uric acid synthesis, and administration of oral calcium or aluminum-based compounds to bind intestinal phosphate and enhance calcium absorption. Intravenous calcium administration can potentially cause calcium-phosphate precipitation in the presence of severe hyperphosphatemia and should be used with extreme caution. Dialysis may be needed in cases of symptomatic hypocalcemia and serum phosphorus levels higher than 10 mg/dL.

Cisplatin has been associated with hypocalcemia. One proposed mechanism of cisplatin's ability to induce hypocalcemia is through hypomagnesemia resulting in a decreased PTH secretion. Other theories include the inhibition of 1,25-dihydroxy vitamin D formation by hypomagnesemia or cisplatin inhibition of mitochondrial function in the proximal renal tubules. Plicamycin (mithramycin) is an antitumor antibiotic that has a major effect on calcium metabolism. It inhibits bone resorption, resulting in lowered serum calcium concentrations within 24-48 h. The inhibitory effect of plicamycin on osteoclast function has made it useful in the treatment of Paget disease of bone and osteoclast-mediated hypercalcemia associated with malignancy when other first-line agents have failed. Plicamycin carries a risk of hepatic and renal toxicity; therefore, it has limited usefulness in treating hypercalcemia of malignancy.

Other agents reported to induce hypocalcemia include dactinomycin, carboplatin, doxorubicin, and cytarabine. Hypocalcemia has been seen following bisphosphonate infusions (zolendronic acid and pamidronate) used to reduce skeletal complications in the treatment and prevention of advanced malignancies involving bone (46).

Serum calcium levels and 25-hydroxy vitamin D levels should be checked prior to and during therapy with bisphosphonates.

HYPOMAGNESEMIA

Hypomagnesemia is a well-known side effect in patients receiving platinum-based chemotherapy. Cisplatin has toxic effects on the kidney, causing morphologic changes and necrosis in the proximal tubule, a major site of magnesium reabsorption. Hypomagnesemia is a frequent complication of cisplatin chemotherapy, affecting up to 90% of patients; 10% of these patients have symptoms of muscle weakness, tremulousness, and dizziness.

Vigorous hydration and the use of osmotic diuretics such as mannitol may prevent renal failure but have little effect on renal magnesium wasting, which can persist for long periods after cisplatin discontinuation.

Carboplatin is a second-generation platinum compound that was developed in an attempt to reduce the side effects of cisplatin. Hypomagnesemia following therapy with carboplatin is seen with increasing frequency and severity at higher doses of carboplatin and can be severe enough to cause clinical symptoms (47).

Oxaliplatin is a third-generation platinum derivative that has become an integral part of various chemotherapy protocols, particularly in advanced colorectal cancer. Oxaliplatin has dose-limiting cumulative sensory neurotoxicity similar to cisplatin (48). Renal toxicity was absent in phase I trials with doses up to 200 mg/m^2 (49). It is felt to carry a much smaller risk, if any, for hypomagnesemia.

■ PITUITARY AND HYPOTHALAMIC DISORDERS

Hypothalamic-pituitary damage leading to single or multiple hormonal deficiencies can occur in patients treated with cranial or craniospinal irradiation or intracranial surgery (Fig. 45-2). Cranial radiotherapy often occurs in patients with leukemia and lymphoma, nonpituitary brain tumors, pituitary tumors, nasopharyngeal carcinoma and skull base tumors (50). The hypothalamus appears to be more radiosensitive than the pituitary gland and may be damaged by lower radiation doses (<40 Gy), but higher radiation doses are likely to damage both hypothalamic and pituitary function. Deficiency of one or more pituitary hormones occurs following irradiation (>40 Gy) of the hypothalamic-pituitary areas in about 90% of patients 5 years after radiation treatment (Fig. 45-3). T-lymphocyte-associated antigen-4 (CTLA-4) antibodies are in clinical trials for melanoma and renal cell carcinoma. Autoimmune hypophysitis has been reported in some patients receiving CTLA-4 blockade (51).

GROWTH HORMONE DEFICIENCY

Growth hormone (GH) deficiency is frequently noted after cranial irradiation. In children, isolated GH deficiency can occur after lower radiation doses, but higher doses may produce panhypopituitarism. This side effect of radiation therapy appears to be dose-dependent. At lower doses (20-24 Gy), the only effect may be an

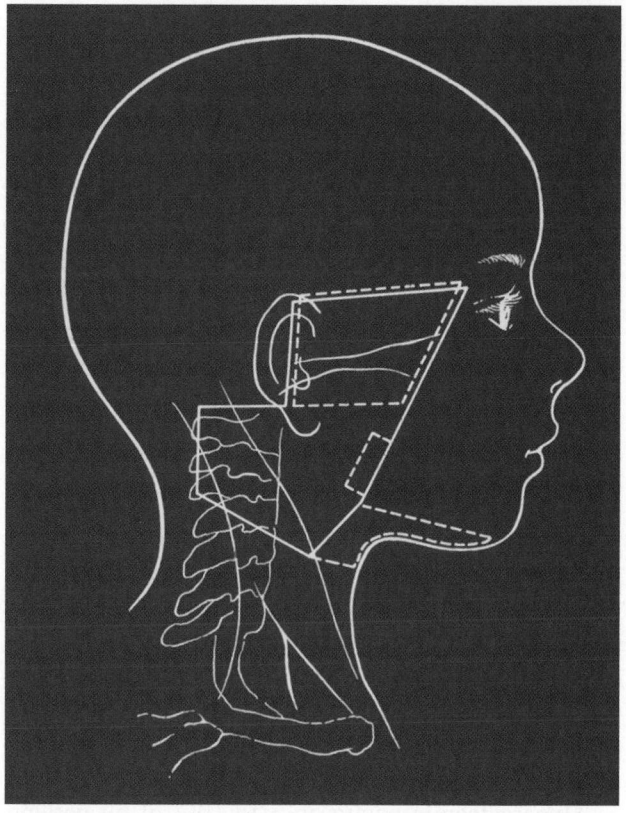

FIGURE 45-2. Mapping of possible radiation ports on a patient exposed during treatment for cancer of the head and neck region.

altered pulsatile secretory pattern. At doses higher than 30 Gy, deficient GH secretion and growth retardation is observed in more than a third of patients (52) (Fig. 45-4).

GH deficiency is also common in adults who have undergone cranial radiation therapy. In adults, GH deficiency is thought to cause decreased bone and muscle mass, fatigue, impaired sense of well-being, lowered exercise capacity, increased volume of adipose tissue, and altered myocardial function. In addition, patients with GH deficiency may have a higher occurrence of atherosclerotic plaques and an increased risk for cardiovascular diseases. GH replacement in these patients can restore normal adipose tissue composition, bone metabolism, quality of life, sense of well-being, lipid profile and cardiac function. Despite the apparent benefits, data about the effect of GH replacement in long-term cancer survivors are still lacking. GH replacement is contraindicated in any patient with an active malignant condition, but it can be initiated in an adult in whom malignant disease has been absent for at least 5 years.

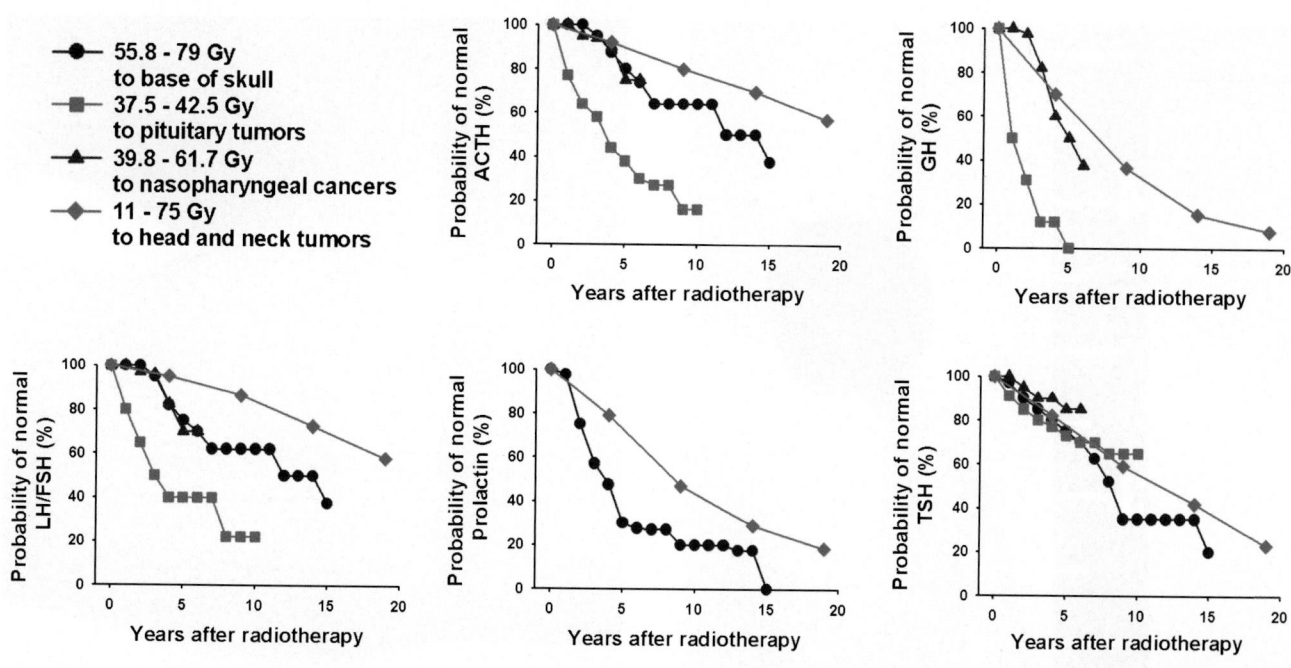

FIGURE 45-3. Probability of normal pituitary hormone secretion over time after radiation exposure to the hypothalamic-pituitary areas. Data from four studies are replotted on this figure. The first set of values (*black circle*) are from Pai et al. (57), in which the patient received 55.8 to 79 Gy to the base of the skull. The second set of values (*red square*) are from Shalet et al. (52), in which patients with pituitary tumors were treated with 37.5 to 42.5 Gy. The third series (*blue triangle*) from Lam et al. (126) shows the effect of radiation treatment for nasopharyngeal carcinoma with 39.8 to 61.7 Gy. The final series (*green diamond*) shows data from Samaan et al. (58), in which 11 to 75 Gy was administered to treat head and neck tumors.

Another treatment reported to result in GH deficiency includes long-term intrathecal opioids; these have about a 15% risk of developing GH deficiency (53).

CENTRAL HYPOTHYROIDISM

Radiotherapy can cause immediate and long-term effects; central hypothyroidism may be a result of the possible effects of brain or head and neck irradiation on hypothalamic and pituitary regulation of thyroid stimulating hormone (TSH) secretion. Fifteen to 20% of patients who had undergone cranial irradiation had diminished TSH secretion at 5 years after the treatment and approximately 35% after 10 years. The combined effect of irradiation on the thyroid gland and pituitary-hypothalamic area is so striking that we suggest routine screening for this group of patients, with measurement of both serum-free thyroxine and TSH concentration at 2- to 4-year intervals.

Chemotherapy may enhance the deleterious effect of radiation. Children with brain tumors (not involving the hypothalamic-pituitary axis) who receive vincristine, carmustine or lomustine, procarbazine, and brain irradiation have a 35% incidence of hypothyroidism compared

with a 10% incidence for patients who undergo brain irradiation alone (54). Bexarotene was found to cause central hypothyroidism in 40% of patients with cutaneous T-cell lymphoma patients (31). Reversible, retinoid X receptor–mediated suppression of TSH secretion is one explanation for this side effect (55). The fact that these patients often require twice the typical doses used to treat other causes of hypothyroidism suggests that bexarotene probably also increases thyroid hormone metabolic clearance (56).

HYPOGONADOTROPIC HYPOGONADISM

Brain surgery and irradiation of the skull carry the potential for hypothalamic-pituitary damage, including hypogonadotropic hypogonadism. Hyperprolactinemia is the most commonly reported hormonal abnormality in patients who have undergone head and neck irradiation, occurring in more than 66% of patients (57,58). Hyperprolactinemia inhibits gonadotropin secretion from the pituitary gland and decreases the responsiveness of the pituitary gland to gonadotropin-releasing hormone, causing secondary hypogonadism. Dopamine agonists could reverse this process, and it may be reasonable to

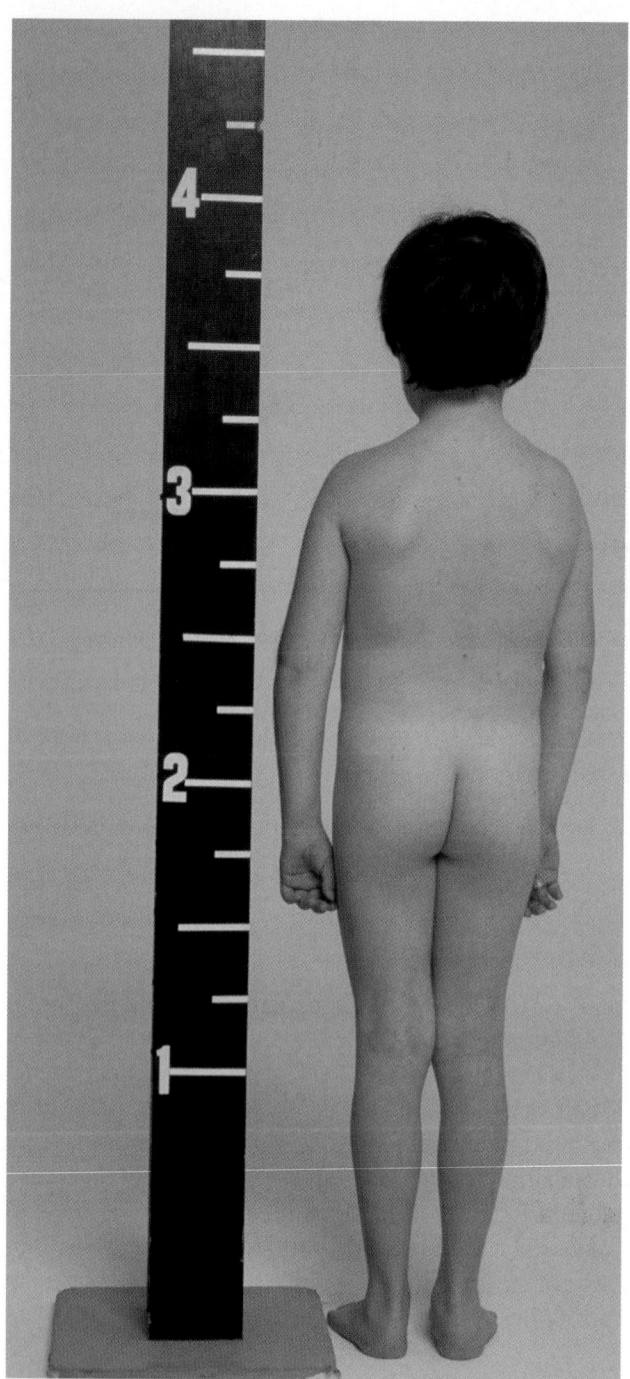

FIGURE 45-4. Patient developed short stature due to growth hormone deficiency from radiation treatment of a brain tumor.

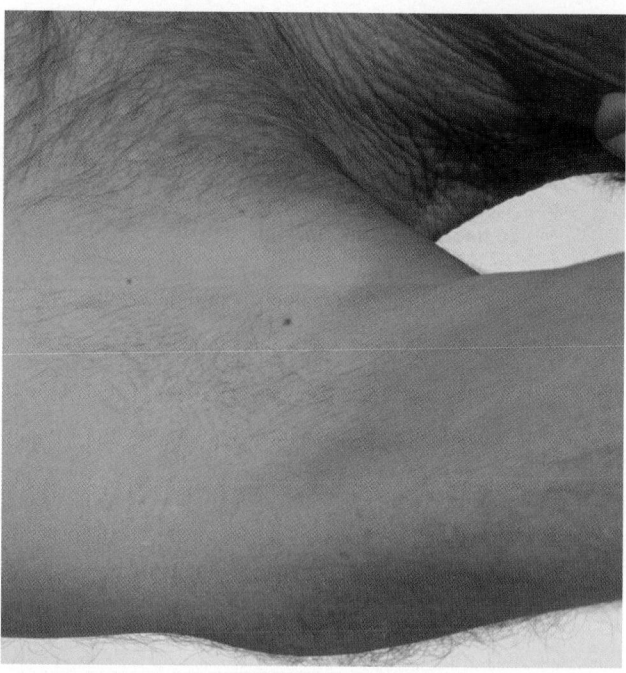

FIGURE 45-5. Loss of axillary hair in a patient who developed secondary hypogonadism after cranial irradiation.

adults, gonadotropin deficiency may cause sex steroid hormone deficiency and infertility (Fig. 45-5). Sex steroid hormone deficiency lowers libido and may have deleterious effects on bone and lipid metabolism.

Early or even precocious puberty has also been reported in patients treated with combined chemotherapy and cranial irradiation for acute lymphoblastic leukemia (ALL) or cranial irradiation for brain tumors. This phenomenon is more common in girls. Coexisting GH deficiency is frequently noted. In a recent study of male cancer survivors (excluding those who had undergone treatment that may have otherwise affected gonadal function), chronic opioid therapy, given in morphine-equivalent daily doses of at least 200 mg daily, was associated with secondary hypogonadism (59).

■ THYROID DISORDERS

THYROID NEOPLASMS

Ionizing radiation is the only well-established etiology of thyroid cancer. Irradiation of the thyroid results in DNA damage, with formation of chromosomal rearrangements involving the intracellular tyrosine kinase of RET fused with another gene product, typically H4 or ELE1, creating RET/PTC1 and RET/PTC3 rearrangements, respectively. There are different types of RET/PTC

proceed with a therapeutic trial if the other anterior pituitary hormone axes are normal. Hypogonadism has been reported in 29% of patients following high-dose conformal fractionated proton-photon beam radiotherapy for tumors at the base of the skull (57). In children, inadequate sexual development, delayed puberty, and absent menarche are significant problems, whereas in rearrangements, with RET/PTC1 and RET/PTC3, accounting for more than 90%. The prevalence of RET/PTC in papillary carcinomas shows significant geographic variation and is approximately 35% in North America. RET/PTC is more common in tumors in children and young adults and in papillary carcinomas associated with radiation exposure (60). A dose-response relationship between radiation exposure and relative risk of thyroid cancer is seen for radiation doses of ≤5 Gy (61). Female sex, age less than 15 years at radiation exposure, and 20 to 30 years postradiation exposure are all associated with increased risk for thyroid cancer. Papillary thyroid carcinomas make up 90% of radiation-induced thyroid cancers; there is a higher incidence of local invasion, multicentric disease, and distant metastasis on presentation in radiation-induced thyroid cancer than there is in sporadic thyroid cancer (62). There is an increased prevalence of thyroid cancer among patients therapeutically irradiated in anatomic locations other than the head and neck because of unintended low-dose radiation exposure to the thyroid gland. Children tend to be more sensitive to these radiation doses (63). Thyroid carcinoma is most evident in long-term survivors of Hodgkin disease and non-Hodgkin lymphoma.

Chemotherapy is not a proven risk factor for thyroid carcinoma despite rare case reports to the contrary. The administration of ^{131}I for diagnostic purposes does not seem to increase the risk of developing carcinoma of the thyroid.

HYPERTHYROIDISM

Radiation-induced hyperthyroidism has been described but is far less common than radiation-induced hypothyroidism.

Radiation-induced silent thyroiditis with transient thyrotoxicosis has been reported in patients treated with radiation therapy. Thyroiditis-induced thyrotoxicosis occurs within 2 years of radiation therapy in most cases; several months later, hypothyroidism occurs. There is an increased risk of Graves disease following radiation therapy. Patients with lymphoma who have been treated with radiation therapy constitute the largest number of patients who have developed Graves disease after-radiation therapy; this raises the possibility of a relationship between the two clinical entities. Patients treated with radiation for nasopharyngeal, breast and/or laryngeal carcinomas may also develop Graves disease. Cytokines have also been reported to lead to Graves disease. IFNα is known to induce the production of autoantibodies and can lead to the occurrence of autoimmune thyroid disease, specifically, autoimmune primary hypothyroidism, transient thyrotoxicosis, or, more rarely, Graves disease. Women have a higher risk of developing autoimmune thyroid disease upon starting IFNα treatment (64). It is important to distinguish the cases in which IFNα induces transient thyrotoxicosis followed by hypothyroidism from the cases in which IFNα induces Graves disease (65). Thyroid scans showing increased homogeneous uptake in the presence of hyperthyroidism are highly suggestive of Graves disease and warrant antithyroid medications (eg, methimazole).

Interleukin-2 treatment alone causes transient hyperthyroidism followed by hypothyroidism in about 50% of patient (66). The mechanism of interleukin-2–induced autoimmune thyroid dysfunction is unclear, although interleukin-2–induced disruption of self-tolerance has been suggested as a mechanism.

HYPOTHYROIDISM

Head and neck irradiation is an important etiology of dysfunction of the thyroid gland. Radiation can induce primary hypothyroidism when given in doses higher than 25 Gy to the region near the thyroid gland (Fig. 45-6); secondary and tertiary hypothyroidism can be seen with doses of 40 Gy or higher to the hypothalamic-pituitary area. Most cases of primary hypothyroidism occur about 5 years after radiation therapy. The probability of hypothyroidism is dose-related and increases with longer duration of follow-up after radiation treatment. In a study of 1677 patients with Hodgkin disease whose thyroid had been irradiated, the risk of thyroid disease

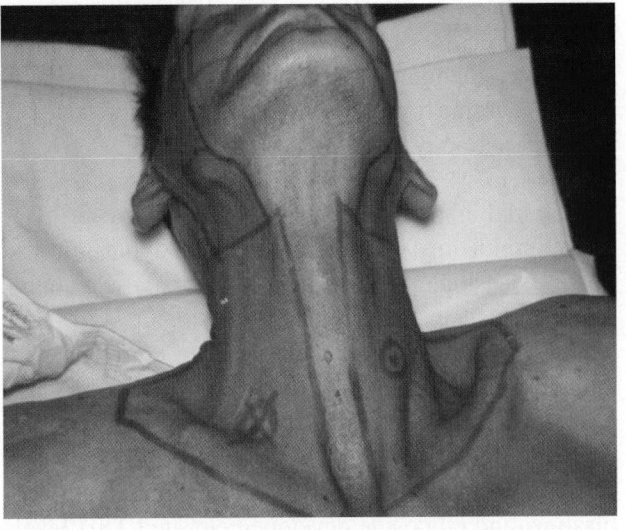

FIGURE 45-6. Mapping of radiation ports on a patient with squamous cell cancer of the head and neck. The patient developed primary hypothyroidism a few years after radiation therapy.

was 52% and 67% after 20 and 26 years of follow-up, respectively. Four hundred eighty-six patients (29%) received thyroxine therapy because of elevated serum TSH concentrations and 27 (2%) had transient elevations of their serum thyrotropin level that were not treated (67).

A significant number of patients develop subclinical hypothyroidism (elevated TSH with normal thyroxine levels) not overt hypothyroidism when less than 40 Gy of radiation are given (68). Multiple factors increase the risk for hypothyroidism including high doses of radiation to the head and neck, combined radiation and surgical treatments, time interval since therapy, and failure to shield midline structures. Other risk factors include thyroid resection during a laryngectomy or disruption of the vascular supply of the thyroid gland during surgery.

The use of ^{131}I may result in thyroid dysfunction. ^{131}I-metaiodobenzylguanidine (MIBG) in the treatment of metastatic pheochromocytoma carries the possibility of inducing primary hypothyroidism and requires the routine use of potassium perchlorate to block the thyroid ^{131}I uptake.

IFNα administration was reported to cause primary hypothyroidism in about 10% of treated patients and was not related to IFN dosage (69). The presence of pretreatment serum antithyroid antibodies in patients treated with IFN therapy increases the risk for the development of IFN-induced thyroid disease. During 6 years of observation after IFN therapy, the absence of thyroid autoantibodies at the end of IFN treatment was found to be a protective factor for the successive development of thyroiditis, whereas the positivity for thyroid antibodies at high titers at the end of IFN treatment was significantly related to chronic subclinical hypothyroidism. IFNα-related thyroid autoimmunity is not a completely reversible phenomenon because some patients may develop chronic thyroiditis especially in the presence of high autoantibody titers.

Interleukin-2 causes painless thyroiditis of acute onset, with initial hyperthyroxinemia followed by primary hypothyroidism. The hypothyroidism may last months but is occasionally permanent; 9% of these patients require replacement thyroid hormone therapy (70).

Patients treated with multiple drug regimens with antineoplastic agents (with or without radiation) also have a higher than normal incidence of primary hypothyroidism. Fifteen percent of patients who received a combination of cisplatin, bleomycin, dactinomycin, vinblastine, and etoposide developed elevated TSH levels with normal free T3 and free thyroxine (T4), compatible with subclinical primary hypothyroidism in contrast to the control group (71).

The expanding use of targeted therapy has been also linked to the development of variety of thyroid abnormalities.

Autoimmune thyroid disease has been seen in 23% of patients receiving alemtuzumab (72). Tyrosine kinase inhibitors are small molecules with variable receptor affinity and block intracellular signaling. Imatinib use was reported in increase levothyroxine requirements in thyroidectomized patients while non-thyroidectomized patients had no significant alterations of their thyroid functions (73). These data suggest that imatinib and maybe tyrosine kinase inhibitors in general may accelerate the clearance of levothyroxine leading to clinical hypothyroidism in patients who are dependent on exogenous supply of levothyroxine(74).

Thyroid dysfunction was reported in 21% of renal cell carcinoma patients receiving sorafenib (75). Prospective studies estimated the risk of thyroid dysfunction to reach 68%; however, only 6% had clinical symptoms requiring thyroid hormone replacement (76). Sorafenib-related thyroiditis has been suggested as a mechanism in some of these patients but it is unclear if this represents an autoimmune process or a manifestation of VGEF blockade affecting thyroid blood supply.

Similarly, thyroid dysfunction was reported in 62% of patients receiving sunitinib including 36% of patients who had persistent elevation of TSH suggestive of primary hypothyroidism especially in patients with longer duration of sunitinib use. Destructive thyroiditis has been suggested as an explanation though some patient became athyrotic on sunitinib after having normal thyroid functions at baseline (77). Other prospective studies found that 27% of patients receiving sunitinib had elevated TSH requiring hormone replacement (78). Some patients were reported to present with thyrotoxicosis phase preceding hypothyroidism which further supports the theory of sunitinib-related destructive thyroiditis leading to hypothyroidism in these patients (79,80). Impaired iodine uptake and inhibition of peroxidase activity were also suggested as potential mechanism to explain hypothyroidism (81,82).

ABNORMALITIES IN THYROID HORMONE-BINDING PROTEINS

Thyroid hormone is preferentially bound to thyroid hormone-binding globulin (TBG) (65-70%), transthyretin (15-20%), and albumin (10-15%) in serum. Multiple factors can affect the levels of these binding proteins and the subsequent levels of measured bound thyroid hormones. In patients with malignancies, changes in sex hormone levels, glucocorticoids, narcotics, nutritional status, and some antineoplastic agents are the major factors affecting the protein-binding properties. Overall, the level of total T3 and T4 may be affected, but in general, the free hormone levels (biologically active) are normal. This effect on TBG synthesis or clearance is usually reversible. Estrogens are known to increase TBG and total thyroid hormone levels, but tamoxifen also causes elevated plasma concentrations of TBG in postmenopausal women with breast cancer after 6 months of therapy. Nonsteroidal aromatase inhibitors (anastrozole and letrozole) are known to lower estrogen levels, but the effect on TBG has still not been fully reported in the literature; when letrozole was given at 2.5 mg per day, however, there was a statistically significant decrease in total T4 but not total T3 levels (83).

Glucocorticoids are frequently used in combination with chemotherapy and are known to suppress TSH secretion and inhibit TBG synthesis. L-asparaginase has been shown to inhibit the synthesis of albumin and TBG, which affects serum thyroid hormone levels (84,85). 5-Fluorouracil increases total T3 and T4 levels and maintains a normal free thyroxine index, suggesting that it increases serum thyroid hormone-binding proteins, resulting in normal thyroid function (86).

Mitotane increases levels of hormone-binding globulins, but the increase in TBG is less remarkable than mitotane's effect on corticosteroid-binding globulin.

■ ADRENAL DISORDERS

PRIMARY ADRENAL INSUFFICIENCY

Mitotane is an insecticide derivative with selective toxicity for both normal and malignant adrenocortical cells. Adrenal insufficiency is commonly seen at the high doses used to treat adrenocortical carcinoma. It also causes a two- to threefold increase in serum levels of cortisol-binding globulin protein (87). Glucocorticoid replacement therapy is needed when mitotane is used; doses higher than usual are required because of the increased levels of binding globulin and enhanced metabolic clearance of dexamethasone by mitotane.

Preapproval animal studies found cases of adrenal necrosis associated with sunitinib use leading the Food and Drug Administration to recommend monitoring adrenal functions in patients receiving sunitinib. However, there was no evidence of adrenal hemorrhage or clinical evidence of adrenal insufficiency on subsequent clinical safety data that involved more than 300 patients receiving sunitinib (88).

SECONDARY ADRENAL INSUFFICIENCY

Prolonged glucocorticoid treatment is the most common cause of adrenal dysfunction in patients with cancer. Secondary (central) adrenal insufficiency may develop after discontinuation of glucocorticoids and can persist for months. This can occur up to 2 years after discontinuation of therapy. Irradiation to the hypothalamic-pituitary region causes deficiency of ACTH with resultant secondary adrenal insufficiency in 19 to 42% of these patients. The median time interval for the development of adrenal insufficiency after therapy is 5 years, but it can occur as early as 2 years after radiotherapy. One microgram cosyntropin stimulation test has been proposed to screen cancer survivors who received >30 Gy of radiation to the hypothalamic and pituitary areas and those with other hypothalamic/hypopituitary endocrinopathies (89).

Prolonged therapy with busulfan was initially reported to cause a reversible clinical syndrome resembling central adrenal insufficiency as evidenced by metyrapone testing (90). No recent reports have corroborated this. Long-term intrathecal opioid therapy for intractable nonmalignant pain (mean duration of treatment, 26.6 ± 16.3 months) resulted in central adrenal insufficiency in 15% of patients when they were tested with insulin-induced hypoglycemia (53).

Megestrol acetate is used to stimulate appetite in patients with cancer, but its prolonged use can lead to a Cushings-like syndrome, and sudden withdrawal of prolonged treatment may result in adrenal insufficiency. Megestrol shows glucocorticoid-like effects with an acute depressing effect on the hypothalamic-pituitary-axis (HPA) and ACTH secretion, leading to central adrenal insufficiency as tested with the 1-μg ACTH stimulation test (91,92). Secondary adrenal insufficiency can be diagnosed by a variety of tests with varying sensitivity and specificity, but in our practices, we tend to frequently use a combination of basal (8 AM) serum cortisol measurements and low-dose (1 μg) cosyntropin stimulation testing. Rarely, insulin-induced hypoglycemia is used to assess the overall cortisol and GH response to hypoglycemia when evaluating patients for panhypopituitarism.

■ GONADAL DISORDERS

Direct radiation exposure and cytotoxic chemotherapeutic agents are common causes of hypogonadism and infertility in cancer survivors. There are considerable differences between female and male gametogenesis,

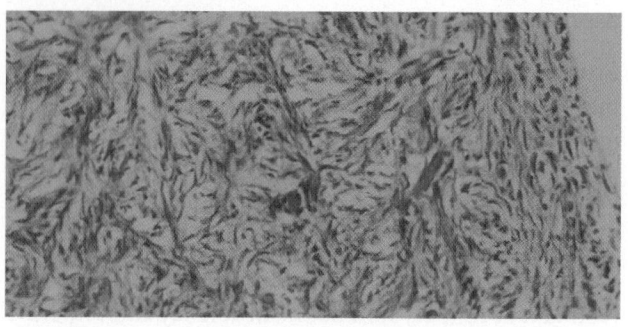

FIGURE 45-7. Hematoxylin and Eosin staining of tissue from an ovarian biopsy showing atrophy of ovarian tissue after cytotoxic chemotherapy.

which results in a variety of effects of the cancer therapy on fertility and gonadal functions.

FEMALE GONADAL DISORDERS

Oogenesis occurs during embryonic life, and oocytes remain quiescent most of their lifespan; it is this property that makes them resistant to the adverse effects of cytotoxic chemotherapy. However, the combination of a limited number of oocytes and the inability to replace damaged ones results in a shortened reproductive period when oocytes have been damaged. The granulosa cells are also susceptible to these cytotoxic drugs as shown by the results of ovarian biopsies performed after chemotherapy (Fig. 45-7). Infertility may occur as a result of either granulosa cell or oocyte impairment.

With advances in cancer treatment, an increasing number of women survive their malignancies to face reproductive disorders. It is of vital importance to discuss fertility issues before radiation or systemic chemotherapy as these modalities carry significant risks for ovarian dysfunction and infertility. The effects of radiation treatment on the ovaries differ according to the patient's age, radiation dose, and field of treatment. With doses as low as 6 Gy, prepubertal girls can experience primary amenorrhea, and women more than 40 years in age can develop ovarian failure and infertility (93,94). Permanent infertility in women less than 40 years of age usually occurs after doses of 20 Gy or higher (93). Fractionated radiation seems to carry less risk for permanent sterility (95). When possible, fractionated radiation should be used with shielding of the gonads, and restricting of radiation fields reduce the risk of ovarian failure. Ovarian transposition (oophoropexy) to the paracolic gutters before pelvic irradiation has been suggested to preserve ovarian function in women less than 40 years of age

with cervical carcinoma less than 3 cm in diameter (96). It can also be used prior to pelvic irradiation in other diseases, including lymphoma. This procedure can be done by either laparotomy or laparoscopy with the intent of preventing radiation but not chemotherapy-induced ovarian failure. Assisted fertilization is often needed after this procedure.

Oocyte cryopreservation has been proposed as a means of preserving fertility in women treated for cancer, but it has been less successful in humans than it has in animal models. Ovarian tissue cryopreservation and transplantation has also been proposed for patients before cancer treatment.

The ethical issues behind these techniques are still being disputed, and there is still the concern of potential disease recurrence from residual disease in autografted ovarian tissues; obtaining unilaminar follicles from cryopreserved, thawed tissue and growing them in vitro has been proposed to reduce this risk of recurrence. The cytotoxic effects of chemotherapeutic agents are seen more in rapidly dividing cells than in cells at rest, which led to the hypothesis that gonadotropin-releasing hormone agonists would suppress the hypothamamic pituitary ovary axis and make the ovaries less susceptible to the cytotoxic effects of chemotherapy. In animal models, gonadotropin-releasing–hormone agonist therapy lowered cyclophosphamide-induced but not radiation-induced ovarian toxicity. Some studies have reported encouraging results of the use of this approach in women with breast cancer, leukemia, and lymphoma (97,98).

In premenopausal women with breast cancer treated with regimens based on cyclophosphamide, methotrexate, and fluorouracil (CMF), the chemotherapy-related amenorrhea rate is 68% (99). Alkylating agents are non–cell-cycle-specific drugs and are generally highly gonadotoxic.

Mechlorethamine is usually used in combination with vincristine, procarbazine, and prednisone, (MOPP), a highly gonadotoxic combination; this makes the exact contribution of mechlorethamine to the gonadotoxicity of MOPP difficult to evaluate.

Chlorambucil appears to have a dose-dependent gonadotoxic effect with infrequent ovarian failure at cumulative doses of 236 mg/m^2 (100,101). Melphalan, busulfan, and cyclophosphamide also carry a high risk of ovarian damage. The estimated odds ratio for ovarian failure with alkylating agents is 3.98 (102).

Procarbazine is also a non–cell-cycle-specific agent. Data regarding its gonadotoxic effects when used alone are unavailable; however, when it was used in combination regimens for Hodgkin disease, gonadal toxicity was higher with procarbazine (103).

The nitrosoureas lomustine and carmustine whether used alone or in combination with other agents have been implicated in gonadal failure in prepubescent patients treated for brain tumors. These patients, however, also underwent craniospinal radiation and procarbazine, making the role of these agents in ovarian failure less clear (104,105).

The extent of cisplatin toxicity in women is less well defined, with an odds ratio of 1.77 (102). Temporary amenorrhea developed in 2 of 12 female patients in whom cisplatin (0.4-0.6 g/m^2) was used in combination with bleomycin and vinblastine to treat ovarian germ cell tumors; the amenorrhea lasted from 12 to 15 months after the cessation of chemotherapy.

Transient and permanent ovarian failure had been reported with etoposide (VP-16) use (106,107).

Antimetabolites are cell-cycle-specific and may exert few toxic effects on the ovaries. As a single agent, doxorubicin has few, if any, adverse effects on ovarian function, although a synergistic effect of the combination of doxorubicin and cyclophosphamide is a concern.

Vinblastine has been known to cause reversible and dose-related amenorrhea when combined with alkylating agents (108).

MALE GONADAL DISORDERS

Spermatogenesis occurs in a continuous cycle of meiosis, mitosis, differentiation, and maturation. Germ cells and spermatogonia, in contrast to Leydig or Sertoli cells, are sensitive to cytotoxic agents. If sufficient germ cells remain after cytotoxic chemotherapy, resumption of spermatogenesis usually occurs; the longer the duration of azoospermia, the lower the likelihood of spermatogenesis recovery (109).

Radiation damage to the gonads is dose-dependent (110). Low-dose testicular irradiation leads to a transient suppression of sperm counts with a recovery time proportional to the radiation dose (111). Permanent infertility was reported after fractionated radiation doses of more than 2 Gy, whereas clinically significant Leydig cell impairment occurs rarely with doses of less than 20 Gy (Fig. 45-8*A* and *B*) (112).

Therapy with alkylating agents such as cyclophosphamide and chlorambucil used as monotherapy may result in reversible but prolonged azoospermia. Chlorambucil also causes azoospermia at cumulative doses of 400 to 800 mg; recovery may take 3 to 4 years after a mean total dose of about 750 mg/m^2 (113).

Cyclophosphamide affects spermatogenesis more than Leydig cell function, causing reduced sperm count with normal testosterone levels.

A high rate of permanent testicular dysfunction has been reported with procarbazine use. Permanent sterility occurred in all 92 patients who received six or more cycles of cyclophosphamide, vincristine, procarbazine, and prednisone (114).

Dose-related impairment of spermatogenesis has been reported during testicular carcinoma treatment with cisplatin, etoposide, and bleomycin (PEB). Azoospermia was present in 19% of the patients who received a low-dose chemotherapeutic regimen (cisplatin 20 mg/m^2 × 5 q3week, etoposide 100 mg/m^2 × 5 q3week, and bleomycin 15 mg/m^2 q1week) compared with 47% of the high-dose-treated patients (cisplatin 40 mg/m^2 × 5 q3week, etoposide 200 mg/m^2 × 5 q3week, and bleomycin 15 mg/m^2 q1week) (115). Only transient oligospermia was reported in 50% of patients treated with methotrexate plus leucovorin (116). The effect of doxorubicin as monotherapy on male gonadal function has not been well studied in humans, but in rats, testicular toxicity can be detected at high doxorubicin doses (117). In patients with Hodgkin disease treated with doxorubicin, bleomycin, vinblastine, and dacarbazine (ABVD), there was no evidence of long-term azoospermia (118). In patients with hairy cell leukemia, IFN seemed to have no significant effect on testicular function (119).

Multiple methods of preventing or reversing infertility in men treated for cancer have been suggested. In rats, fertility can be restored by suppressing testosterone with gonadotropin-releasing hormone (GnRH) agonists or antagonists, either before or after cytotoxic therapy. This approach does not protect the survival of the stem cells in the testes but enhances the ability of the testes to maintain the differentiation of the type A spermatogonia (120). It would be premature to apply this method to everyday clinical practice as the limited data from human trials did not show this proposed benefit.

Semen cryopreservation before starting gonadotoxic therapy followed by assisted fertilization is another strategy to preserve fertility in men with cancer.

In patients with Hodgkin disease, different combination chemotherapies, including methotrexate, vincristine, prednisone, and procarbazine (MOPP); cyclophosphamide, vincristine, prednisone, and procarbazine (COPP); mechlorethamine, vinblastine, prednisolone, and procarbazine (MVPP); and a variety of combinations of chlorambucil, vinblastine, prednisolone plus procarbazine, doxorubicin, and vincristine plus etoposide (ChIVPP/EVA) are known to cause substantial and considerable damage to gonadal function (121-123). Two different combinations, vincristine, epirubicin, etoposide, prednisolone (VEEP); and doxorubicin, bleomycin,

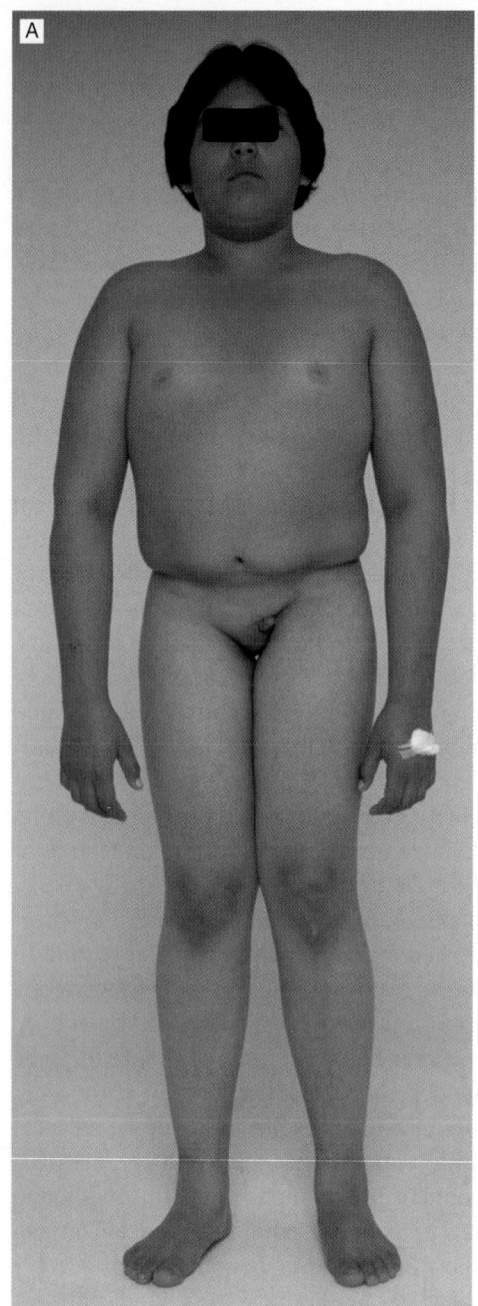

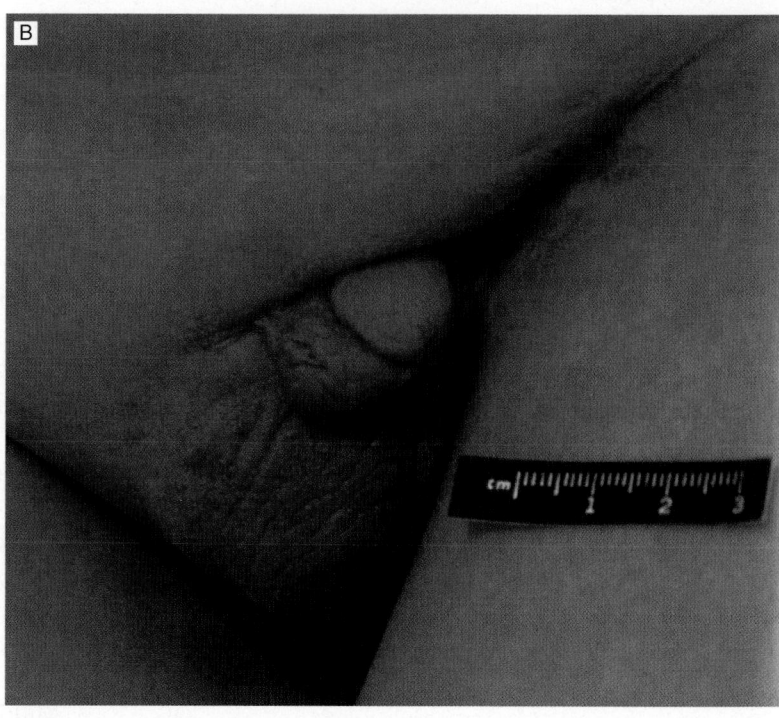

FIGURE 45-8. **A** and **B.** A young male patient after therapeutic irradiation to the left testicle for a testicular tumor. Note the loss of body hair, hypogonadal facial puffiness, decreased muscle mass, and increased body fat. The left testicle was small and firm. This patient was infertile.

vinblastine, and dacarbazine (ABVD) are associated with much lower incidences of gonadal toxicity (124,125).

■ SURVEILLANCE FOR COMPLICATIONS IN CANCER SURVIVORS

Primary care physicians and oncologists should be aware of the major long-term consequences of cancer therapy for early detection and management. Long-term follow-up is frequently needed because many of these complications occur years after treatment and can have subtle clinical presentations.

For long-term cancer survivors who were treated with streptozocin, L-asparaginase, or partial pancreatectomy, screening for the delayed development of diabetes mellitus is recommended.

In children with a history of cranial irradiation or craniospinal irradiation, the growth rate should be assessed at 6-month intervals. A more detailed evaluation, including measurement levels of GH, insulin-like growth factor 1 (IGF-1), insulin-like growth factor binding protein 3, thyroid function tests, and bone-age assessments should be performed where there is evidence of an abnormal growth pattern.

In adults who have undergone head and neck irradiation, clinical monitoring with measurement of serum IGF-1 (if the patient is a candidate for GH replacement) and measuring serum testosterone levels and documenting menstrual history should be undertaken annually for 5 years and then at 5 year intervals for another 10 years (126).

If there is clinical suspicion of partial or complete pituitary failure in patients who have undergone total body or head and neck irradiation, a thorough evaluation of pituitary-hypothalamic function, including assessment of GH levels, thyroid function, adrenal and gonadal axes is appropriate. Dynamic testing may be performed to confirm hormone deficiencies prior to the initiation of replacement therapy. This detailed evaluation can be repeated in the future when there is a clinical presentation of radiation-related hormonal abnormality.

In children who have undergone either cranial or neck irradiation, T4, and TSH measurements should be performed annually for the first 5 years, and every 2 years thereafter. Careful physical examination should be performed annually to detect thyroid nodules, and if any are detected, a more detailed examination should be performed using ultrasound and if necessary, fine-needle aspiration biopsy.

In survivors of childhood malignancies, bone mass may be assessed in the early thirties, an age at which peak bone mass has been attained in most people. If bone mass is normal, no further evaluation is needed beyond the usual recommendations for prevention of osteoporosis.

It is also important to consider the possibility of bone loss in androgen- or estrogen-deficient adults. In those with low bone mass, an active program of calcium and vitamin D supplementation, exercise, and, occasionally, medical therapy (bisphosphonates or recombinant parathyroid hormone) should be combined with periodic assessment of bone mass every 12 to 18 months.

Patients who have been treated with chemotherapeutic agents that cause hypophosphatemia, hypomagnesemia, or hypocalcemia, such as ifosfamide, platinum compounds, fludarabine, or estramustine, are particularly at risk for osteomalacia and should undergo an evaluation of serum calcium, phosphorus, magnesium, alkaline phosphatase, and vitamin D metabolites levels.

Patients who have been treated with aromatase inhibitors should have bone mineral density measurements before and during treatment and should be given calcium and vitamin D. Patients can be given bisphosphonates if deemed necessary.

References

1. Nunez NP, Oh WJ, Rozenberg J, et al. Accelerated tumor formation in a fatless mouse with type 2 diabetes and inflammation. *Cancer Res* 2006;66(10):5469-5476.
2. Tran TT, Medline A, Bruce WR. Insulin promotion of colon tumors in rats. Cancer Epidemiol *Biomarkers Prev* 1996;5(12):1013-1015.
3. Weinstein D, Simon M, Yehezkel E, et al. Insulin analogues display IGF-I-like mitogenic and anti-apoptotic activities in cultured cancer cells. *Diabetes Metab Res Rev* 2009;25(1):41-49.
4. Eckardt K, May C, Koenen M, et al. IGF-1 receptor signalling determines the mitogenic potency of insulin analogues in human smooth muscle cells and fibroblasts. *Diabetologia* 2007;50(12):2534-2543.
5. Home PD, Lagarenne P. Combined randomised controlled trial experience of malignancies in studies using insulin glargine. *Diabetologia* 2009;52(12):2499-2506.
6. Hemkens LG, Grouven U, Bender R, et al. Risk of malignancies in patients with diabetes treated with human insulin or insulin analogues: A cohort study. *Diabetologia* 2009;52(9):1732-1744.
7. Gerullis H, Bergmann L, Maute L, et al. Experiences and practical conclusions concerning temsirolimus use and adverse event management in advanced renal cell carcinoma within a compassionate use program in Germany. *Cancer Chemother Pharmacol* 2009;63(6):1097-1102.
8. Guevremont C, Alasker A, Karakiewicz PI. Management of sorafenib, sunitinib, and temsirolimus toxicity in metastatic renal cell carcinoma. *Curr Opin Support Palliat Care* 2009;3(3):170-179.
9. Radu RG, Fujimoto S, Mukai E, et al. Tacrolimus suppresses glucose-induced insulin release from pancreatic islets by reducing glucokinase activity. *Am J Physiol Endocrinol Metab* 2005;288(2):365E-371E.
10. Avramis VI, Sencer S, Periclou AP, et al. A randomized comparison of native Escherichia coli asparaginase and polyethylene glycol conjugated asparaginase for treatment of children with newly diagnosed standard-risk acute lymphoblastic leukemia: A Children's Cancer Group study. *Blood* 2002;99(6):1986-1994.
11. Whitecar JP, Jr., Bodey GP, Harris JE, et al. L-asparaginase. *N Engl J Med* 1970;282(13):732-734.
12. Whitecar JP, Jr., Bodey GP, Hill CS, Jr., et al. Effect of L-asparaginase on carbohydrate metabolism. *Metabolism* 1970;19(8):581-586.
13. Gillette PC, Hill LL, Starling KA, et al. Transient diabetes mellitus secondary to L-asparaginase therapy in acute leukemia. *J Pediatr* 1972;81(1):109-111.
14. Land VJ, Sutow WW, Fernbach DJ, et al. Toxicity of L-asparginase in children with advanced leukemia. *Cancer* 1972;30(2):339-347.

15. Sadoff L. Patterns of intravenous glucose tolerance and insulin response before and after treatment with streptozotocin (NSC-85998) in patients with cancer. *Cancer Chemother Rep* 1972;56(1):61-69.

16. Schein PS, O'Connell MJ, Blom J, et al. Clinical antitumor activity and toxicity of streptozotocin (NSC-85998). *Cancer* 1974;34(4):993-1000.

17. Broder LE, Carter SK. Pancreatic islet cell carcinoma. II. Results of therapy with streptozotocin in 52 patients. *Ann Intern Med* 1973;79(1):108-118.

18. Okanoue T, Sakamoto S, Itoh Y, et al. Side effects of high-dose interferon therapy for chronic hepatitis C. *J Hepatol* 1996;25(3):283-291.

19. Guerci AP, Guerci B, Levy-Marchal C, et al. Onset of insulin-dependent diabetes mellitus after interferon-alfa therapy for hairy cell leukaemia. *Lancet* 1994;343(8906):1167-1168.

20. Murakami M, Iriuchijima T, Mori M. Diabetes mellitus and interferon-alpha therapy. *Ann Intern Med* 1995;123(4):318.

21. Imagawa A, Itoh N, Hanafusa T, et al. Autoimmune endocrine disease induced by recombinant interferon-alpha therapy for chronic active type C hepatitis. *J Clin Endocrinol Metab* 1995;80(3):922-926.

22. Rhodes CJ, Taylor KW. Effect of human lymphoblastoid interferon on insulin synthesis and secretion in isolated human pancreatic islets. *Diabetologia* 1984;27(6):601-603.

23. Brod SA, Atkinson M, Lavis VR, et al. Ingested IFN-alpha preserves residual beta cell function in type 1 diabetes. *J Interferon Cytokine Res* 2001;21(12):1021-1030.

24. Berruti A, Gorzegno G, Vitetta G, et al. Hypertriglyceridemia during long-term interferon-alpha therapy: Efficacy of diet and gemfibrosil treatment. A case report. *Tumori* 1992;78(5):353-355.

25. Fujiwara H, Umeda Y, Yonekura S. Cerebellar infarction with hypertriglyceridemia during all-trans retinoic acid therapy for acute promyelocytic leukemia. *Leukemia* 1995;9(9):1602-1603.

26. Vahlquist C. Effects of retinoids on lipoprotein metabolism. *Curr Probl Dermatol* 1991;20:73-78.

27. Kanamaru A, Takemoto Y, Tanimoto M, et al. All-trans retinoic acid for the treatment of newly diagnosed acute promyelocytic leukemia. Japan Adult Leukemia Study Group. *Blood* 1995;85(5):1202-1206.

28. Castaigne S, Chomienne C, Daniel MT, et al. All-trans retinoic acid as a differentiation therapy for acute promyelocytic leukemia. I. Clinical results. *Blood* 1990;76(9):1704-1709.

29. Marsden J. Hyperlipidaemia due to isotretinoin and etretinate: possible mechanisms and consequences. *Br J Dermatol* 1986;114(4):401-407.

30. Duvic M, Hymes K, Heald P, et al. Bexarotene is effective and safe for treatment of refractory advanced-stage cutaneous T-cell lymphoma: Multinational phase II-III trial results. *J Clin Oncol* 2001;19(9):2456-2471.

31. Duvic M, Martin AG, Kim Y, et al. Phase 2 and 3 clinical trial of oral bexarotene (Targretin capsules) for the treatment of refractory or persistent early-stage cutaneous T-cell lymphoma. *Arch Dermatol* 2001;137(5):581-593.

32. Vassilopoulou-Sellin R, Samaan NA. Mitotane administration: An unusual cause of hypercholesterolemia. *Horm Metab Res* 1991;23(12):619-620.

33. Raghavan D, Cox K, Childs A, et al. Hypercholesterolemia after chemotherapy for testis cancer. *J Clin Oncol* 1992;10(9):1386-1389.

34. D'Angelo P, Conter V, Di Chiara G, et al. Severe osteoporosis and multiple vertebral collapses in a child during treatment for B-ALL. *Acta Haematol* 1993;89(1):38-42.

35. Baum M, Budzar AU, Cuzick J, et al. Anastrozole alone or in combination with tamoxifen versus tamoxifen alone for adjuvant treatment of postmenopausal women with early breast cancer: First results of the ATAC randomised trial. *Lancet* 2002;359(9324):2131-2139.

36. Nash TJ, Howlett CR, Martin C, et al. Effect of platelet-derived growth factor on tibial osteotomies in rabbits. *Bone* 1994;15(2):203-208.

37. Li B, Boast S, de los Santos K, et al. Mice deficient in Abl are osteoporotic and have defects in osteoblast maturation. *Nat Genet* 2000;24(3):304-308.

38. Fitter S, Dewar AL, Kostakis P, et al. Long-term imatinib therapy promotes bone formation in CML patients. *Blood* 2008;111(5):2538-2547.

39. Berman E, Nicolaides M, Maki RG, et al. Altered bone and mineral metabolism in patients receiving imatinib mesylate. *N Engl J Med* 2006;354(19):2006-2013.

40. Grey A, O'Sullivan S, Reid IR, et al. Imatinib mesylate, increased bone formation, and secondary hyperparathyroidism. *N Engl J Med* 2006;355(23):2494-2495.

41. Seufert J, Ebert K, Muller J, et al. Octreotide therapy for tumor-induced osteomalacia. *N Engl J Med* 2001;345(26):1883-1888.

42. Paglia F, Dionisi S, Minisola S. Octreotide for tumor-induced osteomalacia. *N Engl J Med* 2002;346(22):1748-1749; author reply 1748-1749.

43. Vassilopoulou-Sellin R, Newman BM, Taylor SH, et al. Incidence of hypercalcemia in patients with malignancy referred to a comprehensive cancer center. *Cancer* 1993;71(4):1309-1312.

44. Sakamoto O, Yoshinari M, Rikiishi T, et al. Hypercalcemia due to all-trans retinoic acid therapy for acute promyelocytic leukemia: A case report of effective treatment with bisphosphonate. *Pediatr Int* 2001;43(6):688-690.

45. Miller VA, Benedetti FM, Rigas JR, et al. Initial clinical trial of a selective retinoid X receptor ligand, LGD1069. *J Clin Oncol* 1997;15(2):790-795.

46. Jones SG, Dolan G, Lengyel K, et al. Severe increase in creatinine with hypocalcaemia in thalidomide-treated myeloma patients receiving zoledronic acid infusions. *Br J Haematol* 2002;119(2):576-577.

47. English MW, Skinner R, Pearson AD, et al. Dose-related nephrotoxicity of carboplatin in children. *Br J Cancer* 1999;81(2):336-341.

48. Grothey A. Oxaliplatin-safety profile: Neurotoxicity. *Semin Oncol* 2003;30(4 Suppl 15):5-13.

49. Extra JM, Espie M, Calvo F, et al. Phase I study of oxaliplatin in patients with advanced cancer. *Cancer Chemother Pharmacol* 1990;25(4):299-303.

50. Darzy KH. Radiation-induced hypopituitarism after cancer therapy: Who, how and when to test. *Nat Clin Pract Endocrinol Metab* 2009;5(2):88-99.

51. Blansfield JA, Beck KE, Tran K, et al. Cytotoxic T-lymphocyte-associated antigen-4 blockage can induce autoimmune hypophysitis in patients with metastatic melanoma and renal cancer. *J Immunother* 2005;28(6):593-598.

52. Shalet SM, Clayton PE, Price DA. Growth and pituitary function in children treated for brain tumours or acute lymphoblastic leukaemia. *Horm Res* 1988;30(2-3):53-61.

53. Abs R, Verhelst J, Maeyaert J, et al. Endocrine consequences of long-term intrathecal administration of opioids. *J Clin Endocrinol Metab* 2000;85(6):2215-2222.

54. Ogilvy-Stuart AL, Shalet SM, Gattamaneni HR. Thyroid function after treatment of brain tumors in children. *J Pediatr* 1991;119(5):733-737.

55. Sherman SI, Gopal J, Haugen BR, et al. Central hypothyroidism associated with retinoid X receptor-selective ligands. *N Engl J Med* 1999;340(14):1075-1079.

56. Sherman SI. Etiology, diagnosis, and treatment recommendations for central hypothyroidism associated with bexarotene therapy for cutaneous T-cell lymphoma. *Clin Lymphoma* 2003;3(4):249-252.

57. Pai HH, Thornton A, Katznelson L, et al. Hypothalamic/pituitary function following high-dose conformal radiotherapy to the base of skull: Demonstration of a dose-effect relationship using dose-volume histogram analysis. *Int J Radiat Oncol Biol Phys* 2001;49(4):1079-1092.

58. Samaan NA, Schultz PN, Yang KP, et al. Endocrine complications after radiotherapy for tumors of the head and neck. *J Lab Clin Med* 1987;109(3):364-372.

59. Rajagopal A, Vassilopoulou-Sellin R, Palmer JL, et al. Hypogonadism and sexual dysfunction in male cancer survivors receiving chronic opioid therapy. *J Pain Symptom Manage* 2003;26(5):1055-1061.

60. Nikiforov YE: RET/PTC rearrangement in thyroid tumors. Endocr Pathol 2002;13(1):3-16.

61. Ron E, Lubin JH, Shore RE, et al. Thyroid cancer after exposure to external radiation: A pooled analysis of seven studies. *Radiat Res* 1995;141(3):259-277.

62. Samaan NA, Schultz PN, Ordonez NG, et al. A comparison of thyroid carcinoma in those who have and have not had head and neck irradiation in childhood. *J Clin Endocrinol Metab* 1987;64(2):219-223.

63. Tucker MA, Jones PH, Boice JD, Jr., et al. Therapeutic radiation at a young age is linked to secondary thyroid cancer. The Late Effects Study Group. *Cancer Res* 1991;51(11):2885-2888.

64. Prummel MF, Laurberg P. Interferon-alpha and autoimmune thyroid disease. *Thyroid* 2003;13(6):547-551.

65. Wong V, Fu AX, George J, et al. Thyrotoxicosis induced by alpha-interferon therapy in chronic viral hepatitis. *Clin Endocrinol* (Oxf) 2002;56(6):793-798.

66. Vialettes B, Guillerand MA, Viens P, et al. Incidence rate and risk factors for thyroid dysfunction during recombinant interleukin-2 therapy in advanced malignancies. *Acta Endocrinol* (Copenh) 1993;129(1):31-38.

67. Hancock SL, Cox RS, McDougall IR. Thyroid diseases after treatment of Hodgkin's disease. *N Engl J Med* 1991;325(9):599-605.

68. Smith RE, Jr., Adler AR, Clark P, et al. Thyroid function after mantle irradiation in Hodgkin's disease. *JAMA* 1981;245(1):46-49.

69. Dalgard O, Bjoro K, Hellum K, et al. Thyroid dysfunction during treatment of chronic hepatitis C with interferon alpha: No association with either interferon dosage or efficacy of therapy. *J Intern Med* 2002;251(5):400-406.

70. Krouse RS, Royal RE, Heywood G, et al. Thyroid dysfunction in 281 patients with metastatic melanoma or renal carcinoma treated with interleukin-2 alone. *J Immunother Emphasis Tumor Immunol* 1995;18(4):272-278.

71. Stuart NS, Woodroffe CM, Grundy R, et al. Long-term toxicity of chemotherapy for testicular cancer–the cost of cure. *Br J Cancer* 1990;61(3):479-484.

72. Coles AJ, Compston DA, Selmaj KW, et al. Alemtuzumab vs. interferon beta-1a in early multiple sclerosis. *N Engl J Med* 2008;359(17):1786-1801.

73. de Groot JW, Zonnenberg BA, Plukker JT, et al. Imatinib induces hypothyroidism in patients receiving levothyroxine. *Clin Pharmacol Ther* 2005;78(4):433-438.

74. Dora JM, Leie MA, Netto B, et al. Lack of imatinib-induced thyroid dysfunction in a cohort of non-thyroidectomized patients. *Eur J Endocrinol* 2008;158(5):771-772.

75. Tamaskar I, Bukowski R, Elson P, et al. Thyroid function test abnormalities in patients with metastatic renal cell carcinoma treated with sorafenib. *Ann Oncol* 2008;19(2):265-268.

76. Miyake H, Kurahashi T, Yamanaka K, et al. Abnormalities of thyroid function in Japanese patients with metastatic renal cell carcinoma treated with sorafenib: A prospective evaluation. *Urol Oncol* 2010;28(5):515-519.

77. Desai J, Yassa L, Marqusee E, et al. Hypothyroidism after sunitinib treatment for patients with gastrointestinal stromal tumors. *Ann Intern Med* 2006;145(9):660-664.

78. Wolter P, Stefan C, Decallonne B, et al. The clinical implications of sunitinib-induced hypothyroidism: A prospective evaluation. *Br J Cancer* 2008;99(3):448-454.

79. Grossmann M, Premaratne E, Desai J, et al. Thyrotoxicosis during sunitinib treatment for renal cell carcinoma. *Clin Endocrinol* (Oxf) 2008;69(4):669-672.

80. Faris JE, Moore AF, Daniels GH: Sunitinib (sutent)-induced thyrotoxicosis due to destructive thyroiditis: A case report. *Thyroid* 2007;17(11):1147-1149.

81. Mannavola D, Coco P, Vannucchi G, et al. A novel tyrosine-kinase selective inhibitor, sunitinib, induces transient hypothyroidism by blocking iodine uptake. *J Clin Endocrinol Metab* 2007;92(9):3531-3534.

82. Wong E, Rosen LS, Mulay M, et al. Sunitinib induces hypothyroidism in advanced cancer patients and may inhibit thyroid peroxidase activity. *Thyroid* 2007;17(4):351-355.

83. Bajetta E, Zilembo N, Dowsett M, et al. Double-blind, randomised, multicentre endocrine trial comparing two letrozole doses, in postmenopausal breast cancer patients. *Eur J Cancer* 1999;35(2):208-2013.

84. Garnick MB, Larsen PR. Acute deficiency of thyroxine-binding globulin during L-asparaginase therapy. *N Engl J Med* 1979;301(5):252-253.

85. Heidemann PH, Stubbe P, Beck W. Transient secondary hypothyroidism and thyroxine binding globulin deficiency in leukemic children during polychemotherapy: An effect of L-asparaginase. *Eur J Pediatr* 1981;136(3):291-295.

86. Beex L, Ross A, Smals A, et al. 5-fluorouracil-induced increase of total serum thyroxine and triiodothyronine. *Cancer Treat Rep* 1977;61(7):1291-1295.

87. van Seters AP, Moolenaar AJ. Mitotane increases the blood levels of hormone-binding proteins. *Acta Endocrinol* (Copenh) 1991;124(5):526-533.

88. Goodman VL, Rock EP, Dagher R, et al. Approval summary: Sunitinib for the treatment of imatinib refractory or intolerant gastrointestinal stromal tumors and advanced renal cell carcinoma. *Clin Cancer Res* 2007;13(5):1367-1373.

89. Patterson BC, Truxillo L, Wasilewski-Masker K, et al. Adrenal function testing in pediatric cancer survivors. *Pediatr Blood Cancer* 2009;53(7):1302-1307.

90. Vivacqua RJ, Haurani FI, Erslev AJ. "Selective" pituitary insufficiency secondary to busulfan. *Ann Intern Med* 1967; 67(2):380-387.

91. Meacham LR, Mazewski C, Krawiecki N. Mechanism of transient adrenal insufficiency with megestrol acetate treatment of cachexia in children with cancer. *J Pediatr Hematol Oncol* 2003;25(5):414-417.

92. Raedler TJ, Jahn H, Goedeken B, et al. Acute effects of megestrol on the hypothalamic-pituitary-adrenal axis. *Cancer Chemother Pharmacol* 2003;52(6):482-486.

93. Lushbaugh CC, Casarett GW. The effects of gonadal irradiation in clinical radiation therapy: A review. *Cancer* 1976;37 (2 Suppl):1111-1125.

94. Howard GC. Fertility following cancer therapy. *Clin Oncol (R Coll Radiol)* 1991;3(5):283-287.

95. Thibaud E, Rodriguez-Macias K, Trivin C, et al. Ovarian function after bone marrow transplantation during childhood. *Bone Marrow Transplant* 1998;21(3):287-290.

96. Morice P, Juncker L, Rey A, et al. Ovarian transposition for patients with cervical carcinoma treated by radiosurgical combination. *Fertil Steril* 2000;74(4):743-748.

97. Recchia F, Sica G, De Filippis S, et al. Goserelin as ovarian protection in the adjuvant treatment of premenopausal breast cancer: A phase II pilot study. *Anticancer Drugs* 2002;13(4): 417-424.

98. Blumenfeld Z. Ovarian rescue/protection from chemotherapeutic agents. *J Soc Gynecol Investig* 2001;8(1 Suppl Proceedings):60S-64S.

99. Bines J, Oleske DM, Cobleigh MA. Ovarian function in premenopausal women treated with adjuvant chemotherapy for breast cancer. *J Clin Oncol* 1996;14(5):1718-1729.

100. Freckman HA, Fry HL, Mendez FL, et al. Chlorambucil-Prednisolone Therapy for Disseminated Breast Carcinoma. *JAMA* 1964;189:23-26.

101. Ezdinli EZ, Stutzman L. Chlorambucil Therapy for Lymphomas and Chronic Lymphocytic Leukemia. *JAMA* 1965; 191:444-450.

102. Meirow D, Nugent D. The effects of radiotherapy and chemotherapy on female reproduction. *Hum Reprod Update* 2001;7(6):535-543.

103. Bokemeyer C, Schmoll HJ, van Rhee J, et al. Long-term gonadal toxicity after therapy for Hodgkin's and non-Hodgkin's lymphoma. *Ann Hematol* 1994;68(3):105-110.

104. Ahmed SR, Shalet SM, Campbell RH, et al. Primary gonadal damage following treatment of brain tumors in childhood. *J Pediatr* 1983;103(4):562-565.

105. Clayton PE, Shalet SM, Price DA, et al. Ovarian function following chemotherapy for childhood brain tumours. *Med Pediatr Oncol* 1989;17(2):92-96.

106. Choo YC, Chan SY, Wong LC, et al. Ovarian dysfunction in patients with gestational trophoblastic neoplasia treated with short intensive courses of etoposide (VP-16-213). *Cancer* 1985;55(10):2348-2352.

107. Wong LC, Choo YC, Ma HK. Primary oral etoposide therapy in gestational trophoblastic disease. An update. *Cancer* 1986; 58(1):14-17.

108. Morgenfeld MC, Goldberg V, Parisier H, et al. Ovarian lesions due to cytostatic agents during the treatment of Hodgkin's disease. *Surg Gynecol Obstet* 1972;134(5): 826-828.

109. Meistrich ML, Wilson G, Brown BW, et al. Impact of cyclophosphamide on long-term reduction in sperm count in men treated with combination chemotherapy for Ewing and soft tissue sarcomas. *Cancer* 1992;70(11): 2703-2712.

110. Rowley MJ, Leach DR, Warner GA, et al. Effect of graded doses of ionizing radiation on the human testis. *Radiat Res* 1974;59(3):665-678.

111. Clifton DK, Bremner WJ. The effect of testicular x-irradiation on spermatogenesis in man. A comparison with the mouse. *J Androl* 1983;4(6):387-392.

112. Howell SJ, Shalet SM. Effect of cancer therapy on pituitary-testicular axis. *Int J Androl* 2002;25(5):269-276.

113. Cheviakoff S, Calamera JC, Morgenfeld M, et al. Recovery of spermatogenesis in patients with lymphoma after treatment with chlorambucil. *J Reprod Fertil* 1973;33(1): 155-157.

114. Charak BS, Gupta R, Mandrekar P, et al. Testicular dysfunction after cyclophosphamide-vincristine-procarbazine-prednisolone chemotherapy for advanced Hodgkin's disease. A long-term follow-up study. *Cancer* 1990;65(9): 1903-1906.

115. Petersen PM, Hansen SW, Giwercman A, et al. Dose-dependent impairment of testicular function in patients treated with cisplatin-based chemotherapy for germ cell cancer. *Ann Oncol* 1994;5(4):355-358.

116. Shamberger RC, Rosenberg SA, Seipp CA, et al. Effects of high-dose methotrexate and vincristine on ovarian and testicular functions in patients undergoing postoperative adjuvant treatment of osteosarcoma. *Cancer Treat Rep* 1981;65(9-10): 739-746.

117. Adachi T, Nishimura T, Imahie H, et al. Collaborative work to evaluate toxicity on male reproductive organs by repeated dose studies in rats 9). Testicular toxicity in male rats given adriamycin for two or four weeks. *J Toxicol Sci* 2000;25 Spec No:95-101.

118. Bonadonna G, Santoro A, Viviani S, et al. Gonadal damage in Hodgkin's disease from cancer chemotherapeutic regimens. *Arch Toxicol Suppl* 1984;7:140-145.

119. Schilsky RL, Davidson HS, Magid D, et al. Gonadal and sexual function in male patients with hairy cell leukemia: Lack of adverse effects of recombinant alpha 2-interferon treatment. *Cancer Treat Rep* 1987;71(2):179-181.

120. Meistrich ML, Shetty G. Suppression of testosterone stimulates recovery of spermatogenesis after cancer treatment. *Int J Androl* 2003;26(3):141-146.

121. Whitehead E, Shalet SM, Blackledge G, et al. The effects of Hodgkin's disease and combination chemotherapy on gonadal function in the adult male. *Cancer* 1982;49(3): 418-422.

122. Clark ST, Radford JA, Crowther D, et al. Gonadal function following chemotherapy for Hodgkin's disease: A comparative study of MVPP and a seven-drug hybrid regimen. *J Clin Oncol* 1995;13(1):134-139.

123. Shafford EA, Kingston JE, Malpas JS, et al. Testicular function following the treatment of Hodgkin's disease in childhood. *Br J Cancer* 1993;68(6):1199-1204.

124. Hill M, Milan S, Cunningham D, et al. Evaluation of the efficacy of the VEEP regimen in adult Hodgkin's disease with assessment of gonadal and cardiac toxicity. *J Clin Oncol* 1995;13(2):387-395.

125. Viviani S, Santoro A, Ragni G, et al. Gonadal toxicity after combination chemotherapy for Hodgkin's disease. Comparative results of MOPP vs ABVD. *Eur J Cancer Clin Oncol* 1985; 21(5):601-605.

126. Lam KS, Tse VK, Wang C, et al. Effects of cranial irradiation on hypothalamic-pituitary function–a 5-year longitudinal study in patients with nasopharyngeal carcinoma. *Q J Med* 1991;78(286):165-176.

ONCOLOGIC EMERGENCIES

Sai-Ching Jim Yeung
Ellen F. Manzullo

Oncologic emergencies can result from either the cancer or its treatment. Cancer patients often have immunologic, metabolic, and hematologic defects, which can lead to complex emergency conditions when they present to an emergency center. In addition, emergencies resulting from comorbid conditions also occur in cancer patients. It is important for practitioners who treat patients with cancer to be aware of the various oncologic emergencies so that they can be recognized and treated promptly. This chapter discusses many of these emergencies, including their signs and symptoms, causes, and management.

■ NEUROLOGIC EMERGENCIES

SPINAL CORD COMPRESSION

Spinal cord compression is a serious complication of cancer progression, affecting about 2.5% of cancer patients overall (1). It is not immediately life-threatening unless it involves the first three cervical vertebrae, but involvement in the rest of the spine leads to significant morbidity (2). The spinal cord is compressed at the thoracic vertebrae in 70% of patients, cervical vertebrae in 10% of patients, and lumbar vertebrae in 20% of patients. In 10 to 38% of cases, spinal cord compression occurs at multiple levels (3). Such compression is predominantly due to metastatic tumors, with lung, breast, and prostate cancer comprising 50% of these. Other tumors that commonly metastasize to the spine are multiple myeloma, renal cell carcinoma, melanoma, lymphoma, sarcoma, and gastrointestinal (GI) cancers. The mechanisms by which tumors can appear in the spine are hematogenous spread of tumor cells to the vertebral bodies, metastasis of primary lesions to the posterior spinal elements, and direct extension of paraspinal tumors. Spinal cord compression is caused by epidural metastases in 75% and bony collapse in 25% of cases (4).

The most common presentation of spinal cord compression is back pain, occurring in over 90% of patients. Depending on the location of the tumor in the spinal canal, the pain can be unilateral or bilateral following dermatomal patterns. Patients typically report that their pain is worse when they are supine and better when they are upright. Some patients present with ataxia, which is due to compression of the spinocerebellar tracts. Ataxia can be confused with cerebellar metastasis, overmedication with analgesics, or other disorders. Metastasis to the spinal cord can precede spinal cord compression by weeks or months. The patient may also note sensory symptoms, including numbness or tingling in the toes, which can progress proximally. Preexisting peripheral neuropathy must be differentiated from spinal cord compression and acute worsening of existing symptoms or experienced new numbness or tingling. Motor symptoms are the second most common complaint after pain; difficulty walking, buckling under of the legs, and a feeling of heaviness in the legs are all frequent symptoms. In this case, compression of the spinal cord must be distinguished from dehydration, anemia, and orthostatic hypotension. The last symptoms to appear are autonomic symptoms, such as an inability to urinate, urinary retention, and constipation. Autonomic symptoms are late findings in spinal cord compression and must be distinguished from the effects of chemotherapy, pain medicines, and antihistamines. It is important to remember that the patient may present with intractable pain only, so a high level of suspicion for spinal cord compression is important in treating cancer patients.

The physical examination usually reveals tenderness to percussion over the affected level of the spine, but the spine might not be tender if there is no bone involvement. Other possible findings are urinary retention, decreased rectal sphincter tone, and muscle weakness. The patient might have pain at a referred site; for instance, patients with L1 compression might have pain in the sacroiliac area. Sensory changes are more difficult to diagnose than motor deficits and can either precede or accompany motor effects. The patient might have decreased sensation in the lower extremities, which may ascend to the level of spinal cord involvement with dorsal column deficits, including loss of light touch sensation, proprioception, and position sense. When the cauda equina is compressed, the sensory changes are dermatomal, with loss of sensation in the perineal area, the posterior thigh, or lateral leg.

The differential diagnosis of spinal cord compression includes osteoarthritis, degenerative disk disease, spinal abscess, hematoma/bleeding, hemangioma, chordoma, meningioma, and neurofibroma. A standard x-ray is generally ordered first to analyze the area of the spine within which compression is suspected. However, simple roentgenography yields false-negative results in 10 to 17% of cases, in part because approximately 30 to 50% of the bone must be destroyed before bony lesions can be seen on x-ray films (5). Magnetic resonance imaging (MRI) is the imaging technique of choice today for suspected spinal cord compression (Fig. 46-1).

In the past decades, myelography was the "gold standard" in diagnosing spinal cord compression, but this technique is invasive, time-consuming and painful,

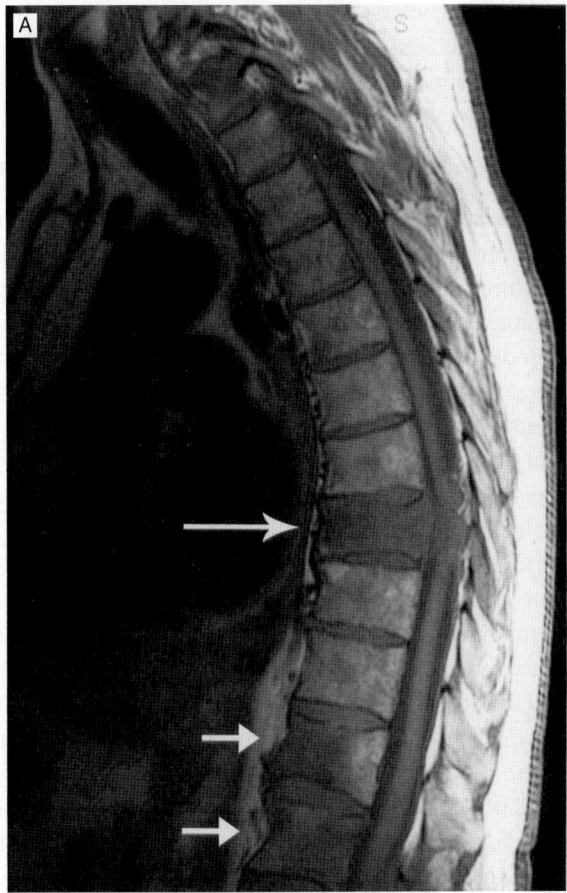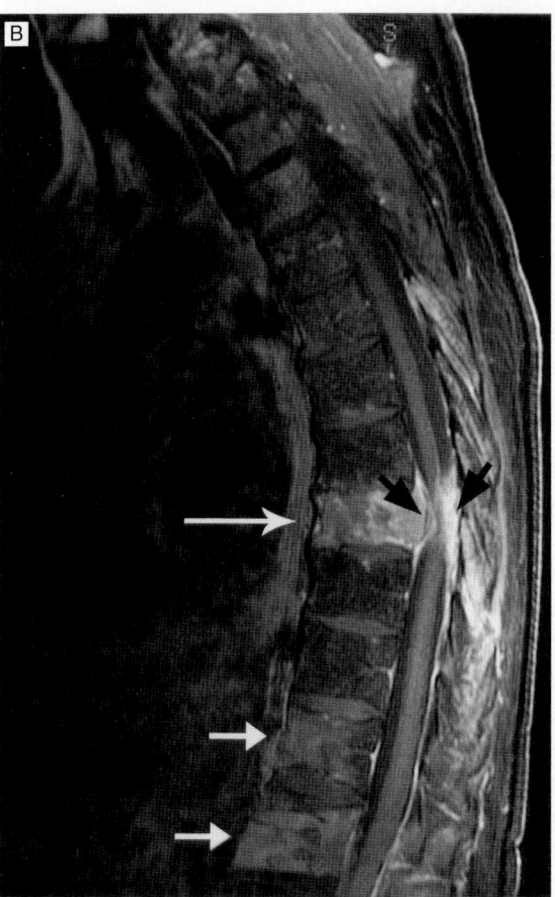

FIGURE 46-1. **A.** Precontrast T1-weighted MR image of thoracic cord compression at the T8 level produced by an epidural tumor from vertebral body metastasis (*large arrow*). Smaller arrows point to other sites of bony metastasis. The patient is a 67-year-old man with melanoma and back pain. **B.** Postcontrast T1-weighted MR image of the same patient. The epidural tumor is visualized better with contrast (*black arrows*). (*Courtesy of Dr. Ashok Kumar, MD Anderson Cancer Center.*)

and requires the use of intrathecal contrast. Patients who are not able to undergo MRI can undergo computed tomography (CT) myelogram, although, like myelography, this technique is more time-consuming and tedious than MRI. Nevertheless, these options are available for use on patients who cannot tolerate MRI because of the presence of cerebral aneurysm clips, cardiac pacemakers, magnetic implants, or severe claustrophobia. For patients with suspected spinal cord compression, physicians should consider imaging the entire spine, as spinal epidural disease is often multifocal. Findings for the whole spine can help the physician optimize the type and extent of therapy needed. For any patient with rapidly progressive neurologic symptoms, diagnostic imaging should be performed on an emergency basis.

Corticosteroid is a temporizing measure to stabilize or even improve neurologic function until definitive treatment. Conventionally, dexamethasone is initially given at 10 to 100 mg intravenously and then 4 to 24 mg every 4 to 6 h (6). The duration of therapy with high-dose glucocorticoids should be minimized to prevent complications of steroid use. Surgery is indicated for recurrent or progressive disease at an area with previous maximal radiotherapy, spinal mechanical instability, an unknown tissue diagnosis of malignancy, or for compression of the spinal cord by bony structure/fragment (2,3). Patchell and colleagues in 2005 reported the first phase III randomized clinical trial comparing the role of decompressive surgery and radiation to radiation alone (7). In this study, patients were initially treated with 100 mg of dexamethasone followed by 24 mg every 6 h and then treated with radiation therapy (30 Gy in 10 fractions) alone or surgery (usually within 24 h) followed by the same course of radiation within 2 weeks of surgery. The percentage of ambulatory patients was significantly higher in the group treated with surgery and radiation compared with radiation alone (84 versus 57%, respectively), so were their duration of ambulation (median 122 versus 13 days) and median survival (126 versus 100 days). Currently, anterior decompression with spinal stabilization is the surgery of choice, allowing removal of the affected vertebral body and stabilization above and below the vertebrae by metal hardware. For paraplegic patients with spinal cord compression, surgery with postoperative radiotherapy maximizes neurologic function and modestly prolongs survival (6). Benefit from decompressive surgery is evident in ambulatory patients with poor prognostic factors for radiotherapy, and in paralyzed patients with a single spinal area of compression, paraplegia less than 48 h, nonradiosensitive tumors, and a expected survival of more than 3 months (8). If surgery is not indicated, radiation therapy can be used for radiosensitive tumors; the most common dosage is 3000 cGy delivered in 10 fractions (3). The incidence of myelopathy, which can occur as a complication of radiation therapy, increases with increasing total dosage of therapy and can appear from months to several years after such therapy is given (9). Palliative radiotherapy is recommended for those with paraplegia longer than 48 h, expected to live for fewer than 3 months, unable to tolerate surgery, and with multiple areas of compression. An ambulatory patient with a stable spine may be considered for radiation treatment only (6). The role of chemotherapy to treat spinal cord compression is not clear. Chemotherapy is occasionally used for chemosensitive tumors, such as those of Hodgkin disease, neuroblastoma, non-Hodgkin lymphoma, germ cell tumors, and breast cancer. Agents reported in the literature for treatment of spinal cord gliomas include temozolomide, irinotecan, cisplatin, and carboplatin (6). Hormonal therapy can benefit some patients with hormone-responsive tumors, such as prostate and breast cancers (5). One of the most important prognostic factors at diagnosis is the patient's neurologic function. Of patients who are ambulatory at the time of presentation, approximately three-fourths will be able to regain their strength with treatment. By contrast, only a small percentage of patients who are paralyzed at the time of presentation are likely to walk again (9). This difference illustrates why it is imperative to diagnose spinal cord compression at an early stage. A scoring system, which is derived from a multivariate survival analysis of 1852 patients who were treated with radiotherapy for spinal cord compression and is based on tumor type, interval between tumor diagnosis and spinal cord compression, other bone or visceral metastases, ambulatory status, and duration of paralysis, can

estimate survival (10). Overall, the median survival following the first episode of spinal cord compression is about 3 months. (1)

INCREASED INTRACRANIAL PRESSURE

Increased intracranial pressure in cancer patients is commonly due to hemorrhage (from thrombocytopenia or tumor bleeding), brain metastasis with vasogenic edema and mass effect, or hydrocephalus due to obstruction of the flow of cerebrospinal fluid (CSF). Increased intracranial pressure can also be caused by tumor treatments, such as radiation therapy and surgery. The normal CSF pressure is less than 10 mm Hg. As intracranial pressure increases, herniation syndromes may develop, including uncal, central, and tonsillar herniation. Uncal herniation is caused by unilateral supratentorial lesions that push brain tissue through the tentorial notch. Signs and symptoms include ipsilateral pupil dilation, decreased consciousness, and hemiparesis, first contralateral and then ipsilateral to the mass. Central herniation involves bilateral supratentorial lesions that displace tissue symmetrically and bilaterally. Signs and symptoms of central herniation include decreased consciousness leading to coma and Cheyne-Stokes respiration, followed by central hyperventilation, midposition unreactive pupils, and posturing. Tonsillar herniation involves increased pressure in the posterior fossa, which forces the cerebellar tonsil through the foramen magnum, thereby compressing the medulla. Signs and symptoms of tonsillar herniation include decreased consciousness and respiratory abnormalities leading to apnea. Headache is the most frequent symptom reported in increased intracranial pressure. Headache is a common symptom in any patient population, but in cancer patients the clinician must always maintain a high index of suspicion for increased intracranial pressure. Headaches due to increased intracranial pressure are typically present on waking in the morning, recur throughout the day, and are increased with Valsalva maneuver; they can be associated with nausea and vomiting, altered mental status, vision changes, seizures, or focal neurologic deficits. On physical examination, the patient might have papilledema, focal neurologic deficits, or a decreased level of consciousness.

The diagnosis of increased intracranial pressure can be ascertained from CT scans of the brain. Noncontrast CT imaging of the brain is superior to MRI in detecting acute hemorrhage (Fig. 46-2).

CT scans with contrast will usually reveal cerebral metastasis and occasionally leptomeningeal disease (LMD). Contrast-enhanced MRI is more sensitive than

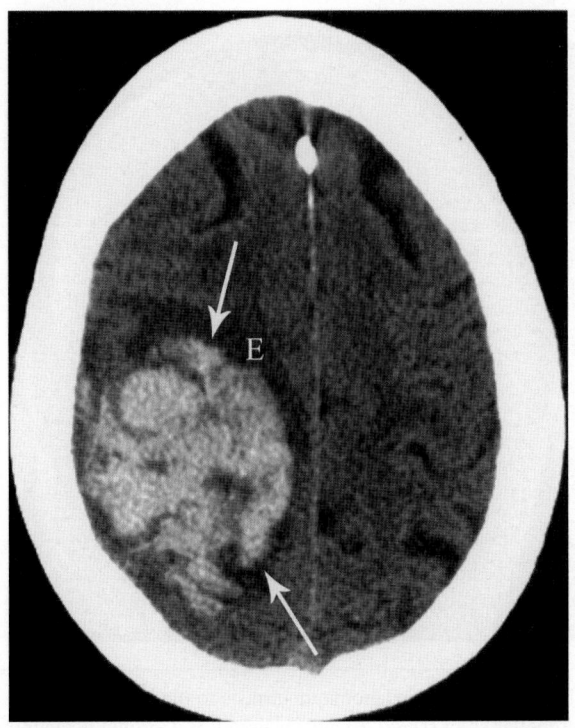

FIGURE 46-2. Acute intracranial hemorrhage within the right frontoparietal lobe (*arrows*) with edema (E) in a 79-year-old woman with ovarian cancer. The hemorrhage was revealed by noncontrast CT imaging. This modality is superior to MRI in detecting acute hemorrhage. (*Courtesy of Dr. Ashok Kumar, MD Anderson Cancer Center.*)

CT in revealing cerebral neoplasms and metastases as small as 3 mm (Fig. 46-3), LMD (Fig. 46-4), and early strokes (Fig. 46-5). Lumbar puncture should not be used to diagnose increased intracranial pressure, as this can lead to brain herniation.

The differential diagnosis of increased intracranial pressure includes bleeding, tumor edema, hydrocephalus, postradiation effects, postradiosurgery effects, brachytherapy-induced changes, benign tumor effects, subdural hematomas, meningitis, encephalitis, and abscess formation.

Brain metastases may develop in 10 to 40% of cancer patients (11,12). LMD occurs in 5% of all patients with cancer (13). Two-thirds to three-quarters of brain metastases are recognized as multiple lesions on MRI. Lung cancer is the neoplasm that most frequently metastasizes to the brain, followed by breast cancer and melanoma. Other cancers that commonly metastasize to the brain are colorectal, kidney, prostate, testicular, and ovarian cancers and sarcomas, although any systemic cancer can metastasize to the brain. Melanomas have the highest propensity to metastasize to the brain, with up to 40% of cases behaving in this manner at some point. Tumors most commonly metastasize to the gray-white junction where the vessels are small and narrow and tumor emboli can be trapped. Eighty percent

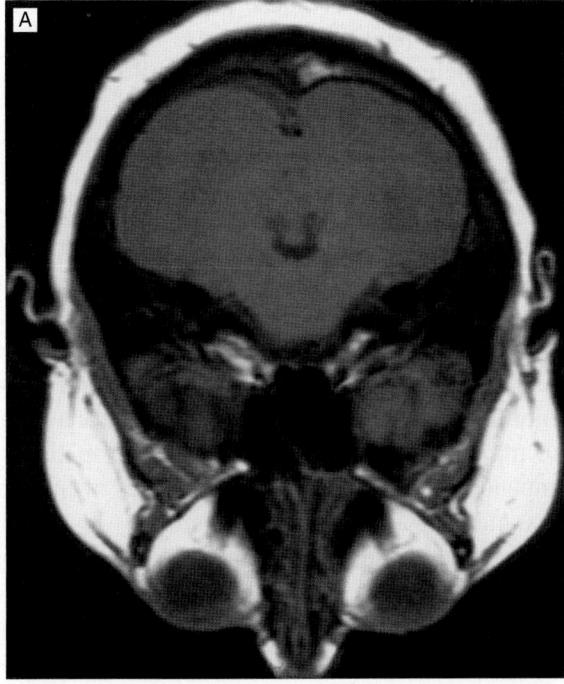

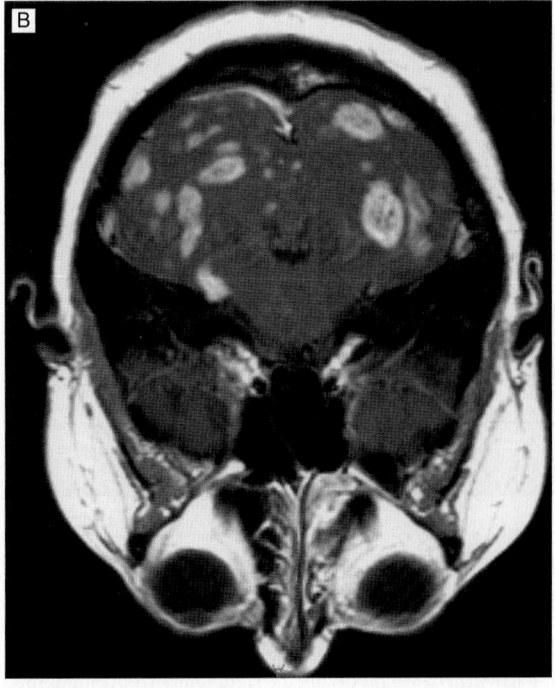

FIGURE 46-3. **A.** Precontrast T1-weighted MR images in a 40-year-old woman with breast cancer and multiple cerebellar metastases. **B.** Postcontrast images of the same patient reveal dramatic enhancement of the cerebellar metastases.

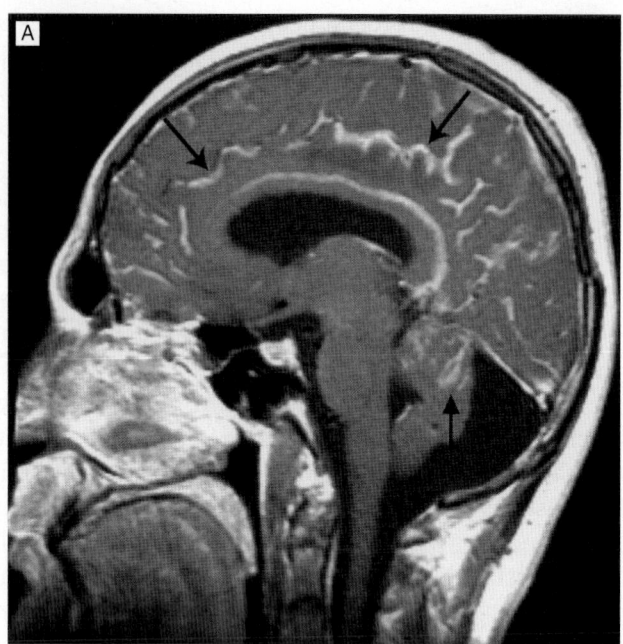
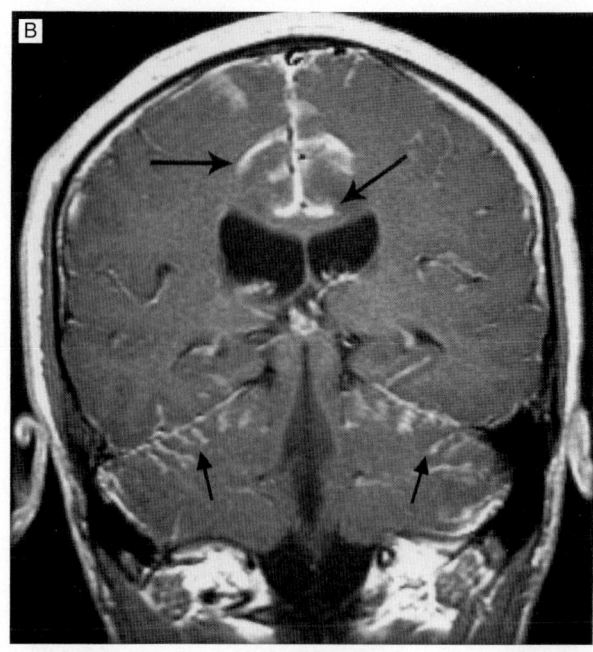

FIGURE 46-4. **A.** Sagittal postcontrast T1-weighted MRI showing subarachnoid spread of melanoma metastasis to the brain in a 29-year-old man. Abnormal enhancement of the cortical sulci (*large arrows*) and cerebellar sulci (*small arrows*) is noted. **B.** Coronal postcontrast T1-weighted MRI in the same patient. (*Courtesy of Dr. Ashok Kumar, MD Anderson Cancer Center.*)

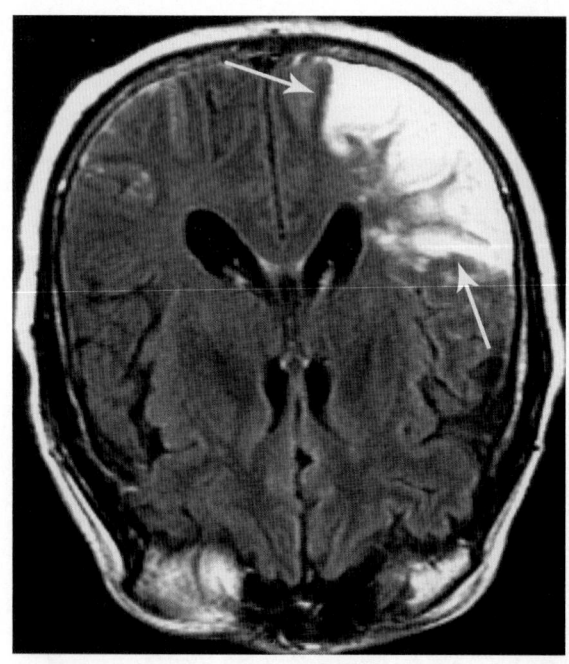

FIGURE 46-5. Acute infarction involving the territory of the right middle cerebral artery in a 58-year-old patient with renal cell carcinoma. MRI (fluid-attenuated inversion recovery [FLAIR] image) demonstrates abnormal thickening, with a T2-weighted increase in signal intensity (*arrows*) involving the right temporo-occipital lobe cortex and subcortical white matter. MRI is more sensitive than CT in detecting early stroke. (*Courtesy of Dr. Ashok Kumar, MD Anderson Cancer Center.*)

of tumors metastasize to the cerebral hemispheres, 15% to the cerebellum, and 5% to the brainstem. Pelvic tumors have an increased propensity to metastasize to the posterior fossa, possibly by means of venous drainage of these tumors through Batson plexus (14). The tumors that are most often hemorrhagic include melanoma, renal cell carcinoma, and choriocarcinoma (15).

The treatment for increased intracranial pressure depends on the underlying etiology. Infectious sources, such as meningitis, should be treated with antibiotics, and brain abscesses should be drained. Hydrocephalus should be treated with surgical shunting or ventriculostomy, and subdural hematomas should be either drained or, if small, monitored under the guidance of a neurosurgeon. Edema associated with brain tumors is initially treated with oral dexamethasone at a dosage of 16 mg/day or 4 mg every 6 h (16). For patients with impending herniation, very large doses of intravenous dexamethasone can be used, initially 40 to 100 mg intravenously and subsequently 40 to 100 mg/day (3). Dexamethasone is the steroid of choice because of its lack of mineralocorticoid effect and therefore minimal effects on blood pressure and electrolytes. Steroid myopathy is a possible complication of corticosteroid use. Steroids may not be needed in asymptomatic brain lesions (17).

For life-threatening edema, mannitol can be used to decrease intracranial pressure in patients with an intact blood–brain barrier. Mannitol is a hyperosmotic agent that can draw fluid out of the brain and into the vessels; its effect can be augmented by the use of diuretics. The recommended dose of mannitol is a 20 to 25% solution at 0.5 to 2.0 g/kg administered intravenously over 10 to 30 min. Mannitol has a rapid onset of action and lasts for hours, but prolonged use can lead to hyperosmolarity and an inadvertent increase in intracranial pressure (3). Hyperventilation can be used to decrease intracranial pressure, but it must be kept within the modest range of a PCO_2 of 25 to 30 mm Hg to prevent acidosis. The onset of action is immediate and its effect will last for several minutes (3).

Radiation therapy can be used to treat brain metastasis. The dosage for whole-brain radiation therapy (WBRT) typically ranges between 20 Gy over 1 week and 50 Gy over 4 weeks. WBRT can increase survival in patients by 3 to 6 months relative to no treatment (16). Increased intracranial pressure should be treated before WBRT is instituted, as radiotherapy can further increase pressure. Common side effects of WBRT are nausea and vomiting, alopecia, headache, hearing loss, loss of taste, and fever. Possible delayed complications of WBRT are progressive leukoencephalopathy with dementia, ataxia, apraxia, and incontinence syndrome, which can mimic normal-pressure hydrocephalus. This dreaded side effect can occur as long as 1 year after therapy, and elderly patients are more susceptible (15,18).

Surgery can be used to treat accessible brain metastases. A stereotactic biopsy can be performed for the patient with multiple brain metastases, which are then generally treated with radiation (19). Surgery is generally not indicated for patients with widespread systemic disease, poor functional status, or tumors in critical or hard-to-access locations (16,19). The experience at the University of Texas MD Anderson Cancer Center (MD Anderson) has been that for select patients with good functional status, even when multiple brain metastases are present, survival time is longer for those patients who have all tumors removed than for those who do not. Consequently, it is common for the neurosurgeons at our institution to remove up to four metastatic lesions at a time (17). Patchell and colleagues found that patients with single brain metastases who underwent WBRT after surgery had longer survival than those who had surgery alone (20).

For patients with brain lesions that are not amenable to surgery, stereotactic radiosurgery can be used in single doses as high as 1400 cGy. This approach is typically used for brain tumors less than 4 cm in diameter and has the benefit of being noninvasive and relatively fast-acting (5,18). Brachytherapy can be used on larger tumors, but this approach requires that radioactive seeds be invasively implanted in the designated area and left for 5 or 6 days, delivering approximately 6000 cGy to the area. One common side effect of brachytherapy is radiation necrosis, which develops in up to 50% of patients 6 months after treatment. This adverse effect can mimic tumor recurrence, is not distinguishable from tumor on MRI, and often requires biopsy to determine the etiology. Positron emission tomography (PET) scanning can be helpful, typically revealing decreased uptake in radiation necrosis and increased uptake in recurrent tumor. Radiation necrosis is not often found after stereotactic radiosurgery, perhaps because of the relatively small size of the irradiated area (18). No treatment exists for radiation necrosis, although the symptoms may respond to corticosteroids.

Chemotherapy can be used in some patients with brain metastasis. Dexamethasone, which is thought to aid in reestablishing the blood–brain barrier, should not be used if possible, so that the selected chemotherapeutic agent(s) can reach the tumor cells. Cancers for which chemotherapy has been used include choriocarcinoma, small cell cancer of the lungs, and breast cancer (16,18,21).

LEPTOMENINGEAL DISEASE

Leptomeningeal disease (LMD) can involve invasion of the brain, the spinal parenchyma, the nerve roots, and blood vessels of the nervous system. The cancers that most commonly result in LMD are breast and lung cancer, melanoma, non-Hodgkin lymphoma, and leukemia. Patients present with a variety of symptoms depending on the location of the leptomeninges affected, but they can include headache, altered mental status, cranial nerve palsies (in about 50% of patients), incontinence, back pain, sensory changes, seizures, isolated neurologic findings, and even a stroke-like presentation (5,9,22). Leptomeningeal metastases occur in 0.8 to 8% of all cases of cancer (5). The mechanism of LMD spread can be hematogenous, as in leukemias, by direct extension or bone marrow metastasis.

The diagnosis of LMD can be difficult to make. CT scans will occasionally be suggestive of LMD. MRI scanning has better sensitivity than CT for detecting LMD, including leptomeningeal enhancement, hydrocephalus, and cortical nodules. However, MRI results are not diagnostic (9). Inflammation of the meninges can also be found in cases of meningitis, trauma, infection, and hematoma formation (23). Lumbar puncture and evaluation of the CSF is the gold standard for diagnosing LMD, although multiple lumbar taps may be required to make the diagnosis, as only 50% of patients will have positive cytologic evidence of LMD on the first CSF evaluation (5,23). CSF findings consistent with LMD include a high opening pressure, low glucose and high protein levels, and a mononuclear pleocytosis (5). Among patients with normal values for CSF protein, glucose, opening pressure, and cytology negative for LMD, fewer than 5% will have LMD (23).

The treatment of LMD can include chemotherapy through an implanted subcutaneous reservoir and ventricular catheter (SRVC) or through lumbar puncture instillation. Lumbar tap administration does not require placement of a catheter, but 10 to 15% of the subarachnoid space might be missed using this technique. Chemotherapeutic agents frequently used are methotrexate and thiotepa. Cytarabine can also be used in patients with leukemias and lymphomas, but it is generally not effective against solid tumors. Radiation therapy is commonly used for localized LMD or in areas of nerve root involvement where intrathecal chemotherapy is not likely to reach adequate concentrations. Fixed neurologic deficits caused by LMD are not likely to improve with therapy, but encephalopathy may (23). The prognosis of patients with LMD is very poor, with a median survival of 3 to 6 months and only a 15 to 25% chance of surviving longer than 1 year (5).

SEIZURES

Seizures are the presenting symptom in 15 to 20% of patients with brain metastases (22). In cancer patients presenting with seizures and metabolic, infectious, and coagulopathic causes should also be considered. The initial laboratory work should include analysis of glucose level, electrolytes, blood urea nitrogen (BUN), creatinine, liver enzymes, calcium, urine analysis, prothrombin time (PT), activated partial thromboplastin time (aPTT), and toxicology screening if indicated (Fig. 46-6).

Patients can have seizures during withdrawal from high-dose, short-acting benzodiazepines (such as alprazolam), alcohol withdrawal, antibiotics (such as the carbapenems), pain medicines (such as meperidine), and many other medicines. The patient's family can be helpful in sorting out the etiology of seizures by providing information about the patient's medications, social history, and preceding symptoms, such as fever or headache. CT without and with contrast is also helpful and can identify increased intracranial pressure, bleeding, or brain metastasis. Electroencephalography (EEG) is also helpful in the evaluation of seizures and can determine whether an epileptic focus is present. Lumbar tap can be helpful if the seizures are believed to be secondary to infection or LMD, but this procedure should not be performed in patients with suspected increased intracranial pressure because of the risk of cerebral herniation.

Status epilepticus occurs when a patient has prolonged seizures lasting more than 30 min or recurrent seizures without full recovery of consciousness between seizures (24,25). Initial care for patients with status epilepticus includes placing the patient in a safe environment, administering 100% oxygen by non-rebreather mask, monitoring with a continuous-pulse oximeter providing suction, and administering intravenous fluids (normal saline). Priority should be placed on protecting the airway and extinguishing the seizure, which can be treated initially with intravenous benzodiazepines (such as diazepam, 0.2 mg/kg at 5 mg/min, up to 10 mg, or lorazepam, 0.1 mg/kg at 2 mg/min, up to 4 mg). For persistent seizures, fosphenytoin or phenytoin can be administered intravenously. Fosphenytoin can be given more rapidly and causes less hypotension than phenytoin, but continuous cardiac and blood pressure monitoring should be instituted during intravenous administration of 15 to 20 mg phenytoin equivalents (PE) per kilogram. Patients with persistent seizures might require intubation and sedation with phenobarbital (20 mg/kg intravenously at 100 mg/min) or other agents, such as pentobarbital or a midazolam drip. At this point, the patient will require careful monitoring and intensive care unit (ICU) care.

It is the general consensus of the American Academy of Neurology that routine use of prophylactic antiepileptic drugs (AEDs) for patients with brain metastases who have not experienced a seizure is not indicated (16). In certain instances prophylactic AEDs should be considered, including cases of metastatic melanoma with more than one brain metastasis, brain metastases involving the motor cortex, and cases involving both brain metastases and LMD. These three conditions have a high propensity for seizure development (5,12,22). Prophylactic AEDs might also be considered for patients in whom the brain metastases and edema are so large that a seizure would increase intracranial pressure, predisposing the patient to cerebral herniation (18).

Once seizures have been controlled, the patient should be placed on an AED. Several drugs can be used, among them phenytoin, carbamazepine, clonazepam, gabapentin, lamotrigine, phenobarbital, primidone, topiramate, and valproate. For many of the newer

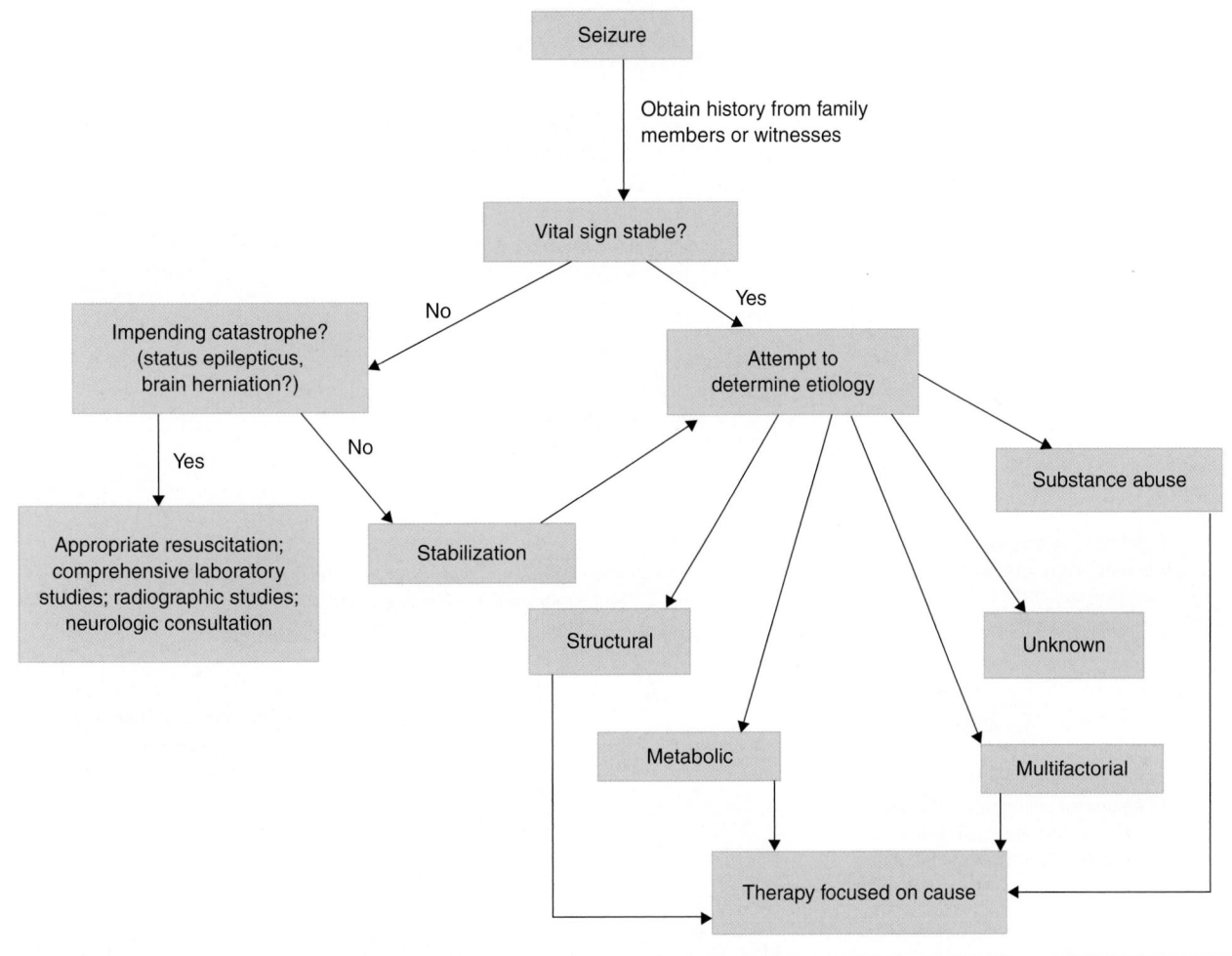

FIGURE 46-6. Algorithm for the evaluation of seizure. (*Adapted from Escalante CP, Hwang JP, Grover TS, et al. Major presenting symptoms. In: Yeung SJ, Escalante CP [eds]: Oncologic Emergencies. Hamilton, Ontario, Canada: BC Decker; 2002, with permission.*)

AEDs, the appropriate serum levels are not monitored. For those medicines in which effective and safe levels have been defined, such as phenytoin, carbamazepine, phenobarbital, and valproate, the levels should be monitored carefully to limit toxic effects and maintain an effective preventive drug concentration.

ALTERED MENTAL STATUS

Altered mental status is a common neurologic complaint in cancer patients, with metabolic encephalopathy being the most common cause (9,15). Altered mental status can range from a slight decrease in normal intellectual functioning to coma. A cancer patient's mental status may change in response to several factors, such as infections, metabolic derangements, bleeding, medications, hypoxemia, cancer therapies, paraneoplastic neurologic syndromes, and intracranial events,

such as brain metastases. Organ failure whether hepatic, renal, adrenal, thyroid, or pulmonary can also produce fluctuations in mental status. The most common metabolic deficiencies causing such alterations are hyponatremia, hypercalcemia, hypoglycemia, and vitamin B_1 deficiency (9). The causes of altered mental status are numerous; an extensive history and physical examination can help to identify the underlying cause and determine appropriate therapy (Fig. 46-7). The differential diagnosis and diagnostic evaluation are beyond the scope of this chapter, but a few entities are unique to cancer patients.

For instance, cancer therapy is a common cause of altered mental status. Many neurologic manifestations, such as dementia, cognitive decline, and encephalopathy, can result from chemotherapy. Table 46-1 highlights some of the common neurologic complications of chemotherapy (5,9,17,26).

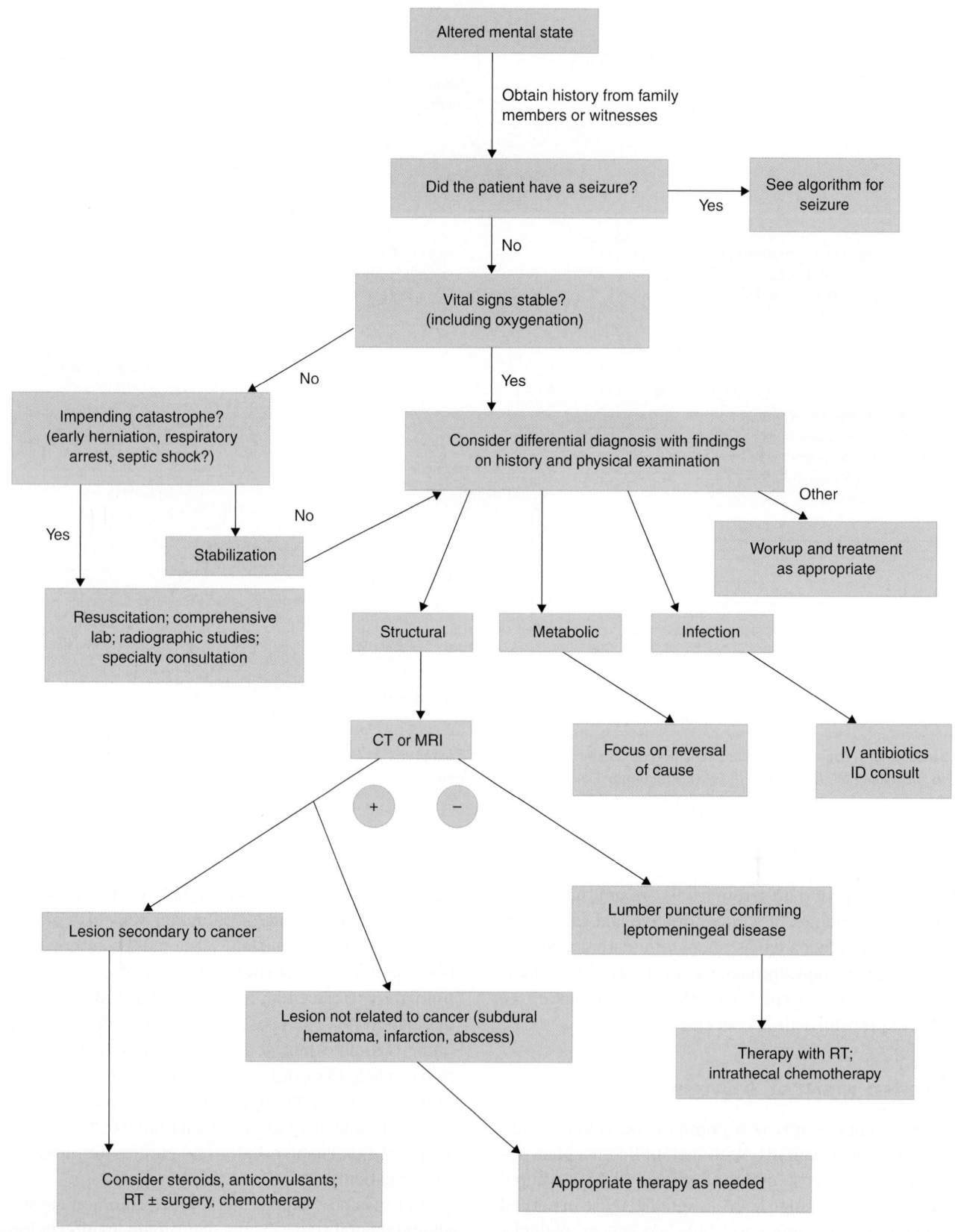

FIGURE 46-7. Algorithm for the evaluation and treatment of altered mental status. CT, computed tomography; ID, infectious disease; IV, intravenous; MRI, magnetic resonance imaging; RT, radiation therapy. (*Adapted from Escalante CP, Hwang JP, Grover TS, et al. Major presenting symptoms. In: Yeung SJ, Escalante CP [eds]: Oncologic Emergencies. Hamilton, Ontario, Canada: BC Decker; 2002, with permission.*)

TABLE 46-1 NEUROLOGIC COMPLICATIONS OF CHEMOTHERAPY

Chemotherapy	Seizure	Neuropathy or Sensory Changes	Encephalopathy	Cerebellar Symptoms	Vascular Events/Stroke	Cognitive/Dementia	Cranial Nerve Palsy	Visual Changes/Loss	Myelopathy	Other
BCNU	+		+		+		+	+		
Busulfan	+									
Cisplatin	+	+	+		+		+		+	Ototoxicity
Cystosine arabinoside		+	+	+						
Dacarbazine	+	+								
Docetaxel		+								
Doxorubicin								+		
Etoposide	+									
Fludarabine		+	+							
5-Fluorouracil		+	+	+						
Gemcitabine		+	+	+			+			
Ifosfamide	+	+	+		+	+	+			
Interferon	+		+			+	+			
Interleukin-2	+		+			+				
L-Asparaginase	+		+		+					
Methotrexate	+	+	+	+	+	+	+	+	+	Gait abnormality
Paclitaxel		+	+							
Procarbazine		+		+						
Tamoxifen		+						+		
Taxol		+								
Tenoposide		+								
Thalidomide		+								
Thiotepa			+							
Vincristine	+	+		+			+	+	+	Vertigo, autonomic neuropathy
Vinorelbine		+								

Radiation therapy can also cause complications, among them leukoencephalopathy, radiation necrosis, and decreased memory and mental functioning. (The preceding section on increased intracranial pressure provides a fuller discussion of the cognitive side effects of radiation therapy.) Other possible causes of cognitive decline are narcotics (commonly prescribed for pain), infections (pneumonia, sepsis, urinary tract infection), and cerebral infarction.

Paraneoplastic syndromes are unique to cancer patients and should be considered in cases of altered mental status. In many instances, the paraneoplastic syndrome will precede the cancer diagnosis. Paraneoplastic syndromes must be differentiated from cancer, the side effects of cancer therapy, and disease progression.

Paraneoplastic cerebellar degeneration is the most common paraneoplastic syndrome; affected patients present with subacute and progressive cerebellar degeneration with ataxia and dysarthria. This syndrome is most commonly found in patients with Hodgkin disease, ovarian and breast cancers, and small cell cancer of the lungs. It can be diagnosed by lumbar puncture, which can reveal pleocytosis, high protein levels, and oligoclonal bands in the CSF. MRI results might initially be normal, but later scans reveal cerebellar atrophy. Anti-Yo antibody is found in some patients' CSF and blood. This syndrome can be debilitating, with only some patients responding to treatment of the underlying tumor (5).

Lambert-Eaton myasthenic syndrome is an autoimmune disorder that involves the presynaptic nerve terminals and is associated with small cell lung cancer. Patients present with weakness, cranial nerve palsies, and autonomic symptoms. Physical examination reveals decreased tendon reflexes and muscle weakness, which, however, improves with use. Neurophysiologic findings and detection of anticholinesterase antibodies are helpful in diagnosing this syndrome, which can improve with treatment of the underlying cancer, administration of corticosteroids, and plasmapheresis (5).

Paraneoplastic opsoclonus-myoclonus syndrome presents as involuntary, erratic eye movements and saccades. This syndrome has been associated with small cell cancer of the lungs and breast cancer. Some patients have anti-Ri antibody. Remissions can occur in response to cancer treatment or spontaneously (5).

Dermatomyositis occurs in 10% of patients with cancer. The cancers with which it is most often associated are lung, ovarian, breast, and stomach cancers. The diagnosis of this disorder typically precedes that of the underlying cancer, but the search for a cancer diagnosis in patients with dermatomyositis is not often revealing. Diagnosis is based on skin changes, elevation of creatinine phosphokinase (CPK), electromyelographic (EMG) changes, and muscle biopsy results revealing myositis. Dermatomyositis responds to treatment of the underlying tumor and to immunosuppressive drugs.

■ CARDIAC EMERGENCIES

CARDIAC TAMPONADE

Tumors involving the heart are much more frequently metastatic than primary. The tumors that most often metastasize to the heart are lung, breast, and GI tract cancers; leukemia; lymphoma; melanoma; and sarcoma. Metastatic involvement of the heart has also been noted in leukemia and lymphoma patients. Certain therapies can also affect the myocardium and cause pericardial disease, especially cyclophosphamide and ifosfamide at high doses, all-*trans* retinoic acid (ATRA), doxorubicin, and radiation therapy (27). Cardiac tamponade occurs when pericardial fluid accumulates and presses on the heart, increasing diastolic pressure in the ventricles and thereby decreasing stroke volume. The patient develops decreased cardiac output and systemic arterial pressure and can present with a shock-like syndrome. Most patients with pericardial effusions report no symptoms, but patients with cardiac tamponade present with shortness of breath, cough, hoarseness, epigastric pain, or chest pain that is made worse by lying down or leaning forward. On examination, the patient typically has distended neck veins, low systemic blood pressure, and low pulse pressure, and can have a pericardial rub or decreased heart sounds. The presence of pulsus paradoxus, which is an inspiratory decline in systolic blood pressure of >10 mm Hg, should be ruled out. Pulsus paradoxus can also occur in chronic obstructive pulmonary disease (COPD), pulmonary embolism, right ventricular infarction, and shock. Chest x-ray often reveals a "water bottle" configuration if the effusion has accumulated slowly, but the cardiac silhouette can appear normal if the effusion accumulates rapidly. Prior chest x-ray images can be useful in determining changes in the size of the cardiac silhouette. The electrocardiogram (ECG) might reveal electrical alternans (a variation of voltage in individual QRS complexes), low-voltage or ST-segment and T-wave changes. Transthoracic echocardiography is the best test to determine whether tamponade exists. If cardiac tamponade is present, echocardiography can help determine whether the effusion is localized or loculated, and it can also aid in planning pericardiocentesis. On echocardiograms, tamponade can be evidenced

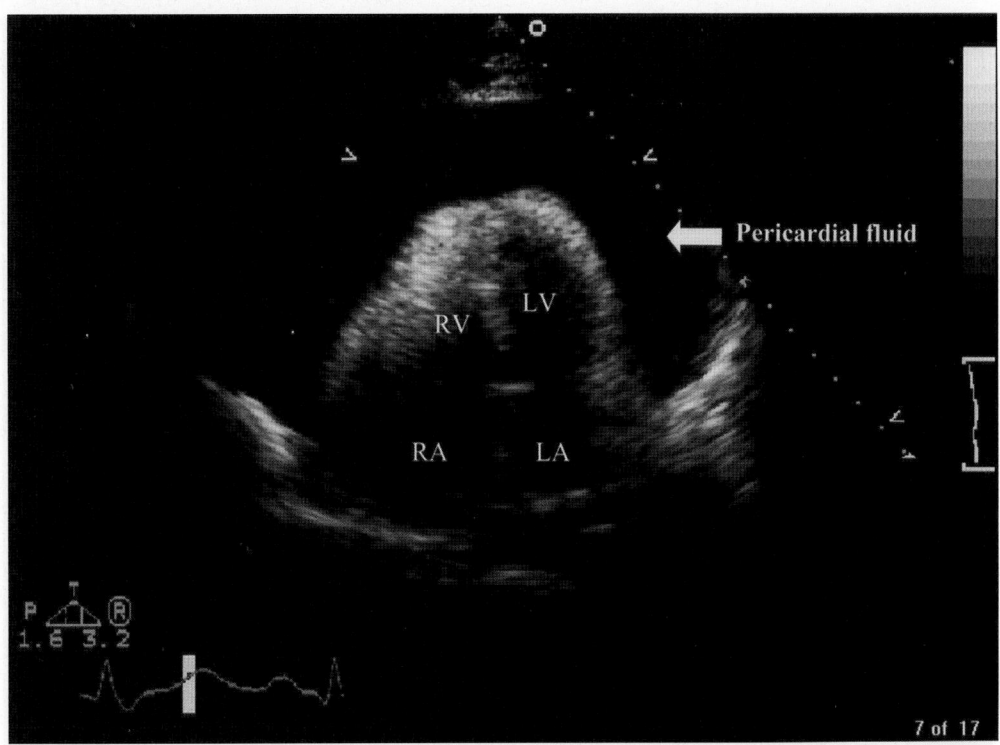

FIGURE 46-8. Two-dimensional echocardiogram in the apical four-chamber view demonstrating a large pericardial effusion. The right ventricle is not well visualized because of acoustic shadowing, which commonly occurs with large effusions. (*Courtesy of Dr. Joseph Swafford, MD Anderson Cancer Center.*)

by collapse of the right ventricle and atria in diastole (Fig. 46-8).

Treatment of tamponade includes the administration of oxygen, intravenous fluids, and vasopressors if necessary. Pericardiocentesis can be performed under ultrasound guidance and is relatively safe. Data collected from 1127 consecutive cases at the Mayo Clinic between 1979 and 2000 revealed a success rate of 97% and a complication rate of 4.7% in patients with significant pericardial effusions (28). At MD Anderson, a drainage catheter is commonly placed in patients with tamponade, with drainage performed daily. When the total volume of fluid drained is less than 50 mL/day, the catheter can be removed. A pericardial window can also be created to prevent reaccumulation of fluid. Radiation therapy and chemotherapy can also be used to prevent reaccumulation of fluid, as can sclerosis of the pericardial sac.

SUPERIOR VENA CAVA SYNDROME

Superior vena cava (SVC) syndrome is characterized by low blood flow from the SVC to the right atrium. Malignancy is by far the most common cause of SVC syndrome, although nonmalignant causes, such as indwelling central venous catheters, aneurysms, and goiters, can also cause this syndrome (2). Lung cancer is the most common malignant neoplasm causing SVC syndrome, but lymphoma, breast and GI cancers, sarcomas, melanomas, prostate cancer, and any mediastinal tumor can also cause this disorder. Among mechanisms that can lead to this syndrome are extrinsic compression by tumor, intrinsic compression by tumor or clot, or fibrosis. Patients may present with headache; dizziness; confusion; swelling of the upper extremities, face, and neck; shortness of breath; and dysphagia. Physical examination often reveals engorgement of veins and collaterals in the upper extremities due to elevated pressure in the venous system.

Diagnosis of SVC syndrome requires imaging. Routine chest x-rays will often reveal mediastinal widening, a right-side chest mass, or a mediastinal mass. CT scanning of the chest using intravenous contrast is an excellent means of delineating the cause of the obstruction and any associated finding (Fig. 46-9). MRI, Doppler ultrasound, and radionuclide venography can be used to exclude the presence of a clot.

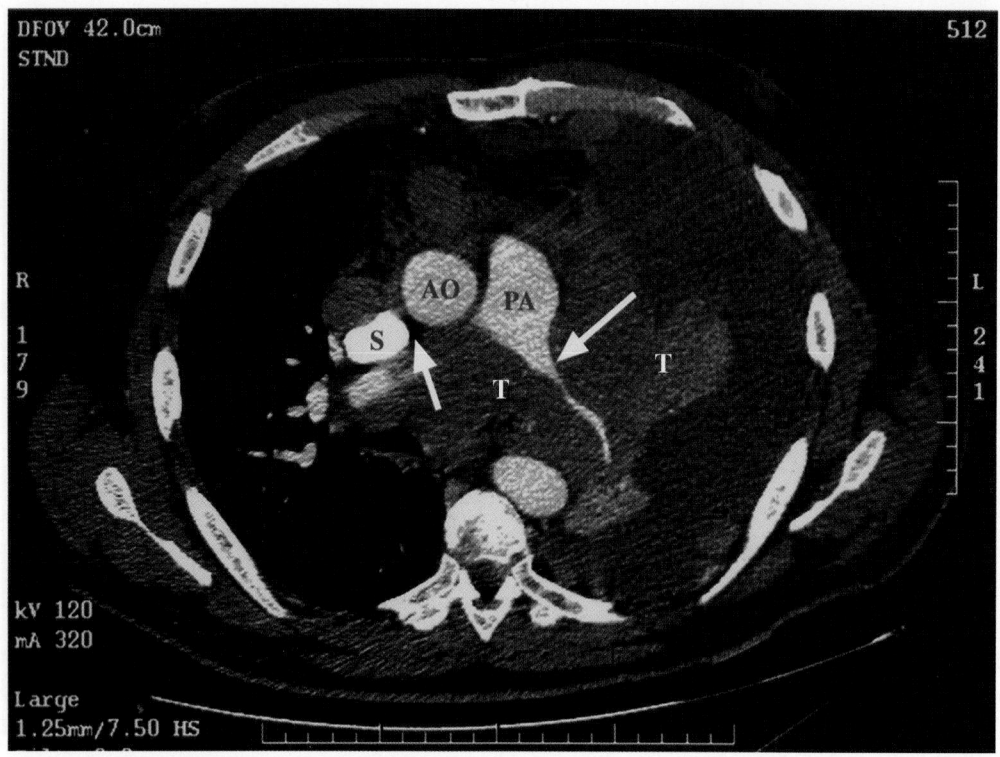

FIGURE 46-9.   CT scan revealing superior vena cava (SVC) syndrome from extrinsic compression of the SVC in a patient with non–small cell lung cancer. Large arrow indicates compression of the left pulmonary artery; small arrow indicates obliteration of the right pulmonary artery. T, tumor; AO, aorta; PA, main pulmonary artery; S, superior vena cava. (*Courtesy of Dr. Joel Dunnington, MD Anderson Cancer Center.*)

The treatment of SVC syndrome depends on the nature of the obstruction. Patients might respond to elevation of the head, corticosteroids if the intracranial pressure is increased, and occasionally diuretics. If thrombosis is present, local lytic therapy or anticoagulation can be used. It is important to obtain a tissue specimen of the tumor if its type is not known, so that it can be treated adequately. For patients with tumors that are chemosensitive, such as small cell lung cancer, chemotherapy can be instituted. Patients with non–small cell lung cancer will often respond to radiation therapy. Intravascular stenting with metallic stents can be used, as can angioplasty. Stent placement has been associated with a faster resolution of symptoms relative to radiation therapy (29) (Fig. 46-10).

MYOCARDIAL ISCHEMIA

Patients with cancer can present to the emergency center with myocardial ischemia. A full discussion of ischemic heart disease is beyond the scope of this chapter, but there are special considerations in cancer patients that should be mentioned.

Many cancer patients have thrombocytopenia due to chemotherapy, radiation therapy, or bone marrow infiltration with tumor. Despite platelet counts in the single or double digits, these patients can still present with acute cardiac syndrome. Although the practitioner might feel uncomfortable giving aspirin to these patients, cardiologists at MD Anderson have found that patients with platelet counts less than $50,000/\mu L$ who have cardiac ischemia and are treated with aspirin have a better 24-h survival rate than those who are not given aspirin.

Certain chemotherapeutic agents can predispose patients to myocardial ischemia, including 5-fluorouracil (5-FU), interferons, and presumably capecitabine, which is a metabolite of 5-FU. Radiation therapy can also be a predisposing factor (27). It is important to consider myocardial ischemia in patients who have undergone any of these therapies, especially those who otherwise have no risk factors for ischemic heart disease.

The cardiac markers troponin, CPK, and CPK-MB are useful in diagnosing myocardial infarction. Cardiac troponins are more sensitive and specific markers for ischemic heart disease than CPK-MB, which can be influenced by skeletal muscle injury; however, cardiac

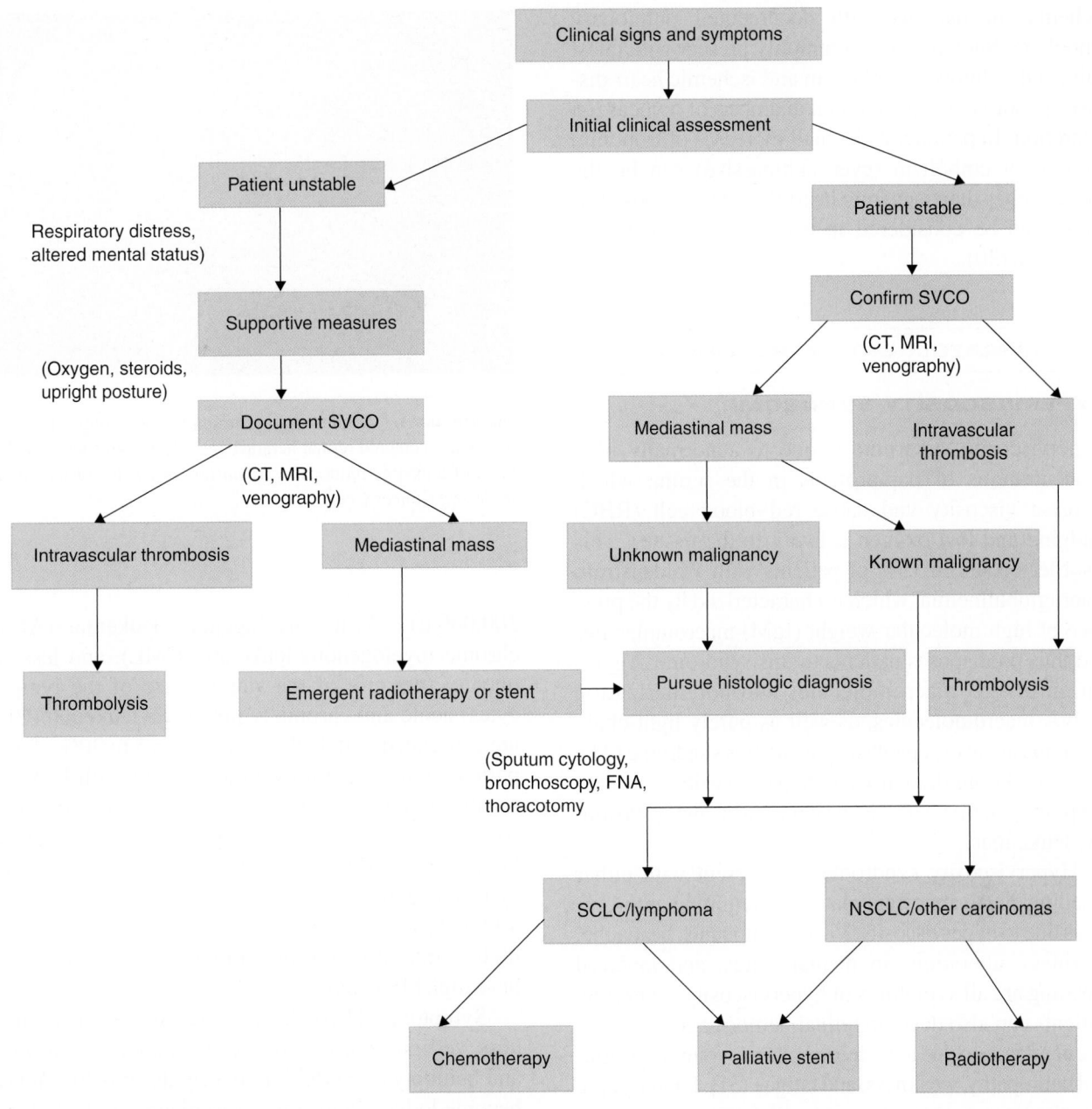

FIGURE 46-10. Algorithms for the diagnosis and management of superior vena cava syndrome. CT, computed tomography; MRI, magnetic resonance imaging; FNA, fine-needle aspiration; NSCLC, non–small cell lung cancer; SCLC, small cell lung cancer; SVCO, superior vena cava obstruction. (*Adapted from Gao S, Shannon VR. Vascular emergencies. In: Yeung SJ, Escalante CP [eds]: Oncologic Emergencies. Hamilton, Ontario, Canada: BC Decker; 2002, with permission.*)

troponin levels can also be raised by chronic renal insufficiency (CRI), cardiomyopathy with severe congestive heart failure, myocarditis, and massive pulmonary embolism. In one small study evaluating 24 patients with submassive pulmonary embolism, troponin levels were higher than normal in five patients (30). In this study, those patients who presented with chest pain and for whom a ventilation/perfusion (V/Q) scan revealed a

high probability of submassive pulmonary embolism were analyzed. High troponin was defined as a level >0.4 μg/L, and myocardial infarction was evidenced by a level >2.3 μg/L. It was found that four of the five patients with submassive pulmonary embolism had slightly elevated troponin levels and the fifth patient had a troponin level of 11.1 μg/L. The study was limited in that it did not investigate the possibility of underlying ischemia in patients with documented pulmonary embolism. Such patients commonly present with chest pain, and pulmonary embolism and ischemic heart disease are both in the differential diagnosis of myocardial infarction. In patients with small increases of troponin, pulmonary embolism (even submassive) can be the cause, rather than ischemic heart disease; this possibility should be considered in patients presenting with chest pain (30).

■ HEMATOLOGIC EMERGENCIES

HYPERVISCOSITY SYNDROME

Hyperviscosity syndrome is due to abnormally high concentrations of paraproteins in the serum, which increase viscosity and cause red blood cell (RBC) sludging and low oxygen delivery to the tissues. This disorder occurs in 15% of patients with Waldenstrom macroglobulinemia, which is characterized by the presence of high molecular-weight (IgM) macromolecules and thus predisposes patients to this syndrome. Aggregation of IgG macromolecules and polymerization of IgA macromolecules, as well as purely light-chain myeloma are also capable of causing this syndrome (31). Other conditions that can cause hyperviscosity syndrome are polycythemia vera, dysproteinemias, and occasionally leukemias.

Hyperviscosity syndrome can present with either bleeding due to abnormal platelet functioning or thrombosis due to hyperviscosity. Visual complaints, headache, dizziness, alterations in mental status, and mucosal bleeding are all symptoms of hyperviscosity syndrome. Patients can also develop retinal hemorrhages, congestive heart failure due to increased plasma volume, peripheral neuropathy, weakness, and fatigue (31). Funduscopic examination can reveal venous dilatation, retinal vein occlusion, or papilledema (Fig. 46-11).

The diagnosis is made on the basis of a high serum viscosity. Normal serum viscosity ranges between 1.4 and 1.8 Ostwald units (relative to water, at 1). Patients start to develop symptoms when serum viscosity exceeds 4.0 Ostwald units (31-33).

The treatment for hyperviscosity syndrome includes the administration of intravenous fluids followed by diuresis. Plasma exchange can decrease symptoms quickly and can be followed by chemotherapy (31).

HYPERLEUKOCYTOSIS

Hyperleukocytosis is typically defined as a white blood cell (WBC) count in the peripheral blood higher than

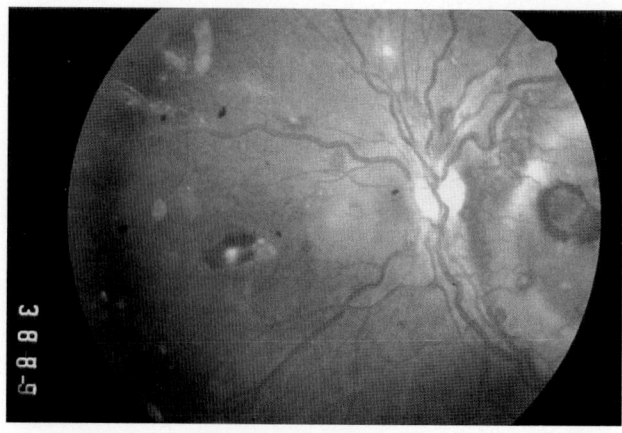

FIGURE 46-11. Funduscopic examination revealing a Roth spot (the white-centered retinal hemorrhage). The Roth spot is the hallmark of leukemic retinopathy. (*Courtesy of Dr. Bita Esmaeli, MD Anderson Cancer Center.*)

100,000/μL. Acute myelogenous leukemia (AML), chronic myelogenous leukemia (CML), and less frequently (because of the smaller size of the lymphocytes) acute and chronic lymphocytic leukemia (CLL) are associated with leukostasis. From 5 to 30% of adult patients with acute leukemias present with leukostasis that requires prompt recognition and initiation of therapy to prevent respiratory failure or intracranial hemorrhage (32). The WBC count in acute lymphocytic leukemia (ALL) typically must be greater than 400,000/μL before leukostasis will develop (3). The highest rate of mortality is in patients with AML who have high blast counts.

Symptoms of hyperleukocytosis are headache, dizziness, vertigo, shortness of breath, altered mental status, and hemoptysis. WBCs are poorly deformable and can become lodged in the microvasculature of the kidneys, lungs, brain, and other organs. The pulmonary and neurologic systems are most critically affected in hyperleukocytosis syndrome. In the lungs, WBCs can get caught in the pulmonary circulation, causing adult respiratory distress syndrome (ARDS), or can mimic pulmonary embolism because of WBC stasis in the pulmonary vasculature, thereby causing a ventilation/perfusion mismatch (33). Patients with the latter condition should not be given diuretics, as this will further increase stasis. Most patients with leukemia are anemic; this condition can offset the WBC elevation, so hyperviscosity is not as common in these patients. It is important not to give these patients blood transfusions unless absolutely necessary, as this treatment can exacerbate hyperleukocytosis and increase the RBC mass without changing the total blood volume (26). Patients can present with decreased mental status, which can be caused by endothelial leakage from the small vessels of the brain or hemorrhage, but other causes of altered mental status should also be considered, including infection, LMD from leukemia, and metabolic sources. Imaging studies, such as CT scan and MRI, as well as lumbar tap should be performed when indicated (3,12).

The treatment of hyperleukocytosis involves lowering the WBC count, which can be accomplished with leukapheresis or chemotherapy. Leukapheresis can lower the WBC count by 30 to 60% from pretreatment levels. These effects can be transient; therefore repeat leukapheresis might be necessary. Patients undergoing leukapheresis should also be monitored closely to prevent tumor lysis syndrome.

THROMBOSIS

Venous thromboembolism (VTE) is influenced by Virchow triad: venous stasis, higher-than-normal coagulability, and intimal injury. Patients with cancer have a high risk of VTE, and up to 15% of patients will develop VTE because of hypercoagulability, the use of central venous catheters, and high stasis (34). Cancer patients can have increased serum viscosity due to dehydration or, less frequently, hyperviscosity syndrome (described previously). Stasis and intimal injury can be caused by numerous events—for example, tumor encroachment on blood vessels or indirect effects of cancer, such as spinal cord compression, brain metastasis, dehydration, or impaired ambulation. Some chemotherapeutic cancer agents can also induce VTE, among them tamoxifen, cisplatin, cyclophosphamide, methotrexate, and 5-FU (34).

Symptoms of pulmonary embolism (PE) include chest pain, shortness of breath, palpitations, fever up to 102°F, and syncope in the case of massive PE. ECG findings can include T-wave inversion in the precordial leads, sinus tachycardia, right bundle branch block, or rightward movement of the QRS axis. Chest roentgenograms can be normal or might reveal a pleural effusion or elevation of the diaphragm on the involved side. Physical examination can reveal tachypnea, tachycardia, and leg edema or erythema in the case of associated deep vein thrombosis.

Diagnosis of PE can be made by V/Q scanning, spiral CT angiography, pulmonary angiography, or MRI (Fig. 46-12).

V/Q scans are noninvasive and the results are useful in patients with a high probability of PE, which can be

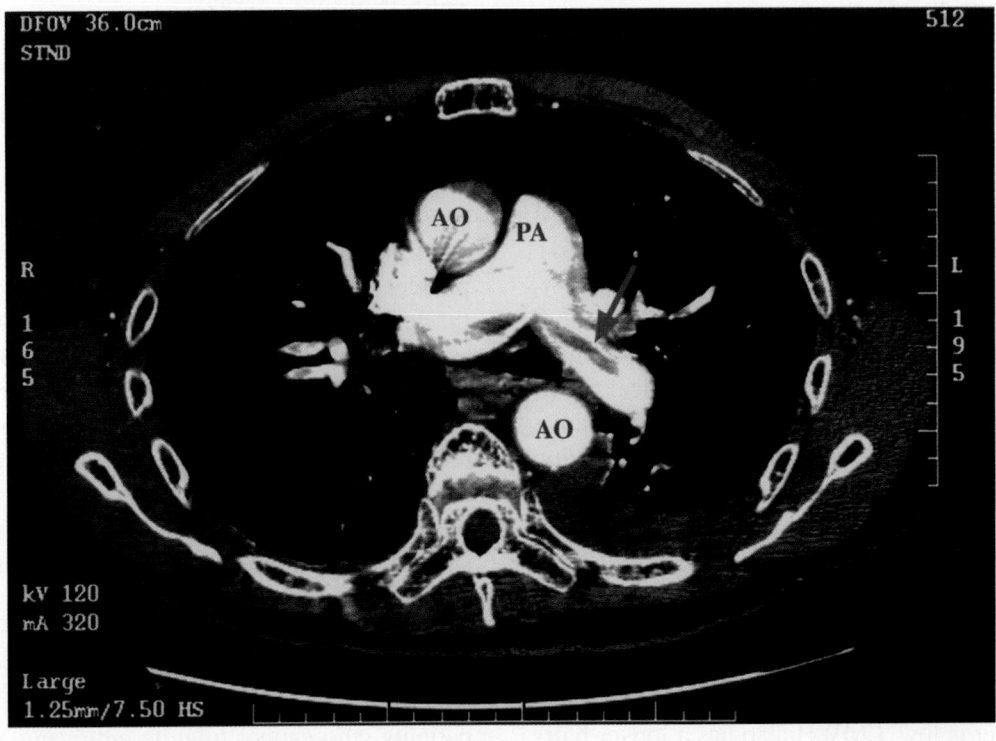

FIGURE 46-12. Spiral CT angiogram in a patient with a saddle pulmonary embolism (*arrow*). AO, aorta; PA, main pulmonary artery. (*Courtesy of Dr. Joel Dunnington, MD Anderson Cancer Center.*)

treated as VTE; normal results on V/Q scans can rule out PE. Clinical suspicion based on the patient's risk factors and results of other tests can guide the clinician regarding the patient's pretest probability of PE. Patients with indeterminate result from V/Q scans who are strongly suspected of having a PE can undergo further testing, such as spiral CT angiography, pulmonary angiography, or MRI. Spiral CT scanning and MRI can detect segmental PE but not necessarily subsegmental PE. Both of these tests are useful in that they give further information about the condition of the lung, such as whether pneumonia is present, tumor size, and impingement on the bronchial airways; this additional information is helpful in determining the cause of the patient's symptoms. Pulmonary angiography remains the gold standard in detecting PE, although it requires more dye than other contrast methods and a greater risk of renal complications. The alveolar-arterial gradient (A-a gradient) from an arterial blood gas (ABG) can serve to corroborate the diagnosis of PE, but a normal A-a gradient does not rule out a PE. The upper limit of normal of an A-a gradient is equal to patient age/4 + 4, but this value can also increase when the patient is supine. In the PIOPED (Prospective Investigation of Pulmonary Embolism Diagnosis) study, ABGs were normal in 14% of patients with preexisting cardiopulmonary disease and in 38% of patients with no underlying cardiopulmonary disease despite the presence of pulmonary emboli (35) (Fig. 46-13).

The diagnosis of peripheral VTE can be made by Doppler ultrasound, impedance plethysmography (IPG), venography, nuclear venogram, or magnetic resonance (MR) venography (Fig. 46-14).

The D-dimer test can also be used in the evaluation of VTE; normal results are associated with a significantly lower likelihood of VTE than high values (34). D-dimer has a high negative predictive value for pulmonary embolism in cancer patients, and a normal D-dimer can be used to exclude pulmonary embolism in cancer patients. Combining D-dimer with clinical symptoms and signs did not substantially change negative predictive value, positive predictive value, sensitivity, or specificity (36). Because D-dimer is commonly high in patients with cancer, an elevated D-dimer is not useful in diagnosing VTE.

First-line treatment for VTE consists of either unfractionated heparin (UFH) or low-molecular-weight heparin (LMWH). LMWH has the advantage that factor Xa levels usually do not have to be monitored because protein binding is low. LMWH also has a longer half-life than UFH and thus can be given less frequently (once or twice per day). The LMWHs enoxaparin,

tinzaparin, and dalteparin are all different and cannot be used interchangeably. Monitoring may be required for patients with obesity and renal insufficiency, because LMWH is cleared by the kidneys. When monitoring is necessary, the Xa level should be measured 4 h after the injection, with a target level ranging from 0.6 to 1.0 IU/mL for twice-daily dosing. For daily dosing, the Xa level should range between 1.9 and 2.0 IU/mL (37). For patients who will be transitioned to warfarin treatment, there should be an overlap of at least 5 days with LMWH.

In a study, 672 cancer patients with VTE were randomized to dalteparin with oral anticoagulation versus dalteparin alone (38). The oral anticoagulation (OA) group was given warfarin and dalteparin 200 IU/kg subcutaneously every day for 5 to 7 days until the international normalized ratio (INR) reached 2 to 3. At that point, dalteparin was discontinued and the warfarin continued for 6 months. In the OA group, the goal INR was 2.5. The dalteparin group was given dalteparin 200 IU/kg subcutaneously every day for 1 month and then 150 IU/kg subcutaneously every day for the remaining 5 months. The patients in the dalteparin group had a lower rate of recurrent VTE at 6 months (8.8%) than those in the OA group (17.4%). There were no significant differences in major or minor bleeding between the two groups. The study investigators concluded that the occurrence of recurrent VTE can be decreased by the use of dalteparin rather than warfarin (38).

Although VTE can often be treated on an outpatient basis, patients not eligible for outpatient treatment are those with active bleeding, major comorbid illnesses, a history of heparin-induced thrombocytopenia, hypertensive emergencies, major surgery or trauma within the previous 2 weeks, recent GI bleeding, stroke or transient ischemic attack, severe renal dysfunction, or a platelet count below 100,000/μL (39). Table 46-2 shows the dosing schedule.

Most patients are treated for at least 3 to 6 months. Patients from whom the central venous catheter has been removed can undergo repeat testing using such techniques as Doppler ultrasound or nuclear venous flow study to determine whether the clot has resolved, so that cessation of anticoagulation therapy may be considered. For patients with small clots at the distal tip, manifested by the inability of the central line to work, tissue plasminogen activator (t-PA) can be given carefully provided that there are no contraindications.

Inferior vena cava (IVC) filters can be used for patients who cannot tolerate anticoagulation therapy. IVC filters do not decrease peripheral edema from deep venous thrombosis (DVT) and, in fact, can serve

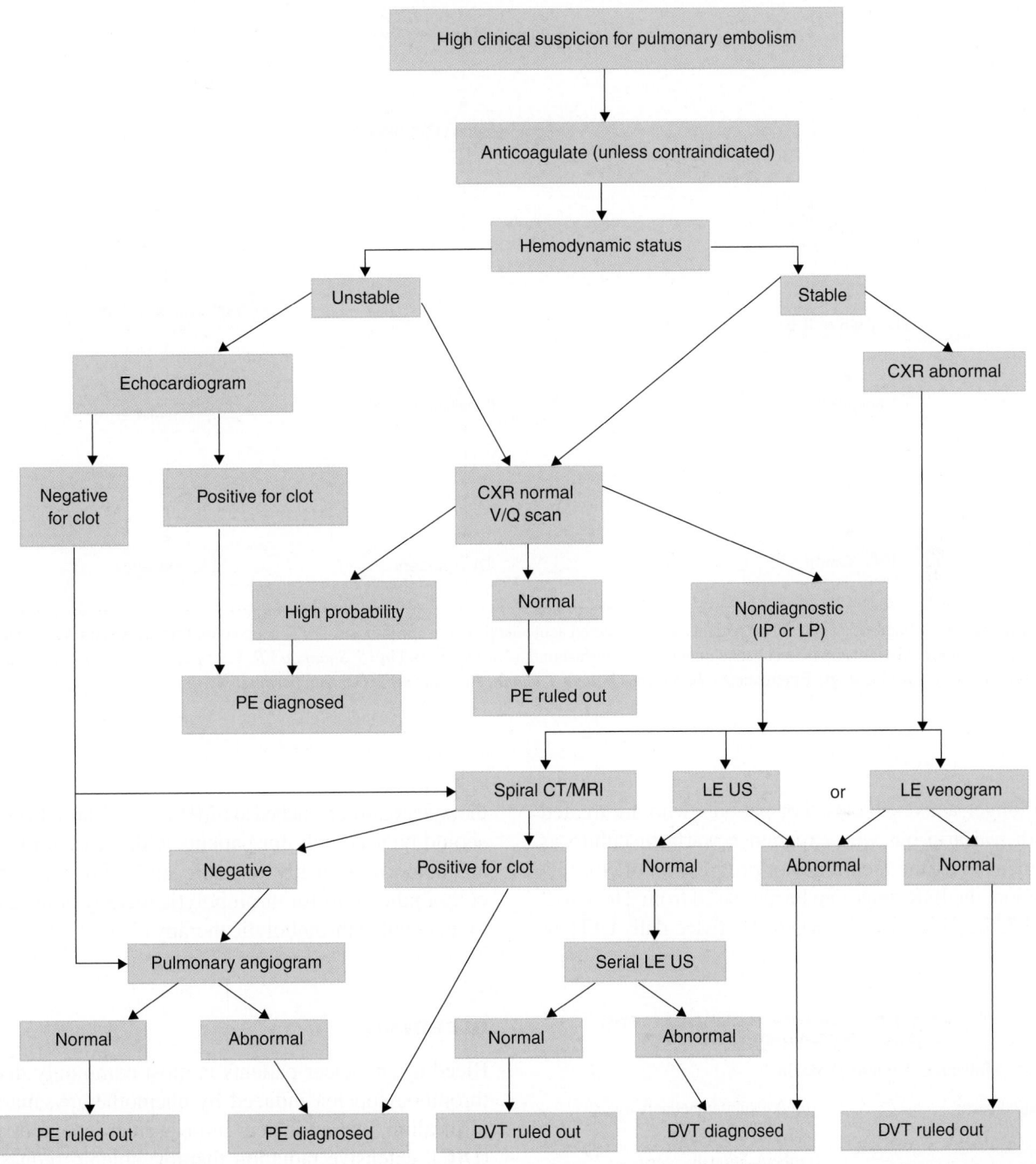

FIGURE 46-13. Suggested algorithm for the evaluation of pulmonary embolism. CXR, chest x-ray; DVT, deep venous thrombosis; IP, intermediate probability; LE US, lower extremity ultrasound; LE venogram, lower extremity venogram; LP, low probability; PE, pulmonary embolism; V/Q scan, ventilation/perfusion scan. (*Adapted from Shannon VR, Ng A. Noninfectious pulmonary emergencies. In: Yeung SJ, Escalante CP [eds]:* Oncologic Emergencies. *Hamilton, Ontario, Canada: BC Decker; 2002, with permission.*)

as a nidus for further clot formation. IVC filters can prevent life-threatening pulmonary emboli. Patients with massive pulmonary emboli may require thrombolysis or embolectomy. See Table 46-3 for a synopsis of the relative and absolute contraindications for thrombolytic therapy and Table 46-4 for thrombolytic doses.

Patients with cancer and VTE should be treated indefinitely if the cancer remains active or for at least 3 to 6 months after resolution of the VTE if the cancer is

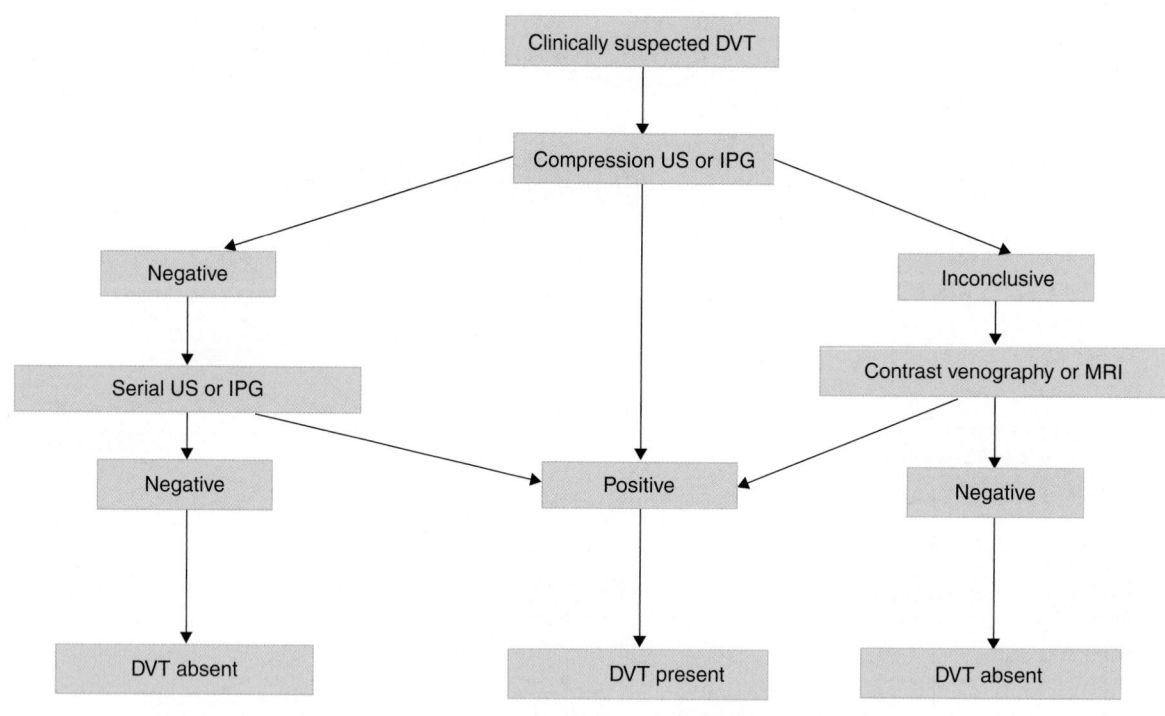

FIGURE 46-14. Diagnostic approach to patients with suspected acute deep venous thrombosis. DVT, deep venous thrombosis; IPG, impedance plethysmography; MRI, magnetic resonance imaging; US, ultrasound. (*Adapted from Gao S, Shannon VR. Vascular emergencies. In: Yeung SJ, Escalante CP [eds]: Oncologic Emergencies. Hamilton, Ontario, Canada: BC Decker; 2002, with permission.*)

no longer active (40,41). For patients who are treated with warfarin but who experience warfarin failure as evidenced by the recurrence or progression of clot formation, the INR range can be increased from 2 to 3, to 3 to 3.5, the patient can be switched to twice-daily UFH, or the patient can be switched to LMWH (42). Thrombectomy should be used only for patients with massive PE who are hemodynamically unstable and who either have contraindications for thrombolytic therapy or have previously failed thrombolytic therapy (34).

TABLE 46-2	HEPARIN DOSAGE SCHEDULE FOR VENOUS THROMBOEMBOLISM
Low-Molecular-Weight Heparin	
Enoxaparin	1 mg/kg subcutaneously every 12 h or 1.5 mg/kg subcutaneously every 24 h
Dalteparin	200 IU/kg subcutaneously every 24 h or in a divided dose every 12 h. Maximum dosage = 18,000 IU.
Tinzaparin	175 *anti*-Xa antibody IU/kg subcutaneously every 24 h
Unfractionated Heparin	80 IU/kg bolus, with a maintenance dose of 18 IU/kg/day. This should be adjusted to keep PTT at 1.5-2.5 X the normal range.

BLEEDING

Bleeding in cancer patients is most commonly due to thrombocytopenia induced by chemotherapy, marrow infiltration, disseminated intravascular coagulopathy (DIC), extensive radiation therapy, splenic sequestration, peripheral destruction, or infection. Thrombocytopenia usually manifest as mucocutaneous bleeding, such as gum oozing, epistaxis, and gynecologic or GI bleeding (34). At MD Anderson, all patients generally receive platelet transfusions if their platelet count falls to 10,000/μL or below. If the patient has active bleeding and the platelet count is between 20,000 and 50,000/μL, a platelet transfusion will also be given. A patient will also receive a platelet transfusion if an invasive procedure is planned and his or her platelet count is below 50,000/μL. The American Society of Clinical

TABLE 46-3	**ABSOLUTE AND RELATIVE CONTRAINDICATIONS TO THROMBOLYSIS**

Absolute Contraindications to Thrombolysis

Major intracranial surgery or trauma within prior 2 months

Cerebrovascular hemorrhage within prior 3-6 months

Active intracranial neoplasm

Major internal hemorrhage within prior 6 months

Severe bleeding diastheses, including those associated with severe liver or renal disease

Relative Contraindications to Thrombolysis

Prolonged cardiopulmonary resuscitation

Pregnancy or postpartum period within prior 10 days

Nonhemorrhagic stroke within prior 2 months

Major trauma or surgery (excluding that of the central nervous system) within prior 10 days

Thrombocytopenia (platelet count <100,000/mm^3)

Hemorrhagic retinopathy

Allergies to thrombolytic agents

Minor surgery to noncompressible vessels within prior 10 days

Tissue biopsy within prior 10 days

Peptic ulceration within prior 3 months

Infective endocarditis/pericarditis

Uncontrolled hypertension (systolic BP ≥200 or diastolic BP ≥110 mm Hg)

Aortic aneurysm

Absolute and relative contraindications to thrombolysis. (Adapted from Shannon VR, Ng A. Noninfectious pulmonary emergencies. In: Yeung SJ, Escalante CP [eds]: Oncologic Emergencies. Hamilton, Ontario, Canada: BC Decker; 2002, with permission.)

Oncology (ASCO) recommends prophylactic platelet transfusions for patients being treated for leukemia and those receiving bone marrow transplants if their platelet counts are below 10,000/μL. Transfusion thresholds may be higher for patients with fever, hyperleukocytosis, a rapid fall in platelet count, coagulation abnormalities, or active bleeding. ASCO recommends that patients

TABLE 46-4	**DOSAGES OF THROMBOLYTICS**

Streptokinase	250,000 IU intravenous load over 30 min, then 100,000 IU/h for 24 h for pulmonary embolism or 72 h for deep vein thrombosis
Urokinase	4400 IU/kg intravenous load over 10 min, then 4400 IU/kg/h for 12 h
Alteplase	100 mg intravenous infusion over 2 h; initiate heparin at the end of alteplase infusion

with chronic stable thrombocytopenia who are not undergoing active treatment, such as those with aplastic anemia and patients with myelodysplastic syndrome (MDS), be monitored and given platelets only for active bleeding, even if their platelet count is below 10,000/μL. For patients with solid tumors, prophylactic platelet transfusions should be given if the platelet counts are below 10,000/μL unless the tumor is necrotic or is located in the bladder and undergoing treatment; in those cases the threshold for transfusion should be 20,000/μL. According to ASCO's guidelines, platelet counts of 50,000/μL should be sufficient for invasive procedures, such as surgery. For lumbar puncture, the platelet count should be above 20,000/μL. Patients with AML commonly receive multiple transfusions and can develop alloimmunization against human leukocyte antigens (HLA). Approximately 25 to 35% of patients with AML will become alloimmunized and refractory to nonhistocompatible platelet transfusions, predominantly through their exposure to leukocytes. Random-donor platelets are derived from pooled platelet concentrates from whole-blood donations, whereas single-donor platelets are obtained from one donor by platelet pheresis. The likelihood of alloimmunization can be decreased by using single-donor platelets, leukocyte-depleted platelets, leukocyte filters, and UV-irradiated platelets. ASCO recommends that patients who are platelet-refractory not receive platelet transfusions unless they are hemorrhaging or HLA-compatible platelets are available (42).

DIC can cause bleeding and thrombosis. DIC should be suspected in a patient who has an unexplained elevation in PT, PTT, or thrombocytopenia with associated bleeding or thrombosis. Although bleeding is most often noted in patients with DIC, it is the thrombosis of small (and occasionally large) blood vessels that leads to the most serious complications (43). Collaborative laboratory findings are high D-dimer and fibrin split product (FSP) levels, low levels of fibrinogen and thrombin-antithrombin III (TAT), or the presence of schistocytes (43). It is important to remember that DIC is a clinical diagnosis based on the entire clinical scenario, and results for these laboratory tests might not be abnormal. Patients can also have mildly abnormal test results in cases of subclinical DIC, and these patients should be monitored closely for conversion to overt DIC.

Tumors can cause DIC, especially adenocarcinomas of the breast, prostate, stomach, lungs, and colon. In this instance, the disorder is believed to be stimulated by mucin produced from these cancers. Leukemia, especially acute promyelocytic leukemia (APL), is associated with DIC in up to 85% of patients because of a tissue factor in APL that has procoagulant activity. Other tumors associated with DIC are melanoma, lymphoma, and ovarian and pancreatic cancers. Other causes of DIC are sepsis, acidosis, extensive burns, the use of Denver catheters or LaVeen shunts in patients with malignant ascites, hemolytic blood transfusion reactions, polycythemia rubra vera, and amniotic fluid embolism (34,43).

Patients who have both DIC and bleeding can present with oozing from multiple sites, such as arterial or venous punctures or the mucous membranes, with GI, or with epistaxis. Thrombotic complications can be visible on the skin in the form of hemorrhagic bullae, acral cyanosis, or even gangrene (43). Microvascular thrombosis most commonly affects the lungs, brain, and kidneys. The patient may develop shortness of breath, pleuritic chest pain, and ARDS. The kidneys can become clogged with microemboli, in which case patients often present with oliguria, anuria, hematuria, or proteinuria. The small vessels of the brain also can receive microemboli, causing strokes, seizures, altered mental status, or coma. As the patient deteriorates, hypotension, acidosis, and hypoxia can develop (43).

The treatment of DIC should focus on reversing the underlying cause or trigger, such as treating an underlying infection. Acidosis, high catecholamine release, vasoconstriction, and corticosteroid use can exacerbate thrombosis associated with DIC (43). Additional therapeutic measures for thrombosis can include heparin administration at 15 U/kg/h by continuous infusion. When the patient is bleeding, blood components (including platelets) can be transfused to correct coagulation abnormalities. Platelet transfusions are indicated to maintain platelet counts of at least 50,000/µL. Cryoprecipitate should only be used for severe hypofibrinogenemia <50 mg/dL, or <100 mg/dL if patient is actively bleeding. Cryoprecipitate can be given at 0.2 bags per kilogram of body weight, and the fibrinogen level should be tested 20 to 60 min after the infusion and every 6 h thereafter until the bleeding has stopped. Fresh frozen plasma (FFP) can be transfused at 10 to 15 mg/kg to correct abnormalities in PT. Other products that might be needed are prothrombin complex, antithrombin concentrates, or washed RBCs. For patients with persistent bleeding, fibrinolytic inhibitors such as epsilon-aminocaproic acid (EACA) can be given. EACA should always be given with heparin to prevent thrombosis; because EACA can cause hypotension, ventricular arrhythmias, and hypokalemia, it should be used with caution. Tranexamic acid is a newer fibrinolytic inhibitor that has fewer side effects and has been used successfully in DIC associated with APL.

■ GENITOURINARY EMERGENCIES

HEMORRHAGIC CYSTITIS

Hemorrhagic cystitis is inflammation or bleeding of the bladder; it can be due to radiation therapy, viral infection, or chemotherapy. Radiation-induced bladder bleeding can present as early as 3 months or as late as 5 years after the termination of radiation therapy (44). Chemotherapeutic agents associated with hemorrhagic cystitis are cyclophosphamide and ifosfamide (because of the liver metabolites secreted during use of these compounds, namely acrolein and chloroacetaldehyde). The mechanism by which cyclophosphamide and ifosfamide metabolites are toxic to the urinary bladder is not known, but they have been implicated as the cause of hematuria in some patients (45). Mesna is a thiol compound that binds acrolein, chloroacetaldehyde, and other metabolites of cyclophosphamide and ifosfamide; when it is administered before the patient receives the chemotherapeutic agents, the incidence of bladder toxicity can be decreased (45). Forced diuresis and adequate hydration complement mesna administration (45).

In addition to radiation therapy and chemotherapy-inducing hemorrhagic cystitis, the BK virus (a polyomavirus) can become activated in immunocompromised patients undergoing bone marrow transplantation and cause hematuria (45).

Treatment of hemorrhagic cystitis involves gentle bladder irrigation to remove any clots and decompress the bladder. Any coagulopathy, such as thrombocytopenia, should be corrected, as should manifestations of DIC, such as low fibrinogen levels or an elevated PT or PTT. For patients with persistent bleeding, prostaglandins E_2 or F_2, 1% alum, or formalin can be instilled. Formalin instillation is painful and requires general or spinal anesthesia. To correct continued bleeding, some patients require surgery, hypogastric artery embolization, or open surgical intervention.

URINARY TRACT OBSTRUCTION

Obstructive uropathy can be secondary to outflow obstruction or impingement on the ureters or kidneys; it can also be due to tumor invasion, radiotherapy-induced changes, or indirect effects of the tumor, such as ascites, lymphadenopathy, or fibrosis. A patient who is unable to urinate should have a small Foley catheter, such as a 14F placed. In patients with benign prostatic hypertrophy (BPH), a coudé catheter can often be inserted more easily (45). The catheter should not be forced, and, if the bladder cannot be accessed, a suprapubic catheter can be used. A lack of residual urine in the absence of severe dehydration usually indicates either obstruction at a more proximal level in the urinary system or acute anuric renal failure. Patients who have residual urine may be unable to urinate because of a mechanical cause, such as BPH, urethral stricture, tumor impingement, or stone obstruction. Other possible causes of acute urinary retention are infection, spinal cord compression, viral radiculomyelitis, postsurgical effects interrupting bladder innervation, or medicines such as pain medications and antihistamines (45). In each case, the underlying disorder should be treated. Patients with BPH can undergo a trial of alpha blockers, such as terazosin, prazosin, doxazosin, or finasteride, a type II 5-alpha–reductase inhibitor. Transurethral resection of the prostate (TURP) can be considered for patients who do not respond to medical treatments.

Laboratory values are also useful in differentiating prerenal, postrenal, and renal failure. Patients with prerenal failure typically have a high ratio of BUN to creatinine of more than 20:1, although upper tract GI bleeding, corticosteroid use, and high protein intake can also increase the BUN-to-creatinine ratio. Acute urinary obstruction can present as flank pain, whereas chronic obstruction is often painless, with patients presenting with anuria or decreased urine output. The tumors most likely to cause ureteral obstruction are cervical, prostate, bladder, ovarian, breast, and GI cancers as well as lymphoma (45). Patients with infected urine and obstruction may also present with symptoms of urosepsis, including fever, confusion, and a high WBC count.

CT scanning of the abdomen is good for evaluating the cause of ureteral obstruction in that it can elucidate the nature of the obstruction. Other tests that can be used are MRI, renal ultrasound, intravenous urography, retrograde pyelography, and radionuclide renography (45). Helical CT scanning of the abdomen has the added benefit of avoiding the use of intravenous contrast. Urinary obstruction can be managed with ureteral stents or percutaneous nephrostomy tubes with or without internal stents; the stents or tubes are typically placed under guidance by interventional radiology. Many patients with stents develop infection, which often requires hospitalization, intravenous antibiotics, and stent replacement. Other possible complications are stent clogging and stent migration. The "double J" stent, which is now most frequently used, is anchored in the bladder and the renal pelvis, so that stent migration is less common than it once was. Open surgical procedures are much less frequently performed now than in the past and are generally reserved for patients in whom endourologic procedures have failed (45).

■ RESPIRATORY EMERGENCIES

AIRWAY OBSTRUCTION

Airway obstruction can be caused by intraluminal tumor growth or compression of the airway by an extraluminal tumor. Rigid or flexible bronchoscopy can be used to both diagnose and treat airway obstruction. Patients with severe respiratory distress and airway obstruction should undergo endotracheal intubation distal to the obstruction before the obstruction is treated. Once the airway has been stabilized, the obstruction can be treated. The methods that can be used to provide expedient relief of airway obstruction include laser treatment, argon plasma coagulation (APC), electrocautery, endobronchial balloon dilation, and stent placement. APC can be achieved through flexible or rigid bronchoscopy at a relatively low cost and degrades the obstructive tissue by increasing its temperature. Electrocautery is also relatively inexpensive and can provide immediate relief of the obstruction, but side effects can include fire, hemorrhage, and electric shock. Rigid bronchoscopy can be used to treat extraluminal tumors by metal or silicone stent placement; this technique is most useful for tracheal or main bronchial disease. Metal stents can promote the growth of granulomatous tissue, whereas silicone stents are more likely to develop mucous plugging and to migrate. Laser therapy can also be used for endobronchial lesions, with the possible side effects of hemorrhage, pneumothorax, and pneumomediastinum. Laser therapy is more expensive than the other techniques and requires a skilled technician. Other methods that can be used for airway obstruction are cryotherapy, brachytherapy, and photodynamic therapy, although in many cases these do not provide rapid relief (29) (Table 46-5).

HEMOPTYSIS

Massive hemoptysis is defined as bleeding into the airway at a rate of 100 to 600 mL/day, although any amount of blood that compromises the airway can be considered massive. Some 7 to 10% of patients with lung cancer will develop massive hemoptysis, which carries a poorer prognosis than massive hemoptysis associated with other cancers (29). In addition to structural abnormalities in the lungs, bleeding can be due to chemotherapy or other medications, sepsis, fungal infections, and thrombocytopenia. Death from this type of hemorrhage usually results from asphyxiation rather than anemia or blood loss.

The most important aspect of managing massive hemoptysis is protecting the airway. If the right lung is affected, the left lung can be selectively intubated through bronchoscopy. Use of a rigid bronchoscope

| TABLE 46-5 | BRONCHOSCOPIC METHODS OF TREATING DYSPNEA FROM TUMOR OBSTRUCTION |

Tumor Type	Tumor Location (I) Intraluminal (E) Extraluminal	Rate of Relief of Dyspnea Symptoms (I) Immediate (D) Delayed	Complications/ Disadvantages	Advantages/Uses
Argon plasma coagulation	I	I		Low cost Ease of use Rapid coagulation
Brachytherapy	I	D	Fistula Hemoptysis	Best used in small epithelial tumors
Cryotherapy	I	D		Less expensive
Electrocautery	I	I	Fire Hemorrhage Shock	Less expensive
Laser	I	I	Bleeding Pneumothorax Pneumomediastinum	Special training; expensive equipment
Photodynamic therapy	I	I	Phototoxicity Hemoptysis Bronchial obstruction due to debris	
Stent placement	I/E	I	Migration of stent	Used in tracheal or main bronchial disease

allows removal of the tumor or clots, whereas flexible bronchoscopy allows access to the more distal airways. If the left lung is affected, the right lung should not be selectively intubated because inadvertent collapse of the right upper lobe can ensue. A single-lumen endotracheal tube is easier to place than a double-lumen tube and allows a larger area for evacuation of blood and clots. The patient should lie on the side of the bleeding lung to promote aeration of the unaffected lung. Any coagulopathy should be corrected, and cough suppressed with codeine or other agents. If a tumor is causing the bleeding and it can be localized, the patient can undergo bronchial artery embolization or tumor resection. If the tumor is unresectable, external beam radiation therapy (EBRT) can be used. If only the location of the bleeding can be determined, a solution of 1:10,000 epinephrine can be injected. Other means of halting bleeding are laser treatment, electrocautery, APC, photocoagulation, balloon tamponade, or iced-saline lavage.

TOXIC LUNG INJURY

ARDS is a serious condition that can be a complication of infection or chemotherapy. ATRA is a chemotherapy used in APL, and it has been found to cause ARDS in 26% of patients starting 2 to 47 days after treatment.

Cytarabine (Ara-C) can cause diffuse lung injury, capillary leakage, and pulmonary edema, usually after 6 days of therapy. These effects can be treated with diuresis and corticosteroids. Bleomycin can cause pulmonary fibrosis and increased sensitivity to intraoperative oxygen administration. Other chemotherapeutic agents that can cause pulmonary edema are mitomycin C, gemcitabine, cyclosporine, interferon, tumor necrosis factor, interleukin 2, and granulocyte macrophage colony-stimulating factor (GM-CSF) (27).

Interstitial lung disease can be caused by bleomycin, carmustine, lomustine, busulfan, cyclophosphamide, methotrexate, doxorubicin, and actinomycin D. Bleomycin toxicity is usually dose-related and most often occurs when the cumulative dose is greater than 450 units. It can be treated with corticosteroids. Busulfan's toxic effects can occur after 3 weeks of therapy, but they sometimes emerge as late as 3 years after treatment. Busulfan toxicity is associated with a high mortality rate, but corticosteroids can be used with some response. Cyclophosphamide complications present differently depending on whether they are early or late. The early-onset effect is pneumonitis, which can be treated with corticosteroids. The late-onset symptoms include a progressive fibrosis that is not responsive to steroids. Methotrexate can also produce pulmonary fibrosis, which can appear from several days to years after treatment. Doxorubicin and actinomycin D can present with pulmonary fibrosis characterized by a "recall" effect after radiation therapy, even in areas of the lung not exposed to radiation (27). Radiation can cause pneumonitis or fibrosis, the occurrence of which is most closely related to the rate of delivery of radiation. Pneumonitis is an acute-phase reaction that occurs 2 to 6 months after irradiation and may respond to corticosteroids. The late-phase response to radiation toxicity, fibrosis of the lungs, does not respond to corticosteroids.

Pulmonary veno-occlusive disease can be caused by bleomycin, mitomycin C, or carmustine. Patients present with shortness of breath, pulmonary hypertension, pleural effusions, or respiratory failure. Patients with this disorder have a poor prognosis.

■ CHEMOTHERAPY-INDUCED EXTRAVASATIONS

Extravasation injuries due to chemotherapy can produce a variety of symptoms ranging from skin irritation to skin ulceration, tissue necrosis, nerve damage, and (rarely) loss of limbs. Vesicant chemotherapy agents, including the alkylating agents (mechlorethamine, cisplatin, mitomycin C), DNA intercalating agents (doxorubicin, daunorubicin), and plant alkaloids (vinblastine, vincristine, vinorelbine), can cause the most severe reactions. Irritant chemotherapy extravasations are generally not severe, causing only pain, erythema, and inflammation at the extravasated site (46).

The goal is to prevent chemotherapy extravasations. The patient should be told to inform the staff of any discomfort, swelling, or erythema over the infusion site. Nursing staff should evaluate the intravenous infusion site carefully by administering intravenous fluids before chemotherapy agents are infused, and they should monitor the patient frequently for any evidence of extravasation. Intravenous lines should be placed carefully; areas that have a poor blood supply or overlie a joint should be avoided. If an extravasation does occur, the infusion should be stopped immediately with the catheter left in place, and the staff should attempt to withdraw any remaining chemotherapy agents. Cold compresses should then be placed on the involved site except when the agents are plant alkaloids, in which case warm compresses should be applied (44,47,48).

Topical dimethylsulfoxide (DMSO) in a 50% solution can relieve extravasations when applied at a volume of 1.5 mL to the site every 6 h for 7 to 14 days. DMSO is commonly used to treat extravasations caused by mitomycin C and the anthracyclines (46-50). For extravasations caused by plant alkaloids (vinblastine, vincristine, vinorelbine) and epidophyllotoxins (etoposide, teniposide), a solution of 150 units of hyaluronidase in 1 to 3 mL of saline can be injected into the needle and subcutaneously around the extravasated site (47,48).

A 0.17-mol/L solution of sodium thiosulfate can be injected into mechlorethamine-induced extravasation sites (2). Sodium thiosulfate is thought to work by creating an alkaline-rich site to which the vesicant binds instead of the skin. The by-product is then excreted in the urine (48). There is some evidence that sodium thiosulfate can also be used for extravasations caused by carmustine, cisplatin, carboplatin, cyclophosphamide, dacarbazine, and oxaliplatin (46). Table 46-6 lists selected chemotherapeutic agents and their antidotes.

If local measures fail to contain symptoms in all patients with anthracycline-induced extravasations, a plastic surgeon should be consulted. Surgery can consist of debridement, excision of dead tissues, and, in severe cases, skin graft placement. In patients with doxorubicin-induced extravasation, the drug remains in the tissue for a long period, perhaps being released by dying or dead cells and spreading over time.

Patients who have had previous extravasation reactions can also experience a "recall reaction" when the same chemotherapy is received later, causing ulcerations or burns to reappear at the previously affected area.

■ METABOLIC EMERGENCIES

SYNDROME OF INAPPROPRIATE ANTIDIURETIC HORMONE SECRETION

Hyponatremia is the most common electrolyte abnormality, present in approximately 2% of hospitalized patients. The syndrome of inappropriate antidiuretic hormone (SIADH) secretion is a paraneoplastic syndrome in which antidiuretic hormone (ADH) is secreted inappropriately from the posterior pituitary gland, despite lower serum osmolality. Typically ADH is secreted in response to hypernatremia, hypotension, or hypoxemia to increase the permeability of the collecting ducts so that water can be reabsorbed and the blood pressure and sodium level restored to normal values. In patients with cancer, a protein similar to ADH, atrial natriuretic factor (ANF), is secreted by the cardiac atria, which increases the renal excretion of sodium. The pituitary gland does not respond to feedback from ANF. Thus SIADH can be characterized by inappropriate ADH secretion despite normal blood volume, with hyponatremia, serum osmolality less than 260 mOsm/L, inappropriate sodium secretion

TABLE 46-6   CHEMOTHERAPEUTIC EXTRAVASATIONS AND THEIR ANTIDOTES

Chemotherapy Agent	Irritant/ Vesicant	Sodium Thiosulfate	DMSO	Hyaluronidase	Cool	Warm
Carboplatin	I	+			+	
Carmustine	I/V	+		+		Dry warm
Cisplatin	I/V	+			+	
Cyclophosphamide	I	+			+	
Dacarbazine	I/V	+				
Dactinomycin	I/V				+	
Daunorubicin	I/V		+		+	
Docetaxel	I				+	Warm soaks
Doxorubicin	I/V		+		+	
Epirubicin	I/V		+		+	
Etoposide	I/V			+		+
Idarubicin	I/V		+		+	
Ifosfamide	I				+	
Mechlorethamine	I/V	+				
Mitomycin C	V		+		+	
Oxaliplatin	I/V	+				
Paclitaxel	I/V			+		
Plicamycin	I/V					
Streptozocin	I/V					
Teniposide	I/V			+		+
Topotecan					+	
Vinblastine	I/V			+		+
Vincristine	I/V			+		+
Vindesine	I/V			+		+
Vinorelbine	I/V			+		+

DMSO, dimethylsulfoxide.

in the urine of greater than 20 mEq/L, and high urine osmolality greater than 100 (51).

SIADH can be caused by various cancers, including small cell lung cancer, pancreatic cancer, and primary brain cancers. Other causes of SIADH are pulmonary infections, postoperative effects, central nervous system disorders (meningitis, stroke, hemorrhage), and chemotherapeutic agents (vincristine, cisplatin, and cyclophosphamide).

Symptoms of SIADH depend on the sodium level and the rate at which the sodium level declines. The patient can present with confusion, seizures, headache, or weight gain without edema. In evaluating hyponatremia, the patient's volume status should be addressed, and the plasma osmolality, urine osmolality, and urine sodium and chloride levels should be determined. Hyponatremia should be distinguished from pseudohyponatremia, in which plasma osmolality is normal (hyperlipidemia, hyperproteinemia) or even high (hypertriglyceridemia, hyperglycemia, and mannitol use).

Most patients with hyponatremia have low serum osmolality, which can be grouped by type: primary sodium loss, primary sodium gain, and primary water gain. Patients with sodium gain present with volume overload, which occurs in congestive heart failure, liver disease, and nephrotic syndrome. Patients with primary sodium loss present with dehydration; sodium deficits can be due to GI loss (nausea, vomiting, diarrhea, bowel obstruction), renal loss (thiazide diuretics), and skin loss (severe burns). Patients with SIADH can also have primary water gain, although other sources of primary water gain (primary polydipsia, decreased solute intake, beer potomania, chronic renal insufficiency, adrenal or thyroid deficiency, or increased ADH secretion in response to pain, nausea, vomiting, or drugs) should be distinguished. Some patients appear to have SIADH based on laboratory test results but actually have a reset osmostat. This adjustment can occur in patients with quadriplegia, tuberculosis, psychosis, chronic illness, volume contraction, encephalitis, malnutrition, or malignancy and in elderly or pregnant patients. Other rare causes of euvolemic hyponatremia are an incomplete pituitary stalk and increased sensitivity to ADH secretion.

Treatment of SIADH involves restricting water to 500 to 1000 mL/day from all sources and treating the underlying disorder. If this combination is not effective, demeclocycline (600-1200 mg/day) can be used in divided doses two to four times per day (51). Patients whose symptoms include coma or seizure can be treated by slow infusion of 3% normal saline; care must be taken not to increase serum sodium by more than 0.5 to 1 mEq/h. Too-rapid correction of serum sodium level can lead to central pontine myelinolysis (Fig. 46-15).

TUMOR LYSIS SYNDROME

Tumor lysis syndrome (TLS) is a result of excessive tumor breakdown, causing hypocalcemia, hyperphosphatemia, hyperkalemia, elevated uric acid, and occasionally acute renal failure. Risk factors for TLS include high tumor burden, chronic renal insufficiency, and certain tumor types (Burkitt lymphoma, lymphoblastic lymphoma, diffuse large cell lymphoma, undifferentiated lymphoma, and leukemia) (2). TLS usually presents during chemotherapy, but it can also occur after radiation therapy, corticosteroid treatment for sensitive tumors, or administration of hormonal agents.

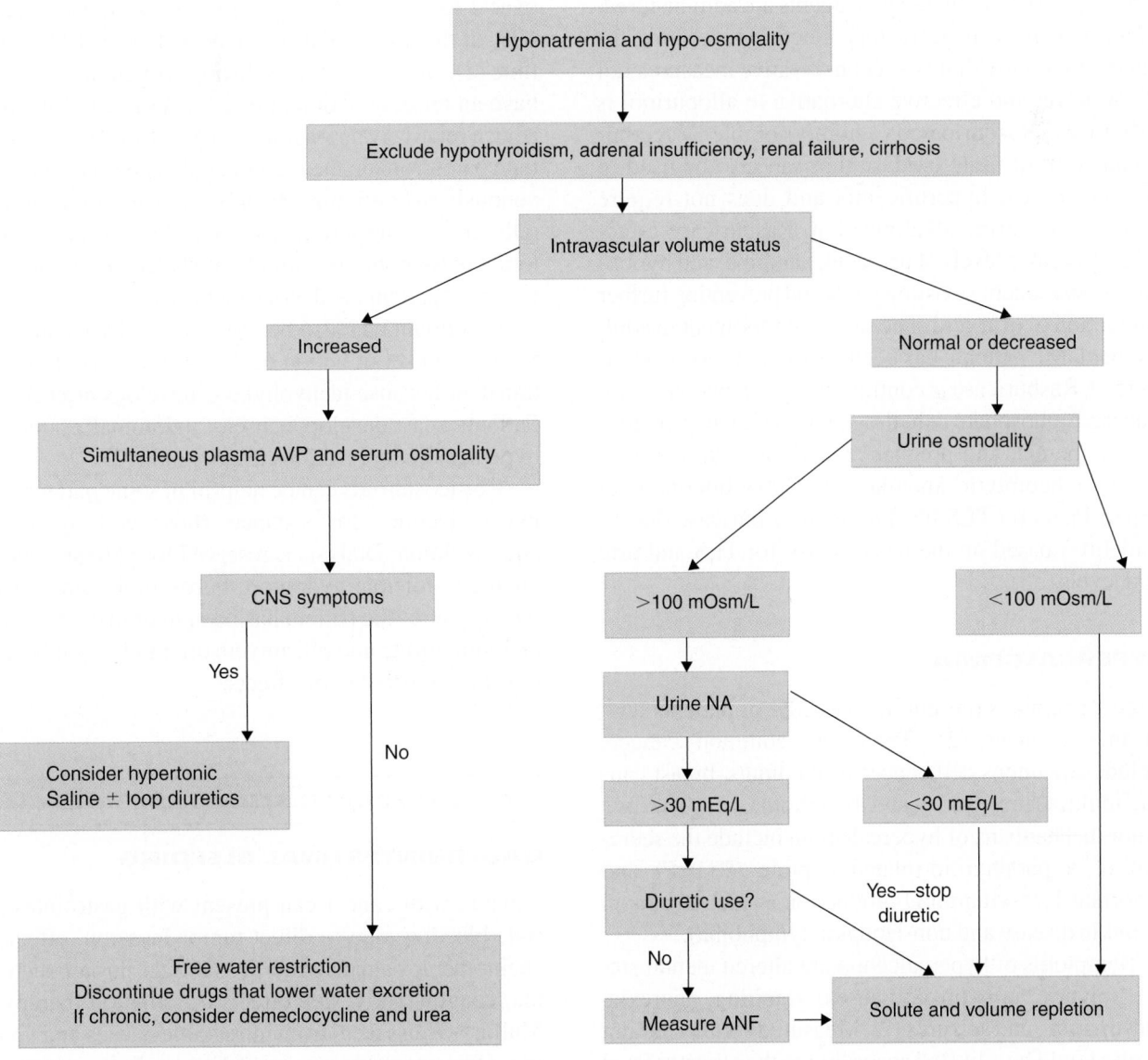

FIGURE 46-15. Algorithm for the evaluation and treatment of hyponatremia. ANF, atrial natriuretic peptide; AVP, arginine vasopressin; CNS, central nervous system. (*Adapted from Yeung SJ, Diaz GL, Gagel RF. Metabolic and endocrine emergencies. In: Yeung SJ, Escalante CP [eds]: Oncologic Emergencies. Hamilton, Ontario, Canada: BC Decker; 2002, with permission.*)

Patients with TLS can present with nausea and vomiting, diarrhea, constipation, low urine output, weight gain, acute renal failure, weakness, cramps, seizures, tetany, or arrhythmias.

Prophylaxis is very important in preventing TLS and consists of intravenous hydration, oral allopurinol (100-600 mg/day), and occasionally alkalinization of the urine with sodium bicarbonate to maintain a urine pH greater than 7.5. Alkalinizing the urine decreases uric acid crystallization in the kidneys. Because allopurinol use is now common before chemotherapy, hyperphosphatemia, rather than hyperuricemia, is now the predominant cause of acute renal failure in TLS. To prevent TLS, patients with leukemia and high WBC counts should be treated with leukapheresis or hydroxyurea before chemotherapeutic agents are administered. Some patients with refractory electrolyte abnormalities might require dialysis if conservative measures fail (2). A newer and effective alternative to allopurinol is rasburicase. Rasburicase is a highly soluble IV recombinant form of urate oxidase that can also be used to prevent or treat hyperuricemia and does not require simultaneous urine alkalinization. Rasburicase effectively decreases levels of uric acid, xanthine, and hypoxanthine by reducing existing pools and preventing further production of uric acid. The safety of this agent in adult and pediatric patients has been verified in several studies (52). Rasburicase is contraindicated in patients with glucose-6-phosphate dehydrogenase deficiency, methemoglobinemia, and pregnancy, and has a known side effect of hemolytic anemia. The 2008 International Expert Panel on TLS has provided rasburicase dosing guidelines based on the level of risk for TLS and uric acid levels (53).

HYPERCALCEMIA

Hypercalcemia is present in 10 to 20% of patients with advanced cancer (2). The most common cancers include squamous cell cancer of the lungs, breast cancer, multiple myeloma, and lymphoma (2). The two major mechanisms of hypercalcemia include the secretion of a parathyroid-related peptide (PTHrP) and abnormal 1,25-vitamin D production (which occurs in Hodgkin disease and non-Hodgkin lymphoma).

Symptoms of hypercalcemia are altered mental status, polyuria, polydipsia, nausea, vomiting, anorexia, constipation, and seizures (2). Measured serum calcium levels should be adjusted according to the albumin level for accurate estimation. A low albumin level should be subtracted from 4, and the difference should be multiplied by 0.8. This product should be added to the serum calcium level to arrive at the estimated calcium. Alternatively, ionized calcium can be measured, which assesses the active calcium in the serum and is more accurate.

The choice of treatment for hypercalcemia depends on the patient's calcium level and symptoms. Calcium is a potent diuretic, and patients with mild hypercalcemia can be treated by intravenous fluids. Patients with a calcium level greater than 14 mg/dL should be treated with additional measures. Patients who have symptoms of hypercalcemia and a calcium level between 12 and 14 mg/dL should also receive additional treatment to lower the calcium level.

Bisphosphonates are the drugs of choice in treating hypercalcemia. Pamidronate can be given intravenously over 2 to 24 h. A 60-mg dose corrects hypercalcemia 60% of the time, and a 90-mg dose does so 100% of the time (2). Bisphosphonates do not work immediately but have an onset of action after 12 to 48 h (2). Zoledronic acid, a relatively new agent, can be infused more rapidly than pamidronate; the recommended dose is 4 mg intravenously over 15 min. Bisphosphonates are useful not only in reducing serum calcium levels but can also help to decrease bone pain and treat skeletal complications in cancer patients with bone metastases (54).

Calcitonin can also be used to treat hypercalcemia; it has an onset of action of 2 to 4 h, but its effects are transient because tachyphylaxis develops after 3 days. Patients may develop nausea, abdominal cramps, or hypersensitivity reactions to calcitonin (2).

Corticosteroids can be helpful in some patients with hypercalcemia—for instance, those with lymphoma and myeloma. Dialysis is reserved for patients who are unable to tolerate hydration. Furosemide can be used, but only after the patient has been hydrated adequately. Gallium nitrate and plicamycin are rarely used because of the high risk of toxic effects.

■ GASTROINTESTINAL EMERGENCIES

GASTROINTESTINAL BLEEDING

Patients with cancer can present with gastrointestinal (GI) bleeding due to direct tumor invasion, effects of chemotherapy agents or corticosteroids, thrombocytopenia, coagulopathy, side effects of radiation therapy, or Mallory-Weiss tears from intractable nausea and vomiting. Other possible causes of GI bleeding are gastritis, peptic ulcer disease, duodenal ulcers, arteriovenous malformations, and diverticulosis. Patients who have undergone bone marrow transplantation can present with GI bleeding as a manifestation of graft-versus-host disease, which typically presents as ulcerations in the small intestine. For patients bleeding from the upper GI tract, a nasogastric tube should be inserted and the tract lavaged with normal saline until the bleeding clears. If the bleeding does not clear, emergent upper GI endoscopy may be considered. Patients with small tumors rarely have significant bleeding, and patients with large tumors tend to ooze and bleed. However, relief of bleeding by endoscopic measures is usually temporary, and these tumors tend to bleed repeatedly. Endoscopic interventions can include electrocoagulation, epinephrine injections, and argon plasma laser treatment. For patients with persistent bleeding, arteriography and embolization is occasionally successful. If all other interventions have failed, surgery can be considered. Patients with bleeding should have any coagulopathy corrected, including deficits in the platelet count, which should be greater than 60,000/µL. Somatostatin or vasopressin can be used to control bleeding of esophageal varices. The patient should receive either an H_2 blocker or a proton pump inhibitor intravenously. Nausea should be controlled using intravenous antiemetics, and the patient should receive nothing by mouth. The patient should

also receive maintenance IV fluid. If hypotensive, the patient should be volume resuscitated with intravenous crystalloid fluid and/or transfusion.

TYPHLITIS

Typhlitis is a syndrome of bowel inflammation, edema, and wall thickening involving the proximal large bowel in patients with neutropenic fever. It commonly affects the cecum but can also affect the ascending colon and occasionally the transverse colon. Typhlitis can occur in conjunction with any cancer but is most common in patients with leukemia (27). The organisms most often isolated in cases of typhlitis are *Clostridium* and gram-negative bacilli (55).

Patients with typhlitis present with fever, pain in the right lower quadrant of the abdomen, and sometimes diarrhea, which may be bloody. The patient with typhlitis is neutropenic, and plain abdominal x-ray films are often inconclusive. The diagnosis of typhlitis is made based on clinical suspicion and CT or MRI findings that reveal bowel inflammation, edema, wall thickening, and possibly air formation or, in severe cases, free air (Fig. 46-16).

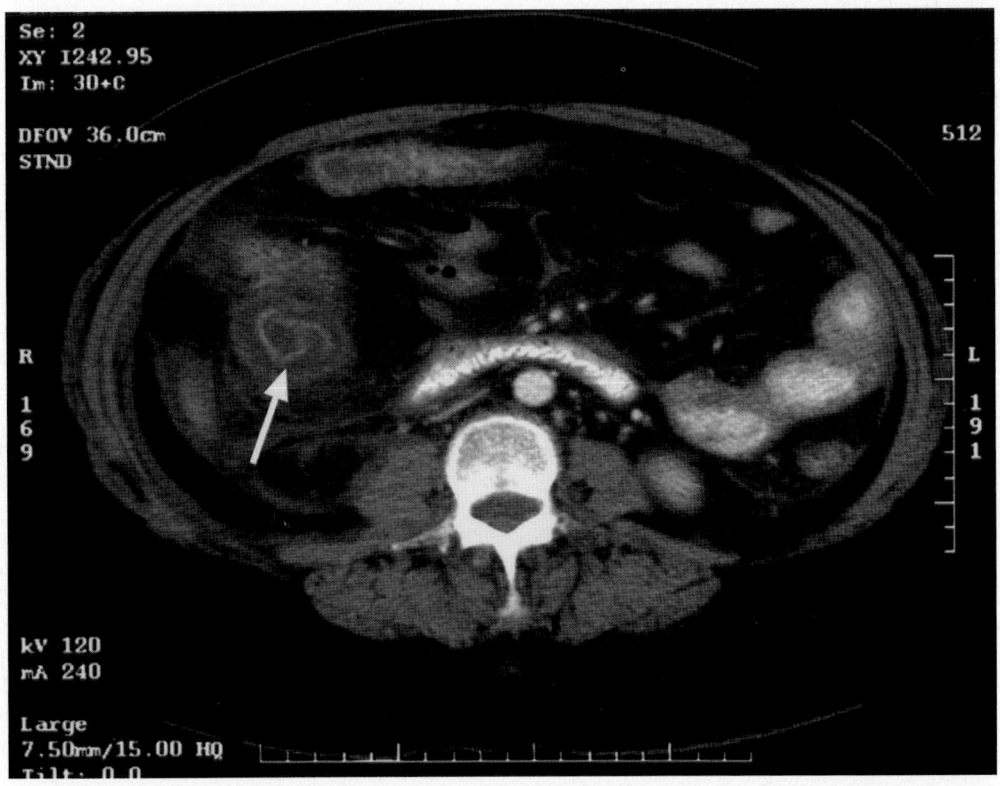

FIGURE 46-16. Inflammation of the cecum and ascending colon in a 45-year-old patient with typhlitis. The arrow points to inflammation and edema of the cecum. (*Courtesy of Dr. Stephanie Mundy, MD Anderson Cancer Center.*)

Typhlitis is managed by bowel rest and intravenous administration of broad-spectrum antibiotics, including anaerobic coverage. Patients rarely require surgery unless they develop intractable bleeding or bowel perforation or do not respond to conservative measures.

References

1. Loblaw DA, Laperriere NJ, Mackillop WJ. A population-based study of malignant spinal cord compression in Ontario. *Clin Oncol (R Coll Radiol)* 2003;15(4):211-217.

2. Krimsky WS, Behrens RJ, Kerkvliet GJ. Oncologic emergencies for the internist. *Cleve Clin J Med* 2002;69(3):209-210, 213-214, 216-217 passim.

3. Quinn JA, DeAngelis LM. Neurologic emergencies in the cancer patient. *Semin Oncol* 2000;27(3):311-321.

4. Saarto T, Janes R, Tenhunen M, et al. Palliative radiotherapy in the treatment of skeletal metastases. *Eur J Pain* 2002;6(5):323-330.

5. Schiff D, Batchelor T, Wen PY. Neurologic emergencies in cancer patients. *Neurol Clin* 1998;16(2):449-483.

6. Vaillant B, Loghin M. Treatment of spinal cord tumors. *Curr Treat Options Neurol* 2009;11(4):315-324.

7. Patchell RA, Tibbs PA, Regine WF, et al. Direct decompressive surgical resection in the treatment of spinal cord compression caused by metastatic cancer: A randomised trial. *Lancet* 2005;366(9486):643-648.

8. George R, Jeba J, Ramkumar G, et al. Interventions for the treatment of metastatic extradural spinal cord compression in adults. *Cochrane Database Syst Rev* 2008;(4):CD006716.

9. Cascino TL. Neurologic complications of systemic cancer. *Med Clin North Am* 1993;77(1):265-278.

10. Rades D, Dunst J, Schild SE. The first score predicting overall survival in patients with metastatic spinal cord compression. *Cancer* 2008;112(1):157-161.

11. Kaal EC, Taphoorn MJ, Vecht CJ. Symptomatic management and imaging of brain metastases. *J Neurooncol* 2005;75(1):15-20.

12. Vecht CJ. Clinical management of brain metastasis. *J Neurol* 1998;245(3):127-131.

13. Chamberlain MC. Leptomeningeal metastasis. *Curr Opin Neurol* 2009;22(6):665-674.

14. Soffietti R, Ruda R, Mutani R. Management of brain metastases. *J Neurol* 2002;249(10):1357-1369.

15. O'Neill BP, Buckner JC, Coffey RJ, et al. Brain metastatic lesions. *Mayo Clin Proc* 1994;69(11):1062-1068.

16. Arnold SM, Patchell RA. Diagnosis and management of brain metastases. *Hematol Oncol Clin North Am* 2001;15(6):1085-1107, vii.

17. Sawaya R. Considerations in the diagnosis and management of brain metastases. *Oncology (Williston Park)* 2001;15(9):1144-1154, 1157-1158; discussion 1158, 1163-1165.

18. DeAngelis LM. Management of brain metastases. *Cancer Invest* 1994;12(2):156-165.

19. Wen PY, Loeffler JS. Brain metastases. *Curr Treat Options Oncol* 2000;1(5):447-458.

20. Patchell RA, Tibbs PA, Regine WF, et al. Postoperative radiotherapy in the treatment of single metastases to the brain: A randomized trial. *JAMA* 1998;280(17):1485-1489.

21. Ewend MG, Carey LA, Morris DE, et al. Brain metastases. *Curr Treat Options Oncol* 2001;2(6):537-547.

22. Davey P. Brain metastases: Treatment options to improve outcomes. *CNS Drugs* 2002;16(5):325-338.

23. Grossman SA, Krabak MJ. Leptomeningeal carcinomatosis. *Cancer Treat Rev* 1999;25(2):103-119.

24. Meierkord H, Boon P, Engelsen B, et al. EFNS guideline on the management of status epilepticus in adults. *Eur J Neurol.* 2010 Mar;17(3):348-55.

25. Miller LC, Drislane FW. Treatment of status epilepticus. *Expert Rev Neurother* 2008;8(12):1817-1827.

26. Demopoulos A, DeAngelis LM. Neurologic complications of leukemia. *Curr Opin Neurol* 2002;15(6):691-699.

27. Shanholtz C. Acute life-threatening toxicity of cancer treatment. *Crit Care Clin* 2001;17(3):483-502.

28. Tsang TS, Enriquez-Sarano M, Freeman WK, et al. Consecutive 1127 therapeutic echocardiographically guided pericardiocenteses: Clinical profile, practice patterns, and outcomes spanning 21 years. *Mayo Clin Proc* 2002;77(5):429-436.

29. Kvale PA, Simoff M, Prakash UB. Lung cancer. Palliative care. *Chest* 2003;123(1 Suppl):S284-S311.

30. Douketis JD, Crowther MA, Stanton EB, et al. Elevated cardiac troponin levels in patients with submassive pulmonary embolism. *Arch Intern Med* 2002;162(1):79-81.

31. Blumenthal DT, Glenn MJ. Neurologic manifestations of hematologic disorders. *Neurol Clin* 2002;20(1):265-281, viii.

32. Majhail NS, Lichtin AE. Acute leukemia with a very high leukocyte count: Confronting a medical emergency. *Cleve Clin J Med* 2004;71(8):633-637.

33. Kaminsky DA, Hurwitz CG, Olmstead JI. Pulmonary leukostasis mimicking pulmonary embolism. *Leuk Res* 2000;24(2):175-178.

34. DeSancho MT, Rand JH. Bleeding and thrombotic complications in critically ill patients with cancer. *Crit Care Clin* 2001;17(3):599-622.

35. Tissue plasminogen activator for the treatment of acute pulmonary embolism. A collaborative study by the PIOPED Investigators. *Chest* 1990;97(3):528-533.

36. King V, Vaze AA, Moskowitz CS, et al. D-dimer assay to exclude pulmonary embolism in high-risk oncologic population: Correlation with CT pulmonary angiography in an urgent care setting. *Radiology* 2008;247(3):854-861.

37. Nazario R, Delorenzo LJ, Maguire AG. Treatment of venous thromboembolism. *Cardiol Rev* 2002;10(4):249-259.

38. Levine MN. Can we optimise treatment of thrombosis? *Cancer Treat Rev* 2003;29(Suppl 2):19-22.

39. Garcia DA, Spyropoulos AC. Update in the treatment of venous thromboembolism. *Semin Respir Crit Care Med* 2008;29(1):40-46.

40. Levine MN. Managing thromboembolic disease in the cancer patient: Efficacy and safety of antithrombotic treatment options in patients with cancer. *Cancer Treat Rev* 2002;28(3):145-149.

41. Lee AY. Treatment of venous thromboembolism in cancer patients. *Thromb Res* 2001;102(6):V195-V208.

42. Schiffer CA, Anderson KC, Bennett CL, et al. Platelet transfusion for patients with cancer: Clinical practice guidelines of the American Society of Clinical Oncology. *J Clin Oncol* 2001;19(5):1519-1538.

43. Bick RL. Disseminated intravascular coagulation: A review of etiology, pathophysiology, diagnosis, and management: Guidelines for care. *Clin Appl Thromb Hemost* 2002;8(1):1-31.

44. Bertelli G. Prevention and management of extravasation of cytotoxic drugs. *Drug Saf* 1995;12(4):245-255.

45. Russo P. Urologic emergencies in the cancer patient. *Semin Oncol* 2000;27(3):284-298.

46. Alley E, Green R, Schuchter L. Cutaneous toxicities of cancer therapy. *Curr Opin Oncol* 2002;14(2):212-216.

47. Dorr RT. Antidotes to vesicant chemotherapy extravasations. *Blood Rev* 1990;4(1):41-60.

48. Kassner E. Evaluation and treatment of chemotherapy extravasation injuries. *J Pediatr Oncol* Nurs 2000;17(3):135-148.

49. Fenchel K, Karthaus M. Cytotoxic drug extravasation. *Antibiot Chemother* 2000;50:144-148.

50. Valks R, Garcia-Diez A, Fernandez-Herrera J. Mucocutaneous reactions to chemotherapy. *J Am Acad Dermatol* 2000;42(4):699.

51. Milionis HJ, Liamis GL, Elisaf MS. The hyponatremic patient: A systematic approach to laboratory diagnosis. *CMAJ* 2002; 166(8):1056-1062.

52. Goldman SC, Holcenberg JS, Finklestein JZ, et al. A randomized comparison between rasburicase and allopurinol in children with lymphoma or leukemia at high risk for tumor lysis. *Blood* 2001;97(10):2998-3003.

53. Coiffier B, Altman A, Pui CH, et al. Guidelines for the management of pediatric and adult tumor lysis syndrome: An evidence-based review. *J Clin Oncol* 2008;26(16):2767-2778.

54. Janjan N. Bone metastases: Approaches to management. *Semin Oncol* 2001;28(4 Suppl 11):28-34.

55. Davila ML. Neutropenic enterocolitis. *Curr Treat Options Gastroenterol* 2006;9(3):249-255.

Palliative Care and Symptom Management

DEFINING PALLIATIVE CARE IN ONCOLOGY

Jessica Masterson
Michael J. Fisch
Commentary: Jeffrey E. Lee

■ CASE VIGNETTE: TRADITIONAL MODEL DEFINING PALLIATIVE CARE

John, a 37-year-old construction foreman, worked long hours to provide for his wife and their two young children. For the past few weeks, John had been experiencing some mild abdominal discomfort that curtailed his appetite, but not enough to slow him down. He noticed he had lost some weight and felt nausea from time to time, but was not concerned. One evening his abdominal pain was the worst he ever felt, and for the first time in his life went to the emergency room. He was worried he had appendicitis; it was the only illness he could think of that could cause such pain. His CT scan revealed a large mass in the head of the pancreas, and soon John would come to learn he had pancreatic cancer.

Upon meeting with an oncologist, he learned his tumor was resectable, and thus his treatment plan would be aimed for cure. This would involve a combination of surgery, radiation, and chemotherapy. It was a lot of information to handle quickly, but John trusted in his care team and soon started on the several month journey of postoperative recovery, radiation, and chemotherapy treatments. During this time, John was unable to work due to the burden of his appointments and the side effects of treatment. He experienced significant fatigue, nausea, and diarrhea. These symptoms often kept him from participating in family activities.

When his course of treatment was completed, John slowly began to feel like himself again and the pulse of his life returned. In five months time, however, he began to experience increasing fatigue and shoulder pain when lifting up his children, something he had never experienced before. Restaging scans showed that he had developed metastatic bone disease. It was explained to John that his disease was no longer curable, and that his prognosis may very well be measured in months. After an extensive discussion with his wife and oncologist, John decided to pursue palliative radiation for his shoulder pain followed by systemic chemotherapy. The radiation treatment helped with his shoulder pain initially, but once John began systemic chemotherapy, his symptom burden exploded. His pain returned and now involved his back and hips as well as his shoulder; he had significant nausea and diarrhea from chemotherapy and his fatigue kept him in bed most of the day. After four weekly treatments of systemic chemotherapy with resultant clinical decline, it was decided that John's disease burden was such that the risks of chemotherapy outweighed its potential benefits. It was at this time that John was referred to palliative care for pain, symptom management, and "end-of-life" care. He was enrolled in hospice within 2 weeks, and died within 5 weeks of his last oncology visit.

■ INTEGRATING PALLIATIVE CARE INTO ONCOLOGY: EVOLVING DEFINITIONS AND MODELS OF CARE

In 1990, the World Health Organization (WHO) began its definition of palliative care with "Palliative Care is the active total care of patients whose disease is not responsive to curative treatment. Control of pain, of other symptoms, and of psychological, social, and spiritual problems is paramount" (1). For a generalist physician, this definition poses little contextual conflict. The general practitioner most often deals with diseases that are chronic from the start, such as dementia or peripheral vascular disease. Their "treatments" are not ever directed at a cure, but rather at controlling the disease to delay or prevent unwanted outcomes that may include pain or other symptoms. In their care of the patient, they do not need to make a distinction between curative and noncurative treatment. In this way, initiating and integrating palliative care does not seem like a frank departure from the original goals of care, but rather a more comprehensive extension of care as more needs arise. For an oncologist, however, the distinction between curative and noncurative treatments is more profound, and this distinction has translated into how palliative care has been perceived and defined within the field of oncology (2). The term "palliative care" is still regarded by many oncologists as synonymous with "terminal care," and this is illustrated by the nonintegrated referral pattern in the case above. A recent study done by Fadul et al at MD Anderson Cancer Center showed that 56% of surveyed medical oncologists and 58% of mid-level providers felt the term "palliative care" was synonymous with hospice and end of life (3). Interestingly, the study goes on to show that medical oncologists are more likely to refer patients at earlier stages of illness to a service named "supportive care" compared with "palliative care" ($p < .0001$). The WHO definition goes on to further state that care that is palliative "neither hastens nor postpones death." Many oncologists use "palliative" chemotherapy in the noncurative setting with the intent of improving overall survival, that is, postponing death. Is chemotherapy in this setting then not really palliative?

For many oncologists, the 1990 WHO definition of palliative care was inadequate in providing a framework for shared goals of care that could encompass all stages of cancer's disease trajectory. Practice patterns reflected this, and palliative care was sought at the end stages of disease, separate from a patient's oncologic care (4,5). Over the next decade, however, the role of palliative care within a cancer patient's treatment plan began to change. The United States saw a tremendous rise in the number of cancer centers with integrated clinical palliative medicine programs (6), with MD Anderson establishing its program in 1999. In 2002, the WHO modified its definition to reflect that palliative care is for patients with "life-threatening illness," rather than just those "whose disease is not responsive to curative treatment" (7). The current working definition of palliative care shared by the National Cancer Institute (NCI) and National Institute of Health (NIH) reflects the paradigm shift regarding palliative care and oncologic care:

Care given to improve the quality of life of patients who have a serious or life-threatening disease. The goal of palliative care is to prevent or treat as early as possible the symptoms of a disease, side effects caused by treatment of a disease, and psychological, social, and spiritual problems related to a disease or its treatment (8).

This definition of palliative care reflects not only the multiple domains of care addressed but also a model of care that is flexible and dynamic, meeting the complex and changing needs of the cancer patient at any point in the disease trajectory. The appropriate time to introduce palliative care into a cancer patient's care plan is specific to an individual patient's needs and goals. As the evolving definition of palliative care suggests, this time may be significantly earlier than the traditional model of integrating at "the end of life."

■ PALLIATIVE CANCER CARE: MEETING CRITICAL NEEDS THROUGH AN INTERDISCIPLINARY TEAM

In 2009, the American Society of Clinical Oncology (ASCO) convened a special task force of palliative care experts to assess the current palliative care needs of oncology patients and to further define the role of palliative care in oncology. From this task force emerged the concept of "Palliative Cancer Care": "the integration into cancer care of therapies that address the multiple issues that cause suffering for patients and their families and impact their life quality" (9). This definition acknowledges two important and interrelated aspects of palliative care for oncology patients. First, there are a variety of needs and issues within the environment of a cancer patient that go beyond the management of tumor burden. Secondly, the end goal of all palliative care interventions is to relieve suffering and improve overall quality of life.

When a patient is diagnosed with cancer, the environment surrounding their life is changed. Time spent at work is now spent in the waiting room, leading to lost wages. A full night's sleep may be interrupted with symptoms of nausea and diarrhea from chemotherapy. Fatigue may dominate the day, leaving responsibilities to fall on the shoulders of friends or family members. Fear and uncertainty may develop as the disease progresses. Patients with advanced cancer experience an average of 13 symptoms while hospitalized, and at least 7 in the outpatient setting (10). These physical, psychosocial, and spiritual needs are recognized by oncologists as crucial aspects in the comprehensive care of their patients. With the complex demands involved in the management of tumor burden, it may be difficult for an oncologist to fully attend to all of these needs. Incorporating palliative care into the care plan of patients with complex needs allows for improved patient and family satisfaction and decreased burden and burnout for the oncologist. A core interdisciplinary team consisting of a physician, nurse, social worker, and chaplain work together to assess and meet the needs of patients and their families (Fig. 47-1).

In the classic 1982 New England Journal of Medicine article "The nature of suffering and the goals of medicine," Eric Cassell defines suffering as "a state of severe distress associated with events that threaten the

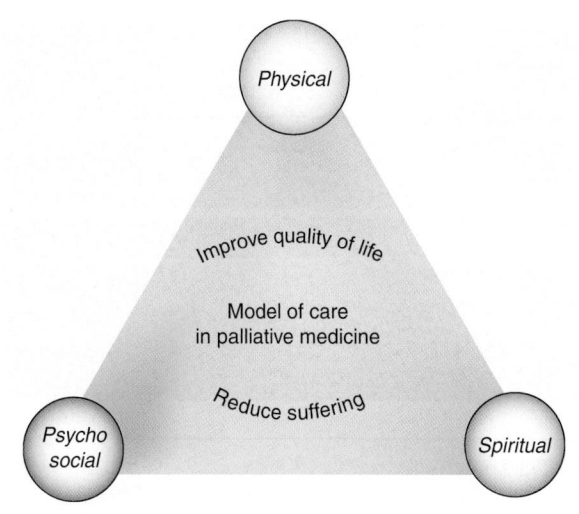

FIGURE 47-2. The comprehensive, interdisciplinary model of palliative care to reduce suffering and improve quality of life. *(Courtesy of Danielle M. Walsh.)*

intactness of the person" (11). In addition to being an interdisciplinary model of care, palliative medicine is also a philosophy of care (12). All assessments and interventions are intended to identify and relieve suffering when present, and to optimize quality of life. What constitutes suffering and defines quality of life is subjective and individual for any given patient. The philosophy of palliative care acknowledges the dependant relationships between the physical, psychosocial, and spiritual aspects of patients and incorporates them into a comprehensive interdisciplinary model of care to address suffering and quality of life (Fig. 47-2).

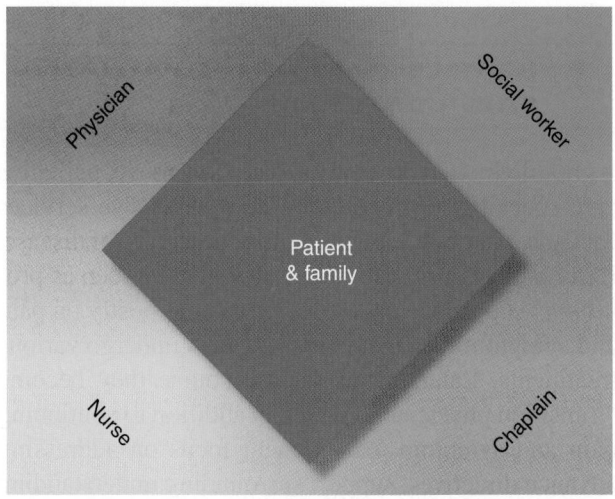

FIGURE 47-1. The core interdisciplinary team who work together to address the physical, psychological, and spiritual needs of the patient with life-threatening disease. *(Courtesy of Danielle M. Walsh.)*

■ CONTINUUM OF CARE: DEFINING NEEDS

The journey of a cancer patient can take various paths. While for many the journey ends with a cure, for others it does not. Approximately 50% of patients diagnosed with cancer will die of complications from their disease. While an individual's journey is unique, there are common turning points encountered: initiation of chemotherapy, progression of disease despite multiple treatment regimens, the last weeks of life. At different points in the trajectory of illness, palliative care can assist in meeting the needs of patients in a way that is appropriate for their stage of disease. A common misconception is that the introduction of palliative care implies treatment goals can no longer be curative or disease-modifying (13). More accurately, palliative care aims to support treatment goals dynamically over the

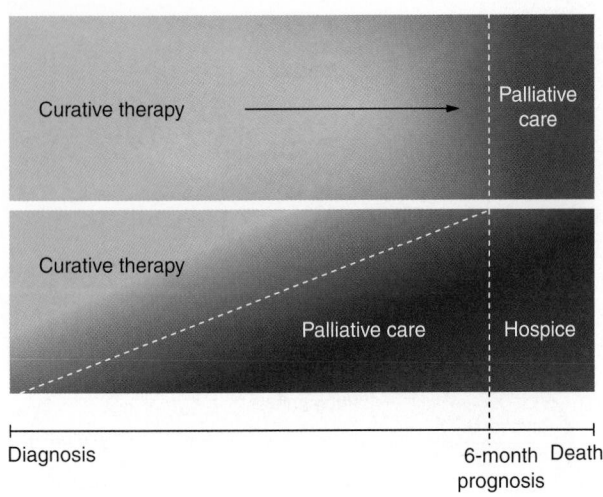

Curative therapy → Palliative care

Curative therapy

Palliative care   Hospice

Diagnosis   6-month Death
                            prognosis

FIGURE 47-3. The top panel represents the model of palliative care as total care of patients whose disease is not responsive to curative treatment. The lower panel illustrates the modern paradigm where palliative care is integrated early in the course of serious illness.

course of illness, meeting changing needs and goals along the way (Fig. 47-3). The key to effective integration of palliative care in oncology is to keep the needs and goals of care clearly defined.

Take the case of John, the 37-year-old construction worker with pancreatic cancer. At diagnosis, the goals of care were for cure, and his treatment plan reflected that. If the need had arisen, a palliative care physician may have assisted with postoperative pain and symptom management from radiation and chemotherapy treatments. Additionally, emotional support and guidance could have been provided for members of his family by the social worker. When his disease became metastatic and incurable, a shared turning point for many patients with cancer, his goals of care shifted. His treatment plan was still aimed at modifying the course of his disease, but no longer aimed for cure. A new constellation of symptoms emerged, now the result of disease burden. In addition to symptom management, psychosocial support surrounding issues of prognosis, code status, and advanced directives could be provided by the interdisciplinary palliative care team, without compromising oncologic goals of care. One of the most difficult turning points in cancer's trajectory, for both patient and provider, is the decision to discontinue all disease-modifying treatments. While in some cases the decision is clear to both patient and provider—the disease is progressing, the patient is too sick to safely receive more treatment—in other cases it is more difficult. There are times when the risks and potential benefits of further treatment are in a balance, and there is no

objective "right" decision. At this time, patients and their families may play a more central role in treatment planning, and be asked to think about goals and values in a way they have never been asked to before. Existential and spiritual concerns may emerge as patients begin to accept the imminence of their own mortality. Spouses and family members may struggle with hopelessness, fear, and grief in anticipation of the loss of their loved one. Palliative care teams are equipped with social workers and chaplains to engage in therapeutic dialogue surrounding these issues and assist in decision making and clarifying goals of care (14). When the decision is made to discontinue therapy, palliative care teams can assist in transitioning patients to hospice care (see below) when appropriate and provide support as provider care relationships change. Table 47-1 describes the domains of needs addressed by palliative care providers.

For John, the referral to palliative care came at the time disease-modifying therapy was discontinued. His wife recalls that the care and treatment planning they provided for John in the last few weeks of his life were incredible, but that the transition of goals and providers was difficult to process so quickly. In addition to helping oncologists meet the complex needs of their patients throughout the trajectory of illness, early integration of palliative care allows for provider continuity at one of the most important turning points in a patient's life. This continuity at the end of life can help to ease a patient's fears of provider abandonment, and can allow them an increased sense of satisfaction, completion, and personal growth (15).

■ HOSPICE: PART OF THE PALLIATIVE CARE CONTINUUM

As highlighted in the case presentation above, palliative care specialist teams provide comprehensive services for cancer patients along the entire trajectory of disease. Early in the course of disease they may be seen as providing "supportive oncology," focusing mostly on pain and symptom management as patients undergo various treatments. Later in the disease course they become "transition physicians," which in addition to continuing pain and symptom management focus on addressing advance directives, support surrounding understanding prognosis, and defining goals of care (Fig. 47-4). Much of this care is performed alongside the treating oncologist in the outpatient setting, described by Meyers and Linder as "simultaneous care" (16). As a patient's disease progresses and performance status declines, it

TABLE 47-1	CONCEPTS AND DOMAINS ADDRESSED BY PALLIATIVE CARE

Physical

Pain

    Somatic

    Visceral

    Neuropathic

Non-pain symptoms

    Fatigue

    Nausea

    Dyspnea

    Anorexia

    Mucositis

        Constipation/diarrhea

        Cognitive impairment

        Emotional distress

        Sleep disturbance

Psychosocial

    Interactions with friends and family

    Giving and receiving help

    Contributing to the community

    Recreation

    Sexual life

    Income

    Respect

    Variety in life

Spiritual

    Meaning and affirmation

    Hope and purpose

    Peace and reconciliation

    Divine forgiveness and support

    Religious rites and sacraments

    Prayer

    Visitation by clergy

End-of-life care

    Terminal symptom management

    Personal hygiene

    Treatment preferences and advanced care planning

    Shared knowledge about prognosis and all important aspects of care

    Transparency in care and decision processes

    Cooperation and communication among providers

    Coordination among caregivers, patients, and families

    Providing the patient with locus of control and loved ones with involvement

    Renewed sense of personhood and meaning

    Closure of personal and community relationships

    Transcendence

    Moment of death

    Grief and bereavement

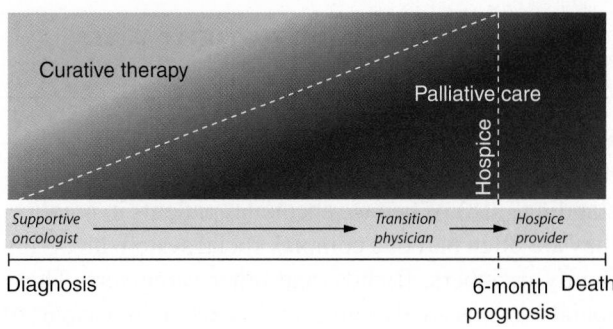

FIGURE 47-4. This model highlights the changing labels that might be used to describe the focus of palliative care physicians over the course of illness.

My cancer is no longer responsive to chemotherapy treatments. I know I have fought the good fight. I now hope to live as well as I can for the remaining time that I have. My cancer will progress along its natural course, and I wish to be as comfortable as possible and free from pain as this inevitably happens. I know that aggressive care measures are not likely to be helpful to me, and may even harm me. I am too sick to travel to the doctor. I don't want to go to the hospital anymore; I wish to remain at home in my last days.

Hospice provides a model of interdisciplinary palliative care for terminally ill patients and their families outside of an acute care setting when a patient's goals of care are that of comfort, and life-prolonging or -sustaining treatments have become burdensome or undesirable. Often confused with a location of care, hospice is rather a philosophy and model of care that can be provided in multiple settings including a patient's home, nursing home, or free-standing facility. Regardless of the site, hospice care represents a continuum of palliative care, and provides pain and symptom management and psychosocial and spiritual support to patients and their families. In addition, the hospice model of care includes trained volunteers, 24-hour clinical support, and bereavement services for families for 1 year following death. All patients regardless of age are eligible to receive the Medicare Hospice Benefit (an additional benefit to Medicare Part A) as long as their physician certifies their prognosis is likely to be 6 months or less if the disease follows its normal course (17). While the physician may suggest that hospice is the most appropriate level of care for a patient, the decision remains in the hands of the patient. Enrolling in hospice requires informed consent and signature of a Medicare hospice benefit election form.

may no longer be desirable or feasible to continue care in the ambulatory or acute care setting. The goals of care may be focused completely on comfort and quality of life, as described by an advanced cancer patient below:

■ FOCUS OF CARE: PATIENT AND FAMILY

Williamson and Noel wrote, "Although the individual is the unit of treatment, the family is the unit of understanding" (18). When we encounter patients in practice, they are often part of a complex social system involving family members, friends, and other caregivers. These social systems are dynamic, and a change in one part of the system can affect all others (18). When a patient is diagnosed with life-threatening illness, a profound stressor is introduced into the social system, which can subsequently be thrown out of balance. In the case of John above, early in the course of his pancreatic cancer treatment he was unable to work or spend significant time with his family due to the burdens of treatment. Such a disruption can lead to increased financial burden, more dependency and responsibility on friends and families, and feelings of isolation. While this can be a time where families pull together and show much strength and courage, for others it becomes a source of profound stress as family roles and behaviors are challenged to change. As patients progress in their illness and become more dependent on those around them, issues such as caregiver burnout, feelings of helplessness and guilt, and anticipatory grief for the dying patient emerge (19). These stresses on the family/caregiver social system can in turn affect the patient, and in a vicious cycle can contribute to increased suffering for all. The impact of terminal illness on a family member's physical and psychologic health has led them to be often referred to as "hidden patients" (20). Recognizing and understanding the functional dynamics and emotional needs of families and caregivers requires considerable skill and cultural competence and are of vital importance in the palliative model of care. Interdisciplinary teams work closely with families and caregivers, counseling on specific strategies for improved communication, healthy coping, and spiritual well-being.

■ ACCESS AND MODELS FOR CARE DELIVERY: OUTPATIENT CARE

In the traditional model of palliative care, the introduction of palliative services occurs late in the trajectory of illness, many times in the last weeks of life. Referral often occurs at times of acute distress such as severe pain, shortness of breath, or failure to thrive, leading to an emergency room visit and subsequent hospital admission. These admissions would lead to a palliative care consultation for expert pain and symptom management as well as discussions surrounding transitioning goals of care and advanced care planning. In some larger medical centers, this care can be provided in specialized tertiary palliative care units devoted to intensive pain and symptom management (21). For those patients that survive the acute admission, many are discharged home with hospice services. For those who were discharged home without hospice, ensuring continuity of care becomes more difficult. In the past, patients receiving palliative care in the acute setting who were discharged home did not have outpatient palliative care follow-up upon discharge; at that time palliative care was defined as "end-of-life" care, and thus there was no need for an outpatient setting. Over the past decade, however, as definitions of palliative care have changed to reflect the concepts of early integration, there has been the establishment of outpatient palliative care clinics in comprehensive cancer centers. The development of the outpatient model of palliative care has been a crucial step in allowing for the successful early integration of palliative care in oncology, and it has improved continuity of palliative care throughout the course of illness.

Outpatient palliative care offers specialist-level interdisciplinary palliative care services as either a single consultation or an ongoing concurrent model of care in collaboration with a patient's primary treating physician (22). These services may be accessed as part of postdischarge follow-up to ensure continuity of care plans initiated in the hospital, as well as by direct referral from outpatient clinics. Pain, symptom management, psychosocial distress, and advanced care planning are just a few of the common needs that may be addressed and followed in the outpatient setting. Table 47-2 lists common reasons for referral to palliative care. In addition, by identifying needs and concerns that unaddressed often lead to crisis, they can help reduce the risk of unnecessary emergency room visits and frequent readmissions (22). Unlike traditional outpatient clinics, successful outpatient palliative care centers are structured to allow for frequent same-day appointments ("drop-ins"), provide spacious, comfortable clinical rooms to accommodate symptomatic patients and accompanying family members, and give access to all interdisciplinary team members (23). In a recent Phase II study investigating the efficacy of an outpatient palliative care intervention in patients with metastatic cancer, patients experienced a statistically significant improvement in a multitude of symptoms and overall care satisfaction, with improvements seen for the duration of the study (4 weeks) (24). The addition of outpatient palliative care services to inpatient consultation and hospice services provides

TABLE 47-2	**COMMON REASONS FOR REFERRAL TO PALLIATIVE CARE**

Cognitive impairment leading to misleading results on symptom assessment

Patient overwhelmed with unexpected bad news about cancer ("hit by a truck," as they say)

Opioid toxicity or phobia, creating poor pain control

Patient too debilitated for systemic chemotherapy, but could benefit from treatment if rehabilitation is achieved

Patient needs immediate anticancer therapy and concomitant intensive symptom management

Complex pain syndrome (neuropathic plus somatovisceral) due to uncontrolled pelvic involvement of tumor

Patient (or family) with magical thinking or extreme denial about health status

Severe chronic dyspnea-triggering anxiety crises and difficult disposition

Patient wants hospice with a link to MD Anderson

Somatization: patient with chronic, stable, and unchangeable levels of extreme symptom expression

Aberrant drug-taking behaviors or known addiction

Patient cannot get hospice care because of special needs or preferences but needs end-of-life care

Primary team wants patient to leave hospital, but patient will not or cannot go

Need to distinguish terminal delirium from potentially reversible delirium (dying from "not quite dying yet")

Indolent, advanced cancer or prolonged survivorship but debilitating psychologic distress

Difficult symptoms compounded by overwhelming family conflict

Difficult symptom control compounded by severe communication barriers (physical or cultural)

One symptom masquerading as another (nausea due to anxiety, fatigue due to pain or depression, pain due to delirium, anxiety due to dyspnea, etc)

Serious medical or psychiatric comorbidities and advanced cancer symptoms in need of careful coordination of care

Particularly high expectations for care or VIP status and some bothersome symptoms

Difficult or surprising acute or chronic complications of cancer treatment

Chronic nonmalignant pain causing distress and confusion in the context of advanced cancer

Acute, reversible medical problems that must be distinguished from chronic cancer problems

Patient's preference (or the preference of the referring doctor) for early integration of palliative care with cancer care

Cancer pain not responding to first-line opioids—hence need opioid dose titration, administration of coanalgesics, and management of expected opioid side effects

Patient who is actively dying and needs suffering management, family counseling, and "peeling back" of care not specifically contributing to comfort at the end of life

accessibility for early integration and a framework for palliative care continuity. This encapsulates the American Society of Clinical Oncology's vision for comprehensive cancer care (9).

■ VISION FOR COMPREHENSIVE CANCER CARE

In 1998, the American Society of Clinical Oncology (ASCO) published the special article "Cancer Care at the End of Life" in which it described the role of the oncologist:

The *oncologists' responsibility to care for their patients in a continuum that extends from the moment of diagnosis throughout the course of the illness. In addition to appropriate anticancer treatment, this includes symptom control and psychosocial support during all phases of care, including those during the last phase of life (25).*

Oncologists have been providing palliative care for their patients for decades. Not long ago, before the explosion in the number of new anticancer agents, palliative care often constituted the majority of cancer care that was provided. Over the past decade, however, the complexity of cancer management and the needs of cancer patients has increased significantly, warranting the need for a team approach to comprehensive cancer care. With a predicted future shortage of oncologists and provider burnout being as high as 60% in oncology communities, the integration of palliative care specialists becomes essential in meeting the growing needs of cancer patients (26,27).

By 2020, the United States and several other countries will have national cancer control plans that include palliative care as a routine part of comprehensive cancer care for all patients. To achieve this vision, ASCO will collaborate with other US and international oncology stakeholders to advocate for the integration of palliative cancer care into existing health care systems and cancer control plans and ensure funding for high-quality care, medications, and ancillary services (9). In addition, ASCO will support oncology fellowship training programs' efforts to incorporate palliative care educational experiences and provide awards for innovative palliative care research. This vision of comprehensive cancer care builds on the belief that quality cancer care "requires access to and the availability of state-of-the-art palliative cancer care rendered by skilled clinicians, buttressed when necessary by palliative care experts" (25).

■ ACKNOWLEDGMENT

The authors would like to thank Danielle M. Walsh for her assistance with figures.

Commentary: Principles of Palliative Care: A Surgeon's Perspective

My patient looked exhausted. He was clearly depressed. I was also frustrated that he was not feeling better by now. A retired pilot, Mr. T had been healthy all his life until 9 months ago, when he became jaundiced and was found to have pancreatic cancer. While there was no evidence for metastasis, Mr. T had a relatively advanced pancreatic cancer that surrounded his superior mesenteric vein and appeared to be attached to his superior mesenteric artery. His care team recommended treatment with combination systemic chemotherapy followed by chemoradiation. Mr. T had tolerated this treatment well; his disease remained stable and his blood level of CA19-9 fell by nearly 90%, both signs of a favorable response to treatment.

The consensus of the patient's care team at that point was that surgery with curative intent was a reasonable treatment goal. I, therefore, operated on him 6 months following his initial diagnosis. The operation required was a large one: a pancreaticoduodenectomy ("Whipple" procedure), along with removal of the right colon and removal and reconstruction of a portion of the superior mesenteric vein. Mr. T made an excellent initial recovery from his surgery, and we were all encouraged that his final pathology report was favorable: all margins were free of tumor, and there was no lymph node spread. Because of a somewhat slow recovery of postoperative gastrointestinal function, I had sent Mr. T back home on supplemental intravenous nutrition, with the expectation that he would be ready to transition away from intravenous nutrition within a few weeks.

Yet here we were in clinic, 3 months following surgery, and Mr. T was still on intravenous nutrition. His appetite was poor. He was tired, weak, discouraged, sleeping poorly, uncomfortable and frustrated over his lack of progress, yet there was no evidence of infection, and his digestion at this point was objectively nearly normal. Unfortunately, his restaging evaluation helped explain at least one big reason for his lack of progress: his CA19-9 level was back up, and his CT scan showed multiple liver metastases. Mr. T's cancer had spread; his condition was now incurable, and his life expectancy likely measured in months. While additional systemic therapy could potentially provide Mr. T with symptomatic improvement and modest survival benefit, he was in no condition to tolerate any meaningful form of chemotherapy.

At this point I consulted our Palliative Care team for assistance with Mr. T's care. The Palliative Care team stopped Mr. T's anti-nausea, prokinetic, and sleeping medications that were contributing to his restlessness and sleep disturbances. They started Mr. T on low-dose long-acting narcotic analgesics, megesterol to mitigate weight loss, mirtazapine for sleep disturbance, anxiety, and depression, and methylphenidate for fatigue and depression. In addition to these recommendations, dietary counseling was provided by our Clinical Nutrition service. Within 2 weeks, Mr. T was much improved. He was off intravenous nutrition. His appetite had picked up, his energy level was better, he was more comfortable, he was sleeping through the night; he was himself again. Mr. T was ready to return home to continue his recuperation, with a plan for reconsideration of systemic therapy after his next restaging evaluation in 2 to 3 months time.

The clear, substantial, and dramatic benefit Mr. T received from Palliative Care consultation is illustrative of my experience with Palliative Care services in the management of my patients. In this situation, input from Palliative Care was extraordinarily helpful to the patient in improving his quality of life at a time when his overall cancer situation was dynamic, difficult, and complex; the patient's cancer had returned while he was still recovering from radical surgery. Symptom management was the single most important aspect of the patient's care at that time, and an essential part of Mr T's comprehensive care. It is worth emphasizing that this example demonstrates just one aspect of the role of Palliative Care in the management of my patients with cancer; the accompanying chapter outlines a vision for even more complete and effective integration of Palliative Care into the management of patients with cancer.

Jeffrey E. Lee

■ RESOURCES

The following is a list of resources for further information on Palliative Cancer Care:

National Cancer Institute. EPEC™ O: Education in Palliative and End-of-Life Care for Oncology. CD-ROM & DVD self study modules at *http://www. cancer. gov/aboutnci/epeco.*

American Cancer Society. When the Focus is on Care: Palliative Care and Cancer. Paperback published by the American Cancer Society.

National Institute of Health, National Institute of Nursing Research. Palliative Care: The Relief You Need When You're Experiencing the Symptoms of Serious Illness. PDF Brochure at: *www. ninr.nih. gov/PalliativeCareBrochure.*

National Comprehensive Cancer Network. Clinical Practice Guidelines for Supportive Care at *www. nccn.org.*

Institute of Medicine National Research Council. Improving Palliative Care for Cancer. Paperback published by the National Academy Press.

References

1. World Health Organization. *Cancer Pain Relief and Palliative Care.* World Health Organization Technical Report Series 804. Geneva, 1990.
2. Van Kleffens T, Van Baarsen B, Hoekman K, et al. Clarifying the term 'palliative' in clinical oncology. *Eur J Cancer Care* 2004;13:263-271.
3. Fadul N, Elsayem A, Palmer JL, et al. Supportive versus palliative care: What's in a name? *Cancer* 2009;115:2013-2021.
4. Ferrell BR. Late Referrals to palliative care. *J Clin Oncol* 2005;23(12):2588-2589.
5. Cheng WW, Willey J, Palmer JL, et al. Interval between palliative care referral and death among patients treated at a comprehensive cancer center. *J Palliat Med* 2005;8: 1025-1032.
6. Task Force on Cancer Care at the End of Life: Cancer care during the last phase of life. *J Clin Oncol* 1998;16(5): 1986-1996.
7. Sepulveda C, Marlin A, Yoshida T, et al. Palliative care: The World Health Organization's global perspective. *J Pain Symptom Manage* 2002;24:91-96.
8. National Cancer Institute Dictionary of Cancer Terms. *http:// www.cancer.gov/dictionary/?CdrID=269448.* Accessed January 16, 2010.

9. Ferris FD, Bruera E, Cherny N, et al. Palliative cancer care a decade later: Accomplishments, the need, next steps–From the American Society of Clinical Oncology. *J Clin Oncol* 2009; 27(18):3052-3058.
10. Portenoy RK, Thaler HT, Kornblith AB, et al. Symptom prevalence, characteristics and distress in a cancer population. *Qual Life Res* 1994;3:183-189.
11. Cassell EJ. The nature of suffering and the goals of medicine. *N Engl J Med* 1982;306:639-645.
12. Hopkins K. Food for life, love and hope: An exemplar of the philosophy of palliative care in action. *Proc Nutr Soc* 2004; 63(3):427-429.
13. Rodriguez KL, Barnato AE, Arnold RM. Perceptions and utilization of palliative care services in acute care hospitals. *J Palliat Med* 2007;10:99-110.
14. Weissman DE. Decision making at a time of crisis near the end of life. *JAMA* 2004;292(14):1738-1743.
15. Byock I. *Dying Well: The Prospect for Growth at the End of Life.* New York: Riverhead Books; 1997.
16. Meyers FJ, Linder J. Simultaneous care: Disease treatment and palliative care throughout illness. *J Clin Oncol* 2003;21(7): 1412-1415.
17. Prince-Paul M. When hospice is the best option: an opportunity to redefine goals. *Oncology* 2009;23(4 suppl nurse ed): 13-17.
18. Williamson DS, Noel ML. Systemic family medicine: An evolving concept. In: Rakel RE, (ed): *Textbook of Family Practice,* 4th ed. Philadelphia, PA: WB Saunders; 1990: 61-79.
19. Andershed B, Ternestedt B. Involvement of relatives in the care of the dying in different care cultures: Involvement in the dark or in the light? *Cancer Nurs* 1998;21:106-116.
20. Kristjanson LJ, Aoun S. Palliative care for families: Remembering the hidden patients. *Can J Psychiatry* 2004; 49:359-365.
21. Von Guten CF. Secondary and tertiary palliative care in US hospitals. *JAMA* 2002;287(7):875-881.
22. Meier DE, Beresford L. Outpatient clinics are a new frontier for palliative care. *J Palliat Med* 2008;11(6): 823-828.
23. Osta BE, Bruera E. Models of palliative care delivery. In: Bruera E, Higginson IJ, Ripamonti C, et al, (eds): *Textbook of Palliative Medicine.* New York: Oxford University Press;2006: 268-269.
24. Follwell M, Burman D, Le LW. Phase II study of an outpatient palliative care intervention in patients with metastatic cancer. *J Clin Oncol* 2009;27(2):206-213.
25. American Society of Clinical Oncology. Cancer care during the last phase of life. *J Clin Oncol* 1998;16(5):1986-1996.
26. Hortobagyi GN. A shortage of oncologists? The American Society of Clinical Oncology Workforce Study. *J Clin Oncol* 2007;25(12):1468-1469.
27. Allegra CJ, Hall R, Yothers G. Prevalence of burnout in the U.S. oncology community: Results of a 2003 survey. *J Oncol Prac* 2005;1:140-147.

PAIN MANAGEMENT AND SYMPTOM CONTROL

Suresh K. Reddy
Gabriel Lopez
Ahmed Elsayem

Patients with cancer develop a number of devastating physical and psychosocial symptoms that may arise during different phases and stages of cancer (1). These patients need optimal control of symptoms in order to continue receiving anticancer treatment as well as to improve their quality of life in advanced stages. They need access to multidisciplinary palliative care services in order to achieve optimal symptom control. Symptoms in patients with advanced incapacitating illness include fatigue, pain, anorexia, nausea, dyspnea, constipation, anxiety, depression, and cachexia (Table 48-1).

■ **PAIN**

Pain is one of the most common symptoms experienced by cancer patients. It was the most common symptom (82%) among patients referred to a palliative care service (2). Pain may be the only symptom before the diagnosis of cancer and may indicate the recurrence and spread of cancer. It can occur both during active treatment as well as in the advanced and terminal stages of cancer. Generally as many as 30 to 50% of patients in active anticancer therapy, and as many as 60 to 90% of those with advanced disease have pain (3-7).

Most pain in cancer is caused by direct involvement of tumor with body structures, most notably neural structures. Pain associated with direct tumor involvement occurs in 65 to 85% of patients with advanced cancer (7). Cancer therapy accounts for pain in approximately 15 to 25% of patients receiving chemotherapy, surgery, or radiation therapy, and 3 to 10% of cancer patients have pain syndromes of the sort commonly observed in the general noncancer population—for example, low back pain secondary to degenerative disk disease.

TABLE 48-1	SYMPTOMS IN ADVANCED CANCER
Pain (80-85%)	
Fatigue (90%)	
Weight loss (80%)	
Lack of appetite (80%)	
Nausea, vomiting (80-90%)	
Anxiety (25%)	
Shortness of breath (50%)	
Confusion/agitation (80%)	

Reproduced, with permission, from Elsayem A, Driver LC, Bruera E. The MD Anderson Palliative Care Handbook. Houston, TX: MD Anderson Cancer Center; 2002.

PATHOPHYSIOLOGY

The pathophysiologic classification of pain forms the basis for therapeutic choices. Pain states may be broadly divided into those associated with ongoing tissue damage (nociceptive) and those resulting from nervous system dysfunction (neuropathic), due either to tissue damage or in the absence of damage in some situations. Nociceptive pain can be of the somatic or visceral type. It results from the activation of nociceptors in cutaneous and deep tissues and is described as well localized aching, throbbing, and gnawing. Visceral pain is caused by activation of nociceptors resulting from distention, stretching, and inflammation of visceral organs. It is described as poorly localized, deep aching, cramping, and as a sensation of pressure. Sometimes it is referred pain, for example, pancreatic cancer pain in the abdomen with referral to back.

Breakthrough pain is a common entity in cancer patients and is defined as "transitory exacerbation of pain that occurs on a background of otherwise stable persistent pain"; it is caused by activity or end-of-dose failure or can occur spontaneously. It tends to be moderate to severe and, according to one study is less than 3 min in duration in 43% of such cases with a frequency of one to four episodes per day (8). Breakthrough pain tends to be an adverse prognosticator for the successful treatment of pain, as per Bruera et al. (9)

ASSESSMENT

It is crucial to assess and monitor the intensity of pain. This can be measured by simply using visual analog scales, verbal scales, numerical scales, or more complex pain questionnaires (10). The most popular tool used generally is a scale of 0 to 10, where 0 is the least pain and 10 is the worst pain. Most instruments and techniques are very reliable for the assessment of the intensity of pain. The assessment can be made more effective by graphic ongoing display of pain and other symptoms in the patient's chart, along with other vital sign monitoring. This forms a basis for outcomes as well as helping to administer appropriate care (Fig. 48-1). Pain assessment should always be done in the context of other symptoms in cancer.

In 1984, the World Health Organization (WHO) proposed a simple analgesic ladder for the pharmacologic management of cancer pain (11). Experience with the adoption of this ladder in several countries worldwide has shown that the simple principle of escalating from nonopioid to strong opioid analgesics is safe and effective (Fig. 48-2). In addition to the WHO guidelines, a number of other guidelines have been published subsequently (12).

PRINCIPLES OF MANAGEMENT

Assess pain syndromes and other symptoms accurately.
Respect and accept the complaint of pain as real.
Treat pain appropriately.
Treat underlying disorder(s).
Address psychosocial issues.
Utilize a multidisciplinary approach.

■ PHARMACOTHERAPY

PRINCIPLES OF PHARMACOTHERAPY

Match drug to pain syndrome.
Have low threshold to prescribe opioids.
Sustained-release formulations for constant pain and short-acting ones for breakthrough pain are commonly used.
Add adjunct medications where appropriate.
The oral route should be the route of choice.
Use the intravenous route for acute titration.
Treat side effects before switching opioids.
Sequential opioid trials should be done, including methadone.
Familiarize yourself with equianalgesic dosing.
Familiarize yourself with the pharmacokinetics of opioids.
Differentiate between tolerance, physical dependence, and addiction.
Be aware of renal failure and analgesic drugs.
Pharmacotherapy is the most simple and very effective way to control cancer pain. The class of medications used includes opioids as well as nonopioids and adjuvant medications.

Referral date:		Referring physician:												
Date:														
Pain	(0-10)*													
Fatigue	(0-10)*													
Nausea	(0-10)*													
Depression	(0-10)*													
Anxiety	(0-10)*													
Drowsiness	(0-10)*													
Shortness of breath	(0-10)*													
Appetite	(0-10)*													
Sleep	(0-10)*													
Feeling of well-being	(0-10)*													
Mini mental state score (0-30)														
Assessment from: Pt/SO/HCP (If SO or HCP – use red ink)														
Total opioid MEDD:_____mg/day														
Staff initials (signature & title below)														

*0 = No symptom/best   10 = Worst imaginable

FIGURE 48-1. Edmonton symptom assessment scale (ESAS). *(Reproduced, with permission, from Elsayem A, Driver LC, Bruera E. The MD Anderson Palliative Care Handbook. Houston, TX: MD Anderson Cancer Center; 2002.)*

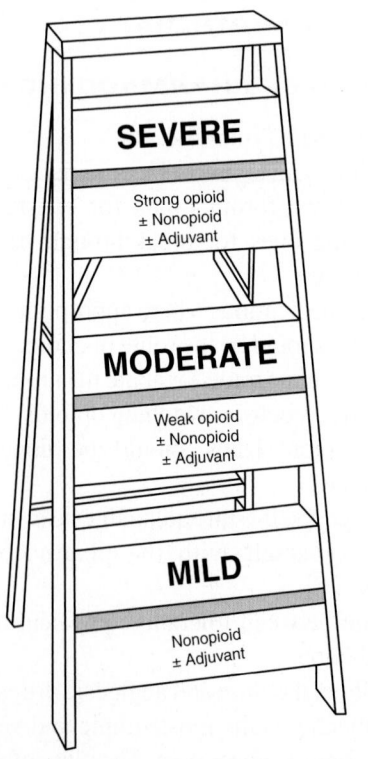

FIGURE 48-2. World Health Organization (WHO) three-step ladder oral analgesic program for managing cancer pain.

OPIOIDS

Opioid medications form the basis for the management of cancer pain regardless of its pathophysiology. Opioids are the drugs of choice for somatic pain, but there is good evidence that they are effective in neuropathic pain also, contrary to earlier belief (13,14).

Opioids are pharmacodynamically classified into pure agonists, mixed agonist–antagonists, and antagonists. As a rule in our practice, only pure agonists are used. Partial agonists and agonist–antagonists are not used because they exhibit a "ceiling effect" and have an unfavorable side-effect profile. Table 48-2 lists the most commonly used opioids in cancer pain with their equianalgesic dose ratios.

LOW-POTENCY OPIOID AGONISTS

This list includes codeine, hydrocodone, and dihydrocodeine, with potency about one-quarter to one-tenth that of morphine sulfate. Indications for drugs from this group include mild to moderate pain not responsive to nonopioids. A good example is mild bone pain and an early visceral pain. They are also occasionally

TABLE 48-2 | **OPIOID ANALGESICS**

Drug	Usual Starting Dosages
Full opioid agonists	
Morphine*	15-30 mg PO q 3-4 h
	30-60 mg PO q 8-12 h
Hydromorphone (Dilaudid)	2-4 mg PO q 4-6 h
Levorphanol (Levo-Dromoran)	2-4 mg PO q 4-6 h
Fentanyl (Duragesic)	25-50 mcg/h TD every 3 days
Codeine	15-30 mg PO q 3-4 h
Oxycodone (Percodan and others)	5-10 mg PO q 3-4 h
Meperedine (Demerol hydrochloride)	75-100 mg IM q 3-4 h
Methadone Hydrochloride (Dolophine)[†]	5-10 mg PO q 3-4 h
Partial agonists and mixed agonists/antagonists[‡]	
Nalbuphine (Nubain)	10 mg IV q 3-4 h
Butorphanol (Stadol)	0.5-2 mg IV q 3-4 h
	1-2 mg SL three times a day
Dezoncine (Dalgan)	10 mg IV q 3-4 h
Pentazocine (Talwin)	50 mg PO q 4-6 h

Equianalgesic Dosing[#]	From Parenteral Opioid to Parental Opioid	From Same Parenteral Opioid to Oral Opioid	From Oral Opioid to Oral Morphine	From Oral Morphine to Oral Opioid
Opioid				
Morphine	1	2.5	1	1
Hydromorphone	5	2	5	0.2
Meperidine	0.13	4	0.1	10
Levorphanol	5	2	5	0.2
Codeine	NA	NA	0.15	7
Oxycodone	NA	NA	1.5	0.7
Hydrocodone	NA	NA	0.15	7

*Morphine can be given as an immediate-release or sustained-release preparation. It is recommended that a relatively rapid onset, short-acting opioid preparation (such as immediate-release morphine) be given to patients who take sustained-release morphine to provide rescue medication for breakthrough pain.

[†]Methadone is 10-15 times more potent than morphine. Expertise is needed to use it.

[‡]This class of drugs is *not* recommended for the management of chronic cancer pain because they will reverse analgesia when coadministered with full opioid agonists and precipitate withdrawal in physically dependent individuals.

[#](1) Take the total amount of opioid that effectively controls pain in 24 h. (2) Multiply by conversion factor in table; give 30% less of the new opioid to avoid partial cross tolerance. (3) Divide by the number of doses per day.

NA, not applicable.

Reproduced, with permission, from Elsayem A, Driver LC, Bruera E. The MD Anderson Palliative Care Handbook. Houston, TX: MD Anderson Cancer Center; 2002.

used for in-between breakthrough pain for patients with constant pain on sustained-release opioids. Drugs in this group are formulated with acetaminophen; hence the dose escalation of these drugs is limited by the maximum allowable dose of acetaminophen. However, formulations without acetaminophen can be prepared by some pharmacies.

HIGH-POTENCY OPIOID AGONISTS

These classes of drugs are used for all pain types.

MORPHINE

Available in short- and long-acting formulations, *morphine* is the standard drug most widely used and is the prototype drug of its class. It is a micro agonist, working in the spinal cord and brain receptors. It is converted to morphine-3-glucoronide and morphine-6-glucoronide (M3G and M6G, respectively) by glucuronyl transferase in the liver. These compounds may contribute to the opioid side effects, mostly excitatory side effects by M3G (15). Caution should be exercised in patients with renal impairment, as these compounds are excreted by the kidney. They are available for oral, rectal, intramuscular, intravenous, and sublingual use as well as in intrathecal preparations. Other strong opioid-class drugs which will be reviewed include oxycodone, hydromorphone, meperidine, fentanyl, and methadone.

OXYCODONE

Once classified as a low-potency opioid when its dosage was limited by its combination with acetaminophen or aspirin, oxycodone is now gaining widespread popularity as an alternative to morphine in the treatment of cancer pain. According to recent studies, oxycodone is $1^1/_2$ times more potent than morphine. It is available only in the oral form in the United States and has a higher bioavailability than morphine. It is available in the sustained-release as well as the short-acting form.

HYDROMORPHONE

Commercially known as Dilaudid (Knoll AG, Listeral, Switzerland), hydromorphone is a useful short-acting opioid that is six to seven times more potent than morphine. It is available for administration via all routes including the neuroaxial route. Hydromorphone is commonly used as a "rescue" agent in patients on longer-acting opioid preparations; a new long acting preparation has recently become available in the United States. Hydromorphone is used as an alternative to morphine when dose-limiting side effects necessitate opioid rotation to a more potent opioid.

MEPERIDINE

Meperidine (Demerol) is a commonly used opioid analgesic throughout the world, but it is not used as often as morphine. In the oral form, its potency is one-tenth that of morphine, which makes it less efficacious in most patients. The increase in dosing to get to morphine's equianalgesic level on a chronic basis is associated with the risk of accumulation of the metabolite normeperidine, produced by the liver. Both compounds cause central nervous system (CNS) excitability and may result in frank convulsions, especially in renally impaired and elderly patients (16). Hence the use of meperidine has been rapidly declining in the cancer patient population.

FENTANYL

Fentanyl is a semisynthetic opioid available in parenteral as well as transdermal form. Its rapid onset and relatively short duration of action make it a good choice for control of acute pain. A sustained-release, transdermal form has been developed and used successfully for stable pain. Each patch is changed every 72 h and hence was found to be convenient in patients whose pain is stable. Oral transmucosal fentanyl has been approved for use in breakthrough pain (17-19).

METHADONE

Methadone is a synthetic opioid that has recently reemerged and is being used beneficially to treat cancer pain. Recent updates (20) and research on the equianalgesic dosing (21,22), lower cost, absence of active opioid metabolites, excellent bioavailability, and possible N-methyl-D-aspartate antagonist action (23) have enabled many to use methadone safely and effectively to treat cancer pain. The potency of methadone seems to be 10 to 15 times that of morphine. Hence caution should be exercised when switching from an opioid to methadone. Methadone is characterized by a long plasma half-life and low cost, making it suitable for most pain syndromes. Close monitoring at the time of commencement is warranted secondary to the cumulative side effects of methadone. The half-life seems to be 15 to 190 h. Drug interactions with methadone involve the same pathway of the cytochrome P-450 system common to antifungals, antiretroviral agents, and selective serotonin reuptake inhibitors (SSRIs) (24). Recent evidence pointed toward methadone causing QTc interval prolongation (25,26). However our prospective study found it to be safe in advanced cancer patients (27).

Opioid medications exhibit a wide interindividual variation, possibly because of differences in intrinsic activity and action at different receptors of different subtypes (28,29). Hence opioid rotation is a worthwhile exercise when dose-limiting side effects are encountered. Some groups treat side effects of opioids before embarking on opioid rotation. But the generally accepted method is to treat side effects before opioid switching. There is no general consensus as to the number of opioid rotations, but in the authors' experience at least two to three opioid rotations, which should include methadone at some stage, need to be attempted.

ADJUVANT MEDICATIONS

These groups of drugs are used mostly in conjunction with opioid medications in cancer pain. The categories include nonsteroidal anti-inflamatory drugs (NSAIDs), tricyclic antidepressants (TCAs), antiepileptic drugs (AEDs), and a miscellaneous group (Table 48-3).

TABLE
48-3

ADJUVANT ANALGESICS
Tricyclic antidepressants
Amitriptyline
Nortriptyline
Doxepin
Doxepram
Antiepileptic drugs
Gabapentin
Topiramate
Levetiracetam
Tiagabine
Oxcarbazepine
Lamotrigine
Felbamate
Local anesthetics
Lidocaine
N-methyl-D-aspartate (NMDA) receptor antagonists
Ketamine
Methadone
Dextromethorphan
Topical analgesics
Capsaicin
Lidocaine patches

Miscellaneous drugs (psychotropic drugs, benzodiazepines, bisphosphonates, steroids, radiopharmaceuticals).

NONSTEROIDAL ANTI-INFLAMMATORY DRUGS

NSAIDs are essentially limited to the inhibitors of the enzyme cyclooxygenase (COX), thus inhibiting the synthesis of prostaglandin, the pain and inflammation mediator. This group is now subdivided into nonspecific COX inhibitors and selective COX-2 inhibitors. The nonselective inhibitors, which are also referred to as NSAIDs, are medications such as ibuprofen and naproxen. However, these drugs continue to cause concern with regard to the integrity of gastric mucosa and alteration in renal function. COX-2 inhibitors block COX-2 enzyme with little effect on COX-1, thereby offering an advantageous effect on the integrity of gastric mucosa and platelet aggregation (30). After initial approval by the US Food and Drug Administration (FDA), rofecoxib (Vioxx), a leading COX-2 inhibitor, has been withdrawn from the market secondary to increasing incidents of heart attacks and strokes (31).

TRICYCLIC ANTIDEPRESSANTS

TCAs are the main group of antidepressants currently being used to treat neuropathic pain syndromes. They probably act by inhibiting reuptake of serotonin and norepinephrine at the nerve endings in the spinal cord as well as in the brain. Recently it has been widely accepted that their action is independent of their mood-altering effects and that they exert either an inherent influence over the nervous system or modulate the opioid pathways (32,33).

TCAs are not universally tolerated, especially at the initiation of therapy, and they often have to be discontinued or decreased due to dose-limiting side effects, most commonly the anticholinergic and sedative effects. Amitriptyline and nortriptyline (which have lower cardiovascular side-effect profiles) are felt to be the most efficacious agents and thus are more often used.

ANTICONVULSANTS

Anticonvulsants (AEDs) are traditionally used in the treatment of diabetic neuropathy, postherpetic neuralgia, trigeminal neuralgia, and similar syndromes with good results (33). These conditions can definitely coexist in cancer patients; however, AEDs are useful in treating brachial and lumbosacral plexopathies (Table 48-4).

Medications such as phenytoin, valproate, carbamazepine, and clonazepam have been used. Owing to concerns over safety and side effects, their use has been strictly limited. Gabapentin has become the "gold standard" and prototypical drug in this category to treat neuropathic pain (34,35). With its wide therapeutic window and a level of efficacy comparable to that of other anticonvulsants, gabapentin is preferred by many clinicians, especially as it does not require the monitoring of blood levels or other clinical tests. Sedation is a noted side effect, which can be reduced by starting therapy at 100 mg tid and adding 100 mg to each dose every second or third day until the desired effect is achieved. If necessary, dose escalation up to 3600 mg/day is recommended. More recently, pregablin has become available as an alternative to gabapentin with similar therapeutic efficacy (36).

Recently newer AEDs are gaining in popularity (see Table 48-4).

MISCELLANEOUS

In refractory pain situations, drugs from other classes have been tried; some have been tried with a good response and others with only a minimal response. They include: psychotropic drugs (37,38), benzodiazepines (39), bisphosphonates (40-42), steroids (in spinal cord compression) (43), lidocaine, intravenous and patch (44-46), ketamine (47,48), capsaicin (49), and radiopharmaceuticals (strontium 89, samarium) (50,51).

TABLE 48-4 | **ANTIEPILEPTIC DRUGS**

Drug	Action	Uses	Dose
Carbamazepine	Anticonvulsant decreases abnormal CNS neuronal activity	Useful for neuropathic pain; hematologic monitoring suggested	Start with 100 mg daily, increase by 100 mg q4day to 500-800 mg/day
Phenytoin	Anticonvulsant decreases abnormal CNS activity	Useful for neuropathic pain; hematologic monitoring suggested	Start with 100 mg/day, increase by 25-50 mg q4day to 250-300 mg/day
Gabapentin	Anticonvulsant decreases abnormal CNS neuronal activity	Useful for neuropathic pain; better toxicity profile	300-3200 mg
Lamotrigine	Treatment of trigeminal analgesia, migraine headaches, diabetic neuropathy	Inhibitor of voltage-gated Na^+ channels, suppresses glutamate release and inhibits serotonin reuptake	25-50 mg/day, increased by 50 mg/week until max 900 mg bid or tid
Topiramate	Treatment of cluster headaches, diabetic neuropathy	Increases CNS GABA levels, blocks AMPA kainite excitatory receptors	200-400 mg/day with bid dosing Start at 25 mg bid increasing 50 mg every week
Oxcarbezapine	Treatment of trigeminal neuralgia, neuropathic pain states	Blockade of voltage-gated Na^+ channels	300-600 mg/day, up to a max 1200-2400 mg/day
Zonisamide	Trials ongoing	Na^+ channel blockade T-type Ca^{2+} channel blockade	
Tiagabine	Neuropathic pain therapeutic effects	GABA reuptake inhibitor	Dosage

Reproduced, with permission, from Elsayem A, Driver LC, Bruera E. The MD Anderson Palliative Care Handbook. Houston, TX: MD Anderson Cancer Center; 2002.

■ STEPS TO TREAT CANCER PAIN

The successful formula to treat cancer pain involves some simple rules. Pain management is governed by factors such as pain syndrome (somatic versus neuropathic), pain severity, previous opioid use, dosing and side effects, the presence of other symptoms such as delirium, anxiety, depression, and preexisting conditions.

PAIN SYNDROME

Pain syndromes in cancer can be somatic, neuropathic, or mixed. Based on the predominance of one versus the other, medications are chosen accordingly. If the pain is predominantly somatic but mild, an NSAID with a mild opioid is initiated. The medication can be advanced to a strong opioid based on the pain's severity. A short-acting opioid may be tried first to test its tolerability; the medication may then be advanced to a sustained-release form once the pain stabilizes. If the pain is predominantly neuropathic, either a TCA or an AED is started, possibly with a mild opioid. Again, titration to a strong opioid is undertaken based on the severity of the pain. Most often cancer pain is of a mixed type, in which case

a balanced analgesic approach involving drugs with different mechanisms of action are chosen.

PAIN SEVERITY

Pain severity will serve as a guide in the decision-making process with regard to choosing a low-potency opioid versus a high-potency drug such as morphine. Most low-potency opioids are less suitable for high-grade pain due to dose limitations and the presence of the ceiling effect or a plateau effect seen with increasing doses. Most cancer pain situations need high-potency opioids. If the patient had an optimal trial with oral opioids, including rotation to a different opioid, or has experienced dose-limiting side effects, an alternative route (eg, intravenous or neuroaxial) may be tried. Pain severity reported on a verbal numerical scale should be interpreted in the context of associated psychosocial symptoms.

IV administration of opioids may be given via patient controlled analgesia (PCA) or as a supplemental intravenous bolus. The PCA dose interval should be not more often than every 30 to 60 minutes. More frequent dosing intervals are appropriate in postoperative settings. PCA dosing should be avoided if delirium is suspected.

OPIOID HISTORY AND SIDE EFFECTS

Patient-to-patient variability in the response to a specific opioid has been widely appreciated and documented (28). Some patients may respond surprisingly well to one opioid after failing or not tolerating others, possibly due to how a given drug acts on different opioid receptors and also owing to genetic factors. This phenomenon will obviously influence drug selection within the same class (28,29).

PREVIOUS OPIOID DOSING AND PHARMACOKINETICS

This reflects the degree of tolerance to opioids, as "opioid naive" patients will obviously require lower doses, at least initially. The "opioid naïve" patient is more likely to experience sedation during the first 3 to 4 days of consistent opioid use after which sedation is reduced and analgesia is maintained. Alternative central stimulatory pathways are recruited to maintain alertness. Opioid-tolerant patients may require stronger opioids from the beginning and also higher than conventional doses.

PRESENCE OF OTHER SYMPTOMS

Sometimes symptoms of delirium, anxiety, and depression may be interpreted as physical pain, and opioid dosages are escalated with worsening of delirium. Hence assessment of these symptoms is mandatory to avoid overdosing of opioids.

■ SIDE EFFECTS OF OPIOIDS

Diminution or elimination of side effects is an important part of effective opioid therapy. With few exceptions, dose readjustment whenever possible should be the first measure in managing adverse reactions. Some of the common opioid side effects are as follows:

Sedation
Nausea and vomiting
Constipation
Cognitive impairment
Urinary retention
Myoclonus
Respiratory depression
Pruritus
Loss of libido

■ NONPHARMACOLOGIC TREATMENT

Many nonpharmacologic approaches are available for the treatment of cancer pain and are widely employed. Adjuvant therapies include such interventions as nerve blocks, neurosurgical procedures, and radiation.

Physical and psychologic modalities for pain control include counseling, psychotherapy, relaxation techniques, massage therapy, music therapy, addressing psychosocial and spiritual needs, and bereavement counseling for family members.

NERVE BLOCKS

A small percentage of patients who fail to respond to oral therapy may be helped with appropriate nerve blocks (Table 48-5).

It is not known which patients might benefit from interventions done earlier in the course of the disease (52,53). Somatic nerve blocks are effective for nociceptive somatic pain in the territory of a root, plexus, or peripheral nerve. Blocks can be short-lasting when a local anesthetic is employed. These temporary blocks have a limited role in cancer pain management but may act as precursors to permanent neurolysis. Examples include root block, brachial plexus block, and psoas compartment block.

Neurolytic blocks generally have a favorable risk-benefit ratio in patients with advanced cancer whose life expectancy is limited. Sympathetic blocks such as celiac plexus block have been demonstrated to be effective for pancreatic cancer pain and other abdominal visceral pain syndromes (54). Contrary to a previous study demonstrating improved survival (55), Wong et al. showed that although pain is better relieved with a celiac plexus block, there was no significant difference in survival or quality of life (56). Occasionally a subarachnoid

TABLE 48-5	USEFUL ANESTHETIC PROCEDURES
Celiac plexus/splanchnic block for abdominal visceral pain, eg, pancreatic cancer pain	
Subarachnoid neurolytic block for extremity and thoracic wall pain in terminally ill patients	
Epidural/intrathecal opioids ± local anesthetic, eg, for neuropathic or plexopathy pain	
Cordotomy for intractable lower extremity pain	
Vertebroplasty (injection of cement into a vertebral body) for metastatic spinal pain involving one or two vertebrae	

Reproduced, with permission, from Elsayem A, Driver LC, Bruera E. The MD Anderson Palliative Care Handbook. Houston, TX: MD Anderson Cancer Center; 2002.

neurolytic block (57) and a neurolytic intercostal block may be employed. The risks of neurologic deficits that may result from these blocks must be weighed against the possible benefits. A recent study by Smith et al. (58), randomizing intrathecal and comprehensive medical management, favored intrathecal opioid therapy and found improved survival in the intrathecal group; however, a number of concerns, particularly about the comprehensive medical management group, were raised (59,60). Perhaps more studies with more carefully selected cohorts are needed to confirm the findings.

Surgical ablation (61) may be accomplished by rhizotomy (section of a nerve root) or dorsal root entry zone lesions. Spinal anterolateral tractotomy or cordotomy, midline myelotomy, and cingulotomy should be reserved for carefully selected cases. Percutaneous cordotomy employed for intractable pain of the lower extremity has been shown to be useful in selected patients (62). Vertebroplasty, which involves injecting cement into metastatic compression fractures, has been employed successfully and is gaining wide popularity (63,64). Radiofrequency lesioning of bone metastasis has recently been shown to be another way of treating bone pain (65).

■ FATIGUE

Fatigue is one of the most common symptoms in cancer patients (66), experienced by 70 to 100% of those receiving cancer treatment (67). The term *fatigue* refers to a subjective sense of decreased vitality in physical and/or mental functioning; it usually occurs in the setting of medical disease. The physical dimension is usually described as a perception of muscle weakness or a tendency to tire rapidly. Physical activity is difficult to sustain and in some cases dyspnea accompanies minimal exertion. Rest or sleep does not return perceived strength or stamina to normal. The mental component is described as lack of interest or motivation in objects or activities. Other symptoms include difficulty in concentrating or maintaining attention. Mood may be flat or depressed. Lethargy or tendency to somnolence may be noted, but there is no need for excessive sleep. Rest or sleep may improve symptoms but does not eliminate them. Fatigue is experienced both during treatment as well as during terminal stages. For patients with advanced cancer, however, fatigue may be a severe symptom that either decreases their capacity for physical and mental work or renders them completely unable to function normally. Fatigue gets worse as the disease progresses toward the end stage. The presence of fatigue may also magnify other symptoms affecting the patient. The causes of fatigue are multifactorial and interrelated. These include problems related to the cancer itself, side effects or toxicities of treatment, underlying systemic pathophysiologic disorders, and other causes (Fig. 48-3).

ASSESSMENT

The severity of fatigue can be measured on a scale of 0 to 10 (where 0 equals no fatigue and 10 equals the worst fatigue imaginable), as in the Edmonton Symptom Assessment System (ESAS) or by other numerical or verbal rating scales (see Fig. 48-1). Like other symptoms in cancer, the assessment of fatigue should focus on the multidimensional aspect. The impact of fatigue on activities, function, and quality of life should be assessed. Laboratory investigations and imaging studies

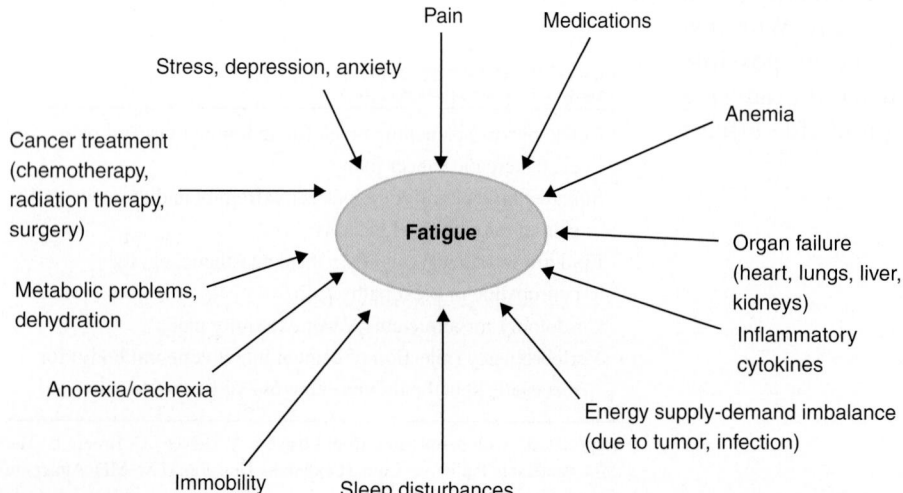

FIGURE 48-3. Multifactorial etiologies of fatigue. *(Reproduced, with permission, from Elsayem A, Driver LC, Bruera E. The MD Anderson Palliative Care Handbook. Houston, TX: MD Anderson Cancer Center; 2002.)*

should be based on indications derived from the patient's history and physical examination.

MANAGEMENT

As with other problematic symptoms in advanced cancer patients, management of fatigue should address possible underlying etiologies as well as the patient's expression of symptoms (68,69).

Underlying problems such as pain, depression, anxiety, stress, and sleep disturbances must be treated. Dehydration should be corrected and an attempt made to treat cachexia in appropriate cases. Medication regimes can be simplified; infections treated; as well as anemia relieved by transfusions or erythropoietin where appropriate (70). Low-dose steroids may alleviate some of the symptoms of fatigue in patients with advanced cancer (71,72). Psychostimulants, such as methylphenidate 5 to 10 mg in the morning and at noon, may be useful if the patient is experiencing concomitant problems such as depression, hypoactive delirium, or drowsiness due to opioids (73-75). Some antidepressants, such as the SSRIs, may improve energy levels in fatigued patients, though their benefit is unproven. Recently there is increasing evidence that cancer patients with hypogonadism who are on chronic opioid therapy may suffer from fatigue (76). Replacement therapy with testosterone may improve fatigue in these patients but needs further study. Bruera et al. showed that patient-controlled methylphenidate administration rapidly improved fatigue and other symptoms (77).

■ DYSPNEA

Dyspnea is defined as the "uncomfortable awareness of breathing" (78). It is described in terms of air hunger, suffocation, choking, or heavy breathing. It is a subjective sensation, associated with and affected by factors such as the location and progression of the tumor, psychosocial phenomena (79), and preexisting chronic lung pathology such as chronic obstructive pulmonary disease (COPD), asthma, and congestive heart failure. The frequency and severity of dyspnea depends on the stage of the disease; it increases in frequency when death is imminent.

Dyspnea as an isolated symptom or in association with other parameters is an adverse prognostic indicator of survival (80,81). Dyspnea is a multidimensional symptom influenced by factors such as anxiety, tumor location, fatigue, and others. It can be caused by a number of clinical conditions, but the causes fall into two main categories: (1) dyspnea with abnormal mechanics of ventilation, for example, cachexia, asthenia, myasthenic syndrome, Eaton-Lambert syndrome, and so on, and (2) dyspnea with normal mechanics of ventilation. This category may be subdivided into respiratory and nonrespiratory causes of dyspnea (Table 48-6).

ASSESSMENT

Dyspnea is a complex symptom caused by various factors, some not well understood. But a thorough history with physical examination and appropriate laboratory and imaging studies should be undertaken to assess it. Some of the factors that contribute to dyspnea include anxiety, phobia, pain, and fatigue.

TREATMENT

The aim of the dyspnea treatment is a subjective improvement in the patient's perception. Treatment involves treating the cause and the symptoms as well as managing psychosocial issues contributing to dyspnea.

Treatment of the Cause

Treatment of the underlying cause is attempted as an initial step: thoracentesis for pleural effusion, blood transfusion for anemia, corticosteroids for lymphangitic carcinomatosis, anticoagulants for pulmonary embolism, and antibiotics for pneumonia where appropriate.

Symptomatic Treatment

Oxygen Therapy

Long-term oxygen therapy has been shown to have beneficial effects on the outcome of patients with COPD (82,83). Crossover trials with cancer patients suffering from dyspnea suggest beneficial effects of oxygen (84,85). Oxygen may be given by nasal cannula and should be humidified whenever feasible. Oxygen treatment toward the end of life may lead to anxiety among family members, who sometimes interpret this as a way of prolonging life and suffering. Counseling of family members with regard to this issue is of paramount importance.

Drug Therapy

A number of pharmacologic agents have been used effectively to relieve dyspnea in terminally ill cancer patients. The major drugs are opioids, corticosteroids, and benzodiazepines. Many studies have found that opioids of different types, doses, and routes of administration are capable of relieving dyspnea (86,87). Nebulized

TABLE 48-6	CAUSES OF DYSPNEA IN CANCER PATIENTS*

Dyspnea with Abnormal Mechanisms of Ventilation	Dyspnea with Normal Mechanisms of Ventilation
☐ Asthenia ☐ Cachexia ☐ Myasthenia gravis ☐ Eaton-Lambert syndrome ☐ Rib fracture ☐ Chest wall deformity ☐ Neuromuscular disease (motor neuron disease)	**Direct effect of the tumor** ☐ Primary or metastatic tumor ☐ Pleural effusion/pericardial infusion ☐ Superior vena cava syndrome ☐ Carcinomatous lymphangitis ☐ Atelectasis ☐ Phrenic nerve palsy ☐ Tracheal obstruction ☐ Tracheal-esophageal fistula ☐ Carcinomatous infiltration of the chest wall (carcinoma en cuirasse) **Effect of therapy** ☐ Postactinic fibrosis ☐ Postpneumectomy ☐ Mitomycin-vinca alkaloid (acute dyspnea syndrome) ☐ Bleomycin-induced fibrosis ☐ Doxorubicin- and cyclophosphamide-induced cardiomyopathy **Not directly related to the tumor or therapy** ☐ Anemia ☐ Ascites ☐ Metabolic acidosis ☐ Fever ☐ Chronic obstructive pulmonary disease ☐ Asthma ☐ Pulmonary embolism ☐ Pneumonia ☐ Pneumothorax ☐ Heart failure ☐ Obesity ☐ Thyrotoxicosis ☐ Psychosocial distress (ie, anxiety, somatization) ☐ Unknown

*The physician is to check off all the causes of dyspnea in a given patient.
Reproduced, with permission, from Elsayem A, Driver LC, Bruera E. The MD Anderson Palliative Care Handbook. Houston, TX: MD Anderson Cancer Center; 2002.

morphine, among other opioids, has shown efficacy in some studies (88-92). Opioids may act by reducing the subjective sensation of dyspnea without reducing respiratory rate or oxygen saturation. They may also cause venodilation of pulmonary vessels, thereby reducing preload to the heart and improving breathing. Corticosteroids are most effective when dyspnea is caused by lymphangitic carcinomatosis or superior vena cava syndrome. They may also play a role if associated COPD or

asthma coexists (93). Benzodiazepines have a limited role in dyspnea except when anxiety and apprehension are underlying causes. Consequently benzodiazepines are commonly used medications for terminal dyspnea in hospice settings. Bronchodilators play a role if dyspnea is caused by bronchospasm. Both nebulized and oral agents are used. In a study by Congleton and Muers, bronchodilators provided significant relief of dyspnea in patients with lung carcinoma and airflow obstruction (94).

Phenothiazines such as chlorpromazine may help in drying secretions and reducing anxiety (95).

General Supportive Measures

A number of measures can be implemented for the support of both the patient and the family. Relaxation techniques or guided imagery provide relief in patients with anticipatory or anxiety-driven dyspnea. Assist devices can be used to minimize muscle effort. Maneuvers such as postural drainage and incentive spirometry can help in special situations.

■ DELIRIUM

Delirium is defined as a transient organic brain syndrome characterized by the acute onset of disordered attention (arousal) and cognition, accompanied by disturbances of psychomotor behavior and perception (96). Delirium is common with progressive disease. It may signal a new and serious medical complication, markedly impair the function and comfort of the patient, and increase the family's distress (97). The prevalence of delirium in hospitalized medical and surgical patients is approximately 10%, and the prevalence in hospitalized cancer patients ranges from 8 to 40% (98-100). Causes of delirium are listed in Fig. 48-4.

CLINICAL FEATURES

The symptoms and signs of delirium fluctuate; therefore, careful attention should be paid to the mental status examination. The diagnosis is established by a new onset of cognitive dysfunction accompanied by a disturbance of arousal or clouding of consciousness. Three clinical variants have been described based on the type of arousal disturbance: hypoalert-hypoactive, hyper-alert-hyperactive, and mixed type (101,102). The presenting features include memory impairment or confusion, dysphoria, hypomania, illusions, hallucinations, and altered arousal state. The criteria for delirium presented in the fourth edition of the *Diagnostic and Statistical Manual of Mental Disorders* (DSM-IV) (103) have been considered the gold standard for its diagnosis. These include impairment in responsiveness and alertness as manifest by fluctuating inability to maintain or shift attention to external stimuli; cognitive dysfunction of recent onset; development of the disturbance over a short period of

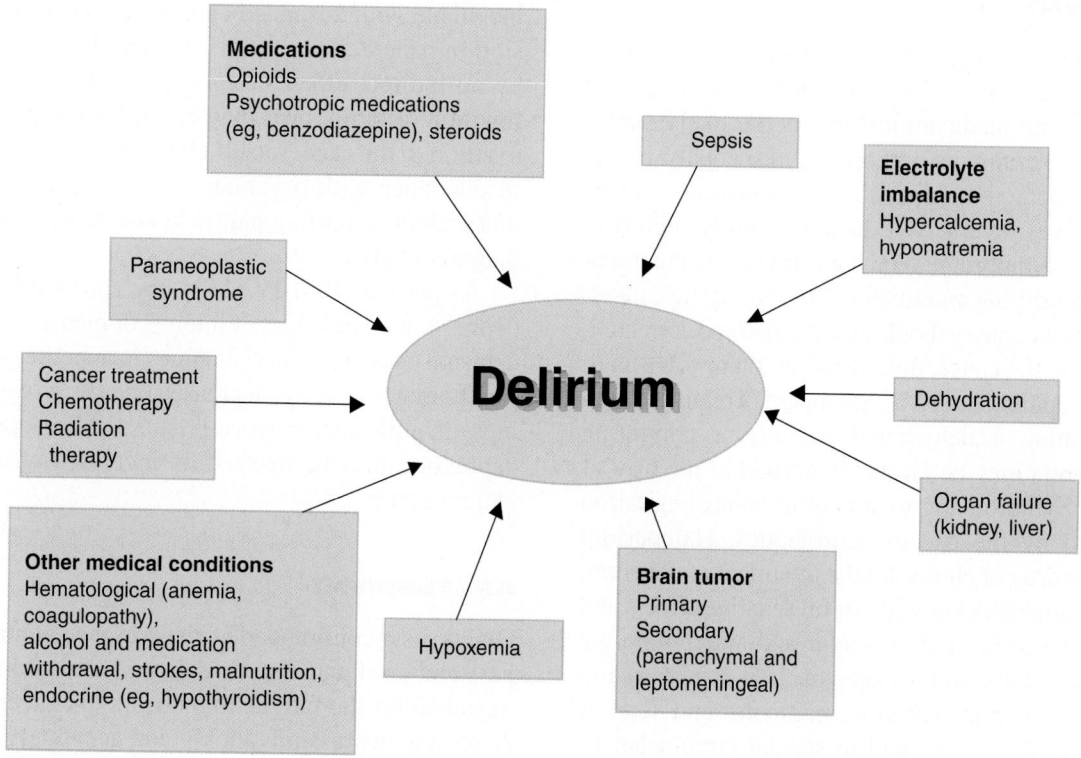

FIGURE 48-4. Causes of delirium in cancer patients.

time; and evidence from history, physical examination, or laboratory findings that are etiologically related to the disturbance.

ASSESSMENT

Delirium is a frequently missed diagnosis and is more often misdiagnosed as insomnia, anxiety, or depression because the presenting symptoms may mimic any of these conditions. Understanding the patient's baseline and listening to the observations of family members and nurses will help pick up the diagnosis of delirium before the condition is florid and out of control. The regular use of a brief and reliable clinical assessment tool such as the Memorial Delirium Assessment Scale (MDAS) may help diagnose more subtle cases of delirium and result in earlier interventions. The cause of the delirium should be investigated, if possible, since the treatment will depend on correction of the cause. The history is of utmost importance, especially when this condition has an acute onset. Medications—particularly opioids, benzodiazepines, some antiemetics and corticosteroids—are frequent causes of delirium. Physical examination may reveal signs of dehydration or increased intracranial pressure. Laboratory examinations may show hypercalcemia, hyponatremia, and renal or hepatic failure.

TREATMENT

If the diagnosis of delirium is suspected, the clinician should act immediately to establish the diagnosis and remove inciting medication if this is the likely cause. Safety is of paramount importance, especially in the agitated (hyperactive) type, since patients may endanger themselves or others. Educating family members and nurses is important. The appropriate management includes identifying and treating the underlying causes. Other reversible causes should be identified and corrected. If opioids are the cause, dosage reduction or rotation to a different opioid should be attempted. Treating infection, hydrating a dehydrated patient, or correcting hypercalcemia may be all that is needed in the way of treatment. Symptomatic treatment to control agitation is achieved by the use of neuroleptics. Haloperidol remains the drug of choice for the treatment of delirium. It is a dopamine blocker with useful sedative effects and a low incidence of cardiovascular and anticholinergic side effects. Haloperidol doses of 1 to 3 mg/day are effective in treating agitation, paranoia, and fear. A higher dose may be needed in special circumstances (104). Sometimes acute dystonias and extrapyramidal side effects are seen with haloperidol, in which case

benztropine can be administered. Newer antipsychotics such as olanzapine (105) are as effective and may be more sedating in the control of agitated patients, but unfortunately they are more expensive. Sometimes a combination of haloperidol and a benzodiazepine is useful. In a study by Brietbart (106), lorazepam alone was ineffective in the treatment of delirium and, in fact, contributed to the worsening of delirium and increased cognitive impairment. In severe cases, consultation with a palliative care physician is important; if, in terminal cases, the condition proves to be refractory to antipsychotic medication, sedation should be considered. Figure 48-5 indicates treatment algorithm for delirium.

■ DEPRESSION

Depression is a common and devastating problem for patients with cancer and other terminal diseases. Major depression can affect from 25 to 35% of cancer patients (107). This prevalence touches 77% in those with advanced disease (108). Pancreatic cancer is more likely to be associated with depression, in which case it will be associated with an even greater loss of appetite, weight loss, and low energy. Thus it can be critically important to diagnose and treat depression early, thereby ameliorating some of the physiologic changes that are inevitable with advanced cancer. The cause of depression in pancreatic cancer is unclear. It may be caused by an indirect effect of cancer on the serotoninergic function of brain, or it may result from a psychologic reaction to the cancer itself (109). Pain has a close correspondence with psychiatric illness. It is very likely that patients reporting pain will also have a psychiatric diagnosis (110).

As per the DSM-IV (111), the cardinal features of depression include loss of interest or pleasure; impaired decision-making ability; changes in appetite, sleep, and psychomotor activity; decreased energy; as well as feelings of guilt and/or worthlessness. Mild episodes of depression may be masked by increased effort on the patient's part.

ASSESSMENT

Diagnosis is confounded by the presence of normal sadness and grief and also by delirium. Anhedonia can be mistaken for the fatigue that occurs in cancer patients. Assessing depression quickly and accurately is important. There are no clear-cut guidelines on assessing depression in terminal cancer patients. A report by

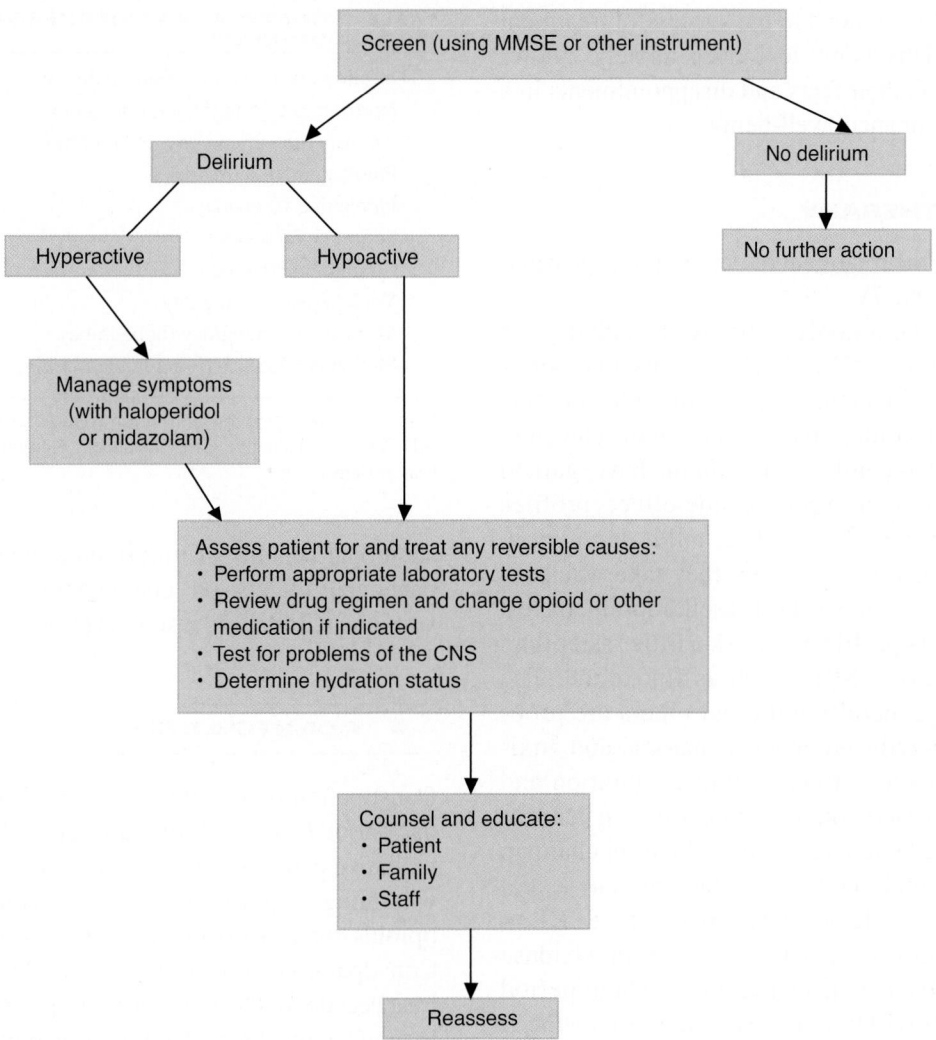

FIGURE 48-5. Algorithm for the assessment and treatment of delirium. *(Reproduced, with permission, from Elsayem A, Driver LC, Bruera E. The MD Anderson Palliative Care Handbook. Houston, TX: MD Anderson Cancer Center; 2002.)*

Fisch et al. (112) suggested the usefulness of a brief two-question assessment of depression in advanced cancer patients, with the primary objective being to measure the quality of life after intervention with fluoxetine and the secondary objective being to assess the reduction in depression. Other validated measures of assessing depression in the primary care setting include the WHO-5 well-being index (113), the PHQ-9 screening test (114), Hamilton Rating Scale for Depression (HAM-D) (115), and the Montgomery Asberg Depression Rating Scale (116) (MADRS). The patient should be evaluated for depressive episodes and substance abuse, family history of depression and suicide, concurrent life stressors, losses secondary to cancer, and availability of social support.

Delirium, particularly in the early stages, is often misidentified as depression and treated as such, with poor effects (117). The key is to diagnose the clinical problem accurately. In doubtful situations, a consultation with a palliative care physician or psychiatrist should be obtained.

TREATMENT

A combination or a balanced approach of supportive psychotherapy and pharmacotherapy is key to the optimal treatment of depression. Individual or group counseling has been shown to be useful. Other methods include relaxation techniques, guided imagery (118), and music therapy (119). Counseling of both patients and their families is crucial to the successful treatment of depression. This helps to reduce anxiety, allows patients to express their fears and disappointments in a "safe" way, and enhances well-being.

PHARMACOTHERAPY

The mainstay of the treatment of depression is pharmacotherapy (Table 48-7).

The agents commonly employed include the newer SSRIs (120), TCAs (121), and psychostimulants (122). The SSRIs fluoxitene hydrochloride, sertraline hydrochloride, paroxetine hydrochloride, citalopram, and recently escitalopram have gained popularity due to their improved side-effects profiles compared with the TCAs. For mild depression, SSRIs are very useful. However, they take weeks to become effective. Some, such as escitalopram, have a lower side-effects profile and work a little faster than the first-generation SSRIs, such as fluoxetine. The side effects are generally mild, but others are problematic, such as reduced appetite, nausea, and anxiety. These effects tend to be of limited duration and have not prevented their application in cancer patients. Other problems arise from their mechanism of action; these include diarrhea, fatigue, and sexual dysfunction (120). If a switch from an SSRI to another medication, especially a monoamine oxidase inhibitor (MAOI), is considered, the washout period of various SSRIs will have to be taken into account. It may therefore be useful to have a patient take SSRIs such as sertraline or escitalopram, which have a shorter washout period than older drugs such as fluoxetine. Our experience has shown methylphenidate to be particularly useful, especially in patients with a limited life expectancy where a few weeks could be too much to ask. Methylphenidate also helps to reduce the symptoms of fatigue, a common problem in cancer patients; this makes it a particularly useful medication (77).

TCAs have been widely used and work faster than SSRIs; however, they have more side effects, some of which (like their anticholinergic effects) can be a major problem for older cancer patients. They do offer additional benefits for patients suffering from neuropathic pain. For that reason, these medications should be started at a low dose and slowly escalated as tolerated. Desipramine and nortriptyline are generally better tolerated than amitriptyline and imipramine in the older population.

Mirtazapine was found to be effective in ameliorating symptoms of depression in cancer patients (123). Some

TABLE 48-7	COMMON ANTIDEPRESSANT DOSAGES
The following are common initial doses:
Nortriptyline 25 mg/day (at bedtime)
Amitriptyline 25 mg/day (at bedtime)
Fluoxetine 10-20 mg/day
Paroxetine 10 mg/day
Sertraline 20 mg/day
Citalopram 20 mg/day
Venlafaxine 37.5 mg/day
Mirtazapine 15 mg/day (at bedtime)
Methylphenidate 5-10 mg in the morning and 5 mg at noon

Reproduced, with permission, from Elsayem A, Driver LC, Bruera E. The MD Anderson Palliative Care Handbook. Houston, TX: MD Anderson Cancer Center; 2002.

additional benefits of mirtazapine may accrue from its beneficial effects on chemotherapy-induced nausea/vomiting (CINV) and insomnia (124).

■ CONSTIPATION

Constipation is the infrequent and difficult passage of hard stool. It is a very common cause of morbidity in the palliative care setting and is thought to affect the overwhelming majority (>95%) of patients consuming opioids for cancer-related pain syndromes (125,126). Constipation can be a difficult condition to assess and treat because of the wide variety of presenting symptoms. Patients may report a feeling of incomplete evacuation, bloating, decreased appetite, or generalized abdominal discomfort or pain. Due to the wide variability in normal bowel movement patterns in individual patients, the diagnosis of constipation can be made only in comparison with an individual's normal pattern (127).

CAUSES

The most common causes of constipation include opioid medication and progressive disease. Other causes include anorexia/cachexia, bowel obstruction, immobility, hypercalcemia, and dehydration. In the palliative care setting, careful attention must be given to the multifactorial nature of constipation. The common causes of constipation are outlined in Table 48-8.

COMPLICATIONS

Although constipation is often overlooked in the setting of other comorbid conditions, it is not necessarily a benign condition; some of the complications of unrelieved constipation can indeed be life-threatening (128).

TABLE 48-8	CAUSES OF CONSTIPATION IN PATIENTS WITH ADVANCED CANCER

Structural abnormalities
   Obstruction
   Pelvic tumor mass
   Radiation fibrosis
   Painful anorectal conditions
      Anal fissure, hemorrhoids, perianal abscess
Drugs
   Opioids
   Agents with anticholinergic actions
      Anticholinergics
      Antispasmodics
      Antidepressants
      Antipsychotics (eg, phenothiazines, haloperidol)
      Antacids (aluminum-containing)
      Antiemetics (eg, ondansetron)
   Diuretics
   Anticonvulsants
   Iron
   Antihypertensive agents
   Anticancer drugs (eg, vinca alkaloids)
Metabolic disturbances
   Dehydration (vomiting, fever, polyuria, poor fluid intake, diuretic use)
   Hypercalcemia
   Hypokalemia
   Uremia
   Diabetes
   Hypothyroidism
Neurologic disorders
   Cerebral tumors
   Spinal cord compression
   Sacral nerve infiltration
   Autonomic failure

Reproduced, with permission, from Elsayem A, Driver LC, Bruera E. The MD Anderson Palliative Care Handbook. Houston, TX: MD Anderson Cancer Center; 2002.

Severe constipation can lead to bowel obstruction, with attendant issues of severe morbidity. In patients who are neutropenic, severe constipation can lead to bacterial transfer across the colon, with bacteremia and sepsis.

DIAGNOSIS

The diagnosis of constipation begins with a careful history of the patient's recent bowel movements. Specific topics to be queried include the date of the last bowel movement, the characteristics of the stool (hard versus soft, loose versus formed, "ribbon-like" versus "pellet-like"), the degree of straining and pain involved, and whether or not the movement felt complete. Related questions include whether or not there was blood in the stool (possibly identifying tumor mass or a hemorrhoid) or an urge to defecate at all (suggesting colonic inertia) (125,127).

After the history, a careful physical examination should include the abdominal examination (distention, firmness, tenderness, the presence or absence of bowel sounds) and a rectal examination. The rectal examination should assess the presence of hard stool in the vault and may reveal the presence of masses, hemorrhoids, fissures, or fistulas. Caution should be exercised in performing a rectal examination on anyone with neutropenia or thrombocytopenia.

In addition to the history and physical examination, a simple "constipation score" (129) may also be obtained. A flat abdominal radiograph of the abdomen is obtained whereby the colon is divided into four quadrants (ascending, transverse, descending, and sigmoid) by drawing a large "X" with the umbilicus in the middle. Each quadrant is assigned a score from 0 to 3 based on the degree of stool in the lumen. A score of zero indicates no stool, a score of 1 indicates less than 50% occupancy, a score of 2 indicates greater than 50% occupancy, and a score of 3 indicates complete occupancy of the lumen with stool. Scores may range from 0 to 12 and score of 7 (or greater) indicates severe constipation (Fig. 48-6).

PREVENTION AND TREATMENT

Prevention of constipation includes patient education on the various reasons for constipation, encouragement of adequate fluid intake, and the prescription of stool softeners and laxatives. In addition, a high degree of vigilance should be maintained regarding the patient's other medications that may cause constipation.

Initial treatment of constipation includes starting the patient on a stool-softening agent (eg, docusate 100-240 mg by mouth twice daily) with a laxative agent (eg, senna 8.6 mg one to two tablets twice daily). Refractory constipation may be managed with lactulose 30 mL by mouth every 6 h until a large bowel movement occurs. Intractable cases may require a bisacodyl suppository, milk-and-molasses enema, or Fleet enema. Proximal impaction may require magnesium citrate. In rare cases where hard stools are present in the vault, manual disimpaction may be necessary. In refractory cases, the opioid antagonist naloxone, given orally, may produce laxation (130-132). Mild opioid withdrawal may be seen with naloxone. Recently methylnaltrexone, given parenterally, has shown promising effects in the treatment of opioid-induced constipation (133-135).

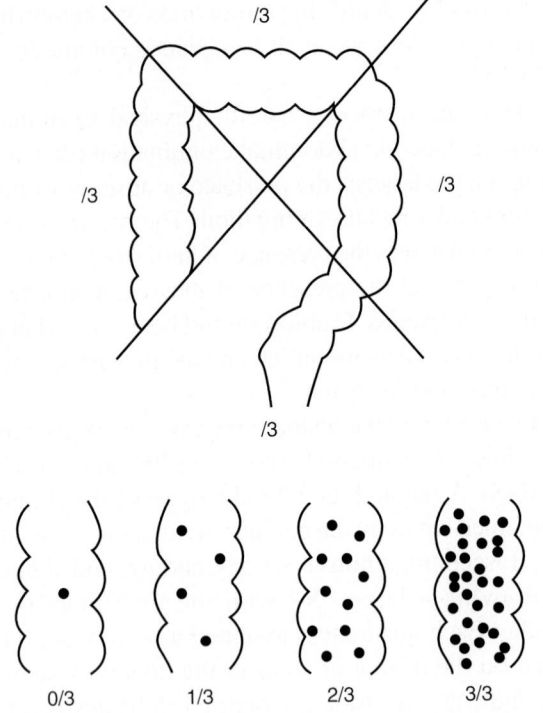

*On a flat abdominal x-ray, draw two diagonal lines intersecting at the umbilicus as shown here. This transects the abdomen into four quadrants corresponding to the ascending, transverse, descending, and rectosigmoid colons. Then, assess the amount of stool in each of the four quadrants using the following scoring system: 0 = no stool; 1 = stool occupying <50% of the lumen of colon; 2 = stool occupying >50% of the lumen; 3 = stool completely occupying the lumen. The total score will therefore range from 0 to 12. A score of 7 indicates severe constipation and requires immediate intervention.

FIGURE 48-6. How to calculate a "constipation score" using a flat abdominal x-ray.

■ CHRONIC NAUSEA

Nausea and vomiting are highly unpleasant symptoms that affect between 40 and 70% of patients in the palliative care setting (136-138). In the cancer setting, nausea is prevalent in patients under the age of 65, females, and patients with breast, stomach, or gynecologic cancers. The etiology of chronic nausea is often multifactorial and could be due to the underlying disease, its treatment, or as a side effect of medications that treat cancer-related pain (eg, opioids). The underlying cause of nausea should be ascertained if possible, and the selection of the antiemetic agent should be tailored to maximize therapeutic value (136). Figure 48-7 lists the common causes of nausea in the cancer setting.

Medication side effects and chronic constipation are the most common causes. As shown in the figure below, the experience of nausea and vomiting is generated as a result of the complex interrelationship between the chemoreceptor trigger zone (CTZ) and the vomiting center (VC). The CTZ can be affected directly by drugs, toxins, or metabolites or may receive afferent impulses from chemoreceptors and mechanoreceptors originating in the gastrointestinal tract, chest, or pelvis, which will subsequently influence the vomiting center. The VC also receives direct input from the cerebral cortex (Fig. 48-8).

ASSESSMENT

The etiology of nausea should be determined if at all possible, since proper management will depend on

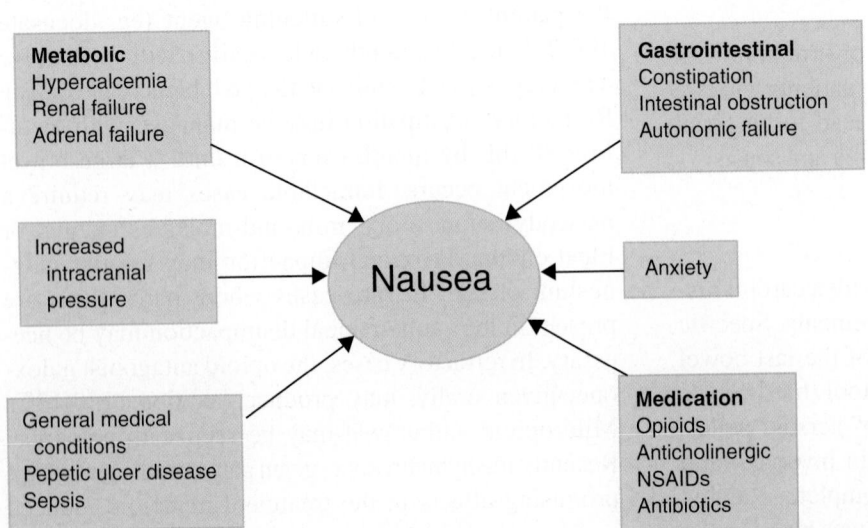

FIGURE 48-7. Causes of nausea. (*Reproduced, with permission, from Elsayem A, Driver LC, Bruera E. The MD Anderson Palliative Care Handbook. Houston, TX: MD Anderson Cancer Center; 2002.*)

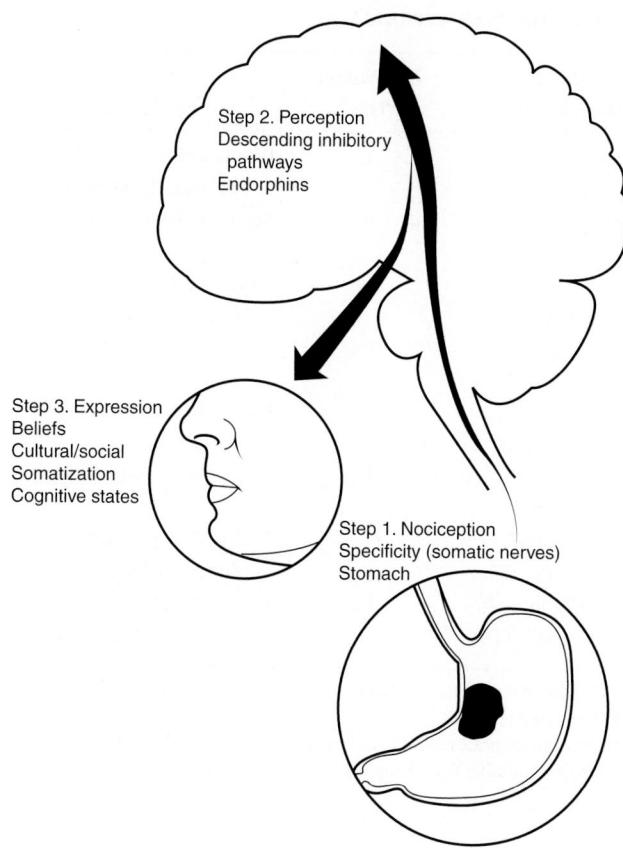

Step 2. Perception
Descending inhibitory
pathways
Endorphins

Step 3. Expression
Beliefs
Cultural/social
Somatization
Cognitive states

Step 1. Nociception
Specificity (somatic nerves)
Stomach

FIGURE 48-8. Vomiting cascade. *(Reproduced, with permission, from Elsayem A, Driver LC, Bruera E. The MD Anderson Palliative Care Handbook. Houston, TX: MD Anderson Cancer Center; 2002.)*

identifying and treating the underlying cause. The assessment of the patient with nausea should be part of the multidimensional approach to assess multiple symptoms simultaneously. It begins by taking a detailed history, including the onset of the nausea, its duration, the frequency of episodes and their severity, all noted on a 0 to 10 scale of ESAS. In addition, since chronic constipation is one of the main causes of nausea, bowel function should also be assessed. The list of medications should be reviewed for possible medication side effects.

The examination of the patient should focus on life-threatening complications related to dehydration, such as hypotension and tachycardia; if present, these should be corrected promptly. It should include an abdominal examination, looking for signs of obstruction or constipation; a CNS examination to rule out raised intracranial pressure; and possibly even a cardiac examination to rule out initial symptoms of a major cardiac event.

Diagnostic tests include serum evaluation of electrolytes, serum calcium, and liver and kidney function tests. Abdominal x-rays may be obtained to gauge the

degree of constipation (see the discussion of constipation). Brain imaging may be considered to assess for new or worsening CNS lesions.

TREATMENT

Correction of the underlying problem should be attempted if a cause can be found. Treating constipation or removing the inciting medication may relieve the nausea if it was caused by any of them. Steroids or radiation may help nausea caused by increased intracranial pressure. If opioids are the cause, adding an antiemetic may help; rarely, opioid rotation may be required.

Pharmacologic therapy should be directed toward the underlying problem. Table 48-9 illustrates the most commonly used antiemetics.

For most chronic, opioid-related nausea, a prokinetic agent such as metoclopramide (10 mg PO/IV/SC every 4-6 h) is helpful. The antidopaminergic properties of haloperidol (1-2 mg PO/IV/SC every 4-8 h) may help to relieve certain forms of refractory nausea. The 5 HT_3 antagonists (eg, ondansetron 4-8 mg PO/IV/ SC) and the neurokin-1 (NK1) receptor antagonist, aprepitant, may ameliorate chemotherapy-related nausea (136,137,139) but are less helpful in chronic nausea. Moreover, these agents are expensive and constipating. Octreotide, a somatostatin analog that reduces gastric motility and secretions, is helpful in nausea caused by intestinal obstruction. Benzodiazepines and anxiolytic agents may help anxiety-provoked nausea. Finally, steroids have been shown to be helpful for nausea both with a direct effect (eg, in certain chemotherapy- or opioid-related problems with nausea) and by an indirect effect (eg, by reducing intracranial pressure in patients with intracranial neoplasms) (138,140). Figure 48-9 is an x-ray of a patient suffering from nausea as a result of constipation, with stool in all quadrants.

■ CACHEXIA

The cachexia syndrome, characterized by a marked weight loss, anorexia, asthenia, and anemia, is invariably associated with the growth of a tumor and leads to a malnutrition status caused by the induction of anorexia or decreased food intake. In addition, the competition for nutrients between the tumor and the host results in an accelerated catabolic state, which promotes severe metabolic disturbances. Cachexia is a complex metabolic syndrome characterized clinically by progressive involuntary weight loss, which can lead to the death of the host. The mechanism is not precisely

ANTIEMETIC MEDICATIONS—DRUGS USEFUL FOR THE TREATMENT OF CHRONIC NAUSEA

Drug*	Main Receptor	Main Indication	Starting PO Dose/Route	Equivalent Price†	Side Effects
Metoclopramide	D2	Opioid-induced, gastric stasis	10 mg q4h PO, SC, IV	1	EPS (akathisia, dystonia, dyskinesia)
Prochlorperazine	D2	Opioid-induced	10 mg q6h PO, IV	3	Sedation, hypotension
Cyclizine	H1	Vestibular causes, intestinal obstruction	25-50 mg q8h PO, SC, PR		Sedation, dry mouth, blurred vision
Promethazine	H1	Vestibular, motion sickness, obstruction	12.5 mg q4h PO, PR, IV	2	Sedation
Haloperidol	D2	Opioid, chemical, metabolic	1-2 mg bid PO, IV, SC	1	Rarely EPS
Ondansetron	5 HT$_3$	Chemotherapy	4-8 mg q8h PO, IV	84	Headache, constipation
Diphenhydramine	H1, Ach	Intestinal obstruction, vestibular, ICP	25 mg q6h PO, IV, SC	0.2	Sedation, dry mouth, blurred vision
Hyoscine	Ach	Intestinal obstruction, colic, secretions	0.2-0.4 mg q4h SL, SC, TD	0.4	Dry mouth, blurred vision, urine retention, agitation

Ach, acetylcholine; D2, dopamine; EPS, extrapyramidal symptoms; H1, histamine; ICP, intracranial pressure; PR, per rectum; SL, sublingual; TD, transdermal.
*Corticosteroids are not included because they vary in dosage and have limited indications (see text).
†Prices are compared to metoclopramide 10-mg tablets orally for 10 days based on the formulary prices at MD Anderson Cancer Center, November 2001.
Reproduced, with permission, from Elsayem A, Driver LC, Bruera E. The MD Anderson Palliative Care Handbook. Houston, TX: MD Anderson Cancer Center; 2002.

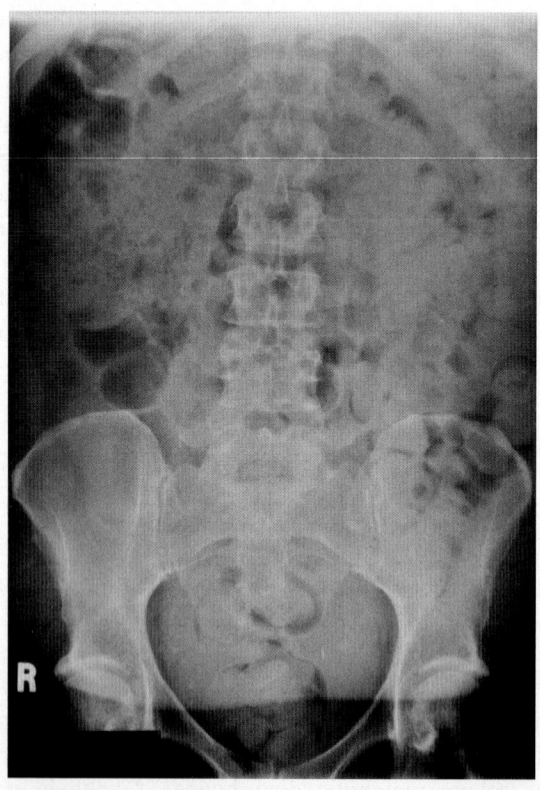

FIGURE 48-9. Constipation x-ray. *(Reproduced, with permission, from Elsayem A, Driver LC, Bruera E. The MD Anderson Palliative Care Handbook. Houston, TX: MD Anderson Cancer Center; 2002.)*

known, but the condition represents abnormalities of carbohydrate, fat, protein, and energy metabolism. Cachexia is found in majority of patients with advanced cancer and is a major contributing factor to death in about 50% of these patients (141). Cachexia leads to diminished appetite, weight loss, severe lethargy, fatigue, and generalized weakness known as asthenia. Patients with this syndrome are prone to have side effects and respond poorly to treatment. Cachexia commonly tends to occur in patients with solid tumors, in children, and in elderly patients. The etiology is multifactorial. It is caused mainly by tumor by-products and host cytokines, such as tumor necrosis factor, proteolysis-inducing factor, lipid-mobilizing factor, and interleukins (Fig. 48-10) (142,143).

In patients with this syndrome, the basal metabolic rate is increased. The liver produces acute-phase proteins that play a role in the inflammatory and antitumor process but draw their energy from muscle breakdown. Glucose turnover is increased and at the same time there is a relative glucose intolerance in the muscle, with insulin resistance. There is suppression of de novo lipogenesis and peripheral activation of lipolysis, whereas central (hepatic) lipogenesis is increased. Whole-body protein turnover is increased and liver protein synthesis is directed toward an increase in the production of

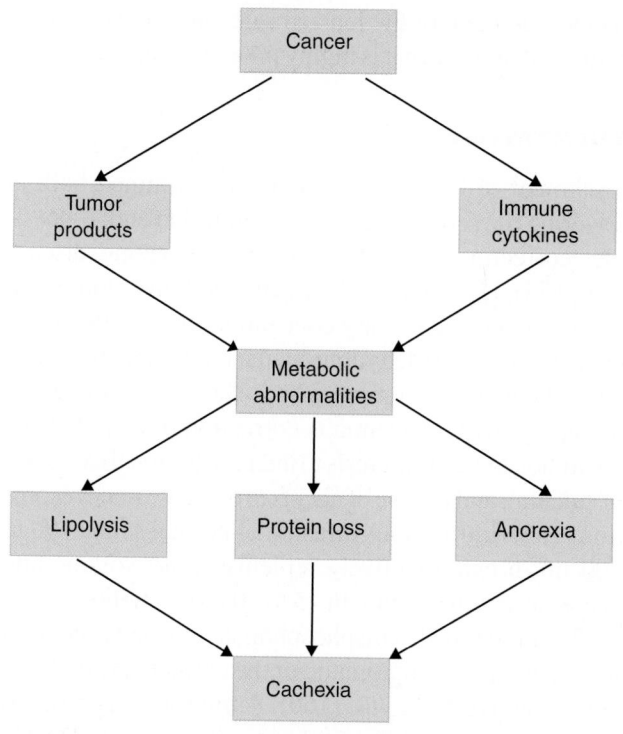

FIGURE 48-10. Mechanism of cachexia. *(Reproduced, with permission, from Elsayem A, Driver LC, Bruera E. The MD Anderson Palliative Care Handbook. Houston, TX: MD Anderson Cancer Center; 2002.)*

acute-phase proteins and lower production of albumin. Thus cachexia is characterized by an *increase* in energy expenditure, protein synthesis (largely acute-phase proteins at the expense of muscle proteins), proteolysis, lipolysis, and glucose turnover; a decrease in muscle proteins and lipogenesis; and an increase in ketone bodies (143).

Feeding of the patient with cancer cachexia was found to increase acute-phase protein production without influencing the rate of albumin synthesis (144). Other contributory factors include nausea, dysphagia, bowel obstruction, or constipation. Sometimes food aversion, depression, and apathy play a role.

ASSESSMENT

The clinical assessment includes a careful history that is focused on nutritional issues and a physical examination. A 5-lb weight loss in the previous 2 months and/or an estimated daily caloric intake of less than 70 cal/kg is a simple diagnostic indicator. Simple and inexpensive tests are available to assess body composition, such as anthropometric measurements, skinfold thickness, arm muscle circumference and area, and weight and body mass index (BMI). Biochemical measurements are also available, such as serum albumin, transferrin, and prealbumin. Careful clinical assessment and laboratory tests, especially serum sodium, are the keystones for diagnosis and effective management. Bioelectrical impedance (BEI) is an easy way to assess both nutritional status and fluid deficits in advanced cancer and should be used more often (145).

MANAGEMENT

The approach to management consists of identifying the etiology and treating the underlying cause. The nutritionist should advise on the dietary options to maximize nutritional intake. Small frequent meals are less intimidating than the usual large three meals a day.

The pharmacologic treatment consists of symptom control of the contributory factors and appetite stimulation. Chronic nausea or early satiety is treated with metoclopramide 10 mg every 4 to 6 h. Appetite stimulants include progestational agents, corticosteroids, cannabinoids, or adjuvant agents. Progestational agents include megestrol acetate; 40 to 120 mg PO qid will improve appetite in up to 80% of patients and induce weight gain in many (146,147). Symptomatic improvement in appetite occurs in less than 1 week; however, weight gain may take several weeks. Appetite stimulation with these agents lasts longer than that resulting from the use of corticosteroids. Caution must be exercised in patients with venous thrombosis, pulmonary embolism, or severe cardiac disease. Corticosteroids may stimulate appetite and decrease nausea (148,149). The effect does not last long. A cannabinoid, dronabinol, is approved for appetite stimulation and is dosed at 2.5 mg PO bid; it may produce concurrent antiemetic effects but may also produce CNS side effects (150). Antidepressants TCAs, and SSRIs may help with appetite in patients with depression. Thalidomide has been studied and has been shown to improve appetite, nausea, and well-being (151). Synthetic and semisynthetic testosterone derivatives have been studied especially in terminal AIDS patients and have been shown to be of benefit in improving appetite and reducing weight loss (152).

Enteral and parenteral forms of nutrition are inappropriate for most patients with advanced cancer (153) other than those who have a starvation component to cachexia, such as severe dysphagia or bowel obstruction. They do not enhance response to antineoplastic therapy or significantly abate its toxicity and do not improve survival or quality of life. They can be burdensome to patients and families and may obstruct transition to a hospice setting.

NONPHARMACOLOGIC THERAPY

Counseling of the patient as well as the family and loved ones is very important in assuring them that they may express their fears and needs and that their concerns will be acted on. In addition, counseling provides a venue to reframe the condition from that of "starving to death" to the more complex one of irreversible (usually) metabolic abnormalities and the futility of pushing nutrition. This reframing can decrease the distress of both patients and families and can maintain the social benefit of mealtimes. Exercise has benefit both for maintaining muscle and reducing depression; leaving the confines of the hospital room and being in sunlight have benefits for mood, depression, and overall sense of well-being.

■ HYPERCALCEMIA

Hypercalcemia is a common life-threatening complication of cancer, affecting 10 to 20% of patients; it is more common in certain cancers such as squamous cell of lung or head and neck, renal cell carcinoma, breast cancer, and multiple myeloma (87-89,154-156). The usual cause of hypercalcemia is humoral secretion of the parathyroid hormone–related protein (PTHrP), and the clinical syndrome mimics hyperparathyroidism biochemically except that the serum PTH is suppressed. Less frequent causes include ectopic production of parathyroid hormone itself. Clinically, the disorder contrasts with primary hyperparathyroidism. Hypercalcemia is abrupt in onset and is often severe; the associated neoplasm is usually obvious. It is usually unnecessary to measure the serum PTHrP levels to confirm the diagnosis; a determination of PTH will rule out intercurrent primary hyperparathyroidism. In multiple myeloma, it is caused by direct activation of bone resorption by cytokines secreted from myeloma cells in the bone marrow. Lymphomas can cause hypercalcemia by a similar local osteolytic mechanism or by conversion of vitamin D to 1,25-dihydroxyvitamin D.

CLINICAL PRESENTATION

Early symptoms are mild and include anorexia, nausea and vomiting, constipation, fatigue, weakness polydipsia, and polyuria (nephrogenic diabetes insipidus). Late symptoms are usually severe and include dehydration, altered mental status, generalized weakness, progressive gastrointestinal symptoms, and cardiac arrhythmias, especially when serum calcium levels rise rapidly. A high index of suspicion is required and the diagnosis is established by measurement of the ionized calcium or the corrected serum calcium since it is highly protein-bound.

TREATMENT

Treatment of hypercalcemia should be aimed both at lowering the serum calcium concentration and, if possible, correcting or decreasing the underlying disease (157,158). Hypercalcemia impairs both the glomerular filtration rate and urinary concentration; with the resultant azotemia and dehydration, the renal route for clearance of calcium is compromised. The mainstay of acute therapy of hypercalcemia is correction of dehydration, institution of saline diuresis to increase the renal excretion of calcium, and the use of agents to decrease bone resorption (159). Intravenous infusion of normal saline 100 to 200 mL/h can effectively replenish fluid volume and decrease serum calcium in 15 to 30% of patients.

Treatment with a bisphosphonate is usually required if the patient is symptomatic or the corrected serum calcium is above 12 mg/dL (160). Pamidronate is given in a dose of 90 mg in 500 mL of normal saline over 2 to 4 h. Pamidronate decreases bone resorption by inhibiting osteoclast activity (161). Renal function should be monitored both before and after pamidronate therapy, since this agent is relatively contraindicated in patients with renal dysfunction. Zoledronic acid has emerged in clinical trials as another bisphosphonate with results superior to those of pamidronate (162). Zoledronic acid is given at a dose of 4 mg over 15 min. The peak effect of bisphosphonates is reached after 5 to 7 days and the dose is repeated at 4-week intervals.

In severe hypercalcemia, rapid lowering of calcium levels may be achieved by subcutaneous administration of calcitonin 100 to 200 units tid for three to six doses (163). Serum calcium should be evaluated 1 day after calcitonin treatment. The other available agents for treatment of acute hypercalcemia are less useful (etidronate disodium, gallium nitrate) or toxic (plicamycin).

■ HYDRATION

"To hydrate or not" is a topic that is brought up many times in a terminal situation, both by health care providers as well as patients and family members. The traditional medical model always supported the maintenance of intravenous fluids in terminal patients (164,165). In one study at a tertiary care teaching hospital, 73 of 106 patients died with an intravenous line running (166). This practice has been challenged by some palliative care providers (167). The negative effect of hydration in terminal patients was based mostly on anecdotal evidence rather than on scientifically tested data (168-170). Other anecdotal evidence, however, pointed to a beneficial effect of hydration in terminal patients (171). Dehydration can lead to delirium, exacerbate opioid side effects, and worsen other symptoms such as constipation, fatigue, and hypercalemia. While many patients die peacefully without parenteral fluids, there is some consensus on the need for individualized management (172,173).

ASSESSMENT

Symptoms of dehydration may include fatigue, confusion/delirium, constipation, and dry mouth. The physical examination may reveal drowsiness or confusion, poor skin turgor, decreased jugular venous pressure, dry mucous membranes, decreased urinary sodium, elevated hematocrit reflecting hemoconcentration, hypernatremia, elevated blood urea nitrogen, and normal creatinine in early dehydration.

MANAGEMENT

The decision to hydrate a patient is based on individual patient assessment and clinical presentation. Principles include the following:

1. Consider a short therapeutic trial of hydration in cases involving confusion.
2. Consider maintenance of hydration in patients with obstruction of the small bowel, especially when their overall quality of life is fair.
3. Consider the disadvantages of hydration, such as maintaining IV/SC lines, issues of care at home and in rural areas, cost, worsening of symptoms in preexisting congestive heart failure.
4. Consider discontinuing hydration if the symptoms worsen.

METHODS OF HYDRATION

The option to hydrate the patient depends on the ability of the patient to take fluids orally. Oral fluid intake is the preferred route due to its ease of administration, low maintenance, and minimal cost involved. However, terminal patients may be unable to take fluids orally, especially if they are confused and drowsy. In that situation, fluids should be given intravenously (if a preexisting long intravenous line is already in place) or subcutaneously (also known as hypodermoclysis or clysis); this last is considered the better option by many palliative care specialists (174-176). Fluids may be administered via clysis as either a bolus or continuous infusion. Advantages of clysis include ease of access to site, suitability for home administration because of its ease and safety, ability to use a single site up to 7 days, and ease of disconnection for the patient's mobility. Methods of administration include normal saline at the rate of 70 to 100 mL/h via continuous infusion for rehydration. For maintenance, two-thirds dextrose and one-third normal saline at the rate of 40 to 80 mL/h, 1000 mL by gravity overnight, or 500 mL bolus twice a day, with each bolus infused over 1 h. On some occasions, hyaluronidase may facilitate fluid absorption (177).

■ COMMUNICATION IN PALLIATIVE CARE

Communication in medical practice and palliative medicine in particular is the key to a successful and satisfactory experience for patients, families, and health care professionals (178,179). There is enough evidence to suggest that the emotional and psychologic needs of a dying patient are of paramount importance (180,181). There are a number of reasons for miscommunication between an advanced cancer patient and a health care professional (182,183). Health care professionals are typically trained to cure and therefore feel stressed when they have to break bad news to their patients. Patients in the western world also try to avoid talk of death and dying. There are no paradigms to help us make the transition from life to death. Some of the major subjects that may call for discussion include diagnosis and prognosis, the natural history of the disease, symptom management, compliance with therapy, hopes and expectations of treatment, planning for the future, transition from curative treatment to palliative care, advance directives and do-not-resuscitate (DNR) orders, hospice care, and end-of-life issues. An honest, sensitive, and compassionate discussion about a poor prognosis sets the stage for an exploration of the emotions, fears, and spiritual needs surrounding the dying process (184). The quality of prognostic discussion has an important influence on the patient's emotional and physical well-being (180,181,185,186).

Communicating a poor prognosis is one of the most difficult ordeals faced by physicians. Multiple factors have been identified as barriers to communicating a poor prognosis. Many physicians find it stressful to give prognostic information and wait to be asked before providing it (182,183,187,188). Physicians are often inaccurate in prognosticating and tend to be overoptimistic in their assessments (184-186,189-191). Patients

| TABLE 48-10 | THE SPIKES PROTOCOL (SETUP/PATIENT'S PERCEPTION/INVITATION/KNOWLEDGE/EMOTIONS/SUPPORT) |

STEP 1: SETTING UP THE INTERVIEW

Goals	*Purpose*
To prepare yourself for the interview	Reflect on the task at hand.
To establish rapport with the patient and put the patient at ease	Arrange for uninterrupted time.
To facilitate information exchange	Decide who should be present.
	Determine whether the patient is ready.
	Sit down when you speak to the patient.
	Have facial tissues handy.
	Maintain eye contact.

STEP 2: FIND OUT THE PATIENT'S PERCEPTION OF THE ILLNESS

Goals	*Purpose*
To determine what the patient understands	Ask open-ended questions; ie, "Tell me what you've been told," or
To assess denial in the patient/family	"I'd like to make sure you understand the reason for the tests."
To promote rapport through listening	Correct misinformation and misunderstanding.
To understand the patient's expectations and concerns	Address denial.
	Address unrealistic expectation.
	Define your role.

STEP 3: GET AN INVITATION TO GIVE INFORMATION

Goals	*Purpose*
To determine how much information the patient wants and when he or she is ready to hear it	Ask "Are you the type of person who wants information in detail?"
To acknowledge that patient information needs may change over time	Explore sources of family concern.
To resolve conflicts with families regarding information disclosure	

STEP 4: GIVING THE PATIENT KNOWLEDGE AND INFORMATION

Goals	*Purpose*
To prepare the patient for the bad news	"Forecast" the arrival of bad news; ie, "I'm afraid I have some bad news..."
To ensure patient understanding	Give the information in small parcels.
	Check periodically for understanding.
	Avoid using medical jargon.
	Address all questions.

STEP 5: RESPONDING TO PATIENT EMOTIONS

Goals	*Purpose*
To address emotional responses	Anticipate emotional reactions.
To facilitate emotional recovery	Resist the temptation to try and make the bad news better than it really is.
To acknowledge our own emotions	Support the patient by using emphatic response to expressions of emotion such as crying.
	Clarify emotions about which you are not sure.
	Validate the patient's feelings.

SUPPORTING THE PATIENT

Be prepared, and have a strategy (escape is not a strategy).	Sit down and get close if you can.
Have someone with you if it will be difficult.	Respond to any emotions with one of the following:
Shift to a supportive role.	Empathic statements
Give the patient time to emote.	Validating statements
Have facial tissue ready.	Exploratory questions

Reproduced, with permission, from Elsayem A, Driver LC, Bruera E. The MD Anderson Palliative Care Handbook. Houston, TX: MD Anderson Cancer Center; 2002.

in the United States now want to be told of their prognosis despite such barriers (192). The myth about harming the patients with disclosure of their prognosis is ill-founded; in fact, it has been shown that patients with cancer often appreciate being told the truth (193).

Most patients who receive bad news are generally satisfied with the communication, but some have criticized the manner in which they were told of their prognosis. About 25% of the patients with advance cancer felt that the diagnosis of their disease was not communicated in a "clear and caring manner" (194). About 22 to 26% of the patients felt that they could have received more information about the poor prognosis (195,196). Patients who are informed by the telephone or in the recovery room after a diagnostic procedure are more likely to have a negative reaction to the discussion than those who are told in the office or in their hospital rooms (197). Another study of patients with cancer confirms the importance of receiving adequate information, related in a caring and hopeful way, with a supportive person present (198).

There are very few trials testing the effectiveness of different strategies in delivering bad news (199). Most recommendations on discussing bad news agree on key features (200). These recommendations can be organized into five categories per the SPIKES protocol as shown in Table 48-10.

■ CONCLUSION

Symptom control continues to be a challenge for oncologists. Cancer-related symptoms, both physical and emotional, arise and evolve across the course of diagnosis, treatment, cure, survivorship, and end of life. While the oncologist faces the challenge of treating the malignancy, the patient faces the challenge of coping with their illness experience, a constant threat to their independence and connectedness to society in this difficult situation. A well-crafted team approach and dedicated members are needed to fulfill the mission of maintaining the integrity of human life and suffering. Palliative and hospice care are established models that deliver such care. There is an urgent need for health care providers to develop a better appreciation of patients' distress beyond physical symptoms. An interdisciplinary team that is able to understand the complex symptomatology and provide compassionate and competent care to the patient and family both during active treatment as well as in advanced stages of the disease is an ideal model.

A good symptom management approach should incorporate appropriate principles to deal with complex symptoms, maintain open dialogue with patients and families, discuss various options—including treatment options, prognosis, future course, and possible symptoms during the treatment process—as well as futility of treatment whenever applicable and palliative care as a viable option. This can ideally be achieved by involving the palliative care team from the time of diagnosis in routine clinical practice as well as clinical trials.

References

1. Curtis EB, Krech R, Walsh TD. Common symptoms in patients with advanced cancer. *J Palliat Care* 1991;7:25-28.
2. Krech RL, Walsh D. Symptoms of pancreatic cancer. *J Pain Sympt Mgt* 1991;6:360-367.
3. Foley KM. Pain syndromes in patients with cancer. In: Bonica JJ, Ventafridda V (eds): *Advances in Pain Research and Therapy*. New York: Raven Press; 1979:59-75.
4. Bonica JJ. Cancer pain. In: Bonica JJ (ed): *The Management of Pain*. Philadelphia, PA: Lea & Febiger; 1990:400.
5. Twycross RG, Fairfield S. Pain in far-advanced cancer. *Pain* 1982;14:303-310.
6. Levin D, Cleeland CS, Dar R. Public attitudes toward cancer pain. *Cancer* 1985;56:2337-2339.
7. Foley KM. The treatment of cancer pain. *N Engl J Med* 1984;313:84-95.
8. Portenoy RK, Hagen NA. Breakthrough pain: Definition, prevalence, and characteristics. *Pain* 1990;41:273-281.
9. Bruera E, MacMillan K, Hanson J, et al. The Edmonton staging system for cancer pain: Preliminary report. *Pain* 1989;37:203-209.
10. Bruera E, Kuehn N, Miller MJ, et al. The Edmonton symptom assessment system: A simple method for the assessment of palliative care patients. *J Palliat Care* 1991;7:6-9.
11. World Health Organization. *Cancer Pain Relief*. Geneva, Switzerland: World Health Organization; 1986.
12. Jacox A, Carr DB, Payne R, et al. *Management of Cancer Pain*. Clinical Practice Guidelines No. 9, AHCPR Publication 94-0592. Rockville, MD: US Department of Health and Human Services, Agency for Health Care Policy and Research; 1994.
13. Raja SN, Haythornthwaite JA, Pappagallo M, et al. Opioids versus antidepressants in postherpetic neuralgia. A randomized, placebo-controlled trial. *Neurology* 2002;59:1015-1021.
14. Rowbotham MC, Twilling L, Davies PS, et al. Oral opioid therapy for chronic peripheral and central neuropathic pain. *N Engl J Med* 2003;348(13):1223-1232.
15. Andersen G, Christrup L, Sjogren P. Relationships among morphine metabolism, pain and side effects during long-term treatment: An update. *J Pain Sympt Mgt* 2003;25(1):74-91.
16. Szeto HH, Inturrisi CE, Houde R, et al. Accumulation of normeperidine, an active metabolite of meperidine, in patients with renal failure of cancer. *Ann Intern Med* 1977;86(6):738-741.
17. Portenoy RK, Payne R, Coluzzi P, et al. Oral transmucosal fentanyl citrate (OTFC) for the treatment of breakthrough pain in cancer patients: A controlled dose titration study. *Pain* 1999;79(2-3):303-312.

18. Tennant F, Hermann L. Self-treatment with oral transmucosal fentanyl citrate to prevent emergency room visits for pain crises: Patient self-reports of efficacy and utility. *J Pain Palliat Care Pharmacother* 2002;16(3):37-44.

19. Portnenoy RK, Taylor D, Messina J, et al. A randomized, placebo-controlled study of fentanyl buccal tablet for breakthrough pain in opioid-treated patients with cancer. *Clin J Pain*. 2006;22(9):805-811.

20. Davis MP, Walsh D. Methadone for relief of cancer pain: A review of pharmakokinetics, pharmacodynamics, drug interactions and protocols of administration. *Support Care Cancer* 2001;9:63-83.

21. Ripamonti C, Groff L, Brunelli C, et al. Switching from morphine to oral methadone in treating cancer pain: What is the equianalgesic dose ratio? *J Clin Oncol* 1998;16(10): 3216-3221.

22. Ripamonti C, de Conno F, Groff L, et al. Equianalgesic dose/ratio between methadone and other opioid agonists in cancer pain: Comparison of two clinical experiences. *Ann Oncol* 1998;9:79-83.

23. Gorman AL, Elliott KJ, Inturrisi CE. The d-and l-isomers of methadone bind to the non-competitive site on the N-methyl-D-asparatate (NMDA) receptor in rat forebrain and spinal cord. *Neurosci Lett* 1997;223:5-8.

24. Tarumi Y, Pereira J, Watanabe S. Methadone and fluconazole: Respiratory depression by drug interaction. *J Pain Sympt Mgt* 2002;23(2):148-153.

25. Krantz MJ, Lowery CM, Martell BA, et al. Effects of methadone on QT-interval dispersion. *Pharmacotherapy* 2005; 25(11):1523-1529.

26. Cruciani RA, Sekine R, Homel P, et al. Measurement of QTc in patients receiving chronic methadone therapy. *J Pain Symptom Manage* 2005;29(4):385-391.

27. Reddy S, Hui D, El Osta B, et al. The effect of oral methadone on the QTc interval in advanced cancer patients: A prospective pilot study. *J Palliat Med* 2010;13(1):33-38.

28. Galer BS, Coyle N, Pasternak GW, et al. Individual variation in the response to different opiods—Report of five cases. *Pain* 1992;49:87-91.

29. Hanks G, Forbes K. Opioid responsiveness. *Acta Anesthesiol Scand* 1997;41:154-158.

30. Lane NE. Pain management in osteoarthritis: The role of COX-2 inhibitors. *J Rheumatol* 1997;24:20-24.

31. Bresalier RS, Sandler RS, Quan H, et al. Cardiovascular events associated with rofecoxib in a colorectal chemoprevention trial. *N Engl J Med* 2005;352(11):1092-1102.

32. Magni G. The use of antidepressants in the treatment of chronic pain: A review of current evidence. *Drugs* 1991;42:730-748.

33. Kolke M, Hoffken K, Olbrich H, et al. Antidepressants and anticonvulsants for the treatment of neuropathic pain syndromes in cancer patients. *Onkologie* 1999;14:40-43.

34. Rowbotham M, Harden N, Stacey B, et al. Gabapentin for the treatment of postherpetic neuralgia: A randomized controlled trial. *JAMA* 1998;280:1837-1842.

35. Backonja M, Beydoun A, Edwards KR, et al. Gabapentin for the symptomatic treatment of painful neuropathy in patients with diabetes mellitus: A randomized controlled trial. *JAMA* 1998;280:1831-1836.

36. Lesser H, Sharma U, LaMoreaux L, et al. Pregabalin relieves symptoms of painful diabetic neuropathy: A randomized controlled trial. *Neurology* 2004;14:63(11):2104-2110.

37. Brietbart W. Psychotropic adjuvant analgesics for pain in cancer and AIDS. *Psychooncology* 1998;7:333-345.

38. Patt R, Propper G, Reddy S. The neuroleptics as adjuvants analgesics. *J Pain Sympt Mgt* 1994;9:446-453.

39. Reddy S, Patt RB. The benzodiazepines as adjuvant analgesics. *J Pain Sympt Mgt* 1994;9:510-514.

40. Thiebaud D, Leyvarz S, von Fliedner V, et al. Treatment of bone metastases from breast cancer and myeloma with pamidronate. *Eur J Cancer* 1991;27:37-41.

41. Berenson JR, Licherstein A, Porter L, et al. Efficacy of pamidronate in reducing skeletal events in patients with advanced multiple myeloma. *N Engl J Med* 1996;334: 488-493.

42. Hortobagyi GN, Theriault RL, Porter L, et al. Efficacy of pamidronate in reducing skeletal complications in patients with breast cancer and lytic bone metastases. *N Engl J Med* 1996;335(24):178.

43. Grant R, Papadopoulos SM, Sandler HM, et al. Metastatic epidural spinal cord compression: Current concepts and treatment. *J Neurooncol* 1994;19:79-92.

44. Nagaro T, Shimizu C, Inoue H, et al. The efficacy of intravenous lidocaine on various types of neuropathic pain. *Masui* 1995;44(6):862-867.

45. Brose W, Cousins M. Subcutaneous lidocaine for the treatment of neuropathic cancer pain. *Pain* 1991;45(2):145-148.

46. Galer BS, Rowbotham MC Perander J, et al. Topical lidocaine patch relieves postherpetic neuralgia more effectively than a vehicle topical patch: Results of an enriched enrollment study. *Pain* 1999;80:533-538.

47. Mercadante S, Lodi F, Sapio M, et al. Long-term ketamine subcutaneous infusion in neuropathic cancer pain. *J Pain Sympt Mgt* 1995;10(7):564-568.

48. Yang CY, Wong CS, Chiang JY, et. Intrathecal ketamine reduces morphine requirements in patients with terminal cancer. *Can J Anaesth* 1996;43(4):379-383.

49. Ellison N, Loprinzi CL, Kugler J, et al. Phase 3 placebo-controlled trial of capsaicin cream in the management of surgical neuropathic pain in cancer patients. *J Clin Oncol* 1997; 15(8):2974-2980.

50. Crawford ED, Kozlowski JM, Debruyne FM, et al. The use of strontium 89 for palliation of pain from bone metastasis associated with hormone-refractory prostate cancer. *Urology* 1994;44:481-485.

51. Serafini AN, Houston SJ, Resche I, et al. Palliation of pain associated with metastatic bone cancer using samarium-153 lexidronam: A double blind placebo-controlled clinical trial. *J Clin Oncol* 1998;16:1574-1581.

52. Arner S. The role of nerve blocks in the treatment of cancer pain. *Acta Anaesthesiol Scand* 1982;74:104-108.

53. Cousins MJ, Bridenbaug PO (eds). *Neural Blockade,* 2nd ed. Philadelphia, PA: Lippincott; 1988.

54. Brown DL, Bulley CK, Quiel EL. Neurolytic celiac plexus block for pancreatic cancer pain. *Anesth Analg* 1987;66:869-873.

55. Lillemoe KD, Cameron JL, Kaufman HS, et al. Chemical splanchnicectomy in patients with unresectable pancreatic cancer. A prospective randomized trial. *Ann Surg* 1993;217(5): 447-455; discussion 456-457.

56. Wong GY, Schroeder DR, Carns PE, et al. Effect of neurolytic celiac plexus block on pain relief, quality of life, and survival in patients with unresectable pancreatic cancer. A randomized controlled trial. *JAMA* 2004;291:1092-1099.

57. Patt RB, Payne R, Farhat GA, et al. Subarachnoid neurolytic block under general anesthesia in a 3-year-old with neuroblastoma. *Clin J Pain* 1995;11(2):143-146.

58. Smith TJ, Staats PS, Deer T, et al. Randomized clinical trial of an implantable drug delivery system compared with comprehensive medical management for refractory cancer pain: Impact on pain, drug-related toxicity, and survival. *J Clin Oncol* 2002;20(19):4040-4049.

59. Davis MP, Walsh D, Lagman R, et al. Randomized clinical trial of an implantable drug delivery system. *J Clin Oncol* 2003;21(14):2800-2801.

60. Ripamonti C, Brunelli C. Randomized clinical trial of an implantable drug delivery system compared with comprehensive medical management for refractory cancer pain: Impact on pain, drug-related toxicity, and survival. *J Clin Oncol* 2003;21(14):2801-2802.

61. Meyerson BA. The role of neurosurgery in the treatment of cancer pain. *Acta Anaesthesiol Scand* 1982;74:109-113.

62. Macalusco C, Foley KM, Arbit E. Cordotomy for lumbosacral, pelvic and lower extremity pain of malignant origin: Safety and efficacy. *Neurology* 1988;38:110.

63. Weill A, Chiras J, Simon JM, et al. Spinal metastases: Indications for and results of percutaneous injection of acrylic surgical cement. *Radiology* 1996;199:241-247.

64. Cotton A, Boutry N, Cortet B, et al. Percutaneous vertebroplasty: State of the art. *Radiographics* 1998;18:311-322.

65. Goetz MP, Callstrom MR, Charboneau JW, et al. Percutaneous image-guided radiofrequency ablation of painful metastases involving bone: A multicenter study. *J Clin Oncol* 2004;22(2):300-306.

66. Stone P, Richards M, Hardy J. Fatigue in patients with cancer. *Eur J Cancer* 1998;34:1670-1676.

67. Jacobsen PB, Hann DM, Azzarello LM, et al. Fatigue in women receiving adjuvant chemotherapy for breast cancer: Characteristics, course, and correlates. *J Pain Sympt Mgt* 1999;18:233-242.

68. Cella D, Peterman A, Passik S, et al. Progress toward guidelines for the management of fatigue. *Oncology* 1998;12:369-377.

69. Portenoy RK, Itri LM. Cancer-related fatigue: Guidelines for evaluation and management. *Oncologist* 1999;4:1-10.

70. Demetri GD, Kris M, Wade J, et al. Quality of life benefit in chemotherapy patients treated with epoetin alfa is independent of disease response or tumor type: Results from a prospective community oncology study. *Oncology* 1998;16:3412-3425.

71. Bruera E, Roca E, Cedaro L, et al. Action of oral methylprednisolone in terminal cancer patients: A prospective randomized double-blind study. *Cancer Treat Rep* 1985;69:751-754.

72. Tannock I, Gospodarowicz M, Meakin W, et al. Treatment of metastatic prostate cancer with low dose prednisone: Evaluation of pain and quality of life as pragmatic indices of response. *J Clin Oncol* 1989;7:590-597.

73. Bruera E, Brenneis C, Paterson AH, et al. Use of methylphenidate as an adjuvant to narcotic analgesics in patients with advanced cancer. *J Pain Sympt Mgt* 1989;4:3-6.

74. Breitbart W, Mermelstein H. An alternative psychostimulant for the management of depressive disorders in cancer patients. *Psychosomatics* 1992;33:352-356.

75. Katon W, Raskind M. Treatment of depression in the medically ill elderly with methylphenidate. *Am J Psychiatry* 1980;137:963-965.

76. Rajagopal A, Vassilopoulou-Sellin R, Palmer JL, et al. Symptomatic hypogonadism in male survivors of cancer with chronic exposure to opioids. *Cancer* 2004;100(4):851-858.

77. Bruera E, Driver L, Barnes EA, et al. Patient-controlled methylphenidate for the management of fatigue in patients with advanced cancer: A preliminary report. *J Clin Oncol* 2003;23:4439-4443.

78. Wasserman K, Casaburi R. Dyspnea and physiological and athophysiological mechanisms. *Annu Rev Med* 1988;39:503-515.

79. Farncombe M. Dyspnea: Assessment and treatment. *Support Care Cancer* 1997;5:94-99.

80. Hardy JR, Turner R, Saunders M, et al. Prediction of survival in a hospital-based continuing care unit. *Eur J Cancer* 1994;30:284-288.

81. Escalante CP, Martin CG, Elting LS, et al. Dyspnea in cancer patients: Etiology, resource utilization, and survival. *Cancer* 1996;78:1314-1319.

82. Anthonisen NR. Long-term oxygen therapy. *Ann Intern Med* 1983;99:519-527.

83. Nocturnal Oxygen Therapy Trial Group. Continuous or nocturnal oxygen therapy in hypoxemic chronic obstructive lung disease. *Ann Intern Med* 1980;93:391-398.

84. Bruera E, De Stoutz N, Velasco-Leiva, et al. The effects of oxygen on the intensity of dyspnea in hypoxemic terminal cancer patients. *Lancet* 1993;342:13-14.

85. Bruera E, Scholler T, MacEachern T. Symptomatic benefit of supplemental oxygen in hypoxemic patients with terminal cancer: The use of the N of 1 randomized control trial. *J Pain Sympt Mgt* 1992;7:365-368.

86. Bruera E, MacEachern T, Ripamonti C, et al. Subcutaneous morphine for dyspnea in cancer patients. *Ann Intern Med* 1993;119:906-907.

87. Bruera E, MacMillan K, Pither J, et al. The effects of morphine on the dyspnea of terminal cancer patients. *J Pain Sympt Mgt* 1990;5:341-344.

88. Cohen MH, Johnston Anderson A, Krasnow SH, et al. Continuous intravenous infusion of morphine for severe dyspnea. *South Med J* 1991;84:229-234.

89. Davis CL, Hodder C, Love S, et al. Effect of nebulised morphine and morphine-6-glucuronide on exercise endurance in patients with chronic obstructive pulmonary disease. *Thorax* 1994;49:393.

90. Farncombe M, Chater S. Gillin A. The use of nebulized opioids for breathlessness: A chart review. *Palliat Med* 1994;8:306-312.

91. Farncombe M, Chater S. Clinical application of nebulized opioids for treatment of dyspnea in patients with malignant disease. *Support Care Cancer* 1994;2(3):184-187.

92. Zeppetella G. Nebulized morphine in the palliation of dyspnea. *Palliat Med* 1997;11(4):267-275.

93. Weir DC, Gove RI, Robertson AS, et al. Corticosteroids trials in nonasthmatic chronic airflow obstruction: A comparison of oral prednisolone and inhaled bechomethasone diproprionate. *Thorax* 1991;45:112-117.

94. Congleton J, Meurs MF. The incidence of airflow obstruction in bronchial carcinoma, its relation to breathlessness, and response to bronchodilator therapy. *Respir Med* 1995;89:291-296.

95. Neil PA, Morton PB, Stark RD. Chlorpromazine—A special effect on breathlessness? *Br J Clin Pharmacol* 1985;19:793-797.

96. Lipowski ZJ. Delirium (acute confusional states). *JAMA* 1987;258(13):1789-1792.

97. Rabins PV. Psychosocial and management aspects of delirium. *Int Psychogeriatr* 1991;3:319-324.

98. Derogatis LR, Morrow GR, Fetting J, et al. The prevalence of psychiatric disorders among cancer patients. *JAMA* 1983;249:751-757.

99. Levine PM, Silberfarb PM, Lipowski ZJ. Mental disorders in cancer patients: A study of 100 psychiatric referrals. *Cancer* 1978;42:1385-1391.

100. Stiefel F, Finsinger R, Bruera E. Acute confusional states in patients with advanced cancer. *J Pain Sympt Mgt* 1992; 7:94-98.

101. Lipowski ZJ. Delirium in the elderly patient. *N Engl J Med* 1989;320:578-582.

102. Liptzin B, Levkoff SE. An empirical study of delirium subtypes. *Br J Psychiatry* 1992;161:843-845.

103. American Psychiatric Association. *Diagnostic and Statistical Manual of Mental Disorders,* 4th ed. Washington, DC: American Psychiatric Association; 1994.

104. Hui D, Bush SH, Gallo LE, et al. Neuroleptic dose in the management of delirium in patients with advanced cancer. *J Pain Symptom Manage.* 2010;39(2):186-196.

105. Voruganti L, Cortese L, Owyeumi L, et al. Switching from conventional to novel antipsychotic drugs: Results of a prospective naturalistic study. *Schizophr Res* 2002;57(2-3):201-208.

106. Briebart W, Marotta R, Platt MM, et al. A double-blinded trial of haloperidol, chlorazepam, and lorazepam in the treatment of delirium in the hospitalized AIDS patients. *Am J Psychiatry* 1996;153:231-237.

107. Derogatis LR, Marrow GR, Fettig J, et al. The Prevalence of psychiatric disorders among cancer patients. *JAMA* 1983: 249;751-757.

108. Wilson KG, Chochinov HM, de Faye B, et al: Diagnosis and management of depression in palliative care. In: Chochinov HM, Breitbart W (eds): *Handbook of Psychiatry in Palliative Care.* Oxford, UK: Oxford University Press; 2000:25-49, 106.

109. Green AI, Austin PV. Psychopathology of pancreatic cancer: A psychobiologic probe. *Psychosomatics* 1993;34:208.

110. Massie MJ, Holland J. The cancer patient with pain: Psychiatric complications and their management. *Med Clin North Am* 1987;71:243.

111. American Psychiatric Association. *Diagnostic and Statistical Manual of Mental Disorders,* 4th ed. Washington, DC: American Psychiatric Association; 1994.

112. Fisch MJ, Loehrer PJ, Kristeller J, et al. Fluoxetine versus placebo in advanced cancer outpatients: A double-blinded trial of the Hoosier Oncology Group. *J Clin Oncol* 2003; 21(10):1937-1943.

113. Bonsignore M, Barkow K, Jessen F, et al. Validity of the five item WHO Well Being Index (WHO-5) in an elderly population. *Eur Arch Psychiatry Clin Neurosci* 2001;251(suppl 2): II27-II31.

114. Kroenke K, Spitzer RL, Williams JB. The PHQ-9: Validity of a brief depression severity measure. *J Gen Intern Med* 2001;16:606-613.

115. Hamilton M. A rating scale for depression. *J Neurol Neurosurg Psychiatry* 1960;23:56-62.

116. Montgomery S, Asberg MA. A new depression scale designed to be sensitive to change. *Br J Psychiatry* 1979;134:382-389.

117. Massie MJ, Popkin MK. Depressive disorders. In: Holland JC (ed): *Psycho-Oncology.* New York: Oxford University Press; 1998:518-540.

118. Holland JC, Morrow G, Schmale A, et al. Reduction of anxiety and depression in cancer patients by alprazolam or by a behavioural technique (abstr). *Proc Am Soc Clin Oncol* 1988;6:258.

119. Vickers AJ, Cassileth BR. Unconventional therapies for cancer and cancer-related symptoms (review). *Lancet Oncol* 2001;2(4):226-232.

120. Vaswani M, Linda FK, Ramesh S. Role of selective serotonin reuptake inhibitors in psychiatric disorders: A comprehensive review. *Prog Neuropsychopharmacol Biol Psychiatry* 2003;27(1):85-102.

121. Nierenberg AA, Papakostas GI, Petersen T, et al. Nortriptyline for treatment-resistant depression. *J Clin Psychiatry* 2003;64(1):35-39.

122. Pereira J, Bruera E. Depression with psychomotor retardation: Diagnostic challenges and the use of psychostimulants. *J Palliat Med* 2001;4(1):15-21.

123. Theobald DE, Kirsh KL, Holtsclaw E, et al. An open-label, crossover trial of mirtazapine (15 and 30 mg) in cancer patients with pain and other distressing symptoms. *J Pain Sympt Mgt* 2002;23(5):442-447.

124. Kast R. Mirtazapine may be useful in treating nausea and insomnia of cancer chemotherapy. *Support Care Cancer* 2001; 9(6):469-470.

125. Sykes NP. Constipation and diarrhoea. In: Doyle D, Hanks GWC, MacDonald N (eds): *Oxford Textbook of Palliative Medicine,* 2nd ed. Oxford, UK: Oxford University Press; 2001:513-526.

126. Mancini I, Bruera E. Constipation in advanced cancer patients. *Support Care Cancer* 1998;6:356-364.

127. Mercadante S. Diarrhea, malabsorption and constipation. In: Berger AM, Portenoy RK, Weismann DE (eds): *Principles and Practice of Supportive Oncology.* Philadelphia, PA: Lippincott-Raven; 1998:191-206.

128. Mercadante S, Casuccio A, Fulfaro F, et al. The course of symptom frequency and intensity in advanced "cancer patients followed at home. *J Pain Sympt Mgt* 2000;20:104-112.

129. Bruera E, Suarez-Almazor M, et al. The assessment of constipation in terminal cancer patients admitted to a palliative care unit: A retrospective review. *J Pain Sympt Mgt* 1994;9: 515-519.

130. Sykes NP. An investigation of the ability of oral naloxone to correct opioids-related constipation in patients with advanced cancer. *Palliat Med* 1996;10:135-144.

131. Latasch L, Zimmerman M, Eberhart B, et al. Oral naloxone antagonizes morphine-induced constipation. *Anesthetist* 1997; 46:191-194.

132. Meissner W, Schimdt U, Hartman M, et al. Oral naloxone reverses opioids-associated constipation. *Pain* 2000;84: 105-109.

133. Yuan CS, Foss JF, O'Connor M, et al. Methylnaltrexone for reversal of constipation due to chronic methadone use: A randomized controlled trial. *JAMA* 2000;283(3):367-372.

134. Stephenson J. Methylnaltrexone reverses opioid-induced constipation. *Lancet Oncol* 2002;3(4):202.

135. Thomas J, Karver S, Cooney GA, et al. Methylnaltrexone for Opioid-Induced Constipation in Advanced Illness. *N Engl J Med.* 2008;358(22):2332-2343.

136. Mannix KA. Palliation of nausea and vomiting. In: Doyle D, Hanks GWC, MacDonald N (eds): *Oxford Textbook of Palliative Medicine,* 2nd ed. Oxford, UK: Oxford University Press; 2001:489-499.

137. Elsayem A, Driver LC, Bruera E. *The MD Anderson Palliative Care Handbook.* Houston, TX: MD Anderson Cancer Center; 2002.

138. Bruera ED, Roca E, Cedaro L, et al. Improved control of chemotherapy-induced emesis by the addition of dexamethasone to metoclopramide in patients resistant to metoclopramide. *Cancer Treat Rep* 1983;67:381-383.

139. de Wit R, Herrstedt J, Rapoport B, et al. Addition of the oral NK1 antagonist aprepitant to standard antiemetics provides protection against nausea and vomiting during multiple cycles of cisplatin-based chemotherapy. *J Clin Oncol.* 2003;21(22): 4105-4111.

140. Mercadante S, Fulfaro F, Casuccio A. The use of corticosteroids in home palliative care. *Support Care Cancer* 2001; 9:386-389.

141. DeWys WD, Begg D, Lavin PT. Prognostic effect of weight loss prior to chemotherapy in cancer patients. *Am J Med* 1980;69:491-499.

142. Tisdale MJ. Loss of skeletal muscle in cancer: Biochemical mechanisms. *Front Biosci* 2001;6:164D-174D.

143. Belizario JE, Katz M, Chenker E, et al. Bioactivity of skeletal muscle proteolysis-inducing factors in the plasma proteins from cancer patients with weight loss. *Br J Cancer* 1991;63(5): 705-710.

144. Barber MD, Fearon KC, McMillan DC, et al. Liver export protein synthetic rates are increased by oral meal feeding in weight losing cancer patients. *Am J Physiol Endocrinol Metab* 2000;279:707E-E714E.

145. Sarhill N, Mahmoud FA, Christie R, et al. Assessment of nutritional status and fluid deficits in advanced cancer. *Am J Hosp Palliat Care* 2003;20(6):465-473.

146. Loprinzi CL, Ellison NM, Schaid DJ, et al. Phase III evaluation of four doses of megestrol acetate as therapy for patients with cancer anorexia and/or cachexia. *J Clin Oncol* 1993; 11:762-767.

147. Feliu J, Gonzales-Baron M, Berrocal A, et al. Usefulness of megestrol acetate in cancer cachexia and anorexia. *Am J Clin Oncol* 1992;15:436-440.

148. Popiela T, Lucchi R, Giongo F. Methylprednisolone as an appetite stimulant in patients with cancer. *Eur J Cancer Clin Oncol* 1989;25:1823-1829.

149. Wilcox J, Corr J, Shaw J, et al. Prednisolone as an appetite stimulant in patients with cancer. *Br Med J* 1984;27:288-290.

150. Sacks N, Hutcheson JR, Watts JM, et al. Case report: The effect of tetrahydrocannabinol on food intake during chemotherapy. *J Am Coll Nutr* 1990;9:630-632.

151. Bruera E, Neumann CM, Pituskin E, et al. Thalidomide in patients with cachexia due to terminal cancer: Preliminary report. *Ann Oncol* 1999;10:857-859.

152. Mulligan K, Schambelan M. Anabolic treatment with GH, IGF-I, or anabolic steroids in patients with HIV-associated wasting. *Int J Cardiol* 2002;85(1):151-159.

153. Bozzetti F, Gavazzi C, Ferrari P, et al. Effect of total parenteral nutrition on the protein kinetics of patients with cancer cachexia. *Tumori* 2000;86:408-411.

154. Mundy GR, Guise TA. Hypercalcemia of malignancy. *Am J Med* 1997;103:134-145.

155. Heys SD, Smith IC, Eremin O, et al. Hypercalcaemia in patients with cancer: Aetiology and treatment. *Eur J Surg Oncol* 1998;24:139-142.

156. Bower M, Brazil L, Coombes R. Endocrine and metabolic complications in advanced cancer. In: Doyle D, Hanks G, MacDonald N (eds): *Oxford Textbook of Palliative Medicine,* 2nd ed. Oxford, UK: Oxford University Press; 1998:709-712.

157. Bilezikian JP. Management of acute hypercalcemia. *N Engl J Med* 1992;326:1196-1203.

158. Bilezikian JP. Hypercalcemia. *Curr Ther Endocrinol Metab* 1994;5:511-514.

159. Kovacs CS, MacDonald SM, Chik CL, et al. Hypercalcemia of malignancy in the palliative care patient: A treatment strategy. *J Pain Sympt Mgt* 1995;10:224-232.

160. Riccardi A, Grasso D, Danova M. Bisphosphonates in oncology: Physiopathologic bases and clinical activity. *Tumori* 2003;89(3):223-236.

161. Gucalp R, Theriault R, Gill I, et al. Treatment of cancer-associated hypercalcemia. Double-blind comparison of rapid and slow intravenous infusion regimens of pamidronate disodium and saline alone. *Arch Intern Med* 1994;154: 1935-1944.

162. Neville-Webbe H, Coleman RE. The use of zoledronic acid in the management of metastatic bone disease and hypercalcaemia. *Palliat Med* 2003;17(6):539-553.

163. Ljunghall S. Use of clodronate and calcitonin in hypercalcemia due to malignancy. *Recent Results Cancer Res* 1989; 116:40-45.

164. Micetich KC, Steinecker PH, Thomasma DC, et al. Are intravenous fluids morally required for a dying patient? *Arch Intern Med* 1983;143:975-978.

165. Siegler M, Weisbard, AJ. Against the emerging stream. Should fluids and nutritional support be discontinued? *Arch Intern Med* 1985;145:129-131.

166. Hamdy RC, Braverman AM. Ethical conflicts in long-term care of the aged. *Br Med J* 1980;280:717.

167. Burge FI. Dehydration and provision of fluids in palliative care. What is the evidence? *Can Fam Physician* 1996;42: 2383-2388.

168. Twycross RG. Symptom control: The problem areas. *Palliat Med* 1993;7:1-8.

169. Andrews M, Bell ER, Smith SA, et al. Dehydration in terminally ill patients. Is it appropriate palliative care? *Postgrad Med* 1993;93:201-208.

170. Sullivan RJ Jr. Accepting death without artificial nutrition or hydration. *J Gen Intern Med* 1993;8:220-224.

171. Yan E, Bruera E. Parenteral hydration of terminally ill cancer patients. *J Palliat Care* 1991;7:40-43.

172. Fainsinger R, Bruera E. The management of dehydration in terminally ill patients. *J Palliat Care* 1994;10:55-59.

173. Berger EY. Nutrition by hypodermoclysis. *J Am Geriatr Soc* 1984;32:199-203.

174. Bruera E, Legris MA, Kuehn N, et al. Hypodermoclysis for the administration of fluids and narcotic analgesics in patients with advanced cancer. *J Pain Sympt Mgt* 1990;5: 218-220.

175. Hays H. Hypodermaclysis for symptom control in terminal cancer. *Can Fam Physician* 1985;31:1253-1256.

176. Fainsinger RL, MacEachern T, Miller MJ, et al. The use of hypodermoclysis for rehydration in terminally ill cancer patients. *J Pain Sympt Mgt* 1994;9:298-302.

177. Constans T, Dutertre JP, Froge E. Hypodermoclysis in dehydrated elderly patients: Local effects with and without hyaluronidase. *J Palliat Care* 1991;7:1012.

178. Cousins N. How patients appraise physicians. *N Engl J Med* 1985;313:1422-1424.

179. Ley P, Bradshaw PW, Kincey JA, et al. Increasing patients' satisfaction with communications. *Br J Soc Clin Psychol* 1976;15:403-413.

180. Kristjanson LJ. Quality of terminal care: Salient indicators identified by families. *J Palliat Care* 1989;5:21-30.

181. Kaplan SH, Greenfield S, Ware JE Jr, et al. Assessing the effects of physician-patient interactions on the outcomes of chronic disease. *Med Care* 1989;27:110S-127S.

182. Houts PS, Yasko JM, Harvey HA, et al. Unmet needs of persons with cancer in Pennsylvania during the period of terminal care. *Cancer* 1988;62:627-634.

183. Saunders JM, McCorkle R. Models of care for persons with progressive cancer. *Nurs Clin North Am* 1985;20:365-377.

184. Maguire P. Barriers to psychological care of the dying. *Br Med J (Clin Res Ed)* 1985;291:1711-1713.

185. Hockley JM, Dunlop R, Davies RJ, et al. Survey of distressing symptoms in dying patients and their families in hospital and the response to a symptom control team. *Br Med J (Clin Res Ed)* 1988;296:1715-1717.

186. Maguire P. Barriers to psychological care of the dying. *Br Med J (Clin Res Ed)* 1985;291:1711-1713.

187. Buckman R. Breaking bad news: Why is it still so difficult? *Br Med J (Clin Res Ed)* 1984;288:1597-1599.

188. Weissman DE. Consultation in palliative medicine. *Arch Intern Med* 1997;157:733-737.

189. McCormick TR, Conley BJ. Patients' perspectives on dying and on the care of dying patients. *West J Med* 1995;163:236-243.

190. Lind SE, DelVecchio-Good MJ, et al. Telling the diagnosis of cancer. *J Clin Oncol* 1989;7:583-589.

191. Christakis NA, Iwashyna TJ. Attitude and self-reported practice regarding prognostication in a national sample of internists. *Arch Intern Med* 1998;158:2389-2395.

192. Christakis NA. Predicting patient survival before and after hospice enrollment. *Hosp J* 1998;13:71-87.

193. Parkes CM. Accuracy of predictions of survival in later stages of cancer. *Br Med J* 1972;2:29-31.

194. Novack DH, Plumer R, Smith RL, et al. Changes in physicians' attitudes toward telling the cancer patient. *JAMA* 1979;241:897-900.

195. Sell L, Devlin B, Bourke, SJ, et al. Communicating the diagnosis of lung cancer. *Respir Med* 1993;87:61-63.

196. Chan A, Woodruff RK. Communicating with patients with advanced cancer. *J Palliat Care* 1997;13:29-33.

197. Seale C. Communication and awareness about death: A study of a random sample of dying people. *Soc Sci Med* 1991;32:943-952.

198. Peter JR, Abrams HE, Ross DM, et al. Presenting a diagnosis of cancer: Patients' views. *J Fam Pract* 1991;32:577-581.

199. Girgis A, Sanson-Fisher RW. Breaking bad news: Consensus guidelines for medical practitioners. *J Clin Oncol* 1995;13:2449-2456.

200. Ptacek JT, Eberhardt TL. Breaking bad news: A review of the literature. *JAMA* 1996;276:496-502.

Long-Term
Survival

PEDIATRIC LONG-TERM FOLLOW-UP

Joann L. Ater
Norman Jaffe
Nita R. Burrer

■ LATE EFFECTS OF CHILDHOOD CANCER AND CANCER TREATMENTS—A GUIDE FOR THE COMMUNITY PROVIDER

The community health care provider will at some point be faced with caring for a survivor of childhood cancer. This may be episodic care or follow-up care for the cancer and treatment. Approximately 1 of every 250 persons living in the United States today has been diagnosed or will be diagnosed with cancer before the age of 20. Prior to 1960, nearly all children diagnosed with cancer died of their disease. Since 1960, however, due to innovative and combined treatment modalities, the rate of survival for childhood cancers has been climbing rapidly. Current estimates are that 80% of all patients diagnosed with cancer who are less than 20 years of age will now be cured. However, many will suffer long-term health sequelae of their cancer and treatment (1-4). This represents a rapidly growing group of individuals who have survived both their cancer and their cancer treatment; currently it is estimated to comprise about 328,600 individuals in the United States (1-4). Many of these patients are followed in one of the 145 clinics, located in the United States and Canada, identified by the Children's Oncology Group (COG) Late-Effects Directory of Services (www.childrensoncologygroup.org). However, many of the 328,600 living survivors of childhood cancer are followed by pediatric practitioners, family practice practitioners, general practitioners, internists, or health clinics at colleges or universities. These practitioners may have little or no experience in managing late effects of childhood cancer and cancer treatment or in addressing cancer survivorship issues.

Over the last 30 years, researchers have identified many potential late effects of childhood cancer and the treatments. Based on this research, the Long-Term Follow-Up Guidelines were developed by committees of experts in the COG. These guidelines were developed as a resource of clinicians who provide ongoing health care to survivors of pediatric malignancies. While these guidelines are written primarily for pediatric oncologists who are familiar with the long-term follow-up needs of this population, they can also assist the community physician. The ideal care is a partnership between the original treating center and the community physicians. Most Long-Term Follow-Up Clinics now try to provide a "Passport for Care" that summarizes the patient's treatment and recommendations for follow-up care (5).

The first intervention for the community physician when managing the long-term survivor of childhood cancer is to obtain an accurate cancer diagnosis, a complete treatment history, a family history of cancer, and information on any known existing late effects. It is often necessary to contact the physician or institution where the child received either treatment or previous late-effect surveillance. The patient and his or her family may or may not be accurate historians; therefore, it is extremely important to obtain copies of the pathology report and treatment record. Communication with the attending oncologist or a copy of the Passport for Care may be invaluable. Only by being aware of the diagnosis, treatments, and family history can proper surveillance be performed (6-9). Late effects of childhood cancer and cancer treatments will vary from patient to patient on the basis of age at the time of diagnosis, treatment regimen, and the patient's underlying genetic predisposition (6). Late effects may be divided into four categories, as outlined below.

The first and most serious late effect is relapse of the original disease either at the primary site or as metastatic disease. The second category of late effect is the development of a treatment-related or genetically induced second primary cancer. The third category of late effects comprises what is generally referred to as treatment effects that persist long after the cancer has been controlled and all treatment has been stopped. The fourth category of late effects is related not to the physiology or biology of the cancer or treatment but rather to the social arena of insurance, employment, adjustment, and physical or esthetic impairment.

■ OVERVIEW OF CHILDHOOD CANCERS

The peak age of cancer incidence in children occurs in early childhood. Infantile cancer is associated with a poor survival rate of about 35% (10). During the childhood and adolescent years, survival rates improve dramatically, approaching 60 to 90%, depending on the type of cancer. The most common type of cancer diagnosed during infancy and childhood is leukemia, followed by lymphoma, malignancies of the central nervous system, neuroblastoma, and Wilms tumor. Cancers in the adolescent are associated with a 77% survival rate, with the most common cancer being Hodgkin disease, followed closely by germ cell tumors.

■ OVERVIEW OF SURVEILLANCE

Generally, patients off active therapy should be followed every 4 to 6 months until the risk of relapse, recurrence, or development of metastatic lesions is minimal. This is usually considered to be 2 to 5 years after treatment has been completed. Normally, the treating oncologist will provide this care. Once the risk of recurrence, relapse, or development of metastasis is minimal,

the patients should be followed yearly for 5 more years and then every 1 to 2 years indefinitely. If late effects are present, then the schedule should be adjusted to accommodate the symptomatology. Should the survivor have children, an opportunity to determine that the offspring are normal and healthy should also be provided.

During the first visit in long-term follow-up, the practitioner should obtain the following information if not already known:

1. Date of diagnosis, diagnosis, stage, grade, site, relapses, and previously diagnosed late effects
2. All treatments received for cancer, including
   a. Chemotherapy: type, route, schedule of administration, and total cumulative doses
   b. Radiation history, including type of field, total dose, and number of fractions
   c. All surgical procedures, including amputation, resection, central access line, and temporary interventions (eg, gastrostomy)
   d. History of blood transfusions and/or blood products
   e. Complication of treatment

SURVEILLANCE FOR RECURRENCE, METASTASIS, AND SECOND PRIMARY NEOPLASM

The most serious late effect is the possibility of recurrence of the primary tumor or the late development of a metastatic lesion. Generally, the oncologist should follow the patient until the likelihood of metastasis, relapse, or recurrence has passed. However, this is not always the case; in fact, the community physician may very well be called on to do disease surveillance during the time of high likelihood of relapse or recurrence. Surveillance during this time should continue with the same testing or diagnostic tools previously used by the oncologist to follow the disease.

Minimally in follow-up, all long-term survivors of childhood cancer who have had chemotherapy should have a yearly hemogram (complete blood count, including differential and platelet count); renal, hepatic, and metabolic profiles; and a urinalysis. For patients with a history of lymphoma, the practitioner providing surveillance should continue previously established methods of investigation for possible recurrence within the first 5 years from diagnosis. These include computed tomography, magnetic resonance imaging, or plain films. Surveillance in patients with a history of a solid tumor should include a chest x-ray to identify metastatic disease (particularly with the sarcomas). For leukemia patients, bone marrow aspiration and lumbar punctures are not indicated for routine surveillance unless there are symptoms of a relapse. Patients who had tumors with markers should continue to have blood drawn to test for those markers (eg, human chorionic gonadotropin, carcinoembryonic antigen, erythrocyte sedimentation rate, etc). Radiographic examination of previously radiated sites should be obtained at 2- to 3-year intervals to identify changes and detect early evidence of any second radiation-induced malignancy.

The previously mentioned Children's Oncology Group's (COG) Long-Term Follow-up Guidelines which are readily available from COG and on its Web site at http://www.childrensoncologygroup.org/disc/LE/default.htm are risk-based guidelines for identifying late effects of therapy and do not provide recommendations for surveillance for primary cancer. Recommendations for surveillance for recurrence of primary cancer should be provided by the original treating pediatric oncologist and ideally included in the patient's Passport for Care that is given to the patient and community physician at the time of the transfer of care.

SURVEILLANCE FOR SPECIFIC LATE EFFECTS RELATED TO TREATMENT MODALITIES

Two-thirds of adult survivors of childhood cancer have at least one chronic health condition and 27% have had a severe condition (grade 3 or 4) related to the previous cancer or treatment. The most common severe and life-threatening (grade 3 and 4) chronic health conditions identified in the national Childhood Cancer Survivor Study (CCSS) were in order of decreasing incidence: major joint replacement, congestive heart failure, second malignant neoplasm, cognitive dysfunction, coronary artery disease, cerebrovascular accident, renal failure, hearing loss, legal blindness or loss of eye, and ovarian failure (4). The goal of surveillance for late effects is to identify and treat them early before they become serious.

Surgery

Most of the surgical late effects are obvious: a missing limb or (known) missing organ. The practitioner should be alert to changes within the surgical site or scar that may require revision or biopsy. The practitioner may also be called on to write a prescription for a prosthesis, assist the patient in acquiring disability documentation and a handicap parking permit, provide a letter to excuse the patient from military service, or initiate an occupational intervention for special needs or other equally obvious physical needs. Prior surgical intervention may also be responsible for surgical menopause, sterility, blindness, hypothyroidism, cognitive impairment, and so on. Secondary problems related to surgical intervention (eg, oophorectomy and premature menopause) include bone loss, osteopenia and osteoporosis, and loss of fertility. In patients who had abdominal surgery, the risk of bowel obstruction due to adhesions continues for many years.

Patients who have had a splenectomy or spleen ablative therapy should be placed on a prophylactic antibiotic, usually penicillin or erythromycin. They should receive prompt medical attention and antibiotics for suspected bacterial febrile illnesses. Pneumococcal vaccine to prevent pneumococcal pneumonia should be given routinely. The generally accepted immunizations schedule for pneumococcal vaccine is every 5 years. Patients who have no functioning spleen should also be vaccinated against hepatitis B and flu and should also receive other routine vaccinations. Finally, patients without functioning spleens should be protected from animal and mosquito bites and should wear a medical alert bracelet identifying them as "asplenic" (11).

Chemotherapy

Long-term and late effects of chemotherapy include damage to the heart, liver, kidneys, lungs, and bone marrow.

Heart

It is widely known that anthracyclines may damage the heart. In view of this, some oncologists administer these drugs over a longer infusion period and limit the total cumulative dose (2,12). In children, cardiotoxicity increases rapidly at a cumulative dose in excess of 450 mg/m^2, but certain individual patients, exquisitely sensitive to this drug, may develop cardiotoxicity at a lower dose. Increased risk factors for anthracycline cardiotoxicity includes younger age (<5 years), larger dose, short infusion period, and possibly malnutrition or undernutrition with altered body habitus for age (12,13). Coadministration of other cardiotoxic drugs (eg, cyclophosphamide or ifosfamide) may also be a factor. Mediastinal radiation may also injure the heart.

The following is a brief list of the major late cardiac complications, which may occur following treatment with the anthracyclines and/or cardiac radiation:

- Congestive heart failure
- Pericardial effusion

- Constrictive pericarditis
- Coronary artery disease
- Myocardial infarction
- Arrythmias

The cardiotoxic effects may become apparent only in later years. Patients who are at risk of developing cardiac toxicity should be monitored yearly for heart problems, preferably with an echocardiogram. Plain chest films and electrocardiograms are also useful. Initially, patients, particularly females, may appear asymptomatic, but they can decompensate rapidly when the body is under stress, as in pregnancy. These patients should be instructed to inform the gynecologist that they may be at risk of developing complications during pregnancy. They should be monitored throughout the pregnancy and the postpartum period for cardiac decompensation. Generally a knowledgeable obstetrician is recommended for such patients.

Rigorous exercise and exercise programs that involve lifting heavy weights should be avoided. Otherwise, physical activity need not be limited unless symptoms are present or there is a decrease in the ejection fraction greater than 10% from baseline. A cardiologist experienced in cardiomyopathy related to anthracyclines should be consulted for symptomatology suggestive of heart failure or a significant change in the ejection fraction. (2,13). Survivors should be encouraged to have a healthy lifestyle with exercise and healthy diet to prevent other known risk factors for cardiovascular disease such as obesity and hyperlipidemia.

Liver

Many chemotherapeutic agents can also place the survivor at the risk of hepatic damage—specifically but not limited to methotrexate, 6-mercaptopurine, and busulfan. Concomitant oncologic therapy with administration of hepatotoxic drugs should be avoided or used minimally if possible. Yearly liver function tests and liver biopsies, if indicated, are necessary to assess the integrity of the liver. Because of blood product administration, cancer patients are also at risk for hepatitis C infection; at some point, therefore, posttreatment testing should be done. These patients should also be immunized for hepatitis B infection. Alcohol and large doses of acetaminophen should be avoided.

Lungs

Busulfan produces diffuse pulmonary fibrosis. A chest x-ray will reveal diffuse interstitial and intra-alveolar infiltrates. These may appear at any time after treatment. This sequelum is associated with progressive deterioration in lung function; commonly called a "busulfan lung," it may also be seen with cyclophosphamide.

Bleomycin may also damage lung tissue. The first indication of lung damage is inspiratory rales, followed by a decrease in oxygen diffusion capacity. Pulmonary function studies will reveal a diffuse interstitial fibrosis, restrictive pulmonary disease, and arterial hypoxemia. A chest x-ray will show a pattern of diffuse interstitial fibrosis with patchy basilar infiltrates. A lung biopsy will show an atypical alveolar cell and fibrinous exudate. A hilar membrane may be present during the acute stage. In the chronic stage, there is diffuse interstitial and intra-alveolar fibrosis (2).

Gonads

Many chemotherapeutic drugs have the potential to cause gonadal failure or impairment. The alkylating agents, particularly cyclophosphamide and ifosfamide, can cause damage to the testes, resulting in sterility or lack of production of testosterone. The risk is greater in the pubescent male. There may also be damage to the ovaries in the pubescent female. This may result in infertility, lack of estrogen, and premature menopause. Patients who received cyclophosphamide or ifosfamide should be evaluated for gonadal failure, loss of testosterone or estrogen, and infertility. This may manifest itself as delayed puberty, amenorrhea, absence of secondary sexual characteristics, and growth retardation in addition to infertility. Levels of follicle-stimulating hormone, luteinizing hormone, and insulin-like growth factor should be determined, semen analysis performed, and a testosterone or estrogen level obtained. In addition, the left wrist should be measured to determine bone age. If the ovaries or testes are damaged due to lack of estrogen or testosterone, there will be impairment of the osteoblastic and osteoclastic processes in addition to infertility. Careful screening to assess osteopenia or osteoporosis may be required (2,14). If there is an indication of gonadal insufficiency, hormone replacement should be instituted. The community practitioner may consult an endocrinologist in managing hormone replacement.

Although cyclophosphamide and ifosfamide may result in infertility, it is never advisable to inform the long-term survivor that infertility is "absolute," since conception may occasionally still occur (2,14). A referral to a fertility expert is always indicated if pregnancy is desired. Several conceptions achieved by "infertile" long-term survivors, both male and female, have been reported. Contraception should always be encouraged when a pregnancy is not a desired outcome of intercourse.

Brain radiation that affects the pituitary gland can also cause gonadal failure.

Kidney

Cisplatin is extremely toxic to the kidneys and may cause lifelong renal insufficiency or frank failure. Assessment of renal function should be routine in patients who have received cisplatin. (It may also cause hearing impairment.)

An outline of several frequently utilized chemotherapeutic agents and their related side effects is presented in Table 49-1. The list is not exhaustive but covers the more common important side effects as well as recommendations for investigation and guidance.

TABLE 49-1	CHEMOTHERAPY FOR LATE EFFECTS		
Chemotherapy Drug	**Target Organ**	**Testing**	**Instruction to Patient**
Actinomycin D	Liver	Chemistry profile, LFT	
Doxorubicin Daunomycin Idarubicin	Heart	Echocardiogram, ECG, CXR, cardiology consult if heart function is abnormal	Consult high-risk obstetrician for pregnancy. Obtain medical clearance prior to beginning a weight-lifting program or a strenuous exercise program. Provide information on cumulative anthracycline dose prior to any surgery or during pregnancy.
Cisplatin	Kidneys	Chemistry profile, electrolytes, urinalysis	Check auditory and kidney function.
Carboplatin	Hearing	Audiogram	Patient may need hearing aid.
	Urinary bladder	Chemistry profile, electrolytes	Kidney function may be vulnerable.
Cyclophosphamide Ifosfamide	Urinary bladder Kidneys	Urinalysis	
	Ovaries	Pelvic examination (female) FSH, LH, estradiol	Infertility may be a problem, especially if patient is male.
	Testes	Sperm count FSH, LH, testosterone If gonadal failure, bone-density scan	
Dacarbazine	Liver	Chemistry profile, LFT	
L-Asparaginase Peg-asparaginase	Liver (rare) Pancreas (rare)	Chemistry profile, LFT	
Methotrexate	Liver	Chemistry profile, LFT	
Nitrogen mustard	Ovaries	Pelvic examination (female), FSH, LH, estradiol, sperm count, FSH, LF, testosterone	Infertility may be a problem, especially if patient is male. Patient may need hormone replacement.
	Testes	If gonadal failure, bone-density scan	
Procarbazine	Liver Kidneys	Chemistry profile, electrolytes, urinalysis, monitor blood pressure regularly	Infertility may be a problem, especially if patient is male. Patient may need hormone replacement.
	Ovaries	Pelvic examination (female) LH, FSH, estradiol	
	Testes	Sperm count, FSH, LF, testosterone If gonadal failure, bone-density scan	
6-Mercaptopurine 6-Thioguanine	Liver	Chemistry profile, LFT	
Vincristine	Liver	Chemistry profile, LFT	
Velban/VP-16	Bone marrow	Hemogram	
Intrathecal chemotherapy	Cognitive impairment	MRI of brain, neuropsychological testing	Cognitive remediation.

CXR, chest x-ray; ECG, electrocardiogram; FSH, follicle-stimulating hormone; LFT, liver function test; LH, luteinizing hormone; MRI, magnetic resonance imaging.

Radiation

The younger the patient when the radiation is administered, the greater the damage that can occur (14). The following is an outline of radiation-induced sequelae, which may affect various sites organs and systems.

Head and Neck

Radiation to the head and neck will cause growth retardation of the involved area. If radiation is administered to the eyes, the bitemporal diameter will be reduced. Radiation administered to the brain may result in a small head. If the pituitary is involved, it may cause absent or delayed sexual maturity, thyroid insufficiency, hypopituitary dwarfism, and diabetes insipidus. These patients preferably should be managed with the assistance of an endocrinologist.

With nasopharyngeal radiation there may be extensive damage to the teeth, mandible and maxillary ridge, sinus cavities, and structures of the mouth and nasopharynx. Vision and hearing may also be affected. Dental radiation predisposes the patient to caries, abnormal tooth growth, and destruction of the hard and soft palates. Dry eyes and skin damage may also occur. Sinus infections may be a major problem. Care must be taken with all dental procedures: hyperbaric oxygen pre- and post-treatment may be required.

Radiation involving the neck affects the thyroid. Careful attention must be paid to the thyroid gland throughout the lifespan looking for a secondary cancer and for hypo- or hyperthyroidism. Damage to the muscles and vascular structures of the neck may occur and patency of the carotid arteries may be affected.

Musculoskeletal Sequelae

- Chest growth disturbances (40% of survivors)
- 70 to 80% of late sequelae
- 15 to 20 Gy results in growth abnormalities
- Growing bone tolerates <20 Gy (likely 15-18 Gy)
- Decreased height, most apparent in children treated at <6 years of age or during adolescence (when fastest growth is occurring)
- Significant scoliosis is uncommon with <35 Gy to spine
- Muscular hypoplasia is common
- Decreased long bone length due to treatment of epiphyseal growth plates
- Delayed or arrested tooth development with >45 to 50 Gy to the mandible

Radiation to the chest may damage the heart, large vessels, and lung. Careful attention must be paid to lung function, cardiac output, and electrical activity of the heart. An echocardiogram, electrocardiogram, and occasionally pulmonary function testing should be performed as follow-up for such patients.

Central Nervous System Sequelae

- Seizures
- Learning disabilities
- Hearing loss (inner ear tolerance is approximately 45 Gy)
- Cognitive dysfunction
- Neuropsychologic dysfunction

Endocrine Sequelae

- Most sensitive to least sensitive: GH > TSH > ACTH > FSH/LH
- Hypothalamus is more sensitive than the pituitary
- 30 Gy results in 30% incidence of decreased GH levels in children

Fertility

- Ovary: 8-9 Gy results in sterility. Older females are more sensitive than younger girls.
- Testicle: 1.5 Gy results in decreased sperm count. Four to six Gy results in complete azospermia. Twenty-four Gy results in decreased testosterone; younger males are more sensitive than men.

Back

Patients who have received radiation to the upper back may also experience damage to the involved area, lungs, and heart; the follow-up care should be the same as for chest radiation. The practitioner should examine adolescents and young adults who have been radiated for a unilateral Wilms tumor and for scoliosis.

Abdomen and/or Pelvis

Radiation involving the abdomen or pelvis may damage organs within the radiation field. Secondary damage may occur from malfunctioning or nonfunctioning organs. If the ovaries are damaged, in addition to infertility, there will be impairment of the osteoblastic and osteoclastic processes because of the lack of estrogen. As described earlier, screening should be implemented for osteopenia or osteoporosis. Fibrosis of the genitourinary tract may occur. This may cause a hydronephrosis, small urinary bladder, and frank kidney damage. If the radiation port involved the femoral arteries, stenosis may develop. Radionecrosis of the femoral head and neck may also occur. Patients treated with prior radiation to the spleen must be treated similarly to those who have undergone surgical splenectomy.

Extremity

Radiation to extremities may result in deformity and growth retardation of the affected limb. All structures, including skin, in the radiation field will be affected. Follow-up care must address skin changes as well as risk of secondary bone or soft tissue cancers.

Miscellaneous Sequelae

- Retinopathy (at >30-50 Gy)
- Secondary tumors
- Skin

Psychosocial Sequelae

Long-term cancer survivors may be subjected to employment discrimination and recruitment into the military forces. An increased incidence of suicide ideation has been reported (15). The possibility of tumor recurrence or development of a new tumor remains a constant threat. However, overall, most survivors are psychologically healthy and report satisfaction with their lives. However, certain groups of childhood cancer survivors are at high risk for psychologic distress, neurocognitive dysfunction, and poor health-related quality of life (HRQOL), especially in physical domains. Risk factors for psychologic distress and poor HRQOL are female sex, lower educational attainment, unmarried status, annual household income less than $20,000, unemployment, lack of health insurance, presence of a major medical condition, and treatment with cranial radiation and/or surgery. Interventions are needed for groups at highest risk for adverse outcomes. Further study of the positive growth that remains despite the trauma of childhood cancer is also needed (16).

■ SUMMARY

Providing surveillance of the sequelae of disease and treatment to the survivor of childhood cancer is a complicated process optimally performed at a comprehensive cancer center by health care providers well versed in follow-up surveillance. If the community physician provides the follow-up care, either episodic or continuing,

there must be a basic understanding of the natural history of the cancer and treatment. Knowledge of the late effects of the disease and the treatments will also help provide psychosocial support to the patient.

References

1. Mariotto AB, Rowland JH, Yabroff KR, et al. Long-term survivors of childhood cancers in the United States. *Cancer Epidemiol Biomarkers Prev* 2009;18:1033-1040.
2. Diller L, Chow EJ, Gurney JG, et al. Chronic disease in the Childhood Cancer Survivor Study cohort: A review of published findings. *J Clin Oncol* 2009;27:2339-2355.
3. Hudson MM, Mertens AC, Yasui, et al. Health status of adult long-term survivors of childhood cancer: A report from the Childhood Cancer survivor Study. *JAMA* 2003;290:1583-1592.
4. Oeffinger KC, Mertens AC, Sklar CA, et al. Chronic health conditions in adult survivors of childhood cancer. *N Engl J Med* 2006;355:1572-1582.
5. Horowitz ME, Fordis M, Krause S, et al. Passport for Care: Implementing the survivorship care plan. *J Oncol Practice* 2009;5:110-112.
6. Bhatia S, Constine LS. Late morbidity after successful treatment of children with cancer. *Cancer J* 2009;15(3): 174-180.
7. Kadan-Lottick NS, Robison LL, Gurney GA, et al. Childhood cancer survivors knowledge about their past diagnosis and treatment. *JAMA* 2002;287:1832-1839.
8. Dickerman JD. The late effects of childhood cancer therapy. *Pediatrics* 2007;119(3):554-568.
9. Plon SE, Malkin D. Childhood cancer and heredity. In: Pizzo PA, Poplack DG (eds): *Principles and Practice of Pediatric Oncology*, 5th ed. Philadelphia, PA: Lippincott, Williams & Wilkins; 2006:14-37.
10. Gurney JC, Bondy M. Epidemiology of childhood cancer. In: Pizzo PA, Poplack DG (eds): *Principles and Practice of Pediatric Oncology*, 5th ed. Philadelphia, PA: Lippincott, Williams & Wilkins; 2006:1-13.
11. American Academy of Pediatrics. Section 1. Active and passive Immunization: Immunocompromised children. In: Pickering LK (ed): *2009 Red Book: Report of the Committee on Infectious Disease*, 28th ed. Elk Grove Village, IL: American Academy of Pediatrics; 2009:72-86.
12. Shankar SM, Marina N, Hudson MM, et al. Monitoring for cardiovascular disease in survivors of childhood cancer: Report from the Cardiovascular Disease Task Force of the Children's Oncology Group. *Pediatrics* 2008;121:e387-396.
13. Gianni L, Herman E, Lipshultz S, et al. Anthracycline cardiotoxicity: From bench to bedside. *J Clin Oncol* 2008;26: 3777-3784.
14. Nandagopal R, Laverdière C, Mulrooney D, et al. Endocrine late effects of childhood cancer therapy: A report from the Children's Oncology Group. *Horm Res* 2008;69(2):65-74.
15. Recklitis CJ, Lockwood RA, Rothwell MA, et al. Suicidal ideation and attempts in adult survivors of childhood cancer. *J Clin Oncol* 2006;24;3852-3857.
16. Zeltzer LK, Recklitis C, Buchbinder D, et al. Psychological status in childhood cancer survivors: A report from the childhood cancer survivor study. *J Clin Oncol* May 10 2009;27(14): 2396-2404.

■ RESOURCES

Childhood Cancer Survivor Long-Term Follow-Up Guidelines, Version 3.0, Children's Oncology Group. Available at: http://www.childrensoncologygroup.org/disc/LE/default.htm. Accessed February 03, 2010.

Cancer Reference Information. ACS 2009. Available at: http://www.cancer.org/docroot/cri/content/cri_2_6x_late_ effects_of_childhood_cancer.asp. Accessed February 03, 2010.

Late Effects of Treatment for Childhood Cancer. Available at: http://www.cancer.gov/cancertopics/pdq/treatment/lateeffects/ HealthProfessional/page2. Accessed February 03, 2010.

The Childhood Cancer Survivor Study. Available at: http://ccss.stjude.org/published-research. Accessed February 03, 2010.

ADULT LONG-TERM FOLLOW-UP

Pamela N. Schultz
Charles J. Stava
Mouhammad Amir Habra
Rena Vassilopoulou-Sellin

CANCER SURVIVOR PREVALENCE AND/OR INCIDENCE

The population of cancer survivors, which numbered over 11 million in 2006 (1), continues to grow as "baby boomers" reach a cancer-prone age (increasing the annual incidence of new cases) and as cancer patients survive longer (increasing the prevalence of cancer survivors).

LITERATURE REVIEW

According to the National Institute of Health's Surveillance, Epidemiology, and End Results (SEER) *Cancer Statistics 1975-2006,* there has been an increase in 5-year relative survival rates; in 1954 the 5-year survival rate for all cancer sites was 35%, but by 2005 this figure had increased to 69.1% (2). Obviously survival rates are dependent on cancer site and the 5-year relative survival rate is not correlated with cancer incidence as illustrated in Table 50-1.

LATE EFFECTS OF CANCER

There has been a gradual appreciation that the life trajectory of individuals diagnosed and treated for cancer can extend far beyond the often limited duration of active therapy. Indeed, both the national Coalition for Cancer Survivorship (NCCS) established in 1986 and the Office of Cancer Survivorship (OCS) established in 1995 have served to highlight the importance of life after cancer treatment. For many malignancies, cancer is now considered a chronic condition with prolonged life expectancy occasionally punctuated by intervals of disease reactivation requiring treatment but also with need to monitor lifelong for the detection and management of potential cancer-related late effects.

Efforts are increasingly directed toward understanding the long-term impact of cancer and cancer therapy, especially as they might affect the quality of life of cancer survivors. There is a robust collection of literature addressing the psychosocial late effects of cancer in survivors of childhood and adult cancers. However, information regarding the lasting medical late effects of cancer and cancer therapy remains limited.

TABLE 50-1	INCIDENCE AND 5-YEAR SURVIVAL RATE BY SPECIFIC CANCER SITE	
Cancer Site	Age-Adjusted Incidence per 100,000 US Population	Survival (%)
Hodgkin lymphoma	2.8	86.0
Testis	5.3	96.6
Cervix	8.0	71.9
Lymphocytic leukemia	3.8	78.8
Brain	6.5	36.2
Oral cavity and pharynx	10.3	61.2
Exocrine pancreas	11.3	5.2
Kidney	14.5	68.0
Non-Hodgkin lymphoma	2.8	86.0
Colorectal	48.2	67.4
Lung	67.6	15.6
Breast	63.8	89.8
Prostate	142.1	100.0

Data from Horner MJ, Ries LAG, Krapcho M, et al (eds). SEER Cancer Statistics Review, 1975-2006. http://seer.cancer.gov/csr/1975_2006/. Updated January 28, 2010. Accessed February 25, 2010.

Several investigators have addressed the presence and complexity of lasting medical effects of cancer throughout the adult lives of childhood cancer survivors (3-5). Stevens et al. (6) reported that 58% of survivors had at least one chronic health problem and 32% had two or more, including second primary cancers. Much less is known about the lasting medical impact of cancer treatment in survivors of adult-onset cancers. Investigators addressing the physiologic late effects of adult cancers (7,8) highlight the paucity of information but emphasize that they are aware that multiple systems are often affected. For example, pelvic surgery can impair fertility, and splenectomy increases susceptibility to bacterial infections. Certain chemotherapy agents and regimens can compromise the health of the cardiac, pulmonary, genitourinary, endocrine, and neurologic systems. Radiotherapy may potentiate these complications and also impair skeletal development and dental health in addition to contributing to the risk of second primary cancers. Combined treatments can increase the number and severity of medical late effects.

Recently attention has been directed toward the impact of cancer treatment on long-term survivors, particularly as it concerns quality of life. In recognition of the challenges facing cancer survivors, the Institute of Medicine and the National Research Council released recommendations for long-term follow-up care and research in this field (9). Several investigators have begun to characterize the physiologic and psychosocial health profiles of survivors of childhood cancers and the psychosocial profiles of survivors of adult cancers. However, there remains a stark paucity of data regarding the physiologic health profile of survivors of adult cancers.

DEFINITION OF *SURVIVOR*

Further complicating the understanding of the impact of cancer treatment on long-term survivors is how one defines the term *survivor*. Survivors groups have emphasized that one who is diagnosed with cancer is a "survivor" from the onset of the diagnosis. How does one differentiate the cancer survivor being treated for active disease from the survivor who has been treated and is free of disease? Traditionally, one's 5-year anniversary after a diagnosis of cancer has been designated an important milestone in survival. Inherent problems exist with this arbitrary definition and the definition could be different based on the underlying malignancy.

■ "LIFE AFTER CANCER CARE" PROGRAM AND SURVIVORSHIP CLINICS

Cancer survivors have unique health needs; however, their antecedent malignancy and/or the often intensive treatments required to achieve cure may affect their long-term health status. At MD Anderson Cancer Center, we have developed the Life after Cancer Care (LACC) program, which focuses on the health of cancer survivors. The LACC clinic was established to give long-term cancer survivors the opportunity to have follow-up medical care targeting diagnosis, appropriate referral and consultation, and treatment of possible long-term effects of previously treated disease. After successful cancer treatment, survivors would inevitably experience other medical conditions that were going untreated or inadequately treated because of the uncertainty of the origin or etiology of subsequent medical conditions. Primary care providers have been reluctant to treat such patients because of concerns about how distant cancer treatment might have affected new medical conditions.

With the emphasis on health care after the acute cancer therapy period, cancer survivorship long-term clinics are emerging as an important mechanism with which to focus on long-term surveillance for disease recurrence, detection and management of potential treatment-related complication and late effects including second malignancies as well as promotion of health. Currently, three well-established clinics are serving breast, prostate, and thyroid cancer survivors at our institution and the emerging date will likely shape the future of clinical care in thyroid cancer survivors.

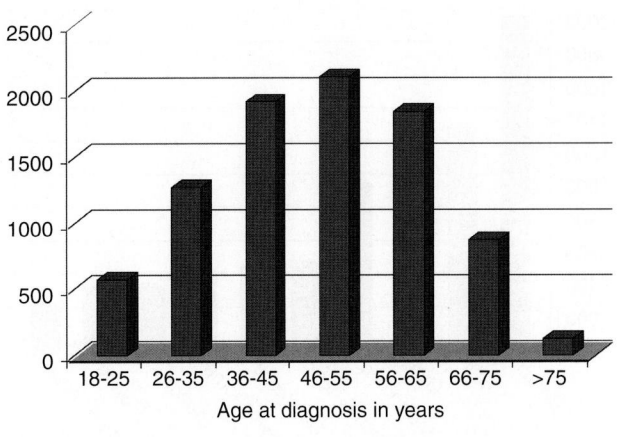

FIGURE 50-1. Age at diagnosis in 8739 adult long-term cancer survivors.

■ TEN THOUSAND CANCER SURVIVORS

Recently there has been increased interest in understanding the long-term effects of cancer and cancer therapy, especially as they may affect the quality of life of cancer survivors. However, information regarding the lasting late effects of cancer and cancer therapy in long-term adult cancer survivors remains limited. Because of this lack of information, the LACC program began a systematic search for living cancer survivors who had been treated at MD Anderson. The inclusion criteria were that they had been diagnosed with cancer, were at least 5 years from their cancer diagnosis, were 18 years or older at diagnosis, had a US address, and at their last contact were free of malignant disease. Surveys were developed to systematically collect health information from such survivors, and the resulting questionnaires were sent out to over 20,000 individuals who met the above criteria. Simultaneously, the survey was made available through the Internet.

Preliminary analyses were initiated after the receipt of the first 6000 entries, 5209 of which included complete information. These responders included 3344 women (64.2%) and 1865 men (35.8%). The response rates were evaluable for the mailed surveys and were reassuringly robust independent of gender (50.8% for women and 50.9% for men) but are possibly underestimated (we could not confirm, for example, that all mailed surveys were received). Cancer survivors therefore appear willing to provide information about their health. Almost one-third of the survivors also provided additional contact information (addresses, telephone numbers), and often voluminous unsolicited comments about their cancer, their health, and their opinions. Additional contact information can be used to update or provide additional information for those willing to participate in that manner.

Data from more than 10,000 survivors are now available for analysis. Complete data are available on 8739 survivors who meet the criteria outlined above. Of the entire sample, 62% are female and 92% are white. The distribution by age at diagnosis is illustrated in

Fig. 50-1 and the mean ± standard deviation (SD) of age at diagnosis was 47.9 ± 14.2 years.

Fifty percent of the survivors were diagnosed between the ages of 18 and 48 years and 25% were diagnosed after the age of 59 years. Male survivors were significantly older at diagnosis than female survivors (50.6 ± 15.1 versus 46.3 ± 13.3 years, $p < .00001$), and Hispanic survivors were significantly younger at diagnosis than white and black survivors (42.9 ± 14.3 versus 48.2 ± 14.1 and 46.9 ± 14.2 years, $p = .00002$).

Approximately 25% of the survivors in our database have lived more than 20 years since their original diagnosis. Figure 50-2 shows the distribution of survivors by time from diagnosis. Ten percent of survivors are at least 30 years from diagnosis.

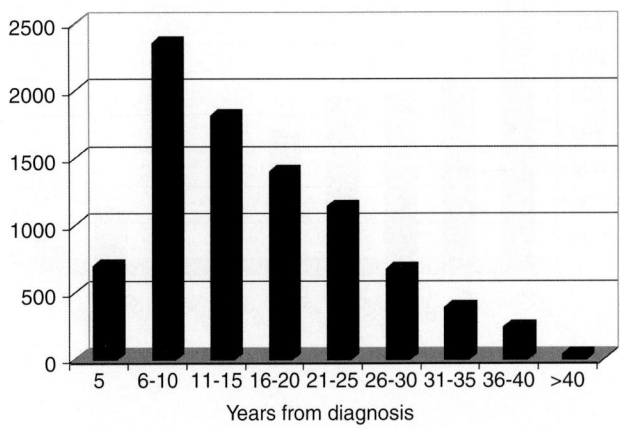

FIGURE 50-2. Distribution of cancer survivors by years from diagnosis.

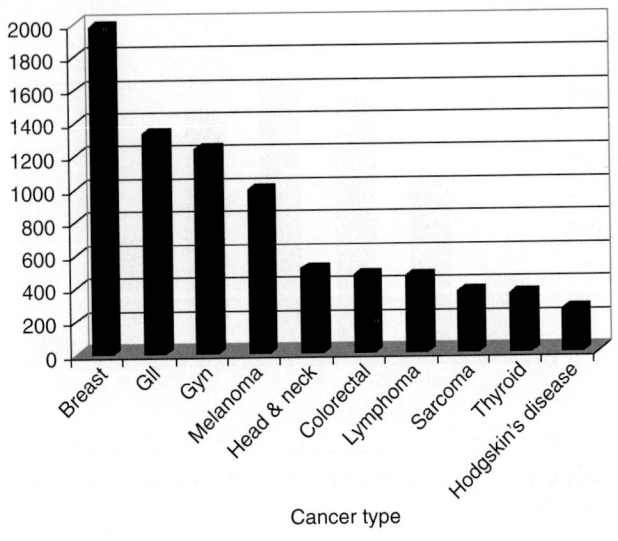

FIGURE 50-3. Distribution of cancer survivors by the 10 most frequent cancer types within the sample of adult survivors.

Breast cancer patients are the most common long-term survivors in our database (1987, or 23%). Figure 50-3 illustrates the distribution of survivors by cancer type.

The gender distribution of cancers—other than breast, gynecologic, prostate, or testicular—is illustrated in Fig. 50-4. This figure illustrates that long-term survivors have similar representation in our database as in the incidence patterns by cancer type.

For instance, the incidence of thyroid cancer is predominantly female and cancer of the head and neck is predominantly male; this is congruent with our database of long-term survivors. Naturally, the distribution of the diagnoses reflects the likelihood of long-term survival with different cancers and patterns that may be unique to MD Anderson referral.

AGE AT DIAGNOSIS AND HEALTH EFFECTS

Survivors were asked to respond to the question "Has cancer affected your overall health?" Interestingly, only 37.4% replied yes to that question, and there were no gender or ethnic differences in their replies. Previously we had reported gender differences in a smaller cohort of survivors (5836) (10). In the larger cohort, univariate analysis indicated that age at diagnosis accounted for the gender variance: females tended to be younger at diagnosis and those who reported that cancer affected their overall health were younger at diagnosis than those who did not report health effects (Fig. 50-5). However when the response to that question was analyzed according to cancer type, it was clear that cancer type affected the survivors' responses. Likewise, those survivors who were most likely to report health effects tended to be younger at diagnosis. Table 50-2 illustrates these findings.

Age at diagnosis seems to be an extremely good predictor of how the survivor experiences long-term survival. When the survivors are grouped according to age at diagnosis, there is the tendency for the survivor to attribute fewer overall health effects from the cancer

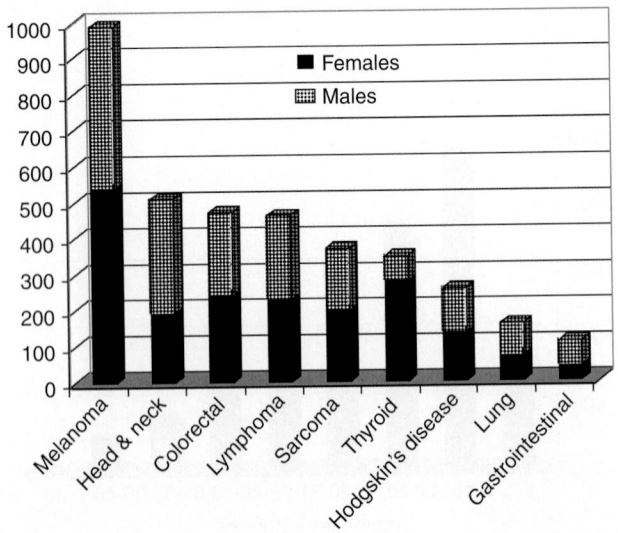

FIGURE 50-4. Distribution of cancer survivors by cancer types and gender.

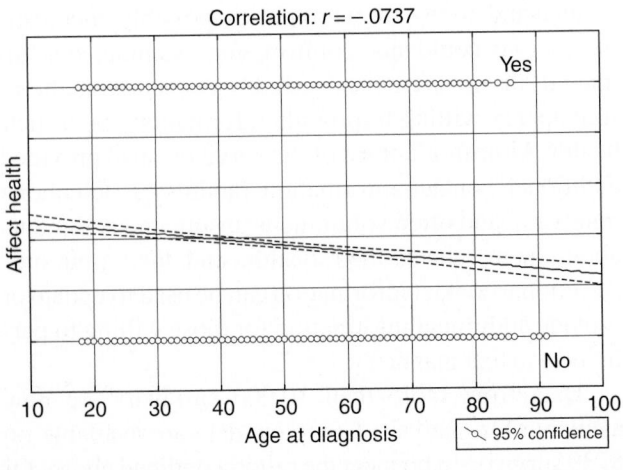

FIGURE 50-5. Inverse correlation between age at diagnosis and self-reported health effects.

TABLE 50-2 | PERCENTAGE OF SURVIVORS WHO RESPONDED "YES" TO "HAS CANCER AFFECTED YOUR HEALTH?"

Cancer Type	Affected Health	Mean Age at Diagnosis in Years
Melanoma	16.7	43.4
Colorectal	31.3	50.2
Gynecologic	31.4	44.5
Breast	35.9	46.5
Genitourinary	36.4	55.5
Sarcoma	39.5	40.5
Head and neck	39.8	50.8
Acute leukemia	45.3	39.8
Thyroid	50.3	35.4
Lung	53.3	55.9
Lymphoma	56.9	46.3
Gastrointestinal	57.0	56.0
Chronic leukemia	60.2	49.3
Hodgkin disease	61.7	30.3

as they age. Of survivors diagnosed between 18 and 40 years of age, 41% report overall health effects from cancer; of those diagnosed between 41 and 65 years of age, 36% reported overall health effects; and of those diagnosed after 65 years of age, 28% reported overall health effects. Perhaps health effects in the older person were less likely to be attributable to cancer effects. It is obvious that aging would have a considerable impact on an individual's perception of his or her health, and this would possibly allow the sequelae of a distant diagnosis and treatment for cancer to be overlooked.

Previously we have reported that specific health effects reported by long-term cancer survivors illustrate a complex interplay between age, gender, cancer type, and cancer treatment as well as ethnicity, race, and social and cultural factors (11-13). For instance, the most frequently reported health effect was arthritis/osteoporosis (1541 survivors, or 26.4%).

Gender was an important variable, as men generally reported fewer specific problems; the most frequently mentioned were heart problems (17.2% of responding men), hearing loss (14.9%), and arthritis/osteoporosis (15.5%). Women generally reported more specific problems; the most frequently mentioned were arthritis/osteoporosis (32.9% of responding women), heart problems (13.9%), and thyroid problems (12.1%). There was a gender difference in the likelihood of reporting any of the specific health problems; for example, women were more likely to report thyroid problems (12.1 versus 6.2%, $p < .00001$) or arthritis/osteoporosis (32.9 versus 15.5%, $p < .00001$). Men, on the other hand, were more likely to report kidney/bladder problems (14.2 versus 9.8%, $p < .00001$) or hearing loss (14.9 versus 9.9%, $p < .00001$). These patterns likely reflect a complex interaction of gender-related cancer diagnoses and comorbidities.

Arthritis/osteoporosis and heart problems were among the most frequently mentioned health problems. The pattern of perceived and reported health problems was different among the cancer types. For example, survivors of Hodgkin disease prominently reported thyroid and lung problems (33.8% of responders with the diagnosis), while a prior diagnosis of lymphoma was associated with frequent mentions of memory loss (14.7%).

NATIONAL HEALTH INTERVIEW SURVEY

A large number of health conditions are reported by the National Health Interview Survey and categorized by age, ethnicity/race, and gender (14). Five of these health conditions were comparable with health conditions reported by our cancer survivor cohort: arthritis symptoms, diabetes, migraine or severe headaches, heart disease, and hearing loss. The frequencies of these conditions in the general population (computed as affected individuals per 1000 people) were compared with their frequencies in our cancer survivor cohort relative to patient age, ethnicity/race, and gender. There were significant differences in the frequencies of the five health conditions between men and women and among ethnic/racial groups. The most common difference in our cancer survivor cohort for all groups analyzed was a statistically significant loss of hearing. Hispanic-American women had significantly more reports of diabetes and African-American men had significantly more reports of heart disease than the race-adjusted national prevalence rates. Whereas apparent differences in the frequency of these health conditions may be the result of the methodology of the questionnaires, prior cancer or cancer therapy may also play a role in the survivors' health profile. For example, the consistent overreporting of hearing loss may be related to ototoxic chemotherapy. Clearly, further detailed analysis is needed in this area. Further research about health comorbidities may provide information about health effects from a past cancer diagnosis.

The importance of the uniqueness of the cancer type was made obvious in two studies from our survey cohort of thyroid cancer survivors and breast cancer survivors. We previously published the thyroid cohort and noted several distinctions (11). Thyroid cancer survivors tended to be significantly younger at diagnosis, were significantly closer to their diagnosis, were significantly more likely to be women, and reported significantly more specific health effects. However, we were impressed by the frequent complaints of symptoms that were reminiscent of thyroid hormone imbalance, and we described these effects as "thyroid dysregulation." Most of the patients in the thyroid cohort usually survive for many years. However, we found that lifetime supplementation of thyroid hormone carried unique problems that compromised the patients' perception of their overall health.

Likewise in another study (15), 291 breast cancer patients (not randomly selected) who completed the original survivor survey agreed to participate in another survey, which included queries about symptoms commonly associated with menopause, including hot flushes, painful sexual intercourse, inability to concentrate, fatigue, and sleep disturbance. Two other items, which pertained to quality of life (QOL) but were not specifically related to menopause, queried the participants about unhappiness and lymphedema. Forty-six percent of these breast cancer survivors indicated that breast cancer had affected their overall health. The number of survivors reporting this was highest among those who had received chemotherapy alone or in combination with radiotherapy. In addition, there were 19 self-reported specific health conditions analyzed by treatment. We thought that increased menopausal symptoms caused by breast cancer might account for the difference in the survivors' QOL compared with that of women in the general population. However, we encountered a problem in differentiating between naturally occurring menopausal symptoms and other physical health problems that affect QOL. In our sample, hot flushes and painful sexual intercourse were obviously related to menopause. Because of the close relationship between these symptoms and the ability to concentrate, fatigue, sleep problems, and general unhappiness, it is difficult to determine whether these represent normal menopausal symptoms or long-term sequelae of cancer treatment. No one would argue that long-term effects of cancer treatment might include cognitive impairment, sleep disturbances, and general unhappiness; however, these conditions are also characteristic of normal menopause, whether or not the patient experiences breast cancer. The relationship among menopausal symptoms, QOL and health effects of cancer treatment is complex. Our study has shown that QOL parameters need to be rigidly defined and that they are time-sensitive or, more specifically, age-specific. There is indication that there are complex interactions between QOL indicators and specific

physiologic consequences of treatment. It is important for menopausal symptoms to be understood within the context of the breast cancer survival and not lost among the QOL/psychosocial issues faced by the cancer survivor. This study reminds us that breast cancer and menopause are independent issues. Further study is necessary to understand these complicated interactions and how to better integrate the issues of aging, long-term cancer survival, and QOL as they relate to the consequences of cancer treatment.

These findings emphasize that cancer survivors should not be lumped into one cohort and that generalizations should not be made about their cancer experience. Cancer type is a major determinant of survival potential. If we are to understand how cancer affects long-term survivors, we should develop studies in which cancer type is matched. Thyroid and breast cancer survivors have unique problems as a result of cancer treatment. Some health effects are clearly related to their cancer, but others are not so clear. Is the fatigue and cognitive impairment a result of too little thyroid hormone replacement, a consequence of normal menopause, or due to their cancer treatment? These questions need further clarification.

ETHNIC AND RACIAL INFLUENCES ON CANCER SURVIVORSHIP

We have previously reported (12) that ethnicity did not appear to be a factor in the self-reporting of health effects overall. However, caution should be exercised, in that ethnic minorities are markedly underrepresented in our database of survivors. In the larger cohort, Asians and Native Americans make up <1% of the survivors, but 48 and 56%, respectively, reported that cancer had affected their overall health.

Previously we have reported that there were significant differences among Caucasians, Hispanics, and blacks in the types of specific health effects they experienced as long-term survivors of cancer (12). We found significant ethnic/racial differences with respect to age at diagnosis, interval since diagnosis, marital status, educational level, insurability, regular medical care, and the effects on family relationships. Differences in health effects probably reflected not only ethnicity/race but also cancer type, gender, type of treatment, and disease stage, to name a few. There was a complex relationship between ethnicity/racial group, family and intimate relationships, and treatment types for survivors of cervical cancer.

Published literature specifically focusing on the impact of ethnic/racial factors in long-term cancer survivors (>5 years from diagnosis) is scarce at best. There are ethnic/racial differences in the incidence and mortality of various cancers (1); these are generally considered to be due to disparities in access to health care and/or the inequities of health care for the poor, resulting in more advanced disease at the time of diagnosis (16); however, other intrinsic factors may also play a role.

It is generally accepted that ethnic/racial factors can (and do) contribute to important disparities in health care access and health outcomes (17-19). A study examining information from the National Survey of Functional Health, Ren et al. (20) reported that race and class discrimination were pervasive and adversely affected the health status of ethnic/racial minorities. Although studies addressing the impact of ethnic/racial differences on health generally relate to diagnosis and treatment-related outcomes (21-26), it is plausible that they may also influence other physiologic and psychosocial aspects of health. In examining the information provided by cancer survivors in our review, we found that, for the most part, cancer survivors had a similar view of the impact or lack thereof of their cancer experience on their physiologic health overall. There were, however, differences with respect to specific health items. For example, African Americans were more likely to report arthritis/osteoporosis than were Caucasian Americans or Hispanic Americans, whereas Hispanic Americans were more likely to report abdominal pain and diabetes mellitus. Such differences in health profile and patterns may be partially related to other ethnic/racial propensities, as demonstrated by Brooks et al. (21) in a study showing that the poor outcomes of African-American women with cervical cancer were associated with preexisting comorbidities. Care must be taken in interpreting these ethnic/racial differences, since race is largely a social and political construct (27).

Grenier and Lipschultz (23) found that African-American childhood cancer patients treated with anthracyclines might be at higher risk for cardiotoxicity; they suggested that this could be true also of adult cancer survivors. We also found a higher incidence of self-reported heart disease in African-American cancer survivors when compared with Caucasian-American or Hispanic-American cancer survivors. Whereas such differences may have a biological basis, socioeconomic parameters may also play a role. It is not clear how powerful one parameter is over the other in influencing these differences. For example, does education and family support have a greater impact on the health of cancer survivors than cancer type and treatment, or vice

versa? Which of these factors is most influenced by ethnicity or race? Clearly, further research in socioeconomically diverse populations is needed.

Ren et al. (20) showed that education was another factor adversely affecting health in Hispanic Americans. Although we found some difference in education among the ethnic/racial groups, this factor did not appear to affect the cancer survivors' perceptions of their overall health except in the Hispanic-American survivor group. Overall, however, the groups were well educated; referral patterns at MD Anderson may have affected these results in our cohort of survivors.

It is generally thought that marital status is closely related to health conditions (28). Unmarried people tend to have higher mortality from all causes, they use more health services, they have more psychologic distress, and their perceptions of their own general health are poorer compared with those of married people. In a study of marriage in survivors of childhood cancers, Rauck et al. (29) found that Caucasian Americans had the lowest divorce rates and that African Americans had the highest ones; Hispanic Americans fell in between. We found differences in health perception among the ethnic/racial groups according to marital status at the time of the survey. We did not consistently find a protective effect of marriage; however, our results suggest that there is a positive correlation between the perception of overall health and the perceived positive impact of the cancer experience on family relationships.

It is clear that socioeconomic, psychologic, and cultural factors interact with the physiologic factors. To better understand these interactions, further research is needed with larger populations that are racially and ethnically diverse.

We reported previously that effects on physiologic health in survivors of cervical cancer appeared to be related to treatment rather than histologic type or ethnic/racial group (12). A consistent finding in analyzing the effect of cancer on family relationships was the differences among the ethnic/racial groups. Hispanic-American survivors were more likely to report that having cancer (especially cervical cancer) had improved their family relationships; clearly, the families of Hispanic-American cancer survivors are affected differently from African-American and Caucasian-American families.

It is clear that ethnicity and race influence the cancer survivor experience. In order to understand these differences, multiculturalism must be incorporated into cancer survivor research. Our present findings point to a significant impact of ethnic/racial influences in the health profiles of cancer survivors. However, non–Caucasian Americans constitute a small minority of the overall cohort. Accordingly, any observations and conclusions must be interpreted with caution and configured with additional research involving much larger populations.

WORK-RELATED ISSUES FOR CANCER SURVIVORS

We analyzed survey information from 4264 long-term survivors of cancer in which survivors were asked to respond to items describing their ability to work, their experience of job discrimination, and their QOL (30). Thirty-five percent of the respondents were working at the time of the survey; significantly more of these individuals were men rather than women and proportionately more were Hispanic Americans than white Americans or African Americans. According to the correlation coefficient ($r = -0.49$, $p < .05$), the younger the survivors were at the time of diagnosis, the more likely they were to be working. Univariate analysis indicated a significant effect of age and cancer type on whether or not the participant was working ($p = .0008$). For most cancer types, workers were significantly younger at diagnosis than individuals who were not working, and they had a significantly higher QOL score than those who were not working. Further correlations regarding the potential influence of other medical and social factors on employment are needed.

Of the survivors working at the time of the survey, 7.3% indicated they had experienced job discrimination; this finding was independent of age, gender, and ethnic/racial group. One participant characterized the job discrimination as originating from coworkers' attitudes toward him as a cancer survivor, whereas another individual indicated that the job discrimination was more age-related than cancer-related. Two survivors described their job experiences in detail. One indicated that the employer in this instance was unsympathetic and resistant to adjusting job responsibilities to accommodate the employee's chronic fatigue. This employee had used all of his "sick time" and "vacation time" over an 8-year period while continuing to work. Another participant reported being suspended from the job on three separate occasions as a result of absences from work during treatment for cancer recurrences. This participant indicated that the employer expressed disbelief over the necessity of taking sick leave.

There were 371 (8.5%) participants who indicated that they were unable to work as a result of the effects of cancer, cancer treatment, or both. Significantly more women reported being unable to work than did men (9.2 versus 7.2%, $p = .02$), and significantly more African Americans reported being unable to work than did white Americans or Hispanic Americans (23.2, 9.7, and 4.3%, respectively). The role of socioeconomic factors in these findings is not clear. The mean age at diagnosis for this group of survivors was 46.3 ± 14.1 years, with a mean time from diagnosis of 19.6 ± 8.6 years. The cancer type did influence the survivors' ability to work. Survivors of melanoma were least likely to report inability to work (3.7%), whereas survivors of gastrointestinal cancers were most likely to be unable to work (20%).

Those who considered themselves unable to work were significantly older at diagnosis. Proportionately, more men were working than unable to work, and proportionately more African Americans were likely to be unable to work than to be working. The distribution of cancer types among those working and the unable-to-work was also different. Cancer types most associated with working status were genitourinary, melanoma, and Hodgkin disease. Cancer types most associated with inability to work were gynecologic, lung, head and neck, gastrointestinal, and colon cancers. Cancer types that were similar proportionately in their association with the ability to work were breast, lymphoma, thyroid, sarcoma, and leukemia.

A reassuring finding is that most cancer survivors do not perceive employment-related problems. Most survivors assimilate back into the workforce with few cancer-related issues. However, for those who do have such issues, little is known about their experiences, because research data for this group is scanty and heterogeneous. Nevertheless, the physical and psychologic impact of cancer as a life-threatening illness is widely accepted, but its impact on society, other than economic, is not well studied or understood. From these results, we know that cancer by type, age, gender, and possibly ethnic/racial group may interact to affect the survivor's ability to work.

INTERNET MESSAGE BOARD FOR CANCER SURVIVORS AND THEIR FAMILIES

As a component of LACC, a message board was created whereby cancer patients and their family members or other loved ones could communicate with and provide support for other patients and families. The message board was accessible to anyone who visited the MD Anderson web page (http://www2.mdanderson.org/sapp/wblacc). It was also monitored, and findings from the postings were used to further clarify the cancer experience and to facilitate support for cancer patients (13).

During the initial 16 months of its creation, 972 individuals logged onto the message board (users) and 284 persons posted 619 messages (posters). The majority of the posters posted only one message (64%), 59 posted two messages (21%), and the rest posted multiple messages. Sixty percent of the posters had cancer and 40% did not. Of those who did not have cancer, 22% identified themselves as spouses of a cancer patient, 69% as other family members, and 9% as non-family members. The majority of the message posters were women (74%); the majority of the posters who identified themselves as cancer patients were also women (72%).

Messages were read and analyzed for content. The most common cancer types represented by the posted messages were breast cancer, gastrointestinal cancer, lung cancer, gynecologic cancer, head and neck cancer, and colon cancer. Forty-seven messages did not indicate a specific cancer type. The most frequent themes were questions about treatment, support, and long-term effects. The pattern of message themes differed between posters who had cancer and those who were posting a message for another person with cancer. For example, whereas the most frequent queries for all posters were about treatment, such queries more frequently came from those without cancer. Of interest, posters posed questions about the long-term effects of cancer significantly more often than did those without cancer. Questions about support and diagnosis appeared to be of similar interest to both groups of posters.

Posters dealing with breast cancer were more likely to post messages about treatment than posters dealing with head and neck cancer. On the other hand, posters dealing with lung cancer were more likely to post messages about support than posters dealing with colon cancer. In general, treatment was the most prominent message theme.

Message board entries reflect yet another aspect of cancer survivors' experience. In general, literature pertaining to health care and the Internet highlights the significance of this resource. However, few data are available about the types of information on which Internet users tend to concentrate. Such information would allow health care providers and educators to develop materials better suited to respond to the needs of consumers and patients.

The concept of using the Internet and message boards for data collection and research has not yet received a great deal of attention within the health care arena. We suggest that continued, systematic analysis of Web site traffic, message content, and utilization patterns may prove promising in clarifying the interests and information needs of patients and their families.

■ CANCER SURVIVORSHIP AND THE FUTURE

The successfully treated cancer patient has much to teach us. Cancer survivorship has become part of the mainstream society, leading to the Institute of Medicine's and the National Research Council's recommendations for the long-term follow-up of cancer survivors and for research in this area. Traditionally cancer research has focused on the diagnosis and treatment of cancer, and appropriately so. We have studied those who have not responded to treatment seeking answers in order to develop better treatments. We should, in our quest to eradicate cancer, look not only to those patients who have succumbed to the disease but also to those who have survived. They provide a living laboratory for the understanding of cancer. We have only scratched the surface in understanding how the survivor of cancer has arrived at long-term survivorship. We have accumulated over 10,000 individual cancer survivors' responses to a survey designed to shed some understanding of the cancer survivors' long-term sequelae of cancer treatment. This survivorship project has raised many questions that need further research. This work requires longitudinal and prospective studies of large numbers of survivors. MD Anderson is poised to lead the cancer survivorship initiative through programs such as the Thyroid Cancer, Breast Cancer, Genitourinary Cancer, and Childhood Cancer Survivorship Clinics.

References

1. American Cancer Society. Cancer Facts & Figures: 2009. http://www.cancer.org/downloads/STT/500809web.pdf. Updated May, 2009. Accessed February 25, 2010.
2. Horner MJ, Ries LAG, Krapcho M, et al (eds). SEER Cancer Statistics Review, 1975-2006. http://seer.cancer.gov/csr/1975_2006/. Updated January 28, 2010. Accessed February 25, 2010.
3. Meadows AT, Hobbie WL. The medical consequences of cure. *Cancer* 1986 Jul 15;58(2 suppl):524-528.
4. Ried H, Zietz H, Jaffe N. Late effects of cancer treatment in children. *Pediatr Dent* 1995 Jul-Aug;17(4):273-284.
5. Marina N. Long-term survivors of childhood cancer. The medical consequences of cure. *Pediatr Clin North Am* 1997 Aug; 44(4):1021-1042.
6. Stevens MC, Mahler H, Parkes S. The health status of adult survivors of cancer in childhood. *Eur J Cancer* 1998 Apr; 34(5):694-698.
7. Loescher LJ, Welch-McCaffrey D, Leigh SA, et al. Surviving adult cancers. Part 1: Physiologic effects. *Ann Intern Med* 1989 Sep 1; 111(5):411-432.
8. Ganz PA. Late effects of cancer and its treatment. *Semin Oncol Nurs* 2001 Nov; 17(4):241-248.

9. Hewitt M, Greenfield S, Stovall E, (eds). *From Cancer Patient to Cancer Survivor: Lost in Transition*, 1st ed. Washington, DC: National Academies; 2006.

10. Schultz PN, Beck ML, Stava C, et al. Health profiles in 5836 long-term cancer survivors. *Int J Cancer* 2003 Apr 20; 104(4): 488-495.

11. Schultz PN, Stava C, Vassilopoulou-Sellin R. Health profiles and quality of life of 518 survivors of thyroid cancer. *Head Neck* 2003 May; 25(5):349-356.

12. Schultz PN, Stava C, Beck ML, et al. Ethnic/racial influences on the physiologic health of cancer survivors. *Cancer* 2004 Jan 1;100(1):156-164.

13. Schultz PN, Stava C, Beck ML, et al. Internet message board use by patients with cancer and their families. *Clin J Oncol Nurs* 2003 Nov-Dec;7(6):663-667.

14. Lethbridge-Cejku M, Rose D, Vickerie J. Summary health statistics for US Adults: National Health Interview Survey, 2004. National Center for Health Statistics. Vital Health Stat 10(228). 2006.

15. Schultz PN, Klein MJ, Beck ML, et al. Breast cancer: Relationship between menopausal symptoms, physiologic health effects of cancer treatment and physical constraints on quality of life in long-term survivors. *J Clin Nurs* 2005 Feb; 14(2): 204-211.

16. Reuben SH. Voices of a Broken System: Real People, Real Problems. President's Cancer Panel. http://deainfo.nci.nih.gov/advisory/pcp/PCPvideo/voices_files/index.html, Updated September, 2001. Accessed February 25, 2010.

17. Ross H. Lifting the unequal burden of cancer on minorities and the underserved. Closing the Gap 2001. http://physiciancareers.kp.org/co/scholarship/downloads/clas_closing_the_gap.pdf. Updated May 04, 2001. Accessed February 25, 2010.

18. Shavers VL, Brown ML. Racial and ethnic disparities in the receipt of cancer treatment. *J Natl Cancer Inst* 2002 Mar 6;94(5):334-357.

19. Rodney P, Rodney ZK, Nu S, et al. Cervical cancer and black women: An analysis of the disparity in prevalence of cervical cancer. *J Health Care Poor Underserved* 2002 Feb; 13(1):24-37.

20. Ren XS, Amick BC, Williams DR. Racial/ethnic disparities in health: The interplay between discrimination and socioeconomic status. *Ethn Dis* 1999 Spring-Summer; 9(2):151-165.

21. Brooks SE, Baquet CR, Gardner JF, et al. Cervical cancer— The impact of clinical presentation, health and race on survival. *J Assoc Acad Minor Phys* 2000; 11(4):55-59.

22. Flores-Luna L, Salazar-Martinez E, Escudero-De los Rios P, et al. Prognostic factors related to cervical cancer survival in Mexican women. *Int J Gynaecol Obstet* 2001 Oct; 75(1): 33-42.

23. Grenier MA, Lipshultz SE. Epidemiology of anthracycline cardiotoxicity in children and adults. *Semin Oncol* 1998 Aug; 25(4 suppl 10):72-85.

24. Grigsby PW, Hall-Daniels L, Baker S, et al. Comparison of clinical outcome in black and white women treated with radiotherapy for cervical carcinoma. *Gynecol Oncol* 2000 Dec;79(3): 357-361.

25. Hamilton AS, Stanford JL, Gilliland FD, et al. Health outcomes after external-beam radiation therapy for clinically localized prostate cancer: Results from the Prostate Cancer Outcomes Study. *J Clin Oncol* 2001 May 1;19(9):2517-2526.

26. Potosky AL, Harlan LC, Stanford JL, et al. Prostate cancer practice patterns and quality of life: The Prostate Cancer Outcomes Study. *J Natl Cancer Inst* 1999 Oct 20;91(20): 1719-1724.

27. Graves Jr, Joseph L. *The Emperor's New Clothes*. Piscataway, NJ: Rutgers University Press; 2001.

28. Ren XS. Marital status and quality of relationships: The impact on health perception. *Soc Sci Med* 1997 Jan; 44(2):241-249.

29. Rauck AM, Green DM, Yasui Y, et al. Marriage in the survivors of childhood cancer: A preliminary description from the Childhood Cancer Survivor Study. Med *Pediatr Oncol* 1999 Jul;33(1):60-63.

30. Schultz PN, Beck ML, Stava C, et al. Cancer survivors. Work-related issues. *AAOHN J* 2002 May; 50(5):220-226.

REHABILITATION

Jack B. Fu
Ki Y. Shin

■ GENERAL PRINCIPLES

Cancer and its treatments are a major cause for impairments and disability. Because cancer treatments have become increasingly successful and have improved survival, there has been an increasing focus on quality of life and, in particular, rehabilitation. Cancer rehabilitation is practiced in outpatient clinics, oncology wards, inpatient rehabilitation units, skilled nursing facilities, nursing homes, long-term acute care centers, palliative care units, and hospices. Common diagnoses addressed include asthenia, deconditioning, hemiplegia, spinal cord injury, peripheral neuropathy, steroid myopathy, lymphedema, bowel/bladder management, limb amputation, and limb dysfunction.

The major goal of cancer rehabilitation is to improve quality of life by minimizing the disability caused by cancer and its treatments and decreasing the "burden of care" needed by cancer patients and their caregivers. The more patients can do for themselves, the more personal dignity they are able to maintain and the less help they require from those around them.

In 1978, Justus Lehmann, supported by the National Cancer Institute (NCI) screened 805 randomly selected cancer patients, identifying multiple problems in the cancer patient population that could be improved by rehabilitation interventions and also multiple barriers limiting the delivery of cancer rehabilitation care (1). More than 20 years later, many of Lehmann's remediable cancer rehabilitation problems as well as barriers to rehabilitation care remain the same (Table 51-1) (1).

In 1980, Dietz categorized cancer rehabilitation into four stages: preventative, restorative, supportive, and palliative (2). Preventative rehabilitation occurs before or immediately after a treatment to prevent loss of function or disability. An example would include preamputation stump care teaching and walker ambulation in a patient with a lower extremity sarcoma. Courneya et al. described a concept called "buffering" where by a cancer patient undergoes exercises and therapies to increase their physical and functional reserves before cancer treatment (3).

Restorative rehabilitation occurs in patients who are believed to be disease free or will have an anticipated relatively stable disease course. A lower extremity sarcoma patient with no known metastatic disease status postamputation undergoing prosthetic rehabilitation would be an example. These first two stages are not

TABLE 51-1	REMEDIABLE REHABILITATION PROBLEMS AND BARRIERS TO DELIVERY OF REHABILITATION CARE	
Remediable Rehabilitation Problems		**Barriers to Delivery of Rehabilitation Care**
Psychological/psychiatric impairments	Lymphedema management	Lack of identification of patient problems
Generalized weakness	Musculoskeletal difficulties	Lack of appropriate referral by physicians unfamiliar with the concept of rehabilitation
Impairments in activities of daily living	Swallowing dysfunction	Patient too ill to participate
Pain	Impaired communication	Patient denies need
Impaired gait/ambulation	Skin management	Cancer prognosis too limited
Disposition/housing issues	Vocational assessments	Rehabilitation unavailable
Neurologic impairments	Impaired nutrition	No financial resources
Vocational assessments	Lymphedema management	
Impaired nutrition		

Data from Lehmann JF, DeLisa JA, Warren CG, et al: Cancer rehabilitation: assessment of need, development, and evaluation of a model of care. Arch Phys Med Rehabil 59:410-9, 1978.

significantly different from conventional nononcologic rehabilitation. Fortunately, as survivorship has increased, restorative rehabilitation has become more prominent. Issues commonly addressed include disability, return to work, and lymphedema management.

Supportive rehabilitation is performed in patients with persistent ongoing disease. A sarcoma patient with known multiple metastasis undergoing chemoradiation treatment is an example.

Palliative rehabilitation is done on patients to reduce discomfort and improve independence in patients with advanced disease. A sarcoma patient with advancing metastatic disease who has failed multiple treatment regimens might require such rehabilitation. The emphasis of palliative rehabilitation is typically to get the patient safely home as soon as possible. The patient likely has limited time to live and the opportunity cost of a lengthy inpatient rehabilitation stay must be taken into consideration. Goals are often simply to get the patient home in a safe environment focusing on family training and transfer training. Higher level goals should be addressed as an outpatient or through home health therapy.

These last two stages are relatively unique to cancer rehabilitation. The typical course for a patient in conventional rehabilitation, for example after a stroke, is continued improvement after the inciting event. However, for the cancer patient with persistent disease the war continues with brief victories followed by declines as the disease progresses (Fig. 51-1) (4).

Multiple studies have established a need for rehabilitation in the cancer patient population (5,6). Furthermore, the functional improvements of cancer rehabilitation patients has been demonstrated in a number of settings, including inpatient (7-10), palliative care (11,12), on a

consultation basis (13), in a hospice setting (14,15), and for outpatients (16). The maintenance of physical activity and exercise has been implicated in increasing survival particularly in breast and colon cancer patients. The mechanism for these findings could be related to levels of insulin/c-peptide and buffering's positive effects on physiological reserves which could allow more treatment (17,18). Cancer rehabilitation physiatrists must also address medical sequelae and complications that are unique to this patient population. It is one of the most challenging aspects of cancer rehabilitation. Good communication between the primary oncology team and the rehabilitation team is crucial. The transfer rate from inpatient rehabilitation to acute care teams is quite high compared to other rehabilitation diagnoses (19).

Rehabilitation goals are accomplished by the efforts of a comprehensive interdisciplinary team of health care professionals, including the rehabilitation physician, rehabilitation nurse, physical therapist, occupational therapist, speech therapist, dietitian, pharmacist, chaplain, social worker, and case manager. Each member of the team has specific expertise in assisting the patient with a care

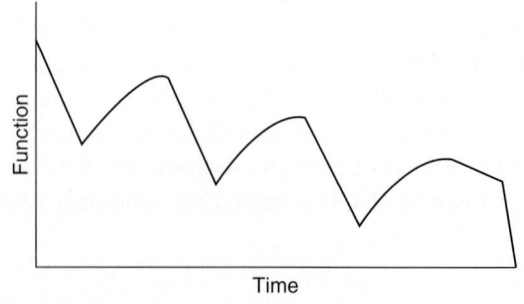

FIGURE 51-1. Function/time graph of cancer patient.

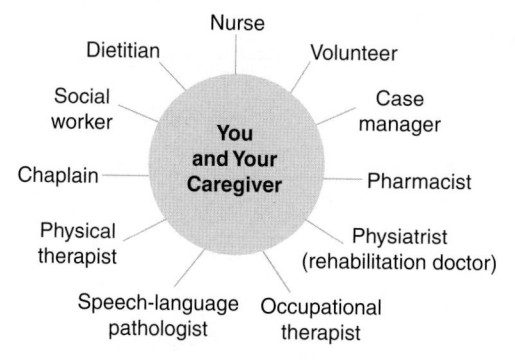

FIGURE 51-2. Rehabilitation team.

plan of maximizing medical stability, function, financial resources, and caregiver involvement for a discharge that is as safe and meaningful as possible (Fig. 51-2).

At the University of Texas MD Anderson Cancer Center (MD Anderson), our cancer rehabilitation practice includes five physical medicine and rehabilitation physicians, a rehabilitation therapy staff of over 60 physical therapy and occupational therapy clinicians, and 8 speech pathologists. Rehabilitation therapists see over 200 inpatients and 50 outpatients per day. The inpatient rehabilitation unit at MD Anderson had 427 admissions from September 2008 to August 2009. A total of 1098 inpatient physical medicine and rehabilitation consultations were performed. Patients included most of the different tumor types seen in the institution, the most common being brain, spine, lung, breast, hematologic, genitourinary, gastrointestinal, and head and neck tumors. The most common inpatient rehabilitation diagnoses included asthenia, gait abnormality, dyspnea, hemiparesis, spinal cord injury, and neurogenic bowel and bladder. Common outpatient rehabilitation diagnoses included lymphedema, myofascial pain, rotator cuff dysfunction, peripheral neuropathy, and low back pain. Inpatient and outpatient electromyograms were performed for neuropathic and myopathic diagnoses and spasticity management.

■ PRACTICAL ASPECTS

When describing a cancer patient's functional status, the Karnofsky Performance Scale is often used. It is the most widely used scale in oncology patients both clinically and in research [20]. It is an easy and quick generalized measurement of a patient's function. Weaknesses of the scale include overgeneralization (unable to measure specific tasks) and poor correlation with cognition (Table 51-2) [21].

In rehabilitation, the outcome scale most often used is the Functional Independence Measure. This multidimensional scale addresses 18 items from a scale of 1 (total assistance) to 7 (complete independence). Items are subdivided into self-care, sphincter control, transfers, locomotion, communication, and social cognition. An aggregate score is also often useful out of a total of 126. Criticisms of the scale include that it is too general and omits items which are important for particular populations such as spinal cord injuries, etc (Fig. 51-3) [22].

TABLE 51-2 | KARNOFSKY SCORE

Condition	Percentage	Comments
A: Able to carry on normal activity and to work. No special care needed.	100	Normal, no complaints, no evidence of disease.
	90	Able to carry on normal activity, minor signs or symptoms of disease.
	80	Normal activity with effort, some signs or symptoms of disease.
B: Unable to work. Able to live at home, care for most personal needs. A varying degree of assistance is needed.	70	Cares for self. Unable to carry on normal activity or to do active work.
	60	Requires occasional assistance, but is able to care for most of his needs.
	50	Requires considerable assistance and frequent medical care
C: Unable to care for self. Requires equivalent of institutional or hospital care. Disease may be progressing rapidly.	40	Disabled, requires special care and assistance.
	30	Severely disabled, hospitalization is indicated although death not imminent.
	20	Hospitalization necessary, very sick, active supportive treatment necessary.
	10	Moribund, fatal processes progressing rapidly.
	0	Dead.

FIM™ Instrument

L e v e l s	7 Complete independence (timely, safely) 6 Modified independence (device)	**No helper**
	Modified dependence 5 Supervision (subject = 100%) 4 Minimal assistance (subject = 75%+) 3 Moderate assistance (subject = 50%+) **Complete dependence** 2 Maximal assistance (subject = 25%+) 1 Total assistance (subject = less than 25%)	**Helper**

Self-care   Admission   Discharge   Follow-up

A.   Eating
B.   Grooming
C.   Bathing
D.   Dressing—upper body
E.   Dressing—lower body
F.   Toileting

Sphincter control
G.   Bladder management
H.   Bowel management

Transfers
I.   Bed, chair, wheelchair
J.   Toilet
K.   Tub, shower

Locomotion
L.   Walk/wheelchair   W Walk / C Wheelchair / B Both
M.   Stairs

Motor subtotal score

Communication
N.   Comprehension   A Auditory / V Visual / B Both
O.   Expression   A Auditory / V Visual / B Both

Social cognition
P.   Social interaction
Q.   Probelm solving
R.   Memory

Cognitive subtotal score

Total FIM™ score

NOTE: Leave no blanks. Enter 1 if patient is not testable due to risk.

FIGURE 51-3.   FIM Score.

Physiatry is a holistic specialty. It views the patient not just from a medical perspective but also functional and social. The primary concern of rehabilitation health care professionals is safety. The first question a physiatrist often asks is, "what is the minimum level of safe function for this patient to be discharged?" That "safe" functional level goal is dependent on what the patient's current functional level, strength, cognition, level of supervision or assistance at home, home conditions (eg, one- versus two-story house), and at times financial resources (to hire help if none is available). Physiatrists must ask detailed social questions to patients and their caregivers above what is typically asked by other health care providers.

Common obstacles confronted are lack of assistance or supervision at home. This often is due to the patient's significant other be required to work during the day, the significant other's inability either physically or mentally (eg, dementia) to care for the patient, or having no one available to care for them.

One of the most practical and simple rehabilitation techniques that an inpatient must learn is to transfer. A transfer is a change in station or position from sitting in bed to standing or from sitting in bed to sitting in a chair. A person must transfer to get into a wheelchair or into a car seat. Patients cannot effectively mobilize until this is accomplished. Depending on the patient's level of disability, a transfer may be done sit to stand, stand and pivot, a sliding board, or with a lift requiring total assistance. After basic transfers are mastered, ambulation may be the next goal to increase mobility. Weakness from paresis, deconditioning, neuropathy, or brain injury can also make self-care difficult. Practical skills such as feeding, grooming, bathing, and dressing are taught or relearned to improve independence (Figs. 51-4, 51-5, and 51-6).

■ TOPICS IN CANCER REHABILITATION

The basic foundations and principles of cancer rehabilitation have been delineated; specific subjects in cancer rehabilitation are presented below. This includes the rehabilitation of patients with brain tumors, lymphedema, disability, spinal cord injuries related to cancer, and cancer-related deconditioning.

Thrombocytopenia, a specific issue unique to cancer rehabilitation, is also described.

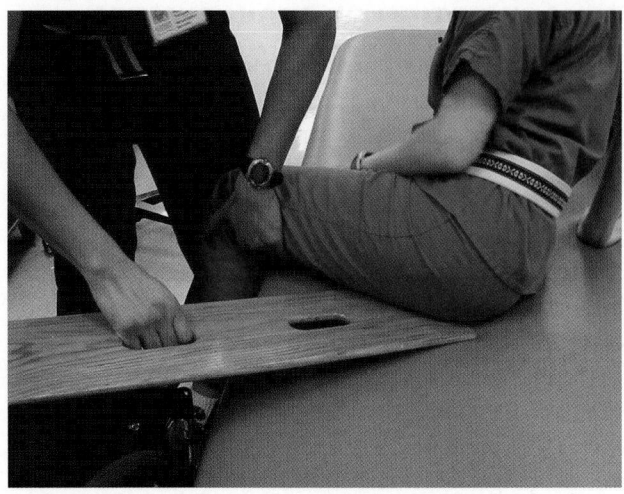

FIGURE 51-4. Sliding-board transfer.

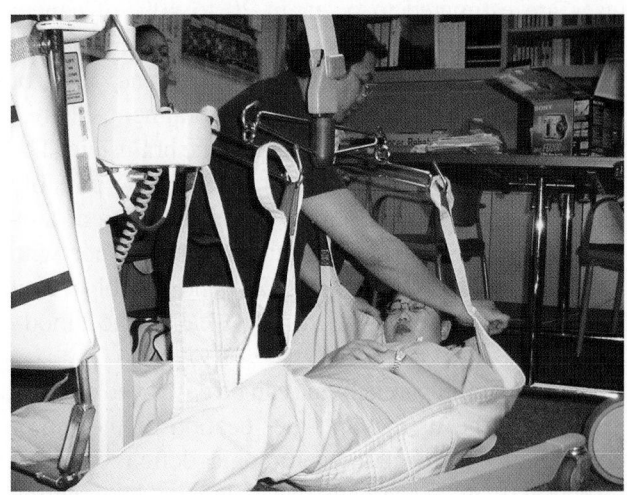

FIGURE 51-5. Lift transfer. Getting on.

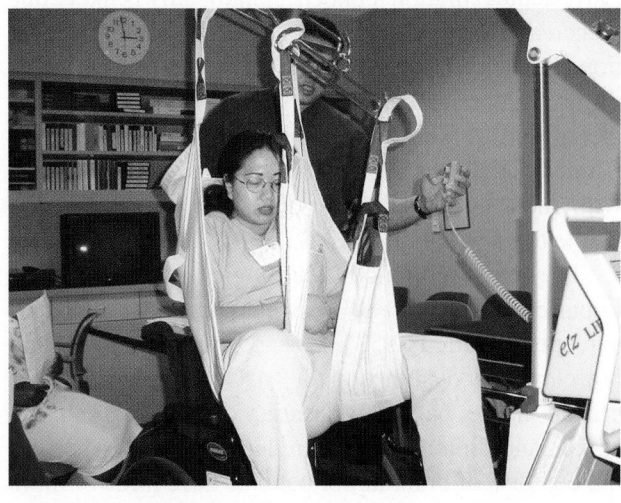

FIGURE 51-6. Lift transfer. Getting up.

REHABILITATION OF BRAIN TUMORS

Primary brain tumors are less than 2% of all malignancies but are the second leading cause of death from neurologic disorders after stroke (23). One-half to two-thirds of intracranial tumors have been reported to be primary tumors (24). Primary brain tumors are classified by cell of origin; the primary system of classification is that of the World Health Organization, which divides tumors into nine categories. The most common categories include tumors that displace brain parenchyma of the intracranial supratentorial compartment. Of these tumors, the most common in adults are the astrocytomas, in particular grade IV astrocytoma otherwise known as glioblastoma multiforme (GBM) (25). The median survival for a GBM patient has been reported between 7 and 17 months (26).

In addition to primary brain tumors, brain metastases are estimated to occur in 20 to 40% of cancer patients. The most common mechanism of metastasis to the brain is through hematogenous spread. Most of the metastases are located in the cerebral hemispheres, followed by the cerebellum and then the brainstem. The incidence of brain tumor metastases is rising possibly due to the increasing length of cancer patient survival (27), increasing ability to diagnose tumor with improved radiographic imaging (28), and possibly recent chemotherapy agents which may weaken the blood–brain barrier (29).

Normal brain parenchyma can be destroyed or compressed by the tumor, and the location of the tumor determines the resultant neurologic deficit. Surgical resection may exacerbate these deficits by creating inflammation and/or peritumoral infarct (30). Radiation treatment has long been an integral part of brain tumor treatments and often results in collateral damage. Early acute radiation leukoencephalopathy is likely due to increased cerebral edema. Late delayed radiation reactions include focal cerebral radiation necrosis (FCRN), diffuse cerebral radiation injury (DCRI), and combined-therapy diffuse white matter injury/leukoencephalopathy. Clinical DCRI has been reported in 2 to 5% of patients with metastases and 19% of 1-year survivors after whole brain radiation (31,32).

The most common neurologic deficits include impaired cognition (80%), weakness (78%), visual-perceptual deficits (53%), sensory loss (38%), and bowel/bladder dysfunction (37%). Other deficits include cranial nerve palsy, dysarthria, dysphagia, aphasia, ataxia, and diplopia which are less common. Approximately 75% of brain tumor patients have three or more neurologic deficits concurrently and 39% have five or more deficits (33). Because of the diverse nature of these neurologic deficits, comprehensive multidisciplinary inpatient rehabilitation is often necessary for these patients. In rehabilitation medicine, the physical impairments that could result in functional deficits are primarily addressed.

Patients who have impairments resulting in functional decline that could affect bed mobility, ambulation, transferring from sitting or lying to a standing position, and/or activities of daily living (ADL) (such as eating, grooming, dressing, bathing, and toileting) can benefit from comprehensive inpatient rehabilitation. Comprehensive cancer rehabilitation services are not widely available for these patients (34). Because of this, many brain tumor patients receive their rehabilitation at general rehabilitation facilities alongside stroke and traumatic brain injury patients. Brain tumor patients have similar efficiencies of improvement when compared to traumatic brain injury, stroke, and between brain tumor types. Lengths of stay tend to be shorter among brain tumor patients possibly secondary to a need to return the patients home sooner given their shorter life expectancies (35-39). However, some notable differences between these populations should be noted, for example physiatrists may need to be cognizant of the continued decline of patients with progressive tumors.

Neurologic Motor Impairment

Motor impairment can be due to hemiparesis, ataxia, and apraxia. Motor impairment may lead to an unsafe gait pattern creating a higher risk for falls and a need for inpatient rehabilitation transfer. In inpatient rehabilitation, the patient will be seen by physical and occupational therapists. Physical therapy would focus on gait and transfers. To address transfers, efforts could be focused on sliding board transfer or stand pivot transfers. With respect to mobility, PT's focus on wheelchair mobility and gait with or without an assistive device (eg, a single point cane, quad cane, rolling walker, hemi-walker). Occupational therapy would focus on problems with activities of daily living. Commonly addressed basic activities of daily living include dressing, bathing, toileting, grooming, eating, etc. The OT and PT are also aware of the cognitive component necessary for mobility and ADLs. Once a patient is functionally safe using an assistive device such as a rolling walker, he or she can be discharged home. Then the patient can continue with outpatient rehabilitation, gradually improving his or her ambulation with an assistive device and further strengthening weakened muscles by way of a progressive resistance exercise program.

The pattern of recovery of muscle strength and function does not always follow the pattern of recovery observed in stroke patients. However, the stroke recovery pattern is often used as a guideline for patients with brain tumors. The recovery of strength occurs in a proximal-to-distal direction, with flaccidity and decreased muscle tone progressing to spasticity and increased muscle tone. The spasticity in the affected limbs can evolve into flexor or extensor synergy patterns. Recovery of muscle movement may plateau at any stage or may progress to isolated coordinated volitional motor movement (40,41).

Several techniques and exercises are used for neuromuscular facilitation in stroke patients. Often, a combination of procedures and techniques from the various programs are used in cancer patients with neuromuscular weakness. Proprioceptive neuromuscular facilitation developed by Kabat, Knott, and Voss relies on several mechanisms such as spiral diagonal movement patterns of the extremities and quick stretch. Brunnstrom movement therapy facilitates the use of the synergy patterns mentioned above as a means of developing voluntary control. Rood proposed that cutaneous sensory stimulation in the form of superficial stroking, tapping, brushing, vibrating, or icing provides facilitatory or inhibitory inputs (42).

In addition to the traditional range-of-motion and strengthening exercises as well as neuromuscular facilitation techniques, functional electric stimulation can also be incorporated into the rehabilitation program for neuromuscular weakness. It uses a low-level electric current that stimulates motor nerves or reflex sensory nerves to produce muscle contraction. The goal of functional electric stimulation is to produce purposeful, functional movements in paretic or paralytic muscles (43).

Sometimes, because of weakness of the ankle dorsiflexors, it is necessary to use an ankle-foot orthosis (AFO) to improve hemiparetic gait. There are two major types of AFOs: the double metal upright AFO attached to an orthopedic shoe and the molded plastic AFO, which is more commonly used. With the plastic AFO, the footplate sits within the shoe and extends upward behind the calf. The advantages of a plastic AFO over a double metal upright AFO include better cosmesis, lighter weight, and the freedom to wear different shoes.

Shoulder subluxation, predominantly inferior, which is caused by the loss of normal motor control of the shoulder stabilizers including the deltoid and supraspinatus muscle, is often seen in the hemiparetic patient (44). It can often be the cause of shoulder pain in hemiplegic patients (45,46). Other possible causes of shoulder pain in this patient population include complex regional pain syndrome, traction injury of the brachial plexus, rotator cuff tendinitis or tear, subacromial or subdeltoid bursitis, adhesive capsulitis, or heterotopic ossification. Diagnosis of glenohumeral subluxation is made through physical examination and radiographic evaluation. The acromiohumeral interval is compared on each side with the arms in an unsupported position during physical examination, and radiographic evaluation is used to quantify the amount of subluxation. Radiographic studies can provide an early evaluation for subluxation with slight gapping of the superior aspect of the glenohumeral joint (47).

Treatment of hemiparetic shoulder subluxation involves proper positioning of the arm, physical modalities, and exercise. The use of an arm sling can help maintain proper positioning and posture during ambulation. However, this is discouraged when the patient is seated, and its overuse may contribute to compromise of superficial blood flow as well as to joint contracture. Arm troughs and lapboards are used while patients are seated (48). Other interventions include biofeedback and functional electric stimulation.

Hemisensory deficit and homonymous hemianopsia may be seen with hemiparesis. Visual or somatic hemineglect is more frequently seen when the nondominant cerebral hemisphere is affected. Hemispatial neglect has a negative effect on sitting balance, visual perception, wheelchair mobility safety awareness, and risk of falling (42). Patients with neglect have difficulty with hygiene and self-care activities on the affected side. Rehabilitation programs must address the issue of hemispatial neglect through focused measures led by speech therapists, occupational therapists, and physical therapists. Family training and education are important in this setting as well.

Ataxia

Cerebellar ataxia may be seen with mass effect within the posterior fossa. Of note, cerebellar ataxia can also be seen in paraneoplastic cerebellar degeneration and with high-dose administration of cytarabine (ara-C) or 5-fluorouracil (5-FU) (49,50). Involvement of the cerebellum can produce intention tremors, dysmetria, and dysdiadochokinesis as patients lose the ability to coordinate the agonist and antagonist muscle groups (51).

The response to pharmaceutical management has been poor; consequently physical and occupational therapy has been the mainstay of treatment for ataxia. This includes the teaching of compensatory techniques for performing basic self-care and occupational activities and the possible use of weighted bracelets or similar devices to help decrease the oscillations. Physical therapy directed at gait training with the use of assistive devices can help improve mobility in ataxic individuals (52).

Aphasia

Depending on its location, a tumor may be associated with deficits in speech, which can vary in severity and type. Often one can diagnose the type of aphasia from a comprehensive neurologic examination, including speech comprehension, fluency, and repetition. These include Broca aphasia, Wernicke aphasia, anomic aphasia, global aphasia, conduction aphasia, and the transcortical motor and sensory aphasias.

A speech pathologist will implement treatment approaches, including melodic intonation therapy, Amer-Ind Code treatment, functional communication treatment, stimulation approach, and PACE (Promoting Aphasics' Communicative Effectiveness) therapy (53).

Cognitive Deficits

Cognitive deficits often are more problematic than motor deficits. They can arise from direct injury to the brain tissue due to the tumor itself, from surgical resection, radiation, chemotherapy, depression/anxiety, as well as medications in particular steroids and anticonvulsants (28). The most often seen deficits include impairments in memory and attention, decreased initiation, and psychomotor retardation (54).

The rehabilitation physician will assess the patient's cognitive status as part of the physical examination. This assessment is needed in order to formulate a rehabilitation program involving speech pathologists. Specific deficits in language and cognition can further be delineated through specific testing performed by a speech pathologist. However, it is sometimes necessary to have formal neuropsychological testing done, especially in cases where the patient wishes to return to work.

Dysphagia

A disruption in the swallowing process can also occur in patients with brain tumors or following craniotomies. It is important to determine, through clinical assessment, whether dysphagia is present, because there is the potential for serious complications such as malnutrition and aspiration pneumonia if dysphagia remains undetected. Often its presence can be established from a history and neurologic examination. If dysphagia is suspected, a speech pathologist is consulted; then daily swallowing therapy and exercises are incorporated into the therapeutic milieu.

Treatments include dietary modifications and dysphagia exercise and facilitation techniques (55). Depending on the results from a clinical swallowing evaluation or videofluoroscopic evaluation, food can be modified to different consistencies, including puree, semisolid, or solid. Liquids may also have to be thickened by using various thickening agents (55).

Exercises and facilitation techniques are employed to aid and strengthen various components of the swallowing process. These include exercises employed for treatment for the lips to facilitate the ability to prevent food or liquid from leaking out of the oral cavity. There are exercises to assist the pharyngeal swallow by improving tongue base retraction. Vocal cord adduction exercises are instituted to strengthen weak cords to prevent aspiration.

Compensatory strategies include proper head and trunk positioning, which for most patients is to be seated upright with head midline, trunk erect, and the neck slightly flexed forward. Other techniques include the chin-tuck method and head turning and tilting during swallowing.

After dysphagia has been identified and measures are implemented for its treatment, regular follow-up to assess for improvement is required. This again can be done through clinical examination or radiographically. If improvement is noted, the diet may be advanced appropriately.

Spasticity

Spasticity is defined as velocity-dependent resistance to passive movement across a joint. It is an abnormality involving increased muscle tone and is one of the positive findings of the upper motor neuron syndrome. Spasticity must be distinguished from soft tissue contractures. Soft tissue contractures result from scar tissue formation and may be the result of a number of causes including uncontrolled spasticity.

Often brain tumors can cause muscle spasticity. This can affect the gait pattern, ADL, and, in severe cases, can cause pain and joint contractures as well as being a detriment to hygiene of the involved areas. Sometimes spasticity may be beneficial, when a patient may use knee extensor spasticity to assist in transferring from a sitting to a standing position. Indications for the treatment of spasticity include the need to decrease pain, improve hygiene, improve gait and transfers, minimize contractures, and improve self-care.

Treatment measures for spasticity include physical and medical interventions. Proper positioning, passive range-of-motion exercises, serial casting, splints, and braces are some of the physical interventions used in treating spasticity. Oral medications may also be used, including tizanidine, dantrolene sodium, and baclofen. Because these medications work systemically, the most common limiting side effects are excessive drowsiness and cognitive changes. Tizanidine or dantrolene is recommended by most clinicians for treating spasticity stemming from primary brain pathology (56). Often because of the cognitive side effects of these oral medications, botulinum toxin injections, phenol injections, or intrathecal baclofen pumps may be useful. These medications act locally but are harder to administer and more invasive.

Bladder Dysfunction

As in stroke patients, bladder incontinence may be present in patients with brain tumors. The causes of bladder incontinence can be multifactorial and include an untreated urinary tract infection, inability to ambulate to the bathroom, and altered cognitive status. If the pontine micturition center is preserved, patients with brain tumors can have upper motor neuron bladder dysfunction, which is characterized by bladder hyperreflexia with reflex or urge incontinence and complete emptying (57). Postvoid residual volumes are generally low in the absence of bladder outlet obstruction. Persistent areflexia and retention may occur with bilateral lesions (57).

Treatment first involves identifying the cause of the bladder dysfunction. Obtaining a urinalysis with cultures and sensitivities and then starting appropriate antibiotics is the treatment for urinary tract infections. Using a bedside commode or a urinal is of benefit for patients who have weakness or inability to safely ambulate to the bathroom. A timed voiding program that has the patient urinate at set times throughout the day, before the bladder can contract, can be of help for patients with hyperreflexic urgency. Anticholinergic medications such as oxybutynin (Ditropan) or tolterodine tartrate (Detrol) can be used for persistent incontinence in this setting of a hyperreflexic detrusor (58). If the patient's blood pressure can tolerate it, a trial of an alpha adrenergic agent (eg, tamsulosin, terazosin) may be useful in reducing urinary resistance in older male patients who are experiencing symptoms of urinary retention.

LYMPHEDEMA

Physiatrists are often asked to assist with the care of lymphedema patients. Malignancy (including breast, melanoma, gynecologic, lymphoma, and urologic cancers) is the number one cause of secondary lymphedema in the United States. The lymphedema can be caused by a combination of the cancer, surgical treatments, and radiation treatments. Breast cancer is the leading cause of upper extremity lymphedema in the United States and develops in 2 to 40% of patients after surgery, radiation, or both (59,60).

The majority of lymphedema cases are diagnosed clinically. The differential diagnosis would include deep venous thrombosis, venous insufficiency, myxedema, lipedema, heart failure, kidney failure, and hypoproteinemia. If difficult to diagnose cases, lymphoscintigraphy is the gold standard.

The treatment of lymphedema typically starts with conservative treatments consisting of manual lymph drainage, compression sleeves, and sometimes pneumatic compression sleeves. Patients are taught a lymphedema regimen to do at home over 1 to 2 sessions by lymphedema-trained physical therapists. Measurements are often taken and the patients are followed up periodically to ensure that they are completing the regimen as prescribed and to measure changes in their lymphedema. Progression of lymphedema can be measured using a number of techniques, including volumetric/circumferential measurements, bioelectric impedance, tonometry, and perometry. In patients with severe or difficult to treat lymphedema, a number of surgical options are available, including microsurgery, liposuction, and debulking procedures.

DISABILITY

Impairment is any loss or abnormality of psychological, physiologic, or anatomic structure or function. Impairments occur at the organ level. An example of impairment includes amputation of a limb, loss of joint function, loss of strength, and loss of endurance. Disability is any restriction or lack (resulting from impairment) of ability to perform an activity in the manner or within the range considered normal for a human being. Disability occurs at the personal level. An example would be an inability to perform basic activities of daily living or inability to walk. Handicap is a disadvantage for a given individual that limits or prevents the fulfillment of a role that is normal (depending on age, sex, and social and cultural factors) for that individual. A handicap occurs at a social level. Examples include lack of access to a public facility because of wheelchair confinement or loss of telemarketing job due to Broca aphasia (61). Disability is related to impairment, it is also subject to modulation by numerous other factors, such that identical types of measured impairments may result in widely different levels of reported disability. Even among individuals without measured impairments, disability may be reported and demonstrated. Impairments and disability evaluations are complicated by the fact that there is a considerable variation between objectively measured impairment and subjectively reported disability. Psychological, social, and behavioral factors must be recognized as significant contributors to the relationship between impairment and disability.

Increasing survivorship among cancer patients has led to an increased focus on disability. Many cancer survivors are unable to work secondary to the effects of chemotherapy, operations, the tumor itself, and symptoms associated with the tumor, including chronic pain and fatigue. The patient may have beaten cancer, but he/she must live with the sequelae of those battles. It has been reported that 38% of cancer survivors are working age (62). Survivors frequently wish to return to work for continued insurance benefits, income, and self-esteem. Quality-of-life assessments show that employed cancer survivors have a higher quality of life. It provides a sense of normalcy and control when cancer takes control away from other aspects of their lives (63). Survivors may report an inability to work for a variety of reasons, including fatigue, physical limitations, emotional problems, changing personal priorities, cognitive deficits, awkward interaction with coworkers, and unsympathetic employers (64).

Yankelovich surveyed 200 supervisors of cancer survivors in two studies. Sixty-six percent of supervisors were concerned about the cancer survivor's ability to work. Prior to the survivor returning to work after cancer treatment, 33% believed the survivor would not be able to handle the job. Thirty-one percent believed the survivor needed to be replaced. After the survivor returned to work 34% of supervisors and 43% of coworkers were less concerned regarding the survivor ability to work. About 50% of supervisors admitted that a cancer diagnosis would affect their decision to hire (65). Ferrell surveyed 662 fellow employees of cancer survivors. Fourteen percent felt that cancer survivors probably would not be able to do their job and 27% of workers felt that they would have to pick up the slack of their cancer survivor colleague (66).

Twenty percent of cancer patients report some cancer-related disability. However, most working cancer patients do return to work after treatment. Seventy-three percent are employed at 1 year and 84% at 4 years. CNS, head and neck, and stage IV hematologic cancer patients had the highest risk of disability. Also, patients who were involved in more physically demanding work, were less educated, female, and of older age were less likely to return to work after treatment. Eighty-seven percent reported that their employer was accommodating (67). Fifty-four percent of employed cancer survivors reported having to adjust their work schedule during their cancer treatment (68). The American With Disabilities Act of 1990 brought legislative protection to cancer survivors with disabilities. It requires employers to make "reasonable accommodation" for employees with disabilities and prevents discrimination in pay, hiring, firing, fringe benefits, and working conditions. It also requires employers to make accommodations for family members who are not an "undue hardship." Accommodations can include extended leave, flexible work schedules, permitting working from home, changing work environment, and allowing rest periods.

If there is uncertainty as to whether a cancer survivor can return to work, several options are available. If the primary concern is energy and endurance, a "weaning schedule" is often done. The cancer survivor's hours are gradually increased each week with the patient reporting any difficulties to the physician. When issues of coordination, strength, or endurance are uncertain, a functional capacity evaluation can be performed by a physical or occupational therapist. The evaluation can be useful for determining tolerance for lifting, bending, squatting, etc. Often, the therapist is able to replicate the duties of the patient and recommend ergonomic or environmental modifications if necessary.

REHABILITATION OF CANCER-RELATED SPINAL CORD INJURY

Spinal cord injury in the cancer patient has several etiologies. These involve primary spinal cord tumor or metastatic lesions. Primary tumors such as meningiomas, neurofibromas, and gliomas are relatively rare, and the majority of tumors involving the spinal cord are metastatic. The metastatic lesions that cause nerve root or spinal cord compression can be paravertebral, extradural, intradural, or intramedullary; however, 95% of metastatic lesions are extradural. These lesions most often originate from primary tumors of the breast, lungs, and prostate. Other tumors that metastasize to the spine include renal, melanoma, myeloma, and thyroid. Most extradural metastases arise from the vertebral body and result in compression of the anterior spinal cord. Approximately 70% of spinal metastases occur in the thoracic spine, which has a smaller ratio of canal-to-cord diameter than the other two spinal segments (69).

Pain that is worse at night and in the supine position is a common clinical presentation. Weakness and sensory loss and the development of bowel or bladder incontinence may indicate spinal cord compromise. Rapid progression of paraparesis over only a few hours indicates arterial compromise by tumor invasion or pressure; slowly evolving symptoms suggest gradual cord impingement and may respond to steroids and radiotherapy (70).

Corticosteroids can alleviate pain and improve neurologic function, and radiation therapy is the treatment of choice with most cases of cord compression. If the tumor involves two or three columns of the spine, spinal stability is of concern; consequently, treatment is aimed toward stabilization of the spinal column. This can be done with cervical orthoses. Sternal occipital mandibular immobilization (SOMI) is well tolerated and provides adequate flexion and extension as well as stability to the lower cervical segments. Philadelphia collars provide stability in flexion and extension for higher levels but do not restrict rotation and lateral bending in the lower cervical segments. The "clamshell" thoracic lumbar-spinal orthosis is used to provide thoracic and lumbar support but may not be an option in patients with friable or intolerant skin following chemotherapy or steroid use. Therefore the Taylor-Knight brace, which limits spinal extension, and the Jewett brace, which limits spinal flexion, can be used to provide thoracic and lumbar support (70).

Surgery is also indicated sometimes with instability and neurologic compromise; indications include pathologic fracture and dislocation, failure of radiation therapy, and rapidly progressing myelopathic signs and symptoms. Surgical stabilization can frequently alleviate the need for external bracing which is an added benefit.

Once spinal stabilization is achieved, comprehensive inpatient rehabilitation can address the impairments, functional limitations, and disabilities associated with spinal cord compression and injury due to cancer. Individuals with nontraumatic spinal cord injuries can achieve significant gains in functional independence measurements during inpatient rehabilitation (10). It has also been suggested that because of the limited prognosis of cancer patients with spinal cord compression, an expedited inpatient rehabilitation stay with the focus on family training and home safety should be emphasized.

Bladder Management

For all cancer patients with neurologic involvement and those with profound deconditioning, it is prudent to check postvoid residuals for signs of bladder dysfunction. This can be performed noninvasively by an ultrasound-mediated bladder scanner or, more accurately, by straight catheterization and measurement postvoid. If the postvoid volumes are 100 to 150 mL or greater, an intermittent catheterization program is initiated.

Tumors involving the spinal cord cause suprasacral neurogenic bladder problems, which typically result in a hyperreflexic detrusor; this is characterized by low urinary volumes, high bladder pressures, and diminished bladder compliance. Incomplete lesions may produce the supraspinal pattern, with urgency and adequate emptying, while patients with complete lesions have reflex incontinence and incomplete voiding due to detrusor-sphincter dyssynergia (57). Some patients have hypocontractile or areflexic bladders, with urinary retention and associated overflow incontinence if the lesion involves the sacral micturition center. Sometimes there is a mixed picture of upper motor neuron dysfunction, hyperreflexic bladder and lower motor neuron dysfunction, and areflexic bladder.

Management of lower motor neuron bladder dysfunction involves the use of a condom catheter for men or an indwelling catheter for women in the situation where sphincter tone is diminished with normal or compromised detrusor tone. When the sphincter tone is competent but the bladder tone diminished, an intermittent catheterization program is instituted. This can frequently be seen in patients with sacral tumors such as chordomas and chondromas.

The management of upper motor neuron bladder dysfunction involves the use of an anticholinergic medication such as oxybutynin to decrease detrusor tone and allow for greater capacity; then an intermittent catheterization program can be instituted.

An intermittent catheterization program first involves daily measurements of postvoid residuals, or the volume of urine left in the bladder after a void. If the postvoid volumes are 100 to 150 mL or greater, the patient is catheterized initially every 4 h. The goal is to have the catheterized volumes not exceed 400 to 500 mL. If the volumes remain consistently below those numbers, the frequency of catheterization can be decreased to every 6 h.

In addition, management of bladder dysfunction in this population involves assessing for urinary tract infections, which can be common. Appropriate antibiotics should be started based on urinalysis, cultures, and sensitivities.

It is important to note that in the cancer population, life expectancy often plays a part in rehabilitation management. Intermittent catheterization is the preferred method of management for the scenarios mentioned above; however, a Foley catheter is sometimes used instead for ease and comfort in those patients with limited prognosis.

Bowel Management

Typically, with lesions above the conus medullaris, an upper-motor-neuron bowel dysfunction is present, with the muscles of the external anal sphincter and pelvic floor becoming spastic. The connection between the spinal cord and the colon remain intact and bowel and stool can be propelled by reflex activity. With lesions below the conus medullaris, an areflexic lower-motor-neuron bowel dysfunction is present, with the myenteric plexus intrinsically moving stool slowly (71).

A complicating matter with cancer patients is opioid-induced constipation. This and other premorbid factors and current bowel function must be ascertained before instituting a bowel program. Often, a plain x-ray of the abdomen is obtained to assess for obstipation before beginning a bowel program. If obstipation is present, suppositories or enemas can be given to clean out the bowels and especially to evacuate the rectal vault.

The goals of a bowel management program are to prevent fecal impaction and to facilitate bowel evacuation on a routine schedule compatible with one's daily activities. This is a logical, structured program based initially on evaluation of the current bowel pattern. A bowel management program begins with a proper diet, which should contain adequate amounts of fluid and fiber in order to create soft bulky stools, which can decrease bowel transit time. Fatty foods can increase transit time. Medication management involves the introduction of a stimulant such as senna. A bisacodyl suppository can be used as an adjunct.

In stepwise fashion, a bowel program begins with an x-ray in order to determine whether evacuation by enemas is necessary; then an appropriate diet is begun, along with stool softeners and/or stimulants. To take advantage of the gastrocolic reflex, the patient is placed on the commode approximately 30 min after a meal, preceded by a bisacodyl suppository 10 min before the patient is placed on the commode. In addition, manual digital stimulation 20 min after suppository insertion can induce the rectocolic reflex (57).

Spasticity

Similar to brain injury, many patients with spinal cord injury suffer from spasticity, which is an abnormality of muscle tone and is velocity-dependent resistance to passive movement across a joint. In addition, they experience muscle flexor spasms, which also respond to the same treatment strategies as those used for spasticity.

Treatment begins with proper positioning and can also involve splinting, casting, stretching, range-of-motion exercises, and the use of medications. In contrast to spasticity originating from brain pathology, spasticity associated with spinal cord injury is treated medically, primarily with baclofen. Tizanidine is also an appropriate choice. In addition, chemical neurolysis, botulinum toxin, and—for severe cases—an intrathecal baclofen pump may be used.

REHABILITATION OF GENERALIZED DECONDITIONING

A common problem in patients with cancer is generalized weakness and deconditioning, which simply means a loss of or decrease in a prior state of conditioning. Often this results from prolonged bed rest. It was stated earlier that many patients admitted to the hospital with cancer develop asthenic symptoms. This is due to the severity of their disease process or prolonged bed rest, which results in a deconditioned state. The role of rehabilitation in this setting is to either help prevent further deconditioning or to "recondition" the deconditioned patient. This is frequently seen in the hematologic and stem cell transplant inpatients at the MD Anderson.

There are three types of muscle fibers. Type I muscle fibers are the slow-twitch oxidative metabolism fibers, which have slow fatigability and are used for prolonged activity. Type IIB fibers are the fast-twitch fibers, which use glycolytic anaerobic metabolism and have rapid fatigability. Type IIA is an intermediate fiber.

Prolonged bed rest can result in muscle weakness. In a classic study by Müller, the muscles of a person on strict bed rest can decrease approximately 1.0 to 1.5% of their initial strength per day, corresponding to approximately a 10 to 20% loss of strength per week (72). Antigravity muscles like the gastrocnemius and back extensor muscles tend to lose strength disproportionately, with larger muscles losing strength more quickly than smaller muscles; handgrip strength is unaffected (73,74). Type I fibers are more affected than type II fibers (75).

These effects on muscles can be counteracted by a daily stretching program, which delays muscle atrophy (76). In addition, daily isometric muscle contractions of 10 to 20% of maximal tension for 10 s can help maintain muscle strength (72). Electric stimulation of muscles can also be used. In general, it may take two or more times as long as the period of immobilization to recover muscle strength (77).

Joint contracture is an abnormal limitation of passive joint range of motion and can be caused by prolonged immobilization. Typical contractures from immobilization include hip flexion, knee flexion, elbow flexion, and internally rotated shoulder contractures as well as ankle plantar flexion contractures. Once they have developed, contractures are treated with range-of-motion exercises. For more severe cases, deep heating followed by range-of-motion exercises and serial casting may be necessary. One goal of nursing and inpatient therapists should be to prevent joint contractures before they occur. Hip flexion contractures can be prevented with the avoidance of an overly soft mattress and lying occasionally in a prone position. Dorsiflexion exercises and footboards can help prevent ankle plantar flexion contractures.

Immobilization can also affect the bones. The Wolff law states that the ratio of formation to resorption is influenced by the stresses to which bones are subjected. The primary stress on most bones is weight bearing, which causes a buildup of bone; a lack of stress on bones leads to a predominance of bone resorption. Weight bearing is eliminated when lying in bed in a supine position and can lead to disuse osteoporosis. This is best treated with preventive measures such as active muscle contraction and active weight-bearing exercises. Exercises conducted in bed are not particularly effective (78). Out of bed to chair activities are encouraged as soon as possible.

There are cardiovascular effects from prolonged bed rest. The first such form of cardiac deconditioning is resting tachycardia. After a period of bed rest, the heart rate can increase by about one-half beat per minute each day for the first 3 to 4 weeks of immobilization (79). In addition, there are decreased diastolic filling times, with resultant decreased myocardial perfusion, decreased stroke volume with submaximal and maximal exercises, decline in cardiac output at submaximal exercise, and deleterious hemodynamic and orthostatic changes (78).

Thrombotic complications, such as the development of deep venous thrombosis and pulmonary embolism, are a risk from immobility. The Virchow triad states that hypercoagulability, endothelial injury, and stasis of blood flow are factors that can contribute to clot formation.

The treatment of the cardiovascular effects is mainly aimed at prevention. Sitting in a chair prevents deterioration of $\dot{V}_{O_2max}$ and orthostatic intolerance. Isometric exercise minimizes decreases in $\dot{V}_{O_2max}$ (80). Cardiovascular deconditioning can be reversed by a progressive increase in activity and regaining an upright posture. Orthostatic intolerance can be helped by range-of-motion exercises, progressive ambulation, abdominal strengthening, and leg exercises to reverse venous stasis. In addition, supportive treatments for orthostatic intolerance include the use of a tilt table, supportive garments, leg stockings, abdominal binders, and medications such as ephedrine, midodrine, and fludrocortisone acetate (Florinef Acetate). Finally, it is essential to prevent deep venous thrombosis. This is done by mobilizing the patient, encouraging ambulation on a continual basis, using external intermittent leg compression devices, and administering low-dose anticoagulation (78).

THROMBOCYTOPENIA

In the cancer population, thrombocytopenia is often seen, especially in patients receiving chemotherapy and/or extensive irradiation, with resulting myelosuppression, bone marrow infiltration, and splenomegaly as well as leukemias and lymphomas. A rehabilitation program or exercise in a thrombocytopenic patient is controversial. The major concern in this situation is the development of an intracranial hemorrhage. With platelet counts over 5000/mm^3, one study found fatal intracranial hemorrhage in only 1 of 92 patients receiving chemotherapy (81).

Hematologic guidelines allow nonresistive activities at platelet counts between 5000 and 10,000/mm^3 and light resistive exercises with counts above 10,000/mm^3, with ambulation allowed with counts above 5000/mm^3 (82). Clinicians must use their own judgment with individual patients. In addition, platelet transfusions with counts below 10,000 should be performed in patients undergoing comprehensive rehabilitation.

References

1. Lehmann JF, DeLisa JA, Warren CG, et al. Cancer rehabilitation: Assessment of need, development, and evaluation of a model of care. *Arch Phys Med Rehabil* 1978;59:410-419.
2. Dietz JH, Jr. Adaptive rehabilitation of the cancer patient. *Curr Probl Cancer* 1980;5:1-56.
3. Courneya KS, Friedenreich CM. Framework PEACE: An organizational model for examining physical exercise across the cancer experience. *Ann Behav Med* 2001;23:263-272.
4. Fu J. *Palliative Rehabilitation: Optimizing Function at End of Life*. American Academy of Physical Medicine & Rehabilitation Medicine Annual Assembly, Austin, Texas, 2009.
5. Houts PS, Yasko JM, Harvey HA, et al. Unmet needs of persons with cancer in Pennsylvania during the period of terminal care. *Cancer* 1988;62:627-634.
6. Morasso G, Capelli M, Viterbori P, et al. Psychological and symptom distress in terminal cancer patients with met and unmet needs. *J Pain Symptom Manage* 1999;17:402-409.
7. Marciniak CM, Sliwa JA, Spill G, et al. Functional outcome following rehabilitation of the cancer patient. *Arch Phys Med Rehabil* 1996;77:54-57.

8. Sliwa JA, Marciniak C. Physical rehabilitation of the cancer patient. *Cancer Treat Res* 1999;100:75-89.

9. Cole RP, Scialla SJ, Bednarz L. Functional recovery in cancer rehabilitation. *Arch Phys Med Rehabil* 2000;81:623-627.

10. McKinley WO, Conti-Wyneken AR, Vokac CW, et al. Rehabilitative functional outcome of patients with neoplastic spinal cord compressions. *Arch Phys Med Rehabil* 1996; 77:892-895.

11. Scialla S, Cole R, Scialla T, et al. Rehabilitation for elderly patients with cancer asthenia: Making a transition to palliative care. *Palliat Med* 2000;14:121-127.

12. Oldervoll LM, Loge JH, Paltiel H, et al. The effect of a physical exercise program in palliative care: A phase II study. *J Pain Symptom Manage* 2006;31:421-430.

13. Sabers SR, Kokal JE, Girardi JC, et al. Evaluation of consultation-based rehabilitation for hospitalized cancer patients with functional impairment. *Mayo Clin Proc* 1999;74:855-861.

14. Yoshioka H. Rehabilitation for the terminal cancer patient. *Am J Phys Med Rehabil* 1994;73:199-206.

15. Cheville A. Rehabilitation of patients with advanced cancer. *Cancer* 2001;92:1039-1048.

16. Porock D, Kristjanson LJ, Tinnelly K, et al. An exercise intervention for advanced cancer patients experiencing fatigue: A pilot study. *J Palliat Care* 2000;16:30-36.

17. Newton RU, Galvao DA. Exercise in prevention and management of cancer. *Curr Treat Options Oncol* 2008;9:135-146.

18. Friedenreich CM, Gregory J, Kopciuk KA, et al. Prospective cohort study of lifetime physical activity and breast cancer survival. *Int J Cancer* 2009;124:1954-1962.

19. Guo Y, Persyn L, Palmer JL, et al. Incidence of and risk factors for transferring cancer patients from rehabilitation to acute care units. *Am J Phys Med Rehabil* 2008;87:647-653.

20. Karnofsky D, Burchenal JH. Clinical evaluation of chemotherapeutic agents in cancer. In: Macleod CM (eds): *Evaluation of Chemotherapy Agents*. New York: Columbia University Press; 1949:191-205.

21. Meyers CA, Weitzner MA. Neurobehavioral functioning and quality of life in patients treated for cancer of the central nervous system. *Curr Opin Oncol* 1995;7:197-200.

22. Meyers CA. Neuropsychological aspects of cancer and cancer treatment. In: Garden FH, Grabois M (eds): *Physical Medicine and Rehabilitation: State of the Art Reviews*. Philadelphia: Hanley & Belfus; 1994:229-241

23. Radhakrishnan K, Bohnen NI, Kurland L. Epidemiology of brain tumors. In: Morantz RA, Walsh JW (eds): *Brain Tumors: A Comprehensive Text*. New York: Marcel Dekker; 1994:1-18.

24. Osborn A. *Diagnostic Neuroradiology*. St. Louis: Mosby; 1994

25. Berger MS, Leibel SA, Bruner JM, et al. Primary cerebral tumors. In: Levin VA (ed): *Cancer in the Nervous System*, 2nd ed. New York: Oxford University Press; 2002:75-134

26. Shawl EG, Seiferheld W, Scott C, et al. Re-examining the radiation therapy oncology group (RTOG) recursive partitioning analysis (RPA) for glioblastoma multiforme (GBM) patients. *Int J Radiat Oncol Biol Phys* 2003;57:S135-S136.

27. Nugent JL, Bunn PA, Jr., Matthews MJ, et al. CNS metastases in small cell bronchogenic carcinoma: Increasing frequency and changing pattern with lengthening survival. *Cancer* 1979;44: 1885-1893.

28. Bell KR, O'Dell MW, Barr K, et al. Rehabilitation of the patient with brain tumor. *Arch Phys Med Rehabil* 1998;79: S37-S47.

29. Greenberg MS. *Handbook of Neurosurgery*. Vol 1. Lakeland: Greenberg Graphics; 1997:240-322.

30. Ulmer S, Braga TA, Barker FG, 2nd, et al. Clinical and radiographic features of peritumoral infarction following resection of glioblastoma. *Neurology* 2006;67:1668-1670.

31. Dropcho EJ. Central nervous system injury by therapeutic irradiation. *Neurol Clin* 1991;9:969-988.

32. DeAngelis LM, Delattre JY, Posner JB. Radiation-induced dementia in patients cured of brain metastases. *Neurology* 1989;39:789-796.

33. Mukand JA, Blackinton DD, Crincoli MG, et al. Incidence of neurologic deficits and rehabilitation of patients with brain tumors. *Am J Phys Med Rehabil* 2001;80:346-350.

34. Meyers CA, Boake C, Levin VA, et al. Symptom management, rehabilitation strategies, and improved quality of life for patients with brain tumors. In: Levin VA (ed): *Cancer in the Nervous System*. New York: Churchill Livingstone; 1996: 449-459.

35. Marciniak CM, Sliwa JA, Heinemann AW, et al. Functional outcomes of persons with brain tumors after inpatient rehabilitation. *Arch Phys Med Rehabil* 2001;82:457-463.

36. Huang ME, Cifu DX, Keyser-Marcus L. Functional outcome after brain tumor and acute stroke: A comparative analysis. *Arch Phys Med Rehabil* 1998;79:1386-1390.

37. Huang ME, Cifu DX, Keyser-Marcus L. Functional outcomes in patients with brain tumor after inpatient rehabilitation: Comparison with traumatic brain injury. *Am J Phys Med Rehabil* 2000;79:327-335.

38. Huang ME, Wartella J, Kreutzer J, et al. Functional outcomes and quality of life in patients with brain tumours: A review of the literature. *Brain Inj* 2001;15:843-856.

39. O'Dell MW, Barr K, Spanier D, et al. Functional outcome of inpatient rehabilitation in persons with brain tumors. *Arch Phys Med Rehabil* 1998;79:1530-1534.

40. Twitchell TE. The restoration of motor function following hemiplegia in man. *Brain* 1951;74:443-480.

41. Sawner K, LaVigne J. *Brunstromm's Movement Therapy in Hemiplegia: A Neurophysiological Approach*, 2nd ed. Philadelphia: Lippincott; 1992.

42. Roth EJ, Harvey RL. Rehabilitation of stroke syndromes. In: Braddom RL (ed): *Physical Medicine and Rehabilitation*. Philadelphia: Saunders; 1996:1053-1099.

43. Kraft GH. New methods for the assessment and treatment of the hemiplegic arm and hand. *Phys Med Rehabil Clin North Am* 1991;2:579.

44. Chaco J, Wolf E. Subluxation of the glenohumeral joint in hemiplegia. *Am J Phys Med* 1971;50:139-143.

45. Calliet R. *The Shoulder in Hemiplegia*. Philadelphia: Davis; 1980.

46. Van Ouwenaller C, Laplace PM, Chantraine A. Painful shoulder in hemiplegia. *Arch Phys Med Rehabil* 1986;67:23-26.

47. Shai G, Ring H, Costeff H, et al. Glenohumeral malalignment in the hemiplegic shoulder. An early radiologic sign. *Scand J Rehabil Med* 1984;16:133-136.

48. Garrison SJ, Rolak LA. Rehabilitation of patients with completed stroke. In: DeLisa JA (ed): *Rehabilitation Medicine, Principles and Practice*, 2nd ed. Philadelphia: Lippincott; 1993:801.

49. Macdonald DR. Neurologic complications of chemotherapy. *Neurol Clin* 1991;9:955-967.

50. Posner JB. Paraneoplastic syndromes. *Neurol Clin* 1991;9: 919-936.

51. Diener HC, Dichgans J. Pathophysiology of cerebellar ataxia. *Mov Disord* 1992;7:95-109.

52. Silver KH, Fishman P, Speed J. Movement disorders. In: O'Young BJ, Young MA, Steins SA (eds): *Physical Medicine and Rehabilitation Secrets*, 2nd ed. Philadelphia: Hanley & Belfus; 2002;182-193.

53. Rao PR. Adult communication disorders. In: Braddom RL (ed): *Physical Medicine and Rehabilitation*. Philadelphia: Saunders; 1996:43-65.

54. Gillis TA, Yadav R, Guo Y. Rehabilitation of patients with neurologic tumors and cancer-related central nervous system disabilities. In: Levin VA (ed): *Cancer in the Nervous System*, 2nd ed. New York: Oxford University Press; 2002: 470-492.

55. Noll S, et al. Rehabilitation of patients with swallowing disorders. In: Braddom RL (ed): *Physical Medicine and Rehabilitation*, 2nd ed. Philadelphia: Saunders; 2000:535-557.

56. Kaplan M. Upper motor neuron syndrome and spasticity. In: Woo BH, Nesathurai S (eds): *The Rehabilitation of People With Traumatic Brain Injury*. Malden: Blackwell Science; 2000:85-99.

57. Cardenas DD, Mayo ME, King JC. Urinary tract and bowel management in the rehabilitation setting. In: Braddom RL (ed): *Physical Medicine and Rehabilitation*. Philadelphia: Saunders; 1996:555-579.

58. Abbott K, Blaustein D. Stroke rehabilitation. In: Nesathurai S, Blaustein D (eds): *Essentials of Inpatient Rehabilitation*. Malden: Blackwell Science; 2000:117-126.

59. Logan V. Incidence and prevalence of lymphedema: A literature review. *J Clin Nurs* 1995;4:213-219.

60. Ozalslan C, Kuru B. Lymphedema after treatment of breast cancer. *Am J Surg* 2004;187:69-72.

61. Wood PH. Appreciating the consequences of disease: The international classification of impairments, disabilities, and handicaps. *WHO Chron* 1980;34:376-380.

62. National Cancer Institute, 2004. http://www.dccps.nci.gov/ocs/prevalence/index.html

63. Frazier LM, Miller VA, Horbelt DV, et al. Employment and quality of survivorship among women with cancer: Domains not captured by quality of life instruments. *Cancer Control* 2009;16:57-65.

64. Chapman SA. The experience of returning to work for employed women with breast cancer. Academy for Health Services Research and Health Policy. Meeting. *Abstr Acad Health Serv Res Health Policy Meet* 2000;17: Unknown.

65. Yankelovich CS. Cerenex survey on cancer patients in the workplace: Breaking down discrimination barriers, 1992.

66. Ferrell BR, Grant MM, Funk B, et al. Quality of life in breast cancer survivors as identified by focus groups. *Psychooncology* 1997;6:13-23.

67. Short PF, Vasey JJ, Tunceli K. Employment pathways in a large cohort of adult cancer survivors. *Cancer* 2005;103:1292-1301.

68. Bradley CJ, Bednarek HL. Employment patterns of long-term cancer survivors. *Psychooncology* 2002;11:188-198.

69. Gilbert RW, Kim JH, Posner JB. Epidural spinal cord compression from metastatic tumor: Diagnosis and treatment. *Ann Neurol* 1978;3:40-51.

70. Garden FH, Gillis TA. Principles of cancer rehabilitation. In: Braddom RL (ed): *Physical Medicine and Rehabilitation*. Philadelphia: Saunders; 1996;1199-1214.

71. Bergman, SB. Bowel management. In: Nesathurai S (ed): *The Rehabilitation of People With Spinal Cord Injury*, 2nd ed. Malden: Blackwell Science; 2000:53-58.

72. Müller EA. Influence of training and of inactivity on muscle strength. *Arch Phys Med Rehabil* 1970;51:449-462.

73. Deitrick JE, Whedon GD, Shorr E. Effects of immobilization upon various metabolic and physiologic functions of normal men. *Am J Med* 1948;4:3-36.

74. Greenleaf JE, Van Beaumont W, Convertino VA, et al. Handgrip and general muscular strength and endurance during prolonged bedrest with isometric and isotonic leg exercise training. *Aviat Space Environ Med* 1983;54:696-700.

75. Appell HJ. Muscular atrophy following immobilisation. A review. *Sports Med* 1990;10:42-58.

76. Baker JH, Matsumoto DE. Adaptation of skeletal muscle to immobilization in a shortened position. *Muscle Nerve* 1988; 11:231-244.

77. Houston ME, Bentzen H, Larsen H. Interrelationships between skeletal muscle adaptations and performance as studied by detraining and retraining. *Acta Physiol Scand* 1979;105:163-170.

78. Buschbacher RM. Deconditioning, conditioning, and the benefits of exercise. In: Braddom RL (ed): *Physical Medicine and Rehabilitation*. Philadelphia: Saunders; 1996:687-707.

79. Taylor HL, Henschel A, et al. Effects of bed rest on cardiovascular function and work performance. *J Appl Physiol* 1949; 2:223-239.

80. Stremel RW, Convertino VA, Bernauer EM, et al. Cardiorespiratory deconditioning with static and dynamic leg exercise during bed rest. *J Appl Physiol* 1976;41:905-909.

81. Gaydos LA, Freireich EJ, Mantel N. The quantitative relation between platelet count and hemorrhage in patients with acute leukemia. *N Engl J Med* 1962;266:905-909.

82. Sayre R, Marcoux B. Exercise and autologous bone marrow transplants. *Clin Manag Phys Ther* 1992;12(4):78-82.

INDEX

Applied Microsoft Power Bi

Bring your data to life!

Third Edition

Teo Lachev

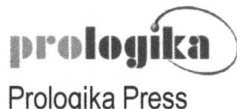

Prologika Press

Applied Microsoft Power BI
Bring your data to life!
Third Edition

Published by:
Prologika Press
info@prologika.com
http://prologika.com

ISBN 13   978-0-9766353-8-3
ISBN 10   0-9766353-8-0

Author: Teo Lachev
Editor: Edward Price
Cover Designer: Zamir Creations

The manuscript of this book was prepared using Microsoft Word. Screenshots were captured using TechSmith SnagIt.

contents

preface

To me, Power BI is the most exciting milestone in the Microsoft BI journey since circa 2005, when Microsoft got serious about BI. Power BI changes the way you gain insights from data; it brings you a cloud-hosted, business intelligence and analytics platform that democratizes and opens BI to everyone. It does so under a simple promise: "five seconds to sign up, five minutes to wow!"

Power BI has plenty to offer to all types of users who're interested in data analytics. If you are an information worker, who doesn't have the time and patience to learn data modeling, Power BI lets you connect to many popular cloud services (Microsoft releases new ones every week!) and get insights from prepackaged dashboards and reports. If you consider yourself a data analyst, you can implement sophisticated self-service models whose features are on a par with organizational models built by BI pros.

Speaking of BI pros, Power BI doesn't leave us out. We can architect hybrid organizational solutions that don't require moving data to the cloud. And besides classic solutions for descriptive analytics, we can implement innovative Power BI-centric solutions for real-time and predictive analytics. If you're a developer, you'll love the Power BI open architecture because you can integrate custom applications with Power BI and visualize data your way by extending its visualization framework.

From a management standpoint, Power BI is a huge shift in the right direction for Microsoft and for Microsoft BI practitioners. Not so long ago, Microsoft BI revolved exclusively around Excel on the desktop and SharePoint Server for team BI. This strategy proved to be problematic because of its cost, maintenance, and adoption challenges. Power BI overcomes these challenges. Because it has no dependencies to other products, it removes adoption barriers. Power BI gets better every week, and this should allow us to stay at the forefront of the BI market. As a Power BI user, you're always on the latest and greatest version. And Power BI has the best business model: most of it it's free!

I worked closely with Microsoft's product groups to provide an authoritative (yet independent) view of this technology and to help you understand where and how to use it. Over more than a decade in BI, I've gathered plenty of real-life experience in solving data challenges and helping clients make sense of data. I decided to write this book to share with you this knowledge, and to help you use the technology appropriately and efficiently. As its name suggests, the main objective of this book it so to teach you the practical skills to take the most of Power BI from whatever angle you'd like to approach it.

Trying to cover a product that changes every week is like trying to hit a moving target! However, I believe that the product's fundamentals won't change and once you grasp them, you can easily add on knowledge as Power BI evolves over time. Because I had to draw a line somewhere, *Applied Microsoft Power BI (Third Edition)* covers all features that were that were released by December 2017.

Although this book is designed as a comprehensive guide to Power BI, it's likely that you might have questions or comments. As with my previous books, I'm committed to help my readers with book-related questions and welcome all feedback on the book discussion forums on my company's web site (http://bit.ly/powerbibook). Consider also following my blog at http://prologika.com/blog and subscribing to my newsletter at http://prologika.com to stay on the Power BI latest.

Bring your data to life today with Power BI!

Teo Lachev
Atlanta, GA

acknowledgements

Welcome to the third revision of my Power BI book! The book added about 20% new content and about that much content was rewritten to keep it up with the ever-changing world of Power BI. Writing a book about a cloud platform, which adds features weekly, is like trying to hit a moving target. On the upside, I can claim that this book has no bugs. After all, if something doesn't work now, it used to work before, right? On the downside, I had to change the manuscript every time a new feature popped up. Fortunately, I had people who supported me.

The book (my ninth) would not have been a reality without the help of many people to whom I'm thankful. As always, I'd like to first thank my family for their ongoing support.

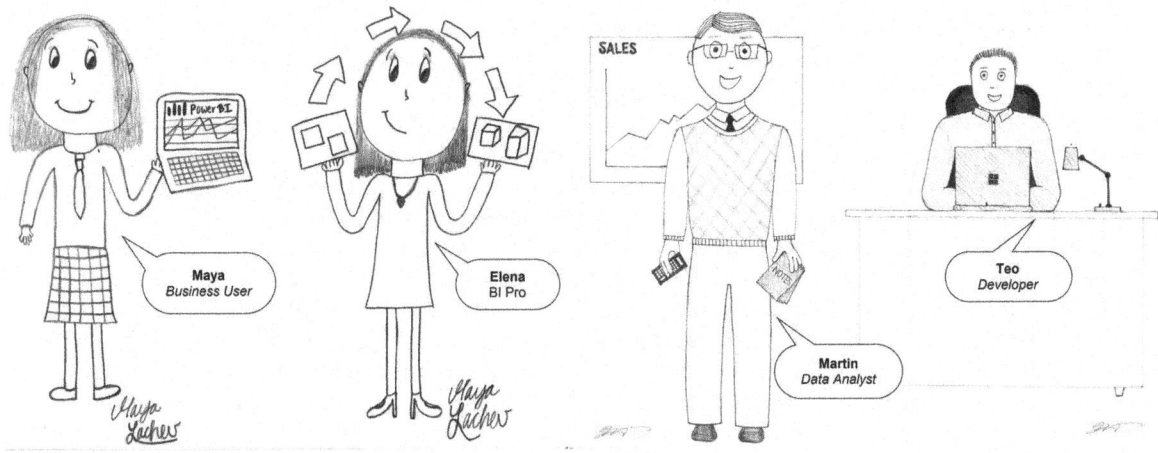

The main personas in the book, as imagined by my 17-year old daughter, Maya, and 14-year old son, Martin.

As a Microsoft Most Valuable Professional (MVP), Gold Partner, and Power BI Red Carpet Partner, I've been privileged to enjoy close relationships with the Microsoft product groups. It's great to see them working together! Special thanks to the Power BI, Analysis Services, and Reporting Services teams.

Finally, thank *you* for purchasing this book!

about the book

The book doesn't assume any prior experience with data analytics. It's designed as an easy-to-follow guide for navigating the personal-team-organizational BI continuum with Power BI and shows you how the technology can benefit the four types of users: information workers, data analysts, pros, and developers. It starts by introducing you to the Microsoft Data Platform and to Power BI. You need to know that each chapter builds upon the previous ones, to introduce new concepts and to practice them with step-by-step exercises. Therefore, I'd recommend do the exercises in the order they appear in the book.

Part 1, *Power BI for Information Workers*, teaches regular users interested in basic data analytics how to analyze simple datasets without modeling and how to analyze data from popular cloud services with predefined dashboards and reports. Chapter 2, *The Power BI Service*, lays out the foundation of personal BI, and teaches you how to connect to your data. In Chapter 3, *Creating Reports*, information workers will learn how to create their own reports. Chapter 4, *Creating Dashboards*, shows you how to quickly assemble dashboards to convey important metrics. Chapter 5, *Power BI Mobile*, discusses the Power BI native mobile applications that allow you to view and annotate BI content on the go.

Part 2, *Power BI for Data Analysts*, educates power users how to create self-service data models with Power BI Desktop. Chapter 6, *Data Modeling Fundamentals*, lays out the ground work to understand self-service data modeling and shows you how to import data from virtually everywhere. Because source data is almost never clean, Chapter 7, *Transforming Data*, shows you how you can leverage the unique query capabilities of Power BI Desktop to transform and shape the data. Chapter 8, *Refining the Model*, shows you how to make your self-service model more intuitive and how to join data from different data sources. In Chapter 9, *Implementing Calculations*, you'll further extend the model with useful business calculations. And, Chapter 10, *Analyzing Data*, shares more tips and tricks to get insights from your models.

Part 3, *Power BI for Pros*, teaches IT pros how to set up a secured environment for sharing and collaboration, and it teaches BI pros how to implement Power BI-centric solutions. Chapter 11, *Enabling Team BI*, shows you how to use Power BI workspaces and apps to promote sharing and collaboration, where multiple coworkers work on the same BI artifacts, and how to centralize access to on-premises data. Chapter 12, *Power BI Premium*, shows how you can achieve consistent performance and reduce licensing cost with Power BI Premium and how to implement on-premises report portals to centralize report management and distribution. Written for BI pros, Chapter 13, *Organizational BI*, walks you through the steps to implement descriptive, predictive, and real-time solutions with Power BI.

Part 4, *Power BI for Developers*, shows developers how to integrate and extend Power BI. Chapter 14, *Programming Fundamentals*, introduces you to the Power BI REST APIs and teaches you how to use OAuth to authenticate custom applications with Power BI. In Chapter 15, *Power BI Embedded*, you'll learn how to report-enable custom apps with embedded dashboards and reports. In Chapter 16, *Creating Custom Visuals*, you'll learn how to extend the Power BI visualization capabilities by creating custom visuals to present effectively any data.

source code

Applied Microsoft Power BI covers the entire spectrum of Power BI features for meeting the data analytics needs of information workers, data analysts, pros, and developers. This requires installing and configuring various software products and technologies. **Table 1** lists the software that you need for all the exercises in the book. Depending on your computer setup, you might need to download and install other components, as I explain throughout the book.

Table 1   The complete software requirements for practices and code samples in the book

Software	Setup	Purpose	Chapters
Power BI Desktop	Required	Implementing self-service data models	6, 7, 8, 9, 10
Visual Studio 2015 (or higher) Community Edition	Required	Power BI programming	14, 15, 16
Power BI Mobile native apps (iOS, Android, or Windows depending on your mobile device)	Recommended	Practicing Power BI mobile capabilities	5
SQL Server Database Engine Developer, Standard, or Enterprise 2012 or later with the AdventureWorksDW database	Recommended	Importing and processing data	6
Analysis Services Tabular Developer, Business Intelligence, or Enterprise 2012 or later edition	Recommended	Live connectivity to Tabular	2, 13
Analysis Services Multidimensional Developer, Standard, Business Intelligence, or Enterprise 2012 or later edition	Optional	Live connectivity to Multidimensional	6
Power BI Report Server Developer or Enterprise	Optional	Importing from SSRS and integrating Power BI with Power BI Report Server	4, 6, 12

Although the list is long, don't despair! As you can see, most of the software is not required. In addition, the book provides the source data as text files and it has alternative steps to complete the exercises if you don't install some of the software, such as SQL Server or Analysis Services.

You can download the book source code from the book page at http://bit.ly/powerbibook. After downloading the zip file, extract it to any folder of your hard drive. Once this is done, you'll see a folder for each chapter that contains the source code for that chapter. The source code in each folder includes the changes you need to make in the exercises in the corresponding chapter, plus any supporting files required for the exercises. For example, the Adventure Works.pbix file in the Ch06 folder includes the changes that you'll make during the Chapter 6 practices and includes additional files for importing data. Save your files under different names or in different folders to avoid overwriting the files that are included in the source code.

 NOTE   The data source settings of the sample Power BI Desktop models in this book have connection strings to databases and text files. If you decide to test the provided samples and refresh the data, you must update some data sources to reflect your specific setup. To do so, open the Power BI Desktop model, and then click the Edit Queries button in the ribbon's Home tab. Select the query that fails to refresh in the Queries pane, and then double-click the Source step in the Applied Steps list (Query Settings pane). Change the server name or file location as needed.

Installing the Adventure Works databases
Some of the code samples import data from the AdventureWorksDW database. This is a Microsoft-provided database that simulates a data warehouse. I recommend you install it on a local or shared SQL Server because importing form a relational database is a common requirement. Again, you don't have to do this (installing a SQL Server alone can be challenging) because I provide the necessary data extracts.

NOTE Microsoft ships Adventure Works databases with each version of SQL Server. More recent versions of the databases have incremental changes and they might have different data. Although the book exercises were tested with the Adventure-WorksDW2012 database, you can use a later version if you want. Depending on the database version you install, you might find that reports might show somewhat different data.

Follow these steps to download the AdventureWorksDW2012 database:

1. Open the Microsoft SQL Server Product Samples Database webpage on Codeplex (http://msftdbprodsamples.codeplex.com).

2. Click the SQL Server 2012 DW tile. The link URL as of the time of this writing is http://msftdbprodsamples.codeplex.com/releases/view/55330. Click the AdventureWorksDW2012 Data File link.

3. When Internet Explorer prompts you, click Run to download the file.

4. Open SQL Server Management Studio (SSMS) and connect to your SQL Server database instance. Attach the AdventureWorksDW2012_Data.mdf file. If you're not sure how to attach a database file, read the instructions at https://msdn.microsoft.com/en-us/library/ms190209.aspx.

Installing the Adventure Works Analysis Services models

In chapters 2 and 13, you connect to the Adventure Works Tabular model, and Chapter 6 has an exercise for importing data from Analysis Services. If you decide to do these exercises, install the Analysis Services models as follows:

1. Open the Microsoft SQL Server Product Samples Database webpage on Codeplex (http://msftdbprodsamples.codeplex.com).

2. Click the SQL Server 2012 DW tile. The link URL as of the time of this writing is http://msftdbprodsamples.codeplex.com/releases/view/55330.

3. Click the "AdventureWorks Multidimensional Models SQL Server 2012" link to download the zip file.

4. Follow the steps in the "Readme for Analysis Services Tutorial on Multidimensional Modeling" section of the of the "SQL Server Samples Readme" document at http://bit.ly/1PwLLP2 to deploy the Adventure Works cube.

5. Back to the SQL Server 2012 DW Codeplex page, download and unzip the "AdventureWorks Tabular Model SQL Server 2012" file.

6. Follow the steps in the "Readme for Adventure Works DW Tabular SQL 2012" section of the of the "SQL Server Samples Readme" document at http://bit.ly/1PwLLP2 to deploy the Adventure Works Tabular model.

7. In SQL Server Management Studio, connect to your Analysis Services instance. (Multidimensional and Tabular must be installed on separate instances.)

8. Expand the Databases folder. You should see the SSAS database.

Reporting errors

Please submit bug reports to the book discussion list on http://bit.ly/powerbibook. Confirmed bugs and inaccuracies will be published to the book errata document. A link to the errata document is provided in the book web page. The book includes links to web resources for further study. Due to the transient nature of the Internet, some links might be no longer valid or might be broken. Searching for the document title is usually sufficient to recover the new link.

Your purchase of APPLIED MICROSOFT POWER BI includes free access to an online forum sponsored by the author, where you can make comments about the book, ask technical questions, and receive help from the author and the community. The author is not committed to a specific amount of participation or successful resolution of the question and his participation remains voluntary. You can subscribe to the forum from the author's personal website http://bit.ly/powerbibook.

Chapter 1

Introducing Power BI

Without supporting data, you are just another person with an opinion. But data is useless if you can't derive knowledge from it. And, this is where Microsoft data analytics and Power BI can help! Power BI changes the way you gain insights from data; it brings you a cloud-hosted, business intelligence and analytics platform that democratizes and opens BI to everyone. Power BI makes data analytics pervasive and accessible to all users under a simple promise: "five seconds to sign up, five minutes to wow!"

This guide discusses the capabilities of Power BI, and this chapter introduces its innovative features. I'll start by explaining how Power BI fits into the Microsoft Data Platform and when to use it. You'll learn what Power BI can do for different types of users, including business users, data analysts, professionals, and developers. I'll also take you on a tour of the Power BI features and its toolset.

1.1   What is Microsoft Power BI?

Before I show you what Power BI is, I'll explain business intelligence (BI). You'll probably be surprised to learn that even BI professionals disagree about its definition. In fact, Forester Research offers two definitions (see https://en.wikipedia.org/wiki/Business_intelligence).

DEFINITION   Broadly defined, BI is a set of methodologies, processes, architectures, and technologies that transform raw data into meaningful and useful information that's used to enable more effective strategic, tactical, and operational insights and decision-making. A narrower definition of BI might refer to just the top layers of the BI architectural stack, such as reporting, analytics, and dashboards.

Regardless of which definition you follow, Power BI can help you with your data analytics needs.

1.1.1   Understanding Business Intelligence

The definition above is a good starting point. but to understand BI better, you need to understand its flavors. First, I'll categorize who's producing the BI artifacts, and then I'll show you the different types of analytical tasks that these producers perform.

Self-service, team, and organizational BI
I'll classify BI by its main users and produced artifacts and divide it into self-service, team, and organizational BI.

- Self-service BI (or personal BI) – Self-service BI enables data analysts to offload effort from IT pros. For example, Maya is a business user and she wants to analyze CRM data from Salesforce. Maya can connect Power BI to Salesforce and get prepackaged dashboards and reports without building a data model. In the more advanced scenario, Power BI empowers analysts to build data models for self-service data exploration and reporting. Suppose that Martin from the sales department wants to analyze some sales data that's stored in a Microsoft Access database or in an Excel workbook. With a few clicks, Martin can import the data from various data sources into a data model (like the one shown in **Figure 1.1**), build reports, and gain valuable insights. In other words, Power BI makes data analytics more pervasive because it enables more employees to perform BI tasks.

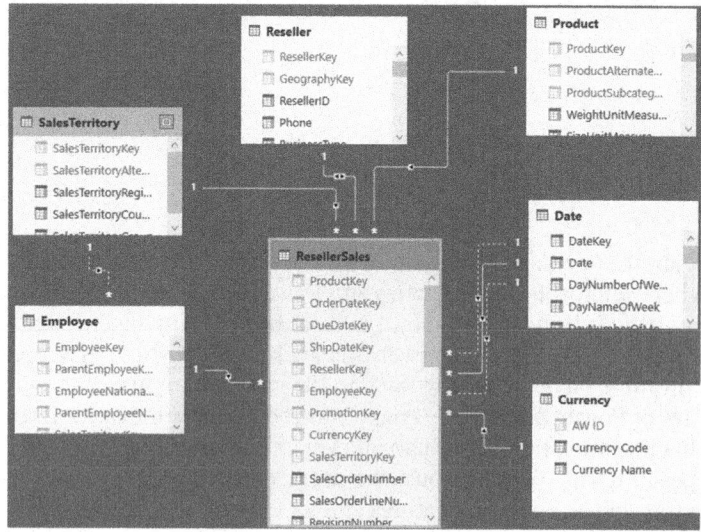

Figure 1.1 Power BI allows analysts to build data models whose features are on par with professional models implemented by BI pros.

- Team BI – Business users can share the reports and dashboards they've implemented with other team members without requiring them to install modeling or reporting tools. Suppose that Martin would like to share his sales model with his coworker, Maya. Once Martin has uploaded the model to Power BI, Maya can go online and view the reports and dashboards Martin has shared with her. She can even create her own reports and dashboards that connect to Martin's model.

- Organizational BI (or corporate BI) – BI professionals who implement organizational BI solutions, such as semantic models or real-time business intelligence, will find that they can use Power BI as a presentation layer. For example, as a BI pro, Elena has developed a Multidimensional or Tabular model layered on top of the company's data warehouse. Elena can install connectivity software on an on-premises computer so that Power BI can connect to her model. This allows business users to create instant reports and dashboards in Power BI by leveraging the existing investment in Analysis Services without moving data to the cloud! Or, if management asks for a real-time dashboard, Elena can write some code to push data to Power BI so that the dashboard updates itself as new data streams in.

 NOTE To learn more about Analysis Services, I covered implementing Analysis Services Multidimensional models in my book "Applied Microsoft Analysis Services 2005" and Tabular models in "Applied Microsoft SQL Server 2012 Analysis Services: Tabular Modeling".

Descriptive, predictive and prescriptive analytics

The main goal of BI is to get actionable insights that lead to smarter decisions and better business outcomes. Another way to classify BI is from a time perspective. Then we can identify three types of data analytics (descriptive, predictive, and prescriptive).

Descriptive analytics is retrospective. It focuses on what has happened in the past to understand the company's performance. This type of analytics is the most common and well understood. Coupled with a good data exploration tool, such as Power BI or Microsoft Excel, descriptive analytics helps you discover import trends and understand the factors that influenced these trends. You do descriptive analytics when you slice and dice data. For example, a business analyst can create a Power BI report to discover sale trends by year. Descriptive analytics can answer questions, such as "Who are my top 10 customers?", "What is the company's sales by year, quarter, month, and so on?", or "How does the company's profit compare against the predefined goal by business unit, product, time, and other subject areas?"

Predictive analytics is concerned with what will happen in the future. It uses machine learning algorithms to determine probable future outcomes and discover patterns that might not be easily discernible based on historical data. These hidden patterns can't be discovered with traditional data exploration since data relationships might be too complex, or because there's too much data for a human to analyze. Typical predictive tasks include forecasting, customer profiling, and basket analysis. Machine learning can answer questions, such as, "What are the forecasted sales numbers for the next few months?", "What other products is a customer likely to buy along with the product he or she already chose?", and, "What type of customer (described in terms of gender, age group, income, and so on) is likely to buy a given product?" Power BI includes several predictive features. Quick Insights applies machine learning algorithms to find hidden patterns, such as that the revenue for a product is steadily decreasing. You can use the Power BI clustering algorithms to quickly find groups of similar data points in a subset of data. You can add time-series forecasting to a line chart to predict sales for future periods. Thanks to the huge investments that Microsoft has made in R, a data analyst can use R scripts for data cleansing, statistical analysis, data mining, and visualizing data. Power BI can integrate with Azure Machine Learning experiments. For example, an analyst can build a predictive experiment with the Azure Machine Learning service and then visualize the results in Power BI. Or, if a BI pro has implemented a predictive model in R or Python and deployed to SQL Server, the analyst can simply query SQL Server to obtain the predictions.

Finally, *prescriptive analytics* goes beyond predictive analytics to not only attempt to predict the future but also recommend the best course of action and the implications of each decision option. Typical prescriptive tasks are optimization, simulation, and goal seek. While tools for descriptive and predictive needs have matured, prescriptive analytics is a newcomer and currently is in the realm of startup companies. The good news is that you can get prepackaged advanced analytics and prescriptive solutions with Cortana Analytics Suite, such as solutions for product recommendations and customer churn. The Microsoft Cortana Analytics Suite is a fully managed big data and advanced analytics suite that enables you to transform your data into intelligent action. The suite includes various cloud-based services, such as Azure Machine Learning for predictive analytics, Stream Analytics for real-time BI, and Power BI for dashboards and reporting. I'll show you some of these capabilities, including the Cortana digital assistant in Chapter 10, and Azure Machine Learning and Stream Analytics in Chapter 13.

1.1.2 Introducing the Power BI Products

Now that you understand BI better, let's discuss what Power BI is. Power BI is a set of products and services that enable you to connect to your data, visualize it, and share insights with other users. Next, I'll introduce you to the Power BI product offerings.

What's behind the Power BI name?
At a high level, Power BI consists of several products (listed in the order they appear in the Products menu on the powerbi.com home page):

■ Power BI (also known as Power BI Service) – A *cloud-based* business analytics service (powerbi.com) that allows you to host your data, reports, and dashboards online and share them with your coworkers. Because Power BI is hosted in the cloud and managed by Microsoft, your organization doesn't have to purchase, install, and maintain an on-premises infrastructure. Microsoft delivers weekly updates to Power BI, so the pace of innovation and improvement will continue unabated. To stay up to date with the latest features, follow the Power BI blog (https://powerbi.microsoft.com/blog/).

- Power BI Desktop – A freely available Windows desktop application that allows analysts to design self-service data models and for creating interactive reports connected to these models or to external data sources. For readers familiar with Power Pivot for Excel, Power BI Desktop offers similar self-service BI features in a standalone application (outside Excel) that updates every month.

- Power BI Premium – Targeting large organizations, Power BI Premium offers a dedicated capacity environment, giving your organization more consistent performance without requiring you to purchase per-user licenses. Suppose you want to share reports with more than 500 users within your organizations and most of these users require read-only access. Instead of licensing each user, you can reduce cost by purchasing a Power BI Premium plan that doesn't require licenses for viewers and gives you predictable performance.

- Power BI Mobile – A set of freely available mobile applications for iOS, Android, and Windows that allow users to use mobile devices, such as tablets and smartphones, to get data insights on the go. For example, a mobile user can view and interact with reports and dashboards deployed to Power BI.

- Power BI Embedded – Power BI Embedded is a collective name for a subset of the Power BI APIs for embedding content. Integrated with Power BI Service, Power BI Embedded let developers embed interactive Power BI reports in custom apps for internal or external users. For example, Teo has developed a web application for external customers. Instead of redirecting to powerbi.com, Teo can use Power BI Embedded to let customers view interactive Power BI reports embedded in his app.

- Power BI Report Server – Evolving from Microsoft SQL Server Reporting Services (SSRS), Power BI Report Server allows you to deploy Power BI data models and reports to an on-premises server. This gives you a choice for deployment and sharing: cloud and/or on-premises. And the choice doesn't have to be exclusive. For example, you might decide to deploy some reports to Power BI to leverage all features it has to offer, such as natural queries, quick insights, and integration with Excel, while deploying the rest of the reports to a Power BI Report Server portal.

 DEFINITION Microsoft Power BI is a data analytics platform for self-service, team, and organizational BI that consists of several products. Although Power BI can access other Office 365 services, such as OneDrive and SharePoint, Power BI doesn't require an Office 365 subscription and it has no dependencies to Office 365. However, if your organization has Office 365 E5 plan, you'll find that Power BI is included in it.

Product usage scenarios

The Power BI product line has grown over time and a novice Power BI user might find it difficult to understand where each product fits in. **Figure 1.2** should help you visualize the purpose of each product at a high level.

1. Power BI Desktop – The Power BI journey typically starts with Power BI Desktop. You can use Power BI Desktop to mash up data from various data sources and create a self-service data model. Or, you can use Power BI Desktop to connect directly to a data source, such as a semantic model, and start analyzing data immediately without importing data and do any modeling.

2. Power BI Report Server – One option to share your Power BI artifacts is to deploy them to on-premises Power BI Report Server. This is a good option if your organization needs an on-premises report portal that hosts not only Power BI reports but also operational SSRS reports and Excel reports.

3. Power BI – Another sharing option is to deploy to Power BI (powerbi.com). This allows you to leverage all features Power BI has to offer but it requires per-user licensing.

4. Power BI Premium – To avoid licensing per user for many users who will only view reports, a larger organization might decide to purchase a Power BI Premium plan. Besides cost savings, Power BI Premium is appealing from a performance standpoint as it offers a dedicated environment just for your organization.

5. Power BI Mobile – Although Power BI reports can render in any modern browser, your mobile workforce can install the Power BI Mobile apps on their mobile devices so that Power BI reports are optimized for the display capabilities of the device.

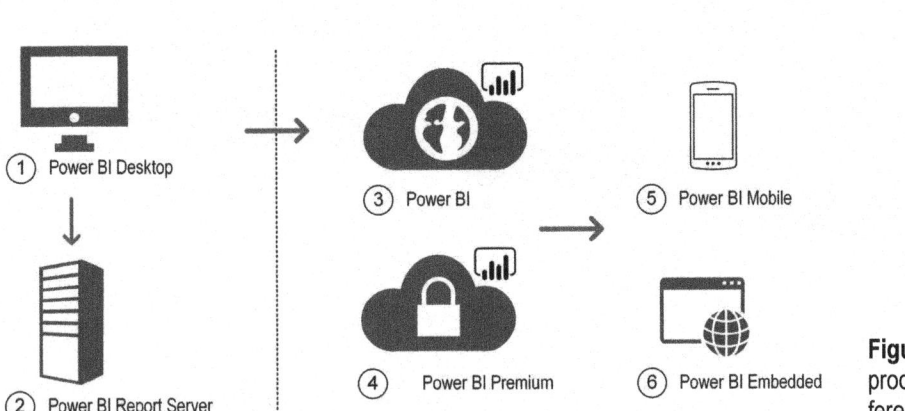

Figure 1.2 How Power BI products can be used for different tasks.

6. Power BI Embedded – A developer can integrate a custom web app with Power BI Embedded to embed Power BI reports, so they render inside the app.

As you could imagine, Power BI is a versatile platform that enables different groups of users to implement a wide range of BI solutions depending on the task at hand.

1.1.3 How Did We Get Here?

Before I delve into the Power BI capabilities, let's step back for a moment and review what events led to its existence. **Figure 1.3** shows the major milestones in the Power BI journey.

Power Pivot
Realizing the growing importance of self-service BI, in 2010 Microsoft introduced a new technology for personal and team BI called PowerPivot (renamed to Power Pivot in 2013 because of Power BI rebranding). Power Pivot was initially implemented as a freely available add-in to Excel 2010 that had to be manually downloaded and installed. Office 2013 delivered deeper integration with Power Pivot, including distributing it with Excel 2013 and allowing users to import data directly into the Power Pivot data model.

 NOTE   I covered Excel and Power Pivot data modelling in my book "Applied Microsoft SQL Server 2012 Analysis Services: Tabular Modeling". If you prefer using Excel for self-service BI, the book should give you the necessary foundation to understand Power Pivot and learn how to use it to implement self-service data models and how to integrate them with SharePoint Server.

The Power Pivot innovative engine, called xVelocity, transcended the limitations of the Excel native pivot reports. It allows users to load multiple datasets and import more than one million rows (the maximum number of rows that can fit in an Excel spreadsheet). xVelocity compresses the data efficiently and stores it in the computer's main memory.

 DEFINITION   xVelocity is a columnar data engine that compresses and stores data in memory. Originally introduced in Power Pivot, the xVelocity data engine has a very important role in Microsoft BI. xVelocity is now included in other Microsoft offerings, including SQL Server columnstore indexes, Tabular models in Analysis Services, Power BI Desktop, and Power BI.

For example, using Power Pivot, a business user can import data from a variety of data sources, relate the data, and create a data model. Then the user can create pivot reports or Power View reports to gain insights from the data model.

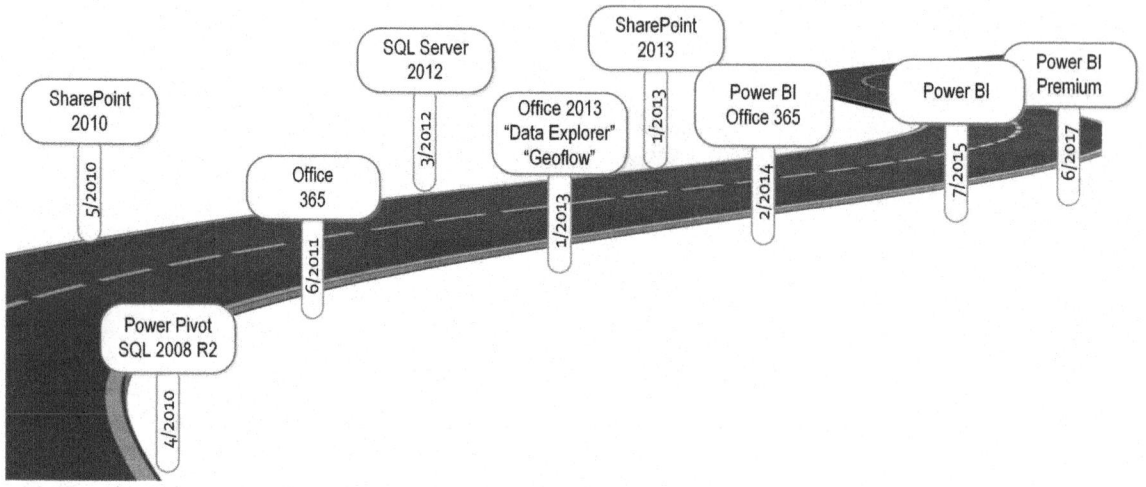

Figure 1.3 Important milestones related to Power BI.

SQL Server

Originally developed as a relational database management system (RDBMS), Microsoft SQL Server is now a multi-product offering. In the context of organizational BI, SQL Server includes Analysis Services, which has traditionally allowed BI professionals to implement multidimensional cubes. SQL Server 2012 introduced another path for implementing organizational models called Tabular. Think of Analysis Services Tabular as Power Pivot on steroids. Just like Power Pivot, Tabular allows you to create in-memory data models but it also adds security and performance features to allow BI pros to scale these models and implement data security that is more granular.

SQL Server includes also Reporting Services, which has been traditionally used to implement paper-oriented standard reports (also referred to as paginated reports). However, SQL Server 2012 introduced a SharePoint 2010-integrated reporting tool, named Power View, for authoring ad hoc interactive reports. Power View targets business users without requiring query knowledge and report authoring experience. Suppose that Martin has uploaded his Power Pivot model to SharePoint Server. Now Maya (or anyone else who has access to the model) can quickly build a great-looking tabular or chart report in a few minutes to visualize the data from the Power Pivot model. Or, Maya can use Power View to explore data in a Multidimensional or Tabular organizational model. Microsoft used some of the Power View features to deliver the same interactive experience to Power BI reports.

In Office 2013, Microsoft integrated Power View with Excel 2013 to allow business users to create interactive reports from Power Pivot models and organizational Tabular models. And Excel 2016 extended Power View to connect to multidimensional cubes. However, Microsoft probably won't enhance Power View in Excel anymore (it's disabled by default in Excel 2016) to encourage users to transition to Power BI Desktop, which is now the Microsoft premium data exploration tool.

SharePoint Server

Up to the release of Power BI, Microsoft BI has been intertwined with SharePoint. SharePoint Server is a Microsoft on-premises product for document storage and collaboration. In SharePoint Server 2010, Microsoft added new services, collectively referred to as Power Pivot for SharePoint, which allowed users to deploy Power Pivot data models to SharePoint and then share reports that connect to these data models.

For example, a business user can upload the Excel file containing a data model and reports to SharePoint. Authorized users can view the embedded reports and create their own reports.

SharePoint Server 2013 brought better integration with Power Pivot and support for data models and reports created in Excel 2013. When integrated with SQL Server 2012, SharePoint Server 2013 offers other compelling BI features, including deploying and managing SQL Server Reporting Services (SSRS) reports, team BI powered by Power Pivot for SharePoint, and PerformancePoint Services dashboards.

Later, Microsoft realized that SharePoint presents adoption barriers for the fast-paced world of BI. Therefore, Microsoft deemphasized the role of SharePoint as a BI platform in SharePoint Server 2016 in favor of Power BI in the cloud and Power BI Report Server on premises. SharePoint Server can still be integrated with Power Pivot and Reporting Services but it's no longer a strategic on-premises BI platform.

Microsoft Excel

While prior to Power BI, SharePoint Server was the Microsoft premium server-based platform for BI, Microsoft Excel was their premium BI tool on the desktop. Besides Power Pivot and Power View, which I already introduced, Microsoft added other BI-related add-ins to extend the Excel data analytics features. To help end users perform predictive tasks in Excel, Microsoft released a Data Mining add-in for Microsoft Excel 2007, which is also available with newer Excel versions. For example, using this add-in, an analyst can perform a market basket analysis, such as to find which products customers tend to buy together.

 NOTE In 2014, Microsoft introduced a cloud-based Azure Machine Learning Service (http://azure.microsoft.com/en-us/services/machine-learning) to allow users to create predictive models in the cloud, such as a model that predicts the customer churn probability. SQL Server 2016 added integration with R and SQL Server 2017 added integration with Python. Azure Machine Learning and R supersede the Data Mining add-in for self-service predictive analytics and Analysis Services data mining for organizational predictive analytics. It's unlikely that we'll see future Microsoft investments in these two technologies.

In January 2013, Microsoft introduced a freely available Data Explorer add-in for Excel, which was later renamed to Power Query. Power Query is now included in Excel 2016 and Power BI Desktop. Unique in the self-service BI tools market, Power Query allows business users to transform and cleanse data before it's imported. For example, Martin can use Power Query to replace wrong values in the source data or to un-pivot a crosstab report. In Excel, Power Query is an optional path for importing data. If data doesn't require transformation, a business user can directly import the data using the Excel or Power Pivot data import capabilities. However, Power BI always uses Power Query when you import data so that its data transformation capabilities are there if you need them. For example, **Figure 1.4** shows that I have applied several steps to cleanse and shape the data in Power Query (called Query Editor in Power BI Desktop).

Another data analytics add-in that deserves attention is Power Map. Originally named Geoflow, Power Map is another freely available Excel add-in that's specifically designed for geospatial reporting. Power Map is included by default in Excel 2016. Using Power Map, a business user can create interactive 3D maps from Excel tables or Power Pivot data models. Power Map is not included in Power BI but you can get some of its capabilities in Power BI when you import the GlobeMap custom visual from Microsoft Store (https://appsource.microsoft.com).

Power BI for Office 365

Unless you live under a rock, you know that one of the most prominent IT trends nowadays is toward cloud computing. Chances are that your organization is already using the Microsoft Azure Services Platform - a Microsoft cloud offering for hosting and scaling applications and databases through Microsoft datacenters. Microsoft Azure gives you the ability to focus on your business and to outsource infrastructure maintenance to Microsoft.

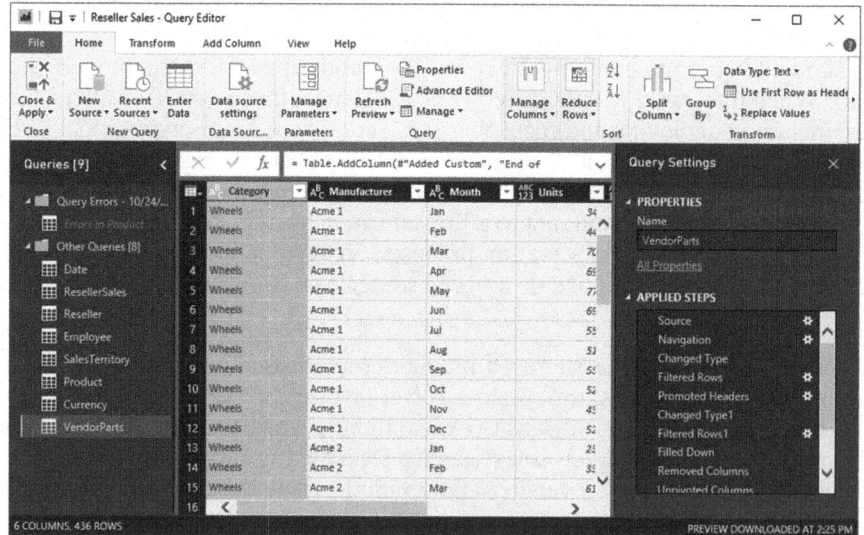

Figure 1.4 A free Excel add-in, Power Map enables you to analyze geospatial data by creating 3D visualizations with Bing maps.

In 2011, Microsoft unveiled its Office 365 cloud service to allow organizations to subscribe to and use a variety of Microsoft products online, including Microsoft Exchange and SharePoint. For example, at Prologika we use Office 365 for email, a subscription-based (click-to-run) version of Microsoft Office, OneDrive for Business, Skype for Business, Dynamics Online and other products. From a BI standpoint, Office 365 allows business users to deploy Excel workbooks and Power Pivot data models to the cloud. Then they can view the embedded reports online, create new reports, and share BI artifacts.

In early 2014, Microsoft further extended SharePoint for Office 365 with additional BI features, including natural queries (Q&A), searching and discovering organizational datasets, and mobile support for Power View reports. Together with the "power" desktop add-ins (Power Pivot, Power View, Power Query, and Power Map), the service was marketed and sold under the name "Power BI for Office 365". While the desktop add-ins were freely available, Power BI for Office 365 required a subscription. Microsoft sold Power BI for Office 365 independently or as an add-on to Office 365 business plans.

Because of its dependency to SharePoint and Office, Power BI for Office 365 didn't gain wide adoption. One year after unveiling the new Power BI platform, Microsoft discontinued Power BI for Office 365. Power BI for Office 365 shouldn't be confused with the new Power BI platform, which was completely rearchitected for agile and modern BI.

Power BI

Finally, the winding road brings us to Power BI, which is the subject of this book. In July 2015, after several months of public preview, Microsoft officially launched a standalone version of Power BI that had no dependencies on Office 365, SharePoint and Microsoft Office. What caused this change? The short answer is removing adoption barriers for both Microsoft and consumers. For Microsoft it became clear that to be competitive in today's fast-paced marketplace, its BI offerings can't depend on other product groups and release cycles. Waiting for new product releases on two and three-year cadences couldn't introduce the new features Microsoft needed to compete effectively with "pure" BI vendors (competitors who focus only on BI tools) who have entered the BI market in the past few years.

After more than a decade working with different BI technologies and many customers, I do believe that Microsoft BI is the best and most comprehensive BI platform on the market! But it's not perfect. One ongoing challenge is coordinating BI features across product groups. Take for example SharePoint, which Microsoft promoted as a platform for sharing BI artifacts. Major effort underwent to extend SharePoint with SSRS in SharePoint integration mode, PerformancePoint, Power Pivot, and so on. But these products are owned by different product groups and apparently coordination has been problematic. For example, after years of promises for mobile rendering, Power View in SharePoint Server still requires Microsoft Silverlight for rendering, thus barring access from non-Windows devices.

Seeking a stronger motivation for customers to upgrade, Excel added the "power" add-ins and was promoted as the Microsoft premium BI tool on the desktop. However, the Excel dependency turned out to be a double-edged sword. While there could be a billion Excel users worldwide, adding a new feature must be thoroughly tested to ensure that there are no backward compatibility issues or breaking changes, and that takes a lot of time. Case in point: we had to wait almost three years until Excel 2016 to connect Power View reports to multidimensional cubes (only Tabular was supported before), although Analysis Services Multidimensional has much broader adoption than Tabular.

For consumers, rolling out a Microsoft BI solution has been problematic. Microsoft BI has been traditionally criticized for its deployment complexity and steep price tag. Although SharePoint Server offers much more than just data analytics, having a SharePoint server integrated with SQL Server has been a cost-prohibitive proposition for smaller organizations. As many of you would probably agree, SharePoint Server adds complexity and troubleshooting it isn't for the faint of heart. Power BI for Office 365 alleviated some of these concerns by shifting maintenance to become Microsoft's responsibility, but many customers still find its "everything but the kitchen sink" approach too overwhelming and cost-prohibitive if all they want is the ability to deploy and share BI artifacts.

Going back to the desktop, Excel wasn't originally designed as a BI tool, leaving the end user with the impression that BI was something Microsoft bolted on top of Excel. For example, navigating add-ins and learning how to navigate the cornucopia of features has been too much to ask from novice business users.

How does the new Power BI address these challenges?
Power BI embraces the following design tenets to address the previous pain points:

- Simplicity – Power BI was designed for BI from the ground up. As you'll see, Microsoft streamlined and simplified the user interface to ensure that your experience is intuitive, and you aren't distracted by other non-BI features and menus.

- No dependencies to SharePoint and Office – Because it doesn't depend on SharePoint and Excel, Power BI can evolve independently. This doesn't mean that business users are now asked to forgo Excel. To the contrary, if you like Excel and prefer to create data models in Excel, you'll find that you can still deploy them to Power BI.

- Frequent updates – Microsoft delivers weekly updates for Power BI Service and monthly updates for Power BI Desktop. This should allow Microsoft to stay at the forefront of the BI market. For example, Microsoft delivered more than 1,000 new features and enhancements since Power BI became generally available, as you can witness at http://aka.ms/pbifeatures!

- Always up to date – Because of its service-based nature, as a Power BI subscriber you're always on the latest and greatest version. In addition, because Power BI is a cloud service, you can get started with Power BI in a minute as you don't have to provision servers and software.

- Free – As you'll see in "Power BI Editions and Pricing" (later in this chapter), Power BI has the best business model: most of it is free! Power BI Desktop and Power BI Mobile are free. Following a freemium model, Power BI is free for personal use and has subscription options that you could pay for if you need to share with other users. Cost was the biggest hindrance of Power BI, and it's now been turned around completely. You can't beat free!

1.1.4 Power BI and the Microsoft Data Platform

No tool is a kingdom of its own and no tool should work in isolation. If you're tasked to evaluate BI tools, consider the Power BI is an integral part of the Microsoft Data Platform that started in early 2004 with the powerful promise to bring "BI to the masses." Microsoft subsequently extended the message to "BI to the masses, by the masses" to emphasize its commitment to democratize. Indeed, a few years after Microsoft got into the BI space, the BI landscape changed dramatically. Once a domain of cost-prohibitive and highly specialized tools, BI is now within the reach of every user and organization!

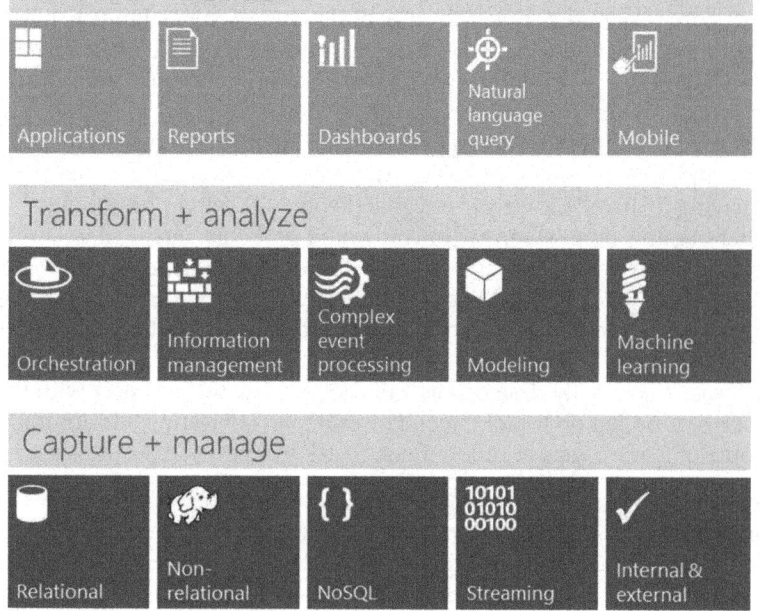

Figure 1.5 The Microsoft Data Platform provides services and tools that address various data analytics and management needs on premises and in the cloud.

Understanding the Microsoft Data Platform

Figure 1.5 illustrates the most prominent services of the Microsoft Data Platform (and there are new cloud services added almost every month!)

 DEFINITION The Microsoft Data Platform is a multi-service offering that addresses the data capturing, transformation, and analytics needs to create modern BI solutions. It's powered by Microsoft SQL Server on premises and Microsoft Azure in the cloud.

Table 1.1 summarizes the various services of the Microsoft Data Platform and their purposes.

Table 1.1   The Microsoft Data Platform consists of many products and services, with the most prominent described below.

Category	Service	Audience	Purpose
Capture and manage	Relational	IT	Capture relational data in SQL Server, Analytics Platform System, Azure SQL Database, Azure SQL Data Warehouse, and others.
	Non-relational	IT	Capture Big Data in Azure HDInsight Service and Microsoft HDInsight Server.
	NoSQL	IT	Capture NoSQL data in cloud structures, such as Azure Table Storage, Cosmo DB, and others.
	Streaming	IT	Allow capturing of data streams from Internet of Things (IoT) with Azure StreamInsight.
	Internal and External	IT/Business	Referring to cloud on your terms, allow connecting to both internal and external data, such as connecting Power BI to online services (Google Analytics, Salesforce, Dynamics CRM, and many others).

Category	Service	Audience	Purpose
Transform and analyze	Orchestration	IT/Business	Create data orchestration workflows with SQL Server Integration Services (SSIS), Azure Data Factory, Power Query, Power BI Desktop, and Data Quality Services (DQS).
	Information management	IT/Business	Allow IT to establish rules for information management and data governance using SharePoint, Azure Data Catalog, and Office 365, as well as manage master data using SQL Server Master Data Services.
	Complex event processing	IT	Process data streams using SQL Server StreamInsight on premise and Azure Stream Analytics Service in the cloud.
	Modelling	IT/Business	Transform data in semantic structures with Analysis Services Multidimensional, Tabular, Power Pivot, and Power BI.
	Machine learning	IT/Business	Create data mining models in SQL Server Analysis Services, Excel data mining add-in, and Azure Machine Learning Service.
Visualize and decide	Applications	IT/Business	Analyze data with desktop applications, including Excel, Power BI Desktop, SSRS Designer, Report Builder, Power View, Power Map.
	Reports	IT/Business	Create operational and ad hoc reports with Power BI, SSRS, and Excel.
	Dashboards	IT/Business	Implement and share dashboards with Power BI and SSRS.
	Mobile	IT/Business	View reports and dashboards on mobile devices with Power BI Mobile.

For more information about the Microsoft Data Platform, please visit https://www.microsoft.com/en-us/server-cloud/solutions/business-intelligence.

About Cortana Analytics Suite

While I'm on the subject of the Microsoft Data Platform, you should know that Microsoft has a much broader vision for building intelligent applications, collectively known as Cortana Analytics Suite (see **Figure 1.6**).

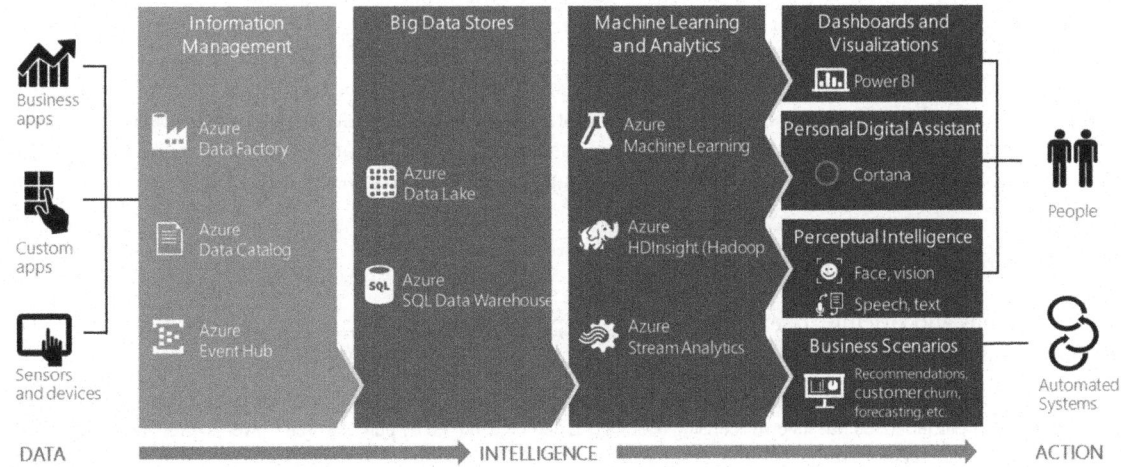

Figure 1.6 Cortana Analytics Suite is a set of tools and services for building intelligence applications.

Cortana Analytics Suite was built on years of Microsoft's research in perceptual intelligence, including speech recognition, natural user interaction, and predictive analytics. The key benefit is Cortana Analytics will let you roll out prepackaged analytics solutions, reducing time to market and project costs over do-it-all-yourself approaches. For example, there will be prepackaged solutions for Sales and Marketing (customer acquisition, cross-sell, upsell, loyalty programs, and marketing mix optimization), Finance and Risk (fraud detection and credit risk management), Customer Relationships Management (lifetime customer value, personalized offers, and product recommendation), and Operations and Workspace (operational efficiency, smart buildings, predictive maintenance, and supply chain).

Cortana Analytics Suite provides services to bring data in so that you can analyze it. For example, you can use Azure Data Factory (a cloud ETL service) so that you can pull data from any source (both relational and non-relational data sources), in an automated and scheduled way, while performing the necessary data cleansing and transformations. As I mentioned, Event Hubs ingests data streams. The incoming data can be persisted in Big Data storage services, such as Data Lake and Azure SQL Data Warehouse.

You can then use a wide range of analytics services from Azure Machine Learning and Stream Analytics to analyze the data that is stored in Big Data storage. This means you can create analytics services and models that are specific to your business needs, such as real time-demand forecasting. The resulting analytics services and models that you create by taking these steps, can then be surfaced as interactive dashboards and visualizations powered by Power BI.

These same analytics services and models can also be integrated with various applications (web, mobile, or rich-client applications), as well as via integrations with Cortana Personal Digital Assistant (demonstrated in Chapter 10). This way, end users can naturally interact with them via speech. For example, end users can be notified proactively by Cortana if the analytics model finds a new data anomaly, or whatever deserves the attention of the business users. For more information about Cortana Analytics Suite, visit http://www.microsoft.com/en-us/server-cloud/cortana-analytics-suite/overview.aspx.

The role of Power BI in the Microsoft Data Platform

In **Table 1.1**, you can see that Power BI plays an important role in the Microsoft Data Platform by providing services for getting, transforming and visualizing your data. As far as data acquisition goes, it can connect to cloud and on-premises data sources so that you can import and relate data irrespective of its origin.

Capturing data is one thing but making dirty data suitable for analysis is quite another. However, you can use the data transformation capabilities of Power BI Desktop (or Power Query in Excel) to cleanse and enrich your data. For example, someone might give you an Excel crosstab report. If you import the data as it is, you'll quickly find that you won't be able to relate it to the other tables in your data model. However, with a few clicks, you can un-pivot your data and remove unwanted rows. Moreover, the transformation steps are recorded so that you can repeat the same transformations later if you're given an updated file.

The main purpose and strength of Power BI is visualizing data in reports and dashboards without requiring any special skills. You can explore and understand your data by having fun with it. To summarize insights from these reports, you can then compile a dashboard. Or, you can build the dashboard by asking natural questions. **Figure 1.7** shows a sample dashboard assembled from existing reports.

1.1.5 Power BI Editions and Pricing

Power BI editions and pricing are explained at https://powerbi.microsoft.com/pricing. As it stands, Power BI is available in three editions: Free, Power BI Pro, and Power BI Premium.

 NOTE These editions apply to Power BI Service (powerbi.com) only. Power BI Desktop and Power BI Mobile are freely available. Power BI Embedded has its own licensing options and can be acquired by purchasing a Power BI Premium plan or Azure Power BI Embedded plan.

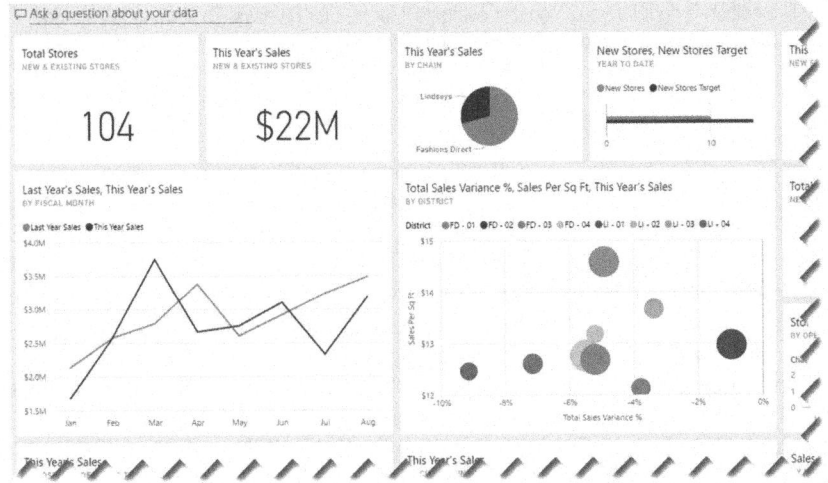

Figure 1.7 Power BI lets you assemble dashboards from existing reports or by asking natural questions.

Understanding the Free edition

The Power BI Free edition is a free offering which include most of the Power BI features, but it's licensed for personal use. "Personal" means that a Power BI Free user can't share artifacts with other users. Power BI veterans would probably recall that Power BI Free had many limitations in the past, including limitations for data refresh, data storage, and data connectivity. After the licensing changes surrounding the release of Power BI Premium in June 2017, Microsoft lifted these limitations so Power BI Free has the same features as Power BI Pro except for sharing and collaboration. Specifically, here are the most significant features that are not available in Power BI Free:

- Dashboard sharing – If you have been using Power BI for a while you might recall that that was the only sharing option available for Power BI Free users. This is no longer the case. A Power BI free user can't share dashboards with other users.

- Workspaces – A Power BI Free user can't create workspaces or be added as a member of a workspace.

- Apps – A Power BI Free user can't create an app (Power BI apps are a mechanism to distribute pre-packaged external or internal content).

- Subscriptions – Power BI supports report subscriptions so that reports are delivered via email to subscribed users when the data changes. Power BI Free users can't create subscriptions.

- Connect to published datasets – This feature allows users to connect Excel or Power BI Desktop to datasets published to Power BI, and create pivot reports. This is conceptually like connecting directly to an Analysis Services semantic model. This feature is not available to Power BI Free users.

 NOTE Microsoft views Power BI Free as an experimental edition for testing Power BI features without requiring a formal approval or on-boarding process. Any user can sign up for Power BI Free using a work email and can keep on using it without time restrictions.

Understanding the Power BI Pro edition

This paid edition has a sticker price of $9.99 per user per month but Microsoft offers discounts so check with your Microsoft reseller. Also, if your organization uses Office 365, you'll find that Power BI Pro is included in the E5 business plan. Power BI Pro offers all the features of Power BI Free, plus sharing and collaboration.

NOTE Not sure if the Power BI Pro edition is right for you? You can evaluate it for free for 60 days. To start the trial period, log in the Power BI portal, click the Settings menu in the top right corner, and then click "Manage Personal Storage". Then click the "Try Pro for free" link.

Understanding the Power BI Premium edition

Think of Power BI Premium as an add-on to Power BI Pro. It requires your organization to commit to a monthly plan. A Power BI Premium plan gives you preconfigured hardware (called a node) that is isolated from other organizations. You can purchase additional nodes to scale out your workload. A Power BI Premium plan has a fixed monthly cost irrespective of how many Power BI Free users you distribute content to. However, every user who will contribute content or change existing content requires a separate Power BI Pro license. Microsoft provides a nice online calculator at https://powerbi.microsoft.com/calculator/ to help you estimate your workload of contributors (Pro users), frequent users, and occasional users. Once you plug in the numbers, the online calculator recommends a Power BI Premium plan. For example, given 1,000 total users (200 Pro users, 350 frequent users, and 450 occasional users), the calculator recommends one node on P1 plan costing 6,993 per month ($1,998/month for the 200 Pro users and $4,995 per month for the 1 P1 node). This is $3,007 less compared to Power BI Pro per-user licensing!

 NOTE From a cost perspective alone, it's obvious that the break-even point between Power BI Pro and Power BI Premium is 500 users. Above that number, Power BI Premium saves money.

From a feature standpoint and compared to Power BI Pro, Power BI Premium adds higher dataset refresh rates (Power BI Pro is limited to a maximum of 8 refreshes per day). Microsoft has promised more Power BI Premium-specific features in the future, such as unlimited dataset size, pin to memory, incremental refresh, read-only replicas, and geo distribution.

Comparing editions and features

Table 1.2 summarizes features so you can compare editions side by side.

Table 1.2 Comparing Power BI editions and features.

Feature	Power BI Free	Power BI Pro	Power BI Premium
Connect to all data sources	Yes	Yes	Yes
Create self-service data models	Yes	Yes	Yes
Publish to web (anonymous access)	No	Yes	Yes
Dashboard sharing	No	Yes (can't share to Power BI Free)	Yes (can share to Power BI Free)
Workspaces	No	Yes	Yes
Organizational apps	No	Yes (can't distribute to Power BI Free)	Yes (can distribute to Power BI Free)
Subscriptions	No	Yes (can't distribute to Power BI Free)	Yes (can distribute to Power BI Free)
Connect Excel and Power BI Desktop to published datasets	No	Yes	Yes
Maximum dataset size	1GB	1GB	1GB
Dataset refresh frequency	8/day	8/day	48/day
Isolation with dedicated capacity	No	No	Yes

1.2   Understanding the Power BI Capabilities

Now that I've introduced you to Power BI and the Microsoft Data Platform, let's take a closer look at the Power BI capabilities. I'll discuss them in the context of each of the Power BI products. As I mentioned in section 1.1, Power BI is an umbrella name that unifies several products: Power BI Service, Power BI Desktop, Power BI Premium, Power BI Mobile, Power BI Report Server, and Power BI Embedded. Don't worry if you don't immediately understand some of these technologies or if you find this section too technical. I'll clarify them throughout the rest of this chapter and the book.

1.2.1   Understanding Power BI Service

At the heart of Power BI is the cloud-based business analytics service referred to as *Power BI* or *Power BI Service*. You use the service every time you utilize any of the powerbi.com features, such as connecting to online services, deploying and refreshing data models, viewing reports and dashboards, sharing content, or using Q&A (the natural language search feature). Next, I'll introduce you to some of Power BI Service's most prominent features.

Connect to any data source
The BI journey starts with connecting to data that could be a single file or multiple data sources. Power BI allows you to connect to virtually any accessible data source, either hosted on the cloud or in your company's data center. Your self-service project can start small. If all you need is to analyze a single file, such as an Excel workbook, you might not need a data model. Instead, you can connect Power BI to your file, import its data, and start analyzing data immediately. However, if your data acquisition needs are more involved, such as when you relate data from multiple sources, you can use Power BI Desktop to build a data model whose capabilities can be on par with professional data models and cubes!

Some data sources, such as Analysis Services models, support live connections. Because data isn't imported, live connections allow reports and dashboards to always be up to date. In the case when you need to import data, you can specify how often the data will be refreshed to keep it synchronized with changes in the original data source. For example, Martin might have decided to import data from the corporate data warehouse and deploy the model to Power BI. To keep the published model up to date, Martin can schedule the data model to refresh daily.

Apps (content packs) for online services
Continuing on data connectivity, chances are that your organization uses popular cloud services, such as Salesforce, Marketo, Dynamics CRM, Google Analytics, Zendesk, and others. Power BI apps (also known as content packs) for online services allow business users to connect to such services and analyze their data without technical setup and data modeling. Apps include a curated collection of dashboards and reports that continuously update with the latest data from these services. With a few clicks, you can connect to one of the supported online services and start analyzing data using prepackaged reports and dashboards. If the provided content isn't enough, you can create your own reports and dashboards. **Figure 1.8** shows a prepackaged dashboard for analyzing website traffic. This dashboard is included in the Power BI Google Analytics app.

Dashboards and reports
Collected data is meaningless without useful reports. Insightful dashboards and reports is what Power BI Service is all about. To offer a more engaging experience and let users have fun with data while exploring it, Power BI reports are interactive. For example, the report in **Figure 1.9** demonstrates one of these interactive features. In this case, the user selected Linda in the Bar Chart on the right. This action filtered the Column Chart on the left so that the user can see Linda's contribution to the overall sales. This feature is called cross highlighting

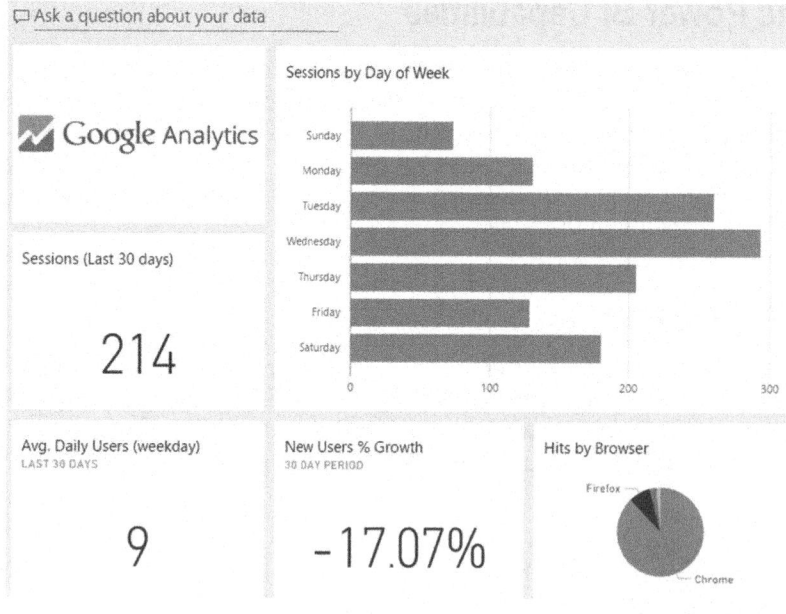

Figure 1.8 Apps allow you to connect to online services and analyze data using prepackaged reports and dashboards.

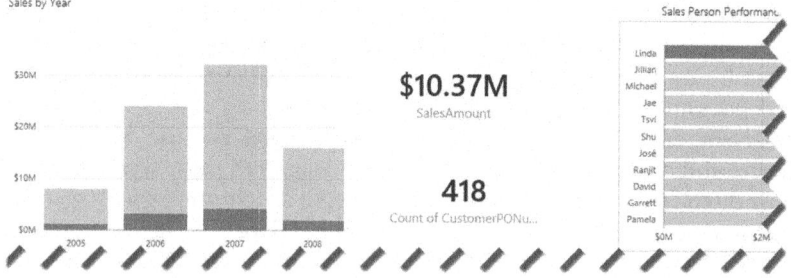

Figure 1.9 Interactive reports allow users to explore data in different ways.

Natural queries (Q&A)

Based on my experience, the feature that excites the users the most is Power BI natural queries or Q&A. End users are often overwhelmed when asked to create ad hoc reports from a data model. They don't know which fields to use and where to find them. The unfortunate "solution" by IT is to create new reports to answer new questions. This might result in a ton of reports that are replaced by new reports and are never used again. However, Power BI allows users to ask natural questions, such as "this year's sales by district in descending order by this year's sales" (see **Figure 1.10**).

Not only can Power BI interpret natural questions, but it also chooses the best visualization! While in this case Q&A has decided to use a Bar Chart, it might have chosen a map if the question was phrased in a different way. And, you can always change the visualization manually if the Power BI selection isn't adequate.

NOTE As of the time of writing this book, Q&A is supported only when data is imported into Power BI, such as when you create a Power BI Desktop model that sources data, and then upload the model to Power BI Service. Q&A is also available when Power BI connects live to Analysis Services Tabular model but not with other data sources that support direct connections. Q&A is also available in the Power BI Mobile iOS apps. Q&A is currently in English only (Spanish language support is in preview).

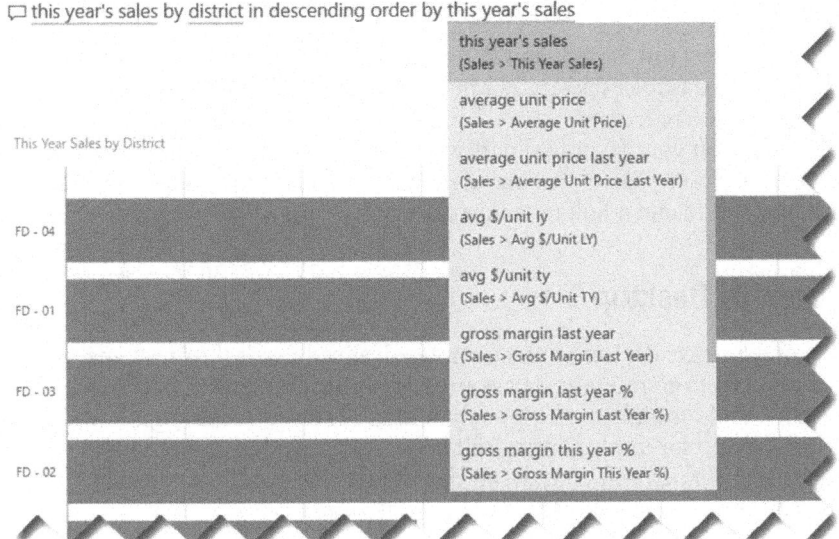

Figure 1.10 Q&A allows users to explore data by asking natural questions.

Sharing and collaboration

Once you've created informative reports and dashboards, you might want to share them with your coworkers. Power BI supports several sharing options but recall that all of them require Power BI Pro or Premium subscriptions. To start, you can share dashboards as read-only with your coworkers. Or you can use Power BI Pro workspaces to allow groups of people to have access to the same workspace content and collaborate on it. For example, if Maya works in sales, she can create a Sales Department workspace and grant her coworkers access to the workspace. Then all content added to the Sales Department workspace will be shared among the group members.

Yet a third way to share content is to create an organizational app. Like an online app that you can use to analyze data from popular online services, you can use a Power BI app to share content from a workspace across teams or even with everyone from your organization. Users can discover and open organizational apps from the Power BI AppSource page (see **Figure 1.11**). In this case, the user sees that someone has published a Reseller Sales app. The user can connect to the pack and access its content as read-only.

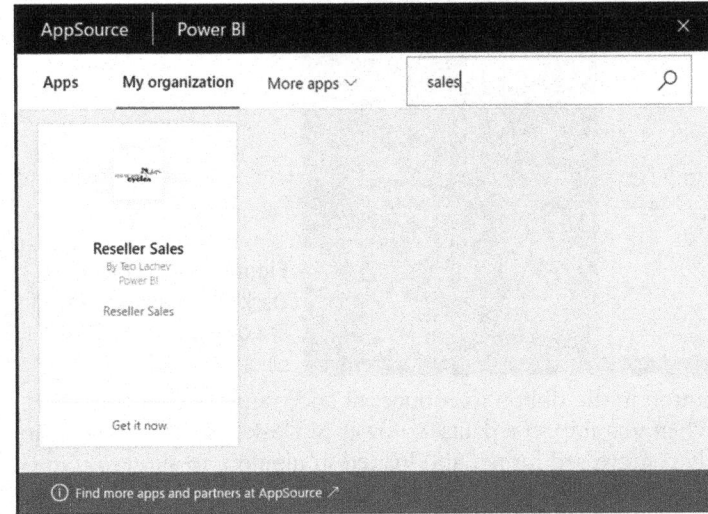

Figure 1.11 Users within your organization can use the Power BI AppSource to discover published external (online services) or internal (organizational) apps.

Alerts and subscriptions

Do you want to be notified when your data changes beyond certain levels? Of course, you do! You can set up as many alerts as you want in both Power BI Service and Power BI Mobile. You can set rules to be alerted when single number tiles in your dashboard exceed limits that you set. With data-driven alerts, you can gain insights and act wherever you're located.

Would you like Power BI to email you your favorite report when its data changes? Just view the report in Power BI Service and subscribe to a report page of interest. Power BI will regularly send a screenshot of that report page directly to your mail inbox and a link to the actual report.

1.2.2 Understanding Power BI Desktop

Oftentimes, data analytics go beyond a single dataset. To meet more advanced needs, business analysts create data models, such as to relate data from multiple data sources and then implement business calculations. The Power BI premium design tool for implementing such models is Power BI Desktop. Power BI Desktop is a freely available Windows app for implementing self-service data models and reports. You can download it for free from https://powerbi.microsoft.com/desktop or from the Downloads menu in Power BI. Windows 10 users can also install Power BI Desktop from Microsoft Store.

Understanding Power BI Desktop features

Before Power BI, data analysts could implement data models in Excel. This option is still available, and you can upload your Excel data models to Power BI. However, to overcome the challenges associated with Excel data modeling (see section 1.1.3), Microsoft introduced Power BI Desktop.

If you are familiar with Excel self-service BI, think of Power BI Desktop as the unification of Power Pivot, Power Query, and Power View. Previously available as Excel add-ins, these tools now converge in a single tool. No more guessing which add-in to use and where to find it! At a high level, the data modelling experience in Power BI Desktop now encompasses the following steps (see **Figure 1.12**).

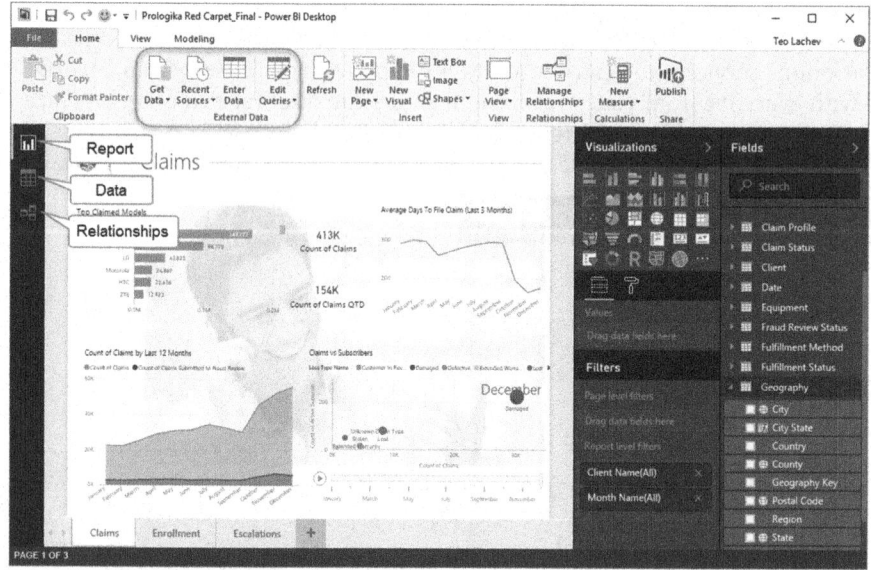

Figure 1.12 Power BI Desktop unifies the capabilities of Power Pivot, Power Query, and Power View.

1. Former Power Query – Use the Get Data button in the ribbon to connect to and transform the data. This process is like using Excel Power Query. When you import a dataset, Power BI Desktop creates a table and loads the data. The data is stored in a highly compressed format and loaded in memory to allow you to slice and dice the data without sacrificing performance. However, unlike Excel, Power BI Desktop allows

you to connect directly to a limited number of fast databases, such as Analysis Services and Azure SQL Data Warehouse, where it doesn't make sense to import the data.

2. Former Power Pivot – View and make changes to the data model using the Data and Relationships tabs in the left navigation bar. This is the former Power Pivot part.

3. Former Power View – Create interactive reports using the Report tab on the left, as you can do using Power View in Excel (version 2013 or higher).

 NOTE Some data sources, such as Analysis Services, support live connectivity. Once you connect to a live data source, you can jump directly to the Report tab and start creating reports. There are no queries to edit and models to design. In this case, Power BI Desktop acts as a presentation layer that's directly connected to the data source.

Comparing design environments

Because there are many Power Pivot models out there, Power BI allows data analysts to deploy Excel files with embedded data models to Power BI Service and view the included pivot reports and Power View reports online. Analysts can now choose which modeling tool to use:

- Microsoft Excel – Use this option if you prefer to work with Excel and you're familiar with the data modelling features delivered by Power Pivot, Power Query, Power View and Power Map.
- Power BI Desktop – Use this free option if you prefer a simplified tool that's specifically designed for data analytics and that's updated more frequently than Excel.

Table 1.3 compares these two design options side by side to help you choose a design environment. Let's go quickly through the list. While Excel supports at least three ways to import data, many users might struggle in understanding how they compare. By contrast, Power BI Desktop has only one data import option, which is the equivalent of Power Query in Excel. Similarly, Excel has various menus in different places that relate to data modelling. By contrast, if you use Power BI Desktop to import data, your data modelling experience is much more simplified.

Table 1.3   This table compares the data modelling capabilities of Microsoft Excel and Power BI Desktop.

Feature	Excel	Power BI Desktop
Data import	Excel native import, Power Pivot, Power Query	Query Editor
Data transformation	Power Query	Query Editor
Modeling	Power Pivot	Data and Relationships tabs
Reporting	Excel pivot reports, Power View, Power Map	Power BI reports (enhanced Power View reports)
Update frequency	Office releases or more often with Office 365 click-to-run	Monthly
Server deployment	SharePoint, Power BI, and Power BI Report Server	Power BI and Power BI Report Server
Power BI deployment	Import data or connect to the Excel file	Deployed as Power BI Desktop (pbix) file
Convert models	Can't import Power BI Desktop models	Can import Excel data model
Upgrade to Tabular	Yes	Yes
Object model for automation	Yes	No
Cost	Excel license	Free

Excel allows you to create pivot, Power View, and Power Map reports from Power Pivot data models. At this point, Power BI Desktop supports interactive Power BI reports (think of Power View reports on steroids) and some of the Power Map features (available as a GlobeMap custom visual), although it regularly adds more visualizations and features.

The Excel update frequency depends on how it's installed. If you install it from a setup disk (MSI installation), you need to wait for the next version to get new features. Office 365 includes subscription-based Microsoft Office (click-to-run installation) which delivers new features as they get available. If you take the Power BI Desktop path, you'll need to download and install updates as they become available. Power BI Desktop is updated monthly so you're always on the latest!

As far as deployment goes, you can deploy Excel Power Pivot models to SharePoint, Power BI Report Server, or Power BI. Power BI Desktop models (files with extension *.pbix) can be deployed to Power BI and Power BI Report Server. Behind the scenes, both Excel and Power BI Desktop use the in-memory xVelocity engine to compress and store imported data.

Power BI Desktop supports importing Power Pivot models from Excel to allow you to migrate models from Excel to Power BI Desktop. Excel doesn't support importing Power BI Desktop models yet, so you can't convert your Power BI Desktop files to Excel data models. A BI pro can migrate Excel data models to Tabular models when organizational features, such as scalability and security, are desirable. Although not officially supported by Microsoft, it's possible to upgrade Power BI Desktop models to Analysis Services Tabular because they share the same schema.

1.2.3 Understanding Power BI Premium

I previously explained that Power BI Premium extends the Power BI Pro capabilities by providing a dedicated environment and ability to reduce licensing cost. Let's take a quick look at some of the most prominent Power BI Premium features.

Understanding shared and dedicated capacity

Like how a Windows folder or network share is used to stored logically related files, a Power BI workspace is a container of logically related Power BI artifacts. A workspace is in a shared capacity when its workloads run on computational resources shared by other customers. Power BI Free and Power BI Pro workspaces always run in a shared capacity. However, in Power BI Premium, a Power BI Pro user with special capacity admin permissions can move a workspace to a premium capacity. Premium capacity is a dedicated hardware provisioned just for your organization.

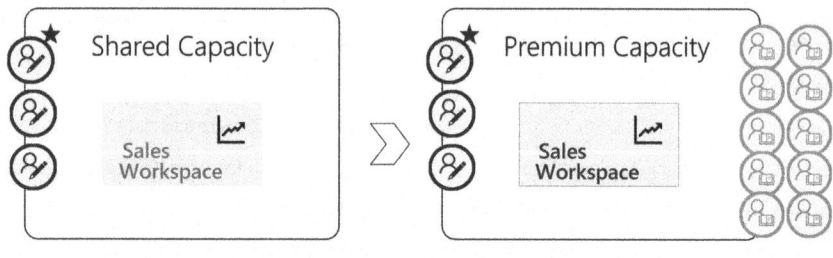

Figure 1.13 The Capacity Admin can move workspaces in and out of dedicated capacity.

In **Figure 1.13**, the Sales workspace was initially created in a shared capacity. Its report performance could be affected by workloads from other Power BI customers. To avoid this, the admin might decide to move it to a premium capacity. Now the workspace is isolated, and its performance is not affected by other organizations that use Power BI. However, it's still dependent on the activity of other premium workspaces in *your* organization and the resourced constraints of the Power BI Premium plan that it's associated with.

The interesting detail is that the admin can move a workspace in and out of the premium capacity at any point of time. For example, increased seasonal workloads may prompt the admin to move some workspaces to a premium capacity for a certain duration and then move them back to shared capacity when the workloads are reduced. You control which workspaces are in what capacity.

Understanding content distribution

Glancing again at **Figure 1.13**, we can see that when the Sales workspace was in a shared capacity, only Power BI Pro members can access its content. Power BI Free users would need to upgrade to Power BI Pro to gain access as members. However, when the workspace is moved to a premium capacity, its content can be shared to Power BI Free users in two ways: dashboard sharing and apps. This is how Power BI Premium helps large organizations reduce Power BI licensing cost and distribute content to many users when only read-only access is sufficient.

1.2.4   Understanding Power BI Mobile

Power BI Mobile is a set of native mobile applications for iOS, Windows and Android devices. You can access the download links from https://powerbi.microsoft.com/mobile. Why do you need these applications? After all, thanks to Power BI HTML5 rendering, you can view Power BI reports and dashboards in your favorite Internet browser. However, the native applications offer features that go beyond just rendering. Although there are some implementation differences, this section covers some of the most compelling features (chapter 4 has more details).

Optimized viewing

Mobile devices have limited display capabilities. The Power BI mobile apps adjust the layout of dashboards and reports, so they display better on mobile devices. For example, by default viewing a dashboard in a phone in portrait mode will position each dashboard tile after another. Rotating the phone to landscape will show the dashboard as it appears in Power BI Service (**Figure 1.14**). You can further tune the mobile layout by making changes to dashboards and reports in a special Phone View layout mode.

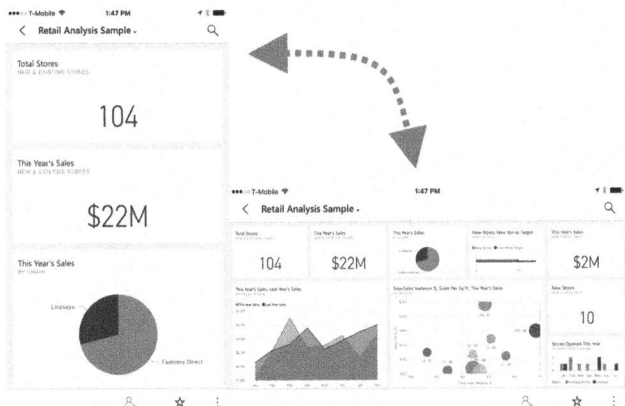

Figure 1.14 Power BI Mobile adjusts the dashboard layout when you rotate your phone from portrait to landscape.

Favorite dashboard tiles

Suppose that, while viewing dashboard tiles on your iPad, you want to put your favorite tiles in one place. You can just tap a tile to mark it as a favorite. These tiles appear in a separate "Favorites" folder. The dashboard tiles displayed on your device are live snapshots of your data. To interact with a tile, just tap it!

Alerts

Instead of going to powerbi.com to set up an alert on a dashboard tile, you can set up alerts directly in your mobile app. For example, **Figure 1.15** shows that I've enabled an iPhone data alert to be notified when this year's sales exceed $23 million. When the condition is met, I'll get a notification and email.

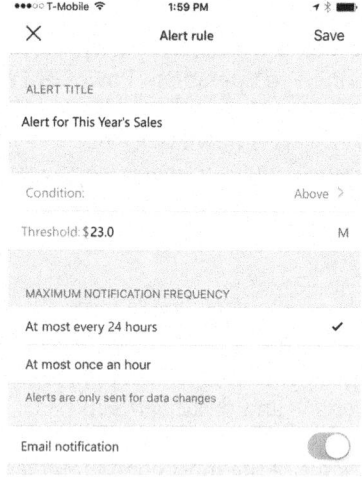

Figure 1.15 Alerts notify you about important data changes, such as when sales exceed a certain threshold.

Annotations

Annotations allow you to add comments (lines, text, and stamps) to dashboard tiles (see **Figure 1.16**). Then you can mail a screen snapshot to recipients, such as to your manager.

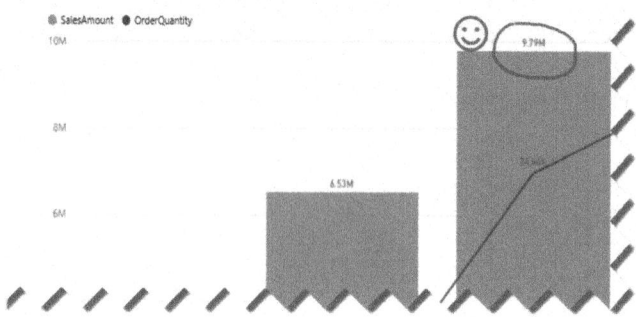

Figure 1.16 Annotations allow you to add comments to tiles and then send screenshots to your coworkers.

Sharing

Like Power BI simple sharing, you can use mobile device to share a dashboard by inviting coworkers to access the dashboard. Dashboards shared by mail are read-only, meaning that the people you share with can only view the dashboard without making changes.

1.2.5 Understanding Power BI Embedded

Almost every app requires some reporting capabilities. Traditionally, developers would either use third-party widgets or embed Reporting Services reports using the Microsoft ReportViewer control. The first approach requires a lot of custom code. The latter limits your users to static (canned) reports. What if you want to deliver the Power BI interactive experience with your apps? Microsoft didn't have a good answer in the past. Enter Power BI Embedded!

Introducing Power BI Embedded features

Power BI Embedded allows developers and Independent Software Vendors (ISV) to add interactive Power BI reports in their custom apps for internal or external users. Because Power BI Embedded uses the same APIs as Power BI Service, it has feature parity with Power BI Service. Suppose Teo has developed an ASP.NET MVP app for external customers. The app authenticates users any way it wants, such as by using Forms Authentication. Teo has created some nice reports in Power BI Desktop that connect directly to an Analysis Services semantic model or to data imported in Power BI Desktop.

With a few lines of code, Teo can embed these reports in his app (see **Figure 1.17**). If the app connects to a multi-tenant database (customers share the same database), the app can pass the user identity to Power BI Embedded, which in turn can pass it to the model. Then, row-level security (RLS) filters can limit access to data.

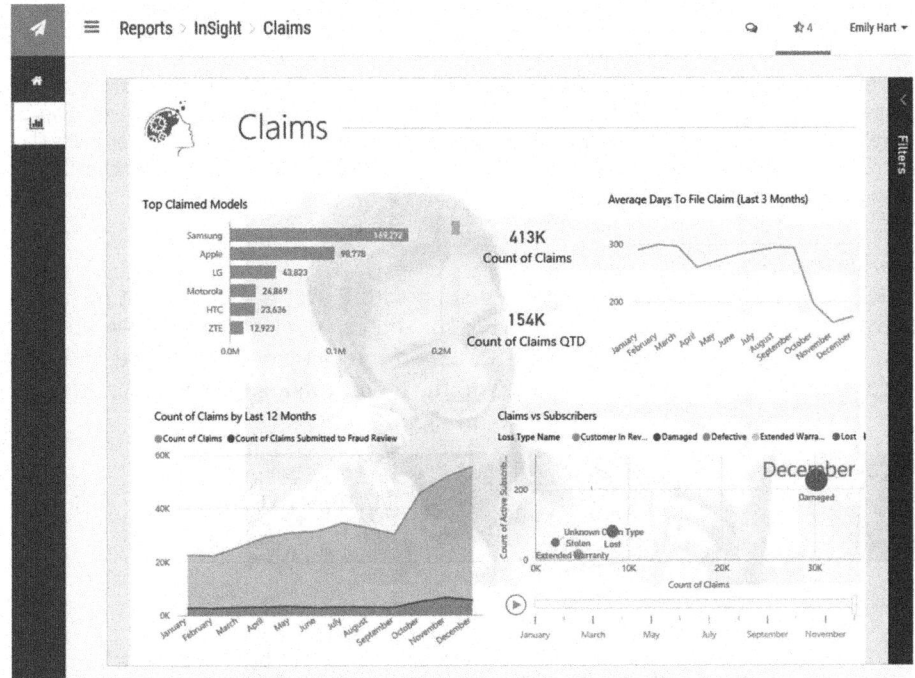

Figure 1.17 Power BI Embedded allows developers to embed Power BI reports in custom applications for internal or external users.

Power BI Embedded is extensible. Teo can use its JavaScript APIs to programmatically manipulate the client-side object model. For example, he can replace the Filters pane with a customized user interface to filter data. Or, can navigate the user programmatically to a specific report page.

About Power BI Embedded licensing

Per-user, per-month licensing is not cost effective for delivering reports to many users. Like Power BI Premium, Power BI Embedded utilizes capacity-based pricing. Power BI Embedded can be acquired by purchasing a Power BI Premium P plans or EM plans. The Power BI Premium P plans give you access to both embedded and service deployments. The EM plans are mostly for embedded deployments.

Power BI Embedded can also be acquired outside Power BI Premium by purchasing an Azure Power BI Embedded plan (https://azure.microsoft.com/pricing/details/power-bi-embedded/). More information about these plans can be found at https://azure.microsoft.com/pricing/details/power-bi-embedded/. I'll also provide more details when I discuss Power BI Embedded in Chapters 12 and 15.

1.2.6 Understanding Power BI Report Server

Many organizations have investments in on-premises reporting with Microsoft SQL Server Reporting Services (SSRS). Starting with SQL Server 2017, SSRS doesn't ship with SQL Server anymore but can be downloaded separately from the Microsoft Download Center as two SKUs:

- Microsoft SQL Server Reporting Services – This is the SSRS SKU you are familiar with that continues to be licensed under SQL Server. It allows you to deploy operational (RDL) reports and SSRS mobile reports but it doesn't support Power BI reports and Excel reports.

- Power BI Report Server – This SKU associates with the strong Power BI brand. It's still SSRS but in addition to operational and mobile reports, it also supports Power BI reports and Excel reports (the latter requires integration with Microsoft Office Online Server). With Power BI Report Server, you have full flexibility to decide what portions of the data and reports you want to keep on-premises and what portions should reside in the cloud.

 NOTE Besides splitting SSRS into two products, decoupling SSRS from SQL Server allows Microsoft to deliver new features faster and be more competitive in the fast-changing BI world. Also, while there is nothing stopping you from deploying Power BI Desktop files and Excel files to SSRS, reports won't render online, and the user will be asked to download and open the file locally. So, when I said that Power BI Report Server supports Power BI and Excel reports I meant that these reports render online, and that their management is integrated in the report portal.

Introducing Power BI Report Server features

As of this time, Power BI Report Server is limited to basic integration with Power BI reports, but Microsoft is actively working to deliver more features every two months or so. You can deploy Power BI Desktop files to the server and then view them online (see **Figure 1.18**). Report interactivity is supported. Power BI reports share the same security model as other items deployed to the report catalog. Power BI reports deployed to Power BI Report Server can also be viewed in Power BI mobile apps.

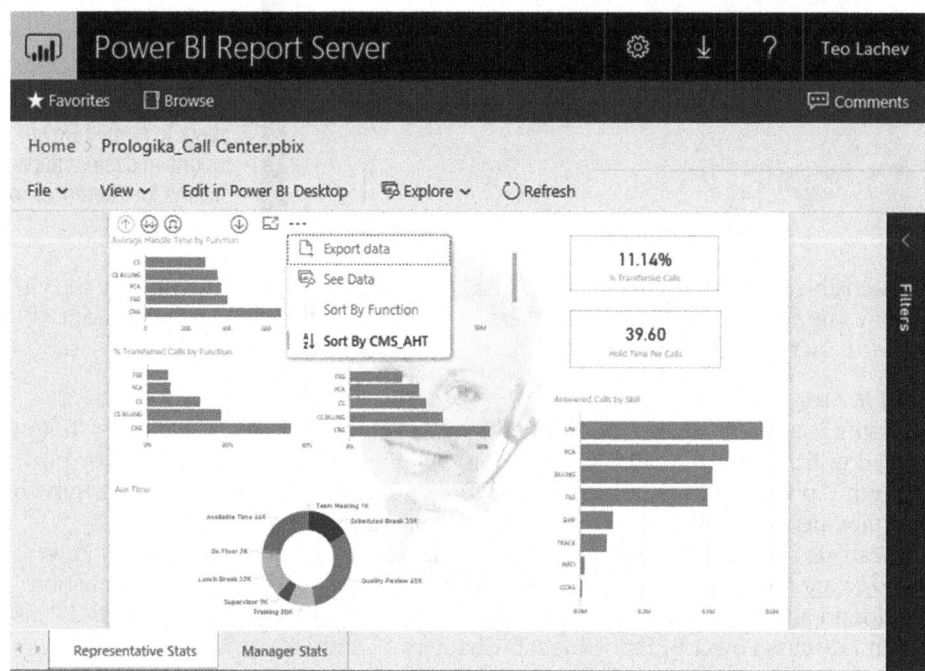

Figure 1.18 Power BI reports render online when deployed to Power BI report server.

The rest of the Power BI Service features, such as Q&A, Quick Insights, Analyze in Excel, subscriptions, data alerts, and others, are not yet supported.

Understanding Power BI Report Server licensing
Power BI Report Server can be acquired in two ways:

- Power BI Premium P Plan – A P plan licenses the same number of on-premises cores as the number of v-cores licensed for cloud usage. Suppose your organization has purchased the Power BI Premium P1 plan. This plan licenses 8 v-cores of a premium capacity in Power BI Service. When you install Power BI Report Server on premises, it will be licensed for 8 cores, giving you a total of 16 licensed cores!

- SQL Server Enterprise with Software Assurance license – Not interested in the cloud yet? You can cover Power BI Report Server under the SQL Server Enterprise licensing model, just as you license SSRS Enterprise Edition.

 NOTE Like Power BI, Power BI Report Server requires Power BI Pro licenses for content creators. For example, if you have 5 report developers that will deploy reports to Power BI Report Server, you would need 5 Power BI Pro licenses (recall that each Power BI license is $9.99 per user, per month). Licensing content creators is honor-based as currently there is no mechanism to ensure that the user is licensed on deploying content to the Power BI Report Server.

1.3   Understanding the Power BI Service Architecture

Microsoft has put a significant effort into building Power BI Service that consists of various Azure services that handle data storage, security, load balancing, disaster recovery, logging, tracing, and so on. Although it's all implemented and managed by Microsoft (that's why we like the cloud) and it's completely transparent for you, the following sections give you a high-level overview of these services to help you understand their value and Microsoft's decision to make Power BI a cloud service.

The Power BI Service is hosted on Microsoft Azure cloud platform and it's deployed in various data centers around the world. **Figure 1.19** shows a summarized view of the overall technical architecture that consists of two clusters: a Web Front End (WFE) cluster and a Back End cluster.

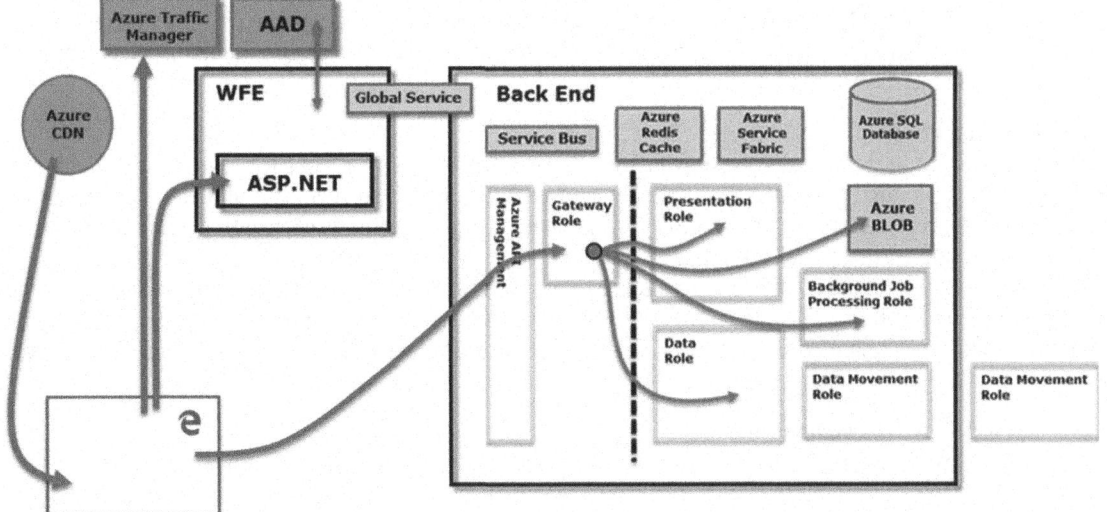

Figure 1.19 Power BI is powered by Microsoft Azure clusters.

1.3.1 The Web Front End (WFE) Cluster

The WFE cluster manages connectivity and authentication. Power BI relies on Azure Active Directory (AAD) to manage account authentication and management. Power BI uses the Azure Traffic Manager (ATM) to direct user traffic to the nearest datacenter. Which data center is used is determined by the DNS record of the client attempting to connect. The DNS Service can communicate with the Azure Traffic Manager to find the nearest datacenter with a Power BI deployment.

> 💡 **TIP** To find where your data is stored, log in to Power BI and click the Help (?) menu in the top-right corner, and then click "About Power BI". Power BI shows a prompt that includes the Power BI version and the data center.

Power BI uses the Azure Content Delivery Network (CDN) to deliver the necessary static content and files to end users based on their geographical locale. The WFE cluster nearest to the user manages the user login and authentication, and provides an access token to the user once authentication is successful. The ASP.NET component within the WFE cluster parses the request to determine which organization the user belongs to, and then consults the Power BI Global Service.

The Global Service is implemented as a single Azure Table that is shared among all worldwide WFE and Back End clusters. This service maps users and customer organizations to the datacenter that hosts their Power BI tenant. The WFE specifies to the browser which Back End cluster houses the organization's tenant. Once a user is authenticated, subsequent client interactions occur with the Back End cluster directly and the WFE cluster is not used.

1.3.2 The Back End Cluster

The Back End cluster manages all actions the user does in Power BI Service, including visualizations, dashboards, datasets, reports, data storage, data connections, data refresh, and others. The Gateway Role acts as a gateway between user requests and the Power BI service. As you can see in the diagram, only the Gateway Role and Azure API Management (APIM) services are accessible from the public Internet.

When an authenticated user connects to the Power BI Service, the connection and any request by the client is accepted and managed by the Gateway Role, which then interacts on the user's behalf with the rest of the Power BI Service. For example, when a client attempts to view a dashboard, the Gateway Role accepts that request, and then sends a request to the Presentation Role to retrieve the data needed by the browser to render the dashboard.

Where is data stored?
As far as data storage in the cloud goes, Power BI uses two primary repositories for storing and managing data. Data that is uploaded from users is typically sent to Azure BLOB storage, but all the metadata definitions (dashboards, reports, recent data sources, workspaces, organizational information, tenant information) are stored in Azure SQL Database.

The working horse of the Power BI service is Microsoft Analysis Services in Tabular mode, which has been architected to fulfill the role of a highly scalable data engine where many servers (nodes) participate in a multi-tenant, load-balanced farm. For example, when you import some data into Power BI, the actual data is stored in Azure BLOB storage, but an in-memory Tabular database is created to service queries.

Analysis Services Tabular enhancements
For BI pros who are familiar with Tabular, new components have been implemented so that Tabular is up to its new role. These components enable various cloud operations including tracing, logging, service-to-service operations, reporting loads and others. For example, Tabular has been enhanced to support the following features required by Power BI:

- Custom authentication – Because the traditional Windows NTLM authentication isn't appropriate in the cloud world, certificate-based authentication and custom security were added.

- Resource governance per database – Because databases from different customers (tenants) are hosted on the same server, Tabular ensures that any one database doesn't use all the resources.

- Diskless mode – For performance reasons, the data files aren't initially extracted to disk.

- Faster commit operations – This feature is used to isolate databases from each other. When committing data, the server-level lock is now only taken for a fraction of the time, although database-level commit locks are still taken and queries can still block commits and vice versa.

- Additional Dynamic Management Views (DMVs) – For better status discovery and load balancing.

- Data refresh – From the on-premises data using a gateway.

- Additional features – Such as the new features added to Analysis Services in SQL Server 2016.

1.3.3 Data on Your Terms

The increasing number of security exploits in the recent years have made many organizations cautious about protecting their data and skeptical about the cloud. You might be curious to know what is uploaded to the Power BI service and how you can reduce your risk for unauthorized access to your data. In addition, you control where your data is stored. Although Power BI is a cloud service, this doesn't necessarily mean that your data must be uploaded to Power BI.

Live connections
In a nutshell, you have two options to access your data. If the data source supports live connectivity, you can choose to leave the data where it is and only create reports and dashboards that connect live to your data. Currently, a subset of the supported data sources supports live connectivity, but that number is growing! Among them are Analysis Services, SQL Server (on premises and on Azure), Oracle, Azure SQL Data Warehouse, and Hadoop Spark.

For example, if Elena has implemented an Analysis Services model and deployed to a server in her organization's data center, Maya can create reports and dashboards in Power BI Service by directly connecting to the model. In this case, the data remains on premises; only the report and dashboard definitions are hosted in Power BI. When Maya runs a report, the report generates a query and sends the query to the model. Then, the model returns the query results to Power BI. Finally, Power BI generates the report and sends the output to the user's web browser. Power BI always uses the Secure Sockets Layer (SSL) protocol to encrypt the traffic between the Internet browser and the Power BI Service so that sensitive data is protected.

NOTE   Although in this case the data remains on premises, aggregated data needed on reports and dashboards still travel from your data center to Power BI Service. This could be an issue for software vendors who have service level agreements prohibiting data movement. You can address such concerns by referring the customer to the Power BI Security document (http://bit.ly/1SkEzTP) and the accompanying Power BI Security whitepaper. Or, you can wait for the next version of Reporting Services that will support deploying Power BI Desktop models to your on-premises report server.

Importing data
The second option is to import and store the data in Power BI. For example, Martin might want to build a data model to analyze data from multiple data sources. Martin can use Power BI Desktop to import the data and analyze it locally. To share reports and allow other users to create reports, Martin decides to deploy the model to Power BI. In this case, the model and the imported data are uploaded to Power BI, where they're securely stored.

To synchronize data changes, Martin can schedule a data refresh. Martin doesn't need to worry about security because data transfer between Power BI and on-premises data sources is secured through Azure Service Bus. Azure Service Bus creates a secure channel between Power BI Service and your computer. Because the secure connection happens over HTPS, there's no need to open a port in your company's firewall.

 TIP If you want to avoid moving data to the cloud, one solution you can consider is implementing an Analysis Services model layered on top of your data source. Not only does this approach keep the data local, but it also offers other important benefits, such as the ability to handle larger datasets (millions of rows), a single version of the truth by centralizing business calculations, row-level security, and others. Finally, if you want to avoid the cloud whatsoever, don't forget that you can deploy Power BI reports to an on-premises Power BI Report Server.

1.4 Power BI and You

Now that I've introduced you to Power BI and its building blocks, let's see what Power BI means for you. As you'll see, Power BI has plenty to offer to anyone interested in data analytics, irrespective of whether you're a content producer or consumer, as shown in **Figure 1.20**.

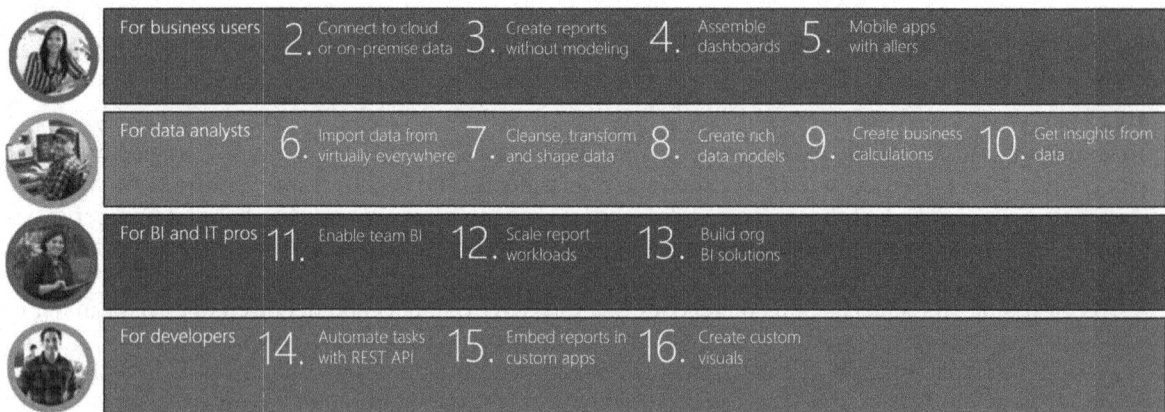

Figure 1.20 Power BI supports the BI needs of business users, analysts, pros, and developers.

By the way, the book content follows the same organization so that you can quickly find the relevant information depending on what type of user you are. For example, if you're a business user, the first part of the book is for you and it has four chapters (chapters 2-5) for the first four features shown in the "For business users" section in the diagram.

1.4.1 Power BI for Business Users

To clarify the term, a business user is someone in your organization who is mostly interested in consuming BI artifacts, such as reports and dashboards. This group of users typically includes executives, managers, business strategists, and regular information workers. To get better and faster insights, some business users often become basic content producers, such as when they create reports to analyze simple datasets or data from online services.

For example, Maya is a manager in the Adventure Works Sales & Marketing department. She doesn't have skills to create sophisticated data models and business calculations. However, she's interested in monitoring the Adventure Works sales by using reports and dashboards produced by other users. She's also a BI content producer because she must create reports for analyzing data in Excel spreadsheets, website traffic, and customer relationship management (CRM) data.

Connect to your data without creating models

Thanks to the Power BI apps, Maya can connect to popular cloud services, such as Google Analytics and Dynamics CRM, and get instant dashboards. She can also benefit from prepackaged datasets, reports, and dashboards, created jointly by Software as a Service (SaaS) partners and Microsoft.

For example, the Dynamics CRM connector provides an easy access to analyze data from the cloud-hosted version of Dynamics CRM. This connector uses the Dynamics CRM OData feed to generate a model that contains the most important entities, such as Accounts, Activities, Opportunities, Products, Leads, and others. Pre-built dashboards and reports, such as the one shown in **Figure 1.21**, provide immediate insights and can be further customized.

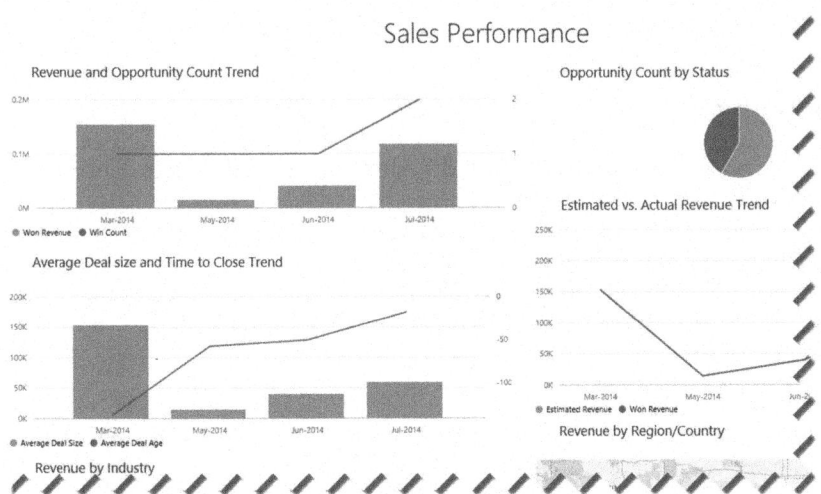

Figure 1.21 The Dynamics CRM app includes prepackaged reports and dashboards.

Similarly, if Maya uses Salesforce as a CRM platform, Power BI has a connector to allow Maya to connect to Salesforce in a minute. Power BI apps support data refresh, such as to allow Maya to refresh the CRM data daily.

Create reports

Power BI can also help Maya analyze simple datasets without data modeling. For example, if Maya receives an Excel file with some sales data, she can import the data into Power BI and create ad hoc reports with a few mouse clicks. The experience is not much different than creating Excel pivot reports.

Create and share dashboards

Maya can easily assemble dashboards from her reports and from reports shared with her by her colleagues. She can also easily share her dashboards with coworkers. For example, Maya can navigate to the Power BI portal, select a dashboard, and then click the Share button next to the dashboard name (see **Figure 1.22**).

Go mobile

Some business users, especially managers, executives, and sales people, would need access to BI reports on the go. These users would benefit from the Power BI Mobile native applications for iPad, iPhone, Android, and Windows. As I explained in section 1.2.4, Power BI Mobile allows users to not only to view Power BI reports and dashboards, but to also receive alerts about important data changes, as well to share and annotate dashboards.

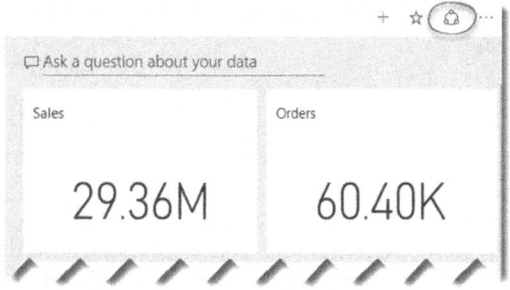

Figure 1.22 Business users can easily share dashboards with coworkers using the Power BI portal or Power BI Mobile.

For example, while Maya travels on business trips, she needs access to her reports and dashboards. Thanks to the cloud-based nature of Power BI, she can access them anywhere she has an Internet connection. Depending on what type of mobile device she uses, she can also install a Power BI app, so she can benefit from additional useful features, such as favorites, annotations, and content sharing.

1.4.2 Power BI for Data Analysts

A data analyst or BI analyst is a power user who has the skills and desire to create self-service data models. A data analyst typically prefers to work directly with the raw data, such as to relate corporate sales data coming from the corporate data warehouse with external data, such as economic data, demographics data, weather data, or any other data purchased from a third-party provider.

For example, Martin is a BI analyst with Adventure Works. Martin has experience in analyzing data with Excel and Microsoft Access. To offload effort from IT, Martin wants to create his own data model by combining data from multiple data sources.

Import and mash up data from virtually everywhere
As I mentioned previously, to create data models, Martin can use Microsoft Excel and/or Power BI Desktop, which combines the best of Power Query, Power Pivot, and Power View in a single and simplified design environment. If he has prior Power Pivot experience, Martin will find Power BI Desktop easier to use and he might decide to switch to it to stay on top of the latest Power BI features. Irrespective of the design environment chosen, Martin can use either Excel or Power BI Desktop to connect to any accessible data source, such as a relational database, file, cloud-based services, SharePoint lists, Exchange servers, and many more.

Figure 1.23 shows the supported data sources in Power BI Desktop. Microsoft regularly adds new data sources and developers can create custom data sources using the Power BI Data Connector SDK.

Cleanse, transform, and shape data
Data is rarely cleaned. A unique feature of Power BI Desktop is cleansing and transforming data. Inheriting these features from Power Query, Power BI Desktop allows a data analyst to apply popular transformation tasks that save tremendous data cleansing effort, such as replacing values, un-pivoting data, combining datasets and columns, and many more tasks.

For example, Martin may need to import an Excel financial report that was given to him in a crosstab format where data is pivoted by months on columns. Martin realizes that if he imports the data as it is, he won't be able to relate it to a date table that he has in the model. However, with a couple of mouse clicks, Martin can use a Power BI Desktop query to un-pivot months from columns to rows. And once Martin gets a new file, the query will apply the same transformations so that Martin doesn't have to go through the steps again.

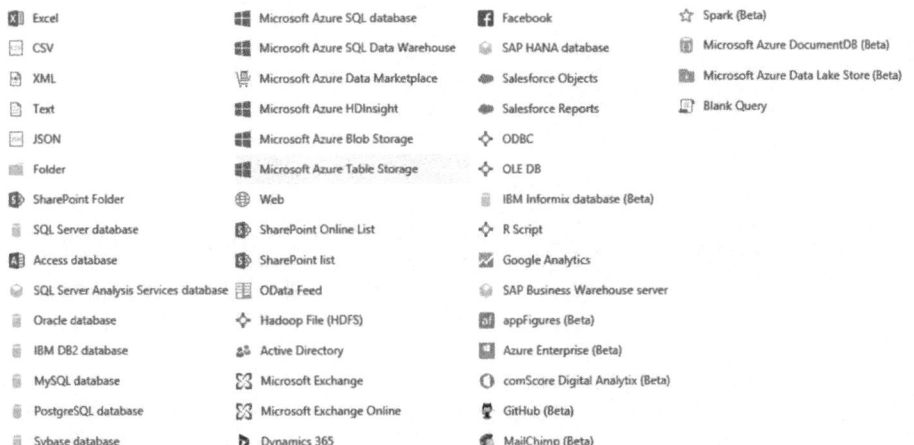

Excel	Microsoft Azure SQL database	Facebook	Spark (Beta)
CSV	Microsoft Azure SQL Data Warehouse	SAP HANA database	Microsoft Azure DocumentDB (Beta)
XML	Microsoft Azure Data Marketplace	Salesforce Objects	Microsoft Azure Data Lake Store (Beta)
Text	Microsoft Azure HDInsight	Salesforce Reports	Blank Query
JSON	Microsoft Azure Blob Storage	ODBC	
Folder	Microsoft Azure Table Storage	OLE DB	
SharePoint Folder	Web	IBM Informix database (Beta)	
SQL Server database	SharePoint Online List	R Script	
Access database	SharePoint list	Google Analytics	
SQL Server Analysis Services database	OData Feed	SAP Business Warehouse server	
Oracle database	Hadoop File (HDFS)	appFigures (Beta)	
IBM DB2 database	Active Directory	Azure Enterprise (Beta)	
MySQL database	Microsoft Exchange	comScore Digital Analytix (Beta)	
PostgreSQL database	Microsoft Exchange Online	GitHub (Beta)	
Sybase database	Dynamics 365	MailChimp (Beta)	
Teradata database	PowerApps Common Data Service (Beta)	Marketo (Beta)	

Figure 1.23 Power BI self-service data models can connect to a plethora of data sources.

Implement self-service data models

Once the data is imported, Martin can relate the datasets to analyze the data from different angles by relating multiple datasets (see **Figure 1.1** again). No matter which source the data came from, Martin can use Power BI Desktop or Excel to relate tables and create data models whose features are on par with professional models. Power BI supports relationships natively with one-to-many and many-to-many cardinality, so Martin can model complex requirements, such as analyzing financial balances of joint bank accounts.

Create business calculations

Martin can also implement sophisticated business calculations, such as time calculations, weighted averages, variances, period growth, and so on. To do so, Martin will use the Data Analysis Expression (DAX) language and Excel-like formulas, such as the formula shown in **Figure 1.24**. This formula calculates the year-to-date (YTD) sales amount. As you can see, Power BI Desktop supports IntelliSense and color coding to help you with the formula syntax. IntelliSense offers suggestions as you type.

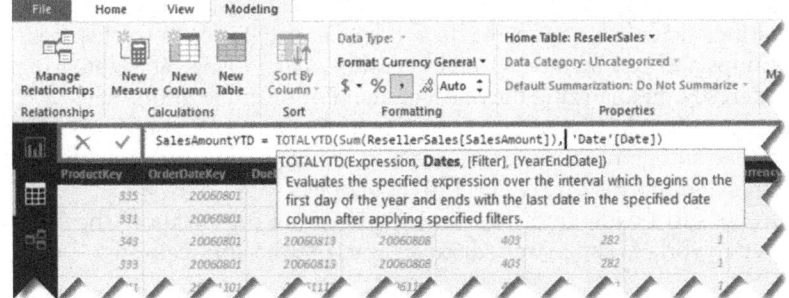

Figure 1.24 Business calculations are implemented in DAX.

Get insights

Once the model is created, the analyst can visualize and explore the data with interactive reports. If you come from using Excel Power Pivot and would like to give Power BI Desktop a try, you'll find that not only does it simplify the design experience, but it also supports new visualizations, including Funnel and Combo Charts, Treemap, Filled Map, and Gauge visualizations, as shown in **Figure 1.25**. And when the Microsoft-provided visualizations aren't enough, Martin can use a custom visual contributed by Microsoft and the Power BI community. To do this, Martin uses the Power BI Desktop "Import from store" feature to navigate to the Microsoft Store (https://appsource.microsoft.com). Then Martin picks a visual and start visualizing data in awesome ways!

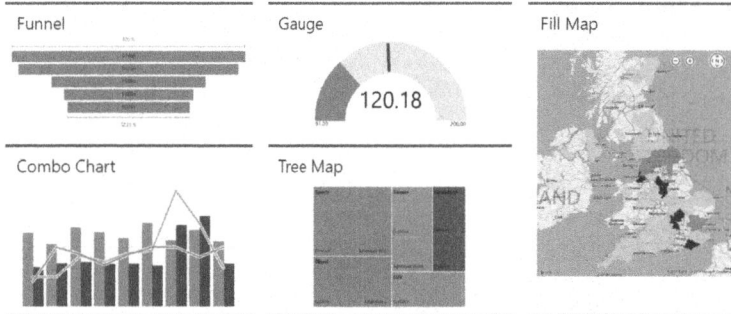

Figure 1.25 Power BI Desktop adds new visualizations.

Once Martin is done with the report in Power BI Desktop, he can publish the model and reports to Power BI, so that he can share insights with other users. If they have permissions, his coworkers can view reports, gain more insights with natural query (Q&A) questions, and create dashboards. Martin can also schedule a data refresh to keep the imported data up to date.

1.4.3 Power BI for Pros

BI pros and IT pros have much to gain from Power BI. BI pros are typically tasked to create the backend infrastructure required to support organizational BI initiatives, such as data marts, data warehouses, cubes, ETL packages, operational reports, and dashboards. IT pros are also concerned with setting up and maintaining the necessary environment that facilitates self-service and organizational BI, such as providing access to data, managing security, data governance, and other services.

In a department or smaller organization, a single person typically fulfills both BI and IT pro tasks. For example, Elena has developed an Analysis Services model on top of the corporate data warehouse. She needs to ensure that business users can gain insights from the model without compromising security.

Enable team BI
Once she provided connectivity to the on-premises model, Elena must establish a trustworthy environment needed to facilitate content sharing and collaboration. To do so, she can use Power BI workspaces. As a first step, Elena would set up groups and add members to these groups. Then Elena can create workspaces for the organizational units interested in analyzing the SSAS model. For example, if the Sales department needs access to the organizational model, Elena can set up a Sales Department group. Next, she can create a Sales Department workspace and grant the group access to it. Finally, she can deploy to the workspace her sales-related dashboards and reports that connect to the model.

If Elena needs to distribute BI artifacts to a wider audience, such as the entire organization, she can create an app and publish it. Then her coworkers can search, discover, and use the app read-only.

Scale report workloads
No one likes to wait for a report to finish. If Elena works for a larger organization, she can scale report workloads by purchasing a Power BI Premium plan. She then decides which workspaces can benefit from a dedicated capacity and promote them to premium workspaces. Not only Power BI Premium delivers consistent performance but also it allows the organization to save on the Power BI licensing cost. Elena can now share out content in premium workspaces to "viewers" by sharing specific dashboards or distributing contents with apps.

Implementing BI solutions
Based on my experience, most organizations could benefit from what I refer to as a classic BI architecture that includes a data warehouse and semantic model (Analysis Services Multidimensional or Tabular mode)

layered on top of the data warehouse. I'll discuss the benefits of this architecture in Part 3 of this book. If you already have or are planning such a solution, you can use Power BI as a presentation layer. This works because Power BI can connect to the on-premises Analysis Services, as shown in **Figure 1.26**.

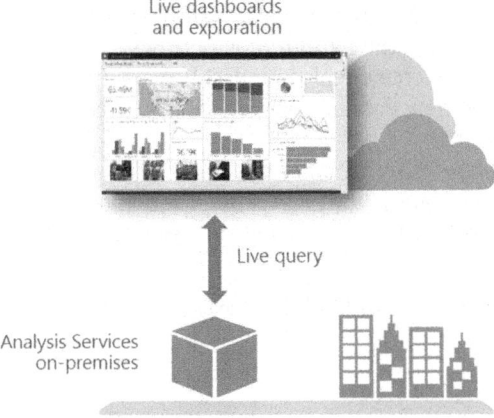

Figure 1.26 Power BI can directly connect to on-premises Analysis Services models.

So that Power BI can connect to on-premises SSAS models, Elena needs to download and install a component called a gateway to an on-premises computer that can connect to the semantic model. The gateway allows Elena to centralize management and access to on-premises data sources. Then Elena can implement reports and dashboards that connect live to Analysis Services and deploy them to Power BI. When users open a report, the report will generate a query and send it to the on-premises model via the gateway. Now you have a hybrid solution where data stays on premises but reports are hosted in Power BI.

If you're concerned about the performance of this architecture, you should know that Power BI only sends queries to the on-premises data source so there isn't much overhead on the trip from Power BI to the source. Typically, BI reports and dashboards summarize data. Therefore, the size of the datasets that travel back to Power BI probably won't be very large either. Of course, the speed of the connection between Power BI and the data center where the model resides will affect the duration of the round trip.

Another increasingly popular scenario that Power BI can help you implement is real-time BI. You've probably heard about Internet of Things (IoT) which refers to an environment of many connected devices, such as barcode readers, sensors, or cell phones, that transfer data over a network without requiring human-to-human or human-to-computer interaction. If your organization is looking for a real-time platform, you should seriously consider Power BI. Its streamed datasets allow an application to stream directly to Power BI with a few lines of code. If you need to implement Complex Event Processing (CEP) solutions, Microsoft Azure Stream Analytics lets you monitor event streams in real time and push results to a Power BI dashboard.

Finally, BI pros can implement predictive data analytics solutions that integrate with Power BI. For example, Elena can use the Azure Machine Learning Service to implement a data mining model that predicts the customer probability to purchase a product. Then she can easily set up a REST API web service, which Power BI can integrate with to display results. If all these BI pro features sound interesting, I'll walk you through these scenarios in detail in Part 3 of this book.

1.4.4 Power BI for Developers

Power BI has plenty to offer to developers as well because it's built on an open and extensible architecture. In the context of data analytics, developers are primarily interested in incorporating BI features in their applications or in providing access to data to support integration scenarios. For example, Teo is a developer with Adventure Works. Teo might be interested in embedding Power BI dashboards and reports in a web application that will be used by external customers. Power BI supports several extensibility options, including apps, real-time dashboards, custom visuals, and embedded reporting.

Automate management tasks

Power BI has a set of REST APIs to allow developers to programmatically manage certain Power BI resources, such as enumerating datasets, creating new datasets, and adding and removing rows to a dataset table. This allows developers to push data to Power BI, such as to create real-time dashboards. In fact, this is how Azure Stream Analytics integrates with Power BI. When new data is streamed, Azure Stream Analytics pushes the data to Power BI to update real-time dashboards.

The process for creating such applications is straightforward. First, you need to register your app. Then you write OAuth2 security code to authenticate your application with Power BI. Then you'd write code to manipulate the Power BI objects using REST APIs. For example, here's a sample method invocation for adding one row to a table:

```
POST https://api.powerbi.com/beta/myorg/datasets/2C0CCF12-A369-4985-A643-0995C249D5B9/Tables/Product/Rows HTTP/1.1
Authorization: Bearer {AAD Token}
Content-Type: application/json
{    "rows":
     [{
          "ProductID":1,
          "Name":"Adjustable Race",
          "Category":"Components",
          "IsCompete":true,
          "ManufacturedOn":"07/30/2014"}
     ]}
```

Microsoft supports a Power BI Developer Center website (https://powerbi.microsoft.com/developers) where you can read the REST API documentation and try the REST APIs.

Embed reports in custom applications

Many of you would like to embed beautiful Power BI dashboards and reports in custom applications. For example, your company might have a web portal to allow external customers to log in and access reports and dashboards. Up until Power BI, Microsoft hasn't had a good solution to support this scenario.

For internal applications where users are already using Power BI, developers can call the Power BI REST APIs to embed dashboard tiles and reports. As I mentioned, external applications can benefit from Power BI Embedded. And, because embedded reports preserve interactive features, users can enjoy the same engaging experience, including report filtering, interactive sorting, and highlighting. I cover these integration scenarios in Chapter 15.

Implement custom visuals

Microsoft has published the required interfaces to allow developers to implement and publish custom visuals using any of the JavaScript-based visualization frameworks, such as D3.js, WebGL, Canvas, or SVG. Do you need visualizations that Power BI doesn't support to display data more effectively? With some coding wizardry, you can implement your own!

Moreover, to speed up development, Microsoft has provided Custom Visual Developer Tools (https://github.com/Microsoft/PowerBI-visuals). You can use whatever tool you prefer to code the custom visual (visuals are coded in TypeScript), such as Microsoft Visual Code or Visual Studio. Custom Visual Developer Tools integrates with Power BI and allows you to test the visual exactly as the end user would use it on a report. When the custom visual is ready, you can publish it to Microsoft AppSource at https://appsource.microsoft.com where Power BI users can search for it and download it.

Power BI is an extensible platform and there are other options for building Power BI solutions outside the scope this book, including:

- Integrate Power BI with Microsoft Flow and PowerApps – For example, in my blog "Going with the Flow" (http://prologika.com/going-with-the-flow/), I explain how a developer can use Microsoft Flow to intercept a Power BI data alert and distribute it to a larger audience.

- Implement custom data connectors – You can extend the Power BI data capabilities by implementing custom data connectors in M language (the programming language of Power Query). To learn more, see the M Extensions GitHub repo at https://github.com/Microsoft/DataConnectors/blob/master/docs/m-extensions.md.

- Implement service apps – I've already discussed how Power BI online services apps can help you connect to popular online services, such as Dynamics CRM or Google Analytics. You can implement new apps to facilitate access to data and to provide prepackaged content. You can contact Microsoft and sign up for the Microsoft partner program which coordinates this initiative.

1.5 Summary

This chapter has been a whirlwind tour of the innovative Power BI cloud data analytics service and its features. By now, you should view Power BI as a flexible platform that meets a variety of BI requirements. An important part of the Microsoft Data Platform, Power BI is a collective name of several products: Power BI, Power BI Desktop, Power BI Premium, Power BI Mobile, Power BI Embedded, and Power BI Report Server. You've learned about the major reasons that led to the release of Power BI. You've also taken a close look at the Power BI architecture and its components, as well as its editions and pricing model.

Next, this chapter discussed how Power BI can help different types of users with their data analytics needs. It allows business users to connect to their data and gain quick insights. It empowers data analysts to create sophisticated data models. It enables IT and BI pros to implement hybrid solutions that span on-premises data models and reports deployed to the cloud. Finally, its extensible and open architecture lets developers enhance the Power BI data capabilities and integrate Power BI with custom applications.

Having laid the foundation of Power BI, you're ready to continue the journey. Next, you'll witness the value that Power BI can deliver to business users.

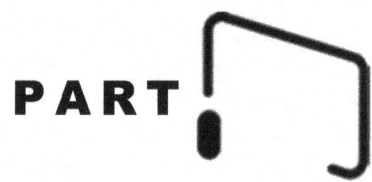

PART

Power BI for Business Users

I f you're new to Power BI, welcome! This part of the book provides the essential fundamentals to help you get started with Power BI. It specifically targets business users: people who use Excel as part of their job, such as information workers, executives, financial managers, business managers, people man-agers, HR managers, and marketing managers. But it'll also benefit anyone new to Power BI. Remember from Chapter 1 that Power BI consists of six products. This part of the book teaches business users how to use two of them: Power BI Service and Power BI Mobile.

First, you'll learn how to sign up and navigate the Power BI portal. You'll also learn how to use apps so that you connect to popular online services. Because business users are often tasked to analyze simple datasets, this chapter will teach you how to import data from files without explicit data modelling.

Next, you'll learn how to use Power BI Service to create reports and dashboards and uncover valuable insights from your data. As you'll soon see, Power BI doesn't assume you have any query knowledge or reporting skills. With a few clicks, you'll be able to create ad hoc interactive reports! Then you'll create dashboards from existing visualizations or by asking natural questions.

If you frequently find yourself on the go, I'll show you how you can use Power BI Mobile to access your reports and dashboards on the go if you have Internet connectivity. Besides mobile rendering, Power BI Mobile offers interesting features to help you stay on top of your business, including data alerts, favorites, and annotations.

As with the rest of the book, step-by-step instructions will guide you through the tour. Most features that I'll show you in this part of the book are available in the free edition of Power BI, so you can start practicing immediately. The features that require Power BI Pro will be explicitly stated.

Chapter 2

The Power BI Service

In the previous chapter, I explained that Power BI aims to democratize data analytics and make it available to any user...BI for the masses! As a business user, you can use Power BI to get instant insights from your data irrespective if it's located on premises or in the cloud. Although no clear boundaries exist, I define a business user as someone who would be mostly interested in consuming BI artifacts, such as reports and dashboards. However, when requirements call for it, business users could also produce content, such as to visualize data stored in Excel files. Moreover, basic data analytics requirements can be met without explicit modeling.

This chapter lays out the foundation of self-service data analytics with Power BI. First, I'll help you understand when self-service BI is a good choice. Then I'll get you started with Power BI by showing you how to sign up and navigate the Power BI portal. Next, I'll show you how to use content packs to connect to a cloud service and quickly gain insights from prepackaged reports and dashboards. If you find yourself frequently analyzing data in Excel files, I'll teach you how to do so without any data modeling.

2.1   Understanding Types of Business Intelligence

Remember that self-service BI enables business users (information workers, like business managers or marketing managers, and power users) to offload effort from IT pros so they don't stay in line waiting for someone to enable BI for them. And, team BI allows the same users to share their reports with other team members without requiring them to install modeling or reporting tools. Before we go deeper in personal and team BI, let's take a moment to compare it with organizational BI. This will help you view self-service BI not as a competing technology but as a completing technology to organizational BI. In other words, self-service BI and organizational BI are both necessary for most businesses, and they complement each other.

2.1.1   Understanding Organizational BI

Organizational BI defines a set of technologies and processes for implementing an end-to-end BI solution where the implementation effort is shifted to IT professionals (as opposed to information workers and people who use Power BI Desktop or Excel as part of their job).

Classic organizational BI architecture
The main objective of organizational BI is to provide accurate and trusted analysis and reporting. **Figure 2.1** shows a classic organizational BI solution.

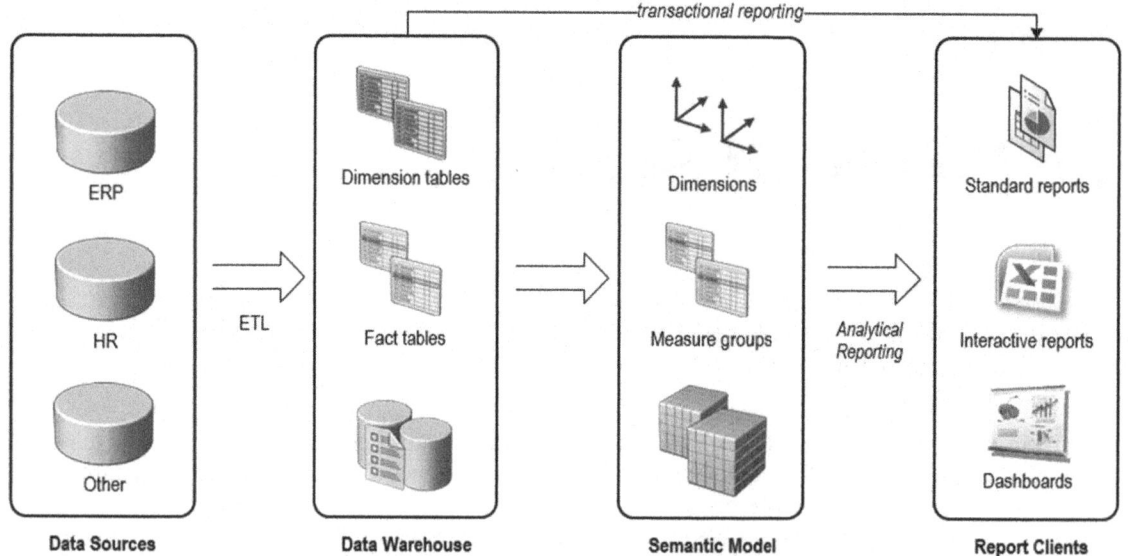

Figure 2.1 Organizational BI typically includes ETL processes, data warehousing, and a semantic layer.

In a typical corporate environment, data is scattered in a variety of data sources, and consolidating it presents a major challenge. Extraction, transformation, and loading (ETL) processes extract data from the original data sources, clean it, and then load the trusted data in a data warehouse or data mart. The data warehouse organizes data in a set of dimensions and fact tables. When designing the data warehouse, BI pros strive to reduce the number of tables to make the schema more intuitive and facilitate reporting processes. For example, an operational database might be highly normalized and have Product, Subcategory, and Category tables. However, when designing a data warehouse, the modeler might decide to have a single Product table that includes columns from the Subcategory and Category tables. So instead of three tables, the data warehouse now has only one table, and end users don't need to join multiple tables.

While end users could run transactional reports directly from the data warehouse, many organizations also implement a semantic model in the form of one or more Analysis Services Multidimensional cubes or Tabular models for analytical reporting. As an information worker, you can use Power BI Desktop, Excel, or another tool to connect to the semantic model and author your own reports so that you don't have to wait for IT to create them for you. And IT pros can create a set of standard operational reports and dashboards from the semantic model.

 NOTE Everyone is talking about self-service BI, and there are hundreds of vendors out there offering tools to enable business users to take BI into their own hands. However, my experience shows that the best self-service BI is empowering users to analyze data from trusted semantic models sanctioned and owned by IT. If the architecture shown in **Figure 2.1** is in place, a data analyst can focus on the primary task, which is analyzing data, without being preoccupied with the data logistics (importing data, shaping data, modeling data). This will require more upfront effort, but the investment should pay for itself in time.

Understanding organizational BI challenges

Although it's well-defined and established, when implementing organizational BI, your company might face a few challenges, including the following:

- Upfront planning and implementation effort – Depending on the data integration effort required, implementing an organizational BI solution might not be a simple task. Business users and IT pros must work together to derive requirements. Most of the implementation effort goes into data logistics processes to clean, verify, and load data. For example, Elena from the IT department is tasked to implement an organizational BI solution. First, she needs to meet with business users to obtain the necessary business knowledge and gather requirements (business requirements might be hard to come by). Then she must identify where the data resides and how to extract, clean, and transform the data. Next, Elena must implement ETL processes, models, and reports. Quality Assurance must test the solution. And IT pros must configure the hardware and software, as well as deploy and maintain the solution. Security and large data volumes bring additional challenges.

- Highly specialized skillset – Organizational BI requires specialized talent, such as ETL developers, Analysis Services developers, and report developers. System engineers and developers must work together to plan the security, which sometimes might be more complicated than the actual BI solution.

- Less flexibility – Organization BI might not be flexible enough to react quickly to new or changing business requirements. For example, Maya from the Marketing department might be tasked to analyze CRM data that isn't in the data warehouse. Maya might need to wait for a few months before the data is imported and validated.

The good news is that self-service BI can complement organizational BI quite well to address these challenges. Given the above example, while waiting for the pros to enhance the organization BI solution, Maya can use Power BI to analyze CRM data or Excel files. She already has the domain knowledge. Moreover, she doesn't need to know modeling concepts. At the beginning, she might need some guidance from IT, such as how to get access to the data and understand how the data is stored. She also needs to take *responsibility* that her analysis is correct and can be trusted. But isn't self-service BI better than waiting?

REAL WORLD   Influenced by the propaganda by vendors and consultants, my experience shows that many organizations get overly excited about the perceived quick gains with self-service BI. Unfortunately, many underestimate the data complexity and integration. After pushing the tool to its limits for some time, they realize the challenges related to data quality and the extent of the transformation required before the data is ready for analysis. Although I mentioned that upfront planning and implementation is a negative for organizational BI, it's often a must and it needs to be done by a pro with a professional toolset. If your data doesn't require much transformation and it doesn't exceed a few million rows (if you decide to import the data), then by all means go ahead with self-service BI. However, if you need to integrate data from multiple source systems, then a self-service BI would probably be a stretch. Don't say I didn't warn you!

2.1.2   Understanding Self-service BI

Self-service BI empowers business users to take analytics into their own hands with guidance from their IT department. For companies that don't have organizational BI or can't afford it, self-service BI presents an opportunity for building customized ad hoc solutions to gain data insights outside the capabilities of organizational BI solutions and line-of-business applications. On the other hand, organizations that have invested in organizational BI might find that self-service BI opens additional options for valuable data exploration and analysis.

REAL WORLD   I led a self-service BI training class for a large company that has invested heavily in organizational BI. They had a data warehouse and OLAP cubes. Only a subset of data in the data warehouse was loaded in the cubes. Their business analysts were looking for a tool that would let them join and analyze data from the cubes and data warehouse. In another case, an educational institution had to analyze expense report data that wasn't stored in a data warehouse. Such scenarios can benefit greatly from self-service BI.

Self-service BI benefits
When done right, self-service BI offers important benefits. First, it makes BI pervasive and accessible to practically everyone! Anyone can gain insights if they have access to and understand the data. Users can import data from virtually any data source, ranging from flat files to cloud applications. Then they can

mash it up and gain insights. Once data is imported, the users can build their own reports. For example, Maya understands Excel, but she doesn't know SQL or relational databases. Fortunately, Power BI doesn't require any technical skills. Maya could import her Excel file and build instant reports.

Besides democratizing BI, the agility of self-service BI can complement organizational BI well, such as to promote ideation and divergent thinking. For example, as a BI analyst, Martin might want to test a hypothesis that customer feedback on social media, such as Facebook and Twitter, affects the company's bottom line. Even though such data isn't collected and stored in the data warehouse, Martin can import data from social media sites, relate it to the sales data in the data warehouse and validate his idea.

Finally, analysts can use self-service BI tools, such as Power BI Desktop and Power Pivot, to create prototypes of the data models they envision. This can help BI pros to understand their requirements.

Self-service BI cautions

Self-service BI isn't new. After all, business users have been using tools like Microsoft Excel and Microsoft Access for isolated data analysis for quite a while (Excel has been around since 1985 and Access since 1992). Here are some considerations you should keep in mind about self-service BI:

- What kind of user are you? – Are you a data analyst (power user) who has the time, desire, and patience to learn a new technology? If you consider yourself a data analyst, then you should be able to accomplish a lot by creating data models with Power BI Desktop and Excel Power Pivot. If you're new to BI or you lack data analyst skills, then you can still gain a lot from Power BI, and this part of the book shows you how.

- Data access – How will you access data? What subset of data do you need? Data quality issues can quickly turn away any user, so you must work with your IT to get started. A role of IT is to ensure access to clean and trusted data. Analysts can use Power BI Desktop or Excel Power Query for simple data transformations and corrections, but these aren't meant as ETL tools.

- IT involvement – Self-service BI might be good, but managed self-service BI (self-service BI under the supervision of IT pros) is even better and sometimes a must. Therefore, the IT group must budget time and resources to help end users when needed, such as to give users access to data, to help with data integrity and more complex business calculations, and to troubleshoot issues when things go wrong. They also must monitor the utilization of the self-service rollout.

- With great power comes great responsibility – If you make wrong conclusions, damage can be easily contained. But if your entire department or even organization uses wrong reports, you have a serious problem! You must take the responsibility and time to verify that your model and calculations can be trusted. Data governance supervised by IT is important. For example, IT can set up a governance committee that meets on a regular basis to review new self-data models and reports, and "certify" them for wider distribution.

- "Spreadmarts" – I left the most important consideration for the CIO for last. If your IT department has spent a lot of effort to avoid decentralized and isolated analysis, should you allow the corporate data to be constantly copied and duplicated?

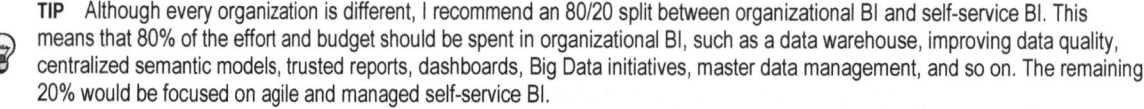 **TIP** Although every organization is different, I recommend an 80/20 split between organizational BI and self-service BI. This means that 80% of the effort and budget should be spent in organizational BI, such as a data warehouse, improving data quality, centralized semantic models, trusted reports, dashboards, Big Data initiatives, master data management, and so on. The remaining 20% would be focused on agile and managed self-service BI.

Now that you understand how organizational BI and self-service BI compares and completes each other, let's dive into the Power BI self-service BI capabilities which benefit business users like you.

2.2   Getting Started with Power BI Service

In Chapter 1, I introduced you to Power BI and its products. Recall that the main component of Power BI is its cloud-hosted Power BI Service (powerbi.com) that enables team BI by letting you share your data and reports with your coworkers. If you're a novice user, this section lays out the necessary startup steps, including signing up for Power BI and understanding its web interface. As you'll soon find out, because Power BI was designed with business users and data analytics in mind, it won't take long to learn it!

2.2.1   Signing Up for Power BI

The Power BI motto is, "5 seconds to sign up, 5 minutes to wow!" Because Power BI is a cloud-based offering, there's nothing for you to install and set up. But if you haven't signed up for Power BI yet, let's put this promise to the test. But first, read the following steps.

Five seconds to sign up
Follow these steps to sign up for the Power BI Service:

1.   Open your browser, navigate to http://powerbi.com, and then click "Sign up free" button in the top right corner or "Start Free" button (see **Figure 2.2**).

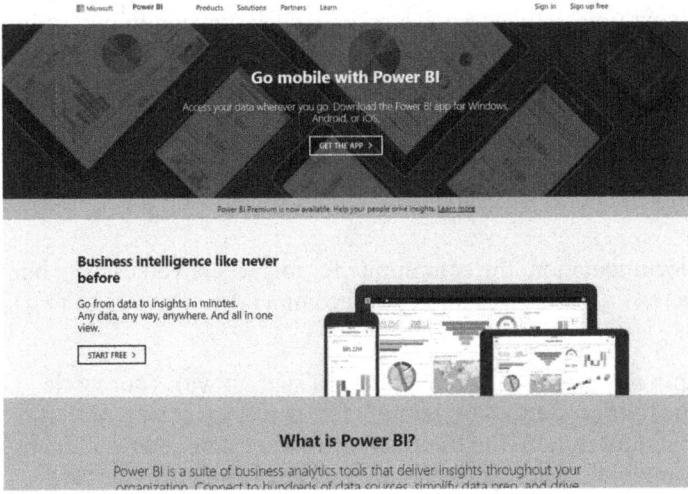

Figure 2.2 This is the landing Power BI web page.

2.   The next page asks you how you want to start with Power BI: download Power BI Desktop so that you can start your BI journey on the desktop, or sign up for Power BI so that you can use the Power BI Service. I'll discuss Power BI Desktop in Part 2 of this book so let's ignore this option for now. Click the "Try free" button to sign up for Power BI Service.

3.   In the Get Started page, enter your work email address. Notice that the email address must be your work email. At this time, you can't use a common email, such as @hotmail.com, @outlook.com, or @gmail.com. This might be an issue if you plan to use Power BI for your personal use. As a workaround, consider registering a domain, such as a domain for your family (some providers give away free domains).

4.   If your organization already uses Office 365, Power BI will detect this and ask you to sign up using your Office 365 account. If you don't use Office 365, Power BI will ask you to confirm the email you entered and then to check your inbox for a confirmation email.

5. Once you receive your email conformation with the subject "Time to complete Microsoft Power BI signup", click the "Complete Microsoft Power BI Signup" link in the email. Clicking on the link will take you to a page to create your account (see **Figure 2.3**).

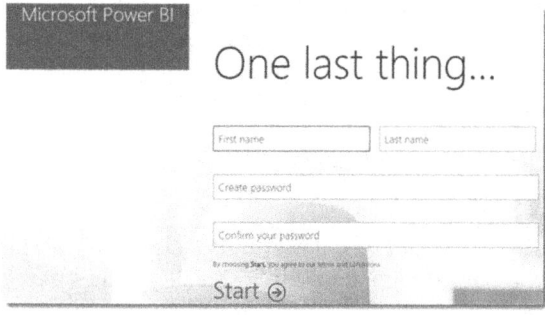

Figure 2.3 Use this page to create a Power BI account to gain access to Power BI Service.

6. You need to provide a name and a password, and then click Start.

This completes the process which Microsoft refers to as the "Information Worker (IW) Sign Up" flow. As I said, this signup flow is geared for an organization that doesn't have an Office 365 tenant.

The main page

After you complete the signup process, the next time you go to powerbi.com, click the Sign In button in the top-right corner of the main page (see **Figure 2.2** again). The main page includes the following menus:

- Products – Explains the Power BI product family and pricing.

- Solutions – Explains how Power BI addresses various data analytics needs.

- Partners – Includes links to the Partner Showcase (where Microsoft partners, such as Prologika, demonstrate their Power BI-based solutions) and to pages to find a partner to help you if you need training or implementation assistance.

- Learn – Includes links to the product documentation, the community forums where you can ask questions, a page to provide feedback to Microsoft, and Power BI blog (I recommend you subscribe to it).

What happens during signup?

You might be curious why you're asked to provide a password given that you sign up with your work email. Behind the scenes, Power BI stores the user credentials in Azure Active Directory (Azure AD). If your organization doesn't have an Office 365 subscription, the Information Worker flow creates a tenant for the domain you used to sign up. For example, if I sign up as teo@prologika.com and my company doesn't have an Office 365 subscription, a prologika.onmicrosoft.com tenant will be created in Azure AD and that tenant won't be managed by anyone at my company. If the domain in the email address matches the tenant, Power BI will add your coworkers to the same tenant when they sign up.

> **NOTE** What is a Power BI tenant? A tenant is a dedicated instance of the Azure Active Directory that an organization receives and owns when it signs up for a Microsoft cloud service such as Azure, Microsoft Intune, Power BI, or Office 365. A tenant houses the users in a company and the information about them - their passwords, user profile data, permissions, and so on. It also contains groups, applications, and other information pertaining to an organization and its security. For more information about tenants, see "What is an Azure AD tenant" at http://bit.ly/1FTFObb.

If your organization decides one day to have better integration with Microsoft Azure, such as to have a single sign-on (SSO), it can synchronize or federate the corporate Active Directory with Azure, but this isn't required. To unify the corporate and cloud directories, the company IT administrator can then take over the unmanaged tenant. I provide more details about managing the Power BI tenant in Chapter 11, but for now remember that you won't be able to upgrade to Power BI Pro if your tenant is unmanaged.

2.2.2 Understanding the Power BI Portal

I hope it took you five seconds or less to sign up with Power BI. (Or at least hopefully it feels quick.) After completing these signup steps, you'll have access to the free edition of Power BI. Let's take a moment to get familiar with the Power BI portal where you'll spend most of your time when analyzing data.

 NOTE Currently, the Power BI portal isn't customizable. For example, you can't rearrange or remove menus, and you can't brand the portal. If these features are important to your organization, your IT department can consider signing up for SharePoint Online and them embed Power BI dashboards and reports inside SharePoint. SharePoint supports a comprehensive set of branding and UI customization features, and you can embed Power BI content on SharePoint pages.

Welcome to Power BI page

Upon signup, Power BI discovers that you don't have any BI artifacts yet. Therefore, it navigates you to the "Welcome to Power BI" page, which is shown in **Figure 2.4**.

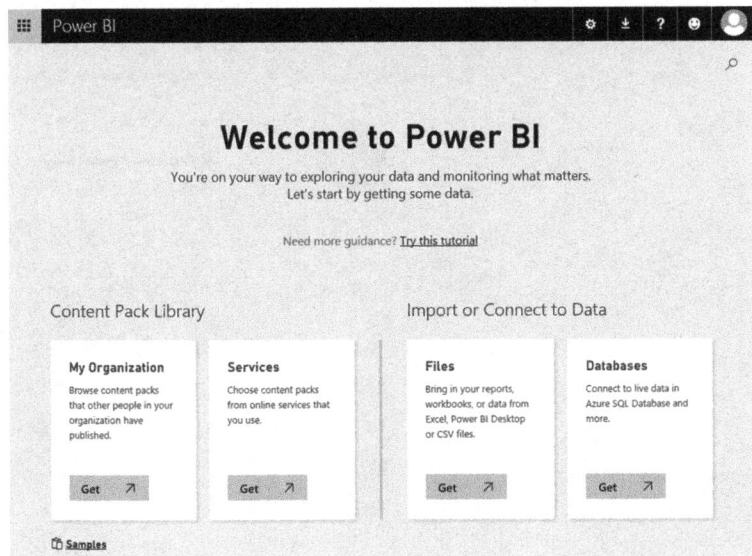

Figure 2.4 The "Welcome to Power BI" page allows you to connect to data and install samples.

Before analyzing data, you need to first connect to wherever it resides. Therefore, the "Welcome to Power BI" page prompts you to start your data journey by connecting to your data. The My Organization tile under the "Content Pack Library" section allows you to browse and use organizational apps (discussed in Chapter 11), if someone within your organization has already published BI content as apps. The Services tile allows you to use Microsoft-provided content packs to connect to popular online services, such as Google Analytics, Salesforce, Microsoft Dynamics CRM, and many more.

The Files tile under the "Import or Connect to Data" section lets you import data from Excel, Power BI Desktop, and CSV files. The Databases tile allows you to connect to data sources that support live connections, such as Azure SQL Database and SQL Server Analysis Services.

 NOTE As you'll quickly discover, a popular option that's missing in the Databases tile is connecting to an on-premises database, such as SQL Server or Oracle. Currently, this scenario requires you create a data model using Power BI Desktop or Excel before you can import data from on-premises databases. Power BI Desktop also supports connecting directly to some data sources, such as SQL Server. Then you can upload the model to Power BI. Because it's a more advanced scenario, I'll postpone discussing Power BI Desktop until Chapter 6.

1. To get some content you can explore in Power BI and quickly get an idea about its reporting capabilities, click the Samples link.

2. In the Samples page, click the "Retail Analysis Sample" tile. As the popup informs you, the Retail Analysis Sample is a sample dashboard provided by Microsoft to demonstrate some of the Power BI capabilities. Click the Connect button. Are you concerned that samples might clutter the portal? Don't worry; it's easy to delete the sample later. To do this, you can just delete the Retail Analysis Sample dataset which will delete the dependent reports.

The Power BI portal

After installing the Retail Analysis Sample, Power BI navigates you to the portal home page, which has the following main sections (see the numbered areas in **Figure 2.5**):

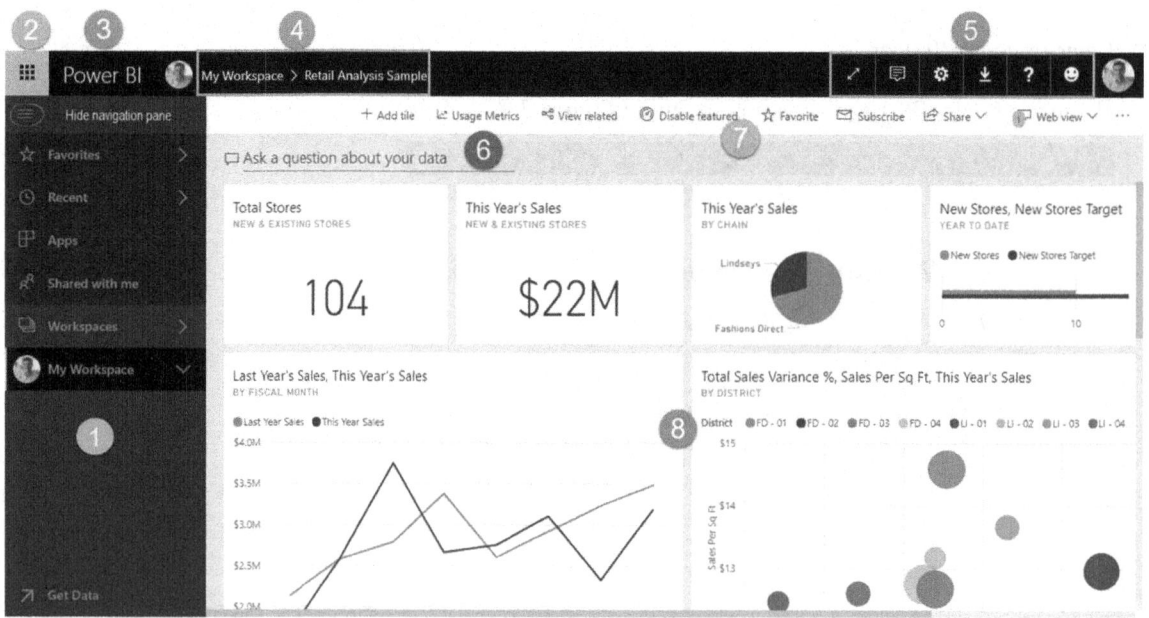

Figure 2.5 The Power BI portal home page

1. Navigation Pane – The navigation pane organizes the content deployed to Power BI.

Starting from the top, you can show/hide the navigation pane by toggling the "Hide the navigation pane" button. You might prefer Power BI to show a specific "featured" dashboard when you open the portal (instead of navigating you to the last dashboard you visited). While you can have one featured dashboard, you can have several favorite dashboards that you can access from the Favorites link. And the Recent link shows a list of the last 20 reports and dashboards that you've visited recently.

Recall from Chapter 1 that apps are for consuming prepackaged content from external online services or from Power BI workspaces. You can click the Apps button to see what external or organizational apps you have installed. If someone has shared dashboards with you, they can be accessed from the "Shared with me" menu.

In Power BI, workspaces can be used to organize and secure content. For example, a Sales workspace can let members of the Sales department create and collaborate on BI content. If you have Power BI Pro subscription, you can access all workspaces you are a member of by clicking the Workspaces menu. Think of My Workspace as your private desk. By default, all BI content you publish to Power BI is deployed to My Workspace. Unless you share content with other users, no one else can see what's in your workspace.

To see the actual published content in a workspace (My Workspace or another workspace you are a member of), simply click on the workspace name or expand it. For example, to see what's inside My

Workspace, expand the down arrow next to it or click My Workspace in the navigation pane. If you expand the workspace, you'll see sections for Dashboards, Reports, Workbooks and Datasets in the navigation pane. If you click the workspace, you'll be navigated to another page where the workspace content is organized in several tabs, as shown in **Figure 2.6**. As your workspace gets busier, you'd probably favor the tabbed interface because it allows you to search for items by name.

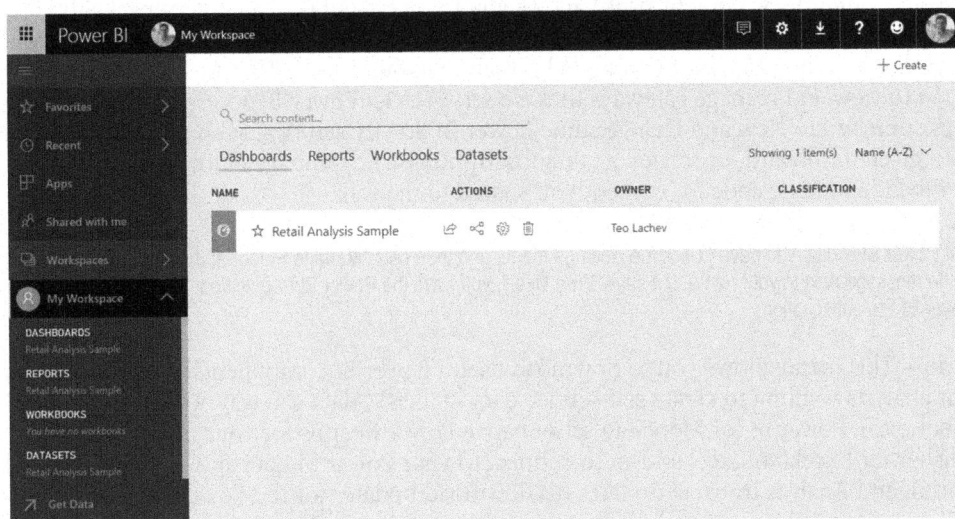

Figure 2.6 The workspace content is organized in several tabs.

The Dashboards tab includes the dashboards that you've developed or that someone shared with you. Similarly, the Reports section contains all reports that are available to you. The Workbooks session brings you to Excel files that you've connected to (yes, Power BI allows you to bring in existing Excel reports). The Datasets section shows all the datasets that you've created or that someone shared with you. If you have a lot of items and you still find it difficult to locate something, use the "Search content" field to search within the content in the corresponding tab. Besides simply clicking the item to open it, you can perform additional tasks from the Actions column, such as to share a dashboard, delete a dashboard, and access the dashboard settings.

Going down the navigation pane, the Get Data button at the bottom brings you to the Get Data page. Like the "Welcome to Power BI" page, the Get Data page allows you to connect to your cloud and on-premises data.

2. Office 365 application launcher – If you have an Office 365 subscription, this menu allows you to access the Office 365 applications you are licensed to use. Doesn't Microsoft encourage you to use Office 365?

3. Power BI home – No matter which page you've navigated to, this menu takes you to the portal home page (see again **Figure 2.5**).

4. Navigation breadcrumb – Displays the navigation path to the displayed content.

5. Application toolbar – Let's explain the available menus starting from the left:

   ■ Enter Full Screen Mode menu – Shows the active content in full screen and removes the Power BI UI (also called "chrome"). Once you're in Full Screen mode, you have options to resize the content to fit to screen and to exit this mode (or press Esc). Another way to open a dashboard in a full screen mode is to append the chromeless=1 parameter to the dashboard URL, such as:

   https://app.powerbi.com/groups/me/dashboards/3065afc5-63a5-4cab-bcd3-0160b3c5f741?chromeless=1

   ■ Notifications menu – Power BI publishes important events, such as when someone shares a dashboard with you or when you get a data alert, to the Power BI Notification Center.

- Settings menu – This menu expands to several submenus. Click "Manage Personal Storage" to check how much storage space you've used (recall that the Power BI Free and Power BI Pro editions have different storage limits) or to start a Power BI Pro 60-day trial. Previously, content packs were used to distribute content to a wider audience, but they are now superseded by apps (more details in Chapter 11). If you have Power BI Pro, the "Create content pack" submenu allows you to create an organizational content pack, while "View content pack" allows you to access published content packs. If you are a Power BI administrator, you can use the Admin Portal to monitor usage and manage tenant-wide settings, such as if users can publish content to web for anonymous access. The "Manage gateways" menu allows you to view and manage gateways that are set up to let Power BI access on-premises data. Use the Settings submenu to view and change some Power BI Service settings, such as if the Q&A box is available for a given dashboard, or to view your subscriptions. The "Manage embed codes" menu is to obtain the embedded iframe code for content you shared to the web.

> **TIP** Not sure what Power BI edition you have? Click the Settings menu, and then click "Manage Personal Storage". At the top of the next page, notice the message next to your name. If it says "Free User", you have the Power BI free edition. If it says "Pro User", then you have Power BI Pro subscription.

- Download menu – This menu allows you to download useful Power BI components, including Power BI Desktop (for analysts wanting to create self-service data models) , data gateways (to connect to on-premises data sources), Power BI for Mobile (a set of native Power BI apps for your mobile devices), Power BI publisher for Excel (an Excel add-in to connect to your Power BI data and to create and publish pivot reports), and Analyze in Excel updates (to download updates for the Power BI Analyze in Excel feature).

- Help and Support menu – Includes several links to useful resources, such as product documentation, the community site, and developer resources.

- Feedback menu – Rate your experience with Power BI on a scale from 1 to 10, submit an idea (new Power BI features are ranked based on the number of votes each idea gets), and submit an issue to community discussion lists.

6. Natural question box (Q&A) – When you select a dashboard and the dashboard uses a dataset that supports natural queries, you can use this box to enter the natural query. For example, you can ask it how many units were shipped in February last year.

7. Context menu – It displays different options depending on the item selected. In the case of dashboard, it gives you access to dashboard-related tasks, such as to add a tile, mark the dashboard a favorite, and share a dashboard with your coworkers. And the ellipsis menu (…) lets you perform additional tasks, such as to print the dashboard or go to the dashboard settings.

8. Content area – This is where the content of the selected item in the navigation pane is shown. For example, if a dashboard is selected, the content pane shows the dashboard tiles.

2.3   Understanding Power BI Content Items

The key to understanding how Power BI works is to understand its three main content items: datasets, reports, and dashboards. These elements are interdependent, and you must understand how they relate to each other. For example, you can't have a report or dashboard without creating one or more datasets. **Figure 2.7** should help you understand these dependencies.

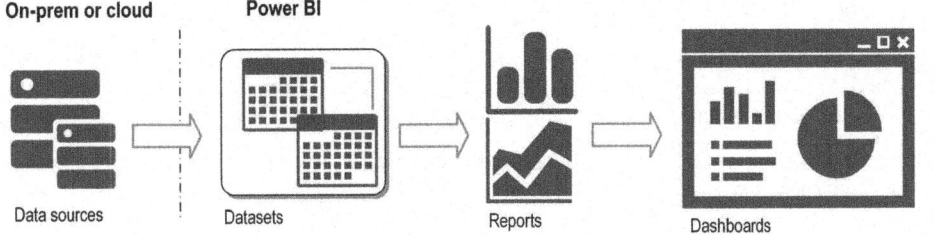

Figure 2.7 The Power BI main content items are datasets, reports, and dashboards.

Data sources Datasets Reports Dashboards

2.3.1 Understanding Datasets

Think of a dataset as a blueprint or a definition of the data that you analyze. For example, if you want to analyze some data stored in an Excel spreadsheet, the corresponding dataset represents the data in the Excel spreadsheet. Or, if you import data from a database table, the dataset will represent that table. Notice in **Figure 2.7**, however, that a dataset can have more than one table. For example, if Martin uses Power BI Desktop or Excel to create a data model, the model might have multiple tables (potentially from different data sources). When Martin uploads the model to Power BI, his entire model will be shown as a single dataset, but when he explores it (he can click the Create Report icon next to the dataset under the Datasets tab to create a new report), he'll see that the Fields pane shows multiple tables. You'll encounter another case of a dataset with multiple tables when you connect to an Analysis Services model.

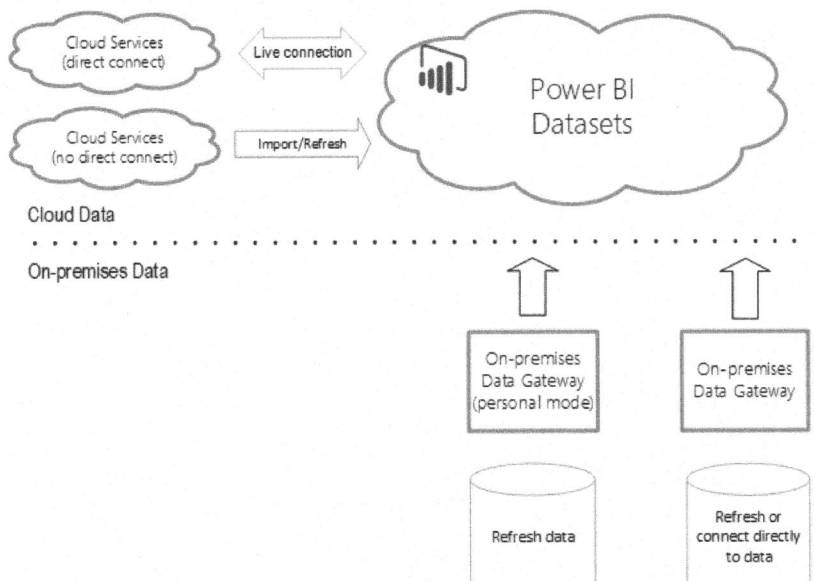

Figure 2.8 Power BI can import data or create live connections to some data sources.

Getting data

Data sources with useful data for analysis are everywhere (see **Figure 2.8**). As far as the data source location goes, we can identify two main types of data sources:

- Cloud (SaaS) services – These data sources are hosted in the cloud and available as online services. Examples of Microsoft cloud data sources that Power BI supports include OneDrive, Dynamics CRM, Azure SQL Database, Azure SQL Data Warehouse, and Spark on Azure HDInsight. Power BI can also access many popular cloud data sources from other vendors, such as Salesforce, Google Analytics, Marketo, and many others (the list is growing every month!).

■ On-premises data sources – This category encompasses all other data sources that are internal to your organization, such as databases, cubes, Excel, and other files. For Power BI to access on-premises data sources, it needs a special connectivity software called a *gateway*.

 DEFINITION A gateway is connectivity software that is installed on premises to enable Power BI to access data in your corporate network. While Power BI can connect to online data sources, it can't tunnel directly into your corporate network unless it goes through a gateway.

Depending on the capabilities and location of the data source, data can be either a) imported in a Power BI dataset or b) left in the original data source without importing it, but it can be accessed directly via a live connection. If the data source supports it, direct connectivity is appropriate when you have fast data sources. In this case, when you generate a report, Power BI creates a query using the syntax of the data source and sends the query directly to the data source. So, the Power BI dataset has only the definition of the data but not the actual data. Not all data sources support direct connections. Examples of cloud data sources that support direct connections include Azure SQL Database, Azure SQL Data Warehouse, Spark on Azure HDInsight, and Azure Analysis Services. And on-premises data sources that support direct queries include SQL Server, Analysis Services, SAP, Oracle, and Teradata. The list of directly accessible data sources is growing in time.

Because only a limited set of data sources supports direct connectivity, in most cases you'll be *importing* data irrespective of whether you access cloud and on-premises data sources. When you import data, the Power BI dataset has the definition of the data *and* the actual data. In Chapter 1, I showed you how when you import data, Microsoft deploys the dataset to scalable and highly-performant Azure backend services. Therefore, when you create reports from imported datasets, performance is good and predictable. But the moment the data is imported, it becomes outdated because changes in the original data source aren't synchronized with the Power BI datasets. Which brings me to the subject of refreshing data.

Refreshing data
Deriving insights from outdated data in imported datasets is rarely useful. Fortunately, Power BI supports automatic data refresh from many data sources. Refreshing data from cloud services is easy because most vendors already have connectivity APIs that allow Power BI to get to the data. In fact, chances are that if you use an app to access a cloud data source, it'll enable automatic data refresh by default. For example, the Google Analytics dataset refreshes by default every hour without any manual configuration.

 TIP OneDrive and SharePoint Online are special locations for storing Excel, Power BI Desktop, and CSV files because Power BI automatically synchronizes changes to these files once every hour.

On-premises data sources are more problematic because Power BI needs to connect to your corporate network, which isn't accessible from outside. Therefore, if you import corporate data, you or IT will need to install a gateway to let Power BI connect to the original data source. For personal use, you can install the gateway in personal mode to refresh imported data without waiting for IT help. For enterprise deployments, IT can centralize data access by setting up the gateway on a dedicated server (discussed in Chapter 11). Besides refreshing data, this installation mode supports direct connections to data sources that supports this connectivity option.

Table 2.1 summarizes the refresh options for popular data sources.

Table 2.1 This table summarizes data refresh options when data is imported from cloud and on-premises data sources.

Location	Data Source	Refresh Type	Frequency
Cloud (Gateway not required)	Most cloud data sources, including Dynamics Online, Salesforce, Marketo, Zendesk, and many others.	Automatic	Once a day
	Excel, CSV, and Power BI Desktop files uploaded to OneDrive, OneDrive for Business, or SharePoint Online	Automatic	Once every hour
On premises (via gateway)	Supported data sources (see https://powerbi.microsoft.com/en-us/documentation/powerbi-refresh-data/)	Scheduled or manual	As configured by you up to 8/day or unlimited with Power BI Premium
	Excel 2013 (or later) Power Pivot data models with Power Query data connections or Power BI Desktop data models	Scheduled or manual	As configured by you up to 8/day or unlimited with Power BI Premium
	Local Excel files via Get Data in Power BI Service	Not supported	

Understanding dataset actions

Once the dataset is created, it appears under the Datasets tab in the workspace content. For example, when you installed the Retail Analysis Sample, Power BI added a dataset with the same name. You can perform several tasks from the Datasets tab (see **Figure 2.9**). Some of these tasks are also available when you click the ellipsis (…) menu next to the dataset name in the navigation pane.

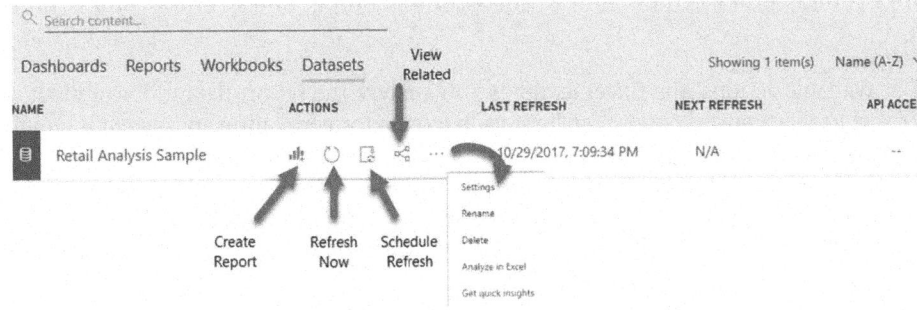

Figure 2.9 The Dataset tab allows you to perform several dataset tasks.

Create Report lets you visualize the data by creating a new report (the subject of the next section). Refresh Now initiates an immediate refresh while Schedule Refresh allows you to schedule the refresh task (refreshing applies to datasets with imported data). Use the View Related icon to find which reports and dashboards use the dataset. More Options (…) opens additional tasks, including accessing the dataset settings, renaming and deleting the dataset, analyzing in Excel, getting quick insights, and setting up data security (not shown in the screenshot). What tasks will be available depends on the data source and how the dataset is configured. For example, the Security menu won't be available if the dataset doesn't have row-level security (RLS) (you need Power BI Desktop to set up RLS). Let's explain these tasks in more detail.

The Settings menu allows you to see how the dataset is configured for refresh, to enable integration with Windows Cortana, and to enter featured Q&A questions. Don't worry if you have existing reports connected to the dataset when you rename it because changing the dataset name won't break dependent reports and dashboards. However, if you delete a dataset, Power BI will automatically remove dependent reports and dashboard tiles that connect to that dataset. Analyze in Excel allows you to create pivot reports in Excel Desktop connected to the dataset. As I mentioned in Chapter 1, Quick Insights runs machine algorithms and auto-generates useful reports that might help you to understand the root cause of data fluctuations. The Security menu allows you to add members to RLS roles.

There are additional properties next to the dataset. The Last Refresh and Next Refresh columns show the dates when the dataset was last refreshed and will be refreshed next respectively. The API Access property is for developers. For example, Power BI supports streaming datasets to allow developers to implement real-time dashboards (discussed in Chapter 13) and such a dataset will be denoted as streaming in the API Access column.

2.3.2 Understanding Reports

Let's define a Power BI report as an interactive view for quick data exploration. Unlike other reporting tools that you might be familiar with and that require report authoring and database querying skills, Power BI reports are designed for business users in mind and they don't assume any technical skills. Reports are the main way to analyze data in Power BI. Reports are found under the Reports section in the left navigation pane (see **Figure 2.10**).

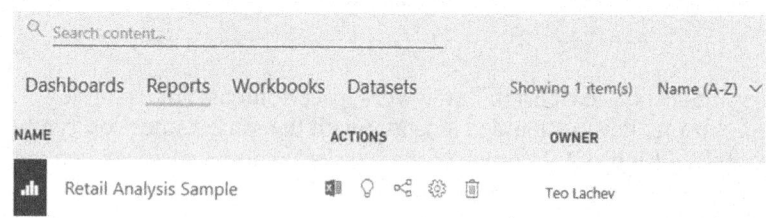

Figure 2.10 The Reports tab lists the reports in the workspace and lets you perform report-related actions.

Understanding report actions
Going through the list of available actions, the Excel icon lets you analyze the report data in Excel pivot reports by connecting Excel to the report dataset. The light bulb icon is for generating and viewing Quick Insights from the report data. The View Related icon shows the dashboards that use content from the selected reports and the dataset the report depends on. Currently, the only available option in the Settings action is to rename the report. And the Delete action removes the report from the workspace. Deleting a report removes any dashboard tiles that came from the report, but keeps the underlying report dataset.

Viewing reports
Clicking the report name in the Reports tab opens the report for viewing. For example, if you click the Retail Analysis Sample report, Power BI will open it in a reading mode (called Reading View) that supports interactive features, such as filtering, but it doesn't allow you to change the report layout. If you have permissions, you can change the report layout by clicking the Edit Report menu on the top of the report (see **Figure 2.11**).

Creating reports
Reports can be created in several ways:

- Creating reports from scratch – Once you have a dataset, you can create a new report by exploring the dataset (the Create Report action in the dataset context menu). Then you can save the report.
- Importing reports – If you import a Power BI Desktop file and the file includes a report, Power BI will import the report and add it to the Reports tab. If you import Excel Power Pivot data models, only Power View reports are imported (Excel pivot and chart reports aren't imported).

NOTE Power BI Service can also connect to Excel files and show pivot table reports and chart reports contained in Excel files. The Excel workbooks you connected to will appear under the Workbooks tab. I'll postpone discussing Excel reports to the next chapter. For now, when I talk about reports I'll mean the type of reports you can create in the Power BI portal.

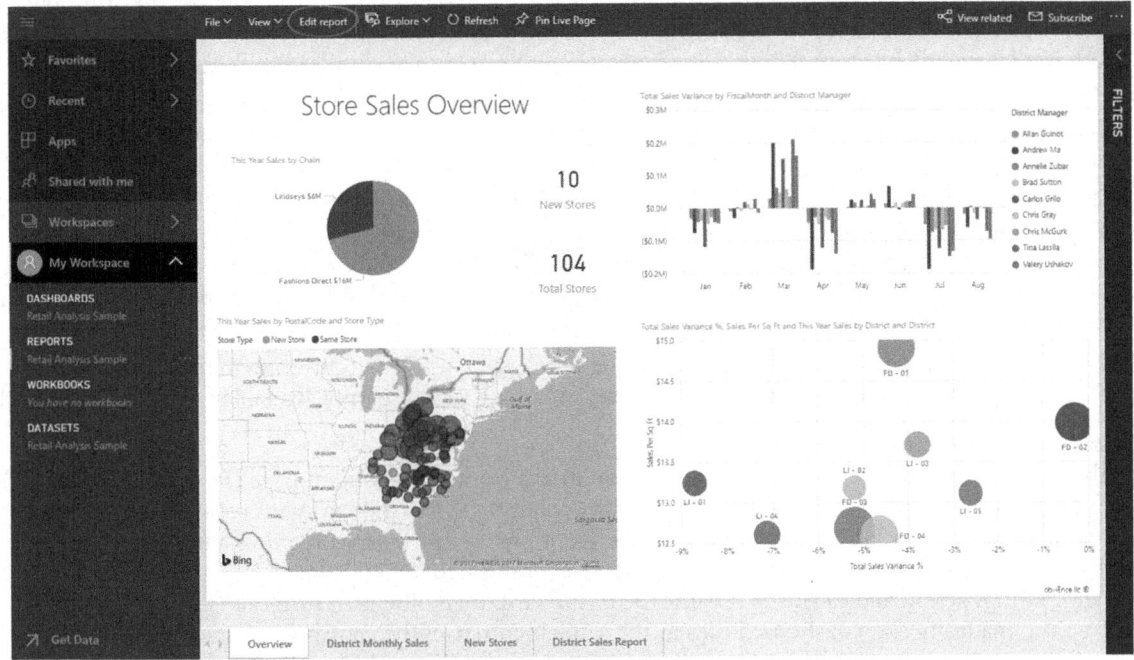

Figure 2.11 A report helps you visualize data from a single dataset.

- Distributing reports – If you use Power BI organizational apps, the reports included in the app are available to you when you install the app.

How reports relate to datasets
Currently, a Power BI report can only connect to and source data from a single dataset only. Suppose you have two datasets: Internet Sales and Reseller Sales. You can't have a report that combines data from these two datasets. Although this might sound like a limitation, you have options:

1. Create a dashboard – If all you want is to show data from multiple datasets as separate visualizations on a single page, you can just create a dashboard.
2. Implement a self-service model – Remember that a dataset can include multiple tables. So, if you need a consolidated report that combines multiple subject areas, you can build a self-service data model using Power BI Desktop or Excel. This works because when published to Power BI, the model will be exposed as a single dataset with multiple tables.
3. Connect to an organizational model – To promote a single version of the truth, a BI pro can implement an organizational data model using Analysis Services. Then you can just connect to the model; there's nothing to build or import. Finally, if all you want is to show data from multiple datasets as separate visualizations on a single page, you can just create a dashboard.

For the purposes of this chapter, this is all you need to know about reports. You'll revisit them in more detail in the next chapter.

2.3.3 Understanding Dashboards

For a lack of a better definition, a dashboard is a summarized one-page view with strategic metrics related to the data you're analyzing. Dashboards convey important metrics so that management can get a high-level view of the business. To support root cause analysis, dashboards typically allow users to drill from summary sections (called tiles in Power BI) down to more detailed reports. Why do you need dashboards if you have dashboard-like reports? There are several good reasons to consider dashboards:

- Combine data from multiple reports and thus from multiple datasets – For example, you might have a report with some sales data and another report with inventory data. A dashboard can combine (but not filter or join) visuals from these two reports. That's why dashboards are available only in Power BI Service and not available in Power BI Desktop, which is limited to a single report per file.

- Expose only certain elements from reports – You might have created a report with many pages, but you want another user to focus only on the most import sections. You can create a dashboard that shows the relevant visuals or entire pages. Remember though that dashboards are not a security mechanism as the user can always click a tile, drill down to the underlying report, and see all the pages.

- Dashboard-specific features – Some Power BI features, such as Q&A (currently in preview for Power BI Desktop), dashboard sharing, data alerts and streaming tiles, are only available at a dashboard level.

Understanding dashboard actions

Dashboards are listed under the Dashboards section in the workspace content page (see again **Figure 2.6**). The first icon to the right of the dashboard name is for sharing the dashboard with someone else (besides this sharing option, Power BI supports other sharing options to distribute content to a larger audience). The View Related action shows you the reports that the dashboard depends on.

The Settings action allows you to rename the dashboard, turn off Q&A, turn on a feature called "tile flow" to automatically align dashboard tiles to the top left corner of the canvas (instead of the default layout to freely position tiles on the dashboard), and change the dashboard classification (classifications are discussed in Chapter 11). And the Delete icon removes the dashboard from the workspace content. Deleting a dashboard doesn't affect the dependent datasets and reports.

Creating dashboards

A dashboard consists of rectangular areas called *tiles*. Dashboard tiles can be created in several ways:

- From existing reports – If you have an existing report, you can pin one or more of its visualizations to a dashboard or even an entire report page! For example, the Retail Analysis Sample dashboard was created by pinning visualizations from the report with the same name. It's important to understand that you can pin visualizations from multiple reports into the same dashboard. This allows the dashboard to display a consolidated view that spans multiple reports and thus multiple datasets.

- By using Q&A – Another way to create a dashboard is to type in a question in the natural question box (see **Figure 2.5** again). This allows you to pin the resulting visualization without creating a report. For example, you can type a question like "sales by country" if you have a dataset with sales and geography entities. If Power BI understands your question, it will show you the most appropriate visualization.

- By using Quick Insights – This powerful predictive feature examines your dataset for hidden trends and produces a set of visualizations. You can pin a Quick Insights visualization to a dashboard.

- From Excel – If you connect to an Excel file, you can pin any Excel range as an image to a dashboard. Or, if you use Analyze in Excel, you can pin the pivot report as an image.

- From Power BI Report Server reports – If your organization uses Power BI Report Server and has enabled Power BI integration, you can pin image-producing report items (charts, gauges, maps) to dashboards as images.

- From other dashboards – Dashboards can be shared via mail or distributed with apps. You can add tile to your dashboard from another dashboard you have access to.

Drilling through content

To allow users to see more details below the dashboards, users can drill into dashboard tiles. What happens when you drill through depends on how the tile was created. For example, if it was created by pinning a report visualization, you'll be navigated to the corresponding report page. Or, if it was created through Q&A, you'll be navigated to the page that has the visualization and the natural question that was asked. Or, if it was pinned from an Excel or SSRS report, you'd be navigated to the source report.

1. In the Power BI portal, click the Retail Analysis Sample dashboard in the Dashboard tab.
2. Click the "This Year Sales, Last Year Sales" surface Area Chart. Notice that Power BI navigates to the "District Monthly Sales" tab of the Retail Analysis Sample report.

That's all about dashboards for now. You'll learn much more in Chapter 4. Now let's get back to the topic of data and practice the different connectivity options.

2.4   Connecting to Data

As a first step in the data exploration journey, you need to connect to your data. Let's practice what we've learned about datasets. Because this part of the book targets business users, we'll practice three data connectivity scenarios that don't require creating data models. It might be useful to refer to **Figure 2.4** or click the Get Data button to see these options. First, you'll see how you can use a Power BI content pack to analyze Google Analytics data. Next, I'll show you how you can import an Excel file. Finally, I'll show you how to connect live to an organizational Analysis Services model.

2.4.1   Using Service Apps

Power BI comes with pre-defined service apps (also known as service content packs) that allow business users to connect to popular online services. Suppose that Maya wants to analyze the Adventure Works website traffic. Fortunately, Power BI includes a Google Analytics app to get her started with minimum effort. On the downside, Maya will be limited to whatever data the app's author has decided to import which could be just a small subset of the available data.

 TIP   If you need more data than what's included in the app, consider creating a data model using Excel or Power BI Desktop that connects to the online service to access all the data. For example, your organization might have added custom fields or tables to Salesforce that you need for analysis. Besides data modeling knowledge, this approach requires that you understand the entities and how they relate to each other. So, I suggest you first determine if the app has the data you need.

To perform this exercise, you'll need a Google Analytics account and you must add a tracking code to the website you want to analyze. Google supports free Google Analytics accounts. For more information about the setup, refer to http://www.google.com/analytics. If setting up Google Analytics is too much trouble, you can use similar steps to connect to any other online service that you use in your organization, if it has a Power BI app. To see the list of the available connectors, click the Get Data link in the navigation bar, and then click the Get button in the Services tile. Alternatively, you can click Apps in the navigation bar, click Get Apps, and then select the Apps tab in the AppSource page.

Connecting to Google Analytics

If Maya has already done the required Google Analytics setup, connecting to her Google Analytics account takes a few simple steps:

1. To avoid cookie issues with cached accounts, I suggest you use private browsing. If you use Internet Explorer (IE), open it and then press Ctrl-Shift-P to start a private session that ignores cookies. (Or right-click IE on the start bar and click "Start InPrivate Browsing".) If you use Google Chrome, open it and press

Ctrl-Shift-N to start an incognito session. (Or right-click it on the start bar and click "New incognito window".)

2. Go to powerbi.com and sign in with your Power BI account. In the Power BI portal, click the Get Data link in the navigation pane.

3. In the Get Data page, click the Get button in the Services tile whose message reads "Choose content packs from online services that you use".

4. In the Services page, search for "Google Analytics", and then click the Google Analytics app. In the popup that follows, click Connect.

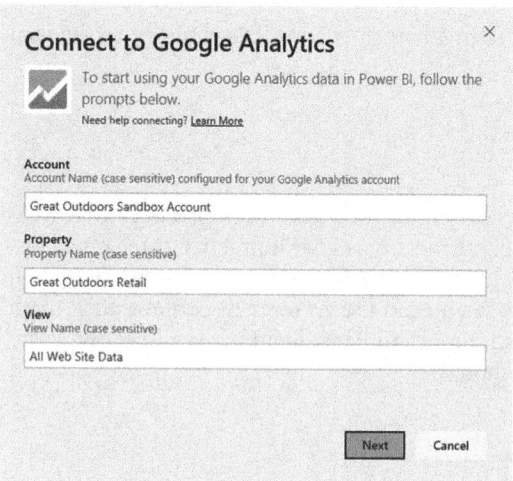

Figure 2.12 As a part of using the Google Analytics app, you need to specify the account details.

5. In the "Connect to Google Analytics" window, specify the Google Analytics details, including account, property, and view. You can get these details by logging into Google Analytics and navigating to the Administration section (Property Settings page). In my case, I'm using a fictitious company provided by Google for testing purposes (see **Figure 2.12**). Click Next.

6. When asked to choose an authentication method, the only option you should see is OAuth. Click Next.

7. In the Google confirmation page that follows, click the Allow button to let Power BI connect to Google Analytics. When asked to authenticate, enter your Google account credentials (typically your Gmail account credentials).

8. Return to the Power BI portal. If all is well, Power BI should display a popup informing you that it's importing your content.

Understanding changes

Like the Retail Analysis Sample, the Google Analytics content pack installs the following content in Power BI:

■ A Google Analytics dataset – A dataset that connects to the Google Analytics data.

■ A Google Analytics report – This report has multiple pages to let you analyze site traffic, system usage, total users, page performance, and top requested pages.

■ A Google Analytics dashboard – A dashboard with pinned visualizations from the Google Analytics report.

That's it! After a few clicks and no explicit modeling, you now have prepackaged reports and dashboards to analyze your website data! If the included visualizations aren't enough, you can explore the Google Analytics dataset and create your own reports. As I previously mentioned, content packs usually schedule an automatic data refresh to keep your data up to date. To verify:

1. In the navigation pane, click My Workspace and then click the Datasets tab. Notice that the Last Refresh column shows you the time when the dataset was last refreshed.

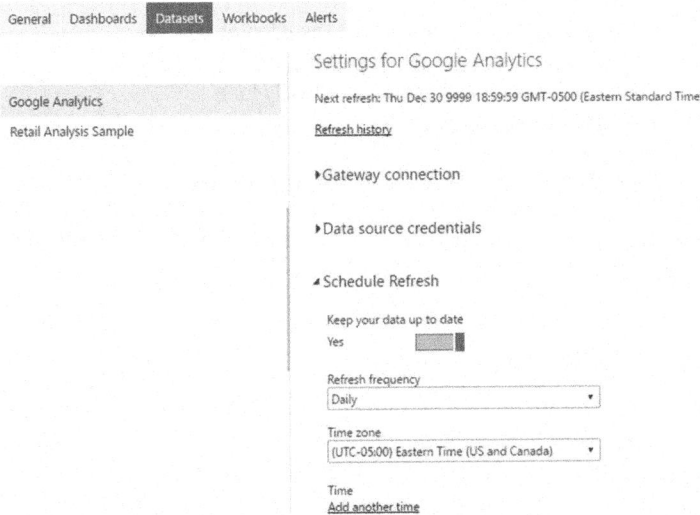

Figure 2.13 The content pack configures automatic daily refresh to synchronize the imported data with the latest changes in the data source.

2. Click the Schedule Refresh action to open the dataset settings page. Notice the app is scheduled for a daily refresh (see **Figure 2.13**).

 NOTE   As you can imagine, thousands of unattended data refreshes scheduled by many users can be expensive in a multi-tenant environment, such as Power BI. This is why Power BI limits you to up to 8 refreshes per day and it doesn't guarantee that the refresh will start exactly at the scheduled time. Power BI queues and distributes the refresh jobs using internal rules. However, the Power BI Premium edition doesn't restrict refresh rate.

3. Expand the "Gateway connection" section. It shows that the content pack connects directly to Google Analytics. That's because both Power BI and Google Analytics are cloud services and no gateway is needed.

2.4.2 Importing Local Files

Another option to get data is to upload a file. Suppose that Maya wants to analyze some sales data given to her as an Excel file. Thanks to the Power BI Get Data feature, Maya can import the Excel file in Power BI and analyze it without creating a model.

Importing Excel data
In this exercise, you will create a dataset by importing an Excel file. You'll analyze the dataset in the next chapter. Start by familiarizing yourself with the raw data in the Excel workbook.

1. Open the Internet Sales.xlsx workbook in Excel. You can find this file in the \Source\ch02 folder of the source code.

2. If Sheet1 isn't selected, click Sheet1 to make it active. Notice that it contains some sales data. Specifically, each row represents the product sales for a given date, as shown in **Figure 2.14**. Also, notice that the Excel data is formatted as a table so that Power BI knows where the data is located.

Date	Product	SalesAmount	OrderQuantity
7/1/2005	Mountain-100 Silver, 44	30599.91	9
7/1/2005	Mountain-100 Black, 38	10124.97	3
7/1/2005	Road-650 Black, 44	1398.1964	2
7/1/2005	Road-650 Red, 52	1398.1964	2
7/1/2005	Road-650 Black, 52	1398.1964	2
7/1/2005	Road-650 Black, 58	2097.2946	3
7/1/2005	Road-150 Red, 56	53674.05	15
7/1/2005	Mountain-100 Black, 48	10124.97	3
7/1/2005	Road-150 Red, 62	78721.94	22
7/1/2005	Mountain-100 Silver, 48	10199.97	3
7/1/2005	Mountain-100 Silver, 42	6799.98	2
7/1/2005	Road-150 Red, 44	82300.21	23
7/1/2005	Road-650 Red, 44	1398.1964	2
7/1/2005	Road-650 Red, 62	699.0982	1

Figure 2.14 The first sheet contains Internet sales data where each row represents the product sales amount and order quantity for a specific date and product.

 TIP The Excel file can have multiple sheets with data, and you can import them as separate tables. Currently, Power BI Service doesn't allow you to relate multiple tables (you need a data model to do so). In addition, Power BI requires that the Excel data is formatted as a table. You can format tabular Excel data as a table by clicking any cell with data and pressing Ctrl-T. Excel will automatically detect the tabular section. After you confirm, Excel will format the data as a table!

3. Close Excel.

4. Next, you'll import the data from the Internet Sales.xlsx file in Power BI. In Power BI, click Get Data.

5. In the Files tile, click the Get button. If you are in the workspace content page, another way to add content is to click the plus (+) sign in the upper-right corner of this page.

6. In the Files page, click "Local File" because you'll be importing from a local Excel file. Navigate to the source code \Source\ch2 folder, and then double-click the Internet Sales file.

7. In the Local File page, click the Import button to import the file (let's postpone connecting to Excel files until the next chapter).

8. Power BI imports the data from the Excel file into the Power BI Service. Once the task completes, you'll see a notification that your dataset is ready. If you click View Dataset, you'll be able to create a report from the dataset but let's not do this now.

Understanding changes

Let's see where the content went:

1. In the navigation pane, click My Workspace (you can also expand My Workspace in the navigation pane).

2. In the workspace content page, click the Datasets tab. A new dataset Internet Sales has been added to the lists of datasets. The asterisk next to the database name denotes that this is a new dataset.

3. Click the Reports tab and notice that there isn't a new report. However, if the Excel had Power View reports, Power BI would import them and add them to the Reports tab.

4. Click the Dashboard tab and notice that there is a new dashboard with the same name as the Excel file (Internet Sales.xlsx). Click the dashboard to open it. Notice that it has a single tile "Internet Sales.xlsx".

5. Click the "Internet Sales.xlsx" tile.

6. Notice that this action opens an empty report (see **Figure 2.15**) to let you explore the data on your own. The Fields pane shows a single table (Internet Sales) whose fields correspond to the columns in the original Excel table. From here, you can just select which fields you want to see on the report. You can choose a visualization from the Visualizations pane to explore the data in different ways, such as a chart or a table.

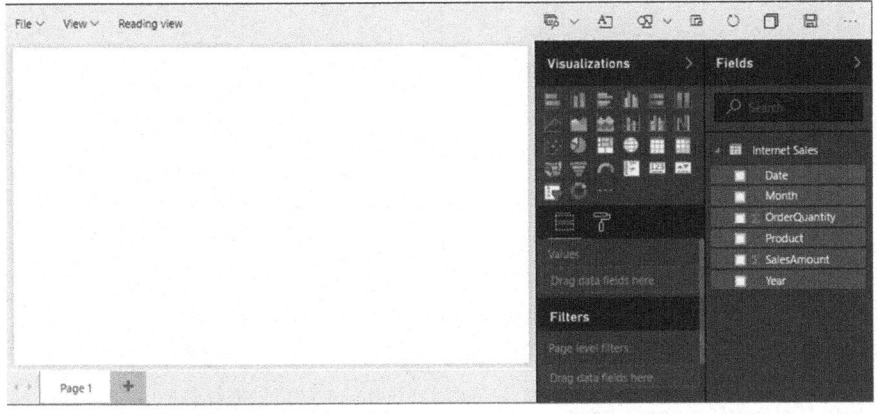

Figure 2.15 The Create Report action lets you create a report from the dataset by dragging fields from the Fields pane.

TIP As I mentioned previously, Power BI can't refresh local Excel files. Suppose that Maya receives an updated Excel file on a regular basis. Without the ability to schedule an automatic refresh, she needs to delete the old dataset (which will delete the dependent reports and dashboard tiles), reimport the data, and recreate the reports. As you can imagine, this can get tedious. A better option would be to save the Excel file to OneDrive, OneDrive for Business, or SharePoint Online. Power BI refreshes files saved to OneDrive every hour and whenever it detects that the file is updated.

2.4.3 Using Live Connections

Suppose that Adventure Works has implemented an organizational Analysis Services semantic model on top of the corporate data warehouse. In the next exercise, you'll see how easy it is for Maya to connect to the model and analyze its data.

Understanding prerequisites

As I explained in the "Understanding Datasets" section, Power BI requires special connectivity software, called *On-premises Data Gateway*, to be installed on an on-premises computer so that Power BI Service can connect to an on-premises Analysis Services. This step needs to be performed by IT because it requires admin rights to Analysis Services. I provide step-by-step setup instructions to install and configure the gateway in Chapter 11 of this book. You can't install the gateway in personal mode on your laptop because in this mode the gateway doesn't support live connections.

Besides setting up the gateway, to perform this exercise, you'll need help from IT to install the sample Adventure Works database and Tabular model (as per the instructions in the book front matter) and to grant you access to the Adventure Works Tabular model.

Connecting to on-premises Analysis Services

Once the gateway is set up, connecting to the Adventure Works Tabular model is easy.

1. In the Power BI portal, click Get Data.
2. In the Get Data page, click the Get button in the Databases pane that reads "Connect to live data in Azure SQL Database and more."
3. In the Databases & More page (see **Figure 2.16**), click the SQL Server Analysis Services tile. In the popup that follows, click Connect. If you don't have a Power BI Pro subscription, this is when you'll be prompted to start a free trial.

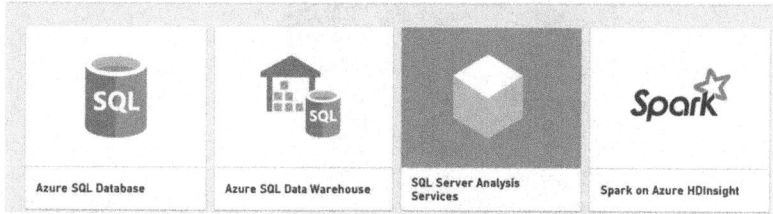

Figure 2.16 Use the SQL Server Analysis Services tile to create a live connection to an on-premises SSAS model.

4. In the SQL Server Analysis Services page that follows, you should see all the Analysis Services databases that are registered with the gateway. Please check with your IT department which one you should use. Once you know the name, click it to select it.

5. Power BI verifies connectivity. If something goes wrong, you'll see an error message. Otherwise, you should see a list of the models and perspectives that you have access to. Select the "Adventure Works Tabular Model SQL 2012 – Model" item and click Connect. This action adds a new dataset to the Datasets tab of the workspace content page.

6. Click the Create Report action to explore the dataset. The Fields lists will show all the entities defined in the SSAS model. From here, you can create an interactive report by selecting specific fields from the Fields pane. This isn't much different from creating Excel reports that are connected to an organizational data model.

7. Click File ⇨ Save and save the report as *Adventure Works SSAS*.

2.5   Summary

Self-service BI broadens the reach of BI and enables business users to create their own solutions for data analysis and reporting. By now you should view self-service BI not as a competing technology but as a completing technology to organizational BI.

Power BI is a cloud service for data analytics and you interact with it using the Power BI portal. The portal allows you to create datasets that connect to your data. You can either import data or you can connect live to data sources that support live connections. Once you have a dataset, you can explore it to create new reports. And once you have reports, you can pin their visualizations to dashboards.

As a business user, you don't have to create data models to meet simple data analytics needs. This chapter walked you through a practice that demonstrated how you can perform basic data connectivity tasks, including using a content pack to connect to an online service (Google Analytics), importing an Excel file, and connecting live to an on-premises Analysis Services model. The next chapter will show you how you can analyze your data by creating insightful reports!

Chapter 3

Creating Reports

In the previous chapter, I showed you how Power BI allows business users to connect to data without explicit modeling. The next logical step is to visualize the data so that you can derive knowledge from it. Fortunately, Power BI lets you create meaningful reports with just a few mouse clicks. A data analyst would typically use Power BI Desktop for report authoring. However, a regular business user might prefer to create reports directly in the Power BI Portal and that's the scenario discussed in this chapter.

I'll start this chapter by explaining the building blocks of Power BI reports. Then I'll walk you through the steps to explore Power BI datasets and to create reports with interactive visualizations directly inside Power BI Service (powerbi.com). Because Excel is such an important tool, I'll show you three ways to integrate Power BI with Excel: importing data from Excel files, connecting to existing Excel workbooks, and creating your own pivot reports connected to Power BI datasets. You can also pin Reporting Services reports to dashboards but I'll postpone this integration scenario to the next chapter. Because this chapter builds on the previous one, make sure you've completed the exercises in the previous chapter to install the Retail Analysis Sample and to import the Internet Sales dataset from the Excel file.

3.1 Understanding Reports

In the previous chapter, I introduced you to Power BI reports. I defined a Power BI report as an interactive visual representation of a dataset. Power BI also supports Excel and SSRS reports. Let's revisit the three report types that you can have in Power BI Service:

- Power BI native reports – This report type delivers a highly visual and interactive report that has its roots in Power View. This is the report type I'll mean when I refer to Power BI reports. For example, the Retail Analysis Sample report is an example of a Power BI report. You can use Power BI Service, Power BI Desktop, and to some extent Excel Power View (deprecated) to create these reports.

- Excel reports – Power BI allows you to connect to Excel 2013 (or later) files and view the included table, pivot and Power View reports. For example, you might have invested significant effort into creating Power Pivot models and reports. Or, a financial analyst might prefer to share an Excel spreadsheet with results from some complex formulas. You don't want to migrate these Excel reports to Power BI Desktop, but you'd like users to view them as they are, and even interact with them! To get this to work, you can just connect Power BI to your Excel files. However, you still must use Excel Desktop to create or modify the reports and data model (if the Excel file has a Power Pivot model).

- Reporting Services reports – SSRS is Microsoft's most customizable reporting tool. If your organization has Power BI Report Server and it's configured for Power BI integration, you can pin report items to Power BI dashboards. For example, a report developer might have implemented a sophisticated map with multiple layers. Now Maya wants to add this map to her dashboard. Maya can open the report and pin the map image as a dashboard tile. When Maya clicks the map, she's navigated to the SSRS report, but Maya needs to be on the corporate network for this to happen.

Most of this chapter will be focused on Power BI native reports but I'll also show you how Power BI integrates with Excel and SSRS reports.

3.1.1 Understanding Reading View

Power BI Service supports two report viewing modes. Reading View allows you to explore the report and interact with it, without worrying that you'll break something. Editing View lets you make changes to the report layout, such as to add or remove a field.

Opening a report in Reading View
Power BI defaults to Reading View when you open a report. This happens when you click the report name in the Reports tab or when you click a dashboard tile to open the underlying report.

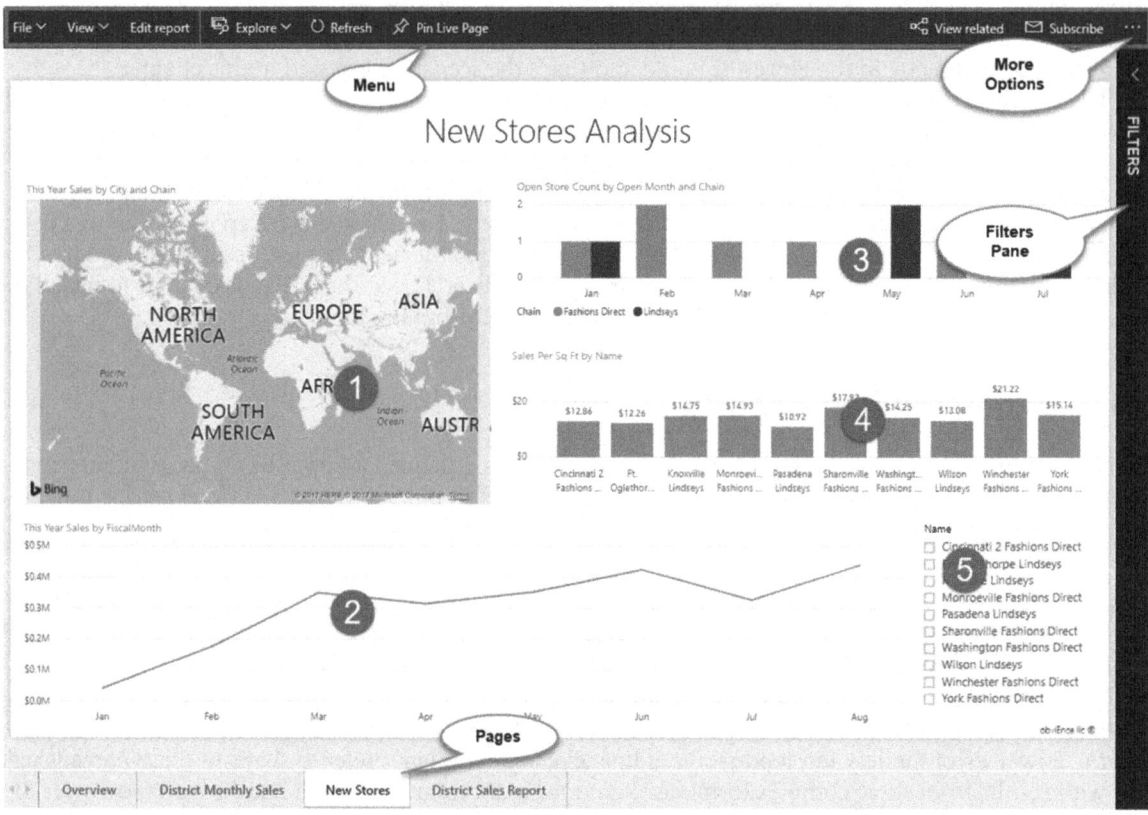

Figure 3.1 Reading View allows you to analyze and interact with the report, without changing it.

1. In the Power BI portal, click My Workspace. In the workspace content page, click the Reports tab and then click the Retail Analysis Sample report to open it in Reading View.
2. On the bottom-left area of the report, notice that this report has four pages. A report page is conceptually like a slide in a PowerPoint presentation – it gives you a different view of the data story. So, if you run out

of space on the first page, you can add more pages, but you must be in Edit Report mode. Click the "New Stores" page to activate it. Notice that the page has five visualizations (see **Figure 3.1**).

Understanding the File menu
Expanding the File menu gives you access to the following features:

- Save as – Creates a new report with a different name in the current workspace.

- Print – Prints the current report page. Printing doesn't expand visualizations to show all the data. In other words, what you see on the screen is what you get when you print the page.

- Publish to web – If the "Publish to web" feature is enabled by the Power BI administrator in the Admin Portal (it is by default) and you're a Power BI Pro user, this feature allows you to publish the report for anonymous access. You'll be given a link that you can send to someone and an embed code (iframe) that you can use to embed the report on a web page, such as in a blog. To find later which reports you've published to the web, go to the Settings menu (the upper-right gear button in the portal), and then click Embed Codes. Be very careful with this feature as you might expose sensitive data to anyone on the Internet!

- Export to PowerPoint – Export the report as a PowerPoint presentation. Each report page becomes a slide and all visualizations are exported as static images.

- Download report – Exports the report and underlying dataset as a Power BI Desktop file. Currently, this feature works only for reports connected to datasets published from Power BI Desktop. Therefore, it's disabled for the Retail Analysis Sample report which you obtained from one of the Power BI samples (the developer has implemented the sample as an Excel Power Pivot model). This menu will also be disabled for the report that you'll later create from the Internet Sales dataset because you created this dataset directly in Power BI Service. As this feature stands, its primary goal is to recover reports and data if the Power BI Desktop file ever gets lost. You can download existing, new, and changed reports, and the underlying datasets can contain imported data or connect directly to the data source.

> **TIP** Instead of relying on users to export reports they've created directly in Power BI Service to Power BI Desktop as a disaster recovery procedure, a better option might be to use Power BI Desktop to connect to the published dataset (Get Data ⇨ Power BI service) and then create the reports. Since you always start with Power BI Desktop, you always have its file in case someone deletes the published reports.

Understanding the View menu
The View menu is for adjusting the report size. The "Fit to page" option scales the report content to best fit the page. "Fit to width" resizes the report to the width of the page. And "Actual size" displays content at full size. For now, let's skip the "Edit report" menu which switches you to Editing View to edit the report.

> **TIP** While I'm on the subject of report sizing, both Power BI Service and Power BI Desktop support predefined and custom page sizes. In Power BI Service, while editing the report, you can use the Visualizations pane (Format tab) to specify a page layout for the selected report page, such as 16:9, 4:3, Cortana, Letter, or a custom size. For example, the District Sales Report page in the Retail Analysis Sample report has Cortana layout which is optimized to be rendered by Windows Cortana. Power BI Desktop supports also specifying a mobile view which optimizes the layout for viewing in a Power BI mobile app.

You can use the View menu to enable the Selection Pane so that you toggle the visibility of report elements. In edit mode, this could be useful to temporarily hide visualizations on a busy report page while you are working on a new visual. If the report has bookmarks (discussed in Chapter 10), you can also enable the Bookmarks pane so that you can tell your data story by navigating to specific bookmarks.

Understanding the Explore menu
Some Power BI visualizations, such as charts, allow you to drill down the data. For example, you might have a column chart that has Country and City fields added to the Axis area. The chart initially shows data

by country. If you select the chart and click Explore ⇨ See Data (or right click a bar and click See Data), you can see the actual data behind the chart (as if you flip the chart to a Table visualization). Similarly, when you toggle Explore ⇨ See Records (or right click a bar and click See Records) and then click a chart bar, you see the actual data behind that bar only. This is also called drilling through data. The rest of the exploration menus fulfill the same role as the interactive features for data exploration when you hover on the chart.

Understanding the Refresh menu

Clicking the Refresh menu refreshes the data on the report. The report always queries the underlying dataset when you view it. The report Refresh menu could be useful if the underlying dataset was refreshed or has a live connection and you want to get the latest data without closing and reopening the report.

Understanding the Pin Live Page menu

You can quickly assemble a dashboard from existing report visualizations. You can also pin entire report pages to a dashboard. This could be useful when the report page is already designed as a dashboard. You can pin the entire page instead of pinning individual visualizations. Although this might sound redundant, promoting a report to a dashboard gives you access to dashboard features, such as Q&A.

Another scenario for pinning report pages is when you want to filter dashboards tiles because dashboards don't have filtering features (the Filter pane is not available). To accomplish this, you can create a report page that has the visualizations you need, add a slicer, and then pin the entire page.

Understanding the Subscribe menu

I've already explained the purpose of the View Related menu. Besides viewing a report interactively (on demand), Power BI lets you subscribe to it. The Subscribe menu is only available in Reading View. It brings you to a window where you can indicate which report pages you want to subscribe to and to manage subscriptions you've created. Once you set up a subscription, Power BI will detect data changes in the underlying report dataset and send you an email with screenshots of the subscribed pages. Subscribed report delivery is a Power BI Pro feature. If a Power BI Free user clicks the Subscribe menu, the user will be informed that this feature is not available unless the user upgrades.

Interacting with visualizations

Although the name might mislead you, Reading View allows you to interact with the report and filter data.

1. Expand the Filters pane on the right of the report. Notice that the report author has added a Store Type filter that filters only new stores. Note also that you can change the filter, such as to show all store types.

2. In the fourth visualization ("Sales Per Sq Ft by Name") on the New Stores page, click the first column "Cincinnati 2 Fashions Direct" (you can hover on the column bar and a tooltip pops up to show the full name). Notice that the other visualizations change to show data only for the selected store. This feature is called *cross filtering* (or *interactive highlighting*), and it's another way to filter data on the report. Cross filtering is automatic, and you don't need to do anything special to enable it. Click the bar again or an empty area in the same chart to show all the data.

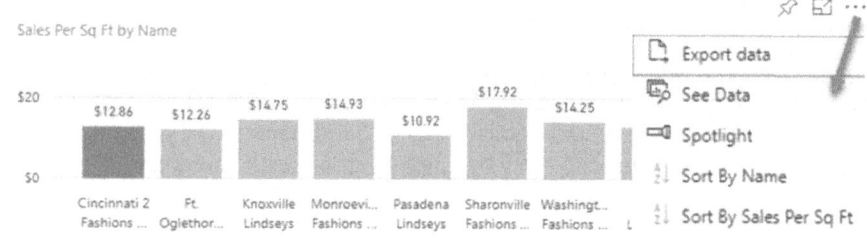

Figure 3.2 You can see how the visualization is sorted and you can change or remove the sort.

3. Hover on the same visualization and notice that Power BI shows an ellipsis menu (More Options) in the top-right corner (see **Figure 3.2**).

4. Notice that you can sort by fields added to the chart. Click "Sort by Name" to sort the chart by the store name in a descending order. If you change the sort, an orange bar will appear to the left of the sorted field. Notice the pin button to the left of the ellipsis menu. It allows you to pin the visualization to a dashboard.

5. On the right of the pin button, there is another button that lets you pop out the visualization in focus mode in case you want to examine its data in more detail. Try it out.

Exporting data

You can export the data behind a visualization in a Comma-Separated Values (CSV) or Excel format.

1. Click Export Data in the More Options menu. In the "Export data" window (see **Figure 3.3**), notice that by default Power BI will export the summarized data as it's aggregated on the chart. The "Underlying data" option lets you export the underlying (detail) data.

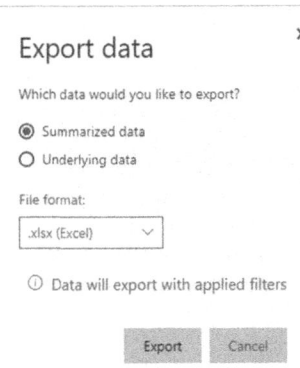

Figure 3.3 You can export the visualization data in Excel or CSV format.

2. Click the Export button and export the chart data as an Excel file. If the report has any filters applied, the exported data will be filtered accordingly.

 TIP Currently, Power BI caps See Records (drillthrough) to 1,000 rows and exporting data to 10,000 rows. There is nothing you can do to change these limits. One workaround is to use the Analyze in Excel feature and drill through a cell in a pivot report. In this case, there is no limit on the number of rows returned.

To wrap up the More Options menu, the See Data option allows you to see the data that the chart is bound to without exporting. Used with bookmarking, the Spotlight option allows you to draw attention to a visual while it fades the other visuals on the page.

Drilling down

Drilling down is a popular data analytics feature that lets you explore data in more detail. For example, the default chart might show sales by country but then you might want to drill down to cities. If the chart had multiple fields or a hierarchy added to the Axis zone (the "Sales per Sq Ft" chart doesn't), you'll also see Explore Data indicators (shown by the red circles at the top of **Figure 3.4**) that fulfill the same role as the corresponding options in the Explore main menu.

Because, by default, Power BI initiates cross filtering when you click a chart element, the indicators allow you to switch to a drill mode. For example, you can click the down arrow indicator (in the top-right corner) to switch to a drill mode, and then click a bar to drill through and see the underlying data. To drill up, just click the up arrow indicator in the top-left corner. Or, you can simply right-click a bar and initiate the same actions from the context menu.

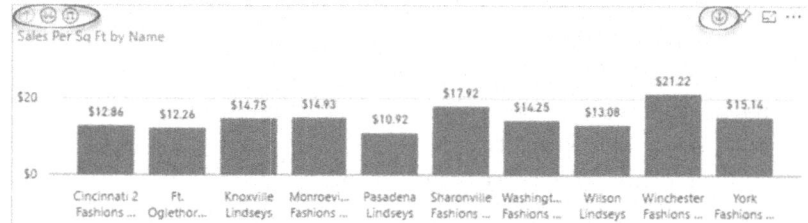

Figure 3.4 You can drill down the next level if the visualization is designed for this feature.

1. If you have a chart with multiple fields in the Axis area, click the double-arrow indicator to go to the next level (the next field you have in the Axis zone). This is the same as Show Next Level in the Explore main menu. For example, if the chart had Country and City fields in the Axis area and you are initially at the Country level, clicking the double-arrow indicator would show the chart data by City as though the Country field isn't in the Axis area. By contrast, clicking the "Expand all down" button (the third one from the group on the left), would drill down all data points to the next level but it'll preserve the parent grouping, such as to show data by city grouped by country.

> **TIP** Some visualizations, such as Column Chart allow you to add multiple fields to specific areas when you configure the chart, such as in the Axis area. So to configure a chart for drilldown, you need to open the report in Editing View and just add more fields to the Axis area of the chart. These fields define the levels that you drill down to. Power BI Desktop allows the modeler to create hierarchies to define useful navigational paths. If hierarchies are defined, you can just drag the hierarchy to the chart axis.

2. Power BI has more interactive features. Hover on top of any column in the chart. Notice that a tooltip pops up to let you know the data series name and the exact measure amount. By default, the tooltip shows only the fields added to the chart. However, you can switch to Editing View and add more fields to the visualization's Tooltips area if you want to see these fields appear in the tooltip.

3.1.2 Understanding Editing View

If you have report editing rights, you can make changes to the report layout. You have editing rights when you're the original report author or when the report is available in a workspace you're a member of and you have rights to edit the content. You have editing rights to all content in My Workspace. You can switch to Editing View by clicking the Edit Report menu.

> **NOTE** Edit mode allows you to make report layout changes only, as you can do in Power BI Desktop. However, it lacks modeling capabilities, such as adding tables, renaming fields, relationships, or calculations. Among all the Power BI products, modeling features are available in Power BI Desktop only. In addition, although creating and editing reports directly in Power BI Service might be convenient for business users, it might not be a best practice. For example, deleting a dataset would delete all related reports and there is no way to restore them. A better, although more advanced option, might be to create reports in Power BI Desktop that connect to published datasets using the Power BI Service data source.

Understanding menu changes

One of the first things you'll notice when you switch to Editing View is that the report menu changes (see **Figure 3.5**). Let's go quickly through the changes. The File menu adds a Save submenu to let you save changes to the report. The View menu adds Show Gridlines, Snap to Grid, and Lock Objects menus. When you enable "Show Gridlines", Power BI adds a grid to help you position items on the report canvas. If "Snap to Grid" is enabled, the items will snap to the grid so that you can easily align them. And when "Lock Objects" is enabled, you can't make layout changes, such as when you're learning Power BI and you want to avoid making inadvertent changes to an existing report. The "Reading view" menu brings you back to opening the report as read-only.

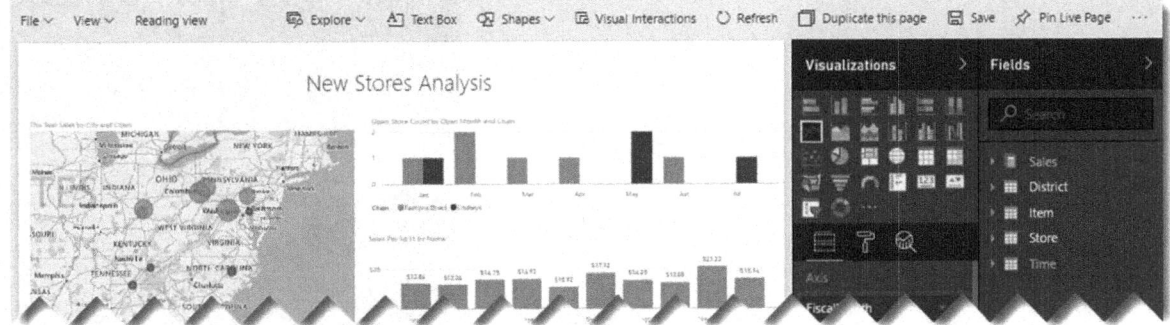

Figure 3.5 The Editing View menu adds links to create text elements and save the report.

Editing View also adds menus on the right side of the report for editing features. Use the Text Box menu to add text boxes to the report which could be useful for report or section titles, or for any text you want on the report. The Text Box menu opens a comprehensive text editor that allows you to format the text and implement hyperlinks. The Shapes menu allows you to add rectangle, oval, line, triangle, and arrow shapes to the report for decorative or illustrative purposes. Currently, you can't add images, such as a company logo. You can use Power BI Desktop to add images.

The Visual Interactions menu allows you to customize the behavior of the page's interactive features. You can select a visual that would act as the source and then set the interactivity level for the other visualizations on the same page. For example, you can use this feature to disable interactive highlighting to selected visualizations. To see this feature in action, watch the "Power BI Desktop November 2015 Update" video at https://youtu.be/ErHvpkyQjSg.

The Duplicate Page menu creates a copy of the current report page. This could be useful if you want to add a new page to the report that has similar visualizations as an existing page, but you want to show different data. The Save menu is a shortcut that does the same thing as the File ⇨ Save menu.

Understanding the Visualizations pane
The next thing you'll notice is that Editing View adds two panes on the right of the report: Visualizations and Fields. Use the Visualizations pane to configure the active visualization, such as to switch from one chart type to another.

 NOTE When you make changes to the Visualizations pane, they are applied to the currently selected (active) visualization. An active visualization has a border around it with resize handles. You need to click a visualization to activate it.

1. If it's not already active, click the "New Stores Analysis" page to select it.
2. Click the "Sales Per Sq Ft by Name" visualization to activate it. **Figure 3.6** shows the Visualizations pane. The Filters section occupies the bottom part of the Visualizations pane, but the screenshot shows it adjacent to the Visualizations pane to accommodate space constraints.

The Visualizations pane consists of several sections. The top section shows the Power BI visualization types, which I'll discuss in more detail in the next section "Understanding Power BI Visualizations". The ellipsis button below the visualizations allows you to import custom visuals from a file or from Microsoft AppSource, or to delete a custom visual you added by mistake. So, when the Power BI-provided visualizations are not enough for your data presentation needs, check AppSource. Chances are that you'll find a custom visual that can fill in the gap!

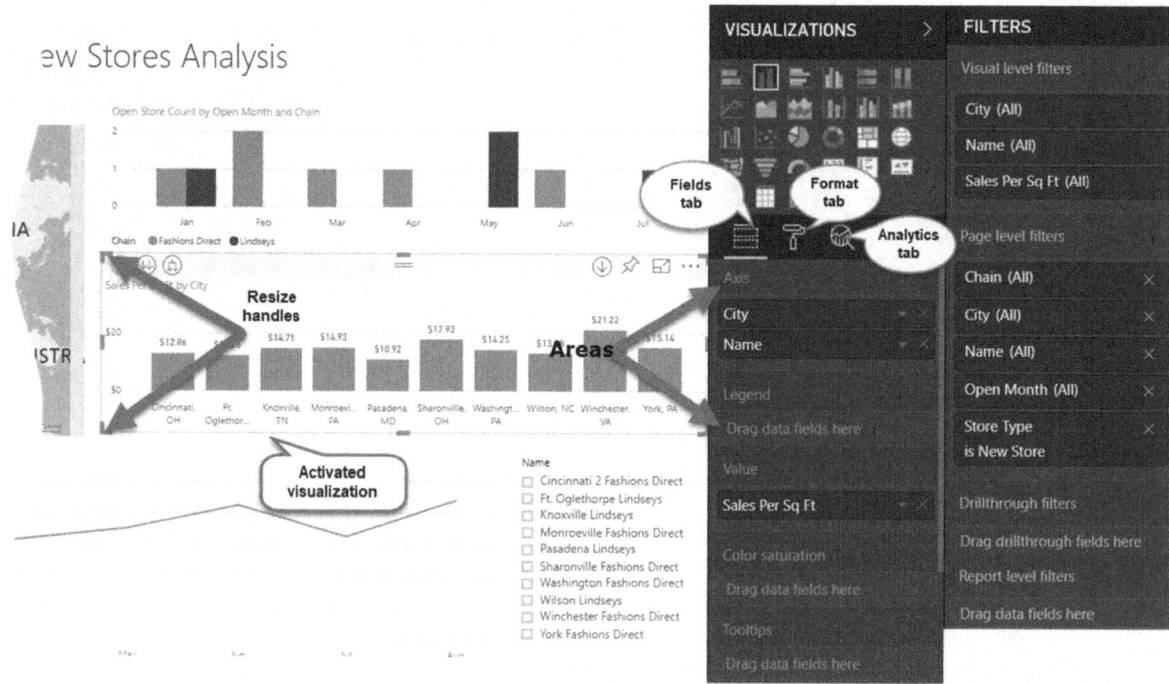

Figure 3.6 The Visualizations pane allows you to switch visualizations and to make changes to the active visualization.

The Fields tab consists of areas that you can use to configure the active visualization, similarly to how you would use the zones of the Excel Fields List when you configure a pivot report. For example, this visualization has the Name field of the Store table added to the Axis area and the "Sales Per Sq Ft" field from the Sales table added to the Value area.

 TIP You can find which table a field comes from by hovering on the field name. You'll see a tooltip pop up that shows the table and field names, such as 'Store'[Name]. This is the same naming convention that a data analyst would use to create custom calculations in a data model using Data Analysis Expressions (DAX).

The Filters section of the Fields tab is for filtering data on the report. Use the "Visual level filters" section to filter the data in the active visualization. By default, you can filter any field that's used in the visualization, but you can also add other fields. For example, the "Visual level filters" has the Name and "Sales per Sq Ft" fields because they are used on the chart. The (All) suffix next to the field tells you that these two fields are not filtered (the chart shows all stores irrespective of their sales).

Use the "Page Level Filters" section to apply filters to all visualizations on the active page. For example, all four visualizations on this page are filtered to show data for new stores (Store Type is "New Store"). The "Drillthrough Filters" is for defining a drillthrough target page, such as in the case where you want to start with a summary view but allow the user to drill to another page to see the details. Finally, filters in the "Report Level Filters" section are applied globally to all visualizations on the report even if they are on different pages.

The Format tab of the Visualizations pane is for applying format settings to the active visualization. Different visualizations support different format settings. For example, column charts support custom colors per category (for tips and tricks for color formatting see https://powerbi.microsoft.com/en-us/documentation/powerbi-service-tips-and-tricks-for-color-formatting), data labels, title, axis labels, and other settings. As Power BI evolves, it adds more options to give you more control over customizing the visual appearance.

Finally, the Analytics tab is for adding features to the visualization to augment its analytics capabilities. For example, Maya plots revenue as a single-line chart. Now she wants to forecast revenue for future periods. She can do this by adding a Forecast line (discussed in more detail in Chapter 10). The analytics features vary among visualization types. For example, table and matrices don't currently support analytics features, a bar chart supports a constant line, while a linear chart supports constant, min, max, average, median, percentile, and forecast lines.

NOTE Do you think that Power BI visualizations are rather basic and they don't support enough customization compared to other tools, such as Excel or SSRS? Remember from Chapter 1 that Microsoft committed to a monthly release cadence, so you might not have to wait long to get a frequently requested feature. But to prioritize your wish, I encourage you to submit your idea or vote for an existing feature at https://ideas.powerbi.com. If you don't want to wait, a web developer in your organization with JavaScript experience can create custom visuals and the last chapter shows how this can be done.

Understanding filter conditions

Revisiting the Filters section, currently Power BI supports three filter types (**Figure 3.7**):

- Basic filtering – Presents a list of distinct values from the filtered field. The number to the right of the value tells you how many times this value appears in the dataset. You can specify which values you want to include in the filter by checking them. This creates an OR filter, such as Product is "AWC Logo Cap" or "Bike Wash – Dissolver". To exclude items, check "Select All" and then uncheck the values you don't need.

- Advanced filtering – Allows you to specify more advanced filtering conditions, such as "contains", "starts with", "is not". In addition, you can chain filters using AND and OR conditions.

- Top N filtering – Filters the top N or bottom N values of the field. You can also drag a data field to the "By value" area and specify an aggregation function. For example, you can drag SalesAmount and specify Top N 10 to return the top 10 products that sold the most.

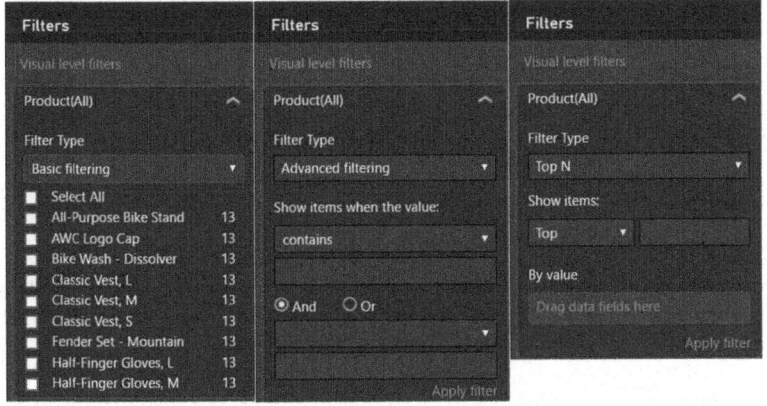

Figure 3.7 Power BI supports three filtering types: Basic, Advanced, and Top N.

Understanding the Fields pane

The Fields pane shows the tables in your dataset. When implementing the Retail Analysis Sample, the author implemented a self-service data model by importing several tables. By examining the Fields pane, you can see these tables and their fields (see **Figure 3.8**). For example, the Fields pane shows Sales, District, Item, and Store tables. The Store table is expanded, and you see some of its fields, such as Average Selling Area Size, Chain, City, and so on. If you have trouble finding a field in a busy Field pane, you can search for it by entering its name (or a part of it) in the Search box.

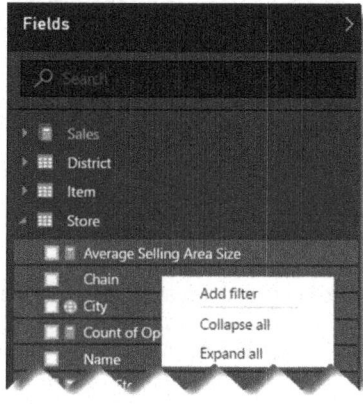

Figure 3.8 The Fields pane shows the dataset tables and fields, and allows you to search the model metadata.

Although you can't preview the data in the Fields pane, Power BI gives you clues about the field content. For example, if the field is prefixed with a calculator icon ▦, such as the "Average Selling Area Size" field, it's a calculated field that uses a formula. Fields prefixed with a globe icon ▦ are geography-related fields, such as City, that can be visualized on a map. If the field is checked, it's used in the selected visualization. If the name of the table has an orange color, one or more of its fields are used in the selected visualization. For example, the Sales and Store tables are orange because they each have at least one field used in the selected visualization.

Each field has an ellipsis menu to the right of the field that allows you to add the field as a filter. If you have selected a visualization, the field will be added as a visual-level filter. For example, if you select a chart on the report and add the City field as a filter, you can filter the chart data by city, such as to show data for Atlanta only. If no visualization is selected, the field will be added as a page-level filter. For example, if you add the City field as a filter but you haven't selected a specific visualization, it'll get added to the "Page level filters" area and you can filter all the visualizations on the page by this field. The "Collapse All" option collapses all the fields so you can see only the table names in the Fields list. And "Expand All" expands all tables so that you can see their fields.

Working with fields

Fields are the building blocks of reports because they define what data is shown. In the process of creating a report, you add fields from the Fields pane to the report. There are several ways to do this:

- Drag a field on the report – If you drag the field to an empty area on the report canvas, you'll create a new visualization that uses that field. If you drag it to an existing visualization, Power BI will add it to one of the areas of the Visualizations pane.

 NOTE Power BI always attempts to determine the right default. For example, if you drag the City field to an empty area, it'll create a map because City is a geospatial field. If you drag a field to an existing visualization, Power BI will attempt to guess how to use it best. For example, assuming you want to aggregate a numeric field, it'll add it to the Value area.

- Check the field's checkbox – It accomplishes the same result as dragging a field. If a visualization is selected on the report, Power BI decides which area on the Fields tab to add the field to.
- Drag a field to a visualization – Instead of relying on Power BI to infer what you want to do with the field, you can drag and drop a field into a specific area of the Fields tab in the Visualizations pane. For example, if you want a chart to create a data series using the "Sales per Sq Ft" field, you can drag this field to the Value area of the Fields tab in the Visualizations pane (see again **Figure 3.6**).

Similarly, to remove a field, you can uncheck its checkbox in the Fields pane. Or, you can drag the field away from the Visualizations pane to the Fields pane. If the field ends up in the wrong area of the Visualizations pane, you can drag it away from it and drop it in the correct area.

TIP   Besides dragging a field to an empty area, you can create a new visualization by just clicking the desired visualization type in the Visualizations pane. This adds an empty visualization to the report area. Then, you can drag and drop the required fields onto the visualization or to specific areas in the Fields tab to bind it to data.

3.1.3   Understanding Power BI Visualizations

You use visualizations to help you analyze your data in the most intuitive way. Power BI supports various common visualizations and their number is likely to grow in time. And because Power BI supports custom visuals, you'll be hard pressed not to find a suitable way to present your data. But let's start with the Power BI-provided visualizations.

 TIP   Need visualization best practices? I recommend the "Information Dashboard Design" book by the visualization expert Stephen Few, whose work inspired Power View and Power BI visualizations. To sum it up in one sentence: keep it simple!

Column and Bar charts
Power BI includes the most common charts, including Column Chart, Bar Chart, and other variants, such as Clustered Column Chart, Clustered Bar Chart, 100% Stacked Bar Chart, 100% Stacked Column Chart, and Ribbon charts. **Figure 3.9** shows the most common ones: column chart and bar chart. The difference between column and bar charts is that the Bar Chart displays a series as a set of horizontal bars. In fact, the Bar Chart is the only chart type that displays data horizontally by inverting the axes, so the x-axis shows the chart values and the y-axis shows the category values.

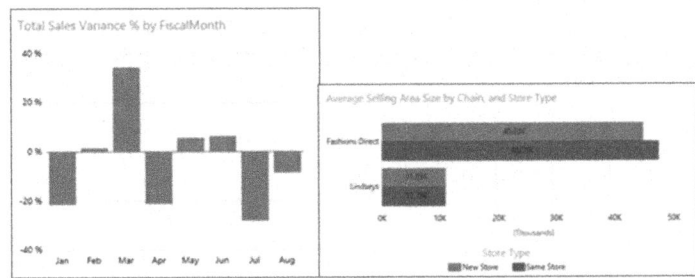

Figure 3.9   Column and bar charts display data points as bars.

Line charts
Line charts are best suited to display linear data. Power BI supports basic line charts and area charts, as shown in **Figure 3.10**. Like a Line Chart, an Area Chart displays a series as a set of points connected by a line with the exception that all of the area below the line is filled in. The Line Chart and Area Chart are commonly used to represent data that occurs over a continuous period. Currently, a single line chart is the only chart type that supports forecasting.

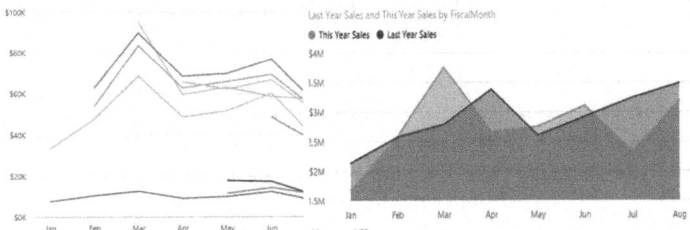

Figure 3.10   Power BI supports line charts and area charts.

Combination Chart

The Combination (combo) Chart combines a Column Chart and a Line Chart. This chart type is useful when you want to display measures on different axes, such as sales on the left Y-axis and order quantity on the right Y-axis. In such cases, displaying measures on the same axis would probably be meaningless if their units are different. Instead, you should use a Combination Chart and plot one of the measures as a Column Chart and the other as a Line Chart, as shown in **Figure 3.11**.

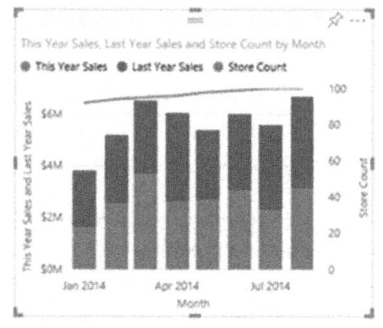

Figure 3.11 A Combo Chart allows you to plot measures on different axes. In this example, the This Year Sales and Last Year Sales measures are plotted on the left Y-axis while Store Count is plotted on the right Y-axis.

Scatter Chart

The Scatter Chart (**Figure 3.12**) is useful when you want to analyze correlation between two variables. Suppose that you want to find a correlation between units sold and revenue. You can use a scatter chart to show Units along the y-axis and Revenue along the x-axis. The resulting chart helps you understand if the two variables are related and, if so how. For example, you can determine if these two measures have a linear relationship; when units increase, revenue increases as well.

A unique feature of the scatter chart is that it can include a Play Axis. You can add any field to the Play Axis, you would typically add a date-related field, such as Month. When you "play" the chart, it animates and bubbles move!

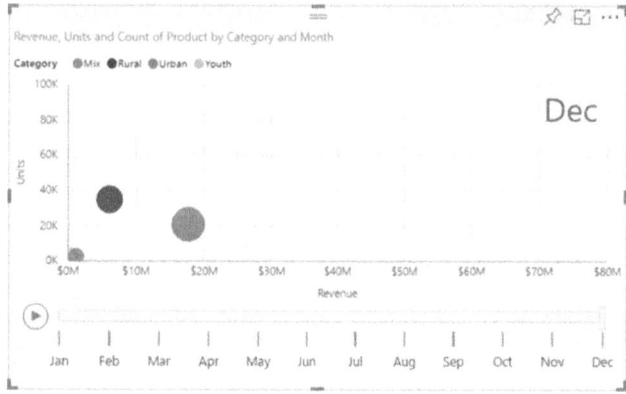

Figure 3.12 Use a Scatter Chart to analyze correlation between two variables.

Shape charts

Shape charts are commonly used to display values as percentages of a whole. Categories are represented by individual segments of the shape. The size of the segment is determined by its contribution. This makes a shape chart useful for proportional comparison between category values. Shape charts have no axes. Shape chart variations include Pie, Doughnut, and Funnel charts, as shown in **Figure 3.13**. All shape charts display each group as a slice on the chart. The Funnel Chart order categories from largest to smallest.

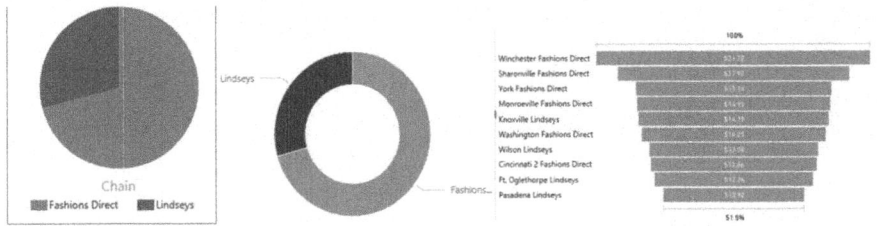

Figure 3.13 Pie, Doughnut, and Funnel charts can be used to display values as percentages of a whole.

Treemap and Waterfall charts

A treemap is a hierarchical view of data. It breaks an area into rectangles representing branches of a tree. Consider the Treemap Chart when you have to display large amounts of hierarchical data that doesn't fit in column or bar charts, such as the popularity of product features. Power BI allows you to specify custom colors for the minimum and maximum values. For example, the chart shown in **Figure 3.14** uses a red color for show stores with less sales and a green color to show stores with the most sales.

Consider a waterfall chart to show a running total as values are added or subtracted, such as to see how profit is impacted by positive and negative revenue reported over time.

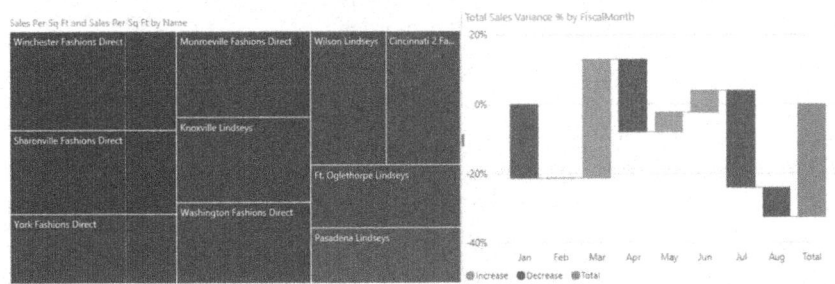

Figure 3.14 Consider Treemap to display large amounts of hierarchical data and Waterfall chart to show a running total as values are added or subtracted.

Table and Matrix visualizations

Use the Table and Matrix visualizations to display text data as tabular or crosstab reports. The Table visualization (left screenshot in **Figure 3.15**) displays text data in a tabular format, such as the store name and sales as separate columns.

Territory	This Year Sal...
DE	$123,446
GA	$332,246
KY	$298,656
MD	$869,726
OH	$2,616,326
Total	**$4,240,401**

Territory	Jan	Feb	Mar	Apr	Total
DE	$22,370	$26,705	$42,784	$31,587	$123,446
GA	$49,898	$82,267	$123,235	$76,846	$332,246
KY	$46,843	$76,086	$107,936	$67,792	$298,656
MD	$149,974	$201,722	$298,310	$219,721	$869,726
OH	$415,579	$622,028	$933,258	$645,461	$2,616,326
Total	**$684,663**	**$1,008,808**	**$1,505,523**	**$1,041,406**	**$4,240,401**

Figure 3.15 Use Table and Matrix visualizations for tabular and crosstab text reports.

The Matrix visualization (right screenshot in **Figure 3.15**) allows you to pivot data by one or more columns added to the Columns area of the Visualization pane, to create crosstab reports. Both visualizations support interactive sorting by clicking a column header, such as to sort stores in an ascending order by name. Matrix supports drilling down from one level to another.

Both visualizations support pre-defined quick styles that you can choose from in the Format tab of the Visualizations pane to beautify their appearance. For example, I chose the Alternating style to alternate the background color of the table rows. These visualizations also support conditional formatting as the Table visual demonstrates. You can access the conditional formatting settings by expanding the dropdown next to the measure in the Values area and clicking "Conditional formatting" and then selecting what will be formatted: background color, font color, or show values as data bars (see **Figure 3.19**).

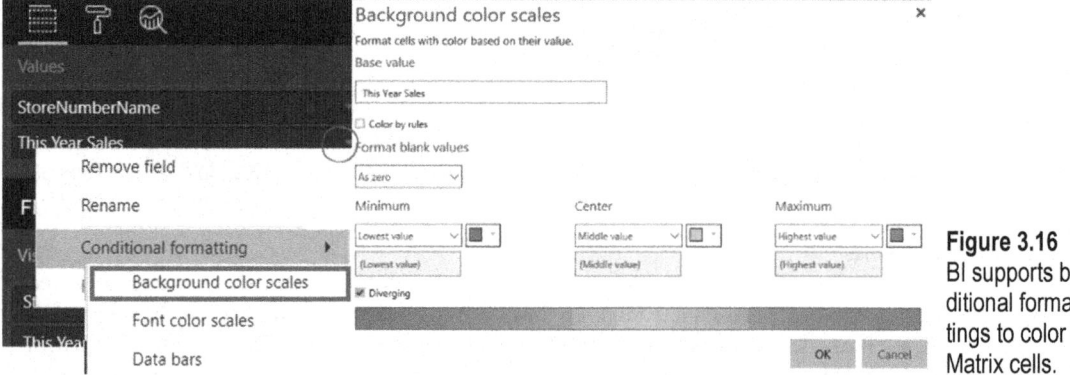

Figure 3.16 Power BI supports basic conditional formatting settings to color Table and Matrix cells.

Then you can let Power BI figure the lowest and highest value for the color range, or enter specific numbers. In **Figure 3.16**, I checked the Diverging setting to have a center zone and specified that cells with low values will be colored in Red and cells with higher values will be colored in Blue. You can also check "Color by rules" to specify more advanced rules and their precedence order.

Map visualizations

Use map visualizations to illustrate geospatial data. Power BI Service includes four map visualizations: Basic Map, Filled Map, ArcGIS, and ShapeMap (currently available as a Power BI Desktop preview feature). **Figure 3.17** shows Basic Map and Filled Map. All maps are license-free and use Microsoft Bing Maps, so you must have an Internet connection to see the maps.

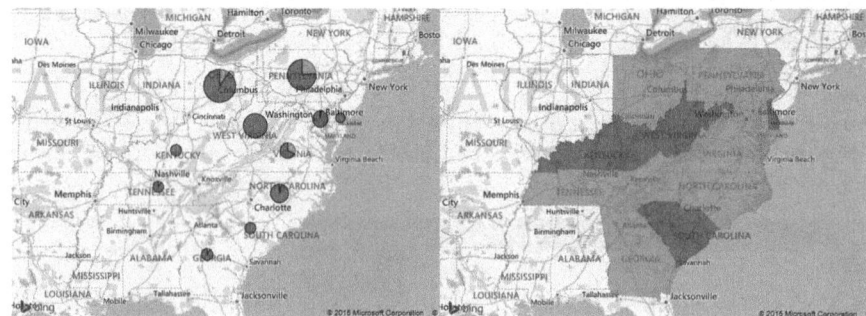

Figure 3.17 Examples of basic maps and filled maps.

You can use a Basic Map (left screenshot in **Figure 3.17**) to display categorical and quantitative information with spatial locations. Adding locations and fields places dots on the map. The larger the value, the bigger the dot. When you add a field to the Legend area of the Visualization pane, the Basic Map shows pie charts on the map, where the segments of the chart correspond to the field's values. For example, each Pie Chart in the Basic Map on the left of **Figure 3.17** breaks the sales by the store type.

As the name suggests, the Filled (choropleth) Map (right screenshot in **Figure 3.17**) fills geospatial areas, such as USA states. This visualization can use shading or patterns to display how a value differs in proportion across a geography or region. You can zoom in and out interactively, by pressing the Ctrl key and using the mouse wheel. Besides being able to plot precise locations (latitude and longitude), they can infer locations using a process called geo-coding, such as to plot addresses.

Like the Filled Map, the Shape Map fills geographic regions. The big difference is that the Shape Map allows you to plug in TopoJSON maps. TopoJSON is an extension of GeoJSON - an open standard format designed for representing simple geographical features based on JavaScript Object Notation (JSON).

The latest addition to the Power BI mapping arsenal is the ArcGIS map. This map type was contributed by Esri, a leader in the geographic information systems (GIS) mapping industry. Now not only can you plot data points from Power BI, but you can also add reference layers! These layers include demographic layers provided by Esri and public web maps, or those published into Esri's Living Atlas (http://doc.arcgis.com/en/Living-Atlas). For example, the map in **Figure 3.18** plots customers in Georgia as bubbles on top of a layer showing the 2016 USA Average Household Income (the darker the state color, the higher the income). For more information about ArcGIS maps, visit http://doc.arcgis.com/en/maps-for-powerbi. Esri also offers a subscription that offers more ArcGIS features, such as global demographics, sat-ellite imagery, and ready-to-use data. More details can be found at http://go.esri.com/plus-subscription.

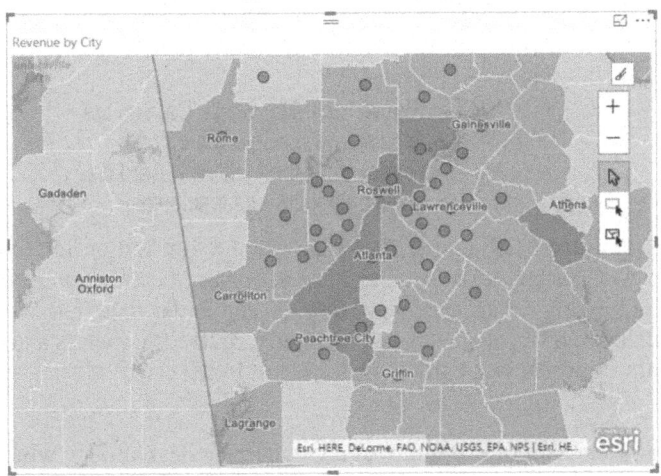

Figure 3.18 This ArcGIS map plots customers in Georgia on top of a layer showing the average household income.

Gauge visualizations

Gauges are typically used on dashboards to display key performance indicators (KPIs), such as to measure actual sales against budget sales. Power BI supports Gauge and KPI visuals for this purpose (**Figure 3.19**) but they work quite differently. To understand this, examine the data shown in the table below the visuals.

CalendarYear	SalesAmount	SalesAmountQuota
2005	$8,065,435	$9,513,000
2006	$24,144,430	$29,009,000
2007	$32,202,669	$38,782,000
2008	$16,038,063	$18,410,000
Total	**$80,450,597**	**$95,714,000**

Figure 3.19 The Gauge and KPI visuals display progress toward a goal.

The Gauge (the left radial gauge on the left) has a circular arc and displays a single value that measures progress toward a goal. The goal, or target value, is represented by the line (pointer). Progress toward that goal is represented by the shaded scale. And the value that represents that progress is shown in bold inside the arc. The Gauge aggregates the source data and shows the totals. It's not designed to visualize the trend of the historical values over time.

By contrast, the KPI visual can be configured to show a trend, such as how the indicator value changes over years. If you add a field to the Trend axis (CalendarYear in this example), it plots an area chart for the historical values. However, the indicator value always shows the last value (in this example, 16 million for year 2008). If you add a field to the "Target goals" area, it shows the indicator value in red if it's less than the target.

Because both visuals show a single scalar value, your users can subscribe for data alerts when these visuals are added to a dashboard. For example, assuming a dashboard tile shows a Gauge visual, Maya can go to the tile properties and create an alert to be notified when the sales exceed 80 million.

Card visualizations
Power BI supports Single Card and Multi Row card visualizations, as shown in **Figure 3.20**.

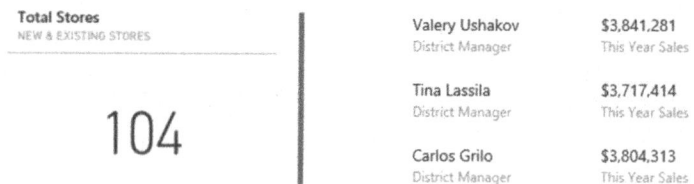

Figure 3.20 The Single Card on the left displays a single value (total stores) while the Multi Row Card displays managers and their sales.

The Single Card visualization (left screenshot in **Figure 3.20**) displays a single value to draw attention to the value. Like gauges, you can set up data alerts on single cards, such as to receive a notification when the number of stores exceed a given value. If you're looking for another way to visualize tabular data than plain tables, consider the Multi Row Card visualization (right screenshot in **Figure 3.20**). It converts a table to a series of cards that display the data from each row in a card format, like an index card.

Slicer
The Slicer visualization isn't really meant to visualize data but to filter data. Unlike page-level filters, which are found in the Filter pane when the report is displayed in Reading View, the Slicer visualization is added on the report so users can see what's filtered and interact with the slicer without expanding the Filter pane. Currently, the slicer filters only visualizations on the same page. Slicer is a versatile visual that supports different configurations depending on the data type of the field bound to the slicer. **Figure 3.21** shows three different slicer configurations.

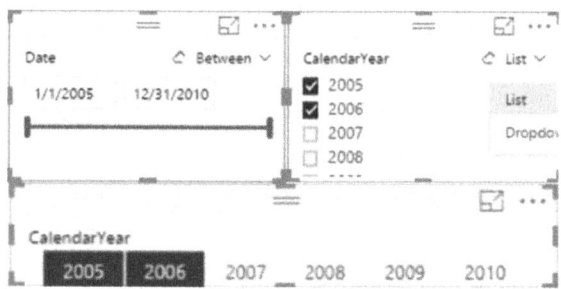

Figure 3.21 Use the Slicer visualization to create a filter that filters all visualizations on the report page.

When you bind the slicer to a field of a Date data type, it becomes a slider (the upper-left configuration). You can either use the sliders to set the dates or pick the date using a calendar. It also supports relative dates expressed as a specified number of last, this, or next periods of time. The configuration on the right shows the slicer in the default vertical configuration where you can check values from a list or pick a single value from a dropdown. By default, the slicer is configured for a single selection but it also supports multi-value selection by holding the Ctrl key and selecting items or by changing the Single Selection property to

Off in the Format tab of the Visualizations pane. You can also configure the slicer for a horizontal layout (the bottom slicer). Slicer supports a Search mode, such as to filter a long list of values as you type. To enable the Search mode, bind the slicer to a text field, expand the ellipsis (…) menu in the top-right corner, and then select Search.

3.1.4 Understanding Custom Visuals

No matter how much Microsoft improves the Power BI visualizations, it might never be enough. When it comes to data presentation, beauty is in the eye of the beholder. However, the Power BI presentation framework is open, and developers can donate custom visuals that you can use with your reports for free!

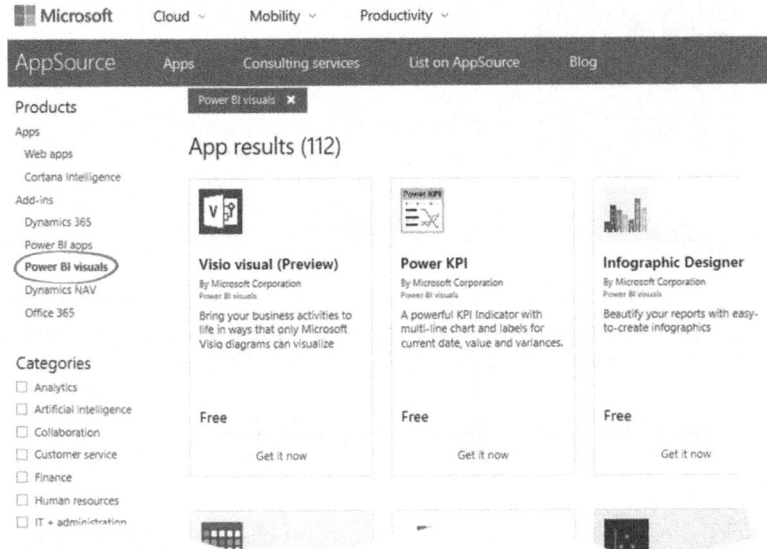

Figure 3.22 In AppSource you can find and download custom visuals contributed by Microsoft and the community.

Understanding AppSource

Custom visuals contributed by the community are available on the Microsoft AppSource site (https://appsource.microsoft.com), as shown in **Figure 3.22**. There you can search and view custom visuals. When you find an interesting visual, click it to see more information about the visual and its author. Custom visuals are contributed by Microsoft and the Power BI community. If you decide to use the visual, click "Get it now" to download the visual and then import it using the ellipsis menu (…) in the Visualizations pane. Visuals are distributed as files with the *.pbiviz extension.

Using custom visuals

Business users can use custom visuals in Power BI Service and data analysts can do the same in Power BI Desktop. To make it even easier for you to add a custom visual, AppSource is integrated with Power BI Service and Power BI Desktop. You can click the ellipsis menu (…) in the Visualizations pane and then click "Import from store" to browse AppSource (only Power BI visuals will show up) and import a visual. Once the visual is imported, it's included in the report and it can be used in that report only. If you decide that you don't need the visual, right-click the visual icon in the Visualizations pane and then click "Delete custom visual".

NOTE Custom visuals are written in JavaScript, which browsers run in a protected sandbox environment that restricts what the script can do. However, the script is executed on every user who renders a report with a custom visual. When it comes to security you should do your homework to verify the visual origin and safety. If you're unsure, consider involving IT to test the visual with anti-virus software and make sure that it doesn't pose any threats. For more information about how you or IT can test the visual, read the "Review custom visuals for security and privacy" document at https://powerbi.microsoft.com/documentation/powerbi-custom-visuals-review-for-security-and-privacy/.

Once you import the visual, you can use it on reports just like any other visual. **Figure 3.23** shows that I imported the Bullet Chart visual and its icon appears at the bottom of the Visualizations pane. Then I added the visual and configured it to show this year sales by store type.

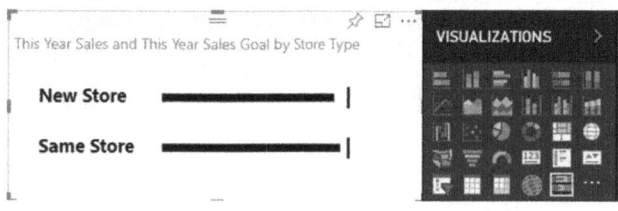

Figure 3.23 The Bullet Chart custom visual is added to the Visualizations pane and can be used on reports.

3.1.5 Understanding Subscriptions

Besides on-demand report delivery where you view a report interactively, Power BI can deliver the report to you once you set up a subscription. Subscriptions let you automate the process of generating and distributing reports. Subscribed report delivery is convenient because you don't have to go to Power BI Service to view the report online. Instead, Power BI sends the report to you. Subscription require a Power BI Pro license. Every Power BI Pro user can create individual subscriptions to report pages, if that the user has rights to view the report.

Creating subscriptions
Creating a subscription takes a few clicks. Open the report in Reading View and click the Subscribe menu. In the "Subscribe to emails" window, select which report page you want to subscribe to. **Figure 3.24** shows the available options for two reports that connect to different dataset types.

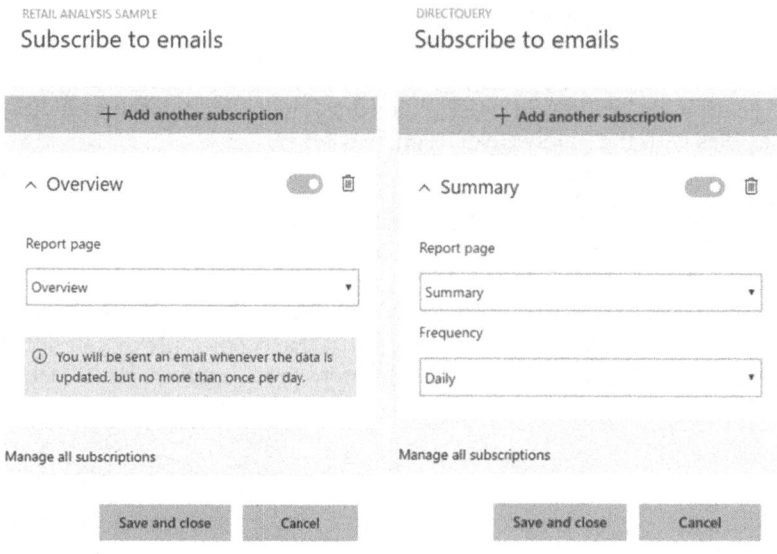

Figure 3.24 When setting up a subscription, specify which page you want to subscribe to and the subscription frequency for DirectQuery reports.

The Retail Analysis Sample report (the screenshot on the left) connects to a dataset with imported data. In this case, you can't specify the subscription frequency. Instead, you'll get an email when the dataset is refreshed, if you haven't gotten an email in the last 24 hours. In other words, the subscription schedule follows the dataset refresh schedule although you get an email at most once a day. The DirectQuery report (the screenshot on the right) connects directly to the data source. In this case, you can specify the mail frequency (Daily or Weekly).

As you know by now, a report can have multiple pages. When you create a subscription, you subscribe to a page in a report. For example, if Maya wants to subscribe to all four pages in the "Retail Analysis Sample" report, she'll have to create four subscriptions. She can do that by clicking "Add another subscription". If the report connects directly to the data source, each subscribed page can have its own frequency for sending mails.

Once you're done configuring your subscriptions, click "Save and close" to save your changes. You'll start receiving emails periodically with screenshots of each page you subscribe to. If you want to temporarily disable a subscription for a given page, turn the slider for that page off. To permanently delete a page subscription, click the trashcan icon next to the page.

Understanding subscription frequency
The subscription schedule (the frequency you receive emails) depends on how the report dataset connects to the source data. **Table 3.1** summarizes the schedule options.

Table 3.1   Schedule options for report subscriptions.

Dataset	Custom schedule interval	Can detect data changes?	Description
Imported data with scheduled refresh	None	No	Follows the dataset refresh schedule. You can't specify a different schedule. You will get an email every time the scheduled refresh happens, if you haven't gotten an email in the last 24 hours.
DirectQuery	Daily or Weekly	No	Power BI checks the data source every 15 minutes. You'll get an email as soon as the next check happens, if you haven't gotten an email in the last 24 hours (if Daily is selected), or in the last seven days (if Weekly is selected).
Live connection to Analysis Services (on premise/cloud)	None	Yes	Power BI checks the data source every 15 minutes and it's capable of detecting if the data has changed. You'll get an email only if the data has changed if you haven't gotten an email in the last 24 hours.
Connected Excel reports	None	Yes	Power BI checks the data source every hour. You'll get an email only if the data has changed if you haven't gotten an email in the last 24 hours.

Managing your subscriptions
As the number of your subscriptions grows, you might find it difficult to keep track of which reports you've subscribed to. Luckily, Power BI lets you view your subscriptions in one place - the Subscriptions tab in the Power BI Settings page (**Figure 3.25**). To get there, click the "Manage all subscriptions" link in the "Subscribe to emails" window.

Alternatively, click the Power BI Settings (cog) menu in the upper-right corner of the Power BI portal and then click Settings. You can see the number of pages you subscribed to for each report. Click the Actions icon if you want to make changes to a given report subscription. This brings you to the "Subscribe to emails" window.

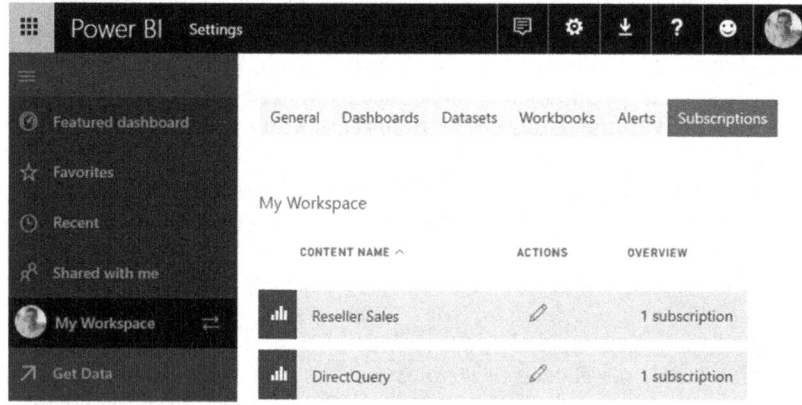

Figure 3.25 Use the Subscriptions tab in the Settings page to view and manage your subscriptions.

Understanding subscription limitations

As of time of writing, Power BI subscriptions have these limitations:

- The only export option is screenshot. You can't receive the page exported to PowerPoint, for example.

- You can create individual subscriptions only. You can't subscribe other users as you can do with Reporting Services data-driven subscriptions.

- You can specify subscription frequency for reports that connect directly to the data source (DirectQuery connections). For other datasets, subscriptions either follow the dataset refresh schedule (for imported datasets), or Power BI determines when to send emails (for datasets connected to Analysis Services or Excel).

- The Power BI admin can't see or manage subscriptions across the tenant.

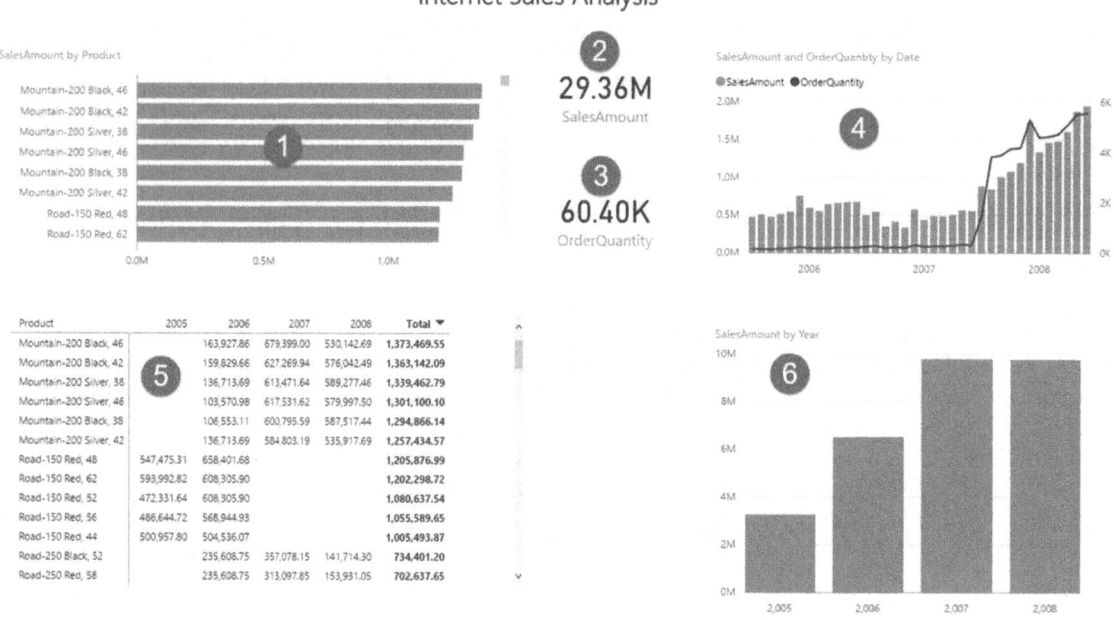

Figure 3.26 The Summary page of the Internet Sales Analysis report includes six visualizations.

3.2　Working with Power BI Reports

Now that you know about visualizations, let's use them on reports. In the first exercise that follows, you'll create a report from scratch. The report will source data from the Internet Sales dataset that you created in Chapter 2. In the second exercise, you'll modify an existing report. You'll also practice working with Excel and Reporting Services reports.

3.2.1　Creating Your First Report

In Chapter 2, you imported the Internet Sales Excel file in Power BI. As a result, Power BI created a dataset with the same name. Let's analyze the sales data by creating the report shown in **Figure 3.26**. This report consists of two pages. The Summary page has six visualizations and the Treemap page (not shown in **Figure 3.26**) uses a Treemap visualization to help you analyze sales by product at a glance. (For an example of a Treemap visualization skip ahead to **Figure 3.28**.)

Getting started with report authoring
One way to create a new report in Power BI is to explore a dataset.

1. In the Power BI portal, expand My Workspace in the navigation pane and then click the Internet Sales dataset. Alternatively, in the navigation pane click My Workspace. In the workspace content page, select the Datasets tab. Click the Create Report icon (⬛) next to the Internet Sales dataset to create a new report that is connected to this dataset.

2. Power BI opens a blank report in Editing View. Expand the View menu and turn on Snap to Grid so that you align easier elements on the report canvas.

3. Click the Text Box menu to create a text box for the report title. Type *"Internet Sales Analysis"* and format as needed. Position the text box on top of the report.

4. Note the Fields pane shows only the table "Internet Sales" because the Internet Sales dataset, which you imported from an Excel file, has only one table.

5. Click the Save menu and save the report as *Internet Sales Analysis*. Remind yourself to save the report (you can press Ctrl-S) every now and then so that you don't lose changes.

 NOTE　Power BI times out your session after a certain period of inactivity to conserve resources in a shared environment. When this happens, and you return to the browser, it'll ask you to refresh the page. If you have unsaved changes, you might lose them when you refresh the page so get in the habit to press Ctrl-S often.

Creating a Bar Chart
Follow these steps to create a bar chart that shows the top selling products.

1. In the Fields pane, check the SalesAmount field. Power BI defaults to a Column Chart visualization that displays the grand total of the SalesAmount field.

2. In the Fields pane, check the Product field. Power BI adds it to the Axis area of the chart.

3. In the Visualizations pane, click the Bar Chart icon to flip the Column Chart to a Bar Chart. Power BI sorts the bar chart by the product name in an ascending order.

4. Point your mouse cursor to the top-right corner of the chart. Click the ellipsis "..." menu and check that the data is sorted by SalesAmount in a descending order. Compare your results with the "SalesAmount by Product" visualization in the upper left of **Figure 3.26**.

5. (Optional) With bar chart selected, select the Format tab in the Visualizations pane. Switch "Data labels" to On to show data labels on the chart.

Adding Card visualizations

Let's show the total sales amount and order quantity as separate card visualizations (items 2 and 3 in **Figure 3.26**) to draw attention to them:

1. Click an empty space on the report canvas outside the Bar Chart to deactivate it.

💡 **TIP** As I explained, another way to create a new visualization is to drag a field to an empty space on the canvas. If the field is numeric, Power BI will create a Column Chart. For text fields, it'll default to a Table. And for geo fields, such as Country, it will default to a Map.

2. In the Field list, check the SalesAmount field. Change the visualization to Card. Position it as needed.

3. Repeat the last two steps to create a new card visualization using the OrderQuantity field.

4. (Optional) Experiment with the card format settings. For example, suppose you want a more descriptive title. In the Format tab of the Visualization pane, switch "Category label" to Off. Switch Title to On. Type in a descriptive title and change its font and alignment settings.

Creating a Combo Chart visualization

The fourth chart in **Figure 3.26** shows how the sales amount and order quantity change over time:

1. Drag the SalesAmount field and drop it onto an empty area next to the card visualizations to create a Column Chart.

2. Drag the Date field and drop it onto the new chart.

3. Switch the visualization to "Line and Stacked Column Chart". This adds a new Line Values area to the Visualizations pane.

4. Drag the OrderQuantity field and drop it on the Line Values area. Power BI adds a line chart to the visualization and plots its values to a secondary Y-axis. Compare your results with the "SalesAmount and Order-Quantity by Date" visualization (item 4 in **Figure 3.26**).

5. To avoid the sharp dip in the last bar of the chart caused by incomplete sales, apply a visual-level filter to exclude the last date. To do so, with the combo chart selected, expand the Date field in the "Visual level filters" area, check "Select All", then scroll all the way down the list, and then uncheck '7/1/2008'.

Creating a Matrix visualization

The fifth visualization (from **Figure 3.26**) represents a crosstab report showing sales by product on rows, and years on columns. Let's build this with the Matrix visualization:

1. Drag the SalesAmount field and drop it onto an empty space on the report canvas to create a new visualization. Change the visualization to Matrix.

2. Check the Product field to add it to the visualization on rows.

3. Drag the Year field and drop it on the Columns zone to see data grouped by years on columns.

4. Resize the visualization as needed. Click any of the column headers to sort the visualization interactively in an ascending or descending order.

5. (Optional) In the Format tab of the Visualizations pane, change the matrix style to Minimal. Change the "Horiz grid" to Off.

6. (Optional) In the Fields tab of the Visualizations pane, expand the drop-down button next to the SalesAmount field in the Values area. Notice that the SalesAmount is aggregated using the Sum aggrega-

tion function but you can choose another aggregation function. In the same drop-down menu, click "Conditional formatting" and experiment with different conditional format settings, such as to color cells with lower values in Red.

 TIP Want to see "Sales Amount" instead of SalesAmount in the Matrix? You can rename column captions to show fields with different names on reports. To do so, just double-click the field name in the Fields tab of the Visualizations pane. Or, right-click the field name in the Fields tab and then click Rename.

Creating a Column Chart visualization

The sixth visualization listed shows sales by year:

1. Create a new visualization that uses the SalesAmount field. Power BI should default to Column Chart.
2. In the Fields pane, check the Year field to place it in the Axis area of the Column Chart.
3. Hover on one of the chart columns. Notice that a tooltip pops up to show Year and SalesAmount. Assuming you want to see the order quantity as well, drag OrderQuantity from the Fields pane and drop it to the Tooltips area of the Fields tab in the Visualizations pane.
4. (Optional) Suppose you want to change the color of the column showing the 2008 data. Switch to the Format tab in the Visualizations pane. Expand Data Colors and turn "Show all" to On. Change the color of the 2008 item.
5. (Optional) Suppose you need a trend line on the chart. Switch to the Analytics tab in the Visualizations pane. Expand the Trend Line section and then click Add. Change the format settings of the trend line as needed.
6. (Optional) Change the chart type to Line Chart. Notice that the Analytics tab adds a Forecast section. Add a forecast line to predict sales for future periods.

Filtering the report

Next, you'll implement page-level and visual-level filters. Let's start by creating a page-level Date filter that will allow you to filter all visualizations on the page by date.

1. Click an empty area on the report canvas to make sure that no visualization is activated.
2. Drag the Date field onto the Page Level Filters area. This creates a page-level filter that filters all visualizations on the activated page.

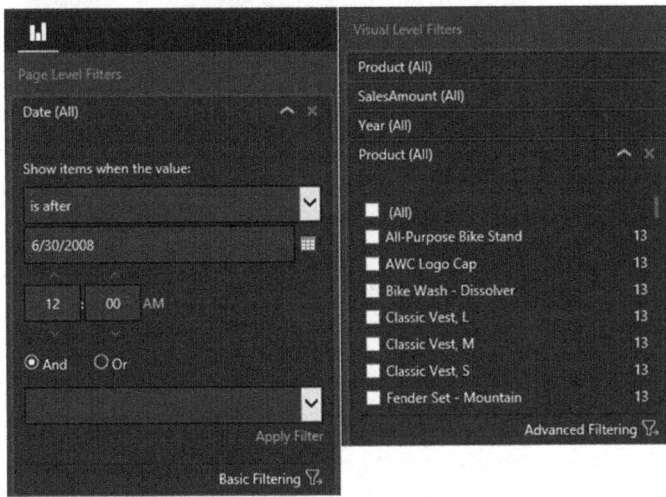

Figure 3.27 The Advanced Filter mode (left screenshot) allows you to specify more complex criteria and multiple conditions for filtering, such as filter dates where the Date field is after June 30th, 2008. The Visual Level Filters area (right screenshot) includes by default all the fields that are used in the visualization.

3. Practice different ways to filter. For example, switch to Advanced Filtering mode and filter out dates after June 30th, 2008, as shown on the left screenshot in **Figure 3.27**.

4. To work with visual-level filters, click the fifth (Matrix) visualization. To practice another way to create a filter besides drag and drop, hover on the Product field in the Fields pane. Then expand the ellipsis menu and click Add Filter.

Because there's an activated visualization, this action configures a visual-level filter. Notice that the Visual Level Filters (see the right screenshot in **Figure 3.27**) already includes the three fields used in the visualization so that you can filter on these fields without explicitly adding them as filters.

Creating a Treemap
Let's add a second page to the report that will help you analyze product sales using a Treemap visualization (see **Figure 3.28**).

1. At the bottom of the report, click the plus sign to add a new page. Rename the page in place to *Treemap*.

2. In the Fields list, check the SalesAmount and Product fields.

3. Change the visualization type to Treemap.

4. By default, Power BI uses arbitrary colors for the tree map tiles. Assuming you want to color the bestselling products in green and worst-selling products in red, drag the SalesAmount field to the Color Saturation area of the Visualizations pane.

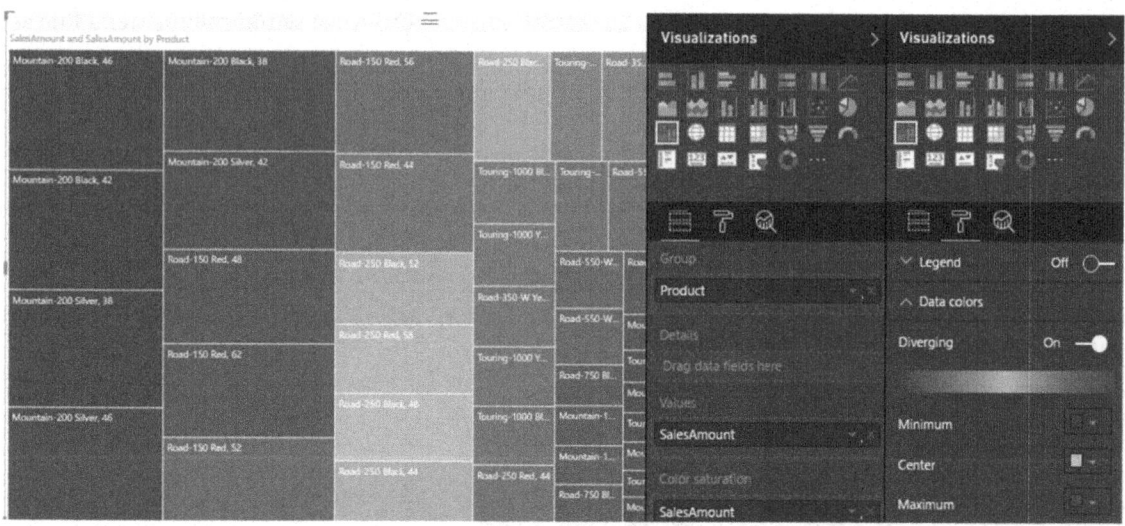

Figure 3.28 The Treemap visualization helps you analyze product sales.

5. In the Format tab of the Visualizations pane, change the Data Colors settings, as shown in **Figure 3.28**. Turning off the Diverging option allows you to specify a color for the values that fall in the middle. You can use the Minimum, Center, and Maximum fields to fine tune the ranges.

6. Save your report.

3.2.2 Getting Quick Insights

Let's face it, slicing and dicing data to perform root cause analysis (RCA) could be time consuming and tedious. For example, a report might show you that sales are increasing or decreasing, but it won't tell you why. Retrospectively, such tasks required you to produce more detailed reports, to explain sudden data fluctuations. And this gets even more difficult if you're analyzing a model created by someone else because you don't know which fields to use and how to use them to get answers. Enter Quick Insights!

Understanding Quick Insights

Power BI Quick Insights gives you new ways to find insights hidden in your data. With a click of button, Quick Insights run various sophisticated algorithms on your data to search for interesting fluctuations. Originating from Microsoft Research, these algorithms can discover correlations, outliers, trends, seasonality changes, and change points in trends, automatically and within seconds. **Table 3.2** lists some of the insights that these algorithms can uncover.

Table 3.2 **This table summarizes the available insights.**

Insight	Explanation
Major factors(s)	Finds cases where a majority of a total value can be attributed to a single factor when broken down by another dimension.
Category outliers (top/bottom)	Highlights cases where, for a measure in the model, one or two members of a dimension have much larger values than other members of the dimension.
Time series outliers	For data across a time series, detects when there are specific dates or times with values significantly different than the other date/time values.
Overall trends in time series	Detects upward or downward trends in time series data.
Seasonality in time series	Finds periodic patterns in time series data, such as weekly, monthly, or yearly seasonality.
Steady Share	Highlights cases where there is a parent-child correlation between the share of a child value in relation to the overall value of the parent across a continuous variable.
Correlation	Detects cases where multiple measures show a correlation between each other when plotted against a dimension in the dataset

By default, Quick Insights queries as much of the dataset as possible in a fixed time window (about 20 seconds). Quick Insights requires data to be imported in Power BI. Quick Insights isn't available for datasets that connect directly to data.

Working with Quick Insights

Let's find what insights we can uncover by applying Quick Insights to the Retail Analysis Sample dataset:

1. In Power BI, expand My Workspace. In the Datasets section, right-click the "Retail Analysis Sample" dataset and click Quick Insights. Alternatively, click My Workspace in the navigation pane. In the workspace content page, select the Datasets tab. Click the ellipsis (…) button to the right of the "Retail Analysis Sample" dataset, and the click "Get quick insights". Or, you can select the Reports tab and click the bulb icon to the right of the "Retail Analysis Sample" report to start Quick Insights.

2. While Power BI runs the algorithms, it displays a "Searching for insights" message. Once it's done, it shows "Insights are ready" message.

3. Click the ellipsis next to the "Retail Analysis Sample" dataset again. Note that the Quick Insights link is renamed to View Insights. Click View Insights.

Power BI opens a "Quick Insights for Retail Analysis Sample" page that shows four auto-generated insights. **Figure 3.29** shows the first report. The "Gross Margin This Year" report has found a correlation between the "Gross Margin This Year" and "Gross Margin Last Year" measures. This is an example of a Correlation insight. As you can see, Quick Insights can really help understand data changes. The refresh button (next to the page title) allows you to rerun the Quick Insight algorithms. Currently, Power BI deactivates them when you close your browser. However, if you find an insight useful, you can click the pin button in the top-right corner to pin to a dashboard. (I discuss creating dashboards in more detail in the next chapter.

Quick Insights for **Retail Analysis Sample** ↻

A subset of your data was analyzed and the following insights were found. **Learn more**

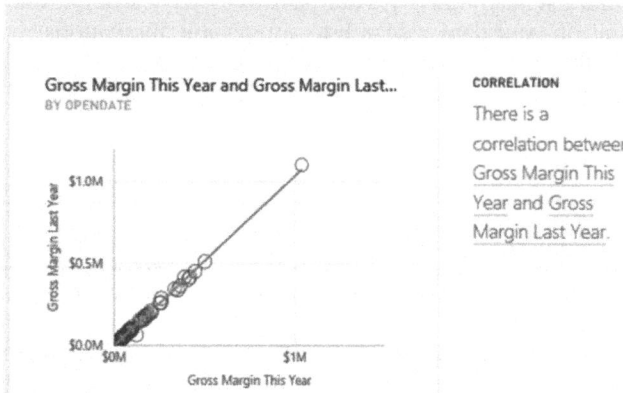

Gross Margin This Year and Gross Margin Last...
BY OPENDATE

CORRELATION

There is a correlation between Gross Margin This Year and Gross Margin Last Year.

Figure 3.29 The first Quick Insight report shows a correlation between two measures.

3.2.3 Subscribing to Reports

In the previous chapter, I walked you through the steps to create the Adventure Works report from an Analysis Services model. Suppose that Maya would like to subscribe to a report so that she receives the report by email when the underlying data has changed.

NOTE You might wonder why not use the Internet Sales report that you just created. Recall that this report imports data from an Excel file and you created it directly in Power BI Service (without using Power BI Desktop). As I explained in section 2.3.1, Power BI can't refresh these type of reports or the included sample reports, such as Retail Analysis Sample. Although you can subscribe to such reports, you won't get an email because there will be nothing to trigger the subscription. If you haven't created the Adventure Works report, fast forward and follow the instructions in section 11.2.3 to deploy the Adventure Works Power BI Desktop model and schedule it for refresh. Then, create and test a subscription to the Adventure Works report.

Creating a subscription
Follow these steps to create a subscription to an existing report.

1. In Power BI Service, expand My Workspace and click the Adventure Works report in the Reports section.
2. Click the Adventure Works report to open it in Reading View. Click the Subscribe menu.
3. In the "Subscribe to emails" window, leave the default settings to subscribe to the first page of the report. Or, if the report has multiple pages and you want to subscribe to them, click the "Add another subscription" button to create more subscriptions, one page at the time.
4. Click "Save and close" to create the subscription.

Receiving reports
When the Analysis Services model is refreshed, you'll get an email with screenshots of all report pages that you subscribed to. Power BI will determine the exact time when this will happen.

TIP If you've subscribed to a report connected to a dataset with imported data and you've scheduled the dataset for refresh, you can manually refresh the dataset to get the email faster. To do so, go to the workspace content page, click the Datasets tab, and then click the "Refresh Now" icon next to the dataset name.

1. Check your mail inbox for an email from no-reply@email.powerbi.com. **Figure 3.30** shows the content of a sample email. The email includes screenshots of all subscribed pages. In this case, I've subscribed to only one page so I get only one screenshot.
2. Suppose you want to open the report and interact with it. Click the "Go to Report" button and Power BI navigates you to the report.
3. Back to the email, click the "Manage subscription" link. This navigates you to the report and opens the "Subscribe to emails" window so that you can review and make changes to your report subscription.
4. In the "Subscribe to emails" window, click the "Manage all subscriptions" link. This navigates you to the Settings page that shows all your subscriptions that exist in the current workspace.

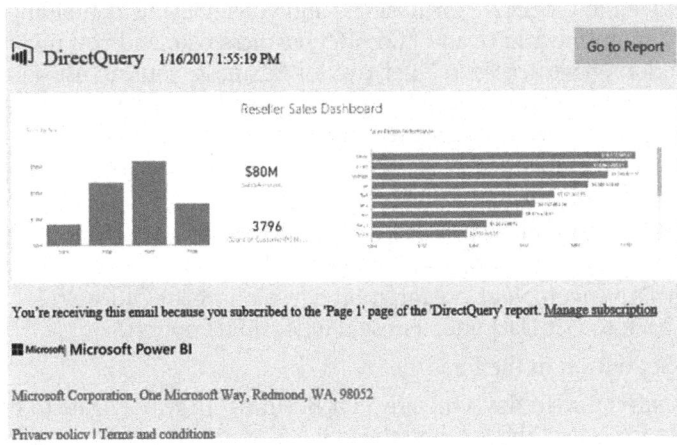

Figure 3.30 The subscription email includes page screenshots, a link to the report, and a link to change the subscription settings.

3.3 Working with Excel Reports

Ask a business user what tools they currently use for analytics and Excel comes on top. Thanks to its integration with SharePoint Online, Power BI can connect to existing Excel table or pivot reports and render them online (without importing the Excel file). In addition, business users can connect Excel desktop to Power BI datasets and create Excel pivot reports, just like they can connect Excel to Analysis Services models. Let's take a more detailed look at these two integration options with Excel.

3.3.1 Connecting to Excel Reports

Before you connect to your Excel reports, you need to pay attention to where the Excel file is stored:

- Excel files stored locally – If the Excel file is stored on your computer, Power BI needs to upload the file before Excel Online can connect to it. Because Excel Online can't synchronize the uploaded version with the local file (even if you set up a gateway), you have to re-upload the file after you make changes if you want the connected reports to show the latest.
- Excel files stored in the cloud – If your Excel file is saved to OneDrive for Business or SharePoint Online, Power BI doesn't have to upload the file because it can connect directly to it. As long as you save changes to the same location in the cloud, Power BI will always show the latest.

OneDrive for Business is a place where business users can store, sync, and share work files. While the personal edition of OneDrive is free, OneDrive for Business requires an Office 365 plan. For example, Maya might maintain an Excel file with some calculations. Or, Martin might give her an Excel file with Power Pivot model and pivot reports. Maya can upload these files to her OneDrive for Business and then add these reports to Power BI, and even pin them to a dashboard!

 NOTE Online Excel reports have limitations which are detailed in the "Bring Excel files in Power BI" article by Microsoft at https://powerbi.microsoft.com/en-us/documentation/powerbi-service-excel-workbook-files. One popular and frequently requested scenario that Power BI still doesn't support is Excel reports connected to Analysis Services although reports connected to Power Pivot data models work just fine. That's because currently SharePoint Online doesn't support external connections, even if you have a gateway set up. This might be a serious issue if you plan to migrate your BI reports from on-premises SharePoint Server to Power BI.

Connecting to Excel

In this exercise, you'll connect an Excel file saved to OneDrive for Business and you'll view its containing reports online. As a prerequisite, your organization must have an Office 365 business plan and you must have access to OneDrive for Business. If you don't have access to OneDrive for Business, you can use a local Excel file. The Reseller Sales.xlsx file in the \Source\ch03 folder includes a Power Pivot data model with several tables. The first two sheets have Excel pivot tables and chart reports, while the third sheet has a Power View report. While all reports connect to an embedded Power Pivot data model, they don't have to. For example, your pivot reports can connect to Excel tables.

1. Copy and save the Reseller Sales.xlsx to your OneDrive for Business. To open OneDrive, click the Office 365 Application Launcher button (the yellow button in the upper-left corner in the Power BI portal) and then click OneDrive. If you don't see the OneDrive icon, your organization doesn't have an Office 365 business plan (to complete this exercise, go back to Get Data and choose the Local File option).

2. In Power BI, click Get Data. Then click the Get button in the Files tile.

3. In the next page, click the "One Drive – Business" tile. In the "OneDrive for Business" page, navigate to the folder where you saved the Reseller Sales.xlsx file, select the file, and then click Connect.

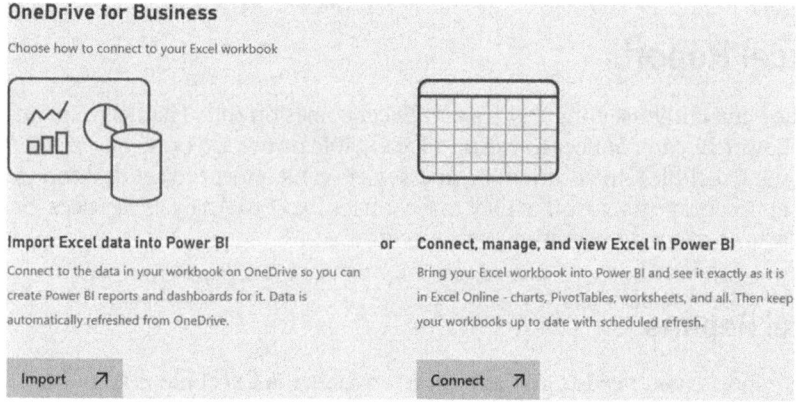

Figure 3.31 When you connect to an Excel file stored on OneDrive for Business, Power BI asks you how you want to work with the file.

Power BI prompts you how to work with the file (see **Figure 3.31**). You practiced importing from Excel in Chapter 2. If you take this path, Power BI will import only the data from the Excel file. If there are any pivot reports in the Excel workbook, they won't be added to Power BI.

 NOTE If you've selected the Local File option in Get Data, the button caption will read "Upload" instead of "Connect". This is to emphasize the fact that Power BI will upload the file to its cloud storage before it connects to it.

4. Click the Connect button to connect directly to the Excel file. Power BI processes the Excel file and notifies you that it's added to your list of workbooks.

Interacting with Excel reports

Excel Online (a component of SharePoint Online) renders the Excel reports in HTML so you don't need Excel on the desktop to view the Excel reports added to Power BI. And not only can you view the Excel reports but you can also interact with them, just as you can do so in Excel Desktop.

1. In the Power BI portal, expand My Workspace. You should see Reseller Sales listed in the Workbooks section. Alternatively, in the navigation pane click My Workspace. In the workspace content page, click the Workbooks tab. You should see Reseller Sales listed. This represents the Excel file that is now available to Power BI.

2. Click the Reseller Sales workbook. Power BI renders the pivot reports and the Power View report online via Excel Online (see **Figure 3.32**).

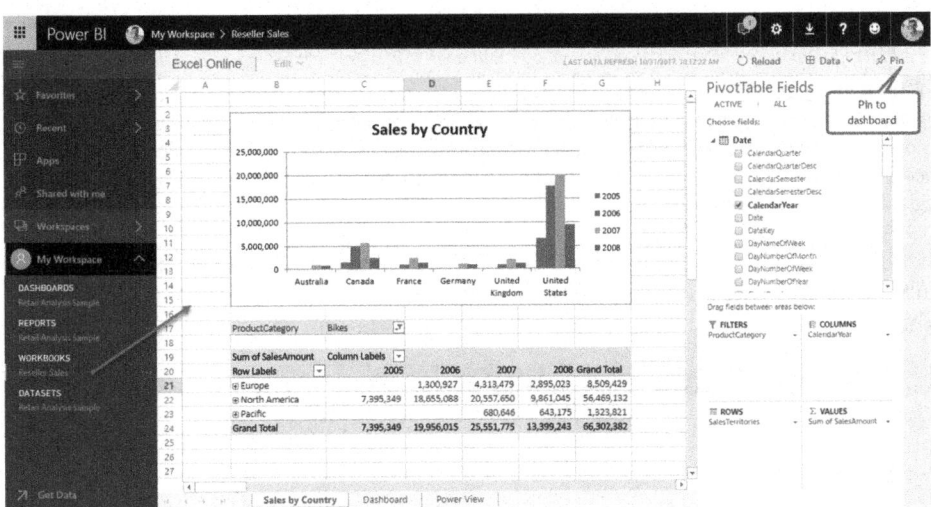

Figure 3.32
Power BI supports rendering Excel reports online if the Excel file is stored in OneDrive for Business.

3. (Optional) Try some interactive features, such as changing the report filters and slicers, and notice that they work the same as they work in SharePoint Server or SharePoint Online. For example, you can change report filters and slicers, and you can add or remove fields.

TIP You can pin a range from an Excel report as a static image to a Power BI dashboard. To do so, select the range on the report and then click the Pin button in the upper-right corner of the report (see again **Figure 3.32**). The Pin to Dashboard window allows you to preview the selected section and prompts you if you want to pin it to a new or an existing dashboard. For more information about this feature, read the "Pin a range from Excel to your dashboard!" blog at https://powerbi.microsoft.com/en-us/blog/pin-a-range-from-excel-to-your-dashboard. Q&A is not available for Excel tiles.

3.3.2 Analyzing Data in Excel

Besides consuming existing Excel reports, business users can create their own Excel pivot reports connected to Power BI datasets. This feature, called Analyze in Excel, brings you another option to explore Power BI datasets (besides creating Power BI reports). For example, Maya knows Excel pivot reports and she wants to create a pivot report that's connected to the Retailer Analysis Sample dataset. She can use the Analyze in Excel feature to connect to her data in Power BI, just like she can do so by connecting Excel to a multidimensional cube. She can then use the Power BI Publisher for Excel add-in to pin her report as an image to a dashboard. Analyze in Excel is a Power BI Pro feature.

Creating Excel reports

Follow these steps to create an Excel report connected to the Retailer Analysis Sample dataset:

1. In Power BI portal, expand My Workspace in the navigation pane. Under the Datasets section, click the ellipsis menu (…) next to the Retail Analysis Sample dataset and then click Analyze in Excel. Alternatively, in the navigation pane click My Workspace. In the workspace content page, click the Datasets tab. Expand the ellipsis (…) menu next to the Retailer Analysis Sample dataset and click Analyze in Excel.

2. You'll be asked to install some updates to enable this feature. Accept to install these updates. They will install a newer version of the MSOLAP OLEDB provider that Excel needs to connect to Power BI. Then your web browser downloads a Retailer Analysis Sample.odc file which includes the connection details to connect Excel to the Power BI dataset.

3. Click the download file. Excel opens and prompts you to enable the connection. Once you confirm the prompt, Excel adds an empty pivot table report connected to the Power BI dataset.

 NOTE As far as Excel is concerned, Analyze in Excel connects to Power BI using the same mechanism as it uses to connect to cubes. Excel parses the dataset metadata and it looks for measures and dimensions. Therefore, if you want to aggregate data you must define explicit measures in the datasets. In other words, the dataset must be created in Power BI Desktop and it must have explicit DAX measures. In fact, Analyze in Excel won't work if you have created the dataset directly in Power BI Service (as you did with the Internet Sales file).

Besides creating ad-hoc Excel pivot reports, another practical benefit of using Analyze in Excel is that it doesn't limit the number of rows when drilling through data (just double-click an aggregated cell in the pivot report to drill through).

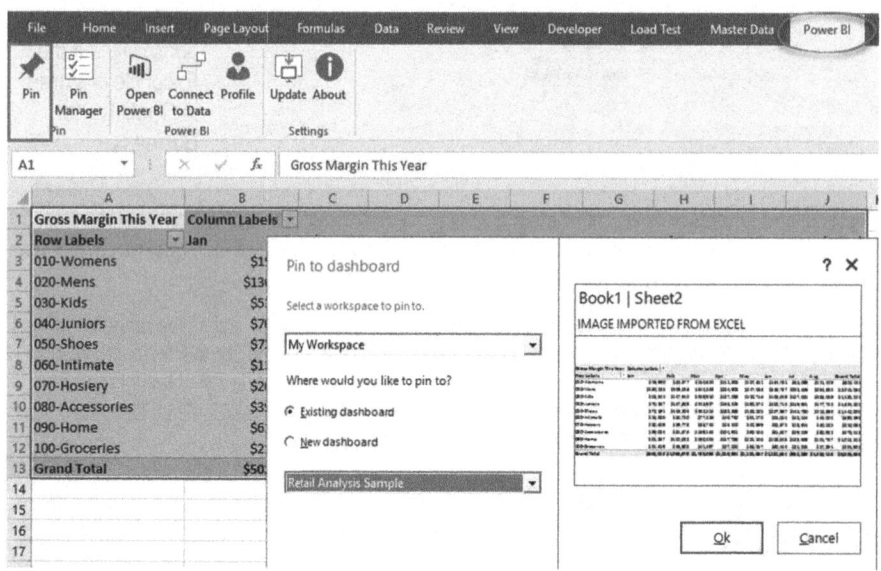

Figure 3.33 Power BI publisher for Excel lets you pin reports to dashboards.

Using Power BI publisher for Excel

If you like Analyze in Excel, consider installing the "Power BI publisher for Excel" add-in. The tool adds the ability to connect to Power BI datasets directly from Excel (without downloading the *.odc file from Power BI portal) and to pin Excel ranges as static images to Power BI dashboards.

1. In Power BI portal, expand the Downloads menu and then click "Power BI publisher for Excel". Run the setup to install the tool.

2. Open Excel. Notice that the add-in adds a Power BI menu to the Excel ribbon (see **Figure 3.33**).

3. Click the "Connect to Data" button. Log in to Power BI and connect to the Retailer Analysis Sample datasets in My Workspace. The publisher will create an empty PivotTable report connected to the dataset.

4. Drag some fields on the report, such as the "Gross Margin This Year" measure (Sales Table) in the Values area, Category (Item table) in the Rows area, and Fiscal Year (Time table) in the Columns area.

5. Let's pin this report to a dashboard. Select the entire report and then click Pin. In the "Pin to dashboard" window, select My Workspace and then select the "Retail Analysis Sample" dashboard.

6. In Power BI Service, open the "Retail Analysis Sample" dashboard and notice that it includes an image of the Excel pivot report. Unlike connecting to an Excel file, you can't open the report online and interact with it. That's because the report was produced on the desktop.

For more information about the Power BI publisher for Excel, read the "Power BI publisher for Excel" article at https://powerbi.microsoft.com/documentation/powerbi-publisher-for-excel.

NOTE To have an interactive report, you might decide to try uploading the Excel workbook to OneDrive or SharePoint Online and using Get Data to connect to the Excel file. However, you'll find that although you'll be able to render the report in Excel Online, you won't be able to interact with it. That's because the report has an external connection to the Power BI dataset. This is the same limitation as with Excel reports connected to Analysis Services.

3.3.3 Comparing Excel Reporting Options

At this point, you might be confused about which option to use when working with Excel files. **Table 3.3** should help you make the right choice. To recap, Power BI offers three Excel integration options.

Table 3.3   This table compares the Power BI options to work with Excel.

Criteria	Import Excel files	Connect to Excel files	Analyze in Excel
Data acquisition	Power BI parses the Excel file, imports data, and creates a dataset.	Power BI doesn't parse and import the data. Instead, Power BI connects to the Excel file hosted on OneDrive or SharePoint Online.	Connects to existing dataset in Power BI
Data model (Power Pivot)	Power BI imports the model and creates a dataset.	Power BI doesn't import the data model.	N/A
Pivot reports	Power BI doesn't import pivot reports.	Power BI renders pivot reports via Excel Online.	Create your pivot reports
Power View reports	Power BI imports Power View reports and adds them to Reports section in the left navigation bar.	Power BI renders Power View reports via Excel Online (requires Silverlight).	N/A
Change reports	You can change the imported Power View reports but the original reports in the Excel file remain intact.	You can't change reports. You must open the file in Excel, make report changes, and upload the file to OneDrive.	You can change reports saved in the Excel file.
Publish reports	Import or create new Power BI reports	Reports are available in the Workbooks tab; you can pin Excel ranges as static images to Power BI dashboards.	Pin Excel ranges as static images to Power BI dashboards
Data refresh	Scheduled dataset refresh (automatic refresh if saved to OneDrive or OneDrive for Business).	Dashboard tiles from Excel reports are refreshed automatically every few minutes.	N/A

Importing Excel files

Use this option when you need only the Excel data and you'll later create Power BI reports to analyze it. As a prerequisite for importing Excel files directly in Power BI Service, the data must be formatted as an Excel table (Power BI Desktop doesn't have this limitation). If the Excel file has Power View reports, Power BI will create a corresponding Power BI report but it won't import any pivot reports. Because data is imported, you'd probably need to set up a data refresh. However, a scheduled refresh is not required if the workbook is saved in OneDrive or SharePoint Online because Power BI synchronizes changes every hour.

Connecting to Excel files

Use this option when you need to bring in existing Excel pivot reports and Power View reports to Power BI. In this case, Power BI doesn't import the data. Instead, it leaves the Excel file where it is and it just connects to it. However, you must upload the file to OneDrive for Business or SharePoint Online. All connected Excel workbooks appears under the Workbooks tab in the workspace content page.

When you open the workbook, you can see its reports online without needing Excel on the desktop. You'll be able to interact with the reports if the data is imported in the Excel workbooks. At this point, external connections are not supported. You can select a range and pin to a dashboard as an image.

Analyze in Excel

Use this option when you want to create your own PivotTable and PivotChart reports connected to datasets published to Power BI Service. If you use Power BI publisher for Excel, you can pin the pivot reports as images to dashboards, just like you can do when connecting to Excel files.

3.4 Summary

As a business user, you don't need any special skills to gain insights from data. With a few clicks, you can create interactive reports for presenting information in a variety of ways that range from basic reports to professional-looking dashboards.

You can create a new report by exploring a dataset. Power BI supports popular visualizations, including charts, maps, gauges, cards, and tables. When those visualizations just won't do the job, you can import custom visuals from Microsoft AppSource.

Because Excel is a very pervasive tool for self-service, BI supports several integration options with Excel. You can import data from Excel tables. To preserve your investment in Excel pivot and Power View reports, save the Excel files in OneDrive for Business and connect to these files to view the included reports in Excel Online. Finally, you can connect Excel to Power BI datasets and create ad-hoc pivot reports.

Now that you know how to create reports, let's learn more about Power BI dashboards.

Chapter 4

Creating Dashboards

In Chapter 2, I introduced you to Power BI dashboards and you learned that dashboards are one of the three main Power BI content items (the other two are datasets and reports). I defined a Power BI dashboard as a summarized view of important metrics that typically fit on a single page. You need a dashboard when you want to combine data from multiple reports (datasets), or when you need dashboards-specific features, such as data alerts or real-time tiles.

This chapter takes a deep dive into Power BI dashboards. I'll start by discussing the anatomy of a Power BI dashboard. I'll walk you through different ways to create a dashboard, including pinning visualizations, using natural queries by typing them in the Q&A box, from predictive insights, and from SSRS reports. You'll also learn how to share dashboards with your co-workers.

4.1   Understanding Dashboards

Like an automobile's dashboard, a digital dashboard enables users to get a "bird's eye view" of the company's health and performance. A dashboard page typically hosts several sections that display data visually in charts, graphs, or gauges, so that data is easier to understand and analyze. You can use Power BI to quickly assemble dashboards from existing or new visualizations.

NOTE   Power BI isn't the only Microsoft-provided tool for creating dashboards. For example, if you need an entirely on-premises dashboard solution, dashboards can be implemented with Excel (requires SharePoint Server or Power BI Report Server for sharing) and Reporting Services (requires SQL Server). While Power BI dashboards might not be as customizable as SSRS reports, they are by far the easiest to implement. They also gain in interactive features, the ability to use natural queries, and even to get real-time updates (when data is streamed to Power BI)!

4.1.1   Understanding Dashboard Tiles

A Power BI dashboard has one or more tiles. Each tile shows data from one source, such as from one report. For example, the Total Stores tile in the Retail Analysis Sample dashboard (see **Figure 4.1**) shows the total number of stores. The Card visualization came from the Retail Analysis Sample report. Although you can add as many tiles as you want, as a rule of thumb try to limit the number of tiles so that they can fit into a single page and so the user doesn't have to scroll horizontally or vertically.

A tile has a resize handle that allows you to change the tile size to one of the predefined tile sizes (from 1x1 tile units up to 5x5). Because tiles can't overlap, when you enlarge a tile it pushes the rest of the content out of the way. If the tile flow setting is enabled, when you make the tile smaller, adjacent tiles "snap in" to occupy the empty space.

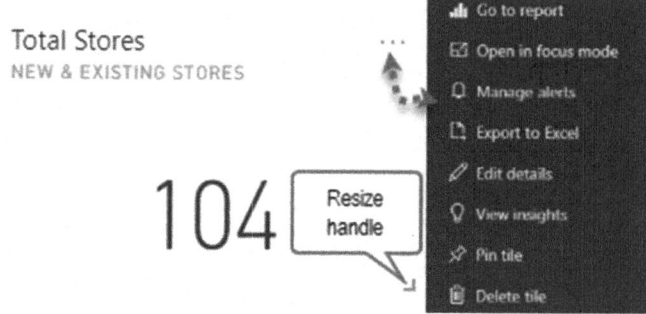

Total Stores
NEW & EXISTING STORES

104 [Resize handle]

Figure 4.1 When you hover on a tile, the ellipsis menu (...) allows you to access the tile settings.

If the tile flow setting is not enabled, Power BI won't reclaim the empty space. To turn on tile flow, open the dashboard, click the ellipsis menu in the upper-right corner of the dashboard (next to the Share button), click Settings, and then slide the "Dashboard tile flow" slider to On. You can move a tile by just dragging it to a new location. You don't need to explicitly save the layout changes you've made to a dashboard when you resize or move its tiles.

Understanding tile actions

When you hover on a tile, an ellipsis menu (...) shows up in the top-right corner of the tile. When you click the ellipsis menu, a context menu pops up with a list of tile-related actions. What actions are included in the menu depends on where the tile came from. For example, if the tile was produced by pinning an Excel pivot report, you won't be able to set alerts, export to Excel, and view insights. Or, if the dataset has row-level security applied, you won't see "View insights" because this feature is not available with RLS.

1. Go to report – By default, when you click a tile, Power BI "drills through" it and navigates you to the underlying source. For example, if the tile is pinned from a report, you'll be taken to the underlying report. Another way to navigate to the report is to invoke "Go to report" from the context menu.

2. Open in focus mode – Like popping out visualizations on a report, this action pops out the tile so that you can examine it in more detail.

3. Manage alerts – A tile pinned from a visualization showing a scalar value (Single Card, Gauge, KPI) can have one or more data alerts, such as to notify you when the number of stores reaches 105.

4. Export to Excel – Exports the tile data to a Comma-separated values (CSV) text file. You can then open the file in Excel and examine the data.

5. Edit details – Allows you to change the tile settings, such as the tile title and subtitle.

6. View insights – Like Quick Insights but targets the specific tile for discovering insights. Power BI will search the tile and its related data for correlations, outliers, trends, seasonality, change points in trends, and major factors automatically, within seconds.

7. Pin tile – Pins a tile to another dashboard. Why would you pin a tile from a dashboard instead of from the report? Pinning it from a dashboard allows you to apply the same customizations, such as the title, subtitle, and custom link, to the other dashboard, even though they're not shared (once you pin the tile to another dashboard, both titles have independent customizations).

8. Delete tile – Removes the 1 from the dashboard.

Some of these actions deserve more attention so I'll explain them next in more detail.

Understanding the focus mode

When you click the "Open in focus mode" button, Power BI opens another page and enlarges the visualization (see **Figure 4.2**). Tooltips allow you to get precise values. If you pop out a line chart, you can also click a data point to place a vertical line and see the precise value of a measure at the intersection of the vertical bar and the line. The Filter pane is available so that you can filter the displayed data by specifying visual-level filters.

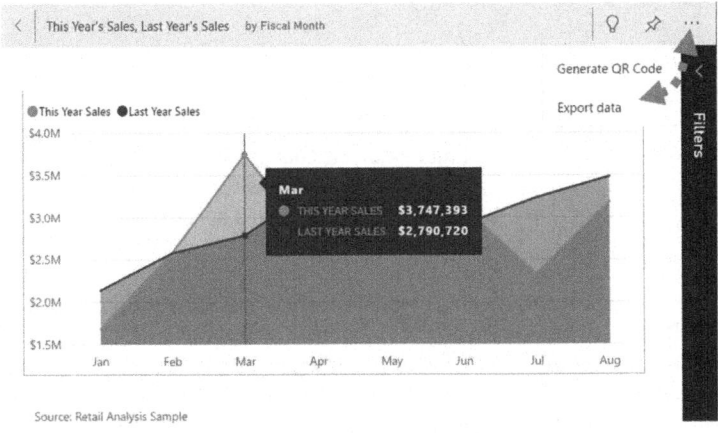

Figure 4.2 The focus mode page allows you to examine the tile in more details, generate a QR code, and export the tile data.

The focus page has an ellipsis menu (...) in the top-right corner. When you click it, a "Generate QR Code" menu appears. A QR Code (abbreviated from Quick Response Code) is a barcode that contains information about the item to which it is attached. In the case of a Power BI tile, it contains the URL of the tile. How's this useful, you might wonder? You can download the code, print it, and display it somewhere or post the image online. When other people scan the code (there are many QR Code reader mobile apps, including the one included in the Power BI iPhone app), they'll get the tile URL. Now they can quickly navigate to the dashboard tile. So QR codes give users convenient and instant access to dashboard tiles.

For example, suppose you're visiting a potential customer and they give you a pamphlet. It starts gushing about all these stats about how great their performance has been. You have a hard time believing what you hear or even understanding the numbers. You see the QR Code. You scan it with your phone. It pops up Power BI Mobile on your phone, and rather than just reading the pamphlet, now you're sliding the controls around in Power BI and exploring the data. You go back and forth between reading the pamphlet and then exploring the associated data on your phone.

Or, suppose you're in a meeting. The presenter is showing some data, but wants you to explore it independently. He includes a QR Code on their deck. He also might pass around a paper with the QR Code on it. You scan the code and navigate to Power BI to examine the data in more detail. As you can imagine, QR codes open new opportunities for getting access to relevant information that's available in Power BI. For more information about the QR code feature, read the blog "Bridge the gap between your physical world and your BI using QR codes" at http://bit.ly/1lsVGJ5.

Understanding tile insights

In the previous chapter, you saw how Quick Insights makes it easy to apply brute-force predictive analytics to a dataset and discover hidden trends. Instead of examining the entire dataset, you can scope Quick Insights to a specific tile. You can do so by clicking the "View insights" action found in the tile's properties and in the upper-right corner of the tile while it's in focus.

Power BI will scan the data related to the tile and display a list of visualizations you may want to explore further. **Figure 4.3** shows two of the Insights visuals for the Total Stores card of the Retail Analysis Sample dashboard. To get even more specifics insights, you can click a data point in the visual, and Related Insights will focus on that data point when searching for insights. If you find a given insight useful, you can hover on the visual and click the pin button to pin it to a dashboard.

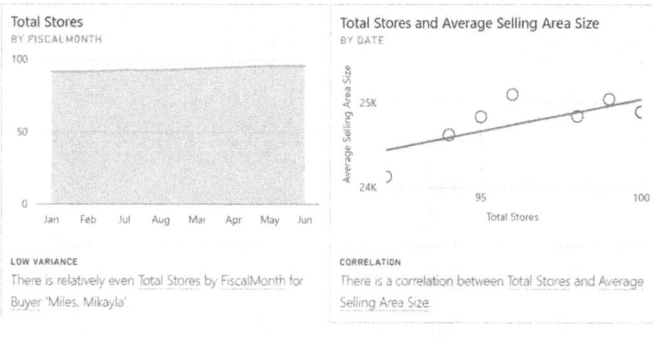

Figure 4.3 Insights applies the same predictive algorithms as Quick Insights but limits their scope to a specific tile.

Understanding data alerts

Wouldn't it be nice to be notified for important data changes, such as when this year's revenue reaches a specific goal? Now you can be with Power BI data alerts! You can create alerts on Single Card, Gauge, and KPI tiles. A tile can have multiple alerts, such as to notify you when the value is both above and below certain thresholds. You can create a data alert in Power BI Service (click "Manage alerts" in the tile properties) or in Power BI Mobile native applications for mobile devices. This brings you to the "Manage alerts" window (see **Figure 4.4**) where you can create one or more alerts.

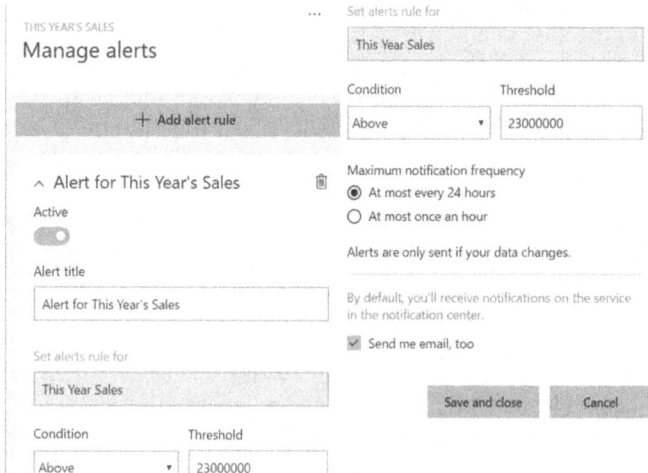

Figure 4.4 When you create an alert, you specify a condition and notification frequency.

Currently, Power BI supports two conditions (Above and Below) and two notification intervals (daily and hourly). By default, you'll get an email when the condition is met in addition to a notification in the Power BI Notification Center. If you have Power BI Mobile installed on your mobile device, you'll also get an in-app notification.

 TIP To view all data alerts that you defined for dashboards in My Workspace, in Power BI Portal expand the Settings menu, click Settings, and then select the Alerts tab. There you can deactivate the alert, edit it, or delete it. Currently, there isn't a way for the tenant admin to see alerts by other users.

Understanding tile details

Additional tile configuration options are available when you click "Edit details" (the fifth option in **Figure 4.1**). It brings you to the "Tile details" window (see **Figure 4.5**). Since report visualizations might have Power BI-generated titles that might not be very descriptive, the Tile Details window allows you to specify a custom title and subtitle for the tile.

Tile details

* Required

Details

☑ Display title and subtitle

Title

| Total Stores |

Subtitle

| New & Existing Stores |

Functionality

☐ Display last refresh time

☐ Set custom link

Link type

◉ External link

○ Link to a dashboard or report in the current workspace

URL *

| |

Open custom link in the same tab?

○ Yes

◉ No

Restore default

Technical Details

[Apply] [Cancel]

Figure 4.5 The Tile Details window lets you change the tile's title, subtitle, and specify a custom link.

As you know by now, clicking a tile brings you to the report where the tile was pinned from. However, if you want the user to be navigated to another report or even a web page, you can overwrite this behavior by checking the "Set custom link" checkbox. Then you can specify if this is an external link (you need to enter the page URL) or a link to an existing dashboard and report in the workspace where your dashboard is in (you can pick the target dashboard or report from a dropdown). You can also configure the link to open in a new browser tab.

 TIP An external link could navigate the user to any URL-based resource, such as to an on-premises SSRS report. This could be useful if you want to link the tile to a more detailed report. Unfortunately, you can't pass the field values as report parameters.

This completes our discussion about tile-related actions. Let's now see what dashboard-relates tasks are available in Power BI.

Understanding dashboard actions

Additional dashboard-related actions are available to you from the menu in the upper-right corner of the dashboard, as shown in **Figure 4.6**. Starting from the left, the "Add tile" menu is yet another way to add a tile to a dashboard. It allows you to add media, such as web content, image, video, and custom streaming data (streamed datasets are covered in Chapter 13).

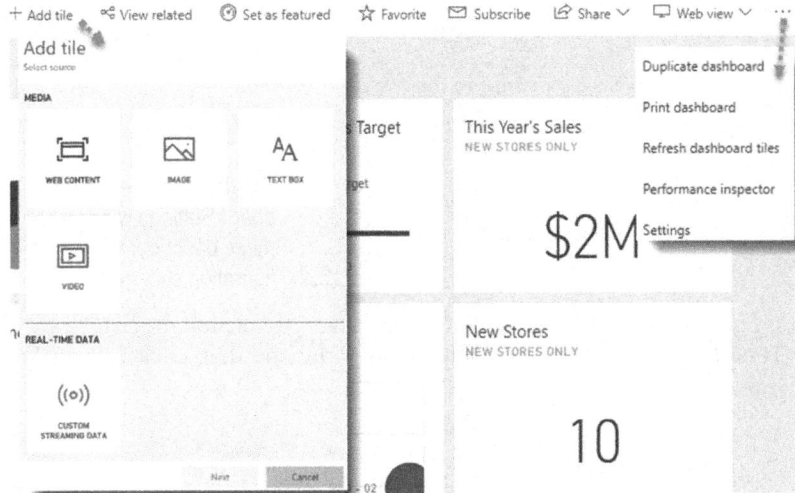

Figure 4.6 Additional actions are available from the menus in the upper-right corner of the open dashboard.

"View related" shows reports (and their related datasets) from which the dashboard tiles originate. "Set as featured" marks the dashboard as featured so that you see this dashboard when you log in to Power BI. If you don't have a featured dashboard, you'll be navigated to the last dashboard you visited. Clicking the Favorite button adds the dashboard to the Favorites section of the Power BI navigation bar.

Like report subscriptions, the Subscribe menu lets you create a dashboard-level subscription to get an email with a snapshot image of the dashboard when Power BI detects that the underlying data has changed. Let's skip the Share button for now. Power BI supports two dashboard views. The default Web view is for large screens. However, when you view dashboards in the Power BI Mobile app on a phone, you'll notice the dashboard tiles are laid out one after another, and they're all the same size. You can switch to Phone view to create a customized view that targets the limited display capabilities of phones. When you're in Phone view, you can unpin, resize, and rearrange tiles to fit the display. Changes in Phone view don't affect the web version of the dashboard.

Clicking the ellipsis menu (…) opens a list of dashboard-related actions. Going quickly through the list, "Duplicate dashboard" clones the dashboard with a new name. Duplicating a dashboard could be useful if you want to retain the existing dashboard customization settings, but make layout changes, such as to add or remove tiles. "Print dashboard" prints the dashboard content exactly as it appears on the screen. By default, Power BI updates the cache for dashboard tiles every fifteen minutes to synchronize them with data changes. You can force a tile refresh by clicking "Refresh dashboard tiles".

No one likes to wait for a report to show up. "Performance inspector" helps you inspect and diagnose why the dashboard loading time is excessive. A window pops up with alerts to help you identify the potential issue and tips about how to fix it. The last action is Settings and it deserves more attention.

Understanding dashboard settings

The Settings menu brings you to the dashboard settings window (see **Figure 4.7**), which is also accessible from the Dashboard tab in the workspace content page. You can rename the dashboard, disable Q&A, and turn on tile flow. If your tenant administrator has enabled data classification (discussed in Chapter 11), you can assign a data classification category to a dashboard. For example, Maya's dashboard might show some sensitive information. Maya goes to the dashboard settings and tags the dashboard as Confidential Data. When Maya shares the dashboard with co-workers, they can see this classification next to the dashboard name.

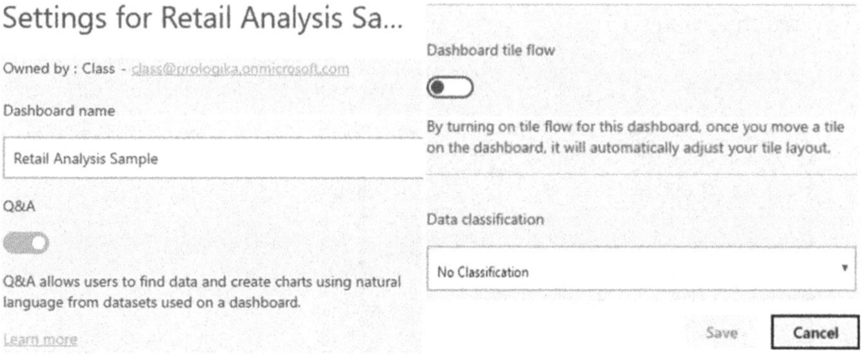

Settings for Retail Analysis Sa...

Owned by : Class - class@prologika.onmicrosoft.com

Dashboard name

| Retail Analysis Sample |

Q&A

Q&A allows users to find data and create charts using natural language from datasets used on a dashboard.

Learn more

Dashboard tile flow

By turning on tile flow for this dashboard, once you move a tile on the dashboard, it will automatically adjust your tile layout.

Data classification

| No Classification | ▾ |

Save   **Cancel**

Figure 4.7 Use the dashboard Settings window to make dashboard-wide configuration changes.

You can also find the same dashboard settings in the Power BI Service Settings page (click the Settings menu in the Power BI Application Toolbar on the upper-right side of the portal and then click Settings), as shown in **Figure 4.8**.

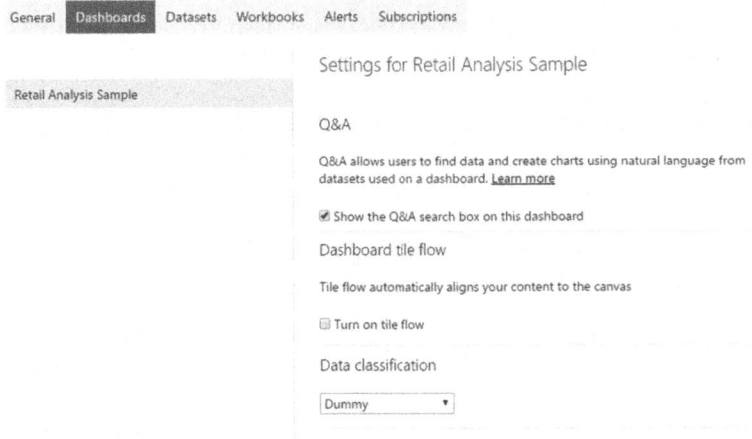

Figure 4.8 Dashboard settings are also available in the Power BI Service Settings page.

4.1.2 Sharing Dashboards

Power BI allows you to share dashboards easily with your coworkers. This type of sharing let other people see the dashboards you've created. Remember that all Power BI sharing options, including dashboard sharing, require the user who shares content to have a Power BI Pro or Power BI Premium license. Shared dashboards and associated reports are ready-only to recipients.

 NOTE Besides simple dashboard sharing, Power BI supports two other sharing options: workspaces and apps. Workspaces allow groups of users to contribute to shared content and apps are for broader content sharing, such as to share content with many viewers who can't make changes. Because these options require more planning, I discuss them in Chapter 11.

Understanding sharing access

Consider dashboard sharing when you need a quick and easy way to share your dashboard. It works only with dashboards; you can't use simple sharing to directly share reports and datasets. When sharing a dashboard with your coworkers, they can still click the dashboard tiles and interact with the underlying reports in Reading View (the Edit Report menu will be disabled). They can't create new reports or make changes to existing reports nor can they make layout changes to the dashboard. When the dashboard author makes changes, the recipients can immediately see the changes. They can access all shared dashboards in the "Shared with me" section of the Power BI navigation pane (see **Figure 4.9**). They can further filter the list of shared dashboards for a specific author by clicking that person's name.

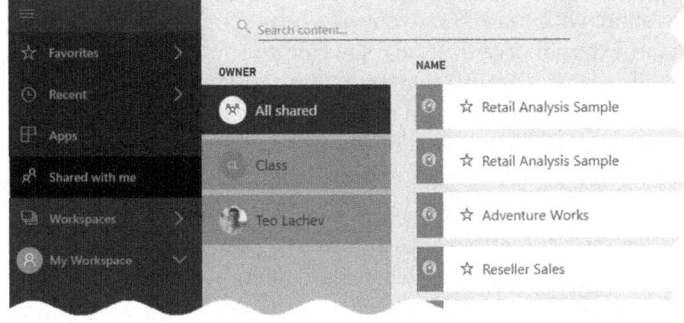

Figure 4.9 Recipients can find shared dashboards in the "Shared with me" section.

Sharing a dashboard

To share a dashboard, click the Share link in the upper-right corner of an open dashboard (see **Figure 4.6** again). This brings you to the "Share dashboard" window, as shown in **Figure 4.10**.

Share dashboard
ADVENTURE WORKS
Share   Access

Recipients will have the same access as you unless row-level security on the dataset further restricts them. Learn more
Grant access to

Martin

Martin ▓▓▓▓▓▓▓▓▓▓▓▓▓▓▓▓▓▓

Include an optional message...

☑ Allow recipients to share your dashboard
☑ Send email notification to recipients
Dashboard Link ⓘ

https://app.powerbi.com/groups/me/dashboards/34ac3937-1b95-4800-8249-e:

Share   Cancel

Share dashboard
ADVENTURE WORKS
Share   Access

The following have access to this dashboard

🔍 Search

NAME	ACCESS
Teo Lachev	Owner
▓▓▓▓▓	Read and reshare ...

Close

Figure 4.10 Use the "Share dashboard" window to enter a list of recipient emails, separated with a comma or semi-colon.

Enter the email addresses of the recipients separated by comma (,) or semi-colon (;). You can even use both. Power BI will validate the emails and inform you if they are incorrect.

 TIP Want to share with many users, such as with everyone in your department? You can type in the email of an Office 365 distribution list or security group. If you are sharing a dashboard from a workspace in a Power BI Premium capacity, you can also share the dashboard with Power BI Free users.

Next, enter an optional message. To allow your coworkers to re-share your dashboard with others, check "Allow recipients to share your dashboard". If you change your mind later and you want to stop sharing, click the Access tab. This tab allows you to stop sharing and/or disable re-shares for each coworker you shared the dashboard with.

By default, the "Send email notification to recipients" checkbox is checked. When you click the Share button, Power BI will send an e-mail notification with a link to your dashboard. When the recipient clicks the dashboard link and signs in to Power BI, the shared dashboard will be added to the "Shared with me" section in the navigation bar. You might not always want the person you share a dashboard with to go through the effort of checking their email and clicking a link just for your dashboard to show up in their workspace. If you uncheck the "Send email notification to recipients" checkbox, you can share dashboards directly without them having to do anything. Now when you click Share, the dashboard will just show up in the other users' " Shared with me" section with no additional steps required on their end.

Sharing with external users

You can share dashboards with people within your organization and external users. For example, if Maya's email is maya@adventureworks.com, she can share with martin@adventureworks.com. If Maya wants to share with Matthew who works for Contoso (an external organization), she can do so by just typing in Matthew's business email address. Matthew will receive a notification with a link to the dashboard (Matthew should save that link as it has important encrypted information attached). When he clicks the link, he'll be asked to sign in to Power BI with his work email (or create a Power BI account if he doesn't have one). In other words, external recipients need to be Power BI users for their organization. From a licensing perspective, external users can gain access to shared content under one of these three options:

- They have a Power BI Pro license in their tenant – If Matthew has a Power BI Pro license in his (Contoso) tenant, that license will propagate to other organizations that share content with him.

- They have a Power BI Pro license in the other organization tenant – If Matthew has a Power BI Pro license in the AdventureWorks tenant, he can see the shared content.

- The workspace is in a Power BI Premium capacity – A premium workspace can share content out to Power BI Free internal and external users. The recipients need not be licensed.

Once Matthew has signed in, he'll see the shared dashboard in the web browser without the Power BI left navigation pane. Like internal sharing, Matthew can drill through tiles and access the underlying reports. All interactive features work but the reports are real-only. Maya can see all the external users who have access to this dashboard and revoke their permission from the Access tab in the "Share dashboard" window. All the external users who have access to this dashboard are marked as "Guest". External sharing works also with Power BI Desktop models that have Row-Level Security (RLS) and with dynamic data security in Analysis Services semantic models because the user email is passed on to the data source.

 NOTE For more information and a step-by-step guide to distributing BI content with Power BI and Azure AD B2B read the "Distribute Power BI content to external guest users using Azure Active Directory B2B" whitepaper at https://aka.ms/powerbi-b2b-whitepaper.

4.2 Adding Dashboard Content

You can create as many dashboards as you want. One way to get started is to create an empty dashboard by clicking the plus sign (+) in the upper-right corner of the workspace content page and then giving the new dashboard a name. Then you can add content to the dashboard. Or, instead of creating an empty dashboard, you can tell Power BI to create a new dashboard when pinning content. You can add content to a dashboard in several ways:

- Pin visualizations from existing Power BI reports or other dashboards
- Pin ranges from Excel Online reports or from Power BI publisher for Excel
- Pin visualizations from Q&A
- Pin visualizations from Quick Insights or Related Insights
- Pin report items from Power BI Report Server reports
- Add tiles from media and streamed datasets (click the "+Add tile" dashboard menu)

I showed in Chapter 3 how to add content from Excel ranges. I mentioned about adding tiles from media in the "Understanding Dashboard Tiles" section. I'll cover streamed datasets in Chapter 13 because they require programming. Next, I'll explain the rest of the options for adding content to dashboards.

4.2.1 Adding Content from Power BI Reports

The most common way to add dashboard content is to pin visualizations from existing reports or dashboards. This allows you to implement a consolidated summary view that spans multiple reports and datasets. Users can drill through the dashboard tiles to the underlying reports.

Pinning visualizations
To pin a visualization to a dashboard from an existing report, you hover on the visualization and click the pushpin button (⚲). This opens the Pin to Dashboard window, as shown in **Figure 4.11**. This window shows a preview of the selected visualization and asks if you want to add the visualization to an existing dashboard or to create a new dashboard. If you choose the "Existing dashboard", you can select the target dashboard from a drop-down list. Power BI defaults to the last dashboard that you open. If you choose a new dashboard, you need to type in the dashboard name and then Power BI will create it for you.

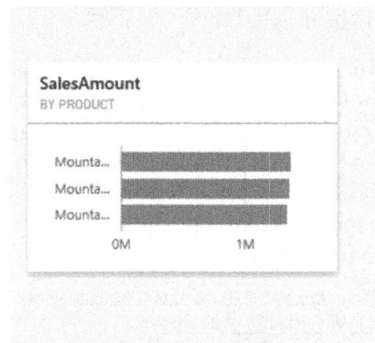

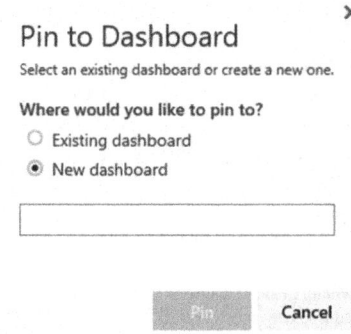

Pin to Dashboard

Select an existing dashboard or create a new one.

Where would you like to pin to?

○ Existing dashboard

◉ New dashboard

[   ]

Pin   Cancel

Figure 4.11 Use the Pin to Dashboard window to select which dashboard you want the visualization to be added to.

Think of pinning a visualization like adding a shortcut to the visualization on the dashboard. You can't make layout changes to the visualization on the dashboard once it's pinned as a dashboard tile. You must make such changes to the underlying report where the visualization is pinned from. Interactive features, such as automatic highlighting and filtering, also aren't available in dashboards. You'll need to click the visualization to drill through the underlying report to make changes or use interactive features.

 TIP When pinning a visualization to a dashboard, you might want to show a subset of its data. You can do this by applying a filter (or a slicer) to the report prior to pinning the visualization. If the visualization is filtered, the filter will propagate to the dashboard.

Pinning report pages

As you've seen, pinning specific visualizations allows you to quickly assemble a dashboard from various reports in a single summary view. However, the pinned visualizations "lose" their interactive features, including interactive highlighting, sorting, and tooltips. The only way to restore these features is to drill the dashboard tile through the underlying report. In addition, when you pin individual visualizations you lose filtering capabilities because the Filtering pane won't be available, and you can't pin slicers.

 NOTE Currently Power BI doesn't support filtering across dashboard tiles when you pin individual visuals from a report. And the Filter pane is not available in dashboards. Cross-tile filtering is a frequently requested feature and it's on the Power BI roadmap.

However, besides pinning specific report visualizations, you can pin entire report pages. This has the following advantages:

- Preserve report interactive features – When you pin a report page, the tile preserves the report layout and interactivity. You can fully interact with all the visualizations in the report tile, just as you would with the actual report. You'll also get all the page visuals including slicers.

- Reuse existing reports for dashboard content – You might have already designed your report as a dashboard. Instead of pinning individual report visualizations one by one, you can simple pin the whole report page.

- Synchronize changes – A report tile is always synchronized with the report layout. So, if you need to change a visualization on the report, such as from a Table to a Chart, the dashboard tile is updated automatically. No need to delete the old tile and re-pin it.

Follow these steps to pin a report page to a dashboard:

1. Open the report in Reading View or Editing View.
2. Click "Pin Live Page" in the top menu.
3. In the "Pin to Dashboard" window, select a new or existing dashboard to pin the report page to, as you do when pinning single visualizations. Now you have the entire report page pinned and interactivity works!

For example, **Figure 4.12** shows the "New Stores Analysis" page from the "Retail Analysis Sample" report that is now pinned to a dashboard.

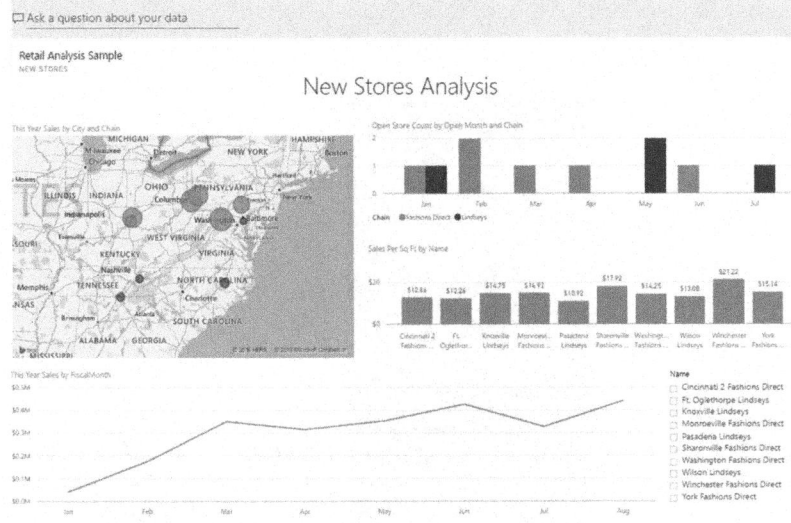

Figure 4.12 You can pin report pages to your dashboards to preserve interactive features, reuse reports as dashboards, and synchronize layout changes.

4.2.2 Adding Content from Q&A

Another way to add dashboard content is to use natural questions (Q&A). Natural queries let data speak for itself by responding to questions entered in natural language, similar to how you search the Internet. The Q&A box appears on top of every dashboard that connects to datasets with imported data.

 NOTE As of the time of writing, natural queries are available only with datasets created by importing data and datasets with direct connections to Analysis Services Tabular models. Also, Q&A currently supports English only (supports for Spanish is currently in preview).

Understanding natural questions
When you click the Q&A box, it suggests questions you could ask about the dashboard data (see **Figure 4.13**). If the dashboard uses content from multiple datasets, there will be suggested questions from all datasets.

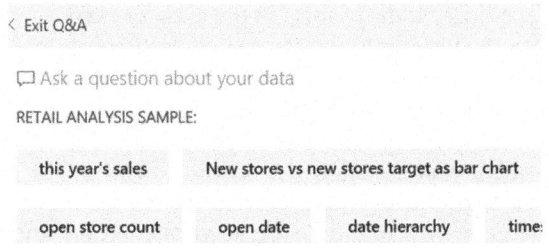

Figure 4.13 The Q&A box has predefined questions which are derived from the dataset metadata.

Of course, these suggestions are just a starting point. Power BI inferred them from the table and column names in the underlying dataset. You can add more predefined questions by following these steps:

1. In Power BI portal, click the Settings (cog) menu in the upper-right corner, and then click Settings.
2. Click the Datasets tab (see **Figure 4.8** again) and then select the desired dataset.
3. In the dataset settings, expand the "Featured Q&A Questions" section.

4. Click "Add a question" and then type a statement that uses dataset fields, such as "sales by country".

Users aren't limited to predefined questions. They can ask for something else, such as "what were this year sales", as shown in **Figure 4.14**.

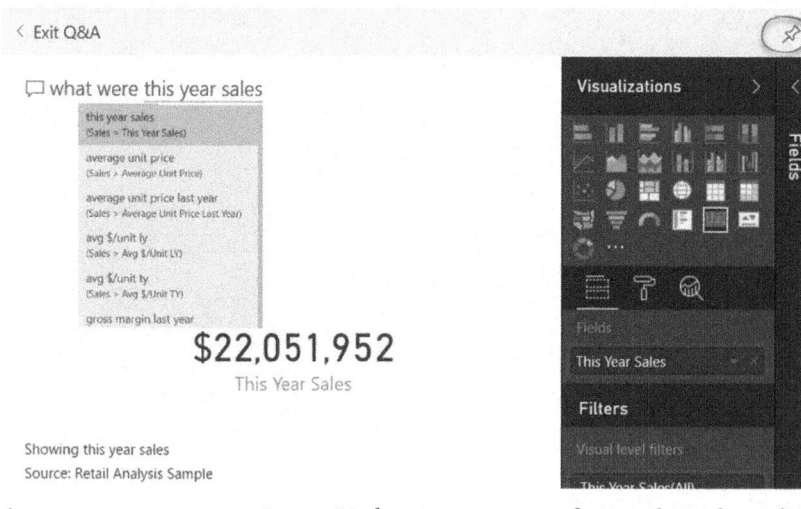

Figure 4.14 The Q&A box interprets the natural question and defaults to the best visualization.

As you type a question, Power BI shows suggestions from a drop-down list. These suggestions correspond to fields in the dataset tables. The drop-down list also shows which table and field correspond to the suggestion. Q&A shows you how it interpreted the question below the visualization. By doing so, Power BI searches the datasets used in the dashboard. So that you can understand which dataset answers your question, Power BI displays the source dataset below the visualization. **Figure 4.14** shows "Source: Retail Analysis Sample" because this question was answered from the Retail Analysis Sample dataset.

Understanding Q&A reports

Power BI attempts to use the best visualization, depending on the question and supporting data. In this case, Power BI has interpreted the question as "Showing this year sales" and decided to use a card visualization. If you continue typing so the question becomes "what were this year sales by product", it would probably switch over to a Bar Chart. However, if you don't have much luck visualizing the data the way you want, you can always use the Visualizations and Fields panes to customize the visualization, as you can do with reports.

In other words, think of Q&A as a way to jump start your data exploration by creating a report that you can customize further, such as changing the color of the lines, adding labels to the axes, or even choosing another visualization type! Once you're done with the visualization, you can click the pushpin button to add the visualization to the dashboard. Once the tile is added, you can click it to drill through into the dataset. Power BI brings you the visualization you created and shows the natural question that was used. If you change the visual and you want to apply the changes to the dashboard, you'd need to pin the visual again. Power BI will add it as a new tile so you might want to delete the previous tile.

So how smart is Q&A? Can it answer any question you might have? Q&A searches metadata, including table, column, and field names. It also has built-in smarts on how to filter, sort, aggregate, group, and display data. For example, the Internet Sales dataset you imported from Excel has columns titled "Product", "Month", "SalesAmount", and "OrderQuantity". You could ask questions about any of those entities. You could ask it to show SalesAmount by Product or by Month, and others. You should also note that Q&A is smart enough to interpret that SalesAmount is actually "sales amount", and you can use both interchangeably.

NOTE Data analysts creating Power BI Desktop and Excel Power Pivot data models can fine tune the model metadata for Q&A. For example, Martin can create a synonym (discussed in Chapter 8) to tell Power BI that State and Province mean the same thing.

4.2.3 Adding Content from Predictive Insights

Recall from the previous chapter that Power BI includes an interesting predictive feature called Quick Insights. When you apply Quick Insights at a dataset level it runs predictive algorithms on the entire dataset to find hidden patterns that might not be easily discernable, such as outliers and correlations. A similar feature can be applied to a dashboard tile to limit the data to whatever is shown in the tile. In both cases, Quick Insights results are available within the current session. Once you close Power BI, they are removed but you can regenerate them quickly when you need them (they only take 20 or so seconds to create).

Adding Quick Insights
To generate Quick Insights at the dataset level, go to the workspace content page, click the Datasets tab, expand the ellipsis menu (…) next to the dataset name, and then click "Get quick insights". Or, click the ellipsis menu (…) next to the dataset name in the navigation bar and then click "Quick Insights". Once Quick Insights are ready, the menu changes to View Insights. You can add one or more of the resulting reports to a dashboard by pinning the visualization (hover on the visualization and click the pin button).

Once the visualization is added to the dashboard it becomes a regular dashboard tile. However, when you click it, Power BI opens the visualization in focus mode so that you can examine it in more detail and apply visual-level filters.

Adding Tile Insights
To generate insights for a specific dashboard tile, hover on the tile, click the ellipsis menu (…) in the upper-right corner of the tile, and then click "View insights". Then click the Related Insights (bulb) icon. This pops up the tile and shows the related insights in the Insights window on the right. You can add one or more of the resulting visualizations you like to a dashboard by pinning the visualization (hover on the visualization in the Insights pane and click the pushpin button).

Like tiles produced by Quick Insights at the dataset level, once a tile insight is added to the dashboard it becomes a regular dashboard tile. When you click it, Power BI opens the visualization in focus so that you can examine it in more detail and apply visual-level filters.

4.2.4 Adding Content from Power BI Report Server

The chances are that your organization uses SQL Server Reporting Services for distributing paginated reports and it's looking for ways to integrate different report types in a single portal. Recall from Chapter 1 that Power BI Report Server extends SSRS and allows you to deploy Power BI reports on an on-premises report server. If your report administrator has configured the Power BI Report Server for Power BI integration, you can add report items to Power BI dashboards. I'll provide general guidance to the administrator about this integration scenario and explain its limitations in Chapter 12. In this section, I'll show you how you can add content from SSRS reports to Power BI dashboards.

Pinning report items
Follow these steps to pin a report item:

1. Open the Power BI Report Server portal, such as http://<servername>/reports. Open a report you want to pin content from. The report's data source(s) must use stored credentials to connect to data (verify this with your report administrator).

2. Click the "Pin to Power BI Dashboard" toolbar button (see **Figure 4.15**). If you don't see this button, the report server is not configured for Power BI integration. If you see it and click it but you get a message that the report is not configured for stored credentials, you need to change the report data sources(s) to used stored credentials instead of other authentication options. Ask your SSRS administrator for help.

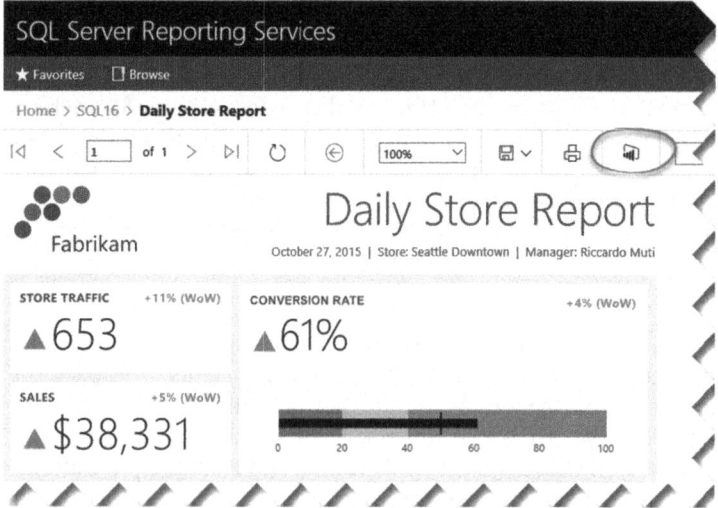

Figure 4.15 If Power BI Report Server is configured for Power BI integration, you can click the "Pin to Power BI Dashboard" toolbar button to pin report items.

3. If you are not already signed in to Power BI, you'll be prompted to do so.

4. The report page background changes to black and the report items you can pin on the current page are highlighted while the items that you cannot pin, will be shaded dark. Currently, you can pin only image-generating report items, including charts, gauges, maps, and images. You can't pin tables and lists. Continuing the list of limitations, the items must be in the report body (you can't pin from page headers and footers).

5. Click the report item you want to add to your Power BI dashboard.

6. In the "Pin to Power BI Dashboard" window (see **Figure 4.16**), choose a workspace, dashboard, and update frequency (Hourly, Daily, or Weekly). The frequency interval specifies how often the dashboard tile will check for changes in the report data.

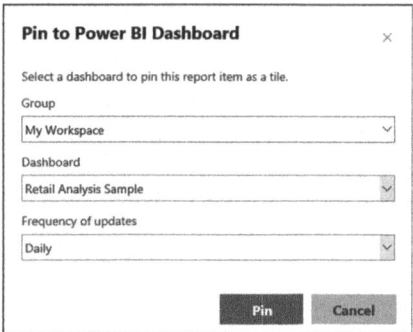

Figure 4.16 When you pin an SSRS item, you can specify the frequency of updates.

7. Click Pin. You should see a Pin Successful dialog. Click the provided link to open the Power BI dashboard.

NOTE Behind the scenes to synchronize changes, the report server creates an individual subscription with the same frequency. You can see the subscription in the Power BI Report Server portal (expand the Settings menu and then click My Subscriptions). It's important to know that the report server doesn't remove the subscription when you remove the tile from the dashboard. To avoid performance degradation to the report server, you must manually remove your unused subscriptions.

Understanding tile changes

Once the report item is pinned to a dashboard, its tile looks just like any other tile except that it's subtitle shows the date and time the tile was pinned or when the report was last refreshed. If you open the tile actions (click the ellipsis menu (…) in the upper-right corner of the tile), you'll see that Power BI Report Server tiles don't have all the features of regular tiles (see **Figure 4.17**). For example, Insights and Focus Mode are not available. Continuing the list of limitations, Q&A is also not available.

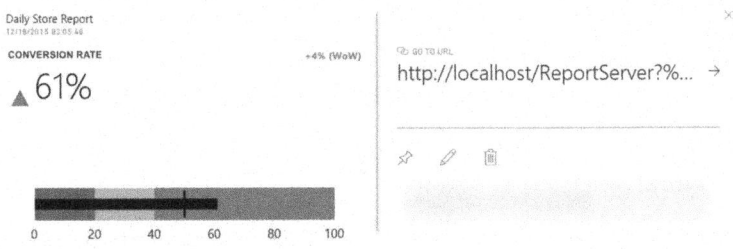

Figure 4.17 The dashboard tile with a pinned report item has a link to the original report.

If you click Tile Details, you can see that the custom link includes the report URL. Consequently, when you click the tile, you'll be navigated to the report in the report portal. However, you must be on your corporate network for this to work. Otherwise, the report server won't be reachable and you'll get an error in your web browser.

TIP Your organization can set up a web application proxy to view Power BI Report Server reports outside the corporate network. The Chris Finlan's "Leveraging Web Application Proxy in Windows Server 2016 to provide secure access to your SQL Server Reporting Services environment" blog has the details at bit.ly/ssrsproxy.

4.3   Working with Dashboards

Next, you'll go through an exercise to create the Internet Sales dashboard shown in **Figure 4.18**. You'll create the first three tiles by pinning visualizations from an existing report. Then you'll use Q&A to create the fourth tile that will show a Line Chart.

4.3.1   Creating and Modifying Tiles

Let's start implementing the dashboard by adding content from a report. Then you'll customize the tiles and practice drilling through the content. Compared to reports, one difference you'll discover is that you can't manually save your changes to dashboard tiles as Power BI saves layout changes automatically every time you make a change (there is no Save menu).

Pinning visualizations

Follow these steps to pin visualizations from the Internet Sales Analysis report that you created in the previous chapter:

1. In the navigation bar, click the Internet Sales Analysis report to open it in Reading View or Editing View.

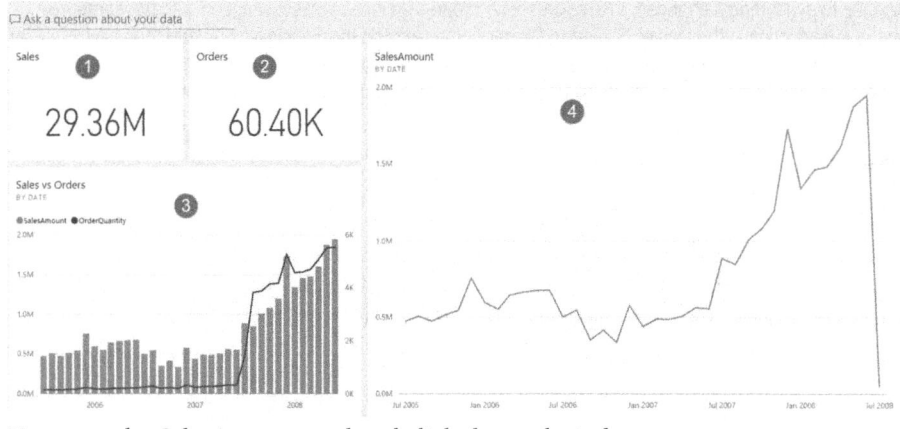

Figure 4.18 The Internet Sales dashboard was created by pinning visualizations and then using a natural query.

2. Hover on the SalesAmount card and click the pushpin button.

3. In the Pin to Dashboard window, select the "New dashboard" option, enter *Internet Sales*, and click Pin.

4.3.2 Creating and Modifying Tiles

Let's start implementing the dashboard by adding content from a report. Then you'll customize the tiles and practice drilling through the content. Compared to reports, one difference you'll discover is that you can't manually save your changes to dashboard tiles as Power BI saves layout changes automatically every time you make a change (there is no Save menu).

Pinning visualizations

Follow these steps to pin visualizations from the Internet Sales Analysis report that you created in the previous chapter:

1. In the navigation bar, click the Internet Sales Analysis report to open it in Reading View or Editing View.

2. Hover on the SalesAmount card and click the pushpin button.

3. In the Pin to Dashboard window, select the "New dashboard" option, enter *Internet Sales*, and click Pin.

This creates a new dashboard named *Internet Sales*. You can find the dashboard in the workspace content page (Dashboards tab). Power BI shows a message that the visualization has been pinned to the Internet Sales dashboard.

4. In the Internet Sales Analysis report, pin also the OrderQuantity Card and the "SalesAmount and Order-Quantity by Date" Combo Chart, but this time pin them to the Internet Sales existing dashboard.

5. In the navigation bar under Dashboards, click the Internet Sales dashboard. Hover on the SalesAmount Card, and click the ellipsis menu (…). Click "Edit details". In the Tile Details window, enter *Sales* as a title.

6. Change the title for the second Card to *Orders*. Configure the Combo Chart tile to have *Sales vs Orders* as a title and *BY DATE* as a subtitle.

7. Rearrange the tiles to recreate the layout shown back in **Figure 4.18**.

Drilling through the content

You can drill through the dashboard tiles to the underlying reports to see more details and to use the interactive features.

1. Click any of the three tiles, such as the Sales card tile. This action navigates to the Internet Sales Analysis report which opens in Reading View.

2. To go back to the dashboard, click its name in the Dashboards section of the navigation bar or click your Internet browser's Back button.

3. (Optional) Pin visualizations from other reports or dashboards, such as from the Retail Analysis Sample report or dashboard.

4. (Optional) To remove a dashboard tile, click its ellipsis (…) button, and then click "Delete tile".

4.3.3 Using Natural Queries

Another way to create dashboard content is to use natural queries. Use this option when you don't have an existing report or dashboard to start from, or when you want to add new visualizations without creating reports first.

Using Q&A to create a chart

Next, you'll use Q&A to add a Line Chart to the dashboard.

1. In the Q&A box, enter "sales amount by date". Note that Power BI interprets the question as "Showing sales amount sorted by date" and it defaults to a Line Chart, as shown in **Figure 4.19**.

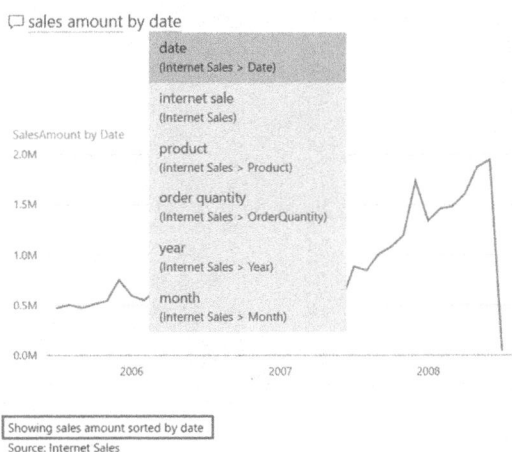 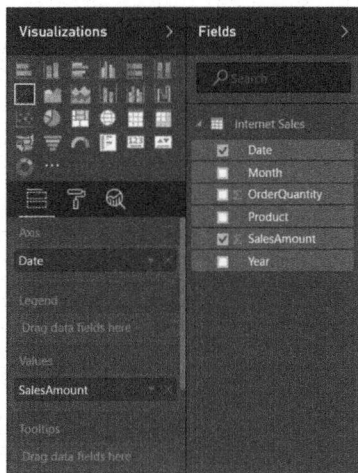

Figure 4.19 Create a Line Chart by typing a natural question.

2. You should also notice that you can use the Visualizations pane to change the visualization. Another way to use a specific visualization is to specify the visualization type in the question. Change the question to "sales amount by date as column chart". Power BI changes the visualization to a Column Chart.

3. (Optional) Practice your reporting skills to customize the visualization using the Visualizations and Fields pane. For example, use the Format tab of the Visualizations pane to turn on data labels.

4. Click the pushpin button to pin the visualization as a new dashboard tile in the Internet Sales dashboard.

Drilling through content

Like tiles bound to report visualizations, Power BI supports drilling through tiles that are created by Q&A:

1. Back in the dashboard, click the new tile that you created with Q&A. Power BI brings you back to the visualization as you left it (see **Figure 4.19**). In addition, Power BI shows the natural question you asked in the Q&A box.

2. (Optional) Use a different question or make some other changes, and then click the pushpin button again. This will bring you to the Pin to Dashboard window. If you choose to pin the visualization to the same dashboard, Power BI will add a new tile to the dashboard.

4.4 Summary

Consider dashboards for displaying important metrics at a glance. You can easily create dashboards by pinning existing visualizations from reports or from other dashboards. Or, you can use natural queries to let the data speak for itself by responding to questions, such as "show me sales for last year". You can drill through to the underlying reports to explore the data in more detail.

You can add content to your dashboards from predictive reports generated by Quick Insights or Related Insights. If your organization has invested in Power BI Report Server, you can pin report items from your reports to Power BI dashboards. Remember that you can also pin ranges from Excel reports and from pivot reports created in Power BI Publisher for Excel, as I showed you in the previous chapter.

Besides using the Power BI portal, you can access reports and dashboards on mobile devices, as you'll learn in the next chapter.

Chapter 5

Power BI Mobile

To reach its full potential, data analytics must not only be insightful but also pervasive. Pervasive analytics is achieved by enabling information workers to access actionable data from anywhere. Mobile computing is everywhere, and most organizations have empowered their employees with mobile devices, such as tablets and smartphones. Preserving this investment, Power BI Mobile enriches the user's mobile data analytics experience. Not only does it allow viewing reports and dashboards on mobile devices, but it also enables additional features that your users would appreciate. It does so by providing native mobile applications for iOS, Android, and Windows devices.

This chapter will help you understand the Power BI Mobile capabilities. Although native applications differ somewhat due to differences in device capabilities and roadmap priorities, there's a common set of features shared across all the applications. I'll demonstrate most of these features with the iPhone native application.

5.1   Introducing Mobile Apps

Power BI is designed to render reports and dashboards in HTML5. As a result, you can view and edit Power BI content from most modern Internet browsers. Currently, Power BI officially supports Microsoft Edge, Microsoft Explorer 10 and 11, the Chrome desktop version, the latest version of Safari for Mac, and the latest Firefox desktop version.

To provide additional features that enrich the user's mobile experience outside the web browser, Power BI currently offers three native applications that target the most popular devices: iOS (iPad and iPhone), Android, and Windows devices. These native applications are collectively known as Power BI Mobile (https://powerbi.microsoft.com/mobile). These apps are for viewing dashboard and reports; you can't use them to make changes. That's understandable considering the limited display capabilities of mobile devices. Next, I'll introduce you briefly to each of these applications.

 TIP Your organization can use Microsoft Intune to manage devices and applications, including the Power BI Mobile apps. Microsoft Intune provides mobile device management, mobile application management, and PC management capabilities from the Microsoft Azure cloud. For example, your organization can use Microsoft Intune to configure mobile apps to require an access pin, control how data is handled by the application, and encrypt application data when the app isn't in use. For more information about Microsoft Intune, go to https://www.microsoft.com/cloud-platform/microsoft-intune.

5.1.1   Introducing the iOS Application

Microsoft released the iOS application on December 18th, 2014, and it was the first native app for Power BI. Initially, the application targeted iPad devices but was later enhanced to support iPhone, Apple Watch, and iPod Touch. Users with these devices can download the Power BI iOS application from the Apple App Store. Realizing the market realities for mobile computing, the iOS app receives the most attention and it's prioritized to be the first to get any new features.

Viewing content

The iOS application supports an intuitive, touch optimized experience for monitoring business data on iPad or iPhone. You can view your dashboards, interact with charts and tiles, explore additional data by browsing reports, and share dashboard images with your colleagues by email. **Figure 5.1** shows the Retail Sales Analysis dashboard in landscape mode on iPhone.

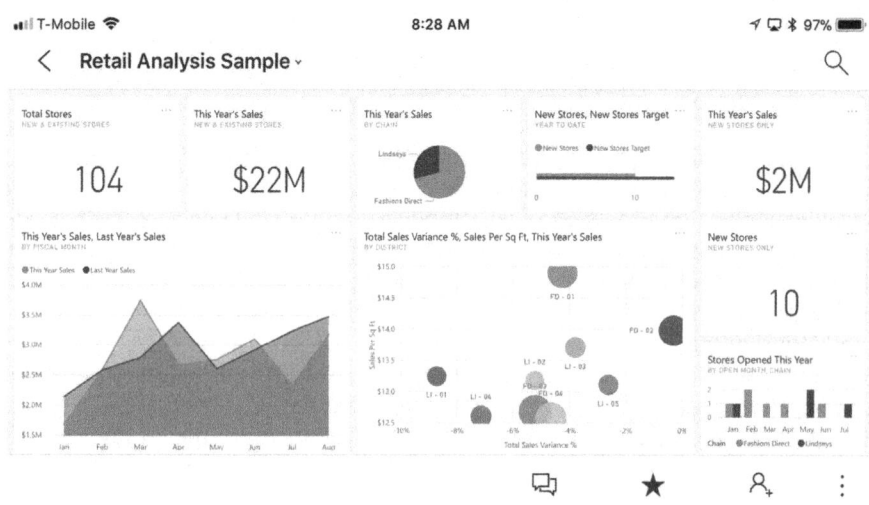

Figure 5.1 The iOS application targets iPad and iPhone devices.

In portrait mode, the app shows dashboard tiles positioned one after another. Remember that if this is not desired, you can go to Power BI Service and open the dashboard in Phone edit view (click the ellipsis button in the upper-right corner of the dashboard and then click Phone in the Edit View section). Then, you can optimize the dashboard layout for portrait mode. Landscape mode lets you view and navigate your dashboards in the same way as you do in the Power BI portal. To view your dashboard in landscape, open it and simply rotate your phone. The dashboard layout changes from a vertical list of tiles to a "Bird's eye" landscape view. Now you can see all your dashboard's tiles as they are in the Power BI portal.

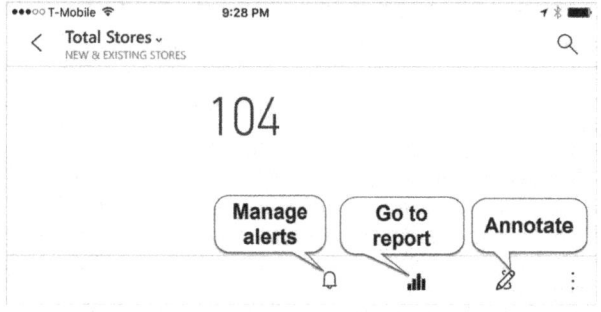

Figure 5.2 The iOS app supports data alerts, drilling through the underlying report, and annotations.

Understanding tile actions

While you're viewing a dashboard with the iPhone app, let's see what happens when you click a tile. Clicking a tile opens it in focus mode (see **Figure 5.2**) as opposed to going to the underlying report in Power BI Service. This behavior applies to all mobile apps. The buttons at the bottom are for the three most common tile actions: create data alerts (remember that alerts are available for Single Card, Gauge, and KPI visuals only), go to the report, and annotate. The same commands are available from the ellipsis menu in the bottom-right corner.

5.1.2 Introducing the Android Application

Microsoft released the Power BI Mobile Android application in July 2015 (see **Figure 5.3**). This application is designed for Android smartphones and Android tablets (Android 5.0 operating system or later) and it's available for download from Google Play Store.

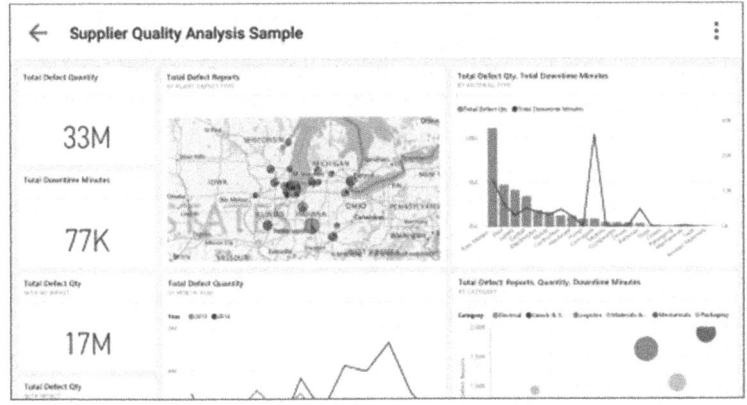

Figure 5.3 The Android application targets Android phones and tablets.

Android users can use this app to explore dashboards, invite colleagues to view data, add annotations, and share insights over email.

5.1.3 Introducing the Windows Application

In May 2015, Power BI Mobile added a native application for Windows 8.1 and Windows 10 devices, such as Surface tablets (see **Figure 5.4**). Microsoft has enhanced the app for Windows 10 phones. You can download the app from Windows Store (search for *Microsoft Power BI*). Your Windows device needs to be running Windows 10 and Microsoft recommends at least 2 GB RAM.

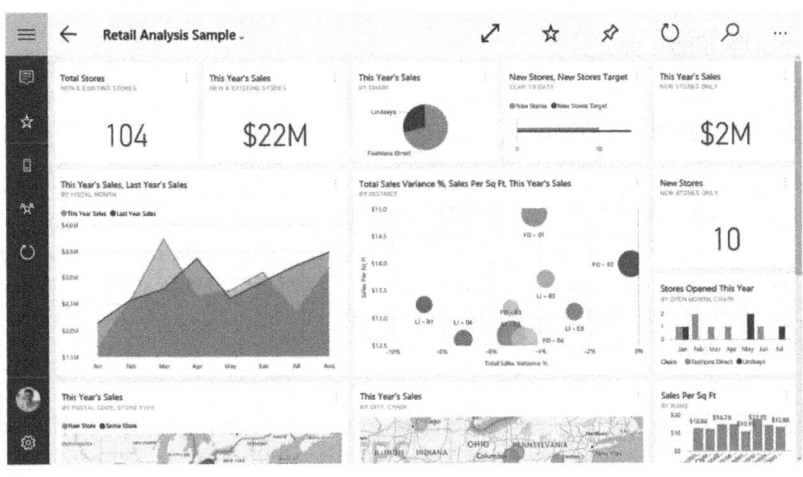

Figure 5.4 The Windows application targets Windows 10 devices and phones.

For the most part, the Windows app has identical features as the other Power BI Mobile apps. One feature that was originally included but Microsoft later removed was annotations. However, the Windows Ink Sketch Tool (only available in touch-enabled devices) has similar features, including taking a snapshot, annotating and sharing. For more information about how to use the Sketch Tool, refer to the "Windows Ink: How to use Screen Sketch" article at http://windowscentral.com/windows-ink-how-use-screen-sketch.

5.2   Viewing Content

Power BI Mobile provides simple and intuitive interface for viewing reports and dashboards. As it stands, Power BI Mobile doesn't allow users to edit the published content. This shouldn't be viewed as a limitation because mobile display capabilities are limited, and mobile users would be primarily interested in viewing content. Next, you'll practice viewing the BI content you created in the previous two chapters using the iPhone native app. As a prerequisite, install the iOS Power BI Mobile app from AppStore.

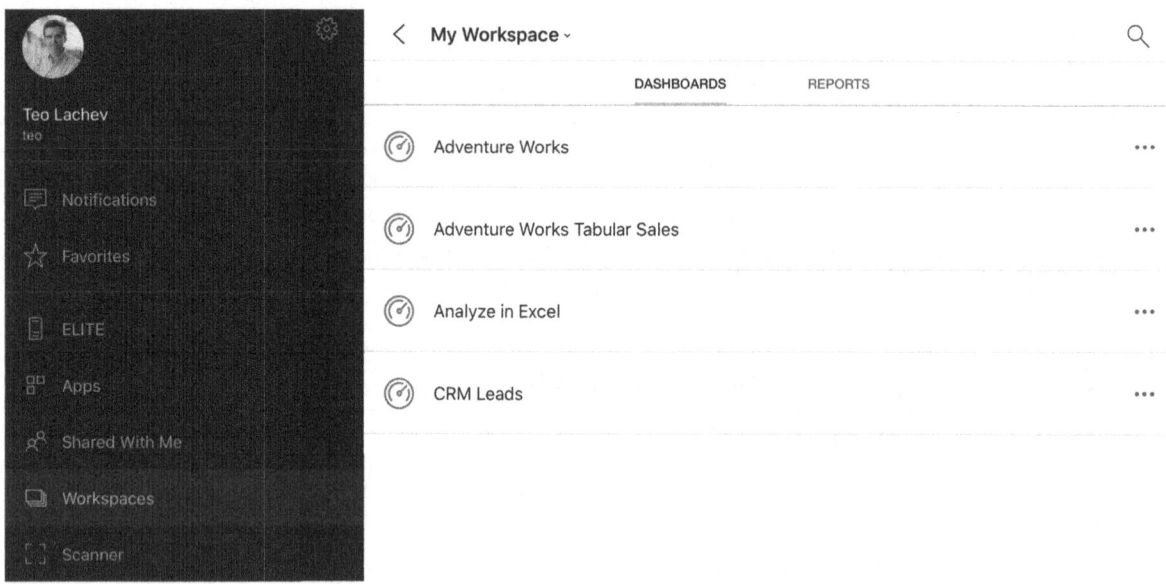

Figure 5.5   The navigation experience of the iPhone app.

5.2.1   Getting Started with Power BI Mobile

When you open the iPhone Power BI app and sign in to Power BI, you'll be presented with a landing page. If you have previously marked dashboards as favorites, the landing page will show a list of these dashboards. Or, if you have subscribed to apps, the landing page will show these apps. Otherwise, the landing page will let you know that you have no apps and encourage you to go to Power BI Service and add apps. When you expand the menu in the top-left corner, you'll see the navigation bar shown in **Figure 5.5**. Let's go quickly through the links starting from the top.

Understanding settings
Clicking the Settings (gear) menu in the top-right corner opens the Settings page (see **Figure 5.6**). The Accounts section allows you to sign in to Power BI. If your organization has installed Power BI Report Server, the "Connect to server" link allows you to add one or more report servers. To do so, you need to provide

the server address, such as https://<ServerName>/reports, and an optional friendly name so you can tell the servers apart.

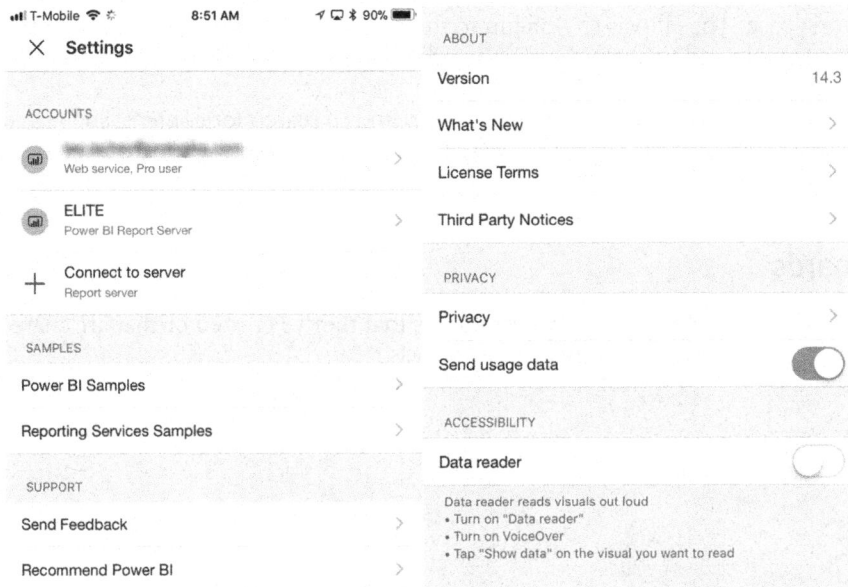

Figure 5.6 The iPhone Settings page allows you to sign it to Power BI, connect to report servers, and control app settings.

The samples section is to view sample Power BI and SSRS reports. Unlike Power BI Service, samples are ready to browse, and you don't have to install them. The Support section has links to send feedback to Microsoft and recommend Power BI to other people via email. The About section shows details about the Power BI app. You can use the Privacy section to read the Microsoft privacy statement and allow the Power BI app to send usage data to Microsoft. Finally, the Accessibility section allows people with accessibility needs to turn on data reader and hear information about visuals.

 TIP Looking for an easy way to demonstrate Power BI content in mobile apps? Currently, there are six dashboards available for VP Sales, Director of Operations, Customer Care, Director of Marketing, CFO, and HR Manager. And, if you connect your mobile app to a Power BI Report Server, you can get Reporting Services samples as well.

Understanding navigation bar

Next, let's explore the navigation menus starting from the top:

- Notifications – Shows the notifications from the Power BI Service Notification Center.
- Favorites – Shows dashboards that you marked as favorites.
- Power BI Report servers – If your organization has integrated Power BI Report Server with Power BI, the next links will show the friendly names of the report server(s) you've added. You can click each link to navigate the report catalog, and to view Power BI reports, SSRS mobile reports and KPIs.
- Apps – Allows you to access your Power BI apps that you have previously installed.
- Shared With Me – Shows the list of dashboards that other people have shared with you.
- Workspaces – Shows the workspaces you are a member of so that you can select a workspace to work with. My Workspace is the default workspace.
- Scanner – This link shows only on mobile phones. It allows you to scan a Power BI QR code so that you can navigate to the report tagged with that code.

Browsing workspace content

Once you select a menu in the navigation bar, the relevant content shows in the right pane. Back to **Figure 5.5**, I've clicked the Workspaces menu, and then I've selected My Workspace. The Dashboards tab lists all dashboards in the selected workspace. The ellipsis (…) menu to the right of the dashboard name allows me to mark the dashboard as a favorite and to share the dashboard with others. And the Reports tab lists all reports hosted in the workspace.

Use the Search button to view most recent content you've visited and to search for content, such as to type "sales" to see all sales-related reports and dashboards. Matches are organized in dashboards, reports, and groups (workspaces) sections.

5.2.2 Viewing Dashboards

Mobile users will primarily use Power BI Mobile to view dashboards that they've created or that are shared with them. Let's see what options are available for viewing dashboards.

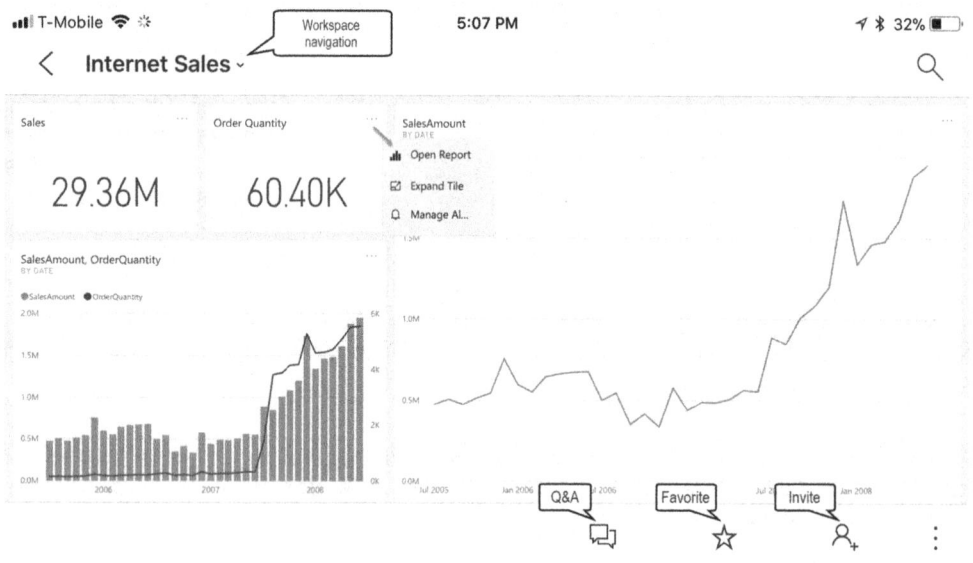

Figure 5.7 The Internet Sales dashboard open in Power BI Mobile.

Working with dashboards

This exercise uses the Internet Sales dashboard that you created in the previous chapter.

1. On your iPhone, open the Power BI app.

2. From the navigation bar, click Workspaces and select My Workspace.

3. In the Dashboards tab, click the Internet Sales dashboard to open it (see **Figure 5.7**). Power BI Mobile renders the dashboard content as it appears in the Power BI portal.

4. Click the Q&A button at the bottom of the page and notice that you can type or speak natural questions. As you type your question, the app shows suggestions just like Power BI Service. Unlike Power BI Service, however, when you submit your question, the app shows not only a report but also narrated quick insights. For example, if you type "sales by year", you'll get a line chart and related insights, such as "There is a correlation between product and internet sales". When you click the insight, it shows it as a visual.

5. Back to the dashboard, if you'd like to mark the dashboard as a favorite, click the Favorite button (star).

6. If you want to share the dashboard with someone else, click the Invite button.

7. Expand the Workspace Navigation dropdown and notice that it shows which workspace the dashboard is located in. The back arrow button lets you navigate backward to the content. For example, if you click it, the mobile app will navigate you to the Internet Sales dashboard. If you click again, you'll be in My Workspace if the Internet Sales dashboard is in this workspace.

Working with tiles

There are additional features specific to tiles. You can click the ellipsis (…) menu to access the most popular actions: drill: Open Report (drill to the underlying report), Expand Tile (opens the tile in focus), Manage Alerts (set up and manage alerts).

1. Click the Sales tile. As you would recall, clicking a tile in Power BI Portal drills the tile through the underlying visualization (which could originate from several sources, including pinning a visual from a report or Q&A). However, instead of drilling through, Power BI Mobile pops the tile out so that you can examine the tile data (see **Figure 5.8**).

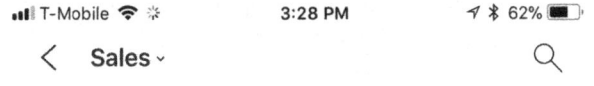

29.36M

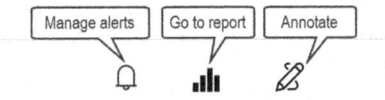

Figure 5.8 Clicking a tile opens the tile in focus mode.

Microsoft refers to this as "focus" mode. Because the display of mobile devices is limited, the focus mode makes it easier to view and explore the tile data. That's why this is the default action when you click a tile.

Understanding tile actions

When a tile is in focus, users can take several actions. You can click "Manage alerts" to create and manage alerts for visualizations that display a single value (Single Card, Gauge, and KPIs). It has the identical settings as in Power BI Service to allow mobile users to create alerts while they are on the go. But when the underlying data meets the condition, you'll get an in-app notification on your phone instead of an email.

The "Go to report" button bring you to the underlying report which the visualization was pinned from. This action opens the report in Reading View (Power BI Mobile doesn't support Editing View). The Reports menu is available only for tiles created by pinning visualizations from existing reports. You won't see the Report menu for tiles created with Q&A.

I'll postpone discussing annotations to the Sharing and Collaboration section.

Examining the data

It might be challenging to understand the precise values of a busy chart on a mobile device. However, Power BI Mobile has a useful feature that you might find helpful.

1. Navigate back to the Internet Sales dashboard and click the line chart.

2. In the line chart, drag the vertical bar to intersect the chart line for Jan 2006, as shown in **Figure 5.9**.

Notice that Power BI Mobile shows the precise value of the sales amount at the intersection. If you have a Scatter Chart (the Retail Analysis Sample dashboard has a Scatter Chart), you can pop out a chart and select a bubble by positioning the intersection of a vertical line and a horizontal line. This allows you to see the values of the fields placed in the X Axis, Y Axis, and Size areas of the Scatter visualization. And for a Pie Chart, you can spin the chart to position the slices so that you can get the exact values.

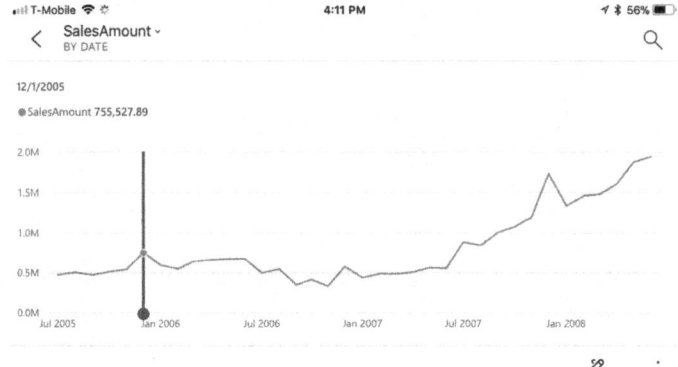

Figure 5.9 You can drag the vertical bar to see the precise chart value.

5.2.3 Viewing Reports

As you've seen, Power BI Mobile makes it easy for business users to view dashboards on the go. You can also view reports. As I mentioned, Power BI Mobile doesn't allow you to edit reports; you can only open and interact with them in Reading View.

TIP As you'll discover, regular Power BI reports don't reflow when you turn your phone in a portrait mode. Unlike dashboards which reflow, reports always render in landscape. However, you can use Power BI Desktop to create a special phone-optimized view for each page on the report. Phone-optimized reports have a special icon in the Reports tab. For more information about how to create phone-optimized report layouts, refer to the "Create reports optimized for the Power BI phone apps" topic at https://powerbi.microsoft.com/documentation/powerbi-desktop-create-phone-report/.

Viewing Power BI reports
Let's open the Internet Sales Analysis report in Power BI Mobile. **Figure 5.10** shows the report.

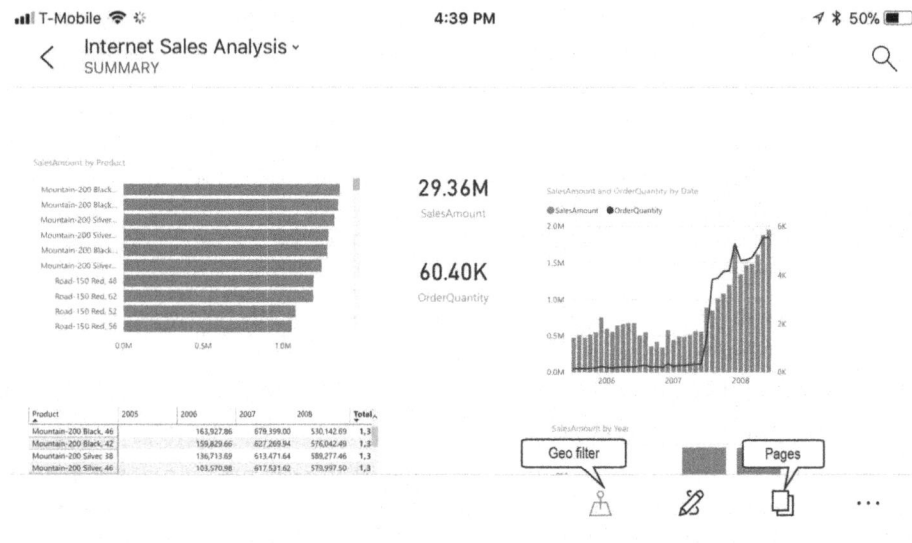

Figure 5.10 Power BI Mobile opens reports in Reading View but supports interactive features.

1. Navigate to your workspace. You can do this by clicking the Back button in the top-left area of the screen.

2. Under the Reports section, click the Internet Sales Analysis report to open it. Power BI Mobile opens the report in Reading View. Notice that you can't switch to Editing View to change the report. You shouldn't view this as a limitation because the small display size of mobile devices would probably make reporting and editing difficult anyway. Although you can't change the report, you can interact with it.

3. Click any bar in the Bar Chart or a column in the Column Chart. Notice that automatic highlighting works, and you can see the contribution of the selected value to the data shown in the other visualizations. However, the other interactive features, such as drilling through or exporting data, are not available.

4. Click a column header in the Matrix visualization and note that every click toggles the column sort order.

5. The Pages button shows you a list of the report pages, so you can navigate to another page. You can also swipe the report to the right or left to go to the next or previous page.

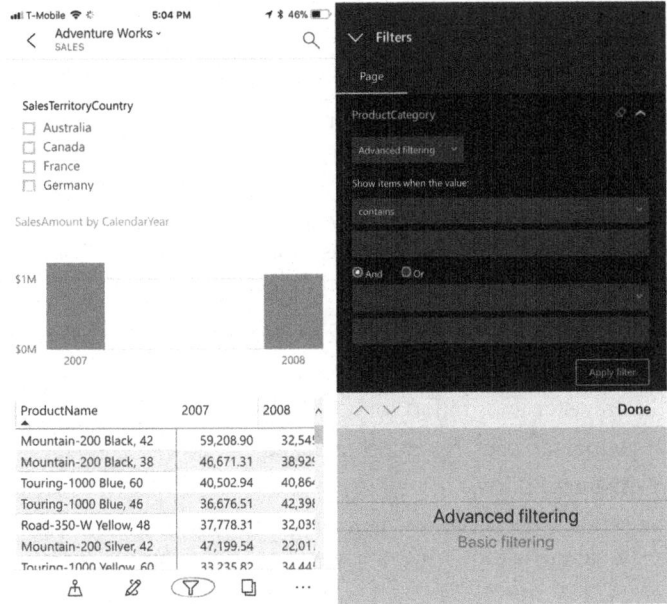

Figure 5.11 Available in phone-optimized report layouts only, the Filters pane lets you apply visual, page, and report filters.

Filtering report data

Examining the icons at the bottom, the first button ("Geo filter") is only available for reports with map visuals. Use it to filter a map to your current location. For example, imagine a sales person visiting customers. He opens a report that shows customer sales by state. He's in Georgia and he only wants to filter the report to show customers in Georgia. He can click Geo filter which will discover his location so that he can filter the map to show only Georgia.

Recall that Power BI reports allow you to specify visual, page, and report filters. You might wonder why the Filter pane is nowhere to be found in the iPhone app. As it turns out, you need a phone-optimized report to get the filtering options. If you use Power BI Desktop to create a phone-optimized layout, then you'll discover that the Filters button is available at the bottom of the report (see **Figure 5.11**). It will bring you to the Filters page that will show the page and report filters. And when you tap a visual on the report, it will also show visual-level filters. As in Power BI, the Filters page supports Basic and Advanced filtering options.

As you'd recall, prefiltering the report content at design time (by setting slicers or filtering options in the Filter pane) preserves the filters when users view the reports. When you view a prefiltered report, the app will show a status bar at the top of the page, notifying you that there are active filters on the report.

Viewing Excel reports

Remember that Power BI allows you to connect existing Excel reports. Let's see what happens when you open an Excel report.

1. Navigate to My Workspace.
2. In the Reports section of the workspace content page, click the Reseller Sales report.

Notice that the report won't open inside the app. Instead, the app informs you that to view an Excel workbook, it must be saved to OneDrive. That's because Excel reports are rendered in Excel Online, which is a cloud service and it's not available in the mobile app. To view the workbook, you must either open the browser and navigate to powerbi.com or save the workbook to OneDrive before you connect to it.

Viewing reports in Power BI Report Server

If your organization uses Power BI Report Server, you can view content from a report server running in native mode. Currently, you can view three types of content:

- Power BI reports – Power BI Report Server allows users to upload Power BI Desktop files to the report catalog. If the file has a report and you have permissions, you can view the report in Power BI Mobile.
- KPIs – Starting with SQL Server 2016 Reporting Services, you can define key performance indicators (KPIs) directly in a SSRS folder (without creating a report). These KPIs will show up in the Power BI mobile apps.
- Mobile reports – A new report type in SQL Server 2016 Reporting Services, mobile reports are optimized for mobile devices. When you navigate to a report folder that has mobile reports, you'll see thumbnail images of the reports. Clicking a report opens it inside the mobile app.

 NOTE Currently, traditional paginated (RDL) Reporting Services reports won't show up in the mobile apps. You can navigate the report catalog but you can't see them.

Before you can access SSRS content, you need to register your report server:

1. In the navigation bar, click Settings. On the Accounts tab click "Connect to server".
2. Fill in the server address, such as http://<servernname/reports.
3. (Optional) Under "Advanced options", give the server a user-friendly name, such as Reporting Services. This is the name you'll see when you click the global navigation button (the yellow home button in the top-left corner).

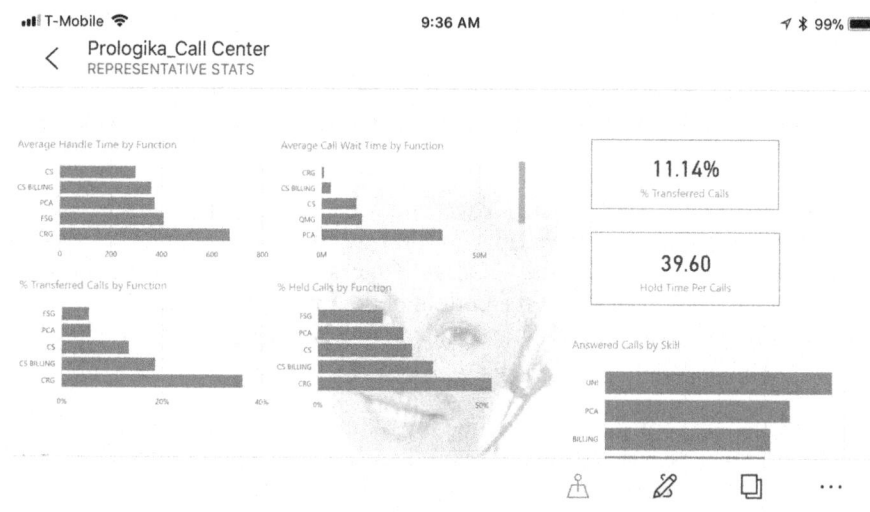

Figure 5.12 Access KPIs, Power BI reports, and mobile reports in your mobile app.

4. Click Connect.

Once you are connected, you can view the reports that you're authorized to access.

5. In the navigation bar, tap your report server.

6. Navigate to the folder as instructed by your administrator. If the folder has Power BI reports, mobile reports, or KPIs, they'll show up in Power BI Mobile. You can tell Power BI reports by a special icon that looks like a column chart.

7. Click a Power BI report. **Figure 5.12** shows a Power BI report that I've previously deployed to Power BI Report Server. It renders online, just like when you view the report in Power BI Service.

> 💡 **TIP** If you mark reports or KPIs as favorites on your Power BI Report Server portal, they'll appear in the Power BI Favorites folder and you can access them by clicking Favorites in the navigation bar.

5.3 Sharing and Collaboration

Power BI Mobile goes beyond just content viewing. It lets mobile workers share BI content and collaborate while on the go. Specifically, they can share dashboards with other users and annotate dashboard tiles and reports. Let's examine these two features in more detail.

5.3.1 Sharing Dashboards

Remember from the previous chapter that Power BI Service allows you to share dashboards with your colleagues by sending email invitations. You can do the same with Power BI Mobile. Both options are interchangeable. For example, if you initiate dashboard sharing in Power BI Service, you can see the sharing settings in Power BI Mobile, and vice versa. Let's share a dashboard but remember that all sharing options require a Power BI Pro license:

1. Back to the Home page, click the Internet Sales dashboard to open it.

2. Click the Invite button 🔗 in the bottom-right corner.

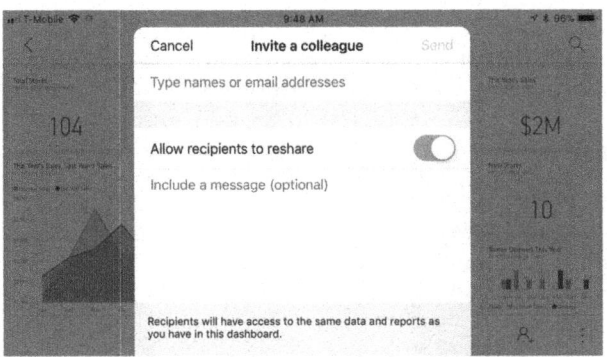

Figure 5.13 Power BI Mobile lets you share dashboards with your coworkers.

This action opens the "Invite a colleague" flyout window (see **Figure 5.13**). You need to enter the recipient email addresses, type in an optional message, and decide if you want them to be able to re-share the dashboards.

5.3.2 Annotating Tiles and Reports

While you're viewing the dashboard content, you might want to comment on some data and then share the comment with your coworkers. For example, after sharing her dashboard with a manager, Maya might ask the manager to formally approve that the data is correct. Her manager can open the dashboard on his mobile device, sign the dashboard, and then send a screenshot to Maya. Annotations allow you to enter text, simple graphics, or a smiley, and then share a screenshot of the annotated content. Annotations aren't saved in the Power BI content. Once you exit the annotation mode, all annotations are lost.

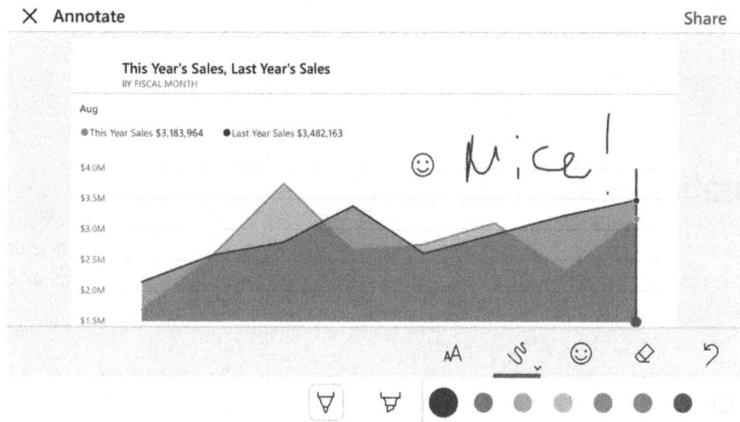

Figure 5.14 You can annotate a tile by typing text, drawing lines, or placing stamps.

Adding annotations

You can annotate dashboard tiles, entire reports, or specific report visualizations. Let's annotate a dashboard tile:

1. With the Retail Analysis Sample dashboard open, click the "This Year's Sales, Last Year's Sales" surface chart to open it in focus mode.

2. Click the Annotate (pencil) button in the bottom-right corner. This switches the tile to annotation mode.

3. Click the Smiley button and then click the first smiley icon to add a smiley to the tile. Position the smiley as shown in **Figure 5.14**.

4. Click the curve icon to the right of the smiley icon, and type some text on the tile. If you make a mistake, you can click the Undo button in the bottom-right corner. The eraser button discards all your annotations.

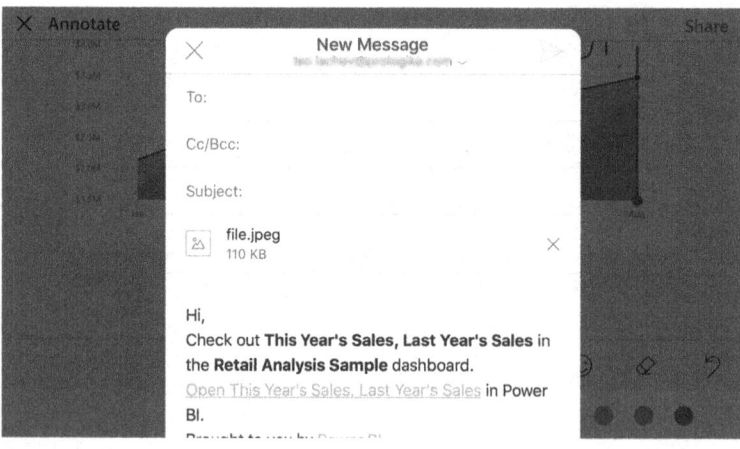

Figure 5.15 You can share screenshots of your annotations with your coworkers by email.

Sharing screenshots

You can send screenshots to your colleagues by a text message or email. Let's send a screenshot of your annotations:

1. In annotation mode, click the Share link in the top right corner of the screen.
2. A flyout window asks you if you want to choose a delivery mechanism. Click Mail or whatever application you use as email client.
3. Power BI Mobile captures a screenshot of the annotated item (tile, report, or specific report visualization), and attaches it to the email (see **Figure 5.15**). It also includes a link to the item. Enter the recipient addresses separated by a semi-colon (;) and click the Send button.

If the recipients have rights to view the annotated item, such as when you've already shared the dashboard with them or you share the same workspace, they can click the link to go straight to the item.

5.4 Summary

Power BI Mobile is a collective name of three native applications for iOS, Android, and Windows devices. Power BI Mobile enriches the data analysis experience of mobile workers. Besides dashboard and report viewing, it allows you to share dashboards and annotate dashboard tiles. You can also create a data alert and get a notification when data meets specific thresholds that you specify.

This chapter concludes our Power BI tour for business users. Power BI has much more to offer than what you've seen so far, but it requires more knowledge. In the next part of the book, you'll see how data analysts (also referred to as power users) can create sophisticated data models to address more complicated data analytics needs.

PART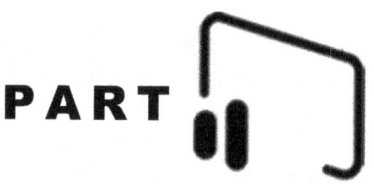

Power BI for Data Analysts

I f you consider yourself a data analyst or power user, welcome! This part of the book teaches you how to implement self-service models with Power BI Desktop. If you're new to self-service data analytics, I recommend you review the first part of the book "Power BI for Business Users" beforehand as it explains important self-service BI and Power BI fundamentals.

As you've seen in the first part of the book, Power BI lets business users perform rudimentary data analysis without requiring data models. However, once the self-service BI path goes beyond apps and one-table datasets, you'll need a data model. Although you can still implement models with Excel, Power BI Desktop is the Power BI premium modeling tool for self-service BI. Packed with features, Power BI Desktop is a free tool that you can download and start using immediately to gain insights from your data.

If you have experience with Excel data modeling, you'll find that Power BI Desktop combines the best of Power Pivot, Power Query, and Power View in a simplified and standalone desktop tool. In this part of the book, I'll introduce you to Power BI Desktop and fundamental data modeling concepts. Next, you'll learn how to connect to data from a variety of data sources, ranging from relational databases, text files, Excel files, and cloud services.

Data quality is a big issue with many organizations and chances are that your data is no exception. Fortunately, Power BI Desktop has features that allow you to cleanse and transform dirty data before it enters your model, so you won't have to rely on someone else to clean the data for you. A self-service data model is rarely complete without important business metrics. Thanks to its Data Analysis Expressions (DAX) language, Power BI Desktop lets you implement sophisticated calculations using Excel-like formulas. Then you can explore your data by creating interactive reports as you can do in Power BI Service.

If you're already a Power Pivot user, you'll undoubtedly breeze through the content of this part of the book (this will be a review with some important new changes). As you'll find out, you can almost seamlessly transfer your Excel data modeling knowledge to Power BI Desktop. Again, that's because the underlying technology is the same. However, with Power BI Desktop, you'll always have the latest Power BI features because Microsoft updates it every month.

Also, know that Power BI Desktop and Analysis Services Tabular share the same foundation – the in-memory xVelocity data engine. Therefore, a nice bonus awaits you ahead. While you're learning Power BI Desktop, you're also learning Analysis Services Tabular. So, if one day you decide to upgrade your self-service model from Power BI Desktop to a scalable organizational model powered by Analysis Services Tabular, you'll find that you already have most of the knowledge. You're now a BI pro!

To practice what you'll learn, the book includes plenty of exercises that will walk you through the steps for implementing a self-service model for analyzing sales data.

Chapter 6

Data Modeling Fundamentals

As a first step to building a data model, you need to acquire the data that you'll analyze and report on. Power BI Desktop makes it easy to access data from a variety of data sources, ranging from relational databases, such as a SQL Server database, to text files, such as a comma-delimited file extracted from a mainframe system. The most common way of bringing data into Power BI Desktop is by importing it from relational databases. When the data isn't in a database, Power BI Desktop supports other data acquisition methods, including text files, cubes, data feeds, and much more. And for some fast databases, Power BI Desktop allows you to connect directly to the data source without importing the data.

In this chapter, you'll learn the fundamentals of self-service data modeling with Power BI Desktop. To put your knowledge in practice, you'll implement a raw data model for analyzing the Adventure Works reseller sales. You'll exercise a variety of basic data import options to load data from the Adventure Works data warehouse, a cube, an Excel workbook, a comma-delimited file, and even from a Reporting Services report. You'll find the resulting Adventure Works model in the \Source\ch06 folder.

6.1   Understanding Data Models

When you work with Power BI Desktop, you create a self-service data model with the data you need to analyze. As a first step, you need to obtain the data. The primary data acquisition option with Power BI Desktop is importing it. This option allows you to load and mash up data from different data sources into a consolidated data model. For example, Martin could import some CRM data from Salesforce, finance data from Excel reports, and sales data from the corporate data warehouse. Once Martin relates all this data into a single model, he can then create a report that combines these three business areas. As you might realize, Power BI Desktop gives you tremendous power and flexibility for creating self-service data models!

Power BI Desktop allows you to import data from a variety of data sources with a few mouse clicks. While getting data is easy, relating data in your model requires some planning on your side to avoid inconsistent or even incorrect results. For example, you might have imported a Customer table and a Sales table, but if there isn't a way to relate the data in these tables, you'll get the same sales amount repeated for each customer. Therefore, before you click the Get Data button, you should have some basic understanding about the Power BI data modeling requirements and limitations. So, let's start by learning some important fundamentals of data modeling. Among other things, they will help you understand why having a single monolithic dataset is not always the best approach and why you should always have a date table.

6.1.1 Understanding Schemas

I previously wrote that Power BI Desktop imports data in tables, like how Excel allows you to organize data into Excel tables. Each table consists of columns, also referred to as *fields* or *attributes*. If all the data is provided to you as just one table, then you could congratulate yourself and skip this section altogether. In fact, as you've seen in Part 1 of this book, you can skip Power BI Desktop and modeling because you can analyze a single dataset directly with Power BI Service. Chances are, however, that you might need to import multiple tables from the same or different data sources. This requires learning some basic database and schema concepts. The term "schema" here is used to describe the table definitions and how tables relate to each other. I'll keep the discussion light on purpose to get you started with data modeling as fast as possible. I'll revisit table relationships in the next chapter.

 NOTE Importing all data as a single table might not require modeling but it isn't a best practice. Suppose you initially wanted to analyze reseller sales and you've imported a single dataset with columns such as Reseller, Sales Territory, and so on. Then you decide to extend the model with direct sales to consumers to consolidate reporting that spans now two business areas. Now you have a problem. Because you merged business dimensions into the reseller sales dataset, you won't be able to slice and dice the two datasets by the same lookup tables (Reseller, Sales Territory, Date, and others). In addition, a large table might strain your computer resources as it'll require more time to import and more memory to store the data. At the same time, a fully normalized schema, such as modeling a product entity with Product, Subcategory, and Category tables, is also not desirable because you'll end up with many tables and the model might become difficult to understand and navigate. When modeling your data, it's important to find a good balance between business requirements and normalization, and that balance is the star schema.

Understanding star schemas

For a lack of better terms, I'll use the dimensional modeling terminology to illustrate the star schema (for more information about star schemas, see http://en.wikipedia.org/wiki/Star_schema). **Figure 6.1** shows two schema types. The left diagram illustrates a star schema, where the ResellerSales table is in the center. This table stores the history of the Adventure Works reseller sales, and each row represents the most atomic information about the sale transaction. This could be a line item in the sales order that includes the order quantity, sales amount, tax amount, discount, and other numeric fields.

Dimensional modeling refers to these tables as *fact tables*. As you can imagine, the ResellerSales table can be very long if it keeps several years of sales data. Don't be alarmed about the dataset size though. Thanks to the state-of-the art underlying storage technology, your data model can still import and store millions of rows!

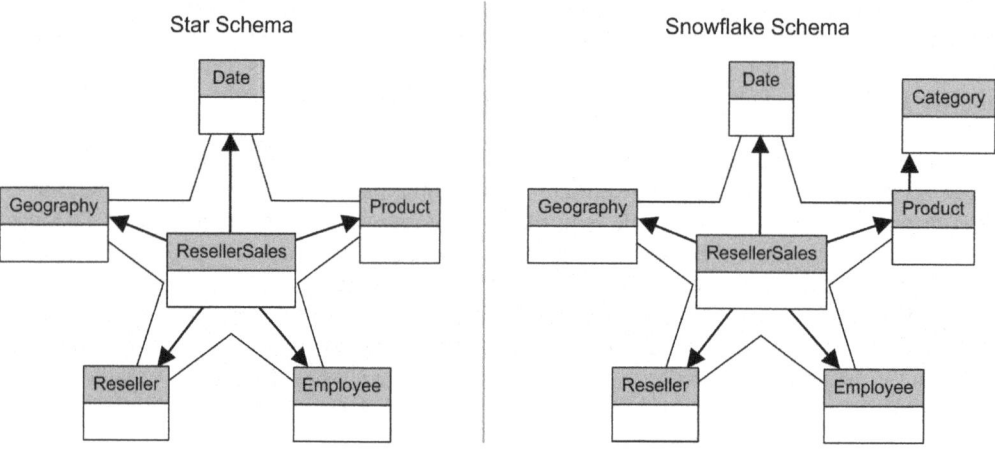

Figure 6.1 Power BI models support both star and snowflake schema types.

The ResellerSales table is related to other tables, called *lookup* or *dimension* tables. These tables provide contextual information to each row stored in the ResellerSales table. For example, the Date table might include date-related fields, such as Date, Quarter, and Year columns, to allow you to aggregate data at day, quarter, and year levels, respectively. The Product table might include ProductName, Color, and Size fields, and so on.

The reason why your data model should have these fields in separate lookup tables, is that, for the most part, their content doesn't need a historical record. For example, if the product name changes, this probably would be an in-place change. By contrast, if you were to continue adding columns to the ResellerSales table, you might end up with performance and maintenance issues. If you need to make a change, you might have to update millions of rows of data as opposed to updating a single row. Similarly, if you were to add a new column to the Date table, such as FiscalYear, you'll have to update all the rows in the ResellerSales table.

Are you limited to only one fact table with Power BI? Absolutely not! For example, you can add an InternetSales fact table that stores direct sales to individuals. In the case of multiple fact tables, you should model the fact tables to share some common lookup tables so that you could match and consolidate data for cross-reporting purposes, such as to show reseller and Internet sales side by side and grouped by year and product. This is another reason to avoid a single monolithic dataset and to have logically related fields in separate tables (if you have this option). Don't worry if this isn't immediately clear. Designing a model that accurately represents business requirements is difficult even for BI pros but it gets easier with practice.

NOTE Another common issue that I witness with novice users is creating a separate dataset for each report, e.g. one dataset for a report showing reseller sales and another dataset for a report showing direct sales. Like the "single dataset" issue I discussed above, this design will lead to data duplication and inability to produce consolidated reports that span multiple areas. Even worse would be to embed calculations in the dataset, such as calculating Profit or Year-to-Date in a SQL view that is used to source the data. Like the issue with defining calculations in a report, this approach will surely lead to redundant calculations or calculations that produce different results from one report to another.

Understanding snowflake schemas

A *snowflake* schema is where some lookup tables relate to other lookup tables, but not directly to the fact table. Going back to **Figure 6.1**, you can see that for whatever reason, the product categories are kept in a Category table that relates to the Product table and not directly to the ResellerSales table. One strong motivation for snowflaking is that you might have another fact table, such as SalesQuota, that stores data not at a product level but at a category level. If you keep categories in their own Category table, this design would allow you to join the Category lookup table to the SalesQuota table, and you'll still be able to have a report that shows aggregated sales and quota values grouped by category.

Power BI supports snowflake schemas just fine. However, if you have a choice, you should minimize snowflaking when it's not needed. This is because snowflaking increases the number of tables in the model, making it more difficult for other users to understand your model. If you import data from a database with a normalized schema, you can minimize snowflaking by merging snowflaked tables. For example, you can use a SQL query that joins the Product and Category tables. However, if you import text files, you won't have that option because you can't use SQL. However, when you use Power BI Desktop, you can still handle denormalization tasks in the Query Editor, or by adding calculated columns that use DAX expressions to accomplish the same goal, such as by adding a column to the Product table to look up the product category from the Category table. Then you can hide the Category table.

To recap this schema discussion, you can view the star schema as the opposite of its snowflake counterpart. While the snowflake schema embraces normalization as the preferred designed technique to reduce data duplication, the star schema favors denormalization or data entities and reducing the overall number of tables, although this process results in data duplication (a category is repeated for each product that has the same category). Demormalization (star schemas) and BI go hand in hand. That's because star schemas reduce the number of tables and required joins. This makes your model faster and more intuitive.

Understanding date tables

Even if the data is given to you as a single dataset, you should strongly consider having a separate date table. A date table stores a range of dates that you need for data analysis. A date table typically includes additional columns for flexible time exploration, such as Quarter, Year, Fiscal Quarter, Fiscal Year, Holiday Flag, and so on. In addition, DAX time calculations, such as TOTALYTD, TOTALQTD, and so on, require a separate date table. A date table must meet several requirements:

- It must have a column of a Date data type.

- It must also have a day granularity, where each row in the table represents a calendar day.

- It must contain a consecutive range of dates you need for analysis, such as starting from the first day with data to a few years in the future. More importantly, a date table can't have gaps (it can't skip days). If it has gaps, DAX time calculations will produce wrong results.

There are many ways to create a date table. You can import it from your corporate data warehouse, if you have one. You can maintain it in an Excel file and import it from there. You can import it from the DateStream feed, as I'll show you in section 6.2.7. You can even generate it in the Query Editor using custom code written in the query language (referred to as "M"), as I'll show you in the next chapter. And you can have more than one date table in your model. This could be useful if you want to aggregate the same fact table by multiple dates, such as order date, ship date, and due date.

 NOTE To avoid requiring date tables, Power BI Desktop is configured to automatically generate date hierarchies (the Auto Date/Time setting in File ⇨ Options and Settings ⇨ Options (Data Load tab) is on). This feature generates a date table with a Year-Quarter-Month-Day hierarchy for *every* date field. This can severely bloat your data model if you have millions of rows and dates with large time spans. To make things worse, time calculations in Quick Measures (discussed in Chapter 9) won't work if this feature is off. If you plan to use Quick Measures, leave it on, but monitor the size of your data model. A best practice is to have a separate date table and write time calculations to use this table.

6.1.2 Introducing Relationships

Once you import multiple tables, you need a way to relate them. If two tables aren't related, your model won't aggregate data correctly when you use both tables on a report. To understand how to relate tables, you need to learn about Power BI relationships.

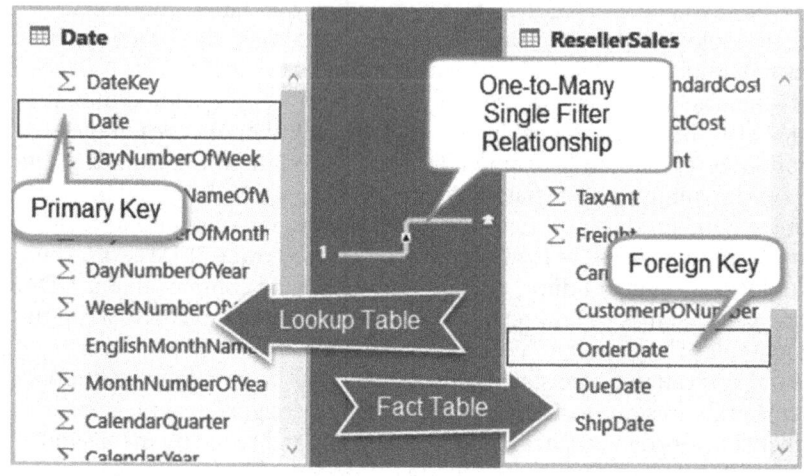

Figure 6.2 The Date column (primary key) in the Date table is related to the matching OrderDate column (foreign key) in the ResellerSales table.

Understanding relationships

In order to relate two tables, there must be schema and data commonalities between the two tables. This isn't much different than joins in relational databases, such as Microsoft Access or SQL Server. For example, you won't be able to analyze sales by product if there isn't a common column between the ResellerSales and Date tables that ties a date to a sale (see **Figure 6.2**).

If the underlying data source has relationships (referential integrity constraints) defined, Power BI Desktop will detect and carry them to the model (this is controlled by the "Import relationships from data sources" setting in File ⇨ Options and setting ⇨ Options ⇨ Data Load under the Current File session). If not, Power BI is capable of auto-detecting relationships using internal rules (this is controlled by the "Autodetect new relationships after data is loaded" setting in the same section). Of course, you can also create relationships manually. It's important to understand that your data model is layered on top of the original data. No model changes affect the original data source and its design. You only need rights to read from the data source so that you can import the data you need.

Understanding keys

Common columns in each pair of tables are called *keys*. A *primary key* is a column that uniquely identifies each row in a table. A primary key column can't have duplicate values. For example, the Date column uniquely identifies each row in the Date table and no other row has the same value. An employee identifier or an e-mail address can be used as a primary key in an Employee table. To join Date to ResellerSales, in the ResellerSales table, you must have a matching column, which is called a *foreign key*. For example, the OrderDate column in the ResellerSales table is a foreign key.

A matching column means a column in the fact table that has matching values in the lookup table. The column names of the primary key and foreign key don't have to be the same (values are important). For example, if the ResellerSales table has a sale recorded on 1/1/2015, there should be a row in the Date table with date in the Date column of 1/1/2016. If there isn't, the data model won't show an error, but all the sales that don't have matching dates in the Data table would appear under an unknown (blank) value in a report that groups ResellerSales data by some column in the Date table.

Typically, a fact table has several foreign keys, so it can be related to different lookup tables. For performance reasons, you should use shorter data types, such as integers or dates. For example, the Date column could be a column of a Date data type. Or if you're importing from a data warehouse database, it might have an Integer data type, with values such as 20110101 for January 1st, 2011, and 20110102 for January 2nd, 2011, and so on.

NOTE Relationships from fact tables to the same lookup table don't have to use the same column. For example, ResellerSales can join Date on the Date column but InternetSales might join it on the DateKey column, for example in the case where there isn't a column of a Date data type in InternetSales. If a column uniquely identifies each row, the lookup table can have different "primary key" columns.

About relationship cardinality

Note back in in **Figure 6.2**, the number 1 is shown on the left side of the relationship towards the Date table and an asterisk (*) is shown next to the Reseller Sales table. This denotes a one-to-many cardinality. To understand this better, consider that one row (one date) in the Date table can have zero, one, or many recorded sales in ResellerSales, and one product in the Product table corresponds to one or many sales in ResellerSales, and so on. The important word here is "many".

Although not a common cardinality, Power BI also supports a one-to-one relationship type. For example, you might have Employee and SalesPerson tables in a snowflake schema, where a sales person is a type of an employee and each sales person relates to a single employee. By specifying a one-to-one relationship between Employee and SalesPerson, you're telling Power BI to check the data cardinality and show an error if the one-to-many relationship is detected on data refresh. A one-to-one relationship also brings additional simplifications when working with DAX calculations, such as to let you interchangeably use the DAX RELATED and RELATEDTABLE functions.

About relationship cross filter direction

Note also that in **Figure 6.2**, there's an arrow indicator pointing toward the ResellerSales table. This indicates that this relationship has a single cross filtering direction between the Date and Reseller tables. In other words, the ResellerSales table can be analyzed using the Date table, but not the other way around. For example, you can have a report that groups sales by any of the fields of the Date table. However, you can't group dates by a field in the ResellerSales table, which is probably meaningless anyway.

Now suppose you want to know how many times a product is sold by date. You might be able to find the answer by counting on a ProductKey field in the ResellerSales table without involving the Product table at all. However, what if you need to find how many times a product model (the ModelName column in the Product table) was sold on a given date? To avoid adding this column to the ResellerSales table, you'd want to count on the ModelName field in the Product table. However, this will cause the relationship direction to reverse. First, you need to follow the Date ⇨ ResellerSales relationship, which is one-to-many (no problems here), but then to get to the Product table, we need to traverse the many-to-one ResellerSales ⇨ Product relationship. Although Power BI Desktop won't show any error, the report will return meaningless results because the relationship filter won't propagate from ResellerSales to Product.

This is where a cross filtering direction set to Both can help. This cross filtering type is commonly referred to as a many-to-many relationship (many products can be sold on a single day and a single product can be sold on many days). It has a double arrow indicator (see **Figure 6.3**).

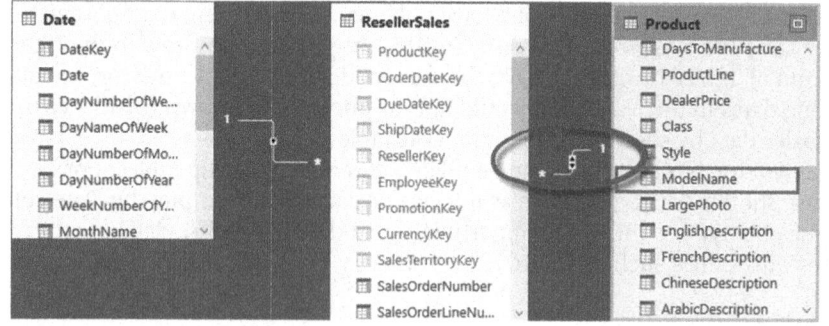

Figure 6.3   The relationship between the ResellerSales and Product table has a cross filtering direction set to Both.

Readers with prior experience in Power Pivot for Excel and Analysis Services Tabular (prior to SQL Server 2016) might recall that these tools didn't support declarative many-to-many relationships. This scenario required custom calculations so that aggregations are computed properly. Interestingly, the many-to-many relationship type (cross filtering set to both) is the default cross filtering type for new relationships in Power BI Desktop.

NOTE   At this point, you might be concerned about the performance overhead associated with bidirectional cross filtering. Rest assured that there isn't any additional performance overhead, so I welcome the decision to set relationship cross filtering to Both by default. There are scenarios, such as relationships to a Date table and closed-looped relationships, which require Single cross filtering, as you'll see in Chapter 8. To learn more about bidirectional cross filtering, read the related whitepaper by Kasper De Jonge at http://bit.ly/2eZUQ2Z.

That's all you need to know about data modeling for now. Next, let's see what options you have for connecting to your data.

6.1.3 Understanding Data Connectivity

In Chapter 2, I mentioned that Power BI supports two options for accessing data: data import and live connections, but this was a simplified statement. Technically, Power BI Service and Power BI Desktop support three options to connect to your data. Let me explain them to you now, because it's important to understand how they differ and when to use each one (if you have a choice). **Figure 6.4** should help you understand their differences.

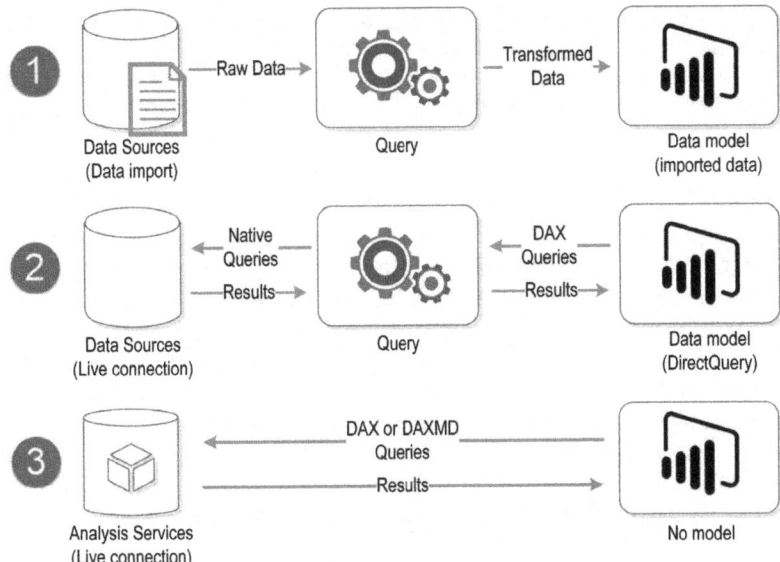

Figure 6.4 Power BI supports three connectivity options.

Importing data

Unless you connect to a single data source that supports direct connectivity, you'll need to import data. This is option 1 in the **Figure 6.4** diagram. What if you need to relate data from a data source that supports direct connections to some other data coming from a data source that doesn't support direct access? You'd still need to import the data and you need to do so from *both* data sources. As it stands, Power BI only supports a live connection to a single data source, and you can't mix "live" and imported data.

When Power BI imports the data, it stores the data in the xVelocity in-memory data engine. The in-memory engine is hosted in an out-of-process Analysis Services instance that is distributed with Power BI Desktop. So that you can pack millions of rows, data is stored in a highly compressed format and loaded in memory when you analyze the data. When you import data, you can transform and clean it before it's loaded into the model. Power BI Desktop always connects to raw data that you import via a connectivity component called a "query". Think of a query as a layer between the raw data and your data model. Yes, the Power BI Desktop query is a successor of Excel Power Query, which you might be familiar with. However, unlike Excel, queries aren't optional when you import data in Power BI Desktop.

> **NOTE** Data analysts experienced with Excel data modelling might know that Excel has at least three ways to import data into a data model – Excel native import, Power Pivot Table Import Wizard, and Power Query. There hasn't been a way in Excel to switch easily from one import option to another without recreating your table, such as from Table Import Wizard to Power Query, to use the Power Query transformation features. To simplify this, in Power BI Desktop, all the data import roads go through queries, which are the equivalent of Power Query in Excel. On the downside, even if you don't transform the data, queries add some performance overhead when extracting the data from the data source.

Unless you use advanced query features, such as query functions to automate importing data from multiple files, each imported table has a corresponding query. So, if you import three tables from a database and then import two files, you'll end up with five queries. A query is your insurance against current and future data quality issues. Even if the data is clean, such as when you load it from a data warehouse, it might still require some shaping later, and the query is the best place to perform these transformations.

Once the data is imported, the data is cached inside the Power BI Desktop file. Data exploration queries are handled internally by Power BI Desktop (or Power BI Service when the model is deployed). In other words, once the data is imported, Power BI Desktop doesn't open connections and query the original data source unless you refresh the data.

 NOTE Similar to Microsoft Office files, a Power BI Desktop file (*.pbix) is an archive zip file. If you rename it to have a zip extension and open it, you'll see that the imported data is stored in the DataModel folder. xVelocity (the storage engine that powers Excel data models), Power BI, Analysis Services Tabular and SQL Server columnstore indexes) uses internal algorithms to compress the data. Depending on the cardinality of the data you import, expect a compression ratio of 5:1 or higher.

Connecting live via DirectQuery

You might decide to connect Power BI Desktop to fast data sources that support direct (live) connectivity and then create reports that send native queries directly to these data sources (no data is cached in the model). This is option 2 in the **Figure 6.4** diagram. Only a subset of the data sources supports direct connectivity. The list includes Analysis Services (on premises or Azure), SQL Server, Oracle, Azure SQL Database, Azure SQL Data Warehouse, Teradata, Amazon Redshift, Spark on Azure HDInsight, Impala, or SAP Hana, but the list is growing as Power BI evolves.

One of the DirectQuery most important limitations is that you can connect live to a *single* data source only. For example, if you connect to a SQL Server database, that's the only data source you can use in your model. As I explained, you can't connect to other data sources live or to import some other data. You can't even connect live to another database in the same server. When you connect live to any of the supported data sources (other than Analysis Services), Power BI Desktop configures xVelocity in a special DirectQuery mode.

With DirectQuery, Power BI Desktop doesn't import any data, and xVelocity doesn't store any data. Instead, xVelocity generates DAX queries that the query layer translates to native queries. For example, if you connect Power BI Desktop to SQL Server with DirectQuery, the model will send T-SQL queries to SQL Server. Note that because Power BI uses the query layer in between, you can still perform basic data transformation tasks, such as column renaming. You can also create DAX calculations with some limitations. For example, DAX time calculations, such as TOTALYTD, are currently not supported with DirectQuery.

 NOTE Compared to importing data, DirectQuery has modeling limitations related to the complexity of auto-generating queries on the fly. To understand all DirectQuery limitations in Power BI Desktop, please read the document "Use DirectQuery in Power BI Desktop" at https://powerbi.microsoft.com/documentation/powerbi-desktop-use-directquery/.

When you connect to a data source that supports DirectQuery and before you load a table, Power BI Desktop will ask you how you want to get data: by importing data or by using DirectQuery (see **Figure 6.5**).

Connection Settings   ×

You can choose how to connect to this data source. Import allows you to
bring a copy of the data into Power BI. DirectQuery will connect live to this
data source.

⦿ Import
○ DirectQuery

Learn more about DirectQuery here

OK

Figure 6.5   When connecting to a data source that supports DirectQuery, you need to decide how to access the data.

In this case, I'm connecting to SQL Server and Power BI Desktop asks me if I want to import the data or use DirectQuery. If I select DirectQuery, Power BI Desktop will auto-generate native queries as I explore data and will show me the results it gets from SQL Server. DirectQuery supports limited modeling capabilities using the Data View and the Fields pane. You can create and manage relationships, rename the metadata (table and column names), and perform basic data transformations.

As I previously said, DirectQuery is currently limited to a single data source. If you attempt to import data from another data source (even if it supports DirectQuery), Power BI Desktop will disallow this. You'll be given a choice to cancel the import process or to switch to a data import mode and import all the data.

If you publish a DirectQuery model to Power BI Service, the dataset needs the Power BI on-premises data gateway to be installed on premises in standard mode (not personal) to connect live to the original data source. If the gateway is not configured, the dataset will be published but it will be disabled (it will show grayed out in the Power BI navigation bar) and you won't be able to use it.

Connecting live to Analysis Services

Finally, a special live connectivity option exists when you connect live to Analysis Services in all its flavors: Multidimensional, Tabular and published datasets using the Power BI Service in Get Data (see option 3 in the **Figure 6.4** diagram). In this case, the xVelocity engine isn't used at all. Instead, Power BI connects directly to Analysis Services. Power BI generates DAX queries when connected to Analysis Services (Multidimensional handles DAX queries through a special DAXMD interop mechanism). There is no additional query layer in between Power BI Desktop and Analysis Services.

In other words, Power BI becomes a presentation layer that is connected directly to the semantic mode, and the Fields pane shows the metadata from the model. This is conceptually very similar to connecting Excel to Analysis Services. When connecting to Analysis Services Tabular, you can create report-level DAX measures in Power BI Desktop on top of the model just like you can create MDX calculations in Excel. The measure formulas will be stored in the Power BI Desktop file and the original model is not affected.

When Power BI discovers that you connect to Analysis Services, it opens the window shown in **Figure 6.6**. The Explore Live option connects you directly to the model.

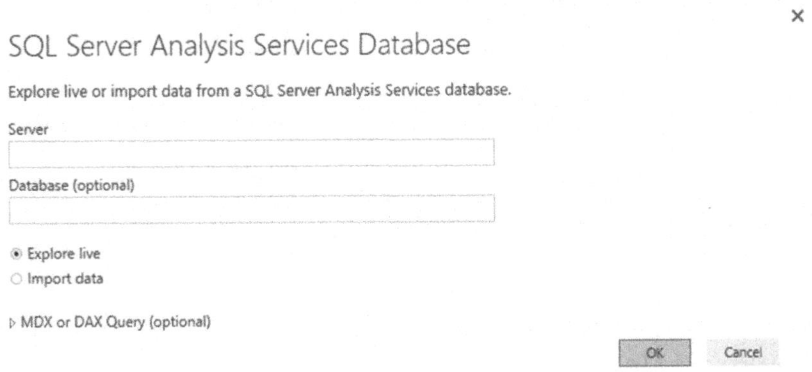

Figure 6.6 When connecting to Analysis Services, Power BI allows you to connect live or import the data.

Like DirectQuery, if you publish a model that connects live to on-premises model, the dataset needs the Power BI on-premises data gateway to be installed in standard mode to connect to Analysis Services. If the connector is not configured, the dataset will be published, but it will be disabled (it will be grayed out in the Power BI navigation bar) and you won't be able to use it.

NOTE Analysis Services is also available as a Platform as a Service (PaaS) Azure service. If you use Azure Analysis Services, you don't need a gateway to connect Power BI reports to Azure Analysis Services. However, you'd still need a gateway to process (refresh) your cloud model from an on-premises data source if this is where the model gets data from.

Table 6.1 summarizes the key points about the three data connectivity options. Because most real-life needs would require importing data, this chapter focuses on this option exclusively. If you plan to connect to live data sources, your experience would be very similar to how you would do this in Power BI Service (refer to the section "Using Live Connections" in Chapter 2).

Table 6.1 This table compares the three connectivity options.

Feature	Data import	Connecting Live (DirectQuery)	Connecting Live (Analysis Services)
Data sources	Any data source	SQL Server (on premises), Azure SQL Database, Azure SQL Data Warehouse, Spark on Azure HDInsight, Azure SQL Data Warehouse, Oracle, Teradata, Amazon Redshift, Impala, SAP Hana	Analysis Services
Usage scenario	When you need data from multiple data sources or a data source that doesn't support DirectQuery	When you connect to a single fast and/or large database that supports DirectQuery and you don't want to import data	When you connect to a single Analysis Services model
Queries for data cleansing (Query Editor)	Available	Available (basic transformations only)	Not available
Connect to multiple data sources	Yes	No	No
Data storage	Data imported in xVelocity	Data is left at the data source	Data is left at the model
Connect to on-premises data from published models	Personal or on-premises gateway is required to refresh data	On-premises gateway is required to connect to data	On-premises gateway is required to connect to SSAS models
Data modeling	Available	Available with limitations	Not available
Relationships	Available	Available with limitations	Not available
Business calculations in a data model	All DAX calculations	DAX calculations with limitations	DAX calculations both in the model and report (usually defined in model)
Data exploration	Handled internally by Power BI Desktop or Power BI Service when the model is deployed without making connections to the original data sources	Power BI Desktop/Power BI Service (published models) autogenerates native queries, sends them to the data source, and shows the results	Power BI Desktop/Power BI Service (published models) autogenerates DAX/DAXMD queries, sends them Analysis Services, and shows the results

6.2   Understanding Power BI Desktop

As I mentioned in Chapter 1, data analysts have two tool options for creating self-service data models. If you prefer Excel, you can continue using the Excel data modeling capabilities and deploy Excel workbooks to Power BI Service, Power BI Report Server, or SharePoint Server. Be aware though that Excel has its own roadmap, so its BI features lag Power BI. By contrast, if you prefer to stay always on the latest BI features, consider Power BI Desktop, which combines the best of Excel Power Pivot, Power Query, and Power View in a standalone, freely available tool that Microsoft updates every month.

6.2.1 Installing Power BI Desktop

Power BI Desktop is available only on Windows operating system, but Mac users have options to run Windows apps. They can configure their MacBooks for dual boot, or run Windows in a virtual environment, such as by using Parallel Desktop for Mac.

Understanding bitness

Power BI Desktop is available as 32-bit and 64-bit Windows installations. The download page determines what version of Windows you have (32-bit or 64-bit) and downloads the appropriate executable. Nowadays, you can't buy a 32-bit computer (not easily, anyway). However, even if you have a 64-bit computer and 64-bit Windows OS, you can still install 32-bit applications. The problem is that 32-bit applications are limited to 2 GB of memory. By contrast, 64-bit computing enables applications to use more than 2 GB of memory. This is especially useful for in-memory databases that import data, such as xVelocity (remember that xVelocity is the storage engine of Power BI Service and Power BI Desktop).

In general, if you have a 64-bit version of Windows, you should install the 64-bit version of any software if a 64-bit version is available. Therefore, the 64-bit version of Power BI Desktop is a better choice. However, although your model on the desktop can grow and grow until it exhausts all the memory, remember that Power BI Pro won't let you upload a file that is larger than 1 GB (Power BI Premium supports files up to 10 GB) so keep this in mind as well if you plan to publish the model.

NOTE   Readers familiar with Excel data modeling might remember that the Office setup installs the 32-bit version of Office by default and getting IT to install the 64-bit version has been a struggle. The Office setup favors the 32-bit version in case you use 32-bit add-ins. Because Power BI Desktop doesn't depend on Office, you can go ahead and install the 64-bit version even if you have the 32-bit version of Office installed.

Understanding availability

You can download Power BI Desktop from https://powerbi.microsoft.com/desktop or from the Downloads menu in Power BI. This option requires you to be proactive and update Power BI Desktop periodically. In addition, you must have local admin rights to install it. Instead, if you have Windows 10, I recommend you install Power BI Desktop from the Windows Store because of the following benefits:

- Automated updates – All data analysts within the company use the latest and greatest version. This avoids the issue of someone attempting to open a model created with more recent version of Power BI Desktop. While Power BI Desktop will automatically upgrade older files, it doesn't support downgrading to a previous version.

- You don't need admin rights – Many corporate users don't have local admin rights to their computers.

- Faster installation – Because you don't have to run a setup, upgrading is much faster.

For more information about Power BI Desktop availability and minimum requirements, check the "Get Power BI Desktop" article at https://powerbi.microsoft.com//documentation/powerbi-desktop-get-the-desktop/.

6.2.2 Understanding Design Environment

Let's get familiar with the Power BI Desktop design environment. **Figure 6.7** shows its main elements numbered in the typical order of steps you'd take to create and refine self-service data models.

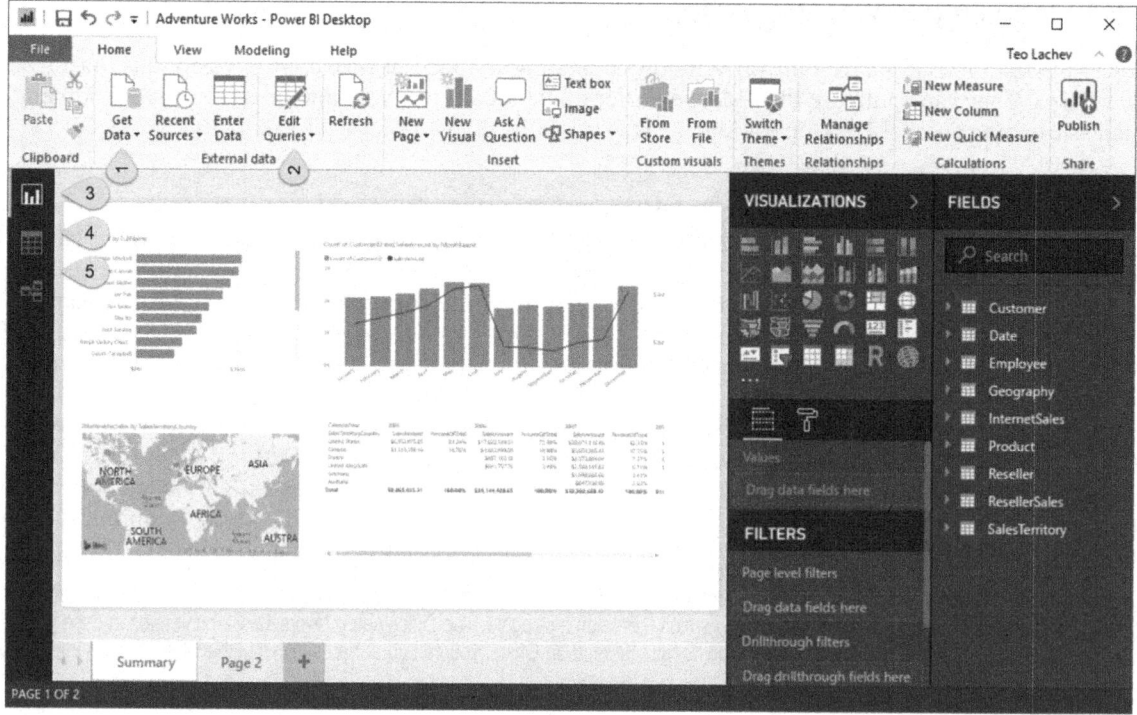

Figure 6.7 Power BI Desktop has five commonly used areas that correspond to the main modeling steps.

Understanding data modeling steps

A typical self-service data modeling workflow consists of the following five main steps (each step refers to the numbers in **Figure 6.7**):

1. Get data – The process starts with connecting to your data by clicking the Get Data button. Remember that when you import the data or use DirectQuery, Power BI Desktop creates a query for each table you import (except when you connect to Analysis Services, in which case there is no query).

2. Transform data – If the data requires cleansing or transformations, click the Edit Queries button to open Query Editor and to modify the existing queries and perform data transformation tasks, such as replacing column values.

3. Explore and refine data – Switch to the Data View to explore and refine the imported data, such as to see what data is loaded in a table and to change column data types. The Data View isn't available when you connect to DirectQuery sources or to Analysis Services. However, in the case of DirectQuery data sources, you can use the Query Editor to perform these tasks.

4. Create relationships – As a part of refining the data model, if you import multiple tables you need to relate them either using the Relationships View or the Manage Relationships button in the ribbon's Home tab. Relationships aren't available when connecting live to Analysis Services.

5. Visualize data – Finally, you build reports to visualize your data by switching to the Report View, which is available with all the data connectivity options.

Visualizations and Fields panes

When the Report tab is active, the Visualizations and Fields panes (on the right) should be familiar to you by now, as you've already worked with them in the first part of the book. The Fields pane shows the model metadata consisting of tables and fields. A field can be a table column or a calculation, such as Sales

YTD. You can also use the Fields pane to create DAX calculations. The Fields pane is available when you're in the Report and Data views.

The Visualizations pane is only available when the Report View is active. It includes Microsoft-provided and custom visualizations. You can click the ellipsis menu (…) below the visualization icons to import custom visualizations from Microsoft AppSource or distributed as files. You can use the Visualizations pane to configure the visual data options and formatting.

6.2.3 Understanding Navigation

Power BI Desktop has a simplified navigation experience using a ribbon interface that should be familiar to you from other Microsoft products, such as Excel. But if you come from Excel data modeling, you'll undoubtedly appreciate the change toward simplicity. There is no more confusion about which ribbon to use and which button to click! By the way, if you need more space, you can minimize the ribbon by clicking the chevron button in the top-right corner or by pressing Ctrl-F1.

Understanding the ribbon's Home tab
The ribbon's Home tab (see **Figure 6.7** again) is your one-stop navigation for common tasks. The Clipboard group allows you to copy and paste text, such as a DAX calculation formula. It doesn't allow you to create tables by pasting data as you can with Excel Power Pivot. However, you can use the Enter Data button in the External Data group to create tables by pasting or entering data. Like other Microsoft Office applications, you can use the Format Painter to copy and apply limited format settings from one selection to another. Let's say you've changed the format settings, such as colors and fonts, of a chart and you want to apply the same settings to another chart. Click the first chart to select it, click the Format Painter button to copy the settings, and then click the other chart to apply the settings.

The External Data group allows you to connect to data (the Get Data button). The Recent Sources button lets you bypass the first Get Data steps, such as when you want to import additional tables from the same database. The Enter Data button allows you to create your own tables by either pasting tabular data or typing in the data manually. The latter could be useful to enter some reference data, such as KPI goals. The Edit Queries button opens a separate Query Editor window so that you can edit queries, if you want to cleanse or transform data. For models with imported data, the Refresh button deletes the data in all tables and re-imports the data. For DirectQuery models, it only refreshes the metadata.

The Insert ribbon group is available when the Report View is active. It allows you to insert new report pages or visuals to a report (alternatively, you can click the visual icon in the Visualizations pane). You can also insert graphical elements, such as text boxes, images, and shapes. The "Ask a Question" button (Q&A is currently in preview) brings Q&A from Power BI Service to the desktop. It creates a report from a natural question you ask! Fulfilling the same role as the ellipsis (…) menu in the Visualizations pane, the "Custom visuals" ribbon group lets you insert custom visuals from Microsoft AppSource or from a file.

You can create a report theme to apply consistent colors to your report, such as corporate colors or seasonal coloring. You specify the color theme by hand in a file described in JavaScript Object Notation (JSON) format. Then, you use the Switch Theme button to import the file. For more information about the color theme specification, read the "Use Report Themes in Power BI Desktop" article at https://powerbi.microsoft.com/documentation/powerbi-desktop-report-themes/. You can also find ready-to-use themes contributed by the community at https://community.powerbi.com/t5/Themes-Gallery/bd-p/ThemesGallery.

The Manage Relationships button allows you to relate tables in your model. The Calculations group is for creating DAX calculations (measures and calculated columns). And the Publish button lets you publish your model to Power BI Service.

Understanding the ribbon's View tab
The ribbon's View tab allows you to optimize the page layout for phone devices. Recall from the previous chapter that the Power BI Mobile apps favor phone-optimized report layouts. Power BI reports typically

have a lot of visualizations and this is fine if users view them on laptops or tablets. But phones have much smaller displays. To avoid excessive scrolling, you can use the Change Layout button to define a layout optimized for phones.

In **Figure 6.8**, I clicked the Change Layout button to switch to a phone layout. Then, I dragged an existing visualization from the Visualizations pane, dropped it to the phone layout, and resized it accordingly. Now when users view this page on their phones, the Power BI native app will detect the phone view and it will apply it. It will also enable report filtering. If there isn't a phone-optimized view, the report will open in the non-optimized, landscape view and the filtering pane will be missing. Note that when you define a phone layout, you can't make changes to the visualizations; you can only resize them. Clicking the Change Layout button one more time toggles to the master layout, as you defined it in the Report View.

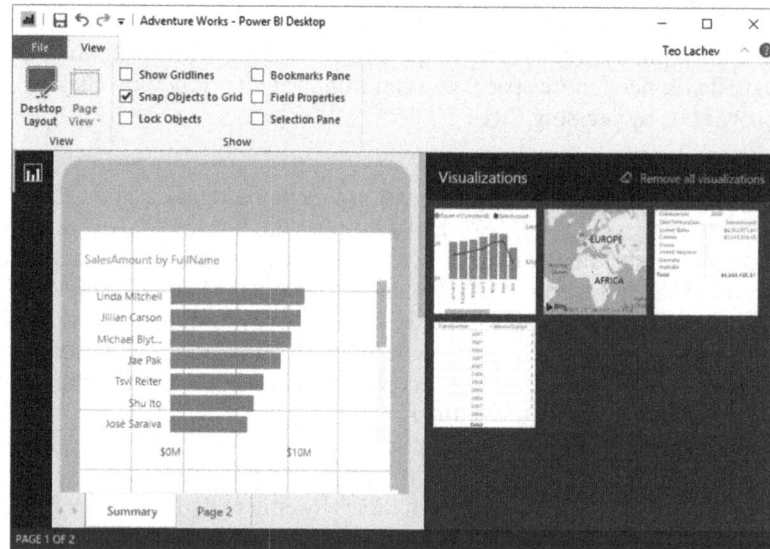

Figure 6.8 Use the Phone Layout to define a phone-optimized views of your report pages.

Continuing the list of menu options, the Page View button zooms the report in desktop layout. It has three options: Fit to Page, Fit to Width, and Actual Size. When checked, the "Show gridlines" shows a grid in the Report View to help you arrange elements on the report canvas. If you want to snap items to the grid to align them precisely, check "Snap objects to grid". When enabled "Lock Objects" prevents you from making accidental changes to visuals on the report.

The Selection pane allows you to toggle the visibility of report elements. This could be useful during design time and it's particularly useful when used together with the Bookmarks Pane. Important for data storytelling, the Bookmarks Pane (bookmarks are currently in preview) lets you capture the current view of a report page, including applied filters and visibility state of the visual, and later go back to that state by clicking the saved bookmark. Finally, when enabled Field Properties opens another pane that lets you enter a description for the field selected in the Fields pane.

 TIP As your data models grow in complexity, users might find it difficult to understand the model metadata, such as which field to use and what's the purpose of a given field or a measure formula. However, you're disciplined to enter informative descriptions, they will show in a tooltip when the user hovers on the field in the Fields list. Now you have a self-documented model!

Understanding the ribbon's Modeling tab

The ribbon's Modeling tab (**Figure 6.9**) allows you to extend and refine your data model. It's available only when the Data View is active.

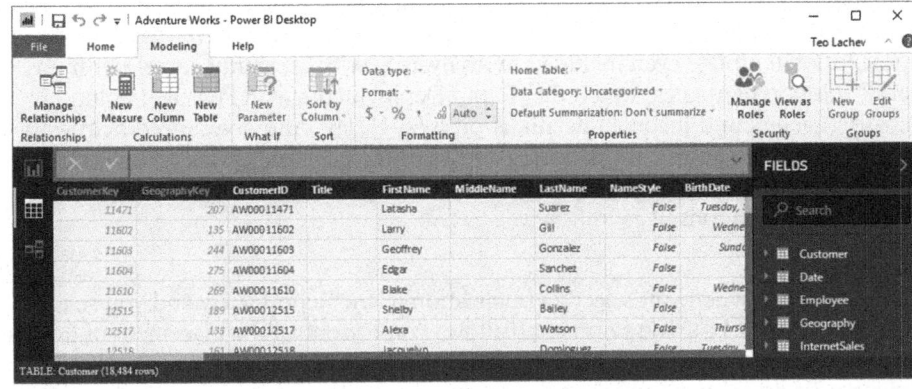

Figure 6.9 The ribbon's Modeling tab is for performing data modeling tasks, such as creating calculations and defining data security.

The Manage Relationships button is available here as well. The Calculations group gives you access to DAX features to create calculated columns, measures, tables, and to define custom sorting. The New Parameter button in the What If ribbon group is for what-if analysis, such as to see how changes to a product discount affects sales. The "Sort by Column" button is for defining custom column sorting, such as to sort a Month Name column by the ordinal month number instead of the default alphanumeric sorting. The Formatting group lets you change the data type and formatting of a table column, such as to format a sales amount with two decimal places. The Properties group is for changing the purpose of specific columns, such as to tell Power BI Desktop that a Country column has a Country category so that a map knows how to plot it. In addition, it allows you to change the default aggregation behavior or a column, such as to mark a Year column as "Don't summarize" since it meaningless to aggregate years as numbers.

The Security group allows you to define data security, also known as Row-Level Security (RLS). Suppose that while Martin can see all the data in the model, Elena can see United States sales. You can define a role that grants Elena rights only to United States in the Sales Territory table. Then, when Elena views the published model, she can see only the data related to the United States as though the other countries don't exist in the model. Finally, the Groups group allow you to define new custom groups, such as to group all European countries in an "European Countries" group so they can be shown as one bar on a chart (groups are discussed in more detail in Chapter 10).

Understanding the ribbon's Help tab

The Help tab includes several useful resources divided into Help, Community, and Resources sections. The Help section includes shortcuts to access guided learning, documentation (Power BI has an excellent documentation!), training videos, support and the About submenu. Use the About button to see the version and monthly release (recall that Power BI Desktop is updated every month!) of the installed Power BI Desktop.

The Community section has shortcuts to the Power BI blog, community forums, samples, report an issue, and submit an idea about improving Power BI. The "Power BI for Developers" button brings you to the Power BI Developer Center, which contains useful resources for developers interested in implementing Power BI-centric solutions. The "Submit an idea" submenu is a shortcut for submitting a suggestion for improving Power BI.

The Solution Templates button in the Resources section navigates to Microsoft AppSource (appsource.microsoft.com) where you can find working end-to-end enterprise-ready Power BI solutions. Suppose your company uses Salesforce.com for customer relationship management. You already know that you can use the Salesforce apps (content packs) in Power BI Service to get prepackaged datasets, reports and dashboards. Or, you can use Power BI Desktop if you want to have more control over what's imported. But what if you work for a large organization and your dataset exceeds the Power BI maximum dataset size (1 GB for Power BI and up to 10 GB for Power BI Premium)? You can use the Salesforce solution template to schedule incremental data extraction from Salesforce to a local SQL Server database or an Azure SQL Database. The solution template even includes an Analysis Services semantic layer! For more information about Power BI solution templates, watch the "Rapid Deployments with Power BI Solution Templates" video by Richard Tkachuk and Justyna Lucznik at bit.ly/2y1J2Hv. And if you need help with implementing the solution templates or Power BI consulting and training, click the Partner Showcase. It brings you to https://powerbi.microsoft.com/partners/ where consulting partners, such as Prologika, demonstrates their Power BI-based solutions.

Understanding the ribbon's Format tab

Two additional tabs become available when you select a visualization in the Report View and you select a visual: Format and Drill tabs (**Figure 6.10**). The Format tab allows you to control the placement of the selected visualization. For example, you might decide to add a background image to a report page that appears behind all visualizations. To do so, you can select the image, expand the Send Backwards button and then click Send to Back. Or, if you want to align specific visualizations, you can hold the Ctrl key to select them one by one, and then use the Align button to align them.

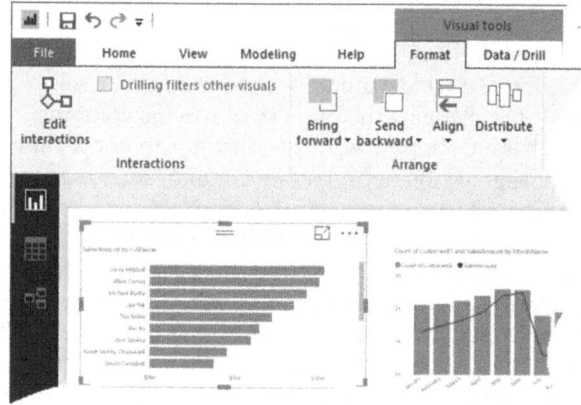

Figure 6.10 The ribbon's Format tab is for controlling placement and interaction behavior of selected visualization.

Like the Power BI Service Visual Interactions menu in report edit mode, the Edit Interactions button controls how visualizations on a report page interact with each other, such as in the case when you want to disable the default cross-highlighting to other charts on the page when you select a category in a chart. When checked, "Drilling filters other visuals" propagates the visual filters to other visuals on the page when you drill down. Let's say you have a report page with multiple charts and visualizations. One of the chart shows Sales by Year and you drill down into 2017 to see the sales by month in 2017. When this checkbox is checked, the drill-down will affect the other visuals so they also show data for just 2017.

Understanding the ribbon's Drill tab

Some visualizations, such as charts, maps and Matrix, allow users to interactively drill down data. For example, if you add Year and Month fields to the chart's Axis area, you can drill down from year to month. However, because by default clicking a chart column invokes the highlighting feature, you can use the buttons in the ribbon's Drill tab (or the indicators in the chart) to tell Power BI Desktop that you want to drill down or up instead (see **Figure 6.11**). Or, you can right-click a bar and then use the context menu.

The See Data button opens a table below the visualization that shows the data behind the visualization at the current aggregation level. By contrast, See Records allows you to drill through to the lowest of level of detail behind a given chart. To do so, click the See Records button, and either click a chart element or right-click it and then click See Records.

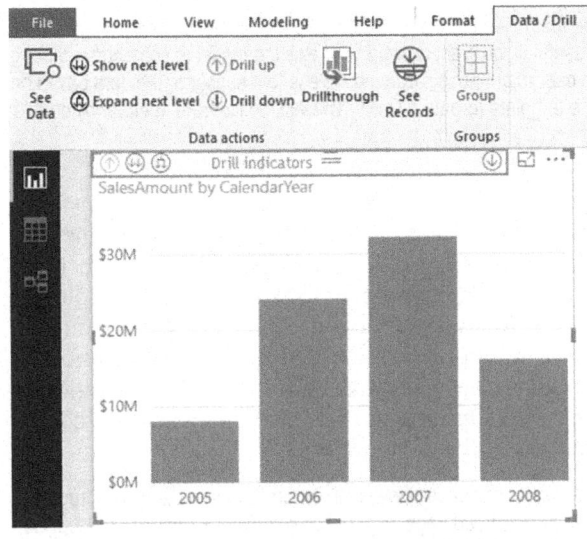

Figure 6.11 The ribbon's Drill tab is to see the levels of detail behind a visualization, such as to drill down.

"Show next level" groups data by the next level. For example, if the Month field shows the name of the month, "Show next level" at the year level would now shows data grouped by each month, so the X-axis will show January to December. "Expand the next level" will group the data by the combination of year and month. In this case, the X-axis will show 2005 January, 2005 February...2005 December, 2006 January, 2006 February...2006 December, and so on.

The Drillthrough button is to drill through another report page that is specifically configured as a drillthrough target. For example, you might want to start with a summary matrix showing sales data by country for a specific date but allow the user to right-click a cell and drill through another page that shows orders for customer for that date and country.

Understanding the File menu

The File menu gives you access to additional tasks. To save space, **Figure 6.12** shows the bottom half of the menu side by side.

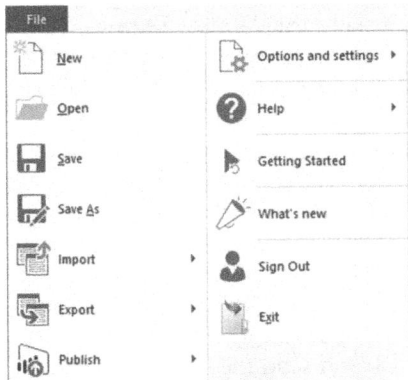

Figure 6.12 Use the Power BI Desktop File menu to work with files and change application settings.

Use the New menu to create a new Power BI Desktop (*.pbix) file and the Open menu to open an existing file. The Save menu saves changes to the current file, and the Save As menu saves the file as another file. If you're transitioning to Power BI Desktop from Excel, the Import menu allows you to import the Excel Power Pivot data model into Power BI Desktop (the reverse is not supported). You can also use the Import menu as another way to import custom visuals into the open Power BI Desktop file. Finally, you can use the Import menu to import an existing Power BI template file.

DEFINITION A Power BI template (.pbit) file includes all the main elements of an existing Power BI Desktop file (report, data model and queries), but not the actual data. This could be useful if you want to send your existing model to someone without giving them access to the data, such as in the case where the user might have restricted access to a subset of the data based on the user's Windows credentials. The user can instantiate the template (create a Power BI Desktop file from it) either by double-clicking on the template file or by using the Import menu.

The Export menu allows you to export your existing model to a Power BI template. The Publish menu is for publishing the data model to Power BI Service (same as the Publish button in the ribbon's Home tab). Remember that although Power BI Desktop can load as much data as it can fit in your computer memory, Power BI Service caps the file size, so be aware of this limitation. If you plan to target larger data volumes, you should consider Analysis Services. When you have an Analysis Services model, your data remains on the server, while you publish only the definitions of your reports and dashboards to Power BI Service, so the dataset size is not an issue. Chapter 13 provides more details when an Analysis Services semantic model could be a better choice than Power BI Desktop. The "Options and settings" menu lets you configure certain program and data source features, as I'll discuss in the next section.

 NOTE Why there is no option to publish to Power BI Report Server? Because Power BI Report Server updates less frequently than Power BI Desktop. This is why the Power BI Report Server download page includes its version of Power BI Desktop. So, there are two Power BI Desktop versions: the untethered version, which will add features at a monthly cadence, and a version locked to Power BI Report Server and updated when a new report server release is available. The unfortunate side effect is that if you want to publish to both Power BI Service and Power BI Report Server, you need to install and keep both versions.

The Help menu fulfills the same role as the Help ribbon tab. The "Get started" menu opens the Power BI Desktop startup screen, which has shortcuts (Get Data, Recent Sources, and recent files), video tutorials, and links to useful resources. If you haven't signed in to Power BI, you can do this right from the startup screen. Signing in to Power BI Desktop helps later when you are publishing to Power BI Service. Continuing the menu list, the "What's new" menu brings you to the Power BI blog to read about the new features in the installed release of Power BI Desktop. The Sign Out menu signs you out of Power BI Service in case you want to sign under another account when you publish the model to Power BI. And the Exit menu closes Power BI Desktop.

Understanding Options and Settings menu
Currently, the "Options and settings" menu has two submenus: Options and Data Source Settings. The Data Source Settings menu lets you change certain security settings of the data sources in the current model (you initially specified these settings when you used Get Data). For example, you can use the Data Source Settings menu to switch from SQL Server Windows authentication to standard authentication (requires a login and password). For data sources that support encrypted connections, such as SQL Server, it also allows you to change the connection encryption settings.

The Options menu brings you to the Options window (see **Figure 6.13**) that allows you to change various program features and settings. I'll cover most of them in appropriate places in this and subsequent chapters but I'd like to explain some now. The Updates tab allows you to configure Power BI Desktop to receive a notification when there's a Power BI Desktop update (enabled by default). Recall that you can install Power BI Desktop from the Windows Store so you are always on the latest. If you experience issues with Power BI Desktop, you can enable tracing from the Diagnostics tab and send the trace to Microsoft. An interesting setting is Preview Features. It allows you to test "beta" features that Microsoft makes available for testing. The goal is to get your feedback to help Microsoft improve these features before enabling them by default.

Like automatic recovery in other Microsoft Office applications, Auto Recovery has settings that allow you to recover your model in the case of an application or operating system crash. Finally, use the Query Reduction tab to disable some interactive settings, such as cross-highlighting, slicer and filter selection.

This could be useful with DirectQuery connections to slow data sources to avoid querying the data source each time you change a filter. Instead, you can set filters and chose when to apply them.

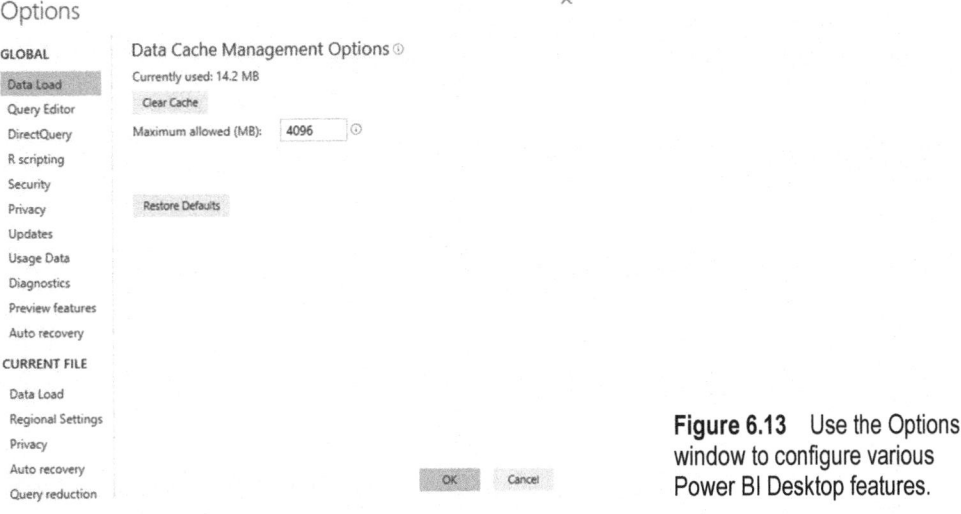

Figure 6.13 Use the Options window to configure various Power BI Desktop features.

Now that I've introduced you to Power BI Desktop and data modeling, let's start the process of creating a self-service data model by getting the data!

6.3   Importing Data

Now let's go back to Martin, who's a data analyst with Adventure Works. Martin realizes that to perform comprehensive sales analysis, he needs data from different data sources. He'll implement a self-service data model and he'll import data from multiple data sources, including data residing in the data warehouse, an Analysis Services cube, flat files, and so on.

6.3.1   Understanding Data Import Steps

Power BI Desktop makes it easy to import data. For those of you who are familiar with Excel data modeling, the process is very similar to using Power Query in Excel. Importing data involves the following high-level steps (you'll repeat for each new data source you use in your model):

1. Choose a data source
2. Connect to the data
3. (Optional) Transform the raw data if needed
4. Load the data into the data model

Choosing a data source

Power BI Desktop can import data from a plethora of data sources with a few clicks and without requiring any scripting or programming skills. You can start the process by clicking the Get Data button in the Power BI Desktop ribbon (or in the splash screen). The most common data sources are shown in the drop-down menu (see **Figure 6.14**), but many more are available when you click the "More..." menu.

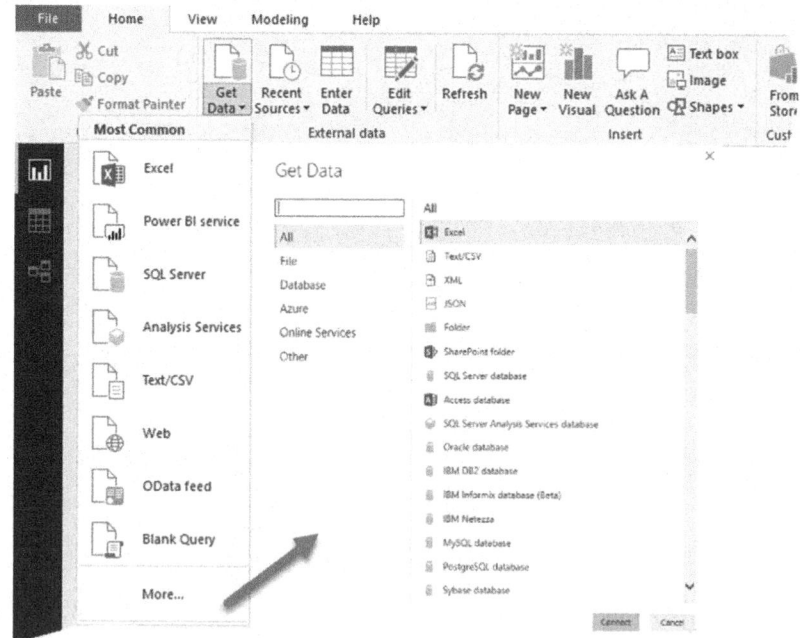

Figure 6.14 Power BI Desktop can connect to a variety of data sources without requiring any scripting or programming.

TIP You might wonder what's the "Power BI service" option and why it has such a prominent place in Get Data. Like Analyze in Excel, which allows you to connect Excel on your desktop to published datasets, the "Power BI Service" option allows you to connect Power BI Desktop to dataset deployed in Power BI Service. Then you can create reports in Power BI Desktop. Why not create reports directly in Power BI Service? One good reason could be that if someone deletes the dataset, Power BI will remove dependent reports, but you could still back up the file if you create them in Power BI Desktop. Another reason is to treat a published dataset as a "semantic layer" so that other users don't have to reimport the same data.

To make it easier to find the appropriate data source, the Get Data window organizes them in File, Database, Azure, Online Services, and Other categories. Table 6.2 summarizes the currently supported data sources, but expect the list to grow because Microsoft adds new data sources on a regular basis.

Table 6.2   This table summarizes the data sources supported by Power BI Desktop.

Data Source Type	Data Sources
File	Excel, CSV, XML, other delimited and fixed-width text files, JSON, a list of files in a Windows or SharePoint folder
Database	SQL Server, Microsoft Access, Analysis Services (Multidimensional, Tabular, PowerPivot workbooks deployed to SharePoint), Oracle, IBM DB2, IBM Informix, IBM Netezza, MySQL, PostgreSQL, Sybase, Teradata, SAP HANA, SAP Business Warehouse, Amazon Redshift, Impala, Google BigQuery, Snowflake, and other ODBC-compliant databases
Azure	SQL Database, SQL Data Warehouse, Analysis Services, Azure Marketplace, HDInsight, Blob Storage, Cosmos DB, Table Storage, HDInsight Spark, Cosmos DB, Data Lake Store
Online Services	Power BI Service datasets, SharePoint Online list, Microsoft Exchange Online, Dynamics CRM Online, Facebook, Github, Google Analytics, Salesforce, appFigures, Azure Enterprise, comScore, GitHub, MailChimp, Marketo, Mixpanel, Planview, Projectplace, Quickbooks Online, SparkPost, Smartsheet, SQL Sentry, SparkPost, Stripe, SweetIQ, Troax, Twillio, tyGraph, Visual Studio Team Services, Webtrends, Zendesk
Other	Vertica, Web, SharePoint list, OData feed, Hadoop File from HDFS, Active Directory, Microsoft Exchange, ODBC, OLEDB, RScript, Spark

It's important to note that every data source requires installing appropriate connectivity software (also called provider or driver). Chances are that if you use Microsoft Office or other Microsoft applications, you already have drivers to connect to SQL Server, Excel files, and text files. If you need to connect to the data sources from other vendors, you need to research what connector (also called driver or provider) is needed and how to install it on your computer. For example, connecting to Oracle requires Oracle client software v8.1.7 or greater on your computer.

 TIP   Because Power BI Desktop borrowed the Power Query features from Excel, you can find more information about the prerequisites related to connectivity in the "Import data from external data sources (Power Query)" document by Microsoft at http://bit.ly/1FQrjF3.

What if you don't find your data source on the list? If the data source comes with an ODBC connector, try connecting to it using the ODBC option. Although the data source might not be officially supported by Microsoft, chances are that you will be able to connect via ODBC. Or, if it comes with an OLE DB driver, try the generic OLE DB connector. Finally, remember that you can create your own connectors using the Power BI Data Connector SDK.

Connecting to data

Once you select your data source you want to connect to, the next step depends on the type of the data source. For example, if you connect to a database, such as SQL Server, you'll see a window that looks like the one in **Figure 6.15**. The only required field is the database server name that will be given to you by your database administrator. You can also specify the database name, but it's not required because you can do this in the next step unless you use the advanced options to specify a custom query.

×

SQL Server database

Server ⓘ

[   ]

Database (optional)

[   ]

Data Connectivity mode ⓘ
● Import
○ DirectQuery

◢ Advanced options
Command timeout in minutes (optional)

[   ]

SQL statement (optional, requires database)

[   ]

☑ Include relationship columns
☐ Navigate using full hierarchy
☐ Enable SQL Server Failover support

[OK]   [Cancel]

Figure 6.15   Connecting to a database requires a server name but additional options are available.

If the Power BI Desktop supports direct connectivity to the data source, you'll be able to specify how you want to access the data: import it in the Power BI Desktop file or connect to it directly using DirectQuery. However, if you have already imported data from the same server or another data source, the DirectQuery option will be disabled. Again, that's because currently DirectQuery supports a single data source only.

Moving to the advanced options, you can specify a command timeout in minutes to tell Power BI Desktop how long to wait before it times out the query. Instead of selecting a table or view in the next step, you can enter a custom SQL statement (also called a native database query). For example, if you need to execute a SQL Server stored procedure, you can enter the following statement:

```
exec <StoredProcedureName> parameter1, parameter 2, ...
```

One caveat about custom SQL statements is that currently, DirectQuery doesn't support them, so you must import tables (or SQL views) if you want to connect live to your data.

If the data source supports referential integrity and you leave "Include relationship column" checked, in the next step (Navigator window) you can let Power BI Desktop preselect the related tables. If you check the "Navigate using full hierarchy", the Navigator window will organize tables in roles and schemas defined in the database (for data sources that support these features). For example, the Adventure-Works2012 database has all sales-related tables in the Sales schema. If this checkbox is checked, the Navigator window will show the database schemas. It'll also show the tables within the Sales schema when you expand it.

There could be additional data source-specific options. For example, if you connect to SQL Server configured to be an Always On Failover Cluster Instance, you can check "Enable SQL Server Failover support" to connect to the secondary replica when a failover occurs.

Specifying credentials

If you connect to a database for the first time, the next step asks you to enter your credentials as instructed by your database administrator. For example, when connecting to SQL Server, you can use Windows credentials (behind the scenes it uses your Windows login) or standard authentication (user name and password).

Power BI Desktop shows the "Access a SQL Server Database" window (see **Figure 6.16**) to let you specify how you want to authenticate. Note the Windows tab allows you specify alternative Windows credentials. This could be useful if the database administrator has given you the credentials of a trusted Windows account. The Database tab lets you use standard authentication.

 TIP Once you've connected to a data source, you don't need to use Get Data to import additional tables. Instead, use the Recent Sources button in the Power BI ribbon. If you need to change the data source credentials or encryption options, use the File ⇨ Options and Settings ⇨ Data Source Settings menu.

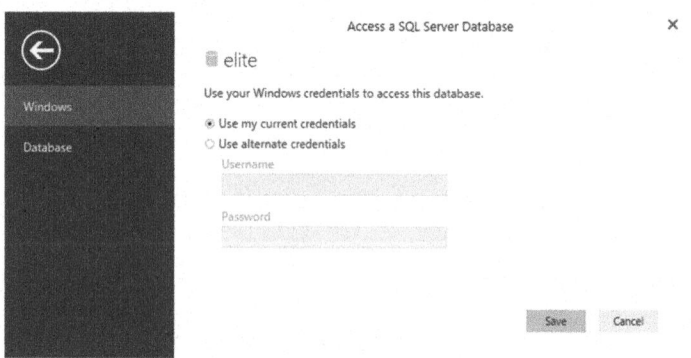

Figure 6.16 SQL Server supports Windows and standard authentication.

If you connect to a data source that is configured for encrypted connections, such as SQL Server, you'll be asked if you want to encrypt the connection while data is imported. If the data source doesn't support encrypted connections, Power BI Desktop will warn you about it.

If the data source has multiple entities, such as a relational database that has multiple tables, or an Excel file with multiple sheets, Power BI Desktop will open the Navigator window (see **Figure 6.17**). Use this window to navigate the data source objects, such as databases and tables, and select one or more tables to import. If the database has many objects, you can search the database metadata to find objects by name. To select a table or a SQL view to import, check its checkbox. The Navigator window shows a preview of the data in the right pane.

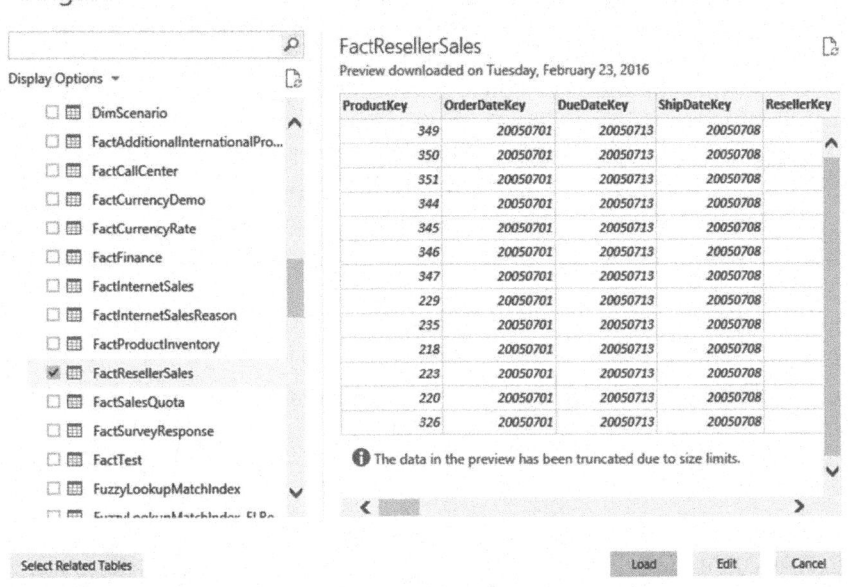

Figure 6.17 The Navigator window allows you to select tables and preview data.

If the database has table relationships (the AdventureWorks databases have relationships), the "Select Related Tables" button allows you to include related tables (if the "Include relationship column" setting was left checked in the previous step) so that you can import multiple tables in one step. There are two refresh buttons. The refresh button in the Navigator left pane, refreshes the metadata. This could be useful if someone makes a definition change, such as adding a column, and you don't want to close the Navigator window to start over. The refresh button on top of the preview pane refreshes the data preview so you can see the latest data changes or the effect of making column changes to the table whose data you're previewing, such as removing, adding, or renaming columns. Again, queries (and everything you do in Power BI Desktop) never make changes to the original data source, so don't worry about breaking something.

The Edit button launches the Query Editor, and this unlocks a whole new world to shape and transform data, such as if you want to replace values, merge data, unpivot columns, and so on. (I'll cover the Query Editor in detail in Chapter 7.) The Load button in the Navigator window adds a new table to the data model and loads it with the data from the selected table. If you click the Edit button to open the Query Editor, you can load the data from the Query Editor window once you're done transforming it.

NOTE Readers familiar with Excel data modeling might know that the Power Pivot Table Import Wizard allows you to filter the data before it's imported. The Navigator window doesn't support filtering. However, you can click the Edit button to edit the query. Among many transformation options, you can apply necessary filtering in the Query Editor, such as removing columns and filtering rows for a given date range.

Next, let's go through a series of exercises to practice importing data from the most common data sources (the ones listed when you drop down the Get Data button), including databases, Excel files, text files, Web, and OData feeds.

6.3.2 Importing from Databases

Nowadays, most corporate data resides in databases, such as SQL Server and Oracle. In this exercise, you'll import two tables from the Adventure Works data warehouse database. The first table, FactResellerSales, represents a fact table and it keeps a historical record of numeric values (facts), such as Sales Amount and Order Quantity. You'll also import the DimDate table from the same database so that you can aggregate data by date periods, such as month, quarter, year, and so on. As a prerequisite, you need to install the Power BI Desktop (read Chapter 1 for installation considerations), and you need to have the Adventure-Works2012 (or later) database installed locally or on a remote SQL Server instance.

 NOTE Installing the AdventureWorks databases too complicated? If you don't have a SQL Server to install the AdventureWorks databases, you can import the FactResellerSales.txt and DimDate.txt files from the \Source\ch06 folder to complete this practice.

Connecting to the database
Follow these steps to import data from the FactResellerSales table:

1. Open Power BI Desktop. Close the splash screen. Click File ⇨ Save (or press Ctrl-S) and then save the empty model as *Adventure Works* in a folder on your local hard drive.

2. Expand the Get Data button in the ribbon and then click SQL Server. This opens the SQL Server Database window.

3. In the Server field, enter the name of the SQL Server instance, such as *ELITE*, if SQL Server is installed on a server called ELITE, or *ELITE\2012* if the SQL Server is running on a named instance 2012 on a server called ELITE. Confirm with your database administrator (DBA) what the correct instance name is. Leave the "Import" option selected. Because you're importing data from multiple sources, you can't use Direct-Query anyway. Click OK.

 TIP If the AdventureWorksDW database is installed on your local computer, you can enter localhost, (local), or dot (.) instead of the machine name. However, I recommend that you always enter the machine name. This will avoid connectivity issues that will require you to change the connection string if you decide to move the workbook to another computer and then try to refresh the data.

4. If this is the first time you connect to that server, Power BI Desktop opens the "Access a SQL Server Database" window to ask you for your credentials. If you have access to the server via Windows security, leave the default "Use my current credentials" option selected. Or if the database administrator (DBA) has created a login for you, select the "Use alternate credentials" option, and then enter the login credentials. Click Connect, and then click OK to confirm that you want to use unencrypted connections.

Loading tables
If you connect successfully, Power BI Desktop opens the Navigator window. Let's load some tables:

1. Expand the AdventureWorksDW2012 database. It's fine if you have an older or later version of the database, such as AdventureWorksDW2014.

2. Scroll down the table list and check the FactResellerSales table. The data preview pane shows the first few rows in the table (see **Figure 6.17** again). Although the Navigator doesn't show row counts, this table is relatively small (about 60,000 rows), so you can go ahead and click the Load button to import it.

If the source table is large and you don't want to import all the data, you might want to filter the data before it's imported (as I'll show you how in the next step) so that you don't have to wait for all the data to load and end up with a huge data model.

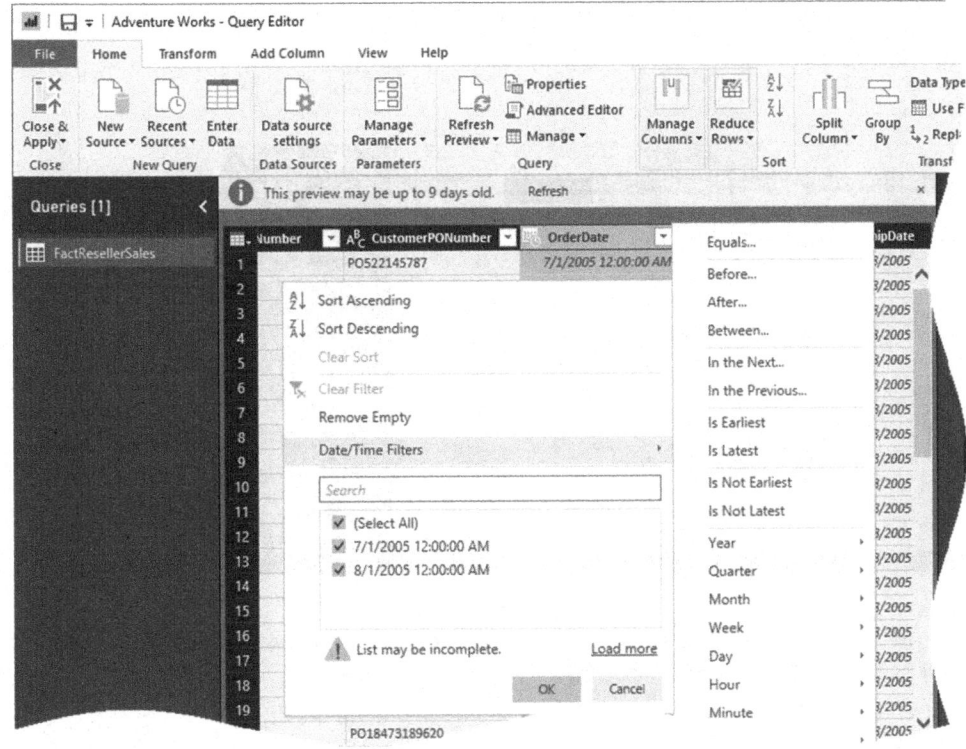

Figure 6.18
Use Query Editor to filter rows and columns.

Filtering data

As a best practice, don't import data you don't immediately need for analysis to avoid a large memory footprint and spending an unnecessary long time to load and refresh the data. The Query Editor makes it easy to filter the data before it's imported. While the Query Editor deserves much more attention (Chapter 7 has the details), let me quickly show you how to filter rows and columns:

1. While you are still in the Navigator window, click the Edit button to open Query Editor in a new window.

2. In the data preview pane, scroll horizontally to the right until you find the OrderDate column.

3. Assuming you want to filter rows by date, expand the drop-down in the OrderDate column header, as shown in **Figure 6.18**. Notice that you can filter by checking or unchecking specific dates. For more advanced filtering options, click the "Date/Time Filters" context menu and notice that you can specify date-related filters, such as After (to filter after a given date) and Between (to filter rows between two dates).

4. You can also remove columns that you don't need. This also helps keep your model more compact, especially with columns that have many unique values because they can't compress well. Right-click a column. Note that the context menu includes a Remove option, which you can use to delete a column. Don't worry if you need this column later; you can always bring back removed columns by undoing the Remove Column step.

> **TIP** A more intuitive option for removing and bringing columns back is Choose Columns. (The Choose Columns button is in the Home ribbon of Query Editor.) It allows you to search columns by name, which is very useful for wide tables. And you can bring columns back by just checking the column name.

5. If you've decided to open the Query Editor, click the "Close & Apply" button in the Query Editor ribbon to import FactResellerSales.

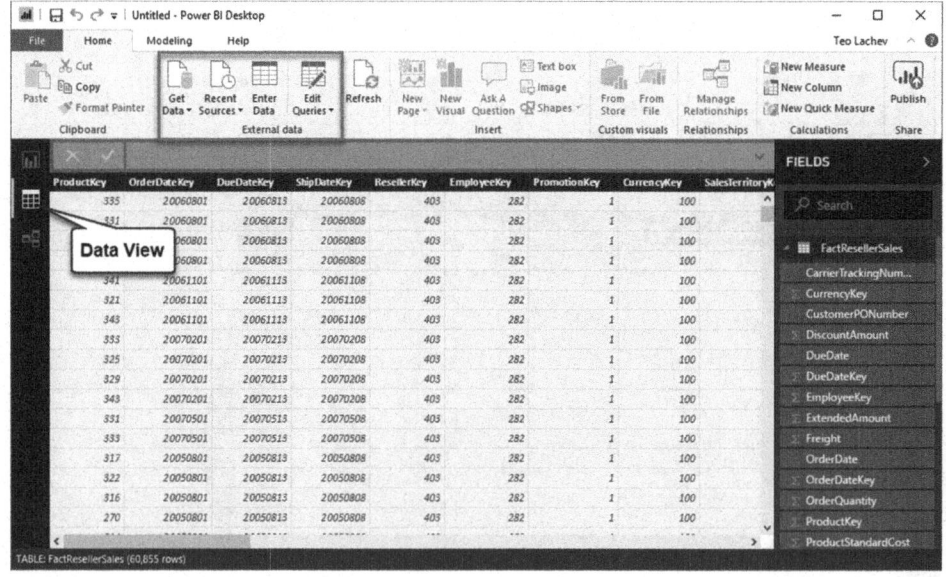

Figure 6.19 The Data View shows the tables in the model and preview of the data.

Understanding changes

Irrespective of which path you took (loading the table from the Navigator or from the Query Editor), Power BI Desktop does the following behind the scenes:

1. It creates a query that connects to the database.

2. It adds a FactResellerSales table to the model.

3. It runs the query to extract the data from the FactResellerSales table in the AdventureWorksDW database.

4. It compresses the data and loads it into the FactResellerSales table inside the model.

5. Power BI Desktop switches to the Data View to show you the new table and read-only view of the loaded data (**Figure 6.19**). The Fields pane shows you the table fields.

Don't confuse the Data View, which represents your data model, with the Query Editor, which represents the query used to load a table in the model. While both show a read-only view of the same data, it comes from different places. The Query Editor opens in another window to show you the source data after all transformations you applied but *before* it's loaded to the data model. The Data View shows the data after it's loaded into the data model. In other words, the Query Editor shows what will happen to the data after you transform it, while the Data View shows what actually happened after the query was applied and data is loaded.

The External Data ribbon group is your entry point for data-related tasks. You already know about the Get Data button. You can use the Recent Sources menu if you need to import another table from the data source that you've already used and if you want to jump directly to the Navigator. The Edit Queries button opens the Query Editor. And the Refresh button reloads all the data so you can get the latest data changes.

 NOTE When you work with Power BI Desktop, the only way to synchronize the imported data with the data source changes is to manually refresh the data. You can do so by clicking the Refresh button to refresh all the tables. Or, you can right-click a table in the Field List and click "Refresh data" to reload only the selected table. Recall that once you publish the model to Power BI, you have the option to schedule an automatic data refresh, such as to reimport all the data on a daily basis.

Importing another table

As I explained at the beginning of this chapter, most models would benefit from a date table. Let's import the DimDate table from the same database:

1. In the External Data ribbon group, expand the Recent Sources button. Click the name of the database server that you specified when you connected to SQL Server. This opens the Navigator window.

2. Expand the AdventureWorksDW2012 node and check the DimDate table. Click the Load button. Power BI adds a table with the same name to the model and to the Fields pane.

   As I pointed out, you should exclude columns you don't need for analysis. You can right-click a column in Data View (or the Field List) and click Delete. Alternatively, you can delete the column in the Data View. In both cases, the Query Editor will add a "Removed Columns" transformation step to the Applied Steps list. However, I prefer to use the Choose Columns transformation so I can see which columns are available and which ones are excluded.

3. Click the Edit Queries button. In the Query Editor, select DimDate in the Queries pane, and then click the Choose Columns button in the Query Editor ribbon's Home tab.

4. Uncheck all columns whose names start with "Spanish" and "French", and then click OK.

5. Click the "Close & Apply" button to apply the query changes and to reload the data. Note that these columns are removed from the DimDate table in the model.

6. Press Ctrl-S to save your data model or click File ⇨ Save. Unless you trust the auto recovery feature, get in a habit to save regularly so you don't lose changes if something unexpected happens and Power BI Desktop shuts down.

6.3.3 Importing Excel Files

Like it or not, much of corporate data ends up in Excel, so importing data from Excel files is a common requirement. If you have a choice, ask for an Excel file that has only the data in an Excel list with no formatting. If you must import an Excel report, things might get more complicated because you'll have to use the Query Editor to strip unnecessary rows and clean the data. In this exercise, I'll show you the simple case for importing an Excel list. In Chapter 7, I'll show you a more complicated case that requires parsing and cleansing an Excel report.

Understanding source data

Suppose that you're given a list of resellers as an Excel file. You want to import this list in the model.

1. Open the Resellers file from \Source\ch06 in Excel (see **Figure 6.20**).

ResellerKey	GeographyKey	ResellerAlternateKey	Phone	BusinessType	ResellerName
1	637	AW00000001	245-555-0173	Value Added Reseller	A Bike Store
2	635	AW00000002	170-555-0127	Specialty Bike Shop	Progressive S
3	584	AW00000003	279-555-0130	Warehouse	Advanced Bike
4	572	AW00000004	710-555-0173	Value Added Reseller	Modular Cycle S
5	322	AW00000005	828-555-0186	Specialty Bike Shop	Metropolitan
6	303	AW00000006	244-555-0112	Warehouse	Aerobic Exercis
7	599	AW00000007	192-555-0173	Value Added Reseller	Associated Bike
8	409	AW00000008	872-555-0171	Specialty Bike Shop	Exemplary C
9	568	AW00000009	488-555-0130	Warehouse	Tandem Bicycle
10	44	AW00000010	150-555-0127	Value Added Reseller	Rural Cycle Em
11	96	AW00000011	926-555-0159	Specialty Bike Shop	Sharp Bikes
12	96	AW00000012	112-555-0191	Warehouse	Bikes and Moto

Figure 6.20 The Resellers file represents a list of resellers and it only has the data, without formatting.

2. Notice that the Excel file includes only data on the first sheet. This Excel list includes all the resellers that Adventure Works does business with. Close Excel.

TIP Consider saving the source text files on a network share. If you import local files and you need to schedule your published dataset to refresh from Power BI Service, you'll be restricted to use a gateway installed on your machine. The chances are that neither Power BI Report Server nor a gateway on another server will be able to reach your local files.

Importing from Excel

Follow these steps to import from an Excel file:

1. With the Adventure Works model open in Power BI Desktop, expand Get Data, and then select Excel.

2. Navigate to the \Source\ch06 folder and double-click the Resellers file.

3. In the Navigator window, check Sheet1. The Navigator parses the Excel data and shows a preview of the data in Sheet1 (see **Figure 6.21**).

As you've seen, importing Excel files isn't much different than importing from a database. If the Excel file has multiple sheets with data, you can select and import them in one step. Power BI Desktop will create a query and a corresponding table for each sheet.

 TIP Don't like "Sheet1" as a table name in your data model? While you can rename the table in the Data View, you can also re-name the query before the data is loaded. Power BI Desktop uses the name of the query as a default table name. While you're still in the Navigator, click the Edit button to open the Query Editor, and then change the query name in the Query Settings pane.

4. Click the Edit button. In the Query Settings pane of the Query Editor, change the query name from Sheet1 to *Resellers*. Click the "Close & Apply" button. Power BI Desktop adds a third table (Resellers) to the data model.

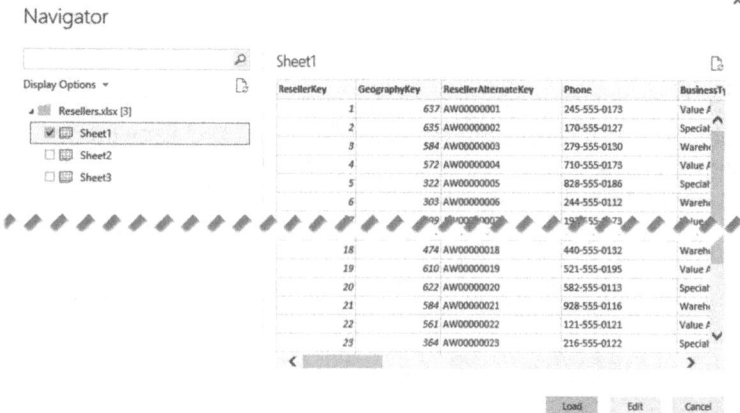

Figure 6.21 The Navigator parses the Excel data and shows a preview.

6.3.4 Importing Text Files

Importing from text files (delimited and fixed-length) is another common requirement. Security and operational requirements might prevent you from connecting directly to a database. In such cases, data could be provided to you as text files. For example, your database administrator might give you a data extract as a file as opposed to granting you direct access to a production database.

Importing from CSV files

Suppose that Adventure Works keeps the employee information in an HR mainframe database. Instead of having direct access to the database, you're given an extract as a comma-separated values (CSV) file. Follow these steps to import this file:

1. Expand the Get Data button and click CSV.
2. Navigate to the \Source\ch06 folder and double-click the Employees file.
3. Because a text file only has a single dataset, Power BI doesn't open the Navigator window. Instead, it just shows you a preview of the data, as shown in **Figure 6.22**.

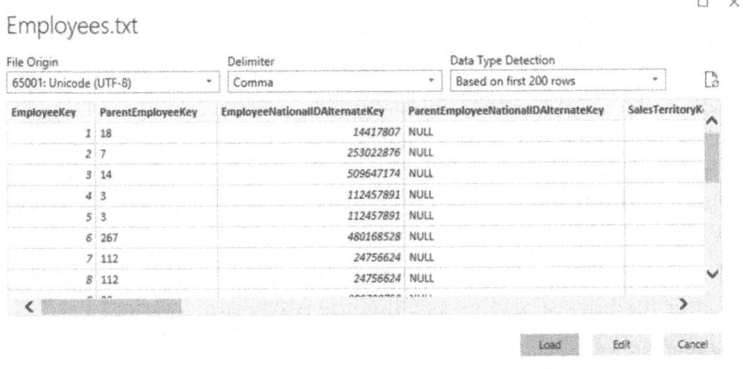

Figure 6.22 When importing from files, Power BI Desktop shows a data preview without opening the Navigator pane.

As you can see, it parses the file content and separates it in columns. Notice Power BI has detected that a comma is used as a column separator. Also notice that by default Power BI parses the first 200 rows in the file to detect the column data types.

NOTE What happens if a column has numeric data in the first 200 rows but some text values, such as "N/A" in rows after that? Power BI will flag the column data type as numeric, but it will fail the import for rows with the inconsistent data types and it will show you which rows have failed. Then, you can use the Query Editor to address the data quality issue, such as by replacing the text values with "null".

4. Click Load to create a new Employees table and to load the data. At this point, the Adventure Works model should have four tables: DimDate, Employees, FactResellerSales, and Resellers.

Importing other formats

You might be given a file format other than CSV. For example, the file might use a pipe character (|) as a column separator. Or you might be a given a fixed-length file format, such as the one I demonstrate with the Employees2.txt file in the \Source\ch06 folder (see **Figure 6.23**).

```
EmployeeID  FirstName  LastName    Title
14417807    Guy        Gilbert     Production Technician - WC60
253022876   Kevin      Brown       Marketing Assistant
509647174   Roberto    Tamburello  Engineering Manager
112457891   Rob        Walters     Senior Tool Designer
```

Figure 6.23 The Employees2 file has a fixed-length format where each column starts at a specific position.

You can use either CSV or Text import options to parse such formats. To make it easier on you, Power BI Desktop will use its smarts to detect the file format. If it's successful, it will detect the delimiters automatically and return a multi-column table. If not, it'll return a single-column table that you can subsequently split into columns using Split Columns and other column tasks in the Query Editor.

NOTE Readers familiar with Power might know that Power Pivot was capable of parsing more complicated file formats using a schema.ini file if it's found in the same folder as the source file. The Power BI Desktop queries don't support schema.ini files.

6.3.5 Importing from Analysis Services

If your organization has invested in SQL Server Analysis Services (SSAS), you have two ways to access Multidimensional or Tabular models:

- Import – Choose this option if you want to mash up data from multiple data sources, including SSAS databases or Power Pivot models deployed to SharePoint. This is especially useful when your model needs the results from business calculations or from KPIs defined in a multidimensional cube or a Tabular model.

- Connect live – Choose this option when you want to create interactive reports connected to an SSAS model without importing the data, just like you would do it in Excel. For this to work, your Power BI Desktop file must not have any other connections or imported data. If you decide to connect live to SSAS, the Data and Relationships views, and the Query Editor are not available. This makes sense because you wouldn't want to have a model on top of another model.

Next, you'll import the Sales Territory dimension data and a key performance indicator (KPI) from the Adventure Works cube. (The book front matter includes steps for installing the Adventure Works cube.)

 NOTE If you don't have an Analysis Services instance with the Adventure Works cube, you can import the DimSalesTerritory CSV file found in the \Source\ch06 folder. Importing DimSalesTerritory won't import the Revenue KPI because it's only defined in the cube and that's OK. When going through subsequent exercises, ignore steps that reference the Revenue KPI.

Connecting to an SSAS database
Start by connecting to the Adventure Works cube as follows:

1. Expand the Get Data button and click Analysis Services to open the "SQL Server Analysis Services Database" window. Remember that Analysis Services supports live connectivity, but it must be the only data source in your Power BI Desktop model. If you combine data from multiple sources, you must import data from *all* data sources. Therefore the "Connect live" option is disabled.

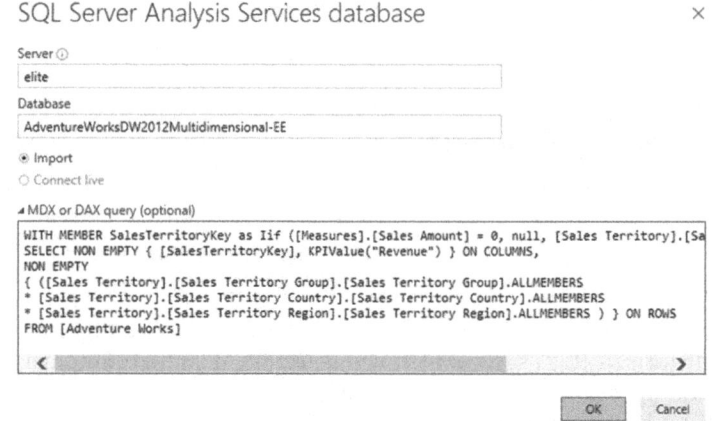

Figure 6.24 Power BI Desktop allows you to import data from SSAS.

If you don't specify a custom query (or leave the Database field empty) and click OK, the Navigator window will pop up, allowing you to select the dimensions and measures. Once you are done, the Navigator window will auto-generate the MDX query for you. However, unlike the MDX Designer included in Excel, the Navigator doesn't let you create calculated members (business calculations in cubes). In this case, we need a simple calculation member that returns the key property of the "Sales Territory Region" dimension attribute so that we can subsequently relate the SalesTerritory table to FactResellerSales. Therefore, we need a custom MDX query that includes a SalesTerritoryKey calculated member.

2. In the "SQL Server Analysis Services Database" window, enter the name of your SSAS database, such as *AdventureWorksDW2012Multidimensional-EE*.

3. In the "MDX or DAX Query" field, enter the MDX query, which you can copy from the \Source\ch06\Queries file. Compare your results with **Figure 6.24**.

4. Click OK. Power BI Desktop shows a data preview window (see **Figure 6.25**).

elite: AdventureWorksDW2012Multidimensional-EE ✕

[Sales Territory Region].[Sales Territory	[Measures].[SalesTerritoryKey]	[Measures].[Sales Amount]
	7	7251555.649
	8	4878300.376
	10	7670721.038
	6	16355770.46
	3	7909009.007
	2	6939374.483
	1	16084942.55
	5	7879655.075
	4	24184609.6
	9	10655335.96

Load   Edit   Cancel

Figure 6.25 The SalesTerritoryKey column returns the key value of the Sales Territory Region attribute which you'll subsequently use as a primary key for creating a relationship.

Renaming metadata
If you click the Load button, you'll end up with "Query1" as a table name and system-generated column names. You can fix this later, but let's refine the metadata before the data is loaded.

1. Click the Edit button.

2. In the Query Settings pane, rename the query from "Query1" to *SalesTerritories*.

3. To rename the columns, double-click the column header of each column, and rename the columns to *SalesTerritoryGroup*, *SalesTerritoryCountry*, *SalesTerritoryRegion*, *SalesTerritoryKey*, and *SalesAmount*.

4. Click the "Close & Apply" button to create and load a new SalesTerritories table.

6.3.6 Importing from the Web

A wealth of information is available on the Web. Power BI Desktop can import tabular data that's accessible by URL. One popular Web-enabled data source is SQL Server Reporting Services (SSRS). Once a report is deployed to a report server, it's accessible by URL, which is exactly what the Web import option requires. Next, I'll show you how to import an SSRS report.

 NOTE   Readers familiar with the Power Pivot import capabilities might recall that Power Pivot supports importing SSRS reports as data feeds. Unfortunately, as it stands, the Power BI Desktop (and Power Query) OData import option doesn't support the ATOM data feed format that SSRS generates. However, the report URL can export the report as CSV, and the output then can be loaded using the Power BI Web import option.

Deploying the report
You can find a sample report named Product Catalog in the \Source\ch06 folder. This report must be deployed to a Reporting Services server that is version 2008 R2 or higher.

 NOTE   If configuring Reporting Services isn't an option, you can import the required data from the AdventureWorksDW database using the custom SQL query I provided in the DimProduct.sql file, or from the \Source\ch06\DimProduct.txt file. The query doesn't return the exact results as the Product Catalog report, and that's okay.

1. Upload the Product Catalog.rdl file from the \Source\ch06 folder to your report server, such as to a folder called *PowerBI* in the SSRS catalog. Please note that the report data source uses the AdventureWorks2012 database (see the book front matter for setup instructions), and you probably need to change the connection string in the report data source to reflect your specific setup.

2. To test that the report is functional, open the Report Manager by navigating to its URL in your Web browser (assuming SSRS is running in native mode).

3. Navigate to the PowerBI folder. Click the Product Catalog report to run the report. The report should run with no errors.

Importing the report

Follow these steps to import the Product Catalog report in the Adventure Works data model:

1. In Power BI Desktop, expand the Get Data button and click Web.

2. In the "From Web" window that pops up, enter the following URL, but change it to reflect your SSRS server URL (tip: if you test the URL in your Web browser, it should execute fine and it should prompt you to download Product Catalog.csv file):

http://localhost/ReportServer?/PowerBI/Product Catalog&rs:Command=Render&rs:Format=CSV

This URL requests the Product Catalog report that's located in the PowerBI folder of my local report server. The Render command is an optimization step that tells SSRS that the requested resource is a report. The Format command instructs the server to export the report in CSV.

3. Click OK. Power BI Desktop shows a preview of the report data.

4. Click the Edit button. In the Query Editor, rename the query to *Products*.

5. Use the Choose Columns feature to remove all the columns whose names start with "Textbox". Click the "Close & Apply" button to load the Products table.

6.3.7 Importing OData Feeds

Power BI Desktop supports importing data from data feeds that use the OData protocol. Initiated by Microsoft in 2007, Open Data Protocol (OData) is a standard Web protocol for querying and updating data. The protocol allows a client application (consumer), such as Power BI Desktop or Excel, to query a service (provider) over the HTTP protocol and then get the result back in popular data formats, such as Atom Syndication Format (ATOM), JavaScript Object Notation (JSON), or Plain Old XML (POX) formats. Power BI can integrate with any OData-compliant provider, including Azure Marketplace, SharePoint, and cloud applications. This makes it possible to acquire data from virtually any application and platform where developers have implemented an OData API. For more information about OData, see http://odata.org.

To demonstrate importing OData feeds, I'll show you another approach to generate a Date table that uses the DateStream feed available on Microsoft Azure Marketplace. The Microsoft Azure Marketplace is an online market for buying and selling datasets exposed as OData feeds. Some of the datasets, such as DateStream, are freely available. Note that this is an optional exercise as it's meant to show you how the OData import works. You won't need the actual data because the data model already has a date table.

Understanding the DateStream feed

Previously, you imported the Date table from the Adventure Works data warehouse. But where do you get a Date table from if you don't have a data warehouse? While a future release of Power BI Desktop might support auto-generating date tables natively, currently this isn't supported. One option is to maintain a date table in Excel and import it from there. Another option is to obtain it from the DateStream feed (http://datamarket.azure.com/dataset/boyanpenev/datestream) available at Microsoft Azure Marketplace.

The DateStream feed is documented at http://datestream.codeplex.com. Developed by Boyan Penev, it was initially designed to be consumed by Power Pivot. However, because it's implemented as an OData feed, it can be integrated with any OData client. DateStream supports localized date calendars, including US and English calendars. If you need to analyze data by time, it also supports time tables at a minute and second grain.

Importing the DateStream feed

Because Microsoft Azure Marketplace requires authentication, you can't use the OData Feed import option. Instead, you need to import using the Microsoft Azure Marketplace option. As a prerequisite, you need to create a marketplace account so that you can authenticate to Microsoft Azure Marketplace. Once you register with Azure Marketplace, you need to go to https://datamarket.azure.com/dataset/boyanpe-nev/datestream and sign up to use the DateStream service (it's free!). Let's import the DateStream feed:

1. In Power BI Desktop, click the Get Data button.
2. In the Get Data window, select the Azure tab. Select Microsoft Azure Marketplace and click Connect.
3. If this is the first time you're connecting to Azure Marketplace, you need to authenticate either using a Microsoft account or an account key.
4. In the Navigator window, expand the DateStream node, and then check the appropriate calendar, depending on your localization requirements. In **Figure 6.26**, I selected BasicCalendarUS. Note that the DateKey column in the data preview shows that dates are formatted in US culture ("mm/dd/yyyy").

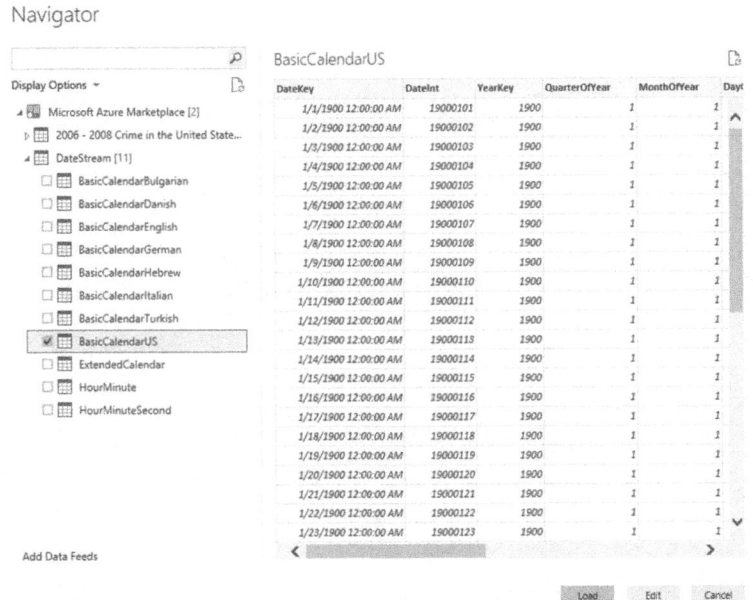

Figure 6.26 The DateStream feed includes localized calendars and time tables.

The feed starts with the year 1900 and goes all the way to 2100. If needed, you can use the Query Editor to filter a smaller range. Just click the Edit button and then apply column filtering to filter the date feed, such as on the YearKey column. And if you need additional columns, such as for fiscal years and quarters, add custom columns in the Query Editor, or add DAX calculated columns in the Data View.

5. Because you won't need this data for the purposes of the Adventure Works data model, click Cancel.

This completes the import process of the initial set of tables that you'll need to analyze the Adventure Works sales. At this point, the Fields list should have six tables: FactResellerSales, DimDate, SalesTerritories, Resellers, Employees, and Products.

6.4   Summary

A Power BI model is a relational-like model and represents data as tables and columns. This chapter started by laying out fundamental data modeling concepts (such as table schemas, relationships, and keys) that you need to understand before you import data. It also explained data connectivity options supported by Power BI Desktop and introduced you to the Power BI premium tool for self-service data modeling.

Next, the chapter explained the data import capabilities of Power BI Desktop. As you've seen, you can acquire data from a wide variety of data sources, including relational and multidimensional databases, Excel files, text files, Web, and data feeds. Once the data is imported in the model, every table is an equal citizen and it doesn't matter where the data came from!

Source data is seldom clean. Next, you'll learn how to use queries to shape and transform raw data when needed.

Chapter 7

Transforming Data

As you've seen, it doesn't take much effort to import data from wherever it might reside. Importing data is one thing, but transforming arbitrary or dirty data is quite another. Fortunately, Power BI Desktop has a query layer that allows you to clean and transform data before it's loaded in the model. Remember that this layer is available when you import data or when you connect live to data sources using the Direct-Query connectivity mechanism. The query layer isn't available when you connect live to Analysis Services.

This chapter explores the capabilities of the Query Editor component of Power BI Desktop. It starts by introducing you to the Query Editor design environment. Next, it walks you through an exercise to practice its basic transformation steps. It also teaches you about its more advanced transformation features that require custom code. Since you won't need the results from these exercises in the Adventure Works model, you'll practice with a new Power BI Desktop file. You can find the finished query examples that you'll do in this chapter in the Query Examples.pbix file located in the \Source\ch07 folder.

7.1   Understanding the Query Editor

The Query Editor is packed with features that let you share and transform data before it enters the data model. The term "transformation" here includes any modification you apply on the raw data. All transformations are repeatable, meaning that if you import another data extract that has the same structure, Power BI Desktop will apply the same transformation steps when you refresh the data.

> **NOTE**   You might have heard of BI pros implementing Extraction, Transformation, and Loading (ETL) processes to clean data in an automated way. Think of the Query Editor (or Excel Power Query) relationship to self-service BI as what ETL is to organizational BI. Although not as flexible and powerful as professional ETL tools, the Query Editor should be able to help when issues with source data require basic to moderate cleansing and shaping. If your data requires more complex integration and transformation steps, such as when integrating data from multiple systems, consider the organization BI architecture (discussed in chapter 2) and plan for dedicated ETL.

7.1.1   Understanding the Query Editor Environment

Before I dive into the Query Editor's plethora of features, let's take a moment to explore its environment. As I mentioned, you launch the Query Editor when you click the Edit Queries button in the Power BI Desktop ribbon's Home tab or when you right-click a table in the Fields pane and then click "Edit Query". The Query Editor opens in a new window, side by side with the Power BI Desktop main window. **Figure 7.1** shows the main elements of Query Editor when you open it in the Adventure Works model that you implemented in the previous chapter.

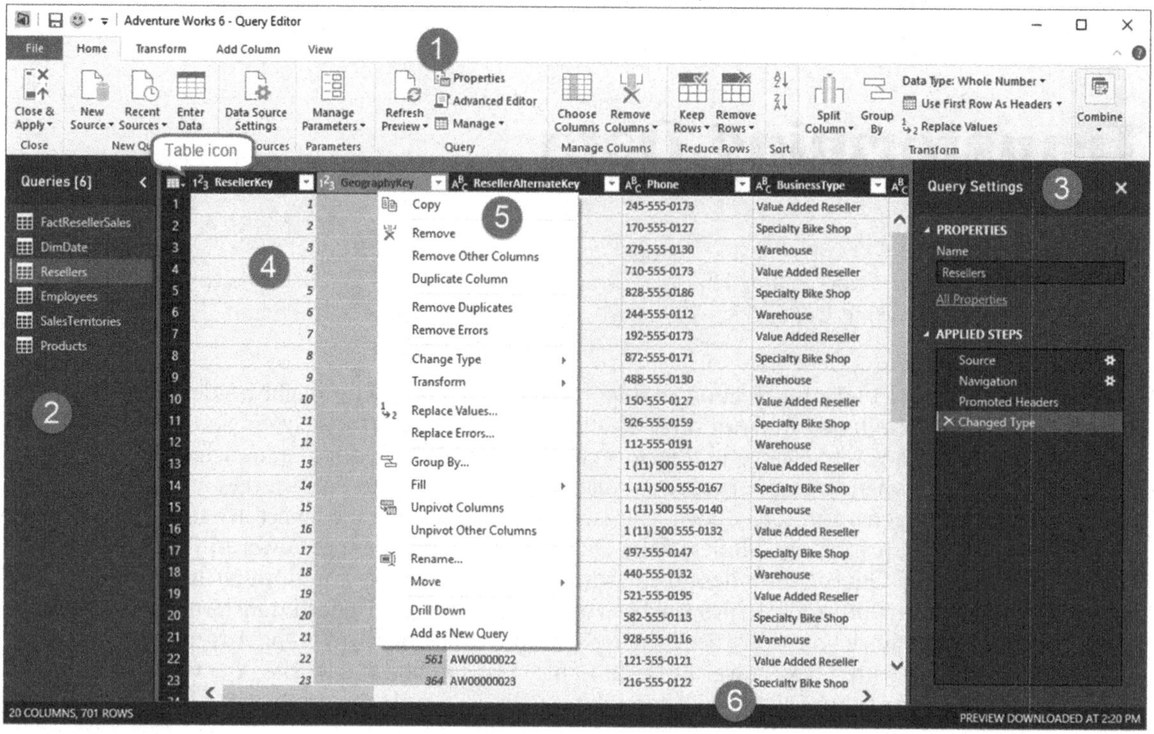

Figure 7.1 The Query Editor opens in a new window to give you access to the queries defined in the model.

Understanding the ribbon's Home tab

The Home tab in the ribbon (see item 1 in **Figure 7.1**) includes buttons for common tasks and some frequently used columns and table-level transformations. Starting from the left, you're already familiar with the Close & Apply button. When expanded, this button has three values, giving you options to close the Query Editor without applying the query changes to the data model (Close menu), to apply the changes without closing the editor (Apply), and both (Close & Apply). If you choose to close the editor without applying the changes, Power BI Desktop will display a warning that pending query changes aren't applied.

> **NOTE** Some structural changes, such as adding a new column, must reload the data in the corresponding table in the data model. Other changes, such as renaming columns, are handled internally without data refresh. Power BI Desktop (more accurately the xVelocity engine) always tries to apply the minimum steps for a consistent model without unnecessary data refreshes.

The New Query ribbon group is another starting point for creating new queries if you prefer to do so while you're in the Query Editor as opposed to Power BI Desktop. The New Source button is equivalent to the Get Data button in the Power BI Desktop's ribbon. The Recent Sources and Enter Data buttons are the Editor Query counterparts of the same buttons in the Power BI Desktop ribbon's Home tab.

The "Data Source Settings" button in the Data Sources ribbon's group brings the "Data Source Settings" window (you can also open it from the Power BI Desktop File ⇨ "Options and settings" ⇨ "Data source settings" menu) allows you to see what data sources are used in the current Power BI Desktop file, as well as change their authentication, encryption, and privacy settings (all these settings that you specified when you connected to the data source the first time). For example, you can go to the properties of a data source to change the authentication properties, such as to switch from Windows to standard authentication that requires a username and password to connect to a database.

NOTE The data source privacy level determines its level of isolation from other data sources. Suppose you import a list of customers that has some sensitive information, such as contact details. To prevent inadvertently sending this information to another data source, such as a data feed, set the data source privacy level to Private. For more information about privacy levels, read the "Power BI Desktop privacy levels" blog at https://docs.microsoft.com/power-bi/desktop-privacy-levels.

The Managed Parameters button is to define query parameters to customize conveniently certain elements of the data models, such as a query filter, a data source reference, a measure definition, and others. For example, a parameter can change the data source connection information so that you refresh data from Production or Testing environments based on the selected parameter value. I'll postpone discussing the Manage Parameters button to the "Using Advanced Feature" section in this chapter.

The ribbon's Query group is to perform query-related tasks. Specifically, the Refresh Preview button refreshes the preview of the query results, such to see a new column that you just added to an underlying table in the database. Not to be confused with the Refresh button in Power BI Desktop's Home ribbon, it doesn't refresh the data in the model. The Properties button opens a Query Properties window (**Figure 7.2**) that allows you to change the query name. Alternatively, you can change the query name in the Query Settings pane or double-click the query in the Queries pane (or right-click and click Rename).

×

Query Properties

Name

Products

Description

☑ Enable load to report

☑ Enable refresh of this query

OK   Cancel

Figure 7.2   Use the Query Properties pane to change the query name, to enable data load to report, and to enable data refresh.

Sometimes, you might not want to load the query data in the data model, such as when you plan to append the query results to another query. If you don't want the query to generate a table in the data model, uncheck the "Unable load to report" checkbox. And, if you don't want to refresh the query results when the user initiates Power BI Desktop table refresh, uncheck "Enable refresh of this query". Continuing the list of Home tab's buttons, the Advanced Editor button gives you access to the query source. Finally, you can use Manage drop-down button to delete, duplicate, and reference a query. These tasks are also available when you right-click a query in the Queries navigation pane.

NOTE Queries are described in a formula language (informally known as "M"). Every time you apply a new transformation, the Query Editor creates a formula and adds a line to the query source. For more information about the query formula language, read "Microsoft Power Query for Excel Formula Language Specification" at http://go.microsoft.com/fwlink/p/?linkid=320633.

The rest of the buttons on the Home tab let you perform common transformations, including removing columns, reducing rows, grouping by and replacing values, and combining queries. We'll practice many of these in the lab exercise that follows.

Understanding the ribbon's Transform tab

The Transform tab (see **Figure 7.3**) includes additional table and column transformations. Many of the column-level transformations from the context menu (see item 5 in **Figure 7.1**) are available when you right-click a column in the data preview pane. And, many of the table-level transformations are available when you expand or right-click the Table icon (▦) in the top-left corner of the data preview pane.

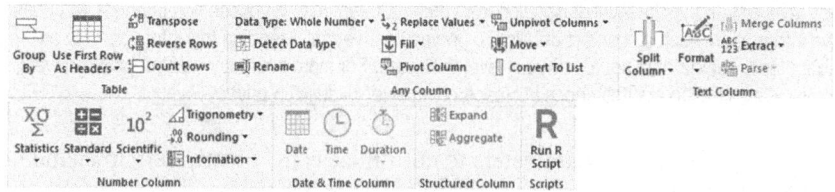

Figure 7.3 The Transform ribbon (split in the screenshot to reduce space) includes many table and column transformations.

Some transformations apply to columns that have specific data types (see the second row in **Figure 7.3**). For example, the Split Column transformation applies only to text columns, while the Rounding transformation applies only to number columns. If you have experience in R and you prefer to use R for data cleansing and shaping, the "Run R Script" is for inserting the R code. To learn about data shaping with R, check the "Data Cleansing with R in Power BI" blog by Sharon Laivand at http://bit.ly/2eZ6f4R.

Understanding the ribbon's Add Column tab

The Add Column tab (see **Figure 7.4**) lets you create custom columns. For example, I'll show you later how you can create a custom column that returns the last day of the month from a date.

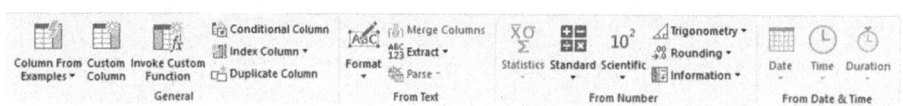

Figure 7.4 Use the Add Column tab in the ribbon to create custom columns.

 NOTE Don't confuse query custom columns with data model calculated columns. Added to the query, query custom columns are created using the Power Query formula language called "M" and they can't reference fields in the data model. On the other hand, calculated columns in the data model are described in DAX and they can reference other fields in the model.

Another interesting variant of a custom column is a conditional column that lets you define different values depending on a condition. For example, like a SWITCH CASE statement in programming languages, you can create a conditional column that examines the product cost and assigns each row in the Product table to a cost band which values Low, Medium, or High (see **Figure 6.5**).

Add Conditional Column

Add a conditional column that is computed from the other columns or values.

New column name

CostBand

	Column Name	Operator	Value ⓘ		Output ⓘ	
If	StandardCost	is less than	10	Then	Low	...
Else If	StandardCost	is less than	20	Then	Medium	
Else If	StandardCost	is greater than or...	20	Then	High	

Add Rule

Otherwise ⓘ

Undefined

OK   Cancel

Figure 7.5 The CostBand conditional column evaluates the ProductCost column and assigns each row to a band.

A very powerful feature awaits you in the "Column From Example" button. As you probably realize, the Query Editor is a great tool, but it might difficult for a novice user to understand which transformation to apply to get the desired result. No worries, you can let Query Editor take a guess! Let's say I want a column that shows the employee's first name and their department, such as "Guy from Production" (see **Figure 7.6**). I selected the Employees table in Query Editor. Next, I expanded "Column From Examples", chose "From Selection", and checked the FirstName and Department columns.

Then, In the first cell of the new Merged column, I typed *Guy from Production* and pressed Ctrl-Enter. Query Editor understood what I want to do and filled in all rows with the desired results. For more information about this excellent feature, read the "Add a column from an example in Power BI Desktop" article at https://powerbi.microsoft.com/documentation/powerbi-desktop-add-column-from-example/.

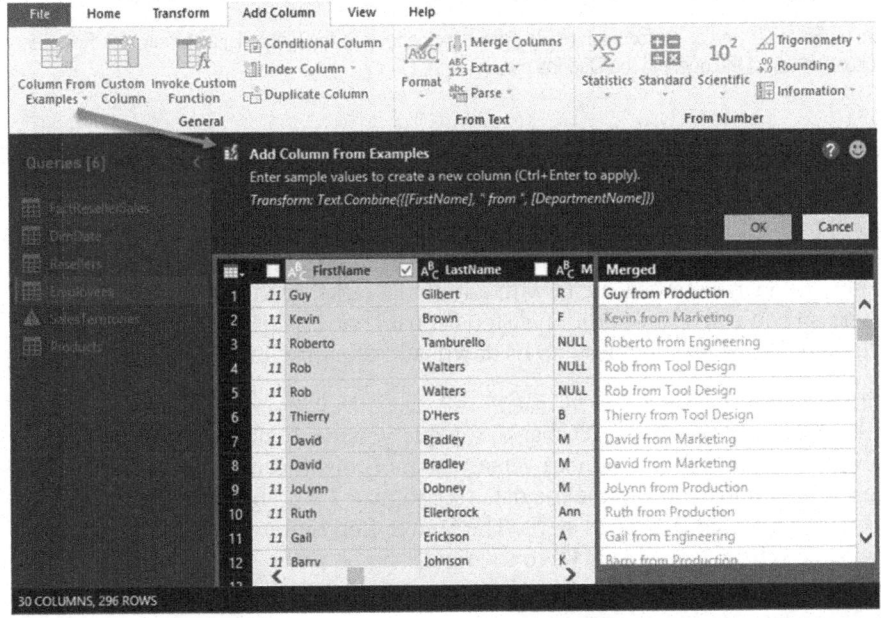

Figure 7.6 You can create custom columns by giving Query Editor an example of the desired outcome.

Understanding the ribbon's View tab

Figure 7.7 shows the ribbon's View tab. The Query Settings button in the Layout group toggles the visibility of the Query Settings pane (item 3 in **Figure 7.1**). The Formula Bar checkbox toggles the visibility of the formula bar that shows you the "M" formula behind the selected transformation step. Checking the Monospace checkbox in the Data Preview tab changes the text font in the Data Preview window (the window that shows the query results) to Monospace. When checked, the "Show whitespace" checkbox shows whitespace and newline characters in the Data Preview window.

Checking the "Always allow" checkbox turns on the "Parameter selection" control, so that users can interact with this widget without having to create a parameter beforehand. The Advanced Editor button does the same thing as the button with the same name (also called Advanced Editor) in the Home tab. It shows the source code of the query and allows you to change it. Finally, clicking the Query Dependencies button shows a diagram that can help visualize the dependencies between data sources and queries.

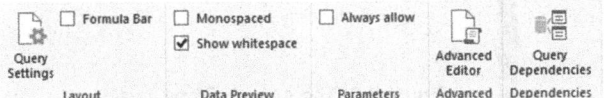

Figure 7.7 The View tab gives you access to the query source.

So, what does this "M" query language do for you anyway? It allows you to implement more advanced data manipulation. For example, Martin needs to load multiple Excel files from a given folder. Looping through files isn't an out-of-box feature. However, once Martin applies the necessary transformations to a single file, he can use the Advanced Editor to modify the query source to define a query function. Now Martin can automate the process by invoking the query function for each file, passing the file path. I'll show you some of these capabilities later in this chapter.

7.1.2 Understanding Queries

I mentioned in the previous chapter that there's a query behind every table you import or access live via DirectQuery (except when you connect live to Analysis Services). The whole purpose of the Query Editor is to give you access to these queries so that you can add additional transformation steps if needed.

 TIP A quick way to navigate to the underlying query for a table is to right-click the table in the Fields list and then click Edit Query. This will open the Query Editor and select the query in the Queries pane.

Understanding the Queries pane

The Queries pane (see item 5 in **Figure 7.1**) shows you all the queries that exist in the Power BI Desktop file. In the Adventure Works model, there are six queries because you've loaded six tables. In general, the number of queries correspond to the number of tables you use in the model, unless you've created queries for other more advanced tasks, such as to merge a query with results from other queries.

You can right-click a query to open a context menu with additional tasks, such as to delete, duplicate, reference (reuse another query so you can apply additional steps), enable or disable load (controls if the query produces a table in the model), move the query up or down, and organize queries in groups.

Understanding the Query Settings pane

As you've seen, the Query Settings pane allows you to change the query name. Renaming the query changes the name of the table in the data model and vice versa. The more significant role of Query Settings is to list all the steps you've applied to load and shape the data (see **Figure 7.8**). The query shown in the screenshot is named Products and it has four applied steps. The Source step represents the connection to the data source. Customizable steps have a cog icon (✿) to the right.

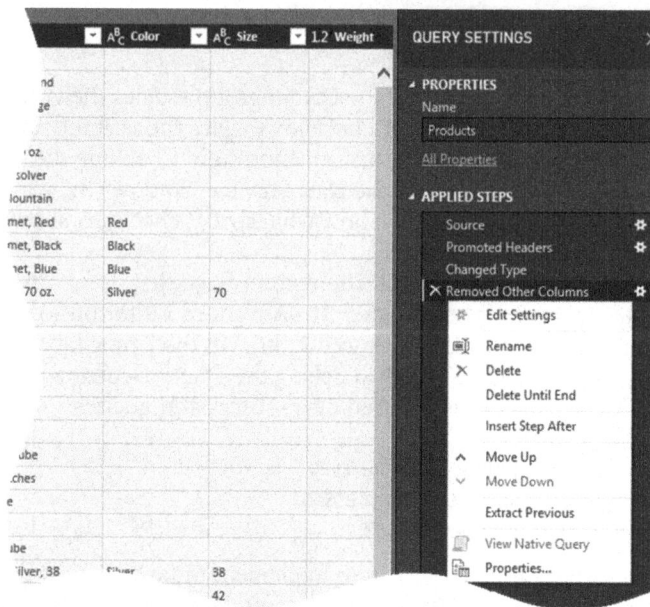

Figure 7.8 The Applied Steps section of Query Setting show all the steps applied to load and shape the data.

For example, when you click this icon for the Source step, a window opens to let you view and change the source settings, such as the name of the file and what delimiter will be used to parse the columns. If the Get Data flow used the Navigator window, such as to let you select a database table or an Excel sheet, the second step would be Navigation so that you can view or change the source table if needed. However, you imported the Products table from an SSRS report, and you didn't use the Navigator window.

Although you didn't specifically do this, Power BI Desktop applied the Promoted Headers step to promote the first row as column headers. Power BI Desktop applies the Change Type step when it discovers that it needs to overwrite the column data types. Finally, you applied the "Removed Other Columns" step when you removed some of the source columns when you imported the Product Catalog report.

You can click a step to select it. If the formula bar is enabled (you can check the Formula checkbox in the ribbon's View tab to enable it), you'll see the query language formula behind the step. In addition, selecting a step updates the data preview to show you how the step affected the source data. When you select a step in the Applied Steps list, the Data Preview pane shows the transformed data after that step is applied. So, you can always go back in the step history to check the effect of every step!

If the step is not needed, click the (X) button that appears to the left of the step name when you hover on it, or press the Delete key to remove a step. The Query Editor will ask you to confirm deleting intermediate steps because there might be dependent downstream steps and removing a prior step might result in breaking changes. You can also right-click a step to get additional options, such as to rename a step to make its name more descriptive, to delete it, to delete the current steps and all subsequent steps, to move the step up or down in the Applied Steps list, and to extract previous steps in a separate query.

7.1.3 Understanding Data Preview

The data preview pane (see item 4 back in **Figure 7.1**) shows a read-only view of the source schema and the data as of the time the query was created, or the data preview was last refreshed. Each column has a drop-down menu that lets you sort and filter the data before it's imported. Icons in the column headers indicate the column data type, such as a calendar icon for Date/Time columns.

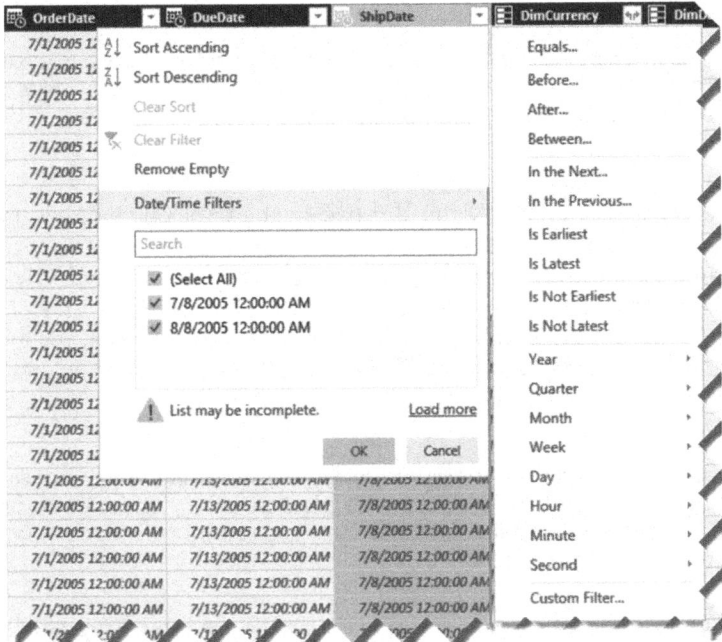

Figure 7.9 The column drop-down allows you to sort and filter the source data before it's loaded in the model

Understanding data filtering
Filtering allows you to exclude rows so you don't end up with more data than you need. The filtering options differ, based on the data type of the column. **Figure 7.9** shows the filtering options available for date/time columns.

NOTE Power BI queries have smarts to push as much processing as possible to some data sources. This is called query folding. For example, if you filter a column in a table that was imported from a relational database, the query would append a WHERE clause and pass it on to the data source. This is much more efficient than filtering the results after all the data is loaded. Filters, joins, groupings, type conversions, and column removal are examples of work that gets folded to the source. What gets folded depends on the capabilities of the source, level of support, internal logic, and the data source privacy level. If a transformation step results in query folding, you can right-click the step in the Applied Steps pane, and then click "View Native Query" to see what query is generated. You can't change the native query that the Query Editor generates.

For example, if I filter the ShipDate column in FactResellerSales for the last year, this will create a new transformation step that will load only the data for last year based on the system date.

TIP Do you want to export the data shown in the preview pane? While waiting for Microsoft to implement the "Export to Excel" feature, you can expand the Table icon in the top-left corner of the preview pane and click "Copy Entire Table". Then you can paste the data in Excel.

Understanding preview caching

The Query Editor status bar (see item 6 in the figure) informs you when the data preview of the selected query was last refreshed. A cached copy of the query preview results is stored on your local hard disk for faster viewing later. You can control the size of the data cache from File ⇨ Options and Settings ⇨ Options (Data Load tab). Because the preview results are cached, the data preview might get out of sync with schema and data changes in the data source. Click the Refresh Preview button to update the data preview.

If the data preview hasn't been refreshed for more than two days, a warning will be displayed above the preview pane. Don't confuse data preview refresh with table refresh in the data model (the Refresh button in the Power BI Desktop ribbon). The data model refresh executes the queries and reloads the data, while the query preview shows you what the data would look like after a step is applied.

NOTE By default, every time you refresh the model, Power BI will refresh the data previews for all queries in the model. This could become expensive with many queries or slow data sources. Try mitigating the performance hit by disabling "Allow data preview to download in the background" option from File ⇨ Options and Settings ⇨ Options (Data Load tab).

Auto-discovering relationships

When you import data from a database that has relationships defined between tables, the query discovers these relationships and adds corresponding columns to let you bring columns from the related tables. For example, if you select FactResellerSales and scroll the data preview pane all the way to the right, you'll see "split" columns for DimCurrency, DimDate (three columns for each relationship), DimEmployee, and all the other tables that FactResellerSales has relationships with in the AdventureWorksDW database. If you click the split button (⁍) in the column header, Query Editor opens a list that allows you to add columns from these tables. This handy feature saves you steps to create custom queries to join tables and to look up values in related tables.

NOTE The relationships in the Query Editor are different than the relationships in the model (discussed in detail in the next chapter). The former result in lookup joins between database tables. The later let you analyze data in one table by another. When you import tables, Power BI Desktop checks for database relationships during the auto-discovery process and it might add corresponding relationships to both the query as split columns and to the data model.

As you've seen, you can also rename columns in the Query Editor and in the Data View interchangeably. No matter which view you use to rename the column, the new name is automatically applied to the other view. However, I encourage you to check and fix the column data types (use the Transform group in the ribbon's Home tab) in the Query Editor so you can address data type issues before your data is loaded.

For example, you might expect a sales amount field to be a numeric column. However, when Query Editor parsed the column, it changed its data type to Text because of some invalid entries, such as "N/A" or "NULL". It would be much easier to fix these data type errors in the Query Editor, such as by using the

Remove Errors, Replace Errors, and Replace Values column-level transformations, than to use DAX formulas in the data model.

7.2 Shaping and Cleansing Data

Suppose that the Adventure Works Finance department gives Martin periodically (let's say every month or year) an Excel file that details accessories and parts that Adventure Works purchases from its vendors. Martin needs to analyze spending by vendor. The problem is that the source data is formatted in Excel tables that the Finance department prepared for its own analysis. This makes it very difficult for Martin to load the data and relate it to other tables that he might have in the model. Fortunately, the Query Editor component of Power BI Desktop allows Martin to transform and extract the data he needs. For the purposes of this exercise, you'll use the Vendor Parts.xlsx file that's located in the \Source\ch07 folder.

7.2.1 Applying Basic Transformations

Figure 7.10 shows the first two report sections in the Vendor Parts file. This format is not suitable for analysis and requires some preprocessing before data can be analyzed. Specifically, the data is divided in sections and each section is designed as an Excel table. However, you need just the data as a single Excel table, similar to the Resellers Excel file that you imported in the previous chapter. Another issue is that the data is presented as crosstab reports, making it impossible to join the vendor data to a Date table in the data model. Further, the category appears only in the first row of every section and each section has a subtotal row that you don't need.

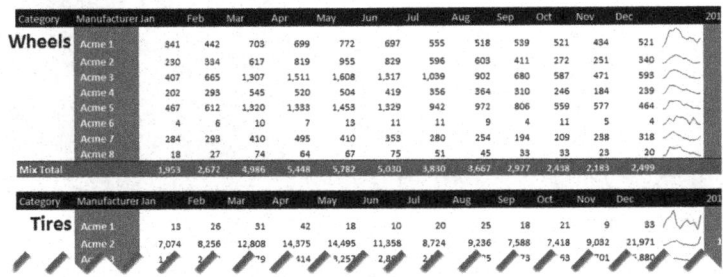

Figure 7.10 The Vendor Parts Excel file includes crosstab reports, which present a challenge for relating this data to other tables in the model.

Exploring source data
Let's follow familiar steps to connect to the Excel file. However, this time you'll launch the Query Editor before you import the data.

1. If the Vendor Parts file is open in Excel, close it so that Excel doesn't lock the file and prevent importing.
2. Open a new instance of Power BI Desktop. Save the file as *Query Examples*.
3. Expand the Get Data menu, and click Excel because you'll import an Excel file.
4. Navigate to the \Source\Ch07 folder and select the Vendor Parts.xlsx file. Then click Open.
5. In the Navigator window, check Sheet1 to select it and preview its data. The preview shows how the data would be imported if you don't apply any transformations. As you see, there are many issues with the data, including mixed column content, pivoted data by month, and null values.
6. Click the Edit button to open the Query Editor.

Removing rows
First, let's remove the unnecessary rows:

1. Right-click the first cell in the Column1 column, and then click Text Filters ⇨ "Does Not Equal" to filter only rows where the text in the first column doesn't equal "Vendor Parts – 2008". The net effect after applying this step is that the "Filtered Rows" step will all rows with that text (in our case only the first row will be excluded).

2. Locate the *null* value in the first cell of Column3, and apply the same filter (Text Filters ⇨ "Does Not Equal") to exclude all the rows that have *null* in Column3.

3. Promote the first row as headers so that each column has a descriptive column name. To do so, in the ribbon's Transform tab, click the "Use First Row as Headers" button. Alternatively, you can expand the table icon (in the top-left corner of the preview window), and then click "User First Row as Headers". Compare your results with **Figure 7.11**.

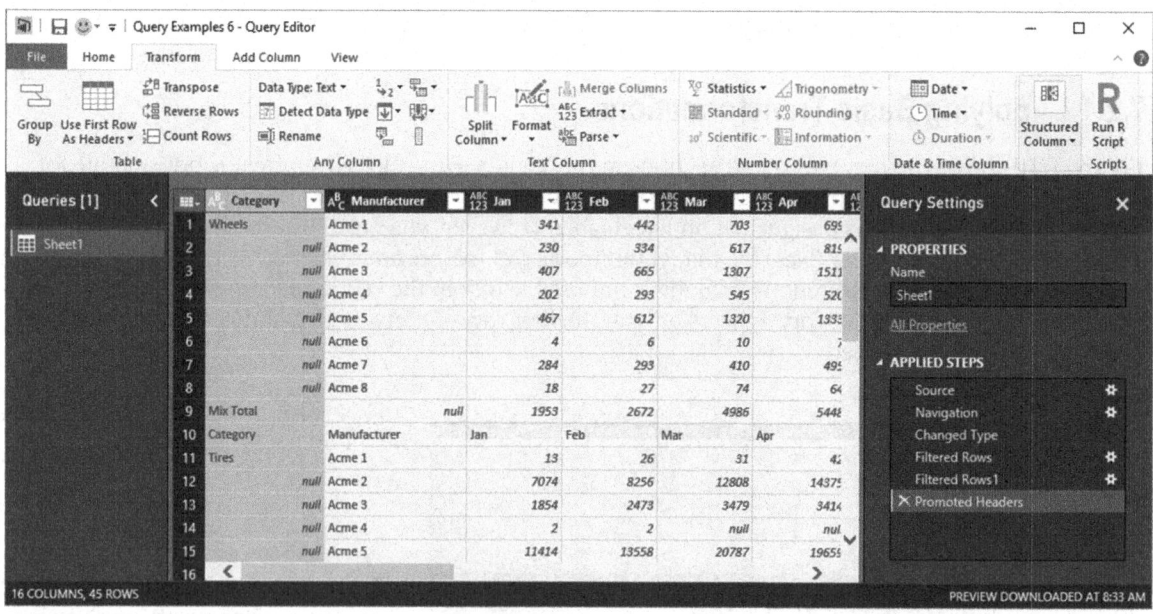

Figure 7.11   The source data after filtering unwanted rows.

4. Note that the first column (Category) has many null values. These empty values will present an issue when relating the table to other tables, such as Product. Click the first cell in the Category column (that says Wheels), and then click the ribbon's Transform tab. Click the Fill ⇨ Down button. This fills the null values with the actual categories.

5. Let's remove rows that represent report subtotals. To do so, right-click a cell in the Category column that contains the word "Category" (should be the first cell in the tenth row). Click Text Filters ⇨ "Does Not Equal" to remove all the rows that have "Category" in the first column.

6. Next, you will need to filter all the rows that contain the word "Total". Expand the column drop-down in the column header of the Category column. Click Text Filters ⇨ "Does Not Contain". In the Filter Rows dialog box, type "Total", and then click OK.

7. Hold the Ctrl key and select the last two columns, Column15 and 2014 Total. Right-click the selection, and then click Remove Columns.

Un-pivoting columns

Now that you've cleansed most of the data, there's one remaining task. Note how the months appear on columns. This makes it impossible to join the table to a Date table because you can't join on multiple columns. To make things worse, as new periods are added, the number of columns might increase. To solve this problem, you need to un-pivot the months from columns to rows. Fortunately, this is very easy to do with the Query Editor!

1. Hold the Shift key and select all the month columns, from Jan to Dec.

2. Right-click the selection, and then click Unpivot Columns. The Query Editor un-pivots the data by creating new columns called Attribute and Value, as shown in **Figure 7.12**.

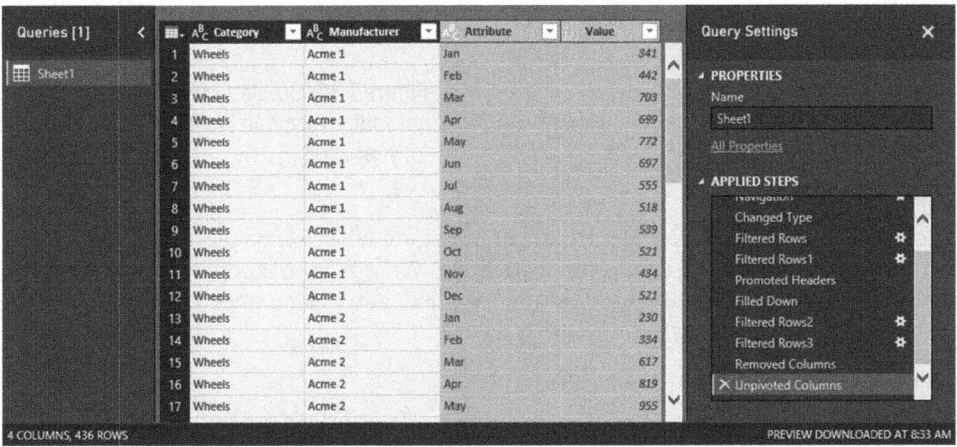

Figure 7.12 The un-pivoted dataset includes Attribute and Value columns.

8. Double-click the column header of the Attribute column, and rename it to *Month*. Rename the Value column to *Units*.

Adding custom columns

If you have a Date table in the model, you might want to join this data to it. As I mentioned, a Data table is at a day granularity. So that you can join to it, you need to convert the Month column to a date. Click the ribbon's Add Column tab, and then click "Custom Column".

1. In the "Add Custom Column" dialog box, enter *FirstDayOfMonth* as the column name. Then enter the following formula (be careful because the "M" query language is case sensitive):

```
=Date.FromText([Month] & " 1, 2008")
```

2. Compare your results with **Figure 7.13**. Click OK to close the "Add Custom Column" window.

This formula converts the month value to the first day of the month in year 2008. For example, if the Month value is Jan, the resulting value will be 1/1/2008. The formula hardcodes the year to 2008 because the source data doesn't have the actual year. If you need to default to the current year, you can use the formula Date.Year(DateTime.LocalNow()). Or, had the year been present in a column, you could simply reference that column in the expression.

> **NOTE** Unfortunately, as it stands the "Add Custom Column" window doesn't have IntelliSense or show you the formula syntax, making it difficult to work with formulas and forcing a "trial and error" approach. If you've made a mistake, the custom column will display "Error" in every row. You can click the Error link to get more information about the error. Then in the Applied Steps pane, click the Settings next to the step to get back to the formula, and try again.

3. Assuming you need the month end date instead of the first date of the month, select the FirstDayOfMonth column in the data preview pane. In the ribbon's Transform tab, expand the Date drop-down button, and then select Month ⇨ "End of Month".

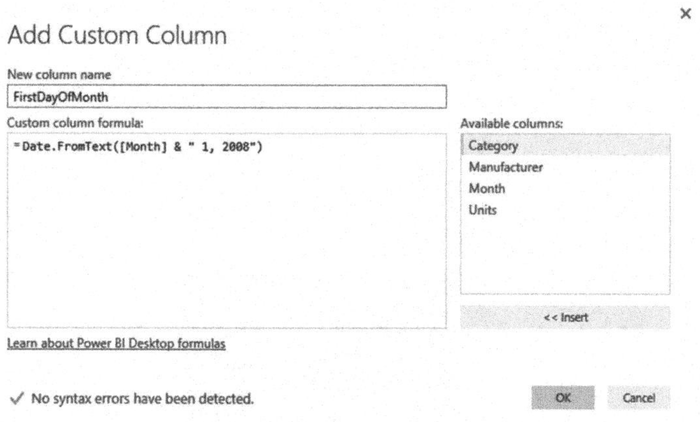

Add Custom Column

New column name

FirstDayOfMonth

Custom column formula:

`=Date.FromText([Month] & " 1, 2008")`

Available columns:

Category
Manufacturer
Month
Units

<< Insert

Learn about Power BI Desktop formulas

✓ No syntax errors have been detected.

OK   Cancel

Figure 7.13 Create a custom column that converts a month to the first day in that month for year 2008.

4. Rename the new column to *Date*.

That's it! With a few clicks you added a dozen steps that will transform and cleanse the source data into a format that is suitable for reporting. But the data is not loaded yet. What you just did was defining the steps that will be executed in the order that are listed in the "Applied Steps" pane once you load or refresh the data.

7.2.2 Loading Transformed Data

As I explained before, you have used the "Close & Apply" button to load the data. Recall that the first option "Close & Apply" closes the Query Editor and applies the changes to the model. You can close the Query Editor without applying the changes, but the model and queries aren't synchronized. Finally, you can choose to apply the changes without closing the Query Editor so that you can continue working on the queries.

Renaming steps and queries
Before loading the data, consider renaming the query to apply the same name to the new table. You can also rename transformation steps to make them more descriptive. Let's rename the query and a step:

1. In the Query Settings pane, rename the query to *VendorParts*. This will become the name of the table in the model.

2. In the Applied Steps pane, right-click the last step and click Rename. Change the step name to *"Renamed Column to Date"*, and click Enter.

3. (Optional) Right-click any of the steps in the Applied Steps pane, and click Properties. Notice that you can enter a description. Then when you hover on the step, the description will show in a tooltip. This is a great way to explain what a step does in more detail.

Loading transformed data
Let's load the transformed data into a new table:

1. Click the Close & Apply button in the ribbon's Home tab. Power BI Desktop imports the data, applies all the steps as the data streams into the model, closes the Query Editor, and adds the VendorParts table to the Fields pane.

2. In the ribbon's Home tab, click the Edit Queries button. This brings you to the Query Editor in case you want to apply additional transformation steps.

3. (Optional) You can disable loading query results. This could be useful if another query uses the results from the VendorParts query and it doesn't make sense to create unnecessary tables in the model. To demonstrate this, open Query Editor, right-click the VendorParts query in the Queries pane, and then uncheck "Enable Load". Accept the warning that follows that disabling the query load will delete the table from the model and break existing reports. Click Close & Apply and notice that the VendorParts table is removed from the Fields list.

> **TIP** Sometimes things go bad, such when an input file is not found in the expected source folder. Power BI doesn't have native capabilities for error handling or branching so the query would just fail. However, with some coding effort, you can handle errors gracefully. Chris Webb demonstrates a possible approach in his "Handling Data Source Errors in Power Query" blog at https://blog.crossjoin.co.uk/2014/09/18/handling-data-source-errors-in-power-query/.

7.3 Using Advanced Features

The Query Editor has much more to offer than just basic column transformations. In this section, I'll walk you through more advanced scenarios that you might encounter so that you handle them yourself instead of asking for help. First, you'll see how you can join and merge datasets. Then I'll show you how query functions can help you automate mundane data processing tasks. You'll find how to use the "M" query language to auto-generate date tables and how to parameterize connections to data sources.

7.3.1 Combining Datasets

As I mentioned previously, if relationships exist in the database, the query will discover these relationships. This allows you to expand a table and reference columns from other tables. For example, if you open the Adventure Works model (Adventure Works.pbix) and examine the data preview pane of the FactResellerSales query, you'll see columns that correspond to all the tables that are related to the FactResellerSales table in the AdventureWorksDW database. These columns show the text "Value" for each row in FactResellerSales and have an expansion button ([↔]) in the column header (see **Figure 7.14**).

When you click the expansion button, the Query Editor opens a window that lists all the columns from the related table so that you can include the columns you want in the query. This is a useful feature, but what if there are no relationships in the data source? As it turns out, if you have matching columns, you can merge (join) queries.

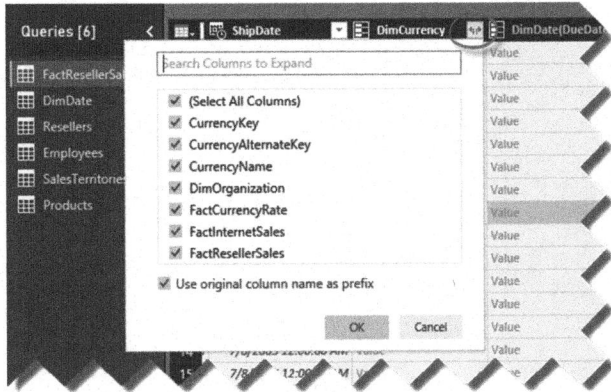

Figure 7.14 Create a custom column that converts a month to a date.

Merging queries

We're back to the Query Examples.pbix file. Suppose you have another query that returns a list of vendors that Adventure Works does business with. Let's import this list.

1. If the Query Editor is closed, click the Edit Queries button in the Power BI Desktop's ribbon to open it. In the Query Editor's Home ribbon, expand Get Data and then click Excel.

2. Navigate to the \Source\ch07 folder and select the Vendor Parts file.

3. In the Navigator window, check the Vendors sheet and then click Load. This creates a Vendors query that load the data from the Vendors sheet in the Excel file.

4. In the Queries pane, make sure the Vendors query is selected. Select the Transform ribbon tab and then click "Use First Row as Headers" button to promote the first row as column headers.

5. Compare your results with **Figure 7.15**.

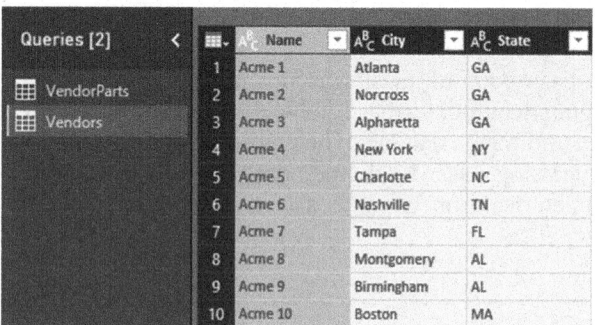

Figure 7.15 The Vendors query returns a list of vendors imported from the Vendors sheet in the Vendor Parts Excel file.

Now I'd like to join the VendorParts query to the Vendors query so that I can look up some columns from the Vendor query and add them to the VendorParts query. If two queries have a matching column(s) you can join (merge) them just like you can join two tables in SQL.

6. In the Queries pane, select the VendorParts query because this will be our base query.

7. In the ribbon's Home tab, click Merge Queries (in the Combine group).

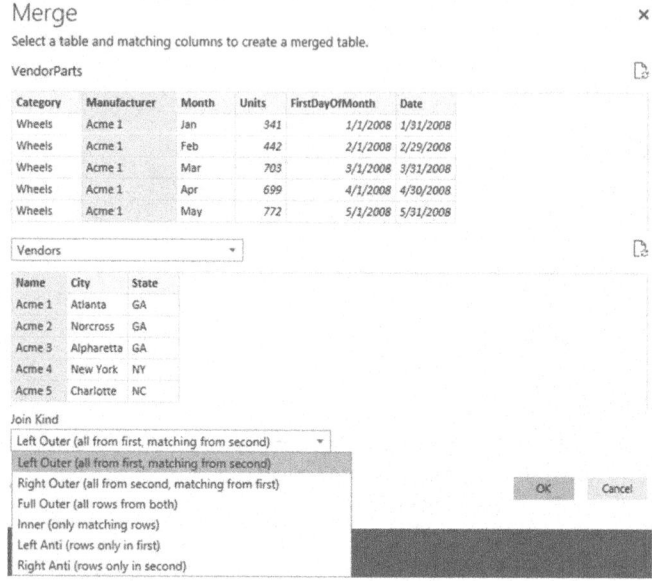

Figure 7.16 You can merge queries by one or more matching columns.

8. Configure the Merge window as shown in **Figure 7.16**. This setup joins the Manufacturer column from the VendorParts query to the Name column of the Vendors query. Notice that the Join Kind list has different types of joins. For example, a Left Outer Join will keep all the rows from the first query and only return the matching values from the second query, or null if no match is found. By contrast, the Inner Join will only return matching rows.

9. Click OK. The Query Editor adds a NewColumn column to the end of the VendorParts query.

10. Click the expansion button in the column header of the new column. Notice that now you can add columns from the Vendors query (**Figure 8.16**). You can also aggregate these columns, such as by using the Sum or Count aggregation functions.

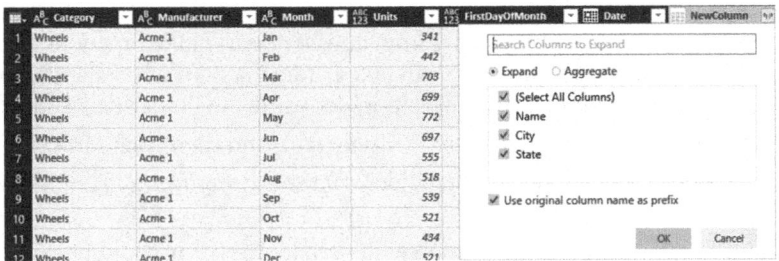

Figure 7.17 Once you merge queries, you can add columns to the source query from the merged query.

Appending queries

Suppose that some time has passed, and Martin gets another Vendors Parts report, for the year 2009. Instead of overwriting the existing data for 2008 in the data model, which will happen if Martin refreshes the data, Martin wants to append the second dataset to the VendorParts table so he can analyze data across several years. If Martin is given a new file occasionally, such as in a month or year, he can use the "Append Queries" feature to append datasets manually. This will work if the dataset format (schema) is the same. To simulate a second dataset, you'll clone the existing VendorParts query.

 TIP If Martin knows that he'd be importing multiple files, instead of appending queries he can just use the Get Data ⇨ Folder data source. I'll demonstrate the Folder data source in "Using Functions" section. The Append Query feature is useful when you want to combine a limited number of datasets, especially if they require different transformations before appending them.

1. In the Queries pane, right-click the VendorParts query, and then click Duplicate. The Query Editor adds a VendorParts (2) query.

2. In the Queries pane, select the VendorParts (2) query. Click the cog icon (✿) to the right of "Added Custom" step, and then change the formula to use year 2009. You do this to simulate that this dataset has data for the year 2009.

=Date.FromText([Month] & " 1, 2009")

3. In the Query Settings pane, rename the VendorsParts (2) query to *VendorParts 2009*.

4. Right-click *VendorParts 2009* and turn off Enable Load because you'll append this query and you don't want it to create a new table when you click Close & Apply.

5. In the Queries pane, select the VendorParts query.

6. In the ribbon's Home tab, click Append Queries (in the Combine group).

7. In the Append window, expand "Table to append" and select the VendorParts 2009 query. Click OK. The Query Editor appends VendorParts 2009 to VendorParts. As a result, the VendorParts query returns a combined dataset for years 2008 and 2009. If two queries have the same columns, you can append them.

 TIP If you need more complicated logic to look up values from another table you might find my blog "Implementing Lookups in Power Query" at http://prologika.com/implementing-lookups-in-power-query/ useful. It demonstrates a query function that uses a range filter for the lookup.

7.3.2 Using Functions

Appending datasets manually can get tedious quickly as the number of files increase. What if Martin is given Excel files every month and he needs to combine 100 files? Or, what if he needs to extract data from many pages in a paged table on a web page? Well, when the going gets tough, you write some automation code, right? If you have a programming background, your first thought might be to write code that loops through files, to check if the file is an Excel file, to load it, and so on. However, the "M" language that Power BI queries are written in is a functional language, and it doesn't support loops and conditional logic. What it does support is functions and they can be incredibly useful for automation.

Using the Folder data source

Think of a query function as a query that can be called repeatedly from another query. Like functions in programming languages, such as C# and Visual Basic, a function can take parameters. To understand how query functions work, we'll create a query that combines some files in folder using the Folder data source.

1. In the Query Editor, expand the New Source button (in the ribbon's Home tab), and then click More.

2. In the Get Data window, click the File tab and select Folder. The Folder data source returns a list of files in a specific folder. Click Connect.

3. In the Folder window, specify the folder path where the Excel source files are located. For your convenience, I saved two Excel files (with same definition) in the \Source\ch07\Files folder. Click OK.

4. A window opens to show a list of files in that folder. Click the "Combine & Edit" button.

5. In the Combine Files window, select Sheet1. Notice that the preview window shows what the data would look like after the files are appended. Notice also that without any transformations, the data will have the same issues that we've addressed in the Vendor Parts query. Click OK.

Query Editor does several things. First, it creates a new query called Files. Then it creates a new query group "Transform File from Files" (see **Figure 7.18**). A query group shows related items together and makes it easier to work with functions. For example, the "Transform File from Files" group has a Sample Query subgroup that shows the definition of one of the files in the source folder. Then, there is a "Transform Sample File from Files" query, which has a dependent function "Transform File from File" (prefixed with *fx*). When you make changes to the "Transform Sample File from Files" query, Query Editor updates the function automatically to match changes to the source file.

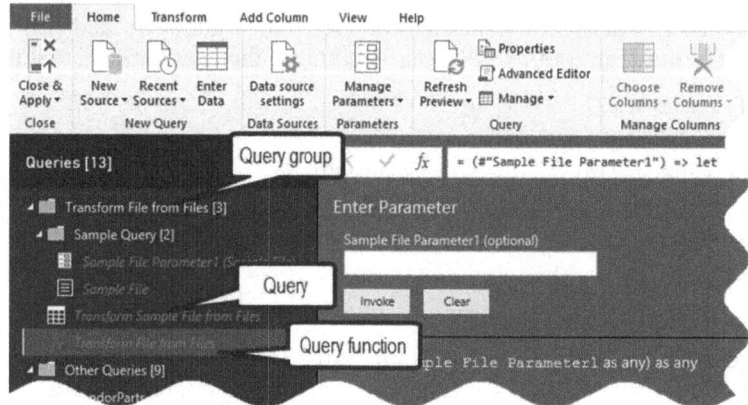

Figure 7.18 A query group facilitates testing query functions.

6. From the View ribbon, click Query Dependencies to visualize how these objects related to each other. Click Close in the Query Dependencies window.

Understanding functions

Let's take a moment to understand how the "Transform File from Files" function works.

1. In the Query Pane, click the "Transform File from Files" function. Notice that it takes a parameter that represents the full path to a file. The Enter Parameter dialog allows you to pass a value for the parameter and test the function. However, in this case the function expects the binary content of the file, which is what the Folder data source creates, so you can't really test the function using the Enter Parameter feature.

2. In the Queries pane, rename the "Transform File from Files" function to *fnProcessFile*.

3. Right-click *fnProcessFile* and click Advanced Editor to see the function source described in the M programming language (see **Figure 7.19**).

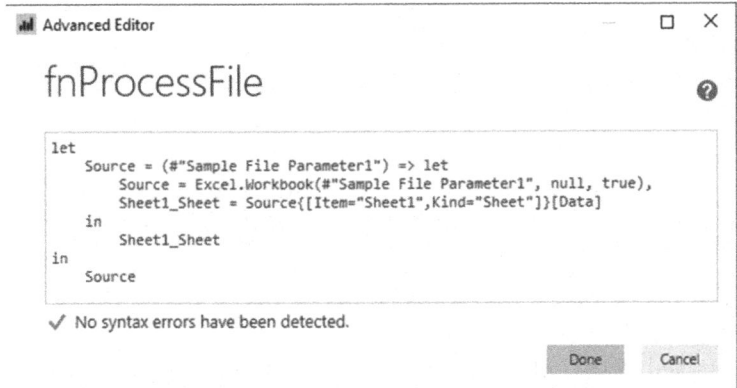

Figure 7.19 The fnProcessFile function takes the file content as an argument and loads the file.

Notice that function takes a parameter called #"Sample File Parameter1" that represents the file binary content. Then it loads Sheet1 from the Excel file.

4. In the Queries pane, click the Files query at the bottom of the list. Note that the second step invokes the fnProcessFile function for each file in the folder.

 TIP Do you want to process only files with a specific file extension? Click the Source step in the Applied Steps pane. In the data preview pane, expand the drop-down in the column header of the Extension column, and select only the file extension(s) you need.

Modifying functions

As useful as the fnProcessFile query function is, it doesn't apply the transformations we did in the Vendor Parts query. Let's fix this now.

1. In the Queries pane, right-click the Vendor Parts query and then click Advanced Editor. Copy all rows starting with Sheet1_Sheet line and ending with the #"Appended Query" line (before the *in* operator).

2. In the Queries pane, right-click the fnProcessFile function and then click Advanced Editor. Replace the content of the function, as shown below.

```
let
    Source = (#"Sample File Parameter1") => let
    Source = Excel.Workbook(#"Sample File Parameter1", null, true),
    Sheet1_Sheet = Source{[Item="Sheet1",Kind="Sheet"]}[Data],
    #"Changed Type" = Table.TransformColumnTypes(Sheet1_Sheet,{{"Column1", type text}, {"Column2", type text}, {"Column3", type any}, {"Column4", type any}, {"Column5", type any}, {"Column6", type any}, {"Column7", type any}, {"Column8", type any}, {"Column9", type any}, {"Column10", type any}, {"Column11", type any}, {"Column12", type any}, {"Column13", type any}, {"Column14", type any}, {"Column15", type any}, {"Column16", type any}}),
    #"Filtered Rows" = Table.SelectRows(#"Changed Type", each [Column1] <> "Vendor Parts - 2008"),
    #"Filtered Rows1" = Table.SelectRows(#"Filtered Rows", each [Column3] <> null),
```

```
    #"Promoted Headers" = Table.PromoteHeaders(#"Filtered Rows1"),
    #"Filled Down" = Table.FillDown(#"Promoted Headers",{"Category"}),
    #"Filtered Rows2" = Table.SelectRows(#"Filled Down", each [Category] <> "Category"),
    #"Filtered Rows3" = Table.SelectRows(#"Filtered Rows2", each not Text.Contains([Category], "Total")),
    #"Removed Columns" = Table.RemoveColumns(#"Filtered Rows3",{"Column15", "2014 Total"}),
    #"Unpivoted Columns" = Table.UnpivotOtherColumns(#"Removed Columns", {"Category", "Manufacturer"}, "Attribute", "Value"),
    #"Renamed Columns" = Table.RenameColumns(#"Unpivoted Columns",{{"Attribute", "Month"}, {"Value", "Units"}}),
    #"Added Custom" = Table.AddColumn(#"Renamed Columns", "FirstDayOfMonth", each Date.FromText([Month] & " 1, 2008")),
    #"Inserted End of Month" = Table.AddColumn(#"Added Custom", "EndOfMonth", each Date.EndOfMonth([FirstDayOfMonth]), type
date),
    #"Renamed Column to Date" = Table.RenameColumns(#"Inserted End of Month",{{"EndOfMonth", "Date"}}),
    #"Merged Queries" = Table.NestedJoin(#"Renamed Column to Date",{"Manufacturer"},Vendors,{"Name"},"NewColumn",Join-
Kind.LeftOuter),
    #"Appended Query" = Table.Combine({#"Merged Queries", #"VendorParts 2009"})
in
    #"Appended Query"
in
    Source
```

3. (Optional) Change the #"Sample File Parameter1" to *FileContent* to describe better its purpose. For your convenience, I provided the source code of the fnProcessFile function in the fnProcessFile.txt file in the \Source\ch07 folder.

4. Click OK to close the Advanced Editor.

5. Notice in the Queries pane that the Files query shows a warning sign.

6. Click the Files query. Click each of the applied steps (unfortunately, there isn't a better way to discover which steps has failed), and find that the issue is with the last step Changed Type. This step is looking for Column1 which the code from Vendor Parts doesn't have. Delete this step.

7. Rename the Files query to *ProcessExcelFiles*.

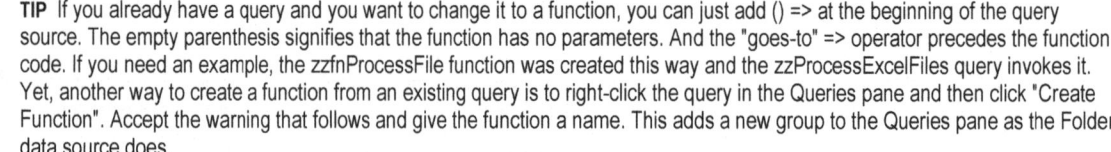

TIP If you already have a query and you want to change it to a function, you can just add () => at the beginning of the query source. The empty parenthesis signifies that the function has no parameters. And the "goes-to" => operator precedes the function code. If you need an example, the zzfnProcessFile function was created this way and the zzProcessExcelFiles query invokes it. Yet, another way to create a function from an existing query is to right-click the query in the Queries pane and then click "Create Function". Accept the warning that follows and give the function a name. This adds a new group to the Queries pane as the Folder data source does.

For each file in the folder, the ProcessExcelFiles query calls the fnProcessFile function. Each time the function is invoked, it loads the file passed as argument and appends the results. So, the function does the heavy work but you need a query to invoke it repeatedly.

NOTE If you expand the drop-down of the Date column in the ProcessExcelFiles results, you'll only see dates for year 2008, which might let you believe that you have data from one file only. This is not the case, but it's a logical bug because year 2008 is hard-coded in the query. If the year is specified in the file name, you can add another custom column that extracts the year, passes it to a third parameter in the fnProcessFile function, and uses that parameter instead of hardcoded references to "2008".

7.3.3 Generating Date Tables

Now that you know about query functions, I'm sure you'll think of many real-life scenarios where you can use them to automate routine data crunching tasks. Let's revisit a familiar scenario. As I mentioned in Chapter 6, even if you import a single dataset, you should strongly consider a separate date table. I also mentioned that there are different ways to import a date table, and one of them was to generate it in the Query Editor. The following code is based on an example by Matt Masson, as described in his "Creating a

Date Dimension with a Power Query Script" blog post (https://mattmasson.com/2014/02/creating-a-date-dimension-with-a-power-query-script/).

Generating dates

The Query Editor has useful functions for manipulating dates, such as for extracting date parts (day, month, quarter), and so on. The code uses many of these functions.

1. Start by creating a new blank query. To do so, in the Query Editor, expand the New Source button (the ribbon's Home tab) and click Blank Query. Rename the blank query to *GenerateDateTable*.

2. In the Queries pane, right-click the GenerateDateTable query and click Advanced Editor.

3. In the Advanced Editor, paste the following code which you can copy from the GenerateDateTable.txt file in the \Source\ch07 folder:

```
let GenerateDateTable = (StartDate as date, EndDate as date, optional Culture as nullable text) as table =>
  let
    DayCount = Duration.Days(Duration.From(EndDate - StartDate)),
    Source = List.Dates(StartDate,DayCount,#duration(1,0,0,0)),
    TableFromList = Table.FromList(Source, Splitter.SplitByNothing()),
    ChangedType = Table.TransformColumnTypes(TableFromList,{{"Column1", type date}}),
    RenamedColumns = Table.RenameColumns(ChangedType,{{"Column1", "Date"}}),
    InsertYear = Table.AddColumn(RenamedColumns, "Year", each Date.Year([Date])),
    InsertQuarter = Table.AddColumn(InsertYear, "QuarterOfYear", each Date.QuarterOfYear([Date])),
    InsertMonth = Table.AddColumn(InsertQuarter, "MonthOfYear", each Date.Month([Date])),
    InsertDay = Table.AddColumn(InsertMonth, "DayOfMonth", each Date.Day([Date])),
    InsertDayInt = Table.AddColumn(InsertDay, "DateInt", each [Year] * 10000 + [MonthOfYear] * 100 + [DayOfMonth]),
    InsertMonthName = Table.AddColumn(InsertDayInt, "MonthName", each Date.ToText([Date], "MMMM", Culture), type text),
    InsertCalendarMonth = Table.AddColumn(InsertMonthName, "MonthInCalendar", each (try(Text.Range([MonthName],0,3))
      otherwise [MonthName]) & " " & Number.ToText([Year])),
    InsertCalendarQtr = Table.AddColumn(InsertCalendarMonth, "QuarterInCalendar", each "Q" & Number.ToText([QuarterOfYear]) & " "
& Number.ToText([Year])),
    InsertDayWeek = Table.AddColumn(InsertCalendarQtr, "DayInWeek", each Date.DayOfWeek([Date])),
    InsertDayName = Table.AddColumn(InsertDayWeek, "DayOfWeekName", each Date.ToText([Date], "dddd", Culture), type text),
    InsertWeekEnding = Table.AddColumn(InsertDayName, "WeekEnding", each Date.EndOfWeek([Date]), type date)
  in
    InsertWeekEnding
in
  GenerateDateTable
```

This code creates a GenerateDateTable function that takes three parameters: start date, end date, and optional language culture, such as "en-US", to localize the date formats and correctly interpret the date parameters. The workhorse of the function is the List.Dates method, which returns a list of date values starting at the start date and adding a day to every value. Then the function applies various transformations and adds custom columns to generate date variants, such as Year, QuarterOfYear, and so on.

Invoking the function

Remember that you need an outer query to invoke the GenerateDateTable function even if don't have to execute it repeatedly. Fortunately, Query Editor can do this for you.

1. In the Queries pane, select the GenerateDateTable function.

2. In the Enter Parameters window (see **Figure 7.20**), enter StartDate and EndDate parameters. Click OK to invoke the function. Query Editor adds an Invoked Function query to wrap the function call.

3. Click the Invoked Function query and notice that it has the desired results. If you want to regenerate the table with a different range of values, simply delete the "Invoked Function" query in the Queries pane, and then invoke the function again with different parameters, or change the query's Source step.

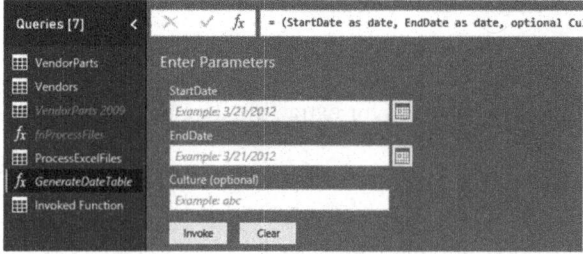

Figure 7.20 Invoke the Generate-DateTable function and pass the required parameters.

7.3.4 Working with Query Parameters

As you've seen, query functions can go a long way to help you create reusable queries. However, sometimes you might need a quick and easy way to customize the query behavior. Suppose you want to change the data source connection to point to a different server, such as when you want to switch from your development server to a production server. Or, you might need a convenient way to pass parameters to a stored procedure. This is where query parameters can help.

A query parameter externalizes certain query settings, such as a data source reference, a column replacement value, a query filter, and others, so that you can customize the query behavior without having to change the query itself. How do you know what query settings can be parameterized? If a step in the Applied Steps pane has a cog icon next to it (has a window that let you change its settings), click it and look for settings that are prefixed with a drop-down A^B_C ▾. If you see it, then that setting can be parameterized.

 TIP Even if you don't see the "abc" drop-down, you can still parameterize they query but you need to change the code manually. My blog "Power BI DirectQuery with Parameterized Stored Procedure" at http://prologika.com/power-bi-directquery-with-parameterized-stored-procedure/ demonstrates how this can done to pass parameters to a stored procedure.

Don't confuse query parameters with what-if parameters (the New Parameter in the Modeling ribbon). The former is for parameterizing queries to the data source. The latter is for parameterizing DAX measures for runtime what-if analysis.

Creating query parameters

Suppose you're given access to a development SQL Server and you have created a model with many tables. Now, you want to load data from another server, such as your production server. This isn't as bad as it sounds because you can click the "Data Source Settings" button found in the Query Editor's Home ribbon group and change the server name. But suppose you want to switch back and forth between development and production environments and you don't want to remember (and type in) the server names (they can get rather cryptic sometimes). Instead, you'll create a query parameter that will let you change the data source with a couple of mouse clicks.

1. To have a test query, in the Query Editor (Home ribbon), expand Get Data and import a table, such as DimProduct, from the AdventureWorksDW database. You can import any table you want. If you don't have access to SQL Server, you can import the \Source\ch07\DimProduct file and then follow similar steps to parameterize the query connection string.

2. In the Home ribbon's tab, click the Manage Parameters button.

3. In the Parameters window, click the New link and create a new parameter (see **Figure 7.21**).

I've created a required parameter named *Server*. The parameter data type is Text. I've decided to choose the parameter value from a pre-defined list that includes two servers (ELITE and MILLENNIA). You can also type in the parameter value or load it from an existing query. The parameter will default to ELITE and the parameter current value is ELITE. Consequently, I'll be referencing the ELITE server in my queries.

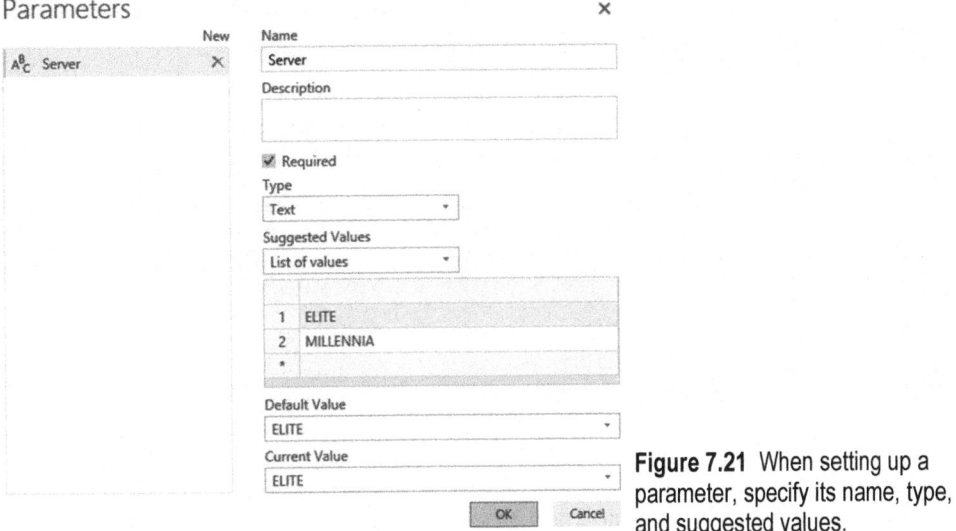

Figure 7.21 When setting up a parameter, specify its name, type, and suggested values.

4. Click OK to create the parameter.

Using query parameters

Now that we have the Server parameter defined, let's use it to change the data source in all queries. The following steps assume that you want to change the server name in all queries that reference the SQL Server. If you want to change only specific queries, instead of using Data Source Settings, change the Source step in the Applied Steps pane for these queries.

1. In the Home ribbon, click the Data Source Settings button.

2. In the Data Source Settings window, select the data source that references your server, and then click the Change Source button. If the data source is SQL Server, the familiar "SQL Server Database" window opens.

3. Expand the drop-down to the left of the server name and choose Parameter. Then expand the drop-down to the right and select the Server parameter (see **Figure 7.22**). Click OK.

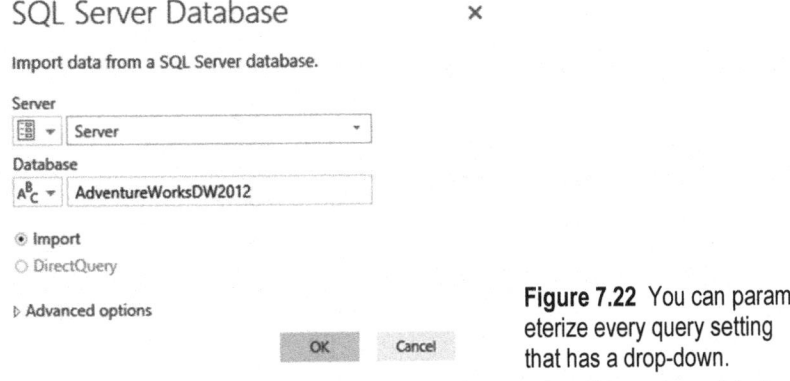

Figure 7.22 You can parameterize every query setting that has a drop-down.

4. In the Query Editor, observe that a new query named Server is added to the query list. By default, the query results won't be loaded in a table, but you can right-click the query and click Enable Load.

5. Besides settings the parameter value in the Query Editor, you can do so directly in Power BI Desktop without having to open Query Editor. In the Power BI Desktop window (Home ribbon's tab), expand the Edit Queries tab and then click Edit Parameters. Notice that you can change the Server parameter.

NOTE Unfortunately, Power BI doesn't expose the query parameters in reports. Therefore, there is no way for the end user viewing a report in Power BI Service or Power BI Report Server to set the query parameter, such as to pass a different value to a stored procedure with DirectQuery connection to SQL Server. You can change query parameters only in Power BI Desktop.

7.4 Summary

Behind the scenes, when you import data, Power BI Desktop creates a query and there's a query for every table you import. Not only does the query give you access to the source data, but it also allows you to shape and transform data using various table and column-level transformations. To practice this, you applied a series of steps to shape and clean a crosstab Excel report so that its results can be used in a self-service data model.

You also practiced more advanced query features. You learned how to join, merge, and append datasets. Every step you apply to the query generates a line of code described in the M query language. You can view and customize the code to meet more advanced scenarios and automate repetitive tasks. You learned how to use query functions to automate importing files. And you saw how you can use custom query code to generate date tables if you can't import them from other places. You can also define query parameters to customize the query behavior.

Next, you'll learn how to extend and refine the model to make it more feature-rich and intuitive to end users!

Chapter 8

Refining the Model

In the previous two chapters, you learned how to import and transform data. The next step is to explore and refine your data model before you start gaining insights from it. Typical tasks in this phase include making table and field names more intuitive, exploring data, and changing the column type and formatting options. When your model has multiple tables, you must also set up relationships to relate tables.

In this chapter, you'll practice common tasks to enhance the Adventure Works model. First, you'll learn how to explore the loaded data and how to refine the metadata. Next, I'll show you how to manage schema and data changes, including managing connections and tables, and refreshing the model data to synchronize it with changes in the data sources. Finally, I'll walk you through the steps needed to set up table relationships so that you can perform analysis across multiple tables.

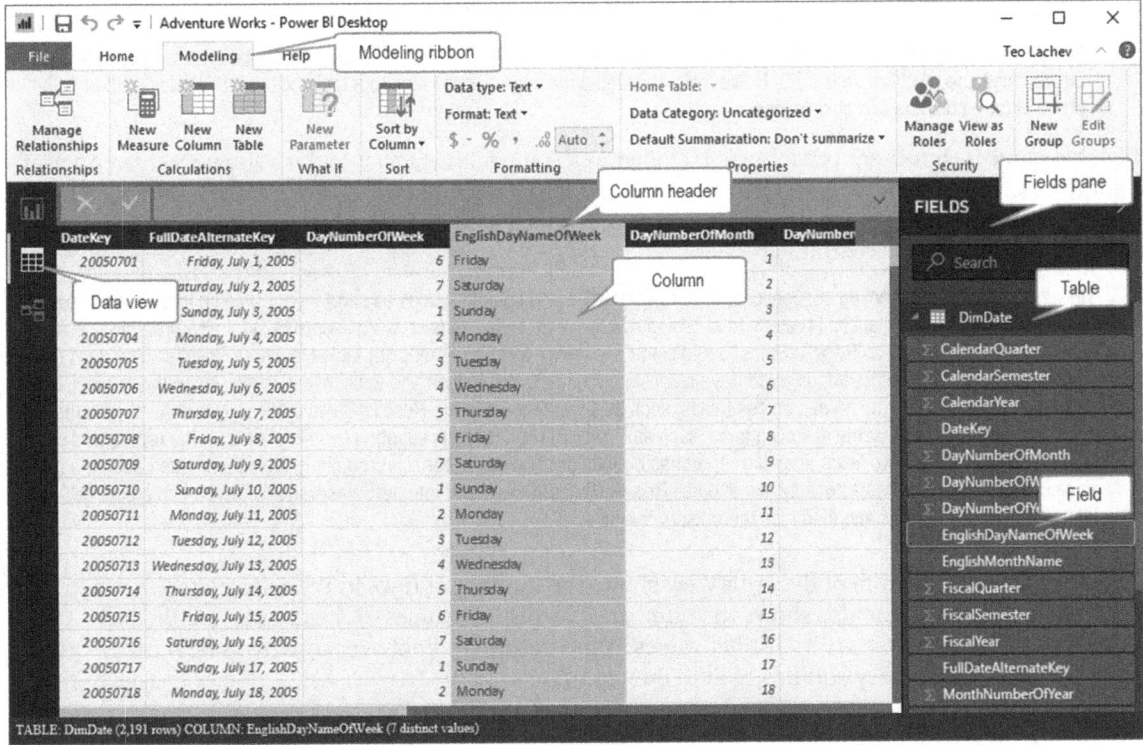

Figure 8.1   In the Data View, you can browse the model schema and data.

8.1 Understanding Tables and Columns

Recall from Chapter 6 that Power BI Desktop supports two data connectivity options: you can either import or connect directly to your data. If you decide to import, Power BI stores imported data in tables. Although the data might originate from heterogeneous data sources, once it enters the model, it's treated the same regardless of its origin. Like a relational database, a table consists of columns and rows. You can use the Data View (only available for models that import data) to explore the table schema and its data, as shown in **Figure 8.1**.

8.1.1 Understanding the Data View

The Power BI Desktop navigation bar (the vertical bar on the left) has three view icons: Report, Data, and Relationships. As its name suggests, the Data View is for browsing the model data. In contrast, the Relationships View only shows a graphical representation of the model schema. And the Report View is for creating visualizations that help you analyze the data. In Chapter 6, I covered how the Data View shows the imported data from the tables in the model. This is different from the Query Editor data preview, which shows the source data and how it's affected by the transformations you've applied.

Understanding tables

The Fields pane shows you the model metadata that you interact with when creating reports. When you select a table in the Fields pane, the Data View shows you the first rows in the table. As it stands, the Adventure Works model has six tables. The Data View and the Fields pane shows the metadata (table names and column names) sorted alphabetically. You can also use the Search box in the Fields pane to find fields quickly, such as type in *sales* to filter all fields whose name include "sales".

 NOTE What's the difference between a column and a field anyway? A field in the Fields pane can be a table column or a calculated measure, such as SalesYTD. However, a calculated measure doesn't map to a table column. So, fields include both physical table columns and calculations.

The table name is significant because it's included in the model metadata, and it's shown to the end user. In addition, when you create calculated columns and measures, the Data Analysis Expressions (DAX) formulas reference the table and field names. Therefore, spend some time to choose suitable names and to rename tables and fields accordingly.

 TIP When it comes to naming conventions, I like to keep table and column names as short as possible so that they don't occupy too much space in report labels. I prefer camel casing where the first letter of each word is capitalized. I also prefer to use a plural case for fact tables, such as ResellerSales, and a singular case for lookup (dimension) tables, such as Reseller. You don't have to follow this convention, but it's important to have a consistent naming convention and to stick to it. While I'm on this subject, Power BI supports identical column names across tables, such as SalesAmount in the ResellerSales table and SalesAmount in the InternetSales table. However, some reporting tools, such as Power BI reports, don't support renaming fields on the report, and you won't be able to tell the two fields apart if a report has both fields. Therefore, consider renaming the columns and adding a prefix to have unique column names across tables, such as ResellerSalesAmount and InternetSalesAmount. Or you can create DAX calculations with unique names and then hide the original columns.

The status bar at the bottom of the Data View shows the number of rows in the selected table. When you select a field, the status bar also shows the number of its distinct values. For example, the English-DayNameOfWeek field has seven distinct values. This is useful to know because that's how many values the users will see when they add this field to the report.

Understanding columns

The vertical bands in a table open in the Data View represent the table columns. You can click any cell to select the entire column and to highlight the column header. The Formatting group in the ribbon's Modeling tab shows the data type of the selected column. Like the Query Editor data preview, Data View is read-only. You can't change the data – not even a single cell. Therefore, if you need to change a value, such as when you find a data error that requires a correction, you must make the changes either in the data source or in the query. I encourage you to make data changes in the query (that's what it is for).

Another way to select a column is to click it in the Fields pane. The Fields pane prefixes some fields with icons. For example, the sigma (Σ) icon signifies that the field is numeric and can be aggregated using any of the supported aggregate functions, such as Sum or Average. If the field is a calculated measure, it'll be prefixed with a calculator icon (▤). Even though some fields are numeric, they can't be meaningfully aggregated, such as CalendarYear. The Properties group in the ribbon's Modeling tab allows you to change the default aggregation behavior, such as to change the CalendarYear default aggregation to "Do not aggregate". This is just a default; you and other users can still overwrite the aggregation type on reports.

The Data Category property in the Properties group (ribbon's Modeling tab) allows you to change the column category. For example, to help Power BI understand that this is a geospatial field, you can change the data category of the SalesTerritoryCountry column to Country/Region. This will prefix the field with a globe icon. More importantly, this helps Power BI to choose the best visualization when you add the field on an empty report, such as to use a map visualization when you add a geospatial field. Or, if a column includes hyperlinks and you would like the user to be able to navigate by clicking the link, set the column's data category to Web URL.

8.1.2 Exploring Data

If there were data modeling commandments, the first one would be "Know thy data". Realizing the common need to explore the raw data, the Power BI team has added features to both the Query Editor and Data View to help you become familiar with the source data.

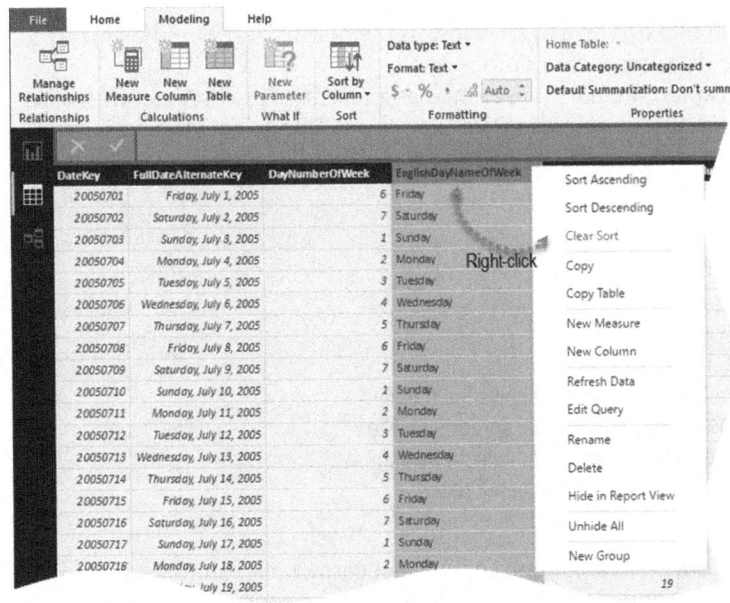

Figure 8.2 You can sort the field content in ascending or descending order.

Sorting data

Power BI doesn't sort data by default. As a result, Data View shows the imported data as it's loaded from the source. You can right-click a column and use the sort options (see **Figure 8.2**) to sort the data. You can sort the content of a table column in an ascending or descending order. This type of sorting is for your benefit, because it allows you to get familiar with the imported data, such as to find what's the minimum or maximum value. Power BI doesn't apply the sorting changes to the way the data is saved in the model, nor does it propagate the column sort to reports. For example, you might sort the EnglishDayNameOf-Week column in a descending order. However, when you create a report that uses this field, the visualization would ignore the Data View sorting changes and it will sort days in an ascending order (or whatever sort order the reporting tool prefers).

When a column is sorted in the Data View, you'll see an up or down arrow in the column header, which indicates the sort order. You can sort the table data by only one column at a time. To clear sorting and to revert to the data source sort order, right-click a column, and then click Clear Sort.

NOTE Power BI Desktop automatically inherits the data collation based on the language selection in your Windows regional settings, which you can overwrite in the Options and Settings ⇨ Option ⇨ Data Load (Current File section). The default collations are case-insensitive. Consequently, if you have a source column with the values "John" and "JOHn", then Power BI Desktop imports both values as "John" and treats them the same. While this behavior helps the xVelocity storage engine compress data efficiently, sometimes a case-sensitive collation might be preferable, such as when you need a unique key to set up a relationship, and you get an error that the column contains duplicate values. However, currently there isn't an easy way to change the collation and configure a given field or a table to be case-sensitive. So you'll need to try to keep the column names distinct.

Custom sorting

Certain columns must be sorted in a specific order on reports. For example, calendar months should be sorted in their ordinal position (Jan, Feb, and so on) as opposed to alphabetically. This is where custom sorting can help. Custom sorting allows you to sort a column by another column, assuming the column to sort on has one-to-one or one-to-many cardinality with the sorted column.

Let's say you have a column MonthName with values Jan, Feb, Mar, and so on, and you have another column MonthNumberOfYear that stores the ordinal number of the month in the range from 1 to 12. Because every value in the MonthName column has only one corresponding value in MonthNumberOfYear column, you can sort MonthName by MonthNumberOfYear. However, you can't sort MonthName by a Date column because there are multiple dates for each month.

Compared to field sorting for data expiration, custom sorting has a reverse effect on data. Custom sorting doesn't change the way the data is displayed in the Data View, but it affects how the data is presented in reports. **Figure 8.3** shows how changing custom sorting will affect the sort order of the month name column on a report.

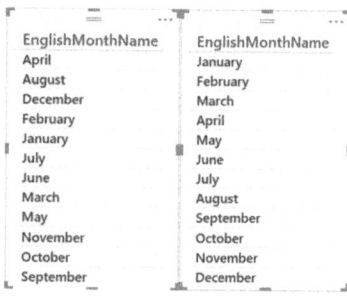

Figure 8.3 The left table shows the month with the default alphabetical sort order while the right table shows it after custom sorting was applied by MonthNumberOfYear.

Copying data

Sometimes you might want to copy the content of a column (or even an entire table) and paste it in Excel or send it to someone. You can use the Copy and Copy Table options from the context menu (see

Figure 8.2 again) to copy the content to Windows Clipboard and paste it in another application. You can't paste the copied data into the data model. Again, that's because the data model is read-only.

The Copy Table option is also available when you right-click a table in the Fields pane. Copying a table preserves the tabular format, so pasting it in Excel produces a list with columns instead of a single column.

8.1.3 Understanding the Column Data Types

A table column has a data type associated with it. In Chapter 6, I mentioned that a query column already has a data type. When a query connects to the data source, it attempts to infer the column data type from the data provider and then maps it to one of the data types it supports. Although it seems redundant to have data types in two places (query and storage), it gives you more flexibility. For example, you can keep the inferred data type in the query but change it in the table.

Currently, there isn't an exact one-to-one mapping between query and storage data types. Instead, Power BI Desktop maps the query column types to the ones that the xVelocity storage engine supports. **Table 8.1** shows these mappings. Queries support a couple of more data types (Date/Time/Timezone and Duration) than table columns.

Table 8.1   This table shows how query data types map to column data types.

Query Data Type	Storage Data Type	Description
Text	String	A Unicode character string with a max length of 268,435,456 characters
Decimal Number	Decimal Number	A 64 bit (eight-bytes) real number with decimal places
Fixed Decimal Number	Fixed Decimal Number	A decimal number with four decimal places of fixed precision useful for storing currencies.
Whole Number	Whole number	A 64 bit (eight-bytes) integer with no decimal places
Percentage	Fixed Decimal Number	A 2-digit precision decimal number
Date/Time	Date/Time	Dates and times after March 1st, 1900
Date	Date	Just the date portion of a date
Time	Time	Just the time portion of a date
Date/Time/Timezone	Date	Universal date and time
Duration	Text	Time duration, such as 5:30 for five minutes and 30 seconds
TRUE/FALSE	Boolean	True or False value
Binary	Binary data type	Blob, such as file content (supported in Query Editor but not in the data model)

How data types get assigned

The storage data type has preference over the source data type. For example, the query might infer a column date type as Decimal Number from the data provider, and this type might get carried over to storage. However, you can overwrite the column data type in the Data View to Whole Number. Unless you change the data type in the query and apply the changes, the column data type remains Whole Number.

The storage engine tries to use the most compact data type, depending on the column values. For example, the query might have assigned a Fixed Decimal Number data type to a column that has only whole numbers. Don't be surprised if the Data View shows the column data type as Whole Number after you import the data. Power BI might also perform a widening data conversion on import if it doesn't support certain numeric data types. For example, if the underlying SQL Server data type is tinyint (one byte), Power BI will map it to Whole Number because that's the only data type that it supports for whole numbers.

Power BI won't import data types it doesn't recognize and won't import the corresponding columns. For example, Power BI won't import a SQL Server column of a geography data type that stores spatial data. If the data source doesn't provide schema information, Power BI imports data as text and uses the Text data type for all the columns. In such cases, you should overwrite the data types after import when it makes sense.

Changing the column data type

As I mentioned, the Formatting group in ribbon's Modeling tab and the Transform group in the Query Editor indicate the data type of the selected column. You should review and change the column type when needed, for the following reasons:

- Data aggregation – You can sum or average only numeric columns.

- Data validation – Suppose you're given a text file with a SalesAmount column that's supposed to store decimal data. What happens if an 'NA' value sneaks into one or more cells? The query will detect it and might change the column type to Text. You can examine the data type after import and detect such issues. As I mentioned in the previous chapter, I recommend you address such issues in the Query Editor because it has the capabilities to remove errors or replace values. Of course, it's best to fix such issues at the data source, but probably you won't have write access to the source data.

 NOTE What happens if all is well with the initial import, but a data type violation occurs the next month when you are given a new extract? What really happens in the case of a data type mismatch depends on the underlying data provider. The text data provider (Microsoft ACE OLE DB provider in this case) replaces the mismatched data values with blank values, and the blank values will be imported in the model. On the query side of things, if data mismatch occurs, you'll see "Error" in the corresponding cell to notify you about dirty data, but no error will be triggered on refresh.

- Better performance – Smaller data types have more efficient storage and query performance. For example, a whole number is more efficient than text because it occupies only eight bytes irrespective of the number of digits.

Sometimes, you might want to overwrite the column data type in the Data View. You can do so by expanding the Data Type drop-down list in the Formatting ribbon group and then select another type. Power BI Desktop only shows the list of the data types that are applicable for conversion. For example, if the original data type is Currency, you can convert the data type to Text, Decimal Number, and Whole Number. If the column is of a Text data type, the Data Type drop-down list would show all the data types. However, you'll get a type mismatch error if the conversion fails, such as when trying to convert a non-numeric text value to a number.

Understanding column formatting

Each column in the Data View has a default format based on its data type and Windows regional settings. For example, my default format for Date columns is MM/dd/yyyy hh:mm:ss tt because my computer is configured for English US regional settings (such as 12/24/2011 13:55:20 PM). This might present an issue for international users. However, they can overwrite the language from the Power BI Desktop's File ⇨ "Options and settings" ⇨ Options ⇨ Regional Settings (Current File section) menu to see the data formatted in their culture.

Use the Formatting group in the ribbon's Modeling tab to overwrite the default column format settings, as shown in **Figure 8.4**.

TIP Unlike changing the column data type, which changes the underlying data storage, changing column formatting has no effect on how data is stored because the column format is for visualization purposes only. As a best practice, format numeric and date columns that will be used on reports using the Formatting group in the ribbon's Modeling tab. If you do this, all reports will inherit these formats and you won't have to apply format changes to reports.

You can use the format buttons in the Formatting ribbon group to apply changes interactively, such as to add a thousand separator or to increase the number of decimal places. Formatting changes apply automatically to reports the next time you switch to the Report View. If the column width is too narrow to show the formatted values in Data View, you can increase the column width by dragging the right column border. Changing the column width in Data View has no effect on reports.

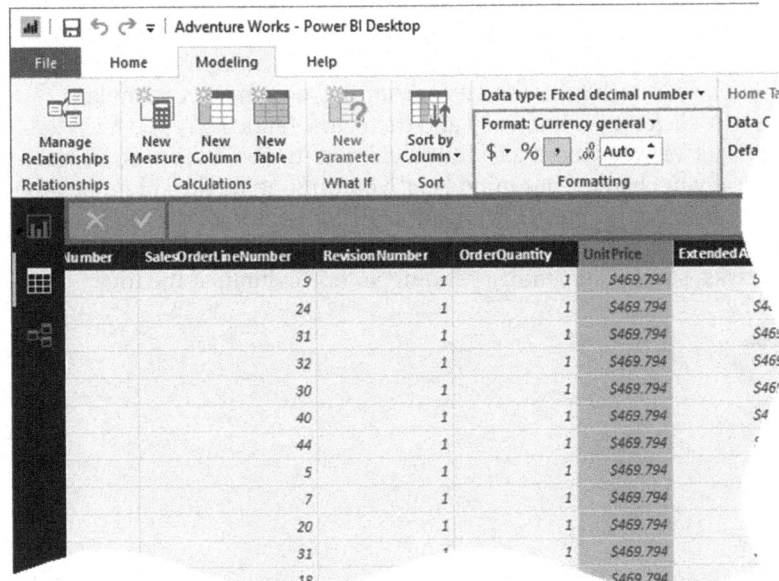

Figure 8.4 Use the Formatting ribbon group to change the column format.

8.1.4 Understanding Column Operations

You can perform various column-related tasks to explore data and improve the metadata visual appearance, including renaming columns, removing columns, and hiding columns.

Renaming columns

Table columns inherit their names from the underlying query that inherits them in turn from the data source. These names might be somewhat cryptic, such as TRANS_AMT. The column name becomes a part of the model metadata that you and the end users interact with. You can make the column name more descriptive and intuitive by renaming the column. You can rename a column interchangeably in three places: Data View, Query Editor, and Fields pane. For example, if you rename a column in the Data View and then switch to the Query Editor, you'll see that Power BI Desktop has automatically appended a Rename Column transformation step to apply the change to the query.

 NOTE No matter where you rename the column, the Power BI "smart rename" applies throughout all the column references, including calculations and reports to avoid broken references. You can see the original name of the column in the data source by inspecting the Rename Column step in the Query Editor formula bar or by looking at the query source.

To rename a column in the Data View, double-click the column header to enter edit mode, and then type in the new name. Or, right-click the column, and then click Rename Column (see **Figure 8.2** again). To rename a column in the Fields pane (in the Data and Report Views), right-click the column and click Rename (or double-click the column).

Removing and hiding columns

In Chapter 6, I advised you to not import a column that you don't need in the model. However, if this ever happens, you can always remove a column in the Data View, Query Editor, and Fields pane. I also recommended you use the Choose Columns transformation in Query Editor as a more intuitive way to remove and add columns. If the column participates in a relationship with another table in the data model, removing the column removes the associated relationship(s).

Suppose you need the column in the model, but you don't want to show it to end users. For example, you might need a primary key column or foreign key column to set up a relationship. Since such columns usually contain system values, you might want to exclude them from showing up in the Fields pane by simply hiding them. The difference between removing and hiding a column is that hiding a column allows you to use the column in the model, such as in hierarchies or custom sorting, and in DAX formulas.

To hide a column in Data View, right-click any column cell and then click "Hide in Report View". A hidden column appears grayed out in Data View. You can also hide a column in the Fields pane by right-clicking the column and clicking Hide. If you change your mind later, you can unhide the column by toggling "Hide in Report View" (see **Figure 8.5**). Or, you can click Unhide All to unhide all the hidden columns in the selected table. Unfortunately, Power BI Desktop doesn't currently support selecting multiple columns, so you must apply column tasks, such as renaming or hiding, to one column at the time.

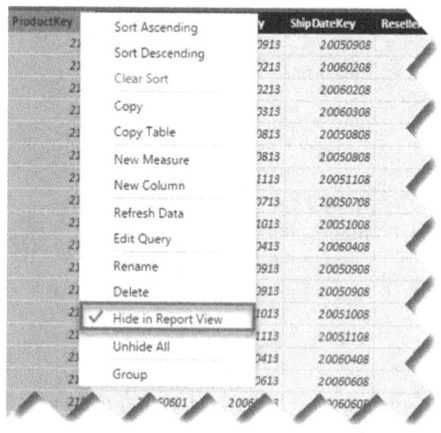

Figure 8.5 Toggle the "Hide in Report View" menu to hide or unhide a column.

The Copy operation allows you to copy the content of the selected columns and paste it in another application, such as in Microsoft Excel. You can't paste the column content inside the Data View because the model is read-only. The Group menu (also available when you right-click a field in the Fields pane) is for creating groups (also called bins or buckets) from the values in the selected column, such as to split the SalesAmount field into 10 equally sized groups. I'll discuss groups in the "Implementing Analytical Features" section later this chapter.

8.1.5 Working with Tables and Columns

Now that you're familiar with tables and columns, let's turn our attention again to the Adventure Works model and spend some time exploring and refining it. The following steps will help you get familiar with the common tasks you'll use when working with tables and columns.

NOTE I recommend you keep on working and enhancing your version of the Adventure Works model. However, if you haven't completed the Chapter 6 exercises, you can use the Adventure Works file from the \Source\Ch06 folder. However, remember that my samples import data from several local data sources, including the Adventure Works cube and the Product Catalog report. If you decide to refresh the data, you need to update all the data sources to reflect your specific setup. To do so, open the Query Editor, and then click the Data Source Settings button in the ribbon's Home tab and click the Change Source button for each data source. Or, double-click the Source step in the Applied Steps section (Query Settings pane) for each data source that fails to refresh. Then, change the server name and database name as needed.

Sorting data

You can gain insights into your imported data by sorting and filtering it. Suppose that you want to find which employees have been with the company the longest:

1. In Power BI Desktop, open the Adventure Works.pbix file that you worked on in Chapter 6.

2. Click Data View in the navigation bar. Click the Employees tab in the Fields pane.

3. Right-click the HireDate column, and then click Sort Ascending. Note that Guy Gilbert is the first person on the list, and he was hired on 7/31/1998.

4. Right-click the HireDate column again, and then click the Clear Sort menu to remove the sort and to revert to the original order in which data was imported from the data source.

Implementing a custom sort

Next, you'll sort the EnglishMonthName column by the MonthNumberOfYear column so that months are sorted in their ordinal position on reports.

1. In the Fields pane, click the DimDate table to select it.

2. Click a cell in the EnglishMonthName column to select this column.

3. In the ribbon's Modeling tab, click the "Sort by Column" button, and then select MonthNumberOfYear.

4. (Optional) Switch to the Report View. In the Fields pane, check the EnglishMonthName column. This creates a Table visualization that shows months. The months should be sorted in their ordinal position.

Renaming tables

The name of the table is included in the metadata that you'll see when you create reports. Therefore, it's important to have a naming convention for tables. In this case, I'll use a plural naming convention for fact tables (tables that keep a historical record of business transactions, such as ResellerSales), and a singular naming convention for lookup tables.

1. Double-click the DimDate table in the Fields pane (or right-click the DimDate table and then click Rename) and rename it to *Date*. You can rename tables and fields in any of the three views (Report, Data, and Relationships).

2. To practice another way for renaming a table, click the Edit Queries button to open the Query Editor. In the Queries pane, select the Employees query. In the Query Settings pane, rename the query to *Employee*. Click the "Apply & Close" button to return to the Data View.

3. Rename the rest of the tables using the Fields pane. Rename FactResellerSales to *ResellerSales*, Products to *Product*, Resellers to *Reseller*, and SalesTerritories to *SalesTerritory*.

Working with columns

Next, let's revisit each table and make column changes as necessary.

1. In the Fields pane (in the Data View), select the Date table. Double-click the column header of the FullDateAlternateKey column, and then rename it to *Date*. In the data preview pane, increase the Date column width by dragging the column's right border so it's wide enough to accommodate the content in the column. Rename the EnglishDayNameOfWeek column to *DayNameOfWeek* and EnglishMonthName to *MonthName*. Right-click the DateKey column and click "Hide in Report View" to hide this column.

2. You can also rename and hide columns in the Fields pane. In the Fields pane, expand the Employee table. Right-click the EmployeeKey column and then click "Hide in Report View". Also hide the ParentEmployeeKey and SalesTerritoryKey columns. Using the Data View or Fields pane, delete the columns EmployeeNationalIDAlternateKey and ParentEmployeeNationalIDAlternateKey because they're sensitive columns that probably shouldn't be available for end-user analysis.

3. Click the Product table. If you've imported the Product table from the Product Catalog report, rename the ProdCat2 column to *ProductCategory*. Increase the column width to accommodate the content. Rename ProdSubCat column to *ProductSubcategory*, ProdModel to *ProductModel*, and ProdName to *ProductName*. Hide the ProductKey column. Using the ribbon's Modeling tab (Data View), reformat the StandardCost and ListPrice columns as Currency. To do so, expand the Format drop-down and select Currency ⇨ $ English (United States). Hide the ProductKey column.

4. Select the Reseller table. Hide the ResellerKey and GeographyKey columns. Rename the ResellerAlternate-Key column to *ResellerID*.

5. Select the ResellerSales table. The first nine foreign key columns (with the "Key" suffix) are useful for data relationships but not for data analysis. Hide them.

6. To practice formatting columns again, change the format of the SalesAmount column to two decimal places. To do so, select the column in the Data View (or in the Fields pane), and then enter 2 in the Decimal Places field in the Formatting group on the ribbon's Modeling tab. Press Enter.

7. Select the SalesTerritory table in the Fields pane. Hide the SalesTerritoryKey column. If you have imported the SalesTerritory table from the cube, rename the SalesAmount column to Revenue and format the Revenue column as Currency ⇨$ English (United States).

8. Press Ctrl-S (or click File ⇨ Save) to save the Adventure Works data model.

8.2   Managing Schema and Data Changes

To review, once Power BI Desktop imports data, it saves a copy of the data in a local file with a *.pbix file extension. The model schema and data are *not* automatically synchronized with changes in the data sources. Typically, after the initial load, you'll need to refresh the model data on a regular basis, such as when you receive a new source file or when the data in the source database is updated. Power BI Desktop provides features to keep your model up to date.

8.2.1   Managing Data Sources

It's not uncommon for a model to have several tables connected to different data sources so that you can integrate data from multiple places. As a modeler, you need to understand how to manage connections and tables, such as to rebind a table to another server when you move from test to production.

Managing data source settings
Suppose you need to import additional tables from a data source that you've already set up a connection to. One option is to use Get Data again. If, you connect to the same server and database, Power BI Desktop will reuse the same data source definition. To see and manage all data sources defined in the current file, expand the Edit Queries button in the ribbon's Home table and then click "Data Source Settings". For example, if the server or security credentials change, you can use the "Data Source Settings" window (see **Figure 8.6**) to update the connection. Recall that you can also open the Data Source Settings window from File ⇨ "Options and settings" ⇨ "Data source settings".

For data sources in the current file, you can select a data source and click the Change Source button to change the server, database, and advanced options, such as a custom SQL statement (the SQL Statement is disabled if you didn't specify a custom query in the Get Data steps). As you can see in **Figure 8.6**, there are drop-downs in front of the server and database fields. Recall from Chapter 7, that you can further simplify data source maintenance by using query parameters instead of typing in names.

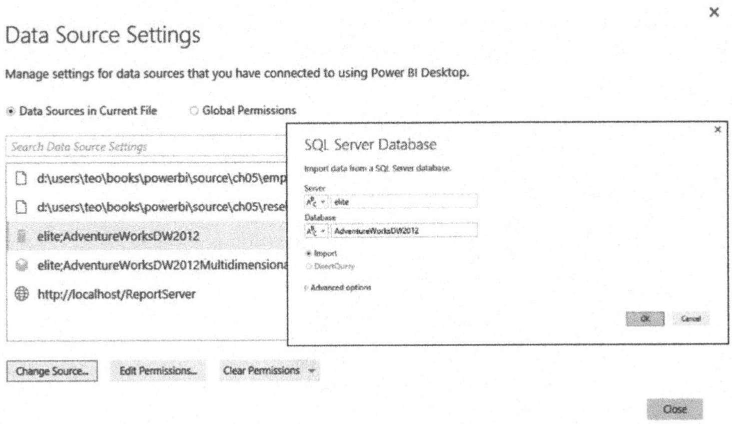

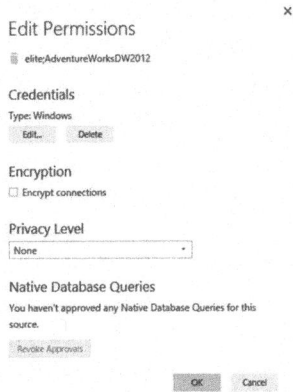

Figure 8.6 Use the "Data Source Settings" window to view and manage data sources used in the current Power BI Desktop file.

Managing sensitive information
Power BI Desktop encrypts the connection credentials and stores them in the local AppData folder on your computer. Use the Edit Permissions button to change credentials (see **Figure 8.7**), such as to switch from Windows to standard security (username and password) or encryption options if the data source supports encryptions.

Figure 8.7 Use the "Edit Permissions" window to change the data source credentials and privacy options.

For security reasons, Power BI Desktop allows you to delete cached credentials by using the Clear Permissions button which supports two options. The first (Clear Permissions) option deletes the cached credentials of the selected data source. For local data sources, this option removes the credentials and privacy settings. For non-local data sources, this option does the same but also removes the data source from the Global Permissions list. The second option (Clear All Permissions) deletes the cached credentials for all data sources in the current file (if the Data Sources in Current File option is selected), or all data sources used by Power BI Desktop (if the Global Permissions option is selected).

Although deleting credentials might sound dangerous, nothing really gets broken and models are not affected. However, the next time you refresh the data, you'll be asked to specify credentials and encryption options as you did the first time you used Get Data to connect to that data source.

Finally, if you used custom SQL Statements (native database queries) to import data, another security feature allows you to revoke their approval. This could be useful if you have imported some data using a custom statement, such as a stored procedure, but you want to prevent other people from executing the query if you intend to share the file with someone else.

Using recent data sources

If you need more tables from the same database, instead of going through the Get Data steps and typing in the server name and database, there is a shortcut: use the Recent Sources button in the ribbon's Home tab (see **Figure 8.8**).

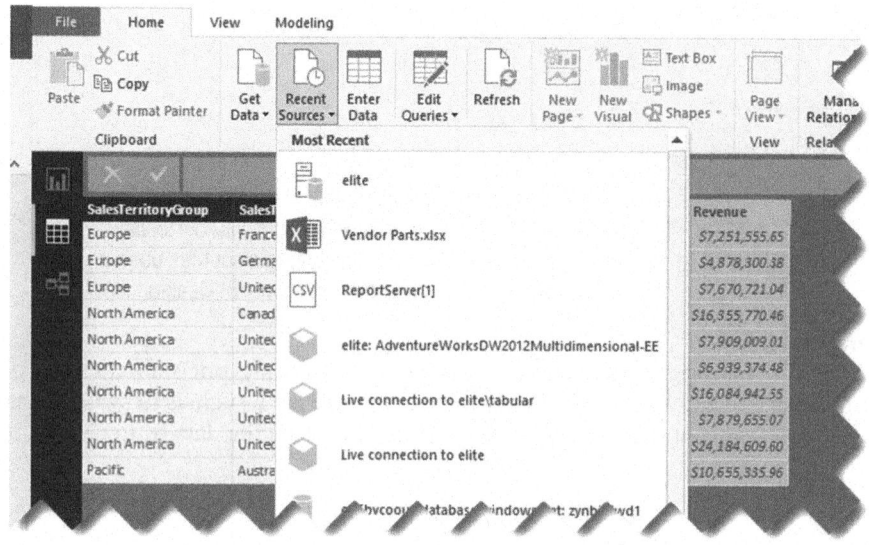

Figure 8.8 Use the Recent Data Sources window to manage the data source credentials and encryption options in one place.

If you connect to a data source that has multiple entities, such as a relational database, when you click the data source in Recent Sources, Power BI Desktop will bring you straight to the Navigator window so that you can select and import another table.

Importing additional tables

Besides wholesale data, the Adventure Works data warehouse stores retail data for direct sales to individual customers. Suppose that you want to extend the Adventure Works model to analyze direct sales to customers who placed orders on the Internet.

NOTE Other self-service tools on the market restrict you to analyzing single datasets only. If that's all you need, feel free to skip this exercise as the model has enough tables and complexity already. However, chances are that you might need to analyze data from different subject areas side by side. This requires you to import multiple fact tables and join them to common dimensions. And this is where Power BI excels because it allows you to implement self-service models whose features are on a par with professional models. I encourage you to stay with me as the complexity cranks up and learn these features so you never say "I can't meet this requirement".

Follow these steps to import three additional tables:

1. In the ribbon's Home tab, expand the Recent Sources button, and then click the SQL Server instance that hosts the AdventureWorksDW database. Or, use Get Data to connect to it.

NOTE If you don't have a SQL Server with AdventureWorksDW, I provide the data in the DimCustomer.csv, DimGeography.csv and FactInternetSales.csv files in the \Source\ch08 folder. Import them using the CSV or TEXT option in Get Data.

2. In the Navigator window, expand the AdventureWorksDW database, and then check the DimCustomer, DimGeorgraphy, and FactInternetSales tables. In the AdventureWorksDW database, the DimGeography

table isn't related directly to the FactInternetSales table. Instead, DimGeography joins DimCustomer, which joins FactInternetSales. This is an example of a snowflake schema, which I covered in Chapter 6.

3. Click the Edit button. In the Queries pane of the Query Editor, select DimCustomer and change the query name to *Customer*.

4. In the Queries pane, select DimGeography and change the query name to *Geography*.

5. Select the FactInternetSales query and change its name to InternetSales. Use the Choose Columns transformation to exclude the RevisionNumber, CarrierTrackingNumber, and CustomerPONumber columns.

6. Click "Close & Apply" to add the three tables to the Adventure Works model and to import the new data.

7. In the Data View, select the Customer table. Hide the CustomerKey and GeographyKey columns. Rename the CustomerAlternateKey column to *CustomerID*.

8. Select the Geography table, and hide the GeographyKey and SalesTerritoryKey columns.

9. Select the InternetSales table, and hide the first eight columns (the ones with "Key" suffix).

8.2.2 Managing Data Refresh

When you import data, Power BI Desktop caches it in the model to give you the best performance when you visualize the data. The only option to synchronize data changes on the desktop is to refresh the data manually.

 NOTE Unlike Excel, Power BI Desktop doesn't support automation and macros. At the same time, there are many scenarios that might benefit from automating data refresh on the desktop. While there is an officially supported way to do so, my blog "Automating Power BI Desktop Refresh" (http://prologika.com/automating-power-bi-desktop-refresh/) lists a few options if you have such a requirement.

Refreshing data

As it stands, Power BI Desktop refresh is simple. You just need to click the Refresh button in the Report View or in the Data View. This executes all the table queries, discards the existing data, and imports all the tables from scratch. If you need to refresh a specific table, right-click the table in the Fields pane (Report View or Data View) and click "Refresh data". Currently, there isn't an option to process only a portion of a table or to refresh data incrementally, such as to process rows where LastUpdateDate is within the last 30 days.

 NOTE Analysis Services Tabular, which also uses xVelocity as a storage engine, supports more processing options, including processing specific partitions of a large table. Consider Tabular when you need a centralized and scalable semantic model that can handle much larger data volumes than Power BI Desktop.

Suppose that you've been notified about changes in one or more of the tables, and now you need to refresh the data model.

1. In Power BI Desktop, click the Data View icon (or the Report View icon) in the navigation bar.

2. In the ribbon's Home tab, click the Refresh button to refresh all tables.

3. Press Ctrl-S to save the Adventure Works data model.

When you initiate the refresh operation, Power BI Desktop opens the Refresh window to show you the progress, as shown in **Figure 8.9**.

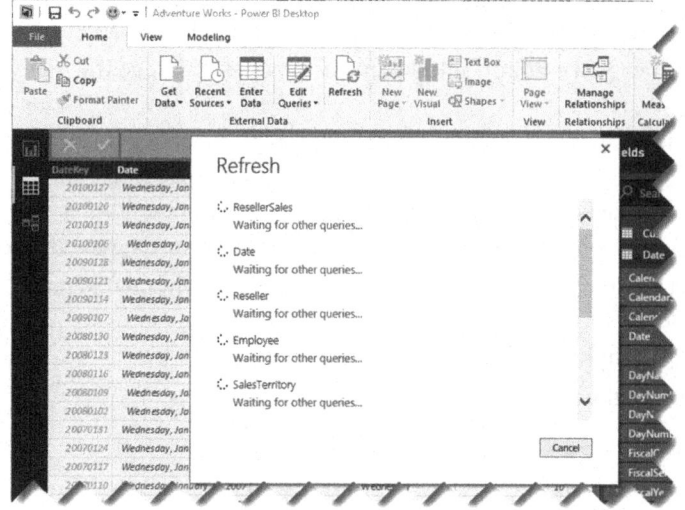

Figure 8.9 Power BI Desktop refreshes tables sequentially and cancels the entire operation if a table fails to refresh.

Power BI Desktop refreshes tables sequentially, one table at the time. The Refresh window shows the number of rows imported. You can't cancel the refresh once it has started.

NOTE Based on usability feedback, Microsoft decided on the sequential data refresh in Power Pivot and Power BI Desktop for easier failure analysis. If a table fails to refresh, the entire refresh operation stops so that the user can more easily identify which table failed.

The xVelocity storage engine can import more than 100,000 rows per second. The actual data refresh speed depends on many factors, including how fast the data source returns rows, the number and data type of columns in the table, the network speed, your machine hardware configuration, and so on.

REAL LIFE I was called a few times to troubleshoot slow processing issues with Analysis Services and Power Pivot. In all the cases, I've found that the external factors impacted the processing speed. In one case, it turned out that the IT department had decided to throttle the network speed on all non-production network segments in case a computer virus takes over.

Troubleshooting data refresh

If a table fails to refresh, such as when there's no connectivity to the data source, the Refresh window shows an error indicator and displays an error message, as shown in **Figure 8.10**. When a table fails to refresh, the entire operation is aborted because it runs in a transaction, and no data is refreshed. At this point, you need to troubleshoot the error.

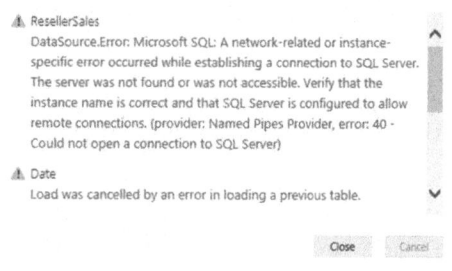

Figure 8.10 If the refresh operation fails, the Refresh window shows which table failed to refresh and shows the error description.

8.3　Relating Tables

One of the most prominent Power BI strengths is that it can help an analyst analyze data across multiple tables. Back in Chapter 6, I covered that as a prerequisite for aggregating data in one table by columns in another table, you must set up a relationship between the two tables. When you import tables from a relational database that supports referential integrity and has table relationships defined, Power BI Desktop detects these relationships and applies them to the model. However, when no table joins are defined in the data source, or when you import data from different sources, Power BI Desktop might be unable to detect relationships upon import. Because of this, you must revisit the model and create appropriate relationships before you analyze the data.

8.3.1　Relationship Rules and Limitations

A relationship is a join between two tables. When you define a table relationship with one-to-many cardinality, you're telling Power BI that there's a logical one-to-many relationship between a row in the lookup (dimension) table and the corresponding rows in the fact table. For example, the relationship between the Reseller and ResellerSales tables in **Figure 8.11** means that each reseller in the Reseller table can have many corresponding rows in the ResellerSales table. Indeed, Progressive Sports (ResellerKey=1) recorded a sale on August 1st, 2006 for $100 and another sale on July 4th 2007 for $120. In this case, the ResellerKey column in the Reseller table is the primary key in the lookup (dimension) table. The ResellerKey column in the ResellerSales table fulfills the role of a foreign key in the fact table.

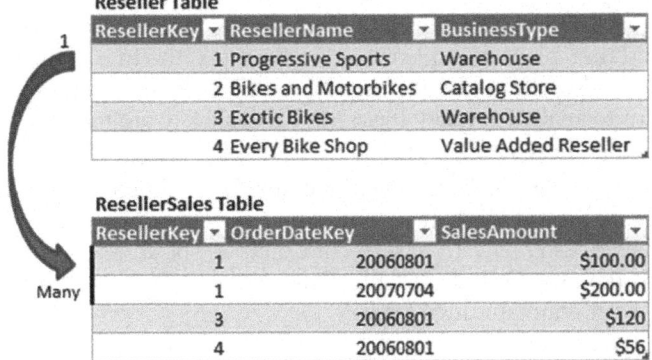

Figure 8.11　There's a logical one-to-many relationship between the Reseller table and the ResellerSales table because each reseller can have multiple sales recorded.

Understanding relationship rules
A relationship can be created under the following circumstances:

- The two tables have matching columns, such as a ResellerKey column in the Reseller lookup table and a ResellerKey column in the ResellerSales table. The column names don't have to be the same but the columns must have matching values. For example, you can't relate the two tables if the ResellerKey column in the ResellerSales table has reseller codes, such as PRO for Progressive Sports.

- The key column in the lookup (dimension) table must have unique values, like a primary key in a relational database. The key column can't have (empty) null values. In the case of the Reseller table, the ResellerKey column fulfills this requirement because its values are unique across all the rows in the table. However, this doesn't mean that all fact tables must join the lookup table on the same primary key. As long as the column is unique, it can serve as a primary key. And some fact tables can use one column while others can use another column. If you attempt to establish a join to a column that doesn't contain unique values in a lookup table, you'll get the following error:

The relationship cannot be created because each column contains duplicate values. Select at least one column that contains only unique values.

Interestingly, Power BI doesn't require the two columns to have matching data types. For example, the ResellerKey column in the Reseller table can be of a Text data type while its counterpart in the fact table could be defined as the Whole Number data type. Behind the scenes, Power BI resolves the join by converting the values in the latter column to the Text data type. However, to improve performance and to reduce storage space, use numeric data types whenever possible.

Understanding relationship limitations

Relationships have several limitations. To start, only one column can be used on each side of the relationship. If you need a combination of two or more columns (so the key column can have unique values), you can add a custom column in the query or a calculated column that uses a DAX expression to concatenate the values, such as =[ResellerKey] & "|" & [SourceID]. I use the pipe delimiter here to avoid combinations that might result in the same concatenated values. For example, combinations of ResellerKey of 1 with SourceID of 10 and ResellerKey of 11 and SourceID of 0 result in "110". To make the combinations unique, you can use a delimiter, such as the pipe character. Once you construct a primary key column, you can use this column for the relationship.

Moving down the list, you can't create relationships forming a closed loop (also called a diamond shape). For example, given the relationships Table1 ⇨ Table2 and Table2 ⇨ Table3, you can't set an active relationship Table1 ⇨ Table3. Such a relationship probably isn't needed anyway, because you'll be able to analyze the data in Table3 by Table1 with only the first two relationships in place. Power BI will let you create the Table1 ⇨ Table3 relationship, but it will mark it as inactive. This brings to the subject of role-playing relationships and inactive relationships.

As it stands, Power BI doesn't support role-playing relationships. A role-playing lookup table is a table that joins the same fact table multiple times, and thus plays multiple roles. For example, the InternetSales table has the OrderDateKey, ShipDateKey, and DueDateKey columns because a sales order has an order date, ship date, and due date. Suppose you want to analyze sales by these three dates. Here are the two most common approaches to handle role-playing lookup tables:

- Reimport the same table – One approach is to import the Date table three times with different names and to create relationships to each date table. This approach gives you more control because you now have three separate Date tables and their data doesn't have to match. For example, you might want the ShipDate table to include different columns than the OrderDate table. On the downside, you increase your maintenance effort because now you must maintain three tables.

- Create calculated tables – Another approach is to create calculated tables by clicking the New Table button in the Modeling ribbon. A calculated table is a table that uses a DAX table-producing formula. Like a calculated column, a calculated table is updated when the model is refreshed and then its results are saved. For example, the DAX formula ShipDate = 'Date' creates a ShipDate calculated table from the Date table. Then you can use the ShipDate just like any other table.

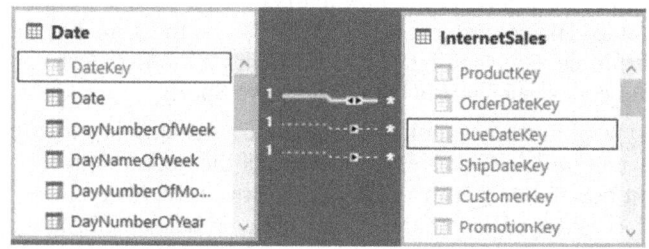

Figure 8.12 Power BI supports only one active relationship between two tables and marks the other relationships as inactive.

REAL WORLD About date tables, AdventureWorksDW uses a "smart" integer primary key for the Date table in the format YYYYMMDD. This is a common practice for data warehousing, but you should use a date field (Date data type). Not only is it more compact (3 bytes vs. 4 bytes for Integer) but it's also easier to work with. For example, if a business user imports ResellerSales, he can filter easier on a Date data type, such as to import data for the current year, than to parse integer fields. And DAX time calculations work if a date column is used as a primary key. That's why in the practice exercises that follow, you'll recreate the relationships to the date table.

Understanding active and inactive relationships

Another approach is to join the three date columns in InternetSales to the Date table. This approach allows you to reuse the same date table three times. However, Power BI supports only one active role-playing relationship. An active relationship is a relationship that Power BI follows to automatically aggregate the data between two tables. A solid line in the Relationships View indicates an active relationship while a dotted line is for inactive relationships (see **Figure 8.12**). You can also open the Manage Relationships window (click the Manage Relationships button in ribbon's Home or Modeling tabs) and inspect the Active flag.

When Power BI Desktop imports the relationships from the database, it defaults the first one to active and marks the rest as inactive. In our case, the InternetSales[DueDateKey] ⇨ DimDate[DateKey] relationship is active because this happens to be the first of the three relationships between the DimDate and FactInternetSales tables that you imported. Consequently, when you create a report that slices Internet dates by Date, Power BI automatically aggregates the sales by the due date.

 NOTE I'll use the TableName[ColumnName] notation as a shortcut when I refer to a table column. For example, InternetSales[DueDateKey] means the DueDateKey column in the InternetSales table. This notation will help you later on with DAX formulas because DAX follows the same syntax. When referencing relationships, I'll use a right arrow (⇨) to denote a relationship from a fact table to a lookup table. For example, InternetSales[OrderDateKey] ⇨ DimDate[DateKey] means a relationship between the OrderDateKey column in the InternetSales table to the DateKey column in the DimDate table.

If you want the default aggregation to happen by the order date, you must set InternetSales [OrderDateKey] ⇨ DimDate[DateKey] as an active relationship. To do so, first select the InternetSales[ShipDateKey] ⇨ DimDate[DateKey] relationship, and then click Edit. In the Edit Relationship dialog box, uncheck the Active checkbox, and then click OK. Finally, edit the InternetSales[OrderDateKey] ⇨ DimDate[DateKey] relationship, and then check the Active checkbox.

What if you want to be able to aggregate data by other dates without importing the Date table multiple times? You can create DAX calculated measures, such as ShippedSalesAmount and DueSalesAmount, that force Power BI to use a given inactive relationship by using the DAX USERELATIONSHIP function. For example, the following formula calculates ShippedSalesAmount using the ResellerSales[ShipDateKey] ⇨ DimDate[DateKey] relationship:

```
ShippedSalesAmount=CALCULATE(SUM(InternetSales[SalesAmount]), USERELATIONSHIP(InternetSales[ShipDateKey],'Date'[Date-Key])
```

Cross filtering limitations

In Chapter 6, I mentioned that a relationship can be set to cross-filter in both directions. This is a great out-of-box feature that allows you to address more advanced scenarios that previously required custom calculations with Power Pivot, such as many-to-many relationships. However, bi-directional filtering doesn't make sense and should be avoided in the following cases:

- When you have two fact tables sharing some common dimension tables – In fact, to avoid ambiguous join paths, Power BI Desktop won't let you turn on bi-directional filtering from multiple fact tables to the same lookup table. Therefore, if you start from a single fact table but anticipate additional fact tables down the road, you may also consider a uni-directional model (Cross filtering set to Single) to keep a consistent experience to users, and then turn on bi-directional filtering only if you need it.

NOTE To understand this limitation better, let's say you have a Product lookup table that has bi-directional relations to ResellerSales and InternetSales tables. If you define a DAX measure on the Product table, such as Count of Products, but have a filter on a Date table, Power BI won't know how to resolve the join: count of products through ResellerSales on that date, or count of products through InternetSales on that date.

- Relationships toward the date table – Relationships to date tables should be one-directional so that DAX time calculations continue to work.
- Closed-loop relationships – As I just mentioned, Power BI Desktop will automatically inactivate one of the relationships when it detects a closed loop, although you can still use DAX calculations to navigate inactive relationships. In this case, bi-directional relationships would produce meaningless results.

 NOTE As a best practice, start with a unidirectional model (Cross Filter Direction = Single) and then turn on cross filtering to Both when needed, such as when you need a many-to-many relationship between tables.

8.3.2 Auto-detecting Relationships

When you create a report that uses unrelated tables, Power BI Desktop can auto-detect and create missing relationships. This behavior is enabled by default, but you can disable it by turning it off from the File ⇨ Options and Settings ⇨ Options menu, which brings you to the Options window (see **Figure 8.13**).

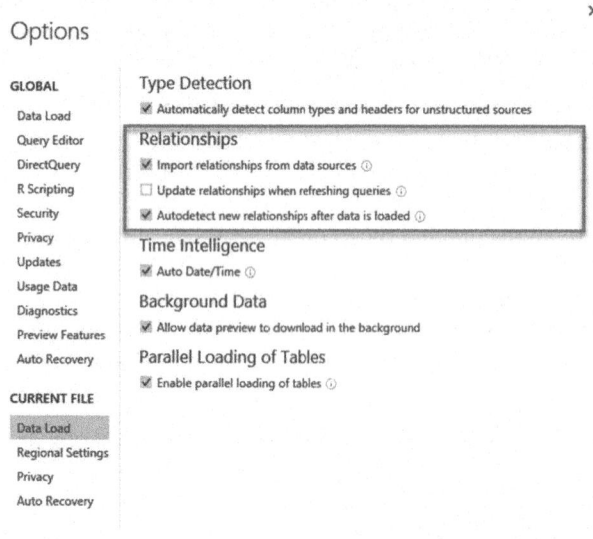

Figure 8.13 You can use the Relationships options in the Data Load section to control how Power BI Desktop discovers relationships.

Configuring relationships detection
There are three options that control how Power BI desktop detects relationships. The "Import relationships from data sources" option (enabled by default) instructs Power BI Desktop to detect relationships from the data source *before* the data is loaded. When this option is enabled, Power BI Desktop will examine the database schema and probe for existing relationships.

The "Update relationships when refreshing queries" option will attempt to discover missing relationships when refreshing the imported data. Because this might result in dropping existing relationships that you've created manually, this option is off by default. Finally, "Autodetect new relationships after data is loaded" will attempt to auto-detect missing relationships *after* the data is loaded. Because this option is on by default, Power BI Desktop was able to detect relationships between the InternetSales and Date tables, as well as between other tables. The auto-detection mechanism uses an internal algorithm that considers column data types and cardinality.

Understanding missing relationships

What happens when you don't have a relationship between two tables and attempt to analyze the data in a report? You'll get repeating values. In this case, I attempted to aggregate the SalesAmount column from the ResellerSales table by the ProductName column in the Product table, but there's no relationship defined between these two tables. If reseller sales should aggregate by product, you must define a relationship to resolve this issue.

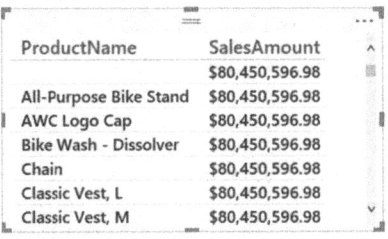

ProductName	SalesAmount
	$80,450,596.98
All-Purpose Bike Stand	$80,450,596.98
AWC Logo Cap	$80,450,596.98
Bike Wash - Dissolver	$80,450,596.98
Chain	$80,450,596.98
Classic Vest, L	$80,450,596.98
Classic Vest, M	$80,450,596.98

Figure 8.14 Reports show repeating values in the case of missing relationships.

Autodetecting relationships

The lazy approach to handle missing relationships is to let Power BI Desktop create them by clicking the Autodetect button in the Manage Relationship window. If the internal algorithm detects a suitable relationship candidate, it creates the relationship and informs you, as shown in **Figure 8.15**.

Manage Relationships

Active	From: Table (Column)	To: Table (Column)
☑	Customer (GeographyKey)	Geography (GeographyKey)
☑	InternetSales (CustomerKey)	Customer (CustomerKey)
☑	InternetSales (DueDateKey)	Date (DateKey)
☐	InternetSales (OrderDateKey)	Date (DateKey)
☐	InternetSales (ShipDateKey)	
☑	Reseller (GeographyKey)	
☑	ResellerSales (DueDateKey)	
☑	ResellerSales (EmployeeKey)	
☐	ResellerSales (OrderDateKey)	
☑	ResellerSales (ResellerKey)	
☐	ResellerSales (ShipDateKey)	Date (DateKey)

Autodetect

Found 1 new relationship(s).

Close

New...   Autodetect...   Edit...   Delete

Figure 8.15 The Autodetect feature of the Manage Relationship window shows that it has detected and created a relationship successfully.

Close

In the case of an unsuccessful detection process, the Relationship dialog box will show "Found no new relationships". If this happens and you're still missing relationships, you need to create them manually.

8.3.3 Creating Relationships Manually

Since table relationships are very important, I'd recommend that you configure them manually. You can do this by using the Manage Relationships window or by using the Relationships View. Because relationships are very important, you can find the Manage Relationships button in the ribbon in all views (Report, Data, and Relationships).

Steps to create a relationship
Follows these steps to set up a relationship:

1. Identify a foreign key column in the table on the Many side of the relationship.
2. Identify a primary key column that uniquely identifies each row in the lookup (dimension) table.
3. In the Manage Relationship window, click the New button to open the Create Relationship window. Then create a new relationship with the correct cardinality. Or you can use the Relationships View to drag the foreign key from the fact table onto the primary key of the lookup table.

Understanding the Create Relationship window
You might prefer the Create Relationship window when the number of tables in your model has grown and using the drag-and-drop technique in the Relationships View becomes impractical. **Figure 8.16** shows the Create Relationship dialog box when setting up a relationship between the ResellerSales and Product tables. Note that if you have imported the Product table from the SSRS Product Catalog report, it will have an empty row with a null value in the ProductKey column. As a mentioned before, a key column can't have a null value. To fix this issue, open Query Editor, expand the drop-down in the ProductKey column header of the Product table, and uncheck the null value.

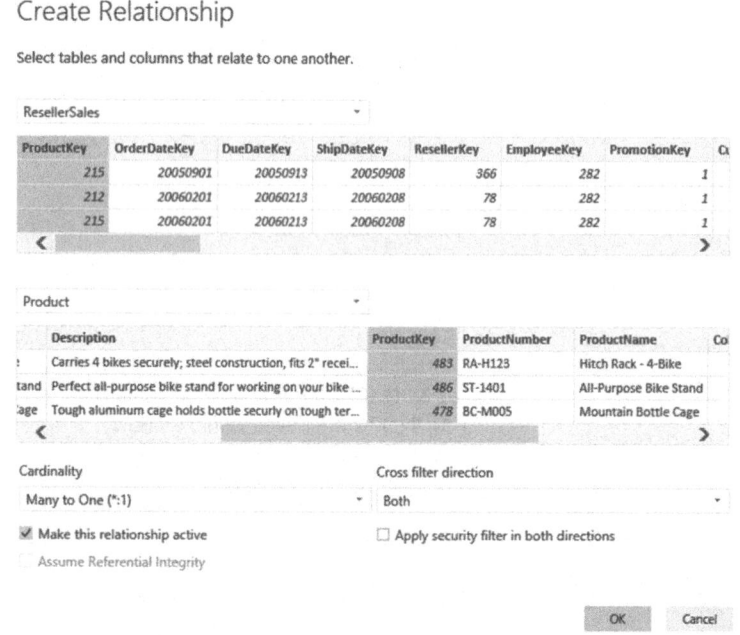

Figure 8.16 Use the Create Relationship window to specify the columns used for the relationship, cardinality and cross filter direction.

When defining a relationship, you need to select two tables and matching columns. The Create Relationships window will detect the cardinality for you. For example, if you start with the table on the many side of the relationship (ResellerSales), it'll choose the Many to One cardinality; otherwise it selects One to Many. If you attempt to set up a relationship with the wrong cardinality, you'll get an error message ("The

Cardinality you selected isn't valid for this relationship"), and you won't be able to create the relationship. And if you choose a column that doesn't uniquely identify each row in the lookup table, you'll get the error message "You can't create a relationship between these two columns because one of the columns must have unique values".

Because there isn't another relationship between the two tables, Power BI Desktop defaults the "Make this relationship active" to checked. This checkbox corresponds to the Active flag in the Manage Relationship window. It also defaults the "Cross filter direction" to Both. The "Assume Referential Integrity" checkbox is disabled because it applies only to DirectQuery. When checked, it auto-generates queries that use INNER JOIN as opposed to OUTER JOIN when joining the two tables. Don't worry for now about "Apply security filter in both direction". I'll explain it when I discuss row-level security (RLS) in the next chapter.

 NOTE   When data is imported, all Power BI joins are treated as outer joins. For example, if ResellerSales had a transaction for a reseller that doesn't exist in the Reseller table, Power BI won't eliminate this row, as I explain in more detail in the next section.

Understanding unknown members

Consider the model shown in **Figure 8.17**, which has a Reseller lookup table and a Sales fact table. This diagram uses an Excel pivot report to demonstrate unknown members, but a Power BI Desktop report will behave the same. The Reseller table has only two resellers. However, the Sales table has data for two additional resellers with keys of 3 and 4. This is a common data integrity issue when the source data originates from heterogeneous data sources and when there isn't an ETL process to validate and clean the data.

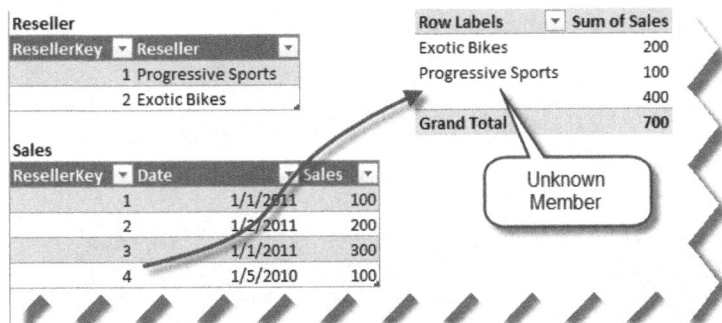

Figure 8.17   Power BI enables an unknown member to the lookup table when it encounters missing rows.

Power BI has a simple solution for this predicament. When creating a relationship, Power BI checks for missing rows in the lookup table. If it finds any, it automatically configures the lookup table to include a special unknown (Blank) member. That's why all unrelated rows appear grouped under a blank row in the report. This row represents the unknown member in the Reseller table.

 NOTE   If you have imported the Product table from the SSRS Product Catalog report in Chapter 6, you'll find that it has a subset of the Adventure Works products. Therefore, when you create a report that shows sales by product, a large chunk of sales will be associated with a (Blank) product.

What about the reverse scenario where there are resellers with no sales and you want to show all resellers irrespective if they have sales or not in the Sales table? Once you add the desired field from the Reseller table to the report, expand the drop-down next to the field in the Fields tab of the Visualizations pane and then click "Show items with no data" in the drop-down menu.

Managing relationships

You can view and manage all the relationships defined in your model by using the Manage Relationships window (see **Figure 8.15** again). In this case, the Manage Relationships window shows that there are 11 relationships defined in the Adventure Works model from which four are inactive, plus one relationship that was just discovered using the Autodiscover feature.

The Edit button opens the Edit Relationship window, which is the same as the Create Relationship window, but with all the fields pre-populated. Finally, the Delete button removes the selected relationship. Don't worry if your results differ from mine. You'll verify the relationships in the lab exercise that follows and will create the missing ones.

8.3.4 Understanding the Relationships View

Another way to view and manage relationships is to use the Relationships View. You can use the Relationships View to:

- Visualize the model schema
- Create and manage relationships
- Make other limited schema changes, such as renaming, hiding, deleting objects

Recall that the Relationships view is available in models with imported data or in models that connect live to data sources, except when connecting live to Analysis Services. One of the strengths of the Relationships View is that you can quickly visualize and understand the model schema and relationships. **Figure 8.18** shows a subset of the Adventure Works model schema open in the Relationships View. Glancing at the model, you can immediately see what relationships exist in the model! If you have a lot of tables, you might find the Reset Layout useful to auto-arrange the tables in a more compact layout.

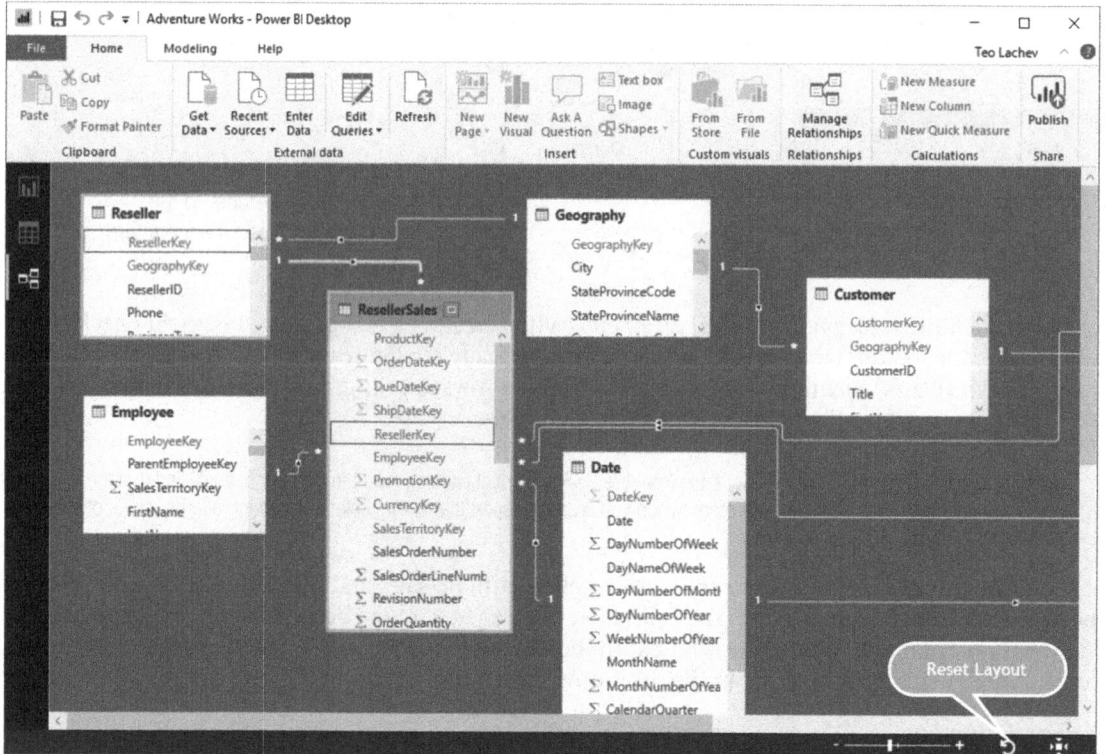

Figure 8.18 The Relationships View helps you understand the model schema and work with relationships.

Making schema changes

You can make limited schema changes in the Relationships View. When you right-click an object, a context menu opens to show the supported operations, as shown in **Table 8.2**.

Table 8.2 This table shows the schema operations by object type.

Object Type	Supported Operations	Object Type	Supported Operations
Table	Delete, Hide, Rename, Maximize, Synonyms	Measure	Delete, Hide, Rename
Column	Delete, Hide, Rename		
Relationship	Delete		

Managing relationships

Speaking of relationships, let's take a closer look at how the Relationships View represents them. A relationship is visualized as a connector between two tables. Symbols at the end of the connector help you understand the relationship cardinality. The number one (1) denotes the table on the One side of the relationship, while the asterisk (*) is shown next to the table on the Many side of the relationship. For example, after examining **Figure 8.18**, you can see that there's a relationship between the Reseller table and ResellerSales table and that the relationship cardinality is One to Many with the Reseller table on the One side of the relationship and the ResellerSales table on the many.

When you click a relationship to select it, the Relationships View highlights it in an orange color. When you hover your mouse over a relationship, the Relationships View highlights columns in the joined tables to indicate visually which columns are used in the relationship. For example, pointing the mouse to the highlighted relationship between the ResellerSales and Reseller tables reveals that the relationship is created between the ResellerSales[ResellerKey] column and Reseller[ResellerKey] (see **Figure 8.18** again).

As I mentioned, Power BI has a limited support of role-playing relationships where a lookup table joins multiple times to a fact table. The caveat is that only one role-playing relationship can be active. The Relationships View shows the inactive relationships with dotted lines. To make another role-playing relationship active, first you need to deactivate the currently active relationship. To do so, double-click the active relationship, and then in the Edit Relationship window uncheck the "Make this relationship active" checkbox. Next, you double-click the other role-playing relationship and then check its "Make this relationship active" checkbox.

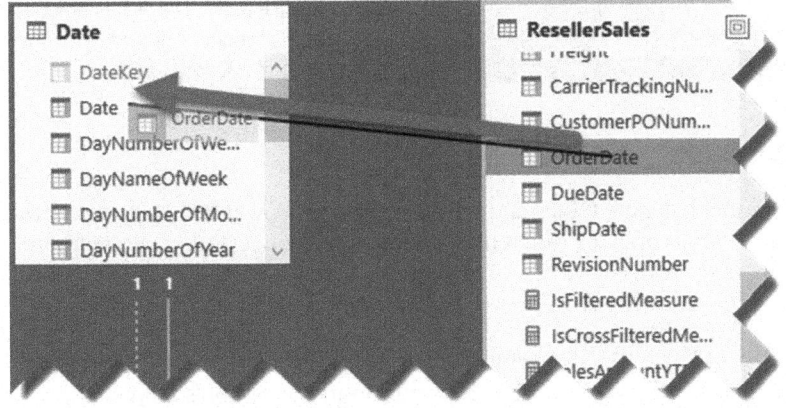

Figure 8.19 The Relationships View lets you create a relationship by dragging a foreign key column onto a primary key column.

A great feature of Relationships View is creating relationships by dragging a foreign key column and dropping it onto the primary key column in the lookup table. For example, to create a relationship between the

ResellerSales and Date tables, drag the OrderDate column in the ResellerSales table and drop it onto the Date column in the Date table. The Relationships View won't allow you to create a relationship in the reverse direction. To delete a relationship, simply click the relationship to select it, and then press the Delete key. Or right-click the relationship line, and then click Delete.

Understanding synonyms

Remember the fantastic Q&A feature that let business users gain insights in dashboards by asking natural queries? The Relationships View allows you to fine tune Q&A by defining synonyms. A synonym is an alternative name for a field. Suppose you want to allow natural queries to use "revenue" and "sales amount" interchangeably. The following steps shows how to define a synonym.

1. In the Relationships View, select the ResellerSales table.

2. In the ribbon's Modeling tab, click the Synonyms button. A Synonyms pane opens. Notice that Power BI Desktop has already defined a synonym "sales amount" for the SalesAmount field.

3. Next to "sales amount", type in *revenue* (see **Figure 8.20**). That's all it takes to define a synonym. Once you deploy your model to Power BI Service or use Q&A in Power BI Desktop, you can use the synonym in in your natural questions, such by typing "revenue by product".

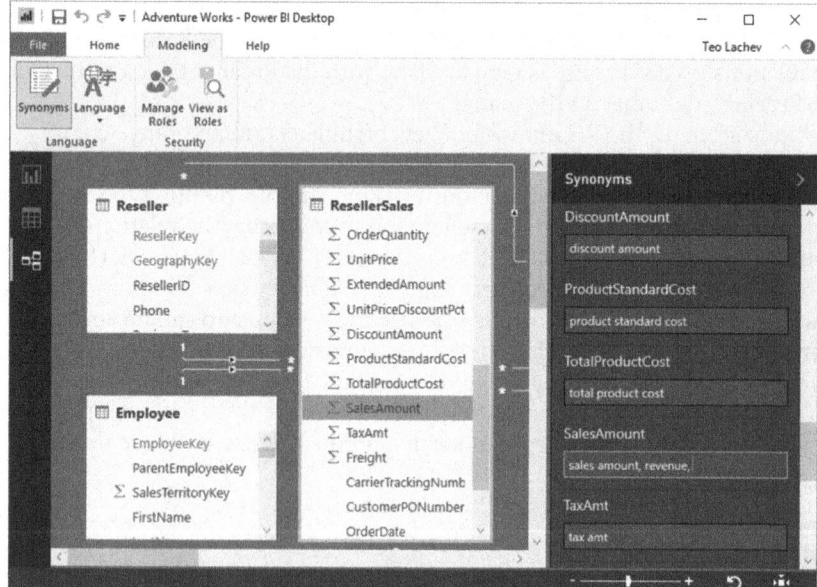

Figure 8.20 The "sales amount" and "revenue" are synonyms for the SalesAmount field.

8.3.5 Working with Relationships

As it stands, the Adventure Works model has nine tables and 11 relationships. Power BI has done a great job auto-detecting relationships. Next, you'll practice different techniques to change and create relationships.

Auto-detecting relationships

Let's see how far you can get by letting Power BI Desktop auto-detect relationships:

1. In the Data View (or Report View), click the Manage Relationships button in the ribbon's Home tab to open the Manage Relationships window.

2. Click the Autodetect button. If there's no relationship between the Customer and Geography tables, the auto-detection finds one new relationship. Click OK. Notice that a relationship Reseller[GeographyKey] ⇨ Geography[GeographyKey] is added. This relationship reflects the underlying snowflake schema consisting of the ResellerSales, Reseller, and Geography tables. The new relationship allows us to analyze reseller sales by geography using a cascading relationship spanning three tables (ResellerSales ⇨ Reseller ⇨ Geography).

 NOTE Usually a byproduct of a snowflake schema, a cascading relationship joins a fact table to a lookup table via another referenced lookup table. Power BI supports cascading relationships that can traverse multiple lookup tables.

Now let's clean up some existing relationships. As it stands, the InternetSales table has three relationships to the Date table (one active and two inactive) which Power BI Desktop auto-discovered from the underlying database. All these relationships join the Date table on the DateKey column. As I mentioned before, I suggest you use a column of a Date data type in the Date table. Luckily, both the Reseller Sales and InternetSales tables have OrderDate, ShipDate, and DueDate date columns. And the Date table has a Date column which is of a Date data type.

3. While still in the Manage Relationships window, delete the two inactive relationships (the ones with an unchecked Active flag) from the InternetSales table to the Date table. You can press and hold the Ctrl key to select multiple relationships and delete them in one step.

4. Delete also the three relationships from ResellerSales to Date: ResellerSales[DueDateKey] ⇨ Date[DateKey], ResellerSales[ShipDateKey] ⇨ Date[DateKey] and ResellerSales[OrderDateKey] ⇨ Date[DateKey].

Using the Manage Relationships window
The Adventure Works model has two fact tables (ResellerSales and InternetSales) and seven lookup tables. Let's start creating the missing relationships using the Manage Relationships window:

 TIP When you have multiple fact tables, join them to common dimension tables. This allows you to create consolidated reports that include multiple subject areas, such as a report that shows Internet sales and reseller sales side by side grouped by date and sales territory.

1. First, let's rebind the InternetSales[OrderDateKey] ⇨ Date[DateKey] relationship to use another set of columns. In the Manage Relationship window, double-click the InternetSales[OrderDateKey] ⇨ Date[DateKey] relationship (or select it and click Edit). If this relationship doesn't exist in your model, click the New button to create it. In the Edit Relationship window, select the OrderDate column (scroll all the way to the right) in the InternetSales table. Then select the Date column in the Date table and click OK.

 NOTE When joining fact tables to a date table on a date column, make sure that the foreign key values contain only the date portion of the date and not the time portion. Otherwise, the join will never find matching values in the date table. If you don't need it, the easiest way to discard the time portion is to change the column data type from Date/time to Date. You can also apply query transformations to strip the time portion or to create custom columns that have only the date portion.

2. Back in the Manage Relationship window, click New. Create a relationship ResellerSales[OrderDate] ⇨ Date[Date]. Leave the "Cross filter direction" drop-down to Single, and click OK.

3. Create ResellerSales[SalesTerritoryKey] ⇨ SalesTerritory[SalesTerritoryKey] and ResellerSales[ProductKey] ⇨ Product[ProductKey] relationships. However, change the "Cross filtering direction" option to *Single* to avoid errors related to ambiguous relationships later on.

4. Click the Close button to close the Manage Relationship window.

Creating relationships using the Relationships View
Next, you'll use the Relationships View to create relationships for the InternetSales table.

1. Click the Relationships View icon in the navigation bar.

2. If this relationship doesn't exist, drag the InternetSales[ProductKey] column and drop it onto the Product[ProductKey] column.

3. Drag the InternetSales[SalesTerritoryKey] column and drop it onto the SalesTerritory[SalesTerritoryKey] column.

4. Click the Manage Relationships button. Compare your results with **Figure 8.21**. As it stands, the Adventure Works model has 11 relationships. For now, let's not create inactive relationships. I'll revisit them in the next chapter when I cover DAX.

5. If there are differences between your relationships and **Figure 8.21**, make the necessary changes. Don't be afraid to delete wrong relationships if you have to recreate them to use different columns.

6. Once your setup matches **Figure 8.21**, click Close to close the Manage Relationships window. Save the Adventure Works file.

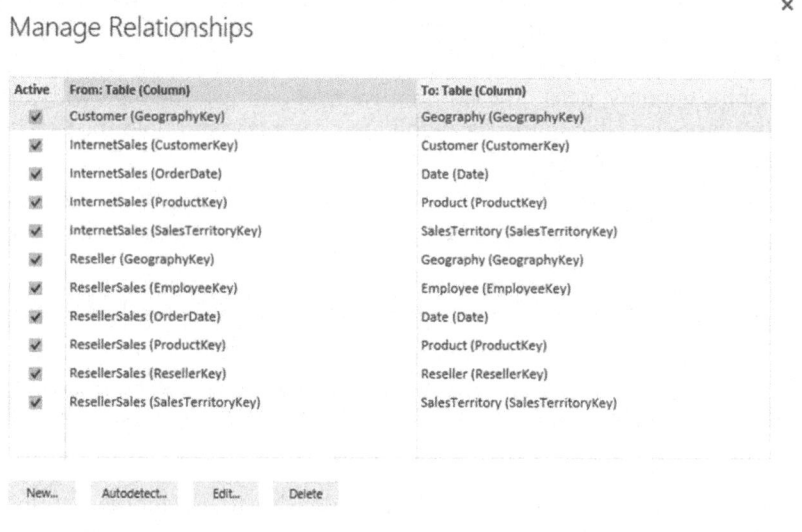

Active	From: Table (Column)	To: Table (Column)
✓	Customer (GeographyKey)	Geography (GeographyKey)
✓	InternetSales (CustomerKey)	Customer (CustomerKey)
✓	InternetSales (OrderDate)	Date (Date)
✓	InternetSales (ProductKey)	Product (ProductKey)
✓	InternetSales (SalesTerritoryKey)	SalesTerritory (SalesTerritoryKey)
✓	Reseller (GeographyKey)	Geography (GeographyKey)
✓	ResellerSales (EmployeeKey)	Employee (EmployeeKey)
✓	ResellerSales (OrderDate)	Date (Date)
✓	ResellerSales (ProductKey)	Product (ProductKey)
✓	ResellerSales (ResellerKey)	Reseller (ResellerKey)
✓	ResellerSales (SalesTerritoryKey)	SalesTerritory (SalesTerritoryKey)

New...   Autodetect...   Edit...   Delete

Close

Figure 8.21 The Manage Relationships dialog box shows 11 relationships defined in the Adventure Works model.

8.4 Implementing Analytical Features

Power BI Desktop has additional modeling capabilities for you to implement end-user features that further enrich the model. This section discusses features that don't require the Data Analysis Expressions DAX experience and are not available in Power BI Service, including hierarchies and data categories.

8.4.1 Working with Hierarchies

A hierarchy is a combination of fields that defines a navigational drilldown path in the model. As you've seen, Power BI allows you to use any column for slicing and dicing data in related tables. However, some fields form logical navigational paths for data exploration and drilling down. You can define hierarchies to group such fields.

Understanding hierarchies

A hierarchy defines a drill-down path using fields from a table. When you add the hierarchy to the report, you can drill down data by expanding its levels. A hierarchy can include fields from a single table only. If you want to drill down from different tables, just add the fields (don't define a hierarchy). A hierarchy offers two important benefits:

- Usability – You can add all fields for drilling down data in one click by adding the hierarchy instead of individual fields.

- Performance – Suppose you add a high-cardinality column, such as CustomerName, to a report. You might end up with a huge report. This might cause unnecessary performance degradation. Instead, you can hide the Customer field and you can define a hierarchy with levels, such as State, City, and Customer levels, to force end users to use this navigational path when browsing data by customers.

Typically, a hierarchy combines columns with logical one-to-many relationships. For example, one year can have multiple quarters and one quarter can have multiple months. This doesn't have to be the case though. For example, you can create a reporting hierarchy with ProductModel, Size, and Product columns, if you wish to analyze products that way.

Once you have a hierarchy in place, you might want to hide high-cardinality columns to prevent the user from adding them directly to the report and to avoid performance issues. For example, you might not want to expose the CustomerName column in the Customer table, to prevent users from adding it to a report outside the hierarchies it participates in.

Understanding in-line date hierarchies

The most common example of hierarchy is the date hierarchy, consisting of Year, Quarter, Month, and Date levels. In Chapter 6, I encouraged you to have a separate Date table so that you can define whatever date-related columns you need and implement DAX time calculations, such as YTD, QTD, and so on. But what if you didn't follow my advice and you want a quick and easy date hierarchy? Fortunately, Power BI Desktop can generate an in-line date hierarchy. All you need to do is add a column of a Date data type to the report. For example, **Figure 8.22** shows that I've added a Date field to the Values area of a Table report. Power BI has automatically generated a hierarchy with levels Year, Quarter, Month, and Day.

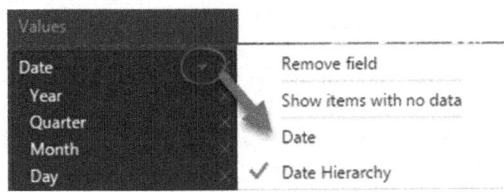

Figure 8.22 Power BI Desktop creates an inline hierarchy when you add a date field to the report.

If you don't want any of the levels, you can delete them by clicking the X button next to the level. And if you want to see just the date and not the hierarchy on the report, simply click the drop-down next to the Date hierarchy and then check the Date field.

> **NOTE** One existing limitation of the automatic in-line date hierarchy feature is that it doesn't generate time levels, such as Hour, Minute, and so on. If you need to perform time analysis, you need to create a Time table with the required levels and join it to the table with the data. Also, keep in mind that in-line hierarchies might increase your model size substantially (see the blog "Power BI Model Size Bloat and Auto Date/Time Tables" by Chris Webb at bit.ly2iKRbZe for more information). To remove them, go to File ⇨ Options and Settings ⇨ Options and uncheck the "Auto Date/Time" setting on the Data Load tab.

Implementing user-defined hierarchies

Follow these steps to implement a Calendar Hierarchy consisting of CalendarYear, CalendarQuarter, Month, and Date levels:

1. In the Fields pane (Report View or Data View), click the ellipsis button next to the CalendarYear field in the Date table, and then click New Hierarchy. This adds a CalendarYear Hierarchy to the Date table.

2. Click the ellipsis button next to the CalendarYear Hierarchy and then click rename. Rename the hierarchy to *Calendar Hierarchy*.

3. Click the ellipsis button next to the CalendarQuarter field and then click Add to Hierarchy ⇨ Calendar Hierarchy.

4. Repeat the last step to add MonthName and Date fields to the hierarchy. If you didn't add the fields in the correct order, you can simply drag a level in the hierarchy and move it to the correct place.

5. The name of the hierarchy level doesn't need to match the name of the underlying field. Click the ellipsis button next to the MonthName level of the Calendar Hierarchy (not to the MonthName field in the table) and rename it to *Month*. Compare you results with **Figure 8.23**.

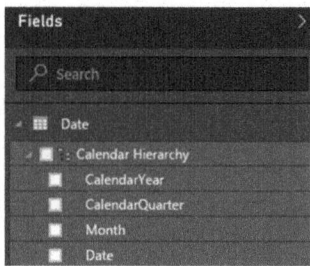

Figure 8.23   The Calendar Year hierarchy includes CalendarYear, CalendarQuarter, Month and Date levels.

6. (Optional) Create a chart report to add the Calendar Hierarchy to the Axis area of the chart. Enable drill-down behavior of the chart and test your new hierarchy.

 TIP   A quick way to create a hierarchy is simply to drag a field and drop onto another within the same table. The resulting hierarchy will have two levels with the lower level corresponding to the field that you dragged.

8.4.2   Assigning Data Categories

When Power BI Desktop imports data, not only does it get the actual data, it also gets additional metadata such as the table and column names, data types, and column cardinality. This information also helps Power BI Desktop to visualize the field when you add it to a report. A data category is additional metadata that you assign to a field to inform Power BI Desktop about the field content so that it can be visualized even better. You assign a data category to a field by using the Data Category drop-down in the ribbon's Modeling tab.

Assigning geo categories

When you expand the Data Category drop-down, you'll find that most of the data categories are geo-related, such as Address, City, Continent, and so on. Actually, when you use a geo-related field on a report, Power BI Desktop tries its best to infer the field content and geocode the field. For example, you add the AddressLine1 field from the Customer table to an empty Map visualization, Power BI Desktop will correctly interpret it as an address and plot it on the map. So, in most cases, specifying a data category is not necessary.

In some cases, however, Power BI might need extra help. Suppose you have a field with abbreviated values such as AZ, AL, and so on. Do values represent states or countries? This is where you'd need to specify a data category. For more information about Power BI geocoding and geo data categories, read my blog "Geocoding with Power View Maps" at prologika.com/geocoding-with-power-view-maps.

TIP Maps show cities in wrong locations? Cities with the same name can exist in different states and countries. If cities end up in the wrong place on the map, consider adding Country, State and City fields (or create a hierarchy with these levels) to the map's Location area and enabling drilling down. When you do this, Power BI will attempt to plot the location within the parent territory. Of course, another solution to avoid ambiguity is to use latitude and longitude coordinates instead of location names.

Configuring navigation links

Sometimes, you might want to show a clickable navigation link (URL) to allow the user to navigate to a web page or another report. For example, the Table visual in **Figure 8.24** shows a list of reseller names and their websites (I fabricated a Website field from the Reseller Name with empty spaces removed). The user can click the website URL to navigate to it in the browser. Assuming you have a field with the links, you can simply assign it to the Web URL data category.

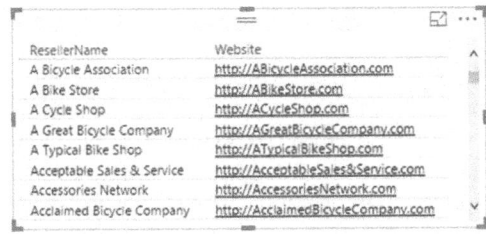

Figure 8.24 Assign the Web URL data category to implement clickable links.

And if you have a field that stores links to images, you can assign the Image URL category to it so that the images show in a Table or Card visuals.

8.5   Summary

Once you import the initial set of tables, you should spend time exploring the model data and refining the model schema. The Data View supports various column operations to help you explore the model data and to make the necessary changes. You should make your model more intuitive by having meaningful table and column names. Revisit each column and configure its data type and formatting properties.

Relationships are the cornerstone of self-service data modelling that involves multiple datasets. You must have table relationships to integrate data across multiple tables.

As Power BI Desktop evolves, it adds more features to address popular analytical needs. Hierarchies let you explore data following natural paths. Data categories help Power BI Desktop interpret the field content. Use quick calculations to implement common measures without writing DAX code. Define forecast lines to implement time series forecasting. Use groups to analyze data across categories that you specify.

You've come a long way in designing the Adventure Works model! Next, let's make it even more useful by extending it with business calculations.

Chapter 9

Implementing Calculations

Power BI promotes rapid personal business intelligence (BI) for essential data exploration and analysis. Chances are, however, that in real life you might need to go beyond just simple aggregations. Business needs might require you to extend your model with calculations. Data Analysis Expressions (DAX) gives you the needed programmatic power to travel the "last mile" and unlock the full potential of Power BI.

DAX is a big topic that deserves much more attention, and this chapter doesn't aim to cover it in depth. However, it'll lay down the necessary fundamentals so that you can start using DAX to extend your models with business logic. The chapter starts by introducing you to DAX and its arsenal of functions. Next, you'll learn how to implement custom calculated columns and measures. I'll also show you how to handle more advanced scenarios with DAX. And you'll create various visualizations to test the sample calculations.

9.1   Understanding Data Analysis Expressions

Data Analysis Expressions (DAX) is a formula-based language in Power BI, Power Pivot, and Tabular that allows you to define custom calculations using an Excel-like formula language. DAX was introduced in the first version of Power Pivot (released in May 2010) with two major design goals:

- Simplicity – To get you started quickly with implementing business logic, DAX uses the Excel standard formula syntax and inherits many Excel functions. As a business analyst, Martin already knows many Excel functions, such as SUM and AVERAGE. When he uses Power BI, he appreciates that DAX has the same functions.

- Relational – DAX is designed with data models in mind and supports relational artifacts, including tables, columns, and relationships. For example, if Martin wants to sum up the SalesAmount column in the ResellerSales table, he can use the following formula: =SUM(ResellerSales[SalesAmount]).

DAX also has query constructs to allow external clients to query organizational Tabular models. As a data analyst, you probably don't need to know about these constructs. This chapter focuses on DAX as an expression language to extend self-service data models. If you need to know more about DAX in the context of organizational BI, you might find my book "Applied Microsoft SQL Server 2012 Analysis Services: Tabular Modeling" useful.

You can use DAX as an expression language to implement custom calculations that range from simple expressions, such as to concatenate two columns together, to complex measures that aggregate data in a specific way, such as to implement weighted averages. Based on the intended use, DAX supports two types of calculations: calculated columns and measures.

9.1.1 Understanding Calculated Columns

A calculated column is a table column that uses a DAX formula to compute the column values. This is conceptually like a formula-based column added to an Excel list, although DAX formulas reference columns instead of cells.

How calculated columns are stored

When a column contains a formula, the storage engine computes the value for each row and saves the results, just like it does with a regular column. To use a techie term, values of calculated columns get "materialized" or "persisted". The difference is that regular columns import their values from a data source, while calculated columns are computed from DAX formulas and saved after the regular columns are loaded. Because of this, the formula of a calculated column can reference regular columns and other calculated columns.

The storage engine might not compress calculated columns as much as regular columns because they don't participate in the re-ordering algorithm that optimizes the compression. So, if you have a large table with a calculated column that has many unique values, this column might have a larger memory footprint.

Understanding row context

Every DAX formula is evaluated in a specific context. The formulas of calculated columns are evaluated for each row (row context). Let's look at a calculated column called FullName that's added to the Customer table, and it uses the following formula to concatenate the customer's first name and last name:

FullName=[FirstName] & " " & [LastName]

Because its formula is evaluated for each row in the Customer table (see **Figure 9.1**), the FullName column returns the full name for each customer. Again, this is very similar to how an Excel formula works when applied to multiple rows in a list, so this should be easy to understand.

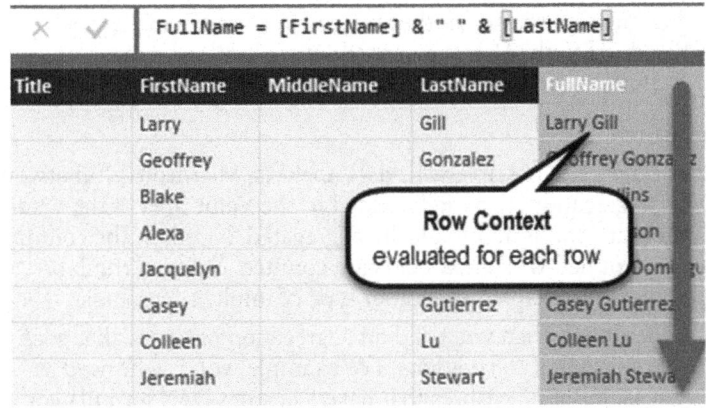

Figure 9.1 Calculated columns operate in row context, and their formulas are evaluated for each table row.

In terms of reporting, you can use calculated columns to group and filter data, just like you can use regular columns. For example, you can add a calculated column to any area of the Visualizations pane.

When to use calculated columns

In general, use a calculated column when you need to use a DAX formula to derive the column values. Because DAX formulas can reference other tables, a good usage scenario might be to look up a value from another table, just like you can use Excel VLOOKUP to reference values from another sheet. For example, to calculate the profit for each line item in ResellerSales, you might need to look up the product cost from the Product table. In this case, using a calculated column might make sense because its results are stored for each row in ResellerSales.

TIP You should be able to implement even this cross-table lookup scenario in the Query Editor either by merging datasets or using query functions (see my blog "Implementing Lookups in Power Query" at http://prologika.com/implementing-lookups-in-power-query/ for an example). Whether to use a DAX calculated column or another approach is a tradeoff between convenience and performance. As a best practice, implement your calculated columns as downstream as possible: in the data source, view, Query Editor, and finally DAX.

When shouldn't you use calculated columns? I mentioned that because calculated columns don't compress, they require more storage than regular columns. Therefore, if you can perform the calculation at the data source or in the model query, I recommend you do it there instead of using calculated columns. This is especially true for high-cardinality calculated columns in large tables because they require more memory for storage. For example, you might need to concatenate a carrier tracking number from its distinct parts in a large fact table. It's better to do so in the data source or in the table query before the data is imported. Continuing this line of thought, the example that I gave for using a calculated column for the customer's full name should probably be avoided in real life because you can perform the concatenation in the query.

Sometimes, however, you don't have a choice. For example, you might need a more complicated calculation that can be done only in DAX, such as to calculate the rank for each customer based on sales history. In these cases, you can't easily apply the calculation at the data source or the query. This is a good scenario for using DAX calculated columns.

9.1.2 Understanding Measures

Besides calculated columns, you can use DAX formulas to define measures. Unlike calculated columns, which might be avoided by using other implementation approaches, measures typically can't be replicated in other ways – they need to be written in DAX. DAX measures are very useful because they are used to produce aggregated values, such as to summarize a SalesAmount column or to calculate a distinct count of customers who have placed orders. Although measures are associated with a table, they don't show in the Data View's data preview pane, as calculated columns do. Instead, they're accessible in the Fields pane. When used on reports, measures are typically added to the Value area of the Visualizations pane.

Understanding measure types
Power BI Desktop supports two types of measures:

- Implicit measures – To get you started as quickly as possible with data analysis, Microsoft felt that you shouldn't have to write formulas for basic aggregations. Any field added to the Value area of the Visualizations pane is treated as an implicit measure and is automatically aggregated, based on the column data type. For example, numeric fields are summed while text fields are counted. You can think of quick calculations that I discussed in the previous chapter as another type of implicit measures.

- Explicit measures – You'll create explicit measures when you need an aggregation behavior that goes beyond the standard aggregation functions and quick calculations. For example, you might need a year-to-date (YTD) calculation. Explicit measures are measures that have a custom DAX formula you specify. **Table 9.1** summarizes the differences between implicit and explicit measures.

Table 9.1   Comparing implicit and explicit measures.

Criterion	Implicit Measures	Explicit Measures
Design	Automatically generated	Manually created
Accessibility	Can be changed on the report	Become a part of the model
DAX support	Standard aggregation formulas only	Can use DAX functions

Implicit measures are automatically generated by Power BI Desktop when you add a field to the Value area of the Visualizations pane. By contrast, you must specify a custom formula for explicit measures. Once the implicit measure is created, you can use the Visualizations pane to change its aggregation function. By contrast, explicit measures become a part of the model, and they can't be changed on the report. Implicit measures can only use the DAX standard aggregation functions: Sum, Count, Min, Max, Average, Distinct-Count, Standard Deviation, Variance, and Median. However, explicit measures can use any DAX function, such as to define a custom aggregation behavior.

Understanding filter context

Unlike calculated columns, DAX measures are evaluated *at run time* for each report *cell* as opposed to once for each table row. DAX measures are always dynamic, and the result of the measure formula is never saved. Moreover, measures are evaluated in the filter context of each cell, as shown in **Figure 9.2**.

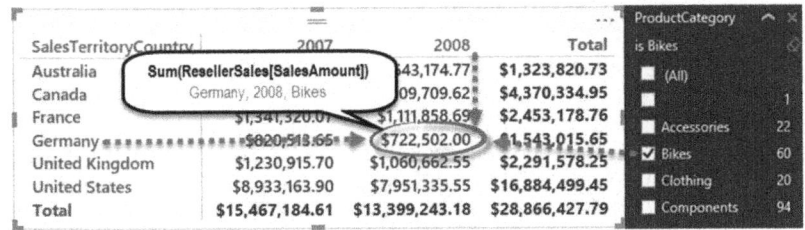

Figure 9.2 Measures are evaluated for each cell, and they operate in filter context.

This report summarizes the SalesAmount measure by countries on rows and by years on columns. The report is further filtered to show only sales for the Bikes product category. The filter context of the highlighted cell is the Germany value of the SalesTerritory[SalesTerritoryCountry] fields (on rows), the 2008 value of the Date[CalendarYear] field (on columns), and the Bikes value of the Product[ProductCategory] field (used as a filter).

If you're familiar with the SQL language, you can think of the DAX filter context as a WHERE clause that's determined dynamically and then applied to each cell on the report. When Power BI calculates the expression for that cell, it scopes the formula accordingly, such as to sum the sales amount from the rows in the ResellerSales table where the SalesTerritoryCountry value is Germany, the CalendarYear value is 2008, and the ProductCategory value is Bikes.

When to use measures

In general, measures are most frequently used to aggregate data. Explicit measures are typically used when you need a custom aggregation behavior, such as for time calculations, aggregates over aggregates, variances, and weighted averages. Suppose you want to calculate year-to-date (YTD) of reseller sales. As a first attempt, you might decide to add a SalesAmountYTD calculated column to the ResellerSales table. But now you have an issue because each row in this table represents an order line item. It's meaningless to calculate YTD for each line item.

As a second attempt, you could create a summary table in the database that stores YTD sales at a specific grain, such as product, end of month, reseller, and so on. While this might be a good approach for report performance, it presents issues. What if you need to lower the grain to include other dimensions? What if your requirements change and now YTD needs to be calculated as of any date? A better approach would be to use an explicit measure that's evaluated dynamically as users slice and dice the data. And don't worry too much about performance. Thanks to the memory-resident nature of the storage engine, most DAX calculations are instantaneous!

NOTE The performance of DAX measures depends on several factors, including the complexity of the formula, your knowledge of DAX (whether you write inefficient DAX), the amount of data, and even the hardware of your computer. While most measures, such as time calculations and basic filtered aggregations, should perform very well, more involved calculations, such as aggregates over aggregates or the number of open orders as of any reporting date, are more intensive.

9.1.3 Understanding DAX Syntax

As I mentioned, one of the DAX design goals is to look and feel like the Excel formula language. Because of this, the DAX syntax resembles the Excel formula syntax. The DAX formula syntax is case-insensitive. For example, the following two expressions are both valid:

=YEAR([Date])
=year([date])

That said, I suggest you have a naming convention and stick to it. I personally prefer the first example where the function names are in uppercase and the column references match the column names in the model. This convention helps me quickly identify functions and columns in DAX formulas, and so that's what I use in this book.

Understanding expression syntax
A DAX formula for calculated columns and explicit measures has the following syntax:

Name=expression

Name is the name of the calculated column or measure. The expression must evaluate to a scalar (single) value. Expressions can contain operators, constants, or column references to return literal or Boolean values. The FullName calculated column that you saw before is an example of a simple expression that concatenates two values. You can add as many spaces as you want to make the formula easier to read.

Expressions can also include functions to perform more complicated operations, such as aggregating data. For example, back in **Figure 9.2**, the DAX formula references the SUM function to aggregate the SalesAmount column in the ResellerSales table. Functions can be nested. For example, the following formula nests the FILTER function to calculate the count of line items associated with the Progressive Sports reseller:

=COUNTROWS(FILTER(ResellerSales, RELATED(Reseller[ResellerName])="Progressive Sports"))

DAX supports up to 64 levels of function nesting, but going beyond two or three levels makes the formulas more difficult to understand. When you need to go above two or three levels of nesting, I recommend you break the formula into multiple measures. This also simplifies testing complex formulas.

Understanding operators
DAX supports a set of common operators to support more complex formulas, as shown in **Table 9.2**. DAX also supports TRUE and FALSE as logical constants.

Table 9.2   DAX supports the following operators.

Category	Operators	Description	Example
Arithmetic	+, -, *, /, ^	Addition, subtraction, multiplication, division, and exponentiation	=[SalesAmount] * [OrderQty]
Comparison	>, >=, <, <=, <>	For comparing values	=FILTER(RELATEDTABLE(Products),Products[UnitPrice]>30))
Logical	||, &&	Logical OR and AND	=FILTER(RELATEDTABLE(Products),Products[UnitPrice]>30 && Products[Discontinued]=TRUE())
Concatenation	&	Concatenating text	=[FirstName] & " " & [LastName]
Unary	+, -, NOT	Change the operand sign	= - [SalesAmount]

Referencing columns

One of DAX's strengths over regular Excel formulas is that it can traverse table relationships and reference columns. This is much simpler and more efficient than referencing Excel cells and ranges with the VLOOKUP function. Column names are unique within a table. You can reference a column using its fully qualified name in the format <TableName>[<ColumnName>], such as in this example:

ResellerSales[SalesAmount]

If the table name includes a space or is a reserved word, such as Date, enclose it with single quotes:

'Reseller Sales'[SalesAmount] or 'Date'[CalendarYear]

When a calculated column references a column from the same table, you can omit the table name. The AutoComplete feature in the formula bar helps you avoid syntax errors when referencing columns. As **Figure 9.3** shows, the moment you start typing the fully qualified column reference in the formula bar, it displays a drop-down list of matching columns. The formula bar also supports color coding, and it colors the function names in a blue color.

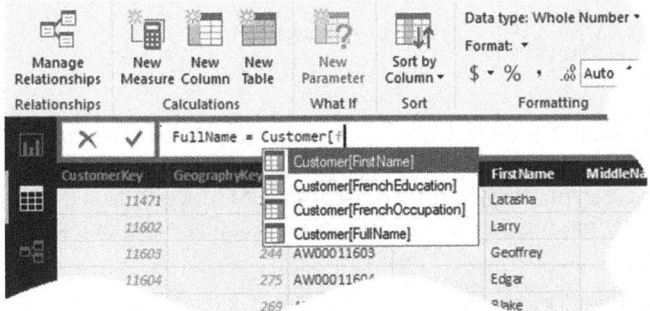

Figure 9.3 AutoComplete helps you with column references in the formula bar.

9.1.4 Understanding DAX Functions

DAX supports over a hundred functions that encapsulate a prepackaged programming logic to perform a wide variety of operations. If you type in the function name in the formula bar, AutoComplete shows the function syntax and its arguments. For the sake of brevity, this book doesn't cover the DAX functions and their syntax in detail. For more information, please refer to the DAX language reference by Ed Price (this book's technical editor) at http://bit.ly/daxfunctions, which provides a detailed description and examples for most functions. Another useful resource is "DAX in the BI Tabular Model Whitepaper and Samples" by Microsoft (http://bit.ly/daxwhitepaper).

Functions from Excel

DAX supports approximately 80 Excel functions. The big difference is that DAX formulas can't reference Excel cells or ranges. References such as A1 or A1:A10, which are valid in Excel formulas, can't be used in DAX functions. Instead, when data operations are required, the DAX functions must reference columns or tables. **Table 9.3** shows the subset of Excel functions supported by DAX with examples.

Aggregation functions

As you've seen, DAX "borrows" the Excel aggregation functions, such as SUM, MIN, MAX, COUNT, and so on. However, the DAX counterparts accept a table column as an input argument instead of a cell range. Since only referencing columns can be somewhat limiting, DAX adds X-version of these functions: SUMX, AVERAGEX, COUNTAX, MINX, MAXX. These functions take two arguments. The first one is a table and the second is an expression.

Table 9.3 DAX borrows many functions from Excel.

Category	Functions	Example
Date and Time	DATE, DATEVALUE, DAY, EDATE, EOMONTH, HOUR, MINUTE, MONTH, NOW, SECOND, TIME, TIMEVALUE, TODAY, WEEKDAY, WEEKNUM, YEAR, YEARFRAC	=YEAR('Date'[Date])
Information	ISBLANK, ISERROR, ISLOGICAL, ISNONTEXT, ISNUMBER, ISTEXT	=IF(ISBLANK('Date'[Month]), "N/A", 'Date'[Month])
Logical	AND, IF, NOT, OR, FALSE, TRUE	=IF(ISBLANK(Customers[MiddleName]),FALSE(),TRUE())
Math and Trigonometry	ABS,CEILING, ISO.CEILING, EXP, FACT, FLOOR, INT, LN, LOG, LOG10, MOD, MROUND, PI, POWER, QUOTIENT, RAND, RANDBETWEEN, ROUND, ROUNDDOWN, ROUNDUP, SIGN, SQRT, SUM, SUMSQ, TRUNC	=SUM(ResellerSales[SalesAmount])
Statistical	AVERAGE, AVERAGEA, COUNT, COUNTA, COUNTBLANK, MAX, MAXA, MIN, MINA	=AVERAGE(ResellerSales[SalesAmount])
Text	CONCATENATE, EXACT, FIND, FIXED, LEFT, LEN, LOWER, MID, REPLACE, REPT, RIGHT, SEARCH, SUBSTITUTE, TRIM, UPPER, VALUE	=SUBSTITUTE(Customer[Phone],"-", "")

Suppose you want to calculate the total order amount for each row in the ResellerSales table using the formula [SalesAmount] * [OrderQuantity]. You can accomplish this in two ways. First, you can add an OrderAmount calculated column that uses the above expression and then use the SUM function to summarize the calculated column. However, a better approach is to perform the calculation in one step by using the SUMX function, as follows:

=SUMX(ResellerSales, ResellerSales[SalesAmount] * ResellerSales[OrderQuantity])

Although the result in both cases is the same, the calculation process is very different. In the case of the SUM function, DAX simply aggregates the column. When you use the SUMX function, DAX will compute the expression for each of the detail rows behind the cell and then aggregate the result. What makes the X-version functions flexible is that the table argument can also be a function that returns a table of values. For example, the following formula calculates the simple average (arithmetic mean) of the SalesAmount column for rows in the InternetSales table whose unit price is above $100:

=AVERAGEX (FILTER(InternetSales, InternetSales[UnitPrice] > 100), InternetSales[SalesAmount])

This formula uses the FILTER function, which returns a table of rows matching the criteria that you pass in the second argument.

Statistical functions

DAX adds new statistical functions. The COUNTROWS(Table) function is similar to the Excel COUNT functions (COUNT, COUNTA, COUNTX, COUNTAX, COUNTBLANK), but it takes a table as an argument and returns the count of rows in that table. For example, the following formula returns the number of rows in the ResellerSales table:

=COUNTROWS(ResellerSales)

Similarly, the DISTINCTCOUNT(Column) function, counts the distinct values in a column. DAX includes the most common statistical functions, such as STDEV.S, STDEV.P, STDEVX.S, STDEVX.P, VAR.S, VAR.P, VARX.S, and VARX.P, for calculating standard deviation and variance. Similar to Count, Sum, Min, Max, and Average, DAX has its own implementation of these functions for better performance instead of just using the Excel standard library.

Filter functions

This category includes functions for navigating relationships and filtering data, including the ALL, ALLEXCEPT, ALLNOBLANKROW, CALCULATE, CALCULATETABLE, DISTINCT, EARLIER, EARLIEST, FILTER, LOOKUPVALUE, RELATED, RELATEDTABLE, and VALUES functions. Next, I'll provide examples for the most popular filter functions.

You can use the RELATED(Column), RELATEDTABLE(Table), and USERELATIONSHIP (Column1, Column2) functions for navigating relationships in the model. The RELATED function follows a many-to-one relationship, such as from a fact table to a lookup table. Consider a calculated column in the ResellerSales table that uses the following formula:

=RELATED(Product[StandardCost])

For each row in the ResellerSales table, this formula will look up the standard cost of the product in the Product table. The RELATEDTABLE function can travel a relationship in either direction. For example, a calculated column in the Product table can use the following formula to obtain the total reseller sales amount for each product:

=SUMX(RELATEDTABLE(ResellerSales), ResellerSales[SalesAmount])

For each row in the Product table, this formula finds the corresponding rows in the ResellerSales table that match the product and then it sums the SalesAmount column across these rows. The USERELATIONSHIP function can use inactive role-playing relationships, as I'll demonstrate in section 9.4.1.

The FILTER (Table, Condition) function is useful to filter a subset of column values, as I've just demonstrated with the AVERAGEX example. The DISTINCT(Column) function returns a table of unique values in a column. For example, this formula returns the count of unique customers with Internet sales:

=COUNTROWS(DISTINCT(InternetSales[CustomerKey]))

When there is no table relationship, the LOOKUPVALUE (ResultColumn, SearchColumn1, SearchValue1 [, SearchColumn2, SearchValue2]...) function can be used to look up a single value from another table. The following formula looks up the sales amount of the first line item bought by customer 14870 on August 1st, 2007:

=LOOKUPVALUE(InternetSales[SalesAmount],[OrderDateKey],"20070801",[CustomerKey],"14870", [SalesOrderLineNumber],"1")

If multiple values are found, the LOOKUPVALUE function will return the error "A table of multiple values was supplied where a single value was expected". If you expect multiple values, use the FILTER function instead.

The CALCULATE(Expression, [Filter1],[Filter2]..) function is a very popular and useful function because it allows you to overwrite the filter context. It evaluates an expression in its filter context that could be modified by optional filters. Suppose you need to add a LineItemCount calculated column to the Customer table that computes the count of order line items posted by each customer. On a first attempt, you might try the following expression to count the order line items:

=COUNTROWS(InternetSales)

However, this expression won't work as expected (see the top screenshot in **Figure 9.4**). Specifically, it returns the count of all the rows in the InternetSales table instead of counting the line items for each customer. To fix this, you need to force the COUNTROWS function to execute in the current row context. To do this, I'll use the CALCULATE function as follows:

=CALCULATE(COUNTROWS(InternetSales))

The CALCUATE function determines the current row context and applies the filter context to the formula. Because the Customer table is related to InternetSales on CustomerKey, the value of CustomerKey for each row is passed as a filter to InternetSales. For example, if the CustomerKey value for the first row is 11602, the filter context for the first execution is COUNTROWS(InternetSales, CustomerKey=11602).

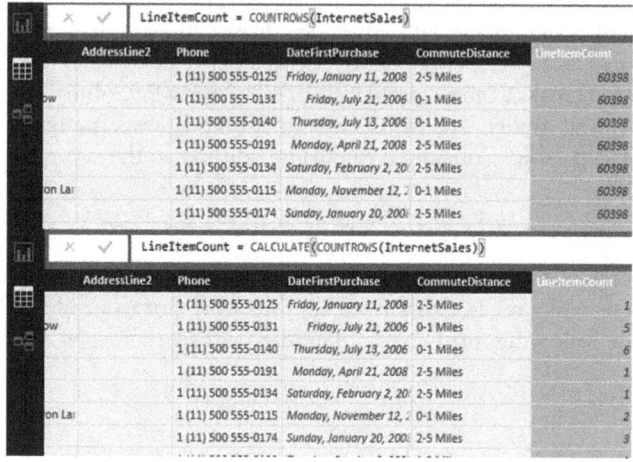

Figure 9.4 This calculated column in the second example uses the CALCULATE function to pass the row context to the InternetSales table.

The CALCULATE function can also take one or more filters as optional arguments. The filter argument can be a Boolean expression or a table. The following expression returns the transaction count for each customer for the year 2007 and the Bikes product category:

=CALCULATE(COUNTROWS(InternetSales), 'Date'[CalendarYear]=2007, Product[ProductCategory]="Bikes")

The following expression counts the rows in the InternetSales table for each customer where the product category is "Bikes" or is missing:

=CALCULATE(COUNTROWS(InternetSales), FILTER(Product, Product[ProductCategory]="Bikes" || ISBLANK(Product[ProductCategory])))

The FILTER function returns a table that contains only the rows from the Product table where ProductCategory="Bikes". When you pass the returned table to the CALCULATE function, it'll filter away any combination of column values that doesn't exist in the table.

 TIP When the expression to be evaluated is a measure, you can use the following shortcut for the CALCULATE function: =MeasureName(<filter>). For example, =[SalesAmount1]('Date'[CalendarYear]=2006)

Time intelligence functions
One of the most common analysis needs is implementing time calculations, such as year-to-date, parallel period, previous period, and so on. The time intelligence functions require a Date table. The Date table should contain one row for every date that might exist in your data. You can add a Date table using any of the techniques I discussed in Chapter 6. DAX uses the Data table to construct a set of dates for each calculation depending on the DAX formula you specify. For more information about how DAX uses a date table, read the blog post, "Time Intelligence Functions in DAX" by Microsoft's Howie Dickerman (http://bit.ly/daxtifunctions).

 NOTE Readers familiar with Excel data modeling might know that you need to explicitly mark a date table. Power BI Desktop doesn't have this feature yet but for time intelligence functions to work, the relationships to the date table must join on a column of a Date data type.

As I mentioned in the previous chapter, Power BI doesn't limit you to a single date table. For example, you might decide to import three date tables so you can do analysis on order date, ship date, and due date. If they are all related to the ResellerSales table, you can implement calculations such as:

SalesAmountByOrderDate = TOTALYTD(SUM(ResellerSales[SalesAmount]), 'OrderDate'[Date])
SalesAmountByShipDate = TOTALYTD(SUM(ResellerSales[SalesAmount]), 'ShipDate'[Date])

DAX has about 35 functions for implementing time calculations. The functions that you'll probably use most often are TOTALYTD, TOTALQTD, and TOTALMTD. For example, the following formula calculates the YTD sales. The second argument tells DAX which Date table to use as a reference point:

= TOTALYTD(SUM(ResellerSales[SalesAmount]), 'Date'[Date])
-- or the following expression to use fiscal years that end on June 30th
= TOTALYTD(SUM(ResellerSales[SalesAmount]), 'Date'[Date], ALL('Date'), "6/30")

Another common requirement is to implement variance and growth calculations between the current and previous time period. The following formula calculates the sales amount for the previous year using the PREVIOUSYEAR function:

=CALCULATE(SUM(ResellerSales[SalesAmount]), PREVIOUSYEAR('Date'[Date]))

There are also to-date functions that return a table with multiple periods, including the DATESMTD, DATESQTD, DATESYTD, and SAMEPERIODLASTYEAR. For example, the following measure formula returns the YTD reseller sales:

=CALCULATE(SUM(ResellerSales[SalesAmount]), DATESYTD('Date'[Date]))

Finally, the DATEADD, DATESBETWEEN, DATESINPERIOD, and PARALLELPERIOD functions can take an arbitrary range of dates. The following formula returns the reseller sales between July 1st 2005 and July 4th 2005.

=CALCULATE(SUM(ResellerSales[SalesAmount]), DATESBETWEEN('Date'[Date], DATE(2005,7,1), DATE(2005,7,4)))

Ranking functions

You might have a need to calculate rankings. DAX supports ranking functions. For example, the RANK.EQ(Value, Column, [Order]) function allows you to implement a calculated column that returns the rank of a number in a list of numbers. Consider the Rank calculated column in the SalesTerritory table (see **Figure 9.5**).

× ✓	Rank = RANK.EQ([Revenue], SalesTerritory[Revenue])					
SalesTerritoryGroup	SalesTerritoryCountry	SalesTerritoryRegion	SalesTerritoryKey	Revenue	Rank	1
North America	United States	Southwest	4	$24,184,609.60	1	
North America	Canada	Canada	6	$16,355,770.46	2	
North America	United States	Northwest	1	$16,084,942.55	3	
Pacific	Australia	Australia	9	$10,655,335.96	4	
North America	United States	Central	3	$7,909,009.01	5	
North America	United States	Southeast	5	$7,879,655.07	6	
Europe	United Kingdom	United Kingdom	10	$7,670,721.04	7	
Europe	France	France	7	$7,251,555.65	8	
North America	United States	Northeast	2	$6,939,374.48	9	
Europe	Germany	Germany	8	$4,878,300.38	10	

Figure 9.5 The RANK.EQ function ranks each row based on the value in the REVENUE column.

The formula uses the RANK.EQ function to return the rank of each territory, based on the value of the Revenue column. If multiple territories have the same revenue, they'll share the same rank. However, the presence of duplicate numbers affects the ranks of subsequent numbers. For example, had Southwest and Canada had the same revenue, their rank would be 1, but the Northwest rank would be 3. The function can take an Order argument, such as 0 (default) for a descending order or 1 for an ascending order.

Creating calculated tables

An interesting Power BI Desktop feature is creating calculated tables using DAX. A calculated table is just like a regular table, but it's populated with a DAX function that returns a table instead of using a query. I mentioned in the previous chapter that a good use for calculated tables is implementing role-playing lookup tables, such as ShipDate, OrderDate, DueDate. You can create a calculated table by clicking the New Table button in the ribbon's Modeling tab. For example, you can add a SalesSummary table (see **Figure 9.6**) that summarizes reseller and Internet sales by calendar year using the following formula:

SalesSummary = SUMMARIZE(ResellerSales, 'Date'[CalendarYear], "ResellerSalesAmount", SUM(ResellerSales[SalesAmount]), "InternetSalesAmount", SUM(InternetSales[SalesAmount]))

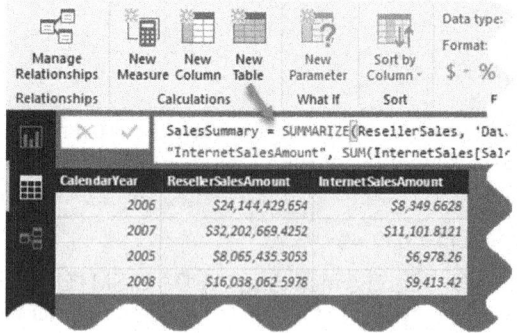

Figure 9.6 You can use the New Table button in the ribbon's Modeling tab to create a calculated table that uses a DAX formula.

This formula uses the SUMMARIZE function which works similarly to the SQL GROUP BY clause. It summarizes the ResellerSales table by grouping by Date[CalendarYear] and computing the aggregated ResellerSales[SalesAmount] and InternetSales[SalesAmount]. Unlike SQL, you don't have to specify joins because the model has relationships from the ResellerSales and InternetSales tables to the Date table.

Now that I've introduced you to the DAX syntax and functions, let's practice creating DAX calculations. You'll also practice creating visualizations in the Report View to test the calculations, but I won't go into the details because you've already learned about visualizations in Chapter 3. If you don't want to type in the formulas, you can copy them from the dax.txt file in the \Source\ch09 folder.

9.2 Implementing Calculated Columns

As I previously mentioned, calculated columns are columns that use DAX formulas for their values. Unlike the regular columns you get when you import data, you add calculated columns after the data is imported, by entering DAX formulas. When you create a report, you can place a calculated column in any area of the Visualizations pane, although you'd typically use calculated columns to group and filter data on the report.

9.2.1 Creating Basic Calculated Columns

DAX includes various operators to create basic expressions, such as expressions for concatenating strings and for performing arithmetic operations. You can use these operators to create simple expression-based columns.

Concatenating text

Suppose you need a visualization that shows sales by employee (see **Figure 9.8**). Since you'd probably need to show the employee's full name, which is missing in the Employee table, let's create a calculated column that shows the employee's full name:

1. Open the Adventure Works file with your changes from the previous chapter.

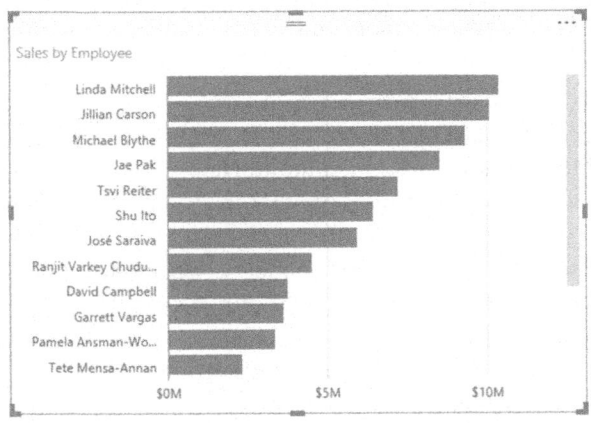

Figure 9.7 This visualization shows sales by the employee's full name.

2. Click the Data View icon in the navigation bar. Click the Employee table in the Fields pane to select it.

3. In the Modeling bar, click the New Column button. This adds a new column named "Column" to the end of the table and activates the formula bar. In the formula bar, enter the following formula:

FullName = [FirstName] & " " & [LastName]

This formula changes the name of the calculated column to *FullName*. Then, the DAX expression uses the concatenation operator to concatenate the FirstName and LastName columns and to add an empty space in between them. As you type, AutoComplete helps you with the formula syntax, although you should also follow the syntax rules, such as that a column reference must be enclosed in square brackets.

4. Press Enter or click the checkmark button to the left of the formula bar. DAX evaluates the expression and commits the formula. Power BI Desktop adds the FullName field to the Employee table in the Fields pane and prefixes it with a special *fx* icon.

Working with date columns

Instead of DAX calculated columns, you can implement simple expression-based columns in table queries. This is the technique you'll practice next.

1. Right-click the Customer table in the Fields pane and then click Edit Query.

2. Add a FullName custom column (in the ribbon's Add Column tab, click Custom Column) to the Customer query with the following formula:

=[FirstName] & " " & [LastName]

3. In the Queries pane, select the Date query. Add the custom columns shown in **Table 9.4** to assign user-friendly names to months, quarters, and semesters.

Table 9.4 Add the following calculated columns in the Date query.

Column Name	Expression	Example
MonthNameDesc	=[MonthName] & " " & Text.From([CalendarYear])	July 2007
CalendarQuarterDesc	="Q" & Text.From([CalendarQuarter]) & " " & Text.From([CalendarYear])	Q1 2008
FiscalQuarterDesc	="Q" & Text.From([FiscalQuarter]) & " " & Text.From([FiscalYear])	Q3 2008
CalendarSemesterDesc	="H" & Text.From([CalendarSemester]) & " " & Text.From([CalendarYear])	H2 2007
FiscalSemesterDesc	="H" & Text.From([FiscalSemester]) & " " & Text.From([FiscalYear])	H2 2007

In case you're wondering, the Text.From() function is used to cast a number to text. An explicit conversion is required because the query won't do an implicit conversion to text, and so the formula will return an error.

4. Click the "Close & Apply" button to apply the changes to the data model.

5. In the Fields pane, expand the Date table, and click the MonthNameDesc column to select it in the Data View. Click the "Sort By Column" button (ribbon's Modeling tab) to sort the MonthNameDesc column by the MonthNumberOfYear column. You do this so that month names are sorted in the ordinal order when MonthNameDesc is used on a report.

6. To reduce clutter, hide the CalendarQuarter, CalendarSemester, FiscalQuarter and FiscalSemester columns in the Date table. These columns show the quarter and semester ordinal numbers, and they're not that useful for analysis.

7. In the Reports tab, create a Bar Chart using the SalesAmount field from the ResellerSales table (add it to Value area) and the FullName field from the Employee table (add it to the Axis area).

8. Hover on the chart and click the ellipsis (…) menu in the upper-right corner. Sort the visualization by SalesAmount in descending order. Compare your results with **Figure 9.7** to verify that the FullName calculated column is working. Save the Adventure Works model.

Performing arithmetic operations

Another common requirement is to create a calculated column that performs some arithmetic operations for each row in a table. Follow these steps to create a LineTotal column that calculates the total amount for each row in the ResellerSales table by multiplying the order quantity, discount, and unit price:

1. Another way to add a calculated column is to use the Fields pane. In the Fields pane, right-click the ResellerSales table, and then click New Column.

2. In the formula bar, enter the following formula and press Enter. I've intentionally misspelled the OrderQty column reference to show you how you can troubleshoot errors in formulas.

LineTotal = [UnitPrice] * (1-[UnitPriceDiscountPct]) * [OrderQty]

This expression multiplies UnitPrice times UnitPriceDiscountPrc times OrderQty. Notice that when you type in a recognized function in the formula bar and enter a parenthesis "(", AutoComplete shows the function syntax. Notice that the formula bar shows the error "Column 'OrderQty' cannot be found or may be used in this expression". In addition, the LineTotal column shows "Error" in every cell (see **Figure 9.8**).

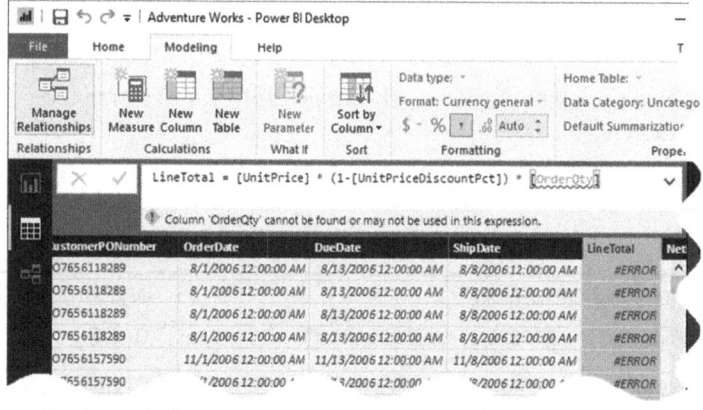

Figure 9.8 The formula bar displays an error when the DAX formula contains an invalid column reference.

3. In the formula bar, replace the OrderQty reference with OrderQuantity as follows:

LineTotal = [UnitPrice] * (1-[UnitPriceDiscountPct]) * **[OrderQuantity]**

4. Press Enter. Now, the column should work as expected.

9.2.2 Creating Advanced Calculated Columns

DAX supports formulas that allow you to create more advanced calculated columns. For example, you can use the RELATED function to look up a value from a related table. Another popular function is the SUMX function, with which you can sum values from a related table.

Implementing a lookup column

Suppose you want to calculate the net profit for each row in the ResellerSales table. For the purposes of this exercise, you'd calculate the line item net profit by subtracting the product cost from the line item total. As a first step, you need to look up the product cost in the Product table.

1. In the Fields pane, add a new NetProfit calculated column to the ResellerSales table that uses the following expression:

NetProfit = RELATED(Product[StandardCost])

This expression uses the RELATED function to look up the value of the StandardCost column in the Product table. Since a calculated column inherits the current row context, this expression is evaluated for each row. Specifically, for each row DAX gets the ProductKey value, navigates the ResellerSales[ProductKey] ⇨ Product[ProductKey] relationship, and then retrieves the standard cost for that product from the Product[StandardCost] column.

2. To calculate the net profit as a variance from the line total and the product's standard cost, change the expression as follows:

NetProfit = [LineTotal] - RELATED(Product[StandardCost])

Note that when the line item's product cost exceeds the line total, the result is a negative value.

Aggregating values

You can use the SUMX function to aggregate related rows from another table. Suppose you need a calculated column in the Product table that returns the reseller sales for each product:

1. Add a new ResellerSales calculated column to the Product table with the following expression:

ResellerSales = SUMX(RELATEDTABLE(ResellerSales), ResellerSales[SalesAmount])

The RELATEDTABLE function follows a relationship in either direction (many-to-one or one-to-many) and returns a table containing all the rows that are related to the current row from the specified table. In this case, this function returns a table with all the rows from the ResellerSales table that are related to the current row in the Product table. Then, the SUMX function sums the SalesAmount column.

2. Note that the formula returns a blank value for some products because these products don't have any reseller sales.

Ranking values

Suppose you want to rank each customer based on the customer's overall sales. The RANKX function can help you implement this requirement:

1. In the Fields pane, right-click the Customer table and click New Column.

2. In the formula bar, enter the following formula:

SalesRank = RANKX(Customer, SUMX(RELATEDTABLE(InternetSales), [SalesAmount]),,,Dense)

This function uses the RANKX function to calculate the rank of each customer, based on the customer's overall sales recorded in the InternetSales table. Similar to the previous example, the SUMX function is used to aggregate the [SalesAmount] column in the InternetSales table. The Dense argument is used to avoid skipping numbers for tied ranks (ranks with the same value).

9.3 Implementing Measures

Measures are typically used to aggregate values. Unlike calculated columns whose expressions are evaluated at design time for each row in the table, measures are evaluated at run time for each cell on the report. DAX applies the row, column, and filter selections when it calculates the formula. DAX supports implicit and explicit measures. An implicit measure is a regular column that's added to the Value area of the Visualizations pane. An explicit measure has a custom DAX formula. For more information about the differences between implicit and explicit measures, see Table 9.1 again.

9.3.1 Implementing Implicit Measures

In this exercise, you'll work with implicit measures. This will help you understand how implicit measures aggregate and how you can control their default aggregation behavior.

Changing the default aggregation behavior
I explained before that by default, Power BI Desktop aggregates implicit measures using the SUM function for numeric columns and the COUNT function for text-based columns. When you add a column to the Value area, Power BI Desktop automatically creates an implicit measure and aggregates it based on the column type. For numeric columns Power BI Desktop uses the DAX SUM aggregation function. If the column date type is Text, Power BI Desktop uses COUNT. Sometimes, you might need to overwrite the default aggregation behavior. For example, the CalendarYear column in the Date table is a numeric column, but it doesn't make sense to sum it up on reports.

1. Make sure that the Data View is active. In the Fields pane, click the CalendarYear column in the Date table. This shows the Date table in the Data View and selects the CalendarYear column.

2. In the ribbon's Modeling tab, expand the Default Summarization drop-down and change it to "Do Not Summarize". As a result, the next time you use CalendarYear on a report, it won't get summarized.

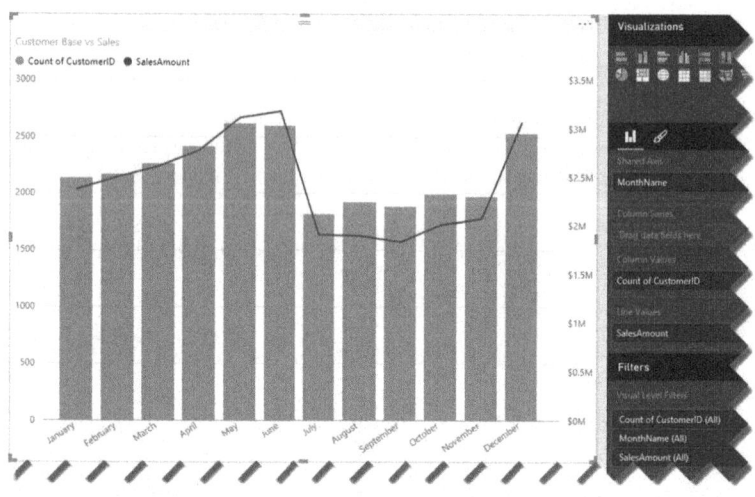

Figure 9.9 Implemented as a combo chart, this visualization shows the correlation between count of customers and sales.

Working with implicit measures
Suppose need to check if there's any seasonality impact to your business. Are some months slower than others? If sales decrease, do fewer customers purchase products? To answer these questions, you'll create the report shown in **Figure 9.9**. Using the Line and Clustered Column Chart visualization, this report

shows the count of customers as a column chart and the sales as a line chart that's plotted on the secondary axis. You'll analyze these two measures by month.

Let's start with visualizing the count of customers who have purchased products by month. Traditionally, you'd add some customer identifier to the fact table and you'd use a Distinct Count aggregation function to only count unique customers. But the InternetSales table doesn't have a CustomerID column, and your chances to get IT to add it to the data warehouse are probably slim. Can you count on the CustomerID column in the Customer table?

 NOTE Why not count on the CustomerKey column in InternetSales? This will work if the Customer table handles Type 1 changes only. A Type 1 change results in an in-place change. When a change to a customer is detected, the row is simply overwritten. However, chances are that business requirements necessitate Type 2 changes as well, where a new row is created when an important change occurs, such as when the customer changes a state. Therefore, counting on CustomerKey (called a surrogate key in dimensional modeling) is often a bad idea because it might lead to overstated results. Instead, you'd want to do a distinct count on a customer identifier that is not system generated, such as the customer's account number.

1. Switch to the Report View. From the Fields pane, drag the CustomerID column from the Customer table, and then drop it in an empty area in the report canvas.

2. Power BI Desktop defaults to a table visualization that shows all customer identifiers. Switch the visualization type to "Line and Clustered Column Chart".

3. In the Visualizations pane, drag CustomerID from the Shared Axis area to the Column Values area.

4. Expand the dropdown in the "Count of CustomerID" field. Note that it uses the Count aggregation function, as shown in **Figure 9.10**.

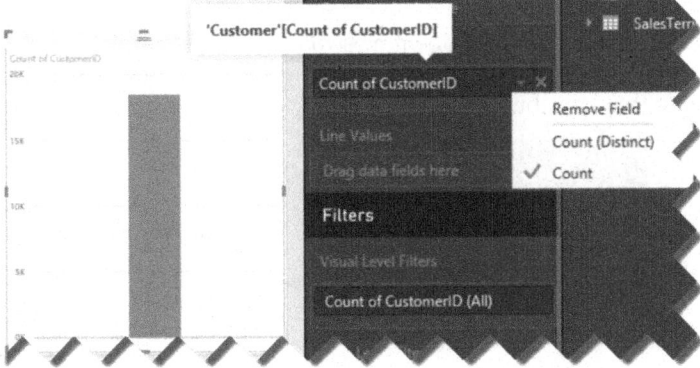

Figure 9.10   Text-based implicit measures use the Count function by default.

5. A product can be sold more than once within a given time period. If you simply count on CustomerID, you might get an inflated count. Instead, you want to count customers uniquely. Change the aggregation function of "Count of CustomerID" to Count (Distinct).

6. (Optional) Use the ribbon's Modeling tab to change the CustomerID default summarization to Count (Distinct) so you don't have to overwrite the aggregation function every time this field is used on a report.

7. With the new visualization selected, check the MonthName column of the Date table in the Fields pane to add it to the Shared Axis area of the Visualizations pane.

At this point, the results might be incorrect. Specifically, the count of customers might not change across months. The issue is that the aggregation happens over the InternetSales fact table via the Date ⇔ InternetSales ⇨ Customer path (notice that the relationship direction changes). Furthermore, the cardinality of the Date and Customer tables is Many-to-Many (there could be many customers who purchased something on the same date, and a repeating customer could buy multiple times). So, in case you skipped the change in the previous chapter (the binning example), make sure that the InternetSales ⇨ Customer relationship is bidirectional in the next step.

8. Switch to the Relationships View. Double-click the InternetSales ⇨ Customer relationship. In the Advanced Options properties of the relationship, change the cross filter direction to Both.

9. Switch to the Report View. Note that now the results vary by month.

10. Drag the SalesAmount field from the InternetSales table to the Line Values area of the Visualizations pane.

Note that because SalesAmount is numeric, Power BI Desktop defaults to the SUM aggregation function. Note also that indeed, seasonality affects sales. Specifically, the customer base decreases during the summer. And as the number of customers decreases, so do sales.

9.3.2 Implementing Quick Measures

As you've started to realize, DAX is a very powerful programming language. The only issue is that there is a learning curve involved. At the same time, there are frequently used measures that shouldn't require extensive knowledge of DAX. This is where "showing values as" and quick measures could help.

Showing value as
A common requirement is to show a value as a percent of total. Fortunately, there is a quick and easy way to meet this requirement.

1. Create a new Table visualization that has SalesTerritoryCountry (SalesTerritory table) and SalesAmount (ResellerSales table) fields in the Values area. Add the SalesAmount field one more time to the Values area.

2. In the Values area of the Visualizations pane, expand the drop-down next to the second SalesAmount field and choose "Show value as". Select "Percent of column total". Compare your results with **Figure 9.11**. Notice that the "%CT SalesAmount" now shows the contribution of each country to the column total.

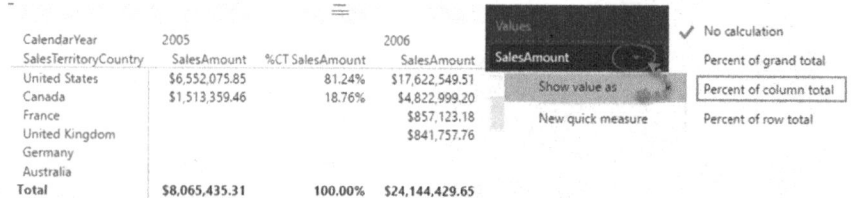

Figure 9.11 The %CT SalesAmount field shows each value as a percent of the column total.

3. (Optional) In the Visualizations pane (Fields tab), double-click the "%CT Sales Amount" field and rename it to *% of Total Sales*.

"Show value as" changes an existing measure in place to show its results as a percentage of a column, row, or grand total. It doesn't create a new measure. Power BI implements this feature internally so don't try to find or change the DAX formula. If you require more control, I'll walk you through implementing an explicit measure in the next section that does the same thing but this time with a DAX formula.

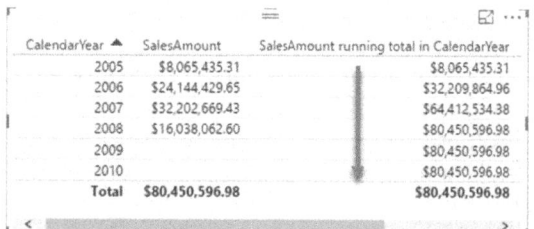

Figure 9.12 The second measure accumulates sales over years and it's produced by the "Running total" quick measure.

Creating quick measures

Before further honing your DAX skills, let's look at another feature that may help you avoid, or at least help you learn DAX. Quick measures are prepackaged formulas for common analytical requirements, such as time calculations, aggregates, and totals. Unlike "show value as", quick measures are implemented as DAX explicit measures, so you can see and change the quick measure formula. Suppose you want to implement a running sales total across years (see **Figure 9.12**).

1. Create a new Table visualization that has CalendarYear (Date table) and SalesAmount (ResellerSales table) fields in the Values area.

2. Right-click the ResellerSales table and click "New quick measure". Alternatively, you expand the drop-down next to the SalesField in the Values area and then click "New Quick Measure".

3. In the "Quick measures" window, expand the Calculation drop-down. Observe that Power BI supports various measure types organized in categories. Select the "Running total" measure under the Totals category.

4. Drag the SalesAmount field from the ResellerSales table to the "Base value" area. Drag the CalendarYear field from the Date table to the Field area. Click OK.

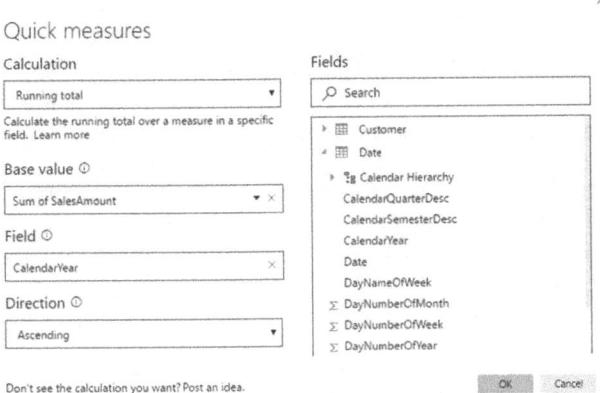

Figure 9.13 Power BI supports various quick measures to meet common analytical requirements.

5. Power BI adds a new "SalesAmount running total in CalendarYear" field to the ResellerSales table in the Fields pane. Click this field. Notice that the formula bar shows the DAX formula behind the measure.

Once you create the quick measure, it becomes just like any explicit DAX measure. You can rename it or use it on your reports. However, you can't go back to the "Quick measures" dialog. To customize the measure, you have make changes directly to the formula, so you still need to know some DAX.

 NOTE Can't get quick measures for time calculations, such as YTD, QTD, and others, to work? As they stand, they rely on auto-generated (in-line) date hierarchies that I introduced in the previous chapter. For more detail about this limitation, read my "Understanding Dates in Power BI Quick Measures" blog at http://prologika.com/understanding-dates-in-power-bi-quick-measures/. Fortunately, as you'll see next, implementing your own time calculations is not that difficult.

9.3.3 Implementing Explicit Measures

Explicit measures are more flexible than implicit measures because you can use custom DAX formulas. Like implicit measures, explicit measures are typically used to aggregate data and are usually placed in the Value area in the Visualizations pane.

TIP DAX explicit measures can get complex and it might be preferable to test nested formulas step by step. To make this process easier, you can test measures outside Power BI Desktop by using DAX Studio. DAX Studio (http://daxstudio.codeplex.com) is a community-driven project to help you write and test DAX queries connected to Excel Power Pivot models, Tabular models, and Power BI Desktop models. DAX Studio features syntax highlighting, integrated tracing support, and exploring the model metadata with Dynamic Management Views (DMVs). If you're not familiar with DMVs, you can use them to document your models, such as to get a list of all the measures and their formulas.

Implementing a basic explicit measure

A common requirement is implementing a measure that filters results. For example, you might need a measure that shows the reseller sales for a specific product category, such as Bikes. Let's implement a BikeResellerSales measure that does just that.

1. In Fields pane (Data View or Report View), right-click the ResellerSales table, and click New Measure.

2. In the formula bar, enter the following formula and press Enter:

BikeResellerSales = CALCULATE(SUM(ResellerSales[SalesAmount]), 'Product'[ProductCategory]="Bikes")

Power BI Desktop adds the measure to the ResellerSales table in the Fields pane. The measure has a special calculator icon in front of it.

 TIP Added a measure to a wrong table? Instead of recreating the measure in the correct table, you can simply change its home table. To do this, click the measure in the Fields pane to select it. Then, in the ribbon's Modeling tab, use the Home Table dropdown (Properties group) to change the table. Because measures are dynamic, they can be anchored to any table.

3. (Optional) Add a map visualization to show the BikeResellerSales measure (see **Figure 9.14**). Add both SalesTerritoryCountry and SalesTerritoryRegion fields from the SalesTerritory table to the Location area of the Visualizations pane. This enables the drill down buttons on the map and allows you to drill down sales from country to region!

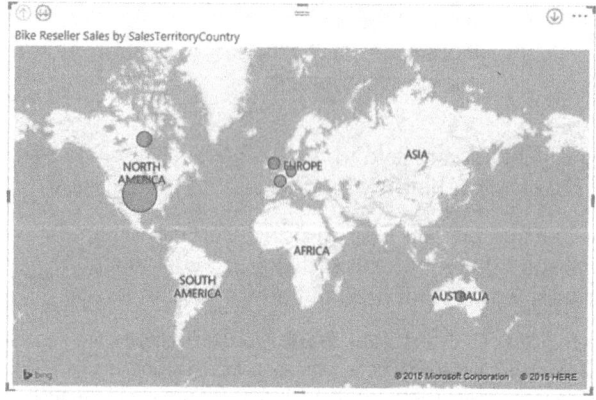

Figure 9.14 This map visualization shows the "Sum of Bike Reseller Sales" measure.

Implementing a percent of total measure

Suppose you need a measure for calculating a ratio of current sales compared to overall sales across countries. Previously, you've used the "show value as" feature. As easy as it was, this feature doesn't give you control over the calculation formula. Next, I'll show you how to implement an explicit measure that accomplishes the same (see **Figure 9.15**).

SalesTerritoryCountry	2005	2006	2007	2008	Total
Australia			2.63 %	4.66 %	1.98 %
Canada	18.76 %	19.98 %	17.55 %	14.90 %	17.87 %
France		3.55 %	7.37 %	8.58 %	5.73 %
Germany			3.41 %	5.52 %	2.47 %
United Kingdom		3.49 %	6.71 %	7.96 %	5.32 %
United States	81.24 %	72.99 %	62.33 %	58.37 %	66.63 %
Total	100.00 %	100.00 %	100.00 %	100.00 %	100.00 %

Figure 9.15 The PercentOfTotal measure shows the contribution of the country sales to the overall sales.

1. Another way to create a measure is to use the New Measure button. Make sure that the Data View is selected. In the Fields pane, click the ResellerSales table.

2. Click the New Measure button in the Modeling ribbon.

3. In the Formula field, enter the following formula:

PercentOfTotal = DIVIDE (SUM(ResellerSales[SalesAmount]), CALCULATE (SUM(ResellerSales[SalesAmount]), ALL(SalesTerritory)))

To avoid division by zero, the expression uses the DAX DIVIDE function, which performs a safe divide and returns a blank value when the denominator is zero. The SUM function sums the SalesAmount column for the current country. The denominator uses the CALCULATE and ALL functions to ignore the current context so that the expression calculates the overall sales across *all* the sales territories.

4. Click the Check Formula button to verify the formula syntax. You shouldn't see any errors. Press Enter.

5. In the Formatting section of the ribbon's Modeling tab, change the Format property to Percentage, with two decimal places.

6. (Optional). In the Report View, add a matrix visualization that uses the new measure (see **Figure 9.15** again). Add the SalesTerritoryCountry to the Rows area and CalendarYear to the Columns area to create a crosstab layout.

Implementing a YTD calculation

DAX supports many time intelligence functions for implementing common date calculations, such as YTD, QTD, and so on. These functions require a column of the Date data type in the Date table. The Date table in the Adventure Works model includes a Date column that meets this requirement. Also remember that for the DAX time calculations to work, relationships to the Date table must use the Date column and not the DateKey column. Let's implement an explicit measure that returns year-to-date (YTD) sales:

1. In the Fields pane, right-click the ResellerSales table, and then click New Measure.

2. In the formula bar, enter the following formula:

SalesAmountYTD =TOTALYTD(Sum(ResellerSales[SalesAmount]), 'Date'[Date])

This expression uses the TOTALYTD function to calculate the SalesAmount aggregated value from the beginning of the year to date. Note that the second argument must reference the column of the Date data type in the date table. It also takes additional arguments, such as to specify the end date of a fiscal year.

3. To test the SalesAmountYTD measure, create the matrix visualization shown in **Figure 9.16**. Add CalendarYear and MonthName fields from the Date table in the Rows area and SalesAmount, and SalesAmountYTD fields in the Values area.

If the SalesAmountYTD measure works correctly, its results should be running totals within a year. For example, the SalesAmountYTD value for 2005 ($8,065,435) is calculated by summing the sales of all the previous months since the beginning of the year 2005. Notice also that the formula works as of *any* date and the date fields don't have to be added to the visual. For example, if the report has a slicer, the user can pick a date, and as any other measure, SalesAmountYTD will recalculate as of that date. This brings a tremendous flexibility to reporting and avoids saving the results of time calculations in the database!

CalendarYear	MonthName	SalesAmount	SalesAmountYTD
2005	July	$489,328.58	$489,328.5787
	August	$1,538,408.31	$2,027,736.8909
	September	$1,165,897.08	$3,193,633.9687
	October	$844,721.00	$4,038,354.965
	November	$2,324,135.80	$6,362,490.7625
	December	$1,702,944.54	$8,065,435.3053
	Total	**$8,065,435.31**	**$8,065,435.3053**
2006	January	$713,116.69	$713,116.6943
	February	$1,900,788.93	$2,613,905.6247
	March	1,455 0.41	$4,0 186.0

Figure 9.16 The SalesAmountYTD measure calculates the year-to-date sales as of any date.

9.4 Implementing Advanced Relationships

Besides regular table relationships where a lookup table joins the fact table directly, you might need to model more advanced relationships, including role-playing, parent-child, and many-to-many relationships. Next, I'll show you how to meet such requirements with DAX.

9.4.1 Implementing Role-Playing Relationships

In Chapter 6, I explained that a lookup table can be joined multiple times to a fact table. The dimensional modeling terminology refers to such a lookup table as a role-playing dimension. For example, in the Adventure Works model, both the InternetSales and ResellerSales tables have three date-related columns: OrderDate, ShipDate, and DueDate. However, you only created relationships from these tables to the OrderDate column. As a result, when you analyze sales by date, DAX follows the InternetSales[OrderDate] ⇨ Date[Date] and ResellerSales[OrderDate] ⇨ Date[Date] paths.

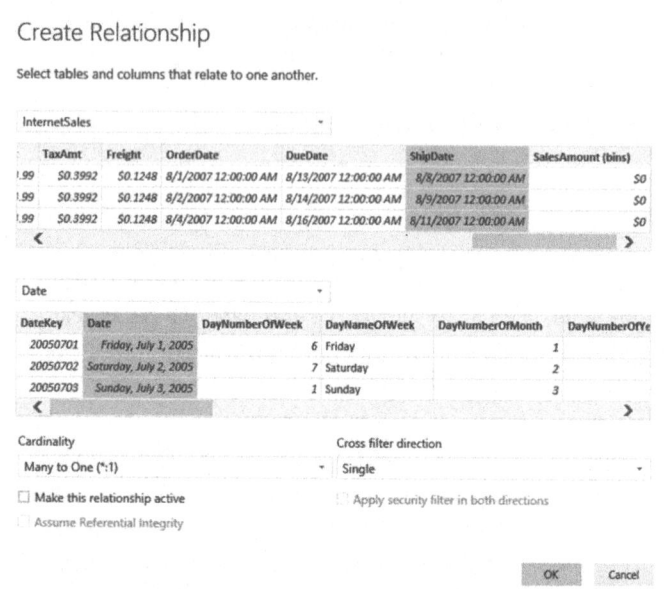

Figure 9.17 The InternetSales[ShipDate] ⇨ Date[Date] relationship will be created as inactive because there is already a relationship between these two tables.

Creating inactive relationships

Suppose that you'd like to analyze InternetSales by the date the product was shipped (ShipDate):

1. Click the Manage Relationships button. In the Manage Relationships window, click New.

2. Create the InternetSales[ShipDate] ⇨ Date[Date] relationship, as shown in **Figure 9.17**. Note that this relationship will be created as inactive because Power BI Desktop will discover that there's already an active relationship (InternetSales[OrderDate] ⇨ Date[Date]) between the two tables.

3. Click OK and then click close.

4. In the Relationships View, confirm that there's a dotted line between the InternetSales and Date tables, which signifies an inactive relationship.

Navigating relationships in DAX

Let's say that you want to compare the ordered sales amount and shipped sales amount side by side, such as to calculate a variance. To address this requirement, you can implement measures that use DAX formulas to navigate inactive relationships. Follow these steps to implement a ShipSalesAmount measure in the InternetSales table:

1. Switch to the Data View. In the Fields pane, right-click InternetSales, and then click New Measure.

2. In the formula bar, enter the following expression:

```
ShipSalesAmount = CALCULATE(SUM([SalesAmount]), USERELATIONSHIP(InternetSales[ShipDate], 'Date'[Date]))
```

The formula uses the USERELATIONSHIP function to navigate the inactive relationship between the ShipDate column in the InternetSales table and the Date column in the Date table.

3. (Optional) Add a Table visualization with the CalendarYear (Date table), SalesAmount (InternetSales table) and ShipSalesAmount (InternetSales table) fields in the Values area. Notice that the ShipSalesAmount value is different than the SalesAmount value. That's because the ShipSalesAmount measure is aggregated using the inactive relationship on ShipDate instead of OrderDate.

9.4.2 Implementing Parent-Child Relationships

A parent-child relationship is a hierarchical relationship formed between two entities. Common examples of parent-child relationships include an employee hierarchy, where a manager has subordinates who in turn have subordinates, and an organizational hierarchy, where a company has offices and each office has branches. DAX includes functions that are specifically designed to handle parent-child relationships.

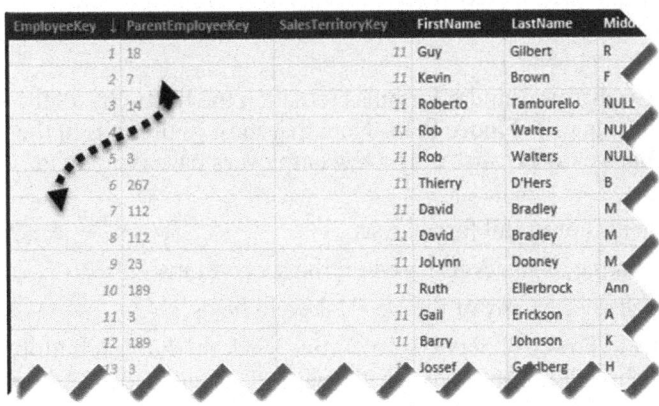

Figure 9.18 The ParentEmployeeKey column contains the identifier for the employee's manager.

Understanding parent-child relationships

The EmployeeKey and ParentEmployeeKey columns in the Employee table have a parent-child relationship, as shown in **Figure 9.18**. Specifically, the ParentEmployeeKey column points to the EmployeeKey column for the employee's manager. For example, Kevin Brown (EmployeeKey = 2) has David Bradley (EmployeeKey=7) as a manager, who in turn reports to Ken Sánchez (EmpoyeeKey=112). (Ken is not shown in the screenshot.) Ken Sánchez's ParentEmployeeKey is blank, which means that he's the top manager. Parent-child hierarchies might have an arbitrary number of levels. Such hierarchies are called *unbalanced* hierarchies.

Implementing a parent-child relationship

Next, you'll use DAX functions to flatten the parent-child relationship before you can create a hierarchy to drill down the organizational chart:

1. Start by adding a Path calculated column to the Employee table that constructs the parent-child path for each employee. For the Path calculated column, use the following formula:

Path = PATH([EmployeeKey], [ParentEmployeeKey])

> **NOTE** At this point, you might get an error "The columns specified in the PATH function must be from the same table, have the same data type, and that type must be Integer or Text". The issue is that the ParentEmployeeKey column has a Text data type. This might be caused by a literal text value "NULL" for Ken Sánchez's while it should be a blank (null) value. To fix this, open the Query Editor (right-click the Employee table and click Query Editor), right-click the ParentEmployeeKey column, and then click Replace Values. In the Replace Value dialog, replace NULL with blank. Then, in the Query Editor (Home ribbon tab), change the column type to Whole Number and click the "Close & Apply" button.

The formula uses the PATH DAX function, which returns a delimited list of IDs (using a vertical pipe as the delimiter) starting with the top (root) of a parent-child hierarchy and ending with the current employee identifier. For example, the path for Kevin Brown is 112|7|2. The rightmost part is the ID of the employee on that row and each segment to the right follows the organizational path.

The next step is to flatten the parent-child hierarchy by adding a column for each level. This means that you need to know beforehand the maximum number of levels that the employee hierarchy might have. To be on the safe side, add one or two more levels to accommodate future growth.

2. Add a Level1 calculated column that has the following formula:

Level1 = LOOKUPVALUE(Employee[FullName], Employee[EmployeeKey], VALUE(PATHITEM([Path],1)))

This formula uses the PATHITEM function to parse the Path calculated column and return the first identifier, such as 112 in the case of Kevin Brown. Then, it uses the LOOKUPVALUE function to return the full name of the corresponding employee, which in this case is Ken Sánchez. The VALUE function casts the text result from the PATHITEM function to Integer so that the LOOKUPVALUE function compares the same data types.

3. Add five more calculated columns for Levels 2-6 that use similar formulas to flatten the hierarchy all the way down to the lowest level. Compare your results with **Figure 9.19**. Note that most of the cells in the Level 5 and Level 6 columns are empty, and that's okay because only a few employees have more than four indirect managers.

4. Hide the Path column in the Employee table as it's not useful for analysis.

5. (Optional) Create an Employees hierarchy consisting of six levels based on the six columns.

6. (Optional) Create a table visualization to analyze sales by any of the Level1-Level6 fields.

7. (Optional) Deploy the Adventure Works model to Power BI Service. To do this, click the Publish button in the ribbon's Home tab, or use the File ⇨ Publish ⇨ "Publish to Power BI" menu. This will add an Adventure Works dataset and Adventure Works report to the navigation bar in the Power BI portal. Once the

model is published, go to Power BI Service (powerbi.com) and test the visualizations you've created. Use your knowledge from Part 1 of this book to explore and visualize the Adventure Works dataset.

```
Level6 = LOOKUPVALUE(Employee[FullName],Employee[EmployeeKey],VALUE(PATHITEM([Path],6)))
```

ne	FullNameFromQuery	Path	Level1	Level2	Level3	Level4	Level5	Level6
Flood	Kathie Flood	112|23|201|13	Ken Sánchez	Peter Krebs	Lori Kane	Kathie Flood		
McAskill	Katie McAskill-White	112|23|186	Ken Sánchez	Peter Krebs	Katie McAskill			
yer	Ken Myer	112|23|214|19	Ken Sánchez	Peter Krebs	Brenda Díaz	Ken Myer		
nchez	Ken Sánchez	112	Ken Sánchez					
l Keil	Kendall Keil	112|23|16|31	Ken Sánchez	Peter Krebs	Taylor Maxwe	Kendall Keil		
iu	Kevin Liu	112|23|214|58	Ken Sánchez	Peter Krebs	Brenda Díaz	Kevin Liu		
omer	Kevin Homer	112|23|27|232	Ken Sánchez	Peter Krebs	Zheng Mu	Kevin Homer		
rown	Kevin Brown	112|7|2	Ken Sánchez	David Bradley	Kevin Brown			
ercrom	Kim Abercrombie	112|23|18|239	Ken Sánchez	Peter Krebs	Jo Brown	Kim Abercrom		
lls	Kim Ralls	112|23|87|74	Ken Sánchez	Peter Krebs	Pilar Ackerma	Kim Ralls		
ly Zimm	Kimberly Zimmerman	112|23|66|238	Ken Sánchez	Peter Krebs	Cristian Petcu	Kimberly Zimm		

Figure 9.19   Use the PATHITEM function to flatten the parent-child hierarchy.

9.4.3 Implementing Many-to-Many Relationships

Typically, a row in a lookup table relates to one or more rows in a fact table. For example, a given customer has one or more orders. This is an example of a one-to-many relationship that most of our tables have used so far. Sometimes, you might run into a scenario where two tables have a logical many-to-many relationship. As you've seen in the case of the Customer distinct count example, handling many-to-many is easy, thanks to the DAX bi-directional relationships. But what if you need to report closing balances (common for financial reporting)?

Understanding many-to-many relationships

The M2M.pbix sample in the \Source\ch09 folder demonstrates a popular many-to-many scenario that you might encounter if you model joint bank accounts. Open it in another Power BI Desktop and examine its Relationship View. It consists of five tables, as shown in **Figure 9.20**. The Customer table stores the bank's customers. The Account table stores the customers' accounts. A customer might have multiple bank accounts, and a single account might be owned by two or more customers, such as a savings account.

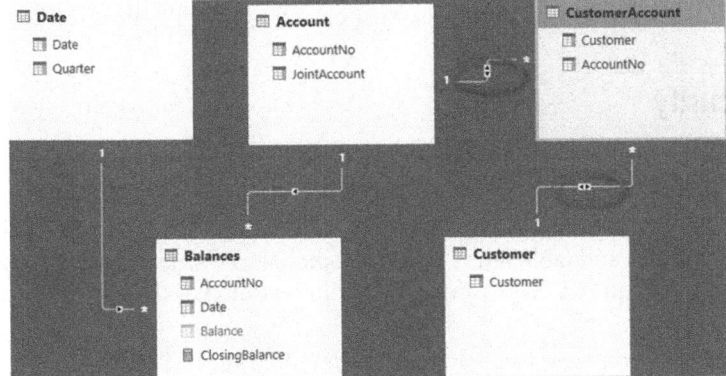

Figure 9.20   The M2M model demonstrates joint bank accounts.

The CustomerAccount table is a bridge table that indicates which accounts are owned by which customer. The Balances table records the account balances over time. Note that the relationships CustomerAccount[AccountNo] ⇨ Account[AccountNo] and CustomerAccount[Customer] ⇨ Customer[Customer] are bi-directional.

Implementing closing balances

If the Balance measure is fully additive (can be summed across all lookup tables that are related to the Balances table), then you're done. However, semi-additive measures, such as account balances and inventory quantities, are trickier because they can be summed across all the tables except for the Date table. To understand this, look at the report shown in **Figure 9.21**.

Quarter	Q1 2011				Q2 2011			Total
Customer	1/1/2011	2/1/2011	3/1/2011	Total	4/1/2011	5/1/2011	Total	
Alice	100	200	300	300				300
Bob	600	700	300	300				300
John	100	200		200				200
Sam		100	100	100	200	50	50	50
Total	700	1000	400	400	200	50	50	50

Figure 9.21 This report shows closing balances per quarter.

If you create a report that simply aggregates the Balance measure (hidden in Report View), you'll find that the report produces wrong results. Specifically, the grand totals at the customer or account levels are correct, but the rest of the results are incorrect. Instead of using the Balance column, I added a ClosingBalance explicit measure to the Balances table that aggregates his account balance correctly. The measure uses the following formula:

ClosingBalance = CALCULATE(SUM(Balances[Balance]), LASTNONBLANK('Date'[Date], CALCULATE(SUM(Balances[Balance]))))

This formula uses the DAX LASTNONBLANK function to find the last date with a recorded balance. This function travels back in time, to find the first non-blank date within a given time period. For John and Q1 2011, that date is 2/1/2011 when John's balance was 200. This becomes the first quarter balance for John, as you can see in the Matrix visualization. He didn't have an account balance for Q2 (perhaps, his account was closed) so the Q2 balance is empty. His overall balance matches the Q1 balance of 200.

9.5   Implementing Data Security

Do you have a requirement to allow certain end users to see only a subset of data that they're authorized to access? For example, as a model author Martin can see all the data he imported. However, when he deploys the model to Power BI Service, he wants Elena to see only sales for a specific geography. This is where the Power BI data security (also known as row-level security or RLS) can help. Data security is a Power BI Pro feature so users who access published secured models must have Power BI Pro licenses.

9.5.1   Understanding Data Security

Data security is supported for models that import data and that connect live to data, except when connecting live to Analysis Services, which has its own security model. At a high level, implementing data security is a two-step process:

- Modeling step – This involves defining roles and table filters inside the model to restrict access to data. Because more involved security scenarios require DAX knowledge for filters, I discuss data security in this chapter.

- Operational step – Once roles are defined, you need to deploy the model to Power BI Service to assign members to roles. Configuring membership is the operational aspect of RLS that needs to be done in Power BI Service.

It's important to understand that data security is only enforced in Power BI Service, that is when the model is deployed and shared with other users who have view-only rights (they don't have Admin or Edit Content permissions to a workspace) to shared content. Such users won't be able to access any data unless they are assigned to a role. However, if you email the Power BI Desktop file to another user and he opens it in Power BI Desktop, data security is *not* enforced, and the user can see all the data.

Understanding roles

A role allows you to grant other users restricted access to data in a secured model. **Figure 9.22** is meant to help you visualize a role.

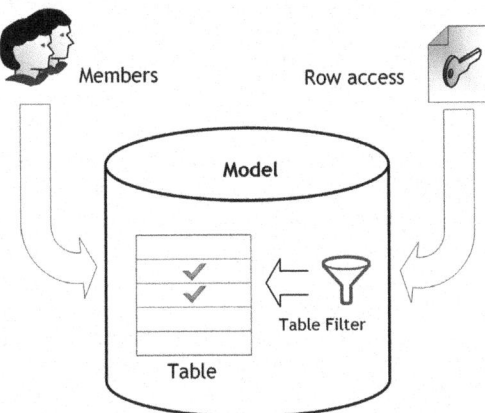

Figure 9.22 A role grants its members permissions to a table, and it optionally restricts access to table rows.

In a nutshell, a role gives its members permissions to view the model data. To create a new role, click the Manage Roles button in the ribbon's Modeling tab. Then click the Create button in the "Manage roles" window and name the role. As I mentioned, after you deploy the model to Power BI Service, you must assign members to the role. You can type in email addresses of individual users, security groups, and workspace groups.

What happens if a user with view-only rights to shared content in Power BI Service attempts to view a report in a secured model, and the user is not assigned to a role, either individually or via a group membership? When they view a report, all report visualizations show errors (see **Figure 9.23**).

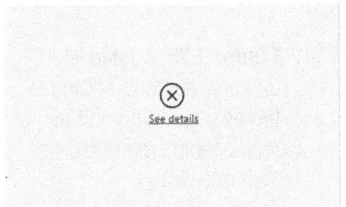

Figure 9.23 If a user with view-only rights is not added to a role when data security is enabled, report visualizations show errors with details "Couldn't load the data for this visual".

Understanding table filters

By default, a role can access all the data in all tables in the model. However, the whole purpose of implementing data security is to limit access to a subset of data, such as to allow Maya to see only sales for the United States. This is achieved by specifying one or more table filters. As its name suggests, a table filter defines a filter expression that evaluates which table rows the role is allowed to see. To set up a row filter in Role Manager, enter a DAX formula next to the table name. The DAX formula must evaluate to a Boolean condition that returns TRUE or FALSE. For example, when the user connects to the published model and the user is a member of the role, Power BI applies the row filter expression to each row in the SalesTerritory table. If the row meets the criteria, the role is authorized to see that row.

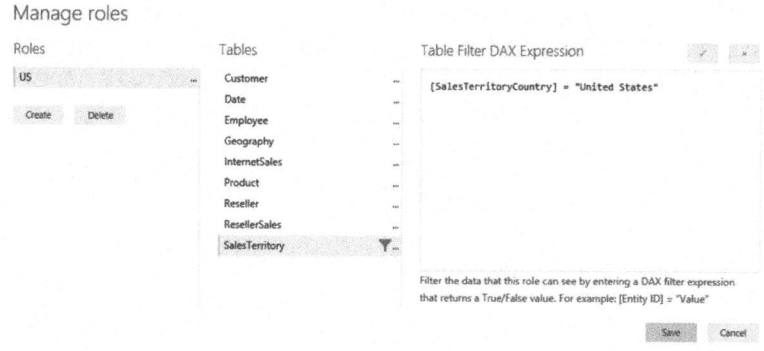

Figure 9.24 This table filter grants the US role access to rows in the SalesTerritory table where SalesTerritoryCountry is United States.

Roles are additive. If a user belongs to multiple roles, the user will get the superset of all the role permissions. For example, suppose Maya is a member of both the Sales Representative and Marketing roles. The Sales Representative role grants her rights to United States, while the Marketing role grants her access to all countries. Because roles are additive, Maya can see data for all countries.

 TIP As it stands, Power BI doesn't support object security to hide entire tables. Even if the table filter qualifies no rows, the table will show in the model metadata. The simplest way to disallow a role from viewing any rows in a table is to set up a table filter with a FALSE() expression. If no table filter is applied to a table, TRUE() is assumed and the user can see all of its data.

How table filters affect related tables

From an end-user perspective, rows the user isn't authorized to view and their related data in tables on the many side of the relationship simply don't exist in the model. Imagine that a global WHERE clause is applied to the model that selects only the data that's related to the allowed rows of all the secured tables.

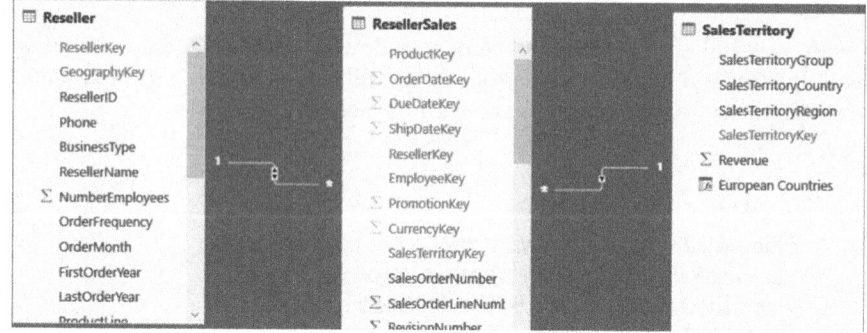

Figure 9.25 A table filter can propagate to related tables depending on the relationship type and cross filter direction.

Given the model shown in **Figure 9.25**, the user can't see any other sales territories in the SalesTerritory table except United States. Moreover, because of the SalesTerritory ⇨ ResellerSales one-to-many relationship, the user can't see sales for these territories in the ResellerSales table or in any other tables that are directly or indirectly (via cascading relationships) related to the SalesTerritory table. In other words, Power BI propagates data security to related tables following the existing one-to-many relationships.

What about the Reseller table? Should the user see only Resellers with sales in the United States? The outcome depends on the relationship cross-filter direction. If it's Single (there is a single arrow pointing from Reseller to ResellerSales), the security filter is not propagated to the Reseller table and the user can see all resellers. To clarify, the user can see the list of all resellers but he can see only sales for the US resellers because sales come from the filtered ResellerSales table. However, if the cross filter direction is Both and the "Apply security filter in both directions" setting (see **Figure 8.16**) is checked, then the security filter propagates to the Reseller table and the user can see only resellers with sales in the United States.

 NOTE If you don't see the "Apply security filter in both directions" checkbox, the feature is probably still in preview. To enable it, check "Enable cross filtering in both directions for DirectQuery" in the File ⇨ Options and settings ⇨ Options menu ("Preview features" tab).

9.5.2 Implementing Basic Data Security

In the exercise that follows, you'll add a role that allows the user to view only the United States. Then, I'll show you how to test the role on the desktop and how to add members to the role after you deploy your model to Power BI Service.

Creating a role
Start by creating a new role in the Adventure Works model.

1. In the ribbon's Modeling tab, click the Manage Roles button.

2. In the Manage Roles window, click the Create button. Rename the new role to *US*.

3. Click the ellipsis button next to the SalesTerritory table, and then click "Add filter…" ⇨ [SalesTerritory-Country] to filter the values in this column.

4. Change the "Table Filter DAX Expression" content with the following formula (see again **Figure 9.24**):

[SalesTerritoryCountry] = "United States"

5. Click Save.

 TIP Consider adding an Open Access role that doesn't have any table filter. This role is for users who need full access to data. Recall that by default a role has unrestricted access unless you defined a table filter.

Testing data security
You don't have to deploy the model to Power BI Service to test the role. Power BI Desktop lets you do this conveniently on the desktop. Recall that you can add yourself to a role in Power BI Desktop (even if you were able to, you'll still gain unrestricted access as a model author). However, you can test the role as though you're a user who is a member of the role.

1. In the ribbon's Modeling tab, click the "View as Roles" button.

2. In the "View as roles" window, make sure that that US role is selected (see **Figure 9.26**). Click OK.

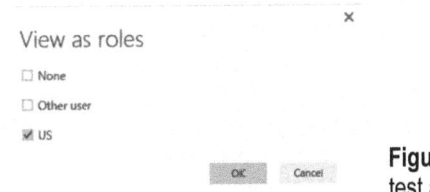

Figure 9.26 The "View as roles" lets you test a role inside Power BI Desktop.

3. You should see a status bar showing "Now viewing report as: US". Create a report that includes the SalesTerritoryCountry column from the SalesTerritory table, such as the one shown in **Figure 9.27**. The report should show only data for US.

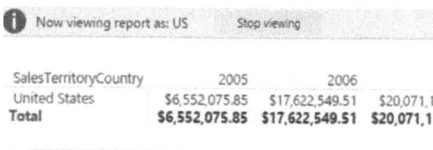

SalesTerritoryCountry	2005	2006	
United States	$6,552,075.85	$17,622,549.51	$20,071,1
Total	**$6,552,075.85**	**$17,622,549.51**	**$20,071,1**

Figure 9.27 The report shows only data for United States.

4. (Optional) Add a Table visualization showing the ResellerName column from the Reseller table. You should see all resellers. However, if you add a measure from the ResellerSales table, you should see only resellers with sales in the USA. If you want to prevent the role to see non-US resellers, change the cross filter direction of the ResellerSales[ResellerKey] ⇨ Reseller[ResellerKey] to Both.

Defining role membership

Now that the role is defined, it becomes a part of the model, but its setup is not complete yet. Next, you'll deploy the model to Power BI Service and add members to the role.

1. In the ribbon's Home tab, click Publish. If prompted, log in to Power BI and deploy the Adventure Works model to My Workspace.

2. Open your browser and navigate to Power BI Service (powerbi.com). Click My Workspace.

3. In the workspace content page, click the Datasets tab. Click the ellipsis button next to the Adventure Works dataset, and then click Security from the drop-down menu.

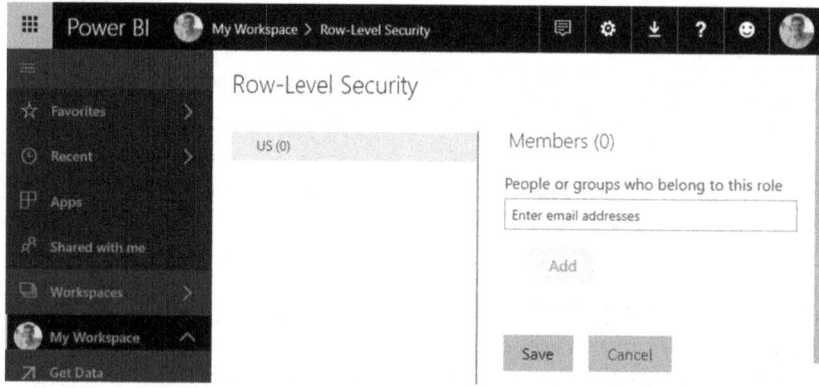

Figure 9.28 You set up the role membership in Power BI Service.

4. In the "Row-Level Security" window, add the emails of individuals or groups who you want to add to the role (**Figure 9.28**). Click Save.

5. (Optional) Create a dashboard that uses visualizations from the Adventure Works report, and share the dashboard with users who belong and don't belong to the role (you and the recipients must have Power BI Pro or Power BI Premium subscriptions). Ask them to view the dashboard and report their results.

6. (Optional) Republish the Adventure Works model. Power BI Desktop will ask you to replace the dataset. In Power BI Service, go to the Adventure Works dataset security settings and notice that the role membership is preserved. That's because the role membership is external to the Adventure Works model and re-publishing the file doesn't overwrite it. However, if you delete the dataset in Power BI Service, you'll lose its role membership.

 NOTE As a model author, you always have admin rights to model so don't be surprised that you see all the data irrespective of your role membership. If you publish the model to a workspace (workspaces are discussed in the next chapter), the workspace administrators and members who can edit content also gain unlimited access.

9.5.3 Implementing Dynamic Data Security

The row filter example securing on a territory that I've just shown you returns a fixed (static) set of allowed rows. This works well if you have a finite set of unique permissions. For example, if there are three regions, you can build three roles. Static filters are simple to implement and work well when the number of roles is relatively small. However, suppose you must restrict managers to view only the sales data of the employees that are reporting directly or indirectly to them. If static filters were the only option, you'd have no choice except to set up a database role for each manager. This might lead to a huge number of roles and maintenance issues. Therefore, Power BI supports dynamic data security.

Understanding dynamic data security

Dynamic security relies on the identity of the interactive user to filter data. For example, if Maya logs in to Power BI as maya@adventure-works.com, you can filter the Employee table to allow Maya to access herself and her subordinates. You need only a single role with the following table filter applied to the Employee table:

PATHCONTAINS(Employee[Path], LOOKUPVALUE(Employee[EmployeeKey], Employee[EmailAddress], USERPRINCIPALNAME()))

This expression uses the USERPRINCIPALNAME() DAX function (specifically added to support Power BI) which returns the user principal name (UPN) in both Power BI Service and Power BI. If you have set up dynamic security with Analysis Services Multidimensional or Tabular, you have probably used the USERNAME() function. However, this function returns the user domain login in Power BI Desktop (see **Figure 9.29**). You can use the WhoAmI.pbix Power BI Desktop file in the \Source\ch09 folder to verify the results.

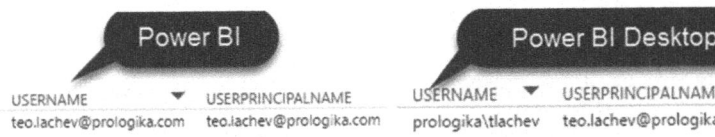

Figure 9.29 USERPRINCIPALNAME() and USERNAME() return different results on the desktop.

To avoid using an OR filter to support both Power BI and Power BI Desktop, use USERPRINCIPAL-NAME() but make sure that the EmailAddress column stores the user principal name (typically but not always UPN corresponds to the user's email address) and not the user's Windows login (domain\login). To explain the rest of the filter, the DAX expression uses the DAX LOOKUPVALUE function to retrieve the value of the EmployeeKey column that's matching the user's login. Then, it uses the PATHCONTAINS function to parse the Path column in the Employee table in order to check if the parent-child path includes the employee key. If this is the case, the user is authorized to see that employee and the employee's related data because the user is the employee's direct or indirect manager.

 NOTE If your computer is not joined to a domain, both USERPRINCIPALNAME() and USERNAME() would return your login (NetBIOS name) in the format MachineName\Login in Power BI Desktop. In this case, you'd have to use an OR filter so that you can test dynamic security in both Power BI Service and Power BI Desktop.

Setting up the test environment

Next, I'll walk you through the steps required to implement dynamic data security for the manager-subordinate scenario. Ideally, you would have two Power BI accounts to test dynamic security in Power BI. Since you're not on the adventure-works domain, start by making changes to the Employee table:

1. In the Adventure Works model, right-click the Employee table in the Fields pane, and then click Edit Query to open the Query Editor.

2. Find the row for Stephen Jiang (EmployeeKey = 272). Right-click the EmailAddress cell for that row and click Copy to copy his email (it should be stephen0@adventure-works.com). In the next step, you'll replace this email with your email address.

3. Right-click the EmailAddress column and then click "Replace Values...". In the Replace Values window, paste the copied email address in the "Value to Find" field. In the "Replace With" field, type in your email address (the one you use to log in to Power BI).

4. (Optional) Right-click the EmailAddress column and then click "Replace Values..." again. In the Replace Values window, enter *amy0@adventure-works.com* in the "Value to Find" field. In the "Replace With" field, type in the email address of someone else in your organization that has a Power BI Pro subscription.

5. In the ribbon's Home tab, click Close & Apply to reload the Employee table.

Creating a new role
Next, you'll create a new role that will filter the Employee table.

1. In the ribbon's Modeling tab, click Manage Roles.

2. In the "Manage roles" window create a new *Employee* role.

3. In the Table section, select the Employee table. Enter the following expression in the "Table Filter DAX Expression" field:

```
PATHCONTAINS(Employee[Path], LOOKUPVALUE(Employee[EmployeeKey], Employee[EmailAddress], USERPRINCIPALNAME()))
```

4. Click the checkmark button in the top right corner of the window to check the expression syntax. If there are no errors, click Save to create the role.

Testing the role
Now that the Employee role is in place, let's make sure it works as expected.

1. In the ribbon's Modeling tab, click "View As Roles".

2. In the "View as roles" window (**Figure 9.30**), check the Employee role to test it as though you're a member of the role.

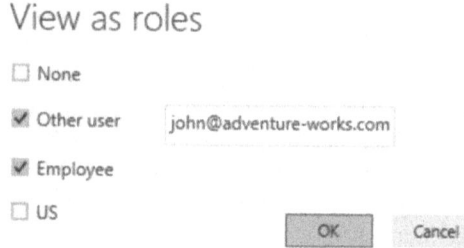

Figure 9.30 The "View as roles" window lets you test specific roles and impersonate users.

3. If you'd like to impersonate another user to test his permissions, check the "Other user" checkbox and type in the user's UPN. As a result, USERPRINCIPALNAME() will return whatever you typed in. Click OK.

	Level1	Level2	Level3	Level4	Level5	Level6
	Ken Sánchez	Brian Welcker	Stephen Jiang			
	Ken Sánchez	Brian Welcker	Stephen Jiang	David Campbell		
	Ken Sánchez	Brian Welcker	Stephen Jiang	Garrett Vargas		
	Ken Sánchez	Brian Welcker	Stephen Jiang	Jillian Carson		
	Ken Sánchez	Brian Welcker	Stephen Jiang	José Saraiva		
	Ken Sánchez	Brian Welcker	Stephen Jiang	Linda Mitchell		
	Ken Sánchez	Brian Welcker	Stephen Jiang	Michael Blythe		
	Ken Sánchez	Brian Welcker	Stephen Jiang	Pamela Ansman-Wolfe		
	Ken Sánchez	Brian Welcker	Stephen Jiang	Shu Ito		
	Ken Sánchez	Brian Welcker	Stephen Jiang	Tete Mensa-Annan		
	Ken Sánchez	Brian Welcker	Stephen Jiang	Tsvi Reiter		

Now viewing report as: Employee, teo.lachev@prologika.com   Stop viewing

Figure 9.31 The "View as roles" window lets you test specific roles and impersonate users.

4. (Optional) Create a Table report that uses the Employees hierarchy (or Level1-Level6 fields), as shown in **Figure 9.31**. Notice that the report lets you access Stephen Jiang and his direct or indirect subordinates.

9.5.4 Externalizing Security Policies

The final progression of data security is externalizing security policies in another table. Suppose that Adventure Works uses a master data management application, such as Master Data Services (MDS), to associate a sales representative with a set of resellers that she oversees. Your task is to enforce a security role that restricts the user to see only her resellers. This would require importing a table that contains the employee-reseller associations.

 REAL LIFE This approach builds upon the factless fact table implementation that I demonstrated in my "Protect UDM with Dimension Data Security, Part 2" article (http://bit.ly/YBcu1d). I've used this approach in real-life projects because of its simplicity, performance, and ability to reuse the security filters across other applications, such as across operational reports that source data directly from the data warehouse.

Implementing the security filter table
A new SecurityFilter table is required to store the authorized resellers for each employee (see **Figure 9.32**).

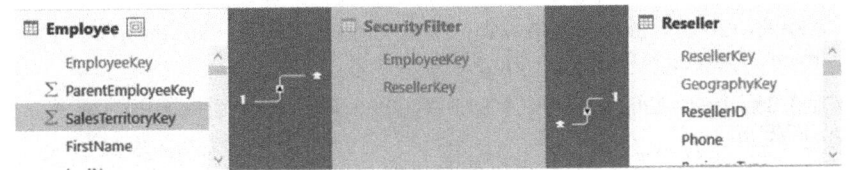

Figure 9.32 The Security-Filter bridge table stores the authorized resellers for each employee.

This table is related to the Reseller and Employee tables. If an employee is authorized to view a reseller, a row is added to the SecurityFilter table. In real life, business users or IT pros will probably maintain the security associations in a database or external application. For the sake of simplicity, you'll import the security policies from a text file (you can also enter the data directly using the Enter Data button in the ribbon's Home tab).

1. In the ribbon's Home tab, click Get Data. Choose CSV.

2. Navigate to the \Source\ch09 folder and select the SecurityFilter.csv file. Click Open.

3. Preview the data and compare your results with **Figure 9.33**. Click Load. Power BI Desktop adds a SecurityFilter table to the model.

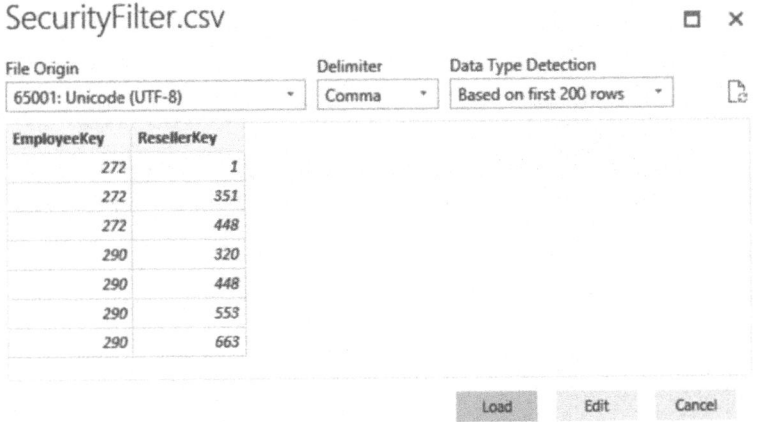

Figure 9.33 The SecurityFilter table specifies the resellers that an employee can access.

4. Because users shouldn't see this table, right-click the SecurityFilter table in the Fields pane (Data View) and click "Hide in Report View".

5. In the Relationships View, double-click the ResellerSales[ResellerKey]⇨Reseller[ResellerKey] relationship. If the "Apply security filter in both directions" checkbox is checked, uncheck it because it will conflict with the new relationships.

6. In the Relationships View, verify that the SecurityFilter[EmployeeKey]⇨Employee[EmployeeKey] and SecurityFilter[ResellerKey]⇨Reseller[ResellerKey] relationships exist and that they are active. If that's not the case, make the necessary changes to create these two relationships.

 REAL LIFE Although in this case the SecurityFilter table is related to other tables, this is not a requirement. DAX is flexible and it allows you to filter tables using the FILTER() function even if they can't be related. For example, a real-life project required defining application security roles and granting them access to any level in an organization hierarchy. The DAX row filter granted the role access to a parent without explicit access to its children. The security table didn't have relationships to the tact table.

Implementing the Reseller role
Next, you'll add a role that will enforce the security policy. Follow these steps to set up a new Reseller role:

1. In the ribbon's Modeling tab, click Manage Roles.

2. In the "Manage roles" window create a new *Reseller* role.

3. In the Table section, select the Reseller table. Enter the following expression in the "Table Filter DAX Expression" field (you can copy it from \Source\ch09\dax.txt file):

CONTAINS(RELATEDTABLE(SecurityFilter), SecurityFilter[EmployeeKey], LOOKUPVALUE(Employee[EmployeeKey], Employee[EmailAddress], USERPRINCIPALNAME())))

Let's digest this expression one piece at a time. As you already know, the LOOKUPVALUE function is used to obtain the employee key associated with the email address. Because the table filter is set on the Reseller table, for each reseller, the CONTAINS function attempts to find a match for that reseller key and employee key combination in the SecurityFilter table. Notice the use of the RELATEDTABLE function to pass the current reseller. The net effect is that the CONTAINS function returns TRUE if there is a row in the SecurityFilter table that matches the ResellerKey and EmployeeKey combination.

Testing the Reseller role
Let's follow familiar steps to test the role:

1. In the ribbon's Modeling tab, click "View As Roles".

2. In the "View as roles" window, check the Reseller role.

3. If you'd like to impersonate another user to test his permissions, check the "Other user" checkbox and type in the user's UPN. As a result, USERPRINCIPALNAME() will return whatever you typed in. Click OK.

4. (Optional) Create a Table report that uses the ResellerName field from the Reseller table. The report should show only the three resellers associated with Stephen.

5. In the Home ribbon, click the Publish button. Deploy the Adventure Works model to Power BI Service. Add members to the Employee and Reseller roles. Ask the role members to view reports and report results.

9.6 Summary

One of the great strengths of Power BI is its Data Analysis Expressions (DAX) language, which allows you to unlock the full power of your data model and implement sophisticated business calculations. This chapter introduced you to the DAX calculations, syntax, and formulas. You can use the DAX formula language to implement calculated columns and measures.

Calculated columns are custom columns that use DAX formulas to derive their values. The column formulas are evaluated for each row in the table, and the resulting values are saved in the model. The practices walked you through the steps for creating basic and advanced columns.

Measures are evaluated for each cell in the report. Power BI Desktop automatically creates an implicit measure for every column that you add to the Value area of the Visualizations pane. You can create explicit measures that use custom DAX formulas you specify.

More complex models might call for role-playing, parent-child, and many-to-many relationships. You can use DAX formulas to navigate inactive relationships, to flatten parent-child hierarchies, and to change the measure aggregation behavior.

Power BI supports a flexible data security model that can address various security requirements, ranging from simple filters, such as users accessing specific countries, to externalizing security policies and dynamic security based on the user's identity. You define security roles and table filters in Power BI Desktop and role membership in Power BI Service.

Chapter 10

Analyzing Data

Up until now in this part of the book, you have seen how a business analyst can implement a self-service model and mash up data from virtually everywhere. This is the ground work required when you don't have an organizational semantic model. Now that the model is complete, let's get some insights from it. After all, the whole purpose of creating a model is to derive knowledge from its data. I've already shown you in the first part of this book how to create meaningful and attractive reports with just a few mouse clicks. But Power BI has more to offer.

In this chapter, I'll walk you through more analytics features for data exploration. With the momentum about machine learning, I'll show you the Power BI predictive features. Finally, I'll demonstrate the Power BI data storytelling capabilities. You'll find the examples in the \Source\ch10 folder. Think of this chapter as tips and tricks for report authoring. However, instead of walking you step by step through the process of creating a report (Chapter 3 covers the fundamentals), this chapter focuses on specific features that deserve more attention. If you need additional practice to hone your report authoring skills, check the excellent Dashboard in a Day (DIAD) material by Microsoft at http://aka.ms/diahanddiad (download the diad.zip file from the diad folder). Microsoft updates the training material monthly to keep up with the latest features!

10.1 Getting More Insights

Let's start with some popular analytical features that I haven't previously covered or haven't covered in sufficient detail, including drilling down and through, custom grouping and binning, conditional formatting, and working with images.

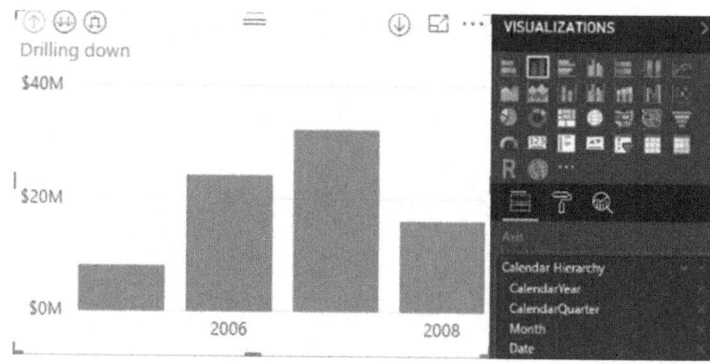

Figure 10.1 Drilling down data using a hierarchy.

10.1.1 Drilling Down and Across Tables

Drilling down data is a common requirement. For example, you might have a chart, matrix, or map that shows some summary information, but you want to explore underlying data in more detail.

Drilling down the same table

As you've learned in Chapter 6 and 8, drilling down the same table can be achieved in two ways:

- Adding the required fields that form the drilldown path to the same area in the Visualizations pane (Data tab)
- Creating a hierarchy and dragging it to the appropriate area in the visualization.

Consider the chart shown in **Figure 10.1** (located on the "Drill data" page in the Adventure Works.pbix file). I added the Calendar Hierarchy to chart axis area. To drill down data in both Power BI Desktop and Power BI Service, use the Data/Drill ribbon, the drill indicators on top of the chart, or right-click and pick an option from the context menu.

Drilling across tables

Consider the matrix in **Figure 10.2**. I've added two fields from different tables in the Rows area. You can start your analysis at the CalendarYear level. Then, you use one of the drill options, such as right-click a year and click "Expand to Next Level" to drill down to SalesTerritoryCountry (from SalesTerritory table). Or, you can right-click a year and then click "Drill Down" to expand only that year.

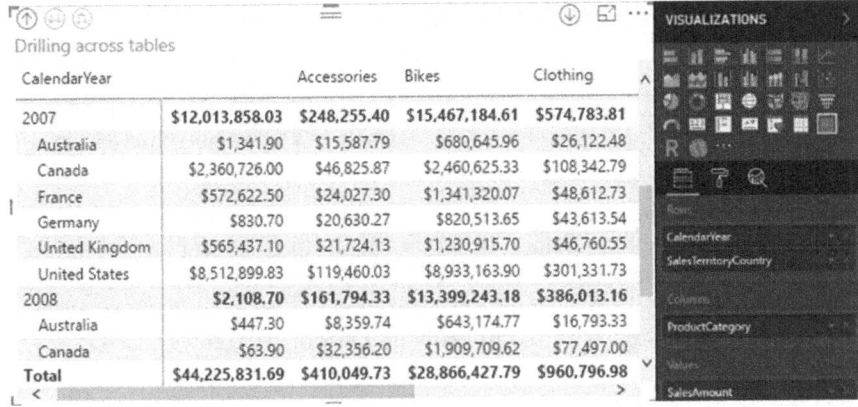

Figure 10.2 Drilling across tables can be achieved by using fields from different tables.

While we're discussing the matrix visual, notice that it defaults to a stepped layout. Fields added to the Rows area are stacked to occupy a single column and reduce horizontal space. However, some report types, such as financial reports, may require fields to appear in separate columns. To configure this layout, go to the Format tab in the Visualizations pane, expand the "Row headers" section, and then turn off "Stepped layout". While you are there, notice that the "Stepped layout indentation" setting lets you control the indentation space for the stepped layout.

TIP You may have a requirement to implement a master-detail report, such as a typical invoice header-details report. Currently, Power BI doesn't have a visual for a freeform layout to position fields at arbitrary locations, so you must resort to Card, Multi-row Card, Table or Matrix visuals. However, cross-highlighting works across Table or Matrix visuals. Therefore, one approach is to use a Table or Matrix for the header and another for the details. Then, you can select a row in the "header" section and see the "details" in the second table or matrix.

10.1.2 Drilling Through Data

Another very popular requirement is drilling through data. For example, you might want to see the transactions (as they are imported) behind a cell, or to drill from a summarized view through another page. Power BI supports two drillthrough options:

- See records – Power BI generates a default drillthrough report which supports limited customization.
- Drillthrough page – You create a drillthrough page and customize it just like any other page.

Using "See Records"

Drilling through a data point on chart, map, or matrix can be accomplished by using the "See Records" feature. While you drill *down* fields in (lookup) dimension tables, you drill *through* measures, such as fields added to the Values area of a chart or matrix. To drill through, right-click a cell and click See Records, or use the same menu in the Data/Drill ribbon. For example, right-click the 2006 bar in the column chart and then click "See Records". Power BI Desktop generates a new tabular report that displays the rows from the ResellerSales table that contribute to the cell value, as shown in **Figure 10.3**.

CalendarYear	CalendarQuarter	Month	Date	OrderQuantity	SalesOrderNumber	CarrierTrackingNumber	Customer
2007	2	May	Tuesday, May 1, 2007	44	SO50270	A828-45A2-8B	PO18676
2007	3	August	Wednesday, August 1, 2007	40	SO51783	B7A2-498C-89	PO18676
2007	4	November	Thursday, November 1, 2007	40	SO57186	EF93-4946-97	PO88451!
2007	3	July	Sunday, July 1, 2007	36	SO51109	0EFE-4639-8E	PO12441
2007	3	August	Wednesday, August 1, 2007	36	SO51783	B7A2-498C-89	PO18676
2007	2	May	Tuesday, May 1, 2007	33	SO50294	F34B-46CA-8D	PO37991!
2007	3	July	Sunday, July 1, 2007	33	SO51089	A635-4BAF-BC	PO16588
2007	4	October	Monday, October 1, 2007	33	SO55241	F7DC-49D7-89	PO16588
2007	4	November	Thursday, November 1, 2007	33	SO57186	EF93-4946-97	PO88451!
2007	3	August	Wednesday, August 1, 2007	32	SO51789	A5AF-4504-83	PO18618
2007	3	September	Saturday, September 1, 2007	32	SO53527	0EBE-4ACB-85	PO17981!
2007	4	December	Saturday, December 1, 2007	32	SO58972	07C8-43BD-85	PO17981!
2007	2	April	Sunday, April 1, 2007	31	SO49843	D3CA-4A51-B6	PO11484

Figure 10.3 "See Records" generates a new report that shows the individual rows from the underlying table.

By default, Power BI adds all text fields from the underlying table and fields from the other tables that are used in the main report. Currently, you can't choose default fields for the drillthrough report. However, you can add additional fields to the generated report with the caveat that your changes are not preserved when you click "Back to Report" to navigate to the main report. Continuing the list of limitations, "See Records" isn't available for DAX explicit measures. It's also currently limited to 1,000 rows and there is no way to increase the limit.

 TIP If you need to see more than 1,000 records, consider "Analyze in Excel" (expand the ellipsis menu next to the dataset name in Power BI Service and then click Analyze in Excel). Then, you can double-click a cell to initiate the default drillthrough action. This approach doesn't limit the detail rows.

Creating drillthrough pages

Do you need more customization over the drillthrough report? You can create your own page(s) as a drillthrough target! Going back to **Figure 10.2**, suppose you want a list of the customer orders behind a given cell. Start by adding a new page to the report that returns the required fields (refer to the "Drill target" page in the Adventure Works file, which is shown in **Figure 10.4**). This page shows detailed information about customer orders. There is nothing special about this page except that the SalesAmount measure came from a different table (InternetSales) than the calling page. I wanted to demonstrate that drilling through data doesn't have to target the same fact table.

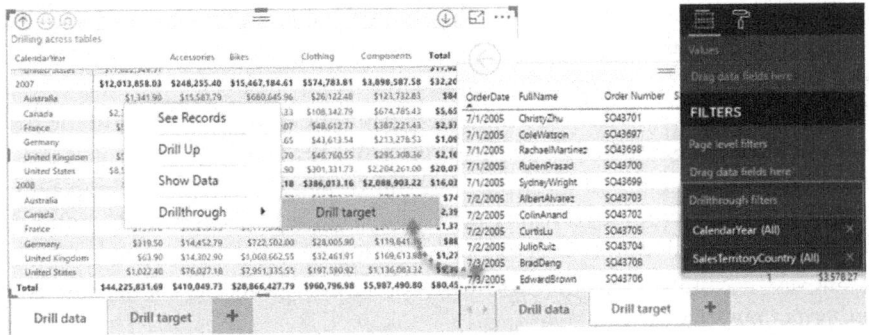

Figure 10.4 Unlike default drillthrough, a custom drillthrough page allows you to define the report layout.

The trick for configuring drillthrough is to add fields to the "Drillthrough filters" area in the Visualizations page. Interestingly, the main page automatically checks if its visual has one of the fields used in the "Drillthrough filters" area. If it does, it automatically enables the Drillthrough context menu. The context menu is activated even if the source page has a subset of the fields used as drillthrough filters. For example, if the Sales visual has only CalendarYear, the drillthrough page would show all customer orders for that year. If it has also SalesTerritoryCountry, the drillthrough page would show orders for that year and for that country. If the Sales visual has none of the fields used for drillthrough filters, then the Drillthrough context menu won't show up. In other words, Power BI automatically matches the source fields and drillthrough filters and this saves you a lot of configuration steps, such as to configure parameters, to check which fields exist, and to pass All to the parameters that don't exist!

Once you add a field to the "Drillthrough filters" area, Power BI automatically adds an image to let you navigate back to the main page. You can use your own image if you don't like the Microsoft-provided one. To configure it as a back button, click the image, go to the image properties in the Format Image pane, expand the Link section, and then set its Type property to Back.

10.1.3 Grouping and Binning

Dynamic grouping allows you to create your own groups, such as to group countries with negligible sales in an "Others" category. In addition to grouping categories together, you can also create bins (buckets or bands) from numerical and time fields, such as to segment customers by revenue or create aging buckets.

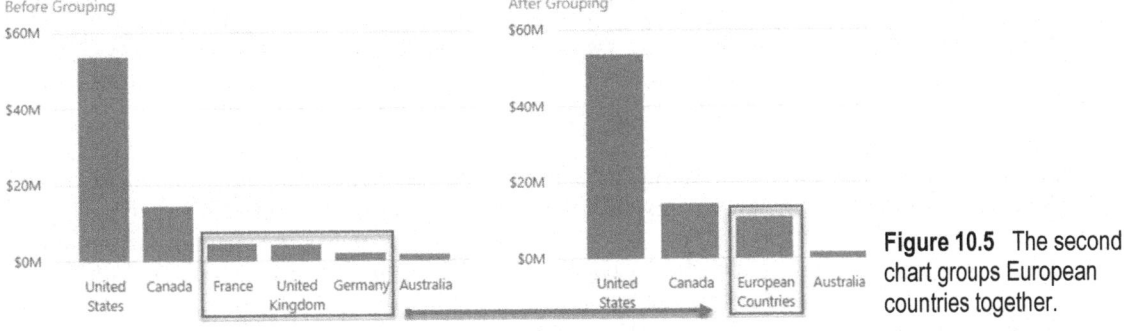

Figure 10.5 The second chart groups European countries together.

Implementing groups
Consider the two charts shown in **Figure 10.5**. The chart on the left displays sales by country. Because European countries have lower sales, you might want to group them together as shown on the right. Follow these steps to implement the group:

1. Create a Stacked Column Chart with SalesTerritoryCountry (SalesTerritory table) in the Axis area and SalesAmount (ResellerSales table) in the Values area.

2. Hold the Ctrl key and click each of the data categories you want to group. Only charts support this way of selecting group members. To group elements in tables or matrices, expand the drop-down next to the field in the Visualizations pane (or click the ellipses button in the Field list), and then click New Group.

3. Right-click any of the selected countries and click Group from the context menu. Power BI Desktop adds a new SalesTerritoryCountry (group) field to the SalesTerritory table. This field represents the group and it's prefixed with a special double-square icon. Power BI Desktop adds the field to the chart's Legend area.

4. In the Fields pane, click the ellipsis (...) button next to SalesTerritoryCountry (group). Click Rename and change the field name to *European Countries*.

5. Click the ellipsis (...) button next to the European Countries field and then click Edit Groups.

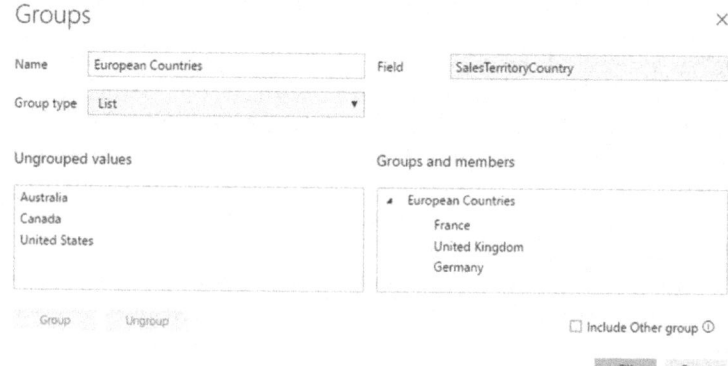

Figure 10.6 Use the Groups window to view the grouped values and control how the ungrouped values are shown.

6. In the Groups window (see **Figure 10.6**), you can change the group name and see the grouped and ungrouped members. If the "Include Other group" checkbox is checked (default setting), the rest of the data categories (Canada and United States) will be grouped into an "Other" group. Leave the "Include Other group" checkbox unchecked so that Canada and United States show as separate data categories. Click OK.

7. Back to the report, remove SalesTerritoryCountry from the Axis area. Add the European Countries field to the Axis area. Compare your report with the right chart shown in **Figure 10.5**.

 TIP Although Power BI Desktop doesn't currently support lassoing categories for as a faster way of selecting many items, you can use the Groups window to select and add values to group. Instead of clicking elements on the chart, right-click the corresponding field in the Fields pane and then click New Group to open the Groups window. Select the values in the "Ungrouped values" (you can hold the Shift key for extended selection) and then click the Group button to create a new group.

Binning data

Besides grouping categories, Power BI Desktop is also capable of discretizing numeric values or dates in equally sized ranges called *bins*. Suppose you want to group customers in different bins based on the customer's overall sales, such as $0-$99, $100-$200, and so on (see the X-axis of the chart shown in **Figure 10.7**). This report counts distinct values of the CustomerID field (Count Distinct aggregation function) in the Customer table which is related to the InternetSales table. This requires following the InternetSales[CustomerKey] ⇨ Customer[CustomerKey] relationship because the SalesAmount field in the InternetSales table will become the "dimension" while the measure (Count of Customers) comes from the Customer table. Follow these steps to create the report:

1. In the Relationships View, if the InternetSales[CustomerKey] ⇨ Customer[CustomerKey] relationship has a single arrow (cross filter direction is Single), double-click it to open Edit Relationship window and change the "Cross filter direction" drop-down to Both. Click OK.

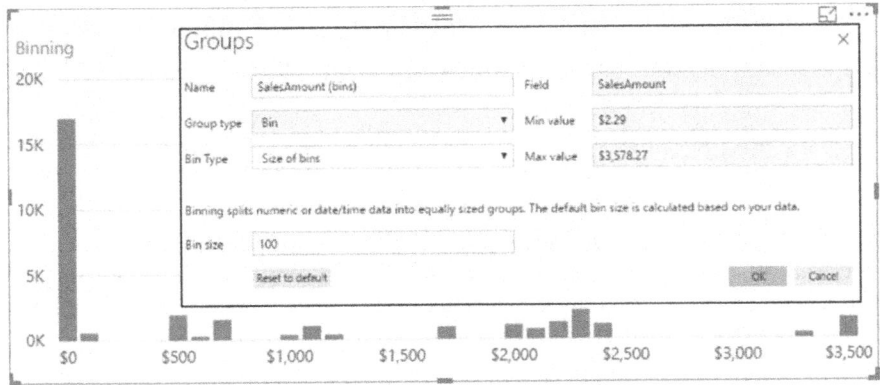

Figure 10.7 This report counts customers in bin sizes of $100 based on the overall sales.

2. Switch to the Report View (or Data View). In the Fields pane, click the ellipsis (…) button next to the SalesAmount field in the InternetSales table and then click New Group.

3. In the Groups window, change the bin size to 100 (you're grouping customers in bins of $100). Given the group a descriptive name, such as *SalesAmount (bins)*, and then click OK.

4. Add a Stacked Column Chart visualization. Add the SalesAmount (bins) field that you've just created to the Axis area of the Visualizations pane (you'll be grouping the chart data points by the new field).

5. Add the CustomerID field from the Customer table to the Value area. Expand the drop-down next to the CustomerID field in the Value area and switch the aggregation to Count (Distinct). Compare your results with **Figure 10.7**.

 TIP The built-in binning feature creates equal bins based on the bin size you specify in the Groups window. If you need more control over the bin ranges, consider either using Query Editor to add a conditional column, as I explained in Section 7.1.1, or creating a separate lookup (dimension) table for the bins and then joining this table to the fact table.

10.1.4 Applying Conditional Formatting

You can apply conditional formatting to change the color of measures in Table and Matrix visuals based on different conditions, such as to color negative numbers in red. Power BI supports conditional formatting expressed as data bars, font, and background colors. The report in **Figure 10.8** uses conditional formatting to emphasize trends (see the "Conditional formatting" tab in Adventure Works.pbix).

FullName	SalesAmountYTD	SalesAmount	NetProfit	OrderQuantity
Amy Alberts	$98,323	$98,323	$56,525	
David Campbell	$674,625	$674,625	$475,513	1,677
Garrett Vargas	$570,416	$570,416	$316,985	2,165
Jae Pak	$1,807,979	$1,807,979	$1,225,418	5,640
Jillian Carson	$1,372,940	$1,372,940	$845,258	4,686
José Saraiva	$1,236,082	$1,236,082	$828,542	3,591
Linda Mitchell	$1,885,942	$1,885,942	$1,327,592	5,214
Lynn Tsoflias	$719,877	$719,877	$352,650	1,853
Michael Blythe	$1,537,712	$1,537,712	$973,242	3,738
Pamela Ansman-Wolfe	$649,827	$649,827	$464,797	1,458
Rachel Valdez	$829,193	$829,193	$516,780	2,816
Ranjit Varkey Chudukatil	$1,374,664	$1,374,664	$954,638	3,940
Shu Ito	$1,076,089	$1,076,089	$677,061	2,805
Stephen Jiang	$249,400	$249,400	$170,542	729
Syed Abbas	$26,580	$26,580	$8,869	79
Tete Mensa-Annan	$837,303	$837,303	$519,799	1,678
Tsvi Reiter	$1,089,001	$1,089,001	$643,538	2,841
Total	**$16,035,954**	**$16,035,954**	**$10,357,748**	**45,097**

Figure 10.8 This report demonstrates data bars, background and foreground conditional formatting, and using rules.

Applying data bars

I used the following steps to configure the SalesAmountYTD column to show data bars.

1. Add a Table with the FullName field (Employee table) and the SalesAmountYTD, SalesAmount, NetProfit, and OrderQuantity measures from the ResellerSales table.

2. In the Visualizations pane (Fields tab), right-click the SalesAmountYTD field and then click Conditional Formatting ⇨ Data Bars. Alternatively, click the ellipsis button (…) next to the SalesAmountYTD field in the Values area to see the Conditional Formatting menu.

3. Accept the default settings in the "Data bars" window (see **Figure 10.9**). Going through them quickly, check "Show bar only" if you want to show only the data bar and not the data. By default, Power BI detects the data range for each cell but if you want to enter a specific range, expand the "Lowest value" (or Highest value) and enter a number for the lowest or highest boundary.

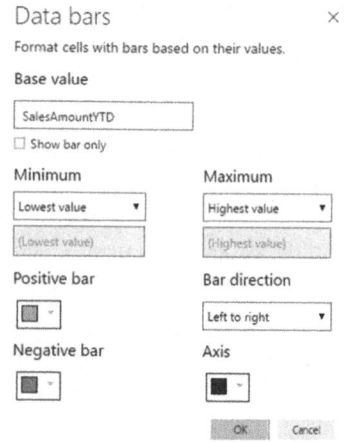

Figure 10.9 Use this window to configure the data bar configuration settings.

4. Click OK. You can now easily see that Linda Mitchel has the highest YTD sales.

Applying color formatting

Back to the report, the SalesAmount measure uses conditional formatting to change its background cell color (Conditional Formatting ⇨ Background Color Scales). And the NetProfit measure changes conditionally the font color (Conditional Formatting ⇨ Font Color Scales). These options have similar settings as the data bars, but they support a diverging option so that you can specify a center value and color. The OrderQuantity measure brings conditional formatting one step further by using rules (the "Color by rules" checkbox is on), as shown in **Figure 10.9**.

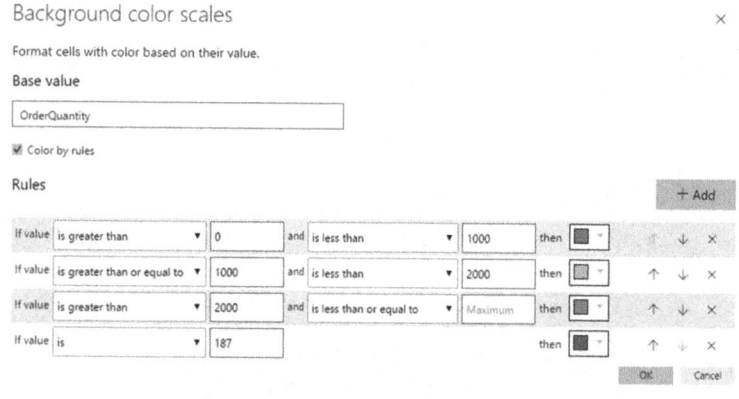

Figure 10.10 Conditional coloring lets you specify rules (the rules below win over rules above).

Specifically, the first three rules specify colors for different data ranges. The last rule checks for a specific value. Rules are evaluated in the order they are defined, and subsequent rules win over. Therefore, although the last rule checks for 187, which falls within the first rule, rows on the report with OrderQuantity = 187 will "win" over the rules above, and these cells will be colored in purple. You can change the rule precedence by clicking the up or down arrows.

10.1.5 Working with Links

You saw in Chapter 4 how you can configure a custom URL for a dashboard tile to navigate the user to a web page, instead of navigating to the report where the visual was pinned from. You can also use links in your reports to implement navigation features.

Implementing static links
You can manually enter the link URL to navigate the user to a specific web page, as demonstrated by the "Working with links" page (see **Figure 10.11**)

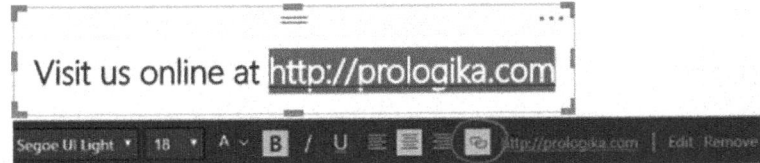

Figure 10.11 Use the Text Box element to specify static links.

I used a text box for the report title (in the Home ribbon, click "Text box" in the Insert ribbon group). As you type the text, you can select the URL portion, and then click the Insert Link button to configure the link. After you publish the file to Power BI Service or Power BI Report Server, users can click the link. This opens another browser window that will navigate them to the web page.

Implementing web URLs
The Table visual on the same page builds upon the visual in the "Drill target" page by allowing the user to click a link next to the order number (see **Figure 10.12**). In real life, such a link can navigate the user to an ERP system to get more information about the order. Follow these steps to implement this scenario:

```
OrderLink = "http://prologika.com?OrderNumber=" & [SalesOrderNumber]
```

OrderDate	FullName	Order Number		SalesOrderLi..	SalesAmount
7/1/2005	ChristyZhu	SO43701		1	$3,399.99
7/1/2005	ColeWatson	SO43697		1	$3,578.27
7/1/2005	RachaelMartinez	SO43698		1	$3,399.99
7/1/2005	RubenPrasad	SO43700		1	$699.0982
7/1/2005	SydneyWright	SO43699		1	$3,399.99
⁀5	AlbertAlvar·	⁀O43703		1	⁀8.27

Figure 10.12 Use the Text Box element to specify static links.

1. To manufacture a link for every order, add a calculated column OrderLink to the InternetSales table with the following DAX formula:

OrderLink = "http://prologika.com?OrderNumber=" & [SalesOrderNumber]

2. Add the OrderLink column to the report. You can now see the URL for every order but it's not clickable.

3. In the Fields pane, click the OrderLink field to select it. In the Modeling ribbon, expand the Data Category drop-down and select Web URL. The link is now clickable, but it might not be desirable to show the URL.

4. With the Table visual selected, select the Format tab in the Visualizations pane, expand the Values area, and then turn on the "URL icon" slider.

5. (Optional) If you don't need a caption for the link column, rename the OrderLink field in the Values area of the Visualizations pane to an empty space (double click the field and then enter an empty space).

 NOTE As of the time of writing, you can't configure links on DAX calculated measures, such as to enable or disable links depending on a report filter, or to make SalesAmountYTD "clickable". Therefore, you must have all the information to construct the link in regular or calculated columns.

10.1.6 Working with Images

A picture is sometimes better than a thousand words. Power BI supports various ways to work with images, ranging from static and web images, image areas, and Visio diagrams. One notable exception are images stored in a database table, which are not supported yet in Power BI.

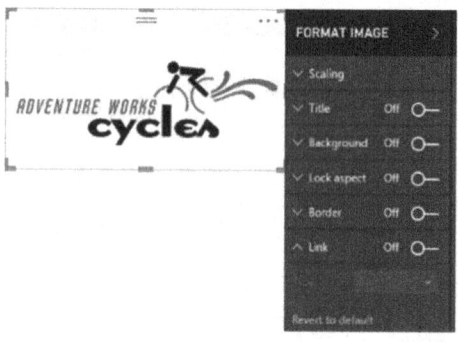

Figure 10.13 Use the Image element to embed company logos, buttons, and report background images.

Working with static images
Static images are typically used for logos, buttons, or report backgrounds. You can use the Image element (Home ribbon) to embed and display an image. Follow these steps to display the Adventure Works logo:

1. In the Home ribbon, click the Image element.

2. Navigate to the \Source\ch10 folder, select the awc.jpg file, and click Open.

3. Position and resize the image as necessary.

When you select the image, you'll see the Visualizations pane is replaced with the Format Image pane (see **Figure 10.13**). Use this pane to set various image options, such as scaling.

 TIP To use an image as a page background, size the image to occupy the entire page. Then, select the image and send it to the back. To do so, click the Format ribbon tab, expand the "Send backward", and then click "Send to back".

Working with image URLs
You could have images stored on a web server or a web page that you may want to show on reports. For example, the Table visual on **Figure 11.10** shows three Power BI-related book images from their respective Amazon pages. Follow these steps to implement such reports:

1. Obtain the image URLs and import them into a table. You can use the calculated column approach I demonstrated for link URLs to construct the image URLs. For this example, I used the "Enter Data" button in the Home ribbon to create a static table with two columns: Book and ImageURL. Then, I entered three rows in that table.

2. In the Fields list, click the ImageURL field to select it.

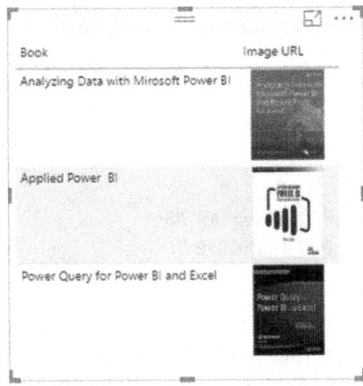

Figure 10.14 Table, Matrix, and Multi-row Card visuals can display images from URLs.

3. In the Modeling table, change the field data category to Image URL.

4. Use Table, Matrix, or Multi-row Card to visualize the images.

Working with image areas

Since the dawn of Internet, web designers have used image areas (called image maps) to create clickable locations in an image. You can use a similar technique to divide an image into clickable areas. Power BI doesn't natively support this feature, but a popular custom visual called Synoptic Panel by SQLBI can be used for this purpose. For example, **Figure 10.15** shows a floor plan where the colored areas are clickable.

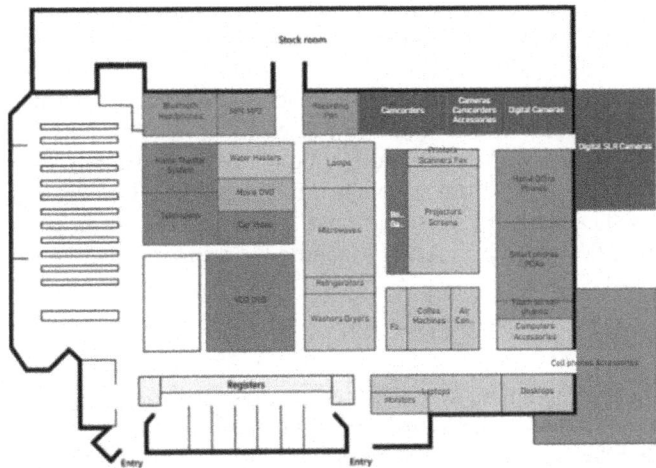

Figure 10.15 Use the Synoptic Panel custom visual to define clickable image areas.

As with the Power BI native visuals, when the user clicks an area, cross-highlighting filters other visualizations on the page. For more information about how to use Synoptic Panel, define image maps, and download a sample Power BI report, go to the product home page at http://okviz.com/synoptic-panel/.

Embedding Visio diagrams

Bringing image maps further, another custom visual (currently in preview) allows you to embed Visio diagrams in your Power BI reports. By using Visio and Power BI together, you can illustrate data as both diagrams and visualizations in one place to drive operational and business intelligence. I demonstrate this integration scenario in the Visio Demo.pbix file (see **Figure 10.16**), but make sure to follow the steps listed on the report to set it up for integration with Visio Online.

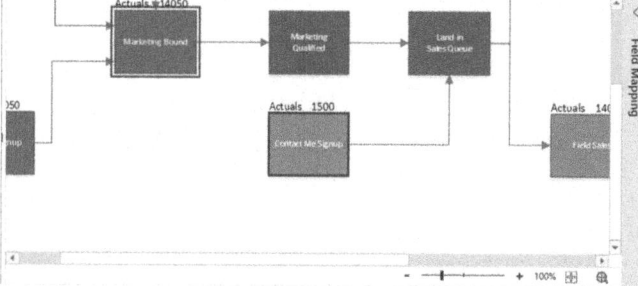

Figure 10.16 The Visio custom visual allows you to add interactive Visio diagrams to your reports.

This report imports data from an Excel file. The data represents different stages in the process of acquiring customers, starting from Trial Signup to Opportunity, like the typical sales funnel in CRM systems. Each stage has Target, Actual, and Gap numbers. The Visio diagram shows how these stages are related. During the process of configuring the custom visual, you specify which fields would be used and whether they will be used to change the shape text or color. Cross-highlighting works so that you can click a Power BI chart bar to zoom in the corresponding Visio shape.

The Visio custom visual requires the Visio file to be saved to Office 365 OneDrive for Business or SharePoint Online. That's because the diagram needs to be rendered online using O365 Visio Online. For more information about how to configure the Visio custom visual, refer to the "Add Visio visualizations to Power BI reports" article by Microsoft at http://bit.ly/powerbivisio.

10.2 Using Predictive Features

Predictive analytics is concerned with what will happen in the future. It uses machine learning algorithms to determine probable future outcomes and discover patterns that might not be easily discernible based on historical data. With all the interest surrounding predictive analytics and machine learning, you may wonder what Power BI has to offer. As you'll discover, they range from simple features that take a few clicks to building integrated solutions with Azure Machine Learning. In this section, we'll focus on the Power BI Desktop predictive features. I'll discuss integrating Power BI with Azure Machine Learning in Chapter 13.

10.2.1 Explaining Increase and Decrease

As you've seen, Power BI Desktop helps you quickly implement sophisticated models for descriptive analytics. But you can slice and dice all day long and still have unanswered questions, such as "Why there is drop in sales for this month?". You've already seen how Quick Insights helps you discover hidden trends in Power BI Service with a few clicks. A similar feature, called Explain Increase/Decrease is available in Power BI Desktop to help you perform root cause analysis (RCA) for unexpected variances.

Using Explain Increase/Decrease
Consider the column chart on page "Explain Decrease and Clustering" in the Adventure Works file (see **Figure 11.13**). As you examine the data, you see a decrease in sales for Q3 of 2016. Instead of trying to narrow down the cause on your own, you'll let Power BI do it. You right-click on the bar and then click Analyze ⇨ Explain the Decrease.

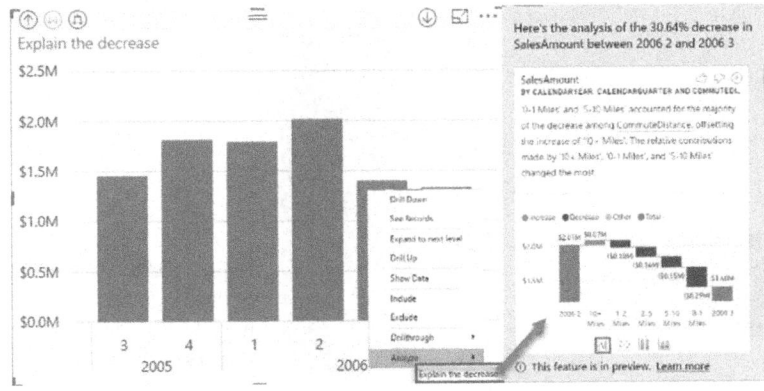

Figure 10.17 Use Explain Increase/Decrease to uncover hidden trends that are not easily discernible.

Power BI applies machine learning algorithms, finds possible insights, ranks them, and shows reports. For example, in this case Power BI has found that the most significant decrease was from customers who don't commute much to work. You can vote a report up and down to help Microsoft tune the algorithms, switch to another visual, or add the visual to the report if you like it.

> **TIP** Do you wonder how I configured the chart to group by year and then quarter? In the Visualizations pane (Format tab), I expanded the X-axis section and then turned off "Concatenate labels".

Understanding limitations
Currently in preview, Explain Increase/Decrease isn't available if the visual has one of these features:

- Filters (top N filters, include/exclude filters, measure filters)
- Non-additive measures and aggregates, non-numeric measures, "show value as" measures
- Categorical columns on X-axis, unless it defines a sort by column that is scalar
- DirectQuery connection (only datasets with imported data are supported at this time)

10.2.2 Implementing Time Series Forecasting

Another common predictive task is forecasting, such as to show revenue over future periods. Power BI Desktop supports basic forecasting capabilities to address such requirements.

Understanding time series forecasting
Time series forecasting produces forecasts over data points indexed in time order. Power BI Desktop uses a built-in predictive algorithm to automatically detect the interval, such as monthly, weekly, or annually. It's also capable of detecting seasonality changes. Currently, forecasting is supported for single series line charts with a continuous (quantitative) axis. You can use the Analytics tab of the Visualization pane (see **Figure 10.18**) to add a forecast line.

You can customize certain aspects of the forecasting model. Change the "Forecast length" setting to specify the number of future intervals to forecast. Change the "Ignore last" setting to exclude a specified number of last points, such as when you know that the last period of data is incomplete. This is especially useful if you know the last month of data is still incomplete. "Confidence interval" lets you control the upper and lower boundaries of the forecasted results.

The Seasonality setting lets you override the automatically detected seasonality trend, such as 3 points if the seasonal cycle rises and falls every 3 months, assuming you're forecasting at the month level. When you hover over the line chart, you can see the exact values of the forecasted value, as well as the upper and lower bands (the shaded area width is controlled by the "Confidence interval" setting).

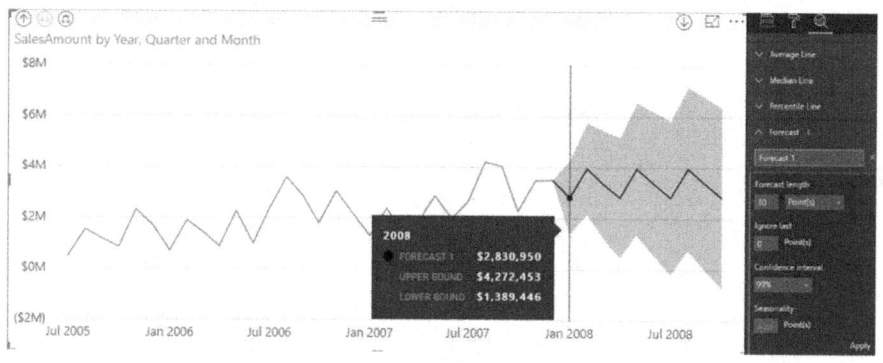

Figure 10.18 Time series forecasting uses a built-in model that supports limited customization.

Implementing forecasting

Follow these steps to implement time series forecasting:

1. Add the "Line Chart" visualization to the report.
2. Add the Calendar Hierarchy from the Date table to the Axis area of the Visualizations pane.
3. Add the SalesAmount field from the ResellerSales table to the Values area.
4. Click twice the "Expand one level down the hierarchy" button in the top-left corner of the chart to navigate to the Month level of the hierarchy.
5. In the Format tab of the Visualizations pane, change the Type setting of the X-Axis section to Continuous. You can only do this if the data type of the field added to the Axis area is Date or Numeric.
6. In the Analytics tab of the Visualizations tab, expand the Forecast section and click the Add link.
7. (Optional) Experiment with the settings to see how they affect the forecasted area in the chart.

10.2.3 Clustering Data

Clustering (also called segmentation) is another way for dynamic grouping (the others are custom groups and binning) that lets you quickly find groups of similar data points in a subset of your data. It uses predictive algorithms to group data points in similar clusters. You must use a scatter chart to detect clusters.

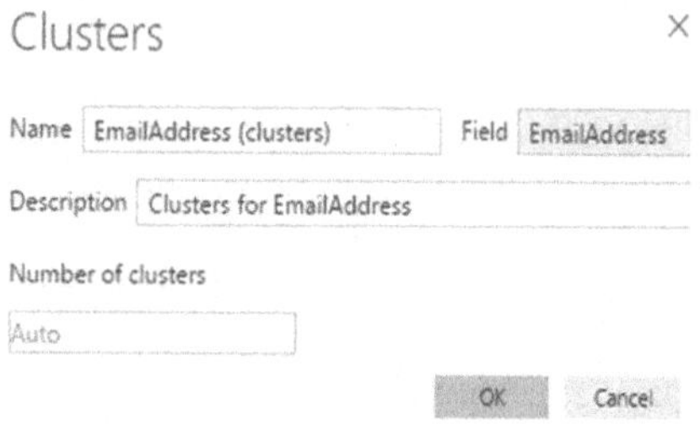

Figure 10.19 By default, Power BI would automatically detect the number of clusters.

Implementing clustering

Follow these steps to detect clusters that group customers by analyzing the correlation between the customer spend and number of items they bought.

1. Add the Scatter visual to an empty area of the report.
2. Add EmailAddress (Customer table) in the Details area, SalesAmount (InternetSales) in the X Axis area, and OrderQuantity (InternetSales table) in the Y Axis area. This configuration will see a correlation between the quantity of the items sold and generated revenue.

3. Hover over the visualization, click the ellipsis (…) menu in the top-right corner, and then click "Automatically find clusters".

4. In the Clusters window (see **Figure 10.19**), leave the default to auto-detect clusters to let Power BI automatically find clusters. Click OK.

Interpreting results

The algorithm finds three clusters and shows them in different colors. After the clustering algorithm runs, it creates a new categorical field called "EmailAddress (clusters)" with the different cluster groups in it. This new field is added to your scatter chart's Legend field.

 NOTE All Power BI charts and maps are high-density visuals that can plot efficiently thousands of points. If you click the information icon in the top left corner, you'll see that the algorithm prioritizes the most significant data points. For more information about how the algorithm works, read the "High Density Sampling in Power BI scatter charts" article at https://powerbi.microsoft.com//documentation/powerbi-desktop-high-density-scatter-charts/.

1. In the Visualizations pane, select the Format tab and turn on "Fill point". Rename the "EmailAddress (clusters)" to *CustomerClusters*. Compare your results with **Figure 10.20**.

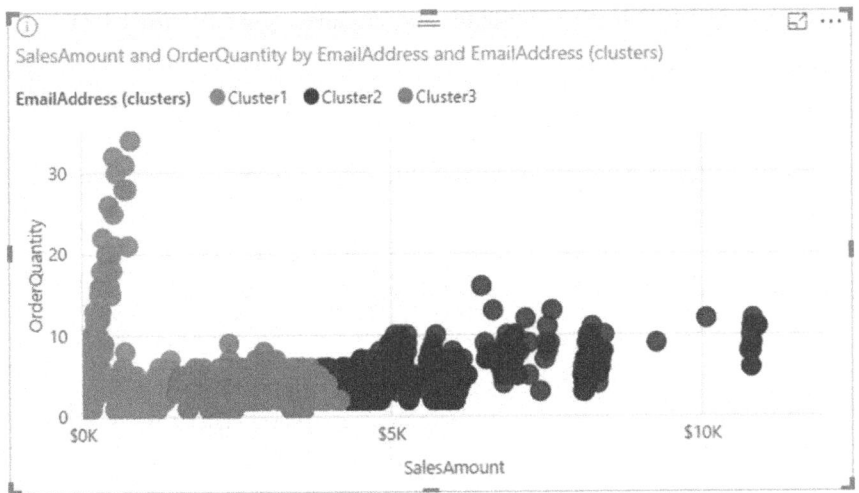

Figure 10.20 Automatic clustering found three clusters.

2. In the Fields pane, click the ellipsis next to CustomerClusters and then click "Edit clusters". This bring you back to the Clusters window where you can review the clusters and make changes, such as to increase the number of clusters. Now you understand that the first cluster (the one with low sales) has 6,230 customers, the second cluster has 1,439 customers, and the third cluster has 3,179 customers. Unfortunately, as it stands Power BI doesn't allow you to compare the cluster characteristics, such as to find similarities or differences between two clusters, nor does it allow you to rename the clusters.

3. (Optional) Create another visualization that uses the new CustomerClusters field. Although you must use a scatter chart to detect clusters, you can then use the clusters just like any other field.

10.2.4 Using R

With all the buzz surrounding R, data analysts might want to preserve their investment in R scripts and reuse them to import, transform, and analyze data with Power BI. Fortunately, Power BI supports R as a data source. The R integration brings the following benefits:

- Cleanse your data – If you prefer to do so, you can use R (instead of or in addition to the Query Editor) to cleanse your data, such as to ensure that all the data points are in place, correct outliers, and normalize to uniform scales. To learn about data shaping with R, check the "Data Cleansing with R in Power BI" blog by Sharon Laivand at http://bit.ly/2eZ6f4R.

- Visualize your R data – Once your R script's data is imported in Power BI, you can use a Power BI visualization to present the data. That's possible because the R data source is not different than any other data source.

- Share the results – You can leverage the Power BI sharing and collaboration capabilities to disseminate the results computed in R with everyone in your organization.

- Operationalize your R script – Once the data is uploaded to Power BI Service, you can configure the dataset for a scheduled refresh, so that the reports are always up to date.

- Reuse your R visualizations – You might use the R ggplot2 package to plot beautiful statistical graphs. Now you can bring these R Visuals into Power BI by using the R script visual in the Visualizations pane. You can also share your R visuals (or use the ones published by the community) at the R Script Showcase (https://community.powerbi.com/t5/R-Script-Showcase/bd-p/RVisuals/). This opens a whole world of new data visualizations! To learn more about how to create R Visuals, read the "Create Power BI visuals using R" blog by David Iseminger at http://bit.ly/2eQ5dHu.

In this exercise, I'll show you how to use R to forecast time series and visualize it (see **Figure 10.21**). The first segment in the line chart shows the actual sales, while the second segment shows the forecasted sales that are calculated in R. Because we won't need the forecasted data in the Adventure Works data model, you'll find the finished example in a separate "R Demo.pbix" file located in the \Source\ch10 folder.

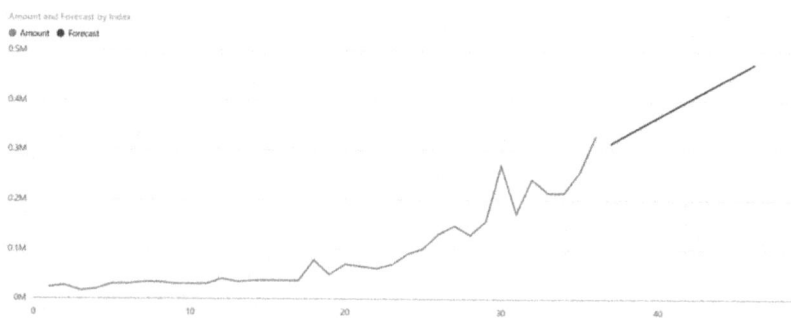

Figure 10.21 This visualization shows actual and forecasted sales.

Getting started with R

R is an open source programming language for statistical computing and data analysis. Over the years the community has contributed and extended the R capabilities through packages that provide various specialized analytical techniques and utilities. Besides supporting R in Power BI, Microsoft invested in R by acquiring Revolution Analytics, whose flagship product (Revolution R) is integrated with SQL Server 2016.

Before you can use the Power BI Desktop R integration, you must install R. Microsoft R Open, formerly known as Revolution R Open (RRO), is an enhanced distribution of R from Microsoft and it's a free open source platform for statistical analysis and data science. For more information about Microsoft R, go to https://aka.ms/microsoft-r-open-docs.

1. Open your web browser and navigate to https://mran.revolutionanalytics.com/download, and then download and install R for Windows.

2. I also recommend that you install RStudio Desktop (an open source R development environment) from http://www.rstudio.com. RStudio Desktop will allow you to prepare and test your R script before you import it in Power BI Desktop.

TIP As I mentioned, you can also use R to visualize your data by using the R visual in the Visualization pane. In this scenario, you can configure Power BI Desktop to use an external IDE, such as R Studio or Visual Studio. For more information about how to do so, read the "Use an external R IDE with Power BI " article at https://powerbi.microsoft.com/documentation/powerbi-desktop-r-ide/.

3. Use the Windows ODBC Data Sources (64-bit) tool (or 32-bit if you use the 32-bit version of Power BI Desktop) to set up a new ODBC system data source AdventureWorksDW that points to the AdventureWorksDW2012 (or a later version) database.

Using R for time series forecasting

Next, you'll create a basic R script for time series forecasting using RStudio. The RStudio user interface has four areas (see **Figure 10.22**). The first area (shown as 1 in the screenshot) contains the script that you're working on. The second area is the RStudio Console that allows you to test the script. For example, if you position the mouse cursor on a given script line and press Ctrl-Enter, RStudio will execute the current script line and it will show the output in the console.

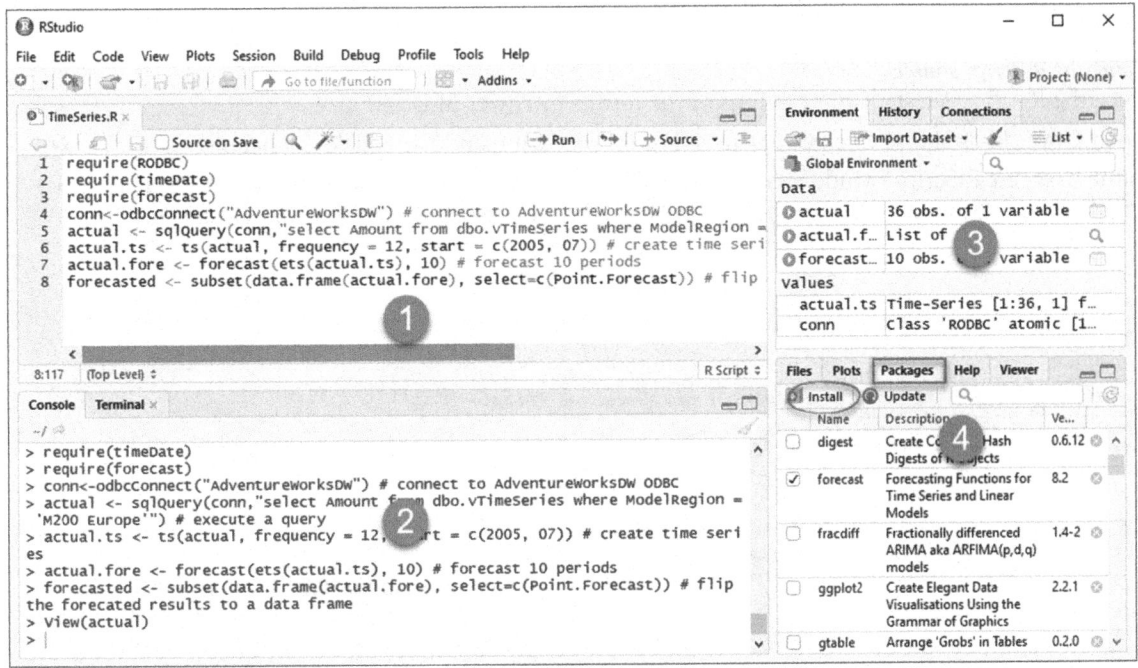

Figure 10.22 Use RStudio to develop and test R scripts.

The Global Environment area (shown as 3 in **Figure 10.22**) shows some helpful information about your script variables, such as the number of observations in a time series object. Area 4 has a tabbed interface that shows some additional information about the RStudio environment. For example, the Packages tab shows you what packages are loaded, while the Plots tab allows you to see the output when you use the R plotting capabilities. Let's start by importing the packages that our script needs:

1. Click File ⇨ New File ⇨ R Script File (or press Ctlr+Shft+N) to create a new R Script. Or, if you don't want to type the R code, click File ⇨ Open File, then open my TimeSeries.R script from the \Source\ch10 folder.

2. In the area 4, select the Packages tab, and then click Install.

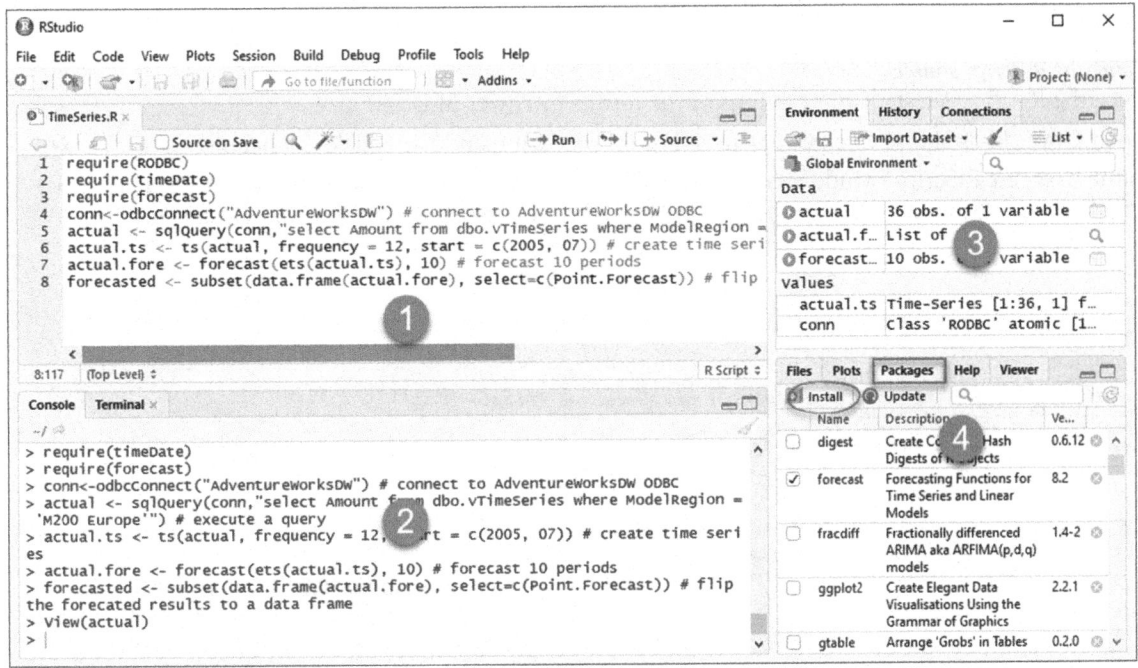

3. In the Install Packages window, enter *RODBC* (IntelliSense helps you enter the correct name), and then click Install. This installs the RODBC package which allows you to connect to ODBD data sources.

4. Repeat the last two steps to install the "timeDate" and "forecast" packages.

Going through the code, lines 1-3 list the required packages. Line 4 connects to the AdventureWorksDW ODBC data source. Line 5 retrieves the Amount field from the vTimeSeries SQL view, which is one of the sample views included in the AdventureWorksDW database. The resulting dataset represents the actual sales that are saved in the "actual" data frame. Like a Power BI dataset, an R data frame stores data tables. Line 6 creates a time series object with a frequency of 12 because the actual sales are stored by month. Line 7 uses the R forecast package to create forecasted sales for 10 periods. Line 8 stores the Point.Forecast column from the forecasted dataset in a data frame.

NOTE As of the time of writing, the R Source data source in Power BI only imports data frames, so make sure the data you want to load from an R script is stored in a data frame. Going down the list of limitations, columns that are typed as Complex and Vector are not imported, and are replaced with error values in the created table. Values that are N/A are translated to NULL values in Power BI Desktop. Also, any R script that runs longer than 30 minutes will time out. Interactive calls in the R script, such as waiting for user input, halt the script's execution.

Using the R Script source
Once the R script is tested, you can import the results in Power BI Desktop.

1. Open Power BI Desktop. Click Get Data ⇨ More ⇨ R Script, and then click Connect.

2. In the "Execute R Script" window (see **Figure 10.23**), paste the R script. Expand the "R Installation Settings" section and make sure that the R installation location matches your R setup. Click OK.

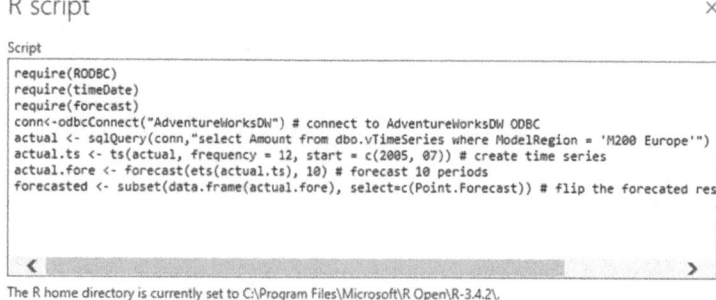

Figure 10.23 Enter the script in "R Script" window to use it as a data source.

3. In the Navigator window, notice that the script imports two tables (actual and forecasted) that correspond to the two data frames you defined in the R script. Click the Edit button to open Query Editor.

4. Click the "actuals" table. With the "actuals" query selected in the Queries pane, click the Append Queries button in ribbon's Home tab.

5. In the Append window, select the "forecasted" table, and then click OK. This appends the forecasted table to the actual table so that all the data (actual and forecasted) is in a single table.

6. Rename the "actual" table to *ActualAndForecast*. Rename the Point.Forecast column to *Forecast*.

7. (Optional) If you need actual and forecasted values in a single column, in the ribbon's Add Column tab, click "Add Custom Column". Name the custom column "Result" and enter the following expression:

```
if [Amount]=null then [Forecast] else [Amount]
```

This formula adds a new Result column that combines Amount and Forecast values into a single column.

8. In the ribbon's Add Column tab, click "Add Index Column" to add an auto-incremented column that starts with 1.

9. In the Home ribbon, click Close & Apply to execute the script and import the data.

10. To visualize the data, create a Line Chart visualization that has the Index field added to the Axis area, and Amount and Forecast fields added to the Values area.

11. (Optional) Deploy the Power BI Desktop file to Power BI Service and schedule the dataset for refresh.

10.3 Data Storytelling

Creating compelling and insightful reports goes a long way toward extracting value from your data. By combining analytics with narrative flow, data storying is the last mile for unlocking the full potential of your data. For a lack of a better definition, data storytelling is a way for communicating data insights that combines three key elements: data, visuals, and natural interfaces, such as Q&A and narratives. So far, our focus has been on the first two. Now you'll see how can you communicate your data story effectively with Power BI.

10.3.1 Asking Natural Questions

In Chapter 4, I showed you how you can ask natural questions at a dashboard level in Power BI Service, such as "Show me sales by year". And in Chapter 5, I showed you how to do the same in the Power BI mobile apps. Wouldn't be nice to do the same in the Power BI Desktop? You can, but make sure to enable first Q&A from File ⇨ Options and Settings ⇨ Options ("Preview features") tab because it's currently a preview feature. Once you do this and restart Power BI Desktop, you should see "Ask A Question" button in the Home ribbon.

Activating Q&A
As of this time, Q&A requires data to be imported. It doesn't work with DirectQuery connections. There are two ways to activate Q&A in Power BI Desktop:

1. Double-click an empty space anywhere on a page.
2. Click the "Ask A Question" button in the Home ribbon's tab.

This adds an empty "Stacked Column Chart" visual and a Q&A area above it that prompts you to ask a question about your data.

Using Q&A
On the desktop, Q&A works the same way as in Power BI Service (see **Figure 10.24**). As you type in your question, it guides you through the metadata fields and visualizes the data.

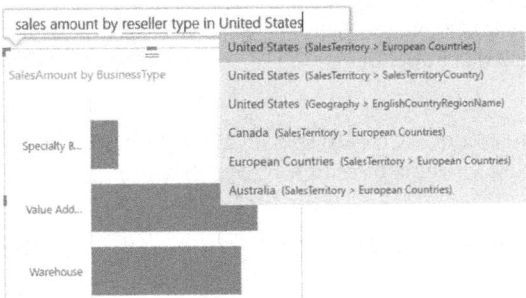

Figure 10.24 As you type your question, Power BI Desktop visualizes the data.

Once you're done with the question, you can use the visual just like any other visuals. Unlike Power BI Service, once you deactivate the visual, such by clicking somewhere else on the page, the Q&A box disappears, and you can't bring it back to see what question was asked.

10.3.2 Integrating with Windows Cortana

To recap, Q&A is available in Power BI Service, Power BI Mobile, and Power BI Desktop. But most of us still use laptops and most of them run Windows. Wouldn't it be nice to integrate data insights from Power BI directly in Windows? This is where Cortana comes in.

Cortana is an intelligent personal assistant that Microsoft included in Windows 10, Windows phones, and Xbox One. Cortana can help you update your schedule and answer questions using information from a variety of places, such as current weather and traffic conditions, sports scores, and biographies. For more information about Cortana's features, read "What is Cortana?" at http://windows.microsoft.com/windows-10/getstarted-what-is-cortana. And, of course, Cortana knows about Power BI. Who doesn't?

Configuring Cortana for Power BI
Follow these steps to integrate Cortana with Power BI:

1. Ensure that you have Windows 10. To check, in Windows press the hotkey Win+R to open the Run dialog, type *winver*, and then press Enter.
2. To find if Cortana is activated, type *Cortana* in the Windows search box (located in the taskbar on the left).
3. In the Search results window, click "Cortana & Search settings". In the Settings window, make sure that the first setting "Cortana can give you suggestions…" is on. If you want Cortana to respond to your voice when you say "Hey Cortana", turn on the "Hey Cortana" setting as well.
4. So that Cortana can reach out to Power BI and access your datasets, you must first add your work or school account to Windows. Right-click the Windows button to the left of the search box in the Windows taskbar, and then click Settings. In the Settings window, click Accounts. In the next window, click "Access work or school".
5. Check if the work email you use to sign in to Power BI is listed (see **Figure 10.25**). If the account is not listed, click the "Add a Microsoft account" link, and then add the account.

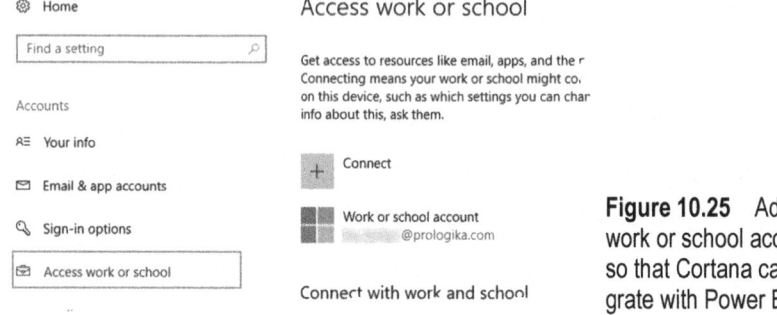

Figure 10.25 Add your work or school account so that Cortana can integrate with Power BI.

Configuring Power BI for Cortana
To get the most out Cortana, you need to add pages to your reports that are specifically optimized for Cortana (also known as Cortana answer cards). You can also use Cortana to search Power BI dashboards and reports by name.

NOTE Why doesn't Cortana just search all datasets when you ask a natural question? When the Power BI integration with Cortana was initially released, Cortana did this. However, Microsoft noticed there were a large percentage of cases where customers were enabling Q&A in Cortana simply to search for reports, without intending to ask natural questions. This was resulting in unexpected Q&A ad-hoc results showing up in Cortana answer lists, leading to user confusion. So, Microsoft decided it would be better to restrict results to Cortana answer cards until Power BI supports configuration settings to allow model authors to explicitly control whether ad-hoc answers should be enabled as well.

Let's start by allowing Cortana to access specific datasets.

1. By default, Power BI datasets are not enabled for Cortana. You need to turn on the Cortana integration for each dataset that you want Cortana to access. Open your web browser and log in to the Power BI portal. In the Application Toolbar at the top-right corner, expand the Settings (gear) menu, and then click Settings.

2. In the Settings page, click the Datasets tab (**Figure 10.26**).

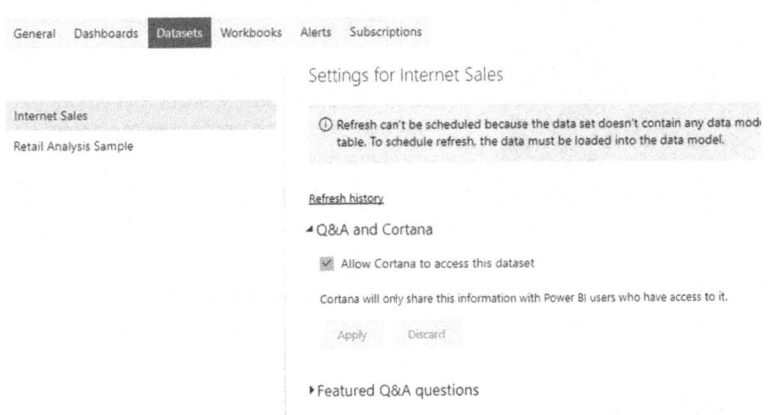

Figure 10.26 Use the Settings page to enable Cortana to access datasets.

3. To enable Cortana for the "Internet Sales" dataset, click that dataset, and then check the "Allow Cortana to access this dataset" checkbox. Click Apply. Now Cortana can access this dataset and its dependent reports and dashboards, but give it some time to discover it and learn about its data.

4. On your desktop, type in the dashboard or report name. Once you see it in the Cortana list, click it and watch it open in a separate browser window.

Creating answer cards

If you want to get more from Cortana, you'd need to create Cortana answer cards. As of this time, Cortana answer cards work only if the dataset is created in Power BI Desktop. They don't work for the Power BI samples or for reports created from datasets that are imported directly in Power BI Service. Let's create quickly a Cortana answer card in Power BI Desktop (you can also do this directly in Power BI Service):

1. Add a new page to your report. Change the page name to *Internet Sales*.

2. Click the gray area outside the report canvas to unselect any visualization you might have selected. Select the Format tab in the Visualization pane to access the page properties.

3. Change the page type to Cortana. Power BI will reduce the page size, so it fits the Cortana window.

4. (Optional) In the Page Information section of the Visualization pane, enter additional synonyms if you want users to search by other phrases, such as *Cortana Sales answer card*. Remember that Cortana requires at least two words for questions.

5. Add and configure some visualizations to that card that you want to see in Cortana (see **Figure 10.27**).

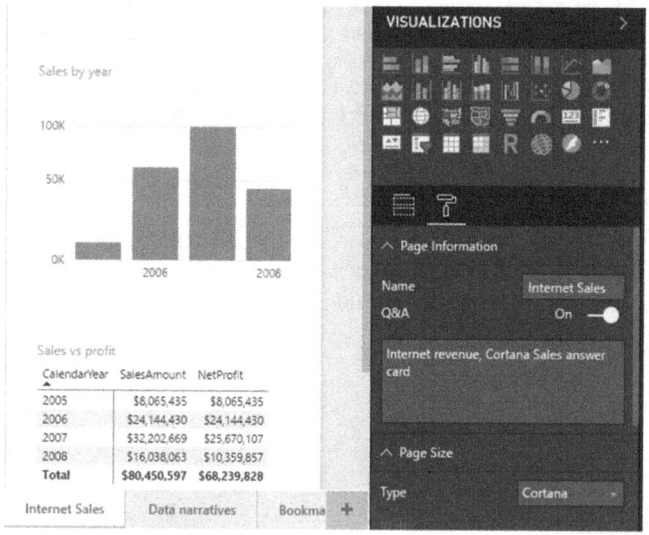

Figure 10.27 Create a Cortana answer card to provide preconfigured reports to Cortana questions.

6. (Optional) To require the user to specify a report filter, add a field to the Page Filters area, change the filter mode to Basic and check "Require single selection". Cortana will only display this report as an answer if the question includes one of the filter items.

7. Deploy the file to Power BI Service and remember to enable Q&A in the dataset settings. Give some time for Cortana to discover and index the card.

Getting data insights with Cortana

Now that the answer card is ready, let's take Cortana for a ride.

1. In the Windows search box, enter the page name or one of synonyms, such as "Internet revenue" or "what's Internet revenue". Cortana should show some matches under the Power BI category. Alternatively, you can say "Hey Cortana" to activate Cortana and dictate your question.

2. Click the match. Cortana shows the answer card as you've designed it (see **Figure 10.28**). Notice that the report includes interactive features, such as cross-highlighting and sorting!

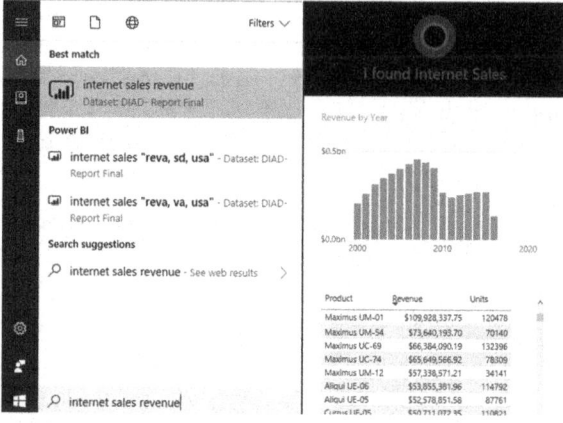

Figure 10.28 Cortana finds Power BI matches to your questions and visualizes your data.

3. (Optional) If you have enabled the answer card for Q&A, you can further explore the data by appending to the card name, such as "Internet revenue for 2010". To further explore an answer, click the "Open in

Power BI" link under the visualization. This opens your Web browser and navigates you to the Power BI Q&A page that is prepopulated with the same question. From here, Q&A takes on.

Can't get enough from Cortana or get it to work at all? Try the "Troubleshoot Cortana for Power BI" article at https://powerbi.microsoft.com/documentation/powerbi-service-cortana-troubleshoot/?

As you can see, Cortana opens new opportunities to enable your business, and your customers' businesses, to get things done in more helpful, proactive, and natural ways.

10.3.3 Narrating Data

Power BI by itself doesn't have data narrating capabilities. But as an open platform, third-party vendors can extend it in versatile ways. Narrative Science has contributed a Narratives for Business Intelligence custom visual that explains the data in natural language. These intelligence narratives bring the following value:

■ Tell stories from your data – Narratives can be generated from any data source.

■ Act as a companion analyst – Dynamic narratives update as you change visualizations.

■ Can be customized and shared – Narratives are updated when you set filters or apply cross-highlighting, extending the context of insights.

Getting started with data narratives
Let's examine the Sales by Year report shown in **Figure 10.29**. The Narratives for Business Intelligence custom visual explains the data. The chart and custom visual aren't connected. I just configured the custom visual the same way I configured the chart.

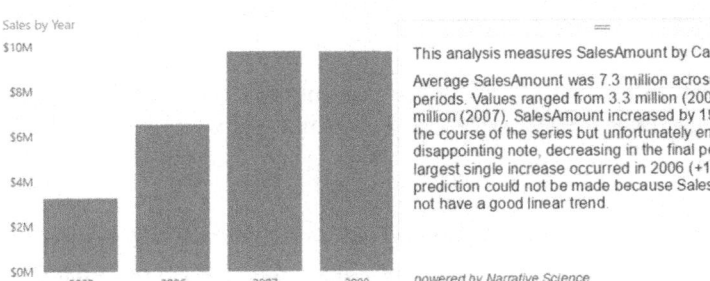

Figure 10.29 The narrative next to the column chart explains the data in the chart.

As you can see, the custom visual explains the data in English. What's not so obvious is that if you filter the report, such as when you set a slicer or cross-filter it from another visual, the custom visual would pick the filter and change the narrative!

Configuring narratives
Configuring the Narratives for Power BI visual is not much different than configuring any other visual:

1. Click the ellipsis (…) in the Visualizations pane, and then click "Import from store". Find and import the Narratives for Business Intelligence visual.

2. Drop the visual on the report canvas. Drag CalendarYear (Date table) to the Dimensions area in the Visualizations pane. Drag SalesAmount (InternetSales table) to the Values area.

3. When the visual asks you "How would you describe your data?", leave the "Continues" data type selected, and then click Write Narrative.

This covers the basics but notice that you can customize the visual behavior by clicking the Settings button. For more information about the Narratives for Business Intelligence visual, refer to the "Narratives for Power BI Solution Overview" article at https://narrativescience.com/Resources/Resource-Library/Article-Detail-Page/narratives-for-power-bi-solution-overview.

10.3.4 Sharing Insights with Bookmarks

Imagine you're working on some an executive report that will provide insights into the sales performance of your organization. You end up with many visualizations on many pages. You're concerned that the message might be lost in the minutia of details. You need a way to communicate the data story step by step. This is where bookmarking can help. In Power BI, effective data storytelling with bookmarking involves three features:

■ Bookmarks – A bookmark is a captured state of a report page that saves the visibility and applied filters, including cross highlighting from other visuals. For example, if Martin wants to start his presentation with the sales for the current year, he can apply a date filter and save the page as a bookmark. However, a bookmark is not a data snapshot. Although the filters are preserved, the visual would still query the underlying dataset because the data is not saved in the bookmark.

■ Visual visibility – Sometimes less is more. When drawing attention to specific visuals, you could hide other visuals on the page. You can configure the visual visibility using the Power BI Selection pane.

■ Spotlight – Instead of hiding visuals, you might decide to fade some away by bringing others to the forefront (in the spotlight).

 NOTE As of this time, bookmarking is a preview feature and it's not enabled by default. Make sure to enable Bookmarks from File ⇨ Options and Settings ⇨ Options (Preview Features tab).

Creating bookmarks
You can create as many bookmarks as needed to communicate a story efficiently. Consider the Bookmarks page in the Adventure Works.pbix file. Suppose you want to start your presentation by showing the USA sales first.

1. Change the Country slicer to "United States".
2. In the View ribbon, check Bookmarks Pane. In the Bookmarks Pane, click Add to create a new bookmark.
3. Double-click "Bookmark 1" and change its name to *USA* (or expand its ellipsis menu and click Rename). Compare your results with **Figure 10.30**.

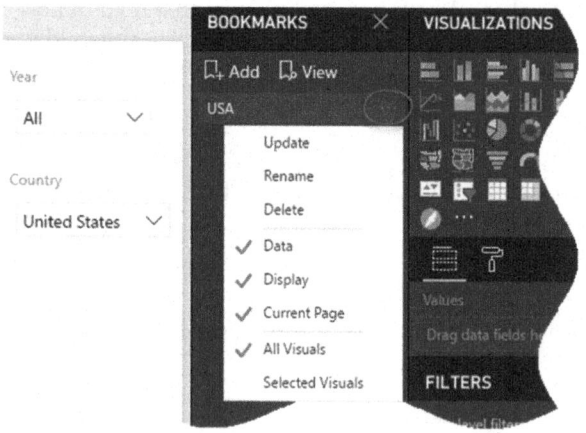

Figure 10.30 The Bookmarks Pane shows all bookmarks defined in the report and let you specify which properties the bookmark saves.

4. To test the bookmark, clear the Country slider to show data for all countries. In the Bookmarks Pane, click the USA bookmark. Notice that the Country slider is filtered for USA.

5. (Optional) Navigate to another report page and then click the USA bookmark. Notice that Power BI navigates to the Bookmarks page. It's helpful to think about the Bookmarks Pane as a Table of Contents (TOC) of your report to help you navigate pages.

6. Click the ellipsis (…) menu next to the USA bookmark in the Bookmarks pane. Notice that you can configure what visual properties get saved in the bookmark. For example, when Data is selected, the data-related properties (filters and slicers) will be saved. The Display property is for saving the "visual" properties, such as visibility and spotlight. And "Current Page" is for the page change that moves users to the page that was visible when the bookmark was added.

By default, a bookmark saves all visuals on the page. However, if you want to save only specific visuals, you can hold the Ctrl key and select them one by one, and then enable the "Selected Visuals" option in the bookmark properties.

Hiding visuals

When you tell your data story, you might prefer to hide some visuals on a busy report so that a bookmark brings attention to the most important visuals. Suppose you want to hide the scatter chart when showing the USA sales.

1. In the View ribbon, check the Selection Pane to add it to the report. The pane lists all the visuals on the page and allows you to change their visibility.

2. Click the eye icon next to the Clusters visual to hide it. Notice that you can also reorder visuals. This could be useful if you have overlapping visuals and you want to change their display order.

3. Expand the ellipsis (…) menu next to the USA bookmark in the Bookmarks Pane and then click Update. This updates the bookmark to reflect the current state of the page, as shown in **Figure 10.31**

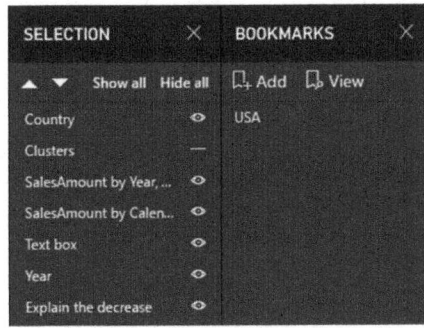

Figure 10.31 Use the Selection Pane to change the visibility of visuals.

4. In the Selection Pane, click "Show all" to show all visuals and clear the Country slider. Add another bookmark and name it *Default*. Drag the Default bookmark before the USA bookmark.

5. Click the Default bookmark and then click the USA bookmark. Notice that the Default bookmark shows all visuals without filters, while the USA bookmark doesn't show the Clusters visual and shows data only for USA.

6. In the Bookmarks Pane, click View. Notice that a slider is added to the bottom of the report that allows you to navigate your bookmarks. The same slider is available when you deploy a report with bookmarks to Power BI Service and view the report. Use the slider to tell your story one step at a time.

7. Click the Exit button in the Bookmarks pane to exit the View mode.

> **TIP** Although frequently used together with bookmarking, the Selection Pane is also useful during report authoring and analysis. For example, when analyzing data on a busy report page, you might want to focus on a specific visual and hide the rest.

Bringing visuals to spotlight

Instead of hiding visuals, you can fade them away by using the Spotlight feature that is available for every visual on the page. Suppose that you want to start your presentation by bringing focus to the "Explain the decrease" column chart.

1. In the Bookmarks Pane, click the Default bookmark.

2. Hover on the column chart, click the ellipsis (…) menu in the top-right corner, and then click Spotlight. The chart stands out while all other visuals fade away in the background.

3. In the Bookmarks pane, click the ellipsis (…) menu next to the Default bookmark and click Update. If you can't find the ellipsis menu, make sure to first click the Exit button to exit the View mode.

Using images to trigger bookmarks

Sometimes, you might want to allow users to click "buttons" to toggle visibility of visuals or to navigate them to different pages. You can use any image to trigger a bookmark.

1. In the Home ribbon, click the Image button and import the On.jpg image from the \Source\ch10 folder.

2. Size and position the image above the "Explain the decrease" chart.

3. Click the image to select it. The Visualizations Pane changes to Format Image pane.

4. Turn on the Link slider. Expand the Link section in the Format Image pane. Expand the Type drop-down and select Bookmark. Recall that the other option (Back) can be used to navigate the user from a drillthrough page to the calling page.

5. Expand the Bookmark drop-down and select the USA bookmark, as shown in **Figure 10.32**.

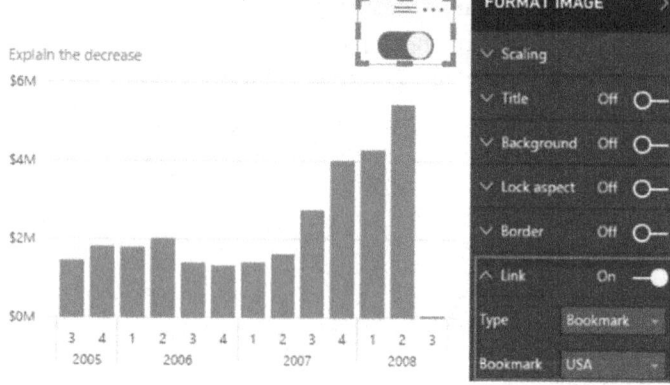

Figure 10.32 Configure an image to act as a button for navigating the user to a bookmark.

6. To test the changes, hold the Ctrl key and click the image. Notice that it navigates you to the USA bookmark.

7. (Optional) Add an "Off" image and position it behind the "On" image. Link the "Off" image to the Default bookmark. Hide the "Off" image in the selection pane and update the Default bookmark. Update the USA bookmark to show the "Off" image and hide the "On" image. The desired effect is to allow the user to toggle the image "button".

10.4 Summary

Power BI is all about bringing your data to life and getting insights to make decisions faster. You can show more details behind a data point by drilling down, drilling across, and drilling through. You can create custom groups and bins. Conditional formatting helps change colors to spot trends easier. You can extend your reports with links that bring users to other systems and display web images.

Power BI doesn't limit you to only descriptive analytics. Use Explain Increase/decrease for root cause analysis. Use time-series forecasting to predict periods in the future. Find data similarities by detecting clusters. And use R scripts for data cleansing, predictive analytics, and custom visuals.

Consider the Power BI data storytelling capabilities to communicate your insights more effectively. Get insights by asking natural questions on the desktop as you do in Power BI Service. Integrate Cortana on your Windows 10 computer with Power BI so that you can ask natural questions as you work without navigating to powerbi.com. Explain the story behind a visual with Narratives for Power BI. Walk your audience through your data story by creating bookmarks.

By now, as a data analyst, you should have sufficient knowledge to implement sophisticated self-service data models. One important task though is publishing your model to Power BI Service and sharing it with your teammates, which I'll discuss in the next chapter.

PART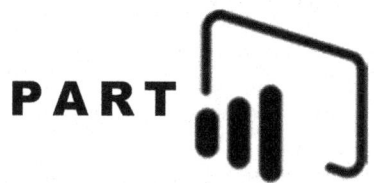

Power BI for Pros

BI and IT pros have much to gain from Power BI. Information technology (IT) pros are concerned with setting up and maintaining the necessary environment that facilitates self-service and organizational BI, such as providing access to data, managing security, data governance, and other services. On the other hand, BI pros are typically tasked to create backend services required to support organizational BI initiative, including data marts and data warehouses, cubes, ETL packages, operational reports, and dashboards.

We're back to Power BI Service now. This part of the book gives IT pros the necessary background to establish a trustworthy and collaborative environment! You'll learn how Power BI security works. You'll see how you can create workspaces and groups to promote team BI where multiple coworkers can work on the same BI artifacts. Finally, you'll learn how to create apps so that you can push BI content to a larger audience and even to the entire company. And you'll discover how the on-premises data gateway can help you centralize data management and implement hybrid solutions where your data remains on premises, but you can still enjoy Power BI interactive reports dashboards and reports that connect to the data via the gateway.

Next, you'll see why Power BI Premium is preferred by larger organizations. You'll understand how to move workspaces to a premium capacity and how to secure them. You'll learn about features that are only available in Power BI Premium. I'll show you how to use Power BI Report Server to implement on-premises report portals for centralizing and managing different types of reports.

I'll show BI pros how to integrate popular organizational BI scenarios with Power BI. If you've invested in on-premises Analysis Services models, you'll see how you can create reports and dashboards connected to these models without moving data to the cloud. If you plan to implement real-time BI solutions, I'll show how you can do that with Azure Stream Analytics and Power BI. And if you're interested in predictive analytics, you'll see how you can integrate Power BI with Azure Machine Learning!

Chapter 11

Enabling Team BI

We all need to share information, and this is even more true with BI artifacts that help an organization understand its business. To accomplish this, an IT department (referred to as "IT" in this book) must establish a trustworthy environment where users have secure access to the BI content and data they need. While traditionally Microsoft has promoted SharePoint for sharing all your documents, including BI artifacts, Power BI doesn't have dependencies on SharePoint Server or SharePoint Online. Power BI has its own sharing and collaboration capabilities! Although these capabilities are available to all users, establishing a cooperative environment should happen under the guidance and supervision of IT. Therefore, I discuss sharing and collaboration in this part of the book.

Currently, Power BI doesn't have all the SharePoint data governance capabilities, such as workflows, taxonomy, self-service BI monitoring, versioning, retention, and others. Although a large organization might be concerned about the lack of such management features now, Power BI gains in simplicity and this is a welcome change for many who have struggled with SharePoint complexity, and for organizations that haven't invested in SharePoint. This chapter starts by laying out the Power BI management fundamentals. Next, it discusses workspaces and groups, and then explains how members of a department or a group can share Power BI artifacts. Next, it shows you how IT can leverage Power BI organizational apps to bundle and publish content across your organization, and how to centralize data management.

11.1 Power BI Management Fundamentals

Recall from Chapter 2 that Power BI makes it easy for users to sign up for Power BI. When the first user signs up, Power BI creates an unmanaged "shadow" tenant (yourcompany.onmicrosoft.com) in Azure AD. It's unmanaged because it's under Microsoft's management, not yours. I refer to this stage as "The Wild West". Everyone can sign up without any supervision. The next progression is to take over the unmanaged tenant in Office 365. This allows the Office 365 admin to manage certain aspects of the user enrollment and enables the Power BI Admin Center. The final step is to federate your organizational Active Directory to Azure Active Directory to achieve a single sign-on between your on-premises AD and Azure Active Directory. To accomplish this, you can use the DirSync tool to synchronize your on-premises AD with Azure, or you can federate (extend) your corporate AD to Azure.

   NOTE If you deploy models with imported data, your data will be stored in a Microsoft data center in a specific geography. When the first user signs up, Power BI will ask the user which country your company is located in. Based on the country selection, Power BI will choose a data center. Unfortunately, once that data center is selected and associated with the tenant, it can't be changed although there are good scenarios to do so, such as a multinational company that prefers a data center closer to where most of the Power BI users will be located. For more information about Power BI data regions, read the "How the Power BI Data Region is selected" blog by Adam Saxton at https://guyinacube.com/2016/08/power-bi-data-region-selected.

11.1.1 Managing User Access

If your tenant is still unmanaged, I strongly suggest you or your system administrator take it over so that it can be actively managed. I said "system administrator" because the takeover process requires knowledge of your organization's domain setup and small changes to the domain registration so that Power BI can verify domain ownership. For more information about the specific takeover steps, refer to the blog "How to perform an IT Admin Takeover with O365" by Adam Saxton at https://powerbi.microsoft.com/en-us/blog/how-to-perform-an-it-admin-takeover-with-o365.

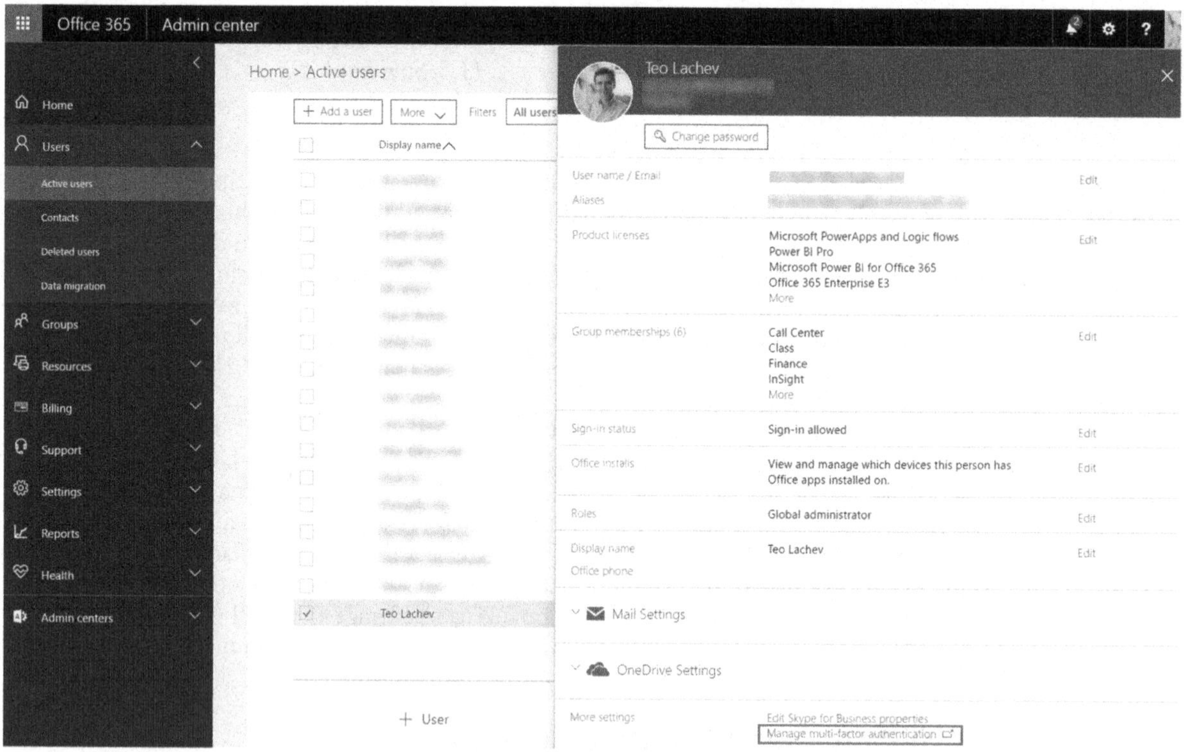

Figure 11.1 The global administrator can manage users and Power BI licenses in the Office 365 Admin Center.

Managing users

Once the admin takeover is completed, the Office 365 global administrator can use the Office 365 Admin Center (https://portal.office.com) to manage users and licenses (see **Figure 11.1**). Another way to navigate to the Office 365 Admin Center is to click the "Office 365 Application Launcher" icon in the top left corner of the Power BI portal and then click the Admin button. Only Office 365 global admins can see the Admin button. Finally, a third option to navigate directly to the "Active Users" section of the Office 365 Admin Center is from the "Manage users" area in the Power BI Admin Portal (discussed in the "Using the Admin Portal" section later in this chapter).

> **TIP** You can promote users to O365 global administrators by clicking Edit next to the Roles item in the user properties and then assigning the user to the "Global administrator" role. This will grant the user rights to manage all aspects of the Office 365 tenant, including Power BI licenses.

Unless you extend or synchronize your on-premises AD, the user chooses a password when the user signs up with Power BI. The Power BI password is independent of the password he uses to log in to the corporate network. As a best practice, it's a good idea to expire passwords on a regular basis. Switching to a managed client gives you a limited control over the password policy, which you can find under the Settings menu in the left toolbar ⇨ "Security & privacy". You can turn on the password expiration policy using the "Days before password expire" setting. You can also specify if the users will be able to reset their passwords.

Managing licenses

From a Power BI standpoint, one important task that the administrator will perform is managing Power BI Pro licenses for internal and external (B2B) users. Users don't need a license to access Power BI Free features. Yet, your organization might have concerns about indiscriminate enrolling to Power BI and uploading corporate data. Solutions can be found in the "Power BI in your organization" document by Microsoft at http://bit.ly/1IY87Qt.

Users contributing Power BI content require a Power BI Pro license. Unless the workspace is in a Power BI Premium capacity, recipients of shared content also require a Power BI Pro license. The Product Licenses section of the user properties (see again **Figure 11.1**) show what licenses the user has. Click the Edit link to grant the user a Power BI Pro license. This of course will entail a monthly subscription fee unless your organization is on the Office 365 E5 business plan which includes Power BI Pro.

Enabling conditional access

The cloud nature of Power BI could be both a blessing and a curse. Users can access Power BI reports and dashboards from anywhere and on any device if they're connected to Internet. However, unless you take additional steps, Power BI security hinges only on the user's password since the user email is not secure. One of the most important steps you can take to enforce an additional level of security is to restrict access to Power BI (and your organization's data) by enabling conditional access.

A multifactor authentication (MFA) is a security configuration that requires more than one method of authentication to verify the user's identity. For example, Office 365 could send an application password to the user's mobile device. The user will have to enter it in addition to the Power BI password when signing in to Power BI. You can enable MFA for all Office 365 services (see the corresponding link in the "More settings" section on the user properties page in **Figure 11.1**) or just for Power BI.

 NOTE Depending on the O365 business plan your organization has, tenant-level MFA might require an additional fee, or it might be included in the plan. For more information about MFA, read the "Getting started with Azure Multi-Factor Authentication in the cloud" article by Kelly Gremban at https://docs.microsoft.com/en-us/azure/multi-factor-authentication/multi-factor-authentication-get-started-cloud.Configuring application-level access (also known as conditional rules) requires a subscription to Azure Active Directory Premium. In addition, it requires a federated or managed Azure Active Directory tenant.

Follow these steps to enable MFA for Power BI only:

1. Open your browser and navigate to portal.azure.com and sign in with your account (you need to be an admin on the tenant).
2. In the left navigation bar, click Azure Active Directory.
3. In your AD organization page, click the Enterprise Applications tab, and then click All Applications.
4. Change the filter on top of the page to Microsoft Applications.
5. Scroll down the list and click Power BI Service (see **Figure 11.2**).
6. In the next page, click the Configure link.

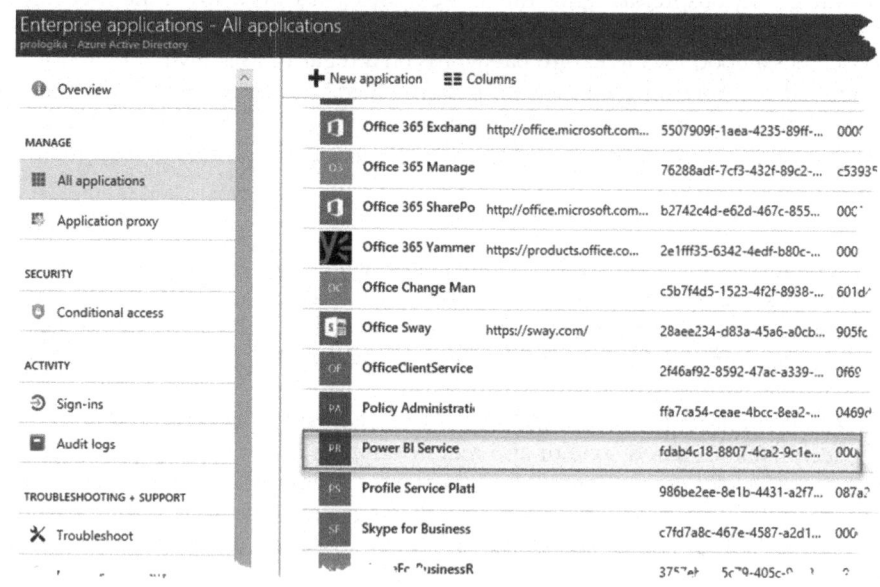

Figure 11.2 Use the Azure Portal to enable MFA for Power BI.

7. In the next page, click Conditional Access and set rules. For more information about how to do this, read the "Conditional Access now in the new Azure portal" article by Microsoft at https://cloudblogs.microsoft.com/enterprisemobility/2016/12/15/conditional-access-now-in-the-new-azure-portal/.

Understanding conditional rules

You can set up the following rules:

■ Require Multi-factor authentication – Users to whom access rules apply will be required to complete multi-factor authentication before accessing the application affected by the rule.

■ Require Multi-factor authentication when not at work – Users trying to access the application from a trusted IP address won't be required to perform multi-factor authentication. Click the link below to enter the trusted IP address ranges that define your work location.

■ Block access when not at work – Users trying to access the application from outside your corporate network will not be able to access the application.

 REAL LIFE I helped a large organization to evaluate and adopt Power BI. One of the first questions their review committee asked was if they can limit access to Power BI only from the corporate network and from approved devices. I didn't have a good answer then. Conditional access can help you meet this requirement.

Once the rules are configured, Azure will apply them when a user attempts to sign in to Power BI. For example, let's say that Elena (Office 365 admin) has configured a conditional access policy requiring MFA for only Power BI. When Maya visits the Office 365 portal to check her email, she can log in (or automatically sign in if the active directory is federated to Azure) without using MFA. But when Maya tries to navigate to Power BI, she'll be asked to complete an MFA challenge irrespective of the device she uses. If the "Block access when not at work" rule is enabled, she can access Power BI only from the corporate network.

 TIP You can secure access to Power BI even further by enabling these conditional access policies alongside Risk Based Conditional Access policy available with Azure AD Identity Protection. Azure Identity Protection detects risk events involving identities in Azure Active Directory that indicate that the identities may have been compromised. For more information, read the "AzureAD Identity Protection adds support for federated identities" at bit.ly/2gwdTGu.

11.1.2 Using the Admin Portal

Power BI provides an admin portal to allow the administrator to monitor Power BI utilization and to control tenant wide settings. To access the Admin Portal, log in to Power BI Service, expand the Settings menu in the top-right corner, and then click Admin Portal.

Understanding portal access

To see the Admin Portal menu, you have a member of one of these roles:

- Office 365 Global Administrator – The Office 365 global administrator can manage all aspects of Office 365, including Power BI.

- Power BI Service Administrator – The Office 365 global administrator can delegate Power BI admin access to other users. Since currently there isn't a user interface for this task, the global administrator would need to run a PowerShell command (before you run the command, install Azure PowerShell from https://docs.microsoft.com/en-us/powershell/).

For example, to grant Martin Power BI Administrator rights to the Adventure Works Power BI tenant, Elena would execute the following command:

Add-MsolRoleMember -RoleMemberEmailAddress "martin@adventureworks.com" -RoleName "Power BI Service Administrator"

Now Martin can access the Power BI Admin Portal, which is shown in **Figure 11.3**. Currently, the portal has five management areas (Usage metrics, Manage Users, Audit logs, Tenant and Capacity settings).

Admin portal

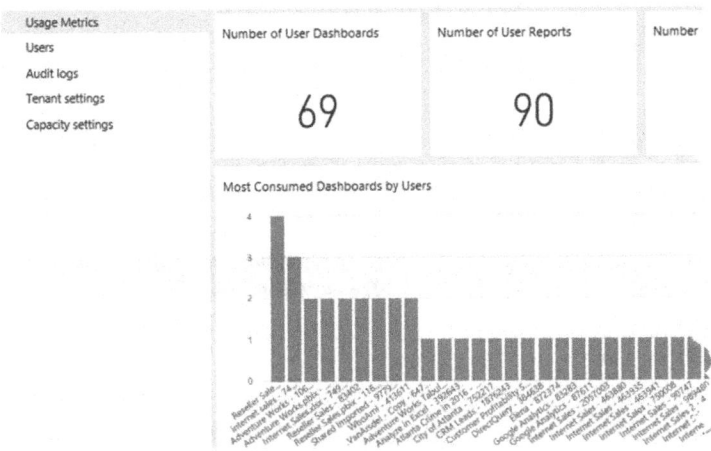

Figure 11.3 Use the Admin Portal to view usage statistics and control tenant wide settings.

Monitoring usage metrics

The "Usage metrics" management area provides insights into the usage of Power BI within your organization. It opens a dashboard that has two sections of tiles:

- User-level information – The top three rows provide usage statistics for individual users, including the total number of dashboards, reports, and datasets, top users with most dashboards and reports, most consumed dashboards, and most consumed content packs.

- Group-level information – The bottom three rows provide the same information but for groups (I'll discuss workspaces and groups in the next section).

The "Usage metrics" is a good starting point to help you understand Power BI utilization but much more is needed to make it useful. I hope Microsoft extends it in the future with additional health monitoring features to help you proactively manage Power BI, such as CPU and memory utilization, data quotas, refresh failures, and others.

Managing users

The second management area (Manage users) includes a shortcut that brings you to the Office 365 Admin Center (see again **Figure 11.1**). Recall that you can use the Office 365 Admin Center to manage users, licenses, and groups.

Auditing logs

The "Audit logs" management area provides another shortcut to the Office 365 portal where you view tenant activity and export the audit logs. I'll discuss auditing user activity in the next section.

Managing tenant settings

Go to the "Tenant settings" section of the Admin Portal to manage tenant-wide settings (see **Figure 11.4**). Many of these settings can be enabled for specific security groups or the entire organization but some, such as dashboard tagging, are organization-level only.

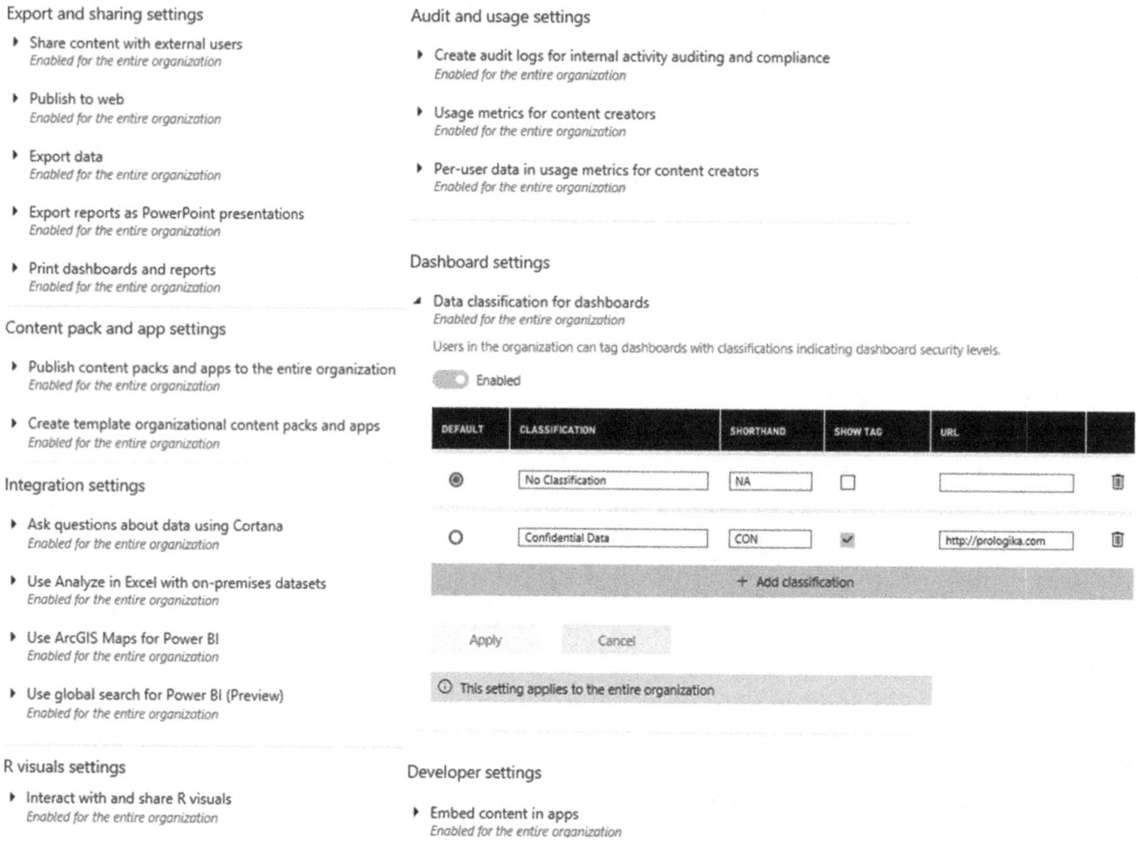

Export and sharing settings

▸ Share content with external users
  Enabled for the entire organization

▸ Publish to web
  Enabled for the entire organization

▸ Export data
  Enabled for the entire organization

▸ Export reports as PowerPoint presentations
  Enabled for the entire organization

▸ Print dashboards and reports
  Enabled for the entire organization

Content pack and app settings

▸ Publish content packs and apps to the entire organization
  Enabled for the entire organization

▸ Create template organizational content packs and apps
  Enabled for the entire organization

Integration settings

▸ Ask questions about data using Cortana
  Enabled for the entire organization

▸ Use Analyze in Excel with on-premises datasets
  Enabled for the entire organization

▸ Use ArcGIS Maps for Power BI
  Enabled for the entire organization

▸ Use global search for Power BI (Preview)
  Enabled for the entire organization

R visuals settings

▸ Interact with and share R visuals
  Enabled for the entire organization

Audit and usage settings

▸ Create audit logs for internal activity auditing and compliance
  Enabled for the entire organization

▸ Usage metrics for content creators
  Enabled for the entire organization

▸ Per-user data in usage metrics for content creators
  Enabled for the entire organization

Dashboard settings

◢ Data classification for dashboards
  Enabled for the entire organization

Users in the organization can tag dashboards with classifications indicating dashboard security levels.

Enabled

DEFAULT	CLASSIFICATION	SHORTHAND	SHOW TAG	URL	
◉	No Classification	NA	☐		🗑
○	Confidential Data	CON	☑	http://prologika.com	🗑
	+ Add classification				

Apply   Cancel

ⓘ This setting applies to the entire organization

Developer settings

▸ Embed content in apps
  Enabled for the entire organization

Figure 11.4 Use the "Manage tenant settings" area to manage important tenant-wide security and functionality settings.

Understanding export and sharing settings

Let's go quickly through these settings. The "Share content with external users" controls whether users can share content to users external to your organization (discussed in more detail in section 11.3.1). By default, Power BI Pro users can share content to both internal and external users, so consider disabling this setting for added data security if not needed. The "Publish to web" setting is even more dangerous. By default, your users will be able to share reports anonymously to anyone on the Internet, such as by embedding reports in blogs! This is *not* the setting you need to share with external users securely. Strongly consider turning this setting off.

The "Export data" setting controls if users would be able to export data from report visualizations. By default, users would be able to export summarized and underlying data. When off, the "Export reports as PowerPoint presentations" disables exporting to PowerPoint (this export option is in the report File menu). Similarly, "Print dashboards and reports" disables the corresponding menus.

Understanding settings for content packs and apps

The "Publish content packs and apps to the entire organization" setting controls the allowed audience when creating organizational content packs and apps (discussed in the "Packaging and Publishing Content" section later in this chapter). If it's off, users can publish content packs to specific groups only.

Unless "Create template organizational content packs and apps" is off, when a user creates an organizational content with imported data they can decide to remove the data and package the content as a template content pack. This works conceptually like Power BI Desktop templates.

Understanding integration settings

When off, the "Ask questions about data using Cortana" setting disables Power BI integration with Cortana. Consequently, a Windows 10 user can't use Cortana to ask Power BI questions on the desktop (they must go to Power BI Service). Recall that the "Analyze in Excel" feature allows users to create pivot reports in Excel Desktop connected to Power BI datasets, just like they'd use Excel to connect to cubes. Users can publish the Excel reports to Power BI Service dashboards. "Analyze in Excel with on-premises datasets" disables this feature for datasets that connect directly to on-premises databases.

When off, "Use ArcGIS Maps for Power BI" removes this visual from the Visualizations pane in Power BI Service and disables usage of this visual. This control exists because ArcGIS maps may use the Esri cloud services that are outside of your Power BI tenant's geographic region. You saw in Chapter 10 how you can use Cortana to get answers from Power BI without navigating to Power BI Service. Behind the scenes, the Cortana integration relies on the Azure Search Service (https://azure.microsoft.com/en-us/services/search/) because of its ranking, error correction, and auto complete capabilities. The "Use global search for Power BI" controls if the Azure Search Service can access Power BI Service.

Understanding R visuals settings

"Interact with and share R visuals" is for custom visuals designed with R. R visuals can be created in Power BI Desktop, and then published to the Power BI service. Unless this setting is off, R visuals behave like any other visual in the Power BI service; users can interact, filter, slice, and pin them to a dashboard, or share them with others.

Understanding audit and usage settings

The "Audit and usage" section controls if Power BI will generate auditing and usage data from user activity. I'll discuss auditing in more detail in the next section but by default Power BI records the user activity which can be monitored in Office 365. I just explained the Usage Metrics tab of the Audit Portal. The next two settings control what usage data Power BI captures that can be analyzed on that tab.

Understanding dashboard settings

When on, "Data classifications for dashboards" lets you tag dashboards. For example, your users might have dashboards that show some sensitive information and they might request a mechanism to inform the users about it. As the administrator, you can use the Admin Portal to create a "Confidential Data" tag. Then, your users can go to the dashboard settings in Power BI Service and select the tag from the "Data classification" dropdown. Once they choose a tag, it'll show next to the dashboard name when the user views the dashboard in the Power BI portal (see **Figure 11.5**).

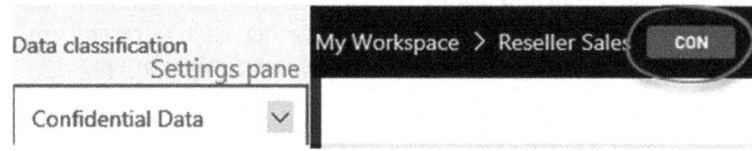

Figure 11.5 Users can use the data classification tags defined in the Admin Portal to tag dashboards.

If you mark a tag as a default tag in the Admin Portal (see again **Figure 11.4**), all new and existing dashboards will show this tag. To avoid this, create a dummy tag, set it as a default tag, and clear the "Show Tag" setting. Also, when setting up a tag, consider providing a tag URL so that users can click on the dashboard tag and learn more about why the dashboard was classified this way.

 NOTE Data classification tags could have been very useful for allowing IT to certify BI content. Unfortunately, every Power BI Pro user can access and change them from the dashboard settings because currently this feature is a tenant-level option. And it's limited to dashboards only.

Understanding developer settings
Developers can call the Power BI REST APIs to support two main scenarios for embedding Power BI content: embedding for internal users and embedding for external customers. The "Embed content in app" setting controls if these REST APIs can be invoked.

11.1.3 Auditing User Activity

Regulatory and compliance requirements are typically met with audit policies. Power BI can log certain user activities, such as creating, editing, printing, exporting, sharing reports and dashboards, and creating groups and content packs (for the full list, see "List of activities audited by Power BI" at http://bit.ly/power-biaudit).

Getting started with Power BI auditing
You can turn on Power BI auditing by flipping the "Create audit logs for internal activity auditing and compliance purposes" setting to On in the Power BI Admin Portal (see again **Figure 11.4**). Be patient though because audit logs can take up to 24 hours to show after you enable them. To see the actual logs, you need to use the Office 365 Admin Center again. A convenient shortcut is available in the "Audit Logs" area of the Power BI Admin Portal and it brings you directly to the "Audit search" page in the Office 365 Admin Center.

 NOTE Auditing is a Power BI Pro feature and auditing events are only available for Power BI Pro users. Users with Power BI (free) licenses will be displayed as Free User when you view the audit logs. In addition, to enable auditing for Power BI, you need at least one Exchange mailbox license in your tenant.

Viewing audit logs
The "Audit log search" page (see **Figure 11.6**) allows you to view and search all Office 365 audit logs. To view only the Power BI logs, expand the Activities drop-down and then select "Power BI activities" or choose specific Power BI activities, such as "Viewed Power BI dashboard". To search logs for a user, start typing in the user name and Power BI will show a drop-down to help you locate the user (you can enter multiple users). You can also subscribe to receive an alert that meets the search criteria.

If the search criteria result matches existing logs, the logs will be shown in the Results pane. You can see the date, the user IP address, user email, activity (corresponds to the items in the Activities drop-down), item (the object that was created or modified because of the corresponding activity) and Detail (some activities have more details). You can click a row to see more details, such as to see if the activity succeeded or failed. You can click the "Export results" to export the results as a CSV file.

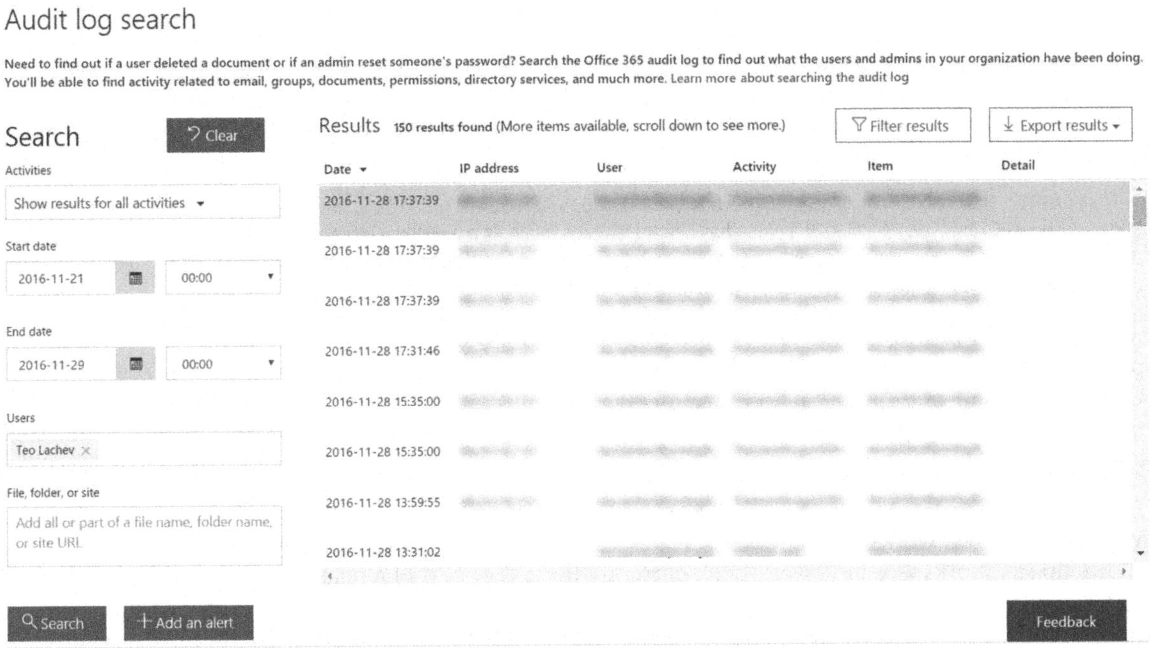

Audit log search

Need to find out if a user deleted a document or if an admin reset someone's password? Search the Office 365 audit log to find out what the users and admins in your organization have been doing. You'll be able to find activity related to email, groups, documents, permissions, directory services, and much more. Learn more about searching the audit log

Search		Results	150 results found (More items available, scroll down to see more.)					⊽ Filter results	↓ Export results ▾
	↻ Clear	Date ▾	IP address	User	Activity	Item	Detail		
Activities		2016-11-28 17:37:39							
Show results for all activities ▾		2016-11-28 17:37:39							
Start date		2016-11-28 17:37:39							
2016-11-21 📅	00:00 ▾	2016-11-28 17:31:46							
End date		2016-11-28 15:35:00							
2016-11-29 📅	00:00 ▾	2016-11-28 15:35:00							
Users		2016-11-28 13:59:55							
Teo Lachev ×		2016-11-28 13:31:02							
File, folder, or site									
Add all or part of a file name, folder name, or site URL									
🔍 Search	+ Add an alert							Feedback	

Figure 11.6 Use the "Audit log search" page to view Office 365 audit logs, including logs for Power BI.

11.2   Collaborating with Workspaces

Oftentimes, BI content needs to be shared within an organizational unit or with members of a project group. Typically, the group members require write access so that they can collaborate on the artifacts they produce and create new content. This is where Power BI workspaces can help. Remember that as with all sharing options, only Power BI Pro users can create workspaces.

For example, now that Martin has created a self-service data model with Power BI Desktop, he would like to share it with his coworkers from the Sales department. Because his colleagues also intend to produce self-service data models, Martin approaches Elena to set up a workspace for the Sales department. The workspace would only allow the members of his unit to create and share BI content.

11.2.1 Understanding Workspaces and Groups

A Power BI workspace is a container of BI content (datasets, reports, and dashboards) that its members share and collaborate on. By default, all the content you create goes to the default workspace called "My Workspace". Think of My Workspace as your private desk – no one can see its content unless you share it.

By contrast, a workspace is shared by all the members. Although Microsoft indicated that they will decouple workspaces from Office 365 groups, currently workspaces rely on Office 365 groups so let's take a moment to understand what an Office 365 group is.

What is a group?

From an implementation standpoint, a group is a record in Azure Active Directory (AAD) that has a shared membership. Office 365 supports multiple group types, such as Office 365 groups, Office 365 distribution lists, security groups, and Exchange distribution lists. To understand why you need Office 365 groups consider that today every Office 365 online application (Exchange, SharePoint, OneDrive for Business, Skype for Business, Yammer, and others) has its own security model, making it very difficult to restrict and manage security across applications. Microsoft introduced groups in Office 365 to simplify this and to foster sharing and collaboration.

 NOTE Conceptually, an Office 365 group is like a Windows AD security group; both have members and can be used to simplify security. However, an Office 365 group has shared features (such as a mailbox, calendar, task list, and others) that Windows groups don't have. Unlike security groups, Office 365 groups can't be nested. To learn more about Office 365 groups, read the "Find help about groups in Office 365" document by Microsoft at http://bit.ly/1BhDecS.

Although Power BI workspaces use Office 365 groups behind the scenes, they don't require an Office 365 plan. However, if you have an Office 365 subscription or if you're an administrator of your organization's Office 365 tenant, you can use both Power BI and the Office 365 portal to create and manage groups. You must use Office 365 to manage some aspects of the group, such as the group description, to see the group email address, and to find which groups a user is a member of.

How workspaces relate to groups

When you create a workspace, Power BI creates a group and vice versa, a group created in Office 365 shows up as a workspace in Power BI. So, currently there is one-to-one relationship between a workspace and a group and you can't have one without the other. A Power BI user can be added to multiple workspaces. For example, **Figure 11.7** shows that besides My Workspace, I'm a member of several other workspaces, which I can access by clicking the Workspaces menu in the navigation bar.

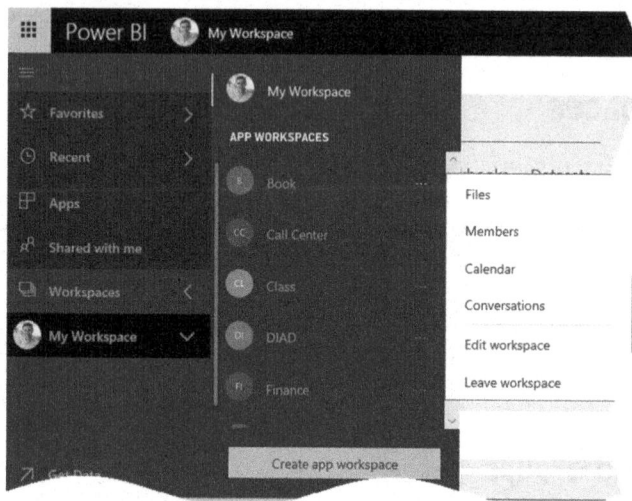

Figure 11.7 A user can belong to multiple workspaces and he can access them by clicking the Workspaces menu.

Currently there isn't a way to move or copy content from one workspace, such as from My Workspace to another. Therefore, it makes sense to create a workspace before you start adding content to Power BI. If you're a Power BI Pro user, think of who you want to share the content with and create a workspace that includes these people. As I said, workspaces typically align with organizational departments.

Understanding collaboration features

Because the primary goal of Power BI workspaces is to facilitate communication and collaboration, they go beyond BI and support collaborative features. Workspaces members can access these features by clicking the ellipsis (…) menu next to the workspace name, as shown in **Figure 11.7**. Alternatively, click the workspace and from the workspace content page, click the ellipsis (…) menu in the top-right corner. Let's review the available collaboration features:

■ Files – Brings you to the OneDrive for Business file storage that's dedicated to the workspace. That's right, a workspace gets its one Power BI storage quota (10 GB with Power BI Pro) and its OneDrive for Business cloud storage. While you can save all types of files to OneDrive, Excel workbooks used to import data to Power BI are particularly interesting. As I mentioned, that's because Power BI automatically refreshes the datasets you import from Excel files stored to OneDrive every ten minutes or when the file is updated.

■ Members – This menu allows you to manage the group membership, such as to view, add, or remove members.

■ Calendar – This brings you to a shared group calendar that helps members coordinate their schedules. Everyone in the group sees meeting invites and other events posted to the group calendar. Events that you create in the group calendar are automatically added and synchronized with your personal calendar. For events that other members create, you can add the event from the group calendar to your personal calendar. Changes you make to those events automatically synchronize with your personal calendar.

■ Conversations – Think of a conversation as a real-time discussion list. The conversations page displays each message. If you use Outlook, conversations messages are delivered to a separate folder dedicated to the group. You can either use Outlook or the conversation page to reply to messages and you can include attachments.

■ Edit workspace – This allows you to change the workspace name and manage membership. You can also delete the workspace. Deleting a workspace deletes all its content so be very careful!

■ Leave workspace – Use this menu if you want to be removed from the workspace.

11.2.2 Managing Workspaces

Currently, any Power BI Pro user can create a workspace. The user who creates the workspace becomes its administrator. The administrator has full control over the workspace, such as adding other users as members, renaming, or deleting the workspace.

Creating workspaces

Creating a workspace only takes a few mouse clicks:

1. Once you log in to Power BI Service, click Workspaces in the navigation bar.
2. Click the "Create app workspace" button (see again **Figure 11.7**).
3. In the "Create an app workspace" window (shown in **Figure 11.8**), enter the workspace name and members, and click Save.

Let's go through these settings in more detail. When creating a workspace, you need to give it a name, such as *Finance*. Every workspace has a unique identifier which Power BI auto-generates from the name. A workspace can have one of the following privacy settings:

■ Private (default) – Only the group members can access the content.

■ Public – Every user can become a member and gain access to the workspace. A public workspace doesn't automatically grant access to everyone. Users still must discover and join its group. One way for users to discover public groups is to use Outlook, as explained in more detail in "Join a group in Outlook" at bit.ly/2fAIQtn.

Create an app workspace

Name your workspace

Finance

Workspace ID

finance

✎ Available

Private - Only approved members can see what's inside ⌄

Members can edit Power BI content
Members can only view Power BI content

Add workspace members

Enter email addresses

Add

teo.lachev@prologika.com   Admin   ⌄ 🗑

finance@prologika.onmicrosoft.com   🗑

Advanced ⌃

Premium ⓘ
⬤ Off

Save   Cancel

Figure 11.8 When creating a workspace, specify the group name, privacy, member access, and membership.

Understanding content security

Next, you need to specify the content permissions for workspace members: edit or only view content. It's important to understand that the content permissions are granted at a workspace level and *not* at the member level. However, admin users always have the rights to create and edit content. It's important to consider content security when you plan your workspaces.

If you select "Members can only view Power BI content", all the members will get read-only rights to the group's content. Now all the members of this group can only view the Power BI dashboards and reports inside the workspace. They can't create or edit content. They can't even view the datasets in the workspace.

If you select "Members can edit Power BI content", all the members will get unrestricted rights to the workspace content, including removing datasets, reports, and dashboards. However, they can't change the workspace membership or delete the workspace.

 NOTE Microsoft views workspaces primarily to let teams collaborate on shared content, so the default option is "Members can edit Power BI content". Unfortunately, this means that the Sales department can't add members from another department as view-only members. To provide read-only access, the Sales department must resort to sharing specific dashboards or publishing an app.

Understanding membership

If you want to add members right away, enter a name or email alias in the "Add workspace members" field. You can separate multiple members with a comma (,) or a semi-colon (;). You can add individual members or Office 365 groups. The chances are that by the time you read this, Office 365 distribution lists and security groups will also be supported as Microsoft promised to unify group membership across Power BI features (more details in my "Power BI Group Security" blog at http://prologika.com/power-bi-group-security/)

Individual users can be added with one of two roles: Admin or Member. Administrators have unrestricted access to the workspace. Members gain permissions according to the content security rights you specify. Don't bother adding Power BI Free users because they won't be able to gain access since sharing is a Power BI Pro feature. They will see the workspace added to their navigation bar, but they will be asked to upgrade to Power BI Pro when they try to access its content. The only way to share content with Power BI Free users is to purchase a Power BI Premium plan and move the workspace to a premium capacity, which is what the Premium slider on the bottom of the window is for (it will be disabled if your organization isn't on Power BI Premium). I'll discuss Power BI Premium in the next chapter.

Once the group is created, a welcome page opens that's very similar to the Get Data page, so that you can start adding content the group can work on.

 NOTE It might take a while for Office 365 to fully provision a group and enable its collaboration features. When the group is ready, the members will receive an email explaining that they've joined the new group. The email includes useful links to get the members started with the collaboration features, including access to group files, a shared calendar, and conversations.

Understanding data security
The main goal of workspaces is to allow all group members to access the same content. When the group members explore datasets with imported data, everyone sees the same data. If Elena creates and publishes the Adventure Works self-service model created by Martin to the Sales workspace, every member will have access to all the data that Martin imported. In other words, Martin and the workspace members have the same access to the data. If Martin has scheduled the Adventure Works model for data refresh, the consumers will also see the new data.

What if you want consumers to have different access rights to the data? For example, you might want Martin to have unrestricted access but want Maya to see data for only a subset of your customers. If you prefer to keep your model in Power BI Desktop, you can extend the model with row-level security (RLS), which I discussed in Chapter 9. Another option is to implement an Analysis Services model that applies data security based on the user identity. Then, in Power BI Service you need to create a dataset that connects live to the Analysis Services model. You can create this dataset by using Get Data in the Power BI Portal (see steps in Chapter 4) or by using Power BI Desktop to create reports and publishing the file to Power BI Service.

There are factors that might influence your decision to choose the implementation path, such as planning for a centralized data model, scalability, and others. But in both cases, when Maya opens the report, her identity will be passed to the model, and she'll get restricted access depending on how the model security is set up. So, users access content in the workspace under their identity. It's helpful to think of two levels of security: workspace security that grants permissions to content and model data security that determines if the user has access to the model and what subset of data they can see (if data security is implemented in the model).

Taking over the workspace administrator
Remember that when you import data, Power BI datasets cache a copy of the data. However, a user can schedule a data refresh to periodically synchronize the Power BI dataset with changes that occur in the data source. What happens if you need to make changes to the data refresh, but this user goes on vacation or leaves the company?

Fortunately, another user can take over maintaining the data refresh. To do so, the workspace member would click the ellipsis button (...) next to the dataset to go to the dataset properties, and then click Schedule Refresh. Then the user clicks Take Over (see **Figure 11.9**) to take ownership of the data refresh and to overwrite the refresh settings if needed.

Disabling workspace creation
One of the benefits (and shortcomings) of workspaces is that any user with Power BI Pro rights can create them without relying on IT. At the same time, IT might want to prevent indiscriminate use of this feature. Currently, the only way to disable creating new groups is to use a PowerShell script that applies a policy to the user Exchange mail account. For more information and the steps required to disable groups across the

board or for specific users, read the "Disable Group creation" document by Microsoft at http://bit.ly/1MvPGF0. I hope that once Microsoft decouples workspaces from Office 365 groups, there will be more oversight and governance options.

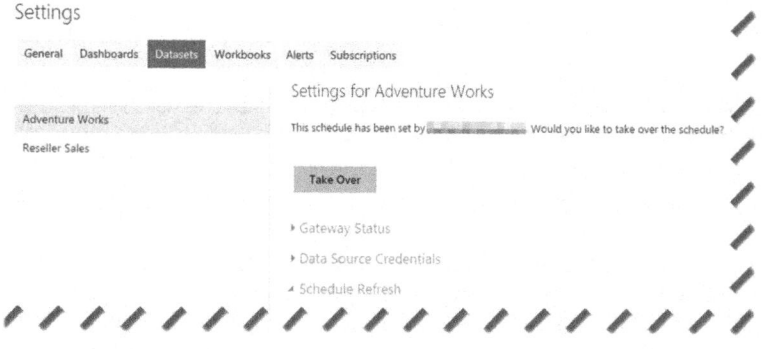

Figure 11.9 A Power BI Pro work-space member can take over the data refresh settings.

11.2.3 Working with Workspaces

We're back to Martin, a data analyst from Adventure Works. Martin approached Elena, who oversees data analytics, to help him set up a workspace for the Sales Department. This workspace will be accessed only by members of his unit, and it'll contain BI content produced by Martin and his colleagues.

 NOTE Unless IT has disabled Office 365 group creation, currently there's nothing stopping Martin from creating a group on his own (if he has a Power BI Pro subscription) and becoming the new group's admin. However, I do believe that someone needs to coordinate groups and workspaces, because creating groups indiscriminately could quickly become as useful as having no groups at all. It would be impossible for IT to maintain security over groups they didn't know existed.

Creating a group
As a first step, you need to create a Sales Department workspace:

1. Open your web browser and navigate to http://powerbi.com. Log in to Power BI Service.
2. In the left navigation bar, click Workspaces, and then click "Create app workspace".
3. In the "Create an app workspace" window, enter *Sales Department* as a workspace name.
4. In the "Add workspace members" field, enter the email addresses of some of your coworkers, or leave the field blank for now. You don't have to add your email because your membership is applied when you create the workspace, and you'll be the workspace admin.
5. Click Save to create the workspace.

In the navigation bar, the Workspaces section now includes the Sales Department workspace.

Uploading content
As you create a group, Power BI opens a "Welcome to the Sales Department group" page so that you can start adding content immediately. Let's add the Adventure Works model (that you previously created) to the Sales Department workspace. Since you're in Power BI Service, the steps that follow show you how to upload the file to Power BI Service by using Get Data. However, you can also publish it directly from Power BI Desktop by clicking the Publish button in the Home ribbon.

1. In the welcome page, click the Get button in the Files section. If you close your web browser and go back to Power BI, make sure that you click Workspaces and select Sales Department so that content is added to this workspace and not to your personal "My Workspace".

2. In the Files page, click Local File.

3. Navigate to the Adventure Works.pbix file you worked on in the previous part of the book, and upload it in Power BI. If you decide to use the one included in the book source, make sure to change the data sources to reflect your setup. To do so, open the file in Power BI Desktop, in the Home ribbon expand Edit Queries, and click "Data source settings". Then verify and change the data source connection strings as needed.

4. Using your knowledge from reading this book, view and edit the existing reports, and create some new reports and dashboards. For example, open the Adventure Works.pbix dashboard. Click the Adventure Works.pbix tile to navigate to the underlying report, and then pin some tiles to the dashboard. Back to the dashboard, delete the Adventure Works.pbix tile, and rename the dashboard to *Adventure Works Sales Dashboard*.

Scheduling data refresh

Once a business user uploads a dataset to the workspace, the user might want to schedule an automatic data refresh to keep a dataset with imported data synchronized with changes to the data source(s). If the dataset imports data from on-premises data sources (data sources hosted on physical or virtual machines side in your corporate network), such as our Adventure Works data model, you need to install a gateway. Recall that if the dataset imports data from cloud services, such as Azure SQL Server Database, then gateway is not needed.

Remember that you can install the gateway in one of two modes: personal and standard. As its name suggests, the personal mode is for your personal use. The idea here is to allow business users to refresh imported data without involving IT. You can install the gateway on your computer or another machine that has access to the data source(s) you want to refresh the data from. Each personal gateway installation is tied to the user who installs it and it can't be shared with other users. By contrast, the standard mode (discussed in section 11.4) is for centralizing access to important on-premises data sources.

 NOTE Currently, Power BI doesn't offer an option to prevent users from installing gateways. The only option might be to set up a software restriction corporate policy as you would restrict installation of other unwanted software. For more information, read the article "Using Software Restriction Policies to Protect Against Unauthorized Software" at bit.ly/restrictsoftware.

If you haven't done so, start with installing the data gateway in personal mode:

1. From the Power BI portal, expand the Downloads menu in the top-right corner, and click Data Gateway. In the next page, click the "Download gateway" button (both gateways are included in the same setup).

2. Once the setup program starts, select "on-premises data gateway (personal mode)" when the setup asks you what type of gateway you want to install. For detailed setup steps, refer to the "Power BI Gateway – Personal" article at https://docs.microsoft.com/en-us/power-bi/personal-gateway.

3. Back in Power BI Service, click the ellipsis (…) button next to the Adventure Works dataset. In the properties window, click Schedule Refresh to open the Settings page (see **Figure 11.10**).

4. The Gateway Status should show that the personal gateway is online on the computer where it's installed.

 NOTE If you use the on-premises data gateway (standard mode) to schedule the refresh, make sure that the data sources in your Power BI Desktop model have the same connection settings as the data sources registered in the on-premises data gateway. For example, if you have imported an Excel file, make sure that the file path in the underlying query matches the file path in the gateway data source. If the connection settings differ, you won't be able to use the on-premises data gateway.

The "Data source credentials" section shows that the credentials are incorrect. Although this might look alarming, it's easy to fix, and you only need to do it once per data source. For added security, Power BI doesn't carry the credentials you used in Power BI Desktop. Connecting to relational databases and cloud services may require a user name and password to authenticate. The only authentication option to connecting to files is Windows authentication.

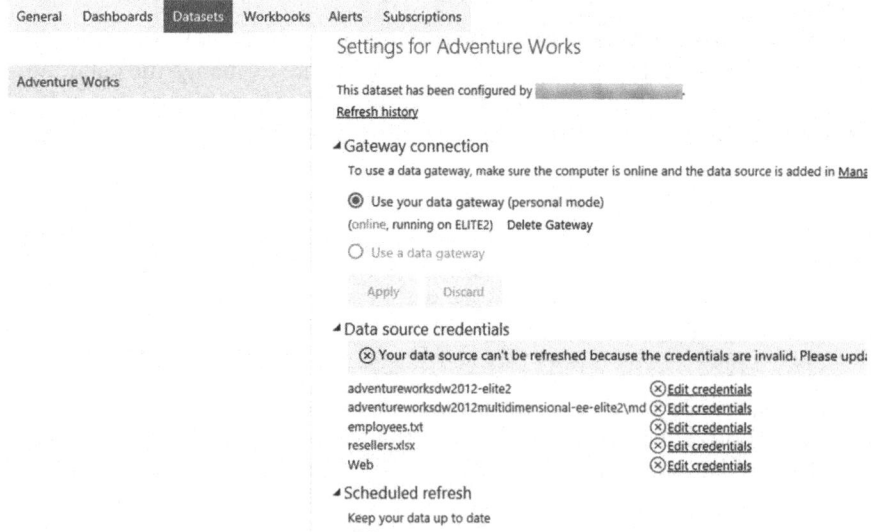

General   Dashboards   Datasets   Workbooks   Alerts   Subscriptions

Settings for Adventure Works

Adventure Works

This dataset has been configured by ⬛⬛⬛⬛⬛.
Refresh history

◢ Gateway connection

To use a data gateway, make sure the computer is online and the data source is added in Man...

⦿ Use your data gateway (personal mode)
(online, running on ELITE2)   Delete Gateway

◯ Use a data gateway

Apply   Discard

◢ Data source credentials

⊗ Your data source can't be refreshed because the credentials are invalid. Please upd...

adventureworksdw2012-elite2	⊗ Edit credentials
adventureworksdw2012multidimensional-ee-elite2\md	⊗ Edit credentials
employees.txt	⊗ Edit credentials
resellers.xlsx	⊗ Edit credentials
Web	⊗ Edit credentials

◢ Scheduled refresh

Keep your data up to date

⦿◯ Off

Figure 11.10   The dataset Settings page allows you to configure data refresh.

5. Click the "Edit credentials" link for each data source, specify the appropriate authentication, and then click the "Sign In" button (see **Figure 11.11**). Power BI will communicate with the gateway to ensure you have permissions to the data source.

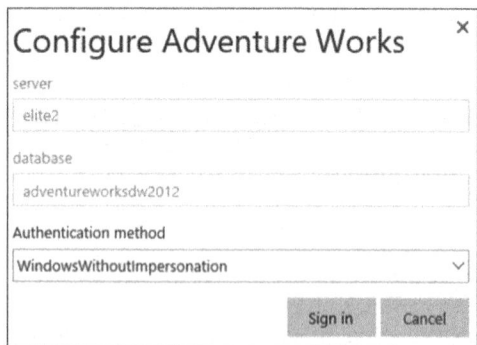

Configure Adventure Works ✕

server

elite2

database

adventureworksdw2012

Authentication method

WindowsWithoutImpersonation ⌄

Sign in   Cancel

Figure 11.11   The first time you configure scheduled data refresh, you need to specify credentials.

6. Turn the "Keep your data up to date" slider to On. Specify the refresh details, including the refresh frequency, your time zone, time of the refresh (you can schedule multiple refreshes per day on specific times), and whether you want refresh failure email notifications. When you're finished, click Apply.

Now the Adventure Works is scheduled for an automatic refresh. When the schedule is up, Power BI will connect to the data gateway, which in turn will connect to all the data sources in the model and will reload the data. Currently, there isn't an option to refresh specific data sources or to specify data source-specific schedules. Once a model is enabled for refresh, Power BI will refresh all the data on the same schedule.

7. (Optional) A few minutes after the schedule is up, go back to the Settings page and click the "Refresh history" link to check if the refresh was successful. If another member in your group has scheduled a dataset refresh, go to the dataset Settings page and discover how you can take over the data refresh when you need to. Once you take over, you can overwrite the data source and the schedule settings.

11.3 Distributing Content

You saw how workspaces foster collaboration across team members. But what if you want to package and publish content to a broader audience, such as across multiple departments or even to the entire organization? Enter Power BI organizational apps. Your users no longer need to wait for someone else to share content and will no longer be left in the dark without knowing what BI content is available in your company! Instead, users can discover and open apps from a single place - the Power BI AppSource page by clicking the Apps link in the navigation bar.

NOTE Organizational apps supersede organizational content packs, which Power BI previously had for broader content delivery. The problem with content packs was that once installed, they lose their package identity and users couldn't tell them apart from other BI content. Organizational content packs are still available (under the Power BI Service Settings menu) but they are deprecated, and I won't discuss them.

11.3.1 Understanding Organizational Apps

In Chapter 2, I explained that Power BI comes with service apps that allow your information workers to connect to a variety of online services, such as Google Analytics, Dynamics CRM, QuickBooks, and many more. Microsoft and its partners provide these content packs to help you analyze data from popular cloud services. Not only do content packs allow you to connect easily to external data, but they also include pre-packaged reports and dashboards that you can start using immediately! Like Power BI service apps, organizational apps let data analysts and IT/BI pros package and distribute BI content within their organization or to external users.

What's an organizational app?

An organizational app is a way for any company to distribute Power BI content to anyone who's interested in it. One of the prominent advantages of apps is that they isolate consumers from changes to content. Let's say Martin creates an app to distribute content from the Sales workspace and Maya installs the app. Now Maya gets a read-only copy of all reports and dashboards included in the app. Martin continues making changes to the workspace content, but Maya only get these changes when Martin republishes the app.

NOTE At this point, apps might not look very appealing. I'd personally preferred the ability to add members to a workspace with different permissions. But besides isolating content changes, Microsoft is planning more features for apps, so they might be even more useful in time.

Here are the most common scenarios for considering apps:

- You plan to distribute read-only content from a workspace, such as a workspace with certified reports to many users, groups, or the entire organization.
- If you're on Power BI Premium, you plan to distribute read-only content to Power BI Free users without incurring additional cost.
- You want to distribute content to users external to your organization.

You can create apps only from shared workspaces (you can't create an app from My Workspace). There is a one-to-one relationship between an app and a workspace. That's because when you create an app from a workspace, it includes *all* content from that workspace. If you want to distribute only specific dashboards and reports, then use dashboard sharing and not apps.

Creating an app

It's easy to create an organizational app and here are the steps (remember that you need to have a Power BI Pro license to create an app):

1. In Power BI Service, click Workspaces, and then click the workspace whose content you want to distribute to other users. In the workspace content page, click the "Publish App" button in the top-right corner.

2. In the Details tab (see **Figure 11.12**), enter a description for the app. You can also specify a background color for the app menu (more on this in a moment).

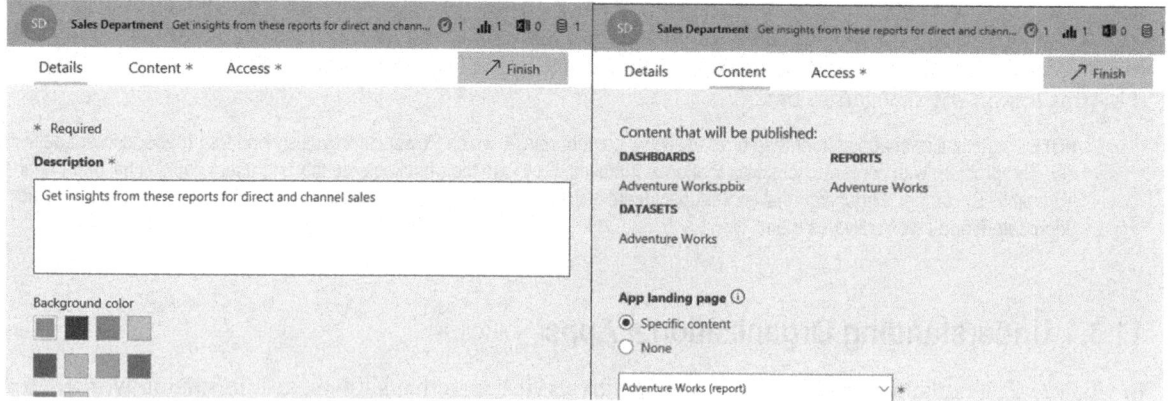

Figure 11.12 An organizational app includes all the workspace content.

3. In the Content tab, notice that all the workspace content will be included in the app. As an optional step, select a specific dashboard or report as a landing page (the default item that the users will see when they click the app).

Understanding content access

Next, you use the Access tab to specify which users will have access to the app. You can publish the app to the entire organization or restrict it to specific individuals or groups. Currently, app distribution supports Office 365 distribution lists and AD groups (with emails) but Microsoft is working on supporting Office 365 groups as well.

Any Power BI Pro user with edit permissions can create an app from a workspace the user belongs to, or update the existing app. Until Microsoft introduces more governance control over apps, this latitude might cause issues with larger organizations that seek more control over who can create and publish apps. The workaround is to have a workspace that is owned only by IT, such as "Certified Reports", and IT is solely responsible for distributing its content out of this workspace after approving content submitted by business users.

Once you specify the recipients, click Publish to publish the app. You'll be given a link that you can distribute to recipients. They can add this link to their browser's favorites to go directly to the app. Of course, they can navigate to the app from within Power BI Service as well. As I mentioned, think of a published app as a snapshot of dashboard and report definitions (not data). Users won't get changes to content until you republish the app. To do so, go to the workspace content page, and click the same button that you used to publish the app, but it should now read "Update App". This will bring you to the same "Publish app" tabbed page and you follow the same steps to republish the app.

Discovering and consuming apps

On the consumer side of things, any Power BI Pro user can consume an app. In addition, if your organization is on Power BI Premium, Power BI Free recipients can also consume apps. If the app is restricted to specific groups, the user must be a member of one or more of these groups. All consumers get read-only access to the content and they can't personalize it or make copies. The recipients can install the app using either one of these options:

1. Open the browser and enter the app link.

2. Click Apps in the Power BI Service navigation bar. If they haven't installed the app yet, they need to click the Get Apps button to navigate to AppSource. Find the app and click "Get it now"

3. Click Get Data and then click the My Organization tile to navigate to AppSource.

The Apps tab in the navigation bar gives the user access to all apps they have installed. When they access the app, they will see the landing page you specified. The recipients can use the app menu to navigate to other content included in the app, as shown in **Figure 11.13**. If they have edit permissions to the app workspace, they can click the pencil icon to update the app.

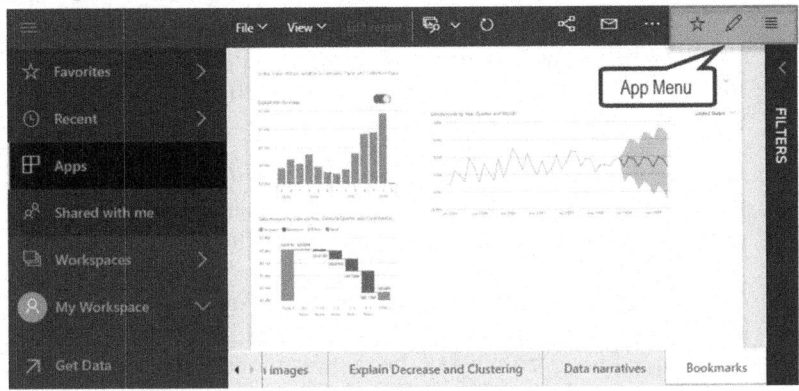

Figure 11.13 Use the app menu to navigate to other content included in the app.

Removing apps
Consumers can remove an app they installed. To do so, they click Apps in the Power BI left navigation bar. In the Apps page, they hover on the app and then click the Trash button to delete the app. An app might also reach the end of its lifecycle and it's no longer needed. Then, a workplace member with edit permissions can remove it. Deleting an app removes the installed app from all consumers. Suppose that the Sales app is outdated, and Elena needs to remove it.

1. In the navigation bar, Elena clicks Workspaces and then she selects the Sales workspace.

2. In the workspace content page, Elena expands the ellipsis (...) menu in the top-right corner and clicks Unpublish App.

3. When Maya clicks Apps in the navigation bar, she notices that the app is gone.

11.3.2 Comparing Sharing Options

To recap, Power BI supports three ways of sharing BI content: simple dashboard sharing, workspaces, and organizational apps. Because having that many options could be confusing, **Table 11.1** summarizes their key characteristics and usage scenarios. Below the table, you'll find some high-level best practices for content sharing.

Table 11.1 This table compares the sharing options supported by Power BI.

	Dashboard Sharing	Workspaces	Organizational Apps
Purpose	Ad hoc dashboard sharing	Team collaboration	Broader content delivery
Discovery	Invitation email or direct sharing to another user's workspace	Workspace content	AppSource (My Organization tab)
Target audience	Selected individuals (like your boss)	Groups (your team)	Anyone who might be interested

	Dashboard Sharing	Workspaces	Organizational Apps
Content permissions	Read-only dashboards and underlying content	Read/edit to all workspace content	Read-only dashboards and reports
Memberships	Individuals, O365 distribution lists, security groups (with email)	Individuals and O365 groups	Individuals, O365 distribution lists, and security groups (with email)
Content isolation	No	No	Yes
Collaboration features	No	Calendar, conversations, files	No
License	Power BI Pro Power BI Free with Power BI Premium	Power BI Pro	Power BI Pro Power BI Free with Power BI Premium

Dashboard sharing

The primary purpose of dashboard sharing is the ad hoc sharing of dashboards and underlying reports by sending an email to selected individuals or direct sharing to their workspace. For example, you might want to share your dashboard with your boss or a teammate. Consumers can't edit the shared dashboards (not even to rearrange tiles).

When the user clicks a tile, they see the underlying content, which could be a Power BI report (if the tile was pinned from a report visual), Excel report (if the tile was pinned from an Excel report), a Reporting Services report (if the tile was pinned from SSRS), Q&A page (if the tile was pinned from Q&A), or a Quick Insight report (if the tile was pinned from Quick Insights). Dashboard sharing allows you to distribute dashboards to Power BI Free users from a Power BI Premium workspace.

Workspaces

Workspaces foster team collaboration and communication. They're best suited for departments or project teams. Currently relying on Office 365 groups, workspaces allow all its members to edit and view the workspace content. Group workspaces are the only option that supports shared communication features, including OneDrive for Business file sharing, a shared calendar, and conversations. They are also the only option that allows members to edit shared content.

Organizational apps

Organizational apps are designed for broader content delivery, such as across groups or even across the entire organization. Consumers discover content packs in Power BI AppSource. Consumers get read-only access to the published content. Apps allow you to distribute content to Power BI Free users from Power BI Premium workspaces.

Best practices

I'd like to provide some best practices around sharing that I harvested from my consulting practice:

- Create workspaces to reflect your organization structure, such Sales, Finance, Customer Care. Allow members to collaborate on self-service BI content in their respective workspace.

- Establish a data governance committee that meets regularly (for example, monthly) to oversee self-service BI and review content submitted for broader sharing. To avoid wrong decision making, discourage users from distributing content on their own.

- Consider creating a Certified workspace for approved reports and dashboards. You don't have to clone datasets to this workspace. Remember that Power BI Desktop includes a Power BI Service data source that allows you to create reports from published datasets. So, you can leave datasets in the original workspaces and create or deploy reports connected to these datasets to the Certified workspace. Share content out of this workspace using apps or specific dashboards.

- Constantly monitor what data your users are importing and what business metrics they are producing. Consider including useful and common entities into an organizational semantic model.
- Encourage self-service BI for what's suited best: agile BI, such as to mash up data from multiple data sources. For most users, the best self-service BI would be an organizational semantic model that delivers a single version of the truth. I discuss pros and cons of self-service BI in Chapter 2.

11.3.3 Working with Organizational Apps

Several departments at Adventure Works have expressed interest in the content that the Sales Department has produced, so that they can have up-to-date information about the company's sales performance. Elena decides to create an organizational app to publish these artifacts to a broader audience.

Creating an organizational app

As a prerequisite, Elena needs to discover if there are any existing Office 365 or security groups that include the authorized consumers. This is an important step from a security and maintenance standpoint. Elena doesn't want the app to reach unauthorized users. She also doesn't want to create a new group if she can reuse what's already in place. Elena needs to be an admin or a member of the Sales Department workspace so that she has access to this workspace.

1. Elena discusses this requirement with the Adventure Works system administrator, and she discovers that there's already a security group for the Finance Department. Since the rest of the users come from other departments, the system administrator recommends Elena creates a security group (or O365 distribution list) for them.
2. If Adventure Works is not on Power BI Premium, Elena ensures that all members have Power BI Pro licenses. This restriction doesn't apply to Power BI Premium, but Elena needs to ensure that the workspace is in a premium capacity to share with Power BI Free users.
3. In Power BI Service, she clicks Workspaces and then she selects the Sales Department workspace. She does this so that, when she creates an app, the app includes the content from this workspace.
4. In the workspace content page, Elena clicks "Publish app".
5. In the "Publish app" page (see **Figure 11.12** again), Elena enters a description. She switches to the Access tab and enters the authorized groups. She clicks Publish.

At this point, the Adventure Works Sales content pack is published and ready for authorized consumers.

Consuming an organizational app

Maya learns about the availability of the Sales app, and she wants to use it. Maya belongs to one of the groups that's authorized to use the app.

1. Maya logs in to Power BI and clicks Apps ⇨ Get Apps.
2. If there are many apps available, Maya uses the search box to search for "sales".
3. Maya discovers the Sales app. She clicks "Get it now". Power BI installs the app. Maya can now gain insights from the prepackaged content.
4. (Optional) Review and practice the different steps of the app lifecycle, such as to make changes to the workspace content and republish the app.

11.3.1 Sharing with External Users

Many organizations share reports with external users for Business to Business (B2B) or Business to Consumer (B2C) scenarios. Consider Power BI Embedded (discussed in Chapter 15), if these reports need to be embedded in an Internet-facing web portal so that they appear as a part of an integrated offering for your external customers. However, Power BI Embedded requires coding effort to extend your app with the Power BI REST APIs and many organizations do not have the time or resources to create a custom app just to distribute Power BI content to their external partners. If all you need is granting some external users access to content inside Power BI Service, you can do so by just sharing it out using dashboard sharing or apps, as you do with internal users. But there are some special considerations though so read on.

Understanding Azure Active Directory

Like using Power BI for internal use, external users need to be authenticated by a trusted authority. To authenticate external users, Power BI relies on Azure Active Directory (AAD). Therefore, the external user needs an AAD account. If the user doesn't have an AAD account, the user will be prompted to create one. **Figure 11.14** shows the high-level flow.

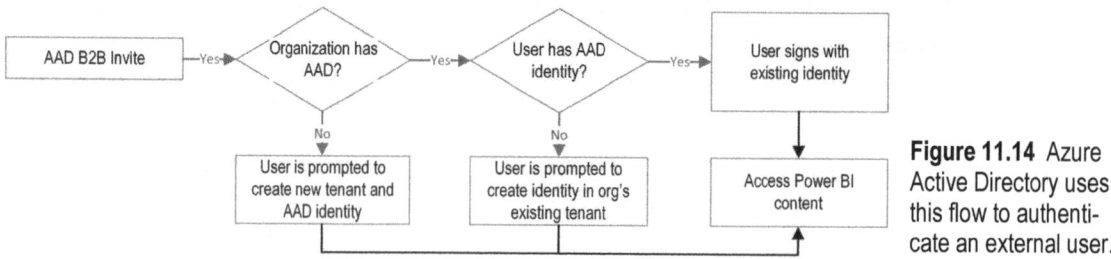

Figure 11.14 Azure Active Directory uses this flow to authenticate an external user.

Let's say Elena from Adventure Works wants to grant Matthew from Prologika access to some Power BI content. Elena creates a workspace to host the external content and then she invites Matthew using one of these options:

- Planned invite – She can go to Azure portal and create a new guest user (Azure Active Directory ⇨ Users and groups ⇨ All users ⇨ New guest user). Elena can also use the Azure Portal to set up policies that control external sharing, such as to turn off invitations and specify which users and groups can invite external users.

- Ad-hoc invite – She can simply share a dashboard or create an app, and then add Matthew's email as a recipient. Elena can use the Tenant Settings in Power BI Admin Portal to control which users and groups can share with external users.

In both cases, Matthew receives an invitation email with a link to the dashboard or app. Because the link contains some important information, Matthew must save that link somewhere, such as by adding it to its browser's favorites. Matthew clicks the link to access the content. Azure AAD checks if Prologika has an AAD tenant. If not, Matthew will be asked to create a new tenant. If a Prologika tenant exists, AAD checks if Matthew has an account in that tenant. If not, he'll be asked to create an account and specify credentials. This is no different than internal users signing up for Power BI. Then, AAD will ask Matthew to sign in with his AAD credentials and grant him access to the shared Power BI content.

NOTE What about the B2C scenario where external users sign in with their personal emails? As of this time, personal accounts are not yet supported, but by the time you read this, Power BI will probably support Microsoft Live ID accounts. As AAD expands support for more identity providers, Power BI will support those in time as well. This doesn't mean that users will be able to sign up for Power BI with their personal emails. Personal emails will be supported to access Power BI content shared with them by other organizations.

Understanding licensing

Power BI licensing for external users is not much different from licensing internal users. In a nutshell, the external user must have a Power BI Pro license to access Power BI content in the sharing tenant. This license can be acquired in one of three ways:

1. The sharing organization is on Power BI Premium – If Adventure Works is on Power BI Premium and the sharing workspace is in a premium capacity, Elena can share content to external users, just like she can share content with internal Power BI Free users.

2. The sharing organization assigns Power BI Pro licenses – Elena can assign one of her organization's Power BI Pro licenses to Matthew.

3. The external organization assigns Power BI Pro licenses – In this case, Matthew has a Power BI Pro license from the Prologika's Power BI tenant. Matthew can bring in his license to all organizations that share content with Prologika.

Understanding data security

Like internal users, external users access content under their identity. If you need to restrict access to data with row-level security (RLS), you have the following options:

- RLS for Power BI models and Azure Analysis Services -- The external user email can be added to the appropriate role to grant the user restricted access to data. Or, the model can obtain the user identity, such as by using the USERPRINCIPALNAME function (see Chapter 9).

- RLS for on-premises SSAS models –Things can get more complicated here because the AAD accounts are not available to the on-premises Active Directory. However, the Power BI data gateway supports a CustomData option that lets you pass the user identity to the model.

For more information about external sharing, read the "Distribute Power BI content to external guest users using Azure Active Directory B2B" whitepaper by Microsoft at https://aka.ms/powerbi-b2b-whitepaper.

11.4 Centralizing Data Management

Because it's a cloud platform, Power BI requires special connectivity software to access on-premises data. You saw in the "Working with Workspaces" section how the data gateway (personal mode) allows end users to refresh datasets connected to on-premises data sources, such as relational databases and files. However, this connectivity mechanism doesn't give IT the ability to centralize and sanction data access. Moreover, in personal mode the gateway is limited to refreshing datasets with imported data, and it doesn't support DirectQuery to on-premises databases. The on-premises data gateway fills in these gaps.

11.4.1 Understanding the On-premises Data Gateway

The On-premises Data Gateway supports the following features:

- Serving many users – Unlike the personal gateway, which serves the needs of individuals, the administrator can configure one or more on-premises gateways for entire teams and even the organization.

- Centralizing management of data sources, credentials, and access control – The administrator can use one gateway to delegate access to multiple databases and can authorize individual users or groups to access these databases.

- Providing DirectQuery access from Power BI Service to on-premises data sources – Once Martin creates a model that connects directly to a SQL Server database, Martin can publish the model to Power BI Service and its reports will just work.

- Cross-application support – Besides Power BI, the On-premises Data Gateway can be used by other applications, including PowerApps, Flow, and Azure Logic Apps.

Comparing gateways

Thanks to Microsoft unifying the gateways, deciding which gateway to use is much simpler. In a nutshell, the personal gateway is meant for a business user who wants to set up automated data refresh without bothering IT by installing the gateway on his computer. By contrast, the On-premises Data Gateway will be used by IT for centralizing data access to both refreshable and DirectQuery data sources. **Table 11.2** compares the two gateways.

Table 11.2 This table compares the two gateways.

	On-premises Data Gateway	On-premises Data Gateway (personal mode)
Purpose	Centralized data management	Isolated access to data by individuals
Audience	IT	Business users
DirectQuery	Yes	No
Data refresh	Yes	Yes
User access	Users and groups managed by IT	Individual user
Data sources	Multiple data sources (DirectQuery and refreshable)	All refreshable data sources
Data source registration	Must register data sources	Registration is not required
High availability	Yes	No

11.4.2 Getting Started with the On-Premises Data Gateway

Next, I'll show you how to install and use the On-Premises Data Gateway. While you can install the gateway on any machine, you should install it on a dedicated server within your corporate network. You can install multiple gateways if needed, such as to assign department-level admin access.

Installing the on-premises data gateway

For your convenience, Microsoft has packaged both gateways in a single installation package. Follow these steps to download the gateway:

1. Remote in to the server where you want to install the gateway. This server should have a fast connection to the on-premises databases that the gateway will access. Verify that you can connect to the target databases.
2. Open the web browser and log in to Power BI Service.
3. In the Application Toolbar located in the upper-right corner of the Power BI portal, click the Download menu, and then click "Data Gateway". You can also access the download page directly at https://powerbi.microsoft.com/gateway/.
4. In the next page, click "Download gateway".
5. Once you download the setup executable, run it. On the "Choose the type of the gateway you need", leave the default option of "On-premises data gateway" selected.
6. Select the installation folder, read and accept the agreement, and then click Install. The gateway installs and runs as a Windows service called "On-premises data gateway service" (PBIEgwService) and its default location is the "C:\Program Files\On-premises data gateway" folder. The setup program configures the service to run under a low-privileged NT SERVICE\PBIEgwService Windows account.

What's interesting about the gateway is that it doesn't require any inbound ports to be open in your corporate firewall. Data transfer between the Power BI service and the gateway is secured through Azure Service Bus (relay communication). The gateway communicates on outbound ports 443 (HTTPS), 5671, 5672,

9350 thru 9354. By default, the gateway uses port 443, which is used for all secure socket layer (SSL) connections (every time users request HTTPS pages). If this port is congested, consider allowing outbound connections through the other outbound ports (my experience has been that port 443 is sufficient). What all this means is that in most cases the gateway should just work with no additional configuration.

 REAL LIFE I helped a large organization to implement a Power BI hybrid architecture to keep their data on premises. In this case, the gateway failed to register after installation. The reason was that this organization used a web proxy server. Had the proxy supported Windows Authentication, we could have solved the issue by just changing the gateway service account to an account that had rights to the proxy. However, their proxy server was configured for Basic Authentication so we had to pass the account password to the proxy. We had to change the gateway configuration file to specify the account credentials. For more technical details, read my "Power BI Hybrid Architecture" blog at http://prologika.com/power-bi-hybrid-architecture.

Configuring the on-premises data gateway

Next, you need to configure the gateway:

1. Once the setup program installs the gateway, it'll ask you to sign in to Power BI.

2. In the next step, leave the default option of "Register a new gateway on this computer". Notice that the second option is to migrate, restore, or take over an existing gateway.

3. Specify the gateway name and a recovery key (see **Figure 11.15**). Save the recovery key in a safe place. Someone might need it to restore the gateway if admin access is lost or the gateway needs to be moved to another server.

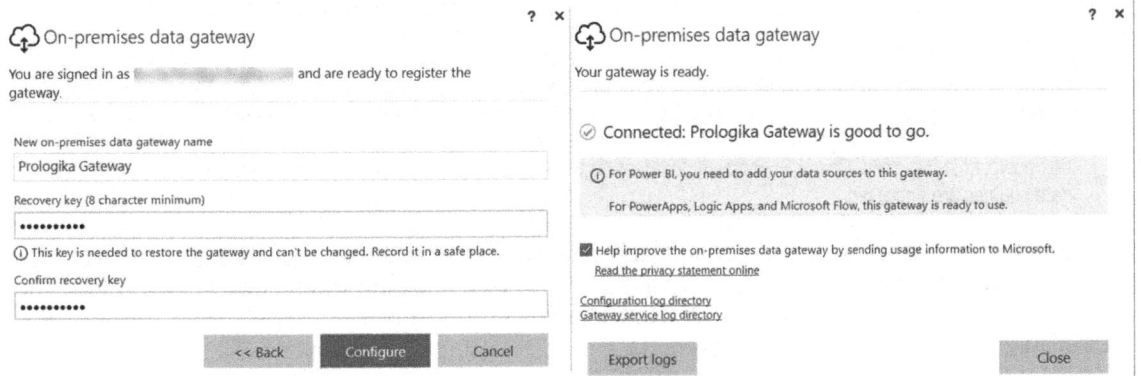

Figure 11.15 When you configure the on-premises gateway, you need to give it a name and provide a recovery key.

4. Click Configure. This registers the gateway with Power BI. You should see a message that the gateway is connected.

Registering data sources

Now that the gateway is connected, it's time to add one or more data sources to the gateway. Note that unlike the Personal Gateway which doesn't require data source registration, the On-premises Data Gateway requires you to register all data sources that the gateway serves. This needs to be done in Power BI Service, as follows:

1. Log in to Power BI Service. Click the Settings menu in the Application Toolbar in the upper-right corner, and then click "Manage gateways".

2. In the Gateways page, select your gateway and notice that you can enter additional gateway settings, such as the department and description. Moreover, you can specify additional administrators who can manage the gateway (the person who installs the gateway becomes the first administrator).

3. Next, add one or more data sources that the gateway will delegate access to. Suppose you want to set up DirectQuery to the AdventureWorksDW2012 database (I'll show how to connect to SSAS in Chapter 13).

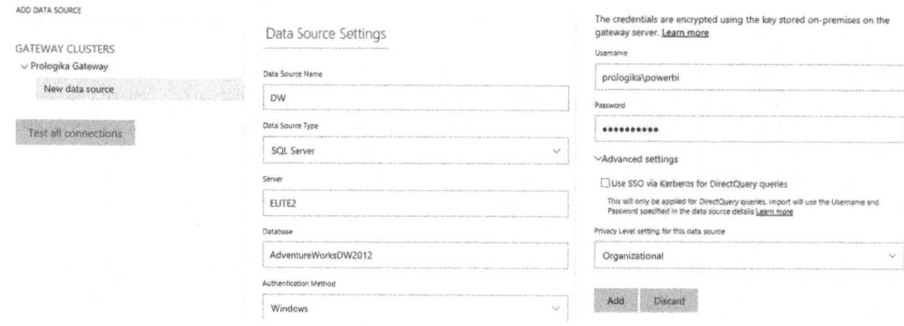

Figure 11.16 The On-Premises Data Gateway can provide access to many databases.

4. In the Gateways page, click "Add Data Source" (see **Figure 11.16**).

5. Fill in the data source settings to reflect your database setup.

6. The Authentication method allows you to specify the credentials of a trusted Windows account or a standard SQL Server login that has access to the database. Remember to grant this account at least read credentials to the database, such by assigning it to the SQL Server db_reader role. Note that all queries from all users will use these credentials to connect to the database, so grant the account only the minimum set of permissions it needs to the SQL Server database. This might result in different data permissions than the permissions a data analyst had when he used Power BI Desktop to connect to SQL Server under *his* credentials.

 NOTE Currently, the only data source that supports passing the user identity via Windows security is Analysis Services. Microsoft is working on enabling this scenario for SQL Server as well. If you are concerned about compromising the communication from Power BI to the gateway, the gateway uses asymmetric encryption to encrypt the credentials so that they cannot be decrypted in the cloud. Power BI sends the credentials to the gateway server, which decrypts the credentials when the data sources are accessed.

7. (Important!) Once you add a data source and click the data source in the Gateways page, you'll see a new Users tab. For an added level of security, all users who will be publishing reports that will connect to this data source, must be added to the Users tab. Note that you need to add *only* the publishers and not the rest of the users who will be just viewing reports.

 TIP If you have issues with the On-premises Data Gateway setup or data source access, you can configure it for troubleshooting. You can find the troubleshooting steps in the "Troubleshooting the On-Premises Data Gateway" article by Adam Saxton at https://docs.microsoft.com/en-us/power-bi/service-gateway-onprem-tshoot.

That's almost all you need to know about the gateway. There are special considerations that apply when connecting to Analysis Services, but I'll discuss them in the next chapter. Let's now put our business user's hat on and see how you can create reports that connect to on-premises data via the gateway.

11.4.3 Using the On-Premises Data Gateway

Once the On-premises Data Gateway is set up and functional, you can use it for setting up automated data refresh and for reports that connect directly to on-premises data sources. In Chapter 2, I showed you how a business user can connect to an on-premises Analysis Services model via the gateway. Next, I'll show you how to use the gateway to connect directly to an on-premises SQL Server database. Except for Analysis

Services, setting up DirectQuery connections to on-premises databases are currently only available in Power BI Desktop, so you must create a data model.

 NOTE The gateway is completely transparent to Power BI Desktop. You never specify a gateway when you connect to a data source in Power BI Desktop. Instead, you connect as usual by entering the server name and database. Only after you publish the Power BI Desktop file, Power BI Service examines the connections and determines which gateway services the data source(s). So, gateways are only for Power BI Service and don't apply to Power BI Desktop.

Connecting directly to SQL Server

Follow these steps to create a simple data model that you can use to test the gateway:

1. Open Power BI Desktop and expand the Get Data button in the ribbon's Home tab. Select SQL Server.
2. In the SQL Server Database prompt, specify the name of the SQL Server instance.
3. In the Navigator Window, expand the database the gateway delegates access to, select one or more tables, and then click Load.
4. In the Connection Settings window, select DirectQuery and click OK to create the dataset.
5. (Optional) Create a report that shows some data.
6. Publish the model to Power BI Service by clicking the Publish button in the ribbon's Home page.

Testing connectivity

Next, test that you can create reports from Power BI Service:

1. Log in to Power BI. In the navigation bar, click My Workspace, and then click the dataset to explore it. Note that it's not enough to see the model metadata showing in the Fields pane because the list comes from the Tabular backend database in the Microsoft data center where the model is hosted. You need to visualize the data to verify that the gateway is indeed functional.
2. In the Fields pane, check a field to create a visualization. If you see results on the report, then the gateway works as expected. You can also use the SQL Server Profiler to verify that the report queries are sent to the SQL Server database.

11.5 Summary

Power BI has comprehensive features for establishing a trustworthy environment. As an administrator, you can use the Office 365 Admin Center to manage users and grant them access to Power BI. You can use the Power BI Admin Portal to monitor utilization and configure tenant-wide settings.

Power BI allows teams to collaborate and share BI artifacts via dashboard sharing, workspaces, and organizational apps. Workspaces allow a team to collaborate on shared Power BI content. Workspaces include collaboration features, such as calendar, files, and conversations, which allow the group to share information. Organizational apps are designed to complement workspaces by letting content producers share their insights with other teams and even with the entire organization. Authorized users can discover apps in Power BI AppSource. When consumers install an app, they can view all the published content, but they can't edit the content and they are isolated from changes to the content. As the content changes, Power BI Pro users can update the app to propagate the changes.

This chapter compared the three sharing and collaboration options and recommended usage scenarios. It also walked you through a few exercises to help you practice the new concepts. Finally, I showed you how the On-premises Data Gateway is positioned to centralize access to on-premises data.

Remember that if your organization is on Power BI Premium, you can distribute content to internal or external viewers for free by sharing specific dashboards or using organizational apps. But Power BI Premium has much more to offer and it's the subject of the next chapter.

Chapter 12

Power BI Premium

As you've seen, Power BI Service is packed with features for both free and paid users. Power BI Pro is a good choice for most smaller to midsize organizations. Larger organizations, however, gravitate towards Power BI Premium for cloud deployments and I'll show you why in this chapter. Not interested in the cloud yet? If your organization is looking for an on-premises report portal for hosting different types of reports, including Power BI reports, Power BI Report Server should warrant your serious interest.

This chapter starts by introducing you to Power BI Premium. I'll discuss its features and I'll compare it with Power BI Service. You'll understand how to save licensing cost when distributing content to users who only need to view it. Although Power BI Report Server has no dependencies on Power BI Premium, it can be licensed under Power BI Premium, so I included essential coverage of this product. Previously, I've shown you how to pin report items from Power BI Report Server and how to view on-premises reports in the Power BI Mobile apps. Now, you'll learn how Power BI Report compares with Power BI Service and SSRS. You'll also learn how to deploy and manage Power BI reports to an on-premises report server.

12.1 Understanding Power BI Premium

Think of Power BI Premium as an add-on to Power BI Pro. It's for organizations requiring predictable performance and scalability, and the ability to distribute content to many "viewers" without requiring per-user licensing. As its name suggests, Power BI Premium is the Power BI most advanced edition for cloud deployments. To recap from Chapter 1 where I compared features and editions side by side, the Power BI Service portfolio includes the following editions:

- Power BI Free – Power BI Free is for personal use. Once Maya signs up for Power BI Free, she can enjoy most of Power BI Service features for free, but she can't share content with other users.

- Power BI Pro – A step above Power BI Free, this edition includes sharing and collaboration and it carries a $9.99 price tag per user, per month. When she upgrades to Power BI Pro, Maya can now share content with other colleagues using any of the three supported options (dashboard sharing, workspaces, and organizational apps). She can also subscribe to reports and create reports from published datasets in Excel or Power BI Desktop.

- Power BI Premium – This edition offers greater scale and performance, flexibility to license by capacity, embedded analytics, and extends Power BI to on-premises so that you can license Power BI Report Server under Power BI Premium.

Let's dive in the Power BI Premium features to understand what they really mean for you.

12.1.1 Understanding Premium Performance

When you use Power BI Free or Power BI Pro, your organization is effectively sharing resources with other organizations. In other words, all your BI content is in shared capacity. This isn't any different than other Software as a Service (SaaS) offerings, such as Salesforce, Amazon Web Services, or other Microsoft Azure services. Microsoft has done its job to scale out report loads across clusters of servers and to enforce restrictions that ensure that hyper active users can't monopolize the shared environment. Examples include restricting the maximum dataset size to 1 GB, limiting the number of dataset refreshes to eight per day, and capping the number of rows when users export or drill through reports. However, the performance of your reports might still be impacted in a shared environment.

Understanding dedicated (premium) capacity

When you purchase Power BI Premium, Microsoft allocates a dedicated capacity (hardware) to your organization. Although some of the cluster resources are dedicated, they are still integrated with Power BI Service, meaning that Power BI Premium doesn't lag in features. To the contrary, since this hardware is yours, Microsoft can safely remove some of the shared limitations. For example, Power BI Premium ups the number of refreshes to 48 per day and increases the dataset size to up to 10 GB. More restrictions will probably go away, and new features will be added, such as incremental refreshes, and geo replication.

Dedicated capacity is completely transparent to end users. They continue to log in to the Power BI Portal as usual. Power BI administrators control which workspaces are in a shared or dedicated capacity. With a mouse click, a workspace can be moved in and out of a dedicated capacity, and this all happens in the background.

Understanding capacity nodes

When you sign up for Power BI Premium (you can start the process from the "Capacity settings" tab in the Admin Portal), you need to decide how much capacity you need, expressed as capacity nodes (or plans), which are listed in **Table 12.1**.

Table 12.1 Power BI provides several capacity nodes.

Node	Total V-cores	Backend Cores	Frontend Cores	Max Page Renders per hour	Max Dataset Size (GB)	Direct Query max connections per second	Price per month
P1	8	4 (25 GB RAM)	4	1201-2400	3	30	$4,995
P2	16	8 (50 GB RAM)	8	2401-4800	6	60	$9,995
P3	32	16 (100 GB RAM)	16	4801-9600	10	120	$19,995
EM1 (EA only)	1	5 (3 GB RAM)	5	1-300	1	5	$625
EM2 (EA only)	2	1 (5 GB RAM)	1	301-600	1	10	$1,245
EM3	4	2 (10 GB RAM)	2	601-1200	1	15	$2,495

Like a virtual machine (VM), a capacity node includes a predefined number of virtual frontend and backend cores (v-cores). The frontend cores are responsible for the user experience (web service, dashboard and report document management, access rights management, scheduling, APIs, uploads and downloads). The backend cores do the heavy lifting (query processing, caching, data refresh, rendering of reports). Each capacity node also reserves a specific amount of memory for the backend cores.

> **NOTE** What's a page render? A page render happens when a report page needs to be refreshed. A page render occurs when the page is initially shown and every time the page is updated because of some user activity, such as applying filters or changing the visual configuration. Typically, multiple queries processed by the backend cores are involved in a page render because every visual sends a query.

Microsoft provides an interactive calculator (https://powerbi.microsoft.com/en-us/calculator/) to help you calculate how much capacity you need. Most organizations start with the P1 capacity node. The embedded (EM) plans are for embedding Power BI content in custom apps (the EM1 and EM2 plans can be acquired only through Enterprise Agreement with Microsoft). You can also acquire Power BI Embedded via the Azure Power BI Embedded (A*) plans (https://azure.microsoft.com/pricing/details/power-bi-embedded/), as I'll discuss in more detail in Chapter 15.

Understanding capacity features

Why do we need so many different capacities? The short answer is to give you the most licensing flexibility to distribute Power BI content to different audiences. **Table 12.2** shows how capacity SKUs differ in terms of content accessibility for different types of users. For example, the P capacities allow all user types to access any Power BI content (in Power BI Portal and embedded in custom apps). By contrast, an EM capacity allows only Power BI Pro users to view reports in Power BI Portal because EM capacities are mostly for embedding reports for third party.

Table 12.2 Understanding capacity features for content distribution.

Capacity	Audience	Power BI Portal	Custom app with embedded content
P capacity	Power BI Pro users	Yes	Yes
	Power BI Free users	Yes	Yes
	External users	Yes	Yes
EM capacity	Power BI Pro users	Yes	Yes
	Power BI Free users	No	Yes
	External users	No	Yes
A capacity	Power BI Pro users	Yes	Yes
	Power BI Free users	No	No
	External users	No	Yes

When you work the calculator, you'll notice that you can purchase more nodes to scale out. When would you scale out by adding more nodes versus scaling up to a higher node? As I mentioned, each node has a specific amount of memory associated with the backend cores. One consideration is the maximum dataset size supported in Power BI Premium compared to the available memory of the smallest node. Currently, all P plans have more memory than the maximum dataset size Power BI Premium supports (up to 10 GB with P1). But in the future, Microsoft might be increasing the maximum dataset size to the point where some datasets may be too large to fit in a smaller node's memory, but if you had purchased a larger node size, they would have fit in the available memory. Conversely, there are reasons why you may want to have multiple smaller capacities rather than one large one, such as to provide isolation between workloads and delegate management to different groups of people.

12.1.2 Understanding Premium Workspaces

Allocating Power BI content to a dedicated (premium) capacity happens at the workspace level. For example, realizing the importance of the Sales workspace, Elena might decide to move to a premium capacity so that it can benefit from Power BI Premium features. If she changes her mind later, she can move it back to a shared capacity.

How workspaces relate to nodes

Figure 14.1 shows a few possible options for assigning workspaces to capacity nodes. In this case, Adventure Works has scaled out Power BI Premium to two P1 nodes and one P2 node. The administrator has allocated some workspaces across the premium nodes, but other workspaces are left in a shared capacity.

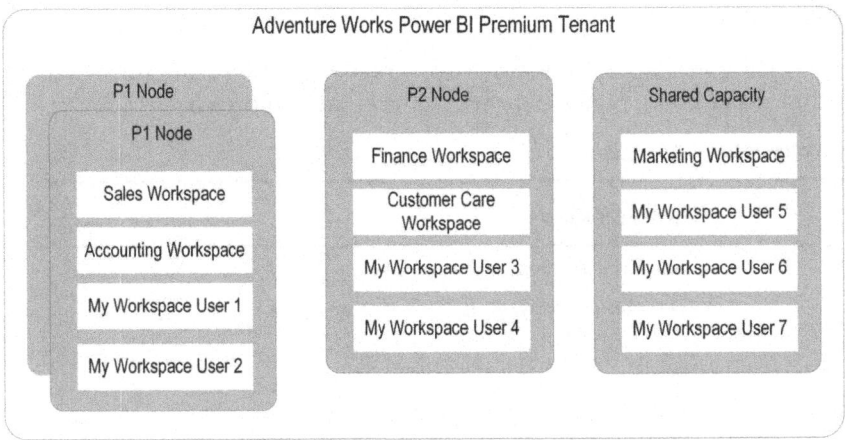

Figure 12.1 The administrator can assign workspaces to premium and shared capacities.

Therefore, the workspaces in a premium capacity would benefit from consistent performance and Power BI Premium features, while non-significant workspaces can remain in a shared capacity. Notice also that personal "My Workspace" workspaces can be in a premium capacity as well.

Sharing content to Power BI free users

A workspace in a shared capacity requires Power BI Pro licenses for any form of sharing (dashboard sharing, workspace membership, or apps). But one of the Power BI Premium benefits is that a premium workspace can share out content to Power BI Free users. There are two options to distribute content to viewers without requiring Power BI Pro licenses:

- Dashboard sharing – Any Power BI Pro member of a premium workspace can share dashboards. Consider this option when you need to share out only specific dashboards and their reports.

- Organizational apps – Any Power BI Pro member of a premium workspace can create an app to distribute all the workspace content to other users, including Power BI Free users.

Power BI Free users can only view shared content. Users contributing content to an app workspace (examples include creating or editing reports and dashboards) still require Power BI Pro licenses.

NOTE From a costing perspective alone, the break-even point between Power BI Pro and Power BI Premium is 500 users, if all users would need access to shared content. That's because licensing 500 users with Power BI Pro costs $5,000 per month, which is the monthly cost of the lowest Premium (P1) plan for one node. Of course, there are other compelling reasons to consider Power BI Premium and there will be even more over time as Microsoft adds more premium features.

12.2 Managing Power BI Premium

Power BI Premium adds security and administration features to let you manage premium workspaces and capacities. The first time you land at the Power BI Admin Portal under "Capacity settings", you will find a "Buy" button, which will redirect you to the Office 365 Admin Portal. There you can purchase a subscription to Power BI Premium and capacity nodes. For more information, read "How to purchase Power BI Premium" at https://docs.microsoft.com/en-us/power-bi/service-admin-premium-purchase.

Note that you must be an Office 365 global admin to buy a capacity. Besides purchasing Power BI Premium, no further management is required in the Office 365 portal. All Power BI Premium management features are accessible from the "Capacity settings" tab in Power BI Admin Portal.

12.2.1 Managing Security

To delegate rights to specific users for managing premium features, Power BI Premium introduces two new security roles (Capacity Admins and Capacity Assignment), as shown in **Table 12.3**.

Table 12.3 Power BI Premium adds two security roles.

Capacity Admin	Capacity Assignment
Add capacity	Assign workspaces to capacity
Assign admins	Grant other Pro users access to their capacity workspace
Granting workspace permissions	
Bulk assign workspaces to capacity	
Remove workspaces from capacity	
Monitor capacity usage	

Understanding Capacity Admin role
Each capacity has its own admins. Capacity administrators can add capacity, assign admins, and assign and remove workspaces. Capacity admins can also grant permissions to a workspace, increase capacity, and monitor logging and auditing. All Office 365 Global admins and Power BI admins are automatically capacity admins of both Power BI Premium capacity and Power BI Embedded capacity. They can grant this right to other people and for *specific* capacities. Assigning a capacity admin to a capacity does not grant him Power BI Admin rights. For example, a capacity administrator can't control tenant settings or access usage metrics. Only Global admins or Power BI admins have access to those items.

Understanding Capacity Assignment role
While Capacity Admin is restricted to a specific capacity, the Capacity Assignment role is even more restricted. It grants Power BI Pro users rights to assign workspaces to a specific capacity. This means members of the Capacity Assignment role can move workspaces from a shared capacity to a dedicated capacity and can also grant other Pro users access to that capacity workspace.

So, if I'm a Pro user and I have assignment permissions, I can create a workspace, give other Pro users access to that workspace, so everyone can collaborate on its content. However, unlike a regular workspace admin, I can move the workspace in and out of a premium capacity at any time. For example, to address peak demand, such to scale with seasonal increases in business, I can move the workspace to a premium capacity, but when the demand drops, I can move it to a shared capacity to free up resources.

12.2.2 Managing Capacities

After you've purchased capacity nodes in Office 365, you can go to the Power BI Admin Portal to set up a new capacity. In the process, you need to specify a capacity size, such as P1, and capacity admins.

Setting up a new capacity

You set up a new capacity in the "Capacity settings" tab of the Power BI Admin Portal (see **Figure 12.2**). The Power BI Premium tab (available if your organization is on Power BI Premium) is for creating and managing Power BI Premium capacities.

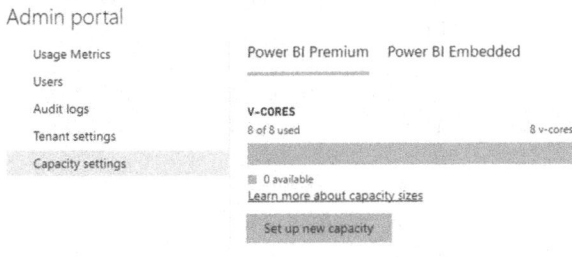

Figure 12.2 Click "Set up new capacity" to create a new capacity.

The Power BI Embedded tab is for managing embedded capacities (they need to be created in the Azure Portal). For example, your organization might not be on Power BI Premium, but it might need to embed reports for third party. After purchasing a Power BI Embedded plan in the Azure Portal, the administrator can manage the embedded capacity under the Power BI Embedded tab, while the Power BI Premium tab will be empty. On the next page, you give the capacity a name, specify its size, and assign capacity administrators. Now Office 365 global administrators, Power BI administrators, and the capacity administrators can see the new capacity in the "Capacity settings" tab, as shown in **Figure 12.3**.

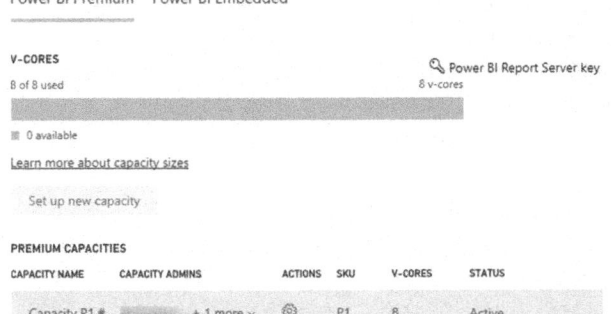

Figure 12.3 The "Capacity settings" tab shows available capacities.

Once the capacity is added, you can access its settings by clicking the Actions (gear) icon next to the capacity name. In the Settings page, you can change the capacity name, see its admins, or delete the capacity.

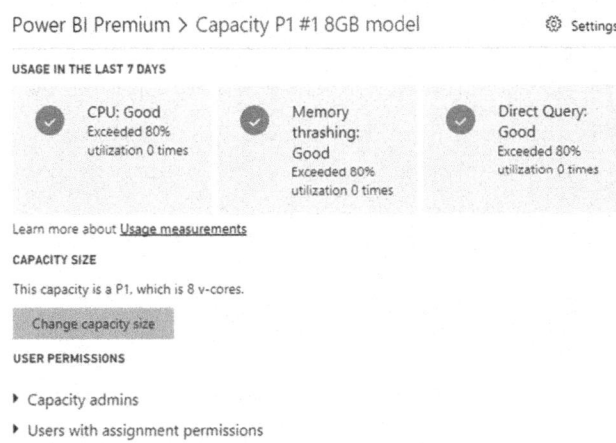

Figure 12.4 You can monitor the capacity utilization and upgrade the capacity.

Managing capacity settings

Going back to the "Capacity settings" page, you can click the capacity name in the Premium Capacities section. This brings you to the page shown in **Figure 12.4**. For each capacity, you can monitor CPU, memory, and Direct Query usage. The CPU indicator monitors the CPU usage of the capacity cores. The Memory indicator monitors the memory pressure of the backend cores. And the Direct Query indicator monitors the number of live connections per second (refer to **Table 12.1** to see the limits per capacity).

Each KPI has three indications, Good (green), Marginal (yellow) and Critical (red). When these metrics are marginal or critical, your users may experience performance degradation, especially during peak load times. You should monitor these metrics and consider upgrading the capacity if you constantly see that it's overutilized.

Power BI admins and Office 365 global admins can use this page to change the capacity size, such as by downgrading or upgrading the capacity depending on the available resources. They can also add or remove users from the Capacity Admin and Capacity Assignment roles.

12.2.3 Assigning Workspaces to Capacities

A workspace can use the Power BI Premium features only if it's assigned to a premium capacity. Power BI Premium supports two ways to do this: bulk assignments and individual assignments.

Understanding bulk assignments

Capacity admins, along with Power BI admins and Office 365 admins, can bulk assign workspaces to a capacity. The bottom half of the "Capacity settings" page shows the available workspaces, including personal workspaces (My Workspace) for every user in the organization. You can use this page to see the workspace admins assigned to each workspace. You can click the "Assign workspaces" button to open the "Assign workspaces" page (see **Figure 12.5**), which gives you three choices for bulk assignment:

- Workspaces by users – Allows you to enter one or more email addresses of specific users and assign their workspaces to a premium capacity.

- Specific workspaces – Allows you to search and assign specific workspaces.

- The entire organization's workspaces – Assigns all app workspaces and personal workspaces (My Workspace) to this capacity. Moreover, future workspaces will be assigned to this capacity because it's now the default capacity.

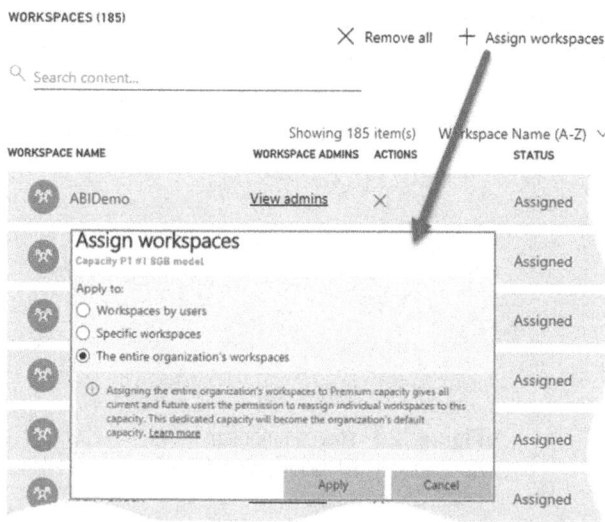

Figure 12.5 Use the "Assign workspaces" page to bulk assign workspaces.

Understanding individual assignments

If you're a workspace admin and you have Capacity Assignments rights to the workspace, you can assign that workspace to a premium capacity. To do this, go to the workspace settings and expand the Advanced section (see **Figure 12.6**). Then move the Premium slider to On and choose one of the existing capacities to which you have Capacity Assignments rights, and then click Save.

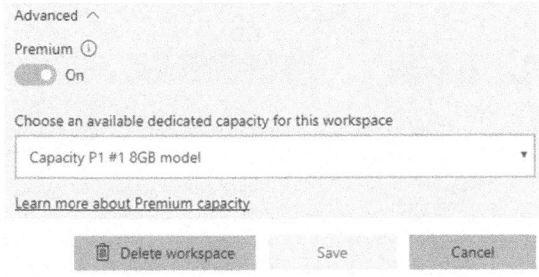

Figure 12.6 Workspace admins with Capacity Assignment can assign a workspace to an existing capacity.

The workspace is now in a premium capacity. You can easily tell which ones of the workspaces you have access to are in a premium capacity because they have a diamond icon, as shown in **Figure 12.7**.

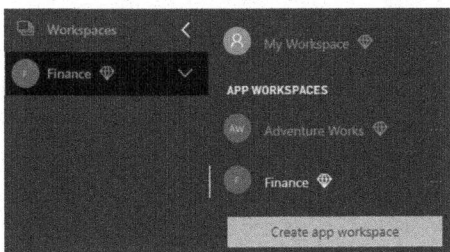

Figure 12.7 Workspaces in a premium capacity have a diamond icon next to their name in the navigation bar.

12.3 Understanding Power BI Report Server

As a cloud SaaS service, Power BI accelerates data analytics, so you can derive insights from your data faster. There isn't much for you and your users to install besides Power BI Desktop and Power BI Mobile apps. But there are cases, such as compliance and security requirements, where on-premises hosting is preferred. Enters Power BI Report Server.

 NOTE I've been privileged to contribute to and witness the evolution and success of Microsoft SQL Server Reporting Services since its debut in 2004. SSRS is Microsoft's most mature and extensible reporting platform and I can't cover its breath of features in one section. Instead, I'll focus on its integration with Power BI reports. Although written a decade ago, my book "Applied Microsoft SQL Server 2008 Reporting Services" should help you learn SSRS. To learn how to integrate Power BI Report Server with Office Online Server to render Excel reports online, read the "Configure your report server to host Excel workbooks using Office Online Server" at https://docs.microsoft.com/en-us/power-bi/report-server/excel-oos.

12.3.1 Understanding Reporting Roadmap

Think of Power BI Report Server as an add-on to Microsoft SQL Server Reporting Services (SSRS). It extends SSRS with Power BI interactive reports and Excel reports. It allows you to set up an on-premises report portal for hosting all popular Microsoft report types: traditional (RDL) reports, mobile reports, Power BI reports, and Excel reports. As far as the reason for the name change, the Power BI name has a strong recognition for modern BI while SSRS has been associated with paginated reports.

Understanding deployment options

With Power BI Report Server, Microsoft delivers on their promise for a unified reporting platform on cloud and premises. For more information about their vision, read the blog "Microsoft Business Intelligence – our reporting roadmap" at https://blogs.technet.microsoft.com/dataplatforminsider/2015/10/29/microsoft-business-intelligence-our-reporting-roadmap. **Figure 12.8** shows how Power BI Report Server fits into the reporting roadmap.

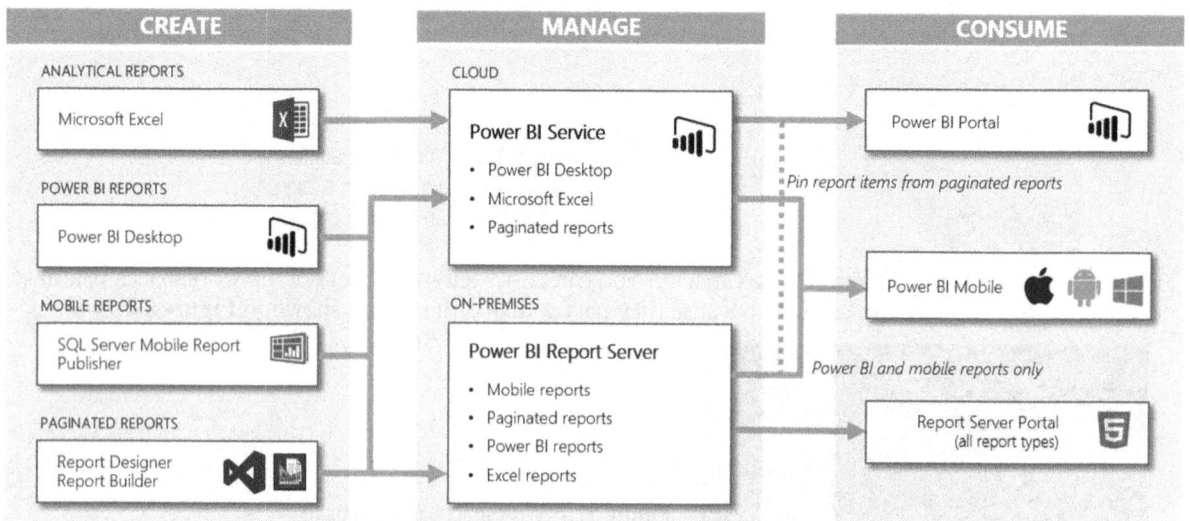

Figure 12.8 The Microsoft roadmap envisions a unified reporting platform delivered in cloud and on premises.

Microsoft BI has four popular report types: analytical Excel reports, Power BI reports, mobile reports (introduced in SSRS 2016), and paginated (RDL) reports. **Table 12.4** shows how these report types can be deployed to the cloud and on premises, and the main limitations.

Table 12.4 How the four main report types integrate with Power BI Service and Power BI Premium

Report Types	Power BI	Power BI Report Server
Excel reports	Pros: Can connect to Excel files. Cons: Excel reports can't connect live to Analysis Services	Pros: Can render Excel reports, including connected live to AS Cons: You need to install Office Online Server. For live connections, Kerberos authentication might be required
Power BI reports	Pros: Natively supported Cons: Power BI Service lacks modeling features	Pros: You can deploy Power BI reports to the report server Cons: Lagging in features compared to Power BI Service
SSRS mobile reports	Pros: Power BI Mobile can display on-premises mobile reports Cons: Can't deploy these reports to Power BI Service	Pros: Natively supported Cons: Difficult to find a good fit for these reports as they as not as interactive as Power BI reports
Paginated reports	Pros: Can pin report items from on-premises report server to Power BI dashboards Cons: Can't be deployed to Power BI Service	Pros: Natively supported, most extensible report type Cons: Power BI Mobile can't display them, pinned report items are exported as images and lose interactivity

Comparing reporting options

If you have used SSRS in the past, you might wonder how Power BI Report Server compares to it and to Power BI Service. **Table 12.5** compares these three products side by side.

Table 12.5 Feature comparison between SSRS, Power BI Report Server, and Power BI Service

	SQL Server Reporting Services	Power BI Report Server	Power BI Service Power BI Premium
Deployment	On-premises	On-premises	Cloud
Excel reports	No	Yes	Yes (no live connections to Analysis Services)
Power BI reports	No	Yes (restricted features)	Yes
SSRS mobile reports	Yes	Yes	No
Paginated (RDL) reports	Yes	Yes	No (can pin report items from Power BI Report Server)
Max imported dataset size	N/A	2 GB	1 GB (Power BI Pro), up to 10 GB (Premium)
Apps	No	No	Yes
Q&A	No	No	Yes
Quick Insights	No	No	Yes
Embedding Power BI reports for third party	No	Planned	Yes
Subscriptions	Paginated reports only	Paginated reports only	Page-level subscriptions for Power BI reports
Data alerts	No	No	Yes (dashboard tiles)
Mobile apps	No	Yes (mobile and Power BI reports)	Yes

To summarize, based on my experience, most organizations gravitate toward cloud deployments, so Power BI Service would be their natural choice. Some organizations prefer on-premises report portals. If you're looking for a report portal that can host all the four main report types in Microsoft BI, then Power BI Report Server is the way to go. One caveat that you need to be aware of if you plan to embed reports for external customers is that the ASP.NET Report Viewer control, which you probably use to embed paginated reports, doesn't support Power BI reports. While waiting for Microsoft to enable the Power BI Embedded APIs in Power BI Report Server, consider configuring the report server for custom security.

 NOTE To give Microsoft credit, embedding Power BI reports in internal web apps is easy and it can be done with iframe, such as <iframe src="https://server/reports/powerbi/ReportName?rs:Embed=true" width="800px" height="600px"></iframe>. However, this approach probably won't work for external users where Windows security is not an option.

12.3.2 Getting Started with Power BI Report Server

Now that you understand at a high level what Power BI Report Server is, let's cover some important considerations of how to acquire and install it. Starting with SQL Server 2017, Microsoft has removed SSRS from the SQL Server setup program so that it can be enhanced more frequently. Similarly, Power BI Report Server is not included in the SQL Server setup.

How to acquire Power BI Report Server
Power BI Report Server can be acquired in one of two ways:

■ Power BI Premium – If your organization has Power BI Premium, Microsoft gives you rights to concurrently deploy Power BI Report Server to the same number of on-premises cores. Let's say you purchased one Power BI Premium P1 node. It gives you eight v-cores. You get also eight on-premises cores to run Power BI Premium Server! If you decide to acquire Power BI Report Server this way, you can obtain the Power BI Report Server product key from the "Capacity settings" page in the Power BI Admin Portal.

■ SQL Server Enterprise license with Software Assurance – If you don't use Power BI Premium or you need more cores, you can license Power BI Report Server under the SQL Server Enterprise Edition license just like you license SSRS. However, your organization needs a Software Assurance (SA) agreement with Microsoft. With this option, you can obtain the product key from the Volume Licensing Service Center at https://www.microsoft.com/Licensing/servicecenter/.

Like SQL Server Developer Edition, Power BI Report Server doesn't require a license for development and testing (during the setup, simply select the Developer edition which doesn't require a product key). It's important to understand that like Power BI Service, every user who deploys reports to the report server must be covered by a separate Power BI Pro license. This is an honor-based system as Power BI Report Server has no checks to enforce this requirement.

Installing Power BI Report Server
Microsoft is actively working on enhancing Power BI Report Server and have committed to a bi-monthly release cadence. To achieve this goal, Power BI Report Server is available as a standalone product that can be downloaded from the Microsoft Download Center at https://aka.ms/pbireportserver. There isn't much to install and configure. Once you acquire the product key (assuming production use), you only need to decide where to install the server and the Report Server Database.

Like SSRS, Power BI Report Server stores report definitions and management settings in a SQL Server database (its default name is ReportServer), and temporary data in another SQL Server database (its default name is ReportServerTempDB). You can install the SQL Server Database Engine on the same machine where the report server is installed. In this case, both products could be covered by the same license. Or, you might decide to host the databases on a separate SQL Server instance (SQL Server 2008 is the minimum lowest version supported). Keep in mind that not all editions of SQL Server can be used to host the database. For example, you can't install Power BI Report Server for production use and have the report database on SQL Server Developer Edition.

Installing Power BI Desktop
Here is something unfortunate for those of us who plan to deploy Power BI reports to both Power BI Service (powerbi.com) and Power BI Report Server. Because Power BI is evolving faster (new features are released every month), Power BI Report Server is lagging Power BI. So, there are two Power BI Desktop versions:

■ Untethered version – Adds features at a monthly cadence and can be downloaded from the Power BI Desktop download page or from Microsoft Store.

■ Power BI Report Server version – This version is locked to Power BI Report Server and updated when a new report server release is available. You can download it from the Power BI Report Server download page. The unfortunate side effect is that if you want to publish to both Power BI Service and Power BI Report Server, you need to install and keep both versions.

You can install both versions side by side because the Power BI Report Server version installs in a separate folder (\Program Files\Microsoft Power BI Desktop RS). Only the Power BI Report Server version has an option to deploy the file to Power BI Report Server (Save as ⇨ Power BI Report Server).

 NOTE Why couldn't the Power BI Report Server just ignore Power BI features it doesn't recognize, so we can have just one Power BI Desktop app? Unfortunately, the PBIX file format doesn't yet have the infrastructure to consistently and reliably do so because it was developed for Power BI Service. Therefore, Microsoft had to resort to Power BI Desktop builds optimized for specific Power BI Report Server.

12.3.3 Understanding Integration with Power BI

In Chapter 4, I showed you how you can pin report items from paginated reports to Power BI dashboards. And in Chapter 5, I showed you how to view Power BI and mobile reports deployed to a report server in Power BI Mobile. You have also the option to deploy Power BI Desktop files to Power BI Reports Server. Let's provide some additional guidance about these three options from a management perspective.

Pinning report items
Your users can pin image-generating report items, such as charts, gauges, maps, and images, to a Power BI dashboard. When the user clicks a dashboard tile that is pinned from a report item, the user is navigated by default to the underlying report (you can change the URL in the tile properties to navigate the user elsewhere). Consequently, the user must be on the corporate network to navigate to the report (the user doesn't have to be on the corporate network to view the tile). However, you can set up a web application proxy to view SSRS reports outside the corporate network. The Chris Finlan's "Leveraging Web Application Proxy in Windows Server 2016 to provide secure access to your SQL Server Reporting Services environment" blog has the details at bit.ly/ssrsproxy.

Pinning report items requires specific configuration steps that are well documented by Microsoft in the "Power BI Report Server Integration (Configuration Manager)" article at bit.ly/2g0vHW0. Microsoft has also done a good job documenting limitations, but I'd like to add a few comments for you to consider before you enable this feature. First, the source reports must use stored credentials. This is because the underlying mechanism for refreshing pinned items rely on individual subscriptions that are scheduled and run unattended with SQL Server Agent. What this limitation means is that when configuring the report data source, you must specify user name and password of a login that has read rights to the data source.

This limitation has been a personal frustration of mine since the early days of SSRS because it's impractical when connecting to data sources that require Windows authentication, such as Analysis Services. For example, it's a common requirement to implement dynamic security in SSAS models to restrict data depending on the user identity. But now you have a predicament because you must store the user credentials and the data security won't work.

 REAL LIFE Power BI Report Server uses individual subscriptions to refresh the Power BI tiles. Because individual subscriptions are associated with the user who pinned the item, Microsoft could have implemented a mechanism to pass the user identity without requiring the password, like how Power BI uses EffectiveUserName.

Continuing the list of limitations, you can't pin tables and matrices, which happen to be the most popular report items. Another thing to watch for is that deleting a dashboard tile with a pinned report item doesn't remove the individual subscriptions. So, if 10 users pin a report item and all users decide that they don't need that tile anymore and delete it from their dashboards, you still have 10 scheduled subscriptions that will continue running on report-specific schedules! Since currently the report server doesn't give the administrator an easy way to view what individual subscriptions exist, it might not be long before your report server starts experiencing performance issues.

Viewing reports in Power BI Mobile
Users can use the Power BI mobile apps to view Power BI reports and SSRS mobile reports. SSRS mobile reports (not to be confused with the Power BI mobile apps) were introduced in SSRS 2016. A BI developer creates them using Microsoft SQL Server Mobile Report Publisher. As I explain in my blog "Choosing a reporting tool" at http://prologika.com/choosing-a-reporting-tool, I have reservations about this report type. In my opinion, besides Power BI reports, it would have been much more useful to support traditional (now referred to as paginated) reports, which is the most popular report type.

Deploying Power BI reports to report server
Only Power BI Report Server supports rendering Power BI reports online. While you can deploy Power BI Desktop files to SQL Server Reporting Services (you can upload any file to the report catalog), when the

end user clicks the report, the Power BI Desktop file is downloaded locally. Consequently, the user needs to have Power BI Desktop installed to view reports. So, you need Power BI Report Server for a better user experience. Next, let's review essential considerations for deploying and managing Power BI reports.

12.3.4 Managing Power BI Reports

As I mentioned, Microsoft has committed to frequent releases of Power BI Report Server. As of this time, the latest release is the October 2017 release. It includes the following features:

- Direct Query connectivity to Analysis Services, SQL Server, Azure SQL Database, Oracle, Teradata, SAP HANA and SAP BW. For an up-to-date list of the supported data sources, refer to the "Power BI report data sources in Power BI Report Server" article at https://docs.microsoft.com/en-us/power-bi/report-server/data-sources.
- Imported datasets with up to 2 GB maximum file size, though the default setting of the MaxFileSizeMb system property is 1 GB (in SSMS, connect to the report server to change it).
- Scheduled data refresh for imported datasets
- Custom visuals are supported

Managing Power BI settings
The administrator can control some settings specific to Power BI by following these steps:

1. Open SQL Server Management Studio. In Object Explorer, expand the Connect drop-down and choose Reporting Services.
2. Enter either the report server machine name or URL address, such as http://<ServerName>/reportserver.
3. Right-click the report server in Object Explorer, and click Properties.
4. In the Server Properties window, select the Advanced tab.

Table 12.6 shows the properties specific to Power BI Report Server.

Table 12.6 Power BI specific settings in Power BI Report Server

Report Types	Default Setting	Purpose
EnableCustomVisuals	True	Enables rendering custom visuals in reports.
EnablePowerBIReportEmbeddedModels	True	Enables reports with imported data
EnablePowerBIReportExportData	True	Allows exporting data from Power BI reports
MaxFileSizeMb	1 GB	Maximum file size for uploaded reports. Default is 1000 MB (1 GB). Maximum value is 2000 MB (2 GB).
ModelCleanupCycleMinutes	15 minutes	Defines how often the model is checked to evict it from memory.
ModelExpirationMinutes	60 minutes	Defines how long until the model expires based on the last time used and is evicted
ScheduleRefreshTimeoutMinutes	120 minutes	Defines how long the data refresh can take for a model before connection expires

These settings allow you to govern certain aspects of Power BI reports. For example, if you don't want to support custom visuals, you can turn off the EnableCustomVisuals setting, or if you want to support 2 GB datasets, you can increase the MaxFileSizeDb setting.

Deploying reports

Remember that you need the Power BI Report Server version of Power BI Desktop to deploy pbix files. This version is available on the Power BI Report Server download page. To deploy a Power BI Desktop file to the report catalog:

1. Open the file in Power BI Desktop. Click Save As ⇨ Power BI Report Server.

2. If this if the first time you connect to the report server, enter the Web Portal address of the report server, such as http://ServerName/reports. Once the address is validated, it will be added to "Recent report servers", so you don't have to type it in every time. If you're unsure about the address, open the Report Server Configuration Manager (not the SSRS Reporting Services Configuration Manager), connect to the server, and check the address in the Web Portal URL tab.

3. Select a folder in the report catalog where you want to publish the file to, and click OK. Another way to upload your file is to navigate to the Power BI Report Server portal and upload it manually.

Back to Power BI Desktop, if you want to open a (*.pbix) file from the report catalog, use the Open ⇨ Power BI Report Server menu.

 NOTE If you try using the latest untethered version of Power BI Desktop to upload the *.pbix file manually to the report catalog, you'd probably be greeted with the "Can't upload this report" error. As the error explains, the reason is that either the file is a newer version or has component parts that are not supported. Instead of starting from scratch, try opening the file in the Power BI Report Server version to ignore the features it doesn't recognize, and then upload the file to the report catalog.

Viewing reports

The whole reason why you'd want to have Power BI Report Server is to view Power BI reports online. "Online" means that reports are rendered in the browser, instead of prompting the user to download the file and open it in Power BI Desktop. End users must have permissions to view reports and Power BI reports share the same security model as other report types. For example, you can add AD groups and individual users to the predefined Browser role to let them view reports in a folder and its subfolders.

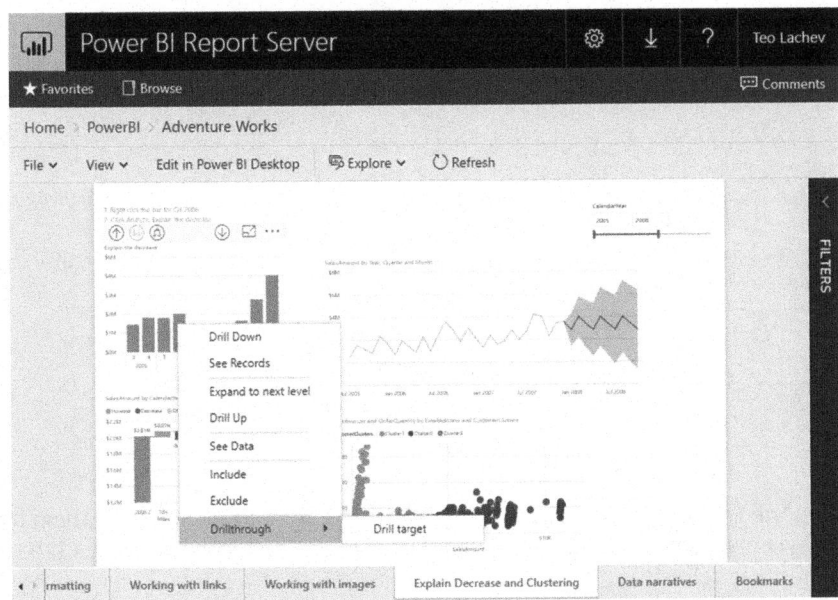

Figure 12.9 Power BI reports render online in the Power BI Report Server portal and preserve their interactive features.

Figure 12.9 shows the Adventure Works report (discussed in the previous chapter) rendered inside the Power BI Report Server portal. The report preserves its interactivity, but the latest features won't work. For example, the bookmarks slider (a preview feature) doesn't show up. One feature that your users gain in Power BI Report Server is ability to post comments. They can click the Comments menu to start a discussion thread regarding the report data. A similar Power BI Service feature is group conversations, but they are at a workspace (not report) level.

Managing data sources

As an IT Pro, you need to manage different aspects of deployed Power BI reports. And one of the most common tasks is managing the report data sources.

1. Hover on any Power BI report and click the ellipsis (…) menu. Click Manage.

2. In the Manage Report page, click Data Sources.

3. Notice that the Data Sources page lists all the data sources in the *.pbix file. However, you can only change the authentication type (not the connection string), as shown in **Figure 12.10**.

If you plan to schedule a model with imported data for automated refresh, you must specify stored credentials in the data sources. That's because the report server will start the refresh operation on its own and there won't be an interactive user to authenticate. You can use either Windows Authentication or Basic Authentication. With the former, you must specify a Windows account that has read rights to the data source. The latter is only available for relational databases, such as SQL Server, and lets you specify the credentials of a login that has read rights to the data.

> **TIP** If your model imports data from files, the connection string needs to reference network shares. If you import local files, open the file in Power BI Desktop, expand the Edit Queries button (Home ribbon) and click "Data source settings". Select the file data source and click Change Source. Then, change the file path to be a UNC file path. For example, instead of referencing C:\PowerBI\Resellers.xlsx, enter \\YourComputerName>\C$\PowerBI\Resellers.xlsx, and upload the file to Power BI Report Server.

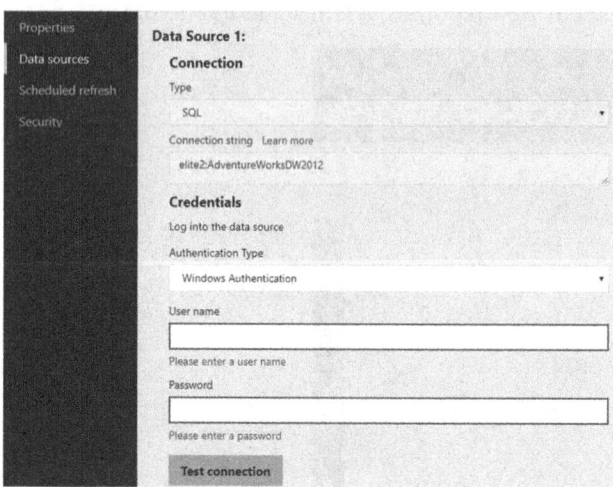

Figure 12.10 You can only change the data source authentication type for published Power BI reports.

Managing scheduled refresh

Like deploying datasets with imported data to Power BI Service, you'd probably want to schedule them for automatic refresh to keep them synchronized with changes to the data sources. Two conditions need to be met before you can schedule automatic refresh:

■ You must change all data sources to use stored credentials before you can schedule a report for automated refresh.

■ The SQL Server Agent service needs to be running on the SQL Server hosting the report database.

Setting up automated refresh requires a refresh plan. Think of a refresh plan as a set of refresh properties related to a specific Power BI report, including a description and schedule. A report can have multiple refresh plans, such as to refresh multiple times per day Monday to Friday, and once per day on weekends.

1. In the Manage Report page, click the "Schedule refresh" tab.

2. Click "New scheduled refresh plan". In the next page, choose between an existing shared schedule or create a report-specific schedule. This works the same way as when you schedule SSRS individual or data-driven subscriptions.

3. Click "Create scheduled refresh plan" to create the plan. Going back to the "Scheduled refresh" page, you should now see the refresh plan (see **Figure 12.11**).

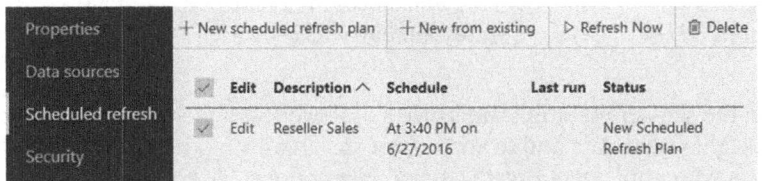

Figure 12.11 A refresh plan specifies how often the report will be refreshed.

4. Check the checkbox preceding the plan name. Notice that you can create a new plan from the one you selected. You can also click "Refresh now" to trigger manual refresh, such as to test the plan.

5. Observe that the Status column says "Started data refresh". After some time, click F5 to refresh the page. If the refresh is still running, the status should read "Refreshing". If all is well, the status should say "Completed Data Refresh". If something goes wrong, it should read "Several errors occurred during data refresh. Please try again later or contact you administrator.". You can click the information icon next to the status to see the errors.

TIP Currently, the report server doesn't have a user interface to show the refresh history. However, the status messages are logged in the SubscriptionHistory table in the ReportServer database. Report refreshes are logged in the ExecutionLog table with RequestType=DataRefresh. You can use the ExecutionLog3 view to monitor the overall status, frequency, and outcome of refreshes for all reports.

12.4 Summary

This chapter focused on two important products in the Power BI portfolio: Power BI Premium and Power BI Report Server. Larger organizations will benefit from the Power BI Premium dedicated capacity that ensures consistent performance and protection from activities of other tenants in Power BI Service. Such organizations can also reduce licensing cost by sharing content of premium workspaces to Power BI Free users by either dashboard sharing or apps. Microsoft is expected to add more features to Power BI Premium to make it ever more appealing.

Power BI Report Server allows you to implement an on-premises report portal to centralize BI assets and manage them in one place. An add-on to SSRS, Power BI Report Server can accommodate the four most popular report types in Microsoft BI: Excel analytical reports, Power BI reports, SSRS mobile reports, and traditional paginated (RDL) reports. Power BI Report Server can be acquired by a Power BI Premium plan or under a SQL Server Enterprise Edition with Software Assurance license. Microsoft has committed to enhancing Power BI Report Server bi-monthly and keeping it up to date with Power BI Service.

Power BI is a part of a much broader Microsoft Data Platform. You've seen how Power BI can integrate with popular cloud services and on-premises report servers. The next chapter will show you how you can create other BI solutions that integrate with Power BI!

Chapter 13

Organizational BI

So far, the focus of this book has been the self-service and team aspects of Power BI, which empower business users and data analysts to gain insights from data and to share these insights with other users. Now it's time to turn our attention to BI pros who implement organizational BI solutions. Back in Chapter 2, I compared self-service and organizational BI at a high level. I defined organizational BI as a set of technologies and processes for implementing an end-to-end BI solution where the implementation effort is shifted to BI professionals.

This chapter shows BI pros how to build common organizational BI solutions. You'll understand the importance of having an organizational semantic layer, and you'll learn how to integrate it with Power BI. Implementing real-time BI solutions is one of the fastest growing BI trends. I'll show you how this can be done using the Power BI real-time API and Azure Stream Analytics Service, while you use Power BI for real-time dashboards. Because predictive analytics is another popular scenario, I'll show you how you can integrate Power BI with predictive models that you publish to Azure Machine Learning.

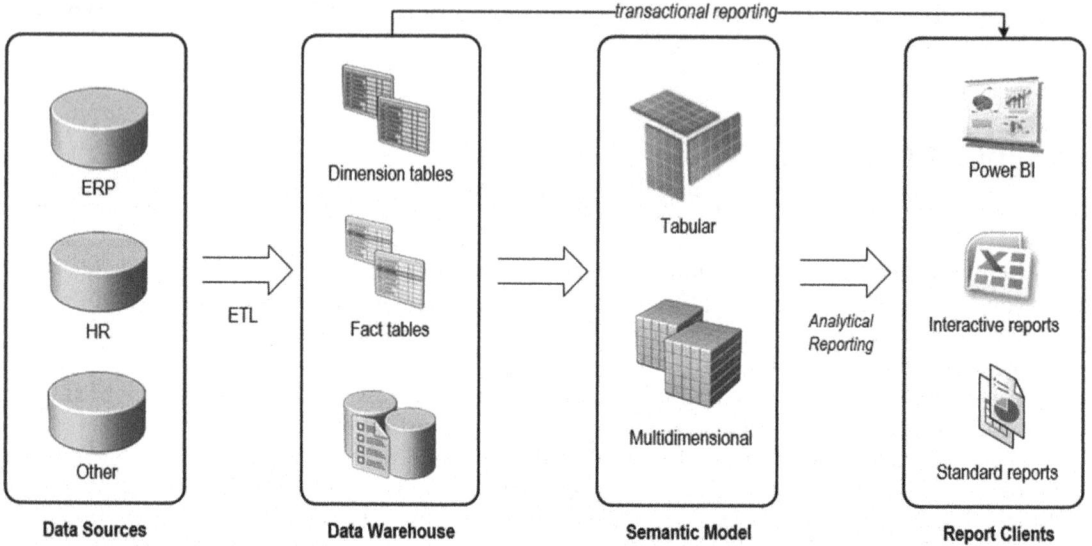

Figure 13.1   Organizational BI typically includes ETL processes, data warehousing, and a semantic layer.

13.1 Implementing Classic BI Solutions

In Chapter 2, I introduced you at a high level to what I refer to as a classic BI solution (see **Figure 13.1**). This diagram should be familiar to you. Almost every organization nowadays has a centralized data repository, typically called a data warehouse or a data mart, which consolidates cleaned and trusted data from operational systems.

> **REAL LIFE** Data warehousing might mean different things to different people. In my consulting practice, I've seen data warehouse "flavors" ranging from normalized operational data stores (ODS) to hub-and-spoke architectures. If they work for you then that's all that matters. I personally recommend and implement a consolidated data repository designed in accordance with Ralph Kimball's dimensional modeling (star schema), consisting of fact and dimension tables. For more information about dimensional modeling, I recommend the book "The Data Warehouse Toolkit" by Ralph Kimball and Margy Ross.

You might not have an organizational semantic layer that sits between the data warehouse and users, and you might not know what it is. In general, semantics relates to discovering the meaning of the message behind the words. In the context of data and BI, semantics represents the user's perspective of data: how the end user views the data to derive knowledge from it. As a BI pro, your job is to translate machine-friendly database structures and terminology into a user-friendly semantic layer that describes the business problems to be solved. In Microsoft BI, the role of this layer is fulfilled by Microsoft BI Semantic Model (BISM).

13.1.1 Understanding Microsoft BISM

Microsoft BISM is a unifying name for several Microsoft technologies for implementing semantic models, including self-service models implemented with Excel Power Pivot or Power BI Desktop, and organizational Microsoft Analysis Services models. From an organizational BI standpoint, BI pros are most interested in Microsoft Analysis Services modeling capabilities.

> **NOTE** Besides the necessary fundamentals, this chapter doesn't attempt to teach you Multidimensional or Tabular. To learn more about Analysis Services, I covered implementing Analysis Services Multidimensional models in my book "Applied Microsoft Analysis Services 2005" and Tabular models in "Applied Microsoft SQL Server 2012 Analysis Services: Tabular Modeling".

Introducing Multidimensional and Tabular
Since its first release in 1998, Analysis Services has provided Online Analytical Processing (OLAP) capabilities so that IT professionals can implement Multidimensional OLAP cubes for descriptive analytics. The OLAP side of Analysis Services is referred to as *Multidimensional*. Multidimensional is a mature model that can scale to large data volumes. For example, Elena can build a Multidimensional cube on top of a large data warehouse with billions of rows, while still providing an excellent response time where most queries finish within a second!

Starting with SQL Server 2012, Microsoft expanded the Analysis Services capabilities by adding a new path for implementing semantic models, where entities are represented as relational-like constructs, such as two-dimensional tables, columns, and relationships. Referred to as *Tabular*, this technology uses the same xVelocity engine that powers Power BI Desktop, Excel Power Pivot, Power BI, and SQL Server columnstore indexes. Although not as scalable as Multidimensional, Tabular gains in simplicity and flexibility. And because Tabular uses the same storage engine, if you know how to create self-service data models in Power BI Desktop or Excel, you already know 90% of Tabular! That's right, while you were learning how to build self-service data models with Power BI Desktop you were also learning how to implement Tabular models.

Understanding implementation paths
Microsoft organizational BISM can be visualized as a three-tier model that consists of data access, business logic, and data model layers (see **Figure 13.2**). The data model layer is exposed to external clients. Clients

can query BISM by sending Multidimensional Expressions (MDX) or Data Analysis Expressions (DAX) queries. For example, Excel can connect to both Multidimensional and Tabular and send MDX queries, while Power BI and Power View send DAX queries.

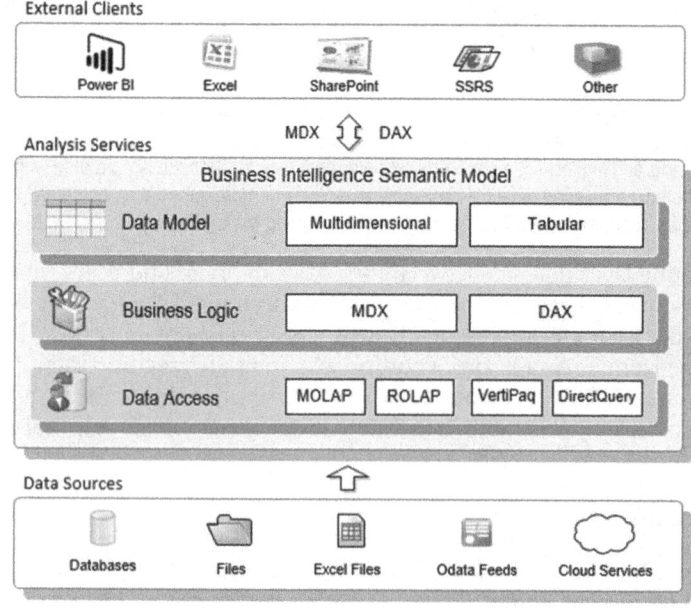

Figure 13.2 BISM has two organizational BI implementation paths: Multidimensional and Tabular.

The business logic layer allows the modeler to define business metrics, such as variances, time calculations, and key performance indicators (KPIs). In Multidimensional, you can implement this layer using Multidimensional Expressions (MDX) constructs, such as calculated members, named sets, and scope assignments. Tabular embraces the same Data Analysis Expressions (DAX) that you've learned about in Chapter 9 when you added business calculations to the Adventure Works model.

The data access layer interfaces with external data sources. By default, both Multidimensional and Tabular import data from the data sources and cache the dataset on the server for best performance. The default multidimensional storage option is Multidimensional OLAP (MOLAP), where data is stored in a compressed disk-based format. The default Tabular storage option is xVelocity, where data is initially saved to disk but later loaded in memory when users query the model.

Both Multidimensional and Tabular support real-time data access by providing a Relational OLAP (ROLAP) storage mode for Multidimensional and a DirectQuery storage mode for Tabular. When a Multidimensional cube is configured for ROLAP, Analysis Services doesn't process and cache the data on the server. Instead, it auto-generates and sends native queries to the database. Similarly, when a Tabular model is configured for DirectQuery, Analysis Services doesn't keep data in xVelocity; it sends native queries directly to the data source. As I mentioned in Chapter 6, the DirectQuery mode of Tabular enables DirectQuery connections in Power BI Desktop.

Understanding the BISM advantages

Having a semantic model is very valuable for organizational BI for the following main reasons:

- Larger data volumes – Remember that Power BI Service currently limits imported files to 250 MB each, including Power BI Desktop models. This size limit won't be adequate for organizational solutions that are typically built on top of corporate data warehouses. By contrast, BISM can scale to billions of rows and terabytes of data!

- Great performance – BISM is optimized to aggregate data very fast. Queries involving regular measures and simple calculations should be answered within seconds even, when aggregating millions of rows!
- Single version of the truth – Business logic and metrics can be centralized in the semantic model instead of being defined and redefined in the database or in reports.

> **REAL WORLD** The BI department of a retail company included some 20 report developers on staff whose sole responsibility was creating operational reports from stored procedures. Over time, stored procedures have grown in complexity, and developers have defined important business metrics differently. Needless to say, operational reports didn't tally. Although the term "a single version of the truth" is somewhat overloaded, a centralized semantic model can get you very close to it.

- Data security – Like row-level security (RLS) in Power BI Desktop, BISM models can apply data security based on the user's identity, such as to allow Maya to only see the data for the customers she's authorized to access.
- Implicit relationships – In the process of designing the semantic layer, the modeler defines relationships between entities, just like a data analyst does when creating a self-service model. As a result, end users don't need to join tables explicitly because the relationships have already been established at design time. For example, you don't have to know how to join the Product table to the Sales table. You simply add the fields you need on the report, and then the model knows how to relate them!
- Interactive data analysis – From an end-user perspective, data analysis is a matter of dragging and dropping attributes on the report to slice and dice data. A "smart" client, such as Power BI, auto-generates report queries, and the server takes care of aggregating data, such as to summarize sales at the year level.
- Good client support – There are many reporting tools, including Power BI, Excel, Reporting Services, and third-party tools, that support BISM and address various reporting needs, including standard reports, interactive reports, and dashboards.

When should you upgrade to organizational BI?
You might have started your BI journey with a self-service model in Excel or Power BI Desktop. Why can't this be your semantic model given that it could be as feature-rich as a Tabular model. At what point should you consider switching to an organizational solution? What would you gain?

> **REAL WORLD** Everyone wants quick and easy BI solutions, ideally with a click of a button. But the reality is much more difficult. I often find that companies have attempted to implement organizational BI solutions with self-service tools, like Power BI Desktop, Excel, or some other third-party tools. The primary reasons are cutting cost and misinformation (that's why it's important to know who you listen to). The result is always the same – sooner or later the company finds that it's time to "graduate" to organizational BI. Don't get me wrong, though. Self-service BI has its important place, as I explain in Chapter 2. But having trusted organizational-level solutions will require the right architecture, toolset, and investment.

You should consider moving to an organizational solution when the following happens:

- Data integration – The requirements call for extracting data from several systems and consolidating data instead of implementing isolated self-service data models.
- Data complexity – You realize that the data complexity exceeds the capabilities of the Power BI Desktop queries. For example, the integration effort required to clean and transform corporate data typically exceeds the simple transformation capabilities of self-service models.
- Data security – Security requirements might dictate leaving data on premises without compromising report performance. This excludes deploying data extracts to the cloud.
- Enterprise scalability – Power BI Desktop and Excel models import data in files. Once you get beyond a few million rows, you'll find that you stretch the limits of these tools. For example, it'll take a while

to save and load the file. It'll take even longer to upload the file to Power BI. By contrast, organizational models must be capable of handling larger data volumes. Just by deploying the model to an Analysis Services instance, you gain better scalability that's boosted by the hardware resources of a dedicated server.

■ Faster data refresh – Unlike the Power BI Desktop sequential data refresh, organizational models support processing tables and partitioned tables in parallel, to better utilize the resources of a dedicated server. Also, to reduce the data load window and to process data incrementally, you can divide large tables in partitions.

■ Richer model – Tabular supports additional features that might be appealing to you, including international translations, drillthrough actions, display folders, and programmatically generating the model schema. Because you'll be using Visual Studio to design your BISM, you can enjoy all the Visual Studio IDE features, including source control integration.

 NOTE What if you have started with Power BI Desktop but want to upgrade to Tabular? Currently, Tabular supports upgrading from Excel Power Pivot only. There's no officially supported upgrade path from Power BI Desktop models. That's because Microsoft updates Power BI Desktop monthly, and it can get ahead of Tabular, which is included in the SQL Server box product and only releases a new version every few years. However, I outlined an unsupported way in my blog "Upgrading Power BI Desktop Models to Tabular" at http://prologika.com/upgrading-power-bi-desktop-models-to-tabular. Use it at your own risk!

Comparing self-service and organizational models

Since you're reading this book, the logical transition path is from Power BI Desktop (or Excel) to Tabular. Then you'll discover that you can seamlessly transition your knowledge to organizational projects. Indeed, an organizational Tabular model has the same foundation as Power Pivot or Power BI Desktop, but it adds enterprise-oriented and advanced features, such as options for configuring security, scalability, and low latency. **Table 13.1** provides a side-by-side comparison between self-service and organizational features.

Table 13.1 This table highlights the differences between self-service and organizational semantic models.

Feature	Self-service Models	Organizational Models
Target users	Business users	Professionals
Environment	Power BI Desktop or Excel	Visual Studio (SSDT)
xVelocity Engine	Out of process (local in-memory engine)	Out of process (dedicated Analysis Services instance)
Size	One file (dataset size limits apply)	Large data volumes, table partitions
Refreshing data	Sequential table refresh	Parallel table refresh, incremental processing (parallel partition refresh starting with SQL Server 2016)
Data transformation	Power Query in Excel, queries in PBI Desktop	Not available (typically ETL processes are in place)
Development	Ad-hoc development	Project (business case, plan, dates, hardware, source control)
Lifespan	Weeks or months	Years

How Power BI Service connects to on-premises Analysis Services

Now that you understand the benefits of an organizational semantic model, let's see how Power BI integrates with Analysis Services. One implementation path leads to hosting your semantic model in the cloud using Azure Analysis Services. In this case, no gateways are needed because Power BI can connect directly to cloud data sources. If operational or other requirements dictate on-premises deployment, Power BI can access on-premises Analysis Services models with the Power BI On-premises Data Gateway.

NOTE Currently, the gateway doesn't support connecting to Tabular in SharePoint integration mode (Power Pivot for SharePoint uses this mode). I hope this limitation is lifted soon so that you can connect Power BI to cubes and to Power Pivot models deployed to SharePoint if you have invested in Power Pivot. Unfortunately, Power BI doesn't support HTTP access to Analysis Services using a special component called data pump (HTTP access to SSAS is discussed in the "Configure HTTP Access to Analysis Services on Internet Information Services (IIS) 8.0" article at https://msdn.microsoft.com/library/gg492140.aspx). So, you can't avoid using a gateway to access on-premises SSAS models.

From the Power BI standpoint, the BISM integration scenario that will inspire the most interest is the hybrid architecture shown in **Figure 13.3**. This architecture will be also appealing for companies that prefer to keep data on premises but want to host only report and dashboard definitions to Power BI. Elena has implemented an Analysis Services Tabular model layered on top of the Adventure Works data warehouse, and she deployed it to an on-premises server. "On premises" could mean any model that is not hosted in Azure Analysis Services, such as a server hosted in the company's data center or on an Azure virtual machine. So that Power BI can connect to the model, Elena installs the On-premises Data Gateway on a machine that can connect to the Analysis Services instance. Elena has granted Maya access to the model.

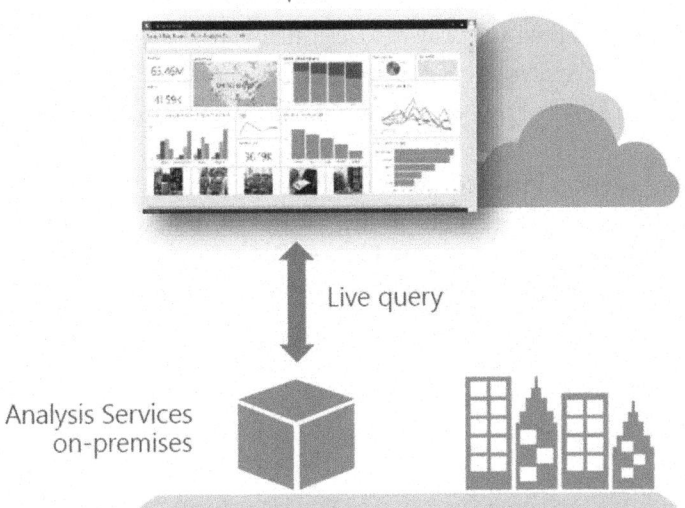

Live dashboards and exploration

Live query

Analysis Services on-premises

Figure 13.3 You can implement a hybrid architecture by connecting Power BI to on-premises Analysis Services models.

Maya logs in to Power BI and uses Get Data to connect to Analysis Services. Maya selects the Adventure Works model. Power BI establishes a live connection. Now Maya can create reports and dashboards, as I demonstrated in Chapter 2. If the model is configured for data security, Maya can only see the data that the model security authorizes her to access. When she explores the data, Power BI auto-generates DAX queries and sends them to the Adventure Works model. The model sends results back. No data is hosted on Power BI!

13.1.2 Understanding Setup Requirements

Because Power BI needs to connect to the on-premises model and pass the user identity, IT needs to take care of certain prerequisites for both on premises and in the cloud. The exact setup steps depend on how your company is set up for Microsoft Azure.

Understanding domain considerations
The following special considerations apply when setting up a gateway data source that connects to SSAS.

1. Analysis Services must be installed on a domain-joined machine. That's because Analysis Services supports only Windows security.

2. The Windows account that you specify in the data source properties of the On-premises Data Gateway, must have admin rights to the Analysis Services instance. That's because behind the scenes the gateway passes the user identity by appending an EffectiveUserName setting to the connection string. This connectivity mechanism requires admin rights.

 NOTE Behind the scenes, the gateway appends a special EffectiveUserName connection setting when it connects to an on-premises SSAS. If Maya connects to the Analysis Services server, then EffectiveUserName will pass Maya's email, such as EffectiveUserName=maya@adventureworks.com. To verify or grant the account admin rights to SSAS, open SQL Server Management Studio (SSMS) and connect to your SSAS instance. Right-click on the instance, and then click Properties. In the Security tab of the Analysis Services Properties page, add the account to the server administrators list.

3. Without special mapping (see next section), the end user and Analysis Services must be on the same domain or trusted domains. For example, if I log in to Power BI as teo@adventureworks.com, Analysis Services must be on the adventureworks.com domain, or on a domain that has a trust relationship.

Checking access

Follow these steps to verify whether the On-premises Data Gateway can delegate the user identity:

1. Make sure that you have administrator access to the Analysis Services instance.

2. Open SQL Server Management Studio (SSMS). In Object Explorer, expand the Connect drop-down, and then click Connect ⇨ Analysis Services.

3. In the "Connect to Server", enter your Analysis Services instance name. Don't click Connect yet.

4. Click Options. In the Additional Connection Parameters tab, enter EffectiveUserName, followed by the Universal Principal Name (UPN) of the user who you want to test (see **Figure 13.4**). Typically, UPN is the same as the user's email address. If you're not sure, ask the user to open the command prompt and enter the following command: whoami /upn.

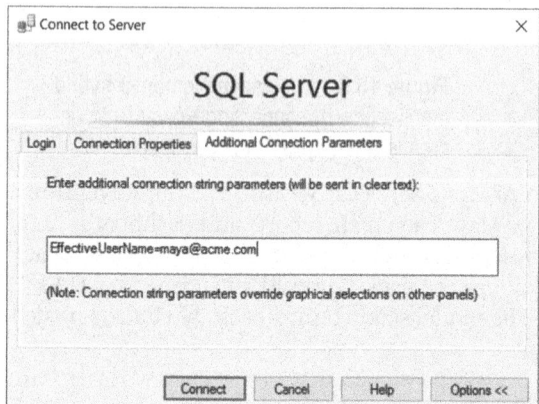

Figure 13.4 Use SSMS to verify if the interactive user will gain access to Analysis Services by passing the EffectiveUserName setting.

5. Click Connect. If you can connect successfully, the gateway should be able to delegate the user identity. If you get an error, see the next section.

Mapping user names

If you get an error, more than likely there isn't a trust relationship between the two domains. For example, Adventure Works might have acquired Acme and the Acme employees might still be on the acme.com domain. This will cause an issue when these employees attempt to connect to Analysis Services and the connection will fail. If you follow the steps to test EffectiveUserName and open SQL Server Profiler to monitor connections to Analysis Services, you'll see the error "The following system error occurred: The user name or password is incorrect."

Fortunately, Power BI has a simple solution. When setting up a data source to Analysis Services in the On-premises Data Gateway, the Users tab has a "Map user names" button, which brings you to the "Map user names" window (see **Figure 13.5**).

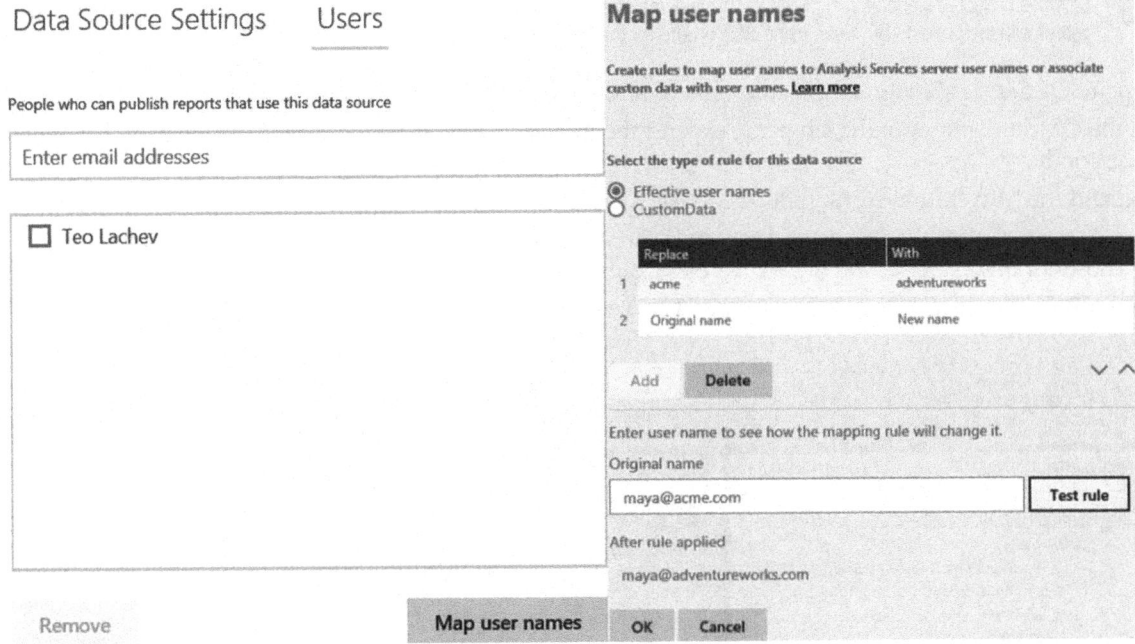

Figure 13.5 Map user names when users and Analysis Services are on different domains.

You can set up a simple mapping rule to replace some text in the user's email, such as to replace "acme" with "adventureworks" if Analysis Services is installed on somedomain.com domain. Make sure to click the Add button to add the rule to the grid. Use "Test rule" to test it by providing a sample email address.

> **TIP** What is the CustomData setting? When USERNAME isn't enough, another option that's less frequently used for dynamic data security is to use the CustomData setting. This option could be useful when you share reports and dashboards with external users. In this case, you can't use EffectiveUserName because there is no Active Directory account for the external user. However, the user identity can be passed under the CustomData option. Then, a row filter can use the CUSTOMDATA DAX function to obtain the identifier. For example, the expression IF(CUSTOMDATA()="<UserIdentity>", TRUE, FALSE) allows the user to see all rows associated with that external user.

13.1.3 Using Analysis Services in Power BI Service

Once you register Analysis Services with the On-Premises Data Gateway, users can go to Power BI and connect live to Analysis Services. However, users still might not be able to connect if they don't have rights to access the Analysis Services models. As you can see, there are multiple levels of security so be patient.

Granting user access

By default, users don't have access to Analysis Services models. To grant users access, you need an Analysis Services database role. For the purposes of this exercise, you'll use SQL Server Management Studio (SSMS) to add users to a role. Let's grant user access to the Adventure Works Tabular model:

 TIP As a best practice, the BI developer should use SQL Server Data Tools (SSDT) to define role membership in the Analysis Services project, instead of using SSMS. This way the role membership becomes a part of the project and can be deployed together with the project. But we're using SSMS here for the sake of simplicity.

1. Open SQL Server Management Studio (SSMS) and connect to the Analysis Services instance.
2. In the Object Explorer in the left pane, expand the Analysis Services instance, and then expand the Databases node.
3. Expand the "AdventureWorks Tabular Model SQL 2012" database, and then expand the Roles folder.
4. The Adventure Works SSAS database includes an Analysts role that grants access to the model. For the purposes of this exercise, you'll use this role. Double-click the Analysts role.
5. In the Role Properties window (see **Figure 13.6**), select the Membership tab and add the users.

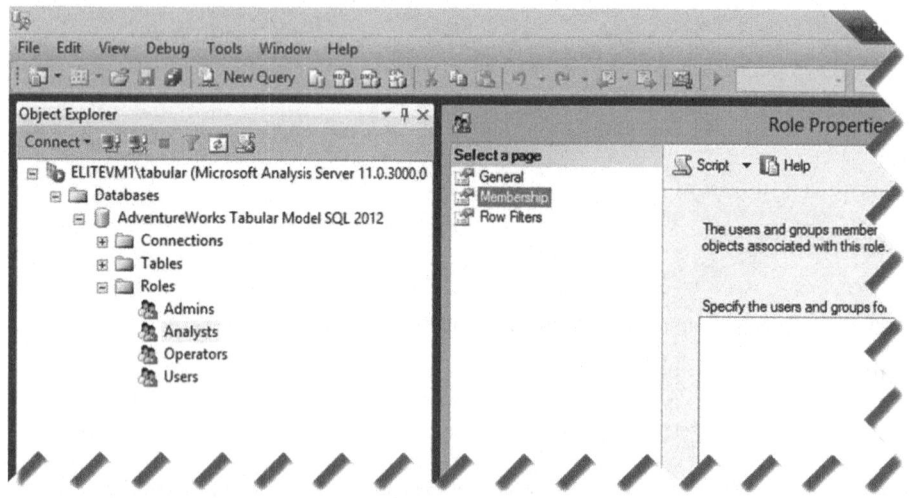

Figure 13.6 You must grant users access to the SSAS model by assigning users to a database role.

Verifying user connectivity

Once you grant the users access to the model, they should be able to run reports in Power BI Service that connect to SSAS. I showed you how they do this back in Chapter 2. From an administrator standpoint, you need to know how to troubleshoot connectivity issues.

Ask the user to go to Power BI Service and connect to SSAS (Get Data ⇨ Databases ⇨ SQL Server Analysis Services). The user will see all the registered gateways (see **Figure 13.7**), even though he might not have rights to access any of the databases. Power BI Service will make the actual connection only when the user selects a gateway and clicks Connect. At this point, the user will only see the SSAS databases they can access on that instance.

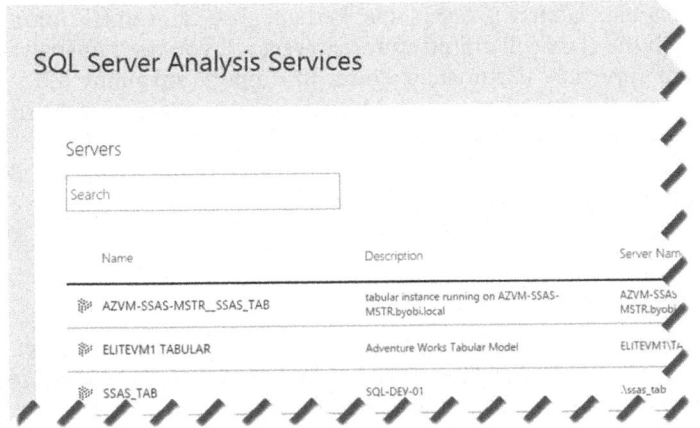

Figure 13.7 Power BI lists all the registered gateways, regardless if the user has permissions to any of the databases hosted on that SSAS instance.

If the connection fails, the best way to verify what identity the user connects under is to use the SQL Server Profiler connected to the SSAS instance. Many events, such as Discover Begin or Query Begin, have a PropertyList element that includes the EffectiveUserName property (see **Figure 13.8**).

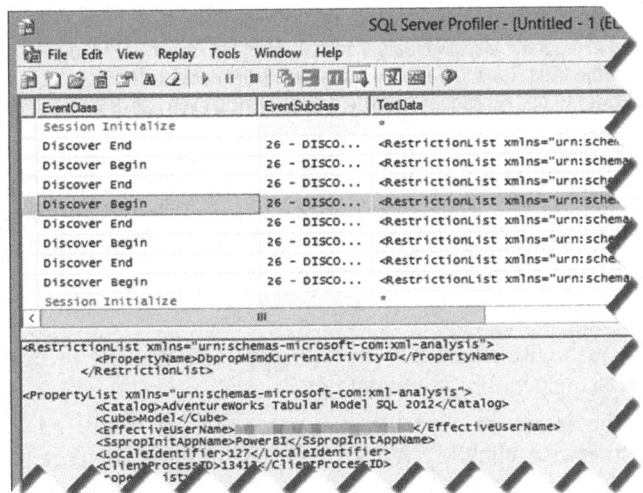

Figure 13.8 The EffectiveUserName property includes the identity of the interactive user.

The EffectiveUserName should match the work email that the user typed to log in to Power BI, such as maya@adventureworks.com. If you need data security, you can set up row filters in your Tabular model to filter the SSAS model data, based on the user identity, just like you can set up roles in Power BI Desktop.

13.2 Implementing Real-time BI Solutions

The growing volume of real-time data and the reduced time for decision making are driving companies to implement real-time operational intelligence systems. You might have heard the term "Internet of Things" (IoT), which refers to sensors, devices, and systems that constantly generate data. Unlike the classic descriptive BI architecture (which is all about analyzing the past), real-time data analytics is concerned about what happens now. For example, Adventure Works might be interested in sentiment analysis, based on customer feedback that was shared on popular social networks, such as Twitter. A descriptive approach would require you to import customer data, transform it, and then analyze it.

But what if you're interested in what customers are saying *now*? Your implementation approach might depend on your definition of "now", and what data latency is acceptable. Perhaps, you can run ETL more often and still address your requirements with the classic BI architecture? However, if you need to analyze data as it streams, then you'll need a different approach. Fortunately, Power BI supports streaming API, that makes it easy to push data to Power BI and show the data in a dashboard that changes as the new data streams in. You can meet more advanced requirements with complex event processing (CEP) solutions. Microsoft StreamInsight, which ships with SQL Server, allows you to implement on-premises real-time BI solutions. And Microsoft Azure Stream Analytics is its cloud-based counterpart.

13.2.1 Using the Streaming API

The simplest way to stream data in Power BI is to use its real-time API – a lightweight, simple way to get real-time data onto a Power BI dashboard. It only takes a few lines of code to write a custom app that programmatically accesses the data as it streams in and then pushes the data to Power BI! For example, you might have a requirement to show call center statistics real-time as calls are handled. The phone system might provide a TCP socket, which your application can connect to and get the data stream. Then your app can push some statistics, such as the count of handled calls, to a Power BI dashboard. Let's cover quickly the implementation steps.

 REAL LIFE Before streaming datasets, a developer had to programmatically create a dataset using the Power BI API (discussed in the next chapter), define a table, and then call the "Add Rows to Table" API to populate the dataset. This approach doesn't require much code and it's still supported but Power BI has subsequently made data streaming even easier with streaming datasets and streaming tiles.

To help you get started with the real-time streaming API, Microsoft has provided a sample C# console app PBIRealTimeStreaming. For your convenience, I included the source code in the \Source\Ch13\Real-time folder. The app pushes the current date and a random integer to the Power BI REST API every second. As a first step to implementing a real-time dashboard, you need to create a streaming dataset.

Implementing a streaming dataset
A streaming dataset is a special dataset that has a push URL attached to it. Your app calls this URL using HTTP POST to push the data. Follow these steps to create a streaming dataset:

1. Log in to Power BI Service. If you want to create the dataset in a specific workspace so it can be shared with other people, navigate to that workspace. Otherwise, click My Workspace to go to the workspace content page.

2. In the upper-right corner, expand the Create menu and then click "Streaming dataset".

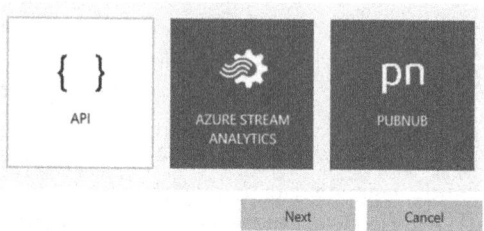

Figure 13.9   Power BI supports API, Azure Streaming Analytics, and Pub-Nub as sources for pushing data into a streaming dataset.

3. On the "Choose the source of your data" page (see **Figure 13.9**), you choose where the streaming data will come from. Currently, Power BI supports the streaming API, Azure Stream Analytics, and PubNub as streaming sources (see **Figure 13.9**). Leave API selected and click Next.

NOTE   What's PubNub? PubNub (https://www.pubnub.com) is a cloud service that allows developers to build real-time web, mobile, and IoT apps. With Power BI's PubNub integration, you can connect your PubNub data streams to Power BI in seconds, to create low latency visualizations on top of streaming data.

4. In the dataset properties page (**Figure 13.10**), enter *Real-time API* as the dataset name. Our dataset will have only two fields: *ts* (DateTime data type) and *value* (Text data type).

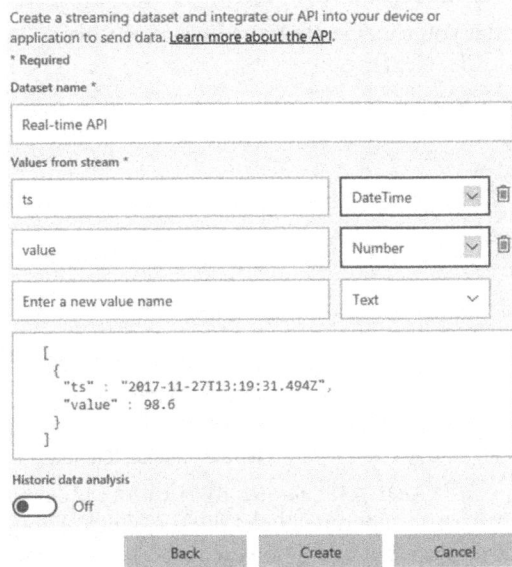

Figure 13.10 Specify the dataset name, fields, and retention policy.

The "Historic data analysis" slide corresponds to the dataset's defaultRetentionPolicy setting. The dataset will store up to 200,000 rows. After that, as new rows come in, old rows will be removed from the dataset. If you turn the slider on, the dataset won't remove old rows and it will grow until its maximum allowed size allowed by Power BI Service.

5. Click Create. The Real-time API dataset is added to the workspace.

The next page (API info on Real-time API) shows the Push URL and different ways to load the dataset (Raw, cURL, and PowerShell). For example, your app can submit the following raw payload to insert the value 98.6 for a specific date in the dataset.

[{"ts" :"2016-12-04T18:17:01.020Z", "value" :98.6}]

6. Copy the Push URL and click Done. You can also get the Push URL later from the dataset properties.

7. Locate the dataset in the Datasets tab and notice that its API Access property shows Streaming.

Implementing a real-time tile
Now that we have a place to store the streamed data, let's visualize it in a real dashboard.

1. Back to the workspace content page, expand the Create menu again and create a new dashboard. Type in *Real-time API* as the dashboard name, and then click Create.

2. In the Real-time API dashboard, click "+Add tile" in the dashboard menu.

3. In the Add Tile page, select the "Custom Streaming Data" source under Real-time Data, and click Next.

4. In the "Add a custom streaming data tile" page, select the Real-time API dataset and click Next. Notice if you don't have a streaming dataset, you can use this page to create one by clicking the "+Add streaming dataset" button.

5. In the "Visualization design" page (**Figure 13.11**), leave the Card visualization preselected. Click "Add value", then expand the Fields dropdown and select the *value* field. You can also show data as various charts or a gauge. Each visualization type requires different fields. For example, if you want to show the streaming data as a line chart, you can bind the timestamp (ts) field to the Axis area and the value field to the Values area. By contrast, the Card visualization can show a single field.

6. Click the Format tab (the one with the pencil icon). Notice that you can specify basic format settings, including display units and the number of the decimal places. Click Next.

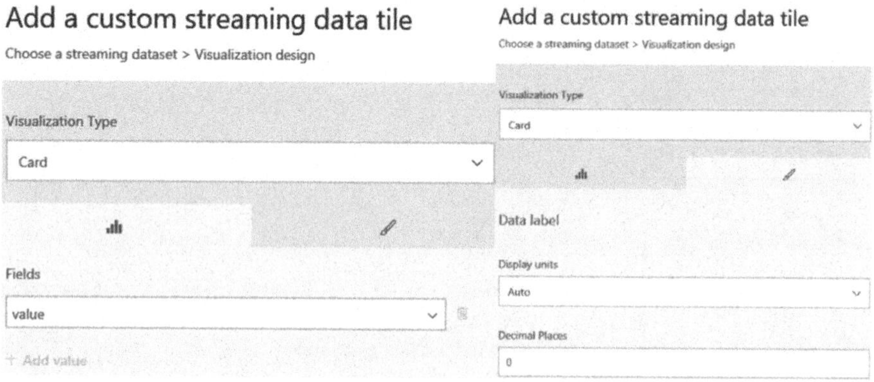

Figure 13.11 When configuring the real-time tile, specify the visualization type and fields to show.

7. In the Tile Details page, enter *Real-time API* as the tile name. Notice that you can specify additional tile properties, such as a Subtitle and URL to navigate the user to a report when he clicks the tile. Click Apply to add the tile to the dashboard. A confirmation message will pop up and will give you an option to create a Phone view for the dashboard, which you can ignore.

Streaming data

The last piece left is to stream the actual data. This is where the PBIRealTimeStreaming sample comes in.

1. Open the PBIRealTimeStreaming.sln solution file in Visual Studio. If you don't have Visual Studio, install the free Visual Studio Community Edition from https://www.visualstudio.com/vs/community.

2. In the Solution Explorer, double-click the Program.cs file.

3. Locate the realTimePushURL variable and replace its value with the Push URL of your dataset.

4. Press Ctrl+F5 to run the application. Switch to Power BI Service and notice that the Real-time API tile updates every second with new data.

Behind the scenes, the sample uses the .NET WebRequest class to create a new POST request for each new row. The sample then sends the request to the dataset Push URL. You now have a real-time dashboard!

13.2.2 Using Azure Stream Analytics

As you've seen, it's easy to meet basic real-time BI needs with the Power BI streaming API. But, what if your solution needs to ingest thousands of events per second and scale on demand. Or, what if you need to aggregate data as it streams in, such as to calculate the average count of calls for a given duration. Such requirements call for a complex event processing (CEP) solution, which you can implement with Azure Stream Analytics.

Understanding Microsoft Azure Stream Analytics

Traditionally, implementing a complex event processing (CEP) solution has been difficult because…well, it's complex, and it requires a lot of custom code. Microsoft sought to change this by introducing Azure Stream Analytics as a fully managed stream-processing service in the cloud. Azure Stream Analytics provides low latency and real-time processing of millions of events per second in a highly resilient service (see its architecture in **Figure 13.12**).

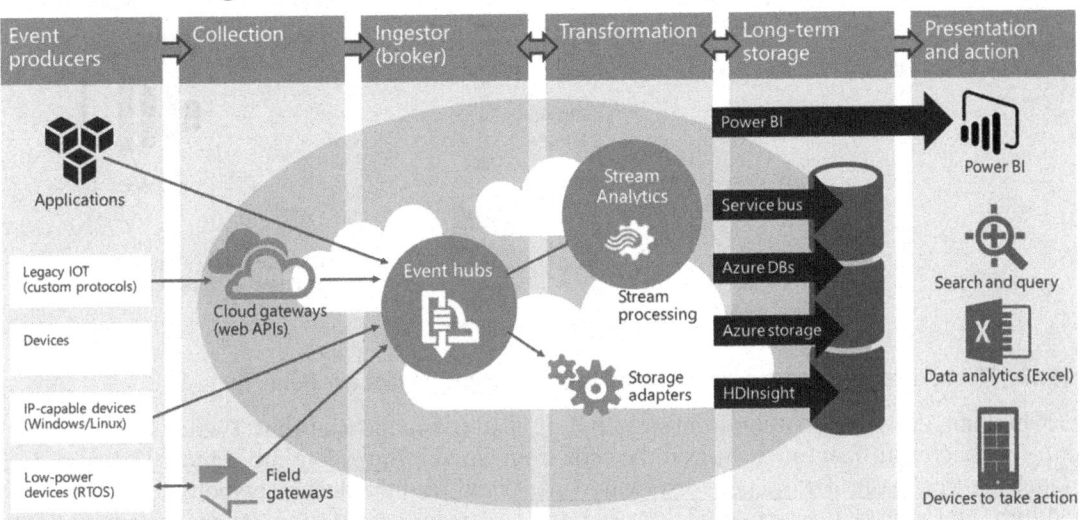

Figure 13.12 Stream Analytics is a cloud-based service and it's capable of processing millions of events per second.

Common real-time BI scenarios that will benefit from Stream Analytics include fraud detection, identity protection, real-time financial portfolio analysis, click-stream analysis, energy smart grid utilization, and Internet of Things (IoT) projects. Stream Analytics integrates with Azure Event Hubs, which is a highly scalable service for ingesting data streams. It enables the collection of event streams at high throughput from a diverse set of devices and services.

For example, Event Hubs is capable of processing millions of events per second via HTTP(S) or Advanced Message Queuing Protocol (AMQP) protocols. Once data is brought into Event Hubs, you can then use Stream Analytics to apply a standing SQL-like query for analyzing the data as it streams through, such as to detect anomalies or outliers. The query results can also be saved into long-term storage destinations, such as Azure SQL Database, HDInsight, or Azure Storage, and then you can analyze that data. Like the Power BI streaming API, Stream Analytics can output query results directly to Power BI streaming datasets, which in turn can update dashboard streaming tiles! This allows you to implement a real-time dashboard that updates itself constantly when Stream Analytics sends new results.

Now that you've learned about real-time BI, let me walk you through a sample solution that demonstrates how Azure Stream Analytics and Power BI can help you implement CEP solutions. Suppose that Adventure Works is interested in analyzing customer sentiment from messages that are posted on Twitter. This is immediate feedback from its customer base, which can help the company improve its products and services. Adventure Works wants to monitor the average customer sentiment about specific topics in real time. **Figure 13.13** shows you the process flow diagram.

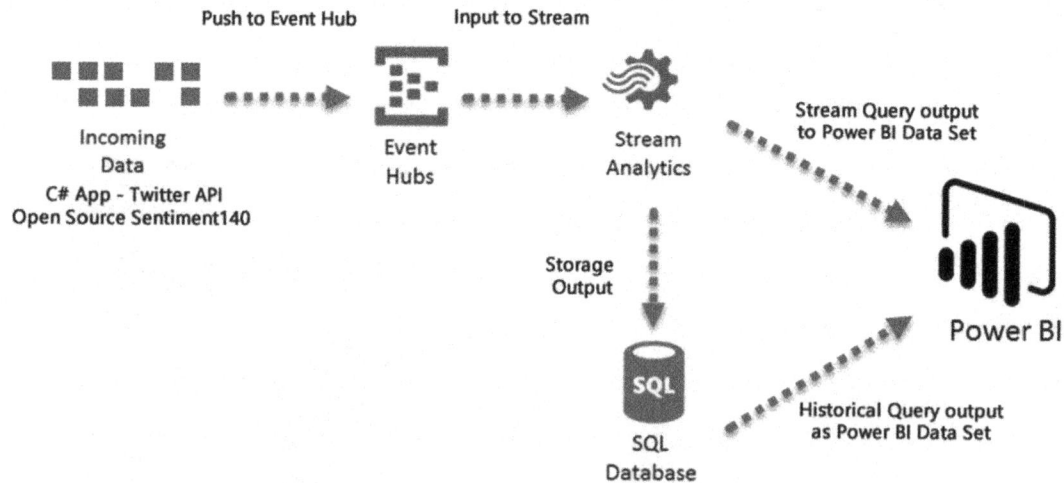

Figure 13.13 This solution demonstrates how you can integrate Stream Analytics with Power BI.

Instead of building the entire solution from scratch, I decided to use the Real-time Twitter sentiment analysis sample by Microsoft. You can download the code from GitHub (https://github.com/Azure/azure-stream-analytics/tree/master/DataGenerators/TwitterClient) and read the documentation from https://github.com/Azure/azure-content/blob/master/articles/stream-analytics/stream-analytics-twitter-sentiment-analysis-trends.md or online at https://azure.microsoft.com/en-us/documentation/articles/stream-analytics-twitter-sentiment-analysis-trends.

NOTE This sample demonstrates how remarkably simple it is to implement CEP cloud solutions with Stream Analytics. You only need to write custom code to send events to Events Hub. By contrast, a similar StreamInsight-based application would require much more coding on your part, as the Big Data Twitter Demo (http://twitterbigdata.codeplex.com) demonstrates. That's because you'd need to write the plumbing code for observers, adapters, sinks, and more.

Understanding the client application

Designed as a C# console application, the client app uses the Twitter APIs to filter tweets for specific keywords that you specify in the app.config file. To personalize the demo for our fictitious bike manufacturer, (Adventure Works), I used the keywords "Bike" and "Adventure". In the same file, you must specify the Twitter OAuth settings that you obtain when you register a custom application with Twitter. For more information about registering an application with Twitter and about obtaining the security settings, read the "Tokens from dev.twitter.com" topic at https://dev.twitter.com/oauth/overview/application-owner-access-tokens.

Note that the client app (as coded by Microsoft) doesn't have any error handling. If you don't configure it correctly, it won't show any output and won't give you any indication of what's wrong. To avoid this and to get the actual error, I recommend that you re-throw errors in every catch block in the EventHubObserver.cs file.

```
catch (Exception ex)
{
    throw ex;
}
```

The application integrates with an open source tool (Sentiment140) to assign a sentiment value to each tweet (0: negative, 2: neutral, 4: positive). Then the tweet events are sent to the Azure Event Hubs. Therefore, to test the application successfully, you must first set up an event hub and configure Stream Analytics. If all is well, the application shows the stream of tweets in the console window as they're sent to the event hub.

Configuring Stream Analytics

The documentation that accompanies the sample provides step-by-step instructions to configure the Azure part of the solution. You can perform the steps using the old Azure portal (https://manage.windowsazure.com) or the new Azure portal (http://portal.azure.com). Instead of reiterating the steps, I'll just emphasize a few points that might not be immediately clear:

1. Before setting up a new Stream Analytics job, you must create an event hub that ingests that data stream.

2. After you create the hub, you need to copy the connection information from the hub registration page and paste it in the EventHubConnectionString setting in the client application app.config file. This is how the client application connects to the event hub.

3. When you set up the Stream Analytics job, you can use sample data to test the standing query. You must have run the client application before this step so that the event hub has some data in it. In addition, make sure that the date range you specify for sampling actually returns tweet events.

4. This is the standing query that I used for the Power BI dashboard:

```
SELECT System.Timestamp as Time, Topic, COUNT(*), AVG(SentimentScore), MIN(SentimentScore),
Max(SentimentScore), STDEV(SentimentScore)
FROM TwitterStream TIMESTAMP BY CreatedAt
GROUP BY TUMBLINGWINDOW(s, 5), Topic
```

This query divides the time in intervals of five seconds. A tumbling window is one of the window types that's supported by both Stream Analytics and SQL Server StreamInsight (read about windowing at https://msdn.microsoft.com/en-us/library/azure/dn835055.aspx). Within each interval, the query groups the incoming events by topic and calculates the event count, minimum, maximum, average sentiment score, and the standard deviation. Because stream analytics queries are described in a SQL-like grammar, you can leverage your SQL query skills.

 NOTE Unlike SQL SELECT queries, which execute once, Stream Analytics queries are standing. To understanding this, imagine that the stream of events passes through the query. As long as the Stream Analytics job is active, the query is active and it's always working. In this case, the query divides the stream in five-second intervals and calculates the aggregates on the fly.

Outputting data to Power BI

A Stream Analytics job can have multiple outputs, such as to save the query results to a durable storage for offline analysis and to display them on a real-time dashboard. **Figure 13.14** shows that I selected Power BI as an output (other input types include SQL Database, Blob Storage, Cosmos DB, Azure Data Lake, and more). Follow these steps to configure Stream Analytics to send the output to Power BI.

 NOTE If Power BI has a dataset and table that have the same names as the ones that you specify in the Stream Analytics job, the existing ones are overwritten. Although you can create a Stream Analytics dataset beforehand, you should let Stream Analytics create it. The dataset will be automatically created when you start your Stream Analytics job and the job starts pumping output into Power BI. If your job query doesn't return any results, the dataset won't be created.

1. In the "Add an output to your job" step, select Power BI. Click the Authorize button to sign in to Power BI.

2. In "Output details" (see again **Figure 13.14**), enter the name of the Power BI dataset and table names. You can send results from different queries to separate tables within the same dataset. If the table with the same name exists, it'll be overwritten.

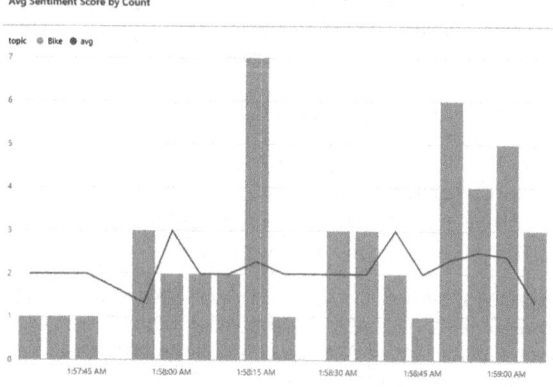

New output _ □ × | **Output details** _ □ ×
TwitterStreamOutput
⚙ Test 🗑 Delete

* Output alias | **Group Workspace**
TwitterStreamOutput ✓ | My Workspace ∨

* Sink ❶ | *** Dataset Name**
Power BI ∨ | TwitterSentimentScore

Authorize Connection
You'll need to authorize with Power BI to
configure your output settings.

⚠ If the dataset or table already exists in your
Microsoft Power BI subscription, it will be
overwritten.

[Authorize]

* Table Name
TwitterSentimentScore

Figure 13.14 Specify Power BI as a sink and then the names of the dataset and table where the results will be loaded.

Creating a real-time dashboard

Now that all the setup steps are behind us, we're ready to have fun with the data:

1. Run the Stream Analytics job. It might take a while for the job to initiate, so monitor its progress on the Stream Analytics dashboard page.

2. Once the job is started, it'll send the query results to Power BI, assuming there are incoming events that match the query criteria. Power BI will create a dataset with the name you specified.

 TIP You can create a streaming tile using the Azure Streaming Analytics dataset type, like what you did in the previous example. This allows you to implement the two most common real-time requirements: 1) showing the latest value and 2) showing values on a line chart over a time window. However, if you want to use another Power BI visual, you can just explore the dataset.

3. Now you log in to Power BI Service and explore the dataset.

4. To show the data in real time, you need to create a dashboard by pinning the report visualization. The dashboard tile in **Figure 13.15** is based on a report visualization that uses a Combo Chart. It shows the count of events as columns and the average sentiment score as a line. Time is measured on the shared axis.

Avg Sentiment Score by Count

topic ● Bike ● avg

Figure 13.15 Power BI updates a real-time dashboard as Stream Analytics streams the events.

5. Watch the dashboard update itself as new data is coming in, and you gain real-time insights from your CEP solution!

13.3 Implementing Predictive Solutions

Predictive analytics (based on data mining and machine learning algorithms) is an increasingly popular requirement. It also happens to be one of the least understood because it's usually confused with slicing and dicing data. However, predictive analytics is about discovering patterns that aren't easily discernible. These hidden patterns can't be derived from traditional data exploration, because data relationships might be too complex or because there's too much data for a human to analyze.

Typical data mining tasks include forecasting, customer profiling, and basket analysis. Data mining can answer questions, such as, "What are the forecasted sales numbers for the next few months?", "What other products is a customer likely to buy along with the product he or she already chose?", and "What type of customer (described in terms of gender, age group, income, and so on) is likely to buy a given product?"

13.3.1 Understanding Azure Machine Learning

Predictive analytics isn't new to Microsoft. Microsoft extended Analysis Services with data mining back in SQL Server 2000. Besides allowing BI pros to create data mining models with Analysis Services, Microsoft also introduced the Excel Data Mining add-in to let business users perform data mining tasks in Excel.

 NOTE With the focus shifting to Azure ML and R, we probably won't see future investments from Microsoft in SSAS Data Mining (and the Excel data mining add-in for that matter) which is currently limited to nine algorithms.

SQL Server 2016 added R Services that allow you to integrate the power of R with your T-SQL code. You've already seen that Power BI includes Quick Insights, time-series forecasting, and clustering as built-in predictive features.

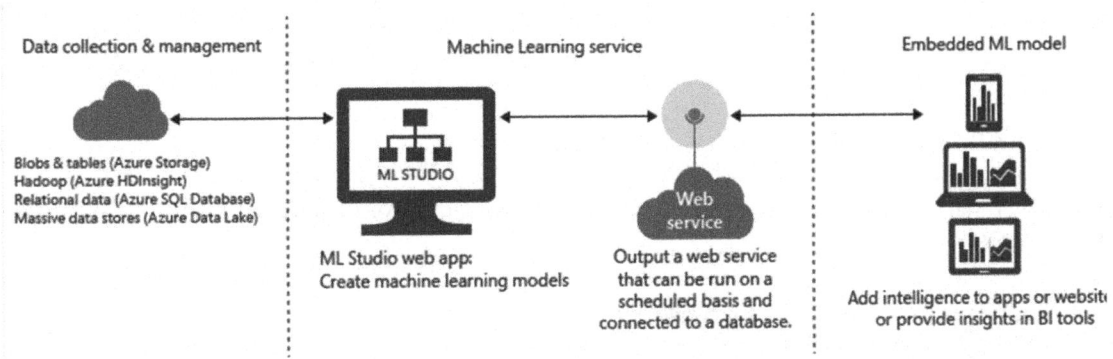

Figure 13.16 The diagram demonstrates a common flow to implement predictive models with AzureML.

Introducing Azure Machine Learning
In 2014, Microsoft unveiled a cloud-based service for predictive analytics called Azure Machine Learning or AzureML, which also originated from Microsoft Research. In a nutshell, Azure Machine Learning makes it easy for data scientists to quickly create and deploy predictive models. The Azure ML value proposition includes the following appealing features:

■ It provides an easy-to-use, comprehensive, and scalable platform without requiring hardware or software investments.

- It supports workflows for transforming and moving data. For example, AzureML supports custom code, such as R or Python code, to transform columns. Furthermore, it allows you to chain tasks, such as to load data, create a model, and then save the predictive results.

- It allows you to easily expose predictive models as REST web services, so that you can incorporate predictive features in custom applications. **Figure 13.16** shows a typical AzureML implementation.

Understanding workflows
Because it's a cloud service, AzureML can obtain the input data directly from other cloud services, such as Azure tables, Azure SQL Database, or Azure HDInsight. Alternatively, you can export on-premises data as a file and upload the dataset to AzureML, or connect directly to an on-premises SQL Server database by using a data gateway.

Then you use ML Studio to build a workflow for creating and training a predictive model. ML Studio is a browser-based tool that allows you to drag, drop, and connect the building blocks of your solution. You can choose from a large library of Machine Learning algorithms to jump-start your predictive models! You can also extend the workflow with your own custom R and Python scripts.

Like Stream Analytics and Power BI, AzureML is an integral component of the Cortana Analytics Suite, although you can also use it as a standalone service. The Cortana Analytics Gallery (http://gallery.cortanaanalytics.com) is a community-driven site for discovering and sharing predictive solutions. It features many ready-to-go predictive models that have been contributed by Microsoft and the analytics community. You can learn more about Azure Machine Learning at its official site (https://azure.microsoft.com/en-us/services/machine-learning) and start using for free!

13.3.2 Creating Predictive Models

Next, I'll walk you through the steps to implement an AzureML predictive model for a familiar scenario. Our bike manufacturer, Adventure Works, is planning a marketing campaign. The marketing department approaches you to help them target a subset of potential customers who are the most likely to purchase a bike. You need to create a predictive model that predicts the purchase probability from some sales data accumulated in the past.

Understanding the historical dataset
To start, you'd need to obtain an order history dataset that you'd use to train the model:

1. In SQL Server Management Studio (SSMS), connect to the AdventureWorksDW2012 database and execute the following query:

```
SELECT
    Gender,YearlyIncome,TotalChildren,NumberChildrenAtHome,
    EnglishEducation,EnglishOccupation,HouseOwnerFlag,
    NumberCarsOwned,CommuteDistance,Region,Age,BikeBuyer
FROM [dbo].[vTargetMail]
```

This query returns a subset of columns from the vTargetMail view that Microsoft uses to demonstrate the Analysis Services data mining features. The last column, BikeBuyer, is a flag that indicates if the customer has purchased a bike. The model will use the rest of the columns as an input to determine the most important criteria that influences a customer to purchase a bike.

 NOTE The Adventure Works Analysis Services Multidimensional cube includes a Targeted Mailing data mining structure, which uses this dataset. The mining models in the Targeted Mailing structure demonstrate how the same scenario can be addressed with an on-premises Analysis Services solution.

2. Export the results to a CSV file. For your convenience, I included a Bike Buyers.csv file in the \source\ch13\AzureML folder.

Creating a predictive model

Next, you'll use AzureML to create a predictive model, using the Bike Buyers.csv file as an input:

1. Go to https://studio.azureml.net and sign in. If you don't have an Azure subscription, you can start a trial subscription, or just use the free version!

2. Once you are in Microsoft Azure Machine Learning (Azure ML) Studio, click New on the bottom of the screen, and then create a dataset by uploading the Bike Buyers.csv file. Name the dataset *Bike Buyers*.

3. Click the New button again and create a new experiment. An Azure ML experiment represents the workflow to create and train a predictive model. When you're done, your experiment will look like the one shown in **Figure 13.17**.

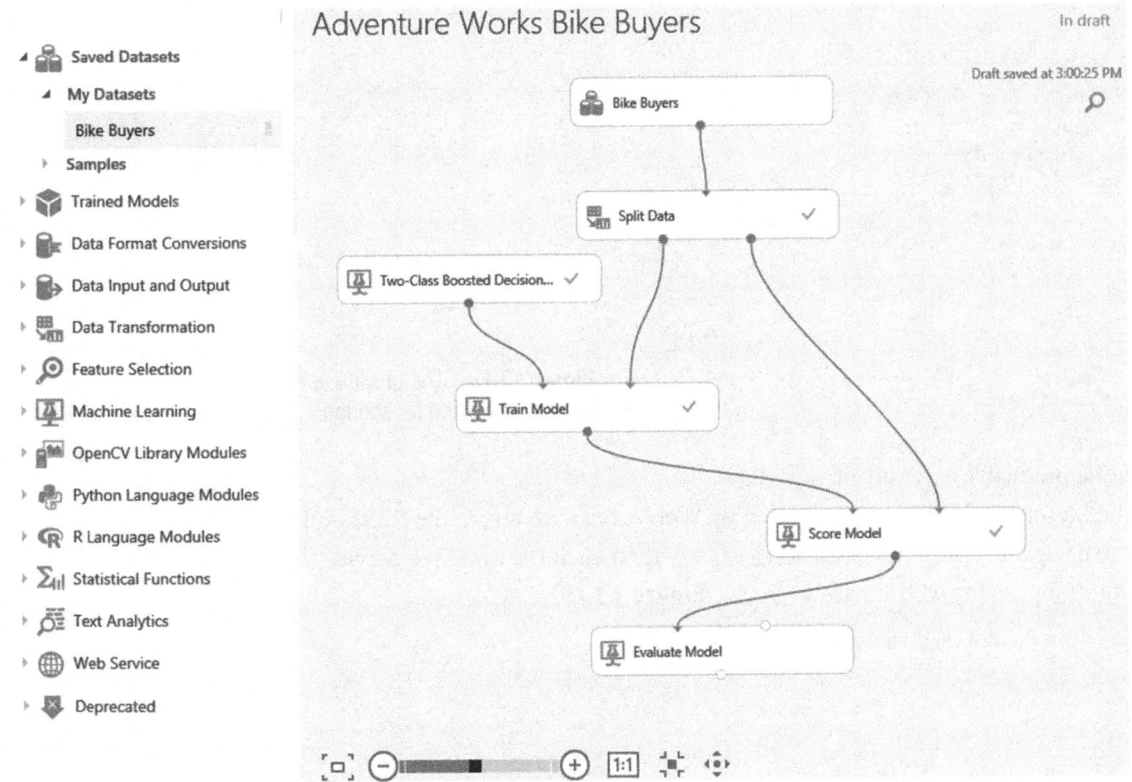

Figure 13.17   The Adventure Works Bike Buyer predictive model.

4. From the Saved Datasets section in the navigation bar, drag and drop the Bike Buyers dataset.

5. Using the search box, search for each of the workflow nodes shown in **Figure 13.17** by typing its name, and then drop them on the workflow. Join them as shown in **Figure 13.17**. For example, to find the Split Data task, type "Split" in the search box. From the search results, drag the Split Data task and drop it onto the workflow. Then connect the Bike Buyer dataset to the Split Data task.

6. The workhorse of the model is the Two-Class Boosted Decision Tree algorithm, which generates the predictive results. Click the Split Data transformation and configure its "Fraction of rows in the first output dataset" property for a 0.8 split. That's because you'll use 80% of the input dataset to train the model and the remaining 20% to evaluate the model accuracy.

Setting up a web service

A great AzureML feature is that it can easily expose an experiment as a REST web service. The web service allows client applications to integrate with AzureML and use the model for scoring. Setting up a web service is remarkably easy.

1. Click the Run button to run the experiment.
2. (Optional) Right-click the output (the small circle at the bottom) of the Evaluate Model task, and then click Visualize to analyze the model accuracy. For example, the Lift graph shows the gain of the model, compared to just targeting all the customers without using a predictive model.
3. At the bottom of the screen, click "Set up Web Service". AzureML creates a new experiment because it needs to remove the unnecessary tasks from the web service, such as the task to train the model. **Figure 13.18** shows the workflow of the predictive experiment after AzureML sets up the web service.

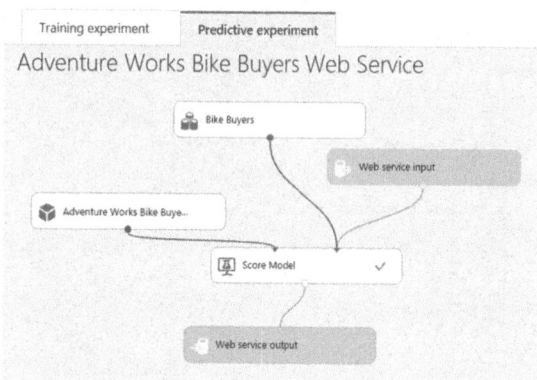

Figure 13.18 The predictive experiment is optimized for scoring.

4. Run the predictive experiment.
5. At the bottom of the screen, click "Deploy Web Service" to create the REST API endpoint.
6. In the navigation bar, click Web Services, and then click the new web service that you just created.
7. AzureML opens the web service page (see **Figure 13.19**).

adventure works bike buyers web service

DASHBOARD   CONFIGURATION

General

Published experiment
View snapshot   View latest

Description
No description provided for this web service.

API key

Default Endpoint

API HELP PAGE	TEST
REQUEST/RESPONSE	Test
BATCH EXECUTION	

Figure 13.19 The web service page allows you to obtain the API key and test the web service.

Your application will use the API key to authenticate against ML. Think of it as a password. Copy the API key because you'll need it later. The Request/Response link is for calling the web service in a singleton manner (one row at a time). The Batch Execution link is for scoring multiple rows in one batch.

> **TIP** The Microsoft Azure ML team has provided an Excel Azure Machine Learning Add-in (bit.ly/2g0oAgc) that allows you to integrate the Azure ML predictive web service with Excel. The add-in supports scoring multiple rows from an Excel range by calling the Azure ML batch API.

8. Click the Request/Response link to see the web service developer documentation and to test the web service. The documentation page includes the web service endpoint, which should look like this following example (I excluded the sensitive information):

https://ussouthcentral.services.azureml.net/workspaces/<...>/execute?api-version=2.0&details=true

The page also shows a simple POST request and response described in JSON (see **Figure 13.20**).

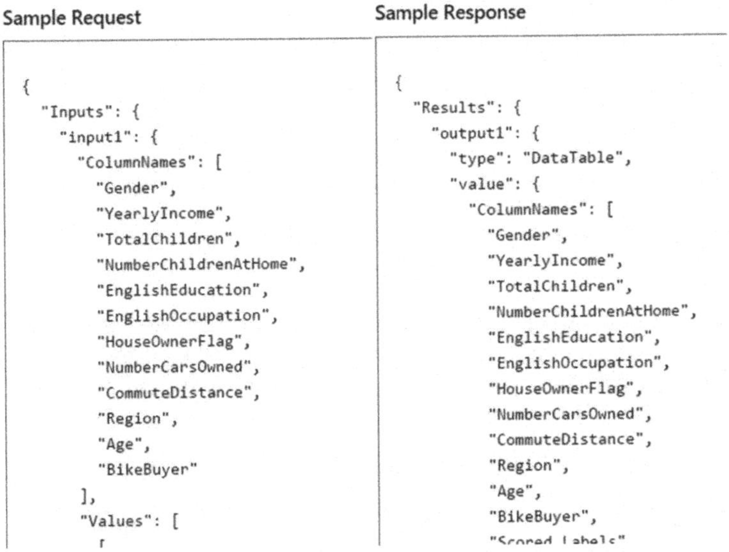

Sample Request

```
{
  "Inputs": {
    "input1": {
      "ColumnNames": [
        "Gender",
        "YearlyIncome",
        "TotalChildren",
        "NumberChildrenAtHome",
        "EnglishEducation",
        "EnglishOccupation",
        "HouseOwnerFlag",
        "NumberCarsOwned",
        "CommuteDistance",
        "Region",
        "Age",
        "BikeBuyer"
      ],
      "Values": [
        [
```

Sample Response

```
{
  "Results": {
    "output1": {
      "type": "DataTable",
      "value": {
        "ColumnNames": [
          "Gender",
          "YearlyIncome",
          "TotalChildren",
          "NumberChildrenAtHome",
          "EnglishEducation",
          "EnglishOccupation",
          "HouseOwnerFlag",
          "NumberCarsOwned",
          "CommuteDistance",
          "Region",
          "Age",
          "BikeBuyer",
          "Scored Labels",
```

Figure 13.20 A simple request and response from the Adventure Works Bike Buyers predictive web service.

Operationalizing the predictive service

While creating a web service is easy, operationalizing it takes more work. For example, you might be interested in automating your predictive solution, such as scheduling your experiment for retraining. Azure ML supports several ways of retraining your models, including retraining programmatically, using PowerShell, or by using Azure Data Factory.

For more information about operationalizing Azure ML models, check the "Azure Machine Learning Web Services: Deployment and consumption" article at https://docs.microsoft.com/en-us/azure/machine-learning/studio/deploy-consume-web-service-guide. Going back to the subject of this book, let's see next how you can derive insights from your predictive models in Power BI.

13.3.3 Integrating Machine Learning with Power BI

Currently, Power BI doesn't include a connector to connect directly to Azure Machine Learning. This leaves you with two integration options:

- Instead of publishing to a web service, save the predictive results to Azure Storage, such as to an Azure SQL Database. Then use Power BI Service's Get Data to visualize the predictive results.

- Publish the predictive model as a web service, and then use Power BI Desktop or Power Query to call the web service.

The second option allows you to implement flexible integration scenarios, such as to call the web service for each customer from a dataset you imported in Power BI Desktop. Moreover, it demonstrates some of the advanced capabilities of Power BI Desktop queries and Power Query. This is the integration option I'll demonstrate next.

EMailAddress	Gender	YearlyIncome	TotalChildren	NumberChi	EnglishEducation	EnglishOccupation	HouseOwner	NumberC.	CommuteDistance	Region	Age	BikeBuyer
jon24@adventur	M	90000	2	0	Bachelors	Professional	1	0	1-2 Miles	Pacific	49	0
eugene10@adve	M	60000	3	3	Bachelors	Professional	0	1	0-1 Miles	Pacific	50	0
ruben35@adven	M	60000	3	3	Bachelors	Professional	1	2	2-5 Miles	Pacific	50	0
christy12@adver	F	70000	0	0	Bachelors	Professional	0	1	5-10 Miles	Pacific	47	0
elizabeth5@adve	F	80000	5	5	Bachelors	Professional	1	4	1-2 Miles	Pacific	47	0
julio1@adventur	M	70000	0	0	Bachelors	Professional	1	1	5-10 Miles	Pacific	50	0
janet9@adventu	F	70000	0	0	Bachelors	Professional	1	1	5-10 Miles	Pacific	49	0
marco14@adven	M	60000	3	3	Bachelors	Professional	1	2	0-1 Miles	Pacific	51	0
rob4@adventure	F	60000	4	4	Bachelors	Professional	1	3	10+ Miles	Pacific	51	0
shannon38@adv	M	70000	0	0	Bachelors	Professional	0	1	5-10 Miles	Pacific	51	0
jacquelyn20@ad	F	70000	0	0	Bachelors	Professional	0	1	5-10 Miles	Pacific	51	0
curtis9@adventu	M	60000	4	4	Bachelors	Professional	1	4	10+ Miles	Pacific	51	0
lauren41@adven	F	100000	2	0	Bachelors	Management	1	2	1-2 Miles	North Am	47	0
ian47@adventur	M	100000	2	0	Bachelors	Management	1	3	0-1 Miles	North Am	47	0
sydney23@adver	F	100000	3	0	Bachelors	Management	0	3	1-2 Miles	North Am	47	0
chloe23@advent	F	30000	0	0	Partial College	Skilled Manual	0	1	5-10 Miles	North Am	36	0
wyatt32@advent	M	30000	0	0	Partial College	Skilled Manual	1	1	5-10 Miles	North Am	36	0
shannon1@adve	F	20000	4	0	High School	Skilled Manual	1	2	5-10 Miles	Pacific	71	0
clarence32@adv	M	30000	2	0	Partial College	Clerical	1	2	5-10 Miles	Pacific	71	0
luke18@adventu	M	40000	0	0	High School	Skilled Manual	0	2	5-10 Miles	Europe	37	0

Figure 13.21 The New Customers Excel file has a list of customers that need to be scored.

Understanding the input dataset

Let's get back to our Adventure Works scenario. Now that the predictive web service is ready, you can use it to predict the probability of new customers who could purchase a bike, if you have the customer demographics details. The marketing department has given you an Excel file with potential customers, which they might have downloaded from the company's CRM system.

1. In Excel, open the New Customers.xlsx file (in \ch13\Machine Learning folder), which includes 20 new customers (see **Figure 13.21**).

2. Note that the last column (BikeBuyer) is always zero. That's because at this point you don't know if the customer could be a potential bike buyer. That's what the predictive web service is for.

The predictive web service will calculate the probability for each customer to purchase a bike. This requires calling the web service for each row in the input dataset by sending a predictive query (a data mining query that predicts a single case is called a singleton query). To see the final solution, open the Predict Buyers.pbix file in Power BI Desktop.

Creating a query function

You already know from Chapter 7 how to use query functions. Like other programming languages, a query function encapsulates common logic so that it can be called repeatedly. Next, you'll create a query function that will invoke the Adventure Works predictive web service:

1. In Power BI Desktop, click Edit Queries to open the Query Editor.

2. In Query Editor, expand the New Source button and click Blank Query. Then in the ribbon's View tab, click Advanced Editor.

3. Copy the function code from the \source\ch13\real-time\fnPredictBuyer.txt file and paste in the query. The query function code follows:

```
1.    let
2.    PredictBikeBuyer = (Gender, YearlyIncome, TotalChildren, NumberChildrenAtHome, EnglishEducation, EnglishOccupation,
      HouseOwnerFlag, NumberCarsOwned, CommuteDistance, Region, Age, BikeBuyer) =>
3.    let
4.    //replace service Uri and serviceKey with your own settings
5.    serviceUri="https://ussouthcentral.services.azureml.net/workspaces/.../execute?api-version=2.0&details=true",
6.    serviceKey="<your service key>"
7.    RequestBody = "
8.    {
9.    ""Inputs"": {
10.   ""input1"": {
11.   ""ColumnNames"": [
12.   ""Gender"", ""YearlyIncome"", ""TotalChildren"", ""NumberChildrenAtHome"", ""EnglishEducation"", ""EnglishOccupation"",
13.   ""HouseOwnerFlag"", ""NumberCarsOwned"", ""CommuteDistance"", ""Region"", ""Age"", ""BikeBuyer""
14.   ],
15.   ""Values"": [
16.   [
17.   """&Gender&""", """&Text.From(YearlyIncome)&""", """&Text.From(TotalChildren)&""", """&Text.From(NumberChildren-
      AtHome)&""", """&EnglishEducation&""", """&EnglishOccupation&""", """&Text.From(HouseOwnerFlag)&""",
      """&Text.From(NumberCarsOwned)&""", """&Text.From(CommuteDistance)&""",
18.   """&Region&""", """&Text.From(Age)&""", """&Text.From(BikeBuyer)&"""
19.   ]]}},
20.   ""GlobalParameters"": {}
21.   }
22.   ",
23.   Source=Web.Contents(serviceUri,
24.   [Content=Text.ToBinary(RequestBody),
25.   Headers=[Authorization="Bearer "&serviceKey,#"Content-Type"="application/json; charset=utf-8"]]),
26.   #"Response" = Json.Document(Source),
27.   #"Results" = Record.ToTable(#"Response")
28.   in
29.   #"Results"
30.   in
31.   PredictBikeBuyer
```

The code in line 2 defines a PredictBikeBuyer function with 12 arguments that correspond to the columns in the input dataset. Remember to update lines 5 and 6 with your web service URI and service key. Then the code creates a request payload described in JSON, as per the web service specification (see **Figure 13.20** again). Notice that the code obtains the actual values from the function arguments. Lines 23-25 invoke the web service. Line 26 reads the response, which is also described in JSON. Line 27 converts the response to a table.

4. Rename the query to *fnPredictBuyer* and save it.

Creating a query

Now that you have the query function, let's create a query that will load the input dataset from the New Customers Excel file, and then call the function for each customer:

1. In Query Editor, expand New Source again and then click Excel.

2. Navigate to New Customers.xlsx and load Table1. Table1 is the Excel table that has the new customers.

3. Rename the query to *PredictedBuyers*.

4. Add a custom column called PredictedScore, as shown in **Figure 13.22**. This column calls the fnPredict-Buyer function and passes the customer demographic details from each row in the input dataset.

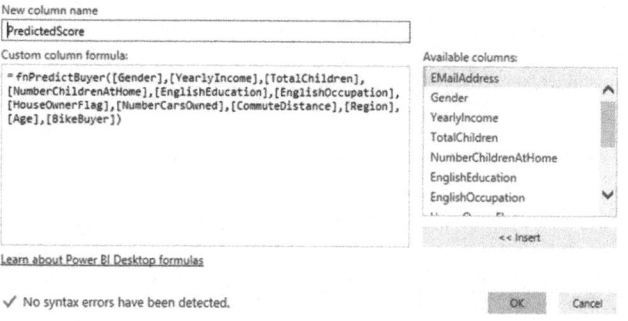

Figure 13.22 The PredictedScore custom column calls the fnPredictBuyer function.

5. The results of the custom column will be a table, which includes other nested tables, as per the JSON response specification (see **Figure 13.23**). You need to click the "expand" button four times until you see "List" showing in the PredictedScore column.

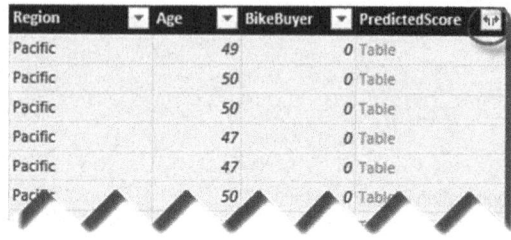

Figure 13.23 Expand the PredictedScore column four times until you get to the list of values.

6. Once you get to the list, add another custom column to get the last value of the list. Because you have 12 input columns, the last value will always be at position 13. This value represents the score:

[PredictedScore.Value.output1.value.Values]{0}{13}

7. The final steps are to rename the column, change the column type to Decimal Number, and remove any errors.

8. Create a table report that shows the customer e-mail and the probability for each customer to purchase a bike, as shown in **Figure 13.24**.

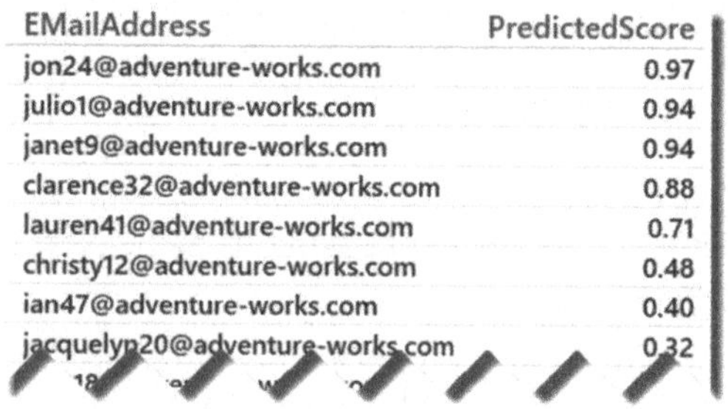

EMailAddress	PredictedScore
jon24@adventure-works.com	0.97
julio1@adventure-works.com	0.94
janet9@adventure-works.com	0.94
clarence32@adventure-works.com	0.88
lauren41@adventure-works.com	0.71
christy12@adventure-works.com	0.48
ian47@adventure-works.com	0.40
jacquelyn20@adventure-works.com	0.32

Figure 13.24 A table report that shows the predicted results.

13.4 Summary

As a BI pro, you can meet more demanding business requirements and implement versatile solutions with Power BI and Azure cloud services. You can preserve the investments you've made in classic BI by integrating Power BI with Analysis Services. This allows you to implement a hybrid scenario, where data remains on premises, and Power BI reports and dashboards connect live to Analysis Services.

If you need to implement real-time solutions that analyze data streams, you'll save significant effort by using the Power BI Streaming API. And, when requirements call for complex event processing (CEP) solutions, Azure Stream Analytics Service will make your task much easier. It's capable of ingesting millions of events per second. You can create a standing query to analyze the data stream and send the results to a real-time Power BI dashboard.

Your Power BI solutions can do more than descriptive analytics. If you need to predict future outcomes, you can implement on-premises or cloud-based predictive models. Azure Machine Learning lets business users and professionals build experiments in the cloud. You can save the predictive results to Azure, or you can publish the experiment as a predictive REST web service. Then Power BI Desktop and Power Query can call the predictive web service so that you can create "smart" reports and dashboards that transcend traditional data slicing and dicing!

Thanks to its open architecture, Power BI supports other integration scenarios that application developers will find very appealing, as you'll see in the next part of this book.

PART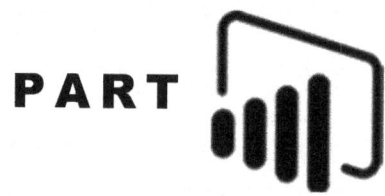

Power BI for Developers

O ne of Power BI's most prominent strengths is its open APIs, which will be very appealing to developers. When Microsoft architected the Power BI APIs, they decided to embrace popular industry standards and formats, such as REST, JSON, and OAuth2. This allows any application on any platform to integrate with the Power BI APIs. This part of the book shows developers how they can extend Power BI and implement custom solutions that integrate with Power BI.

I'll start by laying out the necessary programming fundamentals for programming with Power BI. Once I introduce you to the REST APIs, I'll walk you through the Power BI developer site, which is a great resource to learn and test the APIs. I'll explain how Power BI security works. Then I'll walk you through a sample application that uses the REST APIs to programmatically retrieve Power BI content and to load datasets with application data.

Chances are that your organization is looking for ways to embed insightful BI content on internal and external applications. Thanks to the embedded APIs, Power BI supports this scenario, and I'll walk you through the implementation details of embedding dashboards and reports. Then you'll see how Power BI Embedded makes report embedding even easier.

As you've likely seen, Power BI has an open visualization framework. Web developers can implement custom visuals and publish them to Microsoft Store. If you're a web developer, you'll see how you can leverage your experience with popular JavaScript-visualization frameworks, such as D3, WebGL, Canvas, or SVG, to create custom visuals that meet specific presentation requirements, and if you wish, you can contribute your custom visualizations to the community!

Chapter 14

Programming Fundamentals

Developers can build innovative solutions around Power BI. In the previous chapter, I've showed examples of descriptive, predictive, and real-time BI solutions that use existing Microsoft products and services. Sometimes, however, developers are tasked to extend custom applications with data analytics features, such as to implement real-time dashboards for operational analytics. Because of the open Power BI APIs, you can integrate any modern application on any platform with Power BI!

If you're new to Power BI development, this chapter is for you. I'll start by introducing you to the Power BI REST APIs. To jump start your programming journey, you'll see how to use the Power BI Developer Center to learn and test the APIs. You'll find how to register your custom applications so that they can access the Power BI APIs. I'll demystify one of the most complex programming topics surrounding Power BI programming: OAuth authentication. Finally, I'll walk you through a sample application that demonstrates how a custom application can integrate with the Power BI APIs.

14.1 Understanding Power BI APIs

When Microsoft worked on the Power BI APIs, they adopted the following design principles:

- Embrace industry standards – Instead of implementing proprietary interfaces, the team looked at other popular cloud and social platforms, and decided to adopt already popular open standards, such as Representational State Transfer (REST) programming (https://en.wikipedia.org/wiki/Representational_state_transfer), OAuth authorization (https://en.wikipedia.org/wiki/OAuth), and JavaScript Object Notation (JSON) for describing object schemas and data (https://en.wikipedia.org/wiki/JSON).

- Make it cross platform – Because of the decision to use open standards, the Power BI APIs are cross platform. Any modern native or web application on any platform can integrate with Power BI.

- Make it consistent – If you have experience with the above-mentioned industry specifications, you can seamlessly transfer your knowledge to Power BI programming. Consistency also applies within Power BI so that the APIs reflect the same objects as the ones the user interacts with in the Power BI portal.

- Easy to get started – Nobody wants to read tons of documentation before writing a single line of code. To help you get up to speed, the Power BI team created a Power BI Developer Center site where you can try the APIs as you read about them!

14.1.1 Understanding Object Definitions

As I've just mentioned, one of the design goals was consistency within Power BI. To understand this better, let's revisit the three main Power BI objects: *datasets*, *reports*, and *dashboards*. Please refer to the diagram shown in **Figure 14.1**, which shows their relationships.

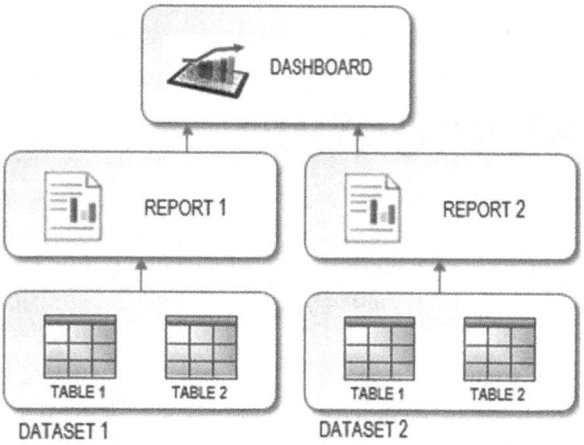

Figure 14.1 The main Power BI objects are datasets, reports, and dashboards.

Understanding dataset definitions

As you might know by now, the dataset object is the gateway to Power BI. A dataset connects to the data, and the other two main objects (reports and dashboards) show data from datasets. Specifically, a report can reference a single dataset. A dashboard can include visualizations from multiple reports, and thus display data from multiple datasets. From a developer standpoint, the dataset object has this JSON definition:

```
{
    "id": "<guid>",
    "name": "<dataset name>",
    "tables": [],
    "relatonships": []
}
```

As you can see, a dataset has a unique identifier of a GUID data type and a name. The JSON name property returns the dataset name you see in the Power BI portal's navigation bar. The *tables* element defines a collection of the dataset tables and the *relationships* element defines the relationships among these tables.

Understanding table definitions

A dataset is just a logical container of your data. The actual data is exposed as tables. When you import the data, a table stores the schema and the cached data. When you use DirectQuery, the table has just the schema. A dataset could have multiple tables, such as when you use Get Data in Power BI Service or Power BI Desktop to import multiple Excel sheets. Each table has a collection of columns. Here's what the JSON definition of a hypothetical Product table might look like (the definition is split into three columns to conserve space):

```
{
 "name": "Product",
 "columns": [
  {
    "name": "ProductID",
    "dataType": "Int64"
  },
```

```
{
    "name": "Name",
    "dataType": "string"
}, {
    "name": "IsCompete",
    "dataType": "bool"
},
```

```
{
    "name": "ManufacturedOn",
    "dataType": "DateTime"
},
{
    "name": "Category",
    "dataType": "string" } ]}
```

The Product table has five columns. Each column has a name and a data type. As far as column data types are concerned, Power BI supports a subset of the Entity Data Model (EDM) data types. but with some restrictions, as shown in **Table 14.1**. If the table has measures, there will be included in a *measures* collection.

Table 14.1 Power BI supports the following subset of EDM data types for table columns.

Data type	Purpose	Restrictions
Int64	A whole integer number	Int64.MaxValue and Int64.MinValue aren't allowed
Double	A decimal number	Double.MaxValue and Double.MinValue are not allowed. NaN isn't supported.
Boolean	A Boolean TRUE/FALSE value	
Datetime	A datetime value	Precision to 3.33 ms
String	A text value	Up to 128K characters

14.1.2 Understanding the REST APIs

Some of the tasks users perform in the Power BI Portal are exposed as Power BI APIs to let developers automate them. Because of the importance of datasets, the initial set of APIs was centered around dataset manipulation. Later, the team added APIs to list and manage groups, dashboards, reports, imported datasets, and gateways. In this section, you'll learn about the capabilities of the existing operations. These operations are fully described in the "Power BI REST API reference" documentation at bit.ly/powerbiapi.

Understanding the verbs
As I mentioned, the Power BI APIs are based on a programming specification for method invocation over HTTP, called Representational State Transfer (or REST for short). Because the same API can serve different purposes, REST supports a set of HTTP verbs to indicate the purpose of the operation. For example, to get the list of existing datasets, you'll use the GET verb. Power BI supports the most common HTTP verbs, as shown in **Table 14.2**.

Table 14.2 Power BI supports four HTTP verbs.

Verb	Operation	Success Response Codes	Error Response Codes
GET	Read	200 (OK)	404 (Not Found) or 400 (Bad Request).
POST	Create	201 (Created)	404 (Not Found), 409 (Conflict) if resource already exists
PUT	Update	200 (OK) (or 204 if not returning any content in response body)	404 (Not Found) if ID is not found
DELETE	Delete	200 (OK)	404 (Not Found) if ID is not found

The HTTP GET operation is used to retrieve a representation of a resource, such as a dataset collection. When executed successfully, GET returns the JSON representation in the response body. POST is used to create a new resource, such as a new dataset. Upon successful completion, it returns the HTTP status 201 and a Location header with a link to the newly created resource.

You typically use the PUT verb to update an existing resource by using the unique identifier of the resource. Upon a successful update, you'll get a response code of 200 (or 204 if the API doesn't return any content in the response body). Finally, given an identifier, DELETE removes the specified resource, such as a given row in a dataset table.

Understanding the dataset operations

The dataset-related operations are centered around the manipulation of datasets and tables, as shown in **Table 14.3**. Using the Power BI Rest API's, you can programmatically create new datasets, and you can add or remove rows to and from the tables in those datasets.

Table 14.3 This table shows the dataset-related operations.

Purpose	Verb	Operation Signature	Purpose
Bind to Gateway	POST	https://api.powerbi.com/v1.0/myorg/datasets/{dataset_id}/BindToGateway	Binds a dataset to data gateway
Create Dataset	POST	https://api.powerbi.com/v1.0/myorg/datasets	Creates a new dataset with a retention policy (None, basicFIFO)
Get Datasets	GET	https://api.powerbi.com/v1.0/myorg/datasets	Lists all datasets
Get Dataset	GET	https://api.powerbi.com/v1.0/myorg/datasets/{dataset_id}	Get definition of a dataset
Get Dataset Refresh History	GET	https://api.powerbi.com/v1.0/myorg/datasets/{dataset_id}	Gets the refresh history of a dataset with imported data and scheduled refresh
Refresh Dataset	POST	https://api.powerbi.com/v1.0/myorg/datasets/{dataset_id}/refreshes	Refreshes a dataset
Take Over	POST	https://api.powerbi.com/v1.0/myorg/datasets/{dataset_id}/takeover	Takes over the dataset ownership

As you can see, the verb indicates the intended action. For example, if I use the GET verb when I call the dataset API, I'll get a list of all the datasets, exactly as they're listed in the Power BI Service navigation bar under My Workspace. If I call the same API with a POST verb, I instruct Power BI to create a new dataset. I can specify an optional *defaultRetentionPolicy* parameter on the call to Create Dataset. It controls the store capacity of the dataset. The retention policy becomes important when you start adding rows to the dataset, such as to supply data to a real-time dashboard. By default, the dataset will accumulate all the rows. However, if you specify defaultRetentionPolicy=basicFIFO, the dataset will store up to 200,000 rows. Once this limit is reached, Power BI will start purging old data as new data comes in (see **Figure 14.2**).

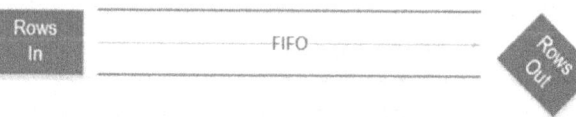

Figure 14.2 The basic FIFO dataset policy stores up to 200,000 rows and removes old data as new data flows in.

NOTE Besides tables, the "Create a dataset" operation also supports specifying relationships programmatically, DAX calculations, and additional modeling properties. This allows you to create datasets programmatically with the same features as in Power BI Desktop. For more information about these features, refer to the "New features for the Power BI Dataset API" blog by Josh Caplan at https://powerbi.microsoft.com/blog/newdatasets.

Understanding the table operations

Table 14.4 shows the existing table-related operations. The Get Tables operation lists all tables in a dataset, while Update Table Schema updates the table definitions, such as to add new columns or tables, or change existing columns.

Table 14.4 This table shows the table-related operations.

Purpose	Verb	Operation Signature	Purpose
Get Tables	GET	https://api.powerbi.com/v1.0/myorg/datasets/<dataset_id>/tables	Lists tables in a dataset
Update Table Schema	PUT	https://api.powerbi.com/v1.0/myorg/datasets/<dataset_id>/tables/<tableName>	Updates dataset table schema

Understanding row operations

Table 14.5 shows operations for adding and deleting data in a dataset table.

Table 14.5 This table shows the row-related operations.

Purpose	Verb	Operation Signature	Purpose
Add Rows	POST	https://api.powerbi.com/v1.0/myorg/datasets/<dataset_id>/tables/<tableName>/rows	Add rows to existing table
Delete Rows	DELETE	https://api.powerbi.com/v1.0/myorg/datasets/<dataset_id>/tables/<tableName>/rows	Removes rows from existing table

Understanding the group operations

Recall that besides My Workspace, users can access other workspaces that they are members of. Therefore, to present the user with all the objects he has access to, a custom app must enumerate not only the user's My Workspace but also all other app workspaces he's a member of. **Table 14.6** enumerates operations for working with groups. Despite the "group" nomenclature, these are workspace-related operations.

Table 14.6 This table shows operations for working with groups.

Purpose	Verb	Operation Signature	Purpose
Add Group	POST	https://api.powerbi.com/v1.0/myorg/groups	Creates new app workspace
Add Group User	POST	https://api.powerbi.com/v1.0/myorg/groups/{group_id}/users	Adds new workspace admin
Delete Group User	DELETE	https://api.powerbi.com/v1.0/myorg/groups/{group_id}/users/{user_emailAddress}	Removes admin user from workspace
Get Groups	GET	https://api.powerbi.com/v1.0/myorg/groups	Lists workspaces user is member of
Get Group Users	GET	https://api.powerbi.com/v1.0/myorg/groups/{group_id}/users	List all workspace members

What if you want to retrieve objects from another workspace that you're a part of through your group membership, such as to list the datasets from the Finance workspace, or to create a new dataset that's shared by all the members of a group? Fortunately, the dataset, dashboard, and report operations support specifying a group. For example, to list all the datasets for a specific group, you can invoke https://api.PowerBI.com/v1.0/myorg/**groups/{group_id}**/datasets, where group_id is the unique group identifier that you can obtain by calling the "List all groups" operation. As it stands, the developer's console doesn't allow you to change the operation signature, so you can't use the group syntax when testing the APIs, but you can use it in your applications.

Understanding the import operations

The import APIs lets you programmatically upload a Power BI Desktop file (*.pbix) or an Excel file to a workspace. This could be useful if you want to automate the deployment process of uploading datasets and reports but remember that organizational apps might be an easier and more flexible option to distribute content to many users. **Table 14.7** shows the import operations.

Table 14.7 This table shows the Imports operations.

Purpose	Verb	Operation Signature	Purpose
Create Import	POST	https://api.powerbi.com/v1.0/myorg/imports	Imports PBIX, Excel, or text file in workspace
Get Imports	GET	https://api.powerbi.com/v1.0/myorg/imports	Lists all objects imported for all imports
Get import by GUID	GET	https://api.powerbi.com/v1.0/myorg/imports/<import_guid>	Lists all objects imported for given import

The "Get Imports" operation lists all files that were imported. For each file, the operation returns when the dataset was created and updated, and the datasets and reports that were included in the file. The "Create Import" operation is for automating the task for importing a file. To call this operation, you must create a "POST" request whose body includes a filePath parameter that points to the file to be uploaded. The actual import operation executes asynchronously.

Understanding the dashboard operations

The dashboard operations allow you to retrieve dashboards and tiles. This is useful if you need to embed dashboards and tiles in a custom app, as I'll cover in the next chapter. **Table 14.8** shows you the dashboard operations.

Table 14.8 This table shows the dashboard-related operations.

Purpose	Verb	Operation Signature	Purpose
Add dashboard	POST	https://api.powerbi.com/v1.0/myorg/dashboards	Creates new dashboard
Clone Tile	POST	https://api.powerbi.com/v1.0/myorg/dashboards/{dashboard_id}/tiles/{tile_id}/Clone	Creates a tile copy and adds it target dashboard
Get Dashboards	GET	https://api.powerbi.com/beta/myorg/dashboards	Lists all dashboards
Get Tiles	GET	https://api.powerbi.com/v1.0/myorg/dashboards/{dashboard_id}/tiles	Lists dashboard tiles except pinned report pages and "model tiles" (default tiles that point to the dataset)

The "Get Dashboards" operation returns a list of dashboards as they appear in the Power BI portal's navigation bar. Every dashboard element in the response body has a GUID identifier, name, and an *isReadOnly* property that indicates whether the dashboard is read-only, such as when it's shared with you by someone else or when you're a member with read-only permissions of a workspace. The "Get Tiles" operation takes the dashboard identifier, and returns a collection of the dashboard tiles. Here's a sample JSON format that describes the "This Year's Sales" tile of the Retail Analysis Sample dashboard:

```
{
    "id": "b2e4ef32-79f5-49b3-94bc-2d228cb97703",
    "title": "This Year's Sales",
    "subTitle": "by Chain",
    "embedUrl": https://app.powerbi.com/embed?dashboardId=<dashboard id>&tileId=b2e4ef32-79f5-49b3-94bc-2d228cb97703,
    "rowSpan": 0,
    "colSpan": 0,
    "reportId": "{report_id}",
    "datasetId": "{dataset_id}"
}
```

From a content embedding standpoint, the most important element is *embedUrl*, because your application needs it to reference a tile.

Understanding the report operations
The report API allows you to retrieve, clone and export reports. **Table 14.9** shows the report operations.

Table 14.9 **This table shows the report-related operations.**

Purpose	Verb	Operation Signature	Purpose
Clone Report	POST	https://api.powerbi.com/v1.0/myorg/reports/{report_id}/Clone	Clones report under new name within the same or another workspace
Delete Report	DELETE	https://api.powerbi.com/v1.0/myorg/groups/{group_id}/reports/{report_id}	Deletes report
Export Report	GET	https://api.powerbi.com/v1.0/myorg/reports/{report_id}/Export	Export report to PBIX file
Get Reports	GET	https://api.powerbi.com/beta/myorg/reports	Lists all reports within workspace
Get Report	GET	https://api.powerbi.com/v1.0/myorg/reports/{report_id}	Get specific report
Rebind Report	POST	https://api.powerbi.com/v1.0/myorg/reports/{report_id}/Rebind	Rebinds report to another dataset

The "Get Reports" operation returns a list of reports as they appear in the navigation bar. Every report element in the response body has a GUID-based identifier (*id*), name, webUrl, embedUrl and dataset identifier. The webUrl link navigates to the report in Power BI Service. The embedUrl link is what you need to embed the report in a custom application. Here's a sample JSON format that describes the Retail Analysis Sample report that you implemented in Chapter 4.

```
{
"id":"22454c20-dde4-46bc-9d72-5a6ea969339e",
"name":"Retail Analysis Sample",
"webUrl":"https://app.powerbi.com/reports/22454c20-dde4-46bc-9d72-5a6ea969339e",
"embedUrl":"https://app.powerbi.com/reportEmbed?reportId=22454c20-dde4-46bc-9d72-5a6ea969339e",
"datasetId": "21354c20-dde4-46bc-9d72-5a6ea969339e "
}
```

Understanding data source operations
The data source-specific operations are listed in **Table 14.10**.

Table 14.10 **This table shows the data source-related operations.**

Purpose	Verb	Operation Signature	Purpose
Get Datasources	GET	https://api.powerbi.com/v1.0/myorg/groups/{group_id}/datasets/{datasetID}/dataSources	dataset_id (the dataset identifier)
Get BoundGatewayDataSources	GET	https://api.powerbi.com/v1.0/myorg/datasets/<dataset_id>/Default.GetBoundGatewayDataSources	dataset_id (the dataset identifier)
Set All Connections	POST	https://api.powerbi.com/v1.0/myorg/datasets/<dataset_id>/Default.SetAllConnections	dataset_id (the dataset identifier)

These operations apply to datasets that use DirectQuery connections. For example, your application can call "Get BoundGatewayDataSources" to obtain the connection string for a DirectQuery dataset and then call "Set All Connections " to change it.

Understanding gateway operations

Finally, there are currently 14 gateway-related operations to manage programmatically on-premises gateways, including listing gateways, setting credentials, adding, updating, and removing data sources, and maintaining users associated with a gateway.

14.1.3 Testing Power BI APIs

Now that you've learned about the Power BI REST APIs, you're probably eager to try them out. But hold off writing code in Visual Studio. As it turns out, Microsoft has integrated the Power BI APIs with Apiary (https://apiary.io) to help you get started with Power BI programming!

Getting started with Apiary

You can access the Power BI REST Apiary in two different ways:

1. Navigate to https://powerbi.docs.apiary.io.
2. From the Power BI REST API reference, click the "Try on Apiary" link on most operations, as shown in **Figure 14.3**).

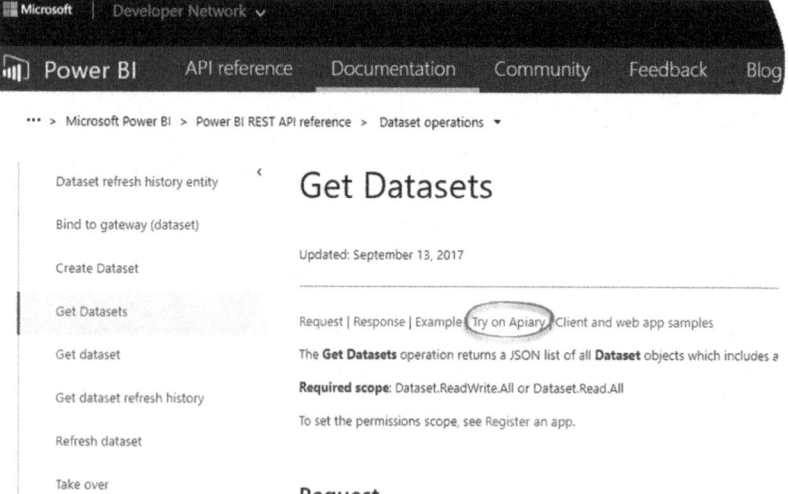

Figure 14.3 Most operations include a "Try on Apiary" link.

Both options navigate you to the Power BI REST API Apiary site, where you can test the APIs.

Testing the APIs

The Apiary includes a testing console where you can try the APIs without writing a single line of code! Currently, Microsoft hasn't updated the Apiary to list the new API names and groups, so finding the right API might take same time (the "Try on Apiary" link will be your best bet). Follow these steps to test the dataset APIs:

1. In Apiary, click the Datasets link in the navigation page to expand the section.
2. Click the Datasets Collection item. This shows you the documentation of the dataset-related APIs.
3. Click "List all Datasets". which corresponds to "Get Datasets" API. The right pane shows an example of the method call, including a sample request and a sample raw JSON response (see **Figure 14.4**).

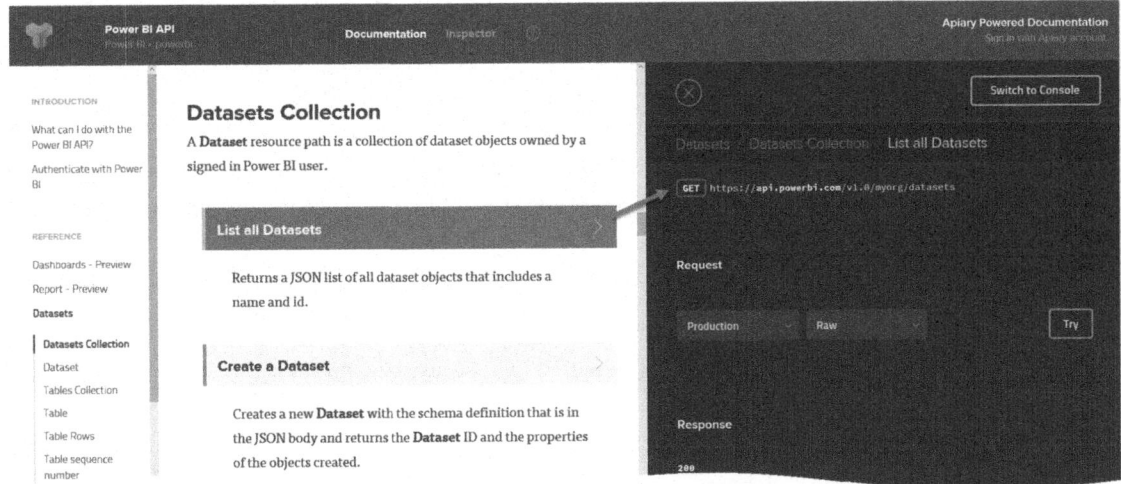

Figure 14.4   The Power BI REST API site shows an example of the method invocation.

4. To get a code example written in your preferred programming language, expand the drop-down menu to the left of the Try button (that says "Raw"), and then select your targeted language, such as C#, Visual Basic, JavaScript, Node.js, and others. The default Raw option shows only the request and response payloads that your application needs to invoke the API and process the results. Another good use of the Raw option is that you copy the Request code, and then use it to make direct method invocations with network tools, such as Fiddler, when you want to test or troubleshoot the APIs.

5. To try the API, click the Try button. This switches you to an interactive console, as shown in **Figure 14.5**.

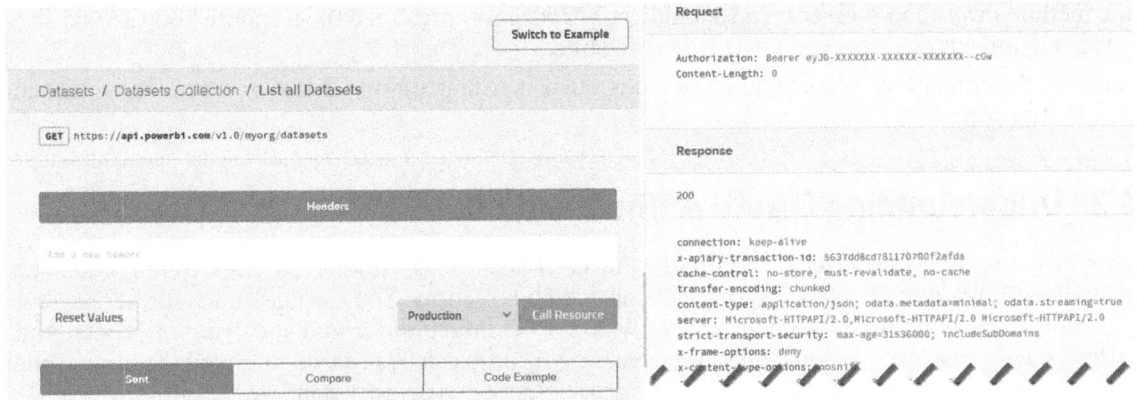

Figure 14.5   The console lets you invoke APIs and shows the request and the response.

6. Click the Get Resource button. If you haven't signed in to Power BI, this is when you'll be asked to do so. That's because all the API calls happen under the identity of the signed user. Next, you'll get the actual request/response pair from the method invocation.

If you examine the request body, you'll see an Authorization header. The obfuscated setting after "Bearer" is where the OAuth authorization token will go with an actual method invocation. The Response pane shows the result of the call. As you know already, the "200" response code means a successful invocation.

Next, the Response section displays the response headers and the response body (not shown in **Figure 14.5**). The response body includes the JSON definition of the dataset collection, with all the datasets in My Workspace.

Working with parameters

Now let's use Apiary to get a list of tables in a dataset:

1. Scroll down the response pane and copy the GUID of the id property of the Retail Analysis Sample dataset.
2. In the navigation pane, click the Tables Collection tab. On the Tables Collection page, click the "List all Tables" link.
3. In the Console pane (see **Figure 14.6**), click the URI Parameters button. This method takes an id parameter, which in this case is the dataset identifier.

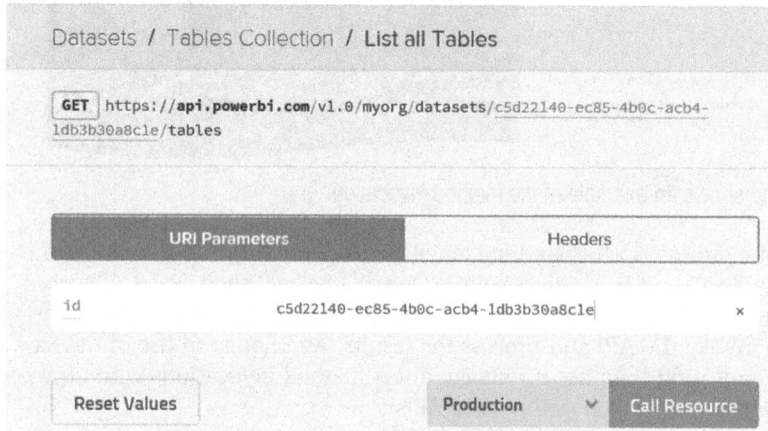

Figure 14.6 The console lets you pass parameters to the method, such as the dataset identifier in this example.

4. Paste the dataset identifier next to the id parameter, and then click Call Resource.
5. If the method invocation succeeds, you should get a "200" response. Then the response body should show the JSON definition of a table collection with five tables.
6. (Optional) Experiment with calling other methods, such as to create a new dataset, create a new table, and add rows to a table.

14.2 Understanding OAuth Authentication

Apiary makes it easy to understand and test the Power BI REST APIs. However, it hides an important and somewhat complex part of Power BI programming, which is security. You can't get much further beyond the console if you don't have a good grasp of how Power BI authentication and authorization works. And security is never easy. In fact, sometimes implementing security can be more complicated than the application itself. The good news is that Power BI embraces another open security standard, OAuth2, which greatly reduces the plumbing effort to authenticate users with Power BI! As you'll see in this chapter and the next one, OAuth2 is a flexible standard that supports various security scenarios.

REAL LIFE Security can get complicated. I once architected a classic BI solution consisting of a data warehouse, cube, and reports for a card processing company. After a successful internal adoption, their management decided to allow external partners to view their own data. One of the security requirements was federating account setup and maintenance to the external partners. This involved setting up an Active Directory subdomain, a web application layer, and countless meetings. At the end, the security plumbing took more effort than the actual BI system!

14.2.1 Understanding Authentication Flows

OAuth2 allows a custom application to access Power BI Service on the user's behalf, after the user consents that this is acceptable. Next, the application gets the authorization code from Azure AD, and then exchanges it for an access token that provides access to Power BI.

Understanding the OAuth parties

There are three parties that are involved in the default three-leg authentication flow:

- User – This is the Power BI user.
- Application – This is a custom native client application or a web application that needs to access Power BI content on behalf of the user.
- Resource – In the case of Power BI, the resource is some content, such as a dataset or a dashboard.

With the three-leg flow, the custom application never has the user's credentials because the entire authentication process is completely transparent to the application. However, OAuth opens a sign-in window so that the user can log in to Power BI. Microsoft refers to the three-leg flow as "user owns the data". In the case when the application knows the user credentials, OAuth2 supports a two-leg flow where the application directly authenticates the user to the resource. The two-leg flow bypasses the sign-in window, and the user isn't involved in the authentication flow. Microsoft refers to the two-leg flow as "application owns the data". I'll demonstrate the two-leg scenario in the next chapter.

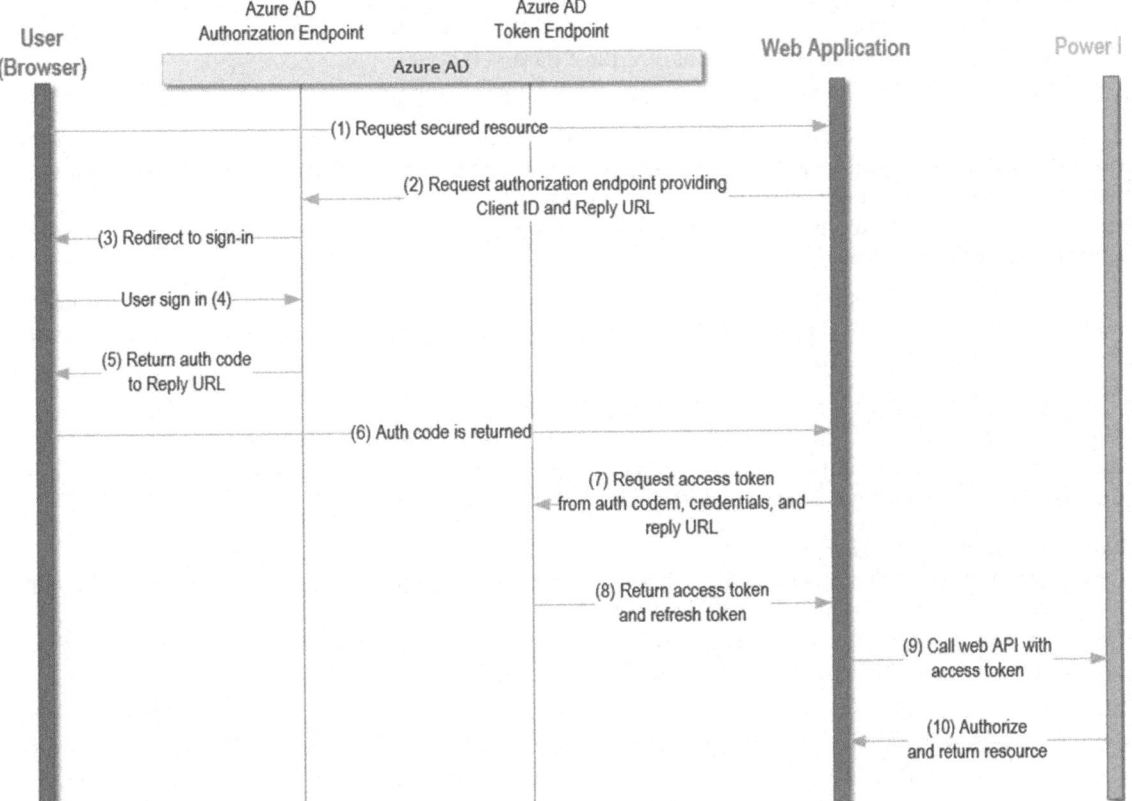

Figure 14.7   This sequence diagram shows the OAuth2 flow for web applications.

Understanding the web application flow

Figure 14.7 shows the OAuth flow for web applications. By "web application", I mean any browser-based application, such as a custom ASP.NET application.

The typical authentication flow involves the following steps:

1. The user opens the Web browser and navigates to the custom application to request a Power BI resource, such as to view a report.

2. The web application calls to and passes the application client ID and Reply URL (AD). Azure Active Directory uses the client ID to identify the custom application. You obtain the client ID when you register your application with Azure AD. The Reply URL is typically a page within your application where Azure AD will redirect the user after the user signs in to Power BI.

3. Azure AD opens the Power BI sign-in page.

4. The user signs in using valid Power BI credentials. Note that the actual authentication is completely transparent to the application. The user might sign in using his Power BI credentials or, if the organization policy requires it, the user might use a smart card to authenticate. Azure AD determines the authentication mechanism depending on the AD corporate policy.

 NOTE The first time the user signs in, he will be asked to authorize the custom app for all the permissions you granted the app when you register it in the Azure AD. To see the authorized custom apps, the user can open the Power BI portal, and then click the Office 365 Application Launcher button (at the top-left corner of the portal) ⇨ "View all my apps". The user can use this menu to remove authorized custom applications at any point, and then see the granted permissions.

5. The Azure AD Authorization Endpoint service redirects the user to the page that's specified by the Reply URL, and it sends an authorization code as a request parameter.

6. The web application collects the authorization code from the request.

7. The web application calls down to the Azure AD Token Endpoint service to exchange the authorization code with an access token. In doing so, the application presents credentials consisting of the client id and client secret (also called a key). You can specify one or more keys when you register the application with Azure AD. The access token is the holy grail of OAuth because this is what your application needs to access the Power BI resources.

8. The Azure AD Token Endpoint returns an access token and a refresh token. Because the access token is short-lived, the application can use the refresh token to request additional access tokens instead of going again through the entire authentication flow.

9. Once the application has the access token, it can start making API calls on behalf of the user.

10. When you register the application, you specify an allowed set of Power BI permissions, such as "View all datasets". Power BI will evaluate these permissions when authorizing the call. If the user has the required permission, Power BI executes the API and returns the results.

Understanding the native client flow

A native client is any installed application that doesn't require the user to use the Web browser. A native client could be a console application, desktop application, or an application installed on a mobile device. **Figure 14.8** shows the OAuth sequence flow for native clients. As you can see, the authentication flow for native clients is somewhat simpler than the flow for web apps.

1. Before making a Power BI API call, the native client app calls to the Azure AD Authorization Endpoint and presents the client id. A native client application probably won't have a redirect page. However, because Azure AD requires a Redirect URI, a native client app can use any URI, as long as it matches the one you specified when you register the app with Azure AD. Or, if you're running out of ideas of what this artificial URI might be, you can use the Microsoft suggested URI for native clients, which is https://login.live.com/oauth20_desktop.srf.

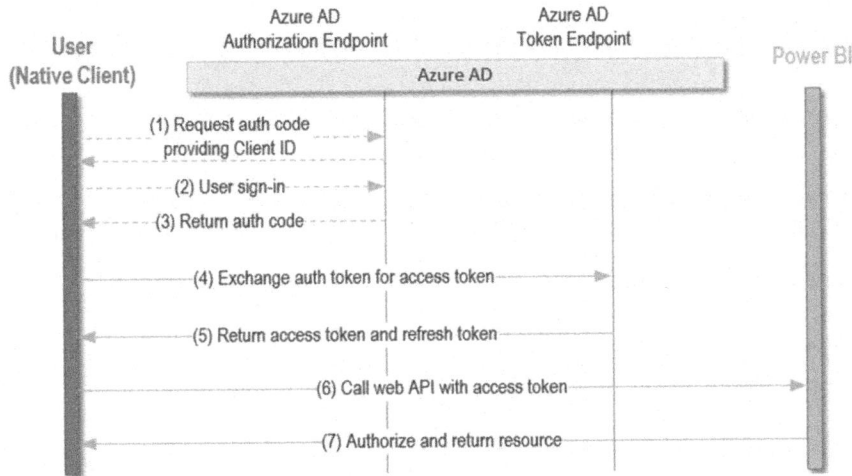

Figure 14.8 This sequence diagram shows the OAuth2 flow for native clients.

The diagram labels:

User (Native Client)
Azure AD Authorization Endpoint
Azure AD Token Endpoint
Azure AD
Power BI

(1) Request auth code providing Client ID
(2) User sign-in
(3) Return auth code
(4) Exchange auth token for access token
(5) Return access token and refresh token
(6) Call web API with access token
(7) Authorize and return resource

2. As with the web application flow, Azure AD will open the Web browser so that the user can sign in to Power BI. Again, the sign-in experience depends on how the organization is set up with Azure AD, but typically the user is asked to enter credentials in the Power BI sign-in page.

3. The Azure AD Authorization Endpoint returns an authorization code. The dotted lines in the **Figure 14.8** represent that this handshake happens within a single call. All a .NET application needs to do is call the *AcquireToken* method of the *AuthenticationContext* class to get the user to sign in, and then acquire the authorization code. In fact, the *AquireToken* method also performs the next step (step 4) on the same call.

4. A handshake takes place between the native client and the Azure AD Token Endpoint to exchange the authorization code for an access token.

5. The Azure AD Token Endpoint returns an access token and a refresh token.

6. The client calls the Power BI resource passing the access token.

7. Power BI authorizes the user and executes the call if the user has the required permissions.

14.2.2 Understanding Application Registration

As a prerequisite of integrating custom applications with Power BI, you must register the app with Azure AD. In the process of registering the application, you specify the OAuth2 details, including the type of the application (web or native client), keys, Redirect URL, and permissions. The easiest way to register a custom application is to use the Power BI registration page. You can also use the Azure Management Portal to register your application, but the process is more involved.

Note that although you can use the Power BI registration page for the initial registration process, you still need to use the Azure Management Portal to make subsequent changes, such as to change the Redirect URL. Next, I'll walk you through the steps to register web and native client applications using the Power BI registration page and Azure Management Portal.

Getting started with registration

The application registration page helps you create a new application in Azure AD that has all the information required to connect to Power BI. Anyone can register a custom application. You can find the Power BI registration page in the Power BI Developer Center, as follows:

1. Open your Web browser, navigate to Power BI Service (http://powerbi.com), and log in.

2. In the Application Toolbar at the top-right corner of the screen, click the Help & Support menu, and then click "Power BI for developers".

3. In the Power BI Developer Center, scroll down the page and then click the "Register your app" link found in the Web section.

4. Or instead of these three steps, you can go directly to the "Register an Application for Power BI" page at https://dev.powerbi.com/apps.

Registering your application using the Power BI registration page

Figure 14.9 shows the app registration page (to preserve space, steps 3 and 4 are shown on the right).

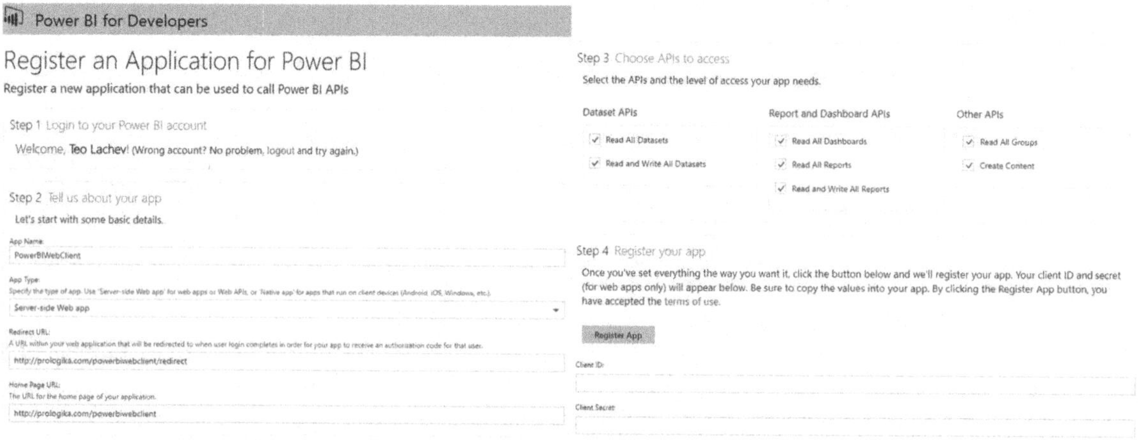

Figure 14.9 Register your custom app in four steps, using the Power BI registration page.

Registering a custom application takes four simple steps:

1. Sign in to Power BI. Specify the app details (see **Table 14.11**).

Table 14.11 This table describes the application registration details.

Setting	Explanation	Example
App Type	Choose "Server-side Web app" for browser-based web apps, and choose "Native app" for an installed application, such a console app	
Redirect URL	The web page where Azure AD will redirect the user after the Power BI sign-in completes	http://localhost:999/powerbiwebclient/redirect (for web apps) https://login.live.com/oauth20_desktop.srf (for native apps)
Home Page URL (web apps only)	The URL for the home page of your application (used by Azure AD to uniquely identify your application)	http://prologika.com/powerbiwebclient

2. Specify which Power BI REST APIs your app needs permissions to call. For example, if the custom app needs to push data to a dataset table, you'll have to check the "Read and Write All Dataset permissions". As a best practice, grant the app the minimum set of permissions it needs. You can always change this later if you need to.

3. Click the Register App button to register your app. If all is well, you'll get back the client ID. For web apps, you'll also get a client secret (also called a key). As I mentioned, your custom web app needs the client secret to exchange the authorization code for an access token.

TIP Because Power BI currently doesn't let you update the registration details (you need to use the Azure Management Portal for this), if you develop a web app I recommend you put some thought in the Redirect URL. Chances are that during development, you would use the Visual Studio Development Server or IIS Express. The Redirect URL needs to match your development setup, such as to include localhost. Once the application is tested, your Azure administrator can use the Azure Management Portal to change your web app and to add a production Redirect URL, such as http://prologika.com/powerbiwebclient/redirect.

Because managing registered applications can't be done in Power BI, next I'll show you how you can use the Azure Management Portal to view, register, and manage custom apps. You must have Azure AD admin rights to your organization's Active Directory to register an application. In addition, although the basic features of Azure Active Directory are free, you need an Azure subscription to use the portal and this subscription must be associated with your organizational account.

Registering web applications using Azure Management Portal
Follow these steps to register a custom web application in the Azure Management Portal:

1. Navigate to the Azure Management Portal (at https://portal.azure.com) and sign in with your organizational account. Again, the account you use must be associated with an Azure subscription.
2. In the navigation bar on the left, select Azure Active Directory. In the next page, click "App registrations" to view the registered applications (see **Figure 14.10**).

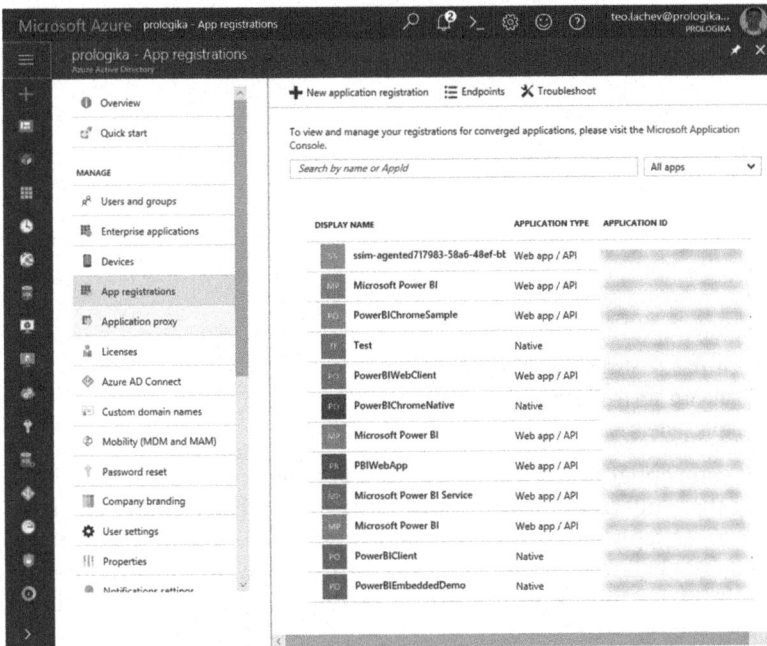

Figure 14.10 Select the "App registrations" tab to view and register custom applications.

3. On the top of the page, click "New application registration" to register a new app.
4. In the Create blade, enter the name of your application, such as *PowerBIWebClient* (see **Figure 14.11**). The name must be unique across the registered application within your organization. Because this is a web application, leave the default type of "Web app / API" selected. Enter the application Sign-on URL (same as "Home Page URL" in the Power BI registration page). This is the address of a web page where users can sign in to use your app, such as http://prologika.com/powerbiwebclient. Azure AD doesn't validate this URL, but it's required. Click Create to create the application. Once Azure creates the app, it adds it to the list of the registered apps.

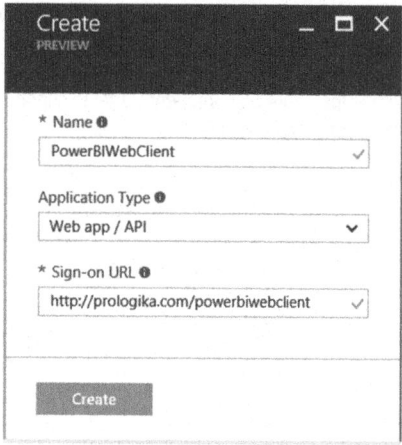

Figure 14.11 Specify the application name, application type (web or native), and sign-on URL.

5. In the app registrations, select the app you just registered to show its settings. The Settings blade is where you can configure the rest of the application registration details. It has Properties, Reply URLs, Owners, "Required permissions", and Keys tabs (see **Figure 14.12**).

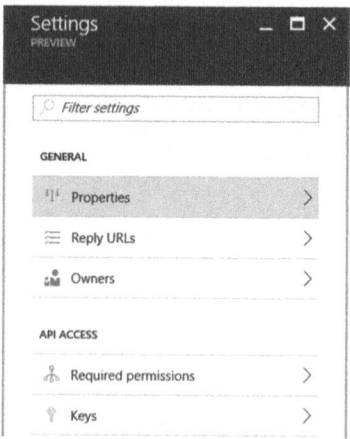

Figure 14.12 Use the Settings blade to configure the rest of the application registration details.

For example, in the Properties tab you can configure if the app has a multi-tenant scope. By default, the application isn't multi-tenant, meaning that only users on your domain can access the app. The "Reply URLs" tab allows you to specify one or more reply URLs (fulfill the same role as the redirect URL in the Power BI registration page) where Azure AD will redirect the user after the user signs in to Power BI. Enter a valid URL, such as http://prologika.com/powerbiwebclient/redirect. The Owners tab lets you register additional owners who can change the app settings.

6. So that Power BI can authorize your application, use the "Required permissions" tab to grant your app permissions to Power BI. To do this, select the "Power BI Service (Microsoft.Azure.AnalysisServices)" API. If you don't see "Power BI Service" in the list of applications, make sure that at least one user has signed up for and accessed Power BI. **Figure 14.13** shows you the permissions that Power BI currently supports or that are currently in preview.

Some of these permissions correspond to the available REST APIs that you see in the Power BI registration page. For example, if the application wants to get a list of the datasets available for the signed user, it needs to have the "View all Datasets" permission. As a best practice, grant the application the minimum permissions it needs.

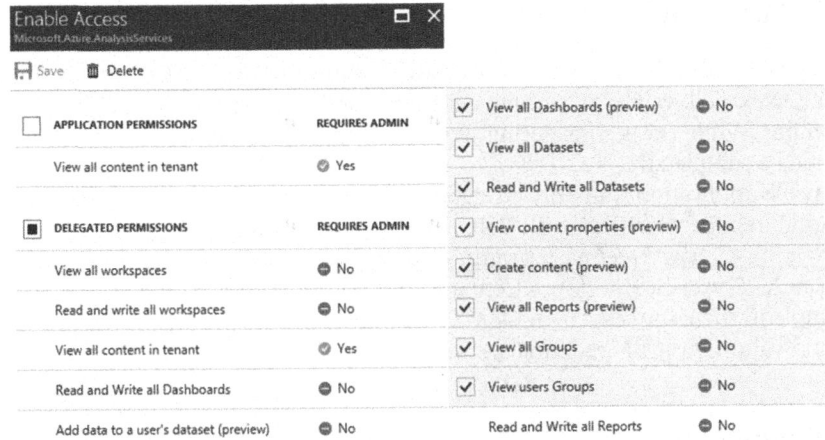

Figure 14.13 You must grant your application permissions to Power BI.

7. Use the Keys tab to create a key(s) (same as the client secret in the Power BI registration page) that you can use as a password when the application exchanges the authorization code for an access token. Currently, the maximum duration for the key validity is two years.

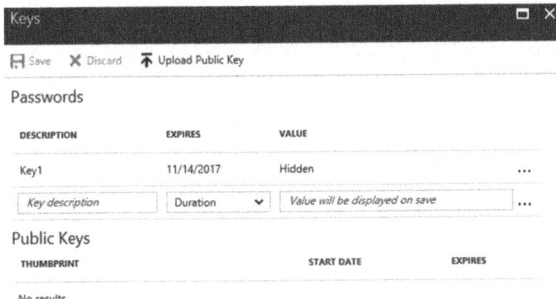

Figure 14.14 Create one or more client keys that your app will use to authenticate with Power BI.

Registering native clients

The native client registration is much simpler. The only required properties are the application name and Redirect URI. As I mentioned, you can use https://login.live.com/oauth20_desktop.srf as a Redirect URI. **Figure 14.15** shows a sample configuration for a native client application. As with registering a web app, you need to grant the native app permissions to Power BI (not shown in **Figure 14.15**).

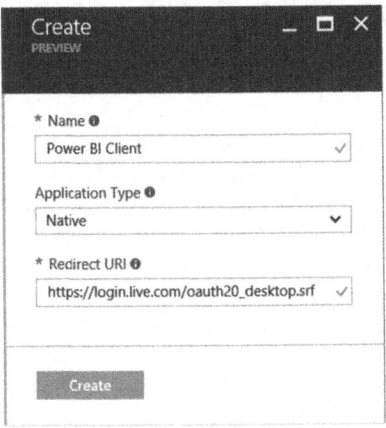

Figure 14.15 Registering a native client application requires a name and Redirect URI.

14.3 Working with Power BI APIs

Now that you know about the Power BI REST APIS and how to configure custom applications for OAuth, let's practice what you've learned. Next, I'll walk you through a sample application that will help you get started with Power BI programming. While I was considering writing a sample from scratch, as it turned out Microsoft has already provided a sample app.

Implemented as a .NET console application, the PBIGettingStarted application demonstrates how a native client can authenticate and integrate with Power BI. You can download it from GitHub at https://github.com/Microsoft/PowerBI-CSharp/tree/master/samples/consoleapp/getting-started-for-dotnet, or by clicking the Sample link on the Power BI Developer Center under the "Client app" section. For your convenience, I included the sample in the \Source\ch14 folder. To run the sample, you'll need Visual Studio 2010 or a higher version (and valid Power BI credentials).

14.3.1 Implementing Authentication

Let's start with understanding how the application uses OAuth2 to authenticate the user before she makes calls to Power BI. As a prerequisite, you'll need to register a native client application in Azure AD.

Configuring the application
Before running the application, you need to change a few class-level variables to reflect your setup.

1. Open the PBIGettingStarted application in Visual Studio.

2. In Solution Explorer, double click Program.cs to open it.

3. Change the following variables:

```
private static string clientID = "<client_id>";
private static string redirectUri = "https://login.live.com/oauth20_desktop.srf";
private static string datasetName = "SalesMarketing";
private static string groupName = "Finance";
```

Replace the *clientID* variable with the Client ID of your application when you register it using either the Power BI registration method or from Azure AD (see **Figure 14.14** again). Replace the redirectUri variable with the Redirect URI of your application or leave it set to https://login.live.com/oauth20_desktop.srf if this is the Redirect URI that you register. One of the tasks that the application demonstrates is programmatically creating a new "SalesMarketing" dataset. If the dataset name isn't what you want, change it accordingly. The application demonstrates working with groups. To try this feature, use Power BI Service to create a workspace group, such as "Finance". Then, change the groupName variable to the name of the group. If you use Power BI Free, which doesn't support groups, you can just skip this part of the application.

Implementing OAuth
Every API invocation calls the *AccessToken* method, which performs the actual authentication. **Figure 14.16** shows the *DatasetRequest* method that is used by all dataset-related examples, such as when the application lists datasets (the *GetDatasets* method). The *DatasetRequest* method creates a web request object as required by the Power BI API specification. It adds an Authorization header with a Bearer property that specifies the access token. In case you're wondering, the access token is a base64-encoded hash that looks like this: "eyJ0eXAiOiJKV1QiLCJhbGciOiJSUzI1N...".

Remember that you need the access token to authenticate successfully with OAuth. The application obtains the token by calling the *AccessToken* method. Line 551 constructs a .NET *AuthenticationContext* class, passing the URL of the Azure AD Token Endpoint and an instance of a *TokenCache* class. I separated the original code to call *AcquireToken* into two lines to illustrate better what happens next. Line 553 calls

AcquireToken. It passes the URL of the resource that needs to be authorized. In your case, the resource is Power BI and its resource URI is https://analysis.windows.net/powerbi/api. The code also passes the Client ID and the redirect URI.

```
543    static string AccessToken()
544    {
545        if (token == String.Empty)
546        {
547            //Get Azure access token
548            // Create an instance of TokenCache to cache the access token
549            TokenCache TC = new TokenCache();
550            // Create an instance of AuthenticationContext to acquire an Azure access token
551            authContext = new AuthenticationContext(authority, TC);
552            // Call AcquireToken to get an Azure token from Azure Active Directory token issuance endpoint
553            AuthenticationResult result = authContext.AcquireToken(resourceUri, clientID, new Uri(redirectUri), PromptBehavior.RefreshSessio
554            token = result.AccessToken;
555        }
556        else
557        {
558            // Get the token in the cache
559            token = authContext.AcquireTokenSilent(resourceUri, clientID).AccessToken;
560        }
561
562        return token;
563    }
593    private static HttpWebRequest DatasetRequest(string datasetsUri, string method, string accessToken)
594    {
595        HttpWebRequest request = System.Net.WebRequest.Create(datasetsUri) as System.Net.HttpWebRequest;
596        request.KeepAlive = true;
597        request.Method = method;
598        request.ContentLength = 0;
599        request.ContentType = "application/json";
600        request.Headers.Add("Authorization", String.Format( "Bearer {0}", accessToken));
601
602        return request;
603    }
604    }
605 }
```

Figure 14.16   The AccessToken method performs the OAuth authentication flow.

When the application calls *AcquireToken*, you'll be required to sign in to Power BI. Once you type in your credentials and Power BI authenticates you successfully, you'll get back an instance of the Authentication-Result class. AuthenticationResult encapsulates important details, including the access token, its expiration date, and refresh token. On line 554, the application stores the access token so that it can pass it with subsequent API calls without going through the authentication flow again. As it stands, the application doesn't use the refresh token flow, but you can enhance it to do so. For example, you can check if the access token is about to expire and then call the authContext.AquireAccessTokenByRefreshToken method.

14.3.2 Invoking the Power BI APIs

Once the application authenticates the interactive user, it's ready to call the Power BI APIs. The next sample demonstrates calling various APIs to create a dataset, adding and deleting rows to and from a dataset table, changing the dataset table schema, and getting the groups that the user belongs to. I'll walk you through the PBIGettingStarted code for creating datasets and loading a dataset table with data.

Creating datasets
A custom application can create a Power BI dataset to store data from scratch. The sample application demonstrates this with the *CreateDataset* method (see **Figure 14.17**). Line 213 constructs the API method signature for creating datasets by using the POST verb. Line 216 calls the *GetDatasets* method (not shown in **Figure 14.17**), which in turn calls the "List all datasets" Power BI API.

```
207     static void CreateDataset()
208     {
209         //In a production application, use more specific exception handling.
210         try
211         {
212             //Create a POST web request to list all datasets
213             HttpWebRequest request = DatasetRequest(String.Format("{0}/datasets", datasetsUri), "POST", AccessToken());
214
215             //Get a list of datasets
216             dataset ds = GetDatasets().value.GetDataset(datasetName);
217
218             if (ds == null)
219             {
220                 //POST request using the json schema from Product
221                 Console.WriteLine(PostRequest(request, new Product().ToDatasetJson(datasetName)));
222             }
223             else
224             {
225                 Console.WriteLine("Dataset exists");
226             }
227         }
228         catch (Exception ex)
229         {
230             Console.WriteLine(ex.Message);
231         }
232     }
```

Figure 14.17   The CreateDataset method demonstrates how to programmatically create a dataset.

Line 221 passes an instance of the Product object, and it serializes the object to the JSON format. As a result, the request body contains the JSON representation of a dataset that has a single table called Product with five columns (ProductName, Name, Category, IsComplete, and ManufacturedOn). Once the call completes, you should see the SalesMarketing dataset in the Power BI Service navigation bar.

At this point, the dataset Product table contains no data. However, I recommend you take a moment now to create a table report for it, and then pin a visualization from the report to a dashboard. This will allow you to see in real time the effect of loading the dataset with data. Next, the code loads some data.

Loading data

The custom application can programmatically push rows to a dataset table. This scenario is very useful because it allows you to implement real-time dashboards, like the one we've implemented with Azure Stream Analytics Service in the previous chapter. The difference is that in this case, it's your application that pushes the data and you have full control over the entire process, including how the data is shaped and how often it pushes data to Power BI. The *AddRows* method demonstrates this (see **Figure 14.18**).

```
375     static void AddRows(string datasetId, string tableName)
376     {
377         //In a production application, use more specific exception handling.
378         try
379         {
380             HttpWebRequest request = DatasetRequest(String.Format("{0}/datasets/{1}/tables/{2}/rows", datasetsUri, datasetId, tableName), "POST", AccessToken());
381
382             //Create a list of Product
383             List<Product> products = new List<Product>
384             {
385                 new Product{ProductID = 1, Name="Adjustable Race", Category="Components", IsCompete = true, ManufacturedOn = new DateTime(2014, 7, 30)},
386                 new Product{ProductID = 2, Name="LL Crankarm", Category="Components", IsCompete = true, ManufacturedOn = new DateTime(2014, 7, 30)},
387                 new Product{ProductID = 3, Name="HL Mountain Frame - Silver", Category="Bikes", IsCompete = true, ManufacturedOn = new DateTime(2014, 7, 30)},
388             };
389
390             //POST request using the json from a list of Product
391             //NOTE: Posting rows to a model that is not created through the Power BI API is not currently supported.
392             //      Please create a dataset by posting it through the API following the instructions on http://dev.powerbi.com.
393             Console.WriteLine(PostRequest(request, products.ToJson(JavaScriptConverter<Product>.GetSerializer())));
394         }
395         catch (Exception ex)
396         {
397             Console.WriteLine(ex.Message);
398         }
399     }
```

Figure 14.18   The AddRows method demonstrates how your custom app can load a dataset table.

On line 380, the code creates the API method signature for creating rows using the POST verb. Then the code creates a list collection with three products. This collection will be used to add three rows to the dataset. On line 393, the code calls the *PostRequest* method and passes the collection (serialized as JSON). This JSON output will be included in the request body. Once this method completes, three rows will be added to the Product table in the *SalesMarketing* dataset. If you watch the Power BI dashboard, you should see its tile data updating in real time. Now you have a real-time BI solution!

14.4 Summary

The Power BI APIs are based on open industry standards, such as REST, JSON, and OAuth. These APIs allow you to automate content management and data manipulation tasks, including creating and deleting datasets, loading dataset tables with data, changing the dataset schema, and determining the user's group membership. You can use the Power BI Developer Center to learn and try the APIs.

As a trustworthy environment, Power BI must authenticate users before authorizing them to access the content. The cornerstone of the Power BI authentication is the OAuth2 protocol. By default, it uses a three-leg authentication flow (user owns the data) that asks the user to sign in to Power BI. As a prerequisite to integrating a custom app with Power BI, you must register the custom app with Azure AD.

The PBIGettingStarted sample app demonstrates how a Windows native client app can authenticate and call the Power BI REST APIs. I walked you through the code that creates a new dataset and loads it with data. This allows you to implement real-time dashboards that display data as the data streams from your application.

Another very popular integration scenario that the Power BI APIs enable is embedding reports in custom applications. This is the subject of the next chapter.

Chapter 15

Power BI Embedded

Because Power BI generates HTML5, users can enjoy insightful reports on any platform and on any device. Wouldn't it be nice to bring this experience to your custom apps? Collectively known as Power BI Embedded, Power BI includes REST APIs that allow you to embed reports and dashboards in any modern web app. This avoids navigating users out of your app and into powerbi.com. Embedded reports preserve their interactive features and offer the same engaging experience as viewing them in Power BI Service. Users can even edit existing reports or create their own reports if you let them do it! Tasked to embed reports in a web portal for external customers? It gets even better thanks to the Power BI Embedded special licensing that lets you embed content for third party without requiring a per-user license!

As with the previous chapter, this is a code-intensive chapter, so be prepared to wear your developer's hat. I'll start by introducing you to the Power BI REST APIs that let you embed dashboards and reports. I'll walk you through some sample code that demonstrates how your intranet and Internet apps can use these features. You can find the sample web applications in the \Source\ch15 folder.

15.1 Understanding Power BI Embedded

Embedded reporting is a common requirement for both internal and external (customer-facing) applications. The subset of the Power BI REST APIs that let developers embed content is known as Power BI Embedded. Because Power BI Embedded has its own licensing model, it's listed as a separate product in the Power BI product portfolio.

NOTE When Microsoft introduced Power BI Premium in June 2017, they also revamped Power BI Embedded. Previously, Power BI Embedded was for embedding content for external users only. It was implemented as a Microsoft Azure Service and it had its own content storage and different APIs. The old Power BI Embedded didn't have feature parity with Power BI Service. This all changed with the new Power BI Embedded. Think of the new Power BI Embedded as Power BI Service with its own licensing model.

15.1.1 Getting Started with Power BI Embedded

The first thing you need to understand about Power BI Embedded is how to acquire it. As a developer, if you have a Power BI Pro license, you can start using the Power BI Embedded APIs right away. If all your users have Power BI Pro subscriptions, they can view the embedded content and you're all set. But from a pure licensing standpoint, things get more complicated when your app services many users, especially Power BI Free internal users or external users. At that point, licensing by user, by month is not practical. So, you need to consider purchasing an embedded capacity to support many users in a cost-efficient way.

Understanding Power BI Embedded capacities

There are two ways to acquire an embedded capacity. If your organization is on a Power BI Premium P plan, you already have everything you need to embed content for both internal and external users. Power BI Premium EM plans are more restrictive. Refer to section 12.1.1 to understand how P, EM, and A plans compare as far as targeting internal and external users.

Another way to obtain an embedded capacity is to purchase an Azure plan. Most smaller companies and Independent Software Vendors (ISV) looking for embedding content to external users only, would gravitate toward the Azure Power BI Embedded plans. The Azure plans can also result in significant cost savings because they allow you to quickly scale up and down, and even pause the capacity, as I'll explain when I walk you through the steps to acquire an Azure embedded capacity! For example, if the most report activity happens within normal working hours, you can scale it down to a lower capacity out-side the peak period.

 REAL LIFE I've helped a few ISVs integrate their apps with Power BI Embedded (see one related Microsoft study at https://pow-erbi.microsoft.com/blog/zynbit-empowers-sales-with-microsoft-power-bi-embedded/). All of them have considered other vendors and third-party libraries for embedding content, but were attracted to Power BI Embedded because of its rich code-free visualizations and very cost-effective licensing model.

Understanding Azure capacity nodes

Like Power BI Premium, an Azure plan represents a capacity node and its associated hardware. Currently, there are size Azure capacity nodes, which are shown in **Table 15.1**.

Table 15.1 Power BI Embedded has six Azure capacity nodes.

Node	Capacity Type	Total V-cores	Memory	Max Page Renders (per hour)	Direct Query connection limits (per sec)	Estimated Price (per month)
A1	Shared	1	3 GB	300	5	$750
A2	Shared	2	5 GB	600	10	$1,500
A3	Dedicated	4	10 GB	1,200	15	$3,000
A4	Dedicated	8	25 GB	2,400	30	$6,000
A5	Dedicated	16	50 GB	4,800	60	$12,000
A6	Dedicated	32	100 GB	9,600	120	$24,000

Estimating how much capacity your app would need isn't an exact science, but the most important factor (especially if your reports will connect live to an external data source) is the hourly distribution of page renders. Like Power BI Premium, a page render happens every time a report page is refreshed. So, if a report has two pages, and the user visits the first page and then the second page, and changes a filter on the second page, there will be three page renders. Exceeding the maximum page renders per capacity won't result in Power BI refusing to render reports, but it will likely degrade the report performance because Power BI will start queuing the report requests.

 TIP You can pause or scale down your Power BI Embedded capacity in the Azure portal to reduce your cost. For example, if the most report activity happens within normal working hours, you can scale it down to a lower capacity outside the peak period.

Purchasing an Azure embedded capacity

To reduce cost during app development and testing, developers can use any Power BI workspace and the workspace doesn't have to be in an embedded capacity. The only requirement is that each developer must be covered with a Power BI Pro license. However, deploying the app to production requires the workspace from which the content is embedded to be in either a Power BI Premium or Power BI Embedded capacity.

If you prefer to acquire Power BI Embedded via an Azure pricing plan, follow these steps to purchase an embedded capacity:

1. Go to https://azure.portal.com and sign in with your work account (needs to be on the same tenant as Power BI). As a prerequisite, you must have previously signed in to Power BI and you must have a subscription associated with that tenant.

2. Click New and search for "Power BI", as shown in **Figure 15.1**. In the search results, select "Power BI Embedded". Don't select "Power BI Workspace Collection" because this is the old Power BI Embedded (Microsoft will support it until July 2018). In the information page, click Create.

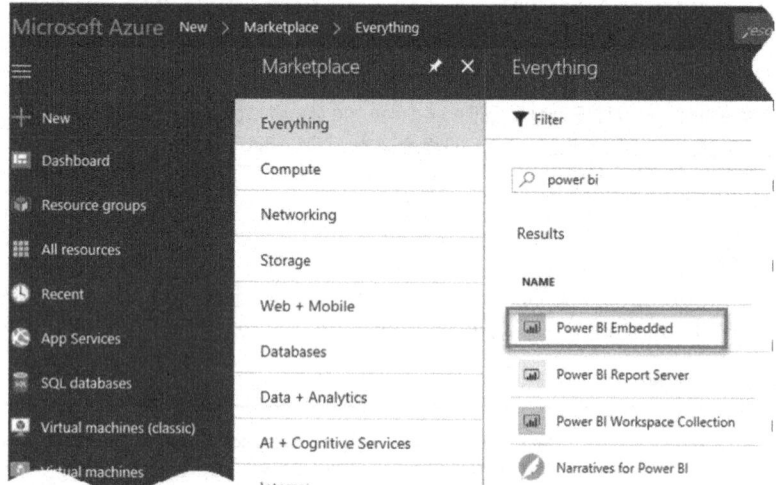

Figure 15.1 Choose Power BI Embedded to purchase an embedded capacity.

3. In the Power BI Embedded page (see **Figure 15.2**), specify the capacity details.

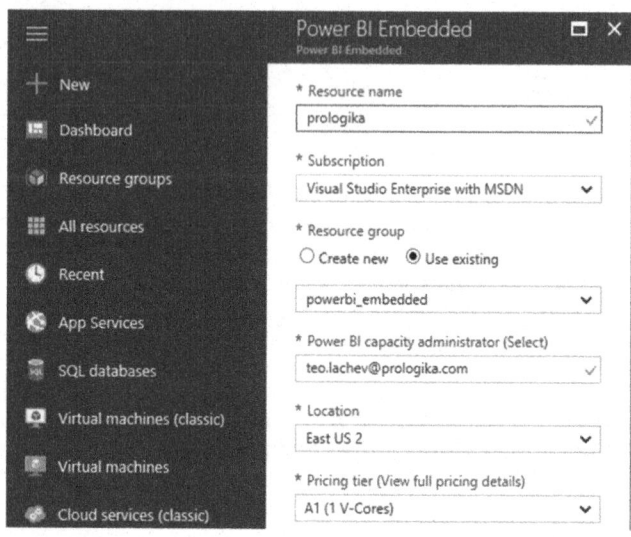

Figure 15.2 Specify the embedded capacity details, including the resource group, administrator, and pricing tier.

Let's explain these settings in more detail:

■ Resource name – Give the capacity a name. This is the name that you'll see in Power BI when you assign a workspace to an embedded capacity so choose a descriptive name.

- Subscription – Chose the subscription that will be billed.
- Resource group – Choose an existing resource group (an Azure resource group represent a logical container for managing related resources).
- Power BI capacity administrator – Specify a default capacity administrator. Later, you can add other capacity admins in the "Capacity settings" page for the embedded capacity in Power BI Admin Portal.
- Location – Associate the data center where the capacity will reside in. The only choice would be the data region where your Power BI tenant resides in.
- Pricing tier – Select one of the six Azure capacity nodes.

4. Click Create to let Azure create the embedded capacity.

5. Now that the capacity is created, go to its properties and notice that you can pause the capacity. You can also scale up and down the capacity from the Scale tab.

Understanding high-level flow for embedding content
Once you have the embedded capacity, you can start writing code to integrate your app with the embedded APIs. In a nutshell, these are the high-level steps to embed Power BI content into your app:

1. Register your app – I've shown you how to register web and native apps in the preceding chapter.

2. Authenticate – You can't go far with anything Power BI unless you take care of security first. You need to call the Power BI APIs to obtain an access token that determines the end-user permissions. Let's skip this step for now. We will revisit it later in this chapter in the content of internal and external apps.

3. Embed Power BI content – Once you have an access token, you can embed specific tiles, reports, or dashboards.

The content that you want to embed in your app needs to reside in a Power BI workspace within your Power BI tenant. Next, I'll provide some considerations that you need to keep in mind when planning your content.

15.1.2 Configuring Workspaces

As with sharing content via the powerbi.com portal, you use Power BI Desktop to create datasets and reports that you plan to embed. Once you are done with the reports, you upload the Power BI Desktop file to a workspace in your Power BI tenant.

Planning content storage
How many workspaces do you need? Consider a custom app that connects to a multi-tenant database and uses Power BI row-level security (RLS) to isolate data among customers. You can provision just one workspace that will host a single Power BI Desktop file.

What if you want to physically separate data by providing each customer with a data extract as a separate (*.pbix) file? Or, to provide customer-specific reports. Then, you might create a workspace per customer and deploy each file to a separate workspace. You'll end up having as many workspaces as customers that you want to support (with all the maintenance headaches to support that many files). It's up to you how you want to organize the content across workspaces. Since you're not charged per workspace, you can have as many as you want.

Assigning a workspace to an embedded capacity
Remember that you must assign a workspace to either a premium or embedded capacity before you go live. The workspace must have a diamond icon next to its name in the Power BI navigation pane. Recall

from Chapter 12 that you can use the Advanced section in the workspace properties to assign the workspace to a premium or embedded capacity. Alternatively, you can use the Capacity settings in the Admin Portal (see **Figure 15.3**).

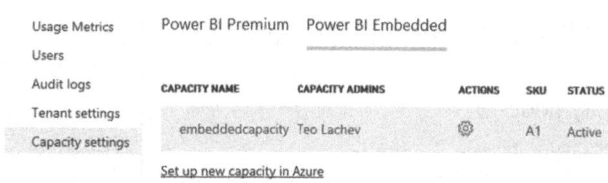

Admin portal

		Power BI Premium	Power BI Embedded			
Usage Metrics						
Users						
Audit logs	**CAPACITY NAME**	**CAPACITY ADMINS**	**ACTIONS**	**SKU**	**STATUS**	
Tenant settings	embeddedcapacity	Teo Lachev	⚙	A1	Active	
Capacity settings						
	Set up new capacity in Azure					

Figure 15.3 The Power BI Embedded tab in the Admin Portal shows workspaces in embedded capacities.

Now that you've learned about Power BI Embedded, let's see what features it supports for embedding content in your custom apps.

15.2 Understanding Embedded Features

Typically, the application presents a list of reports or dashboards to the user, so the user can pick which one to view. Then the application embeds the content in the presentation layer, so that reports and dashboards appear to be a part of the application itself (as opposed to redirecting the user to Power BI).

NOTE When you embed Power BI content in a web app, it's important to understand where you need to write code: server or client. User authentication and content enumeration, such as enumerating dashboards, reports, and tiles, typically takes place on the server, while the actual embedding happens on the client. As discussed in the previous chapter, Microsoft has provided Power BI REST and OAuth APIs that you can call on the server. Microsoft has also provided a Power BI JavaScript library (https://microsoft.github.io/PowerBI-JavaScript/) to reduce the JavaScript code you need to write to embed content on the client.

Microsoft has provided an online Microsoft Power BI Embedded Sample (https://microsoft.github.io/PowerBI-JavaScript/demo/v2-demo/) that shows the client-side code that you need to write to embed reports, dashboards, and tiles, and to add Q&A features in your apps. I'll use this app to demonstrate the capabilities of the embedded APIs and explain what you need to do on the client to embed content.

NOTE It's important to understand that because JavaScript code is not secure, you can't use the JavaScript APIs to overwrite Power BI security. The actual permissions are controlled by an access token that reflects Power BI security (in User Owns Data scenario) or by permissions granted in the embed token (in the App Owns Data scenario). For example, you can't switch a report from Reading View to Editing View if the user doesn't have permissions to edit reports.

15.2.1 Embedding Tiles

Power BI includes dashboard APIs that let you embed specific dashboard tiles in your apps. One benefit of tile embedding is to let the user select which tiles they want to see on a consolidated dashboard provided by your application. This way your app can mimic the dashboard features of Power BI Service. It can allow the user to compile its own dashboards from Power BI dashboard tiles, and even from tiles in different Power BI dashboards!

Understanding implementation steps
At a high level, the embedding tile workflow consists of the following steps (excluding authentication):
- Obtain the tile identifier – You need to gain access programmatically to a dashboard before you get to a tile. So, you'd need to find the dashboards available for the user, and then enumerate the dashboard

tiles. Once the user chooses a tile, then you work with the tile identifier. Typically, the code to authenticate the user and enumerate content will be executed on the server.

- Embed a tile – Embed the tile in your application. This code takes place on the client.
- (Optional) Handle tile interaction – For example, you might want to open the underlying report when the user clicks a tile. This is client-side code.

Selecting the "Embed sample tile" option on the main page of the "The Power BI Embedded Sample" shows a tile embedded on a web page (see **Figure 15.4**).

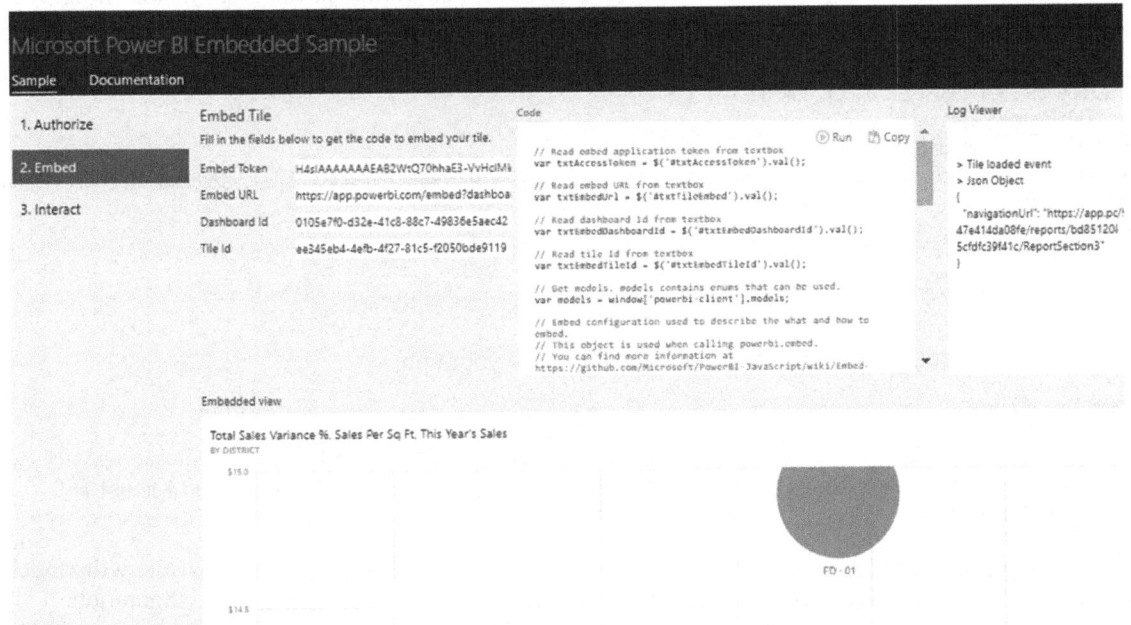

Figure 15.4 You can use the embedded APIs to embed specific dashboard tiles.

Enumerating dashboards

I mentioned in the previous chapter that Power BI includes REST APIs for enumerating dashboards and tiles. Your application can call these APIs to present the users with a list of tiles that they might want to see in your application. The "Get Dashboards" method returns the dashboards available in the user's My Workspace. This method has the following signature:

https://api.powerbi.com/v1.0/myorg/dashboards

Like enumerating datasets, this method supports enumerating dashboards in another workspace by passing the workplace identifier. You can get the workspace identifier by clicking the workspace in the Power BI portal and copying the GUID portion from the URL in the browser address bar. For example, if the workspace identifier of the Finance workspace is e6e4e5ab-2644-4115-96e0-51baa89df249 (you can obtain the workspaces that the user belongs to by calling the "Get Groups" method or from the browser address bar when you navigate to the workspace in the Power BI Portal), you can get a list of dashboards available in the Finance workspace by using this signature:

https://api.powerbi.com/v1.0/myorg/**groups/e6e4e5ab-2644-4115-96e0-51baa89df249**/dashboards

Enumerating tiles

Once you retrieve the list of dashboards, you can present the user with a list of tiles from a specific dashboard by calling the "Get Tiles" method. This method takes an *id* parameter that corresponds to the dashboard identifier, which you obtain from the "Get Dashboards" method, or by copying the GUID portion from the URL in the browser address bar after you click the dashboard to view it. Here is a sample "Get Tiles" method invocation:

https://api.powerbi.com/v1.0/myorg/dashboards/<dashboard_id>/tiles

The result of this method is a JSON collection of all the tiles hosted in that dashboard. The following snippet shows the definition of the "This Year's Sales" tile from the Retail Analysis Sample dashboard:

```
{
"id": "a2e8ee89-d321-4932-b26b-840c770d488d",
"title": "This Year's Sales",
"subTitle": "New & Existing Stores",
"embedUrl": "https://app.powerbi.com/embed?dashboardId=9a9a94b8-07a1-4e70-b29e-9f16dea08afc&tileId=a2e8ee89-d321-4932-b26b-840c770d488d",
"rowSpan": 0,
"colSpan": 0,
"datasetId": "f183dd3c-4474-46c5-9850-88781e02d816"
}
```

The *embedUrl* element is what you need to embed the tile in your app.

Embedding a tile

Once you have the embed URL, the next step it to embed the tile on a web page.

 NOTE Currently, the tile embedded API doesn't support real-time tiles that get updated by pushing rows to a dataset, as I showed you in Chapter 13.

In the most common scenario, you'd probably embed content in a web app. You don't have to write much client-side code if you use the Power BI JavaScript library. Start by creating the embed configuration.

```
// Read embed application token from Model
var accessToken = "@Model.EmbedToken.Token";
// Read embed URL from Model
var embedUrl = "@Html.Raw(Model.EmbedUrl)";
// Read tile Id from Model
var embedTileId = "@Model.Id";
// Read dashboard Id from Model
var embedDashboardId = "@Model.dashboardId";
// Embed configuration used to describe the what and how to embed.
// This object is used when calling powerbi.embed.
// You can find more information at https://github.com/Microsoft/PowerBI-JavaScript/wiki/Embed-Configuration-Details.
var config = {
    type: 'tile',
    tokenType: models.TokenType.Embed,
    accessToken: accessToken,
    embedUrl: embedUrl,
    id: embedTileId,
    dashboardId: embedDashboardId
};
// Get a reference to the embedded tile HTML element
var tileContainer = $('#tileContainer')[0];
// Embed the tile and display it within the div container.
var tile = powerbi.embed(tileContainer, config);
```

The code obtains the OAuth access token from the Model controller (assuming an ASP.NET MVC application). Next, it obtains the tile embed URL, title identifier, and dashboard identifier. It creates an embedded configuration from these properties. Then, the code gets a reference to an HTML DIV element where the tile will be rendered. The actual embedding magic happens with a single (last) line of code. Don't you appreciate how simple this is?

Handling user interaction

Table 15.2 shows the interactive features that JavaScript library supports on the client. One difference between Power BI Service dashboards and embedding tiles in your app is that, by default, clicking a tile doesn't do anything. You need to write code for something to happen, such as to navigate the user to the underlying report (from which the visualization was pinned). On the upside, your custom code has more control over what happens when the end user clicks a tile.

Table 15.2 Embedded tiles support these interactive features.

Interaction	Name	Purpose
Events	tileLoaded	Fires when the tile is fully loaded
	tileClicked	Fires when the tile is clicked

Remember that when the user clicks a tile in Power BI Service it's navigated to the underlying report from which the tile was pinned. You can add a similar feature to your app. Tiles support two events: tileLoaded and tileClicked, that you can handle in JavaScript.

```
// Tile.off removes a given event handler if it exists.
tile.off("tileLoaded");
// Tile.on will add an event handler which prints to Log window.
tile.on("tileLoaded", function(event) {
    Log.logText("Tile loaded event");
});
// Tile.off removes a given event handler if it exists.
tile.off("tileClicked");
// Tile.on will add an event handler which prints to Log window.
tile.on("tileClicked", function(event) {
    // do something here, such as navigate user somewhere
});
```

It's up to you what you want to do when your code intercepts the event. For example, you can show the report from which the tile was pinned.

Filtering tile content

You can pass optional filters in the embed configuration object to filter the tile content. The syntax is the same as the filters you use on reports. There are two types of filters:

- Basic filters – They have a single operation with one or more values, such as Country In ("USA", "Canada").

- Advanced filters – They can have multiple AND and OR conditions, just like when you use advanced filters and configure multiple conditions in the Filters area of the Visualizations pane.

For more information about how to construct filters, refer to the Filters topic at https://github.com/Microsoft/PowerBI-JavaScript/wiki/Filters.

15.2.2 Embedding Dashboards

Besides individual tiles, you can embed entire dashboards deployed to Power BI Service. The sample app demonstrates this feature when you select the "Embed sample dashboard" option. It embeds the Retail Analysis Sample dashboard, which is one of the dashboards included in the Power BI Service samples.

Embedding a dashboard

I've already explained that the "Get Dashboards" API can be used to enumerate dashboards. Once you obtain the dashboard identifier and embedUrl, you can embed the dashboard on the client side using embedded configuration. You need to pass the dashboard embed URL and the dashboard identifier.

```
var config = {
    type: 'dashboard',
    tokenType: models.TokenType.Embed,
    accessToken: txtAccessToken,
    embedUrl: txtEmbedUrl,
    id: txtEmbedDashboardId
};
```

Understanding dashboard interaction

Table 15.3 shows what interactive features are available for dashboards.

Table 15.3 Embedded dashboards support these interactive features.

Interaction	Name	Purpose
Methods	getId	Returns the dashboard identifier
	fullscreen	Opens the dashboard in full screen mode
	exitfullscreen	Exists full screen
Events	tileClicked	Fires when a tile is clicked
	Loaded	Fires when the dashboard is fully loaded
	error	Fires when an error occurs during dashboard loading

Your JavaScript code can call the fullscreen method to show the dashboard in full screen. The following code does this:

```
// Get a reference to the embedded dashboard HTML element
var dashboardContainer = $('#dashboardContainer')[0];
// Get a reference to the embedded dashboard.
dashboard = powerbi.get(dashboardContainer);
// Displays the dashboard in full screen mode.
dashboard.fullscreen();
```

As with tiles, the most interesting event is tileClicked, which is fired when the user clicks a tile. The event argument includes the report URL for embedding (reportEmbedUrl), if the tile was added by pinning a report visual. You need this URL to embed the report.

15.2.3 Embedding Q&A

Recall that users can use natural questions to get insights from data. Wouldn't be nice to add Q&A features to your apps? Of course, it would! The embedded APIs allow developers to add such capabilities in several configurations:

- Show Q&A only – Shows the Q&A box without a predefined question.
- Show Q&A with a predefined question -- Shows a predefined question and the resulting visual.
- Show answer only – This could be useful if your app collects the question from the user and only wants to show a visual that best answers the question.

Embedding Q&A

As a prerequisite, you need to obtain the identifiers of the datasets that you'd want Q&A to use. You can use the "Get Datasets" API. For example, this method returns all datasets within a specified workspace.

https://api.powerbi.com/v1.0/myorg/groups/e6e4e5ab-2644-4115-96e0-51baa89df249/datasets

This code shows the embedded configuration for embedding Q&A with a predefined question.

```
var config= {
    type: 'qna',
    tokenType: models.TokenType.Embed,
    accessToken: txtAccessToken,
    embedUrl: txtEmbedUrl,
    datasetIds: [txtDatasetId],
    viewMode: models.QnaMode[qnaMode],
    question: txtQuestion
};
```

The configuration type is set to 'qna'. The embedUrl has the format https://app.powerbi.com/qnaEmbed?groupId=<groupId>, where groupId is the workspace identifier. Unlike Power BI Service, where Q&A is a dashboard-level feature, embedding Q&A doesn't require a dashboard. Instead, you need to pass the identifiers of one or more datasets in the datasetIds property. Finally, you can use the question property to pass a predefined question, such as "Sales by country for year 2017".

Understanding Q&A interaction

Table 15.4 shows the interactive features for embedded Q&A.

Table 15.4 Embedded Q&A supports these interactive features.

Interaction	Name	Purpose
Methods	setQuestion	Passes a question to Q&A, such as "This year sales"
Events	Loaded	Fires when the Q&A is loaded
	visualRendered	Fires when the question has changed

For example, to change the question, you can call the setQuestion method.

```
// Get a reference to the embedded Q&A HTML element
var qnaContainer = $('#qnaContainer')[0];
// Get a reference to the embedded Q&A.
qna = powerbi.get(qnaContainer);
qna.setQuestion("This year sales")
```

15.2.4 Embedding Reports

For years, Microsoft hasn't had a good story about embedded interactive reporting. If developers wanted to distribute interactive reports with their applications, they had to use third-party components. The good news is that Power BI supports this scenario and even allows users to edit reports! This means that users can enjoy report interactive features, such as filtering and highlighting, and they can change the report layout if your app lets them, such as to reconfigure the visuals. In other words, the embedded APIs have similar feature parity as viewing and editing reports in Power BI Service, although some features that depend on Power BI Service are missing, such as pinning tiles and report pages, and subscribing to report pages.

Enumerating reports

As a first step, you'd probably want to present the user with a list of reports. Your application can call the "Get Reports" API to show a list of reports that the user can access. This signature returns all the reports that are available in the user's My Workspace. It has the following signature:

https://api.powerbi.com/v1.0/myorg/reports

The resulting JSON response is a collection of report elements. Each report element has *id* (report identifier), name, webUrl, embedUrl, and datasetId properties. Here's the definition of the Internet Sales Analysis report:

```
{
    "id":"b605950b-4f18-4eba-9292-82720f215693",
    "name":"Internet Sales Analysis",
    "webUrl":"https://app.powerbi.com/reports/b605950b-4f18-4eba-9292-82720f215693",
    "embedUrl":https://app.powerbi.com/reportEmbed?reportId=b605950b-4f18-4eba-9292-82720f215693,
    "datasetId": "cf6ea374-1d1e-4288-bc41-5e25ccbe4967"}
```

Chances are that your users will share their content. Like the "Get Dashboards" method, the "Get Reports" method supports enumerating reports in another workspace by passing the group identifier. For example, if the group identifier of the Finance workspace is e6e4e5ab-2644-4115-96e0-51baa89df249 (remember that you can obtain the group identifier by calling the "Get Groups" method), you can get a list of the reports available in the Finance workspace by using this signature:

https://api.powerbi.com/v1.0/myorg/**groups/e6e4e5ab-2644-4115-96e0-51baa89df249**/reports

 TIP To show all the reports that the user can access, you need to enumerate the reports in the user's My Workspace and the reports from all the groups (workspaces) that the user belongs to.

Understanding embedded features for reports

Figure 15.5 shows a Power BI report embedded in a web page. Note that the report supports the same features as when you open the report in Reading View in Power BI Service. For example, you can sort data in visualizations that support sorting and they can cross highlight other visuals. The Filters pane is also available. If the report has multiple pages, users navigate through the report pages. Users can also pop out visualizations to examine them in more detail and access more tasks from the ellipsis (…) menu.

Viewing reports

When the user picks a report, client-side JavaScript embeds the report. This is very similar to embedding dashboards and tiles. However, your embedded configuration can specify the default mode (view or edit the report). You can also let the user create a report from scratch.

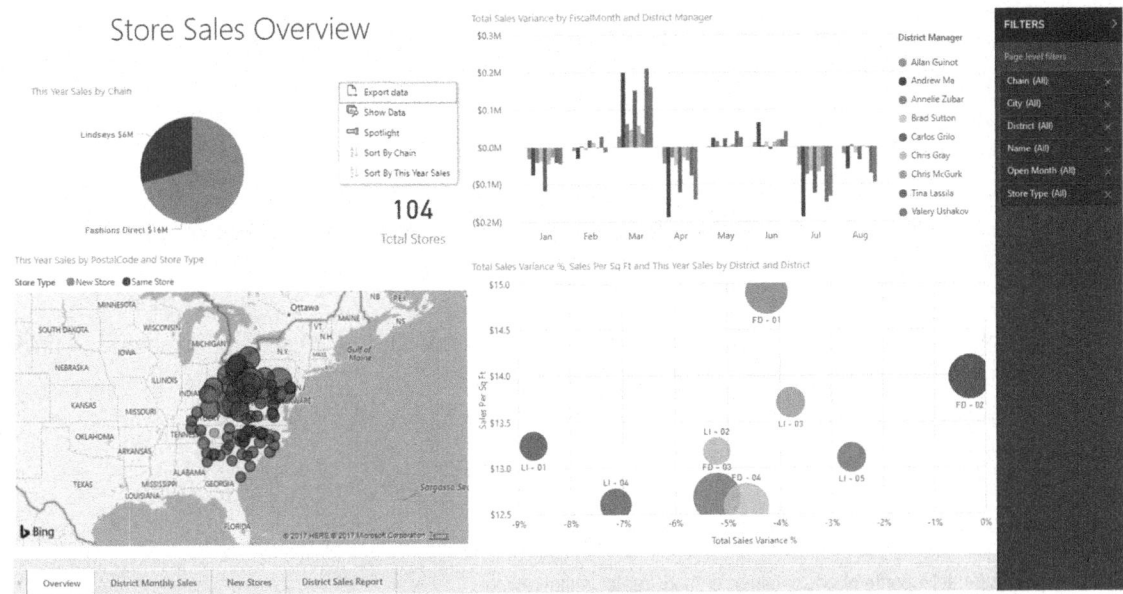

Figure 15.5 Embedded reports preserve their interactive features.

Here is the embedded configuration for embedding reports read only (corresponds to Reading View in Power BI Service).

```
var config= {
  type: 'report',
  tokenType: models.TokenType.Embed,
  accessToken: txtAccessToken,
  embedUrl: txtEmbedUrl,
  id: txtEmbedReportId,
  permissions: permissions,
  settings: {
    filterPaneEnabled: true,
    navContentPaneEnabled: true
  }
};
var embedContainer = $('#embedContainer')[0];
var report = powerbi.embed(embedContainer, config);
```

The embedUrl property has the report embedUrl, which you can obtain from the "Get Reports" API. You also need to set the id property to the report identifier. The settings collection lets you specify if you want the report to include the Microsoft-provided filter pane (filterPaneEnabled setting) and page navigation (setting navContentPaneEnabled to false will hide the page navigation pane).

Editing reports

If the user is authorized to edit the report, the client-side code can alternate between Reading View and Editing View. For example, here is the embedded configuration for switching to Editing View:

```
var config = {
  type: 'report',
  tokenType: models.TokenType.Embed,
  accessToken: txtAccessToken,
```

```
  embedUrl: txtEmbedUrl,
  id: txtEmbedReportId,
  permissions: models.Permissions.All /*gives maximum permissions*/,
  viewMode: models.ViewMode.Edit,
  settings: {
    filterPaneEnabled: true,
    navContentPaneEnabled: true   }};
```

The viewMode property is now set to ViewMode.Edit. As a result, the report now shows the Visualization and Fields panes. The user can make layout changes and save the report if the user has permissions to change the report (the access token controls the user permissions).

Creating reports

If the user has permissions to create reports, the client-side code can call the createReport method to navigate the user to a blank report connected to a given dataset.

```
var embedCreateConfiguration = {
  tokenType: models.TokenType.Embed,
  accessToken: txtAccessToken,
  embedUrl: txtEmbedUrl,
  datasetId: txtEmbedDatasetId,
};
var report = powerbi.createReport(embedContainer, embedCreateConfiguration);
```

In this case the configuration specifies the identifier of the dataset. Power BI responds with a blank report connected to that dataset, just like when you explore the dataset in Power BI Service. The user can save the report in the workspace.

Understanding report interaction

Because reports inspire the most interest, the JavaScript library includes various methods and events to handle user interaction. **Table 15.5** shows the interactive features for embedded reports.

Table 15.5 Embedded reports support these interactive features.

Interaction	Name	Purpose
Methods	getId	Get the report identifier
	getPages, setPage (report or page)	Enumerate or set the active report page
	setFilters, getFilters, removeFilters	Set, get, or remove basic or advanced page-level or report-level filters
	Print	Prints the report
	updateSettings	Updates the report settings that control Filter and Page Navigation pane
	reload, refresh	Reloads (call it after creating a new report to show the new report) or refreshes a report
	Extend Options, Extend Context	Allow you to add custom options to the visual options and content menus
	fullscreen, exitFullscreen	Display report in full screen mode
	switchMode	Switches between Reading View and Editing View
	save, saveAs	Saves the report
Events	pageChanged	Fires when the user navigates to a new page
	dataSelected	Fires when the user selects a visual element, such as clicking a data point
	saveAsTriggered	Fires when the user clicks the Save As menu

Filtering the report data

One interactive feature that you might need is implementing application-level filtering instead of using the Microsoft-provided Filter pane. The following code demonstrates how your app can pass filters.

```
// Instead of a constant, your app would gather the filters
const filter = {
 $schema: "http://powerbi.com/product/schema#basic",
 target: {
  table: "Store",
  column: "Chain"
 },
 operator: "In",
 values: ["Lindseys"]
};
// Get a reference to the embedded report HTML element
var embedContainer = $('#embedContainer')[0];
// Get a reference to the embedded report.
report = powerbi.get(embedContainer);
// Set the filter for the report (you can also filter at page level)
// Pay attention that setFilters receives an array.
report.setFilters([filter])
// Remove the Filter pane but leave page navigation enabled
const newSettings = {
 navContentPaneEnabled: true,
 filterPaneEnabled: false
};
report.updateSettings(newSettings);
```

Like tiles, reports support filtering capabilities. This could be useful when you want to further filter the report content based on some user-specified filter, after the report filters are applied. You can filter on any field in the underlying model, even though the field might not be used in the report itself.

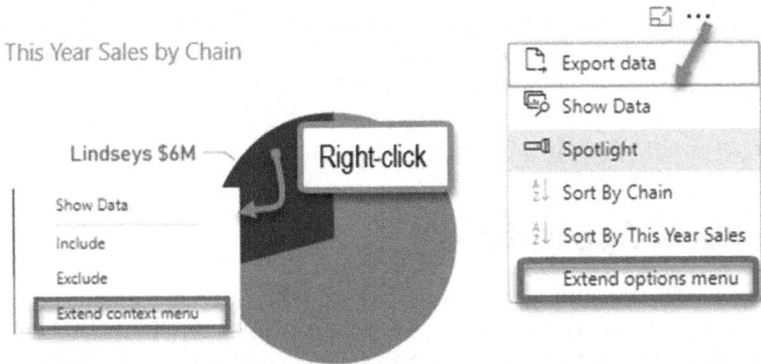

Figure 15.6 You can add your own menu options to the visual options and context menus.

Extending menus

Another interesting option is the ability to extend the following visual menus (see **Figure 15.6**):

■ Th visual options menu that appears when you hover on the visual and click the ellipsis (…) button in the top-right corner.

■ The visual context menu that appears when you right-click a data point, such as a slice in a pie chart.

For example, this code adds a "Extend context menu" submenu to the visual context menu.

```
// The new settings that you want to apply to the report.
const newSettings = {
 extensions: [   {
    command: {
     name: "extension command",
     title: "Extend command",
     extend: {
      // Define visualContextMenu to extend context menu.
      visualContextMenu: {
       // Define title to override default title.
       //You can override default icon as well.
       title: "Extend context menu", } } } } ]};

// Get a reference to the embedded report HTML element
var embedContainer = $('#embedContainer')[0];
// Get a reference to the embedded report.
report = powerbi.get(embedContainer);
// Update the settings by passing in the new settings you have configured.
report.updateSettings(newSettings)
    .then(function (result) {
       $("#result").html(result);
    })
    .catch(function (error) {
       $("#result").html(error);
    });
// Report.on will add an event handler to commandTriggered event which prints to console window.
report.on("commandTriggered", function(event) {
    var commandDetails = event.detail;
    // Do something with the data point
});
```

When the user clicks the menu, the commandTriggered event fires and the JavaScript library passes the data point details, including the data point identity and value. For example, if the user right-clicks the Lindseys slice in the pie chart, the event argument will include "Lindseys" as a data point identity and "$6,393,844" as a data point value. This feature allows you to extend embedded visuals in interesting ways, such as by navigating the user to another system and passing the context of the user action.

15.3 Report-enabling Intranet Applications

Now that you've learned about the Power BI embedding capabilities, let me walk through sample code to help you report-enable your intranet applications. You can use this code to embed Power BI reports in internal applications when your end users already have Power BI licenses. For example, you can use this approach to embed Power BI reports in report portals or Line of Business (LOB) systems, such as SharePoint or Dynamics. If you plan to embed reports in apps for external customers, skip to the next section where I discuss Power BI Embedded. The sample demonstrates the following features:

■ Authenticating users – The sample code shows both a three-leg authentication flow (a Power BI sign-on page opens). Microsoft refers to this authentication type as "user owns data" because the user authenticates with Power BI and content embedding happens under the user identity.

■ Embedding reports – The application shows a list of reports to the end user. Once the user picks a report, the JavaScript code embeds the report on a web page.

15.3.1 Understanding the Sample Application

The book source code includes a sample PBIWebApp ASP.NET application in the \Source\ch15\User Owns Data\ folder. The code is based on Microsoft's sample (https://github.com/Microsoft/PowerBI-Developer-Samples), but I've made changes to it to let you configure which workspace and report you want to embed (the Microsoft version was configured to show the first report in My Workspace). The Microsoft code also includes samples to show how to embed dashboards and tiles.

Registering the application
I mentioned in the previous chapter that any custom application that integrates with Power BI must be registered in Azure Active Directory. Follow the steps in the previous chapter to register PBIWebApp using the settings in **Table 15.6**.

Table 15.6 The registration settings for the PBIWebApp sample.

Setting	Value	Notes
Name*	PBIWebApp	Defines the name of the application
Type	Web app/API	Defines the app type
Home page	http://localhost:13526/	The URL of the home page
Application is multi-tenant	No	The application won't need access to data owned by other organizations
Keys	Auto-generated	Create a key because this is a web app.
Reply URL*	http://localhost:13526/	The redirect page for three-leg authentication (make sure that the port number matches your development setup)
Permissions*	Power BI Service (all permissions)	Grant all Power BI Service permissions

For the sake of completeness, the table lists all settings that you need if you register the application using the Azure Management Portal (the settings you need for the Power BI registration page are suffixed with an asterisk).

Configuring the application
Before you run the application, you need to change a few configuration settings to match your setup.

1. Open the PBIWebApp project file in Visual Studio (version 2015 or higher) from the \User Owns Data\integrate-report-web-app\PBIWebApp folder. If you don't have Visual Studio, you can download and install the free Visual Studio 2017 Community Edition.
2. In Solution Explorer, right-click the project, and then click Properties ⇨ Settings (see **Figure 15.7**).
3. Change the *ClientID* setting to match the client ID of your application that you obtain after you register it.
4. Change the *ClientSecret* setting to match the app key.
5. Change the *WorkspaceName* setting to match one of your workspaces or leave it blank for My Workspace.
6. Change the *ReportName* setting to match one of the reports in the workspace.

15.3.2 Authenticating Users

Intranet applications would typically authenticate users with Windows integrated security. However, Power BI is a cloud application that requires the user to sign in. In the three-leg flow (user owns data) the app navigates the user to the Power BI sign-in page. I explained this flow in detail in the previous chapter.

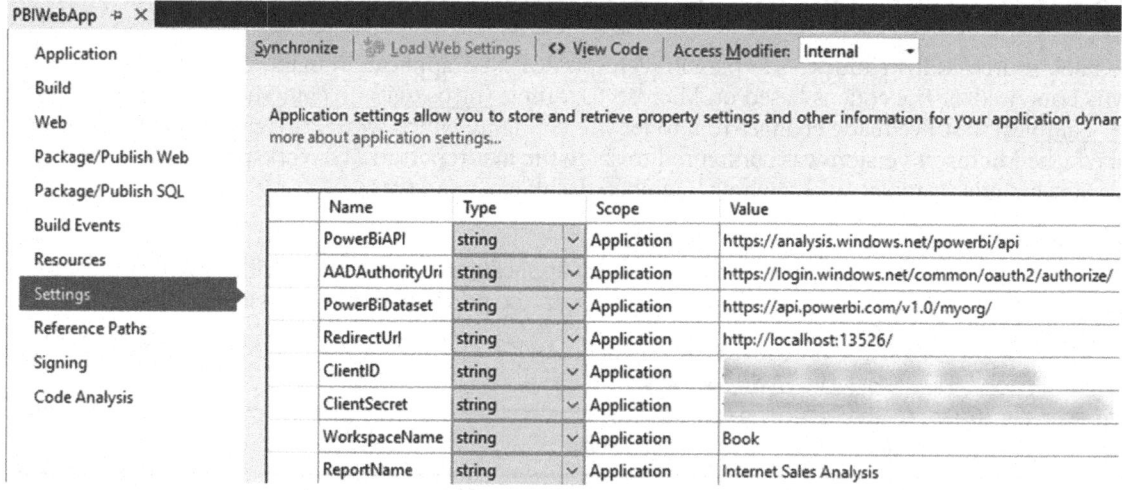

Figure 15.7 Update the PBIWebApp settings to match your setup before you run the application.

Implementing the three-leg flow

When the app starts, the default page shows a Get Report button. When you click it, the page calls the server-side GetAuthorizationCode method, which is shown in **Figure 15.8**.

```
185    public void GetAuthorizationCode()
186    {
187        //NOTE: Values are hard-coded for sample purposes.
188        //Create a query string
189        //Create a sign-in NameValueCollection for query string
190        var @params = new NameValueCollection
191        {
192            //Azure AD will return an authorization code.
193            {"response_type", "code"},
194
195            //Client ID is used by the application to identify themselves to the users that they are requesting permissions from.
196            //You get the client id when you register your Azure app.
197            {"client_id", Settings.Default.ClientID},
198
199            //Resource uri to the Power BI resource to be authorized
200            //The resource uri is hard-coded for sample purposes
201            {"resource", Properties.Settings.Default.PowerBiAPI},
202
203            //After app authenticates, Azure AD will redirect back to the web app. In this sample, Azure AD redirects back
204            //to Default page (Default.aspx).
205            { "redirect_uri", Settings.Default.RedirectUrl}
206        };
207
208        //Create sign-in query string
209        var queryString = HttpUtility.ParseQueryString(string.Empty);
210        queryString.Add(@params);
211
212        //Redirect to Azure AD Authority
213        //  Authority Uri is an Azure resource that takes a client id and client secret to get an Access token
214        //  QueryString contains
215        //      response_type of "code"
216        //      client_id that identifies your app in Azure AD
217        //      resource which is the Power BI API resource to be authorized
218        //      redirect_uri which is the uri that Azure AD will redirect back to after it authenticates
219
220        //Redirect to Azure AD to get an authorization code
221        Response.Redirect(String.Format(Properties.Settings.Default.AADAuthorityUri + "?{0}", queryString));
222    }
```

Figure 15.8 The three-leg flow redirects the user to the Power BI sign-on page.

The application creates a query string that includes the client id, the Power BI API authorization URL, and the Redirect URI that you specified when you registered the application. Line 221 sends the request to the authorization endpoint, which redirects the user to the Power BI sign-on page. Once the user authenticates with Power BI, the user is redirected back to the Default.aspx page (the app Redirect URL is set to the web root URL).

Obtaining the access token

The access token is the cornerstone of every OAuth security flow. Upon successful authentication, the authority passes the authorization code to the redirect Uri you specified. Because in this case, we don't have a redirect page, the Page_Load event in the Default.aspx page is executed. It calls the GetAccessToken method (see **Figure 15.9**).

```
224    public string GetAccessToken(string authorizationCode, string clientID, string clientSecret, string redirectUri)
225    {
226        //Redirect uri must match the redirect_uri used when requesting Authorization code.
227        //Note: If you use a redirect back to Default, as in this sample, you need to add a forward slash
228        //such as http://localhost:13526/
229
230        // Get auth token from auth code
231        TokenCache TC = new TokenCache();
232
233        //Values are hard-coded for sample purposes
234        string authority = Properties.Settings.Default.AADAuthorityUri;
235        AuthenticationContext AC = new AuthenticationContext(authority, TC);
236        ClientCredential cc = new ClientCredential(clientID, clientSecret);
237
238        //Set token from authentication result
239        return AC.AcquireTokenByAuthorizationCode(
240            authorizationCode,
241            new Uri(redirectUri), cc).AccessToken;
242    }
243 }
```

Figure 15.9   The GetAccessToken method extracts the access token from the authorization code.

This method gets the authorization code (passed as a first argument) and creates an AuthenticationContext object. Then it calls AuthenticationContext.AcquireTokenByAuthorizationCode to obtain an AuthenticationResult object, which has the access token, refresh token, and other details, such as the token expiration date. Then the app extracts the access token from AuthenticationResult, and passes it back to the Page_Load event. The Page_Load event caches the token into a session variable to avoid reauthenticating for subsequent page reposts.

 NOTE   Remember that for additional security, the access token has a limited lifespan, and your code needs to catch errors that are caused by expired tokens. This is explained in more detail in the " Configurable token lifetimes in Azure Active Directory" article at https://docs.microsoft.com/azure/active-directory/active-directory-configurable-token-lifetimes. Although PBIWebApp doesn't demonstrate this flow, your code can use the refresh token in the AuthenticationResult object to extend the user session when the access token expires. By default, the access token expires in one hour and the refresh token expires in 14 days. So, instead of caching just the access token, consider caching the entire AuthenticationResult object in a session variable and calling AC.AcquireTokenByRefreshTokenAsync to renew the access token from the refresh token.

15.3.3 Embedding Reports

Once the app obtains the access token, it can embed Power BI content that the user has permissions to access in Power BI Service. The PBIWebApp demonstrates the minimum code you need to write to embed reports in your apps. **Figure 15.10** shows the Internet Sales Analysis report embedded on a web page.

Power BI Embed Report

Basic Sample

First make sure you <u>register your app</u>. After registration, copy <u>Client ID</u> and <u>Client Secret</u> to web.config file.

Select "**Get Report**" to get and embed first report from your Power BI account.

Get Report

Report Name	Internet Sales Analysis
Report Id	546d3ae3-f94b-4f29-8c31-da8c589bc0de
Report Embed URL	https://app.powerbi.com/reportEmbed?reportId=546d3ae3-f94b-4f29-8c31-da8c589bc0de&groupId=22b6f73d-e151-4630-89c4

Embedded Report

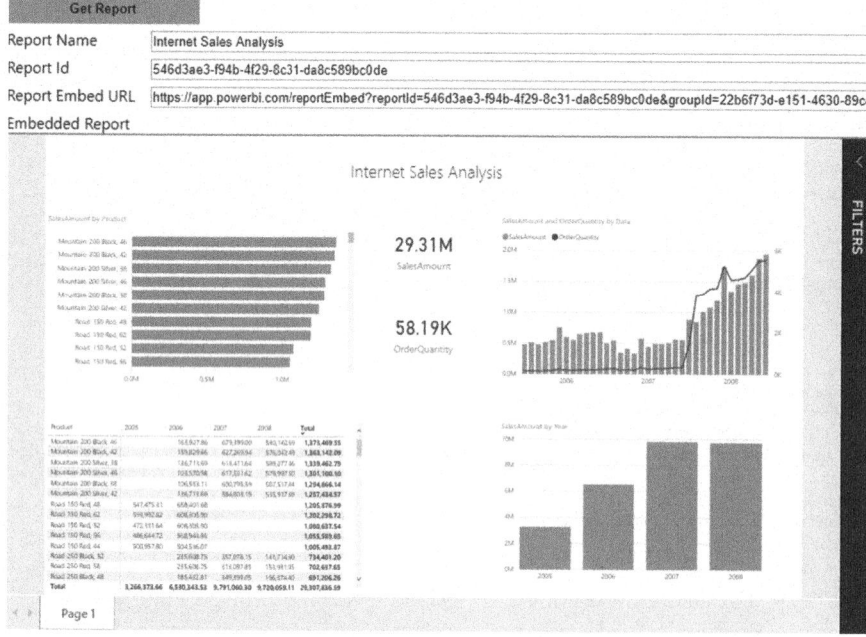

Figure 15.10 PBI-WebApp shows the embedded Internet Sales Analysis report.

Getting reports

The Default.aspx page demonstrates how a custom app can embed a report. As a first step, the app would probably present the user with a list of reports to choose from. But to make things simpler, the sample skips this step and shows the report you specified in the configuration settings. As I mentioned, the ReportName app setting controls which report the app would show and the WorkspaceName setting specifies the workspace where the report is located. The GetReport method (see **Figure 15.11**) demonstrates the server-side code you need to write to obtain the report details required for embedding.

Line 67 checks the value of the WorkspaceName configuration setting. If it's specified, the app gets the workspace identifier by calling the GetWorkspaceId method. This method invokes the "Get Groups" API to retrieve all the user's workspaces and then loops through the workspaces to find a match. Line 70 constructs the "Get Reports" API call in the case where a shared workspace is specified. And line 73 constructs the call for My Workspace (the groups part is missing).

Line 76 creates a web request using the GET verb. Line 80 includes the access token in the payload. Line 83 makes the API invocation and gets the response. Then, the code invokes the method and saves the response as a collection of *PBIReport* objects. Finally, the code enumerates through the collection (not shown in **Figure 15.11**) to obtain the report identifier, name, and the embed URL and show these details on the page.

```
60    //Get a Report. In this sample, you get the first Report.
61    protected void GetReport()
62    {
63        string embedReportUrl;
64        PBIReport report = null;
65        string workspaceId = null;
66
67        if (Settings.Default.WorkspaceName != string.Empty)
68        {
69            workspaceId = GetWorkspaceId(Settings.Default.WorkspaceName);
70            embedReportUrl = String.Format("{0}groups/{1}/reports", baseUri, workspaceId);
71        }
72        else
73            embedReportUrl = String.Format("{0}/reports", baseUri);
74
75        //Configure Reports request
76        System.Net.WebRequest request = System.Net.WebRequest.Create(String.Format(embedReportUrl, baseUri))
77
78        request.Method = "GET";
79        request.ContentLength = 0;
80        request.Headers.Add("Authorization", String.Format("Bearer {0}", accessToken.Value));
81
82        //Get Reports response from request.GetResponse()
83        using (var response = request.GetResponse() as System.Net.HttpWebResponse)
84        {
85            //Get reader from response stream
86            using (var reader = new System.IO.StreamReader(response.GetResponseStream()))
87            {
88                //Deserialize JSON string
89                PBIReports Reports = JsonConvert.DeserializeObject<PBIReports>(reader.ReadToEnd());
```

Figure 15.11   This code demonstrates how to enumerate reports in a workspace.

Embedding the report

Next, you'd need to write client-side JavaScript code that does the actual report embedding by calling the Power BI JavaScript library. Open the markup code of the Default.aspx page (shown in **Figure 15.12**) to see how this works. Line 3 references the Power BI JavaScript library. Line 8 defines an event for window.onload that obtains the previously-generated access token. For demonstration and testing purposes, the app shows the access token on the web page although this presents a security vulnerability. In real life, the client code would obtain the server-generated token and the report details to construct the embedded configuration.

> **NOTE** The transfer of the access token from the server to the client must happen over the HTTPS protocol to prevent a hacker from intercepting the token. It's true that JavaScript code is not secure, but before getting to the access token, the hacker must gain access to the user machine to open the page client-side code. If this happens, you have a much bigger security issue. Recall that all web apps that require authentication must somehow pass the user identity between the client and the server, so OAuth is no less secure than any other LOB web-based app, including Salesforce, Dynamics Online, and internal apps. Moreover, if the hacker obtains the token, he might not be able to do much with it as the token expires in a few minutes.

Line 21 shows the embedded configuration. At minimum, you need to include the access token, report embedUrl, and report identifier. The actual embedding happens with just one line of code (line 34)! This line calls the embed method and passes as arguments the html element where the report will be rendered and the embed configuration.

```
1  <%@ Page Title="Home Page" Language="C#" MasterPageFile="~/Site.Master" AutoEventWireup="true" CodeBehind="Default.aspx.cs" Inheri
2  <asp:Content ID="BodyContent" ContentPlaceHolderID="MainContent" runat="server">
3      <script type="text/javascript" src="scripts/powerbi.js"></script>
4      <script type="text/javascript">
5
6          //This code is for sample purposes only.
7          //Configure IFrame for the Report after you have an Access Token. See Default.aspx.cs to learn how to get an Access Token
8          window.onload = function () {
9              var accessToken = document.getElementById('MainContent_accessToken').value;
10             if (!accessToken || accessToken == "")
11             {
12                 return;
13             }
14             var embedUrl = document.getElementById('MainContent_txtEmbedUrl').value;
15             var reportId = document.getElementById('MainContent_txtReportId').value;
16
17             // Embed configuration used to describe the what and how to embed.
18             // This object is used when calling powerbi.embed.
19             // This also includes settings and options such as filters.
20             // You can find more information at https://github.com/Microsoft/PowerBI-JavaScript/wiki/Embed-Configuration-Details.
21             var config= {
22                 type: 'report',
23                 accessToken: accessToken,
24                 embedUrl: embedUrl,
25                 id: reportId,
26                 settings: {
27                     filterPaneEnabled: true,
28                     navContentPaneEnabled: true
29                 }
30             };
31             // Grab the reference to the div HTML element that will host the report.
32             var reportContainer = document.getElementById('reportContainer');
33             // Embed the report and display it within the div container.
34             var report = powerbi.embed(reportContainer, config);
```

Figure 15.12 The client-side JavaScript code that embeds the report.

15.4 Report-enabling Internet Applications

Many organizations provide reports to their external customers to support both (Business-to-Business) B2B and (Business-to-Consumer) B2C scenarios. In Chapter 11, I showed you that you can use dashboard sharing or apps to share content out to external users. But this approach has some important drawbacks:

- Dependency on Azure Active Directory (AAD) – Every user must have an AAD account.

- Not adequate support for B2C – I mentioned that soon AAD would support Live IDs, such as out-look.com emails, but you'd need to wait for other providers. Yet, many B2C apps allow external customers to authenticate with email addresses of their choice.

- Per-user license – Despite that Power BI offers three licensing options for external users, every user must be covered by a Power BI Pro license.

- Read-only reports – Users are limited to read-only reports. They can't change existing reports or create new reports.

These limitations present challenges for external reporting. An Internet-facing app typically authenticates users with Forms Authentication, by showing a login form to let the users enter application credentials. Then the application verifies the credentials against a profile store, such as a table in a SQL Server database. If you plan many external users, you'd want to avoid registering your users twice: with your application and with Power BI (Azure Active Directory). Power BI Embedded lets you address these challenges in a cost-effective way.

15.4.1 Understanding the Sample Application

To help you get started with Power BI Embedded, Microsoft included another sample "App Owns Data" in the same location (https://github.com/Microsoft/PowerBI-Developer-Samples). For your convenience, the book source includes it in the \Source\ch15\User Owns Data\ folder.

Configuring the app

The Readme file that accompanies the app explains how to configure the app.

1. Register the app as a native app in https://dev.powerbi.com/apps. If you have already registered PBI-WebApp as a web app for the intranet example that I've previously discussed, you can reuse the registration, but you need to make some changes, so read on.

2. There is no need for Reply URL because the app authenticates directly with Power BI. In other words, the app uses the two-leg OAuth flow instead of the three-leg flow (the user is not navigated to the Power BI sign-in page so there is no redirect).

3. Open the web.config file and change the settings listed in **Table 15.7**.

Table 15.7 The configuration settings for the PBIWebApp sample.

Setting	Notes
clientId	The Client ID of the app from the registration (in Azure Portal, this is Application ID)
groupId	The identifier of the workspace where the Power B content is located (get it from the browser address bar after you navigate to the workspace content page in Power BI)
reportId	The identifier of the report to embed (get it from the browser address bar after you open the report)
pbiUsername	The email address of a Power BI user who is added as an admin to the workspace
pbiPassword	The password of the admin user

It's important to understand that the app will authenticate to Power BI using the credentials of a Power BI account on your tenant and then embed the content on behalf of the user. By default, all users would see the same data unless the report is set up for row-level security (RLS).

 NOTE The app stores the password of the admin user in clear text in web.config for the sake of simplicity. This is not a best practice. For your real-life apps, consider storing the password encrypted or retrieve it from Microsoft Key Vault.

4. Deploy a Power BI Desktop file with a report to the workspace. If you want to test dashboard embedding, create a dashboard in Power BI Service. By default, the app shows the first dashboard in the workspace.

5. Recall that when your real-life app is ready to be used by other users, you need to assign the workspace to a premium or embedded capacity.

That's all that's needed to configure the app. Remember that while embedding has a dependency on the Power BI service, there is not a dependency on Power BI for your customers. They do not need to sign up for Power BI to view the embedded content in your app.

Running the app

Let's now take the app for a ride.

1. Open the app in Visual Studio.

2. Right-click the project in Solution Explorer and then click Build. The app should build successfully. If it doesn't, you're probably missing some dependencies. To fix this, right-click the app, click "Manage NuGet Packages", and then install all dependencies the app requires.

3. Press Ctrl-F5 to run the app. On the startup screen, click "Embed Report". You should see your report embedded (see **Figure 15.13**). Take some time to test interactive features to make sure they work.

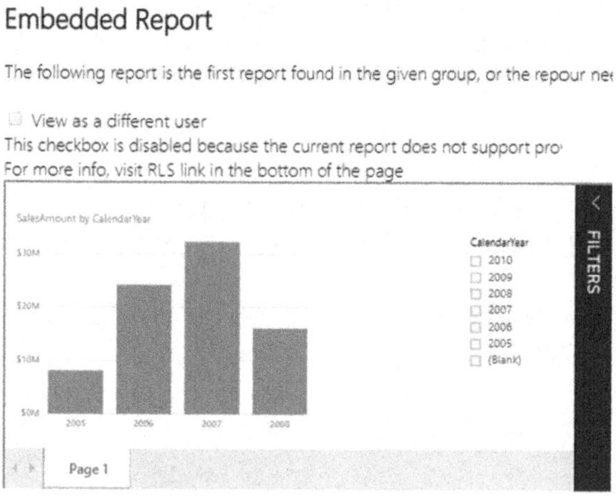

Embedded Report

The following report is the first report found in the given group, or the repour net

☐ View as a different user
This checkbox is disabled because the current report does not support pro'
For more info, visit RLS link in the bottom of the page

Figure 15.13 Use the "App Owns Data" app to see how you can embed Power BI content for external users.

15.4.2 Authenticating Users

Next, let me walk you through some important implementation details to help you understand how the app integrates with Power BI Embedded and how this differs from the intranet app.

Obtaining access token

The app is designed as an ASP.NET MVC application and the server-side code is in HomeController.cs. Because Power BI and Power BI Embedded share the same programming interface, the app calls the same APIs. One difference from the intranet app is authentication. **Figure 15.14** shows how the EmbedReport method handles authentication (the same code is used for embedding dashboards in tiles). Your real-life app should refactor the authentication code in one place.

```
44  // Create a user password cradentials.
45  var credential = new UserPasswordCredential(Username, Password);
46
47  // Authenticate using created credentials
48  var authenticationContext = new AuthenticationContext(AuthorityUrl);
49  var authenticationResult = await authenticationContext.AcquireTokenAsync(ResourceUrl, ClientId, credential);
50
51  if (authenticationResult == null)
52  {
53      result.ErrorMessage = "Authentication Failed.";
54      return View(result);
55  }
56
57  var tokenCredentials = new TokenCredentials(authenticationResult.AccessToken, "Bearer");
```

Figure 15.14 The server-side code in the MVC controller authenticates the user.

Line 45 creates a credential object from the credentials of the admin user that you specified in web.config. Line 49 calls AcquireTokenAsync to authenticate the user. Again, the app authenticates directly with Power BI and uses a trusted account on your domain that has admin access to the workspace. The user is not asked to authenticate with Power BI.

Presumably, your app has previously authenticated the user and now it discovers what reports are available for the user. After the app obtains the access token (line 57), the app calls the familiar APIs to enumerate reports and retrieve the report you specified in web.config.

Obtaining embed token

As you've seen, the intranet sample demonstrates the "User Owns Data" scenario. Once the user authenticates with Power BI, embedding happens under his identity and the access token controls what he can do, such as only view reports or edit and create reports. However, external users are authenticated and authorized by your application, and your application uses a trusted account that has admin access to the workspace. This presents a security issue because you don't want external users to gain more permissions they need and to access content under the admin account.

To further restrict the permissions of the interactive user, your app needs to issue a less-permissive type of token, called an *embed token*. Here is the relevant code:

```
GenerateTokenRequest generateTokenRequestParameters;
generateTokenRequestParameters = new GenerateTokenRequest(accessLevel: "view");
var tokenResponse = await client.Reports.GenerateTokenInGroupAsync(GroupId, report.Id, generateTokenRequestParameters);
```

The *accessLevel* parameter of the GenerateTokenRequest method specifies a view permission to the report. This method takes another *allowSaveAs* argument, which when set to true, allows the user to change the report and save it as another report. The documentation for the GenerateTokenRequest method specifies how to invoke the method for other operations, such as creating reports, Q&A, viewing dashboards, and tiles. The embed token (not the access token) is what your app needs to pass to client-side code to embed content. For example, the client-side code in the EmbedReport.cshtml view uses the embed token to embed the report. The rest of the embedded APIs should be familiar to you by now.

15.4.3 Implementing Data Security

If all users will see the same data on the report, there is no need to propagate the user identity to the data source. However, the chances are that your app would need to restrict access to data for different users. In Chapter 9, I showed you how to implement data security in Power BI Desktop models. Another popular scenario for propagating the user identity is when the report connects to an Analysis Services semantic model.

Using effective identity

Data security is also known as row-level security (RLS). **Figure 15.15** shows the relevant code to handle RLS. Line 82 obtains a reference to the dataset used by the report. Line 83 checks if the dataset supports an effective identity. This will be the case when the Power BI Desktop model has security roles or when you connect live to Analysis Services. Line 84 checks if the dataset supports roles. If RLS is defined in Power BI Desktop, you must pass one or more roles that match the ones in the file. Using roles is optional when you connect live to Analysis Services.

Testing data security

Referring to **Figure 15.13**, you can test RLS by checking "View as a different user" and entering the user name and a comma-separated list of roles. If RLS uses dynamic security, USERNAME() and USERPRINCIPALNAME() will return whatever username your app passes as an effective identity. Typically, this will be the login name that the user enters to authenticate with your app, but it can be whatever is required for dynamic security to work (recall that external users don't sign to Power BI Service, so the username can be anything).

The roles that you pass to the method must exist in the Power BI Desktop file or the Analysis Services semantic model. If the app passes multiple roles, the user will get the superset of all the role permissions. Line 89 creates an effective identity from the user name and the dataset identifier. If you specify roles, they are added to the effective identity. Finally, line 97 obtains an embed token from the effective identity.

```
82  var datasets = await client.Datasets.GetDatasetByIdInGroupAsync(GroupId, report.DatasetId);
83  result.IsEffectiveIdentityRequired = datasets.IsEffectiveIdentityRequired;
84  result.IsEffectiveIdentityRolesRequired = datasets.IsEffectiveIdentityRolesRequired;
85  GenerateTokenRequest generateTokenRequestParameters;
86  // This is how you create embed token with effective identities
87  if (!string.IsNullOrEmpty(username))
88  {
89      var rls = new EffectiveIdentity(username, new List<string> { report.DatasetId });
90      if (!string.IsNullOrWhiteSpace(roles))
91      {
92          var rolesList = new List<string>();
93          rolesList.AddRange(roles.Split(','));
94          rls.Roles = rolesList;
95      }
96      // Generate Embed Token with effective identities.
97      generateTokenRequestParameters = new GenerateTokenRequest(accessLevel: "view", identities: new List<EffectiveIdentity> { rls })
98  }
99  else
100 {
101     // Generate Embed Token for reports without effective identities.
102     generateTokenRequestParameters = new GenerateTokenRequest(accessLevel: "view", allowSaveAs:true);
103 }
104
105 var tokenResponse = await client.Reports.GenerateTokenInGroupAsync(GroupId, report.Id, generateTokenRequestParameters);
```

Figure 15.15   The server-side code to handle row-level security (RLS).

15.5 Summary

Developers can enrich custom applications with embedded BI content. Thanks to the Power BI open architecture, you can report-enable any web-enabled application on any platform! Collectively known as Power BI Embedded, the Power BI embed API are for embedding tiles, dashboard, reports, and Q&A in your apps. You can acquire Power BI Embedded with Power BI Premium or by purchasing an embedded capacity. Embedded reports preserve their interactive features, such as filtering, highlighting, and sorting. Because the Power BI embedded APIs have the same feature parity as Power BI Service, users can view, edit, and create reports. Microsoft has provided JavaScript APIs and a report object model to help you extend your apps with interactive features, such as to handle events resulting from user actions or to extend the Microsoft-provided menus.

One of the most challenging aspects of report-enabling custom applications is security. If you're tasked to report-enable internal business apps and your users have Power BI licenses, your app can pass the user identity to Power BI with OAuth and then call the Power BI embedded APIs. As you saw, OAuth is a flexible security framework that supports different authentication flows. The default three-leg (User Owns Data) flow navigates the user to a sign-on page, so the user owns the data.

External (Internet-facing) apps can avoid registering users twice and benefit from the per-render licensing model of Power BI Embedded. Most apps will use the two-leg authentication (Apps Owns Data) flow, where the app uses a trusted account to authenticate with Power BI but issues a restricted embed token to avoid granting the user admin rights to the workspace.

Besides report-enabling custom applications, the Power BI APIs allow web developers to extend Power BI's visualization capabilities. You can read about custom visuals in the next chapter!

Chapter 16

Creating Custom Visuals

The Power BI visuals can take you far when it comes to presenting data in a visually compelling and engaging way, but there is still room for the occasional requirement that simply cannot be met with the built-in visuals. For example, suppose you want to convey information graphically using a graph that Power BI does not support. Or, you might need a feature that Microsoft currently doesn't have, such as a 3D chart. Fortunately, web developers can extend the Power BI data visualization capabilities by implementing custom visuals. They can do this with open source JavaScript-based visualization frameworks, such as D3.js, WebGL, Canvas, or SVG.

In this chapter, I'll introduce you to this exciting extensibility area of Power BI. I'll start by explaining what a custom visual is and the developer toolset that Microsoft provides for implementing visuals. Then, I'll walk you through the steps of implementing a sparkline visual for showing data trends. Finally, I'll show you how to deploy the custom visual and use it in Power BI. This chapter targets web developers experienced in TypeScript and JavaScript, D3.js and Node.js.

16.1 Understanding Custom Visuals

In Chapter 3, I introduced you to custom visuals from an end user standpoint. You saw that you can click the ellipsis (…) button in the Visualizations pane (both in Power BI Service and Power BI Desktop) and import a custom visual from Microsoft AppSource (https://appsource.microsoft.com). Now let's dig deeper and understand the anatomy of a custom visual before you learn how to implement your own.

16.1.1 What is a Custom Visual?

A custom visual is a JavaScript plug-in that extends the Power BI visualization capabilities. Because the custom visual is dynamically rendered in the Web browser, it's not limited to static content and images. Instead, a custom visual can do anything that client-side JavaScript code and JavaScript-based presentation frameworks can do. As you can imagine, custom visuals open a new world of possibilities for presenting data and new visuals are posted to AppSource every week!

 NOTE BI developers might remember that SSRS has been supporting .NET-based custom report items. They might also recall that SSRS custom report items render on the server as static images with limited interactivity. By contrast, Power BI runs the custom visual JavaScript code on the client side. Because of this, custom visuals can be more interactive. To emphasize this, the sparkline visual (whose implantation I discuss in this chapter) demonstrates animated features, although this might not necessarily be a good visualization practice.

Understanding the custom visual framework

To allow developers to implement and distribute custom visuals, Microsoft provides the following toolset:

1. Support of custom visuals in Power BI reports – Users can create reports with custom visuals in Power BI Service and Power BI Desktop. Reports with custom visuals can also render in Power BI Report Server.

2. Microsoft AppSource – A community site (https://appsource.microsoft.com) that allows developers to upload new Power BI visuals and users to discover and download these visuals. Both Microsoft and the community have donated custom visuals to AppSource.

3. Power BI custom visual developer tools – Custom Visual Developer Tools (https://github.com/Microsoft/PowerBI-Visuals/) that integrate with Power BI to assist developers in debugging and testing the visual code.

Understanding host integration

Power BI has different hosting environments where visuals can be used, including dashboards, reports, Q&A, native mobile applications, and Power BI Desktop. From an end user standpoint, once the user imports a custom visual, the user can use it on a report just like the visualizations that ship with Power BI. In **Figure 16.1**, the last icon in the Visualizations pane shows that I've imported the Sparkline visual and then added it to the report.

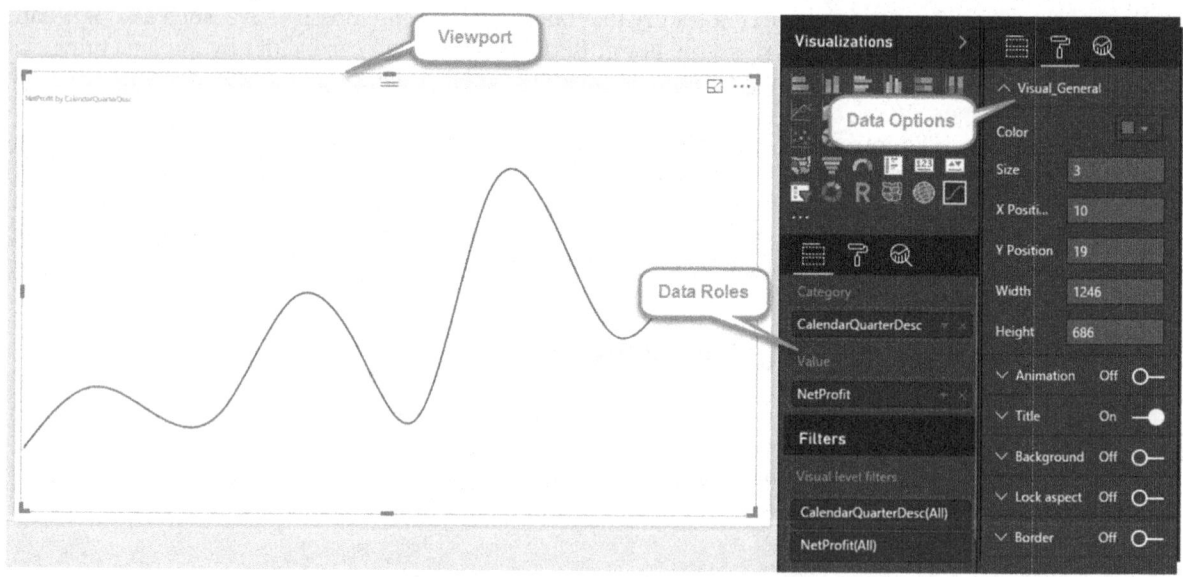

Figure 16.1 The host takes care of the plumbing work required to configure the visual.

When a custom visual is added to a report, the user can specify the size of the visual by dragging its resize handles. The resulting area determines the boundaries of the canvas (also called a viewport) that is available to the visual to draw whatever visualization it creates. When you create a visual, you need to adhere to a specification that determines how the visual interacts with the host environment.

The hosting environment takes care of most of the plumbing work required for configuring the visual. It is the host that takes care of configuring the Fields and Format tabs of the Visualizations pane. The visual simply advertises what capabilities it supports. For example, the Sparkline visual tells the host that it supports one category field and one value field. Once the host discovers this information, it configures the Fields tab of the Visualizations pane accordingly.

The Format tab (shown expanded on the right of the Fields tab in **Figure 16.1**) works in the same way. The visual advertises the formatting options it supports and how they should be presented. However, it is the host that configures the UI (the Format tab). For example, the Sparkline visual tells the host that it supports two properties for formatting the graph: Color (for the line color) and Size (for the line width). It also supports an optional animation feature under the Animation section that controls the delay of each redraw and the duration of how fast the graph is drawn. Given this information, the host configures the Format pane accordingly so that the user can configure these settings.

The host integration adds a slew of additional features that don't require any coding on your part. The host gets the data based on how the Fields tab is configured, and passes the data to the visual. Interactive highlighting, that cross filters the rest of visualizations on the page (when the user selects an element in one visual), also works without any coding. The host also takes care of report-level, page-level and visual-level filters, and adds common settings, such as Tile and Background, in the Format pane.

16.1.2 Understanding the IVisual Interface

As I noted, a custom visual must adhere to a design specification. This specification defines an IVisual interface, which every custom visual must implement. The specification is documented and available at https://github.com/Microsoft/PowerBI-visuals/blob/master/Visual/IVisualApi.md. The IVisual interface defines four key methods, as follows:

- *constructor (options: VisualConstructorOptions)* – when you place a visual on a report, the host calls the *constructor()* method to give the visual a chance to perform some initialization tasks. The host passes an options argument, which among other things includes the viewport height and width. Microsoft recommends that you don't draw the visual in the *constructor* method. Instead, use this method to execute one-time code for initializing the visual, such as to class and style the visual div container.

- *update (options: VisualUpdateOptions): void* – This is the workhorse of the visual. The *update()* method is responsible for drawing the visual presentation. Every time the host determines that the visual needs to be refreshed, such as a result of configuration changes or resizing, the host will call the *update()* method. Similar to the *constructor()* method, the host passes an options parameter.

- *enumerateObjectInstances (options: EnumerateVisualObjectInstancesOptions): VisualObjectInstancesEnumeration* – As I mentioned, the visual is responsible for advertising its capabilities. You can use the *enumerateObjectInstances()* method to return objects that the host discovers to populate the Fields and Formats pane. This method is called for each object defined in the visual capabilities. The host won't display the property if it's not enumerated.

- *destroy(): void* – The host calls this method when the visual is about to be disposed. This typically happens when the visual is removed from the report or the report is closed. The code in *destroy()* should release any resources that might result in memory leaks, such as unsubscribing event handlers.

I'll walk you through implementing IVisual when I discuss the implementation of the Sparkline visual. For now, let's understand what skillset is required to code custom visuals.

16.2 Custom Visual Programming

How do you implement custom visuals and what development tools are available to code and test custom visuals? Microsoft provided a comprehensive toolset to assist web developers to implement custom visuals. In addition, Microsoft published sample visuals, so there is plenty of reference material to get you started.

Creating custom visuals is not that difficult but as with any coding effort, it requires a specific skillset. First, you need to know TypeScript and JavaScript to code custom visuals. To save you coding effort (drawing graphics elements in plain JavaScript is hard), you should also have experience in a JavaScript-based visualization framework, such as Data-Driven Documents (D3.js). However, you can also use other JavaScript-based frameworks if you prefer something else than D3.js, such as SVG or WebGL. Finally, you need to have web developer experience, including experience with HTML, browser Document Object Model (DOM), and Cascading Style Sheets (CSS). You can use an integrated development environment (IDE) of your choice for coding custom visuals, such as Microsoft Visual Studio Code.

To get you started with custom visual programming, let me introduce you to TypeScript – the programming language for coding custom visuals.

16.2.1 Introducing TypeScript

So that they work across platforms and devices, custom visuals are compiled and distributed in JavaScript. But writing and testing lots of code straight in JavaScript is difficult. Instead, for the convenience of the developer, custom visuals are implemented in TypeScript.

What is TypeScript?
When you implement custom visuals, you use TypeScript to define the visual logic and interaction with the host. TypeScript is a free and open source (http://www.typescriptlang.org) programming language, developed and maintained by Microsoft for coding client-side and server-side (Node.js) applications. Its specification (http://www.typescriptlang.org/docs/) describes TypeScript as "a syntactic sugar for JavaSript". Because TypeScript is a typed superset of JavaScript, when you compile TypeScript code you get plain JavaScript. So, why not write directly in JavaScript? Here are the most compelling reasons that favor TypeScript:

- Static typing – TypeScript extends tools, such as Visual Studio, to provide a richer environment for helping you code and spotting common errors as you type. For example, when you use Visual Studio and Power BI Developer Tools you get IntelliSense as you type. And when you build the code, you get compile errors if there are any syntax issues.

- Object-oriented – TypeScript is not only data-typed but it's also object-oriented. As such, it supports classes, interfaces, and inheritance.

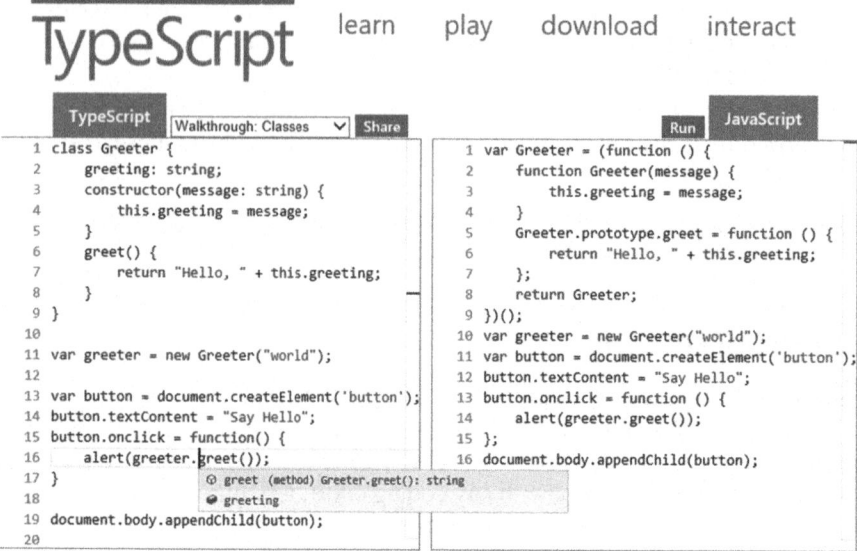

Figure 16.2 The TypeScript Playground allows you to compare TypeScript and JavaScript side by side.

To learn more about what led to TypeScript and its benefits, watch the video "Introducing TypeScript" by Anders Hejlsberg at https://channel9.msdn.com/posts/Anders-Hejlsberg-Introducing-TypeScript. Although he doesn't need an introduction, Anders Hejlsberg is a Microsoft Technical Fellow, the lead architect of C#, and creator of Delphi and Turbo Pascal. Anders has worked on the development of TypeScript.

Comparing TypeScript and JavaScript

To compare TypeScript and JavaScript, here's a short sample from the Typescript Playground site (http://www.typescriptlang.org/Playground), which is shown in **Figure 16.2**.

The TypeScript code on the left defines a Greeter class that has a member variable, a constructor, and a *greet*() method. Notice that the TypeScript window supports IntelliSense. This is possible because TypeScript defines the type of member variables and method parameters. These types are removed when the code is compiled to JavaScript, but can be used by the IDE and the compiler to spot errors and help you code. TypeScript is also capable of inferring types that aren't explicitly declared. For example, it would determine that the *greet*() method returns a string, so you can write code like this:

```
someMethodThatTakesString(greeter.greet());
```

16.2.2 Introducing D3.js

Coding the application flow in TypeScript is one thing but visualizing the data is quite another. Again, using plain JavaScript and CSS to draw graphs would be a daunting experience. Fortunately, there are open-source visualization frameworks that are layered on top of JavaScript. Microsoft decided to adopt the Data-driven Documents (D3.js) framework to implement all the Power BI visualizations, but you are not limited to it if you prefer other JavaScript-based visualization frameworks.

What is D3.js?

As you know, JavaScript is the de facto standard language as a client-side browser language. But JavaScript was originally designed for limited interactivity, such as clicking a button or handling some input validation. As Internet evolved, developers were looking for tools that would enable them to visually present data within Web pages without requiring reposting the page and generating visuals on the server side. There were multiple projects sharing this goal but the one that gained the most acceptance is D3.js.

According to its site (http://d3js.org), "D3.js is a JavaScript library for manipulating documents based on data". Documents in this context refer to the Document Object Model (DOM) that all Web browsers use to manipulate client-side HTML in an object-oriented way. D3 uses other web standards, such as HTML, CSS, and Scalable Vector Graphics (SVG) to bind data to DOM, and then to apply data-driven transformations to visualize the data. The D3.js source code and a gallery with sample visualizations are available on GitHub (https://github.com/mbostock/d3).

Automating visualization tasks with D3.js

To give you an idea about the value that D3.js brings to client-side visualization, consider the bar chart shown in **Figure 16.3**.

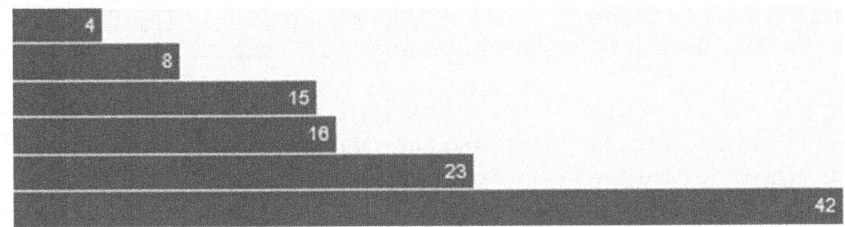

Figure 16.3 Although simple, this bar chart is not easy to update in plain JavaScript and CSS.

The left section in **Figure 16.4** shows how a web developer would implement the same chart using HTML and CSS. The code has one div element for a container, and one child div for each bar. The child DIV elements have a blue background color and a white foreground color.

```
.chart div {
  font: 10px sans-serif;
  background-color: steelblue;
  text-align: right;
  padding: 3px;
  margin: 1px;
  color: white;
}

</style>
<div class="chart">
  <div style="width: 40px;">4</div>
  <div style="width: 80px;">8</div>          d3.select(".chart")
  <div style="width: 150px;">15</div>          .selectAll("div")
  <div style="width: 160px;">16</div>            .data(data)
  <div style="width: 230px;">23</div>        .enter().append("div")
  <div style="width: 420px;">42</div>            .style("width", function(d) { return d * 10 + "px"; })
</div>                                             .text(function(d) { return d; });
```

Figure 16.4   The left section shows the chart definition in HTML/CSS while the right section shows the D3 code.

So far so good. But what if you want to bind this chart dynamically to data, such as when the report is refreshed, or new fields are added? This would require JavaScript code that manipulates DOM to put the right values in the right div element. By contrast, the right section shows how you can do this in D3.js. Let's break it down one line at a time.

First, the code selects the chart element using its class selector (.chart). The second line creates a data join by defining the selection to which you'll join data. The third line binds the data to the selection. The actual data could be supplied by the application as a JavaScript array, which may look like this:

var data = [4, 8, 15, 16, 23, 42];

The fourth line outputs a div element for each data point. The fifth line sets the width of each div according to the data point value. The last line uses a function to set the bar label. Note that you'd still need the CSS styles (shown on the left code section) so that the chart has the same appearance. If you have experience with data-driven programming, such as using ADO.NET, you might find that D3.js is conceptually similar, but it binds data to DOM and runs in the Web browser on the client side. It greatly simplifies visualizing client-side data with JavaScript!

16.2.3 Understanding Developer Tools

Microsoft has provided the Custom Visual Developer Tools (https://github.com/Microsoft/PowerBI-visuals) to help developers implement custom visuals. The toolset includes documentation, tools for testing and packaging your visual, and sample visuals that demonstrate implementation details.

 NOTE   This section is intended to get you introduced and get started with Custom Visual Developer Tools. For more in-depth information, see the reference documentation within the Power BI Visuals repo at https://github.com/Microsoft/PowerBI-visuals. While you're there, look at the tool roadmap at https://github.com/Microsoft/PowerBI-visuals/tree/master/Roadmap.

Getting started with Developer Tools
The Developer Tools consists of a command-line tool (pbiviz) and integration hooks to Power BI Service. The toolset brings the following benefits to developers interested in implementing Power BI visuals:

■ Ability to use external libraries – Because the Developer Tools use the standard typescript compiler, you can bring any external library and use it within your visual. Moreover, a custom visual runs in a sandboxed iframe. This allows you to use specific versions of libraries and global styles, without worrying that you'll break other visuals.

- Your choice of IDE – The Developer Tools doesn't force you into a coding environment. It's implemented as a command-line tool that works across platforms with any IDE of your choice, including Visual Studio, Visual Studio Code, CATS, Eclipse, and so on.
- Integration with Power BI Service – You can add your visual on a report to test and debug it as you code and see how it'll work when a Power BI user decides to use it. You can also turn on a special live preview mode where the visual automatically updates when you make changes to the source.

Configuring the Developer Tools involves the following high-level steps:

1. Follow the installation steps at https://github.com/Microsoft/PowerBI-visuals/tree/master/tools to install NodeJS, the command-line tool (pbiviz), and server certificate. The server certificate is needed to enable the live preview mode for testing the visual in Power BI Service. In this mode, the visual code runs in a trusted https server, so you need to install an SSL certificate (included with the tool) to allow the visual to load in your browser.

2. To view and test your visual, you need to enable this feature in Power BI Service. To do so, log in to powerbi.com, then click the Settings menu in the top-right corner. In the Developer section (General tab), check "Enable developer visual for testing" (see **Figure 16.5**). When checked, this setting adds a special Developer Tools icon to the Visualizations pane.

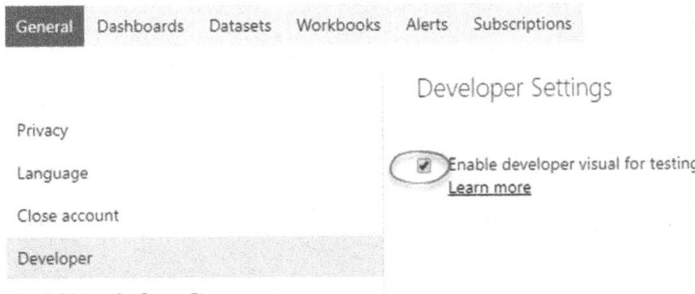

Figure 16.5 Check the "Enable developer visual for testing" checkbox to view and test custom visuals in Power BI Service.

 TIP If you find that the "Enable developer visual for testing" setting doesn't stay enabled after you check it, make sure to follow the installation steps for installing the server certificate.

Creating a new visual

The Developer Tools can generate the folder structure and required dependencies for new visuals. You can create a new project by opening the command prompt, navigating to the folder where you want the project to be created, and typing the following command (replace VisualName with the name of your visual):

```
pbiviz new VisualName
```

This command will create a new project folder with the same name as the VisualName you provided and will then add some files organized in subfolders. **Table 16.1** shows the structure of the project folder and describes the purpose of the most important folders and files.

Table 16.1 This table shows the structure of the project folder.

Item	Purpose	Item	Purpose
.api/	Power BI libraries and interfaces	.gitignore	Lists files to ignore when check in source in GitHub
.vscode/	Settings for launching and debugging custom visuals	capabilities.json	Defines the Data and Format settings of your visual

Item	Purpose	Item	Purpose
assets/	Stores additional information to distribute, such as icon, image, screenshot	package.json	Used by package manager for JavaScript (npm) to manage modules
dist/	Outputs the *.pbiviz file when you package your visual	package-lock.json	Describers the dependency tree and dependencies
node_mod-ules/	Created after you run "npm I", it contains the Node.js librar-ies	pbiviz.json	Main configuration file
src/	The TypeScript code of your visual goes here	tsconfig.json	Specifies compiler options (see bit.ly/2gdlbuv)
style/	CSS styles	tslint.json	Specifies coding rules when compiling source

Once the project is created, the next step is to open the src/visual.ts file in your favorite editor and start coding your visual.

Configuring D3.js types

Recall that Power BI custom visuals are coded in TypeScript - a typed superset of JavaScript. But where do you get the actual type definitions (known as *typings*) from? Instead of installing files containing the typings, the current recommendation is to use *npm @types*. For example, if you target D3.js and you want to install version 3.5.5 (Power BI does not yet support D3 v4) along with its types, you can use the following syntax (see npmjs.com/package/@types/d3).

```
npm install d3@3.5.5 @types/d3@3.5.36 --save
```

Installing dependencies

To test the visual with Power BI Service, you need to install the required dependencies. These dependencies are distributed as Node.js modules. Node.js modules are JavaScript libraries that you can reference in your code. Follow these steps to install the dependencies:

1. Open the Windows Command Prompt as Administrator.
2. Navigate to the folder that has your visual source.
3. Run the following command:

```
npm install
```

 TIP Installing the dependencies results in a node_modules folder whose size exceeds 80 MB! To avoid including the dependencies when you check in your visual to GitHub, add the node_modules folder to the .gitignore file. When sending the code to someone else, don't include the node_modules folder. Other developers can restore node_modules by executing "npm install".

Testing custom visuals

To test the visual, you need to build it and then add it to a report in Power BI Service. Use the pbiviz command-line to build the visual (open the command prompt, navigate to the project folder, then type the command and press Enter).

```
pbiviz start
```

First, the command-line tool builds the visual and notifies you of any errors. If all is well, it packages the visual for testing. Next, it launches an https server that will serve your visual for testing. If there are no errors, the command window should show the following output:

```
info  Building visual...
done  build complete
info  Starting server...
info  Server listening on port 8080.
```

Next, go to powerbi.com. Find a test dataset that will supply the data to the visual and click it to create a new report. Notice that a Developer Tools icon is added to the Visualizations Pane (see **Figure 16.6**).

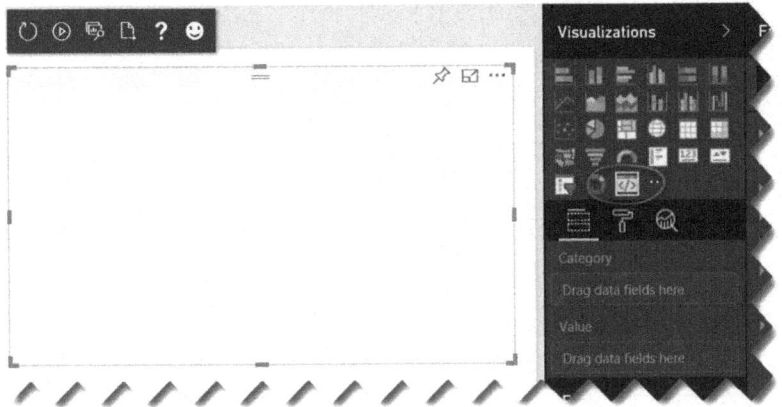

Figure 16.6 Use the Developer Tools icon to test your custom visual in Power BI Service.

When you click this icon, Power BI Service will add a frame to the report canvas and connect it to the visual you're testing (make sure to execute "pbiviz start" before you click the Developer Tools icon. A toolbar appears on top of the frame. **Table 16.2** describes the toolbar buttons.

Table 16.2 This table describes the toolbar buttons for testing custom visuals in Power BI Service starting from left.

Button	Purpose
Reload Visual Code	Manually refresh the visual if auto reload is disabled.
Toggle Auto Reload	When turned on, the visual will automatically update every time you make changes and save the visual file.
Show Dataview	Shows the dataview (actual data) that is passed to the visual's update method.
Export Dataview	Exports the dataview to a JSON format if you want to inspect it further or send it to someone else.
Get Help	Navigates to the tool documentation on GitHub.
Send Feedback	Navigates to GitHub where you can leave feedback.

Debugging custom visuals

You can use the browser debugging capabilities to step through the visual code in Power BI Service. However, you can put breakpoints because the visuals script is entirely reloaded every time the visual is updated and all breakpoints are lost. Instead, use the JavaScript debugger statement.

1. Put a debugger statement somewhere in the visual code that you want the script execution to stop.
2. Start your visual test session as explained before in the "Testing custom visuals" section.
3. Assuming you use Chrome, press F12 to open its developer environment.
4. Perform the task on the report that triggers that code. For example, if you put a breakpoint in the update method, simply resize the visual on the report (this will invoke the update method). If your code is reachable, the execution should stop at the debugger statement (see **Figure 16.7**).
5. Step through the code and examine it. For example, in Chrome you can press F10 to step over to the next line and hover over a variable to examine its value. You can also use the Console tab to test variables, or you can add a variable to the Watch window.

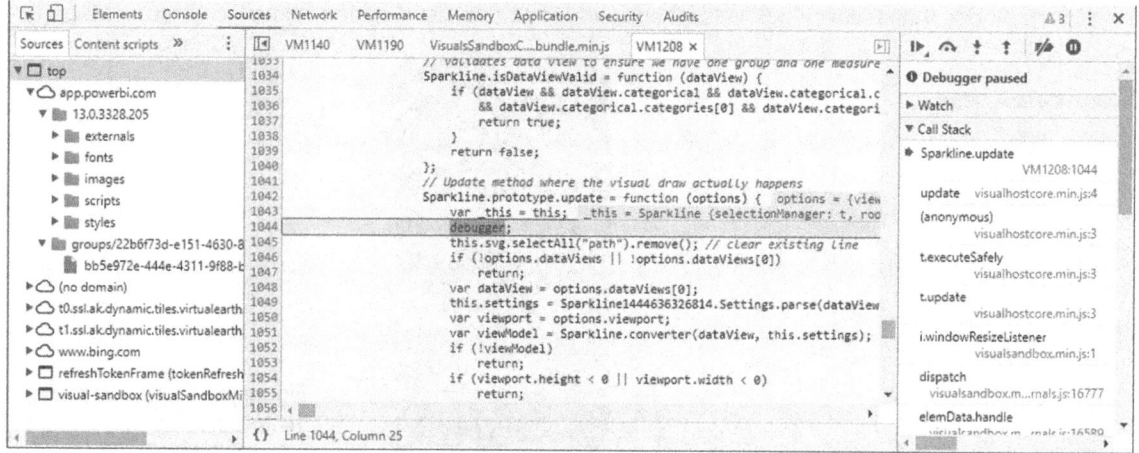

Figure 16.7 Use the browser debugging capabilities to step through your visual code in Developer Tools.

Although you can change variable values while debugging your code, you won't be able to make changes to the visual source in the browser. You need to do so in the IDE you use to code the visual. However, if Auto Reload is turned on, the visual will update in Power BI Service automatically when you save the source file. For more debugging tips, refer to the "PowerBI Visual Tools (pbiviz) – Debugging" article at https://github.com/Microsoft/PowerBI-visuals/blob/master/tools/debugging.md.

Upgrading the Developer Tools
Overtime, Microsoft will upgrade both the Developer Tools and scripts. The roadmap (https://github.com/Microsoft/PowerBI-visuals/blob/master/Roadmap) informs you when a new version is available. You can upgrade your visual by executing these commands:

```
#Update the command-line tool (pbiviz)
npm install -g powerbi-visuals-tools
```

```
#run update from the root of your visual project, where pbiviz.json is located
pbiviz update
```

The first command will download the latest command-line tool from npm, including the updated type definitions and schemas. The second command will overwrite the apiVersion property in your pbiviz.json.

Now that you've learned about programming and testing custom visuals, let me walk you through the implementation steps of the Sparkline visual.

16.3 Implementing Custom Visuals

A sparkline is a miniature graph, typically drawn without axes or coordinates. The term sparkline was introduced by Edward Tufte for "small, high resolution graphics embedded in a context of words, numbers, images". Tufte describes sparklines as "data-intense, design-simple, word-sized graphics". Sparklines are typically used to visualize trends over time, such as to show profit over the past several years. Although other Microsoft reporting tools, such as Excel and Reporting Services include sparkline elements, Power BI doesn't have a sparkline visual. Yet, sparklines are commonly used on dashboards so I hope you'll find my sparkline implementation useful not only for learning custom visuals but also for your real-life projects.

16.3.1 Understanding the Sparkline Visual

Sparklines come in different shapes and forms. To keep things simple, I decided to implement a "classic" smooth line sparkline that is shown in **Figure 16.8**.

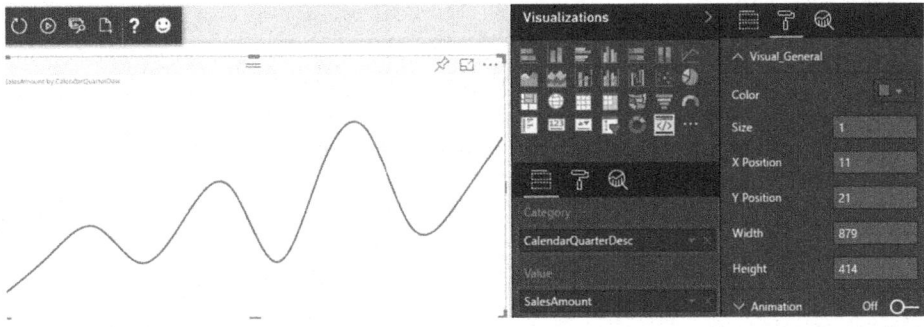

Figure 16.8 You can configure the sparkline using the Data and Format tabs.

Understanding capabilities
Once you import and add the sparkline to a report, you bind the sparkline to data using the Data tab of the Visualization pane. **Figure 16.8** shows that I'm aggregating a SalesAmount field added to the Value area by the CalendarQuarterDesc field, which is added to the Category area. The resulting graph shows how sales fluctuate over quarters. You can use any field to group the data, not just a field from the Date table. The sparkline supports several formatting options to customize its appearance. The General section lets you change the line color and width. The default properties are "steelblue" as a color and one pixel for the line width.

The Animation section lets you turn on an animation effect that draws the line gradually from left to right. Although in general I advise against animations and other visual distractors in real-life reports, I wanted to emphasize the fact that Power BI visuals can support anything clients-side JavaScript can do. If you expand the Animation section, you'll see that you can specify two settings: Duration and Delay. The Duration setting controls how fast the line draws (the default setting is 1,000 milliseconds) and the Delay setting controls the interval between redraws (the default is 3,000 milliseconds).

Understanding limitations
The main limitation of the current implementation is that the sparkline doesn't render multiple times in the same visualization, such as for each product category. This limitation also applies to Microsoft-provided visuals, such as the Gauge visual. Preferably, at some point Power BI would support a repeater visual, like the SSRS Tablix region. This would allow nesting the sparkline into other visualizations, such as a table, that could repeat the sparkline for each row. As Power BI stands now, the only way to implement this feature is to draw the visual for each category value. Although the sparkline doesn't repeat, it could be used to display multiple measures arranged either horizontally or vertically by adding it multiple times on the report.

Another limitation related to the one I've just discussed is that the sparkline supports only a single field in the Category area and a single field in the Value area. In other words, the sparkline is limited to one measure and one group.

16.3.2 Implementing the IVisual Interface

I coded the sparkline using Microsoft Visual Studio Code. Visual Studio Code (https://code.visualstudio.com) is a free source code editor developed by Microsoft for Windows, Linux, and macOS. Think of Visual Studio Code as a light-weight version of Visual Studio, which is specifically useful if you spend most of your time writing client-side JavaScript code. Visual Studio Code includes support for debugging, embedded Git control, syntax highlighting, intelligent code completion, snippets, and code refactoring.

Let's start its implementation with the IVisual interface. Remember that IVisual has four key methods: *constructor()*, *update()*, *enumerateObjectInstances()* and *destroy()*. You can find the project code in the /Source/Ch16/sparkline folder. The sparkline visual code is in the src/sparkline.ts file.

Implementing the constructor() method

Power BI calls the *constructor()* method to give a chance to the visual to initialize itself. Figure 16.9 shows its implementation.

```
112 public constructor(options: VisualConstructorOptions) {
113     this.selectionManager = options.host.createSelectionManager();
114     this.root = d3.select(options.element);
115     this.tooltipServiceWrapper = createTooltipServiceWrapper(options.host.tooltipService,
116                                 options.element);
117
118     this.svg = this.root
119         .append('svg')
120         .classed('sparkline', true)
121         .attr('height', options.element.clientHeight)
122         .attr('width', options.element.clientWidth);
123 }
```

Figure 16.9 The constructor() method initializes the visual.

First, the code creates an instance of the SelectionManager, which the host uses to communicate to the visual user interactions, such as clicking the graph. The sparkline doesn't handle user selection events but it's possible to extend it, such as to navigate to another page or highlight a line segment. Line 114 initializes the D3.js framework with the DOM element that the visual owns, which is passed to the *constructor()* method as a property of the VisualConstructorOptions parameter.

Line 115 is for the tooltip support which I'll explain in section 16.3.3. Line 118 creates a *svg* HTML element and classes it as "sparkline". It's a good practice to create another element instead of using the root in case you need to draw more elements in the future. The code also sizes the *svg* element so that it occupies the entire viewport.

Implementing the update() method

The *update()* method is where the actual work of drawing the graph happens (see **Figure 16.10**). Line 127 removes the existing graph so that redrawing the sparkline doesn't overlay what's already plotted on the canvas and to avoid drawing new lines when the visual is resized.

When the host calls the *update()* method, it passes the data as a dataView object. For example, if you add the CalendarQuarter field to the Category area and SalesAmount field to the Value area, the host will aggregate SalesAmount by quarter and pass the corresponding data representation and the metadata describing the columns under the *options.DataView* object.

The definition of the *DataView* object is documented at https://github.com/Microsoft/PowerBI-visuals/blob/master/Capabilities/DataViewMappings.md. When binding the visual to the CalendarYear and SalesAmount fields, the DataView object might look like the example shown in **Figure 16.11**. Since the sparkline visual supports only one field in the Category area, there is only one element in the *DataView.categorical.categories* array. The values property returns the actual category values, such as Q1 2015. The *identity* property returns system-generated unique identifiers for each category value. The *DataView.categorical.values* property contains the values of the field added to the Value area. Because the sparkline visual supports only one field in the Value area, the values array has only one element.

```
126 public update(options: VisualUpdateOptions) {
127     this.svg.selectAll("path").remove(); // clear existing line
128     if (!options.dataViews || !options.dataViews[0]) return;
129     const dataView: DataView = options.dataViews[0];
130     this.settings = Settings.parse(dataView) as Settings;
131     var viewport = options.viewport;
132     var viewModel: SparklineModel = Sparkline.converter(dataView, this.settings);
133
134     if (!viewModel) return;
135     if (viewport.height < 0 || viewport.width < 0) return;
136     var graph = this.svg;
137
138     // stop animation if graph is animating for update changes to take effect
139     this.stopAnimation();
140     // resize draw area to fit visualization frame
141     this.svg.attr({
142         'height': viewport.height,
143         'width': viewport.width
144     });
145
146     var data = viewModel.data;
147     // X scale fits values for all data elements; domain property will scale the graph width
148     var x = d3.scale.linear().domain([0, data.length - 1]).range([0, viewport.width]);
149     // Y scale will fit values from min to max calibrated to the graph higth
150     var y = d3.scale.linear().domain([Math.min.apply(Math, data), Math.max.apply(Math, data)]).range([0, viewport.height]);
151     // create a line
152     var line = d3.svg.line<number>()
153         .interpolate("basis") // smooth line
154         // assign the X function to plot on X axis
155         .x(function (d, i) {
156             // enable the next line when debugging to output X coordinate
157             // console.log('Plotting X value for data point: ' + d + ' using index: ' + i + ' to be at: ' + x(i) + ' using xScale.');
158             return x(i);
159         })
160         .y(function (d) {
161             // enable the next line when debugging to output X coordinate
162             // console.log('Plotting Y value for data point: ' + d + ' to be at: ' + y(d) + " using yScale.");
163             return viewport.height - y(d); // values are plotted from the top so reverse the scale
164         })
165
166     // display the line by appending an svg:path element with the data line we created above
167     var path = this.svg.append("svg:path")
168         .attr("d", line(data))
169         .attr('stroke-width', function (d) { return viewModel.size })
170         .attr('stroke', function (d) { return viewModel.color });
```

Figure 16.10 The update() method draws the graph.

Working directly with the DataView object is impractical. Therefore, line 132 calls the converter method, which converts the DataView object into a custom object for working with the data in a more suitable format. Using a converter is a recommended pattern since it allows you to organize the data just as you are to draw it, which makes your code focused on the task at hand and not on manipulating the data. For example, in our case the *data* property on line 146 returns the data points as a JavaScript array.

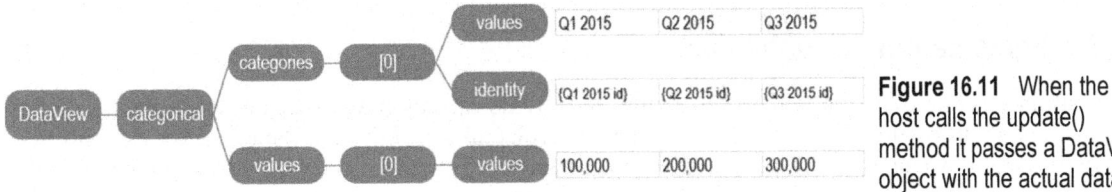

Figure 16.11 When the host calls the update() method it passes a DataView object with the actual data.

The D3.js code starts at line 148. First, the code calibrates the X axis to plot the number of data points. Conveniently, D3.js supports quantitative scaling and the *d3.scale.linear.domain* property scales the X axis to fit the data points. Next, the code calibrates the Y axis to fit the values given the minimum and maximum data point values. Lines 152-164 plot the line. One cautionary note here is that the zero coordinate of the Y axis starts at the top of the viewport. Therefore, line 163 inverts the data point Y coordinate. Line 167 draws the line using the user-specified line width and color.

Animating the graph

If the user turns on the Animate setting, the line constantly redraws itself using a configurable delay and redrawing speed. The code that animates the graph is shown in **Figure 16.12**. Line 186 checks if the animation effect is turned on. If so, it uses the JavaScript *setInterval()* function to call periodically the *redrawWithAnimation()* function.

```
173 function redrawWithAnimation() {
174     var totalLength = (<SVGPathElement>path.node()).getTotalLength();
175     graph.selectAll("path")
176         .data([data]) // set the new data
177         .attr("d", line)
178         .attr("stroke-dasharray", totalLength + " " + totalLength)
179         .attr("stroke-dashoffset", totalLength)
180         .transition()
181         .duration(viewModel.duration)
182         .ease("linear")
183         .attr("stroke-dashoffset", 0);
184 }
185
186 if (viewModel.animate) {
187     this.timer = setInterval(function () {
188         redrawWithAnimation();
189     }, viewModel.delay);
190 }
```

Figure 16.12 The graph supports animated line redrawing by calling repeatedly the redrawWithAnimation function.

D3.js and SVG make the task of animating the graph easy. Line 174 calls the SVG *getTotalLength()* function to calculate the length of the graph. The stroke-dasharray attribute lets you specify the length of the rendered part of the line. The stroke-dashoffset attribute lets you change where the dasharray behavior starts. Then the SVG transition() function is used to animate the path.

Implementing the destroy() method

Remember that the host calls the *destroy()* method to give the visual a chance to release any resources that might result in memory leaks. Our implementation releases the D3.js graph elements. It also releases the timer variable that holds a reference to the timer identifier when the animation effect is used.

```
public destroy(): void {
    this.svg = null;
    this.root = null;
    this.timer = nulll;}
```

16.3.3 Implementing Capabilities

Power BI hosts enumerate the visual's capabilities to provide various extensions. For example, the report host uses this information to populate the Field and Format tabs in the Visualizations pane. For this to work, the custom visual needs to tell Power BI what data and formatting capabilities it supports.

Advertising data capabilities

Figure 16.13 shows how the Sparkline visual advertises its data capabilities. This code is located in the capabilities.json file. The *dataRoles* property informs the host about the field areas the visual is expecting, while the *dataViewMappings* property describes how these fields relate to one another, and informs Power BI how it should construct the Fields tab areas. It can also inform the host about special conditions, such as that only one category value is supported.

```
 1    {
 2      "dataRoles": [
 3        {
 4          "name": "Category",
 5          "kind": 0,
 6          "displayName": "Category"
 7        },
 8        {
 9          "name": "Value",
10          "kind": 1,
11          "displayName": "Value"
12        }
13      ],
14      "dataViewMappings": [
15        {
16          "conditions": [
17            {
18              "Category": { "max": 1 },
19              "Value": { "max": 1 }
20            }
21          ],
22          "categorical": {
23            "categories": {
24              "for": { "in": "Category" },
25              "dataReductionAlgorithm": { "bottom": { "count": 100 } }
26            },
27            "values": {
28              "group": {
29                "by": "Series",
30                "select": [ { "bind": { "to": "Value" } } ]
31              }
32            }
33          }
34        }
35      ],
36      "objects": {
37        "general": {
38          "displayName": "Visual_General",
39          "properties": {
40            "fill": {
41              "type": { "fill": { "solid": { "color": true } } },
42              "displayName": "Color"
43            },
44            "size": {
45              "type": { "numeric": true },
46              "displayName": "Size"
47            }
48          }
49        },
50        "labels": {
51          "displayName": "Animation",
52          "properties": {
53            "show": {
54              "type": { "bool": true },
55              "displayName": "Visual_Show"
56            },
57            "delay": {
58              "type": { "numeric": true },
59              "displayName": "Delay"
60            },
61            "duration": {
62              "type": { "numeric": true },
63              "displayName": "Duration"
64            }
65          }
66        }
67      }
68    }
```

Figure 16.13   The visual describes its data capabilities in the capabilities.jscon file.

On line 2, the Sparkline custom visual uses *dataRoles* to tell Power BI that it needs a Category area for grouping the data and a Value area for the measure. When the host interrogates the visual capabilities, it'll add these two areas to the Fields tab of the Visualizations pane. On line 14, the custom visual uses data-ViewMappings to instruct the host that the Category and Value areas can have only one field. To avoid performance degradation caused by plotting too many data points, line 25 specifies a bottom 100 data reduction condition to plot only the last 100 categorical values. So, if the user adds the Date field from the Date table, only the last 100 dates will be displayed.

Advertising formatting capabilities
Custom visuals are not responsible for implementing any user interface for formatting the visual. Instead, they declare the formatting options they support, and the host creates the UI for them. As it stands, Power BI supports three types of objects:

- Statically bound – These are formatting options that don't depend on the actual data, such as the line color.
- Data bound – These objects are bound to the number of data points. For example, the funnel chart allows you to specify the color of the individual data points.
- Metadata bound – These objects are bound to actual data fields, such as if you want to color all the bars in a series of a bar chart in a given color.

The Sparkline supports additional settings that allow the user to customize its appearance and animation behavior (shown in the right pane in **Figure 16.13**). All the sparkline formatting settings are static. They are grouped in two sections: General and Animation (it might be beneficial to refer to **Figure 16.1** again).

The fill property (line 40) allows the user to specify the line color. The type of this property is color. This will cause the host to show a color picker. The *displayName* property defines the name the user will see ("Color" in this case). The Size property is for the line width and has a numeric data type.

The labels section defines the animation settings. The *show* property (line 53) is a special Boolean property that allows the user to turn on or off the entire section. The *delay* property controls how often the line is redrawn, while the *duration* property controls the speed of redrawing the line.

Providing default values

When the host discovers the visual capabilities, it calls the *IVisual.enumerateObjectInstances()* method to obtain the default values for each setting. And when the user changes a setting, the host calls this method again to push the new property values. This is all handled by the framework. Besides declaring the visual capabilities, you only need to provide default settings. As a best practice, the setting default values are stored in another src\settings.ts file (see **Figure 16.14**).

```
27 module powerbi.extensibility.visual {
28     "use strict";
29
30     import DataViewObjectsParser = powerbi.extensibility.utils.dataview.DataViewObjectsParser;
31
32     export class Settings extends DataViewObjectsParser {
33         public general: GeneralSettings = new GeneralSettings();
34         public labels: LabelsSettings = new LabelsSettings();
35     }
36
37     export class GeneralSettings {
38         public fill: string = "#4682b4";
39         public size: number = 1;
40     }
41
42     export class LabelsSettings {
43         public show: boolean = false;
44         public delay: number = 3000;
45         public duration: number = 1000;
46     }
47 }
```

Figure 16.14 The host calls enumerateObjectInstances to get and set the visual capabilities.

The *fill* general setting in the GeneralSettings class defaults the line stroke to SteelBlue color (#4682b4) and the *size* setting specifies 1pt for the line width. The LabelsSetting section defaults the *show* parameter to false (animation is off by default), and specifies default settings for line redraw delay and duration when the user turns animation on.

Handling tooltips

Tooltips allow users to see the values behind a data point. Follow these to support tooltips:

1. Add tooltipInterfaces.ts, tooltipeService.ts, and tooltipTouch.ts fields from the framework code (https://github.com/Microsoft/powerbi-visuals-utils-tooltiputils) to the src folder.

2. Reference these files in tsconfig.json.

3. In the visual *constructor* method, initiate the tooltipServiceWrapper object (see again Figure 16.9).

4. In the visual *update* method, call addTooltip.

```
this.tooltipServiceWrapper.addTooltip(this.svg.selectAll("path"),
    (tooltipEvent: TooltipEventArgs<number>) => this.getTooltipData(tooltipEvent, dataView, viewport),
    (tooltipEvent: TooltipEventArgs<number>) => null);
```

This method calls your implementation of what the tooltip shows. The sparkline implementation calls a helper function getTooltipeData and passes the tooltipEvent object, the visual dataView and viewport. **Figure 16.15** shows the implementation of the getTooltipData method.

```
213 private getTooltipData(value: any, dataView:DataView, viewport:IViewport): VisualTooltipDataItem[] {
214     var model = Sparkline.converter(dataView, this.settings);
215     var tooltip = <TooltipEventArgs<number>> value;
216     var x = tooltip.coordinates[0];
217     var width = viewport.width;
218     var i = Math.floor((x/width) * model.data.length); // find the closest data point from coordinates
219     var d = model.data[i];
220
221     return [{
222         displayName: dataView.categorical.categories[0].values[i].toString(),
223         value: d.toString()
224     }];
225 }
```

Figure 16.15 The getTooltip method returns what the tooltip should show when the user hovers on the line.

Line 214 obtains the Sparkline model from dataView. Line 216 obtains the coordinates of the hover event. Because the sparkline draws a line, it needs to approximate the nearest data point from the coordinates. This is done in line 218 which divides the x coordinate by the viewport width and multiplies the result by the number of data points. Line 219 retrieves the data point. Line 221 returns a tooltip object with a display name set to the data point category and actual value.

16.4 Deploying Custom Visuals

Once you test the custom visual, it's time to package it, so that your users can start using it to visualize data in new ways. If you want to make the visual publicly available, consider also submitting it to Microsoft AppSource.

16.4.1 Packaging Custom Visuals

Sot that end users can import your custom visual in Power BI Service and Power BI Desktop, you need to package the visual as a *.pbiviz file.

Understanding visual packages
A pbiviz file is a standard zip archive. If you rename the file to have a zip extension and double-click it, you'll see the structure shown in **Figure 16.16**.

resources   File folder
package.json   JSON File

Figure 16.16 A *.pbiviz file is a zip archive file that packages the visual code and resources.

The package.json file is the visual manifest which indicates which files are included and what properties you specified when you exported the visual. The resources folder includes another JSON file. This file bundles the visual code and all additional resources, such as the visual icon from the \assets folder.

Packaging custom visuals
The Custom Visual Developer Tools make it easy to export and package the visual.

1. In Visual Studio Code, open the pbiviz.json file.
2. Fill in the visual properties. **Figure 16.17** shows the settings that I specified for the Sparkline visual.
3. (Optional) Create a visual icon (20x20 pixels) and save it as an icon.png file under the assets/ folder. This is the icon the users see in the Visualizations pane after they import the visual.

```
 1 {
 2   "visual": {
 3     "name": "Sparkline",
 4     "displayName": "Sparkline",
 5     "guid": "Sparkline1444636326814",
 6     "visualClassName": "Sparkline",
 7     "version": "1.2.0",
 8     "description": "",
 9     "supportUrl": "",
10     "gitHubUrl": ""
11   },
12   "apiVersion": "1.9.0",
13   "author": {
14     "name": "",
15     "email": ""
16   },
17   "assets": {
18     "icon": "assets/icon.png"
19   },
20   "externalJS": [
21     "node_modules/d3/d3.min.js",
22     "node_modules/powerbi-visuals-utils-dataviewutils/lib/index.js"
23   ],
24   "style": "style/visual.less",
25   "capabilities": "capabilities.json",
26   "dependencies": "dependencies.json",
27   "stringResources": []
28 }
```

Figure 16.17 Enter information that you want to distribute with the visual in the pbiviz.json file.

4. Open the Command Prompt, navigate to your project and execute the *pbiviz package* command. The last four lines represent the output the command generates.

pbiviz package

info   Building visual...
done   build complete
info   Building visual...
done   packaging complete

This command-line tool packages the visual and saves the pbiviz file under the dist/ folder. If only users within your organization will use the visual, you are done! You just need to distribute the *.pbiviz file to your users so they can import it in Power BI Desktop or Power BI Service.

Publishing to Microsoft AppSource
If you would like to make your visual publicly available, consider submitting it to Microsoft AppSource. To learn more about how to do so:

1. Open your web browser and navigate to Microsoft AppSource (https://appsource.microsoft.com).

2. If you haven't done so already, create an individual or corporate developer account.

3. Click the "List on AppSource" menu.

4. On the next page, scroll all the way down and then click the "Submit Your App" button. This will bring you to a page that will ask you to describe your app.

 NOTE Is your organization concerned about quality and security of visuals published to AppSource? From a personal experience I can tell you that Microsoft follows a strict process to validate submissions. They'll check the custom visual thoroughly for bugs and best practices. Be patient because it will probably take a few cycles for your visual to appear in the gallery.

16.4.2 Using Custom Visuals

Once downloaded, custom visuals can be added to a report in Power BI Service or Power BI Desktop. Your users can add your custom visual to a report by clicking the ellipsis (…) button in the Visualizations pane. They will see options to import a custom visual from a file or from AppSource.

Understanding import limitations

As it stands, Power BI imports the custom visual code into the report. Therefore, the visual exists only within the hosting report that imports the visual. If you create a new report, you'll find that the Visualizations pane doesn't show custom visuals. You must re-import the custom visuals that the new report needs.

 NOTE As a best practice, you should test a custom visual for privacy and security vulnerabilities by using the Microsoft recommendations at https://powerbi.microsoft.com/en-us/documentation/powerbi-custom-visuals-review-for-security-and-privacy. I recommend you compare the TypeScript and JavaScript files to make sure they have the same code and test the JavaScript code with an anti-virus software.

Removing custom visuals

As you can see, users can easily add custom visuals to reports. Fortunately, Power BI makes it easy to remove visuals from a report if you no longer need them. To do so, edit the report, right-click the visual in the Visualizations pane (works in both Power BI Service and Power BI Desktop) and then click "Delete custom visual" (see **Figure 16.18**).

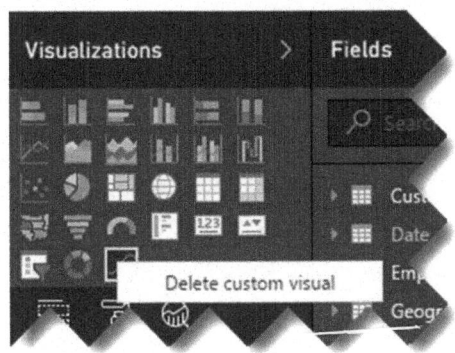

Figure 16.18 Right-click the custom visual to remove it if you no longer need it on the report.

16.5 Summary

The Microsoft presentation framework is open source to let web developers extend the Power BI visualization capabilities and to create their own visuals. Consider implementing a custom visual when your presentation requirements go beyond the capabilities of the Microsoft-provided visuals or the visuals contributed by the community. Custom visuals help you convey information as graphics and images. Any data insights that can be coded and rendered with JavaScript and client-side presentation frameworks, such as D3.js and SVG, can be implemented as a custom visual and used on Power BI reports.

You create custom visuals by writing TypeScript code that implements the Power BI IVisual interface. You can code a custom visual in your IDE of choice. Once the visual is ready and tested, you can export it to a *.pbiviz file, and then import it in Power BI Service or Power BI Desktop. You can also share your custom visuals with the community by submitting them to Microsoft AppSource.

With this chapter, we've reached the last stop of our Power BI journey. I sincerely hope that this book has helped you understand how Power BI can be a powerful platform for delivering pervasive data analytics. As you've seen, Power BI has plenty to offer to all types of users who are interested in BI:

- Information worker – You can use content packs and the Power BI Service Get Data feature to gain immediate insights without modeling.
- Data analyst – You can build sophisticated BI models for self-service data exploration with Power BI Desktop or Excel. And then you can share these models with your coworkers by publishing these models to Power BI or Power BI Report Server.
- BI or IT pro – You can establish a trustworthy environment that promotes team collaboration. And you can implement versatile solutions that integrate with Power BI, such as solutions for descriptive, predictive and real-time BI.
- Developer – Thanks to the Power BI open architecture, you can extend the Power BI visualization capabilities with custom visuals and integrate your apps with Power BI.

Of course, that's not all! Remember that Power BI is a part of a holistic vision that Microsoft has for delivering cloud and on-premises data analytics. When planning your on-premises BI solutions, consider the Microsoft public reporting roadmap at http://bit.ly/msreportingroadmap. Keep in mind that you can use both Power BI (cloud-based data analytics) and the SQL Server box product on-premises to implement synergetic solutions that bring your data to life!

Don't forget to download the source code from http://bit.ly/powerbibook and stay in touch with me on the book discussion list. Happy data analyzing with Power BI!

Appendix A

Glossary of Terms

The following table lists the most common BI-related terms and acronyms used in this book.

Term	Acronym	Description
Analysis Services Tabular		An instance of SQL Server Analysis Services that's configured in Tabular mode and is capable of hosting tabular models for organizational use.
App		A mechanism for packaging and distributing Power BI content.
AppSource		An area in Power BI Service where users can discover apps
Application Programming Interface	API	Connectivity mechanism for programmatically accessing application features
Azure Marketplace		The Windows Azure Marketplace is an online market buying, and selling finished software as a Service (SaaS) applications and premium datasets.
Azure Machine Learning	AzureML	An Azure cloud service to creating predictive experiments
Business Intelligence Semantic Model	BISM	A unifying name that includes both Multidimensional (OLAP) and Tabular (relational) features of Microsoft SQL Server Analysis Services.
Capacity		A set of hardware resources dedicated to Power BI.
Content pack (superseded by apps)		A packaged set of dashboards, reports, and datasets from popular cloud services or from Power BI content (see organizational content pack)
Custom visual		A visualization that a web developer can create to plug in to Power BI or Power BI Desktop
Corporate BI		Same as Organizational BI.
Cube		An OLAP structure organized in a way that facilitates data aggregation, such as to answer queries for historical and trend analysis.
D3.js		A JavaScript-based visualization framework
Dashboard		A Power BI page that can combine visualizations from multiple reports to provide a summary (preferably one-page) view of important business metrics.
Data Analysis Expressions	DAX	An Excel-like formula language for defining custom calculations and for querying tabular models.
Data model		A BI model designed with Power BI Desktop or Analysis Services.
Dataset		The definition of the data that you connect to in Power BI, such as a dataset that represents the data you import from an Excel file.
Descriptive analytics		A type of analytics that is concerned about analyzing history.
DirectQuery		A data connectivity configuration that allows Power BI to generate and send queries to the data source without importing the data.

Dimension (lookup) table		A table that represents a business subject area and provides contextual information to each row in a fact table, such as Product, Customer, and Date.
Extraction, transformation, loading	ETL	Processes extract from data sources, clean the data, and load the data into a target database, such as data warehouse.
Fact table		A table that keeps a historical record of numeric measurements (facts), such as the ResellerSales in the Adventure Works model.
Group		A Power BI group is a security mechanism to simplify access to content.
HTML5		A markup language used for structuring and presenting content on the World Wide Web.
Key Performance Indicator	KPI	A key performance indicator (KPI) is a quantifiable measure that is used to measure the company performance, such as Profit or Return on Investment (ROI).
Measure		A business calculation that is typically used to aggregate data, such as SalesAmount, Tax, OrderQuantity.
Microsoft AppSource		A site where developers can share apps.
Multidimensional		The OLAP path of BISM that allows BI professionals to implement multidimensional cubes.
Multidimensional Expressions	MDX	A query language for Multidimensional for defining custom calculations and querying OLAP cubes.
Office 365		A cloud-hosted platform of Microsoft services and products, such as SharePoint Online and Exchange Online.
OneDrive and OneDrive for Business		Cloud storage for individuals or businesses to uploading, organizing, and storing files.
Online Analytical Processing	OLAP	A system that is designed to quickly answer multidimensional analytical queries to facilitate data exploration and data mining.
On-premises Data Gateway		Connectivity software that allows Power BI to refresh and query directly on-premises data.
OAuthentication	OAuth	Security protocol for authentication users on the Internet
Personal BI		Targets business users and provides tools for implementing BI solutions for personal use, such as PowerPivot models, by importing and analyzing data without requiring specialized skills.
Personal Gateway		Connectivity software that allows business users to automate refresh data from on-premises data sources by installing it on their computers.
Power BI		A data analytics platform for self-service, team, and organizational BI that consists of Power BI Service, Power BI Desktop, Power BI Premium, Power BI Mobile, Power BI Embedded, and Power BI Report Server products.
Power BI Desktop		A free desktop tool for creating Power BI reports and self-service data models.
Power BI Embedded		Power BI APIs for embedding Power BI content in apps for internal and external customers.
Power BI Mobile		Native mobile applications for viewing and annotating Power BI content on mobile devices.
Power BI Portal		The user interface of Power BI Service that you see when you go to powerbi.com.
Power BI Premium		A Power BI Service add-on that allows organizations to purchase a dedicated environment.
Power BI Report Server		An extended edition of SSRS that supports Power BI reports and Excel reports.
Power BI Service		The cloud-based service of Power BI (powerbi.com). The terms Power BI and Power BI Service are used interchangeably.
Power Map		An Excel add-in for 3D geospatial reporting.
Power View		A SharePoint-based reporting tool that allows business users to author interactive reports from PowerPivot models and from organizational tabular models.

Power Pivot for Excel		A free add-in that extends the Excel capabilities to allow business users to implement personal BI models.
Power Pivot for SharePoint		Included in SQL Server 2012, PowerPivot for SharePoint extends the SharePoint capabilities to support PowerPivot models.
Power Query		An Excel add-in for transforming and shaping data.
Predictive analytics		Type of analytics that is concerned with discovering patterns that aren't easily discernible
Questions & Answers	Q&A	A Power BI feature that allows users to type natural questions to get data insights.
Representational State Transfer	REST	Web service communication standard
Row-level Security	RLS	A security mechanism for ensuring restricted access to data.
Self-service BI		Same as Personal BI.
Semantic model		Layered between the data and users, the semantic model translates database structures into a user-friendly model that centralizes business calculations and security.
SharePoint Products and Technologies	SharePoint	A server-based platform for document management and collaboration that includes BI capabilities, such as hosting and managing PowerPivot models, reports, and dashboards.
SQL Server Analysis Services	SSAS	A SQL Server add-on, Analysis Services provides analytical and data mining services. The Business Intelligence Semantic Model represents the analytical services.
SQL Server Integration Services	SSIS	A SQL Server add-on, Integration Services is a platform for implementing extraction, transformation, and loading (ETL) processes.
SQL Server Management Studio	SSMS	A management tool that's bundled with SQL Server that allows administrators to manage Database Engine, Analysis Services, Reporting Services and Integration Services instances.
SQL Server Reporting Services	SSRS	A SQL Server add-on, Reporting Services is a server-based reporting platform for the creation, management, and delivery of standard and ad hoc reports.
Snowflake schema		Unlike a star schema, a snowflake schema has some dimension tables that relate to other dimension tables and not directly to the fact table.
Star schema		A model schema where a fact table is surrounded by dimension tables and these dimension tables reference directly the fact table.
StreamInsight		An Azure cloud service for streaming
Tabular		Tabular is the relational side of BISM that allows business users and BI professionals to implement relational-like (tabular) models.
Team BI		Provides tools to allow business users to share BI solutions that they create with co-workers.
Tile		A dashboard section that can be pinned from an existing report or produced with Q&A.
TypeScript		A typed superset of JavaScript
Visualization		A visual representation of data on a Power BI report, such as a chart or map.
Workspace		A Power BI content area that is allocated for either an individual (My Workspace) or a team
xVelocity		xVelocity is a columnar data engine that compresses and stores data in memory.

index

Increase your BI IQ!

Besides Business Intelligence consulting and implementation services, Prologika offers onsite and online training courses. As with our books, we pride ourselves on delivering applied, under-the-hood training, instead of focusing only on the theoretical aspects of the technology. Check our services, case studies, and training catalog at http://prologika.com.

Applied SQL Server Analysis Services (Multidimensional)

This intensive 4-day class is designed to help you become proficient with Analysis Services (Multidimensional) and acquire the necessary skills to implement OLAP and data mining solutions.

Learn More >>

Applied BI Semantic Model (Tabular and Multidimensional)

Targeting BI developers, this intensive 5-day onsite class is designed to help you become proficient with Analysis Services and acquire the necessary skills to implement Tabular and Multidimensional models.

Learn More >>

Applied SQL Server Reporting Services

This intensive 4-day class is designed to help you become proficient with Microsoft SQL Server Reporting Services and acquire the necessary skills to author, manage, and deliver reports.

Learn More >>

Applied Master Data Services and Data Quality Services

Organizations that invest in master data management and improving the quality of their informational assets will be best positioned to reap ...

Learn More >>

Applied Excel and Analysis Services

This 1-day class is designed to help business users become proficient with using the Excel BI features to analyze corporate data in Analysis Services Multidimensional cubes or Tabular models.

Learn More >>

Applied Power BI

Power BI is a suite of products for personal business intelligence (BI). It brings the power of Microsoft's Business Intelligence platform to business users. At the same time, Power BI lets IT monitor and manage published...

Learn More >>

Applied Power BI Service

Power BI Service (or Power BI 2.0) is a cloud-based business analytics service that gives you a single view of your most critical business data. Monitor the health of your business using a live dashboard...

Learn More >>

Applied MS Visualization Tools

Reporting is an essential feature of every business intelligence solution. One way to extract and disseminate the wealth of information is to author Reporting Services standard reports,...

Learn More >>

Applied MS End-to-End BI

This four-day class is designed to help you become proficient with the Microsoft BI toolset and acquire skills to implement an end-to-end organizational BI solution, including data warehouse, ETL processes, and a semantic model.

Learn More >>

Applied SQL Server Fundamentals

This 2-day instructor led course provides you with the necessary skills to query Microsoft SQL Server databases with Transact-SQL. It teaches novice users how to query data stored in SQL Server data structures.

Learn More >>

Applied MS Visualization Tools

Reporting is an essential feature of every business intelligence solution. One way to extract and disseminate the wealth of information is to author Reporting Services standard reports,...

Learn More >>

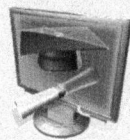

88019731R00233

Made in the USA
Columbia, SC
23 January 2018